Timothy E Welty PharmD

# Pharmacotherapy

## A Pathophysiologic Approach

# Pharmacotherapy

## A Pathophysiologic Approach


Editors

**Joseph T. DiPiro, PharmD**
Associate Professor, College of Pharmacy, University of Georgia;
Associate Clinical Professor of Surgery, Medical College of Georgia,
Augusta, Georgia

**Robert L. Talbert, PharmD**
Professor, College of Pharmacy, University of Texas at Austin, Austin, Texas;
Professor, Departments of Pharmacology and Medicine, University of Texas
Health Science Center at San Antonio, San Antonio, Texas

**Peggy E. Hayes, PharmD**
Associate Professor of Pharmacy and Pharmaceutics, School of Pharmacy,
Virginia Commonwealth University, Medical College of Virginia,
Richmond, Virginia

**Gary C. Yee, PharmD**
Associate Professor, Department of Pharmacy Practice, College of Pharmacy,
University of Florida, J. Hillis Miller Health Center, Gainesville, Florida

**L. Michael Posey**
President, Pharmacy/Association Services, Arlington, Virginia



**Elsevier**
New York • Amsterdam • London

No responsibility is assumed by the publisher for any injury and/or damage to persons or property as a matter of products liability, negligence or otherwise, or from any use or operation of any methods, products, instructions, or ideas contained in the material herein. No suggested test or procedure should be carried out unless, in the reader's judgment, its risk is justified. Because of rapid advances in the medical sciences, we recommend that independent verification of diagnoses and drug dosages should be made. Discussions, views, and recommendations as to medical procedures, choice of drugs, and drug dosages are the responsibility of the authors.

Elsevier Science Publishing Co., Inc.
52 Vanderbilt Avenue, New York, New York 10017

Sole distributors outside the United States and Canada:
Elsevier Science Publishers, B.V.
P.O. Box 211, 1000 AE Amsterdam, the Netherlands



Library of Congress Cataloging-in-Publication Data

Pharmacotherapy : a pathophysiologic approach.

Includes index.
1. Chemotherapy. 2. Physiology, Pathological.
I. DiPiro, Joseph T. [DNLM: 1. Drug Therapy.
WB 330 P5357]
RM263.P52 1988 615.5'8 88-21355
ISBN 0-444-01323-7

Current printing (last digit):
10 9 8 7 6 5 4 3 2 1

Manufactured in the United States of America

*To those pharmacists who had the courage and perseverance to take the early steps that were needed to develop personally and professionally in the clinical practice of pharmacy*

*To our mentors whose vision provided educational and training programs that encouraged professional growth of their students*

*And to our families and faculty colleagues for their efforts and support for our endeavors*

# Contents

# Foreword

Evidence of the maturity of a profession is not unlike that characterizing the maturity of the individual; a child's utterances and behavior typically reveal an unrealized potential for attainment, eventually, of those attributes characteristic of an appropriately confident, independently competent, socially responsible, sensitive, and productive member of society.

Within a period of perhaps 15 or 20 years, we have witnessed a profound maturation within the profession of pharmacy. The utterances of the profession, as projected in its literature, have evolved from mostly self-centered and self-serving issues of trade protection to a composite of expressed professional interests that prominently include responsible explorations of scientific/technological questions and ethical issues that promote the best interests of the clientele served by the profession. With the publication of *Pharmacotherapy: A Pathophysiologic Approach,* pharmacy's utterances bespeak a matured practitioner who is able to call upon unique knowledge and skills so as to function as an appropriately confident, independently competent pharmacotherapeutics expert.

In 1987, the Board of Pharmaceutical Specialties (BPS), in denying the petition filed by the American College of Clinical Pharmacy (ACCP) to recognize "clinical pharmacy" as a specialty, conceded nonetheless that the petitioning party had documented in its petition a specialist who does in fact exist within the practice of pharmacy and whose expertise clearly can be extricated from the performance characteristics of those in general practice. A refiled petition from ACCP requests recognition of "pharmacotherapy" as a Specialty Area of Pharmacy Practice. While the BPS had issued no decision when this book went to press it is difficult to comprehend the basis for a rejection of the second petition.

Within this book one will find the scientific foundation for the essential knowledge required of one who may aspire to specialty practice as a pharmacotherapist. As is the case with any such publication, its usefulness to the practitioner or the future practitioner is limited to providing such a foundation. To be socially and professionally responsible in practice, the pharmacotherapist's foundation must be continually supplemented and complemented by the flow of information appearing in the primary literature. Of course this is not unique to the general or specialty practice of pharmacy; it is essential to the fulfillment of obligations to clients in any occupation operating under the code of professional ethics.

Because of the growing complexity of pharmacotherapeutic agents, their dosing regimens, and techniques for delivery, pharmacy is obligated to produce, recognize, and remunerate specialty practitioners who can fulfill the profession's responsibilities to society for service expertise where the competence required in a particular case exceeds that of the general practitioner. It simply is a component of our covenant with society and is as important as any other facet of that relationship existing between a profession and those it serves.

The recognition by BPS of pharmacotherapy as an area of specialty practice in pharmacy will serve as an important statement by the profession that we have matured sufficiently to be competent and willing to take unprecedented responsibilities in the collaborative, pharmacotherapeutic management of patient-specific problems. It commits pharmacy to an intention that will not be uniformly or rapidly accepted within the established health care community. Nonetheless, this formal action places us on the road to an avowed goal, and acceptance will be gained as the pharmacotherapists proliferate and establish their importance in the provision of optimal, cost-effective drug therapy.

Suspecting that other professions in other times must have faced similar quests for recognition of their unique knowledge and skills, I once searched the literature for an example that might parallel pharmacy's modern-day aspirations. Writing in the *Philadelphia Medical Journal,* May 27, 1899, D. H. Galloway, MD, reflected on the need for specialty training and practice in a field of medicine lacking such expertise at that time. In an article entitled "The Anesthetizer as a Speciality," Galloway commented:

> *The anesthetizer will have to make his own place in medicine; the profession will not make a place for him, and not until he has demonstrated the value of his services will it concede him the position which the importance of his duties entitles him to occupy. He will be obliged to define his own rights, duties and privileges, and he must not expect that his own estimate of the importance of his position will be conceded without opposition. There are many surgeons who are unwilling to share either the credit or the emoluments of their work with any one, and their opposition will be overcome only when they are shown that the importance of their work will not be lessened, but enhanced, by the increased safety and dispatch with which operations may be done. . . .*

It has been my experience that, given the opportunity for one-on-one, collaborative practice with physicians and other health professionals, pharmacy practitioners who have been educated and trained to perform at the level of pharmacotherapeutics specialists almost invariably have convinced the former that "the importance of their work will not be lessened, but enhanced, by the increased safety and dispatch with which" individualized problems of drug therapy could be managed in collaboration with clinical pharmacy practitioners.

It is fortuitous, the coinciding of the release of *Pharmacotherapy: A Pathophysiologic Approach* with ACCP's petitioning of BPS for recognition of the pharmacotherapy specialist. The utterances of a maturing profession as revealed in the contents of this book, and the intraprofessional recognition and acceptance of a higher level of responsibility in the safe, effective, and economical use of drugs and drug products, bode well for the future of the profession and for the improvement of patient care with drugs.

Charles A. Walton, PhD
San Antonio, Texas

# Preface

Twenty years have passed since the term *clinical pharmacy* was applied to the practice of pharmacists whose primary focus includes the patient as well as the drug product. Consequently, the curricula of pharmacy schools have changed dramatically, placing a higher priority on patient-oriented practice. Therefore, there is a continuing need for instructional materials in clinical drug therapy, that is, pharmacotherapy. *Pharmacotherapy: A Pathophysiologic Approach* provides a basis of principles and information that reflects the breadth and depth of knowledge appropriate for today's pharmacy student and practitioner.

The text presents chapters, or primers, on topics such as pharmacokinetics or the use of laboratory tests in infectious diseases, which provide necessary background. The majority of the text is devoted to specific diseases; a concise review of epidemiology, etiology, and a thorough discussion of pathophysiology and clinical symptoms are presented. The sections on treatment attempt to place drug therapy in its proper perspective with other modalities. Accepted drug regimens are presented along with pertinent controversies in drug therapy. In recognition of the importance of adverse drug effects, specific chapters are devoted to these topics.

The pathophysiology sections of the text are the key to imparting a way of thinking for the developing practitioner. Mechanisms of disease processes identified in the beginning of the chapters should lead naturally into identification of possible approaches to treatment. The goal of the text is to present this logical process to the student, not just specific facts about therapy as we know it today. Understanding of pathophysiology and the principles of therapy will allow the student to assess more adequately the place of newly introduced drugs. The number of reference citations has purposely been limited to those of most relevance and value. The overall scope of the text is intended to match the topics likely to be included in most therapeutics courses for Doctor of Pharmacy programs.

*Pharmacotherapy: A Pathophysiologic Approach* is very much a snapshot of the clinical practice of pharmacy in the late 1980s. Production of this text has required the contribution of 155 authors from 60 different universities and institutions. The authors demonstrate a high level of expertise in such diverse areas as cardiology, pulmonology, gastroenterology, nephrology, neurology, psychiatry, oncology, infectious diseases, and nutrition, to name just a few.

The editors recognize that many areas of this text will rapidly become outdated as our understanding of disease processes increases or new therapies are adopted. The challenge for student and practitioner is to integrate information from a variety of sources and form a basis for application in pharmacotherapy, and to be receptive to new information as it appears in the literature or is gained by personal experience.

We are indebted to the efforts of our authors, without whose contributions we would still be talking about a great idea for a textbook. Also, we are very grateful for the efforts of Yale Altman who assisted in the birth of the idea for the text and then convinced us that it was possible to accomplish this task. Finally, we are appreciative of the patience of Barbara Johnson-Schwagerl and the efforts of many others at Elsevier including Allison Essen, Regina Dahir, Philip Schafer, and Kathryn Silverio.

# Contributors

**Paul A. Abraham, MD**
Assistant Professor, University of Minnesota Medical School; Division of Nephrology, Department of Medicine, Hennepin County Medical Center, Minneapolis, Minnesota

**J. V. Anandan, PharmD**
Assistant Director, Department of Pharmacy, Henry Ford Hospital; Adjunct Assistant Professor, College of Pharmacy and Allied Health Professions, Wayne State University, Detroit, Michigan

**David M. Angaran, MS**
Director, Biomedical Research, United Hospital Heart Institute; Associate Professor, University of Minnesota, Minneapolis, Minnesota

**Edward P. Armstrong, PharmD**
Assistant Professor, Department of Pharmacy Practice, College of Pharmacy, University of Arizona, Tucson, Arizona

**Jacqueline R. Barber, PharmD**
Director, Nutrition Support Pharmacy Services, Medical University of South Carolina; Assistant Professor, Colleges of Pharmacy and Medicine, Charleston, South Carolina

**Steven L. Barriere, PharmD**
Clinical Specialist, Infectious Diseases, Department of Pharmaceutical Services; Adjunct Associate Professor of Medicine and Pharmacology, School of Medicine, UCLA Center for the Health Sciences, Los Angeles, California

**Sharyn R. Batey, PharmD**
College of Pharmacy, University of South Carolina, Columbia, South Carolina

**Larry A. Bauer, PharmD**
Associate Professor, School of Pharmacy, University of Washington, Seattle, Washington

**Jerry L. Bauman, PharmD**
Associate Professor of Pharmacy and Instructor of Medicine in Cardiology, Colleges of Pharmacy and Medicine, University of Illinois, Chicago, Illinois

**Terry J. Baumann, PharmD**
Assistant Professor of Pharmacy, Wayne State University; Clinical Coordinator, Henry Ford Hospital, Detroit, Michigan

**Steven F. Bauwens, PharmD**
Associate Professor, University of Wisconsin, Madison, Wisconsin

**Eula D. Beasley, PharmD**
Assistant Professor of Pharmacy Practice, Howard University; Clinical Pharmacist, Washington Hospital Center, Washington, DC

**Rosemary R. Berardi, PharmD**
Associate Professor of Pharmacy, College of Pharmacy; Clinical Pharmacist, Gastroenterology, University Hospital, University of Michigan, Ann Arbor, Michigan

**Joseph S. Bertino, Jr, PharmD**
Assistant Director, Clinical Pharmacy Service, Mary Imogene Bassett Hospital, Cooperstown, New York

**Charles A. Biggio, RPh**
Director of Pharmacy, Eye, Ear, Nose and Throat Hospital, New Orleans, Louisiana

**Larry E. Boh, MS**
Associate Professor (CHS), School of Pharmacy, University of Wisconsin, Madison, Wisconsin

**John A. Bosso, PharmD**
Professor of Clinical Pharmacy and Pediatrics, University of Utah, Salt Lake City, Utah

**Talmadge A. Bowden, Jr, MD**
Professor of Surgery, Medical College of Georgia, Augusta, Georgia

**J. Chris Bradberry, PharmD**
Professor and Head, College of Pharmacy, Section of Pharmacy Practice, University of Oklahoma Health Sciences Center, Oklahoma City, Oklahoma

**Rex O. Brown, PharmD**
Associate Professor of Clinical Pharmacy, University of Tennessee, Memphis, Memphis, Tennessee

**Dianne M. Brundage, PharmD**
Assistant Professor, College of Pharmacy, Medical University of South Carolina, Charleston, South Carolina

**Gilbert J. Burckart, PharmD**
Associate Professor of Pharmacy Practice and Pediatrics, University of Pittsburgh, Pittsburgh, Pennsylvania

**Mark B. Burlingame, PharmD**
Fellow, Department of Pharmacy Practice, College of Pharmacy, University of Florida, Gainesville, Florida

**Henry I. Bussey, PharmD, FCCP**
Assistant Professor of Pharmacy, University of Texas at Austin, Austin, Texas; Assistant Professor of Pharmacology, University of Texas Health Science Center, San Antonio, Texas

**Ed Casabar, PharmD**
Clinical Pharmacist, Barnes Hospital, St. Louis, Missouri

**Judy L. Chase, PharmD**
Oncology Pharmacy Fellow, University of California Medical Center, San Francisco, California

**Linda A. Chiarello, BS, RN, CIC**
Research Scientist, New York State Department of Health, AIDS Epidemiology Program, Albany, New York

**John D. Cleary, PharmD**
Assistant Professor, School of Pharmacy, University of Mississippi, Jackson, Mississippi

**Melody A. Cobleigh, MD**
Associate Professor, College of Medicine, University of Illinois at Chicago, Chicago, Illinois

**Ann C. Collier, MD**
Assistant Professor of Medicine, University of Washington, Harborview Medical Center, Seattle, Washington

**Anthony A. Coniglio, PharmD**
Medical Development Coordinator, E. R. Squibb & Sons, U.S., Princeton, New Jersey

**Joel O. Covinsky, PharmD**
Director of Clinical Research, Marion Laboratories, Inc., Kansas City, Missouri

**Brian L. Crabtree, PharmD**
Assistant Professor, School of Pharmacy, University of Mississippi, Jackson, Mississippi

**William R. Crom, PharmD**
Chief, Clinical Programs, Pharmaceutical Division, St. Jude Children's Research Hospital; Associate Professor, Clinical Pharmacy, University of Tennessee, Memphis, Memphis, Tennessee

**Clarence E. Curry, Jr, PharmD**
Associate Professor of Pharmacy Practice, College of Pharmacy and Pharmacal Sciences, Howard University, Washington, DC

**Christina Dalmady-Israel, PharmD**
Assistant Professor of Pharmacy, Medical College of Virginia, Virginia Commonwealth University, Richmond, Virginia

**Larry H. Danziger, PharmD**
Assistant Professor of Pharmacy Practice, College of Pharmacy, University of Illinois, Chicago, Illinois

**Robin L. Davis, PharmD**
Assistant Professor of Pharmacy, College of Pharmacy, University of New Mexico, Albuquerque, New Mexico

**Jeffrey C. Delafuente, MS**
Associate Professor of Pharmacy and Medicine, Colleges of Pharmacy and Medicine, University of Florida, Gainesville, Florida

**Joseph T. DiPiro, PharmD**
Associate Professor, College of Pharmacy, University of Georgia; Associate Clinical Professor of Surgery, Medical College of Georgia, Augusta, Georgia

**Michael Doukas, MD**
Assistant Professor, College of Medicine, University of Kentucky, Lexington, Kentucky

**Nicky Dozier, PharmD**
Assistant Director of Pharmacy Patient Care Services, University of Texas, M. D. Anderson Hospital and Tumor Institute, Houston, Texas

**Michael N. Dudley, PharmD**
Associate Professor of Pharmacy, University of Rhode Island College of Pharmacy; Adjunct Assistant Professor of Medicine, Brown University, Division of Infectious Diseases and Department of Pharmacy, Roger Williams General Hospital, Providence, Rhode Island

**Mary Lou Ebbert-Sauer, PharmD**
Pharmacy Clinical Coordinator, West Suburban Hospital Medical Center, Oak Park, Illinois

**Steven C. Ebert, PharmD**
Assistant Professor of Pharmacy, School of Pharmacy, University of Wisconsin, Madison, Wisconsin

**Larry Ereshefsky, PharmD**
Professor of Pharmacy, Pharmacology, and Psychiatry, College of Pharmacy, University of Texas at Austin, Austin, Texas; University of Texas Health Science Center, San Antonio, Texas

**W. Gary Erwin, PharmD**
Associate Professor of Clinical Pharmacy, Philadelphia College of Pharmacy and Science; Program Administrator, Geriatric Pharmacy Institute, Philadelphia, Pennsylvania

**Martha P. Fankhauser, MS**
Clinical Assistant Professor, Department of Pharmacy Practice, College of Pharmacy; Department of Psychiatry, College of Medicine, University of Arizona, Tucson, Arizona

**Rebecca S. Finley, PharmD, MS**
Assistant Professor of Clinical Pharmacy, University of Maryland Cancer Center/School of Pharmacy, Baltimore, Maryland

**Richard G. Fiscella, RPh, MPH**
Supervisor/Clinical Instructor, College of Pharmacy, University of Illinois, University of Illinois Eye and Ear Infirmary, Chicago, Illinois

**John Fisher, MD**
Associate Professor of Medicine, Infectious Diseases, Department of Infectious Diseases, Medical College of Georgia, Augusta, Georgia

**George E. Francisco, Jr, PharmD**
Associate Dean, University of Georgia, College of Pharmacy, Athens, Georgia

**William R. Friedenberg, MD**
Hematology Department, Marshfield Clinic, Marshfield, Wisconsin

**Gregory G. Gaar, MD**
Co-Medical Director, Florida Poison Information Center; Clinical Assistant Professor of Pediatrics, College of Medicine, University of South Florida, Tampa, Florida

**Peter Gal, PharmD**
Director, Pharmacy Education and Research, Greensboro AHEC, Moses H. Cone Memorial Hospital; Clinical Associate Professor, School of Pharmacy, University of North Carolina, Chapel Hill, North Carolina

**William R. Garnett, PharmD**
Professor, Department of Pharmacy and Pharmaceutics, Medical College of Virginia, Virginia Commonwealth University, Richmond, Virginia

**Mark A. Gill, PharmD**
Associate Professor of Clinical Pharmacy, School of Pharmacy, University of Southern California, Los Angeles, California

**Anne M. Glynn-Barnhart, PharmD**
Assistant Professor of Clinical Pharmacy, College of Pharmacy, University of Colorado, Denver, Colorado

**Barry R. Goldspiel, PharmD**
Clinical Pharmacist, National Cancer Institute, Bethesda, Maryland

**Edgar R. Gonzalez, PharmD**
Assistant Professor of Pharmacy and Pharmaceutics, Director, Critical Care Pharmacy Services, Medical College of Virginia, School of Pharmacy, Richmond, Virginia

**David R.P. Guay, PharmD, FCP**
Assistant Professor, University of Minnesota College of Pharmacy; Clinical Scientist, Drug Evaluation Unit, Hennepin County Medical Center, Minneapolis, Minnesota

**John G. Gums, PharmD**
Assistant Professor of Pharmacy Practice and Medicine, University of Florida, Gainesville, Florida

**Charles Halstenson, PharmD**
Associate Professor, College of Pharmacy, University of Minnesota; Director, Clinical Research, Drug Evaluation Unit, Hennepin County Medical Center, Minneapolis, Minnesota

**Erkan Hassan, PharmD**
Assistant Professor, Department of Clinical Pharmacy, University of Maryland, Baltimore, Maryland

**David W. Hawkins, PharmD**
Associate Professor and Assistant Dean, College of Pharmacy, University of Georgia; Assistant Dean and Clinical Professor of Family Medicine, Medical College of Georgia, Augusta, Georgia

**Peggy E. Hayes, PharmD**
Associate Professor of Pharmacy and Pharmaceutics, Virginia Commonwealth University, Medical College of Virginia, School of Pharmacy, Richmond, Virginia

**Maria G. Hegland, PharmD**
Clinical Pharmacist, Department of Pharmaceutical Services, University of Chicago Hospitals, Chicago, Illinois

**Karen L. Heim-Duthoy, PharmD**
Assistant Professor, University of Minnesota, College of Pharmacy; Clinical Scientist, Drug Evaluation Unit, Hennepin County Medical Center, Minneapolis, Minnesota

**Paul R. Hutson, PharmD**
Assistant Professor, College of Pharmacy, University of Illinois at Chicago, Chicago, Illinois

**Robert J. Ignoffo, PharmD**
Clinical Professor of Pharmacy, University of California Medical Center, San Francisco, California

**Michael Jann, PharmD**
Clinical Associate Professor, Department of Pharmacology, College of Pharmacy, University of Texas at Austin, Austin, Texas, University of Texas Health Science Center, San Antonio, Texas

**B.L. Kasiske, MD**
Clinical Assistant Professor, University of Minnesota School of Medicine; Division of Nephrology, Department of Medicine, Hennepin County Medical Center, Minneapolis, Minnesota

**William F. Keane, MD**
Professor, University of Minnesota School of Medicine and College of Pharmacy; Co-Director, Drug Evaluation Unit, Division of Nephrology, Department of Medicine, Hennepin County Medical Center, Minneapolis, Minnesota

**H. William Kelly, PharmD**
Associate Professor of Pharmacy and Pediatrics, College of Pharmacy and School of Medicine, University of New Mexico, Albuquerque, New Mexico

**Janet L. Kinney-Parker, PharmD**
College of Pharmacy, University of Arizona, Tucson, Arizona

**William R. Kirchain, PharmD**
Assistant Professor of Pharmacy Practice, School of Pharmacy and Allied Health Professions, Creighton University, Omaha, Nebraska

**Cynthia Kristoff Kirkwood, PharmD**
Research Assistant Professor of Pharmacy and Pharmaceutics, Virginia Commonwealth University, Medical College of Virginia, School of Pharmacy, Richmond, Virginia

**Leroy C. Knodel, PharmD**
Assistant Professor, Department of Pharmacology, University of Texas Health Science Center, San Antonio, Texas

**Jim M. Koeller, MS**
Clinical Associate Professor, College of Pharmacy, University of Texas at Austin, Austin, Texas; Clinical Associate Professor, Pharmacology and Medicine, University of Texas Health Science Center, San Antonio; Oncology Clinical Specialist, Audie L. Murphy Memorial Veterans' Hospital, San Antonio, Texas

**John G. Kuhn, PharmD, FCCP**
Associate Professor, College of Pharmacy, University of Texas at Austin, Austin, Texas

**Tom A. Larson, PharmD**
Associate Professor, College of Pharmacy, University of Minnesota, Minneapolis, Minnesota

**John A. Lazor, PharmD**
Senior Pharmacokineticist, Division of Biopharmaceutics, Food and Drug Administration, Rockville, Maryland

**Mark E. Lehman, PharmD**
Associate Director of Pharmacy Services, Medical College of Virginia Hospital; Assistant Professor, Department of Pharmacy and Pharmaceutics, School of Pharmacy, Virginia Commonwealth University, Richmond, Virginia

**Thomas Leither, MS**
Nephrologist, St. Cloud Clinic of Internal Medicine, St. Cloud, Minnesota

**Thomas P. Lennon, PharmD**
Branch Manager, New England Critical Care, Seattle, Washington

**Timothy S. Lesar, PharmD**
Assistant Director of Pharmacy, Albany Medical Center Hospital, Albany, New York

**R. Leon Longe, PharmD**
Associate Professor, The University of Georgia; Associate Clinical Professor, Medical College of Georgia, Augusta, Georgia

**John A. Mansberger, MD**
Consulting Surgeon, Archbold Medical Center, Thomasville, Georgia

**Gary R. Matzke, PharmD, FCP, FCCP**
Professor, University of Minnesota, College of Pharmacy; Co-Director, Drug Evaluation Unit, Hennepin County Medical Center, Minneapolis, Minnesota

**J. Russell May, PharmD**
Assistant Director of Pharmacy for Clinical Services, Medical College of Georgia Hospital and Clinics; Adjunct Associate Professor, College of Pharmacy, University of Georgia, Augusta, Georgia

**Janet McCombs, PharmD**
Clinical Pharmacy Associate, College of Pharmacy, University of Georgia, Athens, Georgia

**Timothy R. McGuire, PharmD**
Clinical Pharmacy Fellow, University of Florida, Gainesville, Florida

**Katherine A. Michael, PharmD**
Assistant Professor, Medical University of South Carolina, Charleston, South Carolina

**Julie B. Milstein, PhD**
Research Chemist, Office of Epidemiology and Biostatistics, Food and Drug Administration, Rockville, Maryland

**Jay M. Mirtallo, MS**
Clinical Pharmacist, Nutrition Support, Ohio State University Hospitals, Columbus, Ohio

**Timothy Mullenix, MS**
Assistant Professor, College of Pharmacy, University of South Carolina, Columbia, South Carolina

**Christopher P. Murphy, PharmD**
Clinical Pharmacy Coordinator, Bone Marrow Transplantation, Wilford Hall, USAF Medical Center, Lackland Air Force Base, Texas

**Milap C. Nahata, PharmD**
Associate Professor of Pharmacy and Pediatrics, Colleges of Pharmacy and Medicine, Ohio State University and Children's Hospital, Columbus, Ohio

**Warren A. Narducci, PharmD**
Assistant Professor and Chairman, Department of Pharmacy Practice, College of Pharmacy, University of Nebraska, Omaha, Nebraska

**Sven A. Normann, PharmD**
Administrative Director, Florida Poison Information Center, Tampa General Hospital, Tampa, Florida

**Paul R. O'Dea, RPh**
Pharmacist, Jules Stein Eye Institute, University of California at Los Angeles, Los Angeles, California

**John A. Opsahl, MD**
Clinical Assistant Professor, University of Minnesota, School of Medicine and College of Pharmacy; Division of Nephrology, Department of Medicine, Hennepin County Medical Center, Minneapolis, Minnesota

**Michael D. Parr, PharmD**
Assistant Professor, College of Pharmacy, University of Kentucky, Lexington, Kentucky

**L. Michael Posey**
President, Pharmacy/Association Services; Editor, *The Consultant Pharmacist* and *Clinical Laboratory Science*, Arlington, Virginia

**Randall A. Prince, PharmD**
Associate Professor, College of Pharmacy, University of Iowa, Iowa City, Iowa

**Richard J. Ptachcinski, PharmD**
Associate Professor of Pharmacy Practice, University of Pittsburgh, Pittsburgh, Pennsylvania

**Christine M. Quandt, PharmD**
College of Pharmacy, University of Texas, Austin, Texas

**Robert P. Rapp, PharmD**
Professor of Pharmacy, College of Pharmacy, University of Kentucky, Lexington, Kentucky

**Kenneth E. Record, PharmD**
Associate Professor, College of Pharmacy, University of Kentucky, Lexington, Kentucky

**Michael D. Reed, PharmD**
Associate Professor of Pediatrics, Division of Pediatric Pharmacology and Critical Care, School of Medicine, Case Western Reserve University, Department of Pediatrics, Cleveland, Ohio

**Dennis H. Robinson, PhD**
Assistant Professor of Pharmaceutical Sciences, College of Pharmacy, University of Nebraska, Omaha, Nebraska

**Keith A. Rodvold, PharmD**
Assistant Professor, College of Pharmacy, University of Illinois at Chicago, Chicago, Illinois

**Raylene Rospond, PharmD**
Clinical Assistant Professor, Department of Pharmacy, College of Pharmacy, University of Texas at Austin, Austin, Texas; University of Texas Health Science Center, San Antonio, Texas

**John C. Rotschafer, PharmD**
Associate Professor, College of Pharmacy, University of Minnesota, Minneapolis, Minnesota

**Jean A. Rumsfield, PharmD**
Clinical Assistant Professor, University of Illinois at Chicago Health Science Center, Chicago, Illinois

**Nathan J. Schultz, PharmD**
Director of Clinical Pharmacy, Abbott/Northwestern Hospital, Minneapolis, Minnesota

**Arthur A. Schuna, MS**
Clinical Pharmacy Coordinator, William S. Middleton Memorial Veterans' Hospital; Clinical Associate Professor, School of Pharmacy, University of Wisconsin, Madison, Wisconsin

**John Siepler, PharmD**
Department of Pharmacy, University of California, Davis Medical Center, Sacramento, California

**Ember A. Skidmore, PharmD**
Fellow in Geriatrics, Philadelphia College of Pharmacy and Science, Philadelphia, Pennsylvania

**Charles Lee Smith, MD**
Assistant Professor of Medicine, University of Minnesota School of Medicine, Division of Nephrology, Department of Medicine, Hennepin County Medical Center, Minneapolis, Minnesota

**Marie A. Smith, PharmD**
Director of Clinical Affairs, American Society of Hospital Pharmacists, Bethesda, Maryland

**William J. Spruill, PharmD**
Associate Professor, Pharmacy Practice, College of Pharmacy, University of Georgia, Athens, Georgia

**Robert J. Stagg, PharmD**
Assistant Clinical Professor of Pharmacy, University of California Medical Center, San Francisco, California

**Irving Steinberg, PharmD**
Assistant Professor, School of Pharmacy, University of Southern California, Los Angeles, California

**Clinton F. Stewart, PharmD**
Assistant Professor, University of Tennessee, Memphis, Memphis, Tennessee

**Glen L. Stimmel, PharmD**
Professor of Clinical Pharmacy and Psychiatry, Schools of Pharmacy and Medicine, University of Southern California, Los Angeles, California

**Mark A. Stratton, PharmD**
Associate Professor, College of Pharmacy, University of New Mexico, Albuquerque, New Mexico

**Edward Sypniewski, Jr, PharmD**
Assistant Professor of Pharmacy, Medical College of Virginia, Virginia Commonwealth University, Richmond, Virginia

**Robert L. Talbert, PharmD**
Professor, College of Pharmacy, University of Texas at Austin, Austin, Texas; Professor, Departments of Pharmacology and Medicine, University of Texas Health Science Center at San Antonio, San Antonio, Texas

**Teresa A. Tartaglione, PharmD**
Assistant Professor of Pharmacy, University of Washington, Harborview Medical Center, Seattle, Washington

**A. Thomas Taylor, PharmD**
Associate Professor, College of Pharmacy, University of Georgia; Associate Clinical Professor, Department of Family Medicine, Medical College of Georgia, Augusta, Georgia

**Jerry W. Taylor, PharmD**
Associate Professor, School of Pharmacy, University of Mississippi, Jackson, Mississippi

**Kathleen M. Teasley, MS**
Associate Professor, College of Pharmacy, University of Minnesota, Minneapolis, Minnesota

**Mary E. Teresi, PharmD**
Assistant Professor, Division of Clinical Hospital Pharmacy, College of Pharmacy, University of Iowa, Iowa City, Iowa

**Thomas F. Turco, PharmD**
Drug Information Specialist, University of Maryland Medical Services, Department of Pharmacy Services, Baltimore, Maryland

**Wayne M. Turner, PharmD**
Reviewing Pharmacist, Office of Orphan Drug Development, Food and Drug Administration, Rockville, Maryland

**Clarence T. Ueda, PharmD, PhD**
Professor of Pharmaceutical Sciences and Dean, College of Pharmacy, University of Nebraska, Omaha, Nebraska

**Jeanne Hawkins Van Tyle, PharmD, MS**
College of Pharmacy, Butler University, Indianapolis, Indiana

**Beth D. Vejraska, PharmD**
Clinical Pharmacist, Rochester Medical Group Associates, Rochester, New York

**Raman Venkataramanan, PhD**
Associate Professor of Pharmaceutical Sciences, University of Pittsburgh, Pittsburgh, Pennsylvania

**William E. Wade, PharmD**
Assistant Professor, Pharmacy Practice, College of Pharmacy, University of Georgia, Athens, Georgia

**Mary Jane Watson, PharmD**
Medical Research Specialist, Minnesota Clinical Study Center, Minneapolis, Minnesota

**Lynda S. Welage, PharmD**
Program Director, Critical Care, Clinical Pharmacokinetics Laboratory, Millard Fillmore Hospital, Buffalo, New York

**Barbara G. Wells, PharmD**
Associate Professor and Director, Mental Health Pharmacy Programs, College of Pharmacy, University of Tennessee, Memphis, Tennessee

**Dennis P. West, MS, FCCP**
Associate Professor, University of Illinois at Chicago Health Science Center, Chicago, Illinois

**Michael S. Willett, PharmD**
Clinical Pharmacist, Wesley Long Community Hospital, Greensboro, North Carolina

**Michael Z. Wincor, PharmD**
Assistant Professor of Clinical Pharmacy, School of Pharmacy, University of Southern California, Los Angeles, California

**Madolin K. Witte, MD**
Assistant Professor of Pediatrics, Division of Pediatric Pulmonology, Department of Pediatrics, University of Utah Medical Center, Salt Lake City, Utah

**Dabney Yarbrough III, MD**
Professor of Surgery, Director, Burn and Trauma Unit, Medical University of South Carolina, Charleston, South Carolina

**Gary C. Yee, PharmD**
Associate Professor, Department of Pharmacy Practice, University of Florida College of Pharmacy, Gainesville, Florida

**Sharon L. Young, PharmD**
Assistant Professor of Clinical Pharmacy, Philadelphia College of Pharmacy and Science, Philadelphia, Pennsylvania

**Humphrey Z. Zokufa, PharmD**
Research Fellow, College of Pharmacy, University of Minnesota, Minneapolis, Minnesota

# 1 Basic Concepts of Pathophysiology and Pharmacotherapy

# *Chapter 1* / Clinical Pharmacokinetics and Individualization of Drug Therapy

Larry A. Bauer, PharmD

Pharmacokinetic concepts have been used successfully to individualize patient drug therapy. Laboratories routinely measure patient serum or plasma samples for many drugs including antibiotics (aminoglycosides, chloramphenicol), theophylline, antiepileptics (phenytoin, phenobarbital, ethosuximide, carbamazepine), methotrexate, lithium, and antiarrhythmics (lidocaine, procainamide, quinidine, digoxin). With a knowledge of the disease states and conditions that influence the disposition of a particular drug, kinetic concepts can be used to modify doses to produce serum drug concentrations that result in desirable pharmacologic effects but avoid unwanted side effects. The narrow range of concentrations within which the pharmacologic response is produced and the adverse effects prevented in the majority of patients is the therapeutic range of the drug (Table 1.1). Although most individuals experience favorable effects with serum drug concentrations in the therapeutic range, there is much interpatient variability in the effect of a given serum drug concentration. Clinicians should never assume that a serum concentration within the therapeutic range is safe and effective for every patient. The response to the drug, such as number of seizures a patient experiences while taking an antiepileptic agent, should always be assessed when serum concentrations are measured. Commonly used abbreviations are shown in Table 1.2.

## Clinical Pharmacokinetics

Clinical pharmacokinetics is the discipline that describes the absorption, distribution, metabolism, and elimination of drugs in patients requiring drug therapy. When a drug is administered extravascularly to patients, it must be absorbed across biologic membranes to reach the systemic circulation. If the drug is given orally, the drug molecules must pass through the gastrointestinal tract wall where they eventually enter capillaries. In the case of transdermal patches, the drug must penetrate the skin before it enters the vascular system. In general, the pharmacologic effect of the drug is delayed when it is given extravascularly because it takes time for the drug to be absorbed into the body.

After the drug reaches the systemic circulation it can leave the vasculature and penetrate the various tissues or remain in the blood. If the drug remains in the blood it may bind to endogenous proteins such as albumin or $\alpha_1$-acid glycoprotein. In most cases, the binding is reversible and equilibrium exists between protein-bound drug and unbound drug. Unbound drug in the blood provides the driving force for distribution of the agent to body tissues. If unbound drug leaves the bloodstream and distributes to tissue it may become tissue bound, it may remain unbound in the tissue, or, if the tissue can metabolize or eliminate the drug, it may be rendered inactive or be eliminated from the body. If the drug becomes tissue bound, it may bind to the receptor that causes its pharmacologic or toxic effect or to a nonspecific binding site that causes no effect. Again, tissue binding is usually reversible so that the tissue-bound drug is in equilibrium with unbound drug in the tissue.

Certain organs such as the liver and lung possess enzymes that metabolize drugs. The resulting metabolite may be inactive or have a pharmacologic effect of its own. The blood also contains esterases that break ester bonds in drug molecules and render them inactive. Drug metabolism usually occurs in the liver and can be classified in two categories. Phase I reactions generally make the drug molecule more polar and water soluble so that it is prone to elimination by the kidney; the chemical modifications include oxidation, hydrolysis, and reduction. Phase II reactions involve conjugation to form glucuronides, acetates, or sulfates.

Other organs have the ability to eliminate drugs or metabolites from the body. The kidney can excrete drugs by glomerular filtration or by such active processes as proximal tubular secretion. Drugs can also be eliminated via bile produced by the liver or air expired by the lungs.

### *Concepts*

Most drugs follow linear pharmacokinetics. Linear pharmacokinetics exists when serum drug concentrations change proportionally with chronic drug dosing. As an example, if the drug dose were doubled from 300 to 600 mg/d, the patient's serum drug concentration would also double.

When a drug is given by continuous intravenous infusion, serum concentrations increase until an equilibrium is established between the drug dosage rate and the rate of drug elimination. Serum concentrations level off and remain constant when the rate of drug administration equals the rate of drug elimination (Fig. 1.1). For example, if a patient were receiving a continuous intravenous infusion at 40 mg/h, the serum drug concentration would increase until the patient's body was eliminating the drug at 40 mg/h. When serum drug concentrations reach a constant value, steady state is achieved. If the drug is given at intermittent dosage intervals, such as 250 mg every 6 hours, steady state is achieved when the serum concentration-versus-time curves for each dosage interval are superimposable. The amount of drug eliminated during the dosage interval equals the dose.

**Table 1.1** Selected Therapeutic Ranges

| *Drug* | *Therapeutic Range* |
|---|---|
| Digoxin | 0.9–2 ng/mL |
| Lidocaine | 1.5–5 μg/mL |
| Procainamide/*N*-acetyl-procainamide | 10–30 μg/mL |
| Quinidine | 2–5 μg/mL |
| Amikacin | 20–30 μg/mL (peak)<br>< 5 μg/mL (trough) |
| Gentamicin, tobramycin, netilmicin | 5–10 μg/mL (peak)<br>< 2 μg/mL (trough) |
| Chloramphenicol | 10–20 μg/mL |
| Lithium | 0.6–1.4 mEq/L |
| Carbamazepine | 4–12 μg/mL |
| Ethosuximide | 40–100 μg/mL |
| Phenobarbital | 15–40 μg/mL |
| Phenytoin | 10–20 μg/mL |
| Primidone | 5–12 μg/mL |
| Valproic acid | 50–100 μg/mL |
| Theophylline | 10–20 μg/mL |

**Table 1.2** Pharmacokinetic Abbreviations

| *Abbreviation* | *Definition* |
|---|---|
| CL | Clearance |
| $k_0$ | Intravenous infusion rate |
| $C_{ss}$ | Steady-state concentration |
| $D$ | Dose |
| $\tau$ | Dosage interval |
| $F$ | Fracton of drug absorbed into the systemic circulation |
| $Q$ | Blood flow |
| $E$ | Extraction ratio |
| $C_{out}$ | Concentration of drug in blood coming out of an organ |
| $C_{in}$ | Concentration of drug in blood going into an organ |
| $f_b$ | Fraction of drug in the blood that is unbound |
| $f_t$ | Fraction of drug in the tissues that is unbound |
| $CL'_{int}$ | Intrinsic clearance |
| $C_{ss,u}$ | Steady-state concentration of unbound drug |
| $V_D$ | Volume of distribution |
| LD | Loading dose |
| MD | Maintenance dose |
| $V_b$ | Volume of blood |
| $V_t$ | Volume of tissue |
| $t_{1/2}$ | Half-life |
| $A_i$ | *y* intercept of *i*th line |
| $k_i$ | Rate constant for *i*th line |
| $k$ | Elimination rate constant |
| $k_a$ | Absorption rate constant |
| $\alpha$ | Distribution rate constant |
| $\beta$ | Terminal rate constant |
| $V_{D,\beta}$ | $V_D$ during $\beta$ phase of curve |
| $V_{D,ss}$ | $V_D$ at steady state |
| $k_{12}$, $k_{21}$, $k_{10}$ | Microconstants |
| $t'$ | Postinfusion time |
| $T$ | Duration of infusion |
| AUC | Area under serum or blood concentration-versus-time curve |
| AUMC | Area under the first moment curve |
| $C_{last}$ | Last serum or blood concentration |
| $t_{last}$ | Time at which $C_{last}$ was obtained |
| $V_{max}$ | Maximum rate of drug metabolism |
| $K_m$ | Serum concentration at which the rate of metabolism equals $V_{max}/2$ |
| $C_{max}$ | Maximum serum or blood concentration |
| $C_{min}$ | Minimum serum or blood concentration |
| DR | Dosage rate |
| $C_{est}$ | Estimated serum or blood concentration |
| $C_{act}$ | Actual serum or blood concentration |

### Clearance

Clearance (CL) is the most important pharmacokinetic parameter because it determines the steady-state concentration for a given dosage rate. When a drug is given at a continuous intravenous infusion rate equal to $k_0$, the steady-state concentration ($C_{ss}$) is determined by the quotient of $k_0$ and CL ($C_{ss} = k_0/\text{CL}$). If the drug is given as individual doses ($D$) at a fixed dosage interval ($\tau$), the average steady-state concentration ($C_{ss}$) over the dosage interval is given by the equation[1] $C_{ss} = F(D/\tau)/\text{CL}$, where $F$ is the fraction of dose absorbed into the systemic vascular system. The average steady-state concentration over the dosage interval is the steady-state concentration that would have occurred had the same dose been give as a continuous intravenous infusion (e.g., 300 mg every 6 hours at an infusion rate of 50 mg/h).

Physiologically, clearance is determined by blood flow ($Q$) to the organ that metabolizes or eliminates the drug and the efficiency of the organ in extracting the drug from the bloodstream.[2] Efficiency is measured using an extraction ratio ($E$) that is calculated by subtracting the concentration in the blood leaving the extracting organ ($C_{out}$) from the concentration in the blood entering the organ ($C_{in}$) and then dividing the result by $C_{in}$: $E = (C_{in} - C_{out})/C_{in}$. Clearance for that organ is calculated by taking the product of $Q$ and $E$: $\text{CL} = QE$. For example, if liver blood flow equals 1.5 L/min and the drug's extraction ratio is 0.33, hepatic clearance equals 0.5 L/min. Total clearance is computed by summing all of the individual organ clearance values. Clearance changes occur in patients when the blood flow to extracting organs changes or when the extraction ratio changes. Vasodilators like hydralazine increase liver blood flow, whereas congestive heart failure and hypotension can decrease hepatic blood flow. Extraction ratios can increase when enzyme inducers increase the amount of drug-metabolizing enzyme. Extraction ratios may decrease if enzyme inhibitors inhibit drug-metabolizing enzymes or necrosis causes loss of parenchyma.

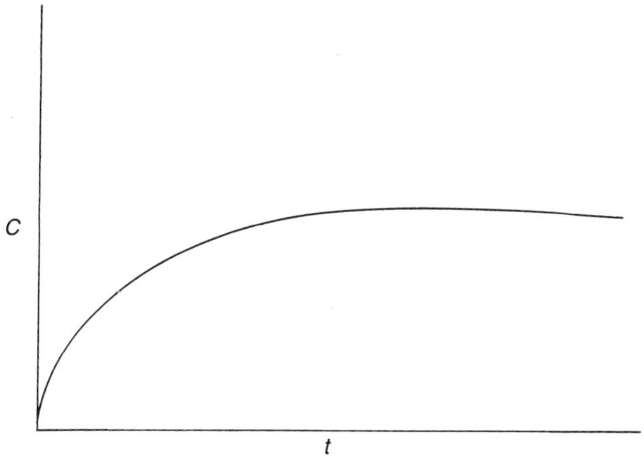

**Figure 1.1** Normal serum concentration–time curve following a continuous IV infusion.

### Intrinsic Clearance

The extraction ratio can also be thought of in terms of unbound drug in the blood ($f_b$), the intrinsic ability of the extracting organ to clear unbound drug from the blood ($CL'_{int}$), and blood flow to the organ ($Q$)[3,4]: $E = f_b\ CL'_{int}/(Q + f_b CL'_{int})$. In this case the clearance equation becomes $CL = Qf_b\ CL'_{int}/(Q + f_b\ CL'_{int})$. Clearance changes occur when blood flow to the clearing organ changes (e.g., shock, congestive heart failure, vasodilators), binding in the blood changes (e.g., protein binding displacement), or intrinsic clearance of unbound drug changes (e.g., enzyme inhibition or induction).

If $CL'_{int}$ is large (i.e., enzymes have a large capacity to metabolize the drug), the product of $f_b$ and $CL'_{int}$ is much larger than $Q$. When $f_b\ CL'_{int}$ is much greater then $Q$, the sum of $Q$ and $f_b CL'_{int}$ in the denominator of the clearance equation almost equals $f_b\ CL'_{int}$: $f_b\ CL'_{int} = Q + f_b\ CL'_{int}$. Substituting this expression in the denominator of the clearance equation and canceling common terms lead to the following expression for drugs with a large $CL'_{int}$: $CL = Q$. In this case the clearance of the drug is equal to blood flow to the organ; such drugs are called "high-clearance" drugs and have large extraction ratios. Propranolol, verapamil, morphine, and lidocaine are high-clearance drugs.

If $CL'_{int}$ is small (i.e., enzymes have a limited capacity to metabolize the drug), $Q$ is much larger than the product of $f_b$ and $CL'_{int}$. When $Q$ is much greater than $f_b CL'_{int}$, the sum of $Q$ and $f_b CL'_{int}$ in the denominator of the clearance equation almost equals $Q$: $Q \approx Q + f_b CL'_{int}$. Substituting this expression in the denominator of the clearance equation and canceling common terms lead to the following expression for drugs with a small $CL'_{int}$: $CL \approx f_b\ CL'_{int}$. In this case, clearance of the drug is equal to the product of the fraction unbound in the blood and the intrinsic ability of the organ to clear unbound drug from the blood; such drugs are known as "low-clearance" drugs and have small extraction ratios. Warfarin, theophylline, diazepam, and phenobarbital are low-clearance drugs.

As previously mentioned the concentration of unbound drug in the blood is probably more important than total (bound + unbound) concentration. The unbound drug in the blood is in equilibrium with the unbound drug in the tissues and reflects the concentration of drug at its site of action. Therefore, the pharmacologic effect of a drug is thought to be proportional to the concentration of unbound drug in the blood. The unbound steady-state concentration ($C_{ss,u}$) can be calculated by multiplying $C_{ss}$ by $f_b$.

The effect that changes in $Q$, $f_b$, and $CL'_{int}$ have on $C_{ss,u}$ and the pharmacologic response of a drug depends on whether the drug is a high- or low-clearance drug. For a high-clearance drug, $CL = Q$. A change in $f_b$ or $CL'_{int}$ does not change CL or $C_{ss}$ ($C_{ss} = k_0/CL$); however, a change in $f_b$ does alter $C_{ss,u}$ ($C_{ss,u} = f_b C_{ss}$) and the pharmacologic response. This type of plasma protein binding displacement drug interaction is the most hazardous because the changes in $C_{ss,u}$ are not reflected in changes in $C_{ss}$. Laboratories usually measure only total concentrations because concentrations of unbound drug are difficult to determine. This makes the interaction hard to detect. If $CL'_{int}$ changes for a high-clearance drug, CL, $C_{ss}$, $C_{ss,u}$, and pharmacologic response do not change. Changes in $Q$ cause a change in CL; changes in $C_{ss}$, $C_{ss,u}$, and drug response are indirectly proportional to changes in CL.

For low-clearance drugs, $CL = f_b CL'_{int}$. A change in $Q$ does not change CL, $C_{ss}$, $C_{ss,u}$, or pharmacologic response; however, a change in $f_b$ or $CL'_{int}$ does alter CL and $C_{ss}$ ($C_{ss} = k_0/CL$). Changes in $CL'_{int}$ cause a proportional change in CL; changes in $C_{ss}$, $C_{ss,u}$, and drug response are indirectly proportional to changes in CL. Altering $f_b$ for low-clearance drugs produces interesting results. A change in $f_b$ alters CL and $C_{ss}$ ($C_{ss} = k_0/CL$). As CL and $C_{ss}$ change in opposite directions with changes in $f_b$, $C_{ss,u}$ ($C_{ss,u} = f_b C_{ss}$) and pharmacologic response do not change with alterations in the fraction of unbound drug in the blood. For example, a low-clearance drug is administered to a patient until steady state is achieved ($CL = f_b CL'_{int}$, $C_{ss} = k_0/CL$). Another drug is administered to the patient that displaces the first drug from plasma protein binding sites and doubles $f_b$ ($f_b$ now equals $2f_b$). CL doubles because of the protein binding displacement ($2CL = 2f_b CL'_{int}$), and $C_{ss}$ decreases by one half because of the change in clearance: $C_{ss}/2 = k_0/2CL$. $C_{ss,u}$ does not change because even though $f_b$ is doubled, $C_{ss}$ decreased by one half: $C_{ss,u} = f_b C_{ss}$. The potential for error in this situation is that clinicians may increase the dose of a low-clearance drug after a protein binding displacement interaction because $C_{ss}$ decreased; however, as $C_{ss,u}$ and the pharmacologic effect do not change, the dose should remain unaltered.

### Volume of Distribution

The volume of distribution ($V_D$) is a proportionality constant that relates the amount of drug in the body to the serum concentration (amount in body $= CV_D$). $V_D$ is used to calculate the loading dose (LD) of a drug that will immediately achieve a desired $C_{ss}$: $LD = C_{ss}V_D$; however, in practice the patient's own $V_D$ is not known at the time the loading dose is administered. In this case an average $V_D$ is assumed and used to calculate a loading dose. As the patient's $V_D$ is almost always different from the average $V_D$ for the drug, a loading dose does not attain $C_{ss}$ but, hopefully, achieves a therapeutic concentration. The numeric value for the volume of distribution is determined by the physiologic volume of blood and tissues and how the drug binds in blood and tissues[5]: $V_D = V_b + (f_b/f_t)V_t$, where $V_b$ and $V_t$ are the volumes of blood and tissues, respectively, and $f_b$ and $f_t$ are the fractions of unbound drug in blood and tissues, respectively.

### Half-Life

Half-life ($t_{1/2}$) is the time required for serum concentrations to decrease by one half after distribution and absorption are complete. It takes the same amount of time for serum concentrations to drop from 200 to 100 mg/L as it does for concentrations to decline from 2 to 1 mg/L. Half-life is important because it determines the time required to reach steady state and the dosage interval. It takes approximately three to five half-lives to reach steady-state concentrations during continuous dosing. In three half-lives, serum concentrations are about 90% of their ultimate steady-state values. As most serum drug assays have about a 10% error, it is difficult to differentiate concentrations that are within 10% of each other. For this reason, many clinicians consider concentrations obtained after three half-lives to be steady-state concentrations. Half-life is also used to determine the dosage interval for a drug. For instance, it may be desirable to maintain maximum steady-state concentrations at 20 μg/mL and minimum steady-state concentrations at 10 μg/mL. In this case it would be necessary to administer the drug every one half-life, as the minimum desirable concentration is one half the maximum desirable concentration. Half-life is a dependent kinetic variable because its value depends on the values of CL and $V_D$.[5] The equation that describes the relationship among three variables is $t_{1/2} = 0.693V_D/\mathrm{CL}$. Changes in half-life can result from a change in either $V_D$ or CL; a change in half-life does not necessarily indicate that CL has changed. Half-life can change solely because of changes in $V_D$.

## *Deterministic Models*

Pharmacokinetic models are useful to describe data sets, predict serum concentrations after several doses or different routes of administration, and calculate pharmacokinetic constants such as CL, $V_D$, and $t_{1/2}$.[6] Two methods have been devised to accomplish these goals. In the first, multiexponential equations are used to describe the data. The other method uses compartmental models that depict the body as one or more discrete compartments to which drug is distributed and/or from which drug is eliminated. In both cases the shape of the serum concentration-versus-time curve determines the number of exponents in the equation or the number of compartments in the model. Hence the term *deterministic model.*

### Exponential Equations

In serum concentration-versus-time graphs concentrations often appear to change according to an exponential equation of the form $C = \Sigma_{i=1}^{n}(A_i\ e^{-k_it})$, where $C$ is the serum concentration at any time $t$ and $A_i$ is the $y$ intercept of the $i$th line with a slope equal to $-k_i/2.303$. CL, $V_D$, and $t_{1/2}$ can easily be calculated using the $A_i$ and $k_i$ values of the individual lines.[7,8]

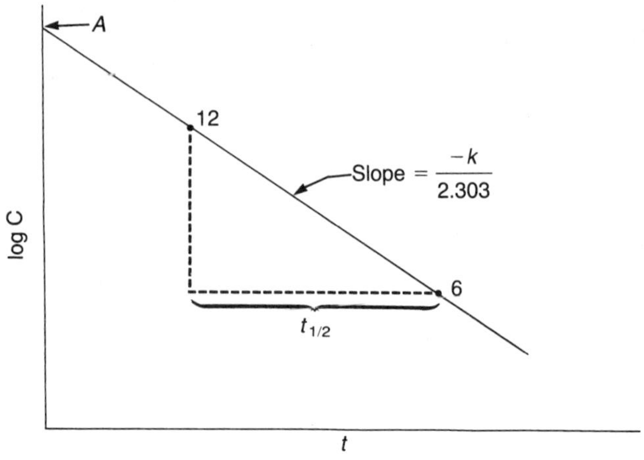


**Figure 1.2** Calculation of the half-life of a drug following intravenous bolus dosing.

*Monoexponential Equations* The simplest situation occurs when the logarithms of the serum concentrations after a single intravenous bolus decline in a straight line with time (Fig. 1.2). In this case the equation that describes the data is $C = Ae^{-kt}$. $A$ is obtained from the graph by extrapolating the line back to the $y$ intercept. The terminal elimination rate constant ($k$) can be computed using the slope of the line: slope $= -k/2.303$. Alternately, $t_{1/2}$ can be obtained from the graph by determining the time it takes for serum concentrations to decrease by one half and the following formula can be used to compute $k$: $k = 0.693/t_{1/2}$. CL and $V_D$ are calculated using the equations $\mathrm{CL} = D/(A/k)$ and $V_D = \mathrm{CL}/k$.[9–11]

More complex situations occur when drugs are given by different routes of administration. When a dose is given extravascularly, serum concentrations usually increase while the drug is being absorbed, reach a maximum concentration ($C_{max}$), and then decline in a straight line when plotted on semilogarithmic coordinates (Fig. 1.3). The multiexponential equation that describes this data set is $C = Ae^{-kt} - Ae^{-k_at}$, where $k$ is the terminal rate constant (slope $= -k/2.303$), $A$ is the $y$ intercept of the terminal slope, $k_a$ is the absorption rate constant, and $t$ is time. This equation represents the difference between two lines. When plotted on semilogarithmic paper, the first line has a $y$ intercept of $A$ and a slope equal to $-k/2.303$. The other line has the same $y$ intercept ($A$) but a slope equal to $-k_a/2.303$. The method of residuals is used to obtain the slopes and intercepts of the two lines (Fig. 1.2). $A$ is determined by extrapolating the terminal slope to the $y$ axis; $k$ can be obtained by calculating the slope or half-life and using the formulas given for the intravenous bolus case. At each time point in the absorption portion of the curve, the concentration value from the extrapolated line is noted and called the extrapolated concentration. For each point the actual concentration is subtracted from the extrapolated concentration to compute the residual concentration. When the residual concentrations are plotted on semilogarithmic coordinates, a line with $y$ intercept equal to $A$ and slope equal to $-k_a/2.303$ is obtained. When these values are calculated, they can be placed into the equation $C = Ae^{-kt} - Ae^{-k_at}$ and used to compute the

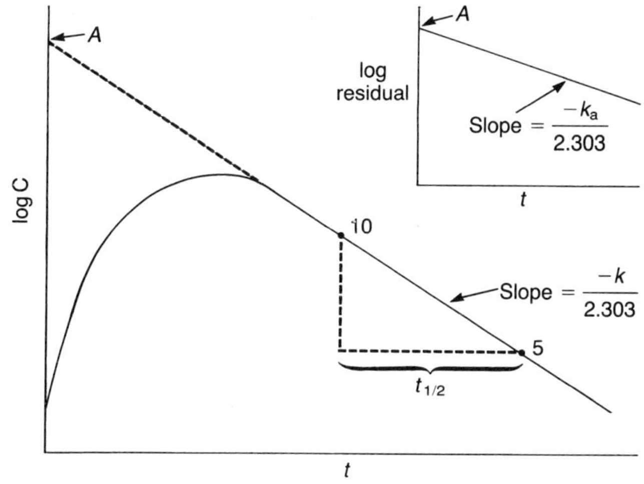


**Figure 1.3** Calculation of the half-life of a drug following oral, intramuscular, or other extravascular dosing route.

serum concentration at any time after the extravascular dose. The slopes and rate constants can also be used to compute CL and $V_D$: CL = $FD/(A/k - A/k_a)$ and $V_D$ = CL/$k$, where $F$ is the fraction of the dose absorbed into the systemic circulation.

***Continuous Intravenous Infusion*** During a continuous intravenous infusion, $C_{ss}$ is achieved after three to five half-lives (Fig. 1.4). $C_{ss}$ is used to calculate CL: CL = $k_0/C_{ss}$. If the infusion is discontinued, $k$ and $t_{1/2}$ can be calculated from the terminal slope. The volume of distribution is computed once CL and $k$ are known: $V_D$ = CL/$k$.

***Multiexponential Equations*** After an intravenous bolus dose, serum concentrations often decline in two or more phases. During the early phase(s), drug leaves the bloodstream, distributes into tissues, and is metabolized and eliminated. Because the drug is leaving the bloodstream through these three mechanisms, serum concentrations decline rapidly. After tissues and blood are in equilibrium, only metabolism and elimination remove drug from the blood. During this terminal phase, serum concentrations decline more slowly. The half-life is measured during the terminal phase by determining the time required for concentrations to decline by one half.

***Biexponential Equations*** For the simplest case the serum concentration-versus-time curve decreases in two phases and is described by the equation $C = Ae^{-\alpha t} + Be^{-\beta t}$, where $\beta$ is computed from the terminal slope (slope = $\beta$/2.303 or $\beta$ = 0.693/$t_{1/2}$) and is called the terminal rate constant, $B$ is the $y$ intercept of the terminal extrapolated line, $\alpha$ is computed from the slope of the residual line, and $A$ is the $y$ intercept of the residual line (Fig. 1.5).

The residual line is calculated as before using the method of residuals. The terminal line is extrapolated to the $y$ axis, and extrapolated concentrations are determined for each time point. As actual concentrations are greater in this case, residual concentrations are calculated by subtracting the

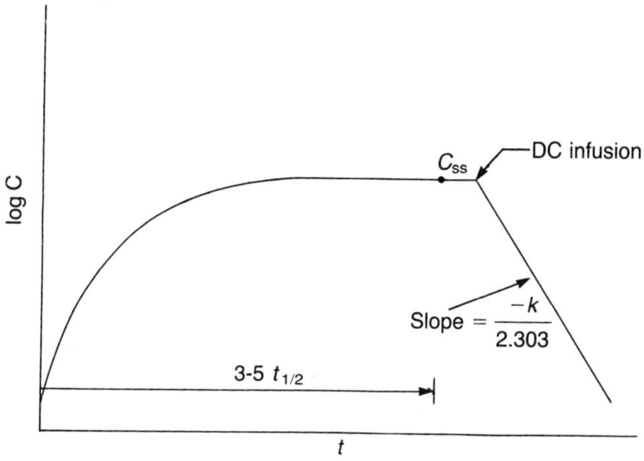


**Figure 1.4** Achievement of steady-state serum concentrations of three to five half-lives of a drug. Note the elimination phase after discontinuance of the infusion.

extrapolated concentrations from the actual concentrations. When plotted on semilogarithmic paper the residual line has a $y$ intercept equal to $A$. The slope of the residual line is used to compute $\alpha$ (slope = $-\alpha$/2.303). With the rate constants $\alpha$ and $\beta$ and the intercepts $A$ and $B$, concentrations can be calculated for any time after the intravenous bolus dose ($C = Ae^{-\alpha t} + Be^{-\beta t}$) or pharmacokinetic constants can be computed (CL = $D/(A/\alpha + B/\beta)$, $V_{D,\beta}$ = CL/$\beta$, $V_{D,ss}$ = $[D(A/A^2 + B/\beta^2)]/(A/\alpha + B/\beta)^2$).

***Volumes of Distribution in Multiexponential Equations*** Two different $V_D$ values are needed as proportionality constants for drugs that require multiexponential equations to describe the serum concentration-versus-time curve. The $V_D$ that is used to compute the amount of drug in the body during the terminal ($\beta$) portion of the curve is called $V_{D,\beta}$ (amount of

**Figure 1.5** Calculation of $\alpha$ and $\beta$ half-lives following intravenous dosing.

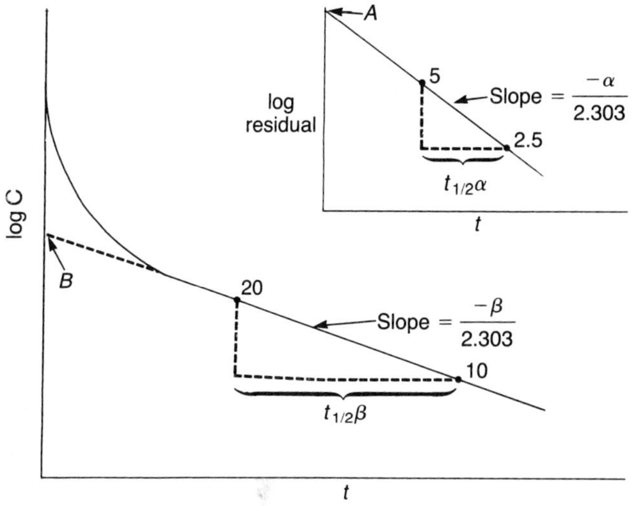

drug in body = $V_{D,\beta}C$). During a continuous intravenous infusion at steady state, $V_{D,ss}$ is used to compute the amount of drug in the body (amount of drug in body = $V_{D,ss}C_{ss}$). $V_{D,ss}$ is also the volume of distribution that can be computed using the physiologic volumes of blood and tissues and the ratio of unbound drug in blood to that in tissues: $V_{D,ss} = V_b + (f_b/f_t)\ V_t$. Because the value of $V_{D,\beta}$ changes when CL changes, $V_{D,ss}$ should be used to indicate if drug distribution changes during pharmacokinetic experiments.

**Compartmental Models**

Compartmental models can also be used to describe pharmacokinetic data sets.[12,13] As mentioned previously, these models depict the body as one or more compartments from which drug is eliminated and/or to which drug is distributed (Fig. 1.6). First-order rate constants, known as microconstants, describe the rate of transfer from one compartment to another. Each compartment also has its own volume of distribution. In all situations, the equations derived from compartmental models are very similar to those derived using intercepts and rate constants.

***One-Compartment Model*** The simplest case uses a single compartment to represent the entire body (Fig. 1.6). Drug enters the compartment by continuous intravenous infusion ($k_0$), absorption from an extravascular site with an absorption rate constant of $k_a$, or intravenous bolus ($D$). After an intravenous bolus, serum concentrations decline in a straight line when plotted on semilogarithmic coordinates. As before, the slope of the line is $-k/2.303$; the half-life can be computed by determining the time required for concentrations to decrease by one half: $t_{1/2} = 0.693/k$. The equation that describes the data is $C = (D/V_D)e^{-kt}$. $V_D$ is calculated by dividing the intravenous dose by the $y$ intercept (the concentration at time zero, $C_0$) of the graph. Clearance is computed by taking the product of $k$ and $V_D$. Once $V_D$ and $k$ are known, concentrations at any time after the dose can be computed: $C = (D/V_D)e^{-kt}$.

When an extravascular dose is given, one-compartment model serum concentrations rise during absorption, reach $C_{max}$, and then decrease in a straight line with a slope equal to $-k/2.303$. The equation that describes the data is $C = [FDk_a/V_D(k_a-k)]\ (e^{-kt} - e^{-k_at})$, where $F$ is the fraction of the dose absorbed into the systemic circulation. The absorption rate constant ($k_a$) is obtained using the method of residuals. The $y$ intercept ($A$) of the terminal phase and the residual line is $A = FDk_a/V_D(k_a-k)$. If $F$ is known, $V_D$ can be calculated using $A$, $k_a$, and $k$. Clearance is computed by taking the product of $k$ and $V_D$.

During a continuous intravenous infusion, the serum concentrations in a one-compartment model change according to the equation $C = (k_0/\mathrm{CL})\ (1 - e^{-kt})$. If the infusion has been running for more than three to five half-lives, the patient will be at steady state and clearance can be calculated: $\mathrm{CL} = k_0/C_{ss}$. When the infusion is discontinued, serum concentrations appear to decline in a straight line when plotted on semilogarithmic paper with a slope of $-k/2.303$. $V_D$ is computed by dividing CL by $k$.

Figure 1.6 Visual representations of one- and two-compartment drug-distribution models.

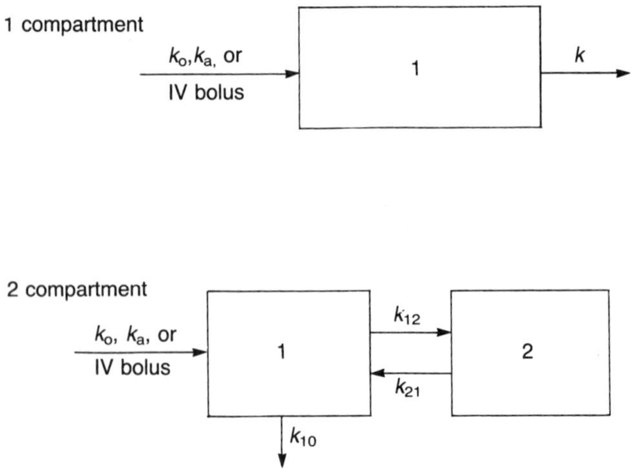


***Multicompartment Model*** After an intravenous bolus dose, serum concentrations decrease as if the drug were being injected into a central compartment that not only metabolizes and eliminates drug, but also distributes drug to one or more other compartments. Of these multicompartment models, the two-compartment model is most commonly encountered (Fig. 1.6). After intravenous bolus injection, serum concentrations decrease in two distinct phases described by the equation:

$$C = \{D(\alpha - k_{21})/V_{D,1}(\alpha - \beta)\}\ e^{-\alpha t} + \{D(k_{21} - \beta)/V_{D,1}(\alpha,\beta)\}e^{-\beta t}$$

where $k_{21}$ is the first-order rate constant and reflects the transfer of drug from compartment 2 to compartment 1 and $V_{D,1}$ is the $V_D$ of compartment 1. As previously explained, $A$, $B$, $\alpha$, and $\beta$ are obtained using the method of residuals. Once these have been computed the following equations are used to calculate kinetic constants:

$$k_{21} = (A\beta + B\alpha)/(A + B)$$
$$k_{10} = \alpha\beta/k_{21}$$
$$k_{12} = \alpha + \beta - k_{21} - k_{10}$$
$$V_{D,1} = D/(A + B)$$
$$V_{D,\beta} = D/[\beta(A/\alpha) + B/\beta]$$
$$V_{D,ss} = V_{D,1}[(k_{21} + k_{12})/k_{21}]$$
$$\mathrm{CL} = V_{D,1}\ k_{10}$$
$$t_{1/2} = 0.693/\beta$$

If serum concentrations of a drug given as a continuous intravenous infusion decline in a biphasic manner after the infusion is discontinued, a two-compartment model describes the data set[14,15] (Fig. 1.7). In this instance the postinfusion concentrations decrease according to the equation $C = Re^{-\alpha t'} + Se^{-\beta t'}$, where $t'$ is the postinfusion time ($t'$ = 0 when infusion is discontinued), and $R$, $S$, $\alpha$, and $\beta$ are determined from the postinfusion concentrations using the method of residuals with the $y$ axis set at $t' = 0$. $R$ and $S$ can be used to compute $A$ and $B$, the $y$ intercepts had the total dose given during the infusion ($D = k_0T$) been given as an intravenous bolus dose

$$A = RD\alpha/k_0(1 - e^{-\alpha T})$$
$$B = SD\beta/k_0(1 - e^{-\beta T})$$

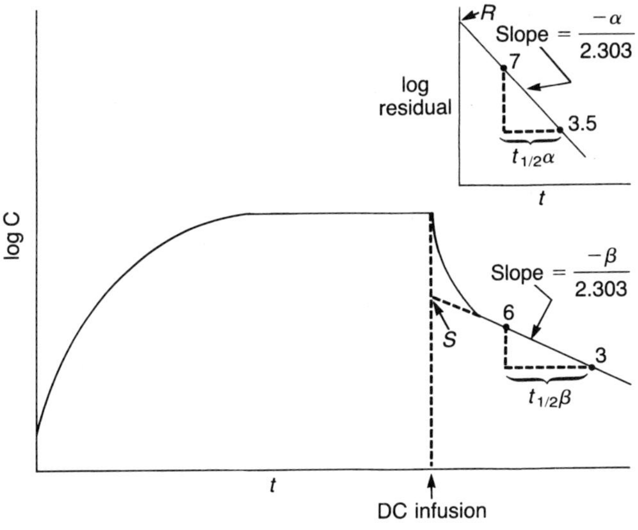


**Figure 1.7** Calculation of $\alpha$ and $\beta$ half-lives following a steady-state infusion.

$T$ is the duration of infusion. Once $A$, $B$, $\alpha$, and $\beta$ are known, the equations for an intravenous bolus are used to compute the pharmacokinetic constants. Often, when a drug is given as an intravenous bolus or continuous intravenous infusion, a two-compartment model is used to describe the data, but when the same agent is given extravascularly a one-compartment model applies.[7] In this case, distribution occurs during the absorption phase, so a distribution phase is not observed.

### Multiple Dosing

Any of these equations can be used to determine serum concentrations after multiple doses. The multiple dosing factor, $(1 - e^{-nK\tau})/(1 - e^{-K\tau})$, where $n$ is the number of doses, $K$ is the appropriate rate constant, and $\tau$ is the dosage interval, is simply multiplied by each exponential term in the equation, substituting the rate constant of each exponent for $K$. Time ($t$) is set at zero at the beginning of each dosage interval. For example, for a single-dose biexponential intravenous bolus

$$C = Ae^{-\alpha t} + Be^{-\beta t}$$

For a multiple-dose biexponential intravenous bolus

$$C = Ae^{-\alpha t}(1 - e^{-n\alpha\tau})/(1 - e^{-\alpha\tau}) + Be^{-\beta t}(1 - e^{-n\beta\tau})/(1 - e^{-\beta\tau})$$

For a single-dose one-compartment intravenous bolus

$$C = (D/V_D)e^{-kt}$$

For a multiple-dose one-compartment intravenous bolus

$$C = (D/V_D)e^{-kt}(1 - e^{-nk\tau})/(1 - e^{-k\tau})$$

### *Noncompartmental Analysis*

Pharmacokinetic constants and serum concentrations after several doses can be calculated without deterministic models.[16–18] This approach requires the measurement of areas under curves. The area under the serum concentration-versus-time curve (AUC) and the area under the first moment curve (serum concentration × time-versus-time curve, AUMC) are determined and used in computations. The trapezoidal rule is among the easiest methods used to calculate areas under curves: area of trapezoid = $[(C_1 + C_2)/2](t_2 - t_1)$ (Fig. 1.8). First the times and serum concentrations are written down in tabular form and the first moments (time multiplied by respective concentration) are calculated:

| *Time (h)* | *Concentration (mg/L)* | *Time × concentration (mg · h/L)* |
|---|---|---|
| 0 | 100 | 0 |
| 0.5 | 80 | 40 |
| 1.0 | 60 | 60 |
| 3.0 | 30 | 60 |
| . | . | . |
| . | . | . |
| . | . | . |
| 7.0 | 7.5 | 52.5 |
| 9.0 | 3.7 | 32.6 |

Individual trapezoids are made for each consecutive time–concentration pair to compute AUC (first trapezoid = [(100 mg/L + 80 mg/L)/2] (0.5 h − 0 h), second trapezoid = [(80 mg/L + 60 mg/L)/2](1 h − 0.5 h), etc) and for each consecutive time–time × concentration pair to compute AUMC (first trapezoid = [(0 mg · h/L + 40 mg · h/L)/2](0.5 h − 0 h), second trapezoid = [(40 mg · h/L + 60 mg · h/L)/2](1 h − 0.5 h), etc). Individual trapezoids for AUC and AUMC, respectively, are added together to compute the AUC and AUMC from $t = 0$ to the time ($t_{last}$) the last serum concentration ($C_{last}$) is obtained ($AUC_{0-t_{last}}$ and $AUMC_{0-t_{last}}$). The following equations are used to calculate the AUC and AUMC from $t_{last}$ to infinity ($\infty$):

**Figure 1.8** Representation of sampling intervals and the trapezoidal rule.

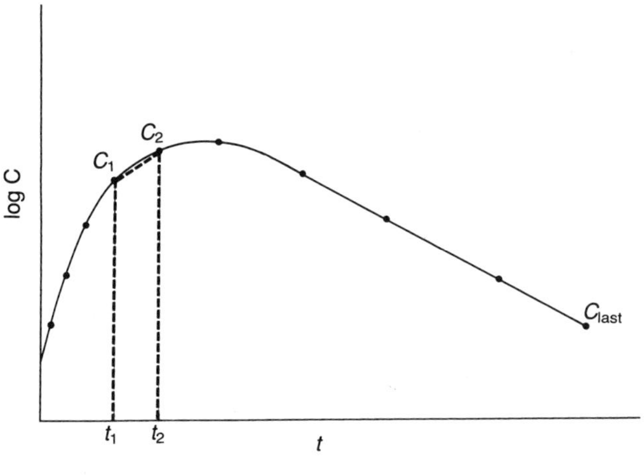

$$\mathrm{AUC}_{t_{last}-\infty} = C_{last}/k$$
$$\mathrm{AUMC}_{t_{last}-\infty} = t_{last}C_{last}/k + C_{last}/k^2$$

Here, $k$ is the terminal rate constant calculated from the slope of the postdistribution serum concentration line or calculated using $t_{1/2}$ (slope $= -k/2.303$ or $k = 0.693/t_{1/2}$). The equations used to compute the total AUC and AUMC from zero to infinity are $\mathrm{AUC}_{0-\infty} = \mathrm{AUC}_{0-t_{last}} + \mathrm{AUC}_{t_{last}-\infty}$ $\mathrm{AUMC}_{0-\infty} = \mathrm{AUMC}_{0-t_{last}} + \mathrm{AUMC}_{t_{last}-\infty}$.

#### Intravenous bolus

After an intravenous bolus dose pharmacokinetic constants are calculated as follows[16,18]:

$$V_{D,\beta} = D/k(\mathrm{AUC}_{0-\infty})$$
$$V_{D,ss} = [D(\mathrm{AUMC}_{0-\infty})]/(\mathrm{AUC}_{0-\infty})^2$$
$$\mathrm{CL} = D/\mathrm{AUC}_{0-\infty}$$
$$t_{1/2} = 0.693/k$$
$$\mathrm{MRT} = \mathrm{AUMC}_{0-\infty}/\mathrm{AUC}_{0-\infty}$$

MRT (mean residence time) is the time the average drug molecule stays in the body.

#### Continuous Intravenous Infusion

After a continuous intravenous infusion, pharmacokinetic constants are computed using the following equations[17,18]:

$$V_{D,\beta} = D/k(\mathrm{AUC}_{0-\infty})$$
$$V_{D,ss} = \{[D(\mathrm{AUMC}_{0-\infty})]/(\mathrm{AUC}_{0-\infty})^2\} - \{(DT)/[2(\mathrm{AUC}_{0-\infty})]\}$$
$$\mathrm{CL} = D/\mathrm{AUC}_{0-\infty}$$
$$t_{1/2} = 0.693/k$$

$T$ is the duration of infusion, $D$ is the total dose infused ($D = k_0T$), and $k$ is calculated from the terminal slope after the infusion has been discontinued.

#### Extravascular Dosing

After an extravascular dose, kinetic constants are computed using similar equations[18]:

$$V_{D,\beta} = FD/k(\mathrm{AUC}_{0-\infty})$$
$$V_{D,ss} = [FD(\mathrm{AUMC}_{0-\infty})]/(\mathrm{AUC}_{0-\infty})^2] - [FD/k_a(\mathrm{AUC}_{0-\infty})]$$
$$\mathrm{CL} = FD/\mathrm{AUC}_{0-\infty}$$
$$t_{1/2} = 0.693/k$$

$k_a$ is the absorption rate constant calculated using the method of residuals and $F$ is the fraction of the dose absorbed systemically.

#### Clearances for Different Routes of Elimination

Clearances for individual organs can be computed if the excretion the organ produces can be obtained. For example, renal clearance can be calculated if urine is collected during a pharmacokinetic experiment. The patient empties his or her bladder immediately before the dose is given. Subsequent urine production is collected until the last serum concentration ($C_{last}$) is obtained. Renal clearance ($CL_R$) is computed by dividing the amount of drug excreted in the urine by $\mathrm{AUC}_{0-t_{last}}$. Biliary and other clearance values are computed in a similar fashion.

#### Multiple Dosing

Serum concentrations after multiple doses can be computed from single-dose data using the principle of superposition.[6] According to the definition of linear pharmacokinetics $C_{ss}$ and $\mathrm{AUC}_{0-\infty}$ change proportionally with dose. Therefore, serum concentration-versus-time curves can be added to or subtracted from each other. For example, if an intravenous bolus dose of 250 mg is administered to a patient and serum concentrations are obtained, the concentration that would occur 6 hours after the third dose (250 mg IV bolus every 8 hours) can be calculated using the data from the single-dose experiment. First, the single-dose curve would be replicated every 8 hours as if no other doses were given (Fig. 1.9). The concentrations contributed from each individual dose would be obtained from the graph at 22 hours (6 hours after the third dose given on an 8-hour schedule) and added together to derive the concentration from all three doses. With this technique, serum concentrations after very complex dosage regimens can be calculated.

Because addition of several concentration curves using superposition can become quite tedious, a mathematical solution has been derived. It assumes that all doses are given after absorption and distribution are complete. The single-dose curve is drawn, the slope of the terminal postabsorption, postdistribution phase is determined (slope $= -k/2.303$), and the terminal phase is extrapolated to determine the $y$ intercept ($B$). The following equation is used to calculate the serum concentration $t$ hours after the $n$th dose ($C_n$) once the serum concentration $t$ hours after the first dose ($C_1$) is known:

$$C_n = C_1 + \{Be^{-k\tau}[(1 - e^{-k\tau(n-1)})/(1 - e^{-k\tau})]e^{-kt}\}$$

$\tau$ is the dosage interval.

### *Bioavailability and Bioequivalence*

The fraction of drug absorbed into the systemic circulation ($F$) after extravascular administration can be calculated after single intravenous and extravascular doses as[19]

**Figure 1.9** Superposition can be used to compute serum concentrations after multiple doses. Serum concentrations from each dose are added together to determine the actual concentration at 22 hours.

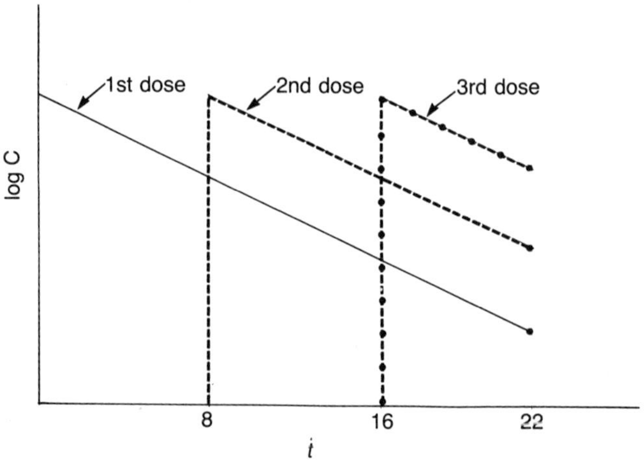

$$F = D_{iv}(AUC_{0-\infty})/D(AUC_{iv_{0-\infty}})$$

$D$ and $D_{iv}$ are the extravascular and intravenous doses, respectively, and $AUC_{iv_{0-\infty}}$ and $AUC_{0-\infty}$ are the intravenous and extravascular AUC, respectively, from time zero to infinity.

When the extravascular dose is administered orally, part of the dose may be metabolized by the liver before it reaches the systemic circulation.[20] This commonly occurs when drugs have a high liver extraction ratio, because after oral administration almost all of the drug must pass through the portal circulation into the liver. For example, if an orally administered drug is 100% absorbed from the gastrointestinal tract but has a hepatic extraction ratio of 0.75, only 25% of the original dose enters the systemic circulation. This "first-pass" effect through the liver is avoided when the drug is given by other routes of administration. The computation of $F$ does not separate loss of oral drug metabolized by the first-pass effect and drug not absorbed by the gastrointestinal tract. Special techniques are needed to determine the fraction of drug absorbed orally for drugs with high liver extraction ratios.

Two different dosage forms of the same drug are considered to be bioequivalent when they produce $AUC_{0-\infty}$, $C_{max}$, and $t_{max}$ values that are neither clinically nor statistically different. When this occurs the serum concentration-versus-time curves for the two dosage forms should be superimposable. Bioequivalence studies have become very important as may expensive drugs have recently become available in generic form. Most bioequivalence studies involve 18 to 25 healthy male volunteers who are given the brand name product and the generic product in a randomized, crossover study design.

### *Steady-State Pharmacokinetics*

Up to this point, pharmacokinetic experiments have involved single-dose trials. It is possible and sometimes desirable to conduct kinetic experiments while the patient is at steady state. Fortunately, if the same dose is administered, the area under the serum concentration-versus-time curve over a dosage interval at steady state ($AUC_{ss}$) is equal to the $AUC_{0-\infty}$ after a single dose. This means that either AUC can be used in any of the noncompartmental model kinetic equations; however, the $AUMC_{0-\infty}$ after a single dose is not equivalent to the AUMC over a dosage interval at steady state.[21] Superposition can be used to construct a single-dose curve from steady-state serum concentrations. The single-dose curve can then be used to compute $AUMC_{0-\infty}$. $AUC_{ss}$ and $AUMC_{0-\infty}$ can be substituted in noncompartmental model equations to compute kinetic constants.

### *Nonlinear Pharmacokinetics*

#### Michaelis–Menten Kinetics

Some drugs do not follow the rules of linear pharmacokinetics. Instead of $C_{ss}$ and AUC increasing proportionally with dose, serum concentrations change more or less than expected (Fig. 1.10). One explanation for the greater-than-expected increase in $C_{ss}$ and AUC after an increase in dose is that the enzymes responsible for the metabolism or elimination of the drug may start to become saturated. When this occurs the maximum rate of metabolism ($V_{max}$) for the drug is approached. This is called Michaelis–Menten kinetics. The serum concentration at which the rate of metabolism equals $V_{max}/2$ is $K_m$. Practically speaking, $K_m$ is the serum concentration at which nonproportional changes in $C_{ss}$ and AUC start to occur when dose is increased. The Michaelis–Menten constants ($V_{max}$ and $K_m$) determine the dosage rate (DR) needed to maintain a given $C_{ss}$: $DR = V_{max}C_{ss}/(K_m + C_{ss})$. Most drugs eliminated by the liver are metabolized by enzymes but still appear to follow linear kinetics. The reason for this disparity is that the therapeutic range for most drugs is well below the $K_m$ of the enzyme system that metabolizes the agent. The therapeutic range is higher than $K_m$ for some commonly used drugs. The average $K_m$ for phenytoin is about 4 $\mu$g/mL. The therapeutic range for phenytoin is usually 10–20 $\mu$g/mL. Most patients experience Michaelis–Menten kinetics while taking phenytoin.

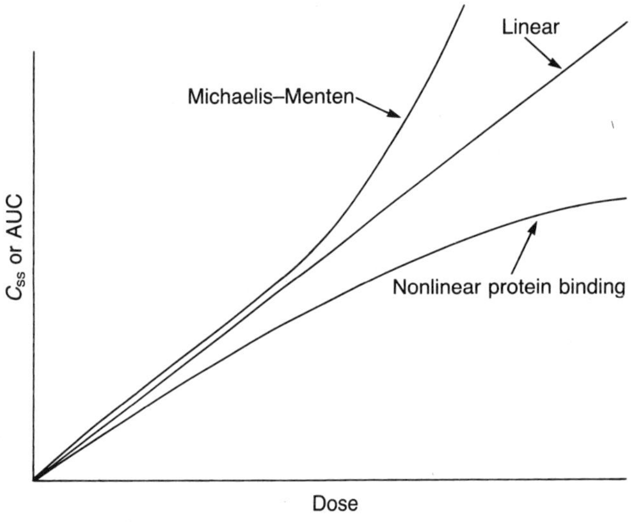


**Figure 1.10** Relationship of dose and $C_{ss}$ or AUC under linear and nonlinear conditions.

#### Nonlinear Protein Binding

Another type of nonlinear kinetics can occur if $C_{ss}$ and AUC increase less than expected after an increase in dose of a low-clearance drug. This usually indicates that plasma protein binding sites are starting to become saturated so that $f_b$ increases with increases in dose (Fig. 1.10). For a low-clearance drug, clearance is dependent on the values of $f_b$ and $CL'_{int}$: $CL = f_bCL'_{int}$. When a dosage increase takes place, $f_b$ increases because nearly all plasma protein binding sites are occupied and no binding sites are available. If $f_b$ increases, CL increases and $C_{ss}$ increases less than expected with the dosage change ($C_{ss} = k_0/CL$); however, $C_{ss,u}$ increases proportionally with dose since it depends on $CL'_{int}$ for low-clearance drugs: $C_{ss,u} = k_0/CL'_{int}$. Valproic acid[22] and disopyramide[23] both follow saturable protein binding pharmacokinetics.

## Individualization of Drug Therapy

Serum drug concentrations are readily available to clinicians. The therapeutic ranges for several drugs have been identified, and it is likely that new drugs will also be monitored using serum concentrations. Although several individualization methods have been advocated for specific drugs, one simple, reliable method is very commonly used. For drugs that exhibit linear pharmacokinetics, $C_{ss}$ changes proportionally with dose. To adjust a patient's drug therapy, a reasonable starting dose is administered for an estimated three to five half-lives. A serum concentration is obtained assuming that it will reflect $C_{ss}$. Independent of the route of administration, the new dose ($D_{new}$) needed to attain the desired $C_{ss}$ ($C_{ss,new}$) is calculated: $D_{new} = C_{ss,new}(D_{old}/C_{ss,old})$, where $D_{old}$ and $C_{ss,old}$ are the old dose and old $C_{ss}$, respectively. To use this method $C_{ss,old}$ *must* reflect steady-state conditions. Often, patients are noncompliant with regard to their drug dosage and, therefore, are not at steady state. This occurs not only in outpatients, but in hospital inpatients as well. Inpatients can spit out oral doses or alter the infusion rates on intravenous pumps after the nurse leaves the hospital room. If $C_{ss,old}$ is much larger or smaller than expected for the $D_{old}$ the patient is taking, one should suspect noncompliance and repeat the serum concentration after another three to five half-lives or change the patient's dose cautiously and monitor for signs of toxicity or lack of effect.

If it is necessary to determine the kinetic constants for a patient, a small kinetic experiment could be conducted in the individual. With the methods outlined under Noncompartmental Analysis and Steady-State Pharmacokinetics, CL, $V_D$, and $t_{1/2}$ can be calculated and used to individualize dose for any drug. Alternatively, several methods for specific drugs have been derived that assume specific kinetic models and clinical situations.

### *Aminoglycosides*

Although aminoglycoside pharmacokinetics follow multicompartment models,[24] a one-compartment model appears sufficient to individualize doses in patients.[25] Aminoglycosides are usually given as short-term intermittent intravenous infusions. When this is the case, kinetic parameters can be calculated at any point in therapy. Serum aminoglycoside concentrations are obtained before a dose ($C_{min}$), after a dose administered as an intravenous infusion of about 1 hour ($C_{max}$), and two or more times prior to the next dose ($C_3$, $C_4$, etc). $C_{max}$, $C_3$, and $C_4$ are plotted on semilogarithmic paper; $t_{1/2}$ and $k$ are obtained from the graph. Assuming a one-compartment model, the following equation is used to compute $V_D$[25]:

$$V_D = [(D/T)(1 - e^{-kT})]/[k(C_{max} - C_{min}\, e^{-kT})]$$

$D$ is dose and $T$ duration of infusion. Once these are known, the dose and dosage interval ($\tau$ can be calculated for any desired maximum $C_{ss}$ ($C_{ss,max}$) and minimum $C_{ss}$ ($C_{ss,min}$):

$$\tau = -\{[\ln(C_{ss,min}/C_{ss,max})]/k\} + T$$
$$D = \tau k V_D C_{ss,max}[(1 - e^{-k\tau})/(1 - e^{-kT})]$$

The dose and dosage interval should be rounded to provide clinically accepted values. This method has also been used to individualize intravenous theophylline dosage regimens.[26]

### *Theophylline*

Theophylline disposition is most accurately described by nonlinear kinetics[27,28]; however, at the usual doses, theophylline acts as if it obeys linear kinetics in the majority of patients. Continuous intravenous infusions of theophylline (or its salt, aminophylline) can be rapidly individualized by determining the patient's clearance.[29] Assuming the patient receives theophylline only by continuous intravenous infusion (previous doses of sustained-release oral theophylline are completely absorbed), two serum theophylline concentrations are obtained 4 or more hours apart. The infusion rate ($k_0$) cannot be changed between the times the concentrations are drawn. With one-compartment model equations, the first ($C_1$) and second ($C_2$) theophylline concentrations are used to calculate theophylline clearance:

$$CL = 2k_0/(C_1 + C_2) + 2V_D(C_1 - C_2)/(C_1 + C_2)(t_2 - t_1)$$

$V_D$ is assumed to be 0.5 L/kg and $t_1$ and $t_2$ are the times at which $C_1$ and $C_2$, respectively, are obtained. Once the clearance is known, $k_0$ can be easily computed for any desired $C_{ss}$: $C_{ss} = k_0/CL$.

This method can probably be applied to other drugs that are administered as continuous intravenous infusions where rapid individualization of drug dosage is desirable.

### *Phenytoin*

Phenytoin doses are very difficult to individualize because the drug follows Michaelis–Menten kinetics, and there is a large amount of interpatient variability in $V_{max}$ and $K_m$. The methods used to individualize phenytoin doses involve rearrangements of the Michaelis–Menten equation (DR = $V_{max}C_{ss}/[K_m + C_{ss}]$ where DR is dosage rate) at steady state so that two or more doses and $C_{ss}$ values can be used to obtain graphic solutions for $V_{max}$ and $K_m$. One rearrangement[30] is DR = $-K_m(\text{DR}/C_{ss}) + V_{max}$. When DR is plotted on the $y$ axis and DR/$C_{ss}$ is plotted on the $x$ axis of Cartesian graph paper, a straight line with a $y$ intercept of $V_{max}$ and slope equal to $-K_m$ is found (Fig. 1.11). To use this method, patients are prescribed an initial phenytoin dose and the $C_{ss}$ is obtained. The phenytoin dose is then changed and a second $C_{ss}$ from the new dose is obtained. Each dose is divided by its respective $C_{ss}$ to derive DR/$C_{ss}$ values. The DR/$C_{ss}$ and $C_{ss}$ values are plotted on the graph to calculate $V_{max}$ ($y$ intercept) and $K_m$ ($-$slope). The steady-state Michaelis–Menten equation can be used to compute $C_{ss}$ for a given DR or a DR for any $C_{ss}$.

### *Computer Programs*

Computer programs that aid in the individualization of therapy are available for many different drugs. The most sophisticated programs use nonlinear regression to fit CL and $V_D$ to actual serum concentrations obtained in a patient.[31] After drug doses and serum concentrations are entered into the computer, nonlinear regression programs

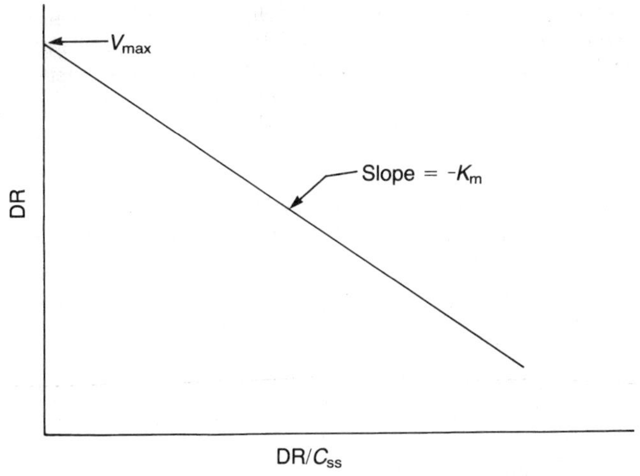


**Figure 1.11** Relationship between dosage rate (DR) and steady-state serum concentrations.

adjust CL and $V_D$ until the sum of the squared error between actual ($C_{act}$) and computer-estimated concentrations ($C_{est}$) is at a minimum ($\Sigma(C_{est} - C_{act})^2$). Once estimates of CL and $V_D$ are available, doses are easily calculated.

Many programs also take into account what the CL and $V_D$ should be on the basis of disease states and conditions present in the patient.[32] Incorporation of expected population-based parameters allows the computer to use a limited number of serum concentrations (one or two) to provide estimates of CL and $V_D$. This type of computer program is called "Bayesian" because it incorporates portions of Bayes' theorem during the fitting routine.[33]

## Summary

The availability of inexpensive, rapidly available serum drug concentrations has changed the way clinicians monitor drug therapy in patients. The therapeutic range for many drugs is known, and it is likely that more drugs will be monitored using serum concentrations in the future. Clinicians need to remember that the therapeutic range is merely an average guideline. Individual patients may respond to smaller concentrations or require concentrations that are much greater to obtain a therapeutic effect. Conversely, patients may show toxic effects at concentrations within or below the therapeutic range. Serum concentrations should never replace clinical judgment.

Three kinetic constants determine the dosage requirements of patients. Clearance determines the maintenance dose (MD = $CLC_{ss}$), volume of distribution determines the loading dose (LD = $V_DC_{ss}$), and half-life determines the time to steady state and the dosage interval. Several methods are available to compute these parameters.

Methods available to individualize drug therapy range from simple mathematical relationships that hold for all drugs that obey linear pharmacokinetics to very complex computer programs that are specific to one drug. New techniques for monitoring serum drug concentrations are available on an experimental basis and may revolutionize clinical pharmacokinetics in the future.

## References


1. Wagner JG, Northam JI, Alway CD, et al. Blood levels of drug at the equilibrium state after multiple dosing. Nature 1965;207:1301–1302.
2. Rowland M, Benet LZ, Graham GG. Clearance concepts in pharmacokinetics. J Pharmacokin Biopharm 1973;1:123–136.
3. Wilkinson GR, Shand DG. A physiological approach to hepatic drug clearance. Clin Pharmacol Ther 1975;18:377–390.
4. Nies AS, Shand DG, Wilkinson GR. Altered hepatic blood flow and drug disposition. Clin Pharmacokin 1976;1:135–155.
5. Gibaldi M, Koup JR. Pharmacokinetic concepts—drug binding, apparent volume of distribution and clearance. Eur J Clin Pharmacol 1981;20:299–305.
6. Gibaldi M, Perrier D. Pharmacokinetics, 2nd ed. New York, Marcel Dekker, 1980.
7. Wagner JG. Model-independent linear pharmacokinetics. Drug Intell Clin Pharm 1976;10:179–180.
8. Wagner JG. Linear pharmacokinetic equations allowing direct calculation of many needed pharmacokinetic parameters from the coefficients and exponents of polyexponential equations which have been fitted to the data. J Pharmacokin Biopharm 1976;4:443–467.
9. Riegelman S, Loo J, Rowland M. Concept of a volume of distribution and possible errors in evaluation of this parameter. J Pharm Sci 1968;57:128–133.
10. Gibaldi M, Nagashima R, Levy G. Relationship between drug concentration in plasma or serum and amount of drug in the body. J Pharm Sci 1969;58:193–197.
11. Gibaldi M, Perrier D. Drug elimination and apparent volume of distribution in multicompartment systems. J Pharm Sci 1972;61:952–954.
12. Riegelman S, Loo JCK, Rowland M. Shortcomings in pharmacokinetics analysis by conceiving the body to exhibit properties of a single compartment. J Pharm Sci 1968;57:117–123.
13. Benet LZ. General treatment of linear mammillary models with elimination from any compartment as used in pharmacokinetics. J Pharm Sci 1972;61:536–541.
14. Gibaldi M. Estimation of the pharmacokinetics parameters of the two compartment open model from post-infusion plasma concentration data. J Pharm Sci 1969;58:1133–1135.
15. Loo JCK, Riegelman S. Assessment of pharmacokinetic constants from postinfusion blood curves obtained after IV infusion. J Pharm Sci 1970;59:53–55.
16. Benet LZ, Galeazzi RL. Noncompartmental determination of the steady state volume of distribution. J Pharm Sci 1979;68:1071–1074.
17. Lee CS, Brater DC, Gambertoglio JG, et al. Disposition kinetics of ethambutol in man. J Pharmacokin Biopharm 1980;8:335–346.
18. Perrier D, Mayersohn M. Noncompartmental determination of the steady state volume of distribution for any mode of administration. J Pharm Sci 1982;71:372–373.

19. Koup JR, Gibaldi M. Some comments on the evaluation of bioavailability data. Drug Intell Clin Pharm 1980;14:327–330.
20. Gibaldi M, Boyes RN, Feldman S. Influence of first pass effect on availability of drugs on oral administration. J Pharm Sci 1971;60:1338–1340.
21. Bauer LA, Gibaldi M. Computation of model independent pharmacokinetic parameters during multiple dosing. J Pharm Sci 1983;72:978–979.
22. Bowdle TA, Patel IH, Levy RH, et al. Valproic acid dosage and plasma protein binding and clearance. Clin Pharmacol Ther 1980;28:486–492.
23. Lima JJ, Boudonlas H, Blanford M. Concentration-dependence of disopyramide binding to plasma protein and its influence on kinetics and dynamics. J Pharm Exp Ther 1981;219:741–747.
24. Schentag JJ, Jusko WJ. Renal clearance and tissue accumulation of gentamicin. Clin Pharmacol Ther 1977;22:364–370.
25. Sawchuk RJ, Zaske DE, Cipolle RJ, et al. Kinetic model for gentamicin dosing with the use of individual patient parameters. Clin Pharmacol Ther 1977;21:362–369.
26. Pancorbo S, Sawchuk RJ, Dashe C, et al. Use of a pharmacokinetic model for individual intravenous doses of aminophylline. Eur J Clin Pharmacol 1979;16:251–254.
27. Sarrazin E, Hendeles L, Weinberger M, et al. Dose-dependent kinetics for theophylline—observations among ambulatory asthmatic children. J Pediatr 1980;97:825–828.
28. Tang-Liu DDS, Williams RL, Riegelman S. Nonlinear theophylline elimination. Clin Pharmacol Ther 1982;31:358–369.
29. Vozeh S, Kewitz G, Wenk M, et al. Rapid prediction of steady state serum theophylline concentrations in patients treated with intravenous aminophylline. Eur J Clin Pharmacol 1980;18:473–477.
30. Ludden TM, Allen JP, Valutsky WA, et al. Individualization of phenytoin dosage regimens. Clin Pharmacol Ther 1977;21:287–293.
31. Koup JR, Killen T, Bauer LA. Multiple-dose nonlinear regression analysis program—aminoglycoside dose prediction. Clin Pharmacokinet 1983;8:456–462.
32. Sheiner LB, Beal S, Rosenberg B, et al. Forecasting individual pharmacokinetics. Clin Pharmacol Ther 1979;26:294–305.
33. Sheiner LB, Beal SL. Bayesian individualization of pharmacokinetics—simple implementation and comparison with non-Bayesian methods. J Pharm Sci 1982;71:1344–1348.

# Chapter 2 / Drug Delivery and Administration

Dennis H. Robinson, PhD, Warren A. Narducci, PharmD, and Clarence T. Ueda, PharmD, PhD

Drugs are delivered in systems that are designed to provide accurate and convenient drug administration, to obtain the desired therapeutic response with minimum side effects, and to maximize patient compliance. In determining the most clinically effective and safe method of drug delivery, three major factors should be considered. First, the most appropriate route of administration depends on whether a local or systemic drug effect is desired. Localized drug administration has the advantage of focusing high concentrations of drug at the desired site of action and minimizing systemic side effects. The systemic approach is used when the target tissue is inaccessible by direct administration or application. Second, the properties of the delivery system frequently dictate by which route the dosage form or device can be given or utilized. Finally, while the desired pharmacologic effect governs the choice of drug used, the physicochemical and pharmacokinetic properties of the drug may restrict its use in only certain dosage forms and/or by specific routes of administration. Other factors that affect the method and route of drug administration include the age and status of the patient, convenience, desired onset time, and duration of drug treatment. Tables 2.1 and 2.2 summarize the principal factors that are known to influence the bioavailability characteristics of a drug and the approach that should be used in the design of a dosage form, respectively. The most common routes of administration are listed in Table 2.3.

An important factor that must not be overlooked in assessing the therapeutic performance of a drug is patient compliance. All attempts that are made to obtain an optimal therapeutic response through the selection of the most desirable drug delivery system and route of administration may be negated if the patient is uncooperative and noncompliant. Further, patient education is important to ensure that the medications are correctly administered and/or applied.[1] Personal factors that may affect patient compliance are summarized in Table 2.4.

Drug delivery systems that are used for systemic and localized drug administration are discussed in the following sections with the aim of addressing the principal factors of the delivery system and associated routes of administration that are known to affect the therapeutic performance of a drug.

## Parenteral Administration

While parenteral drug administration can be interpreted literally to mean giving a drug by any nonoral route, it is most commonly meant to be an injection directly into an internal body compartment or cavity to bypass the protective effects of the skin and mucous membranes. The most common parenteral routes of drug administration are intravenous, intramuscular, and subcutaneous. Other more specialized parenteral routes of administration are listed in Table 2.3. The principal advantages and disadvantages of parenteral drug administration are summarized in Table 2.5.

When a drug is administered parenterally, it is critical that proper injection techniques are used. An improper injection can cause injuries to nerves, muscle, bone, and/or blood vessels. Thus, when an injection is to be self-administered, it is imperative that the patient is properly instructed on the use of the parenteral dosage form and injection procedure.

### *Preparations*

Parenteral drug delivery systems include drug formulations in solution, suspension, or emulsion, or as a drug powder for reconstitution immediately before use. While all products for parenteral drug administration must be sterile and pyrogen free and, in the case of solutions, free of particulate matter, the properties of some preparations are influenced by the route of administration. For example, intraocular, intraspinal, intracisternal, and intrathecal drug administration requires formulations of the highest purity because of the sensitivity of nerve tissue to irritant and toxic substances. Suspensions cannot be administered intravenously because of the possibility of insoluble particles blocking the capillaries. Subcutaneous injections should be isotonic to prevent unnecessary irritation and pain.

Solutions are the most common form of injectable products. Most are aqueous, but they also may be nonaqueous, for example, polyethylene glycol or fixed vegetable oils. Further, some aqueous solutions may contain varying proportions of water-miscible liquids such as propylene glycol or glycerol to increase drug solubility and/or stability. Water-immiscible oils such as sesame, corn, or peanut oil are used as an alternative method to enhance drug solubility or stability or to prolong the rate of drug release to obtain a sustained effect. The ideal parenteral vehicle should be nonirritating, nontoxic, nonsensitizing, and physiologically inert. In addition, it should be easy to purify and sterilize, for example, heat stable.

Parenteral suspensions are prepared with drugs that possess low water solubility. For this type of parenteral preparation, the particle size and size distribution must be carefully controlled to ensure syringability as well as reliable and reproducible drug bioavailability. Further, surfactants and suspending agents are usually added to aid wetting and dispersion of the solid drug.

Parenteral emulsions are usually of the oil-in-water type. An excellent example of this type of preparation is the intravenous lipid emulsion that is used as a source of calories and essential fatty acids for parenteral nutrition. Emulsions

**Table 2.1** Factors That Influence Drug Bioavailability

| | |
|---|---|
| Physicochemical properties of the drug | Physiologic factors |
| Solubility in aqueous and organic solvents | pH |
| pH–solubility profile | Temperature |
| Lipid–water partition coefficient | Surface area |
| $pK_a$ | Surface tension |
| Particle size and size distribution | Volume and composition of biologic fluid |
| Crystalline and polymorphic forms | Disease state |
| Solvation and hydration | Sex |
| Salt form | Age |
| Stability in solid state and solution form | Manufacturing variables |
| Molecular weight | Added diluents |
| Environmental factors | Manufacturing variables, e.g., force of compression |
| Humidity | Manufacturing method |
| Temperature | Packaging |

are not used more widely because of the inherent difficulties in producing stable emulsion drops of the desired size, that is, less than 5 μm.

Unstable drugs are prepared in dry powder form to be reconstituted as a solution or suspension prior to use by the addition of an appropriate diluent such as water for injection, normal saline, or dextrose solution. More detailed information about these and other more specialized parenteral formulations such as total parenteral nutrition, radiopharmaceuticals, and biologicals can be found in the literature.[2–4]

### *Biopharmaceutic Considerations*

Drugs that are administered intravenously are usually injected into a large proximal forearm vein and provide rapid action. The intensity and duration of drug activity depend upon the dose administered, the degree of binding to plasma proteins, the extent of distribution throughout the body, and the rate of elimination by metabolism and/or excretion. Intravenous infusion is commonly used to give drugs with short elimination half-lives.

Intramuscular injections are administered deep into skeletal muscles remote from major nerves and blood vessels. The principal sites of injection are the gluteal (buttocks), deltoid (upper arm), and vastus lateralis (lateral thigh) muscles. Essentially all injectable products can be given intramuscularly including aqueous or oleaginous solutions and suspensions, emulsions, and reconstituted powders. Intramuscular injections form a "depot" in the muscle, and therefore generally produce a slower onset of action and longer duration of effect relative to an intravenous injection. While the extent of drug absorption after intramuscular administration is usually complete, the rate of absorption may vary widely because of the physicochemical properties of the drug, formulation variables, and various physiologic factors such as blood perfusion rate.

Subcutaneous administration is the injection of a small volume (<2 mL) of aqueous solution or suspension into the loose interstitial tissue beneath the skin of the arm, forearm, thigh, abdomen or buttocks. The injection site should be varied when repeated daily dosing is required. Subcutaneous administration should not be confused with the intradermal mode of administration, which involves the injection of a small volume (~0.1 mL) of diagnostic, desensitizing, or immunizing products into the vascular dermis layer of the skin.

Long-acting preparations have been designed for intramuscular administration to provide slow, sustained drug release over an extended period. Most of these preparations act by retarding the rate of drug release and/or dissolution from the finished product via a physical or chemical mechanism.[5]

Some current drug delivery systems that are being investigated as prolonged-release parenterals for site-specific delivery include magnetic and nonmagnetic microspheres, microcapsules, liposomes, multiple emulsions, magnetic emulsions, biocompatible carriers, and prodrugs.[5]

**Table 2.2** Stepwise Approach to Dosage Form Design

1. Select route of administration: systemic or local therapy, chronic or acute treatment, convenience, and patient factors
2. Select dosage form design including drug content, desired release rate, duration of release, and site of release
3. Select method of manufacture
4. Formulate with compatible additives
5. Preliminary in vitro and in vivo evaluations to optimize release
6. In vitro testing
7. In vivo testing
8. Establish quality assurance criteria and validate bioavailability and other clinical testing

### *Therapeutic Considerations*

The most important factors to consider when administering a parenteral medication are the route and injection site, injection volume, needle gauge and length, intended therapeutic effect, and special administration/injection technique to be used.[6] A summary of these factors is provided in Table 2.6.

**Table 2.3** Routes of Drug Administration and Common Dosage Forms

| *Route* | *Site* | *Common dosage form* |
|---|---|---|
| Oral | Mouth, gastrointestinal tract | Solution, suspension, powder, capsule, tablet |
| Sublingual | Under the tongue | Tablet |
| Buccal | Oral mucosa | Tablet lozenge |
| Parenteral | Other than gastrointestinal tract | Solution suspension, implant, device |
| Intravenous | Vein | |
| Intraarterial | Artery | |
| Intraarticular | Joints | |
| Intracisternal | Cerebrospinal column | |
| Intracardiac | Heart | |
| Intradermal | Dermal layer of the skin | |
| Intraspinal | Spinal column | |
| Intraosseous | Bone | |
| Intrasynovial | Joint fluid | |
| Intrathecal | Spinal fluid | |
| Intramuscular | Muscle | |
| Subcutaneous | Beneath the skin | |
| Topical/ transdermal | Skin surface | Ointment, cream, paste, gel, powder, solution, suspension, aerosol, device |
| Intraocular | Eye | Solution, suspension, ointment, insert |
| Intranasal | Nose | Solution, suspension, ointment, aerosol |
| Intrarespiratory | Lung | Solution, suspension, aerosol, inhaler, nebulizer |
| Rectal | Rectum | Solution, ointment, suppository |
| Intravaginal | Vagina | Solution, ointment, foam, tablet, suppository, insert |
| Intrauterine | Uterus | Insert |
| Urethral | Urethra | Suppository |

The most frequent local hazards that occur with parenteral administration include pain at the injection site, infiltration, extravasation and phlebitis after intravenous injection, formation of sterile abscesses from irritating drugs after subcutaneous administration, and the possibility of bleeding and peripheral nerve damage from inappropriately placed intramuscular injections. Each of these adverse effects can be avoided or minimized by using proper injection technique and the utmost caution in the selection and care of the injection site.

The onset and intensity of a drug's pharmacologic effect(s) can be predetermined by selecting the route and method of administration that are best suited for the condition and therapeutic requirements of the patient. An intravenous bolus or infusion provides the most rapid onset of action, but may be undesirable because of the toxicity of the drug or the vehicle, for example, phenytoin and diazepam injections. The subcutaneous route provides a more sustained effect for water-soluble drugs, and intramuscular injections are most appropriate for irritating drugs, aqueous suspensions, and injection volumes greater than 1.5 mL but less than 5 mL. Intramuscular injections usually produce a more rapid onset of effect than subcutaneous injections.

The patient's age and physical condition are major considerations when selecting intravenous and intramuscular injection sites. In elderly, nonambulatory, or emaciated patients, muscle mass is likely to be diminished in the gluteus medius and vastus lateralis. Large intramuscular injections should be administered in the gluteus minimus muscle in these patients. Infants and small children should receive intramuscular injections in their thigh muscles, which are better developed than the gluteal muscles.

With the increasing trend in home health care, self-administration of parenteral medications has become routine, and patient education by pharmacists is essential. Specifically, instruction for site preparation, aseptic technique, injection technique, and self-monitoring of drug therapy is required.

## Infusion

A variety of external and implantable infusion devices are available for long-term controlled drug delivery via subcutaneous, intramuscular, intravenous, and intraperitoneal

**Table 2.4** Factors Contributing to Patient Noncompliance and Compliance

**Factors Contributing to Noncompliance**
Failure to comprehend the importance of therapy
Poor understanding of the instructions
Multiple-drug therapy
Frequency of administration
Duration of therapy
Adverse effects
Fear of becoming drug dependent
Patients may be asymptomatic or the symptoms may subside
Unpleasant taste of medication
Waiting to see the physician or pharmacist
Illness
Cost of the medication
Measurement of medication

**Steps to Improve Patient Compliance**
Identification of risk factors that may contribute to noncompliance
Development of treatment plan with recognition of patient's normal pattern of activities
Designation of specific times of day at which medication is to be taken
Educating the patient—recognition of the need for effective verbal and written communication with the patient
Monitoring therapy

From Gourley DR, Ueda CT: Patient factors that influence dosage form selection, in Banker GS, Chalmers RK (Eds): Pharmaceutics and Pharmacy Practice. Philadelphia, J.B. Lippincott, 1982, p 144, with permission.

routes of administration.[7] Infusion pumps should normally be used only after conventional treatment methods have failed to satisfactorily control the disease or to allow patients greater mobility and freedom. By far, the widest use of infusion devices has been in the treatment of insulin-dependent diabetes.[8,9] Other important uses include the controlled administration of analgesics,[10] anticoagulants,[11] and antitumor agents.[12]

### *Devices*

Originally, infusion devices were large bedside units. Today, portable devices are being used increasingly. Typically, a portable infusion device consists of a refillable drug reservoir with a capacity of 50–100 mL, a rate-controlling pump, an electrical, mechanical, or physical energy source, and a safety mechanism in the event of failure. Future developments in this area include (1) programmed or biofeedback-controlled systems with implantable sensors to meet complicated drug demands, (2) miniaturization of the infusion devices to allow for easier implantation, and (3) administration of a wider range of drugs via alternative routes of administration. The widespread use of infusion devices is presently limited by their high cost and the various patient problems to be discussed.

**Table 2.5** Advantages and Disadvantages of Parenteral Drug Administration

**Advantages**
Drugs can be administered to uncooperative, unconscious, or nauseous patients.
Drugs that are normally ineffective, poorly absorbed, or inactive orally can be effectively administered.
Intravenous route provides immediate onset of drug action when needed during emergency situations.
Other parenteral routes can be used to slow onset of action and/or prolong action of the drug.
Localized and systemic drug effects can be produced depending on the route of administration and product formulation.
Patient compliance problems are largely avoided.
Aside from drug administration the parenteral route can be used to correct patient fluid and electrolyte imbalances, and provide nutrient and caloric requirements.

**Disadvantages**
Parenteral preparations are usually administered by trained personnel.
Strict adherence to aseptic procedures is required.
Some pain is usually inevitable.
Drug effects are difficult to reverse.
Parenteral administration may be inconvenient when frequent dosing is required.

### *Biopharmaceutic Considerations*

Ideally, the flow rate of an infusion device should be adjustable and capable of delivering both a priming dose and a constant zero-order maintenance dose. The subcutaneous route of administration is usually preferred because of the large surface area available for injection sites, ease of access, and low potential for complications; however, the delayed and variable rate of drug absorption from subcutaneous tissue, as seen with insulin, can be a potential problem of this method of drug administration. Although intravenous infusion produces a rapid onset of action, there are significant disadvantages that preclude its widespread use, for example, septicemia and thromboembolism. The intraperitoneal route may be used more extensively in the future because drug absorption from the peritoneal cavity has been shown to be complete and predictable.[9]

### *Therapeutic Considerations*

It is anticipated that the use of portable intravenous and subcutaneous infusion devices will increase as a result of new technologies, improvements in design, and the trend toward ambulatory health care; however, this route of drug administration is not appropriate for all patients. In general, pediatric and geriatric patients are less suited for this form of drug administration than adolescent or adult patients.

Infusion therapy is ideal for the highly motivated patient who has the capability to care for the injection site, to administer the infusion, and to maintain and program the pump. Patient acceptance of an infusion device depends

**Table 2.6** Injection Factors for the Most Common Routes of Parenteral Drug Administration

| *Injection route* | *Tissue* | *Location* | *Typical needle* | *Amount Injected (mL)* | | *Medication commonly administered* |
|---|---|---|---|---|---|---|
| | | | | **Usual** | **Range** | |
| Intraarterial | Artery | Major patent artery in tumor site | Catheter | Q.S.[a] | 10–50 | Antineoplastic agents |
| Intraarticular | Joints | Ankle, elbow, knee, shoulder | 23 G × 1 to 1½ in. | 1 | 0.1–2 | Corticosteroid suspensions |
| | | Hip | 20 G to 22 G × 3 in. | 2 | 2–3 | Corticosteroid suspensions |
| | | Finger and toe | 25 G × 1 in. | | | Corticosteroid suspensions |
| Intracardiac | Myocardium | Left center chest | 18 G to 20 G × 3½ to 4 in. | Q.S. | 1–10 | 1:10,000 aqueous epinephrine |
| | Ventricle | Left center chest | Same | Q.S. | 1–10 | 10% calcium chloride |
| Intradermal | Skin | Ventral midforearm and scapula area of back | 26 G × ⅜ in. | 0.1 | 0.01–0.1 | Antibiotics, tuberculin, and other possible allergens |
| Intramuscular | Deltoid | Triangular muscle of upper arm at shoulder | 23 G to 25 G × ⅝ to 1 in. | 0.5 | 0.5–2 | Absorbed tetanus toxoid, epinephrine in oil, narcotics, sedatives, vitamin $B_{12}$, vaccines, lidocaine hydrochloride |
| | Gluteus medius | Dorsogluteal site | 20 G to 23 G ×1½ to 3 in. | 2–4 | 1–5 | Deep IM and Z-track injections, e.g., iron–dextran complex |
| | Rectus femoris | Medial midthigh | 22 G to 25 G × ½ to 1 in.; common site for infants | 1–2 | 1–3 | Antiemetics, narcotics, sedatives, injections in oil, antibiotics, deep IM and Z-track injections |
| | Gluteus minimus | Ventrogluteal site | 20 G to 23 G × 1½ to 3 in. | 1–4 | 1–5 | |
| | Vastus lateralis | Lateral midthigh | 22 G to 25 G × ⅝ to 1 in.; for infant and pediatric doses 20 G to 23 G × 1½ in. for adults | 1–4 | 1–5 | |
| Intravenous | Basilic and cephalic veins | Back of hand and forearm | 25 G × ⅝ in. for slow injections 19 G to 23 G × 1 to 1½ in. | 1–10 | 0.5–50 | Aminophylline, antibiotics, antineoplastics, vasopressors, vitamins, sugar and electrolyte solutions, corticosteroid solutions |
| Subcutaneous | Fatty layer underlying skin | Lateral upper arms and thighs, abdomen at navel, back, upper hips | 25 G to 27 G × ½ to ⅝ in. | 0.5 | 0.5–1.5 | Aqueous epinephrine solution and suspension, fluid tetanus toxoid, insulins, narcotics, vaccines, vitamin $B_{12}$ |

[a] Q.S., sufficient quantity.

From Newton DW, Newton M: Route, site, and technique: Three key decisions in giving parenteral medication. Nursing 1979;9:18–25, with permission.

largely on perceived benefits, for example, freedom of movement and fewer hospitalizations compared with the risks and inconveniences of carrying a device that requires care and attention to maintain its effectiveness.

An important factor in the selection of an infusion device as an alternative method of drug delivery is drug stability. Very little is known about the stability of drugs in these devices. Consequently, drugs should be assumed to be unstable in an infusion device until stability tests have proven otherwise.

The most common and serious adverse effects from infusion therapy occur at the site of injection. These effects include pain, inflammation, and to a lesser extent, infection. The development of inflammation, particularly with subcutaneous infusion pumps, may affect patient compliance and necessitate removal of the infusion catheter.

## Oral Administration

Oral administration is the most convenient and economic method of systemic drug delivery. Drugs administered orally either exert a local effect on the gastrointestinal system, or are absorbed through the mucosa into the blood and lymphatic circulatory systems and exert a systemic effect. Absorption can occur in the mouth (buccal and sublingual), small intestine, and, to a lesser extent, the stomach and large intestine.

### *Liquid Oral Preparations*

When solid dosage forms are unavailable or inappropriate for oral administration, liquids are the preferred dosage form. The most common liquid oral preparations include aqueous solutions and suspensions. Oil-in-water emulsions and oral aerosols are less commonly used.

Syrups and elixirs are aqueous solutions that are particularly useful for the administration of drugs to pediatric patients. Both are sweetened vehicles that effectively mask drug taste; however, the concentration of sucrose in syrups is high (85% w/v), leaving little water available for drug dissolution. Drugs are usually more soluble in elixirs than in syrups; however, the alcohol content of elixirs may preclude the use of this vehicle in some patients.

Oral suspensions are frequently prepared with drugs that are insoluble, unstable, or unpleasant tasting when in solution. Many oral suspensions are formulated as powders or granules that are reconstituted with purified water prior to dispensing. Oral extemporaneously prepared suspensions can be manufactured by dispersing triturated tablets or the contents of a capsule in simple syrup.

The administration of liquid preparations through a nasogastric (NG) tube may be necessary for some institutionalized patients. The most common type of drug delivered through a nasogastric tube is a suspension or slurry of the drug prepared from a commercial tablet or capsule. Appropriate vehicles for this form of drug administration include diluted syrups (which provide greater viscosity) and purified water.

A number of drug products and dosage forms should not be crushed and administered as a liquid suspension because of local drug toxicity or the characteristics of the dosage form. These products include controlled-release, enteric-coated tablets, drugs with extremely unpleasant tastes or odors, and drugs that are irritating to the mucosal membranes.[13]

Poor patient acceptance and inaccurate drug delivery have restricted the use of oil-in-water emulsions to laxatives and vitamin supplements. Oral aerosol devices can be used for drugs that have limited stability in solutions such as nitroglycerin.

### *Solid Oral Preparations*

Solid oral dosage forms, primarily tablets and capsules, confer greater drug stability and provide a more accurate drug dosage. Nevertheless, they may be less preferable than liquids for some patients such as the pediatric or geriatric patient. Tablets are the most frequently preferred dosage form because they are generally the least expensive delivery system to manufacture and they possess the greatest flexibility in formulation and design.

Buccal and sublingual tablets may be used for local or systemic drug administration. Saliva is usually available to dissolve the drug, and the vascular lining of the buccal cavity and tongue provide sites for drug absorption. Buccal tablets are usually hard, and are designed to dissolve slowly in the buccal cavity or directly on the affected area (e.g., mouth ulcer). They are not to be dissolved under the tongue, chewed, or swallowed. Hot liquids accelerate the dissolution of a buccal tablet. Sublingual tablets are placed under the tongue for rapid drug absorption and onset of action, and usually contain drugs that have poor oral bioavailability characteristics or high hepatic first-pass metabolism.

Chewable tablets are available for patients who have difficulty in swallowing. Frequently, mannitol is used as the tablet base to provide a sweet, pleasant taste, and a cooling sensation within the mouth. Most chewable tablets do not contain disintegrants; therefore, chewing before swallowing is essential to optimize drug bioavailability. Effervescent tablets rely on the reaction between an alkali (e.g., sodium bicarbonate) and an acidic (e.g., tartaric acid) substance to provide rapid disintegration and dissolution of a drug or to improve palatability. It is especially important that effervescent tablets are protected against moisture during storage.

Hard gelatin capsules usually contain between 65 and 1,000 mg of drug and appropriate excipients within a hard gelatin capsule shell. This dosage form is suitable for drugs that are unstable in solution, that cannot readily be compressed, or that have an unpleasant taste or odor; however, they should not be used for extremely water soluble drugs or highly efflorescent or deliquescent compounds. Although the vulnerability of hard gelatin capsules to tampering has resulted in new standards for tamper-resistant packaging, the use of these capsules has increased significantly in the last decade largely because of their relatively good bioavailability characteristics. Release, dissolution, and absorption of a drug are generally more rapid from a capsule than from a tablet.

Soft gelatin capsules contain a liquid solution or suspension in a water-immiscible or water-miscible vehicle such as mineral oil and glycols surrounded by a soft, plasticized, gelatin shell. This one-piece sealed capsule is usually intended for oral use but may also be used for rectal, vaginal, topical, ophthalmic, or otic drug delivery.[14] Soft gelatin capsules are ideal for accurate delivery of drugs in oils and other liquids, but cannot be used for low-molecular-weight compounds or for liquids that dissolve or migrate freely through the capsule.

### *Biopharmaceutic Considerations*

Despite limitations in the design and performance of oral drug delivery systems resulting from intra- and intersubject variation as well as the physiologic constraints and variations within the gastrointestinal tract, the oral route remains the most popular route of drug administration. Drug bioavailability from oral dosage forms in decreasing order is generally solutions > suspensions > oil-in-water emulsions > capsules > tablets > controlled-release capsules and tablets.

Aqueous solutions rapidly reach the duodenum and absorption commences almost immediately. Suspension particles must first dissolve in the gastrointestinal secretions before absorption can occur. Absorption from oral emulsions occurs by pinocytosis and may be relatively rapid, especially if digestible oils are used.

Conventional tablets and capsules must disintegrate in the stomach or small intestine before drug dissolution and absorption can occur. Disintegration, dissolution, and bioavailability are greatly influenced by formulation variables, method of manufacture, and the physicochemical properties of the drug. Many examples of the influence of these factors causing variable drug release, absorption, and bioavailability may be found in the literature relative to the subject of bioequivalence.[15,16]

### *Therapeutic Considerations*

Key factors in selecting the optimal oral dosage form include drug availability, patient age and disease state, environmental conditions, and biopharmaceutic considerations. After the appropriate dosage form has been selected, other factors such as whether the drug should be administered in the presence or absence of food should also be considered.

Pediatric and geriatric patients generally prefer oral liquid dosage forms. Patient-specific doses are more easily administered. Moreover, solid dosage forms are not swallowed very easily by patients in these age groups, a fact that may result in erratic drug absorption, patient noncompliance, and esophageal trauma or irritation.[17] Chewable tablets are an alternative dosage form in these patients, but are not widely available for many drugs and do not mask drug taste as well as flavored liquids. Some components of a liquid vehicle, for example, ethanol, may limit its usefulness in certain patients, including children, diabetics, and persons with peptic ulcer disease.

An alternative route of administration may be required for patients who are unwilling or unable to swallow oral dosage forms. These patients include the blind, comatose, mentally or physically impaired, and those with local gastrointestinal diseases such as peptic ulcer or ulcerative colitis.

The presence of food in the gastrointestinal tract may alter pH, motility, gastric emptying time, and the rate and extent of drug absorption. In general, drugs that cause gastrointestinal irritation should be taken with food. Drugs that should be taken on an empty stomach include those that are acid labile or known to exhibit decreases in their rates and/or extents of absorption when taken with food. A few drugs, for example, anticholinergics, should be taken 15 to 30 minutes before meals so that they can exert their antispasmodic effect prior to food ingestion.[18]

General patient instructions related to oral drug administration include the following:

1. Most tablets and capsules should be swallowed whole with plenty of water.
2. Liquids are preferred for children and elderly patients, but may require special storage precautions to maximize drug stability and prevent accidental poisonings.
3. Specialty oral dosage forms such as sublingual, buccal, and chewable tablets, as well as capsules used as "carriers," that is, those intended to be emptied into food or beverages, require specific and complete patient instructions to ensure optimal drug delivery.
4. Patients should always be given a schedule for taking their medications, with particular reference to meals and nighttime administration.

## Oral Controlled Release

Depending on the desired effect, the rate of drug release from a dosage form may be enhanced or retarded by modifying its design and composition. A controlled-release formulation can delay, prolong, sustain, or target drug delivery. The aim of a controlled-release drug delivery preparation is to maintain drug plasma concentrations for prolonged periods above the minimum effective concentration and below the minimum toxic concentration.

To produce and maintain a constant plasma drug concentration, the rate-limiting step for drug bioavailability must be controlled by the drug delivery system. Further, drug delivery into the body should ideally be at a constant rate and equal to the rate of drug elimination. Few drug delivery systems, however, are able to achieve this ideal situation. Most controlled delivery systems release the drug at a constantly declining, first-order rate. Some potential advantages of controlled-release pharmaceuticals when compared with conventional dosage forms include a reduction in dosing frequency, a decrease in the incidence and/or intensity of adverse effects, greater selectivity of pharmacologic activity, more constant therapeutic effect, and improved patient compliance.[19]

Although various chemical and biologic methods have been employed, physical methods are most commonly used in the design of controlled drug delivery systems.[19] In an attempt to achieve constant plasma concentrations, controlled-release preparations are usually formulated to provide a rapidly available dose to initially establish a therapeutic plasma level, and a controlled-release component to maintain the concentration.

### *Preparations*

Dissolution-controlled systems are usually encapsulated or matrix formulations. Encapsulation methods involve coating drug particles or granules (microencapsulation) with a slowly dissolving wall material. These coated particles can subsequently be formulated into tablets or capsules. Repeat-action capsules can be obtained by coating granules with multiple coats of the same or different wall materials. Alternatively, the rate of dissolution can be controlled by compressing the drug into a slowly dissolving matrix. In these types of controlled-release preparations, drug release rate is influenced by such factors as tablet porosity, surface area, compressional force, soluble additives, and wettability of the delivery system.

Diffusion-controlled systems are either reservoir or matrix devices. In reservoir devices a water-insoluble, semipermeable, polymeric coating surrounds a drug core reservoir. Drug release is governed by Fick's law of diffusion. Matrix systems contain the drug homogeneously dispersed in an inert, insoluble, nondisintegrating matrix consisting of polymeric or fatty materials. In practice, drug release from many oral controlled-release systems is both dissolution and diffusion controlled.

Ion-exchange resins have long been used in attempts to control drug delivery; however, the success with these preparations has been limited largely because of variations in the ionic content of the gastrointestinal tract resulting from diet, pH, water intake, and composition of the gastrointestinal contents. A recent improvement is the Pennkinetic system in which the drug is bound to a nonabsorbable ion-exchange polymer, a portion of which is coated within a semipermeable membrane to provide 12 hours of sustained delivery.[20] Drug molecules are released when displaced by ions from the gastrointestinal fluid. The release of drug from both liquid and solid oral formulations that have been prepared using this approach is reportedly independent of gastrointestinal pH, temperature, and content.

Osmotically actuated dosage forms have been used to deliver drugs via a variety of routes.[21] The oral osmotic system, Oros, consists of an osmotically active drug in a tablet core coated with a semipermeable membrane in which a small delivery orifice has been drilled. When in contact with body fluid, water enters the core because of the osmotic pressure difference across the membrane and dissolves the drug. The increase in hydrostatic pressure inside the tablet core forces the drug in solution out through the orifice. The rate of drug release depends on the rate at which water enters the core, and is essentially independent of the nature of the gastrointestinal environment. Osmotic control provides constant zero-order drug release for approximately 70% of the drug contained in the formulation.

The duration of drug release from oral controlled-release systems is usually restricted by the limited residence time in the vicinity of the absorption site. Hence, attempts have recently been made to prolong the residence time of the drug delivery systems in the gastrointestinal tract through the use of floating and inflatable tablets and capsules, and unfolding multilaminated, hydrodynamic-pressure-controlled, and bioadhesive devices.[22]

### *Biopharmaceutic Considerations*

Once- or twice-daily dosing has emerged as an important emphasis in oral drug delivery; however, without exception, controlled delivery systems do not maximize drug bioavailability and effects. Further, the potential problems inherent in oral controlled release generally relate to interaction among the rate, extent, and location where the dosage form releases the drug, regional differences in gastrointestinal tract physiology and absorption, and the inherent properties of the drug itself. Increased first-pass metabolism, dose dumping, food, and diurnal variation effects may all decrease bioavailability, efficacy, and safety as compared to conventional drug dosage forms.[23] Nevertheless, with the emphasis that has been placed on increasing patient compliance and convenience, controlled drug delivery research will continue to be an important focus of the pharmaceutical industry.

As controlled oral delivery systems must remain at the absorption site for extended periods to slow the apparent absorption rate, factors that influence gastric emptying and intestinal motility will affect drug bioavailability. Attempts to control gastrointestinal transit time and attain site-specific release of a drug at its "absorption window" are alternative approaches that are currently being investigated in the design of controlled oral drug delivery systems.

It is unnecessary to formulate drugs that possess low aqueous solubility or an elimination half-life greater than 10 hours in a controlled-release delivery system because the duration of their pharmacologic effect(s) is inherently long. Other drug properties such as dose size, stability, pH-dependent absorption, first-pass metabolism, or excessive protein binding usually restrict rather than prohibit the formulation of a drug into a controlled-release delivery system.[24]

### *Therapeutic Considerations*

All solid oral controlled-release preparations must be swallowed whole, preferably with a glass of water. Damage to the tablet matrix or other release-controlling mechanism, for example by chewing, can result in potentially serious dose dumping. Some oral controlled-release formulations may be unsuitable for the young or elderly patient because of dose size necessary to sustain therapeutic drug levels. At present, there is controversy over whether solid oral or multiparticulate controlled-release dosage forms provide a more predictable clinical effect. Another potential problem is that coated and matrix tablets may adhere to or become trapped in the folds of the gastrointestinal tract, causing localized irritation, obstruction, and/or ulceration.

## Rectal Administration

The rectal route is used for both local and systemic drug administration. It is an alternative to oral administration in children, the mentally ill, those who are bedridden, or those who have nausea and vomiting. Drugs that cause excessive gastrointestinal irritation or that have a high hepatic first-pass metabolism may be effectively administered rectally. In Anglo-Saxon countries, rectal suppository administration accounts for only 1% to 2% of all drugs that are given for their systemic effects. On the other hand, suppositories account for approximately 15% to 20% of all products used in many European and Latin American countries.[25] When used for their systemic effects, the doses of drugs administered rectally are usually one half to two times the oral dose.

### *Preparations*

Drugs are most commonly administered rectally in solid suppository dosage forms. After insertion, the suppositories dissolve or melt in the rectal secretions, releasing the drug to produce a local effect or to be absorbed through the rectal mucosa to produce a systemic effect. Enemas are solutions or suspensions that can be used for the delivery of drugs locally or systemically, but are most commonly given to stimulate the evacuation of the bowel or to instill radiologic-contrast media.

For rapid and complete drug release from a suppository, lipophilic drugs should be formulated in hydrophilic bases, and water-soluble compounds in lipophilic bases. A variety of natural and synthetic substances of widely differing physical and chemical properties are available for use as suppository bases.[25,26] The ideal suppository basc should melt or dissolve at 37°C and be nonirritating, nontoxic, nonsensitizing, and compatible with a wide range of drugs.

### *Biopharmaceutic Considerations*

The human rectum consists of the terminal 15- to 20-cm segment of the large intestine. It contains approximately 2–3 mL of mucous fluid secretions, pH 7–8, which display no buffering capacity or enzymatic activity. Because of the absence of villi and microvilli, which are present in the small intestine, the available surface area for absorption in the rectum is very limited (200–400 $cm^2$). The luminal pressure, degree of rectal motility, and presence of fecal material affect the extent of dispersion of the dosage form after it has dissolved or melted. These factors are altered with age, trauma, hemorrhoids, or the presence of other diseases.[25]

The availability of drug after rectal administration may be limited by the rate at which the drug is released from the suppository or the absorption rate of the drug across the rectal mucosa. In general, the absorption of drugs from the rectal area is slower, less complete, and more erratic compared with that of drugs given orally. The major source of blood to the rectum is provided by the superior rectal artery. Venous return is via the superior, middle, and inferior hemorrhoidal veins. As the superior hemorrhoid vein drains directly into the portal vein, the extent of hepatic drug metabolism from a first-pass effect increases as the depth of insertion into the rectum increases. The middle and inferior veins drain directly into the general circulation via the iliac vein and vena cava.

### *Therapeutic Considerations*

Cocoa butter and synthetic oil base suppositories should be stored under refrigeration, and warmed in the patient's hands to increase comfort and to facilitate insertion. Polyethylene glycol base suppositories should be moistened with warm tap water prior to insertion for similar reasons. All suppositories should be retained in the rectum for at least 20 to 30 minutes to ensure melting or dissolution of the base, as well as release of the drug from the liquified base. A slight laxative effect may be observed after the use of cocoa butter or synthetic oil base suppositories. With an enema, it is desirable to lubricate the tip of the applicator and warm thecontents in the patient's hands before inserting. Low-volume enemas should be used for children to avoid stimulation of defecation when a systemic effect is desired.

## Topical and Transdermal Administration

Although the multilayered structure and heterogeneous composition of the skin provide an effective barrier to the passage of substances into as well as out of the body, drugs are applied to the skin in various dosage forms for their local and systemic effects. With the exception of drugs that are used for their superficial topical effects (e.g., zinc oxide and sulfur), drugs that are applied to the skin must penetrate to the appropriate skin layer to produce their desired therapeutic effect(s), as summarized in Table 2.7. Of the three main skin layers, stratum corneum, epidermis, and dermis, the principal or rate-limiting barrier for drug absorption through intact skin is the dense, keratinized stratum corneum outer layer. Regional variations in skin drug permeability are due primarily to differences in the structure and thickness of this layer. The target areas for drugs that are applied topically for their "local" effects are the skin surface, stratum corneum, viable epidermis and dermis, and the appendages (e.g., nails, sebaceous and sweat glands, and hair follicles). The presence of an efficient vascular network in the dermis (or corium) enables drugs that penetrate the stratum corneum and viable epidermis to be readily absorbed systemically. Detailed descriptions of the structure, composition, and function of the skin are available in the literature.[27,28]

Improved understanding of the physiology of the skin and the process of percutaneous drug absorption has enabled topically applied drugs to be administered for their systemic effects. Initially, when ointments were applied topically, based on the observations with nitroglycerin,[29] it was noted that systemic drug absorption could be unpredictable because of the variability in skin permeation, imprecise dosage, and unreliable drug delivery.[30] Modern transdermal delivery systems appear to have overcome these problems by controlling the rate of drug release onto the skin surface. With these systems, drug availability is independent of the rate at which the drug permeates the skin into the general circulation.

Assuming that the drug is absorbed in sufficient quantity, transdermal systemic drug delivery offers several advantages. The risks and inconveniences of intravenous therapy are avoided, the variable drug bioavailability that is seen after oral therapy is eliminated, and drugs with narrow therapeutic indices or short biologic half-lives may be ad-

**Table 2.7** Common Drug Treatments and Associated Skin Layers

| *Skin layer* | *Principal structural characteristic* | *Common drug conditions* |
|---|---|---|
| Skin surface | Acid mantle, pH 4.2–5.6 | Antiseptic<br>Antiperspirant<br>Acne<br>Sunburn |
| Stratum corneum (~10 μm) | Densely packed, dead keratinized cells | Emollient<br>Keratolytic<br>Psoriasis<br>Dandruff |
| Viable epidermis (~200 μm) | Four cell layers | Anti-inflammatory<br>Antihistamine<br>Anesthetic<br>Antipruritic |
| Dermis (2,000–5,000 μm) | Fibrous collagen | |
| Capillaries | Reach to within 200 μm of the skin surface | Systemic drug therapy (angina, kinetosis, osteoporosis, menopause, hypertension) |

Modified from Barry BW: Structure, function, diseases and topical treatment of human skin, in Swarbrick J (Ed): Dermatological Formulations: Percutaneous Absorption. New York, Marcel Dekker, 1983, p 32, with permission.

ministered safely and for prolonged periods. As side effects and the frequency of dosing are reduced, patient compliance improves. Rapid termination of drug effect also is possible simply by removing the delivery device from the skin.

### *Preparations*

Topical preparations, as opposed to transdermal drug delivery systems, are used primarily for their local effects and usually contain the following constituents in addition to the active drug: buffer, preservative, cosolvent(s), emulsifying agent, viscosity-enhancing agent, antioxidant, permeation enhancer, and/or propellants. Transdermal drug delivery systems are used exclusively for the production of a systemic effect. They are multiphasic and usually in the form of an adhesive patch.

Liquid dosage forms include low-viscosity solutions, suspensions, and dilute emulsions that are designed to uniformly cover a large area of the body with the medicament. Generally, aqueous vehicles are used for this purpose; however, other solvents such as glycerol may be included in the formulation to promote adhesion of powders to the skin and skin hydration. Ethanol may be added as a cosolvent or to promote a cooling effect.

Semisolids include ointments, creams, gels, and pastes. Ointments are greasy and usually anhydrous, and contain the drug dissolved or suspended in one of four types of bases. Paraffin is the main component of hydrocarbon bases that possess occlusive properties. The water repellent characteristics of a base are enhanced by the inclusion of silicone polymers such as dimethicone. Absorption bases such as anhydrous lanolin are able to absorb water to form water-in-oil (w/o) emulsions. The two remaining types of bases are the water-miscible emulsifying bases and the water-soluble bases. The latter are especially used to incorporate aqueous drug solutions into topical preparations.

Creams are generally water-in-oil emulsions that provide an emollient and cleansing action or oil-in-water emulsions that are used as water-washable bases or vanishing creams. Newer formulations of steroids in fatty alcohol–propylene glycol cream bases have demonstrated superior bioavailability and efficacy.[31] Gels and pastes are not commonly used for topical drug delivery. Drugs can also be administered as solutions, suspensions, foams, or semisolids directly onto the damaged areas as an aerosol. Topical powders are especially useful in drying wound exudates.

All topical preparations should maximize drug availability from the finished dosage form, facilitate easy and uniform application, and adhere to skin while not being too greasy or difficult to remove. The most important factor that influences the rate and extent of percutaneous drug absorption is the occlusive effect of oily vehicles which softens and swells the skin, thereby altering skin permeability dramatically. The general relationship between the type of vehicle and skin hydration and skin permeability is oily base > w/o emulsion > o/w emulsion > powder.

Although numerous designs have been investigated,[32] transdermal drug delivery systems can be classified into four general categories.[33] All are multilayered films with a common backing of drug-impermeable metallic plastic film. To ensure that transdermal systemic drug bioavailability is independent of variations in skin permeability, the rate of drug delivery from the device to the skin surface must be the rate-limiting step in transdermal absorption.

Membrane-moderated systems consist of four layers, with the drug dispersed or suspended in a solid or liquid reservoir compartment. A rate-controlling polymeric membrane of defined drug permeability is covered with a drug-compatible, hypoallergenic adhesive polymer to maintain skin contact. As seen with the scopolamine therapeutic system, ideally the delivery systems should contain a primary dose to rapidly achieve therapeutic plasma concentrations while the membrane controls the availability of the maintenance dose from the reservoir.[12]

Adhesive-diffusion-controlled systems are simplified three-layered devices in which the drug is adsorbed and dissolved in a water-insoluble, polymeric adhesive base that functions as both the drug reservoir and release-control element. The constant thickness of these systems provides diffusion-controlled drug delivery.

Matrix diffusion systems contain the drug homogeneously dispersed in a disk-shaped, crosslinked, hydrophilic polymer matrix of controlled surface area and thickness.[33] Skin contact is maintained by an adhesive rim around the perimeter of the drug matrix; hence, drug does not pass through an adhesive layer.

Microreservoir systems use a combination of the reservoir and matrix dispersion approaches. The drug is dispersed within microscopic aqueous, polymer solution droplets (5–50 μm) that are entrapped in a crosslinked silicone elastomer matrix of controlled thickness and surface area. The rim of adhesive foam pad ensures skin contact.[30]

### *Biopharmaceutic Considerations*

The principal transport mechanism across mammalian skin is passive diffusion. Percutaneous drug absorption is much slower and more selective than gastrointestinal absorption, as the stratum corneum is relatively impermeable to drug molecules. The heterogeneous multilayered structure of the skin provides a complex diffusional barrier to drug transport either through the skin or via hair follicles and sweat glands that act as diffusional shunts. Thus, drug absorption through intact skin can occur via a transepidermal route, which allows drugs to penetrate by intercellular and/or intracellular diffusion through cells of the stratum corneum, and the transappendageal (transfollicular) route, where drugs penetrate by diffusion down hair follicles, in the secretions of the sebaceous and/or eccrine glands.[27,28]

In general, because of their ability to partition into the dead stratum corneum, the transdermal route is considered to be favored by nonelectrolytes that possess both hydrophilic and hydrophobic properties. The transappendageal route is said to be favored by electrolytes, polar molecules, and large molecules such as steroids and antibiotics.[27] Nevertheless, a particular drug will penetrate the skin by the route that offers the least resistance to passive diffusion. Therefore, many physicochemical properties of the drug, dosage form variables, and variations in skin condition determine not only which absorption pathway predominates, but also the rate and extent of percutaneous absorption. Absorption may continually change as the vehicle, skin secretions, and disease state modify the skin barrier.

With the exception of the extremities below the knee or elbow, transdermal systems for the delivery of drug to the systemic circulation may be generally applied to any clean, dry, hairless skin area on the body. The sites used should be varied between applications, avoiding areas where cuts and abrasions are present. Hair that may interfere with the application of the system should be removed by clipping but not shaving. A specifically designed preparation for application behind the ear is the scopolamine therapeutic system.

The rate of drug release from transdermal delivery systems remains constant as long as the diffusion gradient between the system and the skin is maintained. Drug diffusion begins as soon as the system is applied to the skin. After saturation of the binding sites in the skin, constant drug release establishes therapeutically active plasma concentrations. After the transdermal patch is removed, plasma concentrations decrease at a rate determined by the half-life of the drug.[33] As the size of the therapeutic system determines the amount of drug absorbed per unit time, plasma drug concentrations are linearly proportional to the drug-releasing surface of the transdermal system in contact with the skin. The quantity of drug in the reservoir determines the duration of action.

For transdermally administered drugs to be clinically effective, they must be therapeutically potent in daily doses of less than about 2 mg,[27] able to permeate the skin in sufficient quantities to exert systemic effects, nonirritating and nonsensitizing to the skin, and unaffected by enzymes in the epidermis. At present, only a limited number of drugs that meet these criteria have been successfully marketed in a transdermal drug delivery system. They include nitroglycerin,[30] scopolamine,[34] clonidine,[35] estradiol,[36] and isosorbide dinitrate.[33] Evidence of interest in this area, however, is demonstrated by the increasing number of devices and therapeutic agents that are now being investigated for transdermal delivery.

Because of the low skin permeability of most drugs, further research is required before transdermal delivery is a realistic alternative for a wide range of drugs. Future studies should investigate the use of new penetration-enhancing agents, prodrugs, and other techniques such as iontophoresis that have been shown in preliminary studies to promote percutaneous drug absorption.[33]

### *Therapeutic Considerations*

The affected area of the skin should be cleansed thoroughly before the topical preparation is applied. Lotions and emulsions should be shaken before application. Preparations should be applied as a thin film and covered with a sterile occlusive dressing to ensure that the affected skin area remains clean and that the clothing is not stained. Occlusion also enhances percutaneous drug absorption. While drugs are usually distributed rapidly by the capillary network, certain drugs such as corticosteroids remain in the subcutaneous tissues for extended periods.[33] Skin penetration is greatly enhanced when the stratum corneum is damaged. Systemic toxicity can arise when a medication is applied liberally to broken skin or over a large surface area.

Effective adhesion of the transdermal delivery system to the skin surface is critical to maintaining the diffusion gradient that is necessary for drug delivery. Adhesive cover patches may be used over the delivery system so effective contact is ensured for prolonged periods and during daily activities. As transdermal systems deliver the drug at a controlled rate per unit area, most systems are available in more than one size so the dosage of the drug can be varied.

Cutting transdermal devices in an attempt to manipulate the dosage should be avoided, because this may damage the drug reservoir or rate-controlling element or destroy the ability of the device to make effective adhesive contact with the skin surface. Further, as the aluminum-containing backing of transdermal patches may cause arcing when defibrillation is attempted during cardiopulmonary resuscitation, it is recommended that these types of patches be removed before defibrillating.[37] With nitroglycerin patches, it may also be reasonable to consider removing the transdermal delivery system before an electrocardiogram, because mild explosions have been reported.

Although the in vitro release characteristics of nitroglycerin from the four types of transdermal system designs have been observed to be different,[33] human bioavailability studies indicate that when the daily nitroglycerin dose is correlated with the amount released per unit area for each device, the systems are clinically interchangeable.[38,39] Recently, the question has been raised whether transdermal devices provide effective long-term therapy.[40,41] Because nitrate tolerance develops, intermittent use of this system has been suggested to maintain effective angina prophylaxis.[42]

## Ophthalmic Administration

The eye, with its unique structure and function, is an extremely sensitive organ that often requires prompt medical treatment upon injury or in the presence of a disease. Drugs are most commonly applied directly to the eye in the form of eye drops or an ointment. The treatment of diseases of the eye via topical application or systemic administration may be ineffective and/or inefficient because of various factors known to affect the distribution of drugs into the eye (Fig. 2.1).[43]

Ocular injections are used when a drug is unable to penetrate to the desired intraocular site after topical administration, or when it is not possible to obtain a therapeutic concentration of drug in the posterior portion of the eye after direct application. Subconjunctival injections are used in the emergency management of acute infections of the anterior eye. A retrobulbar injection may be used for the treatment of optic nerve damage or for anesthesia prior to surgery.[44] In general, intraocular injections should be avoided because of the dangers and high risks of complications.

### *Preparations*

Ophthalmic drops are usually aqueous, sterile, buffered solutions that frequently contain a preservative and viscosity-enhancing agent. Although the pH of an ophthalmic solution should be in the range 5–9 to avoid corneal damage and pain, it is not essential that it be isotonic, as the solution undergoes rapid dilution after instillation. The eye is able to tolerate an osmotic pressure equivalent to 0.6% to 1.8% (w/v) sodium chloride.

Ophthalmic suspensions may be employed when a drug is insoluble or unstable or when prolonged action is desired. With suspension formulations, drug particle size is critical because it influences the rate and extent of drug absorption as well as patient comfort. Clearly, thorough shaking of all suspensions prior to instillation is essential.

Ophthalmic ointments contain drug that is dissolved or suspended in a petroleum-based vehicle that melts near body temperature. Lanolin may be added to facilitate the inclusion of water-soluble drugs. Ophthalmic ointments are used externally only, and while they may prolong drug release and contact time, they often blur vision and therefore should be limited for use just before bedtime.

Ophthalmic preparations that are intended to be injected must meet all of the requirements for a parenteral solution, for example, sterility.

The relatively frequent dosing required with the present ophthalmic preparations is a major shortcoming of the currently available ophthalmic drug delivery systems. In an attempt to overcome this deficiency and to optimize ophthalmic drug delivery, efforts are being made to reduce ocular drainage using viscosity-enhancing agents, suspensions, emulsions, ointments, or biodegradable and nonbiodegradable inserts or to improve corneal drug penetration using ionophores, ion pairs, liposomes, and prodrugs.[44] For example, in an attempt to reduce drug loss from drainage in the nasolacrimal ducts, the use of soft lenses and soluble and nonbiodegradable ophthalmic inserts have produced an improvement in ocular drug penetration; however, patient acceptance of these drug delivery systems has been poor because they can be uncomfortable and may be dislodged or dispelled.

Attempts to improve ocular absorption have proven to be more successful. For example, dipivalyl epinephrine, a lipophilic prodrug of epinephrine, has been shown to penetrate the cornea approximately 17-fold more readily than epinephrine, and produced a more sustained drug effect with fewer systemic side effects.[45]

### *Biopharmaceutic Considerations*

The human eye is protected by the sclera and cornea, and drug penetration to intraocular target sites is hindered by the presence of various blood–eye "barriers" (Figure 2.1). When drops are instilled in the eye, usually 90% to 99% of the drug is lost because of the limited capacity of the precorneal area (10–20 μL) in comparison with an average drop size of 50 μL.[43,46] This loss is accentuated when the patient blinks or rubs the eyes. Thus, the instillation of multiple drops is wasteful.

Human tears are continuously replaced at a rate of approximately 15% per minute, resulting in limited contact time for drug absorption and rapid dilution of drug concentration. Because of the small volume of medication used, protein binding may significantly decrease absorption, and enzymes located in the tears, cornea, and aqueous humor may extensively metabolize drugs before absorption takes place.

The cornea is a unique biologic barrier consisting of a thick aqueous stroma sandwiched between the lipid epithelium and endothelium layers. Therefore, only drugs that are both hydrophilic and lipophilic can cross the cornea from the external tear chamber into the anterior chamber of the eye by passive diffusion. Further, corneal penetration is greatly affected by the lipid solubility characteristics as well as the

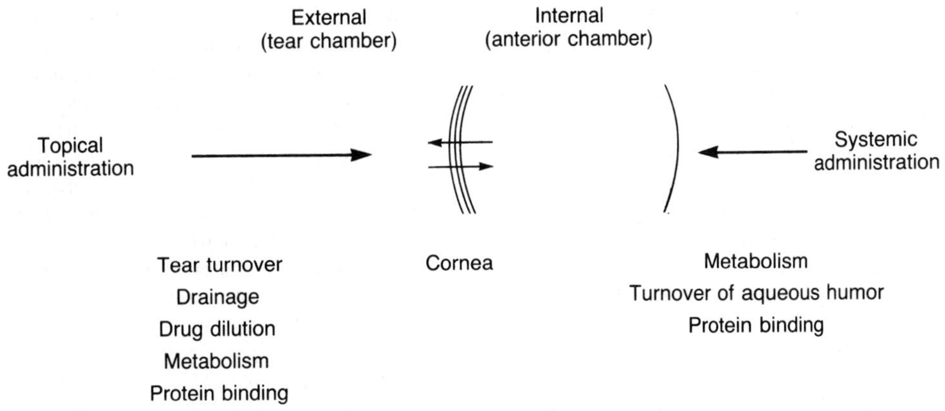


**Figure 2.1** Schematic representation of the sites and factors that influence the effectiveness of a drug in the eye. (From Robinson JR, Goshman LM: Topical drug-delivery systems (eye, ear, nose), in Banker GS, Chalmers RK (Eds): Pharmaceutics and Pharmacy Practice. Philadelphia, J.B. Lippincott, 1982, p 319, with permission).

molecular weight of the drug. Properties of the delivery system also influence corneal penetration, especially when a surfactant is added to decrease surface tension and promote wetting, and when a viscosity-enhancing agent is used to prolong the contact time of the drug.

### *Therapeutic Considerations*

Preserving the sterility of the ophthalmic preparation and the integrity of all its components is of utmost importance. Patients should be instructed to inspect their ophthalmic solutions for cloudiness or discoloration, and to discard the preparation if either exists.

Ideally, someone other than the patient should instill an ophthalmic preparation into the patient's eye to avoid product contamination, ensure accurate drug delivery, and promote compliance. The tip of the drug applicator, that is, the dropper, squeeze bottle, or tube, should never be allowed to come in contact with the eyelid or lashes.

The administration technique for all ophthalmic dosage forms is similar. The solution, suspension, or ointment is instilled in the eye by tilting the head back, gently pulling out the lower lid, and instilling the drops into the pocket formed in the lower lid. A thin ribbon of ointment should be applied in the same manner. The patient should then be instructed to blink gently once or twice to spread the drug product across the eye. If multiple-drug therapy is to be used, the instillation of the drugs should be spaced at least 5 minutes apart to maximize the contact time of each drug in the eye.

Patients receiving ophthalmic drug therapy may experience blurring of their vision as a result of either a drug effect, for example, adrenergics, or the dosage form itself, for example, ointments. Systemic drug absorption of ophthalmic $\beta$-blockers may be a potential problem for patients with cardiovascular and bronchopulmonary diseases, particularly those who have congestive heart failure, bradyarrhythmias, and asthma. Patients with eye trauma should be immediately referred to a physician for emergency medical treatment.

## Respiratory Inhalation Administration

Drug administration by inhalation provides a rapid and convenient means of introducing drugs directly into the respiratory tract for the treatment of bronchopulmonary diseases.[47,48] The main advantages offered by this route and method of administration include the localized delivery of small doses of drug for rapid onset of action and the minimization of systemic side effects; however, patient education about the disease, drug therapy, inhalation devices, and inhalation techniques is essential for optimum therapeutic effect.

### *Preparations*

The ideal inhalation drug delivery device should be portable and easy to operate, and should reproducibly deliver precise doses of drug into the central and peripheral respiratory airways. Essentially three types of delivery devices are used as therapeutic aerosols: nebulizer, pressurized metered-dose aerosol, and dry powder inhaler.[47,49,50]

Nebulizers convert a drug solution into a fine aerosol mist usually using compressed air or oxygen. The patient inhales the aerosol from a mouthpiece or preferably a mask. Because portability is limited, use of a nebulizer is restricted primarily to the treatment of severe bronchopulmonary diseases in the home or hospital.

Pressurized metered-dose aerosols consist of the drug that is either dissolved or suspended in a mixture of liquefied chlorofluorocarbon propellants hermetically sealed within a metal container at high pressures. The mixture may also contain cosolvents, an antioxidant, a dispersant, and a surfactant. Mixtures of propellants are used to produce the desired pressures to aerosolize the drug solution or suspension (approximately 400 kPa at 20°C). Although large doses or repeated inhalations of chlorofluorocarbons may be cardiotoxic, the dose from therapeutic aerosols is generally considered too small to produce adverse effects.[47] The metering chamber, usually 25 to 50 $\mu$L in capacity, is contained in the valve assembly and, when actuated, delivers up to 400 individual metered doses. Patients should be advised that metered-dose aerosols are designed to operate at normal room temperature, and when not in regular use, the devices should be actuated once or twice before use to ensure that the metering chamber is full.

An important adjunct to inhalation therapy in recent years has been the use of spacer attachments that are designed to decrease drug deposition in the oropharyngeal mucosa by allowing more time for the propellant to evaporate and the particle velocity to decrease.[51–53] These auxiliary delivery devices include portable telescopic extension tubes or larger pear- or cone-shaped reservoirs. Further, because as many as 50% of the patients experience difficulty in coordinating actuation of the metered-dose aerosol with inspiration,[52] the reservoir attachments reduce the need for this requirement by the patient.

Dry powder delivery systems are breath-activated inhalation devices such as the Spinhaler or Rotohaler. Micronized solid drug particles are mixed with a more coarse lactose or glucose carrier contained in a hard gelatin capsule. After the capsule is pierced or broken in the delivery device, the powder is then withdrawn from the capsule in a turbulent airstream when the patient inhales. Because dry powder devices are activated when the patient inhales, instruction is relatively simple. The main advantage of dry powder inhalers is that they can be used by patients who lack the coordination necessary to use metered-dose aerosols correctly. The primary disadvantage is local irritation from deposition of the lactose filler on the oropharyngeal mucosa.

### *Biopharmaceutic Considerations*

The lungs provide a multibranching tortuous route for the passage of inhaled drug particles. Further, it is difficult to predict the distribution, deposition, and retention of particles in the lung because the inhaled particle size and velocity change with the distance traveled, the dimensions of the respiratory airways change, and the airway characteristics and patterns of breathing vary between patients and with the disease state. Controversy also still exists as to whether the open- or closed-mouth technique is more effective. The following are important considerations for this route of administration[47–53]:

1. Assuming that the correct inhalation technique is used, aerosol droplet size is probably the most important factor in determining the site of deposition. For optimum deposition in the respiratory airways, the mass median diameter of inhaled particles or droplets should be between 1 and 8 $\mu$m.
2. Even with particles of optimum size distribution and with use of the ideal inhalation technique, only about 10% of the total dose reaches the respiratory airways after oral inspiration. The majority of drug is lost by inertial impaction in the inhalation device or in the mouth and/or oropharyngeal region, where it is then swallowed.
3. Deposition of particles between 1 to 8 $\mu$m occurs by a combination of inertial impaction in the large central airways and gravitational sedimentation in the smaller airways and alveoli. Particles less than 1 $\mu$m are either exhaled or deposited by Brownian diffusion in the alveoli; however, this mechanism of deposition is generally insignificant for therapeutic aerosols. Particles greater than 8 $\mu$m in diameter are deposited by impaction almost exclusively in the oropharynx, and therefore do not reach the lungs.
4. Greater deposition after inhalation occurs with slower inspiration rates (25–30 L/min) and longer breath holding (10 seconds). Directions for the correct use of metered-dose aerosols are given in Table 2.8.

**Table 2.8** Directions for Use of Metered-Dose Aerosols

1. Shake aerosol to homogeneously disperse its contents.
2. Hold aerosol in a vertical position.
3. Exhale fully.
4. Place mouthpiece between the lips.
5. Actuate the inhaler while breathing slowly and deeply.
6. Hold breath for about 10 s or for as long as is possible.
7. If more than one dose is to be administered, wait 1 min before repeating to enable the aerosol to return to thermal equilibrium and the metering chamber to refill.

From Sears MR, Asher MI: Inhaler devices: How to use and which to choose. New Ethicals 1985; 22:43–56, with permission.

### *Therapeutic Considerations*

Dry powder inhalers or metered-dose aerosols fitted with spacers or reservoirs are recommended for the elderly, for the physically and mentally handicapped, for those patients with poor coordination, and for children 3 to 7 years of age. The nebulizer is recommended for patients with severe bronchopulmonary diseases and for young children under 3 years of age. Metered-dose aerosols can be managed by most adults and children over 7 years of age.

Patients receiving polydrug inhalation therapy including sympathomimetic bronchodilators and corticosteroids should be instructed to use the bronchodilator and then the steroid. This regimen enhances the effectiveness of the therapy as a result of increased availability of the steroid at the target site of action, that is, bronchioles and alveoli.

The specific type of bronchopulmonary disease has an impact on the effectiveness of the drug regimen. For example, emphysema patients are able to inhale, but have difficulty exhaling. It is imperative that these patients be instructed to take small, shallow breaths, followed by complete exhalations, prior to drug administration. This technique maximizes air exchange and allows more inhaled particles to reach the small airways.

Provided that the patient's condition is stable and the correct inhalation technique is used, there is little difference in the clinical effects obtained with the various types of inhalation devices; however, a significant limitation of inhalation therapy is that inhaled particles are frequently poorly delivered to diseased, badly ventilated areas. Regardless of the particular device used, maximum therapeutic benefit is possible only when the patient is educated about the disease and the drug therapy program and is instructed in the correct use of the particular inhalation device.

## Intranasal Administration

Administration into the nasal cavity is used primarily to produce local effects; more recently, it has been used to produce systemic effects with drugs that are unstable in the gastrointestinal tract or possess high presystemic hepatic clearances. The nasal cavity is highly vascularized and consists, in part, of the following anatomic regions: (1) central septum, (2) turbinates—projections that extend into the nasal cavity and increase nasal surface area, (3) mucus—a continuous thin liquid layer that traps foreign bodies, and (4) epithelial cilia, which remove foreign bodies by moving the mucus into the nasopharynx. In general, drug absorption after topical nasal administration occurs from the mucosal surfaces in the posterior region of the cavity.

### *Preparations*

The majority of the currently available nasal preparations are isotonic, buffered (pH 5.5–6.5), aqueous solutions that contain a preservative and/or stabilizing agent. These preparations are administered as drops or fine sprays from a plastic dropper bottle, mechanical pump, or aerosol spray container. Suspensions are not normally used owing to the limited amount of water that is available in the nasal passages to dissolve the drug. Additionally, drugs that are insoluble are treated as foreign bodies and are therefore propelled to the back of the throat and swallowed.

Nasal sprays are the preferred form for the delivery of drugs intranasally because of their ability to cover a large surface area with a fine mist. With the increased interest that has been shown in the intranasal route for systemic drug administration,[54] metered-dose mechanical pump nebulizers and metered-dose aerosols are finding increasing use because they allow deeper nasal penetration of the drug solution.

Nasal ointments and gels can be used only for the application of drugs in the anterior regions of the nose.

### *Biopharmaceutic Considerations*

Nasal airflow and nasal valve constriction cause the deposition of most aerosols and fine powders in the anterior area of the nose. For drugs that exhibit a high first-pass effect, intranasal drug administration circumvents the inconveniences of parenteral drug administration. For example, it has been shown with propranolol that the plasma concentrations obtained after intranasal drug administration were comparable to the concentration–time profile obtained after intravenous administration.[55] For some drugs such as insulin, absorption promoters have been used to achieve plasma concentrations similar to those obtained by intravenous and subcutaneous administration.[56,57] Some factors that have been shown to affect plasma drug concentrations after intranasal administration are summarized in Table 2.9.

**Table 2.9** Factors That May Influence Drug Bioavailability After Intranasal Administration

| |
|---|
| Physiologic condition of the nasal passages |
| Rate of mucus flow |
| Infection |
| Atmospheric conditions |
| Formulation factors |
| Drug concentration |
| Volume administered |
| Viscosity |
| pH and tonicity |
| Excipients |
| Administration technique |
| Device used |
| Position of head |
| Droplet size and volume |
| Site of deposition |
| Drug loss, e.g., into the esophagus |

Adapted from Colaizzi JL: Pharmacokinetics of intranasal drug administration, in Chien YW (Ed): Transnasal Systemic Medications. New York, Elsevier, 1985, pp 115–116, with permission.

### *Therapeutic Considerations*

Contamination of nasal preparations occurs routinely as a result of contact of the applicator or dropper with the nasal mucosal surface. Patients should be instructed to wash the tip of the dropper in hot water before replacing it in the bottle. This procedure should also be used with squeeze bottles containing nasal sprays. Before instilling the preparation, the patient should be instructed to inspect the solution for cloudiness or discoloration, and to dispose of the preparation if either exists.

Nasal drops are the preferred dosage form for infants with congestion. Prior to use, parents should clear excessive mucus from the nasal passages of infants using a specially designed nasal bulb syringe.

Rebound congestion, that is, chronic edema of the nasal mucosa, may occur in some patients who use nasal decongestants above the recommended doses for more than 3 to 4 days. Proper use of all nasal preparations is essential to ensure optimum therapeutic effect and to minimize adverse effects.

## Otic Administration

The human ear consists of three distinct anatomic regions: external, middle, and inner ear. Drugs that are instilled in the external ear canal by direct local application are used almost exclusively for their local effects. Agents commonly used as otics include antibiotics, antiinflammatory agents, and anesthetics. Systemic drug administration is necessary for conditions affecting the middle and inner ear.

### *Preparations*

Otic preparations should be manufactured in a nonaqueous, water-miscible vehicle such as glycerol or propylene glycol that will not support bacterial growth and will mix with the cerumen in the ear. The addition of a surfactant is desirable to promote mixing of the solution with the oily secretions of the sebaceous and cerumen glands. Warming of otic solutions, suspensions, and ointments also promotes mixing with these secretions and increases patient comfort. An otic suspension is less desirable than a solution because the particles of the suspension may compact with the ear cerumen.

### *Biopharmaceutic Considerations*

The ideal method of drug administration into the ear canal is direct local application. Because the surfaces of the canal are lined with a thin layer of cerumen, this region is able to tolerate most drugs and chemical substances that may be placed in the ear provided the tympanic membrane is intact. The surfaces of the external ear are essentially extensions of the skin. Therefore, the factors affecting drug absorption in the ear are identical to those governing percutaneous drug absorption if the tympanic membrane is intact. If the membrane is perforated, drug absorption would be similar to that seen across mucous membranes.

### *Therapeutic Considerations*

Before an otic preparation is used, the ear should be thoroughly cleansed, using an ear syringe if necessary. Sharp objects should never be used to remove cerumen. In most cases, 1–4 drops of the otic preparation is instilled in the ear canal. The preparation should remain in contact with the ear canal for a minimum of 15 to 20 minutes. This can be facilitated by gently occluding the ear canal with a cotton plug.

The use of eardrops at extreme temperatures should be avoided. Patients should be instructed to warm the preparation by holding the bottle tightly in their hands prior to instillation. Under no circumstances should an otic preparation be warmed in boiling or very hot water. Patients with fever, severe ear pain, or drainage from the ear should be referred to their physicians.

## Vaginal Administration

The vaginal epithelium is permeable to a wide variety of both organic and inorganic compounds. Therefore, systemic absorption is possible from the vaginal canal. With the exception of extemporaneous formulations of progesterone used for infertility and to maintain pregnancy, drugs that are administered vaginally are used primarily for their local effects. The vaginal route is generally considered inappropriate for the delivery of drugs for their systemic effects because of the influences of the menstrual cycle on the characteristics of the vaginal tissue as well as the composition and volume of the vaginal secretions.

### *Preparations*

Products that are intended to be inserted into the vagina include semisolid vaginal suppositories, vaginal tablets, creams, ointments, gels, liquids, and aerosol foams. Vaginal sponges, rings, foaming tablets, and water-soluble films have been used or are currently being investigated as delivery systems for contraceptive agents.[58] Vaginal applicators are usually required to insert the dosage forms into the vagina.

Vaginal suppositories are usually oval or oblong in shape and weigh approximately 5 g. They are prepared by fusion using a mold or by cold compression. Solid wedge-shaped vaginal tablets are prepared in the same manner as conventional compressed tablets. After insertion, the vaginal preparations soften, melt, or dissolve, and spread over the vaginal surfaces to produce a localized effect. As previously mentioned, systemic drug absorption may also occur after vaginal administration.

In theory, intravaginal controlled-released drug delivery would be an effective means of achieving continuous long-term delivery of therapeutic agents such as progesterone and estradiol, which are poorly absorbed after oral administration because of extensive first-pass hepatic metabolism. Two intravaginal delivery systems that have been investigated for controlled-drug release are vaginal rings and biodegradable microcapsules.

### *Biopharmaceutic Considerations*

The human vagina is a thin-walled fibromuscular cavity 6–8.5 cm in length with a rich blood supply. Numerous microridges on the vaginal epithelium provide a surface structure that is well suited for drug absorption. The vaginal surface is usually covered with a film of moisture.

Drugs are known to be absorbed from the vagina by both active and passive mechanisms. Further, it has been shown that drug absorption is highly dependent upon the physicochemical and pharmacokinetic properties of the drug. For example, most steroids are readily absorbed from the vagina and the extent of absorption is usually greater than that seen after oral administration as a result of a reduction in first-pass effect. Absorption of high-molecular-weight substances such as proteins (including insulin) and nonoxynol-9 has been observed. In addition, therapeutic blood levels of progesterone have been achieved in patients with luteal phase defect after administration of vaginal progesterone suppositories.

Environmental factors within the vagina known to affect the rate and/or extent of drug absorption include the rate of blood perfusion, vaginal pH (which is usually 3.5–4.2 in women of childbearing age), volume and composition of the vaginal secretions, and physiologic status of the vaginal mucosal layer.[59]

### *Therapeutic Considerations*

The primary vaginal dosage forms prescribed include creams, tablets, and suppositories. Foams and jellies are the dosage forms used most often as nonprescription contraceptives. Vaginal drug administration usually requires an applicator, which must be used appropriately to achieve successful drug therapy, especially with anti-infectives and contraceptives.

Tablets and suppositories should be moistened prior to insertion to hasten their mixing with the vaginal mucosa fluid. Local irritation is the most common adverse affect seen with vaginal products, and is usually temporary and tolerable; however, severe cases of vaginal inflammation may occur that could necessitate medical intervention. Spontaneous abortion in pregnant patients receiving vaginal drug therapy has been observed.

Because our knowledge of the effects of drugs administered by this route is limited, it is imperative that complete instructions be given to patients, including administration techniques, possible adverse effects, and the importance of total compliance with the prescribed dosage regimen.

## Intrauterine Administration

As a result of its extensive use in China, intrauterine device (IUD) use now exceeds oral contraceptive use throughout the world.[60] Medicated IUDs are designed to be inserted and retained in the pear-shaped muscular uterus, and to deliver low doses of contraceptives at a controlled rate directly to the endometrium. Therefore, not only are the systemic side effects of synthetic steroids avoided, but the method is simple, readily reversible, and able to deliver drugs with a short biological half-life at a constant rate.

### *Preparations*

Two medicated IUDs that have been extensively studied are Progestasert and Cu-7. The T-shaped Progestasert is a membrane rate-controlled delivery system that delivers 65 $\mu$g of progesterone per day for 1 year. Cu-7 is a polypropylene 7-shaped device that releases 9.87 $\mu$g of copper per day for up to 40 months. Although serious complications are preventable, the main disadvantage of this form of drug delivery is the numerous side effects that can occur with both medicated and nonmedicated IUDs.[61,62] Because of the simplicity of this method and the potential for long-term contraception, however, research continues in an attempt to develop the ideal intrauterine device.[63] Approaches that have been investigated include encapsulated drug delivery devices and biodegradable and nonbiodegradable matrix technologies.[64]

### *Biopharmaceutic Considerations*

The principal reason for using a medicated IUD is to deliver a low dose of drug directly to the target organ. Thus, IUDs are formulated to minimize systemic drug absorption. For example, it has been shown that progesterone is absorbed rapidly by the endometrium to achieve localized effects with minimal systemic side effects.[64] The dynamic changes in size and shape that the uterus undergoes during different phases of the menstrual cycle appear to have little effect on clinical efficacy; however, the lack of structural adaptability may lead to expulsion and uterine bleeding, infection, perforation, and pain.

### *Therapeutic Considerations*

Intrauterine devices are inserted by physicians to ensure proper placement; however, the medical/ethical problems associated with IUD use such as septic abortion and congenital anomalies require a strong emphasis on patient education in the areas of risk/benefit analysis, self-monitoring of therapy, and precautions to ensure safe use of these devices. This method of drug delivery is contraindicated in patients with a history of pelvic inflammatory disease, spontaneous abortions, genital bleeding of unknown etiology, venereal disease, previous ectopic pregnancy, or other uterine abnormalities. Patient package inserts and complete patient instructions are available with these products.

## Innovative Drug Systems

Innovative design of new drug delivery systems has greatly escalated during the last 15 years largely as a result of the high cost of developing new drug entities and the advances that have been made in polymer science and engineering technology. Many of these delivery systems attempt to achieve some level of drug targeting. The following is a brief description of the various approaches that have been used. Additional information is available in the literature.[12,19,32,58,65–71]

### *Prodrugs*

Prodrugs represent a chemical approach to the variety of pharmaceutical problems associated with taste, solubility, stability, absorption, distribution, metabolism, duration of action, and selective pharmacologic effects. After these variables are overcome, the chemically modified compound (prodrug) is biotransformed in the body to the parent compound to elicit a more effective clinical response.

### *Macromolecular Drug Carriers*

Macromolecular drug complexes can be prepared with a wide range of steric and physicochemical properties to facilitate and/or improve drug delivery to receptor sites. Future understanding of transport mechanisms will help make these systems more practical. A variety of carriers have been used including proteins and protein conjugates (albumin, glycoproteins, antibodies, lipoproteins), lectins, hormones, dextran and other polysaccharides, deoxyribonucleic acid, and water-soluble or water-insoluble biodegradable and nonbiodegradable synthetic polymers.

### *Cellular Drug Carriers*

Cellular elements such as erythrocytes, leukocytes, and fibroblasts can be "loaded" with drugs or enzymes for controlled-release or enzyme replacement therapy. The principal advantage of this approach is that the cells are biocompatible and nonantigenic and may be targeted by labeling with immunoglobulins or an external magnet. Because they are unable to diffuse through blood vessels, this application is essentially restricted for use within the circulatory system.

### *Particulate Drug Delivery Systems*

Microcapsules and nanoparticles are small (micrometer and nanometer) particles containing the drug encapsulated within a range of natural or synthetic macromolecular coating materials. They are designed for systemic, localized, or site-specific delivery. Microspheres contain the drug entrapped within a water-soluble or -insoluble carrier. Frequently, ferromagnetic material is included to facilitate magnetically controlled targeting. Presently, however, this approach has limited application, as the magnets that are currently available are unable to create a sufficient magnetic field in deep body cavities.

Liposomes have received more attention as drug carriers than any other carrier system. They are discrete, artificial vesicles composed of one or more concentric lipid bilayers enclosing an equal number of aqueous spaces. Drugs may be encapsulated within either the aqueous or the lipid layers, with selective absorption and distribution theoretically possible by modifying both their size and surface characteristics. Despite problems of instability, liposomes continue to be used as a mechanism to deal with or optimize many drug delivery problems. A variety of multiple emulsions have been developed as carriers of drugs primarily to the lymphatic system. They are formulated either as oil–in water–in oil (o/w/o), water–in oil–in water (w/o/w), or microsphere–in oil–in water (s/o/w) systems. Emulsion instability is often a major problem with these preparations.

### *Controlled Drug Delivery Inserts, Implants, and Devices*

A plethora of modern drug delivery systems proliferate the research and patent literature. The mechanism of drug release may be controlled by dissolution, diffusion, osmosis, pH, or enzyme action. These delivery systems can be designed for insertion into a variety of cavities (ophthalmic, rectal, vaginal, uterus), for localized application to body membranes and tissues (nasal, buccal, skin), or for implantation into subcutaneous and other tissue cavities. Examples of these delivery systems can be found in the literature.[19,65,67,68]

Advances in polymer science and technology have accelerated the interest in controlled-release dosage forms. Alternative routes of administration are being researched. It is anticipated that delivery systems using biofeedback, computer-controlled, complex rate programs will in the future be able to adapt blood levels to circadian or other variations; however, just as there is no ideal drug, there is no ideal drug delivery system or route of administration. The thrust in emphasis on drug delivery system design together with pharmacodynamics will continue in an attempt to optimize drug therapy. Because of their selective application or prohibitive cost, many innovative drug delivery systems will never be widely used or marketed. Many of the issues associated with testing and regulatory approval are just beginning to be addressed. Existing technologies need to be intelligently applied to meet specific clinical needs with products that are cost effective and well received by the patient.

## References


1. Gourley DR, Ueda CT. Patient factors that influence dosage form selection, in Banker GS, Chalmers RK (eds): Pharmaceutics and Pharmacy Practice. Philadelphia, J.B. Lippincott, 1982, pp 131–154.
2. Turco S, King RE. Sterile Dosage Forms, 2nd ed. Philadelphia, Lea and Febiger, 1979.
3. Avis KE. Sterile products, in Lachman L, Lieberman HA, Kanig JL (eds): The Theory and Practice of Industrial Pharmacy, 3rd ed. Philadelphia, Lea and Febiger, 1986, pp 639–677.
4. Avis KE. Parenteral preparations, in Gennaro AR (ed): Remington's Pharmaceutical Sciences, 17th ed. Easton, MD, Mack Publishing, 1985, pp 1518–1541.
5. Leung S-HS, Robinson JR, Lee VHL. Parenteral products, in Robinson JR, Lee VHL (eds): Controlled Drug Delivery: Fundamentals and Applications, 2nd ed. New York, Marcel Dekker, 1987, pp 433–480.
6. Newton DW, Newton M. Route, site, and technique: Three key decisions in giving parenteral medication. Nursing 1979;9:18–25.
7. Franetzki M. Drug delivery by program or sensor controlled infusion devices. Pharm Res 1984;1:237–244.
8. Scott D. Insulin pumps. Patient Manage 1986;15:169–183.
9. Gehres RW, Lasell P, Spencer MR. Insulin infusion pumps. US Pharm 1982;7:62–68.
10. Slattery PJ, Boas RA. Newer methods of delivery of opiates for relief of pain. New Ethicals 1986;23:147–168.
11. Buchwald H, Rohde TD, Schneider PD, et al. Long-term, continuous intravenous heparin administration by an implantable infusion pump in ambulatory patients with recurrent venous thrombosis. Surgery 1980;88:507–516.
12. Heilmann K. Therapeutic Systems, 2nd ed. Stuttgart, Thieme-Stratton, 1984.
13. Mitchell JF. Oral dosage forms that should not be crushed: 1985 revision. Hosp Pharm 1985;20:309–319.
14. Ebert WR. Soft elastic gelatin capsules: A unique dosage form. Pharm Tech 1977;1:44–55.
15. Strom BL. Generic drug substitution revisited. N Engl J Med 1987;316:1456–1462.
16. Riley TN, Ravis WR. Key concepts in drug bioequivalence. US Pharm 1987;12:40–56.
17. Kikendall JW, Friedman AC, Oyewole MA, et al. Pill-induced esophageal injury: Case reports and review of the medical literature. Dig Dis Sci 1983;28:174–182.
18. Bates E, Menkis H, Tiefenbach S, et al. Medication administration and its relationship to meals. Fla J Hosp Pharm 1987;7:51–57.
19. Robinson JR, Lee VHL. Controlled Drug Delivery: Fundamentals and Applications, 2nd ed. New York, Marcel Dekker, 1987.

20. Amsel L. Pennkinetic: A flexible delivery system, in Controlled-Release Drug Delivery and Pennkinetic, Symposium Proceedings. Springfield, IL, Omega Communications, 1983, pp 32–37.
21. Eckenhoff B, Theeuwes F, Urquhart J. Osmotically actuated dosage forms for rate-controlled drug delivery. Pharm Tech 1987;11:96–105.
22. Banakar UV. Innovations in controlled release. Am Pharm 1987;NS27:39–48.
23. Bogentoft C. Oral controlled-release dosage forms in perspective. Pharm Int 1982;3:366–369.
24. Li VHK, Robinson JR, Lee VHL. Influence of drug properties and routes of drug administration on the design of sustained and controlled release systems, in Robinson JR, Lee VHL (eds). Controlled Drug Delivery: Fundamentals and Applications, 2nd ed. New York, Marcel Dekker, 1987; pp 3–94.
25. Roller L. Rectal and vaginal routes of administration. Aust J Hosp Pharm 1980;10:36–40.
26. de Blaey CJ, Polderman J. Rationales in the design of rectal and vaginal delivery forms of drugs, in Ariens EJ (ed): Drug Design. New York, Academic, 1980, Vol 9, pp 237–266.
27. Barry BW. Structure, function, diseases and topical treatment of human skin, in Swarbrick J (ed): Dermatological Formulations: Percutaneous Absorption. New York, Marcel Dekker, 1983, pp 1–48.
28. Flynn GL. Topical drug absorption and topical pharmaceutical systems, in Banker GS, Rhodes CT (eds): Modern Pharmaceutics. New York, Marcel Dekker, 1979, pp 263–327.
29. Elkayam U, Aronow WS. Glyceryl trinitrate (nitroglycerin) ointment and isosorbide dinitrate: A review of their pharmacological properties and therapeutic use. Drugs 1982;23:165–194.
30. Karim A. Transdermal absorption: A unique opportunity for constant delivery of nitroglycerin. Drug Dev Indust Pharm 1983;9:671–689.
31. Ostrenga J, Haleblian J, Poulsen B, et al. Vehicle design for a new topical steroid, fluocinonide. J Invest Dermatol 1971;56: 392–399.
32. Johnson JC. Sustained Release Medications. Park Ridge, IL, Noyes Data Corporation, 1980.
33. Chien YW. Transdermal therapeutic systems, in Robinson JR, Lee VHL (eds): Controlled Drug Delivery: Fundamentals and Applications, 2nd ed. New York, Marcel Dekker, 1987, pp 523–552.
34. Clissold SP, Heel RC. Transdermal hyoscine (scopolamine): A preliminary review of its pharmacodynamic properties and therapeutic efficacy. Drugs 1985;29:189–207.
35. Arndts D, Arndts K. Pharmacokinetics and pharmacodynamics of transdermally administered clonidine. Eur J Clin Pharmacol 1984;26:79–85.
36. Laufer LR, De Fazio JL, Lu JKH, et al. Estrogen replacement therapy by transdermal estradiol administration. Am J Obstet Gynecol 1983;146:533–540.
37. Black CD. Update: Programmed drug delivery system. US Pharm 1983;8:49–65.
38. Chien YW. Pharmaceutical considerations of transdermal nitroglycerin delivery: The various approaches. Am Heart J 1984;108:207–216.
39. Wolff M, Cordes G, Luckow V. In vitro and in vivo release of nitroglycerin from a new transdermal therapeutic system. Pharm Res 1985;2:23–29.
40. Abrams J. The brief saga of transdermal nitroglycerin discs: Paradise lost? Am J Cardiol 1984;54:220–224.
41. Reichek N, Priest C, Zimrin D, et al. Antianginal effects of nitroglycerin patches. Am J Cardiol 1984;54:1–7.
42. Parker JO, Fung H-L. Transdermal nitroglycerin in angina pectoris. Am J Cardiol 1984;54:471–476.
43. Robinson JR, Goshman LM. Topical drug-delivery systems (eye, ear, nose), in Banker GS, Chalmers RK (eds): Pharmaceutics and Pharmacy Practice. Philadelphia, J.B. Lippincott, 1982, pp 312–352.
44. Chiou GCY, Watanabe K. Drug delivery to the eye, in Ihler GM (ed): Methods of Drug Delivery. International Encyclopedia of Pharmacology and Therapeutics, Section 120. New York, Pergamon, 1986; pp 203–212.
45. Kohn AN, Moss AP, Hargett NA, et al. Clinical comparison of dipivalyl epinephrine and epinephrine in the treatment of glaucoma. Am J Ophthalmol 1979;87:196–201.
46. Akers MJ. Ocular bioavailability of topically applied ophthalmic drugs. Am Pharm 1983;NS23:33–36.
47. Lourenco RV, Cotromanes E. Clinical aerosols. I. Characterization of aerosols and their diagnostic uses. Arch Intern Med 1982; 142:2163–2172.
48. Lourenco RV, Cotromanes E. Clinical aerosols. II. Therapeutic aerosols. Arch Intern Med 1982;142:2299–2308.
49. Newman SP. Production of radioaerosols, in Clarke SW, Pavia D (eds): Aerosols and the Lung: Clinical and Experimental Aspects. London, Butterworth, 1984, pp 71–91.
50. Sears MR, Asher MI. Inhaler devices: How to use and which to choose. New Ethicals 1985;22:43–56.
51. Newman SP. Deposition and effects of inhalation aerosols. Lund, Sweden, Rahms i Lund Tryckeri, 1983.
52. McFadden Jr ER. Inhaled Aerosol Bronchodilators. Baltimore, Williams and Wilkins, 1986, p 29.
53. Newman SP. Therapeutic aerosols, in Clarke SW, Pavia D (eds): Aerosols and the Lung: Clinical and Experimental Aspects. London, Butterworth, 1984, pp 197–224.
54. Chien YW. Transnasal Systemic Medications: Fundamentals, Developmental Concepts and Biomedical Assessments. New York, Elsevier, 1985.
55. Hussain AA, Hirai S, Bawarshi R. Nasal absorption of propranolol in rats. J Pharm Sci 1979;68:1196.
56. Colaizzi JL. Pharmacokinetics of intranasal drug administration, in Chien YW (ed): Transnasal Systemic Medications: Fundamentals, Developmental Concepts and Biomedical Assessments. New York, Elsevier, 1985, pp 107–119.
57. Yokosuka T, Omori Y, Hirata Y, et al. Nasal and sublingual administration of insulin in man. J Jpn Diab Soc 1977;20: 146–152.
58. Chien YW. Intravaginal controlled-released drug administration, Novel Drug Delivery Systems. Chien YW (ed): New York, Marcel Dekker, 1982, pp 51–95.
59. Benziger DP, Edelson J. Absorption from the vagina. Drug Metab Rev 1983;14:137–168.
60. Hatcher RA, Guest F, Stewart F, et al. Intrauterine devices, in Contraception Technology, 12th ed. New York, Irvington, 1984, pp 78–105.
61. Edelman DA, Berger GS, Keith LG. Intrauterine Devices and Their Complications. Boston, G.K. Hall and Co., 1979.
62. Zatuchni GI, Goldsmith A, Sciarra JJ. Intrauterine Contraception: Advances and Future Prospects. Proceedings of an International Workshop on Intrauterine Contraception. Philadelphia, Harper and Row, 1985.
63. Chien YW. Intrauterine controlled-release drug administration, in Chien YW (ed): Novel Drug Delivery Systems. New York, Marcel Dekker, 1982, pp 97–147.
64. Chien YW. Implantable therapeutic systems, in Robinson JR, Lee VHL (eds): Controlled Drug Delivery: Fundamentals and Applications, 2nd ed. New York, Marcel Dekker 1987, pp 481–522.
65. Ihler GM. Methods of Drug Delivery. International Encyclope-

dia of Pharmacology and Therapeutics, Section 120. New York, Pergamon, 1986.

**66.** Friend DR, Pangburn S. Site-specific drug delivery. Med Res Rev 1987;7:53–106.

**67.** Poznansky MJ, Juliano RL. Biological approaches to the controlled delivery of drugs: A critical review. Pharmacol Rev 1984; 36:277–336.

**68.** Anderson JM, Kim SW. Recent Advances in Drug Delivery Systems. New York, Plenum, 1984.

**69.** Tirrell DA, Donaruma LG, Turek AB. Macromolecules as drugs and as carriers for biologically active materials. Ann NY Acad Sci 1985;446:1–456.

**70.** Gregoriadis G, Senior J, Postes G. Targeting of Drugs with Synthetic Systems. New York, Plenum, 1986.

**71.** Tomlinson E, Davis SS. Site-Specific Drug Delivery, Cell Biology, Medical and Pharmaceutical Aspects. New York, John Wiley and Sons, 1986.

# Chapter 3 / Pediatrics

Milap C. Nahata, PharmD

Remarkable progress has been made in the management of pediatric patients. Infant mortality declined from 200 per 1,000 births in the nineteenth century to 75 per 1,000 births in 1925 to 11 per 1,000 births in 1984.[1] This success has resulted largely from improvements in identification, prevention, and treatment of common diseases.

Although most marketed drugs are used in pediatric patients, only one fourth of the drugs approved by the Food and Drug Administration have specific indications for use in the pediatric population. Data on the pharmacokinetics, pharmacodynamics, efficacy, and safety of drugs in infants and children are scarce. Lack of this type of information led to such disasters as gray syndrome from chloramphenicol, phocomelia from thalidomide, and kernicterus from sulfonamide therapy. Gray syndrome was first reported in two neonates who died after excessive chloramphenicol doses (100–300 mg/kg/d); the serum concentrations of chloramphenicol immediately before death were 75 and 100 μg/mL. Patients with gray syndrome usually have abdominal distension, vomiting, diarrhea, a characteristic gray color, respiratory distress, hypotension, and progressive shock. Thalidomide is well known for its teratogenic effects. It has been clearly implicated as the cause of multiple congenital fetal abnormalities, particularly limb deformities; it can also cause polyneuritis, nerve damage, and mental retardation. Kernicterus was reported in infants receiving sulfonamides, which displaced bilirubin to cause a hyperbilirubinemia. This results in deposition of bilirubin in the brain and induces encephalopathy in infants.

There is ample evidence that dosage regimens cannot be based simply on body weight or surface area of a pediatric patient extrapolated from adult data. Bioavailability, pharmacokinetics, pharmacodynamics, efficacy, and adverse effects can markedly differ between pediatric and adult patients as well as among pediatric patients because of differences in age, organ function, and disease state. Significant progress has been made in the area of pediatric pharmacokinetics over the last two decades, but few such studies have correlated pharmacokinetics with pharmacodynamics.

Several additional factors should be considered in optimizing pediatric drug therapy. Many drugs widely prescribed for infants and children (e.g., phenobarbital and carbamazepine) are not available in suitable dosage forms. Alteration (dilution or reformulation) of dosage forms intended for adult patients raises questions about the stability and compatibility of these drugs. Because of low fluid volume requirements and limited access to intravenous sites, special methods must be used for the delivery of intravenous drugs to infants and children. As simple as it may seem, administration of oral drugs to young patients continues to be a difficult task for nurses and parents.

Similarly, assuring compliance with drug therapy in pediatric patients poses a special challenge. Finally, the need for additional pharmacologic or therapeutic research brings up the issue of ethical justification for conducting research. The investigators proposing studies and institutional review committees approving human studies must assess the risk/benefit ratio of each study to be fair to a child who is not in a position to accept or reject the opportunity to participate in the research project.

The major objective in this chapter is to highlight important principles of pediatric drug therapy. Specific examples are cited to enhance the understanding.

## Pharmacokinetic Principles

Enormous progress has been made in characterization of drug pharmacokinetics in pediatric patients. Two factors have contributed to this progress: (1) availability of sensitive and specific analytic methods to measure drugs and their metabolites in small volumes of biologic fluids and (2) awareness of the importance of clinical pharmacokinetics in optimization of drug therapy. Absorption, distribution, metabolism, and elimination of many drugs are different in premature infants, full-term infants, and older children.

### *Absorption*

#### Gastrointestinal Tract

Two factors affecting the absorption of drugs from the gastrointestinal tract are pH-dependent passive diffusion and gastric emptying time. Both processes are strikingly different in a premature infant compared with older children and adults. In a full-term infant, gastric pH ranges from 6 to 8 at birth, but declines to 1 to 3 within 24 hours.[2] In contrast, the gastric pH is elevated in premature infants because of immature acid secretion.[3]

Higher serum concentrations of acid-labile drugs such as penicillin,[4] ampicillin,[5] and nafcillin[6] and lower serum concentrations of a weak acid such as phenobarbital[7] in premature infants can be explained by the higher gastric pH. Because of a lack of extensive data comparing serum concentration–time profiles after oral versus intravenous drug administration, differences in the bioavailability of drugs in premature infants are poorly understood. Studies have also shown that gastric emptying is slow in a premature infant.[8] Thus, drugs with limited absorption in adults may be efficiently absorbed in a premature infant because of prolonged contact time with gastrointestinal mucosa.

It is interesting to note the erratic gastrointestinal absorption of chloramphenicol from the oral prodrug chloramphenicol palmitate in premature infants. Because premature infants cannot metabolize the inactive chloramphenicol palmitate to active chloramphenicol in the gastrointestinal tract, the absorption of chloramphenicol is erratic and incomplete.[9]

### Intramuscular Sites

Drug absorption from an intramuscular site may also be altered in a premature infant. Differences in relative blood flow to various muscles, peripheral vasomotor instability, and insufficient muscular contractions in a premature infant compared with older children and adults can influence drug absorption from the intramuscular site. There is no way to predict the net effect of these factors on drug absorption, and specific studies are needed. Phenobarbital has been reported to be rapidly absorbed,[10] whereas diazepam absorption may be delayed.[11]

### Skin

Percutaneous absorption may be substantially increased in newborn infants because of an underdeveloped epidermal barrier (i.e., stratum corneum) and increased skin hydration. The increased permeability can produce toxic effects after the topical use of hexachlorophene soaps and powders,[12] salicylic acid ointment, and rubbing alcohol.[13] Interestingly, a recent study has shown that a therapeutic serum concentration of theophylline can be achieved to control apnea in premature infants of less than 30 weeks' gestation after a topical application of gel containing a standard dose of theophylline.[14] The use of this route of administration may minimize the unpredictability of oral and intramuscular absorption and complications of intravenous drug administration for certain drugs.

## *Distribution*

Drug distribution is determined by the physicochemical properties of the drug itself (e.g., p$K_a$, molecular weight, partition coefficient), and the physiologic factors specific for the patient. Although the physicochemical properties of the drug are constant, the physiologic functions often vary in different patient populations. Some important patient-specific factors include extracellular and total body water, drug protein binding in plasma, and presence of pathologic conditions modifying physiologic function.

Total body water, as a percentage of total body weight, has been estimated to be 94% in the fetus, 85% in premature infants, 78% in full-term infants, and 60% in adults.[15] Extracellular fluid volume is also markedly different in premature infants compared with older children and adults; the extracellular fluid volume may account for 50% of body weight in premature infants, 35% in 4- to 6-month-old infants, 25% in children 1 year of age, and 19% in adults.[15] This conforms to the observed gentamicin distribution volumes of 0.48 L/kg in neonates and 0.20 L/kg in adults.[16] Recent studies have shown that the distribution volume of tobramycin is largest in the most premature infants and decreases with increases in gestational age and birth weight of the infant.[17]

Binding of drugs to plasma proteins is also decreased in newborn infants, because of the decreased plasma protein concentration, lower binding capacity of protein, decreased affinity of proteins for drug binding, and competition for certain binding sites by endogenous compounds such as bilirubin. The plasma protein binding of many drugs, including phenobarbital, salicylates, phenytoin, theophylline, propranolol, lidocaine, penicillin, nafcillin, and chloramphenicol, is significantly less in the neonate than in the adult.[18] The decrease in plasma protein binding of drugs can increase their apparent volumes of distribution. Therefore, premature infants require a larger loading dose than older children and adults to achieve therapeutic serum concentration of such drugs as aminoglycosides,[16,17] phenobarbital,[19] phenytoin,[20] and theophylline.[21]

The consequences of increased concentrations of free or unbound drug in the serum and tissues must be considered. Pharmacologic and toxic effects are directly related to the concentration of free drug in the body. Increases in free drug concentrations may result directly from decreases in plasma protein binding or indirectly from, for example, drug displacement from binding sites. The increased mortality from the development of kernicterus secondary to displacement of bilirubin by sulfisoxazole in neonates has been well documented.[22] On the other hand, because drug bound to plasma proteins cannot be eliminated by the kidney, an increase in free drug concentration may also increase its clearance.[23]

The amount of body fat is substantially lower in neonates compared with adults, and may affect drug therapy. Certain highly lipid-soluble drugs are distributed less in infants than adults. The apparent volume of distribution of diazepam has ranged from 1.4 to 1.8 L/kg in neonates and from 2.2 to 2.6 L/kg in adults.[24]

In recent years, the numbers of mothers breastfeeding their infants has climbed. Thus, certain drugs distributed in breast milk may pose problems for the infants. The American Academy of Pediatrics recommends that amethopterin, bromocriptine, cimetidine, clemastine, cyclophosphamide, ergotamine, gold salts, methimazole, phenindione, and thiouracil should be contraindicated during breastfeeding. Further, metronidazole and radiopharmaceuticals should be temporarily stopped during breastfeeding.[25] It should be noted that these recommendations are based on limited data; other drugs taken over a prolonged period by the mother may also be toxic to the infant. The use of any drug should be avoided by the mother during pregnancy and while breastfeeding.

## *Metabolism*

Drug metabolism is substantially slower in infants compared with older children and adults. There are important differences in the maturation of various pathways of metabolism within a premature infant. For example, the sulfation pathway is well developed but the glucuronidation pathway has not matured in infants.[26] Although acetaminophen metabolism by glucuronidation is impaired in an infant compared with adults, it is partly compensated for by the sulfation pathway.

The tragedy of the chloramphenicol-induced gray baby syndrome in newborn infants is directly related to a decreased metabolism of chloramphenicol by glucuronyl transferases to the inactive glucuronide metabolite.[27] This metabolic pathway appears to be age related[28] and may take several months to a year to fully develop. Evidence for this is the increase in clearance with age up to 1 year.[29]

Metabolism of drugs such as theophylline, phenobarbital, and phenytoin by oxidation is also impaired in newborn infants. The rate of metabolism, however, is more rapid with phenobarbital and phenytoin than with theophylline. Total clearance of phenytoin surpasses adult values by 2 weeks of age, whereas theophylline clearance is not fully developed for several months.[18] Two additional observations should be noted about theophylline metabolism in pediatric patients. First, in premature infants receiving theophylline for the treatment of apnea, a significant amount of its active metabolite caffeine may be present, unlike in older children and adults.[18] Second, theophylline clearance in children 1 to 9 years of age exceeds the values in young infants as well as adults. Thus, a child with asthma often requires markedly higher doses on a weight basis of theophylline compared with an adult.[30] Because of decreased metabolism by oxidation, doses of such drugs as theophylline, phenobarbital, phenytoin, diazepam, amobarbital, tolbutamide, nortriptyline, and mepivacaine should be decreased in premature infants.

### *Elimination*

Drugs and their metabolites are often eliminated by the kidney. The processes of glomerular filtration, tubular secretion, and tubular reabsorption determine the efficiency of renal excretion. These processes may take several weeks to one year after birth to develop fully.[31]

Recent studies in infants have shown that tobramycin clearance during the first postnatal week may increase with an increase in gestational age.[17] Netilmicin studies in infants up to 1 month after birth have suggested that postnatal age is also directly correlated with netilmicin clearance.[29] Thus, premature infants require a lower daily dose of drugs eliminated by the kidney during the first week of life; the dosage requirement then increases with age.

Because of immature renal elimination, chloramphenicol succinate can accumulate in premature infants. Although chloramphenicol succinate is inactive, this accumulation may be the reason for an increased bioavailability of chloramphenicol in premature infants compared with older children.[28] These data indicate that gray baby syndrome may result from an underdeveloped glucuronidation pathway as well as increased bioavailability of chloramphenicol in premature infants.

## Drug Efficacy and Toxicity

Pediatric patients are different inherently from older people, but the differences do not stop there. In addition to pharmacokinetic differences, factors related to drug efficacy and toxicity should be considered. There may be unique pathophysiologic changes in some disease states.

Clinical presentation of chronic asthma differs in a child and an adult.[32] Children present almost exclusively with a reversible extrinsic type of asthma, whereas adults have nonspecific, nonatopic bronchial irritability.[32] This explains the value of adjunctive-hyposensitization therapy in the management of pediatric patients with extrinsic asthma.[33,34]

It is known that the maintenance dose of digoxin is substantially higher in an infant than in an adult. This greater dosage requirement of digoxin in an infant may result partly from a lower binding affinity of receptors in the myocardium and increased digoxin binding sites on neonatal erythrocytes compared with adult erythrocytes.[35]

There is sufficient evidence to suggest that certain adverse effects of drugs are most common in the newborn period, whereas other toxic effects may continue to be important for many years of childhood. Chloramphenicol toxicity is increased in a newborn infant because of immature metabolism and enhanced bioavailability. Similarly, propylene glycol, which is added to many injectable drugs including phenobarbital, digoxin, diazepam, vitamin D, and hydralazine to increase their stability, can cause hyperosmolality in infants.[36] Benzyl alcohol was a popular preservative in intravascular flush solutions until a syndrome of metabolic acidosis, seizures, neurologic deterioration, gasping respirations, hepatic and renal abnormalities, cardiovascular collapse, and death was described in premature infants. A recent study has shown a decline in both mortality and the incidence of major intraventricular hemorrhage after the use of solutions containing benzyl alcohol was stopped in low-birth-weight infants.[37] Tetracyclines are also contraindicated in pregnant women, in nursing mothers, and in children less than 8 years of age because they can cause dental staining and defects in enamelization of deciduous and permanent teeth as well as a decrease in bone growth.[38]

It is interesting that certain drugs may be less toxic in pediatric patients than in adults. Aminoglycosides appear to be less toxic in infants than in adults. In adults, aminoglycoside toxicity has been shown to be related to both peripheral compartment accumulation and the individual patient's inherent sensitivity to these tissue concentrations.[39] Although neonatal peripheral tissue compartments for gentamicin have been reported to closely resemble those of adults with similar renal function,[16] gentamicin is rarely nephrotoxic in infants. This dissimilarity in the incidence of nephrotoxicity implies that newborn infants may have less inherent tissue sensitivity for toxicity than adults.

The differences in efficacy, toxicity, and protein binding of drugs in pediatric versus adult patients raise an important question about the acceptable therapeutic range in children. Therapeutic ranges for drugs are first established in adults and are often directly applied to pediatric patients, but specific studies should be conducted in pediatric patients to define optimal therapeutic ranges of drugs. As an example, a therapeutic range of chloramphenicol peak serum concentration between 10 and 20 μg/mL was established in adults and is widely used in all patients. Experience at my institution as well as a recent study suggests that some children with peak serum chloramphenicol concentrations exceeding 50 μg/mL may exhibit no apparent toxicity.[40]

## Factors Affecting Pediatric Therapy

### *Disease States*

As most drugs are either metabolized by the liver or eliminated by the kidney, hepatic and renal disease are expected to decrease the dosage requirements in patients. Nevertheless, not all diseases require lower doses of drugs; for instance, patients with cystic fibrosis require larger doses of certain drugs to achieve therapeutic concentrations.[41]

### Liver Disease

Because the liver is the main organ for drug metabolism, drug clearance is usually decreased in patients with hepatic disease; however, most studies on the influence of liver disease on dosage requirements have been carried out in adults, and these data may not be extrapolated uniformly to pediatric patients.

Drug metabolism by the liver is dependent on complex interactions among hepatic blood flow, ability of the liver to extract the drug from the blood, drug binding in the blood, and both type and severity of liver disease. Routine liver function tests, such as determination of serum aspartate transaminase, serum alanine transaminase, alkaline phosphatase, and bilirubin levels, have not consistently correlated with drug pharmacokinetics. Furthermore, because of different pathologic changes in various types of liver diseases, patients with acute viral hepatitis may have different abilities to metabolize drugs compared with patients with alcoholic cirrhosis.[42]

On the basis of hepatic extraction characteristics, drugs can be divided into two categories. The first category consists of drugs with a high hepatic extraction ratio, greater than 0.7 (e.g., morphine, meperidine, lidocaine, and propranolol). Clearance of these drugs is affected by hepatic blood flow. A decreased hepatic blood flow in the presence of such disease states as cirrhosis and congestive heart failure is expected to decrease the clearance of drugs with high extraction ratios. The second category comprises drugs that have a low extraction ratio, less than 0.2, and a low affinity for plasma proteins. Metabolism of these drugs (e.g., theophylline, chloramphenicol, and acetaminophen) is influenced mainly by hepatocellular function and not as much by changes in hepatic blood flow or plasma protein binding. A recent report has suggested that theophylline clearance may decrease by 45% in a child with acute viral hepatitis.[43] Because of a lack of specific data on dosage adjustment in liver disease, drug therapy should be closely monitored in pediatric patients to avoid potential toxicity from excessive doses, particularly for drugs with narrow therapeutic indices.

### Renal Disease

Renal failure decreases the dosage requirement of drugs eliminated by the kidney. Once again, because of limited studies, dosage adjustments in pediatric patients are based largely on data obtained in adults. For many important drugs such as aminoglycosides, renal clearance or rate of elimination is directly proportional to the glomerular filtration rate as measured by endogenous creatinine clearance. Serum concentrations should be monitored for drugs with narrow therapeutic indices and eliminated largely by the kidney (e.g., aminoglycosides and vancomycin) to optimize therapy in pediatric patients with renal dysfunction. For drugs with wide therapeutic ranges (e.g., penicillins and cephalosporins), dosage adjustment may be necessary only in moderate to severe renal failure.

### Cystic Fibrosis

Drug therapy in pediatric patients with cystic fibrosis has recently been reviewed.[44] For unknown reasons, these patients require increased doses of drugs including aminoglycosides and penicillins. Studies have reported higher clearance of gentamicin, tobramycin, netilmicin, amikacin, dicloxacillin, cloxacillin, azlocillin, and piperacillin in patients with cystic fibrosis compared with those without this disease; the apparent distribution volume of certain drugs may also be altered in cystic fibrosis.[44] Severity of illness may influence the change in dosage requirements, but this is not certain.

### Other Diseases

Although specific dosage guidelines are not available, pediatric patients with gastrointestinal disease (e.g., celiac disease, gastroenteritis, and severe malabsorption) may require dosage adjustments.[41] Hypoxemia has also been shown to decrease the elimination of amikacin in low-birth-weight infants.[45]

## *Drug Administration*

Drugs are often given by the intravenous route to seriously ill patients. There is a wide variation in flow rates as well as injection sites within a pediatric intravenous set for drug delivery. Effective serum concentrations are expected to be achieved rapidly after drug infusion.

In 1979, a therapeutic drug monitoring service was made available at my institution. Soon thereafter, lower-than-predicted peak and higher-than-predicted trough serum concentrations of aminoglycosides and chloramphenicol were noted. In fact, in some patients, trough exceeded peak serum concentration. Subsequently, several studies demonstrated that the method of drug infusion has a profound influence on peak serum concentration and time to attain peak concentrations of chloramphenicol[46] and tobramycin.[47] This has practical implications for routine therapeutic drug monitoring in that anticipated serum concentrations may be inaccurate, leading to unjustified, costly, and potentially harmful alterations in doses. Proper recommendations for obtaining patient specimens can be made only with the knowledge of drug characteristics and infusion method.

Intravenous drugs can be infused either by an antegrade or a retrograde technique. Drugs are commonly infused in an antegrade fashion. By this method, the doses injected at various sites of the intravenous set (e.g., flashball, Y-site, and a volumetric chamber such as Buretrol) are expected to move directly toward the patient (Fig. 3.1).

In vitro studies with gentamicin and aminophylline have shown that the delivery of these drugs may be delayed substantially depending on the flow rate and injection site.[48] These observations were confirmed with infusion of chloramphenicol succinate[46] and tobramycin.[47]

The time for complete delivery of chloramphenicol succinate in vitro increased with increase in the distance between the drug injection site and the patient, fluid volume of the tubing, and decrease in the flow rate. In pediatric patients, the steady-state peak serum concentrations of both chloramphenicol succinate and chloramphenicol were markedly higher and occurred earlier after injection into the flashball

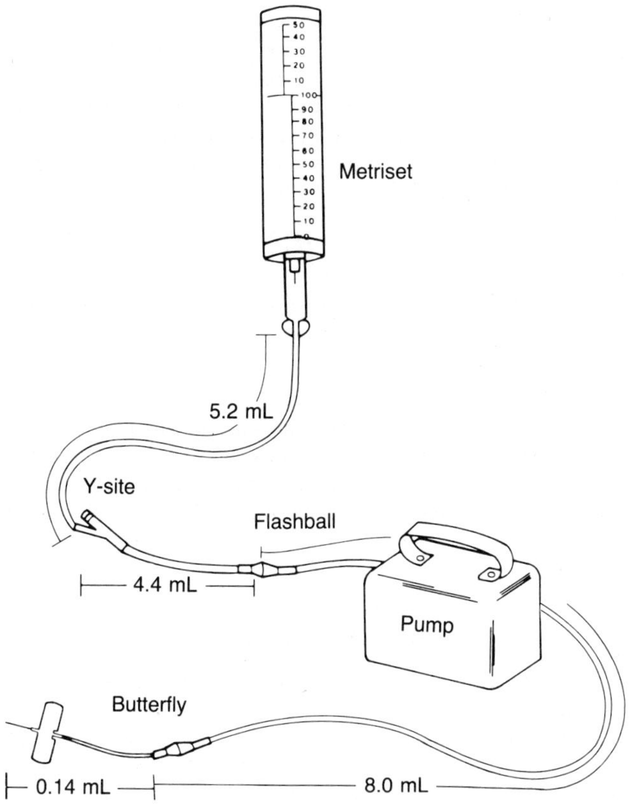


**Figure 3.1** Schematic diagram of an intravenous set with a volumetric chamber (Metriset or Buretrol), Y-site, flashball, and butterfly. Values shown for the various components of the system are volume capacities. *(From Gould T, Roberts RJ: Therapeutic problems arising from the use of intravenous route for drug administration. J Pediatr 1979;95:465–471, with permission.)*

(proximal to patient), compared with the Buretrol (distal to patient) site, at similar flow rates of 7 to 30 mL/h. If the in vitro data for complete delivery were not used for in vivo studies, the total amount of drug delivered to patients would have been affected by these variables.

Because of the delay in drug delivery that occurs at the low flow rates commonly used in newborn infants, in vitro studies were conducted to determine an optimal method for drug infusion.[49,50] In vitro delivery of tobramycin at 2–6 mL/h from IVAC (Model 530), IMED (Model 965), and Auto Syringe pumps was studied.[49] The Auto Syringe was connected to the stopcock at the IVAC–flashball site. It was found that if tobramycin delivery was to be assured within 30 minutes of starting the infusion, Auto Syringe or proximal Y-site of the IMED systems must be used.[49] To determine the clinical relevance of these findings, newborn infants receiving tobramycin at 2–12 mL/h from IVAC–Y-site versus Auto Syringe, IVAC–flashball versus Auto Syringe, or IMED–proximal Y-site versus Auto Syringe were studied.[47] Serum concentrations were highest and occurred earliest after Auto Syringe followed by IMED–Y-site, IVAC–flashball, and IVAC–Y-site.[47]

These studies have clearly demonstrated that the variables of intravenous drug infusion systems (e.g., flow rate, injection site, volume of drug, and fluid volume of the tubing) can markedly affect the serum concentrations of drugs after antegrade infusions into pediatric patients. For example, mean peak serum concentrations of chloramphenicol can be 5 μg/mL higher and occur 1 hour earlier after flashball injection compared with Buretrol injection in infants and children.[46] Similarly, the mean serum concentrations of tobramycin can be 2.3–2.5 μg/mL higher and occur 1.0 to 1.5 hours earlier after Auto Syringe infusion compared with infusions from IVAC systems.[47] These differences can be very important because of the narrow therapeutic indices of chloramphenicol and tobramycin. Furthermore, a lack of knowledge of these variables may result in inappropriate timing and interpretation of blood level data, leading to unnecessary dosage adjustments.

The retrograde infusion method was first described in 1973. This infusion system consists of extension tubing inserted between two four-way stopcocks. When a drug is administered, the stopcock closest to the patient is turned off to the patient end of the system. Diluted drug is then introduced through the stopcock and forced to move in the direction opposite the usual direction of fluid flow (i.e, retrograde, away from the patient). Simultaneously, the distal stopcock is turned off to the pump end of the system, and a syringe is attached to accept displaced maintenance fluid from the extension tubing. This fluid is then discarded. After the drug is introduced into the line, the stopcocks are repositioned to allow normal fluid flow, and the dose infuses at the rate set for the maintenance fluid.

In vitro studies have found this infusion system predictable for delivery of drugs.[50–52] Some practical limitations of the retrograde infusion system exist: (1) certain pumps may not accept this system and (2) the drug volume should not exceed 50% of the volume of the extension tubing to ensure that only displaced maintenance fluid is discarded.[53] The retrograde drug infusion system has not been adequately evaluated in patients.

Specific gravity can also influence drug delivery at slow infusion rates.[54] For example, in vitro studies have indicated that drugs with a specific gravity lower than that of the maintenance fluid may layer at the top of the tubing where delivery would be prolonged by laminar-flow characteristics.[54] Similarly, injections into a filter chamber, Y-site, or T-site with dead space can also prolong drug delivery.

No infusion system is ideal for drug delivery in all institutions. Each hospital can be cognizant of problems of drug delivery and develop specific guidelines for intravenous infusions. At my institution, specific guidelines are provided to the nurses for administration of each drug. These guidelines take into account various infusion rates and provide consistency of delivery with each dose. As long as the time for actual delivery can be anticipated, times to obtain blood samples can be adjusted accordingly to generate meaningful data.

### *Alteration of Dosage Forms*

Many drugs used in pediatric patients are not available in suitable dosage forms. This necessitates dilution of high concentrations of drugs intended for adult patients. Examples of these drugs include atropine, carbamazepine, diazepam, digoxin, epinephrine, hydralazine, insulin, morphine, phenobarbital, and phenytoin. Volumes ranging from 0.001

to 0.1 mL must be measured to dispense these drugs for use in infants. This can obviously be associated with large errors in measurements, and such errors have caused intoxication with digoxin[55] and morphine[56] in infants.

One solution to this problem is to dilute these concentrated products, but such alterations can influence the stability or compatibility of these drugs. Because of a lack of such data, pharmacy departments may justifiably be reluctant to alter dosage forms.

Selection of the appropriate vehicle to dilute the adult dosage forms for use in pediatric patients can also be difficult. Phenobarbital sodium contains propylene glycol in the original product to improve drug stability. As propylene glycol can cause hyperosmolality in infants,[36] further addition of this vehicle may not be wise.

Because of limited access to intravenous sites in pediatric patients, drugs must be administered through the same site; however, data on their compatibility are often missing. Newborn infants often require aminoglycosides for presumed or proven sepsis and calcium gluconate to correct hypocalcemia. Tobramycin and calcium gluconate have been found to be compatible at least during a 1-hour period of administration at the same site.[57]

Administration of oral drugs continues to challenge parents and nurses. Alteration of these drugs by crushing or mixing, refusal of patients to accept the medication, and loss of drug during administration are some factors that can affect pediatric therapy. It is a common practice to mix the medications in applesauce, syrup, ice cream, or other vehicles to make the drugs palatable.

Drug administration into the middle ear, nose, and eye of a child requires special attention. Certain drugs (e.g., sodium valproate and morphine) can be administered rectally to infants who have limited access for intravenous drug administration or if oral drug administration cannot be accomplished.

Transdermal drug delivery can be used in pediatric patients (1) to avoid problems of drug absorption from the oral route and complications from the intravenous route and (2) to maximize duration of effect and minimize adverse effects of drugs. Favorable results with percutaneous theophylline in infants with apnea[14] and with subcutaneous morphine in pediatric patients with cancer[58] form the basis for studies with additional drugs.

### *Medication Compliance*

The issue of medication compliance is more complex in pediatrics than in adults. The parents must appreciate the importance of following the prescribing information. Among the factors that can negatively affect compliance are poor communication between the physician and patient or parent, insufficient prescribing information, lack of understanding about the severity of illness by the patient or parent, fear of side effects, failure of the patient or parent to remember to administer the drugs, inconvenient dosage forms or dosing schedules, and unpalatability of drug products.[59]

## Future Developments

Although tremendous progress has been made in the area of pediatric therapeutics, many questions remain unanswered. The pharmacokinetics of many important drugs have been elucidated, but correlation between pharmacokinetics and pharmacodynamics has not been explored fully. Similarly, effect of disease states, patient characteristics such as genetic status, and protein binding alterations have not been studied for most drugs. Although pharmacokinetics studies are generally conducted once during therapy, data for certain drugs suggest that serum concentrations may change during a typical course of therapy in a patient receiving the same dose. Implications of such changes on patient outcome are unknown.

Finally, there will be a continued need to develop new methods and refine present techniques for measuring drug concentrations in small volumes of various body fluids of pediatric patients. These analytical methods should be easy to use, accurate, precise, sensitive, and specific for measuring drugs in biologic specimens. Although much needs to be learned about the optimization of pediatric therapy, it is encouraging to witness the continued growth in knowledge of this area.

## References


1. Behrman RE, Vaughan VC (eds): Nelson's Textbook of Pediatrics, 12th ed. Philadelphia, W.B. Saunders, 1983, pp 1–90.
2. Avery GB, Randolph JG, Weaver T. Gastric acidity in the first day of life. Pediatrics 1966;37:1005–1007.
3. Agunod M, Yamaguchi N, Lopex R, et al. Correlative study of hydrochloric acid, pepsin, and intrinsic factor secretion in newborns and infants. Am J Dig Dis 1969;14:400–414.
4. Huang NN, High RN. Comparison of serum levels following the administration of oral and parenteral preparations of penicillin to infants and children of various age groups. J Pediatr 1953;42:657–668.
5. Silverio J, Poole JW. Serum concentrations of ampicillin in newborn infants after oral administration. Pediatrics 1973;51: 578–580.
6. O'Connor WJ, Warren GH, Edrada LS, et al. Serum concentrations of sodium nafcillin in infants during the perinatal period. Antimicrob Agents Chemother 1965:220–222.
7. Jalling B. Plasma concentrations of phenobarbital in the treatment of seizures in newborns. Acta Paediatr Scand 1975;64:514–524.
8. Signer E, Fridrich R. Gastric emptying in newborns and young infants. Acta Paediatr Scand 1975;64:525–530.
9. Shankaran S, Kauffman RE. Use of chloramphenicol palmitate in neonates. J Pediatr 1984;105:113–116.
10. Boreus IO. Plasma concentrations of phenobarbital in mother and child after combined prenatal and postnatal administration for prophylaxis of hyperbilirubinemia. J Pediatr 1978;93:695.
11. Morselli PL. Serum levels and pharmacokinetics of anticonvulsants in the management of seizure disorders, in Merkin B (ed): Clinical Pharmacology. Chicago, Year Book Medical Publishers, 1978, p 89.
12. Tyrala FF, Hillman LS, Hillman RE, et al. Clinical pharmacology of hexachlorophene in newborn infants. J Pediatr 1977;91:481–486.

13. McFadden S, Haddow JE. Coma produced by topical application of isopropanol. Pediatrics 1969;43:622–623.
14. Evans NJ, Rutter N, Hadgraft J, et al. Percutaneous administration of theophylline in preterm infant. J Pediatr 1985;107:307–311.
15. Friis-Hansen B. Body water compartments in children: Changes during growth and related changes in body composition. Pediatrics 1961;28:169–181.
16. Haughey DB, Hilligoss DM, Grassi A, et al. Two-compartment gentamicin pharmacokinetics in premature neonates: A comparison to adults with decreased glomerular filtration rates. J Pediatr 1980;96:325–330.
17. Nahata MC, Powell DA, Durrell DE, et al. Effect of gestational age and birth weight on tobramycin kinetics in newborn infants. J Antimicrob Chemother 1984;14:59–65.
18. Roberts RJ. Pharmacologic principles in therapeutics in infants, in: Drug Therapy in Infants. Philadelphia, W.B. Saunders, 1984, pp 3–12.
19. Pitlick W, Painter M, Pippenger C. Phenobarbital pharmacokinetics in neonates. Clin Pharmacol Ther 1978;23:346–350.
20. Painter MJ, Pippenger C, MacDonald H, et al. Phenobarbital and diphenylhydantoin levels in neonates with seizures. J Pediatr 1978;92:315–319.
21. Giacoia G, Jusko WJ, Menke J, et al. Theophylline pharmacokinetics in premature infants with apnea. J Pediatr 1976;89:829–832.
22. Silverman WA, Anderson DH, Blanc WA, et al. A difference in mortality rate and incidence of kernicterus among premature infants allotted to two prophylactic antibacterial regimens. Pediatrics 1956;18:614–624.
23. Odell GB. The dissociation of bilirubin from albumin and its clinical implications. J Pediatr 1959;55:268–279.
24. Morselli PL. Clinical pharmacokinetics in neonates. Clin Pharmacokinet 1976;1:81–98.
25. Committee on Drugs, American Academy of Pediatrics. The transfer of drugs and other chemicals into human breast milk. Pediatrics 1983;72:375–383.
26. Rane A. Basic principles of drug disposition and action in infants and children, in Yaffe JF (ed): Pediatric Pharmacology: Therapeutic Principles in Practice. New York, Grune and Stratton, 1980, pp 7–28.
27. Weiss CF, Glazko AJ, Weston JK. Chloramphenicol in the newborn infant. A physiologic explanation of its toxicity when given in excessive doses. N Engl J Med 1960;262:787–94.
28. Nahata MC, Powell DA. Comparative bioavailability and pharmacokinetics of chloramphenicol after intravenous chloramphenicol succinate in premature infants and older patients. Dev Pharmacol Ther 1983;6:23–32.
29. Kuhn R, Nahata MC, Powell DA, et al. Netilmicin pharmacokinetics in newborn infants. Eur J Clin Pharmacol 1986;29:635–637.
30. Weinberger M, Hendeles L. Theophylline for chronic asthma: Rationale for treatment, product selection, dosage schedule. Pediatr Pharmacol 1983;3:273–285.
31. Loggie JMH, Kleinman LI, Van Maanen EF. Renal function and diuretic therapy in infants and children. Part I. J Pediatr 1975;86:485–496.
32. Leffert FL. The management of chronic asthma. J Pediatr 1980; 97:875–885.
33. Johnston DE. Immunotherapy in children: Past, present, and future. Part I. Ann Allergy 1981;46:1–7.
34. Johnston DE. Immunotherapy in children: Past, present, and future. Part II. Ann Allergy 1981:46:59–66.
35. Kearin M, Kelly JG, O'Malley K. Digoxin "receptors" in neonates: An explanation of less sensitivity to digoxin than in adults. Clin Pharmacol Ther 1980;28:346–349.
36. Glasgow AM, Boeckx RL, Miller MK, et al. Hyperosmolality in small infants due to propylene glycol. Pediatrics 1983;72:353–355.
37. Hiller JL, Benda GI, Rahatzad M, et al. Benzyl alcohol toxicity: Impact of mortality and intraventricular hemorrhage among very low birth weight infants. Pediatrics 1986;77:500–506.
38. Grossman ER, Walchek A, Freedman H. Tetracyclines and permanent teeth: The relation between dose and tooth color. Pediatrics 1971;47:567–570.
39. Schentag JJ, Plaut ME, Cerra FB, et al. Aminoglycoside nephrotoxicity in critically ill surgical patients. J Surg Res 1979;26: 270–279.
40. Shann F, Linnemann V, MacKenzie A, et al. Absorption of chloramphenicol sodium succinate after intramuscular administration in children. N Engl J Med 1985;313:410–414.
41. Kauffman RE, Habersange R. Modification of dosage regimens in disease states of childhood, in Mirkin BL (ed): Clinical Pharmacology and Therapeutics: A Pediatric Perspective. Chicago, Year Book Medical Publishers, 1978, pp 73–88.
42. Roberts RJ. Special considerations in drug therapy in infants, in: Drug Therapy in Infants. Philadelphia, W.B. Saunders, 1984, pp 25–35.
43. Feinstein RA, Miles MV. The effect of acute viral hepatitis on theophylline clearance. Clin Pediatr 1985;24:357–358.
44. Kuhn RJ, Nahata MC. Therapeutic management of cystic fibrosis. Clin Pharm 1985;4:555–565.
45. Myers MG, Roberts JF, Mirhig NJ. Effect of gestational age, birth weight, and hypoxemia on the pharmacokinetics of amikacin in serum of infants. Antimicrob Agents Chemother 1977;11:1027.
46. Nahata MC, Powell DA, Glazer JP, et al. Effect of intravenous flow rate and infection site on in vitro delivery of chloramphenicol succinate and in vivo kinetics. J Pediatr 1981;99:463–466.
47. Nahata MC, Powell DA, Durrell DE, et al. Effect of infusion methods on tobramycin serum concentrations in newborn infants. J Pediatr 1984;104:136–138.
48. Gould T, Roberts RJ. Therapeutic problems arising from the use of intravenous route for drug administration. J Pediatr 1979;95: 465–471.
49. Nahata MC, Powell DA, Durrell DE, et al. Delivery of tobramycin by three infusion systems. Chemotherapy 1984;30:84–87.
50. Leff R, Roberts RJ. Methods for intravenous drug administration in the pediatric patient. J Pediatr 1981;98:631–635.
51. Benzing G, Loggie J. A new retrograde method for administering drugs intravenously. Pediatrics 1973;52:420–425.
52. Eling RF, Brissie EO. Intravenous infusion of drugs by a retrograde technique. Am J Hosp Pharm 1974;31:740–742.
53. Roberts RJ. Intravenous administration of medication in pediatric patients: Problems and solutions. Pediatr Clin North Am 1981;28:23–34.
54. Rajchgot P, Radde IC, MacLeod SM. Influence of specific gravity on intravenous drug delivery. J Pediatr 1981;99:658–661.
55. Berman W, Whitman V, Marks KH, et al. Inadvertent overadministration of digoxin to low birthweight infants. J Pediatr 1978;92:1024.
56. Zenk KE, Anderson S. Improving the accuracy of mini-volume injections. Infusion 1982;(Jan/Feb):7–11.
57. Nahata MC, Durrell DE. Stability of tobramycin sulfate in admixtures containing calcium glyconate. Am J Hosp Pharm 1985;42:1987–1988.
58. Nahata MC, Miser A, Miser J, et al. Analgesic plasma concentrations of morphine in children with terminal malignancy receiving a continuous subcutaneous infusion of morphine sulfate to control severe pain. Pain 1984;18:109–114.
59. Boreus LO. Drug compliance, in Yaffe SJ (ed): Principles of Pediatric Pharmacology. New York, Churchill Livingstone, 1982, pp 176–92.

# Chapter 4 / Geriatrics

W. Gary Erwin, PharmD, and Ember A. Skidmore, PharmD

He that would pass the latter part of life with honor and decency, must when he is young, consider that he shall one day be old and remember when he is old that he was once young.

*Samuel Johnson*

In 1889, Otto von Bismarck of Germany set the arbitrary age of 65 years as the criterion necessary to receive benefits from a social security system. The United States adopted this age for its own social security system in 1935 and thus was born our initial definition of the elderly. Today we recognize that this heterogeneous population of individuals over 65 is not so easily defined. It is clear that chronologic age and physiologic age may be distinct, and that aging, or senescence, in the human organism begins in the mid-twenties and proceeds at varying rates even in individual cells. To better delineate this population, a more acceptable definition based upon age characteristics is available. This definition divides the elderly into the older population, 55+; the elderly, 65+; the aged, 75+; and the very old, 85+.

## Demographics

The number of individuals 65+ is the most rapidly increasing segment of the U.S. population.[1] In 1900, 1 in 25 Americans was 65 or older. In 1984, the proportion had increased to 1 in 8. Currently, those people 65 and older constitute 11.9% of the population; the projection for the year 2040 is 21.7%.

The largest portion of the increase is in the 85+ division, which accounted for 1% of the population in 1985 and is projected to account for 4% of the population in 2040.[2] Average remaining years of life from age 85 has increased by 0.7 year total for men and 1.6 years total for women since 1950.[3] As a result, in 1983, the total life expectancy for 85-year-old men was 90.2 years and for women, 91.6 years. Life expectancy at birth has increased for males from 65.6 years in 1950 to 71.0 years in 1983; for females, from 71.1 years in 1950 to 78.1 years in 1983. Historically, race and gender differentiate life expectancy; white women have the longest projected life span, black men the shortest.

This phenomenon is not limited only to industrialized nations such as the United States. Even among the developing, nonindustrialized nations of the world, the absolute percentage of elderly is increasing, albeit at a slower rate. In 1980, 8.5% of the total world population was 60 or older. By the year 2025, this same age group will constitute 13.7% of the world population.[1]

Gender-specific death rates also contribute to the characteristic makeup of the elderly. In 1983, there were 77 men alive at age 65 for every 100 women alive; at age 85, the ratio was wider, 41 men for every 100 women.[3] There are more single women (widowed) than men in every age group above 55. These differences are further influenced by race; elderly black women are the least likely to be married and the most likely to be widowed. The reverse is true for elderly white men. The average elderly man is married and lives with his spouse; the average elderly woman is widowed and lives alone.

The increase in real numbers and percentages of population for the elderly is due primarily to an increase in the number of annual births before 1920 and after World War II, rather than to an increase in longevity alone. The dramatic rise in the very old population, although a major achievement of disease prevention and improved health care, has vast implications in the areas of public policy because of the high probability of health problems and the need for health and social services for this age group.

## Economic Status

As a group, the elderly have a lower economic status than other adults in our society because of the changes that are often associated with aging: retirement from the work force, death of a spouse, and decline in health. As most elderly have very limited potential to increase income through work, they become reliant upon Social Security benefits supplemented with pensions and assets they have accumulated over their lifetime. This relatively "fixed" income often leaves them economically susceptible to circumstances beyond their control such as the loss of a spouse, deterioration of their health and self-sufficiency, legislation affecting Social Security and Medicare benefits, and inflation.

The elderly as a group have a slightly higher percentage of individuals with incomes below the poverty level (12.4% in 1984) compared with all adults aged 18 to 64 (11.7% in 1984). When considering the percentage of persons close to as well as below the poverty line, the gap widens as 29.1% of the elderly fall into this range, compared with 24.3% of all persons under 65.[1] Age, race, and gender again differentiate the elderly, increasing age, nonwhite race, and female gender being associated with smaller incomes.

## Health Status

Most elderly people view their own health as good. Results of the 1984 National Health Interview Survey showed that 67% of elderly persons living in the community considered their own health as excellent, very good, or good compared with others their own age; only 33% reported their health as fair or poor.[4] A full 60% had no limitation in activity, 29% had some limitations in activity, and 11% were unable to perform their usual activities. As age progresses, disabilities do increase such that by age 85, limitations in activity occur more commonly. Still, 40% of the 85+ age group report no disability. Perceived health status changes little between age groups, with 61% of those over 85 years reporting excellent, very good, or good health. The relatively good health of the majority of elderly who live within the community (95%) contrasts starkly with the health of the minority who reside in long-term-care facilities (5%). This group is much more likely to experience severe limitations in activity and decreased health status.[5]

The elderly individual is more likely to suffer from chronic conditions, the most common being arthritis, hypertension, hearing difficulties, and heart disease.[6] Heart disease is also responsible for more physician office visits, hospital days, and deaths than any other problem experienced by the elderly.[3] The other leading causes of death are cancer and cerebrovascular disease.

Elderly persons have fewer psychiatric problems in terms of incidence, with the exception of the dementias, than other age groups. Cognitive impairment, of which dementia of the Alzheimer type (DAT) is the leading cause, is the primary mental health problem of the elderly. Advancing age correlates most clearly with development of DAT. There is a 10- to 20-fold increase in age-specific prevalence between 60 and 80 years, exceeding 20% by 80 to 85 years.[7] This age-specific prevalence may decline after age 80. Severe cognitive impairment occurs in less than 5% of the 65+ population. Some degree of cognitive impairment is reported in 50% to 75% of patients in long-term-care facilities.

Depression is the other major mental health problem of the elderly. About 5% to 10% of older individuals have a depressive episode at least once during their elderly years.[8] Although individuals 65+ make up only 11.9% of the total population, they are responsible for 25% of the completed suicides in the United States.[9] This figure is questionably low, as many elderly deaths are attributed to natural or accidental causes and the true reason is never ascertained.

## Health Care Consumption

Even though the majority of elderly are relatively healthy, the population as a whole is the greatest consumer of health care resources and accounts for approximately 30% of health care expenditures. In 1984, these expenditures for individuals older than 65 approached $120 billion.[10] Sources of funding included out-of-pocket expenses (25.2%), Medicare (48.8%), and Medicaid (12.8%). Per capita health care expenditures for persons over 65 increased from $2,026 in 1978 to $4,202 in 1984. The largest single expenses for Medicare recipients were hospitalization and physician visits, and for elderly Medicaid recipients, long-term care.

The elderly as a group are the largest consumers of medications, accounting for 30% of medication expenditures. Approximately 75% of all elderly persons are prescribed at least one medication.[11] The number of medications prescribed per person increases with age, such that the 65+ population has a per capita use of 14.2 prescriptions. This polypharmacy is not without consequences, the most important being the contribution to adverse drug reactions. Approximately 4% of all hospital admissions are influenced or caused by adverse drug reactions (ADRs) and there is an increase in age-related ADRs in hospitalized patients.[12]

Provision of long-term care for our nation's sick elderly is a growing concern and expensive responsibility. In 1982, there were approximately 1.7 million long-term-care beds, with an occupancy rate of 91%.[13] By contrast, in 1983, there were approximately 1.1 million acute-care beds, with an occupancy rate of 75%.[3] Approximately 87% of all long-term-care residents are 65+, 71% are 75+, and 36% are 85+. National health care expenditures for hospitals have increased by 34% since 1950.[3] During the same time period, expenditures for nursing homes increased by 453%.[3]

A truism of aging is that a minority of sick elderly consume a disproportionate amount of available health care resources. In 1978, 5.9% of a study group of Medicare recipients died, but they accounted for 27.9% of Medicare expenditures.[14] In 1980, 5% of those individuals older than 65 who resided in the community were institutionalized or died during the year. They accounted for 22% of expenditures for the noninstitutionalized elderly.[15]

In no other single group of patients has the perceived right to health care services versus societal limitations on the availability of funds to pay for these services generated such controversy. The graying of America will have dramatic implications upon health care financing, resource utilization, and governmental spending priorities. The 65+ population, organized by the American Association of Retired Persons into one of the most powerful lobbying and consumer groups in the United States today, will enjoy tremendous influence over those who make decisions concerning these items. The trend toward more 65+ individuals being better educated, financially secure, and professionally oriented will only increase the influence of this population.

## Physiologic Changes With Aging

There is great variation among older individuals as to the manifestation of age-related physical change. The chronologic age of an individual is not nearly as important as the physiologic age. The most accepted theory is that the process of aging does not vary between individuals; rather, the onset, rapidity, and magnitude of the expression of the physical changes caused by the aging process are person specific. Cellular models of aging infer that true aging begins with birth, but most body systems peak in efficiency in the twenties and thirties, and decrease with age thereafter. A quick review is provided; the reader is encouraged to seek expanded information elsewhere.[16,17]

### *The Senses*

Age-related changes affecting sensory capabilities include (1) a decrease in lens transparency and diminution of the power of accommodation (presbyopia); (2) a loss of auditory acuity (presbycusis); (3) a diminished ability to taste sweet, sour, and bitter, but not salty; (4) a generalized decrease in the sensation of touch; and (5) a decreased thirst response with dehydration.

### *Body Composition*

Most older individuals maintain their same body weight until their seventies, when an overall decrease is noted. The body composition, however, changes greatly. On the average, lean body mass decreases and body fat increases as a proportion of total body weight. Extracellular fluid volume, plasma volume, and total body water also decrease with age.

### *Cardiovascular System*

Many clinicians inaccurately attribute changes in the cardiovascular system to age, without defining the changes caused by cardiovascular disease. In fact, early studies determining age-related physiologic changes have questionable validity as researchers did not screen patients for prior occult coronary artery disease. More recent evidence demonstrates no changes in resting or exercise cardiac output with age in healthy, active community dwellers.[18] The one important difference between study populations was that younger patients increased their heart rate to maintain cardiac output with stress, whereas elderly patients increased their stroke volume, thus incorporating the Frank–Starling principle. Left ventricular wall thickness increases with age, as does the collagen content of the arteries and endocardium. Baroreceptor sensitivity declines with aging, increasing the risk of postural hypotension. Finally, myocardial sensitivity to $\beta$-adrenergic stimulation decreases with age.

### *Central Nervous System*

Changes in intellectual function with age are unclear. Controversy exists as to whether there is any true age-related decline in intellect (benign senescent forgetfulness), but cognitive abilities involving speed, unfamiliar material, and complexity of task decrease with age. Reaction time to a positive or negative stimulus is increased in the older individual. Structurally, the brain decreases in weight and volume. The water content of the brain also decreases. There is an increase in the amount of neuritic (senile) plaques and neurofibrillary tangles in the brain but not to the extent seen in patients with DAT.

### *Digestive System*

The greatest amount of change in the aging digestive system occurs within the oral cavity. Loss of teeth and other alterations in dentition affect many elderly individuals. There is a quantitative decrease in saliva flow, making mastication more difficult. Delays in transit time in the esophagus have been implicated in drug-induced ulcerations. Flattening of gastric mucosa and secretory changes have been noted in the normal elderly individual; the clinical importance of these changes is limited mainly to decreased active transport mechanisms for calcium, iron, and vitamin $B_{12}$ absorption. The incidence of histamine-fast achlorhydria increases dramatically for individuals aged 60 to 69, compared with those aged 20 to 29. An age-related component to the chronic constipation that afflicts so many elderly is unclear as many other contributing factors are age dependent. Lastly, the incidence of diverticulum formation in the colon increases with age.

### *Hepatic System*

The hepatic system appears to be the least affected by the aging process even though liver size and weight decline with age. Controversy exists over whether activity of the metabolic enzyme systems of the liver decrease with age; studies of drug metabolism have documented decreased oxidative capacity (phase I reaction)[19] but little or no change in conjugative capacity (phase II reaction).[20]

### *Renal System*

There is a continuous loss of glomeruli with aging, which has significant impact upon renal function. A cross-sectional study in 1950 demonstrated a 46% decline in insulin clearance from ages 20 to 90.[21] In 1976, a longitudinal study demonstrated a similar decline in creatinine clearance but without a concomitant increase in serum creatinine.[22] Most recently, a longitudinal study of healthy men with no underlying renal disease demonstrated a decline in creatinine clearance of 0.75 mL/min/yr.[23] Of particular interest in this study was the finding of three distinct groups, those with significantly decreased creatinine clearance, those with small but significantly decreased creatinine clearance, and those with no decrease in creatinine clearance. Other important physiologic changes in the kidney include decreased renal blood flow, decreased tubular function, and decreased concentrating ability.

### *Endocrine System*

The elderly patient is subject to numerous endocrinopathies. The thyroid gland atrophies with age, resulting in clinical hypothyroidism occurring more frequently in patients older than 50. The aging of the ovaries with the resultant decline in estrogen production and the accompanying osteoporosis is a major health concern in the United States today. The incidence and prevalence of impaired glucose tolerance increase with age, a major contributing factor being decreased glucose-stimulated insulin release.

### *Respiratory System*

Normal aging of the lungs includes decreased total alveolar surface area, loss of elastic recoil, decline in chest wall compliance, and decreased respiratory muscle strength. These produce generally insignificant abnormalities in pulmonary function under normal conditions. These changes do increase the risk of pulmonary disease and compromise pulmonary function when the lungs are stressed.

### *Immune System*

Involution of the thymus gland and alterations in the balance of circulating lymphocytes contribute to impaired humoral and cell-mediated immune responses. This immunosenescence may contribute to the increased susceptibility of the elderly to infectious diseases and cancer and may contribute to pathologic or physiologic aging.[24]

### *Skeletal System*

There is a progressive, linear loss of average skeletal bone mass (osteopenia) with aging, the loss of trabecular mass occurring sooner than that of cortical mass. The loss of trabecular bone affects those areas of the skeleton with greatest trabecular mass: the vertebral bodies and the bones of the wrist and hip. The loss of bone mass is accelerated in postmenopausal women.

### *Integumentary System*

The major gross morphologic changes in the aging skin are dryness, wrinkling, and uneven pigmentation. Dermal thickness decreases, accounting for the paper-thin quality of aged skin. The number of hair follicles decreases with aging, as does the number of melanocytes within each hair bulb, the result being thinner, gray or white hair. Long-term sun exposure can accelerate these age-related changes and is also responsible for a variety of premalignant (actinic keratosis) and malignant (basal and squamous cell carcinomas) lesions commonly seen in the elderly.

## Physiologic Aging Versus Pathologic Aging

The aging process occurs as a continuum with marked individual variability. Senescence reflects the expression of a variety of interacting influences including genetic predisposition and heredity, environmental and social forces, personality traits, and health care habits. There is no single aging process; what is considered as an intrinsic age-related change (physiologic aging) in one individual may be considered a pathologic abnormality associated with age-related illness in another. The result of this complex process is that both chronologic age and standard markers of organ system function are poor predictors of an individual's physiologic age and functional capabilities.

Whether a particular manifestation in an elderly individual represents physiologic aging or a pathologic consequence is often impossible to determine. Intrinsic changes can occur in the presence of good health and without functional deficit. The decline in renal function with aging is such an example. Intrinsic changes can also result in functional deficits. As examples, atrophy of the thyroid gland occurs universally with aging, but not all elderly individuals become clinically hypothyroid. Numbers and function of dopaminergic neurons decrease with aging, but not all elderly individuals develop Parkinson's disease. Other examples of this random and selective progression include (1) benign senescent forgetfulness to DAT, (2) impaired glucose tolerance to non–insulin-dependent diabetes mellitus, (3) osteopenia to osteoporosis, and (4) hyperpigmentation of the skin to proliferative lesions.

One factor that does contribute to some of these occurrences is an organ system's reserve capacity. Under normal conditions, maintenance of normal homeostasis by the aging organ system is not changed. Under physiologic stress, however, the organ system may have lost sufficient function as to be unable to compensate adequately in the maintenance of homeostasis and would therefore demonstrate compromised function. This sequence of events could be viewed as a loss of reserve capacity. For example, if the aged kidney was insulted by a nephrotoxic drug, then renal function would be subject to greater functional deficit because there would be less reserve renal capacity (i.e., fewer remaining functioning nephrons) on which to draw.

Unraveling of the complexities of what constitutes physiologic aging depends upon the longitudinal monitoring of patient populations. The validity of cross-sectional studies of age-related changes is questionable because of the heterogeneity of the elderly population. All confounding factors such as desirable, societal nutritional trends (attainment of lowered serum cholesterol concentrations) and compensatory changes (increase of stroke volume to maintain cardiac output) must be determined by adequate scientific methodology and placed in the proper perspective. The likely result is that precipitous declines in physiologic function in elderly individuals are secondary to pathologic conditions associated with aging rather than to age per se.

## Special Considerations in Geriatric Drug Therapy

The elderly are susceptible to problems associated with drug use because of the influence of aging upon compliance, pharmacodynamics, and pharmacokinetics. Pharmacogeriatrics is the science that evaluates mechanisms of altered drug effects in the elderly secondary to pharmacodynamic and pharmacokinetic changes. An understanding of the interactions between compliance and pharmacogeriatrics is essential to the development of rational drug therapy.

First, the elderly are at great risk for noncompliance. This deviation from a prescriber's planned medical regimen includes omission of doses, errors in frequency of dosing, intentional or unintentional overdosing, taking of medications for the wrong purpose, and taking of medications prescribed for others. Although age alone is a poor predictor of such behavior, other characteristics common to this population are good predictors. Multiple chronic diseases, multiple drugs, and multiple doses, all common in elderly patients, contribute to noncompliance. The most sophisticated pharmacokinetic methodology is of little use in this population if compliance cannot be guaranteed.

Second, with age there may be changes in target organ sensitivity that render the elderly more sensitive to the pharmacologic action of a drug. Simply stated, equal concentrations of drug at receptor sites in young and old individuals produce differing effects. The etiology of such pharmacodynamic changes is unclear but probably relates to altered receptor function or decreased numbers of receptors. Examples of pharmacodynamic changes in the elderly include a greater depression of the central nervous system with similar diazepam concentrations[25] and a decreased production of vitamin K–dependent clotting factors with comparable warfarin concentrations.[26]

Lastly, physiologic changes of aging can greatly affect drug pharmacokinetics (Table 1). An in-depth review is

**Table 4.1** Summary of Physiologic Determinants of Drug Disposition in the Elderly

| *Component of drug disposition* | *Altered physiology* |
|---|---|
| Absorption | Elevated gastric pH |
| | Decreased gastrointestinal blood flow |
| | Decreased active transport mechanisms |
| Distribution | Decreased total body water |
| | Decreased lean body mass |
| | Increased body fat |
| | Decreased serum albumin |
| Metabolism | Decreased liver blood flow |
| | Decreased liver size |
| | Possibly decreased enzymatic activity |
| Excretion | Decreased glomerular filtration rate |
| | Decreased renal blood flow |
| | Decreased tubular function |

beyond the scope of this chapter, and the reader is encouraged to seek out previously published information.[27,28]

A major goal of pharmacogeriatrics is the attainment of a desired steady-state drug concentration within a proven therapeutic range established specifically for the elderly population. If this goal is accomplished, there is a greater potential for beneficial effects than adverse effects. The relevant equation is

$$C_{ss} = \frac{\text{dose} \cdot F}{\text{CL} \cdot \tau} \qquad (1)$$

where $C_{ss}$ is steady-state concentration, CL is clearance, $F$ is bioavailability, and $\tau$ is the dosage interval. The clinician seeks a dose that, when other factors are considered, produces the desired steady-state concentration. Aging can affect this equation in several ways. The bioavailability of a drug can be altered by decreased dissolution or absorption. As mentioned previously, several physiologic changes occur with aging of the gastrointestinal tract that could affect these processes; however, despite these changes, the extent (peak concentration) and rate (time to peak concentration) of absorption of drugs in the elderly patient are not significantly altered, probably because most drugs are absorbed via passive transport. Therefore, altered bioavailability of drugs in the elderly is more dependent upon drug product formulation than the age of the patient.

The most important kinetic variable in Equation (1) is clearance. This biologically independent variable characterizes the ability of body organs to remove a drug from the blood. It is, in theory, the amount of blood from which a drug is completely removed per unit of time. The rate of clearance is determined from the amount of blood that can be delivered to a clearing organ as well as the intrinsic ability of the organ to remove the drug from the blood. Physiologic changes that decrease delivery of blood to an organ, such as a decrease in cardiac output, can decrease the amount of drug cleared; however, these changes in drug delivered may not affect the rate at which the drug is cleared. Clearance is defined in pharmacokinetic terms as

$$\text{CL} = \frac{0.693 \cdot V_D}{t_{1/2}} \qquad (2)$$

where $V_D$ is volume of distribution and $t_{1/2}$ is the elimination half-life. Aging can also affect this equation in several ways. Volume of distribution, a biologically independent variable, can be significantly affected by the changes in body composition that occur with aging. As a result, certain drugs have altered volumes of distribution when used in elderly patients. Lipophilic drugs such as diazepam have a significantly increased volume of distribution[29]; hydrophilic drugs such as acetaminophen have a reduced volume of distribution.[30]

Elimination half-life is a biologically dependent variable dependent upon both clearance and volume of distribution. Aging affects this variable mainly through changes in the intrinsic function of the major drug-clearing organs, the liver and kidney. As stated previously, phase I reactions (oxidation, reduction, hydrolysis) are subject to greater age-related changes than are phase II reactions (conjugation). Drugs with increased volumes of distribution and decreased hepatic clearance secondary to oxidative biotransformation (i.e., diazepam) may have a significantly prolonged half-life in the elderly.[29] Gender and environmental influences such as smoking also contribute to age-related changes in elimination half-life.

Explanation of the effect of age-related changes in renal function upon drug clearance is more difficult. Longitudinal studies have demonstrated a great degree of individuality in changes in renal function. As a result, no prediction of renal function can be made on the basis of age alone. The renal function of each elderly individual must be measured or appropriately estimated using nomograms or equations that take into account the patient's age. Serum creatinine determinations should not be used exclusively as measures of renal function in the elderly because they may overestimate actual functional ability. In general, the otherwise healthy aging kidney is capable of maintaining normal acid–base status, electrolyte balance, and drug clearance. For example, no significant differences in volume of distribution, clearance, or elimination half-life were determined in bacteremic but otherwise healthy young versus old patients receiving gentamicin.[31]

Despite these findings, the aging kidney is at greater risk for nephrotoxicity because it has fewer functioning nephrons; it has lost a portion of its reserve capacity.

The last pharmacokinetic variable substantially affected by aging is protein binding. The two major components of protein responsible for drug binding are serum albumin and $\alpha_1$-acid glycoprotein. With aging, there is a diminished amount of serum albumin and thus the potential for decreased binding of certain drugs with resultant increased plasma free (unbound) fraction. The importance of this increased free fraction is questionable because, although more free drug is available for receptor binding, more free drug is also available for distribution, biotransformation, and excretion. As a result, a new equilibrium in drug disposition is quickly reached; however, with certain drugs (e.g., naproxyn) there may be increased plasma free fraction and decreased total clearance.[32] In these circumstances, it is possible for decreased protein binding to greatly affect pharmacologic activity.

## Summary

The contribution of aging toward health status is an issue that all health care practitioners will eventually face. A thorough understanding of physiologic versus pathologic aging is important but secondary to the larger issue of appropriate drug therapy. Our primary responsibility as pharmacists is still to deliver the right drug to the right patient at the right time and in the right dose. Aging is but another increasingly common, confounding variable in our efforts to meet this responsibility.

## References


1. U.S. Senate Special Committee on Aging. Aging America. Trends and Projections. Washington DC, US Department of Health and Human Services, 1985–1986.
2. Rosenwaite I. A demographic portrait of the oldest old. Milbank Memorial Fund Quarterly/Health and Society 1985;63:187–205.
3. Public Health Service. Health. United States 1985. Hyattsville, MD, US Department of Health and Human Services, 1985, DHHS publication no. (PHS)86-1232.
4. Kovar MG. Aging in the eighties. Preliminary data from the supplement on aging to the National Health Interview Survey, United States, January–June 1984. Advancedata 1986;115:1–6.
5. Ingram DK. Profile of chronic illness in nursing homes, 1973–74. Hyattsville, MD, National Center for Health Statistics, 1977, DHEW publication (PHS) 78-1780 (Vital and Health Statistics; series 13; no. 29).
6. Soldo BJ, Manton KG. Health status and service needs of the oldest old: Current patterns and future trends. Milbank Memorial Fund Quarterly/Health and Society 1985;63:286–319.
7. Special report. Department of Health and Human Services' Task Force on Alzheimer's Disease: Report and recommendations. Neurobiol Aging 1985;6:65–71.
8. Weissman MM, Myers JK. Affective disorders in a US urban community. Arch Gen Psychiatry 1978;35:1304–1311.
9. Sendbuehler J, Goldstein S. Attempted suicide among the aged. J Am Geriatr Soc 1977;25:245–248.
10. Waldo DR, Lazenby HC. Demographic characteristics and health care use and expenditures by the aged in the United States: 1977–1984. Health Care Finan Rev 1984;6:1–29.
11. Kaspar JA. Prescribed medicines: Use, expenditures, and sources of payment. National Health Care Expenditures Study Data Preview no. 9. Washington DC, US Government Printing Office, 1982, DHHS publication no. (PHS) 82-3320.
12. Miller RR. Drug surveillance utilizing epidemiologic methods: A report from the Boston Collaborative Drug Surveillance Program. Am J Hosp Pharm 1973;30:584–592.
13. Sirrocco A. An overview of the 1982 National Master Facility Inventory Survey of Nursing and Related Care Homes. Advancedata 1985;111:1–5.
14. Lubitz J, Prihoda R. The use and costs of Medicare services in the last two years of life. Health Care Finan Rev 1984;5:117–131.
15. Kovar MG. Expenditures for the medical care of elderly people living in the community in 1980. Milbank Memorial Fund Quarterly/Health and Society 1986;64:100–132.
16. Rossman I (ed): Clinical Geriatrics, 3rd ed. Philadelphia, J.B. Lippincott, 1986.
17. Andres R, Bierman EL, Hazzard WR (eds): Principles of Geriatric Medicine. New York, McGraw–Hill, 1985.
18. Rodeheffer RJ, Gerstenblith G, Becker LC, et al. Exercise cardiac output is maintained with advancing age in healthy human subjects: Cardiac dilatation and increased stroke volume compensate for a diminished heart rate. Circulation 1984;69: 203–213.
19. Vestal RE, Norris AH, Tobin JD, et al. Antipyrine metabolism in man: Influence of age, alcohol, caffeine, and smoking. Clin Pharmacol Ther 1975;18:425–432.
20. Greenblatt DJ, Divoll M, Harmatz JS, et al. Oxazepam kinetics: Effects of age and sex. J Pharmacol Exp Ther 1980;215:86–91.
21. Davies DF, Shock NW. Age changes in glomerular filtration rate, effective renal plasma flow and tubular excretory capacity in adult males. J Clin Invest 1950;29:496–507.
22. Rowe JW, Andres R, Tobin JD, et al. The effects of age on creatinine clearance in man: A cross-sectional and longitudinal study. J Gerontol 1976;31:155–163.
23. Lindeman RD, Tobin J, Shock NW. Longitudinal studies on the rate of decline in renal function with age. J Am Geriatr Soc 1985;33:278–285.
24. Weksler ME. Biologic basis and clinical significance of immune senescence, in Rossman I (ed): Clinical Geriatrics, 3rd ed. Philadelphia, J.B. Lippincott, 1986, pp 57–67.
25. Clinical depression of the central nervous system due to diazepam and chlordiazepoxide in relation to cigarette smoking and age: A report from Boston Collaborative Drug Surveillance Program. N Engl J Med 1973;288:277–280.
26. Shephard AMM, Hewick DS, Moreland TA, et al. Age as a determinant of sensitivity to warfarin. Br J Clin Pharmacol 1977;4:315–320.
27. Greenblatt DJ, Sellers EM, Shader RI. Drug disposition in old age. N Engl J Med 1982;306:1081–1088.
28. Pucino F, Beck CL, Seifert RL, et al. Pharmacogeriatrics. Pharmacotherapy 1985;5:314–326.
29. Klotz U, Avant GR, Hoyumpa A, et al. The effects of age and liver disease on the disposition and elimination of diazepam in adult man. J Clin Invest 1975;55:347–359.
30. Divoll M, Abernathy DR, Ameer B, et al. Acetaminophen kinetics in the elderly. Clin Pharmacol Ther 1982;31:151–156.
31. Bauer LA, Blouin RA. Gentamicin pharmacokinetics: Effect of aging in patients with normal renal function. J Am Geriatr Soc 1982;30:309–311.
32. Upton RA, Williams RL, Kelly J, et al. Naproxyn pharmacokinetics in the elderly. Br J Clin Pharmacol 1984;18:207–214.

# Chapter 5 / Pregnancy

Janet McCombs, PharmD

Pregnancy is a normal, natural life event through which most women progress with minimal problems. Modern medicine and the use of updated technology have improved obstetric risks and decreased complications, but they also contribute to new problems such as the teratogenicity of medications. Since the thalidomide tragedy in 1956 and, more recently, the diethylstilbestrol problems, medical practitioners have been more cautious about the recommendation of medication for the pregnant patient.

Most medications have an unknown risk of teratogenicity and fewer than 10 medications have indications for use in pregnancy.[1] Although very little is known about effects on the fetus of most medications, many women ingest drugs during their pregnancy. First, the patient may have an acute or chronic medical problem for which her physician has prescribed a medication. Certainly it would be best to avoid the use of all medications, but the well-being of the mother must also be considered. A mother who is uncomfortable and ill for the duration of the pregnancy is less likely to approach delivery and the newborn with a positive outlook. Second, a patient may take medication before realizing that she is pregnant or before consulting a physician. Third, a patient may assume that because of easy availability, nonprescription medications do not produce toxic effects.

## Diagnosis

Amenorrhea is the first symptom of pregnancy in most patients; however, a woman may also experience morning nausea and vomiting, frequent urination, and tender breasts with enlargement and increased pigmentation of the nipple and areola. Early pregnancy may be confirmed by the presence of human chorionic gonadotropin (HCG), and some HCG assays are sensitive enough to be accurate 7 to 9 days after fertilization. The slide test utilizing latex particles coated with HCG antibody may be completed in 2 minutes but is less accurate than the hemagglutination reaction, which is performed in a test tube. The hemagglutination test takes up to 2 hours to complete but is sensitive enough to detect HCG concentrations as low as 0.5–1 IU. False negatives are often the result of performing the test too early or the result of technical errors, while false positives may result from the high levels of luteinizing hormone (LH) produced in perimenopausal patients, from abnormally high levels of thyroid-stimulating hormone (TSH), or from hormones produced by certain neoplasms. Drugs such as phenothiazines may also cause false positives.[2] Radioimmunoassay (RIA) is a more sensitive and more specific test because it reacts with the $\beta$ subunit of HCG, but this test is inconvenient, expensive, and requires 48 hours to complete. It should be recognized that a positive pregnancy test indicates only a source of HCG and not necessarily pregnancy.

## Normal Course of Pregnancy

The normal duration of human gestation is 267 days from conception or 280 days from the first day of the last menstrual period. Thus, pregnancy usually spans 40 weeks. There are charts and "wheels" developed to aid the practitioner in determining the expected date of confinement (EDC), but Nagele's rule also provides a reasonable estimate. To apply Nagele's rule and calculate the EDC, take the date of the first day of the last menstrual period, subtract 3 months, then add 7 days.[3] (Example: April 21 − 3 months = January 21 + 7 days = January 28.) This method is usually correct to within 2 weeks of delivery and works best with patients who have regular 28-day menstrual cycles.

Gestational age is the number of completed weeks of pregnancy beginning with the first day of the last menstrual period. The product of conception is referred to as an embryo for the first 8 weeks and thereafter is termed *fetus*. The gravidity of a female patient is the total number of pregnancies, including full-term, ectopic, premature, and aborted pregnancies. A gravid patient is pregnant; a primigravida patient is pregnant for the first time and a nulligravida patient has never been pregnant. The parity of a patient refers to the number of deliveries after the twentieth week.

Parity is often further defined for an individual patient by a series of four numbers. In order, these numbers indicate the number of term deliveries, number of premature deliveries, number of aborted and/or ectopic pregnancies, and number of living children. Deliveries involving multiple births add only one parous experience to the mother's obstetric history.

The average weight gain during pregnancy is 24 pounds. Patients gaining 24 pounds or less usually have more success returning to their prepregnancy weight after delivery. Patients who gain more than 24 pounds have usually consumed a diet too high in calories. The gain during the first trimester is about 3 pounds, but during the last 16 weeks, a gain of one pound per week may be expected. Although pregnancy might be considered a good time for controlled weight reduction in the obese patient, this is not recommended because of the possibility of inadequate nutrition for the fetus. Adequate protein intake is especially important during pregnancy as it is essential for fetal development. Normally, a pregnant patient requires an increase of 300 Cal/d, including an additional 30 g of protein. The lactating patient requires an additional 500 Cal daily including 20 g of protein.

During pregnancy, it is common to give vitamin supplements though this may not be necessary for a patient eating a well-balanced diet. An additional 200 mg of elemental iron and 200–400 μg of folic acid are required by many women during pregnancy and are included in most prenatal vitamin products.

## Physiologic Changes in Pregnancy

Many physiologic changes occur in the pregnant patient, altering the use of drugs in this population.

Total blood volume in pregnancy increases 30% to 40% (1,500–1,800 mL). The cellular components increase about 20% and the fluid portion, about 40% to 50%. This disparity may appear as an anemia when the hemoglobin and hematocrit fall in the third trimester. During the second and third trimesters, extravascular volume increases, leading to decreased plasma levels of some drugs.

Serum proteins are often 1–1.5 g lower in pregnancy and the albumin-to-globulin ratio falls by about 50%. Renal function is improved during gestation as the renal plasma flow increases about 30% and the glomerular filtration rate is increased about 50%. Drugs excreted primarily by glomerular filtration could be expected to have an increased rate of excretion. Because of better renal filtration, serum urea, creatinine, and uric acid are decreased in pregnancy.

The cardiovascular system also undergoes several significant changes during pregnancy. Cardiac output increases about 32% because of an increased heart rate of 10–15 beats per minute and an increased stroke volume; however, the blood pressure remains relatively constant during most normal pregnancies.

In the gastrointestinal tract, motility and acidity are decreased. The tone of the bowel is also decreased; thus, symptoms of a hiatal hernia are common and resolve after delivery. The decreased peristalsis of the gastrointestinal tract often leads to constipation in the pregnant patient. Nausea and vomiting in the early weeks of pregnancy may contribute to the decreased absorption of medications, and the decreased motility of the lower gastrointestinal tract may delay the fecal excretion of some drugs.

The metabolism of drugs may be increased or decreased at various stages of gestation, but it is unlikely that this would have a profound effect on the plasma clearance of drugs during pregnancy.[4]

During pregnancy, a hypercoagulable state develops, with higher levels of fibrinogen and factors VII, VIII, IX, and X. The risk of disseminated intravascular coagulation (DIC) is increased during pregnancy, but the incidence of deep vein thrombosis is not increased.

## Drug Effects on the Fetus

Several factors should be kept in mind when considering the effects of drugs on the fetus. The extent to which drugs cross the placenta varies, but many drugs reach concentrations in the fetus of 50% to 100% of the levels in maternal blood. The total concentration of blood protein is less in the fetus and often results in more free drug, especially for drugs that are highly protein bound in the maternal blood. Excretion of medications by the fetus occurs primarily via the fetal liver and the placenta, and clearance may be lower than in adults.

The effects of teratogens are dependent on several factors. The dose reaching the embryo or fetus and the duration of exposure are important considerations. Gestational age at the time of exposure is important as well. It is generally accepted that the first trimester is the most critical time for organ malformation, but other physiologic and functional defects may occur later as may growth retardation. The genotypes of the mother and fetus are significant in determining the amount of drug reaching the fetus because of variations in metabolism (e.g., acetylator status). Other drugs or environmental factors to which exposure occurs simultaneously may also influence teratogenesis.

Teratogens may cause spontaneous abortion, congenital malformations, intrauterine growth retardation, mental retardation, carcinogenesis, and mutagenesis.

Late in pregnancy, effects of medication on labor and delivery should be considered. Very near delivery, the effects on the neonate are important because the medication present in the infant at delivery will have to be metabolized and excreted by the neonate, which may result in prolonged exposure and toxicity.

## Pregnancy-Induced Diseases

Physiologic and functional changes during pregnancy may lead to exacerbation or development of medical problems seen in the nonpregnant patient. Pregnancy often necessitates management different from that in the nonpregnant population.

### *Nausea and Vomiting*

The nausea and vomiting associated with pregnancy are usually mild and referred to as "morning sickness." About half of all pregnant patients experience some degree of nausea and vomiting. The problem usually starts in early pregnancy and lasts 12 to 14 weeks. Nausea is often apparent upon arising but abates as the day progresses. Some women, however, experience nausea throughout the day and in some cases it persists during the entire pregnancy. Severe nausea and vomiting that persist are referred to as hyperemesis gravidarum and may be detrimental to the patient and the fetus. This disorder requires hospitalization with administration of replacement fluids and electrolytes, antiemetics, and sedation. Hyperemesis gravidarum can be a life-threatening problem and must be corrected immediately. The complications associated with this problem include nutritional deficiencies, weight loss, and starvation. Maternal neurologic, renal, retinal, and hepatic damage can also occur and are similar to the changes that occur in starvation.[5,6]

The cause of nausea and vomiting in pregnancy is unknown. Proposed mechanisms include increased levels of hormones during pregnancy and emotional or psychologic factors. As the cause of the nausea is unknown, treatment is directed toward the symptoms. A patient who experiences only early morning nausea may be directed to eat two or three soda crackers when she awakens, then wait 15 or 20 minutes before arising. Dietary management of nausea lasting all day would include small, dry meals high in carbohydrates. Spicy foods and noxious odors should be avoided.

Medication must be considered for patients whose nausea persists in spite of dietary management. Although teratogenic risk cannot be ruled out for any drug, the risk involved with the antiemetic agents currently used for nausea and vomiting during pregnancy seems to be small.[7] Current medications used are the phenothiazines, meclizine, cyclizine, dimenhydrinate, diphenhydramine, doxylamine, and pyridoxine. Bendectin (Merrell Dow; doxylamine 10 mg, pyridoxine 10 mg) was the most widely used agent for morning sickness until its withdrawal from the market by the manufacturer in 1983. Despite lack of evidence associating Bendectin with birth defects, damaging publicity and decreasing patient confidence promoted the decision to stop manufacture of the medication. This tablet had a special coating that delayed activity, making a bedtime dose effective during the morning hours.

The two drugs with the lowest risk for teratogenicity are meclizine and dimenhydrinate.[7] These drugs have also been shown to be efficacious for nausea and vomiting associated with pregnancy.[7] There is conflicting evidence about the teratogenicity of the phenothiazines. Promethazine has been used for quite a number of years with no apparent problems. If promethazine is not effective, prochlorperazine and thiethylperazine may be considered. These more potent phenothiazines have been studied less, but the potential problems caused by poor nutrition may outweigh the risk.

### *Heartburn*

Many patients experience heartburn during the latter half of pregnancy. This usually results from relaxation of the cardiac sphincter and increased pressure in the stomach caused by the enlarging uterus, allowing regurgitation of the stomach contents into the lower esophagus. Dietary management of heartburn should be attempted before drug therapy. Small meals often help alleviate the problem. Elevation of the head of the bed with blocks may help resolve the problem, which occurs when the patient lies down.

Antacids may be used judiciously in patients who do not respond to dietary alterations. Magnesium and/or aluminum hydroxides are usually effective for relieving the pain, and the duration of action is several hours. Sodium bicarbonate has a short duration of action and may lead to rebound symptoms and metabolic alkalosis with long-term use. Use of sodium bicarbonate should be avoided in favor of more effective agents. Medications containing salicylates should be avoided especially in the last trimester. Salicylates may prolong gestation by decreasing prostaglandins and may increase bleeding time because of their antiplatelet activity.[8]

### *Constipation*

Constipation is a common problem in pregnancy and is most likely a result of decreased peristalsis. Patients experiencing constipation should be encouraged to add bulky, high-fiber foods to their diet and increase their fluid intake. Moderate exercise is also helpful in most cases.

Emollient and bulk laxatives are the agents of choice in the pregnant patient. Bulk laxatives are not absorbed and thus would pose less threat to the fetus. Stool softeners such as docusate may be used occasionally. Mineral oil should be avoided as there is possibility of impairment of vitamin K absorption, which could decrease availability to the fetus. The excessive use of any laxative should be avoided as this may promote labor.[9]

### *Hemorrhoids*

Hemorrhoids often develop or worsen in pregnant patients. The cause of hemorrhoids during pregnancy may be the increased pressure of the gravid uterus on the rectum and may be compounded by constipation.

Correction of constipation and regular use of stool softeners are helpful to many patients. Sitting in hot sitz baths two or three times a day for 15 minutes may also make the patient more comfortable. With respect to medications, external products are preferred because many drugs are readily absorbed from the rectal mucosa. External astringent compresses should be tried before other agents. Anal analgesics containing topical anesthetics should be avoided because of possible systemic absorption,[9] and products containing steroids should be used with the same caution as systemic steroids.

### *Coagulation Disorders*

Thromboembolic phenomena are fortunately not common during pregnancy, the incidence being about 0.2% to 0.4%. The mortality associated with thromboembolism may reach 13%, but with adequate anticoagulation this can be reduced to 1% or less.[10]

Another group of pregnant patients who may require anticoagulation are those with a cardiac valve prosthesis.[6] Both patients with a confirmed diagnosis of thromboembolism and those with cardiac valve replacement require treatment.

In the nonpregnant patient, the standard treatment is intravenous heparin followed by maintenance with oral anticoagulants. This protocol cannot be followed in the pregnant patient because neither the warfarin derivatives nor heparin is without risk during pregnancy. The warfarin derivatives pose a very significant risk to the developing fetus[8] and should be avoided during pregnancy. About 30% of pregnancies exposed to oral anticoagulants result in fetal malformations, developmental deficiencies, stillbirths, or hemorrhage.[11] The anticoagulant of choice during pregnancy is subcutaneous heparin though it too has risks. (Risks to the fetus associated with the use of heparin are indirect, such as hemorrhage[8] and the underlying disease requiring anticoagulation.) There have been no reports of congenital defects associated with heparin.[11] The large molecular weight of heparin does not allow it to cross the placenta.[10]

Heparin is also the anticoagulant of choice for use in the pregnant patient because the effect of the medication can be antagonized by administering protamine sulfate. This is advantageous because the onset of labor or the necessity of an operative delivery is not always predictable.

Reproductive-age females who require long-term anticoagulation with oral agents should be counseled about the risks of pregnancy and provided with effective contraception. Conversion from oral anticoagulants to heparin should be considered for those patients desiring pregnancy despite possible indirect maternal and fetal risks from such therapy. Ambulatory patients should be capable of self-administration of subcutaneous heparin and compliant with appointments for follow-up monitoring.

### *Preeclampsia/Eclampsia*

Preeclampsia/eclampsia is a serious obstetric complication that may endanger the lives of the mother and fetus. Preeclampsia is the development of edema, hypertension, and proteinuria after the 20th week of pregnancy. The disease can also occur within 24 hours of delivery or in the presence of trophoblastic disease.[3] Eclampsia involves progression of the symptoms seen in preeclampsia, with the development of seizures or coma.

The incidence of this complication of pregnancy is about 5%[7]; it occurs most often in patients predisposed to hypertension, primigravidas, diabetics, those with essential hypertension, and women carrying multiple pregnancies or molar pregnancies.[9]

The cause of preeclampsia/eclampsia is unknown. Until it is determined, prevention of the condition is not possible, but frequent monitoring of patients and early recognition and treatment may prevent severe forms of the disease. The goal of therapy is to decrease the blood pressure, control convulsions, and deliver a viable infant.

A triad of signs usually occurs in the progression of preeclampsia: the first indication is edema, followed by elevation of blood pressure and lastly proteinuria. Edema, the first symptom of the triad, should be suspected when a patient exhibits a sudden weight gain of 2 pounds or more per week or 6 pounds per month. (Edema may be observed as 1+ pitting edema after 12 hours of bedrest.) Hypertension, the second sign, is defined as a systolic blood pressure increase of at least 30 mm Hg or a reading of 140 mm Hg, or a diastolic blood pressure increase of 15 mm Hg or a reading of 90 mm Hg, on two readings taken at least 6 hours apart. Proteinuria is defined as a concentration of 300 mg of protein per liter over 24 hours or a concentration greater than 1 g per liter in two or more random samples taken 6 hours apart. A patient exhibiting these signs should be treated for mild preeclampsia.

Patients exhibiting mild preeclampsia should be placed on strict bedrest in a lateral recumbent position in a quiet, dark, private room. Diuresis usually begins within 36 to 48 hours with regression of symptoms in 4 to 5 days.

Severely preeclamptic patients usually have systolic blood pressures of 160 mm Hg or greater or diastolic blood pressures of 110 mm Hg or greater despite bedrest. Other problems often seen in these patients include proteinuria greater than 5 g/24 h, oliguria (<400 mL/24 h), cerebral or visual disturbances, pulmonary edema or cyanosis, headache, and epigastric pain. These patients should be started on a regimen of magnesium sulfate to prevent seizures and delivered as soon as possible.

Several different methods of administration of magnesium sulfate have been described.[9] Although both intramuscular and intravenous routes of administration are effective in achieving adequate serum levels, intravenous administration may be preferred for several reasons. First, magnesium sulfate does carry some risk of toxicity and an intravenous infusion may be discontinued immediately should the serum level become too great. Second, the rate of absorption from an intramuscular injection may be variable and erratic because of vascular spasm.[6] Intramuscular administration is also painful and the volume required to achieve a therapeutic dose is large.

One method of administration involves intravenous loading with 4 g of magnesium sulfate followed by intramuscular doses. Another accepted regimen involves intramuscular administration of both a 10-g loading dose and additional 5-g doses at 6-hour intervals. Perhaps the most common routine is to give a loading dose of 4–6 g followed by an infusion of 1–2 g/h controlled by a reliable pump. The 50% solution of magnesium sulfate should be reserved for intramuscular administration, while the 20% solution is most often used intravenously.

It is extremely important that the patient receiving magnesium sulfate be closely monitored for signs of toxicity. The optimum serum level of magnesium for prevention of convulsions is 6–8 mEq/L.[9] At 9–10 mEq/L the patellar reflex becomes hypoactive and may disappear[6]; urine output should be monitored closely because magnesium is excreted only in the urine. Respirations should be at least 12–16/min. Respiratory depression and cardiac conduction abnormalities may occur if the infusion is continued beyond 13–15 mEq/L.[9] The effect of magnesium may be reversed by administration of 1 g of calcium gluconate. An ampule of calcium gluconate should be kept at the bedside of any patient receiving magnesium therapy for preeclampsia. It should be noted that magnesium sulfate is not an antihypertensive; it is given to prevent convulsions and may have mild sedative effects. The patient's reflexes should be checked every 30 minutes. Convulsions not controlled by adequate levels of magnesium sulfate may respond to intravenous diazepam or phenytoin after delivery.

Blood pressure should continue to be monitored frequently. A diastolic reading of 160–180 mm Hg or higher or a systolic reading of 110 mm Hg or greater should be treated with intravenous hydralazine. (Parenteral administration of all medications is preferred in severe preeclampsia and eclampsia.) A dose of 5–10 mg should be given initially, followed by 10 mg every 20 minutes as needed to decrease systolic blood pressure below 100 mm Hg. An intravenous infusion may also be used. It is important not to decrease blood pressure too quickly, to avoid shock. Very often, parenteral hydralazine produces tachycardia, palpitations, flushing, and headache. Propranolol may be useful in opposing the cardiac side effects of hydralazine but should not be used alone.

Diazoxide has been used to decrease blood pressure in pregnant patients[12]; but hypotension often occurs with its use because of the rapid vasodilation. The unpredictability of the initial response is the primary disadvantage of diazoxide, but there are others. Diazoxide causes sodium and water retention and decreases insulin release, which may result in neonatal hyperglycemia. The drug also has a relaxant effect on the uterus that may inhibit labor; thus, the use of diazoxide to control blood pressure in the obstetric patient is best reserved for postpartum hypertension. Diuretics are not recommended for use in preeclampsia/eclampsia. These are useful only for mobilizing edema fluid, which cannot be done effectively without disturbing the patient's electrolyte balance. Ethacrynic acid or furosemide may be used when pulmonary edema is present or likely to develop.

Nitroprusside is not used in the pregnant patient because of lack of experience with the drug in this population and concern over fetal thiocyanate toxicity.[9] It is used only when all other measures fail or when left ventricular failure is present.

In most cases, the response to any treatment is temporary. Labor often begins spontaneously in these patients but, if not, plans for emergency delivery should be made. The only cure for preeclampsia/eclampsia is delivery.

### *Anemias*

The most common anemia during pregnancy results from iron deficiency. Common causes of this deficiency include rapidly recurring pregnancies, abnormal blood loss, and nutritional inadequacies. Hemoglobin values should be expected to drop during pregnancy because of the increase in blood volume with a smaller proportional increase in red blood cell mass. Iron deficiency anemia should be ruled out in pregnancy when the hemoglobin falls below 10 g/dL or the hematocrit is below 30%. Decreased blood levels of serum iron and total iron binding capacity are diagnostic. To prevent the development of iron deficiency anemia in pregnancy, all pregnant patients should receive approximately 200 mg of elemental iron daily.[6] This may be achieved by the administration of ferrous sulfate 300 mg three times a day or ferrous gluconate 600 mg three times daily.

Megaloblastic anemia or pernicious anemia of pregnancy is less common than iron deficiency anemia and is more common in multiparas over age 30. The etiology is a folic acid deficiency secondary to increased requirements during pregnancy. Epileptic patients receiving anticonvulsant therapy are especially at risk for development of this anemia. Folic acid deficiency can be prevented by daily doses of 300 μg per day during pregnancy.[6] Treatment of existing anemia may require daily doses as high as 5–10 mg of folic acid to correct the deficit.

## Chronic Medical Disorders During Pregnancy

### *Diabetes*

Because of the significant metabolic changes during pregnancy, the management of the pregnant diabetic patient differs from that in the prepregnancy state. The White classification of diabetes in pregnancy[13] has been used historically for prognosis and management of the pregnant diabetic. This classification is based on the duration and severity of the disease and remains in use for describing the severity of maternal disease.

When possible, it is best to plan a pregnancy in the diabetic patient, as prevention of complications provides the best management. The patient should be assessed for other risk factors, undergo ophthalmic evaluation and electrocardiography, and have a 24-hour urine collected for creatinine and protein values. The incidence of major congenital abnormalities in diabetics is 6% to 12%, compared with 2% in the normal population.[3] It is especially important that the patient be normoglycemic prior to conception and during the first trimester because the congenital malformations associated with diabetes are related to poor control during the first 8 weeks of gestation.[14] Determination of glycosylated hemoglobin ($A_1C$) prior to conception helps determine the degree of glucose control.

Patients with the highest risk of complications include those with vasculopathy, poor glucose control, a previous stillbirth, and noncompliance. The complications of diabetic pregnancies include fetal macrosomia, polyhydramnios, malformations, and respiratory distress syndrome. Patients with vascular disease are more likely to have a fetus with intrauterine growth retardation. Fortunately, if the neonates do encounter these problems, after early special care, the infants usually develop normally. Diabetic patients now have a 96% to 98% chance of having a healthy child with good prenatal management.[3]

During pregnancy, diabetic patients have an increased risk of hypoglycemia and ketoacidosis. Thus, the goal of therapy in these patients is the avoidance of fasting and postprandial hyperglycemia and hypoglycemia. The quality of maternal glucose control is the best indicator of perinatal risk, and use of the newer home glucose reflectance meters has certainly aided in control. Tests using whole blood determinations of glucose are preferred over urine tests during pregnancy because the renal threshold for glucose is decreased in pregnancy, giving an inaccurate estimate of blood sugar. It has been suggested that glucose be monitored during fasting, before meals, and at bedtime daily. Some physicians also have their patients monitor glucose 1 hour after meals 1 day per week. Evaluation of glycosolated hemoglobin once each trimester helps assess control.

Pregnant patients usually require a diabetic diet of 35 kcal/kg daily, or about 2,200–2,400 Cal. Only intermediate-acting and fast-acting insulins should be used during pregnancy. Long-acting insulins should not be used because of the variable rates of onset and prolonged duration of activity. NPH or Lente insulin combined with regular insulin should be given subcutaneously in two divided doses daily. Optimal management is usually achieved by giving two thirds the total dose before breakfast and the remaining one third before the evening meal. The dose should be adjusted to maintain rigid control; however, there are various opinions in the literature as to what glucose level should be maintained to minimize neonatal morbidity and mortality.[15] About 70% of pregnant patients have increased insulin requirements after the 24th week,[6] making ketoacidosis more likely.

Oral hypoglycemic agents are contraindicated during pregnancy because they cross the placenta and stimulate the fetal pancreas.[9] These agents should be discontinued before conception if at all possible. Should pregnancy occur in a patient taking one of these medications, the drug should be stopped as soon as pregnancy is confirmed and insulin therapy initiated.

Prenatal visits should be scheduled with the patient's internist and obstetrician every 2 weeks during the first half of pregnancy and weekly thereafter. This aids in compliance and early recognition of possible problems.

Glucose intolerance of pregnancy usually develops during the second half of pregnancy in about 2% to 3% of patients.[3] Initially, the patient is placed on a diabetic diet and home glucose monitoring; if this does not control glucose, insulin therapy should be started and the patient managed as a pregnant diabetic.

Tight control should be maintained during labor and delivery to reduce the risk of neonatal hypoglycemia. This may be accomplished by an infusion of 1 L of 5% dextrose injection with 10 units of regular insulin added at a rate of 100 mL/h. Additional glucose or insulin is given to maintain glucose at approximately 100 mg/dL. Another regimen includes intravenous administration of 50 g of glucose every 6 hours, with regular insulin given subcutaneously as needed. In either case, blood glucose should be checked every 1 to 2 hours with a home glucose monitoring system at the bedside.

Epidural anesthesia is acceptable for a diabetic patient if she desires its use. Immediately after delivery of the placenta, insulin requirements drop and remain lower for 24 to 72 hours. During this period, hypoglycemic shock is common and the patient must be monitored closely. Breastfeeding is encouraged in the diabetic patient; lower insulin requirements during lactation are expected.[14]

### *Chronic Hypertension*

Chronic hypertension in pregnancy is described as hypertension present at conception or developing before the twentieth week of gestation. Obstetric patients with chronic hypertension are considered high risk and require close observation during pregnancy with prenatal visits scheduled every 1 to 2 weeks. Hypertensive patients have a greater incidence of decreased fetal weight and fetal growth retardation because of decreased placental function. At delivery, the placenta is small and multiple infarcts may be present. About one third of hypertensive patients have superimposed preeclampsia, which occurs earlier and progresses more rapidly than in otherwise normal pregnancies.[6] These patients have higher maternal and fetal mortality rates and are less responsive to treatment. Abruptio placentae (premature separation of the placenta) occurs more often in patients with vascular disease than in patients with uncomplicated pregnancies. Cerebral hemorrhage is a more common cause of maternal mortality than preeclampsia in these patients. To minimize complications, blood pressure should be controlled during pregnancy. It is common for blood pressure to decrease in the second trimester, and it may be possible to discontinue therapy at this time and reinstate it if necessary.

Given the young age of most pregnant patients, the chronic hypertension seen in these patients is usually mild and with minimal sequelae. Several clinicians agree that a blood pressure slightly higher than acceptable in the nonpregnant patient may be permitted. Mild hypertension should first be treated with bedrest and home monitoring of blood pressure. The patient should have complete bedrest for at least 1 hour at lunchtime and 1 hour in the afternoon in addition to 10 hours of bedrest each night.

Blood pressure not responding satisfactorily to bedrest may be treated with methyldopa. Methyldopa is the most commonly used antihypertensive medication in pregnancy. It is effective, and no fetal or neonatal problems have been reported.[11] The use of methyldopa has been shown to increase fetal survival rates and decrease midtrimester fetal loss.[16]

Propranolol is the second-line drug recommended by some authors. Others prefer hydralazine as a second choice. Reports of intrauterine growth retardation, bradycardia, neonatal respiratory distress syndrome, and hypoglycemia with use of propranolol are found in the literature.[17] The true incidence of these effects is not known. Should it be necessary to use propranolol during pregnancy, when possible the drug should be discontinued 1 to 2 weeks before delivery and the neonate observed closely for adverse effects.

Oral hydralazine is considered by some authors to be less effective than propranolol, but it may be useful in controlling blood pressure if the patient is near delivery.[3] Intravenous hydralazine is the drug of choice for acute exacerbations of hypertension.

Diuretics are to be avoided during pregnancy because these drugs cause a 5% to 10% decrease in plasma volume that may be detrimental to the fetus. Diuretics also cause fluid depletion and electrolyte imbalance and decrease carbohydrate tolerance in the mother. Decreased cardiac output could decrease the uteroplacental blood flow and compromise the fetus.

Reserpine is also avoided during pregnancy because of the possibility of fetal and neonatal bradycardia, congenital abnormalities, and alteration of thermal equilibrium at birth.

Although fetal loss is about 16% in mild hypertension and may reach 40% in severe hypertension,[9] the primary goal of medical management of blood pressure in pregnancy is to prevent maternal complications.

### *Epilepsy*

The incidence of pregnancies complicated by epilepsy is about 0.3% to 0.5%.[9] The primary goal in the management of these patients is prevention of seizures with the fewest possible effects on the fetus. Pregnancy has unpredictable effects on the frequency and severity of seizures. About 40% to 50% of patients experience an exacerbation of the disease, 40% to 50% have no change, and the remaining 5% to 10% see improvement.[18]

Patients with epilepsy, both those taking medication and those on no medication, have a higher incidence of delivering an infant with congenital abnormalities and mental retardation.[18] Though it is difficult to separate the effects of the medication from the effects of the disease, most of the evidence appears to support the anticonvulsants as a cause of congenital problems.[9] The most common anomalies include orofacial clefts, skeletal anomalies, central nervous system malformations, and cardiac abnormalities.[11,18] Mental retardation has also been described. Although teratogenicity does occur with anticonvulsants, the risk of a seizure is considered more likely to be harmful to the fetus.

The American Academy of Pediatrics Select Committee on Anticonvulsants in Pregnancy recommends that a patient who has been seizure free for a number of years undergo a trial of medication withdrawal before becoming pregnant. A patient with recurrent epilepsy on medication should be advised that she has a 90% chance of having a normal child, but that the risk of congenital abnormalities and mental retardation is twice that in the normal population.[19]

Treatment with one medication is preferred when possible to decrease fetal exposure, thus minimizing teratogenic risk. Failure of monotherapy should be followed up by reassessing compliance and evaluation of serum levels with adjustment of dose if necessary. If the first drug does not successfully control seizures, a second drug should be initiated and the first drug gradually withdrawn over 7 days. A third drug may be tried in the same manner. Monotherapy not succeeding with the third drug would indicate a trial with two medications simultaneously.

Serum levels of most anticonvulsants are lower during pregnancy despite maintenance of prepregnancy doses producing therapeutic serum levels.[18] Suggested reasons for decreased serum levels include noncompliance because of fears of teratogenic potential of the medication, inadequate dosage, incomplete absorption secondary to nausea and vomiting, increased hepatic clearance, abnormally rapid excretion, and an increased volume of distribution resulting from passage into fetal tissues. The increased extracellular fluid volume occurring in pregnancy may cause dilutional lowering of serum levels. Anticonvulsant levels should be determined monthly during pregnancy and doses adjusted accordingly.

Requirements of phenytoin are usually increased during pregnancy, but serum levels should be monitored because of individual variation.[9] Teratogenicity, coagulopathy, and vitamin deficiencies occur with the use of phenytoin; however, it is not associated with the neonatal depression and withdrawal reported with other anticonvulsants such as the barbiturates.[20]

The fetal hydantoin syndrome includes craniofacial abnormalities, growth retardation, mental retardation, and limb defects. Many of the congenital malformations are surgically correctable. Phenytoin is probably more teratogenic than phenobarbital, suggesting that phenobarbital should be used in reproductive-age women when possible. In a large percentage of neonates exposed to anticonvulsants, a severe coagulopathy occurs during the first 24 hours after delivery.[21] This is due to a deficiency of the vitamin K–dependent clotting factors, and all exposed infants should be treated with 1 mg vitamin $K_1$ at birth.[18] Cord blood should be sent for clotting studies and, if necessary, additional vitamin K administered. Some physicians give epileptic patients vitamin K 5–10 mg/d orally during the last 6 to 8 weeks of pregnancy as prophylaxis. Prophylaxis of the deficiency is required because treatment may not be successful once there is clinical evidence of bleeding. Folate deficiency also occurs in patients on anticonvulsants and prophylaxis is suggested to prevent megaloblastic anemia.

Phenobarbital is the anticonvulsant of choice in women of childbearing age as there appears to be a much less teratogenic potential than with phenytoin.[19] During pregnancy, higher dosages are usually required to maintain serum levels.[22] The coagulopathy and folate deficiency seen in patients taking phenytoin can also develop with phenobarbital. Neonates exposed to phenobarbital may experience depression at delivery and may experience withdrawal. Withdrawal usually occurs 4 to 7 days after birth; thus, it is likely that it will begin after discharge from the hospital. Parents should be advised to report neuromuscular excitability, hyperactivity or sleep disturbances, excessive crying, tremulousness, or persistent vomiting or diarrhea, as these symptoms may indicate withdrawal. The withdrawal may last 2 to 6 months[23] and may be treated by avoiding excessive stimulation of the infant and sedation with phenobarbital or phenothiazines if necessary.

Phenobarbital is an active metabolite of primidone and thus primidone would be expected to present the same problems.

Carbamazepine has not been fully investigated because of the small number of patients taking this medication alone. There is not yet enough evidence to suggest that this medication be discontinued in pregnant patients or to recommend use of this drug in place of potentially more harmful agents. Serum levels may be decreased during pregnancy, necessitating use of larger doses.

Valproic acid has been associated with cleft palate, renal defects, and neural tube defects, which are often not surgically correctable.[18] Its use should be avoided in women of childbearing age.

Trimethadione is the most potent teratogen in the anticonvulsant class. There is an approximate 83% incidence[5] of major malformations including developmental delays, low-set ears, palatal abnormalities, V-shaped eyebrows, and speech impediments.[18] It should never be used in pregnancy.

### *Asthma*

Approximately 1% of pregnant patients have asthma.[6] The effect of pregnancy on asthma is not predictable; one third of patients experience improvement in their disease, one third worsening, and one third no change.[6] The effect of asthma on pregnancy is generally not a problem in mild cases. Severe asthmatics who have impairment of respiratory function or medical complications may experience an effect on pregnancy outcome.

Of the drugs used to treat asthma in the nonpregnant population, only the iodides are absolutely contraindicated in pregnancy. Iodides cross the placenta and may cause congenital thyroid problems.[11] Cromolyn sodium is not recommended by the manufacturer for use in pregnancy because of lack of evidence confirming safety.

In the patient with mild and/or infrequent attacks, aerosol albuterol, metaproterenol, or isoetharine should be chosen. These drugs seem to have fewer cardiac side effects than isoproterenol and epinephrine. No congenital abnormalities have been reported with these agents.[11]

Patients with more severe or more frequent attacks may receive oral theophylline. Fetal serum levels approximate maternal levels, but no adverse effects have been reported.[11] Oral terbutaline may be added to theophylline if symptoms persist. Metaproterenol has also been used, but there is more experience with use of terbutaline in pregnancy, as it is often used to inhibit preterm labor. Aerosolized steroids are added if necessary to control the frequency and severity of attacks. When oral steroids are required, prednisone and prednisolone are suggested because the fetal serum level appears to be only 10% of the maternal level; other steroids appear in the fetal circulation at greater concentrations.[24]

Severe attacks and status asthmaticus are managed as in the nonpregnant population.

## Treatment of Preterm Labor

Uterine contractions beginning before the thirty-seventh week of gestation are generally considered premature labor.[25] There is some controversy as to the earliest gestational age at which premature labor should be treated. Labor occurring before the twentieth week of amenorrhea usually results in expulsion of an imperfect fetus; inhibition of labor is therefore generally inappropriate before the twentieth week.

Many patients in premature labor may respond to bedrest, hydration, and sedation; however, it is best not to delay pharmacologic treatment too long as the delay may cause treatment to be unsuccessful. Pharmacologic intervention is more successful when the cervix is dilated less than 4 cm and the membranes are intact. Certain maternal and fetal conditions may preclude the use of tocolytic agents (medications that inhibit labor). Although premature rupture of membranes is a contraindication to inhibition of labor, it may be advantageous to administer pharmacologic agents to delay delivery 24–48 hours in order to give glucocorticoids to enhance fetal lung maturity.

Several categories of medications have been used to arrest premature labor.

### *β-Adrenergic Agonists*

The first and most widely used category of drugs is the β-adrenergic drugs. Ritodrine is the only β-adrenergic drug approved in the United States for the treatment of premature labor, but terbutaline and isoxsuprine have also been used.[26] There are currently no data suggesting that one agent is more efficacious or has fewer side effects than another. Isoxsuprine is the least frequently used agent because of the significant tachycardia and hypotension associated with its use.

Before ritodrine was released in 1980, terbutaline was the drug most often used for the inhibition of preterm labor. The efficacy of terbutaline has been demonstrated,[27] and terbutaline is much less expensive.

Terbutaline and ritodrine have very similar side effects. While tachycardia and hypotension occur frequently with the use of these drugs, they are usually less severe than with isoxsuprine. Hypokalemia secondary to a shift of potassium intracellularly occurs in most patients during parenteral drug therapy, but resolves after discontinuation of the infusion. This intracellular shift is not observed during oral therapy. Unless hypokalemia is detrimental to the patient for other medical reasons, no treatment is required.

Hyperglycemia is a common side effect of the β-agonist drugs, but is usually of no consequence unless the patient is diabetic. Diabetic patients should be followed closely and be maintained on an insulin pump with close glucose monitoring.

Pulmonary edema has occurred with β-agonist agents.[28] The incidence of pulmonary edema is greater when the infusion solution is isotonic saline.[29] The fluid of choice is 5% dextrose injection. Some investigators also advocate limiting the fluid intake of the patient to 2,500 mL/24 h. Placing 300 mg ritodrine in 500 mL of 5% dextrose injection to prepare a concentrated solution will help accomplish this goal. The intravenous infusion is usually continued for 12 hours after the contractions cease. Oral medication should be started 30 minutes before the infusion is stopped. The usual dose of oral medication is 10–20 mg every 4 to 6 hours.

Other side effects noted with betamimetic agents include palpitations, tremor, nervousness, angina, and headache.

The effectiveness of prophylactic use of these drugs has not been adequately investigated for prevention of preterm labor in single or twin pregnancies.[25]

### *Magnesium Sulfate*

Though most often used as an anticonvulsant in severe eclampsia, magnesium sulfate is also effective in inhibiting premature labor. Magnesium sulfate probably antagonizes calcium to prevent the actin–myosin interaction, thus reducing uterine activity. Serum magnesium levels of 6–8 mEq/L are effective.[25]

The patient should be observed closely for signs of hypermagnesemia. In addition to monitoring of the patellar reflex, urine output, and respirations, some protocols require serial magnesium levels every 6 hours as an added precaution.

Magnesium sulfate does not alter carbohydrate metabolism and may be the agent of choice in diabetic patients.[25]

Magnesium sulfate crosses the placenta and can produce serum levels comparable to the maternal level.[11] Serious neonatal effects are uncommon unless the treatment fails and delivery occurs during the infusion. Respiratory depression in the mother can be reversed by administration of 10 mL of 10% calcium gluconate; however, this is not effective for reversing neonatal depression.[9]

### *Ethanol*

Ethanol was used extensively in the past to inhibit preterm labor, but its effectiveness is controversial. The recommended dose produces a blood alcohol level of 100–200 mg/dL (legal intoxication is 100–150 mg/dL).[9] The common side effects of nausea, vomiting, restlessness, and depressed consciousness are those associated with overt inebriation. Patients receiving intravenous ethanol may have an impaired gag reflex that may lead to aspiration pneumonitis. Altered carbohydrate metabolism may occur but is more serious in diabetic patients.

Ethanol crosses the placenta and fetal serum concentrations may be equivalent to maternal levels[30]; however, neonatal complications do not occur frequently. Occasionally, fetal lethargy, apnea, hypotonia, and respiratory depression do occur, but these are more often seen in infants born while the infusion is in progress or within 6 to 12 hours after discontinuation.[26]

### *Prostaglandin Synthetase Inhibitors*

Prostaglandins are present in amniotic fluid during labor and delivery but are absent during pregnancy. The production and release of prostaglandins have been postulated as a key factor in the initiation of labor. Thus, it would appear that the prostaglandin synthetase inhibitors would inhibit labor. Oral and rectal indomethacin has been shown to be effective in the treatment of preterm labor[26]; however, the usefulness of this medication has been limited by the serious potential side effects in the fetus. There is a great deal of concern about the possibility of premature closure of the ductus arteriosus and poor cardiopulmonary adaptation after delivery.[26] Maternal side effects appear to be the same as those in the nonpregnant patient.

### *Calcium Channel Blockers*

As calcium is necessary for muscle contraction, it would appear that calcium channel–blocking agents could be useful in the inhibition of premature labor. Two agents, verapamil and nifedipine, have been shown to relax the myometrium in vitro[26]; however, the large doses of verapamil required are not tolerated. Nifedipine has been shown in some studies to be effective in decreasing uterine contractions in severe dysmenorrhea[31] and during prostaglandin-induced abortions.[32] These results would support further investigative studies into the usefulness of nifedipine as a tocolytic agent. No significant side effects have been noted but studies in animals indicate that metabolic alterations in the fetus may occur.

Other agents such as diazoxide, aminophylline, and progesterone have also been suggested for the treatment of preterm labor.[9]

## Induction of Labor

Labor is not usually induced in normal pregnancies as the uterus is the preferred environment for a fetus. Several maternal and fetal conditions exist in which labor should be induced; however, induction is more likely to be successful when the cervix is soft, effaced, partially dilated, and in the center of the vagina.[6] Induction should not be attempted unless an operative delivery would be appropriate should induction fail. Acceptable indications include severe maternal infection, uterine bleeding (usually caused by partial placenta previa or abruptio placentae), preeclampsia/eclampsia or chronic hypertension, diabetes mellitus, maternal renal insufficiency, premature rupture of membranes after the thirty-sixth week, polyhydramnios, evidence of placental insufficiency, isoimmunization, and postdate pregnancy.

Three classes of drugs are effective for stimulating uterine contractions: oxytocin, ergot alkaloids, and prostaglandins. The ergot alkaloids are useful only for pregnancy termination and should not be used to induce labor because of the possibility of violent, sustained uterine contractions that could compromise the fetus or lead to rupture of the uterus. These medications are orally absorbed and are most often used to decrease postpartum or postabortion bleeding.

The available prostaglandins are used only for pregnancy termination because the maternal and fetal effects of these medications are unknown. There is, however, a prostaglandin gel that is being used investigationally for cervical ripening.[33]

Oxytocin is the drug used for the induction of labor and for augmentation of inadequate labor. It may also be used to decrease postpartum bleeding.

Risks and benefits of oxytocin must be considered before administration to the patient as oxytocin has toxic effects. The initial dose is 2 mU per minute by infusion.

The infusion is usually mixed by adding 10 units of oxytocin to 1 L of fluid and must be placed on a pump for accurate dosing. Intravenous infusion is the administration route of choice because the absorption, distribution, and response are more predictable. Intramuscular administration is not recommended for labor induction because the absorption is not consistent and, if the medication needs to be discontinued because of complications or side effects, it cannot be stopped.

The dose may be increased by 2 mU/min every 15 to 20 minutes if needed to achieve adequate contractions. The dose should not exceed 20 mU/min. The goal of treatment is contractions lasting 45 to 60 seconds at intervals of 2 to 3 minutes.

The patient should be attended, and monitoring of uterine contractions (frequency, duration, and force) and fetal heart rate is essential for early recognition and treatment of side effects. It is very important to monitor the force of resting uterine contractions because a resting pressure greater than 15–20 mm $H_2O$ increases the incidence of complications such as uterine rupture, uteroplacental hypoperfusion, and fetal distress from hypoxia.[9] If the resting pressure exceeds this level, the medication should be discontinued. Maternal blood pressure and pulse rate should also be checked frequently.

Side effects of oxytocin are limited if appropriately monitored. Oxytocin does not cross the placenta[9]; the effects on the fetus are indirect effects secondary to the action of the drug on the uterus. The most notable but infrequent side effect is uterine rupture. Oxytocin use can reduce uteroplacental blood flow, resulting in decelerations of fetal heart rate and possible fetal hypoxia. Other side effects observed with oxytocin are maternal hypotension, hypoglycemia, and fluid retention. Oxytocin is structurally very similar to antidiuretic hormone and some fluid retention is unavoidable.

Contraindications to the use of oxytocin include abnormal fetal positions or presentations, cephalopelvic disproportion, repeat cesarean section or other previous uterine surgery, or a firm, closed, uneffaced, posterior cervix. Patients with functional class III or IV heart disease are not good candidates for oxytocin use. Grand multiparas (greater than seven previous deliveries) have a significantly increased risk of uterine rupture when oxytocin is used.

## Pain Control During Labor and Delivery

Painless labor has been reported; however, most patients experience some degree of discomfort during parturition. The amount of pain experienced may be related to several factors. These factors may include the patient's attitude toward the pregnancy and childbirth, her level of endorphins, and adequate educational preparation of the patient.

The perfect agent for analgesia in obstetrics would provide adequate pain relief, not interfere with the progress of labor, and not increase maternal or fetal risk. There is no ideal agent and no routine method for providing pain control during labor and delivery. Each practitioner should present the various alternatives to each patient and assist her in choosing the best analgesic for her.

Systemic analgesics and regional anesthetics are the two methods most often used. Inhalation agents are not used to the extent seen in the past.

### *Systemic Analgesics*

Systemically, the narcotics are the drugs used most often for pain relief in labor. The phenothiazines may be used concurrently with the narcotics but are rarely used alone.

The pharmacologic properties and effects of the narcotics are very similar. These drugs may shorten or prolong labor; the major concern is that of neonatal respiratory depression and should be kept in mind when dosing the patient. The dose should be high enough to decrease the mother's discomfort to a tolerable level and allow her to rest between contractions, but low enough to avoid respiratory depression in the mother and fetus. When these factors are recognized, neonatal respiratory depression is usually mild and transient if it occurs.

The systemic analgesics should be administered parenterally, and many physicians prefer intravenous over intramuscular administration. Gastric motility is significantly decreased during labor and leads to variable absorption of oral medication. Intramuscular administration may result in delayed onset of analgesia and overdosage may be more difficult to manage because of longer duration of activity. Further considerations for narcotic use include the stage of labor and the amount of drug. In general, medication should not be administered to a primagravida patient until contractions are occurring every 2 to 3 minutes and the cervix is dilated 3–4 cm; it may be given slightly sooner to a multiparous patient. If the medication is given too early, it may inhibit or slow the progress of labor, and if given too close to delivery, the neonate may be overly sedated.

Meperidine is the most frequently used agent and is the most accepted narcotic for obstetric analgesia. The usual dose is 50–100 mg every 2 to 3 hours. When intramuscular administration is used, less neonatal depression is observed when delivery occurs within 1 hour of or 4 hours after administration.[34] If delivery is anticipated 2 to 3 hours after administration, intravenous administration is preferred to minimize neonatal depression.

Morphine is an effective analgesic but has been associated with greater neonatal depression than meperidine.[34] After intramuscular administration, the peak usually occurs in 1 to 2 hours, and the duration of effect is 4 to 6 hours. The onset after intravenous administration is about 20 minutes.

Other narcotics used to relieve pain during labor and delivery include pentazocine, alphaprodine, and butorphanol. None of these offers any advantage over meperidine.

Hydroxyzine and the phenothiazines are used frequently in labor patients both alone and as adjuncts to narcotic agents. The phenothiazines are often used for sedation in early labor and to treat nausea and vomiting associated with labor. Toxicity is uncommon, but these drugs lower the seizure threshold and should be used cautiously, if at all, in the preeclamptic or epileptic patient.

The amnestic drugs, ketamine and scopolamine, are no longer popular or recommended for obstetric analgesia.

### *Regional Anesthesia*

Regional anesthesia is preferred by many clinicians and patients because it produces a selective area of anesthesia, it is reversible, the patient is conscious and comfortable, and the neonate is rarely depressed. The disadvantage to the use of these techniques is that they require specially trained personnel for administration and monitoring.

Paracervical blocks are useful during the first stage of labor for decreasing the pain produced by stretching of the cervix. About 5–10 mL of 0.5% lidocaine is injected bilaterally at the junction of the uterosacral ligaments and the cervix. In a primiparous patient, the injections may be administered when contractions are regular and the cervix is dilated 5–6 cm. The injection must be superficial and the dose low to minimize risks. Care must be exercised to prevent injection into the vascular system or fetus. The relief is prompt and lasts about 1 hour. Injections may be repeated if necessary and 75% of patients report successful pain control.[6] Labor may temporarily stop but generally resumes. About 25% of fetuses develop bradycardia and fetal depression, and death can occur if the concentration in fetal tissues becomes too high.[9] Paracervical blocks are useful only during the first stage of labor and must be combined with other blocks for delivery and episiotomy.

Epidural anesthesia requires injection of an anesthetic into the epidural space of the spinal cord. It is preferred because it prevents transmission of painful stimuli but does not interfere with the progress of labor when administration is delayed until labor is well established. The anesthetic may be given by intermittent or continuous injection. The agent preferred for epidural anesthesia is bupivacaine 0.25% to 0.5%.[35] The 0.75% bupivacaine should not be used for obstetric anesthesia. Bupivacaine has a rapid onset and a duration of action of 3 to 10 hours. Chloroprocaine is less acceptable because though it has a short duration of activity, there have been reports of prolonged neural blockade, possibly because of the sodium bisulfite in the solution. Etiodocaine produces a more prolonged and pronounced muscle relaxation that may interfere with the patient's ability to push.

In summary, regional anesthesia is currently the most extensively utilized method of pain control during parturition. This method is both safe and effective and preferable to most patients. The paracervical block has the greatest risk of fetal complications. No reports of fetal death have been directly related to epidural anesthesia.

### *Inhalation Agents*

The inhalation anesthetics are occasionally used during labor. All the agents have been used, but the halogenated agents have been shown to increase bleeding secondary to prolonged uterine relaxation.[9] The anesthetic is combined with oxygen and inhaled during contractions to decrease pain. These agents cause uterine relaxation which may be advantageous when intrauterine relaxations are required for manipulations. The risks include respiratory depression, decreased maternal and fetal oxygenation, and aspiration.

## Lactation Suppression

Lactation is a complex, neuroendocrine-mediated process. Prolactin produced in the hypophysis stimulates the production of milk in breast tissue, whereas oxytocin causes ejection of milk from the nipple.

In the past several years, there has been renewed interest and greater participation in breast-feeding; however, there remain patients who choose not to nurse because of personal preference or working conditions or because their babies are unable to nurse, for example, babies who require intensive care or who have palate abnormalities. These mothers can pump their breasts to establish lactation in the event the baby can later breast-feed. Maternal drug therapy deleterious to the nursing infant would preclude nursing, as would other problems such as inverted nipples not successfully corrected.

Breast engorgement is usually self-limiting, begins about the third to fourth day postpartum, and resolves within 48 to 72 hours. During this time, the breasts are swollen, firm, and tender. Some patients relate severe pain, while others have only mild discomfort. Nondrug treatment includes application of ice packs and binding of the breasts. The patient should be reminded not to express the milk as this will only result in further production.

Two classes of medications have been used to suppress lactation. Hormonal therapy, both androgenic and estrogenic substances, and bromocriptine mesylate have been used effectively.

Although many estrogenic and androgenic substances have been used in the past, the two drugs in this class most often used are chlorotrianisene, a synthetic proestrogen, and a testosterone enanthate/estradiol valerate combination injection. Both are long acting and have a local effect on breast tissue. Chlorotrianisene should be initiated within 8 hours of delivery and the injectable agent, within 1 hour of delivery.

More recently there has been concern over the use of estrogenic substances for postpartum lactation suppression. This concern stems from the hypercoagulable state during the last stages of pregnancy and during parturition. Use of estrogenic agents could possibly potentiate the development of thromboemboli in this population. This has been investigated in the British literature where it was reported that deep vein thromboembolic events were not increased in women less than 25 years of age who had normal vaginal deliveries and received estrogenic medication. The incidence was increased in women over 25 years old and in women undergoing cesarean delivery.[36]

Bromocriptine mesylate inhibits prolactin secretion and thus is useful in the suppression of postpartum breast engorgement and in suppression of milk production after lactation has already been established. Bromocriptine is very effective, but there are a few disadvantages to its use. A dose of 2.5 mg twice daily must be taken for 14 days. The drug should not be initiated until the patient is stabilized, at least 4 hours after delivery, because some women experience hypotension when the drug is started too soon after delivery. Side effects of the medication include headache, nausea, dizziness, and nasal congestion. In the event of rebound lactation after completion of 14 days of therapy, the medication may be administered for an additional 7 days.

## Summary

Medication use in pregnancy is a complex issue, and physicians and pharmacists must work together to provide the patient with the most effective and least potentially harmful medication for her needs. All medication use in pregnancy and during labor and delivery should include patient education and consent.

## References


1. Berlin CM. Pregnancy and childbirth. Presented at National Conference on Women's Health, Bethesda, MD, June 17, 1986.
2. Pavletich KJ, Sause RB. Counseling on use of OTC diagnostic products. Part II. Pregnancy testing. Pharm Times 1982;April: 76–83.
3. Benson RC. Current obstetric and gynecologic diagnosis and treatment, 4th ed. Los Altos, CA, Lange Medical Publications, 1982.
4. Juchau MR, Faustman-Watts E. Pharmacokinetic considerations in the maternal–placental–fetal unit. Clin Obstet Gynecol 1983;26:379–390.
5. DiPalma JR. Drugs for nausea and vomiting of pregnancy. Am Fam Phys 1983;28:272–274.
6. Willson RJ, Carrington ER. Obstetrics and Gynecology, 8th ed. St. Louis, C.V. Mosby, 1987.
7. Leathem AM. Safety and efficacy of antiemetics used to treat nausea and vomiting in pregnancy. Clin Pharm 1986;5:660–668.
8. Collins E. Maternal and fetal effects of acetaminophen and salicylates in pregnancy. Obstet Gynecol 1981;58:57S–62S.
9. Rayburn WF, Zuspan FP. Drug Therapy in Obstetrics and Gynecology, 2nd ed. Norwalk, CT, Appleton-Century-Crofts, 1986.
10. Goldberg E. Anticoagulants in pregnancy, in Niebyl J (ed): Drug Use in Pregnancy. Philadelphia, Lea and Febiger, 1982.
11. Briggs GG, Freeman RK, Yaffe SJ. Drugs in pregnancy and lactation, 2nd ed. Baltimore, Williams and Wilkins, 1986.
12. Nissen JC. Treatment of hypertensive emergencies of pregnancy. Clin Pharm 1982;1:334–343.
13. White P. Pregnancy complicating diabetes. Am J Med 1949; 7:609–616.
14. Gabbe SG. Management of diabetes mellitus in pregnancy. Am J Obstet Gynecol 1985;153:824–828.
15. Leveno KJ, Hauth JC, Gilstrap LC, et al. Appraisal of "rigid" blood glucose control during pregnancy in the overtly diabetic woman. Am J Obstet Gynecol 1979;135:853–862.
16. Redman CWG, Beilin LJ, Bonnar J, et al. Fetal outcome in trial of antihypertensive treatment in pregnancy. Lancet 1976; 2:753–756.
17. Rayburn WF, Lavin JP. Drug prescribing for chronic medical disorders during pregnancy: An overview. Am J Obstet Gynecol 1986;155:565–569.
18. Dalessio DJ. Seizure disorders and pregnancy. N Engl J Med 1985;312:559–563.
19. Committee on Drugs of the American Academy of Pediatrics. Anticonvulsants and pregnancy. Pediatrics 1979;63:331–333.
20. Mirkin BL. Diphenylhydantoin: Placental transport, fetal localization, neonatal metabolism and possible teratogenic effect. J Pediatr 1971;78:329–337.
21. Mountain KR, Hirsh J, Gallus AS. Neonatal coagulation defect due to anticonvulsant drug treatment in pregnancy. Lancet 1970;1:265–268.
22. Lander CM, Edwards VE, Eadie MJ, et al. Plasma anticonvulsant concentrations during pregnancy. Neurology 1977; 27:128–131.
23. Desmond MM, Schwanecke RP, Wilson GS, et al. Maternal barbiturate utilization and neonatal withdrawal symptomatology. J Pediatr 1972;80:190–197.

**24.** Romero R, Berkowitz R. The use of anti-asthmatic drugs in pregnancy, in Niebyl J (ed): Drug Use in Pregnancy. Philadelphia, Lea and Febiger, 1982.

**25.** Gonik B, Creasy RK. Preterm labor: its diagnosis and management. Am J Obstet Gynecol 1986;154:3–8.

**26.** Souney PF, Kaul AF, Osathanondh R. Pharmacotherapy of preterm labor. Clin Pharm 1983;2:29–44.

**27.** Beall MH, Edgar BW, Paul RH, et al. A comparison of ritodrine, terbutaline and magnesium sulfate for the suppression of preterm labor. Am J Obstet Gynecol 1985;153:854–859.

**28.** Guernsey BG, Villarreal Y, Snyder MD, et al. Pulmonary edema associated with the use of betamimetic agents in preterm labor. Am J Hosp Pharm 1981;38:1942–1948.

**29.** Philipsen T, Eriksen PS, Lynggard F. Pulmonary edema following ritodrine–saline infusion in premature labor. Obstet Gynecol 1981;58:304–308.

**30.** Waltman R, Iniquez ES. Placental transfer of ethanol and its elimination at term. Obstet Gynecol 1972;40:180–185.

**31.** Andersson KE, Ulmsten U. Effects of nifedipine on myometrial activity and lower abdominal pain in women with primary dysmenorrhoea. Br J Obstet Gynecol 1978;85:142–148.

**32.** Andersson KE, Ingemarrson I, Ulmsten U, et al. Inhibition of prostaglandin-induced uterine activity by nifedipine. Br J Obstet Gynecol 1979;86:175–179.

**33.** Trofatter KF, Bowers D, Galls SA, et al. Preinduction cervical ripening with prostaglandin $E_2$ (Prepidil) gel. Am J Obstet Gynecol 1985;153:268–271.

**34.** Fisher RL, Lubenow R. Analgesia for labor and delivery. Hosp Ther 1986:38–53.

**35.** Lefevre M. Obstetric anesthesia. Am Fam Phys 1983;27:146–154.

**36.** Jeffcoate TNA, Miller J, Roos RF, et al. Puerperal thromboembolism in relation to the inhibition of lactation by oestrogen therapy. Br Med J 1968;4:19–25.

# Chapter 6 / Drug-Induced Diseases

Wayne M. Turner, PharmD, and Julie B. Milstein, PhD

I will prescribe regimens for the good of my patients according to my ability and my judgment and never do any harm to anyone.

Hippocratic Oath

Hippocrates is given credit for the quotation "first do no harm." We believe that his intent was that no one should intentionally harm another through the use of the knowledge of medicine. Today, with the ever increasing armamentarium of potent pharmaceutical agents, the interpretation of this quote has been expanded to include harming, both intentionally and unintentionally, through the use of medicine or pharmacologic knowledge. It is the unintentional effects of pharmacologic agents that are the focus of this chapter.

Some statistics point to the national impact of drug-induced diseases.

1. The reported incidence of adverse drug reactions (ADRs) varies between 1% and 28%.[1]
2. Of admissions to general hospitals (medical and pediatric), 2% to 5% are attributed to drug-induced diseases.[2,3]
3. Of hospitalized patients, 5% to 30% experience ADRs.[3]
4. Approximately 0.31% of hospital inpatients, or 60,000 to 140,000 people, die because of an ADR.[4]

In fact, the toll of drug-induced diseases on the nation is not known. In 1971, Melmon estimated that one seventh of all hospital days and $3 billion are dedicated to the treatment of drug-induced toxicity.[5] Whatever the toll, it is obviously too great. Each health professional must accept the responsibility of helping to prevent the 70% to 80% of ADRs that are predictable and preventable.[6] Each health professional must also become increasingly knowledgeable of the potential effects of drugs and be prepared to act appropriately whenever confronted with a drug-induced adverse event. It is imperative that the suspicion of drug-induced disease be included in the differential diagnosis of all patients taking medications who present with unexpected disorders. Accurate drug histories must always be documented.

The Food and Drug Administration defines an adverse drug experience as any adverse event associated with the use of a drug in humans, whether or not considered related, including an adverse event occurring with the use of a product in professional practice; an adverse event occurring from drug overdose, whether intentional or accidental; an adverse event occurring from drug abuse; an adverse event occurring from drug withdrawal; or any important failure of expected pharmacologic action.[7]

The World Health Organization defines an adverse drug reaction similarly as any response to a drug that is noxious and unintended and that occurs at doses used in humans for prophylaxis, diagnosis, or therapy of disease, or for the modification of physiologic function.[8]

Adverse drug reactions have been classified in many different ways. In our opinion, the pharmacologic effects of ADRs fall into four categories: (1) side effects, (2) toxic effects, (3) hypersensitivity effects, and (4) idiosyncratic effects. These four categories accommodate the full range of adverse effects that have been observed. Next, these classes of adverse drug reactions are examined; examples are provided where appropriate.

## Side Effects

A *side effect* is defined as a consequence other than the one for which an agent or measure is used; sometimes, it is applied to adverse effects produced by a drug, especially on a system other than the one sought to be benefited by its administration.[9(p 1376)] Though not directly stated, the definition of a side effect implies that the drug was administered at usual therapeutic doses. An individual drug administered at the therapeutic dose not only produces a single effect when it is given to treat a disorder but also produces a range of different effects that are usually part of the drug's pharmacologic action. Side effects are the annoying, usually nonserious, reactions that the patient is expected to complain about: antihistamines cause drowsiness because of their central nervous system (CNS)-depressant effect, theophylline causes nervousness because of its CNS-stimulative effect, and corticosteroids cause weight gain as a result of sodium and water retention as well as effects on carbohydrate and lipid metabolism. Anyone may be susceptible to a particular side effect. Any drug may cause side effects, and prior exposure to the drug is not a prerequisite to experiencing a side effect. When the patient confronts the clinician with a subjective compliant that is associated with the initiation of drug therapy, the clinician must suspect that the complaint may be drug induced and act accordingly (Assessment of Adverse Drug Reactions).

Sublingual nitroglycerin and its association with hypotension is a good example of a side effect. One of the actions of nitroglycerin in relieving anginal attacks is the dilatation of peripheral blood vessels and pooling of venous blood. This effect theoretically decreases the workload (preload and afterload) of the heart, thus decreasing myocardial oxygen consumption and relieving the angina. The dilatation of peripheral blood vessels induced by the nitroglycerin may be sufficient to cause hypotension. Hypotension caused by peripheral dilatation and venous pooling is one of the most common serious side effects of sublingual nitroglycerin.[10]

**Table 6.1** Some Adverse Reactions That May Be Classified as Side Effects

| | |
|---|---|
| Accommodation abnormality | Hallucinations |
| Agitation | Hypotension |
| Arthralgia | Insomnia |
| Bradycardia | Nausea |
| Constipation | Nervousness |
| Dry mouth | Obesity |
| Flatulence | Rhinitis |
| Glossitis | Sinusitis |
| Glycosuria | Twitching |
| | Vertigo |

Rubella vaccine and its association with arthralgia is another good example of a side effect. The most common signs and symptoms of rubella disease include arthralgia. Among adults, particularly women, joint reactions occur so frequently (up to 70%) that they may be considered an expected manifestation of adult infection. Live rubella vaccine causes a milder (or attenuated) infection. Up to 40% of vaccines in large-scale field trials have been associated with joint pain.[11]

Table 6.1 lists some adverse reactions that may be classified as side effects.

## Toxic Effects

*Toxic* is defined as pertaining to, caused by, or of the nature of a poison.[9(p 1191)] Further, a *poison* is defined as any substance that when ingested, inhaled, or absorbed, or when applied to, injected into, or developed within the body, in relatively small amounts, by its chemical action may cause damage to structure or disturbance of function.[9(p 1191)] As with the expectations of pharmacologic side effects, many drugs are also expected to produce certain toxic effects. Toxic effects may occur as a result of usual therapeutic dosing or as a consequence of acute or chronic overdose.

We divide toxic effects into two general categories: overdose effects and effects of direct cellular function alteration.

It is generally accepted that acute and/or chronic overdoses produce adverse effects that are more serious and occur more frequently than the effects of usual therapeutic doses. It is expected that lidocaine overdoses may produce convulsions, that acetaminophen overdose may cause hepatic necrosis, and that digoxin overdose may cause heart block. Drug toxicity associated with an overdose situation is quite clear and the association is well understood.

Direct cellular function alteration or damage is what distinguishes side effects from toxic effects. The alteration of cellular function is, in fact, poisoning of the cell. Therefore, the definition of toxicity fits quite well. An excellent example of the difference between side effects and toxic effects is found in the review of drug-induced alopecia by Harris.[12] The growth of hair is a cyclic process that consists of an active growth phase (anagen), a regression phase (catagen), and a resting phase (telogen). Hair loss usually falls into one of two categories: anagen effluvium (shedding) or telogen effluvium (shedding). Anagen effluvium is typified by drug-induced alopecia associated with antimetabolite therapy. Such therapy causes the anagen hair to stop growing and fall out. In telogen effluvium (associated with heparin, propranolol, and danazol), shedding of normal club hairs follows what is believed to be the premature conversion of anagen hair follicles to telogen follicles. The anagen effluvium effect in this example is a toxic effect. The drug actually poisons the anagen phase of hair growth. The telogen effluvium effect is a side effect in that the drug pharmacologically converts the anagen follicles to telogen follicles, thus causing the alopecia.

Cyclophosphamide and its association with alopecia is another good example of anagen effluvium. Antineoplastic agents have a wide range of toxic effects; however, with the potential life-prolonging benefits of these agents, a greater severity and a greater frequency of effects are more acceptable. Cyclophosphamide is an alkylating antineoplastic agent that is used to treat certain cancers. One of its well-known toxic effects is alopecia (loss of hair). Cyclophosphamide's action in preventing DNA and RNA formation interferes with normal cell division. All rapidly proliferating tissues, such as hair follicles, are most affected by cyclophosphamide's toxic effects.[13]

Influenza vaccine and increased theophylline concentrations constitute an example of a toxic effect caused by an overdose situation. In some cases, a toxic effect of a drug may be caused by its effect on another drug taken at the same time. Case reports suggest that in some patients, the elimination of theophylline may be reduced as much as 50% after influenza vaccination. In one report, symptoms of theophylline excess occurred within 48 hours in two of three patients.[14] In another report, it was shown that the higher the theophylline clearance before vaccination, the greater the degree of clearance depression after vaccination.[15] Thus, although influenza vaccine may not produce the particular toxic effects, in patients receiving theophylline therapy, it may result in a toxic effect of theophylline.

Table 6.2 lists some adverse reactions that may be considered toxic effects.

## Hypersensitivity Effects

*Hypersensitivity* is defined as exhibiting abnormally increased sensitivity or having the specific or general ability to react with characteristic symptoms to application of or

**Table 6.2** Some Adverse Reactions That May Be Classified as Toxic Effects

| | |
|---|---|
| Agranulocytosis | Kidney failure |
| Alopecia | Myopathy |
| Blood dyscrasia | Nephrocalcinosis |
| Convulsions | Necrosis, bone |
| Digitalis intoxication | Neuropathy |
| Ectromelia | Overdose |
| Extrapyramidal syndrome | Paralysis |
| Fertility, decrease | Vitamin toxicity |
| Liver cirrhosis | |

contact with certain substances (allergens) in amounts innocuous to normal individuals.[9(p 707)] These characteristic symptoms range from nonserious rashes and moderately serious wheezes (commonly associated with allergic manifestations) to serious bronchospasm and hypotension associated with anaphylaxis. Some of these hypersensitivity effects may be caused by excipients and stabilizers found in the drug product as well as the active ingredient.

Hypersensitivity to a drug may occur in a few percent to as many as 100% of the population depending on the drug. It may occur with many drugs. Prior exposure to the component is a necessity. Drugs that are proteins, such as vaccines and enzymes, can be expected to be associated with hypersensitivity reactions.[16,17] Hypersensitivity reactions are independent of dose or show an erratic dose–response relationship. In response to the first dose of antigen, a specific IgE antibody is formed. This is facilitated if the drug or its metabolite is bound to a host protein. The antigen–antibody complex then reacts with mast cells to release mediators, especially histamines. These reactions are antagonized by antihistamines, epinephrine, or anti-inflammatory steroids like cortisone. Examples of hypersensitivity reactions include rash in response to ampicillin[18] and hemolytic anemia in response to methyldopa[19] or nomifensine.

All penicillins are cross-sensitizing and cross-reacting. In general, sensitization occurs in direct proportion to the duration and total dose of penicillin received in the past. The responsible antigenic determinants appear to be degradation products of penicillins bound to host proteins. Among those people who are positive reactors to skin tests, the incidence of subsequent penicillin reactions is high and is associated with cell-bound IgE antibodies. The presence of IgG antibodies, in contrast, does not appear to be associated with allergic reactions, except for rare cases of hemolytic anemia. In the United States, 5% to 8% of the population claim a history of penicillin reaction. Of those, about 10% will have an allergic reaction when penicillin is given again. The range of hypersensitivity reactions that may be experienced includes rash, anaphylaxis, serum sickness–type reactions, vasculitis, and hemolytic anemia.

Drug-induced hemolytic anemias are of three types: the penicillin type, the α-methyldopa type, and the "innocent bystander" type. The penicillin type involves the production of immunoglobulin to a hapten (penicillin degradation product) complexed to a protein on the erythrocyte. The erythrocyte is then phagocytosed by macrophages. In the α-methyldopa type, the drug triggers the formation of anti–red cell antibody, probably by inhibiting suppressor-T-cell functions. This antibody is bound to the Rh site on the erythrocyte membrane, and the erythrocyte is phagocytosed by macrophages. In the innocent bystander type of hemolytic anemia, the drug or antigen circulates as part of an antigen–antibody complex. The complex is adsorbed onto the erythrocyte in association with complement, and the erythrocyte is lysed through the complement lytic pathway. Nomifensine and quinidine induce hemolytic anemia of the innocent bystander type.

Table 6.3 lists some adverse reactions that may be considered hypersensitivity effects.

**Table 6.3** Adverse Reaction Terms That May Be Considered Hypersensitivity Effects

| | |
|---|---|
| Allergic reaction | Hypotension |
| Anaphylaxis | Le syndrome |
| Anemia, hemolytic | Pruritus |
| Asthma | Rash |
| Dyspnea | Serum sickness |
| Eosinophilia | Urticaria |
| Erythema multiforme | Vasculitis |

## Idiosyncratic Effects

*Idiosyncrasy* is defined as abnormal susceptibility to some drug, protein, or other agent that is peculiar to the individual.[9(p 722)] This definition encompasses the wide range of effects that occur in certain individuals without logical reason. Although the exact mechanisms by which these reactions arise are usually not known, many of them have been attributed to genetic differences in metabolism of the drug.[20]

These reactions occur generally only in genetically abnormal subjects, and prior exposure is unnecessary. The responses are dose related, and the effect produced is dependent upon the drug and antagonized by specific antagonists.

One example of an idiosyncratic effect is the hemolytic anemia observed with use of sulfonamides. The genetic deficiency of the enzyme glucose-6-phosphate dehydrogenase in erythrocytes causes weaknesses in the cell membrane. Sulfonamides and certain other drugs are capable of affecting the integrity of the cell membrane, causing the cell to hemolyze and resulting in decreased numbers of circulating red blood cells. Blacks, Jews, Greeks, Iranians, and other dark-hued Caucasian groups have been noted to have a greater incidence of this enzyme deficiency.[21] This idiosyncratic effect is also known as primaquine sensitivity. In normal individuals, glucose is metabolized via the enzyme glucose-6-phosphate dehydrogenase. This enzymatic reaction regenerates NADPH, which is required for the reduction of oxidized glutathione and is important in the protection of cellular proteins and enzymes from oxidation. The presence of drugs that can perform these oxidizing activities can result in deranged glucose metabolism and hemolysis of red cell membranes in individuals who have generally low levels of reduced glutathione because of glucose-6-dehydrogenase deficiency. Drugs other than sulfonamides and primaquine known to be associated with this hemolysis include quinine, aspirin, and phenacetin.

Isoniazid, a drug used in the treatment of tuberculosis, may accumulate in some patients because of a reduction in quantity of the acetylating enzyme necessary for biotransformation of this drug. Plasma concentrations determined at a specific time after oral administration fall into two subgroups, depending on whether the subject tested is a slow or rapid inactivator.[22] High acetyl transferase activity results in rapid inactivation of isoniazid and is inherited as an autosomal dominant trait. The average half-life of isoniazid in plasma of rapid inactivators is less than $1\frac{1}{2}$ hours, compared

**Table 6.4** Some Adverse Reactions That May Be Classified as Idiosyncratic Effects

| | |
|---|---|
| Agranulocytosis | Kidney function, abnormal |
| Anemia, hemolytic | Liver function, abnormal |
| Convulsions | Liver necrosis |
| Diarrhea | Nausea |
| Fever | Ulcer, peptic |
| Gastrointestinal disorder | Vomiting |
| Hepatitis | |

with 3 hours for slow inactivators. About half of white and black persons in the United States are slow inactivators and may be more prone to the hepatic toxicity of isoniazid.

A number of other reactions may be idiosyncratic, but have not yet been fully investigated genetically.

Table 6.4 lists some adverse reactions that may be considered idiosyncratic effects.

## Risk/Benefit Analysis

When a drug is approved for marketing, an assessment of its risk/benefit ratio is made based on the known side effects (versus the seriousness of the disorder being treated). The health practitioner must be aware of and make a risk/benefit assessment for each use of the drug in each patient for whom it is prescribed. If the disorder being treated is self-limiting and nonserious, the risk/benefit analysis may warrant the conclusion that the potential occurrence of side effects does not justify the administration of that particular drug in the particular patient at that time. Although the risk/benefit ratio may favor administration of the drug, prevention of side effects may not be possible. The practitioner must inform the patient of possible side effects and give instructions in the event they occur. When an adverse effect is observed, the patient must then participate in the decision to discontinue the drug or reduce the dose to minimize the observed side effects.

## "Influencers" of Adverse Reactions

Often, the occurrence of an adverse effect is influenced by an individual patient characteristic that makes the patient more susceptible to the adverse effect. These patient characteristics usually affect one or more of the processes that influence drug disposition: absorption, distribution, metabolism, and excretion. Here, a knowledge of biopharmaceutics is critical. The characteristic contributing to ADRs in susceptible patients usually affects the metabolism or excretion of the drug, and the adverse effect observed is usually a toxic effect. These types of reactions are different from idiosyncratic reactions, as they usually occur in all patients with these characteristics.

Drug products are approved for marketing only after rigorous testing to characterize how they are handled by the body. A primary problem is that once a drug is marketed it may be used in patients who have influencing characteristics where the ultimate effects of the combination have not been adequately studied. The absorption, distribution, metabolism, and excretion characteristics of a drug in healthy adults are well known and are used to develop the proper dose ranges for the drug before it is marketed. If a drug is influenced by an unusual patient characteristic, its disposition will naturally be affected. If metabolism and/or elimination of a drug is increased or absorption is decreased, the desired therapeutic effect may not be achieved. If absorption of the drug is increased or metabolism and/or elimination is decreased, the probability of a toxic adverse effect is increased.

The following patient characteristics represent the most common "influencers" of adverse effects.

### *Other Drugs or Foods*

Interaction of drug products with other drugs or foods is one of the common causes of adverse effects. Drug interactions are discussed in Chapter 7.

### *Age*

The age of the patient may influence the occurrence of an adverse effect. The experience gained from the use of benoxaprofen in the elderly has recently focused much more attention on drug administration in the geriatric age group than in the past. The normal aging of the liver and kidney may result in decreased metabolism and excretion of some drugs. Accumulation of these drugs in these organs may further damage them, resulting in further accumulation and possibly death because of direct benoxaprofen toxicity.[23] It is imperative that elderly patients be monitored closely and their doses and dosing schedules adequately adjusted to allow more effective and safer administration of drug products. Another example of the effect of age is the immature drug-metabolizing capabilities of the neonate. The quantities of most reductive enzymes, conjugating enzymes, and metabolizing enzymes are substantially lower in the neonate than later in life.[24] Therefore, the half-lives of many drugs are prolonged because of their decreased hepatic clearance. For example, the half-life of digoxin in the neonate is 60 to 107 hours, whereas it is 30 to 60 hours in the adult. The clinician must be aware of this difference and consider hepatic function as well as body weight when dosing neonates.

### *Weight*

Like age, weight plays an important role in the metabolism and excretion of drugs. An interesting example occurred in 1982 when a problem was detected with the use of benzyl alcohol as a preservative in sterile water and normal saline solutions for injection. The use of benzyl alcohol–preserved water and saline solutions to flush intravascular catheters was thought to cause the deaths of 16 preterm neonates weighing less than 2,500 g. It was further reported that changing from the preserved solutions to solutions that did not contain this preservative eliminated the problem.[25] The proposed mechanism for this effect was the metabolism of benzyl alcohol to benzoic acid. The benzoic acid could not be conjugated by the immature liver of the neonates and accumulated causing metabolic acidosis.[26] Interestingly, the problem occurred only in low-birth-weight infants. This points to the need for close monitoring of neonates, especially those of low birth weight, not only for problems associated with the use of drugs but also for problems associated with additives and excipients used in drug products.

### *Sex*

Sex has been demonstrated to be a true influencer of ADRs. An example is the report by Stewart and Cluff that women experience more frequent gastrointestinal reactions to drugs than men.[27] In a study of almost 4,000 patients, there was a statistically significant ($P < 0.001$) difference between the incidence of gastrointestinal reactions in women and in men. This difference may be attributed to differences in gastrointestinal physiology between women and men.

### *Pregnancy*

An important consideration of drug use in pregnancy is the drug's effect on the unborn fetus. The rapidly proliferating cells of the fetus are susceptible to exogenous influences. The best known example of drug-induced fetal problems is the thalidomide disaster in 1961, where exposed infants were born with absent or deformed arms and/or legs (phocomelia). Thalidomide produced malformations in almost all babies of mothers who were exposed to the drug between the thirty-fifth and fiftieth days of pregnancy.[28] A more recent example of a possible teratogen is sodium valproate. Sodium valproate has been associated with fetal neural tube defects.[29] The neural tube is the epithelial tube that develops from the neural plate and forms the central nervous system of the embryo. Defects of the neural tube are associated with the following malformations: spina bifida, myelocele, myelomeningocele, meningocele, and hydrocephalus.

### *Concomitant Diseases*

Certain diseases have profound effects on drug metabolism and hence the ultimate effects of the drug. These disorders may make the patient more sensitive to the normal pharmacologic actions of some drugs. Many drugs cause increases in plasma glucose concentrations and must be used carefully in diabetic or prediabetic patients. Gemfibrozil has been found to cause hyperglycemia and an increased insulin or oral hypoglycemic requirement in some patients.[30] Likewise, other drugs, such as the adrenergic agonists, cause increases in blood pressure and must be used carefully in hypertensive patients. Ritodrine was found to cause blood pressure of 300/120 in a pregnant 32-year-old female.[31]

Patients with heart disease pose a particular problem for health professionals. Certain drugs are particularly dangerous in patients with cardiac problems. Any drug that affects the cardiovascular system must be used with extreme caution in these patients to prevent any life-threatening cardiac arrhythmias. Enflurane[32] and bupivacaine[33] are examples of drugs that are potentially harmful to patients with cardiac disease because of their depressive effect on the myocardium.

Kidney and liver diseases are common causes of drug toxicity. Diseases of both organs decrease drug elimination, hence increasing drug tissue concentrations and adverse effects. Any drug that is eliminated primarily by a renal or hepatic pathway must be monitored closely and the dosage adjusted accordingly in patients with diseases of these organs. This principle can be extended to all of the diseases discussed in this section. Health professionals must be familiar with the effects of the drugs so that they can anticipate problems and make the necessary adjustments when confronted with potentially adverse situations.

### *Assessment of Adverse Drug Reactions*

Adverse reactions in the clinical setting are usually documented because the observing clinician suspects that a drug has caused the adverse effect. That suspicion is usually based on a subjective opinion by the clinician that the drug actually caused the problem. The drug may be known to cause the observed effect and thus the clinician assumes that this is "just another case." Conversely, many times a drug is not considered associated with a particular reaction because the clinician has never heard of the drug causing such a reaction. This may lead to the false hypothesis that another drug caused the problem. Once the clinician suspects that an effect may indeed be drug induced, an objective assessment must be made to determine the most likely causative agent. If only one drug was administered, the task of assessing causality is simple; however, when multiple drugs are involved and administered over different time periods, the task of assessing causality is more complex.

Many authors have studied and published methods for causality assessment.[34–41] These methods range from simple algorithms, with few yes/no responses,[34,35,37] to very complex multilevel statistical rating scales.[40,41] Most methods, however, do agree in the general categorizations used:

1. Temporal sequence. The reaction follows a reasonable temporal sequence after administration of the drug. For example, leukemia that develops 1 day after the first dose of the drug would clearly be temporally unrelated, as would anaphylaxis occurring after 30 days of continuous use. The onset after drug exposure varies with the nature of the reaction; this relationship must be carefully considered.
2. Dechallenge. The reaction abates on stopping the drug or lowering the dosage.
3. Rechallenge. The reaction reappears on repeated exposure to the drug. A negative dechallenge or rechallenge does not necessarily rule out involvement of the drug. Some reactions are irreversible, and thus dechallenge would not be applicable. In some cases, particularly hypersensitivity reactions, the reaction does not always recur with reintroduction of the drug. Often dechallenge and rechallenge are neither practical nor ethical; however, the presence of positive dechallenge and/or rechallenge information lends support to implication of a drug in an ADR.

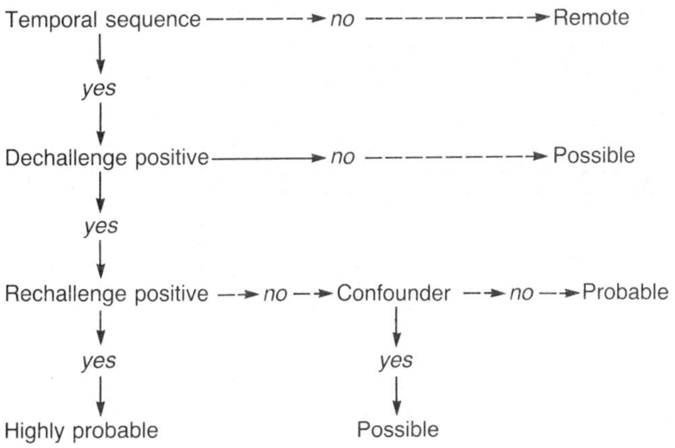


**Figure 6.1** Algorithm used in assessing causality.

4. Confounders. The effect is not caused by the patient's clinical state nor other drugs. For example, if a patient is also on a drug known to cause a specific ADR, the implication of the subject drug in that ADR should be questioned. Pseudomembranous colitis is a known sequela of clindamycin, which selects for the causative toxigenic *Clostridium difficile* organism. Thus, a patient reporting an ADR of colitis must be carefully evaluated for history of antibiotic use. Often, effects of confounding drugs can be differentiated by use of dechallenge and rechallenge information or by time course of drug dosing. An example of disease confounding may exist in a patient exhibiting a manic reaction while on a tricyclic antidepressant. Some patients may become agitated and manic with tricyclic antidepressants, but one should always consider the possibility that the patient in reality has a bipolar depression. Often, the adverse event reported is part of the symptom complex of the disease for which the patient was initially treated with the drug.

Some other categories that may be used in assessing causality follow; however, as they rely on historic documentation, they must be used with caution when dealing with newly approved drugs or when seeking new drug–reaction associations as in a postmarketing surveillance program.

5. Pharmacology. The effect follows a known response pattern for the suspected drug.
6. Literature. The reaction has been previously documented as being associated with the suspect drug.

Each assessment method is valuable in different clinical situations. The simple method is best suited for the busy clinician who must make the quick causality assessment, usually at the bedside. In the simplest algorithm, developed by Jones and used by the FDA, four decision points are used. These decision points correspond to categories 1–4. An algorithm (Fig. 6.1) is used to demonstrate the relationships between these categories and the four probability categories: highly probable, probable, possible, and remote. In multiple-drug situations, each drug must be carried through the algorithm and assessed individually.

The more complex statistical methods are best suited for the clinical study environment. The Kramer method contains up to 57 decision points.[39] The questions asked require access to and knowledge of very detailed medical information. In addition to the information covered in categories 1–4, some other information may be obtained:

How long the drug has been marketed.
Whether there is previous literature documentation.
Whether the event is unusual or follows a known clinical pattern.
Multiple questions related to the time to onset.
Multiple questions related to the evolution of the event and the subsequent withdrawal of the drug.
Relevant laboratory data.

Whatever the method, the causality assessment must objectively determine the most suspect drug. Often, multiple drugs are considered equally suspect. The clinician must then carefully dechallenge and rechallenge with each drug, one by one, to find the culprit. Once the offending drug is determined, it must be removed from the treatment regimen, and it must be clearly documented that the patient has experienced a disorder induced by that drug.

## Need for Postmarketing Surveillance

A primary objective of postmarketing surveillance is to study a drug's efficacy and toxicity under conditions of actual clinical use. Several important differences exist between postmarketing surveillance and premarketing clinical trials[42,43]:

1. A larger patient population is available. Clinical trials are usually severely limited in numbers of recipients and, thus, are not suitable for detecting uncommonly occurring drug-induced diseases.
2. These studies may be open ended in terms of time. Long-term or latent effects that were not detected in clinical trials may appear.
3. The recipient group is not limited to healthy adults. In clinical practice, the drug will probably be used in individuals with diseases or drug exposures that may make them more susceptible to a drug-induced adverse event.
4. The recipient population may include certain classes of patients not studied in clinical trials, such as the elderly, very young children, or pregnant women. These groups may be more susceptible to drug-induced diseases because of differences in metabolism and body size.

Many limitations are associated with postmarketing surveillance systems for drug-induced diseases, some of which include underreporting and selective reporting. Underreporting stems from a number of factors, including barriers to detection of the reaction, attribution of the reaction to the drug, knowledge of where and how to report, and other considerations that affect the reporting of an adverse drug reaction by a health professional.

One study in which reporting of reactions by physicians in a hospital was solicited and improved to an 80% response rate showed that degree of certainty that the adverse event

DEPARTMENT OF HEALTH AND HUMAN SERVICES
PUBLIC HEALTH SERVICE
FOOD AND DRUG ADMINISTRATION (HFN-730)
ROCKVILLE, MD 20857

**ADVERSE REACTION REPORT**
**(Drugs and Biologics)**

Form Approved: OMB No. 0910-0230.

FDA CONTROL NO.

ACCESSION NO.

**I. REACTION INFORMATION**

1. PATIENT ID/INITIALS *(In Confidence)*
2. AGE YRS.
3. SEX
4.-6. REACTION ONSET — MO. DA. YR.

8.-12. CHECK ALL APPROPRIATE:

- ☐ PATIENT DIED
- ☐ REACTION TREATED WITH Rx DRUG
- ☐ RESULTED IN, OR PROLONGED, INPATIENT HOSPITALIZATION
- ☐ RESULTED IN PERMANENT DISABILITY
- ☐ NONE OF THE ABOVE

7. DESCRIBE REACTION(S)

13. RELEVANT TESTS/LABORATORY DATA

**II. SUSPECT DRUG(S) INFORMATION**

14. SUSPECT DRUG(S) *(Give manufacturer and lot no. for vaccines/biologics)*

15. DAILY DOSE

16. ROUTE OF ADMINISTRATION

17. INDICATION(S) FOR USE

18. DATES OF ADMINISTRATION *(From/To)*

19. DURATION OF ADMINISTRATION

20. DID REACTION ABATE AFTER STOPPING DRUG? ☐ YES ☐ NO ☐ NA

21. DID REACTION REAPPEAR AFTER REINTRODUCTION? ☐ YES ☐ NO ☐ NA

**III. CONCOMITANT DRUGS AND HISTORY**

22. CONCOMITANT DRUGS AND DATES OF ADMINISTRATION *(Exclude those used to treat reaction)*

23. OTHER RELEVANT HISTORY *(e.g. diagnoses, allergies, pregnancy with LMP, etc.)*

**IV. ONLY FOR REPORTS SUBMITTED BY MANUFACTURER**

24. NAME AND ADDRESS OF MANUFACTURER *(Include Zip Code)*

24a. IND/NDA. NO. FOR SUSPECT DRUG

24b. MFR CONTROL NO.

24c. DATE RECEIVED BY MANUFACTURER

24d. REPORT SOURCE *(Check all that apply)* ☐ FOREIGN ☐ STUDY ☐ LITERATURE ☐ HEALTH PROFESSIONAL ☐ CONSUMER

25. 15 DAY REPORT? ☐ YES ☐ NO

25a. REPORT TYPE ☐ INITIAL ☐ FOLLOWUP

**V. INITIAL REPORTER *(In confidence)***

26.-26a. NAME AND ADDRESS OF REPORTER *(Include Zip Code)*

26b. TELEPHONE NO. *(Include area code)*

26c. HAVE YOU ALSO REPORTED THIS REACTION TO THE MANUFACTURER? ☐ YES ☐ NO

26d. ARE YOU A HEALTH PROFESSIONAL? ☐ YES ☐ NO

Submission of a report does not necessarily constitute an admission that the drug caused the adverse reaction.

NOTE: Required of manufacturers by 21 CFR 314.80

FORM FDA 1639 (7/86) PREVIOUS EDITION MAY BE USED

**Figure 6.2** FDA Form 1639 for reporting adverse drug effects.

was related to drug therapy, mechanism of reaction, and severity of reaction were major factors in the reporting of reactions.[44]

A more recent study that surveyed physicians who voluntarily reported reactions directly to the FDA indicated that severity of reaction and newness of drug were major factors in reporting of the reaction and that patient attribution of the reaction to the drug was a strong factor in physicians' reporting of less serious reactions.[45]

These factors also result in selective reporting. Koch-Weser et al.[44] stated that only 22% of pharmacologic reactions (classified as side effects in this chapter) were reported, whereas 43% of allergic or idiosyncratic reactions were reported. Wardell et al[42] noted that once a possible reaction has been described, it tends to be more heavily emphasized in spontaneous reporting systems.

Despite these drawbacks, spontaneous postmarketing surveillance systems are currently the most efficient source of early signals of drug-induced diseases.

## Reporting of Adverse Events

In the United States, postmarketing surveillance of approved drugs is performed by FDA. Manufacturers of approved drugs are required by federal regulation (21 CFR §314.80) to submit to FDA reports of adverse events temporally associated with the use of their drugs. The Office of Epidemiology and Biostatistics, FDA, maintains a computerized system of adverse drug reaction case reports for postmarketing surveillance.

With the exception of reporting by pharmaceutical manufacturers, reporting of ADRs to FDA is voluntary. The Joint Commission of Accreditation of Hospitals requires written procedures for the reporting of ADRs within the hospital and encourages hospitals "to report any unexpected or significant adverse drug reactions to the FDA."[46]

Direct reporting by practitioners to FDA's spontaneous reporting system is the most efficient means by which FDA obtains information on new drug–reaction associations. In a comparison of reports received in 1970 with regard to effectiveness and efficiency in identifying new ADRs, direct-to-FDA reports "far exceeded what would have been expected on the basis of their total ADR contribution."[47] A summary of some of these reported reactions can be found elsewhere.[48]

Clinical data submitted in direct-to-FDA spontaneous reports are often more complete than data submitted by drug manufacturers, because the reporting clinician has immediate access to patient charts, records, and discharge summaries. Direct reports may also be more timely than manufacturers' reports, because there is no intervening processing time for the submission of a report. In the spontaneous reporting system, timing is critical for the generation of early warning signals about previously unrecognized, serious adverse reactions.

Increasing numbers of ADR reports are being received by FDA; however, only a very small percentage of these reports are sent directly by pharmacists. ADRs should be reported on the FDA Adverse Reaction Report Form, FDA-1639 (Fig. 6.2), with as much relevant supporting documentation as possible. Small numbers of FDA-1639 forms may be requested from the Office of Epidemiology and Biostatistics, FDA, 5600 Fishers Lane, Rockville, MD 20857, and completed reports may be sent to the same address. Minimum information necessary to evaluate the reaction includes the name of the drug(s); a description of the reaction; the outcome of the reaction (whether the patient required hospital treatment, died, or was permanently disabled); the dates of administration of the drug; and the date of reaction onset. Demographic data important for analysis of aggregate reactions include age, sex, and state of residence of the patient. The basic purpose of FDA's surveillance system is to detect serious and previously unrecognized adverse reactions. Interest is most sharply focused on new chemical entities—drugs marketed within the past three years.

## Summary

Drug-induced adverse effects are divided into four broad categories: side effects, toxic effects, hypersensitivity effects, and idiosyncratic effects. By examining the dose–response relationship, the incidence in the population, and the ability to reverse the reaction, the observer can make some deductions about the nature of the reaction. Important in this evaluation is a knowledge of the pharmacologic action of the drug and its metabolism. Temporal considerations, drug and disease confounding, and dechallenge and rechallenge are among the factors useful in assigning causality.

In evaluation of a drug's effects, there are patient-specific factors that may influence the degree and extent of adverse drug reactions; these include age, sex, liver and kidney function, pregnancy, other drugs, and underlying disease.

Although the extent of the problem cannot be assessed with certainty, unintended adverse effects associated with the use of drugs in clinical practice occur with such frequency that there is a real and continuing need for postmarketing surveillance of drug-associated events.

Pharmacists and other health care professionals are reminded to report to FDA (on Form FDA-1639) reactions of which they are aware. Special emphasis is placed on the reporting of serious reactions (resulting in death or hospitalization) that are not described in the package insert for the drug and on the reporting of those events temporally associated with products during their first 3 years of marketing.

## References

1. Davies DM. Incidence of adverse drug reactions, in: Textbook of Adverse Drug Reactions, 2nd ed. Oxford, Oxford University Press, 1981.
2. Seidl LG, Thornton GF, Cluff LE. Epidemiological studies of adverse drug reactions. Am J Pub Health 1965;55:1170.
3. Cluff LE, Caranasob GJ, Stewart RB. Clinical problems with drugs, in Major Problems in Internal Medicine. Philadelphia, W.B. Saunders, 1975, vol 5.
4. Talley RB, Laventurier MF. Drug-induced illness. JAMA 1974;229:1043.
5. Melmon KL. Preventable drug reactions: Causes and cures. N Engl J Med 1971;284:1361.
6. Manldin RK. Drug-induced diseases, in Herfindal ET, Hirschman JL (eds): Clinical Pharmacy and Therapeutics. Baltimore, Williams and Wilkins, 1975, p 13.
7. Division of Epidemiology and Surveillance, US Food and Drug Administration. Procedure Manual for Processing Drug Experience Reports, 1985.
8. World Health Organization Collaborating Centers for International Drug Monitoring. WHO Publication DEM/NC/84.153 (E), June 1984.
9. Dorland's Illustrated Medical Dictionary, 24th ed. Philadelphia, W.B. Saunders, 1965.
10. Miller RR, Greenblatt DJ (eds): Drug Effects in Hospitalized Patients. New York, John Wiley and Sons, 1976, p 58.
11. Recommendation of the Immunization Practices Advisory Committee (ACIP). Rubella Prevention. MMWR 1984;33:301.
12. Harris PL. Alopecia associated with long term metyrapone use. Clin Pharm 1986; 5:66–86.
13. Gershwin ME, Goetz EJ, Steinberg AD. Cyclophosphamide—use in practice. Ann Intern Med 1974;80:531.
14. Renton KW, Gray JD, Hall RI. Decreased elimination of theophylline after influenza vaccine. Can Med Ass J 1980;123: 288.
15. Meredith CG, Christian CD, Johnson RF. Effects of influenza virus vaccine on hepatic drug metabolism. Clin Pharmacol Ther 1985;37:396.
16. Loelinger EA. Drugs affecting blood clotting and fibrinolysis, in

Dukes MNG (ed): Meyler's Side Effects of Drugs. Amsterdam, Excerpta Medica, 1977, p 177.
17. Hofman B, Lansberg HP. Immunological preparations, in Dukes MNG (ed): Meyler's Side Effects of Drugs. Amsterdam, Excerpta Medica, 1977, vol 8, p 704.
18. Shapiro S, Slone D, Siskind V. Drug rash with ampicillin and other penicillins. Lancet 1969;2:969.
19. Perry HM, Chaplin H, Carmody S. Immunologic findings in patients receiving methyldopa. J Lab Clin Med 1971;78:905.
20. Bourne HN, Roberts JM. Drug receptors and pharmacodynamics, in Katzung BG (ed): Basic and Clinical Pharmacology, 2nd ed. Los Altos, California, Lange Medical Publications, 1984.
21. Kirkman HN. Glucose-6-phosphate dehydrogenase variants and drug-induced hemolysis. Ann NY Acad Sci 1968;151:753.
22. Evans DAP, Manley KA, Mckusick VA. Genetic control of isoniazid metabolism in man. Br Med J 1960;2:485.
23. Prescott LF, Leslie PJ. Side effects of benoxaprofen. Br Med J 1982;284:17830.
24. Cohen MS. Special aspects of perinatal and pediatric pharmacology, in Katzung BG (ed): Basic and Clinical Pharmacology. Los Altos, California, Lange Medical Publications, 1982.
25. Gershanik JJ, Beecher B, George W. Neonatal deaths associated with use of benzyl alcohol—United States. MMWR 1982; 31:290.
26. Kimura ET, Darby TD, Kranse RA. Parenteral toxicity studies with benzyl alcohol. Toxicol Appl Pharmacol 1971;18:60.
27. Stewart RB, Cluff LE. Gastrointestinal manifestations of adverse drug reactions. Am J Dig Dis 1974;19:1.
28. Taussing HB. A study of the German outbreak of phocomelia—the thalidomide syndrome. JAMA 1962;180:1106.
29. Macrae KD. Sodium valproate and neural tube defects. Lancet 1982;2:1283.
30. Konttinem A, Kuisma I, Ralli R. The effect of gemfibrozil on serum lipids in diabetic patients. Am Clin Res 1979;11:240.
31. Gonen R, Sanberg I, Sharf M. Hypertensive crisis associated with ritodrine infusion and betamethasone administration in premature labor. Eur J Obstet Gynecol Reprod Biol 1982;13:129.
32. Chandler S. Isoarrhythmic atrioventricular dissociation during enflurane anesthesia. South Med J 1982; 75:945.
33. Gould DB, Aldrete JA. Bupivacaine cardiotoxicity in a patient with renal failure. Acta Anesthesiol Scand 1983;27:18.
34. Irey NS. Tissue reactions to drugs. Am J Pathol 1976;82: 617–647.
35. Karch FE, Lasagna L. Towards the optimal identification of adverse reactions. Clin Pharmacol Ther 1977;21:247–253.
36. Weber JCP. Storage and retrieval of data on adverse reactions to drugs. Interphase Symposium, Brighton, June, 1980.
37. Turner WM. The Food and Drug Administration algorithm for causality assessment. Drug Info J 1984;18:259–266.
38. Blanc S, Leuenberger P, Berger JP. Judgment of trained observers on adverse drug reactions. Clin Pharmacol Ther 1979;25: 493–498.
39. Hutchison TA, Kramer MS, Leventhal JM. An algorithm for the background assessment of adverse drug reactions—background, description for use and instruction. JAMA 1979;242:623–632.
40. Venulet J, Ciucci A, Bernecker, GC. Standardized assessment of drug–adverse reaction associations—rationale and experience. Int J Clin Pharmacol Ther Toxicol 1980;18:381–388.
41. Naranjo CA, Busto U, Sellers EM. A method for estimating the probability of adverse drug reactions. Br J Clin Pharmacol 1982; 13:112–117.
42. Wardell WM, Tsianco MC, Anavekar SM. Postmarketing surveillance of new drugs—review of objectives and methodology. J Clin Pharmacol 1979;19:85–94.
43. Milstein JB, Faich GA, Hsu JP. Factors affecting physician reporting of adverse drug reactions. Drug Info J 1986;20:151–164.
44. Koch-Weser J, Sidel VW, Sweet RH. Factors determining physician reporting of adverse drug reactions—comparison of 2000 spontaneous reports with surveillance studies at the Massachusetts General Hospital. N Engl J Med 1969;280:20–26.
45. Inman WHW. Postmarketing surveillance of adverse drug reactions in general practice. Search for new methods. Br Med J 1981;282:1131–1132.
46. Joint Commission on the Accreditation of Hospitals. Accreditation manual for hospitals. Chicago, Joint Commission on Accreditation of Hospitals 1985; p 126.
47. Rossi AC, Knapp DE. Discovery of new adverse drug reactions. JAMA 1984;252:1030–1033.
48. Sills JM, Tanner LA, Milstein JB. Food and Drug Administration monitoring of adverse drug reactions. Am J Hosp Pharm 1986;43:2764–2770.

# Chapter 7 / The Basics of Drug Interactions

J. Russell May, PharmD

The term *drug interaction* is used when administration of or exposure to a substance modifies a patient's response to a drug. The substance may be another drug (drug–drug interaction), a food (drug–food interaction), or other substances such as alcohol or tobacco. Although drug interactions are usually thought of as detrimental, some are actually beneficial and are discussed later.

## Magnitude of the Problem

Much has been published on the subject of drug interactions. In 1972, the Boston Collaborative Drug Surveillance Program reported a study of 9,900 patients with 83,200 drug exposures and found 3,600 adverse drug reactions, 234 (6.5%) of which were attributable to drug interactions.[1] Durrence and associates[2] reviewed drug profiles of 1,825 surgical patients and found at least one potential drug interaction in 17% of the patients. A study of nursing home patients revealed that 19% of patients were receiving combinations of drugs with known interactions.[3] A slightly higher percentage, 23%, was found in a similar study of an outpatient clinic population.[4] Borda et al[5] reported that 22% of the adverse reactions on medical wards resulted from drug interactions. Certainly, drug interactions represent a significant challenge for pharmacists.

The magnitude of the problem increases significantly in certain patient populations. One study documented an exponential increase in the incidence of adverse drug interactions in relationship to the number of drugs given.[6] Several population groups have been singled out as having a high potential for drug interactions because of the large number of drugs used. These include the elderly,[7] critical care patients,[8] and patients undergoing complicated surgical procedures.[9]

This chapter focuses on drug interaction concepts. Various types of drug interactions are discussed along with the associated mechanisms and specific examples. Methods are also suggested for managing drug interactions.

## Drug–Drug Interactions

Thousands of drug–drug interactions have been described in the literature, but only a relatively small number are clinically significant. In this section, the three categories of drug–drug interactions—pharmacokinetic, pharmacodynamic, and pharmaceutic—are described and clinically relevant examples are given.

### *Pharmacokinetic Interactions*

A pharmacokinetic interaction may occur by several mechanisms by which one drug alters the absorption, distribution, metabolism, or elimination of another drug, resulting in a change in drug concentration in the body and an altered response. Numerous controlled studies have described various types of pharmacokinetic interactions; however, such controlled trials are typically performed in healthy volunteers and do not always give a true perspective of the potential for an interaction. Data from pharmacokinetic or epidemiologic studies of actual patients are generally more helpful in determining the clinical significance of a pharmacokinetic interaction.

#### Absorption

Absorption interactions result in an increase or decrease in the relative rate of absorption or in the amount of the drug absorbed. A decrease in the rate of absorption may result in failure of a drug to reach a therapeutic concentration even if the total amount of drug absorbed is unchanged. Absorption rate can be slowed by any drug that slows gastric motility, such as anticholinergic drugs (e.g., propantheline) and opiates (e.g., codeine). Because the small intestine provides the largest surface area for absorption, it is the major site of absorption for most orally administered drugs. Any drug that decreases the speed with which another drug passes from the stomach to the small intestine will induce a decrease in absorption rate. On the other hand, drugs that increase gastric motility, such as metoclopramide, can increase the absorption rate. While these agents can produce marked effects on absorption rate, few clinically significant drug–drug interactions have been reported. Interactions resulting in a decrease in the total amount of one drug's absorption are usually more important clinically. Decreases in the amount of drug absorbed may be caused by the formation of insoluble complexes or by changes in gastrointestinal pH. The quantity of drug absorbed may also be affected by agents that decrease gastric motility as described before. Tetracycline's interactions with antacids and dairy products are well known. Divalent or trivalent cations, such as aluminum, calcium, and magnesium, combine with tetracycline to form a nonabsorbable complex, greatly reducing tetracycline serum concentrations. Iron salts affect tetracycline by the same mechanism. These interactions can be prevented by separating administration times by 2 hours.

The absorption of ketoconazole appears to be reduced when the gastrointestinal pH is increased.[10] In the study, a significant reduction in plasma ketoconazole concentrations occurred when it was given concurrently with antacids or cimetidine; however, only a few patients were studied.

Many other absorption interactions have been reported. The clinical importance of most of these is not well documented. Drug–food interactions that affect absorption may be important and are discussed later.

#### Distribution

Two types of distribution interactions are most common: protein binding/displacement interactions and cellular distribution interactions. Once absorbed, drugs are distributed via the blood as both free drug and plasma protein–bound drug. Because only the free or unbound fraction of the drug is active, any change in the percentage bound can lead to a change in a drug's availability to receptor sites and its metabolism and excretion. When two or more highly protein bound drugs are administered concurrently, competitive binding by one may increase the free fraction of the other(s).

Drug–drug interactions in this class are complex and probably in some cases overstated. For example, much has been published about the use of nonsteroidal anti-inflammatory agents (NSAIDs) in combination with warfarin. Many NSAIDs may decrease warfarin's protein binding. The traditional view is that because NSAIDs are highly protein bound, they displace warfarin, thereby increasing its anticoagulant effect; however, a review of the literature reveals that much of the evidence is based on in vitro data, and in vivo studies have downplayed this effect.[11] Other reasons exist for the occasionally observed increase in anticoagulation such as the effect of NSAIDs on warfarin metabolism and their independent effect on hemostasis.[12] Still, caution should be exercised in the administration of any two highly protein bound drugs when one has a narrow therapeutic index.

Interactions involving cellular distribution are unusual but can be clinically significant. Tricyclic antidepressants displace guanethidine from its intracellular site of action,[13] resulting in a markedly reduced antihypertensive effect. This combination should probably be avoided.

#### Metabolism

Many interactions involve the effect of one drug on the metabolism of another drug, and can be clinically important. The metabolic rate may be increased or decreased. Certain drugs, such as barbiturates, are known to induce hepatic enzymes, resulting in a shortened plasma half-life for some drugs. A well-documented and clinically significant example is seen with administration of barbiturates and warfarin[14]; higher-than-usual dosages of warfarin are needed to produce suitable anticoagulation. When a patient stabilized on warfarin discontinues barbiturate therapy, there is a real danger of hemorrhage. Other drugs that may act as enzyme inducers include carbamazepine, phenytoin, rifampin, and phenylbutazone.

Many drugs are metabolized in hepatic microsomes by an enzyme system called the mixed-function oxidase system or the cytochrome $P_{450}$ system. Drugs that inhibit the cytochrome $P_{450}$ system (e.g., cimetidine, influenza vaccine, allopurinol, disulfiram) may affect the metabolic rate of many drugs (e.g., warfarin, theophylline, some benzodiazepines, phenytoin). Drug metabolism rate is affected by genetic background, age, nutritional state, diseases, hormonal state, and endogenous chemicals. Considerable interpatient and intrapatient variation occurs with this type of interaction, making prediction of the extent of the interaction difficult. Cimetidine, a histamine $H_2$-receptor antagonist widely prescribed for the treatment and prevention of gastrointestinal ulcers, has been shown to have inhibitory effects on the cytochrome $P_{450}$ enzyme system. This has resulted in several well-documented drug interactions, for example, cimetidine's effect on the metabolism of theophylline. One study described a 39% mean decrease in theophylline clearance in young healthy volunteers after 2 days of cimetidine therapy.[14] This interaction was later confirmed in case reports.[15–17]

This type of interaction has been reported between influenza vaccine and three drugs (phenytoin, theophylline, warfarin).[18] Like cimetidine, influenza vaccine appears to affect the cytochrome $P_{450}$ system. Meredith and associates[19] studied the effects of influenza vaccine on the metabolism of chlordiazepoxide, theophylline, and lorazepam in healthy male subjects. Only theophylline was affected. Theophylline oxidation was significantly decreased 1 day, but not 7 days, after vaccination.

Given the unpredictability of these reactions, caution is advised in prescribing a drug that affects the $P_{450}$ enzyme system in combination with a drug metabolized via this mechanism.

#### Elimination

Most interactions involving elimination or excretion occur in the kidneys. A change in glomerular filtration rate, tubular secretion, or urine pH can alter the excretion of some drugs. Fortunately, only a handful of these interactions result in clinically relevant changes and some of these are beneficial.

A potentially dangerous interaction in this category is that between diuretics and lithium. Prolonged thiazide therapy has been shown to cause a compensatory increase in proximal tubule reabsorption of sodium, resulting in increased lithium reabsorption as well.[20] This interaction has resulted in serious lithium toxicity.[21]

### *Pharmacodynamic Interactions*

Pharmacodynamic interactions generally fall into four categories on the basis of the effects produced.

#### Antagonistic Effects

These interactions occur when two drugs that have antagonistic pharmacologic effects are given together. For example, a nonspecific $\beta$-adrenergic blocking agent such as propranolol may induce bronchoconstriction because of its effect on the $\beta$ receptors in the bronchi of a patient taking theophylline for bronchodilation. This interaction may also be beneficial as when the opiate antagonist naloxone is given to reverse the effects of opiate analgesics.

#### Synergistic or Additive Therapeutic Effects

When two drugs with similar therapeutic effects are given together, they may interact. For example, coadministration of two central nervous system depressants, such as diazepam for anxiety and chloral hydrate for insomnia, may result in oversedation. Or, administration of a drug that inhibits platelet aggregation (such as aspirin) together with warfarin increases the potential for bleeding.

**Synergistic or Additive Side Effects**

This interaction is similar to the preceding one, except it involves the side effects rather than the therapeutic effects of the drugs. For example, administration of an antihistamine with a skeletal muscle relaxant such as cyclobenzaprine, both of which cause drowsiness, may result in additive sedation. Administering two drugs with anticholinergic side effects, such as disopyramide and a tricyclic antidepressant, may produce intolerable effects.

**Indirect Pharmacodynamic Effects**

In this type of interaction, the pharmacologic effect of one drug indirectly affects another drug's action. Diuretics that decrease body potassium concentrations may alter the therapeutic effects of digoxin and some other antiarrhythmics. The effect of digoxin is enhanced by potassium depletion, whereas the effects of some antiarrhythmics, such as lidocaine and quinidine, are decreased.

### *Pharmaceutic Interactions*

Pharmaceutic interactions occur when two drugs are mixed in the same intravenous fluid, resulting in physical or chemical incompatibility (chemical inactivation or precipitation). Incompatibility can occur for a variety of reasons. For example, drugs known to be alkali labile should not be mixed in intravenous solutions containing aminophylline, which has an alkaline pH. Such drugs include epinephrine, erythromycin gluceptate, and cephalothin sodium.[22] Incompatibility is common with the use of intravenous phenytoin, as crystallization or precipitation may result if the drug's vehicle is altered or the pH lowered.[23–24] Therefore, phenytoin sodium injection should not be mixed in the same intravenous fluid with other drugs.

### *Beneficial Interactions*

Drug–drug interactions are generally thought of as detrimental, but many are actually clinically desirable. Epinephrine is added to some common local anesthetics, such as lidocaine, to produce local vasoconstriction and slow anesthetic absorption; this reduces the risk of lidocaine toxicity and prolongs the localized action of the anesthetic. Carbidopa prevents the metabolism of levodopa by inhibiting dopa decarboxylase, thereby allowing levodopa to cross the blood–brain barrier before it is converted to dopamine. Probenecid inhibits secretion of penicillins into the proximal tubule, thus reducing the rate of penicillin excretion; this combination results in a twofold higher and more prolonged blood penicillin concentration.[25] Trimethoprim and sulfamethoxazole sequentially inhibit two steps in an essential bacterial biosynthetic pathway, resulting in synergistic antibacterial activity.

## Drug–Food Interactions

Administration of drugs with food may result in an interaction that modifies the activity of the drug or the nutritional effect of the food (decreased drug response, increased drug response, or impairment of nutritional status).

**Effect of Food on Drug Absorption**

The most frequently observed type of drug–food interaction affects drug absorption. The primary reason for decreased drug response with drug–food interactions is the effect food has on the absorption of some orally administered drugs. As with drug–drug absorption interactions, the result may be a decreased drug absorption rate or a decreased amount of drug absorbed. Drugs whose absorption may be delayed or reduced by food include most penicillins, tetracycline, digoxin, acetaminophen, levodopa, and aspirin. It may be best for patients to take these medications 1 hour before or 2 hours after meals. Absorption of some drugs, for example, spironolactone[26] and griseofulvin,[27] increases absorption when the drugs are taken with certain foods.

**Pharmacologic Interactions**

Food can interact with drugs in a variety of ways other than that affecting absorption. The most clinically important of these occurs with monoamine oxidase inhibitors (MAOIs). Monoamine oxidase normally metabolizes tyramine in food before it reaches the systemic circulation. If a person is taking a MAOI, large amounts of tyramine may reach the systemic circulation resulting in an excessive pressor effect, which may lead to seriously acute hypertension. Table 7.1 lists foods to be avoided by patients taking MAOIs.

Other examples involve vitamin K and pyridoxine (vitamin $B_6$). Foods rich in vitamin K may antagonize the effect of warfarin. This rarely results in problems if patients avoid the extreme types of food. Examples of vitamin K–rich foods are leafy green vegetables, liver, green tea, tomatoes, and coffee. Pyridoxine can enhance the metabolism of levodopa, decreasing the amount of levodopa available to cross the blood–brain barrier and reach its site of action. Patients taking levodopa should be warned not to eat excessive amounts of pyridoxine-rich foods such as avocados, beans, bacon, beef liver, peas, pork, sweet potatoes, and tuna. Also, many over-the-counter vitamin preparations contain pyridoxine.

**Effect of Drugs on Nutrition**

The most common form of drug-induced nutritional deficiency is mineral depletion in the elderly.[28] Diuretics frequently cause potassium deficiency. This problem can be compounded in patients who also use laxatives frequently. Elderly patients may have an inadequate dietary intake of calcium, magnesium, and zinc, and depletion may be accentuated by some drugs.

**Table 7.1** Foods High in Tyramine

| | |
|---|---|
| Avocados (especially if overripe) | Cola beverages |
| Bananas | Fermented meats (salami, pepperoni, summer sausage) |
| Bean pods | Herring (pickled or dry) |
| Canned figs | Raspberries |
| Cheese (especially aged) | Soy sauce |
| Chicken livers | Wines (especially red) |
| Chocolate | Yeast preparations |
| Coffee | Yogurt |

Many drugs affect a patient's nutritional status indirectly. Drugs that cause nausea, vomiting, gastrointestinal upset, constipation, or diarrhea have an impact on a patient's food intake. As one might guess, this list of drugs is quite long. Oral decongestants, such as phenylpropanolamine and pseudoephedrine, may also result in decreased food intake because they can suppress appetite. Many other drug–food interactions have been reported.

## Ethanol/Tobacco–Drug Interactions

Technically, these interactions should be considered drug–drug interactions but, in the medical literature, they are addressed separately.

### *Tobacco–Drug Interactions*

The effect of smoking on drug metabolism is well established in the medical literature.[29,30] The primary mechanism for this interaction appears to be enhanced drug metabolism resulting from induction of hepatic microsomal enzymes by the constituents of tobacco smoke; however, in many cases, the exact mechanism has not been established. The interaction results in lowered plasma drug concentrations for some drugs (Table 7.2). Of the drugs listed in Table 7.2, the most clinically significant interactions appear to be with the oral contraceptives, other estrogen compounds, and theophylline.

**Table 7.2** Drugs Affected by Tobacco Smoke

| | |
|---|---|
| Antidiabetics, oral | Pentazocine |
| Benzodiazepines | Propoxyphene |
| Chlordiazepoxide | Propranolol |
| Diazepam | Theophylline |
| Chlorpromazine | Tricyclic antidepressants |
| Contraceptives, oral | Amitriptyline |
| Estrogens | Desipramine |
| Heparin | Imipramine |
| Lidocaine | Nortriptyline |

#### Tobacco–Estrogen

Epidemiologic studies indicate that the risk of cardiovascular adverse effects such as stroke, myocardial infarction, and thromboembolism, which are associated with oral contraceptive use, are increased in smokers.[31] The risk increases with age and the number of cigarettes smoked per day. The exact mechanism for this interaction is unclear. Women taking oral contraceptives should not smoke. If they will not stop smoking, they should be encouraged to use alternative birth control methods, such as condoms and contraceptive foam.

#### Tobacco–Theophylline

Smoking significantly affects theophylline pharmacokinetics.[32,33] Smoking stimulates the hepatic metabolism of theophylline, resulting in increased theophylline clearance, a shorter serum half-life, and lower serum concentrations. Some heavy smokers may require as much as two times the usual maintenance dose of theophylline.

### *Ethanol–Drug Interactions*

Several drug interactions involving ethanol are clinically important. Often overlooked and not viewed as the potent drug it actually is, ethanol is involved in both straightforward and complex interactions. The effects of short-term and long-term ethanol consumption on drug metabolism have been studied.[34] Long-term ethanol consumption may increase the clearance of a drug by induction of oxidative metabolism, whereas short-term consumption may decrease clearance. Clearance by hepatic *N*-acetylation appears to increase after just a single drink. Conjugation with glucuronide is inhibited for some drugs in the presence of ethanol. For drugs cleared by multiple pathways, it is not yet possible to estimate the change in total clearance caused by alcohol.

#### Additive Central Nervous System Effects

A dangerous drug interaction may occur when ethanol is combined with other central nervous system (CNS) depressants such as antihistamines, barbiturates, tranquilizers, or other psychotropic drugs. The CNS-depressant effect may be additive or synergistic. With some agents (e.g., benzodiazepines), the interaction involves more than just an additive side effect. Ethanol may increase the absorption[35] and decrease the metabolism[36] of diazepam. Also, patients with alcoholic liver disease may eliminate benzodiazepines more slowly than those with normal liver function.[37]

#### Other Effects

Ethanol interacts with a variety of other drugs. One clinically relevant example is the antagonism by ethanol of the oral antidiabetic agents (e.g., chlorpropamide and tolbutamide), for which several mechanisms are possible. Ethanol itself may produce hypoglycemia.[38] To confuse matters, ethanol may also increase the metabolism of some oral antidiabetics.[39] This action may counteract ethanol's hypoglycemic effect, but it is unpredictable.

Chlorpropamide and possibly other sulfonylureas may also interact with ethanol by producing the "disulfiram reaction" (flushing, hypotension, nausea, tachycardia, vertigo, dyspnea, and blurred vision).[40] Disulfiram, which produces hypersensitivity to alcohol, is used as an alcohol deterrent to help maintain alcohol abstinence. Most believe this reaction occurs because of disulfiram's effect on ethanol metabolism which results in increased production of acetaldehyde; however, other theories exist. Unfortunately, as previously mentioned, other drugs can produce this reaction.

## Treatment

In this section, the steps necessary to identify a drug interaction and management procedures that help to prevent or minimize the adverse effects of a drug interaction are discussed.

## *Identification of Drug Interactions*

The clinician must have a thorough understanding of the pharmacology of the drugs he or she administers to patients in the practice setting, especially pharmacokinetic profiles. This knowledge aids in identifying interactions when they occur and is also helpful in detecting a previously unreported drug interaction.

When a drug interaction is suspected, several pieces of information are necessary to confirm the reaction and identify the offending agents. A complete drug profile provides only part of the picture. Alcohol, food, and tobacco interactions should be ruled out. If a drug interaction is suspected because of a changing laboratory parameter, drug–laboratory test interactions should also be ruled out. Disease state or impaired organ function could be affecting a drug's activity, and a complete medical history is necessary. A thorough description of the response to the suspected interaction should be documented. Finally, a temporal relationship must be established between the reaction and the suspected interacting agents.

The patient-specific information should be compared with the medical literature on drug interactions. Several excellent reference sources are available. As with any drug information question, tertiary sources should be reviewed first (e.g., *Drug Interactions* by Hansten[41]), followed by secondary sources (e.g., *ClinAlert*[42]). If no information is found, a primary literature search may be conducted. It is also helpful to contact the manufacturers of the suspected drugs for any unpublished data.

## *Management and Prevention*

Management of drug interactions usually consists of monitoring specific parameters and then taking the appropriate action. For example, it may be necessary to obtain a serum drug assay or more closely follow a particular laboratory value. In many cases, potentially interacting drugs can be administered concurrently as long as appropriate patient or laboratory assessments are performed.

Steps should be taken to help prevent or minimize the adverse effects of drug interactions. Before initiating drug therapy, risk factors should be identified. For example, is the patient currently receiving any drugs commonly involved in interactions? Other risk factors such as tobacco smoking and alcohol consumption should be documented. The elderly may be at higher risk because of the influence of age on pharmacokinetic parameters. Discontinuing unnecessary drugs certainly will reduce the incidence of interactions.

A formalized drug interaction screening program should be used in all pharmacies. This can be a simple manual system using patient drug profiles and a drug interaction reference book or a computerized system. Because of their growing use in pharmacy, computers can be expected to play a greater role in the screening and analysis of individual drug regimens.

Educating patients about their drug therapy can aid in preventing or minimizing drug interactions. If patients are more attentive to the development of excessive or unexpected responses to their drug therapy, problems may be identified earlier. The use of over-the-counter medications should be discussed with the patient. Interactions with these agents are often overlooked. Finally, patients should be encouraged to ask questions about their drug therapy.

## Summary

A drug's action may be modified by many substances. Drug–drug interactions may be pharmacokinetic, pharmacodynamic, or pharmaceutic in nature. Food may alter a drug's action or a drug may alter nutritional status. Drug interactions with alcohol and tobacco may also occur. Managing drug interactions and establishing methods for preventing them are key components of clinical pharmacy services.

## References


1. Boston Collaborative Drug Surveillance Program. Adverse drug interactions. JAMA 1972;220:1238–1239.
2. Durrence CW, DiPiro JT, May JR, et al. Potential drug interactions in surgical patients. Am J Hosp Pharm 1985;42:1553–1555.
3. Blaschke TF, Cohen SN, Tatro DS. Drug–drug interactions and aging, in Jarvik LF, Greenblatt DJ, Harman D (eds): Clinical Pharmacology in the Aged Patient. New York, Raven, 1981.
4. Stanaszek WF, Franklin CE. Survey of potential drug interaction incidence in an outpatient clinic population. Hosp Pharm 1978;13:255–263.
5. Borda IT, Slone D, Hick H. Assessment of adverse reactions within a drug surveillance program. JAMA 1968;205:645–647.
6. Smith JW, Seidl LG, Cluff LE. Studies on the epidemiology of adverse drug reactions. V. Clinical factors influencing susceptibility. Ann Intern Med 1966;65:629–640.
7. D'Arcy PF. Drug reactions and interactions in the elderly patient. Drug Intell Clin Pharm 1982;16:925–929.
8. Zarowitz B, Conway W, Popvich J. Adverse interactions of drugs in critical care patients. Henry Ford Hosp Med J 1985;33:48–55.
9. Nagashima H. Drug interactions in the recovery room. Int Anesthesiol Clin 1983;21:93–105.
10. Van der Meer JWM, Scheijgrond HW, Heykants J, et al. The influence of gastric acidity on the bioavailability of ketoconazole. J Antimicrob Chemother 1980;6:552–554.
11. O'Callaghan JW, Thompson RN, Russell AS. Combining NSAIDs with anticoagulants: Yes and no. Can Med Assoc J 1984;131:857–858.
12. O'Reilly RA, Trager WF, Motley CH, et al. Stereoselective interaction of phenylbutazone with (12c/13c) warfarin pseudo racemates in man. J Clin Invest 1980;65:746–753.
13. Mitchell JR, Arias L, Oates JA. Antagonism of the antihypertensive action of guanethidine sulfate by desipramine hydrochloride. JAMA 1967;202:973–976.
14. Jackson JE, Powell JR, Wandell M, et al. Cimetidine decreases theophylline clearance. Am Rev Resp Dis 1981;123:615–617.
15. Weinberger MM, Smith G, Milavetz G, et al. Decreased theophylline clearance due to cimetidine. (Lett) N Engl J Med 1981;304:672.
16. Campbell MA, Plachetka JR, Jackson JE, et al. Cimetidine

decreases theophylline clearance: A case report. Ann Intern Med 1981;95:68–69.
17. Fenje PC, Isles AF, Baltodano A, et al. Interaction of cimetidine and theophylline in two infants. (Lett) Can Med Assoc J 1982;126:1178.
18. D'Arcy P. Vaccine–drug interactions. Drug Intell Clin Pharm 1984;18:697–700.
19. Meredith CG, Christian CD, Johnson RFK, et al. Effects of influenza virus vaccine on hepatic drug metabolism. Clin Pharmacol Ther 1985;37:396–401.
20. Peterson V, Hvidts S, Thomsen K, et al. Effect of prolonged thiazide treatment on renal lithium clearance. Br Med J 1974;2:143–145.
21. Mehta BR, Robinson BHB. Lithium toxicity induced by triamterene-hydrochlorothiazide. Postgrad Med J 1980;56:783–784.
22. Trissel LA. Handbook on Injectable Drugs, 4th ed. Bethesda, MD, American Society of Hospital Pharmacists, 1986.
23. Sachtles G. Dilantin for I.V. use. (Lett) Drug Intell Clin Pharm 1973;7:418.
24. Burke WA. I.V. drug incompatibilities—Dilantin. Am J IV Ther 1975;2:16.
25. Weiner IM, Mudge GH. Inhibitors of tubular transport of organic compounds, in Gilman AG, Goodman LS, Rall TW, et al. (eds): The Pharmacological Basis of Therapeutics, 7th ed. New York, Macmillan, 1985, p 923.
26. Melander A, Danielson K, Schersten B, et al. Enhancement by food of canrenone bioavailability from spironolactone. Clin Pharmacol Ther 1977;22:100–103.
27. Crounse RG. Human pharmacology of griseofulvin: The effect of fat intake on gastrointestinal absorption. J Invest Dermatol 1961;37:529–533.
28. Roe DA. Therapeutic significance of drug–nutrient interactions in the elderly. Pharmacol Rev 1984;36:S109–S122.
29. Jusko WJ. Role of tobacco smoking in pharmacokinetics. J Pharmacokinet Biopharm 1978;6:7–39.
30. Vestal RE, Wood AJJ. Influence of age and smoking on drug pharmacokinetics in man—studies using model compounds. Clin Pharmacokinet 1980;5:309–319.
31. Collaborative Group for the Study of Stroke in Young Women. Oral contraceptives and stroke in young women. JAMA 1978;231:718–722.
32. Jusko WJ, Schentag JJ, Clark JH, et al. Enhanced biotransformation of theophylline in marijuana and tobacco smokers. Clin Pharmacol Ther 1978;24:406–410.
33. Hunt SN, Jusko JW, Yurchak AM. Effect of smoking on theophylline disposition. Clin Pharmacol Ther 1976;19:546–551.
34. Lane EA, Guthrie S, Linnoila M. Effects of ethanol on drug and metabolite pharmacokinetics. Clin Pharmacokinet 1985;10:228–247.
35. Hayes SL, Pablo G, Radomski T, et al. Ethanol and oral diazepam absorption. N Engl J Med 1977;296:186–189.
36. Sellers EM, Naranjo CA, Giles HG, et al. Intravenous diazepam and oral ethanol interaction. Clin Pharmacol Ther 1980;28:638–645.
37. Juhl RP, Van Thiel DH, Dittert LW, et al. Alprazolam pharmacokinetics in alcoholic liver disease. J Clin Pharmacol 1984;24:113–119.
38. Baruh S, Sherman L, Kolodny HD, et al. Fasting hypoglycemia. Med Clin North Am 1973;57:1441–1462.
39. Kater RMH, Tobon F, Iber FL. Increased rate of metabolism in alcoholic patients. JAMA 1969;207:363–365.
40. Fitzgerald MG, Gaddie R, Malins JM, et al. Alcohol sensitivity in diabetics receiving chlorpropamide. Diabetes 1962;2:40–43.
41. Hansten PD. Drug Interactions, 5th ed. Philadelphia, Lea and Febiger, 1985.
42. Scheible RM (ed): Clin-Alert. Medford, NJ, Clin-Alert, Inc., 1986.

# Chapter 8 / Drug Therapy in Transplantation

Richard J. Ptachcinski, PharmD, Raman Venkataramanan, PhD, and Gilbert J. Burckart, PharmD

Organ transplantation is now an accepted mode of therapy for diseases that lead to chronic irreversible failure of the kidney, heart, or liver. In 1986, 190 transplant centers in the United States performed more than 8,000 kidney transplant operations. Although the cost of the hospitalization for the transplant procedure varies considerably depending on the organ transplanted and the complications that arise, the hospital bill for initial surgery alone exceeded $300 million for kidney transplants in 1986. With the long-term survival of the transplant recipients, medication costs for immunosuppression become a larger and larger percentage of the overall cost of the transplant procedure. With over 100,000 people enrolled in the End Stage Renal Disease program of the U.S. Medicare system, the numbers of transplants and their costs are expected to increase into the 1990s.

Although kidney transplant operations have become commonplace, the numbers of other solid organ transplants have also increased dramatically since 1980. Ninety heart transplant centers performed 1,427 heart transplants during 1986 at an average cost of $57,000 to $110,000, as compared with approximately $30,000 for a kidney. Forty liver transplant centers did almost 900 operations in 1986 at a much higher cost ($135,000 to $238,000). While the numbers of heart–lung and pancreas transplants are relatively small, 28,000 corneal transplants were performed in 1986. The 1-year patient survival rates are exceptional when compared with the early days of transplantation: 95% for kidneys, 78% for hearts, and 65% for livers in 1986. Although the strides in organ transplantation have been remarkable since 1980, over 10,000 patients remain on waiting lists for kidneys, and as many as 15,000 individuals are estimated to be potential beneficiaries of heart transplantation.[1–3]

The origin of solid organ transplantation is multifaceted. The present success of organ transplant procedures would not be possible if the techniques of vascular anastomosis had not been studied and refined to allow experimental and clinical work. In Europe in 1902, Dr. Alex Carrel published a paper that is the basis for modern techniques of suturing. Mathieu Jaboulay, Carrel's teacher, attempted the first human kidney transplant in 1906 using a pig as a donor. Although this initial trial of transplantation was unsuccessful, Dr. Carrel continued his work in the United States and was awarded the Nobel prize in 1912 for his work with vascular anastomosis.

Interest in kidney transplantation was revived in the early 1950s when several human transplants were conducted without immunosuppression and without long-term success. The understanding of the immune mechanisms of organ rejection was improving rapidly, however, and the first successful kidney transplant with prolonged survival was performed between identical twins in Boston in 1954.

The need for immunosuppression soon became clear, but the means were crude and difficult to control. Total-body irradiation was used on 12 kidney graft recipients in Boston between 1958 and 1962 with only one survivor. Drug therapy offered an alternative to irradiation, and Hitchings and Elion of Burroughs Wellcome had developed 6-mercaptopurine and derivatives for testing. Stimulated by the studies in animals performed by Schwartz and Dameshek, British investigator Roy Calne first used 6-mercaptopurine and later its derivative, azathioprine, to demonstrate that pharmacologic immunosuppression was possible in renal transplantation. Dr. Thomas Starzl further refined these immunosuppressive regimens to routinely include corticosteroids, which significantly improved kidney graft survival and encouraged the practice of organ transplantation in the 1960s.

The 1970s were a quiescent period during which several important things were accomplished for organ transplantation. Methods of tissue typing and organ sharing schemes were developed and improved. The concept of "brain death" was established and would be critical for organ procurement. Most importantly, a drug was developed by Dr. J. Borel at Sandoz, Inc. in Switzerland that would dramatically change the approach to immunosuppression in the 1980s. Cyclosporine (CyA), then called cyclosporin A, had a totally different mechanism of action on the immune system and encouraged the expansion of human organ transplantation to heart, liver, pancreas, and heart–lung.

Immunosuppressive therapy in solid organ transplantation has undergone rapid changes from 1980 to 1987. The objective of the following discussion is not only to review the present immunosuppressive and other pharmacotherapy in current use, but also to provide the conceptual basis for monitoring the continued change that is expected over the next few years in these regimens.

## Mechanism of Action of the Immunosuppressants

The normal immune response to foreign material is incompletely understood. Much of the progress made in understanding the immune system in the past 30 years is due to organ transplantation. Studies in histocompatibility and studies with specific monoclonal antibodies and drugs have provided new insight into the complexity of the immune response to foreign tissue.[4,5]

The lymphoid system is subdivided into two different types of cells. T cells mediate cellular immunity, and B cells are responsible for humoral immunity and the immunoglob-

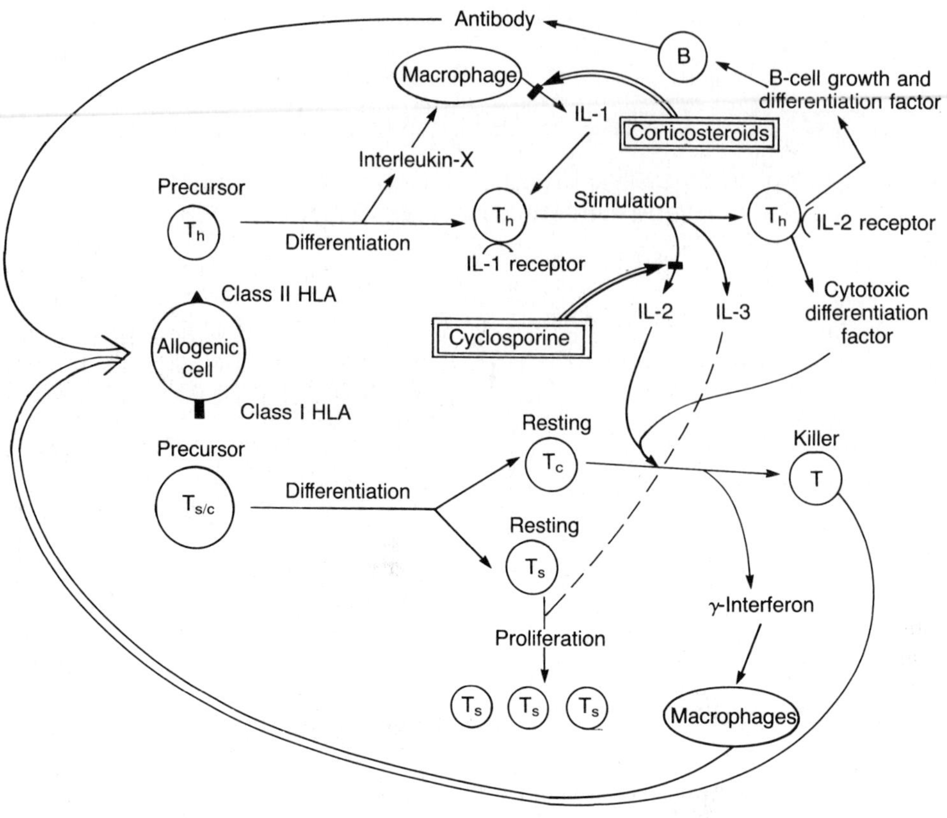


**Figure 8.1** Stimulation of the T-lymphocyte system by an allogenic cell with subsequent attack on the cell by the immune system. Points of blockade of the system by corticosteroids and by cyclosporine are included. HLA, human leukocyte antigens; T, T lymphocyte; $T_h$, helper T lymphocyte; $T_{s/c}$, suppressor/cytotoxic T cell; $T_c$, cytotoxic T cell; $T_s$, suppressor T cell; IL, interleukin; B, B lymphocyte.

ulins. Both types of cells are found in the blood and in peripheral lymphoid tissue. After contact with an antigen, T cells form a clone of cells with immunologic memory for that antigen and provide cellular immune protection. Cellular immune reactions are classically described as delayed hypersensitivity reactions, but are also critically important in graft rejection after organ transplantation. Macrophages bearing the antigen in an immunogenic form on the cell surface come into contact with not only T cells but also B cells, which then form antibody-forming cells. The antibody-forming cells further differentiate into plasma cells which specifically secrete large amounts of antibody in one of the immunoglobulin classes.

Several subsets of T lymphocytes have been identified, and they play a significant role in transplantation immunology. One subset is called a "helper" T cell because, under the proper conditions, it secretes B-cell growth and differentiation factor to help out B cells. Another subset is the "suppressor/cytotoxic" T cell, a multipotential type of lymphocyte. Under the appropriate stimulation, cytotoxic T cells differentiate and proliferate into "killer" T lymphocytes that attack and kill antigenic cells. The interactions between these cells and B cells are complex and are an important part of drug-mediated immunosuppression (see Fig. 8.1).

Plasma cells that have come from the B-cell line can secrete IgD, IgM, IgG, IgA, or IgE. The specific antibody binds to the foreign antigen and causes reactions such as lysis of a red cell, inactivation of a virus, or phagocytosis of a bacteria. Complement frequently plays a role in these antigen–antibody reactions, binding to the complex and facilitating destruction of the antigen. Reexposure to the antigen causes a rapid response, with antibody synthesis and cell proliferation.

Rejection of the transplanted organ begins with recognition of foreign human leukocyte (HLA) antigens or histocompatibility antigens (refer to Fig. 8.1). Class I HLA antigens are virtually on all cell surfaces, whereas class II antigens are on few cells such as B lymphocytes, some monocytes, and activated T lymphocytes. Class I HLA antigens are recognized by receptors on the surface of the suppressor/cytotoxic-T-cell precursor, and these receptors include T3 and T8 proteins. Class II HLA antigens are recognized by receptors on the surface of the helper-T-cell precursor and include T3 and T4 proteins. When monoclonal antibodies are produced against these receptor proteins, the anti-T3 antibody will accordingly immobilize most T lymphocytes, as the T3 protein is shared by helper and suppressor/cytotoxic lymphocytes. More specific activity can be achieved with anti-T4 antibodies, which would inactivate helper lymphocytes, and anti-T8 antibodies, which would immobilize only suppressor/cytotoxic lymphocytes. While macrophage processing of antigenic material is necessary for lymphocyte response to an infectious agent, lymphocytes respond directly to incompatible HLA antigens without macrophage intervention. Macrophages still do play a part in organ transplant rejection, however, because helper T cells activated by class II HLA antigens prompt the release of an intercellular mediator, called a lymphokine, by the lymphocyte. This lymphokine is a macrophage stimulant called interleukin-X, which in turn causes the stimulated macrophage to release another mediator called interleukin-1 (IL-1). The secreted IL-1 stimulates the release of interleukin-2 (IL-2) by stimulated helper T cells, the formation of IL-1 receptors on helper T cells, and the formation of IL-2 receptors on helper T cells and on stimulated suppressor/cytotoxic T cells. Under the influence of IL-1, the helper T cell, which was previously stimulated by the class II HLA antigen, not only secretes IL-2, but also secretes cytotoxic differentiation factor, interleukin-3 (IL-3), and B-cell growth and differentiation factor.

The secretion of IL-2 is a critical step in the process of continuing the immune response and rejecting the transplanted organ. The precursor suppressor/cytotoxic T lymphocytes are uncommitted and can differentiate into clones of either suppressor cells, which suppress the immune response, or cytotoxic cells, which evolve to killer T cells and attack the antigenic material. The form of cell that predominates, either suppressor or cytotoxic T cell, dictates the immune response. IL-2, in conjunction with both the promotion of IL-2 receptors by IL-1 and the elaboration of cytotoxic differentiation factor by stimulated helper T cells, promotes the differentiation and proliferation of cytotoxic T cells. To balance this effect of IL-2, activated helper T cells also elaborate IL-3, also called suppressor cell differentiation/amplification factor, which promotes the clonal expansion of suppressor T cells. Damage to the transplanted organ is produced not only by the direct action of cytotoxic T lymphocytes, which attach to the class I HLA antigens on the cell surface, but also by macrophages, which have been stimulated by the $\gamma$-interferon produced by those cytotoxic T cells.

The classic approach to immunosuppressive drug therapy has been to use cytotoxic agents that kill proliferative cells. Immunosuppression with azathioprine or mercaptopurine results from antimetabolite interference with nucleic acid metabolism at steps that are required for cell proliferation after antigenic stimulation. In this manner these purine analogs destroy stimulated lymphoid cells. These agents have less effect on immunoglobulin synthesis by plasma cells than on nucleic acid synthesis in proliferating cells. In addition to the blockade of the cellular immune response by these cytotoxic purine analogs, the primary and secondary antibody responses can be blocked. An alkylating agent, cyclophosphamide, has been used successfully in renal transplantation but does not share the popularity of azathioprine.

Corticosteroids were first recognized for their lympholytic properties and may have numerous effects on the lymphocyte population. Precursor T cells appear to be sensitive to the lytic effect of corticosteroids, and more subtle actions on intercellular mediators such as the inhibition of IL-1 release from macrophages are part of steroids' broad immunosuppressive actions. Plasma cells appear to be less sensitive to the effect of steroids, but may play a part in long-term immunosuppression by corticosteroids. Steroids not only block the primary immune response, but also decrease previously established immune sensitization with continued use. The catabolism of IgG, the major class of immunoglobulins, is increased with corticosteroids, thereby lowering the effective concentration of specific antibodies. Even the ability of reticuloendothelial macrophages to phagocytize antibody-coated cells is diminished by steroid therapy. The action of the corticosteroids is different from that of the cytotoxic agents, but still represents broad-based immunosuppression of both cellular and humoral immune systems.

The antilymphocytic antibodies in the form of antilymphocytic globulin (ALG) were the first form of immunosuppressive therapy that was selective as anti–T-cell therapy. These antibodies destroy primarily the small peripheral lymphocytes that circulate between blood and lymph. With continued administration, the total pool of T lymphocytes is depleted by cytotoxic destruction assisted by complement, and significant suppression of the cellular immune system can be achieved. Antibodies can also be formed against fetal thymic cells rather than lymphoid cells—antithymocyte globulin (ATG)—and are a very effective anti–T-cell agent. Both ALG and ATG have been limited by the lack of standardization and by significant reactions to these animal-derived products.

Cyclosporine represents a major advance in specific immunosuppressive drug therapy. The inhibition of IL-2 elaboration by stimulated helper-T cells appears to be a major mechanism of cyclosporine's action. Cyclosporine inhibits the clonal differentiation of precursor suppressor/cytotoxic T cells into cytotoxic T cells through its blockade of IL-2. At the same time, IL-3 is not inhibited by cyclosporine, thereby allowing the expansion of the suppressor-T-cell population and increasing the ratio of suppressor to cytotoxic cells in the host. Cyclosporine's inhibition of IL-2 production occurs at the level of messenger RNA transcription, but little is known of its specific receptor. Unlike the cytotoxic drugs and corticosteroids, cyclosporine exerts its effect without killing or lysing any effector cells and is therefore ineffective once antigenic stimulation has already occurred. As the drug is not lymphocytotoxic, discontinuation of cyclosporine is followed by a prompt reversal of its immunosuppressant effect. Cyclosporine has played a significant role in advancing transplantation because it leaves preformed immunity and the humoral immune system intact and thereby reduces some of the infectious complications associated with other immunosuppressants.

An advance in technology has allowed the standardization of an ATG of monoclonal origin produced in the mouse. This monoclonal antibody is directed at the T3 receptor protein on lymphocytes and is very effective at blocking cytotoxic T cells and T-cell function. The T-cell population in peripheral blood decreases after initiation of anti-T3 antibody (OKT3) therapy and increases after discontinuation of therapy.

## Clinical Presentation of Organ Rejection

The diagnosis of graft rejection is frequently difficult in patients after transplantation. This is particularly true when attempting to differentiate renal graft rejection from drug-induced nephrotoxicity or hepatic graft rejection from drug-

**Table 8.1** Drug Interactions Involving Immunosuppresents

| *Interacting Drug* | *Immunosuppressant* | *Effect* |
|---|---|---|
| Modifiers of drug absorption | | |
| Metoclopramide | CyA[a] | Increased CyA concentrations |
| Loperamide | CyA | Decreased CyA concentrations |
| Cholestyramine | CyA | Decreased CyA concentrations |
| Chenodeoxycholic acid | CyA | Increased CyA concentrations |
| Somatostatin | CyA | Decreased CyA concentrations |
| Modifiers of drug distribution | | |
| Cholestyramine | CyA | May increase unbound CyA |
| Lovastatin | CyA | May increase unbound CyA |
| Drug-metabolizing enzyme inhibitors | | |
| Allopurinol | Azathioprine | Decreased elimination |
| Ketoconazole | CyA | Increased CyA concentrations |
| Erythromycin | CyA | Increased steroid concentrations |
| Diltiazem | CyA | Increased CyA concentrations |
| CyA | Steroids | Increased steroid concentrations |
| Oral contraceptives | Steroids | Increased steroid concentrations |
| Drug-metabolizing enzyme inducers | | |
| Phenobarbital | CyA/steroids | Decreased concentrations |
| Phenytoin | CyA/steroids | Decreased concentrations |
| Carbamazepine | CyA | Decreased CyA concentrations |
| Rifampin | CyA/steroids | Decreased concentrations |
| Corticosteroids | CyA | Decreased CyA concentrations |
| Smoking (cigarettes, marijuana) | CyA | Decreased CyA concentrations |
| Nephrotoxic drugs | | |
| Amphotericin B | CyA | Additive nephrotoxicity |
| Aminoglycosides | | |
| Cephalosporins | | |
| Furosemide | | |
| TMP–SMX | | |
| NSAIDs | | |

[a] CyA, cyclosporine (cyclosporin A); TMP–SMX, trimethoprim–sulfamethoxazole; NSAIDs, nonsteroidal anti-inflammatory drugs.

induced hepatotoxicity. Rejection of a transplanted organ is frequently associated with fever, malaise, and graft enlargement. The biochemical changes that occur during graft rejection are those associated with abnormal function of the transplanted organ. Patients with renal allograft rejection have a decreased urine output, accompanied by a rapidly rising serum creatinine, blood urea nitrogen level, and decreased blood flow on renal scan. Liver graft rejection is suspected in patients with an increase in their serum bilirubin, alkaline phosphatase, and serum transaminase concentrations. Rejection in patients after cardiac transplantation may present in a very subtle manner and, only in the later stages, is manifest by changes on ECG and signs of congestive heart failure.

Graft rejection is frequently confirmed by obtaining a graft biopsy. A biopsy specimen with a diffuse infiltrate of lymphocytes is consistent with acute cellular rejection.[6] The absolute usefulness of histologically grading the extent of cellular infiltration is as yet unclear. For example, lymphocytes activated against donor tissue can be grown from biopsy specimens that have no apparent cellular infiltrate. After the diagnosis of rejection has been confirmed, the potential risks and benefits of antirejection therapy must be evaluated.

## Drug Kinetics in Transplant Patients

Organ transplant patients are unique in that they are undergoing a transition from a poorly functioning organ system to normality. Each of the major transplanted organs (kidney, liver, heart) has a significant impact on the disposition of administered drugs, and that altered disposition should be reviewed when monitoring a transplant patient. Drug absorption, distribution, metabolism, and elimination may likewise be undergoing the transition from function associated with organ failure to the normal state. Dosage adjustments and close monitoring in the period of a rapidly changing clinical status are therefore essential in an organ transplant patient.

Successful transplantation should reverse the alteration in drug kinetics observed in patients with liver, kidney, or heart disease. The time course of this change in kinetics is not well defined, however. All transplant patients receive chronic immunosuppressive drug therapy, and two of these drugs (CyA, steroids) can influence the kinetics of coadministered drugs. Table 8.1 lists drugs that are frequently administered to transplant patients that may interact with immunosuppressive agents. Very few studies have been conducted to characterize drug kinetics in transplant patients, but the following is a brief review of the available information in this area.

### *Absorption*

Changes in drug absorption are quite dramatic in liver transplant patients. After a successful liver transplantation, absorption of lipid-soluble compounds such as CyA, vitamin A, and vitamin E is considerably improved. The poor absorption of the lipid-soluble drug CyA improves after successful liver transplantation (from bioavailability of 12% to 26%). Vitamin E deficiency and the neurologic complications associated with liver disease are reversed after successful liver transplantation in pediatric patients. In stable adult liver transplant patients, the concentrations of retinol (1.39 $\mu$g/mL) and tocopherol (8.6 $\mu$g/mL) are similar to those seen in normal healthy subjects (0.72 and 10.2 $\mu$g/mL, respectively), indicating recovery of the ability of the transplanted liver to produce the bile salts needed for fat-soluble-vitamin absorption.[7]

### *Protein Binding*

Table 8.2 summarizes the changes in the concentrations of major drug-binding proteins in renal and liver patients prior to and after transplant surgery.

#### Renal Transplant Patients

Many factors produce changes in serum proteins before and after renal transplantation. After renal transplantation, the abolition of the uremic state, the change from restricted to full diet, and immunosuppressive therapy may influence protein concentrations and drug binding. Marked variations in the concentrations of serum proteins have been reported in renal transplant patients, with low concentrations of albumin, transferrin, and prealbumin and elevated concentrations of acute-phase reactants such as $\alpha_1$-acid glycoprotein (AAG). The protein binding of phenytoin, warfarin, sulfisoxazole, salicylate, morphine, and diazepam increases as evidenced by reduction in the free fraction in plasma after renal transplantation.[8,9] The time course for this binding improvement ranges from 2 to 16 days postoperation. The rapid initial phase of improvement may presumably be related to the removal of endogenous binding inhibitors (i.e., uremic toxins) and is followed by a slower recovery phase related to the presence of newly synthesized albumin.

Lidocaine is a basic drug that is bound to a greater extent in the plasma of uremic patients because of elevated AAG concentrations as compared with normal subjects. After renal transplantation and the resolution of the uremic state, lidocaine binding decreases in comparison with the pretransplant values but remains greater than normal values.[10]

#### Liver Transplant Patients

The serum concentration of albumin in liver transplant patients is frequently lower than that observed in normal subjects.[11] Consequently, the binding of diazepam and salicylic acid, which bind primarily to albumin, is lower in transplant patients than in normal subjects. When compared with that of patients with chronic liver disease, however, the

**Table 8.2** Plasma Proteins in Transplant Patients

| | *Change in proteins*[a] | | | |
|---|---|---|---|---|
| | **Renal transplant** | | **Liver transplant** | |
| *Protein* | **Pre** | **Post** | **Pre** | **Post** |
| Albumin | − | + | − | − |
| $\alpha_1$-Acid glycoprotein | + | + | − | + |
| Transcortin | − | = | − | = |

[a]+, Increased compared with normal subjects; −, decreased compared with normal subjects; =, not different from normal subjects.

binding of both diazepam and salicylic acid is greater in liver transplant patients because of the removal of endogenous binding inhibitors. As acidic drugs bind primarily to albumin, similar results would be expected for such drugs as phenytoin, cephalosporin, furosemide, and warfarin. Studies in liver transplant patients indicate that the concentration of AAG increases after surgery and stays at an elevated level for at least 45 days. Correspondingly, the free fraction of lidocaine in plasma obtained from stable liver transplant patients was lower than the free fraction values observed in plasma from normal volunteers. A significant correlation exists between lidocaine free fraction and AAG concentration ($r = -0.94$) in these patients. Even though the affinity of lidocaine for AAG was reduced in transplant patients, the increased AAG concentration results in increased drug binding. Propranolol also binds to AAG, but no significant difference was observed in the free fraction of propranolol in stable liver transplant patients when compared with normal subjects. An increase in propranolol binding resulting from an increase in AAG concentration is offset by a reduction in albumin concentration, as albumin also contributes to the binding of propranolol. Changes in basic drug–protein binding in liver transplant patients depend on the relative contributions of AAG and albumin to the binding.

### *Elimination (Metabolism and Excretion)*

The oxidative metabolizing capacity of the liver in clinically stable liver transplant patients, as determined by antipyrine kinetics, is similar to that observed in normal subjects. Presently, nothing is known about metabolic pathways such as conjugation and acetylation in transplant patients. In the early postoperative period, liver transplant patients have high concentrations of cyclosporine metabolites in blood which reflects a deficiency in the biliary elimination of those compounds.

## Drug Dosing in Transplant Patients

### *General Considerations*

The preceding discussion provides some basis for the rational dosing of drugs to transplant patients; however, because of multiple factors affecting the kinetics of drugs and the lack of sufficient information on drug kinetics in this patient population, careful monitoring and individualization of therapy are essential.

Renal impairment is common in transplant patients as a result of either poor graft function (for renal transplant patients) or drug-induced nephrotoxicity. Drug dosing in transplant patients with renal failure is difficult as the degree of dysfunction in drug elimination is not easily predictable from common clinical markers of renal function. For example, the clearance of cefotaxime in liver transplant patients was found not to have the same relationship with serum creatinine as observed in other patient populations. While individualized dosing based on plasma concentrations is most appropriate in this situation, therapy must often be initiated without this knowledge, and plasma concentration monitoring is not available for some agents. In these cases, the usual dosing guidelines observed for nontransplant patients with renal failure should be used. The half-life of a renally eliminated drug can be approximated from knowledge of the usual and the anephric drug half-lives, using the percentage of normal creatinine clearance as the guide to extrapolate between the two published half-lives. Table 8.3 lists the usual and anephric elimination half-lives for several drugs used in transplant patients. If hemodialysis or peritoneal dialysis is initiated, drug dosing may have to be adjusted to compensate for drug removed during the dialysis. Once again, the dosing guidelines for the use of drugs in nontransplant patients receiving dialysis should be followed.

Unlike the case in patients with renal failure, no marker is currently available to quantitatively predict hepatic elimination of drugs in transplant patients with liver failure. Drug concentration monitoring in blood or plasma currently remains the best method for dosage adjustment in these patients.

**Table 8.3** Anephric and Normal Elimination Half-lives for Drugs Used in Transplant Patients

| | $T_{1/2}$ (h) | |
|---|---|---|
| ***Drug*** | **Normal** | **Anephric** |
| Ampicillin | 1.2 | 6.3 |
| Carbenicillin | 1.2 | 11.6 |
| Cephalothin | 0.5 | 11.6 |
| Chloramphenicol | 2.3 | 3.5 |
| Digoxin | 40.8 | 86.6 |
| Erythromycin | 1.4 | 5.3 |
| 5-Flucytosine | 2.8 | 99.0 |
| Gentamicin | 2.3 | 34.7 |
| Kanamycin | 2.8 | 69.3 |
| Methicillin | 0.5 | 4.1 |
| Oxacillin | 0.5 | 2.0 |
| Penicillin G | 0.5 | 23.1 |
| Rifampin | 2.8 | 2.8 |
| Sulfamethoxazole | 9.9 | 9.9 |
| Tobramycin | 2.0 | 69.3 |
| Trimethoprim | 11.6 | 34.7 |
| Vancomycin | 5.8 | 231.0 |

## *Specific Agents*

Table 8.4 reviews the dosing and administration of several immunosuppressive drugs.

### Prednisone–Prednisolone

The usefulness of corticosteroids for the prevention and treatment of graft rejection is well established.[12] The first transplants using pharmacologic immunosuppression included therapy with corticosteroids or adrenocorticotropic hormone (ACTH). In the early 1960s the discovery of the immunosuppressive properties of 6-mercaptopurine and azathioprine had a major impact on the success of transplantation. It was rapidly realized that the immunosuppressive combination of azathioprine and low-dose steroids resulted in better graft and patient survival than use of either agent alone. Since that time the combination of corticosteroids with other immunosuppressive agents has been the standard of practice after organ transplantation.

The doses of corticosteroids used to prevent graft rejection vary significantly.[13] Some transplant centers start with high doses of prednisone (200 mg/d orally) that are rapidly tapered over 5 days to 20 mg/d. Other centers start with a prednisone dose of 30 mg/d orally that is slowly tapered (over a period of months) until alternate-day therapy can be used. While there are obvious advantages to using alternate-day steroids for long-term maintenance, patients may be sensitive to even minor changes in their steroid regimen, and aggressive dosage reduction may result in an acute episode of graft rejection.[14] Kahan et al recently compared the clinical courses of two groups of patients following different steroid regimens after renal transplantation.[15] One group received a rapidly tapering steroid regimen with a stepwise decrease in oral prednisone from 1.5 to 0.4 mg/kg/d over 6 days. The second group had a slowly tapered steroid regimen that started at 1.5 mg/kg/d, was 0.57 mg/kg/d at 17 days, and was continued for 30 days. Patients receiving higher doses of steroids (slow taper) had fewer rejection episodes than patients receiving lower doses of steroids. The authors did not report any differences in steroid-related adverse effects between the two groups.

High-dose steroids are the primary treatment for acute graft rejection episodes.[16] The exact dose of steroids required to reverse graft rejection is unknown. Several investigators have evaluated various steroid regimens for the treatment of graft rejection. No significant difference in graft and/or patient survival or in the incidence of toxic effects between treatment regimens has been demonstrated; however, steroid regimens that maintain high doses of steroids for prolonged periods were associated with more steroid-related complications, such as gastrointestinal bleeding, aseptic necrosis, and diabetes mellitus. Unfortunately, published trials comparing high- and low-dose steroids are too few to reach firm conclusions about mortality, graft failure, and the incidence of steroid-induced complications.[16] Steroids have a large number of significant side effects associated with their use, and the lowest dosage possible for maintaining graft function should be administered.

Corticosteroids are involved in several significant drug interactions that may occur in transplant patients (Table 8.1). Concurrent therapy with hepatic enzyme–inducing and –inhibiting agents alters the disposition of corticosteroids. In

**Table 8.4** Dosing and Administration of Immunosuppressants[a]

| *Agent* | *IV dose* | *PO dose* | *Comments* |
|---|---|---|---|
| Azathioprine | Initial: 3–5 mg/kg<br>Maintenance: 1.0–3.0 mg/kg | Initial: 3–5 mg/kg<br>Maintenance: 1.0–3.0 mg/kg | Protect IV solutions from light |
| Antilymphocyte globulin | 10–40 mg/kg for 10–14 d | | Requires central line for infusion<br>Significant batch-to-batch variability |
| Corticosteroids | High dose 250–1,000 mg of methylprednisolone used to treat graft rejection | Initial doses high (>200 mg/d of prednisone), tapered to maintenance doses of 5–15 mg/d<br>Steroids may be discontinued in some patients but this change may precipitate graft rejection in some patients | Corticosteroids should be administered with food or milk to minimize gastrointestinal side effects |
| Cyclosporine | 2–6 mg/kg/d as two or three divided doses<br>Conversion factor from PO to IV dosing is approximately 30% | Initial dose 8–17 mg/kg/d administered as single dose or two divided doses<br>Maintenance dose 2–5 mg/kg/d | Store IV solutions in glass bottles and administer via tubing not containing polyvinyl chloride<br>Administer IV cyclosporine as a slow (2–24 h) infusion |
| $OKT_3$ | 5 MG IV daily for 10–14 d | | Children may receive 2.5 mg IV while some protocols include long IV<br>Administer undiluted over approximately 1 min<br>Premedicate with 200 mg IV hydrocortisone, 25–50 mg diphenhydramine, 325–650 mg acetaminophen<br>Extreme caution is warranted in patients with recent weight gain associated with fluid overload |

[a] Doses stated represent only guidelines; the doses of the agents used may vary significantly according to any transplant center's protocol.

addition, as steroids are capable of inducing hepatic enzymes, therapy with other agents may be affected by the concurrent administration of corticosteroids.

**Monoclonal Antibody (MUROMONAB-CD3 or OKT3)**

OKT3 is a murine monoclonal antibody that reacts with the T3-antigen recognition structure of T lymphocytes.[17] This reaction then blocks both the generation and function of T lymphocytes which are involved in the rejection of a transplanted organ. OKT3 does not affect the nonspecific host defense system and does not cause bone marrow depression.

OKT3 has been compared with high-dose steroids for the treatment of acute graft rejection in renal transplant patients. In one study, OKT3 reversed 94% of the rejection episodes while high-dose steroids reversed 75%.[18] The success of OKT3 in reversing rejection in extrarenal organs has also been encouraging.[1,2] OKT3 appears to be quite useful for the rescue of rejection episodes that are refractory to conventional treatment with high-dose steroids. An appropriate strategy for the treatment of an acute episode of rejection would include use of steroids initially, as they are able to reverse the rejection process in the majority of patients. Patients with steroid-resistant rejection can then be treated with OKT3, which will yield response rates of approximately 75% in this population.

OKT3 is administered as a 5-mg intravenous bolus daily for 10 to 14 days. Methylprednisolone (250–500 mg intravenously) may be administered 6 to 12 hours before, and hydrocortisone (100 mg) is given 30 minutes after, the first dose of OKT3. Acetaminophen (650 mg) and diphenhydramine (50 mg) are frequently given prior to the daily dose of OKT3 to lessen the severity of minor adverse effects (fever, chills). During OKT3 therapy, the doses of other immunosuppressants such as azathioprine, cyclosporine, and steroids are often reduced.[17] Several days before the expected completion of OKT3 therapy, the doses of other immunosuppressants are usually increased to pre-OKT3 levels.

**Cyclosporine**

Cyclosporine (CyA) is a cyclic polypeptide containing 11 amino acids that has dramatically changed the field of transplantation; however, the optimal dose or dosing regi-

**Table 8.5** Summary of Cyclosporine Pharmacokinetics

| |
|---|
| **Absorption** |
| Bioavailability |
| Mean 30% |
| Range <5%–90% |
| Decreased in patients with gastrointestinal disease or diarrhea |
| Increases with increased dosing frequency |
| Increases with time posttransplantation |
| Increases or may not change when administered with food |
| Impaired in patients with liver disease |
| Decreased in patients with a T-tube |
| **Distribution** |
| Extensively distributed throughout the body |
| $V_{SS}$ 4 L/kg |
| Range 0.1–15.5 L/kg |
| Extensively bound to erythrocytes |
| B/P[a] is approximately 2.0; B/P is influenced by |
| Temperature of sample separation |
| Hematocrit |
| Lipoprotein concentration |
| CyA concentration |
| Tissue distribution primarily in liver, pancreas, and lungs |
| Lipoprotein binding |
| HDL 57% |
| LDL 25% |
| VLDL 2% |
| Albumin 10% |
| Unbound fraction 1%–17% |
| **Metabolism** |
| Extensively metabolized by mono- and dihydroxylation and N-demethylation |
| Blood clearance 5 mL/min/kg |
| Range 0.5–15.5 mg/min/kg |
| Clearance decreased in patients with liver disease |
| Clearance (based on body weight) inversely proportional to patient's age |
| Several metabolites have in vitro immunosuppressive activity |
| Concentration range for metabolite 17 (M17) is similar to that of unchanged CyA |
| Metabolite concentrations M17>M1>M18>M21 |
| **Elimination** |
| Urinary excretion |
| <1% of a dose excreted as unchanged CyA |
| <10% of a dose excreted as CyA metabolites |
| Biliary excretion |
| <1% of a dose excreted as unchanged CyA |
| 10%–40% of a dose excreted as CyA and metabolites |
| Enterohepatic cycling of unchanged CyA unlikely; however, CyA metabolites may undergo enterohepatic cycling |

[a] B/P, blood-to-plasma ratio; CyA, cyclosporine (cyclosporin A).

men for CyA that prevents graft rejection with minimal toxicity is not well established. Guidelines for the dosage and administration of CyA are found in Table 8.4. Immunosuppressive regimens at some institutions do not include CyA until 7 to 14 days after transplantation,[19] while in other regimens therapy with CyA is initiated immediately prior to surgery.[20] Immunosuppression with CyA alone has been popular in European transplant centers,[21] although most centers in the United States combine CyA with low-dose corticosteroids. Recently, there has been an increase in the popularity of "triple"- or "quadruple"-drug immunosuppressive therapy, which combines low-dose CyA, corticosteroids, antilymphocytic globulin, and azathioprine.[19] The long-term safety and efficacy of such combinations are still unknown.

The pharmacokinetics of CyA have been extensively evaluated.[22] The kinetics of the drug are highly variable and are dependent on the type of transplant procedure, age, hepatic function, concurrent drug therapy, and other factors.[22] Table 8.5 presents CyA pharmacokinetic parameters and factors that may influence CyA blood concentrations.

CyA blood concentration monitoring is recommended for all patients receiving the drug; however, no well-defined "therapeutic range" for CyA exists. This is due partially to controversies regarding whether blood or plasma is the optimal biologic fluid and whether high-pressure liquid chromatography or radioimmunoassay should be used for monitoring.[23] Generally, patients with very low CyA blood concentrations are at high risk for experiencing graft rejection, while patients with prolonged elevations in their CyA concentrations are most likely to experience drug toxicity. Considerable overlap of the subtherapeutic, therapeutic, and toxic ranges of blood concentrations occurs, however. CyA concentrations should be interpreted cautiously and with reference to the specificity of the drug assay used for the parent CyA compound and its metabolites.

The adverse effects associated with CyA and other frequently used immunosuppressants are presented in Table 8.6.

Therapy with CyA is often complicated by several significant drug interactions. Other drugs may interact with CyA by potentiating the drug's nephrotoxicity, by changing its oral absorption, or by altering (inhibiting or inducing) its hepatic metabolism (see Table 8.1).

**Table 8.6** Adverse Effects Associated With Immunosuppressants[a]

| *Drug* | *Effect* |
|---|---|
| Azathioprine | Infection (viral, bacterial, fungal) |
| | Bone marrow suppression (neutropenia, thrombocytopenia) |
| | Hepatotoxicity |
| Antilymphocyte globulin (ALG) | Infection (viral, bacterial, fungal) |
| | Fever |
| Corticosteroids | Infection (viral, bacterial, fungal) |
| | Sodium and water retention |
| | Gastrointestinal bleeding or irritation |
| Cyclosporine | Infection (primarily viral and fungal) |
| | Nephrotoxicity |
| | Hepatotoxicity |
| | Electrolyte disturbances |
| | Neurologic (tremor, numbness in extremities) |
| | Hirsutism |
| $OKT_3$ | Fever, shortness of breath (primarily with first two doses) |
| | Infection (viral, bacterial, fungal) |
| | Aseptic meningitis |
| | Pulmonary edema (especially in patients with fluid overload) |

[a] These are major side effects associated with treatment with these agents and this is not intended to be a complete list of all adverse effects.

**Azathioprine**

Immunosuppressive regimens that included azathioprine (AZA) were the standard of practice after transplantation from 1963 until 1983. The use of AZA after organ transplantation decreased significantly after the approval of CyA in 1983. Since that time, however, fear of long-term nephrotoxicity from CyA has caused numerous alterations in immunosuppressive regimens utilized throughout the world. The increasing popularity of triple-drug therapy that includes AZA, CyA and prednisone has resulted in a significant increase in the use of AZA after transplantation.[24]

AZA is an imidazolyl derivative of 6-mercaptopurine (6-MP) and is readily metabolized to 6-MP (15–60%) and other metabolites.[25] Therefore, the biologic effects of AZA are due to bone marrow suppression caused by both compounds and the contributions of both AZA and 6-MP must be considered when evaluating the possible effects of transplantation on AZA pharmacokinetics and pharmacodynamics.

The dose of AZA used after transplantation depends on the patient's response to the drug and concurrent immunosuppressive therapy. Initial doses of 2–4 mg/kg/d immediately after transplantation are usually rapidly tapered (over 2–3 days) to a maintenance dose of 1.0–1.5 mg/kg/d.[24,25]

## *Anti-infective Therapy*

Anti-infective (antibacterial, antifungal, antiviral) therapy is part of the routine management of all patients undergoing transplant procedures. Antimicrobial prophylaxis prior to transplantation varies greatly among transplant centers but should follow acceptable guidelines for surgical prophylaxis.[26] The choice of agents generally depends on the type of transplant as different pathogens are encountered in surgical procedures performed above versus below the diaphragm. Surgical prophylaxis is usually discontinued within 48 hours of surgery, although longer regimens are commonly utilized after liver transplantation. Prophylactic anti-infective agents are also used to prevent opportunistic infections (*Pneumocystis carinii* pneumonia, candidiasis, herpes infections) which are common in immunosuppressed patients.[27,28] Table 8.7 lists special concerns that must be considered when choosing or monitoring antibiotic therapy in a patient after transplantation.

A more detailed discussion of the treatment of infections in the immunocompromised host is found in Chapters 89 and 91.

## *Antihypertensive Therapy*

Severe hypertension is a frequent problem after transplantation surgery. While hypertension may be present in some patients prior to transplantation, other patients develop hypertension as a result of changes in fluid balance or as a side effect of immunosuppressive therapy with CyA and steroids.

Antihypertensive therapy after transplantation is based on the step-care approach used in the management of essential hypertension as discussed in Chapter 10 of this text; how-

**Table 8.7** Anti-infective Therapy in Transplantation

| *Antibacterial* | *Use after transplantation* | *Special concerns in transplant patients* |
|---|---|---|
| Antibacterial | | |
| Cefotaxime | Treatment of active infections<br>Prophylactic in liver transplantation | Impaired clearance relative to serum creatinine in patients after orthotopic liver transplantation<br>Nephrotoxicity associated with cephalosporin antibiotics has been reported but is rarely of clinical significance in this population<br>Variable concentrations of desacetyl cefotaxime have been observed in patients after liver transplantation |
| Gentamicin/tobramycin<br>Vancomycin | Treatment of active infections | Impaired clearance relative to serum creatinine in patients after orthotopic liver transplantation |
| Erythromycin | Treatment of active infections (especially *Legionella pneumophila*) | Ototoxicity frequently observed in patients with renal impairment who require high doses of the drug<br>Inhibits the metabolism of CyA,[a] leading to high blood concentrations and possibly nephrotoxicity |
| TMP–SMX | Treatment of active infections<br>Prophylaxis for *Pneumocystis carinii* pneumonia | Elevations in serum creatinine concentrations occur frequently when therapy with TMP/SMX is initiated |
| Antiviral | | |
| Acyclovir | Treatment of active infections caused by herpesvirus<br>Prophylaxis for infections caused by herpesvirus | Acyclovir-induced nephrotoxicity is most prominent in patients with preexisting renal disease or those receiving other nephrotoxic drugs<br>High doses are frequently required in immunocompromised patients |
| Antifungal | | |
| Amphotericin B | Treatment of active infections | Additive nephrotoxicity has been reported in patients concurrently receiving amphotericin B and CyA |
| Ketoconazole | Treatment of active infections | Inhibits the metabolism of CyA, leading to high blood concentrations and possibly nephrotoxicity |

[a] CyA, cyclosporine (cyclosporin A); TMP–SMX, trimethoprim–sulfamethoxazole.

ever, the numerous pharmacologic problems that must be considered when managing hypertension in a patient post-transplantation are briefly described here.

The primary group of diuretics used in transplant patients is the sulfamoyl loop diuretics, such as furosemide and bumetanide. Only a few pharmacokinetic or pharmacodynamic studies of diuretics have been performed in the transplant population. Studies in kidney and liver transplant patients have shown decreased renal clearance and prolonged elimination of furosemide in patients with a poor response to the drug. One study in rats has suggested that furosemide may enhance the nephrotoxicity of CyA; however, the potential for this drug interaction does not preclude the use of furosemide in transplant patients.

$\beta$-Adrenergic blocking drugs are an excellent choice for early antihypertensive therapy in patients posttransplantation. Numerous agents are currently available that have similar pharmacologic activity but differ in receptor specificity and pharmacokinetics. These differences may be of some clinical significance and should be considered when choosing an agent for patients posttransplantation. A comparison of the $\beta$-blocking drugs is presented in Chapter 10.

The use of calcium channel blocking agents (CCBAs) for the control of blood pressure in transplant patients is an important addition to the pharmacologic armamentarium. The kinetics of the individual CCBAs are varied (see Chapter 10) and, depending on the major pathway of elimination or the presence of active drug metabolites, may be altered in transplant patients. Recent reports indicate that diltiazem, nifedipine, and nicardipine increase CyA concentrations in transplant patients.[29] This observation may result from inhibition of the hepatic metabolism of CyA by CCBAs and warrants careful monitoring of CyA concentrations when these drugs are used concurrently.

The angiotensin-converting enzyme inhibitors (captopril and enalapril) are used in some centers to control blood pressure after transplantation. Although these agents are quite effective in reducing blood pressure, the possibility of adverse effects on renal function secondary to these agents in renal transplant patients and/or patients receiving nephrotoxic agents may put some theoretical limitations on the widespread use of these drugs in transplant recipients.

## Summary

Organ transplantation is now a therapeutic option for patients with end-stage kidney, liver, and heart disease. While the surgical and technological problems of organ grafting have largely been addressed, immunosuppressive drug therapy that allows donor-specific immunity for the recipient is still needed. Future improvements in graft and patient survival will result from improved drug therapy and immunosuppression. As new agents are discovered and developed, complex drug regimens combining multiple drugs will take advantage of the beneficial effects of each agent while minimizing its adverse effects.

Drug therapy in organ transplant patients is complicated by a host of factors. Replacement of a kidney, liver, or heart produces dynamic changes in the kinetics of pharmacologic agents. The absorptive process, the protein binding and distribution, and the metabolizing and eliminating capacities for drugs administered to transplant patients undergo rapid changes that could nullify any beneficial effect from the agent. The number of drugs administered to a transplant patient complicates management and results in significant drug–drug interactions. Only an intensive program of monitoring can ensure the optimization of drug therapy and prevent serious adverse drug effects. While a thorough knowledge of the pharmacokinetics of the administered drugs is essential to construction of a monitoring program, the clinical application of kinetics to care of the transplant patient is incomplete. Kinetic measurements are an essential part of the anti-infective monitoring program for an organ transplant recipient, but remain in their infancy for monitoring immunosuppressive agents and are nonexistent for monitoring antihypertensive agents. Clinical measurements and judgment remain the principal methods of drug therapy monitoring in transplant patients, but must be aided by present kinetic knowledge of the agents utilized. The role of the pharmacist in monitoring drug therapy for patients posttransplantation will continue to grow with the number of organ transplant patients and with new immunosuppressive agents.

## References


1. Esquivel CO, Fung JJ, Markus B, et al. OKT3 in the reversal of acute hepatic allograft rejection. Transplant Proc 1987;19:2443–2446.
2. Losman JG. Clinical heart transplantation. Transplant Proc 1987;19:2500.
3. Iwatsuki S, Starzl TE, Gordon RD, et al. Late mortality and morbidity after liver transplantation. Transplant Proc 1987;19:2373–2377.
4. Duran LW, Pease LR. Relating the structure of major transplantation antigens to immune function. Transplantation 1986;41:279–285.
5. Royer HD, Reinherz EL. T lymphocytes: Ontogeny, function and relevance to clinical disorders. N Engl J Med 1987;317:1136–1142.
6. Howry RP, Gurley KE, Clarke Forbes RD. Immune mechanisms in organ allograft rejection. Transplantation 1983;36:391–411.
7. Huang ML, Burckart GJ, Venkataramanan R. Sensitive high-performance liquid chromatographic analysis of plasma vitamin E and vitamin A using amperometric and ultraviolet detection. J Chromatogr 1986;380:331–338.
8. Levy G, Baliah T, Procknal JA. Effect of renal transplantation on protein binding of drugs in serum of donor and recipient. Clin Pharmacol Ther 1976;20:512–516.
9. Dromgoole SH. The effect of uremia and kidney transplantation on the binding capacity of albumin. Clin Chim Acta 1974;52:301–303.
10. Grossman SH, Davis D, Kitchnell BB, et al. Diazepam and lidocaine plasma protein binding in renal disease. Clin Pharmacol Ther 1982;31:350–357.
11. Huang ML, Venkataramanan R, Burckart GJ, et al. Drug binding in liver transplant patients. J Clin Pharm, in press.
12. Hayry P, Ahonen J, Kock B, et al. Glucocorticoids in renal transplantation. Scand J Immunol 1984;19:211–218.
13. Park GD, Bartucci M, Smith MC. High- versus low-dose methylprednisolone for acute rejection episodes in renal transplantation. Nephron 1984;36:80–83.
14. McDonald FD, Hornstein ML, Mayor GB, et al. Effect of alternate day steroids on renal transplant function: A controlled study. Nephron 1976;17:415–429.
15. Kahan BD, Mickey R, Flechner SM, et al. Multivariate analysis of risk factors impacting on immediate and eventual cadaver allograft survival in cyclosporine-treated recipients. Transplantation 1987;43:65–70.
16. Gore SM, Oldham JA. Randomized trials of high-versus-low-dose steroids in renal transplantation. Transplantation 1986;41:319–327.
17. Goldstein G. An overview of orthoclone-OKT3. Transplant Proc 1986;18:927–931.
18. Ortho Multicenter Transplant Study Group: A randomized trial of OKT3 monoclonal antibody for acute rejection of cadaveric renal transplants. N Engl J Med 1985;306:337–342.
19. Heierhoi MH, Sollinger HW, Kalayoglu M, et al. Quadruple immunosuppression in 305 consecutive cadaver renal allografts. Clin Transplant 1987;2:71–74.
20. Rosenthal JT, Hakala TR, Iwatsuki S, et al. Cadaveric renal transplantation under cyclosporine-steroid therapy. Surg Gynecol Obstet 1983;157:309–315.
21. European Multicenter Trial. Cyclosporine A as sole immunosuppressive agent in recipients of kidney allografts from cadaver donors. Lancet 1982;2:57–60.
22. Ptachcinski RJ, Venkataramanan R, Burckart GL. Clinical pharmacokinetics of cyclosporin. Clin Pharmacokinet 1986;11:107–132.
23. Ptachcinski RJ, Burckart GJ, Venkataramanan R. Cyclosporine concentration determinations for monitoring and pharmacokinetic studies. J Clin Pharmacol 1986;26:358–366.

**24.** Canafax DM, Martel EJ, Ascher NL, et al. Two methods of managing cyclosporine nephrotoxicity: Conversion to azathioprine and triple drug therapy with cyclosporine, azathioprine and prednisone. Transplant Proc 1985;17:1176–1177.

**25.** Chan GLC, Canafax DM, Johnson CA. The therapeutic use of azathioprine in renal transplantation. Pharmacotherapy 1987;7: 165–177.

**26.** Kaiser AB. Antimicrobial prophylaxis in surgery. N Engl J Med 1986;315:1129–1138.

**27.** Hughes WT, McNabb PC, Makres TD, et al. Efficacy of trimethoprim and sulfamethoxazole in prevention and treatment of *Pneumocystis carinii* pneumonitis. Antimicrob Agents Chemother 1974;5:289–293.

**28.** Seale L, Jones CJ, Kathpalia S, et al. Prevention of herpesvirus infections in renal allograft recipients of low-dose oral acyclovir. JAMA 1985;254:3435–3438.

**29.** Wagner K, Henkel M, Neumayer HH. Interaction of calcium channel blockers and cyclosporine. Transplant Proc, in press.

# Chapter 9 / General Principles of Toxicology

Sven A. Normann, PharmD, and Gregory G. Gaar, MD

## Incidence of Poisoning

In 1986, 1,098,894 human exposures to toxins were reported to the American Association of Poison Control Centers (AAPCC) National Data Collection System.[1] This represents the largest poisoning data base compiled in the United States. Based on the actual number of reported poisonings and poison center penetrance into their service areas, extrapolated data predict the occurrence of approximately five million poisonings annually in the United States.

Most poisonings are accidental (89.2%); intentional exposures (including suicide and substance abuse and misuse) accounted for 8.1% of cases in 1986. Children under 6 years of age constituted 63.0% of all poisoning cases reported to the AAPCC. Of this group, those under 3 years of age represent 38.8% of total reported poisoning victims. Categories of substances most frequently implicated in poison exposures were cleaning substances, analgesics, plants, and cosmetics.

## Poison Control Centers

Poison control centers first appeared in the United States in the early 1950s. Although the centers were initially developed on a trial basis, the need for a central location for storage and subsequent dissemination of product ingredient information soon became apparent. During the 1960s, poison control centers developed rapidly throughout the United States, and by 1970, there were nearly 600 poison control centers. Great variability in the level of services provided by these centers existed.

In 1958, the AAPCC was formed to serve the rapidly expanding number of poison control centers. Activities of the AAPCC included the development of standards for poison center operation, public education and poison prevention programs, professional education, and data collection. In 1978, to meet a need for standardization for proficiency of operation, the AAPCC issued a set of criteria for regional poison control programs (Table 9.1). Since that time, development and certification of regional poison centers have occurred under the premise that these centers are capable of providing consistently more proficient service than the traditional type of "unregulated" poison center.[2] Today, approximately 32 poison centers have been certified by the AAPCC. As these centers handle more and more of the poisoning calls from consumers and health care professionals, the total number of poison centers in the country continues to decline.

## Roles for Pharmacists in Toxicology

Pharmacists work in a number of areas of toxicology. In poison control centers, they work as poison information specialists, answering calls from consumers and health care professionals. Some centers use pharmacists exclusively, whereas other centers utilize pharmacists in combination with nurses or other health care providers. The AAPCC recently developed an examination for the certification of poison information specialists. Pharmacists and registered nurses demonstrated superior performance on the examination compared with other poison information providers.[3]

In many poison control centers, pharmacists serve in a major clinical and/or administrative capacity. In over 65% of AAPCC-certified regional centers, pharmacists hold such positions as director and assistant director.

Pharmacists, both in traditional hospital pharmacy practice and in clinical roles, make substantial contributions to toxicology and the care of the poisoned patient. Knowledge of the actions, uses, side effects, and pharmacokinetics of drugs and familiarity with the appearance and ingredients of drug products can aid in the correct and rapid identification of an ingested product. Pharmacists are also responsible for maintaining an adequate supply of drugs used in the treatment of the poisoned patient.[4]

Pharmacists in both community and institutional practice play a role in poison prevention. A pharmacist is often the first health professional contacted when an ingestion has occurred. She or he is able to provide immediate first aid information while contacting or referring the patient to the appropriate poison control center. In addition to the utilization and support of child-resistant containers, pharmacists can promote poison prevention by distributing public education materials, preparing mass media materials, and talking to school and civic groups about poisoning and its prevention.

## Information Sources

Poison centers use a number of sources in the evaluation and treatment of exposures. These include basic information resources (such as Poisindex) and other references for specialized information, both primary and secondary.[5]

Poisindex is a computer-generated data base listing and identifying over 400,000 toxic and nontoxic substances. Substances are indexed by brand name, manufacturer's name, generic/chemical name, "street"/slang terminology, botanical/common names, and common misspellings. Management information and treatment protocols are written and

**Table 9.1** General Criteria for Certification of a Regional Poison Control Center

1. Regional poison information service available at all times
2. Regional system for providing comprehensive poisoning care
3. Regional poison data collection and reporting system
4. Outreach health professional education program
5. Outreach health public education program

edited by practicing toxicologists, physicians, clinical pharmacists, and nurses from around the world. This system is believed by many to be the single most valuable toxicology resource. Originally developed on microfiche and updated with new product and treatment data every quarter, the system is now also available on laser disc for use with personal computers and computer tapes for "mainframe" computers. Poisindex is available from Micromedex, Incorporated, a medical information company that also produces other resources such as Drugdex, Emergindex, Identidex, and TOMES. These are useful to pharmacists and poison center personnel as sources of additional information.

Drugdex provides current drug information complete with original references from the scientific literature. The information is comprehensive, covering such topics as dosage forms, side effects, compatibilities, drug interactions, dosing information, and therapeutic indications. Special "consultations" deal in depth with questions that frequently arise with certain drugs. Emergindex is a data base containing clinical information on particular disease states and is aimed at the physician practicing emergency medicine. It deals with pathophysiology, diagnosis, and treatment among other aspects of patient care.

The Identidex system provides rapid identification of tablets and capsules using color, shape, size, and manufacturer's imprint codes. Current slang/"street" terminology is included. TOMES (Toxicology, Occupational Medicine, Environmental Series) includes medical information concerning hazardous materials in industrial settings.

Other "on-line" data bases are available to many poison centers. The pharmacist should have access to these through personal computers or a medical library. Such systems as Medline, Toxline, Chemline, and Toxfile are available for computer searches by topic, author, or title of a particular publication. Numerous privately produced computer programs ("software") containing toxicology information are commercially available.

Primary resources have been defined as journal articles on current topics in toxicology. Original research, case reports, and reviews of pathophysiology, diagnosis, and treatment modalities are included in the resource materials necessary for a library of essential toxicology information.

Secondary resources are generally conceived to be standard textbooks of toxicology, along with primers that aid in the identification of plants and mushrooms, mammalian life, reptiles, amphibians, and fish. Many other texts are available in the local medical library or in the resources of the poison control center. Often used texts are listed in Table 9.2.

**Table 9.2** Textbooks Often Used in Reference to Toxicology

Arena JM: Poisoning–Toxicology–Symptoms–Treatments, 5th ed, 1986.
Dreisbach RH: Handbook of Poisoning, 11th ed, 1986.
Goldfrank LR: Toxicologic Emergencies—A Comprehensive Handbook in Problem Solving, 3rd ed, 1986.
Gosselin RE, Smith RP, Hodge HC: Clinical Toxicology of Commercial Products, 5th ed, 1984.
Grant WM: Toxicology of the Eye, 3rd ed, 1986.
Haddad LM, Winchester JF: Clinical Management of Poisoning and Drug Overdose, 1983.
Klaassen CD, Amdur MO, Doull J: Casarett and Doull's Toxicology: The Basic Science of Poisons, 3rd ed, 1986.
Sax NI: Dangerous Properties of Industrial Materials, 5th ed, 1979.

## General Treatment

### *Supportive Care*

The initial management of all patients is supportive therapy. Prior to any diagnostic procedure, support of the patient's vital signs is imperative to good clinical outcome. The initial vital function to be established is an adequate airway, which, combined with appropriate artificial ventilation, provides the oxygen required for cellular function. Enhancement of circulation with cardiac compressions, if necessary, is also vital in the initial management of any patient. All pharmacists and other health practitioners should learn the appropriate basics of cardiopulmonary resuscitation as taught, for example, by the American Heart Association.

It is also important to support vital signs other than "airway, breathing, and circulation." Many toxins cause fluctuations in body temperature. Phenobarbital can cause hypothermia in children; atropine, on the other hand, can cause extreme hyperthermia. Support of temperature with appropriate warming or cooling devices may be necessary for proper maintenance of cellular aerobic metabolism. Another metabolic parameter to be considered is glucose homeostasis. Any patient comatose upon presentation might be hypoglycemic. Therefore, an immediate bolus of $D_{25}W$ 1–2 mL/kg might be therapeutic. Opiate toxicity is another cause of obtundation; therefore, any comatose person without a specific, determined etiology should receive naloxone as a diagnostic/therapeutic trial. If there is any indication of chronic alcoholism, thiamine should be utilized in a dose of 50 mg intramuscularly initially.

### *Diagnosis/Assessment*

While initial supportive measures are undertaken, a history can be obtained either from the patient (if able to communicate) or from a family member or friend. This is often a prime function of other members of the health care team. The history should include answers to the following questions, among others.

1. What substance was ingested, inhaled, or spilled on skin or in eyes?
2. How much of the toxin was involved?
3. When did the incident occur?
4. What is the age, weight, and general medical condition of the patient?
5. Does the patient have any allergies?
6. What substances were available in the patient's environment?

This information is needed to make the initial diagnosis and therapeutic plan.

Groups of signs and symptoms can be useful in identifying the toxin responsible for a patient's clinical condition. In toxicology, these have been termed *toxidromes*.[6] Some of the most common toxidromes are listed in Table 9.3.[6] Other laboratory data, including electrocardiograms, chemical analyses, and radiologic examinations, are very helpful in identifying the toxic agent responsible.

### *Termination of Exposure*

The therapy employed in termination of exposure obviously depends upon the route of initial exposure. Gastrointestinal tract decontamination is often useful for the ingested toxin, irrigation of skin and eyes is important for dermal or ocular exposure, and immediate removal of the patient from the source of the toxin is vital for inhalation accidents.

Gastrointestinal tract decontamination is often accomplished by emesis. Gastrointestinal lavage ("stomach pumping") is another method.

#### Emesis

Syrup of ipecac is the agent most widely used to terminate exposure to an ingested toxin. This agent works centrally by stimulation of the chemoreceptor trigger zone and locally by irritation of the gastric mucosa. Its effectiveness in producing emesis is very high. Approximately 93% of pediatric patients vomit within 20 to 30 minutes of receiving a single dose of syrup of ipecac. In the remaining 7%, a second dose of ipecac often immediately produces emesis.[7,8]

Efficacy of ipecac in terms of the amount of stomach contents removed is less clear. A number of studies in animals and human volunteers have used small nontoxic quantities of a measurable drug or an inert marker. Extrapolation of these data to the overdose patient is difficult, but it does allow one to conclude that the exact amount of stomach contents removed by induced emesis is dependent on a number of variables, including physical characteristics of the compound (rates of disintegration, dissolution, and absorption), time elapsed since ingestion of toxin, other substances in the stomach (including drugs, food, or alcohol), amount of toxin ingested, and individual characteristics of the patient's gastrointestinal tract.

The disadvantage of syrup of ipecac is that it takes some time before emesis occurs. It must be assumed that the clinical condition of the patient will not change between administration of syrup of ipecac and emesis. Protracted vomiting may also delay administration of activated charcoal.

Absolute contraindications to the induction of emesis and use of syrup of ipecac include the following:

1. Patients who have ingested a caustic agent (strong alkalis, strong acids)
2. Patients who are comatose or have ingested substances that may cause rapid onset of coma
3. Patients who arc seizing or have ingested substances that may cause rapid onset of seizures
4. Patients who have lost their gag reflex and therefore cannot protect their airway

A relative contraindication to the induction of emesis is ingestion of a petroleum distillate such as gasoline or kerosene. In these patients the benefit of removal of the toxin must be weighed against the risk of its aspiration into the lungs.

The dose of syrup of ipecac is 15 mL (one tablespoonful) in infants and children up to the age of 12 years and 30 mL (two tablespoonsful) in patients older than 12 years. It should be pointed out that some poison centers recommend 30 mL for all pediatric patients older than 12 months. A prospective study of 100 patients revealed that those who received 30 mL of syrup of ipecac vomited 10 minutes sooner than those who received only 15 mL. Prolonged episodes of vomiting were not observed.[9] After administration of the ipecac, the patient should be given 8–16 oz of fluid, preferably water or other clear liquid. Milk should be avoided, as it has been shown to delay the onset of emesis.[10]

Problems associated with syrup of ipecac have been minimal considering its widespread use. Cardiotoxic effects related to the alkaloid emetine are reported only with abuse and overuse of the compound itself (as in patients with eating disorders). With recommended dosages, there has been *no* appreciable cardiotoxic effect of syrup of ipecac.[11,12]

Agents used in the past to induce vomiting (salt water, mustard, egg whites, copper sulfate) have been shown to be not only ineffective but potentially harmful. All of them delay appropriate therapy. As an example of a specific harmful effect, a tablespoonful of sodium chloride given to a small child can produce serious hypernatremia. In certain

**Table 9.3** Toxidromes

| |
|---|
| Narcotics |
| Miosis, respiratory depression, hypotension, naloxone reversal if opiates |
| Cholinergics |
| Salivation, lacrimation, urination, defecation, bradycardia, miosis, seizures |
| Anticholinergics |
| Dry skin, tachycardia, flushed appearance, delirium, hyperthermia, coma |
| Tricyclic antidepressants |
| Anticholinergic picture with prolonged QRS duration on ECG rhythm strip |
| Salicylates |
| Mixed respiratory alkalosis and metabolic acidosis, hyperglycemia, fever, anion gap |
| Methanol, ethylene glycol |
| Metabolic acidosis, anion gap, hyperosmolarity, "drunk" in appearance but does not smell of alcohol |

Adapted from Mofenson HC, Greensher J: The unknown poison. Pediatrics 974;54:336–342, with permission.

circumstances, when syrup of ipecac is not readily available and there is no health care facility nearby, then liquid dishwashing soap (not meant for electric dishwashers) has been safely and effectively used. For a further discussion of this topic, see Rodgers and Fort.[13,14]

Apomorphine, although a rapid, effective agent in producing emesis, is rarely used today. Disadvantages associated with its use include parenteral dosage form (excluding its use in the home), difficulty in preparation, and central nervous system (CNS) and respiratory depression. The CNS depression in children is sometimes prolonged and requires the administration of naloxone for reversal.

#### Gastric Lavage

Gastric lavage is the most rapid method of emptying the stomach if a patient is in a health care facility. Obviously, it cannot be used in the home or the prehospital setting; however, with a rapidly acting toxin that might induce seizures or coma prior to the onset of emesis after syrup of ipecac, gastric lavage remains advantageous in that it can be instituted quickly.

Lavage should always be performed with the largest-bore tube available.[15,16] The large size should allow a greater return of tablet or capsule fragments, plant particulate matter, or other matter. Feeding tubes, often used in the pediatric population, do not have adequate internal diameters for appropriate removal of pill fragments or granular toxins; however, if the toxin is purely a liquid, small-bore tubes may be utilized as long as immediate aspiration, not dilution, is performed.

After the tube is positioned, the stomach contents should be aspirated with suction initially prior to any dilution with fluid. This allows immediate removal of the most concentrated toxin. Dilution with its subsequent increase in solvent volume may increase the disintegration/dissolution rate of tablets; this rate is often the rate-limiting step in the absorption process. After the initial aspiration, normal saline is generally recommended as the solution of choice for instillation in lavage. Exotic fluids, such as hypertonic saline, sodium phosphate/biphosphate enema, or even plain tap water, have induced electrolyte imbalances in children.

There is only one absolute contraindication to lavage using a large-bore tube. If the patient has ingested a caustic (either alkali or acid), which might damage the esophageal mucosa, lavage should be avoided as it might result in esophageal rupture or perforation and the subsequent complications.

Caution should be exercised to protect the airway to avoid aspiration during the lavage procedure, especially in a comatose patient or a patient who might seize. As emesis often occurs with passage of a large-bore naso- or orogastric tube, suction should be readily available. Endotracheal intubation with a *cuffed* tube should be performed in a patient who is deeply comatose and nonresponsive and has no gag reflex. Lavage should be performed in the lateral decubitus position if possible.

#### Decontamination of Skin and Eyes

Many toxins can be adsorbed across intact skin and mucous membranes; others, such as caustics, can cause local tissue damage. For this reason, aggression in decontamination is indicated. Exposed skin should be washed immediately with large volumes of soap and water. Running water, such as a shower, may be preferred. Contaminated clothing should be changed.

For ocular exposures, irrigation with copious amounts of water or normal saline is usually indicated. One exception, however, is hydrofluoric acid, for which multiple irrigations may actually increase the likelihood of damage.[17]

### *Reduction of Bioavailability*

When an ingested toxin is not removed from the gastrointestinal tract by emesis induced with syrup of ipecac or by gastric lavage, it is helpful if absorption can be reduced (decreasing bioavailability) so that systemic toxicity might be reduced. In many instances, adsorptive agents can be used without initial therapeutic gastric emptying. Although many agents have been proposed for adsorbing toxins that remain in the gastrointestinal tract, activated charcoal is the most widely accepted.

#### Activated Charcoal

Activated charcoal is a specially prepared compound. Organic matter (often wood pulp) is burned anaerobically. The resulting pure carbon is broken down into small particles. Cleansing procedures follow: acid washing, steam, and oxidizing gas at extremely high temperatures. The result is a very clean compound with a large surface area for adsorption of toxin (standard charcoal has 1,000 $m^2/g$ of weight).

The kinetics of toxin removal by activated charcoal appear to depend upon several factors. The law of mass action is operative, in that increasing doses of charcoal adsorb increasing amounts of toxin.[18] Adsorption is rapid, occurring within the first few minutes of contact, except when food is also present in the gastrointestinal tract. The physical adsorption to charcoal prevents absorption across the mucosa of the gastrointestinal tract into the bloodstream.

Activated charcoal has been shown to be very effective in adsorbing many toxins and has been the subject of several reviews.[18,19] Note that charcoal does *not* adsorb cyanide, ferrous sulfate, lithium, boric acid, DDT, or carbamate insecticides. It should not be used if strong acids or alkalis are ingested.

***Timing*** The timing of administration of activated charcoal is a controversial issue. Frequently, gastric emptying is instituted first in the poisoned patient and is followed by activated charcoal. If emesis is induced with syrup of ipecac, the resultant vomiting may lead to intolerance of the charcoal preparation; however, waiting until emesis ceases delays the administration of charcoal.

Activated charcoal alone (without gastric emptying) may actually be the most effective therapeutic intervention in some situations, especially if it is administered immediately after a toxic exposure.[20] Kulig et al compared two groups of patients treated randomly with either gastric emptying/activated charcoal or charcoal and a cathartic alone. No significant differences in clinical outcome were found between the two groups.[21] In a study of simulated salicylate overdose, Curtis et al[22] showed that activated charcoal/magnesium sulfate ($MgSO_4$) was more effective in reducing salicylate absorption than was ipecac-induced emesis alone or ipecac-induced emesis followed by activated charcoal/$MgSO_4$. When the ingested agents may cause the rapid onset of seizures or coma (e.g., camphor, large amounts of liquid theophylline preparations, propoxyphene, isoniazid), it is more prudent to administer charcoal initially to prevent the complications caused by simultaneous seizures/emesis or coma/emesis.

***Preparations*** Activated charcoal is available as a powder. As such, it is gritty in texture and unpalatable. In an effort to improve its acceptance, it has been mixed with liquid and artificial flavors. Many of these products adsorb to the charcoal, decreasing its ability to adsorb toxins. Several agents have been used to increase the viscosity of the liquid, thus helping to keep the powder in a slurry and mask the texture. Sorbitol, in a 70% solution, adds sweetness without decreasing the efficacy of the compound. The sorbitol solution also acts as an osmotic cathartic so that others do not have to be used. Many preparations are now available in premixed formulations of charcoal in liquid (either water or 70% sorbitol).

***Dosing*** The most common error in administration of activated charcoal is delivery of an inadequate dose. As the law of mass action applies, it has been suggested that charcoal should be given in an amount five to ten times the quantity of the toxin.[18] In light of the fact that the exact quantity of toxin is often not known, at present the recommended dose of charcoal is 20–30 g in children under the age of 12 and 60–100 g in persons older than 12.

Charcoal is most commonly administered in conjunction with a cathartic. Cathartics serve to decrease the chances of inspissated charcoal in the gut and may help to decrease bioavailability further by decreasing transit time and, hence, decreasing time available for absorption of toxin.

***Complications*** There are few complications to the appropriate use of activated charcoal. Emesis often occurs, especially if the compound is given soon after ipecac-induced emesis. Constipation has been reported, but is a rare event when charcoal is given with some type of cathartic. If emesis occurs, aspiration into the tracheobronchial tree, with its subsequent clinical sequelae, is a possibility.[23]

**Cathartics**

It is widely believed that cathartics decrease transit time in the gastrointestinal tract and therefore decrease absorption of toxin by limiting exposure to the mucosa. This hypothesis has never been proven by scientific studies; however, cathartics remain in wide use in the United States. Cathartics may have a place in decreasing transit time of charcoal so that inspissation does not occur; however, care must be taken to choose an agent that is not adsorbed appreciably to the charcoal itself, thereby rendering the charcoal ineffective.

***Preparations*** Sodium sulfate, magnesium sulfate, and magnesium citrate are very commonly used. The sulfate products are given in a dose of 30 g diluted in 300 mL of water for the adult or of 250 mg/kg for the pediatric patient (as a 10% solution). Sorbitol, in a 70% solution, is an osmotic cathartic and is the most effective in rapidly evacuating charcoal from the gut.[24]

***Complications*** The major complications of cathartic therapy are imbalances of fluid and electrolyte status. Continued stooling can lead to marked water loss. Magnesium cathartics should never be used in patients with renal failure, as decreased urinary excretion might lead to magnesium intoxication. Magnesium toxicity has even been observed in a previously healthy patient who received repetitive doses of magnesium citrate.[25] The heavy sodium load often absorbed from sodium sulfate can cause fluid retention, with dire consequences in patients with underlying heart failure or hypertension.

**Other Agents**

Some other agents have been recommended as adsorbents. None is as widely accepted as activated charcoal. One, the "universal antidote," is mentioned only to point out that it has *no* effectiveness and might delay appropriate therapy. The "universal antidote" refers to the outdated practice of mixing 50% burnt toast, 25% tannic acid (tea), and 25% milk of magnesia into one compound.

The diatomaceous earths (fuller's earth and bentonite) have long been used as adsorbents, especially in paraquat or diquat poisoning. Kaolin–pectin has also been used. Because activated charcoal is ubiquitous, its use should be considered in all situations where an adsorbent is needed quickly.

## *Enhancement of Elimination*

**Extracorporeal Removal**

Extracorporeal removal of drugs or toxins from the body can be accomplished by peritoneal dialysis, hemodialysis, or charcoal hemoperfusion.

Peritoneal dialysis is rarely used today although it is widely available. Considered to be less invasive than hemodialysis, peritoneal dialysis is also less effective in that toxin removal across the peritoneal membrane is both slow and inefficient.

Hemodialysis is an efficient procedure in removing drugs/toxins with certain characteristics. The compound must be small enough to cross the dialysis membrane (low molecular weight). It must be water soluble. The proportion of the compound bound to plasma proteins must be relatively small. The volume of distribution must be small, as the only body "compartment" available for dialysis is plasma. These characteristics are described at length by Gwilt and Perrier.[26]

Hemodialysis is the treatment of choice in very few poisonings; the most notable are ethylene glycol, methanol, and diquat. Other agents for which hemodialysis might be useful in certain clinical circumstances are salicylates, phenobarbital, ethanol, lithium, and isopropanol. If they meet the criteria for dialyzability, toxic metabolites are removed in addition to the parent compounds. For an exhaustive list of compounds that are readily removed by hemodialysis, see Winchester et al.[27]

The complications of hemodialysis must be considered. Appropriate arterial and venous access for adequate blood flow is often difficult to obtain in small infants. Electrolyte and fluid imbalances and hypotension can result.

Hemoperfusion removes toxins by passing blood through a column containing either activated charcoal or carbon. Toxic agents adsorb to the charcoal or carbon. Resin hemoperfusion columns are no longer available in the United States. Hemoperfusion is often more effective in toxin removal than is hemodialysis. It is most often used in overdoses of sedative–hypnotics (barbiturates, ethchlorvynol, glutethimide, meprobamate, methaqualone) and theophylline. The risks associated with hemoperfusion include hypotension, hypocalcemia, thrombocytopenia, air embolism, charcoal embolism, and vascular damage secondary to catheter placement. This topic is reviewed extensively by Winchester.[27]

### Forced Diuresis and Urinary pH Changes

Forced diuresis with or without the manipulation of urinary pH is rarely used or recommended for the enhancement of toxin elimination. It was once believed, on a theoretical basis, that "ion trapping" could be used to hasten the elimination of weak acids or bases in the urine. If the toxin was excreted into the urine and there formed an ion, it could not be reabsorbed. Thus, weak acids were to be "trapped" in alkaline urines, and weak bases in acid urines. This procedure was often recommended for salicylate intoxication, phenobarbital intoxication, and poisoning with phencyclidine, amphetamines, and strychnine; however, since the newer treatment modalities became available, manipulation of urinary pH has been found to engender more risks than benefits (small amounts of toxins removed) to the patient. For example, it is very difficult to produce an alkaline urine (pH >7.0) in a pediatric patient. The large amounts of sodium bicarbonate and fluid necessary can lead to hypernatremia and fluid overload. The use of intravenous ammonium chloride to produce an acidic urine in cases of amphetamine or phencyclidine toxicity can actually increase the risk of renal failure in these patients. Already prone to rhabdomyolysis from the toxin, the acidic urine increases deposition of the resulting myoglobin in the renal parenchyma, causing damage.

Forced diuresis was initially thought to increase elimination of toxins by decreasing the time available for reabsorption in the kidney tubule. As many toxins predispose patients to pulmonary edema, the increased fluid load represents a risk that often outweighs the benefits.

As manipulations of both urine volume/flow and urinary pH are associated with risks to the patient, each clinical situation should be carefully evaluated on an individual basis. Other therapeutic modalities, such as multiple-dose activated charcoal or hemodialysis/hemoperfusion, may be more efficacious and safer.

### Multiple-Dose Charcoal

There is evidence in the literature that multiple doses of activated charcoal in the gastrointestinal tract enhance the elimination of several drugs, especially theophylline, phenobarbital, and digitoxin. Although the mechanism of action has still not been described with certainty, kinetic changes evidencing enhanced elimination with this therapeutic modality have been observed.

In patients with prolonged half-lives for theophylline, administration of multiple-dose charcoal significantly reduced the half-life of intravenously administered aminophylline.[28] Thus, it had to be enhancing elimination in some fashion rather than preventing absorption, as 100% of the intravenous preparation is systemically bioavailable. The half-lives of phenobarbital, carbamazepine, and phenylbutazone can all be shortened by using multiple doses of activated charcoal.[29,30] Although these kinetic changes are readily observable, more research is necessary to completely define the role of multiple-dose charcoal in all clinical situations.

It has been proposed that multiple-dose charcoal works by interrupting enterohepatic recirculation (for compounds for which that route of metabolism/elimination is important) or by making the gastrointestinal tract act as a "reverse dialysis" membrane. For a succinct review of these proposed mechanisms of action, see Derlet.[31]

Multiple-dose charcoal is usually delivered in a dosage of 20–60 g every 4 to 6 hours. Initial dosages should be given in conjunction with a cathartic; after the appearance of a "charcoal stool," the charcoal should be given in water to avoid the electrolyte and fluid imbalances caused by massive diarrhea secondary to cathartic overdose.

## *Antidotes*

An *antidote* is a remedy that counteracts the effects of a poison. Few drugs or poisons have specific therapeutic antidotes. As previously discussed, treatment of the poisoned patient involves mainly termination of exposure, reduction of bioavailability of remaining toxin, enhancement of elimination of systemically absorbed product, and supportive care. There are, however, several categories of antidotes that are useful in the management of specific toxins: (1) pharmacologic antagonists, (2) agents that form inert complexes, and (3) miscellaneous agents.

Pharmacologic antagonists exert their action by blockade of specific receptors (naloxone, atropine), by inhibition of conversion of a toxin to a more toxic metabolic product (ethanol), or by enhancement of endogenous detoxification (pralidoxime, *N*-acetylcysteine).

Agents that form inert complexes act by neutralizing the toxic effects of the venom/toxin while allowing it to be easily excreted from the body. Examples are chelating agents such as deferoxamine, dimercaprol, and calcium disodium EDTA; antivenoms; antitoxins; and antibody fragments.

Miscellaneous agents work by a number of mechanisms. For example, pyridoxine is useful in replacing a cofactor depleted by isoniazid overdose. Its administration in this instance can actually stop seizure activity.

For a review of these and other agents, refer to Table 9.2 and numerous publications on this topic.[32–34]

## Summary

Toxicology is an exciting new specialty in the medical and pharmaceutic sciences. New therapeutic interventions are developed and studied daily. The role of the pharmacist in this field varies widely, but, whether in retail practice, hospital dispensing, clinical hospital practice, or administration, *each* pharmacist is involved in some manner with clinical toxicology.

## References


1. Litovitz TL, et al. 1986 Annual report of the American Association of Poison Control Centers National Data Collection System 1987;5:405–445.
2. Manoguerra AS, Temple AR. Observations of the current status of poison control centers in the United States. Emerg Med Clin North Am 1984;2:185–197.
3. Litovitz TL, Klein-Schwartz W, Oderda GM, et al. Poison information providers: An assessment of proficiency. Am J Emerg Med 1984;2:129–137.
4. Troutman W. The pharmacist and poisoning, editorial. Am J Hosp Pharm 1978;35:1351.
5. Veltri JC. Toxicology information resources for poison control centers. Clin Toxicol 1978;12:335–356.
6. Mofenson HC, Greensher J. The unknown poison. Pediatrics 1974;54:336–342.
7. Krenzelok EP, Dean BS. Syrup of ipecac failures: A two-year review of 4306 patients. Vet Hum Toxicol 1985;26:317.
8. Litovitz TL, Klein-Schwartz W, Oderda GM, et al. Ipecac administration in children under one year of age. Pediatrics 1985;76:761–764.
9. Dean BS, Krenzelok EP. Syrup of ipecac: 15 mL versus 30 mL in pediatric poisonings. Clin Toxicol 1985;23:165–170.
10. Varipapa RJ, Oderda GM. Effect of milk on ipecac-induced emesis. N Engl J Med 1977;296:112.
11. Manno BR, Manno JE. Toxicology of ipecac: A review. Clin Toxicol 1977;10:221–242.
12. Rauber A. The cardiac safety of ipecac used as a therapeutic emetic. Vet Hum Toxicol 1978;20:166–168.
13. Rodgers GC, Fort P. Use of dish soap as an emetic in the outpatient management of accidental poisonings. Pediatr Res 1984;18:23A.
14. Rodgers GC, Fort P. Use of liquid dishwashing detergent as an emetic in the outpatient management of poisoning—an update. Vet Hum Toxicol 1985;28:321.
15. Burke M. Gastric lavage and emesis in the treatment of ingested poisons: A review and a clinical study of lavage in ten adults. Resuscitation 1972;1:91–105.
16. Fane LR, Combs HF, Decker WJ. Physical parameters in gastric lavage. Clin Toxicol 1971;4:389–395.
17. McCulley JP, Whiting DW, Petitt MG, et al. Hydrofluoric acid burns of the eye. J Occup Med 1983;25:447–450.
18. Neuvonen PJ. Clinical pharmacokinetics of oral activated charcoal in acute intoxications. Clin Pharmacokinet 1982;7:465–489.
19. Greensher J, Mofenson HC, Picchioni AL, et al. Activated charcoal updated. J Am Coll Emer Phys 1979;8:261–263.
20. Neuvonen PJ, Vartiainen M, Tokola O. Comparison of activated charcoal and ipecac syrup in the prevention of drug absorption. Eur J Clin Pharm 1983;24:557–562.
21. Kulig K, Bar-Or D, Cantrill SV, et al. Management of acutely poisoned patients without gastric emptying. Ann Emerg Med 1985;14:562–567.
22. Curtis RA, Barone J, Giacora N. Efficacy of ipecac and activated charcoal/cathartic: Prevention of salicylate absorption in a simulated overdose. Arch Intern Med 1984;144:48–52.
23. Pollack MM, Dunbar BS, Holbrook PR, et al. Aspiration of activated charcoal and gastric contents. Ann Emerg Med 1981;10:528–529.
24. Krenzelok EP. Gastrointestinal transit times of cathartics combined with charcoal. Ann Emerg Med 1985;14:1152–1155.
25. Jones J, Heiselman D, Dougherty J, et al. Cathartic-induced magnesium toxicity during overdose management. Ann Emerg Med 1986;15:1214–1218.
26. Gwilt PR, Perrier D. Plasma protein binding and distribution characteristics of drugs as indices of their hemodialyzability. Clin Pharmacol Ther 1978;24:154–161.
27. Winchester JF, Gelfand MC, Knepshield JH, et al. Dialysis and hemoperfusion of poisons and drugs—update. Trans Am Soc Artif Intern Organs 1977;23:762–837.
28. Radomski L, Park GD, Goldberg MJ, et al. Model for theophylline overdose treatment with oral activated charcoal. Clin Pharmacol Ther 1984;35:402–408.
29. Neuvonen PJ, Elonen E. Effect of activated charcoal on absorption and elimination of phenobarbitone, carbamazepine and phenylbutazone in man. Eur J Clin Pharmacol 1980;17:51–57.
30. Berg MG, Berlinger WG, Goldberg MJ, et al. Acceleration of the body clearance of phenobarbital by oral activated charcoal. N Engl J Med 1982;307:642–644.
31. Derlet RW, Albertson TE. Activated charcoal—past, present, and future. West J Med 1986;145:493–496.
32. Joe G, McKinney H, Wythe E. Antidotes—1985. CSHP Voice 1985;12:7–10.
33. Meredith T, Caisley J, Volans G. Emergency drugs: Agents used in the treatment of poisoning. Br Med J 1984;289:742–748.
34. Persson H. Aspects on antidote therapy in acute poisoning affecting the nervous system. Acta Neurol Scand 1984;70 (suppl 100):203–213.

# 2 Disorders of Organ Systems

# Section One
# Cardiovascular Disorders

## Chapter 10 / Hypertension

David W. Hawkins, PharmD, and Henry I. Bussey, PharmD, FCCP

Arterial blood pressure is generated by the interplay between blood flow and the resistance to blood flow. It reaches a peak during cardiac systole (systolic pressure) and a nadir at the end of diastole (diastolic pressure).[1,2] Arterial blood pressure is conventionally measured in millimeters of mercury and recorded as systolic pressure over diastolic pressure (e.g., 120/80 mm Hg). The difference between systolic and diastolic pressure, pulse pressure, is an indicator of the tone of arterial walls. The mean arterial pressure is the average pressure throughout the cardiac cycle. Mean arterial pressure (MAP) can be estimated by adding one third of the pulse pressure (PP) to the diastolic blood pressure (DBP): $MAP = \frac{1}{3} PP + DBP$.

Under normal physiologic conditions, the arterial blood pressure stays within narrow limits. It may reach its height during physical or emotional stress and it usually falls to its lowest level during sleep. Blood pressure tends to be lower in women than men, it tends to be higher in blacks than whites, and it rises with age.

Arterial blood pressure can be defined hemodynamically as the product of cardiac output (CO) and total peripheral resistance (TPR): $BP = CO \times TPR$. Cardiac output is the major determinant of systolic pressure while total peripheral resistance largely determines the level of diastolic pressure. In turn, cardiac output is a function of stroke volume, heart rate, and venous capacitance. Factors that increase stroke volume or heart rate may increase cardiac output and, consequently, systolic blood pressure. Venous capacitance affects the volume of blood (or preload) that is returned to the heart through the central venous circulation. Venous dilatation increases venous capacitance and decreases preload and systolic pressure. Contraction of the peripheral veins, of course, would cause the opposite effect.

Total peripheral resistance is regulated chiefly by contraction and dilation of the arterioles. Arteriolar constriction increases peripheral resistance and thus diastolic blood pressure. Other factors that affect intravascular resistance include the elasticity of aortic and arterial walls and blood viscosity.

### Definition

As arterial blood pressure is a continuous variable, it is impossible to define a cutoff point below which the blood pressure is normal and above which the pressure is abnormally high. Nevertheless, evidence from epidemiologic studies clearly indicates a strong correlation between blood pressure and cardiovascular morbidity and mortality.[3,4] The higher the pressure the more likely an individual will experience stroke, myocardial infarction, angina, heart failure, renal failure, or early death from a cardiovascular cause. In addition, large-scale clinical studies have shown that the increased risk of cardiovascular disease and death associated with elevated blood pressure is substantially reduced by interventions that lower blood pressure.[5–7] Moreover, the reduction in risk is proportional to the reduction in blood pressure.

It is therefore reasonable to establish what constitutes high blood pressure based upon epidemiologic and clinical data. Using this approach, hypertension has been defined arbitrarily as a systolic blood pressure greater than 140 mm Hg or a diastolic pressure greater than 90 mm Hg.[8] High blood pressure has been further classified as mild, moderate, or severe based upon the following diastolic blood pressure levels:

| | |
|---|---|
| Mild | 90–104 mm Hg |
| Moderate | 105–114 mm Hg |
| Severe | ≥115 mm Hg |

### Prevalence[1,2]

According to the previously stated definition of high blood pressure, the prevalence of hypertension in the United States is 18.5% in white men, 15.7% in white women, 27.8% in black men, and 28.6% in black women. Because blood pressure increases with age, the prevalence of hypertension in those individuals over 65 years old is approximately 40% in white people and 50% in black people.

## Etiology[3,4,9–11]

Hypertension is a heterogenous disorder that may result from either a specific cause (secondary hypertension) or some underlying pathophysiologic mechanism stemming from an unknown etiology (primary hypertension). About 10% of people who suffer from high blood pressure have secondary hypertension. In most of these, chronic renal disease or renovascular disease is the cause of hypertension. Other conditions that are known to cause secondary hypertension include pheochromocytoma, Cushing's syndrome, primary aldosteronism, and coarctation of the aorta. In some instances, exposure to various exogenous substances may produce hypertension. The most notable of these are estrogens, glucocorticoids, licorice, sympathomimetic amines, nonsteroidal anti-inflammatory agents, and tyramine-containing foods in combination with monoamine oxidase (MAO) inhibitors.

In the vast majority of individuals with high blood pressure, a specific cause of sustained hypertension cannot be found. This hypertension of unknown etiology has been referred to as benign or essential. These terms, however, are misleading and should be replaced by the more appropriate term: primary or idiopathic hypertension. A vigorous search for a single underlying abnormality that eventuates into high blood pressure has led to the discovery of numerous mechanisms that may contribute to the pathogenesis of hypertension.

## Pathophysiology[3,4,9–16]

Multiple factors may contribute to the development of primary hypertension including abnormal neural mechanisms; defects in peripheral autoregulation; disturbances in sodium, calcium, and natriuretic hormone; and malfunctions in either humoral or vasodepressor mechanisms.

### *Neural Components*

Both the central (CNS) and the autonomic nervous systems are intricately involved in the maintenance of arterial blood pressure.

Stimulation of certain areas within the CNS (nucleus tractus solitarius, vagal nuclei, vasomotor center, and the area postrema) can result in either an increase or a decrease in blood pressure. For example, $\alpha$-adrenergic stimulation within the CNS decreases blood pressure through an inhibitory effect on the vasomotor center. Increased angiotensin II, on the other hand, increases sympathetic outflow from the vasomotor center which eventuates in an increase in blood pressure.

Located on the presynaptic surface of sympathetic terminals are a variety of receptors that either enhance or inhibit norepinephrine release. The $\alpha$ and $\beta$ presynaptic receptors play a role in negative and positive feedback to the norepinephrine-containing vesicles located near the neuronal ending. Stimulation of presynaptic $\alpha$ ($\alpha_2$) receptors exerts a negative inhibition on norepinephrine release. Stimulation of presynaptic $\beta$ receptors facilitates further release of norepinephrine.

$\alpha$ and $\beta$ receptors are also located on the surface of effector cells innervated by sympathetic neuronal fibers. Stimulation of postsynaptic $\alpha$ ($\alpha_1$) receptors on arterioles and venules results in vasoconstriction. There are two types of postsynaptic $\beta$ receptors, $\beta_1$ and $\beta_2$. Both types of $\beta$-adrenergic receptors are present in all tissue innervated by the sympathetic nervous system; however, the distribution of $\beta_1$ and $\beta_2$ receptors is such that in some tissue $\beta_1$ receptors predominate and in other tissue $\beta_2$ receptors predominate. Stimulation of $\beta_1$ receptors in the heart results in an increase in heart rate and contractility. When $\beta_2$ receptors in the arterioles and venules are stimulated, vasodilation occurs.

The major negative-feedback mechanism controlling sympathetic activity is the system of baroreceptor reflexes. Baroreceptors are nerve endings lying in the walls of large arteries, especially in the carotid arteries and aortic arch. The baroreceptors respond extremely rapidly to changes in arterial pressure. Baroreceptor impulses are transmitted to the brain stem primarily through the ninth cranial nerve and vagus nerves. In this reflex system, an acute elevation in arterial pressure increases the rate of baroreceptor discharge, which results in vasodilation throughout the peripheral circulatory system and a decrease in heart rate and myocardial contractility. Conversely, low pressure has the opposite effect, causing reflex vasoconstriction and increase in heart rate and force of contraction. These baroreceptor reflex mechanisms may be blunted in elderly individuals.

A pathologic disturbance in any of these neural components that modulate arterial blood pressure could conceivably lead to a sustained elevation in blood pressure. It is reasonable to postulate that the primary defect can occur in any of the four major components: central nervous system, autonomic nerve fibers, adrenergic receptors, or baroreceptors. Also, because they are so physiologically interrelated, a defect in one component may disturb the normal function in another, and the combined abnormalities may then cause hypertension.

### *Peripheral Autoregulatory Components*

Abnormalities in either the renal or tissue autoregulatory processes could cause hypertension. In fact, it seems reasonable to postulate that individuals may first develop a renal defect for sodium excretion and then reset their tissue autoregulatory processes to a higher arterial blood pressure.

Normally, the volume–pressure adaptive mechanism of the kidney works well to maintain a normal blood pressure. When the blood pressure drops, the kidneys adapt by retaining more sodium and water. This leads to plasma volume expansion, which increases blood pressure. Conversely, when blood pressure rises above normal, sodium and water excretion are increased, plasma volume and cardiac output are reduced, and the blood pressure returns to normal.

Local autoregulatory processes operate to maintain adequate tissue oxygenation. When oxygen demand is low, the arteriolar bed is in a relatively constricted state. Peripheral vascular resistance is maintained at a sufficient level to regulate adequate blood flow (flow = pressure/resistance).

An increase in metabolic demand triggers arteriolar vasodilation through autoregulation. This then lowers peripheral vascular resistance to increase blood flow and oxygen delivery.

An initial defect in the renal adaptive mechanism could lead to plasma volume expansion and increase blood flow to peripheral tissues even when blood pressure is normal. To offset the increase in blood flow, local tissue autoregulatory processes would induce arteriolar constriction to raise the peripheral vascular resistance. In time, a thickening of the arteriolar walls may occur, resulting in a sustained elevation in peripheral vascular resistance. An increase in total peripheral vascular resistance is a common underlying problem in patients with primary hypertension.

### *Humoral Mechanisms*

At least two possible humoral abnormalities may be responsible for causing primary hypertension in some individuals. One involves the renin–angiotensin–aldosterone system which has been well described. The other entails the presence of a natriuretic hormone that interferes with sodium transport.

The renin–angiotensin–aldosterone system is important to the regulation of sodium, potassium, and fluid balance, and it significantly influences vascular tone and sympathetic nervous system activity. Of course, all of these factors contribute to blood pressure homeostasis.

Renin is synthesized and stored in the juxtaglomerular cells which are located primarily in the media of the renal afferent arterioles. Several factors are known to control renin release. These can be grouped into intrarenal factors (such as perfusion pressure, catecholamines, angiotensin II) and extrarenal factors (such as sodium, chloride, and potassium).

The juxtaglomerular cell functions as a baroreceptor sensing device in the afferent arteriole. Decreased perfusion pressure leads to an increase in renin secretion and vice versa. The juxtaglomerular apparatus also contains a group of specialized distal tubule cells referred to collectively as the macula densa. The flux of sodium and chloride across the cells influences renin release. A decrease in the amount of sodium and chloride delivered in the distal tubule stimulates renin release.

Angiotensin II has been shown to directly inhibit the release of renin through negative feedback. Catecholamines increase renin release probably by directly stimulating the juxtaglomerular cells through an action involving the formation of cyclic AMP. Both potassium and calcium may also play a direct role in renin release. Decreased serum potassium or intracellular calcium stimulates renin release by the juxtaglomerular cells.

Renin catalyzes the conversion of angiotensinogen to angiotensin I, which is then subsequently converted to angiotensin II by angiotensin-converting enzyme. An increase in circulating angiotensin II can cause an elevation in blood pressure through both pressor and volume effects. The pressor effects of angiotensin II include direct vasoconstriction, stimulation of catecholamine release from the adrenal medulla, and a centrally mediated increase in sympathetic nervous system activity. Angiotensin II also stimulates the release of aldosterone from the adrenal gland, which leads to retention of both sodium and fluid, with a resultant increase in plasma volume and blood pressure. Clearly, any disturbance in the renin–angiotensin–aldosterone system that leads to an increase in any or all of the three components could produce hypertension.

Another humoral factor that may be involved in the development of primary hypertension is the increased concentration of natriuretic hormone. The proposed role of natriuretic hormone is to inhibit $Na^+$, $K^+$-ATPase and, thus, to interfere with sodium transport across cell membranes. It has been suggested that an inherited defect in the kidney's ability to eliminate sodium would cause an increase in extracellular fluid and plasma volume as discussed earlier. This may cause a compensatory increase in the concentration of circulating natriuretic hormone which would increase urinary excretion of sodium and water. This same hormone, however, is also thought to block the active transport of sodium out of arteriolar smooth muscle cells. The increased intracellular concentration of sodium would ultimately lead to increased vascular tone and hypertension.

### *Vasodepressor Mechanisms*

A number of prostaglandins (PGs) and kinins are capable of reducing blood pressure by producing arteriolar dilatation. Two renal prostaglandins ($PGE_2$ and PGA) may also promote the excretion of sodium and water.

It has been postulated that a deficiency in the synthesis of vasodilating prostaglandins and/or an altered kallikrein–kinin system may play a role in the development of primary hypertension.

### *Influence of Dietary Sodium, Calcium, and Potassium on Blood Pressure*

The evidence linking excess sodium to the development of hypertension is based on both epidemiologic studies and clinical experiments. In general, population studies indicate that high salt intake is associated with a high prevalence of stroke and hypertension and low salt intake is associated with a low prevalence of hypertension. Clinical studies have consistently shown that restriction of salt intake in the diet lowers blood pressure in many (but not all) subjects with hypertension. The exact mechanism by which excess sodium leads to hypertension is not known, but it is thought to be linked to the natriuretic hormone hypothesis discussed before. It has been proposed that an increased sodium intake together with an inherited defect in the kidney's ability to excrete sodium leads to a substantial increase in circulating natriuretic hormone. As previously mentioned, natriuretic hormone inhibits intracellular sodium transport which causes increased vascular reactivity and, consequently, a rise in blood pressure.

Altered calcium homeostasis may also play an important role in the pathogenesis of hypertension. The calcium hypothesis states that a lack of calcium in the diet leads to a disturbance in the balance between intracellular and extracellular calcium. This imbalance is characterized by an increased intracellular concentration of calcium which leads to altered vascular smooth muscle function and increased peripheral vascular resistance. Some studies have shown that supplementing the diet with calcium results in a modest decrease in the blood pressure of hypertensive subjects. More research is needed to clarify the role of altered calcium homeostasis in causing hypertension in humans.

The role of potassium fluctuations is also inadequately understood. Potassium depletion may cause an increase in peripheral vascular resistance, but the clinical impact of small changes in the serum potassium concentration is not clearly defined. Furthermore, very limited data have suggested that potassium supplementation is associated with a reduced incidence of stroke, but this issue needs further study before supplementation can be endorsed.

## Clinical Presentation[3,4,9–11]

Patients with uncomplicated, primary hypertension are usually asymptomatic initially. While a complete history and physical examination may help identify concerns that warrant further evaluation, a few basic tests should be performed in all hypertensive patients prior to initiating drug therapy.[8] Hemoglobin and hematocrit, complete urinalysis, serum potassium and creatinine, and electrocardiogram should be performed to determine the severity of vascular disease and to screen for possible causes of hypertension. Total and high-density-lipoprotein cholesterol, plasma glucose, and serum uric acid are indicated to assess other risk factors and to develop baseline data for monitoring drug-induced metabolic changes. As the hypertension progresses, however, symptoms characteristic of cardiovascular, cerebrovascular, or renal disease may occur as the patient develops target organ damage. Patients with secondary hypertension usually complain of symptoms suggestive of the underlying disorder. For example, almost all patients with pheochromocytoma have a history of paraxysmal headaches, sweating, tachycardia, and palpitations occurring singly or in combinations. More than half of the patients with this form of secondary hypertension suffer episodes of orthostatic dizziness or syncope. In primary aldosteronism, hypokalemic symptoms usually manifest including muscle cramps, muscle weakness, and intermittent paralysis or inability to use the proximal leg muscles. Patients who present with hypertension secondary to Cushing's syndrome may complain of weight gain, polyuria, edema, menstrual irregularities, recurrent acne, or muscular weakness.

Frequently, the only sign of primary hypertension is an elevated blood pressure. The rest of the physical examination may be completely normal. Again, as the hypertension progresses, signs of end-organ damage begin to appear. These are chiefly related to pathologic changes in the eye, brain, heart, kidneys, and peripheral blood vessels.

The funduscopic exam may reveal arteriolar narrowing reflective of increased peripheral vascular resistance and/or arteriovenous nicking, which is a consequence of long-standing arteriosclerosis. Retinal hemorrhages and exudates reflect serious vasculitis secondary to high arterial blood pressure indicative of accelerated hypertension. Papilledema in hypertensive patients suggests a malignant stage of high blood pressure requiring rapid treatment. Clinically, the appearance of papilledema or encephalopathy in a patient with hypertension is considered an emergency or crisis situation in which immediate reduction of blood pressure is imperative.

The neurologic examination will reveal gross neurologic deficits in patients with previous cerebral infarcts. A slight hemiparesis with some incoordination and hyperreflexia may also be found upon careful neurologic examination.

Auscultation of the heart may identify an accentuated second heart ($S_2$) sound created by a high intraaortic diastolic pressure, a systolic ejection murmur caused by aortic sclerosis, an $S_4$ gallop rhythm indicative of concentric hypertrophy and decreased ventricular compliance, or an $S_3$ gallop sound secondary to ventricular dilatation in patients with congestive heart failure.

The physical examination may provide clues for diagnosing secondary hypertension. For example, patients with coarctation of the aorta may have diminished or even absent femoral pulses and patients with renal artery stenosis may have an abdominal bruit. Of course, patients with Cushing's syndrome will have the classic physical features (i.e., moon face, buffalo hump, hirsutism, abdominal striae, etc.) that characterize individuals with this endocrine disorder.

Certain routine laboratory tests may help identify patients with secondary hypertension. A low serum potassium before antihypertensive therapy is begun may suggest a primary hyperaldosteronism. The presence of protein, blood cells, and casts in the urine may indicate an underlying parenchymal kidney disease as the cause of hypertension.

More specific laboratory tests are used to diagnose secondary hypertension. These include plasma and urinary catecholamines for pheochromocytoma, plasma and urinary aldosterone levels for primary aldosteronism, and angiography, renal vein renins, and digital subtraction angiography for renovascular disease.

### *Blood Pressure Measurement*

The usual, indirect method of measuring blood pressure is with the sphygmomanometer cuff on the patient's arm at the level of the heart. It is important to use a proper size cuff to avoid overestimating the actual pressure when the cuff is too small and underestimating the actual pressure when the cuff is too large. The inflatable rubber bag should encircle at least 80% of the arm and the width of the cuff should be at least two thirds the length of the upper arm.

Proper technique requires rapid inflation of the cuff to about 30 mm Hg above the point at which the radial pulse disappears and then release at a rate of 2 to 3 mm Hg per second. As the pressure falls, the Korotkoff sounds become audible through a stethoscope applied over the brachial artery in the antecubital fossa. The first sounds consist of clear tapping sounds. Systolic blood pressure should be recorded at the level the first tapping sound is heard. Diastolic blood pressure should be read at the moment all sounds disappear (i.e., at the fifth Korotkoff phase).

It should be emphasized that a single reading of blood pressure elevation does not constitute a diagnosis of hypertension. If the average of three successive readings taken on different days is 140/90 mm Hg or higher, then the patient can be declared hypertensive.

Several factors, in addition to those mentioned previously, may give misleading blood pressure measurements. A falsely high blood pressure may be recorded in elderly patients with a rigid, calcified brachial artery. This has been referred to as pseudohypertension, because the actual pressure as determined by direct intraarterial measurement is much lower than that obtained by the indirect cuff method. The occurrence of an "auscultatory gap" in some patients may result in an erroneous systolic or diastolic measurement. As the cuff pressure falls from the true systolic value, the Korotkoff sound may sequentially disappear (a false diastolic measurement), "reappear" (a false systolic measurement), and then disappear again at the true diastolic value. A third factor that may produce misleading values is an irregular ventricular rate. Because systolic and diastolic pressures may vary from one heartbeat to the next, the correct recording of the patient's blood pressure requires that the highest and lowest systolic and diastolic values be carefully identified and then averaged to yield a "mean" systolic and a "mean" diastolic value. In all instances, it is recommended that the stethoscope bell, rather than the diaphragm, be used. Otherwise, the low-frequency Korotkoff sounds may not be heard clearly and accurately, especially if the patient has faint or "distant" sounds.

### *Natural Course*

Early in the course of primary hypertension, the blood pressure may fluctuate between abnormal and normal levels. This stage of the disease is usually referred to as labile hypertension. It may begin as early as the second decade of life. During this stage, many patients have a hyperdynamic circulation with increased cardiac output and normal or even low peripheral vascular resistance.

As the disease progresses, peripheral vascular resistance increases and patients develop a sustained increase in blood pressure. In most cases the diastolic blood pressure does not exceed 115 mm Hg. Individuals with secondary hypertension are more likely to experience severe elevations in blood pressure. Only a small proportion of patients suffering from primary hypertension develop accelerated or severe hypertension.

The main causes of death in hypertensive subjects are cerebrovascular accidents, cardiovascular events, and renal failure. The probability of premature death from any of these causes increases with increasing systolic or diastolic blood pressure.

There is also a strong correlation between the level of blood pressure and the incidence of stroke, heart attack, heart failure, and renal disease. Hypertension accelerates and aggravates atherosclerosis in both large and medium-sized arteries. It also produces obstructive vascular lesions in small arteries and arterioles.

## Treatment (See Addendum)

The treatment plan for hypertension should always include measures to minimize contributing factors and to reduce other risks. Aggressive dietary and antismoking programs have been shown to reduce cardiovascular events in high-risk groups. Among hypertensive patients screened for the Multiple Risk Factor Intervention Trial (MRFIT) study, those with a modest degree of cholesterol elevation (around 245 mg/dL) were found to have three to four times the relative risk of coronary heart disease of those with a total cholesterol below 183 mg/dL. This risk appeared to be linearly related to the degree of cholesterol elevation throughout this range. Furthermore, smoking was found to at least double the cholesterol-associated risk.

The benefits of treating moderate or severe hypertension with antihypertensive drug therapy are well established. The benefits of pharmacologically treating mild hypertension, however, are less well defined. Although several studies have addressed this issue, questions of study design, patient selection, drug selection, and retrospective subgroup analysis have generated considerable controversy. In short-term studies where cardiovascular mortality is the major endpoint, a large number of patients are needed to detect statistically significant differences between treatment groups, even when the true difference is as large as 25% to 50%. This is especially true if the population contains a large proportion of patients with a relatively low mortality risk because of the absence of other risk factors (i.e., otherwise healthy, young, white females). Furthermore, it is almost impossible to have a truly "untreated" control group because patients who are identified to be "high risk" and are provided close follow-up surveillance may alter their diet and exercise or smoking habits.

The possibility also exists that any drug may provide adverse effects that counteract the beneficial effects of blood pressure reduction. To date, except for the recently published Medical Research Council (MRC) trial, the large studies of drug treatment of mild hypertension have initiated treatment with a diuretic. The MRC trial included randomization to a diuretic, a $\beta$-blocker, or placebo.

Although it is considered to be an unsound scientific practice, the retrospective "rehashing" of these studies has produced conclusions about various subgroups that have been cited to support a number of therapeutic decisions.

The first of the recent large studies of drug treatment was the Hypertension Detection and Follow-up Program (HDFP) reported in 1979.[5] The results of this study were among the most favorable in that the treatment group had a 20.3% reduction in mortality among those patients with diastolic blood pressure of 90–104 mm Hg. Critics, however, pointed out that this impressive percentage reduction in death rate represented a relatively small number of deaths because the 5-year mortality in the "control" group was only 7.7 deaths per hundred patients as compared with 5.9 deaths in the "treatment" group. Additionally, because the greatest reduction in mortality occurred in blacks and patients over 50 years old, some have argued that drug treatment is indicated only in these groups.

Additional studies that followed (such as the Oslo Study, the Australian Therapeutic Trial, and the MRFIT study) failed to demonstrate a significant reduction in mortality.[7,17,18] Although the number of strokes appeared to be reduced by treatment, the number of such events in each separate study was too small to achieve statistical significance. At 10 years of follow-up in the Oslo Study, coronary heart disease mortality was actually higher in the treated group. In the MRFIT study, retrospective analysis found a higher mortality rate in the "treated group" with hypertension and pretreatment ECG abnormalities. These findings have led to the supposition that drug treatment (diuretics) may have contributed to the mortality rate by elevating serum lipids and enhancing atherosclerosis, by precipitating arrhythmias secondary to potassium and/or magnesium depletion, or by other mechanisms.

It was hoped that the MRC trial would help resolve some of the controversy surrounding the treatment of mild hypertension. After enrolling over 17,000 patients and gathering data in excess of 85,000 patient-years of observation, the investigators found no difference in mortality rates.[19] The incidence of stroke, however, was reduced with active treatment, but other cardiovascular events were not. The reduction in the number of strokes appeared to be greater with diuretic therapy than with $\beta$-blocker therapy.

Other concerns generated from retrospective subgroup analysis of data from earlier studies were also supported by some of the subgroup findings of the MRC trial. Just as the MRFIT trial and Oslo study suggested, an increase in premature ventricular contractions and a trend toward excess mortality from coronary events were observed in men given diuretics. Also, while the HDFP study found no benefit of treatment among white women, the MRC trial actually noted an increase in overall mortality with treatment. Major criticisms of the MRC trial include the fact that 44% of men and 37% of women stopped their initially assigned treatment, the dose of diuretic used was excessive, and the dose of $\beta$-blocker (propranolol titrated to a maximum dose of 240 mg/d) was possibly too low, especially for smokers who may metabolize the drug more rapidly.

So, how does one decide which hypertensive patients should be treated and which treatment is appropriate? First, one should not overlook the fact that a successful diet and exercise program together with smoking cessation is likely to be at least as beneficial as drug therapy in patients with mild hypertension, without the associated expense and risk of adverse effects. Such measures should be given an adequate trial and continued if drug therapy is required later. Second, most patients who fail to control their hypertension reasonably soon with nondrug therapy should be started on drug therapy. For blacks, regardless of age, and for white men over 50 years of age, diuretic therapy can be recommended as the initial treatment. Diuretics should be avoided, if possible, in individuals with ECG abnormalities, hypercholesterolemia, diabetes mellitus, or a history of gout. For white women under 50 years of age, both the HDFP study and the MRC trial results generally suggest that treatment of mild hypertension may not be beneficial.

In addition to giving careful consideration to age, sex, race, serum lipids, and ECG abnormalities, one must also take into account concomitant disorders that may interact either positively or negatively with the antihypertensive drug regimen. A differential approach to the management of hypertension is presented later in this chapter.

## *Diuretics*[3,4,14–16,20]

In patients with adequate renal function (i.e., a glomerular filtration rate greater than 30 mL/min), thiazide diuretics appear to be more effective hypotensive agents than loop diuretics such as furosemide. As renal function declines, however, sodium and fluid accumulate and the use of a more potent diuretic is necessary to counter the effects that volume and sodium expansion have on arterial blood pressure.

All thiazide diuretics are equally effective in lowering blood pressure. The major differences between the various thiazides are the serum half-life and the duration of diuretic effect. These differences may not be clinically relevant, however, as the serum half-life of most antihypertensive agents does not correlate with the hypotensive duration of action. Moreover, diuretics may lower blood pressure primarily through extrarenal mechanisms.

### Mechanism of Action

The exact hypotensive mode of action of diuretics is not known. Of course, acutely, diuretics lower blood pressure by causing a diuresis. The reduction in plasma volume and stroke volume associated with a diuresis decreases cardiac output and, consequently, blood pressure. The initial drop in cardiac output produced by the diuresis causes a compensatory increase in peripheral vascular resistance. With continuing diuretic therapy, the extracellular fluid volume and plasma volume return to pretreatment levels and peripheral vascular resistance falls below its pretreatment baseline. It is the reduction in peripheral vascular resistance that accompanies chronic use of diuretics that is responsible for their long-term hypotensive effectiveness.

Evidently, diuretic-induced total body sodium depletion is necessary for blood pressure reduction, because a high dietary sodium intake can reverse the antihypertensive effect and a low salt intake will potentiate the effect of diuretics on blood pressure.[21]

It has been postulated that thiazide diuretics lower blood pressure by mobilizing sodium and water from arteriolar walls. This action would lessen the amount of physical encroachment on the lumen of the vessel created by excessive accumulation of intracellular fluid. Of course, as the diameter of the lumen increases (opens up), there is less resistance to the flow of blood through the vessel (i.e., peripheral vascular resistance drops).

Another postulated hypotensive mechanism of action stems from the possible association between changes in the electrolyte composition of intraarteriolar walls and vascular responsiveness. The alterations in sodium, potassium, calcium, and magnesium intracellular concentrations may decrease vascular response to pressor substances and increase vascular response to depressor substances.

Still another possible antihypertensive mode of action of the thiazide diuretics is direct relaxation of vascular smooth muscle. This theory is based on the known mechanism of action of diazoxide, a chemical closely related to the thiazide diuretics. Diazoxide is a direct vasodilator, and it is possible that the thiazide diuretics exert a similar action.

When diuretics are used in combination with other antihypertensive agents, an additive hypotensive effect is usually observed. This occurs as a result of two independent pharmacodynamic properties. First, it is a well-known pharmacologic principle that when two drugs cause the same effect through different mechanisms of action, their combined use results in an additive or synergistic response. Second, many nondiuretic antihypertensive agents induce salt and water retention which, of course, is counteracted by the concurrent use of a diuretic.

**Side Effects**

The side effects of thiazide diuretics include hypokalemia, hypomagnesemia, hyperuricemia, hyperglycemia, and hypercalcemia. Furosemide may cause the same side effects except that it increases the urinary excretion of calcium and is, in fact, used in the treatment of hypercalcemia.

Potentially, the most serious adverse effect of diuretics is hypokalemia. Severe potassium depletion is associated with ventricular irritability which may result in ventricular ectopy or sudden death. Fortunately, the incidence of severe hypokalemia is low and can be prevented by potassium chloride supplemental therapy or concurrent use of potassium-sparing diuretics.

The clinical importance of diuretic-induced hypokalemia in patients with uncomplicated primary hypertension is quite controversial.[22] There is also considerable debate surrounding the safety and effectiveness of potassium replacement therapy. The administration of potassium supplements may result in hyperkalemia which can also induce cardiac arrhythmias. Several investigators have questioned the etiology of diuretic-induced ventricular ectopy based upon the observation that potassium supplemental therapy does not always correct the arrhythmia. This is in direct contradiction to a number of investigations that clearly show resolution of ventricular ectopy with correction of hypokalemia. More recent studies have shown that magnesium replacement along with potassium supplementation may be necessary to correct diuretic-induced deficits in total body potassium in some patients.

A couple of measures can be taken to help prevent the development of hypokalemia in patients on diuretic therapy. The first measure is the use of low doses of diuretic, such as 12.5–25 mg of hydrochlorothiazide daily or 25 mg of chlorthalidone daily. The propensity for diuretics to cause hypokalemia is dose dependent. A second measure is reduction of the amount of sodium and augmentation of the amount of potassium in the diet. Low-sodium diets alone result in a marked increase in renal conservation of potassium. A number of foods and beverages rich in potassium (e.g., spinach, banana, dried apricots, and orange juice) can be generously incorporated into the diet as a further measure to prevent diuretic-induced hypokalemia. Another source of increased potassium and decreased sodium derives from the use of salt substitutes.

If hypokalemia occurs despite these preventive measures, the use of a potassium chloride supplement or a potassium-sparing diuretic is indicated. Most clinicians prefer potassium chloride when aggressive repletion is indicated. For chronic management of milder degrees of hypokalemia, however, either approach may be employed. Whether a given patient will respond better to potassium chloride or a potassium-sparing diuretic is not predictable; but individual responses may be partially influenced by the ability of potassium-sparing diuretics to conserve magnesium as well.

A variety of potassium supplements are available; some are better tolerated than others. The appropriate use of potassium supplements to correct diuretic-induced hypokalemia calls for the chloride salt, 40–60 mEq of potassium per day, and of course, the patient's compliance with the regimen. One of the sustained-release potassium chloride preparations is generally better tolerated than the liquid preparations.

It may take several months to correct completely a diuretic-induced total body potassium deficit, despite the fact that the serum potassium rapidly returns to normal. It seems prudent to continue the daily supplement of 40–60 mEq for 2 to 3 months while monitoring the serum potassium concentration. In some cases, the same daily dose of potassium chloride can be continued as long as the patient is on diuretics. In other cases, it may be possible to reduce the dosage.

Diuretic-induced hyperuricemia may produce gouty arthritis or uric acid stones, especially in individuals who are predisposed to gout. In patients with no previous history of gout, acute gouty arthritis and nephrolithiasis are extremely unlikely consequences of diuretic-induced hyperuricemia. If some manifestation of gout does occur in a patient who requires diuretic therapy for effective treatment of hypertension, allopurinol or a uricosuric agent can be given to prevent recurrent gouty attacks without compromising the antihypertensive effects of the diuretic.

Exactly how diuretics adversely affect glucose tolerance is not known. In some cases, there appears to be a link among potassium depletion, decreased insulin secretion, and hyperglycemia. In other cases, however, other mechanisms appear to be in operation, as potassium correction fails to reverse the effects diuretics have on the plasma glucose concentration. If diuretic therapy is mandatory for the management of a diabetic hypertensive individual, an appropriate adjustment in the antidiabetic medication may be required. Individuals with impaired glucose tolerance may develop overt diabetes mellitus when placed on diuretic therapy; therefore, diuretics should be avoided if possible. The increase in serum calcium that attends the use of thiazide diuretics is usually insufficient to cause clinically significant hypercalcemia.

### *Central α-Receptor Agonists*[3,4,9–11,14,15,20]

Clonidine, guanabenz, guanfacine, and methyldopa all lower blood pressure primarily by stimulating $\alpha_2$-adrenergic receptors in the brain. Such action leads to a reduction in sympathetic outflow from the vasomotor center in the brain and an associated increase in vagal tone. It is also possible that stimulation of presynaptic $\alpha_2$ receptors peripherally may contribute to the reduction in sympathetic tone. As a consequence of reduced sympathetic activity together with some enhancement of parasympathetic activity, heart rate is decreased, cardiac output decreases slightly, total peripheral resistance is lowered, plasma renin activity is reduced, and baroreceptor reflexes are blunted.

Chronic use of the centrally acting $\alpha$ agonists results in sodium and fluid retention which appears to be most prominent with methyldopa. Low doses of either clonidine, guanfacine, or guanabenz can be used to treat mild hypertension without the addition of a diuretic; however, methyldopa, even at low doses, usually leads to enough sodium and fluid accumulation that tolerance to its hypotensive effect soon develops in the absence of concurrent diuretic therapy.

Sedation and dry mouth are common side effects of these antihypertensive agents. These symptoms may diminish or completely abate with chronic use of low doses. As with other centrally acting antihypertensive drugs, these agents may cause depression.

Abrupt cessation of any antihypertensive agent may lead to rebound hypertension or overshoot hypertension. Rebound hypertension is characterized by a sudden increase in blood pressure to the pretreatment level, whereas overshoot implies an increase in excess of the pretreatment level. In most cases, abrupt withdrawal of antihypertensive therapy leads to a gradual increase in blood pressure. Rebound and overshoot hypertension are rare syndromes. The propensity for these acute withdrawal syndromes is, however, increased in patients requiring large doses of an antihypertensive agent or in patients who require multiple antihypertensive drug therapy.

In addition to the side effects already mentioned, methyldopa may cause rarely hepatitis or hemolytic anemia. A transient elevation in liver function tests is occasionally associated with methyldopa therapy and is clinically unimportant. But a persistent increase in serum transaminases or alkaline phosphatase may herald the onset of a fulminant hepatitis which can be fatal. A Coombs-positive hemolytic anemia occurs in less than 1% of patients receiving methyldopa, although 20% exhibit a positive direct Coombs test without anemia.

One recent pharmaceutical advance that may be associated with fewer side effects and increased compliance is the transdermal delivery system for clonidine. This device, which is applied to the skin and left in place 1 week before being replaced, appears to reduce blood pressure while avoiding the high peak serum drug concentrations that are seen with oral dosing and are thought to contribute to the adverse effects. The disadvantages of this system are cost, a significant incidence of local skin rash or irritation, and a 2- or 3-day delay of onset of effect so that oral medications should be overlapped for this period of time when patch therapy is first started. A similar delay in "offset" of action also may be seen when the patch is removed and the blood pressure returns to pretreatment values over a 2- or 3-day period.

### *Peripheral $\alpha_1$-Receptor Functional Blockers*[3,4,9–11,14,15,20]

Prazosin and terazosin are not direct $\alpha$-receptor blockers like phentolamine and phenoxybenzamine; rather they are functional $\alpha_1$-blockers in that they interfere with the sequence of postreceptor biochemical events that results in vasoconstriction. This action leads indirectly to vasodilation. As the peripheral functional $\alpha_1$-blockers do not alter $\alpha_2$-receptor activity, they do not usually cause reflex tachycardia. Phentolamine and phenoxybenzamine are nonselective $\alpha$-receptor blockers and their use is associated with a substantial increase in heart rate and cardiac output as well as severe postural hypotension. Consequently, these direct $\alpha$-receptor blockers are used only for the treatment of hypertension secondary to a pheochromocytoma, which is a rare epinephrine- or norepinephrine-secreting tumor.

At low doses, prazosin and terazosin may be used as monotherapy in the treatment of mild hypertension. At higher doses, and sometimes with chronic administration of even low doses, fluid and sodium accumulate and concurrent diuretic therapy is then required to maintain the hypotensive efficacy of the $\alpha$-receptor functional blocker.

Even though the antihypertensive effect of these two drugs is achieved through a peripheral mechanism of action, they do cross the blood–brain barrier and may cause CNS side effects such as lassitude, vivid dreams, and depression. The most interesting side effect of functional $\alpha$-blockers is the so-called "first-dose phenomenon." This is characterized by transient dizziness or faintness, palpitations, and even syncope occurring within 1 to 3 hours of the first dose or subsequently after the first increased dose. These episodes are accompanied by orthostatic hypotension and can be obviated by having the patient take the first dose or first increased dose at bedtime. The first-dose phenomenon is dose related; therefore, prazosin or terazosin should be initiated at very low doses. Occasionally, orthostatic dizziness persists with chronic administration despite these precautions. Finally, priapism has been observed in patients with chronic renal failure on hemodialysis.

### *$\beta$-Adrenoceptor Blockers*[3,4,9–11,14,15,20,23]

The hypotensive mechanism of $\beta$-adrenoreceptor blockers ($\beta$-blockers) is not exactly known. Several mechanisms of action have been proposed, but none of them has been shown to be consistently associated with a reduction in arterial blood pressure.

$\beta$-Blockers reduce cardiac output through their negative chronotropic and inotropic effects on the heart. It is reasonable to postulate that drugs that lower cardiac output lower blood pressure, as blood pressure is the product of cardiac output and peripheral vascular resistance; however, even though cardiac output is reduced after both intravenous and oral administration of propranolol therapy, blood pressure falls only when propranolol is given orally. Furthermore, cardiac output falls to the same degree in patients whose blood pressure is not lowered by these drugs as in patients who respond with a fall in blood pressure. Finally, $\beta$-blockers with intrinsic sympathomimetic activity do not reduce cardiac output in the resting state and yet they lower blood pressure.

Another possible explanation of the hypotensive action of $\beta$-blockers is related to a central action. Within the brain there are both $\alpha$ and $\beta$ receptors. Stimulation of $\alpha$-adrenergic receptors causes a reduction in sympathetic outflow from the vasomotor center. It seems plausible that blocking $\beta$-adrenergic receptors in the brain might produce the same effect. All $\beta$-blockers traverse the blood–brain barrier, but the extent to which they enter the brain depends upon their degree of lipophilicity. At one end of the spectrum is propranolol, a highly lipophilic drug; at the other end is atenolol, which is weakly lipophilic. One would therefore expect a much higher concentration of propranolol in the brain than atenolol after equivalent doses of the two drugs are given, and this indeed is the case. Despite this difference in CNS concentrations, there is no difference in their hypotensive effectiveness. Of course, one cannot rule out the possibility that CNS $\beta$-blockade is optimally achieved with atenolol even though it penetrates the blood–brain barrier much more poorly than propranolol.

Blockade of $\beta$ adrenoceptors located on the surface mem-

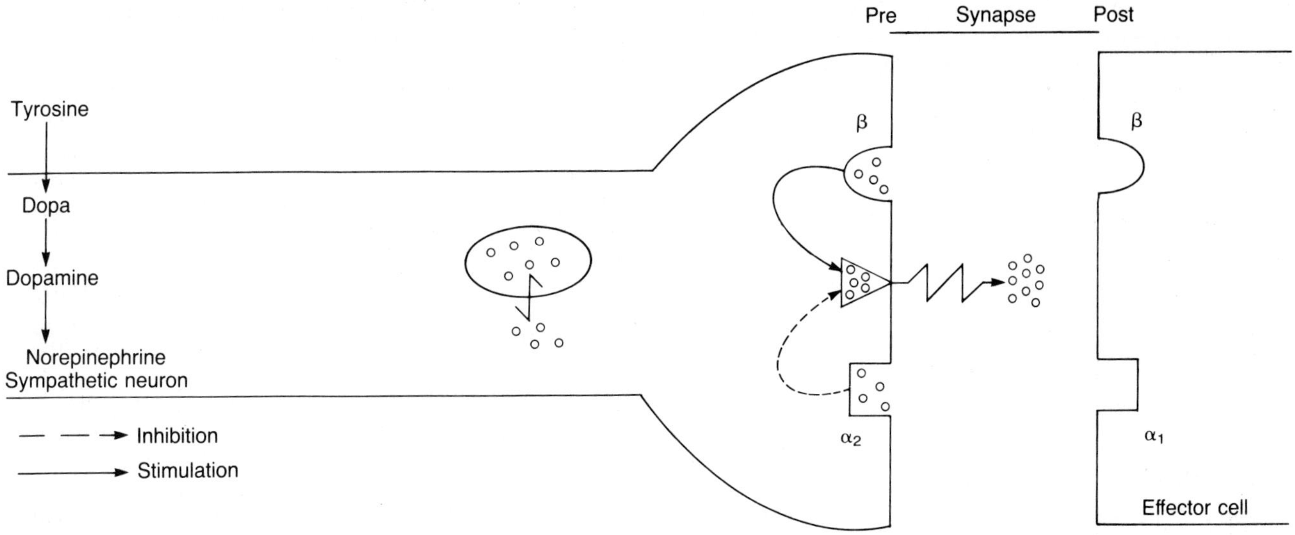


**Figure 10.1** Proposed hypotensive mechanism of action of β-adrenergic blocking agents. Stimulation of a sympathetic neuron triggers the release of norepinephrine into the synapse. Norepinephrine then activates postsynaptic $\alpha_1$ and β receptors of an effector cell. Norepinephrine in the synaptic cleft can also activate presynaptic $\alpha_2$ and β receptors to inhibit or stimulate the further release of norepinephrine. By blocking presynaptic β receptors, β-adrenergic blocking agents interrupt the positive-feedback loop, resulting in a marked decline in the secondary release of norepinephrine.

branes of juxtaglomerular cells leads to a reduction in the release of renin. This, in turn, may result in the attenuation of the renin–angiotensin–aldosterone system, which should reduce blood pressure. Some studies, in fact, have shown a correlation between pretreatment plasma renin activity and reduction in blood pressure by β-blocker therapy. The higher the plasma renin activity the greater the reduction in blood pressure. Other studies, however, have not shown an association between pretreatment plasma renin activity and degree of blood pressure reduction achieved by β-blockers. Furthermore, some β-blockers (e.g., pindolol and acebutolol) lower blood pressure without reducing plasma renin levels. Therefore, alternative or additional mechanisms need to be invoked to account for the antihypertensive effect of β-adrenoceptor blocking agents.

It has been suggested that a peripheral mechanism common to all β-blockers may be responsible for the long-term reduction in blood pressure. The proposed peripheral mechanism involves the possible presence of β adrenoceptors on the surface of sympathetic neuronal endings. Blocking these presynaptic β receptors could lead to a reduction in the release of norepinephrine into the synaptic cleft. This intriguing hypothesis is based upon the theory that norepinephrine release from neuronal endings is regulated to some extent by presynaptic adrenergic feedback loops. Stimulation of presynaptic α ($\alpha_2$) receptors would provoke a negative inhibition on the release of norepinephrine, whereas stimulation of presynaptic β receptors would engender a positive-feedback increase in norepinephrine release (see Fig. 10.1). If presynaptic β receptors do indeed exist, blocking them would interrupt the positive-feedback loop and thus reduce the release of norepinephrine from the neuronal ending. A diminution in the release of norepinephrine from peripheral sympathetic nerve endings should lower blood pressure.

**Pharmacodynamics/Pharmacokinetics**

Even though there are important pharmacodynamic and pharmacokinetic differences among the various β-blockers (Table 10.1), there is no difference in their clinical antihypertensive efficacy. Three pharmacodynamic properties of the β-blockers differentiate them to some extent. The first of these is cardioselectivity. β-Blockers that possess a much greater affinity for $\beta_1$ receptors than $\beta_2$ receptors are said to be cardioselective. $\beta_1$ and $\beta_2$ adrenoceptors are distributed throughout the body, but in certain organs and tissues $\beta_1$ receptors predominate and in other organs and tissues $\beta_2$ receptors predominate. There is a preponderance of $\beta_1$ receptors in the heart and kidney and a preponderance of $\beta_2$ receptors in the lungs, liver, pancreas, and arteriolar smooth muscle. Stimulation of $\beta_1$ receptors produces an increase in heart rate, contractility, and renin release. $\beta_2$-Receptor stimulation results in bronchodilation and vasodilation. β-Adrenergic blockers that bind more avidly to $\beta_1$ receptors than to $\beta_2$ receptors are therefore less likely to provoke bronchospasm and vasoconstriction. Also, because both insulin secretion and glycogenolysis are adrenergically mediated, blockade of $\beta_2$ receptors may reduce either process and cause hyperglycemia or blunt recovery from hypoglycemia, respectively.

At low doses, metoprolol, atenolol, and acebutolol are cardioselective β-blockers. For this reason they may be safer than nonselective β-blockers to use in patients with asthma, chronic obstructive pulmonary disease, peripheral vascular disease, and diabetes; however, it should be

**Table 10.1** Pharmacodynamic and Pharmacokinetic Properties of the β-Adrenoceptor Blocking Agents

| | *Propranolol* | *Nadolol* | *Timolol* | *Metoprolol* | *Atenolol* | *Pindolol* | *Acebutolol* | *Labetolol* |
|---|---|---|---|---|---|---|---|---|
| % Absorbed | 30 | 30 | 75 | 50 | 40 | 100 | 100 | 40 |
| % Protein-bound | 90 | 30 | 10 | 12 | <5 | 57 | 15% | 50 |
| Lipid solubility | 1 | 0.19 | 0.57 | 0.59 | 0.06 | 0.48 | 0.04 | <1 |
| $t_{1/2}$ (h) | 4–6 | 14–24 | 3–4 | 3–4 | 6–9 | 3–4 | 3–4 | 3–5 |
| Elimination | H[a] | R | H/R (20%) | H | R | H/R (40%) | H/R (35%) | H |
| Active metabolite | + | 0 | 0 | 0 | 0 | 0 | + | 0 |
| $\beta_1$ selectivity | 0 | 0 | 0 | + | + | 0 | + | 0 |
| ISA | 0 | 0 | 0 | 0 | 0 | ++ | + | 0 |
| MSA | ++ | 0 | 0 | 0 | 0 | + | + | 0 |
| α-Blockade | 0 | 0 | 0 | 0 | 0 | 0 | 0 | + |

[a] H, hepatic; R, renal; ISA, intrinsic sympathomimetic activity; MSA, membrane-stabilizing activity.

pointed out that cardioselectivity is a dose-dependent phenomenon. At higher doses, metoprolol, atenolol, and acebutolol lose their relative selectivity for $\beta_1$ receptors and block $\beta_2$ receptors as effectively as they block $\beta_1$ receptors. The dose at which cardioselectivity is lost varies from patient to patient.

Another pharmacodynamic difference among the β-blockers is the intrinsic sympathomimetic activity (ISA) that pindolol and acebutolol possess. These two β-blockers are partial β-receptor agonists and are capable therefore of maintaining normal basal sympathetic tone while blocking the effects of excessive adrenergic stimulation. Unlike cardioselectivity, this property is manifested at all dosage levels and varies in significance only with the intrinsic sympathetic tone. When sympathetic tone is low, as it is during resting states, β receptors are partially stimulated. Therefore, resting heart rate, cardiac output, and peripheral blood flow are not reduced when receptors are blocked. Theoretically, pindolol and acebutolol would be less hazardous β-blockers to use in patients with borderline congestive heart failure, sinus bradycardia, or perhaps even peripheral vascular disease; however, clinical studies have not confirmed a clear-cut advantage in patients with the aforementioned disorders.

All β-blockers are capable of exerting a membrane-stabilizing action on cardiac cells if large enough doses are given. It was once thought that this membrane-stabilizing or quinidine-like effect was responsible for the antidysrhythmic effect of β-blockers (see Chapter 12). It is now known that the effectiveness of β-blockers in treating or preventing cardiac dysrhythmias is due primarily to their β-blockade property. The dose of β-blockers required to achieve membrane-stabilizing activity usually greatly exceeds that used in treating hypertension or cardiac arrhythmias.

Pharmacokinetic differences among β-blockers can be found in first-pass metabolism, serum half-lives, degree of lipophilicity, and route of elimination. Propranolol and metoprolol undergo extensive first-pass metabolism. Therefore, the dose required to achieve β-blockade with either drug is quite variable from patient to patient. Atenolol and nadolol, which have relatively long half-lives, are renally excreted and the dosage of each may need to be adjusted in patients with renal insufficiency. Even though the half-lives of the other β-blockers are much shorter, once-daily administration may still be effective. As is the case with most other antihypertensive agents, the serum half-life does not correlate with the drug's hypotensive duration of action. β-Blockers also vary in terms of their lipophilic properties and thus CNS penetration. One might hypothesize that the more water-soluble β-blockers would be less likely to cause CNS side effects, but studies have not adequately tested this hypothesis.

### Side Effects

Most of the side effects of β-blockers represent physiologic consequences of antagonizing β adrenoceptors in various organs and tissues. For example, β-blockade in the myocardium can be associated with bradycardia, atrioventricular conduction abnormalities, and the development of congestive heart failure. Antagonism of $\beta_2$ receptors in the lung may lead to acute exacerbations of bronchospasm in patients with asthma or chronic obstructive pulmonary disease. Blocking $\beta_2$ receptors in arteriolar smooth muscle may aggravate intermittent claudication or Raynaud's phenomenon and it may cause cold extremities as a result of decreased peripheral blood flow. Additionally, an increase of sympathetic tone during periods of acute stress (or hypoglycemia) may result in a significant increase in blood pressure because of unopposed α-receptor–mediated vasoconstriction.

Abrupt cessation of β-blocker therapy may produce unstable angina, myocardial infarction, or even death in patients predisposed to ischemic myocardial events. For this reason, it is always prudent to gradually taper the dose of β-blocker over several days before eventually discontinuing the drug. The acute withdrawal syndrome is felt to be secondary to a combination of factors, including progression of underlying coronary artery disease, hypersensitivity of β-adrenergic receptors, and failure to recognize the need to restrict physical activity upon withdrawal of a drug that decreases myocardial oxygen requirements. The hypersensitivity of β receptors results partly from an increased synthesis of β receptors that occurs in the presence of long-term β-receptor antagonism. In patients without coronary artery disease, abrupt discontinuation of β-blocker therapy may be associated with sinus tachycardia, increased sweating, and generalized malaise.

### *Angiotensin-Converting Enzyme Inhibitors*[3,4,9–11,14,15,20,24]

Currently, there are three angiotensin-converting enzyme (ACE) inhibitors on the U.S. market—captopril, enalapril, and lisinopril. Enalapril is metabolized to enalaprilat, which has a long half-life and duration of hypotensive action, and is therefore given once daily in the treatment of hypertension. Lisinopril has an even longer duration of action but does not require metabolic conversion to exert its effect. Captopril, which has a much shorter half-life than enalapril, is usually administered two to three times daily. Recent studies, however, indicate that once-daily administration of captopril may be adequate for the treatment of hypertension in salt-restricted patients. Furthermore, captopril has been shown to have less of a negative effect on the patient's quality of life. Although there is some concern that such perceptions may be related to centrally mediated mood elevations, this issue deserves further evaluation with all commonly used antihypertensive agents. Whether these agents have significant antiarrhythmic effects is currently under study.

ACE inhibitors block the conversion of angiotensin I to angiotensin II. The latter substance is a potent vasoconstrictor and stimulator of aldosterone secretion. In view of their interference with the renin–angiotensin–aldosterone system, it is easy to understand why ACE inhibitors are effective in hypertensive patients with elevated renin or renin substrate levels; however, they are also effective in hypertensive patients with low plasma renin activity and therefore alternative mechanisms of action may be in operation. Alternative mechanisms include the possible accumulation of bradykinin, a potent vasodilating substance, and stimulation of vasodilatory prostaglandin synthesis. The enzyme that causes degradation of bradykinin is identical to angiotensin-converting enzyme. The role bradykinin plays in the hypotensive action of ACE inhibitors has not been clearly elucidated. When prostaglandin synthesis is inhibited with indomethacin, captopril (but not enalapril) loses its hypotensive effect. This suggests that captopril lowers blood pressure by increasing local vasodilatory prostaglandins. As all these ACE inhibitors are excreted in the urine, an adjustment in dosage may be necessary in patients with renal dysfunction (i.e., creatinine clearance less than 30 mL/min). The absorption of captopril is reduced 30% to 40% by the presence of food in the stomach. Enalapril's absorption is not influenced by food in the gastrointestinal tract.

The most worrisome adverse effects of the ACE inhibitors are neutropenia and agranulocytosis, proteinuria, glomerulonephritis, and angioedema. Fortunately, these serious adverse effects are rare, occurring in less than 1% of patients exposed. Patients with preexisting renal or connective tissue diseases appear to be most vulnerable to the renal and hematologic side effects. Patients with renal artery stenosis are particularly susceptible to developing acute renal failure on ACE inhibitors. A higher incidence of these side effects has been observed when large doses (greater than 200 mg/d) of captopril have been administered.

Approximately 11% of patients who receive captopril develop a skin rash. In most cases the rash is transient and disappears despite continued treatment with the drug. Another fairly common side effect of captopril is a reversible loss of taste or taste disturbance (dysgeusia), which has been reported in about 6% of patients who receive the drug. The higher incidence of skin rash, dysgeusia, and proteinuria with captopril has been attributed to its sulfhydryl group, which is not present on enalapril. Recently, the development of a persistent cough and even asthma has been reported with all three ACE inhibitors.

Acute hypotension may occur at the onset of ACE inhibitor therapy, especially in patients who are severely sodium or volume depleted. It may be necessary to discontinue diuretics and reduce the dosage of other antihypertensive agents before initiating therapy with either captopril, enalapril, or lisinopril. One may also choose to begin ACE inhibitors at the lowest dose possible (2.5 mg enalapril daily or 6.25 mg captopril two or three times daily) and administer the first dose at bedtime.

Finally, hyperkalemia has been observed in patients treated with ACE inhibitors. This propensity for hyperkalemia is seen primarily in patients with renal disease or diabetes mellitus. A uricosuric effect may warrant measures to decrease the risk of uric acid precipitation in patients with hyperuricemia or gout.

### *Vasodilators*[3,4,9–11,14,15,20]

Hydralazine and minoxidil cause direct arteriolar smooth muscle relaxation and therefore vasodilation. They exert little effect, if any, on the venous side of the circulation. By decreasing the amount of systemic pressure in the arterial system, they reduce impedance to myocardial contractility. Hence, hydralazine and minoxidil are also known as afterload-reducing agents and may be used in the management of congestive heart failure.

The reduction in perfusion pressure brought on by direct arteriolar vasodilation activates the baroreceptor reflexes, which results in an increase in sympathetic outflow from the vasomotor center. This leads to an increase in heart rate, cardiac output, and renin release. Consequently, the hypotensive effectiveness of direct vasodilators diminishes in time unless the patient is also taking a sympathetic inhibitor and a diuretic to counteract the compensatory changes created by the baroreceptor reflexes. In older patients, however, baroreceptor mechanisms may be blunted enough that blood pressure may be lowered with vasodilatory therapy without causing sympathetic overactivity.

Direct vasodilator use can precipitate angina in patients with underlying coronary artery disease unless the baroreceptor reflex mechanism is completely blocked. To accomplish this, any sympathetic inhibitor may work, but the $\beta$-adrenergic blocking agents are most effective.

One side effect that is unique to hydralazine is a lupuslike syndrome. This adverse effect is associated with a chronic accumulation of hydralazine and is therefore dose related. The elimination of hydralazine involves hepatic *N*-acetyltransferase activity. As the activity of this enzyme system is predetermined genetically, the rate of acetylation may vary considerably. "Slow" acetylators are especially prone to develop a lupuslike reaction to hydralazine. The syndrome, which is more common in women, seldom progresses to the extent that systemic lupus erythematosus does, and it is reversible upon discontinuation of the drug. By keeping the total daily dose below 200 mg, lupuslike reactions can usually be avoided. Other side effects associated with hydralazine include dermatitis, drug fever, peripheral neuropathy, hepatitis, and vascular headaches.

Because minoxidil is a more potent vasodilator, the compensatory increases in heart rate, cardiac output, renin release, and sodium retention are even more dramatic than those observed with hydralazine. It therefore may be necessary to coadminister a β-adrenergic blocker and a loop diuretic with minoxidil. Other sympathetic inhibitors and thiazide diuretics may prove inadequate in counteracting the minoxidil-induced baroreceptor reflex and intrarenal compensatory mechanisms.

A very troublesome side effect of minoxidil is hypertrichosis. Increased hair growth occurs on the face, arms, back, and chest. This drug-induced hirsutism ceases with discontinuation of the drug. Other minoxidil side effects include pericardial effusion and a nonspecific T-wave change on the electrocardiogram.

### *Calcium Channel Antagonists*[3,4,9–11,14,15,20,25,26]

All three of the currently available calcium channel antagonists (verapamil, diltiazem, and nifedipine) have been shown to be effective antihypertensive agents.

As discussed previously, one of the possible mechanisms for the development of primary hypertension is the increased intracellular concentrations of sodium and calcium. Elevated intracellular calcium increases vascular tone and reactivity and enhances smooth muscle contraction. This results in arteriolar constriction, increased vascular resistance, and hypertension.

By inhibiting the influx of extracellular calcium into the cells of smooth muscles lining arteriolar walls, calcium channel antagonists produce smooth muscle relaxation and vasodilation. Of the three in present use, nifedipine exerts the greatest amount of peripheral vasodilation.

Calcium channel antagonists differ in some of their other pharmacologic effects. For example, verapamil decreases heart rate and slows atrioventricular nodal conduction. These unique properties make it an excellent drug for the treatment of supraventricular tachyarrhythmias. Verapamil also produces a negative inotropic effect that is responsible for its propensity to cause heart failure in subjects with borderline cardiac reserve. Diltiazem also decreases atrioventricular conduction and heart rate, but to a lesser extent than verapamil. Nifedipine, because of its potent peripheral vasodilating effects, causes a baroreceptor-mediated reflex increase in heart rate. It does not alter conduction through the atrioventricular node and it does not decrease myocardial contracility. In fact, it may increase cardiac output in heart failure patients with an increased afterload.

Nifedipine rarely may cause an increase in the frequency, intensity, and duration of angina in association with acute hypotension. This effect may be obviated by the administration of nifedipine with meals. The presence of food in the stomach reduces the rate of nifedipine absorption, which results in a substantially lower peak serum concentration of the drug. Consequently, acute hypotension, which is more likely to be associated with high serum peak nifedipine concentrations, is avoided. Other side effects of nifedipine include dizziness, flushing, headache, peripheral edema, mood changes, and various gastrointestinal complaints.

Diltiazem and verapamil rarely cause cardiac conduction abnormalities such as bradycardia, atrioventricular block, and congestive heart failure. Both can cause anorexia, nausea, peripheral edema, and hypotension. Verapamil causes constipation in about 7% of patients.

### *Postganglionic Sympathetic Inhibitors*[3,4,9–11,14,15,20]

Guanethidine and guanadrel deplete norepinephrine from postganglionic sympathetic nerve terminals and they inhibit the release of norepinephrine in response to sympathetic nerve stimulation.

Hemodynamic studies indicate that the fall in blood pressure produced by postganglionic inhibitors is associated with a reduction in cardiac output and peripheral vascular resistance. Because reflex-mediated vasoconstriction is blocked by these drugs, a much greater hypotensive effect occurs in the upright posture, and postural hypotension is common. The use of postganglionic sympathetic inhibitors is associated with many other unwarranted side effects including impotence, diarrhea, and weight gain. The gastrointestinal side effects occur as a result of unopposed parasympathetic activity.

Long-term norepinephrine depletion leads to postsynaptic receptor supersensitivity. Therefore, the administration of drugs that compete with postganglionic inhibitors for uptake into the nerve terminals (such as tricyclic antidepressants and sympathomimetics) may occasionally provoke acute severe hypertensive episodes.

Because of their potential to cause explosive diarrhea, impotence, and orthostatic hypotension and syncope, the postganglionic sympathetic inhibitors are usually restricted to use in patients with refractory hypertension.

### *Reserpine*[3,4,20]

Reserpine lowers blood pressure through several different mechanisms. It depletes norepinephrine from sympathetic nerve endings and it blocks the transport of norepinephrine into its storage granules. When the nerve is stimulated, less than the usual amount of norepinephrine is released into the synapse. This causes diminution in sympathetic tone with a resulting decrease in peripheral vascular resistance and blood pressure.

Reserpine also depletes catecholamines from the brain and the myocardium. Consequently, the use of reserpine may lead to sedation and depression and decreased cardiac output.

Reserpine is a very-long-acting drug and it may take 2 to 6 weeks before the maximal effect of the drug is realized. Its use is associated with significant sodium and fluid retention and therefore it should be administered in combination with a diuretic.

Reserpine's strong inhibition of sympathetic activity allows increased parasympathetic activity to occur, which is responsible for some of its side effects including nasal stuffiness, increased gastric acid secretion, diarrhea, and bradycardia.

The most important side effect of reserpine, however, is mental depression, which is a consequence of CNS depletion of catecholamines and serotonin. Patients may complain of sadness, loss of appetite, loss of self-confidence, gradual loss of energy, impotence, and early morning awakening. The incidence of reserpine-induced depression is dose related. The problem can be minimized by not exceeding a dose of 0.25 mg daily.

Reserpine is an inexpensive antihypertensive agent and has enjoyed the distinction of being chosen as the sympathetic inhibitor in many of the major clinical trials that have documented the benefit in treating hypertension.

## Differential Approach to the Management of Hypertension

Hypertension is a heterogenous disorder that poses special therapeutic problems in several specific clinical situations. These situations are discussed briefly in this section, which attempts to integrate the pathophysiology of hypertension in certain subgroups of patients with the pharmacology of the various antihypertensive agents. Table 10.2 summarizes some of the key points.

### *Hypertension in Childhood*[4,27,28]

The National Heart, Lung, and Blood Institute recently sponsored the Second Task Force on Blood Pressure Control in Children. That report is recommended for those seeking a more detailed discussion of the area.[28]

In most cases, the factors associated with hypertension in children are identical to those in adults. Hypertensive children often have a family history of high blood pressure. There is, however, one important distinction between hypertension in children and in adults: secondary hypertension is much more common in children than in adults.

Renal disease is the most common cause of secondary hypertension in children. Pyelonephritis, glomerulonephritis, renal artery stenosis, and renal cysts may all produce hypertension in children. Medical or surgical management of the underlying renal disorder usually restores normal blood pressure. Pheochromocytoma and coarctation of the aorta are more often discovered during childhood and are fortunately amenable to corrective surgery. Less common causes of secondary hypertension in children include congenital defects of adrenal steroid synthesis, Wilms' tumor, and neuroblastoma.

Primary hypertension is much more common in children than was once thought. In many young people, primary hypertension is associated with an increased cardiac output and a normal plasma volume and total peripheral vascular resistance. This is often referred to as a hyperdynamic or a hyperkinetic circulatory state. It would seem that this form of hypertension would best be treated with a β-adrenergic blocking agent. An alternative treatment might be clonidine, guanfacine, or guanabenz, which are known to lower serum norepinephrine levels and thus reduce hyperadrenergic activity.

**Table 10.2** Differential Antihypertensive Therapy in Specific Clinical Situations

| | *Advantageous* | *Disadvantageous* |
|---|---|---|
| CHF[a] | ACE inhibitor, diuretic, prazosin, hydralazine | β-blocker, reserpine, verapamil |
| Angina | β-blocker, Ca channel blocker | Hydralazine, minoxidil |
| Elderly | Diuretic, clonidine, Ca channel blocker | β-Blocker |
| Black | Diuretic, clonidine, prazosin, reserpine | β-Blocker as initial therapy |
| Young | β-Blocker, clonidine, prazosin | Diuretic |
| Diabetes | Clonidine, prazosin, ACE inhibitor | β-blocker, diuretic |
| Asthma, COPD | Ca channel blocker | β-Blocker |
| Pregnancy | Methyldopa, clonidine, hydralazine | Diuretic, β-blocker |
| Depression | Prazosin, ACE inhibitor, hydralazine | Methyldopa, reserpine |
| Renal insufficiency | Clonidine, nifedipine, hydralazine, loop diuretic | ACE inhibitor, thiazide diuretic |
| Tachycardia | β-Blocker, clonidine, reserpine | Nifedipine, hydralazine, minoxidil |
| Hyperlipidemia | Prazosin, clonidine, ACE inhibitor | Diuretic, β-blocker |
| Gout/ hyperuricemia | Clonidine, prazosin, Ca channel blocker, ACE[b] | Diuretic, β-blocker, ACE[b] |

[a] CHF, congestive heart failure; ACE, angiotensin-converting enzyme; COPD, chronic obstructive pulmonary disease.

[b] Angiotensin converting enzyme inhibitors may increase urinary clearance of uric acid thereby reducing hyperuricemia but increasing the risk of uric acid deposition in the urine or kidneys.

### *Hypertension in Pregnancy*[9,10,28–31]

Hypertension may present for the first time during pregnancy, or pregnancy may exacerbate preexistent high blood pressure. Classical preeclamptic toxemia of pregnancy presents with proteinuria, edema, and a rise in blood pressure during the third trimester.

There are many gaps in our knowledge concerning the pathophysiology of preeclampsia. The disorder appears to be characterized by extreme vasoconstriction, enhanced vascular reactivity to pressor peptides and amines, and decreased intravascular volume. Other manifestations include decreased glomerular filtration rate, decreased renal blood flow, and decreased urate excretion.

The treatment of hypertension in preeclampsia remains controversial. Diuretics may further contract an already reduced intravascular volume and therefore should probably be avoided. Low-dose methyldopa or clonidine therapy has been used in many cases without producing serious adverse effects on either the mother or the fetus. The use of β-blockers is a little more tenuous because of some reports suggesting adverse effects on the newborn. Oral hydralazine has been used safely and effectively in combination with a sympathetic inhibitor. Of course, nonpharmacologic measures such as bedrest are very important adjuncts to the medical treatment of hypertension in pregnancy. In very mild cases, it may be all that is needed to keep the blood pressure in a safe range.

In acute hypertensive crisis near term, parenteral hydralazine or labetolol may be used to rapidly lower blood pressure without decreasing placental blood flow. Magnesium sulfate is also given if convulsions (eclampsia) seem imminent.

### *Hypertension in the Elderly*[3,9,32–35]

The elderly may present with either isolated systolic hypertension or an elevation in both systolic and diastolic blood pressure. Even though epidemiologic data indicate that cardiovascular morbidity and mortality are more closely related to systolic blood pressure than to diastolic blood pressure, as yet, there is no conclusive evidence that treatment of isolated systolic hypertension causes more good than harm. A double-blind placebo-controlled trial, the Systolic Hypertension in the Elderly Program (SHEP), which addresses the question of therapeutic benefit, is currently in progress.

Systolic hypertension in the elderly is due to arteriosclerotic changes in the media of large arteries, which causes loss of compliance. Some investigators speculate that the cardiovascular morbidity and mortality are secondary to widespread arterial disease and that systolic hypertension is just a marker of the underlying problem. If this is indeed the case, antihypertensive therapy would have only limited usefulness.

The Joint National Committee on Detection, Evaluation, and Treatment of High Blood Pressure recommends that if drug therapy is employed in the treatment of systolic hypertension in the elderly, the systolic blood pressure should be lowered cautiously to the range of 140–160 mm Hg. A goal systolic pressure of less than 140 mm Hg is desirable, but only if it can be achieved without adverse effects.

Elderly patients are usually more sensitive to volume depletion and sympathetic inhibition than their younger counterparts. Therefore, antihypertensive treatment should be initiated with smaller-than-usual dosages. Most authorities agree that the initial drug should be a diuretic. The starting dose should be low (e.g., 12.5 mg of hydrochlorothiazide) and gradually increased, but probably not to the maximum dosage. If diuretic therapy alone does not achieve the desired reduction in systolic blood pressure, a sympathetic inhibitor can be added. Again, it is best to start off with a low dose and slowly increase the dose, if necessary, but avoid excessive doses. In elderly patients with decreased baroreceptor responsiveness, hydralazine may also be used as a second-step agent. Calcium channel blockers should be considered in elderly patients with hypertension and angina, and ACE inhibitors might be preferred for hypertensive patients with congestive heart failure. In contrast to isolated systolic hypertension, the evidence supporting the need for and benefit of treating diastolic hypertension in the elderly is overwhelming. Both the Hypertension Detection and Follow-up Study and the Veterans Administration Cooperative Study found a significant reduction in cardiovascular morbidity and mortality among elderly individuals actively treated with adequate antihypertensive therapy. The pharmacologic management of diastolic hypertension in the elderly should be similar to that previously outlined for systolic hypertension.

### *Hypertension in Blacks*[3,8,20,36]

Hypertension is common in all races, but it affects blacks at a disproportionately higher rate. It is also more severe in blacks than nonblacks. The reasons for the increased prevalence and severity of hypertension in blacks are not fully understood. Differences in electrolyte homeostasis, glomerular filtration rate, sodium excretion and transport mechanisms, plasma renin activity, and blood pressure response to plasma volume expansion have been noted. These differences may help explain the propensity for blacks to develop hypertension, but they do not account for the increased severity of hypertension in blacks as compared with whites. Further investigations in this area are needed.

Although dietary sodium intake is similar in blacks and whites, blacks ingest less potassium and calcium than whites. Supplemental potassium and calcium have both been shown to cause a modest reduction in blood pressure. It would therefore seem reasonable to emphasize the need for increasing the amounts of potassium and calcium in the diet as part of the nonpharmacologic management of hypertension in blacks.

The lower plasma renin activity and increased blood pressure response to sodium and fluid loading observed in blacks suggest a more sodium- and volume-dependent hypertension than exists in nonblacks. Several clinical studies have shown that blacks are hyperresponsive to diuretic therapy, a finding that is entirely consistent with the previously mentioned physiologic observations. These findings also point out the rationale of using diuretic therapy as the initial treatment of hypertension in blacks.

If diuretic therapy alone does not adequately control blood pressure in black hypertensives, then the addition of a sympathetic inhibitor is appropriate. Some clinicians have the misconception that β-blockers are not effective in blacks. Although it is true that β-blockers are inferior to diuretics as the initial treatment, combined β-blocker and diuretic therapy is equally efficacious in hypertensive blacks and whites.

### *Hypertension and Concomitant Disorders*[3,8,13,14,37,38]

When hypertension is associated with other medical problems, the approach to its treatment should reflect proper consideration for the interactions that may occur between the antihypertensive drug regimen and the other disease states. These interactions consist of both positive and negative effects.

For example, if a hypertensive patient also has congestive heart failure, the use of a functional α-blocker or an ACE inhibitor would exert a beneficial effect on both the hypertension and heart failure through their preload- and afterload-reducing properties. On the other hand, the use of β-blockers, verapamil, or reserpine could actually worsen the heart failure in spite of their blood pressure–lowering effects.

Hypertensive patients with angina are excellent candidates for β-adrenergic blocker or calcium channel blocker therapy, as these are effective in the management of both conditions. Hydralazine and minoxidil may aggravate angina unless the baroreceptor reflex mechanism is adequately blocked by sympathetic inhibition.

β-Blockers, even those with $\beta_1$ selectivity, should be avoided in hypertensive patients with asthma, chronic obstructive lung disease, and peripheral vascular disease. On the other hand, calcium channel antagonists may be of added benefit in such patients because of their smooth muscle relaxation effects.

If at all possible, diuretics and β-blockers should not be used to treat the diabetic hypertensive individual. Diuretics cause glucose intolerance through poorly understood mechanisms. β-Blockers may impair insulin secretion and glycogenolysis and delay the compensatory recovery from hypoglycemia episodes. They also mask the symptoms of hypoglycemia (except for sweating which is cholinergically mediated) and thereby eliminate the diabetic's warning of low blood glucose concentration. Additionally, the adrenergic surge associated with severe hypoglycemia may precipitate a hypertensive crisis as a result of the unopposed stimulation of α receptors in the peripheral vascular system.

### *Hypertensive Urgencies and Emergencies*[3,4,8,15,39,40]

Hypertensive urgency is a term used to describe severely elevated arterial pressure without impending complications, such as encephalopathy, severe renal damage, or life-threatening cardiac events. There may be marked retinal arteriolar narrowing, flame-shaped hemorrhages, and fluffy exudates seen on funduscopic examination, but no evidence of papilledema. Such accelerated or severe hypertension should be reduced quickly to stop further vasculitis and to prevent acute target organ damage.

Oral clonidine loading or oral nifedipine has been found to be effective in treating hypertensive urgencies. With oral clonidine loading, 0.2 mg of clonidine is given initially followed by 0.1 mg hourly until the diastolic pressure falls below 110 mm Hg or a total of 0.7 mg of clonidine has been administered. Rapid nifedipine effect is accomplished by having the patient chew a perforated capsule or by puncturing a hole in the capsule and squirting the contents in the mouth. Again, the goal is to lower the diastolic pressure below 110 mm Hg. The initial dose of 10 mg is followed by another 10-mg dose 20 minutes later if necessary. Rapid reduction of diastolic blood pressure below 100 mm Hg should be avoided, as cerebral complications may ensue secondary to decreased cerebral blood flow.

Prazosin and captopril also have been used for initial therapy in hypertensive urgencies. Because the degree and time of response to either agent may be unpredictable in some patients, other agents are usually preferred.

Hypertensive emergencies are life-threatening elevations in blood pressure and require immediate reduction in blood pressure.

Several clinical situations are known to precipitate a hypertensive emergency or crisis. Most of these are cerebrovascular or cardiac events. Encephalopathy, intracerebral hemorrhage, and cerebral infarction in the presence of severe hypertension represent hypertensive emergencies. Severe hypertension in patients with acute aortic dissection, acute left ventricular failure, or acute coronary insufficiency is also an emergency situation. Other types of hypertensive emergencies are those associated with marked increases of blood pressure in patients with a pheochromocytoma or secondary to food or drug interactions in patients receiving MAO inhibitors.

The treatment of hypertensive emergencies can be accomplished with any one of several antihypertensive agents. In the clinical situations just described, one agent may be preferred and another contraindicated.

Nitroprusside is widely considered the agent of choice for the minute-to-minute control of severe hypertension. It is a direct-acting vasodilator that decreases peripheral vascular resistance, but does not increase cardiac output unless left ventricular failure is present. It is usually given as a continuous intravenous infusion at a rate of 0.5–8.0 μg/kg/min. Its onset of hypotensive action is immediate and its effect disappears within 2 to 5 minutes of discontinuation of the infusion. Nitroprusside can be given to treat any hypertensive emergency, but in aortic dissection propranolol should be given first to prevent reflex sympathetic activation. Nitroprusside is metabolized to cyanide and then to thiocyanate and eliminated by the kidneys. When the infusion must be continued longer than 72 hours, serum thiocyanate levels should be measured, and the infusion should be discontinued if the level exceeds 12 mg/dL. Other side effects of nitroprusside include fatigue, nausea, anorexia, disorientation, psychotic behavior, muscle spasms, and, rarely, hypothyroidism. Nitroprusside administration requires constant intraarterial pressure monitoring.

Diazoxide is also a direct-acting arteriolar vasodilator that decreases peripheral resistance, increases cardiac output, and maintains or increases renal plasma flow. Because diazoxide increases plasma volume, it is common practice to give a diuretic concurrently unless the patient is volume depleted. It has quick onset and a duration of action ranging from 4 to 12 hours. Diazoxide occasionally causes overshoot hypotension which can be reversed by pressor agents. To avoid the precipitous fall in pressure that occurs when diazoxide is given as a 300-mg rapid bolus, smaller bolus

Table 10.3 The Antihypertensive Agents

| Drug | Dose range (mg/d) Initial | Dose range (mg/d) Maximum |
|---|---|---|
| **Diuretics** | | |
| Thiazides and related sulfonamide diuretics | | |
| Bendroflumethiazide | 2.5 | 5 |
| Benzthiazide | 25.0 | 50 |
| Chlorothiazide sodium | 250.0 | 500 |
| Chlorthalidone | 25.0 | 50 |
| Cyclothiazide | 1.0 | 2 |
| Hydrochlorothiazide | 25.0 | 50 |
| Hydroflumethiazide | 25.0 | 50 |
| Indapamide | 2.5 | 5 |
| Methyclothiazide | 2.5 | 5 |
| Metolazone | 2.5 | 5 |
| Polythiazide | 2.0 | 4 |
| Quinethazone | 50.0 | 100 |
| Trichlormethiazide | 2.0 | 4 |
| Loop diuretics | | |
| Bumetanide | 0.5 | 10 |
| Ethacrynic acid | 50.0 | 200 |
| Furosemide | 80.0 | 480 |
| Potassium-sparing agents | | |
| Amiloride hydrochloride | 5.0 | 10 |
| Spironolactone | 50.0 | 100 |
| Triamterene | 50.0 | 100 |
| **Adrenergic Inhibitors** | | |
| $\beta$-Adrenergic blockers | | |
| Acebutolol | 400 | 1,200 |
| Atenolol | 25.0 | 100 |
| Metoprolol tartrate | 50.0 | 300 |
| Nadolol | 20.0 | 120 |
| Oxprenolol hydrochloride | 160.0 | 480 |
| Pindolol | 20.0 | 60 |
| Propranolol hydrochloride | 40.0 | 480 |
| Propranolol, long-acting (LA) | 80.0 | 480 |
| Timolol maleate | 20.0 | 60 |
| Central-acting adrenergic inhibitors | | |
| Clonidine hydrochloride | 0.2 | 1.2 |
| Guanabenz acetate | 8.0 | 32 |
| Guanfacine | 1.0 | 3.0 |
| Methyldopa | 500.0 | 2,000 |
| Peripheral-acting adrenergic antagonists | | |
| Guanadrel sulfate | 10.0 | 150 |
| Guanethidine monosulfate | 10.0 | 300 |
| *Rauwolfia* alkaloids | | |
| *Rauwolfia* (whole root) | 50.0 | 100 |
| Reserpine | 0.05 | 0.25 |
| $\alpha_1$-Adrenergic blocker | | |
| Prazosin hydrochloride | 2.0 | 20 |
| Terazosin | 1.0 | 5.0 |
| Combined $\alpha$- and $\beta$-adrenergic blockers | | |
| Labetolol | 200.0 | 1,200 |
| Vasodilators | | |
| Hydralazine hydrochloride | 50.0 | 300 |
| Minoxidil | 5.0 | 100 |
| Angiotensin-converting enzyme inhibitors | | |
| Captopril | 25.0 | 150 |
| Enalapril maleate | 10.0 | 40 |
| Lisinopril | 10 | 80 |
| Slow channel calcium-entry blocking agents | | |
| Diltiazem hydrochloride | 120.0 | 240 |
| Nifedipine | 30.0 | 180 |
| Verapamil hydrochloride | 240.0 | 480 |

doses (50–100 mg every 5 to 10 minutes) or slow infusion over 15 to 30 minutes should be used. Other side effects of diazoxide include nausea, vomiting, tachycardia, hyperglycemia, and hyperuricemia.

Trimethaphan camsylate is a ganglionic blocking agent. It dilates both arterioles and veins, with hypotension potential in the upright position. It reduces cardiac output and renal plasma flow and increases plasma volume. Trimethaphan is particularly useful for treating hypertension in patients with acute aortic dissection. Like nitroprusside, trimethaphan is administered by continuous intravenous infusion which requires constant or frequent intraarterial pressure monitoring. The initial infusion rate is 1 mg/min and the dose can be adjusted up to 10 mg/min. Its onset of action is immediate and its effects disappear within 10 minutes of discontinuation of the infusion. Besides profound orthostatic hypotension, trimethaphan may cause ileus, urinary retention, dry mouth, and visual impairment. Respiratory arrest has been reported at infusion rates greater than 5 mg/min.

Labetolol is a combination nonselective $\beta$-adrenergic and $\alpha$-adrenergic blocker. It reduces blood pressure by decreasing peripheral vascular resistance. It does not significantly affect heart rate of cardiac output. The initial dose is 20 mg by slow intravenous injection over a 2-minute period, followed by repeated injections of 40–80 mg at 10-minute intervals, up to a total dose of 300 mg. Alternatively, the drug can be administered by continuous infusion at an initial rate of 2 mg/min and adjusted according to blood pressure response. Because of its $\alpha$-blocking effects, labetolol can cause orthostatic hypotension. Other side effects include nausea, vomiting, paresthesias, sweating, dizziness, flushing, and headaches.

Hydralazine is an arteriolar vasodilator. It causes a marked reflex tachycardia and an increase in myocardial oxygen demand, which can cause ischemic chest pain in patients with coronary artery disease. Its onset of action ranges from 10 to 30 minutes and its effects last 2 to 4 hours. When given intravenously, 10–20 mg is diluted in 20 mL of 5% dextrose in water ($D_5W$) and administered at a rate of 0.5–1.0 mL/min. Because the hypotensive response is less predictable than with other parenteral agents, its major role is in the treatment of eclampsia or hypertensive encephalopathy associated with renal insufficiency. It has a good track record in the treatment of these two types of hypertensive emergencies.

## Summary

Hypertension is a very common chronic medical disorder. It affects more than 50 million Americans. In more than 90% of cases the etiology of hypertension is unknown. Several pathophysiologic mechanisms have been proposed in the causation of hypertension. These include central and peripheral nervous system abnormalities, autoregulatory dysfunction, renal defects, humoral aberrancies, and deficiencies in various endogenous vasodepressor substances.

Untreated or inadequately controlled hypertension is a major risk factor in the morbidity and mortality of cardiovascular, cerebrovascular, and renovascular diseases. Antihypertensive drug therapy should be individualized according to various patient characteristics and underlying pathophysiologic circumstances. Table 10.3 provides a list of agents currently available for the treatment of hypertension in the United States.

## Addendum

Two important publications occurred while this chapter was in press. The 1988 Joint National Committee Report, which appeared in the May issue of *Archives of Internal Medicine*, provides new recommendations for the detection, evaluation, and management of hypertension. In the April 1, 1988, issue of *JAMA*, the MAPHY study results were presented. This study compared metoprolol and diuretic therapy in men with mild-to-moderate hypertension. The patients treated with metoprolol had a significantly lower rate of cardiovascular and total mortality.

## References

1. Guyton AC. The relationship of cardiac output and arterial pressure control. Circulation 1981;64:1079–1088.
2. Dustan HP. Physiologic regulation of arterial pressure: An overview. Hypertension 1982;4(suppl 3):62–67.
3. Caris TN. A Clinical Guide to Hypertension. Littleton, MA, PSG Publishing, 1985.
4. Kaplan NM. Clinical Hypertension, 4th ed. Baltimore, Williams and Wilkins, 1986.
5. Hypertension Detection and Follow-up Program Cooperative Group. Five year findings of the Hypertension Detection and Follow-up Program. 1: Reduction in mortality of persons with high blood pressure, including mild hypertension. JAMA 1979; 242:2567–2571.
6. Veterans Administration Cooperative Study Group on Antihypertensive Agents. Effects of treatment on morbidity in hypertension. JAMA 1967;202:1028–1034.
7. Management Committee. The Australian therapeutic trial in mild hypertension. Lancet 1980;1:1261–1269.
8. The 1984 Report of the Joint National Committee on Detection, Evaluation and Treatment of High Blood Pressure. Arch Intern Med 1984;144:1045–1057.
9. Genest J, Kuchel O, Hamet P, et al. Hypertension, Physiopathology and Treatment, 2nd ed. New York, McGraw-Hill, 1983.
10. Kincaid-Smith PS, Whitworth JA. Hypertension: Mechanisms and Management. New York, ADIS Health Science Press, 1980.
11. Meyer P. Hypertension mechanisms and clinical and therapeutic aspects. Oxford, Oxford University Press, 1980.
12. Frohlich ED. Mechanisms contributing to high blood pressure. Ann Intern Med 1983;98:709–714.
13. Messerli FH, Ventura HO. Cardiovascular pathophysiology of essential hypertension: A clue to therapy. Drugs 1985;30(suppl 1):25–34.
14. McCarron DA. Management of hypertension: Pathophysiologic and therapeutic perspectives. J Cardiovasc Pharmacol 1984; 6(suppl 6);5:465–545.
15. Chobanian AV. Hypertension. Clin Symposia 1982;34(5):3–32.
16. Sonnenblick EH. Hypertension and hemodynamics: Therapeutic implications. Am J Med 1983;75(4A):1–114.
17. Helgeland A. Treatment of mild hypertension: A five year controlled drug trial. Am J Med 1980;69:725–732.
18. Multiple Risk Factor Intervention Trial Research Group. Multiple risk factor intervention trial. JAMA 1982;248:1465–1477.

19. MRC trial of mild hypertension: Principal results. Br Med J 1985;291:97–104.
20. McMahon FG. Management of Essential Hypertension: The New Low-Dose Era, 2nd ed. Mount Kisco, NY, Futura Publishing, 1984.
21. Houston MC. Sodium and hypertension: A review. Arch Intern Med 1986;146:179–185.
22. Hollenberg NK, Brown RS. Electrolytes and cardiovascular disease. Am J Med 1984;77(5A):1–66.
23. Frishman WH. Clinical Pharmacology of Beta-Adrenoceptor Blocking Drugs, 2nd ed. Norwalk, CT, Appleton-Century-Crofts, 1984.
24. Ferguson RK, Vlasses PH, Rotmensch HH. Clinical applications of angiotensin-converting enzyme inhibitors. Am J Med 1984;77:690–698.
25. Frohlich ED. New concepts in hypertension therapy. Am J Med 1984;77:1–146.
26. Robinson BF. Calcium-entry blocking agents in the treatment of systemic hypertension. Am J Cardiol 1985;55(3):102B–106B.
27. Ingelfinger J. Pediatric Hypertension. Philadelphia, W.B. Saunders, 1982.
28. Report of the Second Task Force on Blood Pressure Control in Children—1987. Pediatrics 1987;79:1–25.
29. Naden RP, Redman CWG. Antihypertensive drugs in pregnancy. Clin Perinatol 1985;12:521–538.
30. Lindheimer MD, Katz AI. Hypertension in pregnancy. N Engl J Med 1985;313:675–680.
31. Brenner BM, Stein JH. Hypertension. New York, Churchill Livingstone, 1981.
32. Gavras H, Gavras I. Hypertension in the elderly. Boston, John Wright–PSG, 1983.
33. Franklin SS. Geriatric hypertension. Med Clin North Am 1983; 67:395–416.
34. O'Malley K, O'Brien E. Management of hypertension in the elderly. N Engl J Med 1980;302;1397–1401.
35. Chobanian AV. Pathophysiologic considerations in the treatment of the elderly hypertensive patient. Am J Cardiol 1983;52: 39D–53D.
36. Hall WD, Saunders E, Shulman NB. Hypertension in blacks: Epidemiology, pathophysiology, and treatment. Chicago, Year Book Medical Publishers, 1985.
37. Kaplan NM. Initial therapy in hypertension. Am J Cardiol 1983; 51:619–660.
38. Frohlich ED. Role of calcium entry-blocking drugs in hypertension. Am J Cardiol 1985;56(16):1H–111H.
39. Drugs for hypertensive emergencies. Med Lett 1985;27:22–24.
40. Cohan JA, Checcio JM. Nifedipine in the management of hypertensive emergencies: Report of two cases and review of the literature. Am J Emerg Med 1985;3:524–530.

# Chapter 11 / Congestive Heart Failure

Joel O. Covinsky, PharmD, and Michael S. Willett, PharmD

Congestive heart failure (CHF) is defined as a pathophysiologic disturbance in which an abnormality of cardiac function results in an inability of the heart to pump blood at a rate commensurate with the metabolic requirements of the body.[1] An estimated four million Americans suffer from chronic CHF. The diagnosis of CHF is associated with a grave prognosis. According to the Framingham study, the 5-year survival of patients with CHF is approximately 50%.[2,3] One of the most disturbing facets of chronic CHF is the observation that approximately half of the deaths occur suddenly and are not due to pump failure.[4,5] Although the reason for sudden death is unknown,[5] many believe arrhythmias are a major contributor and must be considered in any therapeutic plan. Obviously, more information is needed regarding the cause of sudden death and its prevention in patients with CHF if we are going to make any impact on survival in these patients.

CHF is a consequence of a variety of underlying disorders. The disturbance in cardiac function is often due to a disturbance in myocardial contractility[1]; however, not all patients with CHF have disturbances in myocardial contractility. CHF may occur because the normal heart is confronted with an excessive load that exceeds compensatory mechanisms or because ventricular filling or relaxation is impaired. In examination of the mechanical function of the heart, it is important to realize that the pumping action is influenced by two independent systems: those that control contraction and emptying of the heart (inotropic) and those that control myocardial relaxation and filling (lusitropic). The signs and symptoms of CHF can be associated with abnormalities of either or both of these systems. Throughout the 1960s and 1970s, attention focused on alterations in muscular contraction. CHF was viewed in terms of abnormalities in systolic function, specifically, impaired shortening and tension development.[6] Recently, recognition of relaxation abnormalities has begun to receive attention in the literature.[7,8] The development of noninvasive methods to determine ventricular volume, rather than pressure, may allow the clinician to determine whether the patient with CHF exhibits relaxation or contraction abnormalities.[7,9–11] With this information at hand, the clinician can use specific therapeutic interventions directed toward the specific abnormality.

## Pathophysiology/Etiology

The pathophysiology of CHF is associated with five key features (Table 11.1): pressure overload, volume overload, loss of muscle, decreased contractility, and disturbances in filling.[12] Any one or combination of these features may be responsible for the signs and symptoms of CHF. Left ventricular failure is commonly associated with pressure overload caused by systemic hypertension or, less commonly, by outflow obstruction, such as aortic stenosis. In contrast, right ventricular failure frequently develops secondary to left ventricular failure but can be precipitated by pulmonary hypertension.

Volume overload can be caused by several different conditions, including valvular insufficiency; congenital heart anomalies, such as atrial septal defects; and high-output states, such as anemia or thyrotoxicosis. Sustained pressure or volume overload leads to intrinsic changes in cardiac contractility, which often are not reversible. This decline in contractility eventually results in the clinical syndrome of CHF.

Loss of muscle as a cause of CHF is commonly seen in patients with coronary artery disease. Today, this is one of the most common causes of CHF. In the patient who suffers a myocardial infarction, there is irreparable loss of muscle, resulting in a decrease in the pumping capability of the myocardium. In patients who lose more than 40% of their ventricular muscle, irreversible heart failure or cardiogenic shock develops.

In addition to pressure or volume overload, cardiomyopathies may also be responsible for a decrease in the intrinsic contractility of the myocardium. Both mechanical and biochemical changes may be responsible for this loss in contractility. Hypertrophy of the ventricle may produce dramatic changes in compliance, even though each individual muscle unit may have relatively normal passive length–tension relations. Biochemical alterations may be associated with decreases in actinomyosin-ATPase, which releases energy for contraction and influences the velocity of shortening. This change may be mediated by alterations in myosin isozyme activity, decreased oxygen supply, and/or decreased stores of norepinephrine. Alterations in sarcoplasmic reticulum activity may decrease the stores and uptake of calcium, thus affecting contractility. Finally, downregulation of the $\beta$-adrenergic receptors either with aging or with the continued stimulation associated with persistent elevated sympathetic tone may decrease myocardial contractility further.[12–15]

The importance of restricted ventricular filling is receiving new emphasis today. In the past, restrictive filling was considered a problem produced by constrictive pericarditis, pericardial tamponade, or conditions in which a stiff ventricular chamber resisted filling. Examples of the latter include endomyocardial fibrosis, amyloidosis, or a thickened hypertrophied ventricle with decreased compliance. More recently, the association among hypertension, coronary artery disease (especially in diabetics), and reduced ventricular compliance has received more attention, especially in elderly patients. This decreased compliance may be brought about by excessive hypertrophy, scar formation after an

**Table 11.1** Causes of Congestive Heart Failure

| *Pathophysiologic mechanism* | *Etiology* |
|---|---|
| Pressure overload | Left ventricular failure caused by systemic hypertension or outflow obstruction; right ventricular failure caused by pulmonary hypertension |
| Volume overload | Valvular insufficiency, congenital heart abnormalities, high-output states (anemia, thyrotoxicosis) |
| Loss of muscle mass | Coronary artery disease, myocardial infarction |
| Decreased contractility | Cardiomyopathies, ventricular hypertrophy, altered activity of myocardial isozymes or sarcoplasmic reticulum |
| Disturbances in filling | Pericarditis, pericardial tamponade, endomyocardial fibrosis, hypertension, coronary artery disease |

From Covinsky JO: Congestive heart failure. The Consultant Pharmacist 1986(May):47, with permission.

infarct, or changes in myocardial stiffness, presumably secondary to ischemia and the associated disturbances in muscular relaxation. Delayed atrial relaxation may precede clinically apparent alterations in ventricular performance. This disturbance in diastolic function may reduce ventricular filling and result in signs and symptoms of CHF previously assumed to be related primarily to systolic function. At the subcellular level, altered binding and release of calcium may contribute to these diastolic abnormalities.[7,16]

## Compensatory Mechanisms

When the heart fails as a pump, a series of alterations of homeostatic mechanisms occur to compensate for the impaired myocardial contractility. These compensatory mechanisms include (Fig. 11.1) increased preload, ventricular hypertrophy, activation of the sympathetic nervous system, and activation of the renin–angiotensin–aldosterone system. Initially, these mechanisms serve to maintain cardiac output, ensure adequate oxygen delivery to the tissues, and allow the individual to perform normal activities even though endurance may be reduced. Eventually, however, the compensatory mechanisms prove detrimental and the patient's symptoms of CHF worsen. Interestingly, the patient's symptomatology may well reflect the impact that the various compensatory mechanisms have on altering the distribution of the cardiac output.[12]

**Figure 11.1** Compensatory mechanisms in congestive heart failure. PG, prostaglandin; ADH, antidiuretic hormone. *(Adapted from Covinsky JO: Congestive heart failure. The Consultant Pharmacist 1986[May];47, with permission.)*

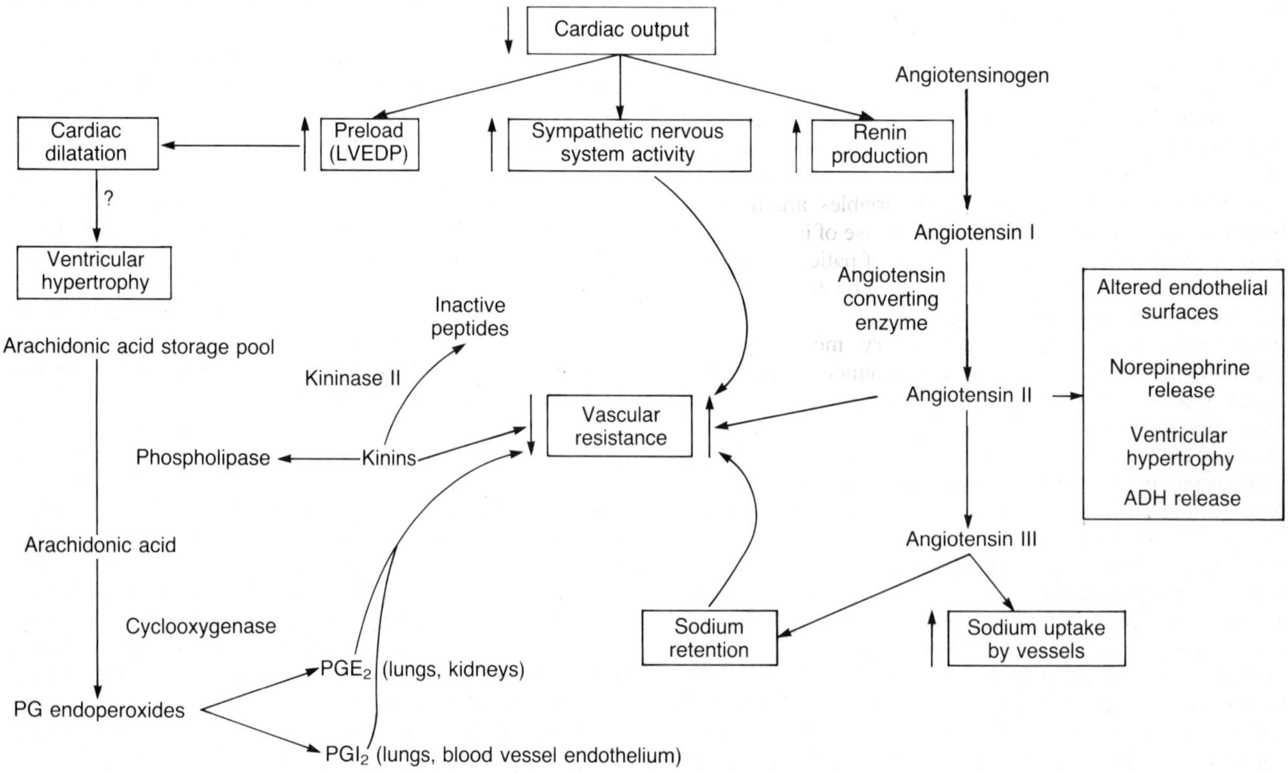

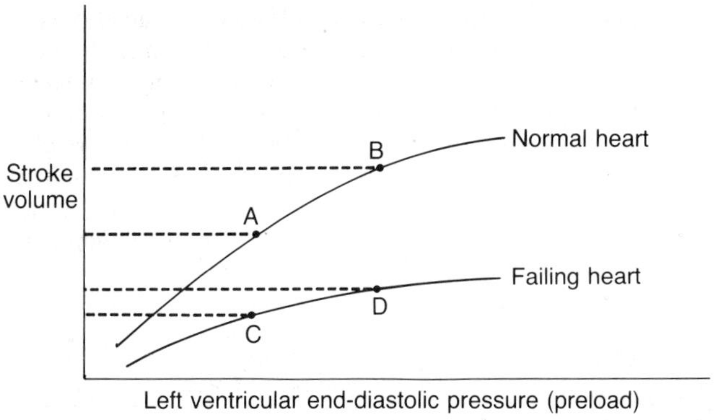


**Figure 11.2** Frank–Starling mechanism: An increase in preload causes the myofibrils to stretch, which results in an increase in the force of contraction as well as an increase in stroke volume. For a given increase in preload, the increase in stroke volume is greater in the normal heart (from A to B) than in the failing heart (from C to D).

To comprehend the compensatory mechanisms that occur in CHF, a fundamental understanding of the determinants of cardiac output and blood pressure is essential. Cardiac output (CO) is the product of heart rate (HR) and stroke volume (SV). HR is regulated by the autonomic nervous system. SV, the amount of blood ejected from the ventricle during systole, is determined by three factors: preload, afterload, and contractility. Preload, the filling pressure of the left ventricle, is approximated by the left ventricle end-diastolic pressure or volume (LVEDP or LVEDV) and is estimated clinically by measuring the pulmonary capillary wedge pressure (PCWP) with a Swan–Ganz catheter. Afterload, or left ventricular wall tension during systole, represents the force that the left ventricle must pump against to eject blood. Afterload is approximated by the systemic vascular resistance (SVR). The contractility of the myocardium is an intrinsic property of the myocardium that allows for alterations in the force and extent of contractions.[17] Finally, blood pressure (BP) is the product of CO and SVR. The interrelationships among these variables are discussed below. A more detailed discussion of the use of invasive hemo dynamic monitoring in the management of patients with acute or severe CHF can be found later in this chapter.

Failure of the myocardium to provide an adequate cardiac output activates several compensatory mechanisms designed to improve myocardial performance. First, in the failing myocardium, the strength with which the ventricle may contract is often reduced. The resultant reduction in ejection fraction causes a decrease in cardiac output (in approximately 70% of these patients) and an increase in residual blood volume within the ventricle at the end of systole. If the atria can continue to deliver blood to the ventricles at the same rate, the end-diastolic volume or pressure (preload) will increase and the ventricle will dilate. The increased length of the cardiac fibers allows an increased force of systolic contraction to be developed according to the Frank–Starling mechanism (Fig. 11.2). In the normal heart, progressive increases in end-diastolic volume and cardiac fiber length continue to provide an increase in contractility and cardiac output; however, in the failing heart, this curve is shifted downward and its slope is not as steep. As a result, similar increases in end-diastolic volume and cardiac fiber length may simply result in congestion without producing additional increases in cardiac output.[17]

With time, myocardial hypertrophy occurs in which the mass of contractile tissue is augmented. Myocardial failure usually develops slowly and generally proceeds by stages in which either the entire heart or the residual viable portion of otherwise damaged heart hypertrophies without failure. Myocardial hypertrophy compensates only temporarily, however, and eventually is inadequate at maintaining an adequate cardiac output.

Also in response to inadequate cardiac output, reflex activation of the sympathetic nervous system and an increase in circulating catecholamines occur. Both centrally and peripherally mediated increases in the sympathetic tone result in vasoconstriction and a reduction in blood supply to those regions of the body most richly endowed with $\alpha$-adrenergic receptors, for example, cutaneous, renal, and splanchnic vascular beds. The magnitude of the response to sympathetic stimulation varies with the posture of the patient. Sympathetic influence on the kidney is greatly reduced in the recumbent position. In contrast, those areas that rely on metabolic circulatory control mechanisms, that is, the coronary and cerebral circulation, receive an increased portion of the cardiac output. These disturbances in autonomic control are not restricted to the sympathetic nervous system. The normal parasympathetic restraint is also reduced, contributing to the commonly observed increase in heart rate. These changes collectively contribute to increased peripheral vascular resistance, increased venous tone, and dramatic changes in renal hemodynamics.

The kidney plays a regulatory role in maintaining an "effective" circulating blood volume. The kidney normally receives about 20% of the cardiac output. This level of perfusion is several times the flow received by other metabolically active organs such as the heart, the liver, and the brain. Accordingly, cardiovascular disturbances that result in a reduction in renal perfusion produce profound changes in renal function and sodium and water retention. Sodium retention is brought about by a number of changes. As cardiac output decreases, and sympathetic tone in the renal vascular bed increases, renal blood flow is diminished. This is interpreted by the kidney as inadequate circulating blood volume. The decrease in glomerular filtration rate is less than the decrease in renal plasma flow. The resultant increase in filtration fraction (the fraction of plasma flowing through the kidney that is filtered into the glomeruli) leads to sodium retention.

In an effort to compensate for this reduction in "effective" blood volume, activation of the renin–angiotensin–aldosterone (RAA) system occurs (Fig. 11.1). Renin is released from the juxtaglomerular cells of the kidney, and this proteolytic enzyme causes the inactive $\alpha_2$-globulin, angiotensinogen, to be converted to angiotensin I. The dipeptidyl carboxypeptidase, angiotensin-converting enzyme, splits the two C-terminal amino acids from the decapeptide, angiotensin I, to form the active octapeptide, angiotensin II. While conversion of angiotensin I to angiotensin II occurs mainly during circulation through the lung, it is important to realize that angiotensin-converting enzyme is a ubiquitous enzyme and is found in many tissues, including the renal cortex.

Angiotensin II is a potent vasoconstrictor with an impact on the peripheral circulation as well as on the renal vasculature.

In addition to its direct effect on the vasculature, angiotensin II appears to work on presynaptic sympathetic nerve endings to cause catecholamine release. The renal vasculature is especially sensitive to angiotensin II. In the kidney, angiotensin II may alter the intrarenal blood flow and increase the flow to the hypertonic renal medulla. This alteration in intrarenal blood flow plays an important role in modifying the excretion of sodium. Circulating angiotensin II is degraded to a heptapeptide, angiotensin III, which stimulates the zona glomerulosa of the adrenal cortex to release aldosterone. Aldosterone, a potent mineralocorticoid, acts on the distal convoluted tubule to enhance sodium reabsorption. Aldosterone may also increase sodium uptake in other vascular beds. The net effect of all these maneuvers is an expansion of the intravascular volume and an increase in both peripheral resistance and return of blood to the heart.

Other vasoactive factors may also contribute to the alteration in peripheral vascular tone and renal function. Arginine vasopressin, an endogenous vasoconstrictor and antidiuretic hormone, is elevated in CHF, presumably in response to inadequate "effective" circulating blood volume. Its exact contribution to peripheral vascular tone and fluid balance in CHF is unclear.

An atrial natriuretic factor (ANF) has been characterized and its activity appears to increase under conditions of volume expansion associated with CHF. ANF normally suppresses renal tubular reabsorption of sodium in response to an expansion of extracellular volume. In CHF patients, the kidney does not respond to ANF with an increase in sodium excretion. Its exact contribution to the process remains under study.

Prostaglandins are synthesized in vascular beds throughout the body. Their exact contribution to homeostasis is also currently under investigation. Prostaglandins of the E series are synthesized in the interstitial and collecting duct cells of the renal medulla. These substances are released into the renal interstitial fluid. Prostaglandin $E_2$ increases intracortical blood flow and induces natriuresis. It is postulated that renal sodium and water excretion is modified by the action of prostaglandins on the renal vasculature. The high concentration of prostaglandins in the renal medulla suggests that they may control medullary circulation. The renal vasoconstrictive response to endogenous norepinephrine and angiotensin II is often poorly sustained. It is postulated that the increased concentration of prostaglandin E–like substances in the renal circulation reverses the vasoconstriction mediated by these other substances. The magnitude of the influence of these prostaglandins in the clinical setting of CHF is only now under investigation. Reduction of the formation of renal prostaglandins in patients with severe CHF may reduce sodium excretion and the ability to respond to diuretic therapy.

## Aggravating or Precipitating Factors

Although CHF may occur in the natural history of organic heart disease, it is prudent to look for certain additional factors that may either aggravate or precipitate cardiac compromise. In the patient with organic heart disease who is active and asymptomatic, CHF does not usually develop suddenly, unless some new problem occurs. The more common causes of abrupt change that may result in cardiac decompensation include (Table 11.2) myocardial infarction, cardiac arrhythmias, pulmonary embolism, rupture of the chordae tendineae, acute pulmonary infection, and sudden emotional turmoil. When CHF develops gradually, it is also important to search for extracardiac factors that may lead to decompensation in the presence of organic heart disease, including anemia, liver disease, renal disease, prostatic obstruction in the elderly male, bacterial endocarditis, acute rheumatic fever in children, endocrine disturbances (i.e., thyrotoxicosis), uncontrolled hypertension, excessive dietary sodium ingestion, and certain drugs that may exacerbate or precipitate CHF (Table 11.3). A systematic search

**Table 11.2** Aggravating and Precipitating Factors in Congestive Heart Failure

| | |
|---|---|
| Myocardial infarction | Anemia |
| Cardiac arrhythmias | Liver disease |
| Pulmonary embolism | Renal disease |
| Rupture of chordae tendineae | Prostatic obstruction |
| Acute pulmonary infection | Bacterial endocarditis |
| Sudden emotional turmoil | Acute rheumatic fever (in children) |
| Uncontrolled hypertension | Excessive dietary sodium intake |
| Endocrine abnormalities (i.e., thyrotoxicosis) | Drugs (see Table 11.3) |
| Medication noncompliance | |

Adapted from Covinsky JO: Congestive heart failure. The Consultant Pharmacist 1986(May):49, with permission.

**Table 11.3** Drugs That May Exacerbate or Precipitate Congestive Heart Failure

Decrease contractility
- Antiarrhythmics (disopyramide, flecainide, and others)
- β-Blockers (propranolol and others)
- Calcium channel blockers (verapamil and others)

Direct cardiac toxins
- Daunomycin
- Doxorubicin

Sodium and water retention
- Androgens
- Diazoxide
- Estrogens
- Excessive licorice (glycyrrhyzic acid)
- Glucocorticoids, especially those with high mineralocorticoid activity (cortisone, hydrocortisone)
- High-sodium-content drugs (carbenicillin disodium)
- Lithium carbonate
- Nonsteroidal anti-inflammatory agents
- Salicylates (high doses)
- Sympatholytic agents (guanethidine, methyldopa)

Osmotic agents
- Albumin
- Mannitol

for these precipitating factors should be made in every patient who presents with CHF, particularly if they are refractory to conventional therapy. Likewise, inquiring into a patient's dietary and medication compliance may identify a noncompliant patient who appears to be refractory to therapy. If properly recognized, the precipitating cause of cardiac decompensation usually can be treated effectively or removed and management of the patient's underlying cardiac disease subsequently improves.

## Clinical Presentation

The clinical manifestations and physical findings of CHF are easily predicted when one understands the pathogenesis of the disease. As mentioned, cardiac output is not dramatically reduced in the initial phase of CHF, and the patient's symptoms result from the presence of the compensatory mechanisms previously described. Most of the symptoms and physical findings of CHF are the result of pulmonary and/or systemic venous congestion and edema formation (Table 11.4). Failure of the heart as a pump results in congestion of blood behind the failing ventricle. Thus, if the left ventricle is functioning inadequately, the congestion occurs in the lungs; whereas when the right ventricle fails, the congestion is found in the systemic circulation. Most patients who have had left-sided CHF for some time, however, present with both pulmonary and systemic congestion.

Backup of blood behind the failing ventricle results in increased venous and capillary hydrostatic pressure, while simultaneously diluting the colloid osmotic pressure. The increased hydrostatic pressure and decreased osmotic pressure cause a redistribution of fluid from the intravascular space to the interstitial space, resulting in the formation of edema. A vicious cycle is set in motion as the already failing heart is not able to accept the increased sodium and water load generated by the kidneys and further cardiac decompensation occurs.

**Table 11.4** Signs and Symptoms of Congestive Heart Failure

| | *Symptoms* | *Signs* |
|---|---|---|
| **Right-Sided Failure** | Abdominal pain<br>Anorexia<br>Bloating<br>Constipation<br>Fluid retention<br>Nausea<br>Vomiting | Ascites<br>Jugular venous distension<br>Hepatojugular reflux<br>Hepatomegaly<br>Peripheral edema<br>Splenomegaly |
| **Left-Sided Failure** | Cough<br>Dyspnea<br>Hemoptysis<br>Orthopnea<br>Tachypnea<br>Paroxysmal nocturnal dyspnea | Bibasilar rales<br>Cheyne–Stokes respirations<br>Pleural effusion<br>Pulmonary edema<br>$S_3$ gallop rhythm |
| **Nonspecific Findings** | Fatigue<br>Mental aberration<br>Nocturia<br>Oliguria (daytime)<br>Weakness | Cardiomegaly<br>Cyanosis<br>Tachycardia |

### *Signs/Symptoms of Left-Sided Congestive Heart Failure*

Pulmonary congestion secondary to left-sided CHF may manifest in patients as dyspnea, orthopnea, paroxysmal nocturnal dyspnea, or cough. Dyspnea on exertion is the most common symptom of CHF. As CHF advances, dyspnea appears with less strenuous activity until eventually it is present even at rest. Orthopnea is usually indicative of more advanced CHF and occurs when the patient assumes a recumbent position. In the recumbent position, blood from the lower extremities and the splanchnic beds redistributes to the lungs, resulting in an elevation of pulmonary venous pressure and subsequent pulmonary congestion. Determining how many pillows a patient sleeps on provides a subjective assessment of the severity of orthopnea. For example, a patient's CHF may be worsening if he or she previously had stable "two-pillow" orthopnea but now needs to sleep on three or four pillows. Paroxysmal nocturnal dyspnea (so-called cardiac asthma) is characterized by severe shortness of breath that generally awakens the patient from sleep in the middle of the night. This is also the result of increased pulmonary vascular congestion that has been allowed to advance until pulmonary edema and bronchospasm develop. Patients with pulmonary congestion may have a cough; if congestion is severe enough, patients may also develop hemoptysis.

Rales (crackles), pleural effusions, and pulmonary edema are also signs of left-sided CHF. A third heart sound, or $S_3$, may be heard in left-sided CHF and results from either an abnormally large diastolic flow into a normal ventricle or normal flow into an abnormal, dilated ventricle. An $S_3$ may also be heard in right-sided CHF. In severe CHF, a patient may develop Cheyne–Stokes respirations, characterized by alternating phases of hyperventilation and apnea.

Depending on the severity of left-sided CHF, a chest roentgenogram (CXR) may reveal the following signs: prominent upper-lobe vessels, reflecting pulmonary venous congestion and redistribution of blood flow from lower to upper lung fields; pleural effusions; septal lines, or Kerley B lines, which are sharp linear densities of interlobular interstitial edema; or a "butterfly pattern" of bilateral perihilar infiltrates consistent with pulmonary edema. When pulmonary vascular congestion is unilateral, it normally occurs on the right side in patients with CHF. It is often difficult to differentiate the vascular changes associated with CHF from pneumonia. Fever, an elevated white blood cell count with a left shift, and an elevated erythrocyte sedimentation rate are more consistent with a pneumonia than CHF and may help in differentiation.

### *Signs/Symptoms of Right-Sided Congestive Heart Failure*

As a result of systemic venous congestion, patients with right-sided CHF may present with a variety of gastrointestinal symptoms including anorexia, abdominal bloating, right-upper-quadrant or epigastric pain, constipation, nausea, and vomiting. They may also complain of fluid retention.

Ankle or pretibial edema, congestive hepatomegaly, splenomegaly, jugular venous distension, and hepatojugular reflux indicate systemic venous congestion and are signs of right-sided heart failure. Ankle and pretibial edema are common findings in ambulatory patients, because fluid tends to accumulate in the dependent portions of the body secondary to the influence of gravity. It should be noted, therefore, that sacral rather than ankle edema may be present in the bedridden patient. Venous congestion may also result in portal hypertension, hepatomegaly, and occasionally ascites. Jugular venous distension (JVD) noted higher than 4 cm above the sternal angle measured while a patient is sitting up at a 45° angle is indicative of right-sided CHF with systemic venous congestion. A positive hepatojugular reflux is elicited by firmly pressing on the patient's liver and noting sustained jugular venous distension as a result.

### *Nonspecific Signs/Symptoms*

Tachycardia and cardiomegaly have obvious causes that have been described earlier. Peripheral cyanosis resulting from compromised respiration, decreased cardiac output, and shunting of blood away from the skin may be apparent. Although nonspecific, weakness and fatigue are commonly found in patients with CHF and are secondary to the altered distribution of the cardiac output. In severe CHF, patients may complain of oliguria during the daytime, secondary to a decreased blood supply to the kidneys. More commonly, however, nocturia occurs as blood is redistributed to the kidneys when the patient is in the supine position. Finally, patients with severe CHF may have alterations in mental status, such as confusion or disorientation, secondary to inadequate blood supply to the brain.

## Assessment of Cardiovascular Disability

Identifying the degree of cardiovascular disability in patients with CHF is important for several reasons: the status of a patient's CHF can be followed longitudinally, the impact of specific therapeutic modalities can be evaluated, and patients can be compared with each other. Several methods are available for assessing cardiovascular disability. The most widely used method is the New York Heart Association (NYHA) Functional Classification System.[18] This system divides patients into four functional classes by relating symptoms to "ordinary" activity. Functional class (FC)-I patients have no limitation of physical activity. FC-II patients have slight limitations; FC-III patients have marked limitations; and FC-IV patients are unable to carry on any physical activity without discomfort and have symptoms even at rest. The system devised by the Canadian Cardiovascular Society (CCS) is more detailed and specific, but is limited to patients with angina pectoris. Finally, a Specific Activity Scale was developed recently by Goldman et al.[19] This system is based on the estimated energy expenditure, termed *mets* or *metabolic equivalents*, required for various activities. It appears to be highly reproducible and a better predictor of exercise tolerance than the NYHA or CCS methods, but is not yet widely used (Table 11.5).[19,20]

## Overview of Treatment

The ultimate goals of therapy are to abolish disabling symptoms, improve the quality of life, and prolong the life of patients with CHF. Thus far, therapy has been successful in alleviating the symptoms of CHF, but has had very little documented impact on the long-term survival of patients with CHF. The principal considerations in the management of CHF include elimination of etiologic factors precipitating CHF, reduction of the workload of the heart, increase of myocardial contractility and performance, decrease in sodium and water retention, and facilitation of myocardial relaxation. Thus, the medical management of CHF includes correction or control of the associated disease states (i.e., hypertension), bedrest (which itself reduces sympathetic tone), a sodium-restricted diet, and specific drug therapy depending on the underlying pathophysiologic problem.

## Treatment of Acute or Severe Congestive Heart Failure

Rapid deterioration of a patient with severe chronic CHF or acute onset of left-sided CHF secondary to such precipitating factors as acute myocardial infarction and malignant hypertension represents a therapeutic challenge requiring aggressive intervention. Such patients frequently present with clinical hypoperfusion and pulmonary edema. Prior to the era of invasive hemodynamic monitoring, the management of these patients was described by the acronym MOSTDAMP. With the advent of afterload-reducing agents, the modified acronym AMOSTDAMP seems more appropriate. Knowledge of this clinical approach along with its applications and limitations is still useful in the emergent management of these patients until invasive hemodynamic monitoring devices can be inserted.

### *AMOSTDAMP*

*A—Afterload Reduction* In the setting of acute or severe CHF, afterload reduction with an agent such as intravenous nitroprusside can be beneficial provided that the mean arterial pressure is above 85 mm Hg. Nitroprusside will dilate both arterial and venous vasculature, and thus can reduce both preload and afterload and subsequently improve cardiac output. Nitrates, such as intravenous nitroglycerin, are known to have consistent venodilating or preload-reducing effects; however, arterial vasodilatory effects are more variable and are dependent on the resting level of SVR. Patients with CHF frequently have elevated resting SVR and often show significant afterload reduction with augmentation of cardiac output with nitrate therapy.[21] These patients are likely to respond to either nitroprusside or nitroglycerin. Patients with myocardial ischemia also may theoretically benefit from the more selective coronary vasodilatory effects

**Table 11.5** Three Methods of Assessing Cardiovascular Disability

| *Class* | *New York Heart Association functional classification* | *Canadian Cardiovascular Society functional classification* | *Specific activity scale* |
|---|---|---|---|
| I | Patients with cardiac disease but without resulting limitations of physical activity. Ordinary physical activity does not cause undue fatigue, palpitation, dyspnea, or anginal pain. | Ordinary physical activity, such as walking and climbing stairs, does not cause angina. Angina with strenuous or rapid or prolonged exertion at work or recreation. | Patients can perform to completion any activity requiring ≥ 7 metabolic equivalents, e.g., can carry 24 lb up eight steps; carry objects that weigh 80 lb; do outdoor work (shovel snow, spade soil); do recreational activities (skiing, basketball, squash, handball, jog/walk 5 mph). |
| II | Patients with cardiac disease resulting in slight limitations of physical activity. They are comfortable at rest. Ordinary physical activity results in fatigue, palpitation, dyspnea, or anginal pain. | Slight limitation of ordinary activity. Walking or climbing stairs rapidly, walking uphill, walking or climbing stairs after meals, in cold, in wind, under emotional stress, or only during the few hours after awakening. Walking more than two blocks on the level and climbing more than one flight of ordinary stairs at a normal pace and under normal conditions. | Patient can perform to completion any activity requiring ≥ 5 metabolic equivalents but cannot and does not perform to completion activities requiring ≥ 7 metabolic equivalents, e.g., have sexual intercourse without stopping, garden, rake, weed, roller skate, dance fox trot, walk at 4 mph on level ground. |
| III | Patients with cardiac disease resulting in marked limitation of physical activity. They are comfortable at rest. Less than ordinary physical activity causes fatigue, palpitation, dyspnea, or anginal pain. | Marked limitation of ordinary physical activity. Walking one to two blocks on the level and climbing more than one flight under normal conditions. | Patient can perform to completion any activity requiring ≥ 2 metabolic equivalents but cannot and does not perform to completion any activities requiring ≥ 5 metabolic equivalents, e.g., shower without stopping, strip and make bed, clean windows, walk 2.5 mph, bowl, play golf, dress without stopping. |
| IV | Patients with cardiac disease resulting in inability to carry on any physical activity without discomfort. Symptoms of cardiac insufficiency or of the anginal syndrome may be present even at rest. If any physical activity is undertaken, discomfort is increased. | Inability to carry on any physical activity without discomfort—anginal syndrome *may* be present at rest. | Patient cannot or does not perform to completion activities requiring ≥ 2 metabolic equivalents. *Cannot* carry out activities listed above (Specific Activity Scale, Class III). |

From Braunwald E: The history, in Braunwald E (Ed): Heart Disease. A Textbook of Cardiovascular Medicine, 3rd ed. Philadelphia, W. B. Saunders, 1988, p 12, with permission.

of intravenous nitroglycerin. Afterload reduction should not be attempted when the mean arterial blood pressure is less than 85 mm Hg, unless combined with an inotropic agent such as dopamine. In any case, continuous blood pressure monitoring with an arterial line is essential in the use of either nitroprusside or nitroglycerin as afterload-reducing agents.

***M—Morphine*** Intravenous morphine is very useful in this setting as it can promptly relieve chest pain and anxiety. Also, intravenous morphine causes peripheral vasodilation that can reduce preload and relieve symptoms associated with pulmonary edema; however, administering morphine in this setting is not without risks, as intravenous morphine can cause respiratory depression or hypotension that could worsen the situation. To minimize these risks, small doses of morphine, such as 2–4 mg, are administered intravenously at a rate of 1 mg per minute. Waiting 15 to 20 minutes between doses allows adequate time to assess response to each dose. Should excessive respiratory depression or hypotension occur, intravenous naloxone can be administered to antagonize morphine's effects.

***O—Oxygen*** Supplemental oxygen can be administered as pulmonary edema frequently results in impaired oxygenation. The route and amount of oxygen are determined by the severity of physical signs and symptoms and arterial blood gas determinations.

***S—Sit up*** Sitting the patient up and possibly hanging the legs over the edge of the bed can relieve the symptoms of pulmonary edema. This maneuver reduces pulmonary congestion by pooling blood in the dependent portions of the body, which decreases venous return and reduces preload.

***T—Tourniquets*** Rotating tourniquets have been utilized to decrease venous return to the heart and relieve symptoms of pulmonary congestion. Tourniquets are applied to three of the four extremities and are rotated every 15 minutes. Their use should be limited to those patients who are not hypotensive.

***D—Digitalis*** Historically, digitalis was included in the management of these patients; however, its relatively weak inotropic effects coupled with its delayed onset and peak effects relative to other intravenous inotropes limit its usefulness. If inotropic support is indicated, intravenous dopamine or dobutamine should be utilized. Digitalis should be reserved for patients who have concomitant supraventricular arrhythmias, such as uncontrolled paroxysmal supraventricular tachycardia or atrial fibrillation.

***A—Aminophylline*** Aminophylline may relieve symptoms of pulmonary edema and bronchospasm by several mechanisms, including direct bronchodilation, positive inotropic and chronotropic effects, decrease in LVEDP (preload) and pulmonary artery pressure, decrease in SVR, and a weak diuretic effect.[22–24] The exact contribution of each of these mechanisms is uncertain and may vary among patients; however, aminophylline can also increase myocardial oxygen consumption and cause tachyarrhythmias and is relatively contraindicated in patients with acute CHF secondary to acute myocardial infarction, as it may extend the size of the infarction or induce arrhythmias.

***M—Mercurial Diuretics*** Historically, mercurial diuretics were used in this setting. Presently, less toxic, faster acting loop diuretics are an important component of the therapy of acute or severe CHF.

***P—Phlebotomy*** Phlebotomizing patients by removing 200–250 mL of blood can decrease venous return and relieve symptoms of pulmonary congestion. Its use should be limited to patients refractory to the preceding measures outlined and is contraindicated in the hypotensive or severely anemic patient.

## *Hemodynamic Monitoring*

### Basic Principles

A notable advance in the management of patients with acute or severe CHF has been the introduction of the Swan–Ganz catheter, a convenient, bedside hemodynamic monitoring device.[25,26] The Swan–Ganz catheter is a long catheter, with a small balloon near its tip, which may be advanced from a peripheral or central vein through the right side of the heart and into the pulmonary circulation. The tip of the catheter is pressure sensitive and records the hydrostatic pressure it encounters within the vascular system. When the balloon is inflated and "wedged" into a pulmonary artery at a level parallel to the left atrium, the catheter tip no longer records pulmonary artery pressure; rather it measures the "down-

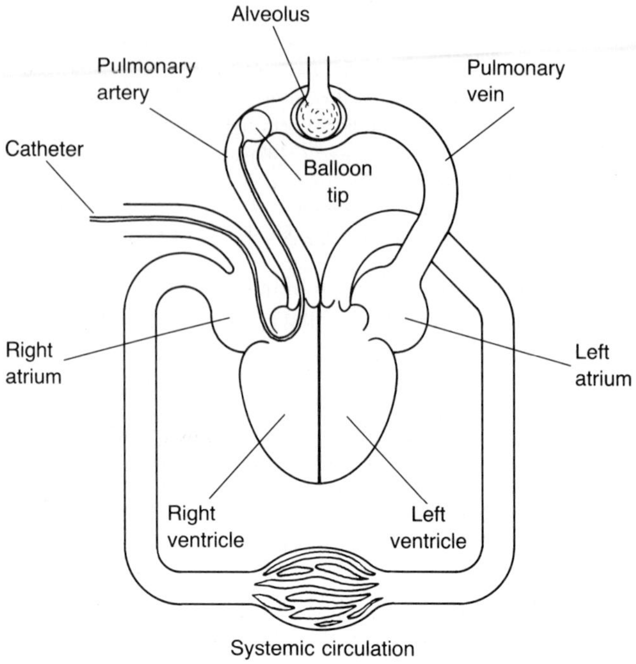


**Figure 11.3** Diagram depicting Swan–Ganz catheter placement. During diastole, the left ventricle, the left atrium, and the pulmonary capillary bed form a common chamber. Thus, "wedging" the balloon tip (inflated) into the pulmonary artery allows measurement of PCWP downstream, which can be used to estimate LVEDP.

stream" pressure, referred to as pulmonary capillary wedge pressure.

During diastole, when the mitral valve is open, the left ventricle, left atrium, and pulmonary venous bed become a continuous chamber. Therefore, the pressure experienced during this time by the left ventricle is transferred to the catheter tip and recorded as the PCWP (Fig. 11.3). The PCWP is therefore essentially equal to the LVEDP. As previously described by the Frank–Starling mechanism, LVEDP usually correlates with the amount of blood returned to the heart in the resting phase.

Some Swan–Ganz catheters are also capable of measuring cardiac output. A lumen that opens approximately 30 cm from the catheter tip is used to inject a known volume of cold solution. A thermistor located just proximal to the catheter tip measures the resultant change in pulmonary artery blood temperature; a small bedside computer then uses this information to calculate right-heart cardiac output, which is usually equal to left-heart cardiac output in all but a few situations, such as isolated right ventricular failure (Fig. 11.4).

### Limitations

When the pulmonary vascular bed, mitral valve, and left ventricle function normally, the pulmonary artery diastolic pressure (PADP), PCWP, mean left atrial pressure, and LVEDP are roughly equivalent. Certain conditions, however, can interfere with the ability of the Swan–Ganz catheter to provide an accurate estimate of the left ventricular filling pressure. For example, in pulmonary hypertension,

$$CO = \frac{(1.08)C_t(60)V_I(T_B - T_I)}{\int_0^T T_B(t)dt}$$

CO = cardiac output (mL/min)

$$1.08 = \frac{pC_p(5\%\ \text{dextrose})}{pC_p(\text{blood})}$$

($p$ = density, $C_p$ = specific heat)

$C_t$ = correction for rise of injectate temperature during injection

60 = seconds/minute

$V_I$ = volume of injectate

$T_I$ = initial injectate temperature (°C)

$T_B$ = initial blood temperature (°C)

$\int_0^t T_B(t)dt$ = integral of blood temperature change (°C-s)

**Figure 11.4** Equation used by the bedside computer for calculation of cardiac output (CO). *(Adapted from Bollish SJ, Foster TS: Swan–Ganz catheter: An important tool for monitoring drug therapy in the critically ill. Hosp Formulary 1980[Feb];105. Courtesy of American Edwards Laboratories.)*

pulmonary vascular resistance increases and PADP no longer equals PCWP. A similar situation occurs in tachycardia, as there is insufficient time for PADP and PCWP to equilibrate. In hypovolemic shock or when positive end-expiratory pressure (PEEP) is administered to ventilator-dependent patients, PCWP may be falsely elevated. In mitral valve disease or markedly reduced ventricular compliance, PCWP and left atrial pressure do not equal LVEDP, and atrial contraction can appreciably increase LVEDP. Therefore, while PCWP can still be used to monitor left ventricular filling pressure, it does not accurately assess left ventricular function. In addition, LVEDP may be disproportionately increased relative to LVEDV in noncompliant ventricles or in ventilator-dependent patients receiving PEEP. Also, drugs like dopamine can increase pulmonary vascular resistance and lead to inaccurate estimates of LVEDP in patients with impaired left ventricular function. Correct placement of the catheter tip at or below the level of the left atrium is also essential for accurate determination of PCWP.[27] Lastly, as stated earlier, measuring the right cardiac output may not accurately reflect left cardiac output in cases of isolated right ventricular failure, such as secondary to pulmonary hypertension.

### Clinical Application

Correlating objective hemodynamic parameters, such as PCWP, to clinical findings is often useful in managing patients with acute or severe CHF (Table 11.6). Normally, the PCWP is between 5 and 12 mm Hg. An optimal PCWP in critically ill patients, such as those with severe CHF, is between 15 and 18 mm Hg. Pulmonary congestion becomes apparent when the PCWP increases above 18 mm Hg. As the PCWP increases, the severity of pulmonary congestion progresses. As discussed before, in patients with severe ischemia where ventricular compliance may be reduced, it may be difficult to predict optimal left ventricular filling pressure because the relationship between PCWP and left ventricular function may be distorted. In any case, these numbers provide a reference point for developing a therapeutic plan.

Cardiac output (CO) or cardiac index (CI) (cardiac output corrected for body surface area) is often useful in characterizing left ventricular performance. A normal resting CI is between 2.7 and 4.3 L/min/m$^2$. Subclinical cardiac depression becomes apparent when the CI is reduced to 2.2–2.7 L/min/m$^2$. Clinically evident CHF often associated with hypoperfusion is apparent when the CI is reduced to 1.8–2.2 L/min/m$^2$. Patients in cardiogenic shock frequently have a CI below 1.8 L/min/m$^2$. These patients often do not survive regardless of their treatment.

### Hemodynamic Subsets as a Guide to Therapy

Utilization of invasive hemodynamic monitoring in patients with acute CHF or severe, refractory CHF allows the clinician to classify patients into hemodynamic subsets (Fig. 11.5).[26] While this classification system was initially created for patients with varying degrees of left ventricular failure complicating an acute myocardial infarction, it is still useful

**Table 11.6** Normal Hemodynamic Variables

| | |
|---|---|
| Mean arterial pressure (MAP) = [SBP + 2(DBP)]/3 | 80–100 mm Hg |
| Pulmonary artery pressure (PAP) | 25/10 mm Hg |
| Mean PAP (MPAP) | 12–15 mm Hg |
| Right atrial pressure (RAP) | 2–5 mm Hg |
| Pulmonary capillary wedge pressure (PCWP) | |
| Normal adults | 5–12 mm Hg |
| Critically ill patients | 15–18 mm Hg |
| Cardiac output (CO) | 4–7 L/min |
| Cardiac index (CI) [CO/BSA] | 2.7–4.3 L/min/m$^2$ |
| Systemic vascular resistance (SVR) = [(MAP − RAP)/CO] × 80 | 800–1200 dyn · s/cm$^5$ |
| Pulmonary vascular resistance (PVR) = [(MPAP − PCWP)/CO] × 80 | 20–120 dyn · s/cm$^5$ |

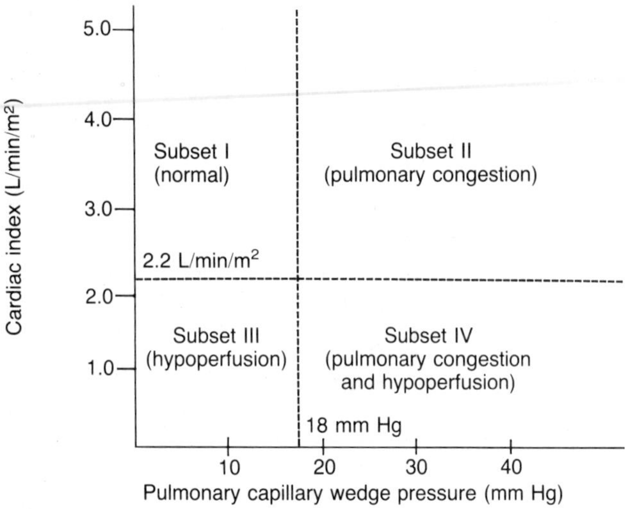


**Figure 11.5** Subsets of CHF patients based on cardiac index and pulmonary capillary wedge pressure. When ventricular compliance is altered, the vertical line may shift right or left, and the relationship between cardiac index and filling pressure (PCWP) becomes distorted. *(Adapted from Forrester JS, et al: Medical therapy of acute myocardial infarction by application of hemodynamic subsets. N Engl J Med 1976;295:1361, with permission.)*

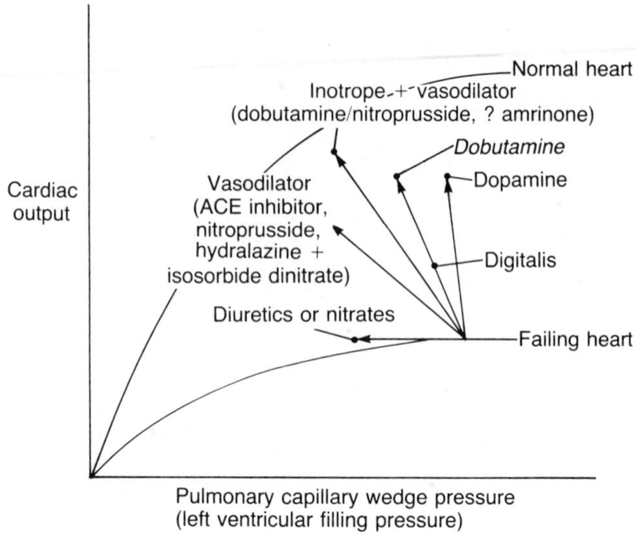


**Figure 11.6** Effects of drugs used in CHF on cardiac output and left ventricular filling pressure. *(Adapted from Cohn JN: Hosp Practice 1984[Aug];19:39, with permission.)*

in the management of patients with acute or severe CHF secondary to other causes. This information coupled with the knowledge of the expected effects of various therapeutic interventions on the Frank–Starling curve (Fig. 11.6) allows the clinician to individualize pharmacotherapy and evaluate responses objectively. Referring to Figure 11.5, patients in subset I have an adequate CI of 2.2 L/min/m$^2$ or greater and no pulmonary congestion with a PCWP less than 18 mm Hg. These patients require no specific therapeutic intervention.

Patients in subset II have an elevated PCWP greater than 18 mm Hg and present with varying degrees of pulmonary congestion depending on how elevated the PCWP is. These patients require diuretics to enhance sodium and water excretion and decrease preload. Should diuretics prove inadequate, venous vasodilators such as nitrates can be used in addition to lower preload. If the calculated SVR (see Table 11.6) is elevated, the patient may benefit from afterload reduction with arterial vasodilators such as hydralazine as well. Alternatively, patients with elevated preload and afterload can be managed with a mixed vasodilator such as prazosin, captopril, or intravenous nitroprusside, which dilates both the arterial and venous circulation.

Patients in subset III present primarily with hypoperfusion, with a CI less than 2.2 L/min/m$^2$ and a PCWP less than 18 mm Hg. If the patient's PCWP is less than 15 mm Hg, judicious administration of fluids can be used to raise the PCWP to 15–18 mm Hg and improve CI by augmenting filling pressure. If this fails to adequately increase CI, intravenous inotropes can be utilized. Extreme caution must be observed if vasodilators are used, as they may excessively lower preload and make the patient hypotensive as a result of inadequate filling pressure.

Patients in subset IV have a CI less than 2.2 L/min/m$^2$ and a PCWP greater than 18 mm Hg and present with both hypoperfusion and pulmonary congestion. This subset of CHF patients requires combination therapy with intravenous inotropes and vasodilators as well as diuretics. When the mean arterial pressure is less than 85 mm Hg, an inotrope that will maintain or raise mean arterial pressure, such as dopamine, should be used. Patients in subset IV with a CI less than 1.8 L/min/m$^2$ and a PCWP greater than 30 mm Hg are in cardiogenic shock and have a high mortality rate despite aggressive therapy.

## Treatment of Chronic Congestive Heart Failure

Specific therapy of chronic CHF can be tailored according to the patient's NYHA functional class (Fig. 11.7). Patients in FC-I have no limitations of physical activity and require no specific treatment. An FC-II patient can be managed initially by restricting physical activity and dietary sodium ingestion. If these measures prove inadequate, either digitalis glycosides or thiazide diuretics can be initiated. If maximal tolerated doses of thiazides fail to improve symptoms adequately, a digitalis glycoside can be added to the thiazide. Conversely, if a digitalis glycoside is chosen first, a thiazide can be added to the patient's regimen. Patients in FC-III require further restriction of physical activity and the addition of a more potent loop diuretic in place of a thiazide diuretic. Currently, such vasodilators as captopril, hydralazine/isosorbide dinitrate, and prazosin are added after loop diuretics fail to control symptoms. Patients with concomitant hypertension and/or ischemic heart disease may be treated with vasodilators earlier and possibly without digitalis glycosides.

Finally, FC-IV patients require aggressive management and are frequently confined to bedrest. They can receive maximally tolerated digoxin doses or be switched to intravenous inotropes such as dopamine or dobutamine. Maximal doses of oral or more frequently intravenous loop diuretics are necessary, possibly in combination with a potassium-

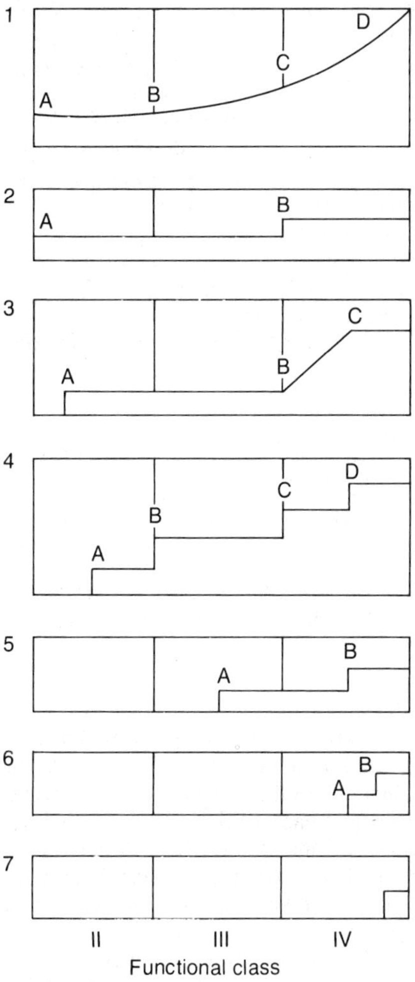


1. Restriction of physical activity
   A. Discontinue exhausting sports and heavy labor
   B. Discontinue full-time work or equivalent activity; introduce rest periods during the day
   C. Confine to house
   D. Confine to bed or chair
2. Digitalis glycoside (if $S_3$ is present)[a]
   A. Usual maintenance dose
   B. Maximum tolerated dose
3. Restriction of sodium intake
   A. Eliminate salt shaker at table (Na = 1.6–2.8 g)
   B. Eliminate salt in cooking and at table (Na = 1.2–1.8 g)
   C. Institute A and B plus low-sodium diet (Na = 0.2–1.0g)
4. Diuretics
   A. Thiazide diuretics (hydrochlorothiazide or others)
   B. Loop diuretics (furosemide or bumetanide)
   C. Loop diuretic plus distal tubular (potassium-sparing) diuretic (spironolactone, triamterene, or amiloride)
   D. Loop diuretic plus thiazide diuretic (metolazone or others) and/or distal tubular diuretic
5. Vasodilators[b]
   A. Angiotensin-converting enzyme inhibitor (captopril or enalapril) or hydralazine plus isosorbide dinitrate
   B. Consider intravenous nitroprusside or nitroglycerin
6. Other inotropic agents
   A. Dopamine or dobutamine
   B. Amrinone
7. Special measures (thoracentesis, paracentesis, dialysis, intraaortic balloon counterpulsation, cardiac transplant)

[a] Presence of an $S_3$ may be less reliable in patients over 60.
[b] Patients with hypertension and/or ischemic heart disease may be treated with vasodilators earlier and possibly without digitalis glycosides.

**Figure 11.7** Overview of treatment of chronic conjestive heart failure. *(Adapted from Covinsky JO: Congestive heart failure. The Consultant Pharmacist 1986[May];50, and Smith TW: Hosp Practice 1984[Aug];19:85, with permission.)*

sparing diuretic or metolazone. Also, if maximal doses of oral vasodilators fail, intravenous vasodilators such as nitroprusside are necessary. In patients refractory to the preceding therapy, special measures may be considered such as physical removal of fluid by thoracentesis, paracentesis, or hemodialysis; temporary circulatory assistance maneuvers, such as intraaortic balloon counterpulsation; implantation of an artificial heart; or cardiac transplantation.

### *Specific Therapeutic Interventions*

A sodium-restricted diet may be instituted to offset the abnormal renal retention of sodium that is observed in patients with CHF. If the ability of the kidney to excrete sodium is not severely compromised, one method to approach normal balance is restriction of the intake of sodium to match excretion. Even though less than 1 g of sodium chloride (NaCl) is required to meet daily physiologic needs, the average American diet contains 10 g of NaCl. Severe salt restriction (less than 500 mg of sodium or 1.3 g of NaCl) results in an unpalatable diet and patients frequently do not comply with such a regimen. Moderate salt intake (2–4 g of NaCl), which can be accomplished by restricting the addition of salt during cooking, is much more acceptable to patients. Patients should also avoid foods that are high in sodium content (Table 11.7). Likewise, clinicians should be aware of drugs that are high in sodium content, such as carbenicillin, and should use low-sodium-content alternatives when possible and practical.

### *Diuretics*

Diuretics are frequently used in patients with CHF who fail to respond satisfactorily to dietary sodium restriction. With respect to use of diuretics in CHF patients, Weber et al have suggested monitoring daily weight before and after diuretic

**Table 11.7** Selected Examples of High-Sodium-Content Foods

| *Food item* | *Amount* | *Sodium content (mg)* |
|---|---|---|
| Meats/fish/cheese | | |
| Bacon | 2 strips | 100 |
| Bologna | 1 slice | 370 |
| Canadian bacon | 1 slice | 537 |
| Cheese, processed | 1 ounce | 300 |
| Chili con carne with beans, canned | 1 cup | 1,354 |
| Corned beef hash, canned | 1 cup | 1,188 |
| Frankfurter | 1 | 495 |
| Ham, baked | $\frac{1}{2}$ cup | 525 |
| Soup, canned | 1 cup | 1,000 |
| Spaghetti and meat balls, canned | 1 cup | 1,220 |
| Breads/crackers | | |
| Corn bread | 1 piece 2 × 2 in. | 332 |
| Crackers, saltines | 5 | 156 |
| Macaroni, noodles, rice, or potatoes cooked with salt | $\frac{1}{2}$ cup | 275 |
| Fruits/vegetables | | |
| Sauerkraut, canned | $\frac{1}{2}$ cup | 880 |
| Vegetables, canned | $\frac{1}{2}$ cup | 300 |
| Beverages | | |
| Buttermilk | 1 cup | 320 |
| Tomato juice | 1 cup | 486 |
| Condiments | | |
| Dill pickles | 1 large | 1,928 |

From Nutritive Value of American Foods in Common Units. Agricultural Handbook No. 456. Agricultural Research Service, 1975.

therapy with the target of inducing a 0.9-kg weight loss per day.[28] Keep in mind that it is easier to mobilize fluid from peripheral edema than ascites.

### Thiazide Diuretics

Thiazide diuretics, such as hydrochlorothiazide, block sodium and chloride reabsorption in the distal convoluted tubule of the nephron and increase fractional excretion of sodium in the kidneys by approximately 5% to 8%. They are usually effective only in patients with mild CHF when the creatinine clearance is greater than 30–40 mL/min. Thiazide diuretics may decrease renal blood flow in patients with reduced creatinine clearance and are less useful in patients with moderate to severe acute CHF.[29,30] Limited data suggest that metolazone may work at lower creatinine clearances than other thiazide diuretics.[31]

### Loop Diuretics

In patients with moderate to severe CHF, potent loop diuretics such as furosemide, bumetanide, or piretanide (an investigational loop diuretic) may be necessary. Ethacrynic acid is a loop diuretic equipotent to furosemide; however, it has a greater tendency to produce ototoxicity and gastrointestinal disturbances. As a result, ethacrynic acid is used less frequently today. Loop diuretics block chloride transport in the ascending limb of the loop of Henle and subsequently can be expected to increase the fractional excretion of sodium approximately 20% to 25%. Loop diuretics in general have a duration of action of approximately 6 hours[30]; however, patients with stable CHF can often be controlled on once- or twice-daily dosing.[32,33]

Until recently, most clinicians believed that the intravenous administration of furosemide always produced a prompt reduction in preload and afterload followed by a rapid diuresis[34–37]; however, a recent report indicates acute worsening of symptoms after rapid and high-dose intravenous furosemide administration in a group of 15 patients with severe chronic CHF.[38] Although the precise mechanism for the deterioration noted in these patients is not fully explained, the authors did describe early activation of the renin–angiotensin system, sympathetic nervous system, and release of arginine vasopressin. As the actual individual hemodynamic parameters of these patients were not provided, it is difficult to determine whether the magnitude of hemodynamic response was similar among the patients.

In the graphic data provided in the aforementioned study,[38] significant variation in individual hemodynamic parameters was noted. Nine of the patients had underlying coronary artery disease and were thought to have "ischemic cardiomyopathy" as a result of multiple previous myocardial infarctions. None had pulmonary edema yet their PCWPs averaged 28 mm Hg. Conceivably these patients may have had lusitropic abnormalities and the dramatic reduction in preload precipitated a reflex activation of the various neurohumoral substances. As the first blood pressure reading in these patients was measured 15 minutes after a 1.5 mg/kg intravenous dose of furosemide, initial hypotension secondary to venodilatation may have been missed. An initial fall in blood pressure would precipitate reflex activation of the renin–angiotensin and sympathetic nervous systems. Additional studies are needed to verify the prevalence of this particular response in patients with chronic CHF.

The authors concluded by stating that "furosemide is a time-honored treatment for heart failure, and this report does not intend to impugn its use when clinically appropriate. Rather, we believe that the systematic study of its effects on patients with heart failure has allowed for a better understanding of how certain therapies interact with the neurohumoral axis, which is already abnormal in patients with this syndrome."[38]

### "Diuretic Resistance"

Occasionally, patients with marked fluid retention do not respond well to oral doses of loop diuretics. Several mechanisms may explain this phenomenon, including marked declines in glomerular filtration rate with inadequate delivery of the loop diuretic to the site of action, avid proximal tubular reabsorption of sodium secondary to decreased effective circulating blood volume, hyperaldosteronism secondary to decreased effective circulating blood volume and activation of the renin–angiotensin–aldosterone system, and patient noncompliance.[30] Serum albumin may also influence the response to diuretics. It may be much more difficult to induce diuresis in patients with a low serum albumin. A common misconception is that CHF patients with significant systemic edema malabsorb loop diuretics. Brater et al demonstrated that bioavailability is no different in patients with CHF than in normal subjects[39–41]; however, they found that while total bioavailability is unaltered, absorption is delayed and peak concentrations are diminished by approximately 50%. Conceivably, this may play a role in diuretic resistance, as diuresing these patients to dry weight returns these pharmacokinetic parameters toward, but not quite to, normal.[41,42]

Several approaches can be tried to manage such diuretic-resistant patients. First, attempts should be made to identify noncompliant patients and educate them on the importance of compliance. Some patients may respond to smaller doses of loop diuretics administered intravenously. The more potent but more costly bumetanide may elicit a response in some patients not responsive to furosemide. In patients who still have marked fluid retention despite large doses of oral or intravenous loop diuretics, addition of metolazone, or other thiazides less commonly, occasionally yields a profound diuretic response. Metolazone is a potent thiazide-like diuretic with an extended duration of action that blocks sodium reabsorption primarily at the distal convoluted tubule but also has secondary effects at the proximal convoluted tubule. It appears that "sequential blockade" along the proximal convoluted tubule, ascending loop of Henle, and distal convoluted tubule with metolazone and a loop diuretic can result in dramatic synergism[30,43,44]; however, sequential blockade with both a potent loop diuretic and a long-acting diuretic can result in severe sodium and potassium depletion; thus, these electrolytes as well as the patient's volume status and renal function must be monitored closely. Another alternative is to add a distal tubule diuretic, such as spironolactone. Finally, prescribing bedrest and adding a peripheral vasodilator or low-dose intravenous dopamine (2–3 μg/kg/min) to the diuretic constitute yet another approach and occasionally result in a markedly enhanced response to the diuretic.

**Adverse Effects**

Patients with CHF are more apt than patients with hypertension to develop severe diuretic-induced hypokalemia. In some patients, it may be difficult to provide adequate potassium supplementation. Patients often find potassium supplements unpalatable and therefore may be noncompliant. Wax-matrix potassium tablets may be a better choice in these patients. Another alternative in place of potassium supplements in these cases is the addition of a potassium-sparing diuretic such as spironolactone, amiloride, or triamterene; however, the potassium-sparing diuretics should not be used in patients with a creatinine clearance less than 40 mL/min as they may develop hyperkalemia. Because ventricular ectopic activity is a common occurrence in patients with severe cardiac dysfunction, the added risk of hypokalemia amplifies the need for close monitoring of the patient's serum potassium.[45] In addition, CHF patients are frequently on a digitalis glycoside, and hypokalemia predisposes these patients to digitalis-induced arrhythmias. Patients should be monitored for other electrolyte abnormalities such as hypomagnesemia, especially if they manifest arrhythmias or have refractory hypokalemia. Correction of the hypomagnesemia may be necessary before correction of the hypokalemia is possible.[46] Table 11.8 summarizes the more common adverse effects of diuretics.

**Table 11.8** Adverse Effects of Diuretics

| | |
|---|---|
| Fluid and electrolyte abnormalities | |
| Hypokalemia | Thiazides, loop diuretics |
| Hyperkalemia | Potassium-sparing diuretics |
| Hyponatremia | |
| Hypercalcemia | Thiazide diuretics |
| Hypomagnesemia | |
| Extracellular volume depletion | Prerenal azotemia |
| Acid–base abnormalities | |
| Metabolic alkalosis | Hypokalemic, hypochloremic; thiazides, loop diuretics |
| Metabolic acidosis | Hyperchloremic; spironolactone, acetazolamide |
| Metabolic abnormalities | |
| Hyperglycemia | Especially thiazides |
| Hyperuricemia | |
| Hyperlipidemia | Especially thiazides |
| Miscellaneous adverse effects | |
| Ototoxicity | Ethacrynic acid; furosemide, less commonly |
| Gynecomastia | Spironolactone |
| Gastrointestinal bleeding | Ethacrynic acid |
| Hypersensitivity reactions | |

## *Cardiac Glycosides*

Historically, cardiac glycosides have been among the most commonly prescribed drugs in the United States. These agents have been considered the cornerstone of treatment of CHF. This time-honored position is currently under careful scrutiny. The cardiac glycosides are, at best, modest inotropic agents and the high incidence of side effects has provided good reason to reexamine the position of these agents in the treatment of CHF.[47] The cardiac glycosides are generally considered in the management of CHF when the patient develops symptoms with moderate activity.[1] The data substantiating the utility of the cardiac glycosides in this setting, however, despite their common usage are controversial.

**Pharmacology of Digitalis**

In 1785, William Withering reported the results of his 9-year study of the effects of digitalis. The study involved 163 patients he personally treated and 46 case histories submitted by his colleagues.[48] Two hundred years later, this report still ranks among the most complete descriptions of the action of digitalis. At the time Withering's report was published, the heart was not thought to be the primary site of functional disease. Withering believed that digitalis exerted its primary effect on the kidney and that the usefulness of the cardiac glycosides in treating dropsy (CHF) was based primarily on their ability to improve renal function. Thus, in modern terms Withering thought that digitalis primarily reduced filling pressure (preload).

In classic modern pharmacology, the subcellular mechanism of digitalis is thought to involve inhibition of the sarcolemmal sodium–potassium ATPase pump. This pump inhibition raises intracellular sodium, which in turn augments sodium–calcium exchange. This enhanced exchange raises intracellular calcium concentrations, which results in calcium-triggered calcium release. Calcium then binds to troponin, removing the inhibition of actin–myosin interaction. As a result, actin and myosin interact, resulting in contraction of the myofibril. Calcium subsequently dissociates and is taken up into the sarcoplasmic reticulum, resulting in relaxation of the myofibril. In short, by increasing intracellular calcium, digitalis is thought to enhance myocardial contractility.[49–51]

Nevertheless, digitalis has several other notable pharmacologic effects. Digitalis augments vagal tone, resulting in increased diastolic filling which can increase stroke volume. Digitalis also blocks the sodium–potassium ATPase pump in the renal tubules which results in a natriuresis. Digitalis has a multiplicity of effects on sympathetic tone[52–54] and plasma renin activity.[55–57]

Currently, most practitioners think primarily of disorders of myocardial contractility when discussing CHF. Consequently, most modern research on digitalis has focused on its ability to improve myocardial contractility. Unfortunately, very few well-designed, controlled studies of the hemodynamic effects of digitalis have been attempted. Of the few studies that do exist, no dramatic improvement in cardiac output has been demonstrated.[58–62] Most of these studies do, however, show a reduction in LVEDP (filling pressure), and this reduction may well result from the impact of digitalis on the kidney and the peripheral circulation.

After more than 200 years, it is interesting to find that recent studies of the cardiac glycosides are beginning to support Withering's original contention that digitalis has a direct effect on the kidney,[63] an effect that results in increased excretion of sodium and water. This effect on the kidney and changes in peripheral vascular tone resulting from complex effects on the autonomic nervous system and plasma renin activity may collectively contribute to the changes in hemodynamics noted in the various controlled clinical studies. In short, classic modern pharmacology has emphasized the effects of digitalis on contractility, whereas the original and now more recent studies suggest the focus of effects of digitalis may be the kidney and the peripheral circulation.

**Pharmacokinetics of Digoxin**

Digoxin is the form of digitalis most frequently prescribed in the United States today. Digoxin is available for oral administration as tablets, capsules, and an elixir. An injectable form is available for intramuscular or intravenous injection. Orally administered digoxin undergoes passive gastrointestinal absorption primarily in the upper small intestine. In patients with normal gastrointestinal function, oral tablets are 70% to 80% absorbed, and the elixir is 75% to 85% absorbed. A formulation of digoxin in a gel solution capsule known as Lanoxicap is available and has a bioavailability of about 90% to 100%.[64] Because of this enhanced bioavailability, the available dosage forms of Lanoxicap contain 80% of the digoxin that the tablets contain (i.e., 0.1 mg Lanoxicap versus 0.125 mg digoxin tablet; 0.2 mg Lanoxicap versus 0.25 mg digoxin tablet). This more expensive dosage form should be reserved for individuals who do not absorb the less expensive tablets sufficiently or reliably.

The intramuscular route is not recommended because it is painful and produces localized muscle damage. In the setting of acute myocardial infarction, intramuscular administration of digoxin may interfere with the assessment of myocardial damage, as this injection causes an increase in serum creatine kinase levels. In a comparison of the various routes of administration, the most rapid increase in plasma concentration is provided by the intravenous route, followed by the oral route and then the intramuscular route.

Digoxin has a distribution half-life of approximately 30 to 60 minutes. Protein binding of digoxin ranges from 20% to 25% in most patients. The drug is extensively tissue bound to skeletal muscle and thus has a very large volume of distribution. The drug is also concentrated in the kidney, central nervous system, and myocardium, but does not distribute significantly into adipose tissue. As a result, digoxin should be dosed on the basis of lean body weight. Elderly patients and chronic renal failure patients have a decreased volume of distribution.[64,65]

Digoxin undergoes some metabolism to more polar, reduced compounds, such as dihydrodigoxin and dihydrodigoxigenin. These compounds are less active or inactive and normally represent less than 10% of the total amount of digoxin excreted in the urine; however, in about 10% of patients, less digoxin may be absorbed initially, delivering more digoxin to the lower intestine where it is more extensively metabolized by the gut flora. These digoxin reduction products may make up 30% to 40% of the total excreted dose. In this subset of patients, administration of erythromycin or tetracycline may dramatically increase bioavailability by altering the gut flora, decreasing the amount of digoxin that is metabolized, and increasing the amount of unmetabolized digoxin that is absorbed.[64,65] Lanoxicap may be more reliably absorbed than conventional tablets in these patients. Enterohepatic recycling of digoxin can be as high as 30%.[66]

Most of digoxin is eliminated unchanged by the kidneys via glomerular filtration and tubular secretion, with some tubular reabsorption at low tubular flow rates. Digoxin's elimination half-life in normal volunteers averages 36 hours. Elderly patients tend to have reduced renal function, and digoxin's elimination half-life averages 48 hours in this patient population. As renal function declines, digoxin's elimination half-life increases, and a greater proportion of digoxin is eliminated nonrenally. Anephric patients rely entirely on nonrenal elimination, and typically have an elimination half-life of about 5 days.[64,65]

A number of drugs can affect digoxin pharmacokinetics, resulting in potentially significant drug interactions. Table 11.9 summarizes the major drug interactions that occur with digoxin. Table 11.10 provides comparative pharmacokinetic parameters for digoxin and digitoxin. Several references

**Table 11.9** Potentially Significant Drug Interactions With Digoxin

| *Drug* | *Mechanism/effect* | *Suggested management* |
|---|---|---|
| Amiodarone | Decreases renal and nonrenal clearance; can increase SDC by 70%–100% | 1. Decrease digoxin dose by 50%<br>2. Monitor[a] |
| Antacids | Decrease oral absorption 25% | Space drugs at least 2 h apart |
| Antimicrobials | | |
| Neomycin, PAS,[b] sulfasalazine | Decrease oral absorption 18%–28%, ? mechanism | 1. Monitor<br>2. Avoid concurrent use if possible |
| Erythromycin, tetracycline | Alter bacterial flora; can increase bioavailability by 40%–100% in patients who extensively metabolize digoxin in the gut | 1. Monitor<br>2. May need to decrease digoxin<br>3. May try capsules<br>4. Avoid concurrent use if possible |
| Rifampin | Increased metabolism; biliary excretion increased up to 50% | 1. Monitor<br>2. May need to increase digoxin |
| Cholestyramine<br>Colestipol | Adsorbs digoxin in gut; decreases oral absorption by 25%; also can decrease enterohepatic recycling | 1. Monitor<br>2. Avoid concurrent use if possible |
| Diltiazem | ? Decreases renal clearance | 1. Monitor |
| Diuretics | Thiazide or loop diuretics induce potassium or magnesium loss, increasing risk of digoxin toxicity | 1. Monitor<br>2. Replace potassium and/or magnesium |
| Kaolin–pectin | Large doses (60 mL) adsorb digoxin and decrease oral absorption ?% | Space drugs at least 2 h apart |
| Metoclopramide | Can increase GI motility; may decrease oral absorption; ? significance | Monitor |
| Propantheline | Anticholinergics can decrease GI motility; may increase oral absorption; ? significance | Monitor |
| Quinidine | Decreases renal and nonrenal clearance; displaces digoxin from tissue binding sites, decreasing $V_D$; ? increase in rate and extent of absorption; can increase SDC 100% | 1. Decrease digoxin dose by 50%<br>2. Monitor |
| Quinine | L-Isomer of quinidine; mechanism similar to that of quinidine; ? magnitude | Monitor |
| Spironolactone | Decreases renal and nonrenal clearance 30%; interferes with some digoxin assays, yielding falsely elevated SDC | Monitor |
| Verapamil | Decreases renal and nonrenal clearance; can increase SDC 70%–100% | 1. Decrease digoxin dose by 50%<br>2. Monitor |

[a] "Monitor" means monitor patient for clinical response and signs and symptoms; measuring serum digoxin concentration (SDC) may be useful.

[b] PAS, *p*-aminosalicylic acid.

Compiled from References 64, 65, 67–69, 71, and 72.

provide in-depth discussions of the clinical significance and management of these drug interactions.[64,65,67–69] Likewise, more comprehensive pharmacokinetic reviews of digoxin can be found elsewhere.[64,65,68–70]

**Pharmacokinetics of Digitoxin**

Digitoxin is the second most frequently prescribed cardiac glycoside in the United States; however, digitoxin is used far less often than digoxin. Digitoxin is 90% to 100% absorbed after oral administration. It is a less polar compound and is approximately 97% plasma protein bound, primarily to albumin. Digitoxin undergoes primarily hepatic metabolism with very limited renal elimination. Digitoxin's elimination half-life is approximately 4 to 6 days regardless of renal function.[65]

**Digoxin Dosing Guidelines**

There is no precise individualized digoxin dosing protocol available that has been extensively validated in CHF patients with varying degrees of renal dysfunction. All patients need to be monitored closely for clinical response and signs and symptoms of toxicity. While digoxin's therapeutic range is frequently quoted as 0.8–2.0 ng/mL, maintenance of serum digoxin concentrations between 0.8 and 1.5 ng/mL may be

**Table 11.10** Comparative Pharmacokinetics of Digoxin and Digitoxin

| | *Digoxin* | *Digitoxin* |
|---|---|---|
| Oral bioavailability | | |
| Tablets | 70%–80% | 90–100% |
| Elixir | 75%–85% | |
| Capsules | 90%–100% | |
| Onset of action | | |
| Oral | 1.5–6 h | 3–6 h |
| Intravenous | 15–30 min | 30–120 min |
| Peak effect | | |
| Oral | 4–6 h | 6–12 h |
| Intravenous | 1.5–3 h | 4–6 h |
| Plasma protein binding | 20%–25% | 97% |
| Half-life (average) | | |
| Normal renal function | 36 h | 4–6 d |
| Elderly | 48 h | 4–6 d |
| Anuric patients | 5 d | 4–6 d |
| Principal route of elimination | Renal | Hepatic |

Compiled from References 64, 65, and 69.

associated with a more reasonable risk-to-benefit ratio.[65] Multiple variables may influence the response to the cardiac glycosides including the nature and the extent of the underlying cardiac problem, other diseases such as hypothyroidism, the relative degree of oxygenation of the myocardium, the serum potassium and magnesium concentrations, and the patient's age and underlying renal function.

If a rapid onset of action is desired, such as in a patient with CHF and uncontrolled atrial fibrillation, rapid digitalization can be accomplished with a loading dose of digoxin ranging from 10 to 15 μg/kg of lean body weight. Loading doses for elderly patients and patients with chronic renal failure should be conservative, starting at 10 μg/kg. The loading dose is divided into two or three fractions administered 6 hours apart. If a rapid onset is not necessary, a maintenance dose of digoxin can be given initially, and a steady-state serum digoxin concentration will be reached in four to five half-lives, or 7 to 10 days, in patients with normal renal function. In the absence of atrial fibrillation with rapid ventricular response, digoxin therapy can frequently be initiated without a loading dose. Adult maintenance doses of digoxin typically range from 0.125 to 0.5 mg daily. Jelliffe devised an equation to estimate the maintenance dose required by CHF patients with varying degrees of renal function. The equation calculates percentage daily digoxin losses to be equal to 14% + [creatinine clearance (mL/min)/5]. In this equation, 14% represents nonrenal digoxin elimination. The other portion represents renal digoxin elimination. The percentage daily digoxin loss is multiplied by the initial loading dose and provides an estimated maintenance dose to replace daily losses.[73]

The Jelliffe equation serves as a rough approximation of initial digoxin requirements, but fails to consider individual differences in nonrenal digoxin elimination as well as varying degrees of renal tubular secretion and reabsorption. Several comprehensive discussions of the application and limitations of more individualized dosing methods can be found elsewhere.[64,69,70]

#### Digitoxin Dosing Guidelines

Because digitoxin has a longer elimination half-life, if a patient is started on a maintenance dose it takes approximately 3 to 4 weeks to reach a steady-state serum concentration without administering a loading dose. Thus, in adults a loading dose of 0.8–1.4 mg of digitoxin can be administered in two or three divided doses at 6- to 8-hour intervals if more immediate action is desired. Adult maintenance doses typically range from 0.1 to 0.2 mg once daily. Reported therapeutic serum digitoxin concentrations range from 10 to 35 ng/mL, with the most commonly reported range being 15–30 ng/mL.[69]

#### Serum Digoxin Concentration Monitoring

As digoxin possesses a narrow therapeutic index, monitoring of serum digoxin concentrations (SDCs) can be of value; however, there is considerable overlap between therapeutic and toxic SDCs measured in patients as a result of highly variable interindividual responses.[64] Thus, knowledge of the indications and limitations of SDC monitoring is essential if safe, rational, cost-effective digoxin therapy is to be provided. To be interpretable, blood for measurement of SDC must be drawn at appropriate times, preferably just prior to a dose or at least 6 to 8 hours after a dose. SDC monitoring may assist in assessing patient compliance; a poor response after usual dosages or unexplained deterioration after an initial good response; the appropriate dose in patients with changing renal function; suspected drug interactions; and suspected digoxin toxicity.[65,69,74] Remember that the diagnosis of digoxin toxicity is based largely on clinical findings, and the usefulness of SDC as a predictor of digoxin toxicity has not been well established.[75]

Another limitation of SDC monitoring is that digoxin assays themselves are subject to interfering substances that can give false readings. For example, digoxin-like immunoreactive substances (DLISs) have been identified in several patient populations, including neonates, pregnant women, hypertensive patients, and patients with renal failure or hepatic failure. These patients have been documented to have detectable SDCs without being on digoxin. CHF patients on digoxin with underlying renal or hepatic failure could conceivably have falsely elevated SDCs because of these interfering substances. Drugs like spironolactone also can cross-react with certain digoxin assays and yield false-positive results. The interfering substances and the magnitude of interference vary from assay to assay. Each clinician should be aware of which digoxin assay his or her institution utilizes and should consult the literature or manufacturer of that assay to obtain a list of interfering substances.[76–78]

#### Digoxin: Clinical Application and Place in Therapy

The value of digoxin in controlling ventricular response in supraventricular tachyarrhythmias such as atrial fibrillation is unquestioned. Therefore, patients with CHF and atrial fibrillation may be a unique subset who respond well to digoxin; however, the role of digoxin in patients with CHF in normal sinus rhythm is unclear. The clinical studies best able to objectively assess the efficacy of digoxin in these patients should have a prospective, double-blind, randomized, placebo-controlled design. Sample size should be large enough to have statistical power. Inclusion criteria should be clearly defined and patients with atrial fibrillation should be excluded. Dosages of concurrent diuretics and vasodilators should be kept constant. Ideally, explicit objective or semi-objective outcomes should be clearly defined and may include such endpoints as clinical signs and symptoms, including presence or absence of an $S_3$ gallop; radiologic evidence of CHF; noninvasive measures of left ventricular function; invasive hemodynamic monitoring; exercise treadmill testing; and mortality.[51,79,80]

Unfortunately, the perfect study is yet to be published. Mulrow et al recently reviewed studies specifically evaluating the efficacy of digoxin in patients with CHF in normal sinus rhythm and found it impossible to draw firm conclusions from most uncontrolled studies.[79] One uncontrolled study by Arnold and Byrd was unique in that all nine patients had deterioration in left ventricular function after digoxin withdrawal; however, the study was uncontrolled and not blinded.[81]

Even the three best designed studies using a placebo-controlled, crossover design suffer from at least one design flaw. Dobbs and colleagues found that 16 of 46 patients clinically deteriorated when switched from digoxin to placebo[60]; however, 13 patients had CHF complicated by atrial fibrillation, and it is impossible to identify whether or not any of these patients clinically deteriorated. In addition, other medications, including diuretics and vasodilators, were not maintained at a constant dosage level throughout the study period. Obviously, diuretics[82–84] and vasodilators[85–91] may each independently alter cardiac hemodynamics in patients with CHF.

A second study, by Fleg and colleagues, evaluated the effects of chronic digoxin use in inpatients and outpatients with CHF.[61] Treatment allocation was not randomized and the study was marred by a 25% dropout rate. Patients withdrawn from digoxin had increases in left ventricular end-diastolic dimension (LVEDD) by echocardiography, meaning left ventricular chamber size increased probably secondary to elevated LVEDP (preload); however, even though LVEDD increased, none of the patients on placebo clinically deteriorated after 3 months. If the data from the study are replotted after removal of the one outlier in the group, an apparent relationship can be demonstrated between elevated LVEDP and LVEDD in patients on placebo and lower LVEDP and LVEDD in patients on digoxin, suggesting that digoxin may reduce preload in CHF.

Finally, Lee and colleagues found that 14 of 25 patients improved on digoxin; but the study had a number of limitations including a 29% dropout rate.[62] Using multivariate analysis, the investigators demonstrated that the presence of an $S_3$ gallop may well be the best predictor of patients who respond to digoxin therapy. Nonresponders either had normal left ventricular ejection fraction at rest, had hypertrophic cardiomyopathy, or were also asymptomatic on placebo. Thus, the presence of lusitropic abnormalities may explain why some patients fail to respond to digitalis. Paradoxically, these patients may actually experience accelerated deterioration in left ventricular performance if given inotropic stimulation.[92–95] More recent, uncontrolled studies have failed to demonstrate long-term benefit from digoxin in CHF patients in normal sinus rhythm, including those patients with an $S_3$ gallop.[96,97]

**Table 11.11** Noncardiac Manifestations of Digitalis Toxicity

| |
|---|
| Gastrointestinal effects |
| Abdominal pain, anorexia, nausea, vomiting |
| Visual effects |
| Hazy vision, photophobia, difficulty with red–green color perception, scotomas, yellow–green vision |
| Central nervous system effects |
| Fatigue, weakness, dizziness, headache, delirium, psychosis |

Compiled from References 98 and 99.

Careful review of the few well-designed scientific studies suggests the need for skepticism regarding the value of long-term digoxin therapy. Patients with CHF presenting with an $S_3$ gallop may benefit from long-term digoxin and deserve a therapeutic trial. Patients older than 60 years of age constitute a special subset with a reduced ability to respond to inotropic stimulation and a higher incidence of side effects and toxicity.[59] In this subset, the risk-to-benefit ratio for administering the cardiac glycosides needs to be carefully reexamined in well-designed prospective studies. Likewise, the comparative value of digoxin versus modern diuretics and vasodilators needs to be addressed. It is hoped that a recently completed, yet unpublished, prospective, randomized, double-blind study comparing digoxin to placebo and milrinone will define whether digoxin has any short- or long-term benefit.

#### Digitalis Toxicity

The prevalence of digoxin toxicity has been estimated to range from 6% to 18%.[98] Signs and symptoms of digitalis toxicity can be divided into two categories: noncardiac and cardiac. While noncardiac symptoms may be very distressing to the patient, the cardiac manifestations are more worrisome as they can be life-threatening. Noncardiac symptoms are often nonspecific and may be difficult to distinguish from underlying CHF. Only 50% of patients with digitalis toxicity have noncardiac symptoms prior to developing arrhythmias.[99] Hyperkalemia in the face of digitalis toxicity is an ominous sign and has been directly correlated with mortality.[100] Noncardiac signs and symptoms are listed in Table 11.11.

Cardiac manifestations consist of a variety of arrhythmias, resulting from enhanced automaticity or slowed conduction. Slowed conduction represents an extension of the vagotonic effects of digitalis. Enhanced automaticity may reflect not only increased intracellular calcium as a result of excessive inhibition of sodium–potassium ATPase, but also increased sympathetic discharge from the CNS.[101] While digitalis can cause virtually any arrhythmia, premature ventricular contractions are most common in adults. Children more commonly present with conduction blocks rather than premature ventricular contractions. Classic digitalis-induced arrhythmias are those involving enhanced automaticity coupled with some type of conduction block such as paroxysmal

**Table 11.12** Common Digitalis-Induced Arrhythmias

| |
|---|
| Ventricular arrhythmias |
| Premature ventricular contractions (PVCs), unifocal PVCs, multifocal PVCs, bigeminy, trigeminy |
| Ventricular tachycardia |
| Atrioventricular (AV) block |
| First degree |
| Second degree (Mobitz type I, or Wenckebach more common) |
| Third degree |
| Atrial arrhythmia with slowed AV conduction or AV block |
| Atrial fibrillation with slow ventricular response |
| Atrial fibrillation with regular ventricular response, representing third-degree AV block with junctional escape |
| Nonconducted premature atrial contractions |
| Paroxysmal atrial tachycardia with 2:1 AV block |
| Sinoatrial arrhythmias |
| Sinus bradycardia |
| Sinus tachycardia |
| Junctional arrhythmias |
| Junctional rhythm |
| Junctional tachycardia |

Compiled from References 102–104.

atrial tachycardia with 2:1 atrioventricular block or atrial fibrillation with a regular ventricular response (representing a junctional escape rhythm).[102–104] Table 11.12 outlines the more common digitalis-induced arrhythmias.[103,104]

Until recently, therapy for digitalis toxicity has been largely supportive involving discontinuation of digoxin; gastric evacuation in acute overdoses; correction of electrolyte abnormalities, particulary hypokalemia and hypomagnesemia; and treatment of symptomatic arrhythmias. Several authors expand on these components of therapy in greater detail.[99,102]

### Digoxin Antibody Fragments for Digitalis Toxicity

A preparation of digoxin-specific antibody fragments called digoxin-immune Fab (Digibind, Burroughs Wellcome) is now available for treatment of life-threatening digoxin or digitoxin overdosage. Digibind has been used in a limited number of patients and has been lifesaving in digitalis-toxic patients with potentially lethal arrhythmias and/or hyperkalemia unresponsive to conventional therapy. After intravenous administration of Digibind, digoxin is bound to the antibodies and inactivated within minutes, and signs and symptoms of digitalis toxicity improve within 30 minutes or less. Adverse effects have been limited to mild increases in CHF or in ventricular rate in patients with atrial fibrillation. In addition, hypokalemia has occurred after rapid reversal of hyperkalemia in patients with low potassium stores. Concern has been raised about the antigenicity of sheep-derived antibodies, but no hypersensitivity reactions have been reported. Digibind is quite expensive and clinical experience with it is limited. In addition, effects of repeated administration are unknown. As a result, Digibind should be reserved

**Table 11.13** Indications for Digibind Administration

| |
|---|
| Life-threatening digoxin or digitoxin toxicity |
| Ventricular tachycardia |
| Ventricular fibrillation |
| Severe bradyarrhythmias |
| Severe sinus bradycardia, second- or third-degree heart block unresponsive to atropine or transvenous pacing |
| Acute digoxin ingestion |
| More than 10 mg digoxin in adults |
| More than 4 mg in children |
| Hyperkalemia (serum potassium > 5 mEq/L) in the setting of digitalis intoxication |

From Digibind, Digoxin Immune Fab (Ovine), package insert. Research Triangle Park, NC, Burroughs Wellcome, 1986, with permission.

for treatment of life-threatening digitalis intoxication as outlined in Table 11.13.[105–108] Specific dosing guidelines can be found in the Digibind package insert.[105]

#### *Intravenous β-Adrenergic Agonists*

In acute or severe CHF, digitalis has limited benefits, and intravenous inotropes are frequently required. Catecholamines like norepinephrine, epinephrine, isoproterenol, dopamine, and dobutamine are known to induce a positive inotropic effect by stimulating myocardial β receptors.[109–113] In addition, catecholamines can stimulate myocardial α-adrenergic receptors also, resulting in a positive inotropic effect with minimal change in heart rate.[114] Table 11.14 compares the relative adrenergic receptor selectivity of the intravenous catecholamines. Table 11.15 provides dosing guidelines and comparative pharmacodynamics of the intravenous catecholamines.

The increase in force of contraction induced by catecholamines characteristically develops very rapidly and is accompanied by a decrease in the duration of contraction. This shortened contraction is due to rapid relaxation of the contraction and is referred to as the "relaxant effect" of adrenergic stimulation. Interestingly, only agents that increase myocardial cyclic AMP, such as the β-adrenergic agonists, possess this ability to shorten the contraction.[115]

From a functional point of view, the relaxant effects of β-adrenergic stimulation are important in facilitating ventricular filling in the face of increased heart rate. The main cardiac effect of the β-adrenergic agonist is to increase the slow inward calcium current by increasing the number of functional calcium channels.[113] In addition, β-adrenergic agonists cause an increase in calcium uptake into the sarcoplasmic reticulum, which also increases the amount of releasable calcium available. This increase in calcium uptake by the sarcoplasmic reticulum not only contributes to the positive inotropic properties, but also explains the relaxant effects of the β-adrenergic agonist. There is some evidence that the latter effect might, in part, result from a decrease in the calcium sensitivity of the contractile proteins.[116,117]

Dopamine and dobutamine are the two most commonly administered catecholamines. Dopamine is a direct- and indirect-acting catecholamine with both α- and β-stimulating

**Table 11.14** Comparative Adrenergic Receptor Selectivity of Intravenous Catecholamines

| *Drug* | $\beta_1$ Inotropic | $\beta_1$ Chronotropic | $\beta_2$ *vasodilation* | $\alpha$ *vasoconstriction* |
|---|---|---|---|---|
| Dopamine[a] | 3+ | 2+ | 2+ | 0–3+ |
| Dobutamine[b] | 3+ | 1+ | 1+ | 1+ |
| Epinephrine | 3+ | 3+ | 3+ | 3+ |
| Isoproterenol | 3+ | 3+ | 3+ | 0 |
| Norepinephrine | 2+ | 1+ | 0 | 3+ |

[a] Dopamine has dose-dependent effects: at low doses (0.5–3 μg/kg/min), dopaminergic effects (renal and mesenteric vasodilation) predominate; at moderate doses (2–10 μg/kg/min), $\beta_1$ effects do; and at high doses (>10 μg/kg/min), $\alpha$ effects predominate.

[b] Dobutamine is a racemic mixture; (−)-isomer has $\alpha$-agonist activity primarily; (+)-isomer has $\beta_1$- and $\beta_2$-agonist activity primarily; this table lists the net effect of the racemic mixture.

properties. $\beta$-Adrenergic stimulation predominates at doses around 5–10 μg/kg/min. At doses above 10 μg/kg/min, $\alpha$-adrenergic stimulation becomes more apparent. At low doses (2–3 μg/kg/min), dopamine stimulates renal dopaminergic receptors, which increases renal cortical blood flow and can augment urine output.[109] If an inotropic agent is needed to maintain arterial pressure, dopamine is the agent of choice. In this setting, an initial dosage of 3–5 μg/kg/min should increase cardiac output and is a reasonable starting point. The infusion rate may be increased every 3 to 5 minutes until the desired effect on blood pressure, perfusion, and cardiac output is obtained. Although dopamine can increase cardiac output, it can also have a number of detrimental effects. First, infusion rates above 4 μg/kg/min dramatically increase the risk of arrhythmias and tend to increase PCWP as well.[110] Dopamine can also increase the heart rate–systolic blood pressure product, an important determinant of myocardial oxygen consumption ($MVo_2$), which can result in myocardial ischemia if oxygen supply is limited. $\alpha$-Adrenergic–mediated vasoconstriction at higher doses also limits dopamine's usefulness. In patients with long-standing CHF, where catecholamine stores may be depleted, the response to dopamine may be reduced initially or after several days of administration.[118]

Dobutamine is a newer inotropic agent that appears to display more selective stimulation of the $\beta_1$-adrenergic receptor[109]; however, dobutamine's pharmacologic effects are more complex than originally suspected. Dobutamine is a racemic mixture. The (−)-isomer is a potent $\alpha$ agonist with weak $\beta_1$- or $\beta_2$-agonist activity. In contrast, the (+)-isomer is a potent $\beta_1$ and $\beta_2$ agonist with minimal $\alpha$ effects.[119,120] Still, the net effect of racemic dobutamine is an increase in cardiac output with a reflex reduction in peripheral vascular tone (SVR). The $\alpha$-agonist properties of the (−)-isomer may explain why dobutamine increases contractility but does not increase heart rate as much as dopamine. Dobutamine does not increase the heart rate–systolic blood pressure product, or $MVo_2$, as much as dopamine. Thus, dobutamine may increase cardiac output at lower oxygen costs than dopamine.[110–112] Dobutamine does not stimulate dopaminergic receptors, but still may increase renal blood flow by improving cardiac output.[110] The combination of dobutamine and low-dose dopamine (2–3 μg/kg/min) increases renal blood flow and urine output in some patients who fail to respond to dobutamine alone.[120]

Both dopamine and dobutamine possess significantly greater inotropic activity than digitalis. Their rapid onset of action, short duration, and thus easy titratability make them preferable agents in the acute management of severe CHF in hospitalized patients, when short-term inotropic support is necessary. While some patients demonstrate sustained hemodynamic improvement with dobutamine,[123] others develop tolerance to the hemodynamic effects after 72 hours.[124] The intermittent short-term administration of dobutamine may be a way to "tune up" some patients with severe, refractory CHF on an outpatient basis. Studies using weekly dobutamine infusions at rates ranging from 1.5 to 15 μg/kg/min infused for 4 to 48 hours have shown sustained

**Table 11.15** Pharmacodynamics of Intravenous Catecholamines

| *Drug* | *Dose*[a] | *HR*[b] | *MAP* | *PCWP* | *CO* | *SVR* |
|---|---|---|---|---|---|---|
| Dopamine | 1–20 μg/kg/min | + | 0/+ | 0/+ | + | 0/+ |
| Dobutamine | 2.5–20 μg/kg/min | + | 0/− | − | + | − |
| Epinephrine | 0.02–0.2 μg/kg/min | + | 0/+ | 0/+ | + | − |
| Isoproterenol | 0.02–0.2 μg/kg/min | + | 0/− | 0/− | + | − |
| Norepinephrine | 2–16 μg/min | Variable | + | + | Variable | + |

[a] Dose represents usual adult dosage range for dopamine, dobutamine, and norepinephrine. Epinephrine and isoproterenol are rarely used in CHF patients and the dose included is a rough approximation.

[b] +, Increase; −, decrease; 0, no change; HR, heart rate; MAP, mean arterial pressure; PCWP, pulmonary capillary wedge pressure; CO, cardiac output; SVR, systemic vascular resistance.

hemodynamic and clinical improvement for weeks to months.[125,126] The impact of this therapy on long-term survival is unknown; hence, the clinical role of this therapy remains to be established.

### *Investigational β-Adrenergic Agonists*

The beneficial effects seen with short-term intravenous dopamine and dobutamine have prompted a search for orally active, longer-acting β-adrenergic agonists for chronic CHF therapy. Table 11.16 lists the β-adrenergic agonists currently being investigated.

#### Levodopa and Dopamine Analogues

Orally administered levodopa has been demonstrated to have beneficial hemodynamic effects in patients with severe CHF.[127] Levodopa is a precursor of dopamine and is converted to dopamine in vivo. Its beneficial hemodynamic effects may result from a positive inotropic effect and/or peripheral vasodilation. Doses of 250 mg four times a day are administered initially to minimize nausea and vomiting. Daily dosage is then titrated up to 1.5–2.0 g four times daily over the next 5 to 7 days. Pyridoxine 50 mg daily appears necessary for adequate conversion of levodopa to dopamine. Other investigational dopamine analogues include ibopamine, propylbutyl dopamine, and dopexamine. Dopexamine is unique in that it appears to stimulate β-adrenergic and dopaminergic, but not α-adrenergic receptors.[128–131]

**Table 11.16** Investigational Adrenergic Inotropes

| | |
|---|---|
| Dopamine analogues | |
| Levodopa | Dopamine precursor, converted to dopamine in vivo |
| Ibopamine | ? Effects similar to levodopa |
| Propylbutyl dopamine | ? Effects similar to levodopa |
| Dopexamine | Dopaminergic, β-agonist, lacks α effects |
| Selective $\beta_1$ agonists | |
| Prenalterol | Withdrawn from clinical trials |
| Xamoterol (Corwin) | |
| TA-064 | |
| Butopamine | Withdrawn from clinical trials |
| Selective $\beta_2$ agonists | |
| Terbutaline | Available orally, not FDA approved |
| Albuterol (Salbutamol) | Available orally, not FDA approved |
| Pirbuterol | Withdrawn from clinical trials |
| Miscellaneous adrenergic agonists | |
| ASL 7022 | $\beta_1$, $\beta_2$, $\alpha_2$ |

Adapted from Colucci WS, Wright RF, Braunwald E: New positive inotropic agents in the treatment of congestive heart failure. Mechanisms of action and recent clinical developments (second of two parts). N Engl J Med 1986;314:350, with permission.

#### Oral β-Adrenergic Agonists

Prenalterol, xamoterol, TA-064, and butopamine are relatively selective $\beta_1$ agonists with positive inotropic properties.[132–137] The ratio of positive inotropic to chronotropic effects may be greater for prenalterol than other β-adrenergic agents[133]; however, one prenalterol trial failed to demonstrate long-term efficacy, and another noted an increase in ventricular arrhythmias in acute myocardial infarction patients receiving prenalterol.[134–138] TA-064 has demonstrated beneficial hemodynamic effects without untoward toxic effects or arrhythmias, but additional studies are needed to fully evaluate its potential and limitations.[136]

Terbutaline, albuterol (salbutamol), and pirbuterol are relatively selective $\beta_2$ agonists.[139–143] These agents appear to possess both inotropic and vasodilatory properties. Long-term studies with terbutaline and albuterol are lacking. In patients with severe CHF refractory to digitalis and diuretics, the addition of pirbuterol can increase cardiac output and decrease PCWP and SVR.[144,145] ASL 7022 is a unique adrenergic agonist that stimulates $\beta_1$, $\beta_2$, and $\alpha_2$ receptors.[146]

Several of the investigational β-adrenergic agonists have been documented to have short-term beneficial hemodynamic effects in some patients with severe CHF. Unfortunately, β-receptor responsiveness may decrease with age[14] as well as after continuous stimulation.[15,147] Thus, hemodynamic tolerance may occur with long-term administration. In addition, as short-term β-adrenergic agonists can precipitate ventricular arrhythmias, the arrhythmogenic potential of long-term β-adrenergic agonist therapy must be carefully assessed. Just recently, pirbuterol was withdrawn from clinical trials because of drug-induced ventricular arrhythmias. Butopamine never did reach extensive clinical trials as a result of its arrhythmogenicity. In addition, in placebo-controlled trials, prenalterol did not demonstrate sustained benefits and was subsequently withdrawn from clinical trials.[148] Clearly, further studies are needed to evaluate the long-term safety and efficacy of β-adrenergic agonists in CHF.

### *Noncatecholamine, Nonglycoside Inotropes: Bipyridine Derivatives*

The bipyridine derivatives are a unique group of inotropic agents that appear not only to increase the force of myocardial contractility but also to produce vascular relaxation. Amrinone is the prototype of this new class of noncatecholamine, nonglycoside cardiotonics. Amrinone was recently released for parenteral use in the United States for the short-term treatment of severe, refractory CHF.[149–152]

#### Amrinone

***Pharmacology*** Amrinone and similar agents are thought to work by selective inhibition of phosphodiesterase fraction III, which causes cyclic AMP to accumulate within myocardial cells.[153–155] Cyclic AMP, an intracellular secondary messenger, increases both the release and the reuptake of calcium within the myocardium. As a result, cyclic AMP influences both the force of contraction and the rate and extent of relaxation of the myocardium.[117] Amrinone's inotropic activity is predicated on adequate stores of cyclic AMP within the myocardium; however, in some patients with severe CHF, cyclic AMP production may be abnormal and myocardial stores may be deficient.[156] As a result, amrinone's inotropic activity may be markedly diminished in these patients. In higher doses, amrinone may alter calcium transport as well.[154,157] As a result of these dose-dependent properties, amrinone displays a biphasic effect on ventricular relaxation time, shortening it at low doses and prolonging it at higher doses.[154] The alterations in calcium transport at higher concentrations may well be a double-edged sword. On one hand, the increased availability of calcium may increase the force of contraction; on the other hand, the interference with the storage of calcium in the myocardial cell may delay relaxation and contribute to the drug's toxic effects.[115] The relative degree of inotropic and vasodilating effects of amrinone seen in an individual patient may vary depending on the dose administered and the underlying disturbance in cardiac function.

***Clinical and Hemodynamic Effects*** The acute hemodynamic effects of amrinone have been studied primarily in NYHA FC-III and FC-IV CHF patients. In most instances, these patients continued to receive cardiac glycosides and diuretics while vasodilators were discontinued. In these studies, amrinone acutely increased cardiac index 30% to 112%, while decreasing pulmonary capillary wedge pressure 16% to 53%, pulmonary vascular resistance 24% to 50%, right atrial pressure 36% to 44% and systemic vascular resistance 28% to 41%. Heart rate and mean arterial pressure usually remained unchanged; however, at higher doses, heart rate may increase and mean arterial pressure may decrease.[150–152,158–161] The etiology of CHF generally does not influence the initial hemodynamic response to amrinone.

Discrepancies in the hemodynamic influence of amrinone have been reported when peak positive rate of left ventricular pressure development (*dP/dt*) has been used as an index of myocardial contractility. Peak positive left ventricular *dP/dt* is dependent on changes in both left ventricular filling pressure and myocardial contractility. Thus, assessment of the inotropic activity of an agent with significant vasodilatory activity such as amrinone is difficult when this parameter is used. Some authors have reported increases in left ventricular *dP/dt* ranging from 21% to 44%[150,159,162] while others have failed to show consistent changes.[163,164] Although Firth et al found that amrinone lacked any effect on contractility, they failed to administer a loading dose and thus may not have achieved adequate amrinone concentrations.[164] These discrepancies have evoked controversy regarding the inotropic potency of amrinone, as some investigators believe amrinone is more of a vasodilator than an inotrope.[163,164]

Amrinone alone has the ability to immediately increase exercise capacity and maximal oxygen consumption in CHF patients.[165,166] This increase in exercise capacity not only is apparent immediately but is sustained in some studies up to 28 weeks.[166] Unfortunately, not all long-term studies have demonstrated continued effectiveness.[167,168] In the largest multicenter double-blind controlled long-term study of oral amrinone, the only difference between the amrinone-treated group and the placebo group was a significantly higher incidence of side effects with amrinone.[168] One concern is that higher doses of amrinone used in some of these studies may have resulted in a significant increase in the rate of ventricular deterioration and mortality.[88,167,169]

The combined inotropic and vasodilatory properties of amrinone may be useful in patients with ischemic heart disease. Amrinone may augment cardiac output in a metabolically efficient manner, resulting in a decrease in $MVo_2$.[170–174] Any increase in $MVo_2$ caused by increased contractility is outweighed by a decrease in ventricular volume. The net result is a decrease in systolic wall tension and a decrease in $MVo_2$, an effect similar to that seen with dobutamine. Early studies in patients with stable ischemic heart disease have been encouraging. Limited data reveal favorable hemodynamic effects when amrinone has been used in left ventricular failure complicating an acute myocardial infarction, but tachycardia can develop at higher doses.[175]

***Comparison With Other Inotropes or Vasodilators*** Amrinone is able to increase cardiac output in a fashion similar to dobutamine[176,177] and dopamine[178]; however, amrinone may produce a more sustained increase in cardiac output than dobutamine.[176] In addition, amrinone does not increase the blood pressure or heart rate and consistently lowers the PCWP and SVR, whereas dopamine may increase heart rate, PCWP, and SVR. Thus, amrinone may improve cardiac output not only by increasing contractility, but also by reducing preload and afterload, an effect like that of the combination of dobutamine and nitroprusside.[179] As amrinone does not increase and may actually decrease blood pressure at higher doses, it should not be used as first-line therapy in the hypotensive patient with low cardiac output.

Limited data are available regarding the concomitant administration of amrinone and other agents. The hemodynamics of amrinone singly and in combination with hydralazine have been studied.[180] Given separately, each drug significantly increases cardiac output; combined administration results in an increase in cardiac output greater than that produced by either agent alone.[180]

Amrinone has also been used in combination with isosorbide dinitrate.[181] This combination resulted in a decrease in right atrial pressure and PCWP greater than that produced by either agent alone. Such a combination would be expected to improve exercise performance.

***Pharmacokinetics*** Amrinone's pharmacokinetics have been studied in healthy volunteers and patients with various degrees of CHF. After intravenous administration, peak plasma amrinone concentrations and maximum hemodynamic effects are reached within 10 minutes. In healthy volunteers, amrinone's volume of distribution averages 1.2 L/kg and its elimination half-life is approximately 2.5 hours. In severe CHF patients, the elimination half-life usually ranges from 5 to 8 hours, but there is considerable interpatient variation and it can be as long as 13 to 15 hours.[152] Amrinone's duration of action ranges from 60 to 90 minutes, compared with less than 10 minutes for dopamine and dobutamine and 3 to 5 minutes for nitroprusside. Because amrinone's duration of action is longer, it may take more time for adverse effects, such as hypotension or tachyarrhythmias, to dissipate after discontinuation of amrinone. Amrinone is metabolized in the liver and conjugated with glucuronic acid, glutathione, or *N*-acetylcysteine. These conjugates and up to 40% of unmetabolized amrinone are eliminated in the urine.[152,182]

***Dosing Guidelines*** An immediate effect is usually desired when using amrinone, and because its elimination half-life is 5 to 8 hours in CHF patients, a loading dose is administered. Therapy can be initiated with an intravenous bolus of 0.75–1.5 mg/kg administered over 3 to 5 minutes. An additional 0.75 mg/kg bolus may be administered in 15 to 30 minutes. Loading doses up to 3.5 mg/kg have been tolerated. The loading dose is followed by a continuous intravenous infusion of 5–10 μg/kg/min. Maintenance infusions may be titrated up to a maximum of 10 mg/kg/d. Doses above 20 mg/kg/d rarely produce additional hemodynamic benefit. An alternative dosing method possibly associated with less hypotension initially is infusion of 40 μg/kg/min over the first hour in place of a bolus dose, followed by a maintenance infusion of 5–10 μg/kg/min.

Amrinone decomposes slowly over 24 hours in dextrose and thus should be administered in saline; however, amrinone may be infused directly into a line containing dextrose, as contact time between amrinone and dextrose would be limited and decomposition negligible. Furosemide should not be administered directly into a line containing amrinone, as the two form a precipitate.[184]

***Adverse Effects*** While the short-term hemodynamic effects are similar for both the oral and the intravenous forms of amrinone, oral amrinone is associated with many more side effects than intravenous amrinone. Oral amrinone's side effect profile coupled with a lack of documented long-term benefit led to its withdrawal from clinical trials. With oral therapy, gastrointestinal side effects occurred in up to 22% of patients and included anorexia, nausea, vomiting, diarrhea, and abdominal pain.[152] Gastrointestinal side effects are much less common with intravenous amrinone.[152,184]

Patients receiving short-term intravenous therapy have a 2.4% incidence of thrombocytopenia,[183,184] whereas oral therapy was associated with thrombocytopenia in 15% to 20% of patients.[152,185,186] The postulated mechanism of amrinone-induced thrombocytopenia is direct, nonimmunologic platelet damage, leading to accelerated platelet removal.[152] Baseline platelet counts should be obtained prior to starting amrinone. Specific guidelines for subsequent platelet count determinations have not been developed, but monitoring platelet counts every 1 to 3 days initially in unstable CHF patients appears reasonable. Should thrombocytopenia or bleeding occur, platelet counts should be monitored daily. The platelet count usually does not fall below 70,000/mm$^3$. Decreasing the dose of amrinone or stopping therapy entirely generally leads to complete reversibility of the thrombocytopenia within 5 to 7 days.[185,186] Patients with baseline thrombocytopenia probably should not receive amrinone. Dobutamine or dopamine, with or without nitroprusside, should be used instead; the choice of agent should be determined by the patient's clinical and hemodynamic status.[187,188] Fever, hypotension, and liver function abnormalities have also been infrequently described with intravenous amrinone.[152,184] More experience is needed to determine the incidence of these side effects.

The incidence of increased ventricular ectopic activity during amrinone administration is quite variable.[165,185] While reports indicate that usual adult dosages of intravenous amrinone have a low arrhythmogenic potential,[184,189] other reports indicate that high doses of oral amrinone therapy may be associated with the high incidence of dangerous ventricular arrhythmias.[167] As arrhythmias are a frequent complication of severe CHF itself, one must be concerned about the potential for increasing that risk with any therapeutic intervention.[189]

***Place in Therapy*** Amrinone is most effective and reasonably well tolerated in normotensive CHF patients with decreased cardiac output, increased SVR, and elevated left ventricular filling pressure; however, at the present time, given amrinone's higher cost and a lack of data indicating clinical superiority over other agents, amrinone should be reserved for patients with acute or severe CHF refractory to dopamine, dobutamine, and/or nitroprusside.[190,191]

As discussed earlier, stores of intracellular myocardial cyclic AMP may be deficient in patients with severe CHF; this may limit amrinone's inotropic activity in some patients.[156] Preliminary evidence suggests that the combination of a $\beta$ agonist, such as dobutamine, and amrinone may act synergistically. Dobutamine may stimulate and increase the synthesis of cyclic AMP and augment the response to amrinone.[192] Thus, combination therapy may offer some advantages in certain situations; however, clinical studies will be needed to clarify this possibility.[152]

**Milrinone**

Milrinone (WIN 47203), an investigational analog of amrinone, is thought to act similarly to amrinone by inhibiting phosphodiesterase F-III. Uncontrolled clinical trials have demonstrated that milrinone has hemodynamic effects similar to those of amrinone, including both inotropic and vasodilatory effects.[194–196] Milrinone's hemodynamic effects are similar to those of dobutamine, with greater decreases in PCWP and a lower $MVo_2$.[197,198] Milrinone also appears comparable to nitroprusside, but produces less hypotension.[197] Milrinone appears to significantly improve ventricular diastolic relaxation and filling.[199] As lusitropic abnormalities may be present in patients with CHF, this improvement in diastolic function may contribute to the beneficial hemodynamic effects seen with milrinone.[199,200]

Milrinone has some potential advantages over amrinone: milrinone is 15 to 30 times more potent than amrinone; oral milrinone is better tolerated than oral amrinone; and oral milrinone appears to have some long-term benefit in terms of sustained hemodynamic effects and improved exercise tolerance.[201–205] Like other inotropes, milrinone has not been documented to impact on survival. A recently completed, yet unpublished clinical trial comparing milrinone with digoxin and placebo, as well as other ongoing clinical trials, will help define milrinone's place in therapy.

### *Investigational Noncatecholamine, Nonglycoside Inotropes*

A host of agents with differing mechanisms of action and varying inotropic and vasodilatory effects are currently under investigation. Fenoximone (MDL 17,043) and piroxi-

**Table 11.17** Investigational Noncatecholamine, Nonglycoside Inotropes

| | |
|---|---|
| **Phosphodiesterase F-III Inhibitors**[a] | |
| Bipyridine derivatives | |
| Milrinone (WIN 47203) | |
| Imidazolone derivatives | |
| Fenoximone (MDL 17,043) | |
| Piroximone (MDL 19,205) | |
| Miscellaneous phosphodiesterase F-III inhibitors | |
| Sulmazole (Vardax, ARL 115 BS) | Withdrawn from clinical trials; also increases sensitivity of contractile proteins to calcium |
| Pimobendane (UD-CG 115 BS) | Mechanism similar to sulmazole |
| UD-CG 212 Cl | |
| OPC-6212 | |
| RO 13-6438 | |
| CI-914 | |
| D 13625 | |
| **Miscellaneous Agents** | |
| Forskolin | Adenylate cyclase activator |
| Bay k 8644 | Slow channel calcium agonist |
| Coenzyme Q10 | Redox component of mitochondrial respiratory chain |
| Berberine | |
| Taurine | |
| DPI 201-106 | α agonist; also increases sensitivity of contractile proteins to calcium |

[a] Although most commonly classified as inotropes, phosphodiesterase inhibitors also possess varying degrees of vasodilatory effects.

Compiled from References 179 and 193.

mone (MDL 19,205) are imidazolone derivatives that inhibit phosphodiesterase and have been extensively studied. Both agents have beneficial acute hemodynamic effects similar to those of dobutamine, amrinone, and milrinone.[206–208] Fenoximone's acute hemodynamic effects are likewise comparable with those of nitroprusside, except that fenoximone produces a greater increase in cardiac output.[209] Fenoximone has significant gastrointestinal side effects and the long-term safety and efficacy of both fenoximone and piroximone have not been clearly established.[210–216]

Sulmazole and pimobendane, two investigational agents, not only inhibit phosphodiesterase but also appear to increase the sensitivity of the contractile proteins to calcium[115,179,217–255]; however, sulmazole has been reported to cause hepatic neoplasms in rats and has been withdrawn from clinical trials. Table 11.17 lists a number of investigational agents. Clinical trials are in progress to evaluate the long-term safety and efficacy of these agents.

## *Vasodilators*

In the mid-1970s the use of vasodilators for the treatment of refractory CHF became popular. Since then, numerous papers have described the value of vasodilators either alone or in combination with inotropic agents.[226–230] The rationale for using vasodilators in CHF relates to their ability to improve cardiac output by reducing the elevated peripheral vascular resistance brought about by the various compensatory mechanisms activated in CHF. Reducing excessive left ventricular filling pressure (preload) with venous vasodilators (i.e., nitrates) or reducing resistance to systolic unloading (afterload) with arterial vasodilators (i.e., hydralazine) has become a part of the everyday management of severe CHF; however, despite the vast literature on the use of vasodilators in CHF, only captopril has received FDA approval for this indication at the present time.

Unfortunately, many of the studies in the literature were poorly designed or uncontrolled. Because of this, results have not been reproducible. In various trials, the presence of confounding variables may have influenced outcome and could explain why some studies have not been reproducible. Examples of such variables include the possible influence of the variation in severity of CHF from trial to trial on outcome; the failure to maintain constant dosages of digitalis and diuretics (resulting in no control of their contribution to outcome); the influence of the posture of the patient at the time of the study on the hemodynamic response produced.[231]

Vasodilators can be categorized by their predominant site of action: venous vasodilators, such as isosorbide and nitroglycerin; arterial vasodilators, such as hydralazine and minoxidil; and mixed venous and arterial vasodilators, such as nitroprusside, prazosin, and angiotensin-converting enzyme (ACE) inhibitors. Table 11.18 lists the available peripheral vasodilators and compares their hemodynamic effects. Each class of vasodilators is discussed here.

### Venous Vasodilators

*Nitrates* Nitroglycerin was the first vasodilator suggested for use in the management of CHF.[232] For years, nitroglycerin has been used intravenously, orally, sublingually, and topically for its venodilating effects which reduce preload. In recent years, it has been recognized that in CHF patients with an elevated SVR and/or severe mitral regurgitation, intravenous nitroglycerin can have significant afterload-reducing properties as well.[21,233] As nitroglycerin also has coronary vasodilatory effects, intravenous nitroglycerin may be preferred over nitroprusside in patients with CHF and concomitant ischemic heart disease.[233,234] An intravenous nitroglycerin infusion can be initiated using an infusion pump at 5–10 μg/min and titrated up in 5 to 10 μg/min increments every 10 minutes to a maximum of 100 μg/min in most cases, although higher dosages have been used. An arterial line and Swan–Ganz catheter are ideal for monitoring hemodynamic response to the drug. Close monitoring of blood pressure and heart rate is necessary to avoid excessive hypotension and tachycardia.

Isosorbide dinitrate is an oral nitrate that has been extensively investigated in CHF.[233,235] Relatively large doses of isosorbide dinitrate are frequently necessary and range from

**Table 11.18** Comparative Pharmacodynamics of Vasodilators

| *Drug* | *Site of action* | *Route* | *Dose* | *Onset* | *Duration* | *HR*[a] | *MAP* | *PCWP* | *CO* | *SVR* |
|---|---|---|---|---|---|---|---|---|---|---|
| Sodium nitroprusside | Arterial and venous | IV infusion | 0.25–3 μg/kg/min (15–200 μg/min) | Seconds | Minutes | 0/+ | − | − | + | − |
| Nitroglycerin | Venous | Sublingual | 0.4–0.6 mg | Minutes | 20–40 min | 0/+ | − | − | Variable | 0/− |
| | Venous | Topical | $\frac{1}{2}$–4 in. | 15 min | 3–6 h | 0/+ | − | − | Variable | 0/− |
| | Venous and arterial | IV infusion | 5–100 μg/min | Seconds | Minutes | 0/+ | − | − | 0/+ | 0/− |
| Isosorbide dinitrate | Venous | Oral | 20–80 mg | 15 min | 3–6 h | 0/+ | − | − | Variable | 0/− |
| Hydralazine | Arterial | Oral | 50–100 mg | 60 min | 6–8 h | 0/+ | − | 0/− | + | − |
| Minoxidil | Arterial | Oral | 5–40 mg | 60 min | 8–24 h | 0/+ | − | 0/− | + | − |
| Prazosin | Arterial and venous | Oral | 2–10 mg | 30–60 min | 6–8 h | 0 | − | − | + | − |
| Captopril | Arterial and venous | Oral | 6.25–50 mg | 15–30 min peak=30–90 min | 8–12 h | 0 | − | − | + | − |
| Enalapril | Arterial and venous | Oral | 2.5–20 mg | 1–2 h peak=4–8 h | 12–24 h | 0 | − | − | + | − |

[a] +, increase; −, decrease; 0, no change; HR, heart rate; MAP, mean arterial pressure; PCWP, pulmonary capillary wedge pressure; CO, cardiac output; SVR, systemic vascular resistance.

20–80 mg every 4 to 6 hours. While isosorbide dinitrate reduces PCWP after the first dose, improvement in exercise capacity is not apparent immediately and becomes evident only after long-term administration. Nitrates do not substantially improve hemodynamics at maximal exercise but can reduce exercise-induced increases in PCWP and can also relieve exertional dyspnea during submaximal exercise. Nitrates allow patients to perform repeated submaximal exercise that can physically condition them and improve their exercise capacity.[233] Thus, nitrates have what is referred to as a "training effect" on patients that results in increased maximal oxygen extraction and improved long-term exercise tolerance.[233,235–237] Nitrate-induced decreases in PCWP may be critically linked to their effects on exercise performance, as vasodilators that do not reduce PCWP do not improve exercise capacity in patients with CHF. Chronic nitrate therapy results in a modest sustained hemodynamic improvement and symptomatic benefit in patients with CHF.[236] Nitroglycerin ointment is another useful nitrate dosage form that can be used in patients with chronic CHF in doses ranging from one-half to 4 in. applied every 4 to 6 hours.[238,239] As oral nitrates and nitroglycerin ointment reduce primarily preload, with minimal effect on afterload or cardiac output, they frequently must be used in combination with other vasodilators and inotropes. Prior to the availability of the ACE inhibitors, hydralazine was the vasodilator most commonly used in combination with nitrates.

***Hemodynamic Tolerance or Attenuation With Nitrates*** While hemodynamic tolerance can occur in some patients on long-term isosorbide dinitrate therapy, it appears that tolerance occurs mainly to its arterial vasodilating effects and not to its venodilating effects.[88] In contrast, hemodynamic tolerance has been reported to the venodilating effects of transdermal nitroglycerin patches, despite high doses and sustained plasma nitroglycerin levels[240]; therefore, both its short- and long-term efficacy in CHF remains unproven. It has been postulated that either a nitrate-free interval, such as removal of the transdermal nitroglycerin patch overnight, or higher dosages of transdermal nitroglycerin may be necessary to overcome the hemodynamic tolerance or attenuation that occurs.[241,242] It is hoped that ongoing clinical trials will define the role of transdermal nitroglycerin patches in the treatment of CHF. Until that time, transdermal nitroglycerin patches cannot be recommended for therapy of chronic CHF.

### Arterial Vasodilators

***Hydralazine*** Hydralazine acts primarily as a systemic arterial vasodilator, with modest changes in preload brought about secondary to improved blood flow.[243] The response to hydralazine is most dramatic in patients with severe CHF associated with aortic or mitral regurgitation, or markedly elevated SVR.[244–246] The left ventricular chamber size, measured by M-mode echocardiography as LVEDD, may be an important factor in determining the hemodynamic and clinical response to hydralazine.[247,248] Patients with an enlarged left ventricle, a thin left ventricular wall, and an

LVEDD greater than 60 mm may represent a unique subset who respond more favorably to hydralazine.[247]

In recent years, the long-term clinical efficacy of hydralazine in CHF has been questioned. Two long-term, double-blind, placebo-controlled studies have demonstrated no significant improvement in exercise capacity compared with placebo.[249,250] In contrast, uncontrolled studies suggest that when hydralazine is combined with nitrates, symptomatic improvement persists.[251,252] Most recently, a long-term, randomized, double-blind, placebo-controlled study demonstrated that the combination of oral hydralazine (300 mg/d) and isosorbide dinitrate (160 mg/d) can improve left ventricular function and survival in chronic CHF patients already taking digoxin and diuretics.[253]

Unfortunately, the use of hydralazine in CHF is complicated by several factors. First, it is extremely difficult to predict what dose of hydralazine is required to produce an effective response.[254] Invasive hemodynamic monitoring is often necessary to determine whether the dosage selected is effective. Second, tolerance may occur with the chronic administration of hydralazine.[234] In addition, the dosages required may be quite high, ranging from 150 to 3,000 mg daily.[247] Hydralazine-induced systemic lupus erythematosus can occur with these higher dosages, particularly in slow acetylators at dosages above 200 mg per day.[255,256] Other adverse effects such as excessive hypotension and reflex tachycardia may precipitate myocardial ischemia and necessitate discontinuation of hydralazine.[257,258]

*Minoxidil* Minoxidil, an arterial vasodilator like hydralazine, has recently been shown to produce sustained hemodynamic effects but failed to improve exercise capacity; however, minoxidil can actually worsen CHF, possibly by causing excessive fluid retention or precipitating ventricular arrhythmias.[259] These adverse effects along with the side effect of hypertrichosis have limited minoxidil's usefulness in the management of chronic CHF.

**Mixed Arterial–Venous Vasodilators**

*Nitroprusside* Sodium nitroprusside is a mixed arterial and venous vasodilator that has proved very useful in the treatment of severe, refractory CHF.[226,227,230] An intravenous nitroprusside infusion is started at 0.25 $\mu$g/kg/min (or approximately 15 $\mu$g/min) using an infusion pump. Dosages may be titrated up in 0.25 $\mu$g/kg/min increments every 5 to 10 minutes as needed and tolerated. In CHF, dosages every 3 $\mu$g/kg/min (approximately 200 $\mu$g/min) are rarely necessary. At these dosages, thiocyanate toxicity is very uncommon, unless infusions are continued for an extended period of time in a patient with renal failure. Both an arterial line and a Swan–Ganz catheter are necessary to adequately monitor response to nitroprusside therapy. Carefully titrated doses of nitroprusside can decrease PCWP and SVR and increase CO without excessive tachycardia or hypotension. These beneficial hemodynamic effects can alleviate signs and symptoms of hypoperfusion and pulmonary congestion. The combination of dopamine or dobutamine with nitroprusside is useful in patients with elevated PCWP and SVR and reduced CO who fail to respond to inotropes or vasodilators alone. If the mean arterial pressure is below 85 mm Hg, nitroprusside must be used with caution and should be combined with an inotrope such as dopamine, which can be titrated to maintain an adequate mean arterial pressure. Unfortunately, sodium nitroprusside can only be administered intravenously and so its use is restricted to short-term therapy of hospitalized CHF patients.[230]

*Prazosin* Prazosin, an $\alpha_1$-receptor antagonist, possesses both arterial and venous vasodilating properties like sodium nitroprusside, and was initially greeted with great enthusiasm as an oral vasodilator for long-term therapy of chronic CHF. Unfortunately, studies evaluating prazosin's efficacy have yielded inconsistent results. Moreover, it appears that hemodynamic and clinical tolerance, or tachyphylaxis, is a significant problem with chronic prazosin administration.[260–270] At one point, it was postulated that prazosin induced its own metabolism, resulting in decreased plasma prazosin concentration over time[269]; however, this hypothesis was refuted by Arnold et al, who noted tachyphylaxis despite increasing plasma prazosin concentrations.[262] Activation of the sympathetic nervous system and renin–angiotensin–aldosterone (RAA) system has been suggested as a reason for delayed tolerance.[270,271] Because activation of the RAA system results in hyperaldosteronism and enhanced sodium and water retention, some have advocated adding spironolactone and/or increasing dosages of diuretics when tachyphylaxis to prazosin occurs. A recent randomized, double-blind, placebo-controlled study showed no difference in left ventricular function or mortality in chronic CHF patients treated with prazosin 20 mg daily compared with placebo.[253] In light of these results as well as the recent FDA approval of captopril for the treatment of CHF, most clinicians have abandoned the use of prazosin. Trimazosin, an investigational analogue of prazosin, may have long-term benefit in CHF patients without producing tachyphylaxis,[272] but further studies are needed to define its role in the treatment of CHF.

*Angiotensin-Converting Enzyme Inhibitors* The ACE inhibitors, captopril and enalapril, are perhaps the two most exciting new vasodilators to be used in the treatment of CHF. By inhibiting ACE and preventing angiotensin II formation, captopril and enalapril reduce both preload and afterload.[273,274] In addition, they can be taken orally and result in both short- and long-term hemodynamic and clinical improvement (improved symptoms and exercise tolerance) as demonstrated in a number of randomized, double-blind, placebo-controlled clinical trials.[85,86,273–278] Recently, the acute hemodynamic effects as well as the long-term clinical efficacy and safety of captopril were assessed in a multicenter cooperative study of 124 patients with CHF refractory to digitalis and diuretics. While this study was not placebo controlled, it did suggest that captopril had a favorable effect on long-term survival of patients with severe CHF.[279] One small, controlled, double-blind crossover study did show a reduced incidence of arrhythmias in NYHA FC-III and FC-IV CHF patients treated with captopril.[276] This reduced frequency of ventricular tachyarrhythmias may result from the reduced circulating levels of norepinephrine or preserved total body stores of potassium.[276]

Steady-state serum sodium concentrations have been shown to be accurate indicators of the degree of activation of the RAA system in CHF patients.[280] In CHF patients, the higher the degree of RAA system activation, the lower the serum sodium concentration. Moreover, hyponatremic patients have a poorer prognosis than patients with a normal serum sodium concentration.[281] Interestingly, hyponatremic patients appear to respond better and survive longer when treated with ACE inhibitors than when treated with other vasodilators.[281]

*Comparative Pharmacokinetics of Captopril and Enalapril* A major difference between captopril and enalapril is in the onset and duration of effects.[274,282–284] Captopril has a rapid onset, 20 to 30 minutes, and a rapid peak effect as well, 30 to 90 minutes. In contrast, enalapril is a prodrug that must be deesterified to the active diacid moiety, enalaprilat (MK-422). As a result, its onset of action occurs within 1 to 2 hours, and its peak effect may be delayed as long as 4 to 8 hours.[284–286] Captopril dosing in CHF patients ranges from 6.25 mg three times daily initially up to a maximum of 50 mg three times daily. Enalapril dosing in CHF patients ranges from 2.5 to 20 mg given twice daily. Enalapril's extended duration of action compared with captopril may allow for single daily dosing in CHF.[284,286] The bioavailability of captopril is reduced 30% to 40% by food: therefore, it should be administered on an empty stomach either 1 hour before or 2 hours after meals. In contrast, the bioavailability of enalapril is not affected by coadministration with food.[284] Elimination of both captopril and enalapril is reduced in renal insufficiency, and dosages of both drugs must be reduced in this setting.[284]

*Adverse Effects of ACE Inhibitors* When captopril was initially released in United States, dosages up to 450 mg daily were frequently used. This dosage led to a relatively high incidence of rash, dysgeusia, neutropenia, and proteinuria, especially in patients with renal impairment.[286] These side effects were thought to be linked to the presence of a sulfhydryl group on captopril. Enalapril, a nonsulfhydryl analogue of captopril, was initially expected to be devoid of these side effects because it lacked the sulfhydryl group; however, compared with the lower dosages of captopril recommended currently (a maximum of 150 mg daily in CHF), the incidence of these side effects is similar for both enalapril and captopril.[286,287] Enalapril may still represent an effective alternative to captopril should a captopril rash develop, as patients have been successfully switched to enalapril in this setting.[288,289] Patients at risk of developing the aforementioned side effects include those receiving greater than 150 mg daily and those with underlying renal impairment or collagen vascular diseases.

The major adverse effect limiting the use of both captopril and enalapril is systemic hypotension.[290] Patients with the lowest initial blood pressure and hyponatremic patients are at greatest risk; 90% of hypotensive episodes occur in patients with severe hyponatremia.[280,290] Patients with normal serum sodium concentrations can also develop hypotension if they have received aggressive diuresis prior to starting the ACE inhibitor.[290] Systemic hypotension can be minimized by starting with small dosages of ACE inhibitors, 6.25 mg of captopril three times daily and 2.5 or 5 mg of enalapril twice daily. Dosages can then be increased every day or two as tolerated. A particular advantage of ACE inhibitors is that unlike most other vasodilators, they do not cause fluid retention and frequently enable patients to reduce their diuretic requirements. In addition, as a result of their inhibitory effects on aldosterone secretion, they can help maintain potassium stores. Hyperkalemia is usually not a problem, unless ACE inhibitors are given concurrently with potassium-sparing diuretics or potassium supplements. When this occurs, especially if renal function deteriorates suddenly, dangerous increases in serum potassium can result.[290,291]

While enalapril's longer duration of action was initially viewed as an advantage over captopril, a recent study indicates that it may actually lead to more prolonged hypotensive episodes, which could compromise cerebral and renal function and lead to greater retention of potassium.[292] Perhaps as more experience is gained with enalapril, lower dosages and/or single daily dosing regimens may be as efficacious and better tolerated. Additional studies are needed to examine this possibility. Lisinopril (MK-521), an investigational lysine analogue of enalaprilat, also possesses an extended duration of action of 24 hours or longer.[293] Whether lisinopril's extended duration of action will prove advantageous or deleterious in CHF patients remains to be determined.

**Place of Vasodilators in Therapy**

Currently, ACE inhibitors and other vasodilators are usually reserved for NYHA FC-III and FC-IV CHF patients not adequately controlled on digitalis and diuretics alone. Although the ACE inhibitors appear to be a logical choice in patients with coexisting systemic hypertension, there currently is no evidence that pretreatment blood pressure predicts a more favorable response to this group of drugs.[294] ACE inhibitors and nitrates also appear to be particularly useful in patients with CHF associated with underlying coronary artery disease.[295] Conceivably, patients with hypertension and/or ischemic heart disease could be treated with vasodilators earlier and possibly even without digitalis glycosides. In certain patients, the combination of nitrates and ACE inhibitors or hydralazine and ACE inhibitors may produce clinical benefits not observed when a single drug is used alone.[296]

In hyponatremic patients, ACE inhibitors may be more beneficial than other vasodilators, but these patients also may have a higher incidence of untoward effects, such as hypotension.[280,290]

Whether or not ACE inhibitors or hydralazine plus nitrates should be used as first-line agents in patients with CHF is unclear at the present time. A recent study demonstrated that the hydralazine/isosorbide dinitrate combination had a favorable effect on left ventricular function and survival in chronic CHF.[253] In contrast, the same study failed to demonstrate any benefit of prazosin over placebo.[253] A study is in progress comparing an ACE inhibitor with the hydralazine/isosorbide dinitrate combination in a similar group of patients. It is hoped that this study will better define the role of ACE inhibitors and hydralazine/isosorbide dinitrate in the treatment of chronic CHF.

### *Calcium Channel Blockers and β-Blockers*

Nifedipine and several of the newer investigational vascular-selective calcium channel blockers such as nicardipine, nitrendipine, felodipine, and isradipine (PN 200-110) have been used as afterload-reducing agents in patients with CHF.[297] These agents represent potentially attractive alternatives in patients with CHF and ischemic heart disease; however, the role of these agents in CHF is still unclear. Verapamil has well-documented negative inotropic effects and can abruptly worsen CHF.[298] Even nifedipine, which acts primarily on the arterial vasculature, can have significant negative inotropic effects and can worsen CHF.[299,300] Consequently, at the present time, caution must be observed when these agents are used in patients with underlying CHF, and they cannot be routinely recommended as afterload-reducing agents in CHF until more studies are available.[301]

In the last few years, with our increasing awareness of the potential diastolic or lusitropic abnormalities in CHF patients, β-blockers and calcium channel blockers have been utilized in certain patient subsets.[94,302] Because the data in this area are so limited, it would be premature to attempt to characterize how these agents may fit into the long-term management of CHF associated with lusitropic abnormalities. The response to β-blockers and calcium channel blockers in this setting still is somewhat unpredictable.[303–305] Most of the studies conducted have been short term, and data concerning the long-term impact on cardiac dynamics remain to be established.

## Summary

CHF is a major clinical and public health problem; moreover, its incidence is expected to increase in the years ahead.[306] Once the clinical syndrome of CHF is present, the mortality rate is extremely high.[3–5,306] Thus, the goals of therapy are not only to relieve symptoms and improve the quality of life, but also to prolong survival. Up to this time, most clinical trials have focused on improving hemodynamics or clinical symptomatology and have not demonstrated improved survival. Although improvement of hemodynamics and clinical symptoms is a desirable objective, it does not necessarily translate into prolonged survival. In fact, some therapeutic modalities may accomplish this objective acutely, but may have deleterious long-term effects and could conceivably decrease survival.[307–309] Another limitation with most clinical studies to date is that sample size is often too small. As a result, such trials lack statistical "power" and may fail to detect a statistically significant difference in mortality even if such a difference actually exists (termed a type II or beta error).

In severe CHF patients, given the limitations of presently available therapeutic modalities, improvement of the quality of life by relief of symptoms may be a realistic endpoint.[115] In light of the extensive myocardial damage that already exists, a heart transplant or artificial heart may be the only hope for prolonging survival in these patients. With the exception of hydralazine/isosorbide dinitrate in chronic CHF patients and possibly captopril in hyponatremic CHF patients with markedly elevated plasma renin activity, none of the drugs has clearly demonstrated the ability to prolong survival in patients with CHF[253,281]; however, the encouraging results obtained with these drugs should provide the impetus for large-scale, multicenter treatment trials. As nearly half of the patients with CHF die suddenly, presumably from arrhythmias, antiarrhythmic agents should also be evaluated prospectively in randomized, double-blind, placebo-controlled trials.[306] A recent uncontrolled trial provides evidence that carefully selected and monitored antiarrhythmic therapy may improve survival in patients with CHF and life-threatening ventricular tachyarrhythmias.[310]

In contrast to patients with severe CHF, the major therapeutic goal in the management of patients with mild CHF is to preserve the myocardium rather than to relieve the symptoms.[115,307] With mild CHF, if the underlying pathophysiologic process can be recognized and its progression halted early before myocardial function deteriorates further, long-term survival may be substantially improved. The type of therapy utilized must be tailored to modify the specific process responsible for that patient's deterioration in cardiac performance (i.e., ACE inhibitor for the patient with hypertension associated with elevated plasma renin activity).[308] Large-scale, multicenter treatment trials will be necessary to demonstrate the impact of any intervention in this group of patients.[306] In patients with mild CHF and minimal symptoms, a placebo control group would be optimal to determine whether any intervention actually influences the long-term outcome. Obviously, progress in improving long-term survival is dependent on a better understanding of the derangements that occur at a subcellular level. Once specific mechanisms can be identified, the future therapy of CHF will be directed at treating the underlying problem rather than attempting to modify the consequences.

## References


1. Braunwald E. Heart failure: Pathophysiology and treatment. Am Heart J 1981;102:486–490.
2. Kannel WB, Castell WP, McNamara PM, et al. Role of blood pressure in the development of congestive heart failure: The Framingham study. N Engl J Med 1972;287:781–787.
3. McKee PA, Castelli WP, McNamara PM, et al. The natural history of congestive heart failure: The Framingham study. N Engl J Med 1971;285:1441–1446.
4. Franciosa JA, Wilen M, Ziesche S, et al. Survival in men with severe chronic left ventricular failure due to either coronary heart disease or idiopathic dilated cardiomyopathy. Am J Cardiol 1983;51:831–836.
5. Wilson JR, Schwartz JS, St. John Sutton M, et al. Prognosis in severe heart failure: Relation to hemodynamic measurements and ventricular ectopic activity. J Am Coll Cardiol 1983;2:403–410.
6. Ross J. Mechanisms of cardiac contraction: What roles for preload, afterload and inotropic state in heart failure? Eur Heart J 1983;4(suppl A):19–28.
7. Smith VE, Katz AM. Inotropic and lusitropic abnormalities in the genesis of heart failure. Eur Heart J 1983;4(suppl A):7–17.

8. Brutsaert DL, Housmans PR, Goethal MA. Dual control of relaxation. Its role in the ventricular function in the mammalian heart. Circ Res 1980;47:637–652.
9. Grossman W, Barry WH. Diastolic pressure volume relations in the disease heart. Fed Proc 1980;39:148–155.
10. Opie LH. Principles of therapy for congestive heart failure. Eur Heart J 1983;4(suppl A):199–208.
11. Firth BG. Southwestern Internal Medicine Conference: Chronic congestive heart failure—the nature of the problem and its management in 1984. Am J Med Sci 1984;288:178–192.
12. Parmley WW. Pathophysiology of congestive heart failure: Am J Cardiol 1985;55:9A–14A.
13. McCall D, O'Rourke RA. Congestive heart failure: I. Biochemistry, pathophysiology and neurohumoral mechanisms. Mod Concepts Cardiovasc Dis 1985;54:55–59.
14. Feldman RD, Limbird LE, Nadeau J, et al. Alterations in leukocyte beta receptor affinity with aging. A potential explanation for altered beta adrenergic sensitivity in the elderly. N Engl J Med 1984;310:815–820.
15. Colucci WS, Alexander RW, Williams GH, et al. Decreased lymphocyte beta-adrenergic receptor density in patients with heart failure and tolerance to the beta-adrenergic agonist pirbuterol. N Engl J Med 1981;305:185–190.
16. Dougherty AH, Naccarelli GV, Gray EL, et al. Congestive heart failure with normal systolic function. Am J Cardiol 1984;54:778–782.
17. Braunwald E, Sonnenblick EH, Ross Jr J. Contraction of the normal heart, in Braunwald E (ed): Heart Disease. A Textbook of Cardiovascular Medicine. 2nd ed. Philadelphia, W.B. Saunders, 1984, pp 423–438.
18. The Criteria Committee of the New York Heart Association. Diseases of the Heart and Blood Vessels: Nomenclature and Criteria for Diagnosis, 7th ed. Boston, Little, Brown, 1973.
19. Goldman L, Hashimoto B, Cook EF, et al. Comparative reproducibility and validity of systems for assessing cardiovascular functional class: Advantages of a new specific activity scale. Circulation 1981;64:1227–1234.
20. Braunwald E. The history, in Braunwald E (ed): Heart Disease. A Textbook of Cardiovascular Medicine, 2nd ed. Philadelphia, W.B. Saunders, 1984, pp 12–13.
21. Goldberg S, Mann T, Grossman W. Nitrate therapy of heart failure in valvular heart disease. Importance of resting level of peripheral vascular resistance in determining cardiac output response. Am J Med 1978;65:161–166.
22. Parker JO, Kelly G, West RO. Hemodynamic effects of aminophylline in heart failure. Am J Cardiol 1966;17:232–239.
23. Murphy GW, Schreiner BR, Yu PN. Effects of aminophylline on the pulmonary circulation and left ventricular performance in patients with valvular heart disease. Circulation 1968;37: 361–369.
24. Sigurd B, Oleson KH. Comparative natriuretic and diuretic efficacy of theophylline ethylenediamine and of bendroflumethiazide during long-term treatment with the potent diuretic bumetanide. Acta Med Scand 1978;203:113–119.
25. Swan HJC, Ganz W, Forrester JS, et al. Catheterization of the heart in man with the use of a flow-directed balloon-tipped catheter. N Engl J Med 1970;283:447–451.
26. Forrester JS, Diamond G, Chatterjee K, et al. Medical therapy of acute myocardial infarction by application of hemodynamic subsets. N Engl J Med 1976;295:1356–1362, 1404–1413.
27. Goldenheim PD, Kazemi H. Cardiopulmonary monitoring of critically ill patients (second of 2 parts). N Engl J Med 1984; 311:776–780.
28. Weber KT, Likoff MJ, Janick JS, et al. Advances in the evaluation and management of chronic heart failure. Chest 1984;85:253–259.
29. Heinemann HO, DeMartini EE, Laragh JH. The mode of action and use of chlorothiazide on renal excretion of electrolytes and free water. Am J Med 1959;26:853–861.
30. Puschett JB. Clinical implications in diuretic selection. Am J Cardiol 1986;57:6A–13A.
31. Dargie HJ, Allison ME, Kennedy AC, et al. High dosage metolazone in chronic renal failure. Br Med J 1972;4:196–198.
32. Hunter KR, Underwood PN. Evaluation of once-daily versus twice-daily bumetanide in heart failure. Postgrad Med J 1975;51(suppl 6):91–95.
33. Exaire JE, Villapando J, Hamdan G, et al. Dosage titration with furosemide in congestive heart failure patients. Angiology 1976;26:665–670.
34. Dikshit K, Vyden JK, Forrester JS, et al. Renal and extrarenal hemodynamic effects of furosemide in congestive heart failure after acute myocardial infarction. N Engl J Med 1973;288: 1087–1090.
35. Bourland WA, Day DK, Williamson HE. The role of the kidney in the early nondiuretic action of furosemide to reduce elevated left atrial pressure in hypovolemic dogs. J Pharmacol Exp Ther 1977;202:221–229.
36. Johnston GD, Hiatt WR, Nies AS, et al. Factors modifying the early vascular effects of furosemide in man: The possible role of renal prostaglandins. Circ Res 1983;53:630–635.
37. Biddle TL, Yu PN. Effect of furosemide on hemodynamics and lung water in acute pulmonary edema secondary to myocardial infarction. Am J Cardiol 1979;43:86–90.
38. Francis CS, Siegel RM, Goldsmith SR, et al. Acute vasoconstrictor response to intravenous furosemide in patients with chronic congestive heart failure. Ann Intern Med 1985; 103:1–6.
39. Brater DC. Disposition and response to bumetanide and furosemide. Am J Cardiol 1986;57:20A–25A.
40. Brater DC, Seiwell R, Anderson S, et al. Absorption and disposition of furosemide in congestive heart failure. Kidney Int 1982;22:171–176.
41. Brater DC, Day B, Burdette A, et al. Bumetanide and furosemide in heart failure. Kidney Int 1984;26:183–189.
42. Vasko MR, Cartwright DB, Knochel JP, et al. Furosemide absorption altered in decompensated congestive heart failure. Ann Intern Med 1985;102:314–318.
43. Marone C, Muggli F, Lahn W, et al. Pharmacokinetic and pharmacodynamic interaction between furosemide and metolazone in man. Eur J Clin Invest 1985;15:253–257.
44. Brater DC, Pressley RH, Anderson SA. Mechanisms of the synergistic combination of metolazone and bumetanide. J Pharmacol Exp Ther 1985;233:70–74.
45. Holland OB, Nixon JV, Kuhnert I. Diuretic-induced ventricular ectopic activity. Am J Med 1981;70:762–768.
46. Henderson RP. Arrhythmias associated with magnesium deficiency. Hosp Ther 1986;11:54–60.
47. Beller GA, Smith TW, Abelmann WT, et al. Digitalis intoxication. N Engl J Med 1971;284:989–997.
48. Withering W. An Account of the Foxglove, and Some of Its Medical Uses: With Practical Remarks on Dropsy and Other Diseases. Birmingham, England, M. Swinney, 1785.
49. Fozzard HA, Sheets MF. Cellular mechanisms of action of cardiac glycosides. J Am Coll Cardiol 1985;5:10A–15A.
50. Katz AM. Effects of digitalis on cell biochemistry: Sodium pump inhibition. J Am Coll Cardiol 1985;5:16A–21A.
51. Braunwald E. Effects of digitalis on the normal and failing heart. J Am Coll Cardiol 1985;5:51A–59A.

52. Gillis RA, Helke CJ, et al. Automatic nervous system actions of cardiac glycosides. Biochem Pharmacol 1978;27:849–856.
53. Garan H, Power Jr WJ. Neurogenic effect of digoxin on vascular resistance during hypotension. Circulation 1977; 56(suppl 3):237.
54. Vatner SF, Higgins CB, Franklin D, et al. Effects of digitalis glycoside on coronary and systemic dynamics in conscious dogs. Circ Res 1979;28:470–479.
55. Churchill PC. Possible mechanism of the inhibitory effect of ouabain on renin secretion from rat renal cortical slices. J Physiol 1979;294:123.
56. Churchill MC, Churchill PC. Separate and combined effects of ouabain in extracellular potassium on renin secretion from rat renal cortical slices. J Physiol 1980;300:105–114.
57. Covit AB, Schaer GL, Sealy JE, et al. Suppression of the renin–angiotensin system by intravenous digoxin in chronic congestive heart failure. Am J Med 1983;75:445–447.
58. Marchionni N, Pini R, Vannucci A, et al. Hemodynamic effects of digoxin in acute myocardial infarction in man: A randomized controlled trial. Am Heart J 1985;109:63–68.
59. Taggart AJ, Johnston GD, McDevitt DG. Digoxin withdrawal after cardiac failure in patients with sinus rhythm. J Cardiovasc Pharmacol 1983;5:229–234.
60. Dobbs SM, Kenyon WI, Dobbs RJ. Maintenance digoxin after an episode of heart failure: Placebo-control trials in outpatients. Br Med J 1977;1:749–752.
61. Fleg JL, Gottlieb SH, Lakatta EG. Is digoxin really important in treatment of compensated heart failure? A placebo-controlled crossover trial in patients with sinus rhythm. Am J Med 1982;73:244–250.
62. Lee DC, Johnson RA, Bingham JB, et al. Heart failure in outpatients: A randomized trial of digoxin versus placebo. N Engl J Med 1982;306:699–705.
63. Hymann AL, Jaques WE, Hymann ES. Observation on the direct effect of digoxin on renal excretion of sodium and water. Am Heart J 1956;52:592–608.
64. Reunig RH, Geraets DR. Digoxin, in Evans WE, Schentag JJ, Jusko WJ (eds): Applied Pharmacokinetics: Principles of Therapeutic Drug Monitoring, 2nd ed. Spokane, WA, Applied Therapeutics, 1986, pp 570–610.
65. Smith TW. Pharmacokinetics, bioavailability and serum levels of cardiac glycosides. J Am Coll Cardiol 1985;5:43A–50A.
66. Caldwell JH, Cline CT. Biliary excretion of digoxin in man. Clin Pharmacol Ther 1976;19:410–415.
67. Hansten PD. Digitalis drug interactions, in Drug Interactions: Clinical Significance of Drug–Drug Interactions, 5th ed. Philadelphia, Lea and Febiger, 1985, pp 273–285.
68. Marcus FI. Pharmacokinetic interactions between digoxin and other drugs. J Am Coll Cardiol 1985;5:82A–90A.
69. Sawyer WT. The digitalis glycosides, in Taylor WJ, Diers-Caviness MH (eds): A Textbook for the Clinical Application of Therapeutic Drug Monitoring. Irving, TX, Abbott Laboratories, Diagnostics Division, 1986, pp 83–96.
70. Vlasses PH, Rocci Jr ML. Digoxin commentary, in Evans WE, Schentag JJ, Jusko WJ (eds): Applied Pharmacokinetics: Principles of Therapeutic Drug Monitoring, 2nd ed. Spokane, WA, Applied Therapeutics, 1986, pp 624–636.
71. Bussey HI, Merritt GJ, Hill EG. The influence of rifampin on quinidine and digoxin. Arch Intern Med 1984;144:1021–1023.
72. Gault H, Longerich L, Dawe M, et al. Digoxin–rifampin interaction. Clin Pharmacol Ther 1984;35:750–754.
73. Jelliffe RW. An improved method of digoxin therapy. Ann Intern Med 1968;69:703–717.
74. Aronson JK. Indications for the measurement of plasma digoxin concentration. Drugs 1983;26:230–242.
75. Ingelfinger JA, Goldman P. The serum digitalis concentration—does it diagnose digitalis toxicity? N Engl J Med 1976;294:867–870.
76. Fitzsimmons WE. Influence of assay methodologies and interferences on the interpretation of digoxin concentrations. Drug Intell Clin Pharm 1986;20:538–542.
77. Valdes R. Endogenous digoxin-like immunoreactive factors: Impact on digoxin measurements and potential physiological implications. Clin Chem 1985;31:1525–1532.
78. Soldin SJ. Digoxin—Issues and controversies. Clin Chem 1986;32:5–12.
79. Mulrow CD, Feussner JR, Velez R. Reevaluation of digitalis efficacy. New light on an old leaf. Ann Intern Med 1984;101: 113–117.
80. Packer M. How should we judge the efficacy of drug therapy in patients with chronic congestive heart failure? The insights of six blind men. J Am Coll Cardiol 1987;9:433–438.
81. Arnold SB, Byrd RC, Meister W, et al. Long-term digitalis therapy improves left ventricular function in heart failure. N Engl J Med 1980;303:1443–1448.
82. Rader BR, Smith WW, Berger AR. Comparison of the hemodynamic effects of mercurial diuretics and digitalis in congestive heart failure. Circulation 1964;29:328–345.
83. McHaffie D, Purcell H, Mitchell-Heggs P, et al. The clinical value of digoxin in patients with heart failure and sinus rhythm. Q J Med 1978;47:401–419.
84. Hutcheon D, Nemeth E, Quinlan D. The role of furosemide alone and in combination with digoxin in the relief of symptoms of congestive heart failure. J Clin Pharmacol 1980;20:59–68.
85. Captopril Multicenter Group. A placebo-controlled trial of captopril in refractory chronic congestive heart failure. J Am Coll Cardiol 1983;2:755–763.
86. Sharpe DN, Murphy J, Coxon R, et al. Enalapril in patients with chronic congestive heart failure: A placebo-controlled, randomized, double-blind study. Circulation 1984;70:271–278.
87. Franciosa JA, Nordstrom LA, Cohn JN. Nitrate therapy for congestive heart failure. JAMA 1978;240:443–446.
88. Leier CV, Huss P, Magorien RD, et al. Improved exercise capacity and differing arterial and venous tolerance during chronic isosorbide dinitrate therapy for congestive heart failure. Circulation 1983;67:817–822.
89. Franciosa JA, Weber KT, Levine TB, et al. Hydralazine in the long-term treatment of chronic heart failure: Lack of difference from placebo. Am Heart J 1982;104:587–594.
90. Colucci WS, Wynne J, Holman BL. Long-term therapy of heart failure with prazosin: Randomized double-blind trial. Am J Cardiol 1980;45:337–344.
91. Markham RV, Corbett JR, Gilmore A, et al. Efficacy of prazosin in the management of chronic heart failure: A 6 month randomized, double-blind, placebo-controlled study. Am J Cardiol 1983;51:1346–1352.
92. Katz AM. A new inotropic drug: Its promises and a caution. N Engl J Med 1978;299:1409–1410.
93. Factor SM, Minase T, Cho S, et al. Microvascular spasm in the cardiomyopathic Syrian hamster: A preventable cause of focal myocardial necrosis. Circulation 1982;66:342–354.
94. Topol EJ, Traill TA, Fortuin NJ. Hypertensive hypertropic cardiomyopathy of the elderly. N Engl J Med 1985;312:277–282.
95. Weisfeldt ML, Scully HE, Frederiksen J, et al. Hemodynamic

determinants of maximum negative *dP/dt* and periods of diastole. Am J Physiol 1974;227:613–621.
96. Gheorghiade M, Beller GA. Effects of discontinuing maintenance digoxin therapy in patients with ischemic heart disease and congestive heart failure in sinus rhythm. Am J Cardiol 1983;51:1243–1250.
97. Aronow WS, Starling L, Etienne F. Lack of efficacy of digoxin in treatment of compensated congestive heart failure with third heart sound and sinus rhythm in elderly patients receiving diuretic therapy. Am J Cardiol 1986;58:168–169.
98. Aronson JK. Digitalis intoxication. Clin Sci 1983;64:253–258.
99. Bhatia SJS. Digitalis intoxication—Turning over a new leaf? West J Med 1986;145:74–82.
100. Bismuth C, Gaultier M, Conso F, et al. Hyperkalemia in acute digitalis poisoning: Prognostic significance and therapeutic implications. Clin Toxicol 1973;6:153–162.
101. Watanabe AM. Digitalis and the autonomic nervous system. J Am Coll Cardiol 1985;5:35A–42A.
102. Elenbaas RM. Congestive heart failure, in Herfindal ET, Hirschman JL (eds): Clinical Pharmacy and Therapeutics, 3rd ed. Baltimore, Williams and Wilkins, 1984, pp 388–392.
103. Chung EK. Digitalis-induced cardiac arrhythmias. Am Heart J 1970;79:845.
104. Fisch C. Digitalis intoxication. JAMA 1971;216:1770.
105. Digibind, Digoxin Immune Fab (Ovine), package insert. Research Triangle Park, NC, Burroughs Wellcome, June 1986.
106. Digoxin antibody fragments for digitalis toxicity. Med Lett 1986;28:87–88.
107. Wenger TL, Butler Jr VP, Haber E, et al. Treatment of 63 severely digitalis-toxic patients with digoxin-specific antibody fragments. J Am Coll Cardiol 1985;5:118A–123A.
108. Cole PL, Smith TW. Use of digoxin-specific Fab fragments in the treatment of digitalis intoxication. Drug Intell Clin Pharm 1986;20:267–270.
109. Goldberg LI. Dopamine: Clinical uses of an endogenous catecholamine. N Engl J Med 1974;291:707–710.
110. Leier CV. Comparative systemic and regional hemodynamic effects of dopamine and dobutamine in patients with cardiomyopathic heart failure. Circulation 1978;58:466–475.
111. Tuttle RR, Millie J. Dobutamine: Development of a new catecholamine to selectively increase cardiac contractility. Circ Res 1975;36:185–196.
112. Leier CV, Unverth DV. Dobutamine. Ann Intern Med 1983;99: 490–496.
113. Reuter H, Scholz H. The regulation of the calcium conductance of cardiac muscle by adrenaline. J Physiol (Lond) 1977;264:49–62.
114. Schuman HJ, Wagner J, Know A, et al. Demonstration in human atrial preparations of alpha-adrenoceptors mediating positive inotropic effects. Naunyn Schmeidebergs Arch Pharmacol 1978;302:333–336.
115. Scholz H. Inotropic drugs and their mechanisms of action. J Am Coll Cardiol 1984;4:389–397.
116. Drummond GI, Severson DL. Cyclic nucleotides and cardiac function. Circ Res 1979;44:145–153.
117. Katz AM. Cyclic adenosine monophosphate effects on the myocardium: A man who blows hot and cold with one breath. J Am Coll Cardiol 1983;2:143–149.
118. Francis GS, Sharma B, Hodge M. Comparative hemodynamic effects of dopamine and dobutamine in patients with acute cardiogenic circulatory collapse. Am Heart J 1982;103:995–999.
119. Ruffolo Jr RR, Yaden EL. Vascular effects of the stereoisomers of dobutamine. J Pharmacol Exp Ther 1983;224:46–50.
120. Ruffolo Jr RR, Spradlin TA, Pollock GD, et al. Alpha and beta adrenergic effects of the stereoisomers of dobutamine. J Pharmacol Exp Ther 1981;219:447–452.
121. Richard C, Ricome JL, Rimailho A, et al. Combined hemodynamic effects of dopamine and dobutamine in cardiogenic shock. Circulation 1983;67:620–626.
122. Liang CS, Sherman LG, Doherty JU, et al. Sustained improvement of cardiac function in patients with congestive heart failure after short-term infusion of dobutamine. Circulation 1984;69:113–119.
123. Applefeld MM, Newman KA, Grove WR, et al. Intermittent, continuous outpatient dobutamine infusion in the management of congestive heart failure. Am J Cardiol 1983;51:455–458.
124. Unverferth DV, Blanford M, Kate RE, et al. Tolerance to dobutamine after a 72 hour continuous infusion. Am J Med 1980;69:262–266.
125. Roffman DS, Applefeld MM, Grove WR, et al. Intermittent dobutamine hydrochloride infusions in outpatients with chronic congestive heart failure. Clin Pharm 1985;4:195–199.
126. Mauro VF, Mauro LS. Use of intermittent dobutamine infusion in congestive heart failure. Drug Intell Clin Pharm 1986;20:919–924.
127. Rajfer SI, Anton AH, Rossen JD, et al. Beneficial hemodynamic effects of oral levodopa in heart failure: Relation to the generation of dopamine. N Engl J Med 1984;310:1357–1362.
128. Dei Cas L, Manca C, Bernardini B, et al. Noninvasive evaluation of the effects of oral ibopamine (SB 7505) on cardiac and renal function in patients with congestive heart failure. J Cardiovasc Pharmacol 1982;4:436–440.
129. Dei Cas L, Bolognesi R, Cucchini F, et al. Hemodynamic effects of ibopamine in patients with idiopathic congestive cardiomyopathy. J Cardiovasc Pharmacol 1983;5:249–253.
130. Fennell WH, Taylor AA, Young JB, et al. Propylbutyldopamine: Hemodynamic effects in conscious dogs, normal human volunteers and patients with heart failure. Circulation 1983;67: 829–836.
131. Brown RA, Farmer JB, Hall JC, et al. The effects of dopexamine on the cardiovascular system of the dog. Br J Pharmacol 1985;85:609–619.
132. Waagstein F, Reiz S, Ariniego R, et al. Clinical results with prenalterol in patients with heart failure. Am Heart J 1981;102: 540–563.
133. Hedberg A, Minnemann KP, Molinoff PB. Differential distribution of beta-1 and beta-2 adrenergic receptors in cat and guinea pig heart. J Pharmacol Exp Ther 1980;213:503–508.
134. Roubin GS, Choong CYP, Devenish-Meares S, et al. Beta-adrenergic stimulation of the failing ventricle: A double-blind, randomized trial of sustained oral therapy with prenalterol. Circulation 1984;69:955–962.
135. Rousseau MF, Pouleur H, Vincent MF. Effects of a cardioselective beta-1 partial agonist (Corwin) on left ventricular function and myocardial metabolism in patients with previous myocardial infarction. Am J Cardiol 1983;51:1267–1274.
136. Thormann J, Kramer W, Kindler M, et al. Analysis of the efficacy of the new cardiotonic agent, TA-064. Am Heart J 1985;110:426–438.
137. Thompson MJ, Huss P, Unverferth DV, et al. Hemodynamic effects of intravenous butopamine in congestive heart failure. Clin Pharmacol Ther 1980;28:324–334.
138. Kirlin PC, Pitt B. Hemodynamic effects of intravenous prenalterol in severe heart failure. Am J Cardiol 1981;47:670–675.
139. Bourdillon FDV, Dawson JR, Foale RA, et al. Salbutamol in treatment of heart failure. Br Heart J 1980;43:206–210.
140. Slutsky R, Hooper W, Gerber K, et al. The effect of terbutaline on left ventricular function and size. (Abstr) Am J Cardiol 1980;45:412.

**141.** Awan NA, Everson MK, Needham KE, et al. Hemodynamic effects of oral pirbuterol in chronic severe congestive heart failure. Circulation 1981;63:96–101.

**142.** Sharma B, Hoback J, Francis GS, et al. Pirbuterol: A new oral sympathomimetic amine for the treatment of congestive heart failure. Am Heart J 1981;102:533–541.

**143.** Awan NA, Needham K, Evenson MK, et al. Therapeutic efficacy of oral pirbuterol in severe chronic congestive heart failure: Acute hemodynamic and long-term ambulatory evaluation. Am Heart J 1981;102:555–563.

**144.** Colucci WS, Alexander RW, Mudge GH, et al. Acute and chronic effects of pirbuterol on left ventricular ejection fraction and clinical status in severe congestive heart failure. Am Heart J 1981;102:564–568.

**145.** Weber KT, Andrews V, Janicki JS, et al. Pirbuterol, an oral beta-adrenergic receptor agonist, in the treatment of chronic cardiac failure. Circulation 1982;66:1262–1267.

**146.** Gorcyznski RJ, Wroble RW. Cardiovascular pharmacology of ASL-7022. II. Mechanisms of inotropic selectivity. J Pharmacol Exp Ther 1982;223:12–19.

**147.** Colucci WS, Wright RF, Braunwald E. New positive inotropic agents in the treatment of congestive heart failure. Mechanisms of action and recent clinical developments (first of two parts). N Engl J Med 1986;314:294–295.

**148.** Weber KT, Janicki JS, Maskin CS. Effects of new inotropic agents on exercise performance. Circulation 1986;73(suppl III): III196–III204.

**149.** Alousi A, Lesher G, Opalka C. Cardiotonic activity or amrinone, WIN 40680 (5-amino-3,4′-bipyridine-6(1*H*)-one). Circ Res 1979;45:666–677.

**150.** Benotti J, Grossman W, Braunwald E, et al. Hemodynamic assessment of amrinone: A new inotropic agent. N Engl J Med 1978;299:1373–1377.

**151.** LeJemtel T, Keun E, Sonnenblick E, et al. Amrinone: A new nonglycoside, nonadrenergic cardiotonic agent effective in the treatment of intractable myocardial failure in man. Circulation 1979;59:1098–1104.

**152.** Mancini D, LeJemtel T, Sonnenblick E. Intravenous use of amrinone for the treatment of the failing heart. Am J Cardiol 1985;56:8B–15B.

**153.** Karlya T, Wille L, Dage R. Biochemical studies on the mechanism of cardiotonic activity of MDL 17043. J Cardiovasc Pharmacol 1982;4:509–514.

**154.** Hayes JS, Bowling N, Boder G, et al. Molecular basis for the cardiovascular activities of amrinone and AR-L57. J Pharmacol Exp Ther 1984;230:124–132.

**155.** Honerjager P, Schafer-Korting M, Reiter M. Involvement of cyclic AMP in the direct inotropic action of amrinone. Naunyn Schmiedebergs Arch Pharmacol 1981;318:112–120.

**156.** Feldman MD, Copelas L, Gwathmey JK, et al. Deficient production of cyclic AMP: Pharmacologic evidence of an important cause of contractile dysfunction in patients with end-stage heart failure. Circulation 1987;75:331–339.

**157.** Parker J, Harper J. Effects of amrinone, a cardiotonic drug, on calcium movements in dog erythrocytes. J Clin Invest 1980;66: 254–259.

**158.** Ward A, Brogden R, Heel R, et al. Amrinone: A preliminary review of its pharmacological properties and therapeutic use. Drugs 1983;26:468–502.

**159.** Cardenas L, Vidauri D. Estudio de los efectos hemodinamicos de diferentes doses de un nuevo inotropico: La amrinone. Arch Inst Cardiol Mex 1979;49:981–986.

**160.** Keung E, LeJemtel T, Ribner H, et al. Amrinone: A new oral agent in the treatment of heart failure. (Abstr) Clin Res 1979; 27:502.

**161.** Wynne J, Malacoif R, Benotti J, et al. Oral amrinone in refractory congestive heart failure. Am J Cardiol 1980;45:1245–1249.

**162.** Jennings K, Glvelt D, Crean P, et al. The clinical cardiovascular pharmacology of amrinone: A selective cardiotonic agent. Acta Cardiol (Brux) 1982;28(suppl):67–73.

**163.** Wilmhurst P, Thompson D, Jenkins B, et al. Haemodynamic effects of intravenous amrinone in patients with impaired left ventricular function. Br Heart J 1983;49:77–82.

**164.** Firth BG, Ratner AV, Grossman ED, et al. Assessment of the inotropic and vasodilator effects of amrinone versus isoproterenol. Am J Cardiol 1984;54:1331–1336.

**165.** Weber K, Andrews V, Janicki J, et al. Amrinone and exercise performance in patients with chronic heart failure. Am J Cardiol 1981;48:164–169.

**166.** Likoff MJ, Weber KT, Andrews V, et al. Amrinone in the treatment of chronic cardiac failure. J Am Coll Cardiol 1984;3: 1282–1290.

**167.** Packer M, Medina, Yushak M. Hemodynamic and clinical limitations of long-term inotropic therapy with amrinone in patients with severe chronic heart failure. Circulation 1984;70: 1038–1047.

**168.** Diabianco R, Shabetai R, Silverman BD, et al. Oral amrinone for the treatment of chronic congestive heart failure: Results of a multicentered randomized double-blind and placebo-controlled withdrawal. J Am Coll Cardiol 1984;4:855–860.

**169.** Sonnenblick E, Mancini DM, LeJemtel TH. New positive inotropic drugs for the treatment of congestive heart failure. Am J Cardiol 1985;55:41A–44A.

**170.** Benotti J, Grossman W, Braunwald E, et al. Effects of amrinone on myocardial energy metabolism and hemodynamics in patients with severe congestive heart failure due to coronary artery disease. Circulation 1980;62:28–34.

**171.** Rude R, Klonar R, Maroko P, et al. Effects of amrinone on experimental acute myocardial ischemic injury. Cardiovasc Res 1980;14:419–427.

**172.** Jentzer J, LeJemtel T, Sonnenblick E, et al. Beneficial effect of amrinone on myocardial oxygen consumption during acute left ventricular failure in dogs. Am J Cardiol 1981;48:75–83.

**173.** Kirk E, LeJemtel T, Nelson G, et al. Mechanisms of beneficial effects of vasodilators and inotropic stimulation in the experimental failing ischemic heart. Am J Med 1978;65:189–196.

**174.** Baim DS. Effects of amrinone on myocardial energetics in severe congestive heart failure. Am J Cardiol 1985;56:16B–18B.

**175.** Taylor SH, Verma SP, Hussain M, et al. Intravenous amrinone in left ventricular failure complicated by acute myocardial infarction. Am J Cardiol 1985;56:29B–32B.

**176.** Klein N, Siskind S, Frishman W, et al. Hemodynamic comparison of intravenous amrinone and dobutamine in patients with chronic congestive heart failure. Am J Cardiol 1981;48: 170–175.

**177.** Benotti JR, McCue JE, Alpert JS. Comparative vasoactive therapy for heart failure. Am J Cardiol 1985;56:19B-24B.

**178.** LeJemtel T, Sonnenblick E. Amrinone: A new noncatecholamine and nonglycoside type cardiac inotropic drug, in Braunwald E (ed): Congestive Heart Failure: Current Research and Clinical Applications. New York, Grune and Stratton, 1982, pp 200–211.

**179.** Colucci WS, Wright RF, Braunwald E. New positive inotropic agents in the treatment of congestive heart failure. Mechanisms of action and recent clinical developments (second of two parts). N Engl J Med 1986;314:349–358.

**180.** Siegel L, Keung E, Siskind S, et al. Beneficial effects of amrinone–hydralazine combination on resting hemodynamics and exercise capacity in patients with severe congestive heart failure. Circulation 1981;63:838–844.

**181.** Bayliss J, Norell M, Canepa-Anson R, et al. Acute haemodynamic comparison of amrinone and pirbuterol in chronic heart failure: Additional effects on isosorbide dinitrate. Br Heart J 1983;49:214–221.

**182.** LeJemtel T, Keung E, Schwartz W, et al. Hemodynamic effects of intravenous and oral amrinone in patients with severe heart failure: Relationship between intravenous and oral administration. Trans Assoc Am Physicians 1979;92:325–333.

**183.** Summary basis of approval: Amrinone. Revised October 11, 1983, submission data to the Food and Drug Administration.

**184.** Treadway G. Clinical safety of intravenous amrinone—a review. Am J Cardiol 1985;56:39B–40B.

**185.** Wilmhurst P, Webb-Peploe M. Side effects of amrinone therapy. Br Heart J 1983;49:447–451.

**186.** Ansell J, Tlarks C, McCue J, et al. Amrinone-induced thrombocytopenia. Arch Intern Med 1984;144:949–952.

**187.** Kullberg MP, Freeman GB, Biddlecome C, et al. Amrinone metabolism. Clin Pharmacol Ther 1981;29:394–401.

**188.** Park GB, Kershner RP, Angelloti J, et al. Oral bioavailability and intravenous pharmacokinetics of amrinone in humans. J Pharm Sci 1983;72:817–819.

**189.** Goldstein RA, Gray EL, Dougherty AH, et al. Electrophysiologic effects of amrinone. Am J Cardiol 1985;56:25B–28B.

**190.** Bottorff MVB, Rutledge DR, Pieper JA. Evaluation of intravenous amrinone: The first of a new class of positive inotropic agents with vasodilator properties. Pharmacotherapy 1985;5:227–235.

**191.** Leier CV. Commentary: Evaluation of intravenous amrinone: The first of a new class of positive inotropic agents with vasodilator properties. Pharmacotherapy 1985;5:235–236.

**192.** Gage J, Strom J, Jordan A, et al. Synergistic effects of beta-adrenergic stimulation with dobutamine and phosphodiesterase inhibition with amrinone on cardiac performance and contractility in chronic heart failure. (Abstr) Clin Res 1985;33:187.

**193.** Klamerus KJ. Current concepts in clinical therapeutics: Congestive heart failure. Clin Pharm 1986;5:481–498.

**194.** Alousi AA, Stankus GP, Stuart JC, et al. Characterization of the cardiotonic effects of milrinone, a new and potent cardiac bipyridine, on isolated tissues from several animal species. J Cardiovasc Pharmacol 1983;5:804–811.

**195.** Borow KM, Come P, Neumann A, et al. Milrinone (WIN 47203): Differentiation of its inotropic and vasodilator effects in humans (Abstr) J Am Coll Cardiol 1984;3:472.

**196.** Sonnenblick EH, Grose R, Strain J, et al. Effects of milrinone on left ventricular performance and myocardial contractility in patients with severe heart failure. Circulation 1986;73(suppl III):III-162–167.

**197.** Monrad ES, Baim DS, Smith HS, et al. Milrinone, dobutamine, and nitroprusside: Comparative effects on hemodynamics and myocardial energetics in patients with severe congestive heart failure. Circulation 1986:73(suppl III): III-168–174.

**198.** Colucci WS, Wright RF, Jaski BE, et al. Milrinone and dobutamine in severe heart failure: Differing hemodynamic effects and individual patient responsiveness. Circulation 1986;73(suppl III):III-175–183.

**199.** Monrad ES, McKay RG, Baim DS, et al. Improvement in indexes of diastolic performance in patients with congestive heart failure treated with milrinone. Circulation 1984;70:1030–1037.

**200.** Grossman W, McLaurin LP, Rolett EL. Alterations in left ventricular relaxation and diastolic compliance in congestive cardiomyopathy. Cardiovasc Res 1979;13:514–519.

**201.** Baim DS, McDowell AV, Cherniles J, et al. Evaluation of a new bipyridine inotropic agent, milrinone, in patients with severe congestive heart failure. N Engl J Med 1983;309:748–756.

**202.** Maskin CS, Sinoway L, Chadwick B, et al. Sustained hemodynamic and clinical effects of a new cardiotonic agent, WIN 47203, in patients with severe congestive heart failure. Circulation 1983;67:1065–1070.

**203.** Kubo SP, Cody RJ, Chatterjee K, et al. Acute dose range study of milrinone in congestive heart failure. Am J Cardiol 1985;55:726–730.

**204.** Monrad ES, Baim DS, Smith HS, et al. Assessment of long-term therapy with milrinone and the effects of milrinone withdrawal. Circulation 1986;73(suppl III):III-205–212.

**205.** LeJemtel TH, Gumbardo D, Chadwick B, et al. Milrinone for long-term therapy of severe heart failure: Clinical experience with special reference to maximal exercise tolerance. Circulation 1986;73(suppl III):III-213–218.

**206.** Crawford MH, Richards KL, Sodums M, et al. Positive inotropic and vasodilator effects of MDL 17043 in patients with reduced left ventricular performance. Am J Cardiol 1984;53:1051–1053.

**207.** Petein M, Levine TB, Cohn JN. Hemodynamic effects of a new inotropic agent, piroximone (MDL 19205), in patients with chronic heart failure. J Am Coll Cardiol 1983;4:364–371.

**208.** Uretsky BF, Generalovich T, Reddy PS, et al. The acute hemodynamic effects of a new agent, MDL 17,043, in the treatment of congestive heart failure. Circulation 1983;67:823–828.

**209.** Amin DK, Shah PK, Hulse S, et al. Comparative acute hemodynamic effects of intravenous sodium nitroprusside and MDL 17043, a new inotropic drug with vasodilator effects, in refractory congestive heart failure. Am Heart J 1985;109:1006–1012.

**210.** Likoff MJ, Martin JL, Andrews V, et al. Long-term therapy with the cardiotonic agent MDL 17043 in chronic cardiac failure. (Abstr) Circulation 1983;68:III-373.

**211.** Kereiakes D, Chatterjee K, Parmley WW, et al. Intravenous and oral MDL 17043 (a new inotropic-vasodilator agent) in congestive heart failure: Hemodynamic and clinical evaluation in 38 patients. J Am Coll Cardiol 1984;4:884–889.

**212.** Rubin SA, Tabak L. MDL 17043: Short- and long-term cardiopulmonary and clinical effects in patients with heart failure. J Am Coll Cardiol 1985;5:1422–1427.

**213.** Uretsky BF, Generalovich T, Verbalis JG, et al. MDL 17043–Therapy in severe congestive heart failure: Characterization of the early and late hemodynamic, pharmacokinetic, hormonal and clinical response. J Am Coll Cardiol 1985;5:1414–1421.

**214.** Uretsky BF, Valdes AM, Reddy PS. Positive inotropic therapy for short-term support and long-term management of patients with congestive heart failure: Hemodynamic effects and clinical efficacy of MDL 17,043. Circulation 1986:73(suppl III):III-219–227.

**215.** Petein M, Levine TB, Cohn JN. Persistent hemodynamic effects without long-term clinical benefits in response to oral piroximone (MDL 19,205) in patients with congestive heart failure. Circulation 1986;73(suppl III):III-230–236.

**216.** Martin JL, Likoff MJ, Janicki JS, et al. Myocardial energetics and clinical response to the cardiotonic agent MDL 17043 in advanced heart failure. J Am Coll Cardiol 1984;4:875–883.

**217.** Thormann J, Schlepper M, Kramer W, et al. Effects of ARL 115-BS (sulmazol), a new cardiotonic agent, in coronary artery disease: Improved ventricular wall motion, increased pump function and abolition of pacing-induced ischemia. J Am Coll Cardiol 1983;2:332–337.

218. Pouleur H, Marechal G, Balasim H, et al. Effects of dobutamine and sulmazol (ARL 115-BS) on myocardial metabolism and coronary, femoral and renal blood flows: A comparative study in normal dogs and in dogs with chronic volume overload. J Cardiovasc Pharmacol 1983;5:861–867.
219. Renard M, Jacobs P, Mols P, et al. The effective plasma concentrations of sulmazol (ARL 115-BS) on hemodynamics in chronic heart failure. Br J Clin Pharmacol 1983;16:313–318.
220. Berkenboom GM, Soboski JC, Depelchin PE, et al. Clinical and hemodynamic observations on orally administered sulmazol (ARL 115-BS) in refractory heart failure. Cardiology 1984;71:323–330.
221. Vincent JL, Goldstein J, Leeman M, et al. Administration of sulmazol in low-output states following cardiac surgery. Chest 1984;86:602–606.
222. Hagemeijer F, Segers A, Schelling A. Cardiovascular effects of sulmazol administration intravenously to patients with severe heart failure. Eur Heart J 1984;5:158–167.
223. Renard M, Jacobs P, Dechamps P, et al. Hemodynamic and clinical response to three-day infusion of sulmazol (ARL 115-BS) in severe congestive heart failure. Chest 1983;84:408–413.
224. Daly PA, Chatterjee K, Viquerat CE, et al. RO13-6438, a new inotrope–vasodilator: Systemic and coronary hemodynamic effects in congestive heart failure. Am J Cardiol 1985;55:1539–1544.
225. Ruegg JC. Effects of new inotropic agents on calcium sensitivity of contractile proteins. Circulation 1986;73(suppl III):III-78–84.
226. Chatterjee K, Parmley WW. The role of vasodilator therapy in heart failure. Prog Cardiovasc Dis 1977;19:301–334.
227. Schwartz AB, Chatterjee K. Vasodilator therapy in chronic congestive heart failure. Drugs 1983;26:148–173.
228. Packer M. Conceptual dilemmas in the classification of vasodilator drugs for severe chronic heart failure. Am J Med 1984: 76(6A):3–13.
229. Miller RR, Palomo AR, Brandon TA, et al. Combined vasodilator and inotropic therapy of heart failure: Experimental and clinical concepts. Am Heart J 1981;102:500–508.
230. Elenbaas RM, Covinsky JO. Approaches to the management of acute, chronic and refractory congestive heart failure. JCE Pharmacy 1979;1:11–39.
231. Ren JH, Unverferth DV, Magorien RD, et al. Postural influences on hemodynamic responses to vasodilating drugs in congestive heart failure. Arch Intern Med 1985;145:641–644.
232. Johnson JB, Blank RC, Cohn JN. Nitrate effects of sublingual administration of nitroglycerin on pulmonary artery pressure in patients with failure of the left ventricle. N Engl J Med 1957; 257:1114–1117.
233. Packer M. New perspectives on therapeutic application of nitrates and vasodilator agents for severe chronic heart failure. Am J Med 1983;74(6B):61–72.
234. Flaherty JT. Comparison of intravenous nitroglycerin and sodium nitroprusside in acute myocardial infarction. Am J Med 1983;74(6B):53–60.
235. Franciosa JA. Isosorbide dinitrate and exercise performance in patients with congestive heart failure. Am Heart J 1985;110: 245–250.
236. Packer M. Vasodilator and inotropic therapy for severe chronic heart failure: Passion and skepticism. J Am Coll Cardiol 1983;2:841–852.
237. Franciosa JA, Goldsmith SR, Cohn JN. Contrasting immediate and long term effects of isosorbide dinitrate on exercise capacity in congestive heart failure. Am J Med 1980;69:559–566.
238. Taylor WR, Forrester JS, Magnusson P, et al. Hemodynamic effects of nitroglycerin ointment in congestive heart failure. Am J Cardiol 1976;38:469–474.
239. Abrams J. Nitroglycerin and long-acting nitrates in clinical practice. Am J Med 1983;74(6B):85–94.
240. Jordan RA, Seth L, Casebolt P, et al. Rapidly developing tolerance to transdermal nitroglycerin in congestive heart failure. Ann Intern Med 1986;104:295–298.
241. Flaherty JT. Clinical relevance of nitrate hemodynamic attenuation. Am Heart J 1986;112:216–220.
242. Armstrong PW, Moffat JA. Tolerance to organic nitrates: Clinical and experimental perspectives. Am J Med 1983; 74(6B):73–84.
243. Chatterjee K, Parmley WW, Massie B, et al. Oral hydralazine therapy for chronic refractory heart failure. Circulation 1976;54:879–883.
244. Greenberg BH, Massie BM, Brundage GH, et al. Beneficial effects of hydralazine in severe mitral regurgitation. Circulation 1978;58:273–279.
245. Greenberg BH, Demots H, Murphy E, et al. Beneficial effects of hydralazine on rest and exercise hemodynamics in patients with chronic severe aortic insufficiency. Circulation 1980;62: 49–55.
246. Wilson JR, St. John Sutton M, Schwartz JS, et al. Determinants of circulatory response to intravenous hydralazine in congestive heart failure. Am J Cardiol 1983;52:299–303.
247. Packer M, Meller J, Medina N, et al. Importance of left ventricular chamber size in determining the response to hydralazine in severe chronic heart failure. N Engl J Med 1980;303: 250–255.
248. Strauer B. Myocardial oxygen consumption in chronic heart disease: Role of wall stress, hypertrophy and coronary reserve. Am J Cardiol 1979;44:730–740.
249. Franciosa JA, Weber KT, Levine TB, et al. Hydralazine in the long-term treatment of chronic heart failure: Lack of difference from placebo. Am Heart J 1982;104:587–594.
250. Weber KT, Andrews V, Kinasewitz GT, et al. Vasodilator and inotropic agents in treatment of chronic cardiac failure. Clinical experience and response in exercise performance. Am Heart J 1981;102:569–577.
251. Massie BM, Kramer B, Haughom F. Acute and long-term effects of vasodilator therapy on resting and exercise hemodynamics and exercise tolerance. Circulation 1981;64:1218–1225.
252. Franciosa JA, Cohn JN. Immediate effects of hydralazine–isosorbide dinitrate combination on exercise capacity and exercise hemodynamics in patients with left ventricular failure. Circulation 1979;59:1085–1097.
253. Cohn JN, Archibald DG, Ziesche S, et al. Effect of vasodilator therapy on mortality in chronic congestive heart failure. N Engl J Med 1986;314:1547–1552.
254. Packer M, Meller J, Medina N, et al. Dose requirements of hydralazine in patients with severe chronic congestive heart failure. Am J Cardiol 1980;45:655–660.
255. Alarcon-Segovia D, Wakim HC, Worthington IW, et al. Clinical and experimental studies on the hydralazine syndrome and its relationship to systemic lupus erythematosus. Medicine 1967;46:1–33.
256. Stratton MA. Drug-induced systemic lupus erythematosus. Clin Pharm 1985;4:657–663.
257. Packer M, Meller J, Medina N, et al. Provocation of myocardial ischemic events during initiation of vasodilator therapy for severe chronic heart failure. Clinical and hemodynamic evaluation of 52 consecutive patients with ischemic cardiomyopathy. Am J Cardiol 1981;48:939–946.
258. Markham RV, Gilmore A, Pettinger WA, et al. Central and regional hemodynamic effects and neurohumoral conse-

quences of minoxidil in severe congestive heart failure and comparison to hydralazine and nitroprusside. Am J Cardiol 1983;52:774–781.
259. Franciosa JA, Jordan RA, Wilen MM, et al. Minoxidil in patients with chronic left heart failure: Contrasting hemodynamic and clinical effects in a controlled trial. Circulation 1984;70:63–68.
260. Awan NA, Miller RR, Mason DT. Comparison of effects of nitroprusside and prazosin on left ventricular function and peripheral circulation in chronic heart failure. Circulation 1978;57:152–159.
261. Packer M, Meller J, Gorlin R, et al. Hemodynamic and clinical tachyphylaxis to prazosin-mediated afterload reduction in severe chronic congestive heart failure. Circulation 1979;59:531–539.
262. Arnold SB, Williams RL, Ports TA, et al. Attenuation of prazosin effect on cardiac output in chronic heart failure. Ann Intern Med 1979;91:345–349.
263. Elkayam U, LeJemtel TH, Mathur M, et al. Marked early attenuation of hemodynamic effects of oral prazosin therapy in chronic congestive heart failure. Am J Cardiol 1979;44:540–545.
264. Desch CE, Magorien RD, Triffon DW, et al. Development of pharmacodynamic tolerance to prazosin in congestive heart failure. Am J Cardiol 1979;44:1178–1182.
265. Colucci WS, Wynne J, Holman BL, et al. Long-term therapy of heart failure with prazosin: A randomized double-blind trial. Am J Cardiol 1980;45:337–344.
266. Colucci WS, Holman BL, Wynne J, et al. Improved right ventricular function and reduced pulmonary vascular resistance during prazosin therapy of congestive heart failure. Am J Med 1981;71:75–80.
267. Harper RW, Claxton H, Middlebrook K, et al. The acute and chronic hemodynamic effect of prazosin in severe congestive cardiac failure. Med J Aust 1980;(suppl):36–38.
268. Higginbotham MB, Morris KG, Bramlet DA, et al. Long-term ambulatory therapy with prazosin versus placebo for chronic heart failure: Relation between clinical response and left ventricular function at rest and during exercise. Am J Cardiol 1983;52:782–788.
269. Markham RV, Corbett JR, Gilmore A, et al. Efficacy of prazosin in the management of chronic congestive heart failure: A six-month randomized, double-blind, placebo-controlled study. Am J Cardiol 1983;51:1346–1352.
270. Rouleau J, Warnica JW, Burgess JH. Prazosin and congestive heart failure: Short- and long-term therapy. Am J Med 1981;71:147–152.
271. Colucci WS, Williams GH, Alexander RH, et al. Clinical, hemodynamic and neuroendocrine effects of chronic prazosin therapy for congestive heart failure. Am Heart J 1981;102:509–514.
272. Weber KT, Kinasewitz GT, West JS. Long term vasodilator therapy with trimazosin in chronic cardiac failure. N Engl J Med 1980;303:242–250.
273. Davis R, Ribner HS, Keung E, et al. Treatment of chronic congestive heart failure with captopril, an oral inhibitor of angiotensin-converting enzyme. N Engl J Med 1979;301:117–121.
274. Cody RJ. Clinical and hemodynamic experience with enalapril in congestive heart failure. Am J Cardiol 1985;55:36A–40A.
275. Kramer BL, Massie BM, Topic RN. Controlled trial of captopril in chronic heart failure: A rest and exercise hemodynamic study. Circulation 1983;67:807–816.
276. Cleland JGF, Dargie HJ, Hodsman GP, et al. Captopril in heart failure. A double-blind controlled trial. Br Heart J 1984;52:530–535.
277. Franciosa JA, Wilen MM, Jordan RA. Effects of enalapril, a new angiotensin converting enzyme inhibitor in a controlled trial in heart failure. J Am Coll Cardiol 1985;5:101–107.
278. Creager MA, Massie BM, Faxon DP, et al. Acute and long-term effects of enalapril on the cardiovascular response to exercise and exercise tolerance in patients with congestive heart failure. J Am Coll Cardiol 1985;6:163–170.
279. Chatterjee K, Parmley WW, Cohn JN, et al. A cooperative multicenter study of captopril in congestive heart failure: Hemodynamic effects and long-term response. Am Heart J 1985;110:439–447.
280. Packer M, Medina N, Yushak M. Relationship between serum sodium concentration and the hemodynamic and clinical responses to converting enzyme inhibition with captopril in severe heart failure. J Am Coll Cardiol 1984;3:1035–1043.
281. Lee WH, Packer M. Prognostic importance of serum sodium concentration and its modification by converting enzyme inhibition in patients with severe chronic heart failure. Circulation 1986;73:257–267.
282. Vlasses PH, Rotmensch HH, Rocci ML, et al. Double-blind comparison of captopril and enalapril in hypertensive patients. Clin Pharmacol Ther 1984;35:280–285.
283. Levine TB, Olivari MT, Garbery U, et al. Hemodynamic and clinical response to enalapril, a long-acting converting enzyme inhibitor, in patients with congestive heart failure. Circulation 1984;69:548–553.
284. Riley LJ, Vlasses PH, Ferguson RK. Clinical pharmacology and therapeutic applications of the new oral converting enzyme inhibitor, enalapril. Am Heart J 1985;109:1085–1089.
285. DiCarlo L, Chatterjee K, Parmley WW, et al. Enalapril: A new angiotensin-converting enzyme inhibitor in chronic heart failure. Acute and chronic hemodynamic evaluations. J Am Coll Cardiol 1983;2:865–871.
286. Vlasses PH, Larijani GE, Conner DP, et al. Enalapril, a nonsulfhydryl angiotensin converting enzyme inhibitor. Clin Pharm 1985;4:27–40.
287. Davies RO, Irvin JD, Kramsch DK, et al. Enalapril: Worldwide experience. Am J Med 1984;77(2A):23–35.
288. Rotmensch HH, Vlasses PH, Ferguson RK. Resolution of captopril-induced rash after substitution of enalapril. Pharmacotherapy 1983;3:131.
289. Navis GJ, DeJong PE, Kallenberg CGM, et al. Absence of cross-reactivity between captopril and enalapril. Lancet 1984;1:1017.
290. Packer M. Is the renin–angiotensin system really unnecessary in patients with severe chronic heart failure: The price we pay for interfering with evolution. J Am Coll Cardiol 1985;6:171–173.
291. Textor SC, Bravo EL, Fouad FM, et al. Hyperkalemia in azotemic patients during angiotensin-converting enzyme inhibition and aldosterone reduction with captopril. Am J Med 1982;73:719–725.
292. Packer M, Lee WH, Yushak M, et al. Comparison of captopril and enalapril in patients with severe chronic heart failure. N Engl J Med 1986;315:847–853.
293. Dickstein K, Aarsland T, Woie L, et al. Acute hemodynamic and hormonal effects of lisinopril (MK-521) in congestive heart failure. Am Heart J 1986;112:121–129.
294. Packer M, Medina N, Yushak M, et al. Hemodynamic patterns of response during long-term captopril therapy for severe chronic heart failure. Circulation 1983;68:803–812.
295. Rouleau JL, Chatterjee K, Benge W, et al. Alterations in left ventricular function and coronary hemodynamics with capto-

pril, hydralazine and prazosin in chronic ischemic heart failure. A comparative study. Circulation 1983;65:671–678.

**296.** Massie BM, Packer M, Hanlon JT, et al. Hemodynamic response to combined therapy with captopril and hydralazine in patients with severe heart failure. J Am Coll Cardiol 1983;2:338–344.

**297.** Colucci WS. Usefulness of calcium antagonists for congestive heart failure. Am J Cardiol 1987;59:52B–58B.

**298.** Colucci WS, Fifer MA, Lorell BH, et al. Calcium channel blockers in congestive heart failure: Theoretical considerations and clinical experience. Am J Med 1985;78(2B):9–17.

**299.** Brooks N, Cattell M, Pidgeon J, et al. Unpredictable response to nifedipine in severe cardiac failure. Br Med J 1980;281:1324.

**300.** Gillmer DJ, Kark P. Pulmonary oedema precipitated by nifedipine. Br Med J 1980;280;1420–1421.

**301.** Josephson MA, Singh BN. Use of calcium antagonists in ventricular dysfunction. Am J Cardiol 1985;55:81B–88B.

**302.** Paulus WJ, Lorrell BH, Craig WE, et al. Comparison of the effects of nitroprusside and nifedipine on diastolic properties in patients with hypertrophic cardiomyopathy: Altered left ventricular loading or improved muscle inactivation? J Am Coll Cardiol 1983;2:876–886.

**303.** Ludbrook PA, Tiefenbrunn AJ, Sobel BE. Acute hemodynamic responses to sublingual nifedipine: Dependence on left ventricular function. Circulation 1982;65:489–492.

**304.** Chew CYC, Hecht HS, Collett JT, et al. Influence of the severity of ventricular dysfunction on hemodynamic responses to intravenously administered verapamil in ischemic heart disease. Am J Cardiol 1981;47:917–922.

**305.** Elkayam U, Weber L, Rose J, et al. Nifedipine versus hydralazine in the treatment of severe heart failure: Evidence for a negative inotropic effect of nifedipine. (Abstr) Circulation 1983;68:III-8.

**306.** Furberg CD, Yusuf S, Thom TJ. Potential for altering the natural history of congestive heart failure: Need for large clinical trials. Am J Cardiol 1985;55:45A–47A.

**307.** LeJemtel TH, Sonnenblick EH. Should the failing heart be stimulated? N Engl J Med 1984;310:1384–1385.

**308.** Oparil S. Pathogenesis of ventricular hypertrophy. J Am Coll Cardiol 1985;5:57B-65B.

**309.** Katz AM. Potential deleterious effects of inotropic agents in the therapy of chronic heart failure. Circulation 1986;73(suppl III):III-184–190.

**310.** Brodsky MA, Allen BJ, Baron D, et al. Enhanced survival in patients with heart failure and life-threatening ventricular tachyarrhythmias. Am Heart J 1986;112:1166–1172.

# Chapter 12 / The Arrhythmias

Jerry L. Bauman, PharmD

The heart has two basic properties: an electrical property and a mechanical property. The synchronous interaction between these two properties is complex, precise, and relatively enduring. The study of the electrical properties of the heart has grown at a slow steady rate, interrupted by salvos of information resulting from paroxysmal scientific breakthroughs. Einthoven's pioneering work allowed graphic electrical tracings of cardiac rhythm and probably represents the first of these breakthroughs. This discovery (of the surface electrocardiogram) has remained the cornerstone of diagnostic tools for cardiac rhythm disturbances; however, one must be aware that prior to the availability of the electrocardiogram, meticulous clinical observation of venous and arterial pulsations provided a relatively sophisticated classification of many cardiac arrhythmias. Recently, intracardiac recordings and programmed cardiac stimulation have led to a wealth of both basic and clinical data. Regarding drug therapy, digitalis and later quinidine were important first steps in achieving effective control of cardiac arrhythmias. Microelectrode and voltage clamp techniques have allowed considerable insight into the electrophysiologic actions and mechanisms of antiarrhythmic drugs. It remains to be seen whether the recent plethora of new drugs will dramatically alter the use of older, first-line therapy.

The purpose of this chapter is to review the principles involved in both normal and abnormal cardiac conduction and to address the pathophysiology and treatment of the more commonly encountered arrhythmias. Certainly, many volumes of complete text could be (and have been) devoted to basic and clinical electrophysiology. Therefore, this chapter briefly addresses those principles necessary for clinical pharmacists.

## Arrhythmogenesis

### *Normal Conduction*

Electrical activity is initiated by the sinoatrial (SA) node and courses through cardiac tissue by a treelike conduction network. The SA node initiates cardiac rhythm under normal conditions because this tissue possesses the highest degree of automaticity or rate of spontaneous impulse generation. The degree of automaticity of the SA node is influenced largely by the autonomic nervous system in that both cholinergic and sympathetic innervation control sinus rate. Most tissues within the conduction system also possess varying degrees of inherent automatic properties[1,2]; however, the rate of spontaneous impulse generation of these tissues is less than that of the SA node. Thus, these latent automatic pacemakers are continuously excited and overdriven by impulses arising from the SA node (primary pacemaker) and do not become clinically apparent.

From the SA node, electrical activity moves in a wavefront through an atrial specialized conducting system and eventually gains entrance to the ventricle via an atrioventricular (AV) node and a large bundle of conducting tissue referred to as the bundle of His. Aside from this AV nodal–Hisian pathway, the atria and ventricles are separated by a fibrous AV ring that does not permit electrical stimulation. The conducting tissues bridging the atria and ventricles are referred to as the junctional areas. Again, this area of tissue (junction) is influenced largely by autonomic input, and possesses a relatively high degree of inherent automaticity (but still less than that of the SA node).[1,2] From the bundle of His, the cardiac conduction system bifurcates into several (usually three) bundle branches: one right bundle and two left bundles. These bundle branches further arborize into a conduction network referred to as the Purkinje system. The conduction system as a whole innervates the mechanical myocardium and serves to initiate excitation–contraction coupling and the contractile process. When a cell or group of cells within the heart is electrically stimulated, a brief period of time follows in which those cells cannot again be excited.[1] This time period is referred to as the refractory period. As the electrical wavefront moves down the conduction system, the impulse eventually encounters tissue refractory to stimulation (recently excited) and subsequently dies out. Then the SA node recovers, fires spontaneously, and begins the process again.

Prior to cellular excitation, an electrical gradient exists between the inside and the outside of the cell membrane.[3] At this time the cell is said to be polarized. In atrial and ventricular conducting tissue, the intracellular space is about 80–90 mV negative with respect to the extracellular environment.[4] The electrical gradient just prior to excitation is referred to as resting membrane potential (RMP) and is the result of differences in ion concentrations between the inside and the outside of the cell. At RMP, the cell is polarized primarily by the action of active membrane ion pumps, the most notable of these being the sodium–potassium pump. For example, this specific pump (in addition to other systems) attempts to maintain the intracellular sodium concentration at 5–15 mEq/L and the extracellular sodium at 135–142 mEq/L; the intracellular potassium concentration at 135–140 mEq/L and the extracellular potassium concentration at 3–5 mEq/L. RMP can be calculated by using the Nernst equation[4–6]:

$$\text{RMP} = -61.5 \log\frac{[\text{ion outside}]}{[\text{ion inside}]}$$

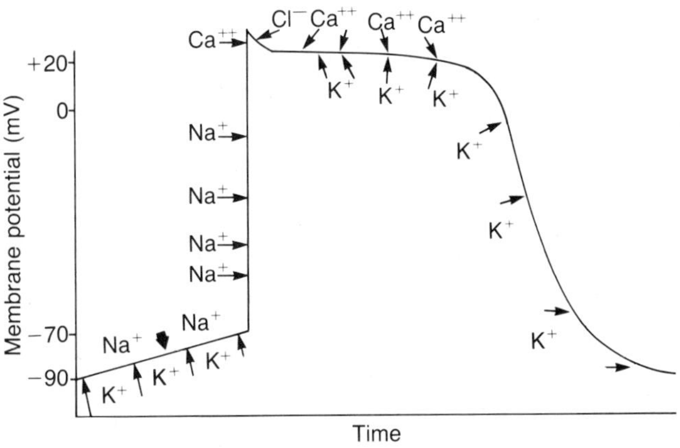


**Figure 12.1** Purkinje fiber action potential showing specific ion flux responsible for the change in membrane potential.

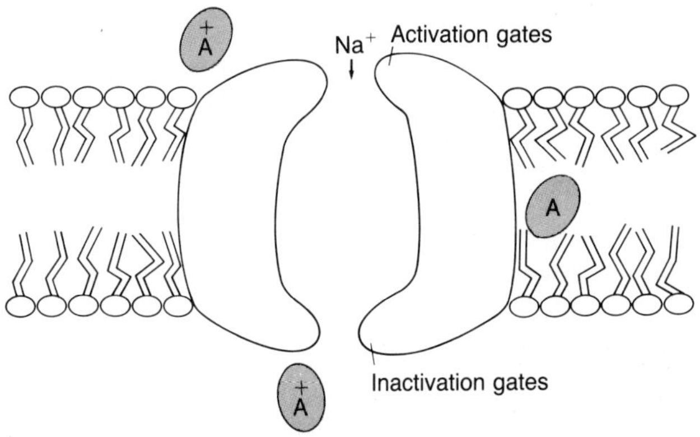


**Figure 12.2** Lipid bilayer, sodium channel, and possible sites of action of the type I agents (A). These drugs may inhibit sodium influx at an extracellular, intramembrane, or intracellular receptor site. Recent evidence points toward an intracellular site of action, the active ionized form interfering with the recovery of channel inactivation.

Electrical stimulation (or depolarization) of the cell results in changes in membrane potential over time or a characteristic action potential curve (Fig. 12.1). The action potential curve results from the transmembrane movement of specific ions and is divided into different phases.[5–7] Phase 0 (rapid depolarization) of atrial and ventricular tissues is due to an abrupt increase in the permeability of the membrane to sodium influx. This rapid depolarization more than equilibrates (overshoot) the electrical potential, resulting in passive chloride influx (initial repolarization) and phase 1. Calcium entry into the intracellular space begins at about −60 mV (during phase 0), causing a slower depolarization. Calcium influx continues throughout phase 2 of the action potential (plateau phase) and is balanced to some degree by potassium efflux. Calcium entrance distinguishes cardiac conducting cells from nerve tissue, and provides the critical ionic link to excitation–contraction coupling and the mechanical properties of the heart as a pump.[4–6] The membrane remains permeable to potassium efflux during phase 3, resulting in cellular repolarization. Phase 4 of the action potential is the gradual depolarization of the cell and is related to a constant sodium leak into the intracellular space balanced by a decreasing (over time) efflux of potassium. The slope of phase 4 depolarization determines, in large part, the automatic properties of the cell.[2] As the cell is slowly depolarized during phase 4, an abrupt increase in sodium permeability is encountered, allowing the rapid cellular depolarization of phase 0. The juncture of phase 4 and phase 0, where rapid sodium influx is initiated, is referred to as the threshold potential of the cell. The level of threshold potential also regulates the degree of cellular automaticity.[2]

Not all cells in the cardiac conduction system rely upon sodium influx for initial depolarization.[7–9] Some tissues depolarize in response to a slower inward ionic current caused by calcium influx. These "calcium-dependent" tissues are found primarily in the SA and AV nodes and possess distinct conduction properties in comparison to "sodium-dependent" fibers. Calcium-dependent cells generally have a less negative RMP (−40 to −60 mV) and a slower conduction velocity. Furthermore, in calcium-dependent tissues, recovery of excitability outlasts full repolarization, whereas in sodium-dependent tissue, recovery is prompt after repolarization. These two types of electrical fibers also differ dramatically in how drugs modify their conduction properties (see later).

Ion conductance across the lipid bilayer of the cell membrane occurs via the formation of membrane pores or "channels" (Fig. 12.2). Selective ion channels probably form in response to specific electrical potential differences between the inside and the outside of the cell (voltage dependent). For example, one theory[10] proposes that electrostatic changes cause rodlike protein subunits lying on the surface of the membrane to flip upright, aggregate, and bind, subsequently forming membrane pores. The membrane itself is composed of both organized and disorganized lipids and phospholipids in a dynamic solgel matrix. During ion flux and electrical excitation, changes in this solgel equilibrium occur and permit the formation of activated ion channels.[11] Besides channel formation and membrane composition, the transmembrane movement of ions is also regulated by intrachannel proteins or phospholipids referred to as gates.[4,5,12] These gates are believed to be positioned strategically within the channel to modulate ion flow (Fig. 12.2). Each ion channel conceptually has two types of gates: an activation gate and an inactivation gate. The activation gate opens during depolarization to allow the ion current to enter or exit the cell and the inactivation gate closes to stop ion movement. Therefore, the activation of SA and AV nodal tissue is dependent upon a slow depolarizing current through calcium channels and gates, whereas the activation of atrial and ventricular tissue is dependent upon a rapid depolarizing current through sodium channels and gates. Sometimes these types of conduction tissues are referred to as slow and fast fibers, respectively.

### *Abnormal Conduction*

Hoffman et al[13] have classified the mechanisms of tachyarrhythmias into two general categories: those resulting from an abnormality in impulse generation, or "automatic" tachycardias, and those resulting from an abnormality in impulse conduction, or "reentrant" tachycardias.

Automatic tachycardias depend upon spontaneous impulse generation in latent pacemakers and may arise by several different mechanisms. Experimentally, chemicals such as digitalis glycosides and catecholamines and conditions such as hypoxemia, electrolyte abnormalities (e.g., hypokalemia), and fiber stretch (cardiac dilatation) may lead to an increased slope of phase 4 depolarization in tissues other than the SA node.[13–15] The increased slope of phase 4 causes increased automaticity of these tissues and competition between the latent pacemaker and the SA node for dominance of cardiac rhythm. If the rate of spontaneous impulse generation of the abnormally automatic tissue exceeds that of the SA node, then an automatic tachycardia may result. These factors which experimentally lead to abnormal automaticity are also known to be arrhythmogenic in clinical situations. Automatic tachycardias have the following characteristics: (1) onset of the tachycardia is not related to an initiating event such as a premature beat, (2) the initiating beat is usually identical to subsequent beats of the tachycardia, (3) the tachycardia cannot be initiated by programmed cardiac stimulation, and (4) the tachycardia often occurs in association with digitalis toxicity, high degrees of sympathetic tone, hypokalemia, and/or severe pulmonary disease.[16]

Triggered automaticity is also a possible mechanism for abnormal impulse generation.[14,15] Triggered automaticity as a cause of atrial or ventricular tachycardias has been demonstrated in the laboratory setting but its role in clinical arrhythmogenesis is not well defined; however, recent research suggests that it may be important in causing several clinical tachycardias.[17] Briefly, triggered automaticity refers to a transient membrane depolarization that occurs during repolarization (early after-depolarization) or after repolarization (delayed after-depolarization) but prior to phase 4 of the action potential.[14,15] After-depolarizations may be related to abnormal calcium and sodium influx during or just after full cellular repolarization. Experimentally, triggered automatic rhythms can be elicited by digitalis and suppressed by calcium channel inhibitors.[15] Triggered automatic rhythms possess some of the characteristics of automatic tachycardias and some of the characteristics of reentrant tachycardias.

As previously mentioned, the impulse originating from the SA node in an individual with sinus rhythm eventually meets previously excited and thus refractory tissue. Reentry is a concept that involves indefinite propagation of the impulse and continued activation of previously refractory tissue.[18,19] There are three conduction requirements for the formation of a viable reentrant focus: two pathways for impulse conduction, an area of unidirectional block (prolonged refractoriness) in one of these pathways, and slow conduction in the other pathway (Fig. 12.3). Usually, a critically timed premature beat initiates reentry. This premature impulse enters both conduction pathways but encounters refractory tissue in one of the pathways at the area of unidirectional block. The impulse dies out because it is still refractory from the previous (sinus) impulse. Although it fails to propagate in one pathway, the impulse may still proceed in a forward direction (antegrade) through the other pathway because of this pathway's relatively shorter refractory period. The impulse may then proceed through a loop of tissue and "reenter" the area of unidirectional block in a backward direction (retrograde). As the antegrade pathway has slow

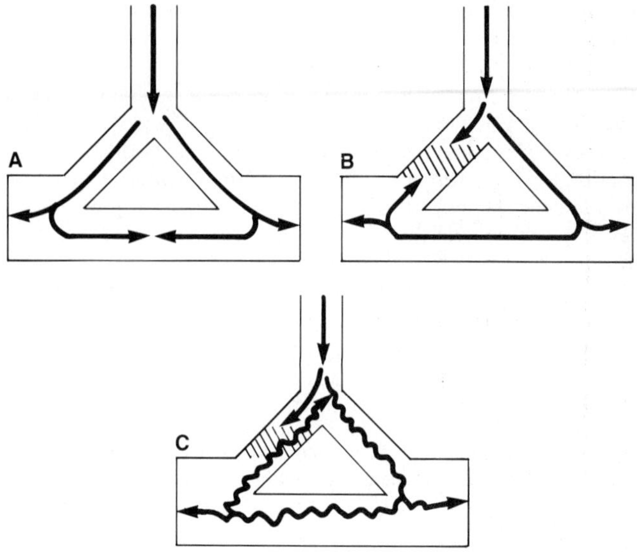


**Figure 12.3** Process of reentry into a loop of tissue. (A) Normal conduction process. (B) Area of unidirectional block caused by prolonged tissue refractoriness. (C) Reentrant loop is formed with necessary ingredients: an area of unidirectional block and a loop of tissue with slowed conduction velocity. *(From Bauman JL: Understanding and treating supraventricular arrhythmias. Clin Pharm 1983;2:313, with permission.)*

conduction characteristics, the area of unidirectional block has time to recover its excitability. The impulse can proceed retrogradely through this (previously refractory) tissue and continue around the loop of tissue in a circular fashion. Thus, the key to the formation of a reentrant focus is crucial conduction discrepancies in the electrophysiologic characteristics of the two pathways. The reentrant focus may excite surrounding tissue at a rate greater than that of the SA node, and a clinical tachycardia results. This model is anatomically determined in that there is only one pathway for impulse conduction with a fixed circuit length. Another form of reentry, referred to as a functional reentrant loop, may also occur.[20] In a functional reentrant focus, the length of the circuit may vary depending on the conduction characteristics of the surrounding tissue. The area in the middle of the loop is continually kept refractory from spreading wavefronts and the impulse chases its tail (so to speak), never preceded by an excitable gap of tissue. Theoretically, reentrant foci may have both anatomic and functional characteristics.[21]

What causes reentry to clinically manifest? Reentrant foci may occur at any level of the conduction system: within the branches of the specialized atrial conduction system, the Purkinje network, and even within portions of the SA and AV nodes. The anatomy of the Purkinje system is felt to provide a suitable substrate for the formation of microreentrant loops and is often used as a model to facilitate the understanding of reentry concepts (Fig. 12.3). Of course, reentry does not usually occur in normal, healthy conduction tissue and therefore various forms of heart disease or conduction abnormalities must usually be present before reentry manifests. In other words, the various forms of heart disease can result in changes in conduction in the pathways of a suitable reentrant substrate.[22] An often used example is reentry occurring as a consequence of ischemic or hypoxic damage: With inadequate cellular oxygen, cardiac tissue resorts to anaerobic glycolysis for ATP production. As high-energy phosphate concentration diminishes, the activity of the transmembrane ion pumps declines and RMP rises. This rise in RMP causes inactivation in the voltage-dependent sodium channel and the tissue begins to assume slow conduction characteristics. If changes in conduction parameters occur in a discordant manner because of varying degrees of ischemia or hypoxia, then a reentry circuit may manifest. Furthermore, an ischemic, dying cell liberates intracellular potassium, which also causes a rise in RMP.[23] In other cases, reentry may occur as a result of anatomic or functional variants in the normal conduction system. Patients, for example, may possess two (instead of one) conduction pathways within the AV node or an anomalous, extranodal AV pathway that possesses electrophysiologic characteristics different from those of the normal AV nodal pathway. Reentry in these cases may occur within the AV node or by encompassing both atrial and ventricular tissue (see later). Reentrant tachycardias have the following characteristics[16]: (1) the onset of the tachycardia is usually related to an initiating event (i.e., premature beat), (2) the initiating beat is usually different in morphology from subsequent beats of the tachycardia, and (3) initiation of the tachycardia is usually possible with programmed cardiac stimulation.

### *Mechanism of Antiarrhythmic Drugs*

In a theoretical sense, drugs may have antiarrhythmic activity by directly altering conduction in several ways. First, a drug may depress the automatic properties of abnormal pacemaker cells. An agent may do this by decreasing the slope of phase 4 depolarization and/or by elevating threshold potential.[13,15,24] If the rate of spontaneous impulse generation of the abnormally automatic foci becomes less than that of the SA node, normal cardiac rhythm can be restored. Second, drugs may alter the conduction characteristics of the pathways of a reentrant loop.[7,19,20] An agent may facilitate conduction (shorten refractoriness) in the area of unidirectional block, allowing antegrade conduction to proceed. On the other hand, an antiarrhythmic may further depress conduction (prolong refractoriness) either in the area of unidirectional block or in the pathway with slowed conduction and a relatively shorter refractory period. If refractoriness is prolonged in the area of unidirectional block, retrograde propagation of the impulse is not permitted, causing a "bidirectional" block. If refractoriness is prolonged in the pathway with slow conduction, antegrade conduction of the impulse is not permitted through this route. In either case, drugs that reduce the discordance and cause a uniformity in conduction properties of the two pathways may suppress the reentrant substrate. According to another theoretically possible mechanism, the drug eliminates the premature impulse that triggers reentry. Relatively little is known regarding drug effects on experimentally induced triggered automaticity.

Antiarrhythmic drugs have specific electrophysiologic actions that alter cardiac conduction in patients with or without heart disease. These actions form the basis for classification of antiarrhythmics into groups of drugs with similar effects (Table 12.1)[25] Type Ia drugs, such as quinidine, procainamide, and disopyramide, slow conduction velocity, prolong refractoriness, and decrease the automatic properties of sodium-dependent (normal and diseased) conduction tissue.[26] Therefore, type Ia agents can be effective in automatic tachycardias by decreasing the rate of spontaneous impulse generation of atrial or ventricular foci. In reentrant tachycardias, these drugs generally depress conduction and prolong refractoriness, transforming the area of unidirectional block into a bidirectional block. Clinically, type Ia drugs are broad-spectrum antiarrhythmics, being effective for both supraventricular and ventricular arrhythmias. The pharmacokinetics of the antiarrhythmic agents are summarized in Table 12.2.

Historically, lidocaine and phenytoin were categorized separately from quinidine-like drugs. This was due to early work demonstrating that lidocaine had distinctly different electrophysiologic actions. In normal tissue models, lidocaine generally had facilitative actions on cardiac conduction

**Table 12.1** Classification of Antiarrhythmic Drugs

| *Type* | *Drug* | *Conduction velocity*[a] | *Refractory period* | *Automaticity* |
|---|---|---|---|---|
| Ia | Quinidine | ↓ | ↑ | ↓ |
| | Procainamide | | | |
| | Disopyramide | | | |
| Ib | Lidocaine | 0/↓ | ↓ | ↓ |
| | Mexiletine | | | |
| | Tocainide | | | |
| Ic | Flecainide | ↓ | 0 | ↓ |
| | Encainide | ↓ | 0 | ↓ |
| II | β-Blockers[b] | ↓ | ↑ | ↓ |
| III | Aminodarone | 0 | ↑ | 0 |
| | Bretylium | | | |
| IV | Verapamil[b] | ↓ | ↑ | ↓ |
| | Diltiazem | | | |

[a] Variables for normal tissue models in ventricular tissue.
[b] Variables for SA and AV nodal tissue only.

**Table 12.2** Pharmacokinetics of Antiarrhythmic Drugs

| *Drug* | *Bioavailability* (%) | *Primary route of elimination*[a] | $V_{D,ss}$ (L/kg) | *Protein binding* (%) | $t_{1/2}$ | *Therapeutic range* ($\mu g/mL$) |
|---|---|---|---|---|---|---|
| Quinidine | 70–80 | H | 2.0–3.5 | 80–90 | 5–9 h | 2–6 |
| Procainamide | 75–95 | H/R | 1.5–3.0 | 10–20 | 2.5–5.0 h | 4–15 |
| Disopyramide | 70–95 | H/R | 0.8–2.0 | 50–80 | 4–8 h | 2–6 |
| Lidocaine | 20–40 | H | 1–2 | 65–75 | 60–180 min | 1.5–5.0 |
| Mexiletine | 80–95 | H | 5–12 | 60–75 | 6–12 h | 0.75–2.0 |
| Tocainide | 90–95 | H | 1.5–3.0 | 10–30 | 12–15 h | 4–10 |
| Flecainide | 90–95 | H | 8–10 | 35–45 | 13–20 h | 0.3–2.5 |
| Encainide[b] | | | | | | |
| Poor | 85–95 | H/R | 2.5–4.0 | 70–80 | 8–11 h | — |
| Extensive | 20–30 | H | | | 1–3 h | |
| Amiodarone | 22–88 | H | 70–150 | 95–97 | 15–100 d | 1.0–2.5 |
| Bretylium | 15–20 | R | 4–8 | Negligible | 5–10 h | 0.5–2.0 |
| Verapamil | 20–40 | H | 1.5–5.0 | 95–99 | 4–12 h | 50 ng/mL |

[a] H, hepatic; R, renal.
[b] Variables for parent compound only (not active metabolites ODE, MODE).

by shortening refractoriness and having little effect on conduction velocity.[27–29] Thus, it was postulated that these agents could improve antegrade conduction, eliminating the area of unidirectional block. Of course, arrhythmias do not usually arise from normal tissue, leading investigators to study lidocaine's and phenytoin's actions in ischemic and hypoxic tissue models. Interestingly, studies have shown these drugs to possess quinidine-like properties in diseased tissues.[28–30] Therefore, it is probable that lidocaine acts similarly to the type Ia drugs in clinical tachycardias. As a result, these drugs have been reclassified as type Ib antiarrhythmics. Furthermore, a new category of type I drugs (type Ic) has been proposed. These agents, such as flecainide and encainide, have some of the electrophysiologic properties of both type Ia and type Ib drugs.[25] Why do agents such as lidocaine exert their major electrophysiologic effects selectively in diseased tissue? The answer is unknown, but some authors have suggested that "intracellular trapping" of lidocaine occurs in ischemic cells because of specific physiochemical properties and receptor binding characteristics of this drug.[31,32] This results in nonuniform drug distribution within the heart and high intracellular concentrations in diseased areas. For phenytoin (but not lidocaine), others have suggested a novel mechanism of action mediated through the central nervous system.[33] For reasons that remain unclear, lidocaine (and structural analogues such as tocainide or mexiletine) are considerably more effective in ventricular arrhythmias than in supraventricular arrhythmias.

Most researchers agree that type I drugs in general exert most of their effects on a subcellular basis by inhibiting the transmembrane influx of sodium. In essence, type I agents can be (but are usually not) referred to as sodium channel inhibitors. These drugs can alter the sodium channel by three possible ways[34]: (1) at an extracellular receptor site, inhibiting sodium entry into the channel, (2) at an intramembrane receptor site, effecting channel integrity, and (3) at an intracellular receptor site, inhibiting sodium entry into the cellular space (Fig. 12.2). Of these possible sites of action, research points toward the type I drugs (in an active, ionized form) gaining entrance into the intracellular space and altering the gating kinetics of the channel.[35] Many feel that these antiarrhythmics interfere primarily with the recovery of the inactivation gate of the fast sodium channel.[25] The type I agents can also be differentiated by characteristics of their binding to the sodium channel at rest or in its active or inactivated state. For example, quinidine has a much higher binding affinity for the sodium channel in its activated state but slowly dissociates from this site, whereas lidocaine has a relatively greater affinity for inactivated channels and rapidly dissociates from its receptor.[36] Further, these actions occur primarily in a use- or frequency-dependent manner.[36]

The β-adrenergic antagonists are classified as type II antiarrhythmic drugs. For the most part, the clinically relevant antiarrhythmic mechanisms of the β-blockers result from their antiadrenergic actions.[37] As the SA and AV nodes are heavily influenced by adrenergic innervation, β-blockers would be most useful in tachycardias in which these nodal tissues are abnormally automatic or are a portion of a reentrant loop. These agents should also be helpful in slowing ventricular response in supraventricular tachycardias by their effects on the AV node. Furthermore, some tachycardias are exercise related or precipitated by states of high sympathetic tone, and β-blockers may be useful in these instances. β-Adrenergic stimulation results in increased conduction velocity, shortened refractoriness, and increased automaticity of the nodal tissues. β-Adrenergic blockers antagonize these effects. Propranolol is often noted to have "local anesthetic" or quinidine-like activity; however, supranpharmacologic concentrations are usually required to elicit this action.[37] In the nodal tissues, β-blockers seem to interfere with calcium entry into the cell by altering catecholamine-dependent channel integrity and gating kinetics. In sodium-dependent atrial and ventricular tissue, β-blockers shorten repolarization somewhat, but otherwise have little effect.

Type III antiarrhythmics include those agents that specifically prolong refractoriness in atrial and ventricular fibers. This class includes bretylium and amiodarone. The mechanisms of action of these two very different drugs remain unclear. They do not seem to be related to inhibition of sodium influx or decreases in conduction velocity or automaticity. Some have postulated an inhibition of potassium conduction as a possible subcellular mechanism.[38] The electrophysiologic actions of bretylium are related to its multifaceted pharmacology.[39] Bretylium is structurally similar to guanethidine and can, likewise, cause an initial increase in catecholamine release from the adrenergic neuron. This action may potentially effect arrhythmogenesis by an indirect mechanism: increase in coronary blood flow and myocardial perfusion that reverses ischemia-related arrhythmias (similar to epinephrine's action in a patient with ventricular fibrillation). After causing catecholamine release, bretylium then causes an uncoupling of autonomic nerve stimulation from the release step, resulting in antiadrenergic effects. Theoretically, bretylium may also be antiarrhythmic by these sympatholytic actions. Nonetheless, bretylium prolongs repolarization, independent of the sympathetic nervous system, and many feel these direct actions account for its clinical effectiveness. Importantly, bretylium increases ventricular fibrillation threshold and seems to have selective antifibrillatory but not antitachycardic effects.[40,41] In other words, bretylium can be effective in ventricular fibrillation, whereas it is rarely effective in ventricular tachycardia. In contrast, amiodarone is effective in most tachycardias. It is clear that amiodarone causes significant prolongation of atrial and ventricular refractoriness, but the underlying subcellular mechanisms are unknown. Theoretically, amiodarone, like type I agents, may interrupt the reentrant substrate by transforming an area of unidirectional block into an area of bidirectional block; however, electrophysiologic studies utilizing programmed cardiac stimulation imply that amiodarone leaves the reentrant loop intact.[42] Rather, it is possible that amiodarone abolishes the premature impulse that usually triggers the reentry process. This is currently an area of controversy. It should be noted that amiodarone also depresses SA and AV nodal conduction by direct (noncompetitive) adrenergic blockade.

The calcium channel blockers (verapamil and diltiazem) compose the type IV antiarrhythmic category. As calcium-dependent tissue and slow channels are found primarily in the SA and AV nodes, one may expect these agents to manifest their activity against tachycardias primarily at these sites. By inhibiting calcium entry into the cell, verapamil and diltiazem slow conduction, prolong refractoriness, and decrease automaticity of the SA and AV nodes. Therefore, these agents are effective in automatic or reentrant tachycardias that arise from or utilize the SA or AV nodes.[43,44] In tachycardias resulting from atrial foci, these drugs can slow ventricular response by slowing AV nodal conduction. Furthermore, as calcium entry seems to be integral to exercise-related tachycardias and/or tachycardias resulting from some forms of triggered automaticity,[45] preliminary evidence shows effectiveness in these types of arrhythmias. One other possibility merits discussion. Disease processes such as ischemia can serve to inactivate the fast sodium channel, allowing calcium-dependent depolarization to predominate. In other words, diseased tissue may acquire, in part, slow fiber characteristics. Therefore, it is conceivable that calcium channel inhibitors may show future potential in some tachycardias arising from atrial or ventricular tissue. The exact site of action of the calcium channel blockers is yet to be determined. In all likelihood, verapamil and diltiazem work at different receptor sites because of their dissimilar chemical structures and pharmacologic actions. Nifedipine does not have significant antiarrhythmic activity because a reflex increase in sympathetic tone counteracts this agent's direct action on the nodes. Calcium antagonists can slightly shorten repolarization in normal sodium-dependent tissue but otherwise have little effect.

## Supraventricular Arrhythmias

The common supraventricular tachycardias that often require drug treatment are (1) atrial fibrillation or atrial flutter, (2) paroxysmal supraventricular tachycardia, and (3) automatic atrial tachycardia. Other common supraventricular arrhythmias that usually do not require drug therapy include premature atrial complexes (PACs), wandering atrial pacemaker, sinus arrhythmia, and sinus tachycardia. As an example, PACs rarely cause symptoms and never cause hemodynamic compromise; therefore, drug therapy is usually not indicated. Likewise, sinus tachycardia is usually the result of underlying metabolic or hemodynamic disorders (such as infection, dehydration, hypotension, etc.), and therapy should be directed at the underlying cause not the tachycardia per se. Of course, there are exceptions to these suggestions. For example, sinus tachycardia may be deleterious in patients after cardiac surgery or myocardial infarction, or with an unusual rhythm termed nonparoxysmal sinus tachycardia, so that antiarrhythmic drugs may be indicated. Stated in another way, although many arrhythmias generally do not require therapy, clinical judgment and patient-specific variables play an important role in this decision. Nevertheless, for the purpose of this discussion, only the tachycardias usually requiring antiarrhythmic drug therapy as previously listed are addressed.

Supraventricular tachycardias may cause a variety of symptoms.[46] Some patients may be totally asymptomatic or complain only of minor palpitations or irregular pulse. In contrast, severe and even life-threatening symptoms can sometimes result. Patients may experience dizziness or acute syncopal episodes associated with the onset of their tachycardia, because of an abrupt drop in cardiac output, blood pressure, and cerebral perfusion. This drop in forward cardiac output occurs because of the rapid ventricular rate with resultant poor ventricular filling and asynchronous AV contraction. Heart failure symptoms may also occur and patients tolerate the tachycardia particularly poorly if preexisting left ventricular dysfunction is present. Furthermore, patients may experience anginal chest pain if underlying coronary obstruction is present, as a result of altered coronary perfusion (low cardiac output) and elevated myocardial oxygen demand (rapid heart rate). More often, patients complain of a choking or pressure sensation during the tachycardia episode that can be confused with angina pectoris. It also should be noted that symptoms such as palpitations and even syncope correlate rather poorly with documented recurrences of the tachycardia.

### *Atrial Fibrillation/Atrial Flutter*

Atrial fibrillation and atrial flutter are common supraventricular tachycardias. These arrhythmias may present as a chronic, established tachycardia, an acute tachycardia, or a self-terminating, paroxysmal tachycardia. Atrial fibrillation is characterized as an extremely rapid (400–600 atrial bpm) and disorganized atrial activation. With this disorganized atrial activity, there is a loss of the contribution of atrial contraction (atrial kick) to forward cardiac output. Supraventricular impulses penetrate the AV conduction system in variable degrees, resulting in an irregular activation of the ventricles and an irregularly irregular pulse. The AV junction will not conduct most of the supraventricular impulses, causing ventricular response to be considerably slower (120–180 bpm). Atrial flutter occurs less frequently than atrial fibrillation, but is similar in its precipitating factors, consequences, and drug therapy approach. This arrhythmia is characterized by rapid (270–330 atrial bpm) but regular atrial activation. The slower and regular electrical activity results in a regular ventricular response and pulse in approximate multiples of 300 bpm (i.e., 1:1 AV conduction = ventricular rate 300 bpm; 2:1 AV conduction = ventricular rate 150 bpm; 3:1 AV conduction = ventricular rate 100 bpm; etc.); however, atrial flutter with varying degrees of AV block or occurring with episodes of atrial fibrillation ("fib-flutter") can cause an irregular ventricular rate and pulse.

It is not yet clear if atrial fibrillation or flutter is the result of abnormal phase 4 automaticity, triggered activity, or reentry.[47,48] Most recent information, including studies concerning tachycardia entrainment, suggest that an atrial reentrant focus is responsible.[49] Some postulate that atrial fibrillation results from multiple atrial reentrant loops and atrial flutter results from a single, dominant reentrant substrate. Atrial fibrillation or flutter usually occurs in association with a form of organic heart disease that causes atrial distension.[47,50] Forms of heart disease that commonly lead to atrial stretch and precipitate atrial fibrillation or flutter include ischemia or infarction, hypertensive heart disease, valvular disorders such as mitral stenosis, congenital abnormalities such as septal defects, and primary myocardial disease such as congestive or obstructive cardiomyopathy. Disorders that cause right atrial stretch and are associated with atrial fibrillation or flutter include acute pulmonary embolus and chronic lung disease resulting in pulmonary hypertension and cor pulmonale. These arrhythmias may also occur in association with states of high adrenergic tone such as thyrotoxicosis, alcohol withdrawal, sepsis, or excessive physical exertion. Established or paroxysmal atrial fibrillation occurring without identifiable heart disease or known precipitating factors is termed "lone" atrial fibrillation. Other states in which patients are predisposed to episodes of atrial fibrillation are the presence of an anomalous AV pathway (i.e., Kent bundle) and sinus node dysfunction (i.e., tachy-brady or sick sinus syndrome). An uncommon familial form has been described.

Patients with atrial fibrillation or flutter may experience the entire range of symptoms associated with other supraventricular tachycardias. As atrial kick is lost with the onset of atrial fibrillation, serious hemodynamic compromise may result in forms of heart disease that rely heavily upon atrial contraction to maintain cardiac output (such as mitral stenosis or hypertrophic obstructive cardiomyopathy). An additional complication of atrial fibrillation is arterial embolization resulting from atrial stasis and poorly adherent mural thrombi. Of course, the most devastating complication in this regard is the occurrence of an embolic stroke.[50] Patients with concurrent mitral stenois or severe dilated heart failure and atrial fibrillation are at particularly high risk for cerebral embolism. In addition, stroke can precede the onset of documented atrial fibrillation, probably as a result of undetected paroxysms prior to the onset of established atrial fibrillation.[51]

The ultimate treatment goals of atrial fibrillation or flutter are the restoration of sinus rhythm and the prevention of further recurrences (Fig. 12.4); however, the methods by which these goals are attained vary and often raise ill-defined areas of controversy. First, consider the patient with new-onset atrial fibrillation or flutter. If presenting symptoms are severe (see earlier), patients may require direct-current cardioversion (DCC) in an attempt to immediately restore sinus rhythm. Atrial flutter often requires relatively low energy levels of countershock, 25–50 W/s, whereas atrial fibrillation often requires higher energy levels, greater than 200 W/s. On the other hand, if tolerable symptoms are present, no such emergency measures are necessary. Type Ia antiarrhythmic agents may restore sinus rhythm but should not be administered initially. These agents may paradoxically increase ventricular response in the absence of drugs that slow AV nodal conduction. Traditionally, this observation has been attributed to the vagolytic action of quinidine, procainamide, or disopyramide despite the fact that only disopyramide displays major anticholinergic side effects. Therefore, a more likely alternative explanation exists: All of these agents slow atrial conduction, decreasing the number of impulses reaching the AV node, and as a result, the AV node paradoxically allows more impulses to gain entrance to the ventricular conduction system (increasing ventricular rate). Because of this phenomenon and the lack of need for immediate restoration of sinus rhythm, drugs that slow conduction and increase refractoriness in the AV node should be used as initial therapy. Traditionally, loading dosages of digoxin have been used because of their time-proven effectiveness and the high incidence of concurrent heart failure. Digoxin is only sometimes effective and often slow in onset; although an initial decrease in ventricular response can be observed within 1 hour of intravenous administration, full control (heart rate $< 100$ bpm) is usually not achieved for 24 to 48 hours. It is uncommon to observe restoration of sinus rhythm with digoxin therapy, although some patients do have spontaneous termination of atrial fibrillation. Recent information implies that a large percentage of patients revert to sinus rhythm if treatment with digoxin is initiated very quickly after the onset of new atrial fibrillation.[52] As can be seen, these two examples are at two ends of the spectrum (i.e., severely symptomatic and asymptomatic or mildly symptomatic) and often patients present somewhere in between. Consequently, clinical judgment is necessary in choosing the proper treatment strategy. For example, intravenous verapamil provides an alternative approach, allowing for a rapid decrease in ventricular rate and symptomatic relief without the need for DCC[53,54]; however, control of ventricular rate with verapamil is often transient, necessitating constant infusion therapy (5–10 mg/h) or rapid institution of oral medication.[54] Nonetheless, if digoxin is chosen for initial therapy in a specific patient, there no longer exists the need to "push" the dosage to toxicity to significantly decrease ventricular response. Oral verapamil or a $\beta$-blocker such as propranolol can simply be added to optimal digoxin therapy. It also should be noted that atrial

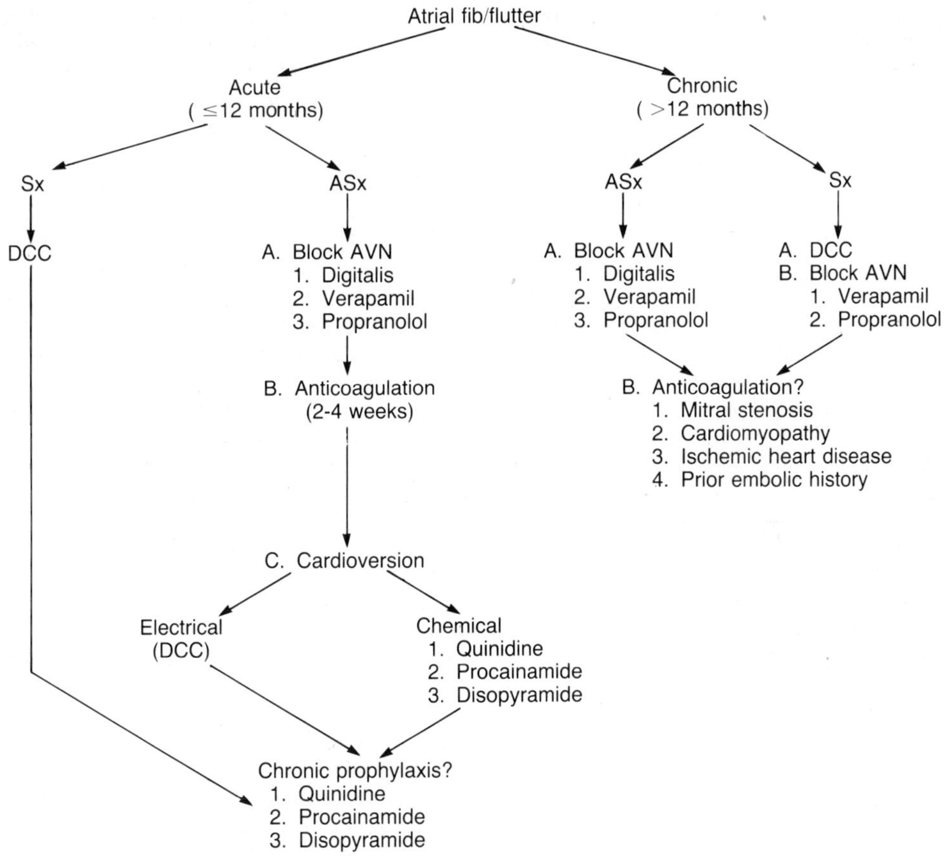


**Figure 12.4** Treatment algorithm for atrial fibrillation or atrial flutter. Sx, symptomatic; ASx, asymptomatic; DCC, direct-current cardioversion. *(From Bauman JL: Understanding and treating supraventricular arrhythmias. Clin Pharm 1983;2:317, with permission.)*

fibrillation or flutter precipitated by states of high adrenergic tone such as thyrotoxicosis is often resistant to digoxin therapy (digoxin slows AV nodal conduction primarily through vagotonic mechanisms), but verapamil or propranolol can be effective in these cases. Patients may present with a slow ventricular response (in the absence of AV nodal blocking drugs) and, thus, do not require therapy with digoxin, verapamil, or propranolol. This type of presentation should alert the clinician to the possibility of preexisting SA or AV nodal conduction disease such as sick sinus syndrome. DCC should not be attempted in these patients without a temporary pacemaker in place (see later).

After treatment with AV nodal blocking agents and a subsequent decrease in ventricular response, the patient should be evaluated for the possibility of restoring sinus rhythm; however, the maintenance of sinus rhythm for a significant length of time is usually not feasible in patients with a history of chronic (longer than 1 year), established atrial fibrillation or those with large atrial size (>45 mm determined by echocardiography).[55,56] Therefore, attempts at cardioversion are unnecessary and these patients can remain in atrial fibrillation treated with AV nodal blocking agents to control ventricular response. Other treatment considerations should be contemplated in these patients. First, long-term therapy with digoxin alone sometimes does not control exercise-related increases in ventricular response and tachycardia symptoms. Usually, verapamil or propranolol can be added; the need for these ancillary agents can be evaluated by treadmill exercise testing. Additionally, as patients with chronic atrial fibrillation are at risk for embolism, long-term warfarin therapy may be needed. Although controversial, atrial fibrillation per se without other risk factors for embolism is usually insufficient cause for chronic anticoagulation. In other words, the risk of long-term warfarin therapy probably outweighs the risk of significant embolism. Instead, the presence of another risk factor for systemic embolism (concurrent with established atrial fibrillation) is an indication for long-term warfarin therapy.[57,58] Common examples of this include those patients with concurrent mitral stenosis, severely depressed left ventricular function, or a history of prior embolism. Of course, only those patients deemed reliable are suitable candidates for chronic anticoagulation.

There are two methods of restoring sinus rhythm in patients with atrial fibrillation or flutter: pharmacologic cardioversion and electrical cardioversion (DCC). The method of choice is a matter of controversy. With pharmacologic cardioversion, the type Ia antiarrhythmic drugs such as quinidine, flecainide, procainamide, or disopyramide can be used. The time-honored method is to begin quinidine therapy; maintenance dosages are sufficient and oral loading schedules are unnecessary. Flecainide, although not yet approved for supraventricular tachycardias, is also quite effective and a suitable alternative to quinidine. The advantage of the drug therapy approach is that an effective agent may be determined in case long-term therapy is required and many feel there is little to lose with a 2- to 3-day trial. The disadvantages of pharmacologic cardioversion are the risk of significant side effects such as drug-induced torsades de pointes,[59] the inconvenience of drug–drug interactions (e.g., digoxin–quinidine), and the generally lesser effectiveness of drugs compared with DCC. The advantages of DCC are that it is quick and more often successful. The disadvantages of DCC are the need for prior sedation/anesthesia and a risk (albeit small) of serious complications such as sinus arrest or ventricular arrhythmias. Recent evidence shows DCC to carry very little risk in patients receiving digoxin without evidence of digitalis toxicity.[60] With either method of cardioversion, many clinicians would premedicate patients with 2 to 4 weeks of warfarin therapy.[58] In theory, the return of sinus rhythm restores an effective atrial contraction that may dislodge poorly adherent thrombi. Anticoagulation prior to cardioversion prevents clot growth or the formation of new thrombi and subsequently allows time for the organization and adherence of those atrial clots that may be present. The effectiveness of this form of prophylactic therapy is controversial and probably not indicated in new-onset atrial fibrillation of less than 1-week duration. A common scenario is for the patient to be discharged on oral warfarin and readmitted to the hospital 2 to 4 weeks later for elective cardioversion.[58]

After sinus rhythm is successfully restored, what chronic medications should the patient receive? In most cases, maintenance digoxin therapy is continued because of underlying ventricular dysfunction and, if atrial fibrillation recurs, ventricular response will be relatively slow. Chronic warfarin therapy in all patients is probably unnecessary. Conflicting data exist regarding the need for long-term type Ia antiarrhythmic drug therapy. Several studies imply that sinus rhythm is maintained for longer periods of time with quinidine therapy, while other studies seem to show that chronic quinidine does not alter recurrences of atrial fibrillation.[61] In any case, the chance of a recurrence after the initial return of sinus rhythm (regardless of quinidine therapy) is very likely.[47] We usually suggest the following approach: Long-term quinidine therapy should not be prescribed after the first episode but is reserved for those patients with a documented recurrence or paroxysmal atrial fibrillation or flutter.[46]

### *Paroxysmal Supraventricular Tachycardia Resulting From Reentry*

Paroxysmal supraventricular tachycardia (PSVT) arising by reentrant mechanisms includes those arrhythmias caused by AV nodal reentry, AV reentry incorporating an anomalous AV pathway, SA nodal reentry, and intraatrial reentry. AV nodal reentry and AV reentry are by far the most common of these tachycardias.

The underlying substrate of AV nodal reentry is the functional or anatomic division of the AV node into two (or more) longitudinal conduction pathways or "dual" AV nodal pathways.[62–64] These two pathways possess key differences in conduction characteristics: one is a fast conducting pathway with a relatively long refractory period (beta or fast pathway) and the other is a slower conducting pathway with a shorter refractory period (alpha or slow pathway). The presence of dual AV nodal pathways does not necessarily imply that the patient will have clinical PSVT. In fact, it is estimated that between 10% and 46% of patients have discernible dual pathways but the incidence of PSVT is considerably lower.[16,65] Sustenance of the tachycardia depends on the critical electrophysiologic discrepancies and the ability of one pathway (usually the slow) to allow repetitive antegrade conduction and the ability of the other pathway (usually the fast) to allow repetitive retrograde conduction. During sinus rhythm, a patient with dual AV nodal pathways conducts supraventricular impulses antegradely through both pathways. Electrical activity reaches the distal common pathway at the level of or above the His bundle and continues to depolarize the ventricles in an antegrade direction. Conduction proceeds via the two pathways but reaches the distal common pathway first through the fast AV nodal route (Fig. 12.5). For this reason, a short PR interval is sometimes observed during sinus rhythm.

PSVT resulting from AV nodal reentry may occur by the following sequence of events. The occurrence of an appropriately timed premature impulse penetrates the AV node, but is blocked in the fast pathway which is still refractory from the previous beat; however, the slow pathway, which has a shorter refractory period, permits antegrade conduction of the premature impulse. By the time the impulse has reached the distal common pathway, the fast pathway has recovered its excitability and now will permit retrograde conduction. The impulse reaches the common proximal pathway, preceded by an excitable gap of tissue, and reenters the slow pathway. A reentrant circuit that does not require atrial or ventricular tissue is completed within the AV node and a tachycardia is thereby initiated (Fig. 12.5). The common form of this tachycardia uses the slow pathway for antegrade conduction and the fast pathway for retrograde conduction. Lown–Ganong–Levine syndrome (LGL) is defined by paroxysms of a narrow QRS tachycardia associated with a short PR interval on surface electrocardiograms (during sinus rhythm) and is commonly due to AV nodal reentry.[66]

AV reentrant tachycardia depends upon the presence of an anomalous or accessory, extranodal pathway that bypasses the normal AV conduction pathway.[62,63] Several different types of accessory pathways have been described, depending on the specific anatomic areas they connect (e.g., atrioventricular bundles or nodoventricular tracts); some are also referred to by eponyms such as the Kent bundle. A Kent bundle is an extranodal AV connection that is associated with the Wolff–Parkinson–White syndrome (WPW).[67] During sinus rhythm (Fig. 12.6) patients with WPW depolarize the ventricles simultaneously through both AV pathways (AV nodal pathway and the Kent bundle), creating a fusion pattern on the early portion of the QRS complex (delta wave).[68] The degree of ventricular "preexcitation" depends on the contribution of antegrade ventricular activation through the accessory pathway. Patients may have an accessory pathway that is not evident on surface electrocardiograms or a "concealed" Kent bundle. The electrocardiographic expression of preexcitation (delta wave) depends on the distance of the accessory pathway from the wavefront of sinus activation and the conduction characteristics of the various structures involved. Also, some accessory pathways

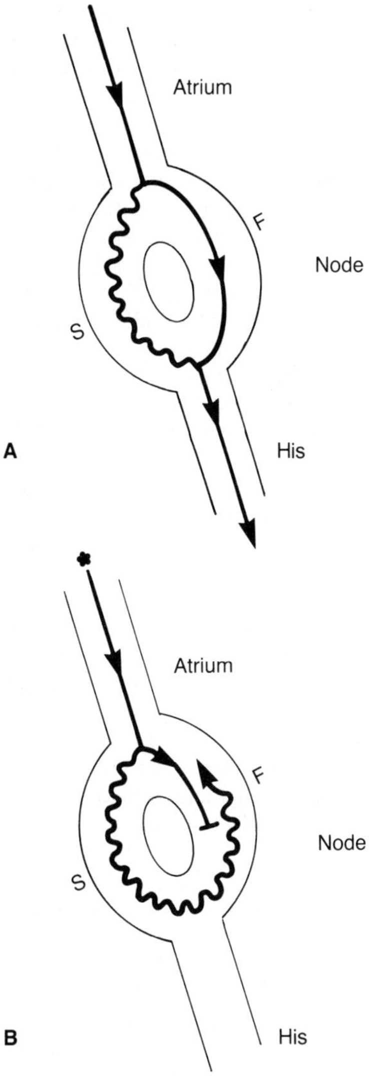


**Figure 12.5** Reentry mechanism of dual-AV-nodal-pathway PSVT. (A) Sinus rhythm: The impulse travels from the atrium through the fast pathway (F) and then to the His–Purkinje system. The impulse also travels through the slow pathway (S) but is stopped when refractory tissue is encountered. (B) Dual-AV-nodal reentry: A critically timed premature impulse (*) is stopped in the fast pathway (because of prolonged refractoriness) but is able to travel antegrade down the slow pathway and retrograde through the fast pathway. *(From Bauman JL: Understanding and treating supraventricular arrhythmias. Clin Pharm 1983;2:314, with permission.)*

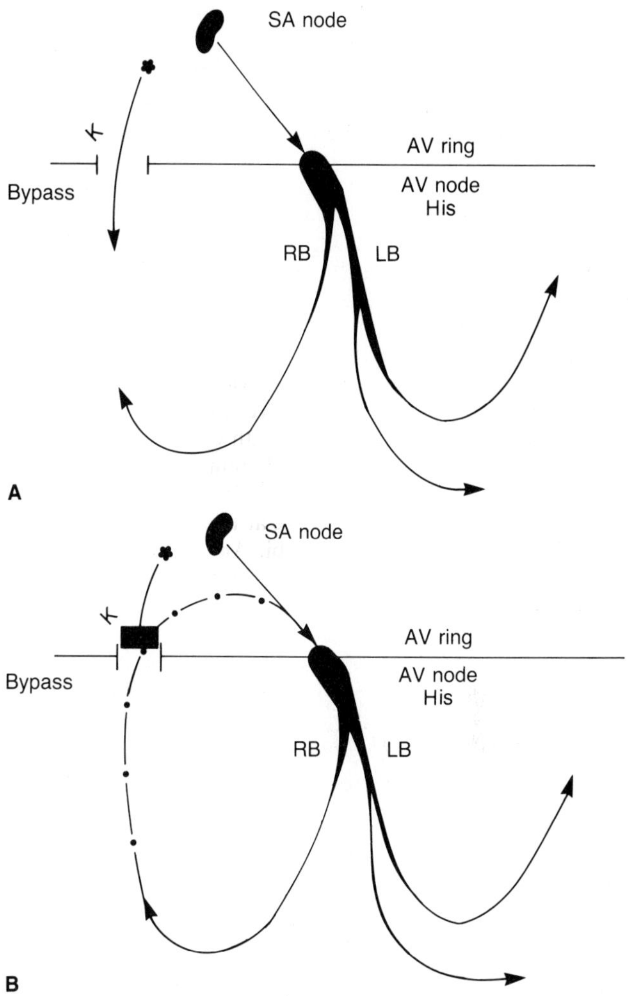


**Figure 12.6** Reentry mechanism for AV-accessory-pathway PSVT in Wolff–Parkinson–White syndrome. (A) Sinus rhythm: The impulse travels from the atrium to the ventricle by two pathways—the AV node and an accessory bypass tract (K, Kent bundle). (B) AV reentry: A critically timed premature impulse (*) is stopped in the Kent bundle (because of prolonged refractoriness) but travels antegrade through the AV node and retrograde through the Kent bundle (—.—). *(From Bauman JL: Understanding and treating supraventricular arrhythmias. Clin Pharm 1983;2:314, with permission.)*

are incapable of antegrade conduction and can accept electrical stimulation only in a retrograde fashion. It should be noted that (similar to patients with dual AV nodal pathways) not all patients with preexcitation resulting from an accessory AV pathway are capable of having clinical PSVT.

Patients with an accessory AV pathway may have two forms of supraventricular tachycardia: PSVT and/or atrial fibrillation or flutter. AV reentrant PSVT occurs by the following sequence of events. Analogous to AV nodal reentry, two pathways (the normal AV nodal pathway and the accessory AV pathway) exist that have different electrophysiologic characteristics. The AV nodal pathway has a relatively slower conduction velocity and shorter refractory period and the accessory pathway has a faster conduction velocity and a longer refractory period. A critically timed premature impulse may block in the accessory pathway because it is still refractory from the previous sinus beat; however, the AV nodal pathway with a relatively shorter refractory period may accept antegrade conduction of the premature impulse. Meanwhile, the accessory pathway may recover its excitability and now allow retrograde conduction. A macroreentrant tachycardia is thereby initiated in which the antegrade pathway is the AV nodal pathway; the distal common pathway is the ventricle; the retrograde pathway is the accessory pathway; and the proximal common pathway is the atrium (Fig. 12.6). This sequence of events (down node, up Kent) is the common variety of

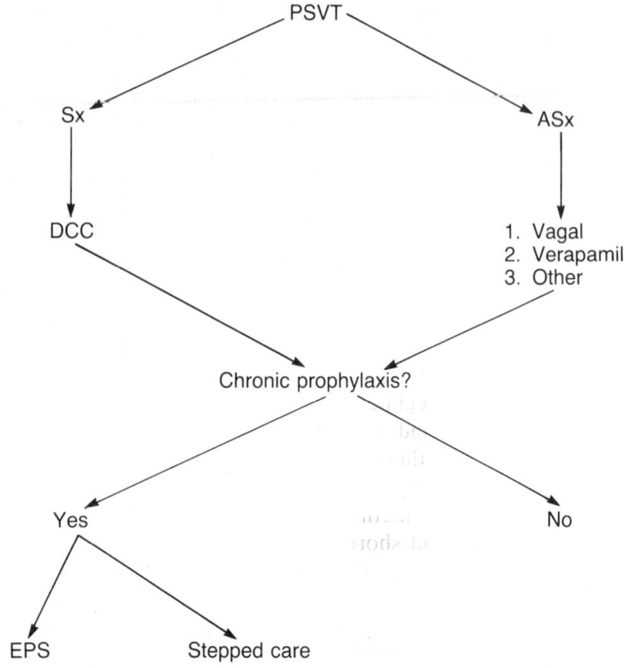


**Figure 12.7** Treatment algorithm for an acute episode of PSVT. Sx, symptomatic; ASx, asymptomatic; DCC, direct-current cardioversion; EPS, electrophysiologic studies. *(From Bauman JL: Understanding and treating supraventricular arrhythmias. Clin Pharm 1983;2:315, with permission.)*

reentry in patients with an accessory AV pathway, resulting in a narrow QRS tachycardia. In the uncommon variety (down Kent, up node), conduction proceeds in the opposite direction, resulting in a wide QRS tachycardia. Patients with WPW can have a second type of tachycardia (other than PSVT), namely, atrial fibrillation or flutter. The mechanism for its occurrence is unknown, but it can be very serious and sudden death is well described. As atrial fibrillation is an extremely rapid atrial tachycardia, conduction can proceed down the accessory AV pathway, resulting in a very fast ventricular response or even ventricular fibrillation.[69] Unlike the AV nodal pathway, the refractory period of the accessory bundle shortens in response to rapid stimulation rates.

Sinus node reentry or intraatrial reentry occurs less commonly and is not as well described as AV nodal or AV reentry.[70] Aside from a characteristic abrupt onset and termination coupled with subtle changes in P-wave morphology, these tachycardias can be difficult to diagnose. Electrophysiologic studies may be necessary to determine the ultimate mechanism of the PSVT.

Both pharmacologic and nonpharmacologic methods have been used to treat patients with PSVT (Fig. 12.7). Drugs used in the treatment of PSVT can be divided into three broad categories: (1) those that directly or indirectly increase vagal tone to the AV node such as edrophonium, vasopressors and digoxin, (2) those that depress conduction through slow, calcium-dependent tissue such as $\beta$-blockers and calcium channel blockers, and (3) those that depress conduction through fast, sodium-dependent tissue such as quinidine, procainamide, disopyramide, and flecainide. Drugs within these categories alter the electrophysiologic characteristics of the reentrant substrate in somewhat different ways so that PSVT cannot be sustained.[71,72] In PSVT caused by AV nodal reentry, type I antiarrhythmic drugs such as procainamide act primarily on the retrograde fast pathway. Digoxin and propranolol may work on either the retrograde fast or the antegrade slow limb. Verapamil prolongs conduction time and increases refractoriness primarily in the slow antegrade pathway of the reentrant loop. In PSVT resulting from AV reentry incorporating an extranodal pathway, type I drugs increase refractoriness in the fast accessory pathway or within the His–Purkinje system. Propranolol, digoxin, and verapamil all act by their effects on the AV nodal (antegrade, slow) portion of the reentrant circuit. Regardless of the mechanism, treatment measures are directed at first terminating an acute episode of PSVT and then (if necessary) preventing symptomatic recurrences of PSVT.

As in any rapid reentrant tachycardia resulting in severe symptoms (syncope, near syncope, anginal chest pain, severe heart failure), synchronized DCC is the treatment of choice. Even at low energy levels (such as 25 W/s), DCC for PSVT is almost always effective in quickly restoring sinus rhythm and correcting severe hemodynamic compromise. Patients with only mild to moderate symptoms usually do not require DCC and nondrug measures that increase vagal tone to the AV node can be utilized first. Carotid sinus massage, valsalva maneuver, ice water facial immersion, induced retching, and other more elaborate vagomimetic measures are often successful in terminating PSVT, although carotid massage and valsalva maneuver are the simplest, least obtrusive, and most frequently used of these techniques.

In the event that these methods fail, intravenous verapamil should be used and is generally considered the drug of first choice. About 80% to 90% of PSVT episodes revert to sinus rhythm within 5 minutes of intravenous verapamil therapy.[44,73] In the remaining group of patients in whom verapamil does not terminate PSVT, the clinician has several treatment options. First, verapamil failure may result in the appearance of severe hemodynamic symptoms because of this agent's negative inotropic and vasodilator properties. If this is the case, then one must quickly resort to DCC. On the other hand, if the patient is tolerating the episode of PSVT well with little or no symptomatology, bed rest and sedatives may be appropriate. Pacing methods or DCC can be used later to terminate PSVT, if the episode does not spontaneously revert to sinus rhythm. Finally, the clinician can attempt alternative drug therapy. Although, there are no firm guidelines regarding which drug to choose next, several concepts (some theoretical) can prove valuable in making this decision.[16,32] Intravenous propranolol should probably not be administered immediately after verapamil because of the possibility of precipitating severe hemodynamic compromise as a result of AV block and/or depressed myocardial contractility. As verapamil works primarily on the antegrade slow pathway of the reentrant circuits, a logical next choice would be a drug that acts on the retrograde fast pathway. Intravenous procainamide is often chosen over the other available type I agents. It should be recognized, however, that because procainamide and verapamil work at different sites in the reentrant loop, these agents may simply offset each other's effects on conduction. In this case, a considerably slower tachycardia that does not easily terminate may result. Furthermore, procainamide can worsen hypotension. An alternative approach is to choose another agent that works on the antegrade slow pathway in an attempt to obtain additive effects with verapamil. Intravenous digoxin exemplifies this strategy and, of course, vagal maneuvers should be periodically repeated. Other agents that indirectly increase vagal tone and have been used in the treatment of PSVT are anticholinesterase inhibitors such as edrophonium and pressor agents such as phenylephrine and metaraminol. Pressors should be titrated to achieve a mild degree of hypertension (150–180 mm Hg systolic) to elicit the baroreceptor-mediated increase in vagal tone. Patients who present with mild hypotension are logical candidates for pressor therapy. Also, several investigational intravenous drugs may prove useful in the future. Esmolol is an ultrashort-acting $\beta$-blocker that has potential advantages over the traditional $\beta$-blockers, primarily in abbreviating the duration of side effects.[74] Adenosine triphosphate (ATP) and adenosine combine the advantages of a very short duration of action and a high degree of effectiveness (90% success rate).[75] These new agents work by depressing calcium influx and/or increasing vagal tone, altering conduction in the antegrade slow pathway.

Once the acute episode of PSVT is terminated, a decision on long-term preventive therapy must follow. Some patients do not require long-term drug therapy; preventive treatment is indicated if (1) frequent episodes occur that necessitate therapeutic intervention (i.e., emergency room visits) or interfere with the patient's life-style or (2) infrequent but severe symptoms occur. Also, effective vagal manuevers can be taught to the patient, obviating the need for chronic drug therapy.

For those patients in whom a preventive drug therapy regimen is deemed necessary, three treatment strategies are available. First, clinicians may use a trial-and-error approach on an ambulatory basis for those patients with frequently recurrent, mildly symptomatic PSVT. Ambulatory electrocardiographic (Holter) recordings or telephonic transmissions of cardiac rhythm (Cardiobeeper) can be used to objectively document the efficacy or failure of drug therapy. How should one choose empiric drug regimens? A combination of digoxin and propranolol is often effective, so that the clinician can try one of these agents first and then add the other drug if monotherapy fails. One may assume that the agent that was successful in terminating the acute episode of PSVT will also provide effective preventive therapy, but actually there is little evidence to support this approach. Indeed, chronic oral verapamil is often ineffective in those patients who responded to intravenous therapy. This is probably due to significant pharmacodynamic and pharmacokinetic differences between the oral and intravenous dosage forms of verapamil coupled with stereoselective first-pass metabolism with the oral racemate.[76] Bauernfeind and co-workers[77] have studied the patterns of drug response in patients with AV reentrant tachycardia that may help the clinician choose empiric therapy. These investigators found a significant concordance of responses between drugs that work on the slow antegrade limb (e.g., propranolol and digoxin), a concordance of drug responses for those agents that act on the fast retrograde limb (e.g., procainamide and quinidine), and a discordance of responses between these two groups of drugs. In other words, if quinidine is effective it is likely that procainamide will also be effective but unlikely that propranolol or digoxin will be effective. These findings imply that there is a "weak link" in the reentrant pathway that is susceptible to drug therapy. The second method in selecting effective long-term therapy is to use the trial-and-error method during hospitalization. In this case, Holter monitoring or telemetry can be used to objectively assess drug efficacy or failure. Initially, all antiarrhythmics should be discontinued and attacks detected and quantified. After this drug-free control period in which the frequency and characteristics of the tachycardia are defined, antiarrhythmic agents are administered in a serial fashion and evaluated for efficacy. It is crucial to determine drug efficacy (abolition of symptomatic PSVT) with consideration to the tachycardia frequency during the control period. Once a seemingly effective regimen is defined, a drug(s) concentration is determined and used as that patient's therapeutic level. Chronic drug therapy is then tailored to match this effective drug concentration.

The trial-and-error methods for determining drug effectiveness have inherent shortcomings. If the PSVT episodes are infrequent, a considerable time period may be consumed before an effective regimen is realized. Also, if the patient has moderate to severe symptoms associated with PSVT, several troublesome episodes may be experienced by the patient before the correct agent(s) is identified. Serial testing of antiarrhythmic agents by invasive electrophysiologic techniques can be a valuable method in determining effective long-term therapy in these patients with sporadic and/or symptomatic PSVT. Basically, the patient's clinical tachycardia is replicated in the laboratory by inserting appropriately timed, premature extra stimuli via a transvenous right heart catheter. The patient is first tapered off of antiarrhythmic therapy, and induction of the tachycardia with premature stimuli by programmed stimulation serves as a control study. Then, over a period of several days specific drugs are administered in a serial fashion and tested for efficacy in preventing the induction of PSVT.[71,72] Inability to induce PSVT or induction of only brief, self-terminating episodes usually predicts that drug regimen will be effective long-term therapy. Electrophysiologic drug testing has several advantages over the trial-and-error methods.[16] First, the actual mechanism of the tachycardia (e.g., PSVT versus ventricular tachycardia or AV reentry versus AV nodal reentry) can be defined. Second, this technique is time efficient and probably cost effective in that an efficacious agent can be determined in a relatively short time. Third, if the patient has PSVT associated with severe symptoms, the tachycardia will be induced in a well-equipped laboratory setting, preventing the potentially serious consequences of PSVT recurrence at home or in a car. Fourth, a patient-specific drug regimen and therapeutic concentration can be identified. Fifth, patients with drug refractory PSVT can be readily identified and appropriate measures can be taken. On the other hand, this is an invasive procedure and although complications are uncommon, candidates for programmed stimulation must be carefully chosen.

### *Automatic Atrial Tachycardia*

Automatic atrial tachycardias such as multifocal atrial tachycardia appear to arise from supraventricular foci that have enhanced automatic properties.[78–80] It is presumed that multifocal atrial tachycardia (sometimes referred to as chaotic atrial tachycardia) is the result of multiple ectopic atrial pacemakers which account for the variable and differing P-wave morphology. Unifocal atrial tachycardia (sometimes referred to as ectopic atrial tachycardia) will have one P-wave morphology different from that of sinus rhythm. In either case, the underlying, precipitating disorder present in the majority of these patients is severe pulmonary disease. Other disease states associated with these arrhythmias include acute infection (pneumonia and sepsis) and dilated congestive cardiomyopathy. As previously referred to, many factors (i.e., electrolyte disturbances, hypoxia, catecholamines, and tissue stretch) may cause an elevated slope of phase 4 depolarization and enhanced automaticity. Clinically, these factors are often present in patients with concurrent pulmonary disease and automatic atrial tachycardia; however, recent information implies that triggered activity may also play a role in the genesis of these tachycardias.[81] Furthermore, digitalis toxicity can result in an automatic atrial tachycardia with AV block.[82]

The first step in the treatment of automatic atrial tachycardia is correction of the underlying, precipitating factors. One should ensure proper oxygenation and ventilation and correct acid–base or electrolyte disturbances. These measures alone may result in the return of sinus rhythm, but in some cases, the tachycardia will persist. Patients with an asymptomatic atrial tachycardia and a relatively slow ventricular response usually require no drug therapy. In symptomatic patients, medical therapy can be tailored either to control ventricular response or to restore sinus rhythm.[79,80] Type I antiarrhythmic drugs such as procainamide and quinidine are occasionally effective in restoring sinus rhythm, presumably because of their ability to decrease the automatic properties of latent pacemakers, but these agents are usually not considered first-line therapy. Direct-current cardioversion is usually ineffective in restoring sinus rhythm.[80] As the underlying disorder is probably enhanced automaticity, programmed stimulation will not replicate the clinical tachycardia so that serial drug testing is of no value. Drugs that slow AV nodal conduction can be used to decrease ventricular response; however, propranolol is usually contraindicated because of the frequent coexistence of severe pulmonary disease or heart failure. Digoxin can be effective but its use is controversial because of its ability to increase the automatic properties of atrial tissue in toxic dosages. Verapamil can also be effective and may now be considered first-line drug therapy.[81] Surprisingly, verapamil seems to decrease ventricular response by altering atrial automaticity and not by slowing AV nodal conduction.[81]

## Ventricular Arrhythmias

The common ventricular arrhythmias include ventricular premature beats (VPBs), ventricular tachycardia (VT), and ventricular fibrillation (VF). Again, these arrhythmias may result in a wide variety of symptoms. VPBs often cause no symptoms or only mild palpitations. VT may be a life-threatening situation associated with hemodynamic collapse or may be totally asymptomatic. VF, by definition, is an acute medical emergency necessitating cardiopulmonary resucitation.

### *Ventricular Premature Beats*

VPBs are very common ventricular rhythm disturbances that occur in patients with or without heart disease. Experimental models have shown that premature ventricular depolarizations may be elicited by abnormal automaticity, triggered activity, or reentrant mechanisms. It has become well known that VPBs can be commonly observed in apparently healthy individuals[83,84]; however, VPBs occurring in overtly normal subjects without discernible heart disease seem to have little if any prognostic significance. In contrast, considerable controversy exists regarding the prognostic significance of VPBs in patients with organic heart disease. VPBs seem to occur more frequently and in more complex forms (see later) in patients with detectable heart disease than in healthy individuals. The prognostic meaning of VPBs has been most well studied in patients with myocardial infarction (acute or remote) with several consistent themes.[85,86] Little is known about the significance of VPBs occurring in association with forms of heart disease (other than ischemic heart disease) such as hypertension, mitral valve prolapse, or primary myocardial disease.

Some investigators have promoted the concept that patients in the acute phase of myocardial infarction may have types of VPBs that are predictive of VF and sudden cardiac death.[87] These types of VPBs are referred to as "warning arrhythmias" and include frequent ectopy (5/min), multiform configuration (different morphology), couplets (two in a row), and R-on-T phenomenon (VPBs occurring during the repolarization phase of the preceding sinus beat in the vulnerable period of ventricular recovery); however, with the use of sophisticated monitoring techniques, it has become apparent that almost all patients have VPBs (often warning arrhythmias) in the acute infarct setting. Furthermore, warning arrhythmias are no more common in patients who experience VF than in those without VF. Therefore, warning arrhythmias observed during acute myocardial infarction are neither a sensitive nor a specific predictive tool in determining which patients will have VF.[88,89] To date, there are no known warning arrhythmias.

On the other hand, recent data strongly imply that VPBs documented in the convalescence period of myocardial infarction do carry prognostic significance.[85,86] VPBs occurring after a myocardial infarction seem to be a risk factor for patient death that is independent of the degree of left ventricular dysfunction or the extent of a coronary atherosclerosis. Lown and Wolf[90] have developed a grading scale for classifying different types of VPBs (Table 12.3). The common assumption is that the higher grades of VPBs imply a higher risk of subsequent arrhythmogenic death. It should be emphasized that this assumption has never been conclusively proven. Ruberman and co-workers[85] have devised a simple classification based upon the significance of simple or benign (infrequent and/or monomorphic) versus complex or malignant (all other types in the Lown classification) forms of VPBs. These investigators found that the presence of complex ventricular ectopy was associated with a higher incidence of cardiac death (but not necessarily arrhythmo-

**Table 12.3** The Lown Grading Scale for Preventricular Contractions

| *Form* | *Grade* |
|---|---|
| No preventricular contractions | 0 |
| Rate < 30/h | 1 |
| Rate > 30/h (unifocal) | 2 |
| Multiform | 3 |
| Couplets | 4a |
| Triplets or more (ventricular tachycardia) | 4b |
| R-on-T phenomenon | 5 |

genic death). One can see that within the controversy of the significance of VPBs is a basic question: Are VPBs simply an unimportant result of underlying structural heart disease or are VPBs an important electrical disorder that should be addressed independently?

Should VPBs be treated with antiarrhythmic drug therapy? As VPBs without associated heart disease in apparently healthy individuals carry little or no risk, drug therapy is unnecessary. Uncommonly, palpitations that are bothersome to the patient occur in association with the VPBs. The clinician should attempt to reassure the patient of the generally excellent prognosis and avoid antiarrhythmic drugs if possible. In patients with acute myocardial infarction, there is little need to direct drug therapy (usually lidocaine) specifically at VPB suppression. Studies have shown that effective prevention of VF in the acute infarct setting may be achieved without the abolition of VPBs. The inability of VPBs (warning arrhythmias) to predict the occurrence of VF coupled with the lack of correlation between a drug's effectiveness in preventing VF and suppressing VPBs form the basis of suggesting lidocaine prophylaxis for all patients with an uncomplicated acute myocardial infarction (see later).[91,92]

A major area of controversy is the treatment of VPBs in patients with associated heart disease (usually postmyocardial infarction). Some suggest aggressive antiarrhythmic drug therapy designed to suppress a large percentage of VPBs, based upon the Lown grading system.[93] The underlying premise of this approach is the attempt to eliminate a risk factor for cardiac death in patients with coronary disease, namely, the presence of complex VPBs; however, others favor a more conservative approach and disregard drug therapy in the absence of significant symptoms. We favor this nonaggressive strategy for the following reasons.[94]

First, the frequency of VPBs is sporadic and extremely variable, making it difficult to determine effective drug therapy. Winkle,[95] by evaluating continuous electrocardiograms (5.5 hours) and VPB frequency, found a marked spontaneous variability that often mimicked drug efficacy or drug-induced aggravation of VPBs. Morganroth and coworkers[96] analyzed the variations in VPB frequency on 24-hour Holter recordings. These investigators estimated that to attribute a reduction in VPB frequency to drug effectiveness instead of spontaneous variability, a decrease in VPB frequency greater than 83% was necessary. Despite this finding, many clinicians and published studies still judge drug efficacy by a 50% reduction in VPB frequency or simply a statistically significant reduction in the number of VPBs by Holter monitors. It is obvious that these criteria do not account for the spontaneous variability in VPB frequency. Other investigators[97] have noted an impressive discordance between the drug concentrations necessary for an 83% reduction in VPB frequency and those necessary to prevent VT or VF. In other words, the high degree of VPB suppression may not be a necessary prerequisite for the successful prevention of VT or VF. When treating a patient with heart disease for complex VPBs, the endpoint of therapy is less than clear and probably does not correlate with abolition of more serious ventricular arrhythmias such as VT or VF.

A second reason for not treating VPBs associated with heart disease is that there is no evidence that this approach significantly reduces the incidence of sudden death, cardiac death, or overall mortality. Although complex VPBs are an independent risk factor for sudden death in patients with coronary disease, there is no information that shows that suppression of these VPBs results in greater longevity. Instead, $\beta$-blockers such as propranolol, metoprolol, and timolol have been shown to significantly decrease mortality from either sudden or other cardiac death after myocardial infarction (but this is not well correlated with VPB suppression). It is likely that sudden death in these individuals often reflects an acute ischemic event not just a primary arrhythmogenic event. It should be noted that a large multicenter study (CAPS trial) is currently in progress that will evaluate the effectiveness of long-term prophylactic antiarrhythmic drugs.

Third, all antiarrhythmic agents currently available have an impressive side effect profile (Table 12.4). A considerable percentage of patients cannot tolerate long-term therapy with these drugs and chances are good that an agent will have to be discontinued because of side effects. In one trial,[98] over 50% of patients had to discontinue long-term procainamide (mostly as a result of a lupuslike syndrome) after myocardial infarction. In another study,[99] disopyramide caused anticholinergic side effects in about 70% of patients. Flecainide and disopyramide may precipitate congestive heart failure in a significant number of patients with underlying left ventricular dysfunction.[100] The new type Ib agents such as tocainide and mexiletine cause neurologic and/or gastrointestinal toxicity in a large percentage of patients.[101] Long-term therapy with amiodarone frequently causes multisystem toxicity, including occasional cases of hepatitis and pulmonary fibrosis.[42,102] Possibly the most frightening adverse effects related to antiarrhythmic drugs are the aggravation of underlying ventricular arrhythmias and the precipitation of new (and life-threatening) ventricular arrhythmias.[59,103] Antiarrhythmic drugs may worsen existing ventricular arrhythmias in 5% to 20% of patients.[103] Also, these agents can cause new VT in patients who only had prior VPBs and have been causally related to out-of-hospital cardiac arrest.[104] Furthermore, torsades de pointes and long QT syndrome are fairly common observations in patients treated with quinidine, procainamide, or disopyramide. Quinidine syncope (torsades de pointes) may occur in 4% to 8% of patients treated with this agent.[105] These data underscore the need to carefully choose those patients who truly require antiarrhythmic drug therapy. In conclusion,

**Table 12.4** Side Effects of Antiarrhythmic Drugs

| | |
|---|---|
| Quinidine | Cinchonism, diarrhea, GI,[a] hypotension, torsades de pointes, aggravation of underlying heart failure, conduction disturbances or ventricular arrhythmias, hepatitis, thrombocytopenia, hemolytic anemia |
| Procainamide | Systemic lupus erythematosus, GI, torsades de pointes, aggravation of underlying heart failure, conduction disturbances or ventricular arrhythmias, agranulocytosis |
| Disopyramide | Anticholinergic symptoms, GI, torsades de pointes, heart failure, aggravation of underlying conduction disturbances and/or ventricular arrhythmias, hypoglycemia, hepatic cholestasis |
| Lidocaine | CNS, seizures, psychosis, sinus arrest, aggravation of underlying conduction disturbances |
| Mexiletine | CNS, psychosis, GI, aggravation of underlying conduction disturbances or ventricular arrhythmias |
| Tocainide | CNS, psychosis, GI, aggravation of underlying conduction disturbances or ventricular arrhythmias, rash/arthralgias, pulmonary infiltrates, agranulocytosis, thrombocytopenia |
| Flecainide, encainide | CNS, blurred vision, dizziness, GI, aggravation of underlying heart failure, conduction disturbances or ventricular arrhythmias |
| Amiodarone | CNS, corneal microdeposits/blurred vision, GI, aggravation of underlying ventricular arrhythmias, torsades de pointes, bradycardia or AV block, bruising without thrombocytopenia, pulmonary fibrosis, hepatitis, hypothyroidism, hyperthyroidism, photosensitivity, blue-gray skin discoloration, myopathy |
| Bretylium | Hypotension, GI |

[a] GI = nausea, anorexia; CNS = confusion, paresthesias, tremor, ataxia, etc.

there is probably insufficient information to justify the routine use of antiarrhythmic drugs in patients with VPBs (simple or complex) associated with organic heart disease.

Occasionally, patients with heart disease and symptomatic VPBs require drug therapy to eliminate bothersome palpitations. None of the currently available agents is clearly superior in efficacy or has less side effects than the others. Amiodarone is extremely effective in suppressing a large percentage of VPBs, but its high degree of toxicity eliminates the possible use of this new drug. Therefore, one should initially choose an agent on an empiric basis with consideration of patient-specific factors; that is, do not first choose disopyramide in patients with preexisting heart failure or urinary difficulties or mexiletine in patients with neurologic problems. Once the decision is made to treat symptomatic VPBs, antiarrhythmics can then be serially tested (by electrocardiographic methods) for the best response and the least side effects. The endpoint of drug therapy in this case should not necessarily be a quantitative reduction in VPB frequency but rather a symptomatic relief of bothersome palpitations.

### *Ventricular Tachycardia*

VT is a wide QRS tachycardia that may acutely occur as a result of metabolic abnormalities, ischemia, or drug toxicity, or chronically recur as a paroxysmal form. On electrocardiographic inspection, VT may appear as either repetitive monomorphic or polymorphic ventricular complexes. The strict definition of VT is three or more repetitive VPBs occurring at a rate greater than 100 bpm. An acute episode of VT may be precipitated by electrolyte abnormalities (hypokalemia), hypoxemia, or digitalis toxicity or during an acute myocardial infarction. In these cases, correction of the underlying precipitating factors usually prevents further recurrences of VT. As an example, if VT occurs during an acute myocardial infarction and is effectively treated, it will probably not reappear on a chronic basis after the infarcted area has healed or ischemia has resolved.[106] This form of acute VT may be due to either enhanced automatic properties of a ventricular focus or reentrant mechanisms within the ischemic ventricle. In contrast, some patients have a chronic recurrent form of VT that is almost always associated with some type of underlying organic heart disease. Common examples are paroxysmal VT associated with idiopathic dilated congestive cardiomyopathy or remote myocardial infarction with a left ventricular aneurysm. Indeed, left ventricular dysfunction and aneurysm formation are risk factors for the development of VT on a recurrent basis after myocardial infarction. In chronic, recurrent VT, microreentry within the distal Purkinje network is presumed to be responsible for the underlying substrate in a large majority of patients.[107] Theoretically, electrophysiologic discrepancies occur as a result of structural damage and heart disease within the ventricular conducting system.

Patients with acute VT associated with a precipitating factor often suffer severe symptoms requiring immediate treatment measures. Chronic recurrent VT may also cause severe hemodynamic compromise but sometimes results in few or no symptoms. Different varieties of VT may occur and require some definition. Sustained VT is that which requires therapeutic intervention to restore a stable rhythm or lasts a relatively long time (usually greater than 30 seconds). Nonsustained VT is that which self-terminates after a brief duration (usually less than 30 seconds). A greater frequency of VT than sinus rhythm (VT is the dominant rhythm) is referred to as incessant VT. Exercise-induced VT is that which occurs during times of high sympathetic tone such as physical exertion. Monomorphic VT has a consistent QRS configuration, whereas polymorphic VT has varying QRS complexes. A very characteristic type of polymorphic VT in which the QRS complexes appear to undulate around a central axis and there is evidence of delayed ventricular repolarization (long QT interval or prominent U waves) is referred to torsades de pointes (see later).

Like other rapid tachycardias, the initial management of an acute episode of VT requires a quick assessment of the patient's status and symptoms. If severe symptoms are present, then DCC should be instituted to immediately restore sinus rhythm. An investigation should be made into possible precipitating factors and these corrected if possible. The diagnosis of acute myocardial infarction should be entertained. If VT is felt to be an isolated electrical event associated with a transient initiating event (such as acute myocardial ischemia or digitalis toxicity), then lidocaine should be administered and continued for 24 to 48 hours or until the patient is stable. In these cases, there may be no need for long-term antiarrhythmic therapy once the precipitating factors are corrected. Nevertheless, the patient should be monitored closely for possible recurrences of VT.

Patients with mild or no symptoms during an acute episode of VT can be initially treated with antiarrhythmic drugs (DCC should be readily available). Lidocaine (loading dose and infusion) is usually considered the drug of choice because of a high degree of effectiveness, quick onset, and ease of administration. In the event that lidocaine fails to terminate the tachycardia, intravenous procainamide (loading dose and infusion) can be tried next. Some feel that procainamide should actually be used prior to lidocaine because (if effective and the patient requires long-term drug therapy) oral procainamide can be used (whereas oral lidocaine cannot). DCC should be instituted if the patient's status deteriorates, VT degenerates to VF, or drug therapy fails. As an alternate to DCC, a transvenous pacing wire can be inserted and VT terminated by overdrive pacing methods. There is basically no reason to allow the patient to remain in VT without intervention even if symptoms are minimal. It has been suggested that bretylium should be used in VT refractory to other drug therapy; however, recent evidence implies that bretylium-like drugs, although effective in VF, are usually ineffective in VT.[46]

The management of the patient with chronic recurrent VT deserves considerable attention. With a few exceptions, patients with documented episodes of recurrent VT should have invasive electrophysiologic studies coupled with serial drug testing. These individuals are at high risk for sudden death so that the trial-and-error approach of finding effective drug therapy is usually not warranted. Electrophysiologic studies utilizing programmed stimulation incorporate the concepts of reentry to replicate the patient's clinical tachycardia in a controlled laboratory setting.[108–110] The patient is admitted to the hospital (often an intensive care setting) and strips of the clinical tachycardia are carefully analyzed. All antiarrhythmic drugs are discontinued and (after the systemic elimination of these drugs) the patient is brought to the electrophysiology laboratory in the nonsedated state. Here a transvenous multipolar catheter, which can both pace the heart and record electrical activity, is inserted into the right heart. Next, attempts to replicate the clinical tachycardia are made by the insertion of early beats and/or pacing methods via programmed stimulation. If replication of the clinical tachycardia is achieved, this initial study (without drug therapy) serves as a control against which subsequent studies on drug therapy can be compared. The electrophysiologist usually uses a protocol of several different grades of programmed stimulation: $S_1$ = continuous pacing train; $S_1,S_2$ = one extra stimuli; $S_1,S_2,S_3$ = two extra stimuli; $S_1,S_2,S_3,S_4$ = three extra stimuli; and rapid ventricular pacing (V burst) at variable rates. Induced VT can then be terminated by programmed stimulation, overdrive pacing, or DCC depending upon the patient's status. Antiarrhythmic drugs are then serially administered and the electrophysiologic study is repeated (at presumed drug steady-state) (Fig. 12.8 and 12.9). If a patient has sustained VT induced during the control study, then the inability to reproduce VT or the induction of only brief, self-terminating episodes of VT (usually less than 10 to 20 beats) generally predicts that that drug will be effective in preventing recurrent episodes on a long-term basis.

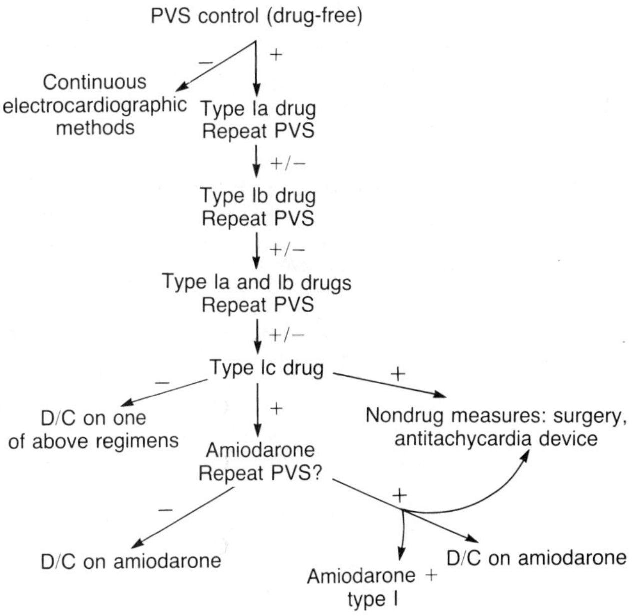


**Figure 12.8** Example of serial drug testing protocol by electrophysiologic testing procedures for a patient with recurrent ventricular tachycardia. PVS, programmed ventricular stimulation; D/C, discharge from hospital; +, VT recurrence or inducible VT; −, no VT recurrence or inducible VT.

Unfortunately (and unlike PSVT), recurrent VT is often refractory to drug therapy and an effective agent can be identified in only 20% to 25% of patients.[111] Therefore, the clinician frequently must search for other therapeutic options or settle for less optimal treatment endpoints. Some feel that a more aggressive grade of stimulation (e.g., $S_2$ induction on control versus $S_4$ induction on drug therapy)

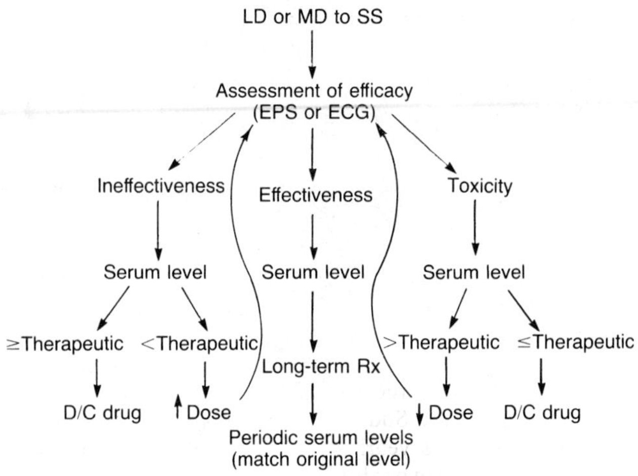


**Figure 12.9** Algorithm for the clinical approach to therapeutic drug monitoring of antiarrhythmic drugs. EPS, electrophysiologic studies; ECG, continuous electrocardiographic monitoring; D/C, discontinue drug. Adapted from reference 131.

will make the clinical tachycardia less likely or that the induction of sustained VT at a considerably slower rate will make the tachycardia better tolerated. Nevertheless, these options are not well studied, and many centers will not consistently rely upon these responses in the electrophysiology laboratory. Sometimes combination therapy is tried for patients refractory to single agents. The combination of a type Ia drug with a type Ib drug (i.e., quinidine and mexiletine) is effective in some patients who are resistant to either drug used alone.[112] In those patients who fail to respond to combination therapy, the clinician still has several therapeutic options, namely, amiodarone, surgical intervention, or antitachycardia devices.

Amiodarone is probably the most effective agent in patients with multiple drug-refractory recurrent VT. Although a matter of controversy, many feel that electrophysiologic drug testing does not predict the clinical efficacy of amiodarone.[113] In other words, a patient may have inducible sustained VT in the laboratory on amiodarone therapy, but have no recurrences of clinical VT on an ambulatory basis. For this reason and in view of the refractory nature of chronic recurrent VT, many patients are empirically treated with long-term amiodarone therapy. As mentioned previously, this drug has a high incidence of side effects (sometimes severe) and should be reserved for those truly refractory cases. Some centers have had excellent results with surgical excision of the VT focus.[114] With the aid of endocardial mapping techniques, such procedures as ventricular aneurysmectomy, encircling ventriculotomy, and cryo or laser ablation can successfully abolish the arrhythmogenic substrate. Also, some patients can benefit from investigational antitachycardia devices such as overdrive pacemakers or implantable defibrillators. These devices sense tachycardia rate and morphology, automatically terminating VT.

Several groups of patients may not require invasive electrophysiologic studies with serial drug testing. Those with exercise-induced VT can be approached with provocative treadmill tests and then testing with antiarrhythmic agents in a serial fashion. In these patients, $\beta$-blockers or calcium antagonists are often effective in preventing exercise-related episodes. Patients with incessant VT (by definition) usually do not have severe symptoms during their tachycardia. As VT dominates cardiac rhythm, it is relatively easy to observe drug response or nonresponse by surface electrocardiographic methods; however, some still utilize programmed stimulation to confirm a good drug response. Similarly, patients with asymptomatic and very frequent (usually many per day) salvos of nonsustained VT can be observed and treated by noninvasive methods. Because of the sporadic nature of ventricular ectopy, the VT should be detected and quantified during a control period prior to drug therapy. However, it should be noted that the treatment of brief episodes of nonsustained VT that is asymptomatic is a matter of controversy.

### *Torsades de Pointes*

Torsades de pointes (TdP) is a rapid form of polymorphic VT (Fig. 12.10) that is associated with evidence of delayed ventricular repolarization (long QT interval or prominent U waves) on surface electrocardiograms.[115] It is important to note that polymorphic VT, occurring in the setting of a normal QT interval, is similar to monomorphic VT in terms of etiology and treatment strategies.[116] TdP may occur in association with hereditary syndromes or as acquired forms.[115] Two well-described heritable forms are Romano–Ward syndrome (long QT, TdP, and high incidence of

**Figure 12.10** Electrocardiographic tracing of quinidine-induced torsades de pointes. Note the characteristic long–short initiating sequence and the polymorphic, wide QRS configuration. *(From Bauman JL, Gallastegui J: Quinidine-induced torsades de pointes. Hosp Ther 1986;11:45, with permission.)*

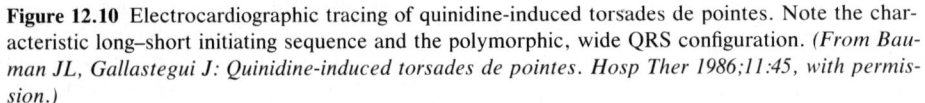

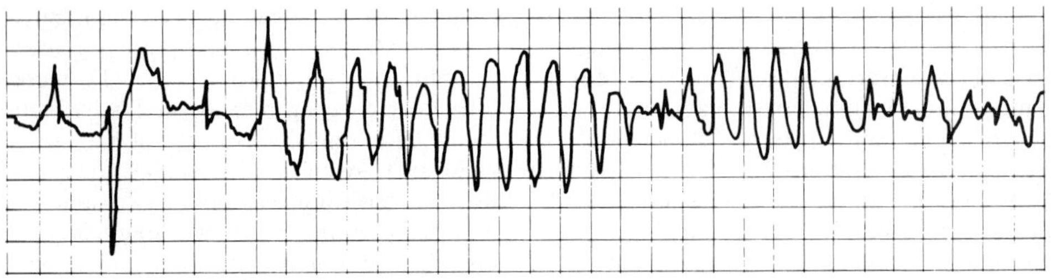

sudden death) and Jervell and Lange–Nielson syndrome (long QT, TdP, high incidence of sudden death and congenital deaf-mutism). Acquired forms of TdP are associated with electrolyte disturbances (hypokalemia or hypomagnesemia), subarachnoid hemorrhage, myocarditis, liquid protein diets, hypothyroidism, or drug therapy (notably phenothiazines, tricyclic or tetracyclic antidepressants, and antiarrhythmics). The type Ia drugs (especially quinidine) are most notorious for precipitating torsades de pointes; type Ib and Ic agents seem to cause torsades de pointes less often. The syndrome often referred to as "quinidine syndrome" is, in most cases, due to drug-induced TdP. Quinidine syncope seems to occur in association with the following factors[59,105]: (1) concurrent digitalis therapy (but not digitalis toxicity or high drug concentrations), (2) low to "therapeutic" quinidine serum concentrations without other evidence of quinidine-related toxicity such as prolonged QRS duration, (3) treatment of atrial fibrillation, (4) concurrent organic heart disease, most commonly ischemic or valvular heart diseases, (5) evidence of mild delayed repolarization prior to quinidine therapy, (6) occurrence usually within 1 week of initiation of quinidine therapy, (7) high incidence of cross-sensitivity (recurrence of TdP) with other type Ia antiarrhythmic agents, (8) frequent coexisting electrolyte disturbances such as hypokalemia or hypomagnesemia, and (9) a characteristic long–short initiating sequence of the episode of TdP. None of these associations, however, are absolute prerequisites to the occurrence of quinidine syncope and TdP.

The electrophysiologic etiology of TdP has not been fully elucidated. It has been suggested that TdP may be a result of discrepancies in ventricular repolarization and inhomogeneous ventricular recovery, allowing the formation of multiple reentrant circuits. Alternatively, recent investigations have suggested that TdP may be a result of triggered activity caused by a delay in ventricular repolarization.

For an acute episode of TdP, most patients require DCC; however, TdP tends to the paroxysmal in nature and often rapidly recurs after countershock. Therefore, after initial restoration of a stable rhythm, therapy designed to prevent recurrences of TdP should be instituted. Almost all antiarrhythmics have been reported to be successful in isolated case reports, but because of the unpredictable and self-terminating nature of TdP, it is difficult to establish a cause-and-effect relationship. Drugs that further prolong repolarization such as intravenous procainamide are absolutely contraindicated. Lidocaine is usually ineffective. It is now well established that preventive therapy should increase heart rate and thereby shorten ventricular repolarization.[115,116] Therefore, the initial treatments (after DCC) include either rapid ventricular pacing (105–120 bpm) or isoproterenol infusion. Preliminary reports suggest (for unclear reasons) that intravenous magnesium sulfate (independent of serum magnesium concentration) may provide valuable adjunctive therapy.[117] All agents that prolong QT interval should be discontinued and exacerbating factors (such as hypokalemia) corrected.

The heritable long-QT syndromes may possibly be caused by a basic derangement in centrally mediated autonomic control of cardiac rhythm. For this reason, propranolol has been shown to prevent recurrences of TdP and prevent sudden death.[118] In refractory patients, phenytoin or permanent pacing techniques have been utilized. In acquired long-QT syndromes, correction of the underlying cause is the key to long-term preventive therapy. No drug agents need be utilized on a chronic basis. In the case of quinidine syncope, type Ia agents should be avoided for the patients' underlying arrhythmias.

### *Ventricular Fibrillation*

VF is total electrical anarchy of the ventricle, resulting in no cardiac output and cardiovascular collapse. Death ensues rapidly if effective treatment measures are not taken. In patients who died suddenly during electrocardiographic monitoring, VF often preceded by VT is the most frequently documented rhythm. Sudden cardiac death accounts for about 400,000 deaths yearly, or 1,000 deaths daily, in the United States. Sudden cardiac death occurs most commonly in patients with ischemic heart disease, primary myocardial disease, WPW, mitral valve prolapse, and occasionally those without associated heart disease.[119] Patients who have sudden cardiac death (not associated with acute myocardial infarction) but survive because of appropriate cardiopulmonary resuscitation often have inducible sustained VT and/or VF during electrophysiologic studies.[120,121] These individuals are at high risk for the recurrence of VT and/or VF. In contrast, patients who have VF associated with acute myocardial infarction (MI) usually have little risk of recurrence. Approximately 50% of patients with acute MI die suddenly prior to hospitalization, presumably as a result of VF. VF associated with acute MI can be subdivided into two types: primary VF and complicated or secondary VF. Primary VF occurs in an uncomplicated MI not associated with heart failure; secondary VF occurs in an MI complicated by heart failure. The time course, incidence, mechanisms, treatment, and complications of these two forms of VF are different.[91,92] For example, about 2% to 11% patients with acute MI suffer primary VF within 24 hours of chest pain, but the risk of VF declines rapidly over time and is very low after the initial 24-hour period.[91,92] Complicated VF does not follow such a predictable time course and may occur in the late infarction period. Moreover, the value of prophylactic lidocaine has been best studied in the prevention of primary VF, with very little information in patients with heart failure complicating the infarction. The premise of prophylactic lidocaine for all patients with uncomplicated MI is based upon the inability to predict which patients are at risk for primary VF, the predictable time course of primary VF (in contrast to complicated VF), and a generally good risk-to-benefit ratio of lidocaine administration in patients without congestive heart failure and altered drug disposition.[91,92] Lie and co-workers[122] performed the classic study showing the effectiveness of lidocaine in preventing primary VF. Although lidocaine significantly reduced the incidence of VF compared with placebo, there was no difference in mortality from VF between the groups. This fact and the effectiveness of rapidly instituted DCC in modern coronary care units with sophisticated monitoring techniques have caused some to reject the notion of prophylactic lidocaine administration for all patients with uncomplicated myocardial infarction. On the other hand, some authors feel that the risk/benefit ratio favors prophylactic lidocaine therapy for 24 to 48 hours, but in a very select group of patients: those with uncomplicated infarcts (without heart failure, bradycardia, or heart block), aged less than 70 years, and presenting within 6 hours of symptoms.[122]

A patient with VF (with or without associated myocardial ischemia) should be managed according to the American Heart Association's recommendations for advanced cardiac life support.[123] Summarizing, DCC should be immediately instituted and repeated (if unsuccessful) prior to drug therapy. If DCC does not restore a stable rhythm, epinephrine (intravenous or endotracheal if a line is not established) should be administered prior to the next DCC. It should be noted that in this case, epinephrine does not act by its direct effect on cardiac conduction. Rather, the vasoconstrictive properties of this agent serve to improve coronary perfusion and thereby cause an indirect improvement in the electrophysiologic characteristics of the heart. Nevertheless, if epinephrine coupled with DCC is unsuccessful, bretylium or lidocaine should be given and DCC repeated as necessary. Bear in mind that the onset of action of bretylium can be delayed (10–20 minutes), presumably because of slow distribution to the myocardium. Procainamide can be tried in the event that the first two agents fail. Sodium bicarbonate can be administered periodically, guided by the analysis of serum pH.

Once the patient is successfully resuscitated, antiarrhythmics should be continued until the patient's rhythm and overall status are stable and then discontinued. If the episode of VF was associated with acute ischemia, long-term antiarrhythmic drugs are probably unnecessary but the patient should be monitored closely for recurrence of VT and/or VF. If, on the other hand, VF was not associated with acute MI (or a known precipitating factor), the patient should probably undergo invasive electrophysiologic studies and (depending upon the results) possibly serial drug testing by programmed stimulation for inducible VT/VF.

## Bradyarrhythmias

For the most part, the symptoms of bradyarrhythmias result from a decline in cardiac ouput. Because cardiac output increases as heart rate increases (to a point), patients experience symptoms in association with hypotension such as dizziness, syncope fatigue, and confusion. If left ventricular dysfunction exists, patients may have an exacerbation of congestive heart failure symptoms. Except in the case of recurrent syncope, these symptoms are often subtle and nonspecific.

### *Sinus Node Dysfunction*

Sinus bradyarrhythmia (heart rate < 60 bpm) is a common finding especially in young, athletically active individuals and usually neither is symptomatic nor requires therapeutic intervention. On the other hand, some patients, particularly the elderly, have sinus node dysfunction. This may be the result of underlying organic heart disease and the normal aging process which, over time, attenuates SA nodal function. Sick sinus syndrome refers to this process resulting in symptomatic sinus bradycardia and/or periods of sinus arrest.[124] Sinus node dysfunction is usually representative of diffuse conduction disease, and accompanying AV block is not uncommon. Furthermore, symptomatic bradyarrhythmias may be accompanied by paroxysmal tachycardias such as atrial fibrillation. Because of diffuse conduction disease, atrial fibrillation sometimes presents with a rather slow ventricular response (in the absence of AV nodal blocking drugs). The occurrence of alternating bradyarrhythmias and tachyarrhythmias is referred to as the "tachybrady syndrome."[124,125] The occurrence of paroxysmal atrial fibrillations in a patient with sinus node dysfunction may be caused by underlying heart disease with atrial dysfunction or atrial escape in response to reduced sinus node automaticity. In fact, as the rate of impulse generation by the sinus node is generally depressed or may fail altogether, other automatic pacemakers within the conduction system may "rescue" the sinus node. These rescue rhythms may present as paroxysmal atrial rhythms or as a junctional escape.

Another reason for paroxysmal bradycardia and sinus arrest not caused directly by sinus node dysfunction is carotid-sinus hypersensitivity.[126,127] Again, this syndrome occurs primarily in the aged with underlying heart disease. Symptoms occur when the carotid sinus is stimulated, resulting in an accentuated baroreceptor reflex. Thus, the patient may experience paroxysmal episodes of dizziness or syncope because of sinus arrest caused by increased vagal tone and sympathetic withdrawal (cardioinhibitory type), drop in systemic blood pressure caused by sympathetic withdrawal (vasodepressor type), or both (mixed cardioinhibitory and vasodepressor types). The diagnosis can be confirmed by performing carotid-sinus massage with electrocardiographic monitoring under controlled conditions.

Treatment of sinus node dysfunction involves the elimination of symptomatic bradycardia and the possibility of managing alternating tachycardias such as atrial fibrillation. In general, the long-term therapy of choice is a permanent ventricular pacemaker. Pacemaker therapy, however, should be reserved for patients with significant symptoms. In other words, the aim of pacing is not to correct electrocardiographic findings but to improve the patient's quality of life. Drugs that are commonly employed to treat supraventricular tachycardias should be used with caution (if at all) in the absence of a functioning pacemaker.[125] Type I agents such as quinidine can suppress the escape or rescue rhythms that appear in severe sinus bradycardia or sinus arrest. These drugs may also transform an asymptomatic patient with bradycardia into a symptomatic case. In addition, drugs that depress SA or AV nodal function such as $\beta$-blockers or calcium channel antagonists may significantly exacerbate bradycardia. Even agents with indirect sympatholytic actions such as $\alpha$-methyldopa or clonidine may worsen sinus node dysfunction. Digitalis use in these patients is controversial but, in most cases, is safe.

Carotid-sinus hypersensitivity can also be treated with permanent pacemaker therapy[126,127]; however, some patients (particularly those with a significant vasodepressor component) still experience syncope or dizziness. In these cases, $\alpha$-adrenergic stimulants such as ephedrine can be tried in addition to the pacemaker.

**Table 12.5** Forms of Atrioventricular Block

| *Type* | *Criteria* |
|---|---|
| First-degree block | Prolonged PR interval (>0.2 s), 1:1 AV conduction |
| Second-degree block | |
| Mobitz I | Progressive PR prolongation until QRS is dropped, 1:1 AV conduction |
| Mobitz II | Random nonconducted beats (absence of QRS), 1:1 AV conduction |
| Third-degree block | AV dissociation, absence of AV conduction |

### *Atrioventricular Block*

Conduction delay or block may occur in any area of the AV conduction system: the AV node, the His bundle, or the bundle branches. AV block is usually categorized into three different types on the basis of surface electrocardiographic findings[128] (Table 12.5). First-degree AV block is 1:1 AV conduction with a prolonged PR interval. Second-degree AV block is divided into two forms: Mobitz I AV block (or Wenckebach periodicity) is less than 1:1 AV conduction with PR intervals that lengthen progressively until a ventricular complex is dropped; Mobitz II AV block consists of intermittent random dropped ventricular beats without progressive PR lengthening. Third-degree AV block is complete heart block where AV conduction is totally absent (AV dissociation). By utilizing intracardiac His-bundle electrocardiograms, the actual site of conduction delay/block can be correlated to the aforementioned diagnosis.[129] First-degree AV block almost always represents prolonged conduction in the AV node. Mobitz I second-degree AV block is also usually due to prolonged conduction in the AV node. Indeed, Wenckebach periodicity is a normal AV nodal response to rapid supraventricular stimulation or high vagal tone. In contrast, Mobitz II AV block is usually due to conduction disease below the AV node (i.e., His bundle). Third-degree AV block may be caused by disease at any level of the AV conduction system: complete AV nodal block, His-bundle block, or trifascicular block. The ventricle will beat independently of the atrium (AV dissociation), and the rate of ventricular activation is determined by the site of AV block. The usual degree of automaticity of ventricular pacemakers progressively declines as impulses move down the conduction system. Therefore, the ventricular escape rate in cases of trifascicular block will be significantly less than that in complete AV nodal block.

AV block may be found in patients without underlying heart disease such as trained athletes or during sleep when vagal tone is high. Also, AV block may be transient where the underlying etiology is reversible as in myocarditis, in myocardial ischemia, after cardiovascular surgery, or as a result of drug therapy. β-Blockers, digitalis, or calcium antagonists may cause AV block, primarily in the AV nodal area. Type I antiarrhythmic agents may exacerbate conduction delays below the level of the AV node (sodium-dependent tissue). In other cases, AV block may be irreversible such as that resulting from acute myocardial infarction, rare degenerative diseases, primary myocardial disease, or congenital forms.

Patients with symptomatic AV block should be treated with the insertion of a ventricular pacemaker.[129,130] Patients without symptoms can usually be followed closely without the need for a pacemaker. As symptoms often correlate with the ventricular rate and the ventricular rate corresponds to the site of block, pacemaker therapy is more often necessary in distal AV blocks such as that occurring in the His bundle or the bundle branches. Patients with acute myocardial infarction and evidence of new AV block often require the insertion of a temporary transvenous pacemaker. AV block more commonly occurs as a complication of inferior wall infarcts because of high vagal innervation at this site, and the coronary blood flow to the nodal areas usually supplies the inferior wall; however, the AV block may be transient, obviating the need for permanent pacing. In patients with chronic AV conduction disturbances, intracardiac recordings (His-bundle electrocardiogram) are sometimes utilized to document the actual site of block and define the potential need for pacemaker therapy.

## References


1. Rosen MR, Wit AL, Hoffman B. Electrophysiology and pharmacology of cardiac arrhythmias. I. Cellular electrophysiology of the mammalian heart. Am Heart J 1974;88:380–385.
2. Vassalle M. Cardiac automaticity and its control. Am J Physiol 1978;233:H625–H634.
3. Page E. The electrical potential difference across the cell membrane of heart muscle. Circulation 1962;26:582–595.
4. Hauswirth O, Singh BN. Ionic mechanisms in heart muscle in relation to the genesis and the pharmacological control of cardiac arrhythmias. Pharmacol Rev 1979;30:5–64.
5. Coraboeuf E. Ionic basis of electrical activity in cardiac tissues. Am J Physiol 1978;234:H101–H116.
6. Weidmann S. Membrane excitation in cardiac muscle. Circulation 1961;24:499–505.
7. Wit AL, Rosen MR, Hoffman BF. Electrophysiology and pharmacology of cardiac arrhythmias. II. Relationship of normal and abnormal electrical activity of cardiac fibers to the genesis of arrhythmias. Am Heart J 1974;88:515–524.
8. Cranefield PF, Wit AL, Hoffman BF. Characteristics of very slow conduction. J Gen Physiol 1972;59:227–246.
9. Trautwein W. Membrane currents in cardiac muscle fibers. Physiol Rev 1973;53:793–835.
10. Baumann G, Mueller P. A molecular model of membrane excitability. J Supramol Struct 1974;2:538–557.
11. Singer SJ, Nicholson GL. The fluid mosaic mode of the structure of cell membranes. Science 1972;175:720–731.
12. Ten Eick RE, Baumgarten CM, Singer DM. Ventricular dysrhythmia: Membrane basis of currents, channels, gates and cables. Prog Cardiovasc Dis 1981;24:157–188.
13. Hoffman BF, Rosen MR, Wit AL. Electrophysiology and

pharmacology of cardiac arrhythmias. III. The causes and treatment of cardiac arrhythmias. Part A. Am Heart J 1975;89: 115–122.

14. Rosen MR, Reder RF. Does triggered activity have a role in the genesis of cardiac arrhythmias? Ann Intern Med 1981;94: 794–801.
15. Wit AL, Rosen MR. Cellular electrophysiology of cardiac arrhythmias, in Josephson ME, Wellens HJJ (eds): Tachycardias: Mechanisms, Diagnosis, Treatment. Philadelphia, Lea and Febiger, 1984, pp 1–27.
16. Bauman JL, Gallastegui J. The diagnosis and treatment of paroxysmal supraventricular tachycardia, in Ornato JP (ed): Cardiovascular Emergencies. New York, Churchill Livingstone, 1986, pp 77–96.
17. Hariman RJ, Holtzman R, Gough WB, et al. In vivo demonstration of delayed after depolarizations as a cause of ventricular rhythms in a day old infarction. J Am Coll Cardiol 1984;3: 478–486.
18. Wit AL, Rosen MR, Hoffman BF. Electrophysiology and pharmacology of cardiac arrhythmias. II. Relationship of normal and abnormal electrical activity of cardiac fibers to the genesis of arrhythmias. B. Reentry section I. Am Heart J 1974; 88:664–670.
19. Wit AL, Rosen MR, Hoffman BF. Electrophysiology and pharmacology of cardiac arrhythmias. II. Relationship of normal and abnormal electrical activity in cardiac fibers to the genesis of arrhythmias. B. Reentry section II. Am Heart J 1974;88:798–806.
20. Allessie MA, Bonke FIM, Schopman FJG. Circus movement in rabbit atrial muscle as a mechanism of tachycardia. III. The "leading circle" concept: A new model of circus movement in cardiac tissue without the involvement of an anatomic obstacle. Circ Res 1977;41:9–18.
21. Wellens HJJ, Brugada P, Farre J. Ventricular arrhythmias: Mechanisms and actions of antiarrhythmic drugs. Am Heart J 1984;107:1053–1058.
22. Gardner PI, Ursell AC, Pham TD, et al. Experimental chronic ventricular tachycardia: Anatomic and electrophysiologic substrates, in Josephson ME, Wellens HJJ (eds): Tachycardias: Mechanisms, Diagnosis, Treatment. Philadelphia, Lea and Febiger, 1984, pp 29–61.
23. Harris AS, Bisteni A, Russell RA, et al. Excitatory factors in ventricular tachycardia resulting from myocardial ischemia. Potassium, a major excitant. Science 1954;119:200–203.
24. Schamroth L. The pathogenesis and mechanism of ventricular arrhythmias. Prog Cardiol 1974;3:75–111.
25. Vaughn Williams EM. A classification of antiarrhythmic actions reassessed after a decade of new drugs. J Clin Pharmacol 1984;24:129–147.
26. Hoffman BF, Rosen MR, Wit AL. Electrophysiology and pharmacology of cardiac arrhythmias. VII. Cardiac effects of quinidine and procainamide B. Am Heart J 1975;90:117–122.
27. Bigger JT, Mandel WJ. Effect of lidocaine on conduction in canine Purkinje fibers and at the ventricular muscle–Purkinje fiber junction. J Pharmacol Exp Ther 1970;172:239–254.
28. Rosen MR, Hoffman BF, Wit AL. Electrophysiology and pharmacology of cardiac arrhythmias. V. Cardiac antiarrhythmic effects of lidocaine. Am Heart J 1975;89:526–536.
29. Kupersmith J, Antman EM, Hoffman BF. In vivo electrophysiological effects of lidocaine in canine acute myocardial infarction. Circ Res 1975;36:84–91.
30. El-Sherif N, Scherlag BJ, Lazzara R, et al. Reentrant ventricular arrhythmias in the late myocardial infarction period. 4. Mechanism of action of lidocaine. Circulation 1977;56:395–402.
31. Benowitz NC, Meister W. Clinical pharmacokinetics of lignocaine. Clin Pharmacokinet 1978;3:177–201.
32. Bauman JL, Curtis RA, Covinsky JO. Effects of antiarrhythmics in ischemic models. Am Heart J 1980;100:947–948.
33. Evans DE, Gillis RA. Effect of diphenylhydantoin and lidocaine on cardiac arrhythmias induced by hypothalamic stimulation. J Pharmacol Exp Ther 1974;191:506–517.
34. Conn HL, Luchi RJ. Some cellular and metabolic considerations relating to the action of quinidine as a prototype antiarrhythmic agent. Am J Med 1964;37:685–699.
35. Glicklich JI, Hoffman BF. Sites of action and active forms of lidocaine and some derivatives on cardiac Purkinje fibers. Am J Cardiol 1978;43:638–651.
36. Hondeghem LM, Katzung BG. Antiarrhythmic agents: The modulated receptor mechanism of action of sodium and calcium channel–blocking drugs. Ann Rev Pharmacol Toxicol 1984;24:387–423.
37. Wit AL, Hoffman BF, Rosen MR. Electrophysiology and pharmacology of cardiac arrhythmias. IX. Cardiac electrophysiology of beta adrenergic receptor stimulation and blockade. Part C. Am Heart J 1975;90:795–803.
38. Steinberg MI, Michelson EL. Cardiac electrophysiologic effects of specific class III substances, in Reiser HJ, Horowitz LN (eds): Mechanisms and Treatment of Cardiac Arrhythmias: Relevance of Basic Studies to Clinical Management. Baltimore, Urban and Schwarzenberg, 1985, pp 263–281.
39. Bigger JT, Jaffe CC. The effect of bretylium tosylate on the electrophysiologic properties of ventricular muscle and Purkinje fibers. Am J Cardiol 1973;223:757–760.
40. Patterson E, Lucchese BR. Bretylium: A prototype for future development of antidysrhythmic agents. Am Heart J 1983;106: 426–431.
41. Bauman JL, Gallastegui J, Prechel D, et al. Bethanidine sulfate in paroxysmal ventricular tachycardia: Toxicity and antifibrillatory actions. Pharmacotherapy 1986;6:184–192.
42. Heger JJ, Prystowsky EN, Jackman WM, et al. Amiodarone. Clinical efficacy and electrophysiology during long-term therapy for recurrent ventricular tachycardia or ventricular fibrillation. N Engl J Med 1981;305:539–545.
43. Antman EM, Stone PH, Miller JE, et al. Calcium channel blocking agents in the treatment of cardiovascular disorders. Part I. Basic and clinical electrophysiologic effects. Ann Intern Med 1980;93:875–885.
44. Sung RJ, Elser B, McAllister RG. Intravenous verapamil for termination of re-entrant supraventricular tachycardia. Ann Intern Med 1980;93:682–689.
45. Wu D, Kow HC, Hung JS. Exercise-triggered paroxysmal ventricular tachycardia. A repetitive rhythmic activity possibly related to after depolarization. Ann Intern Med 1981;95:410–414.
46. Bauman JL. Understanding and treating supraventricular arrhythmias. Clin Pharm 1983;2:312–320.
47. Morris D, Hurst JW. Atrial fibrillation. Curr Probl Cardiol 1980;5:1–51.
48. Josephson ME, Seides SF. Atrial flutter and fibrillation, in: Clinical Cardiac Electrophysiology: Techniques and Interpretations. Philadelphia, Lea and Febiger, 1979, pp 191–210.
49. Waldo AL, Heinthorn RW, Plumb VJ. Atrial flutter—recent observations in man, in Josephson ME, Wellens HJJ (eds): Tachycardias: Mechanisms, Diagnosis, Treatment. Philadelphia, Lea and Febiger, 1984, pp 113–135.
50. Lindsay J, Hurst JW. The clinical features of atrial flutter and their therapeutic implications. Chest 1974;66:114–121.
51. Wolf PA, Dauber TA, Thomas EH, et al. Epidemiologic

assessment of chronic atrial fibrillation and risk of stroke: The Framingham study. Neurology 1978;28:973–977.

52. Weiner P, Bassan MM, Jarchovsky J, et al. Clinical course of acute atrial fibrillation treatment with rapid digitalization. Am Heart J 1983;105:223–227.
53. Klein HO, Panzer H, Di Segni E, et al. The beneficial effects of verapamil in chronic atrial fibrillation. Arch Intern Med 1979; 139:747–749.
54. Barbarash R, Bauman JL, Srebro J, et al. Verapamil infusions in the treatment of atrial tachyarrhythmias. Crit Care Med 1986;14:886–888.
55. Morris JJ, Peter RH, McIntosh HD. Electrical conversion of atrial fibrillation: Immediate and long-term results and selection of patients. Ann Intern Med 1966;65:216–224.
56. Henry WL, Morganroth J, Pearlman AS, et al. Relations between echocardiographically determined left atrial size and atrial fibrillation. Circulation 1976;53:273–279.
57. Levine HJ. Which atrial fibrillation patients should be on chronic anticoagulation? J Cardiovasc Med 1981;6:17–32.
58. Mancini GBJ, Goldberger AL. Cardioversion of atrial fibrillation: Consideration of embolization, anticoagulation, prophylactic pacemaker and long-term success. Am Heart J 1982;104: 617–621.
59. Bauman JL, Bauernfend RA, Hoff JV, et al. Torsades de pointes due to quinidine: Observations in 31 patients. Am Heart J 1984;107:425–430.
60. Mann DL, Maisel AS, Atwood JE, et al. Absence of cardioversion induced ventricular arrhythmias in patients with therapeutic digoxin levels. J Am Coll Cardiol 1985;5:882–890.
61. Resnekov L. Drug therapy before and after electroversion of cardiac dysrhythmias. Prog Cardiovasc Dis 1974;16:531–538.
62. Josephson ME, Kastor JA. Supraventricular tachycardia: Mechanisms and management. Ann Intern Med 1977;87:346–358.
63. Bigger JT, Goldreyer BN. The mechanism of supraventricular tachycardia. Circulation 1970;42:673–688.
64. Denes P, Wu D, Dhingra RC, et al. Demonstration of dual AV nodal pathways in patients with paroxysmal supraventricular tachycardia. Circulation 1973;48:548–555.
65. Denes P, Wu D, Dhingra RC, et al. Dual atrioventricular nodal pathways. A common electrophysiological response. Br Heart J 1975;37:1069–1076.
66. Lown B, Ganong WF, Levine SA. Syndrome of short PR interval, normal QRS complex and paroxysmal rapid heart action. Circulation 1952;5:693–706.
67. Wolff L, Parkinson J, White PD. Bundle branch block with short PR interval in healthy young people prone to paroxysmal tachycardia. Am Heart J 1930;51:685–704.
68. Denes P, Wu D, Amat-Y-Leon F, et al. Determinants of atrioventricular reentrant paroxysmal tachycardia in patients with Wolff–Parkinson–White syndrome. Circulation 1978;58: 415–425.
69. Klein GJ, Bashore TM, Sellers TD, et al. Ventricular fibrillation in the Wolff–Parkinson–White syndrome. N Engl J Med 1979;301:1080–1085.
70. Wu D, Amal-Y-Leon F, Denes P, et al. Demonstration of sustained sinus and atrial reentry as a mechanism of paroxysmal supraventricular tachycardia. Circulation 1975;51:234–243.
71. Bauernfend RA, Wyndham CR, Dhingra RC, et al. Serial electrophysiologic testing of multiple drugs in patients with atrioventricular nodal reentrant paroxysmal tachycardia. Circulation 1980;62:1341–1349.
72. Wu D, Amat-Y-Leon F, Simpson R, et al. Electrophysiological studies with multiple drugs in patients with atrioventricular reentrant tachycardias utilizing an extra nodal pathway. Circulation 1977;56:727–736.
73. Rinkenberger RC, Prystowsky EN, Heger JJ, et al. Effects of intravenous and chronic oral verapamil administration in patients with supraventricular tachycardia. Circulation 1980;62: 996–1010.
74. Abrams J, Allen J, Allen D, et al. Efficacy and safety of esmolol vs. propranolol in the treatment of supraventricular tachycardia: A multicenter double blind clinical trial. Am Heart J 1985;110:913–922.
75. Belhasser B, Pellag A. Acute management of paroxysmal supraventricular tachycardia: Verapamil, adenosine triphosphate or adenosine. Am J Cardiol 1984;54:225–227.
76. Hoon TJ, Bauman JL, Rodvold KA, et al. The pharmacodynamic and pharmacokinetic differences of the D- and L-isomers of verapamil: Implications in the treatment of PSVT. Am Heart J 1986;112:396–403.
77. Bauernfeind RA, Swiryn S, Petropolous AT, et al. Concordance and discordance of drug responses in atrioventricular reentrant tachycardia. J Am Coll Cardiol 1983;2:345–350.
78. Scheinman MM, Basu D, Hollenburg M. Electrophysiologic studies in patients with persistent atrial tachycardia. Circulation 1974;50:266–273.
79. Gillette PC, Garson A. Electrophysiologic and pharmacologic characteristics of automatic ectopic atrial tachycardia. Circulation 1977;56:571–575.
80. Shine KI, Kastor JA, Yurchak AM. Multifocal atrial tachycardia: Clinical and electrocardiographic features in 32 patients. N Engl J Med 1968;279:344–349.
81. Levine JH, Michael JR, Guarnier T. Treatment of multifocal atrial tachycardia with verapamil. N Engl J Med 1985;312:21–25.
82. Lown B, Marcus F, Levine HD. Digitalis and atrial tachycardia with block. A year's experience. N Engl J Med 1959;260: 301–309.
83. Brodsky M, Wu D, Denes P, et al. Arrhythmias documented by 24 hour continuous electrocardiographic monitoring in 50 male medical students without apparent heart disease. Am J Cardiol 1977;39:390–395.
84. Bassett PA, Peter CT, Swan HJC, et al. The frequency and prognostic significance of electrocardiographic abnormalities in clinically normal individuals. Prog Cardiovas Dis 1981;23: 299–318.
85. Ruberman W, Weinblatt E, Goldberg JD, et al. Ventricular premature beats and mortality after myocardial infarction. N Engl J Med 1977;297:750–757.
86. Bigger JT, Fleiss JL, Kleiger K, et al. The relationship between ventricular arrhythmias, left ventricular dysfunction and mortality in the two years after myocardial infarction. Circulation 1984;69:250–258.
87. Lown B, Fakhro AM, Hood WB, et al. The coronary care unit. JAMA 1967;199:156–166.
88. Lie KI, Wellens HJJ, Durrer D. Characteristics and predictability of primary ventricular fibrillation. Eur J Cardiol 1974;1: 379–384.
89. El-Sherif N, Myerburg RJ, Scherlag BJ, et al. Electrocardiographic antecedents of primary ventricular fibrillation. Value of the R on T phenomenon in myocardial infarction. Br Heart J 1976;38:415–422.
90. Lown B, Wolf M. Approaches to sudden death from coronary heart disease. Circulation 1971;44:130–142.
91. Ribner HS, Isaacs ES, Frishman WH. Lidocaine prophylaxis against ventricular fibrillation in acute myocardial infarction. Prog Cardiovasc Dis 1970;21:287–312.

92. Noneman JW, Rogers JF. Lidocaine prophylaxis in acute myocardial infarction. Medicine 1978;57:501–575.
93. Whiting RB. Ventricular premature contractions. Which should be treated? Arch Intern Med 1980;140:1423–1426.
94. Rosen KM, Swiryn SP, Palileo EA, et al. Treatment of asymptomatic ventricular dysrhythmia in patients with ischemic heart disease. Arch Intern Med 1980;140:1419–1421.
95. Winkle RA. Antiarrhythmic drug effect mimicked by spontaneous variability of ventricular ectopy. Circulation 1978;57:1116–1121.
96. Morganroth J, Michelson EL, Horowitz LN, et al. Limitations of routine electrocardiographic monitoring to assess ventricular ectopic frequency. Circulation 1978;58:408–414.
97. Myerburg RJ, Conde C, Sheps DS, et al. Antiarrhythmic drug therapy in survivors of hospital cardiac arrest: Comparison of effects on chronic ventricular arrhythmias and recurrent cardiac arrest. Circulation 1979;59:855–863.
98. Kosowsky BD, Taylor J, Lown B, et al. Long-term procaine amide following acute myocardial infarction. Circulation 1973;47:1204–1210.
99. Bauman JL, Gallastegui J, Strasberg B, et al. Long-term therapy with disopyramide phosphate: Side effects and effectiveness. Am Heart J 1986;111:654–660.
100. Podrid PJ, Schoeneburger A, Lown B. Congestive heart failure caused by oral disopyramide. N Engl J Med 1980;302:614–617.
101. Schrader BJ, Bauman JL. Mexiletine commentary. Pharmacotherapy 1986;6:7–8.
102. Fogoros RN, Anderson KP, Winkle RA, et al. Amiodarone: Clinical efficacy and toxicity in 96 patients with recurrent drug refractory arrhythmias. Circulation 1983;68:88–95.
103. Poser RF, Podrid, Lombardi F, et al. Aggravation of arrhythmia induced with antiarrhythmic drugs during electrophysiologic testing. Am Heart J 1985;110:9–16.
104. Ruskin JN, McGovern B, Garan H, et al. Antiarrhythmic drugs: A possible cause of out-of-hospital cardiac arrest. N Engl J Med 1983;309:1302–1306.
105. Bauman JL, Gallastegui J. Quinidine syncope and torsades de pointes. Cardiol Board Rev 1984;1:54–64.
106. Conley MJ, McNeer JF, Lee KL, et al. Cardiac arrest complicating acute myocardial infarction: Predictability and prognosis. Am J Cardiol 1977;39:7–12.
107. Wellens HJJ, Duren DR, Lie KI. Observations on mechanisms of ventricular tachycardia in man. Circulation 1976;54:237–244.
108. Horowitz LN, Josephson ME, Farshidi A, et al. Recurrent sustained ventricular tachycardia. 3. Role of electrophysiologic study in selection of antiarrhythmic regimens. Circulation 1978;58:986–997.
109. Cameron J, Isner JM, Salem DM, et al. Cardiac electrophysiologic testing: Its role in the selection of antiarrhythmic drug regimens for supraventricular and ventricular arrhythmias. Pharmacotherapy 1985;5:95–107.
110. Josephson ME, Horowitz LN. Electrophysiologic approach to therapy of recurrent sustained ventricular tachycardia. Am J Cardiol 1979;43:631–642.
111. Wellens HJJ, Brugada P, Stevenson LUG. Programmed electrical stimulation of the heart in patients with life-threatening arrhythmias: What is the significance of induced arrhythmias and what is the correct stimulation protocol? Circulation 1985;72:1–7.
112. Greenspan AM, Spielman SR, Webb CR, et al. Efficacy of combination therapy with mexiletine and a type Ia agent for inducible ventricular tachyarrhythmias secondary to coronary artery disease. Am J Cardiol 1985;56:277–284.
113. Bauman JL, Berk SI, Hariman RJ, et al. Amiodarone for sustained ventricular tachycardia: Efficacy, safety and factors influencing long-term outcome. Am Heart J 1987;114:1436–1444.
114. Harken AH, Josephson ME. Surgical management of ventricular tachycardia, in Josephson ME, Wellens HJJ (eds): Tachycardias: Mechanisms, Diagnoses, Treatment. Philadelphia, Lea and Febiger, 1984, pp 475–487.
115. Smith WM, Gallagher JJ. Les torsades de pointes: An unusual ventricular arrhythmia. Ann Intern Med 1980;93:578–588.
116. Soffer J, Dreifus LS, Michelson EL, et al. Polymorphous ventricular tachycardia associated with normal and long QT intervals. Am J Cardiol 1982;49:2021–2029.
117. Tzivoni D, Keren A, Cohen AM, et al. Magnesium therapy for torsades de pointes. Am J Cardiol 1984;53:528–530.
118. Schwartz PJ. Idiopathic long QT syndrome: Progress and questions. Am Heart J 1985;109:399–415.
119. Zipes DP, Heger JJ, Prystowsky EN. Sudden cardiac death. Am J Med 1981;70:1151–1153.
120. Josephson ME, Horwitz LN, Spielman SR, et al. Electrophysiologic and hemodynamic studies in patients resuscitated from cardiac arrest. Am J Cardiol 1980;46:948–955.
121. Ruskin JN, DiMarco JP, Garan H. Out of hospital cardiac arrest. Electrophysiologic observation and selection of long-term antiarrhythmic therapy. N Engl J Med 1980;303:607–613.
122. Lie KI, Wellens HJJ, Van Capelle FJ. Lidocaine in the prevention of primary ventricular fibrillation. N Engl J Med 1974;291:1324–1326.
123. McIntyre KM, Lewis AJ (eds): Abridged Textbook of Advanced Cardiac Life Support. Dallas, American Heart Association, 1983.
124. Ferrer MI. The sick sinus syndrome. Circulation 1973;47:635–647.
125. Talano JV, Euler D, Randall WC, et al. Sinus node dysfunction. An overview with emphasis on autonomic and pharmacologic consideration. Am J Med 1978;64:773–781.
126. Thomas JE. Hyperactive carotid sinus reflex and carotid sinus syncope. Mayo Clin Proc 1969;44:127–139.
127. Sugrue DD, Gersh BJ, Holmes DR, et al. Symptomatic "isolated" carotid sinus hypersensitivity: Natural history and results of treatment with anticholinergic drugs or pacemaker. J Am Coll Cardiol 1986;7:158–162.
128. Kastor JA. Atrioventricular block. N Engl J Med 1975;292:462–465.
129. Narula OS, Shantha N. Atrioventricular block: Clinical concepts and His bundle electrocardiography, in Mandel WJ (ed): Cardiac Arrhythmias. Their Mechanisms, Diagnosis and Management. Philadelphia, J.B. Lippincott, 1980, pp 437–454.
130. Rosen KM, Swiryn S. Bradyarrhythmia—sinus node dysfunction and conduction defects, in Petersdorf RG, Adams RD, Braunwald E, et al. (eds): Harrison's Principles of Internal Medicine. New York, McGraw-Hill, 1983, pp 1365–1372.
131. Berry NS, Bauman JL, Gallastegui JL, et al. Analysis of antiarrhythmic drug concentrations determined during electrophysiologic drug testing in patients with inducible tachycardias. Am J Cardiol 1988;61:922–924.

# Chapter 13 / Ischemic Heart Disease

Robert L. Talbert, PharmD

There is a disorder of the breast, marked with strong and peculiar symptoms, considerable for the kind of danger belonging to it, and not extremely rare, of which I do not recollect any mention among medical authors. The seat of it and sense of strangling and anxiety with which it is attended may make it not improper to be called angina pectoris.
*(Some Account of a Disorder of the Breast—*
*William Heberden, 1768)*

Heberden, in a lecture given in Latin before the Royal College of Physicians of London, vividly described the symptoms of ischemic heart disease and the name *angina pectoris* for this syndrome has been attributed to him.[1] Although Heberden gave an accurate and complete description of this disorder, he had no idea of the origin of the symptoms or of appropriate therapy for the disease. Symptoms similar to those described by Heberden can be found in the writings of Pliny and other authors of antiquity; however, Jenner was the first to suggest during a postmortem examination that angina was due to a morbid change in the heart structure, probably ossification, or some similar disease.[2]

In 1867 Lauder Brunton first described the use of inhaled amyl nitrite to terminate an acute anginal attack, noting an onset of action of 30 to 60 seconds and "simultaneously with the flushing of the face the pain completely disappeared, and did not return."[3] He knew from the experiments of Dr. Gamgee that amyl nitrite reduced blood pressure in animals and humans and that the actions were similar to bleeding, both forms of preload reduction in contemporary terminology. Of interest, Brunton noted that repeated application of amyl nitrite caused less of an effect or that more needed to be used to obtain the same effect; nitrate tolerance was described in the first account of its therapeutic use for angina pectoris. William Murrell provided four reports detailing the use of nitroglycerin to alleviate chest pain in patients with angina in 1879.[4] Additional insight into the mechanism of nitrate action was provided by Francois-Franck, who found that these drugs were coronary vasodilating agents.[2]

After development of the string galvanometer by Ader and, subsequently, the electrocardiograph by Einthoven in 1900, Bousfield published in 1918 the first ECG recording obtained during an attack of angina.[5,6] Although suggested in earlier literature, the diagnosis of myocardial infarction in life and its association with a clot in the coronary artery are credited mainly to Herrick.[7]

The landmark work of Ahlquist in 1948 at the University of Georgia proposed the existence of adrenotropic receptors of different types, the $\alpha$ and $\beta$ receptors.[8] At the time, he thought these receptors to be an abstraction to explain observed responses of tissues produced by chemicals rather than discrete protein entities that would be studied by numerous others and the subject of thousands of future publications. In fact, his observations remained unnoticed for nearly 15 years until Black and Stephenson suggested that $\beta$-blockade should be useful in treating heart disease through reduction of the work of the heart and in treating arrhythmias.[9] Alleyne et al demonstrated that pronethalol, an early $\beta$-blocker, was effective in the treatment of angina, and thus began a revolution in the management of angina culminating in a host of drugs in this category.

In 1967, Professor Fleckenstein discovered a class of drugs that altered the transmembrane flux of calcium and interfered with the energetics of the myocardium and the function of vascular smooth muscle.[10] Initially it was thought these drugs might be $\beta$-blockers, but it was soon realized that entry of calcium though channels in the cell membrane was antagonized and the class of drugs known as calcium channel antagonists or blockers was born. Calcium channel blockers have become valuable agents in the treatment of angina as well as useful tools in gaining a further understanding of cellular physiology and pathophysiology.

## Epidemiology

The syndrome of angina pectoris is reported to occur with an average annual incidence rate (number of new cases per time period/total number of persons in the population for the same time period) of about 1.5% (range 0.1–5/1,000) depending on age, gender, and risk factor profile.[11,12] (see Figs. 13.1 and 13.2). The presenting manifestation in women is more commonly angina, while men more frequently have myocardial infarction as the initial event.[11,13] Estimates of the incidence and prevalence of angina are not entirely accurate because of the waxing and waning of symptoms; angina may disappear in up to 30% of patients with angina that is less severe and of recent onset.[11]

Data from the Framingham study show a prevalence of 5.9% for the 16-year period studied.[11] Others have reported a range of 0.4% in men aged 40–49 years with no ECG changes to 34% in elderly men (60–64 years) with positive ECG findings. The Health Insurance Plan (HIP) of New York found prevalence rates for women and men aged 55 years to be 1.5% and 3.5%, respectively. The natural history of coronary artery disease (CAD) is summarized in Figure 13.3. The risk of developing ischemic heart disease (IHD) is not the same worldwide. Such countries as Japan and France are on the low end of the spectrum, while Finland, Northern Ireland, Scotland, and South Africa have very high rates of IHD.[14]

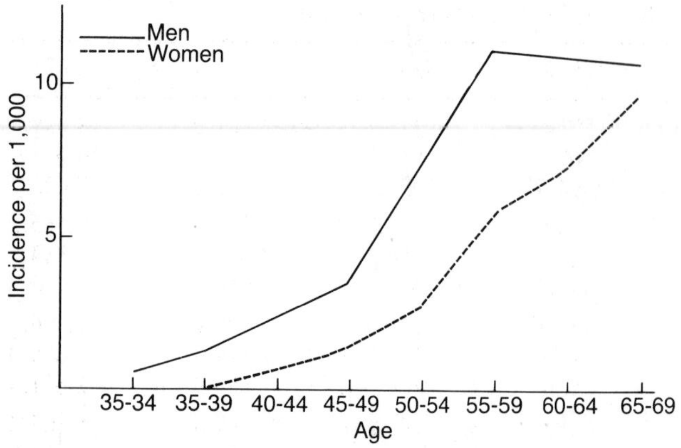


**Figure 13.1** Smoothed average annual incidence of angina pectoris as a presenting complaint. Men and women aged 33 to 69 from the Framingham study. *(From Kannel WB, Feinleib M: Natural history of angina pectoris in the Framingham study. Prognosis and survival. Am J Cardiol 1972;29:157, with permission.)*

**Figure 13.2** Average annual incidence of myocardial infarction (MI) and angina pectoris, by age and sex. *(From Shapiro S, et al: Incidence of coronary heart disease in a population insured for medical care (HIP). Myocardial infarction, angina pectoris, and possible myocardial infarction. Am J Pub Health 1969;59(6):11, with permission.)*

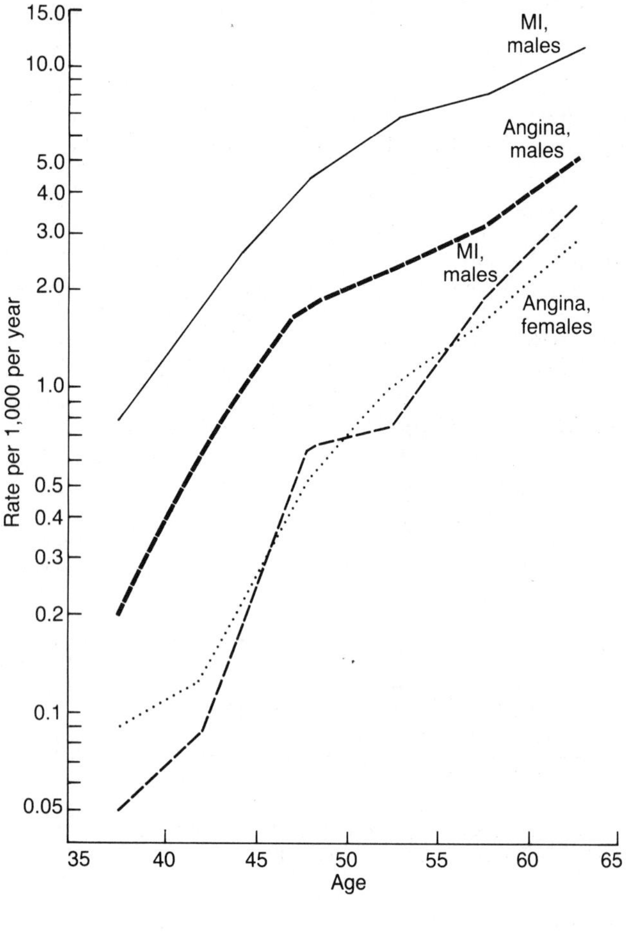


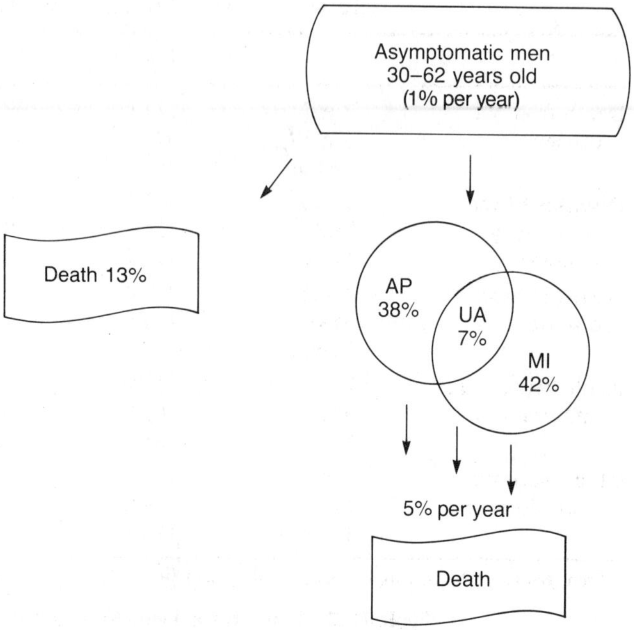


**Figure 13.3** Evolution of ischemic heart disease. AP, angina pectoris; UA, unstable angina; MI, myocardial infarction. *(From Oberman A, et al: Long term results of the medical treatment of coronary artery disease. Angiology 1977;28:161, with permission.)*

Death from IHD continues to be a major contributing source of mortality in this country (see Table 13.1). IHD was responsible for 28.4% of total mortality, acute myocardial infarction (AMI) caused 15.1% of all deaths, and other ischemic heart disease was responsible for 13.4% of total mortality in 1980. Men, regardless of age, are more likely to die from IHD and AMI than women and aging of both sexes is associated with a higher incidence of these afflictions. The disparity in mortality from IHD between men and women decreases with aging, going from about 4.7 times more common in men in their midthirties to 1.9 times more common in very elderly men.

The average annual mortality from angina is 4%; however, the risk of death is related to coronary artery anatomy, age, gender, risk factors present and their gradation, functional class of angina, and the clinical syndrome with which the patient presents.

Angina may be classified according to symptom severity or disability induced (see Table 11.5) or according to a specific activity scale[15] (see Tables 11.5 and 13.2). The latter scale was developed by Goldman and co-workers and may be preferable as it has been shown to be equal to or better than the New York Heart Association and Canadian Cardiovascular Society functional classifications for reproducibility and provides better agreement with treadmill testing.

An important determinant of outcome for the angina patient is the extent of coronary artery obstruction (see Fig. 13.4). As the number of coronary vessels involved and the extent of narrowing (greater than 75% for critical narrowing) in the obstructive process increase, the annual mortality is proportional from 1% to 2% for one-vessel disease, to 2% to 4% for two-vessel disease, to 10% to 12% for three-vessel

**Table 13.1** U.S. Mortality for 1980 by 10-year Increments (per 100,000)

| | | *All ages* | *35–44* | *45–54* | *55–64* | *65–74* | *75+* |
|---|---|---|---|---|---|---|---|
| Death from all causes | Total | 875.8 | 226.3 | 585.8 | 1,343.1 | 2,981.2 | 8,699.2 |
| | Male | 973.8 | 296.9 | 769.3 | 1,811.3 | 4,085.6 | 10,645.6 |
| | Female | 783.2 | 158.2 | 414.3 | 931.8 | 2,135.3 | 7,625.0 |
| Diseases of the circulatory system | Total | 437.2 | 55.4 | 214.6 | 584.3 | 1,513.9 | 5,545.1 |
| | Male | 458.5 | 80.0 | 321.8 | 858.5 | 2,097.5 | 6,314.5 |
| | Female | 417.1 | 31.7 | 114.3 | 343.6 | 1,066.9 | 5,120.4 |
| Ischemic heart disease | Total | 249.0 | 25.9 | 132.3 | 371.5 | 926.4 | 2,990.5 |
| | Male | 136.8 | 48.3 | 217.8 | 579.9 | 1,349.0 | 3,605.0 |
| | Female | 112.2 | 10.3 | 52.4 | 188.5 | 602.7 | 2,651.4 |
| Acute myocardial infarction | Total | 131.9 | 19.4 | 89.9 | 245.2 | 567.5 | 1,302.2 |
| | Male | 161.7 | 32.8 | 149.2 | 386.5 | 839.4 | 1,702.0 |
| | Female | 103.7 | 6.5 | 34.4 | 121.1 | 359.1 | 1,081.5 |
| Other ischemic heart disease | Total | 117.2 | 9.5 | 42.4 | 126.3 | 358.3 | 1,688.4 |
| | Male | 119.8 | 15.5 | 68.6 | 193.4 | 509.6 | 1,903.0 |
| | Female | 114.6 | 3.7 | 18.0 | 67.4 | 243.5 | 1,569.9 |

From World Health Statistics. Geneva, World Health Organization, 1984, pp 178, 180.

**Table 13.2** Criteria for Determination of the Specific Activity Scale Functional Class[a]

| | *Any yes* | *No* |
|---|---|---|
| 1. Can you walk down a flight of steps without stopping (4.5–5.2 mets)? | Go to #2 | Go to #4 |
| 2. Can you carry anything up a flight of 8 steps without stopping (5–5.5 mets)? Or can you:<br>a. Have sexual intercourse without stopping (5–5.5 mets)?<br>b. Garden, rake, weed (5.6 mets)?<br>c. Roller skate, dance fox trot (5–6 mets)?<br>d. Walk at a 4-mph rate on level ground (5–6 mets)? | Go to #3 | Class III |
| 3. Can you carry at least 24 pounds up 8 steps (10 mets)? Or can you:<br>a. Carry objects that are at least 80 pounds (18 mets)?<br>b. Do outdoor work—shovel snow, spade soil (7 mets)?<br>c. Do recreational activities such as skiing, basketball, touch football, squash, handball (7–10 mets)?<br>d. Jog/walk 5 mph (9 mets)? | Class I | Class II |
| 4. Can you shower without stopping (3.6–4.2 mets)? Or can you:<br>a. Strip and make bed (3.9–5 mets)?<br>b. Mop floors (4.2 mets)?<br>c. Hang washed clothes (4.4 mets)?<br>d. Clean windows (3.7 mets)?<br>e. Walk 2.5 mph (3–3.5 mets)?<br>f. Bowl (3–4.4 mets)?<br>g. Play golf—walk and carry clubs (4.5 mets)?<br>h. Push power lawn mower (4 mets)? | Class III | Go to #5 |
| 5. Can you dress without stopping because of symptoms (2–2.3 mets)? | Class III | Class IV |

[a] mets = metabolic equivalents of activity.

From Goldman L, Hashimoto B, Cook F, Loscazo A: Comparative reproducibility and validity of systems for assessing cardiovascular functional class: Advantages of a new specific activity scale. Circulation 1981;64:1228, with permission.

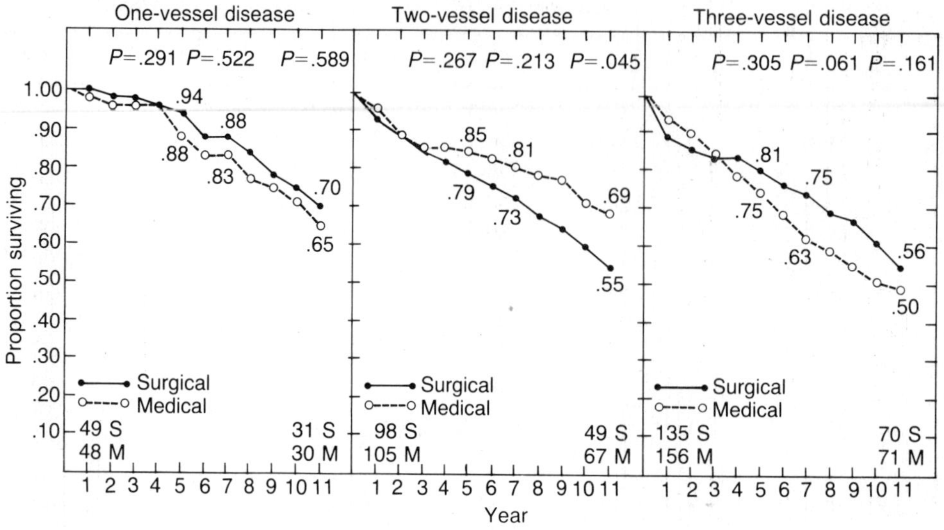


**Figure 13.4** Eleven-year survival rates for patients without left main coronary artery disease who had single-, double-, or triple-vessel disease, from the VA study. M, medical; S, surgical. *(From the Veterans Administration Coronary Artery Bypass Surgery Cooperative Study Group: Eleven-year survival in the Veterans Administration randomized trial of coronary bypass surgery for stable angina. N Engl J Med 1984;311:1335, with permission.)*

involvement. Of particular note, patients with left main artery involvement are at extremely high risk (7%–25% annual mortality) and constitute a unique group for therapeutic consideration.[16,17] The Veterans Administration Coronary Artery Bypass Surgery Cooperative Study Group (CASS) 11-year survival rates are 57% and 58% for medical treatment and surgery groups, respectively.[18] Additional information from subgroup analyses is useful in predicting the outcome of patients managed medically or surgically. Patients at high angiographic risk (three-vessel disease and impaired left ventricular function; see Fig. 13.5) and high clinical risk (defined as at least two of the following: resting ST depression, history of MI, history of hypertension), when combined with angiographic risk considerations, exercise-inducible ischemia resulting in a decline in ejection fraction, and low exercise capacity, constitute a group with a high probability of death if medical management alone is instituted.[18]

**Figure 13.5** Eleven-year cumulative survival for patients without left main coronary artery disease according to angiographic risk, from the VA study. High risk was defined as three-vessel disease plus impaired left ventricular function, and low risk as one-, two-, or three-vessel disease plus normal left ventricular function or one- or two-vessel disease plus impaired left ventricular function. M, medical; S, surgical. *(From the Veterans Administration Coronary Artery Bypass Surgery Cooperative Study Group: Eleven-year survival in the Veterans Administration randomized trial of coronary bypass surgery for stable angina. N Engl J Med 1984;311:1336, with permission.)*

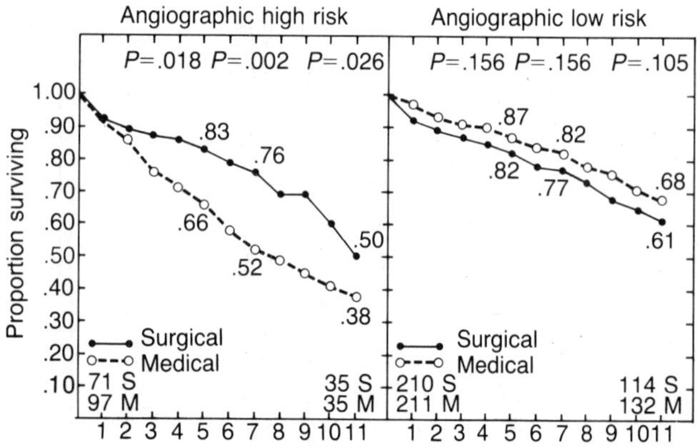


## Pathophysiology[19–21]

IHD has many clinical expressions including the following syndromes: stable exertional angina; unstable (rest, preinfarction, crescendo) angina; silent myocardial ischemia; acute coronary insufficiency; coronary vasomotion or vasospasm associated with atypical, variant, or Prinzmetal's angina; and myocardial infarction. The pathophysiology underlying this disease process is dynamic, evolutionary, and complex. To better understand the rationale for the selection and use of pharmacotherapy for IHD, one must appreciate the importance of the determinants of myocardial oxygen demand ($MVo_2$), regulation of coronary blood flow, the effects of ischemia on the mechanical and metabolic function of the myocardium, and how ischemia may be recognized so that treatment may be instituted.

Ischemia may be defined as lack of oxygen and decreased or no blood flow in the myocardium. In contrast, anoxia, defined as the absence of oxygen in the myocardium, results in continued perfusion with washout of acid by-products of glycolysis, thereby preserving the mechanical and metabolic status of the heart to a greater extent than ischemia for short periods of time.

### *Determinants of Oxygen Demand*

The major determinants of $MVo_2$ are heart rate, contractility, and intramyocardial wall tension. Overall, intramyocardial wall tension is thought to be most important among these three factors. Because the consequences of IHD are due to increased demand in the face of a fixed supply of oxygen in most situations, alterations in $MVo_2$ are critically important in producing ischemia and for interventions intended to alleviate ischemia. $MVo_2$ cannot be directly measured in patients; however, an indirect assessment that correlates reasonably well with $MVo_2$ as determined in experimental animal models is the tension–time index (TTI). This is a measure of the area under the left ventricular (LV) pressure curve. Tension in the ventricle wall is a function of the radius of the LV and intraventricular pressure. These factors are related through Laplace's law, which states that wall stress is related directly to the product of intraventricular pressure and internal radius and inversely to wall thickness multiplied by a factor of 2. Increasing systemic blood pressure or ventricular dilation would increase wall tension and oxygen demand while ventricular hypertrophy would tend to minimize increasing $MVo_2$. Clinical application of these principles has led to the use of the double product, which is heart rate multiplied by systolic blood pressure (DP = HR × SBP). While this is a clinically useful indirect estimate of $MVo_2$, it does not consider changes in contractility (an independent variable), and as only changes in pressure are considered with the double product, volume loading of the LV and increased $MVo_2$ related to ventricular dilation are underestimated.[22]

### *Regulation of Coronary Blood Flow*

Coronary blood flow is influenced by multiple factors; however, the caliber of the resistance vessels delivering blood to the myocardium and $MVo_2$ are the prime determinants in the occurrence of ischemia. The anatomy of the vascular bed will affect oxygen supply and, subsequently, myocardial metabolism and mechanical function.

#### Anatomic Factors

The normal coronary system (Fig. 13.6) consists of large epicardial or surface vessels ($R_1$), which normally offer little intrinsic resistance to myocardial flow, and intramyocardial arteries and arterioles ($R_2$), which branch into a dense capillary network (about 4,000 capillaries per square millimeter) to supply basal blood flow of 60–90 mL/min per 100 g of myocardium (Fig. 13.7). $R_1$ and $R_2$ are in series and total resistance is the algebraic sum; however, in normal circumstances, the resistance in $R_2$ is much greater. Myocardial blood flow is inversely related to arteriolar resistance and directly related to the coronary driving pressure (discussed later). The arterioles dynamically alter their intrinsic tone in response to demands for oxygen and other factors (discussed later); as a result, myocardial oxygen delivery and myocardial oxygen demand are tightly coupled in a rapidly responsive system.

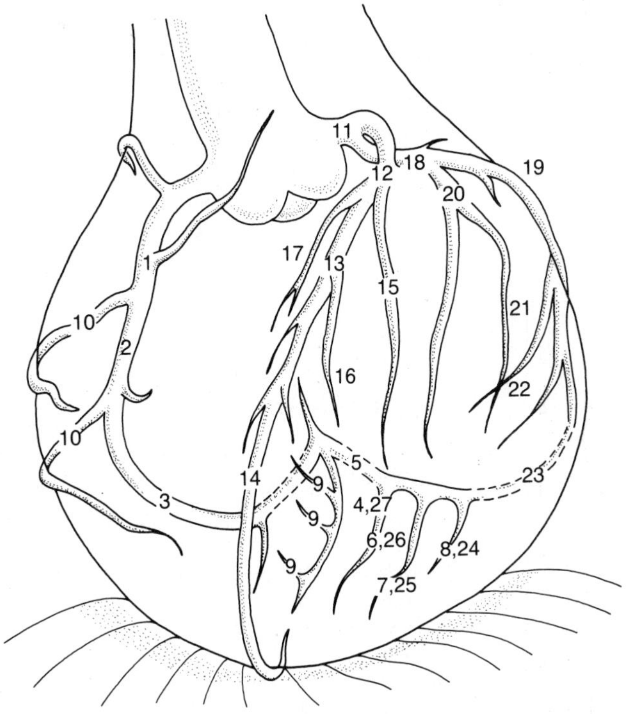


**Figure 13.6** Coronary artery anatomy visualized at angiography, as defined by cooperating centers in the Coronary Artery Surgery Study. (1) Proximal right, (2) midright, (3) distal right, (4) right posterior descending, (5) right posterior lateral segment, (6) first right posterior lateral, (7) second right posterior lateral, (8) third right posterior lateral, (9) inferior septal, (10) acute marginal, (11) left main, (12) proximal left anterior descending, (13) mid left anterior descending, (14) distal left anterior descending, (15) first diagonal, (16) second diagonal, (17) first septal, (18) proximal circumflex, (19) distal circumflex, (20) first obtuse marginal, (21) second obtuse marginal, (22) third obtuse marginal, (23) left atrioventricular, (24) first left posterior lateral, (25) second left posterior lateral, (26) third left posterior lateral, (27) left posterior descending. *(From the Principal Investigators of CASS and their associates: The National Heart, Lung, and Blood Institute coronary artery surgery study (CASS). Circulation 1981;62(Suppl I):I-1, with permission.)*

Atherosclerotic lesions encroaching on the luminal cross-sectional area of the larger epicardial vessels ($R_1$) transform the relationships among $R_1$, $R_2$, and blood flow. As resistance increases in $R_1$ as a result of occlusion, $R_2$ can vasodilate to maintain coronary blood flow (see Fig. 13.7). This response is inadequate with greater degrees of obstruction and the coronary flow reserve afforded by $R_2$ vasodilation is insufficient to meet oxygen demand (also referred to as autoregulation). This scenario is depicted in Figure 13.8 where a linear model is assumed for these effects. It has been determined that this simplistic approach does not account for the complex geometry of atherosclerotic lesions, collateral blood flow, and so on, but it is useful in describing the basic problem. Obviously, the extent of functional obstruction is important in the limitation of coronary blood flow.

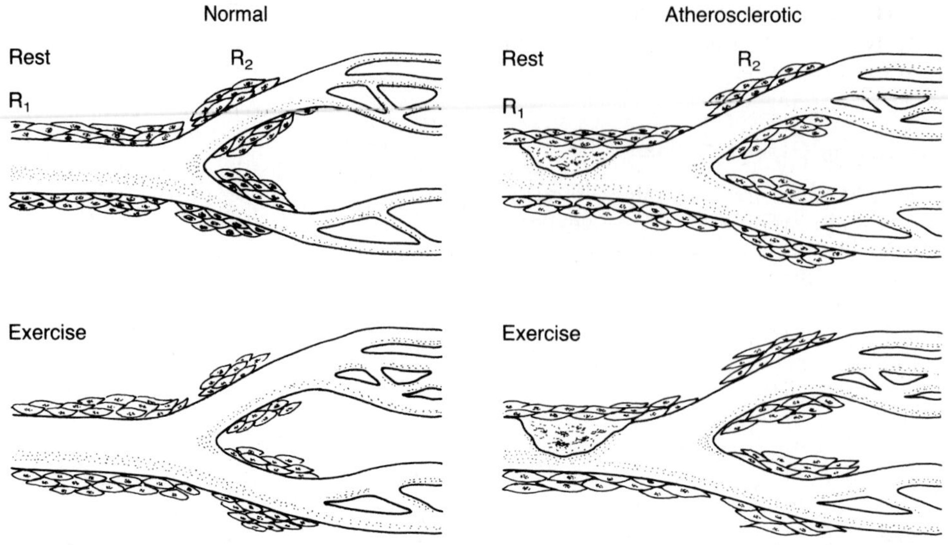


**Figure 13.7** The coronary circulation with large epicardial conductance vessels ($R_1$) that offer little intrinsic resistance to myocardial blood flow and intramyocardial resistance arterioles ($R_2$). Resistance to flow equals $R_1 + R_2$ and $R_2$ resistance is normally much greater than $R_1$; hence flow is equal to the driving pressure across the coronary bed divided by the resistance in $R_2$. Dilatation in $R_2$ normally occurs in response to exercise or increased myocardial oxygen demand. When an atherosclerotic lesion narrows the conductance vessel, the arterioles dilate under resting conditions to prevent ischemia; however, with stress, the vasodilator reserve becomes limited. *(From Epstein SE, Talbot TL: Dynamic coronary tone in precipitation, exacerbation and relief of angina pectoris. Am J Cardiol 1981;48:798, with permission.)*

**Figure 13.8** Influence of degree of stenosis on autoregulatory mechanisms that maintain appropriate levels of myocardial oxygen delivery. As epicardial coronary resistance ($R_1$) increases because of increased stenosis severity, arteriolar resistance ($R_2$) decreases, thereby maintaining total resistance (and thus flow) at normal levels. Once vasodilator reserve of $R_2$ is exhausted, however, further increases in $R_1$ lead to decreases in flow. *(From Epstein SE, et al: Hemodynamic principles in the control of coronary blood flow. Am J Cardiol 1985;56:5E, with permission.)*

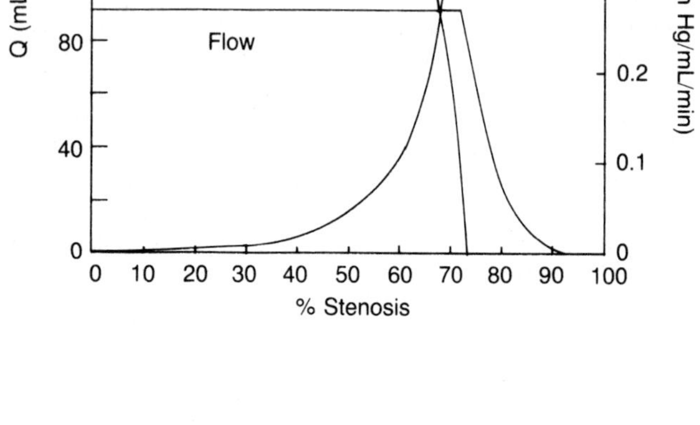

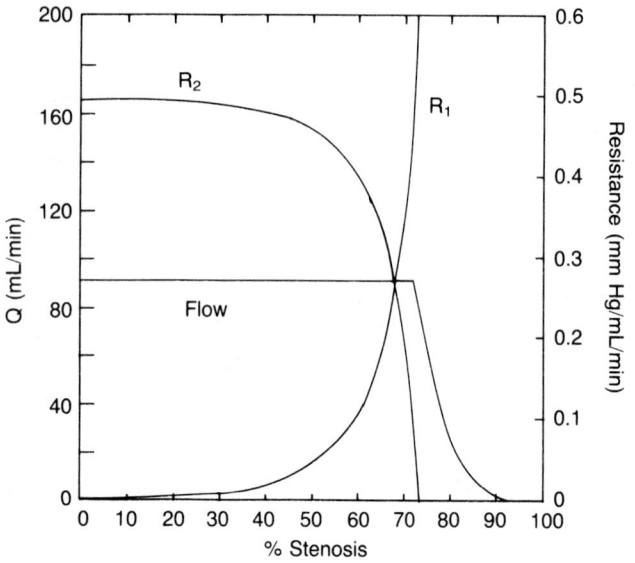


The presence of relatively severe stenosis (80%–85%) may provoke ischemia and symptoms at rest, while less severe stenosis may allow a reserve of coronary blood flow for exertion.[23]

The diameter of the lesion impeding blood flow through a vessel is important but other factors such as length of the lesion and influence of pressure drop across an area of stenosis also affect coronary blood flow and function of the collateral circulation. Resistance to flow in a vessel is directly related to length of the obstructing lesion but resistance is inversely related to the diameter of the vessel to the fourth power. Diameter is, therefore, much more important. As blood flows across a stenotic lesion the pressure drops (energy losses) because of the friction between blood and lesion and the abrupt turbulent expansion as blood emerges from the stenosis. This pressure drop is dynamic and is directly related to flow, giving rise to a resistance that is not fixed, but rather fluctuates as flow is changed. This relationship can dramatically affect collateral blood flow and its response to exercise, resulting in what has been called "coronary steal."[24] A similar situation may also occur with the epicardial or subepicardial vessels "stealing" blood flow from the endocardium in the presence of a stenotic lesion.

Large and small coronary arteries may undergo dynamic changes in coronary vascular resistance and coronary blood flow. Dynamic coronary obstruction can occur in normal vessels and vessels with stenosis in which vasomotion or spasm may be superimposed on a fixed stenosis. While it is possible that these changes may be "active" in small coronary arteries, it is also possible that the observed changes may reflect collapse as a result of poststenotic intraluminal pressure drop or increased intramyocardial compressive forces associated with inadequate ventricular relaxation.

Collateral blood flow exists to a certain extent from birth as native collaterals but persisting ischemia may promote collateral growth as developed collaterals. These two types of collaterals differ in anatomy and in their ability to regulate coronary blood flow. Collateral patency is dependent upon $MVo_2$, flow pressures, and anatomic considerations as discussed previously. Collateral development is highly species dependent and this should be considered when reading experimental literature.

### Factors Extrinsic to the Vascular Bed

Blood flow to the coronary arteries arises from the coronary sinus, and the pressure gradient between the coronary sinus and the coronary arteries determines the perfusion pressure. In a larger sense, perfusion pressure is equal to the difference between the aortic pressure at an instantaneous point in time and the intramyocardial pressure. Coronary vascular resistance is influenced by phasic systolic compression of the vascular bed. The driving force for perfusion is, therefore, not constant throughout the cardiac cycle. Opening of the aortic valve may also lead to a Venturi effect which can slightly decrease perfusion pressure. If perfusion pressure is elevated for a period of time, coronary vascular resistance declines and blood flow increases; however, continued increases in perfusion pressure, within limits, lead to a return of coronary blood flow back toward baseline levels through autoregulation.

Alterations in intramyocardial wall tension throughout the cardiac cycle also impose significant changes in coronary blood flow. Diastole is the period during which coronary artery filling can occur as a result of these pressure differences and little or no coronary blood flow occurs to the left ventricle during systole (Fig. 13.9). The extent of pressure development in the ventricle and heart rate have a major effect on the development of wall tension, time for diastolic coronary artery filling, and myocardial oxygen demand.

Under normal conditions, the average global distribution of blood flow between the epicardial and endocardial layers is about 1:1 at rest and remains approximately even during exercise secondary to autoregulatory changes. Regional disparity of blood flow distribution does exist normally, and these disparities may be magnified in the presence of diseased coronary arteries and with increased cardiac work, as vasodilator reserve in the resistance vessels of the subendocardial layers is exhausted. Factors that favor a reduction in subendocardial blood flow include decreased perfusion pressure resulting from decreased diastolic blood pressure or coronary artery obstruction by atherosclerotic plaques with or without vasomotion, abbreviation of diastole (increased heart rate), and increased intraventricular diastolic pressure (e.g., valvular obstruction to flow).

Extravascular resistance may decrease coronary blood flow, primarily during systole. This effect is much more pronounced in the left compared with the right ventricle. When the effect of increased contractility is separated from the effect of ventricular pressure, about 75% of extravascular resistance is accounted for by passive stretch in equilibrium with ventricular pressure, while only 25% results from active myocardial contraction.

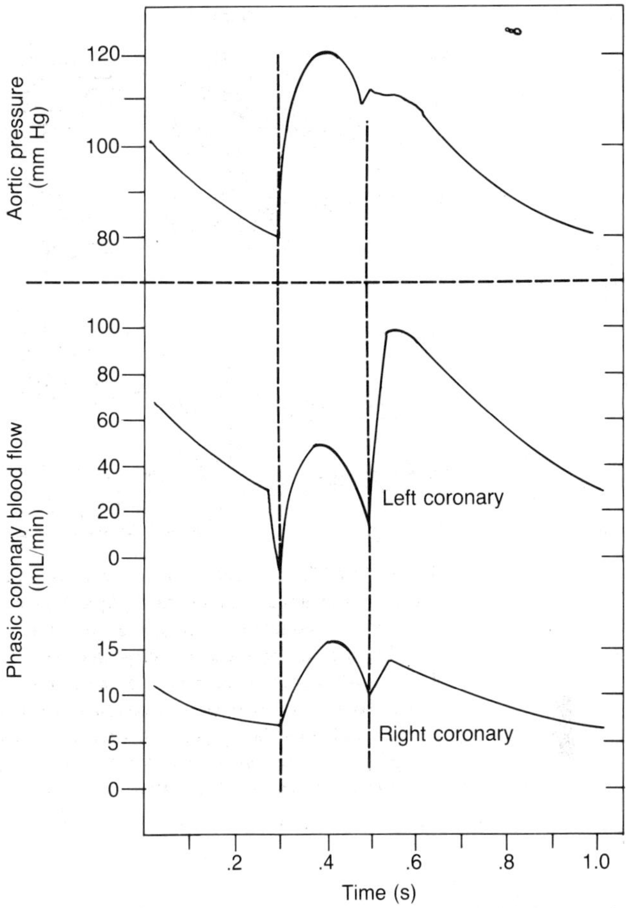


**Figure 13.9** Phasic right and left coronary artery blood flow in relation to aortic blood pressure. *(From Berne RM, Levy MD: Cardiovascular Physiology, 2nd ed, St. Louis, C.V. Mosby, 1972, p. 210, with permission.)*

### Factors Intrinsic to the Vascular Bed

Metabolic factors, myogenic responses, neural reflexes, and humoral substances within the vascular bed of the coronary circulation function in an orchestrated fashion to maintain relative consistency in blood flow to the myocardium in the face of imposed changes in perfusion pressures. Autoregulation, mediated primarily through the effects of myogenic responses and metabolic factors, is thought to be responsible for maintaining regional blood flow in a narrow range, while systemic pressure varies over a range of approximately 50–150 mm Hg.

Myogenic control (also known as the Bayliss effect) of coronary artery tone occurs when the vessel is stretched secondary to an increase in pressure and it contracts to return blood flow to normal. It is thought that the myogenic response to stretching in coronary arteries is a modest one, and that metabolic factors play a much larger role in autoregulation.

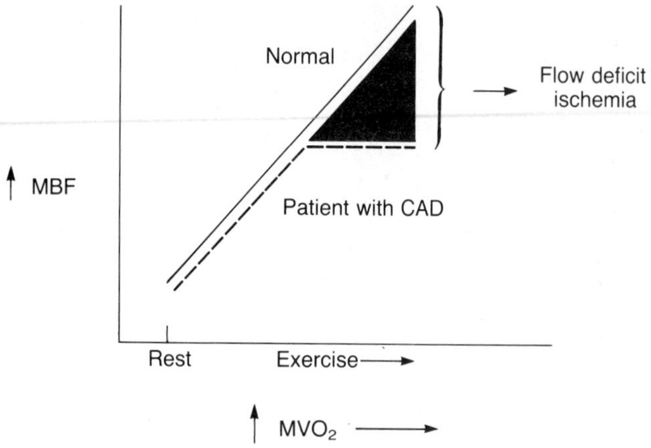


**Figure 13.10** The relation between myocardial oxygen demand ($MVo_2$) and myocardial oxygen supply. In a normal person, myocardial blood flow (MBF) increases in proportion to the increase in $MVo_2$. In a patient with a fixed obstruction resulting from coronary artery disease (CAD) in $R_1$ as shown in Figure 13.7, flow increases with increased oxygen demand until the ceiling for arteriolar dilatation ($R_2$ in Fig. 13.7) is reached. At this time, flow can no longer increase despite the continued increase in myocardial oxygen demand. A flow deficit results, leading to myocardial ischemia and angina pectoris. *(From Epstein SE, Talbot TL: Dynamic coronary tone in precipitation, exacerbation and relief of angina pectoris. Am J Cardiol 1981;48:799, with permission.)*

There are three well-studied metabolic factors that have the ability to modify coronary artery resistance and blood flow at the local level. Basal coronary blood flow meets oxygen demands of 8–10 mL/min per 100 g of myocardium with essentially complete extraction of oxygen from the blood. As cardiac output or mean arterial blood pressure increases, the increased demand for oxygen is met by increasing blood flow (see Fig. 13.10), as little additional oxygen is available from hemoglobin. Decreased oxygen availability causes vasodilation of vascular smooth muscle and relaxation of precapillary sphincters which increase tissue oxygen and help maintain blood flow on a regional basis. It is not known if these changes are due to a direct effect of hypoxia in altering the electromechanical potential of muscle cells (possibly mediated by potassium) or if vasodilating substances are produced locally in response to hypoxia.

These modulating substances for coronary vascular tone include adenosine, prostacyclin, thromboxanes, serotonin, leukotrienes, bradykinins, and potassium. At the present time, adenosine and arachidonate metabolites are considered to play the most important roles.

At perfusion pressures below 60 mm Hg, as the coronary arteries are maximally dilated and the buffering effect of autoregulation has reached its capacity, further reduction in coronary blood flow will decrease perfusion pressure and tissue oxygenation. It is thought that autoregulation works more efficiently in the epicardial layers than in subendocardial layers and this may contribute to coronary steal.

Neural components that participate in the regulation of coronary blood flow include the sympathetic nervous system, the parasympathetic nervous system, coronary reflexes, and, possibly, central control of coronary blood flow. Within the sympathetic system, stimulation of the stellate ganglion elicits coronary vasodilation, which is associated with tachycardia and enhanced contractility. This indirect coronary vasodilation is secondary to increased $MVo_2$ related to the increased heart rate, contractility, and aortic pressure that occur after stellate stimulation. The direct effect of the sympathetic system is $\alpha_1$-mediated vasoconstriction at rest and during exercise. Other receptor types, $\alpha_2$ and $\beta_1$, have little influence on tone, while $\beta_2$ stimulation produces a modest vasodilatory effect. Although coronary atherosclerosis may decrease blood flow secondary to obstruction, severe coronary atherosclerosis and obstruction may also increase the sensitivity of coronary arteries to the effects of $\alpha_1$ stimulation and vasoconstriction.

Vagal stimulation within the parasympathetic system produces a small to moderate increase in coronary blood flow that involves the coronary efferent and afferent parasympathetic components (Bezold–Jarish reflex). Acetylcholine directly causes vasodilation in large and small resistance vessels, with some preferential effect in the vessels supplying the subendocardium. Indirectly, vasoconstriction may result following vagal stimulation as the result of bradycardia and decreased contractility reducing myocardial oxygen demand.

Coronary reflexes have an undetermined role in the regulation of coronary blood flow. On the basis of experimental data, coronary reflexes that may be important include the baroreceptor, the chemoreceptor, the Bezold–Jarish reflex, and the pulmonary inhalation reflex.

### Factors Limiting Coronary Perfusion

During exercise and pacing, as $MVo_2$ increases, coronary vascular resistance can be reduced to about 25% of basal values, which results in a four- to fivefold increase in coronary blood flow. The cross-sectional area can be reduced by about 80% prior to any mechanical or biochemical changes in the myocardium, reflecting a margin of safety for coronary blood flow. The extent of cross-sectional obstruction, the length of the lesion, lesion composition, and the geometry of the obstructing lesion each can all affect flow across coronary arteries with atherosclerosis. Bernoulli's theorem states that the pressure drop across a lesion is directly related to the length of the lesion and inversely related to the radius of the lesion to the fourth power; critical stenosis occurs when the obstructing lesion encroaches upon the luminal diameter and exceeds 70% to 80%. Lesions creating obstruction of 50% to 70% may reduce blood flow; however, these reductions are not consistent and other factors such as vasospasm may be needed for any clinical manifestation to be noted. If the lesion enlarges from 80% to 90%, resistance in that vessel is tripled.[25] Coronary reserve is diminished at about 85% obstruction because of vasoconstriction. Exaggerated responsiveness can be seen when coronary stenosis reaches this critical level and such vasoactive substances as prostaglandins, thromboxanes, and serotonin may play more of a role in the regulation of coronary vascular tone and thrombosis.

Little reserve exists for coronary blood flow and a relatively small reduction of 10% to 20% results in decreased myocardial fiber shortening as the first evidence of abnormal function. The subendocardial layers are affected to a greater extent than the epicardium by ischemia, considering changes in fiber shortening, arteriovenous difference in oxygen saturation, and lactate production. A reduction of 80% gives rise to akinesis and a 95% reduction of coronary blood flow produces dyskinesis during contraction of the ventricles. Although these abnormalities of contraction are associated with transient impaired function, depletion of high-energy-phosphate compounds and ultrastructural changes may last days, even after transient ischemia; this has been referred to as *stunned myocardium*. Regional loss of contractility may impose a burden on the remaining myocardial tissue, resulting in heart failure and, therefore, increased $MVo_2$ and rapid depletion of oxygen stores. Consequently, zones of tissue with marginal blood flow may develop in a lateral or transmural fashion that are at risk of more severe damage if the ischemic episode persists or becomes more severe. Nonischemic areas of myocardium may compensate for the severely ischemic and border zones of ischemia by developing more tension than usual in an attempt to maintain cardiac output. At the cellular level, ischemia and the attendant acidosis are thought to alter calcium release from storage sites such as the sarcolemma and the sarcoplasmic reticulum as well as to inhibit the binding of calcium to troponin, thereby impairing the association of actin and myosin. The clinical correlates of these cellular biochemical events leading to the development of LV or RV dysfunction include an $S_3$, dyspnea, orthopnea, tachycardia, fluctuating blood pressure, transient murmurs, and mitral or tricuspid regurgitation.

Calcium accumulation and overload secondary to ischemia impair ventricular relaxation as well as contraction. This occurs apparently as a result of impaired calcium uptake after systole from the myofilaments, leading to a less negative decline of the pressure in the ventricle over time. Impaired relaxation is associated with enhanced diastolic stiffness, decreased rate of wall thinning, and slowed pressure decay producing an upward shift in the ventricular pressure–volume relationship; put more simply, $MVo_2$ is likely to be increased secondary to increased wall tension. Impairment of both diastolic and systolic function leads to elevation of the filling pressure of the left ventricle.

## Clinical Presentation

### *Symptoms*

The classic symptoms associated with typical chest pain and angina resulting from IHD are listed in Table 13.3. Important aspects of the clinical history for chest pain in patients with angina include the nature or quality of the pain, precipitating factors, duration, pain radiation, and response to nitroglycerin or rest. Because there can be considerable variation in the manifestations of angina, it is more accurate to refer to these symptoms as an anginal syndrome. For some patients

**Table 13.3** Characteristics of Angina Pectoris

| |
|---|
| Quality |
| Sensation of pressure or heavy weight on the chest |
| Burning sensation |
| Feeling of tightness |
| Shortness of breath with feeling of constriction about the larynx or upper trachea |
| Visceral quality (deep, heavy, squeezing, aching) |
| Gradual increase in intensity followed by gradual fading away |
| Location |
| Over the sternum or very near to it |
| Anywhere between epigastrium and pharynx |
| Occasionally limited to left shoulder and left arm |
| Rarely limited to right arm |
| Limited to lower jaw |
| Lower cervical or upper thoracic spine |
| Left interscapular or suprascapular area |
| Duration |
| 0.5–30 min |
| Precipitating factors |
| Relationship to exercise |
| Effort that involves use of arms above the head |
| Cold environment |
| Walking against the wind |
| Walking after a large meal |
| Emotional factors involved with physical exercise |
| Fright, anger |
| Coitus |
| Nitroglycerin relief |
| Relief of pain occurring within 45 s to 5 min of taking nitroglycerin |
| Radiation |
| Medical aspect of left arm |
| Left shoulder |
| Jaw |
| Occasionally right arm |

From Helfant RH, Banka VS: A Clinical and Angiographic Approach to Coronary Heart Disease. Philadelphia, F.A. Davis, 1978, p 47, with permission.

with significant coronary disease, their presenting symptoms may differ from the classic symptoms, yet the symptoms are due to ischemic pain, and these are often referred to as anginal equivalents. Obtaining an accurate and detailed family history is useful in placing symptoms in perspective. Significant positive information would include death, especially any early one, from myocardial infarction as well as the presence of nonfatal myocardial infarction or hypertension, familial lipid disorders, and diabetes mellitus. These are also obviously important in the patient under consideration, as they and smoking are major risk factors for coronary disease. Typical pain radiation patterns include anterior chest pain (96%), left upper arm pain (83.7%), left lower arm pain (29.3%), and neck pain at some time (22%). Pain from other areas is less common. Patients suffering from variant or Prinzmetal's angina secondary to coronary spasm are more likely to experience pain at rest and in the early morning hours, and the pain is not usually brought on by exertion or emotional stress nor relieved by rest; the ECG pattern is that of current of injury with ST elevation rather than depression.[26] It is also important to differentiate the pattern of pain for stable angina from that for unstable angina. The definition of unstable angina is controversial, but includes the presence of one or more of the following: (1) chest pain syndrome of new onset, usually within 1 month and brought on by moderate or minimal exertion; (2) development of crescendo (more severe) pain superimposed on a preexisting pattern of exertion-related angina; or (3) pain at rest. Ischemia may also be painless or "silent" in 60% to 100% of patients depending on the series cited and the patient population.[27] In patients with myocardial ischemia, approximately 70% of the episodes of documented ischemia are painless as determined by ambulatory ECG monitoring, and the ST-segment changes associated with these episodes can be elevation or depression. The mechanism of silent ischemia is unclear, but studies have shown that patients not experiencing pain have altered pain perception and their threshold and tolerance for pain are higher than those of patients who have pain more frequently.[28] Silent ischemia is more common in diabetic patients, perhaps because of their neuropathy and inability to sense pain. The role of altered enkephalin or endorphin concentrations remains to be clarified.

Lastly, it should be recognized that the threshold for pain caused by exertion is fixed in some patients and variable in others and that the amount of exercise or stress necessary to provoke symptoms can change over time. A fixed threshold for the induction of pain or ECG evidence of ischemia means that these indicators of ischemia occur at the same, or nearly so, double rate–pressure product. This is apparently due to at least two factors. Over long periods of time atherosclerosis may progress, leading to more severe stenosis, reduced oxygen supply, and less of an increase in demand to precipitate ischemic symptoms. Once stenotic lesions reach a critical level of about 80% or greater, vasomotion, vasospasm, and thrombotic occlusion become significant factors impairing blood flow to the myocardium. Consequently, anatomic considerations and vasoactive substances may interact to provide an environment amenable to changing thresholds for the production of angina.

There appears to be little relationship between the historic features of angina and the severity or extent of coronary artery vessel involvement. Therefore, one may speculate that severe symptoms might be associated with multivessel disease but no predictive markers exist on a routine basis.

Chest pain may resemble pain arising from a variety of noncardiac sources and the differential diagnosis of anginal pain from other etiologies may be quite difficult based on history alone. Table 13.4 outlines other common problems that may present with episodic chest pain. Although much less common, nonatherosclerotic etiologies of coronary artery disease do exist and they are outlined in Table 13.5.

There are few signs on physical exam to indicate the presence of coronary artery disease and usually only the cardiovascular system reveals any useful information. Elevated heart rate or blood pressure can yield an increased double product and may be associated with angina, and it would be important to correct extreme tachycardia or hypertension if present. Other noncardiac physical findings that suggest significant cardiovascular disease that may be associated with angina include abdominal aortic aneurysms or peripheral vascular disease. A controversial finding is that of a diagonal ear lobe crease, which is said by some to be associated with significant coronary disease. Findings on the cardiac exam that may be seen in patients with coronary artery disease are noted in Table 13.6. During an angina attack these findings may become more prominent or appear, making them more valuable if present.

Other than risk factor screening, there are no specific laboratory tests useful in diagnosing coronary artery disease. Lipid profiling with total cholesterol, high-density-lipoprotein cholesterol, and triglycerides will identify individuals susceptible to atherosclerosis. Of particular importance, total cholesterol concentrations greater than 280 mg/dL are associated with multivessel disease and should be aggressively treated with diet and possibly drug therapy (see Chapter 19). Knowledge of other lipoprotein fractions is useful in selecting appropriate therapy but has little predictive value for IHD. Future trends will undoubtably include nuclear probes for diagnosis of apoprotein abnormalities and these technologies hold great promise. Fasting glucose determinations to exclude diabetes and glucose monitoring for concurrent diabetes should be routine. Cardiac enzymes, creatine phosphokinase, lactate dehydrogenase, and serum aspartate transaminane should all be normal in the angina patient.

Chest x-ray findings of coronary artery calcification are associated with critical stenosis in 90% of patients, but there is little correlation to clinical manifestations. Fluoroscopy has been used in preliminary studies to detect coronary artery calcifications and these seem to be a strong marker for stenosis if patients are less than 50 years old.

### *Diagnostic Tests*

The resting ECG is normal in about one half of patients with angina who are not experiencing an acute attack. Consequently, the ECG is not a reliable predictor of underlying coronary artery disease unless the patient has severe disease or is having an attack. The presence of Q waves indicating myocardial infarction, old or new, or the occurrence of ventricular ectopy can be associated with coronary disease. Most commonly, ST-T-wave changes of various types with or without evidence of Q-wave (transmural) infarction are noted on the ECG. Other nonspecific findings may include conduction abnormalities and premature ventricular depolarizations while LV hypertrophy is uncommon. Typical ST-T-wave changes include depression, T-wave inversion, and ST-segment elevation (described in detail later). Some authors feel that an increased magnitude of P-wave force in lead V is suggestive for ischemia. Isolated minor ST-segment abnormalities have a predictive value of only 8%, but when combined with a positive stress test, the predictive value is increased to 44%.[29] Forms of ischemia other than exertional angina may have ECG manifestations that are different;

**Table 13.4** Differential Diagnosis of Episodic Chest Pain Resembling Angina Pectoris

| | *Duration* | *Quality* | *Provocation* | *Relief* | *Location* | *Comment* |
|---|---|---|---|---|---|---|
| Effort angina | 5–15 min | Visceral (pressure) | During effort or emotion | Rest, nitroglycerin | Substernal radiates | First episode vivid |
| Rest angina | 5–15 min | Visceral (pressure) | Spontaneous (? with exercise) | Nitroglycerin | Substernal radiates | Often nocturnal |
| Mitral prolapse | Minutes to hours | Superficial (rarely visceral) | Spontaneous (no pattern) | Time | Left anterior | No pattern, variable character |
| Esophageal reflux | 10 min to 1 h | Visceral | Recumbency, lack of food | Food, antacid | Substernal epigastric | Rarely radiates |
| Esophageal spasm | 5–60 min | Visceral | Spontaneous, cold liquids, exercise | Nitroglycerin | Substernal radiates | Mimics angina |
| Peptic ulcer | Hours | Visceral, burning | Lack of food, "acid" foods | Foods, antacids | Epigastric substernal | |
| Biliary disease | Hours | Visceral (wax and wane) | Spontaneous, food | Time, analgesia | Epigastric ? radiates | Colic |
| Cervical disc | Variable (gradually subsides) | Superficial | Head and neck movement, palpation | Time, analgesia | Arm, neck | Not relieved by rest |
| Hyperventilation | 2–3 min | Visceral | Emotion tachypnea | Stimulus removal | Substernal | Facial paresthesia |
| Musculoskeletal | Variable | Superficial | Movement palpation | Time, analgesia | Multiple | Tenderness |
| Pulmonary | 30 min + | Visceral (pressure) | Often spontaneous | Rest, time, bronchodilator | Substernal | Dyspneic |

From Christie LG Jr, Conti CR: Systematic approach to the evaluation of angina-like chest pain. Am Heart J 1981;102:897, with permission.

**Table 13.5** Etiologies of Nonatherosclerotic Artery Disease

I. Congenital disorders of the coronary arteries
   A. Anomalous origin of a coronary artery from the pulmonary artery
   B. Anomalous origin of a coronary artery from the aorta or other coronary artery
   C. Coronary arteriovenous fistula
   D. Coronary artery aneurysm
II. Hereditary metabolic derangements with coronary artery involvement
   A. Diseases causing aortic dissection
      1. Marfan's syndrome
      2. Ehlers–Danlos syndrome
   B. Pseudoxanthoma
   C. Gargoylism (Hurler's syndrome)
   D. Homocystinuria
III. Acquired disorders of the coronary arteries
   A. Embolization
   B. Dissection
   C. Syphilitic
   D. Infiltrative
      1. Tumors
      2. Amyloidosis
   E. Connective tissue diseases
      1. Periarteritis nodosa
      2. Rheumatoid arthritis
      3. Systemic lupus erythematosus
   F. Miscellaneous
      1. Irradiation
      2. Chest trauma
      3. Nitrate withdrawal

From Cohn PF (Ed): Diagnosis and Therapy of Coronary Artery Disease, 2nd ed. Boston, Martinus Nijhoff, 1985, p 496, with permission.

**Table 13.6** Cardiac Findings in Patients With Coronary Artery Disease

| *Sign* | *Clinical significance* | *Frequency* |
|---|---|---|
| Abnormal precordial systolic bulge | Left ventricular wall motion abnormality | Not usually present unless patient has sustained a prior myocardial infarction (especially anterior wall) or is experiencing angina at time of examination |
| Decreased intensity of first heart sound | Decrease in left ventricular contractility | Difficult to evaluate in resting state, but can be commonly demonstrated during angina |
| Paradoxical splitting of second sound | Left ventricular wall motion abnormality | Very uncommon, but occasionally noted during angina |
| Third heart sound (ventricular gallop) | Increased left ventricular diastolic pressure, with or without clinical congestive heart failure | Not usually present unless patient sustained an extensive myocardial infarction; may occasionally be present during angina |
| Fourth heart sound (atrial gallop) | Reduced ventricular compliance ("stiff heart") | Common; very common in patients who have sustained a prior myocardial infarction as well as during angina |
| Apical systolic murmur (in absence of rheumatic mitral regurgitation or Barlow's syndrome) | Papillary muscle dysfunction | Not usually present unless patient has sustained a prior myocardial infarction; may occasionally be present during angina |
| Diastolic murmur (in absence of aortic regurgitation) | Coronary artery stenosis | Rare |

From Cohn PF (Ed): Diagnosis and Therapy of Coronary Artery Disease, 2nd ed. Boston, Martinus Nijhoff, 1985, p 101, with permission.

variant angina is associated with ST-segment elevation, while silent ischemia may produce elevation or depression. Significant ischemia is associated with ST-segment depression greater than 2 mm, exertional hypotension, and reduced exercise tolerance.

### Exercise Tolerance Testing

Exercise tolerance (stress) testing (ETT) is useful for a history of equivocal chest pain, for risk stratification, for implementation of medical versus surgical therapy, and for assessment of the efficacy of treatment. The indications for stress testing are given in Table 13.7. False-positive and false-negative tests occur commonly in some populations and a prior knowledge of the patient's history is needed for appropriate interpretation of the ETT. Although some patients have few or no abnormalities at rest, the stress associated with exercise may precipitate angina, elevated ventricular pressures, and symptoms of heart failure or arrhythmias. Exercise may cause oxygen demand to exceed coronary reserve because of increased heart rate (primarily), increased blood pressure, and enhanced inotropic state of the myocardium, all of which are determinants of $MVo_2$. Chest pain in many patients with chronic stable exertional angina occurs at a reproducible double product, reflecting $MVo_2$,[30] and as most of the available oxygen is extracted with each pass of the circulation, coronary blood flow must increase from around 60 mL per 100 g of tissue to 240 mL per 100 g with vigorous exercise or the result is ischemia. Other causes of ischemia must be excluded for the ETT to be valid including the presence of pulmonary disease, anemia, carbon monoxide exposure, and valvular heart disease. ETT is done using graded exercise protocols, because warmup is necessary to prevent early positive tests that underrepresent the patient's capacity for exercise.

**Table 13.7** Indications for Noninvasive Exercise Stress Testing

| |
|---|
| To aid in diagnosis of chest pain |
| To evaluate the prognostic severity of coronary heart disease |
| To evaluate therapy of known coronary heart disease |
| To guide rehabilitation after myocardial infarction |
| To evaluate the benefit of surgical procedures |
| To provide a safety checkup prior to a fitness program |
| To screen high-risk professionals |
| To assess, in part, the risk factor in asymptomatic persons |

From Braunwald E (Ed): Heart Disease. A Textbook of Cardiovascular Medicine. Philadelphia, W.B. Saunders, 1984, p 258, with permission.

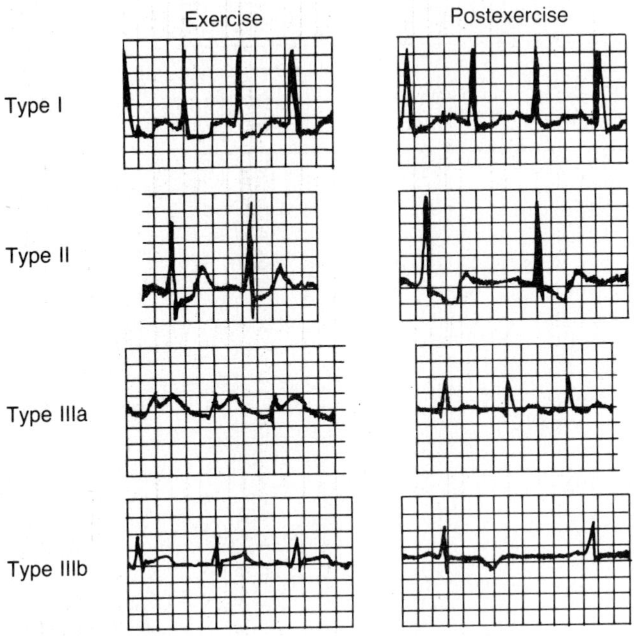


**Figure 13.11** Types of exertional ST-segment displacement: (I) Transient depression during exercise that has virtually disappeared 1 minute after exercise. (II) Depression during exercise that becomes more pronounced after exercise before belatedly returning to normal. (IIIa) ST elevation characteristic of Prinzmetal's angina. (IIIb) ST elevation of modest degree usually caused by dyskinesis or scarring of the left ventricle. *(From Braunwald E: Heart Disease. A Textbook of Cardiovascular Disease, Philadelphia, W.B. Saunders, 1984, p 267, with permission.)*

Although the ETT is insensitive for predicting coronary artery anatomy, it does correlate well with outcome from IHD such as the likelihood of progression to angina, the occurrence of AMI, and cardiovascular death.[31] The consequences of ischemia that can be seen with exercise include pain, arrhythmias, inability to reach or maintain peak levels of work or the occurrence of hypotension during or after exercise, and ST-segment displacement that may be of several different types (see Fig. 13.11). Stress testing can be carried out in a noninvasive laboratory or in an invasive setting such as the cardiac catheterization laboratory. Of the various types of exercise employed, the treadmill is the most common but bicycle ergometry and variable step procedures would be useful for the catherization laboratory and screening of large numbers of patients, respectively. Examples of specific treadmill exercise protocols are given in Table 13.8.

The duration of exercise during an ETT is determined by either open-ended or close-ended tests and by intervening events that may be harmful to the patient such as arrhythmias, hypotension, gait instability, and severe ECG changes. Open-ended testing is most common and could use the following endpoints: (1) exercise to a fixed heart rate; (2) exercise to a variable target heart rate, that is, 90% of that predicted for age; (3) symptom limited by pain or maximal tolerance to fatigue; or (4) attainment of maximal aerobic capacity or maximal oxygen uptake. Endpoint 2 is most commonly used because it balances variability with safety and convenience, which can be problems with endpoints 3 and 4.

A number of biochemical changes and pharmacologic agents can affect the outcome and interpretation of ETT and their effects should be minimized when possible. Hypertension and ventricular outflow obstruction create a pressure overload in the ventricle and cause a false positive. Hypokalemia associated with diuretic use in hypertension or other disease states may also give rise to a false-positive ETT as do Wolff–Parkinson–White syndrome and left bundle branch block. Digitalis glycosides are notorious for their effects on the ECG and they may result in ST-segment depression at rest or during exercise. Other drugs that may result in a false-positive ETT include tricyclic antidepressants and methydopa, although the evidence for their effects is not as convincing.[32] While nitrates and nifedipine are not significant sources of false-positive/false-negative ETT, $\beta$-adrenergic blockers and calcium channel antagonists such as verapamil and diltiazem may obviate the target heart rate concept. In the latter instance, exercise should be continued until ischemia occurs or until exercise intolerance develops.

Non-ECG observations during the ETT that are useful include changes in blood pressure and heart rate and, less commonly, maximal work capacity. During exercise, systolic blood pressure should progressively rise to a peak range of about 160–216 mm Hg; the change in diastolic pressure is age dependent. Failure of the blood pressure to rise reflects inadequate elevation of cardiac output in the face of vasodilation in exercising muscle. Similarly, heart rate should increase with each increment in grade and exercise, reaching a plateau as does oxygen consumption; the capacity for this rise is diminished with age. Abnormal heart rate responses during exercise would be an increment for each stage that is lower than normal and attainment of a plateau at a subnormal intensity of work. Determination of maximal work capacity is cumbersome and not usually used for routine clinical testing; however, it is useful because it correlates with outcome and a low work capacity suggests a greater probability of disease progression and cardiovascular death.

***Prognostic Significance*** Ischemic ST depression that occurs during ETT is an independent risk factor for cardiac events and cardiovascular mortality. The predictive strength of changes in the ST segment is improved when coupled with the presence of four commonly accepted risk factors, namely, positive family history of cardiovascular disease, hypertension, hypercholesterolemia, and cigarette smoking. Sequential risk assessment has shown the annual incidence of coronary events to be 27.8 per 1,000 if ST depression is evident on ETT and one or more risk factors are present. Accordingly, if neither ST depression nor risk factors are present the annual incidence is 2.2 per 1,000 men and if either ST changes or risk factors are present, 3.8 per 1,000 men.[33] In general, the greater the ST depression, the greater the chance of multivessel disease.[34] The presence or absence of ST depression carries significance for the occurrence of coronary heart disease events in other populations, such as those with hypertension and atypical chest pain, as well as in patients who have classical angina with exercise. As discussed previously, abnormal blood pressure and heart rate responses are ominous findings, and ST depression in pa-

**Table 13.8** Three Treadmill Exercise Test Protocols

| | *Stage* | *Speed (mph)* | *Elevation (% grade)* | *Duration (min)* | *Approximate $Vo_2$/kg/min (mL)* |
|---|---|---|---|---|---|
| Bruce test | 1 | 1.7 | 10.0 | 3 | 18.0 |
| | 2 | 2.5 | 12.0 | 3 | 25.0 |
| | 3 | 3.4 | 14.0 | 3 | 34.0 |
| | 4 | 4.2 | 16.0 | 3 | 46.0 |
| | 5 | 5.0 | 18.0 | 3 | 55.0 |
| | 6 | 5.5 | 20.0 | 3 | — |
| | 7 | 6.0 | 22.0 | 3 | — |
| Modified Naughton test | 1 | 2.0 | 0.0 | 3 | 7.0 |
| | 2 | 2.0 | 3.5 | 3 | 10.5 |
| | 3 | 2.0 | 7.0 | 3 | 14.0 |
| | 4 | 2.0 | 10.5 | 3 | 17.5 |
| | 5 | 2.0 | 14.0 | 3 | 21.0 |
| | 6 | 2.0 | 17.5 | 3 | 24.5 |
| | 7 | 3.0 | 12.5 | 3 | 28.0 |
| | 8 | 3.0 | 15.0 | 3 | 31.5 |
| | 9 | 3.0 | 17.5 | 3 | 35.0 |
| | 10 | 3.0 | 20.0 | 3 | 38.5 |
| | 11 | 3.0 | 22.5 | 3 | 42.0 |
| | 12 | 3.4 | 20.0 | 3 | 45.5 |
| | 13 | 3.4 | 22.0 | 3 | 49.0 |
| | 14 | 3.4 | 24.0 | 3 | 52.5 |
| | 15 | 3.4 | 26.0 | 3 | 56.0 |
| Sheffield test[a] (GXT) | 0 | 1.7 | 0.0 | 3 | 8.0 |
| | 1/2 | 1.7 | 5.0 | 3 | 12.0 |
| | 1 | 1.7 | 10.0 | 3 | 18.0 |

[a] Stages 2 through 7 of the Sheffield test are identical to those of the Bruce test.

From Braunwald E (Ed): Heart Disease. A Textbook of Cardiovascular Medicine. Philadelphia, W.B. Saunders, 1984, p 266, with permission.

tients with cardiomegaly suggests the need for more invasive studies as extensive coronary disease is likely.

***Safety*** ETT is considered to be an extremely safe diagnostic test provided that the contraindications to its use are observed (see Table 13.9). The reported mortality rate for ETT is 10/100,000 tests and the rate for morbidity, 24/100,000 tests. Primary ventricular fibrillation occurs in 0.03% and it is most likely to be seen in men with a history of coronary heart disease and exertional hypotension during exercise.[35,36]

Thallium ($^{201}$Tl) myocardial perfusion scintigraphy may be used in conjunction with ETT to detect reversible and irreversible defects in blood flow to the myocardium. $^{201}$Tl, a potassium analogue, is delivered to the myocardium based on blood flow and extraction of the radionuclide by the myocardium cells. Defects in uptake resolving in 2 to 4 hours (up to 24 hours in some instances) are indicative of a redistribution process and reversible ischemia; irreversible defects or "cold spots" indicate myocardial scar resulting from infarction. Stress $^{201}$Tl scintigraphy is useful for improving the sensitivity and specificity of ETT and for overcoming the limitations of ETT in the presence of resting or exercise ECG abnormalities associated with conduction abnormalities, LV hypertrophy, and digoxin. The sensitivity and specificity of ETT and $^{201}$Tl scintigraphy are dependent on the population studied, and Bayesian approaches that consider the pretest probability of coronary artery disease benefit the application of either technique.[37,38]

Radionuclide angiocardiography, usually performed with

**Table 13.9** Contraindications to Exercise Testing

| |
|---|
| Myocardial infarction—impending, acute, or healing |
| Unstable angina pectoris |
| Acute myocarditis or pericarditis |
| Known ominous coronary artery disease pattern |
| Severe hypertension |
| Uncontrolled cardiac arrhythmias |
| Intracardiac conduction block greater than first degree |
| Acute systemic illness |
| Unwillingness to give informed consent |

From Braunwald E (Ed): Heart Disease. A Textbook of Cardiovascular Medicine. Philadelphia, W.B. Saunders, 1984, p 258, with permission.

technetium-99*m*, can be used to measure ejection fraction, regional ventricular performance, cardiac output, ventricular volumes, valvular regurgitation, asynchrony or wall motion abnormalities, and intracardiac shunts. Two methods have been employed, first-pass and equilibrium studies. First-pass radionuclide angiocardiography is based on the appearance of radioactive counts in the heart during the first pass of the radiotracer, whereas count acquisition for equilibrium studies is gated to a physiologic marker, usually the R wave of the ECG. The radioactivity counts from each gate (40–50 milliseconds each), representing a fraction of each cardiac cycle, are summed over time for about 2 minutes. These data are then reformatted into time–activity curves, corrected for background activity; geometric approaches or analysis of changes in count rate can be used to calculate the measurement of interest. Both first-pass and equilibrium studies can be performed at rest or during exercise, the latter being more useful in the detection and quantification of coronary artery disease and the effects of ischemia. Equilibrium studies using this multigated acquisition of radioactivity counts are sometimes referred to as MUGA. Resting and exercise LV performance and markers of ischemia derived from these methods are used along with clinical history and ETT information to aid in diagnosis of IHD and in quantitation of the severity of disease as well as in risk stratification for predicting long-term cardiovascular mortality and morbidity.

Other types of cardiac imaging used to study myocardial infarction and metabolism are available, some for routine use and others primarily for clinical investigation. Technetium pyrophosphate scans are used routinely for detection and quantification of acute myocardial infarction (see Chapter 14). Less commonly available techniques involving positron emission tomography with metabolically important substrates such as oxygen, carbon, and nitrogen are providing insight into the pathogenesis of ischemia. Other metabolic probes utilize radiolabeled fatty acids and glucose to study metabolic processes that may be deranged during ischemia in animals and for investigative purposes in humans.

Echocardiography has become an increasingly useful noninvasive tool in diagnosing the presence of coronary artery disease and assessing its functional consequences. Of the types of echocardiography available, M-mode and cross-sectional or two-dimensional (2-D), 2-D is more commonly used for IHD. Echocardiography has been shown to be useful for direct visualization of lesions in the left main coronary artery and in providing information concerning some of the complications of IHD, including the presence of ventricular aneurysms, and assessing hemodynamic function. Other uses include measurement of ejection fraction and detection of the regional or global LV function abnormalities that occur during ischemic episodes. One recent adaptation of echocardiography that yields accurate estimates of the extent of disease prior to revascularization surgery is epicardial echocardiography; however, it is not commonly available.[39]

### Ambulatory Electrocardiographic (Holter) Monitoring

Ambulatory electrocardiographic monitoring, sometimes referred to as Holter monitoring after the inventor of this method, has been used to record the ECG over variable periods but most commonly for 24-hour recordings. The role of Holter monitoring in the detection of and assessment of treatment of arrhythmias is well established; however, its use in patients with IHD remains controversial.[40] A major consideration in Holter monitoring is the interpretation of ST-segment changes resulting from nonischemic events such as hyperventilation, mechanical artifact, electrolyte disorders, and drug effects. Computer analysis of data derived from ambulatory monitoring has been useful in limiting artifact, thereby separating it from significant ST-segment deviation, and this technologic advance may lead to greater use of this method. At the present time, Holter monitoring appears to be most useful in detecting the presence of ischemia that does not cause pain, silent myocardial ischemia. In patients with documented coronary heart disease, Holter monitoring has shown that about 75% of ischemic episodes are silent, and in well-controlled studies, these events correlate with other markers for ischemia such as ventricular dysfunction or perfusion abnormalities. Both depression and elevation of the ST segment occur during silent ischemia, and ST-segment deviation is not always related to exercise or stress, suggesting that primary alterations in coronary artery tone are responsible. These findings are important, as the total burden of ischemia may be underestimated if reliance is placed on symptomatic complaints, and suggest that therapy for IHD must prevent not only ST-segment changes associated with pain, but also painless episodes not associated with a primary increase in myocardial oxygen demand.

### Cardiac Catheterization and Coronary Arteriography

In 1929, a German physician, Werner Forssmann, inserted a catheter into his right atrium under fluoroscopy to perform the first right heart catheterization in man. Some years later, Sones developed the brachial cutdown approach for selective catheterization in 1962 and Jukins developed the femoral approach in 1967. These two methods are still widely used techniques in cardiac catheterization and coronary angiography and these diagnostic tests have become the "gold standard" with which all noninvasive diagnostic methods are compared. Catheterization and angiography are important in determining the in vivo morphologic characteristics of the coronary circulation as well as the LV performance characteristics. The coronary circulation as visualized by these methods bears a reasonable correlation to the findings seen in postmortem studies, but arteriography may underestimate the physiologic significance as the interpretation of stenosis is based on the assumption that surrounding segments are normal. Coronary angiographic studies allow the detection of as little as 20% narrowing of the arteries involved and a critical stenosis of 75% or greater can almost always be accurately shown. Cardiac catheterization and angiography in patients with suspected coronary artery disease are used diagnostically to document the presence and severity of disease as well as for prognostic purposes. Interventional catheterization is used for thrombolytic therapy in patients with acute myocardial infarction and for the management of patients with significant coronary artery disease to relieve obstruction through percutaneous transluminal coronary angioplasty (PTCA).

The indications for cardiac catheterization and coronary arteriography are listed in Table 13.10. Patients presenting

**Table 13.10** Indications for Diagnostic Cardiac Catheterization

**A. Patients in whom chest pain is the predominant symptom**
1. Chronic chest pain
   a. Severe angina pectoris
   b. Angina that is not severe
   c. Atypical chest pain
2. Unstable angina pectoris
3. Prinzmetal's angina
4. Preoperative evaluation of valvular heart disease
5. Evaluation of recurrent angina after bypass surgery
6. Suspected anomalies of the coronary circulation

**B. Patients in whom chest pain is absent or is not the predominant symptom**
1. Asymptomatic individuals with abnormal ECGs
2. Asymptomatic individuals with normal ECGs
3. Persistent heart failure or shock after a myocardial infarction
4. Unexplained ventricular failure as the predominant symptom
5. Preoperative evaluation of valvular heart disease
6. Intractable ventricular arrhythmias or history of cardiac arrest not associated with recent myocardial infarction
7. Suspected congenital anomalies of the coronary circulation
8. Evaluation of the coronary circulation after bypass surgery

From Cohn PF (Ed): Diagnosis and Therapy of Coronary Artery Disease, 2nd ed, Boston, Martinus Nijhoff, 1985, p 496, with permission.

with chest pain as the predominant symptom may be subdivided according to the severity of pain. The typical patient with severe angina pectoris is a middle-aged man with multiple risk factors who has had typical angina pectoris for years and who is less than optimally controlled with medical management. In this instance, these procedures usually are a prelude to either coronary artery bypass grafting (CABG) to revascularize the myocardium or PTCA to improve blood supply. At the time of catheterization, not only are the site and severity of stenoses determined, but ventricular function is also assessed. Catheterization is performed in patients with less severe angina for intervention purposes as well as for prognostic purposes. If no disease is present or if stenosis is limited to a single lesion, compared with three-vessel disease or left main stenosis, the prognosis is quite different. Left main stenosis carries an average yearly mortality of about 10%, whereas less extensive disease is associated with annual mortality of about 4%. ETT screening prior to catheterization and arteriography is useful in recognizing patients who have left main disease or left main "equivalent" disease. The latter is severe narrowing of the proximal left anterior artery with narrowing in the circumflex trunks. ECG changes during moderate exercise, particularly when occurring with hypotensive responses to exercise, of 2 mm depression or greater are more common with left main stenosis or left main equivalent narrowing. Patients with valvular heart disease may have angina as a result of valvular stenosis imposing a pressure load on the left ventricle, or coronary disease, or both. Catheterization and arteriography may be done after CABG to determine if the graft has closed or if coronary artery disease has progressed.

When chest pain is not the predominant symptom, cardiac catheterizations and arteriography are usually performed after the finding of an abnormal ECG in individuals having an occupation that might endanger public safety, such as an airline pilot or a bus driver. A markedly abnormal ETT that is correlated with more severe disease may prompt cardiac catheterization and arteriography in some instances. Lastly, this procedure is performed under research protocols for high-risk patients, for example, patients with familial hyperlipidemia, for study purposes, and in selected other situations.

Inherent in the decision to perform cardiac catheterization and arteriography is the assumption that the center undertaking this procedure has adequately trained staff to safely complete the procedure. The incidence of complications is related to the expertise and experience of the operators involved and lack of an adequate case load may result in unacceptably high complication rates. Contraindications to cardiac catheterization include the presence of fever, incompetence, overt or latent electrical instability caused by electrolyte or acid–base disorders and drugs, previous reactions to contrast agents used in the procedure, severe involvement of other organ systems (e.g., stroke, cancer), well-established myocardial infarction (between 6 hours and 3 weeks), and bleeding diatheses. The latter contraindication could be related to the use of anticoagulants and, in general, if a patient is on chronic warfarin therapy, heparin should be substituted and then discontinued about 6 hours prior to the procedure. Complications associated with coronary arteriography are provided in Table 13.11.[41,42] Overall, significant complications arise in about 1.8% of patients studied and mortality from the procedure is reported to range from 0.05% to 2.37%, emphasizing how important it is that a well-trained team undertake these procedures.

Prophylactic antibiotics may be indicated for patients with recognized valvular heart disease to prevent infective endocarditis from complicating the procedure. Preoperative anxiolytic and analgesic medications are used conjunctively with patient education and reassurance to allay fear of the

**Table 13.11** Complications of Coronary Arteriography

| *Complication* | *Incidence (%)*[a] | | |
|---|---|---|---|
| | **Overall** | **Brachial** | **Femoral** |
| Death | 0.14 | 0.12 | 0.16 |
| Myocardial infarction | 0.18 | 0.15 | 0.20 |
| Ventricular fibrillation | 0.76 | 0.70 | 0.82 |
| Thrombosis | 0.67 | 1.13 | 0.20 |
| Hemorrhage | 0.09 | 0.05 | 0.14 |
| Pseudoaneurysm | 0.04 | 0.04 | 0.05 |
| Cerebral embolus | 0.09 | 0.08 | 0.09 |
| Contrast reaction | 1.08 | 1.17 | 1.00 |

[a] Number of patients = 89,079.

From Cohn PF, Goldberg S. Cardiac catheterization and coronary arteriography, in Diagnosis and Therapy of Coronary Artery Disease, 2nd ed. Cohn PF (ed): Boston, Martinus Nijhoff, 1985, p 227.

procedure. Other medications that may be used during catheterization and arteriography include intravenous or sublingual nitroglycerin or sublingual nifedipine for chest pain, antiarrhythmic agents for serious ventricular or supraventricular arrhythmias, and vasopressor and positive inotropic drugs to support blood pressure or increase cardiac output as necessary.

Grading of the stenotic lesions observed during arteriography is usually done by eye-reporting the number of vessels involved, the extent or severity of involvement, the location of the stenotic lesion(s), and the geometry of the lesions noted. A standardized grading scale has been developed and is presented in Figure 13.12. Narrowing is graded on a scale from 25% to 100%, and a severity score ranging from 1 to 32 is assigned, as flow is inversely proportional to the fourth power of the radius (Poiseuille's law) rather than directly proportional.

## Treatment

### *Modification of Risk Factors*

Primary prevention of ischemic heart disease through the identification and modification of risk factors prior to the initial morbid event would be the optimal management approach and should result in a significant impact on the prevalence of IHD; however, early recognition of some risk factors may not be possible in all patients, and in others, the patient may not be willing to undertake intervention until overt evidence of coronary disease is apparent. Secondary intervention continues to be more commonly pursued by both health care professionals and patients and it is important to recognize that this type of intervention is effective in reducing subsequent morbidity and mortality. The presence of risk factors in individual patients plays a major role in determining the occurrence and severity of IHD. Risk factors are additive in nature and can be classified as alterable or unalterable. Unalterable risk factors include gender, age, family history or genetic composition, environmental influences such as climate, air pollution, trace metal composition of drinking water, and, to some extent, diabetes mellitus.

**Figure 13.12** The roentgenographic appearance of concentric lesions and eccentric plaques resulting in 25%, 50%, 75%, 90%, and "99%" obstruction as well as complete (100%) occlusion. The column on the right indicates the relative severity of these lesions using a score of 1 for the 25% obstruction and doubling that number as the severity of these obstructions progresses according to the reduction of lumen diameter (left column). *(From Gensini GG: Coronary Arteriography. Mount Kisco, NY, Futura, 1975, with permission.)*

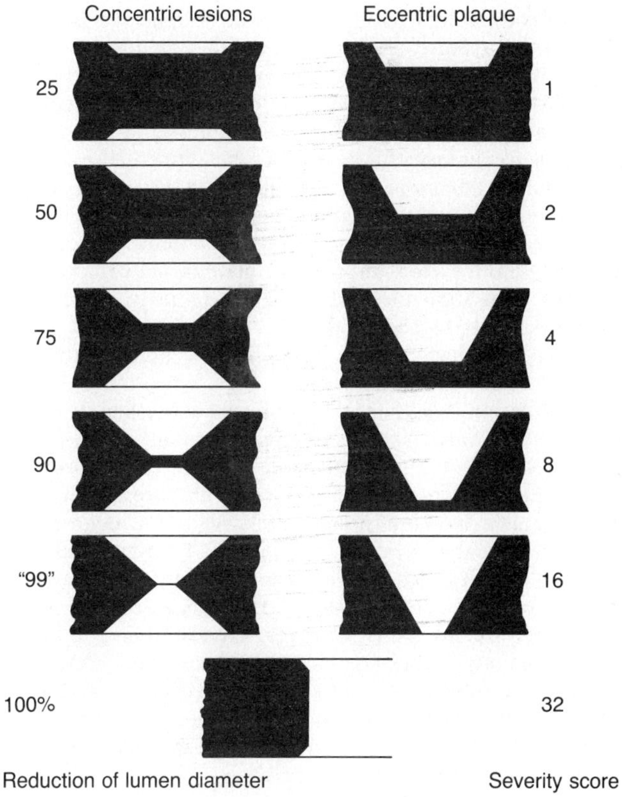

Although it is thought by many that glycemic control that mimics normoglycemia to the degree possible will reduce the complications of diabetes including coronary disease, evidence for this benefit on coronary heart disease is not readily available. Risk factors that can be altered include smoking, hypertension, hyperlipidemia, obesity, sedentary life-style, hyperuricemia, psychosocial factors such as stress and type A behavior patterns, and the use of certain drugs that may be detrimental including estrogens, thiazide diuretics, and $\beta$-adrenergic blocking agents.

Cigarette smoking is common; there are some 50 million regular smokers in this country. The evidence that smokers have a coronary mortality rate two- to threefold higher than that of nonsmokers is unequivocal. Of the 325,000 premature deaths each year caused by smoking, one third are due to coronary heart disease.[43] Risk from smoking is related to the number of cigarettes smoked per day and the duration of smoking; however, even nonsmokers may be affected, as passive smoking has been shown to decrease exercise time in angina pectoris patients. Pipe and cigar smokers are at increased risk compared with nonsmokers but their risk is somewhat less than that of cigarette smokers. The direct effects of cigarette smoke detrimental to patients with angina include the following: (1) Heart rate and blood pressure are elevated by nicotine, which increases $MVo_2$, and impaired myocardial oxygen delivery resulting from the carboxyhemoglobin generated by inhalation of the carbon monoxide in smoke. (2) Carboxyhemoglobin has a negative inotropic effect. (3) Nicotine and carboxyhemoglobin increase platelet adhesiveness and promote aggregation, resulting in thrombotic tendencies. (4) Carboxyhemoglobin lowers the threshold for ventricular fibrillation during ischemia. Similar changes have been noted for marijuana smoking as well. Smoking also accelerates the risk for myocardial infarction, sudden death, cerebrovascular disease, peripheral vascular disease, and hypertension and it reduces high-density-lipoprotein concentrations. Clearly, primary prevention is needed for this risk factor and much of the educational effort to discourage initiation of smoking should be targeted for teenagers. Techniques for cessation of smoking that may be useful include adversive conditioning, group programs, self-help programs, hypnosis, cold turkey, and use of nicotine substitutes (lobeline) or other sources of nicotine (Nicorette chewing gum) for short-term substitution during withdrawal attempts. Cessation of smoking reduces the incidence of coronary events to about one half of that associated with continued smoking, and these benefits are noted within 2 years of cessation.[44]

Hypertension, whether labile or fixed, borderline or definite, casual or basal, systolic or diastolic, at any age regardless of gender, is the most common and a powerful contributor to atherosclerotic coronary vascular disease. Morbidity and mortality increase progressively with the degree of elevation of either systolic or diastolic pressure and no discernible critical value exists (see Chapter 10). Numerous trials have documented the reduction in risk associated with blood pressure lowering; however, most of these studies show that mortality and morbidity reduction is due to fewer strokes and less renal failure and heart failure, and the reduction in coronary heart disease endpoints is not as dramatic. The reasons are unclear but perhaps relate to the multifactorial etiology of IHD.

Hypercholesterolemia is a significant cardiovascular risk factor and risk is directly related to the degree of cholesterol elevation. As with hypertension, no critical value defines risk; rather, risk is incrementally related to the degree of elevation and the presence of other risk factors (see Chapter 19). The role of triglycerides in coronary artery disease remains a controversial issue; however, most would agree that gross elevations, greater than 500 mg/dL, should be treated. In addition to total cholesterol determination, high-density-lipoprotein, low-density-protein and very-low-density-lipoprotein concentration determinations are useful in determining the specific lipid disorder type and for prognostic purposes. Primary intervention with diet therapy has shown mortality to be reduced in some but not all trials and only cholestyramine has been successfully used as a primary pharmacologic intervention in a large trial, the Lipid Research Clinics Program.[45] This program did show that cholestyramine reduced mortality in the high-risk patients studied. Aggressive dietary alteration may result in excessive polyunsaturated fat intake and low serum cholesterol levels but the adverse effects, if any, of these manipulations are not well documented. Secondary intervention in patients with clinically apparent coronary artery disease should be initiated with the intent of correcting abnormal lipid levels or lowering them to the extent possible with nutritional and pharmacologic intervention.

The prevalence of obesity, defined as greater than 20% over ideal body weight, ranges from 7.4% to 17% in men and from 9.6% to 34.7% in women in the United States. Body mass index, weight (kg) divided by height (m) squared, greater than about 32 is associated with an increased mortality ratio compared with individuals of normal body weight and the objective for patients with IHD is to maintain or reduce to a normal body weight. This may be accomplished through dietary modification, exercise, pharmacologic therapy, or surgical therapy. Frequently associated with obesity is a sedentary life-style, and inactivity may contribute to higher blood pressure, elevated blood lipid levels, and greater glucose intolerance in diabetics. Exercise to the level of about 300 kcal three times a week is useful in improving maximal oxygen uptake, improving cardiorespiratory efficiency, promoting collateral artery formation and potential alterations in the risk of ventricular fibrillation and coronary thrombosis, and improving tolerance to stress. Although a regular exercise program may not prevent the occurrence of IHD, participants feel better and their overall cardiovascular risk may be reduced.

Competitiveness, intense striving for achievement, easily provoked hostility, a sense of urgency about doing things quickly and being punctual, impatience, abrupt and rapid speech and gestures, and concentration on self-selected goals to the point of not perceiving and attending to other aspects of the environment are the traits that characterize the behavioral pattern known as type A or coronary prone personality. Although somewhat controversial, type A individuals may have increased cardiovascular risk with risk ratios ranging from insignificant to three times that of a matched population. The mechanism by which personality affects the cardiovascular system is not understood, but may reflect the activity of the sympathetic system and enhanced responsiveness of other stress hormones when compared with non–type A personalities. Asymptomatic hyperglycemia does not appear to be an established risk factor for coronary heart disease, whereas overt diabetes mellitus clearly increases the risk of IHD. Prudent advice would be to control blood glucose concentrations as well as feasible in diabetic patients with the intent of reducing the contribution of diabetes to atherosclerosis and coronary heart disease. Gout or hyperuricemia appears to be indirectly atherogenic, an effect most likely mediated through associated hypertension, hyperlipidemia, and obesity. Attempts at normalizing uric acid levels are rational and may alter the risk of cardiovascular disease.

Alcohol ingestion in small to moderate amounts (<40 g of pure ethanol per day) reduces the risk of coronary heart disease; however, consumption of large amounts (>50 g per day) and binge drinking of alcohol are associated with increased mortality from stroke, malignant neoplasms, and cirrhosis.[46] The mechanisms for the presumed protective effects of alcohol are not known but may be related to increased high-density-lipoprotein levels, impaired platelet function, or associations between the amount of alcohol ingested and personality type. Whatever the relationship, it is well to remember that alcohol drinking is implicated in over 40% of all fatal automobile accidents and consumption of alcohol predisposes to hepatic cirrhosis, the seventh most common cause of death in the United States. With this in mind, it seems illogical to suggest alcohol ingestion as a prophylactic measure for coronary disease but rather that moderation of alcohol consumption, if the preference of the individual, is advisable.

Exogenous administration of estrogens and the use of thiazide diuretics and β-blockers have been shown to elevate serum cholesterol and triglyceride levels; however, a direct association between these drugs and cardiovascular risk has only been shown for estrogens in certain situations. Oral contraceptives in smoking women over the age of 35 years increases the risk of myocardial infarction, stroke, and venous thromboembolism threefold or higher. Alternative forms of contraception and cessation of smoking should be promoted in these patients. The risk for nonsmoking oral contraceptive users under the age of 35 is very small. Men of all ages when exposed to exogenous estrogens have increased risk for cardiovascular disease in general and AMI in particular. Estrogens given to postmenopausal women do not appear to increase relative risk of death compared with nonusers; in particular, risk for users versus nonusers was 0.54 for gynecologically intact women, 0.34 for hysterectomized women, 0.12 for bilaterally oophorectomized women, and 0.37 overall.[47] Others, however, have shown postmenopausal use to be associated with either increased or decreased risk for death from cardiovascular events and the use of postmenopausal estrogens remains a controversy.[48,49] Coffee consumption has also been linked to coronary heart disease and when studies are adjusted for other risk factors, the ingestion of greater than five cups per day by recent history appears to be associated with a relative risk of about 2.5 times that associated with no coffee consumption.[50] Although thiazide diuretics and β-blockers (nonselective without intrinsic sympathomimetic activity) may elevate both cholesterol and triglycerides by some 10% to 20% and these effects may be detrimental, no objective evidence exists from prospective well-controlled studies to support avoidance of these drugs at this time. This controversy is most pertinent in the treatment of mild hypertension and it is discussed in greater detail in Chapter 10.

## *Pharmacologic Management*

### Placebo Effect

Historically, about 30% of anginal syndrome symptoms have responded regardless of the therapy instituted. Examples of these placebo responses include such drug therapies as xanthines, khellin, and vitamin E, as well as surgical procedures such as ligation of the internal mammary artery.[51] These observations stem from two problems inherent in clinical trials undertaken to assess the efficacy of any therapy for angina: (1) adequate trial design incorporating appropriate controls and washout periods and (2) assessment of treatment effects utilizing objective measures of efficacy including improvement in exercise performance, resting and ambulatory ECG improvement in ischemic changes, or other objective tests that address other aspects of myocardial function or metabolism. Pain episode frequency and nitroglycerin consumption are subjective and their use as sole measures of efficacy should be avoided. Objective assessment using ETT has shown that placebo does not provide improvement in patients with exertional angina,[52] substantiating this as a valid means to assess efficacy.

### Nitrate Therapy

Nitroglycerin has a well-documented role in the alleviation of anginal attacks when used as rapidly absorbed and readily available preparations by the oral and intravenous routes (see Table 13.12). Sublingual, buccal, or spray products would be the products of choice for this indication. Prevention of symptoms may be accomplished by the prophylactic use of oral or transdermal products; however, recent concern has been expressed over the long-term efficacy of many of these preparations.

Nitrates have multiple potential mechanisms of action and for a given patient it is not always clear which of these is most important. In general, the major action appears to be indirectly mediated through a reduction of myocardial oxygen demand secondary to venodilation and arterial-arteriolar dilation, leading to a reduction in wall stress from reduced ventricular volume and pressure (see Table 13.13). Systemic venodilation also promotes increased flow to deep myocardial muscle by reducing the gradient between intraventricular pressure and coronary arteriolar ($R_2$) pressure. Direct actions on the coronary circulation include dilation of large and small intramural coronary arteries, collateral dilation, coronary artery stenosis dilation, abolition of normal tone in narrowed vessels, and relief of spasm. It is likely that depending on the underlying pathophysiology, different mechanisms become operative.[53] For example, in the presence of a 60% to 70% stenosis, venodilation and $MVo_2$ reduction are most important; however, with higher grade lesions, direct effects on the coronary circulation and vessel tone are the predominant effects. Although the cellular mechanism of vasodilation by nitrates is not clearly understood, these effects may be mediated by alterations in the activities of prostacyclin or thromboxane $A_2$ or by the

**Table 13.12** Nitrate Products

| | | *Onset (min)* | *Duration (min/h)* | *Initial dose* |
|---|---|---|---|---|
| **Isosorbide dinitrate, sublingual and chewable** | | | | |
| Isosorbide dinitrate (various) | Tablets, sublingual: 2.5 mg | 2–5 | 1–2 | 2.5–5 mg |
| Isonate 2.5 mg SL (Major) | | | | |
| Isordil (Wyeth) | | | | |
| Sorate-2.5 (Trimen) | | | | |
| Sorbitrate (Stuart) | | | | |
| Isosorbide dinitrate (various) | Tablets, sublingual: 5 mg | | | |
| Isonate 5 mg SL (Major) | | | | |
| Isordil (Wyeth) | | | | |
| Sorate-5 (Trimen) | | | | |
| Sorbitrate (Stuart) | | | | |
| Isosorbide dinitrate (various) | Tablets, sublingual: 10 mg | | | |
| Isordil (Wyeth) | | | | |
| Sorbitrate (Stuart) | | | | |
| Onset-5 (Bock) | Tablets, chewable: 5 mg | | | |
| Sorate-5 (Trimen) | | | | |
| Sorbitrate (Stuart) | | | | |
| Isordil (Wyeth) | Tablets, chewable: 10 mg | | | |
| Sorate-10 (Trimen) | | | | |
| Sorbitrate (Stuart) | | | | |
| **Isosorbide dinitrate, oral** | | | | |
| Isosorbide dinitrate (various) | Tablets: 5 mg | 20–40 | 4–6 | 5–20 mg QID |
| Isonage (Major) | | | | |
| Isordil Titradose (Wyeth) | | | | |
| Sorbitrate (Stuart) | | | | |
| Isosorbide dinitrate (various) | Tablets: 10 mg | | | |
| Isonate (Major) | | | | |
| Isordil Titradose (Wyeth) | | | | |
| Sorbitrate (Stuart) | | | | |
| Isosorbide dinitrate (various) | Tablets: 20 mg | | | |
| Isonate (Major) | | | | |
| Isordil Titradose (Wyeth) | | | | |
| Sorbitrate (Stuart) | | | | |
| Isosorbide dinitrate (various) | Tablets: 30 mg | | | |
| Isordil Titradose (Wyeth) | | | | |
| Sorbitrate (Stuart) | | | | |
| Isosorbide dinitrate (various) | Tablets: 40 mg | | | |
| Isordil Titradose (Wyeth) | | | | |
| Sorbitrate (Stuart) | | | | |
| Isosorbide dinitrate (various) | Capsules: 40 mg | | | |
| Isosorbide dinitrate (various) | Tablets, sustained release: 40 mg | | | |
| Isordil Tembids (Wyeth) | | | | |
| Sorbitrate SA (Stuart) | | | | |
| Isosorbide dinitrate (various) | Capsules, sustained release: 40 mg | 1–2 | 4–6 | 40 mg every 8–12 h |
| Dilatrate-SR (Reed and Carnrick) | | | | |
| Iso-Bid (Geriatric Pharm.) | | | | |
| Isordil Tembids (Wyeth) | | | | |
| Isotrate Timecelles (Hauck) | | | | |
| Sorate-40 (Trimen) | | | | |
| **Erythritol tetranitrate** | | | | |
| Cardilate (Burroughs Wellcome) | Tablets, oral or sublingual<br>5 mg (#Cardilate P2B)<br>10 mg (#Cardilate X7A)<br>Tablets, chewable:<br>10 mg (#Cardilate X7A) | 5–30 | 4–6 | 5–10 mg TID |

**Table 13.12** (continued)

| | | | *Onset (min)* | *Duration (min/h)* | *Initial dose* |
|---|---|---|---|---|---|
| **Penterythritol tetranitrate (PETN)** | | | | | |
| PETN (various) | Tablets: 10 mg | | 30 | 4–8 | 10–20 mg TID |
| Pentylan (Lannett) | | | | | |
| Peritrate (Parke–Davis) | | | | | |
| PETN (various) | Tablets: 20 mg | | | | |
| Naptrate (Vortech) | | | | | |
| Pentylan (Lannett) | | | | | |
| Peritrate (Parke–Davis) | Tablets: 40 mg | | | | |
| PETN (various) | Tablets: 80 mg | | | | |
| Duotrate Plateau Caps (Jones Medical) | Capsules, sustained release: 30 mg | | | | |
| Pentritol Tempules (USV) | | | | | |
| Duotrate 45 Plateau Caps (Jones Medical) | Capsules, sustained release: 45 mg | | | | |
| Pentritol Tempules (USV) | Capsules, sustained release: 60 mg | | | | |
| PETN (various) | Capsules, sustained release: 80 mg | | | | |
| PETN (various) | Tablets, sustained release: 80 mg | | | | |
| Peritrate SA (Parke–Davis) | | | | | |
| **Nitroglycerin, intravenous** | | | | | |
| Tridil (American Critical Care) | Injection: 0.5 mg/mL | In 10-mL amps | 1–2 | 3–5 | 5 μg/min |
| Nitrol IV (Rorer) | Injection: 0.8 mg/mL | In 1-, 10-, and 30-mL amps[a] | | | |
| Nitrostat IV (Parke–Davis) | | In 10-mL amps[b] with or without disposable IV infusion set | | | |
| Nitroglycerin (various) | Injection: 5 mg/mL | In 5-, 10-, and 20-mL vials | | | |
| Nitro-Bid IV (Marion) | | In 1-, 5-, and 10-mL vials[c] | | | |
| Nitrol IV Concentrate (Rorer) | | In 10-mL amps[d] | | | |
| Nitrostat IV (Parke–Davis) | | In 10-mL amps[e] with or without disposable IV infusion set | | | |
| Tridil (American Critical Care) | | In 10-mL amps, with or without IV infusion set, and 5-mL vials | | | |
| **Nitroglycerin, sublingual** | | | | | |
| Nitroglycerin (Lilly) | Tablets, sublingual: 0.15 mg (1/400 gr) | | 1–3 | 30–60 | 0.3 mg |
| Nitrostat[f] (Parke–Davis) | | | | | |
| Nitroglycerin (Lilly) | Tablets, sublingual: 0.3 mg (1/200 gr) | | | | |
| Nitrostat[f] (Parke–Davis) | | | | | |
| Nitroglycerin (Lilly) | Tablets, sublingual: 0.4 mg (1/150 gr) | | | | |
| Nitrostat[f] (Parke–Davis) | | | | | |
| Nitroglycerin (Lilly) | Tablets, sublingual: 0.6 mg (1/100 gr) | | | | |
| Nitrostat[f] (Parke–Davis) | | | | | |
| **Nitroglycerin, translingual** | | | | | |
| Nitrolingual (Rorer) | Spray: 0.4 mg per metered dose (200 metered doses) in 13.8 g | | 2 | 30–60 | 0.4 mg |
| **Nitroglycerin, transmucosal** | | | | | |
| Nitrogard (Parke–Davis) | Tablets, buccal controlled release: 1 mg (#P-D) 2 mg (#P-D) 3 mg (#P-D) | | 3 | 3–5 | 1 mg |
| **Nitroglycerin, sustained release** | | | | | |
| Nitroglycerin (various) | Capsules, sustained release: 2.5 mg | | 40 | 4–6 | 2.5 mg TID |
| Nitro-Bid Plateau Caps (Marion) | | | | | |
| Nitrocap T.D. (Vortech) | | | | | |
| Nitroglyn (Schering) | | | | | |
| Nitrolin (Schein) | | | | | |
| Nitrospan (USV) | | | | | |

**Table 13.12** Nitrate Products (continued)

| | | | | Onset (min) | Duration (min/h) | Initial dose |
|---|---|---|---|---|---|---|
| **Nitroglycerin, sustained release,** *continued* | | | | | | |
| Klavikordal (US Ethicals) | Tablets, sustained release: 2.6 mg | | | | | |
| Niong (US Ethicals) | | | | | | |
| Nitronet (US Ethicals) | | | | | | |
| Nitrong (Wharton Labs) | | | | | | |
| Nitroglycerin (various) | Capsules, sustained release: 6.5 mg | | | | | |
| Nitro-Bid Plateau Caps (Marion) | | | | | | |
| Nitrocap 6.5 (Vortech) | | | | | | |
| Nitroglyn (Schering) | | | | | | |
| Nitrolin (Schein) | | | | | | |
| Nitrospan (USV) | | | | | | |
| Klavikordal (US Ethicals) | Tablets, sustained release: 6.5 mg | | | | | |
| Niong (US Ethicals) | | | | | | |
| Nitronet (US Ethicals) | | | | | | |
| Nitrong (Wharton Labs) | | | | | | |
| Nitroglycerin (various) | Capsules, sustained release: 9 mg | | | | | |
| Nitro-Bid Plateau Caps (Marion) | | | | | | |
| Nitroglyn (Schering) | | | | | | |
| Nitrolin (Schein) | | | | | | |
| Nitrong (Wharton Labs) | Tablets, sustained release: 9 mg | | | | | |
| **Nitroglycerin, transdermal** | | | | | | |
| | *Release rate (mg/24 h)* | *Surface area ($cm^2$)* | *Total nitroglycerin content (mg)* | | | |
| Nitro-Dur II 2.5 mg/24 h (Key Pharm) | 2.5 | 5 | 20 | 40–60 | 4–8 | 1 patch |
| Transderm-Nitro 2.5 (Ciba) | 2.5 | 5 | 12.5 | | | |
| Nitrodisc 5 mg/24 h (Searle) | 5 | 8 | 16 | | | |
| Nitro-Dur 5 mg/24 h (Key Pharm) | 5 | 10 | 51 | | | |
| Nitro-Dur II 5 mg/24 h (Key Pharm) | 5 | 10 | 40 | | | |
| NTS 5 mg/24 h (Bolar) | 5 | 10 | 62.5 | | | |
| Transderm-Nitro 5 (Ciba) | 5 | 10 | 25 | | | |
| Nitrodisc 7.5 mg/24 h (Searle) | 7.5 | 12 | 24 | | | |
| Nitro-Dur II 7.5mg/24 h (Key Pharm) | 7.5 | 15 | 60 | | | |
| Nitrodisc 10 mg/24 h (Searle) | 10 | 16 | 32 | | | |
| Nitro-Dur 10 mg/24 h (Key Pharm) | 10 | 20 | 104 | | | |
| Nitro-Dur II 10 mg/24 h (Key Pharm) | 10 | 20 | 104 | | | |
| Nitro-Dur II 10 mg/24 h (Key Pharm) | 10 | 20 | 80 | | | |
| Transderm-Nitro 10 (Ciba) | 10 | 20 | 50 | | | |
| Nitro-Dur II 15 mg/24 h (Key Pharm) | 15 | 30 | 120 | | | |
| NTS 15 mg/24 h (Key Pharm) | 15 | 30 | 120 | | | |
| NTS 15 mg/24 h (Bolar) | 15 | 30 | 120 | | | |
| Transderm-Nitro 15 (Ciba) | 15 | 30 | 75 | | | |
| **Nitroglycerin, topical** | | | | | | |
| Nitroglycerin (various) | Ointment: 2% in a lanolin–petrolatum base | | | 20–60 | 2–8 | $\frac{1}{2}$–1 in. |
| Nitro-Bid (Marion) | | | | | | |
| Nitrol (Rorer) | | | | | | |
| Nitrong (Wharton) | | | | | | |
| Nitrostat (Parke–Davis) | | | | | | |

[a] With lactose.
[b] In 5% alcohol.
[c] With 45 mg propylene glycol per milliliter and 70% ethanol.
[d] In dehydrated alcohol.
[e] With 30% propylene glycol and 30% alcohol.
[f] Stabilized form.

generation of nitric oxide and subsequent stimulation of guanylate cyclase, both with the potential to impair calcium-linked smooth muscle contraction.[54]

Pharmacokinetic characteristics common to the organic nitrates used for angina include a large first-pass effect of hepatic metabolism, short to very short half-lives, large volumes of distribution, high clearance rates, and large interindividual variations in plasma or blood concentrations.[55,56] Pharmacodynamic–pharmacokinetic relationships for the entire class remain poorly defined, presumably as a result of methodologic difficulty in characterizing the parent drug and metabolite concentrations at or within vascular smooth muscle and secondary to counterregulatory or adaptive mechanisms from the drug's effects as well as the occurrence of tolerance. Numerous technical problems limit the generation of reliable pharmacokinetic parameter estimates, including assay sensitivity arterial-venous extraction gradients and, therefore, extrahepatic metabolism; in vitro degradation; drug adsorption to polyvinyl chloride tubing and syringes; potentially saturable metabolism; accumulation of metabolites (some of which are active) with multiple doses; postural and exercise-induced changes in pharmacokinetics; a variety of variables associated with transdermal delivery including delivery system (matrix, membrane-limited, ointment), vehicle used, surface area and thickness of application, site of application, and other skin variables (temperature, moisture content, etc.).

Nitroglycerin concentrations are affected by the route of administration; the highest concentrations are usually obtained with intravenous administration, the lowest with lower oral doses. Peak concentrations with sublingual nitroglycerin appear in 2 to 4 minutes; the oral route produces peaks at about 15 to 30 minutes and the transdermal route, at 1 to 2 hours. The half-life of nitroglycerin is 1 to 5 minutes regardless of route, hence the potential advantage of sustained-release and transdermal products. Transdermal nitroglycerin does produce sufficient concentrations for acute hemodynamic effects to be seen and these concentrations are maintained for long intervals; however, the hemodynamic and antianginal effects are minimal after as little as 1 week on chronic therapy.

Isosorbide dinitrate (ISDN) is metabolized to 2-mono- and 5-monoisosorbide dinitrate; the latter is an active metabolite with a 5-hour half-life and tends to accumulate with chronic dosing. Multiple, larger doses of ISDN lead to disproportionate increases in the area under the plasma time profile, suggesting that metabolic pathways are being saturated or that metabolite accumulation may influence the disposition of ISDN. Little pharmacokinetic information is available for other nitrate compounds.

Nitrate therapy may be used for termination of an acute anginal attack, prevention of effort- or stress-induced attacks, or long-term prophylaxis. Sublingual nitroglycerin 0.3–0.4 mg relieves pain in about 75% of patients within 3 minutes, with another 15% becoming pain free in 5 to 15 minutes.[57] Pain persisting beyond about 30 minutes after the use of two or three nitroglycerin tablets is suggestive of evolving myocardial infarction and the patient should be instructed to seek emergency aid. Patients should be instructed to keep nitroglycerin in the original, tightly closed glass container and to avoid mixing it with other medication, to reduce nitroglycerin adsorption and vaporization. Patients should be counseled that nitroglycerin does not act as an analgesic but rather partially corrects the underlying problem and that repeated use is not harmful or addicting. Patients should also be aware that enhanced venous pooling in the sitting or standing positions may improve the effect as well as the symptoms of postural hypotension and that inadequate saliva may slow or prevent tablet disintegration and dissolution. An acceptable albeit expensive alternative is lingual spray which may be more convenient and has a shelf-life of 3 years compared with 6 months or so for some nitroglycerin tablets.[58]

Chewable, oral, and transdermal products are acceptable for the long-term prophylaxis of angina; however, considerable controversy surrounds their use and it appears that the development of tolerance (discussed later) or adaptive mechanisms limit the efficacy of all chronic nitrate therapy regardless of route. Dosing of the longer acting preparations should be adjusted to provide a hemodynamic response; for example, this may require doses of oral ISDN ranging from 10 to 60 mg as often as every 3 to 4 hours because of tolerance or first-pass metabolism and similar large doses for other products. Nitroglycerin ointment seems to have a duration of up to 6 hours but it is difficult to apply in a cosmetically acceptable fashion over a consistent surface area and response varies depending on epidermal thickness, vascularity, and amount of hair. Percutaneous adsorption of nitroglycerin ointment may occur unintentionally if someone other than the patient applies the ointment and limiting exposure through the use of gloves or some other means is advisable. Peripheral edema may also impair the response to nitroglycerin, as venodilation cannot increase capacitance to a maximum and pooling may be reduced. Transdermal patch delivery systems were approved on the basis of sustained plasma concentrations equivalent to those for other forms of therapy; unfortunately, at the present time no objective evidence exists to support their chronic use.

Methods for subjective assessment of nitrate effect include reduction of the number of painful episodes and the amount of nitroglycerin consumed. Objective assessment includes the resolution of ECG changes at rest, during exercise, or with ambulatory ECG monitoring. As nitrates work primarily through a reduction in $MVo_2$, the double product can be used to optimize the dose of sublingual and oral nitrate products. It is important to realize that reflex tachycardia may offset the beneficial reduction in systolic blood pressure and calculation of the observed changes is necessary. The double product is best assessed in the sitting position and at intervals of 5 to 10 minutes and 30 to 60 minutes after sublingual and oral therapy, respectively. Because of the placebo effect, unpredictable and variable course of angina, numerous pharmacologic effects of nitroglycerin, diurnal variation in pain patterns, and interindividual sensitivity to nitroglycerin, assessment with transdermal and sustained-release products is difficult.[59] ETT provides valuable information concerning efficacy and mechanism of action for nitrates but its use is usually reserved for clinical investigation rather than routine patient care. Most ETT studies have shown nitrates to delay the onset of ischemia (ST-segment changes or initial chest discomfort) at submaximal exercise but the threshold for maximal exercise is unaltered, suggesting that oxygen demand is reduced rather than oxygen supply improved. More sophisticated studies of myocardial function such as wall motion abnormalities and myocardial metabolism could be used to document efficacy; however, these studies are generally used only for investigative purposes.

Adverse effects of nitrates are related most commonly to an extension of their pharmacologic effect and include postural hypotension with associated central nervous system symptoms, headaches and flushing secondary to vasodilation, and occasional nausea from smooth muscle relaxation. If hypotension is excessive, coronary filling may be compromised and myocardial infarction, as well as underfilling of the cerebral circulation and stroke, can result. While reflex tachycardia is most common, bradycardia with nitroglycerin has been reported. Other noncardiovascular adverse effects include rash with all products but particularly with transdermal nitroglycerin, the production of methemoglobinemia with high doses given for extended periods, and measurable concentrations of ethanol and propylene glycol (found in the diluent) with intravenous nitroglycerin.

Tolerance with nitrate therapy was first described by Brunton[3] in the initial use of amyl nitrate for angina; later, it was widely recognized in munition workers who underwent withdrawal reactions during periods of absence from exposure. Studies of nitrate tolerance in humans and animals have not determined the cause; however, at least three possibilities exist. The first mechanism proposes that a critical sulfhydryl group is oxidized at the nitroglycerin receptor, and in animals, work with reducing agents has shown reversal of tolerance.[60–62] Prolonged exposure to nitrates may reduce the availability of sulfhydryl groups from glutathione or other sources that are important for the generation of *S*-nitrosothiol from nitric oxide and the subsequent activation of guanylate cyclase to produce vasodilation.[63] Data on humans and animals suggest that tolerance may be reversed by using sulfhydryl sources such as acetylcysteine, although the clinical application of this information is lacking. Lastly, accumulation of metabolites of nitroglycerin and other nitrates may inhibit activity of the parent compounds or prevent their vascular metabolism necessary for vasodilation.[64] Most of the published controlled trials examining nitrate tolerance have collected information on either ISDN or transdermal nitroglycerin and these studies demonstrate the development of tolerance within as little as 24 hours of therapy.[65,66] While the onset of tolerance is rapid, the offset may be just as rapid and one alternative dosing strategy to circumvent or minimize tolerance is to provide a daily nitrate-free interval of 6 to 8 hours.[67] Interestingly, hemodynamic tolerance does not always coincide with antianginal efficacy but this is not well studied.[68]

For anginal therapy, nitrates may be combined with other drugs, including β-adrenergic blocking agents and calcium channel antagonists. These combinations are usually instituted for chronic prophylactic therapy based on complementary or offsetting mechanisms of action (see Table 13.13). Combination therapy is generally used in patients with more severe symptoms not responding to nitrates alone (nitrates plus β-blockers or calcium blockers) and in patients having an element of vasospasm leading to decreased supply (nitrates plus calcium blockers).

### β-Adrenergic Blocking Agents

Decreased heart rate, decreased contractility, and a slight to moderate decrease in blood pressure with β-adrenergic receptor antagonism reduce $MVo_2$. The predominant receptor type in the heart is the $\beta_1$ receptor and competitive blockade minimizes the influence of endogenous catecholamines on the chronotropic and inotropic state of the myocardium. These beneficial effects may be countered to some measure by the increased ventricular volume and ejection time seen with β-blockade; however, the overall effect of β-blockers in patients with effort-induced angina is a reduction in oxygen demand. The β-blockers do not improve oxygen supply, and in certain instances, unopposed α-adrenergic stimulation after the use of β-blockers may lead to coronary vasoconstriction.[69] For patients with chronic exertional stable angina, β-blockers improve symptoms about 80% of the time and objective measures of efficacy demonstrate improved exercise duration and delay in the time at which ST-segment changes and initial or limiting symptoms occur. β-Blockers do not alter the rate–pressure product (double product) for maximal exercise, therefore substantiating reduced demand rather than improved supply as the major consequence of their actions. Reflex tachycardia from nitrate therapy can be blunted with β-blocker therapy, making this a common and useful combination. Some patients with preexisting LV dysfunction who would

**Table 13.13** Effect of Drug Therapy on Myocardial Oxygen Demand[a]

| | *Heart rate* | *Myocardial contractility* | *LV wall tension* Systolic pressure | LV volume |
|---|---|---|---|---|
| Nitrates | ↑ | 0 | ↓ | ↓↓ |
| β-Blockers | ↓↓ | ↓ | ↓ | ↑ |
| Nifedipine | ↑ | 0 or ↓ | ↓↓ | 0 or ↓ |
| Verapamil | ↓ | ↓ | ↓ | 0 or ↓ |
| Diltiazem | ↓↓ | 0 or ↓ | ↓ | 0 or ↓ |

[a] Calcium channel antagonists and nitrates may also increase myocardial oxygen supply through coronary vasodilation. Diastolic function may also be improved with verapamil, nifedipine, and, perhaps, diltiazem. These effects may vary from those indicated in the table depending on individual patient baseline hemodynamics.

be prone to heart failure may receive digitalis glycosides to maintain cardiac output if β-blockade is necessary for IHD. Although β-blockade may decrease exercise capacity in healthy individuals or in patients with hypertension, it may allow angina patients previously limited by symptoms to perform more exercise and ultimately improve overall cardiovascular performance through a training effect.[70]

Pertinent pharmacokinetics for the β-blockers include half-life and route elimination, which are reviewed in Chapter 10. Drugs with longer half-lives need to be dosed less frequently than those with shorter half-lives; however, disparity exists between half-life and duration of action for several β-blockers (e.g., metoprolol) and this may reflect attenuation of the central nervous system–mediated effects on the sympathetic system as well as the direct effects of this category on heart rate and contractility.[71] Renal and hepatic dysfunction can affect the disposition of β-blockers but these agents are dosed to effect, either hemodynamic or symptomatic, and route of elimination is not a major consideration in drug selection.

Guidelines for the use of β-blockers in treating angina would include the objective of lowering resting heart rate to 50 to 60 bpm and limiting maximal exercise heart rate to about 100 bpm or less. It has also been suggested that exercise heart rate should be no more than about 20 bpm or a 10% increment over resting heart rate with modest exercise. As β-blockade is competitive and circulating catecholamine concentrations vary depending on the intensity of exercise and other factors, and cholinergic tone may be important in controlling heart rate in some patients, these guidelines are general in nature. These effects are generally dose and plasma concentration related, and for propranolol, plasma concentrations of 30 ng/mL are needed for a 25% reduction of anginal frequency.[72] Initial doses of β-blockers should be at the lower end of the usual dosing range and titrated to response as indicated earlier.

There is little evidence to suggest superiority of any β-blocker; however, the duration of β-blockade is dependent partially on the half-life of the agent used and those with longer half-lives may be dosed less frequently.[73–75] Of note, propranolol may be dosed twice a day in most patients with angina and the efficacy is similar to that seen with more frequent dosing.[76,77] The ancillary property of membrane-stabilizing activity is irrelevant in the treatment of angina, and intrinsic sympathomimetic activity appears to be detrimental in patients with rest or severe angina as the reduction in heart rate would be minimized, therefore limiting a reduction in $MVo_2$.[78] Cardioselective β-blockers may be used in some patients to minimize adverse effects such as bronchospasm in asthmatic or chronic obstructive pulmonary disease patients, intermittent claudication, and sexual dysfunction.[79,80] It should be remembered that cardioselectivity is a relative property and the use of larger doses (e.g., metoprolol 200 mg/d) is associated with the loss of selectivity and adverse effects. Post-AMI patients with angina are particularly good candidates for β-blockade, as anginal symptoms may be treated and the risk of post-MI reinfarction and mortality reduced with timolol, propranolol, and metoprolol (see Chapter 14). Combined β-blockade (nonselective) and α-blockade with labetolol may be useful in some patients with marginal LV reserve, and fewer deleterious effects are seen, compared with other β-blockers, on coronary blood flow.[81]

Extension of pharmacologic effect is the underlying reason for many of the adverse effects seen with β-blockade. Hypotension, heart failure, bradycardia and heart block, bronchospasm, peripheral vasoconstriction and intermittent claudication, and altered glucose metabolism are directly related to β-adrenoreceptor antagonism. Patients with preexisting LV dysfunction and those who use other negative inotropic agents are most prone to developing overt heart failure; in the absence of these, heart failure is uncommon (less than 5%). Other drugs that depress conduction are additive to β-blockade and intrinsic conduction system disease predisposes the patient to conduction abnormalities. Altered glucose metabolism is most likely to be seen in insulin-dependent diabetes and β-blockade obscures the symptoms of hypoglycemia except for sweating. One of the more common reasons for discontinuation of β-blocker therapy is related to central nervous system adverse effects of fatigue, malaise, and depression. Although some suggest these effects may be avoided or minimized by the use of hydrophilic rather than lipophilic β-blocking agents, recent evidence suggests differential use may not be possible.[82,83] In a review of prescription use, Avorn et al found antidepressants more commonly used in patients receiving β-blockers with a relative risk of 1.5 to 2 regardless of the type of β-blocker used.[84] Abrupt withdrawal of β-blocker therapy in patients with angina has been associated with increased severity, increased number of pain episodes, and myocardial infarction.[85–89] The mechanism of this effect is unknown but may be related to increased receptor sensitivity or disease progression during therapy that becomes apparent after discontinuation of β-blockade. In any event, tapering of β-blocker therapy over about 2 days should minimize the risk of withdrawal reactions for those patients in whom therapy is discontinued.

β-Adrenoreceptor blockade is effective in chronic exertional angina as monotherapy and in combination with nitrates and/or calcium channel antagonists. After the institution of nitrate therapy, β-blockers are frequently the second line of therapy for patients with inadequate control of symptoms. This is justified based on the pharmacologic interaction between these two classes of drugs, the cost of therapy, and the tolerability of β-blockers. Patients with severe angina, rest angina, or variant angina may be better treated with nitrates and, increasingly, calcium channel blockers.[89,90]

### Calcium Channel Antagonists

Modulation of calcium entry into vascular smooth muscle and myocardium as well as a variety of other tissues is the principal action of the calcium antagonists. The cellular mechanism of these drugs is not completely understood and it differs among the available classes of the phenyalkylamines (verapamil-like), dihydropyridines (nifedipine-like), and benzothiazepines (diltiazem-like).[91] Receptor-operated channels stimulated by norepinephrine and other neurotransmitters and potential-dependent channels activated by membrane depolarization control the entry of calcium and, consequently, the cytosolic concentration of calcium that is responsible for activation of actin–myosin complex leading to contraction of vascular smooth muscle and myocardium.

In the myocardium, calcium entry triggers the release of intracellular stores of calcium to increase cytosolic calcium, whereas in smooth muscle, calcium derived from the extracellular fluid may do this directly. Binding proteins within the cell, calmodulin and troponin, after binding with calcium participate in phosphorylation reactions leading to contraction. Decreased calcium availability, effected by the actions of calcium antagonists, inhibits these reactions.

Direct actions of the calcium antagonists include vasodilation of systemic arterioles and coronary arteries, leading to reduction of arterial pressure and coronary vascular resistance as well as depression of myocardial contractility and conduction velocity of the sinoatrial and atrioventricular nodes (see Chapter 12). Reflex $\beta$-adrenergic stimulation overcomes much of the negative inotropic effect, and depression of contractility becomes clinically apparent only in the presence of LV dysfunction and when other negative inotropic drugs are used concurrently. Verapamil and diltiazem cause less peripheral vasodilation than nifedipine, and, consequently, the risk of myocardial depression is greater with these two agents. Conduction through the atrioventricular node is predictably depressed with verapamil and to some extent with diltiazem, and they must be used with caution in patients with preexisting conduction abnormalities or in the presence of other drugs with negative chronotropic properties. $MVO_2$ is reduced with all of the calcium channel antagonists because of reduced wall tension secondary to reduced arterial pressure and, to a minor extent, depressed contractility (see Table 13.13). Heart rate changes are dependent on the drug used and the state of the conduction system. Nifedipine generally increases heart rate or causes no change, while verapamil and diltiazem cause either no change or decreased heart rate because of the interaction of these direct and indirect effects. In contrast to the $\beta$-blockers, calcium channel antagonists have the potential to improve coronary blood flow through areas of fixed coronary obstruction and by inhibiting coronary artery vasomotion and vasospasm. Beneficial redistribution of blood flow from well-perfused myocardium to ischemic areas and from epicardium to endocardium may also contribute to improvement in ischemic symptoms. Overall, the benefit provided by calcium channel antagonists is related to reduced $MVO_2$ rather than improved oxygen supply based on lack of alteration in the rate pressure product at maximal exercise in most studies performed to date; however, as coronary artery disease progresses and vasospasm becomes superimposed on critical stenotic lesions, improved oxygen supply through coronary vasodilation may become more important.[92]

The three available calcium channel antagonists are characterized by excellent absorption and large, variable first-pass metabolism, resulting in oral bioavailability ranging from about 20% to 50% or greater. Saturation of this effect may occur with verapamil and diltiazem, resulting in greater amounts of drug being absorbed with chronic dosing.[93–95] Nifedipine may have slow or fast absorption patterns and the ingestion of food delays and impairs its absorption.[96–98] This variability in absorption produces fluctuation in the hemodynamic response with nifedipine. Sublingual nifedipine is frequently used to provide a more rapid response; however, the rationale for this application is suspect as little nifedipine is absorbed from the buccal mucosa and the swallowed drug is responsible for the observed plasma concentrations.[99] The presence of severe liver disease, for example, alcoholic liver disease with cirrhosis, has been shown to reduce the first-pass metabolism of verapamil, and this shunting of drug around the liver gives rise to higher plasma concentrations and lower dose requirements in these patients. Interestingly, this effect appears to be stereoselective for the more active isomer of verapamil. Verapamil may also reduce liver blood flow; however, evidence for this reduction is based primarily on experiments in animals. Few data are available regarding the influence of liver disease on the kinetics of nifedipine or diltiazem. These three drugs undergo extensive hepatic metabolism, with little unchanged drug being renally excreted. Nifedipine has no active metabolites, whereas norverapamil possesses 20% or less of the activity of the parent compound. Desacetyldiltiazem has not been studied in humans, but studies in dogs suggest that its potency ranges from 40% to 100% of the parent compound for various cardiovascular effects; the clinical importance of these observations remains to be determined.[100,101] With chronic dosing of verapamil and diltiazem, apparent saturation of metabolism occurs, producing plasma concentrations of each drug higher than those seen with single-dose administration. Consequently, the elimination half-life for verapamil is prolonged and less frequent dosing intervals may be used in some patients. The elimination half-life for diltiazem is also somewhat prolonged, and the half-life of desacetyldiltiazem is longer than that of the parent drug but it is not clear if less frequent dosing may be used. Nifedipine displays no such accumulation; however, it is eliminated via oxidative pathways that may be polymorphic, and slow and fast metabolizers have been described for nifedipine. As oxidative pathways are important for the elimination of these drugs, inhibition or induction by drugs such as cimetidine or rifampin can alter the kinetics and pharmacodynamic response. Conversely, inhibition of hepatic microsomal drug metabolism by diltiazem and verapamil has been demonstrated and interactions with drugs (i.e., theophylline) eliminated through oxidation may be expected.[102,103] Renal insufficiency has little or no effect on the pharmacokinetics of these three drugs. Although disease alterations in kinetics have been described, the most important quantitative alteration is the influence of liver disease on bioavailability and elimination. Altered protein binding as a result of renal disease, decreased protein concentration, or increased $\alpha_1$-acid glycoprotein has been noted but the clinical import of these changes is unknown.

### *Stable Exertional Angina Pectoris*[20,38,104–106]

After the alterable risk factors are assessed and manipulated as discussed previously, the next intervention that could be undertaken is institution of a regular exercise program. Training is possible in many patients with angina and the observed benefits include decreased heart rate and systolic blood pressure as well as increased ejection fraction and duration of exercise.[107,108] Although the mechanism of these effects has been debated, improved overall cardiovascular and muscular condition are probably most important. Obviously, an exercise program should be undertaken with caution and in a graded fashion with adequate supervision.

Nitrate therapy should be the first step in managing acute

attacks for patients with chronic stable angina. The frequency of therapy depends on the number of episodes of chest pain reported by the patient. In general, if angina occurs no more often than once every few days, then sublingual nitroglycerin or the spray or buccal products may be sufficient to allow the patient to maintain an adequate life-style. For episodes of "first-effort" angina occurring in a predictable fashion, nitroglycerin may be used in a prophylactic manner with the patient taking 0.3–0.4 mg sublingually about 5 minutes prior to the anticipated time of activity. Nitroglycerin spray may be useful when inadequate saliva is produced to rapidly dissolve sublingual nitroglycerin or if a patient has difficulty opening the container. Most patients have a response that lasts about 30 minutes or so, but this is subject to interindividual variability. Determination of the appropriate dose for a particular patient can be facilitated by the use of the double product to assess the hemodynamic effect of nitroglycerin. Patient-specific situations may dictate the use of other therapy that may benefit IHD, for example, a $\beta$-blocker for hypertension, and angina may be improved with this intervention; however, most authorities recommend nitrates as the initial therapy of choice. When angina occurs more frequently than once a day, a chronic prophylactic regimen using nitrates or $\beta$-blockers should be considered. Chronic prophylactic therapy with long-acting forms of nitroglycerin (oral or transdermal), isosorbide dinitrate, and pentaerythritol trinitrate may be effective; however, the development of tolerance is a major limitation of their continued effectiveness. As described previously, providing a nitrate-free interval of 6 to 8 hours per day appears to be the most promising approach to maintaining the efficacy of chronic nitrate therapy.[109,110] Oral administration of nitrates is susceptible to a saturable first-pass effect; therefore, larger doses can produce a measurable hemodynamic effect and dose titration should be based on these changes in the double product. There are few well-controlled studies comparing oral or sublingual nitrate efficacy and the choice among these products should be based on familiarity with the preparation, cost, and patient acceptance.

Chronic prophylactic therapy for patients with more than one angina episode per day may also be instituted with $\beta$-adrenergic blocking agents, and in many instances, $\beta$-blockers may be preferable because of less frequent dosing, other properties inherent in $\beta$-blockade (e.g., potential cardioprotective effects, antiarrhythmic effects, lack of tolerance, and antihypertensive effects), and their antianginal effects. In patients who continue to smoke the antianginal efficacy of $\beta$-blockers is reduced, maybe as a result of enhanced hepatic metabolism of drugs eliminated through this route or the effects of smoking on $MVo_2$ and oxygenation.[111] As discussed previously, ancillary properties such as cardioselectivity are useful in patients with concurrent problems but these properties do not contribute to the antianginal efficacy of $\beta$-blockers.[112] The one relevant characteristic is the duration of effect on the double product. Vukovich et al have demonstrated in normal volunteers that nadolol produces a reduction in double product for a longer period compared with several other $\beta$-blockers; however, the intensity of effect (maximal effect) was similar among the drugs tested and was related to dose.[71] In patients with angina, Jones and Mir examined the effects of nadolol, atenolol, and propranolol (regular and sustained-release) on exercise duration.[75] Nadolol increased exercise duration to the greatest extent at the doses used in this study; no difference in efficacy was noted between the two propranolol preparations. In contrast to these studies, other investigators have not detected any significant differences among $\beta$-blockers for the treatment of chronic stable angina.[73,74] The choice of a $\beta$-blocker for angina rests on the dose necessary to achieve the goals outlined for heart rate and double product, individual tolerability and cost. Selective use may incorporate ancillary properties but these are secondary considerations in overall drug product selection. Patients most likely to respond well to $\beta$-blockade are those who have a high resting heart rate and those having a relatively fixed anginal threshold. In other words, their symptoms appear at the same level of exercise or workload on a consistent basis. Symptoms appearing with variable workloads suggest fluctuations in myocardial oxygen supply, perhaps as a result of coronary artery vasomotion, and these patients are more likely to respond to calcium channel antagonists.[104]

Calcium channel antagonists have the potential advantages of improving coronary blood flow through coronary artery vasodilation and of decreasing $MVo_2$ and may be used instead of $\beta$-blockers for chronic prophylactic therapy. They are as effective as $\beta$-blockers and are most useful in patients who have a variable threshold for exertional angina. Calcium antagonists may provide better skeletal muscle oxygenation, resulting in decreased fatigue and better exercise tolerance.[113] Additionally, if contraindications exist to $\beta$-blocker therapy, calcium antagonists can be used safely in many patients. Nifedipine, verapamil, and diltiazem have similar efficacy in the management of chronic stable angina and differences in their electrophysiology, peripheral and central hemodynamic effects, and adverse effect profiles are used in selection of the appropriate agent. Patients with conduction abnormalities and moderate to severe LV dysfunction (ejection fraction <35%) should be treated cautiously with verapamil; nifedipine may be safely used in many of these patients. Diltiazem has significant effects on the atrioventricular node and can produce heart block in patients with preexisting conduction system disease or when other drugs, such as digoxin or $\beta$-blockers, with effects on conduction are used concurrently. Nifedipine may cause excessive heart rate elevation, especially if the patient is not receiving a $\beta$-blocker, and this may offset the beneficial effect it has on $MVo_2$. The hemodynamic effect of calcium antagonists is complementary to $\beta$-blockade; consequently, combination therapy is rational.

Studies examining combination therapy have shown that nifedipine,[114,115] verapamil,[116,117] and diltiazem,[118] when used with $\beta$-blockers, provide objective evidence of improvement by increasing exercise duration and decreasing ECG evidence of ischemia. Recent evidence suggests that the addition of a calcium antagonist to $\beta$-blocker therapy may be more useful than the addition of nitrates,[119] with respect to exercise duration and changes in global and regional ejection fraction in ischemic and nonischemic myocardium. Because both $\beta$-blockers and calcium antagonists have the potential to depress contractility, this combination should be used with care in patients with poor ventricular function; however, in patients with well-preserved ventricular function, the combination is well tolerated.

### *Unstable Angina Pectoris*

Clinical and autopsy studies indicate that most patients who present with unstable angina or acute myocardial infarction have significant underlying coronary atherosclerosis. Precipitation of these acute ischemic syndromes is thought to result from progression of atherosclerosis, acute coronary thrombosis, coronary artery spasm, and platelet aggregation.[120] The interrelationship of these mechanisms is outlined in Figure 13.13. Potential points of intervention in these mechanisms by naturally occurring and pharmacologic means follow the presumed pathogenesis (Fig. 13.14). Unstable angina differs from stable angina in that the primary event is thought to be a reduction in coronary blood flow rather than an increase in $MVo_2$, with corresponding ischemic changes in the ECG occurring prior to changes in heart rate and blood pressure. Initial management of the patient should include bed rest with continuous monitoring, alleviation of emotional stress with reassurance and sedatives, and stabilization with nitroglycerin either sublingually or intravenously, depending on the severity of the situation. Reversible or initiating factors such as anemia, thyroid dysfunction, infection, tachyarrhythmias, or increasing heart failure should be searched for and corrected.[121] Assessment of functional coronary reserve utilizing resting ECG, and, in some instances, a modified ETT, an ambulatory ECG, and a coronary arteriography are useful for risk stratification, prognosis, and planning of long-term treatment.[122] Although the ECG taken without pain is frequently normal, T-wave changes (peaking, pseudonormalization, and inversion) and ST-segment elevation or depression occurring during pain are indicative of severity and location of ischemia. ST-segment elevation without preceding heart rate or blood pressure changes is associated with increased coronary artery tone or spasm. Provocative tests, such as hyperventilation, cold pressor, and ergonovine stimulation, used during arteriography may provide information concerning the relative role of coronary artery spasm in contributing to the effects of coronary atherosclerosis in ischemia.[123] Intravenous nitroglycerin provides a convenient method of titrating the dose and avoids uncertainty concerning drug delivery (Fig. 13.15). Dosing should be started low (1–5 μg/kg/min) and titrated upward to obtain a reduction in systolic blood pressure of at least 15 mm Hg, or to a systolic pressure of 100–110 mm Hg, and to alleviate symptoms. Caution is necessary to avoid hypotension and decreased coronary perfusion pressure as well as excessive heart rate elevation if the patient is not receiving β-blockers. According to the guidelines suggested by Epstein and Palmeri, patients stabilized for 6 to 12 hours without pain on this regimen should receive long-acting nitrates and β-blockers if symptom control is inadequate. Unstable patients with persisting or recurring pain should receive a calcium antagonist and, depending on the response, move on to long-term therapy or intervention with thrombolysis or arteriography. Those undergoing arteriography with no reperfusion may be candidates for percutaneous transluminal coronary angioplasty (PTCA) or coronary artery bypass grafting (CABG). Acutely, heparin may be useful to prevent further thrombosis; aspirin acutely and chronically inhibits platelet aggregation (see Figure 13.15).

Numerous studies have documented the efficacy of nifedipine,[124–127] verapamil,[128–130] and diltiazem[131] in unstable angina and their effects are mediated via inhibition of increased coronary tone and through reduction in $MVo_2$. Calcium antagonists are effective as initial therapy and when used in combination with pretreatment β-blockade. ST-segment elevation appears to respond better than depression to calcium antagonism. Although few comparative studies are available, nifedipine may be the best agent in this

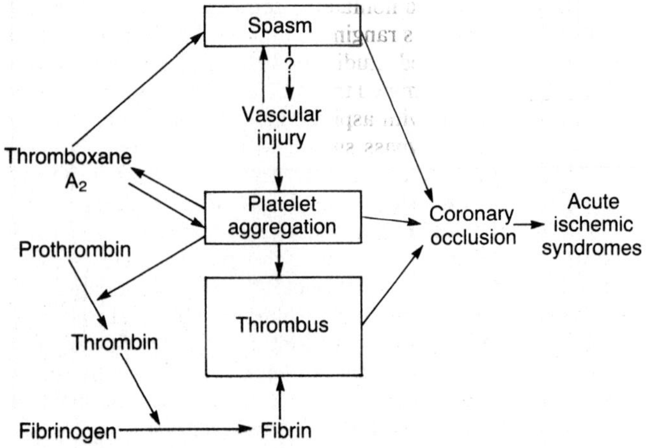


**Figure 13.13** The interrelationship of dynamic mechanisms that may cause or contribute to the clinical presentation of acute ischemic syndromes. *(From Epstein SE, Palmeri ST: Mechanisms contributing to precipitation of unstable angina and acute myocardial infarction: Implications regarding therapy. Am J Cardiol 1984;54:1247, with permission.)*

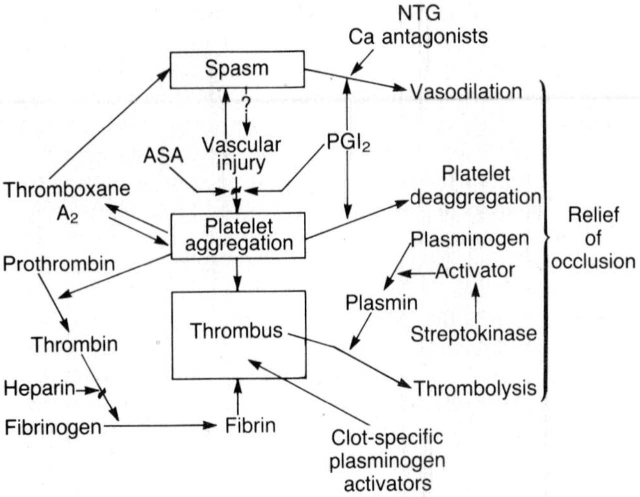


**Figure 13.14** Several possible dynamic mechanisms that may cause acute ischemic syndromes, as well as naturally occurring mechanisms and pharmacologic interventions that may relieve the degree of coronary obstruction. ASA, acetylsalicylic acid; NTG, nitroglycerin. *(From Epstein SE, Palmeri ST: Mechanisms contributing to precipitation of unstable angina and acute myocardial infarction: Implications regarding therapy. Am J Cardiol 1984;54:1247, with permission.)*

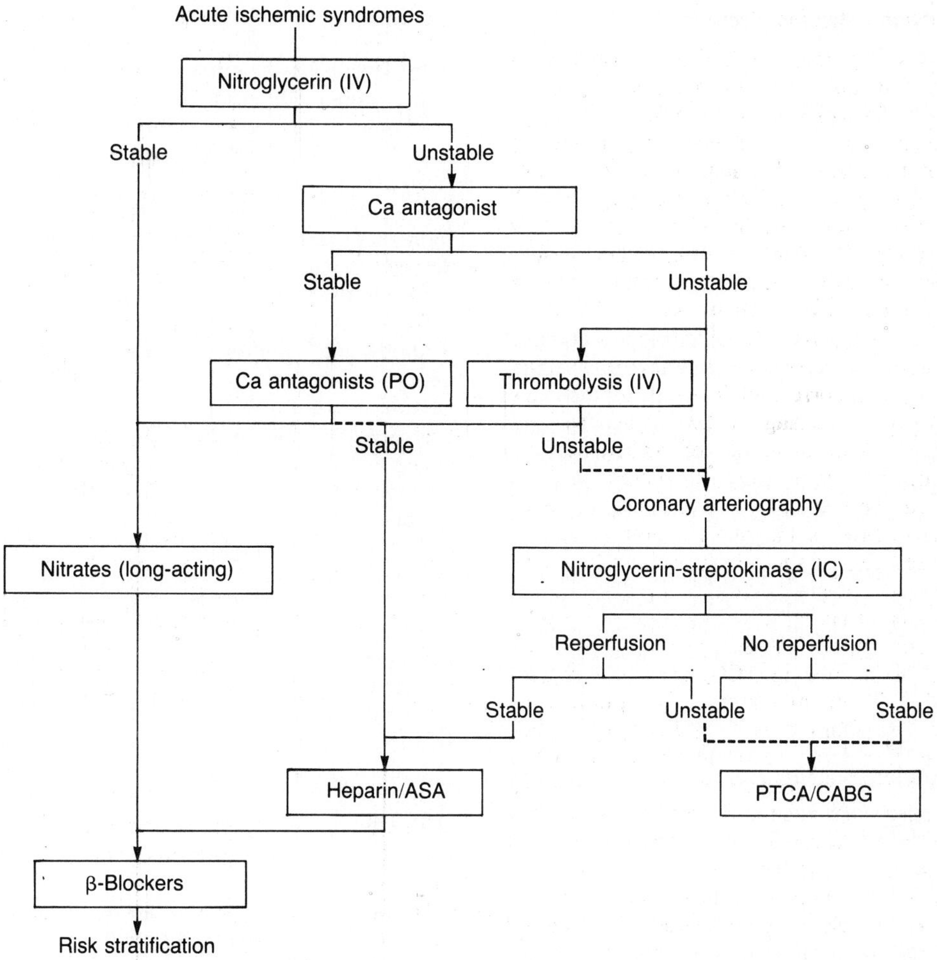


**Figure 13.15** Therapeutic guidelines for managing patients who present with acute ischemic syndromes. ASA, acetylsalicylic acid; CABG, coronary artery bypass graft; IC, intracoronary; IV, intravenous; PO, orally; PTCA, percutaneous transluminal coronary angioplasty. *(From Epstein SE, Palmeri ST: Mechanisms contributing to precipitation of unstable angina and acute myocardial infarction: Implications regarding therapy. Am J Cardiol 1984;54:1250, with permission.)*

situation because it is the most potent coronary artery vasodilator.

The role of β-blockers in unstable angina is controversial.[132] If the patient is currently on β-blocker therapy and intervening complications such as heart failure do not limit their use, the β-blockers may prevent ischemia resulting from tachycardia or increased blood pressure, but concern exists over their effects on coronary artery tone. If the angina worsens because of the potential vasoconstrictive effects of β-blockers, they should be stopped.[133]

Early, uncontrolled studies of anticoagulation for unstable angina and myocardial infarction reported impressive reductions in progression to myocardial infarction; however, these trials had serious design flaws limiting the conclusions that may be drawn. More recently, Telford and Wilson reported that heparin (5,000 units every 6 hours) reduced the development of transmural myocardial infarction as compared with placebo (2% versus 17%) and that atenolol added little to the benefits of heparin in the relatively small numbers of patients in this study.[134] Additional studies are needed to clarify the role of anticoagulation in unstable angina and myocardial infarction.[135] In contrast to the confusion surrounding the use of anticoagulants, antiplatelet therapy with aspirin has unequivocally been shown to reduce the occurrence of mortality and nonfatal infarction in unstable angina by about 50% in doses ranging from 324 to 1,300 mg per day in two well-controlled studies.[136,137] The Canadian multicenter study also examined the effect of sulfinpyrazone alone and in combination with aspirin and found no benefit.

Coronary artery bypass surgery can be performed safely in patients with unstable angina; however, results from the National Cooperative Unstable Angina Study Group show that early or late infarction is not significantly improved by surgery compared with medical therapy.[138–141] This study, which excluded patients with left main stenosis, suggests that most patients should receive intensive medical management initially; however, long term, about 36% of the medically treated patients crossed over to surgery because of inadequate symptom control. Those patients with a previous MI or hypertension, resting ST abnormalities, or ST-segment depression greater than 3 mm on exercise are likely to fail maximal medical therapy (about 3%) and become candidates for surgery, as are those initially controlled patients with high-risk factors including left main stem stenosis and triple or proximal left anterior descending and right coronary stenoses.

PTCA has been used successfully in the management of unstable angina.[142] This procedure involves the insertion of a guidewire and inflatable balloon into the affected coronary artery and enlargement of the lumen of the artery by stretching of the vessel wall.[143] Unfortunately, this may cause atheroma plaque fracture through the stretching of inelastic components and denudation of the endothelium. Consequently, platelet adhesion and aggregation, thrombus formation, and smooth muscle proliferation may give rise to acute occlusion and early or late restenosis. The presence of coronary artery spasm and intraluminal thrombus, common occurrences in unstable angina, increase the hazard of these complications.[144–146] Patients best suited for PTCA are those with recent onset of worsening of angina without a long history of symptoms. Angiographic characteristics associated with these clinical findings that allow the greatest probability of success for PTCA are severe, discrete, proximal lesions in a large epicardial vessel. Candidates for PTCA must also be acceptable for CABG, as a small percentage of procedures result in emergency CABG. After a period of stabilization, patients receive intravenous nitroglycerin with or without calcium channel blockers prior to the procedure and follow-up with heparin acutely and warfarin chronically to prevent coronary thrombosis. Investigations are under way to determine the role for sequential or combination treatment with thrombolytic therapy during PTCA. Initial patency rates average approximately 70% for single-vessel involvement in the hands of experienced operators; however, a restenosis rate of 15% to 30% or higher (e.g., variant angina) in selected patient populations remains a problem.[147,148]

In the event of prolonged chest pain and ischemic ECG changes unrelieved by nitrate therapy or calcium channel antagonists, total occlusion of a coronary vessel may be assumed and steps should be taken to restore blood flow. Thrombolytic therapy given by the intracoronary or intravenous route, either alone or preceding PTCA, has been shown in some centers to be an effective management approach to unstable angina.[149] Thrombolytic therapy for evolving myocardial infarction is further described in Chapter 14. Intraaortic balloon counterpulsation is a mechanical assist device introduced into the femoral artery and advanced to the thoracic aorta. The balloon is triggered by the patient's R wave to inflate in diastole and deflate at the onset of systole, which provides the hemodynamic effects of decreasing systemic vascular resistance and increasing diastolic pressure to improve coronary artery blood flow. Although the balloon pump appears to be effective in patients resistant to medical therapy, this device has a high rate of complications, including thromboembolic episodes and ischemia of lower limbs, and few properly controlled trials exist to evaluate its role in therapy.[150,151] One prospective randomized trial comparing intravenous nitrate therapy and counterpulsation found no difference in symptom control or mortality.[152]

### *Coronary Artery Spasm and Variant Angina Pectoris*[153]

In his original description of variant angina pectoris, Prinzmetal noted the waxing-and-waning course of this syndrome.[26] This has been observed by others and it appears that the most severe symptoms and the greatest risk for mortality and morbidity occur within the first 6 months after the onset of symptoms.[154] After this initial rocky course, spontaneous remissions have been reported to occur, and the cyclic nature of variant angina creates difficulties in assessing the value of any therapeutic intervention.

The merit of any intervention may be assessed by several methods, and a combination of these will most likely provide information for rational decisions concerning therapy. Reduction in symptoms and nitroglycerin consumption as documented by a patient diary can assist the interpretation of objective data obtained from ambulatory ECG recordings. This method may underestimate the number of ischemic episodes because of the variable nature of variant angina, and serial recordings may be of great value. Evidence of efficacy includes the reduction of ischemic events, both depression and elevation of ST segment, which may be symptomatic or asymptomatic, with the latter being overall more common. Additional evidence would be reduced number of attacks of angina requiring hospitalization, absence of myocardial infarction, and sudden death. Ergonovine provocative testing has been suggested by some as a means of determining the effectiveness of therapy; however, not all investigators have found this method to be reliable because of the fluctuating course of variant angina and provocation may be associated with drug-resistant vasospasm and ventricular arrhythmias.

Optimization of therapy includes dose titration using doses sufficiently high to obtain clinical efficacy without unacceptable adverse effects in individual patients. All patients should be treated for acute attacks and maintained on prophylactic treatment for 6 to 12 months after the initial episode. The occurrence of serious arrhythmias during attacks is associated with a greater risk of sudden death and these patients should be treated more aggressively and for prolonged periods.[155] In patients without arrhythmias who become asymptomatic and remain so several months after treatment has been instituted, withdrawal of therapy may be safe after first ascertaining that disease activity is quiescent.[156,157] Aggravating factors such as alcohol consumption and cigarette smoking should be eliminated when treatment is instituted.[158,159]

Nitrates have been the mainstay of therapy for acute attacks of variant angina and coronary artery spasm for many years. Most patients respond rapidly to sublingual nitroglycerin or isosorbide dinitrate; however, intravenous and intracoronary nitroglycerin may be very useful for patients not responding to sublingual preparations. In particular, vasospasm provoked by ergonovine may require intracoronary nitroglycerin. Other nitrate products including intravenous isosorbide dinitrate and nitroglycerin ointment have been shown to be effective for acute attacks of variant angina.[160,161] The efficacy of chronic nitrate therapy has not been extensively investigated in variant angina; however, isosorbide dinitrate (ISDN) in doses of 40–120 (mean 65) mg per day has been shown to decrease anginal frequency by 50% in 71% of the patients treated by Hill et al.[162] They found ISDN to be similar in efficacy to nifedipine as did Ginsburg et al, but nifedipine was better tolerated in the latter study.[163] Waters et al found nitrates to be less effective than calcium antagonists for improving survival without infarction.[164] As calcium antagonists may be more effective, have few serious adverse effects in effective doses, and can be given less frequently than nitrates, some consider them to be the agents of choice for variant angina.

Nifedipine, verapamil, and diltiazem are equally effective as single agents for the initial management of variant angina and coronary artery spasm. Dose titration is important to maximize the response with calcium antagonists. Comparative trials, which are few in number, do not reveal significant differences among these three drugs for variant angina.[165,166] In patients unresponsive to calcium antagonists alone, nitrates may be added with a good response. Combination nifedipine–diltiazem or nifedipine–verapamil therapy has been reported to be useful in patients unresponsive to single-drug regimens.[166,167] This is probably rational as, at the cellular level, the drugs have different receptors, but the verapamil–diltiazem combination should be used cautiously because of their potential additive effects on contractility and conduction.

β-Adrenergic blockade has little or no role in the management of variant angina according to most authorities.[69,89,133,168,169] Although not all studies report increased painful episodes of variant angina with the addition of β-blockers they may induce coronary vasoconstriction and prolong ischemia as documented by continuous ECG monitoring.

Other approaches to therapy have attempted modification of α-adrenergic tone with α-antagonists such as phentolamine, phenoxybenzamine, and prazosin.[170] The overall response to α-blockers is variable and long-term results are discouraging. Anticholinergic agents have also been used to diminish enhanced parasympathetic activity leading to stimulation of sympathetic nerves and coronary vasospasm; however, only parenteral atropine has been studied and the role for chronic therapy is undetermined. Because of its α-blocking properties, labetalol may be useful but very little information is available.[81] Adverse effects limit the utility of amiodarone and perhexilene and only small numbers of patients with variant angina have been treated with these agents. Plexectomy, surgical interruption of the sympathetic innervation of the heart, with and without CABG has been reported to benefit a few patients.

Agents that modify platelet aggregation and arachidonic acid metabolism have undergone preliminary clinical trials and, as sole interventions, dramatic responses have not been seen.[171] Aspirin has not been as effective in variant angina as in unstable angina, perhaps reflecting differences in the underlying pathophysiology. The roles of thromboxane synthesis inhibition, thromboxane receptor antagonism, prostacyclin, lipoxygenase inhibition, and ticlopidine are being clarified in ongoing studies, but they do not occupy a major place in therapy at the present time. Dietary supplementation with fish oil can influence lipid levels, platelet aggregation, and possibly cardiovascular mortality, but as most of the available studies are either in animals or of an epidemiologic nature, routine use cannot be recommended for the prevention or treatment of variant angina.[172]

### *Silent Myocardial Ischemia*[27,40,173,174]

The objective in the treatment of silent myocardial ischemia is to reduce the total number of ischemic episodes, both symptomatic and asymptomatic, regardless of the direction of ST-segment shift. Studies by Gottlieb et al and Assey et al in patients with unstable angina and exercise-induced ischemia demonstrate that silent ischemia is common and associated with a high risk for myocardial infarction and sudden death when compared with painful episodes of ischemia.[175,176] Although the underlying mechanisms for silent ischemia are continuing to be defined, increased physical activity, activation of the sympathetic nervous system, increased cortisol secretion, increased coronary artery tone, and enhanced platelet aggregation may be additive in lowering the threshold for ischemia. Tofler et al have shown that platelet aggregation is increased in the morning hours (7–11 AM) corresponding to circadian rhythms noted for the peak frequency of ischemia, acute myocardial infarction, and sudden death.[177–179] Silent ischemia is associated with ST-segment elevation or depression and frequently occurs without antecedent changes in heart rate or blood pressure, suggesting that this form of ischemia is due to primary reduction in oxygen supply in many instances, while at other times in the same patient oxygen demand is increased prior to the onset of ischemia. Regardless of the exact mechanism, there is increasing concern that painless ischemia carries considerable risk for further damage to the myocardium, arrhythmogenesis, and sudden death, and because it is apparently very common in some settings, major emphasis should be placed on its management. A consensus has not been reached for the most appropriate method of detecting and quantifying the magnitude of silent ischemia; however, ambulatory electrocardiographic monitoring is felt by many to be the most useful tool at the present time. The initial step in management is to modify the major risk factors for IHD—hypertension, hypercholesterolemia, and smoking—and data from the MRFIT show these interventions to be useful in patients with silent ischemia.[180] In a subset of the study population who had abnormal baseline exercise ECG responses, the special intervention group had a 57% reduction in coronary heart disease death (22.2/1,000 versus 51.8/1,000) and a reduction in sudden death resulting from cessation of smoking and lowering of blood pressure and cholesterol, compared with the usual care group.

Several studies with β-blockers have shown improvement in the number of ischemic episodes, primarily ST-segment depression and those associated with effort, compared with placebo; however, this benefit is not seen with all β-blockers. Post-MI patients and those with a high level of sympathetic nervous system activity are perhaps the best candidates for β-blocker therapy. Reductions in number and duration of ischemic episodes have been noted with β-blockers that are nonselective and cardioselective; however, compared with nifedipine, their intrinsic sympathomimetic activity has been found to be detrimental in patients with severe angina[78] or to be useful only in limiting effort angina while little affecting asymptomatic ischemia.[181] Perhaps because it does not alter coronary artery tone compared with other β-blockers, labetalol has been shown to reduce the number of episodes of ST-segment depression (3.4 versus

1.5) and the duration of ischemia (80 versus 22 minutes) compared with placebo.[81,182]

Calcium channel antagonists alone and in combination have been shown to be effective in reducing symptomatic and asymptomatic ischemia.[128,181,183,184] Subramanian et al compared verapamil (360 mg/d) and propranolol (240 mg/d) alone and in combination and found the number of ST segments depressed more than 1 mm to be decreased by either single agent compared with placebo; however, the combination produced a further reduction. The maximum depth of ST depression was significantly reduced with the combination but unaffected by the drugs singly. In patients with variant angina, Johnson et al found that verapamil 240–480 mg/d in a 9-month study reduced the number of ST-segment deviations per week to 7.7 from 33.1 during the placebo phases.

Nitrates, given by various routes, have demonstrated efficacy for silent ischemia; this is related to their effects on $MVo_2$ as well as coronary artery vasodilation and redistribution of myocardial blood flow.[160,185,186] In addition to the studies cited previously, early uncontrolled trials by Oakley et al using propranolol (480 mg/d) and nifedipine (60 mg/d) set the stage for acceptance of combination therapy as effective.[187] In a well-controlled study by Dargie et al using nifedipine 30 or 60 mg/d, propranolol 240 or 480 mg/d, or a combination, the combination was demonstrated to be more effective in reducing the area of ST-segment depression and the number of ST-depression episodes, compared with placebo or with either drug alone.[188] They also noted little benefit from using the higher dose of propranolol.

Other pharmacologic approaches using intravenous aspirin, prostacyclin, and ticlopidine have not shown promising results in the available studies.[173] Surgical intervention using CABG does not appear to be warranted in asymptomatic patients without left main stem disease, severe three-vessel disease, or poor ventricular function, and data from the Coronary Artery Surgery Study show no improvement in survival for these patients. The role for PTCA remains controversial in silent ischemia and, for the present, it should be reserved for patients with discrete, severe proximal lesions in the left anterior descending coronary artery.

### *Coronary Artery Bypass Grafting*

After the introduction of saphenous vein graft replacement for severely occluded coronary arteries by Favorolo in 1967, CABG became an accepted and commonly used alternative approach to the management of IHD.[189] The objectives in performing CABG are twofold: (1) reduce the number of symptomatic anginal attacks and improve the life-style of the patient and (2) reduce the mortality associated with coronary artery disease. Surgery is effective in providing pain relief in large numbers of patients, with about 70% to 95% being pain free at 1 year and 46% to 55% being pain free at 5 years. This compares favorably with medical management, where only about 30% are free of symptoms at 5 years. The second objective is met in certain patients and has been addressed in three large, well-controlled trials of bypass surgery.[18,190,191] These three studies, the Veterans Administration (VA) study, the European Cooperative Surgery Study (ECSS), and the Coronary Artery Surgery Study (CASS), are not directly comparable, as the inclusion and exclusion criteria for entry into each study were different and patients were followed for different periods of time. They have also been criticized for not being representative of the general population who may be candidates for surgery and for crossover of medically managed patients to the surgical group. Consequently, the validity of generalizing the results from these studies to routine practice has been questioned but these studies are useful in providing a basis for decisions concerning surgery. Tables 13.14, 13.15, and 13.16 summarize survival at various time intervals and for several subgroups from each of these studies. In general, those patients who have left main stem stenosis of greater than 70%, proximal stenosis of the left anterior descending artery greater than 70% to 75%, poor left ventricular function, or severe three-vessel disease are most likely to have improved survival with surgical therapy. A notable exception to these observations is the lack of difference in any subgroup for CASS, and although trends suggesting improved survival were observed, no significant ($P<0.05$) differences were found. This is probably related to patient selection, with patients in CASS having less severe disease compared with patients in the other studies. In addition to survival, other aspects that have been evaluated include exercise capacity, evidence of ischemia, need for drugs to treat angina, and quality of life, including employment status. Exercise capacity may be improved early after CABG; however, at 5 years no significant difference was noted between the medical and surgical groups in CASS and ECSS. The need for nitrates and $\beta$-blockers is clearly reduced by surgery, with only 30% of CABG patients requiring chronic medication, whereas 70% of their medical counterparts received anginal drugs. CASS has shown employment status after surgery to be more dependent on pretreatment status than any effect induced by the treatment, and about 70% of patients are employed before and after surgery.

Indications for bypass surgery should not be rigidly defined although general recommendations can be made on the basis of available data.[104] Indications may be based on symptoms, coronary anatomy, ventricular function, or high-risk clinical variables. Patients whose life-style is unacceptably limited because of symptoms despite optimum medical treatment or who are unable to tolerate drug therapy because of side effects are considered to be candidates. Regardless of symptoms, patients with significant stenosis (>50%–70%) of the left main coronary artery, patients with triple-vessel disease, where the proximal left anterior descending coronary has greater than 70% stenosis, or patients with poor left ventricular function should be considered. High-risk clinical variables include early positive (>1.5-mm depression) exercise test, fall in ejection fraction greater than 5% on exercise, large exercise-induced wall motion abnormality, and large or multiple thallium perfusion defects. In patients 65 years of age or older, surgical benefit is greatest in high-risk patients, 62% surviving compared with 33% in the medical group at the 6-year follow-up; significant improvement was also seen overall (surgical 79% versus medical 64%). Corresponding differences were also noted in chest pain.[192] Left main stem disease or left main equivalent (combined proximal left anterior descending and proximal left circumflex) coronary disease clearly benefit from surgical intervention.[193,194] Mortality is related to the severity of stenosis in this situation and perioperative mortality is also increased. Survival at 3 years

**Table 13.14** Veterans Administration Coronary Artery Bypass Surgery Study Survival Rates (%)

| | *5 yr* | | *7 yr* | | *11 yr* | |
|---|---|---|---|---|---|---|
| | M[a] | S | M | S | M | S |
| All patients | 78 | 83 | 70 | 77[f] | 57 | 58 |
| All non-LMD[b] | 80 | 82 | 72 | 77 | 58 | 58 |
| 1 vessel | 88 | 94 | 83 | 88 | 65 | 70 |
| 2 vessels | 85 | 79 | 81 | 73 | 69[f] | 55 |
| 3 vessels | 75 | 81 | 63 | 75 | 50 | 56 |
| Impaired LVF[c] | 73 | 80 | 63 | 74[f] | 49 | 53 |
| Normal LVF | 90 | 85 | 84 | 80 | 71 | 64 |
| Angio Hi risk[d] | 66 | 83[f] | 52 | 76[f] | 38 | 50[f] |
| Angio Lo risk | 87 | 82 | 82 | 77 | 68 | 61 |
| Clinical risk—Hi[e] | 63 | 86[f] | 52 | 72 | 36 | 49[f] |
| Clinical risk—Mid | 80 | 82 | 71 | 79 | 61 | 62 |
| Clinical risk—Lo | 93[f] | 82 | 88 | 81 | 73 | 63 |

[a] M, medically treated patients; S, surgically treated patients.
[b] All patients without left main stem coronary artery disease.
[c] Left ventricular function; impaired LVF was global ejection fraction < 50% or minimal hypokinesis or akinesis of 25%–75% of the heart border or greater.
[d] Angiographic high-risk patients are those with three-vessel disease and impaired LVF.
[e] Two or more of the following: resting ST-segment depression; history of MI; history of hypertension.
[f] $P < 0.05$.

in the surgical group averages about 85% to 90%, while in the medical group survival is significantly lower, about 60% to 70%. In left main equivalent disease, survival at 5 years in CASS was reported to be 85% in the surgical group versus 55% in the medical group, and those patients with ejection fraction less than 50% showed the greatest improvement in survival (69% versus 26%). Similiar trends have been noted in patients with three-vessel disease and abnormal ventricular function, with 4-year survival rates of 89% and 55% in the surgical and medical groups, respectively.[195]

Operative mortality is reported to range from 1% to 3% and is related to the number of vessels involved and perioperative ventricular function. Patients in CASS with one-, two-, or three- vessel disease had operative mortalities of 1.4%, 2.1%, and 2.8%, respectively. The relationship to left ventricular ejection fraction follows a similar trend, with ejection fractions of greater than 50%, 20% to 40%, and less than 20% having operative mortality rates of 1.9%, 4.4%, and 6.7%, respectively. Perioperative infarction averages

**Table 13.15** European Coronary Surgery Study Group Survival Rates (%)

| | *5 yr* | | *8 yr* | |
|---|---|---|---|---|
| | M[a] | S | M | S |
| All patients | 83.6 | 92.4[d] | 79.9 | 88.6[d] |
| LMD[b] | 67.9 | 85.7 | 63.6 | 81.7 |
| 2 vessels | 88.2 | 91.2 | 87.4 | 85.0 |
| 3 vessels | 82.4 | 94.0[d] | 76.7 | 91.8[d] |
| LAD negative | 92.1 | 93.3 | 88.0 | 62.1 |
| LAD positive | 82.0 | 92.7[d] | 78.7 | 87.8[d] |
| ETT with ST ↓ >1.5 mm[c] | 79.0 | 91.7[d] | 76.5 | 89.6[d] |

[a] M, medically treated patients; S, surgically treated patients.
[b] LMD, left main stem coronary artery disease; LAD, left anterior descending coronary artery disease.
[c] ST-segment depression greater than 1.5 mm on exercise tolerance testing.
[d] $P < 0.05$.

**Table 13.16** Coronary Artery Surgery Study Survival Rates (%)[a]

| | *1 yr* | | *5 yr* | |
|---|---|---|---|---|
| | M[b] | S | M | S |
| All patients | 98 | 98 | 90 | 92 |
| 1 vessel | 99 | 98 | 93 | 96 |
| 2 vessels | 99 | 98 | 94 | 95 |
| 3 vessels | 98 | 99 | 89 | 93 |
| Group A[c] | 99 | 98 | 95 | 96 |
| Group B | 98 | 100 | 85 | 96[d] |
| Group C | 96 | 99 | 89 | 89 |
| All EF < 0.5 | 99 | 99 | 84 | 92[d] |
| EF < 0.5 + 1 vessel | 100 | 100 | 81 | 100 |
| EF < 0.5 + 2 vessels | 100 | 100 | 88 | 92 |
| EF < 0.5 + 3 vessels | 97 | 98 | 80 | 90[d] |

[a] Ejection fraction (EF) > 0.5 with 1, 2, and 3 vessels; no significant differences noted in any group.
[b] M, medically treated patients; S, surgically treated patients.
[c] Group A: angina and ejection fraction > 0.5. Group B: angina and ejection fraction < 0.5. Group C: free of angina after MI.
[d] $P < 0.1$ trend toward significant difference. No significant differences were noted in any subgroup analysis for 1 or 5 years.

5% depending on the sensitivity of the method for assessment, and occurrence of an infarct reduces long-term survival. Neurologic dysfunction is relatively common postoperatively in CABG patients, but many of the deficits are clinically insignificant and resolve with time. Fatal brain damage occurs in 0.3% to 7%, stroke in about 5%, and ophthalmologic defects in 25% but only 3% have clinically apparent field defects. Peripheral nerve lesions (12%) and brachial plexopathy (7%) have also been reported. Other complications include constrictive pericarditis (0.2%), cellulitis at the site of vein graft, and mediastinal infections.

Graft patency influences the success for symptom control and survival, and the mechanism for graft in early occlusion is probably different from that associated with late closure. Early occlusion is related to platelet adhesion and aggregation, whereas late occlusion may be related to endothelial proliferation and progression of atherosclerosis. Patency of grafts early after CABG is reported to range from 88% to 97% in at least one graft and 58% to 81% in all grafts at 1 year.[196] Long-term patency based on the CASS Montreal Heart Institute experience suggests that 60% to 67% of all grafts remain patent at 5 to 11 years. Antiplatelet therapy has been demonstrated to improve early and late patency rates and should probably be used in all patients who do not have any contraindications. Chesebro et al used aspirin 325 mg three times daily and dipyridamole 100 mg four times daily to reduce the late development of vein graft occlusions from 27% in the placebo group to 16% in the treated group at 12 months.[197] Using a dose of 100 mg of aspirin alone, Lorenz et al found 90% of grafts patent compared with 68% for the placebo-treated patients.[198] Late graft closure is related to elevated lipid levels and the progression of atherosclerosis in the grafted vessels as well as the native circulation.[199] Elevated levels of very-low-density lipoproteins, low-density-lipoproteins, and low-density lipoprotein apoprotein B correlated to disease progression and graft closure. This process has recently been shown to be delayed by institution of lipid-lowering therapy (colestipol and niacin) in CABG patients; this should be considered if excessive elevations of cholesterol occur in the bypass patient.[200]

Internal mammary artery grafts are preferred by some surgeons; however, the acceptance of this type of graft has been slow. Recent evidence demonstrates better survival rates, as well as fewer postoperative infarctions and recurrent episodes of angina, with the internal mammary artery graft compared with saphenous vein grafts.[201,202]

Valvular heart disease can coexist with coronary heart disease although this is relatively uncommon with rheumatic valve disease (usually the mitral valve) and more common with aortic stenosis and regurgitation.[20] Angina may occur in 35% to 65% of patients with aortic stenosis or regurgitation and, if severe, may be the cause of angina in the absence of coronary artery disease. Patients being evaluated for possible CABG should also be evaluated for valvular disease to determine if valve replacement needs to be performed along with bypass grafting.

### *Percutaneous Transluminal Coronary Angioplasty[142]*

Since its introduction into clinical cardiology by Gruentzig in 1977, PTCA has gained rapid acceptance as a safe and effective means of managing coronary artery disease.[203] It has been estimated that the number of procedures performed in this country during 1984 was about 63,000, nearly double that for 1983. The proposed mechanisms for reduced stenosis with PTCA include (1) compression and redistribution of the atherosclerotic plaque; (2) embolization of plaque contents; (3) aneurysm formation; and (4) disruption of the plaque and arterial wall with distortion and tearing of the intima and media, leading to denudation of the endothelium, platelet adhesion and aggregation, thrombus formation, and smooth muscle proliferation.[142,143] Of these mechanisms, the last one is felt to be the most important, but the others may contribute to opening of the lesions in some situations.

The indications for PTCA are outlined in Table 13.17 based on the recommendations of Vlietstra and Holmes.[142] It should be noted that only about 10% to 20% of all patients with coronary artery disease are candidates for PTCA.[20] Recently, O'Neill et al reviewed the status of PTCA used alone or in conjunction or sequentially with thrombolysis for acute myocardial infarction[204–206]; this topic is also discussed in Chapter 14.

Assessment of outcome with PTCA can be based on several clinical and functional factors. It is important to remember that the success of PTCA depends on the experience of the operator; the complicating factors for the patient, including the number of vessels to be dilated, and the technical advances in the equipment used (e.g., steerable and low-profile catheters). The initial success rate for immediate opening of stenotic lesions averages 80% to 90% in experienced hands and there is usually a significant reduction in the amount of stenosis. Mortality at 1 year is 1% and 3% for single-vessel disease and multiple-vessel involvement, respectively, reflecting the good prognosis associated with this degree of coronary artery disease. At 6 years, survival is 98% and 92% for single and multiple disease, respectively.[207] Most patients remain event free (no death, MI, or CABG) for extended periods (74 months). Symptomatic status, as measured by the New York Heart Association classification, is improved in many patients. Gruentzig

**Table 13.17** Coronary Anatomic Indications for PTCA

| |
|---|
| Widely accepted |
| Single-vessel disease |
| Proximal subtotal stenosis |
| Recent total occlusion |
| Multivessel disease |
| Severe (70% or more) |
| Subtotal stenoses in two or three major vessels (if complete revascularization is possible) |
| Severe (70% or more) subtotal stenoses in one major vessel and moderate (50%–69%) stenoses in other vessels |
| Restenosis |
| Evolving |
| Occlusion during acute myocardial infarction |
| Angina after coronary artery bypass grafting |
| Operation is relatively contraindicated |
| Revascularization is likely to be incomplete |

From Vlietstra RE, Holmes DR Jr: PTCA. Philadelphia, F.A. Davis, 1987, p 52, with permission.

et al found that prior to PTCA 84 of 133 patients were in NYHA Class III or IV, but after PTCA only 8 of 133 remained in these classes. Before PTCA, 97% of his patients had positive ETTs and after PTCA 2 of 61 with single-vessel disease and 7 of 30 with multiple-vessel disease continued to have positive ETTs. Exercise capacity was also improved with only 47% reaching their predicted capacity before PTCA and 78% doing so after PTCA. Restenosis is noted in about 30% of patients at 6 months and two thirds of these patients have angina associated with restenosis. A few late restenotic events occur, but most restenosis occurs within the first 6 months. Factors that predict restenosis include little improvement (<5%) in ejection fraction after PTCA, continuing wall motion abnormalities, and positive exercise thallium scintigraphy. Antiplatelet therapy may be useful in reducing or preventing restenosis but conclusive studies are not yet available. Factors increasing the likelihood of failure or complications with PTCA include female gender, age greater than 60 years, duration of angina greater than 6 months, operator experience with fewer than 50 cases, eccentric stenosis, stenosis severity greater than 90%, calcified stenosis, intraluminal thrombus, involvement of branch vessels, and stenosis located on acute bend in vessel.[142]

The overall complication rate based on PTCA Registry data is 21.1%.[208] Coronary occlusion, dissection, or spasm occurs in 10.4% of patients, while myocardial infarction occurs in 5.5%. Prolonged angina and ventricular tachycardia or fibrillation occur in 6.9% and 2.3%, respectively. Mortality was reported to be 0.9% overall and high-risk events for mortality included ventricular arrhythmias and myocardial infarction. The frequency of urgent CABG because of complications should be less than 5%.

During PTCA, patients are usually heparinized to prevent immediate thrombus formation during the procedure and systemic anticoagulation is continued up to 24 hours. Calcium antagonists may also be given to prevent coronary artery spasm during PTCA; some centers also administer antiplatelet therapy prior to PTCA. After PTCA, calcium antagonists are given for 2 to 4 weeks to prevent coronary artery spasm and for their other anti-ischemic effects. Some authors believe they may also prevent restenosis; however, this has not been conclusively demonstrated. Long-term warfarin has not been shown to be useful in preventing restenosis and it is not recommended unless another indication exists.[209] Antiplatelet therapy with aspirin with or without dipyridamole is also recommended for 1 year after PTCA to delay or prevent restenosis.[210] Experimental data suggest that sulfinpyrazone may also be useful as antiplatelet therapy in PTCA.[211]

## References


1. Heberden W. Some account of a disorder of the breast. Med Tran R Coll Phy Lond 1772;2:59–67.
2. Matthews MB. Historical background, in Julian DG (ed): Angina Pectoris, 2nd ed. New York, Churchill Livingstone, 1985, pp 3–12.
3. Brunton TL. On the use of nitrate of amyl in angina pectoris. Lancet 1867;2:628–629.
4. Murrell W. Nitroglycerine as a remedy for angina pectoris. Lancet 1879;2:80, 113, 151, 225.
5. Bousfield G. Angina pectoris: Changes in electrocardiogram during paroxysm. Lancet 1918;2:457–458.
6. Cooper JK. Electrocardiography 100 years ago: Origins, pioneers, and contributors. N Engl J Med 1986;315:461–464.
7. Herrick JB. Clinical features of sudden obstruction of the coronary arteries. JAMA 1912;59:2015–2020.
8. Ahlquist RP. A study of the adrentropic receptors. Am J Physiol 1948;153:583–600.
9. Black JW, Stephenson JS. Pharmacology of a new adrenergic β-receptor-blocking compound (nethalide). Lancet 1962;2:311–314.
10. Fleckenstein A. Calcium Antagonism in Heart and Smooth Muscle. Experimental Facts and Therapeutic Prospects. New York, John Wiley and Sons, 1983.
11. Kannel WB, Feinleib M. Natural history of angina pectoris in the Framingham study: Prognosis and survival. Am J Cardiol 1972;29:154–163.
12. Greig M, Pemberton J, Hay I, et al. A prospective study of the development of coronary heart disease in a group of 1202 middle-aged men. J Epidem Community Health 1980;34:23–30.
13. Rossouw JE, Weich HFH, Steyn K, et al. The prevalence of ischaemic heart disease in three rural South Africa communities. J Chron Dis 1984;37:97–106.
14. Stamler J, Liu K. The benefits of prevention, in Kaplan NM, Stamler J (eds): Prevention of Coronary Heart Disease. Philadelphia, W.B. Saunders, 1983, pp 188–207.
15. Goldman L, Hashimoto B, Cook F, et al. Comparative reproducibility and validity of systems for assessing cardiovascular functional class: Advantages of a new specific activity scale. Circulation 1981;64:1227–1234.
16. Harris PJ, Behar VS, Conley MJ, et al. The prognostic significance of 50% coronary stenosis in medically treated patients with coronary artery disease. Circulation 1980;62:240–248.
17. Silverman KJ, Grossman W. Angina pectoris. Natural history and strategies for evaluation and management. N Engl J Med 1984;310:1712–1717.
18. Veterans Administration Coronary Artery Bypass Surgery Cooperative Study Group. Eleven-year survival in the Veterans Administration randomized trial of coronary bypass surgery for stable angina. N Engl J Med 1984;311:1333–1339, 1339–1345.
19. Braunwald E (ed): Heart Disease. A Textbook of Cardiovascular Medicine. Philadelphia, W.B. Saunders, 1984.
20. Cohn PF (ed): Diagnosis and Therapy of Coronary Artery Disease, 2nd ed. Boston, Martinus Nijhoff, 1985.
21. Berne RM, Rubio R. Coronary circulation, in Berne RM, Sperelakis N, Geiger ST (eds): Handbook of Physiology, Section 2, The Cardiovascular System. Bethesda, MD, American Physiological Society, 1979, p 897.
22. Vinten-Johansen J, Barnard RJ, Buckberg GD. Left ventricular $O_2$ requirements of pressure and volume loading in the normal canine heart and inaccuracy of pressure-derived indices of $O_2$ demand. Cardiovasc Res 1982;16:439–477.
23. Quyyumi AA. Mechanisms of angina pectoris, in Fox KM (ed): Ischaemic Heart Disease. Boston, MTP Press Limited, pp 91–121.
24. Epstein SE, Cannon RO III, Talbot TL. Hemodynamic prin-

ciples in the control of coronary blood flow. Am J Cardiol 1985;56:4E–10E.
25. Arnett EN, Isner JM, Redwood DR, et al. Coronary artery narrowing in coronary artery disease: Comparison of cineangiographic and necropsy findings. Ann Intern Med 1979;91: 350–356.
26. Prinzmetal M, Kennamer R, Merliss R, et al. Angina pectoris. I. A variant form of angina pectoris. Am J Med 1959;27:375–388.
27. Cohen P (ed): Silent Myocardial Ischemia. New York, Marcel Dekker, 1986.
28. Glazier JJ, Chierchia S, Brown MJ, et al. Importance of generalized defective perception of painful stimuli as a cause of silent myocardial ischemia in chronic stable angina pectoris. Am J Cardiol 1986;58:667–672.
29. Joy M, Trump DW. Significance of minor ST segment and T-wave changes in the resting electrocardiogram of asymptomatic subjects. Br Heart J 1981;45:48–55.
30. Gobel FL, Nordstrom LA, Nelson RR, et al. The rate-pressure product as an index of myocardial oxygen consumption during exercise in patients with angina pectoris. Circulation 1978;57:549–556.
31. Ellestad MH. Stress Testing Principles and Practice, 3rd ed. Philadelphia, F.A. Davis, 1986, p 175.
32. Linhart JW, Laws JG, Satinsky JD. Maximum treadmill exercise electrocardiography in female patients. Circulation 1974;50:1173–1178.
33. Bruce RA. In McDonald L (ed): Early Recognition of Coronary Artery Disease. Amsterdam, Excerpta Medica, 1978.
34. Weiner DA, McCabe Ch, Ryan TJ. Prognostic assessment of patients with coronary artery disease by exercise testing. Am Heart J 1983;105:749–755.
35. Rochmis P, Blackburn H. Exercise tests. A survey of procedures, safety, and litigation experience in approximately 170,000 tests. JAMA 1971;217:1061–1066.
36. Bruce RA, Cohen PF. Exercise testing, in Cohen PF (ed): Diagnosis and Therapy of Coronary Artery Disease, 2nd ed. Boston, Martinus Nijhoff, 1985, pp 135–167.
37. Soufer R, Zaret BL. Nuclear cardiology, in Cohen PF (ed): Diagnosis and Therapy of Coronary Artery Disease, 2nd ed. Boston, Martinus Nijhoff, 1985, pp 191–218.
38. Cohen PF, Braunwald E. Chronic ischemic heart disease, in Braunwald E (ed): Heart Disease. A Textbook of Cardiovascular Medicine, 2nd ed. Philadelphia, W.B. Saunders, 1984, pp 1334–1383.
39. McPherson DD, Hiratzka LF, Lambeth WC, et al. Delineation of the extent of coronary atherosclerosis by high-frequency epicardial echocardiography. N Engl J Med 1987;316:304–309.
40. Singh BN, Nademanee K, Figueras J, et al. Hemodynamic and electrocardiographic correlates of symptomatic and silent myocardial ischemia: pathophysiologic and therapeutic implications. Am J Cardiol 1986;56:3B–10B.
41. Adams DF, Fraser DB, Adams HL. The complications of coronary arteriography. Circulation 1973;48:609–618.
42. Kennedy JW, Registry Committee of the Society for Cardiac Angiography. Complications associated with cardiac catheterization and angiography. Cathet Cardiovasc Diagn 1982;8:5–11.
43. Aronow WS, Kaplan NM. Smoking, in Kaplan NM, Stamler J (eds): Prevention of Coronary Heart Disease. Philadelphia, W.B. Saunders, 1983, pp 51–60.
44. Kannel WB. Update on the role of cigarette smoking in coronary heart disease. Am Heart J 1981;101:319–328.
45. Lipid Research Clinics Program. The Lipid Research Clinics Coronary Primary Prevention Trial Results. I. Reduction in incidence of coronary heart disease. JAMA 1984;251:351–64.
46. Blackwelder WC, Yano K, Rhoads GG, et al. Alcohol and mortality: The Honolulu heart study. Am J Med 1980;68:164–169.
47. Bush TL, Cowan LD, Barrett-Connor E, et al. Estrogen use and all-cause mortality. Preliminary results from the Lipid Research Clinics Program follow-up study. JAMA 1983;249: 903–906.
48. Stamper MJ, Willett WC, Colditz GA, et al. A prospective study of postmenopausal estrogen therapy and coronary heart disease. N Engl J Med 1985;313:1044–1049.
49. Wilson PWF, Garrison RJ, Castelli WP. Postmenopausal estrogen use, cigarette smoking, and cardiovascular morbidity in women over 50. The Framingham study. N Engl J Med 1985;313:1038–1049.
50. LaCroix AZ, Mead LA, Liang KY, et al. Coffee consumption and the incidence of coronary heart disease. N Engl J Med 1986;315:977–982.
51. Benson H, McCallie DP, Jr. Angina pectoris and the placebo effect. N Engl J Med 1979;300:1424–1429.
52. Khurmi NS, Bowles MJ, Kohli RS, et al. Does placebo improve indexes of effort-induced myocardial ischemia? An objective study in 150 patients with chronic stable angina pectoris. Am J Cardiol 1986;57:907–911.
53. Conti CR. Nitrate therapy for ischaemic heart disease. Eur Heart J 1985;6(suppl A):3–11.
54. Zelis R. Mechanisms of vasodilation. Am J Med 1983;74(6B): 3–12.
55. Curry SH, Aburawi SM. Analysis, deposition and pharmacokinetics of nitroglycerin. Biopharm Drug Dispos 1985;6:235–280.
56. Bogaert MG. Clinical pharmacokinetics of glyceral trinitrate following use of systemic and topical preparations. Clin Pharmacokinet 1987;12:1–11.
57. Horowitz LD, Herman MV, Gorlin R. Clinical response to nitroglycerin as a diagnostic test for coronary artery disease. Am J Cardiol 1972;29:149–153.
58. Parker JO, Vankoughnett FA, Farrell B. Nitroglycerin lingual spray. Clinical efficacy and dose-response relation. Am J Cardiol 1986;57:1–5.
59. Zeller FP, Klamerus KJ. Controversies in the use of transdermal nitroglycerin systems. Clin Pharm 1987;6:605–616.
60. Needleman P, Johnson EM. Mechanism of tolerance development to organic nitrates. J Pharmacol Exp Ther 1973;184:709–715.
61. Needleman P, Jakshik B, Johnson EM. Sulfhydryl requirement for relaxation of vascular smooth muscle. J Pharmacol Exp Ther 1973;187:324–331.
62. Moffat JP, Armstrong PW, Marks GS. Investigations into the role of sulfhydryl groups in the mechanism of action of the nitrates. Can J Physiol Pharmacol 1982;60:1261–1266.
63. Winniford MD, Kennedy PL, Wells PJ. Potentiation of nitroglycerin-induced coronary dilation by *N*-acetylcysteine. Circulation 1986;73:138–142.
64. Fung H. Pharmacokinetic determinants of nitrate action. Am J Med 1984;76(6A):22–26.
65. Parker JO, Vankoughnett KA, Farrell B. Comparison of buccal nitroglycerin and oral isosorbide dinitrate for nitrate tolerance in stable angina pectoris. Am J Cardiol 1985;56:724–728.
66. Thadani U, Hamilton SF, Olsen E, et al. Transdermal nitroglycerin patches in angina pectoris: dose titration, duration of effect, and rapid tolerance. Ann Intern Med 1986;105:485–492.
67. Flaherty JT. Hemodynamic attenuation and the nitrate-free

interval. Alternative dosing strategies for transdermal nitroglycerin. Am J Cardiol 1985;56:32I–37I.

68. Kenedi P, Giebeler B. Antianginal efficacy of long-term nitrate therapy. Z Kardiol 1983;72(suppl 3):233–238.

69. Forman MD, Robertson RM. Current treatment of coronary spasm. Advantages and disadvantages of beta blockers, in Conti CR (ed): Coronary Artery Spasm. Pathophysiology, Diagnosis and Treatment. New York, Marcel Dekker, 1986, pp 273–295.

70. Pratt CM, Welton DE, Squires WG, Jr, et al. Demonstration of training effect during chronic β-adrenergic blockade in patients with coronary artery disease. Circulation 1981;64:1125–1129.

71. Vukovich RA, Foley JE, Brown B, et al. Effect of β blockers on exercise double product (SBP × HR). Br J Clin Pharmacol 1979;7(suppl 2):167S–172S.

72. Alderman EL, Davies RO, Crowley JJ, et al. Dose response effectiveness of propranolol for the treatment of angina pectoris. Circulation 1975;51:964–975.

73. Thadani U, Davidson C, Singleton W, et al. Comparison of five β-adrenoreceptor antagonists with different ancillary properties during sustained twice daily therapy in angina pectoris. Am J Med 1980;68:243–250.

74. Miller LA, Crawford MH, O'Rourke RA. Nadolol compared to propranolol for treating chronic stable angina pectoris. Chest 1984;86:189–193.

75. Jones GR, Mir MA. Comparison of antianginal efficacy of one conventional and three long acting β-adrenoreceptor blocking agents in stable angina pectoris. Br Heart J 1981;46:503–507.

76. Thadani U, Parker JO. Propranolol in angina pectoris: Comparison of therapy given two and four times daily. Am J Cardiol 1980;46:117–123.

77. Beller GA, Bittar N, Goelho JB, et al. Double-blind, placebo-controlled trial of propranolol given one, twice and four times daily in stable angina pectoris; A multicenter study using serial exercise testing. Am J Cardiol 1984;54:37–42.

78. Quyyumi AA, Wright C, Mockus L, Fox KM. Effect of partial agonist activity in β blockers in severe angina pectoris: A double blind comparison of pindolol and atenolol. Br Med J 1984;289:951–953.

79. Shub C, Vlietstra RE, McGoon MD. Selection of optimal drug therapy for the patient with angina pectoris. Mayo Clin Proc 1985;60:539–548.

80. Smith PJ, Talbert RL. Sexual dysfunction with antihypertensive and antipsychotic agents. Clin Pharm 1986;5:373–384.

81. Prida XE, Hill JA, Feldman RL. Systemic and coronary hemodynamic effects of combined α- and β-adrenergic blockade (Labetalol) in normotensive patients with stable angina pectoris and positive exercise stress test responses. Am J Cardiol 1987;59:1084–1088.

82. Gengo FM, Huntoon L, McHugh WB. Lipid-soluble and water-soluble β blockers. Comparison of CNS depressant effects. Arch Intern Med 1987;147:39–43.

83. Kirk CA, Cove-Smith R. A comparison between atenolol and metoprolol in respect to central nervous system side effects. Postgrad Med J 1983;59(suppl 3):161–163.

84. Avorn J, Everitt DE, Weiss S. Increased antidepressant use in patients prescribed β blockers. JAMA 1986;255:357–360.

85. Shiroff RA, Mathis J, Zelis R, et al. Propranolol rebound—a retrospective study. Am J Cardiol 1978;41:778–780.

86. Goldstein RE, Corash LC, Tallman JF Jr, et al. Shortening platelet survival time and enhanced heart rate responses after abrupt withdrawal of propranolol from normal subjects. Am J Cardiol 1981;47:1115–1122.

87. Rangno RE, Nattel S, Lutterodt A. Prevention of propranolol withdrawal mechanisms by prolonged small dose propranolol schedule. Am J Cardiol 1982;49:828–833.

88. Lindenfeld J, Crawford MH, O'Rourke RA, et al. Adrenergic responsiveness after abrupt propranolol withdrawal in normal subjects and in patients with angina pectoris. Circulation 1980;62:704–711.

89. Parodi O, Simonetti I, L'Abbate A, Maseri A. Verapamil versus propranolol for angina at rest. Am J Cardiol 1982;50: 923–928.

90. Winniford MD, Fulton KL, Corbett JR, et al. Propranolol–verapamil versus propranolol–nifedipine in severe angina pectoris of effort: A randomized, double-blind, crossover study. Am J Cardiol 1985;55:281–285.

91. Godfraind T. Classification of calcium antagonists. Am J Cardiol 1987;59:11B–23B.

92. Chaitman BR, Wagniart P, Pasternac A, et al. Improved exercise tolerance after propranolol, diltiazem, or nifedipine in angina pectoris: Comparison at 1,3, and 8 hours and correlation with plasma drug concentration. Am J Cardiol 1984;53:1–9.

93. Hamann SR, Blouin RA, McAllister RG, Jr. Clinical pharmacokinetics of verapamil. Clin Pharmacokinet 1984;9:26–41.

94. Smith MS, Verghese CP, Shand DG, et al. Pharmacokinetic and pharmacodynamic effects of diltiazem. Am J Cardiol 1983;51:1369–1374.

95. Chaffman M, Brogden RN. Diltiazem: A review of its pharmacological properties and therapeutic efficacy. Drugs 1985;29: 387–454.

96. Foster TS, Hamann SR, Richards VR, et al. Nifedipine kinetics and bioavailability after single intravenous and oral doses in normal subjects. J Clin Pharmacol 1983;23:161–170.

97. Hirasawa K, Shen WF, Roubin G, et al. Effect of food ingestion on nifedipine absorption and haemodynamic response. Eur J Clin Pharmacol 1985;28:105–107.

98. Sorkin EM, Brogden RN. Nifedipine: A review. Drugs 1985;30:182–274.

99. McAllister RG, Jr. Kinetics and dynamics of nifedipine after oral and sublingual doses. Am J Med 1986;81(6A):2–5.

100. Yabana H, Nagao T, Sato M. Cardiovascular effects of the metabolites of diltiazem in dogs. J Cardiovasc Pharmacol 1985;7:152–157.

101. Rovei V, Gomeni R, Mitchard M, et al. Pharmacokinetics and metabolism of diltiazem in man. Acta Cardiol 1980;35:35–45.

102. Renton KW. Inhibition of hepatic microsomal drug metabolism by the calcium channel blockers diltiazem and verapamil. Biochem Pharmacol 1985;34:2549–2553.

103. Carrum G, Egan JM, Abernathy DR. Diltiazem treatment impairs hepatic drug oxidation: Studies of antipyrine. Clin Pharmacol Ther 1986;40:140–143.

104. Dargie HJ. Investigation and management of chronic stable angina, in Fox KM (ed): Ischaemic Heart Disease. Boston, MTP Press, 1987, pp 149–217.

105. Lorimer AR. Medical management, in Julian DG (ed): Angina Pectoris, 2nd ed. New York, Churchill Livingstone, 1985, pp 164–187.

106. Kloster FE, Bristow JD. Management of stable and unstable angina, in Connor WE, Bristow JD (eds): Coronary Heart Disease. Prevention, Complications, and Treatment. Philadelphia, J.B. Lippincott, 1985, pp 231–250.

107. Redwood DR, Rosing DR, Epstein SE. Circulatory and symptomatic effects of physical training in patients with coronary artery disease and angina pectoris. N Engl J Med 1972;286: 959–965.

108. Amsterdam EA, Wilmore JH, DeMaria AN. Exercise in Car-

diovascular Health and Disease. New York, Yorke Medical Books, 1977, pp 313.
109. Parker JO, Farrell B, Lahey KA, et al. Effect of intervals between doses on the development of tolerance to isosorbide dinitrate. N Engl J Med 1987;316:1440–1444.
110. Parker JO. Drug therapy: Nitrate therapy in stable angina pectoris. N Engl J Med 1987;316:1635–1642.
111. Deanfield J, Wright C, Krikler S, et al. Cigarette smoking and the treatment of angina pectoris with propranolol, atenolol and nifedipine. N Engl J Med 1984;310:951–954.
112. Prida XE, Feldman RL, Hill JA, et al. Comparison of selective and nonselective $\beta_1$ and $\beta_2$, $\beta$-adrenergic blockade on systemic and coronary hemodynamic findings in angina pectoris. Am J Cardiol 1987;60:244–248.
113. Roubin GS, Sadick NA, Anderson SD, et al. Effect of propranolol and verapamil on oxygen utilization, acidosis and fatigue during exercise in stable angina pectoris. Am J Cardiol 1987;60:249–254.
114. Lynch P, Dargie H, Krikler S, et al. Objective assessment of antianginal treatment: A double blind comparison of propranolol, nifedipine and their combination. Br Med J 1980;281:184–187.
115. Tweddel AC, Beattie JM, Murray RG, et al. The combination of nifedipine and propranolol in the management of patients with angina pectoris. Br J Clin Pharmacol 1981;12:229–233.
116. Winniford MD, Huxley RL, Hillis D. Randomised double blind comparison of propranolol alone and a propranolol–verapamil combination in patients with severe angina of effort. J Am Coll Cardiol 1983;1:492–498.
117. Johnston DL, Lesoway R, Humen DP, et al. Clinical and haemodynamic evaluation of propranolol in combination with verapamil, nifedipine and diltiazem in exertional angina pectoris: A placebo-controlled, double-blind, randomised, crossover study. Am J Cardiol 1985;55:680–687.
118. Kenny J, Kiff P, Holmes J, et al. Beneficial effects of diltiazem and propranolol, alone and in combination, in patients with stable angina pectoris. Br Heart J 1985;53:43–46.
119. Nesto RW, White HD, Wynne J, et al. Comparison of nifedipine and isosorbide dinitrate when added to maximal propranolol therapy in stable angina pectoris. Am J Cardiol 1987;60:256–271.
120. Epstein SE, Palmeri ST. Mechanisms contributing to precipitation of unstable angina and acute myocardial infarction: Implications regarding therapy. Am J Cardiol 1984;54:1245–1252.
121. Oliva PB. Unstable rest angina with ST segment depression: Pathophysiologic considerations and therapeutic considerations. Ann Intern Med 1984;100:424–440.
122. Butman S, Piters KM, Olson HG, et al. Early exercise testing in unstable angina: Angiographic correlation and prognostic value. J Am Coll Cardiol 1983;1:638.
123. Fragasso G, Davies GJ, Chierchia S, et al. Relative roles of preload increase and coronary constriction in ergonovine-induced myocardial ischemia in stable angina pectoris. Am J Cardiol 1987;60:238–243.
124. Muller JE, Turi ZG, Pearle DL, et al. Nifedipine and conventional therapy for unstable angina pectoris: A randomized, double-blind comparison. Circulation 1984;69:728–739.
125. Water DD, Theroux P, Szlachcic J, et al. Provocative testing to assess the efficacy of treatment with nifedipine, diltiazem, and verapamil in variant angina. Am J Cardiol 1981;48:123–130.
126. Moses JW, Wertheimer JH, Bodenheimer MM, et al. Efficacy of nifedipine in rest angina refractory to propranolol and nitrates in patients with obstructive coronary artery disease. Ann Intern Med 1981;94:425–429.
127. Gerstenblith G, Ouyang P, Achuff SC, et al. Nifedipine in unstable angina. N Engl J Med 1982;306:885–889.
128. Parodi O, Maseri A, Simonetti I. Management of unstable angina by verapamil: A double-blind crossover study in the CCU. Br Heart J 1979;41:167–174.
129. Parodi O, Simonetti I, Michelassi C, et al. Comparison of verapamil and propranolol therapy for angina pectoris at rest: A randomized multiple-crossover, controlled trial in the coronary care unit. Am J Cardiol 1986;57:899–906.
130. Mehta J, Pepine CJ, Day M, et al. Short term efficacy of oral verapamil in rest angina. Am J Med 1981;71:977–982.
131. Theroux P, Taeymans Y, Morissette D, et al. A randomised study comparing propranolol and diltiazem in the treatment of unstable angina. J Am Coll Cardiol 1985;5:717–722.
132. Singh BN, Nademanee K. $\beta$-Adrenergic blockade in unstable angina pectoris. Am J Cardiol 1986;57:992–994.
133. Kern MJ, Ganz P, Horowitz JD, et al. Potentiation of coronary vasoconstriction by $\beta$-adrenergic blockade in patients with coronary artery disease. Circulation 1983;67:1178–1185.
134. Telford A, Wilson C. Trial of heparin versus atenolol in prevention of myocardial infarction in the intermediate coronary syndrome. Lancet 1981;1:1225–1228.
135. Meade TW (ed). Anticoagulants and Myocardial Infarction. A Reappraisal. New York, John Wiley and Sons, 1984.
136. Lewis HD, Davis JW, Archibald DA, et al. Protective effect of aspirin against acute myocardial infarction and death in men with unstable angina. N Engl J Med 1983;309:396–405.
137. Cairns JA, Gent M, Singer J, et al. Aspirin, sulfinpyrazone, or both in unstable angina. Results of a Canadian multicenter trial. N Engl J Med 1985;313:1369–1375.
138. Unstable Angina Pectoris Study Group. Unstable angina pectoris national cooperative study group to compare medical and surgical therapy. I. Report of protocol and patient population. Am J Cardiol 1976;37:896–902.
139. Unstable Angina Pectoris Study Group. Unstable angina pectoris national cooperative study group to compare medical and surgical therapy. II. In-hospital experience with initial follow-up results in patients with one, two and three vessel disease. Am J Cardiol 1978;42:839–848.
140. Unstable Angina Pectoris Study Group. Unstable angina pectoris national cooperative study group to compare medical and surgical therapy. III. Results in patients with S-T elevation during pain. Am J Cardiol 1980;45:819–824.
141. Unstable Angina Pectoris Study Group. Unstable angina pectoris national cooperative study group to compare medical and surgical therapy. IV. Results in patients with left anterior descending coronary artery disease. Am J Cardiol 1981;48:517–524.
142. Vlietstra RE, Holmes DR, Jr (eds). PTCA. Percutaneous Transluminal Coronary Angioplasty. Philadelphia, F.A. Davis Company, 1987.
143. Faxon DP, Sanborn TA, Haudenschild CC. Mechanism of angioplasty and its relation to restenosis. Am J Cardiol 1987;60:5B–9B.
144. Bresnahan DR, Davis JL, Holmes DR, Jr, et al. Angiographic occurrence and clinical correlates of intraluminal coronary artery thrombus: Role of unstable angina. J Am Coll Cardiol 1985;6:285–289.
145. Corcos T, David PR, Bourassa MG, et al. Percutaneous transluminal angioplasty for the treatment of variant angina. J Am Coll Cardiol 1985;5:1046–1054.
146. Mabin TA, Holmes DR, Jr, Smith HC, et al. Intracoronary thrombus: Role in coronary occlusion complicating percutaneous transluminal coronary angioplasty. J Am Coll Cardiol 1985;5:198–202.

147. Williams DO, Riley RS, Singh AK, et al. Evaluation of the role of coronary angioplasty in patients with unstable angina. Am Heart J 1981;102:1–9.
148. DeFeyter PJ, Serruys PW, Van der Brand M, et al. Emergency coronary angioplasty in unstable angina. N Engl J Med 1985;313:342–346.
149. Melzer RS, Van der Brand M, et al. Sequential intracoronary streptokinase and transluminal angioplasty in unstable angina with evolving myocardial infarction. Am Heart J 1982;104: 1109–1111.
150. Weintaub RM, Voukydis PC, Aroesty JM, et al. Treatment of preinfarction angina with intraaortic balloon counterpulsation and surgery. Am J Cardiol 1974;34:809–814.
151. Langou RA, Geha AS, Hammond GL, et al. Surgical approach for patients with angina pectoris: Role of the response to initial medical therapy and intraaortic balloon pumping in perioperative complications after aortocoronary bypass graft. Am J Cardiol 1978;42:629–633.
152. Flaherty JT, Becker LC, Weiss JL, et al. Results of a randomised trial of intraaortic balloon counterpulsation and intravenous nitroglycerin in patients with acute myocardial infarction. J Am Coll Cardiol 1985;6:434–446.
153. Conti CR (ed). Coronary Artery Spasm. Pathophysiology, Diagnosis, and Treatment. New York, Marcel Dekker, 1986.
154. Waters DD, Bouchard A, Theroux P. Spontaneous remission is a frequent outcome of variant angina. J Am Coll Cardiol 1983;2:195–199.
155. Miller DD, Waters DD, Szlachcic J, et al. Clinical characteristics associated with sudden death in patients with variant angina. Circulation 1982;66:588–592.
156. Rosenthal SJ, Ginsburg R, Lamb IH, et al. Efficacy of diltiazem for control of symptoms of coronary arterial spasm. Am J Cardiol 1980;46:1027–1032.
157. Shick EC, Liang CS, Heupler FA, et al. Randomized withdrawal from nifedipine: Placebo-controlled study in patients with coronary spasm. Am Heart J 1982;104:690–697.
158. Sato A, Taneichi Y, Sekine I, et al. Prinzmetal's variant angina induced only by alcohol ingestion. Clin Cardiol 1981;4:193–195.
159. Freedman SB, Richmond DR, Kelly DT. Long-term follow-up of verapamil and nitrate treatment for coronary artery spasm. Am J Cardiol 1982;50:711–715.
160. Distante A, Maseri A, Severi S, et al. Management of vasospastic angina at rest with continuous infusion of isosorbide dinitrate. Am J Cardiol 1979;44:533–539.
161. Salerno JA, Previtali M, Medici A, et al. Treatment of vasospastic angina pectoris at rest with nitroglycerin ointment: A short-term controlled study in the coronary care unit. Am J Cardiol 1981;47:1128–1133.
162. Hill JA, Feldman RL, Pepine CJ, et al. Randomized double-blind comparison of nifedipine and isosorbide dinitrate in patients with coronary arterial spasm. Am J Cardiol 1982;49: 431–438.
163. Ginsburg R, Lamb IH, Schroeder JS, et al. Randomized double-blind comparison of nifedipine and isosorbide dinitrate therapy in variant angina pectoris due to coronary artery spasm. Am Heart J 1982;103:44–48.
164. Waters DD, Miller DD, Szlachcic J, et al. Factors influencing the long-term prognosis of treated patients with variant angina. Circulation 1983;68:258–265.
165. Winniford MD, Johnson SM, Mauritson DR, et al. Verapamil therapy for Prinzmetal's variant angina: Comparison with placebo and nifedipine. Am J Cardiol 1982;50:913–918.
166. Kimura E, Kishida H. Treatment of variant angina with drugs: A survey of 11 cardiology institutes in Japan. Circulation 1981;63:844–848.
167. Waters DD, Szlachcic J, Theroux P, et al. Ergonovine testing to detect spontaneous remissions of variant angina during long-term treatment with calcium antagonist drugs. Am J Cardiol 1981;47:179–184.
168. Robertson RM, Bernard Y, Carr RK, et al. Exacerbation of vasotonic angina pectoris by propranolol. Circulation 1982;65: 281–285.
169. Tilmant PY, LaBlanche, JM, Thieuleux FA, et al. Detrimental effects of propranolol in patients with coronary arterial spasm countered by combination with diltiazem. Am J Cardiol 1983;52:230–233.
170. Tzivoni D, Schuger C. Potential therapy for coronary artery spasm, in Conti CR (ed): Coronary Artery Spasm. Pathophysiology, Diagnosis, and Treatment. New York, Marcel Dekker, 1986, pp 297–308.
171. Mehta JL, Crea F. Drug therapy of spontaneously occurring myocardial ischemia directed at modification of platelet function and arachidonic acid metabolism, in Conti CR (ed): Coronary Artery Spasm. Pathophysiology, Diagnosis, and Treatment. New York, Marcel Dekker, pp 309–328.
172. Zeller FP, Spears C. Fish oil: Effectiveness as a dietary supplement in the prevention of heart disease. Drug Intell Clin Pharm 1987;21:584–589.
173. Hill JA, Pepine CJ. Treatment of silent myocardial ischemia. Cardiol Clin 1986;4:685–696.
174. Pepine CJ, Hill JA. Management of the total ischemic burden in angina pectoris. Am J Cardiol 1987;59:7C–12C.
175. Gottlieb SO, Weisfeldt ML, Ouyang P, et al. Silent ischemia as a marker for early unfavorable outcomes in patients with unstable angina. N Engl J Med 1986;314:1214–1219.
176. Assey ME, Walters GL, Hendrix GH, et al. Incidence of acute myocardial infarction in patients with exercise-induced silent myocardial ischemia. Am J Cardiol 1987;59:497–500.
177. Muller JE, Stone PH, Turi ZG, et al. Circadian variation in the frequency of onset of acute myocardial infarction. N Engl J Med 1985;313:1315–1322.
178. Muller JE, Ludmer PL, Willich SN, et al. Circadian variation in the frequency of sudden cardiac death. Circulation 1987;75: 131–138.
179. Tofler GH, Brezinski D, Schafer AI, et al. Concurrent morning increase in platelet aggregability and the risk of myocardial infarction and sudden cardiac death. N Engl J Med 1987;316: 1514–1518.
180. Multiple Risk Factor Intervention Trial Research Group. Exercise electrocardiogram and coronary heart disease mortality in the Multiple Risk Factor Intervention Trial. Am J Cardiol 1985;55:16–24.
181. Cocco G, Strozzi C, Chu D, et al. Therapeutic effects of pindolol and nifedipine in patients with stable angina pectoris and asymptomatic resting ischemia. Eur J Cardiol 1979;10:59–69.
182. Quyyumi AA, Wright C, Mockus L, et al. Effects of combined $\alpha$- and $\beta$-adrenoceptor blockade in patients with angina pectoris. A double blind study comparing labetalol with placebo. Br Heart J 1985; 53:47–52.
183. Subramanian VB, Bowles MJ, Davis AB, et al. Combined therapy with verapamil and propranolol in angina pectoris. Am J Cardiol 1982;49:125–132.
184. Johnson SM, Mauritson DR, Willerson JT, et al. A controlled trial of verapamil for Prinzmetal's variant angina. N Engl J Med 1981;304:862–866.
185. Schang JJ Jr, Pepine CJ. Transient asymptomatic ST-segment

depression during daily activity. Am J Cardiol 1977;39:396–402.
186. Cohn PF. Total ischemic burden: Effect of vasoactive agents. Am Heart J 1988;115:215–219.
187. Oakley GDG, Fox KM, Dargie HJ, et al. Objective assessment of therapy in severe angina. Br Med J 1979;1:1540.
188. Dargie HJ, Lynch PG, Krikler D, et al. Nifedipine and propranolol: A beneficial drug interaction. Am J Med 1981;71:676–682.
189. Favaloro RG. Saphenous vein autograft replacement of severe segmental coronary artery occlusion. Ann Thorac Surg 1968;5:334–339.
190. European Coronary Surgery Study Group. Long-term results of prospective randomised study of coronary artery bypass surgery in stable angina pectoris. Lancet 1982;2:1173–1180.
191. CASS Principal Investigators and their Associates. Coronary Artery Surgery Study (CASS): A randomized trial of coronary artery bypass surgery. Survival data. Circulation 1983;68:939–950.
192. Gersh BJ, Kronmal RA, Schaff HV, et al. Comparison of coronary artery bypass surgery and medical therapy in patients 65 years of age or older. N Engl J Med 1985;313:217–224.
193. Chaitman BR, Fisher LD, Bourassa MG, et al. Effect of coronary artery bypass surgery on survival patterns in subsets of patients with left main coronary artery disease. Am J Cardiol 1981;48:765–777.
194. Chaitman BR, Davis KB, Kaiser GC, et al. The role of coronary artery bypass surgery for "left main equivalent" coronary disease: The Coronary Artery Surgery Study Registry. Circulation 1986;74(suppl III):17–25.
195. Vigilante GJ, Weintraub WS, Klein LW, et al. Improved survival with coronary bypass surgery in patients with three-vessel coronary disease and abnormal left ventricular function. Am J Med 1987;82:697–702.
196. Bourassa MG, Fisher LD, Campeau L, et al. Long-term fate of bypass grafts: The Coronary Artery Surgery Study (CASS) and Montreal Heart Institute experiences. Circulation 1985; 72(suppl V):71–78.
197. Chesebro JH, Fuster V, Elveback LR, et al. Effect of dipyridamole and aspirin on late vein-graft patency after coronary bypass operations. N Engl J Med 1984;310:209–214.
198. Lorenz RL, Weber M, Kotzur J, et al. Improved aortocoronary bypass patency by low-dose aspirin (100 mg daily). Lancet 1984;1:1261–1264.
199. Campeau L, Enjalbert M, Lesperance J, et al. The relation of risk factors to the development of atherosclerosis in saphenous-vein bypass grafts and the progression of disease in the native circulation. N Engl J Med 1984;311:1329–1332.
200. Blankenhorn DH, Nessim SA, Johnson RL, et al. Beneficial effects of combined colestipol–niacin therapy on coronary atherosclerosis and coronary venous bypass grafts. JAMA 1987;257:3233–3240.
201. Loop FT, Lytle BW, Cosgrove DM. Influence of the internal mammary artery graft on 10-year survival and other cardiac events. N Engl J Med 1986;314:1–6.
202. Cameron A, Kemp HG, Jr, Green GE. Bypass surgery with the internal mammary artery graft: 15 year follow-up. Circulation 1986;74(suppl III):30–36.
203. Gruentzig AR, Myler RK, Hanna ES, et al. Coronary transluminal angioplasty (abstr). Circulation 1977;56(suppl III):84.
204. O'Neill WW, Topol EJ, Fung A, et al. Coronary angioplasty as therapy for acute myocardial infarction: University of Michigan experience. Circulation 1987;76(suppl II):79–87.
205. O'Neill WW, Timmis GC, Bourdillon PD, et al. A prospective randomized clinical trial of intracoronary streptokinase versus coronary angioplasty for acute myocardial infarction. N Engl J Med 1986;314:812–818.
206. Erbel R, Pop T, Hendrichs K, et al. Percutaneous transluminal coronary angioplasty after thrombolytic therapy: A prospective controlled randomized trial. J Am Coll Cardiol 1986;8:485–495.
207. Gruentzig AR, King SB III, Schlumpf M, et al. Long-term follow-up after percutaneous transluminal coronary angioplasty. The early Zurich experience. N Engl J Med 1987;316:1127–1132.
208. National Heart, Lung and Blood Institute PTCA Registry: Percutaneous transluminal coronary angioplasty. University of Pittsburgh, Data Coordinating Center, November 1983.
209. Thornton MA, Gruentzig AR, Hollman J, et al. Coumadin and aspirin in prevention of recurrence after transluminal coronary angioplasty: A randomized study. Circulation 1984;69:721–727.
210. Holmes DR Jr, Vlietstra RE, Smith HC, et al. Restenosis after percutaneous transluminal angioplasty (PTCA): A report from the PTCA registry of the National Heart, Lung and Blood Institute. Am J Cardiol 1984;53:77C–81C.
211. Faxon DP, Sanborn TA, Haudenschild CC, et al. Effect of antiplatelet therapy on restenosis after experimental angioplasty. Am J Cardiol 1984;53:72C–76C.

# Chapter 14 / Acute Myocardial Infarction: Diagnosis and Treatment

Edgar R. Gonzalez, PharmD, and Edward Sypniewski, Jr, PharmD

Myocardial infarction (MI) is necrosis of heart muscle caused by an imbalance between oxygen supply and demand in the myocardium. Most myocardial infarctions result from severe narrowing of one or more of the coronary arteries. Factors that have been implicated in the pathogenesis of MI include atherosclerotic plaque rupture and spasm.[1] Myocardial infarction can occur in the absence of coronary artery narrowing, but in the presence of excessive myocardial oxygen demand, for example, in the setting of cocaine abuse. The diurnal pattern of acute MI, which peaks from six o'clock in the morning to noon, suggests that other factors may be involved.[2]

Myocardial infarction occurs most commonly at rest or during moderate activity.[1] Nonetheless, the combination of severe stress and fatigue has been incriminated as a precipitant of acute MI. The prompt recognition that infarction is occurring is critical because deaths associated with acute MI are due primarily to electrical instability and occur suddenly and prior to hospitalization.[1] The importance of prompt attention to symptoms of myocardial ischemia is highlighted by observations that the likelihood of ventricular fibrillation (VF) is 15 times greater during the initial hour after the onset of symptoms than during the subsequent 12 hours.[3] Furthermore, the likelihood of successful myocardial salvage is greatest during the first three hours after the onset of symptoms.[3,4] Any unnecessary delays in treatment place the patient at risk for life-threatening complications and increase the long-term mortality rate post-MI.[5]

Suspicion of acute MI is based on the patient's symptoms and medical history. If the history is consistent with the diagnosis of acute MI, the patient must be treated accordingly. Reduction in mortality is the major goal of therapy in acute MI. Survival after MI depends on the amount of myocardium remaining and the occurrence of post-MI complications. Management of acute MI is designed to relieve pain and anxiety, to recognize and control life-threatening arrhythmias, to limit infarct size, and to prevent complications. The management of acute myocardial infarction represents an important aspect of clinical practice, with significant implications in terms of lives and health-care dollars.[6] Because the duration of ischemia equates with the extent of myocardial damage, it is imperative that clinicians learn to recognize and treat patients with acute MI.

## Epidemiology

Acute MI is a common and serious illness that accounts for 500,000 deaths annually in the United States.[6] The incidence of MI is thought to be over 1.5 million cases per year, or roughly 1 out of every 160 persons. Approximately 50% of patients with acute MI die within the first few hours from electrical instability leading to VF.[3] Mortality among acute MI victims ranges from 10% to 15% in the first year, and is 3% to 4% per year thereafter.[2] Almost half of these patients die from out-of-hospital VF. The development of coronary intensive care units (CICUs) has afforded a clinical setting in which optimum patient surveillance and care can be provided.[7] Care of post-MI patients in the CICU has decreased mortality from fatal arrhythmias; unfortunately, death from reinfarction or cardiogenic shock has not significantly changed.[8]

## Pathophysiology

Atherosclerotic coronary artery disease (CAD) is the major underlying cause of myocardial infarction. As an atherosclerotic plaque builds along the wall of the coronary artery, lumen diameter and consequently blood and oxygen supply to the myocardium decrease. The degrees of cardiac muscle damage can be divided into zones of ischemia, myocardial injury, and, lastly, infarction (Fig. 14.1). Ischemia occurs when the imbalance between oxygen demand and supply exceeds a critical level. Infarction occurs after prolonged ischemia, usually greater than 30 minutes in duration, and results in irreversible damage to the myocardium.[9] The infarction may be further pathologically divided into two types: a transmural infarct (Q-wave MI), which extends throughout the full thickness of the myocardial wall, and an epicardial or subendocardial infarct (non–Q-wave MI), in which part of the myocardial wall is damaged. The infarcted area will become fibrous scar tissue within a few weeks of the acute MI. The scarred portion of myocardial wall will not function as viable cardiac muscle. It will, instead, display dyskinetic, hypokinetic, or akinetic motion which will compromise cardiac output. An aneurysm may also form in the area of infarction.

Patients who have greater than 50% occlusion of the left mainstem coronary artery or greater than 70% occlusion of one of the major coronaries are at greatest risk for developing ischemia which may lead to infarction (Fig. 14.2). Occlusion of the right coronary artery or the left circumflex artery results in inferior-posterior wall infarction. Infarction of the right ventricle occurs in 24% to 37% of the patients with inferior-posterior wall myocardial infarction.[10] Occlusion of the left mainstem coronary artery or the left anterior descending artery causes anterior wall infarction.

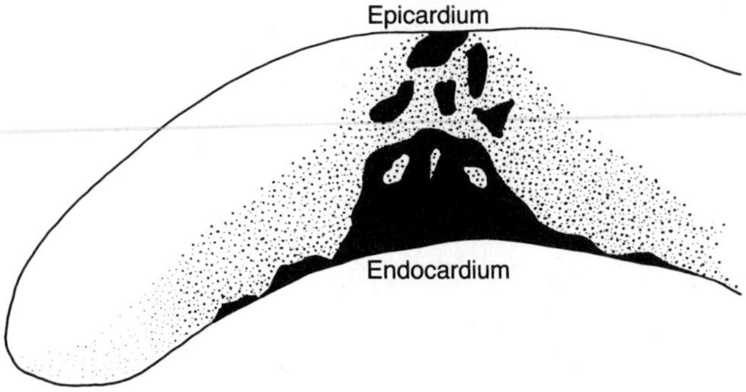


**Figure 14.1** Common cone-shaped pattern of myocardial injury and ischemia associated with transmural infarction. Dark solid zone represents areas of necrosis. Dotted areas indicate zones of injured but still viable myocardium. *(From Stapleton JF: Essentials of Clinical Cardiology. Philadelphia, F.A. Davis, 1983, p 256, with permission.)*

Although CAD is the underlying disease state associated with myocardial infarction, it alone does not cause the acute event.[11] Several mechanisms have been postulated ranging from advanced atherosclerotic disease producing coronary stenosis to the theory of thrombus formation within an area of atheromatous plaque fixation, which has been most widely accepted.[10] More than 85% of MIs are thought to be caused by thrombus formation superimposed on significant atherosclerotic lesions in the coronary arteries. Coronary vasospasm associated with thrombus formation has also been implicated to a lesser degree.[11] Factors implicated in precipitating acute MI are hypoxia, emotional stress, physical exertion, exposure to cold environment, meals, hypoglycemia, hemorrhage, anaphylactic or hypersensitivity reaction, direct myocardial injury or trauma, and drugs.[12] Drugs associated with initiating acute MI include catecholamines, vasodilators, and ergot alkaloids.[12]

## Clinical Presentation

Patients with acute MI may have typical, atypical, or no clinical symptoms. The classic symptoms of myocardial ischemia include pressurelike substernal heaviness or chest pain, diaphoresis, nausea, shortness of breath, and a sense of impending doom.[2] The pain and pressure may radiate to the arms, the back between the scapulae, the neck, or the jaw. Vomiting and diarrhea may also be observed. Nausea and vomiting occurring during myocardial ischemia are believed to be associated with inferior wall infarction; however, recent laboratory and clinical data suggest that cardiac vomiting is associated with larger infarcts and not with infarction of any particular region of the heart.[13] Prodromal symptoms consistent with unstable angina occur in 10% to 15% of patients.[14]

Classic symptoms of acute MI occur in approximately 54% of patients.[15] Approximately 25% of acute MI patients present with atypical symptoms (i.e., indigestion, syncope, shock, pulmonary edema, lethargy, embolic events).[16] Approximately 25% are asymptomatic or cannot give a history.[16] Painless MI occurs most commonly in women, older men, and diabetics.[16,17]

Unlike anginal pain which subsides within minutes, acute MI pain generally lasts 30 minutes to several hours, responding to medical management (i.e., nitroglycerin, morphine) of its own accord or with the occurrence of malignant arrhythmias and sudden cardiac death (SCD). Chest pain associated

**Figure 14.2** Coronary arteries: blood supply to the heart.

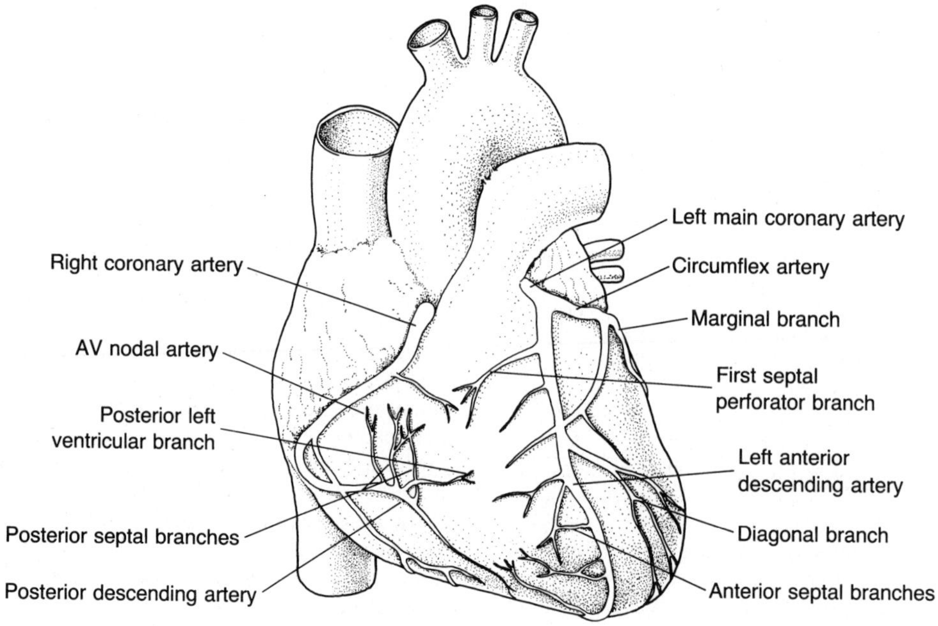

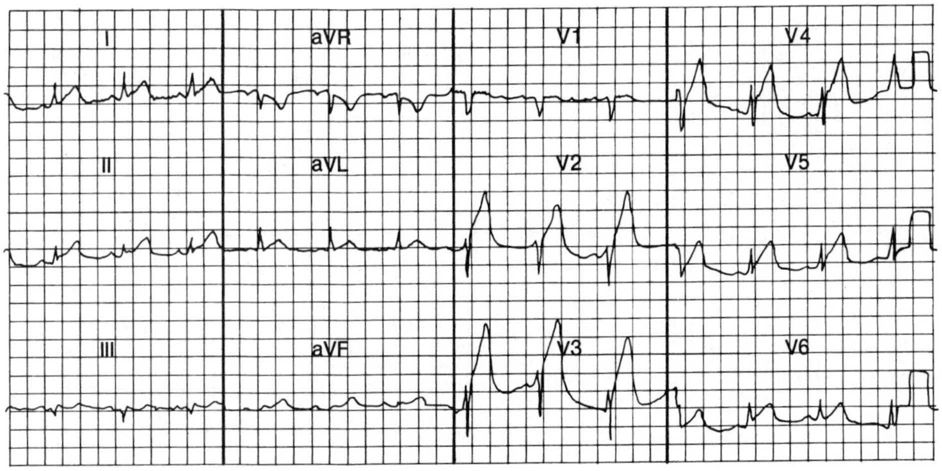


**Figure 14.3** Hyperacute changes with anterior myocardial infarction. Note ST-segment elevation and peaked T waves in leads $V_2$ through $V_5$. *(From Ornato JP (Ed): Cardiovascular Emergencies. New York, Churchill Livingstone, 1986, p 4, with permission.)*

with acute MI can be differentiated from pain that is noncardiac (see Table 13.7) in origin through careful analysis of the patient's past and presenting medical history. Although nitroglycerin will relieve anginal pain, it can also relieve pain associated with dysfunction of the upper gastrointestinal tract and biliary tree.

A low-grade fever is not uncommon during the acute MI, and may continue for several days afterward. Leukocytosis ranging from 12,000/mm$^3$ to 15,000/mm$^3$ can occur and may last 3 to 7 days after the infarct. The patient may be either hypertensive or hypotensive. Hypotension may be caused by one or more of the following: drug administration (nitroglycerin, morphine), hypovolemia, pump failure. Anxiety, apprehension, and chest discomfort lead to shallow, rapid breathing.

The patient's chief complaint and history are invaluable in establishing a diagnosis of MI. A detailed history may help to differentiate myocardial ischemic pain from noncardiac chest pain. Precipitating factors should be identified, and the patient's medication history and compliance should be assessed. Evidence of coronary risk factors may be present, such as retinopathy from hypertension or diabetes, and xanthomas or xanthelasmas from hyperlipidemia. The presence of other factors such as smoking and diabetes should also be determined.

### *Twelve-Lead Electrocardiogram*

The twelve-lead electrocardiogram (ECG) plays an integral role in the evaluation of patients with suspected myocardial infarction. The ECG is diagnostic in 65% to 81% of patients with acute MI who are seen for evaluation of chest pain.[16,18] Patients may have either tachycardia or bradycardia; the latter usually coincides with inferior wall infarction secondary to ischemia within the area of the conduction system. The earliest ECG findings in acute MI are symmetric peaking of the T waves with ST-segment elevation ("hyperacute changes") (Fig. 14.3).[16] These changes are transient, and resolve within minutes to hours. Afterward, the ST segment remains elevated, the T waves invert, and there may be loss of R-wave force or the development of pathologic Q waves ("acute changes") (Fig. 14.4).[16]

The presence of pathologic Q waves on the ECG tracing has led to the description of "Q-wave" and "non–Q-wave" infarction.[19] Significant Q waves are represented by a deepening of the wave equivalent to about one third the size of the QRS complex and a 1-mm (0.04-second) widening of the wave.[20] Insignificant Q waves are often observed in leads I, II, $V_5$, and $V_6$.[20] Although Q waves are more commonly seen in transmural (full-thickness) infarcts, they cannot be used to distinguish between pathologic subendocardial and transmural infarction.[21,22] Phibbs[21] suggests that Q waves are unrelated to clinical outcome. In contrast, Zelma[19] observed that non–Q-wave infarction identified patients with low (4%) in-hospital mortality when compared with the in-hospital mortality (15%) of patients with Q-wave infarctions. Long-term mortality rates for Q-wave and non–Q-wave MI are similar.

### *Serum Enzyme Studies*

Myocardial necrosis causes the release of three intracellular enzymes—creatine kinase (CK), aspartamine aminotransferase (AST), and lactic acid dehydrogenase (LDH)—into the systemic circulation (Fig. 14.5). Serum levels of these enzymes may be elevated after an acute MI; however, cardiac enzyme studies are of limited value in the initial diagnosis of acute MI.[16]

Creatine kinase is a dimeric enzyme that catalyzes the transfer of high-energy phosphate groups and is found predominantly in tissues that consume large amounts of energy.[23] The two isomers of CK are M (for muscle) and B (for brain). The CK-MM isoenzyme is dominant in adult skeletal muscle; CK-BB is found predominantly in central nervous system tissue; myocardial CK is approximately 85% MM and 15% MB.[23] CK-MB is the "gold standard" enzyme for assessing the occurrence and extent of an acute MI.[23] An increase in both total CK and percentage of CK-MB

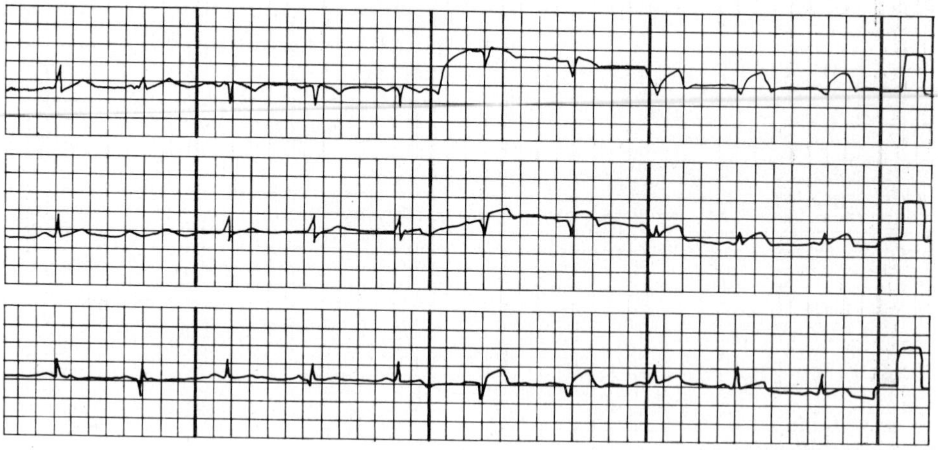

**Figure 14.4** Acute changes with anterior myocardial infarction. Note significant Q waves, ST-segment changes, and initiation of T-wave inversion in leads $V_1$ through $V_4$. *(From Ornato JP (Ed): Cardiovascular Emergencies. New York, Churchill Livingstone, 1986, p 5, with permission.)*

isoenzyme reflects myocardial tissue damage. The peak serum level of total serum CK is also indicative of the extent of the infarction. Release of CK from the myocardium into the serum occurs within the first 6 to 24 hours of acute MI and may be elevated to a two- to threefold increase or greater. Elevated CK levels normalize 48 to 72 hours postinfarction.

Because CK-MM is found in skeletal muscle, any type of physical trauma (i.e., intramuscular injection, cardioversion, cardiopulmonary resuscitation, surgery, heavy exercise) will elevate total CK concentration in blood. Therefore, evaluation of enzyme elevation is dependent not only on total serum CK but also on the increase in the CK-MB fraction above baseline. Blood is routinely drawn every 8 hours during the first 24 to 48 hours after acute MI to measure total CK and CK-MB fractions. Serial CK-MB measurements after acute MI result in 100% sensitivity and 98% specificity for MI.[23] The excretion of CK in the presence of renal insufficiency may be delayed.

**Figure 14.5** Temporal changes in serum enzyme concentrations after an acute myocardial infarction. *(From Stapleton JF: Essentials in Clinical Cardiology. Philadelphia, F.A. Davis, 1983, p 266, with permission.)*

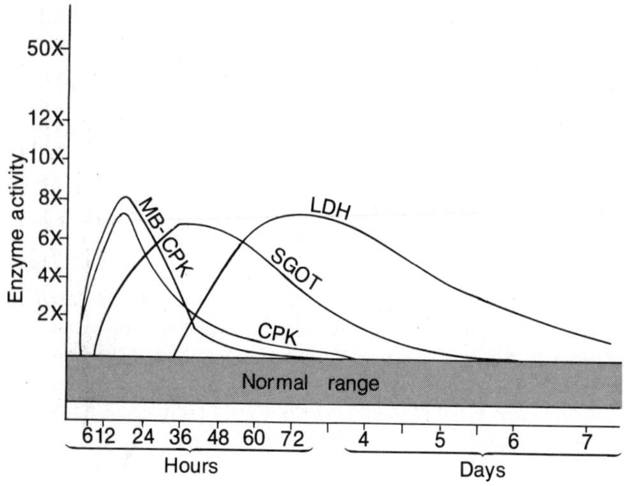


Lactic acid dehydrogenase catalyzes the reversible reduction of pyruvate to lactate during glycolysis. The enzyme consists of polypeptide chains that comprise five isoenzymes labeled $LDH_1$ through $LDH_5$. $LDH_1$ predominates in erythrocytes, kidneys, brain, stomach, and pancreas. $LDH_1$ and, to a lesser extent, $LDH_2$ predominate in heart muscle; skeletal muscle and liver contain mostly $LDH_5$. Normally, serum levels reflect a higher percentage of $LDH_2$ than $LDH_1$. During infarction, $LDH_1$ is released from the myocardial cells secondary to injury, resulting in an increase in total serum LDH and a "flip" in the isoenzyme ratio causing the percentage of $LDH_1$ to be greater than that of $LDH_2$. The elevation of total LDH is observed 48 to 72 hours postinfarction, with 80% of the patients exhibiting a "flip" in the isoenzyme ratio.[24] Concentrations of LDH isoenzymes are considerably more specific than total LDH concentration, and provide a useful diagnostic indicator in patients presenting more than 24 hours after the onset of symptoms.[23]

Serum aspartamine aminotransferase levels peak between the first and second days after acute MI. Because either the CK or LDH level is abnormal during the periods when the AST level is elevated post-MI, the incremental benefit of an AST assay in diagnosis is small; therefore its routine use is discouraged.[23]

In summary, although in the past acute MI has been diagnosed based on the presence of two of three clinical features[25] (ischemic chest pain, new abnormal Q waves or ST-segment changes, or abnormally elevated cardiac enzymes), recent observations[26] suggest that the CK-MB isoenzyme should be the primary determinant for patients admitted to the hospital within 48 to 72 hours of symptoms. Patients presenting after this time period should have a serum analysis for total LDH and, more specifically, $LDH_1$ isoenzyme.

### *Radionuclide Studies*

After diagnosis of acute MI, various noninvasive and invasive studies are performed to determine the exact cause of infarction and extent of myocardial injury. Radionuclide scintigraphy with either technetium-99*m* pyrophosphate or thallium-201 is safe and noninvasive. Both scans can be used to determine the presence of MI in patients whose ECG tracing and serum enzyme determinations are not conclusive in the diagnosis of infarction. In addition, both scans provide a quantitative assessment of the location and extent of myocardial tissue damage and can be performed at the patient's bedside in the CICU.

Technetium-99*m* pyrophosphate is injected into the systemic circulation and localizes in areas of necrosis but does not accumulate to any significant degree in ischemic or reversibly damaged myocardial cells.[27] After myocardial intracellular damage, calcium influx into the cell increases. Technetium-99*m* pyrophosphate complexes with the calcium and enters the damaged cells.[28] Zones of infarction appear as darkened areas or "hot spots" on scintigrams taken 2 to 3 hours after injection of the radionuclide. This scan, when used, is most often performed 2 to 3 days after the infarction.

Perfusion imaging utilizing thallium-201 can be used to assess the extent of infarcted myocardium within several hours of the acute event. After injection of thallium-201 into the systemic circulation, this potassium analogue is quickly taken up by living myocardium. Areas of viable myocardium will transport the thallium-201 intracellularly, whereas dead tissue will not.[29,30] Therefore, scintigraphic interpretation of thallium-201, unlike technetium-99*m*, results in deficits in uptake or "cold spot" imaging. Usually, 100% of the infarcts are detected provided the scan is performed within 6 hours of infarction.[31]

Advantages of thallium-201 over other radionuclides include its low-energy radiation and long shelf life and the rapidity with which an acute MI can be identified and assessed after onset of symptoms.[29]

Coronary angiography and ventriculography aid in the assessment of underlying coronary artery disease for future management, and depict the functional damage suffered by the infarcted myocardium. Assessment of the location and degree of CAD via coronary angiography is essential in the decision-making process regarding the options of percutaneous transluminal coronary angioplasty (PTCA) and coronary artery bypass graft (CABG) surgery.

## Prognosis

The incidence of death after an acute myocardial infarction is highest during the first several hours after onset of symptoms. It is therefore imperative that correct diagnosis and appropriate therapy be instituted without delay. If the infarction occurs outside the hospital setting, immediate transport to a hospital emergency department for management is essential.[5] Once acute therapy has been instituted and the patient has been stabilized he or she should then be transferred to the CICU for close observation and medical management.

Approximately 50% of hospitalized MI patients develop complications.[32] Two general classes of complications have been defined: (1) electrical (arrhythmias) and (2) mechanical (pump failure). ECG monitoring and prompt recognition and treatment of electrical complications have reduced the in-hospital mortality from MI. Unfortunately, a similarly favorable trend has not been observed with MI-associated pump failure despite advances in hemodynamic monitoring and inotropic support. Left ventricular failure with subsequent pulmonary congestion is the primary cause of in-hospital death from MI.

Of the 500,000 patients hospitalized yearly for acute MI, 400,000 patients survive to hospital discharge.[33] The major mortality risk is within the first 6 months of hospitalization; death is equally distributed between sudden and nonsudden cardiac events.[33,34] Approximately 10% of patients die within the first year of their MI, 5% die within the second year, and 3% to 4% die each year thereafter.[33] The major determinants of death in post-MI patients are the extent of jeopardized myocardium and the degree of electrical instability. Anterior infarction, early left ventricular failure, late significant arrhythmias, and poor left ventricular ejection fraction are the major predictors of poor prognosis.[33]

## Treatment

### *General Measures*

The major goals in the management of acute MI are to reduce post-MI complications and mortality by reversing myocardial ischemia and limiting infarct size. The most important therapeutic interventions in the management of acute MI center on reestablishing a balance between oxygen supply and demand. Myocardial oxygen consumption is decreased through reductions in contractility, heart rate, and myocardial wall tension. Tissue oxygenation can be increased through the administration of oxygen and the reperfusion of occluded coronary arteries.

Supportive care and close monitoring of the patient are essential in reducing the risk of MI-related complications. Patients are continuously monitored with regard to vital signs, electrocardiogram, and clinical symptomatology. Continuous electrocardiographic monitoring for about 72 hours after the acute event is recommended because arrhythmias are most likely to occur during this period. A venous access line is inserted for the administration of medications. A flow-directed, balloon-tipped (Swan–Ganz) catheter may be inserted into the pulmonary artery to assess right atrial pressure (RAP), right ventricular pressure (RVP), pulmonary artery pressure (PAP), and pulmonary capillary wedge pressure (PCWP) (Fig. 14.6).[35–37] Candidates for Swan–Ganz catheterization would have evidence of hypoperfusion or pulmonary congestion. An indwelling arterial catheter is helpful in measuring systemic blood pressure and obtaining arterial blood gases (ABGs).

### *Medical Management*

#### Oxygen

During acute MI, hypoxemia results from venoarterial intrapulmonary shunting and ventilation perfusion defects.[37] Administration of oxygen reduces hypoxemia and increases

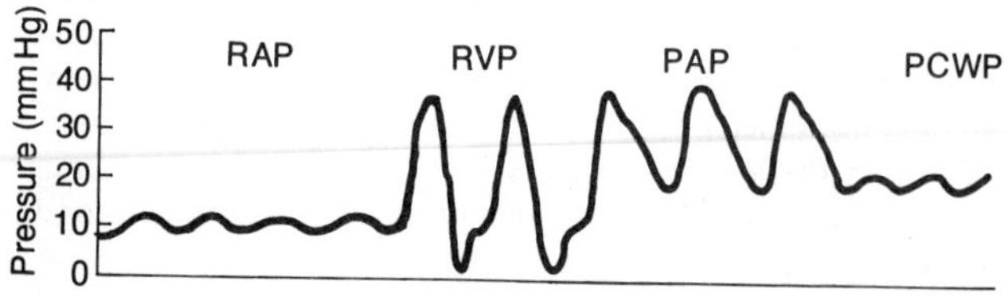


**Figure 14.6** Swan–Ganz catheter pressure waveforms during insertion over time. RAP, right atrial pressure; RVP, right ventricular pressure; PAP, pulmonary artery pressure; PCWP, pulmonary capillary wedge pressure. *(From Ornato JP (Ed): Cardiovascular Emergencies. New York, Churchill Livingstone, 1986, p 119, with permission.)*

oxygen delivery to ischemic tissues by maximizing the arterial oxygen tension. Oxygen is administered by nasal prongs for the first 24 to 48 hours at a flow rate of 3 to 4 L/min. Endotracheal intubation and positive airway pressure mechanical ventilation should be used if adequate oxygenation (oxygen saturation ≥90%) cannot be maintained by mask. High-level, continuous positive airway pressure will improve tissue oxygenation and reduce the spontaneous respiratory effort without compromising cardiac output in acute MI patients with left ventricular dysfunction.[37,38]

### Analgesics

Pain control is often the most pressing need of patients experiencing acute MI. Pain and apprehension induce hyperactivity of the sympathetic nervous system which leads to tachyarrhythmias and increases in myocardial oxygen consumption. Effective treatment of pain depresses this neuronal surge and reduces myocardial oxygen demand, both of which may prevent deleterious consequences.[37] Morphine sulfate is the drug of choice because of its efficacy, rapid onset of action, and sedative properties, which decrease anxiety. In addition to its analgesic effect, morphine increases venous capacitance and relieves pulmonary edema; morphine's potent vasodilatory effects also reduce systemic vascular resistance.[39] Morphine reduces pain and decreases myocardial oxygen demand in patients with acute MI. Initial doses range from 2 to 5 mg intravenously every 5 to 15 minutes as needed until pain is controlled or the patient experiences side effects. Maintenance doses of 4 to 8 mg every 4 to 6 hours may be required for sustained analgesia. If intravenous access is not available, morphine may be given subcutaneously in a dose of 10 to 15 mg.[40] Hypotension and bradycardia which appear to be vagally mediated may occur after morphine administration.[41] These cardiovascular side effects are more pronounced in fluid-dependent patients and patients with increased systemic vascular resistance; hypotension may be attenuated by keeping patients in a supine position.[42] If bradycardia and hypotension develop, atropine should be administered.[42] Other side effects observed with morphine include respiratory and central nervous system (CNS) depression, vomiting, and constipation. Myocardial infarction–related nausea and vomiting respond readily and safely to intravenous prochlorperazine 2.5 mg.[43]

Meperidine 25 to 75 mg by slow intravenous injection every 2 to 3 hours as needed for pain control is a suitable alternative in morphine-intolerant patients. Meperidine's anticholinergic effect counteracts the heightened vagal tone in acute MI patients with either bradycardia or nausea. Tachycardia is a potential adverse effect of meperidine administration. Excessive narcosis and respiratory depression can occur with all narcotics.

Should a patient develop respiratory or CNS depression from either morphine or meperidine, naloxone, an opiate antagonist, may be given. Doses range from 0.4 to 2 mg intravenously as needed for reversal of respiratory depression. The duration of naloxone's effect in patients varies considerably from a few minutes to several hours. Careful observation is recommended between administrations of the antagonist to avoid narcotic withdrawal. Nalbuphine hydrochloride is a fully synthetic opioid analgesic with mixed narcotic agonist and antagonist effects. Results of one study comparing the hemodynamic effects of nalbuphine and morphine in patients with acute MI indicate that nalbuphine relieves pain and reduces myocardial oxygen demand without producing hypotension.[44] Nalbuphine 10 mg is administered intravenously every 3 to 6 hours as needed for pain relief. Although nalbuphine and butorphanol do not appear to significantly alter systemic hemodynamics, increased systemic vascular resistance and myocardial oxygen demand may occur with agonist–antagonist narcotics, and they should be used with caution in acute MI.

The persistence of pain over several hours is a bad prognostic sign, usually indicative of continued myocardial ischemia and necrosis. In this setting, nitroglycerin may effectively relieve refractory chest pain. Nitroglycerin decreases myocardial oxygen demand by reducing intramyocardial wall tension. Patients with signs and symptoms of pulmonary edema derive the most benefit from intravenous nitroglycerin administration. Nitroglycerin is further discussed under Vasodilators.

### Sedation

Anxiety may have deleterious effects on the cardiovascular system, especially in patients with acute MI. The treatment of anxiety should aim to reduce not only the somatic complaints but also the adrenergic hyperactivity present in MI patients.[45] Three groups of medications can be used to treat cardiac symptoms and anxiety disorders post-MI. Antidepressant drugs lower psychic anxiety, but do not suppress adrenergic response. In contrast, $\beta$-adrenergic blockers suppress adrenergic tone, but do not affect psychic anxiety. Benzodiazepines can be used to relax the patient and theoretically decrease catecholamine outpouring secondary to stress.[45] Benzodiazepines also appear to produce experimental coronary vasodilation by potentiating adenosine activity.[46] Alprazolam and diazepam have shown to be effective in decreasing anxiety and catecholamine levels in acute MI patients.[45]

### Vasodilators

Vasodilators are used to decrease intramyocardial wall tension by reducing preload and afterload, to augment stroke volume, and to enhance coronary blood flow (Table 14.1). Generalized sympathetic vasoconstriction is a useful compensatory mechanism for maintaining systemic pressure and coronary perfusion in cardiogenic shock. However, excessive vasoconstriction decreases cardiac output and increases myocardial oxygen demand. By decreasing this reflex vasoconstriction, vasodilator drugs can reduce ventricular wall stress and myocardial oxygen demand, and improve cardiac output. The primary effects of these agents appear to be related to their peripheral actions on arterial and venous beds. By dilating the arterial resistance bed, vasodilators reduce systemic vascular resistance (SVR), with a resultant increase in stroke volume. Vasodilating drugs, which also reduce venous tone, decrease venous return to the heart and lower the pulmonary capillary wedge pressure (PCWP). In summary, vasodilators correct the hemodynamic abnormalities present during left ventricular dysfunction and may restore the balance between myocardial oxygen supply and demand.

The use of vasodilators is limited by their potential to produce hypotension in patients with pump failure. These agents produce a triphasic response: (1) at low dosages, cardiac output increases and PCWP decreases with little change in arterial pressure; (2) at moderate dosages, cardiac output increases, PCWP decreases, and arterial pressures decrease or remain unchanged; and (3) at high dosages, cardiac output, PCWP, and arterial pressure all decrease.[47] Vasodilators should be avoided in patients with a PCWP less than 12 mm Hg. Hemodynamic measurements obtained by Swan–Ganz catheterization should be followed closely in all patients receiving vasodilator therapy, particularly when concomitant diuretic therapy is employed. Nitroglycerin is the preferred vasodilator because of its rapid onset of action and preferential dilation of the venous system, coronaries, and collateral vessels. Indications for nitroglycerin administration in acute MI are recurrent chest pain, hypertension, and left ventricular failure. Sublingual nitroglycerin 0.3 to 0.4 mg every 5 minutes as needed for chest discomfort and nitroglycerin ointment 1 to 2 in. every 4 to 6 hours are the most commonly administered nitrate formulations used in acute MI. Both hypotension and tachycardia are contraindications to the administration of nitrates. Side effects that may be encountered are headache, hypotension, tachycardia, and paradoxical bradycardia. Nitrate-induced hypotension responds readily to fluid replacement therapy.

Intravenous nitroglycerin is an effective adjunct in the management of unstable angina and cardiogenic shock associated with MI. It is administered by continuous intravenous infusion at 10 to 20 μg/min and increased by 5 to 10 μg/min every 5 to 10 minutes until the desired hemodynamic or clinical response occurs. Low doses (30–40 μg/min) produce predominantly venodilation; high doses (250 μg/min) lead to arteriolar dilation as well.[48] The combination of nitroglycerin and an inotrope (dopamine or dobutamine) produces marked hemodynamic improvements while reducing the risk of ischemic damage.[49] Overall, patients with the most severe degree of left ventricular failure have the most beneficial hemodynamic effects. Potential complications of intravenous nitroglycerin include reversible hypotension and bradycardia, hypoxemia caused by increased pulmonary ventilation–perfusion mismatch, methemoglobinemia, and headache. In general, the drug has been well tolerated.

Sodium nitroprusside is a potent peripheral vasodilator with effects on both arterial and venous smooth muscle. Its rapid onset and short duration of action make it a suitable agent in hemodynamically unstable situations. Numerous studies have reported improvement in left ventricular function, tissue perfusion, cardiac output, and clinical status in patients with low-output states and high systemic vascular resistance refractory to dopamine.[50] Nevertheless, nitroprusside should not be routinely used in patients who develop a PCWP >20 mm Hg within the first 9 hours after acute myocardial infarction because it may adversely affect outcome.[51]

The recommended dosing range is 0.5 to 5 μg/kg/min, but higher doses (up to 10 μg/kg/min) may be needed. The major complication of nitroprusside is hypotension. Patients should be monitored for signs of cyanide or thiocyanate toxicity. Cyanide toxicity is detected by the presence of metabolic acidosis; thiocyanate toxicity manifests as confusion, hyperreflexia, and convulsions. Thiocyanate levels above 12 mg/dL are suggestive of thiocyanate toxicity.[52] Low-dose infusions (<3 μg/kg/min) shorter than 72 hours rarely lead to toxicity.

Recent studies have suggested a difference between nitroglycerin and nitroprusside relative to their effects on myocardial blood flow.[53] Nitroglycerin has a greater dilatory effect on collateral capacitance vessels. Nitroprusside has a greater dilatory effect on arteriolar resistance vessels. Therefore, nitroglycerin is less likely to produce coronary steal. Furthermore, nitroprusside has a greater propensity to lower coronary perfusion pressure when compared with nitroglycerin.[54]

In summary, nitroglycerin is the intravenous vasodilator of choice in acute MI. Its systemic vasodilatory effects increase cardiac output and lower oxygen consumption. Nitroglycerin's venodilatory action increases blood supply to ischemic areas as compared with nitroprusside.[55]

### β-Adrenergic Blockers

A number of clinical trials[56–58] have been performed to assess the usefulness of acute intravenous β-adrenergic blocker administration on reduction of mortality and infarct size. The latter is discussed under Limitation of Infarct Size.

Two large trials[57,58] totaling more than 19,000 patients have addressed the issue of acute intravenous β-blocker administration followed by short-term oral therapy in the acute MI setting. The Metoprolol in Acute Myocardial Infarction (MIAMI) trial[58] was a multicenter double-blinded placebo-controlled randomized study in which 2,877 patients with suspected or definite myocardial infarction received 5 mg of metoprolol intravenously every 2 minutes for a total of 15 mg within 24 hours of onset of symptoms. Patients were randomized into the study after arrival at the coronary care unit. After intravenous dosing, patients received oral metoprolol 100 mg every 6 hours for the first 2 days beginning 15 minutes after the last intravenous injection. The dose was then decreased to 100 mg every 12 hours for the remaining 13 days of the study. The cumulative mortality for all patients at the conclusion of the 15-day trial was 123 (4.3%) deaths in the treatment group compared with 142 (4.9%) deaths in the placebo group. This difference did not reach statistical significance. Mortality in patients with definite MI was 120 of 2,028 in the metoprolol group versus 137 of 2,099 in the placebo group. High-risk patients in MIAMI were found to benefit, whereas other subgroups did not benefit.

The most recent and largest multicenter trial was conducted by the First International Study of Infarct Survival

**Table 14.1** Inotropes and Vasoactive Agents

| Drug and Usual Dose | Receptor specificity | | | | | Pharmacologic effect | | | | | Hemodynamic effect | | | | | Comments |
|---|---|---|---|---|---|---|---|---|---|---|---|---|---|---|---|---|
| | α | $\beta_1$ | $\beta_2$ | Dop | Sm Msc | VD | VC | INT | CHT | RBF | MAP | PCWP | CO | SVR | UO | |
| Norepinephrine (Levophed) IV 2–12 μg/min | ++++ | ++ | — | — | — | — | ++++ | + | ++ | ↓ | ↑ | ↑ | ↕ | ↑ | ↓ | Decreased peripheral perfusion<br>Painful extravasation<br>Arrhythmias<br>Angina |
| Dopamine (Inotropin) | | | | | | | | | | | | | | | | Arrhythmias, headache, hypertension, decreased peripheral perfusion, painful extravasation |
| 2–5 μg/kg/min | | + | | ++++ | — | + | | ++ | + | | | | | | | |
| 6–10 μg/kg/min | | ++++ | ++ | + | | + | | +++ | ++ | ↕ | ↑ | ↑ | ↕ | ↕ | ↕ | |
| 10–20 μg/kg/min | +++ | ++++ | + | | | | +++ | +++ | +++ | | | | | | | |
| Dobutamine (Dobutrex) 2.0–15.0 μg/kg/min | + | ++++ | ++ | — | — | ++ | + | +++− | ++ | ↑ | ↕ | ↓ | ↑ | →↓ | ↑ | Headache, palpitation, hypotension |

| | | | | | | | | | | | | | | | | |
|---|---|---|---|---|---|---|---|---|---|---|---|---|---|---|---|---|
| Amrinone (Inocor) 0.75 mg/kg 5–10 µg/kg/min | — | — | ? | — | — | ++ | — | +++ | +++ | ↑ | ↕ | ↓ | ↑ | ↕ | ↑ | Thrombocytopenia, nausea, flulike syndrome, arrhythmias, hypotension |
| Nitroprusside (Nipride) 0.5–10 µg/kg/min | — | — | — | — | ++++ A=V | — | — | — | — | ↕ | ↓ | ↓ | ↕ | ↓ | ↕ | Hypotension, nausea, abdominal pain, tremor, headache, confusion |
| Nitroglycerin 5–300 µg/min | — | — | — | — | ++++ A<V | — | — | — | — | ↕ | ↓ | ↓ | ↕ | →↓ | ↕ | Headache, tachycardia, hypotension, nausea |
| Hydralazine (Apresoline) 5–10 mg IV bolus | — | — | — | — | A ++++ | — | — | — | — | ↑ | ↓ | → | ↑ | ↓ | ↑ | Hypotension, headache, reflex tachycardia, angina |

$\alpha$, $\alpha$-adrenergic; $\beta_1$, $\beta_1$-adrenergic; $\beta_2$, $\beta_2$-adrenergic; DOP, dopaminergic; Sm Msc, smooth muscle; VD, vasodilation; VC, vasoconstriction; INT, inotropic; CHT, chronotropic; RBF, renal blood flow; MAP, mean arterial pressure; PCWP, pulmonary capillary wedge pressure; CO, cardiac output; SVR, systemic vascular resistance; UO, urine output.

From Ornato JP (Ed): Cardiovascular Emergencies, New York, Churchill Livingstone, 1986, p 123, with permisison.

**Table 14.2** Acute β-Adrenergic Blocker Administration to Limit Infarct Size

| *Study* | *Drug* | *Start of treatment (h)* | *No. of patients* | *Results (CK-MB release)* |
|---|---|---|---|---|
| Peter [62] | Propranolol | | | |
| | 0.1 mg/kg IV | <4 | 37 | Decreased w/propranolol |
| | 320 mg/d PO | 4–12 | 58 | No difference |
| Yusef [63] | Atenolol | | | |
| | 5 mg IV | <12 | 477 | Decreased w/atenolol |
| | 100 mg/d PO | | | |
| Hjalmarson (Goteborg)[64] | Metoprolol | | | |
| | 15 mg IV | <12 | 936 | Decreased w/metoprolol |
| | 200 mg/d PO | >12 | 424 | No difference (used LDH 1 + 2 rather than CK-MB) |
| Sederholm (International Collaborative Study Group)[65] | Timolol IV × 24 h | <4 | 144 | Decreased w/timolol |
| | 20 mg/d PO | | | |
| Roberts (MILIS)[66] | Propranolol | | | |
| | 0.1 mg/kg IV | <8 | 124 | No difference |
| | 20–200 mg/d PO | 8–18 | 113 | No difference |

From Rackley CE (Ed): Advances in Critical Care Cardiology. Philadelphia, F.A. Davis, 1986, p 34, with permission.

(ISIS-1) Collaborative Group.[57] A total of 16,207 patients were randomized to receive 5 to 10 mg of atenolol, in 5-mg intravenous doses, or placebo within a mean of 5 hours of onset of suspected MI. Oral dosing in the treatment group followed, with 100 mg of atenolol per day as either a single dose or divided every 12 hours for a total of 7 days. Mortality occurred in 313 of 8,037 (3.89%) atenolol-treated patients and 365 of 7,990 (4.57%) control patients. The beneficial effect of atenolol in decreasing the incidence of mortality was statistically significant ($2P<0.04$).

In summary, all of the smaller trials evaluating the beneficial effect of acute, short-term β-adrenergic blockade have not significantly altered mortality. The ISIS-1[57] study has been the largest and only study to show significant benefit with atenolol.

### *Limitation of Infarct Size*

Of great importance in the management of acute MI is the ability to limit the size or "zone" of infarction because infarct size correlates directly with incidence of mortality.[59] It takes approximately 4 to 6 hours after ischemia for irreversible injury of the myocardium to occur. Reperfusion of this "zone of ischemia" within a 3- to 4-hour period after the initiation of the ischemic episode may reduce the area of infarction and subsequent myocardial damage. A number of studies in humans have been performed to assess the efficacy of β-adrenergic blocking agents, calcium antagonists, thrombolytic agents, and hyaluronidase in limiting infarct size.

#### β-Adrenergic Blockers

The primary mechanism of the beneficial effect of β-adrenergic blocking agents in reducing the size of the infarction is believed to be through a reduction in myocardial oxygen consumption by suppression of catecholamine levels and redistribution of collateral blood flow to areas of ischemia.[60,61] A number of clinical studies in humans have been performed[62–66] utilizing serum enzyme analysis (CK-MB) to assess reduction in infarct size. The results of these trials are presented in Table 14.2. The reader is also referred to a more comprehensive review published by Yusef et al.[56] Patient tolerance to acute administration of β-adrenergic blockade has been very good. Overall, the literature[62–65] supports the use of β-blockers in the acute setting. Treatment is successful if begun within 4 to 6 hours of the onset of symptoms. The extent of infarct size reduction based on CK-MB release ranges from 10% to 30%.[62–65] Contradictory results indicating failure of β-blockers to decrease cellular CK-MB release appear to be related to delayed initiation of therapy.[66] Contraindications to the use of β-blockers in the acute setting include heart block greater than first degree, bradycardia, hypotension, and high left ventricular filling pressures (PCWP > 24 mm Hg).

#### Calcium Channel Blockers

There are several potentially beneficial effects supporting the use of calcium blocking agents during or immediately after acute MI. The negative inotropic and chronotropic effects of both diltiazem and verapamil may decrease myocardial oxygen demand as observed with β-adrenergic blockers, thereby limiting infarct size. Also, the vasodilating properties of the calcium channel blockers may enhance collateral blood flow to the area of ischemia as well as block any vasospastic component contributing to the acute MI. Finally, the calcium channel blocking agents may protect the ischemic myocardial cells from the damaging influx of calcium that occurs during the infarction.

Although calcium channel blocking agents have proven to be effective in treating angina they have not been shown to be beneficial in limiting infarct size.[67–69] The Nifedipine Angina Myocardial Infarction Study (NAMIS)[67] was the first multicenter placebo-controlled trial to assess nifedipine 20 mg every 4 hours, starting 4.6 ± 0.1 hours after the onset of chest pain for 14 days. A total of 171 patients with either threatened MI or early acute MI were admitted into the study. No significant difference in size of infarction, as assessed by CK-MB serum levels, between the two groups was noted. A startling observation was that the nifedipine-treated group exhibited a higher incidence of mortality (7.9% versus 0% in the control group) during the 2-week study period. Long-term mortality at 6-month follow-up was not statistically significant between the nifedipine and placebo groups.

The Norwegian Nifedipine Multicenter Trial[68] randomized 277 patients to receive either nifedipine 10 mg five times a day or placebo. Unlike the NAMIS trial, randomization occurred within 12 hours of onset of symptoms. Treatment on the average was initiated within 5.5 ± 2.9 hours of symptoms and nifedipine was administered for 6 weeks. Results showed no difference in CK-MB release or 6-week mortality between the two groups.

Lastly, the Danish Multicenter Study Group[69] randomized 100 patients to receive verapamil 0.1 mg/kg intravenously followed by 120 mg orally three times a day or placebo for 6 months. Patients were randomized within 4 hours of onset of symptoms of acute MI. As with the nifedipine trials, no difference in CK-MB release was observed.

### Thrombolytic Agents

The prognosis after infarction is closely related to the amount of functional myocardium remaining. Efforts over the past decade to limit infarct size pharmacologically, by reducing myocardial oxygen demand, have generally met with disappointment. The more appealing possibility of acutely restoring blood flow has become a reality with thrombolytic therapy. The goals of thrombolytic therapy with streptokinase, urokinase, or tissue plasminogen activator are to lyse coronary thrombi during the early phase of acute MI, to limit infarct size by reperfusing jeopardized myocardium, and to reduce morbidity and mortality. Patients with recent onset of chest pain (usually less than 6 hours) and with persistent ECG abnormalities indicative of an evolving transmural acute MI are candidates for thrombolytic therapy.[70] Patients with recent stroke, recent surgery, cardiopulmonary resuscitation, age over 65, blood pressure 180/110 mm Hg or greater, pregnancy, active bleeding, intracranial neoplastic disease, uncontrolled hypertension, or bleeding diathesis should not receive thrombolytic therapy.[71,72]

Streptokinase, a protein elaborated by $\beta$-hemolytic streptococci, forms a complex with plasminogen that acts to convert additional circulating plasminogen to plasmin. Activation is rapid, and plasmin formation occurs promptly after streptokinase administration. Plasmin, a nonspecific proteolytic enzyme, lyses fresh fibrin clots and digests clotting factors V and VIII, prothrombin, and fibrinogen. Degradation of fibrin and fibrinogen leads to the formation of fibrin split products (FSPs), which inhibit further clotting. The combination of fibrinogen depletion and formation of FSPs gives rise to a systemic lytic state. Additional beneficial effects of streptokinase include reductions in plasma viscosity[73,74] and systemic vascular resistance.[75] Intracoronary streptokinase is initiated with a 10,000- to 30,000-unit bolus, followed by an infusion of 2,000 to 4,000 units per minute. Clot lysis generally occurs within 30 minutes after initiation of the infusion and requires an average of 65,000 units of streptokinase. The infusion is continued for 30 to 60 minutes after successful reperfusion or until a predetermined maximal dose of streptokinase (150,000–500,000 units) has been given. Intravenous streptokinase is administered at a dose of 750,000 to 1.5 million units over 30 to 60 minutes. After streptokinase, patients receive full-dose, intravenous heparin for 24 to 72 hours. Hydrocortisone 100 mg and diphenhydramine 25 mg may be given intravenously before treatment to decrease adverse immunologic reaction to streptokinase, although their value is unproven.

Urokinase is an enzyme produced by human renal tubular cells. It directly activates the conversion of plasminogen to plasmin without binding to plasminogen or other bloodborne products. Urokinase may be used in patients with hypersensitivity to streptokinase or with high antibody titers for *Streptococcus* sp. Urokinase costs approximately five times more than streptokinase[76] and does not offer any therapeutic advantages. Three units of urokinase is approximately equivalent to one unit of streptokinase. Thrombolytic doses of urokinase produce an excess of plasmin, which leads to a systemic lytic state.[76,77]

Unlike streptokinase and urokinase, tissue-type plasminogen activator (t-PA) has minimal affinity for free, circulating plasminogen. Tissue-type plasminogen activator produces clot-selective thrombolysis by activating fibrin-bound plasminogen; t-PA's activity is dose dependent.[78] Pharmacologic doses of t-PA activate circulating plasminogen, resulting in systemic fibrinogenolysis and the appearance of a modest systemic lytic state.[78–80] The short half-life of t-PA, approximately 10 minutes, does not ensure prompt reversal of hemostatic abnormalities.[79,80] This process depends upon the replenishment of fibrinogen and the elimination of fibrinogen breakdown products.[79] Tissue plasminogen activator is generally well tolerated. Hematoma and prolonged bleeding at the site of injection are the most commonly reported adverse effects; their frequency is similar to that observed with streptokinase.[78–80] The optimal dose of t-PA remains to be determined. The major disadvantages of t-PA include moderate hemostatic defect, the need for prolonged administration (3 hours) and concurrent heparin therapy, and the 10- to 20-fold increase in cost of drug therapy alone compared with streptokinase.

Approximately 86% of patients with acute transmural MI have total occlusion of the involved coronary artery.[81] Early treatment reestablishes flow in the infarct-related coronary artery in 60% to 90% of patients treated with intracoronary streptokinase and in 35% to 62% of patients treated with intravenous streptokinase.[82] The two largest trials with intravenous streptokinase, GISSI and ISIS-2, demonstrated 20% and 33% reductions in mortality, respectively.[83,84] In contrast to intravenous streptokinase, the experience with t-PA is considerably less in patient numbers but greater with respect to angiographic catheterization.[85] Preliminary studies with t-PA are encouraging.[78,85] A consistent 70% to 75%

infarct vessel patency rate has been observed with intravenous t-PA, despite changes in dosing patterns and preparation.[85] In the treatment of acute myocardial infarction, intravenous infusions of t-PA produce reperfusion rates similar to those observed with intracoronary streptokinase.[78,79,82]

Clinical experience provides little support for the contention that t-PA is superior to intravenous streptokinase in acute MI when administered within the first 3 hours of onset of symptoms.[79,80,86] Beyond 3 hours after symptom onset, t-PA appears to be superior to streptokinase in reperfusing infarct-related arteries.[85,87] The incidence of reocclusion does not differ between intravenous streptokinase (18%) and intravenous t-PA (23%).[79]

Successful reperfusion is indicated by sudden relief of chest pain, resolution of ST-segment elevation, or onset of reperfusion tachyarrhythmias. These occur in 15% of patients, but do not usually require treatment. Bleeding complications with either route of administration are relatively frequent (23%–47%), but only 5% of patients require blood transfusions.[82] Bleeding complications can be minimized by closely monitoring the patient's coagulation profile, avoiding drugs that affect hemostasis, waiting for the partial thromboplastin time to decline to two to three times control before heparin is administered (except for t-PA–treated patients), and avoiding excess venipuncture.

Successful thrombolytic therapy in acute MI depends on more than just the ability to reperfuse the occluded coronary artery. Prevention of reocclusion and subsequent salvage of infarcted myocardium should reduce morbidity and mortality after thrombolytic therapy. Thrombolytic therapy may be thought of as a bridge to definitive therapy, including PTCA and CABG, to prevent reocclusion and minimize residual stenosis. Clinical trials that assess these factors will ultimately determine the role of thrombolysis in acute MI.

### Hyaluronidase

Hyaluronidase, an enzyme obtained from bovine testicular or microbial sources, reduces myocardial necrosis on the basis of several animal models of acute MI.[59] The mechanism of action of hyaluronidase is unclear; the enzyme enhances the influx of nutrients and the efflux of metabolic waste products, and retards edema formation. An advantage of this agent, if proven effective, is the absence of any detectable hemodynamic action and lack of adverse effects except for rare allergic reactions. Clinical trials in which hyaluronidase was administered 6 to 9 hours after the onset of symptoms failed to show a reduction in infarct size and mortality in acute MI patients.[59]

### Percutaneous Transluminal Coronary Angioplasty

This nonsurgical, invasive technique provides an alternative mechanical method for recanalizing an occluded coronary artery. Preliminary data from acute MI patients show a high initial reperfusion rate and improved prognosis, even in patients who had failed pharmacologic thrombolysis.[3,88,89] Although several studies[90–92] support the role of PTCA immediately after streptokinase, two studies[93,94] show no clear advantage of emergent (less than 3 days) PTCA over delayed (10 days) PTCA in patients treated with t-PA. A major limitation of PTCA is that it requires a skilled team, a fully staffed catheterization laboratory, and a surgical team on standby for emergent coronary artery bypass graft surgery. Potential complications of PTCA include catheter-induced occlusions caused by dissection, spasm, or subintimal hematoma and residual stenosis.

### Coronary Artery Bypass Grafting

Over the last two decades, the option of CABG has become a viable alternative in the treatment of not only unstable angina but also acute MI. A number of studies[95–99] have supported the role of CABG in acute MI intervention. The development of coronary angiography has provided a method to "map out" diseased coronary vessels. Coronary artery bypass surgery restores blood flow to areas of ischemia by "bypassing" the totally or partially occluded vessels, thereby preventing further infarction. In so doing, viable myocardium may be spared from irreversible damage. This surgery is often reserved for those patients who have greater than 50% occlusion of the left mainstem coronary artery, patients with multiple vessel disease, patients with distal coronary artery atherosclerotic plaques that cannot be reached with PTCA, and patients who fail the initial PTCA procedure. The surgery consists of anastomosis of the saphenous vein from the aortic root to an area of the coronary artery distal to the obstruction. Another procedure involves the use of the internal mammary artery (IMA). The distal portion of the IMA is ligated and anastomosed to the distal portion of the coronary artery as just described.

Revascularization in a large number of MI patients was described by Dewood's group.[96] Seven hundred and one patients underwent CABG surgery within 24 hours of the acute MI. The mortality rate for all patients, which included 440 patients with transmural infarction and 261 patients with nontransmural MI, was 4.4% (31/701). The presence of cardiogenic shock before surgery was associated with over 50% of in-hospital mortality in the transmural infarct group, which displayed an initial mortality of 5.2%. In addition, in-hospital mortality was higher in transmural MI patients with three-vessel coronary artery disease (9%) versus single-vessel (2.3%) and two-vessel (4.4%) disease. Also, transmural MI patients with early surgical revascularization (<6 hours from onset of symptoms) had a lower mortality rate (3.8%) than those whose surgery was performed later (>6 hours from onset of symptoms) (8.0%) ($P = 0.05$, $\chi^2$). Total mortality in the transmural group rose from 5.2% to 12.5% over the 10-year study period. A smaller trend in mortality was observed in the nontransmural MI patients, for whom mortality rose from 3.0% to 6.5% during an 8-year follow-up.

Hochberg and associates[99] also noted a similar trend with respect to mortality and left ventricular function. Post-MI patients with low ejection fractions (<50%) exhibited a higher incidence of in-hospital death (22%) compared with those with higher ejection fractions (0%).

In summary, CABG provides a viable alternative in the management of the acute MI patient. Surgery is a consideration in patients in whom thrombolytic therapy is not an option or in whom PTCA cannot be performed or has failed. The incidence of mortality in most patients is lower than that observed in the acute MI patient population (15%). Patients with compromised cardiac function (low ejection fraction, cardiogenic shock) are at a much higher risk of mortality. It

**Table 14.3** β-Adrenergic Blocker and Mortality Reduction in Post-MI Patients

| *Trial* | *No. of patients* | *β-blocker* | *Mortality (%)* Control | Intervention | *P value* |
|---|---|---|---|---|---|
| Multicenter International Study[100] | 3,053 | Practolol 400 mg/d | 8.2 | 6.3 | 0.051 |
| Norwegian Multicenter Study[101] | 1,884 | Timolol 20 mg/d | 16.2 | 10.4 | 0.0003 |
| BHAT[102] | 3,738 | Propranolol 180–240 mg/d | 9.8 | 7.2 | 0.005 |
| Julian[103] | 1,456 | Sotalol 320 mg/d | 8.9 | 7.3 | 0.32 |
| Taylor[104] | 1,103 | Oxprenolol 80 mg/d | 10.2 | 9.5 | 0.78 |
| Goteborg Metoprolol Trial[105] | 1,395 | Metoprolol 200 mg/d | 17.2 | 13.2 | 0.043 |

From Rackley CE (Ed): Advances in Critical Care Cardiology. Philadelphia, F. A. Davis, 1986, p 35, with permission.

is these latter patients, however, who have incurred the most damage to the myocardium and may have the most to gain from surgical revascularization, provided that surgery is performed within a short period (6–8 hours) of onset of symptoms.

### *Post–Myocardial Infarction/Post-Reperfusion Management*

#### Bed Rest

Patients should limit their activities to bed rest during the first 24 hours after the acute event. This is done to decrease cardiac workload (myocardial oxygen consumption) during the healing process after an acute MI and to prevent extension or reinfarction. Activities over the next few days should begin gradually, starting with personal hygiene and in-bed range-of-motion exercises. Patients may begin ambulating 4 to 5 days post-MI. The gradual introduction of activities may decrease the requirement for anticoagulation in this patient population.

#### Diet

At first, a clear liquid diet is instituted for several days during the convalescence period. This diet may require less shunting of blood to the gastrointestinal tract and lower the overall metabolic requirements of the body. Afterward, an appropriate diet (e.g., low-cholesterol, low-sodium, diabetic diet) may be started.

#### Stool Softeners

Once patients are on an appropriate diet, stool softeners are often employed to decrease isometric stress associated with defecation. Either docusate sodium (Colace) 100 mg or docusate calcium (Surfak) 240 mg once or twice a day is satisfactory in emulsifying the stool.

#### β-Adrenergic Blockers

A number of well-controlled oral trials evaluating the long-term efficacy of β-adrenergic blockade in decreasing the incidence of mortality after acute MI have been published[100–105] (Table 14.3). A comprehensive review of all of the trials is also available.[56] All of these studies were double-blinded placebo-controlled randomized evaluations involving large numbers of patients. Oral β-blocking agents were begun a few days to a few weeks after the acute MI. Duration of follow-up ranged from several months to 3 to 4 years, although a majority of the studies were completed within 1 to 2 years.[56] Results indicated that a reduction in mortality was observed in all of the studies,[56,100–105] reaching statistical significance ($P<0.05$) in the timolol,[92] propranolol,[102] and metoprolol[105] trials. The overall reduction in risk of death was approximately 20%.[56]

In addition, the timolol study group[101] observed a 34% decrease in reinfarction rate with drug therapy when compared with placebo. If results from all of the current studies are combined,[56] the risk of reinfarction is reduced by approximately 25% in patients receiving long-term β-blockers.

In summary, the long-term use (1–4 years) of β-adrenergic blockade post-MI is well tolerated[56] and of significant benefit to patients with respect to reduction of both reinfarction and death. Patients with congestive heart failure (CHF) without peripheral hypoperfusion (Killip class II and III) that were enrolled in the β-Blocker Heart Attack Trial[106] experienced a similar decrease (27%) in total mortality compared to those patients without CHF (25%). However, patients with preexisting CHF experienced a 47% reduction in sudden death versus 13% in patients without preexisting heart failure. Candidates for post-MI β-blocker therapy include patients who have hypertension, preexisting heart failure, and/or angina post-MI and do not have contraindication to these agents.

#### Calcium Channel Blockers

As mentioned previously, none of the calcium channel blocker studies[67–69,107] have showed any benefit in decreasing mortality. A recent study by Gibson et al[108] evaluated the effectiveness of diltiazem in reducing the rate of reinfarction in patients with non–Q-wave MI. This multicenter, double-blinded study consisted of 576 patients who were randomized to receive either drug treatment or placebo within 24 to 72 hours of onset of infarction. Diltiazem 90 mg every 6 hours or placebo was continued for 14 days. Reinfarction, defined as a secondary increase in CK-MB during the study period, was observed in 15 of 287 (5.2%) diltiazem-treated patients compared with 27 of 289 (9.3%) control patients ($P=0.0297$); however, 61% of the diltiazem patients were receiving concurrent $\beta$-adrenergic blocker therapy and 80% were also receiving long-acting nitrates. No difference in mortality between the two groups was observed during the 14-day study period. Patients with non–Q-wave acute MI who have early postinfarction angina or angina associated with ECG changes are at high risk of reinfarction and death. This subset of patients appears to have more myocardium in jeopardy and will therefore benefit from prophylactic therapy with diltiazem 90 mg every 6 hours.[109]

Further studies are needed to continue to assess the benefit of calcium channel blocking agents in reducing post-MI reinfarction, sudden death, and long-term mortality.

### Antiplatelet Agents

Two major trials have addressed the use of antiplatelet agents in the post-MI patient.[110,111] The Persantine–Aspirin Reinfarction Study (PARIS)[110] randomized 2,026 survivors of myocardial infarction in double-blind fashion to three groups: dipyridamole 75 mg with aspirin 324 mg three times a day, aspirin 324 mg once daily, and placebo. Each of the two drug groups comprised 810 patients; the placebo group consisted of 406 patients. Patients entered the study after being discharged from the hospital; the enrollment period ranged from 8 weeks to 60 months. Follow-up averaged 41 months. Mortality was decreased by 18% in the aspirin group and 16% in the dipyridamole–aspirin group; when compared with placebo, these changes did not achieve statistical significance. Analysis of the data showed that patients who entered the study within 6 months of their MI had the largest percentage decrease in both total and coronary mortality.

A second dipyridamole–aspirin reinfarction study (PARIS II)[111] enrolled patients who had recently experienced an MI (range 4 weeks to 4 months). A total of 3,128 patients were randomized to receive either dipyridamole 75 mg with aspirin 330 mg three times a day or placebo. Follow-up was a minimum of 1 year, with an average of 23.4 months. The incidence of nonfatal reinfarction plus death from an acute cardiac event was statistically significantly decreased by 30% at 1 year and 24% at the conclusion of the study in the dipyridamole–aspirin group. In addition, coronary mortality was reduced by 20% at 1 year and 6% at the end of the study in the treated group compared with the placebo group. Total mortality in the treatment group was decreased by 11% and 3% at 1 year and the end of the study, respectively.

Several studies have evaluated aspirin with or without dipyridamole for maintenance of bypass graft patency in CABG patients. Recommendations for aspirin (975 mg/d) with dipyridamole (225 mg/d) in three divided doses for the post-CABG patient originate from the study by Chesebro et al.[112] A total of 407 post-CABG patients were randomized to either the treatment regimen or placebo. Patients received dipyridamole 100 mg four times a day for 2 days prior to surgery as well as a single dose 1 hour after surgery. Then dipyridamole and aspirin, in the doses mentioned before, were started 7 hours after the operation. A median 12-month (range 11–18 months) follow-up with vein-graft angiography noted an 11% occlusion rate in the treated group as compared with a 25% rate in the placebo group ($P<0.05$). The ACCP–NHLBI National Conference on Antithrombotic Therapy[113] supports Chesebro's findings. Aspirin 100 mg daily may be used to reduce the incidence of post-CABG reocclusion. A review of the literature[113] reports only one study supporting the efficacy of monotherapy with aspirin in maintaining graft patency. This study by Lorenz et al[114] was limited by a small patient population and a short (4-month) study duration.

### Anticoagulants

Although the use of anticoagulants in acute MI remains controversial, they may be used to prevent systemic and pulmonary embolus formation as well as to halt the progression of the infarction.[115,116] Most patients with uncomplicated acute MI will not require a full anticoagulation, because the low incidence of embolus formation does not outweigh the risks of anticoagulation.

All acute MI patients who are at bedrest should receive "minidose" heparin, 5,000 units subcutaneously every 12 hours to decrease the risk of clot formation. Specific patient populations that are predisposed to thrombus formation with resultant embolization should be fully anticoagulated. This group includes patients who are markedly obese, have a ventricular aneurysm, are in cardiogenic shock, have a history of thrombophlebitis, or have a history of arterial or venous embolism. In addition, patients with transmural anterior myocardial infarction have a 30% to 40% incidence of developing left ventricular thrombi. Anticoagulation of these patients early in the course of therapy will prevent cerebrovascular accident (CVA).[115] Patients with inferior wall myocardial infarction do not usually exhibit left ventricular thrombus formation with resultant CVA. Only those patients with accompanying heart failure, atrial arrhythmias, large acute MI, old anterior wall infarction, or apical dyskinesis or akinesis should be anticoagulated. A two-dimensional echocardiogram can be used to assess the presence of left ventricular thrombi. Oral anticoagulation should be continued for 3 to 6 months after hospital discharge.

The incidence of hemorrhagic side effects from anticoagulation in patients with acute MI ranges from 3% to 7%. Death as a result of hemorrhage is 2% to 4% in warfarin-treated patients and less than 1% in patients receiving heparin.[115] Cerebrovascular accident occurs in 2% to 3% and pulmonary embolus in 1% to 2% of post-MI patients. On the basis of these observations, only those patients at high risk, as described earlier, should be fully anticoagulated. Heparin, which selectively inhibits the intrinsic clotting cascade, is the anticoagulant of choice. An intravenous loading dose of 5,000 units followed by a continuous infusion of approximately 1,000 units per hour is usually employed. The partial thromboplastin time (PTT) should be checked no earlier than 12 hours after the initial bolus. Earlier evaluation of PTT may yield extremely high values because of the effect of the initial 5,000-unit bolus. The infusion rate may be titrated by increments of 100 to 200 units per hour so that PTT is maintained 1.5 to 2 times the control. Side effects of hemorrhage (including cerebral bleed) and thrombocytopenia should be carefully monitored. Contraindications are a history of hemorrhage, severe diabetes, uncontrolled hypertension, vasculitis, and blood dyscrasias.

### *Electrolyte Abnormalities*

Electrolyte abnormalities, most notably hypokalemia and hypomagnesemia, should be identified and corrected. These electrolyte abnormalities can precipitate malignant ventricular arrhythmias in patients with ischemic, hypertrophied, or dilated hearts.

Hypokalemia is the most common electrolyte abnormality encountered in clinical practice, occurring in 23% to 40% of patients treated with thiazide diuretics.[116] When loop and thiazide diuretics are used in combination the incidence increases to approximately 100%.[117] Hypokalemia is present in 9% to 25% of patients with acute MI and may predispose these patients to ventricular fibrillation.[118] Ornato and colleagues[119] found a 49% incidence of hypokalemia in their out-of-hospital cardiac arrest victims. Fifty-five percent of all hypokalemic sudden death victims were receiving diuretics without potassium supplementation; hypokalemia occurred in 13% of victims receiving diuretics plus potassium supplementation. Fortunately, hypokalemia is significantly ($P<0.001$) less common in uncomplicated acute MI patients (11%) compared with sudden death victims (50%).[120] Nonetheless, hypokalemia should be sought and corrected in the acute MI setting. We recommend giving 10 mEq of potassium chloride diluted in 100 mL $D_5W$ over 60 minutes. This dosage can be repeated as necessary, rechecking the serum potassium every hour until it measures 4.0 to 4.5 mEq/L.[121]

The role of magnesium in cardiac disease is well known.[122,123] Magnesium deficiency is associated with a high frequency of cardiac arrhythmias, symptoms of cardiac insufficiency, and sudden cardiac death.[117,122–124] Experimental and clinical studies show that magnesium and potassium metabolism are closely linked.[122,125] Hypomagnesemia, often accompanied by hypokalemia, is usually caused by diuretics.[125,126] Transient hypomagnesemia not induced by renal magnesium loss has been observed in patients with acute myocardial infarction.[127] Because hypomagnesemia can precipitate refractory ventricular fibrillation and can hinder the replenishment of intracellular potassium, it must be corrected if present. One or two grams of magnesium sulfate (2–4 mL of a 50% solution) is diluted in 100 mL of $D_5W$ and administered over 60 minutes.[121] Magnesium supplementation is relatively safe and reduces the incidence of postinfarction ventricular arrhythmias.[124]

### *Post–Myocardial Infarction Complications*

Approximately 50% of hospitalized acute MI patients develop complications. Two general classes of complications have been defined: (1) electrical (arrhythmias) and (2) mechanical (pump failure). ECG monitoring, prompt recognition, and treatment of electrical complications has reduced the in-hospital mortality from acute MI. Unfortunately, a similarly favorable trend has not been observed with acute MI-associated pump failure despite advances in hemodynamic monitoring and inotropic support. Left ventricular failure with subsequent pulmonary congestion is the primary cause of in-hospital death from acute MI. Other rare complications are rupture of the myocardial wall, septum, or papillary muscle and formation of a left ventricular aneurysm, which can lead to a mural thrombus with embolization into the pulmonary or systemic arterial system and pericarditis.[128,129]

#### **Arrhythmias**

Arrhythmias are the most common complication of patients with acute MI. Premature ventricular complexes (PVCs) and ventricular tachycardia not only cause hemodynamic compromise and increase myocardial oxygen consumption but can also degenerate to life-threatening ventricular fibrillation. Ventricular fibrillation has an incidence of 11% and a mortality rate of almost 50%. In addition, about 60% of the ventricular fibrillation episodes occur within 4 hours of symptoms of acute MI and 80% occur within 12 hours. One of the difficulties in preventing this malignant arrhythmia is that it can occur without any "warning arrhythmias" such as frequent or multifocal PVCs. Part of the arrhythmogenicity observed in acute MI patients is thought to be the result of a stress-related increase in the levels of circulating catecholamines whose direct action on adrenergic receptors can be blocked by the administration of $\beta$-adrenergic antagonists. Two $\beta$-adrenergic blocking drugs, metoprolol and propranolol, have been shown to significantly reduce the incidence of ventricular fibrillation in post-MI patients.[130,131] Metoprolol can be instituted after admission of an acute MI patient into the emergency department. Doses of 5 mg are given by slow intravenous push at 5-minute intervals to a total of 15 mg. An oral regimen is then initiated at a dose of 50 mg twice a day. An alternative agent is propranolol, in a dose of 0.1 mg/kg via slow intravenous push divided into three equal doses. The oral maintenance regimen is 180 to 320 mg per day, given in divided doses. Side effects related to $\beta$-blocker administration that should be monitored include bradycardias, atrioventricular conduction delays, and hypotension. Cardiovascular decompensation to cardiogenic shock after $\beta$-adrenergic blocker therapy is rarely observed.[132,133] Contraindications to the use of $\beta$-adrenergic blocking agents include bradyarrhythmias, greater-than-first-degree heart block, conduction delays, hypotension, overt congestive heart failure, and lung disease caused by bronchospasm.

Symptomatic ventricular tachycardia and ventricular fibrillation should be initially managed by synchronous cardioversion and defibrillation, respectively, before drug therapy is started. Lidocaine is the drug of choice in the management of ventricular arrhythmias such as PVCs, asymptomatic ventricular tachycardia, or ventricular fibrillation unresponsive to defibrillation. Many patients receive prophylactic lidocaine during the first 24 hours post-MI, although the reductions in morbidity and mortality have not been shown to be significant.[134] A loading dose of 1 mg/kg is given by intravenous push and is followed by a continuous infusion of 1 to 4 mg/min (20–50 $\mu$g/kg/min). Because of the relatively short distribution half-life ($t_{1/2}$= 6–8 minutes), a second bolus equal to 0.5 mg/kg is given 10 to 15 minutes after the initial bolus. Intravenous boluses of 0.5 mg/kg can be continued at 10- to 15-minute intervals to a total dose of 3 mg/kg if the arrhythmia persists after the first two boluses. Because lidocaine undergoes hepatic metabolism and is a low-extraction drug, alterations in liver blood flow caused by cardiogenic shock, congestive heart failure, hepatic failure, and negative inotropes ($\beta$-adrenergic blocking drugs) all increase the 90-minute half-life of lidocaine. Based on these observations, maintenance infusion rates should be carefully titrated. Central nervous system toxicity, observed as disorientation, is associated with plasma levels above the therapeutic range of 1 to 5 $\mu$g/mL. Heart block and worsening of arrhythmias can occur in patients with underlying heart disease and are not related to either therapeutic or toxic lidocaine serum levels. Some patients with acute MI can tolerate plasma concentrations in the "toxic" range (5–8 $\mu$g/mL). This is thought to be a result of in vivo stress-mediated release of $\alpha_1$-acid glycoprotein during acute MI which binds lidocaine in the systemic circulation.

Procainamide is a second-line agent in the management of ventricular tachycardia. Infusion of a loading dose of 1 g at a rate not faster than 20 to 50 mg/min, followed by a continuous infusion of 2 to 6 mg/min, is recommended. Primary side effects include a proarrhythmic effect and hypotension; the latter is related to the rate of procainamide administration.

Bretylium tosylate is a second-line antiarrhythmic for the treatment of refractory ventricular fibrillation and can be used as a third-line agent for symptomatic ventricular tachycardia. A 5 mg/kg intravenous bolus is given followed by a maintenance infusion of 2 to 4 mg/min. If conversion of the arrhythmia is unsuccessful, a second bolus of 10 mg/kg can be given 30 minutes after the initial bolus dose. Hypotension, nausea, and vomiting may be observed after bretylium administration.

Sinus bradycardia and tachycardia are often observed after acute MI. Transient bradycardia (heart rate < 60) is often observed after inferior wall myocardial infarction and may exert a "protective effect" on the myocardium by decreasing myocardial oxygen demand.[135] If the patient develops symptoms such as hypotension or escape rhythms, atropine should be administered in a dose of 0.5 to 1.0 mg by slow intravenous push to achieve a heart rate greater than 60 beats per minute. This dose may be repeated as needed to maintain the desired rate. Doses of atropine less than 0.5 mg may further depress heart rate through a centrally mediated vagal stimulating effect.[136] It is recommended that asymptomatic bradycardias not be treated because the risk of increasing heart rate with the resultant increase in myocardial oxygen consumption may lead to further ischemia and infarction. If the bradyarrhythmia is refractory to atropine administration, electrical pacing is the management of choice. In life-threatening bradyarrhythmias, in which pacing has not yet been instituted, isoproterenol may be given by intravenous infusion at a rate of 0.5 to 10 $\mu$g/min.

Atrioventricular (AV) block, usually in the form of first-degree heart block, can occur and degenerate to second- or third-degree block. Therapy is the same as for bradyarrhythmias. First-degree block and second-degree Mobitz type I should respond to atropine and isoproterenol if needed. Second-degree Mobitz type II and third-degree heart block may require insertion of a temporary pacemaker.

Atrial tachyarrhythmias associated with acute MI are not uncommon, with incidences of sinus tachycardia and atrial fibrillation/flutter of approximately 30% and 20%, respectively. Atrial tachyarrhythmias should be treated only if ventricular response is unacceptably high or, as with bradyarrhythmias, the patient exhibits hemodynamic compromise. Ventricular response can be controlled by the use of digoxin, $\beta$-adrenergic blocking agents, or calcium channel blocking drugs.

Although cardioversion and drug therapy are used as the initial treatments of cardiac arrhythmias secondary to acute MI, electrolyte abnormalities (hypokalemia, hypomagnesemia) and acid–base disturbances should be sought and corrected if present.

### Cardiogenic Shock

The incidence of cardiogenic shock in patients with acute myocardial infarction is approximately 15%. Management of hypotension centers on determination of the cause. Hypotension resulting from hypovolemia can easily be corrected by repletion of intravascular volume with either crystalloid or colloid. Right ventricular infarction may lead to depressed left ventricular cardiac output as a result of low left ventricular filling pressures. Left ventricular infarction associated with greater than 50% destruction of the myocardium will lead to depressed cardiac output and cardiogenic shock (pump failure). Only 10% to 30% of patients with cardiogenic shock after acute MI survive this complication. Of the survivors, 50% die within the following 2 years.

Clinical signs and symptoms of cardiogenic shock are hypotension with systolic blood pressure less than 80 mm Hg, depressed cardiac index (<1.8 L/min/m$^2$), high left ventricular filling pressures (PCWP > 18 mm Hg), little (<20–30 mL/h) or nonexistent urine output, and bibasilar rales. Insertion of a Swan–Ganz catheter will not only aid in the initial cardiovascular assessment of the patient but also serve as a guide in the therapy of these patients. Once the catheter is in place, an evaluation of the patient's hemodynamic state can be compared with the Forrester subset classification[47] so that appropriate pharmacologic interventions can be employed (Table 14.4).

The goals of medical management of cardiogenic shock are to (1) optimize left ventricular filling pressure, (2) minimize the impedance to left ventricular ejection, and (3) maximize contractility without excessively increasing myocardial oxygen demand. Therapeutic agents used to remedy acute pump failure include diuretics, positive inotropic agents, and vasodilators (Table 14.4).

Treatment of subset II is directed primarily at reducing PCWP. Diuretics are the cornerstone of therapy because they can be given by rapid intravenous administration with few adverse effects. In the cardiogenic shock patient, intravenous diuretics exert two distinctly important effects. The immediate effect is an increase in venous capacitance, redistributing blood away from the lungs and decreasing pulmonary capillary pressures.[137] The second effect is to increase sodium and water excretion by the kidneys. Loop diuretics produce renal vasodilation which may increase their natriuretic effect.[138] The resultant diuresis decreases both intravascular volume and left ventricular volume and filling pressure.

Overzealous diuresis should be avoided because excessive reductions in left ventricular filling pressure may worsen cardiac output. Diuretic-induced electrolyte abnormalities should be identified and promptly corrected. To minimize electrolyte abnormalities and to prevent the risk of subopti-

**Table 14.4** Hemodynamic Classification and Relationship to Clinical Presentation and Percent Mortality Based on Hemodynamic Signs

| | | |
|---|---|---|
| CI > 2.2 | SUBSET I<br>Normal hemodynamics<br>Mortality = 3% | SUBSET II<br>Pulmonary congestion<br>Rales present<br>Mortality = 9% |
| CI < 2.2 | SUBSET III<br>Peripheral hypoperfusion<br>Rales absent<br>Mortality = 23% | SUBSET IV<br>Pulmonary congestion<br>Rales present<br>Peripheral hypoperfusion<br>Mortality = 51% |
| | PCWP < 18 | PCWP > 18 |

CI, cardiac index (L/min/$m^2$); PCWP, pulmonary capillary wedge pressure (mm Hg).

From Ornato JP (Ed): Cardiovascular Emergencies, New York, Churchill Livingstone, 1986, p 123, with permission.

mal cardiac filling pressures, the smallest effective dose of the diuretic should be employed. The patient's hemodynamic parameters and urine output should guide subsequent diuretic administration. If diuretics are ineffective and acute ischemia is present, topical or intravenous nitroglycerin might provide added preload reduction.

The finding of isolated peripheral hypoperfusion (Subset III) is of major prognostic importance because of the high mortality associated with it. These patients present with hypovolemia and/or bradycardia. The goal of therapy is to improve the cardiac index and to reverse the hypoperfusion while minimizing myocardial oxygen expenditure. Initial volume therapy should consist of 100–250 mL of normal saline or 5% albumin administered intravenously over 5 to 10 minutes with appropriate hemodynamic intake and output monitoring. A small group of patients in subset III have a normal stroke volume but a slow heart rate. Temporary transvenous pacing may restore cardiac output, but the increase in myocardial oxygen demand outweighs the marginal increase in cardiac output at rates beyond 90 to 100 beats per minute.[139]

Subset IV carries the highest mortality. The goal of therapy is the simultaneous improvement of CI and PCWP.[139] The choice of therapy lies between inotropic agents and peripheral vasodilators[140] (Table 14.1). Vasodilators are usually better because they impact more favorably on myocardial oxygen demand; however, when severe hypotension is present, a positive inotropic effect will prevent further circulatory collapse. The ideal inotropic agent must maintain or improve myocardial contractility while minimizing oxygen demand. Because no such agent exists, this is best accomplished by careful titration of combined therapy with inotropic and vasodilator drugs (Table 14.1). For example, the combined use of dobutamine (mean 7.7 μg/kg/min) and nitroglycerin (average 267 μg/min) is effective in both decreasing left ventricular (LV) filling pressures and significantly improving cardiac index in patients with severe LV failure resulting from acute MI.[141] In addition, dopamine (7.5 μg/kg/min) with concurrent dobutamine (7.5 μg/kg/min) administration results in substantial hemodynamic improvement when compared to doses of 15 μg/kg/min of either agent alone in patients with cardiogenic shock.[142] If all of the preceding actions are performed without significant effect in decreasing pulmonary congestion and unacceptably low cardiac output, insertion of a left ventricular assist device, such as the intraaortic balloon pump (IABP) for counterpulsation, should be considered.

## Cardiac Rehabilitation

Once the patient has survived the acute event and is well on the way to convalescence, several steps must be taken so that rehabilitation is performed in a safe and effective manner. Patients should increase activity gradually while they are in the hospital, as mentioned previously. A graded exercise program can be implemented with the help of an exercise physiologist. An exercise tolerance test should be performed to assess patients still at risk of developing another MI and those patients should be treated aggressively.

Patients should receive psychological and sexual counseling so that they feel comfortable about returning to their normal lifestyles. Modifiable risk factor management is very important. Smoking should be curtailed. Hypertension, hyperglycemia, hypercholesterolemia, obesity, and stress modification should all be addressed if necessary. Finally, acute MI patients should be counseled with regard to their discharge prescriptions and over-the-counter medication use by a pharmacist.

## Summary

Myocardial infarction is one of the most common reasons for hospitalization in the Western world. The acute mortality rate in hospitals is about 15%; approximately 10% of patients die during the first year after their acute MI. Short- and long-term survival depends on the extent and location of the coronary obstructive lesions and the prompt correction of post-MI complications. Prompt recognition that infarction is occurring is critical because deaths associated with acute MI are due to electrical instability and occur suddenly and prior to hospitalization.[1] The importance of prompt attention to symptoms of myocardial ischemia is highlighted by observations that the likelihood of ventricular fibrillation is 15 times greater during the initial hour after the onset of symptoms than during the subsequent 12 hours.[3] Furthermore, the likelihood of successful myocardial salvage is greatest during the first 3 hours after the onset of symptoms.[3,4] Any unnecessary delays in treatment place the patient at risk for life-threatening complications and increase the long-term mortality rate post-MI.[5] Supportive care and close monitoring of the patient are essential in reducing the risk of MI-related complications. The presence or absence of mechanical, electrical, ischemic, and vascular abnormalities provides the necessary information to institute appropriate medical and/or surgical treatment.

## References


1. Alpert JS, Braunwald E. Acute myocardial infarction: Pathological, pathophysiological, and clinical manifestations, in Braunwald E: Heart Disease, 2nd ed. Philadelphia, W.B. Saunders, 1984, p 1262.
2. Muller JE, Stone PH, Turi ZG, et al. Circadian variation in the frequency of acute myocardial infarction. N Engl J Med 1985; 313:1315–1322.
3. Anonymous. Myocardial infarction, in Jaffe AS (ed): Textbook of Advanced Cardiac Life Support. Dallas, American Heart Association, 1987, pp 11–26.
4. Fine DG, Weiss AT, Sapoznikov D, et al. Importance of early initiation of intravenous streptokinase therapy for acute myocardial infarction. Am J Cardiol 1986;58:411–417.
5. Turi ZG, Stone PH, Muller JE, et al. Implications for acute intervention related to time of hospital arrival in acute myocardial infarction. Am J Cardiol 1986;58:203–209.
6. Hlatky MA, Cotugno HE, Mark DB, et al. Trends in physician management of uncomplicated acute myocardial infarction, 1970 to 1987. Am J Cardiol 1988;61:515–518.
7. Killip T, Kimball JT. Treatment of myocardial infarction in a coronary care unit. Am J Cardiol 1967;20:457–464.
8. Sobel BE, Braunwald E. The management of acute myocardial infarction, in Braunwald E: Heart Disease, 2nd ed. Philadelphia, W.B. Saunders, 1984, p 1301.
9. Epstein SE, Palmeri ST. Mechanisms contributing to precipitation of unstable angina and acute myocardial infarction: Implications regarding therapy. Am J Cardiol 1984;54:1245–1252.
10. Rackley CE, Russell Jr RO, Mantle JA, et al. Right ventricular infarction and function. Am Heart J 1981;101:215–218.
11. Maseri A, L'Abbate A, Baroldi G, et al. Coronary vasospasm as a possible cause of myocardial infarction. A conclusion derived from the study of "preinfarction" angina. N Engl J Med 1978;299:1271–1277.
12. Zeller FP, Bauman JL. Current concepts in clinical therapeutics: Acute myocardial infarction. Clin Pharm 1986;5:553–572.
13. Herlihy T, McIvor ME, Cummings CC, et al. Nausea and vomiting during acute myocardial infarction and its relation to infarct size and location. Am J Cardiol 1987;60:20–22.
14. Alonzo AM, Simon AB, Feinleib M. Prodromata of myocardial infarction and sudden death. Circulation 1975;52:1056.
15. Zarling EJ, Sexton H, Milnor P. Failure to diagnose acute myocardial infarction. JAMA 1983;250:1177.
16. Ornato JP. Computer-assisted diagnosis of chest pain, in Ornato JP (ed): Cardiovascular Emergencies. New York, Churchill Livingstone, 1986, pp 1–24.
17. Kannel WB, Abbott RD. Incidence and prognosis of unrecognized myocardial infarction: An update on the Framingham Study. N Engl J Med 1984;311:1144.
18. Rude RE, Poole WK, Muller JE, et al. Electrocardiographic and clinical criteria for recognition of acute myocardial infarction based on analysis of 3,697 patients. Am J Cardiol 1983;52: 936.
19. Zelma MJ. Q wave, S-T segment, and T wave myocardial infarction. Am J Med 1985;78:391–398.
20. Dubin D. Rapid Interpretation of EKG's, 3rd ed. Tampa, FL, Cover Publishing Co, 1982, pp 215–217.
21. Phibbs B. "Transmural" versus "subendocardial" myocardial infarction: An electrocardiographic myth. J Am Coll Cardiol 1983;1:561.
22. Spodick DH. Q-wave infarction versus ST-infarction. Nonspecificity of electrocardiographic criteria for differentiating transmural and nontransmural lesions. Am J Cardiol 1983;51:913.
23. Lee TH, Goldman L. Serum enzyme assays in the diagnosis of acute myocardial infarction. Recommendations based on qualitative analysis. Ann Intern Med 1986;105:221–233.
24. Roberts R. Diagnostic assessment of myocardial infarction based on lactate dehydrogenase and creatine kinase isoenzymes. Heart Lung 1981;10:486–506.
25. Hypertension and coronary artery disease. Classification and criteria for epidemiological studies. WHO Tech Ser 1959;168:3.
26. Roberts R. The two out of three criteria for the diagnosis of infarction: Is it passe? Chest 1984;86:511–513.
27. Schelbert HR, Ingwall JS, Sybers HD, et al. Uptake of infarct-imaging agents in reversibly and irreversibly injured myocardium in cultured fetal mouse heart. Circ Res 976;39: 860–868.
28. Buja LM, Parkey RW, Dees JH, et al. Morphologic correlates of technetium-99m stannous pyrophosphate imaging of acute myocardial infarction in dogs. Circulation 1975;52:596–607.
29. Wackers FJT, Schoot JB, Sokole EB, et al. Noninvasive visualization of acute myocardial infarction in man with thallium-201. Br Heart J 1975;37:741–744.
30. Pohost GM, Zir LM, Moore RH, et al. Differentiation of transiently ischemic from infarcted myocardium by serial imaging after a single dose of thallium-201. Circulation 1977;55: 294–302.
31. Wackers FJT, Sokole EB, Samson G, et al. Value and limitations of thallium-201 scintigraphy in the acute phase of myocardial infarction. N Engl J Med 1976;295:1–5.
32. Rude RE. Acute myocardial infarction and its complications. Cardiol Clin 1984;2:163–171.
33. Moss AJ. Prognosis after myocardial infarction. Am J Cardiol 1983;52:667–669.
34. Moss AJ, Davis HT, DeCamilla J, et al. Ventricular ectopic beats and their relation to sudden and nonsudden cardiac death after myocardial infarction. Circulation 1979;60:998–1003.
35. Swan HJC, Ganz W, Forrester J, et al. Catheterization of the heart in man with use of a flow-directed balloon-tipped catheter. N Engl J Med 1970;283:447–451.
36. Hoffman EW. Basics of cardiovascular hemodynamic monitoring. Drug Intell Clin Pharm 1982;16:657–664.

37. Gonzalez ER, Meyers DG. Assessment and management of cardiogenic shock, in Ornato JP (ed): Cardiovascular Emergencies. New York, Churchill Livingstone, 1986, pp 115–137.
38. Rasanen J, Vaisanen IT, Heikkila J, et al. Acute myocardial infarction complicated by left ventricular dysfunction and respiratory failure: The effects of continuous positive airway pressure. Chest 1985;278–360.
39. Lee G, DeMaria AN, Amsterdam EA, et al. Comparative effect of morphine, meperidine, and pentazocine on cardiopulmonary dynamics in patients with acute myocardial infarction. Am J Med 1976;60:341–355.
40. Stapleton JF. Essentials of Clinical Cardiology. Philadelphia, F.A. Davis, 1983, p 269.
41. Semenkovich CF, Jaffe AS. Adverse effects due to morphine sulfate—Challenge to previous clinical doctrine. Am J Med 1985;79:325–330.
42. Alderman EL. Analgesics in the acute phase of myocardial infarction. JAMA 1974;229:1646–1648.
43. Wasserberger J, Ordog GJ, Lau JC, et al. Intravenous prochlorperazine for the rapid control of nausea and vomiting in acute myocardial infarction. Ann Emerg Med 1987;5:153–156.
44. Lewis JR. Evaluation of new analgesics: Butorphanol and nalbuphine. JAMA 1980;243:1465–1467.
45. Hoehn-Saric R, McLeod DR. Cardiac symptoms and anxiety disorders: Contributing factors and pharmacologic therapy. Am J Cardiol 1987;60:68J–73J.
46. Barker PH, Clanachan AS. Inhibition of adenosine accumulation into guinea pig ventricle by benzodiazepines. Eur J Pharmacol 1982;78:241–244.
47. Forrester JS, Waters DD. Hospital treatment of congestive heart failure: Management according to hemodynamic profile. Am J Med 1978;65:173.
48. Herling IM. Intravenous nitroglycerin: Clinical pharmacology and therapeutic considerations. Am Heart J 1984;108:141.
49. Swan NA, Evenson MK, Needham KE, et al. Effect of combined nitroglycerin and dobutamine infusion in left ventricular dysfunction. Am Heart J 1983;106:35.
50. Parmley WW, Chatterjee K, Charuzi Y, et al. Hemodynamic effects of noninvasive systolic unloading (nitroprusside) and diastolic augmentation (external counterpulsation) in patients with acute myocardial infarction. Am J Cardiol 1974;33:810.
51. Cohn JN, Franciosa JA, Francis GS, et al. Effect of short-term infusion of sodium nitroprusside on mortality rate in acute myocardial infarction complicated by left ventricular failure. N Engl J Med 1982;306:1129–1135.
52. Cohn JN, Burke LP. Drugs five years later: Nitroprusside. Ann Intern Med 1979;91:752.
53. Chiarello M, Gold HK, Leinbach RC, et al. Comparison between the effects of nitroprusside and nitroglycerin on ischemic injury during acute myocardial infarction. Circulation 1976;54:766.
54. Flaherty JT. Comparison of intravenous nitroglycerin and sodium nitroprusside in acute myocardial infarction. Am J Med 1983;74(6B):53.
55. Roberts R. Intravenous nitroglycerin in acute myocardial infarction. Am J Med 1983;74(6B):45.
56. Yusef S, Peto R, Lewis J, et al. Beta-blockade during and after myocardial infarction: An overview of the randomized trials. Prog Cardiovasc Dis 1985;27:335–371.
57. ISIS-1 (First International Study of Infarct Survival) Collaborative Group. Randomized trial of intravenous atenolol among 16,027 cases of suspected acute myocardial infarction: ISIS-1. Lancet 1986;1:57–65.
58. The MIAMI Trial Research Group. Metoprolol in acute myocardial infarction (MIAMI). A randomized placebo-controlled international trial. Eur Heart J 1985;6:199–226.
59. Campbell CA, Przylenk K, Kloner RA. Infarct size reduction: A review of the clinical trials. J Clin Pharmacol 1986;26:317–329.
60. Mueller HS, Ayres SM. Propranolol decreases sympathetic necrosis activity reflected by plasma catecholamines during evolution of myocardial infarction in man. J Clin Invest 1980; 65:338–346.
61. Pitt B, Crown P. Effect of propranolol in regional myocardial blood flow in acute ischemia. Cardiovasc Res 1970;4:176–179.
62. Peter T, Norris RM, Clarke ED, et al. Reduction of enzyme levels by propranolol after acute myocardial infarction. Circulation 1978;57:1091–1095.
63. Yusuf S, Sleight P, Rossi P, et al. Reduction in infarct size, arrhythmias and chest pain by early intravenous beta-blockade in suspected acute myocardial infarction. Circulation 1983; 67(suppl I):1–32.
64. Hjalmarson A, Herlitz J. Limitation of infarct size by beta blockers and its potential role for prognosis. Circulation 1983; 67(suppl I):1–68.
65. International Collaboration Study Group. Reduction of infarct size with the early use of timolol in acute myocardial infarction. N Engl J Med 1984;310:9.
66. Roberts R, Croft C, Gold HK, et al. Effect of propranolol on myocardial infarct size in a randomized blinded multicenter trial. N Engl J Med 1984;311:218.
67. Sirnes PA, Overskeid K, Pedersen TR, et al. Evolution of infarct size during the early use of nifedipine in patients with acute myocardial infarction: The Norwegian Nifedipine Multicenter Trial. Circulation 1984;70:638–644.
68. Muller JE, Morrison J, Stone PH, et al. Nifedipine therapy for patients with threatened and acute myocardial infarction: A randomized, double-blind, placebo-controlled comparison. Circulation 1984;69:740–747.
69. Danish Multicenter Study Group. Verapamil in acute myocardial infarction. Eur Heart J 1984;5:516–528.
70. Gersh BJ. Role of thrombolytic therapy in evolving myocardial infarction. Mod Concepts Cardiovasc Dis 1985;54:13–17.
71. Health and Public Policy Committee—American College of Physicians. Thrombolysis for evolving myocardial infarction. Ann Intern Med 1985;103:463–469.
72. Gold HK, Leinbach RC. Thrombolysis in acute myocardial infarction. Chest 1988;93:10S–12S.
73. Arntz R, Heitz J, Shafer H, et al. Hemorheology in acute myocardial infarction: Effects of high dose intravenous streptokinase. Circulation 1985;72(Part II):III–417.
74. Jan KM, Reinhart W, Chien S, et al. Altered rheological properties of blood following administration of tissue plasminogen activator and streptokinase in patients with acute myocardial infarction. Circulation 1985;72(Part II):III–417.
75. European Cooperative Study Group. Streptokinase in acute myocardial infarction: Extended report on the European Cooperative Trial. Acta Med Scand 1981;suppl 648:7–57.
76. Laffel GL, Braunwald E. Thrombolytic therapy. A new strategy for the treatment of acute myocardial infarction (first of two parts). N Engl J Med 1984;311:710–717.
77. Smith B, Kennedy JK. Thrombolysis in the treatment of acute transmural myocardial infarction. Ann Intern Med 1987;106: 414–420.
78. Crabbe SJ, Cloninger CC. Tissue plasminogen activator: A new thrombolytic agent. Clin Pharm 1987;6:373–386.
79. Sherry S. Recombinant tissue plasminogen activator ($r^+$-PA): Is it the thrombolytic agent of choice for an evolving acute myocardial infarction. Am J Cardiol 1987;59:984–989.

80. Rich MW. TPA: Is it worth the price? Am Heart J 1987;114: 1259–1261.
81. DeWood MA, Spores J, Hensley GR, et al. Coronary arteriographic findings in acute transmural myocardial infarction. Circulation 1983;68(suppl I):I-39–I-49.
82. Schwartz DE, Yamaga CC. Thrombolysis for evolving myocardial infarction. Ann Intern Med 1985;103:463–469.
83. Gruppo Italiano per lo Studio Della Streptochinasi Nell'Infarcto Miocardio (GISSI). Effectiveness of intravenous thrombolytic treatment in acute myocardial infarction. Lancet 1986;1:397–401.
84. ISIS Steerring Committee. Intravenous streptokinase given within 0–4 hours of onset of myocardial infarction reduced mortality in ISIS-2. Lancet 1987;1:502.
85. Topol EJ. Advances in thrombolytic therapy for acute myocardial infarction. J Clin Pharmacol 1987;27:735–745.
86. Verstraete M, Bernard R, Borg M, et al. Randomised trial of intravenous recombinant tissue-type plasminogen activator versus intravenous streptokinase in acute myocardial infarction. Lancet 1985;1:842–847.
87. TIMI Study Group. The thrombolysis in myocardial infarction (TIMI) trial: Phase I finding. N Engl J Med 1985;312:932–936.
88. Holmes DR, Smith HC, Vlietstra RE, et al. Percutaneous transluminal coronary angioplasty alone or in combination with streptokinase therapy, during acute myocardial infarction. Mayo Clin Proc 1985;60:449–456.
89. Rutherford BD, Hartzler GO, McConahay DR. Direct balloon angioplasty in acute myocardial infarction without prior use of streptokinase. J Am Coll Cardiol 1986;7:149A.
90. Fung AY, Lai P, Topol EJ, et al. Value of percutaneous transluminal coronary angioplasty after unsuccessful intravenous streptokinase therapy in acute myocardial infarction. Am J Cardiol 1986;58:686–691.
91. Sutton JM, Taylor GJ, Mikell FL, et al. Thrombolytic therapy followed by early revascularization for acute myocardial infarction. Am J Cardiol 1986;57:1227–1231.
92. Suryapranata H, Serruys PW, de Feyter PJ, et al. Coronary angioplasty immediately after thrombolysis in 115 consecutive patients with acute myocardial infarction. Am Heart J 1988; 115:519–529.
93. Topol EJ, Califf RM, George BS, et al. A randomized trial of immediate versus delayed elective angioplasty after intravenous tissue plasminogen activator in acute myocardial infarction. N Engl J Med 1987;317:581–588.
94. Guerci AD, Gerstenblith G, Brinker JA, et al. A randomized trial of intravenous tissue plasminogen activator for acute myocardial infarction with subsequent randomization to elective coronary angioplasty. N Engl J Med 1987;317:1613–1618.
95. Jones EL, Waites TF, Craver JM, et al. Coronary bypass for relief of persistent pain following acute myocardial infarction. Ann Thorac Surg 1981;32:33–43.
96. DeWood MA, Spores J, Berg R, et al. Acute myocardial infarction: A decade of experience with surgical reperfusion in 701 patients. Circulation 1983:68(suppl II);II-8–II-16.
97. Phillips SJ, Kongtahworn C, Skinner JR, et al. Emergency coronary artery reperfusion: A choice therapy for evolving myocardial infarction. J Thorac Cardiovasc Surg 1983:86;679–688.
98. Nunley DL, Grunkemeier GL, Teply JF, et al. Coronary artery bypass operation following acute complications of myocardial infarction. J Thorac Cardiovasc Surg 1983:85:485–491.
99. Hochberg MS, Parsonnett V, Gielchinsky I, et al. Timing of coronary revascularization after acute myocardial infarction: Early and late results in patients revascularized within seven weeks. J Thorac Cardiovasc Surg 1984;88:914–921.
100. Multicenter International Study. Reduction in mortality with long-term beta-adrenoreceptor blockade: A multicenter international study. Br Med J 1977;2:49.
101. Norwegian Multicenter Study Group. Timolol-induced reduction in mortality and reinfarction in patients surviving acute myocardial infarction. N Engl J Med 1981;304:801–807.
102. Beta-Blocker Heart Attack Trial Research Group. A randomized trial of propranolol in patients with acute myocardial infarction. 1. Mortality results. JAMA 1982;247:1707–1714.
103. Julian DG, Prescott RJ, Jackson FS, et al. A controlled trial of sotalol for one year after myocardial infarction. Lancet 1982;1: 1142.
104. Taylor SH, Silke B, Ebbutt A, et al. A long-term prevention study with oxprenolol in coronary heart disease. N Engl J Med 1982;307:1293–1301.
105. Goteborg Metoprolol Trial in Acute Myocardial Infarction. Mortality and causes of death. Am J Cardiol 1984;53:90.
106. Chadda K, Goldstein S, Byington R, et al. Effect of propranolol after acute myocardial infarction in patients with congestive heart failure. Circulation 1986;73:503–510.
107. Pearle DL. Calcium antagonists in acute myocardial infarction. Am J Cardiol 1988;61:22B–25B.
108. Gibson RS, Boden WE, Theroux P, et al. Diltiazem and reinfarction in patients with non–Q-wave myocardial infarction. N Engl J Med 1986;315:423–429.
109. Gibson RS, Young PM, Boden WE, et al. Prognostic significance and beneficial effect of diltiazem on the incidence of early recurrent ischemia after non-Q-wave myocardial infarction: Results from the Multicenter Diltiazem Reinfarction Study. Am J Cardiol 1987;60:203–209.
110. Persantine–Aspirin Reinfarction Study Research Group. Persantine and aspirin in coronary heart disease. Circulation 1980; 62:449–461.
111. Klimt CR, Knatterud GL, Stamler J, Meier P. Persantine–aspirin reinfarction study. Part II. Secondary coronary prevention with persantine and aspirin. J Am Coll Cardiol 1986;7:251–269.
112. Chesebro JH, Fuster V, Elveback LR, et al. Effect of dipyridamole and aspirin on late vein-graft patency after coronary bypass. N Engl J Med 1984;310:209–214.
113. Stein PD, Collins JJ, Kantrowitz A. Antithrombotic therapy in mechanical and biological prosthetic heart valves and saphenous vein bypass grafts. Chest 1986;89(suppl):46S–53S.
114. Lorenz RL, Weber M, Kotzur J, et al. Improved aortocoronary bypass patency by low-dose aspirin (100 mg daily). Effects of platelet aggregation and thromboxane formation. Lancet 1984;1:1261–1264.
115. Kaplan K. Prophylactic anticoagulation following acute myocardial infarction. Arch Intern Med 1986;146:593–597.
116. Morgan DB, Davidson C. Hypokalemia and diuretics: An analysis of publications. Br Med J 1980;280:905–909.
117. Hollifield JW. Potassium and magnesium abnormalities: Diuretics and arrhythmias in hypertension. Am J Med 1984;77: 28–32.
118. Kafka S, Langevin L, Armstrong PW. Serum magnesium and potassium in acute myocardial infarction. Arch Intern Med 1987;147:465–469.
119. Ornato JP, Gonzalez ER, Starke H, et al. Incidence and causes of hypokalemia associated with cardiac resuscitation. Am J Emerg Med 1985;3:503–506.
120. Salerno DM, Asinger RW, Elsperger J, et al. Frequency of hypokalemia after successfully resuscitated out-of-hospital cardiac arrest compared with that in transmural acute myocardial infarction. Am J Cardiol 1987;59:84–88.

121. Ornato JP, Gonzalez ER. Refractory ventricular fibrillation. Emerg Decisions 1986;4:35–41.
122. Dyckner T, Wester PO. Magnesium in cardiology. Acta Med Scand 1982;661(suppl):27–31.
123. Ebel H, Gunther T. Role of magnesium in cardiac disease. J Clin Chem Clin Biochem 1983;21:249–265.
124. Rasmussen HS, Norregard P, Lindeneg O, et al. Intravenous magnesium in acute myocardial infraction. Lancet 1986;1:234–235.
125. Whang R, Flink EB, Dyckner T, et al. Magnesium depletion as a cause of refractory potassium repletion. Arch Intern Med 1985;145:1686–1689.
126. Whang R, Oei TO, Aikawa JK, et al. Predictors of clinical hypomagnesemia. Arch Intern Med 1984;144:1794–1796.
127. Rasmussen HS, Aurup P, Hojberg S, et al. Magnesium and acute myocardial infarction. Arch Intern Med 1986;146:872–874.
128. Feneley MP, Chang VP, O'Rourke MF. Myocardial rupture after acute myocardial infarction: Ten year review. Br Heart J 1983;49:550–556.
129. Shapira I, Isakov A, Burke M, et al. Cardiac rupture in patients with acute myocardial infarction. Chest 1987;92:219–223.
130. Ryden L, Arniego R, Arnman K, et al. A double-blind trial of metoprolol in acute myocardial infarction: Effects on ventricular tachyarrhythmias. N Engl J Med 1983;308:614–618.
131. Norris RM, Brown MA, Clarke ED, et al. Prevention of ventricular fibrillation during acute myocardial infarction by intravenous propranolol. Lancet 1984;2:883–886.
132. Mueller H, Ayres SM, Religi A, et al. Propranolol in the treatment of acute myocardial infarction. Circulation 1974;49:1078–1081.
133. Chadda K, Goldstein S, Byington R, et al. Effect of propranolol after acute myocardial infarction in patients with congestive heart failure. Circulation 1986;73:503–510.
134. Wyman MG, Gore S. Lidocaine prophylaxis in myocardial infarction: A concept whose time has come. Heart Lung 1983;12:358–361.
135. Wagner GS. Arrhythmias in acute myocardial infarction. Med Clin North Am 1984;68:1061.
136. Kottmeier CA, Gravenstein JS. The parasympathomimetic activity of atropine and atropine methylbromide. Anesthesiology 1961;29:1125–1133.
137. Biddle TL, Paul NY. Effect of furosemide on hemodynamic and lung water in acute pulmonary edema secondary to myocardial infarction. Am J Cardiol 1979;43:86.
138. Kilcoyne MM, Schmidt DH, Cannon PJ. Intrarenal blood flow in congestive heart failure. Postgrad Med J 1975;51(suppl 6):54.
139. Berkley CE, Russell RO, Mantle JA, et al. Cardiogenic shock. Recognition and management. Cardiovasc Clin 1975;7:251.
140. Gunnar RM, Leab HS, Scanlon PJ, et al. Management of acute myocardial infarction and accelerating angina. Prog Cardiovasc Dis 1979;22:1.
141. Awan NA, Evenson MK, Needham KE, et al. Effect of combined nitroglycerine and dobutamine infusion in left ventricular dysfunction. Am Heart J 1983;106:35–40.
142. Richard C, Ricome JL, Rimailho A, et al. Combined hemodynamic effects of dopamine and dobutamine in cardiogenic shock. Circulation 1983;67:620–626.

# Chapter 15 / The Cardiomyopathies

Christina Dalmady-Israel, PharmD

The definition of cardiomyopathy has undergone many changes in the last few decades. Today, the term still leads to confusion and is not used uniformly by all clinicians. In the strictest sense, *cardiomyopathy* refers only to primary myocardial disorders of unknown cause and, therefore, would not include heart disease resulting from hypertensive, ischemic, valvular, arterial, congenital, or pericardial disorders; however, the term is more commonly utilized to denote nonspecific heart muscle disease of any etiology.[1–6]

Two classifications are used to differentiate the distinct clinical entities that constitute this group of disorders (Table 15.1). On an etiologic basis, primary cardiomyopathies are, by definition, the "true" cardiomyopathies, and consist of myocardial disease of unknown cause. Secondary cardiomyopathies are conditions in which the causative agent or disease process has been identified. The second classification, based on pathophysiology and clinical presentation, categorizes these disorders as dilated, hypertrophic, or restrictive/obliterative cardiomyopathies.[1,2,6–8] This latter classification is more useful clinically and allows the selection of therapy on the basis of pathophysiology. The distinction between these disorders is not absolute, however, and there is some overlap (Figure 15.1).

The cardiomyopathies were at one time considered rare diseases; however, they are now being recognized as relatively common disorders and major causes of morbidity and mortality. In fact, in some underdeveloped countries, these disorders may account for 30% or more of all deaths related to heart disease.[1,2,8,9]

## Dilated (Congestive) Cardiomyopathy

This disorder was formerly known as congestive cardiomyopathy because it was usually detected only in the presence of florid congestive heart failure.[1] Detection is now possible prior to the onset of congestive symptoms, and the term *dilated cardiomyopathy* properly reflects the hallmark of the disease, which is dilation of the ventricles. Dilated cardiomyopathy is also characterized by poor systolic function [ejection fraction (EF) $< 0.40$], and increased end-diastolic and end-systolic ventricular volumes.[1,2,5,6]

### *Pathophysiology*

The etiology of primary dilated cardiomyopathy is, by definition, unknown; however, this syndrome may constitute a final common pathway for myocardial damage produced by a variety of toxic, metabolic, or infectious agents.[1,6] These factors, many of which are associated with secondary cardiomyopathies, include systemic hypertension, excess alcohol consumption, pregnancy or puerperium, and infection.[1,2,7] Unlike hypertrophic cardiomyopathy, familial transmission of dilated cardiomyopathy is rare.[2]

One of the most accepted theories suggests that this disorder is the sequela of immune-mediated acute myocarditis. Active myocarditis produces an acute form of dilated cardiomyopathy, which may evolve into a chronic form of the disease.[5,6,9–11] In the United States, myocarditis is usually of viral etiology, with coxsackievirus B being the virus most frequently implicated; however, almost every infectious agent is capable of producing myocarditis, and many other viruses including echovirus, coxsackievirus A, adenovirus, and influenza have been associated with myocarditis.[9,12] Worldwide, myocarditis caused by the protozoan *Trypanosoma cruzi* (Chagas' disease) is one of the leading causes of secondary dilated cardiomyopathy.[9]

In practice, it is extremely difficult to establish an unequivocal diagnosis of myocarditis, as antibody titers and a definitive histologic confirmation by endocardial biopsy depend on the duration of illness.[10] To date, there have been only a few observations of a transition from myocarditis to dilated cardiomyopathy, and almost no evidence to suggest prior viral infections in patients with proven cardiomyopathy.[8,10]

Another proposed etiologic factor in the pathogenesis of primary dilated cardiomyopathy is increased sympathetic activity.[13,14] Heart failure has been associated with depleted myocardial catecholamine stores, "downregulation" of myocardial $\beta$ receptors,[13,15] and elevated serum catecholamine concentrations.[13] Contrary to the traditional belief that increased sympathetic activity is a compensatory response needed to support a failing heart, this "adaptive" response may actually be harmful.[13] It is not known, however, whether elevated serum catecholamine concentrations mark the severity of the disease or cause its progression.[13–15]

Nutritional deficiency has been suggested as a cause of idiopathic dilated cardiomyopathy because of the prevalence of this heart disorder in underdeveloped countries; however, selenium deficiency is the only nutritional factor that has been associated with this form of heart disease.[5] Dilated cardiomyopathy associated with selenium deficiency is rare in the Western world but may appear in areas of the United States where selenium concentrations are low.[5]

Alcoholic cardiomyopathy is the most common of the secondary dilated cardiomyopathies.[7–9,12] Acute and chronic depression of myocardial contractility caused by the ingestion of large quantities of alcohol for many years may eventually lead to dilated cardiomyopathy.[8–12] Prognosis is poor in patients who continue to drink, with a 40% to 50% mortality in 3 to 6 years, whereas abstinence may halt the progression of the

**Table 15.1** Classification of Cardiomyopathies

| *Dilated* | *Hypertrophic* | *Restrictive* |
|---|---|---|
| Primary | Primary | Primary |
| Secondary | Secondary | Secondary |
| Alcoholic | Hypertensive | Amyloidosis |
| Peripartum | Ischemic | Löffler's endocarditis |
| Viral | | Endomyocardial fibrosis |
| Toxic | | Sarcoidosis |
| | | Hemochromatosis |

disease or even reverse it.[12] Although alcoholic cardiomyopathy frequently appears in association with thiamine deficiency, this nutritional deficiency has not been identified as a cause of this disorder.[12] Nevertheless, these patients should receive adequate thiamine supplementation.

Peripartum cardiomyopathy is another form of secondary dilated cardiomyopathy and occurs in women during the last month of pregnancy or within the first few months after delivery.[16] Females presenting with this disorder are usually black, multiparous, over the age of 30, and living in impoverished conditions.[6,7,12] The etiology is unknown, but may be related to a preexisting cardiomyopathy that was not recognized prior to pregnancy. The mortality for peripartum cardiomyopathy ranges from 25% to 50%. Most deaths occur during the first 3 months postpartum. Prognosis and risk during subsequent pregnancies are related to achievement of a normal heart size after the initial episode.[6]

Other factors associated with secondary dilated cardiomyopathy include doxorubicin, radiation, dactinomycin, cyclophosphamide, lead, arsenic, and cobalt.[9,12]

### *Clinical Presentation*

Symptoms usually develop gradually in patients with dilated cardiomyopathy. Left ventricular dilation may be present for months or even years prior to the onset of symptoms.[7,8,11,12] The first manifestations of the disease are usually signs and symptoms of left and right ventricular failure[2]; however, patients may present with syncope, palpitations, or cardiac arrest as the initial symptoms.[9] Dyspnea on exertion is the most common symptom, and as the disease progresses, additional symptoms ensue, including orthopnea, paroxysmal nocturnal dyspnea, and dyspnea at rest.[5,6,9] Chest pain is experienced by 10% of patients, and may present in the absence of coronary artery disease.[2] Signs of right ventricu-

**Figure 15.1** Types of cardiomyopathy. *(Modified from Hurst JW, Logue RB, Schlant RC, Wenger NK (Eds): The Heart, 4th ed. New York, McGraw–Hill, and Goodwin JF: The frontiers of cardiomyopathy. Br Heart J 1982;48:3, with permission.)*

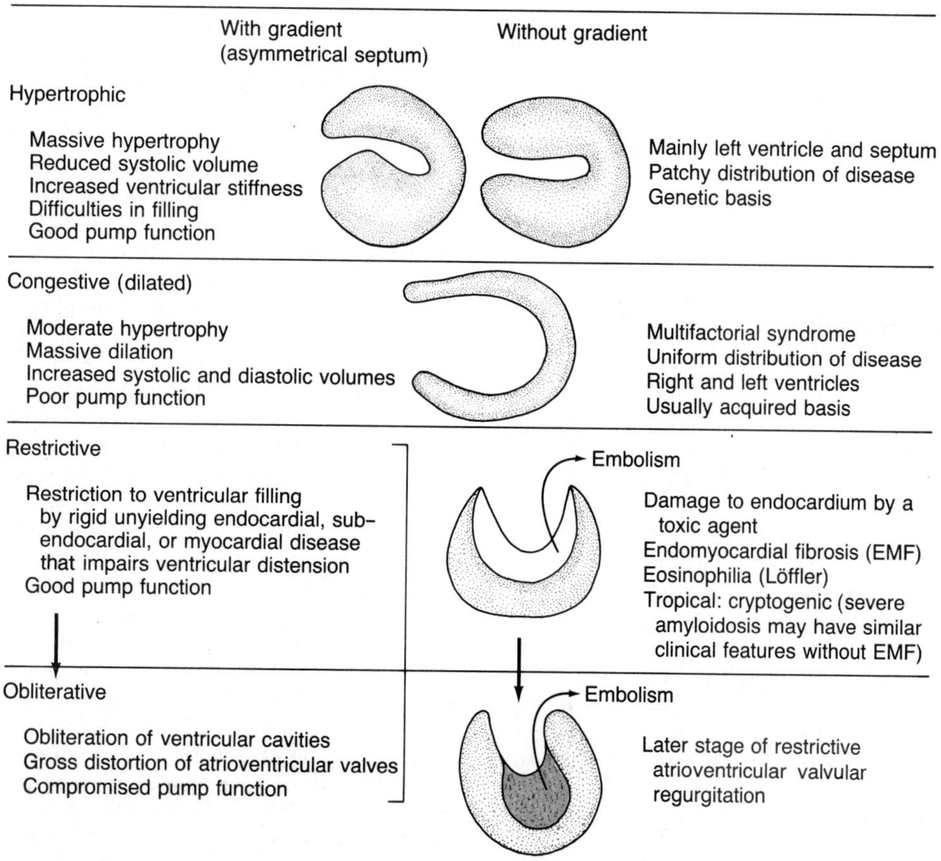

lar failure such as edema, ascites, and hepatomegaly are seen frequently in late stages of the disease.[6] Embolic phenomena such as pulmonary emboli and stroke are also common later in the disease course.[8,9]

Arrhythmias are common in patients with dilated cardiomyopathy and often provide the first clue that the disease is present.[2,9,17,18] The incidence of ventricular tachycardia is reported to range from 43% to 93% and is not correlated with severity of left ventricular dysfunction[17,18]; however, the presence of ventricular ectopy may be a harbinger of sudden death in patients with dilated cardiomyopathy.[17,18]

Supraventricular arrhythmias are also common in dilated cardiomyopathy, especially in alcoholic cardiomyopathy.[18] Atrial fibrillation is present at diagnosis in 11% to 20% of patients, and will develop in an additional 5% during the next 5 years. The presence of supraventricular arrhythmias is associated with an increased risk of thromboembolic complications, especially in patients with hypokinetic or dyskinetic left ventricles.[18]

### *Diagnosis*

The diagnosis of dilated cardiomyopathy is basically one of exclusion, and this disease is usually detected when patients present with congestive symptoms.[1]

Physical exam reveals cardiac enlargement and signs of congestive heart failure. Patients with biventricular failure have distended jugular veins, pulmonary rales, and narrow pulse pressure indicative of decreased stroke volume. Third and fourth heart sounds are commonly present. Mitral or tricuspid regurgitation contributes to the reduction of forward ejection fraction.[6,7,9]

Electrocardiographic findings are usually nonspecific. Sinus tachyarrhythmias or atrial fibrillation, ventricular arrhythmias, diffuse nonspecific ST-T wave abnormalities, and intraventricular conduction defects may be present.[6–15] Left bundle branch block is seen in as many as 40% of patients with dilated cardiomyopathy. Chest x-ray shows cardiomegaly, and M-mode echocardiography reveals increased end-diastolic and end-systolic volumes.[2,5,8] Poor systolic function and decreased ejection fraction (<40%) are observed on two-dimensional echo. Angiography may confirm the diagnosis of dilated cardiomyopathy and may reveal ventricular thrombi.[2,5,8]

Hemodynamic studies show that cardiac output is moderately or severely reduced both at rest and during exercise. Left ventricular end-diastolic, left atrial, and pulmonary capillary wedge pressures are usually elevated, and if right heart failure is present, right ventricular end-diastolic pressure is also elevated.[2,5,8]

Endomyocardial biopsy is not done routinely for diagnostic purposes; however, it does serve to exclude other conditions such as endomyocardial fibrosis, myocarditis, and infiltrative diseases. Histologic evidence of active inflammation is reported to exist in 10% to 65% of patients with dilated cardiomyopathy[10]; however, the likelihood of a positive biopsy depends mostly on the time of the sample with relation to the onset and duration of the illness. If symptoms have existed for less than 4 weeks the likelihood of a positive biopsy is closer to 90%.[10]

### *Natural History/Prognosis*

Much is yet to be learned about the natural history of dilated cardiomyopathy. Once the disease is clinically apparent, prolonged survival is unusual.[2,11] Prognosis is related to the degree of left ventricular dysfunction.[6,11,18,19] Unfortunately, most patients are not diagnosed until they develop symptoms of left ventricular impairment.[6,18] Mortality rates range from 43% to 88% at 2 years, and the majority of patients die within 4 years of diagnosis.[6,11,19] Sudden death accounts for 20% to 45% of all deaths.[5,11,19] Clinical and hemodynamic parameters that have been associated with poor prognosis include age greater than 55 years at diagnosis, a cardiothoracic index greater than 0.55, left ventricular ejection fraction less than 20%, cardiac index less than 3 $L/min/m^2$, and left ventricular end-diastolic pressure above 20 mm Hg.[6,19] Although ventricular arrhythmias are common, their prognostic significance and their correlation with sudden death remain controversial.[19] Left ventricular hypertrophy may be associated with a better prognosis. In patients with equivalent degrees of chamber enlargement, survival has been reported to be longer in those patients with a greater degree of left ventricular hypertrophy. Patients with a higher degree of hypertrophy may compensate better for the increased wall stress resulting from left ventricular enlargement.[6,8,12,20]

### *Treatment*

Specific therapy for dilated cardiomyopathy is not available as the cause of the myopathic process is unknown. Therapy is aimed at improving symptoms, although there is no convincing evidence that therapy improves prognosis.[7–9]

Conventional therapy is, for the most part, similar to that recommended for congestive heart failure and includes salt restriction, diuretics, digitalis, and vasodilators.[1–9] (Please refer to Chapter 11.)

Nondrug therapy includes removal of any causative toxins and avoidance of smoking and alcohol. Strenuous exercise should be avoided, and activity should be restricted in those patients who develop symptoms with exercise.[2] Prolonged, strict bed rest has been reported to decrease heart size and improve prognosis; however, it is usually not feasible and its benefit remains controversial.[8]

The use of $\beta$-adrenergic blocking agents in the treatment of dilated cardiomyopathy is also extremely controversial.[9,13,21] Most patients with cardiac failure demonstrate an increase in sympathetic nervous activity to compensate for depressed myocardial function.[13,15,21,22] $\beta$-Blockers may reduce this compensatory response and, therefore, have generally been contraindicated in the face of congestive heart failure. The rationale for their use is based on the theory of increased sympathetic activity as an etiologic factor in dilated cardiomyopathy. It has been postulated that a decrease in heart rate may reduce the energy demand on the heart, improve diastolic filling, and thus increase stroke volume.[23]

Clinical studies evaluating the use of $\beta$-blockers in dilated cardiomyopathy have yielded inconsistent results. These studies are difficult to compare because of differences in $\beta$-blocking agents and doses utilized, severity of disease,

**Table 15.2** β-Blockers in Dilated Cardiomyopathies

| *Author* | *N* | *Duration (mo)* | *Drug/dose (mg/d)* | *Outcome* |
|---|---|---|---|---|
| Waagstein et al, 1975[23] | 7 | 2–12 | Practolol 100–800 | Symptomatic improvement after 1 month of therapy |
| | | | Alprenolol 100 | Increased exercise tolerance<br>Decreased heart size |
| Swedberg et al, 1979[24] | 24 | 6–62 | Metoprolol 50–200 | Improved survival rate (83%, 66%, 52% at 1, 2, 3 yr) compared with 13 retrospective controls (46%, 19%, 10% at 1, 2, 3 yr) |
| Swedberg et al, 1980[25] | 28 | 6–62 | Metoprolol 50–200 | Improvement in systolic and diastolic function |
| | | | Alprenolol 50–200 | 15/28 increased in functional class |
| | | | Propranolol 80–120 | 12/28 unchanged |
| | | | Practolol 200 | 1/28 decreased in functional class |
| Swedberg et al, 1980[22] | 15 | On β-blockers 6–50 mo | Metoprolol 50–150 | Withdrawal caused deterioration in all patients |
| | | Withdrawal 7–119 d | Alprenolol 200 | 6 decreased in clinical function |
| | | | Propranolol 120 | 7 decreased in diastolic function |
| | | | Practolol 80 | All changes reversed on readministration of β-blocker |
| Anderson et al, 1985[27] | 50 | 19 (mean) | Metoprolol 25–100 | β-Blockade showed trend in decreasing mortality and increasing exercise capacity<br>By intention to treat no difference was observed |
| Ikram and Fitzpatrick, 1981[28] | 15 | 1 | Acebutolol 400 | Decreased left ventricle size; increased ejection fraction<br>Decrease in exercise time; should not be used routinely |
| Currie et al, 1984[26] | 10 | 1 | Metoprolol 100–200 | No symptomatic or hemodynamic improvement |

concomitant medications, length of study, and type of cardiomyopathy (Table 15.2).

Most of the favorable reports with propranolol and metoprolol stem from a group of investigators in Sweden. In a series of mostly uncontrolled, nonrandomized clinical trials, they reported clinical and hemodynamic improvement,[21–25] deterioration upon withdrawal of the β-blocker,[22,23] and improved 3-year survival with β-blockade.[13,22,25] These observations have not been confirmed in adequately controlled trials. Other authors have also reported beneficial effects with β-blockade.[13,21,26]

From these reports, it has been suggested that patients with significant tachycardia may achieve the most benefit from treatment with β-adrenergic blockers. The efficacy of these agents, however, does not seem to depend entirely on the presence of a markedly increased heart rate.[9] Metoprolol is the agent most commonly used in these trials.[13,25,27] The use of partial agonists is of interest as it has been postulated that agents with intrinsic sympathomimetic activity (ISA) may prevent excess depression of contractility and would therefore have less potential for causing negative hemodynamic effects; however, these agents may inhibit the receptor "upregulation" seen with other β-blockers and may be less effective in terms of antiarrhythmic activity.[13] One such agent, acebutolol, was shown to decrease maximum exercise tolerance and ventricular function[28]; however, the patient population studied was not comparable to that evaluated in the Swedish trials.

Most of the unfavorable reports with β-blockers have emphasized the negative hemodynamic effects caused by these agents. The studies are, for the most part, based on short-term use, and the reported hemodynamic changes are moderate and may not be clinically significant. Nevertheless, the risk of acute cardiac decompensation is always present when using these drugs.[13,26,28]

The use of β-blockers in the treatment of dilated cardiomyopathy continues to be controversial. Because of the heterogeneous nature of this disorder, further studies must be undertaken to determine if there is a subset of patients who will benefit from β-adrenergic blockade.

The effects of calcium channel blockers in dilated cardiomyopathy have been even less clear-cut (Table 15.3). Many of these patients have abnormalities in diastolic function in addition to systolic dysfunction.[15] The rationale for the use of these agents is related to the association of decreased diastolic compliance with increased intramyocardial calcium in animal models.[9] Nifedipine is the most widely studied agent in this group, and has been shown to reduce

**Table 15.3** Treatment Modalities for Dilated Cardiomyopathies

| |
|---|
| Nonpharmacological therapy |
| Remove toxins; stop alcohol intake and smoking; limit exercise |
| Conventional therapy |
| Digoxin, diuretics, vasodilators |
| Other modalities |
| β-blockers |
| Calcium antagonists |
| Angiotensin converting enzyme inhibitors |
| Inotrope infusions |
| Antiarrhythmics |
| Anticoagulants |
| Immunosuppressants |
| Cardiac transplantation |

filling pressures and increase cardiac index.[29] Improvement, however, may depend on the severity of underlying left ventricular dysfunction. In addition, doses higher than 20 mg every 6 to 8 hours may result in a clinically apparent negative inotropic effect, and pulmonary edema has been reported with nifedipine in patients with severe heart failure. Adequate trials of verapamil and diltiazem in this population are lacking, but it appears that the negative inotropic effect of verapamil may limit its use in the treatment of dilated cardiomyopathy.[29]

Vasodilators have also been utilized in the treatment of dilated cardiomyopathy. Sustained functional and hemodynamic improvement has been demonstrated with nitrates, hydralazine, hydralazine–nitrate combinations, prazosin, and captopril.[2,30–32]

Arrhythmias in dilated cardiomyopathy are refractory to drug therapy with conventional and investigational agents, and no clear guidelines exist for the administration of antiarrhythmics in this condition.[5,33] Sudden death has been reported to occur despite slowing or improvement of the arrhythmia while on therapy, and these agents have not been shown to improve survival.[5,33] Antiarrhythmics should be used to treat symptomatic or serious arrhythmias, and selection should take into consideration the avoidance of drugs that depress myocardial contractility. Disopyramide should be avoided,[2,5] whereas quinidine, procainamide, and mexiletine have been recommended.[5] (Please refer to Chapter 12.)

The frequency of systemic arterial embolism and pulmonary embolism in patients with dilated cardiomyopathy is reported to range from 18% to 80%.[34] Oral anticoagulation is indicated in patients with atrial fibrillation or prior thrombotic events. Anticoagulants should also be considered in patients with moderate to severe dilated cardiomyopathy, generalized ventricular hypokinesis, or mural thrombi because of the high risk of systemic embolization.[9,16,34] Many authors recommend that anticoagulation be instituted in all patients unless clear-cut contraindications exist.[2,5,16]

Immunosuppressive therapy (prednisone alone or in combination with azathioprine) has been utilized in the treatment of dilated cardiomyopathy if there is evidence of myocardial inflammation. Corticosteroids may have a role in patients with cardiomyopathy secondary to inflammatory disease such as sarcoidosis,[6] and may be of some value in postviral cardiomyopathy if the duration of heart failure is short.[1,35] The use of these agents is controversial, and, although some patients have shown a favorable response, steroids have not been shown to influence the course of disease.[5]

In cases in which the cardiomyopathy remains refractory to medical therapy, cardiac transplantation may be the only alternative. Three-year survival posttransplantation has been reported to be 70%; however, patient selection criteria and the availability of donors severely limit this option.[6,8]

## Hypertrophic Cardiomyopathy

Hypertrophic cardiomyopathy comprises a spectrum of diseases characterized by left ventricular hypertrophy, disproportionate hypertrophy of the interventricular septum, myocardial fiber disarray, and variable degrees of left ventricular outflow tract obstruction (Fig. 15.1).[2,36–39] By definition the etiology is unknown; therefore, the hypertrophy associated with this type of cardiomyopathy is not secondary to a cardiovascular or systemic disease that places a hemodynamic burden on the left ventricle.[7,40]

This disease entity was first described in 1869, but did not receive clinical recognition until the late 1950s. Since then, it has been referred to by a number of different names, most of which allude to the dynamic outflow tract obstruction that was originally thought to be the most characteristic feature. Although hypertrophic cardiomyopathy is the appropriate designation for this spectrum of diseases, many other terms continue to be used in clinical practice today. These include idiopathic hypertrophic subaortic stenosis (IHSS), hypertrophic obstructive cardiomyopathy (HOCM), and muscular subaortic stenosis.[36,41]

Hypertrophic cardiomyopathy occurs less frequently than the dilated variety, although the exact prevalence is unknown. This form of cardiomyopathy is genetically transmitted with an autosomal dominant pattern and linkage to the HLA system has been demonstrated.[2,8,42] Almost half of the first-degree relatives of patients with hypertrophic cardiomyopathy are found to have evidence of the disease. This cardiomyopathy occurs primarily in young adults, with an average age at presentation of 26 years; however, it may occur at any time from birth to the seventh and eighth decades.[8,40]

Wide interpatient variation exists in the clinical course and prognosis of hypertrophic cardiomyopathy. The clinical spectrum of this disorder ranges from patients who are asymptomatic to those who present with severe heart failure.[43]

### *Etiology*

The primary features of this disease are the hypertrophied left ventricle, impaired diastolic function, and myocardial fiber disarray. Many theories exist with regard to the etiology of these features; however, the exact cause remains to be determined. Abnormal sympathetic stimulation resulting from either excessive production of catecholamines or increased responsiveness of the heart to circulating

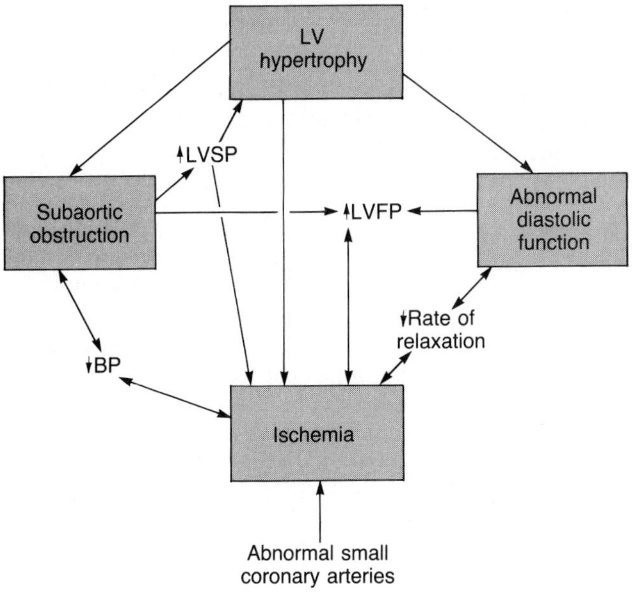


**Figure 15.2** Pathophysiologic and hemodynamic interrelations among left ventricular (LV) hypertrophy, subaortic obstruction, diastolic dysfunction, and myocardial ischemia in hypertrophic cardiomyopathy. The symptoms in any given patient reflect the complex interactions among these pathophysiologic mechanisms. LVSP, left ventricular systolic pressure; LVFP, left ventricular filling pressure; BP, blood pressure. *(From Maron BJ, et al: Hypertrophic cardiomyopathy: Interrelations of clinical manifestations, pathophysiology, and therapy. N Engl J Med 1987;316:845, with permission.)*

catecholamines[1,7,8,15,40,44–46] has been proposed as an etiologic mechanism of hypertrophic cardiomyopathy. Other proposed mechanisms include calcium overload,[8,15] impaired adenosine-mediated autoregulation of the heart,[47] abnormal atrioventricular conduction, and collagen abnormalities.[8]

## *Pathophysiology*

The pathophysiology of hypertrophic cardiomyopathy is complex and involves the interrelation of several disease components including left ventricular hypertrophy, subacute obstruction, diastolic dysfunction, and myocardial ischemia. Each of these components, alone or in combination, is responsible for the hemodynamic and clinical manifestations associated with this disorder; however, the relative contribution of each pathophysiologic mechanism varies among patients[37] (Fig. 15.2).

### Left Ventricular Hypertrophy

Increased myocardial mass and extreme left ventricular hypertrophy are the hallmarks of this cardiomyopathy. The pattern of hypertrophy is distinctive and differs from that seen with secondary hypertrophy in that there is usually a disproportionate thickening of the interventricular septum when compared with the left ventricular free wall.[1,8,15,37,39] The ratio of the thickness of the interventricular septum to that of the left ventricular free wall usually exceeds 1.3.[2,8] This feature is not present in all individuals with hypertrophic cardiomyopathy; however, at one time it was thought to be characteristic of this disease. The use of the term *asymmetric septal hypertrophy (ASH)* stems from this belief. It is now known that a concentric pattern of hypertrophy occurs in 2% to 20% of patients.[1,8,37,40]

Myocardial fiber disarray, although also not pathognomonic for this disease, is considered a sensitive histologic marker.[2,8,41,48] The bizarre and disorderly array of muscle fibers is usually found in the septum, but may sometimes affect the free wall. This abnormal architecture may result in a reduction in the effective mechanical force of the myocardium. This type of disarray may be observed in normal hearts as well as in other disease states; however, the disorganization occurs to a far greater extent in hypertrophic cardiomyopathy.[8,41,48]

### Diastolic Dysfunction

The most characteristic pathophysiologic abnormality of this cardiomyopathy is diastolic dysfunction. Decreased compliance (distensibility) and prolonged relaxation of the ventricle lead to impaired diastolic filling of the hypertrophied ventricle.[8,37,44,47,49,50] In turn, abnormalities in compliance may be related to myocardial cell disorganization or increased ventricular mass. Increased left ventricular filling pressure, along with elevated left atrial, pulmonary venous, and pulmonary capillary wedge pressures, eventually leads to congestive symptoms despite normal systolic function.[8,37,41]

### Systolic Function and Outflow Tract Obstruction

The left ventricle of patients with hypertrophic cardiomyopathy has often been described as "hypercontractile," because as much as 75% to 80% of the stroke volume may be ejected during the first third of systole.[8,15,37] This apparent hypercontractility is probably an artifact, and the left ventricle is better described as "hyperdynamic."[15,37,39,44,47,49]

Another feature of hypertrophic cardiomyopathy that has been the source of considerable controversy over the years is outflow tract obstruction.[1,2,37,40,41,44,51] In the early 1960s, most patients were observed to have loud systolic murmurs that were invariably associated with an intraventricular pressure gradient upon cardiac catheterization. The angiograms also suggested that outflow tract obstruction was caused by systolic apposition of the anterior mitral leaflet and the hypertrophied septum.[37,41] The advent of the echocardiogram in the 1970s confirmed the association of systolic anterior motion of the mitral valve (SAM) with the generation of a pressure gradient.[40,41] This obstruction was thought to be the most important feature of the disease and the cause of clinical symptoms, and is the origin of the terms *idiopathic hypertrophic subaortic stenosis* and *hypertrophic obstructive cardiomyopathy*.[1,2,37]

Some authors believe that SAM represents a true mechanical obstruction to left ventricular outflow, and is responsible for the outflow tract gradient observed in some of these patients.[8,37,40,52] Opposing this view are those who argue that a true obstruction cannot be present if 75% to 80% of the stroke volume is ejected early in systole. These authors believe the gradient to be incidental and the consequence of obliteration of the left ventricular cavity because of continued contraction of a hypertrophied muscle on a small, virtually empty ventricle.[1,8,37,41,51] In this case, SAM is thought to occur as a result of distortion and obliteration of the left ventricular cavity.

Outflow tract obstruction, when it does occur, is dynamic and fluctuates spontaneously. It is also influenced by factors that affect the force of left ventricular contraction, ventricular volume (preload), and ventricular afterload.[37,52] Interventions that increase contractility, such as digoxin, exercise and $\beta$ agonists, and those that decrease preload or afterload, such as the Valsalva maneuver and nitrates, cause an increase in obstruction. Conversely, factors that increase preload ameliorate the systolic gradient. $\beta$-Blockers that decrease myocardial contractility and measures such as squatting, sustained handgrip, or phenylephrine administration, which increase arterial pressure, are used to diminish the gradient and serve as aids in diagnosis.[37,41,52]

It is now recognized that obstruction and pressure gradients are not always present. In fact, only about 25% of patients have gradients at rest; some develop a gradient after provocation, while others show no gradient at rest or after provocation. The importance of these subgroups is unknown as there is no correlation between the presence and magnitude of outflow tract gradient and symptoms or mortality.[1,37,41,51]

### Myocardial Ischemia

Many patients with hypertrophic cardiomyopathy experience chest pain, in the absence of significant atherosclerotic coronary artery disease. Several mechanisms may explain this observation. Increased myocardial mass and high left ventricular pressures, common in this disorder, increase myocardial oxygen requirements at rest and with exertion.[37,53] Furthermore, the hypertrophied ventricle may compress large intramyocardial coronary arteries during systole, thus increasing coronary vascular resistance. Narrowing of small intramural coronary arteries may also contribute to myocardial ischemia in patients with hypertrophic cardiomyopathy.[37,53]

This may result in a vicious cycle where development of myocardial ischemia further increases left ventricular filling pressures which, in turn, may lead to further ischemia.[37]

## *Clinical Presentation*

The clinical manifestations of hypertrophic cardiomyopathy vary tremendously and may range from absence of symptoms to incapacitating heart failure. The classic "triad" of symptoms associated with this disorder consists of dyspnea, chest pain, and syncope, all of which may be exacerbated by exertion.[8,44,48,51]

Dyspnea is the most common symptom and is due largely to elevated diastolic filling pressure resulting from abnormal diastolic function secondary to ventricular hypertrophy.[2,8,37,48,51] Chest pain is also common and frequently occurs in the absence of significant coronary artery disease. Younger patients often present with syncope or presyncope, which is usually attributed to rhythm disturbances,[1,37,40] but has also been associated with sudden decreases in stroke volume.[48]

Sudden death is the most worrisome feature of hypertrophic cardiomyopathy and may be the first manifestation of disease.[40,44] The annual mortality from sudden death is high in children and adolescents (6%), with a reported overall incidence of sudden death between 2% and 4%.[18,37]

The mechanisms responsible for sudden death have not been fully identified. Patients with hypertrophic cardiomyopathy have a high incidence of conduction abnormalities and arrhythmias, and acute hemodynamic changes are therefore frequently proposed as the precipitants of sudden death.[1,18,37,40] The cause of ventricular arrhythmias is unknown, but has been attributed to myocardial fiber disarray, elevated intraventricular pressures, and myocardial ischemia.[37] Ventricular tachycardia appears to be the arrhythmia most predictive of sudden death. Atrial fibrillation is common later in the course of the disease, and is usually associated with an increase in symptoms and a poor prognosis.[7] Other features that may predict an increased incidence of sudden death include young age (14 years or less),[18,40,43,54] family history of sudden death,[1,40,43,54] and exercise.[18,43]

The progression of symptoms in hypertrophic cardiomyopathy is variable. The disease may progress gradually after the onset of symptoms and many patients may show an improvement or stabilization of symptoms with time.[2,7] Sudden death may occur at any time during the disease course, however, and is not related to symptoms.[18] Severe functional limitation is seen only in approximately 20% of patients.[7,18] In rare cases, hypertrophic cardiomyopathy may progress to left ventricular dilation and may mimic dilated cardiomyopathy with congestive symptoms that indicate severe widespread disease.[2,7] Gradients usually disappear with the appearance of congestive heart failure.

## *Diagnosis*

Patients without gradients may have a normal physical exam with the exception of a loud S4 and a left ventricular lift,[8] whereas patients with outflow tract obstruction usually have more significant physical findings.

The hallmark of obstructive hypertrophic cardiomyopathy is a harsh diamond-shaped systolic murmur heard along the left sternal border, in the fourth or fifth intercostal space radiating to the apex.[2] The murmur usually intensifies with maneuvers that enhance contractility or reduce preload or afterload and decreases with maneuvers that decrease contractility or increase preload or afterload.[36,41] The arterial pulse shows a rapid upstroke and rapid decline and there is a palpable atrial beat.[1]

Chest x-ray usually reveals left ventricular and left atrial enlargement[44] and left ventricular hypertrophy; widespread deep Q waves and left atrial abnormalities characteristically appear on the echocardiogram.[44]

The mainstay of diagnosis is M-mode echocardiography, which classically reveals left ventricular hypertrophy, disproportionate septal thickening, septal hypokinesis, reduced systolic diameter of the left ventricle, narrowing of the left ventricular outflow tract, SAM, and midsystolic closure of the aortic valve.[1,8,41,44] Angiography may reveal many of the same findings as echocardiography; however, in some cases the angiogram may have a normal appearance.[50]

Hemodynamic evaluation will often reveal elevated left

ventricular diastolic pressure.[7] A subaortic systolic pressure gradient is also noted if obstruction is present, and may be induced in some patients by the infusion of isoproterenol, inhalation of amyl nitrite, or the Valsalva maneuver.[8,37]

### *Treatment*

Treatment for hypertrophic cardiomyopathy is directed at the improvement of symptoms, the prevention of sudden death, and the arrest of disease progression.[1,2,37,40,44] Treatment must be tailored to the individual patient because of the variable progression and manifestations of this disorder. Most therapeutic modalities involve the reduction of ventricular contractility, the increase of ventricular volume or arterial pressure to decrease outflow tract obstruction, and the avoidance of drugs that increase obstruction (Table 15.4). All therapeutic agents should be used with caution to prevent systemic hypotension, hypovolemia, and vasodilation, all of which would worsen symptoms.

Positive inotropes including digitalis preparations should be avoided as they would tend to increase contractility, thus leading to an increase in outflow tract obstruction. The exception is the patient who has atrial fibrillation with a rapid ventricular rate.[1,2,8] Cardioversion should be attempted immediately when atrial fibrillation develops to avoid the loss of atrial contribution to ventricular filling. Patients with advanced disease evidenced by left ventricular dilation and systolic dysfunction, but no evidence of obstruction, may also benefit from digitalis; however, these patients seem to respond poorly to all therapeutic interventions and are also poor surgical candidates.[2,8]

$\beta$-Blockers have been the cornerstone of treatment for patients with obstructive disease. Initially, these agents were shown to ameliorate symptoms by decreasing systolic pressure gradients and myocardial contractility.[2,44] Propranolol has little effect on intraventricular pressure gradients at rest, but will limit increases in pressure after exercise. Subsequently, $\beta$-adrenergic antagonists have been reported to increase left ventricular distensibility and enhance left ventricular filling.[8,15,44,55] $\beta$-Blockers appear to have a greater effect on anginal symptoms and syncope than on dyspnea. In patients without obstruction, the response to these drugs is unpredictable and variable and they should be used with caution.[2,38]

$\beta$-Blockers may suppress atrial and ventricular arrhythmias, but the use of additional antiarrhythmics is usually required.[52] Furthermore, the $\beta$ antagonists have not been shown to have any effect on sudden death,[2,40] and their effect on prognosis has yet to be established.[40,55]

**Table 15.4** Treatment Modalities for Hypertrophic Cardiomyopathies

| |
|---|
| Avoid vasodilation, hypovolemia, hypotension |
| Do not use digoxin (except in atrial fibrillation) |
| $\beta$-Blockers |
| Calcium antagonists |
| Amiodarone |
| Anticoagulants |
| Surgery |

Propranolol is the $\beta$-blocker most frequently employed in the treatment of hypertrophic cardiomyopathy, with doses ranging from 40 mg four times daily to greater than 500 mg/d. Although improvement in exercise capacity is reported, the mean time to improvement may be prolonged.[41,56]

Calcium channel blockers provide an alternative to treatment with $\beta$-blockers. The rationale for the use of this therapeutic class is based on the theory that altered calcium kinetics are responsible for diastolic filling abnormalities and the hyperdynamic state of the left ventricle.[40,44,57] Calcium antagonists have been reported to improve symptoms, enhance exercise capacity, and improve diastolic relaxation and left ventricular filling, but have not been shown to have an effect on sudden death.[1,15,58–61]

Both verapamil and nifedipine have been reported to improve symptoms, increase exercise capacity, and improve diastolic function[57–59,62]; however, each has also been associated with deleterious effects.[57,63,64] Caution should be exercised when using verapamil because of its potent negative inotropic effects, and it should be avoided in patients with evidence of pulmonary venous hypertension.

The negative inotropic effect of nifedipine is less than that observed with verapamil; however, its potent vasodilator activity may precipitate hemodynamic compromise. Diltiazem has also been reported to have beneficial effects, although further studies are needed to evaluate its effect.[65]

The use of amiodarone in the treatment of hypertrophic cardiomyopathy is promising. This antiarrhythmic has been successful in reducing the frequency of supraventricular and ventricular arrhythmias, and, in contrast to other therapeutic agents, amiodarone has been reported to reduce the incidence of sudden death and prolong survival.[40,66–69] Nevertheless, at this time it is necessary to determine if the suppression of ventricular arrhythmias produced by amiodarone can be maintained and if the effect on survival can be confirmed. Arrhythmias are controlled within 1 week of amiodarone administration in dosages of 600–800 mg/d. This response can usually be maintained with the daily administration of 200–400 mg/d.[67] The minimum effective dose needed to control arrhythmias should be used as a maintenance dose because of the high incidence of dose-related side effects associated with the use of amiodarone. Electrocardiograms should be reevaluated at 3- to 6-month intervals and the dosage adjusted by 50–200 mg depending on the absence or presence of arrhythmias. If arrhythmias persist at a dosage of 400 mg/d, addition of another antiarrhythmic is recommended.[18,67] Propranolol may be used in combination with amiodarone, but patients with sinoatrial or atrioventricular conduction disturbances should be monitored closely. Verapamil should not be used as an adjunct to amiodarone.[18]

Anticoagulation is recommended in all patients with atrial fibrillation, in the absence of any existing contraindications.[44] If amiodarone is added to a patient's therapeutic regimen, the prothrombin time must be monitored closely, and the warfarin dose may have to be decreased by half.[70] Infective endocarditis occurs in less than 10% of patients, and prophylaxis is recommended.[7]

Therapeutic interventions have traditionally sought to decrease left ventricular obstruction; however, with the recognition of left ventricular hypertrophy as the hallmark of the disease and the lack of correlation between obstruction and symptoms, it appears that future efforts should focus on the regression of hypertrophy.[51]

Surgical options include myotomy and myectomy, which reduce outflow tract obstruction and provide symptomatic and functional improvement in 70% of patients.[71] Operative mortality ranges from 7% to 16% and there is no evidence that the surgery prevents progression of disease.[2,44,71] Surgery is indicated in patients with severe symptoms and high-grade obstruction who are refractory to medical treatment.[40,41]

## Restrictive/Obliterative Cardiomyopathies

The restrictive and obliterative cardiomyopathies are the least frequently encountered of all the cardiomyopathies.[2,8,44] These disorders were viewed as two distinct entities until it was discovered that the obliterative form is a later stage of restrictive cardiomyopathy resulting from endomyocardial fibrosis.[1,2,44,72]

In contrast to the dilated and hypertrophic cardiomyopathies, the etiology of these cardiomyopathies is usually known, with the exception of primary disorders which constitute a minority of the cases.[8] Secondary restrictive cardiomyopathy is usually the result of myocardial fibrosis, hypertrophy, or infiltration associated with various disease states. These include eosinophilic endomyocardial disease (Löffler's endocarditis), endomyocardial fibrosis, and amyloidosis.[44] Less frequently, infiltrative diseases such as sarcoidosis, hemochromatosis, glycogen and mucopolysaccharide deposition, and neoplastic processes can lead to this cardiomyopathy.[2,44]

The endocardium appears to react in a similar fashion to a variety of irritants, producing an exudative reaction that leads to fibrosis and thrombosis with changes in the small intramyocardial vessels. Eventually, the myocardium is scarred, and fibrous tissue and thrombi progressively obliterate the ventricular cavity and increase the resistance to ventricular filling.[1]

### *Pathophysiology*

The hallmark of restrictive cardiomyopathy is abnormal diastolic function. In this disorder, the rigid ventricular walls impede ventricular filling and impair diastolic distension, while systolic function is usually normal. Some impairment of systolic function, as well as distortion of the atrioventricular valves, may be seen in obliterative cardiomyopathy.[1,7,8]

### *Clinical Presentation*

Common symptoms include dyspnea on exertion, fatigue, peripheral edema, and, in some cases, chest pain. Signs of right ventricular heart failure such as independent edema, ascites, and hepatomegaly may result from persistently elevated venous pressures. Jugular venous pressure is usually elevated and does not fall normally, or it may rise with inspiration (Kussmaul). Third and fourth heart sounds are common.[2,8]

### *Diagnosis*

The physical exam is nonspecific and may reveal the signs and symptoms discussed in the previous paragraph. The electrocardiogram may show enlargement of one or more of the heart chambers and low-voltage, conduction, and rhythm abnormalities.[2] The echocardiogram may show thickening and increased mass of the left ventricle. Systolic function is usually preserved and the left ventricular ejection is usually normal.[2,8] Transvenous endocardial biopsy is important for the identification of infiltrative causes such as amyloidosis, hemochromatosis and sarcoidosis.[7,8] The ventricular pressure recording in this disorder shows a characteristic "square root" sign, manifested by deep and rapid early decline in ventricular pressure at the onset of diastole, with a rapid rise to an early plateau in early diastole.[8]

### *Clinical Course*

Information regarding the natural history of this group of cardiomyopathies is scarce because of their rare occurrence. Survival beyond 5 years is uncommon once the disease process is recognized clinically by the presence of pulmonary congestive symptoms; however, this may vary depending on the specific cause.[2]

### *Treatment*

Available therapy (Table 15.5) for the restrictive and obliterative cardiomyopathies is unsatisfactory. The underlying pathologic process is usually one of infiltration or fibrosis, and response of these processes to corticosteroids and immunosuppressive therapy has been largely unsuccessful.[1,2,44]

Treatment of the congestive symptoms is only partly successful because systolic function is usually maintained until late stages of the disorder. The high filling pressures necessary to adequately preload the heart also add to the difficulty of treating the disease. The use of diuretics or vasodilators may precipitate hypotension.[1,44] Digitalis has been used to treat systolic dysfunction, but it must be used with caution.[2] The calcium channel blockers may improve myocardial relaxation and reduce filling pressures; however, data evaluating these agents in the treatment of restrictive cardiomyopathy are limited.[44] Anticoagulants may help prevent arterial embolism and the formation of ventricular thrombi.[44]

Surgical intervention includes resection of the endomyocardial fibrous tissue and thrombus and replacement of the atrioventricular valves.[1] Although satisfactory reports have followed surgery, the long-term prognosis is uncertain and surgical mortality is quite significant.[1,44]

**Table 15.5** Treatment Modalities for Restrictive/Obliterative Cardiomyopathies

| |
|---|
| Steroids/immunosuppressants |
| Digitalis |
| Calcium antagonists |
| Anticoagulants |
| Surgery |

## Summary

The cardiomyopathies comprise a group of cardiac disorders that have baffled clinicians for years. The etiology of the dilated and hypertrophic forms is, for the most part, unknown and many theories exist regarding the pathogenesis of these disorders. Treatment is directed primarily at the improvement of clinical symptoms and, to this date, is still largely unsatisfactory.

The dilated cardiomyopathies are characterized by a large dilated ventricle and congestive symptoms that may respond to conventional treatment. Adjunct therapy often includes antiarrhythmics and anticoagulants. The use of $\beta$-blockers and calcium channel antagonists has created considerable controversy and further studies are needed to substantiate their role in the therapy of dilated cardiomyopathy. The agents that appear to hold the most promise in the treatment of this dilated cardiomyopathy are the angiotensin-converting enzyme inhibitors.

The hypertrophic cardiomyopathies are characterized by left ventricular and septal hypertrophy, diastolic dysfunction, and variable degree of outflow tract obstruction. Although these patients may also present with congestive symptoms, positive inotropes should be avoided. Symptoms may improve with the use of $\beta$-blockers or calcium channel antagonists, and amiodarone has been shown to improve survival in this patient population.

The restrictive/obliterative cardiomyopathies are the least common of the cardiomyopathies and are usually secondary to the infiltrative process. Relief of congestive symptoms is limited as systolic function is usually normal. Therapy often includes immunosuppressants and/or surgery.

## References

1. Goodwin JF. The frontiers of cardiomyopathy. Br Heart J 1982; 48:1–18.
2. Miller DH, Borer JS. The cardiomyopathies. A pathophysiological approach to therapeutic management. Arch Intern Med 1983;143:2157–2162.
3. Report of the WHO/ISFC task force on the definition and classification of cardiomyopathies. Br Heart J 1980;44:672–673.
4. Maron BJ, Epstein SE. Hypertrophic cardiomyopathies: A discussion of nomenclature. Am J Cardiol 1979;43:1242–1244.
5. Johnson RA, Palacios I. Dilated cardiomyopathies of the adult. N Engl J Med 1982;307:1051–1058.
6. Orie JE, Liedtke AJ. Cardiomyopathy. 1. Dilated (congestive) type. Postgrad Med 1986;79:83–91.
7. Wynne J, Braunwald E. The cardiomyopathies and myocarditides, in Braunwald E, Isselbacher KJ (eds): Harrison's Principles of Internal Medicine, 11th ed. New York, McGraw-Hill, 1987, pp 998–1004.
8. Wynne J, Braunwald E. The cardiomyopathies and myocarditides, in Braunwald E (ed): Heart Disease. A Textbook of Cardiovascular Medicine, 4th ed. Philadelphia, W.B. Saunders, 1984, pp 1399–1456.
9. Stern TN. Dilated cardiomyopathy: Current concepts. Compr Ther 1986;12:57–62.
10. Dec GW, Palacios IF, Fallon JT, et al. Active myocarditis in the spectrum of acute dilated cardiomyopathies. N Engl J Med 1985;312:885–890.
11. Fuster V, Gersh BJ, Giuliani ER, et al. The natural history of idiopathic dilated cardiomyopathy. Am J Cardiol 1981;47:525–531.
12. Johnson RA, Palacios I. Dilated cardiomyopathies of the adult. N Engl J Med 1982;307:1119–1126.
13. Fisher ML, Plotnick GD, Peters RW, et al. Beta-blockers in congestive cardiomyopathy. Conceptual advance or contraindication. Am J Med 1986;80(suppl 2B):59–66.
14. Bristow MR. The adrenergic system in heart failure. N Engl J Med 1984;311:850–851.
15. Opie LH, Walpoth B, Barsacchi R. Calcium and catecholamines: Relevance to cardiomyopathies and significance in therapeutic strategies. J Mol Cell Cardiol 1985;17:21–34.
16. Homans DC. Peripartum cardiomyopathy. N Engl J Med 1985; 312:1432–1437.
17. Meinertz T, Hofmann T, Kasper W, et al. Significance of ventricular arrhythmias in idiopathic dilated cardiomyopathy. Am J Cardiol 1984;53:902–909.
18. McKenna WJ, Krikler DM, Goodwin JF. Arrhythmias in dilated and hypertrophic cardiomyopathy. Med Clin North Am 1984; 68:983–1000.
19. Costanzo-Nordin MR, O'Connell JB, Engelmeier RS, et al. Dilated cardiomyopathy: Functional status, hemodynamics, arrhythmias and prognosis. Cathet Cardiovasc Diagn 1985;11: 445–453.
20. Franciosa JA, Wilen M, Ziesche S, et al. Survival in men with severe chronic left ventricular failure due to either coronary heart disease or idiopathic dilated cardiomyopathy. Am J Cardiol 1983;51:831–836.
21. Alderman J, Grossman W. Are beta adrenergic-blocking drugs useful in the treatment of dilated cardiomyopathy? Circulation 1985;71:854–857.
22. Swedberg K, Hjalmarson A, Waagstein F, et al. Adverse effects of beta-blockade withdrawal in patients with congestive cardiomyopathy. Br Heart J 1980;44:134–142.
23. Waagstein F, Hjalmarson A, Varnauskas E, et al. Effect of chronic beta adrenergic receptor blockade in congestive cardiomyopathy. Br Heart J 1975;37:1022–1036.
24. Swedberg K, Hjalmarson A, Waagstein F, et al. Prolongation of survival in congestive cardiomyopathy by beta-receptor blockade. Lancet 1979;2:1374–1376.
25. Swedberg K, Hjalmarson A, Waagstein F, et al. Beneficial effects of long term beta-blockade in congestive cardiomyopathy. Br Heart J 1980;44:117–133.
26. Currie PJ, Kelly MJ, McKenzie A, et al. Oral beta-adrenergic blockade with metoprolol in chronic severe dilated cardiomyopathy. J Am Coll Cardiol 1984;3:203–209.
27. Anderson JL, Lutz JR, Gilbert EM, et al. A randomized trial of low-dose beta-blockade therapy for idiopathic dilated cardiomyopathy. Am J Cardiol 1985;55:471–475.
28. Ikram J, Fitzpatrick D. Double-blind trial of chronic oral beta blockade in congestive cardiomyopathy. Lancet 1981;2:490–492.
29. Baughman KL. Calcium channel blocking agents in congestive heart failure. Am J Med 1986;80(suppl 2B):46–50.
30. Smucker ML, Sanford CF, Lipscomg KM. Effects of hydralazine on pressure–volume and stress–volume relations in congestive heart failure secondary to idiopathic cardiomyopathy. Am J Cardiol 1985;56:690–695.

31. Unverferth DV, Mehegan JP, Magorien RD, et al. Regression of myocardial cellular hypertrophy with vasodilator therapy in chronic congestive heart failure associated with idiopathic dilated cardiomyopathy. Am J Cardiol 1983;51:1392–1398.
32. Agostoni PG, De Cesare N, Doria E, et al. Afterload reduction: A comparison of captopril and nifedipine in dilated cardiomyopathy. Br Heart J 1986;55:391–399.
33. Poll DS, Marchlinski FE, Buxton AE, et al. Sustained ventricular tachycardia in patients with idiopathic dilated cardiomyopathy: Electrophysiologic testing and lack of response to antiarrhythmic drug therapy. Circulation 1984;70:451–456.
34. Kyrle PA, Gossinger H, Glogar D, et al. Prevention of arterial and pulmonary embolism by oral anticoagulants in patients with dilated cardiomyopathy. Thromb Haemost 1985;54:521–523.
35. Mason JW, Billingham ME, Ricci DR. Treatment of acute inflammatory myocarditis assisted by endomyocardial biopsy. Am J Cardiol 1979;44:303–309.
36. Maron BJ, Bonow RO, Cannon III RO, et al. Hypertrophic cardiomyopathy. Interrelations of clinical manifestations, pathophysiology, and therapy. N Engl J Med 1987;316:780–789.
37. Maron BJ, Bonow RO, Cannon III RO, et al. Hypertrophic cardiomyopathy. Interrelations of clinical manifestations, pathophysiology, and therapy. N Engl J Med 1987;316:844–852.
38. Hirota Y, Furubayashi K, Kaku K, et al. Hypertrophic nonobstructive cardiomyopathy: A precise assessment of hemodynamic characteristics and clinical implications. Am J Cardiol 1982;50:990–997.
39. Pouleur H, Rousseau M, van Eyll C, et al. Force–velocity–length relations in hypertrophic cardiomyopathy: Evidence of normal or depressed myocardial contractility. Am J Cardiol 1983;52:813–817.
40. McKenna WJ, Goodwin JF. The natural history of hypertrophic cardiomyopathy. Curr Probl Cardiol 1981;6:1–26.
41. Epstein SE, Henry WL, Clark CE, et al. Asymmetric septal hypertrophy. Ann Intern Med 1974;81:650–680.
42. Darsee JR, Heymsfield SB, Nutter DO. Hypertrophic cardiomyopathy and human leukocyte antigen linkage. N Engl J Med 1979;300:877–882.
43. Koga Y, Itaya K, Toshima H. Prognosis in hypertrophic cardiomyopathy. Am Heart J 1984;108:351–359.
44. Orie JE, Liedtke AJ. Cardiomyopathy. 2. Hypertrophic and restrictive/obliterative types. Postgrad Med 1986;79:95–106.
45. Soufer R, Wohlgelernter D, Vita NA, et al. Intact systolic left ventricular function in clinical congestive heart failure. Am J Cardiol 1985;55:1032–1036.
46. McKenna WJ, England D, Deanfield JE, et al. Arrhythmia in hypertrophic cardiomyopathy. I: Influence on prognosis. Br Heart J 1981;46:168–172.
47. Watt AH. Hypertrophic cardiomyopathy: A disease of impaired adenosine-mediated autoregulation of the heart. Lancet 1984;1: 1271–1273.
48. Landmark K. Hypertrophic cardiomyopathy. Acta Pharmacol Toxicol 1986;58(suppl 2):169–174.
49. Manyari DE, Paulsen W, Boughner DR, et al. Resting and exercise left ventricular function in patients with hypertrophic cardiomyopathy. Am Heart J 1973;105:980–987.
50. Topol EJ, Traill TA, Fortuin NJ. Hypertensive hypertrophic cardiomyopathy of the elderly. N Engl J Med 1985;312:277–283.
51. Criley JM, Siegel RJ. Has "obstruction" hindered our understanding of hypertrophic cardiomyopathy? Circulation 1985;72: 1148–1154.
52. Glancy DL, Shepherd RL, Beiser GD, et al. The dynamic nature of left ventricular outflow obstruction in idiopathic hypertrophic subaortic stenosis. Ann Intern Med 1971;75:589–592.
53. Maron BJ, Wolfson JK, Epstein SE, et al. Intramural ("small vessel") coronary artery disease in hypertrophic cardiomyopathy. J Am Coll Cardiol 1986;8:545–557.
54. Frank MJ, Watkins LO, Prisant LM, et al. Potentially lethal arrhythmias and their management in hypertrophic cardiomyopathy. Am J Cardiol 1984;53:1608–1613.
55. Alvares RF, Goodwin JF. Non-invasive assessment of diastolic function in hypertrophic cardiomyopathy on and off beta adrenergic blocking drugs. Br Heart J 1982;48:204–212.
56. Frank MJ, Abdulla AM, Watkins LO, et al. Long term medical management of hypertrophic cardiomyopathy: Usefulness of propranolol. Eur Heart J 1983;4(suppl 4):155–164.
57. Chaterjee K, Raff G, Anderson D, et al. Hypertrophic cardiomyopathy—Therapy with slow channel inhibiting agents. Prog Cardiovasc Dis 1982;25:193–210.
58. Bonow RO, Rosing DR, Bacharach SL, et al. Effects of verapamil on left ventricular systolic function and diastolic filling in patients with hypertrophic cardiomyopathy. Circulation 1981; 64:787–796.
59. McGoon MD, Vlietstra RE, Holmes DR, et al. The clinical use of verapamil. Mayo Clin Proc 1982;57:495–510.
60. Hanrath P, Schluter M, Sonntag F, et al. Influence of verapamil therapy on left ventricular performance at rest and during exercise in hypertrophic cardiomyopathy. Am J Cardiol 1983; 52:544–548.
61. Bonow RO. Effects of calcium-channel blocking agents on left ventricular diastolic function in hypertrophic cardiomyopathy and in coronary artery disease. Am J Cardiol 1985;55:172B–178B.
62. Lorell BH, Paulus WJ, Grossman W, et al. Modification of abnormal left ventricular diastolic properties by nifedipine in patients with hypertrophic cardiomyopathy. Circulation 1982; 65:499–507.
63. Fedor JM, Stack RS, Pryor DB, et al. Adverse effects of nifedipine therapy on hypertrophic obstructive cardiomyopathy. Chest 1983;83:704–706.
64. Perrot B, Danchin N, Terrier de la Chaise A. Verapamil: A cause of death in a patient with hypertrophic cardiomyopathy. Br Heart J 1984;51:352–354.
65. Suwa M, Hirota Y, Kawamura K. Improvement in left ventricular diastolic function during intravenous and oral diltiazem therapy in patients with hypertrophic cardiomyopathy: An echocardiographic study. Am J Cardiol 1984;54:1047–1053.
66. McKenna WJ, Harris L, Perez G, et al. Arrhythmia in hypertrophic cardiomyopathy. II: Comparison of amiodarone and verapamil in treatment. Eur Heart J 1983;4(suppl 4):57–65.
67. McKenna WJ, Harris L, Rowland E, et al. Amiodarone for long-term management of patients with hypertrophic cardiomyopathy. Am J Cardiol 1984;54:802–810.
68. Leman RB, Gillette PC, Zinner AJ. Resolution of congestive cardiomyopathy caused by supraventricular tachycardia using amiodarone. Am Heart J 1986;112:622–624.
69. McKenna WJ, Oakley CM, Krikler MD, et al. Improved survival with amiodarone in patients with hypertrophic cardiomyopathy and ventricular tachycardia. Br Heart J 1985;53:412–416.
70. McKenna WJ. Arrhythmia and prognosis in hypertrophic cardiomyopathy. Eur Heart J 1983;4(suppl F):225–234.
71. Maron BJ, Epstein SE, Morrow AG. Symptomatic status and prognosis of patients after operation for hypertrophic obstructive cardiomyopathy: Efficacy of ventricular septal myotomy and myectomy. Eur Heart J 1983;4(suppl F):175–185.
72. Siegel RJ, Shah PK, Fishbein MC. Idiopathic restrictive cardiomyopathy. Circulation 1984;70:165–169.

# Chapter 16 / Primary Pulmonary Hypertension

John A. Lazor, PharmD

Pulmonary hypertension is an elevation of the pulmonary arterial pressures. Most commonly it is defined as an elevation of the pulmonary arterial systolic pressure greater than 30 or 35 mm Hg or a mean pulmonary arterial pressure greater than 20 or 25 mm Hg.[1–6] The NIH Registry accepts patients with resting mean pulmonary arterial pressures greater than 25 mm Hg or greater than 30 mm Hg with exercise.[7]

Pulmonary hypertension was recognized as a disease entity as early as the turn of the century. Ever since the right heart catheterization was first implemented in 1929, interest has grown in the cardiopulmonary circulation. There was a rapid rise in the recognition of this disease process with the introduction of cardiac catheterization in humans in the 1940s. With supportive data from such catheterizations, Dresdale et al published the first detailed account of primary pulmonary hypertension in 1951.[8]

Primary pulmonary hypertension is one of two broad classifications of pulmonary hypertension; the other is secondary pulmonary hypertension. By strict definition, the diagnosis of primary pulmonary hypertension can be made if the cause of the increased pressure in the pulmonary circulation is not known. It is a diagnosis of exclusion. Other terms used interchangeably with primary pulmonary hypertension include idiopathic pulmonary hypertension and unexplained pulmonary hypertension. Secondary pulmonary hypertension exists when there is an identifiable etiology that can be linked to the increased pulmonary arterial pressure.

The incidence of primary pulmonary hypertension is about 1% to 2% of patients who undergo a right heart catheterization.[9,10] The disease is found at autopsy in 1% of the patients having cor pulmonale.[11] It is found primarily in females between the ages of 20 and 30 years, but it can occur as early as a few days after birth through the seventh decade of life. Up until adolescence the occurrence is equal in males and females, but thereafter affected females outnumber males 2.5–4.0:1.[1,4,10] This female preponderance declines in older age groups.[11]

Three histopathologic types of primary pulmonary hypertension have been identified.[12–14] The most common is thromboembolic and occurs in 56% of the cases. The incidence of primary plexogenic pulmonary arteriopathy is 28% and this is the second most common histopathologic type. The third morphologic subtype is pulmonary veno-occlusive disease.

In the strictest sense, the diagnosis of primary pulmonary hypertension should be reserved for elevated pulmonary pressures without a known etiology. This is in contrast to the vast number of reports of primary pulmonary hypertension associated with a host of disease states. The diagnosis of primary pulmonary hypertension can be made with certainty based on the criteria listed in Table 16.1.[15]

## Normal Pulmonary Circulation

The normal pulmonary circulatory network is a high-flow, low-resistance, high-capacitance system.[3,4,16,17] The average systolic and diastolic pressures in the pulmonary artery are about 22 and 10 mm Hg, respectively. The mean pressure is about 15 mm Hg. The pulmonary arteriovenous pressure gradient is only about 6–10 mm Hg.

The precapillary pulmonary arteries are thin-walled, distensible, elastic vessels. Dilatation of the pulmonary arteries and recruitment of additional circulatory pathways result in an increase in capacitance of the pulmonary vascular bed. This increased capacitance contributes to the maintenance of the low-resistance system and prevents the elevation of pulmonary pressures in response to large increases in blood flow. Normally, the pulmonary vasculature can accommodate increases of cardiac output of 2.5 to 3 times normal before pulmonary pressures rise.[18]

Vascular resistance is determined by the ratio of pressure change to flow. According to Poiseuille's law (Fig. 16.1), resistance increases with increases in vessel length and blood viscosity and with small decreases in vessel radius.[3,17] If blood flow remains constant, a rise in pulmonary vascular resistance will result in an elevation in pulmonary artery pressure. Factors that affect pulmonary vascular resistance include the total mass of the lung tissue, extramural compression of the vessels, and the cross-sectional area of the pulmonary arteries and arterioles.

## The Right Ventricle and the Pulmonary Circulation

The right ventricle of the heart is a thin-walled, low-pressure chamber.[19] In comparison to the left ventricle, it is twice as distensible and its stroke volume is two times as sensitive to changes in ejection pressure or afterload. The right ventricle provides the necessary volume to the left ventricle to maintain cardiac output. The right ventricle can accommodate increases in blood flow without its systolic pressure rising above 40 mm Hg because of the pulmonary circulation's normally low resistance.

The efficiency of the right ventricle is dependent on its preload, afterload, heart rate, and contractility.[20] An increase in pressure or resistance of the pulmonary vascular bed increases the right ventricular afterload. As right ven-

**Table 16.1** Criteria Needed for the Diagnosis of Primary Pulmonary Hypertension With Certainty

| |
|---|
| 1. Pulmonary arterial pressure elevation with a normal pulmonary wedge pressure |
| 2. No secondary cardiac or pulmonary disease |
| 3. Pulmonary angiography does not demonstrate any local pulmonary vascular abnormalities |
| 4. Other causes of pulmonary hypertension have been eliminated by histologic means |
| 5. Characteristic microscopic signs are present in the pulmonary vasculature |

From Riedel M, Widimsky J: Symposium on primary pulmonary hypertension. Cor Vasa 1982;24(6):464, with permission.

tricular afterload or impedance increases, the right ventricular ejection fraction decreases. Because the right ventricle is a thin-walled muscle, its ability to overcome an increased afterload is limited. The right ventricle attempts to compensate with an increase in its contractility, although it is not sufficient to overcome the increased afterload.[21]

Another compensatory mechanism is an increased preload of the right ventricle.[20] As mean pulmonary artery pressure increases, right ventricular end-diastolic volume increases, with a more than proportional increase in end-diastolic pressure. A chronic elevation of pulmonary vascular pressure leads to right ventricular hypertrophy. To overcome the increased pulmonary vascular resistance and pressure to maintain cardiac output, the systolic pressure of the right ventricle may equal the systemic pressure.

The volume overload of the right ventricle may reduce its coronary blood flow. This decrease in blood supply, in combination with an increased myocardial oxygen consumption resulting from increased right ventricular pressures, could lead to ischemia of the right ventricle.[22] Myocardial cell damage in addition to the fluid overload contributes to the development of right heart failure or cor pulmonale.

The cardiac output is reduced because of the inability of the right ventricle to provide the needed outflow to ensure adequate filling of the left ventricle. Cardiac output may also be decreased because of a decrease in left ventricular compliance. In the normal heart, the interventricular septum is curved concave to the left. With chronic elevations in right ventricular volume and pressure the septum can reverse, causing the reduction of left ventricular compliance.[23] As a result, left ventricular end-diastolic volume and pressure increase. Left ventricular failure can develop in addition to right heart failure with long-standing and severe pulmonary hypertension. The interactions of elevated pulmonary arterial pressure and cardiac function are illustrated in Figure 16.2.

**Figure 16.1** Poiseuille's law. *The denominator of the rearrangement to determine resistance can be modified by multiplying by the variable *k* (altered number of vessels).

$$Q = \frac{\pi (P_i - P_0) r^4}{8 \eta l}$$

where $Q$ = flow
$P_i - P_0$ = pressure difference
$r$ = radius
$\eta$ = viscosity
$l$ = length

$$R = \frac{(P_i - P_0)}{Q} = \frac{8 \eta l}{\pi r^4 (k)^*}$$

where $R$ = resistance

## Pathophysiology

The elevation in pulmonary arterial pressure may be caused by a single alteration in the normal physiologic process or it may be the result of a combination of factors. Pulmonary hypertension can occur secondary to an increase in blood flow.[2,17,24,25] Changes in blood flow in the pulmonary circulation are reflective of changes in cardiac output. Intracardiac shunts can also increase pulmonary blood flow. The pulmonary hypertension caused by the shunts of atrial septal defects is delayed in onset, whereas the pulmonary hypertension resulting from ventricular septal defects is developed more rapidly.[4] As mentioned previously, a normal pulmonary circulatory system can adapt to rather large increases in blood flow without creating a significant increase in pulmonary artery pressure. It may, however, be possible that increased shear stress caused by the increased flow can result in endothelial damage and lead to changes in endothelial cell function.[26] This vascular effect may augment the development of pulmonary hypertension. The term *hyperkinetic pulmonary hypertension* has been applied to those circumstances in which the pulmonary hypertension is the result of an increased blood flow.

An increased blood volume can also be a determinant for an elevated pulmonary arterial pressure.[3,17] The pulmonary blood volume is influenced by the balance between the output of the two ventricles and the distensibility of the pulmonary vasculature. An increase in pulmonary blood volume, and therefore pressure, results from a decline in left ventricular output (right ventricular output remains constant) and the absence of adequate pulmonary vessel recruitment.

Increased blood viscosity is a third mechanism in the development of pulmonary hypertension.[2,3,17,27] Some factors contributing to an increased viscosity include agglutination of red cells, immunologic reactions involving white cells, platelet aggregates, and an increase in red cell mass. Polycythemia, with an elevation in hematocrit to 50% to 55%, can result in a 30% to 50% rise in transpulmonary arteriovenous pressure gradient at a constant flow.[3]

There can be a passive rise in pulmonary arterial

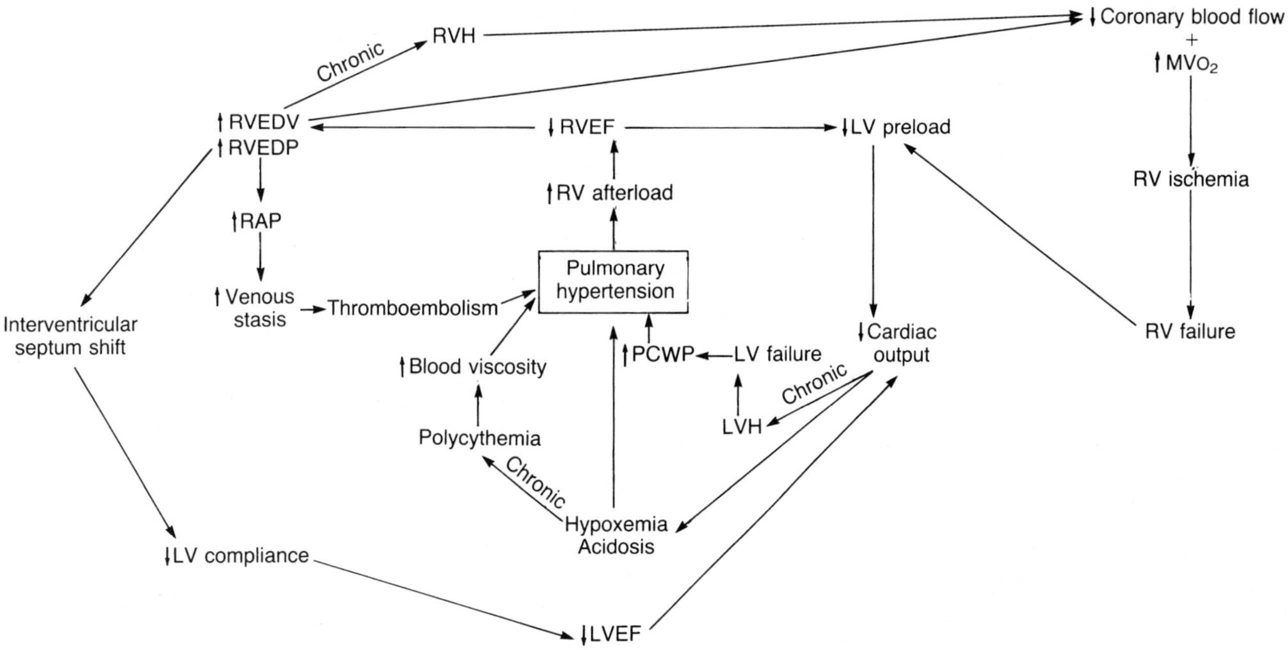


**Figure 16.2** Interactions between pulmonary hypertension and the cardiovascular system. RV, right ventricle; LV, left ventricle; EF, ejection fraction; EDP, end-diastolic pressure; EDV, end-diastolic volume; RVH, right ventricular hypertrophy; LVH, left ventricular hypertrophy; PCWP, pulmonary capillary wedge pressure; RAP, right atrial pressure. *(Adapted from Perkin RM, Anas NG: J Pediatr 1984;105(4):511–521, with permission.)*

pressure.[4,6] Pulmonary hypertension can result as a compensatory mechanism in response to an elevation in pulmonary venous pressure. An increase in left ventricular pressure can also lead to a passive rise in the pulmonary arterial pressure. As the left ventricular pressure rises, the pressure in the left atrium increases, thereby causing an increase in elevated pulmonary venous and capillary pressures. The response to the rise in postcapillary pressures results in pulmonary hypertension. Independent of any pressure change of the left ventricle, an increased left atrial pressure can passively cause an increase in pulmonary artery pressure.

Another mechanism responsible for the development of pulmonary hypertension is a reduction in the size of the pulmonary vascular bed.[2,17,28] As the effective arterial bed decreases, resistance to blood flow increases. About one half to two thirds of the total cross-sectional area of the pulmonary vascular bed must be destroyed before pulmonary pressure rises. The size of the pulmonary vascular bed can be reduced by (1) a direct loss of vessels such as a pneumonectomy, (2) obstruction of the arterial bed, (3) vasoconstriction, and (4) vascular remodeling or structural changes. Table 16.2 summarizes the mechanisms of pulmonary hypertension.

## Causes

### *Hypoxia*

Vasoconstriction reduces the cross-sectional area of the pulmonary vascular bed. It is the most common underlying cause of increased pulmonary arterial resistance.[6] The small pulmonary arteries and arterioles are the main sites of vasoconstriction and increased resistance. Pulmonary hypertension results from this increase in pulmonary vascular resistance.

Alveolar hypoxia and arterial hypoxemia are both considered important stimuli for the induction of pulmonary vaso-

**Table 16.2** Mechanisms of Elevated Pulmonary Arterial Pressures

1. Reduction in surface area of pulmonary vascular bed
   a. Functional (vasoconstriction)
   b. Structural
2. Increase in pulmonary blood flow
3. Increase in blood volume
4. Increase in blood viscosity
5. Increase in pulmonary vascular resistance (secondary to reduction in pulmonary vascular bed or increased blood viscosity)

constriction; however, pulmonary vascular sensitivity is greater to alveolar hypoxia.[29] This response of the pulmonary vasculature contrasts with the dilatation of most blood vessels upon exposure to decreased oxygen. The alveolar $PaO_2$ must be 60 mm Hg or lower to cause vasoconstriction. The pulmonary arteries in the size range 200–300 $\mu$m are the major reactors to hypoxia. These hypoxic effects are accentuated in the presence of acidemia.[2,28]

The mechanism of the pulmonary vascular constriction caused by low oxygen tension is unknown. A direct effect of the pulmonary vascular smooth muscle may occur or the response may be mediated by a vasoactive substance.

It has been proposed that humoral mediators are released from mast cells, neuroepithelial bodies, or autonomic nerve endings in response to hypoxia. The vasoconstrictive substances have included histamine, serotonin, angiotensin II, norepinephrine, prostaglandins, and leukotrienes.[26,30–32] In addition, a direct effect of hypoxia on endothelial cell function may cause an imbalance in the products of the arachidonate pathway.[29] The end products such as thromboxane and prostacyclin may function as modulators of pulmonary vascular tone. Pulmonary hypertension may result from both a decreased production of vasodilators and an excess production of vasoconstrictors such as thromboxane. Thromboxane $A_2$ may also precipitate platelet aggregation, which may be a contributing factor in pulmonary hypertension.

Another proposed intermediate in the hypoxia-induced vasoconstriction of pulmonary vascular smooth muscle is increased entry of slow-channel calcium.[33–35] This transmembrane flux of calcium has been implicated in both the direct and the mediator mechanisms of vascular constriction.

Chronic hypoxia can lead to the development of polycythemia and to structural changes in the pulmonary vessels.[29] Muscularization of small, normally nonmuscular arteries occurs. Smooth muscle hypertrophy and hypoplasia develop in the normally muscular pulmonary arteries. On the basis of the rat model, the most affected area is the immediate precapillary vessel that lies in the alveolar wall.[36] The pericyte and its derivative, the intermediate cells, proliferate and develop into mature smooth muscle.[37] Arteriolar muscularization and medial hypertrophy are the first structural changes.[12] These are followed by cellular intimal thickening with a gradual transition to concentric-laminar intimal fibrosis. These structural changes of the pulmonary arteries and arterioles lead to narrowing of the lumen of the pulmonary vessels. As the disease progresses, plexiform lesions can also form. Plexiform lesions form in small muscular pulmonary arteries near their origin from a larger parent vessel. This lesion consists of focal medial disruptions and aneurysm-like dilatations. At one time the plexiform lesion was considered a pathognomonic feature of primary pulmonary hypertension, but it can occur in secondary pulmonary hypertension and be absent at autopsy in patients with primary pulmonary hypertension. These structural changes contribute to the development and the maintenance of pulmonary hypertension through obstruction of the pulmonary vessel. Alterations in pulmonary vascular reactivity also result from this evolution of fixed pulmonary structural changes.[38,39]

The development of pulmonary hypertension secondary to pulmonary vasoconstriction induced by hypoxia is seen in such disease states as chronic obstructive pulmonary disease,[40,41] bronchitis, emphysema,[27,42] and adult respiratory distress syndrome.[43] The hypoventilation syndromes, which include pickwickian syndrome, sleep apnea,[44,45] and pharyngeal–tracheal obstruction,[3] can progress to the development of pulmonary hypertension. Pulmonary hypertension can also exist with the neuromuscular disorders of myasthenia gravis and poliomyelitis.[4] Kyphoscoliosis can lead to pulmonary vasoconstriction through hypoxia or secondary to anatomic compression of the pulmonary vessels.[3] In the late stages of cystic fibrosis, hypoxia can lead to pulmonary hypertension.[46] Hypoxia is involved in the mechanism of thromboembolism-induced elevations of pulmonary arterial pressure.[47] It is also a component of the multifactorial etiology of pulmonary hypertension in collagen vascular disorders.[48]

Pulmonary hypertension can emerge as a result of hypoxic vasoconstriction in individuals living in high altitudes.[4] Symptoms may become evident particularly in those who return to high altitude after being at sea level for a period of time.

### *Pulmonary Embolism*

As mentioned previously, obstruction of the pulmonary arterial bed causes a decrease in the size of the vascular bed, increasing resistance to flow. Pulmonary thromboemboli, as well as thrombi in situ, can cause obstruction of the precapillary pulmonary vessels.[47,49,50] This obstruction, along with vasoconstriction induced by hypoxia, contributes to the development of pulmonary hypertension. In most patients the embolic episodes are symptomatic but go undiagnosed. Silent thromboembolism is the most malignant cause of thromboembolic pulmonary hypertension because it is rarely diagnosed before irreversible anatomic changes occur. It is estimated that 80% of acute pulmonary thromboembolic events result in pulmonary hypertension. The acute process is more related to the vasoconstrictive mechanism as opposed to direct vascular obstruction. Recurring pulmonary emboli can result in pulmonary hypertension that is more related to obstruction or reduction in the cross-sectional area of the pulmonary vascular bed.

Other embolic events such as tumor emboli[51–53] and fat emboli[54,55] can lead to precapillary obstruction and cause a rise in pulmonary arterial pressure. In patients with a history of intravenous drug abuse, embolization of foreign bodies such as cellulose filter material can cause an elevated pulmonary arterial pressure.[56,57]

### *Schistosomiasis*

Although not endemic in the United States, schistosomiasis is a common cause of chronic pulmonary hypertension worldwide.[4,17,25] The ova of the parasite *Schistosoma mansoni* lodge in the pulmonary arterioles. Inflammatory lesions are produced that obstruct the pulmonary arterioles, producing pulmonary hypertension.

### *Collagen Vascular Disease*

Pulmonary complications of systemic lupus erythematosus (SLE) occur in 50% to 70% of patients.[58–63] The development of pulmonary hypertension is rare but the reported incidence is increasing. Raynaud's phenomenon is present in 75% of those patients with SLE and pulmonary hypertension. Raynaud's phenomenon coexists in as many as 30% of those patients diagnosed as having primary pulmonary hypertension.[64] Pulmonary hypertension has been reported to occur in as few as 1% to 4% to as many as 30% of the cases of systemic sclerosis.[65–67] The incidence increases to about 50% in those patients with the CREST variant.[25] An increased pulmonary arterial pressure has also been demonstrated in mixed connective tissue disease,[48,68] rheumatoid arthritis,[69,70] Sjögren's syndrome,[71] dermatomyositis,[72] polymyositis,[73] and Whipple's disease.[74]

The etiology of pulmonary hypertension in these disease entities is multifaceted. Proposed hypotheses include pulmonary fibrosis, arteritis, thrombosis and embolism possibly related to the lupus anticoagulant[75,76] and platelet dysfunction, vasospasm, hypoxic vasoconstriction, and the disposition of immune complexes resulting in endothelial injury. Myocardial dysfunction was suggested as the mechanism of increased pulmonary arterial pressure in a patient with digital Raynaud's phenomenon because a rise in pulmonary capillary wedge pressure occurred.[77] With few exceptions, pulmonary hypertension develops in collagen vascular disorders secondary to a reduction in the size of the pulmonary vascular bed or to vasoconstriction.

### *External Compression*

Compression of the lung parenchyma and small pulmonary vessels by chest wall abnormalities can increase the pulmonary vascular resistance. A small number of patients with kyphoscoliosis develop pulmonary hypertension.[4] The contributing mechanism is external pulmonary compression by the scoliosis component of the disease entity.

### *Drug Induction*

An epidemic of pulmonary hypertension occurred in Austria, the Federal Republic of Germany, and Switzerland starting in 1967 and lasting until 1972. There was a geographic and temporal relation to the marketing of the drug aminorex fumarate.[78,79] Pulmonary hypertension developed in 1% to 2% of those persons who had taken aminorex. Seventy-one of 92 patients studied from 1967 to 1973 gave a positive history of aminorex intake preceding the onset of their symptoms. Aminorex resembles epinephrine and amphetamine in chemical structure and was used as an appetite suppressant. Histologic examination of the pulmonary arteries revealed changes ranging from medial hypertrophy to the development of plexiform lesions. Attempts to duplicate the plexogenic pulmonary arteriopathy in animals after chronic administration have failed, but marked and transient increases in pulmonary arterial pressure and pulmonary arterial resistance have occurred after the acute administration.

Another anorectic drug that has been implicated as a causative agent of pulmonary hypertension is fenfluramine.[80,81] Fenfluramine is a phenylethylamine, not chemically related to the aminooxazoline aminorex. A postulated mechanism of fenfluramine-induced pulmonary hypertension is an increased pulmonary vascular resistance. Fenfluramine depletes 5-hydroxytryptophan stores, resulting in an increase in serotonin which leads to pulmonary arteriolar and venous vasoconstriction.

Propylhexedrine hydrochloride is a third sympathomimetic that has been suggested to cause an elevated pulmonary arterial pressure.[82] Although a definitive causal relationship has not been established, the patient reportedly had taken the drug as an anorectic for a period of 8 years. In patients with intravenous propylhexedrine abuse, postmortem examinations have demonstrated right ventricular hypertrophy and evidence of pulmonary hypertension.

Intravenous pentazocine abuse has resulted in pulmonary hypertension. Open-lung biopsies have demonstrated areas of alveolar destruction, intravascular and perivascular granulomas, and fibrosis. Pulmonary vascular granulomatosis is thought to be secondary to microembolization of the tablet fillers, cellulose or talc.[56,57]

Esophageal sclerotherapy has been associated with pulmonary hypertension.[83,84] Sodium morrhuate and sodium tetradecyl sulfate are used to control variceal hemorrhaging. These agents can enter the systemic circulation when administered endoscopically. Two patients have been reported recently who experienced dyspnea and hypoxemia and had chest x-ray findings indicative of pulmonary edema after sclerotherapy. These agents have caused a 2- to 2½-fold increase in pulmonary arterial pressure from baseline in a small number of patients. In addition, pulmonary hypertension has been demonstrated in sheep after the administration of these agents. A possible mechanism involves the mediation of prostaglandins because the response was ablated when the sheep were pretreated with indomethacin.

Hydralazine has been implicated in causing pulmonary hypertension.[85] Ironically, as will be discussed later, this drug is used in the treatment of pulmonary hypertension. The patient reportedly had signs and symptoms consistent with systemic lupus erythematosus. The elevated pulmonary arterial pressure was thought to be secondary to the drug-induced lupus syndrome.

Oral contraceptive agents have been associated with pulmonary hypertension.[86] In a review of six patients who developed pulmonary hypertension while taking oral contraceptives from 6 months to 5 years, three patients may have had potential predisposing factors. One patient had SLE, one patient had a brother who died at the age of 14 years from primary pulmonary hypertension, and a third patient had mildly elevated pulmonary arterial pressures after closure of a patent ductus arteriosus. None of the patients had evidence of thromboembolic events. Intimal proliferation of the pulmonary arterial tree was noted on autopsies of three patients who died. There have been previous reports of vascular lesions developing in the pulmonary artery in association with the administration of female reproductive steroids. The role of female hormones has also been alluded to in cases of pulmonary hypertension caused by pregnancy as will be discussed later.

Two recent case reports have implicated mitomycin C[87] and protamine[88] as etiologic agents of pulmonary hypertension. Pulmonary toxicity of mitomycin C can present as acute interstitial pneumonitis, interstitial fibrosis, and diffuse alveolar damage. The postulated mechanism of mitomycin C–induced pulmonary hypertension is intercapillary thrombi and endothelial proliferation of the pulmonary artery. The endothelial changes are thought to be the result of an immunologic phenomenon. Protamine-induced pulmonary hypertension may be mediated by prostaglandins. Thromboxane $B_2$ reportedly increased tenfold after the acute administration of protamine. There was an elevation in 6-ketoprostaglandin $1\alpha$ as well, indicative of a possible compensatory vasodilatory response.

**Diet**

Pulmonary hypertension developed in patients after the ingestion of tainted rapeseed oil that was illegally sold for cooking oil in Spain.[89,90] Exposure to toxic levels of oleoanilide in the rapeseed oil led to fever, dyspnea, cough, skin rash, a spectrum of gastric and neurologic symptoms, eosinophilia, and interstitial pneumonitis. Right ventricular enlargement and elevated pulmonary arterial pressures developed. The alkaloid fulvine, found in bush tea (*Crotalaria fulva*), is believed to be the cause of pulmonary veno-occlusive disease in patients in the West Indies. Another alkaloid, monocrotaline, extracted from the seeds of the shrub *Crotalaria spectabilis*, has produced pulmonary hypertension in various animal species. Monocrotaline is converted by the liver to dehydromonocrotaline. It is this compound that is responsible for the development of medial hypertrophy of the small pulmonary arteries, interstitial fibrosis, and plexiform lesions. The intravenous administration of monocrotaline to rats resulted in alterations in pulmonary arterial smooth muscle responsiveness.[91] Early in the development of pulmonary hypertension, the pulmonary arterial vessels exhibited enhanced responsiveness to contractile agonists, but as the pulmonary hypertension progressed, the responsiveness to those agonists decreased. The pulmonary arterial smooth muscle also showed a decreased responsiveness to vasorelaxants. Additional evidence for diet-induced pulmonary hypertension comes from a case report of the disease being produced in a Tanzanian patient who consumed an herbal remedy that contained the seeds of *Crotalaria laburnoides*.[15]

### *Portal Hypertension and Liver Disease*

Pulmonary hypertension is seen in less than 1% of the patients with portal hypertension.[92,93] In most cases, the interval between the diagnosis of portal hypertension and the first manifestation of pulmonary hypertension ranges from 2 to 15 years. Portal–systemic shunting may increase the risk of developing pulmonary hypertension.[93–95] Histologic findings of the pulmonary vasculature include medial hypertrophy, concentric-intimal proliferation, and plexiform lesions affecting the small pulmonary arteries. One postulated mechanism is thromboembolism to the lungs from the portal, splenic, or mesenteric venous system through the portacaval shunt. A second proposed mechanism is the high blood flow resulting from an increased cardiac output associated with portal hypertension and cirrhosis. In addition, the development of pulmonary hypertension in chronic liver disease may be mediated by a humoral substance.[96,97] A vasoconstrictor agent normally destroyed by a functioning liver may be responsible for the increase in pulmonary vascular resistance. Examples of such a substance include prostaglandin $F_2$ or serotonin. Serotonin escapes hepatic inactivation because of overproduction or metastases beyond the liver in the carcinoid syndrome and causes pulmonary vasoconstriction.[92] In addition to portal hypertension and cirrhosis,[98–99] pulmonary hypertension has been associated with hepatocarcinoma,[100] chronic active hepatitis,[101] and portal vein thrombosis.[102–103]

### *Pregnancy*

Pulmonary hypertension has developed with pregnancy and the immediate postpartum period.[104] Pregnancy can exacerbate pulmonary hypertension, but it is not well understood if the pregnant state can cause pulmonary hypertension. The disease may initially manifest during pregnancy secondary to the hemodynamic alterations that occur in response to pregnancy. Female hormones are thought to play a role, but their exact part in the development of pulmonary hypertension is unknown.

Plasma volume increases progressively throughout pregnancy until about the 34th week.[105] The blood volume may exceed that of a nonpregnant woman by 40%. Cardiac output averages 7 L/min secondary to a rise in stroke volume and an increase in heart rate.[106] Pregnancy in a normal patient generates a marginal increase in pulmonary arterial pressure because the pulmonary vasculature is able to accommodate the increase in blood flow. In patients with pulmonary hypertension, resulting from a high pulmonary vascular resistance, there is no way to compensate for the increase in volume. Excessive pulmonary arterial pressures then develop.

Late in pregnancy, cardiac output may diminish secondary to the pressure put on the vena cava and aorta by the uterus. At delivery, this pressure is removed and cardiovascular collapse may occur secondary to a sudden increase in venous return and subsequent right ventricular dilatation and failure. This postpartum sudden change in blood flow is also influenced by blood being delivered to the maternal circulation by uterine contractions. The maternal mortality is about 38%, occurring from the third month of pregnancy to 14 days postpartum.[105]

### *Familial Trait*

Fourteen families with 52 patients who had pulmonary hypertension have been reported in the North American literature.[107] Recently, a family with six deaths attributable to the disease in two generations was reported. An autosomal dominant pattern has been identified with a female-to-male predominance of 2:1. There seems to be a variable expression of the gene, ranging from infrequent within some families to widely differing frequencies in others. A wide range of survival has been seen, from sudden death to 27 years.

### *Postcapillary Causes*

As mentioned previously, pulmonary arterial pressure can increase in response to postcapillary or pulmonary venous pressure elevations. An increase in pulmonary venous pressure can occur with aortic valve disease, left ventricular failure, and mitral valve disease. Also, elevated left atrial pressures and pulmonary venous obstruction can lead to a passive increase in pulmonary arterial pressure.

Severe pulmonary hypertension in aortic stenosis is rare. A review of 151 cases revealed severe pulmonary hypertension (pulmonary arterial systolic pressure ≥60 mm Hg) in 17 patients.[108] The incidence of moderate pulmonary hypertension (pulmonary arterial systolic pressure = 45 mm Hg) in patients with symptomatic aortic stenosis has been reported to be 4%.[109] When pulmonary hypertension is present in association with aortic stenosis, it may reflect associated mitral valve disease, poor left ventricular function, or preexisting pulmonary disease, although isolated cases can occur.

One of the common causes of increased pulmonary venous pressure is mitral stenosis. If the pulmonary artery-to-left atrial pressure gradient exceeds 12 mm Hg mitral valve disease should be suspected.[4] In certain patients the pulmonary arterial pressures increase more than proportionally to the increased pulmonary venous pressure. This elevation in pulmonary arterial pressure is known as *reactive pulmonary hypertension*. It is suggested that the reason the pulmonary arterial pressure increases beyond what is seen in passive hypertension is the decreased vascular reactivity of the precapillary vessels. The decrease in reactivity is due to structural changes of medial hypertrophy and intimal proliferation.[110]

The left atrial pressure can rise independently of any changes in the aortic or mitral valve or in the left ventricle. This can occur in diseases that mimic mitral stenosis such as atrial myxoma or atrial thrombus. Cardiac myxomas occur most frequently in the atria, with involvement being three times more prevalent in the left than the right.[111] When the myxoma is located in the left atrium the left atrial pressure is elevated. This increased pressure is transmitted retrograde through the pulmonary vascular system to produce pulmonary arterial hypertension. The tumor itself may cause obstruction of blood flow or it may interfere with the function of the mitral valve leaflets. Myxoma of the right atrium can produce pulmonary hypertension secondary to the production of tumor emboli that result in obstruction of the pulmonary vascular bed.

Obstruction of the pulmonary vascular bed results in the development of pulmonary hypertension. This is the mechanism in pulmonary veno-occlusive disease.[12–14] Pulmonary veno-occlusive disease is one of three pathologic categories of primary pulmonary hypertension (the other two being plexogenic pulmonary arteriopathy and recurrent pulmonary thromboembolism). This entity is a rare cause of pulmonary hypertension. Fewer than three dozen cases have been reported. Pulmonary veno-occlusive disease is usually a disease of younger people but cases have been reported in middle-aged and elderly patients.[112] A viral cause and an immunologic cause have been proposed but the definitive etiologic factor is not known.[113] Fibrous narrowing or occlusion of the pulmonary veins leads to the obstruction of pulmonary blood flow and the development of pulmonary arterial hypertension. As is found in patients with mitral valve disease, reactive pulmonary hypertension occurs in pulmonary veno-occlusive disease.[4]

### *Catecholamines*

Norepinephrine increases pulmonary vascular resistance through α-adrenergic stimulation. The endothelial cell of the pulmonary vasculature is responsible for inactivation of norepinephrine. The normal lung extracts 17% to 30% of the norepinephrine that passes through its circulation.[26] Patients with pulmonary hypertension lack this ability to metabolize norepinephrine in the pulmonary vasculature, thereby creating elevated norepinephrine blood levels.[114,115] Baseline pulmonary and radial arterial norepinephrine concentrations correlated with pulmonary vascular resistance, pulmonary arterial pressure, and the pulmonary arterial–pulmonary capillary wedge pressure difference.

Pharmacologic reductions in pulmonary vascular resistance do not restore the pulmonary extraction of norepinephrine. What is not known is whether this pulmonary inactivation of norepinephrine is the cause of the vasoconstriction or a result of endothelial cell dysfunction from vascular remodeling. If the latter is correct, are the increased norepinephrine concentrations leading to further damage to the pulmonary vasculature?

Although it has not been confirmed, an increased serum copper level has been linked to the sympathetic nervous system and pulmonary hypertension.[116] The intravenous infusion of copper sulfate in sheep resulted in an increase in pulmonary vascular resistance which was inhibited by α-adrenergic blockade. In seven patients with pulmonary hypertension, the mean serum copper level was 206 μg/dL as compared with 131 μg/dL in normal people. Dopamine β-hydroxylase is a copper-dependent enzyme that acts as a catalyst in the formation of norepinephrine from dopamine. Theoretically, elevated serum copper should potentiate the activity of this enzyme, leading to an increased synthesis of norepinephrine and the development of pulmonary vasoconstriction and pulmonary hypertension.

### *Sepsis*

Pulmonary hypertension can develop in patients with sepsis. Sepsis was associated with a significant degree of resistance to flow in the pulmonary circulation in 22 of 37 septic patients.[117] The presence of pulmonary hypertension was unrelated to oxygen saturation or acid–base imbalance. Various mechanisms have been proposed to explain the pulmonary vasoconstriction seen in patients with severe bacterial infections, including the release of vasoactive amines and the stimulation of the autonomic nervous system. Pulmonary vascular embolization with platelet, leukocyte, or fibrin microemboli may be another factor.[4]

### *Sickle Cell Disease*

Pulmonary hypertension is one of the cardiovascular complications of sickle cell anemia.[4,11] The sickling of a red blood cell causes it to become rigid and results in obstruction

**Table 16.3** Causes of/Associations With Pulmonary Hypertension

I. Precapillary
- A. Hypoxia/hypoxemia
  1. Pulmonary diseases with ventilation complications
  2. Central hypoventilation disorders
  3. Congenital heart disease
  4. Autoimmune diseases
  5. Neuromuscular diseases
  6. Pulmonary embolism
  7. Hematologic disease
  8. High altitude
  9. Cystic fibrosis
- B. Obstruction of pulmonary vascular bed
  1. Pulmonary embolism
  2. Autoimmune diseases
  3. Parasitic disease
  4. Anatomic restriction
- C. Familial trait
- D. Pregnancy
- E. Diet
- F. Drugs
- G. Liver disease/portal hypertension
- H. Congenital heart disease
- I. Hematologic disease
- J. Catecholamines
- K. Sepsis

II. Postcapillary
- A. Pulmonary venous obstruction
- B. Mitral valve disease
- C. Aortic valve disease
- D. Left ventricular failure
- E. Elevated left atrial pressure

of capillary blood flow. Hypoxemia, secondary to a decreased red blood cell–oxygen affinity, may lead to pulmonary vascular vasoconstriction. The deoxygenation can also increase blood viscosity. These three manifestations of sickle cell disease may all contribute to the development of pulmonary hypertension in these patients.

Table 16.3 provides an overview of the conditions that have been associated with pulmonary hypertension.

## Clinical Presentation

### *Symptoms*

Patients do not seek medical attention until after the early stages of pulmonary hypertension. The pulmonary arterial pressure is usually about two times normal before symptoms appear. The onset of symptoms is insidious, but progression can be rapid. The most common chief complaints of the patient with pulmonary hypertension are dyspnea, especially with exertion, and fatigue. These are associated with the reduction in cardiac output. Paroxysmal nocturnal dyspnea and orthopnea are not experienced unless pulmonary venous congestion is also involved. Dizziness and syncope occur secondary to dysrhythmias or to cerebral hypoperfusion. Cerebral hypoperfusion has also been attributed to symptoms of anxiety, depression, agitation, and psychosis. Both bradyarrhythmias and ventricular tachyarrhythmias with palpitations have been described. Among 101 patients with primary pulmonary hypertension, 27 patients had a total of 34 types of arrhythmias.[118] The most common, representing 70% of the total, were sinus tachycardia, sinus bradycardia, and first-degree atrioventricular block. One can experience angina or atypical chest pain. The chest pain may result from ischemia of the right ventricular subendocardium or from the stretching of the adventitia of the pulmonary artery; however, these two hypotheses have been disputed when it was found that there were no differences between the frequency and type of chest pain in patients with normal pulmonary pressures and those with varying degrees of pulmonary hypertension.[119] An unproductive cough may develop and the patient may develop hoarseness believed to be caused by the compression of the left recurrent laryngeal nerve by the dilated pulmonary artery.[120] This cardiovocal syndrome is referred to as Ortner's syndrome.[121] With chronic pulmonary hypertension, symptoms of right heart failure and possibly left heart failure develop. In the later stages, cyanosis and hemoptysis can occur.

### *Physical Examination*

The physical examination reveals an increased jugular venous distension with a giant "a" wave reflecting a high right ventricular filling pressure. As the disease progresses to the development of tricuspid regurgitation, a "v" wave may be noted. The carotid pulse is normal or depressed, indicating a low cardiac output. A right ventricular, left parasternal heave is present, implying high right ventricular outflow impedance or right ventricular hypertrophy. Peripheral edema occurs secondary to venous congestion. With right ventricular failure, an enlarged liver may be palpable. Ascites and jaundice may be noted with hepatic congestion. In addition, a hepatojugular reflex may be elicited.

What is heard on auscultation of the lungs depends on the underlying etiology of the pulmonary hypertension. In primary pulmonary hypertension the lungs are usually clear, but the respiratory rate is increased. On cardiac auscultation, a split second heart sound is heard with a prominent pulmonic component. At the second left intercostal space an early systolic ejection click is present followed by a pulmonic ejection murmur. When the pulmonary pressure approaches the systemic pressure, an early diastolic murmur of pulmonic regurgitation or insufficiency is heard. Right-sided third and fourth heart sounds are noted. With severe pulmonary hypertension, a holosystolic murmur implies tricuspid regurgitation.

### *Chest Roentgenogram*

The findings on a chest x-ray vary depending on the etiology of the pulmonary hypertension. Increased pulmonary arterial pressure is reflected by a dilated pulmonary arterial trunk with constricted smaller arteries giving the appearance of a pruned vascular tree. The right descending pulmonary artery is greater than 16 mm. On the left lateral projection, a greater than 16- to 18-mm (normal and diseased parenchyma, respectively) width of the left descending pulmonary artery also signifies elevated pressures.[122,123] The mean pulmonary arterial pressure is correlated with the hilar thoracic index and the hilar width. A hilar thoracic index of 36% is associated with a mean pulmonary arterial pressure greater than 20 mm Hg.[124] The cardiothoracic ratio may also be increased in pulmonary hypertension, but it is more indicative of right heart failure rather than an elevated pulmonary arterial pressure.[125] The chest x-ray demonstrates right ventricular enlargement. If the pulmonary hypertension is severe or of long duration, right atrial enlargement secondary to triscuspid regurgitation is noted. The chest x-ray is a useful tool to detect the presence or absence of pulmonary hypertension, although the accuracy of quantifying the elevated pressure is not good.

### *Electrocardiogram*

The ECG findings of pulmonary hypertension are those indicative of right ventricular hypertrophy and right axis deviation.[126] Symmetric and tall "p" waves greater than 2.5 mm denote right atrial hypertrophy seen in severe and advanced cases. The ECG is a specific instrument in detecting right ventricular hypertrophy, but it lacks sensitivity. It cannot detect mild to moderate right ventricular hypertrophy in earlier stages of pulmonary hypertension.

### *Echocardiogram*

Various echocardiographic techniques are utilized to assess the presence of pulmonary hypertension. These procedures are used to evaluate cardiac function and to detect changes in cardiac dimensions such as chamber size and the interventricular septum. They are also used in evaluation of the function of the pulmonic, mitral, and tricuspid valves. Continuous-wave echocardiography is capable of measuring high blood flow velocities.[127] In addition to the continuous-wave echocardiogram, other ultrasound techniques that are used include the M-mode echocardiogram,[128] two-dimensional echo,[129] and the pulsed Doppler echocardiogram.[130] The echocardiogram is not a sensitive procedure, but it is rather specific.[131]

Attempts are being made to quantify the degree of pulmonary pressure elevation by these noninvasive ultrasound tests. Using the two-dimensional echo, the right ventricular systolic pressure ranged from 60 to 118 mm Hg when the ventricular septum was straight or curved toward the left ventricle at end systole.[132] The pulsed Doppler method resulted in a correlation between the right ventricular preejection period/acceleration time index ratio and pulmonary arterial pressure.[130] Pulmonary arterial pressure and total pulmonary vascular resistance were associated with measurements of pulmonary artery peak flow and the acceleration time index using pulsed Doppler echocardiography.[133] Continuous-wave echocardiography has related the pulmonary regurgitant flow velocity to the pulmonary arterial pressure.[127,134] It also may provide a noninvasive estimate of the pulmonary arterial systolic pressure from calculations of the right ventricular-to-right atrial pressure gradient. In addition, tricuspid regurgitation can be identified, especially when the pulmonary arterial pressure exceeds 50 mm Hg.

Echocardiography is useful in combination with the left ventricular systolic time interval in evaluating patients with pulmonary hypertension.[135] This provides an estimate of the overall cardiac–cardiovascular performance of which the pulmonary vascular resistance is probably a major determinant.

Echocardiography is a noninvasive tool that can be utilized for the initial evaluation of pulmonary hypertension. It is best used for qualitative purposes rather than quantitative determinations of the pulmonary arterial pressures. Echocardiography may be employed to follow a clinical course and there is a potential for its use in monitoring patients' response to therapy.[136]

### *Heart Catheterization and Angiography*

The definitive diagnosis of pulmonary hypertension cannot be made without confirming the elevation of the pulmonary arterial pressure. This can be validated by a right heart catheterization or through the insertion of a Swan–Ganz catheter. The information obtained from these procedures includes measurements of right atrial pressure, right ventricular pressure, pulmonary arterial pressure, and pulmonary capillary wedge pressure. Cardiac output can also be determined. The resistance of the pulmonary vasculature is calculated from the pressure and flow data obtained by established relationships as indicated in Table 16.4. Table 16.5 provides normal hemodynamic values of the cardiopulmonary system.

Pulmonary capillary wedge pressure (PCWP) is a reflection of the left ventricular end-diastolic pressure, provided there is no pulmonary venous obstruction or left atrial or mitral valve disease. When the PCWP value is questionable, a left heart catheterization can evaluate the left-sided functions.

Radionuclide angiography is utilized to assess chamber size and function, valvular function, and vessel abnormalities. It can be used to detect the presence of shunts responsible for an increased flow. Right heart function is assessed by the radionuclide techniques of gated blood pool scanning, first-pass imaging, and thallium-201 scanning.[18]

The information obtained from a heart catheterization and angiography is helpful in determining an etiology for the pulmonary hypertension. An elevation of the PCWP in association with an increased pulmonary arterial pressure is evidence for the existence of a secondary cause of pulmonary hypertension. An elevated PCWP and left ventricular end-diastolic pressure with an increased pulmonary arterial pressure is suggestive of pulmonary hypertension caused by left ventricular dysfunction. A normal left ventricular end-diastolic pressure with an increased PCWP and pulmonary arterial pressure illustrates the cause of pulmonary hypertension as being related to the mitral valve, the left atrium, or the pulmonary venous system. In pulmonary veno-occlusive disease the pulmonary arterial pressure is elevated with an increased, decreased, or normal PCWP. Difficulty in wedging the catheter suggests the presence of pulmonary veno-occlusive disease.[112] The pulmonary arterial pressure is increased in primary pulmonary hypertension, but the PCWP is normal.

The degree of elevation of pressures in the right side of the heart reflects the severity of the disease. Right heart chamber pressures are usually not elevated in the early stages of pulmonary hypertension. Initial catheterizations demonstrate elevated pressures, however, because patients usually

**Table 16.4** Hemodynamic Relationships Used in the Evaluation of Pulmonary Hypertension

| | |
|---|---|
| $CI = CO/BSA$ | $L/min/m^2$ |
| $SVI = CI/HR$ | $mL/m^2$ |
| $PVR = \frac{MPAP - PCWP}{CO} \times 80$ | $dynes\text{-}s\text{-}cm^{-5}$ |
| $SVR = \frac{MAP - MRAP}{CO} \times 80$ | $dynes\text{-}s\text{-}cm^{-5}$ |
| $TPR = \frac{MPAP}{CO} \times 80$ | $dynes\text{-}s\text{-}cm^{-5}$ |
| $LVSWI = \frac{(MAP - PCWP) \times CI \times 0.0136}{HR}$ | $g\text{-}m/m^2$ |
| $RVSWI = \frac{(MPAP - MRAP) \times CI \times 0.0136}{HR}$ | $g\text{-}m/m^2$ |

CI = cardiac index
CO = cardiac output
BSA = body surface area
SVI = stroke volume index
HR = heart rate
PVR = pulmonary vascular resistance
MPAP = mean pulmonary arterial pressure
PCWP = pulmonary capillary wedge pressure
SVR = systemic vascular resistance
MAP = mean arterial pressure
MRAP = mean right arterial pressure
TPR = total pulmonary vascular resistance
LVSWI = left ventricular stroke work index
RVSWI = right ventricular stroke work index

do not seek medical attention until symptoms are present, which is not until the later stages of development. Severe or chronic pulmonary hypertension is reflected by increased right ventricular and right atrial pressures. The prolonged retrograde pressure buildup can contribute to tricuspid regurgitation, which is suspected with high right atrial pressures and can be diagnosed by angiography.

Radiopaque materials are used in pulmonary angiography to visualize the pulmonary vasculature. Pulmonary angiography is used to detect pulmonary emboli and congenital or acquired lesions of the pulmonary vessels. In pulmonary hypertension, pulmonary angiography demonstrates a dilated pulmonary trunk and main branches with marked tapering of peripheral small arteries. Angiography is not without risk in patients with pulmonary hypertension, especially in those patients with high pulmonary arterial pressures. Deaths have been reported after angiography in patients with severe pulmonary hypertension.[9] To minimize complications it is recommended to use selective instead of complete angiography and to inject a small quantity (5–10 mL) of contrast medium into the pulmonary artery.

### *Lung Biopsy*

The role of the lung biopsy in pulmonary hypertension is to determine the nature and the extent of pulmonary vascular changes. In primary pulmonary hypertension, the main reason a lung biopsy is undertaken is to try to establish a cause by identifying the types of vascular structural change. The determination of the severity of the structural changes is usually the motive for the lung biopsy in patients with secondary pulmonary hypertension.

The procedure must be an open-lung biopsy, which carries the added risk of anesthesia.[137,138] The specimens obtained from a needle biopsy or transbronchial biopsy are too small and do not contain enough vessels to be of value. The biopsy specimen should be 2.5 × 2.0 × 1.0 cm in an adult. In most instances, a specimen of this size is representative of the lung as a whole. Multiple biopsy sites are therefore usually not necessary. There are instances in which the pulmonary pathology may be different in various areas of the lung, however. The fear of employing the lung biopsy in these cases is that a single biopsy may yield misleading or incomplete information concerning the pulmonary vascular bed as a whole.

Pulmonary vascular damage can be assessed by identifying the involved lesions and estimating the number and size of the vessels affected. Vessel wall damage ranges from reversible lesions, such as medial hypertrophy and arteriole muscularization, to those lesions associated with a poor prognosis, such as fibrinoid necrosis and the plexiform lesion. It is not uncommon to find a combination of lesions present in the biopsy specimen.

**Table 16.5** Normal Hemodynamic Values (at Rest) of the Cardiopulmonary Circulatory System

| | |
|---|---|
| MAP | 80–100 mm Hg |
| MPAP | 12–15 mm Hg |
| PAP | 15–30/4–12 mm Hg |
| RAP | 2–5 mm Hg |
| RVP | 15–30/0–8 mm Hg |
| MLAP | 2–12 mm Hg |
| LVP | 90–140/5–12 mm Hg peak-systolic/ end-diastolic |
| PCWP | 8–12 mm Hg |
| CI | 2.5–4.5 L/min/m$^2$ |
| SVI | 30–50 mL/min |
| SVR | 800–1,200 dynes-s-cm$^{-5}$ |
| PVR | 20–120 dynes-s-cm$^{-5}$ (< 250 dynes-s-cm$^{-5}$) |
| TPR | 205 dynes-s-cm$^{-5}$ |
| LVSWI | 44–68 g-m/m$^2$ |
| RVSWI | 4–8 g-m/m$^2$ |

MAP = mean arterial pressure
MPAP = mean pulmonary arterial pressure
PAP = pulmonary arterial pressure
RAP = right atrial pressure
RVP = right ventricular pressure
MLAP = mean left atrial pressure
LVP = left ventricular pressure
PCWP = pulmonary capillary wedge pressure
CI = cardiac index
SVI = stroke volume index
SVR = systemic vascular resistance
PVR = pulmonary vascular resistance
TPR = total pulmonary vascular resistance
LVSWI = left ventricular stroke work index
RVSWI = right ventricular stroke work index

## Prognosis

Patients with primary pulmonary hypertension usually have a poor prognosis. The average life span is about 3 years after the onset of symptoms, but the range is a few months to 15 to 20 years.[9,11] There are a few reports of spontaneous regression.[139] The cause of death in the majority of cases is right heart failure. In a study of 80 cases from the Mayo Clinic, sudden death occurred in 45% of the patients with the plexogenic subtype of primary pulmonary hypertension.[16] This was 2.5 times more frequent than those cases with an underlying thromboembolic component to their disease. Mortality and survival have been associated with physiologic prognostic indicators. In one study, the best single predictor of survival was the stroke volume index.[140] Poor prognosis was associated with a stroke volume index less than 17 mL/beat/m$^2$. In the same study, the best measured predictor of survival was the right atrial pressure. Poor prognosis was associated with a right atrial pressure greater than 10 mm Hg. Other parameters were significantly different between survivors and nonsurvivors, including, for the nonsurvivors, lower cardiac index, higher systemic resistance, and higher pulmonary vascular resistance. There was no significant difference in pulmonary arterial pressure between the two groups. A comparison of survivors and nonsurvivors in 113 cases of primary pulmonary hypertension resulted in a significantly lower cardiac index, right ventricular work index, and $Pa_{O_2}$ in those patients who died.[141] Total pulmonary vascular resistance was significantly higher in the nonsurvivors. In a retrospective analysis of 34 cases, initial hemodynamic values were evaluated in relation to survival time.[142] Cardiac output was directly related to survival. The longer the survival, the lower were the pulmonary arterial resistance, systemic vascular resistance, and right ventricular end-diastolic pressure. In all these reports the degree of pulmonary arterial pressure elevation was not a prognostic indicator.

## Treatment

It is beyond the scope of this chapter to discuss the current therapeutic alternatives for the varied causes of secondary pulmonary hypertension. In these conditions therapy is aimed at correction of the underlying cause and at palliation of the symptoms associated with pulmonary hypertension.[143] This section is directed specifically at the treatment of primary pulmonary hypertension.

The therapeutic endpoint of pulmonary hypertension has been in question.[144] Because pulmonary hypertension is defined as an elevated pulmonary arterial pressure, should treatment be directed at its reduction? Recall that an elevated pulmonary arterial pressure was not considered a useful prognostic indicator. Instead of focusing on pulmonary pressures should therapy be directed at those parameters that have been significantly different in the nonsurviving population? These questions remain unanswered as evident in the variable indices used to evaluate therapeutic efficacy.

If the reduction in pulmonary vascular resistance is used as a guide to therapy, care must be taken to assess that the reduction was due to pulmonary vascular dilatation rather than a passive reduction secondary to additional recruitment of pulmonary vessels as a result of an increased pulmonary blood flow.[145] A reduction in pulmonary driving force across the vascular bed is reflective of vasodilatation. An ideal response has been suggested to be an increase in cardiac output, a decrease in pulmonary vascular resistance to a greater magnitude than a fall in systemic vascular resistance, and a fall in pulmonary arterial pressure. The increase in cardiac output with a fall in systemic vascular resistance maintains systemic blood pressure.

Another concern in monitoring therapeutic effect is the spontaneous variabilities in the pulmonary arterial pressure and the pulmonary resistance in patients with primary pulmonary hypertension. Patients with the highest total pulmonary resistance have the most variation. It has been suggested that to determine a drug effect in a patient, a mean reduction in pulmonary resistance of 36% or a mean reduction in pulmonary arterial pressure of 22% is required.[146]

Therapeutic agents should be assessed by their acute administration in a controlled environment such as a cardiac catheterization laboratory. This is necessary not only to quantify the pharmacodynamic response, but to be able to provide adequate patient care in the event of a drug-induced adverse effect. It must be emphasized that a response to one drug does not necessarily predict the response to another.

Similarly, the acute effects do not reflect the results of chronic therapy. Changes in response during chronic therapy may result from the progression of disease or the development of tolerance. In a review of 117 patients with primary pulmonary hypertension, 33 of 53 patients benefited from chronic vasodilator treatment (3 months or longer) when pulmonary vascular resistance was lowered acutely by 33% or more.[39] Chronic treatment was of benefit to only 4 of 64 patients having acute reductions in resistance less than 30%. Although patients have benefited from chronic vasodilator therapy, overall outcome has not been affected by long-term vasodilator therapy.[147]

In addition to the correction of hemodynamic parameters, consideration should be given to the alleviation of clinical symptoms in the patient. As the presenting symptom is commonly dyspnea on exertion, the patient's response should be assessed during exercise as well as at rest.

Other ideal objectives of therapy are the eventual regression of right ventricular hypertrophy and the reversal of pulmonary vascular structural changes. Ultimately, therapeutic interventions should have a positive impact on survival.

## *Vasodilator Agents*

As an extrapolation from the therapy of systemic hypertension and the afterload reduction of left heart failure, the vasodilator class of drugs is used most frequently.[148] An important element of vasodilator therapy is the assumption that vasoconstriction is a component of pulmonary hypertension. The experiential use of vasodilators in this disease state consists mostly of anecdotal reports.

The pharmacodynamic response to these drugs is extremely variable. Outcomes differ widely among drugs as well as within patients. The variability in treatment results probably occurs for a number of reasons. The differing aspects of patients include age, etiologic factors of pulmonary hypertension, severity of disease, degree of pulmonary vascular remodeling, and pulmonary vascular reactivity. In addition, as previously discussed, the therapeutic endpoint determines success or failure of an agent.

Vasodilator drugs are known to cause deleterious effects in patients with pulmonary hypertension.[145] If systemic vascular resistance is reduced without an increase in pulmonary blood flow, cardiac output declines with a resultant decrease in systemic blood pressure. Systemic hypotension can lead to myocardial ischemic damage, resulting in a further reduction in cardiac output. It can also contribute to the development of arrhythmias and right ventricular failure. Other mechanisms that have been implicated in precipitating right heart failure are an exacerbation of pulmonary hypertension, salt and water retention, and negative inotropicity.

The vasodilator agents may augment pulmonary hypertension by causing a reflex sympathetic stimulation leading to an increase in cardiac output. An increase in blood flow in an unreactive pulmonary vascular bed will worsen existing pulmonary hypertension.

The vasodilatation of pulmonary vessels in poorly ventilated areas of the lung can lead to hypoxemia. Usually the increase in cardiac output compensates for this increased ventilation/perfusion mismatch; however, if there is no increase in cardiac output a clinically evident hypoxemia may develop. Hypoxemia may also develop in patients with pulmonary hypertension associated with congenital disease. Vasodilators may increase a right-to-left intracardiac shunt, resulting in a decrease in blood oxygenation. Patients with long-standing pulmonary hypertension with elevated right atrial pressures can develop hypoxemia as a result of the opening of a patent foramen ovale.

The choice of vasodilator is basically left to trial and error. It depends on the beneficial response and the adverse effects that are exhibited. Patient convenience and compliance constitute a third consideration in the selection process.

### Acetylcholine

Acetylcholine was one of the first agents used as a vasodilator for the treatment of pulmonary hypertension. As acetylcholine is rapidly hydrolyzed by acetylcholinesterase and butyrylcholinesterase, it has to be administered directly into the pulmonary artery for effect. The disadvantage is the need for pulmonary artery catheterization. But the advantage is a lack of systemic vasodilation because of its rapid metabolism. Acetylcholine has been used to reduce pulmonary arterial pressure and pulmonary vascular resistance in doses of 0.5–8 mg/min.[16] The response has been variable and transient. Patients may respond to a greater degree if their pressure elevation is moderate, rather than normal or high. The lack of response with high pressures may be reflective of severe disease with loss of vascular reactivity. The effect is more pronounced with hypoxia-induced pulmonary hypertension. Acetylcholine has a potential role in the acute testing of vascular reactivity. But it is impractical for treatment because of its required route of administration secondary to its degradation pattern.

### $\alpha$-Adrenergic Antagonists

***Tolazoline*** The use of tolazoline was included in the first description of primary pulmonary hypertension by Dresdale et al.[8] Trials with the drug used intravenous doses from 10 to 75 mg with variable results.[144] Tolazoline has also been used orally but with little or no success.[149] The limitations of tolazoline are its short duration of action and its inconvenience for long-term therapy. It also causes dilatation of the systemic vascular system.

***Phentolamine*** Phentolamine is a more potent $\alpha$-adrenergic blocking agent than tolazoline.[10] As with tolazoline, variable responses to phentolamine have been reported. Minimal hemodynamic effects at rest, but symptomatic improvement with a marked increase in exercise tolerance, have been noted. Response has also been seen after 7 months of oral therapy with 50 mg every 3 hours while awake.[150] Phentolamine 0.3 mg/min intravenously was assessed in three patients.[151] A favorable response was seen in two patients with a reduction in pulmonary arterial pressure and resistance and an increase in cardiac output. In the third patient pulmonary vascular resistance increased with a subsequent reduction in cardiac output. This patient presumably was at a later stage in the disease process and therefore lacked pulmonary vascular reactivity.

Orthostatic hypotension is a common side effect. Phentolamine and tolazoline can cause a cardiac stimulation that is greater than a reflex response to systemic vasodilation.[152,153]

It is associated with an increased sympathetic stimulation resulting in a rapid decline of clinical status. Chest tightness, flushing, increased dyspnea, arrhythmias, and elevations in pulmonary arterial pressure and heart rate occur.

### β-Adrenergic Agonists: Isoproterenol

The administration of isoproterenol has produced both beneficial and unfavorable results. Favorable acute hemodynamic changes after intravenous or intrapulmonary artery administration were maintained with sublingual therapy for 2 to 6 years.[153–156] As the duration of isoproterenol's action is brief, administration of doses ranging from 5 to 20 mg every 1½ to 2 hours may be required. With chronic therapy, evidence exists for the progression of disease despite continued beneficial symptomatic relief.[155] After administration of isoproterenol 2 μg/min into the pulmonary artery, pulmonary arterial pressure rose 40% in one patient with a 52% increase in cardiac output.[157] Aggravation of clinical symptoms along with angina resulted. The patient exhibited a similar response after the sublingual administration of 15 mg. Adverse effects of tremor, palpitations, and headache are commonly encountered side effects. Tolerance to isoproterenol may develop because of a reduction in the β-receptor population and may be overcome by the administration of larger doses.[158] The side effect profile along with the need for frequent administration limits the use of isoproterenol. Other β agonists have not been of benefit in pulmonary hypertension.[159]

### Direct-Acting Vasodilator Agents: Diazoxide

The incremental dosing of diazoxide into the pulmonary artery to a total dose of 600 mg has resulted in reductions in pulmonary arterial pressure and pulmonary vascular resistance with an increase in cardiac output.[160,161] Complete resolution of symptoms occurred after oral therapy of 300 mg every day.[160] Other favorable results have been seen with oral doses ranging from 400 to 600 mg per day.[162] The authors suggested that the dose should be sufficient to maintain a serum concentration of diazoxide of 75–100 μg/mL. As with other vasodilators the response to diazoxide is variable and unsuccessful interventions can occur. Adverse reactions to diazoxide have consisted of death, worsening pulmonary hypertension, asystole, atrioventricular block, nausea, vomiting, sodium and water retention, hirsutism, postural hypotension, and diabetes.[163–165] This wide range of adverse effects has removed diazoxide as a first-line vasodilator agent for the treatment of pulmonary hypertension.

### Nitrates/Nitroprusside

***Nitroglycerin*** The theoretical advantage of using nitrates is that with doses that affect the pulmonary vasculature there are minimal direct effects on the arterial resistance vessels.[166] Nitrates decrease systemic venous capacitance. A reduction in venous return to the right side of the heart may lead to a decrease in pulmonary blood flow and therefore a decrease in pulmonary arterial pressure. Nitroglycerin can be administered intravenously, enabling the dose to be titrated to the desired outcome. With its fast elimination rate, a hemodynamic adverse event can be rapidly reversed.

Pearl et al used intravenous nitroglycerin at doses ranging from 24 to 300 μg/min in nine patients with pulmonary hypertension and normal left ventricular filling pressures.[167] Eight of nine patients showed an increase in cardiac index and a decreased pulmonary vascular resistance. Mean pulmonary arterial pressure decreased in six of nine patients with doses of 24 to 120 μg/min. In the same study, the acute administration of topical nitroglycerin was evaluated in four patients and resulted in similar hemodynamic changes. In addition, five of six patients receiving chronic topical nitroglycerin therapy had improvements in their symptoms. In all patients systemic arterial pressure and resistance decreased, but only one patient developed symptomatic hypotension which occurred at an intravenous dose of 8 μg/kg/min. As a result the authors suggest limiting the dose of nitroglycerin to 4 μg/kg/min.

Intravenous nitroglycerin has been used successfully to reduce pulmonary hypertension postoperatively. A dose of 50 μg/min/$m^2$ resulted in a 30% reduction in mean pulmonary arterial pressure and a 48.4% reduction in pulmonary vascular resistance index in patients who underwent valve replacement for mitral valve stenosis.[168] There were no significant changes in mean systemic arterial pressure after an 18.8% reduction in systemic vascular resistance index with a 25.5% increase in cardiac index. The use of nitroglycerin has also been successful in preventing pulmonary hypertension after an anatomic correction of transposition of the great vessels in a 6-month-old patient.[169] Mean pulmonary arterial pressure and pulmonary vascular resistance were reduced after a 20-minute infusion of nitroglycerin 1 μg/kg/min in four patients.[170] Cardiac output increased but systemic vascular resistance and pressure were reduced in all four patients.

Besides affecting the systemic arterial system at times, nitroglycerin can have other adverse hemodynamic effects. After the administration of nitroglycerin and nitroprusside in 14 patients with pulmonary hypertension and chronic obstructive pulmonary disease, a reduction in preload resulted in a decrease in cardiac output and a reduction in arterial oxygen tension.[171] Systemic hypoxemia can occur when blood is shunted toward poorly ventilated alveoli, causing a ventilation/perfusion mismatch. Paradoxic exacerbation of pulmonary hypertension occurred in a 15-year-old girl after the administration of 200 μg of nitroglycerin.[172] The events were best explained by an initial increase in pulmonary vascular resistance, resulting in an increase in the pulmonary arterial pressure. The cardiac output decreased in response which led to an increase in systemic vascular resistance.

***Isosorbide Dinitrate*** Isosorbide dinitrate was evaluated in 11 patients with pulmonary hypertension secondary to chronic obstructive pulmonary disease.[173] The doses ranged from 25 to 40 mg. Pulmonary arterial pressure decreased, but there was also a reduction in cardiac output and systemic arterial pressure. The peak drug effect was seen 45 minutes after the dose with a pulmonary arterial systolic reduction of 10 mm Hg. Isosorbide dinitrate 10 mg sublingually in combination with prazosin produced an acute fall in pulmonary vascular resistance.[174] Improvement was sustained for 3 months with prazosin 1 mg four times daily and isosorbide dinitrate 5 mg four times daily. The cardiothoracic ratio decreased from 0.49 to 0.40 and there was a marked reduction in "s" waves on the ECG. Isosorbide 10 mg sublingually was the only one of six agents that reduced both pulmonary arterial pressure and pulmonary vascular resistance.[149] There was no change in cardiac output and systemic blood pressure decreased, however. Cardiac output may have failed to increase because of a decrease in venous return caused by the drug.

***Nitroprusside*** Nitroprusside has the same advantage of nitroglycerin in that an adverse reaction should reverse quickly secondary to its short half-life and to its intravenous administration. Nitroprusside (50 $\mu$g/min) reduced the mean pulmonary arterial pressure in six patients with an acute exacerbation of chronic obstructive pulmonary disease and pulmonary hypertension.[175] Pulmonary vascular resistance decreased only slightly and there was no change in cardiac index. Mean arterial pressure and systemic vascular resistance also declined. Nitroprusside was successful in reducing pulmonary hypertension perioperatively in a 3-year-old girl at a dose of 3 $\mu$g/kg/min.[176] Pulmonary arterial pressure decreased during repair of a ventricular septal defect.

### Hydralazine

There are numerous experimental accounts of the use of hydralazine in pulmonary hypertension. Hydralazine is thought to be effective because of its direct vasodilatory action. Its activity may be prostaglandin mediated; however, there is some evidence to suggest that this may not be the case.[149] Indomethacin has been administered concurrently with hydralazine without blocking the hemodynamic effects induced by hydralazine. This result suggests that a prostaglandin mediator is not responsible for hydralazine's activity in the pulmonary vasculature. The average overall beneficial response to hydralazine is an increase in cardiac output and a decrease in pulmonary and systemic vascular resistance. The effects on mean pulmonary arterial pressure are variable. Rubin and Peter studied four patients with primary pulmonary hypertension before the administration of hydralazine 50 mg every 6 hours and after 48 hours.[177] Total pulmonary vascular resistance decreased at rest and with exercise. This reduction was not accompanied by a decline in pulmonary arterial pressure. The hemodynamic effects persisted for 3 to 6 months after the continuous administration of 50–75 mg four times daily. During this period, the patients' clinical conditions improved. Although pulmonary arterial pressure remains unchanged, hydralazine has been shown to have a beneficial effect in patients with right ventricular failure. After the oral administration of hydralazine 50 mg every 6 hours, right ventricular end-diastolic pressure was reduced with an increase in cardiac output and stroke volume.[178] The change in right ventricular end-diastolic pressure was inversely correlated to the change in stroke volume ($r$ = .78) and correlated with a reduction in total pulmonary resistance ($r$ = .73). The increased stroke volume with a reduced right ventricular end-diastolic pressure suggests improved emptying of the right ventricle. The reduced right ventricular end-diastolic pressure and decreased pulmonary resistance illustrate a decrease in the afterload of the right ventricle. A reduced right ventricular afterload caused by hydralazine was also suggested by Lupi-Herrera and others.[179] A positive response was seen after the acute administration of 0.33 mg/kg infused into the pulmonary artery. Hydralazine prevented the increase in pulmonary arteriolar resistance during exercise as well. The beneficial hemodynamic response persisted in five patients 8 months later. This was in contrast to six patients who did not respond to the acute administration of hydralazine. The authors suggested that hydralazine can reduce pulmonary arteriolar resistance in those patients diagnosed with pulmonary hypertension of unknown cause if the following baseline parameters exist: pulmonary arterial pressure less than 60 mm Hg; pulmonary arteriolar resistance less than 15 units/m$^2$; and pulmonary resistance/systemic resistance ratio less than 0.7. The use of hydralazine has been shown to be beneficial in patients with pulmonary hypertension caused by interstitial lung disease.[180] In 12 of 13 patients, 0.33 mg/kg hydralazine injected into the pulmonary artery produced favorable hemodynamic changes along with increases in arterial and mixed venous $O_2$ saturation.

Improved alveolar and mixed venous $O_2$ tensions were also demonstrated in 14 patients with pulmonary hypertension associated with chronic obstructive pulmonary disease.[181] Hydralazine was administered orally as 50 mg every 6 hours. Hemodynamically there was no change in pulmonary arterial pressure and a nonsignificant decrease in total pulmonary resistance. But with exercise, mean pulmonary arterial pressure decreased 12% and there was a 28% decrease in total pulmonary resistance. Cardiac index increased both at rest and during exercise. Other experiences have demonstrated that hydralazine does not increase exercise capacity in patients with chronic obstructive pulmonary disease.[182]

The intravenous administration of 0.15 and 0.30 mg/kg hydralazine in 26 patients with pulmonary hypertension of unknown etiology and associated with cor pulmonale and pulmonary embolism did not cause a significant change in pulmonary arteriolar resistance or pressure.[183] A reduction in systemic vascular resistance resulted that was correlated with hydralazine plasma concentration. Maintenance oral therapy from 9 to 36 months did not seem to have an effect on the patients' symptoms or mortality.

As with other vasodilators, hydralazine is not without its detrimental effects.[184–186] Exacerbation of pulmonary hypertension with clinical deterioration can occur with elevations in pulmonary arterial pressure. This is associated with an increase in cardiac output and decrease in systemic vascular resistance without a concomitant decrease in pulmonary vascular resistance. An elevated pulmonary arterial pressure induced by hydralazine can result in an increase in right ventricular stroke work index. Hydralazine can produce symptomatic hypotension which can lead to death by decreasing systemic vascular resistance to a much greater extent than pulmonary arteriolar resistance. Hydralazine caused a 5% to 19% decrease in pulmonary vascular resistance with a slightly larger decrease (15%–25%) in systemic vascular resistance in a study by Hermiller et al.[149] Systemic blood pressure dropped 10% to 17% despite a rise in cardiac index of 28%. Pulmonary arterial pressure was not affected. Hydralazine can also cause a decline in arterial $O_2$ saturation which can lead to an irreversible cardiovascular collapse.[187]

**Prostaglandins**

In an attempt to find a vasodilator agent that is selective for the pulmonary circulatory system, prostaglandins have been investigated in recent years. The two major prostaglandins that have been evaluated in pulmonary hypertension are prostacyclin ($PGI_2$) and prostaglandin $E_1$ ($PGE_1$). Prostacyclin is an arachidonic acid metabolite that is secreted by vascular endothelial cells. It has both vasodilatory and platelet antiaggregatory properties. Unlike most prostaglandins it is not metabolized by the lungs.

The theoretical advantages of prostacyclin are its potency as a vasodilator, the ability to titrate the dose to the desired hemodynamic effect, and the ability to discontinue an infusion to rapidly reverse unwanted effects. The half-life of prostacyclin is 2 to 3 minutes. In seven patients with primary pulmonary hypertension, prostacyclin was infused for 15 minutes in doses ranging from 2 to 12 ng/kg/min (mean = 5.7 ng/kg/min).[188] Prostacyclin reduced the pulmonary vascular resistance in a dose-dependent manner. Mean pulmonary arterial pressure decreased in six of seven patients. Cardiac output increased greater than 40% which was due to a 40% increase in stroke volume. Mean systemic arterial pressure decreased greater than 5 mm Hg in three patients. Although the hemodynamic profile improved, the frequency of side effects was high. Six patients developed a headache; four patients had nausea with vomiting in two patients; five patients had cutaneous flushing; two patients had symptomatic hypotension; and one patient had diplopia at 6 ng/kg/min. Three patients had sustained reductions in total pulmonary resistance on a continuous prostacyclin infusion of 8 to 10 ng/kg/min for 24 to 48 hours. Mild nausea and headache were the only adverse effects reported during this period.

Guadagni et al also witnessed a dose-related reduction in pulmonary vascular resistance and systemic resistance accompanied by an increase in cardiac output in four patients.[189] The doses ranged from 2 to 16 ng/kg/min. The ratio of pulmonary to systemic vascular resistance remained constant in three of four patients, suggesting that $PGI_2$ did not exhibit a preferential dilation of the pulmonary vasculature. As above, side effects of prostacyclin were quite evident. Symptomatic hypotension occurred in three of four patients. All patients experienced nausea at infusion rates greater than 8 ng/kg/min. The ECG of one patient revealed widening of the QRS complex at an infusion rate of 16 ng/kg/min.

A continuous intravenous infusion of $PGI_2$ was maintained for 7 months in one patient with postpartum pulmonary hypertension.[190] Hemodynamic improvement and an increase in exercise tolerance were seen throughout this period. The infusion was initially titrated to 4 ng/kg/min and after 2 months the rate was up to 20 ng/kg/min.

Prostacyclin has been used in children with congenital heart disease. Doses were titrated to maxima of 4 to 36 ng/kg/min in one series of five infants, but larger doses up to 66 ng/kg/min have been reported.[191] Two of five infants with idiopathic pulmonary hypertension and meconium aspiration–induced pulmonary hypertension benefited from the infusion of $PGI_2$. Systemic hypotension was encountered in two other infants.

Prostacyclin caused a dose-dependent reduction in pulmonary vascular resistance in 20 children (mean age = 3 years) with congenital heart disease.[192] The dose range was 5 to 20 ng/kg/min. This decrease was seen in patients breathing air and 100% oxygen. There was no difference in the hemodynamic parameters resulting from the 20 ng/kg/min $PGI_2$ and the breathing of 100% oxygen, but prostacyclin had an additional vasodilatory effect when added to oxygen therapy.

The acute effects of intravenous prostacyclin were compared with the oral and intravenous effects of hydralazine in seven patients with primary pulmonary hypertension.[193] Incremental doses of prostacyclin began at 2 ng/kg/min and were increased every 15 minutes to 12 ng/kg/min or less if the systemic blood pressure decreased by more than 30%. Four patients received 20 mg of intravenous hydralazine and three patients each received total oral doses of 100, 200, and 250 mg administered in divided doses. Both drugs caused significant increases in cardiac output and decreases in systemic arterial pressure. Neither caused a significant reduction in the pulmonary arterial pressure. There was a greater percent decrease in total pulmonary resistance with prostacyclin compared with that with hydralazine (−46% vs −32%).

Prostacyclin has also been compared with the sublingual administration of nifedipine in children and young adults with primary pulmonary hypertension.[194] The nine patients ranged in age from 9 months to 23 years. Five of nine patients responded to prostacyclin (10–40 ng/kg/min) administration. All five patients also demonstrated a response to nifedipine (0.5–2 mg/kg). None of the remaining four patients responded to either drug. Both drugs produced a greater fall in pulmonary arterial pressure in younger patients than in older ones. The study also demonstrated that hemodynamic changes induced by prostacyclin parallel those caused by nifedipine.

Because of its short duration of action, prostacyclin has been advocated as the preferred drug in the evaluation of pulmonary vascular reactivity in pulmonary hypertension. It has been proposed that patients who have a greater than 20% fall in total pulmonary vascular resistance with prostacyclin 8 ng/kg/min are more likely to respond favorably to long-term vasodilator therapy.[195] Before this can become an accepted practice, further studies comparing acute versus chronic vasodilator administration need to be done. The side effect profile of prostacyclin may limit this proposal.

Prostaglandin $E_1$ has been tried as an alternative for a selective pulmonary arterial vasodilator. About 85% to 95% of $PGE_1$ is inactivated during one passage through the pulmonary circulation.[196] This high rate may protect the cardiovascular system from systemic vasodilation while allowing for a reduction in pulmonary vascular resistance. Unfortunately, for the most part, this potential selectivity has not been seen when $PGE_1$ has been used to treat pulmonary hypertension. As opposed to prostacyclin, $PGE_1$ has only mild platelet antiaggregatory effects.[197]

Twenty patients with pulmonary hypertension resulting from mitral valve disease demonstrated significant reductions in pulmonary arterial pressure and total pulmonary resistance, and increases in cardiac index and heart rate, after the administration of $PGE_1$.[198] Total peripheral resistance fell 25% with significant reductions in aortic pressures. Systemic side effects occurred such as flushing of the facial skin and nausea.

Ten patients responded well to a 30-minute infusion of

$PGE_1$ of 20 ng/kg/min with only a minimal reduction in systemic arterial pressure.[199] As the dose was increased to 40 ng/kg/min in nine patients, there was a reduction in systemic pressure and a slight decrease in arterial oxygenation. Side effects of facial flushing, headache, and malaise occurred at this higher dose. $PGE_1$ did not inhibit vasoconstriction induced by hypoxia in seven healthy subjects at this higher dose, although the side effects previously mentioned still occurred. Doses of $PGE_1$ up to 150 ng/kg/min have been used in combination with norepinephrine in five patients with refractory heart failure and pulmonary hypertension after mitral valve replacement.[200] An 11-year-old boy received 30 ng/kg/min directly into the pulmonary artery after the lack of response to 10 ng/kg/min.[196] Mean pulmonary arterial pressure decreased while systemic blood pressure was maintained.

It seems as though the systemic effects of $PGE_1$ are more prominent at infusion rates of 40 ng/kg/min or greater. A possible explanation for the loss of $PGE_1$'s selectivity for the pulmonary vasculature may be that at higher doses the rate of pulmonary clearance is exceeded, especially in the pulmonary vasculature that may have damaged endothelial cell function.[196]

An analog of prostacyclin, ZK 36-374, has been investigated in the dog.[201] It has advantages over its parent compound in that it has a longer half-life (13 minutes when given intravenously) and it can be administered orally. During hypoxic vasoconstriction, ZK 36-374 reduced pulmonary arterial pressure and pulmonary vascular resistance. There was no significant effect on cardiac output, aortic blood pressure, or arterial blood gases. Compared with prostacyclin, ZK 36-374 reduced pulmonary vascular resistance to a greater extent. ZK 36-374 also resulted in a smaller fall in aortic pressure. The dose of ZK 36-374 used was 0.4 μg/kg/min. ZK 36-374 has been used in humans in peripheral vascular disease.[202] Doses of 0.5–4 ng/kg/min have resulted in a 15% reduction in aortic pressure and a 34% decline in pulmonary vascular resistance. Side effects, including headaches, nausea, and abdominal pain, have been noted at doses of 8 ng/kg/min. In addition, ZK 36-374 has been shown to reduce platelet aggregation in humans.

### Calcium Channel Antagonists

The calcium channel antagonists are active in vasospastic disease states and have been shown to have a direct effect on the pulmonary circulation. The potential advantages of using these agents in pulmonary hypertension are the ability to administer them orally and their prolonged duration of action as compared with some other vasodilators. Calcium channel blockers should be of benefit in those cases of pulmonary hypertension caused by vasoconstriction and if the vasoconstriction is mediated by the intracellular interaction of calcium with myofibrillar elements within the vascular smooth muscle. The administration of calcium channel antagonists may lead to pulmonary vascular relaxation by blocking the influx of extracellular calcium and thereby impeding the excitation–contraction coupling.[34] In contrast, other vasodilators that affect the pulmonary circulatory system may act on the intracellular calcium pool. Most evidence that supports the efficacy of calcium channel antagonists in the treatment of pulmonary hypertension is found in hypoxia-induced vasoconstriction. Of the three calcium antagonists commercially available, nifedipine has sparked the most interest.

***Nifedipine*** Nifedipine appeared to be a more effective pulmonary arterial vasodilator than verapamil or diltiazem in the acute treatment of pulmonary hypertension induced experimentally in dogs.[203] This difference in response may have resulted from the administration of equimolar rather than equipotent doses of these agents.

Camerini et al reported the successful management of primary pulmonary hypertension in a 34-year-old female.[204] After 20 mg sublingually, the pulmonary vascular resistance decreased 54% and the pulmonary arterial pressure decreased 14%. A 40% reduction in systemic vascular resistance accompanied a 90.3% increase in cardiac output. Furthermore, the improvement was maintained over a 3-month period. Nifedipine failed to reduce pulmonary arterial pressures in nine patients with primary pulmonary hypertension after the acute administration of 10–20 mg sublingually[205]; however, nifedipine did cause a reduction in total pulmonary resistance with an increase in right ventricular ejection fraction of 18%. The percent increase in right ventricular ejection fraction was correlated to the percent decrease in total pulmonary resistance after nifedipine ($r$ = .79).

Six patients underwent long-term therapy with nifedipine 40–120 mg per day and reported symptomatic improvement after 4 to 14 months of therapy.[205] Response was lost in one patient after 6 months of therapy. It is unclear whether this was due to the progression of disease or to a loss of nifedipine effect. A sustained beneficial effect of nifedipine in the treatment of primary pulmonary hypertension has also been reported by others.[206–211]

Nifedipine has been shown to blunt an exercise-induced increase in pulmonary arterial pressure, but may not increase the duration of exercise in some individuals.[206] Kennedy et al demonstrated a decrease in mean pulmonary arterial pressure at rest and with exercise while patients were hypoxic.[212] The pulmonary vascular resistance index was decreased to a greater extent during exercise (44% versus 27% reduction). Right ventricular stroke volume decreased both at rest and with exercise, indicating that nifedipine reduced the work load on the right ventricle.

Nifedipine has shown beneficial hemodynamic responses in patients who have developed pulmonary hypertension secondary to chronic obstructive pulmonary disease.[212–214] In a study that consisted of nine patients with chronic obstructive pulmonary disease, two patients with pulmonary embolism, and two patients with pulmonary fibrosis, nifedipine 20 mg sublingually induced a fall in pulmonary vascular resistance that was correlated to the pulmonary vascular resistance before therapy.[215] This suggests that the more severe the vasoconstriction, the greater will be the effect of nifedipine. Simonneau and others also suggested that the more severe the hypoxic vasoconstriction, the greater the effect of nifedipine on the pulmonary circulation.[216] The reduction in pulmonary vascular resistance was inversely correlated with the initial arterial $Po_2$. In contrast, Hamet et al reported no benefit of acute or chronic nifedipine administration in chronic obstructive pulmonary disease.[217]

The acute administration of nifedipine has been successful

in pulmonary hypertension caused by systemic sclerosis.[218] Tolerance, however, developed in one patient within 12 hours, with subsequent doses having no effect.[219] A rapid attenuation of response to nifedipine was also reported by Wood et al in a patient with primary pulmonary hypertension.[220] In both cases, a dramatic hemodynamic improvement occurred after the first dose, but it was not sustained after subsequent doses.

In a comparison with hydralazine, nifedipine appeared to be a more specific pulmonary arterial vasodilator in acute drug testing.[221] Nifedipine also had a more balanced effect in relation to pulmonary and systemic vascular beds. Rich et al also demonstrated that nifedipine possesses a greater pulmonary specificity than hydralazine.[222] In contrast to hydralazine, nifedipine reduced pulmonary arterial pressure and in two of seven patients pulmonary resistance decreased to a greater degree than systemic resistance.

The adverse effects of nifedipine in the treatment of pulmonary hypertension have included the development of peripheral edema, which required the use of a diuretic agent, pulmonary edema, systemic flushing, increase in dyspnea resulting from a decrease in arterial oxygen saturation, acute right ventricular failure, hypotension and sinus arrest, and a decrease in cardiac output.[223–228] Death has occurred after the acute administration and as late as 54 hours after starting chronic therapy.[229,230] The pulmonary edema and right ventricular failure have been thought to occur secondary to the negative inotropic effect imparted by nifedipine. The change in systemic arterial oxygen tension arises from an increase in pulmonary flow to underventilated areas of the lung inducing a deterioration in ventilation/perfusion matching. Flushing, hypotension, and peripheral edema are secondary to the peripheral vasodilatory effect of nifedipine.

***Diltiazem*** The experience with diltiazem is not as extensive as that with nifedipine. Kamabara et al reported a successful outcome in a 22-year-old given an initial dose of 10 mg intravenously followed by 30 mg orally three times daily.[231] The patient experienced symptomatic improvement and after 11 months there was no longer any evidence of right ventricular strain on ECG. Echocardiography demonstrated a decrease in right ventricular enlargement and the cardiothoracic ratio was decreased on the chest x-ray. The acute administration of diltiazem 0.25 mg/kg plus an infusion of 1.4 μg/kg/min resulted in hemodynamic improvement in four of five patients with pulmonary hypertension.[232] Mean pulmonary arterial pressure significantly decreased at rest, but there was little change in total pulmonary resistance. Cardiac output was reduced slightly, 3%. Diltiazem caused a significant decrease in total pulmonary resistance with exercise. Systemic blood pressure decreased with a reduction in systemic vascular resistance both at rest and with exercise. In this small study, diltiazem provided no evidence of adversely altering ventilation/perfusion distribution or arterial oxygenation.

***Verapamil*** The benefits of verapamil in diminishing hypoxic pulmonary hypertension have been demonstrated in the animal model, but it did not promote the regression of pulmonary vascular changes as did nifedipine.[233] Theoretically, verapamil should be more advantageous than nifedipine because it has less effect on the systemic vasculature, but the therapeutic outcome of pulmonary hypertension in humans is variable. Landmark et al studied the effects of injection of verapamil 0.15 mg/kg into the pulmonary artery in 12 patients.[234] Overall, the mean pulmonary arterial pressure decreased with no change in pulmonary arteriolar resistance. There was a small but insignificant decrease in cardiac output. Some patients demonstrated an increase in pulmonary arteriolar resistance as a result of a marked negative inotropic effect. Three patients had a large decrease in pulmonary arteriolar resistance with a reduction in pulmonary arterial pressure and an increase in cardiac index.

Verapamil was administered into the pulmonary artery of an 8-year-old girl at a dose of 17.5 mg.[235] Pulmonary vascular resistance decreased 40% with a reduction in pulmonary arterial pressure from 70/50 to 35/25 mm Hg. There was no change in cardiac index. After 7 months of verapamil 40 mg orally every 6 hours, there was a further reduction in pulmonary pressure and resistance, and cardiac index increased from 3.29 to 4.42 L/min/m$^2$. Sustained benefit with verapamil was also seen in a patient with progressive systemic sclerosis.[236] The administration of verapamil 120 mg orally three times daily increased exercise tolerance and reduced pulmonary vascular resistance for 1 year. Packer et al reported sustained hemodynamic and clinical improvement after 3 months in one patient who received verapamil 120 mg orally every 6 hours.[237] The same authors also provided evidence for detrimental effects of verapamil. After the acute intravenous administration of 10 mg verapamil right ventricular filling pressure increased 50%, indicating a direct depressant effect on the right ventricular function. One patient had severe hypotension and a cardiac arrest. Dyspnea occurred in two patients. It was experienced in one patient during a reduction in systemic vascular resistance and associated chest pain. The other occurrence was the result of a decrease in systemic arterial oxygen saturation from 85% to 79%.

Additional adverse effects associated with verapamil and pulmonary hypertension have included the development of a junctional rhythm and the reduction of left ventricular stroke work index with an increase in left ventricular filling pressure.[228]

***Other Calcium Channel Antagonists*** Nisoldipine appeared to be a more potent vasodilator than nifedipine and bepridil when the comparative effects were evaluated in experimentally induced pulmonary hypertension in dogs.[238] Nisoldipine increased cardiac output by 22% to 25%, decreased pulmonary vascular resistance by 39% to 48%, and decreased pulmonary arterial pressure 23%. Unfortunately, nisoldipine was responsible for a significant decrease in $Po_2$ and pH with an increase in $Pco_2$. As with other vasodilators, nisoldipine's shortcoming, in addition to its effect on arterial blood gases, is the lack of selectivity for the pulmonary vascular bed.

Bepridil was ineffective in altering the hemodynamic variables in hypoxic vasoconstriction. Its administration was associated with a dose-dependent reduction in cardiac output and elevation in pulmonary vascular resistance.

Nitrendipine was evaluated in rats under intermittent hypoxic conditions.[239] Nitrendipine 10 mg/kg prevented the acute increase in right ventricular pressure caused by hypoxia. Chronic administration of nitrendipine 10 mg/kg given twice daily for 30 days reduced right ventricular hypertrophy and reduced pulmonary vascular remodeling that is caused by hypoxia. Whether nitrendipine has pulmonary selectivity in pulmonary hypertension in humans needs to be determined. Based on its structural similarity to nifedipine and its beneficial activity in systemic hypertension, strong evidence exists that nitrendipine will lack the needed pulmonary vascular selectivity.

Felodipine is a type II calcium antagonist like nifedipine that possesses strong vascular effects.[240] Felodipine has a selective action on smooth muscle in arteriolar resistance vessels. Arnman et al reported two cases of primary pulmonary hypertension in which felodipine was administered.[241] One patient received felodipine 12.5 mg orally three times daily, and beneficial responses were seen at 3 and 18 months. Felodipine 6.25 mg six times daily resulted in a reduction of systemic pressure with a resultant increase in cardiac output. Right ventricular systolic pressure and pulmonary arterial pressure were unaffected. Felodipine has been evaluated in patients with chronic obstructive lung disease. Pulmonary and systemic vascular resistances were reduced 20% and 35%, respectively, during continuous infusion of felodipine in 10 patients.[242] Cardiac output increased 28%. Pulmonary vascular pressures remained unchanged but felodipine resulted in a smaller increase in pulmonary pressure with exercise. Overall, felodipine lowered pulmonary vascular resistance along with producing a reduction in arterial oxygenation. Felodipine was administered for 3 to 5 months in nine patients with chronic obstructive lung disease.[243] The dose administered was either 5 mg three times daily or 10 mg twice daily. The most notable effect on pulmonary vascular resistance was seen with exercise. Pulmonary vascular resistance reduced 30% with exercise as compared with a 10% reduction at rest. The systemic vascular resistance decreased 19% at rest and 30% with exercise. Again, there was a moderate decline in arterial oxygenation. The most common side effect was edema of the lower extremities. Five patients experienced sustained facial flushing. Hypotension, dizziness, weakness, sleepiness, and transient tachycardia have also been reported.

### Angiotensin-Converting Enzyme Inhibitors: Captopril

The rationale for using captopril in the treatment of pulmonary hypertension stems from the hypothesis that pulmonary vasoconstriction is induced by angiotensin II. Angiotensin II is formed from angiotensin I by a hydrolase enzyme that occurs in the lung. The potentiation of the formation of bradykinin, a potent vasodilator, from kininogen is another possible mechanism. In addition, captopril has been demonstrated to be of benefit in both systemic hypertension and left ventricular failure.

There are both positive and negative reports on the efficacy of captopril in pulmonary hypertension. The first account of the use of captopril in primary pulmonary hypertension was by Horowitz et al.[244] Cardiac output increased with a reduction in pulmonary vascular resistance and systemic vascular resistance after the administration of 6 mg orally. The patient became less cyanosed and dyspnea decreased at rest, but gross right heart failure persisted after 16 days of treatment. Captopril was discontinued and the patient died 8 days later. Four of five patients responded to captopril during 4 days of therapy at doses ranging from 6.25 to 150 mg orally three times daily.[245] The reduction in mean pulmonary arterial pressure paralleled angiotensin II concentrations ($r = .91$). Right ventricular ejection fraction increased from 39.5% to 59.8% and left ventricular ejection fraction increased from 57.3% to 72.5%. The two youngest patients noticed clinical improvement while one patient developed symptomatic hypotension. The acute administration of captopril 25 mg reduced mean pulmonary arterial pressure, pulmonary vascular resistance, and right ventricular stroke work index in two patients.[246] One of these patients remained asymptomatic while receiving 25 mg orally three times daily. The other patient developed hypotension after 2 weeks, necessitating the discontinuance of the drug.

Captopril is beneficial in some patients with pulmonary hypertension caused by collagen vascular disease. In four of six patients total pulmonary resistance decreased 26% with an increase in cardiac output of 37%.[247] There was no change in mean pulmonary arterial pressure. Captopril had an equal vasodilatory effect on both the systemic and pulmonary vasculature. Captopril was deemed successful in a patient with pulmonary hypertension resulting from the CREST syndrome.[248] Captopril 200 mg twice daily for 1 month increased the right ventricular ejection fraction from 5% to 20% with a concomitant increase in left ventricular ejection fraction from 41% to 62%. The patient died a couple of months later after the deterioration of cardiac function.

Captopril successfully altered the hemodynamic parameters in patients with pulmonary hypertension and chronic obstructive pulmonary disease.[249] The beneficial effect of captopril in this disease state has also been reported to occur only with the coadministration of oxygen.[250] Deleterious effects occurred in one of three patients with chronic obstructive pulmonary disease treated with captopril 50 mg.[251]

The chronic administration of captopril in doses of 75 to 100 mg every 8 hours was assessed by Leier et al.[252] In contrast to the sporadic reports of the success of captopril in pulmonary hypertension, the major hemodynamic parameter that was affected in this population was a reduction in the mean systemic blood pressure. Other parameters were not affected at rest or with exercise after three months of therapy. Three patients developed hoarseness and a nonproductive cough that went away after captopril was stopped. After the acute administration of captopril in these same patients, pulmonary-to-systemic ratios of vascular resistance and blood pressure rose significantly secondary to unaltered pulmonary parameters and reductions in systemic vascular resistance and systemic blood pressure. The lack of captopril effect was also suggested by Rich et al.[253] No significant effect was seen in four patients in cardiac output, pulmonary arterial pressure, and pulmonary vascular resistance at rest or with exercise.

### Miscellaneous Agents

Diethylcarbamazine is a leukotriene synthesis inhibitor. Leukotrienes have been suggested as mediators in hypoxic pulmonary vasoconstriction. Diethylcarbamazine reversibly inhibited acute and chronic pulmonary hypertension induced by hypoxia in the rat.[254]

Serotonin released from platelet aggregates may contribute to pulmonary hypertension. Ketanserin is a quinazoline derivative that acts as an antagonist of serotonin receptors in blood vessels, platelets, and bronchial tissue. Cardiac output was improved and mean pulmonary arterial pressure, along with pulmonary and systemic vascular resistance, was reduced in dogs pretreated with ketanserin before the administration of an endotoxin infusion.[255] Ketanserin was given intravenously to 10 patients at the Mayo Clinic with primary pulmonary hypertension.[256] Both pulmonary and systemic vascular resistance decreased by 18%. Mean pulmonary arterial pressure declined 10%. There was a slight increase in cardiac output. In contrast, ketanserin's only effect in seven patients with hypoxic pulmonary hypertension was a reduction in systemic arterial pressure.[217]

### *Anticoagulation*

Adjunct therapy with anticoagulants is indicated for a known thromboembolic cause of pulmonary hypertension.[257] Anticoagulants are also indicated in those patients who are at risk for the development of deep-vein thrombosis.[158] Included are those patients with pulmonary hypertension who developed venous stasis from right heart failure and those patients who are inactive secondary to the debilitating nature of the disease.

The use of anticoagulation therapy in primary pulmonary hypertension is controversial. Anticoagulation therapy does not appear to cause hemodynamic or symptomatic improvement, or cause a regression of disease[4,11]; however, in reports of the spontaneous regression of primary hypertension, anticoagulation may have been responsible for its reversal.[139]

Those who favor the use of anticoagulants in primary pulmonary hypertension fear missing the diagnosis of thromboembolism in these patients. At times it may be difficult to distinguish between thromboembolic and primary pulmonary hypertension on clinical grounds.[5] In addition, organized thrombi may be confused with the plexogenic lesion as they occasionally resemble one another.[14] Additional support for the use of anticoagulation therapy comes from the retrospective analysis of 80 cases of primary pulmonary hypertension in which it was discovered that thromboembolic disease was the underlying cause for the elevated pulmonary arterial pressure in 56% of the cases.[14] Furthermore, it has been suggested that anticoagulation improves survival in idiopathic pulmonary hypertension, although there is no supportive evidence from hemodynamic improvement.[49]

The risk-to-benefit ratio for anticoagulation therapy needs to be considered in each patient and therapy should be avoided in those patients with specific contraindications.

### *Oxygen*

The use of supplemental oxygen is directed toward the palliation of symptoms related to hypoxia and the alleviation of hypoxic pulmonary vasoconstriction. The administration of high oxygen breathing decreased pulmonary vascular impedance and pulmonary arterial resistance in 10 patients with pulmonary arterial hypertension.[258] This was associated with a decrease in plasma norepinephrine concentrations. The postulated mechanism may be an indirect effect of oxygen on the vessels through an attenuation of sympathetic nerve tone. Recent support for the use of oxygen came from a report of 16 patients with chronic obstructive pulmonary disease and pulmonary hypertension.[259] Oxygen was administered 15 to 18 hours a day. The authors reported a reversal of the progression of pulmonary hypertension in 12 of 16 patients, but that normalization of pulmonary aterial pressure was rare. The Nocturnal Oxygen Therapy Trial compared the effects of administering oxygen for greater than 18 hours per day with nocturnal treatment (12 hours) in patients with chronic hypoxemia.[260] Overall mortality in the nocturnal group was 1.94 times that in the continuous group (longer than 18 hours per day). From this study it was suggested that patients who might benefit from continuous oxygen therapy are those with hypoxemia ($Pa_{O_2}$ less than 55 mm Hg), edema, high hematocrits (greater than 55%), and P pulmonale on ECG.

In contrast, there is little evidence that oxygen produces hemodynamic or clinical benefits in patients with primary pulmonary hypertension without hypoxemia[145]; however, a beneficial response was seen in a 14-year-old with primary pulmonary hypertension.[261] The inhalation of oxygen of 2 L/min for 8 hours at night resulted in clinical improvement. A confounding factor in this case is the administration of medications during this period. There are other reports of little or no benefit with oxygen therapy.[10,149] The administration of oxygen may be detrimental by inducing vasoconstriction and thereby decreasing cardiac output in patients with pulmonary veno-occlusive disease.[145]

Although oxygen therapy has been of little or no benefit in the treatment of primary pulmonary hypertension, supplemental oxygen should not be withheld in those patients with arterial hypoxemia.

### *Heart–Lung Transplant*

As can be seen from the inconsistent responses to medical management, the treatment of pulmonary hypertension is a challenge. A last alternative to the medical palliation of symptoms is the cardiopulmonary transplant. The clinical experience of the combined heart–lung transplant began in 1968, in a 2-month-old infant.[262] Seventeen patients have undergone the procedure at Stanford University from 1981 to 1983.[263] Ten had the diagnosis of Eisenmenger's syndrome and seven had the diagnosis of primary pulmonary hypertension. Twelve of the patients have remained well between 1 and 33 months. Rejection had occurred in 6 of 12 patients and infections had developed in 9 patients. A major complication of the transplant is what is called reimplantation response. It consists of pulmonary edema and resolves in 3 weeks with fluid restriction and diuretics. Three factors have been identified for the success of the cardiopulmonary transplant[264]: preliminary laboratory experience with the procedure in primates, cyclosporin A, anatomic and physiologic advantages of the combined heart–lung transplant. The greatest limitation of the transplant program is a lack of suitable donors. The advantage of cardiopulmonary transplantation in primary pulmonary hypertension is that all diseased pulmonary tissue is removed.

## Summary

Pulmonary hypertension is defined as an elevation of the pulmonary arterial pressure. It can be classified as either primary or secondary pulmonary hypertension. If the etiology is known, the diagnosis is secondary hypertension. An unexplained elevation in pulmonary arterial pressure is assigned the diagnosis of primary pulmonary hypertension.

The reason for an elevated pulmonary arterial pressure may be multifactorial, but the major underlying mechanism is vasoconstriction of the pulmonary arterial vessels induced by hypoxia. This vasoconstrictive process leads to structural changes or remodeling of the pulmonary vascular bed, eventually resulting in a loss of vascular reactivity.

Disease states that have been associated with pulmonary hypertension include aortic and mitral valve disease, left ventricular failure, thromboembolic disease, diseases producing hypoxia and hypoxemia, cardiac myxomas, pulmonary veno-occlusive disease, collagen vascular disease, hepatic disease, sepsis, sickle cell disease, and a parasite infestation. Pulmonary hypertension has also been drug and diet induced and has been affiliated with congenital heart disease and pregnancy.

Symptoms of primary pulmonary hypertension do not present until the disease is in its advanced stages, making the prognosis extremely poor. Whereas the treatment of secondary pulmonary hypertension is directed at correcting the known etiology, treatment of primary pulmonary hypertension has been aimed at reversing or inhibiting the pulmonary arterial vasoconstriction. The vasodilator class of drugs has received the most attention in recent years. The results have been extremely variable. What remains to be established is a consensus as to what hemodynamic alteration constitutes a therapeutic effect. At the present time, it is thought that a beneficial outcome is reflected in an increase in cardiac output associated with a decrease in pulmonary vascular resistance to a greater extent than a reduction in systemic vascular resistance. An accompanying decrease in pulmonary arterial pressure is most ideal but it is not essential.

Selection of a vasodilator agent is based on trial and error. The problem with the current vasodilator agents is a lack of specificity for the pulmonary vasculature. Their effects on the systemic vasculature may produce deleterious results. It is for this reason that the vascular response induced by these agents should be assessed in a controlled environment such as a cardiac catheterization laboratory.

Without an established medical cure for primary pulmonary hypertension, the heart–lung transplant can be considered a viable alternative in the therapeutic armamentarium.

## References


1. McGoon MD, Edwards WD. Primary pulmonary hypertension: Current status. Modern Concepts Cardiovasc Dis 1985;54(6):29–33.
2. Rubin ED. Pulmonary vascular disease and cor pulmonale, in Rubinstein E, Federman D (eds): Scientific American Medicine. New York, Scientific American, Inc, 1983, ch XIX, pp 1–8.
3. Grossman W, Alpert JS, Braunwald E. Pulmonary hypertension, in Braunwald E (ed): Heart Disease: A Textbook of Cardiovascular Medicine. Philadelphia, W.B. Saunders, 1984, pp 823–848.
4. Alpert JS, Irwin RS, Dalen JE. Pulmonary hypertension. Curr Probl Cardiol 1981;5(10):1–39.
5. Hughes JD, Rubin LJ. Primary pulmonary hypertension, an analysis of 28 cases and a review of the literature. Medicine 1986;65(1):56–72.
6. Goldstein RA. Pulmonary hypertension. Postgrad Med 1985;78(6):109–114.
7. Weir EK. Diagnosis and management of primary pulmonary hypertension, in Weir EK, Reeves JT (eds): Pulmonary Hypertension. Mount Kisco, Futuro Publishing Co, 1984, pp 115–168.
8. Dresdale DT, Schultz M, Michtom RJ. Primary pulmonary hypertension. I. Clinical and hemodynamic study. Am J Med 1951;11:686–705.
9. Widimsky J. Primary pulmonary hypertension: A review. Cor Vasa 1982;24(5):309–317.
10. Fishman AP, Pietra GG. Primary pulmonary hypertension. Annu Rev Med 1980;31:421–431.
11. Rich S, Brundage BH. Primary pulmonary hypertension: Current update. JAMA 1984;251(17):2252–2254.
12. Edwards WD, Edwards JE. Clinical primary pulmonary hypertension, three pathologic types. Circulation 1977;56(5):884–888.
13. Rich S, Pietra GG, Kieras K, et al. Primary pulmonary hypertension: Radiographic and scintigraphic patterns of histologic subtypes. Ann Intern Med 1986;105:499–502.
14. Bjornsson J, Edwards WD. Primary pulmonary hypertension: A histopathologic study of 80 cases. Mayo Clin Proc 1985;60:16–25.
15. Riedel M, Widimsky J. Symposium on primary pulmonary hypertension. Cor Vasa 1982;24(6):464–471.
16. Peter RH, Rubin L. The pharmacologic control of the pulmonary circulation in pulmonary hypertension. Adv Intern Med 1984;29:495–520.
17. Rounds S, Hill NS. Pulmonary hypertensive diseases. Chest 1984;85(3):397–405.
18. Niederman MS, Matthay RA. Cardiovascular function in secondary pulmonary hypertension. Heart Lung 1986;15(4):341–351.
19. Weber KT, Janicki JS, Shroff SG, et al. The right ventricle: Physiologic and pathophysiologic considerations. Crit Care Med 1983;11(5):323–328.
20. Sibbald WJ, Driedger AA. Right ventricular function in acute disease states: Pathophysiologic considerations. Crit Care Med 1983;11(5):339–345.
21. Stein PD, Sabbah HN, Mazzilli M, et al. Effect of chronic pressure overload on the maximal rate of pressure fall of the right ventricle. Chest 1980;78(1):10–15.
22. Dubiel JP, Dubiel JS, Horzela T. Myocardial blood flow and right coronary artery hemodynamics in patients with pulmonary hypertension. Cor Vasa 1980;22(4):258–266.

23. Kieffer RW, Hutchins GM, Moore GW, et al. Reversed septal curvature, association with primary pulmonary hypertension and Shone syndrome. Am J Med 1979;66:831–835.
24. Pittman DE. Primary pulmonary hypertension, case report and discussion of the literature. Angiology 1979;30(11):756–767.
25. Scully RE, Mark EJ, McNeely BU. Case records of the Massachusetts General Hospital. N Engl J Med 1985;313(16): 1003–1012.
26. Barst RJ, Stalcup SA. Endothelial function in clinical pulmonary hypertension. Chest 1985;88(suppl):216S–220S.
27. Wallis PJW, Wedzicha JA, Empey DW. Treatment of pulmonary hypertension in chronic bronchitis and emphysema. Br Med J 1985;290(6461):70.
28. Haltman RB. Pulmonary heart disease: Pathophysiology, diagnostic signs, and therapy. Postgrad Med 1979;66(3):58–71.
29. Thompson BT, Hales CA. Hypoxic pulmonary hypertension: Acute and chronic. Heart Lung 1986;15(5):457–465.
30. Ekici E, Olgunturk R, Ilhan M, et al. Possible relationship between pulmonary hypertension and prostaglandins. Prostaglandin Med 1981;7(1):71–77.
31. Das UN. Possible role of prostaglandins in the pathogenesis of pulmonary hypertension. Prostaglandin Med 1980;4:163–170.
32. Rengo F, Trimarco B, Chiariello M, et al. Histamine and hypoxic pulmonary hypertension, a quantitative study. Cardiovasc Res 1978;12(2):752–757.
33. Packer M. Therapeutic application of calcium channel antagonists for pulmonary hypertension. Am J Cardiol 1985;55(3): 196B–201B.
34. Michael JR, Selinger S, Parham W, et al. Use of calcium channel blockers in hypoxic lung disease. Chest 1984;88 (suppl):260S–263S.
35. Kennedy TP, Michael JR, Summer W. Calcium channel blockers in hypoxic pulmonary hypertension. Am J Med 1985;78 (suppl 2B):18–26.
36. Hurewitz AN, Bergofsky EH. Pathogenetic mechanisms in chronic pulmonary hypertension. Heart Lung 1986;15(4):327–335.
37. Reid LM. Structure and function in pulmonary hypertension, new perceptions. Chest 1986;89:279–288.
38. Samet P, Bernstein WH. Loss of reactivity of the pulmonary vascular bed in primary pulmonary hypertension. Am Heart J 1963;66(2):197–199.
39. Reeves JT, Groves BM, Turkevich D. The case for treatment of selected patients with primary pulmonary hypertension. Am Rev Respir Dis 1986;134(2):342–346.
40. Louridas G, Kakoura M, Patakas D, et al. Pulmonary hypertension and respiratory failure in the development of right ventricular hypertrophy in patients with chronic obstructive airway disease. Respiration 1984;46:52–60.
41. Keller CA, Shepard JW, Chun DS, et al. Pulmonary hypertension in chronic obstructive pulmonary disease, multivariate analysis. Chest 1986;90(2):185–192.
42. Williams IP, Boyd MJ, Humberstone AM, et al. Pulmonary arterial hypertension and emphysema. Br J Dis Chest 1984; 78(3):211–216.
43. Snow RL, Davies P, Pontoppidan H, et al. Pulmonary vascular remodeling in adult respiratory distress syndrome. Am Rev Respir Dis 1982;126:887–892.
44. Hurst DL. Pulmonary hypertension and sleep apnea. N Engl J Med 1977;296(11):631.
45. Podszus T, Bauer W, Maayer J, et al. Sleep apnea and pulmonary hypertension. Klin Wochenschr 1986;64:131–134.
46. Perkin RM, Anas NG. Pulmonary hypertension in pediatric patients. J Pediatr 1984;105(4):511–522.
47. Alpert JS, Godtfredsen J, Ockene IS, et al. Pulmonary hypertension secondary to minor pulmonary embolism. Chest 1978;73(6):795–797.
48. Alpert MA, Goldberg SH, Singsen BH, et al. Cardiovascular manifestations of mixed connective tissue disease in adults. Circulation 1983;68(6):1182–1193.
49. Fuster V, Steele PM, Edwards WD. Primary pulmonary hypertension: Natural history and the importance of thrombosis. Circulation 1984;70(4):580–587.
50. Dantzker DR, Bower JS. Partial reversibility of chronic pulmonary hypertension caused by pulmonary thromboembolic disease. Am Rev Respir Dis 1981;124(2):129–131.
51. Fanta CH, Compton CC. Microscopic tumour emboli to the lungs: A hidden cause of dyspnoea and pulmonary hypertension. Thorax 1980;35(10):794–795.
52. Willett IR, Sutherland RC, O'Rourke MF, et al. Pulmonary hypertension complicating hepatocellular carcinoma. Gastroenterology 1984;87(5):1180–1184.
53. Chakeres DW, Spiegel PK. Fatal pulmonary hypertension secondary to intravascular metastatic tumor emboli. Am J Roentgenol 1982;139(5):997–1000.
54. Hagley SR. The fulminant fat embolism syndrome. Anaesth Intensive Care 1983;11(2):162–166.
55. Xiansheng C, Wagenvoort CA. Soft tissue contusion and pulmonary hypertension. Eur J Respir Dis 1986;68:384–387.
56. Houck RJ, Bailey GL, Daroca PJ, et al. Pentazocine abuse, report of a case with pulmonary arterial cellulose granulomas and pulmonary hypertension. Chest 1980;77(2):227–230.
57. Farber HW, Falls R, Glauser FL. Transient pulmonary hypertension from the intravenous injection of crushed, suspended pentazocine tablets. Chest 1981;80(2):178–182.
58. Perez HD, Kramer N. Pulmonary hypertension in systemic lupus erythematosus: Report of 4 cases and review of the literature. Semin Arthritis Rheum 1981;11(1):177–181.
59. Gladman DD, Sternberg L. Pulmonary hypertension in systemic lupus erythematosus. J Rheumatol 1985;12(2):365–367.
60. Asherson RA, Hackett D, Gharani AE, et al. Pulmonary hypertension in systemic lupus erythematosus: A report of three cases. J Rheumatol 1986;13:416–420.
61. Quismorio FP, Sharma O, Koss M, et al. Immunopathologic and clinical studies in pulmonary hypertension associated with systemic lupus erythematosus. Semin Arthritis Rheum 1984;13(4):349–359.
62. Schwartzberg M, Lieberman DH, Getzoff B, et al. Systemic lupus erythematosus and pulmonary vascular hypertension. Arch Intern Med 1984;144(3):605–607.
63. Asherson RA, Mackworth-Young CG, Boey ML. Pulmonary hypertension in systemic lupus erythematosus. Br Med J 1983;287(6398):1024–1025.
64. Salerni R, Rodnan G, Leon D, et al. Pulmonary hypertension in the CREST syndrome variant of progressive systemic sclerosis (scleroderma). Ann Intern Med 1977;86(4):394–399.
65. Barst RJ, Ratner SJ. Sarcoidosis and reactive pulmonary hypertension. Arch Intern Med 1985;145:2112–2114.
66. Ungerer RG, Tashkin DP, Furst D, et al. Prevalence and clinical correlates of pulmonary arterial hypertension in progressive systemic sclerosis. Am J Med 1983;75(1):65–74.
67. Stupi AM, Steen VD, Owens GR, et al. Pulmonary hypertension in the CREST syndrome variant of systemic sclerosis. Arthritis Rheum 1986;29(4):515–525.
68. Wiener-Kronish JP, Solinger AM, Warnock ML, et al. Severe pulmonary involvement in mixed connective tissue disease. Am Rev Respir Dis 1981;124(4):499–503.
69. Kay JM, Banik S. Unexplained pulmonary hypertension with pulmonary arteritis in rheumatoid disease. Br J Dis Chest 1977;71(1):53–59.

70. Asherson RA, Morgan SH, Hackett D, et al. Rheumatoid arthritis and pulmonary hypertension, a report of three cases. J Rheumatol 1985;12:154–159.
71. Fox RI, Howell FV, Bone RC, et al. Primary Sjögren's syndrome: Clinical and immunopathologic features. Semin Arthritis Rheum 1984;14:77–105.
72. Caldwell IW, Aitchison JD. Pulmonary hypertension in dermatomyositis. Br Heart J 1956;18:273–276.
73. Bunch TW, Tancredi RG, Lie JT. Pulmonary hypertension in polymyositis. Chest 1981;79(1):105–107.
74. Morrison DA, Gay RG, Feldshon D, et al. Severe pulmonary hypertension in a patient with Whipple's disease. Am J Med 1985;79(2):263–267.
75. Asherson RA, Morgan SH, Harris N. Pulmonary hypertension and chronic lupus erythematosus: Association with the lupus anticoagulant. Arthritis Rheum 1985;28(1):118.
76. Anderson NE, Ali MR. The lupus anticoagulant, pulmonary thromboembolism and fatal pulmonary hypertension. Ann Rheum Dis 1984;43(5):760–763.
77. Ohar JM, Robichaud AM, Fowler AA, et al. Increased pulmonary artery pressure in association with Raynaud's phenomenon. Am J Med 1986;81:361–362.
78. Widgren S. Pulmonary hypertension related to aminorex intake (histologic, ultrastructural, and morphometric studies of 37 cases in Switzerland). Curr Top Pathol 1977;64:1–64.
79. Gurtner HP. Aminorex and pulmonary hypertension, a review. Cor Vasa 1985;27:160–171.
80. McMurray J, Bloomfield P, Miller HC. Irreversible pulmonary hypertension after treatment with fenfluramine. Br Med J 1986;292:239–240.
81. Douglas JG, Munro JF, Kitchen AF, et al. Pulmonary hypertension and fenfluramine. Br Med J 1981;283(6296):881–883.
82. Cameron J, Waugh L, Loadsman T, et al. Possible association of pulmonary hypertension with an anorectic drug. Med J Aust 1984;140(10):595–597.
83. Glauser FL, Fairman RP, Monroe P, et al. Transient pulmonary hypertension associated with esophageal sclerotherapy. Chest 1984;86(5):658–659.
84. Hammond B, Fairman RP, Monroe P, et al. The pulmonary hypertension of sclerosing agents is prevented by cyclooxygenase inhibitors. Am J Med Sci 1985;290(3):98–101.
85. Asherson RA, Benbow AG, Speirs CT, et al. Pulmonary hypertension in hydralazine induced systemic lupus erythematosus: Association with C4 null allele. Ann Rheum Dis 1986;45: 771–773.
86. Kleiger RE, Boxer M, Ingham RE, et al. Pulmonary hypertension in patients using oral contraceptives, a report of six cases. Chest 1976;69:143–147.
87. McCarthy JT, Staats BA. Pulmonary hypertension, hemolytic anemia, and renal failure, a mitomycin-associated syndrome. Chest 1986;89:608–611.
88. McIntyre RW, Flezzani P, Knopes KO, et al. Pulmonary hypertension and prostaglandins after protamine. Am J Cardiol 1986;58(9):857–858.
89. Garcia MC, Posada De La Paz M, Diaz de Rojas F, et al. Pulmonary hypertension after toxic rapeseed oil ingestion. J Am Coll Cardiol 1984;4(2):443.
90. Garcia-Dorado D, Miller DD, Garcia EJ, et al. An epidemic of pulmonary hypertension after toxic rapeseed oil ingestion in Spain. J Am Coll Cardiol 1983;1(5):1216–1222.
91. Altiere RJ, Olson JW, Gillespie MN. Altered pulmonary vascular smooth muscle responsiveness in monocrotaline-induced pulmonary hypertension. J Pharmacol Exp Ther 1986;236(2): 390–395.
92. Lebrec D, Capron JP, Dhumeaux D, et al. Pulmonary hypertension complicating portal hypertension. Am Rev Respir Dis 1979;120(4):849–856.
93. Krowka MJ, Cortese DA. Pulmonary aspects of chronic liver disease and liver transplantation. Mayo Clin Proc 1985;60:407–418.
94. Lockhart A. Pulmonary arterial hypertension in portal hypertension. Clin Gastroenterol 1985;14(1):123–139.
95. Cohen MD, Rubin LJ, Taylor WE, et al. Primary pulmonary hypertension: An unusual case associated with extrahepatic portal hypertension. Hepatology 1983;3(4):588–592.
96. Pare PD, Chin-Yan C, Wass H, et al. Portal and pulmonary hypertension, with microangiopathic hemolytic anemia. Am J Med 1983;74(6):1093–1096.
97. Bernthal AC, Eybel CE, Payne JA. Primary pulmonary hypertension after portacaval shunt. J Clin Gastroenterol 1983;5(4): 353–356.
98. Morrison EB, Gaffney FA, Eigenbrodt EH. Severe pulmonary hypertension associated with macronodular (postnecrotic) cirrhosis and autoimmune phenomenon. Am J Med 1980;69(4): 513–519.
99. Chun PKC, San Antonio RP, Davia JE. Laennec's cirrhosis and primary pulmonary hypertension. Am Heart J 1980;99(6): 779–782.
100. Brisbane JV, Howell DA, Bonkowsky HL. Pulmonary hypertension as a presentation of hepatocarcinoma. Report of a case and brief review of the literature. Am J Med 1980;68(3):466–469.
101. Chronic active hepatitis and pulmonary hypertension. (Clinicopathologic Conference) Am J Med 1977;63(4):604–613.
102. Saunders JB, Constable TJ, Heath D. Pulmonary hypertension complicating portal vein thrombosis. Thorax 1979;34(2):281–283.
103. Flemale A, Sabot JP, Popijn M, et al. Pulmonary hypertension associated with portal thrombosis. Eur J Resp Dis 1985;66(3): 224–228.
104. Dawkins KD, Burke CM, Billingham ME, et al. Primary pulmonary hypertension and pregnancy. Chest 1986;89:383–388.
105. Feijen HWH, Hein PR, Van Lakwijk-Vondrovicova EL. Primary pulmonary hypertension and pregnancy. Eur J Obstet Gynecol Reprod Biol 1983;15(3):159–164.
106. Nelson DM, Main E, Crafford W, et al. Peripartum heart failure due to pulmonary hypertension. Obstet Gynecol 1983; 62(3 suppl):58S–63S.
107. Lloyd JE, Primm RK, Newman JH. Familial primary pulmonary hypertension: Clinical patterns. Am Rev Respir Dis 1984;129(1):194–197.
108. Basu B, Cherian G, Krishnaswami S, et al. Severe pulmonary hypertension in advanced aortic valve disease. Br Heart J 1978;40(11):1310–1313.
109. Riegel N, Ambrose JA, Mindich BP, et al. Isolated aortic stenosis with severe pulmonary hypertension. Cathet Cardiovasc Diagn 1985;11(2):181–185.
110. Widimsky J. Pulmonary precapillary hypertension in mitral valve disease. Cor Vasa 1983;25(1):17–27.
111. Factor SM, Reichel J. Primary pulmonary hypertension. Am Heart J 1980;99(6):789–798.
112. Glassroth J, Woodford DW, Carrington CB, et al. Pulmonary veno-occlusive disease in the middle-aged. Respiration 1985; 47:309–321.
113. McDowell PJ, Summer WA, Hutchins GM. Pulmonary veno-occlusive disease. Morphological changes suggesting a viral cause. JAMA 1981;246(6):667–671.
114. Sole MJ, Drobac M, Schwartz L, et al. The extraction of circulating catecholamines by the lungs in normal man and in

patients with pulmonary hypertension. Circulation 1979;60(1): 160–163.
**115.** Zaloga GP, Chernow B, Fletcher JR, et al. Increased circulating plasma norepinephrine concentrations in noncardiac causes of pulmonary hypertension. Crit Care Med 1984;12(2): 85–89.
**116.** Ahmed T, Sackner MA. Increased serum copper in primary pulmonary hypertension: A possible pathogenic link? Respiration 1985;47:243–246.
**117.** Sibbald WJ, Patterson NAM, Holliday RL, et al. Pulmonary hypertension in sepsis. Measurement by the pulmonary arterial diastolic–pulmonary wedge pressure gradient and the influence of passive and active factors. Chest 1978;73(5):583–591.
**118.** Kanemoto N, Sasamoto H. Arrhythmias in primary pulmonary hypertension. Jpn Heart J 1979;20(6):765–775.
**119.** Zimmerman D, Parker BM. The pain of pulmonary hypertension. Fact or fancy? JAMA 1981;246(20):2345–2346.
**120.** Wilmshurst PT, Webb-Peploe MM, Conker RJ. Left recurrent laryngeal nerve palsy associated with primary pulmonary hypertension and recurrent pulmonary embolism. Br Heart J 1983;49(2):141–143.
**121.** Nakao M, Sawayawa T, Samukawa M, et al. Left recurrent laryngeal nerve palsy associated with primary pulmonary hypertension and patent ductus arteriosus. J Am Coll Cardiol 1985;49(2):141–143.
**122.** Tatum VD, Light RW. Approach to the diagnosis of secondary pulmonary hypertension: The chest roentgenogram as a diagnostic tool. Heart Lung 1986;15(4):352–357.
**123.** Phipps B, Wong B, Chang CHJ, et al. Unexplained severe pulmonary hypertension in the older age group. Chest 1983;84(4):399–402.
**124.** Chetty KG, Brown SE, Light RW. Identification of pulmonary hypertension in chronic obstructive pulmonary disease from routine chest radiographs. Am Rev Respir Dis 1982;126(2): 338–341.
**125.** Kanemoto N, Furuya H, Etoh T, et al. Chest roentgenograms in primary pulmonary hypertension. Chest 1979;76(1):45–49.
**126.** Kanemoto N. Electrocardiogram in primary pulmonary hypertension. Eur J Cardiol 1981;12:181–193.
**127.** Berger M, Haimowitz A, Vantosh A, et al. Quantitative assessment of pulmonary hypertension in patients with tricuspid regurgitation using continuous wave Doppler ultrasound. J Am Coll Cardiol 1985;6:359–365.
**128.** Zeiher AM, Bonzel T, Wollschlager H, et al. Noninvasive evaluation of pulmonary hypertension by quantitative contrast M-mode echocardiography. Am Heart J 1986;111:297–306.
**129.** Berger BC, Walinsky P, Carey P. Primary pulmonary hypertension: M-mode and two-dimensional echocardiographic findings. Cathet Cardiovasc Diagn 1983;9(2):187–195.
**130.** Isobe M, Yazaki Y, Takaku F, et al. Prediction of pulmonary arterial pressure in adults by pulsed Doppler echocardiography. Am J Cardiol 1986;57:316–321.
**131.** Reeves JT, Groves BM. Approach to the patient with pulmonary hypertension, in Weir EK, Reeves JT (eds): Pulmonary Hypertension. Mount Kisco, Futuro Publishing Co. 1984, pp 1–44.
**132.** Shimada R, Takashirta A, Nakamura M. Noninvasive assessment of right ventricular systolic pressure in atrial septal defect. Analysis of the end-systolic configuration of the ventricular septum by two-dimensional echocardiography. Am J Cardiol 1984;53:1117–1123.
**133.** Martin-Duran R, Lariman M, Trugeda A, et al. Comparison of Doppler-determined elevated pulmonary arterial pressure with pressure measured at cardiac catheterization. Am J Cardiol 1986;57:859–863.
**134.** Masuyama T, Kodama K, Kitabatake A, et al. Continuous wave Doppler echocardiographic detection of pulmonary regurgitation and its application to noninvasive estimation of pulmonary artery pressure. Circulation 1986;74(3):484–492.
**135.** Leier CV, Sahar D, Hermiller JB, et al. Combining left ventricular systolic time intervals and M-mode echocardiography in the evaluation of primary pulmonary hypertension in women. Clin Cardiol 1985;8:166–172.
**136.** Hecht SR, Berger M, Berdoff RL, et al. Use of continuous-wave Doppler ultrasound to evaluate and manage primary pulmonary hypertension. Chest 1986;90:781–783.
**137.** Wagenvoort CA. Lung biopsy specimens in the evaluation of pulmonary vascular disease. Chest 1980;77(8):614–625.
**138.** Wagenvoort CA. Lung biopsy findings in secondary pulmonary hypertension. Heart Lung 1986;15(5):429–450.
**139.** Fujii A, Rabinovitch M, Matthews EC. A case of spontaneous resolution of idiopathic pulmonary hypertension. Br Heart J 1981;46(5):574–577.
**140.** Rich S, Levy PS. Characteristics of surviving and nonsurviving patients with primary pulmonary hypertension. Am J Med 1984;76(4):573–578.
**141.** Kanemoto N, Sasamoto H. Pulmonary hemodynamics in primary pulmonary hypertension. Jpn Heart J 1979;20(4):395–405.
**142.** Rozkovec A, Montanes P, Oakley CM. Factors that influence the outcome of primary pulmonary hypertension. Br Heart J 1986;55:449–458.
**143.** Peil ML, Rubin LJ. Therapy of secondary pulmonary hypertension. Heart Lung 1986;15(5):450–456.
**144.** Rich S, Martinez J, Lam W, et al. Reassessment of the effects of vasodilator drugs in primary pulmonary hypertension: Guidelines for determining a pulmonary vasodilator response. Am Heart J 1983;105(1):119–127.
**145.** Packer M. Vasodilator therapy for primary pulmonary hypertension. Limitations and hazards. Ann Intern Med 1985;103(2): 258–270.
**146.** Rich S, D'Alonzo GE, Dantzker DR, et al. Magnitude and implications of spontaneous hemodynamic variability in primary pulmonary hypertension. Am J Cardiol 1985;55:159–163.
**147.** Rich S, Brundage BH, Levy PS. The effect of vasodilator therapy on the clinical outcome of patients with primary pulmonary hypertension. Circulation 1985;71(6):1191–1196.
**148.** Franciosa JA, Fischer HA. Right ventricular unloading. Lessons from the left. Ann Intern Med 1981;95(5):647–648.
**149.** Hermiller JB, Bambach D, Thompson MJ, et al. Vasodilators and prostaglandin inhibitors in primary pulmonary hypertension. Ann Intern Med 1982;97:480–489.
**150.** Ruskin JN, Hutter AM. Primary pulmonary hypertension treated with oral phentolamine. Ann Intern Med 1979;90:772–774.
**151.** Gould L, Chokshi AB, Patel S, et al. Hemodynamic evaluation of vasodilator therapy in primary pulmonary hypertension. Am Heart J 1981:102:300.
**152.** Fennell WH, Farmer JA, Graf RH. Unanticipated response to alpha-adrenergic blockade in pulmonary hypertension. Chest 1982;81(1):128–129.
**153.** Cohen ML, Kronzon I. Adverse hemodynamic effects of phentolamine in primary pulmonary hypertension. Ann Intern Med 1981;95(5):591–592.
**154.** Lupi-Herrera E, Bialostozky D, Sobrino A. The role of isoproterenol in pulmonary artery hypertension of unknown etiology (primary). Short- and long-term evaluation. Chest 1981;79(3):292–296.
**155.** Shettigar UR, Hultgren HN, Specter M, et al. Primary pulmo-

nary hypertension. Favorable effect of isoproterenol. N Engl J Med 1976;295(25):1414–1415.
156. Pietro DA, LaBresh KA, Shulman RM, et al. Sustained improvement in primary pulmonary hypertension during six-years of treatment with sublingual isoproterenol. N Engl J Med 1984;310(16):1032–1034.
157. Elkayam U, Frishman WH, Yoran L, et al. Unfavorable hemodynamic and clinical effects of isoproterenol in primary pulmonary hypertension. Cardiovasc Med 1978;3:1177–1180.
158. McLeod AA, Jewitt DE. Drug treatment of primary pulmonary hypertension. Drugs 1986;31:177–184.
159. Palevsky HI, Fishman AP. Vasodilator therapy for primary pulmonary hypertension. Annu Rev Med 1985;36:563–578.
160. Klinke WP, Gilbert JAL. Diazoxide in primary pulmonary hypertension. N Engl J Med 1980;302(2):91–92.
161. Honey M, Cotter L, Davies N, et al. Clinical and haemodynamic effects of diazoxide in primary pulmonary hypertension. Thorax 1980;35(4):269–276.
162. Wang SWS, Pohl JEF, Rowlands DJ, et al. Diazoxide in treatment of primary pulmonary hypertension. Br Heart J 1978;40:572–574.
163. Buch J, Wennevold A. Hazards of diazoxide in pulmonary hypertension. Br Heart J 1981;46(4):401–403.
164. Hall DR, Petch MC. Remission of primary pulmonary hypertension during treatment with diazoxide. Br Med J 1981;282 (6270):1118.
165. Rubino JM, Schroeder JS. Diazoxide in treatment of primary pulmonary hypertension. Br Heart J 1979;42(3):362–363.
166. Packer M, Halpern JL, Brooks KM, et al. Nitroglycerin therapy in the management of pulmonary hypertensive disorders. Am J Med 1984;76(6A):67–75.
167. Pearl RG, Rosenthal MH, Schroeder JS, et al. Acute hemodynamic effects of nitroglycerin in pulmonary hypertension. Ann Intern Med 1983;99(1):9–13.
168. Ziskind Z, Pohoryles L, Mohr R, et al. The effects of low-dose intravenous nitroglycerin on pulmonary hypertension immediately after replacement of a stenotic mitral valve. Circulation 1985;72(supp II):164–169.
169. Damen J, Hitchcock JF. Reactive pulmonary hypertension after a switch operation. Successful treatment with glyceryl trinitrate. Br Heart J 1985;53(2):223–225.
170. Zaloga GP, Chernow B, Holt MR, et al. Effect of vasodilators on pulmonary vascular resistance in patients with pulmonary hypertension. Clin Pharm 1983;2:265–268.
171. Brent BN, Berger HJ, Matthay RA, et al. Contrasting acute effects of vasodilators (nitroglycerin, nitroprusside, and hydralazine) on right ventricular performance in patients with chronic obstructive pulmonary disease and pulmonary hypertension: A combined radionuclide–hemodynamic study. Am J Cardiol 1983;51:1682–1689.
172. Hoit B, Gregoratos G, Shabetai R. Paradoxical pulmonary vasoconstriction induced by nitroglycerin in idiopathic pulmonary hypertension. J Am Coll Cardiol 1985;6(2):490–492.
173. Danahy DT, Tobis JM, Aronow WS, et al. Effects of isosorbide dinitrate on pulmonary hypertension in chronic obstructive pulmonary disease. Clin Pharmacol Ther 1979;25(5):541–548.
174. Kanemoto N, Imaoka C, Goto Y. A case of primary pulmonary hypertension treated with prazosin and isosorbide dinitrate. Jpn Heart J 1984;25(6):1085–1089.
175. Cerda E, Esteban A, De La Cal MA, et al. Hemodynamic effects of vasodilators on pulmonary hypertension in decompensated chronic obstructive pulmonary disease. Crit Care Med 1985;13(4):221–223.
176. Faraci PA, Rheinlander HF, Cleveland RJ. Use of nitroprusside for control of pulmonary hypertension in repair of ventricular septal defect. Ann Thorac Surg 1980;29(1):70–73.
177. Rubin LJ, Peter RH. Oral hydralazine therapy for primary pulmonary hypertension. N Engl J Med 1980;302(2):69–73.
178. Rubin LJ, Handel F, Peter RH. The effects of oral hydralazine on right ventricular end-diastolic pressure in patients with right ventricular failure. Circulation 1982;65(7):1369–1373.
179. Lupi-Herrera E, Sandoval J, Seoane M, et al. The role of hydralazine therapy for pulmonary arterial hypertension of unknown cause. Circulation 1982;65(4):645–650.
180. Lupi-Herrera E, Seoane M, Verdejo J. Hemodynamic effect of hydralazine in interstitial lung disease patients with cor pulmonale. Chest 1985;87(5):564–573.
181. Keller CA, Shephard Jr JW, Chun DS, et al. Effects of hydralazine on hemodynamics, ventilation, and gas exchange in patients with chronic obstructive pulmonary disease and pulmonary hypertension. Am Rev Respir Dis 1984;130(4):606–611.
182. Dal Nogare AR, Rubin LJ. The effects of exercise capacity in pulmonary hypertension secondary to chronic obstructive pulmonary disease. Am Rev Respir Dis 1986;133:385–389.
183. McGoon MD, Seward JB, Vlietstra RE, et al. Haemodynamic response to intravenous hydralazine in patients with pulmonary hypertension. Br Heart J 1983;50(6):579–585.
184. Packer M, Greenberg B, Massie B, et al. Deleterious effects of hydralazine in patients with pulmonary hypertension. N Engl J Med 1982;306(22):1326–1331.
185. Tuxen DU, Powles ACP, Mathur PN, et al. Detrimental effects of hydralazine in patients with chronic air-flow obstruction and pulmonary hypertension. A combined hemodynamic and radionuclide study. Am Rev Respir Dis 1984;129(3):388–395.
186. Kronzon I, Cohen M, Winer HE. Adverse effect of hydralazine in patients with primary pulmonary hypertension. JAMA 1982;247(22):3112–3114.
187. Laine JF, Slama M, Petitpretz P, et al. Danger of vasodilator therapy for pulmonary hypertension in patent foramen ovale. Chest 1986;89:894–895.
188. Rubin LJ, Groves BM, Reeves JT, et al. Prostacyclin-induced acute pulmonary vasodilation in primary pulmonary hypertension. Circulation 1982;66(2):334–338.
189. Guadagni DN, Ikram H, Maslowski AH. Haemodynamic effects of prostacyclin ($PGI_2$) in pulmonary hypertension. Br Heart J 1981;45:385–388.
190. Higenbottam T, Wheeldon D, Wells F, et al. Long term treatment of primary pulmonary hypertension with continuous intravenous epoprostenol (prostacyclin). Lancet 1984;1(8385): 1046–1047.
191. Kaapa P, Koiuisto M, Ylikorkala O, et al. Prostacyclin in the treatment of neonatal pulmonary hypertension. J Pediatr 1985;107(6):951–953.
192. Bush A, Busst C, Booth K, et al. Does prostacyclin enhance the selective pulmonary vasodilator effect of oxygen in children with congenital heart disease? Circulation 1986;74(1):135–144.
193. Groves BM, Rubin LJ, Frosolono MF, et al. A comparison of the acute hemodynamic effects of prostacyclin and hydralazine in primary pulmonary hypertension. Am Heart J 1985;110: 1200–1204.
194. Barst RJ. Pharmacologically induced pulmonary vasodilation in children and young adults with primary pulmonary hypertension. Chest 1986;89:497–503.
195. Rozkovec A, Stradling J, Minty K, et al. Hydralazine in pulmonary hypertension. N Engl J Med 1982;307(19):1214–1215.

**196.** Swan PK, Tidballs J, Duncan AW. Prostaglandin $E_1$ in primary pulmonary hypertension. Crit Care Med 1986;14(1):72–73.

**197.** Watkins WD, Peterson MB, Crone RK, et al. Prostacyclin and prostaglandin $E_1$ for severe idiopathic pulmonary artery hypertension. Lancet 1980;1(8177):1083.

**198.** Szczeklik J, Dubiel JS, Mysik M, et al. Effects of prostaglandin $E_1$ on pulmonary circulation in patients with pulmonary hypertension. Br Heart J 1978;40(12):1397–1401.

**199.** Naeije R, Melot C, Mols P, et al. Reduction in pulmonary hypertension by prostaglandin $E_1$ in decompensated chronic obstructive pulmonary disease. Am Rev Respir Dis 1982; 125(1):1–5.

**200.** D'Ambra MN, LaRaia PJ, Philbin DM, et al. Prostaglandin $E_1$. A new therapy for refractory right heart failure and pulmonary hypertension after mitral valve replacement. J Thorac Cardiovasc Surg 1985;89(4):567–572.

**201.** Archer SL, Chesler E, Cohn JN, et al. ZK 36-374, a stable analog of prostacyclin, prevents acute hypoxic pulmonary hypertension in the dog. J Am Coll Cardiol 1986;8(5):1189–1194.

**202.** Kaukinen S, Ylitalo P, Pessi T, et al. Hemodynamic effects of iloprost, a prostacyclin analog. Clin Pharmacol Ther 1984;36(4):464–469.

**203.** Young TE, Lundquist LJ, Chesler E, et al. Comparative effects of nifedipine, verapamil, and diltiazem on experimental pulmonary hypertension. Am J Cardiol 1983;51(1):195–200.

**204.** Camerini F, Alberti E, Klugman S, et al. Primary pulmonary hypertension: Effects of nifedipine. Br Heart J 1980;44:352–356.

**205.** Rubin LJ, Nicod P, Hillis LD, et al. Treatment of primary pulmonary hypertension with nifedipine. A hemodynamic and scintigraphic evaluation. Ann Intern Med 1983;99(4):433–438.

**206.** Olivari MT, Levine TB, Weir EK. Hemodynamic effects of nifedipine at rest and during exercise in primary pulmonary hypertension. Chest 1984;86(1):14–19.

**207.** Saito D, Haraoka S, Yoshida H, et al. Primary pulmonary hypertension improved by long term oral administration of nifedipine. Am Heart J 1983;105(6):1041–1042.

**208.** DeFeyter PJ, Kerkkamp HJJ, DeJong JP. Sustained beneficial effect of nifedipine in primary pulmonary hypertension. Am Heart J 1983;105(2):333–334.

**209.** Lunde P, Rasmusser K. Long-term beneficial effect of nifedipine in primary pulmonary hypertension. Am Heart J 1984; 108(2):415–416.

**210.** Douglas Jr JS. Hemodynamic effects of nifedipine in primary pulmonary hypertension. J Am Coll Cardiol 1983;2(1):174–179.

**211.** Wise Jr JR. Nifedipine in the treatment of primary pulmonary hypertension. Am Heart J 1983;105(4):693–694.

**212.** Kennedy TP, Michael JR, Huang CK, et al. Nifedipine inhibits hypoxic pulmonary vasoconstriction during rest and exercise in patients with chronic obstructive pulmonary disease. Am Rev Respir Dis 1984;129(4):544–551.

**213.** Sturani C, Bassein L, Schiavina M, et al. Oral nifedipine in chronic cor pulmonale secondary to severe chronic obstructive pulmonary disease (COPD). Short- and long-term hemodynamic effects. Chest 1983;84(2):135–142.

**214.** Muramoto A, Caldwell J, Albert RK, et al. Nifedipine dilates the pulmonary vasculature without producing symptomatic systemic hypotension in upright resting and exercising patients with pulmonary hypertension secondary to chronic obstructive pulmonary disease. Am Rev Respir Dis 1985;132:963–966.

**215.** Garzaniti N, Allaf EL, D'Orio U, et al. Hemodynamic effects of nifedipine on secondary pulmonary hypertension in man. Acta Cardiol 1985;40(2):207–215.

**216.** Simonneau G, Escourrou P, Duroux P, et al. Inhibition of hypoxic pulmonary vasoconstriction by nifedipine. N Engl J Med 1981;304(26):1582–1585.

**217.** Hamet A, Kral B, Chernohorsky D. Comparative effects of oxygen, nifedipine, and ketanserin in hypoxic pulmonary hypertension. Cor Vasa 1985;27(6):406–411.

**218.** Ocken S, Reinitz E, Strom J. Nifedipine treatment for pulmonary hypertension in a patient with systemic sclerosis. Arthritis Rheum 1983;26(6):794–796.

**219.** Fudman EJ, Kelling Jr DG. Transient effect of nifedipine on pulmonary hypertension of systemic sclerosis. J Rheumatol 1985;12:1191–1192.

**220.** Wood BA, Tortoledo F, Luck JC, et al. Rapid attenuation of response to nifedipine in primary pulmonary hypertension. Chest 1982;82(6):793–794.

**221.** Fisher J, Borer JS, Moses JW, et al. Hemodynamic effects of nifedipine versus hydralazine in primary pulmonary hypertension. Am J Cardiol 1984;54(6):646–650.

**222.** Rich S, Ganz R, Levy PS. Comparative actions of hydralazine, nifedipine, and amrinone in primary pulmonary hypertension. Am J Cardiol 1983;52(8):1104–1107.

**223.** Bartra AK, Segall PH, Ahmed T. Pulmonary edema with nifedipine in primary pulmonary hypertension. Respiration 1985;47:161–163.

**224.** Aromatorio GJ, Uretsky B, Reddy PS. Hypotension and sinus arrest with nifedipine in pulmonary hypertension. Chest 1985;87(2):265–267.

**225.** Melot C, Naeije R, Mols P, et al. Effects of nifedipine on ventilation/perfusion/matching in primary pulmonary hypertension. Chest 1983;83(2):203–207.

**226.** Kastanos N, Estopa P, Rodriguez-Roisen, et al. Hydralazine in pulmonary hypertension. N Engl J Med 1982;307(19):1215.

**227.** Krol RC, Evans AT, Albright DP, et al. Primary pulmonary hypertension, nifedipine, and hypoxemia. Ann Intern Med 1984;100(1):163.

**228.** Packer M, Medina N, Yushak M. Adverse hemodynamic and clinical effects of calcium channel blockade in pulmonary hypertension secondary to obliterative pulmonary vascular disease. J Am Coll Cardiol 1984;4(5):890–901.

**229.** Dalal JJ, Griffiths BE, Henderson AH. Primary pulmonary hypertension: Effects of nifedipine. Br Heart J 1981;46:230–231.

**230.** Farber HW, Karlinsky JB, Faling LJ. Fatal outcome following nifedipine for pulmonary hypertension. Chest 1983;83(4):708–709.

**231.** Kambara H, Fujimoto K, Wakabayashi A, et al. Primary pulmonary hypertension: Beneficial therapy with diltiazem. Am Heart J 1981;101(2):230–231.

**232.** Crevey BJ, Dantzker DR, Bower JS, et al. Hemodynamic and gas exchange effects on intravenous diltiazem in patients with pulmonary hypertension. Am J Cardiol 1982;49(3):578–583.

**233.** Stanbrook HS, Morris KG, McMurty IF. Prevention and reversal of hypoxic pulmonary hypertension by calcium antagonists. Am Rev Respir Dis 1984;130(1):81–85.

**234.** Landmark K, Refsum AM, Simonsen S, et al. Verapamil and pulmonary hypertension. Acta Med Scand 1978;204(4):299–302.

**235.** Malcic I, Richter D. Verapamil in primary pulmonary hypertension. Br Heart J 1985;53(3):345–347.

**236.** O'Brien JT, Hill JA, Pepine CJ. Sustained benefit of verapamil in pulmonary hypertension with progressive systemic sclerosis. Am Heart J 1985;109(2):380–382.

**237.** Packer M, Medina N, Yushak M, et al. Detrimental effects of verapamil in patients with primary hypertension. Br Heart J 1984;52(1):106–111.

**238.** Archer SL, Yankuvich RD, Chesler E, et al. Comparative

effects of nisoldipine, nifedipine, and bepridil on experimental pulmonary hypertension. J Pharmacol Exp 1985;233(1):12–17.
**239.** Michael JR, Kennedy TP, Buescher P, et al. Nitrendipine attenuates the pulmonary vascular remodeling and right ventricular hypertrophy caused by intermittent hypoxia in rats. Am Rev Respir Dis 1986;133:375–379.
**240.** Singh BN, Baky S, Nademanee K. Second-generation calcium antagonists: Search for greater selectivity and versatility. Am J Cardiol 1985;55:214B–221B.
**241.** Arnman K, Ryden L, Smedgard P, et al. Felodipine in primary pulmonary hypertension, report of two cases. Acta Med Scand 1984;215(3):275–280.
**242.** Bratel T, Hedenstierna G, Nyquist O, et al. The effect of a new calcium antagonist, felodipine, on pulmonary hypertension and gas exchange in chronic obstructive lung Disease. Eur J Respir Dis 1985;67:244–253.
**243.** Bratel T, Hedenstierna G, Nyquist O, et al. Long-term treatment with a new calcium antagonist, felodipine, in chronic obstructive lung disease. Eur J Respir Dis 1986;68:351–361.
**244.** Horowitz JD, Brennan JB, Oliver LE, et al. Effects of captopril (SQ14,225) in a patient with primary pulmonary hypertension. Postgrad Med J 1981;57(664):115–116.
**245.** Ikram H, Maslowski AH, Nichols MG, et al. Haemodynamic and hormonal effects of captopril in primary pulmonary hypertension. Br Heart J 1982;48(6):541–545.
**246.** Hughes GS, Porter RS. Captopril and primary pulmonary hypertension. Ann Intern Med 1983;99(4):569.
**247.** Niarchos AP, Whitman HH, Goldstein JE, et al. Hemodynamic effects of captopril in pulmonary hypertension of collagen vascular disease. Am Heart J 1983;104(4, pt 1):834–838.
**248.** Prouse PJ, Lahiri A, Gumpel JM. The CREST syndrome—Successful reduction of pulmonary hypertension by captopril. Postgrad Med J 1984;60(708):672–674.
**249.** Bertoli L, Lo Cicero S, Buenardo I, et al. Effects of captopril on hemodynamics and blood gases in chronic obstructive lung disease with pulmonary hypertension. Respiration 1986;49: 251–256.
**250.** Boschetti E, Tantucci C, Cocchieri M, et al. Acute effects of captopril in hypoxic pulmonary hypertension. Respiration 1985;48:296–302.
**251.** Kastanos N, Miro RE, Agusti-Vidal A. Captopril in pulmonary hypertension. Br Heart J 1983;49(5):513–514.
**252.** Leier CV, Bambach D, Nelson S, et al. Captopril in primary pulmonary hypertension. Circulation 1983;67(1):155–161.
**253.** Rich S, Martinez J, Lam W. Captopril as treatment for patients with pulmonary hypertension, problem of variability in assessing chronic drug treatment. Br Heart J 1982;48(3):272–277.
**254.** Morganroth ML, Stenmark KR, Morris KG, et al. Diethylcarbamazine inhibits acute and chronic hypoxic pulmonary hypertension in awake rats. Am Rev Respir Dis 1985;131(4):488–492.
**255.** Meuleman TR, Hill DC, Port JD, et al. Ketanserin prevents platelet aggregation and endotoxin-induced pulmonary vasoconstriction. Crit Care Med 1983;11(8):606–611.
**256.** McGoon MD, Vlietstra RE. Vasodilator therapy for primary pulmonary hypertension. Mayo Clin Proc 1984;59:672–677.
**257.** Cohen M, Edwards W, Fuster V. Regression in thromboembolic type of primary pulmonary hypertension during 2½ years of antithrombotic therapy. J Am Coll Cardiol 1986;7:172–175.
**258.** Haneda T, Nakajima T, Shirato K, et al. Effects of oxygen breathing on pulmonary vascular input impedance in patients with pulmonary hypertension. Chest 1983;83(3):520–527.
**259.** Weitzenblum E, Sautegeau A, Ehrhart M. Long-term oxygen therapy can reverse the progression of pulmonary hypertension in patients with chronic obstructive pulmonary disease. Am Rev Respir Dis 1985;131(4):493–498.
**260.** Nocturnal Oxygen Therapy Trial Group. Continuous or nocturnal oxygen therapy in hypoxemic chronic obstructive lung disease, a clinical trial. Ann Intern Med 1980;93(3):391–398.
**261.** Nagasaka Y, Akutsu H, Lee YS, et al. Longterm favorable effect of oxygen administration on a patient with primary pulmonary hypertension. Chest 1978;74(3):299–300.
**262.** Cooley DA, Bloodwell RD, Hallman GL. Organ transplantation for advanced cardiopulmonary disease. Am Thorac Surg 1969;8:30–42.
**263.** Jamieson SW, Stinson EB, Oyer PE. Heart–lung transplantation for irreversible pulmonary hypertension. Ann Thorac Surg 1984;38(6):554–562.
**264.** Reitz BA, Wallwork JL, Hunt SA, et al. Heart-lung transplantation, successful therapy for patients with pulmonary vascular disease. N Engl J Med 1982;306(10):557–564.

# Chapter 17 / Peripheral Vascular Disease

Christine M. Quandt, PharmD

The term *peripheral vascular disease* (PVD), in its broadest sense, applies to disease of any of the blood vessels outside the heart and thoracic aorta and to disease of the lymph vessels. Although this term includes cerebrovascular and hypertensive vascular disease, these two topics are discussed in other sections. The other major area included in this term is peripheral vascular disease of the extremities, which can be divided into two distinct systems: (1) venous disorders such as acute deep vein thrombosis and its complications of pulmonary embolism and postthrombotic syndrome, and (2) peripheral arterial disease resulting from occlusion and arterial vasospasm. In this chapter we concentrate on peripheral arterial disease; Chapter 20 is devoted to acute thromboembolic disorders. Because there are several distinct peripheral vascular diseases, epidemiology, pathophysiology, clinical presentation, and treatment are oriented to the particular disease. A general review of the structure and function of the normal vascular system and its reactive changes is presented first to aid in the understanding of the specific peripheral vascular disorders.

## Structure/Function of the Normal Vascular System

The vascular system consists of varying histologic portions of five component parts: endothelium, basement membrane, elastic tissue, collagen, and smooth muscle.[1] The endothelium is the lining of the luminal surface of the entire vascular system and functions to regulate the flow of blood in and out of the vessel lumen. Endothelial cells have several important functions including the active transport of circulating substances through their cytoplasm. When blood vessel endothelium is damaged, platelets adhere to the exposed intima, aggregate, and serve as a nidus for clot formation. Endothelial cells, however, can inhibit clotting, in part, by regulating synthesis of prostacyclin ($PGI_2$), a vasodilator and inhibitor of platelet function.

Basement membrane is a dense sheath that is adjacent to the external surface of endothelial cells and serves as a transport barrier and support structure. The basement membrane contains a ground substance that is a mixture of mucopolysaccharides, protein–polysaccharide complexes, and glycoproteins which retain large amounts of water and provide a gelatinous medium for transport of materials. Elastic tissue encircles the wall just outside the endothelium and basement membrane. It is also found in the media and adventitia of all vessels except the terminal arterioles, capillaries, and small venules and allows for expansion of the vessel. The internal elastic lamella is prominently affected by nearly all pathologic changes that involve the vascular system.

Another important component of the vessel walls is collagen. In normal vessels it is present in the media and adventitia and is involved in all reactions of vessels to injury. Collagen is highly resistant to stretching and functions to prevent overdistension of the vessels. The fifth component is smooth muscle, which is the actively contracting element of the vascular system. Arterial metabolism is dependent mainly on smooth muscle cells. These are the major connective tissue-forming cells of the vascular wall, producing elastic tissue, collagen, mucopolysaccharides, and myosin. Smooth muscle cells can metabolize glucose, synthesize fatty acids, cholesterol, phospholipids, and triglycerides, and facilitate the entry of lipoproteins into the cell. Several catabolic enzymes such as mixed-function oxidases, fibrinolysins, and lysosomal hydrolases are also present. This function and the proliferative nature of smooth muscle cells are important factors in the reaction of arterial walls to injury and atherogenesis.[2,3]

The structural organization of the vessel wall consists of three well-defined layers: the intima, the media, and the adventitia (Fig. 17.1). The intima is a single continuous layer of endothelial cells and associated basement membrane. It is delineated on its outer surface by a perforated tube of elastic tissue, the internal elastic lamella. This structure is especially prominent in the large elastic arteries and medium-caliber muscular arteries, but is not seen in capillaries. The media consists of only one cell type, the smooth muscle cell. These cells are surrounded by small amounts of collagen and elastic tissue. The media is delineated on the luminal side by internal elastic lamina, and on the abluminal side by a less continuous sheet of elastic tissue, the external elastic lamella. The outer portion is nourished by small blood vessels (vasa vasorum) in the adventitia, and the inner layers receive nutrients from the lumen. The outer layer of the vascular wall is the adventitia. This layer contains a mixture of collagen, elastic fibers, smooth muscle fibers, and fibroblasts. This outer coat also contains nerve fibers, the vasa vasorum, and lymphatics that nourish the vessel wall and remove metabolic waste products.

The vascular system can be divided into elastic arteries, muscular arteries, arterioles, capillaries, veins, and lymphatics. Elastic arteries, such as the aorta and major pulmonary arteries, contain large amounts of elastic tissue. The walls of these arteries distend and increase their elastic tension with systole. During diastole, the elastic fibers recoil, helping to propel the blood distally and maintain flow.

Smooth muscle cells predominate in muscular arteries such as the renal, superior mesenteric, and femoral arteries. These arteries regulate peripheral flow and supply organs

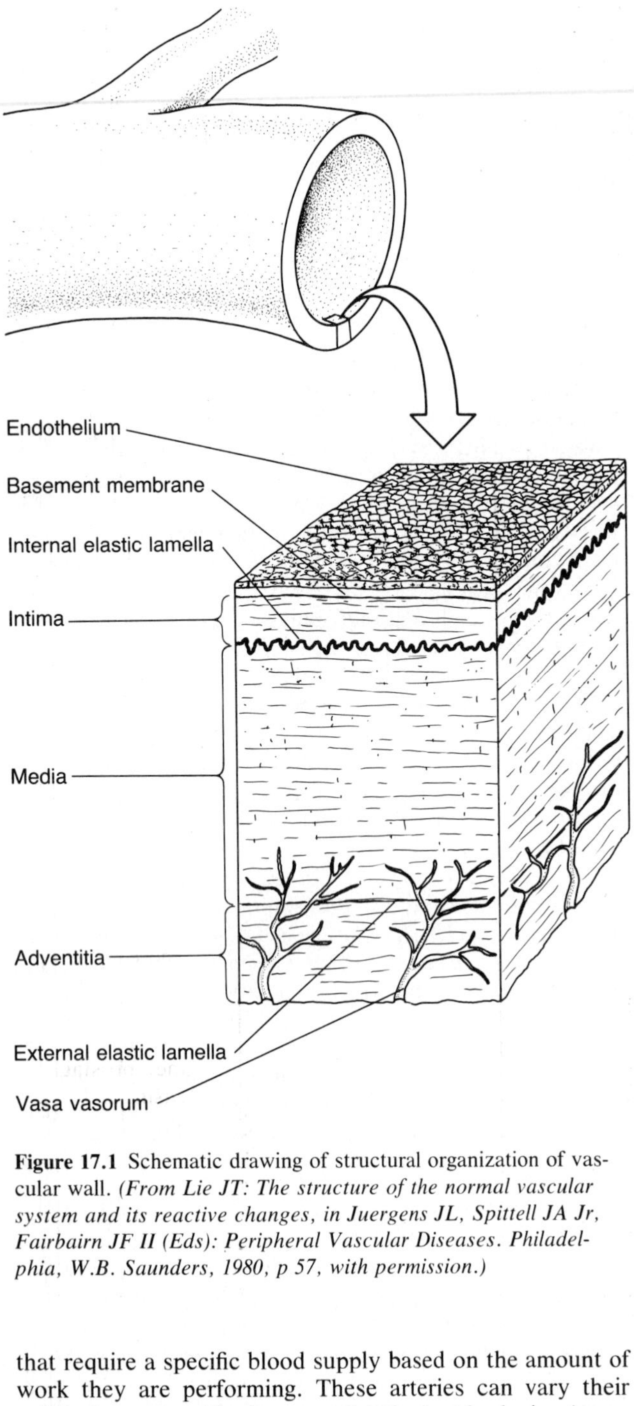


**Figure 17.1** Schematic drawing of structural organization of vascular wall. *(From Lie JT: The structure of the normal vascular system and its reactive changes, in Juergens JL, Spittell JA Jr, Fairbairn JF II (Eds): Peripheral Vascular Diseases. Philadelphia, W.B. Saunders, 1980, p 57, with permission.)*

that require a specific blood supply based on the amount of work they are performing. These arteries can vary their caliber by contracting (vasoconstriction) and relaxing (vasodilation), so that a given cardiac output can be allocated to various tissues depending on their current needs. Thus, muscular arteries function as resistance vessels and are major regulators of systemic blood pressure.

Arterioles are branches of the muscular arteries that differ structurally and functionally from small arteries only by their size. Because of their large number, arterioles form the most important class of resistance channels in the vascular system. Capillaries are blood vessels that have a diameter similar to that of a red blood cell.

Veins are considerably larger than their associated arteries. Their structure reflects both the low pressure of this system and their reservoir function. The walls of the veins are thinner and the media contains fewer smooth muscle cells, collagen, and elastic fibers. Smooth muscle cells are responsible largely for the vasoconstrictive activity of the veins which is seen mainly in the small peripheral veins in the skin. The larger veins can actively constrict during acute changes in pressure, but they passively dilate with slow increases in pressure. The lymphatic channels are the simplest parts of the vascular system. The intima consists of endothelial cells and a few collagen and muscle fibers.

## Reactive Changes of the Vascular System

The arteries are not static structures, but rather they change in response to various physical and chemical stimuli, react to injury, and undergo structural alterations throughout growth and aging.[1]

The major change that occurs with normal aging is a slow, continuous symmetric increase in the intimal thickness, especially in the large elastic arteries. This process results from a gradual accumulation of smooth muscle cells (which presumably migrate from the media), diffuse connective tissue, and an accumulation of sphingomyelin and cholesterol. This diffuse age-related thickening is to be distinguished from discrete raised fibromuscular plaques, a characteristic feature of atherosclerosis. After the sixth decade, the intima also becomes more collagenized and there is a loss of cellular constituents and granular degeneration of elastic fibers. The rate of aortic intimal thickening is more prominent in men and accelerated in patients with hypertension.[4] Structural change in small arteries and arterioles differs somewhat from that in systemic vessels in that there is progressive fibrotic thickening of the adventitia and media, with little intimal change. These changes are closely linked to hypertension and diabetes mellitus.

In the normal arterial wall, lipid content, mainly cholesterol and phospholipid (especially sphingomyelin), also progressively increases with age. Phospholipid synthesis rises with age followed by a compensatory increase in all phospholipases except sphingomyelinase. Accumulations of cholesterol and low-density lipoprotein (LDL) appear to be derived from the plasma. Functionally, these changes result in increased rigidity of arteries. The larger arteries may become dilated, elongated, and tortuous, and aneurysms may form in areas of degenerating arteriosclerotic plaques.

The veins also undergo age-related changes. Phlebosclerosis, also called hyperplastic phlebitis, refers to thickening of the veins. It appears to be age related and is particularly prominent in veins of the lower extremity that are subject to stasis and increased luminal pressure.[5]

## Physiology of Limb Blood Flow

Blood flow to the limbs is controlled by arterial blood pressure and resistance to flow, which is provided by the physical characteristics of blood vessels and of the blood itself. There are two major components to resistance: the

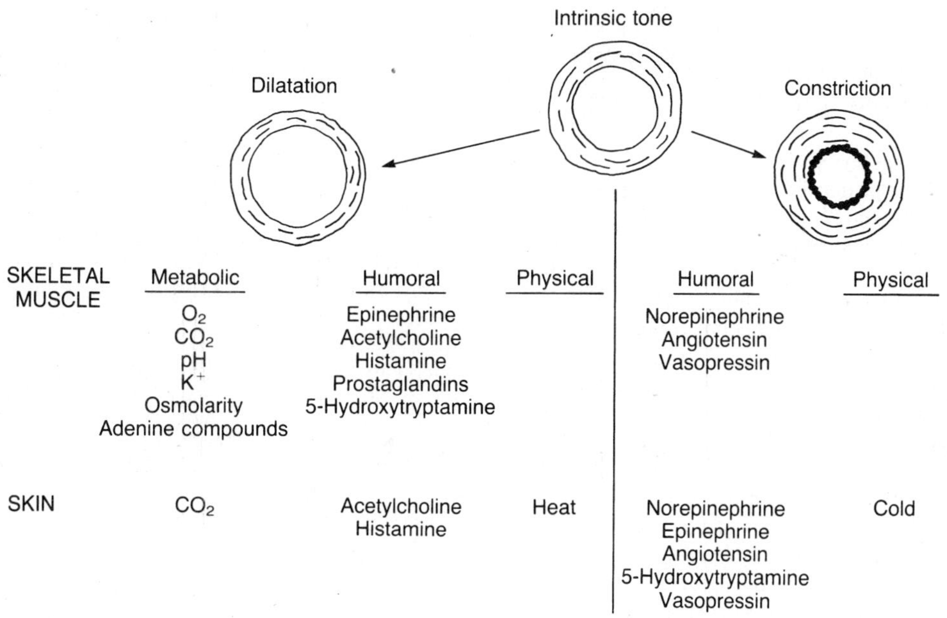


**Figure 17.2** Active changes in vascular diameter are caused by local and nervous mechanisms. Local control includes intrinsic, metabolic, humoral, and physical factors, and the relative importance of each of these varies for different tissues and for different vessels within the same tissue. This figure identifies actions of local factors that can alter arterial diameter in skeletal muscle and skin. *(From McGrath MA, Verhaeghe RH, Shepherd JT: The physiology of limb blood flow, in Juergens JL, Spittell JA, Fairbairn JF (Eds): Peripheral Vascular Diseases. Philadelphia, W.B. Saunders, 1980, p 84, with permission.)*

viscosity of the blood and the tube factor or hindrance, based on size, shape, smoothness, branching, and other aspects of the vessel wall itself. The law governing the flow of fluids through cylindrical tubes is Poiseuille's equation, which simply states that for a given vessel, the resistance to flow is proportional to the viscosity of the fluid and inversely proportional to the fourth power of the radius. Active changes in the radius of the resistance vessels in the limbs are caused by local and neurogenic mechanisms.[1]

### Local Control

Local control of limb blood flow includes intrinsic, metabolic, humoral, and physical factors. The relative importance of each of these varies for different tissues and for different vessels within the same tissue. Intrinsic smooth muscle tone appears to be directly influenced by changes in the wall tension, which in turn is determined by intravascular pressure. A decrease in intravascular pressure and wall tension would result in spontaneous activity of the smooth muscle cells, and an increase in intravascular pressure would have the opposite effect.

The intrinsic myogenic activity is modified by chemical changes in the resistance vessels which adjust blood flow in response to local metabolic needs. Usually, contraction of the limb muscles causes marked increases in blood flow to the limbs (active hyperemia). Similar increases are seen after temporary arrest of circulation to the limbs (reactive hyperemia). Metabolic factors play an important role in controlling blood flow to skeletal muscles. The accumulation of metabolic products such as carbon dioxide, potassium, phosphate, and adenosine during exercise, an increase in the osmolality of venous effluent, or a change in pH causes direct vasodilation of peripheral vessels (Fig. 17.2). The humoral factors that cause dilation of skeletal muscle vessels include epinephrine, acetylcholine, histamine, prostaglandins, and serotonin. Norepinephrine, angiotensin, and vasopressin cause vasoconstriction. In the skin, epinephrine causes vasoconstriction because there is a preponderance of $\alpha$-adrenergic receptors in cutaneous vessels, in contrast to skeletal muscle vessels which have both $\alpha$ and $\beta$ receptors. Epinephrine has a greater affinity for $\beta_2$ receptors in skeletal muscle resistance vessels, and thus causes vasodilation.

Such physical factors as local temperature also control blood flow to extremities. Low temperatures can cause vasoconstriction or vasodilation depending on the thermal state of the body. Application of heat to an extremity dilates the blood vessels. This vasodilation is enhanced by increasing the temperature of the body as a whole.

### Neural Control

The skin of the hands and feet is innervated by sympathetic fibers that mediate reflex changes in vessel tone. Alterations in activity of these fibers under central control cause large fluctuations in the flow to all fingers simultaneously. Temperature changes alter the sympathetic outflow to the skin. Exposure of the body to cold augments the vasoconstrictor tone, whereas an increase in body temperature decreases tone. The circulation in the skin also plays an essential role in thermal homeostasis. Arteriovenous anastomoses, which are numerous in fingers and toes, favor heat dissipation. Sweat glands cause local production of bradykinin, and consequently vasodilation, when stimulated by sympathetic cholinergic nerves.

Changes in the diameter of resistance vessels in skeletal muscle are influenced primarily by sympathetic adrenergic nerves, which are abundant in small arteries and arterioles. Sympathetic nerve fibers to muscle are of two types: vasoconstrictor fibers, whose activity is mediated by the release of norepinephrine, and vasodilator fibers, whose activity is mediated through the release of acetylcholine.[6] Although vessels in both the skin and muscles are innervated by sympathetic fibers, the vasomotor centers controlling these vessels can function independently. In reflex control of body temperature, only the vessels to the skin are involved, whereas with alterations in position, the reflex changes are confined to the vessels in the muscles.

## Peripheral Arterial Disorders

Peripheral vascular disease of the arteries can be generally classified as obstructive and vasospastic. Examples of an obstructive abnormality include arteriosclerosis obliterans and thromboangiitis obliterans (Buerger's disease). Raynaud's disease is the most common example of a vasospastic disorder.

### *Arteriosclerosis Obliterans*

Arteriosclerosis obliterans, also called atherosclerosis obliterans (ASO), is a chronic occlusive arterial disease of the aorta, particularly the terminal portion of the abdominal aorta and its major branches to the extremities. This disease also involves the large and medium-sized arteries of the extremities, especially the iliofemoral and popliteal arteries and, in the lower leg, the posterior tibial artery at the ankle and the anterior tibial artery at its origin. Arteriosclerosis obliterans is considered to be a segmental disease, with significant variation in its extent.

### *Epidemiology*

Arteriosclerosis obliterans occurs primarily in men between the ages of 50 and 70. The disease generally affects women after age 60, perhaps in part because of a menopausal loss of the protective effect of estrogen and an increased incidence of diabetes mellitus in women of this age.[7] It appears that diet, particularly hyperlipoproteinemia, may be an important risk factor for this disease just as it is in general atherosclerosis. Diabetes mellitus significantly increases the prevalence and severity of this disease. One study demonstrated that ASO was 11 times more frequent and developed 10 years earlier in diabetics compared with nondiabetics.[7] Other risk factors important in the pathogenesis of ASO include hypertension and cigarette smoking.

### *Pathophysiology*

The primary lesion in ASO is an intimal plaque, which progressively narrows and, in many cases, leads to complete occlusion of these arteries. The histopathologic changes are essentially identical to those of atherosclerotic occlusive disease of the visceral and cerebral arteries.[8] The primary physiologic disturbance is obstruction of blood flow through large arteries and, therefore, ischemia of those tissues of the extremity supplied by these arteries. The degree of ischemia is proportional to (1) the proximal limit of the occluding process, (2) the patency of collateral blood vessels, and (3) the rapidity of occlusion development. The ischemia produced by the obstruction may be increased by arteriolar constriction from any cause. If the occlusion is not too extensive, dilation may improve the circulation. Obstruction of the large arteries decreases the pressure and blood flow in smaller arteries distal to the obstruction, and thrombosis and gangrene may result. Peripheral occlusive arterial disease is often associated with increased blood viscosity, hyperfibrinogenemia, and a relatively high hematocrit.[8]

### *Clinical Presentation*

Unless there is an acute arterial occlusion such as a thrombosis, the signs and symptoms of arteriosclerosis obliterans have a gradual onset. The most common symptom is intermittent claudication, which is described as pain, cramping, numbness, or weakness in certain muscles that develops only during exercise. The distress is quickly relieved by rest without change in position. Intermittent claudication is caused by inadequate blood supply to a muscle(s) stressed by exercise. The distance a person is able to walk before the pain develops varies with the extent and severity of arterial occlusion. It is usually unilateral at first, may become bilateral with time, and is often worse in one of the extremities if both are involved.[8] The location of the involved muscle group may predict the most proximal level of occlusion. For example, claudication of the calf muscles suggests occlusion of the popliteal artery or higher; claudication of the hip indicates disease low in the aorta or in the iliac artery.

Another important group of symptoms includes pain at rest, paresthesias, and numbness. These symptoms are usually the result of more severe ischemia of tissues and a more advanced form of the disease resulting from multiple levels of occlusion or obstruction of collateral vessels. It is usually felt in the digits but may be noted in the foot and lower leg as well. Ulceration and gangrene are common when the disease reaches this stage. Pain caused by ischemic neuropathy is another clinical feature of arteriosclerosis obliterans, especially in diabetic patients. This pain may be continuous or paroxysmal and may be described as a series of sharp pains or the sensation of electric shocks. A sensation of numbness, coldness, or burning may also occur. When diabetics with a neuropathy develop ulcers the lesions are often painless.

The physical findings in arteriosclerosis of the extremities are for the most part indistinguishable from those seen in other occlusive arterial diseases. Impairment of arterial pulsations, often noted by palpation, is the most important and consistent physical finding. Others include systolic

**Table 17.1** Factors in the Differential Diagnosis of Three Types of Peripheral Vascular Disease

| *Factor* | *Thromboangiitis obliterans* | *Arteriosclerosis obliterans* | *Raynaud's phenomenon* |
|---|---|---|---|
| Age at onset of symptoms | < 40 yr | > 40 yr | < 40 yr |
| Sex | Predominant in males | Predominant in males | Predominant in females |
| Calcification of involved arteries | Absent | Present in 85% | — |
| Initial ischemic manifestations | One lower extremity | Lower extremities, unilateral or bilateral | Both upper extremities |
| Superficial phlebitis in nonvaricose veins | Frequent | Absent | Absent |
| Hyperlipidemia | Rare | Present in 40% of patients < 60 yr | Rare |

bruits over the involved arteries, color and temperature changes in the skin of the extremity, edema, and hypoesthesia and hyporeflexia in patients with severe ischemic neuropathy.

### *Diagnosis*

The diagnosis of arteriosclerosis obliterans is often made on the basis of a good history and physical exam. Sophisticated laboratory studies and diagnostic tests are rarely necessary to establish the diagnosis of atherosclerosis of the extremities; however, routine laboratory tests such as blood chemistry, electrocardiography, and x-ray studies may be needed to determine whether there is an associated disease and to determine prognosis and therapy. The magnitude of arterial occlusion can be assessed simply by measuring the extremity blood pressure at rest and after exercise to the point of claudication. This can be done using a Doppler probe or by a variety of plethysmographs. Arteriography is rarely necessary to establish the diagnosis, but is usually used prior to operation to precisely localize the disease. The clinical differentiation of arteriosclerosis obliterans from other types of occlusive peripheral arterial diseases is given in Table 17.1.

### *Treatment*

The goals of therapy in patients with ASO are to arrest progress of the disease, improve blood flow, relieve pain, and treat ulceration and gangrene. Progression of the disease can be prevented by control of hyperlipoproteinemia, control of any associated disease, and tobacco abstinence. For patients who have severe ischemia manifested by rest pain, ulceration, and gangrene, rest of the extremity is an important adjunct of treatment. If the pain is severe narcotics and other pain medications may be necessary. It is important to take meticulous care of the extremities and avoid even minor trauma as it may lead to ulceration. In these patients, ulceration is usually treated with local care, medical management, including antibiotics if necessary, and surgical amputation.

Arterial surgery and angioplasty are the best methods of improving blood flow. Direct arterial surgery utilizing endarterectomy, prosthetic bypass graphs, or vein-patch arterioplasty may be effective in bypassing or removing areas of stenosis but should be reserved for patients with severe and disabling symptoms.[8] Transluminal angioplasty is very effective for occlusion of the aortoiliac segments. The long-term patency of this procedure for arteries below the groin is not very good; however, angioplasty may be used when short-term improvements in blood flow are necessary to heal ulcers. Lumbar sympathectomy may be useful in patients with mild ischemia rest pain.

Another effective method of improving blood flow to the extremities is to increase collateral flow. This can be accomplished by a warm environmental temperature; avoidance of vasoconstriction caused by drugs, cold, and tobacco; elevation of the head of the bed 12–16 in.; and exercise. A daily exercise training program is very effective in patients with mild or moderate intermittent claudication. Important features of a successful exercise program are (1) repetitive daily walks to 75% of the claudication distance with intermittent periods of rest (1–2 min), (2) weekly increase in walking time and distance, (3) continuation of this program, as cessation results in loss of improvement. Various vasodilating drugs have been used in patients with obstructive arterial disease; however, the results have been disappointing. Dilating the vessels distal to the obstruction will not increase local blood flow unless the collateral blood vessels dilate. Raising the systemic blood pressure has been shown to be an effective method of increasing collateral flow. Most vasodilators decrease systemic pressure and can therefore increase collateral vascular resistance.[9] In some cases, vasodilation in other areas of the body without diseased vessels may actually "steal" flow from the affected area. Therefore, vasodilators are of no value in treating arteriosclerosis obliterans.

There is current controversy regarding the use of $\beta$-blockers in PVD patients with concurrent coronary artery disease or hypertension. A number of case reports have been published indicating that these agents can cause or worsen the symptoms of intermittent claudication.[10–12] By reducing systemic blood pressure these agents could decrease blood flow through stenotic arteries or collateral vessels. A nonselective β-blocker may attenuate epinephrine-induced vasodilation during exercise by blocking $\beta_2$ receptors in peripheral vessels. Controlled trials using both selective and nonselective agents have produced mixed results in patients with peripheral vascular disease. A few studies have demonstrated an increase in muscle blood flow and symptomatic improvement when β-blockers were withdrawn.[13,14] Hiatt et al,[15] however, demonstrated that calf blood flow was not affected by either propranolol or metoprolol compared with placebo in patients with mild to moderate occlusive peripheral vascular disease, and there was no difference in symptoms of claudication. These reports are flawed by problems with study design, and conclusive statements regarding the use of β-blockers in patients with PVD are difficult to make. Until more data are available, these agents should be used with caution, especially in patients with vasospastic peripheral vascular disease.

Recently, pentoxifylline has been shown to be of benefit in patients with chronic occlusive arterial disease. In a double-blind multicenter trial of 128 patients, pentoxifylline in doses up to 1,200 mg/d was significantly more effective than placebo in increasing both the initial and the absolute claudication distances. With regard to the subjective parameters, only incidence of paresthesias showed a significantly greater reduction in the pentoxifylline group compared with the placebo group.[16] This drug reduces blood viscosity and arterial blood flow by improving erythrocyte (RBC) flexibility. Many patients with intermittent claudication have been shown to have a marked decrease in their RBC flexibility. Pentoxifylline has also been shown to decrease fibrinogen levels, probably by interfering with its synthesis, as well as inhibit platelet aggregation, increase the release of prostacyclin, and inhibit phosphodiesterases.[17,18] Pentoxifylline is also used to prevent postoperative rethrombosis after vascular surgery for arterial occlusive disease. This drug has been shown to be superior to the combination of acetylsalicylic acid and dipyridamole in maintaining vascular patency in these patients over a 6-month period.[19]

Other forms of therapy that show promise in patients with peripheral occlusive disease include the use of antithrombotic agents and prostaglandin therapy. There is no definitive evidence that antithrombotic therapy significantly modifies the clinical manifestations and natural history of arteriosclerosis obliterans. A few reports suggest beneficial effects of anticoagulant and antiplatelet agents in these patients, but there are few clinical trials.

Hess et al[20] reported a statistically significant decrease in disease progression with a combination of aspirin and dipyridamole, compared with a placebo, and a slight decrease with aspirin alone. Recent evidence suggests that ticlopidine, an investigational antiplatelet agent, may improve claudication and healing of ischemic ulcers in patients with chronic arterial insufficiency.[21,22] Low-dose regional thrombolytic therapy is sometimes used as an alternative to surgical treatment in acute and chronic arterial occlusion, especially in those patients who are considered to be high surgical risks.[23,24] Prostaglandins $E_1$ ($PGE_1$) and $I_2$ ($PGI_2$, prostacyclin) are potent vasodilators and inhibitors of platelet aggregation that have been shown to improve claudication distance, relieve pain, and promote ulcer healing in patients with peripheral arterial disease resulting from obstruction and vasospasm.[25–27]

## Thromboangiitis Obliterans (Buerger's Disease)

Thromboangiitis obliterans is a disease involving nonatheromatous lesions of the arteries, veins, and nerves that usually occurs in young males and frequently leads to nonhealing ulcers and gangrene. The exact pathogenesis is unknown, but there seems to be a relationship with tobacco smoking or chewing. These patients may have an abnormal cellular or humoral immune response to type I and III collagens. This disease usually starts in the smaller arteries of the hands and feet, in contrast to the segmental disease of medium and large arteries seen with arteriosclerosis obliterans. Typical clinical features include a superficial, migratory, nodular phlebitis, associated with cutaneous erythema, and tenderness. Cold sensitivity of the hands occurs in about 50% of these patients. One of the most common symptoms of Buerger's disease is instep claudication with exercise, which is promptly relieved by rest. Physical findings of intense rubor of the feet, absent foot pulses in the presence of a normal femoral and popliteal pulse, and reduction or absence of the radial and/or ulnar pulse are strongly suggestive of thromboangiitis obliterans.

The only effective treatment is complete abstinence from tobacco. If this is not done, the disease progresses and amputation is usually the only method of controlling the severe rest pain and ulceration.

### *Raynaud's Disease*

The first description of cold-induced digital ischemia presumably caused by arterial vasospasm was made in 1862 by Maurice Raynaud. This condition, which is limited to the skin, usually accompanied by cyanosis, rubor, pain, or paresthesias, and associated with gangrene, came to be termed Raynaud's syndrome. More than a century later, the pathogenesis, diagnosis, and treatment are still unclear.

#### Epidemiology

The prevalence of Raynaud's syndrome in the general population is unknown. This disease affects predominantly women, with a ratio of women to men of 5 to 1.[28] Raynaud's disease usually begins in the early decades of life. One study found that 60% of patients had disease onset before the age of 30, and 81% before age 40.[29] Men with Raynaud's syndrome generally present at an older age, and have a much higher incidence of associated atherosclerosis, which accounts for their symptoms when compared with women.

One interesting group of patients with Raynaud's symptoms comprises those whose occupations involve routine use of vibratory equipment or frequent exposure to cold temperature. Forty to 90% of loggers and 50% of miners using vibratory equipment have been diagnosed with Raynaud's syndrome.[30,31] Heredity may also play a role in the development of this disease.[28]

**Pathophysiology**

Two primary mechanisms may produce Raynaud's syndrome. Either a primary increase in the constrictive force of the arterial wall or a decrease in the intraluminal pressure associated with obstruction may cause a sudden cessation of blood flow in small arteries upon exposure to cold or emotional stress.[32] In most patients both mechanisms contribute to the symptoms. Young women with idiopathic or primary Raynaud's syndrome usually exhibit the purest form of vasospasm. These patients have normal digital arterial blood pressure between attacks. Older male patients usually have secondary Raynaud's syndrome involving both a vasospastic and obstructive disease. In these patients a normal vasoconstrictive stimulus acting on an arterial bed with reduced intraluminal pressure is sufficient to cause arterial closure. Initially these patients may demonstrate pure vasospasm, but later they develop obstruction as underlying autoimmune processes cause damage to the arterial wall. The mechanism of vasospastic arterial occlusion in the absence of luminal arterial obstruction is unknown. Data suggest that cold increases the $\alpha$-adrenergic responsiveness of the digital vessels by increasing release of norepinephrine, decreasing norepinephrine degradation, and possibly increasing receptor sensitivity.[33] Patients with Raynaud's disease may have an increase in adrenergic vasomotor tone, or may have an exaggerated response to endogenous hormones. Local mediator abnormalities such as decreased prostacyclin or increased thromboxane production have also been suggested, along with altered blood viscosity and abnormal serum proteins. Raynaud's syndrome is generally associated with other systemic disorders, especially connective tissue disorders such as scleroderma, systemic lupus erythematosus, and mixed connective tissue disease.

**Clinical Presentation**

The digital color changes are a common manifestation of this disease. A classic attack begins with a sudden loss of arterial blood flow, causing blanching. Next, a small quantity of blood enters the capillary and venous system and desaturates, and the digits become cyanotic. The third phase of the attack involves vasodilation, causing rubor. Not all patients exhibit a triphasic color change; many demonstrate only pallor or cyanosis, during which the digits turn absolutely white. At first only the tips of the fingers of both hands are involved; later the more proximal parts of the fingers are affected. In the late stages the color change may extend back to involve the rest of the hands. Symptoms are worse in the cold season and less severe in warm weather. Pain is not a prominent symptom during the attack or in the interval between attacks. Paresthesias are common during the attack and consist of numbness, tingling, burning, or a feeling of tightness. Slight swelling of the involved fingers may occur but only during attacks.

**Diagnosis**

Because of the episodic nature of Raynaud's attacks, the only absolute requirement for diagnosis is a history of digital pallor or cyanosis induced by exposure to cold or emotional stimuli, especially if the symptoms are bilateral and occur without evidence of secondary cause. This history can be confirmed by measuring digital temperature recovery time after brief immersion of the hand in ice water. The digital temperature of normal subjects returns to baseline within 15 minutes, while patients with Raynaud's have a prolonged recovery time. The disease should have existed long enough for any secondary cause to have become evident before a final diagnosis of Raynaud's disease is made.

All patients should have a complete history and physical exam, with special emphasis on signs and symptoms of connective tissue disease. Routine laboratory tests should include a complete blood count, erythrocyte sedimentation rate, chemistry profile, antinuclear antibody, urinalysis, and hand radiography. Hand arteriography may sometimes be used in assessing the relative roles of vasospastic and occlusive disease, but is rarely used to establish a diagnosis. Digital plethysmography is often used to follow the course of the disease or to evaluate the response to therapy.[32]

**Treatment**

General considerations for treatment include avoidance of cold temperatures, tobacco, emotional situations, and certain drugs. These patients should dress warmly, wear lined gloves, and use styrofoam coasters when handling iced drinks. Large meals and long periods of standing should be avoided as they both reduce peripheral circulation. Drugs that may cause vasoconstriction such as birth control pills, $\beta$-adrenergic blockers, and ergotamine preparations should not be used.

Therapy for Raynaud's phenomenon is aimed at increasing the patient's digital blood flow and consists of behavioral and drug therapy. Behavioral therapy such as biofeedback has been used in recent years primarily to lessen the severity of the attacks. The goal with these techniques is to self-regulate the nervous system and reduce vasoconstrictive autonomic tone. Biofeedback is accomplished with the use of a thermoprobe or thermistor attached to the person's finger or hand, which relays skin temperature information back to the patient. The patient can then concentrate further on raising the peripheral temperature.[34]

Drugs that have been used in Raynaud's disease include sympatholytic agents, calcium channel blockers, and direct-acting vasodilators. Experience with nonselective $\alpha$-adrenergic blockers such as phenoxybenzamine and tolazoline is fairly extensive, but the focus in recent years has been on selective $\alpha$-blockers such as prazosin. Phenoxybenzamine in oral doses of 10–20 mg two to three times a day and tolazoline 25–50 mg three to four times a day have been shown to be effective in improving skin blood flow and symptomatic relief of Raynaud's symptoms, but their long-term use is hampered by frequent side effects such as postural hypotension, tachycardia, impotence, and sodium and water retention.[35] Prazosin, in doses of 2–6 mg/d, has been used with greater success because this drug is a selective $\alpha_1$-receptor blocker, and therefore appears to cause less tachycardia. Waldo[36] reported clinical improvement in 50% of patients with moderate to severe Raynaud's disease; however, this study was not controlled. In a double-blind placebo-controlled trial of 24 patients, prazosin 1 mg three times daily showed a significant improvement in number and severity of attacks compared with a placebo. Finger skin temperature and laser Doppler estimated finger blood flow also revealed a significant improvement with prazosin.[37] The most common side effects in this study were dizziness with standing and transient palpitations, but these effects never prompted patients to withdraw from the study. The overall response rate was 60%; however, only two patients (8.3%) had complete relief with prazosin.

Other sympatholytic agents that have been used for Raynaud's disease include reserpine, guanethidine, and methyldopa. These agents have shown significant improvement in selected patients and are generally much more effective than direct-acting vasodilators.[35] Unfortunately, full benefit is often prevented by unpleasant and sometimes severe side effects that limit dose. Good results are sometimes obtained by combining two sympatholytic agents, such as guanethidine 10 mg/d and prazosin 1 mg twice daily, to decrease adverse effects and provide greater therapeutic benefit.[38] Intraarterial administration of reserpine, 0.5–1.0 mg diluted in 2.5 mL of normal saline, has been suggested as a means of delivering the drug directly to arterial adrenergic sites while avoiding some of the systemic side effects. This method has been shown to be effective, especially in severe cases with digital ulcers.[32] The benefit, however, is usually short-lived and repeated injections present a cumulative risk of arterial damage. Intraarterial reserpine may be indicated for patients with severe Raynaud's phenomenon accompanied by digital infarction.[35] Direct-acting vasodilators such as niacin, papaverine, isoxsuprine, and cyclandelate have not consistently demonstrated significant improvement and are felt to be of no value in the treatment of Raynaud's phenomenon.[9]

Several investigators have studied the effectiveness of calcium channel blockers in patients with Raynaud's phenomenon. Only one study has been done using verapamil in doses of 40–80 mg four times daily. No difference was noted between the placebo- and verapamil-treated patients in the number or severity of attacks, the subjective evaluation of effectiveness, or the digital systolic blood pressure during cold exposure.[38] Diltiazem 30–60 mg three times daily was evaluated in three clinical trials. Only two of these were double-blinded; however, they consistently reported an improvement in patients' subjective assessment of disability and in the frequency of attacks.[39] In one of these trials, which was double-blind and placebo controlled, no objective evidence of improvement in digital blood flow was noted.[40]

Nifedipine has been used in doses of 10–20 mg three times daily for patients with Raynaud's disease.[39,41,42] Many of these patients demonstrated a statistically significant decrease in the frequency of vasospastic attacks and a moderate to marked alleviation of their symptoms. There was some variability in response; patients without underlying vascular disease appeared to respond better, whereas patients with scleroderma responded less well. Despite improvement in the number and severity of attacks, no changes were detected in digital perfusion pressure when nifedipine and placebo were compared.

Another therapeutic intervention for Raynaud's disease is surgical sympathectomy. Benefit from this procedure is inconsistent; generally, the greater the severity of disease, the lesser the degree of success.[35] Lumbar sympathectomy appears to produce a higher incidence of permanent denervation and better results than the cervicodorsal sympathectomy technique. Sympathectomy, particularly in the upper extremity, should be performed only when conservative measures fail to control symptoms.

Current investigational treatment measures include infusion of $PGE_1$ and $PGI_2$, plasmapheresis, and the serotonin receptor antagonist, ketanserin.[36,43] Preliminary data suggest subjective and objective improvements with plasmapheresis, which may result from changes in blood viscosity, alterations in platelet function, removal of unknown toxic substances, or transfusion of absent blood factors. By preventing vasoconstriction and platelet aggregation caused by serotonin, ketanserin shows promise for the treatment of Raynaud's disease associated with connective tissue disorders, especially scleroderma.

## Summary

Peripheral vascular disease as discussed in this chapter includes disorders of peripheral arteries (excluding the heart and thoracic aorta) and the venous system. This group of distinct disorders and syndromes is a common cause of morbidity and mortality, can affect any vessel, is often due to an atheroma, and is frequent in the middle-aged and elderly. A common symptom of peripheral vascular disease is pain of various types, while changes in vascular filling, limb volume, skin color, and temperature are among the most important signs.

The appropriate approach to patients with suspected peripheral vascular disease is to identify the system involved (arterial, venous, or lymphatic), estimate the degree of disability, and determine if special diagnostic tests are needed. Several simple noninvasive methods have been developed to detect, localize, and functionally quantify the disorder, and advances have also been made in vascular imaging techniques. Therapy of peripheral vascular disease depends upon the specific disorder, but includes elimination or minimization of risk factors, pharmacologic and nonpharmacologic therapy, and surgery and radiology, including bypass grafting and percutaneous angioplasty.

## References


1. Lie JT. The structure of the normal vascular system and its reactive changes, in Juergens JL, Spittell JA, Fairbairn JF (eds): Peripheral Vascular Diseases. Philadelphia, W.B. Saunders, 1980, pp 51–81.
2. Ross R, Glomset JA. Atherosclerosis and the arterial smooth muscle cell. Science 1973;180:1332–1339.
3. Ross R. The pathogenesis of atherosclerosis—an update. N Engl J Med 1986;314:488–500.
4. Wilens SL. The nature of diffuse intimal thickening of arteries. Am J Pathol 1951;27:825–839.
5. Stein AA, Rosenblum I, Leather R. Intimal sclerosis in human veins. Arch Pathol 1966;81:548–551.

6. Barker WF. Physiology and pathogenesis, in Gaspar MR, Barker WF (eds): Peripheral Arterial Disease. Philadelphia, W.B. Saunders, 1981, pp 38–76.
7. Dry TJ, Hines EA. The role of diabetes in the development of degenerative vascular disease: With special reference to the incidence of retinitis and peripheral neuritis. Ann Intern Med 1941;14:1893–1941.
8. Juergens JL, Bernatz PE. Atherosclerosis of the extremities, in Juergens JL, Spittell JA, Fairbairn JF (eds): Peripheral Vascular Diseases. Philadelphia, W.B. Saunders, 1980, pp 253–293.
9. Coffman JD. Vasodilator drugs in peripheral vascular disease. N Engl J Med 1979;300:713–717.
10. Fogoros R. Exacerbation of intermittent claudication by propranolol. (Lett) N Engl J Med 1980;302:1089.
11. Gokal R, Dorman T, Ledingham J. Peripheral skin necrosis complicating beta-blockade. Br Med J 1979;1:721–722.
12. Rodger J, Sheldon C, Lerski R, et al. Intermittent claudication complicating beta-blockade. Br Med J 1976;1:1125.
13. Ingram D, House A, Thompson G, et al. Beta-adrenergic blockade and peripheral vascular disease. Med J Aust 1982;1: 509–511.
14. Smith R, Warren D. Effect of $\beta$-blocking drugs on peripheral blood flow in intermittent claudication. J Cardiovasc Pharmacol 1982;4:2–4.
15. Hiatt WR, Stoll S, Nies AS. Effect of $\beta$-adrenergic blockade on the peripheral circulation in patients with peripheral vascular disease. Circulation 1985;72:1226–1231.
16. Porter JM, Carter BS, Lee BY, et al. Pentoxifylline efficacy in the treatment of intermittent claudication: Multicenter controlled double-blind trial with objective assessment of chronic occlusive arterial disease patients. Am Heart J 1982;104:66–72.
17. Gastpar H, Ambrus JL, Ambrus CM, et al. Study of platelet aggregation in vivo. III. Effect of pentoxifylline. J Med 1977;8: 191–197.
18. Takamatsu S, Sato K, Takamatsu M, et al. Changes in haematological and blood chemical parameters after treatment of aged arteriosclerotic patients with pentoxifylline. Pharmatherapeutica 1979;2:165–172.
19. Lucas MA. Prevention of post-operative thrombosis in peripheral arteriopathies. Pentoxifylline vs. conventional antiaggregants. A six-month randomized follow-up study. Angiology 1984;443–449.
20. Hess H, Mietaschk A, Deichsel G. Drug-induced inhibition of platelet function delays progression of peripheral occlusive arterial disease. A prospective double-blind arteriographically controlled trial. Lancet 1985;1:415–419.
21. Katsumura T, Mishima Y, Kamiya K, et al. Therapeutic effect of ticlopidine, a new inhibitor of platelet aggregation, on chronic arterial occlusive diseases, a double-blind study versus placebo. Angiology 1982;33:357–367.
22. Katsumura T. Therapeutic effect of ticlopidine for ischemic leg ulcers. Agents Actions 1984;15(suppl):167–172.
23. Hess H, Ingrisch H, Mietaschk A, et al. Local low-dose thrombolytic therapy of peripheral arterial occlusions. N Engl J Med 1982;307:1627–1630.
24. Jelalian C, Mehrhof A, Cohen IK, et al. Streptokinase in the treatment of acute arterial occlusion of the hand. J Hand Surg 1985;10:534–538.
25. Pardy BJ, Lewis JD, Eastcott HHG. Preliminary experience with prostaglandins $E_1$ and $I_2$ in peripheral vascular disease. Surgery 1980;88:826–830.
26. Fernandez NA, Rosenberg V, Lee M, et al. Prostaglandin $E_1$ in obstructive peripheral vascular disease. Mount Sinai J Med 1983;50:213–217.
27. Hirai M, Nanki M, Nakayama R. Hemodynamic effects of intravenous $PGE_1$ on patients with arterial occlusive disease of the leg. Angiology 1985;36:407–413.
28. Spittell JA. Raynaud's phenomenon and allied vasospastic disorders, in Juergens JL, Spittell JA, Fairbairn JF (eds): Peripheral Vascular Diseases. Philadelphia, W.B. Saunders, 1980, pp 555–583.
29. Blain A, Coller FA, Carver GB. Raynaud's disease. A study of criteria for prognosis. Surgery 1951;29:387–397.
30. Chatterjee DS, Petrie A, Taylor W. Prevalence of vibration-induced white finger in fluorspar mines in Weardale. Br J Ind Med 1978;35:208–218.
31. Taylor W, Pelmear PL. Raynaud's phenomenon of occupational origin. An epidemiological survey. Acta Chir Scand 1976;465 (suppl):27–32.
32. Porter JM, Rivers SP, Anderson CJ, et al. Evaluation and management of patients with Raynaud's syndrome. Am J Surg 1981;142:183–189.
33. Vanhoutte PM, Janssens WJ. Thermosensitivity of cutaneous vessels and Raynaud's disease. Am Heart J 1980;100:263–265.
34. Sedlacek K. Biofeedback for Raynaud's disease. Psychosomatics 1979;20:538–541.
35. Harper FE, LeRoy EC. Raynaud's phenomenon: An update on treatment. J Cardiovasc Med 1982;7:282–288.
36. Waldo R. Prazosin relieves Raynaud's vasospasm. JAMA 1979; 241:1037.
37. Wollersheim H, Thien T, Fennis J, et al. Double-blind, placebo-controlled study of prazosin in Raynaud's phenomenon. Clin Pharmacol Ther 1986;40:219–225.
38. Kinney EI, Nicholas GG, Gallo J, et al. The treatment of severe Raynaud's phenomenon with verapamil. J Clin Pharmacol 1982; 22:75–76.
39. Smith CR, Rodeheffer RJ. Raynaud's phenomenon: Pathophysiologic features and treatment with calcium-channel blockers. Am J Cardiol 1985;55:154B–157B.
40. Vayssairat M, Capron L, Fiessinger JH, et al. Calcium channel blockers and Raynaud's disease. (Lett) Ann Intern Med 1981; 95:243.
41. Smith CD, McKendry RJ. Controlled trial of nifedipine in the treatment of Raynaud's phenomenon. Lancet 1982;2:1299–1301.
42. Rodeheffer RJ, Rommer JA, Wigley F, et al. Controlled double-blind trial of nifedipine in the treatment of Raynaud's phenomenon. N Engl J Med 1983;308:880–883.
43. Roald LK, Seem E. Treatment of Raynaud's phenomenon with ketanserin in patients with connective tissue disorders. Br Med J 1984;289:577–579.

# Chapter 18 / Stroke

J. Chris Bradberry, PharmD

Stroke is a syndrome and is a major manifestation of cerebrovascular disease. Stroke refers to the sudden onset of a focal neurologic deficit. Cerebrovascular disease refers to any type of pathophysiologic vascular disease of the brain. This vascular pathology can include any abnormality of the vessel, blood flow, or quality of the blood. Abnormalities of the vessel include many processes such as developmental defects, arteritis, aneurysm, hypertensive disease, and atherosclerosis. Blood flow can be affected by disease of the vessel and also by thrombotic or embolic processes. The changes in the brain that these abnormalities can produce are either a decrease in blood flow, termed *ischemia*, or bleeding. Ischemia can be present with or without brain tissue infarction. When a stroke occurs, the neurologic manifestations produced are the result of the location of insult in the brain and the extent of ischemia, infarct, or hemorrhage. A stroke may show varied manifestations, reversible and irreversible, ranging from hemiplegia to sensory deficits. Hemiplegia may or may not be accompanied by other manifestations. It is a challenge for the clinician to accurately diagnose a particular lesion because of these variations in presentation; however, a good clinical examination can aid in locating a lesion as well as in helping to determine if the stroke is ischemic or hemorrhagic in nature. The advent of computerized axial tomography (CAT or CT scan) has been of tremendous importance in the diagnosis and assessment of stroke. Results of the CAT scan must be known prior to therapy of certain stroke syndromes with anticoagulants or platelet antiaggregating agents. Although the causes of stroke are many, this chapter centers on the most common types of stroke, with further emphasis on ischemic cerebrovascular disease and pharmacotherapy and cardiogenic embolic stroke and pharmacotherapy. Hemorrhagic and other more unusual forms are deemphasized.

## Epidemiology and Etiology

Figure 18.1 outlines the causes of stroke.

Since the 1940s, cerebrovascular disease death rates have declined in the United States.[1] This prompted the American Heart Association to issue a special statement on risk factors in 1971.[2] At that time, major risk factors for ischemic stroke were identified as transient ischemic attacks, cerebral infarction, hypertension, cardiac abnormalities, and other consequences of atherosclerosis and diabetes mellitus.

Since that statement, mortality from stroke has continued to decline.[3,4] In fact, during the mid-1970s the rate of decline in mortality from cerebrovascular causes was far greater than that from cardiovascular disease. The reasons for this decline are not clear, but evidence would suggest that this decline in mortality from cerebrovascular disease and ischemic stroke, in particular, may be related to more effective treatment of hypertension. Nevertheless, other factors have also undoubtedly contributed to this decline and, in 1984, the Stroke Council of the American Heart Association issued an updated review of risk factors.[5]

General population studies show that atherothrombotic infarction is the most common type of stroke, representing almost 66% of the reported cases.[4,6] Therefore, the majority of strokes are caused by ischemia and infarction secondary to disease of the small and medium-sized arteries. Cerebral embolism causes stroke 5% to 14% of the time, although these data indicate cases for which there is a recognized embolic source. Hemorrhage into the brain tissue and subarachnoid hemorrhages account for 14% to 20% of all strokes. In 1985 the AHA estimated that in the United States more than 156,000 people died from a stroke, and that 1,930,000 people survived a stroke.[7] Stroke is the third leading cause of death in the United States even though mortality is declining. It is estimated that 500,000 people are affected every year by a stroke.

One of the major impacts of stroke is the resultant disability in up to 50% of patients hospitalized for cerebrovascular disease. The economic impact is estimated to be as high as $8 billion annually.[7] Obviously, with this impact both economically and emotionally, stroke is one of the most devastating diseases in this country. Prevention is of primary importance and proper prevention requires correction of risk factors in persons at highest risk. As noted earlier, there is evidence, although not absolute, to show that improved treatment, specifically of hypertension, may decrease death from stroke. The risk factors for stroke are shown in Table 18.1 and are divided into groups on the basis of their relationship to stroke.[5,8]

### *Single Risk Factors*

With regard to single risk factors, it is clear that stroke incidence is related to increasing age, with doubling of stroke rates each decade after 55.[9] Stroke generally has a 30% higher incidence in men than women. There is a higher death rate in blacks than whites and this may be a result of the increased incidence of hypertension in the black population. Environmental factors, such as a high-sodium diet, may also play an important role in the increased stroke rate in blacks.[10] Diabetes mellitus contributes independently to atherothrombotic brain infarction and the risk is greater in women than men.[11] An individual with a prior stroke has a high risk of developing a recurrent stroke.[9] Carotid bruits are evidence of increased risk of stroke; however, asymptomatic carotid bruits have been a controversial topic with regard to

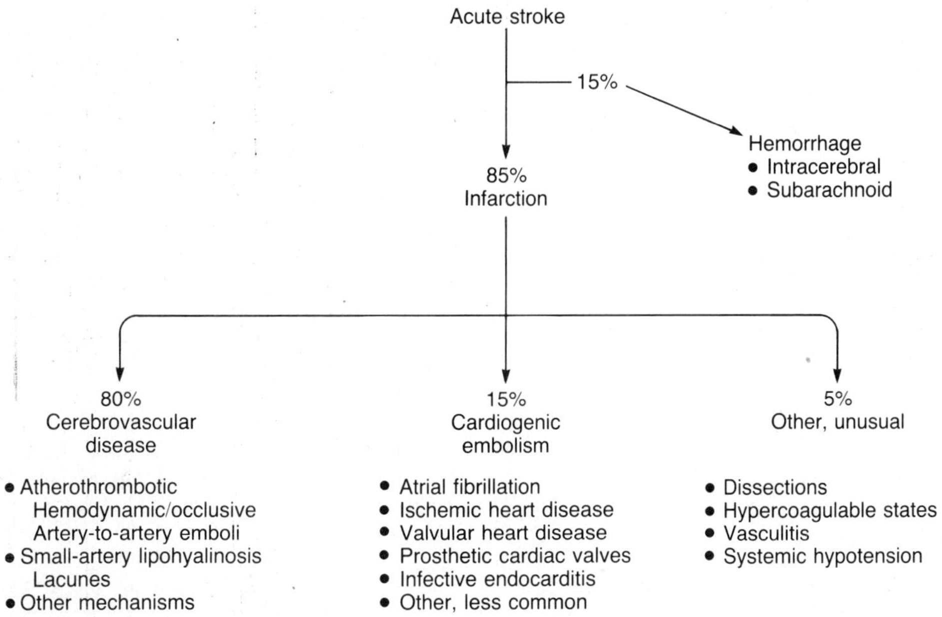


**Figure 18.1** A general framework for conceptualizing the causes of stroke. The precise mechanisms are controversial. *(From Sherman DG, Dyken ML, Fisher M, et al: Cerebral embolism. Chest 1986;89(suppl 2):835, with permission.)*

treatment. In asymptomatic individuals, a carotid bruit is an indication of a generalized atherosclerotic disease and does not necessarily indicate that a cerebral infarction will occur in the cerebral territory supplied by the affected carotid.

Of the treatable single risk factors identified, hypertension is the major predisposing factor for stroke and is strongly related to atherothrombotic brain infarction as well as cerebral hemorrhage.[12] The Framingham study indicated that there is a direct relationship between elevation of blood pressure and stroke risk.[13] There does not seem to be a gender difference in the risk for hypertensive patients, and elevated systolic pressure appears to be closely associated with stroke. The risk does not decrease with age; however, with effective treatment, the elderly have a reduction in stroke as great as or greater than that of the younger population. This was noted by the Hypertension Detection and Follow-up Program in 1982[14] and strongly suggested in the Framingham study. Impaired cardiac function is the next most important single treatable risk factor for stroke. Individuals with cardiac diseases such as coronary heart disease, congestive heart failure, left ventricular hypertrophy, and arrhythmias, and specifically atrial fibrillation, have more than twice the stroke risk as compared with those with normal cardiac function.[8] Atrial fibrillation is strongly correlated with embolic stroke and those patients with nonrheumatic atrial fibrillation have a fivefold increase in stroke frequency over those without fibrillation.[15,16]

Transient ischemic attacks (TIAs) are defined as episodes of focal ischemic neurologic deficit lasting less than 24 hours. The neurologic deficit produced depends on the thrombotic or embolic activity in the particular arterial supply to the brain. TIAs precede an ischemic stroke in about 60% of cases, and 35% of untreated patients will develop a stroke within 5 years of a TIA. TIAs precede 10% of strokes from all causes. The greatest risk for stroke is early, within the first few weeks of the TIA, with about 20% occurring within the first month after the TIA and 50% within the first year after the TIA.[17] TIAs as risk factors are also influenced by other stroke risk factors; therefore, treatment of other risk factors may influence the occurrence of stroke in patients with TIAs. Another treatable risk factor is elevated hematocrit. Several studies[18–20] including data from the Framingham study[21] point to the relationship between increased hematocrit and decreased cerebral blood flow and stroke. Stroke in patients with elevated hematocrits has been attributed to decreased collateral flow caused by increased blood viscosity.[22] Sickle cell disease patients also appear to have an increased incidence of stroke. One study[20] of hospitalized patients showed that 17% of sickle cell disease patients had one or more strokes. Those patients with sickle cell disease had a 1 in 20 rate of stroke and 4 of 227 with sickle cell trait developed stroke.[20] Stroke in middle-aged men has been shown to correlate significantly with a maternal history of stroke.[23]

Risk factors that are less well documented but treatable are now briefly reviewed. Hyperlipidemia and hypercholesterolemia may contribute to stroke. Study results are conflicting[24,25]; however, increased lipids and cholesterol are risk factors for atherosclerosis, which is related to stroke. Cigarette smoking and alcohol consumption have been reported as having unclear contributions to stroke; however, no recent reports have offered additional insights.[1,26] Alcohol intake was reviewed in 230 patients with stroke. It was found in men that heavy alcohol consumption (>300 g/wk) is an independent risk factor, but similar conclusions cannot be made for women on the basis of this study.[26] Twelve years of follow-up of the 7,872 male subjects originally enrolled in the Honolulu Heart Program

**Table 18.1** Risk Factors in Stroke

- Single risk factors
  - Well-documented risk factors
    - Treatment not feasible or value not established
      - Age and gender
      - Familial factors
      - Race
      - Diabetes mellitus
      - Prior stroke
      - Asymptomatic carotid bruits
    - Treatable
      - **Hypertension**
      - Cardiac disease
      - Transient ischemic attacks
      - Elevated hematocrit
      - Sickle cell disease
  - Less well-documented risk factors
    - Treatment not feasible or value not established
      - Geographic location
      - Season and climate
      - Socioeconomic factors
    - Treatable but value not established
      - Elevated blood cholesterol and lipids
      - Cigarette smoking
      - Alcohol consumption
      - Oral contraceptive use
      - Physical inactivity
      - Obesity
- Multiple risk factors
  - Framingham profile
    - Systolic blood pressure
    - Serum cholesterol
    - Glucose tolerance
    - Cigarette smoking
    - Electrocardiogram
    - Left ventricular hypertrophy
  - Paffenbarger and Williams criteria
    - Cigarette smoking
    - Systolic blood pressure
    - Low ponderal index
    - Body height
    - A parent dead
    - Not a varsity athlete

From Dyken ML, Wolf PA, Barnett HJM, et al: Risk factors in stroke—A statement for physicians by the Subcommittee on Risk Factors and Stroke of the Stroke Council. Stroke 1984;15:1106, with permission.

have shown that those who continued to smoke during follow-up had the highest risk of stroke.[26] Smokers had two to three times the risk of stroke compared with nonsmokers, and a four- to sixfold increase in stroke risk compared with those who had never smoked. It was also shown that cessation of smoking had significant benefits in reducing stroke risk. An association between the use of oral contraceptives as an independent risk factor and the incidence of stroke is not certain, and other risk factors for stroke such as coexisting hypertension, history of migraine, age greater than 35 years, cigarette smoking, diabetes, and hyperlipidemia are important.[5]

### *Multiple Risk Factors*

Data from two studies[8,27] have defined cerebrovascular risk profiles consisting of multiple risk factors. The Framingham study determined five factors: elevated systolic blood pressure, elevated serum cholesterol, glucose intolerance, cigarette smoking, and left ventricular hypertrophy by ECG. These factors, if present, can be used to identify the 10% of the population who will have one third of the strokes. Interestingly, various combinations of factors have been studied, including low ponderal index (height in inches/cube root of weight in pounds), and risk can vary four- to eightfold depending on the number of multiple risk factors present. The most important single factor, however, was found to be elevated blood pressure.

The treatable single risk factors should be vigorously addressed, and when risk factors occur in combination, therapy should be initiated aggressively, with particular emphasis on hypertension.

## Pathophysiology of Acute Stroke

The vascular anatomy of the brain with blood flow from the heart is shown in Figure 18.2. The reader may also refer to the diagrams of the brain territory supplied by the middle cerebral artery (Fig. 18.3), the anterior cerebral artery (Fig. 18.4), and the vertebral–basilar system (Fig. 18.5).

The large majority of acute strokes result either from ischemic infarction or from inadequate blood flow, while only 15% result from intracranial hemorrhage. Although exact pathophysiologic mechanisms are controversial, Figure 18.5 describes the anatomical basis of stroke. Using this schema, the pathophysiology of acute stroke is discussed.

### *Cerebrovascular Disease*

#### Atherothrombotic Disease

Atherosclerosis of brain arteries is a process similar to that found in other extracranial vessels. It is generally held that the atherosclerotic process occurs in parallel fashion throughout the body, although the severity may be slightly less in arteries of the brain than in such arteries as the aorta, the arteries of the extremities, and the coronary arteries. Atherosclerosis and subsequent plaque formation result in arterial narrowing or occlusion and constitute the most common cause of aortocranial stenosis. Thrombosis is most likely to occur in areas where plaque has caused the greatest narrowing of the vessel. Formation of a blood clot superimposed on atherosclerotic plaque may cause significant stenosis of large extracranial arteries or the deep penetrating intracerebral arteries. Additional factors such as blood hypercoagulability and increased platelet counts and hematocrit may also contribute to clotting and sludging of blood flow. Embolism can produce a stroke when a clot, plaque, or platelet aggregate breaks off into the circulation and blocks an artery. When atherosclerotic plaque ulcerates and pieces embolize distally, the emboli are called artery-to-artery emboli. Other embolic phenomena are discussed under Cardiogenic Embolism. Platelets play an important role in thrombosis and loss of integrity of the endothelial surface of

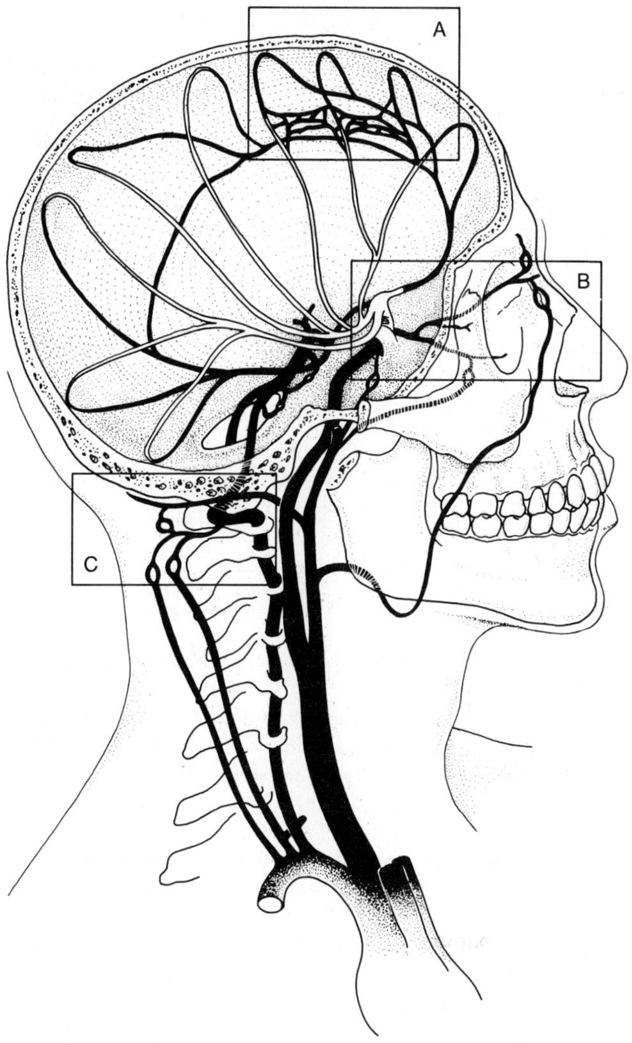


**Figure 18.2** Arrangement of the major arteries of the right side carrying blood from the heart to the brain. Also shown are vessels of collateral circulation that may modify the effects of cerebral ischemia (*A–C*). Not shown is the circle of Willis, which also provides a source for collateral circulation. (*A*) The anastomotic channels between the distal branches of the anterior and middle cerebral artery, termed *borderzone* or *watershed anastomotic channels*. Note that they also occur between the posterior and middle cerebral arteries and the anterior and posterior cerebral arteries. (*B*) Anastomotic channels occurring through the orbit between branches of the external carotid artery and the ophthalmic branch of the internal carotid artery. (*C*) Wholly extracranial anastomotic channels between the muscular branches of the ascending cervical arteries and the muscular branches of the occipital artery that anastomose with the distal vertebral artery. Note that the occipital artery arises from the external carotid artery, thereby allowing reconstitution of flow in the vertebral artery from the carotid circulation. *(From Braunwald E, Isselbacher KJ, et al (Eds): Harrison's Principles of Internal Medicine, 11th ed. New York, McGraw–Hill, 1987, p 1931, with permission.)*

the arterial wall, even if the defect is minor, and platelet activation can lead to formation of a thrombus. This endothelial damage can result from trauma or from diseases such as atherosclerosis and, when this occurs, vessel collagen can be exposed to the blood. This exposed collagen acts as a trigger mechanism to activate the platelets. This activation results in release of adenine diphosphate (ADP) from the platelets, which in turn causes platelets to aggregate. Aggregation is consolidated by coagulation factors, red blood cells, and formation of a fibrin network. Other factors are also produced including thromboxane $A_2$, which promotes platelet aggregation and vasoconstriction. This is balanced by the production of prostacyclin ($PGI_2$) by the vessel endothelium. Prostacyclin is a vasodilator and inhibitor of platelet aggregation. This thrombus may continue to increase in size until the entire lumen of the vessel is blocked, or pieces of the thrombus may break off and embolize into more distal areas. The process of atherosclerosis, as indicated above, results in plaque formation, which stimulates platelet aggregation. Atherosclerosis itself is initially seen as a fatty streak on the vascular wall. This fatty streak starts as a deposition of lipids in the endothelial cells of the vessel wall. This process may regress, remain stable, or progress. If the process continues, yellow fatty, fibrous plaques are formed. Again, if there is progression, an atheromatous lesion may form and hemorrhage into the plaque, and subintimal necrosis, loss of intimal integrity, ulcer formation, or calcification may occur.[28–31] The atherosclerotic process is variable and the ischemic consequences resulting from this process depend on two factors: (1) adequacy of blood flow and collateral circulation and (2) embolism.[32] These factors determine the outcome of any individual ischemic event. To produce a low-blood-flow state leading to ischemia, the blood pressure must be reduced distal to the stenosis or occlusion and, usually, the carotid lumen must be reduced 75% in diameter.[33,34] Impaired collateral circulation to the affected area is also critical. The collateral circulation is composed of a network of arteries on the surface of the brain and those of the circle of Willis.

The most common sites for the atherosclerotic process to occur are at the bifurcation of the common carotid siphon, the origin of the common carotid artery from the aorta; at the bifurcation of the internal carotid artery into the anterior and middle cerebral arteries; and in the circle of Willis at the proximal segments of the anterior, middle, and posterior cerebral arteries (Fig. 18.6).[35]

## Cerebral Ischemia

Cerebral ischemia can be divided into focal and general (or global) ischemia. Global ischemia is associated with lack of collateral blood flow, and irreversible brain damage occurs in a short period of time (4–8 minutes).[36] In focal ischemia, however, there remains some degree of collateral circulation; therefore, this may allow for survival of brain cells and reversal of neuronal damage after periods of ischemia. Because of this potential for recovery, focal ischemia is considered treatable in some cases. The pathophysiologic characteristics of focal ischemia may be reviewed in terms of cerebral ischemia thresholds, metabolic derangements, and microcirculatory changes.[37]

***Cerebral Ischemia Thresholds*** Normal cerebral blood flow (CBF) in humans is about 53 mL per 100 g per minute. Reductions in CBF in the range 15–18 mL/g per minute result

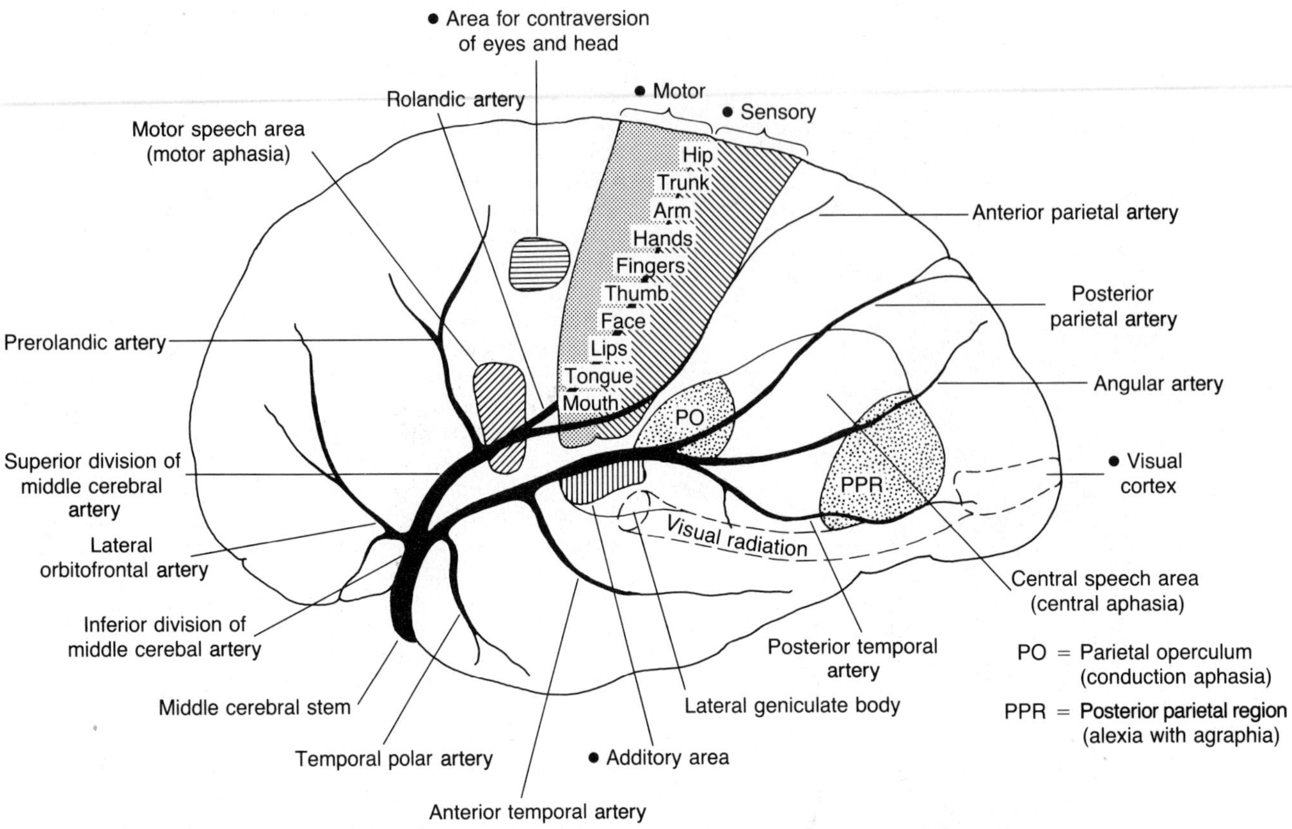


**Figure 18.3** Diagram of a cerebral hemisphere, lateral aspect, showing the branches and distribution of the middle cerebral artery and the principal regions of cerebral localization. Note the bifurcation of the middle cerebral artery into a superior and an inferior division. *(From Braunwald E, Isselbacher KJ, et al (Eds): Harrison's Principles of Internal Medicine, 11th ed. New York, McGraw–Hill, 1987, p 1936, with permission.)*

**Figure 18.4** Diagram of a cerebral hemisphere, medial aspect, showing the branches and distribution of the anterior cerebral artery and the principal regions of cerebral localization. *(From Braunwald E, Isselbacher KJ, et al (Eds): Harrison's Principles of Internal Medicine, 11th ed. New York, McGraw–Hill, 1987, p 1937, with permission.)*

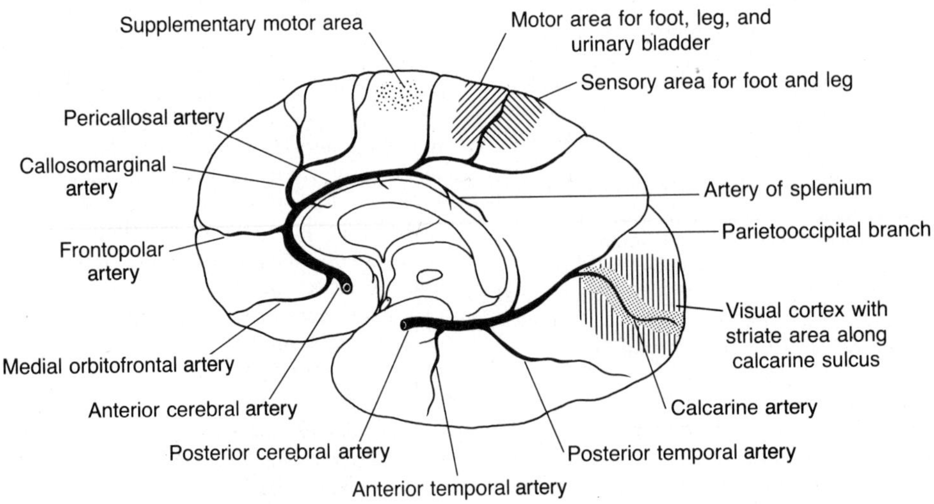

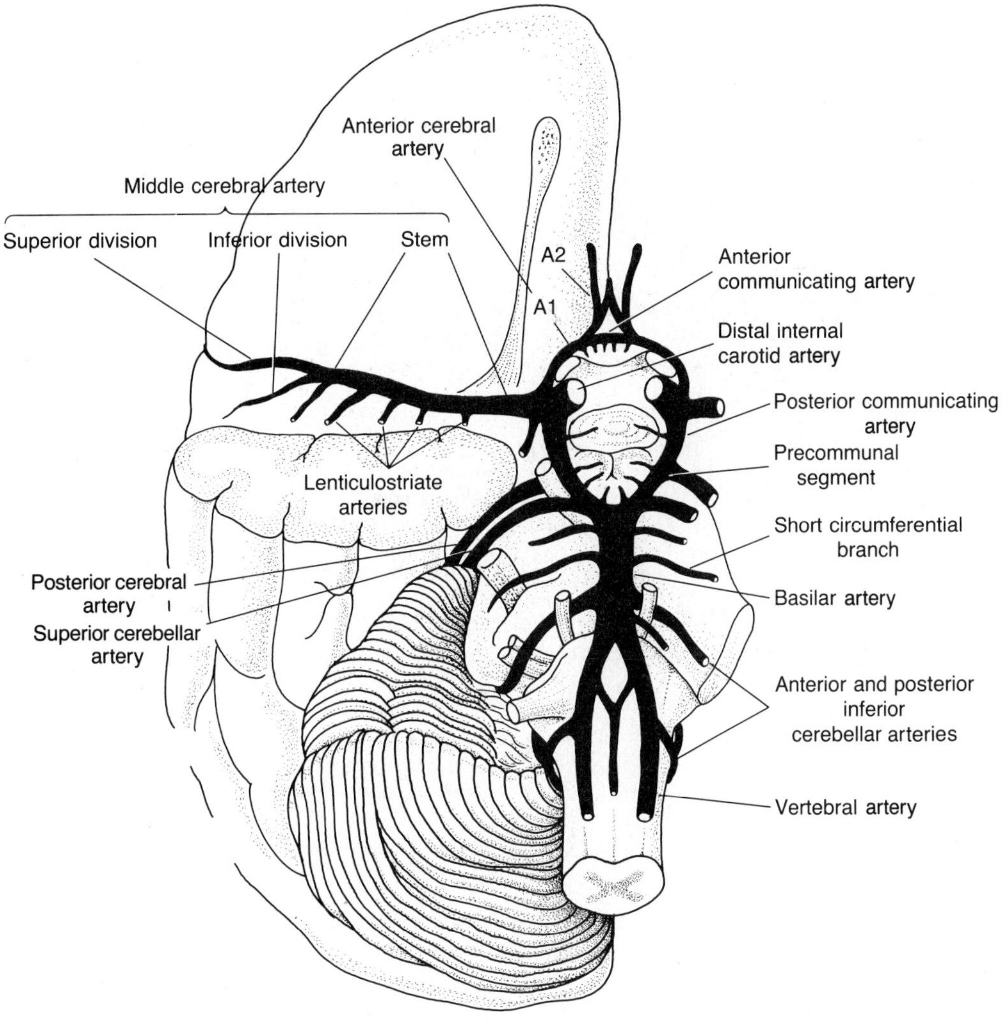


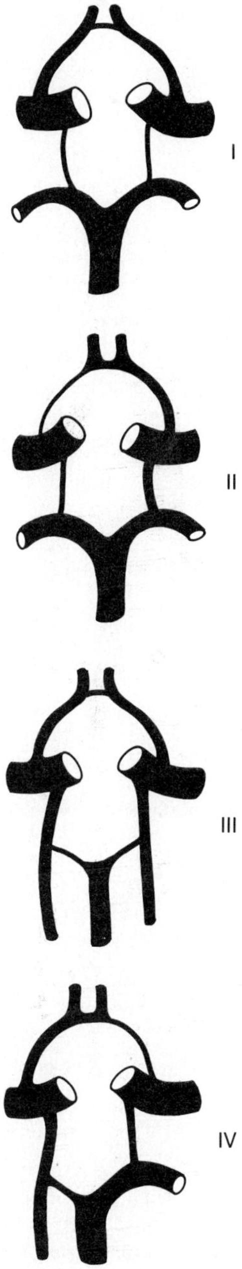


**Figure 18.5** Diagram of the brain stem, cerebellum, inferior right frontal lobe, and temporal lobe transected. Principal branches of the vertebrobasilar arterial system are pictured. Small branches of the vertebral and basilar arteries that penetrate the medulla and pons are not pictured. The stem of the middle cerebral artery with its small, deep penetrating lenticulostriate arteries and the circle of Willis with its small, deep penetrating branches are pictured. Roman numerals I, II, III, and IV represent some of the possible variations of the circle of Willis resulting from atresia of one or more of its arterial components. Great variability in infarct size and location occurs when the basilar or vertebral arteries, or one of their penetrating branches, occlude because of variation in arterial anatomic location and available collateral circulation. Thus the stroke syndromes produced are often atypical or incomplete, or merge with one another. *(From Braunwald E, Isselbacher KJ (Eds): Harrison's Principles of Internal Medicine, 11th ed. New York, McGraw–Hill, 1987, p 1932, with permission.)*

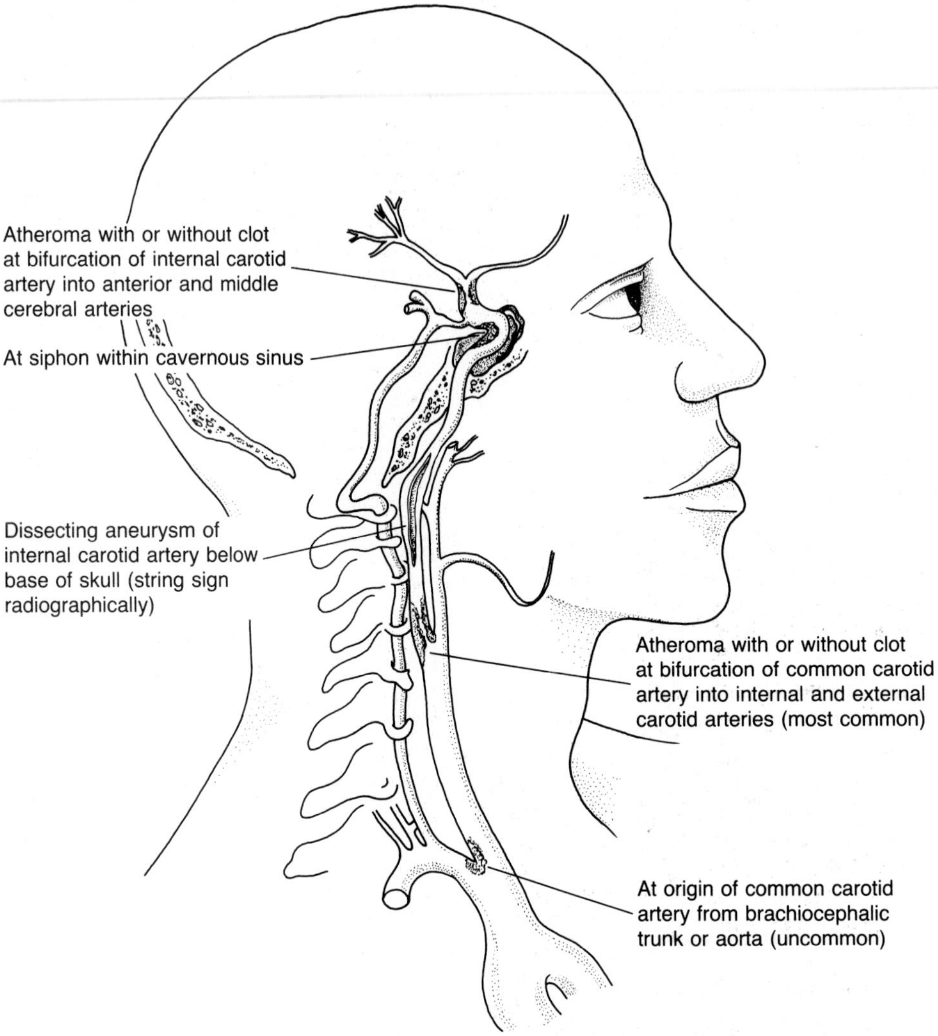


**Figure 18.6** Common sites of atherosclerotic disease in the aortocranial circulation. *(From The Ciba Collection of Medical Illustrations. Ciba Foundation, 1982, vol 1 pt II, p 55, with permission.)*

in abnormal brain electrical activity. At a flow of 10 mL/100 g per minute alterations in intracellular calcium and extracellular potassium homeostasis occur. Also, free fatty acids are released, and adenosine triphosphate (ATP) is depleted. A severe intracellular acidosis ensues in cells in the ischemic area. CBF of 10 mL per 100 g per minute results in failure of ionic regulation and is thought to result in rapid irreversible damage to neurons.[37] The CBF range between electrical failure and ionic failure is thought to be enough to maintain cell function for a time, possibly up to 4 hours, and recovery might be possible in acute focal ischemia, provided adequate collateral flow could supply basic energy requirements. Clinical outcome, as noted earlier, is dependent upon the severity and duration of the decreased CBF.

***Metabolic Derangements*** When the CBF decreases to 10 mL/100 g per minute, accumulation of lactic acid, depletion of ATP, and increase in intracellular calcium may be seen (Fig. 18.7). Extracellular potassium increases because of a failure of the ATP-dependent sodium–potassium pump. This rise in extracellular $K^+$ depolarizes the neuronal membrane which in turn stimulates the opening of the voltage-dependent calcium channels, and an influx of calcium into the intracellular space occurs. Calcium cannot be pumped out normally because of the failure of the ATP-dependent calcium transport system and, in addition, calcium is not taken up normally by the endoplasmic reticulum. This unbalanced intracellular increase in calcium is thought to result in the production of free fatty acids from membrane phospholipids. This loss of phospholipid decreases the integrity of the cell, and the permeability of the cell membranes increases and further impairs calcium homeostasis. Accumulation of free fatty acids, including arachidonic acid, results in oxidation via cyclooxygenase and lipoxygenase pathways, producing prostaglandins, leukotrienes, and, possibly, free radicals.[37] Thromboxane $A_2$ is a potent vasoconstrictor, leukotrienes affect membrane permeability, and free radicals can attack cell membranes.[37] All of these actions can lead to further

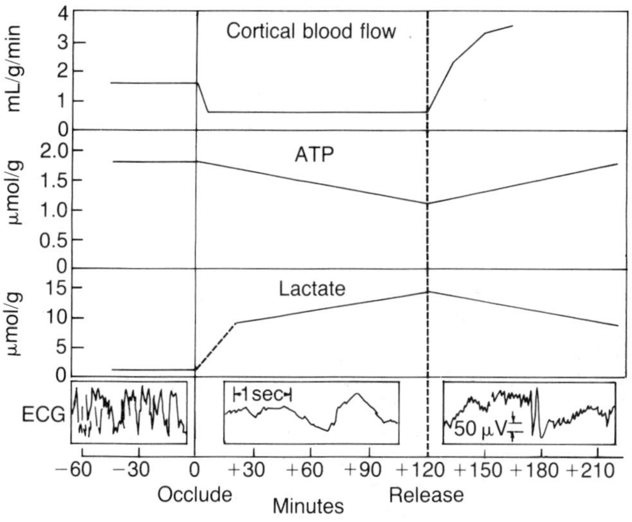


**Figure 18.7** Metabolic derangements in cerebral ischemia. *(From Meyer FB, Sundt TM, Yanagihara T, et al: Focal cerebral ischemia: Pathophysiologic mechanisms and rationale for future avenues of treatment. Mayo Clin Proc 1987;62:38, with permission.)*

intracellular acidosis and increasingly impair cell function. Ischemia and the subsequent production of intracellular acidosis can have devastating effects on the brain cell. These effects include glial edema and denaturation of proteins. Focal ischemia is associated with preserved but marginal CBF, and continued glucose delivery in the face of ischemia promotes anaerobic glycolysis with the production of lactic acidosis. This continues to worsen the intracellular acidosis.

***Microcirculatory Changes and Edema*** At the time of occlusion, blood viscosity and resistance to flow are increased,[38] and blood flow is further slowed as ischemia develops. Soon after this, an ischemia-induced arterial spasm occurs,[39] possibly as a result of the aforementioned increased extracellular potassium or increased intracellular calcium or both. It is not clear why vasospasm of the microcirculation occurs and it is also not clear if this impaired vascular filling is the primary determinant of neuronal damage. In any case, damage to the endothelium of the vessels occurs.

***Ischemia Edema*** Swelling is one of the primary responses of brain tissue to acute injury. An early or intracellular phase and a late or extracellular phase occur. The early phase involves primarily the glial cells surrounding the vessel itself, suggesting a defect in vascular permeability, possibly enhanced by lactic acidosis. The primary difficulty caused by the glial edema is that collateral flow is decreased as a result of the "squeezing down" on the collateral circulation. The late phase or extracellular phase occurs hours to days after vessel occlusion and is probably a result of ischemic damage to vessel endothelial tissue. Movement of plasma into the extracellular space results in increased intracranial pressure. Brain herniation can result from the increased pressure. In animals, there are regional differences in brain tissue vulnerability to ischemia and some tissues may be more or less resistant to ischemic damage than other tissues.[40] Some investigators postulate that these differences may result from the greater number of calcium channels in those tissues that are most vulnerable.[37]

### Lacunar Infarcts

Occlusion of the small arterial branches of the circle of Willis and of the anterior, middle, and posterior cerebral and basilar arteries can result in infarcts deep in the cerebral hemispheres and brain stem. These are small arteries with diameters in the range 100–400 $\mu$m and their occlusion results in small infarcts 2–15 $\mu$m in diameters. The term *lacunar* or *lacune* refers to the small cavity left after necrotic tissue has been removed. The pathophysiology of these infarcts is somewhat different from that of infarcts closer to the surface of the brain. About 10% of all strokes are a result of lacunar infarcts and these infarcts account for one out of seven cerebral infarcts. Arterial hypertension is closely related to the occurrence of lacunar infarcts. The pathophysiology of the small arteries has been described as being a degenerative process in the media of the artery, leading to vessel occlusion.[41,42] The degenerative occlusive process may be, on occasion, histologically different in appearance compared with the atherosclerotic process affecting extracranial and other larger intracranial arteries and may, in fact, circumscribe portions of the involved artery. Microatheroma (plaque) may also be found in the proximal portions of the arterial branches. These different occlusive processes probably account for the multiple types of clinical presentations of lacunar infarcts. The patient's clinical presentation will reflect which small arterial branches are involved in the occlusive process. For example, the lenticulostriate artery is often involved and the most common lacunar syndrome results from an infarct in the internal capsule of the brain and a pure motor hemiparesis is seen.

### Transient Ischemic Attacks

TIAs of cerebral origin are episodes of temporary focal cerebral dysfunction of vascular origin in which the onset is rapid, is of variable duration, and lasts from a few seconds up to 24 hours. The most common duration is a few seconds up to 5 to 10 minutes. Between attacks there may be no neurologic abnormality. The clinical manifestation reflects the territory of the artery involved and usually occurs in the carotid system or in the vertebrobasilar system or both. TIAs have great significance in that they herald an impending stroke. Threatened stroke is a term used to describe any prestroke syndrome, such as TIAs, or patients who have had small or minor strokes or progressing or evolving stroke, and are at further risk for a major stroke. TIAs precede stroke in 60% of cases, with risk for stroke increasing from about 6% the first year after a TIA to a 5-year cumulative risk of 35% to 50%. The pathophysiology of TIAs involves the atherosclerotic process, thrombus formation, and low CBF. It is from the cerebral thrombus that small microemboli, in the form of platelet aggregates and cholesterol crystals, break off and travel to distal areas and lodge, producing the ischemic attack. Cerebral or cerebellar artery thrombosis is most commonly responsible for TIAs. Low flow will also result in a TIA when the CBF is sufficiently reduced in stenosed arteries. Other causes include emboli from the heart caused by valvular disease or endocardial damage and increased blood viscosity from conditions such as polycythemia. Polycythemia is an uncommon cause of TIA.

### *Cerebral Embolism*

Any region of the brain can be affected by embolism; however, the area or territory of the middle cerebral artery is commonly involved. Embolism may result from pieces or fragments of an arterial thrombus that have broken off or from a heart valve vegetation. Occasionally, an embolus may form from an ulcerated atheromatous plaque. Other forms of embolism such as air, fat, or tumor cells occur only rarely. Cerebral embolism from bacterial sepsis occurs frequently, but bacterial emboli large enough to produce a stroke are infrequent. After breaking off from a thrombus or heart valve vegetation, an embolism usually circulates until it is too large to traverse the arterial lumen. The point of occlusion may be at a bifurcation or other narrowed area. Both hemispheres of the brain appear to be equally affected. Hemorrhagic infarction frequently occurs in the embolic process because of the reperfusion of blood into the ischemic tissue, causing hemorrhage, and the area of the middle cerebral artery is often the involved site. The size of the embolus may vary from large to very small; in fact, the embolus may be so small that it produces no infarct or produces an infarct so small that it cannot be detected by diagnostic studies or even at autopsy.

That cerebral embolism has a rapid onset and is not usually preceded by a TIA is evidence of thrombotic disease. This rapid onset is problematic because there is less time for collateral circulation to develop as in cerebral thrombosis. As a result, embolic strokes are often functionally devastating. Cerebral embolism may result from heart disease. It is currently recognized that cardiogenic embolism accounts for 6% to 23% of all ischemic strokes.[43] Embolism has been associated with many types of heart disease, and the following discussion focuses on the most common types. (See Table 18.2.)

**Table 18.2** Major Causes of Cardiogenic Cerebral Embolism

| | |
|---|---|
| Nonvalvular atrial fibrillation | 50% |
| Coronary heart disease | 20% |
| Myocardial infarction | |
| Rheumatic heart disease | 15% |
| Mitral stenosis ± atrial fibrillation | |
| Prosthetic cardiac valves | 10% |
| Other | 5% |
| Cardiomyopathy | |
| Cardiac tumors | |
| Septic endocarditis | |
| Nonbacterial thrombotic endocarditis (marantic) | |
| Congenital heart disease | |
| Venous clots/intracardiac shunt (paradoxic emboli) | |
| Mitral annulus calcification | |
| Calcific aortic stenosis | |
| Mitral valve prolapse | |

From Easton JD, Hart RG, Sherman DG, et al: Diagnosis and management of ischemic stroke. Part 1. Threatened stroke and its management. Curr Prob Cardiol 1983;8:20, with permission.

#### Cardiogenic Embolism

***Atrial Fibrillation*** Chronic atrial fibrillation (AF) is the most common cause of cardiogenic embolism and is the most common sustained dysrhythmia. The incidence of AF increases with age such that 2% to 5% of patients over 60 years have AF. Patients with nonvalvular atrial fibrillation have about the same stroke risk as patients who experience a TIA. Atrial fibrillation enhances the development of left atrial thrombi and arterial embolism. The most common site (75%) in which left atrial thrombi form in patients with nonvalvular AF (NVAF) is the atrial appendage rather than the atrial wall. Patients with AF and valvular disease have thrombi both on the atrial wall and on the appendage in equal incidence. Factors involved in the pathogenesis of atrial thrombus formation in patients with AF include increased left atrial pressure and outflow obstruction. Mitral value obstruction can enhance left atrial stasis similar to that seen in AF alone. Enlargement of the left atrium occurs in AF and the incidence of thrombus formation increases with left atrial enlargement. Damage to the atrial endothelial surface could also induce thrombus formation and initiate AF. Such disorders as rheumatic heart disease, myocardial infarction, and pericarditis can also initiate AF by involvement of the sinoatrial node and change the atrial endothelial surface such that thrombus formation is enhanced. The risk of stroke in patients with AF is high and 20% to 35% of all patients with AF will have an embolic stroke of clinical significance.[44] The risk of stroke in those with AF is six times that of the general population, and those at greatest risk are those patients with AF and rheumatic valvular disease. The risk for development of systemic embolism for these individuals is 17 times that of the general population.[45] The largest group of patients comprises those with NVAF; their rate of systemic embolism is around 35% and their stroke risk is six times that of the general population.[45,46] Even those patients with idiopathic AF have an increased rate of embolism of 7% in the first year, and up to 14% at 5 years of AF.[47] It also appears that patients with paroxysmal AF are at risk and that patients who develop AF could possibly have the highest rate of embolus formation soon after the onset of AF. Recurrence of embolism is frequent. Up to 50% of patients who develop one embolus develop another.[17] Additionally, changing the rhythm by cardioversion increases the rate of embolus occurrence, and about 2% of these patients develop an embolus the first few days after cardioversion of AF to normal sinus rhythm.[48]

Ischemic heart disease and ischemic stroke share the same risk factors and most patients with TIAs and stroke die from myocardial infarction. In myocardial infarction the primary cause of emboli is mural thrombus formation in the left ventricle. Thrombus formation is thought to be started by platelet adherence to and deposition on the damaged (infarcted) akinetic or dyskinetic endocardial surface.[49] There is also an inflammatory white cell response in the damaged area secondary to the tissue infarction. Additionally, the infarcted area may develop into an aneurysmal region where fibrin accumulation can occur. Mural thrombus formation depends on the size and location of the infarct. Thrombus formation and the presence of apical akinesis or dyskinesis are seen almost exclusively in anterior myocardial infarctions. Aneurysms occur most frequently in the apex region of the heart. About 50% to 60% of patients with aneurysm formation in the left ventricle develop a mural thrombus.[49] Most of these mural thrombi develop within the first week of the acute myocardial infarction (AMI) and patients who have mural thrombi as evidenced by echocardiography after AMI are most probably those patients at risk for eventual embolization. The overall incidence of systemic emboli in patients who suffer an AMI is around 5% to 6% and is similar to the incidence in those patients who develop a left ventricular aneurysm. Therefore, of the 50% to 60% of patients with an aneurysm who develop a mural thrombus only 5% to 6% develop a systemic embolus.

***Valvular Heart Disease*** Thromboembolism is commonly found in patients with valvular heart disease and in those with prosthetic heart valves. Thrombus formation in patients with valvular disease or prosthetic valves most often occurs in the left ventricle or on the prosthetic valve. Thrombi can also form, but with a lower incidence, in the left atrium. Mitral stenosis is also associated with an increased risk of thromboembolism.

In valvular heart disease, those patients with mitral stenosis and those with mitral stenosis combined with incompetence of the mitral valve have a thromboembolic event rate of 15% to 20%. Up to 16% of these events may be fatal.[50,51] Patients with only mitral incompetence are at less risk than those with mitral stenosis and the embolic rate is approximately 3%, although this rate may be higher in patients with a severe form of mitral incompetence. Prolapse of the mitral valve appears to carry a very low risk of embolism. The risk of embolism also appears to be low in patients with aortic valve disease. Additional factors that increase risk for systemic embolism in patients with valvular disease are atrial fibrillation, increased left atrial size, and history of a previous embolic event. Atrial fibrillation is the most important single risk factor, and as noted previously, thrombus formation is rare in patients with a normal sinus rhythm. Atrial fibrillation is closely associated with mitral valve disease and emboli may develop shortly after fibrillation develops. Enlargement of the left atrium usually occurs with mitral valve disease. It is felt that left atrial enlargement predisposes to atrial fibrillation. Therefore, there is an indirect relationship between left atrial enlargement and embolism. Recurrent embolic events can occur in up to 20% of mitral stenosis patients with previous embolic history. The mortality rate is quite high in this group of patients and may reach 42%.[51]

***Prosthetic Heart Valves*** Thrombus formation on these valves, whether aortic or mitral valves, is related to the production of turbulence in blood flow by the valve and the thrombogenic potential of the valve material. The three valves currently used are the Starr–Edwards ball valve, the Bjork–Shiley disk valve, and bioprosthetic or biologic valves. The incidence of embolism for these valves is given in Table 18.3. The early Starr–Edwards valve used in the 1960s may have a higher embolic rate than those used in recent years. This may be a result of improved operative procedures and valve factors, as well as patients who have less severe disease and better atrial and ventricular function.

**Table 18.3** Approximate Rates of Thromboembolism From Different Prosthetic Valves

| | ***Events per 100 patient-years*** | |
|---|---|---|
| ***Valve type*** | **Aortic** | **Mitral** |
| Starr–Edwards | 2.0–4.0 | 2.0–5.0 |
| Bjork–Shiley | 1.0–3.0 | 1.0–5.0 |
| Bioprosthetic valves[a] | 0.5–2.0 | 3.0–4.0 |

[a] Patient groups not always anticoagulated.

From Chesebro JH, Ezekowitz M, Badimon L, et al: Intracardiac thrombi and systemic thromboembolism: Detection, incidence, and treatment. Annu Rev Med 1985;36:585, with permission.

The embolism rate with the Bjork–Shiley valve is similar to that with the Starr–Edwards valve; however, a newer material, pyrolytic carbon, in the disk of the valve is less thrombogenic and the embolism rate is lower. The bioprosthetic valves have a different design, a central flow design. This design produces less turbulence in blood flow, and the biologic material (i.e., porcine valve) is less thrombogenic. Thromboembolism occurs less frequently than with the other valves. Other risk factors include atrial fibrillation, large left atrium, inadequate anticoagulation, and a previous embolic event. The overall risk of neurologic deficit with prosthetic valve–induced embolism is high. For instance, data from follow-up of the Starr–Edwards ball valve show that 85% of systemic emboli entered the cerebral circulation and 50% of these emboli resulted in a neurologic deficit, with 10% of all embolic events being fatal.[52]

***Infective Endocarditis*** Emboli may result from bacterial vegetations that can form in infective endocarditis. Arterial emboli are one of the most frequent complications of this disease. Major cerebral emboli have been observed in nearly one third of patients with endocarditis, with the middle cerebral artery and its branches being most frequently involved. The highest frequency of major embolic events occurs in association with infections on the left side of the heart that produce large, mobile vegetations from *Hemophilus parainfluenzae*, or slow-growing fastidious, gram-negative bacilli, fungi (*Aspergillus*), and *Streptococcus viridans*. Emboli from the right side of the heart, as seen in intravenous drug abusers, are often caused by staphylococcal organisms and can produce clinical manifestations of pulmonary emboli. There is another type of endocarditis, called marantic endocarditis, in which sterile thrombi are present on the valves. This condition is seen most often in patients with mucin-secreting adenocarcinomas. This process is nonbacterial and the vegetations are composed mainly of platelets and fibrin. The term *marantic* refers to old and debilitated; however, this thromboembolic process can occur in the young and nondebilitated.

### *Unusual and Other Causes of Infarction*

There are a number of other causes of cerebral infarction, and these are listed in Table 18.4.

**Table 18.4** Unusual Causes of Infarction

| | |
|---|---|
| Venous thrombosis | Contraceptive steroid use |
| Systemic hypotension | Polycythemia |
| Arteriography | Idiopathic thrombocytosis |
| Carotid occlusion | Dissecting aortic aneurysm |
| Arteritis | Hypercoagulable states |
| Moyamoya disease | |

### *Intracranial Hemorrhage*

Hemorrhage is the third most frequent cause of stroke. Approximately 15% of cases of stroke are due to intracranial hemorrhage. The more frequent causes of stroke from intracranial hemorrhage are hypertensive intracerebral hemorrhage, ruptured saccular aneurysms, hemorrhage associated with bleeding disorders, and arteriovenous malformations (AVMs).

Hypertensive intracerebral hemorrhage occurs generally when the blood pressure is significantly elevated. The bleeding occurs in the brain tissue as a result of the rupture of an artery. This allows for an extravasation of blood into the brain tissue which forms a mass. This mass damages the tissue and continues to enlarge as bleeding continues. Brain tissue is pushed, displaced, and compressed and brain functions may be impaired. The larger the hemorrhage, the greater the displacement of tissue. Escape of blood into the ventricles of the brain can occur, and when this happens, the spinal fluid becomes bloody. The cerebrospinal fluid may remain clear if the hemorrhage is small or at a distance from the ventricular system. The extravascular blood undergoes changes such as phagocytosis, and the mass gradually shrinks; after 2 to 6 months, only discoloration is left at the site. Hemorrhagic infarcts, discussed earlier, are due primarily to the reflow or reperfusion of ischemic tissue, with resultant bleeding into the tissue. In hypertensive hemorrhage, the vessels most often involved are the penetrating arteries in the putamen and internal capsule and parts of the white matter, including the frontal lobe, thalamus, pons, and cerebellar hemisphere. Causes of intracranial hemorrhage are listed in Table 18.5.

## Clinical Presentation/Diagnosis

### *Atherothrombotic Disease*

Thrombosis of cerebral vessels produces variable clinical manifestations as compared with embolic disease or intracranial hemorrhage. In a large percentage of cases (>50%), the stroke is preceded by one or more transient ischemic attacks. If the evolving thrombosis involves the internal carotid and middle cerebral arteries, then such focal symptoms as mono- or hemiplegia, mono- or hemiparesthesia, blindness in one eye, and speech disturbance may occur. If the vertebrobasilar system is involved, such symptoms as dizziness, diplopia, numbness, impaired vision, and dysarthria may occur. Usually these attacks are short-lived and resolve in less than 10 minutes. The stroke itself most often develops suddenly as a single attack, or it may show an intermittent or stuttering progression pattern over hours to days. Additionally, a patient may suffer a partial stroke, improve for several hours, then develop full paralysis of one or more parts of the body; other parts become paralyzed in a stepwise manner until the stroke is completed. When the thrombosis produces a developing involvement over hours, days, or weeks, it is called stroke in evolution or progressing stroke. Interestingly, the majority (60%) of cerebral thrombotic strokes occur at rest while sleeping or after arising.[17] Headache may occur, but is often absent; when present, it may occur several days prior to the other symptoms of the stroke.

Diagnosis consists of evaluation of the clinical presentation and laboratory findings. In addition to the clinical presentation just discussed, laboratory evaluation can include tests such as cerebral arteriography, CAT scan, radioactive brain scan study (such as a technetium scan), x-rays

**Table 18.5** Causes of Intracranial Hemorrhage

- Hypertensive intracerebral hemorrhage
- Lobar hemorrhage of undetermined cause and intracerebral hemorrhage associated with congophilic angiopathy (analyzed)
- Ruptured saccular aneurysm, giant aneurysm, or mycotic aneurysm
- Ruptured angioma
- Hemorrhagic disorders: leukemia, aplastic anemia, thrombocytopenic purpura, liver disease, complication of anticoagulant therapy, hyperfibrinolysis, hypofibrinogenemia, hemophilia, Christmas disease
- Trauma, including posttraumatic apoplexy
- Hemorrhage into primary and secondary brain tissue
- Hemorrhagic infarction, arterial or venous
- Inflammatory disease of the arteries and veins
- Miscellaneous rare types: after vasopressor drugs, upon exertion, during arteriography, during painful urologic examination, as a late complication of early-life carotid occlusion, complication of carotid–cavernous arteriovenous fistula, with anoxemia, migraine, teratomatous malformations (acute inclusion body encephalitis produces xanthochromia and up to 2,000 red blood cells or more in the cerebrospinal fluid; acute necrotizing hemorrhagic encephalopathy may be associated with up to 100 red blood cells in the cerebrospinal fluid; tularemia and snake venom poisoning may cause bloody cerebrospinal fluid).

From Braunwald E, Isselbacher KJ, et al (Eds): Harrison's Principles of Internal Medicine, 11th ed. New York, McGraw-Hill, 1987, p 1952, with permission.

of the head, electroencephalogram, echocardiography, Doppler studies, digital subtraction angiography, and lumbar puncture (LP). The definitive test for arterial occlusion or narrowing is arteriography; however, this procedure carries a neurologic risk itself and should be used if the diagnosis of vascular disease is not clear or if vascular surgery is a possibility, such as in carotid TIA patients. When it is performed, transfemoral angiography is usually the procedure of choice as compared with the direct carotid puncture procedure.[17] The CAT scan in cerebral thrombosis usually shows an area of decreased attenuation or hypodense lesion in the infarcted area. The CAT scan is often normal, however, during the first 24 to 48 hours after the thrombotic infarction. The CAT scan is extremely useful in excluding tumors and identifying intracranial hemorrhage both of which dictate different treatment modalities.

Radioisotopic brain scans can be helpful and show infarcts earlier than CAT scans. Skull x-rays are usually not helpful and the electroencephalogram is of limited value as is the lumbar puncture (LP), as the findings are usually normal. Noninvasive techniques like Doppler flow studies and Doppler scanning have been developed but have some disadvantages with consistent differentiation of stenosis from occlusion and detection of distal atherosclerosis.

Digital subtraction angiography (DSA) is a recent addition and it holds significant promise as a diagnostic tool. Arterial injection of contrast medium in DSA currently provides better imaging of the cerebral vasculature than does intravenous administration, which gives imperfect detail.

Other new diagnostic imaging techniques include positron emission tomography (PET), which can give an image of dynamic physiology after injection of positron-emitting isotopes, and magnetic resonance imaging (MRI). MRI is a noninvasive imaging technique that, unlike CAT and PET, does not require x-rays or istopes. These techniques are very promising advances and as they become more refined their place in diagnosis will become clear.[53,54]

### Lacunar Infarcts

The clinical presentation varies depending on the perforating cerebral arteries involved. The most frequently occurring lacunar syndrome is pure motor hemiparesis, which is due to an infarct in the posterior portion of the internal capsule. This infarct results from occlusion of a middle or posterior cerebral perforating artery. The manifestations of the pure motor hemiparesis syndrome are hemiparesis or hemiplegia of the arm, leg, face, and trunk. In addition, a mild dysarthria occurs without sensory or consciousness alterations or visual field defects. The different parts of the body involved in the stroke display the same degree of weakness. This is in contrast to a stroke in the cortical region involving the middle or anterior cerebral artery where there is usually an unequal degree of weakness of the affected parts of the body.

Diagnosis is usually based on clinical evaluation of the patient after careful neurologic examination. A CAT scan can provide evidence of the infarction if performed within about 7 to 10 days of the event; however, infarcts smaller than 2 mm may be missed.

### Transient Ischemic Attacks

Most TIAs last 5 to 10 minutes, and those lasting one or more hours may be a result of embolism rather than ischemia or atherosclerosis. An ischemic event that lasts longer than 24 hours but completely resolves in a short period (up to 3 weeks) is termed a *reversible ischemic neurologic defect* (RIND). A TIA resulting from a carotid system lesion and anterior cerebral artery involvement manifests as weakness in the opposite leg and shoulder. If the anterior cortical branches of the middle cerebral artery are involved, a sensory and motor loss results in the contralateral face, arm, and hand. If the ischemia is in the dominant hemisphere, a nonfluent (Broca's) aphasia usually is present. Ischemia occurring in the posterior portions of the middle cerebral artery often produces contralateral sensory loss and homonymous hemianopia (defective vision or blindness affecting the right halves or the left halves of the visual fields of the two eyes). If there is posterior middle cerebral artery involvement in the dominant hemisphere, a fluent aphasia is likely to occur. Ischemia of the lenticulostriate arteries may result in findings that involve motor and sensory defects in the arms, legs, face, and trunk as noted in the discussion of lacunar infarcts. Clinical manifestations of TIAs arising from ischemia in the vertebrobasilar circulation are numerous. Vertigo and ataxia are seen in ischemia affecting cerebellar and vestibular areas. Bilateral weakness of the extremities indicates that the corticospinal nerve tracts are involved as they cross the brain stem.

Diagnosis of a TIA is difficult because the episode is usually over before the patient can be examined. Therefore, the diagnosis is really made on the basis of the patient's recollection of the symptoms. Table 18.6 shows the symptoms of TIAs. There are many singular symptoms or events that can be confused with TIAs and usually are not TIAs. Some of these events are fainting, convulsions, loss of consciousness, dizziness, spots before the eyes, dysarthria, imbalance and falling, and headache. Diagnostic studies may indicate the presence of vascular disease; however, history is the key to the diagnosis of a TIA. Proper attention to the history is important because treatment of TIAs is important in stroke prevention.

Laboratory studies in the diagnosis of TIA should rule out blood or other disorders that may produce decreased cerebral blood flow. Routine studies include erythrocyte sedimentation rate, complete blood count, platelet count, blood chemistry, urinalysis, coagulation profile, and syphilis (serology). To reveal systemic disease in selected patients, serum protein electrophoresis, antinuclear antibody titers, blood and plasma viscosities, plasma fibrinogen, and cerebral spinal fluid (CSF) examination may be performed. Embolism of cardiac origin should be a consideration in every patient with a single TIA. In these cases a 12-lead ECG should be performed to test for recent myocardial infarction and/or dysrhythmias such as atrial fibrillation. Other laboratory tests include a chest x-ray to exclude heart enlargement or disease of the valves. In patients suspected of having TIAs of embolic origin, echocardiography is an important diagnostic tool. Two-dimensional "echo" is indicated in patients with cerebral ischemia who have evidence of cardiac disease such as AF, enlarged heart, and mitral valve prolapse. The yield of thrombus detection in the hearts

**Table 18.6** Symptoms of Transient Ischemic Attacks

| | |
|---|---|
| Carotid system TIAs | |
| Unilateral weakness—usually hemiparesis | |
| Unilateral sensory complaints—numbness, paresthesia | |
| Aphasia—language comprehension, output or both | |
| Monocular visual loss (amaurosis fugax) | |
| Vertebrobasilar system TIAs | |
| Motor deficit—especially if bilateral | |
| Sensory complaints—especially if bilateral | |
| Simultaneous, bilateral visual complaints | |
| Diplopia | Only in combination, not as isolated symptoms |
| Vertigo | Only in combination, not as isolated symptoms |
| Dysarthria[a] | Only in combination, not as isolated symptoms |
| Ataxia without weakness | Only in combination, not as isolated symptoms |
| Dysphagia | Only in combination, not as isolated symptoms |
| Either carotid or vertebral TIAs | |
| Severe dysarthria[a] | |
| Homonymous visual complaints | |
| Isolated symptoms rarely resulting from TIAs | |
| Vertigo, dizziness | |
| Diplopia | |
| Loss of consciousness | |
| Confusion | |
| Bilateral leg weakness, falling spells | |

[a] Often difficult to distinguish from nonfluent dysphasia on the basis of history.

From Easton JD, Hart RG, Sherman DG, et al: Diagnosis and management of ischemic stroke. Part 1. Threatened stroke and its management. Curr Prob Cardiol 1983;8:13, with permission.

of these patients is 10% to 20%. The lower limit of clot size that is detected accurately by echocardiography is 2–3 mm. As mentioned earlier, cerebral angiography should be performed only in selected patients, and patients who have had a carotid TIA should be studied with angiography as soon as reasonably possible because of the high risk of cerebral infarction in these patients.

**Table 18.7** Clinical Features Suggestive of Cardiogenic Brain Embolism

| | |
|---|
| **Primary Features** |
| Abrupt onset of maximal deficit |
| Presence of a potential embolic source |
| Infarct involving the cerebral cortex or cerebellum |
| Previous ischemic events in other vascular territories |
| **Secondary Evidence** |
| Hemorrhagic infarct by CAT |
| Absence of occlusive cerebrovascular disease by cerebral angiography or reliable noninvasive imaging |
| Angiographic evidence of vanishing occlusions |
| Evidence of embolism to other organs |
| Cardiac thrombi demonstrated by echocardiography, catheterization, cardiac CAT or MRI |

From Sherman DG, Dyken ML, Fisher M, et al: Cerebral embolism. Chest 1986;89(suppl 2):845, Table 2, with permission.

### *Cerebral Embolism/Cardiogenic Embolism*

Cardiogenic brain embolism is the major cause of cerebral embolism and the brain is involved in approximately 70% of all emboli from the heart, whereas systemic or noncerebral nervous system emboli often go unrecognized. Cardiogenic brain embolism accounts for 6% to 23% of all ischemic strokes. The clinical diagnosis is based upon a variety of findings as shown in Table 18.7. The onset is characteristically abrupt, often occurring in an awake patient.[43]

A stuttering course may be seen in about 10% of patients. This represents a distal lodging of emboli. Most cardiogenic emboli that go to the brain lodge in the middle cerebral artery (MCA) or one of its branches. Vertebrobasilar or anterior cerebral artery emboli occur less frequently (<10%) than MCA emboli. Cardiogenic embolism may be suspected when there are multifocal neurologic findings. Seizure or headache at the onset of the stroke is not as useful an indicator as once thought.[43] Cardiogenic embolism should be considered when the following conditions are present: age less than 50, sudden onset of maximal neurologic deficit, prior cortical infarct, past history of valvular heart disease or myocardial infarct, and atrial fibrillation or congestive heart failure. Laboratory studies in those with suspected cardiogenic brain embolism may include two-dimensional echocardiography to assess the presence of left ventricular thrombi and mitral valve dysfunction. Echo does not reliably indicate atrial thrombi. The ECG may indicate a dysrhythmia such as AF.

The new technique of MRI may prove to be useful in the study of embolism of the heart, and recent studies to detect atrial thromboembolism with CAT are under way.[53]

### *Intracranial Hemorrhage*

Usually the clinical manifestations of intracranial hemorrhage have an abrupt onset and changes generally occur over minutes to hours (up to 24 hours). This gradual evolution depends primarily on the bleeding rate and accounts for the time range for the neurologic deficit to become maximal. The neurologic physical findings vary with the site of bleeding and the size of the bleed. The majority of patients lose consciousness, and many die without recovering awareness.

Typically, the patient with spontaneous intracerebral hemorrhage may experience head pain and dizziness prior to losing consciousness. In the case of hypertension-related external capsule (putaminal) hemorrhage, the patient quickly develops signs of hemiplegia and loss of consciousness.

Conjugate deviation of the eyes to the side opposite the affected limbs is commonly seen. If the lesion becomes larger, compression of the upper brain stem produces deepening coma and the patient has dilated and fixed pupils, Babinski signs, bilateral motor hypertonus, and irregular respirations.[55]

In the case of internal capsule (thalamic) hemorrhage the onset is similar to that for putaminal hemorrhage; however, if the patient is still alert a homonymous hemianopia may be seen because of optic nerve involvement in the internal capsule. The location of this hemorrhage produces a variety of gaze disturbances including defective vertical and lateral gaze, fixed downward deviation of the eyes, and unequal pupils. The reader is referred to other sources for discussion of other types of intracranial hemorrhage.[55]

In the diagnosis of hypertensive intracerebral hemorrhage the sudden onset and quick evolution of the physical findings are important. Headache occurs at the onset in approximately 50% of the cases, whereas the occurrence of headaches in thromboembolism is less than 25%. Neck rigidity is common and the funduscopic examination of the eye may reveal periarteriolar hemorrhages and decreased arteriolar size. Convulsions are common as is vomiting, and a history of hypertension is an important clue. Generally, the immediate prognosis for intracerebral hemorrhage is extremely poor, with up to 70% of patients dying in a few days.[55]

Important laboratory findings include blood in the cerebrospinal fluid and evidence of bleeding on the CAT scan. CAT is the diagnostic procedure of choice in assessing intracranial hemorrhage. It is extremely sensitive in detection of blood in very small amounts and is extremely useful in the differential diagnosis of hemorrhage versus infarction.

## Treatment

### *General Therapeutic Considerations*

The therapeutic approach to patients with cerebrovascular disease involves multiple phases, including preventative measures against stroke and vascular disease in general, supportive and medical management during the acute phase of a stroke, measures necessary to mitigate the pathologic or atherothrombotic process, and appropriate rehabilitative and physical therapy programs during the poststroke period.

Prevention of cerebrovascular disease is the most important aspect of therapeutic management, and elimination and/or management of the risk factors discussed earlier under Epidemiology and Etiology are required. Control of hypertension, hyperlipidemia, obesity, cigarette smoking, and tobacco use as well as other risk factors for atherothrombotic disease is essential to the overall care of the patient with cerebrovascular disease. In the patient with hypertension who has atherosclerotic cerebrovascular disease or who has developed an ischemic infarction, care must be taken to avoid drug-induced or other hypotensive episodes. In general, preservation of the systemic circulation in acute stroke and avoidance of orthostatic changes is also advised. The treatment goal should be normotension.

### *Specific Therapeutic Considerations*

As indicated earlier, the focus of this chapter is on ischemic stroke, and the following discussion emphasizes this condition; however, therapeutic management of some of the other types of cerebrovascular disease covered in this chapter is discussed briefly.

### *Ischemic Cerebrovascular Disease*

#### Anticoagulation Therapy

This mode of therapy was the first to gain acceptance in ischemic cerebrovascular disease, and because this therapy has been used for some time, some conclusions can be drawn about the usefulness of anticoagulation in various types of ischemic cerebrovascular disease. A number of studies have been made with heparin and coumarin derivatives over the past 25 years; however, criticisms of poor design, wrong diagnosis, and inadequate number of patients for comparative purposes have limited the acceptance of these studies.

The following is a brief review of anticoagulation therapy in TIA, progressing stroke, and completed stroke.

***Transient Ischemic Attacks*** Four randomized prospective studies (summarized in Table 18.8) comparing patients on anticoagulation therapy with control subjects showed no significant difference in the occurrence of stroke or death.[56] Only one of the four studies was double-blinded; all had small numbers of patients and three studies had short follow-up periods. Although weak, data from these studies indicate that the rate of recurrence of TIAs is reduced. Definite conclusions regarding anticoagulation cannot be stated on the basis of these studies. Six nonrandomized studies have been reported and no reduction was shown in mortality; however, one study did show a decreased incidence of TIAs and one showed a decrease in recurrence of TIAs. It appears from the literature that anticoagulation does not decrease mortality in TIA patients, but it may reduce the rate of recurrence of TIAs and subsequent ischemic infarction.[56]

***Progressing Stroke (Stroke-in-Evolution)*** Three randomized and three nonrandomized studies strongly suggest that

**Table 18.8** Randomized Trials of Anticoagulant Therapy in Transient Ischemic Attack

| *Study* | *No. of patients* | *Mean follow-up (mo)* | *TIA (%)* | *Stroke (%)* |
|---|---|---|---|---|
| Veterans Cooperative | | | | |
| Neurology 1961;11;132–134 | | | | |
| Control | 15 | 13 | 53 | 0 |
| Treated | 22 | 9 | 4.5 | 4.5 |
| Baker et al | | | | |
| Neurology 1966;16:841–847 | | | | |
| Control | 20 | 20 | 50[a] | 25 |
| Treated | 24 | 18 | 11[a] | 5.6 |
| Pearce et al | | | | |
| Lancet 1965;1:6–9 | | | | |
| Control | 20 | 11 | 45 | 10 |
| Treated | 17 | 11 | 59 | 5.9 |
| Baker et al | | | | |
| Neurology 1962;12:823–835 | | | | |
| Control | 30 | 41 | 46.7 | 13.3 |
| Treated | 30 | 38 | 33.3 | 6.7 |

[a] First month only.

From Quandt CM, Talbert RL, De los Reyes RA: Current concepts in clinical therapeutics: Ischemic cerebrovascular disease. Clin Pharm 1987;6:301, with permission.

anticoagulation is of benefit in this condition.[56] Although these studies are strongly suggestive, they are not conclusive because of flaws in study design. There were only slight differences in mortality in the treated groups (most patients were heparinized); however, there were favorable trends reported in the prevention of stroke progression. It appears that although conclusive statements cannot be made, if anticoagulants are of benefit, it would be in the acute phase of a progressing stroke.

***Completed Stroke*** Seven randomized studies have addressed anticoagulation therapy in completed stroke.[56] These studies showed no difference between treatment and control groups in the incidence of recurrent stroke or death. There is also a risk of major bleeding in patients treated for several months with anticoagulation therapy. Therefore, the risk of anticoagulation therapy in completed stroke outweighs any benefits obtained, and based on the best studies to date, anticoagulation generally should not be used.

The risk of hemorrhage is highest in patients with ischemic cerebrovascular disease when anticoagulation therapy lasts longer than 4 weeks. Compared with other indications for anticoagulation, anticoagulation for stroke is associated with a greater risk of hemorrhagic complications.[56,57] Although intensity of therapy and type of reagents used in laboratory testing were the source of some of the differences in European and North American studies, hemorrhagic complications are still the major risk in anticoagulated patients with ischemic cerebrovascular disease.

***Recommendations*** It is recommended that anticoagulation not be routinely used in patients with TIAs and not be used at all in patients with completed stroke.[58] The use of anticoagulation in progressing stroke is still controversial; however, individual judgment must be used in this situation when intracerebral hemorrhage has been ruled out by CAT scan. Short-term anticoagulation may be useful in TIA patients who refuse surgery for a surgically correctable lesion, who are not surgical candidates for whatever reason, or who are awaiting surgery. Patients who remain symptomatic with TIAs and on aspirin therapy who do not have surgical disease may be candidates for anticoagulation. If anticoagulation is used, careful monitoring is required and heparin should be administered acutely by continuous infusion to a target partial thromboplastin time of 1.5 times control value. If warfarin is to be used to continue chronic anticoagulation, it should overlap with heparin for approximately 5 days to obtain warfarin antithrombotic activity. By maintaining partial thromboplastin (using rabbit brain thromboplastin) and prothrombin times at 1.5 times control values, a slightly less intensive anticoagulation effect is obtained with a decreased incidence of bleeding without a decrease in efficacy.

### Antiplatelet Therapy

Antiplatelet agents have been studied for use in ischemic cerebrovascular disease for a number of years; the proposed mechanism of action is an alteration in blood platelet aggregation, thus inhibiting the formation of thrombi in arterial vessels. Several antiplatelet agents have been used; however, aspirin is the only agent with convincing clinical effects.

***Aspirin*** Aspirin (acetylsalicylic acid) was found in the early 1970s to prevent amaurosis fugax (monocular visual loss); subsequently, in a retrospective study, aspirin was

**Table 18.9** Randomized Trials of Aspirin in Cerebral Ischemia

| *Study*[a] | *No. of patients* | *Ischemic stroke (%)* | *Stroke or death (%)* |
|---|---|---|---|
| Canadian Cooperative N Engl J Med 1978;299: 53–59 | | | |
| All patients | | | |
| ASA 325 mg QID | 144 | 15.3 | 18.1 |
| Placebo | 139 | 14.4 | 21.6 |
| SP 200 mg QID | 146 | 18.6 | 24.4 |
| ASA + SP | 156 | 9.6 | 13.7 |
| Male patients | | | |
| ASA 325 mg QID | 98 | 14.3 | 17.4 |
| Placebo | 91 | 16.5 | 24.2 |
| SP 200 mg QID | 115 | 21.8 | 29.6 |
| ASA + SP | 102 | 5.9 | 11.8 |
| Fields et al Stroke 1977;8:301–314 | | | |
| ASA 325 mg QID | 88 | 4.6 | 6.8 |
| Placebo | 90 | 11.1 | 15.6 |
| Fields et al Stroke 1978;9:308–318 | | | |
| ASA 325 mg QID | 65 | 3.1 | 12.3 |
| Placebo | 60 | 13.3 | 13.3 |
| Bousser et al Stroke 1983;14:4–14 | | | |
| ASA 330 mg TID | 198 | 8.6 | 13.6 |
| Placebo | 204 | 15.2 | 17.7 |
| ASA 330 mg TID + DP 75 mg TID | 202 | 8.9 | 11.4 |
| Sorenson et al Stroke 1983;14:15–22 | | | |
| ASA 1,000 mg daily | 101 | 16.8 | 20.8 |
| Placebo | 102 | 10.8 | 16.7 |

[a] ASA, aspirin; SP, sulfinpyrazone; DP, dipyridamole.

Modified from Quandt CM, Talbert RL, De los Reyes RA. Current concepts in clinical therapeutics: Ischemic cerebrovascular disease. Clin Pharm 1987;6:300, with permission.

shown to decrease the number of TIAs without affecting the death rate.[59–61] The Aspirin in Transient Ischemic Attack Study was then initiated to study this potential beneficial effect on TIAs.[62] This multicenter study compared the use of 650 mg twice daily with placebo. Only patients with carotid system TIAs were enrolled in the study. In the analysis of the study, when deaths not caused by stroke were excluded, there was a significant difference in favor of the aspirin-treated group in preventing stroke. The study was small and short, and the definite conclusion that aspirin prevents stroke could not be made. The Canadian Cooperative Study Group was then formed and published its results in 1978.[63] This study involved treatment of 585 patients with one or more cerebral or retinal ischemic attacks. These patients were randomized to aspirin, sulfinpyrazone, and placebo. The average follow-up was 26 months and the aspirin dose was 325 mg four times daily and sulfinpyrazone 200 mg four times daily. For the overall study group, aspirin reduced the risk of TIA, stroke, or death by 19%. If only stroke or death was considered, aspirin reduced the risk of these by 31%. Interestingly, there was no significant benefit shown for women in this study.[64] Sulfinpyrazone did not show any risk reduction for TIA. Other randomized trials have been done and all show statistically significant differences between aspirin and placebo for some ischemic events.[62,63] Table 18.9 summarizes the randomized trials of aspirin. The doses of aspirin used in ischemic cerebrovascular disease studies have ranged from 1.0 to 1.5 g per day. The controversy now is over the appropriate dose of aspirin. Although low doses of aspirin (≤325 mg/d) have been shown to be effective in other conditions such as protection against myocardial infarction in unstable angina patients, prevention of coronary bypass shunt thrombosis, and prevention of thrombosis in arteriovenous shunts of chronic hemodialysis patients, the effectiveness of low doses in preventing stroke is just now being determined. The latest study to address the low-dose issue is the United Kingdom Transient Ischemic Attack/Aspirin Trial (UKTIA).[65] This is the first large study to evaluate low dose versus high dose (300 mg versus 1,200 mg per day). Between July 1979 and September 1985, 2,435 patients were enrolled in the study. All patients had experienced at least one TIA or mild ischemic stroke within 3 months of entry. The mean age was 60, and 75% of patients were male. Patients were randomly assigned to three groups. One group received 1,200 mg aspirin daily, the second group received 300 mg daily, and the third group received placebo. The dose ranges were selected somewhat arbitrarily, and patients were followed an average of 4 years. Preliminary results that have been reported indicate that the incidence of stroke, myocardial infarction, or sudden death was the same in both aspirin-treated groups and 20% lower (statistically significant) than the incidence in the placebo-treated groups. The risk of cerebral infarction alone was 11% higher in the placebo group, although this was not statistically significant. When women were considered separately in the study, no significant differences were found between aspirin and placebo in risk for cerebral infarction or other major vascular event. The investigators note, however, that the number of women in the study was small. Side effects were less frequent with the lower dose of aspirin (29%) as compared with the 1,200-mg dose (39%) and were least frequent in the placebo group (24%). Therefore, the lower dose of aspirin in this study was just as effective as the higher dose but had fewer side effects.

The antiplatelet effects of aspirin are theoretically responsible for aspirin's beneficial antithrombotic effects in TIAs. Aspirin inhibits platelet aggregation by irreversible inactivation of the enzyme cyclooxygenase which, in platelets, prevents conversion of arachidonic acid to thromboxane $A_2$ ($TXA_2$), which is a powerful vasoconstrictor and stimulator of platelet aggregation. Platelets remain impaired for their life span (5–7 days) after exposure to aspirin. Aspirin also inhibits prostacyclin activity in the smooth muscle of vascular walls. Prostacyclin ($PGI_2$) inhibits platelet aggregation, and the vascular endothelium can synthesize prostacyclin such that the platelet antiaggregating effect is maintained. The suppression of $PGI_2$ production by aspirin has been found to be dose and duration related; the higher the dose, the longer the cyclooxygenase production is suppressed. Therefore, the lower the aspirin dose, the less effect on prostacyclin. The optimal dose of aspirin is still under study, but it should be the dose that inhibits $TXA_2$ with the least amount of prostacyclin inhibition. It has been shown that an aspirin dose of 325 mg per day will inhibit $TXA_2$, but will not significantly inhibit $PGI_2$ production.[65] There is probably a point at which lower doses of aspirin do not completely block $TXA_2$, and recent studies indicate the lowest effective dose may be in the range 40–80 mg/d.[66,67] Other potential mechanisms of antithrombotic action of aspirin are currently under investigation.

Pharmacodynamically, as aspirin is converted to salicylate during the normal metabolic process, the ratio of salicylate to aspirin may be important as salicylate may prevent aspirin inhibition of $PGI_2$. Whether or not this proves to be clinically relevant remains to be shown in clinical studies. The interaction can be minimized by using low doses and sustained-release preparations.

***Dipyridamole*** This drug has weak inhibiting properties in vitro on platelet aggregation and it also inhibits platelet phosphodiesterase. Clinical studies have not yielded supportive data for the use of this drug in ischemic cerebrovascular disease.[68,69]

***Sulfinpyrazone*** This agent has been studied in several trials for ischemic cerebrovascular disease. Sulfinpyrazone, like aspirin, produces an inhibition of cyclooxygenase; however, this inhibition is reversible, whereas the aspirin inhibition is not. The drug has metabolites that also have inhibitory effects on cyclooxygenase. Clinical studies have found no beneficial effect for sulfinpyrazone in the treatment of ischemic cerebrovascular disease.[70]

***Recommendations*** Clinical trials have shown the beneficial effects of aspirin in men in prevention of secondary TIAs as well as in producing a decrease in major vascular events. The National Conference on Antithrombotic Therapy in 1986 recommended an aspirin dose of 1 g per day for patients with TIAs.[58] With the more recent evidence from the UK-TIA trial and other studies, a lower dose of aspirin is appropriate. A dose of 300 mg per day (5-grain tablet) is effective in preventing TIAs and stroke and results in a lower incidence of side effects. An enteric-coated product may be better tolerated by some individuals, and further study is needed to determine if this dosage form has therapeutic advantages.

**Surgical Therapy**

The purpose of surgery in ischemic cerebrovascular disease is to prevent the occurrence of cerebral infarctions and TIAs. Generally, the goal of a surgical procedure is to remove the source of occlusion and/or embolus and, hopefully, to increase cerebral blood flow to an ischemic area.

Carotid endarterectomy (CEA) is the most common surgical procedure used for occlusive cerebrovascular disease. This procedure has been popularized since its introduction over 30 years ago. CEA involves exposing the carotid artery in the neck and removing the occlusive atheromatous plaque usually at the carotid bifurcation. The indications have generally been considered to be TIAs and mild completed stroke in the presence of ulcerated or highly stenotic (>75%) plaque.[17] Other indications such as asymptomatic bruits and progressing stroke are controversial; however, there are few data to support the benefit of surgery in these patients.[71] CEA is not indicated in patients with permanent deficits from moderate to severe completed strokes. Although technique varies from institution to institution, the morbidity and mortality should be less than 5% to provide an acceptable risk-to-benefit ratio.[17] For patients with a complete occlusion of an extracranial vessel, CEA is usually unsuccessful, and these patients may be considered for an extracranial–intracranial (EC–IC) bypass procedure.[72] The most common EC–IC bypass procedure is anastomosis of the superficial temporal artery to a branch of the middle cerebral artery. This can augment blood flow to the brain by bypassing the stenotic or occluded artery. The clinical efficacy of this procedure has been disputed by a recent large international trial; however, a recent editorial review of that trial indicates that certain subsets of patients may benefit from this procedure.[73,74] In any event, further well-controlled studies are needed to clarify this point.

**Investigational Therapy**

Investigational therapy for prevention of TIAs and stroke includes thromboxane synthetase inhibitors, such as imidazole and dazoxiben, and ticlopidine, which has platelet antiaggregatory effects as well as other less clear mechanisms.[58,75] Therapy to improve or reverse the effects of an acute stroke includes prostacyclin and the calcium channel blocking agents nimodipine and nicardipine.[76–78] These agents are currently being tested in clinical trials. Another agent, naloxone, has been studied in ischemic cerebrovascular disease; however, controlled trials have failed to show beneficial effects and further study is required before the opiate antagonists can be recommended.

### *Cerebral Embolism of Cardiac Origin*

In patients with cardiogenic brain embolism, immediate anticoagulation should be considered as approximately 12% of such patients have a second embolic stroke within 2 weeks.[43] In nonhypertensive patients with small to moderate stroke, heparin should be given 24 hours after stroke onset without a loading dose so that a less intensive anticoagulation effect is obtained. The PTT should be no greater than 1.5 times the control value using rabbit brain thromboplastin. Before heparin is started, however, a CAT scan should document the absence of spontaneous hemorrhagic transformation. Anticoagulation should be maintained with warfarin at a prothrombin time of 1.5 times the control value. In patients who develop hemorrhagic transformation after embolic stroke, anticoagulation should be postponed 8 to 10 days.

The role of platelet antiaggregating agents in this situation is not clear. Obviously, prevention of the embolic event is the best therapy, and those patients at high risk for cardiogenic embolism, such as patients with atrial fibrillation or mechanical or prosthetic valves, should be treated with prophylactic chronic anticoagulation with warfarin.

### *Intracranial Hemorrhage*

General medical management and supportive therapy are indicated in the patient with this condition. This condition, as noted earlier, has a generally poor prognosis. Preventative therapy of intracranial bleeding is possible in the case of hypertension, where blood pressure can be controlled by diet and/or medication. Surgical management in the acute or early stage of the event is removal of the clot by aspiration or evacuation; this treatment is usually beneficial only in those patients whose hemorrhage is near the surface of the brain and who are not comatose. Cerebellar hemorrhage, on the other hand, is often amenable to surgery within the first 2 days of onset.

Corticosteroids and, more recently, dexamethasone have been used in the treatment of cerebral edema resulting from primary intracerebral hemorrhage. A recent study has shown no beneficial effect; in fact, a harmful effect (infection and diabetic complications) was seen.[79] Therefore, the use of dexamethasone in this condition should be reconsidered. The use of mannitol and other osmotic agents to reduce edema around the hemorrhage is appropriate, provided systemic hypotensive and hypertensive episodes are avoided. The use of mannitol is guided by maintaining the serum osmolality and arterial pressure. Generally, 125 mL of 20% mannitol can be administered every 4 hours until the serum osmolality is raised between 300 and 310 mosm per liter. Cerebral vasospasm in subarachnoid hemorrhage can be severe and therapeutic efforts to prevent or treat the vasospasm have been disappointing. Reserpine, kanamycin, isoproterenol, aminophylline, and nitroprusside have all failed in this condition. Recently, dopamine (3–6 $\mu$g/kg/min) has been used, but there is a risk of rebleeding. Barbiturate coma has been used to reduce intracranial pressure resulting from intracerebral hemorrhage when pressure reduction with dopamine or mannitol has not been successful. Further research is needed in the treatment of cerebral vasospasm and the resulting increased intracranial pressure.[80,81]

## References


1. Abbott RD, Yin Y, Reed DM, et al. Risk of stroke in male cigarette smokers. N Engl J Med 1986;315:717–720.
2. Kannel WB, Blaisdell FW, Gifford R, et al. Risk factors in stroke. Stroke 1971;2:423.
3. Gillum RF. Cerebrovascular disease morbidity in the United States, 1970–1983—Age, sex, region, and vascular surgery. Stroke 1986;17:656–661.
4. Garraway WM, Whisnant JP, Furlan AJ, et al. The declining incidence of stroke. N Engl J Med 1979;300:449.
5. Dyken ML, Wolf PA, Barnett HJM, et al. Risk factors in stroke—A statement for physicians by the Subcommittee on Risk Factors and Stroke of the Stroke Council. Stroke 1984;15: 1105–1111.
6. Kurtzke JF. Epidemiology of cerebrovascular disease, in Cerebrovascular Survey Report for Joint Council Subcommittee on Cerebrovascular Disease. National Institute of Neurological and Communicative Disorders and Stroke and National Heart and Lung Institute (revised). Rochester, Whiting Press, 1980, pp 135–176.
7. Anonymous. 1986 Stroke Facts. American Heart Association, Dallas, 1985.
8. Wolf PA, Kannel WB, Verter J. Current status of risk factors for stroke. Neurol Clin 1983;1:317.
9. Robins M, Baum HM. The National Survey of Stroke Incidence. Stroke 1981;12(supp 1):1–45.
10. Heyman A, Karp HR, Heyden S, et al. Cerebrovascular disease in the biracial population of Evans County, Georgia. Arch Intern Med 1971;128:949.
11. Schoenberg BS, Schoenberg DS, Pritchard DA, et al. Differential risk factors for completed stroke and transient ischemic attacks (TIA): Study of vascular diseases (hypertension, cardiac disease, peripheral vascular disease) and diabetes mellitus, in Duvoisin RC (ed): Transactions of the American Neurological Association. New York, Springer, 1980, vol 105, p 165.
12. Wolf PA. Hypertension as a risk factor for stroke, in Whisnant JP, Sandok B (eds): Cerebral Vascular Diseases. New York, Grune and Stratton, 1975, pp 105–112.
13. Kannel WB, Wolf PA, Verter J, et al. Epidemiologic assessment of the role of blood pressure in stroke: The Framingham study. JAMA 1970;214:301.
14. Hypertension Detection and Follow-up Program Cooperative Group. Five year findings of the Hypertension Detection and

Follow-up Program. III. Reduction in stroke incidence among persons with high blood pressure. JAMA 1982;247:633.
15. Kannell WB, Abbott RD, Savage DD, et al. Epidemiologic features of chronic atrial fibrillation: The Framingham study. N Engl J Med 1982;306:1018.
16. Weinfeld FD (ed): The National Survey of Stroke. Stroke 1981;12(suppl I):1–91.
17. Easton JD, Hart RG, Sherman DG, et al. Diagnosis and management of ischemic stroke. Part 1. Threatened stroke and its management. Curr Probl Cardiol 1983;8:1–80.
18. Tohgi J, Yamanouchi H, Murakami M, et al. Importance of the hematocrit as a risk factor in cerebral infarction. Stroke 1978;9: 369.
19. Thomas DJ, Marshall J, Russell RWR, et al. Effect of haematocrit on cerebral blood flow in man. Lancet 1977;2:941.
20. Portnoy BA, Herion JC. Neurological manifestations in sickle-cell disease, with a review of the literature and emphasis on the prevalence of hemiplegia. Ann Intern Med 1972;76:643.
21. Kannel WB, Gordon T, Wolf PA, et al. Hemoglobin and the risk of cerebral infarction: The Framingham study. Stroke 1972;3: 409.
22. Harrison MJG, Pollock S, Kendall BE, et al. Effect of haematocrit on carotid stenosis and cerebral infarction. Lancet 1981;2: 114.
23. Welin L, Svardsudd K, Wilhelmsen L, et al. Analysis of risk factors for stroke in a cohort of men born in 1913. N Engl J Med 1987;317:521–526.
24. Dyer AR, Stamler J, Paul O, et al. Serum cholesterol and risk of death from cancer and other causes in three Chicago epidemiological studies. J Chronic Dis 1981;34:249.
25. Mathew NT, Davis, Meyer JS, et al. Hyperlipoproteinemia in occlusive cerebrovascular disease. JAMA 1975;232:262.
26. Gill JS, Zezulka AV, Shipley MJ, et al. Stroke and alcohol consumption. N Engl J Med 1986;315:1042–1046.
27. Paffenbarger RS, Williams JL. Chronic disease in former college students. V. Early precursors of fatal stroke. Am J Public Health 1967;57:1290.
28. Grady PA. Pathophysiology of extracranial cerebral artery stenosis. A critical review. Stroke 1984;15:224–234.
29. Nerem RM. Arterial fluid dynamics and interactions with the vessel walls, in Schwartz CJ, Wertheisen NT, Wolf S (eds): Structure and Function of the Circulation. New York, Plenum, 1981, vol 2, pp 719–835.
30. Pessin MS, Hinton RC, Davis KR, et al. Mechanisms of acute carotid stroke. Ann Neurol 1979;5:152–157.
31. Gunning AJ, Pickering GW, Robb-Smith AHT, et al. Mural thrombosis of the carotid artery and subsequent embolism. Q J Med 1964;33:155–195.
32. Kistler JP, Ropper AH, Heros RC. Therapy of ischemic cerebral vascular disease due to atherothrombosis. N Engl J Med 1984;311:27–34.
33. DeWeese JA, May AG, Lipchick EO, et al. Anatomic and hemodynamic correlations in carotid artery stenosis. Stroke 1970;1:149–157.
34. Fisher M. Occlusion of the internal carotid artery. Arch Neurol Psychiatry 1951;65:346–377.
35. Tolle JF. Cerebrovascular Disorders, 3rd ed. New York, Raven, 1984:214–230.
36. Ames A, Wright RL, Kowada M, et al. Cerebral ischemia. II. The no-reflow phenomenon. Am J Pathol 1968;52:437–453.
37. Meyer FB, Sundt TM, Yanagihara T, et al. Focal cerebral ischemia: Pathophysiologic mechanisms and rationale for future avenues of treatment. Mayo Clin Proc 1987;62:35–55.
38. Sundt TM, Davis DH. Reactions of cerebrovascular smooth muscle to blood and ischemia: Primary versus secondary vasospasm, in Wilkins RH (ed): Cerebral Arterial Spasm. Baltimore, Williams and Wilkins, 1980, pp 244–250.
39. Sundt TM, Waltz AG. Cerebral ischemia and reactive hyperemia: Studies of cortical blood flow and microcirculation before, during, and after temporary occlusion of middle cerebral artery of squirrel monkeys. Circ Res 1971;28:426–433.
40. Matsumoto M, Hatakeyama T, Yanagihara T. Combination of cerebral blood flow measurement and immunohistochemical technique in cerebral ischemia. (Abstr) Stroke 1986;17:137.
41. Mohr JP. Lacunes. Stroke 1982;13:3–11.
42. Fisher CM. Capsular infarcts. The underlying vascular lesions. Arch Neurol 1979;36:65–73.
43. Sherman DG, Dyken ML, Fisher M, et al. Cerebral embolism. Chest 1986;89(supp 2):82S–98S.
44. Friedman GD, Loveland DB, Ehrlich SP. Relationship of stroke to other cardiovascular disease. Circulation 1968;38:533–541.
45. Wolf PA, Dawber TR, Thomas E, et al. Epidemiologic assessment of chronic atrial fibrillation and risk of stroke: The Framingham study. Neurology 1978;28:972–977.
46. Hinton RC, Kistler JP, Fallon JT, et al. Influence of etiology of atrial fibrillation on incidence of systemic embolism. Am J Cardiol 1977;40:509–513.
47. Bharucha NE, Wolf PA, Kannel WB, et al. Epidemiological study of cerebral embolism: The Framingham study. (Abstr) Ann Neurol 1981;10:105.
48. Bjerkelund CJ, Orning OM. The efficacy of anticoagulant therapy in preventing embolism related to D.C. electrical conversion of atrial fibrillation. Am J Cardiol 1969;23:208–216.
49. Chesebro JH, Ezekowitz M, Badimon L, et al. Intracardiac thrombi and systemic thromboembolism: Detection, incidence, and treatment. Ann Rev Med 1985;36:579–605.
50. Abernathy WS, Willis PW. Thromboembolic complications of rheumatic heart disease. Cardiovasc Clin 1973;5:131.
51. Askey JM, Berstein S. The management of rheumatic heart disease in relation to systemic arterial embolism. Prog Cardiovasc Dis 1960;3:220.
52. Fuster V, Pumphrey CW, McGoon MD, et al. Systemic thromboembolism in mitral and aortic Starr–Edwards prosthesis: A long term follow-up. Circulation 1982;66(suppl 1):1–157.
53. DeWitt LD. Clinical use of nuclear magnetic resonance imaging in stroke. Curr Concepts Cerebrovasc Dis (Stroke) 1985;20:25–29.
54. Ter-Pogossian MM, Raichle ME, Sobel BE. Positron emission tomography. Sci Am 1980;243:174.
55. Barnett HJM. Cerebrovascular disease, in Wyngarden JB, Smith LD (eds): Cecil Textbook of Medicine, 16th ed. Philadelphia, W. B. Saunders, 1982, pp 2066–2073.
56. Byers JA, Easton JD. Therapy of ischemic cerebrovascular disease. Ann Intern Med 1980;93:742–756.
57. Levine MN, Raskob G, Hirsh J. Risk of haemorrhage with long term anticoagulant therapy. Drugs 1985;30:444–460.
58. Dalen JE, Hirsh J. American College of Chest Physicians and the National Heart, Lung, and Blood Institute National Conference on Antithrombotic Therapy. Arch Intern Med 1986;146: 462–472.
59. Harrison MJG, Marshall J, Meadows JC, et al. Effect of aspirin in amaurosis fugax. Lancet 1971;2:743–745.
60. Mundall J, Quintero P, von Kaulla KN, et al. Transient monocular blindness and increased platelet aggregability treated with aspirin. Neurology 1972;22:280–285.
61. Dyken ML, Kolar OJ, Jones FH. Differences in the occurrence of carotid ischemic attack associated with antiplatelet aggregation therapy. Stroke 1973;4:732–736.
62. Fields WS, Lemak NA, Frankowski RF, et al. Controlled trial of aspirin in cerebral ischemia. Stroke 1977;8:301–306.

**63.** The Canadian Cooperative Study Group. A randomized trial of aspirin and sulfinpyrazone in threatened stroke. N Engl J Med 1978;299:53–59.

**64.** Kelton JG, Hirsh J, Carter CJ, et al. Sex differences in the antithrombotic effects of aspirin. Blood 1978;52:1073–1076.

**65.** Merz B. Multicenter study indicates one aspirin can do the job of four in preventing stroke. JAMA 1987;257:2134–2135.

**66.** Weksler BB, Tack-Goldman K, Subramanian A, et al. Cumulative inhibitory effect of low-dose aspirin on vascular prostacyclin and platelet thromboxane production in patients with atherosclerosis. Circulation 1985;71:332–340.

**67.** Merz B. Why a little aspirin is better than a lot. JAMA 1987;257: 2135.

**68.** Acheson J, Danta G, Hutchinson EC. Controlled trial of dipyridamole in cerebral vascular disease. Br J Med 1969;1:614–615.

**69.** The American–Canadian Cooperative Study Group. Persantine aspirin trial in cerebral ischemia. Part II. End point results. Stroke 1985;16:406–415.

**70.** Barnett HJM, Gent M, Sackett DL. The Canadian Cooperative Study Group: A randomized trial of aspirin and sulfinpyrazone in treated strokes. N Engl J Med 1978;299:53–59.

**71.** Chambers BR, Norris JW. Outcome in patients with asymptomatic bruits. N Engl J Med 1986;315:860–865.

**72.** Chater N, Popp AJ. Microsurgical vascular bypass for occlusive cerebrovascular disease: Current status, in Thompson RA, Green JR (eds): Advances in Neurology. 1977, vol 16, pp 121–132.

**73.** EC/IC Bypass Study Group. Failure of extracranial–intracranial arterial bypass to reduce the risk of ischemic stroke. Results of an international randomized trial. N Engl J Med 1985;313:1191–1200.

**74.** Reiman AS. The extracranial–intracranial arterial bypass study. What have we learned? N Engl J Med 1987;316:809–810.

**75.** Gordon JL. Overview: Pharmacology of ticlopidine. Agents Action 1984; (suppl 15:Quo Vadis?)108–115.

**76.** Huczynski J, Kostha-Trabka E, Sotowska W, et al. Double-blind controlled trial of the therapeutic effects of prostacyclin in patients with completed ischaemic stroke. Stroke 1985;16:810–814.

**77.** Philips JW, DeLong RE, Rowner JK. The effects of nifedipine and felodipine on cerebral blood flow during anoxic episodes. Stroke 1986;17:229–234.

**78.** Gelmers HS, Goetz FC, Sutherland DER, et al. A controlled trial of nimodipine in acute ischemic stroke. N Engl J Med 1988;318:203–207.

**79.** Poungvarin N, Bhoopat W, Viriyavejakul A, et al. Effects of dexamethasone in primary supratentorial intracerebral hemorrhage. N Engl J Med 1987;316:1229–1233.

**80.** Aitkenhead A. Cerebral protection. Br J Hosp Med 1986; 35:(May):290–297.

**81.** Cook DA. The pharmacology of cerebral vasospasm. Pharmacology 1984;29:1–16.

# Chapter 19 / Hyperlipidemia

Robert L. Talbert, PharmD

Cholesterol and triglycerides are transported in the bloodstream as lipoproteins.[1] Plasma lipoproteins are spherical particles with a surface that consists largely of phospholipid, free cholesterol, and protein, and a core that consists mostly of triglyceride and cholesterol ester (see Fig. 19.1). Abnormalities of plasma lipoproteins can result in a predisposition to coronary artery disease, pancreatitis, xanthomas, or neurologic disease. Evidence accumulated over the last three decades has linked elevated total and low-density-lipoprotein cholesterol (LDL-C) and reduced high-density-lipoprotein cholesterol (HDL-C) to the development of coronary heart disease. Premature coronary atherosclerosis, leading to the manifestations of ischemic heart disease (see Chapter 13), is the most common and significant consequence of hyperlipidemia.

## Epidemiology

Total cholesterol and LDL-C increase throughout life in men and women, representing an atherogenic pattern characteristic of Western society (see Fig. 19.2). Data from the Framingham study and other studies demonstrate that the risk for developing cardiovascular disease is related to the degree of cholesterol elevation in a graded, continuous fashion.[2,3] Hypercholesterolemia is additive to the other risk factors for coronary heart disease including cigarette smoking, hypertension, diabetes, and electrocardiographic abnormalities (see Fig. 19.3). Comparison of the United States with other countries has shown similar relationships for total cholesterol and LDL-C, and an inverse relationship for HDL-C, to coronary artery disease mortality (see Fig. 19.4). On a positive note, the U.S. mortality rate is midway among the countries studied and this country has had the greatest decline in coronary artery disease mortality (35%–40%) in men and women over the last 10 years compared with other countries.[4] LDL-C and the ratio of LDL-C/HDL-C have also been used to assess risk but their use adds little information to total cholesterol alone unless the HDL-C is abnormally high or low. HDL-C has been shown to be protective for the occurrence of coronary heart disease and an inverse relationship exists between coronary heart disease and HDL-C levels (see Fig. 19.5). Two fractions of HDL-C occur, $HDL_2$-C and $HDL_3$-C, and it is thought that $HDL_2$ is more important for prevention of cardiovascular disease. Elevated triglycerides may cause pancreatitis but their relationship to coronary heart disease is much weaker than that of cholesterol and most studies have not found a significant relationship between triglycerides and the prevalence of coronary heart disease.[5]

The prevalence of various types of lipid and lipoproteinemic disorders and other characteristics is listed in Table 19.1. The frequency of heterozygotes with familial hypercholesterolemia is minimally 1 in 500 and may be as common as 1 in 100 in some populations (white Afrikaaners in Johannesburg, South Africa), making this inherited disease one of the most common single-gene disorders affecting humans.[6]

## Lipoprotein Metabolism and Transport

Cholesterol and triglycerides, as the major plasma lipids, are essential substrates for cell membrane formation and provide a source of free fatty acids. Hyperlipidemia is defined as an elevation of one or more of the following: cholesterol, cholesterol esters, phospholipids, triglycerides.[7] Hyperlipoproteinemia describes an increased concentration of the lipoprotein macromolecules that transport lipids in the plasma. The density of plasma lipoproteins is determined by their relative content of protein and lipid; density, composition, and electrophoretic mobility have been used to divide lipoproteins into four classes (see Table 19.2). LDLs have been further divided into $LDL_1$, or intermediate-density lipoproteins (density, 1.006–1.019 g/mL), and $LDL_2$ (1.019–1.063 g/mL). $LDL_2$ is the major LDL component in plasma. HDLs have been subfractionated into $HDL_2$ (density, 1.063–1.125 g/mL) and $HDL_3$ (1.125–1.21 g/mL). Fluctuations in HDLs are usually due to alterations in the levels of $HDL_2$. The characteristics of the protein constitutents of lipoproteins, known as apolipoproteins, are listed in Table 19.3.

Chylomicrons, large triglyceride-rich particles, are formed from dietary fat solubilized by bile salts in intestinal mucosal cells. They are normally not present in the plasma after a fast of 12 to 14 hours and are catabolized by lipoprotein lipase (LPL) in vascular endothelium (activated by apolipoprotein C-11) and hepatic lipase (HL) to form chylomicron remnants (see Fig. 19.6). During the catabolism of nascent chylomicrons to remnants, triglyceride is converted to free fatty acids and apolipoprotein A-I, A-II, C-I, C-II, and C-III and phospholipids are transferred to HDLs. Apolipoprotein E and cholesteryl ester are transferred to chylomicrons from HDL. Chylomicron remnants are then taken up by the liver and bind to hepatic apolipoprotein B and E receptors. Hepatic very-low-density-lipoprotein (VLDL) synthesis is regulated in part by diet and hormones and is inhibited by uptake of chylomicron remnants in the liver. VLDL is catabolized by LPL and HL to form LDLs, and in the process, apolipoproteins C and E are transferred to HDLs. VLDL triglycerides are the major triglyceride carriers in plasma.

LDLs, the major cholesterol carrier, are derived mostly

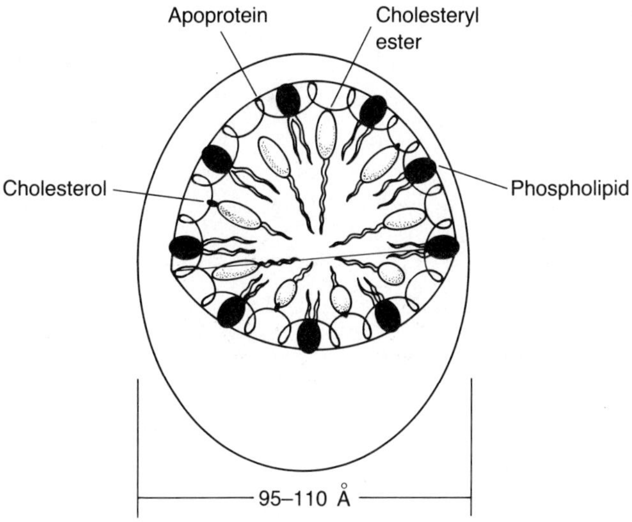


**Figure 19.1** Schematic of a high-density-lipoprotein particle. The protein is represented as having a helical structure and forming the outer 110-Å shell of the particle. The polar head groups of phospholipids are shown interacting with the helices of the protein. Cholesteryl esters are drawn such that the cholesterol moiety interacts with the fatty acyl chains of the phospholipids. *(From Jackson RL, Morrisett JD, Gotto AM, Jr: Lipoprotein structure and metabolism. Physiol Rev 1976;56:276, with permission.)*

from VLDL catabolism but in patients with homozygous familial hypercholesterolemia, direct synthesis may occur. LDLs are catabolized through interaction of cell surface receptors, internalization and degradation, and receptor-independent mechanisms (see Fig. 19.7). Increased intracellular cholesterol resulting from LDL catabolism inhibits the activity of 3-hydroxy-3-methylglutaryl coenzyme A reductase (HMG-CoA reductase), the rate-limiting enzyme for intracellular cholesterol biosynthesis (see Fig. 19.8).

**Figure 19.2** Mean plasma concentrations of total, low-density-lipoprotein (LDL), and high-density-lipoprotein (HDL) cholesterol by age and sex for whites (Lipid Research Clinics random sample). *(From Tyroler HA: An overview of Lipid Research Clinics (LRC) epidemiologic studies as background for the LRC Coronary Primary Prevention Trial. Am J Cardiol 1984;54:15C, with permission.)*

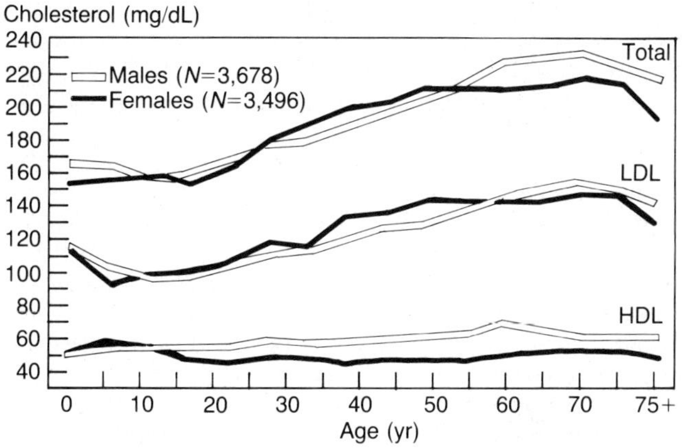


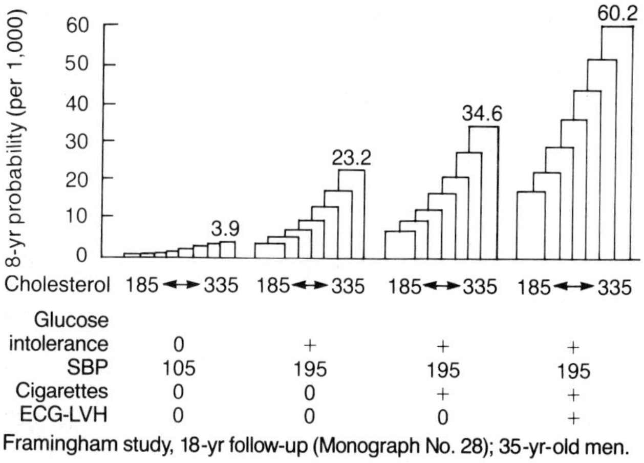


**Figure 19.3** Risk of cardiovascular disease according to serum cholesterol at specified levels of other risk factors. ECG-LVH, electrocardiographic evidence of left ventricular hypertrophy; SBP, systolic blood pressure. *(From Kannel WB. High-density lipoproteins: Epidemiologic profile and risks of coronary artery disease. Am J Cardiol 1983;52:10B.)*

HDLs are derived from liver and gut synthesis as well as from chylomicron and VLDL catabolism. HDLs accept cholesterol from tissue and are the substrate for lecithin:cholesterol acyltransferase (LCAT), which catalyzes the conversion of free cholesterol and lecithin to cholesterol ester and lysolecithin, respectively. Apolipoprotein A-1 is one of the major lipoprotein components of HDLs and its production is increased by estrogens, leading to higher HDL levels in women and in individuals receiving estrogen. These processes serve to rid peripheral tissue (e.g., coronary arteries) of excessive amounts of cholesterol; thus, the protective effect noted with increasing HDL levels is increased by estrogens and so is higher in women than men. Several excellent reviews of lipoprotein metabolism are available for further review.[1,7–9]

Early work by Fredrickson et al helped define hyperlipoproteinemia in terms of specific lipoprotein and apoprotein disorders and establish some of the inheritance traits of these disorders.[10] They classified abnormal lipoprotein disorders into six categories; this scheme, shown in Table 19.4, is still commonly used today for the phenotypical description of hyperlipidemia. More recently, it has become apparent that specific genetic defects with disrupted protein, cell, and organ function give rise to several disorders within each family of lipoproteins (Tables 19.1 and 19.5). In other words, an elevated cholesterol does not necessarily equate to familial hypercholesterolemia or type IIa, as cholesterol may also be elevated in other lipoprotein disorders and the lipoprotein pattern does not describe the underlying genetic defect. The preceding discussion has focused on primary or genetic hyperlipoproteinemia and it should be remembered that secondary forms exist and several drugs may also elevate lipid levels (Table 19.6). These secondary forms of hyperlipidemia should be initially managed by correcting the under-

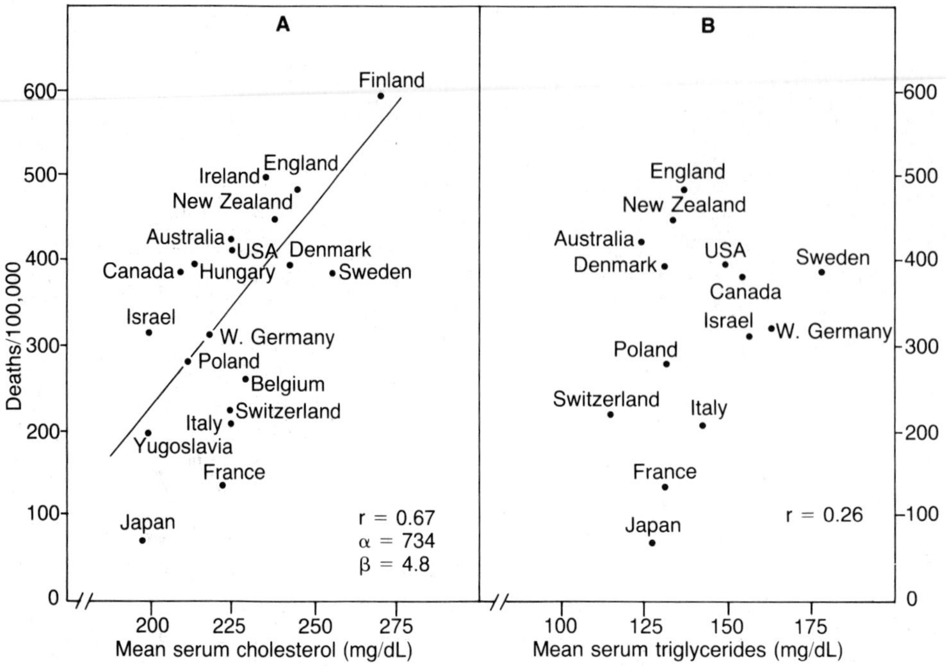


**Figure 19.4** Coronary artery disease mortality rate versus serum cholesterol (A) and triglyceride concentrations (B) in men. NS, not significant; $\alpha$, intercept; $\beta$, slope. *(From Simons L.A.: Interrelations of lipids and lipoproteins with coronary artery disease mortality in 19 countries. Am J Cardiol 1986;57:8G, with permission.)*

lying abnormality, including modification of drug therapy when appropriate.

Familial hypercholesterolemia is the best understood of the primary hyperlipoproteinemia disorders and this stems from the Nobel prize–winning work of Goldstein and Brown in their characterization of LDL receptor (LDL-R) function and importance.[11,12] This receptor is characterized by (1) a selective elevation in the plasma level of LDL; (2) deposition of LDL-derived cholesterol in tendons (xanthomas) and arteries (atheromas); and (3) inheritance as an autosomal dominant trait, with homozygotes more severely affected than heterozygotes. Homozygotes (prevalence 1 in 1,000,000) have severe hypercholesterolemia (650–1,000 mg/dL), with the early appearance of cutaneous xanthomas and fatal coronary heart disease generally before the age of 20. The primary defect in familial hypercholesterolemia is the inability to bind LDL to the LDL-R or, rarely, a defect of internalizing the LDL-R complex into the cell after normal binding. This leads to lack of LDL degradation by cells and unregulated biosynthesis of cholesterol, with total cholesterol and LDL-C being inversely proportional to the deficit in LDL receptors. Heterozygotes have only about one half of the normal number of LDL receptors while homozygotes have essentially no functional LDL receptors. This is illustrated in Figure 19.9, which relates the number of receptors to the fractional catabolic rate for LDL.

**Figure 19.5** Incidence of coronary heart disease by high-density-lipoprotein (HDL) cholesterol level. Framingham study, exam 11; men and women 50–79 years old. Trends significant at $P < 0.01$. *(From Kannel WB: Am J Cardiol 1983;52:10B, with permission.)*

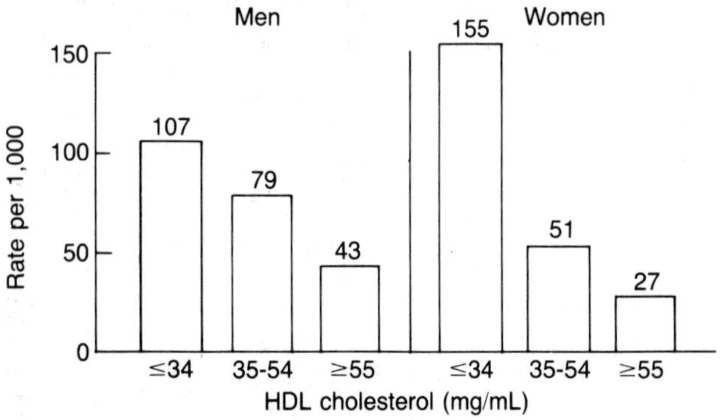


Familial lipoprotein lipase deficiency is characterized by massive accumulation of chylomicrons and a corresponding increase in plasma triglycerides, or a type I lipoprotein pattern. VLDL concentration is normal. The presenting manifestations include repeated attacks of pancreatitis and abdominal pain, eruptive cutaneous xanthomatosis, and hepatosplenomegaly beginning in childhood. Symptom severity is proportional to dietary fat intake and, consequently, to the elevation of chylomicrons. LPL is normally released from vascular endothelium or by heparin and hydrolyzes chylomicrons and VLDL (Fig. 19.6). Diagnosis is based on low or absent enzyme activity with normal human plasma or apolipoprotein C-II, a cofactor of the enzyme. Accelerated atherosclerosis is not associated with this disease. Type V (VLDL + chylomicrons) is characterized by abdominal pain, pancreatitis, eruptive xanthomas, and peripheral poly-

**Table 19.1** Disorders of Lipoprotein and Lipid Metabolism

| *Name of disease* | *Prevalence* | *Mode of inheritance* | *Mutant gene product* | *Chromo-somal location* | *Expression* | | |
|---|---|---|---|---|---|---|---|
| | | | | | **Altered DNA structure** | **Disturbed protein function** | **Disrupted cell and organ function** |
| Abetalipopro-teinemia | ~50 cases reported | Autosomal recessive | Unknown | Unknown | Unknown | Unknown | Lack of synthesis and/or secretion of apoprotein B prevent formation of chylomicrons, VLDL, and LDL. This leads to decreased vitamin E transport, which in turn causes neurologic and retinal abnormalities. Heterozygotes have normal plasma levels of apoprotein B |
| Familial hypo-betalipopro-teinemia | 7 cases reported | Autosomal recessive | Unknown | Unknown | Unknown | Unknown | Homozygotes have a syndrome similar to abetalipoproteinemia. Heterozygotes have one half of the normal levels of apoprotein B in plasma and are asymptomatic. |
| Tangier disease | 26 cases reported | Autosomal recessive | Unknown | Unknown | Unknown | Unknown | Decreased synthesis and increased catabolism of the apoprotein components (ApoA-I and ApoA-II) of HDL. As a result, HDL is absent from plasma and other lipoproteins are abnormal. Cholesteryl esters accumulate in reticuloendothelial cells, causing tonsillar enlargement, splenomegaly, and neuropathy. |
| Familial lipoprotein lipase deficiency | ~100 cases reported | Autosomal recessive | Lipoprotein lipase | Unknown | Unknown | Absent enzyme activity | Accumulation of substrate (chylomicrons) in plasma produces hypertriglyceridemia, pancreatitis, and eruptive xanthomas of skin. |

**Table 19.1** Disorders of Lipoprotein and Lipid Metabolism (continued)

| *Name of disease* | *Prevalence* | *Mode of inheritance* | *Mutant gene product* | *Chromosomal location* | *Expression* | | |
|---|---|---|---|---|---|---|---|
| | | | | | **Altered DNA structure** | **Disturbed protein function** | **Disrupted cell and organ function** |
| Apolipoprotein C-II deficiency | ~25 cases reported | Autosomal recessive | Apolipoprotein C-II (activator of lipoprotein lipase) | Unknown | Unknown | Decreased enzyme activity (lipoprotein lipase) caused by absence of activator | Accumulation of chylomicrons and VLDL in plasma produces hypertriglyceridemia, pancreatitis, and eruptive xanthomas of skin. |
| Familial type 5 hyperlipoproteinemia | Uncommon, but not rare | Autosomal dominant | Unknown | Unknown | Unknown | Unknown | Accumulation of chylomicrons and VLDL in plasma produces hypertriglyceridemia, pancreatitis, and eruptive xanthomas of skin. |
| Familial lecithin:cholesterol acyltransferase (LCAT) deficiency | 26 cases reported | Autosomal recessive | Plasma LCAT | 16 (long arm) | Unknown | Absent enzyme activity | Accumulation of substrate (free cholesterol) in plasma and tissues leads to anemia, cataracts, proteinuria, and renal failure. |
| Familial type 3 hyperlipoproteinemia (dysbetalipoproteinemia) | ~1 per 10,000 | Susceptibility inherited as autosomal recessive trait; expression requires other genetic or environmental factors | Apoprotein $E^D$ | Unknown | Missense mutation (arginine → cysteine) | Abnormal protein structure | Deficient binding of apoprotein $E^D$ to hepatic lipoprotein receptors causes plasma accumulation of chylomicron and VLDL remnants. Hyperlipidemia and atherosclerosis result. |
| Familial hypercholesterolemia, three allelic types | Receptor-negative type: ~1 per 1,000,000. Receptor-deficient type: ~1 per 500. Internalization type: rare | Autosomal dominant | LDL receptor | Unknown | Unknown | Absent or defective receptor activity (homozygotes); half-normal receptor activity (heterozygotes) | Deficient receptor-mediated endocytosis causes LDL to accumulate in plasma and prevents body cells from using cholesterol. Hypercholesterolemia and atherosclerosis result. |

| | | | | | | | |
|---|---|---|---|---|---|---|---|
| Cerebrotendinous xanthomatosis | 53 cases reported | Autosomal recessive | Hepatic sterol hydroxylase [(?) 24-hydroxylase or 26-hydroxylase)] | Unknown | Unknown | Deficient enzyme activity | Reduced synthesis of cholic and chenodeoxycholic acids secondary to hydroxylase deficiency leads to compensatory increase in synthesis of cholesterol and cholestanol, which deposit in tissues. |
| Sitosterolemia with xanthomatosis | 16 cases reported | Autosomal recessive | Unknown | Unknown | Unknown | Unknown | Increased intestinal absorption and decreased excretion of plant sterols (sitosterol and campesterol) and cholesterol lead to sterol deposition in tissues. |
| Phytanic acid storage disease (Refsum's disease) | ~100 cases reported | Autosomal recessive | Phytanic acid $\alpha$-hydroxylase | Unknown | Unknown | Absent enzyme activity | Accumulation of substrate (phytanic acid) causes retinitis pigmentosa, ataxia, and peripheral neuropathy. |

From Stanbury JB, Wyngaaren JB, Fredrickson DS, Goldstein JL, Brown MS (Eds): Introduction, in The Metabolic Basis of Inherited Disease, 5th ed. New York, McGraw–Hill, 1983, pp 46–47, with permission.

**Table 19.2** Composition of Lipoprotein Isolated From Normal Subjects

| Lipoprotein class[a] | Density range (g/mL) | Electrophoretic mobility | Composition (wt %) Protein | Triglyceride | Cholesterol Free | Cholesterol Ester | Phospholipid |
|---|---|---|---|---|---|---|---|
| Chylomicrons | <0.94 | Origin | 1–2 | 85–95 | 1–3 | 2–4 | 3–6 |
| VLDL | 0.94–1.006 | Prebeta | 6–10 | 50–65 | 4–8 | 16–22 | 15–20 |
| LDL | 1.006–1.063 | Beta | 18–22 | 4–8 | 6–8 | 45–50 | 18–24 |
| HDL | 1.063–1.21 | Alpha | 45–55 | 2–7 | 3–5 | 15–20 | 26–32 |

[a] VLDL, very-low-density lipoprotein; LDL, low-density lipoprotein; HDL, high-density lipoprotein.

From Schaefer EJ, Levy RI: Pathogenesis and managment of lipoprotein disorders. N Engl J Med 1985;312:1301, with permission.

neuropathy. Symptoms may occur in childhood but usually the disorder is expressed at a later age. The risk of atherosclerosis is increased with this disorder. These patients are commonly obese, hyperuricemic, and diabetic; alcohol intake, exogenous estrogens, and renal insufficiency tend to be exacerbating factors.[1,13]

Patients with familial type III hyperlipoproteinemia (also called dysbetalipoproteinemia or beta VLDL) develop the following clinical features after age 20: xanthoma striata palmaris (yellow discolorations of the palmar and digital creases); tuberous or tuberoeruptive xanthomas (bulbous cutaneous xanthomas); severe atherosclerosis involving the coronary arteries, internal carotids, and abdominal aorta. A defective structure of apoliproprotein E does not allow normal hepatic surface receptor binding of remnant particles derived from chylomicrons and VLDL. Although homozygosity for the defective allele is common (1 in 100), only 1 in 10,000 express the full-blown picture, and interaction with other genetic or environmental factors or both is needed to produce clinical disease.[14]

Type IV hyperlipoproteinemia is common and occurs in adulthood, primarily in patients who are obese, diabetic, and hyperuricemic and do not have xanthomas. It may be secondary to alcohol ingestion and can be aggravated by stress, estrogens, oral contraceptives, thiazides, or $\beta$-blockers. Two genetic patterns occur in type IV hyperlipo-

**Table 19.3** Characteristics and Functions of Apolipoproteins[a]

| Apolipoprotein | Lipoprotein density class | Approximate plasma concentration (mg/dL) | Approximate molecular weight | Reported functions |
|---|---|---|---|---|
| A-I | Chylomicrons, HDL | 120 | 28,300 | Cofactor with LCAT, structural role in HDL |
| A-II | Chylomicrons, HDL | 35 | 17,400 | Cofactor with HL, structural role in HDL |
| A-IV | Chylomicrons, 1.21B | 15 | 46,000 | ? |
| ApoLp (a) | LDL, HDL | 10 | 900,000 | ? |
| B-100 | VLDL, LDL | 100 | 250,000 | Binding protein–cell receptor, structural role in VLDL and LDL |
| B-48 | Chylomicrons | Trace | 120,000 | Structural role in chylomicrons |
| C-I | Chylomicrons, VLDL, HDL | 7 | 6,300 | Cofactor with LCAT |
| C-II | Chylomicrons, VLDL, HDL | 4 | 8,800 | Cofactor with LPL |
| C-III | Chylomicrons, VLDL, HDL | 13 | 8,800 | Inhibitor with LPL chylomicron remnant uptake |
| D | HDL | 6 | 32,500 | ? |
| E2–E4 | Chylomicrons, VLDL, HDL | 5 | 37,000 | Binding protein–cell receptor |
| F | HDL | 2 | 30,000 | ? |
| G | HDL | — | 72,000 | ? |
| H | Chylomicrons, 1.21B | 10 | 43,000 | Cofactor with LPL |

[a] LCAT, lecithin:cholesterol acyltransferase; HL, hepatic lipase; LP, lipoprotein lipase. 1.21B refers to 1.21 g/mL per milliliter of infranate or lipoprotein-free fraction. Other abbreviations are explained in Table 19.2.

From Schaefer EJ, Levy RI: Pathogenesis and management of lipoprotein disorders. N Engl J Med 1985;312:1301, with permission.

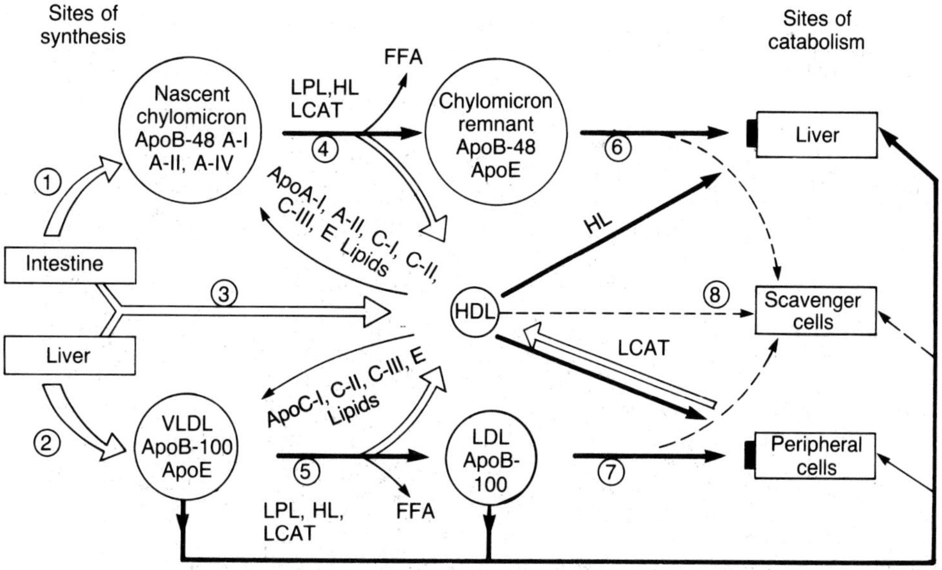


**Figure 19.6** A conceptual overview of lipoprotein metabolism. LPL, lipoprotein lipase; HL, hepatic lipase; LCAT, lecithin:cholesterol acytransferase; Apo, apolipoprotein; FFA, free fatty acid; HDL, high-density lipoprotein; LDL, low-density lipoprotein; VLDL, very-low-density lipoprotein. Open arrows, synthetic pathways; closed arrows, catabolic pathways. *(From Schaefer EJ, Levy RI: Pathogenesis and management of lipoprotein disorders. N Engl J Med 1985;312:1302, with permission.)*

**Figure 19.7** Sequential steps in the LDL receptor pathway in cultured mammalian cells. HMG-CoA reductase, 3-hydroxy-3-methylglutaryl coenzyme A reductase; ACAT, acyl coenzyme-A:cholesterol acyltransferase. *(From Stanbury JB, Wyngaarden JB, Fredrickson DS, Goldstein JL, Brown MS (Eds): The Metabolic Basis of Inherited Disease, 5th ed. New York, McGraw–Hill, 1983, p 687, with permission.)*

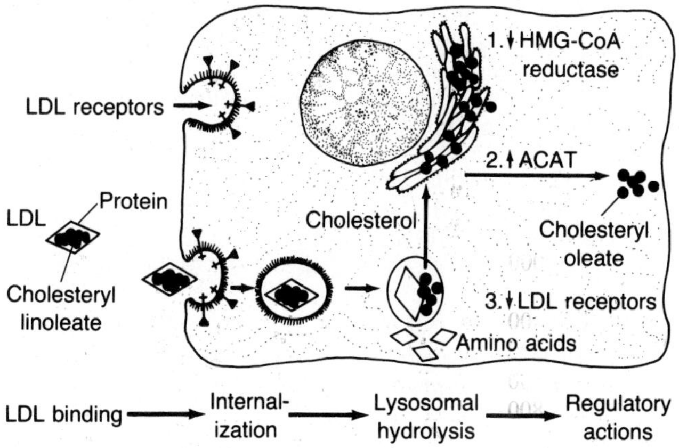


**Figure 19.8** Biosynthetic pathway for cholesterol. The rate limiting enzyme in this pathway is 3-hydroxy-3-methylglutaryl coenzyme A reductase (HMG-CoA reductase).

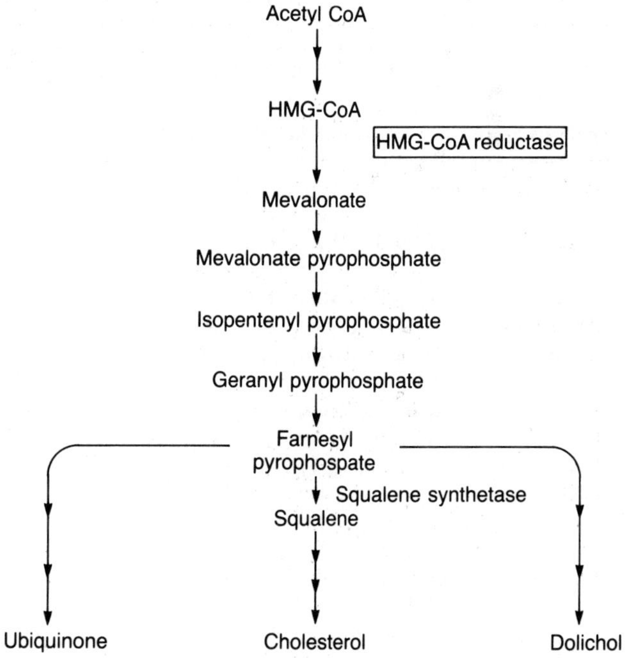

**Table 19.4** Fredrickson–Levy–Lees Classification of Hyperlipoproteinemia

| | | *Approximate mean lipid elevation*[1,11] | |
|---|---|---|---|
| *Type* | *Lipoprotein Elevation* | **Cholesterol (mg/dL)** | **Triglycerides (mg/dL)** |
| I | Chylomicrons | 324 | 3,316 |
| IIa | LDL[a] | 368 | 148 |
| IIb | LDL + VLDL | 354 | 135 |
| III | LDL ($LDL_1$) | 441 | 694 |
| IV | VLDL | 251 | 438 |
| V | VLDL + chylomicrons | 373 | 2,071 |

[a] Heterozygotes for familial hypercholesterolemia.

proteinemia: familial hypertriglyceridemia, which does not carry a great risk for premature coronary artery disease, and familial combined hyperlipidemia, which is associated with increased risk of cardiovascular disease.

Rare forms of lipoprotein disorders may include abnormal LDL or deficiencies in chylomicrons, VLDL, LDL, and HDL (Tables 19.1 and 19.5). The disturbed protein function in these diseases is not usually known and the consequences are given in Table 19.1. Most of these rare lipoprotein disorders do not result in premature atherosclerosis, except for familial lecithin:cholesterol acyltransferase (LCAT) deficiency, cerebrotendinous xanthomatosis (CTX), and sitosterolemia with xanthomatosis. Their treatment consists of dietary restriction of plant sterols (sitosterolemia with xanthomatosis), chenodeoxycholic acid (CTX), or, potentially, blood transfusion (LCAT deficiency).

## Patient Evaluation

Once hyperlipidemia is suspected, two major components of the evaluation are the history/physical examination and the laboratory investigations. A complete history and physical exam should assess the following: presence or absence of cardiovascular risk factors, e.g., smoking, hypertension, diabetes, and obesity; existence of family history of lipid disorders; presence or absence of secondary causes of hyperlipidemia (Table 19.6); presence or absence of xanthomas, abdominal pain or history of pancreatitis, renal or liver disease, or vascular disease.

Measurement of plasma cholesterol, triglyceride, and HDL-C levels after a 12-hour or longer fast is important, as triglycerides may be elevated in nonfasted individuals. Two determinations with the patient on a stable diet and weight and in the absence of acute illness are needed to obtain a reliable baseline.[15] If the physical examination and history are insufficient to diagnose a familial disorder, then agarose-gel lipoprotein electrophoresis is useful in determining which class of lipoproteins is affected.[1,10] If the triglyceride levels are below 400 mg/dL and neither type III hyperlipidemia nor chylomicrons are detected by electrophoresis, then one can calculate VLDL and LDL cholesterol concentrations: VLDL-C = triglyceride/5; LDL-C = total cholesterol − (VLDL-C + HDL-C).

Because total cholesterol is comprised of cholesterol derived from LDL, VLDL, and HDL, determination of HDL-C is useful when total plasma cholesterol is elevated. HDL-C concentration and the ratio of LDL-C/HDL-C can be used to assess the degree of risk and necessity of treatment in patients with elevated total cholesterol.[16] Strong evidence supports an inverse correlation with HDL-C concentration and the risk of coronary artery disease.[5,17] HDL-C may be elevated by moderate alcohol ingestion (less than 2 drinks per day), physical exercise, smoking cessation, weight loss, oral contraceptives, phenytoin, and terbutaline. Of these, only exercise and smoking cessation could be recommended as interventions for hyperlipoproteinemia.

Plasma cholesterol values are about 3% lower than serum values, but more importantly, large interlaboratory and intralaboratory differences have been described for the determination of cholesterol, HDL, and lipoprotein electrophoresis results.[15] Familarity with the method employed by local laboratories is useful for interpretation of reported values. The normal range of lipid concentrations represents a population mean plus or minus two standard deviations and does not define the risk of disease. Currently, blood cholesterol levels exceeding 200 mg/dL for men and women aged 20–29 years place these individuals at moderate risk for coronary heart disease, and greater than 220 mg/dL is considered to be high risk.[16] Reference values for plasma cholesterol and triglyceride concentrations from the Lipid Research Clinics Program are given in Table 19.7.[18]

## Treatment

### *Recommendations*

Based on a careful review of the genetic, experimental pathologic, and epidemiologic evidence relating to the relationship between blood cholesterol levels and coronary heart disease, the Consensus Conference convened by the NIH has made the following recommendations concerning the treatment of hypercholesterolemia:

1. Individuals with high-risk blood cholesterol levels (>90th percentile) should be placed on intensive dietary intervention and, if the response is inadequate, appropriate drugs should be added to the treatment regimen.
2. Adults with moderate-risk blood cholesterol levels (75th–90th percentiles) should be intensively treated with dietary means, especially if additional risk factors are present; only a small proportion should require drug treatment.
3. All Americans (except children less than 2 years of age) should alter their diet to contain no more than 30% total calories as fat, reduce saturated fat to less than 10% of total calories, and reduce total daily cholesterol intake to 250–300 mg or less.
4. Maintain ideal body weight and correct obesity by calorie restriction.
5. Special attention should be given to individuals with hypercholesterolemia and concurrent risk factors.

**Table 19.5** Lipoprotein Disorders

| *Increased chylomicrons (type I and V HLP)*[a] | *Increased VLDL (type IV HLP)* | *Increased beta VLDL (type III HLP)* | *Increased LDL (type II HLP)* | *Abnormal LDL* | *Chylomicron, VLDL, and LDL deficiency* | *HDL deficiency* |
|---|---|---|---|---|---|---|
| Familial hypertriglyceridemia[b] | Familial hypertriglyceridemia[b] | Apolipoprotein E2 phenotype[c] | Familial hypercholesterolemia[d] | Betasitosterolemia[b] | Abetalipoproteinemia[e] | Hypoalphalipoproteinemia[b] |
| Familial combined hyperlipidemia[b] | Familial combined hyperlipidemia[b] | Apolipoprotein E variants[c] | Familial combined hyperlipidemia[b] | Hyperapobetalipoproteinemia[b] | Hypobetalipoproteinemia[e] | Apolipoprotein A-I variants[c] |
| Lipoprotein lipase deficiency[f] | Apolipoprotein C-III DNA polymorphism[c] | Apolipoprotein E deficiency[e] | | Cerebrotendinous xanthomatosis[f] | Normotriglyceridemic abetalipoproteinemia[e] | Tangier disease[c] |
| Lipoprotein lipase inhibitor[f] | | Hepatic lipase deficiency[f] | | | | HDL deficiency with planar xanthomas[b] |
| Apolipoprotein C-II deficiency[e] | | | | | | Apolipoprotein A-I and C-III deficiency[e] |
| Abnormal apolipoprotein C-III sialylation[c] | | | | | | LCAT deficiency[f] |
| Apolipoprotein E4 phenotype[c] | | | | | | Fish eye disease[b] |

[a] HLP, hyperlipoproteinemia. Other abbreviations are explained in Tables 19.2 and 19.3.
[b] Unknown defect.
[c] Apolipoprotein abnormality.
[d] Receptor abnormality.
[e] Apolipoprotein deficiency.
[f] Enzyme abnormality.

From Schaefer EJ, Levy RI: Pathogenesis and management of lipoprotein disorders. N Engl J Med 1985;312:1305, with permission.

**Table 19.6** Secondary Forms of Hyperlipoproteinemia

| *Disease induced* | *Drug induced* |
|---|---|
| **Endocrine/metabolic** | Alcohol |
| Diabetes mellitus | Progestins |
| von Gierke's disease | Thiazide diuretics |
| Lipodystrophies | β-Blockers |
| Cushing's syndrome | Glucocorticoids |
| Sexual ateliotic dwarfism | |
| Acromegaly | |
| Hypothyroidism | |
| Anorexia nervosa | |
| Werner's syndrome | |
| Acute intermittent porphyria | |
| **Renal** | |
| Uremia | |
| Nephrotic syndrome | |
| **Hepatic** | |
| Primary biliary cirrhosis | |
| Acute hepatitis | |
| Hepatoma | |
| **Immunologic** | |
| Systemic lupus erythematosus | |
| Monoclonal gammapathies | |
| **Stress induced** | |

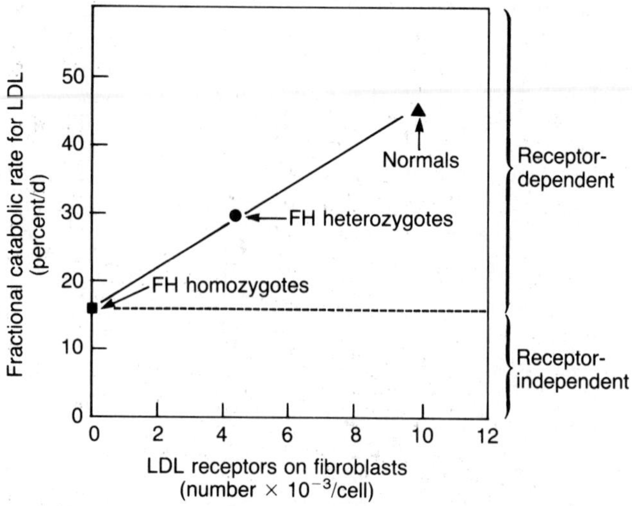


**Figure 19.9** Relation between the fractional catabolic rate (FCR) for plasma LDL and the number of LDL receptors on fibroblasts in patients with familial hypercholesterolemia (FH). The values for the fractional catabolic rate were derived from studies of the turnover of $^{125}$I-labeled apo-LDL in the plasma of 6 normal subjects, 6 FH heterozygotes, and 11 FH homozygotes. The number of LDL receptors per cell was calculated from experiments in which maximal $^{125}$I-labeled LDL binding was measured at 4°C in actively growing fibroblasts deprived of LDL for 48 h. *(From Stanbury JB, Wyngaarden JB, Fredrickson DS, Goldstein JL, Brown MS (Eds): The Metabolic Basis of Inherited Disease, 5th ed. New York, McGraw–Hill, 1983, p 687, with permission.)*

**Table 19.7** Reference Values for Plasma Cholesterol and Triglyceride Concentrations (mg/dL)

| | *Cholesterol* | | | *Triglyceride* | |
|---|---|---|---|---|---|
| *Age (yr)* | **50th percentile** | **75th percentile** | **90th percentile** | **50th percentile** | **95th percentile** |
| Men | | | | | |
| <20 | 155 | 170 | 185 | <80 | <150 |
| 20–24 | 165 | 185 | 205 | 100 | 200 |
| 25–29 | 180 | 200 | 225 | 115 | 250 |
| 30–34 | 190 | 215 | 240 | 130 | 265 |
| 35–39 | 200 | 225 | 250 | 145 | 320 |
| 40–44 | 205 | 230 | 250 | 150 | 320 |
| 45–69 | 215 | 235 | 260 | 140 | 290 |
| >70 | 205 | 230 | 250 | 135 | 260 |
| Women | | | | | |
| <20 | 160 | 175 | 190 | <75 | <130 |
| 20–24 | 170 | 190 | 215 | 90 | 170 |
| 25–34 | 175 | 195 | 220 | 90 | 170 |
| 35–39 | 185 | 205 | 230 | 95 | 195 |
| 40–44 | 195 | 215 | 235 | 105 | 210 |
| 45–49 | 205 | 225 | 250 | 110 | 230 |
| 50–54 | 220 | 240 | 265 | 120 | 240 |
| ≥55 | 230 | 250 | 275 | 125 | 250 |

From Rifkind BM, Segal P: Lipid Research Clinics Program reference values for hyperlipidemia and hypolipidemia. JAMA 1983;250:1870, 1871, with permission.

The target cholesterol values should be 180 mg/dL for adults 30 years or younger and 200 mg/dL for individuals aged 30 years or older.[16] The guidelines for children suggest intervention with counseling, diet, and/or drugs and regular follow-up for all children above the 75th percentile (approximately 170 mg/dL).

Recommendations for treatment of hypertriglyceridemia have also been provided in a Consensus Conference statement and include the following[19]:

1. No changes are recommended, other than those specified for general dietary alterations under cholesterol, when triglyceride levels are less than 250 mg/dL.
2. Triglyceride levels in the range 250–500 mg/dL may be a marker for genetic forms of hyperlipoproteinemia and dietary intervention is the primary approach; however, drugs may have a role in those not responding to diet alone. Normocholesterolemic individuals with borderline hypertriglyceridemia who have no risk factors or family history need no specific treatment.
3. Frank hypertriglyceridemia (>500 mg/dL) is associated with pancreatitis and lowering of triglycerides by diet and, if necessary, by drugs is indicated.

It is important to remember that lipoprotein pattern types I, III, IV, and V are associated with hypertriglyceridemia and these primary lipoprotein disorders should be excluded prior to application of the suggested guidelines.

### *Management*

Many clinicians believe that reduction of elevated levels of cholesterol in patients with hypercholesterolemia should lessen the risk for coronary heart disease. Results from numerous epidemiologic studies are consistent with this concept. Without doubt, hypercholesterolemia increases the risk for coronary heart disease; however, until recently proof of the lipid hypothesis—reduction of elevated cholesterol reduces risk—was lacking. In 1984 the results of the Lipid Research Clinics Coronary Primary Prevention Trial (LRC-CPPT) unequivocally demonstrated a reduction in coronary heart disease, death, and nonfatal myocardial infarction in a large number of asymptomatic men with primary hypercholesterolemia.[20,21] The investigators found that for every 1% reduction in cholesterol, an approximately 2% reduction in coronary heart disease was seen. This study provides a strong rationale for attempting to lower plasma cholesterol and LDL in patients with hyperlipoproteinemia. Results from two other studies show that secondary intervention, not just primary intervention as in the LRC-CPPT, can reduce the angiographic progression and severity of coronary artery disease and reduce progression of lesions or formation of new atheroma in native or bypass grafts of patients who have undergone coronary venous bypass grafting.[22,23] These studies and others provide a rational basis for instituting therapy for hyperlipidemia either prior to the first cardiovascular event (primary intervention) or after a morbid event such as myocardial infarction (secondary intervention).

### *Dietary Therapy*

The objectives of dietary therapy are to progressively decrease the intake of total fat, saturated fatty acids, and cholesterol and to achieve a desirable body weight. The rationale for using the low-fat, low-cholesterol diet for the treatment of hypercholesterolemia is based on the following principles: (1) It represents a reasonable extension of the diet recommended for the general public. (2) It progressively decreases the major cholesterol-raising constitutents of the diet. (3) It precludes large intakes of polyunsaturated fats. (4) It facilitates weight reduction by removing foods of high caloric density.[7] The phased dietary approach recommended by the American Heart Association is outlined in Table 19.8.

Many patients with hyperlipidemia may be managed with dietary therapy alone, obviating the need for drugs.[7,15,24] Diet is considered to be the cornerstone of treatment with hyperlipidemia and the use of a dietitian for patient counseling is recommended. Several cookbooks with recipes generally suitable for implementing an alternate diet as part of the phased diet approach have been published.[25] The basic rationale for reducing dietary cholesterol, saturated fat, and excessive calories is based on the overproduction of VLDL and, subsequently, LDL, with its deposition in peripheral tissues resulting from excessive intake of the precursors for lipoprotein synthesis.[26] It has been estimated that the pre-

**Table 19.8** American Heart Association Phased Diet for Hypercholesterolemia

| | |
|---|---|
| **Phase I** | 30% of total calories as fat, 55% as carbohydrate, and 15% as protein. The fat should contain approximately equal amounts of saturated, monounsaturated, and polyunsaturated fatty acids; i.e., each should contribute about 10% of total calories. Complex carbohydrates should constitute the major source of total carbohydrates. Cholesterol intake should be below 300 mg/d. |
| **Phase II** | 25% of calories as fat (with equal amounts of the three types of fatty acids), 60% as carbohydrate, and 15% as protein; cholesterol, 200–250 mg/d. |
| **Phase III** | 20% of calories as fat (with equal amounts of the three types of fatty acids), 65% as carbohydrate, and 15% as protein; cholesterol, 100–150 mg/d. |

From Gotto AM Jr, Bierman EL, Connor WE, et al: Recommendations for treatment of hyperlipidemia in adults. Circulation 1984;69:1073A, with permission.

**Table 19.9** Summary of Studies on Dietary Therapy

| *Study* | *N* | *Duration (yr)* | *Therapy* | *Design* | *Δ Cholesterol (%)* | *Outcome* |
|---|---|---|---|---|---|---|
| Survey | | | | | | |
| Western Electric[28] | 1,900 | 20 | Diet | Survey | — | Dietary cholesterol associated with serum cholesterol and CHD[a] risk |
| Ireland–Boston[29] | 1,001 | 20 | None | Survey | — | Dietary fatty acids and cholesterol weakly related to the development of CHD |
| Primary intervention | | | | | | |
| Anti-Coronary Club[30] | 1,277 | 6 | Diet | Control Group | −13.1 | Significant reductions noted in coronary events in the diet-treated group |
| Los Angeles[31] | 846 | 8 | Diet | Randomized, double-blind | −12.7 | No significant difference in sudden death or myocardial infarction; however, combining all primary and secondary endpoints, incidence rates were 47.7% and 31.3% for control and experimental groups |
| MRFIT[35] | 12,886 | 7 | Diet, smoking, hypertension | Randomized | −5 | No significant difference in total or CHD mortality in SI versus UC groups |
| Oslo[33,34] | 1,232 | 5 | Diet, smoking | Randomized | −19.7 | Incidence of fatal and nonfatal MI and sudden death was 47% lower in intervention group; benefit maintained for 3.5 yr after completion of study |
| UK-HDPP[36] | 9,734 | 5.5 | Diet, smoking, hypertension | Control group | −4.1 | Only 4% reduction in overall CHD risk but angina and chest pain significantly reduced in intervention group |
| Belgian-HAPA[37] | 19,409 | 6 | Diet, smoking, hypertension, weight control, exercise | Control group | — | Total mortality, coronary incidence, and nonfatal MI all significantly reduced in intervention group |

| | | | | | | |
|---|---|---|---|---|---|---|
| Finland[32] | 581 | 12 | Diet | Crossover | −15.4 | Cholesterol-lowering diet reduced CHD mortality by 53% in men only |
| Secondary intervention | | | | | | |
| Leiden[46] | 39 | 2 | Diet | Longitudinal | −10.1 | Angiographic coronary lesion growth correlated with total/HDL cholesterol |
| MRC[45] | 393 | | Diet | Randomized | −22 | No significant differences for soya bean oil–treated group compared with control |
| Morrison[40] | 100 | 12 | Diet | Control group | −26.6 | At 12 yr, 38% of diet group but none of control group survived |
| Bierebaum[44] | 200 | 5 | Diet | Matched control group | −24 | Diet group had significantly fewer recurrent MIs and mortality was reduced |
| Nelson[39] | 175 | $>3$ | Diet | Control group | −11.8 | Mortality was 10% in group with decreased cholesterol but 32% in those quitting diet or no change |
| Research Committee[42] | 264 | 3 | Diet | Randomized | −15.2 | No significant differences between low-fat and normal diets |
| Hood[41] | 458 | 75 | Diet | Control | −16 | Lower mortality in strict diet group |
| Rose[43] | 80 | 2 | Diet | Randomized | −19.9 | Corn oil was not significantly different from control |
| Lyon[38] | 470 | 5 | Diet | Matched control | — | Recurrent MI and death were four times more common in low-cholesterol-diet group |

[a] cHD, Coronary heart disease; MRFIT, Multiple Risk Factor Intervention Trial; SI, special intervention; UC, usual care; UK-HDPP, United Kingdom Heart Disease Prevention Project; HDPP, Heart Disease Prevention Project.

dicted total change in plasma cholesterol after institution of the phased diet would be reductions of 18, 39, and 53 mg/dL with phases I, II, and III, respectively, if the diet were strictly followed.[27] A review of studies in which dietary intervention was instituted for hyperlipidemia shows the average reduction to be about 15% (see Table 19.9) If the baseline value of plasma cholesterol were 275 mg/dL, then a reduction of about 40 mg/dL to 235 mg/dL would be a realistic expectation with the phase III diet in a compliant patient. Some individuals are more responsive to dietary therapy than others and deviation from the preceding predictions can be expected. Depending on the response to diet, the patient may be advanced until the target cholesterol level is reached. Each phase of the diet should be maintained for a minimum of 4 weeks; however, the optimal response may not be seen for 6 or more months. Long-term counseling of the patient and family to encourage diet compliance and education about the risks and benefits that can be derived from diet modification and life-style changes is important.[10,15] Various trials of dietary intervention are summarized in Table 19.9; overall, reduction of cholesterol and saturated fat intake leads to a reduction of coronary heart disease. This seems to be true regardless of the time of intervention, primary versus secondary, and diet modification works adjunctively with other risk factor interventions, such as cessation of smoking and treatment of hypertension.

### *Drug Therapy*

Several excellent reviews on the treatment of hyperlipidemia and the adverse effects of the drugs used have been published recently.[1,7,15,47–51] Although many efficacious lipid-lowering drugs exist, none is effective in all lipoprotein disorders, and all such agents are associated with some adverse effects.[51] Lipid-lowering drugs can be broadly divided into agents that decrease the synthesis of VLDLs and LDLs, agents that enhance VLDL clearance, agents that enhance LDL catabolism, agents that decrease cholesterol absorption, agents that elevate HDL, or agents that have some combination of these characteristics (see Table 19.10). Drugs of choice for each lipoprotein phenotype and alternate agents are given in Table 19.11. Various drug products and their dosing and costs are listed in Table 19.12.

Treatment of type I hyperlipoproteinemia is directed toward reduction of chylomicrons derived from dietary fat with the subsequent reduction of plasma triglycerides. Total daily fat intake should be no more than 20–25 g per day. Secondary causes of hypertriglyceridemia (Table 19.6) should be excluded, or if present, the underlying disorder should be treated appropriately. Type V hyperlipoproteinemia also requires a stringent fat component of dietary intake; in addition, drug therapy is outlined in Table 19.11 if the response to diet alone is inadequate. Medium-chain triglycerides, which are absorbed without chylomicron formation, may be used as a dietary supplement for caloric intake if needed.

Primary hypercholesterolemia (familial hypercholesterolemia, familial combined hyperlipidemia, type IIa hyperlipoproteinemia) is treated with the bile acid sequestrants, cholestyramine and colestipol. The primary action of both agents is to bind bile acids in the intestinal lumen, with concurrent interruption of enterohepatic circulation of bile acids and markedly increased excretion of acidic steroids in

**Table 19.10** Effects of Drug Therapy on Lipids and Lipoproteins

| *Drug* | *Mechanism of action* | *Effects on lipids* | *Effects on lipoproteins* | *Comment* |
|---|---|---|---|---|
| Cholestyramine and cholestipol | ↑ LDL catabolism | ↓ Cholesterol | ↓ LDL<br>↑ VLDL | Problem with compliance; binds many coadministered drugs |
| Niacin | ↓ LDL and VLDL synthesis | ↓ Triglyceride and cholesterol | ↓ VLDL, ↓ LDL, ↑ HDL | Problems with patient acceptance; good in combination with bile acid resins |
| Dextrothyroxine sodium | ↑ LDL catabolism | ↓ Cholesterol | ↓ LDL | Caution in patients with heart disease |
| Clofibrate | ↑ VLDL clearance | ↓ Triglyceride and cholesterol | ↓ VLDL and LDL, ↑ HDL | Possible long-term toxicity; only modest effects on cholesterol |
| Neomycin sulfate | ↓ Cholesterol absorption | ↓ Cholesterol | ↓ LDL | Potentially ototoxic and nephrotoxic |
| Probucol | ↑ LDL clearance | ↓ Cholesterol | ↓ LDL and HDL | Lowers HDL; modest efficacy |
| Gemfibrozil | ↑ VLDL clearance<br>↓ VLDL synthesis | ↓ Triglyceride and cholesterol | ↓ VLDL<br>↑ ↓ LDL, ↑ HDL | Similar to clofibrate; long-term toxicity may be less than that of clofibrate |
| Lovastatin | ↑ LDL catabolism | ↓ Cholesterol | ↓ LDL | May be highly effective in familial hypercholesterolemia |

From Perry RS: Contemporary recommendations of evaluating and treating hyperlipidemia. Clin Pharm 1986;5:119, with permission.

**Table 19.11** Lipoprotein Phenotype and Recommended Drug Treatment

| *Lipoprotein phenotype* | *Drug of choice* | *Combination therapy* | *Alternative agents* |
|---|---|---|---|
| I | Not indicted | — | — |
| IIa | Cholestyramine or colestipol | Lovastatin<br>Niacin<br>Neomycin | Niacin<br>Lovastatin<br>Neomycin<br>Probucol<br>Sitosterol<br>*p*-Aminosalicylic acid (PAS) |
| IIb | Niacin<br>Gemfibrozil | Cholestyramine or colestipol | Cholestyramine or colestipol<br>Clofibrate |
| III | Niacin<br>Gemfibrozil | | Clofibrate |
| IV | Niacin<br>Gemfibrozil | Gemfibrozil<br>Niacin | Clofibrate |
| V | Niacin<br>Gemfibrozil | | Clofibrate<br>Oxandrolone<br>Norethisterone<br>Fish oils |

the feces. This decreases the bile acid pool size and stimulates hepatic synthesis of bile acids from cholesterol. Depletion of the hepatic pool of cholesterol results in an increase in cholesterol biosynthesis and an increase in the number of LDL receptors on the hepatocyte membrane (see Fig. 19.10). The increased number of LDL receptors stimulates an enhanced rate of catabolism from plasma and lowers LDL levels.[48] Patients with homozygous familial hypercholesterolemia genetically lack the ability to increase synthesis of LDL receptors and bile acid resins are generally ineffective. The increase in hepatic cholesterol biosynthesis may be paralleled by increased hepatic VLDL production and, consequently, bile acid resins may aggravate hypertriglyceridemia in patients with combined hyperlipidemia.[52] Gastrointestinal complaints of constipation, bloating, epigastric fullness, nausea, and flatulence are most commonly reported[51]; however, with long-term therapy, patients tolerate these drugs well, as noted in the LRC-CPPT and the study of Brensike et al[20–22] (see Table 19.13). These adverse effects can be managed by increasing the fluid intake, modifying the diet to increase bulk, and using stool softeners. The other major limiting complaint is the gritty texture and bulk of these resins and these problems may be minimized by mixing the powder with orange drink or juice.[53]

**Table 19.12** Comparison of Drugs Used in the Treatment of Hyperlipidemia

| *Drug* | *Manufacturer* | *Dosage form* | *Usual daily dose* | *Maximum daily dose* | *Monthly cost*[a] ($) |
|---|---|---|---|---|---|
| Cholestyramine (Questran) | Mead Johnson | 4-g packets<br>Bulk powder | 8 g TID | 32 g | 135.65<br>61.29 |
| Colestipol hydrochloride (Colestid) | Upjohn | 5-g packets<br>Bulk powder | 10 g BID | 30 g | 59.44<br>57.06 |
| Niacin | Various | 50-, 100-, 250-, and 500-mg tablets; 125-, 250-, and 500-mg capsules | 2 g TID | 9 g | 4.57—386.06 |
| Probucol (Lorelco) | Merrell Dow | 250-mg tablets | 500 mg BID | 1 g | 38.95 |
| Dextrothyroxine sodium (Choloxin) | Flint | 1-, 2-, 4-, and 6-mg tablets | 6 mg/d | 8 mg | 26.75 |
| Neomycin sulfate | Various | 500-mg tablets | 1 g BID | 2 g | 11.94–68.63 |
| Clofibrate (Atromid-S) | Ayerst | 500-mg capsules | 1 g BID | 2 g | 32.00 |
| Gemfibrozil (Lopid) | Parke–Davis | 300-mg capsules | 600 mg BID | 1.5 g | 41.63 |
| Lovastatin (Mevacor) | Merck | 20-, 40-, and 80 mg tablets | 20–40 mg | 80 mg | 37.50–75.00[b] |

[a] Average wholesale cost based on 1987 Redbook.
[b] Estimated cost.

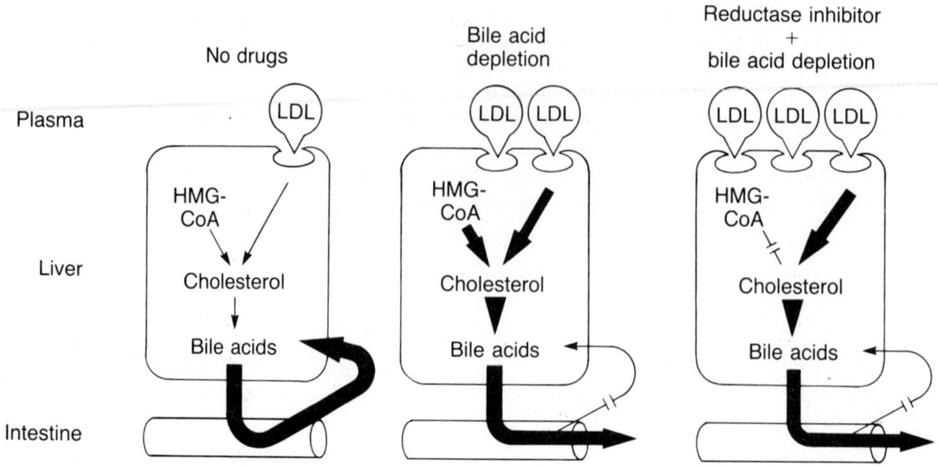


**Figure 19.10** Function of the hepatic low-density lipoprotein (LDL) receptor with pharmacologic intervention, with the addition of a bile acid sequestrant, and with the combined use of bile acid sequestrant and an HMG-CoA reductase inhibitor. *(From Gotto AM Jr: Treatment of hyperlipidemia. Am J Cardiol 1986;57:14G, with permission.)*

Other potential adverse effects include impaired absorption of fat-soluble vitamins A, D, E, and K, hypernatremia and hyperchloremia, gastrointestinal obstruction, and reduced bioavailability of acidic drugs such as coumarin anticoagulants, digitoxin, nicotinic acid, thyroxine, acetaminophen, hydrocortisone, hydrochlorothiazide, loperamide, and possibly iron.[51] Hyperchloremic metabolic acidosis, hypernatremia, and gastrointestinal obstruction have been reported almost exclusively in children and malabsorption of fat-soluble vitamins is probably most common with high doses (e.g., 30 g of cholestyramine per day) of the bile acid resins. Drug interactions may be avoided by alternating administration times, with an interval of 6 hours or greater between the bile acid resin and other drugs. Colestipol and cholestyramine have comparable side effects; however, colestipol may have better palatability as it is odorless and tasteless.[53]

Niacin (nicotinic acid) may also be used in primary hypercholesterolemia in combination with bile acid sequestrants or as monotherapy for this disorder and others (Table 19.11). Niacin reduces the hepatic synthesis of VLDL which in turn leads to a reduction in the synthesis of LDL. Factors responsible for decreased production of VLDL include inhibition of lipolysis with a decrease in free fatty acids in plasma, decreased hepatic esterification of triglycerides, and

**Table 19.13** Adverse Effects of Cholestyramine

| | *Lipid Research Clinics*[20] | | *Brensike et al*[22] | |
|---|---|---|---|---|
| *Adverse effect* | **Cholestyramine (%) [N=1,906]** | **Placebo (%) [N=1,920]** | **Cholestyramine (%) [N=59]** | **Placebo (%) [N=57]** |
| Abdominal pain | 7 | 7 | 3.4 | 0 |
| Belching/bloating | 6 | 9 | 5.1 | 5.3 |
| Constipation | 4 | 8 | 5.1 | 3.5 |
| Diarrhea | 8 | 4 | | |
| Gas | 12 | 12 | 5.1 | 7 |
| Heartburn | 7 | 12 | 5.1 | 0 |
| Nausea | 4 | 3 | NR[a] | NR |
| Vomiting | 3 | 2 | NR | NR |
| Drowsiness | NR | NR | 8.5 | 1.8 |
| Itching | NR | NR | 1.7 | 0 |
| Leg cramps | NR | NR | 8.5 | 1.8 |
| Nervousness | NR | NR | 8.5 | 5.3 |
| Rash | NR | NR | 1.7 | 0 |
| Weakness | NR | NR | 5.1 | 0 |

[a] NR, not reported or recorded in study.

From Knodel LC, Talbert RL: Adverse effects of hypolipidaemic drugs. Med Toxicol 1987;2:12, with permission.

**Table 19.14** Adverse Effects of Nicotinic Acid (Niacin)

| | Coronary Drug Project[55] | | Knopp et al[56] | |
|---|---|---|---|---|
| *Adverse effect* | **Nicotinic acid (%) [N=1,073)**[b] | **Placebo (%) [N=2,695]** | **Nicotinic acid CR**[a] **[N=37]** | **Nicotinic acid SR [N=34]** |
| Stomach pain | 13.9 | 7.9 | 9 | 21 |
| Any gastrointestinal complaint | 25.7 | 20.1 | >30[c] | >100[c] |
| Flushing | 92.0 | 4.3 | 100 | 82 |
| Itching | 48.9 | 6.2 | | |
| Urticaria | 7.2 | 1.5 | 8 | 3 |
| Other types of rash | 19.8 | 5.9 | 3 | 3 |
| Pain or burning on urination | 2.9 | 1.2 | | |
| Frequent urination | 3.9 | 2.1 | | |
| Decreased appetite | 4.1 | 1.5 | 3 | 15 |
| Weight loss | 2.7 | 0.9 | | |
| Increasing sweating | 3.4 | 1.8 | | |
| Need for gout medication | 11.4 | 6.1 | | |
| Ichthyosis | 3.1 | 0.8 | | |
| Acanthosis nigricans | 3.6 | 0.7 | | |
| Any dermal abnormality | 26.3 | 15.8 | | |
| Sexual dysfunction (male) | | | >3[c] | >22 |
| Dry skin | | | 5 | 12 |
| Worsening psoriasis | | | 0 | 3 |
| Body odor | | | 3 | 3 |
| Increased body hair | | | 0 | 3 |
| Tiredness | | | >3[c] | >24 |

[a] CR, conventional release; SR, sustained release.
[b] Significantly different from placebo, $P < 0.01$.
[c] Significantly different from nicotinic acid SR, $P < 0.05$.

From Knodel LC, Talbert RL: Adverse effect of hypolipidaemic drugs. Med Toxicol 1987;2:21, with permission.

a possible direct effect on the hepatic production of apolipoprotein B. The complementary action of niacin and bile acid resins to increase the excretion and decrease the absorption of sterols may account for the additive effects of this combination in hyperlipemia.[54] Niacin also increases HDL by reducing its catabolism. The principal use of niacin is in mixed hyperlipemia or as a second-line agent in combination therapy for hypercholesterolemia. It is also considered to be the first-line agent or an alternative for the treatment of hypertriglyceridemia.[19]

The typical adverse effects of niacin are given in Table 19.14, based on the Coronary Drug Project (CDP) and the study of Knopp et al.[55,56] Niacin has many adverse drug reactions that occur commonly; fortunately, most of the symptoms and biochemical abnormalities seen do not require discontinuation of therapy. Cutaneous flushing and itching appear to be prostaglandin mediated and can be reduced by aspirin 325 mg given shortly before niacin ingestion. Flushing seems to be related to rising plasma concentrations of niacin, and taking the dose with meals and slowly titrating the dose upward may minimize these effects.[54] Potentially important laboratory abnormalities occurring with niacin therapy include elevated liver function tests, hyperuricemia, and hyperglycemia. With less than 3 g per day the degree of liver function test elevation is generally not marked and often transient, and a temporary reduction in dosage frequently corrects the problem. Preexisting gout and diabetes may be exacerbated by niacin and these patients should be monitored more closely and their medication titrated appropriately. Niacin is contraindicated in patients with active liver disease. Dry eyes and other ophthalmologic complaints are also occasionally noted.[57] Concomitant alcohol and hot drinks may magnify flushing and pruritus with niacin and should be avoided at the time of ingestion. Clonidine may inhibit niacin-induced vasodilation, thus inhibiting skin flushing.

Probucol, neomycin, and dextrothyroxine have also been used as alternative drugs for primary hypercholesterolemia; however, their utility is limited by detrimental changes in lipoproteins, adverse effects, and lack of efficacy. Fractional catabolism of LDL and increased biliary excretion of cholesterol reduce both LDL and HDL with probucol. The decrease in HDL levels seen with probucol is due to decreased synthesis of apolipoprotein A-I and decreased lipoprotein lipase activity.[48] VLDL levels are unaffected by probucol. Probucol reduces total and LDL cholesterol by

8% to 21% and reduces HDL concentrations by up to 26%.[47,48] This undesirable effect of probucol on HDL, which may adversely affect coronary heart disease risk, as well as its propensity to increase the QT interval relegate probucol to at least a second-line drug.[51,58] Neomycin reduces the absorption of cholesterol from the small intestine and it is a second-line drug for use in patients with primary hypercholesterolemia who are unable to take bile acid sequestrants. Early in therapy, 38% to 80% of patients experience increased stool frequency or diarrhea with neomycin but this usually resolves in 1 to 3 weeks of therapy. Although neomycin is ototoxic and small amounts are absorbed (3%–5%), producing measurable plasma concentrations, at doses of 2 g/day or lower for up to 3 years no toxicity has been reported.[51] Neomycin may increase the absorption of digoxin, enhance the hypoprothrombinemic effects of warfarin, and interact synergistically with other nephrotoxic drugs and neuromuscular blocking agents. Dextrothyroxine can no longer be recommended for the treatment of hyperlipemia based on the CDP experience in which dextrothyroxine-treated patients experienced a higher mortality rate if ventricular ectopy was present at the initiation of therapy.[59]

Lovastatin (formerly known as mevinolin) is a fermentation product derived from *Aspergillus terreus* that inhibits 3-hydroxy-3-methylglutaryl coenzyme A (HMG-CoA) reductase, interrupting the conversion of HMG-CoA to mevalonate, the rate-limiting step in de novo cholesterol biosynthesis (see Fig. 19.8). Metabolic studies with lovastatin in normal volunteers and patients with hypercholesterolemia suggest reduced synthesis of LDL cholesterol and enhanced catabolism of LDL mediated through LDL receptors as the principal mechanisms for lipid-lowering effects.[60] Total cholesterol and LDL cholesterol are reduced by 30% or more on average when added to dietary therapy, with the effects being more pronounced in nonfamilial hypercholesterolemia than in familial hypercholesterolemia. Combination therapy with bile acid sequestrants and lovastatin is rational, as LDL receptor numbers are increased leading to greater degradation of LDL cholesterol, intracellular synthesis of cholesterol is inhibited, and enterohepatic recycling of bile acids is interrupted (see Fig. 19.10). The addition of colestipol to lovastatin results in further reductions of total and LDL cholesterol of 28% to 46% compared with lovastatin alone.[61] In doses of 20 mg twice daily, lovastatin produces reductions in total and LDL cholesterol of about 22% to 39%.[62] Twice-daily dosing appears to provide a greater reduction in lipid levels than once-daily dosing. Diarrhea, abdominal pain, constipation, and flatulence (all less than 5%) seem to be the most common complaints. A significant elevation in transaminase levels has been noted but in less than 2% of patients. Lens opacities have been reported to be due potentially to lovastatin; however, in the age groups studied, these abnormalities are common and tend to wax and wane with time irrespective of drug therapy.

Combined hyperlipoproteinemia (type IIb) may be treated with niacin or gemfibrozil to lower LDL cholesterol without elevating VLDL and triglycerides. Niacin is the most effective agent and may be combined with a bile acid sequestrant. Cholestyramine or colestipol alone in this disorder may elevate VLDL and triglycerides and their use as single agents for treating combined hyperlipoproteinemia should be avoided.[50,52] Gemfibrozil as a single agent is effective in reducing VLDL but a reciprocal rise in LDL may occur and total cholesterol values may remain relatively unchanged.[50] Gemfibrozil reduces the synthesis of VLDL and, to a lesser extent, apolipoprotein B, with a concurrent increase in the rate of removal of triglyceride-rich lipoproteins from plasma. Plasma HDL concentrations may rise 10% to 15% or more with gemfibrozil. As it is a fibric acid derivative of clofibrate, there has been concern that detrimental effects and adverse effects similar to those observed with clofibrate would occur; however, recent evidence from the Helsinki Heart Study has shown no significant differences between gemfibrozil and placebo.[51,63] Gastrointestinal complaints occur in 3% to 5% of patients, rash in 2%, dizziness in 2.4%, and transient elevations in transaminase levels and alkaline phosphatase in 4.5% and 1.3%, respectively. Similar to clofibrate, gemfibrozil may enhance the formation of gallstones associated with an increase in the lithogenic index; however, the rate is low (0.6%) and similar to that seen with placebo in the Helsinki Heart Study. Gemfibrozil may potentiate the effects of oral anticoagulants, as does clofibrate, but this is not well documented.

Type III hyperlipoproteinemia may be treated with clofibrate, niacin, or gemfibrozil. According to Illingworth,[48] clofibrate is the drug of choice for this disorder; however, given the lack of data supporting its efficacy in altering cardiovascular mortality in the major studies on hypercholesterolemia and its numerous, well-documented and serious adverse effects, it is reasonable to consider niacin or gemfibrozil prior to the use of clofibrate. Clofibrate increases the activity of lipoprotein lipase and reduces to a lesser extent the synthesis or secretion of VLDL from the liver into the plasma. Clofibrate is less effective than gemfibrozil or niacin in reducing VLDL production. Data from the CDP[55] and the World Health Organization (WHO)[64] trials with clofibrate have provided detailed information concerning adverse effects of clofibrate (see Table 19.15). The most disturbing aspects are its potential to induce gallstones (4.7% with clofibrate, 0.54% with placebo), promote ventricular ectopy, and potentially cause gastrointestinal malignancy, causing a greater overall mortality than placebo alone (WHO).[51] A myositis syndrome of myalgia, weakness, stiffness, malaise, and elevations in creatinine phosphokinase and aspartate aminotransaminase is seen with clofibrate and it seems to be more common in patients with renal insufficiency. Enhanced hypoprothrombinemic and hypoglycemic effects are reported to occur when clofibrate is given to patients on coumarin anticoagulants and sulfonylurea compound, but the mechanisms for these interactions are not well understood. Rifampin, a hepatic enzyme inducer of oxidative pathways, may induce the metabolism of clofibrate but the long-term consequences are unknown.

Two fibric acid derivatives (clofibrate and gemfibrozil) are approved in the United States; however, several others are under development or are being used in Europe. These include benzafibrate, fenofibrate, and ciprofibrate.[48] Diprofidrate and fenofibrate appear to be the most useful, both reducing LDL cholesterol by 20% to 25% in heterozygous familial hypercholesterolemia. Compactin, a fungal derivative similar to lovastatin, has been investigated in Japan and at least one of its derivatives is undergoing investigation in the United States. Activated charcoal in doses of 8 g three time daily has been shown to reduce total and LDL choles-

**Table 19.15** Adverse Effects of Clofibrate[a]

| | *Coronary Drug Project*[55] | | *Committee of Principal Investigators (WHO)*[64] | |
|---|---|---|---|---|
| *Adverse effect* | **Clofibrate (%) [N=1,065]** | **Placebo (%) [N=2,695]** | **Clofibrate (%) [N=5,331]** | **Placebo (%) [N=5,296]** |
| Sexual dysfunction | 14.1** | 10.0 | 1.1** | 0.6 |
| Difficulty swallowing capsule | 1.5** | 0.5 | NR[b] | NR |
| Increased appetite | 5.3** | 3.1 | 0.4 | 0.1 |
| Weight gain | NR | NR | 1.9** | 0.8 |
| Indigestion | NR | NR | 6.0** | 4.6 |
| Intestinal hurry | NR | NR | 3.2* | 2.4 |
| Increased anticoagulant use | 13.7** | 10.0 | NR | NR |
| Ventricular diastolic gallop | 14.6** | 11.7 | NR | NR |
| Palpable spleen | 2.4** | 1.1 | NR | NR |
| Hepatomegaly | 19.7** | 15.9 | NR | NR |
| Cholelithiasis | 3.0** | 1.3 | NR | NR |
| Cholecystectomy | NR | NR | 1.1*** | 0.5 |
| Drug-dependent diabetes | | | 2.4 | 1.9 |
| Mortality | | | | |
| All causes | | | 3.0* | 2.4 |
| Cancer | | | 0.57/1,000 yr* | 0.21/1,000 yr |
| All causes but heart disease | | | 2.0 | 1.5 |

[a] Values significantly different from placebo: *$P < 0.05$, **$P < 0.01$, ***$P < 0.001$.
[b] NR, not reported.

From Knodel LC, Talbert RL: Adverse effects of hyperlipidaemic drugs. Med Toxicol 1987;2:16, with permission.

terol by 25% and 41%, respectively in short-term trials.[65] The mechanism for this effect is postulated to be bile acid sequestration and binding of dietary cholesterol. Numerous epidemologic and normal volunteer studies have found that diets high in ω-3 polyunsaturated fatty acids, most commonly eicosapentaenoic acid, reduce cholesterol, triglycerides, LDL cholesterol, and VLDL cholesterol and may elevate HDL cholesterol.[66,67] The effects of fish oil on lipoprotein metabolism are mediated through a reduction in VLDL production and suppression of VLDL apolipoprotein B.[68] In patients with hypertriglyceridemia, either phenotype type IIb or type V, a diet high in ω-3 fatty acids given for 4 weeks reduced cholesterol 27% and 45% and triglyceride 64% and 79% in type IIb and type V patients, respectively.[69] A diet high in eicosapentaenoic acid (EPA) given to hyperlipidemic hemodialysis patients resulted in significant decreases in cholesterol and triglycerides for up to 13 weeks.[70] Fish oil supplementation may be most useful in patients with hypertriglyceridemia; however, its role in treatment is continuing to be defined. Potential complications of fish oil supplementation such as thrombocytopenia and bleeding disorders have been noted, especially with high doses (EPA 15–30 g/d), and well-controlled trials are needed to determine the specific polyunsaturated acids and the safe, effective doses to be used before their use may be broadly recommended.[71]

### *Other Therapies*

Partial ileal bypass has been used in severe heterozygous and homozygous familial hypercholesterolemia; however, it is ineffective in the latter case. Ileal bypass removes the site of bile acid reabsorption, depleting the bile acid pool and increasing the catabolism of cholesterol.[72] Portacaval shunts have been used to decrease the formation of LDL cholesterol and reductions of 10%–20% have been reported.[73] Plasma exchange combined with niacin was found to reduce plasma cholesterol levels by about 50% in homozygous familial hypercholesterolemia over 5 years and coronary atherosclerosis did not progress as documented by angiography.[74] Combined liver and heart transplantation in a 6-year-old girl with homozygous familial hypercholesterolemia reduced total and LDL cholesterol concentrations from 1,079 and 988 mg/dL to 302 and 184 mg/dL, prior to and after surgery, respectively.[75] Liver transplantation replaced the missing LDL receptors and enhanced catabolism and reduced lipoprotein synthesis in this patient.

## Summary of Major Studies

Three primary and five secondary prevention trials have been performed to determine if lowering of cholesterol prevents coronary heart disease (CHD) and these are summarized in Table 19.16. All studies were double-blinded, randomized, placebo-controlled studies lasting 5 or more years, except the CDP using dextrothyroxine, which was terminated early because of adverse effects on CHD mortality. In the Edinburgh study, 180 patients were also given warfarin; the patients remained blinded while the physicians were aware of the treatment group allocation. The Helsinki

**Table 19.16** Randomized Drug Trials of Cholesterol Lowering and Coronary Heart Disease[a]

| Trial | Drug therapy | Years of follow-up | Treatment group *N* | Treatment group Mean total-C[b] | Treatment group Number of CHD cases[c] | Control group *N* | Control group Mean total-C[b] | Control group Number of CHD cases[c] | Reduction in CHD incidence (%)[d] |
|---|---|---|---|---|---|---|---|---|---|
| Primary prevention | | | | | | | | | |
| LRC-CPPT[20] | Cholestyramine | 7 | 1,906 | 251 | 155 | 1,900 | 276 | 187 | 18.9 |
| WHO[64] | Clofibrate | 5 | 5,331 | 224 | 167 | 5,296 | 244 | 208 | 20.9 |
| Helsinki Heart Study[63,80] | Gemfibrozil | 5 | 2,050 | 247 | 56 | 2,031 | 273 | 84 | 34.1 |
| Secondary prevention | | | | | | | | | |
| Newcastle[76] | Clofibrate | 5 | 244 | 227 | 54 | 253 | 253 | 85 | 43.8 |
| Edinburgh[77] | Clofibrate | 6 | 350 | 227 | 59 | 367 | 263 | 79 | 26.1 |
| CDP[55] | Clofibrate | 5 | 1,103 | 235 | 309 | 2,789 | 251 | 839 | 9.5 |
| CDP[55,78] | Niacin | 5 | 1,119 | 226 | 287 | 2,789 | 251 | 839 | 19.8 |
| CDP[59] | Dextrothyroxine | 3 | 1,013 | 226 | 197 | 2,715 | 255 | 449 | −12.2 |

[a] CHD, coronary heart disease; LRC-CPPT, Lipid Research Clinics Coronary Primary Prevention Trial; CDP, Coronary Drug Project.
[b] Annual posttreatment levels of total cholesterol.
[c] Definite nonfatal myocardial infarction or CHD death.
[d] Calculated by subtracting odds ratio from unity and multiplying by 100%.

Modified from Lipid Research Clinics Program: The Lipid Research Clinics Coronary Primary Prevention Trial Results. II. The relationship of reduction in incidence of coronary heart disease to cholesterol lowering. JAMA 1984;251:372, with permission.

Heart Study results have not been reported; however, the drug is at least a safe agent in that few differences in adverse effects have been noted between placebo and gemfibrozil.

Total cholesterol and LDL cholesterol were reduced an average of 13.4% and 20.3%, respectively, by cholestyramine in the LRC-CPPT, and the reduction of lipid levels was related to the amount of drug ingested (e.g., 1 or 2 packets, 5.4% reduction in total cholesterol, versus 5 or more packets, 19.0% reduction). The prescribed dose of cholestyramine was 24 g or 6 packets per day. The cholestyramine group experienced a 19% reduction in risk ($P < 0.05$) of the primary endpoint—definite CHD death and/or definite nonfatal myocardial infarction—reflecting a 24% reduction in definite CHD death and a 19% reduction in nonfatal myocardial infarction. Other endpoints were reduced by 25%, 20%, and 21% for new positive exercise tests, angina, and coronary bypass surgery, respectively. Death from all causes was not significantly reduced by cholestyramine secondary to more accidents and violence in this group. The mean decreases in total and LDL cholesterol in the cholestyramine group were 8% and 12% relative to levels in placebo-treated men, providing evidence that for every 1% reduction in cholesterol, a 2% decline in CHD mortality can be realized.

The cooperative trial sponsored by WHO used clofibrate 1.6 g/d in high-risk men (upper third of cholesterol distribution) and compared this group with a similar high-risk group given placebo and a low-risk group (lower third of cholesterol distribution). Cholesterol was reduced an average of 9% (range 7%–11% for the three study centers in the clofibrate-treated group). Clofibrate reduced nonfatal myocardial infarctions (MIs) by 25%; CHD was reduced by 20%, primarily because of the reduction of nonfatal MIs. Fatal MI was similar in the two high-cholesterol groups and all-cause mortality was higher ($P < 0.05$) in the clofibrate-treated group. Mortality from gastrointestinal malignancy was seen more commonly with clofibrate and the cholecystectomy rate for gallstones was also significantly higher.

In the secondary intervention trials, clofibrate (1.5 g/d) in the Newcastle study significantly reduced mortality (11.1% versus 19.0%) from sudden deaths (9 versus 21 patients in clofibrate and placebo groups, respectively) but not from MI or congestive heart failure. Nonfatal MIs averaged 11.9% with clofibrate versus 18.2% in the placebo group ($P < 0.055$). Clofibrate (1.6–2 g/d) in the Edinburgh trial was less impressive, with no significant effect on the occurrence of fatal or nonfatal MI or overall mortality.[76,77]

Niacin in the CDP significantly reduced definite, nonfatal MI compared with placebo (10.1% vs 13.9%), whereas clofibrate did not reduce death from any cause, nonfatal or fatal MI, or coronary death at the 5-year follow-up. Clofibrate did increase the rate of definite or suspected fatal or nonfatal pulmonary embolism or thrombophlebitis compared with placebo (5.8% versus 3.6%) after adjusting for baseline characteristics for total follow-up. Other findings with clofibrate that occurred more frequently than with placebo included intermittent claudication, arrhythmias, palpable spleen, cholelithiasis (including cholecystectomy), and use of anticoagulants. Skin reactions, gastrointestinal complaints, and use of gout medication were more common with niacin than with placebo. The 5-year total mortalities were 20.0% for clofibrate and 20.9% for placebo. The 5-year total mortality for niacin was 21.2%. Recently, a long-term follow-up of the CDP has shown a reduction in total mortality with niacin that occurred 9 years after the drug had been stopped.[78] The mechanism for this effect is unclear. Gemfibrozil decreased cardiac events in the Helsinki Heart Study; however, this reduction was due primarily to a reduction in nonfatal myocardial infarction.[79,80]

## Conclusion

Hypercholesterolemia is unequivocally linked to increased risk for coronary heart disease morbidity and mortality. Reductions in elevated total and LDL cholesterol reduce CHD mortality. Hypertriglyceridemia has not been conclusively associated with increased cholesterol levels; however, severely elevated triglyceride levels can produce pancreatitis. Cholestyramine and niacin have been shown to decrease nonfatal MI and CHD death. Evidence for these beneficial effects for other lipid-lowering drugs is not currently available.

Initial therapy for any lipoprotein disorder is dietary restriction of fat and cholesterol and a modest increase in polyunsaturated fat intake. Hypercholesterolemia is best treated initially with a bile acid sequestrant and combination or alternative agents include lovastatin and niacin. Hypertriglyceridemia may be treated with niacin, gemfibrozil, or clofibrate and, when considering the side effect profile of each, gemfibrozil may be the best initial choice.

## References


1. Schaefer EJ, Levy RI. Pathogenesis and management of lipoprotein disorders. N Engl J Med 1985;312:1300–1310.
2. Kannel WB, Castelli WB, Gordon T. Cholesterol in the prediction of atherosclerotic disease. New perspectives based on the Framingham study. Ann Intern Med 1979;90:85–91.
3. Pooling Project Research Group. Relationship of blood pressure, serum cholesterol, relative weight and ECG abnormalities to incidence of major coronary events: Final report of the Pooling Project. J Chron Dis 1978;31:201–306.
4. Simons LA. Interrelations of lipids and lipoproteins with coronary artery disease mortality in 19 countries. Am J Cardiol 1986;57:5G–10G.
5. Castelli WP, Doyle JT, Gordon T, et al. HDL-cholesterol and other lipids in coronary heart disease: The Cooperative Lipoprotein Phenotyping Study. Circulation 1977;55:767–772.
6. Goldstein JL, Schbott HG, Hazzard WR, et al. Hyperlipidemia in coronary heart disease. II. Genetic analysis of lipid levels in 176 families and delineation of a new inherited disorder, combined hyperlipidemia. J Clin Invest 1973;52:1544–1568.
7. Gotto Jr AM, Bierman EL, Conner WE, et al. Recommendations for treatment of hyperlipidemia in adults. Circulation 1984;69:1065A–1090A.
8. Brown MS, Kovanen PT, Goldstein JL. Regulation of plasma cholesterol by lipoprotein receptors. Science 1981;212:628–635.
9. Mahley RW, Innerarity TL. Lipoprotein receptors and cholesterol homeostasis. Biochem Biophys Acta 1983;737:197–222.
10. Fredrickson DS, Levy RI, Lees RS. Fat transport in lipoproteins. An integrated approach to mechanisms and disorders. N Engl J Med 1967;276:34–44, 94–104, 148–156, 215–225, 273–281.
11. Goldstein JL, Brown MS. Familial hypercholesterolemia, in Stanbury JB, Wyngaarden JB, Fredrickson DS, et al (eds): The Metabolic Basis of Inherited Disease, 5th ed. New York, McGraw–Hill, 1983, pp 672–712.
12. Brown MS, Goldstein JL. Receptor-mediated control of cholesterol metabolism. Science 1976;191:150–154.
13. Nikkila EA. Familial cholesterol lipase deficiency and related disorders of chylomicron metabolism, in Stanbury JB, Wyngaarden JB, Fredrickson DS, et al. The Metabolic Basis of Inherited Disease, 5th ed. New York, McGraw–Hill, 1983, pp 622–642.
14. Brown MS, Goldstein JL, Fredrickson DJ. Familial type 3 hyperlipoproteinemia (dysbetalipoproteinemia), in Stanbury JB, Wyngaarden JB, Fredrickson DS, et al (eds): The Metabolic Basis of Inherited Disease, 5th ed. New York, McGraw–Hill, 1983, pp 655–671.
15. Council on Scientific Affairs. Dietary and pharmacologic therapy for the lipid risk factors. JAMA 1983;250:1873–1879.
16. Consensus Conference. Lowering blood cholesterol to prevent heart disease. JAMA 1985;253:2080–2086.
17. Gordon T, Castelli WP, Hjortland MC, et al. High density lipoprotein as a protective factor against coronary heart disease. Am J Med 1977;62:707–714.
18. Rifkin BM, Segal P. Lipid Research Clinics Program reference values for hyperlipidemia and hypolipidemia. JAMA 1983;250: 1869–1872.
19. Consensus Conference. Treatment of hypertriglyceridemia. JAMA 1984;251:1196–1200.
20. Lipid Research Clinics Program. The Lipid Research Clinics Coronary Primary Prevention Trial Results. I. Reduction in incidence of coronary heart disease. JAMA 1984;251:351–364.
21. Lipid Research Clinics Program. The Lipid Research Clinics Coronary Primary Prevention Trial Results. II. The relationship of reduction in incidence of coronary heart disease to cholesterol lowering. JAMA 1984;251:365–374.
22. Brensike JF, Levy RI, Kelsey SF, et al. Effects of therapy with cholestyramine on progression of coronary arteriosclerosis: Results of the NHLBI Type II Coronary Intervention Study. JAMA 1984;69:313–324.
23. Blankenhorn DH, Nessim SA, Johnson RL, et al. Beneficial effects of combined colestipol–niacin therapy on coronary atherosclerosis and coronary venous bypass grafts. JAMA 1987;257:3233–3240.
24. Grundy SM, Bilheimer D, Blackburn H, et al. Rationale of the diet–heart statement of the American Heart Association: Report of the nutrition committee. Circulation 1982;65:839A–854A.
25. Connor WE, Connor SL. The dietary treatment of hyperlipidemia. Rationale, technique and efficacy. Med Clin North Am 1982;66:485–518.
26. Grundy SM. AHA special report. Recommendations for the treatment of hyperlipidemia in adults. A joint statement of the Nutrition Committee and the Council on Arteriosclerosis of the American Heart Association. Arteriosclerosis 1984;4:445A–468A.
27. Hegsted DM, McGandy RB, Myers ML, et al. Quantitative effects of dietary fat on serum cholesterol in man. Am J Clin Nutr 1965;17:281–295.
28. Shekelle RB, Shyrick AM, Paul O, et al. Diet, serum cholesterol, and death from coronary disease: The Western Electric Study. N Engl J Med 1981;304:65–70.
29. Kushi LH, Lew RA, Stare FJ, et al. Diet and 20-year mortality from coronary heart disease. The Ireland–Boston Diet-Heart Study. N Engl J Med 1985;312:811–818.
30. Christakis G, Rinzler SH, Archer HS, et al. The Anti-Coronary Club. A dietary approach to the prevention of coronary heart

disease—A seven year report. Am J Public Health 1966;56:299–314.
31. Dayton S, Pearce ML, Hasimoto S, et al. A controlled clinical trial of a diet high in unsaturated fat in preventing complications of atherosclerosis. Circulation 1969;40(suppl II):1–63.
32. Miettinen M, Turpeinen O, Karvonen MN, et al. Effect of cholesterol-lowering diets on mortality from coronary heart disease and other sources. Lancet 1972;2:835–838.
33. Hjermann I, Velve Byre K, Holme I, et al. Effect of diet and smoking interventions on the incidence of coronary heart disease. Report from the Oslo Study Group of a randomized trial in healthy men. Lancet 1981;2:1303–1310.
34. Hjermann I, Holme I, Leren P. Oslo Study Diet and Antismoking Trial. Results after 102 months. Am J Med 1986;80(2A):7–11.
35. Multiple Risk Factor Intervention Trial Research Group. Multiple risk factor intervention trial. Risk factor changes and mortality results. JAMA 1982;248:1465–1477.
36. Rose G, Tunstall-Pedoe HD, Heller RF. UK Heart Disease Prevention Project. Incidence and mortality results. Lancet 1983;1:1062–1065.
37. Kornitzer M, DeBacker G, Dramaix N, et al. Belgian Heart Disease Prevention Project. Incidence and mortality results. Lancet 1983;1:1066–1070.
38. Lyon TP, Yankley A, Gofman JW, et al. Lipoproteins and diet in coronary heart disease. Calif Med 1956:84:325–328.
39. Nelson AM. Treatment of atherosclerosis by diet: Part I. Results in patients followed from 36 to 72 months. Northwest Med 1956;55:643–649.
40. Morrison LM. Diet in coronary atherosclerosis. JAMA 1960;173:884–888.
41. Hood B, Sanne H, Örndahl G, et al. Long-term prognosis in essential hypercholesterolemia: Effect of strict diet. Acta Med Scand 1965;178:161–173.
42. Research Committee. Low-fat diet in myocardial infarction. Lancet 1965;2:501–504.
43. Rose GA, Thomson WB, Williams RT. Corn oil in treatment of ischaemic heart disease. Br Med J 1965;1:1531–1533.
44. Bierebaum ML, Green DP, Flurina A, et al. Modified-fat dietary management of the young male with coronary disease. JAMA 1967;202:1119–1123.
45. Medical Research Council. Controlled trial of soya-bean oil in myocardial infarction: Report of a research committee to the Medical Research Council. Lancet 1968;2:693–700.
46. Arntzenius AC, Kromhout D, Barth JD, et al. Diet, lipoproteins, and the progression of coronary atherosclerosis. The Leiden Intervention Trial. N Engl J Med 1985;312:805–811.
47. Perry RS. Contemporary recommendations for evaluating and treating hyperlipidemia. Clin Pharm 1986;5:113–127.
48. Illingworth DR. Lipid-lowering drugs. An overview of indications and optimum therapeutic use. Drugs 1987;33:259–279.
49. The Expert Panel. Report of the National Cholesterol Education Program Expert Panel on detection, evaluation, and treatment of high blood cholesterol in adults. Arch Intern Med 1988;148:36–69.
50. Brown WV, Goldberg IJ, Ginsberg HN. Treatment of common lipoprotein disorders. Prog Cardiovasc Dis 1984;27:1–20.
51. Knodel LC, Talbert RL. Adverse effects of hypolipidaemic drugs. Med Toxicol 1987;2:10–32.
52. Crouse JR, III. Hypertriglyceridemia: A contraindication to the use of bile acid binding resins. Am J Med 1987;83:243–248.
53. Shaefer MS, Jungnickel PW, Jacobs EW, et al. Acceptability of cholestyramine or colestipol combinations with six vehicles. Clin Pharm 1987;6:51–54.
54. Kane JP, Malloy MJ, Tun P, et al. Normalization of low-density-lipoprotein levels in heterozygous familial hypercholesterolemia with a combined drug regimen. N Engl J Med 1981;304:251–258.
55. Coronary Drug Project Research Group. Clofibrate and niacin in coronary heart disease. JAMA 1975;231:360–381.
56. Knopp RH, Ginsbery J, Algers JJ, et al. Contrasting effects of unmodified and time-release forms of niacin on lipoproteins in hyperlipidemic subjects: Clues to the mechanism of action of niacin. Metabolism 1985;34:642–650.
57. Hoeg JA, Maher MB, Dou E, et al. Normalization of plasma lipoprotein concentrations in patients with type II hyperlipoproteinemia by combined use of neomycin and niacin. Circulation 1984;70:1004–1011.
58. Dujovne CA, Atkins F, Wong B, et al. Electrocardiographic effects of probucol: A controlled perspective clinical trial. Eur J Clin Pharmacol 1984;26:735–739.
59. Coronary Drug Project Research Group. The Coronary Drug Project: Findings leading to further modifications of its protocol with respect to dextrothyroxine. JAMA 1972;220:996–1008.
60. Krukemyer JJ, Talbert RL. Lovastatin: A new cholesterol lowering agent. Pharmacotherapy 1987:198–210.
61. Illingworth DR. Mevinolin plus colestipol in therapy for severe heterozygous familial hypercholesterolemia. Ann Intern Med 1984;101:598–604.
62. Lovastatin Study Group II. Therapeutic response to lovastatin (mevinolin) in nonfamilial hypercholesterolemia. A multicenter study. JAMA 1986;256:2829–2834.
63. Helsinki Heart Study Ethical Committee. Safety as a factor in lipid-regulating primary prevention trials: The Helsinki Heart Study Intern Report, in Wood C (ed): Further Progress with Gemfibrozil. International Congress and Symposium Series No. 87. London, Royal Society of Medicine Servies Limited, 1986, pp 51–61.
64. Committee of Principal Investigators (WHO). A co-operative trial in the primary prevention of ischaemic heart disease using clofibrate. Br Heart J 1978;40:1069–1118.
65. Kuusisto P, Manninen V, Vapaatalo H, et al. Effect of activated charcoal on hypercholesterolaemia. Lancet 1986;2:366–367.
66. Herold PM, Kinsella JE. Fish oil consumption and decreased risk of cardiovascular disease: A comparison of findings from animal and human feeding trials. Am J Clin Nutr 1986;43:556–598.
67. Ballard-Barbash R, Callaway CW. Marine fish oils: Role in prevention of coronary artery disease. Mayo Clin Proc 1987;62:113–118.
68. Nestel PJ, Connor WE, Reardson MF, et al. Suppression by diets rich in fish oil of very low density lipoprotein production in man. J Clin Invest 1984;74:82–89.
69. Phillipson BE, Rothrock DW, Connor WE, et al. Reduction of plasma lipids, lipoproteins, and apoproteins by dietary fish oils in patients with hypertriglyceridemia. N Engl J Med 1985;312:1210–1216.
70. Hamazaki T, Nakazawa R, Tateno S, et al. Effects of fish oil rich in eicosapentaenoic acid on serum lipid hyperlipidemic haemodialysis patients. Kidney Int 1984:26:81–84.
71. Simopoulos AP. Summary of the conference on the health effects of polyunsaturated fatty acids in seafoods. J Nutr 1986;116:2350–2354.
72. Spengel FA, Jadhav A, Duffield RGM, et al. Superiority of partial ileal bypass over cholestyramine in reducing cholesterol in familial hypercholesterolemia. Lancet 1981;2:768–770.
73. Starlz TE, Chase HP, Ahrens EH, et al. Portacaval shunt in patients with familial hypercholesterolemia. Ann Surg 1983;198:273–283.

74. Thompson GR. Plasma exchange for hypercholesterolaemia. Lancet 1981;1:1246–1248.
75. Bilheimer DW, Goldstein JL, Grundy SM, et al. Liver transplantation to provide low-density lipoprotein receptors and lower plasma cholesterol in a child with homozygous familial hypercholesterolemia. N Engl J Med 1984;311:1658–1664.
76. Group of Physicians of the Newcastle upon Tyne Region. Trial of clofibrate in the treatment of ischaemic heart disease. Br Med J 1971;4:767–775.
77. Research Committee of the Scottish Society of Physicians. Ischaemic heart disease: A secondary prevention trial using clofibrate. Br Med J 1971;4:775–784.
78. Canner PL, Bierge KG, Wenger NK, et al. Fifteen year mortality in Coronary Drug Project patients: Long-term benefit with niacin. J Am Coll Cardiol 1986;8:1245–1255.
79. Manninen V. The gemfibrozil study. Acta Med Scand 1985; 701(suppl):83–89.
80. Frick MH, Elo O, Haapa K, et al. Helsinki Heart Study: Primary-prevention trial with gemfibrozil in middle-aged men with dyslipidemia. N Engl J Med 1987;317:1237–1245.

# Chapter 20 / Thromboembolic Disorders

Keith A. Rodvold, PharmD, Christine M. Quandt, PharmD,
and William R. Friedenberg, MD

Venous thromboembolism (venous thrombosis and pulmonary embolism) is a serious and potentially fatal disorder that most often occurs in bedridden hospitalized patients, but may also affect otherwise healthy ambulatory individuals. Pulmonary embolism is responsible for greater than 50,000 deaths per year in the United States.[1] This fatality rate is particularly tragic because it develops in the absence of any established life-threatening conditions in one fourth to one half of these patients. Pulmonary embolism arises from thrombi in the deep venous system, usually of the lower extremities. Venous thrombosis can involve the superficial large veins, deep veins of the calf, and deep veins above the knee (popliteal and proximal veins). It appears that the larger leg veins (those above the knee) are the most common source of those pulmonary emboli that reach clinical attention (see Fig. 20.1). Thrombosis of the deep calf vein is a less serious disorder than proximal vein thrombosis because the thrombi are generally smaller in patients with calf vein thrombosis and are less frequently associated with clinical disability or major complications including pulmonary embolism.

The clinical diagnosis of venous thrombosis and pulmonary embolism is notoriously unreliable; therefore, clinicians faced with suspected thromboembolism have two major responsibilities: confirming the diagnosis and choosing the most appropriate treatment. In general, treatment is started on clinical presentation, and the decision to continue or discontinue treatment is then based on the results of confirmatory diagnostic testing.

## Etiology

Several risk factors for venous thromboembolism have been identified. These include obesity, heart disease (especially congestive heart failure), trauma, paralysis, malignancy (particularly of the pancreas, lungs, or gastrointestinal system), pregnancy, surgery, estrogen use, and some blood dyscrasias. These are summarized in Table 20.1. With malignancy the incidence of venous thromboembolism is increased threefold.[2] The overall incidence of thrombi in patients who undergo major surgical procedures is 30% to 35%. This incidence increases in hip surgery. Fatal pulmonary embolism has been reported in 4% to 7% of patients after emergency hip surgery, and in 0.3% to 1.7% of patients after elective hip surgery.[3,4]

The fate of a given venous thrombus depends on its size and the balance between factors that either promote its extension or lead to its removal. Extension may occur if there is significant endothelial damage, tissue injury, or stasis. Fibrinolysis, digestion of fibrin by leukocytes, or embolization will lead to removal of the thrombus. Complete spontaneous lysis is uncommon with large venous thrombi, in contrast to small asymptomatic calf vein thrombi, which often spontaneously dissolve. Clinically silent pulmonary embolism occurs in approximately 50% of patients with documented proximal venous thrombosis (as determined by perfusion lung scanning) at the time of presentation.[5] Patients with proximal vein thrombosis have larger and more frequent pulmonary emboli compared with patients with calf vein thrombosis.[6] Approximately 70% of patients with symptomatic pulmonary embolism have concurrent asymptomatic venous thrombosis, usually involving the proximal veins. Most fatal pulmonary emboli arise from proximal-vein thrombi.

## Pathophysiology

Venous thromboembolism arises by three fundamental mechanisms: vascular injury, venous stasis, and hypercoagulability.[7] Veins react to noxious stimuli in a stereotypic fashion. Mechanical or chemical injury to the intima of vessel walls provokes an inflammatory response (phlebitis) that leads to local hemostasis and formation of an intraluminal clot. Vascular injury is an important etiologic mechanism after trauma or surgery. Venipuncture, indwelling cannulas and catheters, and chemical irritation by infused or injected agents such as potassium or hypertonic glucose may also result in thrombophlebitis.

### *Stasis*

Venous stasis, or altered blood flow in the deep veins of the lower limbs, plays a key role in the initiation of venous thrombi. Venostasis may result from ineffective venous emptying of the veins from prolonged bed rest, venous insufficiency or varicose veins, venous obstruction because of a tumor, massive obesity, late-stage pregnancy, an arterial anomaly, low systemic blood flow from shock, hypovolemia or severe myocardial infarction. Even short periods of stasis can cause hypoxia and endothelial damage to venous valves, creating a setting in which platelets and procoagulants can interact[8]; thrombi may then form in the pockets of these valves. In addition, a decrease in blood flow prevents activated clotting factors from being diluted by nonactivated blood, prevents their hepatic clearance, and prevents mixing of activated clotting factors with their inhibitors.[5]

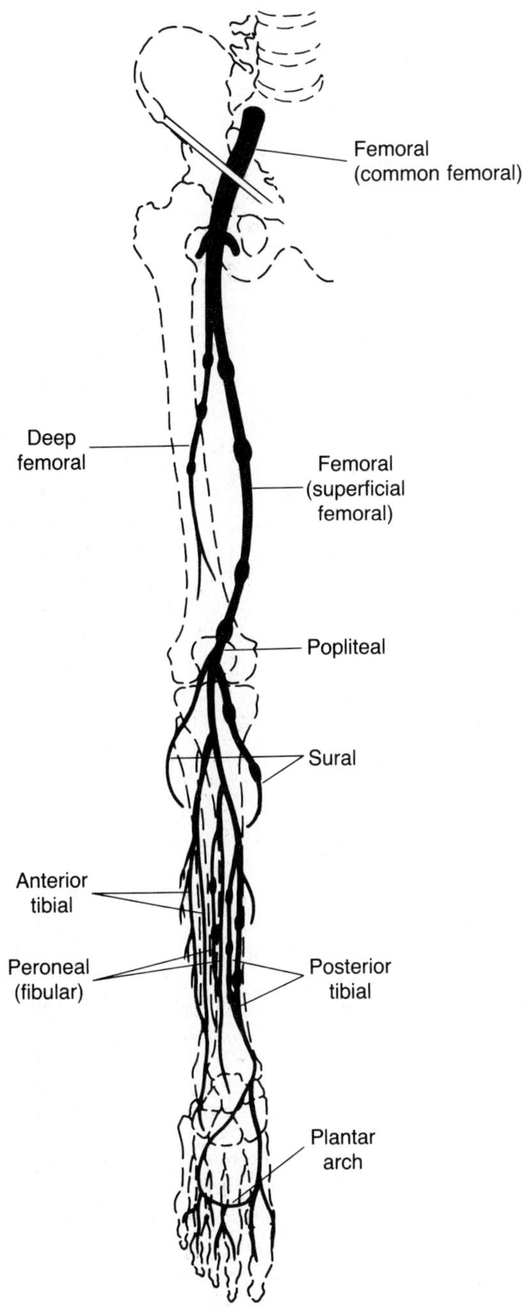


**Figure 20.1** Anatomy of deep veins of lower extremity. *(From Kazimer FJ, Juergens JL: Venous thrombosis and obstructive disease of the veins, in Juergens JL (Ed): Peripheral Vascular Diseases. Philadelphia, W.B. Saunders, 1980, p 733, with permission.)*

### *Activation of Coagulation*

The coagulation cascade, involving a chain of enzymatic reactions that result in the formation and polymerization of fibrin, can be activated by platelet adhesion and aggregation or by the release of tissue thromboplastin or collagen during surgery or trauma. Other conditions that can cause hypercoagulable states include malignancy, pregnancy, and antithrombin III or protein C deficiency[9] (see Table 20.1).

The blood coagulation process can be activated by intrinsic or extrinsic pathways. In the intrinsic pathway all necessary clotting factors are present in the circulating blood.[10] This pathway is initiated when blood comes into contact with a foreign surface. Factor XII, under the influence of kallikrein and high-molecular-weight kininogen, is converted to its active form, XIIa, which in turn converts factor XI into XIa (Fig. 20.2). Factor XIa then activates factor IX. Factor IXa together with factor VIII, calcium, and phospholipid activates factor X.

The extrinsic pathway is activated by tissue thromboplastin, a tissue factor released after vessel damage. Tissue thromboplastin combines with and activates factor VII to form a complex that activates factor X. The extrinsic and intrinsic pathways meet at this point and continue along a common pathway to convert prothrombin to thrombin. Next, thrombin converts fibrinogen to fibrin and activates factor XII, which stabilizes the fibrin polymers.

Blood coagulation is modified by a number of negative-feedback loops and by other mechanisms that tend to limit thrombus formation. The most important of these are prostacyclin synthesis, the activation of protein C, fibrinolysis, and the presence of antithrombin III. Prostacyclin, a potent vasodilator and inhibitor of platelet aggregation, is synthesized in the vessel wall in response to thrombin generation or endothelial injury. Thrombin can also combine with its endothelial cofactor thrombomodulin and transform protein C into activated protein C. Activated protein C inactivates factors VIIIa and Va and initiates fibrinolysis. Newly discovered protein S is a cofactor for activated protein C and is

**Table 20.1** Risk Factors Predisposing to Thromboembolism

| |
|---|
| Inherited risk factors |
| Antithrombin III deficiency |
| Protein C deficiency |
| Protein S deficiency |
| Dysfibrinogenemia |
| Disorders of plasminogen and plasminogen activation |
| Acquired risk factors |
| Lupus anticoagulant |
| Nephrotic syndrome |
| Paroxysmal nocturnal hemoglobinuria |
| Cancer |
| Stasis—congestive heart failure, myocardial infarction, cardiomyopathy, constrictive pericarditis, anasarca |
| Advancing age |
| Estrogen therapy |
| Sepsis |
| Immobilization |
| Stroke |
| Polycythemia rubra vera |
| Inflammatory bowel disease |
| Obesity |
| Prior thromboembolism |

From the Consensus Development Panel: Prevention of Venous Thrombosis and Pulmonary Embolism. JAMA 1986;256:744–749, with permission.

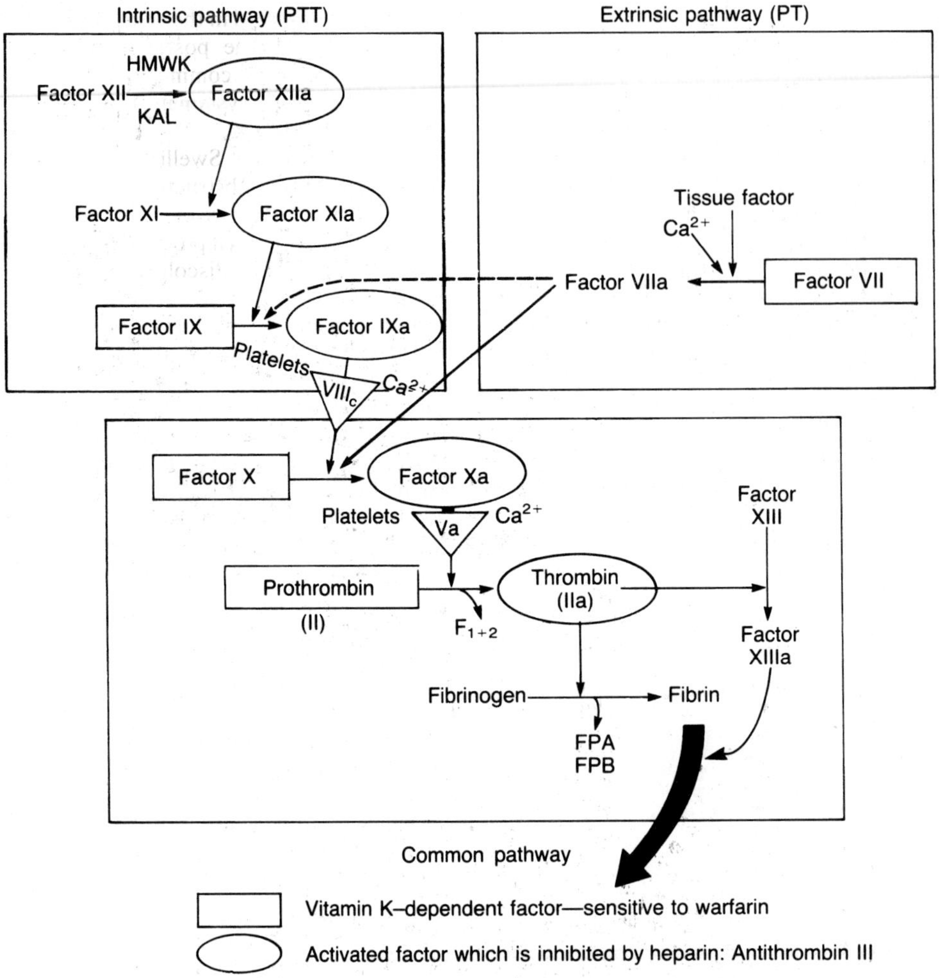


**Figure 20.2** The coagulation cascade. HMWK, high-molecular-weight kininogen; KAL, kallikrein. *(From Stead RB: Clinical pharmacology, in Goldhaber SZ (Ed): Pulmonary Embolism and Deep Venous Thrombosis. Philadedlphia, WB Saunders, 1985, p 100, with permission.)*

required for the anticoagulant action of protein C.[11] The fibrinolytic system involves the conversion of plasminogen to plasmin, which cleaves fibrin into soluble fragments and degrades fibrinogen into fibrin degradation products. Antithrombin III is a plasma protein that inhibits thrombin activity by forming a covalent complex with it.[10] Patients who are congenitally deficient in antithrombin III, protein C, or protein S are at increased risk of thromboembolic disease.[12,13]

### *Venous Thrombosis/Pulmonary Embolism*

Venous thrombi are composed predominantly of fibrin and red blood cells and a smaller number of platelets and leukocytes. The majority of thrombi form in valve cusp pockets or bifurcations of the lower extremities, especially the calf. The six major sites of origin of thrombi are (1) the external iliac vein, just above the inguinal ligament; (2) the common femoral vein; (3) the deep femoral vein; (4) the popliteal vein; (5) the posterior tibial veins; and (6) the intramuscular veins of the calf, particularly the soleal veins[14] (see Fig. 20.1). The major consequences of deep-vein thrombi (DVTs) include compromised blood flow to the lower extremity, destruction of the venous architecture, and embolization. Venous valves are destroyed when valvular endothelium is involved with thrombus organization and vein recanalization.[9] This may result in abnormal venous circulation and venous hypertension.

When venous thrombi dislodge from the site of formation, they flow through the venous system to the pulmonary arterial circulation. About 15% to 20% of venous thrombi in the legs embolize to the lungs.[9] These emboli most often originate from proximal veins in the leg (above the knee). Calf vein thrombi embolize less often and are usually of minor consequence; however, up to 30% propagate to sites above the knee where they are more likely to embolize.[15] An embolism occluding more than one third of the major pulmonary arterial flow is often associated with acute right ventricular failure and sudden death.[16] A large embolus in the main pulmonary artery or one of its primary branches may also cause sudden death. Small emboli are more likely to lodge in more peripheral areas of the lung and often cause no clinically significant pulmonary effects.

The cardiac and pulmonary status of the patient prior to an embolic event plays an important role in the morbidity and mortality. Occlusion of a pulmonary vessel results in acute mechanical obstruction of blood flow, reflex or humoral vasoconstriction, and bronchoconstriction. If the right ventricle is compromised, this increase in vascular resistance may result in heart failure. A preexisting lung abnormality, such as infection or pulmonary edema, increases the likelihood of pulmonary infarction. Even a small embolus in a patient with a compromised pulmonary reserve may be fatal.

A late sequela of DVT is a symptom complex known as postthrombotic syndrome. The symptoms range from leg swelling with discomfort to debilitating pain and ulceration. These symptoms are usually due to either proximal occlusion of the venous system or valvular incompetence.

## Clinical Presentation

The most important point to remember when evaluating the signs and symptoms of acute venous thrombosis is that they are not specific and may result from a variety of other diseases (see Table 20.2 for the differential diagnosis of DVT). Pain and tenderness are common complaints, although their severity usually has no relation to the size or extent of thrombosis. With calf vein thrombosis, the pain and tenderness are usually localized to the calf, but may also extend along the anterior and medial aspects of the thigh and into the groin. Patients with proximal-vein thrombosis are more likely to have diffuse pain, although it may be localized to the calf, thigh, or buttock. Patients with suspected DVT should be examined in the horizontal position with the knees slightly flexed. The posterior tibial, peroneal, popliteal, superficial femoral, common femoral, and iliac veins should be palpated in a systematic fashion. Pain and tenderness located in regions other than those just mentioned suggest another diagnosis.[17] Swelling may also occur as a result of edema caused by obstruction of large proximal veins or by inflammation of perivascular tissues.

**Table 20.2** Differential Diagnosis of the Clinical Features of Deep-Vein Thrombosis

| |
|---|
| Pain and/or tenderness |
| Muscle strain or trauma |
| Muscle tear |
| Direct muscle or leg trauma |
| Spontaneous muscle hematoma |
| Arterial insufficiency |
| Neurogenic pain |
| Ruptured Baker's cyst |
| Arthritis of the knee or ankle joint or achilles tendonitis |
| Varicose veins |
| Pregnancy |
| Oral contraceptive use |
| Leg swelling |
| Compression of the iliac vein |
| Postphlebitic syndrome |
| Leg immobilization |
| Leg inflammation |
| Lymphedema |
| Lipedema |
| Self-induced edema |

Adapted from Hirsh J, et al: Clinical features and diagnosis of venous thrombosis. J Am Coll Cardiol 1986;8:114B–127B, with permission.

Other signs and symptoms of DVT include Homan's sign, a palpable cord, or discoloration. Discomfort in the upper calf on forced dorsiflexion of the foot (Homan's sign) is both insensitive and nonspecific, being present in less than one third of patients with documented thrombosis and in 50% of patients who do not have DVT.[17] A palpable cord is an uncommon sign of DVT, and may be difficult to differentiate from a venous cord resulting from edema or hemorrhage of the calf muscle. A palpable cord noted in the subcutaneous area of the extremity is compatible with superficial phlebitis. In patients with DVT, the leg may occasionally be pale, cyanotic, or a reddish purple color. Rarely, the leg may be diffusely red, hot, and tender as a result of marked perivascular inflammation, and this may be difficult to differentiate from cellulitis. With obstructive iliofemoral vein thrombosis the leg is often very painful, with marked swelling, cyanosis, and multiple petechial hemorrhages (phlegmasia cerulea dolens). The differential diagnosis of venous thrombosis must include muscle strain or trauma, arterial insufficiency, other inflammatory conditions such as arthritis, cellulitis, lymphangitis, vasculitis, myositis, ruptured Baker's cyst, varicose veins, and pregnancy (see Table 20.2).

Pulmonary embolism presents in a variety of ways depending on the size, location, and number of emboli and the patient's underlying condition. These include (1) transient dyspnea and tachypnea; (2) the syndrome of pulmonary infarction or atelectasis, which includes pleuritic chest pain, cough, hemoptysis, pleural effusion, and pulmonary infiltrates on chest x-ray; (3) right-ventricular failure with severe dyspnea and tachypnea; and (4) cardiovascular collapse with hypotension, syncope, and coma.[18] The most common signs and symptoms are tachypnea, rales, pleuritic chest pain, dyspnea, apprehension, and cough.

## Diagnosis

### *Venous Thrombosis*

Clinical evaluation of a patient with venous thromboembolism involves obtaining a complete medical history and a careful physical exam. The medical history is important in establishing predisposing factors that lead to the diagnosis; as previously mentioned, physical findings are nonspecific and unreliable. The diagnosis of venous thrombosis and embolism depends largely upon objective tests. Venography is the gold standard for the diagnosis of deep-vein thrombosis. This test is used to outline the deep venous system of the legs by injecting radiopaque contrast medium into the dorsal foot vein. Ascending venography is used to visualize the deep veins of the calf, the popliteal vein, the femoral vein, and in most patients the external and common iliac veins; however, iliac venography may be needed if the external and common iliac veins are not visualized by the ascending technique or if the inferior vena cava is to be outlined.[17] With this technique, contrast medium is injected directly into the common femoral vein, given by intraosseous injection, or given by retrograde injection by means of a catheter passed through the right atrium and inferior vena cava. The femoral vein puncture is the simplest and most widely used technique, although retrograde catheterization is sometimes used to also visualize the internal iliac system or when combined with pulmonary angiography. Complications of venography include pain during or after injection of the contrast medium, fat emboli (with the intraosseous technique), allergy to contrast medium, and superficial phlebitis.

Iodine-labeled-fibrinogen leg scanning is a method commonly used for detecting DVT. After intravenous injection of radiolabeled fibrinogen, the radioactive tracer tags fibrin as it is incorporated into an existing or growing thrombus. The local accumulation of radioactivity is then detected with an isotope detector. Fibrinogen scanning is used for screening patients who are at risk for developing DVT or as a complement to impedance plethysmography to confirm or exclude the diagnosis of venous thrombosis. Advantages of this technique include minimal invasiveness and over 90% sensitivity in detecting acute calf vein thrombosis.[17] The disadvantages are that this technique requires at least 24 to 48 hours to establish a definitive diagnosis, it is insensitive for proximal or pelvic vein thrombosis, and false positives are common in any area of inflammation or increased fibrin deposition.

Impedance plethysmography (IPG) is a noninvasive technique for measuring volume changes in the legs. This technique is performed with the patient supine and the legs elevated 20–30°, the knees slightly flexed, and the ankle elevated 8–15 cm above the knee. A pneumatic cuff is applied to the midthigh and inflated to 45 cm $H_2O$, thereby occluding venous return. After a predetermined period of time, the cuff is deflated and the change in electrical resistance resulting from changes in blood volume distal to the cuff is detected by four circumferential calf electrodes connected to the plethysmograph, which contains a strip chart recorder. Measurements are made of the total increase in resistance during cuff inflation and of the decrease in blood volume within 3 seconds of cuff release. These measurements are plotted on a special graph and results are reported as normal or abnormal based on whether they fall above or below a discriminant line developed by Hull et al.[19] Impedance plethysmography has a sensitivity and specificity of 94% based on correlation with 2,561 venograms.[20] A recent cost analysis of diagnostic tests used in patients with symptomatic DVT revealed that the combined approach of impedance plethysmography and leg scanning is essentially as effective as, and more cost effective than, venography.[21]

Other noninvasive tests used in the diagnosis of venous thrombosis include Doppler ultrasonography, air cuff and strain gauge plethysmography, and radioisotope techniques using technetium. The venous Doppler exam depends on sound waves being reflected from moving cells. Because the Doppler probe detects velocity of blood flow, the trained ear will recognize abnormal flow patterns produced by obstruction of the underlying veins. Doppler ultrasound is a sensitive method for detecting proximal-vein thrombosis, but is less sensitive for calf vein thrombosis. Air cuff and strain gauge plethysmography relies on the same principle as impedance plethysmography; however, other techniques are used to quantify the changes in blood volume.

Several radioisotope techniques have been used as an adjunct in the diagnosis of venous thrombosis, including radionuclide venography with various tracers. Radionuclide venography is used primarily for thrombosis in the thigh, particularly the iliac veins, where sensitivity and specificity approach 100%. This test is unreliable for calf and popliteal vein thrombosis.[17]

### *Pulmonary Embolism*

Patients with suspected pulmonary embolism (PE) should have an electrocardiogram, chest x-ray, and arterial blood analysis, as well as other more specific diagnostic tests such as pulmonary angiography and lung scanning (Fig. 20.3). Pulmonary angiography is the reference standard for diagnosing pulmonary embolism. A positive diagnosis is made if there is a constant intraluminal filling defect seen on multiple films or if sharp cutoffs are seen in vessels greater than 2.5 mm in diameter.[18] This technique may have insufficient sensitivity to detect small emboli, and it is associated with morbidity and mortality rates of 4% and 0.2%, respectively, because of the complications of hypotension, arrhythmias, endocardial or myocardial injury, cardiac arrest, and hypersensitivity reactions.[22] Pulmonary angiography should not be used in patients with severe chronic pulmonary hypertension or severe cardiac or respiratory decompensation. Therefore, pulmonary angiography should probably be reserved for patients with moderate probability or indeterminate lung scans that make the diagnosis of pulmonary embolism by lung scan equivocal.

The lung scan is the diagnostic examination most often utilized for patients with suspected pulmonary embolism. Perfusion lung scanning usually involves the use of techne-

**Figure 20.3** Diagnostic algorithm for patients with suspected pulmonary embolism (PE). *V–Q*, ventilation–perfusion; IPG, impedance plethysmography. *(From Hirsch J, Hull RD, Raskob GE: Diagnosis of pulmonary embolism. J Am Coll Cardiol 1986;8:134B, with permission.)*

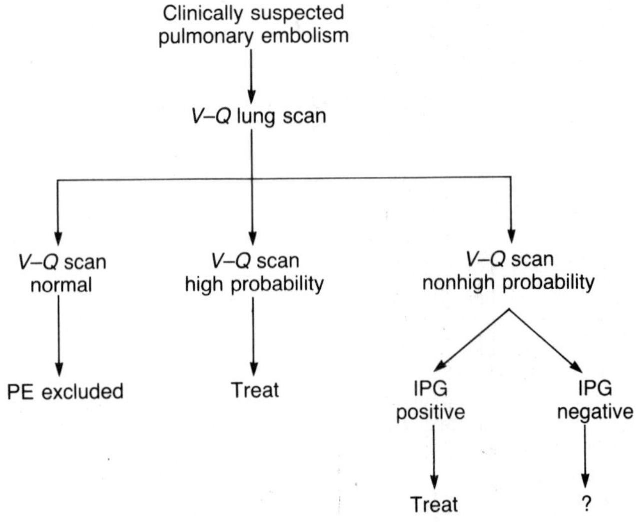

tium-99$m$-macroaggregated albumin or albumin microspheres. The perfusion technique utilizes the lungs as a filter to remove intravenously injected particulate matter. Injected particles are thoroughly mixed within the right heart chambers so that distribution is uniform and these particles remain trapped within the pulmonary vasculature; thus, gamma counters can be used to record areas of lung perfusion. The perfusion scan cannot distinguish between disturbances in pulmonary blood flow from PE and from other causes; therefore, it is nonspecific. The specificity can be improved by using ventilation–perfusion lung scanning. Ventilation imaging employs the principle that ventilation is preserved in areas of reduced perfusion resulting from pulmonary embolism (ventilation–perfusion mismatch), whereas ventilation is abnormal when perfusion defects are caused by the physiologic response to primary lung disease (ventilation–perfusion match). Ventilation scans involve either inhalation of radioactive gases or, much less frequently, intravenous injection of a diffusable radioactive gas dissolved in saline. In patients who undergo ventilation–perfusion lung scanning, the correlation between a scan showing a high probability of PE and the presence of PE on angiography is greater than 90%. Conversely, a normal lung scan will usually exclude the possibility of clinically significant pulmonary embolism.

## Treatment

The main objectives of treating venous thrombosis are (1) to prevent the development of pulmonary embolism, (2) to prevent the postphlebitic syndrome, (3) to reduce morbidity from the acute event, and (4) to achieve these objectives with a minimum of adverse effects and cost. Thus, successful treatment of DVT should prevent extension of the thrombus, prevent embolism to the lungs, and restore patency to the venous circulation, while maintaining normal venous valve function. General management of DVT includes bed rest, with the heels elevated above the heart to enhance venous return, and administration of analgesics for pain. For pulmonary embolism, oxygen should be given and, if necessary, patients should be mechanically ventilated. Definitive management of acute DVT and PE includes anticoagulation, thrombolytic therapy, embolectomy, or inferior vena caval (IVC) interruption.

### *Heparin*

Heparin, which was described by McLean as a medical student in 1916, is the mainstay for the prevention and treatment of venous thromboembolism.[23] Heparin is a complex mucopolysaccharide that is extracted either from porcine gastrointestinal sources or from beef lung. Commercially available heparin is a heterogeneous mixture of polymers ranging from 5,000 to 50,000 in molecular weight, with varying antithrombotic activity. Apparently, a small and distinct fraction of the heparin molecule is responsible for most of its anticoagulant effect. Anticoagulant therapy with heparin is complicated by the chemical and pharmacologic heterogeneity of the product, which accounts for some of the inter- and intraindividual differences in anticoagulant

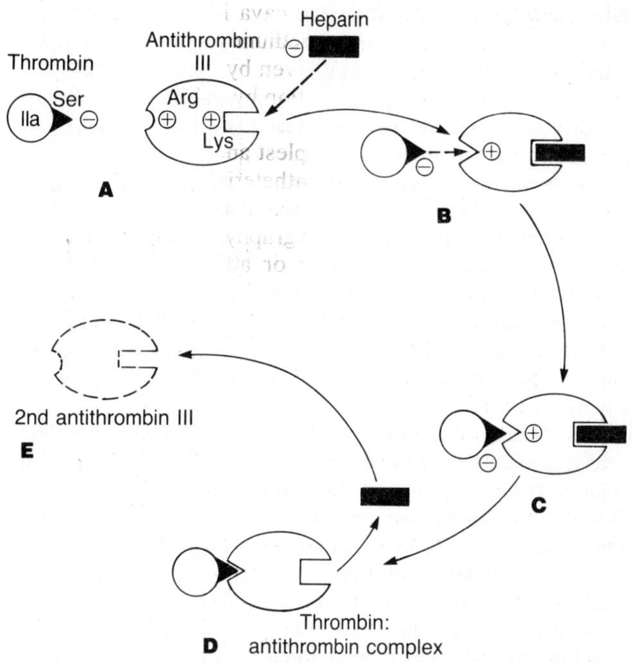


**Figure 20.4** Mechanism of action of heparin. Heparin interacts with antithrombin III, which catalyzes the formation of thrombin:antithrombin complexes. Heparin and antithrombin also inactivate factors XIIa, XIa, and Xa by a similar mechanism. *(From Stead RB: Clinical pharmacology, in Goldhaber SZ (Ed): Pulmonary Embolism and Deep Venous Thrombosis. Philadelphia, W.B. Saunders, 1985, p 101, with permission.)*

response.[9] The rationale for using heparin is to prevent further coagulation and propagation of the thrombus and to prevent recurrent DVT and PE. Heparin does not alter a formed thrombus; rather, it allows the body's natural lytic mechanisms to dissolve the previously formed clot. The anticoagulant function of heparin is thought to depend upon its ability to bind to and catalyze antithrombin III (AT-III) or heparin cofactor, a circulating anticoagulant that neutralizes the proteolytic activities of several clotting factors that have a serine residue at their enzymatically active site.[24] These activated clotting factors include factors XII, XI, X, and IX, kallikrein, and thrombin (see Fig. 20.4). The lack of a readily available direct chemical assay for heparin has limited available pharmacokinetic data. Few carefully designed prospective evaluations of the disposition of heparin in patients are available. No data are available on the rate and extent of absorption of heparin after oral administration; the total amount of heparin required to achieve the same degree of anticoagulant effect over the same time period does not appear to differ whether the agent is administered by intravenous, subcutaneous, or intrapulmonary routes.[25] Some studies have demonstrated significantly lower peak plasma heparin concentrations or decreased anticoagulant effects from the calcium salts; other investigators have failed to find significant differences between sodium and calcium salts.[26,27]

Heparin is distributed primarily throughout the vascular system, and the apparent volume of distribution quantitatively resembles that of plasma or blood volume (mean $V_D$ =

60 mL/kg; range: 40–100).[28] The apparent volume of distribution is directly related to body weight, and it has been suggested that heparin doses for obese patients should be based on ideal body weight.[29] The volume of distribution of heparin varies widely between individual patients, and does not seem to correlate with specific diseases states. The metabolism and excretion of heparin are complex, but involve primarily the metabolic processes of depolymerization and desulfation. Enzymes likely involved in heparin degradation include heparinases and desulfatases.

The anticoagulant activity of heparin in plasma decreases exponentially with time after intravenous administration; however, the half-life increases with increasing dose. The biologic half-life of heparin in humans after a single intravenous injection has been reported to range from 0.4 to 2.5 hours.[28] Heparin clearance ranges from 0.25 to 2 mL/min/kg, and has been found to be related to both total body weight and ideal body weight.[28] Up to a tenfold range in heparin half-life has been reported within individual studies involving the administration of large doses. The interpatient variability in heparin clearance is reported to be 6- to 12-fold. The disappearance of the anticoagulant activity follows nonlinear pharmacokinetics and it has been described by a combination of a saturable and a linear mechanism.[30,31] Heparin elimination is not influenced by renal and hepatic dysfunction.

Patients with pulmonary embolism have shorter heparin elimination half-lives and more rapid total clearances than patients treated for venous thrombosis. Hirsh et al[32] reported a 600% range in heparin clearance in 20 patients with thromboembolic diease. Four of these patients treated for PE had higher mean clearances than did the 16 patients with DVT. This observation was supported by investigators who have recommended larger heparin doses for patients with pulmonary emboli. Elliott and colleagues[33] prospectively evaluated 31 patients, however, and reported no significant differences in dosage requirements between patients with PE and DVT. Similarly, White et al[34] investigated the relationship between heparin dosage requirements and the presence or absence of thromboembolic disease. Although they also reported no significant difference in heparin dosage requirements between patients with PE and DVT, patients with verified thromboembolic diseases required significantly larger mean heparin doses (25 U/kg/h) than did patients without thromboembolic disease (15 U/kg/h). Cipolle et al[35] found a correlation between the time delay from onset of symptoms to initiation of treatment and the heparin dosage requirements of 20 patients with thromboembolic disorders. These data indicate that patients with acute thromboembolic disorders have rapid clearance rates and require larger heparin doses to ensure adequate antithrombotic activity.

### Therapeutic Indications

Anticoagulation with heparin is indicated in patients with a thrombus extending above the popliteal vein because of the high incidence of PE and postphlebitic syndrome in these patients. Patients with symptomatic calf vein thrombosis should receive heparin, as recent studies have shown a higher incidence of recurrent DVT in proximal veins in non-anticoagulated patients compared with anticoagulated patients; however, there are no definitive recommendations in asymptomatic cases of calf vein thrombosis that are detected by routine postoperative leg scanning. Patients with superficial thrombophlebitis should not receive anticoagulation. Heparin is clearly indicated for patients with documented pulmonary embolism. Heparin is also used for the prevention of venous thromboembolism.

Heparin therapy is contraindicated in patients who are hypersensitive to the drug, who are actively bleeding, or who have hemophilia, thrombocytopenia, intracranial hemorrhage, bacterial endocarditis, active tuberculosis, ulcerative lesions of the gastrointestinal tract, severe hypertension, threatened abortion, or visceral carcinoma. Heparin should be withheld during and after surgery of the brain, eye, or spinal cord and should not be administered to patients undergoing lumbar puncture or regional anesthetic block. The drug should be used only when clearly indicated in pregnant women, despite its apparent lack of transfer across the placenta.[36]

### Clinical Efficacy

Heparin pharmacodynamic indices of efficacy and safety are the prevention of thrombosis and the absence of hemorrhagic episodes caused by excessive anticoagulation. The evidence that heparin is effective as an anticoagulant is well documented. In one evaluation of heparin for the treatment of PE in 114 patients, 5 out of the 19 control patients died as a result of the embolism and another 5 had a nonfatal recurrence. An 8% recurrence rate was observed among patients given heparin. In an appraisal of anticoagulation therapy for PE in 458 patients, 92% survived, as compared with 42% of the patients in whom anticoagulants were withheld because of medical contraindications.[37]

High rates of embolism and mortality are seen with venous thromboembolism not treated with anticoagulants. Zero to 5% of patients treated with adequate doses of intravenous heparin develop clinical evidence of recurrence, and the likelihood of fatal embolism during treatment is very low. There is good experimental evidence and persuasive clinical information that the risk of recurrence during treatment is greatest when the coagulation test results are consistently below the therapeutic range. Basu et al found that recurrence of venous thromboembolism, based on clinical diagnosis, was related to an activated partial thromboplastin time (APTT) less than 1.5 times the normal rate on two or more consecutive days during continuous intravenous heparin therapy.[38] In a study by Wilson et al using more objective diagnostic criteria, the same trend was observed in patients being monitored with coagulation tests.[39]

### Administration/Monitoring

Heparin has traditionally been initiated with an intravenous bolus injection (i.e., 5,000–10,000 units) and followed by an intravenous continuous infusion (i.e., 1,000 units per hour) or intermittent injections (i.e., 5,000 units every 4–6 hours). To date, the most efficient method for providing patients with rapid and effective heparin anticoagulation is for the clinician to consider heparin pharmacokinetic and pharmacodynamic data to determine individual initial dosages, systematically monitor anticoagulation studies, and then make quantitative dosage adjustments as indicated. Thus, doses based on body weight are recommended (see Fig.

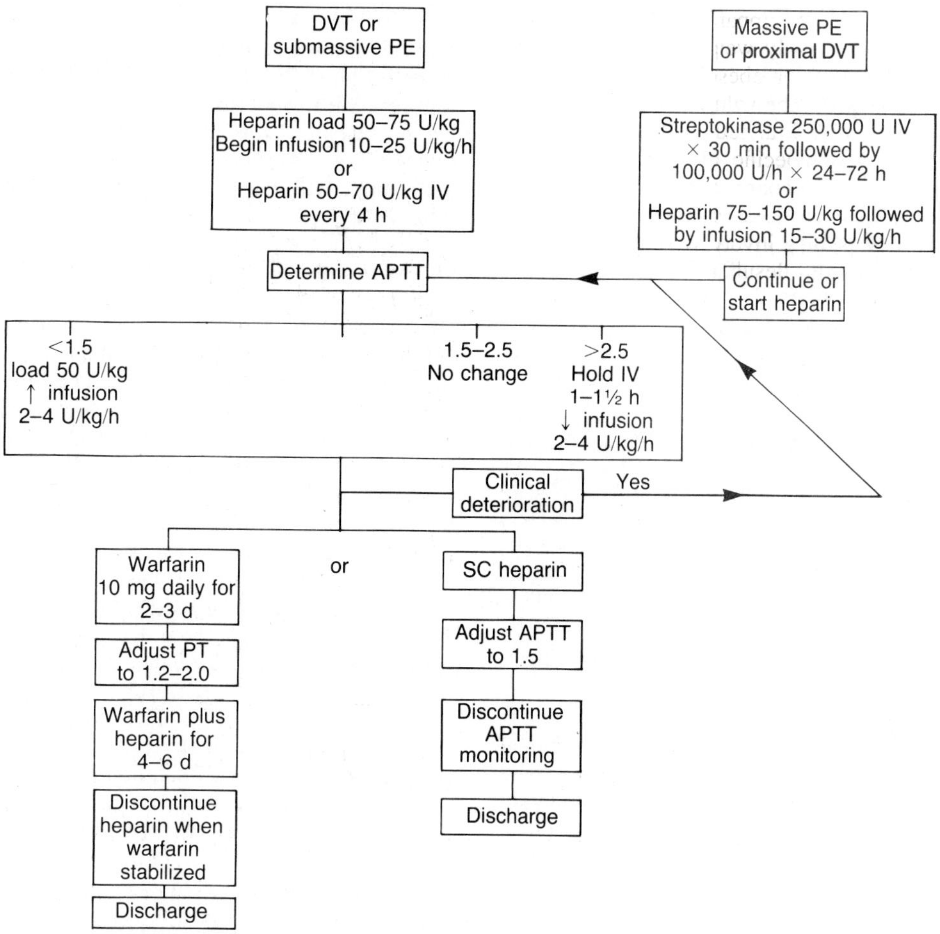


**Figure 20.5** Algorithm for the acute management of pulmonary embolism (PE) and deep-vein thrombosis (DVT). *Note:* If heparin is initiated before the diagnosis of massive PE or proximal DVT is confirmed, it should be discontinued before initiating thrombolytic therapy. *(Adapted from Carter BL, Jones ME, Waickman LA: Pathophysiology and treatment of deep-vein thrombosis and pulmonary embolism. Clin Pharm 1985;4:282, with permission.)*

20.5): a loading dose of 50–150 U/kg and an initial infusion rate of 10–30 U/kg/h.[9,28]

It is imperative that blood samples for coagulation tests (i.e., APTT) used to make heparin dosage adjustments be carefully timed. This requires that after beginning the heparin infusion or after any dosage change, the clinician wait at least 6 hours (preferably 8 hours) to draw samples for coagulation tests to assess the effect of the heparin dose. Samples collected too early are often misleading, resulting in inappropriate dosage alteration, and frequently start a costly cycle of "dosage change–coagulation test–another dosage change–another coagulation test" in a clinically stable patient. It is often most efficient to wait until steady-state conditions exist to monitor coagulation and make dosage alterations. The risk of bleeding is minimal during the first 48 hours of heparin therapy (in patients without identified risk factors), and coagulation tests are helpful primarily to ensure adequate heparinization.

When a continuous infusion is not feasible, heparin can be administered by intermittent intravenous injections. Heparin half-life ranges from 0.4 to 2.5 hours; therefore, every-4-hour dosing intervals are appropriate for most patients. Coagulation tests are best performed 3.5 to 4 hours after the heparin injection. It is imperative to time and document carefully both the injection and the sample for the coagulation test. The heparin dosage is considered adequate when the coagulation test collected 3.5 hours after an intravenous injection is in the therapeutic range for that test (i.e., APTT 1.5 to 2.5 times baseline).

Once a heparin dose has been determined that produces the desired degree of anticoagulation, daily monitoring of coagulation tests for minor dosing adjustments is indicated. Large variations in subsequent coagulation tests necessitate investigations to ensure that the patient's condition has not dramatically changed (i.e., extension or recurrence of the thromboembolic event). Additionally, before dosages are dramatically altered on the basis of fluctuating coagulation test results, the clinician must be certain that the prescribed heparin dose is being administered accurately and that blood samples are being collected and assayed appropriately. If substantial heparin dosage changes are made, the new therapy needs to be monitored in a manner similar to the initial heparin therapy.

Coagulation tests should be performed prior to the initiation of heparin therapy (1) to establish the patient's baseline APTT value which assists in determining the endpoint for heparin therapy and (2) to establish a baseline prothrombin time (PT) as a guide for later oral anticoagulation with warfarin. Additional necessary baseline laboratory parameters include quantitative platelet count prior to heparinization, every 2 or 3 days during therapy, and after the discontinuation of therapy, to determine the risk for thrombosis and/or hemorrhage from heparin-associated thrombocytopenia. Hemoglobin and hematocrit measurements are indicated prior to heparinization and every 1 to 2 days while the patient is receiving heparin, to identify the presence of bleeding. These laboratory parameters are especially useful in determining the existence of occult bleeding, such as retroperitoneal hemorrhage. Sputum and stool should be examined daily for the presence of blood.

Patients should be examined twice daily for signs of bleeding including intravenous catheter sites, hematomas, and ecchymosis. Intramuscular injections should not be administered to patients receiving therapeutic heparinization. Additionally, invasive procedures that can be rescheduled should not be performed on heparinized patients.

The signs and symptoms of pulmonary embolism should be monitored every shift for 1 to 2 days followed by daily monitoring for changes in dyspnea, apprehension, cough, pleuritic chest pain, and hemoptysis. Additionally, repeat arterial blood gases and lung scans and/or perfusion–ventilation studies may be indicated to assess progress of antithrombotic therapy. Similarly, patients being treated for venous thrombosis should be initially monitored twice daily and then daily for changes in pain, limb circumference, swelling, and tenderness.

In addition to the laboratory and clinical parameters just mentioned, clinicians must be aware of other practical concerns in patients receiving heparin. Hattersley et al reported that the four most common errors associated with heparin therapy were (1) lack of precision of pumps being used to infuse heparin, (2) interruption in the continuous infusion, (3) errors in preparation of the solution containing the heparin dose, and (4) errors in charting the dose administered.[40] For the intravenous administration of continuous-infusion heparin, reliable volumetric infusion pumps should be used. Every effort should be made not to interrupt the continuous infusions. During a 1-hour interruption, the APTT can fall from 60 seconds (therapeutic) to less than 40 seconds; hence interruptions in the infusion longer than 30 to 60 minutes may require an additional bolus injection in addition to restarting the infusion.

Finally, to properly interpret a coagulation test, it is essential to know the actual rate of heparin infusion. Failure to adequately document and chart heparin infusion rates can lead to potentially serious errors. The importance of this problem is exemplified by the Boston Collaborative Drug Surveillance Program, which involved 2,656 heparinized patients. The actual heparin doses received could not be determined in 30% of the patients because of inadequate drug administration records.[41]

#### Laboratory Monitoring

The APTT has become the most popular test for monitoring heparin therapy largely because of its suitability for use in routine clinical laboratories, the rapidity with which it can be performed, and its reproducibility.[42] The APTT is a global test that measures the resultant activity from the balance between activators and inhibitors of the intrinsic and common pathways of the coagulation system. Platelet-poor plasma is activated by contact agents in the presence of phospholipid and then recalcified. The APTT uses the generation of a fibrin clot as its endpoint. The APTT reacts similarly with heparin derived from bovine lung and porcine mucosa. There are two major disadvantages to using APTT to monitor heparin therapy: it is unable to distinguish between the anticoagulant activity of heparin and several clotting factor deficiencies, and the instrumentation used requires that the APTT be performed in a laboratory.

Clinicians try to balance prevention of unwanted clotting and increased risk of hemorrhage by keeping the degree of anticoagulation within the therapeutic range (APTT between 1.5 and 2.5 times control or baseline). Normal adult control values vary among laboratories and range from about 28 to 42 seconds. Although there are no prospective controlled studies, some observational studies offer qualitative evidence that monitoring is useful. In the absence of randomized studies, evidence of a correlation between elevated APTT and risk of hemorrhage is suggestive but not conclusive. Similarly, the association between subtherapeutic APTT values and recurrent thrombosis is suggested but not firmly established.[38] In addition, there have been no studies of optimal timing of APTT determinations in monitoring patients on heparin therapy.

#### Adverse Effects

Hemorrhage is the adverse effect of greatest concern with anticoagulant therapy. The risk of major bleeding (bleeding requiring blood transfusion or discontinuation of the anticoagulant) with therapeutic doses of heparin for the treatment of thromboembolic disease has been reported to range from 1% to 33%, although most studies have reported a frequency between 2% and 5%.[43,44] The most frequently encountered bleeding episodes include melena, hematomas, and hematuria, which occur in 2% to 3% of patients.[44] Less common are ecchymosis, epistaxis, and hematemesis, which occur in 0.5% to 1.2% of patients.

The incidence of hemorrhagic complications is thought to be related to the dose, the method of administration, the duration of heparin therapy, and several patient-related factors. Several studies have shown that the risk of bleeding sharply increases as the dose increases and with administration of heparin by intermittent bolus as compared with continuous infusion. Exceeding the normal values of "therapeutic" coagulation tests has been suggested to be predictive of these hemorrhagic complications. Conti et al, however, reported that 84.7% of patients experiencing major bleeding episodes had "therapeutic" activated coagulation times.[45] Mant et al found that neither heparin dose nor APTT results could be related to bleeding complications.[46] Overall, prophylactic low-dose heparin (5,000 units subcutaneously every 12 hours) is not associated with increased risk of major hemorrhage, and the risk of minor bleeding is very low. In

**Table 20.3** Indicators of Risk for Bleeding Among 2,656 Hospitalized Patients Receiving Heparin Sodium

| | *Relative risk for bleeding*[a] | |
|---|---|---|
| *Comparison* | **Minimal and moderate (*n* = 203)** | **Major (*n* = 35)** |
| Sex (F *v* M) | 1.5 (1.1, 1.9)[b] | 2.1 (1.1, 4.0) |
| Age | | |
| 40–59 *v* <40 | 0.9 (0.7, 1.3) | 2.3 (0.6, 8.7) |
| >60 *v* <40 | 1.1 (0.8, 1.5) | 3.1 (0.8, 11.4) |
| Dose, U/kg per dose | | |
| 50–99 *v* <50 | 2.0 (1.2, 3.1) | 1.3 (0.4, 4.3) |
| >100 *v* <50 | 3.2 (2.0, 5.1) | 2.6 (0.8, 8.2) |
| Frequency (every 2 h or every 3 h *v* other) | 0.4 (0.1, 1.5) | 0 |
| Aspirin (used *v* not used) | 1.5 (1.1, 2.0) | 2.4 (1.1, 5.1) |
| Survival (died[c] *v* survived; died this admission) | 1.6 (1.0, 2.6) | 4.0 (2.0, 8.2) |
| Alcohol, drinks per day (>5 or binge *v* ≤5) | 0.7 (0.3, 1.5) | 6.9 (2.2, 21) |
| BUN, mg/dL (≥50 *v* <50) | 1.0 (0.7, 1.7) | 2.0 (0.9, 4.5) |

[a] This is the ratio of "daily risks" between the comparison groups, as derived from a Cox life-table analysis. Each relative risk is adjusted for the effects of all other indicators listed, as well as for interhospital variation and duration of therapy.
[b] Numbers in parentheses are the 90% confidence intervals for the relative risk. These theoretical values of relative risk are consistent with the observed values at a one-sided *P* value of 0.05.
[c] Excluding deaths caused by hemorrhage.

From Walker AM, Jick H: Predictors of bleeding during heparin therapy. JAMA 1980;244:1211, with permission.

general, the risk of bleeding not only varies with the dose but also increases with the length of heparin therapy. The 7-day cumulative risk of bleeding during heparin therapy is 9.1%. Also, this cumulative risk increases with the length of therapy, and by 3 weeks of continuous heparin therapy, bleeding occurs in nearly 20% of patients.

The risk of bleeding is also influenced by several patient-related factors. In an extensive review of 2,656 patients, Walker and Jick identified numerous risk factors associated with both major and minor bleeding episodes in nonsurgical patients.[41] These investigators determined the relative weight of each of these factors as a determinant of heparin bleeding risk (Table 20.3). When bleeding occurs during heparin therapy, it is often related to preexisting hemostatic effects (uremia, drug-related defects in platelet aggregation, thrombocytopenia, liver disease) or to invasive procedures (cutdowns, arterial punctures, thoracenteses) and to patient factors such as gender and age. Women have approximately a twofold greater risk of bleeding than their male counterparts. This gender difference is further exaggerated when advanced age is examined as an additional risk factor.

Minor bleeding from an excess of heparin can usually be controlled by discontinuing the drug. For major bleeding or the threat of significant hemorrhage, specific therapy is warranted. Blood transfusion will correct massive blood loss, but is not a specific antidote. Protamine sulfate remains the drug of choice for reversal of heparin effect. Protamine combines quickly with heparin to form salts that are devoid of anticoagulant effect of heparin. One milligram of protamine sulfate neutralizes approximately 90 USP units of beef lung heparin or 115 USP units of mucosal heparin. Protamine is administered in a milligram amount equivalent to half the last dose of heparin if given after that dose. An excess of protamine can itself produce an anticoagulant effect. The drug, administered intravenously, is given slowly and carefully over a 3-minute period to diminish the incidence and severity of toxic reactions, which include hypotension, vasodilation, bradycardia, and dyspnea.

Other adverse effects of heparin therapy are thrombocytopenia and osteoporosis. Two distinct platelet phenomena are associated with the administration of heparin. A slight decrease in circulation platelets is almost universal; it is transient and is most likely due to a temporary sequestration of platelets that is of no clinical importance. The second effect is a rare but severe thrombocytopenia that occurs between the 2nd and 21st days after drug administration, is independent of dose or route, and most likely has an immunologic basis. Although the reported incidence has varied from less than 1% to 30%, the probable frequency is 1% to 2%.[44,47] Thrombocytopenia seems to be more frequent with beef lung heparin; however, switching to porcine mucosa heparin is not recommended because of the high incidence of cross-sensitivity between products. Careful monitoring of platelet counts (every 2–3 days) can minimize the risk of heparin-associated thrombocytopenia. There is little information on osteoporosis secondary to heparin therapy. This adverse effect has been rarely reported and is generally found in patients receiving in excess of 20,000 U/d for 6 months or longer.[44,48]

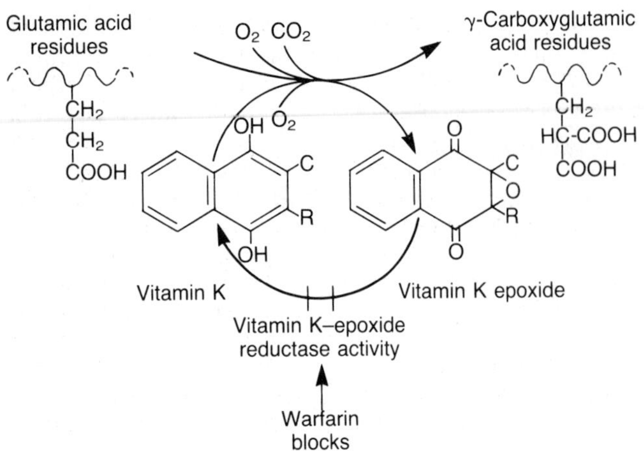


**Figure 20.6** Interactions between vitamin K and warfarin. Warfarin and other vitamin K antagonists inhibit the reduction of vitamin K epoxide to vitamin K by the enzyme vitamin K–epoxide reductase. The oxidation–reduction cycle between the two forms of vitamin K is linked in some unknown way to the γ-carboxylation of glutamic acid residues on vitamin K–dependent coagulation factors II, VII, IX, and X. *(From Hirsh J, Genton E, Hull R (Eds): Venous Thromboembolism. New York, Grune and Stratton, 1981, p 189, with permission.)*

## *Warfarin*

The coumarin derivative warfarin was synthesized at the University of Wisconsin in 1948 (the name warfarin being derived from the Wisconsin Alumni Research Foundation). Warfarin is the most useful of the vitamin K antagonists because of its predictable clinical effects, including onset of action and long duration of effect.

The pharmacologic effects of warfarin include anticoagulation and antithrombotic action. The mechanisms by which warfarin accomplishes these effects include prevention of the formation of γ-carboxyglutamic acid residue (by blocking the carboxylation system) and release of certain proteins that are deficient in γ-carboxyglutamic acid (see Fig. 20.6).[49] Six vitamin K–dependent proteins are involved in the coagulation system (factors II, VII, IX, and X and proteins C and S).

The inhibition of coagulation factors and the indirect anticoagulation of warfarin occurs 12 to 24 hours after oral administration. This is approximately at the same time that depression of protein C and factor VII occurs. In contrast, antithrombotic effects of warfarin may not occur until 2 to 7 days following the initiation of therapy. The in vivo antithrombotic effect occurs after a steady state has been achieved between the decrease in the rate of synthesis and the rate of disappearance of existing clotting factors in the system. The half-lives of the vitamin K–dependent clotting factors are 6, 24, 40, and 60 hours for factor VII, IX, X, and II, respectively. Factor VII concentrations decrease first and account for the initial change in the prothrombin time (PT).

### Pharmacokinetics

Warfarin is commercially available as a racemic mixture of the enantiomers *R*- and *S*-warfarin which exhibit differing pharmacokinetic and pharmacodynamic characteristics. After oral administration, warfarin is well absorbed, with peak plasma concentrations appearing at 60 to 90 minutes.[50] Warfarin is extensively protein bound (97.4%–99.99%), principally to albumin, with the *R*-enantiomer having greater binding than *S*-warfarin. When protein binding is taken into account, the *S*-enantiomer has an inherent potency approximately eight times greater than the *R*-enantiomer.[51,52] Warfarin is stereoselectively oxidized by hepatic microsomal enzyme systems to hydroxy metabolites and then reduced to alcohols which are renally excreted.

Warfarin is a capacity-limited binding-sensitive drug, which has a low intrinsic clearance and low unbound fraction. Protein binding determines the unbound drug fraction available for metabolism and explains the linear relationship observed between warfarin's total clearance and the unbound fraction in plasma. In addition, warfarin isomers have different rates of elimination. Mean (range) half-lives for the *R*- and *S*-isomers are 45.4 (37.4–88.6) and 33 (21.2–42.6) hours.[50,53]

Plasma clearance of warfarin is increased in patients with renal insufficiency.[54] More unbound fraction of warfarin is available for metabolism in patients with renal failure.[55] In addition, there is the potential for the renally excreted active alcohol metabolites to accumulate. However, these alterations have not increased warfarin's pharmacologic responsiveness in patients with renal failure.

### Therapeutic Indications/Clinical Efficacy

Warfarin effectively prevents recurrent thromboembolic complications following the acute treatment of DVT or PE with heparin therapy. The rationale for this indication was derived from the studies of Coon and co-workers which showed a protective effect of anticoagulant therapy for the first 4 months after hospital discharge.[56,57] Beyond this time, the potential beneficial effects of anticoagulation must be weighted against the risk of bleeding complications. The incidence of serious bleeding complications while receiving warfarin ranges from 2.4% to 10% in most series.[58] The risk of recurrent thromboembolic disease is highest in those patients with previous episodes of the same phenomenon. Thus, warfarin administration is indicated for 3 to 6 months for initial episodes of DVT or PE and for 12 months for long-term anticoagulation of recurrent venous thromboembolism.

In several studies, Hull et al have searched for a suitable alternative strategy for managing patients with long-term anticoagulation.[59–61] The clinical efficacy of fixed-low-dose subcutaneous heparin, adjusted-dose subcutaneous heparin, and "less intensive" warfarin therapy (prothrombin times ranging from 1.2 to 1.8 times control or baseline values) has been evaluated in patients initially treated with a continuous intravenous infusion of heparin for 10 to 14 days. These studies demonstrate that adjusted-dose heparin and less intense warfarin therapy are as effective as conventional warfarin therapy for treating proximal-vein thrombosis. The risk of hemorrhage is significantly greater with conventional warfarin therapy. Fixed-low-dose heparin is not effective for treating proximal-vein thrombosis. Hull et al also performed a cost-effectiveness analysis for the various approaches to long-term treatment of proximal venous thrombosis.[62] They concluded that the less intense warfarin therapy was the most cost-effective and that oral therapy was preferred by the majority of patients.

Adjusted-dose subcutaneous heparin is an acceptable alternative to warfarin therapy, particularly in high-risk patients (i.e., pregnancy) and those who cannot have their coagulation tests (PT) monitored on a continuing basis.[9,63] Administration of warfarin during pregnancy should be avoided because of the risk of fetal embryopathy during the first trimester, central nervous system and ocular abnormalities in the second or third trimester, and risk of hemorrhage at the time of delivery. Although heparin is considered the anticoagulant of choice during pregnancy because it does not cross the placenta, the risk of spontaneous abortion and premature labor is still possible.[63,64]

All of the contraindications listed above for heparin apply to warfarin as well. Relative contraindications for warfarin therapy include severe hepatic or renal disease, vitamin K deficiency, chronic alcoholism, and a requirement for intensive salicylate therapy.

#### Drug Administration/Monitoring

Warfarin can be initiated at any time during heparin treatment and should be initiated as soon as it becomes apparent that oral anticoagulation will be used. Initiation of warfarin should occur before intravenous heparin is discontinued to prevent a break in the level of anticoagulation. The "overlapping period" of heparin and warfarin should be 2 to 6 days because of the delayed onset of warfarin's effect and the hypercoagulable state occurring after heparin is discontinued.[9,65] Self et al demonstrated that the number of hospitalization days and the days of heparin therapy are decreased when warfarin is administered within 24 hours of initiating heparin therapy.[66,67]

It must be emphasized that warfarin dosages must be individualized by monitoring PT closely and examining the patient for evidence of bleeding. The initiation of oral warfarin therapy with small doses of approximately 10 mg/d for 3 to 4 days is generally agreed to be less toxic than administration of large loading doses (i.e., 50–75 mg).[68] Administration of a large loading dose places the patient at risk of hemorrhage and may precipitate the potentially serious dermatologic reaction (necrosis).[53]

PT should be performed prior to the initiation of warfarin therapy for the following purposes: (1) screening for preexisting coagulation disorders; (2) evaluating the effect, if any, that heparin therapy may have on PT[69]; and (3) establishing the patient's individual baseline value to determine the therapeutic endpoint of warfarin therapy from a laboratory standpoint (i.e., PT ratio between 1.2 and 2.0 using rabbit brain thromboplastin).[70] PT should be monitored every 24 to 48 hours after warfarin therapy is initiated and until the PT results have stabilized (i.e., PT ratios that are similar for 2 or 3 consecutive days with the same warfarin dosage) or until a maintenance dose is determined. Alterations in warfarin dosage during the initial establishment of a maintenance dosage should be made in small increments to prevent excessive changes in the PT. A patient's discharge from the hospital need not be delayed because the PT has not stabilized; the patient can easily be monitored as an outpatient with frequent PT determinations.

A patient's initial maintenance dosage requirements should not be considered as absolute requirements. Careful follow-up and weekly monitoring of PT is required during the first 4 weeks of therapy after discharge from the hospital (Fig. 20.7). A number of "outpatient" factors including changes in diet, exercise, clinical state, social habits, and compliance frequently alter maintenance dose requirements. Once a stable therapeutic warfarin dose has been attained, PT can be monitored less frequently (i.e., once monthly).

Porter et al have suggested a number of specific factors that may contribute to the explanation of a patient's unusual response to warfarin.[53] These include: (1) inaccurate laboratory results; (2) alterations in the anticoagulant response because of drug–drug interactions, change in nutritional status, or altered receptor site sensitivity to warfarin (i.e., hereditary resistance); (3) alterations in drug administration or patient compliance; and (4) abnormal product performance or use of products from various manufacturers.

A number of pharmacokinetic techniques that are intended to predict warfarin maintenance dose requirements have been suggested.[50,53] In addition, Bayesian forecasting and computer-assisted programs applicable to patient specific data bases may be useful in predicting warfarin dosage; however, further evaluations are necessary. Warfarin prediction techniques may not be clinically applicable because of interpatient variability and differences between laboratory techniques.

#### Laboratory Monitoring

Although there is considerable controversy regarding reagents, technique, and exact definitions of the therapeutic range, the PT test appears to be useful in monitoring treatment with oral anticoagulants.[42,53,70] Previous recommendations for therapeutic anticoagulation in the United States has been 1.5 to 2.5 times the laboratory control value of PT. This suggested PT ratio (patient:laboratory control value) has been shown to be clinically successful but is associated with a high risk of bleeding. Current recommendations suggest maintaining the PT ratio between 1.2 and 2.0 (using rabbit brain thromboplastin). This level of anticoagulation is equivalent to two times the prolongation of the PT using human brain thromboplastin international normalized ratio (INR) or an INR of 2.0 to 3.0 using rabbit brain thromboplastin. It must be emphasized that the minimum level of effective anticoagulation varies with individual thromboplastins.

It is important to recognize the effect that heparin has on PT when heparin and warfarin therapy are "overlapped." It has been shown that heparin increases PT results.[69,71,72] Whereas the effects are minimal, PT will decrease once heparin therapy is discontinued requiring further adjustment to warfarin maintenance doses.

#### Adverse Effects

As with heparin, the major toxic effect of warfarin is hemorrhage. Bleeding during anticoagulation does not always correlate with the PT ratio; however, the majority of bleeding episodes occur when the PT is excessively prolonged. The overall frequency of hemorrhagic complications has ranged from 2.5% to 27%.[56,58] Bleeding complications are proportional to the intensity of anticoagulation and are increased by the presence of risk factors. Treatment of

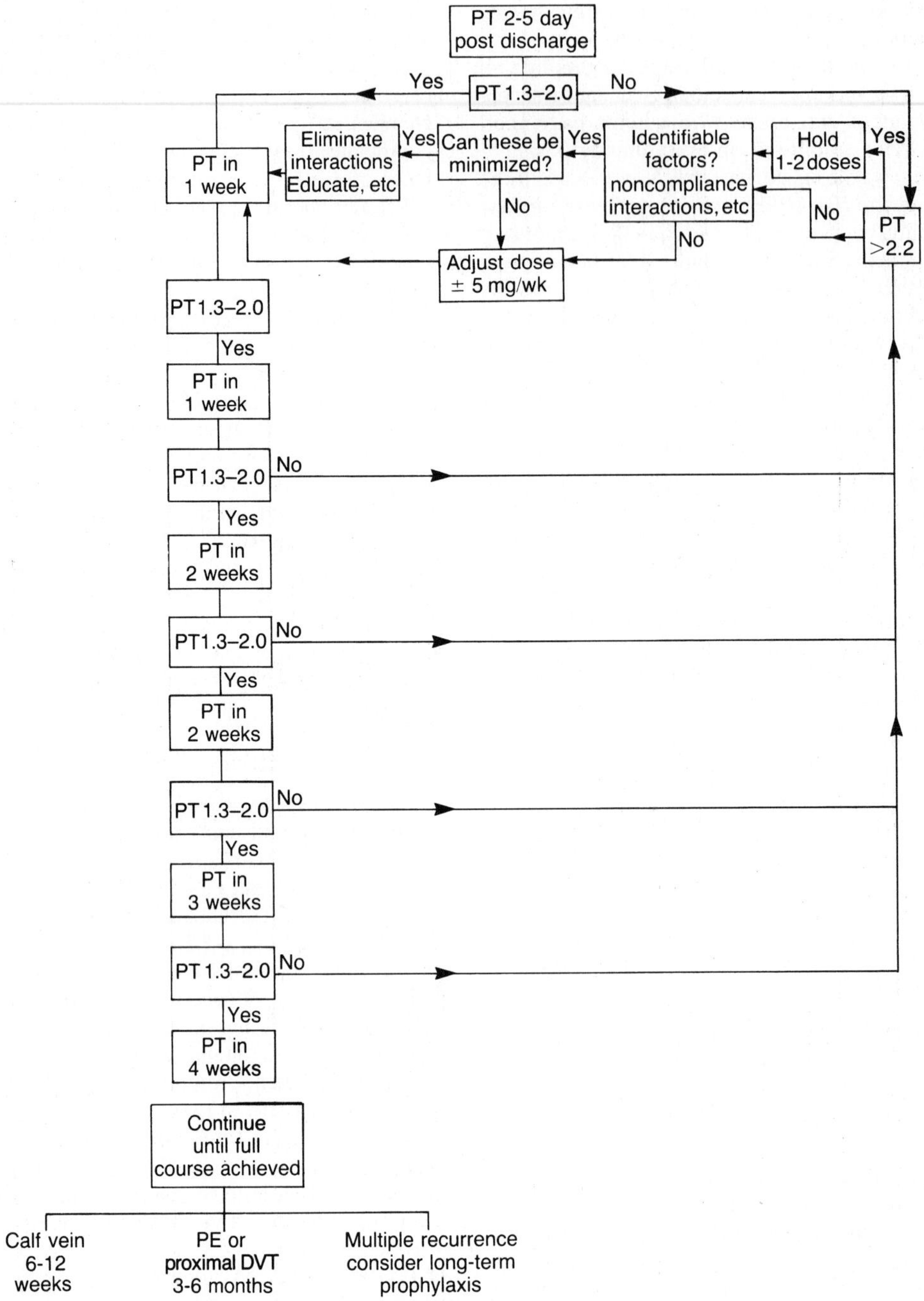


**Figure 20.7** Algorithm for management of long-term warfarin therapy after hospital discharge. *(From Carter BL, Jones ME, Waickman LA: Pathophysiology and treatment of deep-vein thrombosis and pulmonary embolism. Clin Pharm 1985;4:289, with permission.)*

bleeding in patients on warfarin depends on (1) the clinical severity of bleeding, including the rate of hemorrhage and the location; (2) the extent to which the PT is prolonged; (3) the expected duration of anticoagulant therapy; and (4) the initial indication for anticoagulation.

Minor bleeding with a prolonged PT may merely require interruption of warfarin therapy, with or without administration of fresh-frozen plasma, until the PT has returned to the therapeutic range. Major life-threatening bleeding requires immediate treatment with enough fresh-frozen plasma to correct the PT to normal. If the risk of hemorrhage outweighs the need for long-term anticoagulation with warfarin, vitamin K (phytonadione) may be administered parenterally. A dose of 25 mg administered subcutaneously or intramuscularly will usually reverse the effects of warfarin in 6 to 12 hours. Patients who will be returned to warfarin should receive smaller doses of phytonadione of approximately 1–5 mg.

Warfarin-induced skin necrosis and purple-toe syndrome are rare side effects of warfarin.[73,74] Both side effects are unrelated to the intensity of anticoagulation and may be the result of a direct toxic effect. The most commonly involved sites of warfarin-induced skin necrosis are the thigh, breast, and buttocks. It occurs within the first 10 days of therapy, and women are more likely to experience this effect than men. Purple-toe syndrome usually occurs 3 to 8 weeks after warfarin is begun and causes the toe to be painful; the color blanches with pressure and fades with elevation. It is recommended that warfarin be discontinued for this adverse reaction; however, discoloration may persist for weeks to months.

**Drug Interactions**

There are more drug–drug interactions reported for warfarin than for any other drug. Current use of warfarin with prescription or over-the-counter medications must routinely be considered as a cause of increased or decreased anticoagulant effect. Mechanisms responsible for these interactions[75] involve (1) reduced vitamin K availability; (2) reduced warfarin absorption; (3) changes in warfarin protein binding; (4) effects upon warfarin's metabolism; (5) changes in receptor affinity for warfarin; (6) reduction in vitamin K–dependent clotting factor levels; and (7) independent effect on hemostatic metabolism (Fig. 20.8). Close monitoring of the patient's response with additional PT determinations may be indicated whenever other medications are initiated or discontinued.

**Patient Education**

Safe and efficient warfarin therapy requires careful patient selection, cooperation of the patient, and patient education. Areas that need to be included in patient education are outlined in Table 20.4. It is also important that patients inform health care professionals (i.e., physician, dentist, nurse) that they are taking warfarin. It may be useful for patients to carry an identification card or a MEDALERT bracelet stating that they are receiving warfarin.

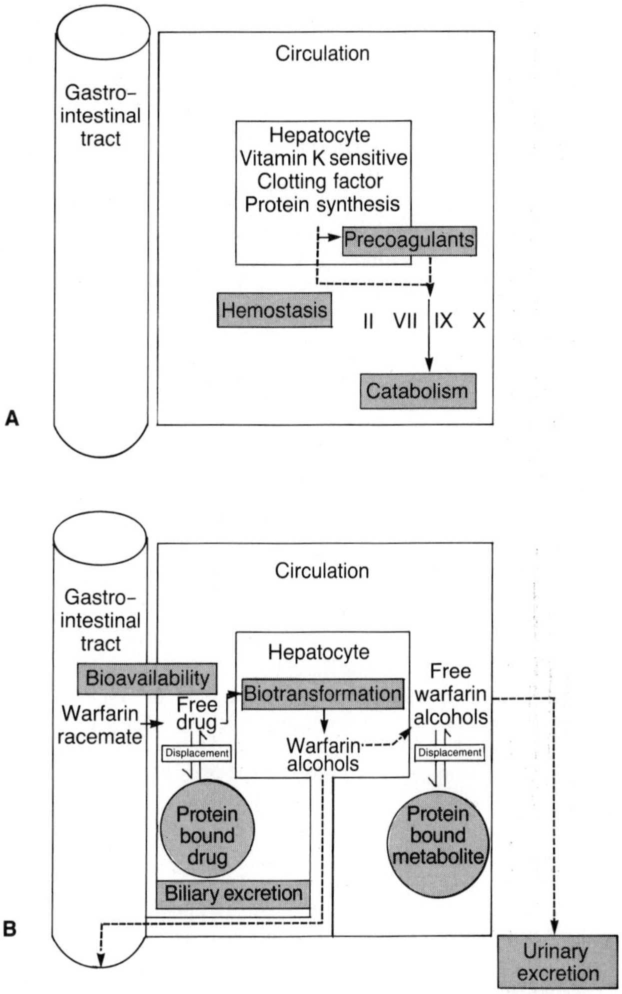


**Figure 20.8** Pharmacodynamic and pharmacokinetic drug interactions with coumarin anticoagulants. (A) Mechanisms of pharmacodynamic interactions, i.e., pharmacologic actions of coumarins that may be altered by other drugs affecting clotting factor synthesis or the hemostatic process. (B) Mechanisms of pharmacokinetic interactions, i.e., interactions in which the absorption, biotransformation, or disposition of coumarin anticoagulants may be altered. *(From MacLeod SM, Seller EM: Pharmacodynamic and pharmacokinetic drug interactions with coumarin anticoagulants. Drugs 1976;11:463, with permission.)*

## *Thrombolytic Therapy*

The advantages of thrombolytic therapy are rapidity and complete removal of a pathologic intraluminal thrombus or embolus that has not been dissolved by spontaneous fibrinolysis. The disadvantage is that the risk of bleeding is somewhat higher than in anticoagulant therapy. At present, two fibrinolytic agents are available, streptokinase (SK) and urokinase (UK). The availability of the more fibrin-specific agent, tissue-type plasminogen activator (TPA), may overcome some of the disadvantages of SK and UK.

All of these agents are proteins with enzymatic activity that directly (UK, TPA) or indirectly (SK) activate endogenous plasminogen to form plasmin (Fig. 20.9), which actually lyses the clot (Table 20.5). Streptokinase is an antigenic, nonenzymatic protein isolated from group C $\beta$-hemolytic streptococci. It combines with plasminogen in vivo to form an active streptokinase–plasminogen complex that converts both free and fibrin–fibrinogen absorbed plasminogen to the active proteolytic enzyme, plasmin. Urokinase is a nonantigenic enzyme isolated from human urine or fetal kidney tissue culture that directly converts plasminogen to plasmin. Plasmin lyses the fibrin clot and also causes degradation of fibrinogen and coagulation factors V, VIII, and XIII.

Tissue plasminogen activator binds specifically to fibrin as a result of the "surface assembly" of TPA and plasminogen on the fibrin surface. Fibrin increases the local plasminogen concentration, which increases the interaction between TPA and its substrate and results in direct activation of plasminogen, with formation of plasmin on the fibrin surface. Tissue plasminogen activator should allow for better controlled, localized activation of fibrinolysis, preferentially at the site of the actual clot, without depletion of fibrinogen.[76]

**Table 20.4** Information for the Patient on Warfarin

1. *Need for strict compliance.* The importance of taking warfarin and other medications as directed and of following instructions regarding prothrombin times and follow-up office visits must be stressed.
2. *Side effects.* The sites and signs of bleeding as well as instructions on when and where to call if bleeding occurs should be reviewed.
3. *Dietary instruction.* The patient should be told that no major dietary restrictions are necessary; however, no abrupt changes in dietary habits should be made. Rarely, diets with excessive quantities of vitamin K have interfered with warfarin therapy.
4. *Frequent prothrombin times.* The patient needs to be aware of the required monitoring of prothrombin times and why this is necessary. Some patients question the need for continued monitoring of warfarin, and this issue is best addressed early in the course of treatment.
5. *Drug interactions.* The patient should be informed that other drugs can greatly influence the effect of warfarin and should be told not to start or stop medications without first asking the physician. It may be useful to make specific recommendations regarding the use of common nonprescription drugs, e.g., antacids, analgesics, and cold products.

Adapted from Carter BL, Jones ME, Waickman LA: Pathophysiology and treatment of deep-vein thrombosis and pulmonary embolism. Clin Pharm 1985;4:292,293, with permission.

**Figure 20.9** Fibrinolysis during thrombolytic therapy. Urokinase and streptokinase activate the fibrinolytic system and convert plasminogen to the active enzyme plasmin, which then lyses a fresh fibrin clot. *(From Sharma GVRK, Cella G, Parisi AF, Sasahara AA: Thrombolytic therapy. N Engl J Med 1982;306:1269, with permission.)*

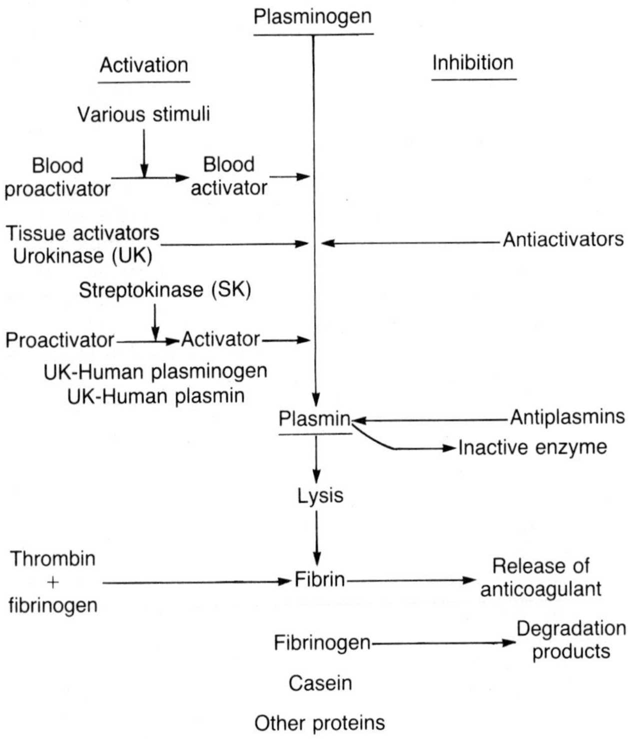


### Therapeutic Indications

The clinical indications for thrombolytic therapy have been defined by the Food and Drug Administration (Table 20.5).[77,78] Although these agents have been investigated in numerous other clinical applications, the small number of patients studied does not permit any conclusions to be drawn, and therefore no clinical recommendation can be made.

Guidelines for selection of patients for systemic thrombolytic therapy should be based on the presence of an appropriate clinical indication. This should include a documented diagnosis of thromboembolism and evidence that the thrombus is of recent origin (within the last 7 days). Relative contraindications and precautions are summarized in Table 20.6.[79]

### Clinical Efficacy

Two controlled trials, one comparing urokinase with heparin[80] and a second comparing urokinase with streptokinase,[81] were performed to define the role of thrombolytic therapy in the treatment of PE. These two trials, in which 327 patients with angiographically confirmed pulmonary embolism were studied, showed that compared with heparin, thrombolytic therapy produced (1) greater resolution of pulmonary emboli; (2) greater improvement of the abnormal hemodynamic status of the right heart and pulmonary circulation; (3) greater reperfusion of the original pulmonary perfusion defects; and (4) maximal clot resolution and general improvement in patients with the largest pulmonary emboli. However, no difference in mortality rate was found between patients given heparin and those given thrombolytic therapy. The incidence of bleeding complications was nearly double for thrombolytic therapy compared with heparin therapy.

A further potential advantage to the use of thrombolytic therapy is a reduction in long-term effects of PE. Sharma et al have shown better improvement in pulmonary capillary

**Table 20.5** Comparison of Streptokinase, Urokinase, and Tissue Plasminogen Activator

| *Feature* | *Streptokinase* | *Urokinase* | *Alteplase, recombinant (tissue plasminogen activator)* |
|---|---|---|---|
| Source | Group C streptococci | Human fetal kidney tissue culture; human urine | Chinese hamster ovary cell culture |
| Half-life | "Fast" 11–13 min<br>"Slow" 83 min | 11–16 min | "Fast" 4.4 min<br>"Slow" 26.5 min |
| Stability | Room temperature | 4°C | Room temperature |
| Antigenicity | Yes | No | No |
| Pyrogenicity | Minimal | None | No |
| Indications | Pulmonary embolism<br>Deep-vein thrombosis<br>Arterial thrombosis<br>Occluded access shunts<br>Acute transmural myocardial infarction | Pulmonary embolism<br>Occluded access shunts | Acute myocardial infarction |
| Cost[a] | $400.00[b] | $2,100.00[c] | $2,300.00[d] |

[a] Cost is the "charge to patient" including distribution fees and manufacturing cost.
[b] Based on a dosage of 250,000 units (bolus) and an infusion of 100,000 U/h for 24 hours.
[c] Based on a dosage for a 154-pound patient, bolus of 4,400 U/kg and infusion of 4,400 U/kg/h for 12 hours.
[d] Approximate cost to pharmacy for 100-mg dose.

Adapted from Sharma GVRK, Cella G, Parisi AF, Sasahara AA: Thrombolytic therapy. N Engl J Med 1982;306:1269, with permission.

blood volume and perfusion at both 2 weeks and 1 year in a streptokinase-treated group when compared with a heparin-treated group.[82] If these physiologic alterations can be shown to be clinically significant in future studies, thrombolytic therapy may become the preferred treatment in patients with PE.

In patients with extensive DVT, it is suggested that thrombolytic therapy may be associated with a reduction in the incidence of the postphlebitic syndrome, particularly if treatment is given soon after the development of symptoms. The incidence of postphlebitic syndrome and normal venograms after DVT may be reduced with streptokinase therapy compared with heparin; however, not all studies demonstrate these findings favoring thrombolytic therapy.[83]

**Table 20.6** Contraindications to Thrombolytic Therapy

| |
|---|
| Absolute contraindications |
| Active internal bleeding |
| Cerebrovascular process, disease, or procedure within 2 months |
| Relative contraindications |
| Conditions requiring fibrin strands and plugs for normal hemostasis or healing (fibrinolysis is usually contraindicated within 10 days of onset of these conditions) |
| Major surgery, organ biopsy, puncture of noncompressible blood vessel |
| Postpartum period |
| Cardiopulmonary resuscitation during presence of rib fractures |
| Thoracentesis, paracentesis, lumbar puncture |
| Recent serious trauma |
| Potentially serious bleeding |
| Uncontrolled coagulation defects |
| Uncontrolled severe hypertension |
| Pregnancy |
| Other conditions deemed potential bleeding risks |

From Sharma GVRK, Cella G, Parisi AF, Sasahara AA: Thrombolytic therapy. N Engl J Med 1982;306:1271, with permission.

### Drug Administration

Safe and effective administration of either drug is best accomplished with continuous intravenous infusion in a precise manner. Although no schedule for optimal dosage in thrombolytic therapy has been established, most investigators recommend the dosage schedule used in the large NIH clinical trials for the treatment of PE.[84–86]

For streptokinase, the initial loading dose of 250,000 units in normal saline or 5% dextrose in water is administered over 30 minutes. Maintenance therapy consists of 100,000 units per hour for 24 to 72 hours. For PE, results from the major studies favor 24 hours of administration. Infusions for DVT have been continued for up to 120 hours, but continuation beyond 72 hours does not generally provide additional benefit. Intravenous administration of a bolus followed by intravenous infusion results in a systemic lytic state (decreased fibrinogen and increased fibrin degradation products) in more than 90% of patients.

Urokinase is given in a loading dose of 4,400 units per kilogram of body weight in normal saline over 10 minutes. Maintenance therapy consists of 4,400 units per kilogram per hour for a total of 12 hours. The total volume of fluid administered should not exceed 200 mL. In one study the drug was administered for 24 hours, but no additional benefit was demonstrated after 12 hours.[81]

Thrombolytic therapy should not be considered a substi-

**Table 20.7** Laboratory Monitoring for Thrombolytic Therapy

| | |
|---|---|
| Tests | |
| | Whole-blood euglobulin lysis time, or |
| | Thrombin time, or |
| | Partial thromboplastin and prothrombin times, or |
| | Fibrin(ogen) degradation products |
| Time of testing | |
| | Before therapy |
| | Detect and correct coagulation defects (by means of thrombin, partial thromboplastin, and prothrombin times) |
| | Determine baseline or control for fibrinolysis [any of the above tests; euglobulin lysis time or fibrin(ogen) degradation products if patient has been receiving heparin] |
| | During therapy (3–4 h after start) |
| | Use same test(s) used for establishing baseline or control |
| | After therapy |
| | Use partial thromboplastin time if heparin therapy is to begin |

From Sharma GVRK, Cella G, Parisi AF, Sasahara AA: Thrombolytic therapy. N Engl J Med 1982;306:1275, with permission.

tute for anticoagulant therapy. Once thrombolytic therapy is discontinued and the thrombin time or APTT has fallen to less than twice the normal values (usually in 2–4 hours), continuous heparin should be given for 7 to 14 days.

### Laboratory Monitoring/Treatment Guidelines[84,85]

Laboratory monitoring of thrombolytic therapy is used simply to determine whether some degree of systemic fibrinolysis has been established. As long as some degree of lysis is established, vigorous dissolutions of clots can be expected, provided that the fibrin clots are fresh. Simple but adequate laboratory monitoring for safe and effective administration of thrombolytic therapy is outlined in Table 20.7.

The two most sensitive tests for fibrinolysis are whole-blood euglobulin lysis time and thrombin time. If they are unavailable, APTT and PT can be used. Whatever test is selected, it should be performed prior to the administration of thrombolytic therapy and after 3 to 4 hours of thrombolytic treatment. As long as the test values during thrombolytic infusion are prolonged beyond the control value (except the euglobulin lysis time, which should be shortened), it can be assumed that systemic lysis has been established.

Concurrent treatment guidelines to minimize local and major hemorrhage of patients receiving thrombolytic therapy are summarized in Table 20.8.

### Adverse Effects

Hemorrhage, allergy, and fever are the three major types of adverse reaction that have been reported with streptokinase or urokinase.[87–89] Current studies indicate that the most disturbing and common side effect is bleeding, causing thrombolytic therapy to be discontinued in 5% to 25% of patients. In the latest clinical trials, however, the incidence of major bleeding complications has been only about 5%, based on patient treatment evaluations submitted to pharmaceutical manufacturers during continuing surveillance periods requested by the Food and Drug Administration.

In response to the question of bleeding complications, Sharma and Sasahara reported their experience with almost 100 patients who were given thrombolytic agents.[90] Twenty-nine percent had minor oozing, 10% had major bleeding, and 4% required replacement transfusion. No deaths were attributable to bleeding. Their figures are considerably lower than those reported in the two trials sponsored by the NIH.[80,81] They believe that careful attention to local hemostasis, close patient observation, and avoidance of unnecessary invasive procedures were responsible for their low incidence of serious bleeding.

Minor bleeding or oozing at cutaneous puncture sites can be controlled locally with pressure dressings. In cases of serious bleeding, thrombolytic therapy should be discontinued. Because of the very short half-life of these agents, lytic activity stops promptly. If blood replacement is indicated, whole blood or blood products (packed red cells, fresh-frozen plasma, or cryoprecipitate) may be given and should rapidly reverse the hemostatic alterations. In situations where uncontrolled bleeding unresponsive to blood component therapy must be rapidly corrected, ε-aminocaproic acid (EACA) may be administered in 5-g doses.

Allergic or hypersensitivity reactions associated with streptokinase include urticaria, itching, flushing, nausea, headache (12%), and transient elevation or decrease of systolic blood pressure (2%). Anaphylaxis (1.3%–2.5%) has ranged in severity from minor breathing difficulty to bronchospasm, periorbital swelling, or angioneurotic edema. Although urokinase is considered to be nonantigenic, relatively mild allergic reactions have been rarely reported.

With streptokinase, the frequency of temperature increase greater than 1.5°F is 30%, but only 3.5% have temperatures greater than 104°F. Febrile episodes with urokinase have occurred in approximately 15% of patients.

Both allergic and febrile reactions may be treated with antihistamines at the time of detection. Acetaminophen is very effective for treating temperature increases. Corticosteroids have also been useful for prophylaxis of adverse reactions.

**Table 20.8** Clinical Guidelines for Patient Treatment

| | |
|---|---|
| 1. | Minimize physical handling of patient |
| 2. | Discontinue parenteral medications |
| 3. | Substitute appropriate oral medications |
| 4. | Minimize invasive procedures, including needle punctures |
| 5. | Apply compression bandages at sites of vessel puncture |
| 6. | Avoid concurrent anticoagulation |
| 7. | Avoid concurrent use of platelet-active drugs, aspirin-containing compounds (erosive), antiplatelet agents, and dextran |

Adapted from Sharma GVRK, Cella G, Parisi AF, Sasahara AA: Thrombolytic therapy. N Engl J Med 1982;306:1274, with permission.

### *Surgical Therapy*

Surgery for acute DVT has been regarded with skepticism and remains controversial. Initial enthusiasm has waned because of reports of early thrombosis and poor objective documentation of long-term results. The main purpose for iliofemoral thrombectomy is to reduce the incidence of PE and to prevent the postthrombotic syndrome, which is reported to occur in 50% of patients treated with heparin.[91] Currently, thrombectomy is considered only in patients with acute DVT and severe limb ischemia (phlegmasia cerulea dolens), as many of these patients progress to venous gangrene with loss of a limb. Ideally, the patient should have a thrombectomy, with adjuncts of heparin infusion through an indwelling catheter and pneumatic segmental compression of the leg, within 2 to 3 days of onset of symptoms before the clot adheres to the vein wall.[91]

Another surgical approach to control DVT and prevent thromboembolism is interruption of the inferior vena cava through insertion of mechanical filters. In recent years, there has been a great deal of enthusiasm for transvenous umbrellas or filters, which are usually placed in either an infrarenal or a suprarenal position through a venotomy. This procedure is performed under local anesthesia with radiographic control. The most common indications for placement of a transvenous filter include absolute contraindication for anticoagulant therapy, major bleeding on anticoagulation for embolism or venous thrombosis, recurrent thromboembolism while receiving anticoagulation therapy, and postembolectomy.[91] Surgical procedures considered for patients with chronic DVT include venous reconstruction procedures, such as vein bypass grafts, valvuloplasty, and autologous vein valve transplantation. These procedures are reserved for patients with postthrombotic syndrome who fail routine medical therapy including support stockings, leg elevation and wound care, and surgical therapy consisting of ligation of the perforator vessels.[92] Finally, pulmonary embolectomy is sometimes performed in patients with massive pulmonary embolism. Reported mortality rates for this procedure are very high; however, an emergency embolectomy may be lifesaving in a few patients. Surgical embolectomy may be performed in a patient with refractory or recurrent cardiac arrest who cannot be stabilized long enough to receive aggressive medical management or in the patient who is clearly failing with aggressive medical therapy.

### *Prevention of Venous Thromboembolism*[93,94]

#### Nonpharmacologic Elimination of Stasis

All pharmacologic techniques of postoperative prophylaxis of DVT and PE have potential serious side effects. Many studies have been performed using nonpharmacologic methods to decrease stasis and decrease the incidence of thromboembolic phenomenon but without the cost or side effects of drug use. Three major modes of nonpharmacologic prophylaxis are compression stockings, electrical stimulation of calf muscles, and intermittent compression of calf muscles.

Standard elastic compression stockings (TED, Tubigrip) have been used to prevent postoperative DVT with conflicting results. Early studies that demonstrated a statistically significant benefit relied upon a clinical diagnosis of DVT which is not as accurate as utilizing $^{125}$I-fibrinogen scanning. Studies using the latter technique have not shown any benefit. TED stockings (thromboembolism deterrent) have a graded pressure; the pressure is highest at the ankle and progressively decreases to the upper thigh. The stocking is manufactured in different sizes in both length and circumference to conform to different-size individuals. Although many studies using these stockings have shown some benefit, DVT has developed in 11% to 23% of patients.[95]

Other investigators have used electrical stimulation of calf muscles to prevent DVT. This technique requires the placement, over calf muscles, of skin electrodes that induce muscle contractions by repeated electrical stimulation. Patient acceptance is poor because of the associated discomfort and in most studies there is a reduction in DVT compared with controls; however, DVT occurs frequently even with stimulation.

Intermittent calf muscle compression has become increasingly popular. Multiple studies of intraoperative compression have shown benefit; few studies of pre- and postoperative compression exist. Intermittent calf muscle compression is frequently begun at the time of surgery or in the immediate postoperative period and may be continued until the patient is fully ambulatory. In some cases these devices can be worn under partial casts.

The best technique for preventing DVT is to ambulate the patient as soon as possible in the postoperative period. As some patients may not be capable of being ambulated early and prophylactic anticoagulation is contraindicated (neurosurgical techniques), nonpharmacologic techniques may be the only prophylaxis therapy available. All these patients should be monitored carefully for clinical signs of DVT and/or PE. If the patient is at high risk, $^{125}$I-fibrinogen scanning, impedance plethysmography, and/or Doppler studies may be used to detect DVT before PE develops.

#### Pharmacologic Counteraction of Blood Coagulability

Currently there is substantial evidence based on 34 randomized trials involving 6,163 patients that low-dose heparin can prevent DVT and PE after general abdominal, thoracic, and urologic surgery (Table 20.9).[94] In these patients, 5,000 units of heparin should be given subcutaneously every 12 hours for the first 7 days after surgery. This regimen is ineffective in reducing the incidence of DVT in patients undergoing total hip replacement. Evidence suggests that these patients should receive subcutaneous heparin adjusted to maintain the APTT in the high–normal range.[96] Low-dose heparin has also been effective in reducing the incidence of DVT after myocardial infarction.[97] The use of prophylactic heparin after myocardial infarction should be reserved for high-risk patients with one of the following conditions: age greater than 70 years, large acute myocardial infarction, heart failure or shock, necessity for immobilization beyond 3 days, or previous DVT or PE.

Combinations (Embolex) of dihydroergotamine (0.5 mg) and heparin (5,000 units) have also been used in prophylactic regimens based on the rationale that changes in blood coagulation and stasis in deep veins contribute to the pathogenesis of DVT.[98] Dihydroergotamine has been shown to increase the velocity of venous flow in the major veins of the legs by selectively constricting the capacitance vessels of the limbs while exerting little effect on resistance vessels. There have been a number of trials using this combination in a variety of patient populations. In general, the addition of dihydroergotamine reduced the incidence of DVT by approximately 50% compared with heparin alone.

The efficacy of low-molecular-weight fractions of heparin in preventing DVT has also been studied. In a randomized double-blind study of 359 patients, there was a significantly lower incidence of DVT in the low-molecular-weight heparin group compared with the unfractionated group.[99]

To recommend an approach to prophylaxis, one can examine the studies conducted to date and make biologically plausible assumptions in situations in which uncertainty persists. Each individual patient's risk for venous thrombosis must be weighed against the risks associated with a particular prophylactic maneuver.

**Table 20.9** Effectiveness of Low-Dose Heparin in the Prevention of Postoperative Deep-Vein Thrombosis[a]

| | | *Frequency of thrombosis (%)* | | |
|---|---|---|---|---|
| ***Patient population*** | ***No. of patients*** | **Controls** | **Low-dose heparin** | **Value** |
| General surgery | 125 | 5 | 6 | NS |
| General surgery | 50 | 63 | 26 | <0.05 |
| Gynecology | 110 | 29 | 4 | <0.01 |
| General surgery | 97 | 27 | 13 | <0.05 |
| Neurosurgery | 100 | 34 | 6 | <0.005 |
| Gynecology, malignancy | 185 | 12 | 15 | NS |
| Urology | 52 | 25 | 21 | NS |
| General surgery | 105 | 10 | 8 | NS |
| General surgery | 209 | 15 | 1 | <0.001 |
| General surgery | 820 | 16 | 4 | <0.05 |
| General surgery | 150 | 42 | 14[b] | <0.003 |
| | | | 8[c] | <0.001 |
| Abdominal surgery | 199 | 27 | 12 | <0.007 |
| General surgery | 194 | 36 | 13 | <0.005 |
| Urology | 59 | 46 | 21 | NS |
| General surgery | 1292 | 25 | 8 | <0.005 |
| Thorax surgery | 183 | 51 | 28 | <0.005 |
| General surgery | 120 | 51 | 9 | <0.0005 |
| General surgery | 78 | 42 | 8 | <0.001 |
| General surgery | 200 | 41 | 8 | <0.001 |
| General surgery | 50 | 63 | 26 | <0.05 |
| Urology | 47 | 36 | 9 | <0.05 |
| Abdominal surgery | 112 | 20 | 5 | <0.05 |
| Abdominal surgery | 242 | 17 | 7 | <0.05 |
| General surgery | 160 | 43 | 15 | <0.05 |
| Gynecology | 55 | 14 | 0 | <0.05 |
| Thoracic surgery | 38 | 44 | 15 | <0.05 |
| General surgery | 251 | 24 | 1 | <0.001 |
| General surgery | 108 | 21 | 7 | <0.05 |
| General surgery, urology | 178 | 36 | 13 | <0.001 |
| General surgery | 154 | 44 | 7 | <0.001 |
| Urology | 65 | 58 | 12 | <0.01 |
| General surgery | 100 | 20 | 6 | <0.05 |
| Gynecology | 57 | 23 | 6 | <0.05 |
| Abdominal surgery | 124 | 33 | 165 | <0.05 |
| Abdominal surgery | 44 | 33 | 0 | <0.02 |
| Abdominal surgery | 88 | 14 | 0 | <0.01 |

[a] The $^{125}$I-fibrinogen test was used to detect deep-vein thrombosis.
[b] In total, three doses of low-dose heparin.
[c] Low-dose heparin for 5 days.

Adapted from Kakkar VV, Adams PC: Preventive and therapeutic approach to venous thromboembolic disease and pulmonary embolism: Can death from pulmonary embolism be prevented? J Am Coll Cardiol 1986;8(suppl): 148B, with permission.

In addition, the major conclusions of the National Heart, Lung, and Blood Institute and the National Institutes of Health Office of Medical Applications of Research consensus panel are as follows[100]:

1. Regimens recommended for prevention of DVT and PE include low-dose heparin, adjusted-dose heparin, dextran, and warfarin. Low-dose warfarin, external pneumatic compression, and gradient elastic stockings, alone or in combination with heparin or heparin plus dihydroergotamine, are also effective in decreasing DVT, which the panel considers to be an indicator of their effects on PE. Aspirin has not been shown to be beneficial.
2. None of the preventive measures are ideal, but most are relatively simple to use; complications are generally minor; and the need for laboratory monitoring is minimal.
3. Effective prophylactic regimens differ according to the type of patient at high risk. Prophylactic therapy should be tailored according to the patient's disease and degree of risk.
4. In some groups of patients, more than one effective prophylactic regimen is available.
5. DVT and PE in high-risk patients can be significantly reduced by prophylactic regimens, which should be used more extensively.

## Summary

Venous thromboembolism has been the target of intensive research in recent years. The disorder is an important source of morbidity and mortality owing to complicating pulmonary embolism in patients on both medical and surgical wards. A major problem in the care of these patients has always been diagnosis. Many patients are asymptomatic, and both false-positive and false-negative diagnoses are common. Significant progress has been made in recent years in diagnostic procedures, identification of high-risk groups, and therapeutic management, although studies are needed to better define the role of thrombolytic therapy in acute DVT and PE. Most clinicians agree, however, that management of venous thromboembolism is ideally achieved through prophylactic approaches rather than by allowing thromboembolism to occur.

## References


1. Moses KM. Pulmonary thromboembolism, in Braunwald E, Isselbacher KJ, Petersdorf RG, et al (eds): Harrison's Principles of Internal Medicine, 11th ed. New York, McGraw–Hill, 1987, pp 1105–1111.
2. Coon WW, Coller FA. Some epidemiologic considerations of thromboembolism. Surg Gynecol Obstet 1959;109:487–501.
3. Gallus AS, Hirsh J. Prevention of venous thromboembolism. Semin Thromb Hemost 1976;2:232–290.
4. Hirsh J. Advances in Antithrombotic Therapy. Wilmington, DE, E.I. du Pont de Nemours, Inc, 1984, pp 3–19.
5. Hirsh J, Hull RD, Raskob GE. Epidemiology and pathogenesis of venous thrombosis. J Am Coll Cardiol 1986;8:104B–113B.
6. Hull RD, Hersh J, Carter CJ, et al. Pulmonary angiography, ventilation lung scanning, and venography for clinically suspected pulmonary embolism with abnormal perfusion lung scan. Ann Intern Med 1983;98:891–899.
7. Virchow RLK. Gesammelte Abhandlungen zur Wissenschaftlichen, in Thrombose und Emboli. Berlin, Hamm-Grotesche Buchhandlung, 1862, vol V, p 219.
8. Hamer JD, Malone PC, Silver IA. The $Po_2$ in venous valve pockets: Its possible bearing on thrombogenesis. Br J Surg 1981;68:166–170.
9. Carter BL, Jones ME, Waickman LA. Pathophysiology and treatment of deep-vein thrombosis and pulmonary embolism. Clin Pharm 1985;4:279–296.
10. Vermylen J, Verstraete M, Fuster V. Role of platelet activation and fibrin formation in thrombogenesis. J Am Coll Cardiol 1986;8:2B–9B.
11. Walker FJ. Regulation of activated protein C by a new protein. J Biol Chem 1980;255:5521–5524.
12. Comp PC, Nixon RR, Cooper MR, et al. Familial protein S deficiency is associated with recurrent thrombosis. J Clin Invest 1984;74:2082–2088.
13. Egeberg O. Inherited antithrombin deficiency causing thrombophilia. Thromb Diath Haemorrh 1965;13:516–530.
14. Kazmier FJ, Juergens JL. Venous thrombosis and obstructive diseases of the veins, in Juergens JI, Spittell JA, Fairbairn JF (eds): Peripheral Vascular Diseases. Philadelphia, W.B. Saunders, 1980, pp 731–755.
15. Menzoian JO, Sequeira JC, Doyle JE, et al. Therapeutic and clinical course of deep vein thrombosis. Am J Surg 1983;146:581–585.
16. Smith GT, Dammin GJ, Dexter J. Postmortem arteriographic studies of the human lung in pulmonary embolization. JAMA 1964;188:135–151.
17. Hirsh J,Hull RD, Raskob GE. Clinical features and diagnosis of venous thrombosis. J Am Coll Cardiol 1986;8:114B–127B.
18. Hirsh J, Hull RD, Raskob GE. Diagnosis of pulmonary embolism. J Am Coll Cardiol 1986;8:128B–136B.
19. Hull R, van Aken WG, Hirsh J, et al. Impedance plethysmography using the occlusive cuff technique in the diagnosis of venous thrombosis. Circulation 1976;53:696–700.
20. Wheeler HB. Diagnosis of deep vein thrombosis. Review of clinical evaluation and impedance plethysmography. Am J Surg 1985;150;7–13.
21. Hull R, Hirsh J, Sackett DL. Cost effectiveness of clinical diagnosis, venography, and noninvasive testing in patients with symptomatic deep-vein thrombosis. N Engl J Med 1981; 304:1561–1566.
22. Mills SR, Jackson DC, Older RA, et al. The incidence etiologies and avoidance of complications of pulmonary angiography in a large series. Radiology 1980;136:295–299.
23. McLean J. The thromboplastic action of cephalia. Am J Physiol 1916;41:250–257.
24. Rosenberg RD. Actions and interactions of heparin and antithrombin III. N Engl J Med 1975;292:146–150.
25. Wright CJ, Jaques LB. Heparin via the lung. Can J Surg 1979;22:317–319.
26. Thomas DP, Sagar S, Tamatakis JD, et al. Plasma heparin

levels after administration of calcium and sodium salts of heparin. Thromb Res 1976;9:241–248.
27. Low J, Biggs JC. Comparative plasma heparin levels after subcutaneous sodium and calcium heparin. Thromb Haemost 1978;40:397–406.
28. Cipolle RJ, Rodvold KA. Heparin, in Evans WE, Schentag JJ, Jusko WJ (eds): Applied Pharmacokinetics. San Francisco, Applied Therapeutics,1986, pp 903–943.
29. Beermann B, Lahnborg G. Pharmacokinetics of heparin in healthy and obese subjects and in combination with dihydroergotamine. Thromb Haemost 1981;45:24–26.
30. McAroy TJ. Pharmacokinetic modeling of heparin and its clinical implications. J Pharmacokinet Biopharm 1979;7:331–354.
31. deSwart CAM, Nijmeyer B, Ruelofs JMM, et al. Kinetics of intravenously administered heparin in normal humans. Blood 1982;60:1251–1258.
32. Hirsh J, VanAken WG, Gallus AS, et al. Heparin kinetics in venous thrombosis and pulmonary embolism. Circulation 1976;53:691–695.
33. Elliott CT, Michocki RJ, Brown R, et al. Heparin requirements in pulmonary embolism and venous thrombosis: A prospective study. J Clin Pharmacol 1982;22:102–109.
34. White TM, Bernene JL, Marino AM. Continuous heparin infusion requirements: Diagnostic and therapeutic implications. JAMA 1979;241:2717–2720.
35. Cipolle RJ, Seifert RD, Neilan BA, et al. Heparin kinetics: Variables related to disposition and dosage. Clin Pharmacol Ther 1981;29:387–393.
36. Hall JG, Pauli RM, Wilson KM. Maternal and fetal sequelae of anticoagulation during pregnancy. Am J Med 1980;68:122–139.
37. Pollack EW, Sparks FC, Barker WF. Pulmonary embolism: An appraisal of therapy in 516 cases. Arch Surg 1973;107:66–68.
38. Basu D, Gallus A, Hirsh J, et al. A prospective study of the value of monitoring heparin treatment with the activated partial thromboplastin time. N Engl J Med 1972;287:324–327.
39. Wilson JE, Bynum LJ, Parkey RW. Heparin therapy in venous thromboembolism. Am J Med 1981;70:808–816.
40. Hattersley PG, Mitsouka JC, King JG. Sources of error in heparin therapy. Arch Intern Med 1980;140:1173–1175.
41. Walker AM, Jick H. Predictors of bleeding during heparin therapy. JAMA 1980;244:1209–1212.
42. Suchman AL, Griner PF. Diagnostic uses of the activated partial thromboplastin. Ann Intern Med 1986;104:810–816.
43. Kelton JG, Hirsh J. Bleeding associated with antithrombotic therapy. Semin Hematol 1980;17:259–291.
44. Wessler S, Gitel SN. Pharmacology of heparin and warfarin. J Am Coll Cardiol 1986;8:10B–20B.
45. Conti S, Daschbach M, Blaisdell FW. A comparison of high-dose versus conventional-dose heparin therapy for deep vein thrombosis. Surgery 1982;92:972–980.
46. Mant MJ, O'Brian BD, Thong KL, et al. Haemorrhagic complications of heparin therapy. Lancet 1977;1:1133–1135.
47. King DJ, Kelton JG. Heparin-associated thrombocytopenia. Ann Intern Med 1984;100:535–540.
48. Griffith GC, Nichols G, Asher JD, et al. Heparin osteoporosis. JAMA 1965;193:91–94.
49. Stenflo M, Suttie JW. Vitamin K–dependent formation of gamma-carboxyglutamic acid. Annu Rev Biochem 1977;46: 157–172.
50. Sawyer WT. Warfarin, in Mungall D (ed): Applied Clinical Pharmacokinetics. New York, Raven, 1983, pp 187–222.
51. Yacobi A, Levy G. Protein binding of warfarin in serum of humans and rats. J Pharmacokinet Biopharm 1977;5:123–131.
52. Toon S, Trager WF. Pharmacokinetic implications of stereoselective changes in plasma-protein binding. Warfarin/sulfinpyrazone. J Pharm Sci 1984;73:1671–1673.
53. Porter RS, Sawyer WT, Lowenthal DT. Warfarin, in Evans WE, Schentag JJ, Jusko WJ (eds): Applied Pharmacokinetics. San Francisco, Applied Therapeutics, 1986, pp 1057–1104.
54. Backmann K, Shapiro R, Mackiewicz J. Warfarin elimination and responsiveness in patients with renal dysfunction. J Clin Pharmacol 1977;17:292–299.
55. Yacobi A, Udall JA, Levy G. Serum protein binding as a determinant of warfarin body clearance and anticoagulant effect. Clin Pharmacol Ther 1976;19:552–558.
56. Coon WW, Willis PW, Symon MJ. Assessment of anticoagulant treatment of venous thromboembolism. Ann Surg 1969;170:559–568.
57. Coon WW, Willis PW. Recurrence of venous thromboembolism. Surgery 1973;73:823–827.
58. Levine MN, Raskob G, Hirsh J. Risk of hemorrhage with long term anticoagulant therapy. Drugs 1985;30:444–460.
59. Hull R, Delmore T, Genton E. Warfarin sodium versus low-dose heparin in the long-term treatment of venous thrombosis. N Engl J Med 1979;301:855–858.
60. Hull R, Delmore T, Carter C. Adjusted subcutaneous heparin versus warfarin sodium in the long-term treatment of venous thromboembolism. N Engl J Med 1982;306:189–194.
61. Hull R, Hirsh J, Jay R, et al. Different intensities of oral anticoagulant therapy in the treatment of proximal-vein thrombosis. N Engl J Med 1982;307:1676–1681.
62. Hull RD, Raskob GE, Hirsh J, et al. A cost-effectiveness analysis of alternative approaches for long-term treatment of proximal venous thrombosis. JAMA 1984;252:235–239.
63. Merril LK, VerBurg DJ. The choice of long-term anticoagulants for the pregnant patient. Obstet Gynecol 1976;47:711–714.
64. Tawes RL, Kennedy PA, Harris EJ, et al. Management of deep venous thrombosis and pulmonary embolism during pregnancy. Am J Surg 1982;144:141–145.
65. Wessler S, Gitel SN. Warfarin. From bedside to bench. N Engl J Med 1984;311:645–652.
66. Westblom TU, Marienfeld RD. Prolonged hospitalization because of inappropriate delay of warfarin therapy in deep venous thrombosis. South Med J 1985;78:1164–1167.
67. Self TH, Bauman JH, Brown JR, et al. Concurrent initiation of heparin and warfarin therapy. Am Heart J 1981;102:470–471.
68. O'Reilly RA, Aggeler PM. Studies on coumarin anticoagulant drugs. Initiation of warfarin therapy without a loading dose. Circulation 1968;38:169–177.
69. Talbert RL, Hersh MR. Effect of heparin on prothrombin time. Clin Pharm 1982;1:204.
70. Hirsh J, Deykin D, Poller L. "Therapeutic range" for oral anticoagulant therapy. Chest 1986;89(suppl):115–155.
71. Lutomski DM, Djuric PE, Draeger RW. Warfarin therapy: The effect of heparin on prothrombin times. Arch Intern Med 1987;432:433.
72. Sawyer WT, Raasch RJ. Effect of heparin on prothrombin time. Clin Pharm 1984;3:192–194.
73. McGehee WG, Klotz TA, Epstein DJ, et al. Coumarin necrosis associated with hereditary protein C deficiency. Ann Intern Med 1984;101:59–60.
74. Lebsack CS, Weibert RT. "Purple toes" syndrome. Postgrad Med 1982;71:81–84.
75. Serlin JH, Breckenridge AM. Drug interactions with warfarin. Drugs 1983;25:610–620.
76. Verstraete M, Collen D. Pharmacology of thrombolytic drugs. J Am Coll Cardiol 1986;8:33B–40B.

77. Abbott Laboratories. Abbokinase package insert. Chicago, IL, January 1984.
78. Hoechst-Roussel Pharmaceuticals Inc. Streptase package insert. Somerville, NJ, April 1982.
79. Consensus Development Panel. Thrombolytic therapy in thrombosis: A National Institutes of Health Consensus Development Panel. Ann Intern Med 1980;93:141–144.
80. A Cooperative Study. Urokinase pulmonary embolism trial phase I results. JAMA 1970;214:2163–2172.
81. A Cooperative Study. Urokinase–streptokinase embolism trial phase 2 results. JAMA 1974;229:1606–1613.
82. Sharma GVRK, Burleson VA, Sasahara AA. Effect of thrombolytic therapy on pulmonary-capillary blood volume in patients with pulmonary embolism. N Engl J Med 1980;303:842–845.
83. Elliott MS, Immelman DJ, Jeffrey P, et al. A comparative randomized trial of heparin versus streptokinase in the treatment of acute proximal venous thrombosis: An interim report of a prospective trial. Br J Surg 1979;66:838–843.
84. Marder VJ. Guidelines for thrombolytic therapy of deep-vein thrombosis. Prog Cardiovasc Dis 1979;21:327–332.
85. Shafer KE, Santoro SA, Sobel BE, et al. Monitoring activity of fibrinolytic agents: A therapeutic challenge. Am J Med 1984;76:879–886.
86. Comer JB, Emanuelsen KL, Drezner AD, et al. Developing guidelines for thrombolytic therapy. Am J Hosp Pharm 1984;41:2374–2377.
87. Marder VJ. The use of thrombolytic agents: Choice of patient, drug administration, laboratory monitoring. Ann Intern Med 1979;90:802–808.
88. Bell MR, Meed AG. Guidelines for the use of thrombolytic agents. N Engl J Med 1979;301:1266–1270.
89. Sharma GVRK, Cella G, Parisi AF, et al. Thrombolytic therapy. N Engl J Med 1982;306:1268–1276.
90. Sharma GVRK, Sasahara AA. Thrombolytic therapy. (Lett) N Engl J Med 1981;304:361.
91. Young AE, Thomas ML, Browse NL. Comparison between sequelae of surgical and medical treatment of venous thromboembolism. Br Med J 1974;4:127–135.
92. Greenfield LF, Alexander EL. Current status of surgical therapy for deep vein thrombosis. Am J Surg 1985;150:64–70.
93. Goldhaber SZ. Prevention of venous thromboembolism, in Goldhaber SZ (ed): Pulmonary Embolism and Deep Venous Thrombosis. Philadelphia, W.B. Saunders, 1985, pp 135–157.
94. Kakkar VV, Adams PC. Preventive and therapeutic approach to venous thromboembolic disease and pulmonary embolism: Can death from pulmonary embolism be prevented? J Am Coll Cardiol 1986;8(suppl):146B–158B.
95. Barnes RW, Brand RA, Clarke W, et al. Efficacy of graded-compression antiembolism stockings in patients undergoing total hip arthroplasty. Clin Orthop Rel Res 1978;132:61.
96. Leyuraz PR, Richard J, Bachmann F, et al. Adjusted versus fixed-dose subcutaneous heparin in the prevention of deep-vein thrombosis after total hip replacement. N Engl J Med 1983;309:954–958.
97. Wray R, Mauer B, Shillingford J. Prophylactic anticoagulant therapy in the prevention of calf-vein thrombosis after myocardial infarction. N Engl J Med 1973;288:815–817.
98. Multicenter Trial Committee. Dihydroergotamine–heparin prophylaxis of postoperative deep vein thrombosis. A multicenter trial. JAM 1984;251:2960–2966.
99. Kakkar VV, Djazaeri B, Fok J, et al. Low-molecular-weight heparin and prevention of postoperative deep vein thrombosis. Br Med J 1982;284:375–379.
100. Anonymous. Prevention of venous thrombosis and pulmonary embolism. JAMA 1986;256:744–749.

# Section Two
# Respiratory Disorders

## Chapter 21 / Asthma

H. William Kelly, PharmD, and Robin L. Davis, PharmD

Bronchial asthma is a common disease of children and adults. Although its clinical manifestations have been known since antiquity, asthma is a disease that still defies precise definition. The word *asthma* is of Greek origin and means "panting." More than 2,000 years ago, Hippocrates used the word asthma to describe episodic shortness of breath; however, the first detailed clinical description of the asthmatic patient was made by Aretaeus in the second century.[1] Since that time asthma has been used to describe any disorder with episodic shortness of breath or dyspnea; thus, the terms *cardiac asthma* and *bronchial asthma* have been used to delineate the etiologies of the dyspnea. These terms are now obsolete and asthma refers to a disorder of the respiratory system characterized by episodes of difficulty in breathing.

The Committee on Diagnostic Standards of the American Thoracic Society[2] defined asthma as "a disease characterized by an increased responsiveness of the trachea and bronchi to a variety of stimuli and manifested by widespread narrowing of the airways that changes in severity either spontaneously or as a result of therapy." More recently, a committee of the American Thoracic Society has attempted to clarify the definition by further defining "reversibility" and "airway obstruction."[3] They defined reversibility as "a significant improvement in measurement(s) of airway obstruction greater than 1.65 times the coefficient of variation of the test(s) used to assess reversibility of the airways." Airway obstruction was characterized as (1) "presence of a significant obstructive ventilatory abnormality in tests of ventilatory mechanics" and (2) "presence of associated periodic cough, tightness, wheezing, or dyspnea."

The lack of a more precise definition for asthma is attributed to our lack of knowledge of the precise pathogenic defect that results in the clinical syndrome we recognize as asthma. Thus, the definition represents a description of the clinical symptoms of asthma without a delineation of etiology. The current definition does allow for the important heterogeneity of the clinical presentation of asthma. New technologies have added substantially to our understanding of the interrelationships of immunology, biochemistry, and physiology to the clinical presentation of asthma, and further research may yet uncover a single cellular defect in asthma. Until such time, asthma will continue to defy exact definition.

### Epidemiology

The lack of a precise uniform definition has hampered epidemiologic research in asthma. As recently as the 1950s, the definition required the presence of allergy, which is clearly not the case now. As a result there are no definitive population-based figures that have used uniform diagnostic criteria to estimate the incidence or prevalence of asthma. Despite this limitation, a number of epidemiologic surveys of asthma have been published.

In 1979, the National Institute of Allergy and Infectious Diseases (NIAID) Task Force on Asthma and Other Allergic Diseases estimated that more than 9 million persons (about 4% of the population) suffered from asthma and as many as 7% of all Americans have had asthma.[4] The estimated economic cost of asthma in the United States in 1979 was $2.4 billion.[5] Asthma was responsible for 6,786,000 physician office visits and more than 2 million hospital days.[5] Asthma was the cause of an estimated 1,872 deaths and a significant contributing factor in an additional 4,401 others. Childhood asthma is a major cause of school absenteeism. Children with asthma have absentee rates 24% higher than overall absentee rates.[6]

Dodge and Burrows[7] recently reported results from the Tucson Epidemiologic Study of lung diseases, a prospective population-based survey. A population-based study for the community of Tecumseh, Michigan, confirmed the Tucson results showing 50% of all subjects had an age of onset younger than 10 years.[8] Both studies suggest that asthma below the age of 15 occurs primarily in boys, whereas older asthmatics are more commonly female.[7,8]

### Natural History

Weiss and Speizer[9] recently reviewed the long-term follow-up studies of patients with asthma published since 1952. They noted that a number of the studies had serious methodologic problems. Many of the studies were retrospective and either clinic or hospital based, leading to possible bias in patient selection. In these studies, the definition of asthma was often unclear and physiologic tests of airway reactivity were not performed. Population-based controls were used in only one study. Despite these limitations, some conclusions about the natural history of asthma can be made. Between 30% and 70% of children with asthma markedly improve or become symptom free by early adulthood; chronic disease persists in about 30% of patients. Although asthmatic patients who develop the disease in childhood are more likely to have remissions, patients who present at an early age have a poorer prognosis.

Martin et al[10] reported that 60% of patients who were symptom-free as adults continued to exhibit bronchial hyperreactivity to inhaled histamine challenges. Data from the Tucson Epidemiologic Study confirmed the findings of the previous studies.[11] They reported a 28.7% remission rate that was highest in the age group 10–19 years (65%) and lowest in the subjects 40–49 years old (6%). Subjects with less frequent attacks and normal pulmonary functions on initial assessment had increased remission rates. In addition, smokers had the lowest remission and highest relapse rates.

All of the follow-up studies indicate that death from asthma is relatively rare. These studies are described in a recent review.[12] The published mortality statistics for the United States from 1978 to 1980 indicate a mortality rate of 0.3 per 100,000 persons aged 5–34 years.[9] The overall mortality from asthma is estimated at 2,000 deaths per year in the United States.[13] This is consistent with the death rates found in Canada, Australia, West Germany, and England and Wales.[13]

Although death from asthma is a relatively rare event, studies of the cause and prevention of death from asthma have presented disturbing results. A recent prospective study of asthma deaths carried out by the British Thoracic Society indicated that 86% of the deaths were preventable.[14] Most deaths from asthma occur outside of the hospital; death is rare after hospitalization.[13] The most common cause of death from asthma is inadequate assessment of the severity of airway obstruction by the patient or physician and inadequate therapy.[13] This was found to be true in deaths of hospitalized patients as well as outpatients; thus the key to prevention of death from asthma as advocated by the British Thoracic Society and others is education of the patients as well as the clinicians caring for them.

## Pathophysiology

Although a specific cellular defect has not yet been discovered, new technologies have substantially advanced our understanding of the pathogenesis of asthma. Hyperreactivity of the airways to physical, chemical, and pharmacologic stimuli is the hallmark of asthma.[15] Bronchial hyperreactivity also occurs in some patients with chronic bronchitis and allergic rhinitis, though to a lesser degree.[16] Normal healthy subjects may also develop a transient increased bronchial reactivity after viral respiratory infections or exposure to ozone[16]; however, the degree of reactivity is quantitatively greater in asthmatic patients than in other groups who demonstrate hyperreactivity. Bronchial reactivity of the general population fits a unimodal distribution that is skewed toward increased reactivity.[9] Patients with clinical asthma represent the extreme end of the distribution. The degree of bronchial hyperreactivity within asthmatics correlates with the clinical course of their disease.[16] Patients with mild symptomatology or in remission demonstrate lower levels of reactivity though still greater than the normal population.

Much of the recent research on the pathogenesis of asthma has focused on explaining airway hyperreactivity. A number of excellent reviews and symposia have highlighted new discoveries and summarized the current state of knowledge of this expanding area of research.[15–19]

### *Pathology*

Our knowledge of the pathological changes in asthma is based primarily on autopsy findings in patients who have died of asthma and more rarely on autopsies in asthmatics who have died of other causes. The intact lungs of the autopsy patients are hyperinflated because of air trapping from widespread mucus plugging. The histologic examination is characterized by three findings (Fig. 21.1): (1) marked hypertrophy and hyperplasia of the airway smooth muscle, (2) increased airway wall thickness caused by an exudative inflammatory reaction and edema, and (3) mucous gland hypertrophy and mucus hypersecretion.[20]

#### Bronchial Smooth Muscle

The smooth muscle of the airways does not form a uniform coat around the airways but is wrapped around in a connecting network that is best described as a spiral arrangement.[21] The muscle contraction displays a sphincteric action that is capable of completely occluding the airway lumen. The airway smooth muscle extends from the trachea through the respiratory bronchioli. When expressed as percentage of wall thickness, the smooth muscle represents 5% of the large central airways and up to 20% of the wall thickness in the bronchioles.[20] Total smooth muscle mass decreases rapidly past the terminal bronchioles to the alveoli so the contribution of smooth muscle tone to airway diameter in this region is relatively small.[22] In the large airways of asthmatics, smooth muscle may account for 11% of the wall thickness.[20]

Airway smooth muscle contraction in vivo is measured indirectly by determining the flow of air into and out of the patient. The difficulties in using changes in airflow as a measurement of smooth muscle contraction have been delineated elsewhere.[16,22] The relationship between airway diameter and flow is dictated by Poiseuille's law[23]

$$\Delta P = 8nl/\pi r^4$$

where $n$ = viscosity of the air, $l$ = length of the tube, $r$ = radius of the tube, and $\Delta P$ = drop in pressure. Since resistance is equal to $\Delta P$ divided by airflow, a twofold change in airway diameter would produce a 16-fold change in airflow resistance. It is possible that the increased smooth muscle mass of the asthmatic airways is important in magnifying and maintaining bronchial hyperreactivity in chronic asthma[16,19]; however, it appears that the hypertrophy and hyperplasia are secondary processes caused by chronic stimulation and are not the primary cause of bronchial hyperreactivity.[16,19,20]

The airway is innervated by parasympathetic, sympathetic, and nonadrenergic inhibitory nerves (Fig. 21.2). The

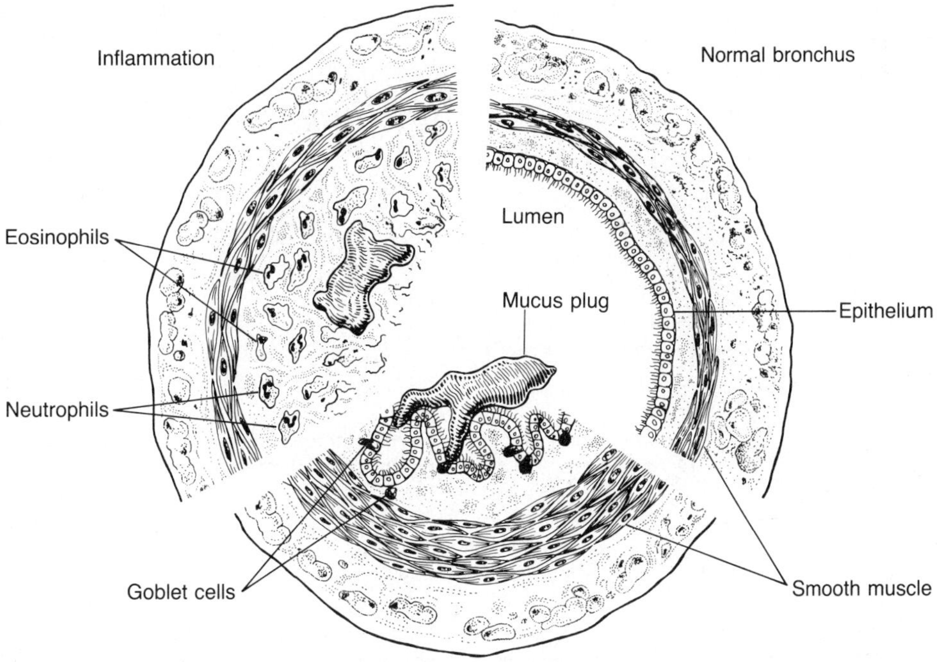


**Figure 21.1** Representative illustration of the pathology found in the asthmatic bronchus compared with a normal bronchus (upper right). Each section demonstrates how the lumen is narrowed. Edema of the basement membrane, mucus plugging, smooth muscle hypertrophy, and constriction contribute (lower section). Inflammatory cells producing epithelial desquammation fill the airway lumen with cellular debris and expose the airway smooth muscle to other mediators (upper left).

normal resting tone of human airway smooth muscle is maintained by vagal efferent activity.[19] Maximum bronchoconstriction mediated by vagal stimulation occurs in the small bronchi and is absent in the small bronchioles.[16] The nonmyelinated "C fibers" of the afferent system lie immediately beneath the tight junctions between epithelial cells lining the airway lumen.[16] These endings probably represent the irritant receptors of the airways. Stimulation of these irritant receptors by mechanical stimulation, chemical and particulate irritants, and pharmacologic agents such as histamine produces reflex bronchoconstriction.[16,19,23]

The sympathetic innervation of the airway smooth muscle is sparse.[16] Stimulation of the innervated sympathetic nerves produces bronchodilation. In addition, all of the airway smooth muscle contains noninnervated $\beta_2$-adrenergic receptors that produce bronchodilation.[23] There is some evidence for $\alpha$-adrenergic receptors in the major resistant airways. Stimulation of these receptors produces bronchoconstriction that is enhanced by pretreatment with histamine.[16] The importance of these receptors in asthma is unknown.

One theory on the pathogenesis of bronchial hyperreactivity was that asthma represented a relative $\beta$-adrenergic blockade.[24] The demonstration of a $\beta$-adrenergic defect in asthmatic patients has been inconsistent,[15,23] and the production of $\beta$-blockade in normal subjects is insufficient, by itself, to cause bronchial hyperreactivity. Recent studies have suggested the existence of a nonadrenergic inhibitory system in the trachea and bronchi. Stimulation of this system leads to bronchodilation.[23] The exact neurotransmitter is unknown.

**Mucus Production**

The mucociliary system is the lungs' primary defense mechanism against irritants and infectious agents. Mucus is composed of 95% water and 5% glycoproteins and is produced by bronchial epithelial glands and goblet cells.[20,21] The lining of the airway consists of a continuous aqueous layer that is controlled by active ion transport across the epithelium where water moves toward the lumen along the concentration gradient. Catecholamines and vagal stimulation enhance the ion transport and fluid movement.[25] Mucus transport is dependent on the viscoelastic properties of the mucus. Mucus that is either too watery or too viscous will not be optimally transported. The exudative inflammatory process and the sloughing of epithelial cells into the airway lumen adversely affect mucociliary transport. The bronchial glands are increased in size and the goblet cells are increased in size and number in asthma, suggesting increased mucus production.[20]

Expectorated mucus from patients with asthma tends to have a high viscosity. The mucus plugs in the airways of patients who die in status asthmaticus are tenacious and tend to be connected by mucous strands to the goblet cells.[21] Asthmatic airways may also become plugged with epithelial and inflammatory cell casts. Although it is tempting to speculate that patients died from asthmatic attacks because of mucous plugging resulting in irreversible obstruction, there is no direct evidence for this. Autopsies of asthmatics who died from other causes have shown similar pathology.[13]

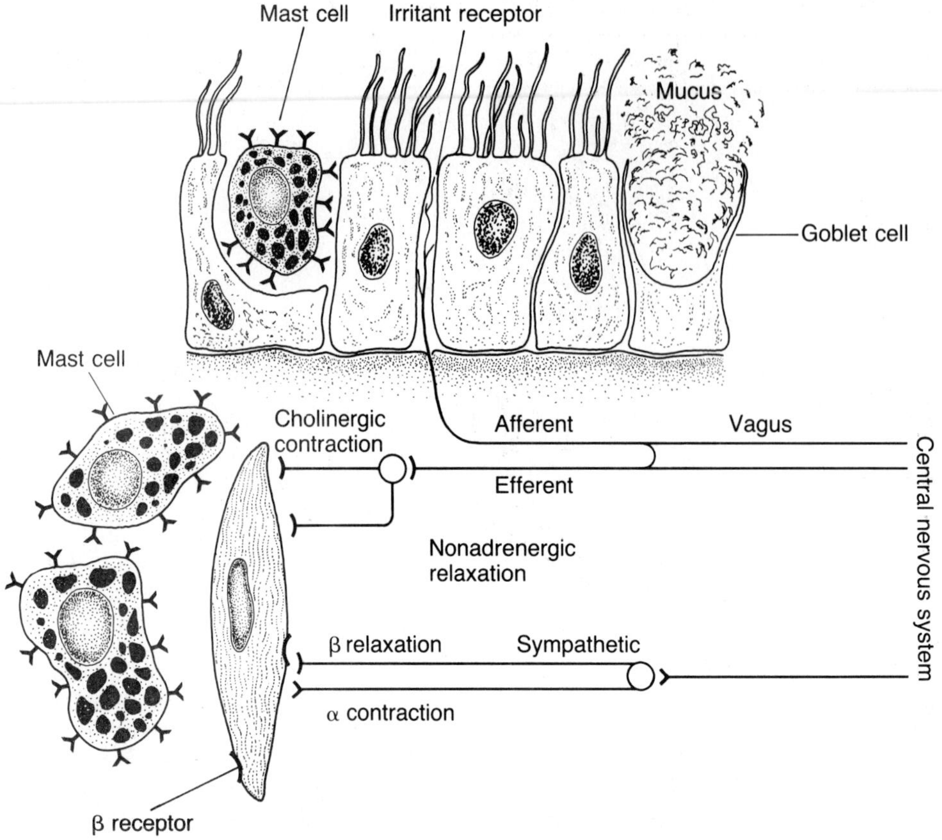


**Figure 21.2** Innervation of the airways by the sympathetic, cholinergic, and nonadrenergic inhibitory systems. Mast cell concentration increases from the epithelial lumen to the submucosa.

In addition, some subjects who have died of sudden severe asthma did not show the characteristic mucus plugging on necropsy.[21]

### Inflammation

The inflammatory reaction appears to be the key mechanism to explain the pathologic changes seen in asthma. In addition, inflammation of the airways and the release of mediators of inflammation appear to be necessary for the development and maintenance of bronchial hyperreactivity.[15,16,20] Inflammation of the airways is associated with epithelial cell damage and increased mucosal permeability.[20] This improves access of noxious stimuli from the lumen to the airway smooth muscle, submucosal mast cells, and the cholinergic irritant receptors located in the junction between cells.[15,19] The epithelial damage and turnover leads to hypertrophy of the basement membrane.[20] Inflammation can also account for mucus hypersecretion.[20] Therefore, recent research on the pathogenesis of bronchial hyperreactivity has focused on inflammation and the mediators of the inflammatory process. Table 21.1 lists a number of identified mediators, their origin, and pathophysiologic processes with which they are associated.[17,18,26]

While our understanding of the complex interactions involved in the inflammatory process is still incomplete, the central role of inflammation in producing or increasing bronchial hyperreactivity appears clear. In human asthma, the inflammation could be caused by IgE-mediated release of mast cell mediators in allergic asthma and by release of mast cell or neutrophil mediators in nonallergic asthma. In addition, neutrophils may also play an important role in allergic asthma. Damage to epithelial cells is also associated with the release of cell wall–bound phospholipids and the production of arachidonic acid metabolites.[26] Figure 21.3 outlines arachidonic acid metabolism by the cyclooxygenase and lipoxygenase pathways and the resultant mediators. With the increased awareness of the role of inflammation in the pathogenesis of asthma, it becomes apparent that therapy directed solely at bronchospasm is incomplete and that attempts to minimize inflammation are an important aspect of asthma therapy.

## *Etiology*

The heterogeneity of asthma appears most obvious when listing the diverse triggers of bronchospasm in asthmatic subjects (Table 21.2). In the past, a good deal of the confusion concerning the definition and etiology of asthma centered on the inclusion of the various triggering events as the etiology. Thus, asthma has been variously defined as an allergic, an emotional, and an infectious disease; however, it has become clear that asthma is first a lung disease, and specific triggering events have relative degrees of impor-

**Table 21.1** The Pathologic Process and Source of Mediators Implicated in the Pathogenesis of Asthma

| *Mediator* | *Source* | *Pathologic Effect* |
|---|---|---|
| Histamine | Tissue, mast cells, circulating basophils | Bronchospasm, mucosal edema, mucus secretion ($H_2$) |
| Leukotrienes | | |
| $LTC_4$, $LTD_4$, $LTE_4$ } SRS-A[a] | Mast cells, eosinophils, neutrophils, basophils, macrophages | Bronchospasm, mucosal edema, mucus secretion, decreased mucus transport |
| $LTB_4$ | Airway epithelium, neutrophils, eosinophils, macrophages | Chemotaxis and adhesion of neutrophils and eosinophils, causing cellular infiltration |
| Eosinophil chemotactic factor of anaphylaxis (ECF-A) | Mast cell | Eosinophil infiltration |
| Neutrophil chemotactic factor (NCF) | Mast cell | Neutrophil infiltration |
| Hydroxyeicosatetraenoic acids | | |
| 15-HETE | Airway epithelium | Stimulation of production of LTB by mast cells |
| 5-HETE | Neutrophils | Neutrophil chemotaxis augments IgE-mediated histamine release |
| 12-HETE | Platelets | Chemotaxis |
| 5,12-diHETE | Neutrophils | Chemotaxis |
| Prostaglandin-generating factor of anaphylaxis (PGF-A) | Mast cell | Induction of production of HETEs and prostaglandins |
| Prostaglandins | | |
| $PGD_2$ | Mast cells | Bronchospasm, constriction of pulmonary artery, mucus secretion |
| $PGF_{2\alpha}$ | Many cell types | Bronchospasm, mucus secretion, constriction of microvasculature |
| Thromboxane | Lung parenchyma, platelets | Bronchospasm, constriction of pulmonary arterioles |
| $PGE_2$ | Many cell types | Mucus secretion, smooth muscle relaxation |
| $PGI_2$ | Lung parenchyma | |
| Major basic protein | Eosinophil granules | Epithelial cell damage and exfoliation, inhibition of mucociliary clearance |
| Bradykinin | Mast cells, circulating plasma precursors | Bronchospasm, mucosal edema |
| Adenosine | Mast cells, tissue epithelium | Increase in mast cell mediator release, bronchospasm |
| Peroxides | Mast cells | Epithelial damage and desquamation |
| Superoxide anions | Eosinophils, neutrophils | |

[a] SRS-A, slow releasing substance of anaphylaxis; LT, leukotriene; PG, prostaglandin; HETE, hydroxyeicosatetraenoic acid.

tance from patient to patient. Epidemiologic studies support the concept of a genetic predisposition to the development of asthma.[9] The mode of genetic transmission is not known and is most likely multifactorial.[6] Studies of occupational asthma and the induction of hyperreactivity in healthy individuals emphasize the effect of environment on the development of asthma.[9,17,18] Asthma is still frequently classified according to its predominant trigger; however, it should be emphasized that this method of classification is at best arbitrary and that many patients respond to a number of stimuli. Indeed it is the uniform increased responsiveness to challenge with the nonspecific stimuli methacholine, histamine, and exercise that is often used to define and diagnose asthma.

**Allergic Asthma**

An allergic component can be demonstrated in 35% to 55% of asthmatic patients and this may be higher in childhood asthma.[6,9,15] The allergens (Table 21.2) that provoke asthma are airborne and evoke the asthmatic response through the classical allergic pathway depicted in Figure 21.4. The role of allergy in the etiology of asthma has been controversial and asthma has been considered an allergic disease by many. Although the allergic reaction plays an important role in the atopic asthmatic patient, atopy is not necessary for the development of asthma and not all atopic individuals develop asthma; however, up to 40% of patients with hay fever

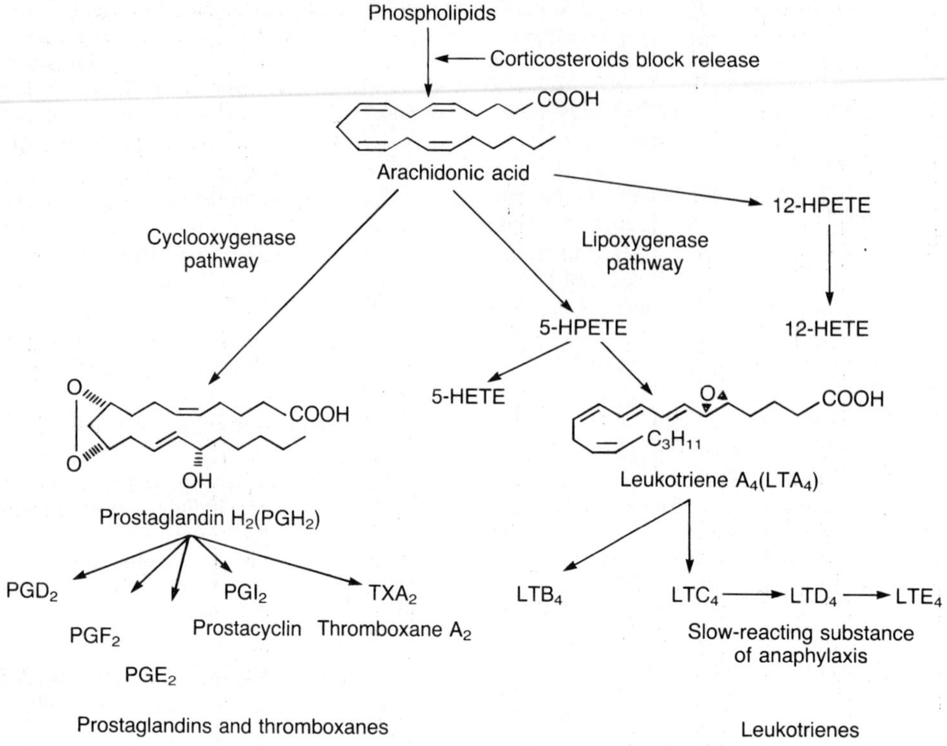


**Figure 21.3** Eicosanoid formation. Prostaglandins and thromboxanes are formed from the metabolism of arachidonic acid via the cyclooxygenase pathway, whereas leukotrienes are formed via the lipoxygenase pathway. Corticosteroids inhibit eicosanoid formation by inhibiting the release of arachidonic acid from membrane phospholipids.

will develop some airway hyperreactivity (though less than asthmatics) during their allergen season.[6]

When allergic asthmatics are given an inhalational challenge with an allergen to which they are sensitized, the patients demonstrate an early asthmatic reaction (Fig. 21.5). The reaction is characterized by a drop in pulmonary functions that reaches maximum intensity in 10–20 minutes and reverses spontaneously by 60–120 minutes.[27] In addition, many subjects experience a late asthmatic reaction (Fig. 21.5) that begins 4 hours after the challenge, reaches maximum intensity in 6 to 8 hours, is often more severe than the early response, and may last as long as 24 hours. The late asthmatic reaction (LAR) has engendered renewed interest from many researchers who believe that it is the pathogenetic mechanism for inducing and maintaining bronchial hyperreactivity in atopic asthmatics.[27] Subjects who experience a LAR demonstrate increased responsiveness to methacholine, histamine, and exercise that may last up to 6 weeks, whereas subjects who experience only the early response demonstrate no increased bronchial reactivity.[27,28] The degree of hyperresponsiveness and its duration correlate with the intensity of the LAR.

The LAR is associated with increased serum concentrations of neutrophil and eosinophil chemotactic factors and the influx of neutrophils and eosinophils into the tissue as well as the degranulation of mast cells. The LAR is associated with greater degrees of obstruction in small airways and air trapping than occur in the early response. The early response is easily blocked or reversed with inhaled $\beta_2$-adrenergic agents and blunted or blocked with methylxanthines, anticholinergics, and oral $\beta_2$-adrenergics. The LAR is not prevented by pretreatment with any of these bronchodilators and often does not respond as well as the early response. Corticosteroid pretreatment does not alter the early response but prevents the LAR, whereas pretreatment with cromolyn sodium blocks both responses.

Clinically, allergic asthmatics develop increased bronchial hyperreactivity with increased exposure to allergens during a pollen season. Avoidance of the pollen or prophylaxis with cromolyn sodium prevents the increased bronchial hyperreactivity.[27,29] Studies have shown that long-term therapy with both cromolyn sodium and corticosteroids reduces bronchial hyperreactivity.[28,29] In contrast, long-term therapy with $\beta_2$-adrenergics and methylxanthines has not been associated with similar decreases in bronchial hyperreactivity.[27]

### Exercise-Induced Asthma

During vigorous exercise pulmonary function in asthmatic patients, as measured by forced expiratory maneuvers, increases during the first few minutes but then begins to decrease after 6 to 8 minutes (Fig. 21.6). A drop in pulmonary function greater than 10% to 15% of the baseline (preexercise) value defines exercise-induced asthma (EIA).[30,31] Most studies suggest that 70% to 90% of all

**Table 21.2** Representative List of Agents and Events Triggering Asthma

| *Trigger* | *Mechanism* |
|---|---|
| Respiratory infection | |
| Respiratory syncytial virus (RSV), rhinovirus, influenza, and parainfluenza, *Mycoplasma* pneumonia | Inflammation and epithelial damage sensitizing cholinergic irritant receptors; virus-induced relative $\beta$ blockade possibly contributes |
| Allergens | |
| Airborne pollens (grasses, trees, weeds), house dust, animal danders, dust mites, insect parts, fungal spores, foods | IgE-mediated mast cell mediator release |
| Exercise | Hyperventilation with loss of water and cooling of the airways and mast cell mediator release |
| Occupational stimuli | |
| Animal handlers, antibiotic drug manufacturing, bakers (flour dust), woodworkers, spice and enzyme workers | IgE-mediated mast cell release |
| Plastic workers (anhydrides), printers (arabic gum), chemical workers (azo dyes, anthraquinone, ethylenediamine, toluene diisocyanates, meat wrappers (heated polyvinyl chloride), plastics and rubber workers (formaldehyde, western red cedar, dimethylethanolamine) | Airway epithelial damage, increased permeability and sensitization of irritant receptors |
| Environment | |
| Cold air, ozone, sulfur dioxide, nitrogen dioxide | Unknown (irritation?); epithelial damage and neutrophil infiltration |
| Emotions | |
| Anxiety, fatigue, stress, laughter | Parasympathetic stimulation; augments preexisting event, generally not a primary event |
| Drugs | See text for discussion |

asthmatics experience EIA.[30] The exact pathogenesis of EIA is unknown; however, heat loss or water loss from the central airways appears to play an important role.[31] EIA is more easily provoked in cold, dry air; warm, humid air can blunt or block it.[15]

A number of studies have demonstrated increased plasma histamine concentrations during EIA, suggesting a role for the mast cell in the pathogenesis. Recent investigations demonstrating a rise in neutrophil chemotactic factor in asthmatics with EIA but not in healthy individuals or asthmatics without EIA confirm the involvement of mediator release in EIA.[31,32] In addition, pretreatment with cromolyn sodium, a drug that stabilizes mast cells, inhibits EIA and inhibits the associated rise in neutrophil chemotactic factor.[30,31] A small number of patients with EIA will have a late response similar to the LAR associated with a secondary rise in neutrophil chemotactic factor.[32]

A refractory period with EIA lasts up to 3 hours after exercise. During this period, repeat exercise of the same intensity either produces no decrease in pulmonary functions or a drop less than 50% of the initial response.[31] The refractory period is thought to be caused by an acute depletion of mast cell mediators and the time required for their repletion.[29] Isocapnic hyperventilation with cold air is not associated with a refractory period.[29] Patients with known refractoriness to exercise will still respond to histamine so that acute hyporesponsiveness of airway smooth muscle does not appear to be a factor.[31]

EIA is believed to be a reflection of the increased hyperreactivity of asthmatics. There is a correlation, though not complete, between EIA and reactivity to histamine and methacholine.[30] Other patient groups with increased airway reactivity (postviral infection, cystic fibrosis, hay fever) show bronchoconstriction after exercise to a lesser degree (5%–10%) than asthmatics (20%–40%).[30] Asthmatics will not always demonstrate the same sensitivity. During periods of remission, they often have a decreased sensitivity to the same degree of exercise; however, a number of children and adults with EIA are otherwise normal, without symptoms or abnormal pulmonary function.

### Miscellaneous Factors

Agents and events that are known to trigger asthma are listed in Table 21.2. Respiratory tract infections are a common cause of asthma exacerbations. Well-controlled investigations have demonstrated that viral infections and not bacteria are primarily responsible for exacerbation of asthma.[9,15] The mechanism is unknown, but is presumably caused by epithelial damage and inflammation in the airway mucosa.

Ozone and sulfur dioxide, common components of air pollution, have been used to induce hyperreactivity in animals. Exposure to 0.2 ppm ozone for 2 to 3 hours can induce bronchoconstriction and increase bronchial reactivity in asthmatics.[15] Sulfur dioxide in the ambient atmosphere is highly irritating, but it is not known how it induces bronchoconstriction. Pretreatment with cromolyn sodium will block the obstruction, implicating mast cell involvement.[15]

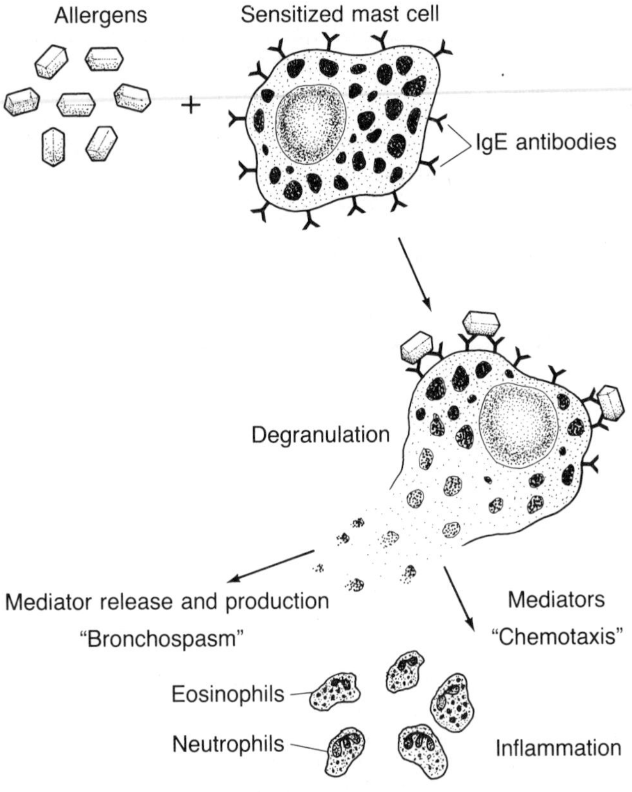


**Figure 21.4** IgE-mediated allergic response. Allergens produce steric changes in a mast cell, leading to the spillage of granules with preformed mediators as well as initiating production of other mediators of anaphylaxis through the lipoxygenase pathway.

Asthma produced by repeated prolonged exposure to industrial inhalants is a significant health problem. It has been estimated that occupational asthma accounts for 2% of all asthmatic persons.[18] Persons with occupational asthma have the typical symptoms of asthma with cough, dyspnea, and wheeze. Typically, the symptoms are related to work with improvement on weekends and vacations. In some instances, symptoms may persist even after termination of exposure.[18]

Emotions and stress rarely precipitate attacks of asthma, but more commonly worsen an attack in progress.[6,15] Bronchoconstriction from psychologic factors appears to be primarily mediated through excess parasympathetic input. Atropine has been shown to block experimental psychogenic bronchoconstriction.[16] It is most important to emphasize to patients and to parents of asthmatic children that asthma is not an emotional disease; however, calming influences and relaxation techniques may benefit the patient who becomes severely emotionally distraught during asthma attacks.

### *Pulmonary Physiology in Asthma*

A complete analysis of pulmonary physiology and the pathophysiology in asthma is beyond the scope of this chapter, so the interested reader should refer to several reviews.[15,22,33,34]

As stated previously, changes in airway diameter are measured indirectly by resistance to airflow or more simply by documenting changes in expiratory spirograms. The total lung capacity (TLC) correlates with the patient's size and gender, and standard values are available. The residual volume (RV) is the amount of air left in the lung to keep the airways open at the end of a forced expiratory maneuver and is obtained by subtracting the forced vital capacity (FVC) from the TLC. The peak expiratory flow rate (PEFR) and forced expiratory volume in 1 second ($FEV_1$) are the tests used most frequently to assess severity of bronchoconstriction and response to therapy. The forced expiratory flow between 25% and 75% of the forced vital capacity ($FEF_{25-75}$), which is also called the maximal midexpiratory flow rate, is calculated from the time taken to deliver the middle 50% of the FVC.

The FVC is determined by TLC and RV. TLC is dependent on the elastic properties of the lung and chest wall.[34] Elastic recoil is decreased and TLC is increased during acute asthma attacks.[33] The hyperinflation is seen on chest roentgenogram and at autopsy. The hyperinflation is also attributed to airway closure at higher lung volumes caused by inflammation, edema, bronchoconstriction, and mucus plugging, which is reflected in an increased RV and a reduced FVC.

The $FEV_1$ and PEFR reflect primarily changes in the diameter of the large central airways. The central airways represent the major resistance to airflow in the lungs because of their minimal cross-sectional area compared with the bronchi less than 2 mm in diameter.[22,34] Because the small peripheral airways constitute a small fraction of overall resistance to airflow, tests that reflect total resistance (i.e., $FEV_1$ and PEFR) are insensitive to abnormalities in small airways. Another disadvantage to the $FEV_1$ and PEFR is that they are highly dependent on the effort of the patient. Despite this, the $FEV_1$ is the most useful lung function test used to evaluate patients and therapy and has been shown to be the best test for evaluation of bronchodilators. An improvement of 15% to 20% in $FEV_1$ after administration of a bronchodilator is said to reflect significant reversibility.[22,33,34]

During an acute attack of asthma, $FEV_1$, PEFR, and FVC are all decreased. Most patients become asymptomatic when the $FEV_1$ reaches 60% of their predicted normal value and substantially impaired at a level less than 40% of predicted.[22] A change of 20% has a noticeable subjective effect in the range of 30% to 70% of predicted.[22] Asymptomatic patients often demonstrate a 15% to 20% improvement in $FEV_1$ after bronchodilator administration despite normal baseline values, and this can be used to help in the diagnosis; however, a failure to respond acutely to a bronchodilator does not rule out the diagnosis of asthma or reversible airway disease.

Tests of flow at low lung volumes (e.g., $FEF_{25-75}$) are less influenced by respiratory effort and reflect flow caused by elastic recoil of the airways.[34] They are more sensitive to changes in smaller airways; however, their coefficient of variation is greater and larger changes (30%–40% for $FEF_{25-75}$) are required to be significant.[22] During acute asthma attacks, $FEF_{25-75}$ shows the greatest degree of impairment followed by $FEV_1$ and FVC and PEFR. After the asthma attack, the $FEF_{25-75}$ may continue to show significant impairment of flow for weeks in the otherwise asymptomatic patient. The RV:TLC ratio is another sensi-

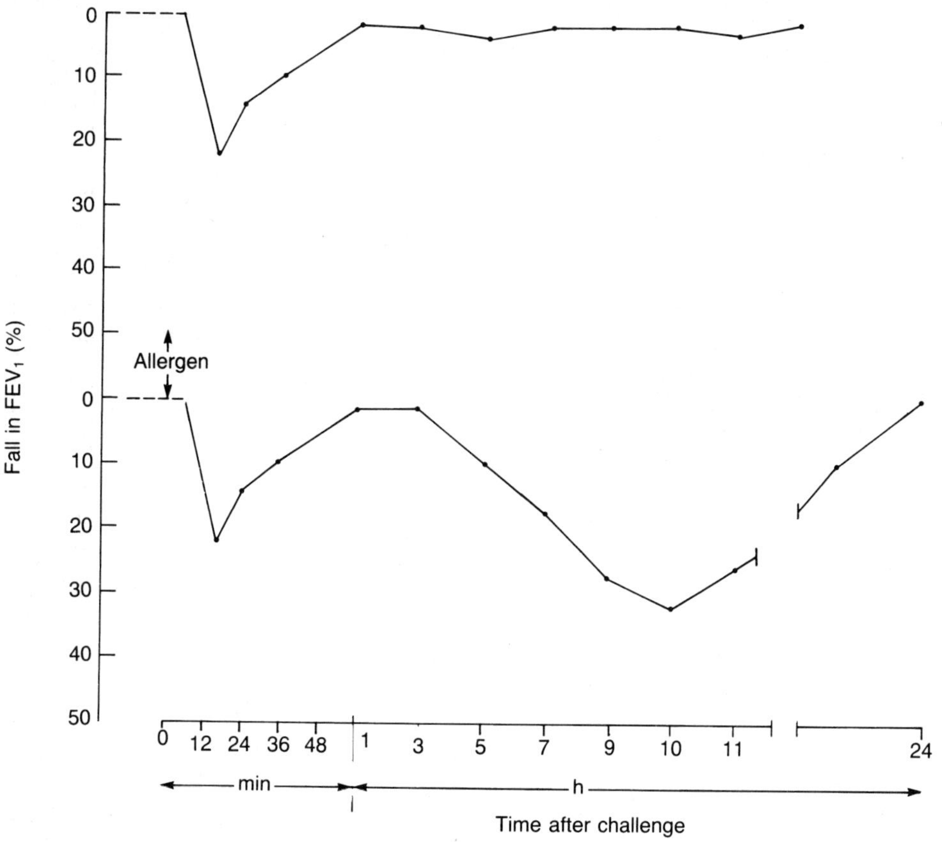


**Figure 21.5** Patterns of response to inhaled antigen. The upper curve represents the early asthmatic response and the lower curve, the dual response. Patients may also exhibit only a late asthmatic response. The late response may be milder or more intense than the early response, but is longer in duration.

tive test of small airway function that is frequently used for long-term follow-up of chronic asthma as a reflection of obstruction from inflammation.[22] In general, during acute asthma attacks, tests of small peripheral airway disease are of limited value because of the lack of correlation with clinical symptoms of obstruction and central airway narrowing interfering with the tests.[33]

### *Blood Gas Measurement*

Gas exchange at the alveoli–capillary interface is dependent on ventilation ($V_a$) or the mechanical properties of the lung, perfusion ($Q$), the flow of blood, and diffusion of gases across the membrane. Studies of diffusion capacity in acute asthma indicate that it is slightly increased or unchanged.[33] Arterial hypoxia is common during acute asthma attacks and is caused by significant derangements in $V_a/Q$ relationships.[33,34] Though diffuse, the airway narrowing during asthma attacks results in large abnormalities in the distribution of ventilation. Perfusion abnormalities appear to be secondary to changes in ventilation. The normal response to alveolar hypoxia is active vasoconstriction to shunt blood flow to better ventilated areas.[34] Unfortunately, the $V_a$ and $Q$ are not perfectly matched in acute asthma. This may in

**Figure 21.6** Typical responses to exercise in a normal subject and an asthmatic subject. Note the initial bronchodilation. PEFR, peak expiratory flow rate.

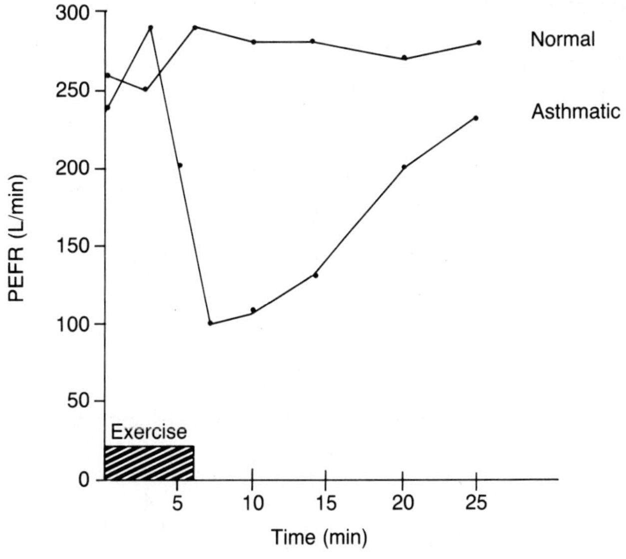

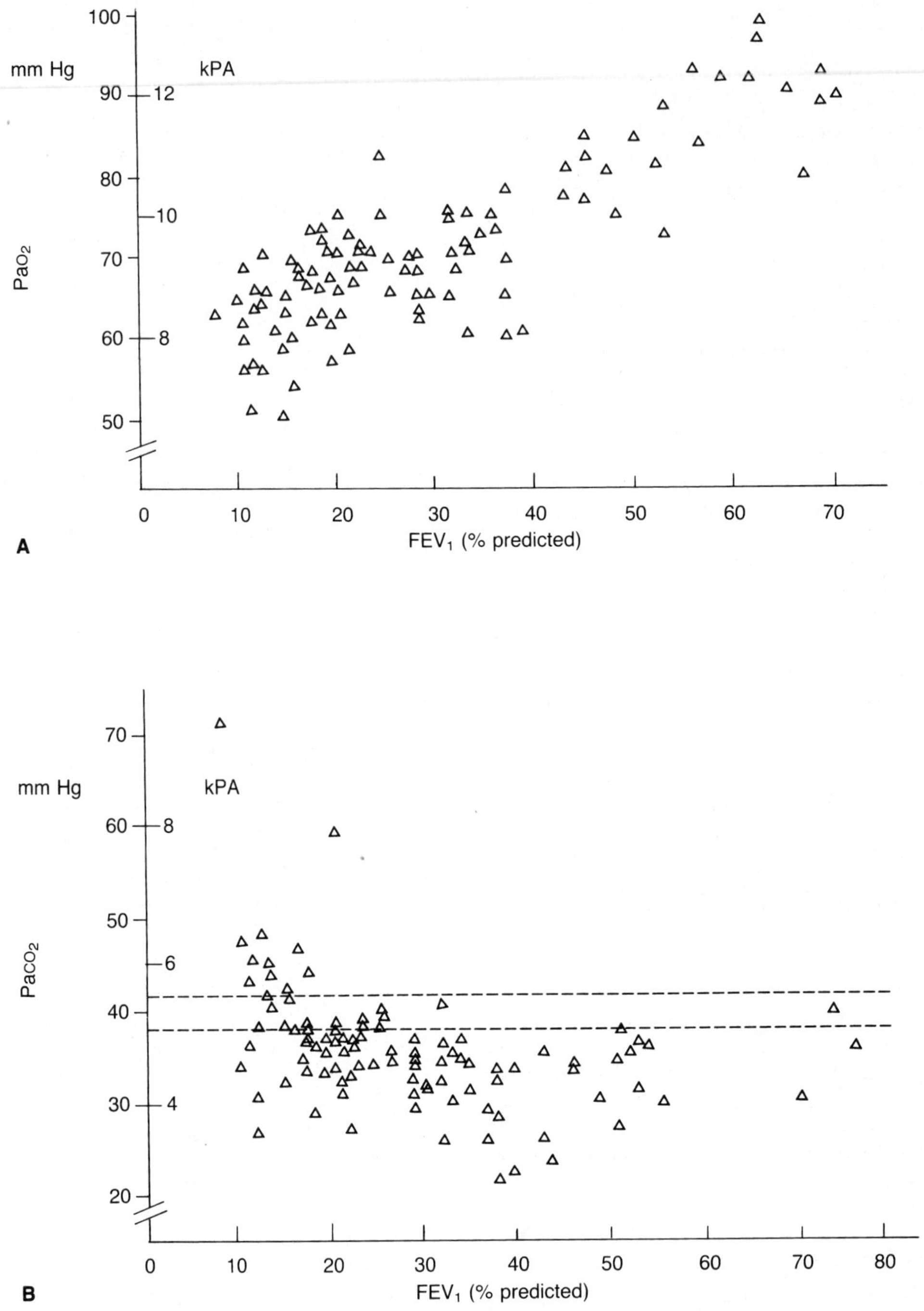


**Figure 21.7** Effect of increasing airway obstruction on arterial $Pao_2$ (A) and $PaCo_2$ (B). The dashed lines show the normal range of $PaCO_2$. *(From McFadden ER Jr, Lyons HA: Arterial blood gas tension in asthma. N Engl J Med 1968;278:1029, with permission.)*

part be caused by the increased vascular resistance produced by the lung hyperinflation.[34] Figure 21.7 demonstrates the effect of increasing airway obstruction on arterial blood gases.

When lungs initially become obstructed, patients demonstrate a marked respiratory drive that is thought to be caused by stimulation of the irritant receptors because it is not obliterated by correcting the hypoxemia.[34] As a result, the asthmatic tends to "blow off" carbon dioxide and the arterial carbon dioxide concentration decreases (Fig. 21.7). Unfortunately, the patient is forced to breathe at higher lung volumes because of air trapping. This requires the use of accessory respiratory muscles. When the respiratory muscles begin to fatigue, the patient will retain carbon dioxide.

## Clinical Presentation

Classic asthma is characterized by episodic dyspnea associated with wheezing; however, the clinical presentation of asthma is as diverse as the number of triggering events. Although wheezing is the characteristic symptom of asthma, the medical literature is replete with the warning that "not all that wheezes is asthma." A wheeze is a high-pitched, whistling sound created by turbulent airflow through an obstructed airway so that any condition that produces significant obstruction can result in wheezing as a symptom. In addition, "all of asthma does not wheeze" is an equally justifiable warning. Patients may present with a chronic persistent cough as their only symptom.[35]

The diagnosis of asthma is based primarily on a good history of recurrent episodes of dyspnea and/or wheezing. The patient may complain of a feeling of tightness in the chest or sometimes a burning sensation. The patient may have a family history of atopy or asthma or have symptoms of allergic rhinitis. A history of exercise or cold air precipitating the dyspnea or an association of increased symptoms during specific allergen seasons would also point to asthma.

In the older child and adult patient in whom spirometric evaluations can be performed, abnormal pulmonary function tests that improve 15% or more after bronchodilator administration help to confirm the diagnosis. Failure of pulmonary function to improve acutely does not necessarily rule out asthma. Patients with long-standing disease or substantial inflammation may require an intensive prolonged course of bronchodilators and corticosteroids before reversibility is detected.[33] If baseline spirometry is normal, challenge testing with exercise, histamine, or methacholine can be used to elicit bronchial hyperreactivity. The histamine and methacholine are inhaled in increasing concentrations until the patient's $FEV_1$ drops at least 20% from the baseline.[29] Standard procedures for performing and interpreting challenge tests have been published elsewhere.[36] Patients with significant symptomatology should not be challenged because of their increased sensitivity and need not be challenged for diagnostic purposes.[29,36] Spirometry and bronchoprovocation have been shown to be more reliable indicators of bronchial hyperreactivity than history of wheezing and physical exam.[37]

Studies for atopy such as serum IgE and eosinophils are not necessary to make the diagnosis of asthma, but they may help differentiate asthma from chronic bronchitis in adults. Clinically, this distinction is often difficult to make. Some patients with chronic bronchitis may have a reversible component and some patients with long-standing severe chronic asthma may have significant irreversible damage and obstruction. Very high eosinophil counts may point to the diagnosis of aspergillosis or other hypereosinophilic syndromes. Skin testing is of no value in diagnosing asthma, but may be useful in identifying etiologic triggers.

In small infants unable to perform spirometry, the diagnosis is more difficult. They may demonstrate hyperinflation on the chest roentgenogram. Radiologic exam is helpful in ruling out other causes of wheezing (e.g., foreign body aspiration, parenchymal lung disease, cardiac disease, and congenital anomalies). In place of pulmonary function tests, the parents should be given a diary card to record symptoms and precipitating events.[38]

## Treatment

The prevention of severe life-threatening attacks and the normalization of activity within the patient's lifestyle are the primary goals in the therapy of asthma. A more ideal goal (although more difficult to realize) is normalization of the patient's lung function. Toward these goals, every effort should be made to decrease the patient's baseline hyperreactivity and prevent it from increasing.

The mainstay of the management of asthma is drug therapy. There are numerous books, symposia, and reviews detailing the basic pharmacology and clinical efficacy of the various pharmacologic agents used in asthma.[39–44] In this section, the therapy of specific clinical presentations of asthma are outlined and controversies in therapy are discussed.

### *Exercise-Induced Asthma*

A number of the drugs used to treat asthma inhibit EIA.[45] It is now well recognized that inhalation of one of the long-acting, $\beta_2$-selective adrenergics just before exercise provides the maximum protection against EIA.[30,31] Inhalation of terbutaline, albuterol, or fenoterol provides maximum protection for 2 hours after inhalation and varying degrees of protection for 4 hours, depending on the patient and the intensity of exercise.[30,45] For all of the sympathomimetic aerosols the duration of protection against EIA is shorter than the duration of bronchodilation.[46] Orally administered $\beta_2$-adrenergics inhibit EIA, but to a lesser extent than when given by inhalation, even at doses that provide equivalent degrees of bronchodilation.[45]

Theophylline inhibits EIA in a concentration-dependent fashion, with maximum inhibition at serum concentrations $\geq 15\ \mu g/mL$.[47] Theophylline appears to produce the same degree of inhibition of EIA as oral $\beta_2$-adrenergics.[48] Either would be useful in young children who are unable to use a metered-dose inhaler (MDI) appropriately. Theophylline and oral $\beta_2$-adrenergics given together produce an additive inhibition.[48] Cromolyn sodium administration before exercise inhibits EIA to the same degree as theophylline and also produces an additive effect with $\beta_2$-adrenergics.[30,49] The degree and duration of inhibition with cromolyn are dose dependent, but the inhibition usually lasts only 1.5 to 2 hours.

The effect of anticholinergic agents is highly variable, producing significant inhibition in some patients and no effect in others.[31] Currently, the data are too inconsistent to recommend anticholinergics for EIA. The acute administration of oral or inhaled corticosteroids prior to exercise has no effect on EIA[30,31]; however, continuous therapy with an inhaled corticosteroid for a 4-week treatment period has been shown to significantly decrease the degree of EIA in children.[50] This is consistent with other trials showing decreased bronchial hyperreactivity with chronic steroid administration.[16,29] Antihistamines have a highly variable and weak inhibitory effect on EIA. The calcium channel–blocking agents nifedipine and verapamil have a moderate inhibitory effect on EIA.[51]

Breathing warm humidified air can prevent or significantly decrease EIA.[15,31] Patients should not be discouraged from exercising. Regular exercise has been shown to increase fitness and tolerance to EIA. Indoor sports and activities, particularly swimming, are preferable, but a large number of asthmatic athletes participate in a wide variety of sports. Most of the aerosol $\beta_2$-adrenergic agents have been approved by the International Olympic Committee for use before competition.

### *Chronic Asthma*

Preventive therapy for asthma is by necessity defined by the severity of illness. Therapy is a cooperative agreement between the clinician and the patient, and education is the cornerstone of any therapeutic plan. The patient must chronically live with asthma and must make constant decisions concerning the disease and the quality of life. There is no question that the majority of asthmatics can have their disease well controlled by various treatment regimens. But at what cost? Each patient is an individual and needs to be treated accordingly. As a result, emphasis has been placed on patient education and the development of self-management programs.[17,52] These programs allow the patients more control in the decision-making process and thus more control of their lives. Self-management programs have successfully improved patient outcome and decreased the cost of asthma care.[52]

Bernstein[53] recently described a stepwise approach to the therapy of asthma not too dissimilar to the therapeutic approaches used in other chronic diseases. In the therapy of asthma, it is imperative that a logical general approach be developed. The specifics of the approach may differ between practitioners or between patients, but haphazard switching or changing of therapies must be avoided. Table 21.3 is a general outline that allows flexibility for individualization.

#### Mild Chronic Asthma

Patients with mild symptoms are those who have only occasional bouts of acute mild bronchospasm or cough that does not require hospitalization but does interfere with normal activity or work and causes school absenteeism. These patients are best treated with one of the newer $\beta_2$-adrenergic aerosols. These preparations are convenient, rapid acting, highly effective bronchodilators that have minimal toxicity by the inhaled route.[46] The aerosol $\beta_2$-adrenergics are the most effective agents for preventing EIA and reversing acute attacks of bronchospasm.[17,40,48] Care should be taken to ensure that the patient can use the metered-dose canisters appropriately to derive optimal benefit.[46] Patients should have the appropriate technique (Table 21.4) demonstrated to them and rechecked periodically. For patients unable to coordinate the actuation of the inhaler with inhalation, there are various tube-spacer devices available that enhance the lung deposition and efficacy of the drugs.[46] In patients who are able to use the appropriate technique with the inhalers, spacer devices do not significantly improve the efficacy.[46]

**Table 21.3** Stepwise Approach to the Treatment of Asthma

| *Degree of Asthma* | *Treatment* |
|---|---|
| Health | No treatment |
| Mild intermittent/ exercise-induced | BA[a] |
| Moderate chronic | T or C + BA + SA? |
| Severe | T + C + SA + BA +AC? |
| | T + SS + BA |
| Acute<br>FEV$_1$ < 50% predicted<br>pH = 7.35<br>Pa$CO_2$ = 30–35 mm Hg<br>Pa$O_2$ = 60 mm Hg | BA + SS? |
| Status asthmaticus<br>pH = 7.35<br>Pa$CO_2$ = 40–45 mm Hg<br>Pa$O_2$ = 60 mm Hg<br>*or*<br>Respiratory failure<br>pH ≤ 7.25<br>Pa$CO_2$ ≥ 50 mm Hg<br>Pa$O_2$ ≤ 50 mm Hg | IA + BA<br>+<br>SS + AC?<br>+<br>IB?<br>+<br>V |

[a] BA, $\beta$-adrenergic aerosols; T, theophylline; C, cromolyn; SA, steroid aerosols; AC, anticholinergics; SS, systemic steroids; IA, intravenous aminophylline; IB, intravenous $\beta$-adrenergics; V, mechanical ventilation; ?, controversial treatment.

The available sympathomimetic agents are listed in Table 21.5. Albuterol, terbutaline, fenoterol, and bitolterol all provide acceptable selectivity, with comparable durations of action. Clinically, there is no apparent advantage or difference for any of these four preparations when given in equipotent doses.[46] Young infants unable to use the canisters can usually be easily controlled with an oral $\beta_2$-adrenergic agonist.[38] For mild intermittent symptoms in infants and children, oral $\beta_2$-adrenergic agonists are preferred over

**Table 21.4** Instructions for Inhalation of Metered-Dose Aerosols

| |
|---|
| Shake canister thoroughly |
| Place mouthpiece between the lips, making sure that the teeth and tongue are out of the way |
| Breathe out steadily |
| Activate the canister while taking a *slow*, deep breath |
| Hold the breath at full inspiration for 5–10 s |
| Wait at least 1 min before the next inhalation from the canister |

**Table 21.5** Relative Selectivity, Potency, and Duration of Action of the $\beta$-Adrenergic Agonists

| | *Selectivity* | | | *Duration of action* | | |
|---|---|---|---|---|---|---|
| *Agent* | $\beta_1$ | $\beta_2$ | $\beta_2$ *potency*[a] | **Bronchodilation** | **Protection** | *Oral activity* |
| Isoproterenol | ++++ | ++++ | 1 | 0.5–2 | 0.5–1.0 | No |
| Metaproterenol | +++ | +++ | 10 | 3–4 | 1–2 | Yes |
| Isoetharine | ++ | +++ | 6 | 0.5–2 | 0.5–1.0 | No |
| Albuterol | + | ++++ | 2 | 4–8 | 2–4 | Yes |
| Bitolterol | + | ++++ | 5 | 4–8 | 2–4 | No |
| Fenoterol | + | ++++ | 2 | 4–8 | 2–4 | Yes |
| Terbutaline | + | ++++ | 4 | 4–8 | 2–4 | Yes |
| Carbuterol | + | ++++ | 2 | 4–8 | 2–4 | Yes |

[a] Relative molar potency; 1 = most potent.

theophylline because they are equally effective yet lack serious CNS toxicity, are more palatable, and do not require the measurement of serum concentrations.[38,48,54]

### Moderate Chronic Asthma

As indicated in Table 21.4, there is not a well-defined stepwise difference between the levels of asthma severity but a continuum that is defined both by the severity of symptoms and the ability of the first line of therapy to control symptoms. A patient with moderate asthma may have mild symptoms that are persistent or may be symptom free between attacks; however, the attacks are of such severity that they require visits to the emergency room or hospitalization to break. If the patients are seasonal atopic asthmatics, they may have symptoms only during a specific allergen season. Regardless, this group of patients is defined by their need for continuous medication for symptom control and prevention of hospitalization even if only for part of the year.

In patients with occupational asthma and seasonal allergic asthma, avoidance of the triggering factor has been shown to decrease symptomatology and bronchial hyperreactivity.[55] Many atopic asthmatics develop sensitivity to a number of allergens, causing their seasonal asthma to become perennial.[27] In the past these patients have been encouraged to move away from the factors that trigger their asthma. While the patient may initially improve, he or she will usually develop sensitivities to new local allergens and symptoms will return in 1 to 2 years.[17,18] The role of immunotherapy in the atopic asthmatic is still controversial and has yet to be proven efficacious in asthma.[17,18,39]

The current choices for the chronic therapy of moderate asthma include cromolyn sodium and theophylline with or without an inhaled $\beta_2$-adrenergic.[38,39,53,54]

***Cromolyn Versus Theophylline*** Table 21.6 is a summary of the studies comparing theophylline and cromolyn. Historically, the debate over theophylline or cromolyn as primary therapy has been international.[47,48,54] In the relatively short-term studies that have been completed, cromolyn and theophylline have been shown to be equally efficacious as primary drugs for mild to moderate chronic asthma.[47,56]

*Theophylline therapy requires serum concentration monitoring to assure attainment of theraputic concentrations and prevent toxicity*. Because of the large interpatient variability in the clearance of theophylline,[47] sustained-release tablets (SRTs) have simplified chronic theophylline therapy by decreasing the number of doses required per day and improving patient compliance.[47] Unfortunately, there exist significant differences of unknown clinical importance in absorption characteristics between products as well as inconsistent absorption of the same product within the same patient.[47,57,58]

Theophylline is intrinsically more toxic than cromolyn or the $\beta_2$-adrenergic agonists, but most of the more serious toxicities can easily be avoided by monitoring serum concentrations.[47,58] There is increasing concern over the more subtle central nervous system effects of theophylline, including hyperactivity and learning disability in already minimally impaired children.[59] Theophylline therapy is less expensive than cromolyn therapy.

Cromolyn is given more frequently (every 4–6 hours) than SRTs, but once controlled, patients can often be maintained on three times daily dosing.[56] Cromolyn is not a bronchodilator and may take up to 4 to 6 weeks before maximum improvement is seen, although most patients demonstrate a significant effect within 2 weeks.[56] Initial administration of cromolyn with a $\beta_2$-adrenergic aerosol provides a more rapid response because of the bronchodilation. Although the need for two drugs might be perceived as a disadvantage, moderate asthmatics often require supplemental $\beta_2$-adrenergics whether on theophylline or cromolyn.[54,56]

Cromolyn is the only drug that inhibits the early and late asthmatic responses to inhaled antigen in atopic asthmatics.[27] Prolonged therapy with cromolyn and steroids, but not theophylline or $\beta_2$-adrenergics, decreases bronchial hyperreactivity and prevents the usual increase in bronchial hyperreactivity seen during the allergy season in atopic asthmatics.[27,55,60,61] In the only relatively short-term (3 months) trial comparing cromolyn with theophylline, the decreased bronchial hyperreactivity produced by cromolyn did not translate into an improved therapeutic effect over theophylline.[61] More studies are needed to evaluate the significance of reducing bronchial hyperreactivity in asthma therapy.

***$\beta_2$-Adrenergic Agonists*** The role of continuous $\beta_2$-adrenergic agonists as first-line drugs for moderate asthma is still

**Table 21.6** Summary of Comparisons of Cromolyn With Theophylline[a]

| *Study* | *Design* | *N* | *Treatment period* | Clinical efficacy: **Symptom score** | **Pulmonary function** | **Bronchodilator PRN use** | *Adverse side effects* |
|---|---|---|---|---|---|---|---|
| Hambleton et al Lancet 1977;1:381 | Rand, DB CO | 28 | 4 wk | C < T < C + T | C = T ≤ C + T | C = T = C + T | C = T = C + T |
| Edmunds et al Br Med J 1980;281:842 | Rand, DB, CO, PC | 30 | 4 wk | P < T < C | P < T = C | P < T = C | P = T = C |
| Glass et al Arch Dis Child 1981;56:648 | Rand, DB, CO, PC | 16 | 8 wk | P = C = T | ND | P = T = C | P = C < T |
| Newth et al Aust NZ J Med 1982;12:232 | Rand, DB | 26 | 8 wk | T < C = C + T | C = T = T + C[b] | C = T < C + T | C < T = C + T |
| Furukawa et al Pediatrics 1984;74:453 | Rand, DB, parallel | 40 | 3 mo | C = T | C = T[c] | C = T | C < T |
| Springer et al J Allergy Clin Immunol 1985;76:64 | Rand, DB, CO | 13 | 4 wk | C = T | C = T | C = T | C = T[d] |

[a] C, cromolyn; T, theophylline; Rand, randomized; DB, double-blind; CO, crossover; PC, placebo-controlled; ND, not done.
[b] Used exercise tolerance as measure because children (1–6 yr) were too young for spirometry.
[c] C produced significant decrease in bronchial hyperreactivity from baseline period theophylline.
[d] C produced significantly less difficulty with visual–spatial planning than theophylline in children with low IQ scores.

not defined. The $\beta_2$-adrenergic aerosols provide an excellent supplement to either theophylline or cromolyn therapy.[46] Not enough comparative studies have been completed for an accurate assessment, although the $\beta_2$-adrenergics have been used for years in Europe as first-line drugs. The development of tolerance that occurs with the use of all of the $\beta_2$-adrenergics is a concern but has yet to be proven clinically important.[48,62] Home nebulizers for delivering aerosol $\beta_2$-adrenergics are being used with increasing frequency. This is a useful alternative (although more expensive) to oral administration in young children or infants unable to coordinate the metered-dose canisters. Objective dose–response studies have failed to demonstrate any advantage of nebulizers and/or intermittent positive pressure breathing (IPPB) over metered-dose canisters.[46,62] Older patients unable to use the metered-dose aerosols optimally respond as well to the metered-dose canister with a tube spacer as to a nebulizer.[46] The higher dosages of $\beta_2$-adrenergics used in nebulizers are misleading because 90% of the dose is lost in the apparatus and air.[46]

***Anticholinergics*** The introduction of ipratropium bromide onto the U.S. market in 1987 as a metered-dose inhaler increased interest in the role of anticholinergic agents for chronic therapy.[63] The ultimate place of these drugs in asthma therapy will be determined after more study and experience. The $\beta_2$-adrenergics are generally more effective than anticholinergics in protecting against bronchospasm induced by histamine, prostaglandin, bradykinin, irritant, antigen, cold air, and exercise.[63] Anticholinergics are more effective against psychogenic and $\beta$ blockade–induced bronchospasm.[63] Anticholinergics appear to be more useful than $\beta_2$-adrenergics in patients with bronchitis and emphysema, whereas the $\beta_2$-adrenergics are more potent in asthma.[63] It should be emphasized, however, that each class of drugs is an effective bronchodilator in each disease. The anticholinergics appear to produce a more variable response in asthma than the $\beta_2$-adrenergics, but this may be only a dosing phenomenon.[63] Anticholinergics produce an additive bronchodilator response in combination with $\beta_2$-adrenergics.[63]

### Severe Chronic Asthma

Severe chronic asthma is defined by the need for continuous or frequent intermittent corticosteroids for symptom control. These patients frequently demonstrate significant residual pulmonary function abnormalities and require chronic bronchodilator therapy for control of symptoms. Short lapses in compliance with the treatment regimen can lead to hospitalization with life-threatening asthma attacks. The most severely ill patients may frequently require hospitalization for acute attacks of asthma despite compliance with maximum dosages of long-term medications. In this sense, they are not unlike the "brittle diabetics" who need only a small insult to tip the balance. They are in the greatest danger of death from asthma and present the greatest challenge to the clinicians caring for them. Clinicians are often forced to assess the risk:benefit ratio of the therapeutic plan, as a number of drugs may be used at their maximum recommended dosages. Fortunately, this is a relatively small percentage of all asthmatics.

Asthmatic patients who cannot be controlled with maxi-

**Table 21.7** Adverse Effects of Chronic Systemic Glucocorticoid Administration

| |
|---|
| Hypothalamic–pituitary–adrenal suppression |
| Growth retardation |
| Skeletal muscle myopathy |
| Osteoporosis fractures |
| Aseptic necrosis of bone |
| Pancreatitis |
| Pseudotumor cerebri |
| Psychiatric disturbances |
| Sodium and water retention |
| Hypokalemia alkalosis |
| Hypertension |
| Skin striae |
| Impaired wound healing |
| Inhibition of leukocyte and monocyte function |
| Subcutaneous tissue atrophy |
| Glaucoma |
| Posterior subcapsular cataracts |
| Moon facies |
| Central redistribution of fat |

mum dosages of cromolyn and/or bronchodilators must be treated with chronic corticosteroids. The mechanism of action and use of corticosteroids in asthma have been recently reviewed.[64,65] Actions useful in treating asthma include (1) increasing the number of $\beta$-adrenergic receptors, improving the receptor responsiveness to $\beta$-adrenergic stimulation, and restoring and preventing tolerance induced with chronic administration of $\beta$-adrenergics; (2) reducing mucus production and hypersecretion; and (3) inhibiting all levels of the inflammatory response, the latter being the most important in the therapy of asthma.[64]

Corticosteroids act through the production of new proteins; therefore, the time required for a particular effect is dependent upon the time required for synthesis of the particular mediator of the response. $\beta$-Receptor density increases within 4 hours of corticosteroid administration.[64] Improved responsiveness to $\beta$-agonists occurs within 2 hours. Reversal of seasonally increased nonspecific bronchial hyperreactivity requires at least 1 week of therapy.[64] Reactivity to EIA decreases after 4 weeks of therapy.[31,64] Although single doses do not inhibit the early asthmatic response to antigen challenge, continued therapy for 1 week partially suppresses the response.[64]

The therapeutic and toxic effects of corticosteroids in asthma are dose and duration dependent. Adverse effects of chronic systemic glucocorticoid therapy are listed in Table 21.7. Because short-term (1–2 weeks) high-dose steroids (1–2 mg/kg/d methylprednisolone) do not produce serious toxic effects, corticosteroids are ideally given in a short burst followed by maintenance bronchodilator and/or cromolyn treatment with long periods between corticosteroid treatment. Short-burst steroid therapy is often effective in reducing hospitalizations in moderate asthmatics. In patients who require long-term corticosteroids for control of asthma not controlled by other means, the lowest possible dose required to control symptoms is the goal of therapy. Clinicians often sacrifice complete control of the patient's symptoms to avoid toxicity.

Methods of decreasing systemic corticosteroid toxicity include alternate-day therapy and topical inhaled corticosteroids. With alternate-day steroid therapy, the drug-free day allows the adrenal axis to recover and decreases the inhibitory effect on white blood cell function. Patients who require 30 to 40 mg of prednisone daily usually cannot be well controlled on alternate-day therapy. Patients requiring smaller doses may also have increased problems on the off day. Posterior subcapsular cataracts are not avoided by alternate-day therapy.[64,65] If the alternate-day dose is too high, continued suppression on the day off will occur.

The inhaled corticosteroids (triamcinolone acetonide, beclomethasone dipropionate, flunisolide, and budesonide) have high topical anti-inflammatory effects and are metabolized to less active substances when absorbed.[64] All are equally effective. As with systemic corticosteroid therapy, the lowest dose required to control symptoms is the appropriate dose. Daily aerosol corticosteroid administration often produces greater control than alternate-day corticosteroids.[66] The combination can be used for further improvement. Aerosol corticosteroids may allow the systemic dose to be lowered in the severe steroid-dependent asthmatic. Optimal dosing of aerosol corticosteroids has not been thoroughly investigated. A number of patients may be controlled with twice-daily dosing, but a recent investigation demonstrated an improved asthma response with decreased systemic effects by giving the same total daily dose four times daily as opposed to twice daily.[66]

Inhaled corticosteroids produce dose-dependent suppression of the adrenal cortex, but much less than systemic corticosteroids.[64] Measurable adrenal suppression occurs at beclomethasone dipropionate dosages greater than 800 $\mu$g daily.[66] Local adverse effects of aerosol corticosteroids include dose-dependent oropharyngeal candidiasis and dysphonia. The dysphonia appears to result from a local steroid-induced myopathy of the vocal cords. The use of a spacer device can decrease oropharyngeal deposition and decrease the incidence and severity of local side effects.[66]

Guidelines for converting a patient from oral to aerosol corticosteroids are listed in Table 21.8. Regardless of the type of corticosteroid therapy, bronchodilator and/or cromolyn therapy should be used in conjunction to allow a decrease in the corticosteroid dose required to control symptoms. Cromolyn appears to be less effective than bronchodilators in reducing the corticosteroid dosage in patients with more severe asthma.[66] High-dose systemic steroids should be administered to all steroid-dependent asthmatics during acute attacks. Aerosol corticosteroids are not effective in acute asthma attacks.[64,66] There is no evidence that the use of corticosteroids in the moderate asthmatic will induce a state of steroid dependence. In fact, most of the evidence demonstrating a decrease in bronchial hyperreactivity with steroid therapy implies just the opposite.

### *Emergency Room Treatment of Acute Asthma*

Acute attacks of asthma vary widely in their severity and response to therapy. To treat an asthma attack appropriately, an accurate assessment of the severity of obstruction is necessary. A brief history of the attack should include

**Table 21.8** Schedule for Converting Asthmatics Dependent on Oral Steroids to Aerosol Corticosteroids

| *Treatment* | *Duration* |
|---|---|
| Start high-dose AC[a] (after a preliminary week of high-dose prednisone if severely obstructed) | 2 wk |
| Convert prednisone to alternate morning: wean prednisone dose by one-half to 1 tablet every 2 weeks | 4 mo |
| Continue high-dose AC while establishing need to resume prednisone and minimum prednisone requirement | 2 mo |
| Reduce AC to ≤1,000 μg/day (continuing minimum prednisone required); observe and adjust AC dose up or down to meet individual minimum AC dose requirements | 6 mo |

[a] AC, aerosol corticosteroid.

From Toogood JH, Jennings B, Baskerville SC: Aerosol corticosteroids. In Weiss EB, Segal MS, Stein M (Eds): Bronchial Asthma: Mechanisms and Therapeutics, 2nd ed. Boston: Little, Brown, 1985, p 700, with permission.

precipitating factors and the duration of time the patient has been experiencing difficulty. A history of the patient's long-term medication intake and compliance should include any drugs taken before coming to the emergency room or clinic. Also, a history of the therapy required to reverse previous attacks helps determine the therapy and likelihood of a response. Clinical assessment of the severity of obstruction is poor. Wheezing requires rapid air movement through narrow airways. In very severe obstruction, the amount of air movement may not be enough to produce wheezing. Wheezing may then become more prominent with effective therapy. The use of accessory muscles (retractions), pulse rate, and pulsus paradoxus (fluctuation of systolic pressure > 10 mm Hg between inspiration and expiration) tend to correlate with the degree of obstruction. Objective measures of airway obstruction such as forced expiratory flow rates ($FEV_1$ or PEFR) are needed.[18,33] Peak flow meters are frequently used to obtain these measurements, although patients with severe obstruction may not be able to register a measurable peak flow and the forced maneuver may worsen bronchospasm. The gold standard for assessing the severity of obstruction is blood gases. All patients who do not respond to the initial management of the acute attack and require more intensive therapy and hospitalization must have a blood gas measurement to assess accurately the severity of the attack. Chest roentgenograms are of little value unless there are signs of a localized obstruction suggesting pneumonia or sputum impaction.

Inhaled bronchodilators are the first line of therapy. Drugs and dosages are listed in Table 21.9. Numerous studies have compared β-adrenergic agonists with theophylline and the combination for therapy of acute bronchospasm. The data in these studies show that the β-adrenergic agonists provide greater bronchodilation than theophylline, and inhaled β-adrenergics produce equivalent bronchodilation with fewer side effects than systemic administration.[48,67] Historically, epinephrine was the first drug used in acute attacks of asthma, but aerosol administration of the newer $\beta_2$-adrenergic agents may be safer. The combination of theophylline and $\beta_2$-adrenergics has not been shown to be significantly better than the $\beta_2$-adrenergics alone in higher dose.[48,67] The data on the toxicity of the combination remain controversial. In patients with preexisting cardiac disease or chronic obstructive lung disease, the combination increases the incidence of arrhythmias, primarily premature ventricular contractions (PVCs), over the use of β-adrenergics alone.[48] In asthmatics without heart disease, the combination does not increase the number of PVCs.[48] Patients who do not respond to the aerosol $\beta_2$-adrenergics or who respond only for a short period of time are given an appropriate loading dose of theophylline orally or intravenously depending on the severity of their attack. (Table 21.9)

The anticholinergics administered by aerosol can also be used, although they are second-line therapy. The response to anticholinergics is slower in onset and less consistent than that with $\beta_2$ agonists.[63] Studies comparing these two groups of drugs have shown β agonists to be superior to[68,69] or equal to[70,71] anticholinergic drugs for the treatment of acute asthma.

Steroid-dependent asthmatic patients should be started on a short burst of oral steroids if they respond well to bronchodilators and are not to be admitted to a hospital. Patients who have deteriorated over several days and respond well to initial treatment but still have residual symptoms may be kept from hospitalization or a return to the emergency room with a 1-week course of corticosteroids.

### *Status Asthmaticus*

Status asthmaticus refers to acute severe asthma that does not respond to usual therapy and constitutes a medical emergency. Patients with acute severe obstruction require oxygen to decrease the hypoxemia from the $V_a/Q$ mismatching that will be aggravated by the bronchodilator therapy. Hypoxemia aggravates bronchial hyperreactivity and cardiac arrhythmias.[18]

Signs of impending respiratory failure are shown in Table 21.10. Figure 21.8 represents the way in which a patient progresses to respiratory failure. Refractory hypoxemia despite oxygen therapy and an absolute $Paco_2 \geq 55$ torr with acidosis ($pH \leq 7.2$) are indications for artificial ventilation.[18,72] Ventilation of asthmatics is difficult because of the increased pulmonary resistance and is fraught with complications. Asthmatics have a higher incidence of pneumothorax, pneumonia, hypoventilation, and endotracheal tube malfunction than nonasthmatics on ventilators.[72] Because asthmatics are struggling to breathe, they often have a more difficult time coordinating with the ventilator and will require sedation with parenteral benzodiazepines or morphine. If sedation fails, the patient should be paralyzed with pancuronium. Pancuronium has the advantage over *d*-tubocurarine or gallamine of not causing histamine release, but there are reports of serious cardiac arrhythmias with simultaneous administration of pancuronium and aminophylline.[72]

Because of the tachypnea and lack of intake, the patients may be somewhat dehydrated. Patients should be adequately hydrated, but not given excess fluids.[17] In patients

**Table 21.9** Dosages of Medications for Acute Severe Asthma

| *Medication* | *Dosage* Pediatric | Adult |
|---|---|---|
| **Sympathomimetics** | | |
| Subcutaneous | | |
| Epinephrine 1:1,000 (1 mg/mL) | 0.01 mg/kg up to 0.5 mg every 20 min for 3 doses | 0.3–0.5 mg every 20 min for 3 doses |
| Sustained-action susphrine 1:200 (5 mg/mL) | 0.005 to 0.01 mL/kg every 6–20 h as needed | 0.5–0.75 mg every 6–10 h as needed |
| Terbutaline (1 mg/mL) | 0.01 mg/kg every 20 min for 3 doses, then every 2–6 h as needed | 0.25–0.5 mg every 20 min for 3 doses, then every 2–6 h as needed |
| Aerosol | | |
| Isoproterenol | | |
| 1:400 (2.5 mg/mL)<br>1:200 (5 mg/mL)<br>1:100 (10 mg/mL) | 0.05–0.1 mg/kg diluted to 3–5 mL with normal saline every 20 min for 3 doses, then every 2–4 h as needed | 1–2.5 mg in 3–5 mL normal saline nebulized every 20 min for 3 doses, then every 2–4 h as needed |
| Isoetharine 0.1–1.0% | 0.1–0.2 mg/kg every 20 min for 3 doses, then every 2–4 h as needed | 3–10 mg every 20 min for 3 doses, then every 2–4 h as needed |
| Metaproterenol 5% (50 mg/mL), 15-mg unit dose | 0.25–0.5 mg/kg every 2–4 h as needed, maximum 15 mg | 0.3 mL (15 mg) in 3–4 mL normal saline every 2–4 h as needed |
| Terbutaline<br>Injection (1 mg/mL)<br>Nebulizer solution (10 mg/mL) | 0.1–0.3 mg/kg every 20 min for 3 doses, then every 2–4 h as needed | 5–10 mg undiluted every 20 min for 3 doses then every 2–4 h as needed |
| Albuterol (5 mg/mL) | 0.05–0.15 mg/kg every 20 min for 3 doses, then every 2–4 h as needed | 2.5–5 mg every 20 min for 3 doses, then every 2–4 h as needed |
| Fenoterol 0.5% (5 mg/mL) | 0.05–0.15 mg/kg every 20 min for 3 doses, then every 2–4 h as needed | 2.5–5 mg every 20 min for 3 doses then every 2–4 h as needed |
| Intravenous | | |
| Isoproterenol 1:5,000 (0.2 mg/mL) | 0.1 μg/kg/min, increase at 15-min intervals by 0.1 μg/kg/min as necessary until heart rate greater than 180–200/min | 0.08–1.7 μg/kg/min as necessary for response |
| **Corticosteroid** | | |
| Methylprednisolone | 1–2 mg/kg every 4–6 h for 24–48 h or severe symptoms abate, then reduce to 1–2 mg/kg every 12–24 h | 100–200 mg initially, then 100 mg every 6 h for 24–48 h, then 100 mg every 12 h |
| Hydrocortisone | 4 mg/kg every 4–6 h for 24–48 h, then reduce | 200–400 mg every 6 h for 24–48 h, then 20 mg every 12 h |
| **Anticholinergics** | | |
| Aerosol | | |
| Atropine $SO_4$ Unit dose 0.2% (1 mg) 0.5% (2.5 mg) | 0.05–0.075 mg/kg every 4–6 h as needed | 0.025 mg/kg or 2.5–5 mg every 4–6 h as needed |
| Ipratropium bromide 0.025% | 250 μg every 4–6 h as needed | 250–500 μg every 4–6 h as needed |
| **Methylxanthines** | | |
| Aminophylline (80% theophylline) | | |
| Loading Doses | Infuse over 20 min | |
| No previous theophylline | 9 mg/kg | |
| Previous theophylline in last 12 h | 6 mg/kg | |
| Previous sustained-release in last 12 h | 3 mg/kg | |
| If theophylline concentration is known a 1 mg/kg theophylline dose will produce approximately a 2 μg/mL increase in serum concentration | | |

**Table 21.9** Dosages of Medications for Acute Severe Asthma (continued)

| *Medication* | Pediatric | | Adult | |
|---|---|---|---|---|
| Infusion rates (to achieve a mean concentration of 15 $\mu$g/mL) | | | | |
| | 1–6 mo | 0.5 mg/kg/h | <50 yr (smokers) | 0.9 mg/kg/h |
| | 6 mo–1 yr | 1.00 mg/kg/h | >50 yr | 0.6 mg/kg/h |
| | 1–9 yr | 1.50 mg/kg/h | COLD | 0.6 mg/kg/h |
| | 10–16 yr | 1.20 mg/kg/h | CHF | 0.5 mg/kg/h |

These are only suggested starting doses; final rates must be determined by serum theophylline concentration monitoring.

with acidosis, sodium bicarbonate may be started at a dose titrated to a blood pH of about 7.25. It should be noted that the pH will not rise appreciably unless the lungs eliminate the carbon dioxide produced.[72] All patients should be started on intravenous aminophylline at appropriate doses with theophylline serum concentrations monitored and dosages adjusted to maintain serum concentration of 15–20 $\mu$g/mL.[72] Aminophylline improves the contractility of the fatigued diaphragm, which may be an added benefit for preventing respiratory failure.[47,72] The inhaled $\beta_2$-adrenergics should be continued and the dosing frequency increased. Higher dosages can be given with careful monitoring of the heart rate. The initial tachycardia caused by obstruction and hypoxemia should not discourage the use of inhaled $\beta_2$-adrenergics. The aerosol $\beta_2$-adrenergics have documented efficacy in acute severe asthma with $FEV_1$ less than 30% of predicted and an initial $PaCO_2 \geq 55$ torr.[48] Edmunds and Godfrey compared inhaled albuterol with intravenous albuterol alone, in combination, or in combination with intravenous aminophylline in severe acute asthma in children. The combination of inhaled albuterol and intravenous aminophylline produced the optimal effect compared to either drug alone with the least toxicity.[73]

Anticholinergic agents may be added to the $\beta_2$-adrenergic nebulization or given immediately afterward. All patients with severe acute asthma should be started on systemic corticosteroids at a dose equivalent to 1–2 mg/kg of methylprednisolone intravenously every 4 to 6 hours until severe symptoms cease and then decreased to 1–2 mg/kg methylprednisolone daily.[64,72] All corticosteroids are equally effective but differ in side effects. Available data indicate that the response to corticosteroids in acute severe asthma is delayed for at least 6 hours.[72] Patients are then carefully monitored clinically with blood gases and pulmonary functions if possible.

Every attempt should be made to avoid mechanical ventilation of asthmatics. In an attempt to prevent mechanical ventilation, a number of authors recommend the use of intravenous isoproterenol; however, these studies failed to demonstrate clearly a reduction in the proportion of patients requiring mechanical ventilation.[72] Complications of intravenous isoproterenol include severe tachycardia, increased $V_a/Q$ mismatching, arrhythmias, and myocardial ischemia.[72] Intravenous isoproterenol should not be used in a patient with a history of serious heart disease.

A more selective $\beta_2$-adrenergic agent such as albuterol or terbutaline intravenously may be more appropriate than isoproterenol. Intravenous albuterol has demonstrated efficacy in severe asthma[48,72]; however, comparisons with isoproterenol have not been made. Continuous inhalation of $\beta_2$-adrenergics to avoid systemic toxicities should also be evaluated.[74]

**Table 21.10** Signs of Impending Respiratory Failure in Status Asthmaticus

| |
|---|
| FVC < 10 mL/kg, $FEV_1$ < 0.5–1.0 L, PEFR < 100 L/min |
| Little or no response to bronchodilators in 1–2 h |
| Altered consciousness |
| Central cyanosis with $O_2$ administration of $Pao_2$ < 50 mm Hg |
| $Paco_2$ of 50–55 mm Hg with adequate therapy |
| Rising $Paco_2$ of 5–10 mm Hg/h with therapy |
| Pneumothorax or pneumomediastinum |
| Pulsus paradoxus > 20 mm Hg |

### *$\beta_2$-Adrenergic Agonists and Theophylline*

Tachyarrhythmias are well-known toxic effects of excessive serum theophylline concentrations, and tachycardia is the dose-limiting toxicity of the $\beta_2$-adrenergic agonists.[47,48] Myocardial ischemia has occurred in children and young adults receiving intravenous isoproterenol for status asthmaticus.[48] Animal studies show a synergistic cardiotoxicity consisting of ectopic atrial and ventricular beats, ventricular tachyarrhythmias, ventricular fibrillation, and myocardial ischemia with combined theophylline and $\beta_2$ agonists.[46,75] A large number of deaths have recently been reported in New Zealand after the widespread use of combined $\beta_2$-adrenergic agonists and theophylline; however, this increase in deaths has been disputed and, if real, has been attributed to delays in patients seeking medical attention and physicians initiating corticosteroid therapy.[76]

Clinical investigations of the combination of $\beta$-adrenergic agonists and theophylline in acute asthma are inconclusive and have yielded conflicting results,[48,77,78] showing that the addition of intravenous aminophylline to subcutaneous epinephrine increased or had no effect on cardiac arrhythmias; however, these studies were limited by short baseline and monitoring periods. Others have shown that the improvement in obstruction and hypoxia from combination therapy resulted in a decrease in ectopic activity, seen by continuous Holter monitoring.[48] Studies of long-term administration

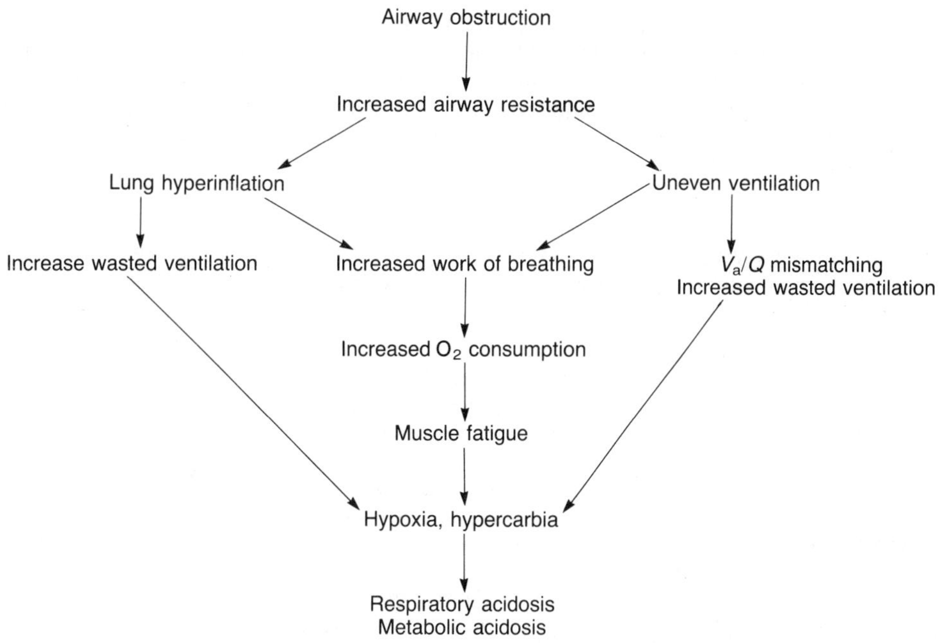


**Figure 21.8** Schematic of pathophysiology in acute severe asthma.

using 24-hour Holter monitoring have shown an increased frequency of arrhythmias from the combination in patients with preexisting arrhythmias and cardiac disease, and no changes to clinically insignificant increases in premature ventricular contractions in patients without preexisting heart disease.[48,79]

Except for the increase in deaths in one study from New Zealand (which has been disputed), there has not been an increase in asthma deaths despite the increasing use of the combination of $\beta_2$-adrenergics and theophylline.[13] The newer $\beta_2$-adrenergics have clearly demonstrated less cardiac stimulation than isoproterenol, particularly when used by the aerosol route.[62] The potential for serious adverse effects would be minimized with the use of a $\beta_2$ selective agonist administered by the aerosol route. Patients on combined therapy should be monitored for dysrhythmia.[74]

### *Miscellaneous Therapies*

Antihistamines have had a controversial role in asthma therapy. Earlier fears that their drying effects would worsen asthma have not been proven. Indeed, most studies of short- and long-term administration of antihistamines in asthma have demonstrated a small improvement of symptoms and pulmonary function tests or no effect.[80] Although antihistamines are generally not helpful in asthma, they are not contraindicated. They are useful adjunctive therapy for the patient with allergic rhinitis and asthma.

Ketotifen (a benzocyclohepathiophene derivative) is a potent antihistamine with in vitro antianaphylactic, SRS-A inhibition, and mast cell–stabilizing properties undergoing extensive clinical testing.[80] Although initial trials suggested efficacy equivalent to cromolyn for EIA and antigen-induced asthma, recent controlled trials have shown that ketotifen's activity is due primarily to its powerful antihistaminic effect.[80] As such, ketotifen has a modest effect in asthma and does not appear to be an important addition to asthma therapy.

Calcium ion flux has a central role in smooth muscle contraction and membrane stabilization.[17,51] Relaxation of airway smooth muscle can be produced by calcium channel antagonists with doses 1,000 times those required for vasodilation,[51] but they do not cause significant bronchodilation in vivo.[71] Verapamil and nifedipine have only modest effects on EIA and histamine-induced bronchospasm. There is a possibility that calcium channel blockers may potentiate the effect of other drugs used for asthma,[81] but current evidence does not support the use of calcium channel antagonists in the treatment of asthma.

The use of expectorants has not been demonstrated to be beneficial in asthma, although mucolytic therapy to assist removal of impacted mucus plugs in a large bronchus has been life-saving in a few instances. Adequate hydration is usually all that is required. In acute asthma, the large negative intrathoracic pressures coupled with mediator-induced capillary permeability may predispose to pulmonary edema that will worsen oxygenation so that excessive hydration should be avoided.[72] Theophylline and $\beta_2$-adrenergics both increase fluid secretion, decreasing the viscosity of mucus, and corticosteroids decrease mucus production. In addition, the $\beta_2$-adrenergics directly stimulate ciliary beating.

## Summary

Asthma is a complicated disease with a multitude of clinical presentations. The exact defect in asthma has not been defined; it may be that asthma is a common presentation of a heterogenous group of diseases. Asthma is defined and characterized by excessive reactivity of the bronchial tree to a wide variety of noxious stimuli. The reaction is characterized by bronchospasm, excessive mucus production, and inflammation. The central role of inflammation in inducing and maintaining bronchial hyperreactivity is now becoming widely appreciated and studied.

The goal of asthma therapy is to normalize the patient's life as much as possible and to prevent chronic irreversible lung changes. Drugs are the mainstay of asthma therapy. The goal of drug therapy is to use the minimum amount that will control the disease completely. In chronic asthma, therapy should be aimed at both bronchospasm and inflammation to produce the best results. Patients should be diligently followed and monitored for drug toxicities. Although death from asthma is an uncommon event, the most common cause of death is underassessment of the severity of obstruction by either the patient or the clinician and then undertreatment. A cornerstone of any therapy is education and the realization that most asthma deaths are avoidable.

## References


1. Rosenblatt MB. History of bronchial asthma, in Weiss EB, Segal MS, Stein M (eds): Bronchial Asthma: Mechanisms and Therapeutics, 2nd ed. Boston, Little, Brown, 1976, pp 5–17.
2. American Thoracic Society Committee on Diagnostic Standards. Definitions and classification of chronic bronchitis, asthma, and pulmonary emphysema. Am Rev Respir Dis 1962;85:762.
3. Scientific Assembly on Allergy and Clinical Immunology subcommittee. Definition of asthma. ATS News 1982:5.
4. NIAID Task Force Report. Asthma and Other Allergic Diseases, DHEW (National Institutes of Health) publication No. 79-387, May 1979.
5. Tenth Report of the Director, National Heart, Lung and Blood Institute. Vol 3, Lung Disease, 1984. US Dept of Health and Human Services. NIH publication No. 84-2358.
6. Siegel SC, Rachelefsky GS. Asthma in infants and children: Part 1. J Allergy Clin Immunol 1985;76:1–14.
7. Dodge RR, Burrows B. The prevalence and incidence of asthma and asthma-like symptoms in a general population sample. Am Rev Respir Dis 1980;122:567–575.
8. Broder I, Higgins MW, Matthews KP, et al. Epidemiology of asthma and allergic rhinitis in a total community, Tecumseh, Michigan: III. Second survey of the community. J Allergy Clin Immunol 1974;53:127–138.
9. Weiss ST, Speizer FE. The epidemiology of asthma: Risk factors and natural history, in Weiss EB, Segal MS, Stein M (eds): Bronchial Asthma: Mechanics and Therapeutics, 2nd ed. Boston, Little, Brown, 1985, pp 14–23.
10. Martin AJ, Landau LI, Phelan PO. Lung function in young adults who had asthma in childhood. Am Rev Respir Dis 1980;122:609–616.
11. Bronnimann S, Burrows B. Natural history of asthma. Chest 1985;87 (suppl):214–215.
12. Benatar SA. Fatal asthma. N Engl J Med 1986;314:423–429.
13. Alberts WM, Moser KM. Asthma: Complications and death, in Weiss EB, Segal MS, Stein M (eds): Bronchial Asthma: Mechanisms and Therapeutics, 2nd ed. Boston, Little, Brown, 1985, pp 938–949.
14. Research Committee for the British Thoracic Association. Death from asthma in two regions of England. Br Med J 1982; 285:1251–1255.
15. McFadden ER. Pathogenesis of asthma. J Allergy Clin Immunol 1984;73:413–424.
16. Boushey HA, Holtzman MJ, Sheller JR, et al. State of the art: Bronchial hyperreactivity. Am Rev Respir Dis 1980;121:389–413.
17. Goldstein RA (ed). Advances in the diagnosis and treatment of asthma. Chest 1985;87 (suppl)1:1–113.
18. Mason R (ed). Twenty-seventh Annual Aspen Lung Conference. Chest 1985;87 (suppl):151–226.
19. Nadel JA, Sheppard D. Mechanisms of bronchial hyperreactivity in asthma, in Weiss EB, Segal MS, Stein M (eds): Bronchial Asthma: Mechanisms and Therapeutics, 2nd ed. Boston, Little, Brown, 1985, pp 30–36.
20. Hogg JC. The pathology of asthma. Chest 1985;87 (suppl):152–153.
21. Lopez-Vidriero MT, Reid L. Pathologic changes in asthma, in Asthma, 2nd ed. London, Chapman and Hall, 1983, pp 79–98.
22. Menendez R, Kelly HW. Pulmonary-function testing in the evaluation of bronchodilator agents. Clin Pharm 1983;2:120–128.
23. Leff A. Pathophysiology of asthma bronchoconstriction. Chest 1982;82 (suppl):13–21.
24. Szentivanyi A. The beta-adrenergic theory of the atopic abnormality in bronchial asthma. J Allergy 1968;42:203–232.
25. Nadel JA, Davis D, Phipps RJ. Control of mucus secretion and ion transport in airways. Annu Rev Physiol 1979;41:369.
26. Robinson C, Holgate ST. New perspectives on the putative role of eicosanoids in airway hyperresponsiveness. J Allergy Clin Immunol 1985;76:140–144.
27. Cockcroft DW. Mechanism of perennial allergic asthma. Lancet 1983;2:253–255.
28. Rocklin RE, Findley SR. Immunologic mechanisms and recent advances in asthma, in Weiss EB, Segal MS, Stein M (eds): Bronchial Asthma: Mechanisms and Therapeutics, 2nd ed. Boston, Little, Brown, 1985, pp 41–51.
29. Hargreave FE, O'Byrne PM, Ramsdale EH. Mediators of airway responsiveness, and asthma. J Allergy Clin Immunol 1985;76:272–276.
30. Godfrey S. Exercise-induced asthma, in Asthma, 2nd ed. London, Chapman and Hall, 1983, pp 57–78.
31. Anderson SD. Exercise-induced asthma: The state of the art. Chest 1985;87 (suppl):191–195.
32. Lee TH, Nagakura T, Paplageorgioun N, et al. Exercise-induced late asthmatic reactions with neutrophil chemotactic activity. N Engl J Med 1983;308:1502–1505.
33. Woolcock AJ. The pathophysiology of asthma, in Weiss EB, Segal MS, Stein M (eds): Bronchial Asthma: Mechanisms and Therapeutics, 2nd ed. Boston, Little, Brown, 1985, pp 180–192.
34. Pride NB. Physiology, in Asthma, 2nd ed. London, Chapman and Hall, 1983, pp 12–56.
35. Corrao WM, Braman SS, Irwin RS. Chronic cough as the sole presenting manifestation of bronchial asthma. N Engl J Med 1979;300:633–637.
36. Specter S. Bronchial provocation tests, in Weiss EB, Segal MS, Stein M (eds): Bronchial Asthma: Mechanisms and Therapeutics, 2nd ed. Boston, Little, Brown, 1985, pp 360–386.

37. Pratter MR, Hingston DM, Irwin RS. Diagnosis of bronchial asthma by clinical evaluation: An unreliable method. Chest 1983;84:42–47.
38. Tabachnik E, Levison H. Infantile bronchial asthma. J Allergy Clin Immunol 1981;67:339–347.
39. Sheffer AL, Rachelefsky GS. Asthma '84: Pharmacologic update. J Allergy Clin Immunol 1985;76(2):1–408.
40. Buckle DR, Smith H (eds). Development of Anti-Asthma Drugs. Boston, Butterworths, 1984.
41. Jenne JS, Murphy SA (eds). Asthma Therapy: Theory and Practice. New York, Marcel Dekker, in press.
42. Svedmyr N, Simonsson BG. Drugs in the treatment of asthma. Pharmacol Ther(B) 1978;3:397–440.
43. Bailey WC (ed). Symposium on asthma: Clin Chest Med 1984;5:555–736.
44. Middleton E, Reed CE, Ellis EF. Allergy: Principles and Practice, 2nd ed. St. Louis, C.V. Mosby, 1983.
45. Anderson S, Seale JP, Ferris L, et al. An evaluation of pharmacotherapy for exercise-induced asthma. J Allergy Clin Immunol 1979;64:612–624.
46. Kelly HW. New $\beta_2$-adrenergic agonist aerosols. Clin Pharm 1985;4:393–404.
47. Hendeles L, Weinberger M. Theophylline: A state of the art review. Pharmacotherapy 1983;3:2–44.
48. Kelly HW. Controversies in asthma therapy with theophylline and the $\beta_2$-adrenergic agonists. Clin Pharm 1984;3:386–395.
49. Sly MR. Beta-adrenergic drugs in the management of asthma in athletes. J Allergy Clin Immunol 1984;73(2):680–685.
50. Henriksen JM, Dahl R. Effects of inhaled budesonide alone and in combination with low-dose terbutaline in children with exercise-induced asthma. Am Rev Respir Dis 1983;128:993–997.
51. Barbero LJ, Anderson WH, Weiss EB. Calcium and its role in the asthmatic process, in Weiss EB, Segal MS, Stein M (eds): Bronchial Asthma: Mechanisms and Therapeutics, 2nd ed. Boston, Little, Brown, 1985, pp 776–791.
52. Green LW, Goldstein RA, Parker SR. Workshop proceedings on self-management of childhood asthma. J Allergy Clin Immunol 1983;72(2):519–526.
53. Bernstein IL. Treatment decisions of asthma based on a paradigm of clinical severity. J Allergy Clin Immunol 1985;76:357–365.
54. Rachelefsky GS, Siegel SC. Asthma in infants and children—treatment of childhood asthma: Part II. J Allergy Clin Immunol 1985;76:409–425.
55. Hargreave FE, Sterk PJ, Ramsdale EH, et al. Inhalation challenge tests and airway responsiveness in man. Chest 1985;87 (suppl):202–206.
56. Godfrey S. The relative merits of cromolyn sodium and high-dose theophylline therapy in childhood asthma. J Allergy Clin Immunol 1980;65:97–104.
57. Szefler SJ. Theophylline and its fickle unpredictability of absorption. Ann Allergy 1985;55:580–583.
58. Menendez R, Kelly HW. Theophylline therapy. J Asthma 1983;20:455–466.
59. Springer C, Goldenberg B, BenDov I, et al. Clinical, physiologic, and psychologic comparison of treatment by cromolyn or theophylline in childhood asthma. J Allergy Clin Immunol 1985;76:64–69.
60. Lowhagen O, Rak S. Modification of bronchial hyperreactivity after treatment with sodium cromoglycate during pollen season. J Allergy Clin Immunol 1985;75:460–467.
61. Furukawa CT, Shapiro GG, Bierman CW, et al. A double-blind study comparing the effectiveness of cromolyn sodium and sustained-release theophylline in childhood asthma. Pediatrics 1984;74:453–459.
62. Nelson HS. Beta-adrenergic therapy, in Middleton E, Reed CE, Ellis EF (eds): Allergy: Principles and Practice, 2nd ed. St Louis, C.V. Mosby, 1983, pp 511–527.
63. Gross NJ, Skorodin MS. State of the art: Anticholinergic, antimuscarinic bronchodilators. Am Rev Respir Dis 1984;129: 856–870.
64. Morris HG. Mechanisms of action and therapeutic role of corticosteroids in asthma. J Allergy Clin Immunol 1985;75:1–13.
65. Kaliner M. Mechanisms of glucocorticosteroids action in bronchial asthma. J Allergy Clin Immunol 1985;76:321–329.
66. Toogood JH, Jennings B, Baskerville JC. Aerosol corticosteroids, in Weiss EB, Segal MS (eds): Bronchial Asthma: Mechanisms and Therapeutics. Boston, Little, Brown, 1985, pp 698–713.
67. Fanta CH, Rossing TH, McFadden ER. Treatment of acute asthma. Is combination therapy with sympathomimetics and methylxanthines indicated? Am J Med 1986;80:5–10.
68. Cook JJ, Ferguson DM, Dawson HP. Ipatropium and fenoterol in the treatment of acute asthma. Pharmatherapeutica 1985;4: 383.
69. Karpel JP, Appel D, Breidbart D, et al. A comparison of atropine sulfate and metaproterenol sulfate in the emergency treatment of asthma. Am Rev Respir Dis 1986;133:727–729.
70. Ward MJ, Fenten PH, Roderick WH, et al. Ipatropium bromide in acute asthma. Br Med J 1981;282:598.
71. Leahy BC, Gomm SA, Allen SC. Comparison of nebulized salbutamol with nebulized ipatropium bromide in acute asthma. Br J Dis Chest 1983;77:159–163.
72. Sybert A, Weiss EB. Status asthmaticus, in Weiss EB, Segal MS (eds): Bronchial Asthma: Mechanisms and Therapeutics. Boston, Little, Brown, 1985, pp 808–837.
73. Edmunds AT, Godfrey S. Cardiovascular response during severe acute asthma and its treatment in children. Thorax 1981;36: 534–540.
74. Robertson CF, Smith F, Beck R, et al. Response to frequent low doses of nebulized salbutamol in acute asthma. J Pediatr 1985;106:673–674.
75. Nicklas RA, Whitehurst VE, Donohue RF, et al. Concomitant use of beta adrenergic agonists and methylxanthines. J Allergy Clin Immunol 1984;73:20–21.
76. Chapman KR, Rebuck AG. Therapeutic problems in the cardiac–hypertensive–diabetic patient, in Weiss EB, Segal MS, Stein M (eds): Bronchial Asthma: Mechanisms and Therapeutics, 2nd ed. Boston, Little, Brown and Company, 1985, pp 843–849.
77. Rossing TH, Fanta CH, McFadden ER, et al. A controlled trial of the use of single versus combined-drug therapy in the treatment of acute episodes of asthma. Am Rev Respir Dis 1981; 123:190.
78. Siegel D, Sheppard D, Gelb A, et al. Aminophylline increases the toxicity but not the efficacy of acute exacerbations of asthma. Am Rev Resp Dis 1985;132:283.
79. Kelly HW, Menendez R, Voyles W. Lack of significant arrhythmogenicity from chronic theophylline and beta-2-adrenergic combination therapy in asthmatic subjects. Ann Allergy 1985; 54:405.
80. Eiser NM. Histamine antagonists and asthma. Pharmacol Ther 1982;17:239–250.
81. Lever AMC, Corris PA, Gibson GT. Nifedipine enhances the bronchodilator effect of salbutamol. Thorax 1984;39:576–578.

# Chapter 22 / Chronic Obstructive Lung Disease

Mark A. Stratton, PharmD

*Chronic obstructive lung disease* (COLD) is a term used to describe patients with chronic bronchitis, emphysema, or both, with evidence of pulmonary obstruction. This term evolved in the late 1950s and early 1960s. Before this time there was not a consensus definition of COLD. The terms *chronic obstructive pulmonary disease* (COPD) and *chronic obstructive airway disease* (COAD) are synonymous with COLD. For the purposes of this chapter, COLD is defined with modification from Petty's definition as follows[1]: an all-inclusive and nonspecific term referring to a progressive condition with chronic cough and sputum production with exertional dyspnea and a significant reduction in pulmonary function without an identifiable cause such as tuberculosis or tumor. Additionally, these patients frequently show minimal reversibility with bronchodilators and at autopsy have significant damage to airways or alveoli or both.

The spectrum of COLD most commonly includes the subsets chronic bronchitis and emphysema. While these two conditions can be defined separately, most patients with COLD have components of both; however, for improved understanding, it is helpful to know the definitions of chronic bronchitis and emphysema and the pathophysiologic characteristics of each. The first definitions of chronic bronchitis and emphysema published by the American Thoracic Society are still applicable with modification.[2] *Chronic bronchitis* is defined as a condition associated with excessive tracheobronchial mucus production sufficient to cause cough with expectoration of at least 30 mL sputum per 24 hours for 3 months of the year for more than 2 consecutive years. Classically, *emphysema* was defined on histologic exam at autopsy as distension of the air spaces distal to the terminal bronchioles with destruction of alveolar septa. Obviously diagnosis at autopsy is of little value; thus, the physical findings and laboratory tests described here help differentiate the predominant emphysematous patient from the predominant chronic bronchitic patient.

## Epidemiology

Accurate estimates of the prevalence of chronic bronchitis, emphysema, and ultimately COLD are difficult to obtain because of the changing definitions of these conditions over the past two decades; however, one fact consistent among surveys is that deaths attributable to COLD rose from 22% to 28% between 1968 and 1978, while during the same time there was an 18% to 22% decline for all causes of death and a 23% decline in deaths caused by heart disease. The group with the highest increase in deaths from COLD during this period was white women. These data reveal that deaths from COLD are the most rapidly increasing of the top 10 leading causes of death in the United States. In 1977, COLD was responsible for 45,000 deaths, accounting for 2.5% of all deaths in the United States. By 1981, it was estimated that COLD was responsible for 60,000 deaths, representing 3.0% of all deaths in the United States.[3,4] These numbers probably underestimate the actual number of deaths from COLD.

In 1980, chronic respiratory diseases were the fourth leading cause of limitation of major activity and the sixth leading cause of premature retirement for disability. The incidence of COLD increases with age and is higher in men than women and in whites than nonwhites.[4] The incidence of chronic bronchitis was reported to be 32.7/1,000 in 1970, 33.0/1,000 in 1978, and 36.1/1,000 in 1980. For emphysema, the incidence was 6.6/1,000 in 1970, 9.7/1,000 in 1978, and 11.4/1,000 in 1980.[3] The ratio of men to women is higher for emphysema than chronic bronchitis. Of concern is that the incidence of women with chronic bronchitis or emphysema increased during the decade, because of the increased number of women smokers.

The most recent data assessing the economic impact of COLD are from 1979 when the cost was $6.5 billion; $2.3 billion of this was for health care and the remainder for costs related to disability and premature retirement.[4]

Of the numerous risk factors (Table 22.1) associated with the development of chronic bronchitis and emphysema, clearly cigarette smoking is the most common. The median risk ratio for smokers versus nonsmokers to develop chronic bronchitis is 5.3 for males and 4.2 for females. Although the risk is lower in pipe and cigar smokers, these people have a higher incidence than nonsmokers. Of interest is the fact that not all smokers who have equal smoking histories develop the same degree of pulmonary impairment, suggesting that other physiologic or environmental factors contribute to the degree of lung dysfunction in smokers.[3,4]

Age is an additional risk factor for the development of COLD. While age alone is a slight risk factor for the development of chronic bronchitis, it is a significant factor in pulmonary obstruction. This may in part result from the natural aging process of lung tissue.

Gender is also considered a risk factor in that men have an increased risk for COLD. The reason for this is most likely that more men smoke than do women, although the number of female smokers is increasing. Thus, it is likely that gender may not prove to be as significant a risk factor in the future.

Existing impaired lung function has also been identified as a risk factor for the development of COLD. Individuals with existing impairment experience a greater decline in lung function over time than their counterparts with normal pulmonary function.

Reduced lung function and deaths from COLD are higher

**Table 22.1** Risk Factors for the Development of COLD

| *Major* | *Minor* |
|---|---|
| Smoking | Air pollution |
| Age | Alcohol |
| Male sex | Race |
| Existing impaired lung function | Nutritional status |
| | Family history |
| Occupation | Socioeconomic status |
| $\alpha_1$-Antitrypsin deficiency | Respiratory tract infections |
| | Bronchial reactivity |

than expected for individuals in numerous occupations, such as coal miners (brown lung disease), workers in glass or ceramic industries exposed to silica dust, workers exposed to cotton dust or grain dust, workers exposed to toluene diisocyanate, and workers exposed to asbestos. Numerous other possible occupational risk factors exist. A confounding factor for identifying occupational hazards is they primarily affect blue-collar workers who have a higher incidence of cigarette smoking and possibly live in areas of higher air pollution. Cigarette smokers have a higher incidence of pulmonary dysfunction than their nonsmoking counterparts in jobs where they are exposed to coal dust, cotton dust, asbestos, and silica.[4]

It is unclear whether or not air pollution alone is a significant risk factor for the development of COLD; however, in individuals with existing pulmonary dysfunction, significant air pollution worsens symptoms. In individuals with normal pulmonary function, whether smokers or not, there are as yet insufficient data to suggest that air pollution contributes to the development of COLD.

$\alpha_1$-Antitrypsin deficiency has been clearly defined as a genetic factor that contributes significantly to the risk of developing COLD, specifically emphysema. The protease inhibitor (Pi) phenotypes with the highest incidence of COLD are the homozygous PiZ and, to a lesser extent, the heterozygous PiMZ individuals. The homozygote patients have the lowest level of the protease inhibitor, $\alpha_1$-antitrypsin, which normally inhibits trypsin and other proteases from destroying normal lung tissue.

Other less clearly defined familial factors may be genetic or environmental. Children and spouses of smokers have an increased risk of developing significant pulmonary dysfunction.

## Pathophysiology

Both chronic bronchitis and emphysema can exist without evidence of obstruction, but by the time dyspnea is present, obstruction is always demonstrable. Chronic bronchitis and emphysema frequently coexist, with one predominating over the other. The pathophysiology of each type of COLD is described separately for clarity.

### *Chronic Bronchitis*

As described earlier, chronic bronchitis is characterized by excessive tracheobronchial mucus secretion with cough. This excessive production of mucus results from hyperplasia and hypertrophy of mucus-producing glands and goblet cells caused by continued bronchial irritation. The extent of hypertrophy and hyperplasia can be quantified using the Reid index. This index is the ratio of bronchial gland to bronchial wall. When the index is low the glands are small; when the index is high the glands are enlarged. The index is a statistically reliable method to diagnose chronic bronchitis morphologically, but it is of little practical value in daily practice. This excessive secretion of mucus is not thought to contribute significantly to airways obstruction.

Additional morphologic changes occur in the bronchi, including increased smooth muscle, cartilage atrophy, inflammation characterized by leukocytic and lymphocytic infiltration, and loss of cilia.[5–7] More distal in the noncartilaginous or membranous bronchioles, inflammation also exists with mucus production and narrowing of the lumen. Additionally there is fibrosis, tortuosity, and irregularity of these smaller airways. Autopsies have shown that chronic bronchitis patients have a larger population of airways less than 0.4 mm in diameter compared with nonbronchitic patients. This is thought to be a result of the previously mentioned morphologic changes. Recently, airway hyperreactivity has also been considered to contribute significantly to the airway narrowing seen in chronic bronchitis.[6]

The lung damage produced by smoking or exposure to other chronic irritants has long been considered to begin in the small airways. Airways less than 2 mm in diameter contribute only 10% to 20% of normal resistance to airflow, because the total cross-sectional area of these airways is much greater than that of larger airways. Therefore, by the time obstruction is detected by pulmonary function tests, extensive damage has occurred. As chronic bronchitis progresses over several years, the changes in small airways begin to impair ventilation ($V$) while perfusion ($Q$) remains fairly adequate, resulting in a $V/Q$ imbalance and hypoxemia. The hypoxemia leads to pulmonary hypertension with subsequent right ventricular failure (cor pulmonale). The persistent hypoxemia also stimulates erythropoiesis with resultant secondary polycythemia and increased blood viscosity, with its attendant complications of mental confusion or thrombotic stroke.

An additional component of chronic bronchitis is repeated respiratory infections. These patients are predisposed to repeated infections due to mucus stagnation and plugging as well as lack of cilia or ciliary movement to clear mucus. The most frequent pathogens are viral, with the respiratory syncytial virus considered to be the most common. Bacteria are less common pathogens and may follow a viral infection. The most common bacterial pathogens include *Streptococcus pneumoniae* and *Hemophilus influenzae*. These are not the only bacteria that act as pathogens, and thus the host's condition and environment must be considered when searching for a pathogen in a patient with chronic bronchitis with a suspected respiratory infection. The signs of infection usually consist of an increase in the volume of sputum, a thickening of the sputum, and a change in color. Fever or other objective evidence of infection need not be present.

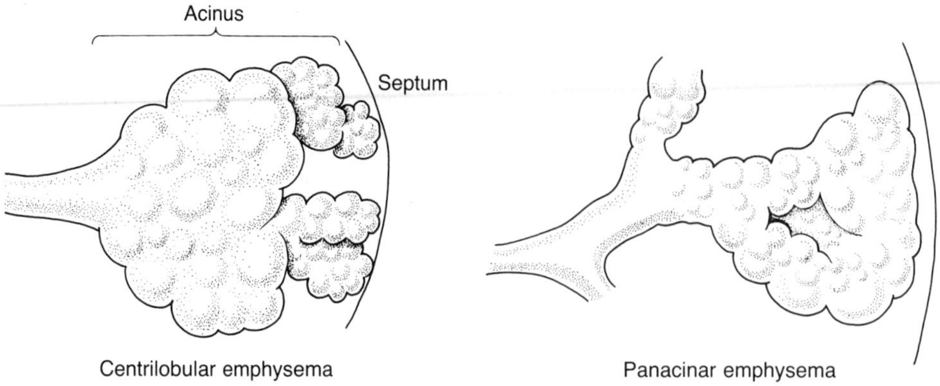


**Figure 22.1** In centrilobular emphysema the terminal bronchioles are involved. In panacinar emphysema the entire acinus is involved.

Repeated respiratory infections in the chronic bronchitis patient can cause severe acute exacerbations in pulmonary status and can contribute significantly in accelerating the decline in pulmonary function tests secondary to the inflammation-induced fibrosis of bronchi and bronchioles.

### *Emphysema*

Emphysema refers specifically to involvement of the acinus. The acinus is the unit of the lung responsible for gas exchange. It consists of three levels—respiratory bronchioles, alveolar ducts, and alveolar sacs—in that order proceeding distally. In a simplistic sense then, emphysema is a condition in which there is destruction of walls within the acinus such that the surface area for gas exchange is diminished.[6]

Several types of emphysema have been described and deserve comment:

1. *Proximal acinar emphysema*. This type includes the centrilobular emphysema (i.e., central lobes of the acinus) characteristically seen in cigarette smokers, especially in the upper lobes, and the simple pneumoconiosis of coal workers. This type of emphysema is confined largely to the proximal portion of the acinus, with the respiratory bronchioles being particularly affected (Fig. 22.1).
2. *Panacinar emphysema*. The entire acinus is involved in this type. It is found in those genetically susceptible individuals who possess the homozygous PiZ phenotype (i.e., 1%–2% of all emphysema patients). These patients have a deficiency of protease inhibitors ($\alpha_1$-antitrypsin) such that proteases are allowed to destroy the alveolar walls of the acinus. This type usually involves the entire lung field (Fig. 22.1).
3. *Distal (paraseptal) emphysema*. As the term suggests, this type of emphysema is associated with the distal portion of the acinus. It is seen as a consequence of spontaneous pneumothorax in young adults.
4. *Irregular emphysema*. This type of emphysema is produced as a consequence of trauma to lung tissue.

Our understanding of the pathogenesis of centrilobular emphysema (the most common type) extends from an understanding of the panacinar emphysema associated with protease inhibitor deficiency states. In centrilobular emphysema specifically caused by smoking, an imbalance develops between the protective protein inhibitors and the proteases from activated neutrophils and mast cells. Cigarette smoke causes a macrophage alveolitis and a respiratory bronchiolitis. The macrophages are chemotactic for neutrophils. Both the macrophages and neutrophils release a greater amount of elastase in response to smoke in smokers than in nonsmokers. The excessive amount of elastase released breaks down elastin, a protein integral to the structural integrity of alveolar walls. Women are less likely to experience this imbalance possibly because of a protective effect of estrogens, which may stimulate synthesis of protease inhibitors. Cigarette smoke is also thought to impair the synthesis of elastin.[8] Protease inhibitor (Pi) phenotype M patients are particularly susceptible to these effects of cigarette smoke.[3]

The destruction of the surface area for gas exchange within the acinus results in a loss of elastic recoil. This loss of elastic recoil permits compression of distal airways during expiration; thus, an obstructive pattern is seen in pulmonary function tests. The exact changes in pulmonary function tests are described later. In cigarette smokers with centrilobular emphysema, the respiratory bronchiolitis leads to narrowing of these terminal bronchioles.[9]

In addition to a reduction in elastic recoil, loss of alveolar walls results in a loss of the capillary network essential to adequate perfusion, resulting in not only a decrease in ventilation (*V*) but also a loss in perfusion (*Q*). Thus, the *V*/*Q* ratio is maintained better than in chronic bronchitis.[10] Therefore, while predominant emphysematous patients experience greater dyspnea than predominant chronic bronchitis patients, the former are better able to preserve gas exchange because their respiratory centers are more responsive to hypoxia. The net result of this on other physiologic systems is less cor pulmonale and less polycythemia than seen in the predominant chronic bronchitic.

## Clinical Presentation

By the time a patient with chronic bronchitis and/or emphysema presents with obstructive airway disease, the diagnosis is rapidly made often by simply observing the patient's

**Table 22.2** Clinical features of COLD

| | ***Predominant emphysema*** | ***Predominant chronic bronchitis*** |
|---|---|---|
| Age | 60–69 | 50–59 |
| Dyspnea | Severe | Mild |
| Cough | After dyspnea starts | Before dyspnea starts |
| Sputum | Scanty, mucoid | Copious, purulent |
| Bronchial infection | Less frequent | More frequent |
| Respiratory insufficiency episode | Often terminal | Repeated |
| Chest film | Increased diameter<br>Flattened diaphragms | Increased bronchovascular markings, large heart |
| $Pa_{CO_2}$ (mm Hg) | 35–40 | 50–60 |
| $Pa_{O_2}$ (mm Hg) | 65–75 | 45–60 |
| Hematocrit (%) | 35–45 | 50–60 |
| Pulmonary hypertension | | |
| Rest | None to mild | Moderate to severe |
| Exercise | Moderate | Worsens |
| Cor pulmonale | Rare | Common |
| Diffusion capacity | Decreased | None to slightly decreased |

Adapted from Ingram RH: Chronic bronchitis, emphysema, and airways obstruction. In Petersdorf RG, Adams RD, Braunwald E, et al (Eds): Harrison's Textbook of Internal Medicine. New York, McGraw–Hill, 1983, p 1548.

breathing pattern. The clinical features are presented in Table 22.2. Again, as described previously, while the majority of patients with COLD have components of both chronic bronchitis and emphysema, it is best to describe the physical examination of each constituent condition separately.

## *Clinical Features*

### Chronic Bronchitis

The patient presenting with predominant chronic bronchitis is often overweight and has an impressive history of productive cough and increasing dyspnea on exertion. By history the cough has been increasing in frequency and duration. The predominant chronic bronchitic patient is also referred to classically as the "blue bloater" (type B) inasmuch as they tend to retain carbon dioxide because of a decreased responsiveness of the respiratory center to hypoxemia and ultimately hypercarbia. They commonly have peripheral edema from cor pulmonale and usually have a normal or only slightly increased respiratory rate at rest. In the case of advanced disease the anteroposterior diameter of the chest is often increased, resulting in the classical "barrel chest" appearance. This need not always indicate advanced disease, as it is a normal part of the aging process. Percussion of the chest is resonant, and the breath sounds are distant on auscultation. Rhonchi and wheezes are frequently heard and change in location as the patient breathes deeply or coughs. A rapid assessment of obstruction can be achieved by placing the stethoscope over the trachea and instructing the patient to forcefully expire. If forced expiration lasts longer than 4 seconds it correlates with obstruction in pulmonary function tests.

In the predominant chronic bronchitic one may not easily note the use of the scalene or sternocleidomastoid muscles of the neck to assist respiration unless severe obstruction is present.

As the degree of obstruction worsens and the arterial oxygen tension ($Pa_{O_2}$) continues to drop, pulmonary hypertension from vasoconstriction ensues. This leads to right ventricular strain and ultimately cor pulmonale. On physical examination this is manifest by jugular venous distension, hepatomegaly, hepatojugular reflux, and peripheral edema. Conventional cardiac examination may be difficult if a barrel chest is present; however, by palpating the epigastric area, a heave may be felt or even seen in thin patients and auscultation of the area may reveal a gallop rhythm suggestive of right ventricular hypertrophy.

In the face of chronic hypoxemia, cyanosis of the lips, mucous membranes, or extremities can be seen. Clubbing of the fingers is rarely seen in chronic bronchitis. The cyanosis worsens during the night, frequently because of chronic oxygen desaturation secondary to sleep apnea. Sleep apnea has recently become an area of increasing study in patients with COLD and it may play a much greater role than previously understood in the pathogenesis of disease, especially with respect to cor pulmonale.

### Emphysema

The patient presenting with predominant emphysema is characteristically older than the chronic bronchitic patient. The chief complaint is often increasing dyspnea, even at rest, with minimal cough. These patients have been classically referred to as "pink puffers" (type A) because of the obvious tachypnea and flushed appearance, as their respiratory centers are quite responsive to hypoxemia as a stimulus to breath.

These patients are frequently thin in physical stature. They present with "pursed lip" breathing. This maneuver is to compensate for loss of elastic recoil so that they can exhale a larger volume of air. They also are tachypneic at rest and often sit with their chests forward and hands resting on the knees, as this position requires the least energy for breathing. Frequently, the patient uses accessory muscles of the chest and neck to assist in the work of breathing. Percussion of the chest is hyperresonant and auscultation reveals diminished breath sounds with rhonchi and minimal wheezes. Excursion of the diaphragms is limited because of persistent hyperinflation of the lungs.

Hypoxemia is not a significant problem in the predominant emphysema patient until late in the disease state. As a result, cor pulmonale is not as common a problem as seen in the predominant chronic bronchitic until the terminal stages.

## *Diagnostic Tests*

### Pulmonary Function

Measurements of pulmonary function by objective means are considered essential in any patient with COLD to determine the severity of the disease, its responsiveness to therapeutic agents, and the prognosis. Provided the patient is compliant and the instrumentation used is reliable, vital information can be obtained easily and in most instances inexpensively.

The conventional displacement spirometers are acceptable for everyday office use to measure lung volumes and flow rates. The tidal volume or the volume of air inhaled and exhaled during normal breathing can be measured. Functional residual capacity (FRC) is the amount of air left after normal exhalation. Vital capacity (VC) is the amount of air moved during maximal inhalation and exhalation. Residual volume (RV) is the volume of air left after maximal exhalation. Total lung capacity (TLC) is the vital capacity plus the residual volume (Fig. 22.2).

In the predominant chronic bronchitic the VC is decreased, the RV is increased, and the TLC is often normal. In the predominant emphysematous patient the VC is decreased while the RV is increased more than in chronic bronchitis and the TLC is usually increased.

**Figure 22.2** Spirogram of a normal breathing pattern.

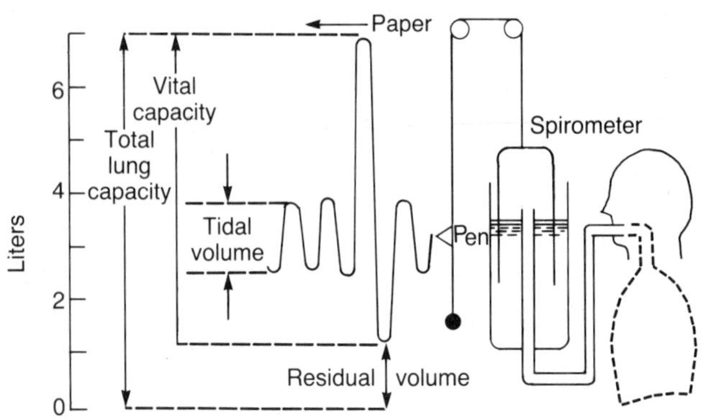


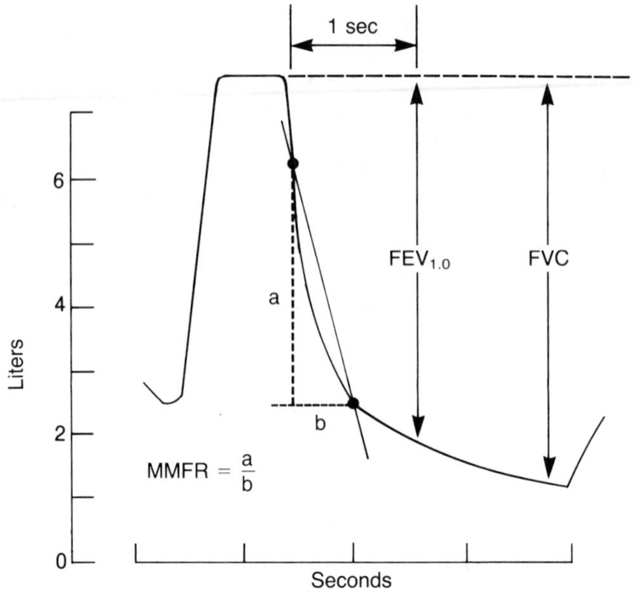


**Figure 22.3** Forced expiratory spirogram.

Forced expiration techniques using conventional displacement spirometers can be enlisted to measure lung volumes and air flow rates (Fig. 22.3). The forced expiratory volume in 1 second ($FEV_1$) is the most commonly measured, although other measures are of equal importance when assessing a patient with COLD. The forced vital capacity (FVC) is used in conjunction with the $FEV_1$. The $FEV_1$/FVC ratio expressed as a percentage is helpful in determining the degree of obstruction. If it is less than 80%, obstruction is present. The forced expiratory flow over the middle 50% of the expiratory curve (MMFR, $FEF_{25-75\%}$, or $FEF_{50\%}$) is helpful specifically in the predominant emphysema patient because it represents the elastic recoil of the lung.

In patients with chronic bronchitis and/or emphysema leading to COLD there are reductions in $FEV_1$, FVC, $FEV_1$/FVC%, and $FEF_{25-75}$. One can easily understand in a situation of predominant chronic bronchitis how flow rates are decreased. What is less easy to understand is how the predominant emphysema patient exhibits these similar decreases in flow rate. The primary defect in emphysema is loss of elastic recoil (i.e., elasticity of the lung parenchyma) such that there is a reduction in pressure, producing airflow. This loss of pressure then results in decreases in flow rates. An additional factor contributing to airflow obstruction in predominant emphysema is the presence of bronchiolitis.

The majority of patients with mixed disease usually experience exertional dyspnea when the $FEV_1$ is less than 50% predicted and have dyspnea at rest when the $FEV_1$ is less than 25% predicted. Patients with predominant chronic bronchitis experience carbon dioxide retention and cor pulmonale when the $FEV_1$ is greater than 25% of predicted values, but the predominantly emphysematous patient does not experience these complications until the $FEV_1$ is less than 25% of predicted value.

A major criticism of the conventional displacement spirometer is that it measures changes only in airways greater than 2.0 mm in diameter. In an effort to detect changes in

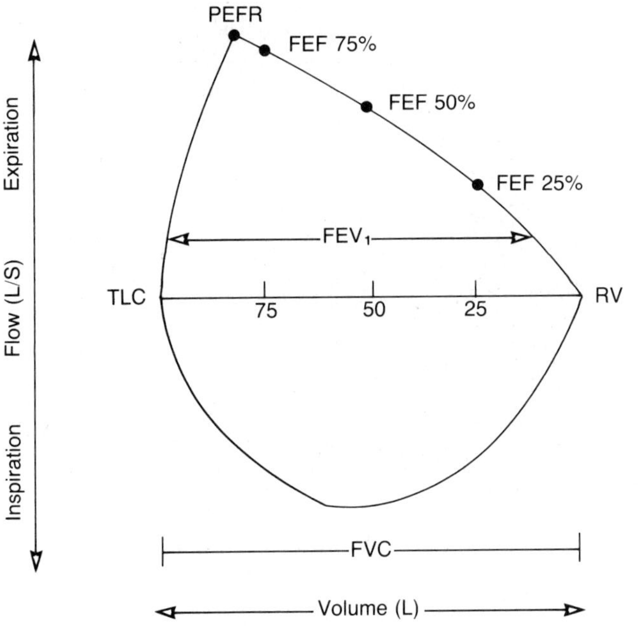


**Figure 22.4** Flow volume loop (normal).

smaller airways before significant clinical symptoms are present, newer techniques have been developed. One such technique is flow–volume spirometry in which flow rate and volume are measured simultaneously (Fig. 22.4 and 22.5). This allows measurement of the $FEF_{75-85\%}$, which provides a sensitive index of obstruction of smaller airways. This requires spirometers more sophisticated than those routinely available for everyday office practice. Although wedge spirometers are currently available, this type of measurement is usually done in a pulmonary function lab with experienced technicians. The closing volume is another measurement that seems to be a sensitive test of small airway disease. Its value as a routine test has yet to be determined.

**Figure 22.5** Flow volume loops of an obstructive and a restrictive pattern.

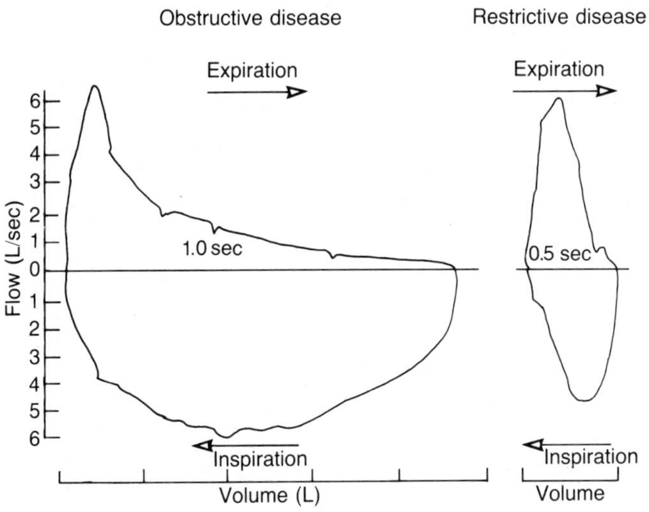


Many portable nondisplacement spirometers are on the market but have yet to be standardized to provide a reliable tool for pulmonary function testing in everyday practice. Additionally, peak expiratory flow rate (PEFR) can also be readily measured with inexpensive but unreliable equipment. The PEFR is often said to represent the poor man's $FEV_1$. These tools may, however, be of assistance in routine screening of large populations.

Measurement of diffusion capacity using carbon monoxide ($D_{CO}$) can help distinguish predominant bronchitis from emphysema. In emphysema, the diffusion capacity is diminished because of loss of surface area available for gas diffusion. In bronchitis the diffusion capacity is normal or only slightly decreased.

The reader is referred to more extensive reviews of pulmonary function tests by Menendez and Kelly[11] and Cherniack.[12]

### Arterial Blood Gases

Just as pulmonary function tests are essential for determining the severity and prognosis of patients with COLD, so are arterial blood gases. Arterial blood gases should be determined at rest and after exercise. The predominant chronic bronchitic is characterized as having a low arterial oxygen tension ($Pa_{O_2}$ = 45–60 mm Hg) and an elevated arterial carbon dioxide tension ($Pa_{CO_2}$ = 50–60 mm Hg). The predominantly emphysematous patient has by comparison a higher $Pa_{O_2}$ and usually normal $Pa_{CO_2}$ with similar degrees of pulmonary dysfunction. In the predominant chronic bronchitic patient the initial abnormality is a decrease in the $Pa_{O_2}$. The major cause of this hypoxemia is an underventilation (*V*) of acini relative to the perfusion (*Q*) of the area. This low *V*/*Q* ratio progresses over a period of several years, resulting in a consistent decline in the $Pa_{O_2}$. For reasons that are not entirely understood, the predominant chronic bronchitic loses the ability to increase the rate or depth of respiration in response to persistent hypoxemia. This decreased ventilatory drive may have its origin in either abnormal peripheral or central respiratory receptors. This relative hypoventilation subsequently leads to hypercapnia and again the respiratory centers do not respond to the persistently increased $Pa_{CO_2}$.

These changes in $Pa_{O_2}$ and $Pa_{CO_2}$ are subtle and progress over a period of many years; as a result the pH is usually near normal because the kidneys compensate by retaining bicarbonate. If an acute change occurs such as might be seen in an acute pneumonia with impending respiratory failure, the $Pa_{CO_2}$ may rise sharply, temporarily resulting in a primary respiratory acidosis until the kidney can compensate (24–72 hours later) or the acid–base defect is corrected by mechanical ventilation.

The persistent hypoxia leads to pulmonary vascular constriction and cor pulmonale. The hypoxemia and hypercarbia lead to an increase in 2,3-diphosphoglyceric acid (2,3-DPG) and a shift in the oxyhemoglobin dissociation curve to the right. This results in a decrease in the affinity of hemoglobin for oxygen, allowing more oxygen to be released to tissues in which the $Pa_{O_2}$ is lowest. Hypoxemia also stimulates erythropoiesis which leads to the secondary polycythemia common in the predominant chronic bronchitic.

Compared to the predominant chronic bronchitic, the

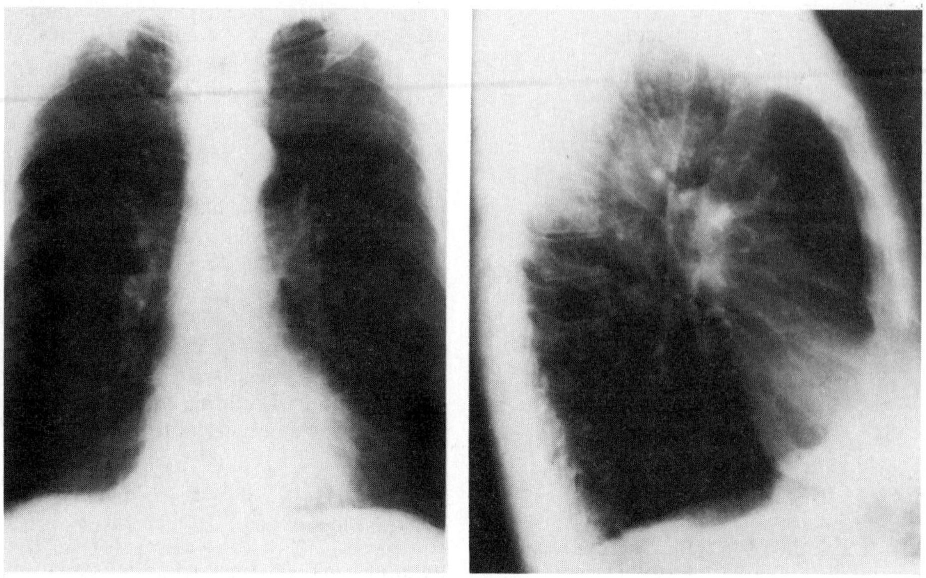

**Figure 22.6** Characteristic emphysematous lungs. Note flattened diaphragms, loss of peripheral vascular markings, and a bullous lesion in the right lower lobe on the posteroanterior view (left), and increased retrosternal airspace on the lateral view (right).

predominantly emphysematous patient can maintain a near-normal $Pa_{O_2}$ in the face of the declining pulmonary function, until the terminal stages, because ventilation (*V*) and perfusion (*Q*) decrease proportionately. These individuals have normal or excess responsiveness of peripheral and central respiratory receptors to hypoxemia or hypercarbia. This helps to explain why the predominant emphysematous patient does not develop cyanosis, cor pulmonale, or polycythemia until the end stages of the disease process.

### Chest Roentgenogram

A chest roentgenogram (posteroanterior and lateral views) is most useful in the diagnosis of the predominant emphysematous patient. The characteristic findings include flattened diaphragms that move less than 3 cm between inspiration and expiration, loss of peripheral vascular markings, bullous lesions, and increased retrosternal air space (Fig. 22.6). All these findings indicate extensive air trapping consistent with severe emphysema. Whether the dimensions of the thoracic cage itself are truly increased is a matter of controversy; it may be that the cage appears large because of the loss of physical mass in the rest of the body. In the predominant chronic bronchitic, the only changes are increased bronchovascular markings in the lower lung field and an increased cardiac silhouette in the presence of right ventricular failure with prominent pulmonary arteries.

### Electrocardiogram

The electrocardiogram is helpful in COLD patients only when cor pulmonale failure develops. Common findings are right-axis deviation, a Q wave in R in $V_1$, an S wave in $V_5$ or $V_6 \geq 7$ mm, and tall peaked P waves in lead II.

### Other Laboratory Tests

***Hematology*** In the predominant chronic bronchitic, the hemoglobin and hematocrit are elevated secondary to erythropoiesis caused by hypoxemia. In exacerbations of chronic bronchitis, the white cell count may or may not rise and a left shift may or may not be present.

***Sputum*** Examination of sputum is helpful in exacerbations of chronic bronchitis to identify potential bacterial pathogens that may have precipitated the exacerbation. It is important to ensure that what is examined microscopically is truly sputum and not saliva. Sputum is identified by the presence of alveolar macrophages and saliva, by squamous epithelial cells. Many laboratories have developed scoring systems to help clinicians assess the adequacy of the sputum sample being examined. Sputum should also be examined for eosinophils to rule out an allergic component to the obstructive picture.

***$\alpha_1$-Antitrypsin Assay*** This test is particularly useful in patients under 40 who present with emphysema and obstructive lung disease. Markedly low levels may detect a PiZ phenotype. Moderately low levels may detect other Pi phenotypes who may be more predisposed to emphysema caused by smoking than the general population.

## *Course/Prognosis*

The clinical course and prognosis of patients with chronic bronchitis and/or emphysema with obstructive pulmonary disease are marked by variable morbidity and mortality. Little is known of the early natural history of COLD, but it probably is characterized by slowly deteriorating pulmonary function for several years before clinical illness is appreciated by patients. Much more is known of the prognosis and clinical course once symptomatology has become evident.

The predominant emphysematous patient's progress is characterized by progressive dyspnea without exacerbations precipitated by increased sputum production, as is characteristic of the predominant chronic bronchitic. The predominant emphysematous patient's terminal event is often characterized by rapidly progressive cor pulmonale and intractable hypercapnia leading to respiratory arrest. The usual course of a patient with predominant bronchitis is one characterized by increasing frequency of exacerbations of acute pulmonary insufficiency precipitated by bronchitis. This is accompanied by progressive decline in pulmonary function, with the chronic complications (previously described) of cor pulmonale, hypercapnia, and polycythemia. Exacerbations of bronchitis are characterized by increased mucopurulent sputum and frequently lead to acute respiratory failure (described later) from which the patient rapidly recovers with appropriate antibiotics and other therapies. These episodes tend to increase in severity and frequency until intractable cor pulmonale and hypercapnia occur.

Mean rate of decline of $FEV_1$ appears to be the most useful objective tool to assess the course of COLD. The rates of decline in prospective follow-up studies of patients with initially abnormal $FEV_1$'s or $FEV_1/FVC$ ratios followed for 3 to 16 years revealed a decline in the $FEV_1$ of 44 to 75 mL per year; however, there was considerable variability. The rate of decline in $FEV_1$ for normal patients from age alone was 24 mL per year.[13–15] In any study assessing rate of decline, an appropriate observation period is essential. In the study reporting a rate of decline in $FEV_1$ of 44 mL per year the observation period was only 3 years.[13] This may be too short to project rate of decline throughout the life of the patient, because during the first year many patients improve their pulmonary function with pharmacologic agents. In longer studies the rate of decline of $FEV_1$ is greater and linear.[14,15] Rate of decline of blood gases has not been shown to be a useful parameter to assess progression of the disease.

In terms of functional capacity, the predominant bronchitic shows more physical impairment at a higher $FEV_1$ than the predominant emphysematous patient because of the comparatively worse arterial blood gases. Most people with mixed disease are not able to perform extremely vigorous activity once the $FEV_1$ falls below 1.5 L, but they can work. Once the $FEV_1$ falls below 1.0 L their ability to perform the usual daily activities becomes impaired.

The survival rate in patients with COLD is related to the initial level of impairment in the $FEV_1$ and possibly to the degree of reversibility with bronchodilators. Other factors, including age, resting pulse, perceived physical disability, diffusing capacity, cor pulmonale, and blood gas abnormalities, contribute. A rapid decline in pulmonary function tests indicates a poor prognosis. Also, people living at high altitudes have a reduced survival rate.[15] Median survival is approximately 10 years when the $FEV_1$ is 1.4 L, 4 years when the $FEV_1$ is 1.0 L, and about 2 years when the $FEV_1$ is 0.5 L.[15]

As of yet, it is not clear that treatment with pharmacologic agents improves survival; however, these agents do improve the quality of life, probably reduce hospitalizations, and may prevent some premature deaths. The only intervention shown to improve survival rate is oxygen therapy (to be discussed in greater detail later).[15] Smoking cessation leads to decreased symptomatology and appears to slow the rate of decline of pulmonary function, even after significant abnormalities in pulmonary function tests have been detected ($FEV_1/FVC < 60\%$).[14]

### *Acute Respiratory Failure*

The diagnosis of acute respiratory failure in COLD is definitively made on the basis of an acute change in the arterial blood gases. Defining acute respiratory failure as a $Pa_{O_2}$ less than 50 mm Hg or a $Pa_{CO_2}$ greater than 50 mm Hg would often be incorrect and inadequate because these values may not represent a significant change from a patient's baseline values. A more precise definition is an acute drop in $Pa_{O_2}$ of 10 to 15 mm Hg or any acute increase in $Pa_{CO_2}$ that decreases the serum pH to 7.30 or less.[16] Additional acute clinical manifestations include restlessness, confusion, tachycardia, diaphoresis, cyanosis, hypotension, irregular breathing, miosis, and unconsciousness.[17]

The most common cause of acute respiratory failure in COLD is acute exacerbation of bronchitis with an increase in the volume and viscosity of sputum. This serves to worsen obstruction and further impair alveolar ventilation, resulting in worsening hypoxemia and hypercapnia.

Additional causes of acute respiratory failure in COLD are pneumonia, pulmonary embolism, left ventricular failure, pneumothorax, and central nervous system depressants.

## Treatment

Therapy of the patient with COLD is multifaceted. The goals of therapy include improvement of the chronic obstructive state, treatment and prevention of acute exacerbations, reduction of the rate of progression of the disease, improvement of physical and psychologic well-being of the patient so that daily activities can be resumed, reduction in days lost from work, and reduction in hospitalizations.

The long-standing opinion that COLD is associated with irreversible obstruction has allowed pharmacotherapy to be largely empiric. This opinion, however, has recently been challenged by the Intermittent Positive Pressure Breathing Group.[18] The data reported from these studies suggest that many individuals with COLD do obtain some degree of improvement in their obstruction from bronchodilators. It also appears that a single test of reversibility using an inhaled sympathomimetic followed by pulmonary function tests is not adequate to assess whether patients with COLD will benefit from bronchodilators. Even if a positive response is not detected, these patients deserve an adequate therapeutic trial of pharmacologic agents for the following reasons: (1) while objective tests may not reveal a response, possibly because of the sensitivity of the equipment, a subjective improvement may occur; (2) some patients may respond to inhaled sympathomimetics on one occasion and not on another; (3) the response to bronchodilators may require prolonged administration; (4) patients may respond to methylxanthines or sympathomimetics via nonbronchodilator mechanisms; and (5) patients not responding in initial tests with sympathomimetics may respond to methylxanthines or anticholinergics.

The question of whether to use a methylxanthine or a sympathomimetic first has no clear answer. The decision should be based on patient compliance, response, and side effects. It is not the purpose of this chapter to provide an exhaustive review of the pharmacology of all bronchodilators but all available agents will be put into perspective.

### *Methylxanthines*

Early studies suggested methylxanthines produced bronchodilation through inhibition of phosphodiesterase, thus preventing the enzymatic breakdown of adenosine 3′,5′-cyclic monophosphate (3′,5′-AMP). More recently this proposed mechanism has been questioned because to exert this effect concentrations of methylxanthines much higher than those obtainable in clinical practice are required.[19] Numerous other mechanisms have been proposed to explain the mechanism of bronchodilation and other respiratory effects, including (1) inhibition of calcium ion influx into smooth muscle; (2) prostaglandin antagonism; (3) stimulation of endogenous catecholamines; (4) adenosine receptor antagonism; and (5) inhibition of release of mediators from mast cells and leukocytes.[19,20] Nonbronchodilator respiratory effects that may be useful to the patient with COLD include (1) improved diaphragmatic strength and reduction of fatigue; (2) stimulation of mucociliary clearance; and (3) improved central respiratory response to hypoxemia (especially helpful in patients with a significant sleep apnea component to their disease).[19,20]

The most common methylxanthine in use in clinical practice is theophylline (1,3-dimethylxanthine). Numerous reliably absorbed sustained-release theophylline preparations are currently available. These have the advantages of improving patient compliance and achieving more consistent serum concentrations over rapid-release theophylline and aminophylline preparations; however, caution must be used in switching from one sustained-release preparation to another, as there are considerable variations in sustained-release characteristics.[19]

Aside from aminophylline there is no need to use the various other complexes of theophylline. There is no indication for rectal suppositories of theophylline or aminophylline or intramuscular administration. Dissolution from rectal suppositories is inconsistent, absorption from intramuscular injections is unreliable, and the injections are painful.

Aminophylline, USP is the complex of ethylenediamine and theophylline dihydrate (contains 80% anhydrous theophylline).[20] Aminophylline has increased water solubility over theophylline, thus is commonly used for parenteral administration. Parenteral administration is indicated for severe acute decompensation or if the patient is unable to take oral medications. During acute exacerbations, patients should be administered loading doses of intravenous aminophylline in order to achieve therapeutic serum theophylline concentrations rapidly. The usual elimination half-life of 8–12 hours in COLD patients would require 40–60 hours (5 half-lives) before steady-state serum concentrations would be reached with maintenance dosing only.[20] The loading dose is based on actual body weight.[20] The recommended loading doses of intravenous aminophylline are 6 or 9 mg/kg for patients who have not taken any theophylline in the previous 24 hours or 3 mg/kg if they have taken sustained-release theophylline within the past 24 hours or rapid-release theophylline within the past 12 hours.

If serum concentration measurements are readily available, one can use the average distribution volume ($V_d$) of 0.5 L/kg for theophylline in adults to estimate whatever loading dose is required to produce the desired increment in serum theophylline concentration:

$$\frac{\text{Loading dose}}{V_d} = \text{Serum level increment}$$

or

$$\frac{1\ \text{mg/kg}}{0.5\ \text{L/kg}} = 2\ \text{mg/L}$$

The administration rate should not exceed 25 mg/min to avoid cardiac arrhythmias or cardiovascular collapse.

The desired therapeutic range is 10 to 20 μg/mL. As most COLD patients are elderly and often have a rapidly changing clinical status that can affect theophylline clearance, it is prudent to aim for levels in the range of 10 to 15 μg/mL in order to minimize the likelihood of toxicity. The infusion is best accomplished with a controlling device and the dose is based on ideal body weight. Initial intravenous maintenance dose recommendations for acute exacerbations of COLD with pneumonia or ventricular failure are 0.45 to 0.7 mg/kg/h of aminophylline. One may wish to initiate therapy at the upper end of this range if the patient is a smoker because of the increased clearance induced by smoking. Factors in COLD patients that decrease theophylline clearance leading to reduced maintenance dose requirements include age, bacterial or viral pneumonia, left or right ventricular failure, liver dysfunction, hypoxemia from the acute decompensation, and drugs such as cimetidine, erythromycin, and ciprofloxacin. Maintenance dose recommendations for these conditions have been proposed (Table 22.3). These recommendations are strictly starting points and serum theophylline concentrations must be obtained to guide further therapy. The conditions described are dynamic and as they worsen or improve so will the clearance of theophylline.

Serum concentrations should be obtained 12 to 24 hours after the initiation of therapy and adjustments made accordingly. The reason for this early time is that if the patient has a clearance much lower than anticipated, the dose can be reduced before the patient becomes toxic, and if the clearance is much higher than anticipated, modest elevations in dose can be made. The serum concentration should be obtained every 24 hours thereafter until the patient is stable.

**Table 22.3** Maintenance Doses of Aminophylline in Exacerbations of COLD

| | |
|---|---|
| Age (>50 yr) | 0.6–0.7 mg/kg/h |
| Bacterial or viral pneumonia | 0.45–0.7 mg/kg/h |
| Left or right ventricular failure | 0.45–0.7 mg/kg/h |
| Liver disease (total bilirubin > 1.5 mg/dL) | 0.2–0.25 mg/kg/h |

Attempting to make adjustments in dose in order to attain a desired concentration using first-order pharmacokinetic equations is fraught with error. Theophylline is metabolized by microsomal enzymes to three major metabolites: 1,3-dimethyluric acid, 1-methyluric acid, and 3-methylxanthine.[20] Each metabolic pathway is potentially saturable. This results in the nonlinear kinetics of theophylline witnessed in acute overdoses. Apparent nonlinearity may occur as a result of physiologic changes that occur during therapy of acute exacerbations. Diminished hemodynamics due to either right or left ventricular failure could result in hepatic congestion and decreases in theophylline clearance. Thus each patient's physiologic character should be carefully monitored and the serum theophylline concentrations obtained if there are any significant changes. There are other pharmacologic interventions; there is no need in COLD to push theophylline to toxicity.

Serum theophylline concentrations above 20 μg/mL are associated with nausea and vomiting and those above 35 to 40 μg/mL with arrhythmias and seizures. In the elderly with exacerbations of COLD, these values should not be used to judge the likelihood of toxicity. Nausea is a common complication in patients with concentrations greater than 15 μg/mL, and seizures and atrial tachyarrhythmias have been reported with serum concentrations of 20 to 30 μg/mL. The seizures and arrhythmias are quite refractory to conventional treatment.

Once the patient is stabilized and serum concentrations are reasonably consistent, one can switch to oral therapy with a sustained-release theophylline preparation. The oral dose is calculated from the 24-hour intravenous theophylline dose. The total 24-hour dose can then be divided in thirds or in half depending upon desired interval and strength of preparation available.

The oral sustained-release preparation can be initiated at the time the intravenous solution is stopped. Follow-up trough concentrations should be obtained several days after initiation of therapy to ensure the appropriateness of the dose and dosing interval for the selected product. Afterward it should not be necessary to routinely monitor serum concentrations unless the patient's disease worsens or toxicity is suspected.

### *Sympathomimetics*

Sympathomimetics either alone or in combination with theophylline have been the cornerstone of pharmacotherapy for COLD. There remains little doubt that combination therapy, when individually designed, can produce additive bronchodilatory effects. While numerous sympathomimetics are currently available in the U.S. market, it is most desirable to use the newer agents with greater $\beta_2$ selectivity and longer duration of action. These agents include albuterol, bitolterol, and terbutaline. $\beta_2$ selective sympathomimetics cause bronchodilation by stimulating the enzyme adenyl cyclase to increase the formation of 3′,5′-AMP. Additionally, like the theophylline, they improve mucociliary clearance. Although shorter-acting and less selective $\beta$ agonists are still widely used (i.e., metaproterenol, isoetharine, isoproterenol) it is difficult to advocate their continued use because of the shorter duration of action and increased cardiostimulatory effects.

The preferred route of administration of the selective $\beta_2$ agonist is an issue that has prompted considerable research in the past several years. The decision on route is based on the comparative efficacy and toxicity of the parenteral, oral, and inhalation routes. The accumulated data suggest that the inhalation route is preferred in terms of both efficacy and toxicity.[21–23] The inhalation route is equal if not superior to the parenteral route and is unquestionably superior to the oral route in bronchodilating effect. The inhalation route consistently has shown fewer cardiostimulatory effects and other systemic effects (i.e., hand tremor) than either the parenteral or oral route. Indepth reviews on these newer agents and routes of administration are available.[19,24]

The objective in therapy with inhaled $\beta_2$ agonists is to provide relatively small doses to the affected airways, to achieve the desired pharmacologic effect with minimal systemic toxicity. The remaining issue is determination of the method of inhaling bronchodilators that best achieves this objective: (1) use of a metered-dose inhaler; (2) use of a metered-dose inhaler with a spacer; or (3) use of a powered nebulizer to deliver the medication. Regardless of which technique is used, the most critical factor is proper technique. Although the usual doses and intervals can be obtained from several sources, the dose and frequency should be individually adjusted to the patient's needs and tolerance. At this time it is not clear if COLD patients with extremely poor inspiration effort on aerosolized $\beta_2$ agonists receive additional benefit or simply greater toxicity by the addition of an oral $\beta_2$ agonist.

Metered-dose inhalers (MDIs) are convenient for the mobile patient and are quite adequate when used appropriately. (A description of appropriate technique is provided in Chapter 21.) The greatest problems are inappropriate technique and overuse. Thus, patient education and reinforcement are critical. Spacer devices improve aerosol delivery from MDIs in patients unable to adequately coordinate MDI actuation with inhalation (i.e., elderly COLD patients). The use of these devices is currently seeing increasing popularity. The wet nebulization method should be reserved for those with the most debilitated lung function. This method of delivery has been considered superior to the MDI, but it is not yet known whether it is superior to use of the MDI with a spacer.[19] When a wet nebulizer is used, the bronchodilator is diluted with 2 to 3 mL of normal saline. This provides treatment for approximately 10 minutes. A T-tube is necessary to prevent excessive loss of drug and diluent. As with the MDI, the inspiration must be slow and deep. The patient should try to hold each inspiration for 3 to 5 seconds. Exhalation should be through the nose. It may be desirable to use more diluent to further moisten secretions and promote their expectoration, but this will alter the delivered dose because the dead volume (the volume of liquid left in the nebulizer following the treatment) remains the same but contains less drug.

### *Corticosteroids*

The efficacy of corticosteroids either in acute exacerbations of COLD or in a chronic state had been a controversial issue until 1980, at which time a study published by Albert et al[25] established the efficacy of corticosteroids in COLD patients with acute exacerbations. The patients, who were on standard therapy of methylxanthines and sympathomimetics, were randomly allocated to receive either placebo or methylprednisolone (IV) 0.5 mg/kg every 6 hours for 72 hours. The steroid-treated group showed greater improvement in pulmonary function tests than the placebo group.

The use of steroids in the chronic COLD patient is less clearly established. Mandella et al[26] have reported a positive response to methylprednisolone 32 mg/d in only 8 of 40 patients studied. In attempts to determine patient characteristics to assess which patients would most likely benefit from steroid administration, it appears that a significant eosinophilia (>300/mm$^3$), eosinophils on sputum examination, and significant response on pulmonary function tests to sympathomimetics are the best predictors.

Corticosteroids produce significant side effects; therefore, many clinicians follow the axiom that as soon as a decision is made to initiate therapy, a similar plan should be made to stop therapy as soon as is feasibly possible. Objective parameters should be followed to substantiate drug use. The anti-inflammatory mechanisms whereby corticosteroids exert their beneficial effect in COLD include (1) reduction of capillary permeability to decrease mucus; (2) inhibition of release of proteolytic enzymes from leukocytes; and (3) inhibition of prostaglandins. These effects are accomplished because of the ability of steroids to be transported into the nucleus of the cell and stimulate RNA synthesis, leading to the desired effect.

The decision to use corticosteroids is usually made in situations of acute exacerbations in which the patient is deteriorating or not improving as expected in the face of adequate methylxanthine and sympathomimetic and/or anticholinergic therapy. Patients taking chronic oral steroid presenting in acute distress should be started on parenteral steroids immediately. Therapy is initiated with methylprednisolone (or its equivalent) 0.5–1.0 mg/kg intravenously every 6 hours. Three to six hours or longer is generally required for a beneficial pharmacologic effect to be observed.

As soon as the patient's symptoms have stabilized, he or she can be switched to 40–60 mg of prednisone daily. The oral dose is largely empiric. A short- to intermediate-acting corticosteroid is preferred to minimize suppression of the hypothalamic–pituitary–adrenal (HPA) axis. If possible, the patient should stop steroids in 7 to 14 days. Therapy extending beyond 2 to 4 weeks with supraphysiologic doses begins to suppress the HPA axis. If therapy needs to be prolonged, the ideal is to achieve the lowest possible effective dose with a minimal likelihood of HPA axis suppression (i.e., prednisone 7.5 mg day). The dose should be given once per day in the morning to mimic the normal diurnal variation of endogenous cortisol secretion. If possible, the patient should be moved to an alternate-day schedule, shown by Blair and Light[27] to be just as effective as daily therapy in COLD patients. This is accomplished by raising one day's dose while decreasing the alternate day's dose. If a patient requires continuous steroid therapy, hospitalization may be diminished by giving short bursts of higher doses of oral prednisone during periods of worsening clinical status. Conversion to aerosol steroids would be preferred to further minimize HPA axis suppression, but data from Shim and Williams[28] suggest that not only do less than 50% of people with COLD respond at all to aerosolized steroids, but those who do respond do so less than when they were on oral steroids. This may represent inadequate dosing from the ventilation abnormalities.

### *Anticholinergics*

The use of anticholinergic agents has increased in use in this country over the past decade. The only agents currently available in the United States are atropine and ipratropium bromide. When given via the inhaled route, anticholinergics produce bronchodilation by competitively inhibiting cholinergic receptors in bronchial smooth muscle. This activity blocks acetylcholine, with the net effect being a reduction in cyclic guanosine monophosphate (GMP). Cyclic GMP normally acts to constrict bronchial smooth muscle. Effects on mucociliary clearance are at this time unclear.[29,30]

Several studies have demonstrated the effectiveness of inhaled anticholinergics in patients with COLD.[31–34] Also, the anticholinergic agent was compared with an inhaled sympathomimetic and in all these studies, anticholinergic agents were found to produce greater improvements in pulmonary function tests than sympathomimetic agents. The use of the two together has been found to have an additive bronchodilator effect. These studies have illustrated the importance of the cholinergic system as a mediator of bronchial tone in COLD patients.

Atropine can be administered via either a hand held nebulizer or a jet nebulizer using the parenteral or ophthalmic solution. The dose of atropine is initiated at 0.025 mg/kg to 0.05 mg/kg. The solution is diluted with 2 to 4 mL of saline for administration. The duration of effect is approximately 4 hours. Absorption can be substantial, and patients should be monitored for signs of toxicity after several doses.[35] Atropine is usually administered earlier in an acute setting.

Ipratropium bromide is available in an MDI and is three to five times more potent on muscarinic receptors than atropine.[19] It provides a peak effect in 1.5 to 2 hours and has a duration of 4 to 6 hours.[36] Systemic absorption is minimal as it has a quaternary structure.[36] Oxitropium bromide is a newer agent being studied in Europe that appears to be even more potent and have a longer duration of action.

When inhaled anticholinergic agents are used with inhaled sympathomimetics, the sympathomimetic should be used first because of its more rapid onset.[31] As with all inhaled agents, the appropriate technique of administration cannot be overemphasized.

### *Long-Term Oxygen*

While long-term oxygen has been used for many years in patients with advanced COLD, it was not until 1980 that data became available documenting the benefits of such therapy. At that time, the Nocturnal Oxygen Therapy Trial Group published their data comparing nocturnal oxygen therapy (NOT) (12 h/d) with continuous oxygen therapy (COT)[37] (average of 20 h/d). The patients were followed for at least 12 months. The results revealed a mortality rate in the NOT group nearly twice that of the COT group. Statistical estimates of the COT group suggest that COT may add 3.25 years to a COLD patient's life.[38] The decline in mortality with oxygen therapy was further substantiated in 1981 in a study by the British Medical Research Council which compared 15 hours of oxygen per day versus no supplemental oxygen in COLD patients.[39] Additional data from the Nocturnal Oxygen Therapy Trial Group revealed that COT patients had fewer (but statistically insignificant) hospitalizations, improved quality of life and neuropsychologic function, reduced hematocrits, and decreased pulmonary vascular resistance. Whether oxygen therapy consistently improves exercise tolerance or sleep is a matter of controversy.

Before patients are considered for long-term oxygen therapy, they should be stabilized in the outpatient setting for 1 month and pharmacotherapy should be optimized. Once this is accomplished, long-term oxygen therapy should be instituted if either of two conditions exists:

1. A resting $Pao_2$ less than 55 mm Hg
2. Evidence of right ventricular failure, polycythemia, or impaired neuropsychiatric function with a $Pao_2$ less than 60 mm Hg

Oxygen therapy may also be used during exercise in those patients who show serious hypoxemia during episodes of increased activity and during the night in those patients who have nocturnal hypoxemia.

The most practical means of administering long-term oxygen is the nasal cannula, which provides 24% to 28% oxygen. The goal is to raise the $Pao_2$ above 60 mm Hg. Caution should be used in those patients known to retain carbon dioxide to not raise the $Pao_2$ so high that they depress their respiratory drive. Patient education about flow rates and avoidance of flames is of the utmost importance.

Currently, three different oxygen delivery systems are available. The conventional liquid oxygen and compressed oxygen are quite bulky, but smaller, portable tanks are available to permit the patient more mobility. The newest method of oxygen delivery is the oxygen concentrator; these devices separate the nitrogen from room air and concentrate the oxygen. These may prove to be the most convenient and ultimately the cheapest method of oxygen delivery. Currently the disadvantages are that they require a continuous electrical supply, thus necessitating a backup system, and they are somewhat noisy.

### *Antibiotics*

Treatment with antibiotics is reasonable therapy in COLD patients who exhibit signs suggestive of bronchial infection, such as increased sputum, increased viscosity of sputum, and/or a change in sputum color. Therapy should be initiated within 24 hours to prevent unnecessary hospitalization. It is also important to prevent an accelerated rate of decline in pulmonary function from irritation and mucous plugging. Perhaps as many as one third of infections are viral. A bacterial infection may follow these initial viral infections. An initial sputum Gram stain may be helpful in determining the need for oral antibiotic therapy; however, given the difficulty of obtaining an appropriate sputum in the outpatient setting, this may not always be practical. Early in the stage of infectious exacerbations patients need not have fever, chills, or a leukocytosis. Sputum cultures, initially, are of little practical value.

The bacterial organisms usually responsible for exacerbations are *Streptococcus pneumoniae* and *Hemophilus influenzae*. Oral ampicillin or amoxicillin are considered the agents of choice in patients not allergic to penicillins. Other acceptable alternatives include tetracyclines, cephalosporins, or co-trimoxazole. Therapy should be continued for at least 7 to 10 days. If the patient deteriorates or does not improve hospitalization may be required and more aggressive attempts should be made to identify potential pathogens responsible for the exacerbation. Parenteral antibiotics may then be required.

### *Immunotherapy*

A empiric recommendation has been that all patients with COLD should receive one dose of pneumococcal vaccine. This recommendation has no objective support and has recently been questioned by Williams and Moser.[40] Regardless, it is currently a standard of practice. At this time, repeated vaccination does not appear to be necessary. COLD patients should also receive a yearly influenza vaccination. If a patient has been exposed to influenza before vaccination, a course of amantadine may be considered.

### *Respiratory Stimulants*

The roles of acetazolamide and progesterone in COLD patients have been investigated for the past 25 years. Acetazolamide, a carbonic anhydrase inhibitor, may exert a beneficial effect by increasing cerebral blood flow, decreasing cerebrospinal fluid bicarbonate, and increasing the responsiveness of central respiratory centers to hypoxemia and hypercarbia.[19] It may be especially useful in COLD patients who are alkalotic as a result of diuretic therapy. Alkalosis depresses the respiratory drive. Acetazolamide does not work when the arterial pH is below 7.35. The exact role of acetazolamide has not been determined nor has the dose or duration of therapy.

Progesterone shares an equally unsure role in patients with COLD and its effectiveness is controversial.[19] Originally, this agent was promoted to be of benefit as a respiratory stimulant in patients with Pickwickian syndrome with sleep apnea; however, it more consistently shows benefit in awake patients than in those asleep.[19]

### *Complications*

#### Cor Pulmonale

Diuretics have been the mainstay of therapy for cor pulmonale. The greatest concern with diuretics is hypokalemic metabolic alkalosis. The hypokalemia may be exacerbated by concomitant use of $\beta$ agonists or corticosteroids. Digitalis glycosides have no role in the treatment of cor pulmonale. The decision to use diuretics must be based on the risk/benefit ratio. If only peripheral edema exists without hepatic congestion, the risk of diuretics may exceed benefit. If hepatic congestion is evident, judicious use of diuretics is certainly indicated.

Recently, research into the treatment of cor pulmonale has been directed at reducing the force against which the right ventricle has to work by dilating the pulmonary vasculature. One method is to remove a primary cause of pulmonary hypertension (i.e., hypoxia) This can be improved by raising the $PaO_2$ above 60 mm Hg. Pharmacologically, hydralazine and nifedipine have been most extensively examined. At this time, data are insufficient to offer guidelines for the role of these agents in COLD patients with cor pulmonale.

#### Polycythemia

Polycythemia secondary to chronic hypoxemia in COLD patients can be improved by either oxygen therapy or periodic phlebotomy if oxygen is not sufficient. Continuous oxygen therapy was shown by the Nocturnal Oxygen Therapy Trial Group to reduce hematocrits.[37] If the hematocrit is above 55% to 60% and the patient is experiencing central nervous system effects suggestive of sludging from the high blood viscosity, then acute phlebotomy is indicated. Long-term oxygen can then be used to help keep the hematocrit lower.

### *Controversies*

#### Expectorants and Mucolytics

Water has been and continues to be the expectorant of choice in COLD patients. Adequate hydration is safe and effective compared with saturated solutions of potassium iodide, ammonium chloride, or guaifenesin. While these agents may promote expectoration, they require such large doses that they are frequently associated with undesirable side effects.

The use of the mucolytic agent acetylcysteine to aid the clearance of mucus has been a matter of controversy for some time. There is no question that it is effective as a mucolytic, but it is irritating via the inhaled route which can cause further narrowing of the airways. It is for this reason that inhaled acetylcysteine fell into disfavor. If it is used via this route, it should always be preceded by an inhaled sympathomimetic. Recently, attention has been focused on the oral and intravenous routes of administration.[19] Although these routes appear to have a beneficial effect as a mucolytic, there have not been sufficient studies to determine their place in therapy.

#### Intermittent Positive Pressure Breathing

IPPB has, for more than 30 years, been a method of delivery of aerosolized medications in patients with COLD. While some patients experience subjective benefit, IPPB is not without risk, especially in patients with predominant emphysema. It can produce bronchospasm and also cause pneumothorax when used improperly. As a means of delivering bronchodilators, it is no more effective than compressor-driven nebulizers.[41] If IPPB is to be used at all, it should be so in patients whose $FEV_1$ values are less than 750 mL and who are too weak to comply with other measures to promote bronchial drainage.[19]

### *Acute Respiratory Failure*

Acute respiratory failure is an emergency situation. When it occurs in a patient with COLD, all pharmacologic maneuvers should be optimized initially and low-flow oxygen delivered. If these agents fail to stabilize or improve the patient's condition, intubation and mechanical ventilation must be considered. This is an extremely difficult decision. Ideally, severe COLD patients should be involved in the decision to intubate. Preferably, this decision should be made before an acute event occurs. If a decision is made to mechanically ventilate because of impending respiratory failure, it is important that ventilator settings not be adjusted to return the patient to normal values; rather, settings should be adjusted to achieve the patient's baseline values in a stable state. This will facilitate weaning from the ventilator. Maintaining the physical strength and nutritional status of the patient is vital in aiding the weaning procedure. Physical therapy and a nutritional intake of 3,000 kilocalories per day are advised. If mechanical ventilation persists beyond 5 to 7 days, the patient should be switched to a tracheostomy to prevent erosion and to facilitate feeding.

Extubation can be considered if the patient's arterial blood gases have reached baseline and are maintained on an $FiO_2$ of 40% or less and a tidal volume of 400 mL or less. Once this is achieved, the following parameters can be measured to allow a reasonable prediction of successful extubation: a minute ventilation of less than 10 L/min and the ability to double this on command; a low spontaneous respiratory rate of 20/min or less; and the ability to achieve an inspiratory force of greater than −20 cm of water. At this point, with the patient alert and willing to comply, a T-tube should be used for 30 minutes with 40% oxygen while the patient is observed for excessive fatigue. Blood gases, respiratory rate, pulse, and general appearance are evaluated. If this is successful, extubation can be attempted and the patient closely observed on oxygen via nasal cannula or mask. Again, blood gases, respiratory rate, pulse, and general appearance are monitored. Intermittent mandatory ventilation (IMV) is another method of weaning before extubation. The reader is referred to a more in-depth discussion of this topic by Petty.[17]

### *Other Aspects of Management*

Narcotics and benzodiazepines should be avoided in COLD patients because they depress respiration. Some have found diphenhydramine useful as an anxiolytic or sedative but there has not been an objective analysis of the effectiveness or safety of this agent in COLD patients.

The role of chest physiotherapy and breathing retraining cannot be overlooked. These topics are beyond the scope of this chapter. The reader is referred to discussions by Hodgkin et al[5] and Miller and Geumei[19] for in-depth information.

## Summary

Chronic obstructive lung disease is indeed a multifaceted disease process. The obstructive process is a result of the progression of chronic bronchitis and emphysema. Most people with COLD have both processes. The most common cause is cigarette smoking. The key to decreasing the incidence of this disease is education to prevent people from starting to smoke and to stop those who do smoke.

The therapeutic management involves numerous medications, oxygen, and physiotherapy. Unfortunately, the pharmacologic management is still largely empiric with methylxanthines, sympathomimetics, corticosteroids, and anticholinergics forming the foundation of therapy. These agents, especially methylxanthines and corticosteroids, are not without considerable toxicity. Therefore, embarking on a pharmacologic plan requires weighing the risk/benefit ratio carefully and having a comprehensive plan to assess subjectively and objectively the efficacy and toxicity of the chosen therapy.

## References


1. Petty TL. Definitions, clinical assessment, and risk factors, in Petty TL (ed): Chronic Obstructive Pulmonary Disease. New York, Marcel Dekker, 1985, pp 1–30.
2. American Thoracic Society. Definitions and classifications of chronic bronchitis, asthma, and pulmonary emphysema. Am Rev Respir Dis 1962;85:762–769.
3. Tuckman MS, Khoury MS, Cohen BH. The epidemiology of COPD, in Petty TL (ed): Chronic Obstructive Pulmonary Disease. New York, Marcel Dekker, 1985, pp 43–92.
4. Higgens M. Epidemiology of COPD: State of the art. Chest 1984;85:3S–8S.
5. Hodgkin JE, et al. Diagnosis and differentiation, in Hodgkin JE (ed): Chronic Obstructive Pulmonary Disease: Current Concepts in Diagnosis and Comprehensive Care. Park Ridge, IL, American College of Chest Physicians, 1979, p 5–34.
6. Thurlbeck WM. Chronic airflow obstruction: Correlation of structure and function, in Petty TL (ed): Chronic Obstructive Pulmonary Disease. New York, Marcel Dekker, 1985, pp 129–202.
7. Mitchell RS, Petty TL. Chronic obstructive pulmonary disease (COPD), in Mitchell RS, Petty TL (eds): Synopsis of Clinical Pulmonary Disease. St Louis, C.V. Mosby, 1982, pp 97–113.
8. Kimbel P. Proteolytic damage and emphysema pathogenesis, in Petty TL (ed): Chronic Obstructive Pulmonary Disease. New York, Marcel Dekker, pp 105–127.
9. Robins AG. Pathophysiology of emphysema. Clin Chest Med 1983;4:413–420.
10. Macklem PT. The pathophysiology of chronic bronchitis and emphysema. Med Clin North Am 1973;57:669–679.
11. Menendez R, Kelly HW. Pulmonary-function testing in the evaluation of bronchodilator agents. Clin Pharm 1983;2:120–128.
12. Cherniack RM. Pulmonary function testing, in Mitchell RS, Petty TL (eds): Synopsis of Clinical Pulmonary Disease. St. Louis: C.V. Mosby, 1982, pp 20–33.
13. Anthonison NR, Wright SC, Hodgkin JE. Prognosis in chronic obstructive pulmonary disease. Am Rev Respir Dis 1986;133: 14–20.
14. Petty TL, Good JT, White DP. Long-term follow-up of a random population observed for the prevalence and outcome of COPD, in Petty TL (ed): Chronic Obstructive Pulmonary Disease. New York, Marcel Dekker, 1985, pp 93–103.
15. Burrows B. Cause and prognosis in advanced disease, in Petty TL (ed): Chronic Obstructive Pulmonary Disease. New York, Marcel Dekker, 1985, pp 31–42.
16. Ingram RH. Chronic bronchitis, emphysema, and airways obstruction, in Petersdorf RG, Adams RD, Braunwald E, et al (eds): Harrison's Textbook of Internal Medicine. New York, McGraw-Hill, 1983, pp 1545–1553.
17. Petty TL. Acute respiratory failure in COPD, in Petty TL (ed): Chronic Obstructive Pulmonary Disease. New York, Marcel Dekker, 1985, pp 389–410.
18. Anthonisen NR, Wright EC, Hodgkin JE, et al. Bronchodilator response in chronic obstructive pulmonary disease. Am Rev Respir Dis 1986;133:814–819.
19. Miller WF, Geumei AM. Respiratory and pharmacological therapy in COPD, in Petty TL (ed): Chronic Obstructive Pulmonary Disease. New York, Marcel Dekker, 1985, pp 205–338.
20. Bukowskyj M, Nakatsu K, Munt PW. Theophylline reassessed. Ann Intern Med 1984;101:63–73.
21. Shim CS, Williams MH. Bronchodilator response to oral aminophylline and terbutaline versus aerosol albuterol in patients with chronic obstructive pulmonary disease. Am J Med 1983;75:697–701.
22. Larsson S, Svedmyr N. Bronchodilating effect and side effects of $\beta_2$-adrenoceptor stimulants by different modes of administration. Am Rev Respir Dis 1977;116:861–869.
23. Shim C, Williams MH. Bronchial response to oral versus aerosol metaproterenol in asthma. Ann Intern Med 1980;93:428–431.
24. Kelly HW. New $\beta_2$-adrenergic agonist aerosols. Clin Pharm 1985;4:393–404.
25. Albert RK, Martin TR, Lewis SW. Controlled clinical trial of methylprednisolone in patients with chronic bronchitis and acute respiratory insufficiency. Ann Intern Med 1980;92:753–758.
26. Mandella LA, Manufreda J, Warren CPW, et al. Steroid response in stable chronic obstructive pulmonary disease. Ann Intern Med 1982;96:17–21.
27. Blair GP, Light RW. Treatment of chronic obstructive pulmonary disease with corticosteroids. Chest 1984;86:525–528.
28. Shim CS, Williams MH. Aerosol beclomethasone in patients with steroid-responsive chronic obstructive pulmonary disease. Am J Med 1985;78:655–658.
29. Pavia D, Bateman JRM, Sheahan NF, et al. Clearance of lung secretions in patients with chronic bronchitis: Effect of terbutaline and ipratropium bromide aerosols. Eur J Respir Dis 1980;61:245–253.
30. Matthys H, Hundenborn J, Daikeler G, et al. Influence of 0.2 mg ipratropium bromide on mucociliary clearance in patients with chronic bronchitis. Respiration 1985;48:329–339.
31. Gross NJ, Skorodin MS. Role of the parasympathetic system in airway obstruction due to emphysema. N Engl J Med 1984;311: 421–425.
32. Passamonte PM, Martinez AJ. Effect of inhaled atropine or metaproterenol in patients with chronic airway obstruction and therapeutic serum theophylline levels. Chest 1984;85:610–615.
33. Marini JJ, Lakshminarayan S, Kradjan WA. Atropine and terbutaline aerosols in chronic bronchitis. Chest 1981;80:285–291.
34. Ashutosh K, Lang H. Comparison between long-term treatment of chronic bronchitic airway obstruction with ipratropium bromide and metaproterenol. Ann Allergy 1984;53:401–416.
35. Kradjan WA, Smallridge RC, Davis R, et al. Atropine serum concentrations after multiple inhaled doses of atropine sulfate. Clin Pharmacol Ther 1985;38:12–15.
36. Massey KL, Gotz VP. Ipratropium bromide. Drug Intell Clin Pharm 1985;19:5–12.
37. Nocturnal Oxygen Therapy Trial Group. Continuous or nocturnal oxygen therapy in hypoxemic chronic obstructive lung disease. Ann Intern Med 1980;93:391–398.
38. Petty TL. Long-term outpatient oxygen therapy, in Petty TL

(ed): Chronic Obstructive Pulmonary Disease. New York, Marcel Dekker, 1985, pp 375–388.

**39.** Medical Research Council Working Party. Long-term domiciliary oxygen therapy in chronic hypoxic cor pulmonale complicating chronic bronchitis and emphysema. Lancet 1981;1:681–685.

**40.** Williams JH, Moser KN. Pneumococcal vaccine and patients with chronic lung disease. Ann Intern Med 1986;104:106–109.

**41.** The Intermittent Positive Pressure Breathing Trial Group. Intermittent positive pressure breathing therapy of chronic obstructive pulmonary disease. Ann Intern Med 1983;99: 612–620.

# Chapter 23 / Respiratory Distress Syndrome in the Newborn

Peter Gal, PharmD

Respiratory distress syndrome (RDS) in the neonate is a major source of neonatal morbidity and mortality. Acute forms of RDS include hyaline membrane disease (HMD) and transient tachypnea of the newborn (TTN). Chronic forms of RDS include chronic pulmonary insufficiency of prematurity (CPIP), bronchopulmonary dysplasia (BPD), and Wilson–Mikity syndrome. Each of these is discussed separately.

## Hyaline Membrane Disease

### *Pathophysiology*

Hyaline membrane disease (HMD), perhaps more appropriately called surfactant deficiency respiratory distress syndrome, is common in neonates below 36 weeks' gestation; the incidence increases as the gestational age decreases (Fig. 23.1).[1] Pulmonary surfactant, containing phospholipids, functions to stabilize the air-filled alveolus against the collapsing forces of surface tension at the air–liquid interface.[1] Thus, surfactant deficiency results in atelectasis and impaired gas exchange. Alveolar transudation of protein-rich fluids forms a hyaline membrane, giving rise to the name *hyaline membrane disease*.[1] Surfactant is secreted primarily by type II alveolar cells, which are sufficiently abundant and differentiated by 35 weeks' gestation to make HMD unlikely. Before 35 weeks' gestation, the risk of HMD, as well as the severity of the disease, increases as a consequence of (1) the immaturity of the alveolar lining cells, (2) impaired surfactant production, (3) impaired release of surface-active phospholipids, and (4) death of many cells responsible for surfactant production.[2]

Several problems associated with acute fetal or intrapartum stress worsen the severity of HMD, possibly as a consequence of further compromising the limited pulmonary blood supply and causing the death of an already limited number of type II alveolar cells. Chronic intrauterine stress, on the contrary, lowers the risk of HMD by promoting lung maturation, perhaps by increasing endogenous glucocorticoid concentrations. The factors influencing the incidence and severity of HMD are summarized in Table 23.1.

### *Clinical Presentation*

Clinically, a premature infant with HMD may appear normal at birth, although often evidence of intrapartum depression or asphyxia is present. During the first few hours after birth, these newborns develop early signs of respiratory failure (i.e., forceful intercostal retractions, use of accessory neck muscles, expiratory grunting, paradoxical seesaw respirations, gradually increasing oxygen requirements, and tachycardia). Pallor or cyanosis may develop. Fluid retention, edema, and oliguria are common in the first 48 hours.

A characteristic chest x-ray film (Fig. 23.2) shows a reticulogranular (ground glass) pattern to the peripheral lung fields, along with clearly defined large airways (air bronchograms) resulting from the presence of air in the large airways and the collapse of air spaces around the large airways.[4]

A number of neonatal disorders may mimic and be indistinguishable from HMD (Table 23.2). By far, the most important is sepsis caused by group B $\beta$-hemolytic streptococcus, pneumococcus, or gram-negative bacilli. Sepsis accounted for 8% of consecutively admitted infants with RDS during a recent 1-year study.[3] All neonates with suspected HMD should be evaluated for sepsis. Antibiotics should be used until sepsis can be ruled out or a full therapeutic course is completed.

Once HMD has occurred and ventilatory assistance is required, the morbidity is substantial, and death occurs in up to 25% of neonates between 28 and 35 weeks' gestation. Mortality increases to about 50% of neonates between 26 and 28 weeks' gestation.[1] Those with a gestation of 30–35 weeks typically have improved pulmonary function and spontaneous diuresis 3 to 4 days after birth. The more immature newborns often have a more complicated course because of secondary lung damage and complications of immaturity, such as intrapulmonary and periventricular hemorrhage and patent ductus arteriosus (PDA). Complications from ventilator therapy may result in a prolonged, complex clinical course.[1–5]

### *Treatment*

Prevention, or minimization of the severity, of HMD is the most important goal of therapy. Several interventions can provide substantial benefit to the newborn. These can be divided into the four categories listed in Table 23.3.

Management of the premature infant during labor and delivery to prevent hypoxia and hypothermia is critical to limiting the severity of RDS. This involves preventing or minimizing maternal hypotension and hemorrhage, supplying adequate warmth to the newborn at delivery to maintain normal body temperature, and providing supplemental oxygen as needed to maintain adequate oxygenation.[1]

In some cases, particularly with premature infants, delaying delivery to allow time for lung maturation should be considered. Helpful in this decision is measurement of the

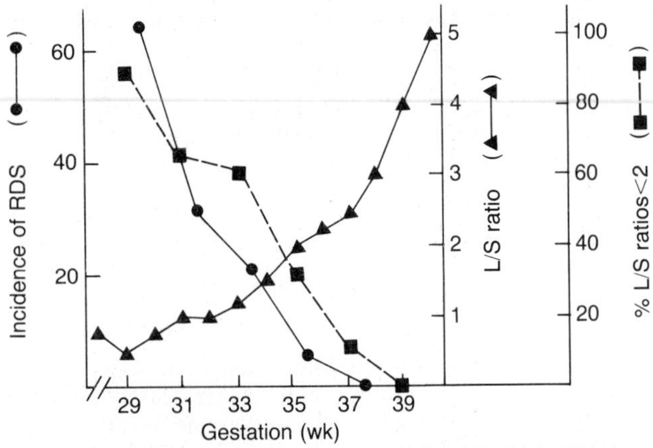


**Figure 23.1** Comparison of the frequency of RDS with lecithin/sphingomyelin (L/S) ratio in amniotic fluid and with gestational age. *(From Farrell PM, Avery ME: Hyaline membrane disease. Am Rev Resp Dis 1975;111:657, with permission.)*

lecithin/sphingomyelin (L/S) ratio in amniotic fluid (Fig. 23.1). An L/S ratio above 2 is generally considered compatible with relatively mature lung function.[1] L/S values below 2 are associated with a risk of RDS of approximately 50%, compared with a risk below 1% when L/S ratios are greater than 2. Other phospholipids (e.g., disaturated lecithin and phosphatidylglycerol) determined in amniotic fluid also show promise as being predictive of lung maturation.[5]

In cases where the L/S ratio is below 2, tocolytic agents (agents inhibiting labor) can reduce the risk of RDS. While several tocolytics are available and have been used clinically (Table 23.4), the $\beta_2$ sympathomimetics are the best studied and should currently be considered the agents of choice. Promising results have also been noted with the calcium channel blockers.[6,7] As different $\beta_2$ agonists are equally effective provided comparable doses are used, drug selection should be based on the convenience of the dosing schedule and cost. Most patients are started in the hospital on an intravenous regimen, then converted to oral therapy once labor is stopped. The lower gestational age limit for labor inhibition is considered to be about 20 weeks.[6] Therapy is continued until the etiology for preterm labor (e.g., urinary tract infection) is resolved or until the fetus is sufficiently mature to be safely delivered (e.g., L/S ratio becomes greater than 2).

Tocolytics are generally started when frequent contractions are noted, although preterm labor may be overdiagnosed in up to 70% of cases using this approach. Ideally, the diagnosis of premature labor should be made only when regular contractions are accompanied by progressive cervical dilation and/or effacement; however, waiting for cervical changes will reduce the likelihood of successful inhibition of labor and thus compromise the fetus.[7,8]

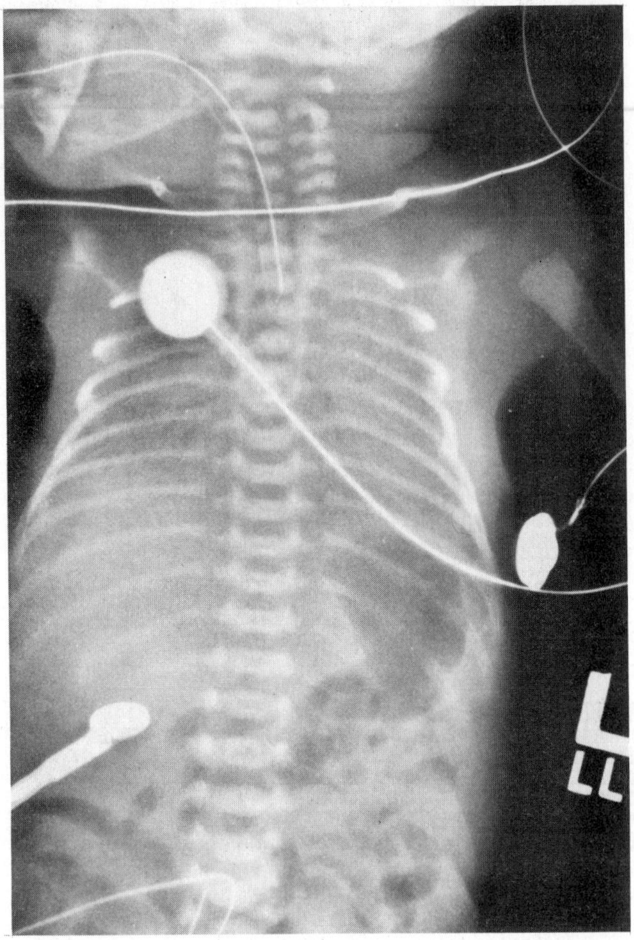

**Figure 23.2** Chest x-ray demonstrating hyaline membrane disease with ground glass appearance and air bronchograms.

**Corticosteroids**

Since 1972, corticosteroids (e.g., betamethasone 12 mg daily for two doses or dexamethasone 5 mg every 12 hours for four doses) have been given at least 24 hours prenatally to a pregnant mother under 32 weeks' gestation to accelerate lung maturation and prevent RDS in the infant.[9,10] Two mechanisms by which lung maturation is enhanced by corticosteroids are increased production of surfactant[10] and acceleration of the normal rise in antioxidant enzymes, for

**Table 23.1** Factors Affecting Severity and Incidence of Respiratory Distress Syndrome

| |
|---|
| Perinatal asphyxia or hypoxia |
| Cold stress |
| Prematurity |
| Failure of closure of the patent ductus arteriosus |
| Diabetes mellitus in mother |
| Acidosis |

**Table 23.2** Differential Diagnosis of Hyaline Membrane Disease

| |
|---|
| Pneumonia—especially group B streptococcus |
| Spontaneous pneumothorax |
| Transient tachypnea of the newborn |
| Congenital cyanotic heart disease |
| Hypoplastic lungs |
| Diaphragmatic hernia |

**Table 23.3** Methods of Preventing, or Minimizing the Severity of, Hyaline Membrane Disease

| |
|---|
| Initiate maternal and neonatal care during labor and delivery to minimize hypoxia and optimize the time for delivery |
| Delay premature delivery (e.g., with tocolytics) to allow more lung maturation |
| Promote (e.g., with prenatal steroids) lung development and surfactant formation |
| Provide exogenous surfactant |

example, superoxide dismutase, catalase, and glutathione peroxidase, which protect lungs against damage from $O_2$ free radicals.[11] Several studies have observed a reduction in RDS with the use of antenatal corticosteroids[12–14]; however, more recent studies have noted that the benefits may be limited to a small population (i.e., white, female infants of 30–32 weeks' gestation).[12] Overt toxicity from antenatal steroids appears to be minimal, prompting some authors to speculate that use of corticosteroids to prevent RDS is warranted for all mothers with pregnancies less than 34 weeks.[14–16] Others[15] feel that the relative benefits are inadequate to justify routine antenatal corticosteroid use. While the appropriate role of antenatally administered corticosteroids remains controversial, the benefit to some subgroups of patients remains clear. The problem is that gestational age by dates and ultrasound are sometimes erroneous, making prenatal identification of this subgroup uncertain. As the relative short- and long-term risks of treatment appear minimal and the consequences of RDS are great, prenatal use of corticosteroids appears warranted.

### Surfactant

Administration of lung surfactant at delivery to neonates with surfactant deficiency RDS is currently under investigation and has met with very favorable initial results.[17–22] Different sources, for example, sheep, bovine, rabbit, and human surfactants, have all been used successfully in human or animal models. While routine use of surfactant cannot yet be advised on the basis of these preliminary studies, it is likely that more frequent use of tracheal instillation of surfactant is inevitable. Compared with control groups, surfactant-treated patients had significantly improved oxygenation, lower oxygenation requirements, fewer episodes of pneumothorax and interstitial emphysema, and lower mortality.[17–20] One controversial complication of surfactant replacement that requires more study is the opening of the ductus arteriosus, which is believed to be associated with prompt improvement of ventilation with a concurrent drop in pulmonary resistance.[17,18,21] On the basis of their favorable but limited experience with this approach, some authors advocate early ductal closure using indomethacin in conjunction with surfactant.[21] If PDA proves to be a common problem, this approach is physiologically sound and will likely enhance future clinical results with tracheal instillation of surfactant.

**Table 23.4** Drugs Used for Inhibiting Preterm Labor

| |
|---|
| β-Adrenergic agonists (ritodrine, terbutaline) |
| Magnesium sulfate |
| Isoxsuprine hydrochloride |
| Calcium channel blockers |
| Ethanol |

### Mechanical Ventilation

Once HMD has occurred, treatment has been directed primarily toward improving ventilation through oxygen supplementation, use of continuous distending pressure, oxygenation through mechanical ventilation, control of acidosis, and prevention of fluid overload and pulmonary edema.

A comprehensive review of ventilator management is beyond the scope of this chapter; however, several excellent sources are available.[23]

In general, oxygen supplementation should maintain the arterial partial pressure of oxygen ($Pao_2$) above 50 mm Hg.[24] Continuous $Pao_2$ monitoring with transcutaneous monitors can facilitate this in a noninvasive manner. Mechanical ventilation is added by some authors when the percentage inspired oxygen ($Fio_2$) and $Paco_2$ exceed 50 mm Hg and the $Pao_2$ is below 50 mm Hg. Terms used in ventilator adjustment are listed in Table 23.5. Adjustment of ventilator settings on the basis of arterial blood gases is summarized in Table 23.6. Further issues of ventilator management are discussed later.

Acidosis is associated with a number of physiologic effects that increase the severity of RDS, including increased pulmonary vascular resistance, impaired synthesis of surfactant, reduced cardiac output, and depressed ventilation. Consequently, measures that reduce the risk of acidosis, for example, prevention of hypoxemia, hypotension, excessive blood loss through venipuncture or bleeding, and minimization of oxygen consumption through careful temperature control, are critical. Correction of metabolic acidosis with sodium bicarbonate or 0.3 M tromethamine (THAM)[24] is recommended when blood pH falls below 7.25.

Pulmonary edema is a prominent feature of RDS. Clinically, the severity of RDS is correlated to the presence of factors that cause pulmonary edema. This is not unexpected, as excess fluid in the alveolar and interstitial spaces impairs pulmonary gas exchange, lowers lung compliance, and reduces functional residual capacity. Prevention of fluid overload and pulmonary edema is critical in minimizing the risk of opening the ductus arteriosus and creating a need for high ventilator pressures and oxygen requirements because of stiff lungs.[25]

Positive end expiratory pressure (PEEP) is beneficial in pulmonary edema because it redistributes fluid in airspaces and improves respiratory gas exchange. It does not, however, reduce lung water content.[26] Oliguria is well recognized during the early stages of RDS. An abrupt diuresis occurs during the recovery phase of RDS. Heaf et al[27] recently showed that pulmonary function improved immediately after the onset of diuresis. This diuretic phase was thought to represent the removal of alveolar or interstitial lung water. The association of diuresis with improvement in RDS prompted several investigators to study furosemide for mobilizing lung edema and improving RDS. In general, studies have not justified the routine use of furosemide for

**Table 23.5** Glossary of Terms for Ventilator Management

| | | | |
|---|---|---|---|
| Et | Expiratory time: in the ventilatory cycle, the amount of time devoted to exhalation | PEEP | Positive end expiratory pressure: positive pressure at the end of exhalation; designed to prevent alveoli from collapsing during expiration |
| It | Inspiratory time: in the ventilatory cycle, the amount of time devoted to inspiration | PIP | Peak inspiratory pressure: the maximum level of pressure achieved by the ventilator during inspiration |
| I:E | Ratio of inspiratory time to expiratory time: in a normal, spontaneously breathing patient, 1:1.5 | IMV | Intermittent mandatory ventilation: mode of ventilation designed to deliver a preset inspiratory rate; continuous flow of gas is available for patient's spontaneous breaths |
| $Paco_2$ | Partial pressure of carbon dioxide present in arterial blood: normal is 34–45 mm Hg | $Fio_2$ | Fraction (percentage) of inspired oxygen |
| $Pao_2$ | Partial pressure of oxygen present in arterial blood: normal level for adults is 80–100 mm Hg; normal level for infants is 60–100 mm Hg | | |

Prepared by Rene Mize, BS, RRT, Assistant Director, Department of Respiratory Therapy, Moses H. Cone Memorial Hospital, Greensboro, NC.

treatment of infants with RDS.[28,29] However, all of the studies had serious limitations, including inadequate definition of RDS (leading to a nonuniform patient population); frequent timing of doses coincident with the time for expected spontaneous diuresis and improved lung functions; and selection by most researchers of too low furosemide doses (1 mg/kg), as 2 mg/kg appears necessary for most RDS cases.[29] The potential but uncertain benefits of furosemide must be weighed against the risks, which include the following: promotion of prostaglandin synthesis may cause an increased incidence of patent ductus arteriosus, which could worsen the RDS; if neonates have inadequate right atrial venous return, diuresis may be detrimental, and electrolyte imbalance may result from furosemide-induced diuresis.[28,30,31] More studies are required to determine the potential value of diuretics.

## Transient Tachypnea of the Newborn

Transient tachypnea of the newborn (TTN), also known as "wet-lung disease," is a syndrome associated with tachyp-

**Table 23.6** Ventilator Response to Arterial Blood Gases[a]

| *pH* | *$Pao_2$* | *$Paco_2$* | *Response* | *Possible complications* |
|---|---|---|---|---|
| Normal, high, or low | Low (<50 mm Hg) | Normal | ↑ $Fio_2$ | Oxygen toxicity |
| | | Normal to high | ↑ PIP | Barotrauma, overdistension, ↓ cardiac output |
| | | Normal | ↑ PEEP | Barotrauma, ↑ $Paco_2$, ↓ cardiac output |
| | | Normal | ↑ It | Barotrauma, ↑ $Paco_2$, ↓ cardiac output |
| | High (>80 mm Hg) | Normal to high | ↓ $Fio_2$ | Hypoxemia |
| | | Normal to low | ↓ PIP | ↑ $Paco_2$, atelectasis |
| | | Normal to high | ↓ PEEP | Hypoxemia, atelectasis |
| | | Normal to high | ↓ It | Hypoxemia |
| Low (<7.25) | Low to normal | High (>45 mm Hg) | ↑ PIP | Barotrauma, overdistension, ↓ $Paco_2$ |
| | Low, normal, high | | ↓ PEEP | Hypoxemia, atelectasis |
| | Normal to high | | ↓ It | Hypoxemia |
| | Low, normal, high | | ↑ IMV | ↑ $Paco_2$ (secondary ↓ Et) |
| | Normal | Low | ↓ PIP | Hypoxemia, atelectasis |
| | Normal | | ↓ IMV | ↑ $Paco_2$ |

[a] Assume that there are no other causes for abnormality (i.e., misplaced or obstructed endotracheal tube).

Prepared by Rene Mize, BS, RRT, Assistant Director, Department of Respiratory Therapy, Moses H. Cone Memorial Hospital, Greensboro, NC.

nea (up to 120 respirations per minute), retractions of the intercostal muscles, grunting, and occasionally mild cyanosis, appearing in the first few hours of life. This disease follows a benign course, usually requiring short-term oxygen but rarely needing ventilatory assistance. Typically, TTN affects term newborns. The neonates do not have a common history providing clues to patients at risk.[2]

## Chronic Pulmonary Insufficiency of Prematurity

This relatively new syndrome of respiratory distress in neonates with birth weights under 1,250 g has become increasingly prominent in intensive care nurseries. The neonates have no respiratory distress in the first few days of life.[32] Beginning on days 4 to 7, neonates develop increasing oxygen requirements, apneic spells, slowly rising $Pa_{CO_2}$, and radiographic changes consistent with hyaline membrane disease and pulmonary edema. Continuous distending airway pressure or mechanical ventilation, with their attendant hazards, may become necessary. Usually, gradual improvement is noted by 3 to 4 weeks and most infants are well by 2 months, barring complications from ventilatory support. The potential value of diuretics in this syndrome is unknown; however, as pulmonary edema plays a role, studies are warranted. Clinically, we have observed substantial benefit coinciding with initiation of daily or alternate-day furosemide in patients with continuing respiratory distress and tachypnea. Other possible pathophysiologic mechanisms include a gradual depletion of surfactant stores, resulting in a surfactant deficiency state (thus raising the possible role of instillation of surfactant into the lungs), and a reduced lung volume and atelectasis resulting from recurrent respiratory muscle and diaphragmatic fatigue. Theophylline may be beneficial because of its bronchodilator effect as well as its ability to increase contractility and decrease fatigability of the diaphragm and intercostal muscles.[33] The potential benefits of other bronchodilators, for example, $\beta$ agonists, are also worthy of study, as increased pulmonary resistance is present in many preterm infants.[34] These interventions are speculative.

## Bronchopulmonary Dysplasia

### *Pathophysiology*

Bronchopulmonary dysplasia (BPD) is associated with a variety of factors, including positive pressure and oxygen toxicity in neonates receiving mechanical ventilation,[35,36] prematurity, vitamin E deficiency, pulmonary air leak syndromes, and genetic factors. More recently, BPD has been recognized in neonates with acute lung injury not requiring mechanical ventilation or high concentrations of inspired oxygen (some authors refer to this as the Wilson–Mikity syndrome). BPD has also been reported in neonates without acute lung injury, but managed with mechanical ventilation (e.g., treatment of recurrent apnea).[36] BPD develops commonly in neonates below 30 weeks' gestation with HMD whose pulmonary function, rather than improving in the first week of life, worsens to the point that prolonged ventilator support at high oxygen concentrations and pressures, often complicated by recurrent pulmonary air leaks, is required.[35]

### *Clinical Presentation*

Clinically, infants with BPD have hyperinflated chests, require prolonged supplemental oxygen, fail to grow, and have hyperreactive airways. The clinical course is often complicated by cor pulmonale, persistent patent ductus arteriosus, recurrent infections, and hyperreactive airway disease. Radiologically, the disease was originally reported to progress in four stages: stage 1 is indistinguishable from HMD; stage 2 involves complete opacification of lung fields; stage 3 involves cystic changes in the lungs and hyperinflation; and stage 4 involves further cystic changes, pulmonary fibrosis, hyperinflation, and cardiomegaly. This orderly progression of radiologic changes is now considered uncommon and hyperinflation is the predominant abnormality.[37]

Attempts to prevent BPD have focused on (1) prevention and effective treatment of HMD, (2) management of pulmonary edema through use of furosemide, (3) minimization of pressure support in assisted mechanical ventilation, and (4) use of antioxidant therapy (vitamin E). Vitamin E's utility in the prevention of oxygen-related toxicity is discussed later.

### *Treatment*

Treatment of BPD requires supplemental oxygen sufficient to keep the $Pa_{O_2}$ above 60 mm Hg.[36] Several months of oxygen supplementation is often necessary. A more controversial area of therapy is the use of diuretics, bronchodilators, and corticosteroids.

#### Diuretics

Diuretics appear to be beneficial in periods of worsening respiratory distress often associated with an acute increase in pulmonary edema or cor pulmonale. Diuretics can improve clinical signs of respiratory distress, increase lung compliance, and decrease total airway resistance.[38,39] The pulmonary benefits appear to last only 1 to 2 hours, and may be related to pharmacologic actions other than diuresis.[30,40] Long-term use of furosemide does not seem warranted[37]; however, intermittent use in the face of worsening respiratory distress is beneficial. Alternate-day furosemide (1–2 mg/kg) has been clinically helpful in some of our infants, without the apparent electrolyte problems or reduced effectiveness that results from tolerance to daily furosemide therapy.[41] Studies comparing daily to alternate-day furosemide in neonates are unavailable. Combined therapy using spironolactone and hydrochlorothiazide has shown promise in early studies. During maintenance therapy with this combination, Kao et al demonstrated reduced airway resistance and increased airway conductance and dynamic pulmonary compliance.[38] These findings require further confirmation.

#### Bronchodilators

Studies using plethysmography or pneumotachography have shown increased airway resistance in neonates with BPD. Bronchodilator therapy provides potential benefit in these neonates.[42–45] Although bronchodilators are purported to be ineffective in infants because of inadequate bronchiolar smooth muscle, BPD patients develop swelling and hypertrophy of bronchiolar smooth muscle and thus develop sufficient muscularity to respond to bronchodilators.[44–46] An additional benefit of theophylline may be its effects on intercostal muscles and the diaphragm to increase contractility and to decrease fatigability,[33,45] respiratory center stimulation, and diuresis.[45] Because the work of breathing is increased in BPD patients and infants already have greater vulnerability to respiratory muscle fatigue,[37] theophylline may offer important advantages. Its long-term use, however, must be weighed against the risk of toxicity, discussed under Apnea. Aerosolized $\beta$ agonists may also provide substantial benefits.[42,43] We have had dramatic clinical responses with aerosolized terbutaline 0.5 to 2 mg every 4 to 6 hours in some cases poorly responsive to theophylline. The appropriate dose of aerosolized $\beta$ agonist in extubated neonates may be markedly lower than the doses required during intubation, as over half the dose may be lost in the tubing, with the greatest losses occurring with the smallest endotracheal tube.[47]

#### Corticosteroids

Corticosteroid therapy has been used in a limited number of studies with favorable short-term results.[48,49] Short-term use of steroids results in rapid improvement of lung compliance and weaning from ventilator support within 72 hours in patients previously making little ventilatory progress after weeks of intubation. Despite these initial benefits, long-term use of corticosteroids has not shortened the length of hospital stay or mortality from BPD.[48,49] Additionally, the benefits (even short-term) must be weighed against acute and chronic toxic effects. Some studies have noted an increased incidence of infection,[49] and postnatal steroid therapy has been associated with diminished T cells and more frequent infections at 5 years of age.[50] More research is required before this mode of therapy can be widely accepted; however, the preliminary results are encouraging.

## Ventilator Management

The frequent need for ventilatory support in RDS is associated with a variety of complications, many of which have serious sequelae or are life-threatening. These complications are listed in Table 23.7. Only those areas where pharmacologic intervention is involved are discussed further in this chapter. More extensive discussions of all aspects are presented elsewhere.[36,51]

**Table 23.7** Effects of Intubation and Ventilation

| |
|---|
| Bronchopulmonary dysplasia (BPD) |
| Air leak syndromes (e.g., pneumothorax, interstitial emphysema, pneumomediastinum) |
| Retrolental fibroplasia (RLF) |
| Central nervous system hemorrhage |
| Subglottic stenosis |
| Defective dentition (particularly maxillary incisors) |

## Management of Ventilated Infant

### *Use of Sedatives and Muscle Relaxants*

Prevention of ventilator toxicity secondary to barotrauma involves using the lowest possible airway pressures and can often be minimized by use of sedatives or muscle relaxants. For example, pneumothorax, a common complication of ventilator support, is strongly associated with breathing against the ventilator.[52] Capturing the infant's own respiratory rate is helpful (this usually requires more than 50 breaths per minute); however, sedation or paralysis is usually needed to allow optimal ventilator manipulation without neonatal resistance. The selection of a sedative or muscle relaxant is controversial as each treatment has important clinical benefits and toxic effects. Approaches differ in each center based on clinicians' experiences with the various options and their interpretation of the literature. The approach discussed next represents this author's and may differ from that used in many centers. In general, only intravenous drugs are recommended until proper gastrointestinal function is established. The advantages and disadvantages of each option are also discussed; dosing recommendations are given in Table 23.8.

#### Pancuronium

In several studies pancuronium (Pavulon)-induced paralysis has been used to reduce ventilator fighting and the consequent complications. These studies have demonstrated a reduction in the duration of oxygen support needed for infants with HMD[53]; reduced periods of hypoxia and hyperoxia[54]; lower incidence of pneumothorax[55,56] (not confirmed in other studies[53]); and reduced intracranial pressure and cerebral blood flow associated with a decreased incidence of intraventricular hemorrhage.[54,57] While these findings are encouraging, they are not consistent across studies.[55,58] Additionally, the toxic effects and hazards of treatment with pancuronium are substantial. These include acute hypoventilation (19 of 35 neonates with HMD),[55,59] increased ventilator pressure support needs,[57] and possibly increased massive intracranial hemorrhage,[59] perhaps caused by acute increases in blood pressure and heart rate.[60] Excessive edema and fluid and electrolyte problems occur in all paralyzed neonates.

Another consideration is the risk of masking seizure activity,[61,62] thus allowing it to go untreated. Neonates receiving pancuronium should be given concurrent prophylactic phenobarbital as electroencephalographic seizure activity has been noted in 13 of 16 paralyzed neonates[61] without clinically noticeable symptoms. Twitching, which may be misinterpreted as a seizure, often occurs when the pancuronium is stopped. Some authors feel that the risks of pancuronium outweigh any possible benefits, whereas others are strong proponents. One issue not discussed in literature on neonates, but commonly known for adults, is the need for adjunctive sedatives in paralyzed patients. It is likely that the feeling of paralysis is stressful and terrifying in the neonate. The only patients in whom the risk/benefit ratio currently favors pancuronium are the 15% of premature infants with HMD in whom an elevated intracranial pressure is documented. Other less hazardous agents, for example, phenobarbital and morphine, may suffice even in this situation.[58,63]

#### Phenobarbital

Phenobarbital, alone or in combination with a benzodiazepine, provides sedation as well as several other possible

**Table 23.8** Guidelines for Sedation and Muscle Relaxation in Neonates Requiring Mechanical Ventilation

| *Drug* | *Dose* | *Comments* |
|---|---|---|
| Phenobarbital | 20 mg/kg IV for 4 doses, then 5–10 mg/kg/d | Keep plasma concentration above 60 μg/mL; avoid hypotension by administering doses slowly (i.e., ≥15 min) |
| Lorazepam | 0.1–0.4 mg/kg IV every 3–6 h prn | Short duration of effect; use as adjunct to phenobarbital |
| Diazepam | 0.1–1.0 mg/kg IV every 6 h prn | Risk excess accumulation in neonates because of long half-life; may cause phlebitis; use as adjunct to phenobarbital |
| Morphine | 0.1–0.2 mg/kg IV every 3–6 h prn | May be preferred for short postoperative therapy, because it also produces analgesia; monitor blood pressure for hypotension and decrease dose if it occurs |
| Pancuronium | 0.01–0.03 mg/kg IV prn | Dosing requirements gradually increase with continuous therapy; monitor closely for sudden drop on $Pa_{O_2}$ within minutes of a dose—either increase PIP or discontinue drug if this occurs; must administer phenobarbital to a concentration of 40 μg/mL to minimize risk of undetected seizures and provide sedation |
| Chloral hydrate | 25–50 mg/kg PO every 4–6 h prn | Only oral form available; may cause GI irritability, vasodilation, hypotension, respiratory depression, and direct hyperbilirubinemia |

beneficial, but controversial, effects. These include reduced intracranial pressure,[64] possibly a lower incidence of intraventricular hemorrhage,[65] and a reduction in the central nervous system sequelae from asphyxia common in this population.[66,67] Sedation is rarely achieved unless plasma concentrations exceed 60 μg/mL.[67,68]

Of concern in the use of this regimen are the potential hazards to brain growth[69] and the prolonged half-life, which results in the persistence of high plasma concentrations several days after the drug is stopped. Concerns about the cardiovascular toxicity of phenobarbital appear ill founded and probably reflect the effects of propylene glycol when the product is administered by rapid intravenous push.[67] No cardiovascular toxicity is seen when a 20 mg/kg dose is given over 5 minutes.[70] We currently utilize plasma concentrations of 40 μg/mL and then add a benzodiazepine (usually lorazepam) if more sedation is needed; however, the use of plasma phenobarbital concentrations above 40 μg/mL is not widely advocated.

**Morphine**

Morphine has been used in some circumstances for sedation and respiratory depression in ventilated neonates. While it appears effective, hypotension, decreased gastrointestinal motility, and physiologic dependence with prolonged use are important risks relegating morphine to a second- or third-line drug in our nursery except in neonates who also have the component of pain (e.g., postsurgery). One advantage of morphine is its rapid reversibility with narcotic antagonists.

**Benzodiazepines**

Diazepam has been used by some clinicians to sedate neonates although literature supporting its use in neonates is lacking. While the therapeutic index is wide, accumulation of diazepam and its active metabolite, *N*-desmethyldiazepam, may occur with repeated doses and may result in severe hypotonia.[71] An additional disadvantage of intravenous diazepam is the propensity for producing phlebitis which can be reduced but not eliminated by slow administration.

We have preferred lorazepam as an adjunct to phenobarbital because it has a lower risk for accumulation than diazepam (its half-life is shorter; 28–65 hours for lorazepam[72] versus 40–400 hours for diazepam[73]). Although the available literature on use of lorazepam in neonates is limited,[72] our experience in over 50 patients has shown it to be a safe, effective sedative that clinically lasts 2 to 4 hours. The doses we use clinically range from 0.1 to 0.4 mg/kg every 2 to 6 hours depending on clinical response and desired level of sedation.

**Chloral Hydrate**

Chloral hydrate has been an effective, relatively safe sedative in children and has been used by some clinicians for neonates. It is metabolized in the liver to the active metabolite trichlorethanol, which has an average half-life of 37 hours; however, doses of 25 to 50 mg/kg result in only 1 to 2 hours of sedation. The major disadvantages of chloral hydrate are that it must be given orally and it can cause gastrointestinal irritation. Other reported toxic effects include vasodilation, hypotension, respiratory depression, cardiac arrhythmias,[74] and direct hyperbilirubinemia.[75]

### *Oxygen Toxicity and Vitamin E*

Oxygen toxicity is also a major problem in ventilated premature infants. Oxygen toxicity may begin either directly via oxidation of tissue or indirectly through autoregulatory effects on blood flow.[62] Three important problems associated with oxygen therapy and hyperoxia are (1) BPD, (2) retrolental fibroplasia (RLF) or retinopathy of prematurity (ROP), and (3) pontosubicular necrosis.[76]

Vitamin E, an antioxidant, has been studied for prevention

of BPD and RLF. Controlled studies of the use of vitamin E in prevention of BPD have failed to demonstrate any benefits.[76] This is not surprising in light of the multiple factors associated with BPD. Further, vitamin E plays only a secondary role to the antioxidant system by terminating lipid peroxidation reactions previously initiated by $O_2$ radical attack on polyunsaturated membrane lipids. Its protective effect in animal studies requires the presence of vitamin E deficiency with normal lung antioxidant enzymes. The existence of normal vitamin E concentrations with a deficiency of pulmonary enzyme activity was shown to leave animals hypersusceptible to pulmonary $O_2$ toxicity.[11] Animal studies with primary antioxidant enzymes, for example, superoxide dismutase, are more encouraging.[11] The value of vitamin E in the prevention of ROP is more controversial. Different doses administered by different routes have been used in several studies, in some of which plasma concentration monitoring was employed to determine doses. Some studies report favorable results, whereas others show no benefit.[63,64] Nevertheless, the risk/benefit ratio does not favor routine use of vitamin E at the doses recommended for RLF prevention, especially if serum concentration measurements are unavailable.[77–79] Toxic effects associated with vitamin E include increased intracranial hemorrhage, creatinuria, decreased platelet aggregation, impaired wound healing, potentiation of vitamin K deficiency coagulopathy, hepatomegaly, and impaired fibrinolysis.[65] In addition, increased incidences of bacterial sepsis and necrotizing enterocolitis in premature infants were associated with sustained serum vitamin E concentrations above 4.5 mg/dL.[78,79] Finally, the drug must be given intramuscularly and may cause local tissue damage. An intravenous vitamin E formulation (E-Ferol) resulted in unexplained hypotension, thrombocytopenia, renal dysfunction, hepatomegaly, cholestasis, ascites, metabolic acidosis, and several deaths.[80]

### *Adjuncts to Promotion of Weaning from and Prevention of Mechanical Ventilation*

Neonates who do not readily wean from ventilatory support after apparent resolution of HMD often are found to develop a PDA. Closure of the PDA using indomethacin or surgery is critical in preventing a prolonged course of ventilatory support and its adverse sequelae.[81]

Many neonates are difficult to wean from low levels of ventilatory support because of the unacceptable accumulation of carbon dioxide when extubation is attempted.[82–84] These neonates generally require below 35% inspired oxygen and have peak inspiratory pressures below 24 cm water and intermittent mandatory ventilation rates below 20 breaths per minute.[84] These cases respond extremely well to theophylline, and can usually be extubated within 24 hours of initiating therapy. The low ventilatory requirements relate in part to easy fatigability of the intercostal muscles and diaphragm and the lack of additional intercostal muscles to recruit for assisting with ventilation. Serum theophylline concentrations must exceed 8 μg/mL to promote contractility and reduce fatigue of respiratory muscles. Additional benefits may be gained by increasing theophylline concentrations up to at least 20 μg/mL. Neonates under 1,000 g often require serum theophylline concentrations of 25 to 30 μg/mL to prevent $Paco_2$ from rising above 60 mm Hg (personal observation). The desired serum theophylline concentration must be individually determined on the basis of clinical response (i.e., prevention of $CO_2$ accumulation and apnea) and toxic effects (e.g., tachycardia, agitation, feeding intolerance). In premature infants without lung disease, early use of theophylline can prevent the need for intubation,[85] even in those patients without apnea. A protocol for dosing theophylline to prevent intubation or promote ventilator weaning is given in Table 23.9.

## Neonatal Apnea

Neonatal apnea has been defined differently by a variety of investigators; most investigators now accept cessation of breathing more than 20 seconds, or less than 20 seconds if accompanied by bradycardia (<100 beats per minute), cyanosis, or pallor.[86–88] The use of continuous $Pao_2$ monitoring with transcutaneous oxygen monitors may further modify the definition to presence of apnea or bradycardia of any duration that causes a decline in $Pao_2$. Apneic episodes occur in up to 25% of neonates with birth weights below 1800 g[89] and 84% of neonates with birth weights below 1000 g.[90]

**Table 23.9** Caffeine Citrate and Theophylline Dosing in Neonates

| *Use* | *Group[a]* | *Loading dose[b] (mg/kg)* | *IV or PO Maintenance dose[c] (mg/kg)* | *Target serum concentration (μg/mL)* |
|---|---|---|---|---|
| Caffeine citrate | | | | |
| Apnea/bradycardia | | 20 (= 10 mg/kg caffeine) | 5.0 daily | 4–20 |
| Theophylline | | | | |
| Apnea/bradycardia (central or obstructive) | A | 6 | 1.5 every 12 h | 4–20 |
| | B | 6 | 2.5 every 12 h | |
| Ventilator weaning and prevention of intubation | A | 10 | 3.0 every 12 h | 8–20 |
| | B | 10 | 5.0 every 12 h | 8–20 |

[a] Group A = asphyxia, congestive heart failure, renal failure; Group B = others.
[b] May repeat loading doses to obtain adequate clinical response.
[c] Doses should be adjusted according to serum concentrations. Measurement of serum concentrations after the initial loading dose and just before the fifth maintenance dose allows adjustments based on trends in the changed serum concentrations with minimal risk of excessive accumulation to toxicity. Repeat levels in 2 to 3 days to confirm predicted values.

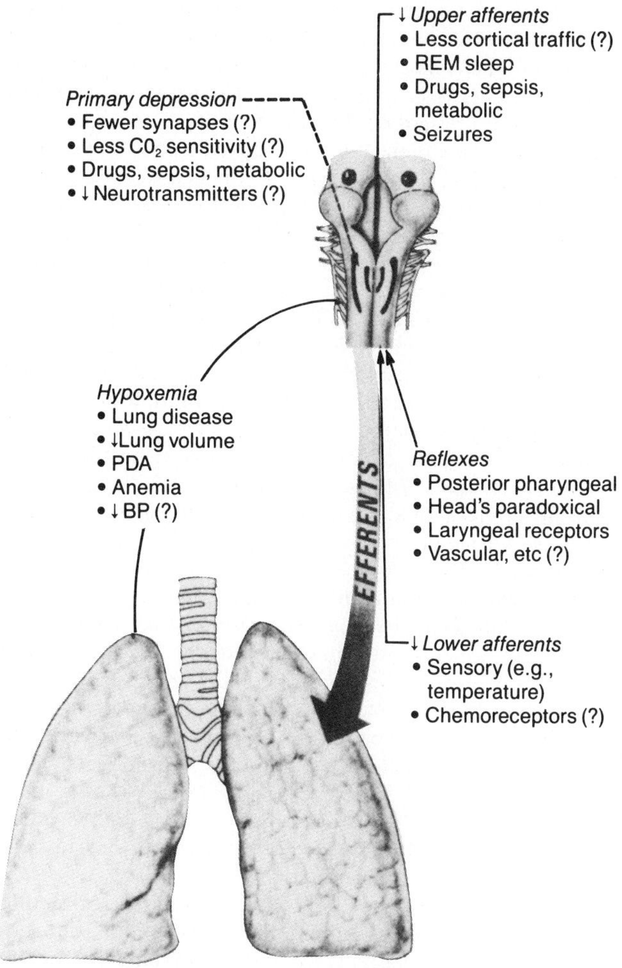


**Figure 23.3** Etiologies for apnea in neonates. *(From Kattwinkel J: Pediatrics 1977;90:342, with permission.)*

The etiology may be primary (caused by prematurity) or secondary (a variety of causes) (Fig. 23.3 and Table 23.10) and must often be resolved before apnea can be stopped. Thus, closure of a PDA, replacement of blood, treatment of sepsis, establishment of a neutral thermal environment, or removal of reflexive stimuli such as a continuous nasogastric tube may rapidly resolve apparently intractable apnea.

Three types of apnea have been identified: (1) central apnea, defined as the absence of airflow and respiratory efforts; (2) obstructive apnea, defined as the absence of airflow with respiratory effort present; and (3) mixed apnea, defined as an initial cessation of airflow and respiratory effort with a return of respiratory effort without airflow in the latter part of the episode.[88] Current systems for monitoring apnea, using chest wall leads that measure the frequency of breathing movements and concurrent continuous recordings of heart rate with ECGs, have been shown to provide inadequate documentation of the frequency of severe apneic episodes.[91] This monitoring system is particularly inadequate for documenting obstructive apneic episodes, as chest wall movements continue and bradycardia may be the only presentation.[92]

The pathophysiology of primary apnea is uncertain. Possible causes of central apnea include an immature central nervous system, resulting in insufficient respiratory drive,[93,94] decreased activity of protective respiratory reflexes,[95] and diaphragmatic fatigue.[96] Possible causes of obstructive apnea include decreased tone of the genioglossus muscle, allowing the tongue to obstruct the posterior oropharynx,[97] and nasal obstruction resulting from secretions or nasogastric tubes.[98]

**Table 23.10** Common Causes of Apnea in Newborns

| |
|---|
| Infection (sepsis, pneumonia, meningitis, necrotizing enterocolitis) |
| Patent ductus arteriosis |
| Periventricular hemorrhage |
| Seizures |
| Metabolic imbalance (hypocalcemia, hypoglycemia, acidosis, hyponatremia) |
| Anemia, hypotension (hypoxemia) |
| Drugs that lower CNS sensitivity to $Paco_2$ |
| Temperature problems (hypothermia, hyperthermia) |
| Stimulation of reflexes (diving reflex, posterior pharyngeal reflex, laryngeal receptors) |
| Gastroesophageal reflux |
| Positioning (neck flexion) |
| REM sleep |
| Gastroesophageal reflux |

The consequences of recurrent neonatal apnea may result from the physiologic changes that occur during apneic episodes: hypoxemia,[99,100] hyperoxemia,[100] and increased cerebral blood flow.[86] Autopsy studies of neonates with prolonged apnea and cyanosis revealed diffuse neuronal loss in the cerebral cortex, leukomalacia in periventricular watershed zones, and subcortical leukomalacia.[101] These findings support several of the clinical consequences associated with recurrent apneas: mental retardation, hearing loss, spastic diplegia, and sudden infant death.[102–107] Prevention of recurrent apnea is essential in minimizing the risks for these adverse outcomes.

Treatment of apnea involves the removal or resolution of secondary causes and the use of several methods to reduce the work of breathing and to stimulate breathing (Table 23.11).

The most common and effective approach is administration of methylxanthines (theophylline or caffeine) to prevent recurrent episodes of apnea. These drugs markedly reduce apneic episodes in more than 85% of neonates, although total abolition of apnea is sometimes not achieved.[108] The benefits of methylxanthines in central as well as obstructive and mixed types of apnea have been described.[109] The mechanism of action of methylxanthines is unknown, but several possibilities have been proposed.[110] The most likely mechanisms are a central stimulant effect increasing central inspiratory drive and chemoreceptor sensitivity to hypoxemia and improved contractility and fatigability of the diaphragm and inspiratory muscles.[110] Another potential benefit is decreased cerebral blood flow.[111]

The therapeutic benefits and toxic effects of theophylline and caffeine are similar,[112] and arguments to promote one over the other are generally based on personal biases. Both drugs can be used with relative safety provided plasma concentrations are carefully monitored along with clinical

**Table 23.11** Treatment of Neonatal Apnea

| | |
|---|---|
| 1 | Evaluate and correct secondary causes (e.g., sepsis, hypoxemia, PDA, anemia) |
| 2 | Set environmental temperature to lower limit of neutral thermal environment |
| 3 | Remove nasogastric tube; reduce feeding volumes |
| 4 | If apnea continues, try continuous stimulation with oscillating air or water bed |
| 5 | If apnea continues, treat with theophylline or caffeine with increasing doses, if necessary, to the upper limit of the therapeutic range |
| 6 | If apnea continues, nasal continuous positive airway pressure |
| 7 | If apnea continues (optional), try doxapram before intubation |
| 8 | Institute mechanical ventilation using intermittent positive pressure ventilation |

manifestations of toxicity (Table 23.12).[113] Neither drug has been associated with long-term adverse sequelae.[114,115]

Theophylline has been used for apnea of prematurity since 1973.[116] Because of its relative safety and efficacy, it has become the most commonly used drug in newborn intensive care units.[117] Theophylline concentrations required to eliminate apnea may be as low as 3 to 4 μg/mL, and approximately 60% of apneic episodes were eradicated in neonates achieving these plasma concentrations.[118,119] Several therapeutic ranges have been suggested for theophylline in neonates, most approximating the 6–11 μg/mL range recommended by Shannon et al[120] on the basis of a small clinical trial and the 7–14 μg/mL range estimated by Aranda et al[121] on the basis of differences in theophylline–protein binding in adults (56.4%) versus neonates (36.4%). The absolute therapeutic range is uncertain; and compelling data arguing against an increase in plasma theophylline concentrations to at least 20 μg/mL in the absence of clinical signs of toxicity are lacking. Some patients require plasma concentrations near 20 μg/mL to eradicate apneic episodes.[110,122,123] Another concern is the conversion of theophylline to caffeine, resulting in caffeine accumulation and toxicity.[122–124] This concern is based on extremely weak evidence, as plasma caffeine concentrations rarely exceed plasma theophylline concentrations and are in the low therapeutic range (e.g., below 10 μg/mL) for caffeine in neonates.[124] Caffeine concentrations up to 50 μg/mL have been observed to be safe, with only transient jitteriness occurring between 50 and 84 μg/mL.[110] Nevertheless, an additive toxicity of theophylline and caffeine, as suggested by some authors,[122] cannot be ruled out.

**Table 23.12** Toxic Effects of Methylxanthines

| |
|---|
| Central nervous system |
| Jitteriness |
| Irritability |
| Agitation |
| Seizures |
| Cardiac |
| Tachycardia (> 180 beats/min) |
| Gastrointestinal tract |
| GI irritation (especially via oral route) |
| Feeding intolerance |
| Metabolic |
| Hyperglycemia |
| Possible associated toxicities |
| Patent ductus arteriosus (increased risk) |
| Necrotizing enterocolitis |
| Diuresis and dehydration |
| Hyponatremia (resulting from increased $Na^+$ renal excretion) |

Theophylline dosing in neonates must be individualized to obtain an acceptable clinical response at a safe plasma concentration. This requires consideration of the intended use of theophylline (e.g., ventilator prevention or weaning versus apnea)[125] as well as the clinical characteristics known to alter theophylline clearance in neonates (i.e., asphyxia and postnatal age).[126] Most importantly, serum theophylline concentrations should guide dosing adjustments.[125,126] A suggested dosing protocol for both theophylline and caffeine is provided in Table 23.9.

Unlike children and adults in whom methylxanthines are mainly metabolized, in the newborn both theophylline and caffeine are primarily renally cleared.[127,128] The half-lives of theophylline and caffeine average 20–30 and 80–100 hours, respectively.[110] The volume of distribution is about 0.8 L/kg for both drugs.[110] Plasma clearances vary markedly for both drugs. Theophylline clearance may range from 3.3 to 38.0 mL/kg/h,[126] and caffeine clearance ranges from 2.5 to 16.8 mL/kg/h.[110] It is likely that clearance is largely influenced by renal function, as both drugs are eliminated primarily unchanged in the urine of newborns.

The duration of apnea and bradycardia does not seem to be shortened by methylxanthine therapy.[129] Consequently, therapy should be continued for several days after apnea and bradycardia have been eliminated on therapy. Alternatively, as central nervous system maturity is sufficient by 34 weeks in most neonates, to minimize further risks of apnea, treatment could be continued until this age is reached. Once the drug is stopped, apnea monitors should continue to be used for several days until subtherapeutic serum methylxanthine concentrations are expected.[115] Caffeine is eliminated very slowly from the neonate (half-life = 80–100 hours) and concentrations as low as 3 to 4 μg/mL can abolish apnea.[130]

Doxapram has been used in a limited number of neonates with apnea unresponsive to theophylline.[131–134] Although apneic spells were significantly reduced within a few hours of adding doxapram to theophylline, the toxic effects of doxapram (e.g., decreased seizure threshold, jitteriness, liver toxicity, hyperthermia, gastrointestinal irritation) dictate that more research be conducted before advocating its widespread use. Because it is equal, but not superior, to aminophylline alone in comparative studies, its use should be restricted as an adjunct to methylxanthines. The usual dose is 2.5 mg/kg/h as a continuous intravenous infusion. Clinical benefits are lost rapidly when the infusion is stopped.

When mechanical ventilation is required to prevent further apneic episodes, a methylxanthine should be continued at the maximum tolerable serum concentrations (e.g., 15–20 μg/mL) to allow extubation at the earliest possible time.

An important consideration in neonates with apnea unresponsive to stimulants is whether seizures are the cause of apnea. A clinical clue is the presence of prolonged apnea

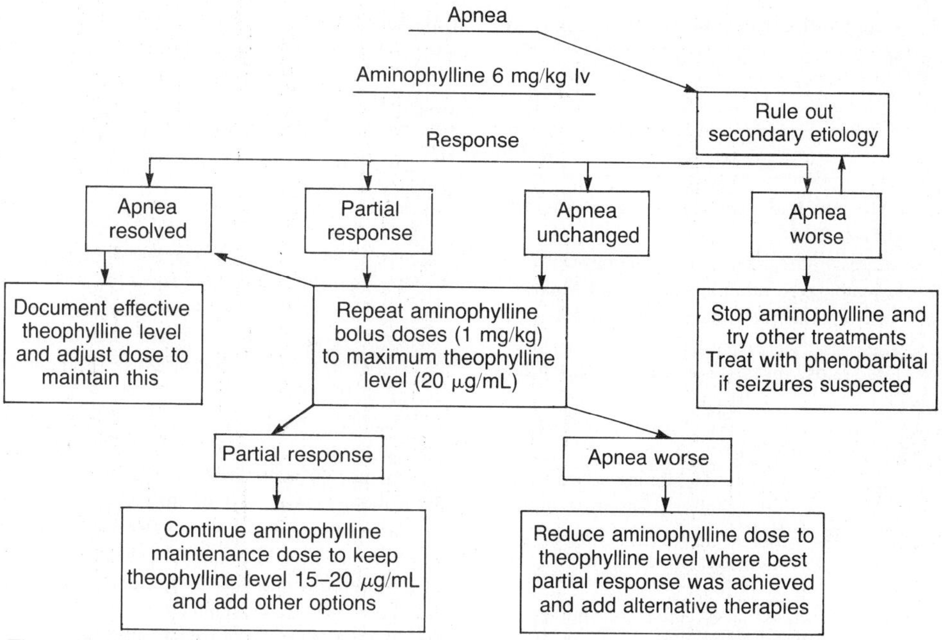


**Figure 23.4** Algorithm for methylxanthine (theophylline) use in treatment of neonatal apnea.

without bradycardia or even with increased heart rate.[135] If transcutaneous oxygen monitoring is used, the gradual return of $Pao_2$ to baseline without the hyperoxia typically seen with apneic episodes may also be a clue to seizure activity. Such cases may be made worse by methylxanthines and may respond clinically to phenobarbital. If seizures are suspected, a neurologic workup should be considered and phenobarbital therapy initiated with loading doses of 20 mg/kg intravenously followed by two 10 mg/kg boluses if needed for continued apnea. Serum phenobarbital concentrations should exceed 40 μg/mL before an inadequate therapeutic response is recorded.[136] While some risk of worsening apnea also exists, these patients have already failed theophylline therapy and likely will be intubated if phenobarbital is ineffective. Careful selection of cases will minimize this risk.

Monitoring clinical response requires careful recordkeeping by nursing staff regarding the presence of apnea, bradycardia, color changes, reduction in $Pao_2$ on transcutaneous oxygen monitoring, and type of stimulation required for recovery of apnea. A bedside flow sheet recording each apneic episode, whether bradycardia occurred and how low the heart rate dropped, the duration of apnea and bradycardia, whether apnea or bradycardia is associated with feedings, whether apneic episodes are self-resolved or require stimulation and the type of stimulation required (e.g., mild, moderate, vigorous, oxygen), and any color changes or fall in oxygenation can provide a great deal of information, especially when partial responses occur. Assessment of response requires close scrutiny of the bedside apnea flow sheet. While a complete response is obvious—no more apnea—partial responses may be more subtle. Manifestations of partial response include reduction in total number of episodes of apnea and bradycardia, no change in frequency of apnea but shorter duration of spells, no change in frequency of apnea but less stimulation required to recover from the spells (e.g., from vigorous to mild stimulation), and any combination of these responses. The opposite subtle patterns, that is, increased duration or frequency of apnea or more vigorous stimulation required to resolve apneic spells, can be used to detect theophylline toxicity or possibly exacerbation of subtle seizures presenting as apnea (one clue to subtle seizures is apnea without bradycardia or with increasing heart rate). An algorithm of response patterns and suggested clinical actions is given in Figure 23.4.

For patients with persisting apnea, the risk of sudden infant death syndrome (SIDS) may be increased.[137] These patients often are placed on home apnea monitors and exhibit abnormalities on pneumograms.[137] The use of theophylline improves pneumogram abnormalities felt to place infants at risk for SIDS.[137] Identification of effective theophylline concentrations and careful follow-up monitoring of serum concentrations are critical. As the rate of change in theophylline elimination with increasing postnatal age is unknown, frequent measurement of serum theophylline concentrations and appropriate adjustment of dose are prudent.

## Summary

Neonates suffer from a variety of pulmonary disorders ranging from mild illness to severe, life-threatening respiratory distress. Pharmacologic management of these disorders is rapidly changing. The most dramatic changes include the use of antenatal therapy (steroids or tocolytics) to promote fetal lung maturation, administration of surfactant at delivery to prevent surfactant deficiency respiratory distress syndrome, use of bronchodilators to treat previously unrecognized bronchospasm, and aggressive use of methylxanthines to minimize the time needed for mechanical ventilation, thereby reducing the risks of pulmonary air leak syndrome and chronic lung disease.

With the advent of newer techniques for monitoring blood

gases and testing pulmonary function, medical advances in the area of neonatal pulmonary medicine are likely to occur rapidly, with exciting pharmacologic interventions and realistic therapeutic endpoints.

## References


1. Farrell PM, Avery ME. Hyaline membrane disease. Am Rev Resp Dis 1975;111:657–66.
2. Stahlman MT. Acute respiratory disorders in the newborn, in Avery GB (ed): Neonatology: Pathophysiology and Management of the Newborn. Philadelphia, JB Lippincott, 1981; pp 371–397.
3. Boyle RJ, Oh W. Respiratory distress syndrome. Clin Perinatol 1978;5:283–297.
4. Lew CD, Ramos AD, Platzer ACG. Respiratory distress syndrome. Clin Chest Med 1980;1:197–309.
5. Avery ME, Taeusch HW. Hyaline membrane disease, in Avery ME, Taeusch HW (eds): Schaffer's Diseases of the Newborn. Philadelphia, W.B. Saunders, 1984; pp 133–147.
6. Caritis SN. Treatment of preterm labour. A review of options. Drugs 1983;26:243–261.
7. Souney PF, Kaul AF, Osathanondh R. Pharmacotherapy of preterm labor. Clin Pharm 1983;2:29–44.
8. Caritis SN, Carson D, Greenbod D, et al. A comparison of terbutaline and ethanol in the treatment of preterm labor. Am J Obstet Gynecol 1982;142:183–190.
9. Liggins GC, Howie RN. A controlled trial of antepartum glucocorticoid treatment for prevention of the respiratory distress syndrome in premature infants. Pediatrics 1972;515.
10. Beck JC, Johnson JWC. Maternal administration of glucocorticoids. Clin Obstet Gynecol 1980;23:93–113.
11. Frank L, Sosenko IRS. Development of lung antioxidant enzyme system in late gestation: Possible implications for the prematurely born infant. J Pediatr 1987;9–14.
12. Collaborative Group on Antenatal Steroid Therapy. Effect of antenatal dexamethasone administration on the prevention of respiratory distress syndrome. Am J Obstet Gynecol 1981;141: 276–287.
13. Sepkowitz S. Prenatal corticosteroid therapy to prevent respiratory distress syndrome. J Pediatr 1984;105:338–339.
14. Avery ME. The argument for prenatal administration of dexamethasone to prevent respiratory distress syndrome. J Pediatr 1984;104:240.
15. Levy DL. Maternal administration of dexamethasone to prevent RDS. J Pediatr 1984;105:339–340.
16. Collaborative Group on Antenatal Steroid Therapy. Effects of antenatal dexamethasone administration in the infant: Long-term follow-up. J Pediatr 1984;104:259–267.
17. Morley CJ, Miller N, Bangham AD, et al. Dry artificial lung surfactant and its effects on very premature babies. Lancet 1981;1:64–69.
18. Enhorning G, Shennan A, Possmayer F, et al. Prevention of neonatal respiratory distress syndrome by tracheal instillation of surfactant: A randomized clinical trial. Pediatrics 1985;76: 145–153.
19. Gitlin JD, Soll RF, Parad RB, et al. Randomized trial of exogenous surfactant for the treatment of hyaline membrane disease. Pediatrics 1987;79:31–37.
20. Ikegami M, Agata Y, Elkady T, et al. Comparison of four surfactants: In vitro surface properties and responses of preterm lambs to treatment at birth. Pediatrics 1987;79:38–46.
21. Fujiwara T, Adams FH. Surfactant for hyaline membrane disease. Pediatrics 1980;66:795–798.
22. Lawson EE. Exogenous surfactant therapy to prevent respiratory distress syndrome. J Pediatr 1987;110:492–493.
23. Carlo WA, Martin RJ. Principles of neonatal assisted ventilation. Pediatr Clin North Am 1986;33:221–237.
24. Corbet A, Adams J. Current therapy of hyaline membrane disease. Clin Perinatol 1978;5:299–315.
25. Hallman M, Gluck L. Respiratory distress syndrome—Update 1982. Pediatr Clin North Am 1982;29:1057–1075.
26. Bland RD. Edema formation in the newborn lung. Clin Perinatol 1982;9:593–611.
27. Heaf DP, Belik J, Spitzer AR, et al. Changes in pulmonary function during the diuretic phase of respiratory distress syndrome. J Pediatr 1982;101:103–107.
28. Green T. The use of diuretics in infants with respiratory distress syndrome. Semin Perinatol 1982;6:172–180.
29. Yeh TF, Raval D, John E, et al. Renal response to furosemide in preterm infants with respiratory distress syndrome during the first three postnatal days. Arch Dis Child 1985;60:621–626.
30. Yeh TF, Shibli A, Lev ST, et al. Early furosemide therapy in premature infants (<2000 gm) with respiratory distress syndrome: A randomized controlled trial. J Pediatr 1984;105:603–609.
31. Green TP, Thompson TR, Johnson DA, et al. Furosemide promotes patent ductus arteriosus in premature infants with respiratory distress syndrome. N Engl J Med 1983;308:743–748.
32. Avery ME, Taeusch HW. Bronchopulmonary dysplasia and other persistent pulmonary dysfunctions, in Avery ME, Taeusch HW (eds): Schaffer's Diseases of the Newborn. WB Saunders, Philadelphia, 1984, pp 148–154.
33. Murciano D, Aubier M, Lecocguic Y, et al. Effects of theophylline on diaphragmatic strength and fatigue in patients with chronic obstructive pulmonary disease. N Engl J Med 1984;311:349–353.
34. Rio MGD, Gerhardt T, Hehre D, et al. Effect of a beta-agonist nebulization on lung function in neonates with increased pulmonary resistance. Pediatr Pulmonol 1986;2:287–291.
35. Fox WW, Shutack JG. Positive pressure ventilation: Pressure and time-cycled ventilators, in Avery ME, Taeusch HW (eds): Schaffer's Disease of the Newborn. Philadelphia, WB Saunders, 1984; pp 133–147.
36. Korones SB. Complications, in: Avery ME, Taeusch HW (eds): Schaffer's Diseases of the Newborn. Philadelphia, W.B. Saunders, 1984; pp 133–147.
37. O'Brodovich HM, Mellins RB. Bronchopulmonary dysplasia. Am Rev Respir Dis 1985;132:694–709.
38. Kao LC, Warburton D, Cheng MH, et al. Effect of oral diuretics on pulmonary mechanics in infants with chronic bronchopulmonary dysplasia: Results of a double-blind crossover sequential trial. Pediatrics 1984;74:37–44.
39. Kao LC, Warburton D, Sargent CW, et al. Furosemide acutely decreases airways resistance in chronic bronchopulmonary dysplasia. J Pediatr 1983;103:624–629.
40. Patel H, Yeh TF, Jain R, et al. Pulmonary and renal responses to furosemide in infants with stage III–IV bronchopulmonary dysplasia. Am J Dis Child 1985;139:917–919.
41. Aranda JV, Chemtoh S, Laudignon N, et al. Furosemide and vitamin E. Pediatr Clin North Am 1986;33:583–602.
42. Cunningham MD, Desai NS. Methods of assessment and findings regarding pulmonary function in infants less than 1000 grams. Clin Perinatol 1986;13:299–313.

43. Sosulki R, Abbasi S, Bhutani VK, et al. Physiologic effects of terbutaline on pulmonary function of infants with bronchopulmonary dysplasia. Pediatr Pulmonol 1986;2:269–273.
44. Kao LC, Warburton D, Platzker AGC, et al. Effect of isoproterenol inhalation on airway resistance in chronic bronchopulmonary dysplasia. Pediatrics 1984;73:509–514.
45. Bancalari E, Gerhardt T. Bronchopulmonary dysplasia. Pediatr Clin North Am 1986;33:1–23.
46. Rooklin AR, Moomjian AS, Shutack JG. Theophylline therapy in bronchopulmonary dysplasia. J Pediatr 1979;95:882–885.
47. Ahrens RC, Ries RA, Popendorf W, et al. The delivery of therapeutic aerosols through endotracheal tubes. Pediatr Pulmonol 1986;2:19-26.
48. Avery GB, Fletcher AB, Kaplan M, et al. Controlled trial of dexamethasone in respirator-dependent infants with bronchopulmonary dysplasia. Pediatrics 1985;75:106–111.
49. Schick JB, Goetzman BW. Corticosteroid response in chronic lung disease of prematurity. Am J Perinatol 1983;1:23–27.
50. Gunn T, Reece ER, Metrakos K. Depressed T cells following neonatal steroid treatment. Pediatrics 1981;67:61–67.
51. Harris TR. Physiologic principles, in Goldsmith JP, Karotkin EH (eds): Assisted Ventilation of the Neonate. W.B. Saunders, Philadelphia, 1981, pp 18–48.
52. Greenough A, Morley C, Davis J. Interaction of spontaneous respiration with artificial ventilation in preterm babies. J Pediatr 1983;103:769–773.
53. Pollitzer MJ, Reynolds EO, Shaw DG, et al. Pancuronium during mechanical ventilation speeds recovery of lungs of infants with hyaline membrane disease. Lancet 1981;1:346–348.
54. Finer NN, Tomney PM. Controlled evaluation of muscle relaxation in the ventilated neonate. Pediatrics 1981;67:641–646.
55. Greenough A, Wood S, Morley CH, et al. Pancuronium prevents pneumothoraces in ventilated premature babies who actively expire against positive pressure inflation. Lancet 1984;1:1–3.
56. Stark AR, Bascom R, Frantz ID. Muscle relaxation in mechanically ventilated infants. J Pediatr 1979;93:439–443.
57. Perlman JM, Goodman S, Kreusser KL, et al. Reduction in intraventricular hemorrhage by elimination of fluctuating cerebral blood-flow velocity in preterm infants with respiratory distress syndrome. N Engl J Med 1985;312:1353–1357.
58. Ment LR. Prevention of neonatal intraventricular hemorrhage. N Engl J Med 1985;312:1385–1387.
59. Runkle B, Bancalari E. Acute cardiopulmonary effects of pancuronium bromide in mechanically ventilated new-born infants. J Pediatr 1984;104:614–617.
60. Cabal LA, Siassi B, Artal R, et al. Cardiovascular and catecholamine changes after administration of pancuronium in distressed neonates. Pediatrics 1985;75:284–287.
61. Goldberg RN, Goldman SL, Ramsay ER, et al. Detection of seizure activity in the paralyzed neonate using continuous monitoring. Pediatrics 1982;69:583–586.
62. Coen RW, McCutchen CB, Wermer D, et al. Continuous monitoring of the electroencephalogram following perinatal asphyxia. J Pediatr 1982;100:628–630.
63. Kilchevsky ES, Wung JT. Pancuronium risks. Pediatrics 1985;75:653.
64. Wimberly PD, Lou HC, Pedersen H, et al. Hypertensive peaks in the pathogenesis of intraventricular hemorrhage in the newborn: Abolition by phenobarbitone sedation. Acta Paediatr Scand 1982;71:537–542.
65. Donn SM, Roloff DW, Goldstein GW. Prevention of intraventricular haemorrhage in preterm infants by phenobarbitone. Lancet 1981;1:215–217.
66. Svenningsen NW, Blennow G, Lindroth M, et al. Brain-oriented intensive care treatment in severe neonatal asphyxia. Arch Dis Child 1982;57:176–183.
67. Gal P. Phenobarbital and primidone, in Taylor WJ, Cavineness MHD (eds): A Textbook for the Clinical Application of Therapeutic Drug Monitoring. Irving, TX, Abbott Laboratories, Diagnostic Division, 1986; pp 237–252.
68. Pippenger CE, Rosen TS. Phenobarbital plasma levels in neonates. Clin Perinatol 1975;2:111–115.
69. Diaz J, Schain RJ, Bailey BG. Phenobarbital-induced brain growth retardation in artificially reared rat pups. Biol Neonate 1977;32:77–82.
70. Donn SM, Goldstein GW, Roloff DW. Prevention of intraventricular hemorrhage with phenobarbital therapy: Now what? Pediatrics 1986;77:779–781.
71. Langslet A, Meberg A, Bredesen JE, et al. Plasma concentrations of diazepam and N-desmethyldiazepam in newborn infants after intravenous, intramuscular, rectal, and oral administration. Acta Paediatr Scand 1978;67:699–703.
72. Deshmulch A, Wittert W, Schnitzler E, et al. Lorazepam in the treatment of refractory neonatal seizures. Am J Dis Child 1986;140:1042–1044.
73. Morselli PL, Franco-Morselli R, Bossi L. Clinical pharmacokinetics in newborns and infants. Clin Pharmacokinet 1980;5:485–527.
74. Laptook AR, Rosenfeld CR. Chloral hydrate toxicity in a preterm infant. Pediatr Pharmacol 1984;4:161–165.
75. Muraskas J, Lambert GH, Ayuste O, et al. Neonatal direct hyperbilirubinemia associated with chloral hydrate dosage. Pediatr Res 1987;2:239.
76. Phelps DL. Neonatal oxygen toxicity—Is it preventable? Pediatr Clin North Am 1982;29:1233–1240.
77. Phelps DL. Vitamin E and retrolental fibroplasia in 1982. Pediatrics 1982;70:420–425.
78. Sobel S, Gueriguian J, Troendle G, et al. Vitamin E in retrolental fibroplasia. N Engl J Med 1982;306:867.
79. Lemons JA, Maisels MJ. Vitamin E—How much is too much? Pediatrics 1985;76:625–627.
80. Martone WJ, Williams WW, Mortensen ML. Illness with fatalities in premature infants: Association with an intravenous vitamin E preparation, E-Ferol. Pediatrics 1986;78:591–600.
81. Bhat R, Fisher E, Raju TNK, Vidyasager D. Patent ductus arteriosus: Recent advances in diagnosis and management. Pediatr Clin North Am 1982;29:1117–1135.
82. Harris MC, Baumgart S, Rooklin AR, et al. Successful extubation of infants with respiratory distress syndrome using aminophylline. J Pediatr 1983;103:303–305.
83. Viscardi RM, Faix RG, Nicks JJ, et al. Efficacy of theophylline for prevention of post-extubation respiratory failure in very low birth weight infants. J Pediatr 1985;107:469–472.
84. Gal P, Ravenel SD, Boer HR. Extubation of infants with respiratory distress syndrome using aminophylline. J Pediatr 1984;104:485–486.
85. Gal P, Culhane MM, Mize R, et al. Theophylline to prevent intubation of premature neonates. Drug Intell Clin Pharm (abstract)(in press).
86. Rigatto H. Apnea. Pediatr Clin North Am 1982;29:1105–1116.
87. Little GA, Ariagno RB, Beckwith B, et al. Prolonged infantile Apnea: 1985. Pediatrics 1985;76:129–131.
88. Kelly DH, Shannon DC. Neonatal and infantile apnea, in Advances in Perinatal Medicine. Milunsky A, Friedman E, Gluck L (eds); New York, Plenum, 1981; pp 1–44.
89. Kattwinkel J. Neonatal apnea. Pathogenesis and therapy. Pediatrics 1977;90:342–347.
90. Alden ER, Mandelkorn T, Woodrum DE, et al. Morbidity and

mortality of infants weighing less than 1000 grams in an intensive care nursery. Pediatrics 1972;50:40–45.

91. Southall DP, Levitt GA, Richards JM, et al. Undetected episodes of prolonged apnea and severe bradycardia in preterm infants. Pediatrics 1983;72:541–551.
92. van Someren V, Stothers JK. A critical dissection of obstructive apnea in the human infant. Pediatrics 1983;71:731–735.
93. Gerhardt T, Bancalari E. Apnea of prematurity. I. Lung function and regulation of breathing. Pediatrics 1984;74:58–62.
94. Henderson-Smart DJ, Pettigrew AG, Campbell DJ. Clinical apnea and brain-stem neural function in preterm infants. N Engl J Med 1983;308:353–357.
95. Gerhardt T, Bancalari E. Apnea of prematurity: II. Respiratory reflexes. Pediatrics 1984;74:63–66.
96. Gerhardt T, Bancalari E. Chestwall compliance in full term and premature infants. Acta Paediatr Scand 1980;69:359–364.
97. Dransfield DA, Spitzer AR, Fox WW. Episodic airway obstruction in premature infants. Am J Dis Child 1983;137:441–443.
98. Wilkinson AR. Adverse effects of nasogastric feeding tubes and the management of recurrent apnea. Arch Dis Child 1983; 57:161.
99. Hiatt IM, Hegyi T, Indyk L, et al. Continuous monitoring of $po_2$ during apnea of prematurity. J Pediatr 1981;98:288–291.
100. Peabody JL, Neese AL, Philip AGS, et al. Transcutaneous oxygen monitoring in aminophylline-treated apneic infants. Pediatrics 1978;62:698–701.
101. Perlman JM, Volpe JJ. Episodes of apnea and bradycardia in the preterm newborn: Impact on cerebral circulation. Pediatrics 1985;76:333–338.
102. Nelson KB, Ellenberg JH. Neonatal signs as predictors of cerebral palsy. Pediatrics 1979;64:225–232.
103. McDonald A. Cerebral palsy in children of very low birth weight. Arch Dis Child 1963;38:579–588.
104. Deykin E, Bauman ML, Kelly DH, et al. Apnea of infancy and subsequent neurologic, cognitive, and behavioral status. Pediatrics 1984;73:638–645.
105. Bennett FC, Chandler LS, Robinson NM, et al. Spastic diplegia in premature infants. Am J Dis Child 1981;135:732–737.
106. Abramovich SJ, Gregory S, Slemick M, et al. Hearing loss in very low birthweight infants treated with neonatal intensive care. Arch Dis Child 1979;54:421–426.
107. Anagnostakis D, Papazissis G, Messaritakis J, et al. Hearing loss in low-birth-weight infants. Am J Dis Child 1982;136:602–604.
108. Aranda JV, Turmen T. Methylxanthines in apnea of prematurity. Clin Perinatol 1979;6:87–108.
109. Roberts JL, Mathew OP, Thach BT. The efficacy of theophylline in premature infants with mixed and obstructive apnea and apnea associated with pulmonary and neurologic disease. J Pediatr 1982;100:968–971.
110. Aranda JV, Grondin D, Sasyniuk BI. Pharmacologic considerations in the therapy of neonatal apnea. Pediatr Clin North Am 1982;28:113–133.
111. Rosenkrantz TS, Oh W. Aminophylline reduces cerebral blood flow velocity in low-birth-weight infants. Am J Dis Child 1984; 138:489–491.
112. Brovard C, Moriette G, Murat I, et al. Comparative efficacy of theophylline and caffeine in the treatment of idiopathic apnea in premature infants. Am J Dis Child 1985;139:698–700.
113. Howell J, Clozel M, Aranda JV. Adverse effects of caffeine and theophylline in the newborn infant. Semin Perinatol 1981; 5:359–369.
114. Gunn TR, Metrakos K, Riley P, et al. Sequelae of caffeine treatment in preterm infants with apnea. J Pediatr 1979;94:106–109.
115. Nelson RM, Resnick MB. Long-term outcome of premature infants treated with theophylline. Semin Perinatol 1981;5:370–373.
116. Kuzemko JA, Paaka J. Apneic attacks in the newborn treated with aminophylline. Arch Dis Child 1973;48:404–406.
117. Willis S (ed): Use of theophylline in infants. FDA Drug Bulletin 1985;15:16–17.
118. Milsap RL, Krauss AN, Auld PAM. Oxygen consumption in apneic premature infants after low-dose theophylline. Clin Pharmacol Ther 1980;28:536–540.
119. Myers T, Milsap RL, Krause AN, et al. Low-dose theophylline therapy in idiopathic apnea of prematurity. J Pediatr 1980;96: 99–103.
120. Shannon DC, Gotay F, Stein IM, et al. Prevention of apnea and bradycardia in low-birthweight infants. Pediatrics 1979;55: 589–594.
121. Aranda JV, Sitar DS, Parsons WD, et al. Pharmacokinetic aspects of theophylline in premature newborns. N Engl J Med 1976;295:413–416.
122. Boutroy MJ, Vert P, Royer RJ, et al. Caffeine, a metabolite of theophylline during the treatment of apnea in the premature infant. J Pediatr 1979;94:996–998.
123. Boutroy MJ, Vert P, Monin P, et al. Methylation of theophylline to caffeine in premature infants. Lancet 1979;1:830.
124. Brazier JL, Renaud J, Ribon B, et al. Plasma xanthine levels in low birthweight infants treated or not treated with theophylline. Arch Dis Child 1979;54:194–199.
125. Gal P, Gilman JT. Concerns about the Food and Drug Administration guidelines for neonatal theophylline dosing. Ther Drug Monit 1986;8:1–3.
126. Gilman JT, Gal P, Levine RS, et al. Factors influencing theophylline disposition in 179 newborns. Ther Drug Monit 1986;8:4–10.
127. Tserng KY, Takieddine FN, King KC. Developmental aspects of theophylline metabolism in premature infants. Clin Pharmacol Ther 1983;33:522–528.
128. Grygiel JJ, Birkett DJ. Effect of age on patterns of theophylline metabolism. Clin Pharmacol Ther 1980;28:456–462.
129. Sims ME, Yau G, Rambhatla S, et al. Limitations of theophylline in the treatment of apnea of prematurity. Am J Dis Child 1985;139:567–570.
130. Banagale RC. Effect of serum caffeine level on pneumocardiogram of premature infants treated for apnea with theophylline. Med Hypotheses 1982;9:639–642.
131. Barrington KJ, Finer NN, Peters KL, et al. Physiologic effects of doxapram in idiopathic apnea of prematurity. J Pediatr 1986; 108:125–129.
132. Weesner KM, Boyle RJ. Successful management of central sleep hypoventilation in an infant using enteral doxapram. J Pediatr 1985;106:513–515.
133. Eyal F, Alpan G, Sagi E, et al. Aminophylline versus doxapram in idiopathic apnea of prematurity: A double-blind controlled study. Pediatrics 1985;75:709–713.
134. Alpan G, Eyal F, Sagi E, et al. Doxapram in the treatment of idiopathic apnea of prematurity unresponsive to aminophylline. J Pediatr 1984;104:634–637.
135. Fenichel GM, Olson BJ, Fitzpatrick JE. Heart rate changes in convulsive and non-convulsive neonatal apnea. Ann Neurol 1980;7:577–582.
136. Gal P, Toback J, Boer HR, et al. Efficacy of phenobarbital monotherapy in treatment of neonatal seizures—Relationship to blood levels. Neurology 1982;32:1401–1404.
137. Hunt CE, Brovillette RT, Hanson D. Theophylline improves pneumogram abnormalities in infants at risk for sudden infant death syndrome. J Pediatr 1983;103:969–974.

# Chapter 24 / Drug-Induced Pulmonary Diseases

H. William Kelly, PharmD

The manifestations of drug-induced pulmonary disease span the entire spectrum of pathophysiologic conditions of the respiratory tract. As with most drug-induced diseases, the pathologic changes are nonspecific. Therefore, the diagnosis is often difficult and in most cases is based on exclusion of all other possible causes. In addition, the true incidence of specific drug-induced pulmonary diseases is difficult to assess as a result of the pathologic nonspecificity and the interaction between the underlying disease state and the drugs.

Considering the physiologic and metabolic capacity of the lung, it is surprising that drug-induced pulmonary disease is not more common. The lung is the only organ of the body that receives the entire circulation. In addition, the lung contains a heterogeneous population of cells capable of various metabolic functions, including N-alkylation, N-dialkylation, N-oxidation, reduction of N-oxides, and C-hydroxylation.

Evaluation of epidemiologic studies on adverse drug reactions provides a perspective on the importance of drug-induced pulmonary disease in the general population. In a 2-year prospective survey of a community-based general practice, 41% of 817 patients experienced adverse drug reactions.[1] Four patients, or 0.5% of the total respondents, experienced adverse respiratory symptoms. Respiratory symptoms occurred in 1.2% of patients experiencing adverse drug reactions. A more recent surveillance study in 3,181 general pediatric outpatients receiving 4,244 courses of drug therapy reported adverse reactions in 473 (11.1%) of the courses.[2] Of these, only 200 were considered definite or probable. Gastrointestinal symptoms, skin reactions, and central nervous system symptoms made up 96.5% of the reactions, with respiratory symptoms included with all other reactions.

Adverse pulmonary reactions would appear to be uncommon in the general population, but they are among the most serious reactions, often requiring intervention. This is illustrated in studies of adverse reactions requiring hospitalization. In a study of 270 adverse reactions leading to hospitalization from two populations, 3.0% were respiratory in nature.[3] Of the reactions considered to be life-threatening, 12.3% were respiratory. An early report on death caused by drug reactions from the Boston Collaborative Drug Surveillance Program indicated that 7 of 27 drug-induced deaths were respiratory.[4] This was confirmed in a follow-up study in which 6 of 24 drug-induced deaths were respiratory in nature.[5]

This chapter is arranged according to the clinical presentation of the respiratory illness. The pathophysiologic mechanism and usual clinical presentation of the most important agents in each disease group are discussed. Tables listing all the agents that have been associated with each disease and their relative frequency complement the discussions. Secondary literature references (i.e., review articles and book chapters) are used to expedite referencing and to provide the reader with a bibliography of reviews on the subject. The interested reader is encouraged to seek out the reviews and the primary literature on this interesting and complex subject.

## Apnea

Apnea may be induced by central nervous system depression or respiratory neuromuscular blockade (Table 24.1). Patients with chronic obstructive airway disease, alveolar hypoventilation, and chronic carbon dioxide retention have an exaggerated respiratory depressant response to narcotic analgesics and sedatives. In addition, the injudicious administration of oxygen in patients with carbon dioxide retention can remove their hypoxic ventilatory drive, producing apnea.[6] Although the benzodiazepines are touted as causing less respiratory depression than barbiturates, they may produce a profound additive or synergistic effect when taken in combination with other respiratory depressants.

Prolonged apnea may follow the administration of any of the neuromuscular blocking agents after surgery. Respiratory failure has occurred after local spinal anesthesia. Apnea from respiratory paralysis and rapid respiratory muscle fatigue has followed the administration of polymyxin and aminoglycoside antibiotics.[6–8] Ventilatory failure from the polymyxins occurred primarily in patients with renal failure as a result of the accumulation of excessive serum concentrations.[7] The mechanism appears to be related to the complexation of calcium and its depletion at the myoneural junction. Intravenous calcium chloride has been variably effective in reversing the paralysis.[7,8]

The aminoglycosides competitively block neuromuscular junctions. This has resulted in life-threatening apnea when neomycin, gentamicin, streptomycin, or bacitracin has been administered in the peritoneal and pleural cavities.[6–8] The aminoglycosides produce an additive blockade and ventilatory paralysis with curare or succinylcholine and in patients with myasthenia gravis or myasthenic syndromes.[7] Intravenous administration of aminoglycosides has resulted in respiratory failure in babies with infantile botulism. The treatment consists of ventilatory support and an anticholinesterase (neostigmine or edrophonium).[7,8]

## Asthma

Bronchoconstriction is the most common drug-induced respiratory problem. Bronchospasm can be induced by a wide variety of drugs through a number of disparate pathophysi-

**Table 24.1** Drugs That Induce Apnea

| | |
|---|---|
| **Central nervous system depression** | |
| Narcotic analgesics | F[a] |
| Barbiturates | F |
| Benzodiazepines | I |
| Other sedatives and hypnotics | I |
| Tricyclic antidepressants | R |
| Ketamine | R |
| Promazine | R |
| Anesthetics | R |
| Antihistamines | R |
| Alcohol | I |
| Fenfluramine | R |
| L-Dopa | R |
| Oxygen | R |
| **Respiratory muscle dysfunction** | |
| Aminoglycoside antibiotics | I |
| Polymyxin antibiotics | I |
| Neuromuscular blockers | I |
| Quinine | R |
| Digitalis | R |

[a] Relative frequency of reactions: F, frequent; I, infrequent; R, rare.

ologic mechanisms (Table 24.2). For a more in-depth discussion, refer to recent reviews on this subject.[9,10] Regardless of the pathophysiologic mechanism, drug-induced bronchospasm is almost exclusively a problem of patients with preexisting bronchial hyperreactivity (see Chapters 21 and 22).[10] By definition, all patients with nonspecific bronchial hyperreactivity experience bronchospasm if given sufficiently high doses of cholinergic or anticholinesterase agents. Severe asthmatics with a high degree of bronchial reactivity may wheeze after inhalation of a number of particulate substances, such as cromolyn (by Spinhaler) or corticosteroids, presumably through direct stimulation of the central airway irritant receptors. Other pharmacologic mechanisms for inducing bronchospasm include $\beta_2$-receptor blockade and nonimmunologic histamine release from mast cells and basophils.[10] A wide variety of agents are capable of producing bronchospasm through IgE-mediated reactions.[9,10] These drugs can become a significant occupational hazard for pharmacists, nurses, and pharmaceutical industry workers.[6,8,10]

## *Aspirin*

### Epidemiology

Aspirin-induced asthma was first recognized in 1902 shortly after the introduction of aspirin.[10] Aspirin sensitivity or intolerance occurs in 4% to 20% of all asthmatics.[11] The frequency of aspirin-induced bronchospasm increases with age. Patients older than 40 have a frequency approximately four times that of patients under 20.[11] The frequency increases to 14% to 23% in patients with nasal polyps.[11]

### Clinical Presentation

The classic description of the aspirin-intolerant asthmatic includes the triad of severe asthma, nasal polyps, and aspirin intolerance. The typical patient experiences intense vasomotor rhinitis beginning during the third or fourth decade of life.[12] Over a period of months, nasal polyps begin to appear, followed by severe asthma exacerbated by aspirin. Bronchospasm typically begins within minutes to hours of ingestion of aspirin and is associated with rhinorrhea, flushing of the head and neck, and conjunctivitis.[12] The reactions are severe and often life-threatening.

A number of epidemiologic studies using aspirin challenges have now shown that a large number of aspirin-sensitive asthmatics do not fit the classic "aspirin triad" picture and that not all patients with asthma and nasal polyps develop sensitivity to aspirin.[13] Indeed, in most cases, aspirin-sensitive asthmatics are indistinguishable clinically from the general population of asthmatics except for their intolerance to aspirin and other nonsteroidal anti-inflammatory agents (NSAIAs). There is a predominance in women over men, but there is no evidence for a genetic or familial predisposition.[12,13]

### Pathogenesis

Aspirin-induced asthma is correctly classified as an idiosyncratic reaction in that the pathogenesis is still unknown. Patients with aspirin intolerance have increased plasma histamine concentrations and elevated peripheral eosinophil counts after ingestion of aspirin.[13,14] All attempts to define an immunologic (immunoglobulin- or T lymphocyte–mediated) mechanism have been unsuccessful. Chemically similar drugs such as salicylamide and choline salicylate do not cross-react, whereas a large number of chemically dissimilar NSAIAs do produce reactions.[13,14] Table 24.3 lists the analgesics that do and do not cross-react with aspirin.

The currently accepted hypothesis is that aspirin intolerance is integrally related to inhibition of cyclooxygenase. This is supported by the following evidence: (1) all NSAIAs that inhibit cyclooxygenase cross-react with aspirin; (2) the degree of cross-reactivity is proportional to the potency of cyclooxygenase inhibition; and (3) each patient with aspirin sensitivity has a threshold dose for precipitating bronchospasm that is specific for the degree of cyclooxygenase inhibition produced, and, once established, the dose of another cyclooxygenase inhibitor needed to induce bronchospasm can be estimated.[14]

The mechanism by which cyclooxygenase inhibition produces bronchospasm in susceptible individuals is unknown. Blockade of cyclooxygenase may deprive the bronchi of prostaglandin $E_2$, which stabilizes mast cells and relaxes bronchial smooth muscle.[14] Inhibition of cyclooxygenase may divert arachidonic acid metabolism through the lipoxygenase pathway, leading to the excess production of leukotrienes (LTs) $C_4$ and $D_4$.[11,14] $LTC_4$, $LTD_4$, and $LTE_4$ produce bronchospasm and promote histamine release from mast cells.[14] Although these mechanisms provide an attractive explanation, they have not been proven and they do not explain why only a small number of asthmatic patients react to aspirin and NSAIAs.

### Desensitization

Patients with aspirin sensitivity can be desensitized. The ease of desensitization correlates with the sensitivity of the patient.[13] Highly sensitive patients who initially react to less than 100 mg of aspirin require multiple rechallenges to

**Table 24.2** Drugs That Induce Bronchospasm

| | | | |
|---|---|---|---|
| Anaphylaxis (IgE-mediated) | | Anaphylactoid mast cell degranulation | |
| Penicillins | F[a] | Narcotic analgesics | I |
| Sulfonamides | F | Ethylenediamine | R |
| Serum | F | Iodinated-radiocontrast media | F |
| Cephalosporins | F | Platinum | R |
| Bromelin | R | Local anesthetics | I |
| Cimetidine | R | Steroidal anesthetics | I |
| Papain | F | Iron–dextran complex | I |
| Pancreatic extract | I | Pancuronium bromide | R |
| Pituitary snuff | F | Cyclooxygenase inhibition | |
| Psyllium | I | Aspirin | F |
| Subtilase | I | Nonsteroidal anti-inflammatory agent | F |
| Tetracyclines | I | Phenylbutazone | I |
| Allergen extracts | I | Acetaminophen | R |
| L-Asparaginase | F | Pharmacologic effect | |
| Pyrazolone analgesics | I | β-Adrenergic receptor blockers | I-F |
| Direct airway irritation | | Cholinergic stimulants | F |
| Acetate | R | Anticholinergics | F |
| Bisulfite | F | α-Adrenergic agonists | R |
| Cromolyn | R | Unknown mechanism | |
| Marijuana | I | Hydrocortisone | R |
| *N*-Acetylcysteine | F | Isoproterenol | R |
| Precipitating IgG antibodies | | Monosodium glutamate | I |
| L-Methyl dopa | R | Piperazine | R |
| Carbamazepine | R | Tartrazine | R |
| (pituitary snuff) | F | Sulfinpyrazone | R |
| Spiramycin | R | Zinostatin | R |

[a]Relative frequency of reactions: F, frequent; I, infrequent; R, rare.

**Table 24.3** Cross-Reactivity Between Aspirin and Other Analgesics and Anti-inflammatory Agents

| *Cross-reactive drugs* | *Drugs with no cross-reactivity* |
|---|---|
| Indomethacin | Dextropropoxyphene |
| Tolmetin | Salicylamide |
| Fenoprofen | Sodium salicylate |
| Ketoprofen | Choline salicylate |
| Ibuprofen | Benzydamine |
| Naproxen | Chloroquine |
| Flurbiprofen | Corticosteroids |
| Diclofenac | Acetaminophen[a] |
| Noramidopyrine | Phenacetin[a] |
| Diflunisal | |
| Sulindac | |
| Mefenamic acid | |
| Flufenamic acid | |
| Phenylbutazone | |
| Oxyphenbutazone | |
| Sulfinpyrazone | |
| Tartrazine | |

[a] A very small percentage (≈6) of aspirin-sensitive patients react to acetaminophen and phenacetin.

produce desensitization.[13] Desensitization usually persists for 2 to 5 days after discontinuance, with full sensitivity reestablished by 7 days.[13] Cross-desensitization has been established between aspirin and all NSAIAs tested to date. Because patients may experience life-threatening reactions, desensitization should be attempted only in a controlled environment by personnel with expertise in handling these patients. In addition, there have been reports of patients who have failed to maintain a desensitized state despite continued aspirin administration.[13] The chronic asthma symptoms have markedly improved in a number of aspirin-sensitive asthmatics who have undergone desensitization.[13,14] The explanation for this is not clear.

It has been reported that up to 80% of aspirin-sensitive asthmatics have an adverse reaction to the yellow azo dye tartrazine (FD&C Yellow No. 5), which is widely used for coloring foods, drinks, drugs, and cosmetics[11,12]; however, those studies reporting high cross-reactivity were poorly controlled and often used only subjective criteria.[11,15] In double-blind placebo-controlled trials using pulmonary function testing, sensitivity to tartrazine has proven to be a rare event.[15] Tartrazine sensitivity appears to occur only in aspirin-intolerant patients at a prevalence of 1% to 15%.[11,15]

Reactions to other azo dyes have been reported much less frequently than reactions to tartrazine.[15] Positive reactions to sodium benzoate, a food preservative, have been reported as high as 23% in aspirin-sensitive individuals.[11] Acetaminophen is a weak inhibitor of cyclooxygenase. As such, a small number of aspirin-sensitive asthmatics, approximately 6%, experience reactions to acetaminophen.[11] For most aspirin-sensitive asthmatics, acetaminophen is a safe alternative to aspirin.

#### Treatment

Therapy for aspirin-sensitive asthmatics takes one of two general approaches: desensitization or avoidance. It should be pointed out that avoidance of triggering substances seldom alters the clinical course of the patient's asthma. The therapy for the patient's asthma is nonspecific, although some authors feel that cromolyn should be tried in all aspirin-sensitive asthmatics.[12] Many of these patients require chronic steroid therapy to control the asthma. The respiratory symptoms can be decreased, but not prevented, by pretreatment with antihistamines and cromolyn.[13]

### *β-Blockers*

β-Adrenergic receptor blockers constitute the other large class of drugs that can be hazardous to the asthmatic. Even the more cardioselective agents—acebutolol, atenolol, and metoprolol—have been reported to cause asthma attacks.[10] Asthmatics may take nonselective and $\beta_1$-selective blockers without incident for long periods; however, the occasional reports of fatal asthma attacks resistant to therapy with β agonists should provide ample warning of the dangers inherent in β-blocker therapy.[10]

If a patient with bronchial hyperreactivity requires β-blocker therapy, one of the relatively selective $\beta_1$-blockers (acebutolol, atenolol, metoprolol) should be used at the lowest possible dose. Two newer agents in testing, pafenolol and betaxolol, appear to possess greater cardioselectivity than currently marketed drugs.[16,17] Fatal status asthmaticus has occurred with the topical administration of the nonselective timolol maleate ophthalmic solution for the treatment of open-angle glaucoma.[18] Early investigations with ophthalmic betaxolol suggest that it is well tolerated even in timolol-sensitive asthmatics.[19]

### *Sulfites*

#### Epidemiology

Six asthmatics with a history of severe life-threatening asthmatic reactions after restaurant meals and wine were discovered to have sensitivity to the food preservative potassium metabisulfite.[15] Sulfites have been used for centuries as preservatives in wine and food. As antioxidants, they prevent fermentation by contaminating organisms in wine and discoloration of fruits and vegetables. Until recently, sulfites had been given generally-recognized-as-safe (GRAS) status by the Food and Drug Administration (FDA).[20] Sensitive patients react to concentrations ranging from 5 to 100 mg, amounts that are routinely consumed by anyone eating in a restaurant. Anaphylactic or anaphylactoid reactions to sulfites in nonasthmatics are extremely rare. In the general asthmatic population, reactions to sulfites are uncommon. Approximately 5% of steroid-dependent asthmatics demonstrate a sensitivity to sulfiting agents, but the prevalence is only around 1% in non–steroid-dependent asthmatic patients.[21,22]

#### Pathogenesis

The mechanism by which sulfites induce asthma is still unknown. The inhalation of 1 to 5 ppm sulfur dioxide produces bronchoconstriction in all asthmatics through direct stimulation of afferent parasympathetic irritant receptors.[20] When $SO_2$ comes into contact with water, it forms $H_2SO_3$, which dissociates to $H^+$ and $HSO_3^-$. Whether $SO_2$ or $HSO_3^-$ is the asthmagenic stimulus is unknown. Upon oral ingestion of metabisulfites, less than 10% of all asthmatics develop bronchospasm. It has therefore been postulated that sulfite-sensitive asthmatics have an inability to clear a sulfite load normally and the sulfite accumulates.[20] At the air–fluid surface of the bronchial mucosa, $HSO_3^-$ ions associate with water to form $H_2SO_3$ and $SO_2$. A reduced concentration of sulfite oxidase enzyme compared with normals has been demonstrated in a group of sulfite-sensitive asthmatics.[20] There has been no correlation between sulfite sensitivity and sensitivity to cyclooxygenase inhibitors.

A number of pharmacologic agents contain sulfites as preservatives and antioxidants. Table 24.4 lists the drugs used to treat asthma that currently contain sulfites. The FDA has urged the labeling of food and drugs containing sulfites. In addition, labeling is required on packaged foods that contain sulfites at 10 ppm or more, and sulfiting agents will no longer be allowed on raw fruits and vegetables (excluding potatoes) intended for sale.

Recent studies have demonstrated that aerosolization of bronchodilator solutions of isoproterenol and isoetharine can produce sulfur dioxide concentrations of 0.1 to 6 ppm.[15,21,22] These are sufficient to produce asthma attacks in sensitive individuals. The concentration of sulfite in metaproterenol aerosol appears insufficient to produce bronchospasm.[22] There are no sulfites in terbutaline solution for injection. Sulfites are not used in the metered-dose inhalers. Concern over the production of bronchospasm in the rare patient after isoproterenol inhalation has focused on the rapid induction of tachyphylaxis or the production of β-blockade by isoproterenol metabolites.[9,10] There is no direct evidence supporting either mechanism. The recent recognition of the sulfite content in some isoproterenol solutions may add another more plausible explanation.

### *Contrast Media*

Most other drugs produce bronchospasm through irritation or as part of an anaphylactic or anaphylactoid reaction. Iodinated radiocontrast materials are the most common of the latter reactions, occurring in 2% to 8% of all contrast medium infusions. Fatalities occur as frequently as 1 in 3,000 procedures for cholangiography.[23] These reactions are associated with increased plasma histamine concentrations, although the mechanism of the histamine release is unknown. Patients with previous reactions have an increased incidence on second exposure (35%–60%). Pretreatment with prednisone and antihistamines reduces the rate of recurrence to 9%.[21]

**Table 24.4** Sulfite-Containing Drugs Used to Treat Asthma

| *Contain sulfites* | *Contain no sulfites* |
|---|---|
| **Oral bronchodilators** | |
| Metaproterenol syrup | Metaproterenol tablets |
| | Albuterol syrup tablets |
| | Terbutaline tablets |
| **Aerosol bronchodilators** | |
| Metaproterenol 5% solution (multidose) | Metaproterenol unit dose |
| Isoproterenol (Isuprel, Breon; Dispos-a-Med, Parke–Davis) | Albuterol metered dose |
| | Terbutaline metered dose |
| Isoetharine (Breon; Parke–Davis; Roxane) | Metaproterenol metered dose |
| Epinephrine (Micronefrin, Bird) | Isoproterenol (Aerolone, Lilly) |
| | Epinephrine (Vaponefrin, Fisons) |
| **Injectable Bronchodilators** | |
| Epinephrine (Adrenalin, Parke–Davis; Epi-Pen, Center; Ana-Kit, Hollister–Stier) | Epinephrine (Susphrine [Berlex]) |
| | Terbutaline |
| **Injectable corticosteroids** | |
| Dexamethasone acetate (MSD; Hyrex; Kea Pharm) | Betamethasone $NaPO_4$ [Organon] |
| | Dexamethasone $NaPO_4$ |
| Dexamethasone $NaPO_4$ (Elkins–Sinn; MSD; Hyrex) | Hydrocortisone Acetate [Upjohn] |
| | Hydrocortisone sodium succinate |
| Hydrocortisone acetate (MSD) | Methylprednisolone |
| Hydrocortisone $NaPO_4$ (MSD) | Triamcinolone |
| Prednisolone $NaPO_4$ | |

## Pulmonary Edema

Pulmonary edema may result from the failure of any of a number of homeostatic mechanisms. The most common cause of pulmonary edema is an increase in capillary hydrostatic pressure because of left ventricular failure. Excessive fluid administration in compromised and noncompromised cardiovascular patients is the most frequent cause of iatrogenic pulmonary edema. Besides hydrostatic forces, other homeostatic mechanisms that may be disrupted include the osmotic and oncotic pressures in the vasculature, the integrity of alveolar epithelium, interstitial pulmonary pressure, and the interstitial lymph flow.[22] The edema fluid in cardiogenic pulmonary edema contains a small amount of protein, whereas noncardiogenic pulmonary edema fluid has a high protein concentration.[22] This indicates that noncardiogenic pulmonary edema results primarily from disruption of the alveolar epithelium.

The clinical presentation of pulmonary edema includes persistent cough, tachypnea, dyspnea, tachycardia, rales on auscultation, hypoxemia from ventilation–perfusion imbalance and intrapulmonary shunting, widespread fluffy infiltrates on chest roentgenogram, and decreased lung compliance (stiff lungs). Noncardiogenic pulmonary edema may progress to hemorrhage; cellular debris collects in the alveoli and is followed by hyperplasia and fibrosis with a residual restrictive mechanical defect.[22]

### *Narcotics*

The most common drug-induced noncardiogenic pulmonary edema is produced by the narcotic analgesics[6,8] (Table 24.5). Narcotic-induced pulmonary edema is most commonly associated with intravenous heroin use but has also occurred with morphine, methadone, meperidine, and propoxyphene.[6,8,24] There have also been two reported cases associated with the use of the opiate antagonist naloxone.[25] The mechanism is unknown but may be related to hypoxemia or similar to the neurogenic pulmonary edema associated with cerebral tumors or trauma.[8] Initially thought to occur only with overdoses, most evidence now supports the theory that narcotic-induced pulmonary edema is an idiosyncratic reaction to usual as well as high doses.[24]

Patients may be comatose with depressed respirations or dyspneic and tachypneic. They may or may not have other signs of narcotic overdose. Symptomatology varies from cough and mild crepitations on auscultation with characteristic radiologic findings to severe cyanosis and hypoxemia even with supplemental oxygen. Symptoms may appear within minutes of intravenous administration, but may take up to 2 hours, particularly after oral methadone.[24] Hemodynamic studies in the first 24 hours have demonstrated normal pulmonary capillary wedge pressures in the presence of pulmonary edema.

Clinical symptoms generally improve within 24 to 48 hours and radiologic clearing occurs in 2 to 5 days, but abnormalities in pulmonary function tests may persist for 10 to 12 weeks. Therapy consists of naloxone administration, supplemental oxygen, and ventilatory support if required.

### *Other Drugs*

Noncardiogenic pulmonary edema has also been associated with the oral and intravenous administration of ethchlorvynol.[24,25] A parodoxical pulmonary edema has been reported in a few patients after hydrochlorothiazide ingestion.[6,8] This phenomenon has not been reported with any

**Table 24.5** Agents That Induce Pulmonary Edema

| | | | |
|---|---|---|---|
| Cardiogenic pulmonary edema | | | |
| Excessive intravenous fluids | F[a] | Sodium diatrizoate | R |
| Blood and plasma transfusions | F | Hypertonic intrathecal saline | R |
| Corticosteroids | F | $\beta_2$-Adrenergic agonists | I |
| Phenylbutazone | R | | |
| Noncardiogenic pulmonary edema | | | |
| Heroin | F | Oxygen | I |
| Methadone | I | Nitrofurantoin | R |
| Morphine | I | Dextran 40 | R |
| Propoxyphene | R | Fluorescein | R |
| Ethchlorvynol | R | Amitriptyline | R |
| Chlordiazepoxide | R | Colchicine | R |
| Salicylate | R | Nitrogen mustard | R |
| Hydrochlorothiazide | R | Epinephrine | R |
| Triamterene + hydrochlorothiazide | R | Metaraminol | R |
| Leukoagglutinin reactions | R | Bleomycin | R |
| Iron–dextran complex | R | Iodide | R |
| Methotrexate | R | Cyclophosphamide | R |
| Cytosine arabinoside | R | VM-26 | R |

[a] Relative frequency of reactions: F, frequent; I, infrequent; R, rare.

other benzothiazide diuretics. Acute pulmonary edema has rarely followed the injection of high concentrations of contrast medium into the pulmonary circulation during angiocardiography.[8] Rare occurrences of pulmonary edema have followed the intravenous administration of bleomycin, cyclophosphamide, and vinblastine.[8]

The selective $\beta_2$-adrenergic agonists terbutaline and ritodrine have been reported to induce pulmonary edema when used as tocolytics.[8] This has never occurred with their use in asthma, even in inadvertent overdosage. This reaction may result from excess fluid administration used to prevent the hypotension from $\beta_2$-mediated vasodilation or the particular hemodynamics of pregnancy.

Excessive salicylate intake has been associated with pulmonary edema. It has usually occurred with inadvertent or intentional overdoses. Patients usually show other effects of salicylate intoxication, including tinnitus, respiratory alkalosis followed by metabolic acidosis, pyrexia, and disorientation.[22] The serum salicylate concentrations are often greater than 45 mg/dL, although some cases have been associated with concentrations in the usual therapeutic range.[24]

## Pulmonary Eosinophilia

Pulmonary infiltrates with eosinophilia (Loeffler's syndrome) have been associated with nitrofurantoin, *para*-aminosalicylic acid, methotrexate, sulfonamides, tetracycline, chlorpropramide, phenytoin, and imipramine[8] (Table 24.6). The disorder is characterized by fever, nonproductive cough, dyspnea, cyanosis, bilateral pulmonary infiltrates, and eosinophilia in the blood.[6] Lung biopsy has revealed perivasculitis with infiltration of eosinophils, macrophages, and proteinaceous edema fluid in the alveoli. The symptoms and eosinophilia generally respond rapidly to withdrawal of the offending drug.

Sulfonamides were first reported as causative agents in users of sulfanilamide vaginal cream.[6] *para*-Aminosalicylic acid frequently produced the syndrome in tuberculosis patients treated with this agent.[6] There have been nine reported cases associated with sulfasalazine use in inflammatory bowel disease.[25] The drug most frequently associated with this syndrome now is nitrofurantoin.[6–8,24] Nitrofurantoin-induced lung disorders appear to be more common in postmenopausal women. There is no apparent correlation between duration of drug exposure and severity or reversibility of the reaction.[7] Although there are anecdotal reports that steroids are beneficial, the usual rapid improvement after discontinuation of the drug brings their utility into question.

A few cases of pulmonary eosinophilia have been reported in asthmatics treated with cromolyn.[6,8] The significance of this is unknown in light of the occasional spontaneous occurrence of pulmonary eosinophilia in asthmatic patients. Cases of acute pneumonitis and eosinophilia have been reported to occur with phenytoin and carbamazepine therapy.[25] The patients have had other symptoms of hyper-

**Table 24.6** Drugs That Induce Pulmonary Infiltrates With Eosinophilia (Loeffler's Syndrome)

| | | | |
|---|---|---|---|
| Nitrofurantoin | F[a] | Phenytoin | R |
| *para*-Aminosalicylic acid | F | Mephenesin | R |
| Sulfonamides | I | Tetracycline | R |
| Penicillins | I | Procarbazine | R |
| Methotrexate | I | Cromolyn | R |
| Imipramine | I | Niridazole | R |
| Chlorpropamide | R | Gold salts | R |
| Carbamazepine | R | | |

[a] Relative frequency of reactions: F, frequent; I, infrequent; R, rare.

sensitivity, including fever and rashes. The symptoms of dyspnea and cough subside after discontinuation of the drug. Corticosteroids may hasten the recovery.

## Oxygen Toxicity

Because of its similarity to pulmonary fibrosis, oxygen-induced lung toxicity is briefly reviewed. More extensive reviews on this topic have recently been published.[26–28]

### Pathophysiology

Oxygen-induced lung damage is well recognized and the pathologic features have been systematically characterized. These are generally separated into the acute exudative phase and the subacute or chronic proliferative phase. The acute phase consists of perivascular, peribronchiolar, interstitial, and alveolar edema with alveolar hemorrhage and necrosis of pulmonary endothelium and type I epithelial cells.[27] The proliferative phase consists of resorption of the exudates and hyperplasia of interstitial and type II alveolar lining cells. Collagen and elastin deposition in the interstitium of alveolar walls then leads to thickening of the gas exchange area and the fibrosis.[27]

### Etiology

Fractional concentration of inspired oxygen ($Fio_2$) and duration of exposure are both important determinants of the severity of damage. Normal human volunteers can tolerate 100% oxygen at sea level for 24 to 48 hours with minimal to no damage.[26] Oxygen concentrations lower than 50% are well tolerated even for extended periods.[26] Inspired oxygen concentrations between 50% and 100% carry a substantial risk of lung damage and the duration required is inversely proportional to the $Fio_2$.[26] Underlying disease states may alter the relationship.

### Clinical Presentation

The earliest manifestation is substernal pleuritic pain from tracheobronchitis.[28] The onset of toxicity follows an asymptomatic period and presents as cough, chest pain, and dyspnea. Early symptoms are usually masked in ventilator-dependent patients. The first noted physiologic change is a decrease in pulmonary compliance caused by reversible atelectasis. Then decreases in vital capacity occur, followed by progressive abnormalities in carbon monoxide–diffusing capacity (DLco).[28] Decreased inspiratory flow rates, reflected in the need for high inspiratory pressures in ventilator-dependent patients, occur as the $Fio_2$ requirement increases. The patient's lungs become progressively stiffer as the ability to oxygenate becomes more compromised.

### Pathogenesis

The biochemical mechanism of the tissue damage that occurs during hyperoxia is the increased production of highly reactive, partially reduced oxygen metabolites.[28] These oxidants are normally produced in small quantities during cellular respiration and include the superoxide anion ($O_2^-$), hydrogen peroxide ($H_2O_2$), the hydroxyl radical ($OH\cdot$), singlet oxygen ($^1O_2$), and hypochlorous acid (HOCl).[27] Oxygen free radicals are normally formed in phagocytic cells to kill invading microorganisms, but they are also toxic to normal cell components. The oxidants produce toxicity through destructive redox reactions with protein sulfhydryl groups, membrane lipids, and nucleic acids.[28]

Because the oxidants are products of normal cellular respiration, an antioxidant defense system is in place to prevent tissue destruction. The antioxidants include superoxide dismutase, catalase, glutathione peroxidase, ceruloplasmin, and α-tocopherol (vitamin E). Antioxidants are ubiquitous in the body. Hyperoxia produces toxicity by overwhelming the antioxidant system. There is experimental evidence that a number of drugs and chemicals produce lung toxicity by increasing production of oxidants and/or by inhibiting the antioxidant system.

## Pulmonary Fibrosis

A large variety of drugs have been associated with chronic pulmonary fibrosis with or without a preceding acute pneumonitis (Table 24.7). The cancer chemotherapeutic agents make up the largest group and have been the subject of numerous recent reviews.[29–31] Although the mechanisms by which all of the drugs produce pneumonitis and/or fibrosis are not known, the clinical syndrome, pulmonary function abnormalities, and histopathology present a relatively homogeneous pattern.[31] The histopathologic picture closely resembles oxidant lung damage and in some experimental cases oxygen enhances the pulmonary injury.[31]

The lung damage following ingestion of the contact herbicide paraquat classically resembles hyperoxic lung damage. Hyperoxia accelerates the lung damage induced by paraquat. Lung toxicity from paraquat occurs after oral administration in man and aerosol administration and inhalation in experimental animal models.[32] The pulmonary specificity of paraquat results in part from its active uptake into lung

**Table 24.7** Agents That Induce Pneumonitis and/or Fibrosis

| | | | |
|---|---|---|---|
| Oxygen | F[a] | Azathioprine, 6-mercaptopurine | R |
| Radiation | F | Chlorambucil | R |
| Bleomycin | F | Melphalan | R |
| Busulfan | F | Lomustine and semustine | R |
| Carmustine | F | Zinostatin | R |
| Hexamethonium | F | Procarbazine | R |
| Paraquat | F | Sulfasalazine | R |
| Amiodarone | F | Phenytoin | R |
| Mecamylamine | I | Gold salts | R |
| Pentolinium | I | Pindolol | R |
| Cyclophosphamide | I | Imipramine | R |
| Practolol | I | Penicillamine | R |
| Methotrexate | I | Phenylbutazone | R |
| Mitomycin | I | Chlorphentermine | R |
| Nitrofurantoin | I | Fenfluramine | R |
| Methysergide | I | | |

[a]Relative frequency of reactions: F, frequent; I, infrequent; R, rare.

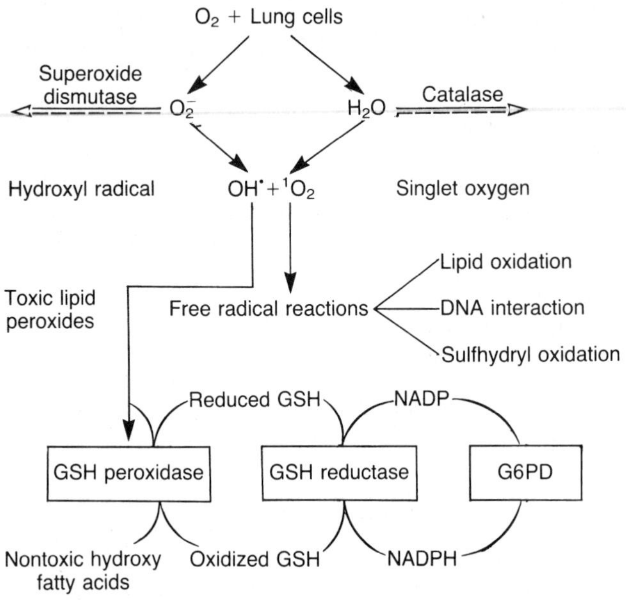


**Figure 24.1** Schematic of the interaction between oxygen radicals and the antioxidant system. GSH, glutathione; G6PD, glucose-6-phosphate dehydrogenase.

tissue. Paraquat readily accepts an electron from NADPH and is then rapidly reoxidized, forming superoxide and other oxygen radicals.[32] The toxicity may be a result of NADPH depletion (Fig. 24.1) and/or excess oxygen free radical generation with lipid peroxidation. Treatment with exogenous superoxide dismutase has had limited and conflicting results.[32]

A number of furans have been shown to produce oxidant injury to lungs.[32] Occasionally, patients with acute nitrofurantoin lung toxicity progress to a chronic reaction, leading to fibrosis, and rarely a patient may develop chronic toxic effects without an antecedent acute reaction. Like paraquat, nitrofurantoin undergoes cyclic reduction and reoxidation that may produce superoxide radicals or deplete NADPH. In addition, nitrofurantoin inhibits glutathione reductase, an enzyme involved in the glutathione antioxidant system (Figure 24.1).

### *Antineoplastics*

A number of cancer chemotherapeutic agents produce pulmonary fibrosis. In an excellent review, Cooper et al[31] listed six predisposing factors for the development of cytotoxic drug-induced pulmonary disease: (1) cumulative dose, (2) increased age, (3) concurrent or previous radiotherapy, (4) oxygen therapy, (5) other cytotoxic drug therapy, and (6) preexisting pulmonary disease. Drugs that are directly toxic to the lung would be expected to show a dose–response relationship. Dose–response relationships have been established for bleomycin, busulfan, and carmustine (BCNU).[24] Bleomycin and busulfan exhibit threshold cumulative doses below which a very small percentage of patients exhibit toxic effects, but carmustine shows a more linear relationship.[32] Older patients appear to be more susceptible, possibly as a result of a decrease in the antioxidant defense system.

Excessive gamma irradiation produces a pneumonitis and fibrosis thought to be caused by oxygen radical formation.[25] Evidence for synergistic toxicity with radiation exists for bleomycin, busulfan, and mitomycin.[25] Hyperoxia has shown synergistic toxicity with bleomycin, cyclophosphamide, and mitomycin.[25] Carmustine, mitomycin, cyclophosphamide, bleomycin, and methotrexate all appear to show increased lung toxicity when they are part of multiple-drug regimens.

### *Nitrosoureas*

Carmustine is associated with a high incidence of pulmonary toxicity (20%–30%).[31] The lung pathology generally resembles that produced by bleomycin and busulfan. Unique to carmustine is the finding of fibrosis in the absence of inflammatory infiltrates. Carmustine preferentially inhibits glutathione reductase, the enzyme required to regenerate glutathione, thus reducing glutathione tissue stores.[31,32] Patients present with dyspnea, tachypnea, and nonproductive cough that may begin within a month of initiation of therapy but may not develop for as long as 3 years.[29] The cumulative dose has ranged from 580 to 2,100 mg/m$^2$.[29] The disease is usually slowly progressive, with a mortality rate from 15% to greater than 90%,[25] but rapid progression and death within a few days occur in a small percentage of patients.[31] Corticosteroids do not appear to be effective in reducing damage. Other nitrosoureas, lomustine and semustine, have also been reported to produce lung damage in patients receiving unusually high doses.[31]

### *Bleomycin*

Bleomycin is the best studied cytotoxic pulmonary toxin. Because of its lack of bone marrow suppression, pulmonary toxicity is the dose-limiting toxicity of bleomycin therapy. Bleomycin-induced pulmonary disease is often used to produce animal models for interstitial pneumonitis and pulmonary fibrosis. The cumulative dose above which the incidence of toxicity significantly increases is 450 to 500 units[29,31]; however, rapidly fatal pulmonary toxicity has occurred with doses as small as 100 units.[31]

Experimentally, bleomycin generates superoxide anions, and the lung toxicity is increased by radiation and hyperoxia.[31] Pretreatment with superoxide dismutase and catalase reduces toxicity in experimental animals.[31] Bleomycin also oxidizes arachidonic acid, which may account for the marked inflammation.[31] Bleomycin may also affect collagen deposition by its stimulation of fibroblast growth.[31] Combination of bleomycin with other cytotoxic agents, particularly regimens containing cyclophosphamide, may predispose patients to pulmonary damage. Radiotherapy and high inspired concentrations of oxygen significantly enhance the development of bleomycin lung toxicity.[31]

There are two distinct clinical patterns of bleomycin pulmonary toxicity. Chronic progressive fibrosis is the most common; acute hypersensitivity reactions occur infrequently.[31] Patients present with cough and dyspnea. The first physiologic abnormality seen is a decreased carbon monoxide–diffusing capacity.[31] Chest radiographs show a bibasilar reticular pattern, and gallium scans show marked uptake in the involved lung.[31] Chest radiographic changes lag behind pulmonary function abnormalities. Spirometry tests before each bleomycin dose are not predictive of toxicity. The DLco is the most sensitive indicator of bleomycin-induced lung disease. Although it is not absolutely predictive, a drop of 20% or greater in the DLco after therapy is considered an indication for using alternative therapies.[31] Corticosteroid therapy appears to be helpful in patients with acute pneumonitis, although there have been no controlled trials.[31] Patients with chronic fibrosis would be less likely to respond.

Mitomycin is an alkylating antibiotic that produces pulmonary fibrosis at a frequency of 3% to 12%.[29–31] The mechanism is unknown, but oxygen and radiation therapy appear to enhance the development of toxicity.[29] The clinical presentation and symptoms are the same as for bleomycin. The mortality rate is about 50%. Early withdrawal of the drug and administration of corticosteroids appear to significantly improve the outcome.

### *Alkylating Agents*

A number of alkylating agents have been associated with pulmonary fibrosis. Busulfan was the first cytotoxic agent reported to cause pulmonary fibrosis in 1961.[31] The incidence of clinical toxicity is around 4%, although subclinical damage is apparent in up to 46% of patients at autopsy. The mechanism of toxicity is unknown; however, epithelial cell damage that triggers the arachidonic acid inflammatory cascade may be the initiating event.[31] The clinical presentation is insidious, with 4 years being the average duration of therapy before onset of symptoms.[30] Patients present with low-grade fever, weight loss, weakness, dyspnea, cough, and rales.[30] Pulmonary function tests initially show abnormal diffusion capacity followed by a restrictive pattern (low vital capacity). The histopathologic findings are nonspecific. The prognosis is one of slow progression with a mean survival of 5 months after diagnosis.[31] Although there is no direct dose-dependent correlation, patients receiving less than 500 mg do not develop the syndrome without concomitant radiation or other pulmonotoxic chemotherapeutic agents.[31] There are anecdotal reports of beneficial responses to corticosteroids, but no controlled studies have been done.

Cyclophosphamide infrequently produces pulmonary toxicity. There have been more than 20 well-documented cases reported to date. In animal models there is some evidence that cyclophosphamide may produce reactive oxygen radicals. High oxygen concentrations produce synergistic toxicity with cyclophosphamide. The duration of therapy before onset of symptoms is highly variable, and there may be a delay of several months between onset of symptoms and discontinuation of drugs.[25] Cyclophosphamide may potentiate carmustine lung toxicity. Clinical symptoms usually consist of dyspnea on exertion, cough, and fever. Inspiratory crackles and the bibasilar reticular pattern typical of cytotoxic drug-induced radiographic changes are present. Histopathologic changes are also nonspecific. Approximately 60% of patients recover. There have been anecdotal reports of benefit from steroids, but there have also been reports of death despite corticosteroid administration.

Chlorambucil, melphalan, and uracil mustard have also been associated with pulmonary fibrosis. Of the alkylating agents, only nitrogen mustard and thiotepa have not been reported to cause fibrotic pulmonary toxicity.[29]

### *Antimetabolites*

Methotrexate was first reported to induce pulmonary toxicity in 1969.[31] The pulmonotoxic response to methotrexate is unique in that discontinuation is not always necessary and reinstitution of the drug may not produce recurrence of symptoms.[8] Methotrexate pulmonary toxicity most commonly appears to result from hypersensitivity.[8] Pulmonary edema and eosinophilia are common and fibrosis occurs only in 10% of the patients who develop acute pneumonitis.[31] Systemic symptoms of chills, fever, and malaise are common before the onset of dyspnea, cough, and acute pleuritic chest pain.[29,30] Methotrexate has also been associated with granuloma formation.[31]

The prognosis of methotrexate-induced pulmonary toxicity is good, with a 1% or less mortality rate.[31] Pulmonary toxicity has followed intrathecal as well as oral administration, and has occurred after single doses as well as long-term daily administration.[31] Numerous anecdotal reports have claimed dramatic benefit from corticosteroid therapy.

Rarely, azathioprine and its major metabolite 6-mercaptopurine have been reported to produce an acute restrictive lung disease. Procarbazine, a methylhydrazine more commonly associated with Loeffler's syndrome, has rarely been associated with pulmonary fibrosis. The vinca alkaloids, vinblastine and vindesine, have been reported to produce severe respiratory toxicity in association with mitomycin. The incidence with the combination is 39% and may represent a true synergistic effect between these agents.[31]

### *Noncytotoxic Drugs*

Pulmonary fibrosis associated with the ganglionic blocking agent hexamethonium was first reported in 1954.[8] Patients developed extreme dyspnea after several months on the drug. Pathologic findings were consistent with bronchiectasis, bronchiolectasis, and fibrosis.[8] This phenomenon has occasionally occurred with the use of the other ganglionic blockers, mecamylamine and pentolinium.[8]

In 1959 Moore[33] reported radiographic changes characteristic of diffuse pulmonary fibrosis in 87% of 31 patients who had taken phenytoin for 2 years or longer. Since then studies have been conflicting. If phenytoin does produce chronic fibrosis, it would appear to be a relatively rare event.

Gold salts (sodium aurothiomalate) used in the treatment of rheumatoid arthritis have produced pulmonary fibrosis with cough, dyspnea, and pleuritic pain 5 to 16 weeks after institution of therapy.[25] Pulmonary function tests show a restrictive defect and patients generally have an eosinophilia. The reactions improve upon discontinuation of the gold therapy and promptly recur on reexposure. The pulmonary deficit may not completely improve.

### *Amiodarone*

The newest agent associated with pulmonary fibrosis is amiodarone, a benzofuran derivative used for supraventricular and ventricular arrhythmias.[34] The duration of amiodarone therapy before onset of symptoms has ranged from 4 weeks to 6 years.[25,34] The estimated incidence is 1 in 1,000–2,000 treated patients per year. The clinical course is variable, ranging from acute onset of dyspnea and rapid progression into severe respiratory failure and death to slowly developing exertional dyspnea over a few months. Patients generally improve upon discontinuation of the drug.[34] The majority of patients were taking maintenance doses greater than 400 mg daily.[34] Routine pulmonary function tests do not appear to be predictive in identifying patients at risk. Clinical findings include exertional dyspnea, nonproductive cough, weight loss, and occasionally low-grade fever.[25,34] Radiographic changes are nondiagnostic and consist of diffuse bilateral interstitial changes consistent with a pneumonitis. Pulmonary function abnormalities include hypoxia, restrictive changes, and diffusion abnormalities.

The mechanism of amiodarone-induced pulmonary toxicity is unknown. Amiodarone is an amphiphilic molecule that contains both a highly apolar aromatic ring system and a polar side chain with a positively charged nitrogen atom.[34] Amphiphilic drugs characteristically produce a phospholipid storage disorder in the lungs of humans and experimental animals.[33] Chlorphentermine, an anorectic, is the prototype amphiphilic compound. The mechanism is currently believed to be the inhibition of lysosomal phospholipases.[33] The inflammation and fibrosis are thought to be a late finding resulting from nonspecific inflammation following the breakdown of phospholipid-laden macrophages.[34]

In a review of 39 cases, 9 patients died and the rest had resolution of abnormalities after withdrawal of the drug.[34] Some patients have had resolution with just a lowering of the dose, and therapy has been reinstituted at lower doses without problems in others. Of the patients who died, one half received corticosteroids. There have been reports of a protective effect with prophylactic corticosteroids and other reports of patients developing amiodarone lung toxicity while on corticosteroids.[25] At this time any benefit of corticosteroids is unclear, as most patients improve with cessation of the drug.

## Miscellaneous Pulmonary Toxicity

A number of drugs may produce serious pulmonotoxic effects as part of a more generalized disorder. The pleural thickening, effusions, and fibrosis that occur as an extension of the retroperitoneal fibrotic reactions of methysergide and practolol or as part of a drug-induced lupus syndrome are the most common examples (see Table 24.8).

**Table 24.8** Drugs That May Induce Pleural Effusions and Fibrosis

| | | | |
|---|---|---|---|
| Idiopathic | | | |
| Methysergide | F[a] | Methotrexate | R |
| Practolol | F | Nitrofurantoin | R |
| Pindolol | R | | |
| Resulting from drug-induced lupus syndrome | | | |
| Procainamide | F | Trimethadione | R |
| Hydralazine | F | Sulfonamides | R |
| Isoniazid | R | Phenylbutazone | R |
| Phenytoin | R | Streptomycin | R |
| Mephenytoin | R | Ethosuximide | R |
| Griseofulvin | R | Tetracycline | R |

[a]Relative frequency of reactions: F, frequent; I, infrequent; R, rare.

Methysergide therapy for prophylaxis of poorly controlled migraine headache occasionally results in pulmonary toxicity associated with pleural effusions. The patients develop pleural pain, dyspnea, and fever. Chest radiography reveals a uniform hazy shadowing over the lower lung fields and a loud pleural rub is heard on auscultation.[8] The mechanism is unknown and most patients improve with discontinuation of the drug.

One case report of pleural and pulmonary fibrosis has been reported in a patient taking pindolol, a $\beta$ blocker, structurally similar to practolol, an agent known to produce fibrosis.[35]

Acute pleuritis with pleural effusions and fibrosis is a prominent manifestation of drug-induced lupus syndrome. Procainamide is associated with the largest number of pulmonary reactions, with 46% of patients with the lupus syndrome developing pulmonary complications.[7] Symptoms include pleuritic pain and fever with muscle and joint pain. Chest radiographs show bilateral pleural effusions and linear atelectasis. Patients have a positive antinuclear antibody (ANA) test. Symptoms usually resolve within 6 weeks of drug withdrawal.[7]

Hydralazine is the next most common cause of lupus syndrome. Most patients who develop pleuropulmonary manifestations have antecedent symptoms of generalized lupus.[7] Other drugs that produce the lupus syndrome include isoniazid and phenytoin. Phenytoin can also produce hilar lymphadenopathy as part of a generalized pseudolymphoma or lymphadenopathy syndrome.[6,8]

## References


1. Martys CR. Adverse reactions to drugs in general practice. Br Med J 1979;2:1194–1197.
2. Kramer MS, Hutchinson TA, Flegel KM, et al. Adverse drug reactions in general pediatric outpatients. J Pediatr 1985;106:305–310.
3. Levy M, Kewitz H, Altwein W, et al. Hospital admissions due to adverse drug reactions: Comparative study from Jerusalem and Berlin. Eur J Clin Pharmacol 1980;17:25–31.
4. Shapiro S, Slone D, Lewis GP, et al. Fatal drug reactions among medical inpatients. JAMA 1971;216:467–472.
5. Porter J, Jick H. Drug-related deaths among medical inpatients. JAMA 1977;237:879–881.
6. Kilburn KH. Pulmonary disease induced by drugs, in Fishman AP (ed): Pulmonary Diseases and Disorders. New York, McGraw-Hill, 1980, pp 707–724.

7. Lippman M. Pulmonary reactions to drugs. Med Clin North Am 1977;61:1353–1367.
8. Brewis RAL. Respiratory disorders, in Davies DM (ed): Textbook of Adverse Drug Reactions, 2nd ed. New York, Oxford University Press, 1981, pp 154–178.
9. Ribon A, Parikh S. Drug-induced asthma: Review. Ann Allergy 1980;44:220–4.
10. Fisher HK. Drug-induced asthma syndromes, in Weiss EB, Segal MS, Stein M (eds): Bronchial Asthma: Mechanisms and Therapeutics, 2nd ed. Boston, Little, Brown, 1985, pp 938–949.
11. Settipane GA. Aspirin and allergic diseases: Review. Am J Med 1983;74(suppl 6a):102–109.
12. Szczeklik A. Analgesics, allergy and asthma. Br J Clin Pharmacol 1980;10:401–405.
13. Stevenson DD. Diagnosis, prevention, and treatment of adverse reactions to aspirin and nonsteroidal antiinflammatory drugs. J Allergy Clin Immunol 1984;74:617–622.
14. Szczeklik A, Gryglewski RJ. Asthma and antiinflammatory drugs: Mechanisms and clinical patterns. Drugs 1983;25:533–543.
15. Simon RA. Adverse reactions to drug additives. J Allergy Clin Immunol 1984;74:623–630.
16. Lofdahl E-G, Marlin GE, Svedmyr N. Pafenolol, a highly selective $\beta_1$-adrenoceptor–antagonist, in asthmatic patients: Interactions with terbutaline. Clin Pharmacol Ther 1983;33:1–9.
17. Riddell JG, Shanks RG. Effects of betaxolol, propranolol, and atenolol on isoproterenol-induced $\beta$-adrenoceptor responses. Clin Pharmacol Ther 1985;38:554–559.
18. Fraunfeder FT, Barker AF. Respiratory effects of timolol. N Engl J Med 1984;311:1441.
19. Dunn TL, Gerber MJ, Shen AS, et el. The effect of topical ophthalmic instillation of timolol and betaxolol on lung function in asthmatic subjects. Am Rev Respir Dis 1986;133:264–268.
20. New sulfite regulations. FDA Drug Bulletin 1986;16:17–18.
21. Bush RK, Taylor SL, Busse W. A critical evaluation of clinical trials in reactions to sulfites. J Allergy Clin Immunol 1986; 78:191–202.
22. Stevenson DD, Simon RA. Sulfites and asthma. J Allergy Clin Immunol 1984;74:469–472.
23. Greenberger PA. Contrast under reactions. J Allergy Clin Immunol 1984;74:600–605.
24. Shanies HM. Noncardiogenic pulmonary edema. Med Clin North Am 1977;61:1319–1337.
25. Cooper JAD, White DA, Matthay RA. Drug-induced pulmonary disease. Part 2: Noncytotoxic drugs. Am Rev Respir Dis 1986; 133:488–505.
26. Deneke SM, Fanburg BL. Normobaric oxygen toxicity of the lung. N Engl J Med 1980;303:76–86.
27. Frank L, Massaro D. Oxygen toxicity. Am J Med 1980; 69:117–126.
28. Jackson RM. Pulmonary oxygen toxicity. Chest 1985;88:900–905.
29. Weiss RB, Muggia FM. Cytotoxic drug-induced pulmonary disease: Update 1980. Am J Med 1980;68:259–266.
30. Batist G, Andrews JL. Pulmonary toxicity of antineoplastic drugs. JAMA 1981;246:1449–1453.
31. Cooper JAD, White DA, Matthay RA. State of the art: Drug-induced pulmonary disease. Part 1: Cytotoxic drugs. Am Rev Respir Dis 1986;133:321–340.
32. Kehrer JP, Kacew S. Systematically applied chemicals that damage lung tissue. Toxicology 1985;35:251–293.
33. Moore MT. Pulmonary changes in hydantoin therapy. JAMA 1959;171:1328–1333.
34. Rakita L, Sobol SM, Mostow N, et al. Amiodarone pulmonary toxicity. Am Heart J 1983;106:906–914.
35. Musk AW, Pollard JA. Pindolol and pulmonary fibrosis. Br Med J 1979;2:581–582.

# Section Three
# Gastrointestinal Disorders

## *Chapter 25* / Gastroesophageal Reflux

Lynda S. Welage, PharmD

Gastroesophageal reflux is the retrograde movement of gastric contents from the stomach into the esophagus. In 1935, Asher Winkelstein alluded to this condition and its consequences. Winkelstein described a new clinical entity, "peptic esophagitis," that resulted from the digestive action of gastric juice on the esophageal mucosa.[1] The actual term *reflux esophagitis* was not introduced until the 1940s by Allison,[2] and since that time reflux esophagitis has referred to inflammation of the esophagus secondary to refluxed material.

By definition, gastroesophageal reflux must precede the development of reflux esophagitis. The reflux of noxious gastric material into the esophagus may also lead to a multitude of other complications, including asymptomatic reflux, hyperplasia of the esophageal epithelial lining (hyperplastic reflux), esophageal strictures, esophageal ulcers, and Barrett's esophagus.[3,4]

Richter et al proposed that the pathogenesis of gastroesophageal reflux is related to the complex balance between defense mechanisms and aggressive factors.[5] To design rational therapeutic treatment regimens, it is therefore important to understand both the normal protective mechanisms and the aggressive factors that may contribute to or promote gastroesophageal reflux. Gastric acid, pepsin, bile acids, pancreatic enzymes, and prostaglandins are considered to be aggressive factors and may promote esophageal damage upon reflux into the esophagus. Normal defense mechanisms include anatomic factors, lower esophageal sphincter, esophageal clearing, mucosal resistance, gastric emptying, gastric distension, and volume of gastric material. Rational therapeutic regimens in the treatment of gastroesophageal reflux are designed to maximize normal defense mechanisms and/or attenuate the aggressive factors.

### Pathophysiology

It is clear that numerous mechanisms normally prevent gastroesophageal reflux. The body of the esophagus lies within the negative-pressure thoracic cavity, while the abdominal cavity has a positive pressure gradient. Without natural defense mechanisms the pressure gradients would favor continual reflux of gastric material into the esophagus. This pathway of least resistance (reflux) would be further accentuated after any increase in intraabdominal pressure, such as bending over, coughing, or eating.[4,6] Numerous defense mechanisms that prevent gastroesophageal reflux have been postulated over the years.

In the 1940s and 1950s anatomic factors were considered to be of primary importance in the prevention of gastroesophageal reflux. Proposed anatomic factors can be categorized into valvular mechanisms, extrinsic compression, intraabdominal esophageal segment, mucosal choke, and spiral stretch mechanisms.[7] Disruptions of the normal anatomic barriers, such as a sliding hiatal hernia, were considered the primary etiology of gastroesophageal reflux and esophagitis.[5–7] It was suggested that the presence of hiatal hernia was diagnostic of esophageal reflux[6]; however, it was later found that numerous patients with hiatal hernia did not have symptoms of esophageal reflux, and patients with esophageal reflux did not always have hiatal hernias. In a series of 1,011 patients, Palmer showed that of the 786 patients who were found to have a hiatal hernia only 23.9% had esophagitis and 4.3% had esophageal strictures. He also found that 225 patients had esophagitis without the presence of a hiatal hernia.[8] More recently, DeMeester et al extensively studied 102 patients who had symptoms of gastroesophageal reflux and found that 53 patients had endoscopic evidence of a sliding hiatal hernia.[9] Gastroesophageal reflux was identified in 83% of the patients with hiatal hernia and 43% of the patients without hiatal hernia. Patients who had gastroesophageal reflux and a hiatal hernia had significantly decreased lower esophageal sphincter pressures, and decreased esophageal clearing ability while in a supine position.

From these studies there appears to be an association between the presence of a hiatal hernia and gastroesophageal reflux; however, no cause-and-effect relationship has been documented. Anatomic factors are still considered by some authors to be of major importance in the prevention of reflux, but the diagnosis of hiatal hernia is currently considered a separate entity with which gastroesophageal reflux may or may not simultaneously occur.

In the 1950s, Ingelfinger and associates demonstrated the

**Table 25.1** Agents That Affect Lower Esophageal Sphincter Pressure (LES)

| *Decrease LES* | *Increase LES* |
|---|---|
| Secretin | Gastrin |
| Cholecystokinin | Pentagastrin |
| Glucagon | Prostaglandin $F_{2\alpha}$ |
| Prostaglandins $E_1$, $E_2$, $A_2$ | Norepinephrine |
| Isoproterenol | Phenylephrine |
| Phentolamine | Bethanechol |
| Atropine | Methacholine |
| Theophylline | Edrophonium |
| Caffeine | Betazole |
| Gastric acidification | Gastric alkalinization |
| Fat meal | Protein meal |
| Chocolate | Metoclopramide |
| Smoking | |
| Ethanol | |

From Castell DO: The lower esophageal sphincter. Physiologic and clinic aspects. Ann Intern Med 1975;83:390–401, with permission.

presence of the lower esophageal sphincter (LES) in humans.[10] A physiologic sphincter had been hypothesized since 1822, and supported by observations that food tended to be held up in the lower esophagus.[6] The LES was not demonstrated until the development of pressure-recording devices.[6] The lower esophageal sphincter is a manometrically defined high-resting-pressure zone.[11,12] This sphincter is normally in a tonic state, preventing the reflux of gastric material from the stomach, but relaxes upon swallowing to permit the free passage of food into the stomach.[11]

Physiologic control of the lower esophageal sphincter has been extensively studied but remains controversial. Sphincter control appears to be a complex system related to the intrinsic smooth musculature, autonomic innervation, and gastrointestinal hormones.[11,12] It has been shown that numerous hormones, pharmacologic agents, and interventions may increase or decrease lower esophageal sphincter pressures (see Table 25.1).[11]

Resting pressures of the lower esophageal sphincter range from 15 to 35 mm Hg above gastric baseline pressure, and vary with manometric methodology.[3,4] In the 1960s and 1970s an incompetent lower esophageal sphincter was considered to be the primary mechanism of gastroesophageal reflux.[13] Patients with gastroesophageal reflux usually have decreased basal lower esophageal sphincter pressures, frequently less than 10 mm Hg and often less than 6 mm Hg.[3] Although a correlation exists between lower esophageal sphincter pressures and the propensity to reflux, it is important to realize that there is a significant overlap between pressure values of normal healthy individuals and those of patients with gastroesophageal reflux.[13,14]

Individuals with gastroesophageal reflux may have a hypotonic lower esophageal sphincter as demonstrated by low resting sphincter pressures; however, individuals with apparently normal lower esophageal sphincter resting pressures may experience reflux secondary to transient decreases in sphincter tone.[4,15] The exact mechanisms by which transient decreases in sphincter tone develop is unclear, but swallowing, esophageal distension, vomiting, belching, and retching have been shown to cause relaxation of the lower esophageal sphincter. A transient decrease in sphincter pressure is not always associated with gastroesophageal reflux. The propensity to develop gastroesophageal reflux secondary to transient decreases in lower esophageal sphincter pressure is probably dependent on numerous factors including degree of sphincter relaxation, efficacy of esophageal clearance, patient position, gastric volume, and intragastric pressure.[4]

As previously stated, a decrease in lower esophageal sphincter pressure resulting from any of the previously mentioned causes is not always associated with gastroesophageal reflux. It has also been shown that individuals who experience decreases in sphincter pressures and subsequently reflux do not always develop esophagitis. The other natural defense mechanisms (esophageal clearance, mucosal resistance, and gastric factors) must be evoked to explain this phenomenon.

The symptoms and/or severity of damage produced by gastroesophageal reflux are partially dependent upon the duration of contact between the gastric contents and the esophageal mucosa.[16] This contact time is dependent on the rate at which the esophagus clears the noxious material and the frequency of reflux. The esophagus is cleared by primary peristalsis in response to swallowing, secondary peristalsis in response to esophageal distension, and gravitational effects. Swallowing may also contribute to esophageal clearance by increasing salivary flow. Saliva may buffer the residual gastric material on the surface of the esophageal mucosa.

Decreased esophageal clearance has been observed in some patients who have symptomatic gastroesophageal reflux. This decrease in esophageal clearance is marked by a defect in esophageal emptying and/or a decrease in the amplitude of esophageal peristalsis.[5,16,17] Gastroesophageal reflux may contribute to decreased clearing and decreased lower esophageal sphincter pressures, both of which can potentiate further reflux. Defective esophageal clearance may be both a primary event and a secondary consequence in gastroesophageal reflux.

Gravity assists in esophageal clearance when a patient is in an upright position. DeMeester et al found that individuals who have symptomatic reflux with an upright posture experience primarily excessive acid exposure secondary to an increased frequency of reflux episodes.[18] Because esophageal clearance is impaired during sleep, excessive acid exposure, in symptomatic patients in the supine position, is due primarily to an increase in duration of reflux episodes (decreased clearance). The patient's awareness of heartburn during sleep may be impaired and this may contribute to the extended duration of acid exposure while recumbent.[18,19]

Within the esophageal mucosa and submucosa there are few mucus-secreting glands. The mucus secreted by these glands may contribute to the protection of the esophagus. Overall, information regarding mucosal resistance is lacking. In theory mucosal resistance may be related not only to esophageal mucus, but also to epithelial cell turnover, nitrogen balance, and tissue prostaglandins.[4–6] A negative nitrogen balance has been suggested to be a factor in the susceptibility of animals to develop esophagitis.[4]

Delayed gastric emptying can also contribute to gastroesophageal reflux. An increase in gastric volume may increase both the frequency of reflux and the amount of gastric fluid available to be refluxed.[4] Gastric volume is related to

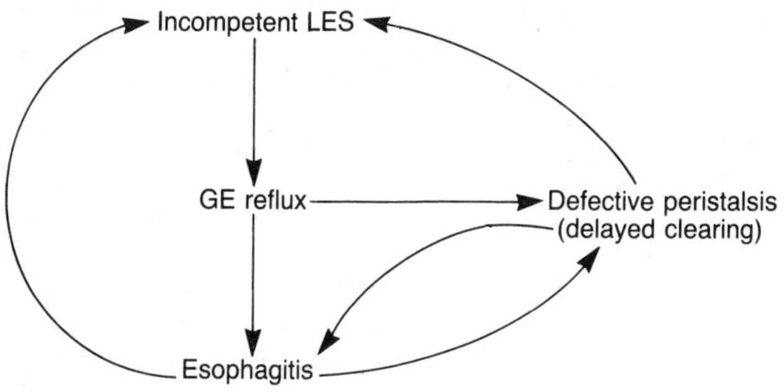


**Figure 25.1.** Schematic representation of the classic concept of the pathogenesis of gastroesophageal (GE) reflux disease and various cyclic mechanisms of potential importance. LES, lower esophageal sphincter.

the volume of material ingested, rate of gastric secretion, rate of gastric emptying, and amount and frequency of duodenal reflux into the stomach.[4] Factors that increase gastric volume and/or decrease gastric emptying are often associated with gastroesophageal reflux. This in part explains the prevalence of postprandial gastroesophageal reflux. Fatty foods may increase postprandial reflux by increasing gastric volume, delaying the gastric emptying rate, and decreasing the lower esophageal sphincter pressure.[20] Delayed gastric emptying of liquid–solid meals has been shown in approximately 41% of patients with symptoms of gastroesophageal reflux.[21]

As previously discussed the tendency for reflux depends on a complex balance of natural defense mechanisms and aggressive mechanisms. The composition and volume of the refluxate are the most important aggressive factors in determining the consequences of gastroesophageal reflux. In animals it has been shown that acid has two primary effects when it is refluxed into the esophagus. First, if the pH of the refluxate is less than 2.0, esophagitis may develop secondary to protein denaturation. Pepsin is activated at this pH and may also cause esophagitis. Alkaline esophagitis refers to esophagitis induced by the reflux of bilious and pancreatic fluid.[4] The term *alkaline esophagitis* may be a misnomer in that the refluxate may be either weakly alkaline or acidic in nature. Bile acids have both a direct irritant effect on the esophageal mucosa and an indirect effect of increasing hydrogen ion permeability of the mucosa.[22] The combination of acid, pepsin, and bile has been shown to be a potent refluxate in producing esophageal damage.[4,22]

The pathophysiology of gastroesophageal reflux is a complex, cyclic system. Reflux is a common occurrence in most individuals; however, reflux esophagitis does not always result. The development of severe reflux and its subsequent complications (esophagitis, strictures, or Barrett's esophagus) is dependent on numerous factors. Patients with symptomatic reflux may have decreased lower esophageal sphincter pressures, decreased esophageal clearing, and/or delayed gastric emptying which predisposes them to gastroesophageal reflux. The reflux of noxious substances into the esophagus and the development of esophagitis may also cause a further decrease in esophageal clearance and lower esophageal sphincter pressure, thus creating a vicious cycle (Fig. 25.1).[5] It is difficult, if not impossible, to determine which event occurred first in a given patient. Did gastroesophageal reflux lead to the noted changes or did the noted changes produce the reflux? Overall, treatment is designed to minimize gastroesophageal reflux and thus its consequences.

## Clinical Presentation

The hallmark symptom of gastroesophageal reflux and esophagitis is heartburn, or pyrosis. It is classically described as a substernal sensation of warmth or burning that may radiate to the neck.[23] It is waxing and waning in character, and is often aggravated by activities that potentiate gastroesophageal reflux (i.e., supine position, bending over). Heartburn is a common complaint of both healthy individuals and patients. Otto et al found that 36% of a healthy hospital employee population experienced heartburn at least once a month, and 7% experienced reflux symptoms on a daily basis.[24] Excluding obstetrical patients, there appears to be no sex- or age-related changes in the incidence.

Other symptoms that may occur secondary to gastroesophageal reflux and esophagitis include regurgitation, water brash, dysphagia, odynophagia, and hemorrhage.[14,23,25] These symptoms are less specific and may occur in other esophageal disorders such as esophageal diverticulum, achalasia, obstruction, esophageal spasm, esophageal infections, scleroderma, and malignancy.[26] Regurgitation is the effortless movement of food or liquid from the esophagus into the mouth; it is frequently associated with gastroesophageal reflux. In contrast, dysphagia (difficulty swallowing) and odynophagia (pain on swallowing) are less common and usually signify a more severe disease. Chronic blood loss may occur in esophagitis; however, acute blood loss is rare. Other symptoms that can result from reflux are wheezing, asthma, and bronchitis.[23,27]

The severity of the symptoms of gastroesophageal reflux does not usually correlate with the degree of esophagitis, but it does correlate with the duration of reflux.[14]

Numerous factors and conditions have been associated with the potentiation of reflux and its symptomatology. Factors that decrease LES pressure (Table 25.1) predispose patients to gastroesophageal reflux. Various foods aggravate esophageal reflux. Some of these foods cause a decrease in LES pressure; other foods such as spicy foods, orange juice, tomato juice, and coffee may precipitate symptomatic reflux by direct mucosal irritation.[24] Pregnancy, chalasia, and scleroderma are conditions in which reflux is common. The incidence of daily heartburn has been reported to be as high as 25% during pregnancy.[24] There are many postulated reasons for the increased incidence of heartburn during pregnancy including hormonal effects on esophageal muscle, lower esophageal sphincter tone, and physical factors resulting from an enlarging uterus.[24]

## Diagnosis

The most useful tool in the diagnosis of gastroesophageal reflux is the clinical history, including both presenting symptoms and associated risk factors. Patients presenting with classic symptoms of reflux do not usually require invasive esophageal evaluation; however, esophageal studies should

**Table 25.2** Diagnostic Tests for Gastroesophageal Reflux Disease

| | $N^a$ | ***Sensitivity* (%)** | ***Specificity* (%)** |
|---|---|---|---|
| Tests that indicate reflux potential | | | |
| Hiatal hernia | | — | — |
| Lower esophageal sphincter pressure (< 10 mm Hg) | 6 | 58 | 84 |
| Tests that indicate esophageal damage | | | |
| Acid perfusion (Bernstein) test | 7 | 79 | 82 |
| Endoscopy (greater-than-grade I esophagitis) | 2 | 68 | 96 |
| Mucosal biopsy | 5 | 77 | 91 |
| Barium esophagram (double contrast) | 1 | 60 | 93 |
| Tests that show reflux | | | |
| Barium esophagram | 3 | 40 | 85 |
| Standard acid reflux test | | | |
| Basal | 3 | 40 | 99 |
| Loading | 8 | 84 | 83 |
| Gastrointestinal scintiscanning | 3 | 61 | 95 |
| Prolonged pH monitoring | 5 | 88 | 98 |

[a] Number of studies from which sensitivity/specificity was calculated.

From Richter JE, Castell DO: Gastroesophageal reflux. Pathogenesis, diagnosis and therapy. Ann Intern Med 1982;97:93–103, with permission.

be used as a tool to guide the diagnosis of gastroesophageal reflux in patients when (1) the diagnosis is uncertain or presentation is atypical, (2) the patient fails to respond to treatment, (3) the possibility of associated disease exists (i.e., peptic ulcer disease), or (4) the symptomatology includes dysphagia or bleeding.[28]

The numerous diagnostic tests used to diagnose esophageal reflux can be categorized on the basis of their ability to detect (1) potential for esophageal reflux, (2) esophageal damage, and (3) presence of reflux. In 1982 Richter et al reviewed the specificity and sensitivity of the various diagnostic studies (Table 25.2).[5] Each of the tests currently available has some limitation associated with it: lack of specificity or sensitivity, difficult to perform, invasive or expensive. The first diagnostic procedure performed generally is a barium esophagram. This test provides information regarding esophageal structure and therefore is used primarily to rule out other possible diagnoses (strictures, ulcers).[28] The use or lack of use of the other diagnostic procedures is dependent on the patient's symptoms and the diagnostic facilities available.

Patients who present with atypical chest pain often require both cardiac and esophageal evaluations. The diagnosis is complicated because esophageal pain may cause electrocardiographic abnormalities, and both esophageal and cardiac disorders may occur simultaneously. In establishing a diagnosis of esophageal disease in these patients, it is crucial to document the production of chest pain simultaneously with an esophageal abnormality.[29]

## Treatment

Therapeutic modalities in the treatment of gastroesophageal reflux are targeted at reversing the various pathophysiologic abnormalities. Therapy is directed at augmenting normal defense mechanisms that may prevent reflux and/or decreasing the aggressive factors that potentiate reflux or mucosal damage. Treatment is categorized into the following modalities: life-style changes, pharmacologic interventions, and surgical interventions. Stepwise treatment, as shown in Table 25.3, is the most frequently utilized approach.[5]

The initial modality generally used in the treatment of gastroesophageal reflux is noninvasive life-style modifications. These modifications include elevation of the head of the bed, dietary changes, cessation of smoking, avoidance of tight clothing, and, if possible, discontinuation of drugs that may promote reflux. Elevation of the head of the bed 6–8 in. is a simple maneuver that significantly improves esophageal acid clearance.[30] Recommended dietary changes include the

**Table 25.3** Therapeutic Approach to Gastroesophageal Reflux Disease

| |
|---|
| Phase 1 |
| Elevation of head of the bed |
| Dietary modifications |
| Decrease or stop smoking |
| Avoid potentially harmful medications |
| Antacids or alginic acid |
| Phase 2 |
| $H_2$ antagonist (cimetidine or ranitidine) |
| Bethanechol |
| Metoclopramide |
| Future agent: sucralfate |
| Phase 3 |
| Antireflux surgery |

Adapted from Richter JE, Castell DO: Gastroesophageal reflux. Pathogenesis, diagnosis and therapy. Ann Intern Med 1982;97:93–103, with permission.

avoidance of foods that may decrease lower esophageal sphincter pressure (fats, chocolate, alcohol, peppermint, and spearmint) and foods that may have a direct irritant effect on the esophageal mucosa (spicy foods, orange juice, tomato juice, and coffee). As studies on volunteers have shown an augmentation of lower esophageal sphincter pressure after a protein-rich meal, many physicians recommend a protein-rich, low-fat diet.[20] Other dietary recommendations designed to minimize reflux potential by decreasing gastric volume include eating of small meals and avoidance of eating immediately prior to retiring to bed. Weight reduction in obese patients is also recommended based on empiric observations that this maneuver tends to decrease symptoms.

Pharmacologic agents used to treat gastroesophageal reflux include agents that decrease gastric acidity (antacids, histamine $H_2$ antagonists), provide mucosal protection (alginic acid, sucralfate), increase lower esophageal sphincter pressure (bethanechol, metoclopramide), or promote gastric emptying (metoclopramide).

Antacids are the mainstay of treatment in the management of gastroesophageal reflux. These agents are used primarily because of their acid-neutralizing ability. These agents also increase lower esophageal sphincter pressure and thus decrease reflux secondary to their alkalinization properties.[31] Originally, the ability to increase lower esophageal sphincter pressure was thought to be gastrin mediated; however, Higgs and associates observed that serum gastrin levels were not altered by gastric alkalinization.[31]

While antacids are commonly used to treat gastroesophageal reflux and esophagitis, documentation of their efficacy in placebo-controlled clinical trials is lacking. Graham et al compared liquid antacid (80 mEq per dose) taken seven times a day with placebo in a double-blind trial involving 32 patients.[32] After 5 weeks of therapy, both treatment groups showed significant improvement in heartburn frequency, severity, and degree of esophagitis, when compared with baseline. There was no significant difference in response between placebo and antacid-treated patients. The authors point out that a larger population may need to be studied to demonstrate antacid's ability to alter the natural history of the disease.

An antacid combination product, containing alginic acid, sodium bicarbonate, aluminum hydroxide, and magnesium trisilicate (Gaviscon), is frequently used in the treatment of gastroesophageal reflux. Unlike antacids, this product is not a potent neutralizing agent and does not enhance lower esophageal sphincter pressure.[33] The alginic acid component forms a highly viscous solution that floats on the surface of the gastric contents. This viscous solution may act by mechanically impairing reflux, or by coating the esophagus, thus preventing mucosal contact of the irritants in reflux material.[34] Stanciu et al and others have shown that antacid–alginic acid tablets significantly decrease the number of reflux episodes.[33,35] Stanciu and Bennett also found that the percentage of time in which esophageal pH is less than 4 was significantly decreased by the antacid–alginic acid product.[35] These results disagree with those of Johnson and DeMeester who found that the alginic acid–antacid product did not decrease esophageal acid exposure.[30]

Several studies have compared the efficacy of the combination product (alginic acid–antacid) with that of antacids alone. In a crossover trial involving 44 patients, Chevrel compared the efficacy of alginic acid–antacid liquid (Gaviscon) with that of an aluminum–magnesium antacid.[36] Eighty-three percent of the patients receiving the combination product had subjective improvement (good to very good) in symptoms, compared with a 23% response rate with the antacid. Similarly, in another double-blind crossover trial by Barnardo et al, a significant advantage of the combination product was demonstrated when compared with the antacid component without the alginic acid–alginate.[34] In contrast, Graham et al found no difference in symptomatic or endoscopic response between patients treated with alginic acid–containing antacid tablets (Gaviscon) and an aluminum–magnesium antacid.[37] Overall, these studies demonstrate that the combination product (Gaviscon) usually relieves symptoms associated with reflux; however, similar to antacids, the true pharmacologic efficacy of this product needs to be further explored.

Conservative management including both life-style modifications and antacids (with or without alginic acid) is often clinically effective in the treatment of gastroesophageal reflux and is therefore considered first-line therapy. Patients who fail to respond to conservative treatment or develop intolerable adverse effects may be treated with other pharmacologic agents as indicated in Table 25.3 as stage II of treatment.

Bethanechol is a cholinergic agent that has been shown to increase lower esophageal sphincter pressure[38,39] and improve esophageal acid clearance.[38] Esophageal pH studies have demonstrated that bethanechol significantly decreases recumbent acid exposure, but has no effect on upright acid exposure.[30]

Farrell et al conducted a double-blind crossover trial comparing bethanechol (25 mg four times a day) with placebo in 20 patients who were refractory to antacid therapy.[40] Bethanechol treatment was superior to placebo in decreasing both reflux symptomatology and as-needed antacid usage. The efficacy of bethanechol compared with high-dose antacids has been evaluated in two separate double-blind controlled studies, yielding conflicting results.[41,42] In a 4-week trial involving 44 patients, Thanik et al demonstrated that bethanechol plus antacids was significantly superior to placebo plus antacids in both symptomatic response (50% versus 13.6%) and endoscopic healing (45.5% versus 13.6%).[41] In contrast, Saco and collegues failed to document any symptomatic or endoscopic benefit of bethanechol plus antacids versus placebo plus antacids after 8 weeks of therapy.[42] Saco et al demonstrated that individuals with normal lower esophageal sphincter pressures responded better to medical therapy than individuals with decreased sphincter pressures.[42] Two major reasons for the disparate results are (1) the increase in the duration of treatment in the Saco trial may account for an increase in antacid response, and (2) the results of the Saco trial may be biased because more patients in the antacid group had normal lower esophageal sphincter pressures compared with individuals in the antacid plus bethanechol group. Bethanechol has also been shown effective in the management of reflux in pediatric patients.[43,44]

The recommended adult dosage regimen of bethanechol is 25 mg given orally four times a day. Oral bethanechol is generally well tolerated but abdominal cramps, urinary frequency, malaise, blurred vision, and diarrhea are adverse

**Table 25.4** Double-Blind Trials Comparing Cimetidine or Ranitidine With Placebo

| *Reference* | *Number of patients* | *$H_2$-antagonist daily dose* | *Improvement* | | |
|---|---|---|---|---|---|
| | | | **Symptomatic** | **Endoscopic** | **Histologic** |
| 48 | 94 | Cimetidine 1.2 g | Yes | No | — |
| 49 | 22 | Cimetidine 1.0 g | Yes | Yes | Yes |
| 50 | 20 | Cimetidine 1.6 g | No | Yes | No |
| 51 | 34 | Cimetidine 1.6 g | Yes | No | Yes |
| 52 | 20 | Cimetidine 1.6 g | No | No | — |
| 53 | 24 | Cimetidine 1.6 g | No | Yes | Yes |
| 54 | 46 | Ranitidine 300 mg | Yes | Yes | Yes |
| 55 | 284 | Ranitidine 300 mg | Yes | Yes | — |
| 56 | 73 | Ranitidine 300 mg | Yes | Yes | — |
| 57 | 36 | Ranitidine 300 mg | Yes | Yes | Yes |

effects that may rarely occur. A theoretical disadvantage of bethanechol is that it may increase gastric acid secretion secondary to its cholinergic properties. This property has not hindered its efficacy in the treatment of gastroesophageal reflux, but should be considered in the treatment of a patient who has both gastroesophageal reflux and duodenal or gastric ulcer disease.

The histamine $H_2$ antagonists decrease gastric acid secretion, which is beneficial in the treatment of gastroesophageal reflux.[5] Decreasing gastric acid secretion results in a less irritating refluxant. Neither ranitidine nor cimetidine alters lower esophageal sphincter pressure, esophageal clearance, or gastric emptying.[5,45–47]

Numerous placebo-controlled studies have been performed evaluating the efficacy of the $H_2$ antagonists (cimetidine or ranitidine) in the treatment of gastroesophageal reflux.[48–57] As shown in Table 25.4 the majority of these studies indicate symptomatic improvement with $H_2$-antagonist therapy.

To date three major studies have compared $H_2$ antagonists and antacid therapy. Petrokubi and Jeffries found cimetidine 300 mg four times a day to be both endoscopically and symptomatically superior to a standard antacid regimen, in a double-blind crossover trial involving patients with reflux disease secondary to scleroderma.[58] Furman et al also found cimetidine (300 mg four times a day) more effective than antacids in decreasing the frequency and severity of heartburn[59]; however, in a crossover trial, Grove and associates found no significant difference between ranitidine (150 mg twice a day) and antacids in symptomatic response.[60]

In a double-blind trial, Thanik et al found that cimetidine 300 mg four times a day or bethanechol 25 mg four times a day improved both symptomatic and endoscopic parameters[61]; however, there was no significant difference between the two treatment regimens.

Limited studies address the efficacy of $H_2$ antagonists in preventing recurrence of reflux disease. Bright-Asare and associates found that neither cimetidine 300 mg twice a day nor cimetidine 400 mg at bedtime was significantly superior to placebo in preventing recurrence over the 12-month study period.[62] There was a slight tendency for the twice-daily regimen to be more effective than the once-daily regimen, suggesting that higher doses should be studied. Sontag et al did a similar study comparing ranitidine 150 mg twice daily and ranitidine 150 mg at bedtime with placebo in preventing recurrence.[63] Again, there was a trend for the twice-daily regimen to be more effective; however, no significant differences were seen between active treatment and placebo.

To date the literature demonstrates that both cimetidine and ranitidine are effective in the treatment of gastroesophageal reflux. Based on the mechanism of action, one would predict that new (famotidine) and future (nizatidine) $H_2$ antagonists will also be effective in the treatment. If one chooses to use an $H_2$ antagonist, one should consider potential adverse reactions and drug interactions, efficacy, compliance, and cost in selection of the appropriate agent for a given patient. Comparative efficacy trials among the $H_2$ antagonists are currently unavailable.

Metoclopramide is a dopamine antagonist that increases lower esophageal sphincter pressure.[64,65] Stanciu and Bennett found that the rise in lower esophageal sphincter pressure was dose related until maximum tone is obtained.[65] The authors also demonstrated that the action of metoclopramide on the lower esophageal sphincter was inhibited by atropine, but was not altered in vagotomized patients. This suggests that metoclopramide may act through an intramural cholinergic neuromuscular pathway.[65] McCallum et al demonstrated that 20 mg of metoclopramide produced a greater increase in lower esophageal sphincter pressure than either 10 mg of metoclopramide or 25 mg of bethanechol.[66]

Conflicting reports exist concerning the effect of metoclopramide on esophageal peristalsis and esophageal clearance. Two studies have shown an increase in amplitude of esophageal peristaltic waves[64,65]; however, other authors have not been able to substantiate these results.[67]

Numerous studies have documented the ability of metoclopramide to accelerate gastric emptying in gastroesophageal reflux patients.[68,69] Fink et al demonstrated that 10 mg of oral metoclopramide significantly increased gastric emptying of a solid–liquid meal in reflux patients with delayed gastric emptying, as well as in patients with normal gastric emptying rates.[68] Behar and Ramsby found that antral contractility was reduced in patients with esophagitis, and both antral contractility and gastric emptying were significantly improved after a single 15-mg dose of metoclopramide.[69]

On the basis of its ability to increase lower esophageal sphincter pressure and improve gastric emptying, metoclopramide may be useful in the treatment of gastroesophageal reflux. A small double-blind crossover trial comparing metoclopramide (10 mg three times a day) with placebo demonstrated no significant difference in symptomatic improvement.[70] Paull and Grant also found no significant difference between placebo and metoclopramide (10 mg four times a day) in symptomatic response rates.[71] In 1977, McCallum et al demonstrated that metoclopramide (10 mg four times a day) was superior to placebo as measured by symptomatic response.[72] In 1983, McCallum and associates again demonstrated that metoclopramide was significantly more effective than placebo in relieving the symptoms of reflux[73]; however, endoscopic and histologic improvement was not significantly different between the two treatment groups. A double-blind trial comparing cimetidine (300 mg four times a day) and metoclopramide (10 mg four times a day) with placebo showed that metoclopramide and cimetidine significantly improved symptomatic response rates compared with placebo.[74] These authors also demonstrated that there was no significant difference in endoscopic response.

In a double-blind placebo-controlled trial, Fuchs and Bartolomeo demonstrated the efficacy of a single 20-mg dose of oral metoclopramide in preventing heartburn and regurgitation induced by a provocative test meal.[75]

A limiting factor with metoclopramide therapy may be the high incidence of adverse effects. Taylor evaluated the safety of this agent in 269 gastroesophageal reflux patients who had participated in a multicenter trial.[76] Dosage regimens ranged from 10 to 50 mg/d. Forty-eight percent of the participants experienced adverse effects and seventeen percent of the population withdrew from the study because of adverse reactions. Most commonly reported adverse reactions were somnolence (9%), nervousness (9%), fatigue (8%), dizziness (5%), weakness (3%), depression (2%), diarrhea (2%), and rash (2%). Other possible adverse reactions include anxiety, insomnia, and extrapyramidal reactions.[5]

Sucralfate is a nonabsorbable aluminum salt of sucrose octasulfate that is effective in the treatment of duodenal ulcer disease.[77] While the precise mechanism of action is unclear, local mucosal protection is achieved. Known properties include binding to inflamed tissue, formation of a barrier to prevent back-diffusion of acid and pepsin, inhibition of pepsin activity, and binding of bile salts.[77,78] On the basis of these mucosal protective properties, sucralfate may be effective in the treatment of gastroesophageal reflux. Elsborg et al studied the efficacy of a sucralfate granulate (1 g four times daily) in 18 patients with esophagitis.[78] After 12 weeks of treatments 94% of the patients demonstrated healing by endoscopy. Inflammatory changes seen on histologic examination disappeared in 60% of the cases after 12 weeks of therapy. During the course of treatment there was also a significant decrease in reflux episodes. This study indicates that sucralfate may be a promising agent in the treatment of gastroesophageal reflux disease; however, well-controlled trials are needed to determine both its efficacy and its role in the management of esophagitis.

Surgical intervention is indicated when (1) the patient fails to respond to conservative and pharmacologic treatment modalities, (2) strictures are present, (3) major bleeding occurs, and (4) pulmonary complications exist.[14] Surgical procedures include Nissen, Belsey Mark IV, and Hill operations. These surgical techniques increase resting pressure of the lower sphincter.[5,14] In approximately 80% of patients, this procedure yields improvement in lower esophageal sphincter pressure, decreased number of reflux episodes, and thus symptomatic relief.[79] Complications include recurrent reflux, obstruction, gastric ulcers, and fistula formation.[14]

## Summary

Gastroesophageal reflux and subsequent esophagitis constitute a common entity that classically presents as heartburn. The pathophysiology of reflux is complex, involving both aggressive factors (acid, pepsin, bile acids, pancreatic enzymes, prostaglandins) and defense mechanisms (anatomic factors, lower esophageal sphincter pressure, esophageal clearance, gastric emptying); however, an understanding of the pathophysiology allows the design of rational therapeutic regimens. The treatment of gastroesophageal reflux currently involves a multidisciplinary stepwise approach.

## References

1. Winkelstein A. Peptic esophagitis. A new clinical entity. JAMA 1935;104:906–909.
2. Allison PR. Peptic ulcer of the esophagus. J Thorac Surg 1946; 15:308–317.
3. Navab F, Texter EC. Gastroesophageal reflux. Pathophysiologic concepts. Arch Intern Med 1985;145:329–333.
4. Dodds WJ, Hogan WJ, Helm JF, et al. Pathogenesis of reflux esophagitis. Gastroenterology 1981;81:376–394.
5. Richter JE, Castell DO. Gastroesophageal reflux. Pathogenesis, diagnosis and therapy. Ann Intern Med 1982;97:93–103.
6. Jamieson GG, Duranceau AC. The defense mechanisms of the esophagus. Surg Clin North Am 1983;63:787–799.
7. Dodds WJ, Hogan WJ, Miller WN. Reflux esophagitis. Dig Dis 1976;21:49–67.
8. Palmer ED. The hiatus hernia esophagitis–esophageal stricture complex. Am J Med 1968;44:566–579.
9. DeMeester TR, Lafontaine E, Joelsson RE, et al. Relationship of a hiatal hernia to the function of the body of the esophagus and gastroesophageal junction. J Thorac Cardiovasc Surg 1981;82:547–558.
10. Sanchez GC, Kramer P, Ingelfinger FJ. Motor mechanisms of the esophagus, particularly of its distal portion. Gastroenterology 1953;25:321–332.
11. Castell DO. The lower esophageal sphincter. Physiologic and clinical aspects. Ann Intern Med 1975;83:390–401.
12. Pope CE II. Pathophysiology and diagnosis of reflux esophagitis. Gastroenterology 1976;70:445–454.
13. Robinson MG. Management of reflux esophageal disease. Am J Med 1984;77(suppl 5B):106–110.
14. Pope CE II. Gastroesophageal reflux disease (reflux esophagitis), in Sleisinger MH, Fordtran JS (eds): Gastrointestinal Disease: Pathophysiology, Diagnosis, Management, 3rd ed. Philadelphia, W. B. Saunders, 1983, pp 449–476.
15. Dodds WJ, Dent J, Hogan WJ, et al. Mechanisms of gastro-

esophageal reflux in patients with reflux esophagitis. N Engl J Med 1982;307:1547–1552.
16. Stanciu C, Bennett JR. Oesophageal acid clearing: One factor in the production of reflux oesophagitis. Gut 1974;15:852–857.
17. Helm JF. Esophageal acid clearance. J Clin Gastroenterol 1986; 8(suppl):5–11.
18. DeMeester TR, Johnson LF, Joseph GL, et al. Patterns of gastroesophageal reflux in health and disease. Ann Surg 1976; 184(4):459–470.
19. Orr WC, Robinson MG, Johnson LF. Acid clearance during sleep in the pathogenesis of reflux esophagitis. Dig Dis Sci 1981;26:423–427.
20. Nebel OT, Castell DO. Inhibition of the lower oesophageal sphincter by fat: A mechanism for fatty food intolerance. Gut 1973;14:270–274.
21. McCallum RW, Berkowitz DM, Lerner E. Gastric emptying in patients with gastroesophageal reflux. Gastroenterology 1981; 80:285–291.
22. Safaie-Shirazi S, DenBesten L, Zike WL. Effect of bile salts on the ionic permeability of the esophageal mucosa and their role in the production of esophagitis. Gastroenterology 1975;68:728–733.
23. Frazier JL, Fendler KJ. Current concepts in the pathogenesis and treatment of reflux esophagitis. Clin Pharm 1983;2:546–557.
24. Nebel OT, Fornes MF, Castell DO. Symptomatic gastroesophageal reflux: Incidence and precipitating factors. Dig Dis 1976; 21:953–956.
25. Behar J. Reflux esophagitis. Pathogenesis, diagnosis, and management. Arch Intern Med 1976;136:560–566.
26. Goff JS. Diagnosis and evaluation of esophageal disorders. Ear Nose Throat 1984;63:19–26.
27. Barish CF, Wu WC, Castell DO. Respiratory complications of gastroesophageal reflux. Arch Intern Med 1985;145:1882–1888.
28. Whelan G. Management of gastro-oesophageal reflux. Aust NZ J Med 1982;12:90–96.
29. Castell DO. Esophageal chest pain. Am J Gastroenterol 1984; 79:969–971.
30. Johnson LF, DeMeester TR. Evaluation of elevation of the head of the bed, bethanechol, and antacid foam tablets on gastroesophageal reflux. Dig Dis Sci 1981;26:673–680.
31. Higgs RH, Smyth RD, Castell DO. Gastric alkalinization: Effect on lower-esophageal sphincter pressure and serum gastrin. N Engl J Med 1974;291:486–490.
32. Graham DY, Patterson DJ. Double-blind comparison of liquid antacid and placebo in the treatment of symptomatic reflux esophagitis. Dig Dis Sci 1983;28:559–563.
33. Malmud LS, Charkes ND, Littlefield J, et al. The mode of action of alginic acid compound in the reduction of gastroesophageal reflux. J Nucl Med 1979;20:1023–1028.
34. Barnardo DE, Lancaster-Smith M, Strickland ID, et al. A double-blind controlled trial of "Gaviscon" in patients with symptomatic gastro-oesophageal reflux. Curr Med Res Opin 1975;3:388–391.
35. Stanciu C, Bennett JR. Alginate/antacid in the reduction of gastro-oesophageal reflux. Lancet 1974;1:109–111.
36. Chevrel B. A comparative crossover study on the treatment of heartburn and epigastric pain: Liquid Gaviscon and a magnesium–aluminium antacid gel. J Int Med Res 1980;8:300–302.
37. Graham DY, Lanza F, Dorsch ER. Symptomatic reflux esophagitis: A double-blind controlled comparison of antacids and alginate. Curr Ther Res 1977;22:653–658.
38. Miller WN, Ganeshappa KP, Dodds WJ, et al. Effect of bethanechol on gastroesophageal reflux. Dig Dis 1977;22:230–234.
39. Farrell RL, Roling GT, Castell DO. Stimulation of the incompetent lower esophageal sphincter. A possible advance in therapy of heartburn. Dig Dis 1973;18:646–650.
40. Farrell RL, Roling GT, Castell DO. Cholinergic therapy of chronic heartburn. A controlled trial. Ann Intern Med 1974;80: 573–576.
41. Thanik KD, Chey WY, Shah AN, et al. Reflux esophagitis: Effect of oral bethanechol on symptoms and endoscopic findings. Ann Intern Med 1980;93:805–808.
42. Saco LS, Orlando RC, Levinson SL, et al. Double-blind controlled trial of bethanechol and antacid versus placebo and antacid in the treatment of erosive esophagitis. Gastroenterology 1982;82:1369–1373.
43. Strickland AD, Chang JHT. Results of treatment of gastroesophageal reflux with bethanechol. J Pediatr 1983;103:311–315.
44. Euler AR. Use of bethanechol for the treatment of gastroesophageal reflux. J Pediatr 1980;96:321–324.
45. Freeland GR, Higgs RH, Castell DO. Lower esophageal sphincter response to oral administration of cimetidine in normal subjects. Gastroenterology 1977;72:28–30.
46. Denis P, Galmiche JP, Ducrotte P, et al. Effect of ranitidine on resting pressure and pentagastrin response of human lower esophageal sphincter. Dig Dis Sci 1981;26:999–1002.
47. Wallin L, Madsen T, Boesby S. Gastro-oesophageal function in normal subjects after oral administration of ranitidine. Gut 1983;24:154–157.
48. Behar J, Brand DL, Brown FC, et al. Cimetidine in the treatment of symptomatic gastroesophageal reflux. Gastroenterology 1978;74:441–448.
49. Brown P. Cimetidine in the treatment of reflux oesophagitis. Med J Aust 1979;2:96–97.
50. Ferguson R, Dronfield MW, Atkinson M. Cimetidine in the treatment of reflux oesophagitis with peptic stricture. Br Med J 1979;25:472–474.
51. Fiasse R, Hanin C, Lepot A, et al. Controlled trial of cimetidine in reflux esophagitis. Dig Dis Sci 1980;25:750–755.
52. Greaney MG, Irvin TT. Cimetidine for the treatment of symptomatic gastro-oesophageal reflux. Br J Clin Pract 1981;35:21–24.
53. Wesdorp E, Bartelsman J, Pape K, et al. Oral cimetidine in reflux esophagitis: A double blind controlled trial. Gastroenterology 1978;74:821–824.
54. Hine KR, Holmes GKT, Melikian V, et al. Ranitidine in reflux oesophagitis: A double-blind placebo controlled study. Digestion 1984;29:119–123.
55. McCallum RW, Eshelman F, Nardi R, et al. A double-blind multicenter trial to compare the efficacy of ranitidine and placebo in the short-term treatment of chronic gastroesophageal reflux disease. Gastroenterology 1984;86(5 part 2):1179.
56. Sherbaniuk R, Wensel R, Bailey R, et al. Ranitidine in the treatment of symptomatic gastroesophageal reflux disease. J Clin Gastroenterol 1984;6:9–15.
57. Wesdorp E, Dekker W, Klinkenberg-Knol EC. Treatment of reflux oesophagitis with ranitidine. Gut 1983;24:921–924.
58. Petrokubi RJ, Jeffries GH. Cimetidine versus antacid in scleroderma with reflux esophagitis: A randomized double blind controlled study. Gastroenterology 1979;77:691–695.
59. Furman D, Mensh R, Winan G, et al. A double-blind trial comparing high dose liquid antacid to placebo and cimetidine in improving symptoms and objective parameters in gastroesophageal reflux. Gastroenterology 1982;82(5 part 2):1062.
60. Grove O, Bekker C, Jeppe-Hansen MG, et al. Ranitidine and high dose antacid in reflux oesophagitis: A randomized, placebo-controlled trial. Scand J Gastroenterol 1985;20:457–461.
61. Thanik K, Chey WY, Shak A, et al. Bethanechol or cimetidine

in the treatment of symptomatic reflux esophagitis: A double-blind control study. Arch Intern Med 1982;142:1479–1481.

62. Bright-Asare P, Behar J, Brand DL, et al. The effects of long term maintenance cimetidine therapy on gastroesophageal reflux disease. Gastroenterology 1982;82(5 part 2):1025.

63. Sontag S, Vlahcevic R, Orr W, et al. Ranitidine versus placebo in longterm treatment of gastroesophageal reflux. Gastroenterology 1985;88(5 part 2):1595.

64. Dilawari JB, Misiewicz JJ. Action of oral metoclopramide on the gastroesophageal junction in man. Gut 1973;14:380–382.

65. Stanciu C, Bennett JR. Metoclopramide in gastroesophageal reflux. Gut 1973;14:275–279.

66. McCallum RW, Kline MM, Curry N, et al. Comparative effects of metoclopramide and bethanechol on lower esophageal sphincter pressure in reflux patients. Gastroenterology 1975;68:1114–1118.

67. Behar J, Biancani P. Effect of oral metoclopramide on gastroesophageal reflux in the post-cibal state. Gastroenterology 1976;70:331–335.

68. Fink SM, Lange RC, McCallum RW. Effect of metoclopramide on normal and delayed gastric emptying in gastroesophageal reflux patients. Dig Dis Sci 1983;28:1057–1061.

69. Behar J, Ramsby G. Gastric emptying and antral motility in reflux esophagitis: Effect of oral metoclopramide. Gastroenterology 1978;74:253–256.

70. Venables CW, Bell D, Eccleston D. A double-blind study of metoclopramide in symptomatic peptic oesophagitis. Postgrad Med J 1973;(suppl, July):73–76.

71. Paull A, Grant AK. A controlled trial of metoclopramide in reflux oesophagitis. Med J Aust 1974;2:627–629.

72. McCallum RW, Ippoliti AF, Cooney C, et al. A controlled trial of metoclopramide in symptomatic gastroesophageal reflux. N Engl J Med 1977;296:354–357.

73. McCallum RW, Fink SM, Winnan GR, et al. Metoclopramide in gastroesophageal reflux disease: Rationale for its use and results of a double-blind trial. Am J Gastroenterol 1984;79:165–172.

74. Bright-Asare P, El-Bassoussi M. Cimetidine, metoclopramide, or placebo in the treatment of symptomatic gastroesophageal reflux. J Clin Gastroenterol 1980;2:149–156.

75. Fuchs B, Bartolomeo RS. Prevention of meal-induced heartburn and regurgitation with metoclopramide in patients with gastroesophageal reflux. Clin Ther 1982;5:179–185.

76. Taylor DM. Evaluation of the safety of metoclopramide in patients with gastroesophageal reflux disease. Clin Ther 1984;7:28–32.

77. Siepler JK, Mahakain K, Trudeau WT. Current concepts in clinical therapeutics: Peptic ulcer disease. Clin Pharm 1986;5:128–142.

78. Elsborg L, Beck B, Stubgaard M. Effect of sucralfate on gastroesophageal reflux in esophagitis. Hepatogastroenterology 1985;32:181–184.

79. Brand DL, Eastwood IR, Martin D, et al. Esophageal symptoms, manometry and histology before and after antireflux surgery: A long term follow up study. Gastroenterology 1979;76:1393–1401.

# Chapter 26 / Peptic Ulcer Disease and Zollinger–Ellison Syndrome

Rosemary R. Berardi, PharmD

## Peptic Ulcer Disease

Peptic ulcer disease (PUD) refers to a group of ulcerative disorders of the upper gastrointestinal tract that appear to require acid and pepsin for their formation. An ulcer differs from an erosion in that it extends through the submucosa into the muscularis mucosae or deeper (Fig. 26.1). True (chronic) peptic ulcers are distinguished from acute ulcers (i.e., drug-induced ulcers) by their depth, etiology, clinical presentation, and tendency to recur. The most frequently occurring ulcers are gastric and duodenal, although ulcers occasionally develop in the distal esophagus and the jejunum. The Zollinger–Ellison syndrome may also be considered a cause of PUD.

Chronic peptic ulcers represent a major health problem in terms of human suffering and cost to society. Both direct costs (i.e., hospital care, physician costs, drug costs) and indirect costs (i.e., lost productivity at work) are incurred as a result of this disease. It has been estimated that 10% to 15% of all Americans will develop PUD during their lifetime. More than 400,000 patients with a diagnosis of peptic ulcer were hospitalized in the United States in 1978.[1] Although overall hospitalizations and mortality related to ulcer disease have declined during the last decade, it is not certain whether this decrease is due to the reduced incidence of new ulcer cases or the combined influence of changes in diagnostic practices, more effective treatment, and fewer serious manifestations of the disease.

### *Epidemiology*

#### Duodenal Ulcer

The absolute incidence of duodenal ulcer is difficult to determine and varies with geographic region. Estimates for the United States suggest that about one-half million new cases of duodenal ulcer occur yearly. An additional four to eight million Americans suffer from active or recurrent disease. The reported decrease in overall peptic ulcer–related hospitalizations results almost exclusively from a reduction in hospital admissions for duodenal ulcer, as evidenced by a decline of 43% in the hospitalization rate over the period 1970 to 1978.[1] Duodenal ulcer is about two to three times more common in men; however, the male-to-female ratios for hospitalization and mortality appear to suggest a recent increase in the proportion of women with duodenal ulcer. Race, occupation, and sociologic factors do not appear to correlate with the incidence of duodenal ulcer.

#### Gastric Ulcer

Gastric ulcers appear to occur less frequently than duodenal ulcers. The total number of patients in the United States with a gastric ulcer is unknown; however, more than 100,000 patients are hospitalized each year with a chronic benign gastric ulcer. The hospitalization rate for gastric ulcer has not changed significantly.[1] The reasons for this lack of change are not known; it may reflect a different pathogenesis for gastric and duodenal ulcer, new treatments more specific for duodenal ulcer, or occurrence of gastric ulcers in older patients with other diseases that require hospitalization. Gastric ulcers rarely develop before the age of 40; incidence peaks between ages 55 and 65, approximately 10 years later than for duodenal ulcer. The incidence is approximately the same for men and women.

### *Etiology*

A number of factors have been postulated to play a role in the etiology of PUD and may be important considerations in determining the risk of ulcer recurrence.

#### Cigarette Smoking

There is strong epidemiologic evidence that suggests an association between cigarette smoking and peptic ulceration. Cigarette smoking is associated with an increased frequency of both gastric and duodenal ulcers and the risk may be proportional to the amount smoked.[2,3] Smoking impairs duodenal ulcer healing, but it is unknown whether it affects the healing rate of gastric ulcers.[4] Cigarette smoking has been shown to be an important risk factor in duodenal ulcer recurrence.[5] The specific reasons why cigarette smoking influences ulcer formation, healing, and recurrence remain unclear, but possible mechanisms include accelerated gastric emptying, increased basal acid secretion, decreased pancreatic bicarbonate secretion, and reflux of duodenal contents. Death rates from peptic ulcers are higher among patients who smoke than among nonsmokers, although it is not known whether this apparent increase in mortality reflects

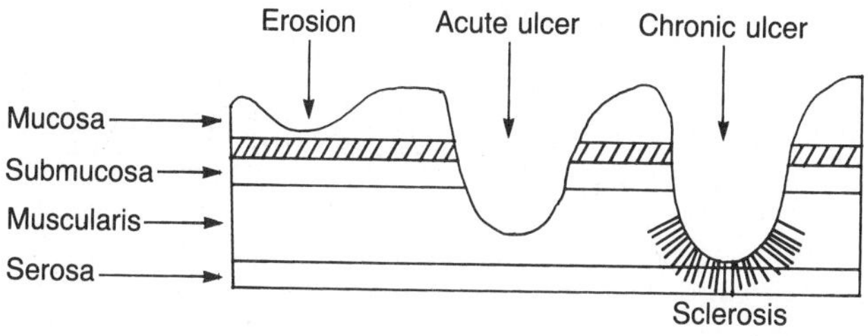


**Figure 26.1** Morphologic distinction between erosions and acute and chronic ulcers. *(From Brook FP: Dig Dis Sci 1985;30(suppl): 15S–29S, with permission.)*

severe ulcer disease or the cardiac and pulmonary sequelae of smoking. There are no satisfactory data on an association between cigar or pipe smoking and ulcer occurrence.

**Alcohol**

Although high alcoholic consumption is associated with acute gastric mucosal lesions and upper gastrointestinal bleeding, there is insufficient evidence to indicate that alcohol is an important factor in the pathogenesis of gastric or duodenal ulcers[6]; however, alcoholic cirrhosis of the liver is associated with an increased incidence of duodenal ulcers (see Chapter 31).

**Diet**

Certain foods, beverages, and spices may cause dyspepsia, but there are no convincing data to indicate that consumption of any of these dietary products is associated with an increased incidence or recurrence of peptic ulcer. Although coffee, decaffeinated coffee, cola beverages, beer, and milk are stimulants of acid secretion, they do not appear to cause ulcers. Beverage restrictions and bland diets do not alter the frequency or severity of ulcer recurrence. Patients should be advised to be moderate in their consumption of alcohol and caffeine and to avoid those foods that bring on ulcer symptoms.

**Drugs**

The relationship between ulcer disease and drug consumption is clouded by statistic, epidemiologic, and pathophysiologic problems. Additionally, gastric and duodenal ulcers must be differentiated, as a drug may affect only one site. No studies to date have adequately described the incidence of drug-related ulcer disease.

***Aspirin*** Aspirin and other salicylates damage the gastric mucosa, precipitate upper gastrointestinal bleeding, and appear to cause gastric ulcers.[7] Numerous mechanisms whereby aspirin and salicylates damage the mucosa have been suggested, the most important of which is their ability to inhibit prostaglandin synthesis. Thus, protective mechanisms are disturbed, allowing acid, pepsin, or bile to produce mucosal damage. Gastric ulcers tend to occur more frequently in patients receiving prolonged low (1 g/d) doses[8] and in those taking large (2.4 g/d) doses of aspirin.[7,9] A dose–response effect appears to exist for both short- and long-term aspirin ingestion.

The relationship between aspirin and duodenal ulcer is less certain. Aspirin preparations influence the incidence of ulcers, with a decreased incidence reported in users of enteric-coated aspirin products[7,10]; however, gastric ulcer occurrence is reported to be as high in those taking buffered aspirin as in those taking regular aspirin.[7,10] Preliminary studies indicate that prostaglandins may be effective in preventing gastric mucosal injury induced by aspirin and other nonsteroidal anti-inflammatory agents.[11]

***Nonsteroidal Anti-inflammatory Drugs*** Nonsteroidal anti-inflammatory drugs (NSAIDs) are often used as aspirin substitutes, and, like aspirin, they inhibit prostaglandin synthesis. While indomethacin and phenylbutazone are potent irritants of the gastrointestinal tract, the newer NSAIDs appear to cause less upper gastrointestinal toxicity.[12] Although the frequency of dyspeptic symptoms and gastrointestinal bleeding may be less with the newer agents, there is no conclusive evidence linking these effects with a decreased incidence of gastric ulcer.

***Corticosteroids*** The effect of corticosteroids on the incidence of ulcer disease is controversial and remains unresolved, primarily because studies were retrospective, concurrent medications were not identified, and radiography was often used instead of endoscopy to detect ulcer occurrence. The administration of steroids for more than 30 days or a total prednisone-equivalent dose in excess of 1 g has been associated with an increased risk of ulcers,[13] whereas others report an increased incidence in less time and with any steroid dose.[14] Although the evidence obtained from these retrospective reviews is inadequate to support firm conclusions, it is likely that corticosteroids cause ulcers and that the risk varies not only with dose and duration, but also with age, sex, nutrition, underlying diseases, and route of administration.

**Associated Diseases**

Certain diseases have been associated with an increased incidence of peptic ulcer, although some of these associations have been based on inconclusive evidence (Table 26.1) The increased incidence of ulcers in patients with rheumatoid arthritis is thought to be related to the ulcerogenic action of aspirin. Peptic ulcers may occur less frequently in patients with pernicious anemia and associated atrophic gastritis, hypertension, and Addison's disease.[15]

**Genetic Factors**

Peptic ulcer disease is thought to be a group of heterogeneous disorders with multiple genetic and environmental causes. First-degree relatives of patients with duodenal or gastric ulcers are at increased risk of developing the same type of ulcer. The gene for blood group O is associated with about a 30% increase in duodenal ulcer incidence compared with other blood groups. Hyperpepsinogenemia I, multiple endocrine neoplasia type I, systemic mastocytosis, and amyloidosis type IV have also been associated with duodenal ulcers.

**Psychologic Factors**

The importance of psychologic factors and stress in the genesis of ulcer disease remains controversial. Although clinical observation supports the belief that many ulcer

**Table 26.1** Chronic Diseases Associated With an Increased Incidence of Peptic Ulcer

| |
|---|
| Definite association |
| Gastrinoma and multiple endocrine tumors, type I |
| Probable association |
| Chronic pulmonary disease |
| Chronic renal failure |
| Cirrhosis of the liver |
| Renal stones |
| Rheumatoid arthritis (because of aspirin therapy) |
| Systemic mastocytosis |
| Basophilic leukemia |
| Association claimed, firm evidence lacking |
| Crohn's disease |
| Carcinoma of the lung |
| Coronary heart disease |
| Cystic fibrosis |
| Chronic pancreatitis |
| Small-bowel resection |
| Hyperparathyroidism |
| Polycythemia vera |
| α-Antitrypsin deficiency |
| Myasthenia gravis |
| Cushing's disease |

patients are excessively affected by stressful life events, scientific studies have failed to support a cause-and-effect relationship.[15] Psychologic factors may be of major importance in predisposing selected patients to PUD and in determining the degree of pain or disability that results from an ulcer in any one patient.

## Gastric Physiology

### Acid Secretion

***Chemical Mediators*** Three major endogenous substances stimulate the parietal cell to secrete acid: acetylcholine, gastrin, and histamine. Acetylcholine is released by postganglionic vagal neurons; gastrin is released from the gastric mucosal antral G cells, and histamine is released by mast cells located in the lamina propria. The parietal cell contains specific receptors for acetylcholine, gastrin, and histamine (Fig. 26.2). Blockade of these receptors inhibits acid secretion and forms the basis for drug therapy. A large number of endogenous chemical messengers inhibit acid secretion. These agents include somatostatin, calcitonin, glucagon, dopamine, vasoactive intestinal peptide, and prostaglandins.[16]

***Second Messengers*** It is likely that there are two second messengers within the parietal cell that regulate acid secretion: intracellular cyclic AMP and intracellular free calcium.[16] Histamine is thought to stimulate the production of cyclic AMP by the parietal cell and intracellular calcium ions are thought to mediate the cholinergic and gastrin response (Figure 26.2).

***Proton Pump*** The secretion of acid by the parietal cell into the gastric lumen occurs against a concentration gradient and requires an active energy-dependent process. Through a series of intracellular events, cyclic AMP and calcium activate hydrogen/potassium adenosine triphosphatase (ATPase) enzyme, which stimulates the proton pump located in the apical membrane of the parietal cell. This action catalyzes a one-to-one exchange of intracellular hy-

**Figure 26.2** Stimulants of acid secretion and sites of action of antiulcer drugs. H, histamine; ACh, acetylcholine; Antichol, anticholinergic; Gas, gastrin; Som, somatostatin; Gas-ant, gastrin antagonist. *(From Bertaccini G, Coruzzi G: Dig Dis Sci 1985;30(suppl):43S–51S, with permission.)*

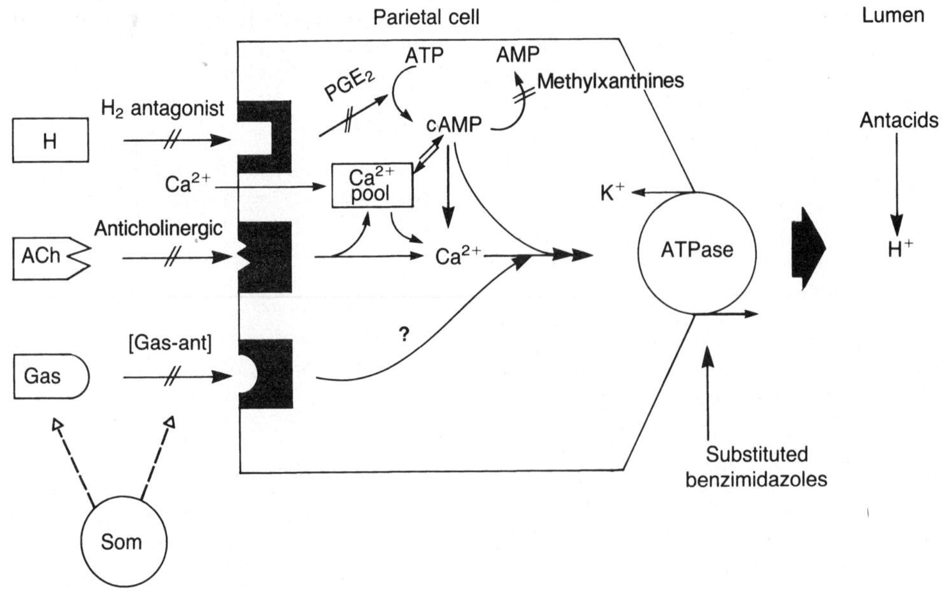

drogen ions for luminal potassium ions (Fig. 26.2). The hydrogen/potassium ATPase proton pump is probably the terminal step in acid secretion.[16]

***Regulation of Acid Secretion*** Basal secretion, or basal acid output (BAO), reflects a continuous fasting gastric acid secretion under the control of vagal stimulation, gastrin, and histamine. Normal BAO is approximately 2–5 mEq/h. Duodenal ulcer patients appear to have an elevated nocturnal BAO thought to be related to the circadian rhythm of histamine.

Maximum acid output (MAO) represents the sum of four 15-minute acid output measurements after an injection of pentagastrin, betazole, or histamine and is an indirect estimator of the parietal cell mass (total number of gastric parietal cells). Peak acid output (PAO) represents the sum of the two highest acid outputs (multiplied by 2) after stimulation. Normal MAO is approximately 20–40 mEq/h. Basal, maximum, and peak acid outputs vary with age, sex, and health status. The ratio of BAO/MAO or PAO represents the fraction of the parietal cell mass that is functional under basal conditions. A higher-than-normal ratio of BAO/MAO indicates that a patient has a basal hypersecretory state such as Zollinger–Ellison syndrome.

***Phases of Stimulated Acid Secretion*** Stimulated acid secretion can be divided into three phases: cephalic, gastric, and intestinal (Table 26.2). Each stage has different mechanisms of stimulation and inhibition.

The cephalic phase is initiated by the sight, smell, and taste of food and is mediated by vagal stimulation of the parietal cells, producing the release of acetylcholine, and the antral G cells, releasing gastrin. The gastric phase results from stimuli acting within the stomach. Two mechanisms stimulate the parietal cell to secrete acid in this phase: gastric distension, which activates vagal nerves in the gastric wall, and the chemical constituents of food (amino acids and peptides), which are mediated by gastrin release. The increased acid response provides a negative-feedback mechanism by suppressing gastrin output.

Chyme in the small intestine stimulates the intestinal phase of gastric acid secretion by either a neurohumoral stimulus or the effect of circulating amino acids. Intraluminal acid, fat, and hyperosmolar solutions inhibit gastric secretion during the intestinal phase. Inhibition of gastric acid secretion by intestinal acid is mediated by secretin. Fats inhibit acid secretion through the release of various gut hormones, including cholecystokinin and gastric inhibitory peptide. The method by which hyperosmolar duodenal contents suppress acid secretion is not known.

**Pepsin Secretion**

The chief cells in the stomach secrete pepsinogen, which is converted to pepsin by gastric acid at an optimal pH of 1.8–3.5. The rate of pepsinogen secretion is usually directly proportional to the rate of acid secretion. Pepsinogens I and II differ in their mucosal distribution and cellular origin. Although most patients with duodenal ulcers have normal pepsinogen secretion rates, ulcer patients with high levels of pepsinogen I have been described.

**Mucosal Defense**

The term "cytoprotection" refers to the ability of the gastroduodenal mucosa to protect itself from autodigestion. Factors believed to be important in mucosal defense include mucus secretion, bicarbonate secretion, mucosal blood flow, and rapid cellular repair after injury. Although the precise mechanisms of cytoprotection are not known, the maintenance of normal mucosal integrity has been linked to mucosal production of prostaglandins.[17,18]

***Mucus Secretion*** Mucus is continuously secreted onto the surface of the gastric and duodenal mucosa and is thought to have two major functions: lubrication and the formation of an "unstirred" layer that impedes hydrogen ion back-diffusion (the permeability of hydrogen ions from the stomach lumen into the gastric mucosa). The extent to which mucus alters the susceptibility of individuals to ulceration is unknown.

***Bicarbonate Secretion*** Bicarbonate is secreted by the gastric and duodenal mucosa, the pancreas, and the biliary system. Most gastric bicarbonate remains trapped within the mucus layer where it is thought to play an important role in maintaining mucosal defense. A small quantity reaches the lumen and is neutralized by hydrogen ions. The balance between stimulation and inhibition of mucosal bicarbonate appears to be an important factor in the pathogenesis of ulcer disease.

***Blood Flow*** Decreased blood flow that results in local ischemia has been linked to the development of stress-related mucosal lesions (stress ulcers); however, it is not

**Table 26.2** Phases of Acid Secretion

| *Phase* | *Stimulus* | *Total stimulation (%)* |
|---|---|---|
| Basal | Endogenous | 15 |
| Cephalic | Sight, smell, and taste of food, mediated by vagus nerve | 30 |
| Gastric | Food in stomach causes distension and stimulation of gastrin by amino acids | 50 |
| Intestinal | Digested food in jejunum | 5 |

known whether a reduction in mucosal blood flow also contributes to the pathogenesis of PUD.

*Epithelial Cell Restoration* Gastrointestinal surface epithelial cells have a rapid turnover rate and, when injured, migrating gastric pit cells are immediately available to restore the damaged surface epithelium.

*Prostaglandins* Prostaglandins are produced by the gastrointestinal mucosal cells and have numerous effects on the gastrointestinal tract, including maintenance of mucosal integrity. This cytoprotective effect seems to result from the prostaglandins' increasing mucus and bicarbonate secretion, increasing mucosal blood flow, and enhancing epithelial cellular repair.[17,18]

## *Pathophysiology*

Peptic ulcers are thought to develop because of an imbalance between aggressive factors (acid, pepsin, bile salts) and defensive factors (mucus, bicarbonate, blood flow, epithelial cell restoration, prostaglandins). Although environmental factors may contribute to the pathogenesis of gastric and duodenal ulcers, the importance of these factors in individual patients is difficult to determine because numerous pathogenic mechanisms may be involved.

### Duodenal Ulcer

Most duodenal ulcers occur in the first part of the duodenum (duodenal bulb). Pathophysiologic abnormalities producing duodenal ulcer are complex, but are thought to be related to an absolute or relative increase in duodenal acidity.[15,17] Most patients with duodenal ulcers have normal acid secretory rates; however, duodenal ulcers develop in some individuals because of pathophysiologic defects leading to high rates of acid secretion. These abnormalities include increased parietal and chief cell mass, increased basal secretory drive (high ratio of BAO to MAO), and increased foot-stimulated acid secretion. Accelerated gastric emptying may be an important factor leading to a relative increase in acidification of the duodenal bulb. Cigarette smoking is thought to impair pancreatic bicarbonate secretion and may be a factor in smoking-related duodenal ulcer, although the significance of mucosal defense mechanisms remains unclear. Infectious agents, such as *Campylobacter pylori*, have been hypothesized as pathogenic factors.[19]

### Gastric Ulcer

Most benign gastric ulcers and aspirin-associated gastric ulcers are located in the antrum of the stomach, on the lesser curvature, just distal to the acid-secreting mucosa. In contrast to duodenal ulcer, patients with gastric ulcers have normal or reduced rates of gastric acid secretion.[17,20]

Although the pathophysiology of gastric ulcer is not fully elucidated, most research suggests defects in antral–pylorus–duodenal motility. Abnormal motility patterns permit duodenal contents to reflux into the stomach with resultant damage to the gastric mucosa. Delayed gastric emptying can increase exposure of acid, pepsin, and refluxed duodenal contents to the gastric mucosa. It appears that bile salts and pancreatic secretions damage the gastric mucosa and allow back-diffusion of hydrogen ions. This action is thought to result in ulcer formation.[20]

The gastric mucosal barrier may also be damaged by drugs such as aspirin and nonsteroidal anti-inflammatory agents whose mechanism is probably related, in part, to prostaglandin inhibition. Thus, evidence supports the importance of primary defects in gastric mucosal resistance and/or direct gastric mucosal injury as the most important elements in the pathogenesis of gastric ulcer.

## *Clinical Presentation/Diagnosis*

### Symptoms

Epigastric pain is the classic and most frequent symptom of duodenal ulcer. The pain is often described as burning or gnawing but can present as a vague discomfort, abdominal fullness, or cramping. Characteristically, the pain occurs 1 to 3 hours after meals and is usually relieved by food or antacids. About 50% to 80% of patients report being awakened with pain at night. Other dyspeptic symptoms, such as belching, bloating, and distension, occur in 40% to 70% of patients.[15]

The severity of symptoms varies from patient to patient, with discomfort lasting up to a few weeks followed by a symptom-free period or remission lasting from weeks to years. Pain does not always correlate with the presence or absence of ulcer craters. From 15% to 44% of symptom-free patients have been found to have a duodenal ulcer at endoscopy, whereas 4% to 39% of endoscopically proven healed ulcer patients have reported persistent symptoms.[15] Changes in the character of the pain may indicate the presence of complications.

Epigastric pain is also the most common symptom in patients with gastric ulcer; however, the pain is much less typical and unpredictable than in duodenal ulcer. Food may precipitate or accentuate the pain and antacids appear to provide less consistent relief. Weight loss is a common finding in patients with either benign or malignant gastric ulcers.[20]

### Physical Examination

The physical examination generally reveals epigastric tenderness, which usually occurs between the umbilicus and the xiphoid process and less commonly radiates to the back. This sign is neither a specific nor a sensitive indicator of duodenal or gastric ulcers. The development of complications associated with PUD (i.e., obstruction, perforation, and hemorrhage) may become evident on physical examination. Unusual findings may be present when duodenal ulcers are associated with hypersecretory states such as Zollinger–Ellison syndrome (see Zollinger–Ellison Syndrome).

### Laboratory Tests

Measurement of gastric acid secretion is not necessary for most patients with uncomplicated duodenal or benign gastric ulcer. Acid secretory studies and a fasting serum gastrin concentration are recommended in those patients unresponsive to therapy and/or cases in which gastrinoma or other hypersecretory states are suspected.

### Endoscopy/Radiography

Duodenal ulcers should be distinguished from other peptic diseases, and benign gastric ulcers must be distinguished from malignant gastric ulcers. The clinical presentations of these disorders do not allow differentiation on the basis of symptoms. Therefore, the diagnosis depends upon radiographic and/or endoscopic findings. Routine single-barium-contrast techniques can detect 30% of peptic ulcers, whereas it is possible to detect approximately 60% of ulcers using double-contrast radiography. Fiber-optic endoscopy detects more than 90% of peptic ulcers and permits direct inspection, biopsy, and visualization of superficial erosions and sites of active hemorrhage. Because of lower cost, greater availability, and perhaps greater safety, many physicians believe that radiography should remain the initial diagnostic procedure in evaluating most patients with suspected peptic ulcer; however, if an accurate diagnosis of peptic ulcer disease is warranted, endoscopy is the diagnostic procedure of choice.

### Clinical Course

The natural history of PUD is characterized by a variable but high tendency for spontaneous ulcer healing. Nevertheless, rapid and frequent ulcer recurrences can be expected in patients after initial healing of both gastric and duodenal ulcers. Symptoms usually appear in clusters with intermittent asymptomatic periods that last a few months to a few years. Two thirds of patients with duodenal ulcers can expect to have their disease subside over a 10- to 15-year period.[15] About 10% of all ulcer patients experience complications from their ulcer disease. Mortality in patients with gastric ulcer is slightly higher than in patients with duodenal ulcer and the general population.[20] Although the effectiveness of treatment for healing and prevention of ulcers is well documented, there is no evidence that ulcer treatment positively affects the natural history of the disease.

## *General Treatment*

The ultimate goals in peptic ulcer treatment are relief of pain, healing of the ulcer, and prevention of ulcer recurrences. In the past, treatment consisted primarily of dietary maneuvers, antacids, and anticholinergics. Today, treatment is based on major technologic developments (i.e., fiber-optic endoscopy, $H_2$-receptor antagonists) and on scientific information obtained during the last 20 years.

A number of studies have demonstrated the strong relationship between cigarette smoking and ulcer frequency, impaired ulcer healing, and ulcer recurrence.[2–5] Patients should be advised to stop smoking cigarettes. Although there is no evidence that alcohol is related to ulcer pathogenesis, it does damage the ulcer mucosa and may cause gastritis.[6] Patients with peptic ulcers should be advised to eliminate or at least decrease alcohol intake. Because salicylate-containing compounds, nonsteroidal anti-inflammatory drugs, and corticosteroids may damage the mucosa, they should be avoided especially during the time an active ulcer is present. Dietary restrictions have not been shown to enhance ulcer healing; however, patients should be advised to avoid those beverages and foods that aggravate their symptoms.

## *Drug Treatment*

Medical therapy has been directed primarily at either neutralizing or inhibiting the aggressive pathogenic factors of acid and pepsin. Only recently have serious attempts been made to develop agents that enhance mucosal defense. At present, only antacids, the $H_2$ receptor antagonists—cimetidine (Tagamet, Smith Kline & French), ranitidine (Zantac, Glaxo), famotidine (Pepcid, Merck Sharp & Dohme), and nizatidine (Axid, Lilly)—and sucralfate (Carafate, Marion) have been approved by the Food and Drug Administration (FDA) for use in healing ulcers. The $H_2$ receptor antagonists currently represent the cornerstone in antiulcer therapy. Although these agents are considered generally safe and effective, recent findings on the physiologic regulation of acid secretion and mucosal defense mechanisms have prompted the investigation of new compounds in the United States, Europe, and Japan.

Ulcer trials are complicated by the variability in ulcer-healing rates in placebo-treated patients, which range from 20% to 80% in a 4- to 8-week period. Such factors as geographic location, smoking, alcohol and aspirin ingestion, antacid consumption, study duration, method and frequency of confirming ulcer healing (i.e., radiology versus endoscopy), and presence or absence of ulcer symptoms may influence reported healing and recurrence rates.

Drugs used to treat peptic ulcers may be classified according to their sites and mechanisms of action (Table 26.3).

### Agents That Neutralize Gastric Acid

*Antacids* Antacids reduce gastric acidity by neutralizing secreted gastric acid. The ulcer-healing effects of antacids may also result from their inactivation of pepsin and bile acids. Antacid preparations vary widely in their neutralizing capacity (Table 26.4). Their therapeutic efficacy appears to depend upon the dose of antacid used, and the timing of administration in relationship to meals. Antacids are effective for only 30 minutes when taken in the fasting state. Meals provide a buffering effect for about 1 hour and prolong the duration of antacid-neutralizing effects (Fig. 26.3) for an additional 2 hours. This information forms the basis for dosing antacids 1 and 3 hours after meals.

In general, when given in sufficient doses on a regular schedule, antacids appear to heal ulcers; however, because of the potential side effects (e.g., diarrhea, constipation) and inconvenience, the $H_2$ antagonists and sucralfate have replaced high-dose antacid therapy as the primary therapeutic modality for treating peptic ulcers. Although antacids are often recommended as needed for ulcer pain relief, the "symptomatic" action of antacids has been challenged.[21]

*Duodenal Ulcer* Early studies did not support the duodenal ulcer-healing efficacy of antacids, probably because of inadequate neutralizing doses. Peterson et al[22] were the first to use high-dose or "intensive" antacid therapy. A regimen of 144 mEq of neutralizing capacity 1 and 3 hours after meals and at bedtime (>1,000 mEq/d) healed 78% of patients with duodenal ulcer compared with 44% in the placebo group at the end of 4 weeks. Diarrhea occurred in two thirds of the antacid-treated patients and an aluminum antacid had to be alternated with the magnesium/aluminum-containing antacid. Similar studies with high-dose antacids have confirmed these findings and have shown antacid at this dose to be

**Table 26.3** Drugs Used in the Treatment of Peptic Ulcer

| *Drug classification* | *Example* |
|---|---|
| Agents that neutralize gastric acid | Antacids[a] |
| Antisecretory agents | |
| Anticholinergics | Tertiary/quaternary ammonium compounds |
| $H_2$-receptor antagonists | Cimetidine[a] |
| | Ranitidine[a] |
| | Famotidine[a] |
| | Nizatidine[a] |
| Substituted benzimidazoles | Omeprazole |
| Tricyclic antidepressants | Trimipramine |
| | Doxepin |
| Antimuscarinic agents | Pirenzepine |
| Gastrin antagonists | Proglumide |
| Corticohypothalamic agents | Sulpiride |
| Other experimental agents | Somatostatin |
| | Calcium channel blockers |
| Agents that enhance mucosal defense | |
| Sulfated disaccharides | Sucralfate[a] |
| Colloidal bismuth | Tripotassium dicitrato bismuthate |
| Licorice extract | Carbenoxolone |
| Antisecretory agents that also enhance mucosal defense | |
| Prostaglandins | Misoprostol |
| | Enprostil |
| | Arbaprostil |
| Agents that alter gastric emptying | |
| Dopamine antagonists | Metoclopramide |
| | Domperidone |

[a] Approved for use in the United States.

comparable to cimetidine in promoting duodenal ulcer healing.[23] Several studies report duodenal ulcer healing with low-dose (175 mEq/d) antacid tablets[24] and medium-dose (400 mEq/d) antacid liquids.[25] Until further studies confirm low-dose antacid therapy, it is unwise to assume that these doses are efficacious in healing duodenal ulcers.

*Gastric Ulcer* Although antacids have been used to treat benign gastric ulcer, results of studies are conflicting.[23,26] Hollander et al[26] compared calcium carbonate with placebo and observed that 45% of patients and 27% of the placebo group healed in 6 weeks. Other investigators have failed to confirm the efficacy of antacids in healing gastric ulcers.[23]

***Antacid Compounds***

*Sodium Bicarbonate* Sodium bicarbonate has an immediate onset of action, but its duration is very short. Sodium and bicarbonate ions are readily absorbed and promote fluid retention and systemic alkalosis. Although widely used for dyspeptic symptoms, sodium bicarbonate is not recommended for long-term use in the treatment of peptic ulcers.

*Calcium Carbonate* Despite its rapid onset and prolonged effect, calcium carbonate may produce acid rebound as well as systemic complications related to the absorption of calcium. Long-term use of calcium-containing antacids is generally not recommended.

*Magnesium Hydroxide* Magnesium hydroxide has a slower onset and a more prolonged duration of action than either sodium bicarbonate or calcium carbonate. Other magnesium compounds include magnesium oxide, magnesium carbonate, and magnesium trisilicate. Overall, the effects and side effects of magnesium oxide and carbonate are similar to those of magnesium hydroxide. Magnesium trisilicate has a slow onset of action and is considered a weak antacid.

*Aluminum Hydroxide* Aluminum hydroxide possesses a relatively low neutralizing capacity. The phosphate salt has very little antacid activity.

*Magaldrate* Magaldrate is hydroxymagnesium aluminate, a complex that dissociates into magnesium and aluminum ions in the presence of hydrochloric acid. Its effects resemble those of other magnesium/aluminum-containing antacids, but it is thought to have fewer gastrointestinal side effects because it contains less magnesium per unit of weight than other aluminum/magnesium antacid combinations.

***Combination Antacids*** Commercially available mixtures of antacids are prescribed in an attempt to maximize antacid-neutralizing properties and to minimize the undesirable effects of each component. Magnesium/aluminum-containing antacids are preferred because of their increased neutralizing capacity, duration of action, and reduced adverse effects.

**Table 26.4** Relative Potency of Selected Antacid Products

| *Product* | *Form* | *Acid-neutralizing capacity (mEq/30 mL or mEq/tablet)* |
|---|---|---|
| High-potency Al/Mg hydroxides | | |
| Delcid (Lakeside) | Liquid | 252 |
| Riopan ES Plus (Ayerst) | Liquid | 180 |
| Maalox TC (Rorer) | Liquid | 170 |
| Mylanta II (Stuart) | Liquid | 152 |
| Gelusil II (Parke–Davis) | Liquid | 144 |
| Mylanta II (Stuart) | Tablet | 23 |
| Gelusil II (Parke–Davis) | Tablet | 21 |
| Regular-potency Al/Mg hydroxides | | |
| Riopan Plus (Ayerst) | Liquid | 90 |
| Maalox (Rorer) | Liquid | 81 |
| Mylanta (Stuart) | Liquid | 76 |
| Gelusil (Parke–Davis) | Liquid | 72 |
| Riopan Plus (Ayerst) | Tablet | 14 |
| Mylanta (Stuart) | Tablet | 11 |
| Gelusil (Parke–Davis) | Tablet | 11 |
| Aluminum hydroxide | | |
| Alternagel (Stuart) | Liquid | 96 |
| Amphogel (Wyeth) | Liquid | 60 |
| Amphogel (Wyeth) | Tablet | 8/16 |
| Aluminum carbonate | | |
| Basaljel (Wyeth) | Liquid | 69 |
| Aluminum phosphate | | |
| Phosphaljel (Wyeth) | Liquid | 12 |
| Calcium carbonate | | |
| Titralac (Riker) | Liquid | 120 |
| Tums (Norcliff Thayer) | Tablet | 10 |

**Figure 26.3** Mean gastric pH after a meal with or without antacid given 1 and 3 hours after meals. *(From Sleisenger MH, Fordtran JS (Eds): Gastrointestinal Diseases: Pathophysiology, Diagnosis, Management. Philadelphia, W.B. Saunders, 1983, p717 with permission.)*

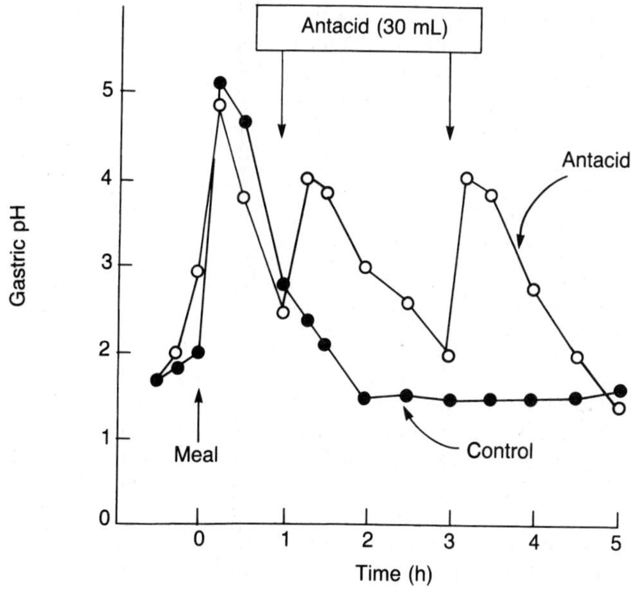


*Other Compounds*

*Simethicone* Simethicone is an antifoaming agent used when gastric distress is associated with gas formation. Although possibly effective for reducing flatulence and bloating, simethicone does not have antacid or antiulcer properties.

*Alginic Acid* Alginic acid is converted to sodium alginate, which is thought to "float" on top of the gastric contents and reduce the irritating effect of gastric acid during periods of gastroesophageal reflux. Alginic acid has no role in the treatment of gastric or duodenal ulcers.

*Adverse Effects*

*Gastrointestinal Effects* The most common side effects of antacids are diarrhea and constipation. Magnesium salts produce a dose-related osmotic diarrhea.[27] The frequency of diarrhea is 60% to 70% when more than 1,000 mEq of antacid is used per day, as compared with less than 20% for low doses (<300 mEq/d). Severe diarrhea could lead to dehydration and electrolyte imbalance. Constipation tends to occur with large doses of aluminum or calcium salts. Diarrhea usually predominates with high doses of magnesium/aluminum-containing antacid combinations. Theoretically, antacids that are similar in potency, but contain less magnesium, should cause less diarrhea. Gastrointestinal side effects can be minimized by alternating magnesium/aluminum with aluminum-containing antacids. Bowel frequency and stool consistency can be determined by adjusting the dose of each antacid preparation.

*Phosphorus Depletion* All aluminum-containing antacids (except aluminum phosphate) form insoluble salts with dietary phosphorus and thereby reduce phosphorus absorption. If aluminum hydroxide antacids are taken in high doses for long periods of time, and/or if dietary phosphate intake is low (e.g., malnutrition, alcoholics), hypophosphatemia may result and the administration of phosphate supplements may be required.[21,28] The phosphorus-lowering action of aluminum hydroxide may be beneficial in renal failure patients with hyperphosphatemia.

*Cation Absorption* Approximately 5% to 10% of the magnesium in magnesium hydroxide can be absorbed, but hypermagnesemia rarely occurs in patients with normal renal function. As significant renal insufficiency (creatinine clearance <30 mL/min) may impair magnesium excretion, magnesium-containing antacids should be avoided in these patients. Aluminum absorption occurs in individuals ingesting antacids and may result in high plasma concentrations in patients with renal failure. The clinical importance of this finding remains to be determined. Hypercalcemia can occur in patients with normal renal function taking calcium carbonate doses greater than 20 g/d. If renal function is impaired, hypercalcemia may develop with doses of 4 g/d.[21,28] Although sodium is readily absorbed from the gastrointestinal tract, most antacid preparations have been reformulated to contain clinically insignificant amounts of sodium.

*Alkalosis* All antacids, to some degree, promote metabolic alkalosis. The development of alkalosis depends upon the irreversibility of the reaction of gastric acid with the antacid and upon the degree of impaired renal function. For example, sodium bicarbonate and calcium carbonate react almost irreversibly with gastric acid, but normal renal function usually prevents perpetuation of the alkalosis.

*Milk–Alkali Syndrome* The milk–alkali syndrome occurs when a high calcium intake combines with systemic alkalosis. Calcium is usually provided by ingestion of large amounts of milk or calcium-containing antacids. The alkalosis may be produced by absorbable antacids (i.e., sodium bicarbonate) or by prolonged vomiting. The main features of this syndrome include hypercalcemia, alkalosis, renal stones, and elevated blood urea nitrogen and creatinine concentrations.

*Acid Rebound* Acid rebound is defined as a sustained hypersecretion of gastric acid after an antacid has emptied from the stomach. Only calcium-containing antacids have been reported to have this effect. The specific mechanism of action is not known but may be related to hypercalcemia and gastrin release. For this reason, calcium carbonate should not be used to treat patients with PUD.

***Drug Interactions*** Antacids can alter the absorption and/or excretion of many drugs when administered concomitantly. The magnitude of the drug interaction may depend on the antacid dose and the type of antacid salt (i.e., aluminum hydroxide versus magnesium hydroxide). Mechanisms by which antacids cause drug interactions include elevation of gastric pH leading to a change in drug dissolution, adsorption of drugs, complexation of drugs, and a change in urinary pH that either increases or decreases renal excretion of drugs. Most drug interactions can be avoided by separating the administration of antacids from that of other oral drugs by at least 1 to 2 hours. Even in situations when no drug interaction has been documented, it is advisable when possible to avoid administering antacids simultaneously with other medications. Drugs that can interact with antacids include tetracycline, warfarin, digoxin, iron, aspirin, quinidine, and isoniazid. A more comprehensive review of specific antacid–drug interactions and their mechanisms is presented elsewhere.[29]

***Product Formulation*** Antacids are available in several dosage forms and in various potencies. Although antacid tablets are convenient, liquid preparations are thought to be more effective because of a smaller particle size and larger surface area. Similarly, antacid effectiveness should also be greater if tablets are chewed rather than swallowed intact. Antacid tablets and liquids vary widely in their potency (Table 26.4) and palatability. Although sodium bicarbonate and calcium carbonate are the most potent antacids, their potential for adverse effects limits their use on a long-term basis. Compliance with antacid regimens may be enhanced by selecting a high-potency antacid and by determining the patient's taste preference.

**Antisecretory Agents**

***Anticholinergics*** The traditional anticholinergic drugs include tertiary ammonium compounds like atropine and quaternary ammonium compounds such as propantheline (Probanthine, Searle), which have both antimuscarinic and ganglion-blocking activity. These agents reduce acid secretion by blocking acetylcholine receptors on the parietal cell (Fig. 26.2). Therapeutic doses of anticholinergic drugs have been shown to reduce basal acid secretion by 50% and maximal acid output by 30% to 40%. This reduction in acid secretion is less than that achieved with the $H_2$-receptor antagonists.[21] For most patients, the optimal ulcer-healing dose usually induces anticholinergic effects (i.e., dry mouth, blurred vision, constipation, urinary retention, tachycardia, and delayed gastric emptying); however, there are large individual variations in the degree of gastric acid inhibition and sensitivity to these drugs. Very few well-controlled clinical trials have documented the efficacy of anticholinergic agents in healing ulcers, and their value as a sole therapeutic agent remains unproven. Today, the classical anticholinergics have been replaced by more potent antisecretory agents and by drugs that selectively block specific muscarinic receptors.

There is evidence that supports the use of anticholinergic agents in combination with other antiulcer drugs.[30,31] The combination of an anticholinergic and an $H_2$-receptor antagonist may suppress acid secretion to a greater extent than either drug alone, as both histamine and acetylcholine receptors on the parietal cells are blocked. This synergistic action may benefit those patients who require high doses of $H_2$ antagonists (i.e., patients with Zollinger–Ellison syndrome) and may permit lowering of the dose of each agent.[32]

***$H_2$-Receptor Antagonists*** $H_1$ receptors mediate the effect of histamine on smooth muscle of the gastrointestinal tract

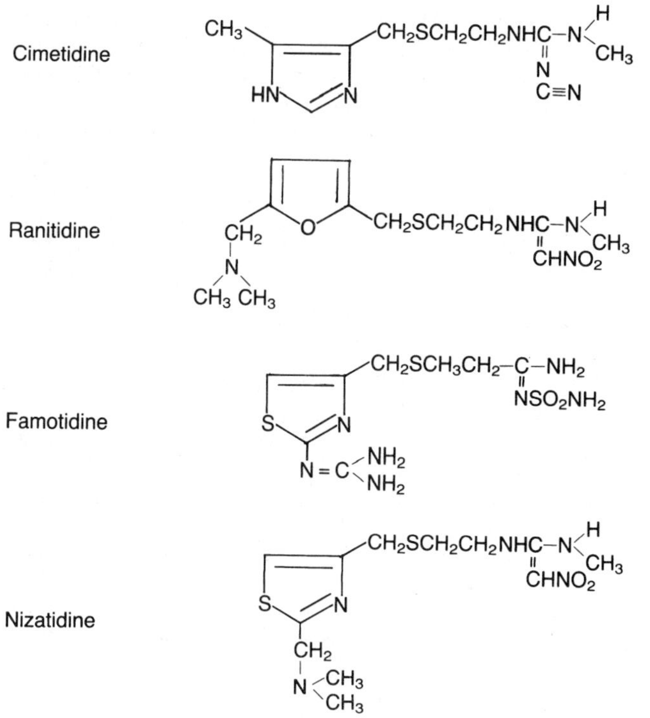


**Figure 26.4** Chemical structures of the $H_2$-receptor antagonists.

and are blocked by $H_1$ antagonists (antihistamines). $H_2$ receptors mediate the action of histamine on gastric parietal cells, heart, uterus, and T lymphocytes and are blocked by $H_2$ antagonists. This action at the site of the parietal cell is believed to inhibit gastric acid secretion through the reduction of intracellular cyclic AMP (Fig. 26.2). Two early $H_2$ antagonists, burimamide and metiamide, were abandoned primarily because of toxic effects. The third, cimetidine, contains an imidazole ring, with a modified cyanoguanidine side chain. The ring structure is not essential for $H_2$-blockade, as ranitidine has a furan ring and famotidine and nizatidine have a thiazole structure (Fig. 26.4).

The development of the $H_2$-receptor antagonists introduced a new era in the treatment of peptic ulcer disease, and today they represent the most important class of drugs available. At present, only cimetidine, ranitidine, famotidine, and nizatidine are available for use in the United States. The major differences among these agents are potency and specificity. Efficacy and safety appear to be similar for all four compounds, although less is known about famotidine and nizatidine.[33]

*Cimetidine* Cimetidine (Tagamet, Smith Kline & French) is thought to inhibit basal and stimulated gastric acid secretion by competitively inhibiting the action of histamine on parietal cell $H_2$ receptors. This reduction in gastric acid output results from a decrease in both acid concentration and volume. Although there is no direct correlation between blood cimetidine concentrations and gastric pH, minimum therapeutic concentrations should exceed 0.5–1.0 $\mu$/mL.

Cimetidine is well absorbed from the gastrointestinal tract, with peak plasma concentrations occurring 90 to 120 minutes after oral administration. Most of the drug is excreted in the urine unchanged, with a small amount metabolized to the hydroxymethyl and sulfoxide metabolites. Because the elimination half-life of cimetidine may be prolonged in patients with renal failure and in severe liver disease, the total daily dose should be reduced by half in these patients. As hemodialysis may remove small amounts of the drug, patients should receive their dose of cimetidine after dialysis.[34]

The effectiveness of cimetidine in healing duodenal ulcers has been documented extensively.[23,35–38] Comparative trials show healing rates similar to those obtained with high-dose antacids.[23] Controlled trials in Europe using 1 g (200 mg three times daily and 400 mg at bedtime) and those in the United States using 1.2 g (300 mg four times daily) of cimetidine daily have shown that 75% to 85% of duodenal ulcers heal during a 4- to 6-week treatment period, with placebo healing rates varying from 30% to 60%. U.S. trials tend to report a higher placebo healing rate than European trials, perhaps because of increased consumption of antacids for pain relief.[37,38]

Results from recent dosing studies emphasize the importance of suppressing nocturnal acid secretion. It appears that nocturnal acidity accounts for more than 80% of the variation in ulcer-healing rates produced by different dosing regimens, while daytime suppression of acid secretion is responsible for less than 1%. This may be related to the finding that duodenal ulcer patients appear to have an elevated nocturnal BAO. Controlled clinical trials confirm that cimetidine 400 mg twice daily or as a single bedtime dose of 800 mg is as effective in healing duodenal ulcers as previous dosage regimens.[39] These new regimens represent a potential advantage in terms of patient compliance, decreased adverse effects, and drug interactions.

The effect of cimetidine on the healing of gastric ulcers has been evaluated in a number of controlled clinical trials.[23,40] Most studies show an increased incidence of healing with rates of approximately 75% to 80% at 6 weeks versus 35% to 40% for placebo groups. Cimetidine, in a daily dose of 1.2 g (300 mg four times daily) or 800 mg at bedtime, is approved in the United States for the treatment of gastric ulcer. It appears that nocturnal dosing is also effective in the treatment of gastric ulcer.

The overall incidence of adverse effects in patients receiving cimetidine is reported to be 4.5%, of which the most frequent are gastrointestinal (2.1%) and central nervous system (1.2%) effects. Mental confusion, disorientation, agitation, hallucinations, and seizures have been associated with cimetidine treatment, especially in the elderly and in patients with renal and/or liver dysfunction. Less frequently occurring adverse reactions include skin rash, headache, tiredness, and dizziness. Mild increases in serum creatinine and hepatic transaminase concentrations commonly occur with therapy, but usually are not associated with renal or liver dysfunction and will return to baseline when the drug is discontinued. Cimetidine has been associated with a few cases of leukopenia, thrombocytopenia, anaphylaxis, interstitial nephritis, and hepatitis.[41]

Endocrine effects, including gynecomastia, impotence, and galactorrhea, have been reported in patients receiving long-term high doses of cimetidine (e.g., Zollinger–Ellison syndrome) and are thought to be a dose-related antiandrogen effect of the drug.[42] These conditions are uncommon with usual therapeutic doses and reverse upon cessation of ther-

**Table 26.5** Potential Drug Interactions With $H_2$-Receptor Antagonists

| *Drug* | *Mechanism* | *Significance* | *Comment* |
|---|---|---|---|
| Antacids | Unknown | May reduce bioavailability of $H_2$ antagonists | Avoid simultaneous use |
| Ketoconazole | Elevation of gastric pH, decreased absorption of ketoconazole | Decreased serum concentration of ketoconazole | Possible failure of ketoconazole therapy; give ketoconazole at time of lowest gastric pH |
| Procainamide | Decreased renal tubular secretion | Increased serum procainamide and NAPA concentrations | Occurs with cimetidine and to a leser extent with ranitidine; check serum concentrations and reduce procainamide dose, if necessary |
| Theophylline | Hepatic microsomal enzyme inhibition | Increased serum theophylline concentration, possible toxicity | Significant with cimetidine, possibly ranitidine; check serum concentration and reduce theophylline dose, if necessary |
| Phenytoin | Hepatic microsomal enzyme inhibition | Increased serum phenytoin concentration, possible toxicity | Significant with cimetidine; check serum concentration and reduce phenytoin dose, if necessary |
| Warfarin | Hepatic microsomal enzyme inhibition | Prolonged prothombin time, bleeding | Significant with cimetidine, possibly ranitidine; check prothrombin time; reduction in warfarin dose may be necessary |
| Propranolol | Hepatic microsomal enzyme inhibition, possible decreased liver blood flow | Bradycardia | Significant with cimetidine; reduction in propranolol dose or use of β-blockers that are eliminated primarily renally (nadolol, atenolol) may be necessary |
| Lidocaine | Hepatic microsomal enzyme inhibition, possible decreased liver blood flow | Possible lidocaine toxicity | Significant with cimetidine; reduction in lidocaine dose may be necessary |
| Benzodiazepines | Hepatic microsomal enzyme inhibition | Increased sedation seen primarily in elderly and/or patients with hepatic disease | Significant with cimetidine; reduction in benzodiazepine dose or use of agents that do not undergo phase I hepatic metabolism (oxazepam, lorazepam) may be necessary |
| Calcium channel blockers | Hepatic microsomal enzyme inhibition | Hypotension, dizziness seen primarily with nifedipine, possibly diltiazem | Significant with cimetidine, to a lesser extent with ranitidine; reduction in calcium channel blocker dose may be necessary |
| Metronidazole | Hepatic microsomal enzyme inhibition | Increased serum metronidazole concentration | Significant with cimetidine; questionable pharmacodynamic effect |

apy. Cimetidine elevates blood prolactin concentrations when given intravenously but not when given orally.

Cimetidine interacts with other drugs by several proposed mechanisms. Cimetidine may (1) bind reversibly to the cytochrome $P_{450}$ mixed-function oxidase system and decrease the hepatic clearance of drugs that undergo phase I metabolism, (2) possibly decrease hepatic blood flow and reduce the hepatic clearance of high-extraction drugs for which blood flow is important, (3) alter the bioavailability of orally administered drugs as a consequence of increasing gastric pH, and (4) decrease renal clearance by inhibiting renal tubular secretion. Table 26.5 lists some of the most important potential cimetidine–drug interactions and their possible mechanisms. Adverse effects have been reported with theophylline, warfarin, phenytoin, lidocaine, propranolol, and nifedipine. Doses of interacting drugs may need to be reduced when patients are treated concomitantly with cimetidine. For some drugs, such as theophylline and phenytoin, there appears to be a correlation between the dose of cimetidine and the degree of metabolic inhibition.[43,44] Thus, the lower, once-a-day dosage regimens may reduce the potential magnitude of cimetidine–drug interactions. Drugs that are metabolized in the liver by glucuronidation (e.g., lorazepam and oxazepam) are not affected by cimetidine. Because cimetidine and other $H_2$ antagonists are thought to have little effect on liver blood flow, the significance of this potential mechanism is questionable. The reader is referred to several reviews for a more comprehensive discussion of drug interactions with $H_2$-receptor antagonists.[45–48]

*Ranitidine* Like cimetidine, ranitidine (Zantac, Glaxo) represents a modification of the histamine molecule (Fig. 26.4). In comparison with cimetidine, ranitidine has a longer antisecretory effect thought to be related to its increased potency (4–10 times that of cimetidine on an equimolar basis).

Ranitidine is well absorbed from the small intestine and has a pharmacokinetic profile similar to that of cimetidine. Because of the prolonged elimination half-life in patients with impaired renal function, the frequency of the oral dose (150 mg) should be increased to 24 hours when the creatinine clearance is less than 50 mL/min. In hemodialysis patients, the dose of the drug should coincide with the end of dialysis. The reduced bioavailability of ranitidine after oral administration suggests a high first-pass effect and requires reduction of the intravenous dose.[49]

The ulcer-healing effects of ranitidine have been investigated extensively. In most clinical trials, the healing rate for duodenal ulcer, after 4 to 6 weeks of treatment with 100 to 150 mg twice daily, has ranged from 70% to 90% and is similar to those rates achieved with cimetidine.[50,51] A single bedtime dose of 300 mg has been confirmed to heal uncomplicated duodenal ulcers at least as effectively as the 150-mg twice-daily dosage regimen.[52]

Gastric ulcer-healing rates with ranitidine are similar to those obtained with cimetidine and vary based on the length of the treatment period.[53] Prolonging treatment from 4 to 8 weeks appears to increase ulcer healing from approximately 60% to more than 90%, suggesting that gastric ulcers tend to heal more slowly than duodenal ulcers.

In general, many of the adverse effects reported with cimetidine have also been reported with ranitidine. Minor side effects include headaches, which are usually mild and resolve with continued therapy. As with cimetidine, transient increases in hepatic transaminases and serum creatinine concentrations have been observed. Intravenous doses of ranitidine 50–100 mg four times daily have been associated with significant liver transaminase elevations.[54] Although the CNS effects that occur with cimetidine have been reported in fewer patients receiving ranitidine, it is difficult to conclude that there is a significant difference in incidence between the two drugs. Ranitidine appears to lack antiandrogenic activity, presumably because it does not bind to androgen receptors. Zollinger–Ellison patients requiring high doses of $H_2$ antagonists could benefit from ranitidine therapy.[32]

Ranitidine differs from cimetidine in its binding affinity and in the manner in which it binds to cytochrome $P_{450}$. In general, recommended doses of ranitidine are not associated with clinically significant effects on hepatic drug metabolism.[47,48] This would seem to favor the use of ranitidine in patients who are taking drugs that are metabolized by the mixed-function oxidase system. Ranitidine can alter drug absorption through its effects on gastric pH, and it can decrease the renal clearance of procainamide but to a lesser extent than does cimetidine.

*Famotidine* Famotidine (Pepcid, Merck Sharp & Dohme), an $H_2$-receptor antagonist with a thiazole ring structure (Fig. 26.4), is about 40–60 times more potent than cimetidine and 12–15 times more potent than ranitidine on an equimolar basis. The drug is absorbed orally, with renal excretion being the major route of elimination. The daily dose of famotidine should be reduced in patients with impaired renal function.[55,56] The pharmacokinetics of famotidine are similar to those of cimetidine and ranitidine.

Clinical trials have shown famotidine 20 mg twice daily or 40 mg at bedtime to be as effective as standard doses of cimetidine and ranitidine for healing duodenal and gastric ulcers.[56–57] Famotidine is well tolerated, with the most common adverse effects reported to be headache and gastrointestinal symptoms. Unlike cimetidine, high doses do not cause antiandrogenic effects in men, and therapeutic doses do not appear to affect the pharmacokinetics of drugs that undergo hepatic elimination[56,58] and renal tubular secretion.[59]

*Nizatidine* Nizatidine (Axid, Lilly), another thiazole derivative (Fig. 26.4), has an antisecretory potency similar to that of ranitidine. Unlike cimetidine, ranitidine, and famotidine, the oral bioavailability of nizatidine exceeds 90%. A dose of 150 mg twice daily or 300 mg at bedtime appears to be as effective as ranitidine 150 mg twice daily or 300 mg at bedtime when used orally to heal duodenal or gastric ulcers.[60] A dosage reduction should be considered in patients with renal dysfunction. Adverse effects are similar to those reported with ranitidine and famotidine. Nizatidine does not interfere with hepatic microsomal enzymes.[61]

Several new long-acting compounds are in the early stages of investigation. These agents differ from previous $H_2$ antagonists in that they do not competitively inhibit histamine at the $H_2$ receptor. Instead, they bind tightly to the receptor, thereby altering both the pharmacokinetic and the pharmacodynamic features of the drug.[62]

***Substituted Benzimidazoles*** The substituted benzimidazoles, or so-called "proton pump" inhibitors, are a new class of antisecretory agents that act by a novel and different mechanism. These agents react covalently with hydrogen/potassium ATPase, resulting in a complete and irreversible inhibition of gastric acid secretion (Fig. 26.2). Omeprazole, the prototype compound, produces a profound and long-acting suppression of gastric acid, the effects of which persist 3 days or longer. Clinical trials indicate that a bedtime dose of 20–60 mg of omeprazole heals 60% to 100% of duodenal ulcers within a 2- to-4-week period.[63,64] Oral doses of up to 180 mg/d have been used to treat patients with Zollinger–Ellison syndrome who are resistant to $H_2$-receptor antagonists.[63,65,66] Because of its profound effect on gastric acid, it is not known whether omeprazole increases the risk of gastric cancer in humans. The drug's potential clinical value cannot be assessed until the results of toxicologic studies are known.

***Tricyclic Antidepressants*** The tricyclic antidepressants doxepin (Sinequan, Roerig; Adapin, Pennwalt) and trimipramine (Surmontil, Wyeth) are undergoing clinical investigation for the treatment of gastric and duodenal ulcers. Their mechanisms of action in peptic ulcer disease are complex and most likely include $H_2$-receptor blockade and an anticholinergic-like effect. Controlled clinical trials suggest that trimipramine, in daily doses of 25–50 mg, is more effective than placebo and may be as effective as cimetidine in the short-term treatment of duodenal ulcer.[67] Although the use of trimipramine in gastric ulcer looks promising, additional studies are needed to confirm its efficacy. Clinical trials indicate that doxepin in daily doses of 50–150 mg/d may also be efficacious in healing duodenal ulcers[67]; however, additional well-controlled, double-blind studies are needed to confirm these preliminary claims. Drowsiness and anticholinergic effects appear to be the most frequently reported adverse effects and tend to limit the use of the tricyclic antidepressants as first-line agents. Trimipramine and doxepin may be effective in those patients who are otherwise unresponsive to conventional antiulcer therapy.

***Antimuscarinic Agents*** Pirenzepine, an antimuscarinic agent, has a structure similar to that of the tricyclic antidepressants but its antidepressant effects are negligible because it does not cross the blood–brain barrier. Pirenzepine inhibits gastric acid secretion similar to the traditional anticholinergic agents, but it appears to have a higher affinity for the muscarinic receptors located in the gastric mucosa. Doses of 100–150 mg/d have been shown to heal gastric and duodenal ulcers but are reported to cause dry mouth and blurred vision. Lower doses of 50–75 mg/d are associated with a decreased incidence of adverse effects, but do not appear to be as effective.[67] Although pirenzepine has fewer side effects than the classic anticholinergics, it does not seem capable of challenging the $H_2$ antagonists as first-line agents.

***Other Antisecretory Agents*** Several other antisecretory agents have been investigated for use in the treatment of peptic ulcer disease, but they remain experimental. Proglumide, a gastrin antagonist, is thought to inhibit gastrin stimulation of parietal cells. Sulpiride, a corticohypothalamic agent, has produced conflicting results in a small number of patients. Somatostatin may heal ulcers by way of its inhibitory effects on acid, pepsin, and gastrin release. The development of more selective and longer lasting somatostatin analogs may produce useful therapeutic agents in the future. The use of calcium channel blockers as inhibitors of gastric acid secretion is being studied in experimental animals.

### Agents That Enhance Mucosal Defense

Agents that enhance mucosal defense differ from those drugs previously discussed in that they heal gastric and duodenal ulcers without suppressing gastric acid secretion. Although their specific ulcer-healing mechanisms of action are not fully understood, they are thought to act by (1) adhering to the ulcer base and forming a protective barrier against acid, pepsin, and bile salts and/or (2) altering the gastromucosal barrier through cytoprotective properties. The compounds tested most extensively include sucralfate, colloidal bismuth (tripotassium dicitrato bismuthate), and carbenoxolone. Only sucralfate is approved for the treatment of duodenal ulcers in the United States.

***Sucralfate*** Sucralfate (Carafate, Marion), an aluminum hydroxide salt of sulfated sucrose, is a nonabsorbable substance that, when exposed to acid, becomes a viscous adhesive. Sucralfate binds electrostatically to positively charged protein molecules in the ulcer crater, forming a protective barrier that inhibits back-diffusion of hydrogen ions and pepsin. The resulting substance is thought to bind more effectively at pH values less than 4.0. Although the drug has a greater affinity for damaged mucosa, binding to normal mucosa does occur. Binding to the ulcer site appears to last up to 6 hours after oral administration. Of unknown importance is sucralfate's adsorption of bile acids. There is evidence that the drug stimulates prostaglandin synthesis in the mucosa and that this contributes to ulcer healing.[68] After oral administration, 3% to 5% of the drug is absorbed, with the majority of the administered dose being excreted unchanged in the feces. A small amount of the absorbed drug is excreted unchanged in the urine.[69]

The efficacy of sucralfate in the short-term treatment of duodenal ulcer has been established by numerous placebo-controlled studies and comparative studies with cimetidine.[69] The dose of sucralfate used in most of these studies was 1 g four times daily 30 to 60 minutes before meals and at bedtime. Compliance is thought to be important, as maximal drug binding may be related to pH and sucralfate may bind with dietary protein if taken with meals.

Van Deventer et al[70] compared the rates of duodenal ulcer healing after concurrent administration of sucralfate and cimetidine. The healing rates achieved at 4 and 8 weeks with combination therapy did not differ significantly from those achieved with either drug alone. Although it appears that combination therapy with these two agents is not incompatible, additional studies are required to verify a trend toward early ulcer healing. A disadvantage of sucralfate is its relatively complicated dosage schedule and the possibility of poor patient compliance. The results of a study by Brandstaetter et al[71] suggest that sucralfate, 2 g twice daily (before breakfast and at bedtime) is as effective as the conventional dose (1 g four times daily) in healing duodenal ulcers.

A limited number of studies have shown sucralfate to be effective for the treatment of gastric ulcer[69] and in protection of the gastric mucosa from aspirin-induced mucosal damage.[72] Additional studies are required to confirm these findings.

Because only a small percentage of sucralfate is absorbed, adverse effects occur infrequently and are rarely serious. Constipation occurs in about 2% of patients receiving the drug. Other adverse effects occur in fewer than 1% of patients and include nausea, metallic taste, and dry mouth.[69]

The concomitant administration of sucralfate with drugs such as phenytoin or digoxin may reduce their bioavailability; however, the clinical importance of this potential interaction has not been determined. Because sucralfate may potentially bind drugs in the gastrointestinal tract, it is recommended that administration of other drugs be separated from that of sucralfate by 1 to 2 hours.

***Colloidal Bismuth*** The mechanism of action of colloidal bismuth is believed to be similar to that of sucralfate. Although colloidal bismuth has been shown to be effective against *Campylobacter pylori,* the precise role of bacteria in the etiology of peptic ulcer disease is unclear. A number of studies, primarily in England, have shown the drug to be comparable to cimetidine in healing peptic ulcers.[73] Side effects appear to be minimal, with no reported signs of bismuth-induced neurotoxicity. Potential drawbacks to bismuth therapy include dosing frequency, a darkening of the feces, tongue, and teeth, and an unpleasant odor and taste to the liquid dosage form. This latter problem may be overcome if the tablet proves as effective as the liquid dosage form.

***Carbenoxolone*** Carbenoxolone is a synthetic derivative of licorice root that has been shown to accelerate gastric and duodenal ulcer healing without affecting gastric secretion.[74] Although its precise mechanism of action is not known, it appears to enhance mucosal defense by increasing mucus production and increasing the life span of gastric epithelial cells. The ulcer-healing properties of carbenoxolone may be mediated by prostaglandins. Approximately 25% of patients treated with the drug exhibit aldosterone-like effects such as fluid retention, hypokalemia, and hypertension. Because of these adverse effects, it is unlikely that the drug will be investigated in the United States.

#### Antisecretory Agents That Also Enhance Mucosal Defense

Naturally occurring prostaglandins are produced by gastrointestinal mucosa cells and have numerous effects on the gastrointestinal tract. They appear to play a role in endogenous protective mechanisms and against injury by noxious agents. Patients with chronic peptic ulcer have been reported to have deficiencies of gastrointestinal prostaglandins, which has led to the use of these agents in the treatment of ulcer disease.

Naturally occurring prostaglandins inhibit acid secretion when administered intravenously, but are relatively inactive when taken by mouth, presumably because of inactivation by prostaglandin dehydrogenases. The synthetic analogues are effective when taken orally, and cause inhibition of both basal and stimulated acid production (Fig. 26.2). Unfortunately, the doses required for acid inhibition sometimes result in diarrhea, the mechanism of which is uncertain. Most prostaglandins, when given in lower doses that do not affect acid secretion, appear to retain some of their ability to prevent or heal peptic ulcers. The specific mechanism of this cytoprotective action remains unclear, but has been postulated to include stimulation of gastrointestinal mucus production, stimulation of gastric bicarbonate, and increased mucosal blood flow.[18,75]

Prostaglandins under investigation include misoprostol (Searle), arbaprostil (Upjohn), and enprostil (Syntex). Misoprostol, a synthetic analogue of prostaglandin $E_1$, has been shown to promote duodenal ulcer healing in acid inhibitory doses of 200 $\mu$g four times daily, but not in doses of 50 $\mu$g four times daily.[76] Diarrhea occurred in 13% of the patients given the 200 $\mu$g dose versus 5% in the placebo-treated group. High-dose (200 $\mu$g) misoprostol appears to be as effective as cimetidine in healing gastric and duodenal ulcers.[77]

Arbaprostil, a prostaglandin $E_2$ analogue, is also undergoing clinical testing for treatment of peptic ulcers. In doses of 100 $\mu$g four times daily, the drug appears to heal duodenal ulcers as compared with placebo. Therapeutic doses of arbaprostil were reported to produce diarrhea in 34% of patients as compared with 4% on placebo.[78] Controlled clinical trials are underway to document the efficacy of enprostil and other synthetic prostaglandins for use in treating gastric and duodenal ulcer.[79] Preliminary results suggest that enprostil is effective in antisecretory doses but that, as with other prostaglandins, diarrhea remains a problem.

Initial studies indicate that several of the prostaglandin E analogues significantly improve gastric and duodenal ulcer healing. The healing rates appear similar to those for high-dose antacids, $H_2$ antagonists, and sucralfate. Of concern is the high incidence of diarrhea associated with ulcer-healing doses and their potential abortive effects on the pregnant uterus. In addition, most agents require multiple daily doses. Because of these reasons and the unknown effects of long-term prostaglandin use, it is possible that these agents will not become first-line drugs for treating peptic ulcers. They may, however, be likely agents for treating that fraction of patients in whom mucosal defense mechanisms appear to play a predominant role (i.e., aspirin-induced ulcers, acute stress-related mucosal injury).

#### Agents That Alter Gastric Emptying

Gastric ulcer is thought to be related to several pathogenic mechanisms, including delayed gastric emptying. A delay in gastric emptying is postulated to prolong the contact time between gastric acid and the gastric mucosa. Metoclopramide, a dopamine antagonist, accelerates gastric emptying and may be of value in treating gastric ulcer. Domperidone, a newer dopamine antagonist, seems to be equally as potent as metoclopramide and has the additional advantage of causing fewer side effects because it does not cross the blood–brain barrier. Controlled clinical trials must be conducted to determine whether motility-altering agents have a role in the treatment of peptic ulcers.

### *Prevention of Ulcer Recurrence*

Peptic ulcer disease is a chronic disorder characterized by ulcer recurrence. Although geographic variations in recurrence rates exist, duodenal ulcer recurrence has been reported to occur in up to 80% of patients within 12 months of full-dose antiulcer drug therapy.[15] Gastric ulcers also tend to recur, but less is known about their recurrence rate. Ulcer recurrence after initial treatment with colloidal bismuth may be less common than after treatment with $H_2$-receptor antagonists.[80] Such factors as patient noncompliance, cigarette smoking, and aspirin or NSAID use are associated with higher ulcer recurrence rates.

The prevention of ulcer recurrence is an important objective in the medical management of peptic ulcer disease and may warrant placing the patient on either intermittent full-dose ulcer-healing therapy or continuous low-dose maintenance therapy. Patients who relapse within 3 to 6 months of initial therapy and/or have severe symptoms may require continuous low-dose maintenance therapy. Prevention against recurrence appears to last only as long as drug treatment is continued, as up to 90% recurrence has been reported after discontinuation of maintenance therapy.[80]

At present, cimetidine, ranitidine, famotidine, and nizatidine are indicated for prevention of duodenal ulcer. Ranitidine 150 mg at bedtime appears to be at least as effective as cimetidine 400 mg at bedtime and, based on the results of two well-controlled clinical trials, may be superior to cimetidine.[81,82] A bedtime dose of cimetidine 300 mg/d is often prescribed, but there are no controlled clinical trials to support this dose. A maintenance dose of famotidine 20 mg or nizatidine 150 mg at bedtime appears to be equally effective to the standard doses of cimetidine and ranitidine. Sucralfate is currently being investigated for the prevention of duodenal ulcer recurrence and may be as effective as the $H_2$-receptor antagonists.[80] Higher doses of the $H_2$-receptor antagonists or sucralfate may also be effective in preventing gastric ulcer recurrence.[80] Very little is known about the role of omeprazole, prostaglandins, and other investigational agents with respect to prevention of recurrence.

Although the $H_2$-receptor antagonists enjoy an excellent safety profile, the duration of maintenance therapy should be limited to 1 year because of unknown long-term consequences. The prolonged use of gastric secretory inhibitors, as a result of their pharmacologic inhibition of gastric secretion, may hypothetically cause gastric cancer. Several mechanisms have been proposed including the formation of carcinogenic nitroso compounds or hypergastrinemia-induced gastric tumors; however, experimental and clinical evidence does not appear to support this hypothesis.

## *Recommendations*

Antacids, $H_2$-receptor antagonists, and sucralfate appear to heal most duodenal and gastric ulcers in 6 to 8 weeks. In most patients, the initial drug of choice must then be based on factors other than efficacy. High-dose antacids are associated with diarrhea and other potentially undesirable adverse effects. New dosing regimens for the $H_2$-receptor antagonists permit a single bedtime dose, which appears to be as effective as the multiple daily doses for most patients. The adverse effect profiles of ranitidine, famotidine, and nizatidine are similar when used in usual therapeutic doses. Although ranitidine, famotidine, or nizatidine may be preferred in patients on drugs that are known to interact with cimetidine, appropriate dosage adjustments and patient monitoring can minimize potential cimetidine–drug interactions. In addition, the dose-dependent nature of certain cimetidine–drug interactions may reduce the magnitude of the interaction. Although sucralfate's potential for adverse effects is low, the drug must be administered four times a day and compliance may be a problem.

### Duodenal Ulcer

The treatment of choice for patients with an initial duodenal ulcer is a single oral bedtime dose of either cimetidine (800 mg), ranitidine (300 mg), famotidine (40 mg), or nizatidine (300 mg). More frequent daily doses (cimetidine 400 mg twice daily or 300 mg four times daily, ranitidine 150 mg twice daily, famotidine 20 mg twice daily, nizatidine 150 mg twice daily) should be used to treat those patients who do not respond to once-daily dosing and/or who have frequent daytime ulcer pain. Alternatively, sucralfate (1 g four times daily) can also be tried. Treatment should continue for at least 4 to 6 weeks at which time the patient should be reevaluated. If the ulcer is still present, treatment may be continued for a total of 12 to 15 weeks. For most patients, there is no therapeutic advantage to combining antiulcer medications. Antacids (15–30 mL) may be used along with other agents when needed for additional ulcer pain relief. When antacids are used in conjunction with other antiulcer drugs, the doses of each drug should be separated by at least 1 hour to avoid impairing the absorption of the $H_2$-antagonists or the binding of sucralfate. About 20% of duodenal ulcer patients do not heal with conventional therapy and require combination therapy and/or further diagnostic procedures. Poor compliance with the treatment program should be considered.

### Gastric Ulcer

Cimetidine (300 mg four times daily), ranitidine (150 mg twice daily), famotidine (20 mg twice daily), or nizatidine (150 mg twice daily) may be used to treat patients with benign gastric ulcer. Drug therapy should be continued until the ulcer heals or for a maximum of 15 weeks. Endoscopy or radiography is usually used to follow the healing process and a biopsy is performed to ensure that the ulcer is benign. Patients whose ulcers do not heal should be considered for combination antiulcer therapy or for surgery.

### Ulcer Recurrences

A recurrence of ulcer symptoms usually requires another course of full-dose therapy. Once ulcer healing occurs, the choice between intermittent full-dose treatment and maintenance therapy depends upon patient-specific factors. Maintenance therapy with a single bedtime dose of cimetidine 400 mg, ranitidine 150 mg, famotidine 20 mg, or nizatidine 150 mg appears to keep a majority of ulcers healed and patients symptom free.[82] Frequent relapsers and those in whom the disease is severe may require surgical intervention.

## *Complications*

***Hemorrhage*** Hemorrhage may be the first manifestation of a chronic peptic ulcer and occurs in approximately 15% to 20% of patients.[83] One bleeding episode appears to increase the chance of a second. Bleeding from a peptic ulcer may be insidious or may present as melena and/or hematemesis. In most patients, hemorrhage responds satisfactorily to gastric lavage and medical management. The treatment of upper gastrointestinal bleeding is discussed in Chapter 27.

***Perforation*** Perforation of peptic ulcers into the peritoneal cavity occurs in 5% to 10% of ulcer patients.[83] Most perforations are preceded by ulcer symptoms that intensify. The pain of perforation is usually sudden and severe, with mortality being higher for gastric than duodenal ulcers.

***Penetration*** Penetration occurs when an ulcer burrows into an adjacent structure rather than open freely into a cavity. The pain is usually chronic, rather than sudden, with hemorrhage occurring in one third of the patients. Duodenal ulcers may penetrate the pancreas, biliary tract, or liver.

***Obstruction*** Gastric outlet obstruction occurs in fewer than 5% of hospitalized patients with peptic ulcer.[83] Symptoms usually occur over several months and include nausea, vomiting, and weight loss.

***Intractability*** A diagnosis of intractability implies that medical therapy has failed. A refractory ulcer occurs when periods of remission become shorter and relapses become longer, and when the severity of pain becomes progressively more severe and of longer duration. Many factors are responsible for intractability including smoking, aspirin and NSAIDs, inadequate treatment, and noncompliance.

### *Surgery*

Failure to respond to medical treatment is the most common cause for surgical intervention. Surgical procedures performed for peptic ulcer include vagotomy with pyloroplasty or vagotomy with antrectomy. Vagotomy inhibits vagal stimulation of gastric acid and may be of three types: truncal, selective, or parietal cell. A truncal or selective vagotomy frequently results in postoperative gastric dysfunction and requires a pyloroplasty or antrectomy to facilitate gastric drainage. When an antrectomy is performed, the remaining stomach is anastomosed with the duodenum (Billroth I) or with the jejunum (Billroth II). A vagotomy is not necessary when an antrectomy is performed for gastric ulcer. Although surgery for peptic ulcer is effective, postoperative consequences do occur and include recurrent ulceration, postvagotomy diarrhea, dumping syndrome, and anemia.

## Zollinger–Ellison Syndrome

Zollinger–Ellison syndrome is characterized by gastric acid hypersecretion and recurrent peptic ulceration from a gastrin-producing tumor (gastrinoma). More than 90% of the gastrinomas are located in the pancreas, with the remaining tumors occurring in the duodenum and other sites. From one half to two thirds of patients with gastrinomas have metastases to various sites including regional lymph nodes, liver, and spleen. Although the true incidence of Zollinger–Ellison syndrome is not known, it is thought to occur in up to 1% of patients with duodenal ulcer disease.[32,84]

### *Clinical Presentation*

The most frequent clinical manifestation is peptic ulcer, with from 90% to 95% of patients developing an ulcer sometime during the course of their disease. Ulcers are usually single but may be multiple. They occur most often in the duodenum, but may involve the stomach or jejunum. Diarrhea is present in approximately one third of the patients and results from mucosal inflammation caused by large amounts of hydrochloric acid entering the duodenum. Steatorrhea, which is less common, is caused by inactivation of pancreatic lipase and precipitation of bile acids. Vitamin $B_{12}$ malabsorption may result from reduced intrinsic factor activity.

### *Diagnosis*

The diagnosis of Zollinger–Ellison syndrome should be suspected in patients with a compatible clinical history and evidence of gastric acid hypersecretion. Two thirds of patients have a BAO that exceeds 10 mEq/h. Basal acid output is often more than 60% of MAO because the parietal cell mass is already being stimulated by excessive endogenous gastrin. A fasting serum gastrin concentration is the most specific and reliable method of establishing the diagnosis. In normal subjects and patients with duodenal ulcer, fasting serum gastrin concentrations are approximately 60 pg/mL and usually do not exceed 150 pg/mL. Marked fasting serum gastrin concentrations (>1,000 pg/mL) along with endoscopic findings usually confirm the diagnosis. Several provocative tests (i.e., secretin, calcium, and test meals) are used in those patients without striking hypergastrinema.[84]

### *Treatment*

Medical therapy is based upon the presence or absence of peptic ulcers, diarrhea, and a gastrinoma, which may be malignant. The $H_2$ receptors cimetidine, ranitidine, and famotidine have all been associated with ulcer healing, improvement in symptoms, and decreased gastric acid output.[84–86] The effective dose of each drug is determined by the amount that will maintain gastric acid output at less than 10 mEq/h, as this level has been associated with ulcer healing.[84] Drug requirements appear to increase progressively in some patients and must be continued indefinitely. Although cimetidine doses larger than 12 g/d have been used, gynecomastia and impotence have been reported in men with the long-term use of doses greater than 2.4 g/d.[42] Ranitidine (given in oral doses up to 6 g/d) and famotidine (given in oral doses up to 0.8 g/d) are more potent agents and appear to be devoid of antiandrogen effects. Thus, they may be preferred in treatment of patients with hypersecretory states. Alternatively, the addition of an anticholinergic drug (i.e., propantheline, isopropamide, pirenzepine) may augment and prolong acid inhibition and permit use of lower doses of the $H_2$ antagonist.[32] Recent studies indicate that omeprazole is effective in treating Zollinger–Ellison syndrome, but additional information is needed to evaluate its relationship to gastric cancer.[63,65,66] Drugs such as proglumide, somatostatin, and prostaglandin analogues are also being investigated.

Total gastrectomy is considered the treatment of choice in those patients who do not respond to medical management; however, there is no evidence that this procedure provides protection from tumor growth or metastasis. Patients with metastatic gastrinoma require tumor resection or treatment with chemotherapeutic agents. Drugs such as streptozotocin, 5-fluorouracil, and doxorubicin have been reported to be effective in some patients.[32,84] Chemotherapy is not effective in reducing acid secretory effects and associated ulcer disease.

## Summary

At present, the effectiveness of antacids, $H_2$ antagonists, and sucralfate in the treatment of peptic ulcer is well documented, but there is no evidence that these drugs alter the natural history of the disease. As efficacy and safety appear comparable, the treatment of choice should be based on individual patient factors and the cost of drug therapy. Single bedtime doses of the $H_2$ antagonists have been shown to heal gastric and duodenal ulcers and may enhance compliance. Maintenance therapy should be reserved for those patients with severe symptoms and/or frequent relapses. Cessation of cigarette smoking may accelerate ulcer healing and decrease ulcer recurrence.

As more is learned about the physiologic regulation of acid secretion and the cytoprotective properties of the gastromucosal barrier, new antiulcer agents will be developed; however, safety rather than increased potency and efficacy will probably be the deciding factor in determining future drug therapy for peptic ulcer disease.


## References


1. Elashoff JD, Grossman MI. Trends in hospital admissions and death rates for peptic ulcer in the United States from 1970 to 1978. Gastroenterology 1980;78:280–285.
2. Sonnenburg A, Muller-Lissner SA, Vogel E, et al. Predictors of duodenal ulcer healing and relapse. Gastroenterology 1981;81: 1061–1067.
3. Friedman GD, Siegelaub AB, Seltzer CC. Cigarettes, alcohol, coffee and peptic ulcer. N Engl J Med 1974;290:469–473.
4. Korman MG, Hansky J, Merrett AC, et al. Ranitidine in duodenal ulcer: Incidence of healing and effect of smoking. Dig Dis Sci 1982;27:712–715.
5. Sontag S, Graham DY, Belsito A, et al. Cimetidine, cigarette smoking, and recurrence of duodenal ulcer. N Engl J Med 1984;311:689–693.
6. Geokas MC. Ethanol, the liver, and the gastrointestinal tract. Ann Intern Med 1981;95:198–211.
7. Graham DY, Smith JL. Aspirin and the stomach. Ann Intern Med 1986;104:390–398.
8. Aspirin Myocardial Infarction Study Research Group of the National Heart, Lung and Blood Institute. A randomized, controlled trial of aspirin in persons recovered from myocardial infarction. JAMA 1980;243:661–669.
9. Silvoso GR, Ivey KJ, Butt JH, et al. Incidence of gastric lesions in patients with rheumatic disease on chronic aspirin therapy. Ann Intern Med 1979;91:517–520.
10. Lanza FL, Royer GL, Nelson RS. Endoscopic evaluation of the effects of aspirin, buffered aspirin, and enteric-coated aspirin on gastric and duodenal mucosa. N Engl J Med 1980;303:136–138.
11. Silverstein FE, Kimmey MB, Saunders DR, et al. Gastric protection by misoprostol against 1300 mg of aspirin: An endoscopic study. Dig Dis Sci 1986;31(suppl):137S–41S.
12. Strand LJ. Upper gastrointestinal effects of newer nonsteroidal antiinflammatory agents, in Pfeiffer CJ (ed): Drugs and Peptic Ulcer II: Pathogenesis of Ulcer Induction Revealed by Drug Studies in Humans and Animals. Boca Raton, FL, CRC Press, 1982, pp 7–24.
13. Conn HO, Blitzer BL. Nonassociation of adrenocorticosteroid therapy and peptic ulcer. N Engl J Med 1976;294:473–479.
14. Messer JM, Reitman D, Sacks HS, et al. Association of adrenocorticosteroid therapy and peptic-ulcer disease. N Engl J Med 1983;309:21–24.
15. Soll AH, Isenberg JI. Duodenal ulcer disease, in Sleisenger MH, Fordtran JS (eds): Gastrointestinal Disease: Pathophysiology, Diagnosis, Management. Philadelphia, W.B. Saunders, 1983, pp 625–672.
16. Feldman M. Gastric secretion, in Sleisenger MH, Fordtran JS (eds): Gastrointestinal Disease: Pathophysiology, Diagnosis, Management. Philadelphia, W.B. Saunders, 1983, pp 541–558.
17. Richardson CT. Pathogenetic factors in peptic ulcer disease. Am J Med 1985;79(suppl 2C):1–7.
18. Hawkey CJ, Rampton DS. Prostaglandins and the gastrointestinal mucosa: Are they important in its function, disease, or treatment. Gastroenterology 1985;89:1162–1188.
19. Dooley CP, Cohen H. The clinical significance of *Campylobacter pylori*. Ann Intern Med 1988;108:70–79.
20. Richardson CT. Gastric ulcer, in Sleisenger MH, Fordtran JS (eds): Gastrointestinal Disease: Pathophysiology, Diagnosis, Management. Philadelphia, W.B. Saunders, 1983, pp 672–707.
21. Peterson WL, Richardson CT. Pharmacology and side effects of drugs used to treat peptic ulcer, in Sleisenger MH, Fordtran JS (eds): Gastrointestinal Disease: Pathophysiology, Diagnosis, Management. Philadelphia, W.B. Saunders, 1983, pp 708–725.
22. Peterson WL, Sturdevant RAL, Franki HD, et al. Healing of duodenal ulcer with an antacid regimen. N Engl J Med 1977;297: 341–345.
23. Ippoliti AF, Sturdevant RAL. Cimetidine versus intensive antacid therapy for peptic ulcer disease. Gastroenterology 1978;74: 393–395.
24. Lam I. Treatment of duodenal ulcer with antacid and sulpiride. Gastroenterology 1979;76:315–320.
25. Bianchi Porro G, Parente F, Lazzaroni M, et al. Medium-dose antacids versus cimetidine in the short-term treatment of duodenal ulcer. J Clin Gastroenterol 1986;8:141–145.
26. Hollander D, Harlan J. Antacids versus placebo in peptic ulcer disease treatment. JAMA 1973; 266:1181–1185.
27. Strom M. Antacid side-effects on bowel habits. Scand J Gastroenterol 1982;17(suppl 75):54–55.
28. Herzog D, Holtermuller KH. Antacid therapy—changes in mineral metabolism. Scand J Gastroenterol 1982;17(suppl 75): 56–62.
29. Ritschel WA. Antacids, in Antacids and Other Drugs in GI Diseases. Hamilton, Ill., Drug Intelligence, 1984, pp 42–124.
30. Feldman M, Richardson CT, Peterson WL, et al. Effect of low-dose propantheline on food-stimulated gastric acid secretion: Comparison with an "optimal effective dose" and interaction with cimetidine. N Engl J Med 1977;297:1427.
31. Londong W, Londong V, Prechtl R, et al. Interactions of cimetidine and pirenzepine on peptone-stimulated gastric acid secretion in man. Scand J Gastroenterol 1980;15(suppl 66):105.
32. Jensen RT, Gardner JD, Raufman JP, et al. Zollinger–Ellison syndrome: Current concepts and management. Ann Intern Med 1983;98:59–75.
33. Siepler JK, Mahakian K, Trudeau ST. Current concepts in clinical therapeutics: Peptic ulcer disease. Clin Pharm 1986;5: 128–142.

34. Somogyi A, Gugler R. Clinical pharmacokinetics of cimetidine. Clin Pharmacokinet 1983;8:463–495.
35. Gray GR, McKenzie I, Smith IS, et al. Oral cimetidine in severe duodenal ulceration. A double-blind controlled trial. Lancet 1977;1:4–7.
36. Bodemar G, Walan A. Cimetidine in the treatment of active duodenal and prepyloric ulcers. Lancet 1976;2:161–164.
37. Binder HJ, Cocco A, Crossley RJ, et al. Cimetidine in the treatment of duodenal ulcer. A multicenter double-blind study. Gastroenterology 1978;74:380–388.
38. Collen MJ, Hanan MR, Maher JA, et al. Cimetidine versus placebo in duodenal ulcer therapy. Six-week controlled double-blind investigation without any antacid therapy. Dig Dis Sci 1980;25:744.
39. Valenzuela JE, Dickson B, Dixon W, et al. Efficacy of a single nocturnal dose of cimetidine in active duodenal ulcer: Results of a United States multicenter trial. Postgrad Med Custom Commun 1985;(Nov):35–41.
40. Ciclitira PJ, Machell RJ, Farthing MJ, et al. A controlled trial of cimetidine in the treatment of gastric ulcer, in Burland WL, Simkins MA (eds): Cimetidine. Amsterdam, Excerpta Medica, 1977, pp 283–286.
41. Sawyer D, Conner CS, Scalley R. Cimetidine: Adverse reactions and acute toxicity. Am J Hosp Pharm 1981;38:188–197.
42. Jensen RT, Collen MJ, Pandol SJ, et al. Cimetidine-induced impotence and breast changes in patients with gastric hypersecretory states. N Engl J Med 1983;308:833–837.
43. Cohen IA, Johnson CE, Berardi RR, et al. Cimetidine–theophylline interaction: Effects of age and cimetidine dose. Ther Drug Monit 1985;7:426–434.
44. Bartle WR, Walker SE, Shapero T. Dose-dependent effect of cimetidine on phenytoin kinetics. Clin Pharmacol Ther 1983;33: 649–655.
45. Somogyi A, Gugler R. Drug interactions with cimetidine. Clin Pharmacokinet 1982;7:23–41.
46. Nazario M. The hepatic and renal mechanisms of drug interactions with cimetidine. Drug Intell Clin Pharm 1986;20:342–348.
47. Powell JR, Donn KH. Histamine $H_2$-antagonist drug interactions in perspective: Mechanistic concepts and clinical implications. Am J Med 1984;77(suppl 5B):57–84.
48. Kirch W, Hoensch H, Janisch HD. Interactions and non-interactions with ranitidine. Clin Pharmacokinet 1984;9:493–510.
49. Roberts CJC. Clinical pharmacokinetics of ranitidine. Clin Pharmacokinet 1984;9:211–221.
50. Walt RP, Trotman IF, Frost R, et al. Comparison of twice daily ranitidine with standard cimetidine treatment of duodenal ulcer. Gut 1981;22:319–322.
51. Lishman AH, Record CO. Ranitidine in the management of duodenal ulceration: Controlled and open comparison with cimetidine, in Misiewicz JJ, Wormsley KG (eds): The Clinical Use of Ranitidine. Oxford, Medicine Publishing Foundation, 1982, pp 163–167.
52. Conlin-Jones DG, Ireland A, Gear P, et al. Reducing overnight secretion of acid to heal duodenal ulcers: Comparison of standard divided dose of ranitidine with a single dose administered at night. Am J Med 1984;77(suppl 5B):116–122.
53. Wright JP, Marks IN, Mee AS, et al. Ranitidine in the treatment of gastric ulcer. S Afr Med J 1982;61:155–158.
54. Cohen A, Fabre L. Tolerance to repeated intravenous doses of ranitidine HCl and cimetidine HCl in normal volunteers. Curr Ther Res 1983;34:475–482.
55. Takabatake T, Ohta H, Maekawa M, et al. Pharmacokinetics of famotidine, a new $H_2$-antagonist, in relation to renal function. Eur J Clin Pharmacol 1985;28:327–331.
56. Berardi RR, Tankanow RM, Nostrant TT. Comparison of famotidine with cimetidine and ranitidine. Clin Pharm 1988; 7:271–284.
57. Texter ED (ed): Famotidine: Clinical applications of a new $H_2$-receptor antagonist. Am J Med 1986;81(suppl 4B):1–64.
58. Somerville KW, Kitchingman GA, Langman MJS. Effect of famotidine on oxidative drug metabolism. Eur J Clin Pharmacol 1986;30:279–281.
59. Opsahl JA, Abrahams PA, Halstenson CE, et al. Renal function after famotidine administration. (Abstr) Clin Pharmacol Ther 1986;39:218.
60. Bianchi Porro G, Keohane PP, eds. Nizatidine in peptic ulcer disease. Scand J Gastroenterol 1987;22(suppl 136):1–88.
61. Secor JW, Speeg KV, Meredith CG, et al. Lack of effect of nizatidine on hepatic drug metabolism. Br J Clin Pharmacol 1985;20:710–713.
62. Buyniski JP, Cavanagh RL, Pircio AW, et al. in Melchiorre C, Gianella M (eds): Highlights in Receptor Chemistry. Amsterdam, Elsevier, 1984, pp 195–213.
63. Clissold SP, Campoli-Richards DM. Omeprazole: A preliminary review of its pharmacodynamic and pharmacokinetic properties, and therapeutic potential in peptic ulcer disease and Zollinger–Ellison syndrome. Drugs 1986;32:15–47.
64. Cooperative Study. Omeprazole in duodenal ulceration: Acid inhibition, symptomatic relief, endoscopic healing, and recurrence. Br Med J 1984;289:525–528.
65. Delchier JC, Soule JC, Mignon M, et al. Effectiveness of omeprazole in seven patients with Zollinger–Ellison syndrome resistant to histamine $H_2$-receptor antagonists. Dig Dis Sci 1986;31:693–699.
66. McArthur KE, Collen MJ, Maton PN, et al. Omeprazole: Effective, convenient therapy for Zollinger–Ellison syndrome. Gastroenterology 1985;88:939–944.
67. Berardi RR, Caplan NB. Agents with tricyclic structures for treating peptic ulcer disease. Clin Pharm 1983;2:425–431.
68. Ligumsky M, Karmski F, Rochmilewitz D. Sucralfate stimulation of gastric PGEs synthesis: Possible mechanism to explain its effective cytoprotective mechanism. (Abstr) Gastroenterology 1984;86:1164.
69. Brogden RN, Heel RC, Speight TM, et al. Sucralfate: A review of its pharmacodynamic properties and therapeutic use in peptic ulcer disease. Drugs 1984;27:194–209.
70. Van Deventer GM, Schneidman D, Walsh JH. Sucralfate and cimetidine as single agents and in combination for treatment of active duodenal ulcers. Am J Med 1985;79(suppl 2C):39–44.
71. Brandstaetter G, Kratochvil P. Comparison of two sucralfate dosages (2 g twice a day versus 1 g four times a day) in duodenal ulcer healing. Am J Med 1985;79(suppl 2C):36–38.
72. Tesler MA, Lim ES. Protection of gastric mucosa by sucralfate from aspirin-induced erosions. J Clin Gastroenterol 1981;3 (suppl 2)171–175.
73. Hamilton I, O'Connor HJ, Wood NC, et al. Healing and recurrence of duodenal ulcer after treatment with tripotassium dicitrato bismuthate (TDB) tablets or cimetidine. Gut 1986;27: 106–110.
74. Grossman MI, Kurata JH, Rotter JI, et al. Peptic ulcer: New therapies, new diseases. Ann Intern Med 1981;95:609–627.
75. Konturek SJ, Pawlik W. Physiology and pharmacology of prostaglandins. Dig Dis Sci 1986;31(suppl):6S–19S.
76. Nicholson PA. A multicenter international controlled comparison of two dosage regimes of misoprostol and cimetidine in the treatment of duodenal ulcer in out-patients. Dig Dis Sci 1985;30(suppl):171S–177S.
77. Shield MJ. Interim results of a multicenter international comparison of misoprostol and cimetidine in the treatment of

outpatients with benign, gastric ulcers. Dig Dis Sci 1985;30 (suppl):178S–184S.
78. Vantrappen G, Janssens J, Popiela T, et al. Effect of 15 R methyl PGE2 (arbaprostil) on the healing of duodenal ulcer. Gastroenterology 1982;83:357–363.
79. Carling L, Unge P, Almstrom C, et al. Enprostil and cimetidine: Comparative efficacy and safety in patients with duodenal ulcer. Scand J Gastroenterol 1987;22:325–331.
80. Berardi RR, Savitsky ME, Nostrant TT. Maintenance therapy for prevention of recurrent peptic ulcers. Drug Intell Clin Pharm 1987;21:493–501.
81. Silvis SE. Final report on the United States multicenter trial comparing ranitidine to cimetidine as maintenance therapy following healing of duodenal ulcer. J Clin Gastroenterol 1985;7: 482–487.
82. Gough KR, Bardhan KD, Crowe JP, et al. Ranitidine and cimetidine in prevention of duodenal relapse: A double-blind, randomized, multicentre, comparative trial. Lancet 1984;2: 659–662.
83. Walker C. Complications of peptic ulcer disease and indications for surgery, in Sleisenger MH, Fordtran JS (eds): Gastrointestinal Disease: Pathophysiology, Diagnosis, Management. Philadelphia, W.B. Saunders, 1983, pp 725–738.
84. Wolfe MM, Jensen RT. Zollinger–Ellison syndrome: Current concepts in diagnosis and management. N Engl J Med 1987;317: 1200–1209.
85. Jensen RT, Collen MJ, McArthur KE, et al. Comparison of the effectiveness of ranitidine and cimetidine in inhibiting acid secretion in patients with gastric hypersecretory states. Am J Med 1984;77(suppl 5B):90–105.
86. Howard JM, Chremos AN, Collen MJ, et al. Famotidine, a new, potent, long-acting histamine $H_2$-receptor antagonist: Comparison with cimetidine and ranitidine in the treatment of Zollinger–Ellison syndrome. Gastroenterology 1985;88:1026–1033.

# Chapter 27 / Upper Gastrointestinal Bleeding

John Siepler, PharmD

Upper gastrointestinal bleeding (UGIB) is a condition in which bleeding occurs in the upper portion of the gastrointestinal tract, usually from a lesion located in the esophagus, stomach, or duodenum. Upper gastrointestinal bleeding may be a complication of peptic ulcer disease or esophageal varices.

In peptic ulcer disease an ulcer erodes into a blood vessel and then bleeds into the lumen of the digestive tract. Esophageal varices result when collateral blood circulation bypasses the liver in a patient with liver disease, resulting in portal hypertension. Vessels then become engorged in the esophagus; these are called esophageal varices. Stress-related mucosal lesions may also cause upper gastrointestinal bleeding. Patients susceptible to stress ulcers include those with sepsis, severe pulmonary disease, or burns or multiple traumas. Other causes of upper gastrointestinal bleeding include erosions from feeding or nasogastric tubes and Mallory–Weiss tears (in patients who experience excessive emesis or retching). Drug therapy is not the primary treatment for either of these causes, so this chapter focuses on the treatment of upper gastrointestinal bleeding as a complication of peptic ulcer disease, bleeding esophageal varices in a patient with severe liver disease, portal hypertension, and stress ulcers.

## Epidemiology

In one recent study, severe, active bleeding was seen in only 32 of 174 admissions for UGIB over $3\frac{1}{2}$ years.[1] The results of this study suggest that UGIB as a severe complication of peptic ulcer disease is a relatively rare occurrence. The overall mortality for massive hemorrhage from peptic ulcer is about 10%. This complication occurs in about 25% of patients and is the most common cause of mortality in this group.[2] The incidence of esophageal variceal bleeding is about the same as that of peptic ulcer bleeding.

The severity of stress ulcers varies from superficial erosions of the stomach and duodenum to deep ulcers producing life-threatening hemorrhage. Mucosal lesions occur almost immediately upon initiation of stress. Whereas early reports suggest a frequency of about 10%, lesions will occur in up to 90% of severely stressed patients.[3] In addition to burn patients, those patients with head injury, medical conditions serious enough to warrant admission to an intensive-care unit, and those patients who have survived major surgery are also thought to be at risk for development of stress ulcers. The incidence of severe bleeding in these stressed patients may be much lower. Some authors have suggested that less than 10% of these stressed patients will have serious bleeding episodes.[4]

The clinical presentation of the patient with UGIB is similar regardless of etiology. The chief complaint will be a history of bright red emesis or of coffee-ground-appearing emesis. The patient may have a history of peptic ulcer disease and/or alcoholic liver disease, but the source of bleeding cannot be differentiated without further diagnostic intervention. The patient may be hypotensive from blood loss and will usually be nontender on abdominal palpation. Even patients who bleed from a peptic ulcer will usually be otherwise asymptomatic.

## Pathophysiology

### *Peptic Ulcer Disease*

Bleeding occurs in patients with peptic ulcer disease when an ulcer or lesion erodes into a blood vessel or when generalized gastritis is so severe that oozing of blood occurs. These lesions can be classified as Forrest class I, II, or III. Forrest class I lesions are those that are actively bleeding. These lesions are classified further into lesions that are spurting or oozing venous blood. In a Forrest class II lesion, a blood vessel is visible at the base of the ulcer crater when viewed endoscopically. Patients with Forrest class I and II lesions have an increased incidence of rebleeding compared with those with Forrest class III lesions. The remaining lesions are grouped as Forrest class III.

The specific reason for the occurrence of a bleeding episode in a patient with peptic ulcer disease is unknown, but it is thought that the peptic ulcer patient whose disease is more severe (more frequent recurrences after cessation of treatment) is at greater risk for this complication. Frequently, the bleeding occurs in association with the ingestion of aspirin or other nonsteroidal anti-inflammatory agents. In a recent study, lesions in 35% of the patients admitted for UGIB over $2\frac{1}{2}$ years were associated with ingestion of drugs of this class.[5] Bleeding is said to occur in greater frequency in the fall and winter months; but experience at the University of California–Davis suggests that the frequency of bleeding has been greater in the summer months.[6]

The bleeding episode may occur frequently without classic peptic ulcer symptoms because of the buffering action of the blood. Often, the first symptom is a bloody emesis or emesis of clots. Some patients notice a dark, tarry, or black stool as the first hint of bleeding. If the bleeding is a slow ooze or trickle, weakness and anemia can be the first symptoms of UGIB. In any event, bleeding peptic ulcers can be serious as mortality rates as high as 35% have been reported.[5]

### *Esophageal Varices*

Patients with liver disease have an increased pressure in the portal vein that supplies the liver. The source of the portal blood is the gastrointestinal tract, and the only outlet for this blood is the liver. In advanced alcoholic cirrhosis, and other types of cirrhosis as well, the fibrosis of the liver causes the resistance of blood flow in the portal system to increase, and as a result, the pressure in the portal system is elevated. This increase in pressure in the portal system is called portal hypertension.

When significant portal hypertension develops, the blood bypasses the liver through collateral vessels. The collateral vessels pass through the hemorrhoidal and esophageal veins, which become engorged with blood at higher-than-normal pressures. These engorged veins located in the lower part of the esophagus are called esophageal varices. The presence of esophageal varices in an alcoholic or any patient with liver disease is consistent with portal hypertension. Occasionally, through some unknown stimulus, these veins bleed into the gastrointestinal tract.

## Clinical Presentation

When a patient presents with upper gastrointestinal bleeding, the cause of bleeding is unknown. Only half of alcoholic patients bleed from esophageal varices.[1] Nevertheless, when the patient with UGIB is admitted to the emergency room or clinic, an adequate history must be taken. The hospital or clinic pharmacist must pay particular attention to a drug history at this time and focus specifically on ulcerogenic drugs. The patient may not consider aspirin a drug and may not mention taking aspirin in a conventional drug history. Other contributing factors are important at this time such as a history of peptic ulcer disease or alcoholic liver disease. The proper mode of treatment involves three stages: (1) stabilization of the patient, (2) diagnosis of the cause of the bleeding episode, and (3) specific treatment of the bleeding lesion.

Upon admission, an intravenous line is inserted, laboratory samples are drawn, and the patient is typed and cross-matched for several units of blood. Intravenous normal saline (0.9%) is given at a rapid rate until vital signs are stable. If the patient does not stabilize, intravenous pressors may be used. Dopamine is frequently administered for pressure stabilization; however, dopamine increases blood flow to the organs that are bleeding and may supply more blood to the bleeding lesion than other pressors. Additionally, a large-bore nasogastric tube is placed, and the stomach is lavaged with large amounts of water or saline. Sterile saline is not necessary at this point. Also, attempts to use iced saline to cut down blood flow to the mucosa and to decrease bleeding have not proven effective. For this reason, and because it may slow the clearing of clots from the stomach, the use of ice during stabilization is discouraged.

## Diagnosis

Once the patient is stable, diagnosis may take place. Despite the most careful history, a precise diagnosis cannot be made until endoscopy. Several studies have shown that even in alcoholic patients who are suspected of having esophageal varices, only about 50% of these patients actually bleed from these varices. The remainder bleed from peptic ulcers and other lesions.[1,6] The recommended diagnostic scheme is shown in Table 27.1.

**Table 27.1** Diagnostic Scheme in Upper Gastrointestinal Bleeding

1. Stabilize patient hemodynamically
   - Stabilize blood pressure
   - Start an intravenous line ($D_5LR^a$ or 0.9% NaCl)
   - Use pressors if necessary
2. Insert large-bore nasogastric tube (large enough to lavage with water or saline): Lavage until clear (to aid diagnosis with endoscope)
3. Obtain medical history
   - Obtain drug history
   - Identify any previous bleeding episodes and possible causes
4. Conduct physical examination
5. Perform endoscopy
6. Treatment initiation depends on diagnosis

[a] 5% dextrose in lactated Ringer's solution.

A physical examination should be performed as soon as possible. Particular attention must be given to the patient's pulse rate and character, the presence or absence of neck vein distension, and the state of peripheral capillary perfusion. Further attention in the examination must be placed on the abdomen. The presence of ascites, spider nevi, or hepatosplenomegaly is significant in the alcoholic patient. When examining the rectum, tarry stools may suggest chronic bleeding that pre-existed this severe episode. Bright red blood without obvious cause (e.g., hemorrhoids) may result from massive upper gastrointestinal bleeding and rapid transit through the alimentary canal.

A large bore nasogastric tube is inserted and manual irrigation of the stomach begun once the diagnosis is certain. If the return from the tube becomes clear, the tube is removed and the patient sedated and an endoscopy performed. The purpose of the endoscopy is to determine the source of the bleeding. The diagnostic accuracy of early endoscopy is greater than 90%[7] and considered crucial to progressing to the next step of therapy. An experienced physician may perform therapeutic endoscopy using bipolar electrocautery, laser photocoagulation, or heater probe.

## Treatment

Treatment depends on the cause of the bleeding. The patient with bleeding esophageal varices demands a different treatment scheme than the patient who presents as a complication of peptic ulcer disease.

### *Esophageal Varices*

When esophageal varices are established as the source of bleeding, treatment is centered on two principles: (1) local injection of the varices (sclerotherapy), and (2) reduction of portal pressure with vasopressin.

**Sclerotherapy**

Injection of the varices is performed via esophageal sclerotherapy. Esophageal sclerotherapy has been performed for at least 20 years. Development of the flexible fiberoptic endoscope and long-needle injectors that fit down one of the channels of the scope has allowed sclerotherapy to become popular among gastroenterologists. In sclerotherapy, a specific sclerosant liquid is injected through an endoscope into the varix by the gastroenterologist. While other sclerosant solutions have been used in other countries, the solutions used in the United States have been limited to sodium tetradecyl sulfate (Sotradecol) and sodium morrhuate. In experiments in animals, additions to these solutions have been found to be more effective than use of the solutions alone; however, a trial in humans has yet to show superiority of one solution to another. The most popular of these additions is a mixture of 50% dextrose, cephalothin, and alcohol. Comparative studies have been conducted and indicate similar efficacy for sodium morrhuate and sodium tetradecyl sulfate, but sodium morrhuate appears to form ulcers at the injection site more frequently than sodium tetradecyl sulfate.[9]

Efficacy of injection sclerotherapy remains controversial. Several researchers have attempted to use sclerotherapy to obliterate varices from patients who are not actively bleeding. The success of this practice depends on the assumption that the obliterated varices will be less likely to bleed than those not injected.

The selection of patients for injection sclerotherapy is critical. To date, no trial has supported an association between the life expectancy of an alcoholic with esophageal varices and injection sclerotherapy. Therefore, injection sclerotherapy cannot be recommended for prophylaxis of bleeding in patients with esophageal varices. Patients who receive injection sclerotherapy on an emergency basis (immediately upon stabilization) rather than an urgency basis (within 24 hours), however, have lower transfusion requirements and better chances of survival.[6]

Few clinicians question the theory that esophageal varices stop bleeding acutely, but several researchers have had difficulty in proving this theory. Recently in a large multicenter study conducted in California, researchers found that mortality and rebleeding rates were greater among patients randomly selected to receive sclerotherapy than in those who did not have sclerotherapy. This study had two limitations, however. The researchers delayed as much as 1 day after initial presentation to enter the patient into the study, which excluded many of the most critically ill patients who died earlier. Also, unequal numbers of patients were entered into the study by different institutions. Some hospitals had larger samples of nonsclerotherapy patients, and other hospitals had larger samples of sclerotherapy patients. This tended to skew the data regarding survival, favoring the nonsclerotherapy group.[10]

As in many areas with conflicting data, some clinicians believe that injection sclerotherapy is effective. The best advice may be that if the gastroenterologists at the institution where the patient presents are experienced in injection sclerotherapy, then the procedure is probably worth trying. If these practitioners are not experienced in sclerotherapy, the best step may be to use vasopressin and wait for the bleeding to stop. Patients who stop bleeding after receiving sclerotherapy are admitted to the intensive care unit for observation for at least 3 days. Data from the University of California at Davis Medical Center have shown that rebleeding occurs within 3 days in 75% of the patients who present with upper gastrointestinal bleeding. Vasopressin is not indicated in patients whose bleeding stops with sclerotherapy.[9]

**Vasopressin**

Antidiuretic hormone, vasopressin (Pitressin), has been used for treatment of esophageal variceal bleeding for at least 20 years. Early researchers used intermittent, intravenous doses of vasopressin in an effort to lower portal pressure to stop bleeding of varices.[11] Later, intraarterial vasopressin was introduced as the treatment of choice for esophageal variceal bleeding. This treatment requires the patient to be stable enough for transport to radiology and to undergo angiography of the splanchnic arterial system. Under angiography, a catheter is placed into the splanchnic arterial bed close to the bleeding lesion. An infusion of vasopressin 0.2–0.4 U/min is started and continued until the patient stops bleeding. Among the common side effects of this therapy are bradycardia and electrolyte abnormalities.[11]

In the mid-1970s, investigators found that in animals the use of intravenous vasopressin was as effective in lowering portal pressure as intraarterial vasopressin. By the late 1970s, intravenous vasopressin had replaced intraarterial delivery as the most common therapy for esophageal varices. Intravenous vasopressin therapy is initiated with an infusion of 30–40 U over 30 to 40 minutes and is followed by a 0.4-U/min infusion. The infusion is continued until 24 hours after bleeding cessation. The infusion dose is then decreased by half and administered for 12 hours and then halved again and administered for another 12 hours. A study conducted at Stanford University and other area hospitals randomly selected patients and divided them into two groups. Patients in one group received vasopressin and patients in the second group received a placebo.[12] These researchers found no significant differences in the amount of blood transfused or survival rates between the two groups. This study was plagued by the same problem that limited the sclerotherapy study mentioned earlier. The effort to allow all patients to sign a consent form meant that the mean time between arrival in the emergency room and entry into the study was about 1.5 days. As a result, the most critically ill patients (and those most likely to benefit from drug treatment) died within the 36-hour period. Despite the negative nature of this study, vasopressin remains the most common treatment for patients with bleeding esophageal varices.

**Nonpharmacologic Treatment**

The most popular of the nonpharmacologic treatments, which are primarily local therapies, is the Sengstaken–Blakemore tube. This tube is designed to compress the varices mechanically and stop bleeding. This form of treatment has never been evaluated scientifically and is prone to such complications as spontaneous bacterial peritonitis, perforation of the esophagus, and resultant esophageal stricture. Therefore, use of the Sengstaken–Blakemore tube cannot be recommended.

Surgery is another form of therapy for bleeding esophageal varices. Various operations are designed to lower the portal pressure by shunting blood around the liver. The problem is that these operations are complicated and require that the patient be stable, which is often not the case with patients who are bleeding acutely. Postoperative follow-up of these patients reveals that they often suffer from hepatic encephalopathy. Nevertheless, such surgical procedures may prolong life in patients with portal hypertension who are stable and considered relatively good risks.

#### Summary

Esophageal variceal bleeding is a catastrophic event that carries a high mortality. The patient who does not die from bleeding often dies from other complications of alcoholic liver disease. Pharmacologic treatment modalities include local injection sclerotherapy and intravenous administration of vasopressin. Despite advances in care for critically ill patients, mortality rates remain near 25% for patients with acutely bleeding esophageal varices.

### *Bleeding Peptic Ulcers*

Therapeutic trials designed to determine the effectiveness of drug treatment for peptic ulcer disease bleeding have concentrated on drugs used to treat peptic ulcers. Acid secretion suppression with $H_2$-receptor antagonists and buffering with antacids are the cornerstones of treatment for this disorder, and these drugs are also used to treat acute bleeding as a result of peptic ulcer disease.

Conventional therapy aimed at reducing gastric acid is of two forms, each with a different pharmacologic mechanism. Antacids buffer the acid produced in the stomach, and histamine $H_2$-receptor antagonists prevent that acid from being produced by the parietal cells. Conventional schemes of dosing require that these two drugs be given on an intermittent basis, with antacids administered orally or via nasogastric tube 8 to 24 times daily (every 1–3 hours), or cimetidine and ranitidine administered intravenously to four times daily. This regimen leads to periods of good acid secretory control (right after the dose is given) and periods of poor acid secretory control (right before the next dose is due). Current treatments for peptic ulcer–induced gastric bleeding require constant acid secretion suppression in an effort to stabilize the clot that has formed, to stop the bleeding episode in the ulcer crater. In vitro studies show that the clot is more stable in gastric juice that has a pH of 7.[13] Therefore, the goal of treatment is creation of a gastric pH of 7. An alternative to conventional dose regimens is one that produces a smooth and constant acid secretion control. Constant infusions of $H_2$-blockers produce this smooth, constant, acid secretion control. Three regimens are available that control acid secretion and thus treat this type of bleeding: (1) oral antacids given at frequent dosage intervals (as often as hourly): (2) $H_2$-receptor antagonists administered in conventional intravenous drip regimens once every 6 hours (cimetidine and ranitidine) or once every 12 hours (famotidine); and (3) $H_2$-blockers administered via constant intravenous infusions.

Titration of intragastric pH with antacids was introduced by Pruitt and colleagues in the early 1970s.[3] Hourly administration of antacids with pH determinations made before each scheduled dose are designed to follow the effect of antacids on gastric pH. If the pH is less than 7, the antacid dose is doubled and monitoring is continued hourly.

In the early 1970s, the development of histamine $H_2$-receptor antagonists was a significant pharmacologic achievement.[14] The drug that reached the market first, cimetidine, was quite effective at eliminating gastric acid for 4 to 5 hours after an oral dose. When given intravenously, the intragastric pH recedes into the acidic range after about 4 to 5 hours. In the United States, a dose of 300 mg given intravenously every 6 hours is the standard intravenous dose for cimetidine.

In late 1979, ranitidine was synthesized. This drug differs from cimetidine by having a furan ring instead of an imidazole ring in its structure. Ranitidine is 4 to 10 times more potent than cimetidine on a milligram-to-milligram basis.[15] When given in intermittent intravenous administrations, the recommended dose of 50 mg of ranitidine has a duration of action similar to that of cimetidine.[16]

Recently, Frank et al[16] published a comparison study of intermittent intravenous cimetidine in 300- and 400-mg doses and ranitidine at a 50-mg dose. The results clearly show that all three doses have similar effects on intragastric pH and similar duration of effect. Peterson and Richardson[17] produced similar results, except for the period 5 to 8 hours after the dose, in which the ranitidine response appeared to flatten out at an intragastric pH of 4. In this study, cimetidine 300 mg produced an intragastric pH of about 2 at the same time after the dose.[17]

This pharmacodynamic anomaly explains cimetidine's apparent failure to control intragastric pH better than antacids. If the intragastric pH testing is done near the time the next dose is due, usually 6 hours after the last dose was given, very little of the drug remains in the stomach, and the intragastric pH is usually acidic. Some patients, however, have responses out of the normal range. Therefore, frequent testing (at least every 3 hours) of intragastric pH is essential to ensure that the patient responds effectively to the drug therapy.

#### Constant Infusions

Alternative-dose regimens for $H_2$ blockers have been used for several years. In 1975, Siepler et al[18] used constant-infusion metiamide to demonstrate effective acid control in a patient who had Zollinger–Ellison syndrome. Recently, Peterson and Richardson[13] compared the intragastric pH response of duodenal ulcer patients to intermittent and constant-infusion cimetidine. These researchers found that cimetidine 300 mg every 6 hours produced peak pH responses of about 5 to 6 immediately after the dose, but this response decreased to an intragastric pH of about 2 to 3 by the end of the 6-hour dosage interval. In contrast, a bolus of cimetidine 300 mg followed by a 50-mg/h infusion of cimetidine produced an intragastric pH that remained in the range 4–5. Addition of an antacid at a rate of 30 mL/h (0.5 mL/min) raised that response to 6–7. Doses of 100 mg/h plus antacids were necessary to achieve a pH response that was uniformly above 7.

Ostro et al[19] studied the responses of patients in an intensive care unit to several doses of intravenous cimetidine given by constant infusion or intermittent injection. These researchers found a pH response similar to that found by Peterson and Richardson[9]—a smoother and more uniform pH response was obtained in the patients receiving constant infusions.

Fewer studies evaluating the intragastric pH response to ranitidine have been published, but we recently evaluated the intragastric pH response of patients receiving total parenteral nutrition and either cimetidine or ranitidine via constant infusions. Two hundred and seventy courses of therapy were studied over a 1-year period. A mean pH for the day was obtained and recorded on a data sheet by the pharmacist. When patients were on constant infusion, the daily pH variance was never greater than 1. The mean daily ranitidine dose was 227 mg, and the mean cimetidine dose was 1,235 mg. The mean pH for all patients was 5 and was sustained for the 7 days during which data were collected. No attempt was made to attain a pH of 7 as Peterson and Richardson did. Clearly, the intragastric pH response to cimetidine and ranitidine is much more smooth with constant infusions than with intermittent dosing. Clinical experience with constant infusion is almost uniform in patients with upper gastrointestinal bleeding, in whom previous studies using intermittent $H_2$-receptor antagonists have produced questionable results.[20]

In 1979, Bauer[21] used constant-infusion cimetidine in patients admitted with episodes of upper gastrointestinal bleeding. By administering a dose of 400 mg followed by a constant-infusion dose of 150 mg/h for 4 hours decreasing to 75 mg/h for the duration of therapy, Bauer allowed the patients to stabilize before surgery to correct the bleeding lesion. For this reason, a comparison of more conventional intermittent-dose cimetidine therapy is not possible. It remains, however, an early attempt using constant-infusion cimetidine.

Clinical studies remain the cornerstone of the evaluation of efficacy of a certain form of drug therapy for the treatment of upper gastrointestinal bleeding.[22–26] All patients in these studies had signs of active hemorrhage. Efficacy criteria differed between studies but generally included the need for emergency surgery or transfusion, the incidence of cessation of acute bleeding, the rate of rebleeding, and the rate of mortality. Most of these patients had peptic ulcer–related hemorrhage, although some patients with variceal bleeding were included in some of the studies.

Controlled comparison studies of intravenous cimetidine reveal that this $H_2$-blocker offers no consistent, significant advantage over placebo with regard to cessation of acute bleeding, rebleeding, or need for surgery[22,23]; however, a slight but statistically significant reduction in mortality was noted subsequent to cimetidine therapy in patients with gastric ulcers.[22] The trend toward clinical improvement among patients with gastric ulcers was also noted in studies of intravenous ranitidine therapy. In a recent study conducted by Nowak et al,[24] ranitidine-treated patients required fewer transfusions than gastric ulcer patients who received placebos. Other studies comparing cimetidine and ranitidine also reveal no significant differences between the groups studied.[25,26]

Continuous infusion of cimetidine has been shown in one recent study to be associated with a lower mortality than intermittent dosing.[5] Siepler showed that 94 patients receiving intravenous cimetidine at 50 mg/h had a lower mortality rate than a matched group of patients who received intermittent doses of cimetidine every 6 hours. Two differences between this study and others were the inclusion of only severe upper gastrointestinal bleeders and the lack of a strict control group. All patients included were admitted to an intensive care unit immediately after being stabilized in the emergency room. Current studies are assessing therapy for this subgroup of patients, who may benefit from drug therapy more than less ill patients.

While no study conclusively shows the efficacy of cimetidine or ranitidine in the treatment of upper gastrointestinal bleeding, conventional therapy continues to employ one of the three $H_2$-blockers in these patients. After stabilization, a loading dose of cimetidine (300 mg), ranitidine (50 mg), or famotidine (20 mg) is given followed by a constant infusion that is titrated (with the addition of antacids if necessary) to produce an intragastric pH of 7. The initial infusion dose currently recommended is cimetidine 50 mg/h, ranitidine 8 mg/h, or famotidine 1.7 mg/h. If the intragastric pH is not controlled with the starting dose, the dose should be doubled. Treatment should continue for at least 3 days. If the patient rebleeds during this period, alternative therapy such as surgery must be considered. Studies have shown that 75% of patients who rebleed do so within 3 days of the initial bleed.

### *Stress-Ulcer Prophylaxis*

As with upper gastrointestinal bleeding, acid secretion suppression is used as the primary form of therapy for patients who require stress-ulcer prophylaxis. Two forms of acid suppression—buffering with antacids and prevention of secretion with $H_2$ blockers—are discussed here.

Attempts to decrease the incidence of stress-related mucosal lesion (SRML) by decreasing gastric acid date back many years. As long as 10 years ago, antacid titration was used in an attempt to control complications from SRML. McAlhaney et al[27] gave antacids on an hourly basis to burn patients in increasing doses that were dependent on the intragastric pH. With a desired intragastric pH endpoint of 7, McAlhaney et al found that these frequent high doses of antacids prevented development of SRML. They also found that 25% of the control patients, who did not receive antacids, and only 4% of the antacid-treated patients required transfusions.

Priebe et al[28] compared the effectiveness of hourly titrations of antacids on intragastric pH with the pH control produced by cimetidine (300 mg intravenously every 6 hours, with the initial dose increased if the goal of intragastric pH is not achieved). These researchers found that hourly titrations of antacid were more effective at keeping the intragastric pH in the desired range than cimetidine, it being given on a less frequent basis. Priebe et al also reported a greater frequency of intragastric fluid testing positive for blood in the cimetidine-treated group. This test, however, was much too sensitive for clinical relevance as the mere presence of a Salem Sump tube often produces small erosions in the stomach that can produce positive results if Hemoccult is used to test for blood in gastric juice.

The need for blood transfusions is a better indicator of significant gastric bleeding in these patients at risk for

SRML, and in the Priebe study,[28] only one patient had a significant upper gastrointestinal bleed that was probably related to SRML. This study is therefore significant primarily in its finding that hourly antacid titration of intragastric pH is more effective at controlling intragastric pH than is intravenous cimetidine given on an intermittent basis.

Zinner et al[29] also compared antacid titration with intravenous cimetidine and placebo infusions. The results of this study also indicated that hourly titrations of antacids were more effective at maintaining the intragastric pH in an acceptable range.

Each of these studies increases the basic understanding of the pharmacotherapy of stress-ulcer prophylaxis. One clear trend is the finding that frequent (hourly) dosing of a drug designed to eliminate acid is superior to administration at greater dosage intervals. Although the lengths of activity of these two drugs depend on two different mechanisms, it is clear that the one given on an hourly basis (antacids) is more effective at maintaining intragastric pH in an acceptable range than the one given at 6-hour intervals.

Despite the evidence that cimetidine in conventional doses produces less than uniform control of intragastric pH, several studies demonstrate that cimetidine is effective in preventing progression and development of complications of SRML. Studies conducted by Halloran et al[30] as well as Peura et al[31] have shown that cimetidine is effective at preventing both the development of SRML and the complications from those gastric lesions.

Studies have also been conducted on ranitidine. Vandenberg et al[32] administered ranitidine 50 mg intravenously followed by a constant infusion of 0.2 mg/kg/h or placebo to treat patients who were at risk for the development of gastrointestinal bleeding from acute gastric mucosal lesions. These researchers found that despite a wide range of pH control, three patients in the placebo group and one patient in the ranitidine group developed a serious gastrointestinal bleed.

## Summary

It is difficult to make conclusions on the basis of these studies. It appears that maintenance of intragastric pH in a neutral range (3.5–7) decreases the incidence of stress-related mucosal lesions in critically ill patients. Most complications of stress ulcers are related to bleeding. Bleeding, however, is quite rare in studies; severe bleeding was seen in very few patients in the trials conducted. While the need for prophylactic therapy is questionable, the efficacy shown for $H_2$ blockers in controlled studies suggests that selective use of stress-ulcer prophylaxis is indicated.[30,31]

## References


1. Krejs GJ, Litle KH, Westergaard H, et al. Laser photocoagulation for the treatment of acute peptic ulcer bleeding. N Engl J Med 1987;316:618–621.
2. Crohn BB. The need for aggressive therapy in massive upper gastrointestinal hemorrhage. JAMA 1954;151:626–627.
3. Czaja AJ, McAlheny JC, Pruitt BA. Gastric acid secretion and acute gastroduodenal disease after thermal injury. Arch Surg 1976;111:243–6.
4. Day SB, MacMillan BF, Altheimer WA. Curlings Ulcer, an Experiment of Nature. Springfield, IL, Charles C. Thomas; 1972, pp 183–184.
5. Siepler JK. A dosage alternative for H-2 receptor antagonists. Clin Ther 1986;8(suppl A):24–33.
6. Sprio H. Complications of peptic ulcer disease, in Clinical Gastroenterology, 2nd ed. New York, Macmillan, 1979.
7. Jones FA, King WE. A study of acute gastric ulcers causing hemorrhage. Aust Ann Med 1953;2:179–182.
8. Forest JAH, Finlayson MPC, Milman J, et al. Endoscopic diagnosis of active bleeding. Dig Dis Sci 1977;23:237–240.
9. Prindiville T, Trudeau W. A comparison of immediate vs. delayed bleeding varices. Gastroenterol Endosc 1986;32:385–388.
10. Larson AW, Cohen H, Zweiban B, et al. Acute esophageal variceal sclerotherapy: Results of a randomized trial. JAMA 1986;155:497.
11. Siepler JK. Esophageal variceal bleeding. US Pharm-Hosp Ed 1979;24:H8–H11.
12. Choskier M, Grossman RJ, et al. A controlled comparison of intra-arterial and intravenous vasopressin. Gastroenterology 1979;77:540.
13. Peterson WL, Richardson CT. Sustained fasting achlorhydria: A comparison of two medical regimens. Gastroenterology 1985; 88:666.
14. Black JW, Duncan WAM, Durant GJ, et al. Definition and antagonism of histamine $H_2$ receptors. Nature 1972;236:499–508.
15. Birner BD, Conner C, Sawyer D, et al. Ranitidine: A new $H_2$ receptor antagonist. Clin Pharm 1982;1:499–508.
16. Frank WD, Peace K, Watson M, et al. Duration of action of three doses of cimetidine and ranitidine. Clin Pharmacol Ther 1987;40:665–672.
17. Peterson WL, Richardson CT. Intravenous cimetidine and two regimens of ranitidine to reduce fasting gastric acidity. Ann Intern Med 1986;104:505–507.
18. Siepler JK, Bombeck CT, Donahue PE, et al. Zollinger–Ellison syndrome. Ill Med J 1978;153:282–284.
19. Ostro MJ, Russel JA, et al. Control of gastric pH with cimetidine: Boluses vs primed infusions. Gastroenterology 1985;89: 532.
20. Siepler JK, Nishikawa R, Mondragon K, et al. Constant infusion cimetidine and ranitidine. Drug Intell Clin Pharm, in press.
21. Bauer H. Cimetidine in the preoperative treatment of acute bleeding gastroduodenal lesions. Munch Med Wochenschr 1979;121:1085–1089.
22. Barer D, Oglivie A, Henry D. Cimetidine and tranexaminic acid in the treatment of upper gastrointestinal bleeding. N Engl J Med 1983;308:1571–1575.
23. Zuckerman G, Welch R, Douglas S, et al. Controlled trial of medical therapy for active gastrointestinal bleeding and prevention of rebleeding. Am J Med 1984;76:361–366.
24. Nowak A, Saldinski C, Gorka Z, et al. Ranitidine in the treatment of acute upper gastrointestinal haemorrhage. Hepato-Gastroenterology 1981;28:267–269.
25. Falk A, Farle N, Haglund U, et al. Histamine $H_2$ receptor antagonists in gastroduodenal haemorrhage. Scand J Gastroenterol 1985;20(suppl 110):95–100.

26. Thompson ABR, Maguire T, Wensel RH, et al. Ranitidine vs. cimetidine in the management of acute gastrointestinal tract bleeding. J Clin Gastroenterol 1984;6:295–299.
27. McAlhaney JC, Czja AJ, Pruitt BA. Antacid control of complications from acute gastroduodenal disease after burn. J Trauma 1976;16:648–655.
28. Priebe HJ, Skillman JJ, Bushnell LS, et al. Antacid vs. cimetidine in preventing acute gastroduodenal bleeding: A randomized control trial. N Engl J Med 1980;302:426–429.
29. Zinner MJ, Zuidema GD, Smith PL, et al. The prevention of upper gastrointestinal tract bleeding in patients in an intensive care unit. Surg Gynecol Obstet 1981;153(2):214–220.
30. Halloran LG, Zfass AM, Gale WE, et al. Prevention of active gastroduodenal complications after severe head trauma: A controlled trial of cimetidine prophylaxis. Am J Surg 1980;139: 44–48.
31. Peura DA, Johnson LF. Cimetidine for prevention and treatment of gastroduodenal mucosal lesions in patients in an intensive care unit. Ann Intern Med 1985;103:173–176.
32. Vandenberg B, Van Blansenstein M. The prevention of stress-induced upper gastrointestinal bleeding by ranitidine in critically ill patients, in Misiewicz JJ, Wormsley KG (eds), The Clinical Use of Ranitidine. London, Medicine Publishing Co, 1985; pp 263–268.

# Chapter 28 / Inflammatory Bowel Disease

Joseph T. DiPiro, PharmD, L. Michael Posey, and Talmadge A. Bowden, Jr, MD

Two forms of idiopathic inflammatory bowel disease (IBD) are of primary concern to the pharmacy clinician: ulcerative colitis, a mucosal inflammatory condition confined to the rectum and colon, and Crohn's disease, a transmural inflammation of gastrointestinal mucosa that may occur in any part of the gastrointestinal tract. The etiologies of both conditions are unknown, but they may have a common pathogenetic mechanism.

In this chapter, these conditions are discussed separately but compared and contrasted when appropriate. Antibiotic-associated colitis (covered in Chapter 81) and other forms of drug- or chemical-induced inflammatory gastrointestinal diseases are not discussed here.

Ulcerative colitis was first identified in 1875[1] and was for many years thought to be a condition of North Americans and Europeans. Today its reported incidence is rising in many parts of the world, with increasing recognition of the disorder as distinct from infectious diarrhea. Crohn's disease, described initially in 1932,[2] was originally thought to be a disease of the ileum. Experience has taught that the disease, sometimes incorrectly called regional enteritis, may occur in any portion of the gastrointestinal tract.

The patterns of clinical presentation of IBD can vary widely. Patients may have a single acute episode that resolves and does not recur, but most patients experience acute exacerbations after periods of remission. With more severe disease, prolonged illness may occur.

Although IBD is expressed primarily in the gastrointestinal tract, it should be recognized as a systemic disease. IBD may be associated with arthritis, uveitis, liver disease, and other complications.

The cause of inflammatory bowel disease is not known; therefore, effective therapy has been difficult to define. For Crohn's disease, no true cure exists, whereas for ulcerative colitis a true cure is achieved by proctocolectomy. Treatment for IBD has changed little over the past 25 years. Sulfasalazine was first used in the early 1940s and steroids were introduced in 1948. Immunosuppressive agents, antibiotics, and nutritional support with hyperalimentation offer help in the management of complications, but the natural progression of these diseases has remained unchanged.

## Epidemiology

At least one million Americans are believed to have inflammatory bowel disease, with 15,000 to 30,000 new cases diagnosed annually.[3] Two key studies, one in Baltimore, Maryland,[4] and the other in Rochester, Minnesota,[5] established a generally accepted incidence for ulcerative colitis of 3 to 6 per 100,000 and a prevalence of 35 to 70 cases per 100,000 Americans. Crohn's disease was believed to have an incidence of 2 to 4 and a prevalence of 20 to 40 per 100,000 people; however, the incidence of Crohn's disease appears to be increasing since those 1960s-era studies. The increase is believed to be real, not just increased awareness or better diagnosis.[3]

Both sexes are affected equally,[3] although some studies have shown slightly greater numbers of women with the disease.[6] Both ulcerative colitis and Crohn's disease have bimodal distributions in age of initial presentation. The peak incidence occurs in the second or third decade of life, but infants and the elderly may present with either disorder. Significantly increased incidences (four to five times normal) have been observed in North American Jews, while blacks and orientals have a relatively low incidence of occurrence.

## Etiology

While the exact etiology of ulcerative colitis and Crohn's disease is unknown, similar factors are believed responsible for each condition (Table 28.1).

***Infectious Theories*** Despite many years of searching, no causative infectious agent has been identified. The infectious theory has always been attractive because the mucosal inflammation produced is very similar to that caused by invasive microbial pathogens. Bacteria-free filtrate, extracted from colonic ulcerations or Crohn's disease tissues, has been shown to produce symptoms in animal models, leading to speculation about viruses, a cytopathic agent, or L-forms of bacteria as causes.[6,7] Current research focuses on viruses, viroids, protozoans, and mycoplasmas.[3]

***Host Factors*** Genetics and altered host susceptibility are two other proposed theories. Cases have been identified in monozygotic twins and families.

Crohn's disease may result from infectious invasion during periods of reduced host immunologic status. Still under study is the possibility that patients with certain HLA genotypes may have increased incidence of Crohn's disease.[6,7]

***Immunologic Mechanisms*** An immunologic basis for ulcerative colitis and Crohn's disease is supported by a number of experimental observations.

1. Intrarectal instillation of dinitrochlorobenzene into sensitized rabbits produces a mild colonic inflammation similar to the human condition.

**Table 28.1** Proposed Etiology for Inflammatory Bowel Disease

| | |
|---|---|
| Infectious agents | Immune defects |
| Viruses | Altered host susceptibility |
| L-forms of bacteria | Immune-mediated mucosal damage |
| *Mycobacteria* | Psychologic factors |
| *Chlamydia* | Stress |
| Endotoxins | Emotional or physical trauma |
| Genetics | Occupation |
| Metabolic defects | Environmental factors |
| Connective tissue disorders | Diet |
| Genetic disorders | |

Compiled from References 3, 6, and 7.

2. Circulating lymphocytes in patients with either condition are cytotoxic through an antibody-dependent mechanism.
3. Antigen–antibody complexes (thought to be antibody–complement complexes), present in Crohn's disease patients, can produce a chronic proctitis in rabbits.

Nevertheless, conclusive support for an immunologic mechanism is lacking at this time.[6,7]

***Psychologic Factors*** Mental health changes appear to correlate with remissions and exacerbations, especially of ulcerative colitis, but psychologic factors overall are not thought to be a major etiologic factor. Most rigorous studies have concluded that no connection can be made between stress-inducing events and disease symptoms.[6,7]

***Diet*** Changes in diet by people in industrialized countries where Crohn's disease is more common have not been consistently associated with the disease. Studies of increased intake of refined sugars or chemical food additives and reduced fiber intake have been conflicting for patients with Crohn's disease.

Much promising research into the etiology of these conditions relates to immune-mediated intestinal damage. Investigators are looking at relationships between various different potential causes, such as interactions between antibodies and activated lymphocytes or enteric organisms, lymphocytes, and mucosal epithelial cells.[3]

## Pathophysiology

Ulcerative colitis and Crohn's disease differ in pathophysiology in two general respects: anatomic sites and depth of involvement of mucosal layers. There is, however, overlap between the two conditions, with a small fraction of patients showing features of both diseases. Confusion can occur, particularly when the inflammatory process is limited to the colon. Table 28.2 compares pathologic distinctions between the two diseases.

### Ulcerative Colitis

Confined to the colon and rectum, ulcerative colitis affects primarily the mucosa and the submucosa. In some instances a short segment of terminal ileum may be inflamed; this is referred to as "backwash ileitis." The histopathology of ulcerative colitis is similar to that of other inflammations of the colon such as that caused by infectious agents. Unlike Crohn's disease, the deeper longitudinal muscular layers, serosa, and regional lymph nodes are not usually involved.[6] As inflammation is usually confined to the mucosa and submucosa, fistulas, perforation, or obstruction are uncommon.

The primary lesion occurs in the crypts of the mucosa (crypts of Lieberkuhn) in the form of a crypt abscess. Here, frank necrosis of the epithelium occurs; it is usually visible only with microscopy but may be seen grossly when coalescence of ulcers occurs. Extension and coalescence ulcers may surround areas of uninvolved mucosa. These islands of mucosa are called pseudopolyps. Other typical ulceration patterns include a "collar-button ulcer," which results from extensive submucosal undermining at the ulcer edge.[6,8] The extensive mucosal damage seen in ulcerative colitis can result in significant diarrhea and bleeding.

Ulcerative colitis can be accompanied by complications that may be local (involving the colon) or systemic (not directly associated with the colon). With either type the complications may be mild, serious, or even life-threatening.

Local complications occur in the majority of ulcerative colitis patients. Relatively minor complications include hemorrhoids, anal fissures, or perirectal abscesses. These complications are more likely to be present during active colitis. Enteroenteric fistulas are rare.

A major complication is toxic megacolon, a severe condition that occurs in 1% to 3% of ulcerative colitis patients. With toxic megacolon, ulceration extends below the submucosa, sometimes even reaching the serosa. Vasculitis, swelling of the vascular endothelium, and thrombosis of small arteries occur; involvement of the muscularis propria causes loss of colonic tone which leads to dilatation and potential perforation.[6] Colonic perforation, however, may occur with or without toxic megacolon, and is a greater risk with the first attack.

Another major local complication is massive colonic hemorrhage. Although rectal bleeding is common, massive hemorrhage occurs infrequently. Colonic stricture, sometimes with clinical obstruction, may also complicate ulcerative colitis. Finally, the risk of colonic carcinoma is much greater in patients with ulcerative colitis as compared with the general population. It appears that the risk of colon cancer is related to the duration of colitis and to the extent of colonic involvement and increases at a rate of 2% per year after the first 8 to 10 years. After 20 years, the chances of having a colonic malignancy are greater than 20%.

The inflammatory response seen in IBD has also been blamed for the "systemic" complications seen in both Crohn's disease and ulcerative colitis and summarized here.

***Hepatic Complications*** Approximately 7% of patients with ulcerative colitis have subclinical evidence of liver disease.[9] This complication usually manifests as mild elevations of alkaline phosphatase or serum transaminases. The histopa-

**Table 28.2** Comparison of the Clinical and Pathologic Features of Crohn's Granulomatous Colitis and Ulcerative Colitis

| *Feature* | *Crohn's colitis* | *Ulcerative colitis* |
|---|---|---|
| Intestinal | | |
| Malaise, fever | Common | Uncommon |
| Rectal bleeding | Intermittent about 50% | Common |
| Abdominal tenderness | Common | May be present |
| Abdominal mass | Very common (especially with ileocolitis) | Not present |
| Abdominal pain | Very common | Unusual |
| Abdominal wall and internal fistulas | Very common | Rare |
| Endoscopic | | |
| Rectal disease | About 20% | Almost 100% |
| Diffuse, continuous symmetric involvement | Uncommon | Very common |
| Aphthous or linear ulcers | Common | Rare |
| Friability | Rare | Rare |
| Radiologic | | |
| Continuous disease | Rare | Very common |
| Ileal involvement | Very common | Rare |
| Asymmetry | Very common | Rare |
| Strictures | Common | Rare |
| Fistulas | Very common | Rare |
| Pathologic | | |
| Discontinuity | Common | Rare |
| Rectal involvement | Rare | Common |
| Intense vascularity | Rare | Common |
| Ileal involvement | Common | Nonexistent |
| Transmural involvement | Common | Rare |
| Lymphoid aggregates | Common | Uncommon |
| Crypt abscesses | Rare | Very common |
| Granulomas | Common | Rare |
| Linear clefts | Common | Rare |
| Surgical treatment | Subtotal or total colectomy, rectum frequently preserved | Proctocolectomy with ileostomy |

From Ramming KP: Diseases of the rectum and colon, in Sabiston DC (Ed): Essentials of Surgery. Philadelphia, W. B. Saunders, 1987, with permission.

thology may appear as one of a number of presentations, including pericholangitis, fatty infiltration, chronic active hepatitis, postnecrotic cirrhosis, amyloidosis, or sclerosing cholangitis. Resolution of the colonic disease may not improve the liver disease.

***Arthritis*** Up to one fourth of patients with IBD experience arthritis.[9] The severity of this complication appears to be related to the severity of disease and usually subsides with control of intestinal inflammation. Arthritis in these patients may be migratory and usually involves the larger joints. Rheumatoid factor is typically negative. Occasionally, patients may have ankylosing spondylitis, which may be progressive and unresponsive to treatment.

***Ocular Complications*** Patients with IBD may have uveitis or iritis which may be characterized during the acute phase by blurred vision, eye pain, and photophobia. In about one half of patients this may be bilateral.

***Dermatologic and Mucosal Complications*** Aphthous mouth ulcerations, erythema nodosum (noted by raised, tender erythematous swellings), and pyoderma gangrenosum (noted by cutaneous ulceration) occur in about 5% of patients with IBD. These manifestations tend to be more prominent during active disease.[10]

### Crohn's Disease

Crohn's disease is best characterized as a transmural inflammatory process. The terminal ileum is the most common site of the disorder (14%–30%), but it may occur in any part of the gastrointestinal tract. About two thirds of patients have some colonic involvement, and 15% to 25% of patients have only colonic disease.[7] Patients often have normal bowel separating segments of diseased bowel.

Regardless of the site, bowel wall destruction is extensive and the intestinal lumen is often narrowed. The mesentery becomes first thickened and edematous and then fibrotic. Ulcers tend to be deep and elongated and extend along the longitudinal axis of the bowel, at least into the submucosa. The "cobblestone" appearance of the bowel wall results from deep mucosal ulceration intermingled with nodular submucosal thickening.

Complications of Crohn's disease may involve the intestinal tract or organs unrelated to it. Small-bowel stricture and subsequent obstruction is a complication that may require surgery. Fistula formation is common and occurs much more frequently than with ulcerative colitis.[7,11] Fistulas often occur in the areas of worst inflammation where loops of bowel have become matted together by fibrous adhesions. Fistulas may connect two segments of the gastrointestinal tract (enteroenteric fistula), the intestinal tract with skin (enterocutaneous fistula), or the intestinal tract with the bladder (enterovesicular fistula). Crohn's disease fistulas almost always require surgical treatment.

Bleeding with Crohn's disease is usually not as severe as with ulcerative colitis, although patients with Crohn's disease may have hypochromic anemia. Also, as with ulcerative colitis, the risk of carcinoma is increased but not as great as with ulcerative colitis.

Systemic complications of Crohn's disease are common, and similar to those found with ulcerative colitis. Arthritis, iritis, skin lesions, and liver disease often accompany Crohn's disease. With Crohn's disease, however, the severity of arthritis does not appear to parallel the severity of the intestinal disease.

## Clinical Presentation/Diagnosis

### Ulcerative Colitis

Although a typical clinical picture of ulcerative colitis can be described, there is a very wide range of presentation. Symptoms may range from mild abdominal cramping with frequent small-volume bowel movements to profuse diarrhea. Most patients with ulcerative colitis experience intermittent bouts of illness after varying intervals with no symptoms. Only a small percentage of patients have continuous unremitting symptoms or have a single acute attack with no subsequent symptoms.

Complex disease classifications are generally not used in clinical practice for ulcerative colitis. The arbitrarily determined distinctions of "mild," "moderate," and "severe" disease are generally used, and these are determined largely by clinical signs and symptoms. Mild disease has been defined as less than four stools daily without anemia, tachycardia, weight loss, or hypoalbuminemia, and severe disease as greater than six stools daily with the signs just listed.[6]

Two thirds of patients with ulcerative colitis have mild disease.[10] Occasionally, the mild form may progress to severe disease. Systemic signs/symptoms of the disease (e.g., arthritis, uveitis, pyoderma gangrenosum) may be present in these patients and, in fact, may be the reason the patient seeks medical attention. Patients with mild disease are believed to be at lower risk of colon cancer. Moderate disease is observed in one fourth of patients.[10] These patients have more prominent abdominal discomfort and usually present with diarrhea as the major complaint. They may be noted to have a low-grade fever.

With severe disease the patient is usually found to be in acute distress, has profuse bloody diarrhea, and often has a high fever with leukocytosis and hypoalbuminemia. Often the patient is dehydrated and therefore may be tachycardic and hypotensive. This presentation may have a sudden onset with rapid progression.

The diagnosis of ulcerative colitis is made on clinical suspicion and confirmed by biopsy, stool examinations, sigmoidoscopy or colonoscopy, and barium radiographic contrast studies. The presence of extracolonic manifestations such as arthritis, uveitis, and pyoderma gangrenosum may also aid in establishing the diagnosis.

### Crohn's disease

As with ulcerative colitis, the presentation of Crohn's disease is highly variable. A single episode may not be followed by further episodes, or the patient may experience continuous, unremitting disease. Because the symptoms may be confusing, an average of three years between the onset of complaints and the initial diagnosis has been reported. The patient typically presents with diarrhea and abdominal pain. Hematochezia occurs in about one half of the patients with colonic involvement and much less frequently when there is no colonic involvement. Commonly, a patient may first present with a perirectal or perianal lesion. The diagnosis should be suspected in children with growth retardation.

The course of Crohn's disease is characterized by periods of remission and exacerbation. Some patients may be free of symptoms for years, while others experience chronic problems in spite of medical therapy.

As in ulcerative colitis the diagnosis of Crohn's disease involves a thorough evaluation using laboratory, endoscopic, and radiologic testing to detect the characteristic features of the disease.

Because of similarities that may exist between ulcerative colitis and Crohn's disease a definitive diagnosis cannot be made in up to 15% of cases, even with pathologic specimens in hand.

## Treatment

### *Overview*

Treatment for inflammatory bowel disease centers on agents used to lessen the inflammatory process (anti-inflammatory agents). Salicylates, corticosteroids, and immunosuppressive agents such as azathioprine are commonly used to treat active disease and, under certain conditions, to lengthen remission from disease. In addition to the use of anti-inflammatory agents, surgery is sometimes performed when active disease is not adequately controlled. For most patients with inflammatory bowel disease, nutritional considerations are also very important as these patients are often malnourished. Finally, a variety of therapies may be used to address complications or symptoms of inflammatory bowel disease. For example, antidiarrheals may be used in some patients, although these are generally to be avoided in ulcerative colitis because they may contribute to the development of toxic colonic dilatation. Antimicrobial agents may be used in conjunction with surgery when abscesses are present. Iron may be required, particularly with ulcerative colitis where blood loss from the colon can be significant.

### *Goals*

To properly treat inflammatory bowel disease, the clinician must have a clear concept of realistic therapeutic goals for each patient. These goals may relate to resolution of acute inflammatory processes, to resolution of attendant complications (e.g., fistulas, abscesses), to alleviation of systemic manifestations (e.g., arthritis), to maintenance of remission from acute inflammation, or to surgical palliation or cure. The approach to the therapeutic regimen differs considerably with varying goals as well as with the two diseases, ulcerative colitis and Crohn's disease.

In determining goals of therapy and selecting therapeutic regimens it is important to understand the natural history of inflammatory bowel disease when untreated.[12] This knowledge is necessary to estimate the value of therapeutic regimens. Admittedly, there is relatively little information on the natural history of inflammatory bowel disease, and most of it is derived from placebo-controlled trials. Since the first recognition of these clinical syndromes, virtually all patients have received some therapeutic measures.

Some types of acute ulcerative colitis are self-limited. With mild to moderate acute colitis, without systemic symptoms, 20% of patients may experience improvement in their disease within a few weeks; however, a small percentage of patients may go on to experience more serious disease. With severe colitis, improvement without treatment cannot be expected. For instance, the response to medical management of toxic megacolon is poor and surgery is usually required. When remission of ulcerative colitis is induced, it is likely to last at least 1 year with medical therapy. In the absence of medical therapy, one half to two thirds of patients are likely to relapse within 9 months.[12] In some reports, remission rates with placebo have approached those with active treatments.

A considerable number of patients with active Crohn's disease may achieve remission without drug therapy. In two large trials, 26% and 42% of ambulatory patients on placebo achieved remission.[13,14] Once remission is achieved, two thirds to three fourths of patients remain in remission up to 2 years without drug therapy.[12] The implication of these data is that up to 40% of patients with active Crohn's disease improve in 3 to 4 months with observation alone, and that most patients remain in remission without medical intervention. These observations apply more to mild or moderate disease and not to severe disease.

### *Nutritional Support*

Proper nutritional support is an important aspect of the treatment of patients with inflammatory bowel disease, not because specific types of diets are often useful in alleviating the inflammatory conditions but because patients with moderate to severe disease are often malnourished. The patient with inflammatory bowel disease may be malnourished because of decreased nutrient intake (anorexia or when eating causes exacerbation of symptoms), because the inflammatory process results in significant malabsorption, or because of the catabolic effects of the disease process. Malabsorption may occur in the patient with Crohn's disease with inflammatory involvement of the small bowel where many nutrients are absorbed, and also in patients who have undergone multiple small-bowel resections with subsequent reduction in absorptive surface.

A number of specific diets have been tried in attempts to improve the condition of patients with inflammatory bowel disease, but none has gained widespread acceptance. With each individual it is helpful to eliminate specific foods that exacerbate symptoms. This elimination process must be conducted cautiously, as patients have been known to exclude a wide range of nutritious products without adequate justification. Many patients with inflammatory bowel disease, although not the majority, have lactase deficiency; therefore, diarrhea may be associated with milk intake. In these patients, avoidance of milk generally improves the patient's symptoms.

The nutritional needs of the majority of patients can be adequately addressed with enteral supplementation. Patients who have severe disease may require a course of parenteral nutrition to attain a reasonable nutritional status or in preparation for surgery. With either route of nutrient administration, patients require protein and caloric supplemention, recognizing that there is an increased requirement for both with malnourishment. Consideration should be given to adequate lipid administration, not only for caloric value but also in recognition of depleted peripheral fat stores in many inflammatory bowel disease patients and the greater potential for fatty acid deficiency. These patients generally require vitamin and mineral supplementation.

Parenteral nutrition is an important component of the treatment of severe Crohn's disease or ulcerative colitis. The use of parenteral nutrition allows complete bowel rest in patients with severe ulcerative colitis, which may alter the need for proctocolectomy. Parenteral nutrition has also been valuable in Crohn's disease as remission may be achieved in about one half of patients.[15] In some patients, the disease may worsen when parenteral nutrition is stopped. Patients with enterocutaneous fistulas of various etiologies have been reported to benefit from parenteral nutrition.[15] Parenteral nutrition may also be valuable in children or adolescents with growth retardation associated with Crohn's disease, but surgery is usually necessary with severe disease.

### *Surgery*

Surgical procedures have an established place in the treatment of inflammatory bowel disease. Although surgery (proctocolectomy) is curative for ulcerative colitis, this is not the case for Crohn's disease. Surgical procedures involve resection of segments of intestine that are affected, as well as correction of complications (e.g., fistulas, abscesses).

For ulcerative colitis, colectomy may be performed when the patient has disease uncontrolled by maximum medical therapy or when there are complications of the disease such as colonic perforation, toxic dilatation (megacolon), uncontrolled colonic hemorrhage, or colonic strictures. Colectomy may be indicated in patients with long-standing disease (greater than 8–10 years), as a prophylactic measure against the development of cancer and in patients with premalignant changes (severe dysplasia) on surveillance mucosal biopsies. The most common surgical procedures include proctocolectomy, after which the patient is left with a permanent ileostomy, and abdominal colectomy, with removal of the mucosa of the rectum and anastamosis of an ileal pouch to the anus. The risk from surgery in these patients is relatively low if the operations are performed on a nonemergency basis.

The indications for surgery with Crohn's disease are not as well established as they are for ulcerative colitis, and surgery is usually reserved for the complications of the disease. A recognized problem with intestinal resection for Crohn's disease is that the rate of recurrence is high. Surgery may be appropriate in well-selected patients who are documented to continue to have severe or incapacitating disease in spite of aggressive medical management. The surgical procedures performed include resections of the major intestinal areas of involvement. In some patients with severe rectal or perineal disease, diversion of the fecal stream is performed with a colostomy. Other indications for surgery include the finding of colon cancer, inflammatory mass, or intestinal perforations.

### *Drug Therapy*

Drug therapy plays an integral part in the overall regimen for inflammatory bowel disease patients. It is important to emphasize that none of the drugs used for inflammatory bowel disease are curative; at best they serve to control the disease process. Therefore, a reasonable goal of drug therapy is resolution of disease symptoms such that the patient can carry on normal daily functions. The major types of drug therapy used in inflammatory bowel disease include anti-inflammatory agents (e.g., sulfasalazine and corticosteroids), immunosuppressive agents (e.g., azathioprine and 6-mercaptopurine), antibiotics (metronidazole), and other agents used investigationally such as immune enhancers (e.g., levamisole or BCG) and mast cell stabilizers (cromolyn sodium).

Sulfasalazine, an agent that combines a sulfonamide (sulfapyridine) antibiotic and 5-aminosalicylic acid (5-ASA, mesalamine) in the same molecule, has been used for many years to treat inflammatory bowel disease. The agent has a unique route of disposition in the body that relates to its effectiveness in treating inflammatory bowel disease (Fig. 28.1). When administered orally, sulfasalazine is absorbed intact from the small bowel. Most of the drug is then excreted unchanged in the bile where it then progresses to the colon. In the colon, sulfasalazine is cleaved by gut bacteria to sulfapyridine (which is mostly reabsorbed and excreted in the urine) and 5-ASA (which mostly remains in the colon and is excreted in stool). When given by mouth, however, both sulfapyridine and 5-ASA are absorbed in the small bowel and excreted primarily in the urine.

The mechanism of action of sulfasalazine has been debated for many years. The active component of sulfasalazine is believed to be 5-ASA, which has local anti-inflammatory effect on the lumen of the intestine; however, other mechanisms are still considered.[16] One theory holds that 5-ASA's main beneficial effect is inhibition of prostaglandins.[17] Alternative theories suggest that sulfasalazine inhibits the migration of inflammatory cells into the bowel wall.[18] The use of 5-ASA, administered alone rectally or orally in the form of a prodrug, has been shown effective and is gaining acceptance, particularly for ulcerative colitis.

Corticosteroids and adrenocorticotropic hormone (ACTH) have been widely used for the treatment of ulcerative colitis and Crohn's disease. There has been a long-standing controversy as to the relative merits of corticosteroids versus ACTH; however, most clinicians currently prefer corticosteroids.[19] Although ACTH is administered parenterally, corticosteroids may be given parenterally, orally, and/or rectally. The exact mechanism of action of corticosteroids is not known but is believed to involve modulation of the immune system.

Immunosuppressive agents such as azathioprine and 6-mercaptopurine (the active form of azathioprine) are sometimes used for the treatment of Crohn's disease. These agents are generally reserved for cases that are refractory to azathioprine and steroids, and may be associated with serious adverse effects such as lymphomas or pancreatitis. The agents are usually used in conjunction with sulfasalazine and/or steroids and must be used for long periods of time (up to 6 months) before benefits may be observed.[20] The proper role for these agents in the treatment of ulcerative colitis has not been determined, and there is little justification for their use.

Antimicrobial agents, particularly metronidazole, are frequently used in attempts to control Crohn's disease. Metronidazole has been demonstrated to be of value in some patients with active Crohn's disease, particularly that involving the perineal area or fistulas.[21] The mechanism of metronidazole's effect on Crohn's disease has not been determined but is theorized to relate to interruption of a bacterial role in the inflammatory process. Although other antimicrobial agents have been studied, none has gained as much attention as metronidazole.

Other agents that have been investigated for treatment of inflammatory bowel disease include mast cell stabilizers, such as cromolyn sodium, and bile salt sequestrants, such as cholestyramine. These agents have not resulted in consistent improvements in patients with inflammatory bowel disease and cannot be recommended for use.

Drug treatment is differentiated by the type of inflammatory bowel disease, as well as by the extent of disease, principal site of inflammation, and degree of severity, because the approaches to treatment and prevention of acute inflammation can be quite different. The data employed to support the use of an agent in one type of disease, or even in a subset of a specific type of IBD, should not be used to justify use under other conditions.

#### **Ulcerative Colitis**

***Mild to Moderate Disease*** The majority of patients with active ulcerative colitis are considered to have mild to moderate disease. These patients are generally ambulatory and do not require parenteral medications. The first line of drug therapy for the patient with mild to moderate colitis is oral sulfasalazine, while for proctitis the preferred therapy is rectally administered steroids. The value of sulfasalazine for treatment of ulcerative colitis has been documented in early studies that compared the agent with placebo.[22,23] From these reports and others it has been recognized that usually 4 g, and up to 8 g, of sulfasalazine per day is required to attain control of active inflammation. There does not appear to be an increased rate of response with increased dosage over 4 g per day. Even with the use of adequate doses, patient improvement usually takes 2 to 3 weeks and some-

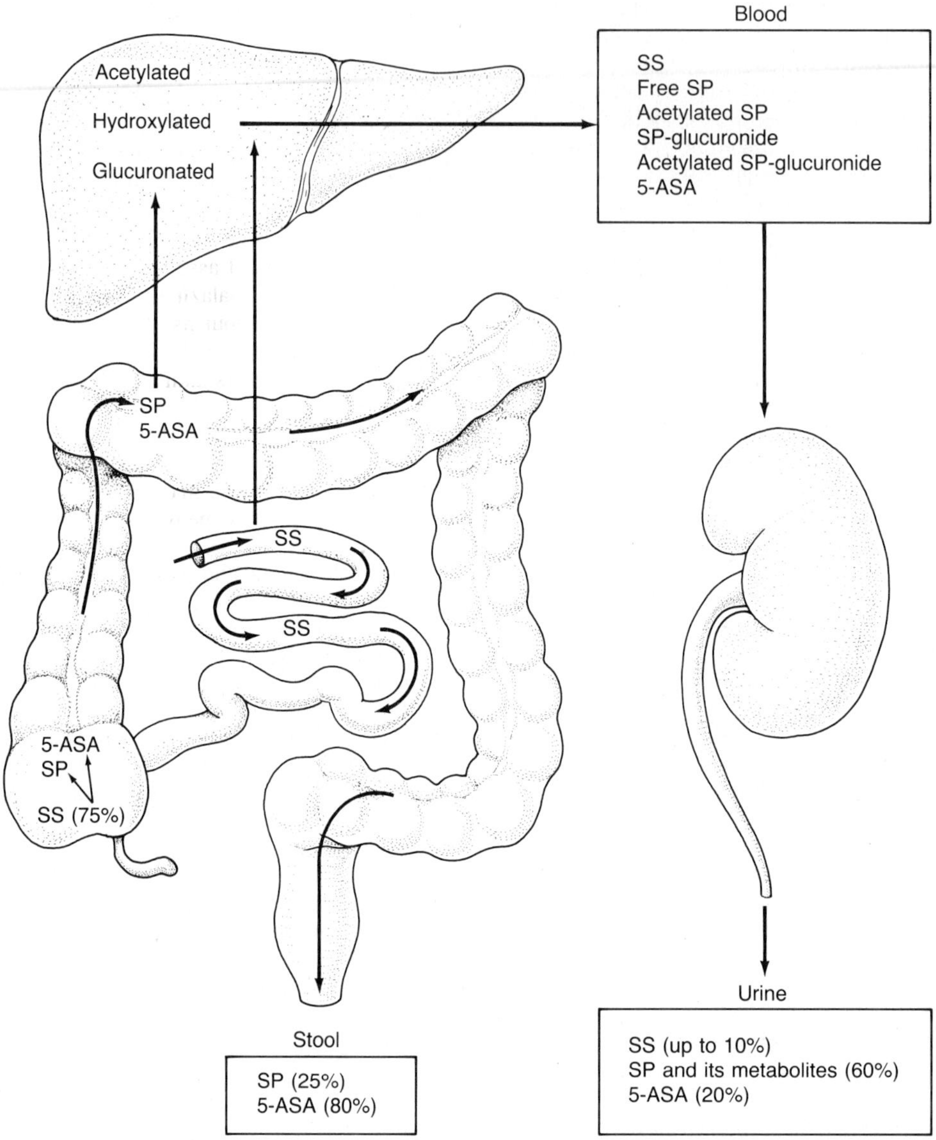


**Figure 28.1** Metabolic pathway of sulfasalazine. Numbers in parentheses indicate percentages of administered dose normally absorbed, metabolized, or excreted. SS, sulfasalazine; SP, sulfapyridine; 5-ASA, 5-aminosalicylic acid. *(From Das KM: Pharmacotherapy of inflammatory bowel disease. Part 1. Sulfasalazine. Postgrad Med 1983;74:143, with permission.)*

times up to 4 weeks. The dosage of sulfasalazine that can be given is usually limited by the patient's tolerance of the agent; most adverse effects of sulfasalazine are dose related.[24] Sulfasalazine therapy should be instituted at 500 mg per day and increased every few days to 4 g or the maximum tolerated (up to 8 g per day).

Steroids have a place in the treatment of moderate to severe ulcerative colitis. Oral steroids (usually up to 1 mg/kg per day of prednisone equivalent) may be used for patients who do not have an adequate response to sulfasalazine. Prednisone dosages in the range 40–60 mg/d have been superior to regimens of 20 mg/d in producing remission.[25] Overall, steroids and sulfasalazine appear to be equally efficacious; however, the response to steroids may be evident sooner.[26,27] The use of oral steroids as initial therapy for mild to moderate ulcerative colitis should be avoided, mainly because of the known risks of steroid use. If steroids are used to attain remission, tapered drug withdrawal should be accomplished to minimize steroid exposure.

Rectally administered steroids or 5-ASA can be used as initial therapy for ulcerative proctitis or distal colitis. With these agents, local actions are believed to be responsible for drug effects. In a trial of 86 patients with mild to moderate colitis who received rectal hydrocortisone or 5-ASA, the latter agent was found superior (93% remission rate).[28] In some patients, combined use of oral sulfasalazine and rectal steroids or rectal 5-ASA may provide advantages.

The choice of rectally administered steroid has been a

subject of debate as there is varying potential for systemic steroid absorption with different products. Although many steroids have been administered rectally, certain agents such as betamethasone-17-valerate, beclomethasone dipropionate, and prednisolone-21-phosphate have been used in attempts to reduce systemic steroid effects. Betamethasone-17-valerate appears to result in less adrenal suppression compared with prednisolone-21-phosphate.[29] Systemic side effects may be the least severe with beclomethasone dipropionate as this agent is rapidly metabolized by the gut wall and liver.[30,31] With whatever product is used rectally, the systemic effects are less severe than those of oral steroids of the same equivalent dose. Most patients do not experience adrenal suppression from rectal steroids. The use of rectal steroids may often result in reduction of the required oral dose. Other agents such as azathioprine, 6-mercaptopurine, and metronidazole have no defined role in the treatment of active ulcerative colitis.

***Severe Disease*** The patient with uncontrolled severe colitis or incapacitating symptoms requires hospitalization for effective management. Under these conditions, the patient often receives nothing by mouth to put the bowel at rest; therefore, most medication is given by the parenteral route. With severe colitis, there is a much greater reliance on parenteral steroids and surgical procedures. Sulfasalazine has not been proven beneficial for treatment of severe colitis. The reason for this may relate to rapid elimination of sulfasalazine from the colon with diarrhea, thereby not allowing sufficient time for gut bacteria to cleave the molecule.[32] Overall, it is very difficult to evaluate drugs in this setting, as patients with severe disease almost always receive additional medications including steroids. In one trial, sulfasalazine was not of added benefit when combined with steroids.[33]

Steroids have been valuable in the treatment of severe disease, because the use of these agents may allow some patients to avoid colectomy. A trial of steroids is warranted (up to 2 weeks in some circumstances) in most patients before proceeding to colectomy, unless the condition is grave or rapidly deteriorating. In one trial of 87 patients with severe colitis, the use of intravenous steroids and parenteral nutrition resulted in remission in 60% of patients, with only 5% of those requiring colectomy after 6 weeks.[34] The dose of steroid generally used is 1 mg/kg of prednisone equivalent daily, although some patients may require much less or much more for satisfactory control. With higher doses, however, steroid side effects may limit drug benefits. The length of the medical trial before consideration of surgery is open to debate. When steroids must be used it is well recognized that they may mask such complications as intra-abdominal sepsis. Steroids also increase surgical risk, particularly infectious risk, if an operation is later required. After a colectomy is performed, steroids should no longer be required for the disease; however, they must be withdrawn gradually (usually over 3–4 weeks) to avoid hypoadrenal crisis from adrenal suppression.

ACTH has been used as an alternative to steroids. Although some investigators have suggested that ACTH is more effective than steroids for inflammatory bowel disease, more recent trials have not supported this.[35,36] ACTH is probably equivalent in efficacy to steroids but no relative added benefits can be demonstrated.

***Maintenance of Remission*** Once remission from active disease has been achieved, the goal of therapy is to maintain remission. The major agent used for maintenance of remission is sulfasalazine (usually 2 g per day); steroids usually do not have a role. The value of sulfasalazine in preventing recurrences has been documented in placebo-controlled trials. Misiewicz and associates[37] found that one fourth of patients taking sulfasalazine (2 g daily) had a relapse within 1 year, while three fourths of patients taking placebo had a relapse. A similar result was obtained by Davies and Rhodes[38] with patients taking sulfasalazine for periods up to 1.4 years.

A major question about the use of sulfasalazine for maintenance of remission with ulcerative colitis is the duration of the preventive regimen. In one trial, the rate of recurrence of acute colitis was the same with placebo or sulfasalazine after 1 year.[39] In another trial, the rate of recurrence was much greater with placebo compared with sulfasalazine for periods of 6 months to 3 years after a year of remission.[40] The efficacy of sulfasalazine appears to be related to dose administered, up to a point. In a trial to assess the effect of daily dosage on recurrence, patients received 1, 2, or 4 g of sulfasalazine per day. The recurrence rates were 33%, 14%, and 9%, respectively. The 4 g/d regimen resulted in intolerable side effects in about one fourth of patients.

Steroids do not have a role in the maintenance of remission with ulcerative colitis as they have been demonstrated to be ineffective.[36,41] Steroids should be gradually withdrawn after remission is induced (over 3–4 weeks). If they are continued the patient will be exposed to steroid side effects without likelihood of benefits. For patients who require chronic steroid use, there is a strong justification for colectomy.

### Crohn's Disease

Management of Crohn's disease often proves more difficult than that of ulcerative colitis, partly because of the greater variation of presentation with Crohn's disease. The disease may be found to involve any segment of the gastrointestinal tract, from mouth to anus, and may involve other visceral structures and soft tissues through fistulization. There is a greater reliance on drug therapy with Crohn's disease, as resection of all involved intestine may not be possible and recurrence after surgery is frequent. Also, it is more difficult to evaluate the published literature with this disease because there is a large diversity in presentation and trial groups may involve widely differing patients.

***Active Crohn's Disease*** The goal of treatment for active Crohn's disease is to achieve remission; however, in many patients reduction of symptoms, so that the patient may carry out normal activities, or reduction of the steroid dose required for control is a significant accomplishment. In the majority of patients, active Crohn's disease is treated with sulfasalazine or steroids.

The role of sulfasalazine in the treatment of active Crohn's disease is accepted but not as well established as its role in the treatment of ulcerative colitis. It appears that sulfasalazine is more effective when Crohn's disease involves the colon[13] and in patients who have not undergone surgery for their disease.[42] In these circumstances, sulfasalazine has been reported to be as effective as prednisone.[13,43] It appears reasonable to initiate a trial of sulfasalazine in patients with mild to moderate Crohn's disease, particularly when the colon is involved. A course of steroids would be appropriate in patients who cannot be controlled on sulfasalazine. When a patient is maintained on steroids, however, there appears to be no benefit from the addition of sulfasalazine.[33]

Steroids are frequently used for the treatment of active Crohn's disease, particularly with more severe presentations. In the National Cooperative Crohn's Disease Study[13] prednisone was documented to be significantly more effective than placebo in achieving remission. In this trial, the prednisone doses were 0.25 mg/kg/d for mild disease, 0.5 mg/kg/d for moderate disease, and 0.75 mg/kg/d for severe disease. Prednisone was found to be effective for disease limited to the small bowel.

The European Cooperative Crohn's Disease Study group examined the effectiveness of 6-methylprednisolone and/or sulfasalazine.[14] They reported that the steroid provided a better overall response than sulfasalazine for treatment of active disease. The combination of steroid and sulfasalazine was more effective in previously untreated patients or in those with disease localized to the colon.

Steroids are preferred for treatment of severe Crohn's disease, mainly because these agents may be given parenterally and response to therapy may occur sooner. Once remission is achieved, however, it may prove difficult to reduce steroid dosage without reintroduction of active disease.

Metronidazole may be useful in some patients with Crohn's disease, particularly in patients with colonic involvement or those with perineal disease. In most patients, metronidazole would be added to sulfasalazine or steroid therapy. In one trial, metronidazole was not significantly different from placebo in terms of clinical response scores; however, about one half of patients on metronidazole had significant improvement.[44] In a comparative trial with sulfasalazine, metronidazole was found to be as effective, and more effective in patients with colonic disease. Metronidazole has also been reported effective in noncomparative trials for treatment of Crohn's disease with perineal involvement.[45] The role for metronidazole is not fully defined. It may deserve a trial as adjunctive therapy for patients with colonic or perineal disease where satisfactory control is not gained with sulfasalazine, or in attempts to reduce steroid dosage.

The immunosuppressive agents (azathioprine and 6-mercaptopurine) are generally limited in use to patients not achieving adequate response to standard medical therapy, or to reduce steroid doses when toxic doses are required. In trials examining the use of azathioprine, beneficial effects have not been demonstrated, although these trials have had significant flaws.[13,46] The major benefits of azathioprine may be in allowing reduction of the steroid dosage.[47,48] Also, treatment with azathioprine may need to be continued up to 6 months to observe a response.[20] 6-Mercaptopurine may have advantages over azathioprine for adjunctive treatment of Crohn's disease.[49] In one trial of patients already receiving sulfasalazine or prednisone, 6-mercaptopurine was compared with placebo.[50] Significant improvements were noted in the 6-mercaptopurine group, mainly in decreasing steroid requirement and in healing fistulas. One problem noted with 6-mercaptopurine was that greater than 3 months was required to observe a response in 32% of patients.

***Maintenance of Remission*** Prevention of recurrence of disease is clearly more difficult with Crohn's disease than with ulcerative colitis. There is no regimen that is consistently effective in maintaining remission from Crohn's disease. Sulfasalazine has been studied in controlled trials for prevention of recurrence of Crohn's disease. In a trial of 120 patients, one fourth of patients on placebo and sulfasalazine experienced a recurrence within the first year of the regimen.[13] Sulfasalazine, therefore, cannot be recommended for prevention of acute Crohn's disease. Steroids also have no place in the prevention of recurrence of Crohn's disease, as these agents do not appear to alter the long-term course of the disease.[51] Prednisone (0.5 mg/kg/d) has been compared with placebo for patients who have achieved remission from Crohn's disease. In a 2-year trial of 274 patients, relapses were observed in 25% of patients in placebo and drug groups in the first year and in 40% of patients in both groups by the end of 2 years.[13] The ineffectiveness of prednisone in preventing recurrence did not seem to be related to the method by which remission was obtained (medical or surgical). In other trials, long-term steroid use has been beneficial in the maintenance of remission.[14]

Azathioprine has been studied as an adjunctive agent for the treatment and prevention of Crohn's disease. Although there are not many data to suggest that the agent is of benefit in preventing recurrences, it has been useful in allowing reduction of the steroid dose.[47,48] This agent should be reserved for patients who cannot tolerate dosages of steroids required to control their disease and who are not good surgical candidates.

## *Selected Complications*

### Toxic Megacolon

Toxic megacolon or "toxic colonic dilatation" is a serious complication of inflammatory bowel disease that occurs in about 1% or 2% of patients with ulcerative colitis. As described before, the patient with toxic megacolon is usually severely ill with fever, abdominal pain and distension, decreased bowel sounds, and often dehydration. Immediate and aggressive measures are required to minimize mortality.

The treatment required for toxic megacolon includes general supportive measures to maintain vital functions, consideration for early surgical intervention, and drugs (steroids and antimicrobials). Aggressive fluid and electrolyte management is often required as these patients may be severely dehydrated. Fluids and electrolytes may be lost through vomiting, diarrhea, and nasogastric intubation, as well as through fluid accumulation in the bowel. When the patient has lost significant amounts of blood (through the rectum), blood replacement may also be necessary. Opiates and anticholinergics should be discontinued as these agents enhance colonic dilatation, thereby increasing the risk of bowel perforation.

Steroids in high dosages should be administered intravenously to reduce acute inflammation. Doses as high as 2 mg/kg/d of prednisone equivalent have been recommended (generally administered as hydrocortisone).[6] The duration of steroid administration is not certain; however, most clinicians continue the high-dose steroids up to 2 weeks after improvement is observed and then reduce the dosages (approximately 0.5–1 mg/kg/d) for a few additional weeks. Antimicrobial regimens that are effective against enteric aerobes and anaerobes (e.g., aminoglycoside with clindamycin or metronidazole) should be administered from the time of diagnosis and should be continued until patient improvement is assured. The duration of the antimicrobial regimen (often up to 2–3 weeks) should be determined considering that there may be significant intraabdominal contamination with signs and symptoms hidden by steroid effects.

Surgical intervention, mainly an abdominal colectomy with formation of an ileostomy, is an important consideration in patients with toxic megacolon and prevents death in some patients. Early surgical intervention in these patients may result in a reduced mortality rate. In most cases in which colectomy is performed in the face of toxic megacolon, there is a significant risk of operative complications, including postoperative infection.

### Systemic Manifestations

The common systemic manifestations of inflammatory bowel disease include arthritis, anemia, skin manifestations such as erythema nodosum and pyoderma gangrenosum, uveitis, and liver disease. Certain of these associated problems may be related to the inflammatory process and we emphasize that these diseases are not limited to the gastrointestinal tract. For some of these manifestations, specific therapies can be instituted, while for others, treatment that is used for the gastrointestinal inflammatory process also addresses the systemic manifestations.

Anemia may be a common problem where there is significant blood loss from the gastrointestinal tract. When the patient can consume oral medication, ferrous sulfate should be administered. If the patient is not able to take oral medication, parenteral iron (iron dextran) may be given; however, this product is associated with frequent allergic reactions. Patients who have significantly depressed hematocrits may require blood transfusion. Anemia may also be related to malabsorption of vitamin $B_{12}$ or folic acid, so these may also be required.

There are no consistently recommended therapies for liver disease, skin manifestations, or uveitis associated with inflammatory bowel disease. Some reports suggest that these manifestations are worse during exacerbations of the intestinal disease and that measures improving intestinal disease will improve these systemic manifestations. Unfortunately, this association has not consistently been demonstrated. For arthritis associated with inflammatory bowel disease, aspirin or other nonsteroidal anti-inflammatory agents may be beneficial as would be steroids.

## *Special Considerations*

### Pregnancy

Pregnancy, either the occurrence or consideration of, may cause significant concerns in the patient with IBD. Questions arise as to fertility in patients with IBD, the effect of pregnancy on the disease course, the effect of the disease on the outcome of pregnancy, and the effects of the drugs used in IBD on the fetus.[52]

It does not appear that patients with IBD are less fertile than women in general.[6,53] The rate of normal childbirth is similar to that for healthy populations. Some studies have noted, however, a greater rate of spontaneous abortions in patients with IBD. It does not appear that pregnancy affects the course of IBD. Patients who are pregnant experience recurrence rates similar to those of nonpregnant females. Also, there is no justification for therapeutic abortion with IBD as termination of the pregnancy has not been observed to improve the disease.

Steroids and sulfasalazine should be administered during pregnancy with the same guidelines that would be applied to the nonpregnant patient.[6,53] Steroids given systemically do not appear to be detrimental to the fetus. Sulfasalazine is generally well tolerated; however, there has been suggestion of increased frequency of congenital abnormalities when it is given during pregnancy.[54] Interestingly, sulfasalazine has also been reported to cause decreased sperm counts in males.[55] This effect is reversible on discontinuation of the drug. Immunosuppressive drugs (azathioprine and 6-mercaptopurine) may be associated with fetal deformities in humans; however, they have been used without detriment in some patients.[53]

Overall, receiving drug therapy for IBD is not a contraindication for pregnancy, and most pregnancies are well managed in patients with these diseases. The indications for medical and surgical treatment are similar to those in the nonpregnant patient. If a patient has an initial bout of IBD during pregnancy, a standard approach to treatment should be initiated.

### Adverse Drug Reactions to Agents Used for Treatment of IBD

Drug intolerance often limits the usefulness of agents used to treat inflammatory bowel disease. Many patients who are receiving sulfasalazine, corticosteroids, metronidazole, azathioprine, or 6-mercaptopurine experience some undesired effects. In some cases, these adverse effects can be significant and require discontinuation of the therapy. Knowledge of the common or important adverse reactions will assist in avoiding or minimizing their effects.

Sulfasalazine is often associated with adverse drug effects and these effects may be classified as either dose related or idiosyncratic. Dose-related side effects usually include gastrointestinal disturbances such as nausea, vomiting, diarrhea, or anorexia, but may also include headache and arthralgia.[33,56] These adverse reactions tend to occur more commonly on initiation of therapy and decrease in frequency as therapy is continued. Patients may experience these adverse effects at the commonly used dosages. One approach to the management of these reactions is to discontinue the agent for a short period and then reinstitute therapy at a reduced dosage. Some have suggested that the rate of adverse effects may be related to the concentration of free sulfapyridine in serum, suggesting that the sulfa portion of the molecule is responsible for the adverse effects.[17]

Non–dose-related adverse effects include rash, fever, or hepatotoxicity most commonly (20%–50% of patients), as well as relatively uncommon but serious reactions such as agranulocytosis, pancreatitis, thrombocytopenia, and toxic epidermal necrolysis.[57] For most patients with idiosyncratic reactions, sulfasalazine must be discontinued. In some patients who have experienced allergic reactions to sulfasalazine, a desensitization procedure can be instituted. By gradually increasing sulfasalazine dosage over weeks to months, patient tolerance has been improved.[58] Most of the idiosyncratic reactions observed with sulfasalazine are similar to those with the class of sulfonamides in general.

Adverse reactions of corticosteroids have been well recognized and may occur when corticosteroids are used for any indication. There is a greater potential for adverse effects when corticosteroids are used for the treatment of inflammatory bowel disease, however, because high doses must often be used for extended periods. In the National Cooperative Crohn's Disease Study, 50% of patients receiving high-dose steroid therapy experienced side effects as did one third of the patients on the lower dose regimens for prophylaxis.[33] The well-appreciated adverse effects of corticosteroids include hyperglycemia, hypertension, osteoporosis, fluid retention and electrolyte disturbances, myopathies, psychosis, and reduced resistance to infection. In addition, corticosteroid use may cause adrenocortical suppression. Specific regimens for withdrawal of corticosteroid therapy have been suggested.[59] To minimize corticosteroid effects, clinicians have used alternate-day steroid therapy; however, some patients do not do well on the days when no steroid is given. For most patients, a single daily corticosteroid dose suffices, and divided daily doses are unnecessary.

Immunosuppressants such as azathioprine and 6-mercaptopurine have a significant potential for adverse reactions. Azathioprine causes bone marrow suppression and has been associated with lymphomas (in renal transplant patients) and pancreatitis. 6-Mercaptopurine causes adverse reactions similar to azathioprine; however, there are fewer reports of lymphomas with this agent. With 6-mercaptopurine, pancreatitis usually occurs within 1 month of initiating therapy and recurs if the patient is rechallenged.[60]

Most patients receiving metronidazole for Crohn's disease tolerate the agent fairly well; however, mild adverse effects occur frequently. They commonly include paresthesias and reversible peripheral neuropathy, metallic taste, urticaria, and glossitis.[21,61] Other effects include a disulfiram-like reaction if alcohol is ingested in conjunction.

### *Assessing Success*

The success of regimens to treat inflammatory bowel disease is judged primarily by the patient's own assessment of the disease process and the ability to function in normal activities. Regimens that result in subjective patient improvement (without significant adverse effects) are usually considered successful. Objective measures, such as number of stools per day, may be applied to the disease process; however, these measures are not consistently valuable. There are no routinely used laboratory tests that serve as reliable markers of the disease process. Endoscopic or radiographic examination of the intestinal tract allows more precise assessment of the disease process by the clinician. In most patients, a satisfactory evaluation of the disease progress can be obtained by direct patient inquiry.

## References


1. Wilks S, Moxon W. Lectures on Pathological Anatomy, 2nd ed. London, J. and A. Churchhill, 1875.
2. Crohn BB. Granulomatous diseases of the large and small bowel. A historical survey. Gastroenterology 1967;52:767.
3. Kraft SC. Modern clinical aspects of inflammatory bowel disease. Radiol Clin North Am 1987;25:213–224.
4. Monk M, Mendeloff AI, Siegel CI, et al. An epidemiological study of ulcerative colitis and regional enteritis among adults in Baltimore: II. Social and demographic factors. Gastroenterology 1969;56:847–857.
5. Sedlack RE, Nobrega FT, Karland LT, et al. Inflammatory colon disease in Rochester, Minnesota, 1935–1964. Gastroenterology 1972;62:935–941.
6. Cello JP. Ulcerative colitis, in Sleisenger MH, Fordtran JS (eds): Gastrointestinal Disease. Philadelphia, W.B. Saunders, 1983, pp 1122–1168.
7. Donaldson RM Jr. Crohn's disease, in Sleisenger MH, Fordtran JS (eds): Gastrointestinal Disease. Philadelphia, W.B. Saunders, 1983, pp 1088–1121.
8. Lichenstein JE. Radiologic–pathologic correlation of inflammatory bowel disease. Radiol Clin North Am 1987;25:3–24.
9. Greenstein A, Janowitz H, Sachar D. The extra-intestinal complications of Crohn's disease and ulcerative colitis: A study of 700 patients. Medicine 1976;55:401.
10. Edwards FC, Truelove SC. The cause and prognosis of ulcerative colitis. I. Short term prognosis. Gut 1964;4:299.
11. Glick SN. Crohn's disease of the small intestine. Radiol Clin North Am 1987;25:25–45.
12. Janowicz HD. The "natural history" of inflammatory bowel disease and therapeutic decisions. Am J Gastroenterol 1987;82: 498–503.
13. Summers RW, Switz DM, Sessions JT, et al. National Cooperative Crohn's Disease Study: Results of drug treatment. Gastroenterology 1979;77:847–869.
14. Malchow H, Ewe K, Brandes JW, et al. European Cooperative Crohn's Disease Study (ECCDS): Results of drug treatment. Gastroenterology 1984;86:249–266.
15. Clouse RE, Rosenberg IH. Intensive nutritional support, in Sleisenger MH, Fordtran JS (eds): Gastrointestinal Disease. Philadelphia, W.B. Saunders, 1983, pp 1831–1850.
16. Klotz U, Maier K, Fischer C, et al. Therapeutic efficacy of sulfasalazine and its metabolites in patients with ulcerative colitis and Crohn's disease. N Engl J Med 1980;303:1499–1502.
17. Das KM, Eastwood MA, McManus JPA, et al. Adverse reactions during salicylazosulfapyridine therapy and the relation

with drug metabolism and acetylator phenotype. N Engl J Med 1973;289:491–495.
18. Sack DM, Peppercorn MA. Drug therapy of inflammatory bowel disease. Pharmacotherapy 1983;3:158–176.
19. Peppercorn MA. Role of corticotropin therapy in ulcerative colitis: The controversy continues. Gastroenterology 1983;85: 472–475.
20. Ginsburg AL. The azathioprine controversy. Dig Dis Sci 1981;26:364–371.
21. Jakobovits J, Schuster MM. Metronidazole therapy for Crohn's disease and associated fistulae. Am J Gastroenterol 1984;79: 533–540.
22. Baron JH, Connell AM, Lennard-Jones JE, et al. Sulfasalazine and salicylazosulphadimidine in ulcerative colitis. Lancet 1962;1:1094–1096.
23. Dick AP, Grayson MJ, Carpenter RG, et al. Controlled trial of sulfasalazine in the treatment of ulcerative colitis. Gut 1964;5: 437–441.
24. Das KM. Pharmacotherapy of inflammatory bowel disease. Part 1. Sulfasalazine. Postgrad Med 1983;74:141–151.
25. Powell-Tuck J, Brown RL, Lennard-Jones JE. A comparison of oral prednisone given as single or multiple daily doses for active proctocolitis. Scand J Gastroenterol 1975;13:833–837.
26. Lennard-Jones JE, Longmore AJ, Newell AC, et al. Assessment of prednisone, salazopyrin, and topical hydrocortisone hemisuccinate used as outpatient treatment for ulcerative colitis. Gut 1960;1:217–222.
27. Truelove SC, Watkinson G, Draper G. Comparison of corticosteroid and sulphasalazine therapy in ulcerative colitis. Br Med J 1962;2:1708–1711.
28. Campieri M, Lanfranchi GA, Bazzocchi G, et al. Treatment of ulcerative colitis with high dose 5-aminosalicylic acid enemas. Lancet 1981;2:270–271.
29. Anonymous. Multicentre trial. Betamethasone-17-valerate and prednisolone-21-phosphate retention enemata in proctocolitis. Br Med J 1971;3:84–86.
30. Kumana CR, Seaton T, Meghi M, et al. Beclomethasone dipropionate enemas for treating bowel disease without producing Cushing's syndrome or hypothalamic–pituitary suppression. Lancet 1982;1:579–582.
31. Bansky G, Buhler H, Stamm B, et al. Treatment of distal ulcerative colitis with beclomethasone enemas: High therapeutic efficacy without endocrine side effects. Dis Colon Rectum 1987;30:288–292.
32. Azad Khan AK, Truelove SC. Circulating levels of sulphasalazine and its metabolites and their relation to the clinical efficacy of the drug in ulcerative colitis. Gut 1980;21:706–710.
33. Singleton JW, Law DH, Kelley ML, et al. National Cooperative Crohn's Disease Study: Adverse reactions to study drugs. Gastroenterology 1979;77:870–882.
34. Truelove SC, Willoughby CP, Lee EG, et al. Further experience in the treatment of severe attacks of ulcerative colitis. Lancet 1978;2:1086–1088.
35. Kaplan HP, Portnoy B, Binder HJ, et al. A controlled evaluation of intravenous adrenocorticotropic hormone and hydrocortisone in the treatment of acute colitis. Gastroenterology 1975;69:91–95.
36. Powell-Tuck J, Bucknell NA, Lennard-Jones JE. A controlled comparison of corticotropin and hydrocortisone in the treatment of severe proctocolitis. Scand J Gastroenterol 1977;12: 971–975.
37. Misiewicz JJ, Lennard-Jones JE, Connell AM, et al. Controlled trial of sulphasalazine in maintenance therapy for ulcerative colitis. Lancet 1965;1:185–188.
38. Davies PS, Rhodes J. Maintenance of remission in ulcerative colitis with sulphasalazine or a high-fibre diet: A clinical trial. Br Med J 1978;1:1524–1525.
39. Riis P, Anthonisen P, Wulff HR, et al. The prophylactic effect of salazosulphapyridine in ulcerative colitis during long-term treatment: A double-blind trial on patients symptomatic for one year. Scand J Gastroenterol 1973;8:71–75.
40. Dissanayake PS, Truelove SC. A controlled therapeutic trial of long-term maintenance treatment of ulcerative colitis with sulphasalazine (salazopyrin). Gut 1973;14:923–926.
41. Lennard-Jones JE, Misiewicz JJ, Connell AM, et al. Prednisone as maintenance treatment for ulcerative colitis in remission. Lancet 1965;1:199–9.
42. Anthonisen P, Baraby F, Folkenborg O, et al. The clinical effect of salazosulphapyridine (salazopyrin) in Crohn's disease. Scand J Gastroenterol 1974;9:549–554.
43. Van Hees PA, Van Lier HJ, Van Elteren PH, et al. Effect of sulphasalazine in patients with active Crohn's disease: A controlled double-blind study. Gut 1981;22:404–409.
44. Blichfeldt PER, Blomhoff JP, Myhre E, et al. Metronidazole in Crohn's disease: A double-blind cross-over trial. Scand J Gastroenterol 1978;13:123–127.
45. Berstein LH, Frank MS, Brandt LJ, et al. Healing of perineal Crohn's disease with metronidazole. Gastroenterology 1980;79: 357–365.
46. Rhodes J, Bainton D, Beck P, et al. Controlled trial of azathioprine in Crohn's disease. Lancet 1971;2:1273–1276.
47. Willoughby JMT, Kumar Praveen J, Beckett J, et al. Controlled trial of azathioprine in Crohn's disease. Lancet 1971;2:294.
48. Rosenberg JL, Levin B, Wall AJ, et al. A controlled trial of azathioprine in Crohn's disease. Dig Dis Sci 1975;20:721.
49. Korelitz BI. Pharmacotherapy of inflammatory bowel disease. Part 3. 6-Mercaptopurine. Postgrad Med 1983;74:165–172.
50. Present DH, Korelitz BI, Wisch N, et al. Treatment of Crohn's disease with 6-mercaptopurine: A long term, randomized, double-blind study. N Engl J Med 1980;302:981–987.
51. Allen R, Steinberg DM, Williams JA, et al. Crohn's disease involving the colon: An audit of clinical management. Gastroenterology 1977;73:723–732.
52. Donaldson RM. Management of medical problems in pregnancy—inflammatory bowel disease. N Engl J Med 1986;312: 1616–1619.
53. Baiocco P. Pregnancy and inflammatory bowel disease, in Korelitz BI, Sohn N (eds): Inflammatory Bowel Disease. Orlando, Harcourt Brace Jovanovich, 1985, pp 91–95.
54. Willoughby JMT, Truelove SC. Ulcerative colitis and pregnancy. Gut 1980;21:469.
55. Toovey S, Hudson E, Hendry WF, et al. Sulfasalazine and male infertility: Reversibility and possible mechanism. Gut 1981;22: 445–451.
56. Taffet SL, Das KM. Sulfasalazine: Adverse effects and desensitization. Dig Dis Sci 1983;28:833–842.
57. Goldman P, Peppercorn MA. Sulfasalazine. N Engl J Med 1975;293:20–23.
58. Korelitz BI, Present DH, Rubin PH, et al. Desensitization to sulfasalazine after hypersensitivity reactions in patients with inflammatory bowel disease. J Clin Gastroenterol 1984;6:27–31.
59. Byyny RL. Withdrawal from glucocorticoid therapy. N Engl J Med 1976;295:30–32.
60. Haber CJ, Meltzer SJ, Present DH, et al. Nature and course of pancreatitis caused by 6-mercaptopurine in the treatment of inflammatory bowel disease. Gastroenterology 1986;91:982–986.
61. Duffy LF, Daum F, Fisher SE, et al. Peripheral neuropathy in Crohn's disease patients treated with metronidazole. Gastroenterology 1984;88:681–684.

# Chapter 29 / Nausea and Vomiting

A. Thomas Taylor, PharmD

Nausea and vomiting are common complaints among most individuals. Because of the variable etiologies of these problems, management may be quite simple or detailed and complex, essentially innocuous or associated with therapy-induced adverse reactions. For these reasons, this chapter provides an overview of nausea and vomiting, two multifaceted subjects.

## Etiology

Nausea is usually defined as the inclination to vomit or as a feeling in the throat or epigastric region alerting an individual that vomiting is imminent. Vomiting is defined as the ejection or expulsion of gastric contents through the mouth, often requiring a forceful event. Both of these conditions may occur transiently with no other associated signs or symptoms; however, these conditions may also be only part of a more complex clinical presentation.

Nausea and vomiting may be associated with a variety of clinical presentations. In addition to numerous gastrointestinal diseases, either or both may accompany cardiovascular, infectious, neurologic, or metabolic disease processes. Nausea and/or vomiting may also be a feature of such conditions as pregnancy or may follow operative procedures or administration of certain medications such as cancer chemotherapy. Psychogenic etiologies of these symptoms may be present, especially in young women having an underlying emotional disturbance. Anticipatory etiologies may be involved, as in patients who have previously received cytotoxic chemotherapy. Specific etiologies associated with nausea and vomiting are presented in Table 29.1.[1]

In addition to identifying problems associated with nausea and vomiting, it is important to address specific related medical problems. For example, nausea and/or vomiting may occur in as many as 70% of patients with inferior myocardial infarction or diabetics with ketoacidosis. As many as 80% to 90% of patients with Addison's disease in its crisis phase, patients with acute pancreatitis, or patients with acute appendicitis may present with nausea and vomiting.

Drug-induced nausea and vomiting have been of particular interest, especially when caused by cytotoxic agents. The reasons for this awareness include the increasing number of patients receiving cytotoxic treatment and the number of agents implicated. Included in Table 29.2 are specific cytotoxic agents categorized by their emetogenic potential. Although some agents may have greater emetogenic potential than others, combinations of agents, high doses, clinical settings, psychologic conditions, prior treatment experiences, and unusual stimuli to sight, smell, or taste may alter a patient's response to a drug treatment. Not only are nausea and vomiting unpredictable, but they may be unavoidable and potentially devastating to the continued delivery of care. Indeed, some patients may experience these problems so intensely that chemotherapy may be postponed or discontinued.

In addition to the emetogenic potential of various cytotoxic regimens, a variety of other common etiologies have been proposed for the development of nausea and vomiting in cancer patients. These are presented in Table 29.3.[2]

The etiology of nausea and vomiting may vary with the age of the patient. For example, vomiting in the newborn during the first day of life suggests upper digestive tract obstruction or an increase in intracranial pressure. Other illnesses associated with vomiting in children include pyloric stenosis, duodenal ulcer, stress ulcer, adrenal insufficiency, septicemia, or diseases of the pancreas, liver, or biliary tree. Also, hepatocellular failure seen in Reye's syndrome may lead to profound cerebral edema followed by persistent emesis. One of the most common etiologies of vomiting in children, however, is viral gastroenteritis caused by rotavirus. Vomiting in infants may also be associated with something as simple as overfeeding, rapid feeding, inadequate burping, or lying down too soon after feeding. It should be recognized that these types of vomiting are usually indicative of minor problems and may be altered by changing the approach to feeding.

## Pathophysiology

Although the exact neurologic pathways that control vomiting are still somewhat undetermined, this act probably involves interactions between the gastrointestinal tract and the central nervous system (CNS). Within the CNS, the vomiting center (VC) is found in the reticular formation, as is the chemoreceptor trigger zone (CTZ), located in the postrema of the fourth ventricle. Various visceral afferent and efferent pathways are probably also involved in the vomiting process. In addition to these commonly mentioned sites of activity, two important sites within the hypothalamus have been identified, the satiety center and the feeding center. Both centers are believed to be involved in the regulation of food intake, possibly through cholecystokinin[1]; however, the extent to which these sites are involved in the control of nausea and vomiting is unknown.

Emesis appears to occur by direct or indirect stimulation of the vomiting center. Stimuli are transmitted to this center from the gastrointestinal tract, the cerebral cortex, the labyrinthine apparatus, and the adjacent CTZ; however, not all stimuli of vomiting follow the same pathway. Cytotoxic

**Table 29.1** Specific Etiologies of Nausea and Vomiting

| | |
|---|---|
| Gastrointestinal mechanisms | Neurologic processes |
| Mechanical gastric outlet obstruction | Midline cerebellar hemorrhage |
| Peptic ulcer disease | Increased intracranial pressure |
| Gastric carcinoma | Migraine headache |
| Pancreatic disease | Vestibular disorders |
| Motility disorders | Head trauma |
| Gastroparesis | Metabolic disorders |
| Drug-induced gastric stasis | Diabetes mellitus (diabetic ketoacidosis) |
| Chronic intestinal pseudoobstruction | Addison's disease |
| Postviral gastroenteritis | Renal disease (uremia) |
| Irritable bowel syndrome | Psychogenic causes |
| Postgastric surgery | Self-induced |
| Idiopathic gastric stasis | Anticipatory |
| Anorexia nervosa | Therapy-induced causes |
| Intraabdominal emergencies | Cytotoxic chemotherapy |
| Intestinal obstruction | Radiation therapy |
| Acute pancreatitis | Theophylline preparations (intolerance, toxic) |
| Acute appendicitis | Anticonvulsant preparations (toxic) |
| Acute pyelonephritis | Digitalis preparations (toxic) |
| Acute cholecystitis | Opiates |
| Acute cholangitis | Drug withdrawal |
| Acute viral hepatitis | Opiates |
| Acute gastroenteritis | Benzodiazepines |
| Viral gastroenteritis | Miscellaneous causes |
| Salmonellosis | Pregnancy causes |
| Shigellosis | Any swallowed irritant (foods, drugs) |
| Staphylococcal gastroenteritis (enterotoxins) | Noxious odors |
| Cardiovascular diseases | Operative procedures |
| Acute myocardial infarction | |
| Congestive heart failure | |
| Shock and circulatory collapse | |

Partially adapted from Hanson JS, McCallum RW: The diagnosis and management of nausea and vomiting: A review. Am J Gastroenterol 1985;80:210–218, with permission.

drugs, for example, appear to stimulate primarily the CTZ, while the gastrointestinal tract and the cerebral cortex may have a less important role. The primary pathway of pregnancy-associated vomiting also appears to be through stimulation of the CTZ.[3]

Anticipatory nausea and vomiting may be elicited either by specific stimuli associated with the administration of noxious, often cytotoxic, agents or by the anxiety associated with such treatments. Many patients demonstrate both types. The most often accepted theory for this pattern of conditioning is that by repeated pairing of chemotherapy and its aftereffects, previously neutral stimuli such as odors, sounds, and settings acquire the ability to elicit nausea and vomiting.[4,5] These types of stimuli should be expected to be more troublesome in patients receiving agents with the greatest inherent emetogenic potential.

The act of vomiting is forceful, requiring the coordinated contractions of abdominal musculature, the pylorus and the antrum, a raised gastric cardia, and diminished lower esophageal sphincter pressure, as well as esophageal dilatation.[6] Vomiting is not simple regurgitation, an act in which the gastric or esophageal contents rise to the pharynx because of pressure differences brought about by such events as an incompetent lower esophageal sphincter.

## Clinical Presentation

Included in the gastrointestinal etiologies of nausea and vomiting are a variety of specific disorders associated with mechanical obstruction, motility changes, and infectious diseases of the vital organs within the abdominal cavity. Although each of these conditions may vary in onset, duration, and severity of symptoms, each is nevertheless a potential source of nausea and vomiting that may need to be addressed. In this regard, attention to other simultaneous signs and symptoms should be helpful in making an accurate diagnosis and evaluation of a specific patient. Additional knowledge of a patient's gastrointestinal history, with particular emphasis on the presence of abdominal pain or discomfort, diarrhea, and blood from the upper or lower gastrointestinal tract, should always be appreciated. Knowledge of the patient's tolerance of food is important. Also, the timing of these symptoms in relation to meals as well as the consistency, content, and odor of the vomitus may be characteristic findings in certain patient types. Other signs and symptoms that may be helpful in understanding a specific clinical presentation include concomitant findings such as fever, weight loss, a description of precipitating

**Table 29.2** Emetogenic Potential of Cytotoxic Chemotherapy

| *Most emetogenic* | *Moderate* | *Least emetogenic* |
|---|---|---|
| Amsacrine | Azacytidine | Asparaginase |
| Cisplatin | Etoposide | Bleomycin |
| Cyclophosphamide | Mitomycin C | Busulfan |
| Dacarbazine | Procarbazine | Chlorambucil |
| Dactinomycin | Thiotepa | Cytarabine |
| Daunorubicin | | Diaziquone |
| Doxorubicin | | Estramustine |
| Hexamethylmethamine | | Floxuridine |
| Mechlorethamine | | Fluorouracil |
| Mitoxantrone | | Hydroxyurea |
| Nitrosoureas | | Melphalan |
| Streptozocin | | Mercaptopurine |
| | | Methotrexate |
| | | Teniposide |
| | | Thioguanine |
| | | Vinca alkaloids |

factors, a complete history of recent medication use, and the history or presence of myalgias, behavioral or visual changes, headache, or pain outside the abdomen.

As it would be impossible to discuss all clinical settings in which the presence of nausea and vomiting might be a pertinent finding, these processes are presented as they might occur together and also as "simple" or "complex" in presentation. Defined here, the term *simple* applies to those episodes of nausea and/or vomiting described by one of the following criteria: (1) occur occasionally and are generally self-limited or relieved by the minimal use of antiemetic methods or medications; (2) account for little patient deterioration such as fluid–electrolyte imbalances, pain, or noncompliance with prescribed therapies; or (3) are not related to the administration of or exposure to noxious agents. Conversely, the term *complex* is used when describing a patient's clinical course as including symptoms that (1) are not adequately or readily relieved by the administration of a single antiemetic method or medication; (2) lead to progressive patient deterioration secondary to fluid–electrolyte imbalances, pain, or noncompliance with prescribed therapies; or (3) are caused by noxious agents or psychogenic events.

Psychogenic vomiting is often related to sexual or marital disturbances, health problems of friends or family members, or deeper emotional strains. Pertinent features of this condition may include a family history. Episodes may be induced by meals, are recurrent, generally have no accompanying nausea, and may be suppressed by the patient. Often these events are not noted to be important to the patient. Unless associated with anorexia nervosa, appetite is usually normal. Many of these conditions subside with reductions in stress.

**Table 29.3** Nondrug Etiologies of Nausea and Vomiting in Cancer Patients

| |
|---|
| Fluid and electrolyte abnormalities |
| Hypercalcemia |
| Volume depletion |
| Water intoxication |
| Adrenocortical insufficiency |
| Bowel obstruction, peritonitis |
| Metastases to the central nervous system |
| Brain |
| Meninges |
| Hepatic metastases |
| Uremia |
| Infections (septicemia, local) |
| Radiation therapy |

Adapted from Frytak S, Moertel CG: Management of nausea and vomiting in the cancer patient. JAMA 1981;245:393–396, with permission.

## Treatment

Most episodes of nausea and vomiting occur in relation to one of the conditions or processes listed in Table 29.1 and decrease in frequency, duration, and severity as the underlying process resolves; however, during the resolution of each underlying problem, it may be desirable to combat specific symptoms such as nausea and vomiting.

Although many approaches to the treatment of nausea and vomiting have been suggested, antiemetic drugs are most often recommended. These agents represent a variety of pharmacologic and chemical classes as well as dosage regimens and routes of administration. In addition, over-the-counter and prescription drugs are often used. With so many treatment possibilities available, factors that enable the clinician to discriminate among various choices must be recognized. These factors include (1) the suspected etiology of the symptoms; (2) the frequency, duration, and severity of the episodes; (3) the ability of the patient to use oral, rectal, injectable, or transdermal topical medications; and (4) the success of previous antiemetic medications. For example, many antiemetics are commercially available as oral agents. Provided a patient can and will adhere to oral dosing, a suitable and effective agent can often be selected; however, for certain other patients, oral medications may be inappropriate because of their inability to retain any appreciable oral ingestions. In these patients, certainly rectal or injectable routes of administration might be preferred. Information concerning commonly available antiemetic preparations is compiled in Table 29.4.

Many of the clinical settings in which an individual initially experiences nausea and vomiting may be at home or outside formal medical settings. For these symptoms, patients may choose from a lengthy list of commercial products. While suitable for occasional "simple" nausea and vomiting, these agents are often abandoned by the patient as symptoms continue or become progressively worse. As the patient's condition warrants, prescription medications may be chosen, possibly as single-agent therapy or in combination. For most conditions, a single-agent antiemetic is preferred; however, in patients in whom single-agent therapy has failed or in those receiving highly emetogenic chemotherapy, multiple-agent regimens are usually recommended. Numerous combinations have been employed through clinical investigation and practice.

The treatment of simple nausea and vomiting usually requires minimal therapy. Many patients may self-medicate with a variety of over-the-counter (OTC) products and avoid medical care. Others will require prescription antiemetic medications to relieve minor episodes of nausea and vomiting. Products available for self-medication include antacids; antihistamine–anticholinergic agents such as buclizine, cyclizine, meclizine, dimenhydrinate, and diphenhydramine; and phosphorated carbohydrate solutions. Agents requiring physician prescription include antihistaminic–anticholinergic drugs not available OTC and phenothiazine agents. These latter agents include benzquinamide, dimenhydrinate, diphenhydramine, hydroxyzine, prochlorperazine, promethazine, and trimethobenzamide. Both OTC and prescription drugs useful in the treatment of simple nausea and vomiting are usually effective in small, infrequently administered doses. Side effects and toxic effects in these settings are also usually minimal.

The management of complex nausea and vomiting may require aggressive drug therapy, possibly with more than one antiemetic. For patients with complex symptoms, effective combinations may include two of the following drugs: benzquinamide, chlorpromazine, dimenhydrinate, droperidol, hydroxyzine, prochlorperazine, promethazine, thiethylperazine, trimethobenzamide. In combination, each of these drugs is usually prescribed in small-to-moderate dosage regimens, approaching symptom control through different pharmacologic mechanisms while avoiding untoward effects caused by high doses. For patients receiving highly emetogenic chemotherapy, antiemetic regimens may include as many as five drugs (see Combination Antiemetic Protocols).

## *Antiemetic Agents*

Since the early 1980s, many antiemetic agents have been more rigorously studied than in previous years. Moreover, with the increasing use of highly emetogenic chemotherapeutic agents, numerous single- and multiple-agent antiemetic clinical trials have been reported in the medical and pharmaceutical literature.

Variables that may affect the assessment of antiemetic trials have also been addressed.[7] In broad terms, there may be variability in patients, emetic stimuli, antiemetic drugs, and study design. More specifically, in evaluating such studies, close attention should be paid to pretreatment variables as well as the types of patients studied. The onset, duration, and frequency of symptoms should be fairly compared as should the various etiologic situations. Anticipatory nausea and vomiting require careful evaluation because this condition may often be refractory to antiemetic drugs.[8,9] Another patient factor that should be considered is age. Age-related responsiveness has been noted particularly in studies in which the greatest efficacy of $\Delta^9$-tetrahydrocannabinol (THC) was reported among younger patients.[10–12]

Other variables that appear to affect patient response to antiemetic therapy and therefore influence the overall interpretation of study results include the setting in which nausea and vomiting occur. For example, inpatients may tolerate chemotherapy better than outpatients, perhaps because of more security in the inpatient environment. The presence of stress or depression as well as the lack of social support may adversely affect patient response.[13,14] Dosage, schedule, and route of administration of each antiemetic agent may greatly influence beneficial as well as toxic effects. Unfortunately, many clinical trials to date have not adequately addressed the pharmacodynamic issues of these drugs. Therefore, efficacy is difficult to compare because of the wide variety of studied protocols.

Research protocols concerning the use of antiemetic drugs have varied tremendously. As these agents are required in controlling the symptoms produced by one or more etiologic factors, study designs have been quite different, especially through investigator approach to randomization, blinding, placebo control, crossover, sample size, and methods of evaluating efficacy and toxicity.

In general, the clinician should evaluate the patient's condition and determine the need for antiemetic treatment of an existing condition or prophylactic therapy to prevent or lessen anticipatory nausea and vomiting episodes, as in the patient requiring cytotoxic drugs. Once this decision, along with the complete and overall medical evaluation, has been made, the selection process may proceed.

### Antacids

Although not often discussed in the recent literature on this subject, various antacids may be sought by patients, particularly those experiencing "simple" nausea and vomiting. In this setting, single or combination OTC antacid products, especially those containing magnesium hydroxide, aluminum hydroxide, and/or calcium carbonate, may provide sufficient relief, primarily through gastric acid neutralization. Patients responding to small and occasional doses of antacids probably do not have significant pathology; however, it is not uncommon for patients with significant gastrointestinal disease to self-medicate with larger and continued doses of antacids.

Common antacid dosage regimens for the relief of nausea and vomiting include one or more small doses of single- or multiple-agent products. Although antacid therapy may be aggressively applied for the treatment of known ulcer disease, OTC products sought by patients are usually taken in

**Table 29.4** Common Antiemetic Preparations

| *Drug* | *Adult dosage regimen* | *Dosage form/route* |
|---|---|---|
| **Over-the-Counter Products** | | |
| Antacids (various) | 15–30 mL every 2–4 h prn | Oral suspension |
| Buclizine (Bucladin-S) | 50 mg BID | Tablet |
| Cyclizine (Marezine) | 50 mg every 4–6 h prn | Tablet, IM |
| Dextrose, levulose, phosphoric acid (Emetrol) | 15–30 mL every 1–3 h prn | Oral liquid |
| Dimenhydrinate (Dramamine) | 50–100 mg every 4–6 h prn | Tablet, oral liquid |
| Diphenhydramine (Benadryl) | 12.5–25 mg every 4–6 h prn | Capsule, oral liquid |
| Meclizine (Bonine, Antivert) | 25–50 mg every 24 h prn | Tablet, chewable tablet |
| **Prescription Products** | | |
| Benzquinamide (Emete-Con) | 25–50 mg every 3–4 h prn | IM, IV |
| Chlorpromazine (Thorazine) | 10–25 mg, every 4–6 h prn | Sustained-released capsule, tablet, oral liquid concentrate, oral syrup, IM, IV, rectal suppository |
| Dexamethasone (Decadron) | 10 mg prior to chemotherapy; repeat with 4–8 mg | IV |
| Diazepam (Valium) | 2–5 mg every 3 h (oral) | Tablet |
| Dimenhydrinate (Dramamine) | 50–100 mg every 4 h prn | IM, IV |
| Diphenhydramine (Benadryl) | 12.5–50 mg every 4–6 h prn | Oral liquid, capsule, IM, IV |
| Diphenidol (Vontrol) | 25–50 mg every 4 h prn | Tablet |
| Dronabinol (Marinol) | 5–7.5 mg/m$^2$ every 3–4 h prn after chemotherapy | Capsule |
| Droperidol (Inapsine) | 2.5–5.0 mg every 4–6 h prn | IM, IV |
| Fluphenazine (Prolixin) | 1.25 mg every 6–8 h prn | Tablet, IM |
| Haloperidol (Haldol) | 1–5 mg every 12 h prn | Tablet, oral liquid concentrate, IM, IV |
| Hydroxyzine (Vistaril, Atarax) | 25–100 mg every 6 h prn | Capsule oral suspension. IM |
| Lorazepam (Ativan) | 0.5–4.0 mg prior to procedure | IV |
| Methylprednisolone (Solu-Medrol) | 125–500 mg every 6 h × 1–2 doses prior to chemotherapy | IV |
| Metoclopramide (Reglan) | 1–2 mg/kg every 2 h × 2 and every 3 h × 3 | IV |
| Perphenazine (Trilafon) | 8–32 mg/d divided prn | Tablet, repeat-action tablet, oral liquid concentrate, IM, IV |

**Table 29.4 Continued**

| *Drug* | *Adult dosage regimen* | *Dosage form/route* |
|---|---|---|
| Prochlorperazine (Compazine) | 5–10 mg TID/QID prn (oral, injectable)<br>2.5–25 mg TID/QID prn (rectal) | Sustained-release capsule, tablet, oral syrup, rectal suppository, IM, IV |
| Promazine (Sparine) | 25–50 mg every 4–6 prn | Tablet, oral syrup, oral liquid concentrate |
| Promethazine (Phenergan) | 12.5–50 mg every 4–6 h prn | Tablet, oral syrup, IM, IV, rectal suppository |
| Scopolamine (Transderm Scop) | 0.5 mg every 72 h prn | Transdermal patch |
| Thiethylperazine (Torecan) | 10 mg TID | Tablet, IM, rectal suppository |
| Triflupromazine (Vesprin) | 20–30 mg/d (oral) | Oral suspension IM |
| Trimethobenzamide (Tigan) | 250 mg TID/prn QID (oral)<br>200 mg, TID/QID prn (rectal) | Capsule, IM, IV, rectal suppository |

response to acute and sporadic nausea and vomiting. Common commercial products usually supply sufficient ingredients to allow a range of approximately 40–180 mEq of acid-neutralizing capacity.[15–17]

Potential adverse effects from antacids are usually related to the presence of magnesium, aluminum, or calcium salts. Specifically, it should be noted that osmotic diarrhea from magnesium and constipation from aluminum and calcium salts may be of concern to patients, particularly those self-medicating or using high and frequently administered antacid doses. Generally, however, when used occasionally for acute episodic relief of nausea and vomiting, antacids do not produce the serious problems sometimes noted with these products.

### Antihistaminic–Anticholinergic Agents

The antihistaminic–anticholinergic category of antiemetic drugs potentially includes a variety of agents: benzquinamide, buclizine, cyclizine, dimenhydrinate, diphenhydramine, hydroxyzine, meclizine, promethazine, pyrilamine, scopolamine, and trimethobenzamide. These agents appear to interrupt various visceral afferent pathways that stimulate nausea and vomiting. And although these agents may be appropriate in the treatment of "simple" symptomatology, when used alone each has had considerable difficulty in proving greater-than-placebo efficacy in patients with more "complex" complaints such as those caused by cytotoxic chemotherapy. Specifically, patients experiencing motion sickness or other labyrinth-induced symptoms may benefit adequately from these agents.[18]

Typical dosage regimens of antihistaminic–anticholinergic agents usually include the oral administration of small-to-moderate doses one to several times each day. When used for their depressant effects on labyrinth excitability, these agents have been shown to produce variable safety and efficacy. In addition, neither the antihistaminic nor the anticholinergic potency appears to correlate well with the ability of these agents to prevent or treat the nausea and vomiting associated with motion sickness. Their precise mechanisms of action are to date unknown. The most useful antiemetic agent for motion sickness prophylaxis appears to be scopolamine, particularly when given 1 to 2 hours prior to symptom-producing exposures.[19]

Adverse reactions that may be apparent with the use of the antihistaminic–anticholinergic agents include primarily drowsiness or confusion, blurred vision, dry mouth, urinary retention, and possibly tachycardia, particularly in elderly patients. Also, as doses are increased or are more frequently administered, patients with narrow-angle glaucoma, prostatic hypertrophy, and asthma will be at greater risk of complications from the anticholinergic effects of these drugs.

### Phenothiazines

The most widely prescribed antiemetic agents through the years have been the phenothiazines, most specifically chlorpromazine, fluphenazine, perphenazine, prochlorperazine, promazine, promethazine (although most like an antihistamine in its antiemetic activity), thiethylperazine, and triflupromazine. These agents appear to block dopamine receptors, most likely in the CTZ. Some investigators have found the phenothiazines to demonstrate greatest efficacy when compared with placebo and less efficacy when compared with other more potent antiemetics.[20–22]

Phenothiazines are marketed in an array of dosage forms, none of which appears to be more efficacious than another; however, there are perhaps some important generalizations concerning their use in overall clinical practice. These agents may be most practical for long-term treatment and are inexpensive in comparison to newer drugs, with the exception of slow-release products which may be too costly and of no established clinical advantage. Little distinguishing information is available in the present literature concerning the efficacy of rectal preparations. Rectal administration is most preferred in patients in whom parenteral administration is impractical or oral medications cannot be retained and are therefore ineffective. In many patients, low doses of phenothiazine drugs may not be effective, while larger doses may produce unacceptable risks.[2]

Phenothiazines are most useful in patients with "simple" nausea and vomiting or in those receiving mildly emetogenic doses of chemotherapy; however, problems associated with these drugs include troublesome and potentially dangerous side effects, including extrapyramidal reactions, hypersensitivity reactions with possible liver dysfunction, marrow aplasia, and excessive sedation. If relief of symptoms is provided and side effects are absent or acceptable, these drugs should be continued. Conversely, failure to achieve adequate antiemetic efficacy during the first course of chemotherapy should most often prompt the clinician to search for more acceptable agents, possibly combination therapies.[21–23]

### Cannabinoids

Tetrahydrocannabinol (THC), although initially faced with unique legal and political controversies, has demonstrated success as an antiemetic agent.[24] This success has even been shown in certain patients in whom other regimens have failed.[25,26] The exact site of activity at which THC exerts its antiemetic effects is unknown and does not appear to be the CTZ.[27] Dronabinol, $\Delta^9$-THC, has recently been marketed in the United States and is indicated solely for nausea and vomiting resulting from cytotoxic therapies. Effective use of dronabinol most often requires the maintenance of adequate blood levels and therefore it should be administered every 4 to 6 hours, beginning the night before chemotherapy. Failure to premedicate adequately may likely result in vomiting.

Although potent antiemetics, the cannabinoids have been associated with certain potentially undesirable features and are not equally effective against all stimuli nor all doses of the same stimuli. Some investigators have suggested that it is necessary to develop significant side effects from THC, even a "high," to realize antiemetic efficacy. Therefore, it should be expected that the major side effects of these agents are dysphoria, including episodes of anxiety, fear, confusion, hallucinations, and time distortion. Depending on the severity of these effects, doses should be lowered or discontinued. Other investigators have claimed that older patients or those having had no previous marijuana experience were most likely to develop dysphoria. This point has not been fully confirmed; however, once dysphoria clears, there appear to be no late sequelae.[24,28]

### Butyrophenones

Two butyrophenone compounds have antiemetic activity, haloperidol and its congener droperidol. Each agent blocks dopaminergic stimulation of the CTZ. Although each agent is effective in relieving nausea and vomiting, droperidol has been used most often, particularly in perioperative and obstetric settings.

Given by injection, usually intravenously, droperidol has been documented as safe and effective, even in ambulatory cancer patients.[29–32] Depending on the reason for droperidol's use, its optimal dosage range may vary considerably. For example, preoperative doses may range from 2.5 to 10 mg, while dosage regimens during cytotoxic chemotherapy have been documented as low as 0.5–2.5 mg by intermittent injection to as great as 1.0–1.5 mg/h by intravenous infusion.[29,33–35] Although the optimal antiemetic dose of droperidol for patients receiving chemotherapy is not well established, many patients benefit from small doses, particularly when combined with other antiemetic drugs.

Adverse reactions resulting from the use of the butyrophenone compounds include primarily sedation and the possibility of dystonic reactions. Although dystonia may occur after the initial dose, some patients may experience this problem later in therapy. Injectable diphenhydramine usually rapidly resolves these extrapyramidal reactions.[33]

### Corticosteroids

Corticosteroids have demonstrated antiemetic efficacy since the initial recognition that patients receiving prednisone as part of their Hodgkin's disease protocol appeared to develop less nausea and vomiting than those treated with protocols excluding this agent. This is of particular interest because the alkylating agents often employed in such protocols rank high in emetogenicity, especially mechlorethamine and cyclophosphamide. Other corticosteroids that have shown efficacy include methylprednisolone and dexamethasone. The exact mechanism by which corticosteroids provide antiemetic activity is unknown; however, the inhibition of prostaglandin synthesis has been postulated and questioned.[36,37] Such mechanism theories are most appealing in light of the known high emetogenic potential of prostaglandins themselves; however, because of their numerous metabolic effects, a single site of steroid antiemetic activity may be difficult to locate or assess. In addition to the antiemetic benefits of corticosteroids, other desirable effects include increased appetite and an elevation of mood or feelings of well-being. Depending on the patient and the drug regimen, these effects may be the primary considerations for corticosteroid preferences.

Quite a variety of dosages have been employed in corticosteroid antiemetic clinical trials. Variations in drug, dosage regimen, and route of administration plague the unraveling of the clinical literature. Although studies utilizing steroids in both single-agent and multiple-agent protocols have demonstrated acceptable efficacy, their exact ranking among antiemetic alternatives is not clear for patients receiving cytotoxic chemotherapy. For patients with "simple" nausea and vomiting, steroids are generally considered unacceptable. As with other conditions, steroids should be employed only when the benefit-to-risk ratio is sufficient to warrant a medication with such complex and potentially deleterious effects.

Benefits from corticosteroids have been quite variable. Of the corticosteroids studied, the use of dexamethasone has been best defined. In clinical trials, dexamethasone has been compared with metoclopramide and prochlorperazine.[38–40] During therapy with mildly to moderately emetogenic agents, dexamethasone appeared to be comparable to metoclopramide and superior to prochlorperazine when each was used alone; however, metoclopramide has shown greater efficacy when studied in patients receiving highly emetogenic regimens, especially those including cisplatin. Methylprednisolone has been compared with metoclopramide and thiethylperazine. Benefit appeared greater for methylprednisolone than thiethylperazine and comparable to typical metoclopramide doses of less than 2 mg/kg.[41–44]

Dosage regimens vary widely among steroid antiemetic protocols. When used alone, dexamethasone has often been administered injectably as a single dose of 8–20 mg prior to chemotherapy and followed by oral doses of 4–12 mg up to 24 hours after completion of chemotherapy. Variations in the dosage regimens of other steroid protocols have been fewer. Usually, methylprednisolone has been administered prior to chemotherapy in a dose of 250 mg. After chemotherapy, up to four subsequent doses have been given.

Adverse effects of corticosteroids used in the preceding types of settings may include changes in mood ranging from anxiety to euphoria. Other reported effects are headache, metallic taste, abdominal discomfort, and itchy throat.[36]

### Benzodiazepines

Benzodiazepines are among the therapeutic alternatives in the treatment of anticipatory nausea and vomiting. The most often prescribed agent in this pharmacologic class is lorazepam, usually administered intravenously for its amnestic effects. Dosage regimens include one dose prior to cytotoxic chemotherapy and multiple doses after each treatment. Although some patients may appreciate their lack of recall of having received chemotherapy, others may find it uncomfortable and unacceptable. These latter patients refuse lorazepam for subsequent treatments; however, acceptability of this feature of one's care may be highly dependent upon the overall severity of symptoms. Maher has reported the use of lorazepam and a phenothiazine with improvement in anticipatory and chemotherapy-induced symptoms.[45] Others believe this combination requires additional study because of the increased risk of respiratory and CNS depression.

As a benzodiazepine, lorazepam may display an array of pharmacologic activities including sedation, hypnosis, anxiolysis, and muscle relaxation in doses of 0.5–4.0 mg, with little change in a patient's respiratory or cardiovascular function; however, other effects on the central nervous system such as disorientation, hallucinations, incontinence, and amnesia appear directly related to dose escalation.[46,47] Diazepam has also been used as an antiemetic and vestibular depressant. Doses are similar to those useful in anxiety.

### Metoclopramide

Procainamide's congener, metoclopramide, has been studied for its antiemetic effects. Its ability to block the dopaminergic receptors centrally in the CTZ as well as peripherally makes it an agent with documented and promising efficacy. Peripherally, metoclopramide increases lower esophageal sphincter tone, aids gastric emptying, and accelerates transit through the small bowel, possibly through the release of acetylcholine.

Although used in Europe for the management of motion sickness, metoclopramide is presently used in the United States for the treatment of "complex" nausea and vomiting in response to chemotherapy administration, again most often cisplatin. For such patients, it has been employed in multiagent combination protocols; however, it has shown efficacy as a single therapy. Alone or in combination, metoclopramide has demonstrated significant efficacy in high doses (1–2 mg/kg intravenously), with one dose administered approximately 30 minutes prior to chemotherapy. Up to four subsequent doses are usually given at 2-hour intervals after chemotherapy.

Because the adverse reactions to metoclopramide include extrapyramidal effects, intravenous diphenhydramine 25–50 mg should be prophylactically administered or provided on-call for its anticipated need. Other adverse effects produced by metoclopramide include restlessness, drowsiness, fatigue, nausea, and diarrhea.[48,49]

### Miscellaneous Agents

A final group of antiemetic preparations available to patients complaining of nausea and vomiting necessitates some mention. First, the phosphorated carbohydrate solutions (mixtures of fructose, dextrose, and phosphoric acid) are available OTC and may be administered in 15- to 30-mL doses as often as every 3 hours or as needed. As one might predict from quick assessment of the ingredients, these solutions are intended only for mild and infrequent symptoms. Because of the inability of these agents to relieve significant symptoms, they should not be used in patients with "complex" problems, especially those receiving chemotherapy. Adverse reactions to these solutions are most often noted as abdominal pain or diarrhea as a consequence of large doses of fructose or as lack of control in diabetic patients because of the dextrose included in the formulations; however, with the use of small doses, most patients experience little benefit or adversity.

Another agent that has received comparatively little attention in the antiemetic literature is diphenidol. Although this agent inhibits the CTZ as well as conduction in vestibular–cerebellar pathways and is indicated in most references for the management of nausea and vomiting associated with surgery, malignant neoplasms, antineoplastic chemotherapy, radiation sickness, infectious diseases, and labyrinthine disturbances, it should be used extremely cautiously. Diphenidol should be used only when there is a clear and unquestionable benefit potential. Even though an oral agent, this product should be utilized only in a hospital or under comparable conditions.

The primary reason for the somewhat drastic measures required for the use of diphenidol is its adverse reaction profile. Auditory and visual hallucinations, disorientation, and confusion have been reported and are the usual warnings against its use. These problems may be even more pronounced in elderly patients or those with declining renal function, as approximately 90% of diphenidol is excreted in the urine. Lastly, diphenidol should be avoided in female patients during pregnancy or lactation as well as in children weighing less than 50 pounds.

Pyridoxine has also been cited as an antiemetic agent; however, its efficacy has not been accepted beyond that of a placebo and probably has little place in the approach to "simple" or "complex" symptoms. In patients in whom it may offer benefit, its beneficial mechanism has been suggested to be restoration of depleted pyridoxine body stores.

Domperidone, a peripheral dopamine blocker, is an investigational agent presently under study for its usefulness as an antiemetic, primarily for patients receiving cytotoxic chemotherapy. Most often administered intravenously, domperidone doses have usually ranged from 1 to 40 mg in single or repeated doses. Patients receiving a variety of cytotoxic regimens have been evaluated using several research methods. The eventual utility of this compound is impossible to predict. Although excellent response has been noted in certain patients, those receiving nitrogen mustard–containing regimens appear to have had less than optimal results. The possible benefit of this drug in other clinical settings is unknown.

### Combination Antiemetic Protocols

The management of nausea and vomiting may include various combinations of known antiemetic drugs. Most often these combination protocols are reserved for patients whose symptoms are complex, especially those receiving anticancer chemotherapy. Such combinations may include as few as two or as many as five antiemetic agents, each in moderate-to-high doses. It should be recognized that these multiagent regimens are usually carefully administered by experienced personnel in a hospital or specialty clinic setting. Although oral agents may be used, most of these regimens utilize the intravenous route of administration and require fairly continuous patient assessment and feedback for evaluation of efficacy and side effects. As an increasing number of patients may require such regimens, careful monitoring should be developed and employed to eliminate possibly severe adverse reactions.

The primary goal of combination antiemetic regimens is to select beneficial agents that have different pharmacologic mechanisms as well as toxic effects that are not considered additive or synergistic. These protocols may affect the vomiting center, the CTZ, the cerebral cortex, and/or the peripheral mechanisms that mediate nausea and vomiting.[52] Combinations often include metoclopramide, diphenhydramine, and dexamethasone. Other agents that may be added to the regimen include droperidol, diazepam, thiethylperazine, secobarbital, pentobarbital, chlorpromazine, and prochlorperazine. From this list of possible combinations, it should be apparent that the state-of-the-art multiagent antiemetic protocol has not been well defined. Nevertheless, studies utilizing metoclopramide-based injectable regimens appear to have a high degree of efficacy in preventing nausea and vomiting, even in patients receiving cisplatin.[50–52]

### Antiemetic Use During Pregnancy

More than one half of pregnant women experience nausea and vomiting, or hyperemesis gravidarum.[53] And because drugs may influence embryonic development most during the first 2 months of pregnancy, there has been much interest in the potential maternal and fetal benefits and risks of the antiemetic agents during this early phase.[54] Included in the list of agents that have commonly been prescribed are the phenothiazines (prochlorperazine and promethazine), the antihistaminic–anticholinergic agents (dimenhydrinate, diphenhydramine, meclizine, and scopolamine), metoclopramide, pyridoxine, and, until recently, Bendectin. Bendectin, a combination of doxylamine succinate and pyridoxine hydrochloride, is no longer commercially available. Although not reviewed here, it has been included in other reference material.[55] By its removal, the most studied antiemetic during pregnancy is no longer a part of the treatment for this commonly troublesome condition.

Although many women experience nausea and vomiting during pregnancy, the etiology of hyperemesis gravidarum is not well understood. Numerous mechanisms have been proposed. Additionally, the severity of symptoms may vary greatly. In its most severe state, hyperemesis gravidarum may result in volume contraction, starvation, and electrolyte abnormalities; however, as a mild condition, it may be self-limiting and intermittent and may respond favorably to placebo. The efficacy of antiemetics has been questioned while the importance of specific management plans has been addressed. These plans have included emphasis on fluid and electrolyte management, vitamin supplements, and efforts aimed at reducing psychosomatic complaints.[56,57]

Evaluation of teratogenicity of products administered during the first trimester of pregnancy is of great importance, particularly in patients with a condition with such variability in its presentation; however, proof of teratogenicity varies among animals and humans. In animals, tests of this nature are performed in the laboratory, may vary with animal strain and breed, and may not be good predictors of human experience. Conversely, the clinical laboratory of patient care is the testing ground for agents used in humans. From this setting, case reports and often retrospective epidemiologic reports document the outcome of these human experiences.

Teratogenicity is a major consideration for the use of antiemetic drugs during pregnancy and is the primary factor that dictates this condition's drug of choice. Therefore, both the benefit/side effect profiles for the mother and the potential fetal risks deserve discussion. Of the agents commonly used, those that have demonstrated teratogenicity in animals include diphenhydramine, meclizine, prochlorperazine, and thiethylperazine[58–60]; however, in humans meclizine has not been shown to have these same effects. Most authors presently do not recommend metoclopramide because its use during pregnancy requires further study. Also, its primary benefit in nonpregnant patients with nausea and vomiting has been in association with cancer, chemotherapy and high intravenous dosing. Presently, meclizine is considered to be the drug of choice for the treatment of nausea and vomiting during pregnancy.[61] Dimenhydrinate and promethazine should be considered as second and third choices, respectively, with prochlorperazine and thiethylperazine being considered only if symptoms are severe and cannot be controlled by adequate trials of one of the first three choices.

### Antiemetic Use in Children

In general, antiemetic studies have included primarily adult patients; however, nausea and vomiting in children present unique problems that deserve mention. There are perhaps more uncertainties concerning drug and dosage selection as well as the appropriateness of combination regimens for use in children. One apparent finding is that children may not require or tolerate the same milligram-per-kilogram doses of drugs commonly used in adults. Striking examples of this include the use of metoclopramide. During the 1960s and 1970s this drug was given as an antiemetic to European children with gastroenteritis. From these populations followed numerous reports citing extrapyramidal reactions at cumulative daily doses less than 2.0 mg/kg.[62,63] It is now appreciated that these side effects should be anticipated in children and may occur at intravenous doses as low as 0.5 mg/kg given as repeated doses as often as four times a day. Also, it is interesting that differences in drug disposition, including plasma metoclopramide concentrations, probably do not explain the occurrence of dystonia.[64]

Dosage regimens and anticipated outcome of other antiemetic drugs in children are also quite interesting compared with adults. Phenothiazines appear to be more likely to produce neuromuscular reactions, particularly dystonias, in this age group than in adults, especially when administered during acute viral illnesses such as chicken pox, measles, and gastroenteritis. Also, these agents probably increase the risk of developing hepatotoxicity in children with Reye's syndrome. For these reasons the phenothiazines should be reserved for patients with prolonged vomiting in whom the benefit-to-risk ratio has been examined carefully. Promethazine may be the best agent in this class as its activity is most like that of the antihistamines rather than the phenothiazines.

The antihistaminic–anticholinergic agents also present some difficulty in selection depending on the exact age of the child. For example, the use of benzquinamide, buclizine, cyclizine, and scopolamine is not recommended in children under the age of 12. Dimenhydrinate, however, has been used in children at doses that differ by age for those less than 2 years, those 2 to 6 years, and children 6 to 12 years. Interestingly, trimethobenzamide may be used in children orally or rectally but is not recommended for injection. When chosen, it should be prescribed according to weight. Trimethobenzamide is also not recommended by any route for premature or newborn infants. The butyrophenones, haloperidol and droperidol, have been used in children but not usually in those younger than 2 to 3. In children over the age of 3, most patients studied have received droperidol in the preoperative setting as an adjunct to general anesthesia. Fewer children, comparatively, have received droperidol during chemotherapy. Diphenidol, an agent associated with significant adverse effects, is usually not prescribed in children and is not recommended in patients weighing less than 50 pounds. Parenteral lorazepam, although perhaps useful in adults, is not generally recommended for patients younger than 18. Likewise, dronabinol is not indicated for children as it has been studied most in patients older than 12. And, finally, corticosteroids are often included in the anticancer regimens received by children but are not generally utilized as antiemetics in this age group.

### *Nonpharmacologic Management*

Nonpharmacologic management of nausea and vomiting may include a variety of dietary, physical, or psychologic changes consistent with the etiology of symptoms. For patients with "simple" complaints, perhaps resulting from excessive or disagreeable food or beverage consumption, avoidance or moderation in dietary intake may be preferable. Patients suffering symptoms of systemic illness may improve dramatically as their underlying condition resolves. And, finally, patients in whom these symptoms result from labyrinthine changes produced by motion may benefit quickly by assuming a stable physical position. Patients troubled by anticipatory nausea and vomiting are often the recipients of chemotherapy. It should be appreciated that it is not uncommon for patients to fear these symptoms so much that subsequent chemotherapy is refused. Many of these patients are lost for follow-up and lack continued care.

The variables associated with the development of anticipatory nausea and vomiting have been studied. Included in investigator findings has been the high association of cisplatin therapy as well as the severity of postchemotherapy vomiting and the duration of the patient's worst nausea.[9] Although many believe antiemetic and antianxiety agents are most successful in treating these patients, others have been disappointed. Various techniques involving relaxation have been reported. These techniques include hypnosis, behavior modification, and guided mental imagery.[65–67] Presently, the efficacy of such nonpharmacologic approaches remains untested in most patients and requires further evaluation. Nevertheless, it is apparent that prevention of these symptoms is extremely important. This may be accomplished through supportive care coupled with potent prophylactic antiemetic regimens prior to chemotherapy treatment.

The management of psychogenic vomiting is greatly dependent on nonpharmacologic methods. Pharmacologic approaches, although not well studied in this setting, may exhibit only minimal benefit, if any. Surgery, such as gastroenterostomy, is of no value. The most likely beneficial interventions are psychologic; however, even these therapies may require in-depth follow-up as the ultimate problems are complex and intertwined in the relationships of the patient and individuals with whom he or she often associates.

## Summary

The approach to the diagnosis and management of nausea and vomiting depends on the clinical setting in which these problems occur. Only with a clear understanding of these settings can therapeutic plans involving nonpharmacologic as well as pharmacologic approaches be adequately developed. In treating an individual patient, a systematic approach should be initially prescribed; alterations should be based on follow-up assessments. These initial and follow-up management protocols should always take into consideration the uniqueness of the patient, with attention to the specific details of the prescribed regimen as well as the unique clinical setting in which it occurs.

## References


1. Hanson JS, McCallum RW. The diagnosis and management of nausea and vomiting: A review. Am J Gastroenterol 1985;80: 210–218.
2. Frytak S, Moertel CG. Management of nausea and vomiting in the cancer patient. JAMA 1981;245:393–396.
3. Midwinter A. Vomiting in pregnancy. Practitioner 1971;206: 743–750.
4. Redd WH. Control of nausea and vomiting in chemotherapy patients: Four effective behavioral methods. Postgrad Med 1984;75:105–113.
5. Eyre HJ, Ward JH. Control of cancer chemotherapy-induced nausea and vomiting. Cancer 1984;54:2642–2648.
6. Feldman M. Nausea and vomiting, in Sleisenger MH, Fordtran JS (eds): Gastrointestinal Disease. Philadelphia, W.B. Saunders, 1983, pp 160–177.
7. Olver IN, Simon RM, Aisner J. Antiemetic studies: A methodological discussion. Cancer Treat Rep 1986;70:555–563.
8. Moher D, Arthur AZ, Peter JL. Anticipatory nausea and/or vomiting. Cancer Treat Rev 1984;11:257–264.
9. Morrow GR. Prevalence and correlates of anticipatory nausea and vomiting in chemotherapy patients. J Natl Cancer Inst 1982;68:585–588.
10. Sallan SE, Zinberg NE, Frei E III. Antiemetic effect of delta-9-tetrahydrocannabinol in patients receiving cancer chemotherapy. N Engl J Med 1975;293;795–797.
11. Sallan SE, Cronin C, Zelen M, et al. Antiemetics in patients receiving chemotherapy for cancer: A randomized comparison of delta-9-tetrahydrocannabinol and prochlorperazine. N Engl J Med 1980;302:135–138.
12. Chang AE, Shilling DJ, Stillman RC, et al. Delta-9-tetrahydrocannabinol as an antiemetic in cancer patients receiving high dose methotrexate: A prospective randomized evaluation. Ann Intern Med 1979;91:819–824.
13. Carey MP, Burish TG, Brenner DE. Delta-9-tetrahydrocannabinol in cancer chemotherapy: Research problems and issues. Ann Intern Med 1983;99:106–114.
14. Broadhead WE, Kaplan BH, James SA, et al. The epidemiologic evidence for a relationship between social support and health. Am J Epidemiol 1983;117:521.
15. Dutro MP, Ammerson AB. Comparison of liquid antacids. N Engl J Med 1980;302:967.
16. Fordtran JS, Morawski S, Richardson C. In vitro and in vivo evaluation of antacids. N Engl J Med 1973;288:923.
17. Seipler JK, Mahakian K, Trudeau WT. Current concepts in clinical therapeutics: Peptic ulcer disease. Clin Pharm 1986;5: 128–142.
18. Maule WF, Perry MC. Management of chemotherapy-induced nausea and emesis. AFP 1983;27:226–234.
19. Wood CD. Antimotion sickness and antiemetic drugs. Drugs 1979;17:471–479.
20. Edmunds SJ, Prys RC. Pharmacology of drugs used in neuroleptanalgesia. Br J Anaesthesia 1970;42:207–216.
21. Wampler G. The pharmacology and clinical effectiveness of phenothiazines and related drugs for managing chemotherapy-induced emesis. Drugs 1983;25(suppl):35–51.
22. Lucas VS. Phenothiazines as antiemetics, in Lazlo J (ed): Antiemetics and Cancer Chemotherapy. Baltimore, Williams and Wilkins, 1983, pp 93–107.
23. Stoudemire A, Cotanch P, Lazlo J. Recent advances in the pharmacologic and behavioral management of chemotherapy-induced emesis. Arch Intern Med 1984;144:1029–1033.
24. Anderson PO, McGuire GG. Delta-9-tetrahydrocannabinol as an antiemetic. Am J Hosp Pharm 1981;38:639–646.
25. Lazlo J, Lucas VS. Synthetic cannabinoids, in Lazlo J (ed): Antiemetics and Cancer Chemotherapy. Baltimore, Williams and Wilkins, 1983, pp 116–128.
26. Herman TS, Einhorn LH, Jones SE, et al. Superiority of nabilone over prochlorperazine as an antiemetic in patients receiving cancer chemotherapy. N Engl J Med 1979;300:1295–1297.
27. Shannon HE, Martin WR, Silcox D. Lack of antiemetic effects of delta-9-tetrahydrocannabinol in apomorphine-induced emesis in the dog. Life Sci 1978;23:49–54.
28. Neidhart JA, Gagen M. Experimental antiemetic agents (other than cannabinoids and metoclopramide), in Lazlo J (ed): Antiemetics and Cancer Chemotherapy. Baltimore, Williams and Wilkins, 1983, pp 142–163.
29. Jacobs AJ, Deppe G, Cohen CJ. A comparison of the antiemetic effects of droperidol and prochlorperazine in chemotherapy with cisplatinum. Gynecol Oncol 1980;10:55–57.
30. Grossman B, Lessin LS, Cohen P. Droperidol prevents nausea and vomiting from *cis*-platinum. N Engl J Med 1979;301:47.
31. Mehrota S, Rosenthal CJ, Barile B, et al. A comparison between droperidol and prochlorperazine in combination with trimethobenzamide as antiemetics for antineoplastic combination chemotherapy. (Abstr) Proc Am Assoc Cancer Res/Am Soc Clin Oncol 1981;22:417.
32. Wilson J, Weltz D, Solimando D, et al. Continuous infusion droperidol. Antiemetic therapy for *cis*-platinum toxicity. (Abstr) Proc Am Assoc Cancer Res/Am Soc Clin Oncol 1981;22:421.
33. Cersosimo RJ, Bromer R, Hoffer S, et al. The antiemetic activity of droperidol administered by intramuscular injection during cisplatin chemotherapy: A pilot study. Drug Intell Clin Pharm 1985;19:118–121.
34. Paladine W, Price L, Sokol G, et al. Antiemetic trial of droperidol. Proc Am Soc Clin Oncol 1980;21:381.
35. Brown RE, Gregg RE, Hood JC. Droperidol treatment of streptozotocin-induced nausea and vomiting. Drug Intell Clin Pharm 1982;16:775–776.
36. Cersosimo RJ, Karp DD. Adrenal corticosteroids as antiemetics during cancer chemotherapy. Pharmacotherapy 1986;6:118–127.
37. Curry SL, Rine J, Whitney CW, et al. The role of prostaglandins in the excessive nausea and vomiting after intravascular cisplatinum therapy. Gynecol Oncol 1981;12:89–91.
38. Cognetti F, Pinnaro P, Carlini P, et al. Randomized open crossover trial between metoclopramide and dexamethasone for the prevention of cisplatin-induced nausea and vomiting. Eur J Cancer Clin Oncol 1984;20:183–187.
39. Aapro MS, Plezia PM, Alberts DS, et al. Double-blind crossover study of the antiemetic efficacy of high-dose dexamethasone versus high-dose metoclopramide. J Clin Oncol 1984;2: 466–471.
40. Markman M, Sheidler V, Ettinger DS, et al. Antiemetic efficacy of dexamethasone. Randomized, double-blind, crossover study with prochlorperazine in patients receiving cancer chemotherapy. N Engl J Med 1984;311:549–552.
41. Kolaric K, Roth A. Methylprednisolone as an antiemetic in patients on *cis*-platinum chemotherapy. Results of a controlled randomized study. Tumori 1983;69:43–46.
42. Giaconne G, Donadio M, Musella R, et al. Comparison of methylprednisolone and metoclopramide in the prophylactic treatment of cisplatin-induced nausea and vomiting. Tumori 1984;70:237–241.

**43.** Schallier D, Van Belle S, De Greve J, et al. Methylprednisolone as an antiemetic drug. A randomized double-blind study. Cancer Chemother Pharmacol 1985;14:235–237.

**44.** Ell C, Konig HJ, Brockmann P, et al. Antiemetic efficacy of moderately high-dose metoclopramide in patients receiving varying doses of cisplatin. Controlled comparison with combination of methylprednisolone and metoclopramide. Oncology 1985;42:354–357.

**45.** Maher J. Intravenous lorazepam to prevent nausea and vomiting associated with cancer chemotherapy. Lancet 1981;1:91–92.

**46.** Lazlo J. Oral lorazepam to improve tolerance of cytotoxic therapy. Lancet 1981;1:1316–1317.

**47.** Meyer M, Long AM, Natale RB, et al. Phase I, II and III trials of a new antiemetic agent—Lorazepam. Proc Am Soc Clin Oncol 1983;2:88.

**48.** Gralla RJ. Metoclopramide: A review of antiemetic trials. Drugs 1983;25(suppl):63–73.

**49.** Schyulze-Delriev K. Metoclopramide. Gastroenterology 1979; 77:768–779.

**50.** Fortner CL, Finley RS, Grove WR. Combination antiemetic therapy in the control of chemotherapy-induced emesis. Drug Intell Clin Pharm 1985;19:21–24.

**51.** Plezia PM, Alberts DS, Kessler J, et al. Immediate termination of intractable vomiting induced by cisplatin combination chemotherapy using an intensive five-drug antiemetic regimen. Cancer Treat Rep 1984;68:1493–1495.

**52.** Strum SB, McDermed JE, Lauer D, et al. Control of acute-onset and delayed-onset chemotherapy-induced nausea and emesis with metoclopramide-based regimens. Intern Med Specialist 1985;6:104–112.

**53.** Järnfelt-Samsioe A, Samsioe G, Velinder GM. Nausea and vomiting in pregnancy—a contribution to its epidemiology. Gynecol Obstet Invest 1983;16:221–229.

**54.** Tuchmann-Duplessis H. Drugs and xenobiotics as teratogens. Pharmacol Ther 1984;26:273–344.

**55.** Leathem AM. Safety and efficacy of antiemetics used to treat nausea and vomiting in pregnancy. Clin Pharm 1986;5:660–668.

**56.** Fairweather DV. Nausea and vomiting during pregnancy. Obstet Gynecol Annu 1978;7:91–105.

**57.** Mellencamp E, Wang RI. The patient with nausea. III. Cancer, pregnancy, or surgery. Drug Ther 1977;7:49–54.

**58.** Schardein JL. Drugs as Teratogens. Cleveland, CRC Press, 1976, pp 5, 130.

**59.** Shepard TH. Catalog of Teratogenic Agents, 4th ed. Baltimore, Johns Hopkins University Press, 1983.

**60.** Nishimura H, Tanimura T. Clinical Aspects of Teratogenicity of Drugs. New York, Elsevier, 1976, pp 212, 241.

**61.** American Medical Association Department of Drugs. AMA Drug Evaluations, 5th ed. Littleton, Mass., Publishing Sciences, 1983, pp 515–522.

**62.** Low LCK, Goel KM. Metoclopramide poisoning in children. Arch Dis Child 1980;55:310–312.

**63.** Casteels-Van Daele M, Jaeken J, Van Der Schueren P, et al. Dystonic reactions in children caused by metoclopramide. Arch Dis Child 1970;45:130–133.

**64.** Bateman DN, Craft AW, Nicholson E, et al. Dystonic reactions and the pharmacokinetics of metoclopramide in children. Br J Clin Pharmacol 1983;15:557–559.

**65.** Lyles JN, Burish TG, Knozely MG, et al. Efficacy of relaxation training and guided imagery in reducing the aversiveness of cancer chemotherapy. J Consult Clin Psychol 1982;50:509–524.

**66.** Morrow GR, Morrell C. Behavioral treatment for the anticipatory nausea and vomiting induced by cancer chemotherapy. N Engl J Med 1982;307:1476–1480.

**67.** Redd WH, Andresen GV, Minagawa RY. Hypnotic control of anticipatory emesis in patients receiving cancer chemotherapy. J Consult Clin Psychol 1982;50:14–19.

# Chapter 30 / Diarrhea and Constipation

R. Leon Longe, PharmD, and Joseph T. DiPiro, PharmD

## Diarrhea

The best description of diarrhea is a troublesome discomfort that is sometimes fatal. Usually, diarrheal episodes begin abruptly and subside within 1 or 2 days without treatment. This review focuses primarily on noninfectious diarrhea, with only minor reference to infectious diarrhea (see Chapter 81). Diarrhea is often a symptom of a disease outside of the gut and not all possible causes can be covered. This chapter presents a basic understanding toward management.

To understand diarrhea, one must arrive at a reasonable definition of the condition, but the literature is extremely variable on this. Simply stated, diarrhea is abnormal frequency and liquidity of fecal discharge compared with the patient's normal stools. Frequency and consistency are variable within an individual and between individuals. For example, some individuals may defecate as many as three times a day but others only two or three times a week. A Western culture diet usually produces a daily stool weighing between 100 and 300 g, depending on the amount of nonabsorbable materials (mainly carbohydrates). Patients with serious diarrhea have a stool in excess of 300 g per day; however, a subset of cases describe frequent small, watery passages. Another exception is the vegetable fiber–rich diet (e.g., some Eastern cultures such as African), which normally produces stools of more than 300 g a day.

Diarrhea may be a specific disease associated with the intestines or secondary to a disease outside the intestines. For instance, bacillary dysentery directly affects the gut, whereas diabetes mellitus may cause secondary diarrheal episodes. Furthermore, diarrhea may be divided into acute or chronic. Infectious diarrhea is often acute; diabetic diarrhea is chronic. Whether acute or chronic, diarrhea shares some common pathophysiologic causes that facilitate identification of specific treatments.

### *Epidemiology*

The epidemiology of diarrhea is different in developed (e.g., United States) versus underdeveloped countries (e.g., Tanzania).[1] In the United States, diarrheal illnesses usually are not reported to the Centers for Disease Control unless associated with an outbreak, unusual organism, or unusual condition. For example, recently, acquired immune deficiency syndrome (AIDS) has been identified with protracted diarrheal illness. Some populations are particularly affected and records are kept as a public health concern. Diarrhea is a major problem in day-care centers and nursing homes, probably because early childhood and senescence along with environmental conditions are risk factors. However, an exact epidemiologic profile in the United States is not available through the Centers for Disease Control or published literature.

In the United States viral and bacterial organisms account for most of the infectious diarrhea. Common bacterial organisms are *Shigella, Salmonella, Campylobacter, Staphylococcus,* and *Escherichia coli.* Acute viral infections are attributed mostly to Norwalk and rotavirus groups.

In developing cultures acute diarrhea is reported to kill five million children annually.[2] The World Health Organization (WHO) estimates that between 744 million and 1 billion diarrheal attacks occur annually in the world's children. These findings are associated with poor sanitation, poor nutrition, and age less than 5 years, especially infancy. The leading cause is invasion by infectious organisms (e.g., parasites, cholera).

### *Pathophysiology*

In the fasting state, 9 L of intestinal fluid enters the proximal small intestine each day.[3] Two liters of this fluid is ingested with the diet; the remainder comes from internal secretions. Because of meal content, duodenal chyme is usually hypertonic. By the time chyme reaches the ileum, osmolality is adjusted to equal that of plasma, with almost all dietary fat, carbohydrate, and protein absorbed; ileal chyme is reduced to approximately 1 L/d entering the colon. The electrolyte profile of ileal chyme per liter is normally sodium 140 mEq, potassium 8 mEq, chloride 60 mEq, and bicarbonate 70 mEq. In the normal state, the colon absorbs 900 mL, thus reducing chyme to 100 mL water loss daily. Fecal electrolyte content (mEq/L) is sodium 40, chloride 15, potassium 90, and bicarbonate 30.

From the preceding description, one can visualize diarrhea as an imbalance in absorption and secretion of water and electrolytes. In normal volunteers, small intestine water has a maximum rate of absorption. If the small intestine absorption capacity is exceeded, chyme overloads the colon, resulting in diarrhea. In humans, the colon absorptive capacity is about 5 L daily.[3] Colonic fluid transport is critical to water and electrolyte balance. In simplistic terms, diarrhea could be modeled as a seesaw with absorption on one end and secretion on the other. If these processes are equally weighed, one has a normal bowel movement. But if absorption is decreased or secretion is increased beyond normal, diarrhea results. Normally the absorption of water and electrolytes exceeds secretory fluxes. One should understand the mechanisms at work controlling water, electrolyte, and glucose movements.

Water passively moves across the gut after the movement

of solutes such as sodium.[4] The intestinal mucosa is semipermeable and allows selective solute and solvent movements. For instance, the proximal intestine rapidly makes meal content isotonic. In the small intestine absorption occurs predominately in the villous cells and secretion in the cryptic cells. In the colon, chyme may be hypertonic; this is partly explained by bacterial metabolism of carbohydrates into absorbable solutes. Unabsorbed carbohydrates are metabolized into volatile fatty acids that can be absorbed across the colon.

Electrolyte transport, like water transport, is handled by villi (absorption) and crypt (secretion) cells. Sodium is the principal ion absorbed and chloride is the primary ion secreted. In both absorption and secretion, an active $Na^+$, $K^+$-ATPase pump mechanism creates an electrical cell imbalance leading to ion exchange. Because of membrane lipophilic properties, specific carriers proteins are also involved in sodium transport. Two classes of protein systems are known. One system carries both sodium and chloride; the other links sodium with glucose or amino acids (e.g., glycine). In addition, studies in animals have identified a one-to-one exchange of $Na^+$ for $H^+$ and a one-to-one exchange of $Cl^-$ for either $OH^-$ or $HCO_3^-$ as another NaCl absorption mechanism.

Paracellular pathways are another major route of ion movement. As ions, monosaccharides, and amino acids are actively transported, an osmotic pressure is created, drawing water and electrolytes across the intestinal wall. This pathway accounts for very large amounts of ion transport. Glucose plays an important role through this pathway, stimulating sodium absorption.

Absorption and secretion are also influenced by gut motility.[5] The length of time in which luminal content is in contact with epithelium is under neural and hormonal control. As a general rule, the longer the transit time the greater the absorption. Neurohormonal substances also regulate membrane permeability.[6]

Four general pathophysiologic mechanisms have been identified that disrupt water and electrolyte balance, leading to diarrhea. Understanding these four mechanisms is the basis of diagnosis and therapy: (1) a change in active ion transport by either decreased sodium absorption or increased chloride secretion; (2) alteration in intestinal motility; (3) increase in luminal osmolarity; (4) increase in tissue hydrostatic pressure. These mechanisms have been related to four broad clinical diarrheal categories: secretory, osmotic, exudative, and altered intestinal transit, respectively.

Secretory diarrhea occurs when a stimulating substance either increases secretion or decreases absorption of large amounts of water and electrolytes. Substances that cause excess secretion include vasoactive intestinal peptide (VIP) from a pancreatic tumor, unabsorbed dietary fat in steatorrhea, laxatives, hormones (e.g., secretin), bacterial toxins, and excessive bile salts. Many of these agents stimulate intracellular cyclic AMP and inhibit $Na^+$, $K^+$-ATPase, leading to increased secretion. Also, many of these mediators inhibit ion absorption simultaneously. Clinically, secretory diarrhea is recognized by large stool volumes (>1 L/d) with normal ionic contents and osmolality about equal to that of plasma. Fasting does not change the stool volume.

Poorly absorbed substances retain intestinal fluids, causing osmotic diarrhea. This mechanism can be seen with malabsorption, lactose intolerance, divalent ions (e.g., antacids), or poorly soluble carbohydrate (e.g., lactulose). As a poorly soluble solute is transported the gut adjusts the osmolality to that of plasma; in so doing water and electrolytes flux into the lumen. The loss of sodium and water is less than with some diarrheal mechanisms. Clinically, osmotic diarrhea is distinguishable because it stops when the patient fasts.

Inflammatory gut diseases discharge mucus, serum proteins, and blood into the gut. At times bowel movements may consist only of mucus, exudate, and blood. Exudative diarrhea probably affects other absorptive, secretory, or motility functions to account for the large stool volume. For example, ulcerative colitis diarrhea stops when ileal content is diverted through an ostomy.

Altered intestinal motility causes diarrhea by three mechanisms: reduction of contact time in the small intestine, premature emptying of the colon, bacterial overgrowth. Chyme must be exposed long enough for normal absorption and secretion. If contact time is decreased, diarrhea occurs. Intestinal resection or bypass surgery and drugs (e.g., metoclopramide) can cause this type of diarrhea. Increased exposure time also may allow fecal bacterial overgrowth. A characteristic small intestine diarrheal pattern is described as rapid, small, coupling bursts of waves. These waves are inefficient, do not allow absorption, and rapidly dump chyme into the colon. Once in the colon, chyme may overwhelm the colonic capabilities to absorb water or a diseased colon may not function properly.

## *Diagnosis*

The diagnosis of diarrhea is divided into acute and chronic diarrheal disorders. Usually, most acute diarrheal episodes subside with 72 hours of onset. Chronic diarrhea is frequent attacks over two to three extended periods. If diarrhea persists or if gross blood is present, an extensive workup is justified.

### History/Physical Examination

Onset and duration differentiate acute and chronic diarrhea. With acute diarrhea, the patient complains of abrupt onset of frequent, watery, loose stools, flatulence, malaise, and abdominal pain. Pain should be evaluated for duration, location, and character. Intermittent periumbilical or lower right quadrant pain with cramps and audible bowel sounds is characteristic of small intestinal disease. When pain is present in large intestinal diarrhea, it may be described as a griping, aching sensation with tenesmus (straining ineffective and painful stooling); pain is localized to the hypogastric region, right or left lower quadrant, and sacral region. Depending upon the specific etiology, fever, vomiting, and muscle aches may also be complaints. In chronic diarrhea, previous bouts, associated weight loss, anorexia, and chronic weakness are significant findings. Certain diarrheal diseases are associated with specific ages. For example, diarrhea from colon cancer is found with advancing age, while diarrhea from viral gastroenteritis is largely a childhood condition.

Americans who have traveled abroad recently may have traveler's or parasitic diarrhea. Environmental conditions such as the recent ingestion of bacteria-contaminated foods

**Table 30.1** Drug-Induced Diarrhea

| | |
|---|---|
| Laxatives | |
| Antacids (magnesium-containing) | |
| Antibiotics | Cholinergics |
| Clindamycin | Bethanechol |
| Tetracyclines | Metaclopramide |
| Sulfonamides | Neostigmine |
| Any broad-spectrum antibiotic | |
| Antihypertensives | Cardiac agents |
| Reserpine | Quinidine |
| Guanethidine | Digitalis |
| Methyldopa | Digoxin |
| Guanabenz | |
| Guanadrel | |

identifies "food poisoning" as a possible etiology. A careful dietary history may identify offending foods (e.g., dairy products with lactose intolerance). With AIDS as a potential cause, a sexual history cannot be overlooked. Recent gastrointestinal surgery may cause a "dumping syndrome."

A medication history is extremely important in identifying drug-induced diarrhea (Table 30.1). For example, numerous agents (including antibiotics and other drugs) have been associated with pseudomembranous colitis. Self-inflicted laxative abuse for weight loss is in vogue and must be considered. Neurotic or psychotic behavior leads to laxative abuse. Drug side effects (e.g., quinidine) frequently present as diarrhea.

Stool characteristics are very important. A description of the frequency, volume, consistency, and color provides diagnostic clues. For instance, diarrhea originating in the small intestine may present as copious, watery or fatty (greasy), and foul-smelling stool; may contain undigested food particles; and may be free of gross blood. Colonic diarrhea appears as small, pasty, and sometimes bloody or mucoid movements. Rectal tenesmus with only flatus accompanies large intestine diarrhea.

In diarrhea, physical examination of the abdomen may reveal hyperperistalsis with borborygmi (growling stomach sounds) and generalized or local tenderness. A rectal examination detects masses or possibly fecal impaction, a common cause of diarrhea in the elderly. The state of hydration should be assessed by checking skin turgor and mouth mucosal moisture. Physical signs of systemic disease (e.g., diabetic neuropathy) should be identified. If the patient presents with hypotension, tachycardia, or absent radial pulse or stupor, severe dehydration is present. Fever is strongly suggestive of an infectious cause.

#### Laboratory and Endoscopic Tests

Special testing is reserved for diagnosing unexplained diarrhea, especially in chronic situations.[7,8] Stool studies include examination for parasites and ova, blood, mucus, fat, osmolality, pH, electrolyte analysis, and cultures. Total daily stool volume is also determined. Besides stool studies, direct endoscopic visualization and biopsy are used to diagnose certain conditions such as colitis. Radiographic studies are helpful in neoplastic and inflammatory conditions.

#### Prognosis

Most diarrhea is self-limiting, subsiding within 72 hours; however, infants, young children, the elderly, and debilitated persons are at risk of morbid and mortal events in prolonged or voluminous diarrhea. These groups are at risk of water, electrolyte, and acid–base disturbances, and, potentially, cardiovascular collapse and death.

### *Prevention*

Acute diarrheal illness often occurs in day-care centers and nursing homes.[9] Isolation techniques are needed to prevent spread among these populations and health care workers. Hidden dietary sources, such as sorbitol in dietetic products or "Chinese food dumping" syndrome, should be identified and avoided; milk allergy is also a cause.[10] If diarrhea is secondary to another illness, controlling the primary condition is the most important prevention. Antibiotics and bismuth subsalicylate have been routinely advocated for preventing traveler's diarrhea, along with special care with respect to drinking water and fresh vegetables.

### *Treatment*

If prevention is not successful and diarrhea occurs, the therapeutic goals are (1) to prevent *excessive* water, electrolyte, and acid–base disturbances; (2) to provide symptomatic relief; (3) to treat curable causes; and (4) to manage secondary disorders causing diarrhea. Clinicians must clearly understand that diarrhea, like a cough, may be a body defense mechanism for ridding itself of harmful substances or pathogens. The correct therapeutic response is not always to stop all diarrhea at all costs!

Management of the diet is a first priority. As a general rule most clinicians recommend stopping solid foods for 24 hours and avoiding dairy products. In osmotic diarrhea these maneuvers may control the problem. If the mechanism is secretory, the diarrhea may persist. When nausea or vomiting is mild, an easily digestible low-residue diet is administered for 24 hours. If vomiting is present and cannot be controlled with antiemetics (see Chapter 29), nothing is taken by mouth. As the number of bowel movements decreases, a bland diet may be begun. Research evidence shows that feeding should continue in children with acute bacterial diarrhea.[11] Children who were fed had less morbidity and mortality, whether or not they were given oral rehydration fluids. Studies are not available in the elderly or other risk groups to determine the value of continued feeding in bacterial diarrhea.

Iatrogenic and surreptitious causes should be sought. Overzealous laxative use in the elderly, whether self- or physician-prescribed, is a common cause of diarrhea and must be identified and discontinued.[12] In the nursing home, up to four to six laxative agents are commonly prescribed on an as-needed basis, leading to diarrhea. Community practitioners often encounter elderly patients who falsely believe a daily bowel movement is essential for good health. Besides antibiotics and laxatives, numerous other drugs induce diarrhea and should be discontinued or the dosage reduced.[13]

Repletion and maintenance of water and electrolytes are the primary concerns until the diarrheal episode ends. Parenteral and enteral routes are used to supply water and

**Table 30.2** Oral Rehydration Solutions

| | *WHO-ORS*[a] | *Lytren (Mead Johnson)* | *Pedialyte (Ross)* | *Rehydralyte (Ross)* | *Resol (Ross)* | *Infalyte (Pennwalt)* |
|---|---|---|---|---|---|---|
| Osmolality (mOsm/L) | 333 | 220 | 249 | 304 | 269 | 251 |
| Carbohydrates[b] (g/L) | 20 | 20 | 25 | 25 | 20 | 20 |
| Calories (cal/L) | 77 | 85 | 100 | 100 | 80 | 77 |
| Electrolytes (mEq/L) | | | | | | |
| Sodium | 90 | 50 | 45 | 75 | 50 | 50 |
| Potassium | 20 | 25 | 20 | 20 | 20 | 20 |
| Chloride | 80 | 45 | 35 | 65 | 50 | 40 |
| Citrate | — | 30 | 30 | 30 | 34 | — |
| Bicarbonate | 30 | — | — | — | — | 30 |
| Calcium | — | 4 | — | — | 4 | — |
| Magnesium | — | 4 | — | — | 4 | — |
| Sulfate | — | 4 | — | — | — | — |
| Phosphate | — | 5 | — | — | 5 | — |

[a] World Health Organization Oral Rehydration Solution.
[b] Carbohydrate is glucose.

electrolytes. If vomiting is not present and dehydration is not severe, enteral feeding is the less costly and preferred method. In the United States many commercial oral rehydration preparations are available (Table 30.2). Some of these products have been criticized as worsening diarrhea by drawing water into the gut by hypertonicity[14]; however, U.S. physicians continue to hospitalize and intravenously correct these deficits for severe dehydration (Chapters 81 and 103). In developing countries, the World Health Organization Oral Rehydration Solution (WHO-ORS) has saved the lives of millions of children (Table 30.2).

During diarrhea, the small intestine retains its ability to actively transport monosaccharides such as glucose that actively carry sodium with water and other electrolytes passively. Because the WHO-ORS has a high sodium concentration, U.S. physicians have been reluctant to use it in well-nourished children. This attitude could be changing as controlled comparative studies describe more favorable results with WHO-ORS than parenteral fluids.[15] As amino acids promote sodium transport and may act as an antisecretory agent, researchers have added glycine to ORS in an attempt to create a "super-ORS." Reports to date, however, have been disappointing as glycine seems to cause an osmotic diarrhea and diuresis in the experimental concentrations.[16] Another promising research oral solution is made from hyposmotically active substrates such as rice, providing long-chain molecules and eluting glucose without increasing stool or urine outflow. These starch solutions may reach 5%, a concentration that would cause osmotic diarrhea with glucose.

Various drugs have been used to treat diarrheal attacks (Table 30.3). These drugs are grouped into several categories: antimotility, adsorbents, antisecretory compounds, antibiotics, enzymes, and intestinal microflora. In most instances, these drugs are not curative but palliative in nature.

Opiates and opioid derivatives (1) delay the transit of intraluminal content and/or (2) increase gut capacity, thus prolonging contact and absorption. Enkephalins, endogenous opioid substances, have been reported to regulate fluid movement across the mucosa by stimulating absorptive processes. Most opiates act through peripheral and central mechanisms, except for loperamide (Imodium, Jansen Pharmaceutical), which is primarily peripheral.[17] Loperamide is antisecretory; it inhibits the calcium-binding protein calmodulin, which is believed to control chloride secretion.[18,19] Although many studies support this mechanism, in an experiment in normal subjects, Schiller et al questioned loperamide's antisecretory mechanism as the important antidiarrheal control.[20]

Loperamide was comparable to bismuth subsalicylate (Pepto-Bismol, Norwich Pharmaceutical) for treatment of traveler's diarrhea.[21] Persons receiving loperamide passed fewer unformed stools compared with those receiving bismuth subsalicylate, and shigellosis was not significantly prolonged. Limitations of the opiates are addiction potential (a real concern with long-term use) and worsening of diarrhea in selected infectious diarrhea.

Adsorbents have been used for many years for symptomatic relief (Table 30.3). These products, many not requiring a prescription, are nontoxic but their effectiveness has not been demonstrated. Absorbents are nonspecific in their action; they adsorb nutrients, toxins, drugs, and digestive juices. Coadministration with other drugs may reduce their bioavailability. Portnoy and associates,[22] comparing kaolin–pectin suspension and diphenoxylate liquid (Lomotil, Searle Pharmaceutical) in acute childhood diarrhea, did not demonstrate relief. The FDA OTC review panel report recommends only polycarbophil (Mitrolan, A. R. Robins) as an effective adsorbent. Polycarbophil absorbs 60 times its weight in water and can treat both diarrhea and constipation.

*Lactobacillus* preparations have been prescribed to replace colonic microflora secondary to antibiotic overkill. A controversial treatment form, seeding the gut with this organism supposedly restores intestinal functions and suppresses the growth of pathogenic microorganisms; however, a dairy product diet containing 200–400 g of lactose or dextrin is equally effective in recolonization. Again, clinical studies validating this clinical use are lacking.

Anticholinergic drugs block vagal tone and prolong gut transit time (Table 30.3). They are available in combination

**Table 30.3** Selected Antidiarrheal Preparations

| | *Dose form* | *Adult dose* |
|---|---|---|
| Antimotility | | |
| Diphenoxylate | 2.5 mg/tablet<br>2.5 mg/5 mL | 5 mg QID; do not exceed 20 mg/d |
| Loperamide | 2 mg/capsule<br><br>1 mg/5 mL | Initially 4 mg, then 2 mg after each loose stool; do not exceed 16 mg/d |
| Paregoric | 2 mg/5 mL (morphine) | 5–10 mL 1–4 times daily |
| Opium tincture | 5 mg/mL (morphine) | 0.6 mL QID |
| Atropine | 0.3, 0.4, 0.6 mg/tablet | 0.4–0.6 mg every 4–6 h |
| Absorbents | | |
| Kaolin–pectin mixture | 0.98 g kaolin + 21.7 mg pectin per 5 mL | 30–120 mL after each loose stool |
| Polycarbophil | 500 mg/tablet | Chew 2 tablets QID or after each loose stool; do not exceed 12 tablets a day |
| Antisecretory (bismuth subsalicylate) | 300/mg tablet<br><br>525 mg/30 mL | Two tablets or 30 mL every 30 min as needed up to 8 doses per day |
| Enzymes (lactase) | 1,250 neutral lactase units per 4 drops | 3–4 drops taken with milk or dairy product |
| | 3,300 FCC lactase units per tablet | 1 or 2 tablets as above |
| Bacterial replacement (*Lactobacillus acidophilus, L. bulgaricus*) | | 2 tablets or 1 granule packet 3 to 4 times daily; give with milk, juice, or water |

in many nonprescription products and as single entities. Their value in controlling diarrhea is questionable and limited by side effects. To stop diarrhea, clinicians have been falsely taught to dose anticholinergics until they decrease salivary and sweat secretion. Despite anticholinergic side effects in 54% of test subjects, Reves et al[23] failed to prove effectiveness of mepenzolate bromide (Cantil, Merrell Dow) in acute infectious diarrhea. Glaucoma, selected heart diseases, and obstructive uropathies are relative contraindications to use of anticholinergic agents.

Many acute diarrheas are caused by infectious agents, which have a strong secretory component. Agents directed at blocking copious fluid flow are highly desirable in secretory diarrheas. For this reason, bismuth subsalicylate suspension has been best studied. When 30 mL of this suspension was given every 30 minutes for eight doses, the number of unformed stools decreased in the first 24 hours in active infection.[24] Use of bismuth subsalicylate to prevent traveler's diarrhea has also been studied. Bismuth subsalicylate tablets (1.05 or 2.1 g versus placebo twice daily) reduced the incidence of diarrhea in 231 volunteers and caused only minor undesirable complaints (taste, constipation, nasuea).[25]

The commercially available bismuth subsalicylate product contains multiple components that might be toxic if given excessively to prevent or treat diarrhea. For instance, the active ingredient is the salicylate component, which may interact with anticoagulants or cause effects of salicylism (tinnitus, nausea, and vomiting). Bismuth toxicity is another potential problem at excessive doses, but clinical problems are rarely encountered. Despite these potential problems, bismuth subsalicylate can be effective and safe in treatment and prevention of traveler's diarrhea with proper dosing.

The role of antibiotics is controversial and is reviewed in Chapter 81. Antibiotics are curative if the organism is susceptible, but most infectious diarrheas are self-limiting and are treated with supportive therapy. In traveler's diarrhea, antibiotic prophylaxis (for example, with tetracycline and co-trimoxazole) has been effective but the fear of antibiotic resistance should be considered.

### *Controversies in Drug Management*

Numerous experimental drugs have been proposed to control diarrhea. Phenothiazines, $\beta$-blockers, nonsteroidal anti-inflammatory drugs, calcium channel blockers, somatostatin, and $\alpha$-adrenergic agonists are only a few agents under investigation in either animals or humans.

Nifalatide is an enkephalin analogue that significantly delayed the onset of castor oil–induced diarrhea and decreased the stool frequency in 72 normal men; dizziness and dry mouth were the most frequent side effects.[26] Enkephalinase inhibitors (e.g., acetorphan) offer another therapeutic alternative.[27] In the search for proabsorption/antisecretory drugs, lidamidine, a prototype $\alpha_2$-adrenergic agonist, has been compared with loperamide and found to counter diarrhea by either promoting absorption or preventing secretion.[28] With lidamidine, a clonidine analogue, hypotension is a limiting dose-related problem. Prostaglandin inhibitors, aspirin and its analogues, and indomethacin are safe and effective in childhood gastroenteritis; studies in animals support indomethacin in enteropathogen secretory states such as with *Vibrio cholerae*.[29,30]

Vaccines are a new therapeutic frontier in controlling infectious diarrheas, especially in developing countries.[2] Cholera vaccine affords some protection but is not totally effective and does not prevent transmission. Oral shigella vaccine has been proven to be effective under field conditions, but requires five doses with repeat booster doses, limiting its practicality in developing nations. With approximately 1,500 serotypes for *Salmonella*, a vaccine still is not available. In the United States, rotavirus vaccine would protect many infants and children, and a vaccine is presently under development.

### *Summary*

In the United States, diarrhea is most often a minor discomfort, not life-threatening and usually self-limited. Children and the elderly are groups at high risk for severe complications of acute diarrhea. Usually, a diagnosis can be made on the basis of the history and physical examination, with extensive diagnostic tests reserved for chronic diarrhea.

Management centers upon preventing excessive water and electrolyte losses, providing symptomatic relief, treating curable causes, and managing secondary disorders causing diarrhea. Acute diarrhea is usually self-limiting and is managed with supportive therapy. Chronic diarrhea is managed by identifying (if possible) and treating the cause or at least supportively managing each diarrheal episode.

## Constipation

Constipation is a very common problem as evidenced by the tremendous dollar volumes spent on laxatives and the prominence they have gained in the advertising media and on the shelves of retail outlets. In 1982, $386 million was spent on OTC laxatives and cathartics.[31] Currently, more than 100 laxative products are available OTC[32] and a few are available on prescription.

Most treatments for constipation are initiated by the patient, often without consultation from a health professional. Constipation continues to be a frequent problem in the United States, primarily because of the inadequate diets of many people. Another unfortunate problem is that many people have misconceptions about normal bowel function, thinking that daily bowel movements are required for health and well-being. Others believe that the lack of a daily bowel movement contributes to the accumulation of toxic substances or is associated with various somatic complaints. These misconceptions lead to the inappropriate use of laxatives by the general public.

Constipation does not have one consistently used definition. When using the term *constipation*, the lay public or health care professionals may be referring to several difficult-to-quantify variables: bowel movement frequency, stool size or consistency, such symptoms as a feeling of incomplete defecation. Stool frequency is most often used to describe constipation. The frequency of bowel movements that may be used to determine constipation is not well established, but it has been determined that normal subjects pass at least three stools per week. In one study of more than 1,400 people in Great Britain, 99% of subjects had a bowel movement more than twice weekly but not more than three times daily.[33] In an older population, 95% of men and 90% of women had a bowel movement from once every 2 days to twice daily.[34] A study of 115 healthy men showed mean (±SD) stool frequency to be 27.6 ± 9.5 hours.[35]

In addition to misconceptions about "normal" bowel function that lead to consideration of constipation, constipation may be caused by a wide range of diseases (e.g., diseases of the gastrointestinal tract, endocrine or metabolic derangements), drugs, or improper diets. Evaluation of the patient complaining of constipation requires a thorough history to determine the nature and frequency of bowel movements and dietary habits, and may include physical and laboratory assessments to evaluate the possibility of underlying diseases. The proper treatment of constipation requires alteration of diet to include a greater quantity of fiber, correction of diseases that may be responsible, and elimination (if possible) of drugs that may cause constipation. Once these factors have been considered, judicious use of selected laxative products is sometimes required.

Constipation requires treatment (not necessarily with drug therapy), mainly because it is usually uncomfortable for the patient, but also because it is associated with more serious diseases. Constipation associated with inadequate dietary fiber may worsen hemorrhoidal disease by the passage of infrequent, relatively hard stool. With some causes of constipation the loops of bowel may become dangerously dilated, with risk of perforation or infarction. Also, some studies have shown that constipation is associated with a greater risk of colon and rectal cancer, particularly in women.[36,37]

### *Etiology*

In dealing with the constipated patient, one should recognize that constipation is not a disease but a symptom of an underlying disease or problem. Approaches to treatment of constipation should begin with attempts to determine its cause, and the causes are varied. There may be disorders of the gastrointestinal tract (e.g., irritable bowel syndrome or diverticulitis), metabolic disorders (e.g., diabetes), or endocrine disorders (e.g., hypothyroidism). Commonly, constipation results from a diet low in fiber or from use of constipating drugs such as opiates. Finally, it is believed that constipation may sometimes be psychogenic in origin. Each of these causes is discussed.

Constipation is a frequent problem in the elderly, probably the result of improper diets (low in fiber and liquids), diminished muscular strength (abdominal wall), and, possibly, diminished physical activity. In addition, diseases that may cause constipation, such as colon cancers and diverticulitis, are more common with increasing age.

#### Gastrointestinal Disorders

Gastrointestinal disorders are a common cause of constipation. The most frequent gastrointestinal causes of constipation are disorders of the large bowel, but diseases of the upper gastrointestinal tract (such as gastroduodenal obstruction from ulceration or cancer) may also be responsible. The most common colonic disorders causing constipation are irritable bowel syndrome and diverticulitis. Irritable bowel syndrome may be associated with constipation, diarrhea, or both. In these patients, objective findings of disease are often absent, but colonic motility is usually abnormal.

Anal and rectal diseases associated with pain on defecation may cause constipation. Hemorrhoids, anal fissures, or ulcerative proctitis may all result in painful elimination and inhibition of the urge to defecate. The result may be a decreased frequency of bowel movements.

Constipation may be an indication of obstruction of the colon. The colon may become obstructed from tumors that originate in the lumen of the colon or from organs or structures adjacent to the colon. Also, constipation may result from hernias, volvulus of the bowel (torsion or twisting of a loop of intestine), or a variety of diseases (syphilis, tuberculosis, helminthic infections, or lymphogranuloma venereum) that may all cause stricture of the lumen of the colon.

Neurologic disorders of the gastrointestinal tract may also be a cause of constipation. The most prominent neurologic disorder of the gastrointestinal tract resulting in constipation is Hirschsprung's disease, also called aganglionosis. With this disorder there is a congenital absence of neurons to the terminal segments of the bowel. The disorder is usually diagnosed by rectal biopsy and manometric studies of the rectum.

#### Metabolic and Endocrine Disorders

Many metabolic and endocrine disorders affect bowel function. Examples include diabetes mellitus with associated neuropathy, which may affect multiple segments of the gastrointestinal tract and result in an atonic colon, uremia, and hypokalemia. Hypothyroidism and panhypopituitarism may result in inhibited bowel function. In fact, for some cases of hypothyroidism the presenting symptom is constipation or bowel obstruction. Other disorders such as pheochromocytoma may cause constipation, as catecholamines inhibit gastrointestinal smooth muscle activity. Hypercalcemia (from any cause) and enteric glucagon excess may also result in inhibited bowel function.

#### Pregnancy

Constipation is a frequent problem during pregnancy, possibly resulting from complex factors that include depressed gut motility, increased fluid absorption from the colon, decreased physical activity, and dietary changes.[38] Dietary factors include inadequate fluid intake, low dietary fiber, and the use of iron salts (see Chapter 5).

#### Neurogenic Constipation

In addition to peripheral neurologic disorders that may cause constipation, central nervous system disorders may also be responsible. The central nervous system is an important component in gastrointestinal regulation, either through gastrointestinal reflexes or through coordination of other organs of the body. In addition, the central nervous system modifies gastrointestinal function in response to conscious effort or emotional stimuli. Many diseases of the central nervous system can therefore affect gastrointestinal function. Trauma to the brain (particularly the medulla) or spinal cord may result in inhibited bowel function as may central nervous system tumors. Also, cerebrovascular accidents and Parkinson's disease may cause inhibited bowel function.

#### Psychogenic Constipation

The term *psychogenic constipation* has variable acceptance among experts in the field as objective evidence for its existence is slim; however, it has been recognized that bowel habits, particularly those developed early in life, may relate to chronic constipation. Ignoring or postponing the urge to defecate may cause blunting of the colonic and rectal response and may possibly lead to prolonged retention of stool. People in certain occupations, such as truck drivers, may be particularly predisposed to this problem. Finally, patients with psychiatric diseases often have constipation. In many instances improvement in constipation is observed with the onset of psychotherapy.

#### Drug-Induced Constipation

Drugs that inhibit the neurologic or muscular function of the gastrointestinal tract, particularly the colon, may result in constipation. A large number of drugs have such properties (Table 30.4). The majority of cases of drug-induced constipation are caused by opiates, various agents with anticholinergic properties, and antacids containing aluminum or calcium. With most of the agents listed, the inhibitory bowel effects are dose dependent, with larger doses clearly causing constipation more frequently.

Opiates have been known for their gastrointestinal inhibitory effects at least as long as they have been known as analgesics. Clearly, opiates used to treat diarrhea have considerable antimotility effects. Opiates have effects on all segments of the bowel, but effects are most pronounced on the colon. The major mechanism of opiate action has been proposed to be prolongation of intestinal transit time by causing spastic, nonpropulsive contractions.[39] An additional, contributory mechanism of action may be by increasing electrolyte absorption.[40]

**Table 30.4** Drugs Causing Constipation

| |
|---|
| Analgesics |
| Inhibitors of prostaglandin synthesis |
| Opiates |
| Anticholinergics |
| Antihistamines |
| Antiparkinsonian agents (e.g., benztropine or trihexaphenidyl) |
| Phenothiazines |
| Tricyclic antidepressants |
| Antacids containing calcium carbonate or aluminum hydroxide |
| Barium sulfate |
| Clonidine |
| Diuretics (non–potassium sparing) |
| Ganglionic blockers |
| Iron preparations |
| Muscle blockers (*d*-tubocurarine, succinylcholine) |
| Polystyrene sodium sulfonate |

All opiate derivatives are associated with constipation, but the degree of intestinal inhibitory effects seems to differ between agents. Orally administered opiates appear to have greater inhibitory effects than parenterally administered agents; oral codeine is well known as a potent antimotility agent. Orally administered enkephalins (endogenous opiate-like polypeptides) are recently established antimotility agents.

Agents with anticholinergic properties inhibit bowel function by parasympatholytic actions on innervation to many regions of the gastrointestinal tract, particularly the colon and rectum. Many types of drugs possess anticholinergic action (Table 29.4), and these agents are used commonly in hospitalized and nonhospitalized patients.

### *Clinical Presentation*

The patient presenting with constipation (usually with abdominal discomfort and distension) should be questioned and examined; constipation may vary in implication from minor discomfort in the otherwise healthy adult to a symptom of colon cancer or other serious diseases. A basis for evaluation and treatment should be a thorough history including questions about the nature of the "constipation." It is important to ascertain whether the patient perceives the problem as infrequent bowel movements, stools of insufficient size, a feeling of fullness, or difficulty and pain on passing stool. The patient should be asked about the frequency of bowel movements and the chronicity of constipation. Constipation occurring recently in an adult may indicate significant colon pathology such as malignancy; constipation present since early infancy may be indicative of neurologic disorders. The patient should also be carefully questioned about usual diet and laxative regimens. Does the patient have a diet consistently deficient in high-fiber items and containing mainly highly refined foods? What laxatives or cathartics has the patient used to attempt relief of constipation? With these questions it should be recognized that laxative abusers frequently deny laxative use. Finally, the patient should be questioned about other concurrent medications, with interest toward agents that might cause constipation.

In most patients complaining of constipation caused by inadequate dietary fiber, a thorough physical examination is not required once it is established that constipation (1) is not a chronic problem, (2) is not accompanied by signs of significant gastrointestinal disease (such as rectal bleeding), and (3) does not cause severe discomfort. In these circumstances the patient may be referred directly to the first-line therapies for constipation described under Treatment (mainly bulk-forming laxatives and dietary fiber with occasional use of saline or stimulant laxatives). Certain patients, however, require a full examination by a physician to determine the cause of constipation. Patients may then have a series of examinations, proctoscopy, sigmoidoscopy, colonoscopy, or barium enema to determine the presence of colorectal pathology. Also, tests (such as thyroid function studies) may be performed to determine the presence of metabolic or endocrine disorders.

### *Treatment*

The proper management of constipation may require a number of different modalities; however, the basis for therapy should be dietary modification. The major dietary change should be an increase in the amount of fiber consumed daily. In addition to dietary management, if necessary and where possible, patients should be encouraged to alter other aspects of their life-style to some extent. Important considerations would be to encourage the patient to obtain adequate exercise (achieved even by brisk walking after dinner) and to adjust bowel habits so that a regular and adequate time is made to respond to the urge to defecate. Another general measure is to increase fluid intake. This is generally recommended and believed beneficial, although there is little objective evidence of benefit.

If an underlying disease is recognized as the cause of constipation, obviously attempts should be made to correct it. Gastrointestinal malignancies may be excised through a surgical resection. Endocrine and metabolic derangements should be corrected by the appropriate methods. For example, when hypothyroidism is the cause of constipation, cautious institution of thyroid-replacement therapy is the most important treatment measure.

As discussed earlier, many drug substances may cause constipation. After determination of a patient's prescription and nonprescription drug therapy, potential drug causes of constipation should be identified. If the patient is consuming medications well known to cause constipation, consideration should be given to alternative agents. For some medications (such as antacids) nonconstipating alternatives exist. If no reasonable alternatives exist to the medication thought to be responsible for constipation, consideration should be given to lowering the dose. If a patient must remain on constipating medications, then more attention must be paid to general measures for prevention of constipation, as discussed next.

#### Dietary Modification and Bulk-Forming Agents

The most important aspect of the therapy for constipation for the majority of patients is dietary modification to increase the amount of fiber consumed. Fiber, the portion of vegetable matter not digested in the human gastrointestinal tract, increases stool bulk, retention of stool water, and rate of transit of stool through the intestine.[41] The result of fiber therapy is an increased frequency of defecation. Also, fiber has been shown to decrease intraluminal pressures in the colon and rectum, which is thought to be beneficial for diverticular disease and irritable bowel syndrome. The specific physiologic effects of fiber are not well understood.

Patients should be advised to include at least 14 g of crude fiber in their daily diets.[42] Dietary fiber may be consumed either as foods or as medicinal products specifically used for their fiberlike properties.[41] Fruits, vegetables, and cereals have the highest fiber content. Bran, a by-product of milling of wheat, is often added to foods to increase fiber content. Raw bran is generally 40% fiber. Medicinal products, often called "bulk-forming agents," such as psyllium hydrophillic colloids (e.g., Effersyllium), methylcellulose (e.g., Cologel), or polycarbophil (Mitrolan) have properties similar to those of dietary fiber and may be taken as tablets, powders, or granules (Table 30.5).

A trial of dietary modification with high-fiber content

**Table 30.5** Dosage Recommendations for Laxatives and Cathartics

| *Agent* | *Recommended dose* |
|---|---|
| **Agents That Cause Softening of Feces in 1–3 d** | |
| Bulk-forming agents | |
| Methylcellulose | 4–6 g/d |
| Polycarbophil | 4–6 g/d |
| Psyllium | Varies with product |
| Emollients | |
| Docusate sodium | 50–360 mg/d |
| Docusate calcium | 50–360 mg/d |
| Docusate potassium | 100–300 mg/d |
| Lactulose | 15–30 mL orally |
| Sorbitol | 30–50 g/d orally |
| Mineral oil | 15–30 mL orally |
| **Agents That Result in Soft or Semifluid Stool in 6–8 h** | |
| Bisacodyl | 5–15 mg orally<br>10 mg rectally |
| Phenolphthalein | 30–270 mg orally |
| Cascara sagrada | Dose varies with formulation |
| Senna | Dose varies with formulation |
| **Agents That Cause Watery Evacuation in 1–3 h** | |
| Magnesium citrate | 18 g in 300 mL water daily |
| Magnesium hydroxide | 2.4–4.8 g orally |
| Magnesium sulfate | 10–30 g orally |
| Sodium phosphates | Varies with salt used |

should be continued for at least 1 month before effects on bowel function are determined. Most patients begin to notice effects on bowel function 3 to 5 days after beginning a high-fiber diet, but some patients may require a considerably longer time. When beginning fiber therapies, the patient should be cautioned that abdominal distension and flatus may be particularly troublesome in the first few weeks, particularly with bran.[43] In most patients, these problems resolve with continued use.

Bulk-forming laxatives have few side effects and minimal systemic effects. The only major caution in the use of bulk-forming laxatives is that obstruction of the esophagus, stomach, small intestine, and colon has been reported when the agents have been consumed without fluid. So, these products should not be used without adequate fluids or in patients with intestinal stenosis.

### Surgery

In a small percentage of patients presenting with complaints of constipation, surgical procedures are necessary. Surgery is usually necessary with most colonic malignancies and with gastrointestinal obstruction from a number of causes. In each case, the involved segment of intestine may be resected or revised to allow flow of gastrointestinal contents through an enterostomy or through the anus. Surgery may be required in some endocrine disorders causing constipation, such as pheochromocytoma, which requires removal of an adrenal tumor.

### Drug Therapy

The traditional classification system for laxatives and cathartics, by suspected mode of action, has not been very useful; the mode of action of many products is not clearly understood.[44,45] In general, most agents work by promoting some of the mechanisms involved in diarrhea, including active electrolyte secretion, decreased water and electrolyte absorption, increased intraluminal osmolarity, and increased hydrostatic pressure in the gut. Laxatives convert the intestine from primarily an organ that absorbs water and electrolytes to an organ that secretes water and electrolytes.[45] The various types of laxatives are discussed in this section. The agents are divided into three general classifications: (1) those causing softening of feces in 1 to 3 days (bulk-forming laxatives, docusates, and lactulose); (2) those that result in soft or semifluid stool in 6 to 8 hours (diphenylmethane derivatives and anthraquinone derivatives); and (3) those causing watery evacuation in 1 to 3 hours (saline cathartics, castor oil, and polyethylene glycol–electrolyte lavage solution).[46]

***Emollient Laxatives*** These surfactant agents, docusate in its various salts, work by facilitating mixing of aqueous and fatty materials within the intestinal tract. They may increase water and electrolyte secretion in the small and large bowel.[47] These products are generally given orally, although docusate potassium has also been used rectally. These products result in a softening of stools within 1 to 3 days.

Emollient laxatives are not effective in treating constipation but are used mainly to prevent constipation. They may be helpful in situations where straining at stool should be avoided, such as after recovery from myocardial infarction, with acute perianal disease, or after rectal surgery. It is unlikely that these agents would be very effective in preventing constipation if major causative factors (e.g., heavy opiate use, uncorrected pathology, inadequate dietary fiber) are not concurrently addressed.

Although docusates are generally safe, a few adverse effects have been noted. They may increase the intestinal absorption of agents administered concurrently and alter toxic potential. Danthron, a laxative previously used in combination with docusates, has been noted to be hepatotoxic when there is increased absorption.[48,49]

***Lubricants*** Mineral oil is the only lubricant laxative in routine use. This agent, obtained from petroleum refining, acts by coating stool and allowing easier passage. It inhibits colonic absorption of water, thereby increasing stool weight and decreasing stool transit time. Mineral oil may be given orally or rectally in a dose of 15–45 mL. Generally, the effect on bowel function is noted after 2 or 3 days of use.

Mineral oil is helpful in situations similar to those suggested for docusates: to maintain a soft stool and avoid straining for relatively short periods of time (a few days to 2 weeks); however, it possesses a much greater potential for adverse effects and its use should be relatively limited. Mineral oil may be minimally absorbed systemically and cause a foreign-body reaction in lymphoid tissue. Also, in debilitated or recumbent patients, mineral oil may be aspirated causing lipoid pneumonia.[50,51] For this reason it should not be used just before bedtime. The agent has been reported to decrease the absorption of fat-soluble vitamins (A, D, E, and K) with chronic use by causing retention in the gastrointestinal tract. Finally, even when given orally, mineral oil may leak from the anal sphincter, causing pruritus and soiling of clothing.

***Lactulose*** This agent is a disaccharide used orally or rectally. It is metabolized by colonic bacteria to low-molecular weight acids, resulting in an osmotic effect whereby fluid is retained in the colon. The fluid retained in the colon lowers the pH and increases colonic peristalsis. Lactulose is generally not recommended as a first-line agent for the treatment of constipation because it is much more costly and not necessarily more effective than such agents as milk of magnesia.[52] It may be justified as an alternative for acute constipation and has been found useful particularly in elderly patients. Occasionally, the use of lactulose may result in flatulence, cramps, diarrhea, and electrolyte imbalances. Sorbitol, a monosaccharide, is occasionally used as a laxative, exerting its effect by osmotic action.

***Diphenylmethane Derivatives*** The two commonly used agents in this class are bisacodyl and phenolphthalein. The actions of these agents are believed to be primarily on the colon. Bisacodyl stimulates the mucosal nerve plexus of the colon; the mechanism of action of phenolphthalein is poorly understood (possibly it inhibits active glucose absorption and sodium absorption, resulting in fluid accumulation in the colon by osmotic action). The dose of these agents effective in various individuals appears to vary greatly. A dose that causes no effects in one patient may result in excessive cramping and fluid evacuation in others. With phenolphthalein, a small portion of the dose undergoes enterohepatic recirculation, which may result in a prolonged laxative action.

These agents are not recommended for daily use on a regular basis. Their use is acceptable intermittently (every few weeks) to treat intermittent constipation or as bowel preparation before diagnostic procedures in which cleansing of the colon is necessary. These agents may sometimes cause severe abdominal cramping as well as significant fluid and electrolyte imbalances with chronic use. These agents should not be used for patients in whom appendicitis is a possibility (as perforation of the appendix may result) or during pregnancy or lactation. Finally, the patient taking phenolphthalein-containing laxatives should be cautioned that it may turn urine pink.

***Anthraquinone Derivatives*** The agents in this class are cascara sagrada, sennosides, danthron, and casanthrol. These agents are metabolized by gut bacteria to their active compounds, but the exact mechanisms of action are not understood. Effects are limited to the colon, and stimulation of Auerbach's plexus may be involved. Recommendations for the use of these agents are similar to those for the diphenylmethane derivatives. In most cases, intermittent use is acceptable; daily use should be strongly discouraged.

Most of the concerns with the use of diphenylmethane derivatives (bisacodyl and phenolphthalein) apply to the anthraquinone derivatives. In addition, the anthraquinone derivatives may cause melanosis coli, an accumulation of dark pigment, mainly in the cecum and rectum, that is evident after 4 to 13 months of use. A pathologic effect of melanosis coli has not been demonstrated, and it appears reversible after use of anthraquinones has been discontinued for 3 to 6 months.

***Saline Cathartics*** Saline cathartics are composed of relatively poorly absorbed ions such as magnesium, sulfate, phosphate, and citrate, which produce their effects primarily by osmotic action to retain fluid in the gastrointestinal tract. Magnesium has been shown to stimulate the secretion of cholecystokinin, a hormone that causes stimulation of bowel motility and fluid secretion. These agents may be given orally or rectally. A bowel movement may result 0.5 to 3 hours after oral doses and 5 to 15 minutes after rectal administration.

These agents should be used primarily for acute evacuation of the bowel, which may be necessary before diagnostic examinations, after poisonings, and in conjunction with some anthelminthics to eliminate parasites. Such agents as milk of magnesia (an 8% suspension of magnesium hydroxide) may be used occasionally (every few weeks) to treat constipation in otherwise healthy adults. Saline cathartics should not be used on a routine basis to treat constipation. With fecal impactions the enema formulations of these agents may be helpful.

As with most laxatives, these agents may cause fluid and electrolyte depletion. Also, magnesium or sodium accumulation may occur when magnesium-containing cathartics are used in patients with renal dysfunction or when sodium phosphate is used in patients with congestive heart failure.

*Castor Oil* Castor oil is metabolized in the gastrointestinal tract to an active compound, ricinoleic acid, which stimulates secretory processes, decreases glucose absorption, and promotes intestinal motility, primarily in the small intestine. Castor oil usually results in a bowel movement within 1 to 3 hours of administration. Because the agent has such a strong purgative action it should not be used for the routine treatment of constipation.

*Glycerin* This agent is usually administered as a 3-g suppository and exerts its effect by osmotic action in the rectum. As with most agents given as suppositories, the onset of action is usually less than 30 minutes. Glycerin is considered a very safe laxative, although it may occasionally cause rectal irritation. Its use is acceptable on an intermittent basis for constipation, particularly in children.

*Polyethylene Glycol–Electrolyte Lavage Solution* Over the past few years, whole-bowel irrigation with polyethylene glycol–electrolyte lavage solution (PEG–ELS) has become popular.[53] Four liters of this solution is administered over 3 hours to obtain complete evacuation of the gastrointestinal tract. The primary use of this solution is before diagnostic procedures requiring colon cleansing or colorectal operations. The solution is not recommended for the routine treatment of constipation and its use should be avoided in patients with intestinal obstruction.

*Other Agents* Tap-water enemas may be used to treat simple constipation. The administration of 200 mL of water by enema to an adult often results in a bowel movement within one-half hour. Soapsuds are no longer recommended for use in enemas as their use may result in proctitis or colitis.

**Recommendations**

The basis for treatment and prevention of constipation should be bulk-forming agents in addition to dietary modification to increase dietary fiber.[54] A variety of products are available that provide adequate bulk. Whichever agent is chosen, it should be used daily and continued indefinitely in most patients, particularly those with chronic constipation. Some bulk-forming agents are available in combination with diphenylmethane or anthraquinone derivatives. Generally, these combinations should be avoided because the added agents should not be used routinely.

For most nonhospitalized persons with acute constipation, the infrequent use (less than every few weeks) of most laxative products is acceptable; however, before more potent laxative/cathartics are used, relatively simple measures may be tried. For example, acute constipation may be relieved by the use of a tap-water enema or a glycerin suppository. A second line of treatment, if an enema or glycerin suppository is not effective, would be the use of low doses of diphenylmethane or anthraquinone derivatives or saline laxatives (such as milk of magnesia). If laxative treatment is required for longer than 1 week, the person should be advised to consult a physician to determine if there is an underlying cause of constipation that requires treatment with agents other than laxatives.

For some bedridden or geriatric patients, or others with chronic constipation, bulk-forming laxatives remain the first line of treatment, but the use of more potent laxatives may be required relatively frequently. When other than bulk-forming laxatives are used, they should be administered in the lowest effective dose and as infrequently as possible to maintain regular bowel function (more than three stools per week). Agents that may be used in these situations include diphenylmethane and anthraquinone derivatives, milk of magnesia, and lactulose. Mineral oil should be avoided, particularly in the bedridden patients, because of the risk of aspiration and lipoid pneumonia. Some patients with chronic constipation may present with fecal impactions. Before vigorous oral laxatives can be used, the impaction needs to be removed using mechanical methods, including tap-water or saline enemas and digital extraction.

In the hospitalized patient without gastrointestinal disease, constipation may be related to the use of general anesthesia and/or opiate substances. Most orally or rectally administered laxatives may be used. For prompt initiation of a bowel movement, a tap-water enema or glycerin suppository is recommended, or milk of magnesia.

With infants and children constipation may occur commonly. The approach to the treatment of constipation in young persons should consider neurologic, metabolic, or anatomic abnormalities when constipation is a persistent problem. When not related to an underlying disease, the approach to constipation is similar to that in an adult. Dietary modification should be considered, with the administration of bulk-forming laxatives in children and infants consuming solid foods. For acute constipation in most age groups, a tap-water enema or glycerin suppository may be helpful. Occasional use of milk of magnesia or anthraquinone derivatives in low doses is justified for acute constipation.

### *Prevention*

For certain groups of patients, such as those recovering from myocardial infarction or rectal surgery, straining at defection is to be avoided. For these patients, the basis of preventive therapy should be the use of bulk-forming laxatives. In addition to these products, the use of docusate has become popular, although its effectiveness is debated. In pregnant patients, constipation may result because of alterations in anatomy or iron supplementation. As described earlier, bulk-forming laxatives and docusates should be the first line of prevention.

### *Laxative Abuse Syndrome*

Misconceptions about normal bowel patterns and the effect of laxatives have contributed to a syndrome of laxative abuse that is relatively common in the United States. The availability of laxatives as chocolates or gums conveys to the public that the use of these agents is without adverse consequences. Abuse of laxatives has occurred traditionally in the person trying to maintain daily bowel function, but more recently has extended to others who use laxatives for the purpose of controlling weight. In either case, the consistent abuse of strong laxatives and cathartics may lead to serious illness.

Laxative abuse for the purpose of maintaining daily bowel

function begins with misconceptions about the frequency, quantity, or consistency of stools. With the use of strong purgatives, the colon may be so thoroughly cleansed that a bowel movement may not occur normally until a few days later. This delay reinforces the need for more purgatives and the cycle of laxative dependence is begun. Eventually the patient may require daily laxatives to maintain bowel function.

The laxative abuser may present with contradictory findings of diarrhea and weight loss.[55,56] In addition, long-term abusers of laxatives tend to have vomiting, abdominal pain, lassitude and weakness, thirst, edema, and bone pain (caused by osteomalacia). With prolonged use of laxatives a number of serious illnesses may arise. These include fluid and electrolyte imbalances (including acid–base imbalances and hypokalemia), protein-losing gastroenteropathy with hypoalbuminemia, and syndromes resembling colitis.

The determination of laxative abuse syndrome can be difficult as many laxative abusers vigorously deny laxative use. Middle-aged women tend to be the most common laxative abusers, and often, the abuser is a health care provider. The chronic laxative abuse problem should be addressed by a combination of measures, including psychiatric evaluation, dietary modification with reliance on bulk-forming laxatives, and specific guidelines to the patient for the withdrawal of stimulant laxatives.

A variation of laxative abuse is seen in persons who use them as a method of weight loss.[57] It appears from the medical literature and daily news sources that this type of abuse is on the increase. Treatment of patients who abuse laxatives in this way has proved very difficult.

### *Summary*

Constipation is a very common problem in our society mostly because the average person's diet has inadequate fiber. Although improper diet is the major cause of constipation, various underlying diseases, such as gastrointestinal cancers, neurologic or metabolic disorders, or use of constipating drugs, are important and relatively frequent causes of constipation.

The primary treatment of constipation should be to correct underlying disease, if present, and to increase the dietary fiber. Dietary fiber can be increased by consumption of high-fiber-content foods or by use of bulk-forming laxatives. Stronger laxatives (diphenylmethane and anthraquinone derivatives, and saline laxatives) should be reserved for infrequent use in constipation more difficult to treat. Unlike many of the diseases described in this text, new drugs are not being developed to treat constipation, as new agents would not be expected to change the approach to the treatment of constipation.

## References


1. Nelson JD. Etiology and epidemiology of diarrheal diseases in the United States. Am J Med 1985;78(suppl 6B):76–80.
2. Rohde JE. Selective primary health care: Strategies for control of disease in the developing world. XV. Acute diarrhea. Rev Infect Diseases 1984;6:840–854.
3. Ooms L. Alterations in intestinal fluid movement. Scand J Gastroenterol 1983;84(suppl):65–77.
4. Keusch GT, Donowitz M. Pathophysiological mechanisms of diarrhoeal diseases: Diverse aetiologies and common mechanisms. Scand J Gastroenterol 1983;84(suppl):33–43.
5. Read NW. Speculations on the role of motility in the pathogenesis and treatment of diarrhoea. Scand J Gastroenterol 1983; 84(suppl):45–63.
6. Gyr K. Infectious diarrhoea and gastrointestinal hormones: Potential therapeutic implications. Scand J Gastroenterol 1983; 84(suppl):135–140.
7. Johnson DA, Cattau EL. Stool chemistries in patients with unexplained diarrhea. Am Fam Physician 1986;33:131–134.
8. Shiau YF, Feldman GM, Resnick MA, et al. Stool electrolyte and osmolality measurements in the evaluation of diarrheal disorders. Ann Intern Med 1985;102:773–775.
9. Haskins R, Kotch J. Day care and illness: Evidence, costs and public policy. Pediatrics 1986;77(suppl):951–958.
10. Babb RR. Coffee, sugars, and chronic diarrhea. Tx-Diet 1984;75:82–87.
11. Anonymous. Feeding during diarrhea. Nutr Rev 1986;44:102.
12. Slugg PH, Carey WD. Clinical features and follow-up of surreptitious laxative users. Cleve Clin Q 1984;51:167–171.
13. George WL. Antimicrobial agent–associated colitis and diarrhea: Historical background and clinical aspects. Rev Infect Dis 1984;6(suppl 1):S208–S213.
14. Brown JD. Oral rehydration therapy for diarrhea. Milit Med 1985;150:577–581.
15. Santosham M, Burns B, Nadkarni V, et al. Oral rehydration therapy for acute diarrhea in ambulatory children in the United States: A double-blind comparison of four different solutions. Pediatrics 1985;76:159–166.
16. Vesikari T, Isolauri E. Glycine supplemented oral rehydration solutions for diarrhoea. Arch Dis Child 1986;61:372–376.
17. Turnberg LA. Antisecretory activity of opiates in vitro and in vivo in man. Scand J Gastroenterol 1983;84:79–83.
18. Sandu BK, Milla PJ, Harries JT. Mechanisms of action of loperamide. Scand J Gastroenterol 1983;84:85–92.
19. Merritt JE, Brown BL, Tomlinson S. Loperamide and calmodulin. (Lett) Lancet 1982;283.
20. Schiller LR, Santa CA, Morawski SG, et al. Mechanism of the antidiarrheal effect of loperamide. Gastroenterology 1984;86: 1475–1480.
21. Johnson PC, Ericsson CD, DuPont HL, et al. Comparison of loperamide with bismuth subsalicylate for the treatment of acute travelers' diarrhea. JAMA 1986;255:757–760.
22. Portnoy BL, DuPont HL, Pruitt D, et al. Antidiarrheal agents in the treatment of acute diarrhea in children. JAMA 1976;236: 844–846.
23. Reves R, Bass P, DuPont HL, et al. Failure to demonstrate effectiveness of an anticholinergic drug in the symptomatic treatment of acute travelers' diarrhea. J Clin Gastroenterol 1983;5:223–227.
24. DuPont HL, Sullivan P, Pickering LK, et al. Symptomatic treatment of diarrhea with bismuth subsalicylate among students attending a Mexican university. Gastroenterology 1977; 73:715–718.
25. Steffen R, DuPont HL, Heusser R, et al. Prevention of traveler's diarrhea by the tablet form of bismuth subsalicylate. Antimicrob Agents Chemother 1986;29:625–627.
26. Ryan J, Leighton J, Kirksey D, et al. Evaluation of an enkeph-

alin analog in men with castor oil–induced diarrhea. Clin Pharmacol Ther 1986;39:40–42.

27. Lecomte JM, Costentin J, Vlaiculescu A, et al. Pharmacological properties of acetorphan, a parenterally active "enkephalinase" inhibitor. J Pharmacol Exp Ther 1986;237:937–944.
28. Sninsky CA, Davis RH, Clench MH, et al. Effect of lidamidine hydrochloride and loperamide on gastric emptying and transit of the small intestine. Gastroenterology 1986;90:68–73.
29. Gots RE, Formal SB, Giannella RA. Indomethacin inhibition of *Salmonella typhimurium, Shigella flexneri*, and cholera-mediated rabbit ileal secretion. J Infect Dis 1974;130:280–284.
30. Burke V, Gracey M. Reduction by aspirin of intestinal fluid-loss in acute childhood gastroenteritis. Lancet 1980;1329–1330.
31. Glaser M, Chi J. Thirty-fifth annual report on consumer spending. Drug Top 1983;July 4:18–20.
32. Curry CE. Laxative products, in Handbook of Nonprescription Drugs, 6th ed. Washington, DC, American Pharmaceutical Association, 1983, pp 69–82.
33. Connell AM, Hilton C, Irvine G, et al. Variation of bowel habits in two population samples. Br Med J 1965;2:1095–1099.
34. Milne JS, Williamson J. Bowel habits in older people. Gerontol Clin 1972;14:56–60.
35. Rendtorff RC, Kashgarian M. Stool patterns of healthy adult males. Dis Colon Rectum 1969;10:222–228.
36. Bjelke E. Epidemiologic studies of cancer of the stomach, colon and rectum. Scand J Gastroenterol 1974;9(suppl):31.
37. Wynder EL, Shigematsu T. Environmental factors of cancer of the colon. Cancer 1967;20:1520.
38. Anderson AS. Dietary factors in the aetiology and treatment of constipation during pregnancy. Br J Obstet Gynaecol 1986;93: 245–249.
39. Sandgren JE, McPhee MS, Greenberger NJ. Narcotic bowel syndrome treated with clonidine. Ann Intern Med 1984;101:331–334.
40. Schiller LR, Davis GR, Santa Ana CA, et al. Mechanism of antidiarrheal action of codeine. Gastroenterology 1981;80:1275.
41. Dwyer JT, Goldin B, Gorbach S, et al. Drug therapy reviews: Dietary fiber and fiber supplements in the therapy of gastrointestinal disorders. Am J Hosp Pharm 1978;35:278–287.
42. DeVroede G. Constipation: Mechanisms and management, in Sleisenger MH, Fordtran JS (eds): Gastrointestinal Disease, 2nd ed. Philadelphia, W.B. Saunders, 1983, pp 288–308.
43. Almy TP, Howell DA. Diverticular disease of the colon. N Engl J Med 1980;302:324–331.
44. Donowitz M. Current concepts of laxative action: Mechanisms by which laxatives increase stool water. Clin Gastroenterol 1979;1:77–84.
45. Binder HJ, Donowitz M. A new look at laxative action. Gastroenterology 1975;69:1001–1005.
46. Brunton LL. Laxatives, in Goodman LS, Gilman AG (eds): The Pharmacologic Basis of Therapeutics, 7th ed. New York, Macmillan, 1985;994–1003.
47. Moriarity KJ, Kelly MJ, Beetham R, et al. Studies on the mechanism of action of dioctyl sodium sulphosuccinate in the human jejunum. Gut 1985;26:1008–1013.
48. Tolman KG, Hammar S, Sannella JJ. Possible hepatotoxicity of doxidan. Ann Intern Med 1976;84:290–292.
49. Anonymous. Safety of stool softeners. Med Lett 1977;19:45–46.
50. Forbes G, Bradley A. Liquid paraffin as a cause of oil aspiration pneumonia. Br Med J 1958;2:1566–1568.
51. Schneider L. Pulmonary hazard of the ingestion of mineral oil in the apparently healthy adult: A clinicoroentgenologic study. N Engl J Med 1949;240:284–291.
52. Anonymous. Lactulose for constipation. Med Lett 1980;22:2–4.
53. Michael KA, DiPiro JT, Bowden TA, et al. Whole-bowel irrigation for mechanical colon cleansing. Clin Pharm 1985;4: 414–424.
54. Tedesco FJ, DiPiro JT. Laxative use in constipation. Am J Gastroenterol 1985;80:303–309.
55. Scully RE, Mark EJ, McNeely BU. Case records of the Massachusetts General Hospital. N Engl J Med 1985;313:1341–1346.
56. Oster JR, Materson BJ, Rogers A. Laxative abuse syndrome. Am J Gastroenterol 1980;74:451–458.
57. Beumont PJV, George GCW, Smart DE. "Dieters" and "vomiters and purgers" in anorexia nervosa. Psychological Med 1976;6:617–622.

# Chapter 31 / Alcoholic Liver Disease

William R. Kirchain, PharmD, and Mark A. Gill, PharmD

Alcoholic liver disease is one of the most prevalent drug-induced liver diseases seen by clinicians worldwide. In the United States, 20,000 deaths per year are thought to result from the end stages of this disease.[1] The health costs of alcoholic liver disease range in the millions of dollars.[1] It is an ancient disease; in fact, some of the earliest descriptions of cirrhosis resulted from observation of the livers of alcoholics.[2] Almost all clinical practitioners must at times deal with some aspect of alcoholic liver disease. Alcoholic liver disease is also important as a model for the treatment of most other drug-induced forms of liver disease.

## Epidemiology

The exact incidence of all forms of alcoholic liver disease is difficult to obtain. There are observations of particular expressions of alcoholic liver disease that are of value. In the United States approximately 11,000 persons die each year from the complications of alcoholic cirrhosis. Alcoholic hepatitis occurs in 29% of all male alcoholics and 47% of all female alcoholics.[3] It is also interesting to note that overall deaths from alcohol have not changed significantly from the numbers estimated in an article published in 1785 (93/100,000 now versus 66/100,000 then).[3]

## Clinical Presentation

Most patients with alcoholic liver disease present initially with alcoholic hepatitis. These patients suffer from malaise, anorexia, nausea and vomiting, and fever. Unlike many other types of hepatitis, alcoholic hepatitis has a mortality rate of 10% to 30%. Although rare, some patients may not experience any symptoms of hepatitis at all and present instead with one of the complications of cirrhosis, such as ascites or hepatic encephalopathy. Most patients with alcoholic liver disease have been long-term drinkers of 10 or more years and ingest on average 80 or more grams of alcohol per day.

## Pathophysiology

Although some controversy still remains, alcoholic liver disease can be viewed as a progressive chronic condition with four basic stages (Fig. 31.1). The initial lesion, steatosis or fatty metamorphosis, may begin as early as the first drink.[4,5] If the pattern of heavy alcohol use is continued, these lesions become necrotic, inducing a mild inflammatory reaction called alcoholic hepatitis or steatonecrosis.[5,6] In some cases, these lesions lead to a third stage involving fibrotic changes of cirrhosis.[6] The endpoint of the disease is hepatic failure and death.

Many theories have been put forth to explain the toxic effect of alcohol on the liver. Originally, a great deal of attention was paid to possible adulterants or contaminants in the alcohol consumed by those with liver disease.[7] Another popular theory held that alcoholic liver disease is primarily a nutritional deficit.[4] Most alcoholics do have serious nutritional deficits and the treatment of alcoholic liver disease often includes nutritional replenishment, but the severity of the disease is not related to the degree of deficit.[8]

The best explanation of alcoholic liver disease is founded on an understanding of how alcohol is metabolized in the liver. When alcohol is ingested, it is metabolized in the liver and pancreas via alcohol dehydrogenase to acetaldehyde, which in turn is, via the mixed-function oxidase system, broken down to acetic acid.[9] This simple reaction series has tremendous cellular consequences. Both the conversion of alcohol to acetaldehyde and the mixed-function oxidase system require NADH–$NAD^+$ or NADPH–$NADP^+$ conversions. This increases the ratio of NADH to $NAD^+$, which increases fatty acid synthesis and triglyceride accumulation within the cell.[9] Concurrently, the production of lactic acid increases, which can lead to increased collagen production. The increase in lactic acid can also decrease the pH slightly, decreasing uric acid excretion.[9] Continued use of alcohol appears to induce the mixed-function oxidase system. This increase in lipid synthesis, along with a decrease in oxidation of fatty acids perhaps caused by acetaldehyde, leads directly to steatosis, the first lesion of alcoholic liver disease.[6]

Steatosis is a lesion characteristic of, although not exclusive to, alcoholic liver disease. When seen at biopsy, the hepatocytes are filled with large lipid-containing vesicles.[2] The pattern of steatosis induced by alcohol is largely centrilobular.[6] This pathologic change is easily reversed by abstinence from alcohol, and little functional impairment is usually encountered.[4]

The next major pathologic event in the progression of alcoholic liver disease is steatonecrosis or alcoholic hepatitis (Table 31.1). Lysis and necrosis of the fat-filled hepatocytes induce the immune system and there is an apparent alteration of cell-mediated immunity leading to an increased rate of damage.[10] This event is also marked by the development of the alcoholic hyaline or Mallory body.[11] Even at this stage of disease many patients can avoid the eventual sequelae by abstinence, though the cellular structure may never return to normal.[12] If there is no continued insult to the liver, a resolution of symptoms can be anticipated in 3 to 8 months.[12]

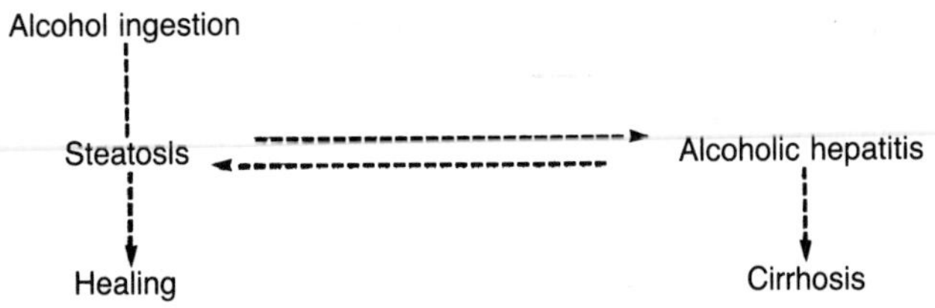


**Figure 31.1** Progression of alcoholic liver disease.

Cirrhosis leading to hepatic failure and its complications is the terminal event in alcoholic liver disease. Cirrhosis is primarily the result of fibrotic changes that distort the architectural integrity of the liver. This is generally accompanied by a loss of parenchymal mass and a concurrent loss of liver function. It is these changes in structure and decreases in function that result in the signs and symptoms of alcoholic cirrhosis, such as portal hypertension or bleeding abnormalities.

### *Portal Hypertension and Ascites*

Portal hypertension in alcoholic liver disease is the direct result of increased mechanical resistance to blood flow through the liver.[13] In individuals with no cirrhosis, the normal liver blood flow is roughly 1–1.5 L/min at a pressure of only 4–6 mm Hg.[13] As the flow is inhibited by the distorted liver architecture in cirrhotic patients, the pressure rises not only in the liver but along the gastrointestinal tract and in the spleen as well. The manifestations then of portal hypertension are primarily the result of low-pressure vessels handling high-pressure loads. To cope with this pressure, blood is diverted into a large number of minor small collateral vessels. This collateral flow is very prominent in the azygous and subclavian veins through the lower esophagus, the abdominal wall, and between the spleen and the left renal vein. Esophageal and abdominal varices often develop; these can rupture and sometimes lead to life-threatening hemorrhage. Splenomegaly is also a common feature, occasionally requiring splenectomy.

Another significant complication of portal hypertension is ascites. Ascites results from the higher pressures of portal hypertension coupled with an increased porosity in the liver sinusoids and an increase in intrahepatic interstitial fluid.[13] The lymphatic system of the liver is able to handle a great deal of excess fluid, but some leakage into the peritoneal cavity still occurs.[14] The amount of fluid leaked into the peritoneal cavity can become quite large over time, leading to mechanical problems with many body systems. The increased intraabdominal pressure acting on the diaphragm can, by affecting thoracic pressure, decrease transmural filling pressure of the heart, increase right atrial pressure, and decrease venous return to the right ventricle.[15] The increased pooling of blood associated with portal hypertension leads to a sequestration of blood in the spleen which, along with the sequestration of fluid in the peritoneum, leads to a relative decrease in renal arteriolar perfusion. This induces the release of renin which may lead to the increased ability of cirrhotics to reabsorb sodium (and water). Renin levels are in fact higher in cirrhotic patients.[16,17] Because cirrhosis is often accompanied by a decrease in the hepatic production of albumin the serum oncotic pressure is also decreased, thus reducing the ability of the body to retain fluid in the vascular space.[6]

**Table 31.1** Signs and Symptoms of Alcoholic Hepatitis

| *Symptom* | % | *Sign* | % |
|---|---|---|---|
| Anorexia | 87 | Hepatomegaly | 91 |
| Nausea | 77 | Ascites | 73 |
| Weakness | 77 | Spider angiomas | 65 |
| Jaundice | 70 | Splenomegaly | 38 |
| Weight loss | 59 | | |
| Fever | 36 | | |

### *Esophageal and Gastric Varices*

Portal hypertension causes pooling of blood in both the spleen and the mesenteric veins and arteries. This causes engorgement of the small capillaries along the entire gastrointestinal tract. These overfilled blood vessels are much easier to rupture than normal vessels. Concurrently there is a breakdown in the gastric mucosa, leading to increased damage from acid and pepsin in the stomach and esophagus caused by an apparent direct toxic effect of alcohol on the mucosal surface.[2]

### *Decreased Liver Function*

Along with the effects of the mechanical problems of cirrhosis there is a progressive loss of basic hepatocyte function because of an overall loss of parenchymal mass.[6] There is generally a decrease in protein synthesis and utilization of available substrates. A loss of enzymes leads to a decrease in the liver's ability to handle both drugs and endogenous toxins, which begin to accumulate. A decrease in serum albumin leads to a decrease in the protein binding of certain drugs and a decrease in the serum oncotic pressure.[8] Vitamin K–dependent coagulation factors (II, VII, IX, X) synthesized by the liver slowly diminish, resulting in an increased frequency of bleeding problems.[2] The ability of the hepatic transaminases to detoxify ammonia is decreased. Ammonia, octopamine, mercaptans, phenols, methanethiols, and other by-products of metabolism begin to accumulate.[18]

Along with this decrease in transamination there is an apparent increase in ammonia production in the gut (Table 31.2).[19] The catabolism induced by the decrease in albumin leads to an increase in aromatic amino acids at a rate 24 times the production of branched-chain amino acids.[20]

### *Hepatic Encephalopathy*

The incidence of hepatic encephalopathy may be much greater than generally perceived. In one study only 15% of patients with chronic liver disease but without a diagnosis of encephalopathy could pass a standardized psychometric test.[21] The cause of hepatic encephalopathy is not known; several factors, such as increased blood levels of ammonia and aromatic amino acids, have been associated with the

**Table 31.2** Urea Breakdown Rate in Normal Individuals Versus Cirrhotics

| | *N* | *Fractional gut urea breakdown* | *Urea-nitrogen synthesis rate* | *Urea-nitrogen breakdown (mmol/h)* | *Nitrogen balance (mmol/h)* | *BUN (mmol/L)* |
|---|---|---|---|---|---|---|
| Normal individuals | 10 | 0.17 ± 0.08 | 26.1 ± 3.8 | 4.5 ± 0.3 | 7.0 ± 5.9 | 10.8 ± 3.7 |
| Cirrhotic patients | 14 | 0.26 ± 0.08 | 22.1 ± 6.8 | 5.7 ± 0.5 | 12.5 ± 7.0[a] | 8.8 ± 1.4 |

[a] Significantly different from normal individuals.

Adapted from Hansen BA, Vilstrap H: Increased intestinal hydrolysis of urea in patients with alcoholic cirrhosis. Scand J Gastroenterol 1985;20:346, with permission.

development of hepatic encephalopathy. Elevated ammonia levels have long been associated with hepatic encephalopathy. It is unclear if this elevation is the actual cause of the encephalopathic symptomatology. As stated earlier there is also a tremendous change in the relative levels of aromatic amino acids in the encephalopathic patient.[22] It is theorized that these aromatic amino acids may either work directly as, or stimulate the production of, false neurotransmitters in the central nervous system.[18]

Finally, the patient with cirrhosis is at risk of developing hepatic carcinoma.[6,23] In fact, simply having alcoholic liver disease increases the risk of developing hepatomas significantly.[23]

## Treatment

The most important treatment for drug-induced liver disease is the discontinuance of drug exposure. It cannot be overemphasized that patients with alcoholic liver disease must stop drinking. With continued exposure to alcohol, hepatic damage will progress. With discontinuation of alcohol exposure, many patients improve dramatically. Steatosis often resolves within weeks, and alcoholic hepatitis within a few months, of the last drink.[12]

### *Alcoholic Hepatitis*

After the discontinuation of alcohol the therapy for alcoholic liver disease is primarily symptomatic. In alcoholic hepatitis glucocorticosteroids are sometimes used during the acute phase; the rationale is to decrease the inflammatory response to the alcoholic hyaline and other antigenic substances present.[24] There is not a clear body of evidence that glucocorticoid therapy reduces the overall morbidity of alcoholic hepatitis patients. A few studies have shown benefits in highly selected patient populations, but even these do not always show a statistically significant response (Table 31.3).[25–27] Regardless of treatment, many patients do not survive severe bouts of the disease (survival rate 22%–45%).[27] Those who do survive often develop cirrhosis in 3 to 5 years.[20]

### *Cirrhosis*

The treatment of cirrhosis is again symptomatic, directed at the particular manifestations in the particular patient. If the patient shows signs of nutritional deficiency it should be corrected. Deficiencies in folate, thiamine, and vitamin C are very common and often severe.[8] Additionally, potassium, phosphorus, magnesium, and iron can be quite low in these patients.[8] Replacement of iron should be done with particular caution in cirrhotic patients, as often liver iron stores are higher than normal despite low serum concentrations, and hemochromatosis can develop.[6] Vitamin K injections can sometimes help regenerate clotting factors, but as cirrhosis worsens the response to vitamin K lessens. Replenishment of serum protein can be very difficult in cirrhotic patients who often require protein restriction, but adequate calories should be given.

### *Ascites*

Ascites is primarily an accumulation of fluid; therefore, the objective in treating ascites should be removal of the fluid. In practice this is not often an easy task. Table 31.4 summarizes the stepwise treatment of ascites. The increase in fluid in the peritoneal cavity causes a relative decrease in intravascular volume. The kidney responds by retaining sodium; sodium restriction is then the first step in treating ascites.[36] Most patients with ascites require 1 g of sodium per day, which essentially means no added salt and no salted foods. This is usually accompanied by a concurrent restriction of fluid intake to a few hundred milliliters per day. Patients who are not hospitalized generally find this a difficult regimen. As the ascites begins to resolve, the amount of sodium can sometimes be increased to a more tolerable 2 to 3 g, and the amount of fluid intake increased upward to a liter per day. The overall fluid loss per day induced by any therapy should not exceed 1–2 L.[37] Because ascitic fluid mobilizes at a rate of only 1–2 L/d, diuresis that is too brisk can lead to problems of relative dehydration and a potentially fatal hepatorenal syndrome.[37] Hepatorenal syndrome is a progressive, fatal loss of renal function in the face of severe hepatic dysfunction. The onset of hepatorenal syndrome is insidious and often unrecognized. A slow but continuous rise in serum creatinine and blood urea nitrogen eventually progresses to complete failure of the kidneys. The patient must then deal not only with a failed liver but also with all the problems associated with acute renal failure. Drug dosing can become extremely difficult in these patients, often requiring extensive use of blood levels and sophisticated pharmacokinetic methods. Paracentesis or diuretic therapy can be used to deplete the volume of ascites with equal efficacy when sodium and fluid restriction fail to produce

**Table 31.3** Studies of Steroid Therapy for Alcoholic Hepatitis

| | | | | *Mortality (%)* | | |
|---|---|---|---|---|---|---|
| *Reference* | *Agent* | *Dosage* | *Total duration (d)* | **Placebo group** | **Steroid group** | **Comments** |
| 28 | MePr[a] | 1 g | 3 | 57 | 63 | A[b] |
| 29 | Pred | 40 mg | 28 | 40 | 6 | B |
| 30 | MePr | 80 mg | 7 | 47 | 50 | A |
| 31 | Pred | 40 mg | 44 | 100 | 29 | C |
| 32 | Pred | 40 mg | 42 | 35 | 37 | D |
| 33 | Pred | 40 mg | 32 | 19 | 4 | A |
| 34 | Pred | 40 mg | 23 | 31 | 50 | D,E |
| 35 | Pred | 40 mg | 60 | 40 | 10 | F |

[a] MePr, methylprednisolone; Pred, prednisone.
[b] A. No difference in healing rates between the two groups.
B. Severely ill patients did much better on steroid therapy; patients with milder disease did about the same in both groups.
C. Some deaths may have resulted from complications of feeding procedures rather than alcoholic hepatitis.
D. Serum albumin levels were higher in the steroid-treated group after treatment.
E. Increased incidence of fungal infections in the steroid-treated group.
F. This was a long-term study of 5 to 12 years; survival is for the first year only. For both groups, the average survival was 3 years.

adequate diuresis.[36] Another technique that can be employed involves dialytic ultrafiltration and reinfusion of ascitic fluid.[38] This procedure is similar to kidney dialysis, but only ascitic fluid from the peritoneal cavity is filtered. Many patients who continue to develop ascites and those who do not respond to diuretics or paracentesis receive a LeVeen or peritoneovenous shunt. Even this does not always prevent ascites from recurring; 30% of patients with a LeVeen shunt in place may later again develop ascites[39] (Fig. 31.2).

Diuretic therapy for ascites is effective in most patients; the process is slow. Patients may require as long as 35–40 days of continuous therapy before the ascites has resolved.[36] The drugs most frequently used are the potassium-sparing diuretics, because of the ability of spironolactone in particular to inhibit the action of aldosterone in the kidney tubule. It is believed that ascites causes a relative decrease in intravascular volume that stimulates the aldosterone-mediated retention of sodium and water in the kidney.[37] The dose of spironolactone required ranges from 100 to 400 mg/d and is usually not effective without concurrent sodium and water restriction.[2,37] The onset of the diuretic effect with spironolactone is slow, 2 to 3 days in some cases, and loop diuretics such as furosemide are sometimes added to increase the rate of weight loss. Spironolactone is a competitive inhibitor of aldosterone in the distal segment of the renal tubule. Aldosterone causes the reabsorption of sodium from the peritubular fluid and the concurrent excretion of potassium. The amount normally presented to the distal tubule is small and inhibiting this reabsorption produces only a mild increase in sodium and water excretion. Again, the rate of weight loss should not exceed 1–2 L/d. As with all patients on diuretics,

**Table 31.4** Treatment of Ascites

| *Therapy* | *Goal* |
|---|---|
| 1. Sodium and water restriction | Loss = 1–2 L/d (weight loss = 1–2 kg) |
| *If inadequate response after 3–5 d, add* | |
| 2. Mild diuretic (spironolactone) 100–400 mg/d | As above |
| *If inadequate response after 4–7 d, add* | |
| 3. Loop diuretic (furosemide) 40–120 mg/d | As above |
| *If inadequate response after 30–60 d, add* | |
| 4. Peritoneal dialysis with reinfusion | As above |
| *or* | |
| 5. Peritoneovenous shunt | As above |

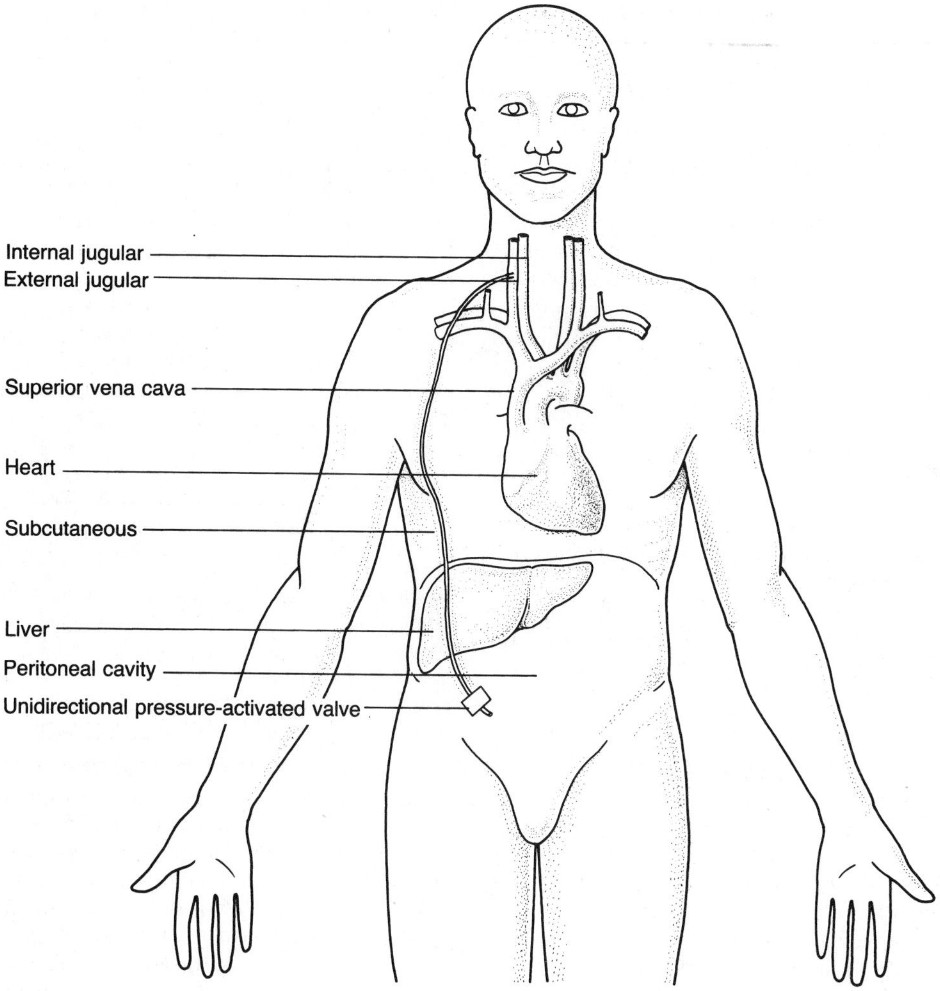


**Figure 31.2** Placement of peritoneovenous shunt or LeVeen shunt.

serum electrolytes must be monitored carefully during therapy and signs of dehydration (orthostatic blood pressure changes, changes in heart rate, decreased urine output) must be carefully monitored.

### *Portal Hypertension*

The therapy for portal hypertension is directed at reducing flow to the portal bed. Operative procedures such as splenectomy or portacaval shunts attempt to do this mechanically.[13] Drug therapy with propranolol has also been used in doses of 40–180 mg/d with some success. In one study, propranolol was shown superior to placebo in preventing rebleeding in patients with esophageal varices. The propranolol dose used was the dose sufficient to decrease the blood pressure by 25 mm Hg.[40] Sclerotherapy by direct application of ethanolamide or other agents is often used to treat esophageal varices. Ulcers that develop after therapy are a serious complication of this procedure.[13] Alternatively, an intravenous infusion of vasopressin at 0.2–0.6 unit per minute can be used to treat acutely bleeding varices.[13] Vasopressin increases the contractility of smooth muscles, particularly the small arterioles of the splanchnic, coronary, pancreatic, and mesenteric beds. Patients must then be monitored for adverse effects resulting from the decreased perfusion of these areas. Coronary and venous thrombosis can occur along with arrhythmias secondary to ischemia. Increases in blood pressure are possible as are severe vascular headaches and angina. It is prudent to have any patient treated with vasopressin monitored by electrocardiogram. Vasopressin can also be administered intraarterially into the superior mesenteric artery. This technique is usually reserved for varices that do not respond to intravenous infusions. Ice water gavage can also be used to slow bleeding; surgery is often required in severe cases.[13]

### *Hepatic Encephalopathy*

Most patients with hepatic encephalopathy respond to some type of protein restriction. The source and types of amino acids in the diet may also be important, as aromatic amino acids, already higher than normal in many cirrhotics, can be utilized in the central nervous system to produce false neurotransmitters.[8] This ratio of aromatic to branched-chain amino acids can be reversed by the use of feedings high in branched-chain amino acids.[18] Vegetable sources of protein that are high in branched-chain amino acids can often aid in this therapy by increasing the amount of fiber in the diet. This increase in fiber can also decrease total urea production in the colon and increase fecal urea excretion.[41] Regardless of the source of amino acid, the total amount of amino acids should initially be restricted to about 20 g protein per day; this can be increased as the patient's symptoms improve. Therapies that reduce the blood ammonia level appear to be effective in the management of hepatic encephalopathy that does not respond to protein restriction alone. Cirrhotic patients have a higher rate of urea breakdown in the gastrointestinal tract than do normal individuals (Table 31.2).[19] Lactulose, a nonabsorbed disaccharide, decreases this rate of urea breakdown and thus decreases the ammonia in the blood derived from the gut.[21] The exact mechanism is unclear, but an increased frequency of stools per day appears to be an important component of lactulose's action. The goal should be two to three stools per day. Lactulose is broken down in the colon to acetic, lactic, and formic acids and to carbon dioxide.[21] It has been shown to increase relative concentrations of *Lactobacillus* and other fermentative bacteria in the colon and to inhibit the proteolytic enzymes of many bacteria. By decreasing the pH in the colon, lactulose also reduces the ability of ammonia to diffuse across the gut wall.

Neomycin given orally is also used to change colonic flora and decrease blood ammonia. The disadvantage with neomycin is that it is partially absorbed, causing ototoxicity and nephrotoxicity.

The endpoint of therapies directed at hepatic encephalopathy is an overall increase in the cognitive ability of the patient from baseline. If the patient is comatose, a return to consciousness is the goal. It is sometimes difficult in patients with milder forms of hepatic encephalopathy to detect changes resulting from therapy. In these patients, improvements in the mental status exam, electroencephalogram, and asterixis are sometimes used.[22] Simple bedside psychomotor exams, such as serial signatures, nine-number connection tests, or drawing a familiar simple figure (a star, a house), can also be of assistance.

## Summary

Alcoholic liver disease is often a frustrating disease for the clinician. There are few direct therapies, and symptomatic treatment often does not work or works poorly. The overall success of therapy depends ultimately on the patient. If the patient can stop drinking there is a chance of recovery. If the patient does not stop drinking, the disease is usually fatal.

## References


1. Anonymous. World Health Statistics. Geneva, World Health Organization, 1984.
2. Conn HO. Cirrhosis, in Schiff L (ed): Diseases of the Liver, 4th ed. Philadelphia, J.B. Lippincott, 1975, pp 833–939.
3. Heckler MM. Fifth special report to the U.S. Congress on alcohol and health from the Secretary of Health and Human Services. Bethesda, Md., National Institute on Alcohol Abuse and Alcoholism, 1983, pp 45–68.
4. Klatskin G. Alcohol and its relationship to the liver. Gastroenterology 1961;41:443–451.
5. Iseri OA, Lieber CS, Gottlieb LS. The ultrastructure of the fatty liver induced by prolonged ethanol ingestion. Am J Pathol 1966;48:535–538.
6. Zimmerman HJ. Hepatoxicity, in: The Adverse Effects of Drugs and Other Chemicals on the Liver. New York, Appleton-Century-Crofts, 1978, pp 122–144.
7. Mallory FB. Phosphorus poisoning and alcoholic cirrhosis. Am J Pathol 1933;9:551–560.
8. Mills PR, Shenkin A, Anthony RS, et al. Assessment of nutritional status and in vivo immune responses in alcoholic liver disease. Am J Clin Nutr 1983;38:849–859
9. Steinmetz PR, Balko C. Liver adaptation and injury in alcoholism. N Engl J Med 1973;288:356–362.
10. Sorrell MF, Leevy CM. Lymphocyte transformation and alcoholic liver injury. Gastroenterology 1972;63:1020–1025.
11. Harinsuta U, Zimmerman HJ. Alcoholic steatonecrosis. Gastroenterology 1971;60:1036–1046.
12. Galambos JT. Natural history of alcoholic hepatitis. Gastroenterology 1972;63:1026–1035.
13. Reynolds TB, Campra TL. Portal hypertension. Postgrad Med J 1983;59(suppl 4):55–63.
14. Guyton AC. The lymphatic system, interstitial fluid dynamics and special fluid systems, in: Basic Human Physiology. Philadelphia, W.B. Saunders, 1977:316–327.
15. Guazzi M, Polese A, Magrini F, et al. Negative influences of ascites on the cardiac function of cirrhotic patients. Am J Med 1975;59:165–170.
16. Chaimovitz C, Sylman P, Alroy G, et al. Mechanism of increased tubular sodium reabsorption in cirrhosis. Am J Med 1972;52:198–202.
17. Schroeder ET, Fich RH, Smulyan H, et al. Plasma renin levels in hepatic cirrhosis. Am J Med 1970;49:186–191.
18. Fischer JE. Amino acids in hepatic coma. Dig Dis Sci 1982;27: 97–101.
19. Hansen BA, Vilstrup H. Increased intestinal hydrolysis of urea in patients with alcoholic cirrhosis. Scand J Gastroenterol 1985; 20:346–350.
20. Gilberstadt SJ, Gilberstadt H, Zieve L, et al. Psychomotor performance defects in cirrhotic patients without overt encephalopathy. Arch Intern Med 1980;140:519–521.
21. Crossley IR, Williams R. Progress in the treatment of chronic portasystemic encephalopathy. Gut 1984;25:85–98.
22. Atterbury CE, Maddrey WC, Conn HO. Neomycin–sorbitol and lactulose in the treatment of acute portal-systemic encephalopathy: A controlled, double-blind clinical trial. Am J Dig Dis 1978;23:398–406.
23. Fischer RL, Sheuer PJ, Sherlock S. Primary liver cell carcinoma: Alcohol and chronic liver disease. Gut 1974;15:343.
24. Edmunson HA, Peters RL, Reynolds TB, et al. Sclerosing hyaline membrane necrosis of the liver in the chronic alcoholic. Ann Intern Med 1963;59:646–673.
25. Helman RA, Temko MH, Nye SW, et al. Alcoholic hepatitis:

Natural history and evaluation of prednisolone therapy. Ann Intern Med 1971;74:311–321.
26. Wells R. Prednisolone and testosterone proprionate in cirrhosis of the liver. Lancet 1960;2:1416–1419.
27. Porter HP, Simon FR, Pope CE, et al. Corticosteroid therapy in severe alcoholic hepatitis. N Engl J Med 1971;284:1350–1355.
28. Theodossi A, Eddleston ALWF, Williams R. Controlled trial of methylprednisolone therapy in severe acute alcoholic hepatitis. Gut 1982;23:75–79.
29. Helman RA, Temko MH, Nye SW, et al. Alcoholic hepatitis, natural history and evaluation of prednisone therapy. Ann Intern Med 1971;74:311–321.
30. Shumaker JB, Resnik RH, Galambos JT, et al. A controlled trial of 6-methylprednisolone in acute alcoholic hepatitis. Am J Gastroenterol 1978;69:443–449.
31. Lesesne HR, Bozymski EM, Fallon HJ. Treatment of alcoholic hepatitis with encephalopathy, comparison of prednisone with caloric supplements. Gastroenterology 1978;74:169–173.
32. Campra JL, Hamlin EM, Kirshbaum RJ, et al. Prednisone therapy of acute alcoholic hepatitis, report of a controlled trial. Ann Intern Med 1973;79:625–631.
33. Maddrey WC, Boitnott JK, Bedine MS, et al. Corticosteroid therapy of alcoholic hepatitis. Gastroenterology 1978;75:193–199.
34. Blitzer B, Mutchnick MG, Joshi PH, et al. Adrenocorticosteroid therapy in alcoholic hepatitis, a prospective, double-blind randomized study. Am J Dig Dis 1977;22:477–484.
35. Schlichting P, Juhl E, Poulson H, et al. Alcoholic hepatitis superimposed on cirrhosis, clinical significance and effect of longterm prednisone therapy. Scand J Gastroenterol 1976;11:305–312.
36. Quintero E, Arroyo V, Bory F, et al. Paracentesis versus diuretics in the treatment of cirrhotics with tense ascites. Lancet 1985;2:611–612.
37. Sherlock S. Ascites formation in cirrhosis and its management. Scand J Gastroenterol 1970;5(suppl 7):9–15.
38. Raju SF, Achord JL. The effects of dialytic ultrafiltration and peritoneal reinfusion in the management of resistant ascites. Am J Gastroenterol 1984;79:308–312.
39. Smadja C, Franco D. The LeVeen shunt in the elective treatment of intractable ascites in cirrhosis. Ann Surg 1985;201:488–493.
40. Lebrec D, Poynard T, Hillon P, et al. Propranolol for prevention of recurrent gastrointestinal bleeding in patients with cirrhosis. N Engl J Med 1981;305:1371–1374.
41. Weber FL, Minco D, Fresard KM, et al. Effects of vegetable diets on nitrogen metabolism in cirrhotic subjects. Gastroenterology 1985;89:538–544.

# Chapter 32 / Drug-Induced Liver Disease

William R. Kirchain, PharmD, and Mark A. Gill, PharmD

The number of drugs associated with adverse reactions involving the liver is extensive (Table 32.1). Between 1980 and 1985, the National Library of Medicine recorded more than 400 articles addressing some type of liver disease associated with drug therapy. Chronic liver disease and cirrhosis are a significant cause of death in the United States, resulting in 20,000 to 30,000 deaths per year.[1] Adverse drug reactions are at most only part of the morbidity and mortality of liver disease on a global or national level. For an individual patient, however, liver disease is usually a profound life-changing disease. The liver's function impacts almost every other organ system in the body. It is important to know basic patterns of drug-related pathology and toxicity to adequately assess adverse reactions when they occur. It is also important to understand how and when to monitor for these reactions in day-to-day patient care and clinical research situations.

## Hepatic Physiology and Function

For most drugs taken orally, the liver is the entrance to the systemic circulation. Blood laden with newly absorbed chemicals flows via the superior mesenteric vein into the liver's portal vein (Fig. 32.1).[2] Once in the sinusoidal portions of the liver, these chemicals are either actively or passively taken up by the hepatocytes. This "first-pass" effect causes the liver to be the first organ exposed to potentially toxic substances.[3] In addition, any drug undergoing enterohepatic recirculation first passes through the liver.

For most metabolized compounds, the hepatocytes that absorb these drugs are the primary site of biotransformation. These cells have a tremendous capacity for metabolizing substrates. It has been estimated that 1 $cm^3$ of tissue in the average liver contains greater than 20 $m^2$ of rough endoplasmic reticulum.[4] This, however, also predisposes them to damage from compounds that become more, rather than less, toxic after the phase I reactions of biotransformation (Fig. 32.2). These bioactivated compounds are often directly toxic to the organelles of the hepatocytes, leading to cell damage.[4,5] For example, valproic acid becomes toxic to the hepatocyte only after it has been converted to $\Delta^4$-valproic acid by cytochrome $P_{450}$.[6]

Along with its metabolic role, the liver serves as a primary storage organ for many substrates. Apparently, certain toxins also concentrate in the liver, leading to selective adverse reactions.[2,7] Vitamin A, which is stored in the space of Disse, can, over time and in high doses, lead to marked hypertrophy and fibrosis. Similarly, amiodarone, which has a very long residence time in the liver, can induce phospholipidosis within the lysosomal bodies of the hepatocyte.

In addition to their metabolic role, the hepatocytes produce bile and are connected to the bile canalicular system. Drugs even partially excreted via this system may cause a decrease in either bile production or bile flow through the system.[4,8,9] Estrogens, for example, can reduce bile salt–dependent flow, thus decreasing the excretion of bile and causing congestion. This congestion in turn leads to the formation of cholestatic lesions in the liver. Cholestatic lesions are often characterized by bile plugs within the biliary capillaries seen at biopsy.

There are anatomic and physiologic divisions in the microstructure and macrostructure of the liver that control the development of the different patterns of hepatic damage. Hepatocytes are in constant contact with other hepatocytes, the perisinusoidal space, and a biliary capillary (Fig. 32.3).[4] The hepatocytes are then arranged around an axis consisting of a central vein, a portal venule, a bile ductule, and lymph vessels that grow outward from a small triangular field called an acinus. This acinar arrangement can be divided physiologically into three zones (Fig. 32.4). Moving from the axial terminal branch toward the central vein, the primary function of the hepatocyte shifts from respiration to biotransformation and storage.[2,5] The hepatocytes in zone 1, the best oxygenated zone, tend to have higher concentrations of the enzymes of respiration, particularly glucose-6-phosphatase and the Kreb's cycle enzymes. These cells tend to be more resistant to nutritional and circulatory disease. The hepatocytes in zone 3 tend to have higher concentrations of NAD and NADP lipoamide reductase (a diaphorase), a higher rate of fatty acid production, and glycogen stores.[2]

Necrotic lesions then develop in patterns correlating with both the type of toxic compound and the position of the most sensitive hepatocytes. For example, a bioactivated compound that requires a specific enzyme, such as isoniazid, tends to produce lesions in areas of the acinus where acetylation is a predominant function.[10] The lesions associated with acetaminophen overdose tend to occur in zone 3, where there is a higher rate of redox reactions.[11]

If the liver parenchyma is continually exposed to periods of acute cell damage and necrosis, nonfunctional fibrous tissue will begin to replace functional hepatocytes.[2,12] Because of the liver's tremendous capacity, small fibrotic changes can usually be tolerated without significant reduction in function. As these changes continue, the architectural integrity of the organ degenerates; when these changes are accompanied by nodular regenèration, cirrhosis ensues.[2]

The cirrhotic liver can take many forms depending on the rate of nodular regeneration and the extent of the initial necrotic process (Table 32.2).[5] Cirrhosis can develop after only one exposure to a drug, but usually is a result of months to years of exposure.[13,14]

**Table 32.1** Monitoring Hepatotoxic Drugs[a]

| *Drug/class* | *Type of reaction* | *Monitoring parameter* |
|---|---|---|
| Anti-infectives | | |
| Penicillins | Idiosyncratic | Signs/symptoms of hepatic disease |
| Cephalosporins | Idiosyncratic | Signs/symptoms of hepatic disease |
| Erythromycins | Idiosyncratic | Signs/symptoms of hepatic disease |
| Tetracycline | Predictable[b] | Bilirubin, GGTP, alkaline phosphatase, AST |
| Sulfonamides | Idiosyncratic | Signs/symptoms of hepatic disease |
| Isoniazid | Idiosyncratic[c] | Signs/symptoms of hepatic disease |
| Nitrofurantoin | Idiosyncratic | Signs/symptoms of hepatic disease |
| Ketoconazole | Idiosyncratic | AST, ALT, LDH, bilirubin |
| Griseofulvin | Predictable | Bilirubin, GGTP, alkaline phosphatase |
| Antineoplastic agents | | |
| Asparaginase | Predictable | Bilirubin, GGTP, alkaline phosphatase, AST |
| Carmustine | Predictable | Bilirubin, GGTP, alkaline phosphatase, AST |
| Chlorambucil | Predictable | Bilirubin, GGTP, alkaline phosphatase, AST |
| Cyclophosphamide | Idiosyncratic | Bilirubin, GGTP, alkaline phosphatase |
| Dacarbazine | Idiosyncratic | Bilirubin, GGTP, alkaline phosphatase, AST |
| Daunorubicin | Idiosyncratic | Signs/Symptoms of hepatic disease |
| Methotrexate | Predictable[d,e] | AST, ALT, LDH, bilirubin |
| Mercaptopurine | Predictable[d] | Bilirubin, GGTP, alkaline phosphatase, AST |
| Mithramycin | Predictable | AST, ALT, LDH |
| Thioguanine | Predictable | Bilirubin, GGTP, alkaline phosphatase, AST |
| Vinblastine | Idiosyncratic | Signs/symptoms of hepatic disease |
| Cardiovascular agents | | |
| Amiodarone | Predictable[d,e] | AST, ALT, LDH |
| Thiazide diuretics | Idiosyncratic | Signs/symptoms of hepatic disease |
| Disopyramide | Idiosyncratic | Signs/symptoms of hepatic disease |
| Hydralazine | Idiosyncratic | Signs/symptoms of hepatic disease |
| Methyldopa | Idiosyncratic | Signs/symptoms of hepatic disease |
| Procainamide | Idiosyncratic | Signs/symptoms of hepatic disease |
| Quinidine | Idiosyncratic | Signs/symptoms of hepatic disease |
| Anti-inflammatory agents | | |
| Acetaminophen | Predictable[d,f] | AST, ALT, LDH, bilirubin |
| Aspirin | Predictable[d] | AST, ALT, LDH, bilirubin |
| Phenylbutazone | Predictable | AST, ALT, LDH, bilirubin |
| Sulindac | Idiosyncratic | AST, ALT, LDH, bilirubin |
| Other nonsteroidals | Idiosyncratic | Signs/symptoms of hepatic disease |
| Gold sodium thiomalate | Predictable | Bilirubin, GGTP, alkaline phosphatase, AST |
| Penicillamine | Idiosyncratic | Bilirubin, GGTP, alkaline phosphatase |
| Anticonvulsants | | |
| Carbamazepine | Idiosyncratic | Signs/symptoms of hepatic disease |
| Phenobarbital | Idiosyncratic | Signs/symptoms of hepatic disease |
| Phenytoin | Idiosyncratic | Signs/symptoms of hepatic disease |
| Valproic acid | Predictable | AST, ALT, LDH, bilirubin |
| Antidepressants/antipsychotics | | |
| Chlorpromazine | Predictable | Bilirubin, GGTP, alkaline phosphatase, AST |
| Desipramine | Idiosyncratic | Signs/symptoms of hepatic disease |
| Fluphenazine | Predictable | Bilirubin, GGTP, alkaline phosphatase, AST |
| Haloperidol | Predictable | Bilirubin, GGTP, alkaline phosphatase, AST |
| Imipramine | Predictable | Bilirubin, GGTP, alkaline phosphatase, AST |
| Thioridazine | Predictable | Bilirubin, GGTP, alkaline phosphatase, AST |
| Contraceptives and androgenic steroids | | |
| Danazol | Predictable | AST, ALT, LDH, bilirubin |
| Diethylstilbestrol | Idiosyncratic | Signs/symptoms of hepatic disease |
| Ethinyl estradiol | Idiosyncratic | Signs/symptoms of hepatic disease |
| Ethynodiol diacetate | Idiosyncratic | Signs/symptoms of hepatic disease |
| Fluoxymesterone | Predictable | Bilirubin, GGTP, alkaline phosphatase, AST |

Table 32.1 Monitoring Hepatotoxic Drugs[a] (continued)

| *Drug/class* | *Type of reaction* | *Monitoring parameter* |
|---|---|---|
| Contraceptives and androgenic steroids (continued) | | |
| Methandrostenolone | Predictable | Bilirubin, GGTP, alkaline phosphatase, AST |
| Methyltestosterone | Predictable | Bilirubin, GGTP, alkaline phosphatase, AST |
| Oxymetholone | Predictable | Bilirubin, GGTP, alkaline phosphatase, AST |
| Tamoxifen | Idiosyncratic | Signs/symptoms of hepatic disease |
| Testosterone | Predictable | Bilirubin, GGTP, alkaline phosphatase, AST |
| Gastrointestinal agents | | |
| Cimetidine | Idiosyncratic | Signs/symptoms of hepatic disease |
| Ranitidine | Idiosyncratic | Signs/symptoms of hepatic disease |
| Antidiabetic agents | | |
| Acetohexamide | Idiosyncratic | Signs/symptoms of hepatic disease |
| Chlorpropamide | Idiosyncratic | Signs/symptoms of hepatic disease |
| Glibenclamide | Idiosyncratic | Signs/symptoms of hepatic disease |
| Tolazamide | Idiosyncratic | Signs/symptoms of hepatic disease |
| Tolbutamide | Idiosyncratic | Signs/symptoms of hepatic disease |
| Anesthetics | | |
| Enflurane | Predictable[d] | AST, ALT, LDH, bilirubin |
| Halothane | Predictable[d] | AST, ALT, LDH, bilirubin |
| Vitamins and minerals | | |
| Vitamin A | Predictable[d] | AST, ALT, LDH, bilirubin |
| α-Tocopherol | Predictable | Bilirubin, GGTP, alkaline phosphatase, AST |
| Iron salts | Predictable[f] | AST, ALT, LDH, bilirubin |
| Nicotinic acid | Idiosyncratic | Signs/symptoms of hepatic disease |

[a] Laboratory assays can be obtained every 2 to 4 weeks during the period of peak onset for a given reaction. Groups at higher risk may require more intensive monitoring. In clinical drug trials, usually one or two samples are assayed for serum enzymes each week during the study and one sample, 1 to 2 months after the end of the study. GGTP, γ-glutamyltransferase; AST, aspartate transaminase; ALT, alanine transaminase; LDH, lactate dehydrogenase.

[b] Toxicity related to intravenous doses, greater than 1.5 g/d.

[c] AST, ALT, LDH, and bilirubin may need to be monitored regularly in patients older than 35 or younger than 15.

[d] Dose related; risk increases with increasing dosages.

[e] A biopsy after 6 to 12 months of therapy and periodic indocyanine green or sulfobromophthalein excretion determinations have also been recommended.

[f] Most commonly seen in cases of accidental and intentional overdose.

## Aging and Hepatotoxicity

There are very few data on specific increase or decrease in susceptibility to drug-induced liver injury with increasing age, but a few observations are important. As the normal liver ages hepatic blood flow decreases as much as 30% by age 65.[15] This decrease in liver blood flow has been shown to increase the bioavailability of highly extractable drugs, such as labetolol, propranolol, lidocaine, and chlormethiazole.[16] The risk of hepatotoxicity is apparently greater in persons 70 or older, according to data from the United Kingdom. There, 5% of all adverse reactions in persons 70 or older are related to the liver, whereas only 2% of all adverse reactions in children (0–14 years old) are related to the liver.[17] The potential mortality from hepatotoxic reactions is also higher in the elderly who often have concurrent decreases in renal or cardiac function. Neoplastic disease, in general, and hepatocellular carcinomas are also more common in the elderly than in younger patients.[17]

## Patterns of Drug-Induced Liver Disease

There are two primary types of drug-induced liver disease, predictable reactions and idiosyncratic or nonpredictable reactions. Predictable reactions usually can be explained by a toxic dose–response relationship. Occasionally, a genetic or an acquired abnormality in a particular metabolic pathway must coexist for a predictable reaction to take place. Predictable reactions usually are associated with relatively high rates of occurrence. Idiosyncratic reactions, on the other hand, tend to occur without association to particular blood concentrations or specifically identified metabolic abnormalities. Idiosyncratic reactions are rare and are sometimes described as a type of liver hypersensitivity to a drug.

### *Centrolobular Necrosis*

Centrolobular necrosis is often a dose-related, predictable reaction secondary to such drugs as acetaminophen; however, it can also be associated with idiosyncratic reactions,

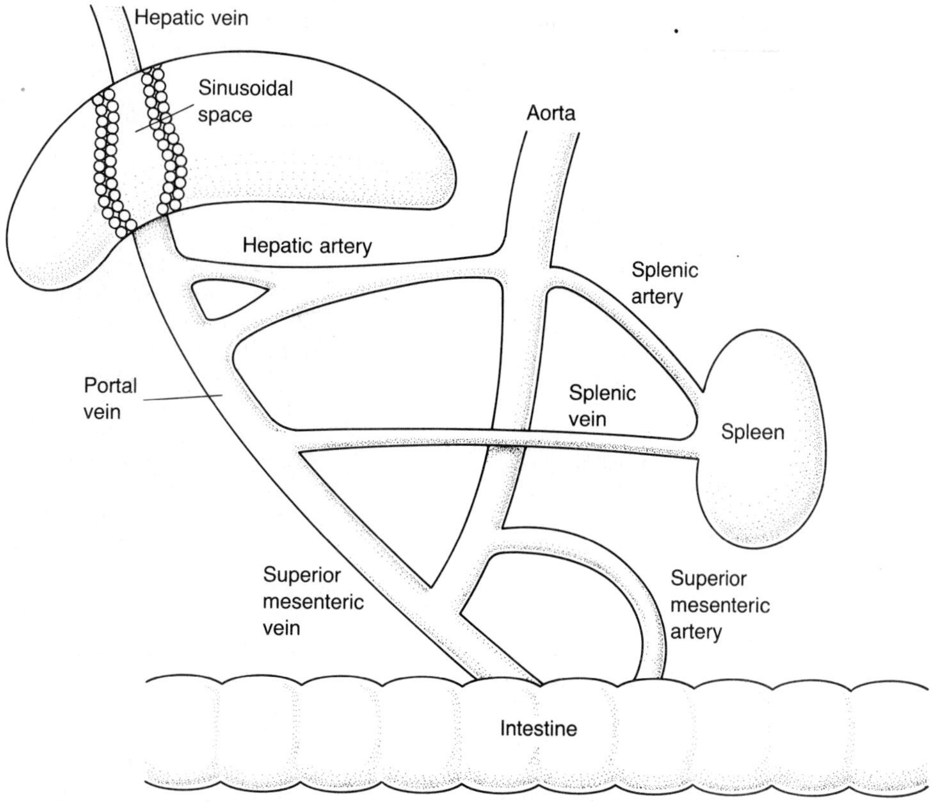


**Figure 32.1** Diagram of hepatic blood flow. The interconnections of the hepatic circulatory system are important in understanding the physiology and pathology of the liver. All substances taken orally pass through the liver via the superior mesenteric vein and hepatic artery. These are low-pressure, low-speed systems that allow for the extraction of substrates from the blood by the hepatocytes.

such as those caused by halothane.[18,19] Also called direct or metabolite-related hepatotoxicity, centrolobular necrosis is usually the result of the production of a toxic metabolite. The process whereby a nontoxic parent compound is converted into a toxic metabolite is termed *bioactivation*. Bioactivation of hepatically cleared compounds is a very important concept. Drugs cleared by the cytochrome $P_{450}$ system are often associated with a bioactivated toxic process.

When taken in overdose, acetaminophen is bioactivated to a toxic intermediate (Fig. 32.2). When the liver's glutathione stores are depleted and there are no longer sulfhydryl groups available to detoxify this metabolite, it begins to react directly within the hepatocyte.[20,21] This process can be accelerated by the induction of hepatic metabolism. Alcoholics commonly have an induced microsomal enzyme system and are much more susceptible to acetaminophen toxicity.[22,23] Theoretically, other inducers of hepatic metabolism might also predispose a patient to acetaminophen toxicity. Phenobarbital, for example, increases the clearance of acetaminophen by 69% and could increase the likelihood of acetaminophen toxicity.[24] Acetaminophen also illustrates how hepatic lesions often become symptomatic late in the process of the disease. Classically, acetaminophen's toxicity is thought to occur in four stages.[20,21] During the first hours after ingestion some patients report mild symptoms of nausea and vomiting, but no elevations of the commonly measured liver enzymes are observed. Not until 40 to 50 hours after ingestion does the pattern of centrolobular necrosis cause elevations in the liver enzymes. Recent investigations have shown that glutathione-*S*-transferase does show elevations very early, but is not commonly determined by most laboratories.[20,21,25]

To avoid the hepatic damage caused by the bioactivation of acetaminophen, acetylcysteine is often given orally to patients who have overdosed. The usual dose is 140 mg/kg body weight every 4 to 6 hours for 48 to 72 hours. Acetylcysteine does not reverse damage that has already occurred; it provides additional sulfhydryl groups to replace the spent stores of glutathione. These sulfhydryl groups are then available for conjugation of the toxic metabolite produced by the cytochrome $P_{450}$ system.[20,21]

Halothane produces centrolobular necrosis in patients who have been exposed to the drug more than once. There is no dose–response relationship associated with halothane exposure, but there is a correlation between the extent of liver damage and the number of times the patient has been anesthetized with halothane.[19] The overall incidence of

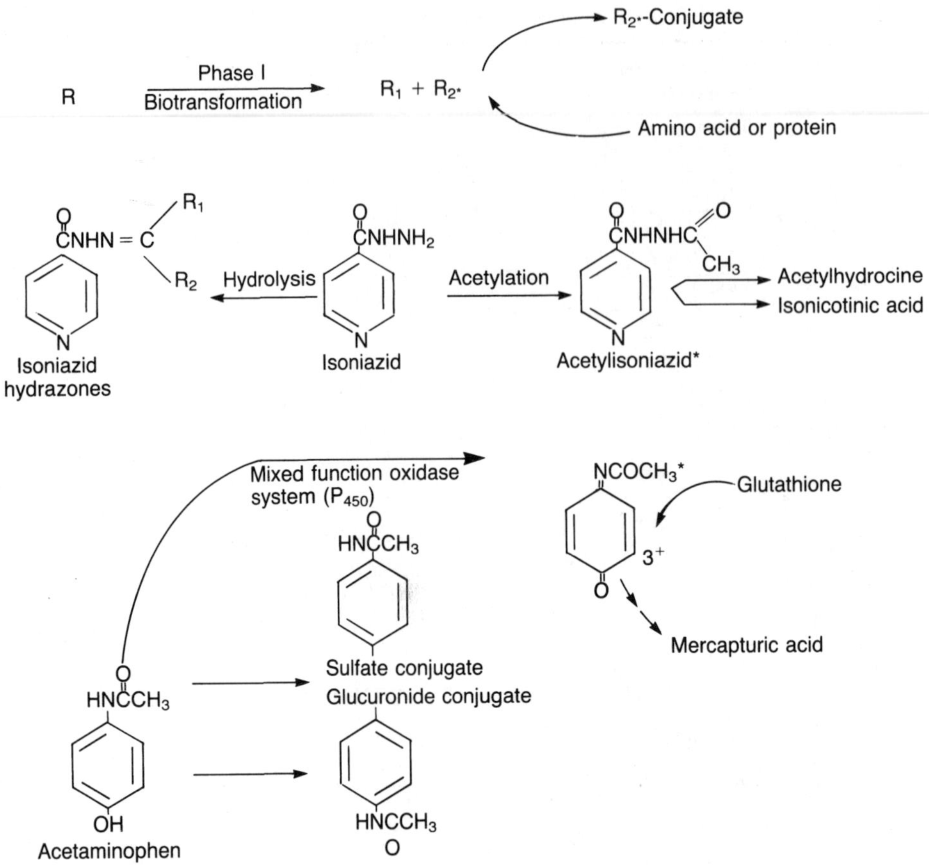


**Figure 32.2** Bioactivation. Usually during a phase I reaction, a drug (R) is converted to an intermediate compound that is intrinsically toxic to the hepatocyte or the canaliculi. Isoniazid is thought to be activated by acetylation, acetaminophen by the mixed-function oxidase system (cytochrome $P_{450}$).

halothane-induced hepatic disease has been estimated at one in several thousand.[26] Halothane is metabolized by both oxidative and reductive pathways. Trifluoroacetic acid is its major oxidative metabolite; the products of reduction include several chlorinated ethylenes and trifluorocarbene.[27] Along with these identifiable compounds, several intermediates may also be produced, including a reactive metabolite that can bind to macromolecules in the hepatocyte and cause disruption of the normal metabolic processes.[28]

Patients suffering from centrolobular necrosis tend to present in one of two ways depending on the extent of necrosis. Mild drug reactions, involving only small amounts of parenchymal tissue, may be detected as asymptomatic elevations in the serum transaminases. When the reaction is diagnosed at this stage, most patients recover with minimal cirrhosis and thus minimal chronic liver impairment. More severe forms of centrolobular necrosis are usually accompanied by nausea, vomiting, upper abdominal pain, and jaundice. These patients can progress rapidly into both complete hepatic and renal failure and require intensive supportive care.[21] Those who survive this initial period often go on to develop chronic liver failure secondary to cirrhosis.

### *Steatonecrosis*

Steatonecrosis is the accumulation of large amounts of microvesicular fat within the hepatocyte. Drugs or their metabolites that cause steatonecrosis do so by affecting fatty acid oxidation within the mitochondria of the hepatocyte. Hepatic vesicles become engorged with fatty acids, eventually disrupting the homeostasis of the hepatocyte. Alcohol is the most common of all drugs that produce steatonecrotic changes in the liver. When alcohol is converted into acetaldehyde the synthesis of fatty acids is increased.[29] When the hepatocyte has become completely engorged with microvesicular fat it often breaks open, spilling its contents into the blood. If enough hepatocytes break open, an inflammatory response is induced. If the offending agent is withdrawn before significant numbers of hepatocytes become necrotic, the process is completely reversible without long-term sequelae.[30] From this point of view, steatonecrotic reactions are the most reversible of all drug-induced liver diseases.

Steatonecrosis is often a concentration-related phenomenon. Tetracycline has been shown to produce steatonecrosis and steatosis in vitro and in vivo.[30,31] The lesions are characterized by large vesicles of fat found diffusely through-

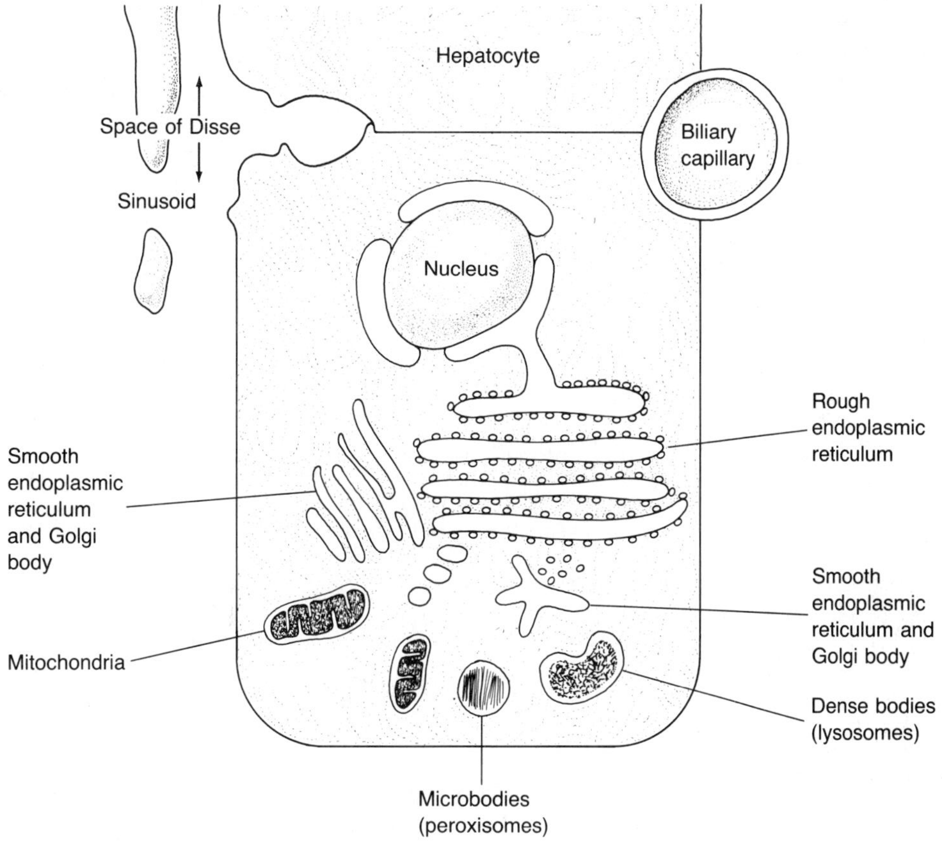


**Figure 32.3** A typical hepatocyte is in constant contact with the hepatic blood, another hepatocyte, and a biliary capillary. There always are large amounts of endoplasmic reticulum, along with many mitochondria and microbodies, in each hepatocyte.

out the liver. This is typical of most steatonecrotic drug reactions in the liver. The development of this reaction is thought to be related to the high concentrations achieved when tetracycline is given intravenously and in doses greater than 1.5 g/d.[32,33] One of the first reports of this reaction related the fatal outcome of several patients given tetracycline intravenously to treat pelvic inflammatory disease.[32] The mortality of tetracycline steatonecrosis is very high (70%–80%) and those who do survive often develop cirrhosis.

Valproic acid can also produce steatonecrosis through the process of bioactivation. Cytochrome $P_{450}$ converts valproic acid to $\Delta^4$-valproic acid. $\Delta^4$-Valproic acid is a potent inducer of microvesicular fat accumulation.[6,34] Estimates of the incidence of this reaction range from 1 in 500 to 1 in 37,000 depending on age and concomitant therapy.[34–36] Phenobarbital, as stated earlier, can induce the cytochrome $P_{450}$ system and has been shown to increase $\Delta^4$-valproic acid production.[6] Caution is therefore appropriate when the two drugs are given together to control epilepsy.

Patients experiencing steatonecrosis may present with hepatomegaly as their only complaint. This is particularly true in cases of mild steatonecrosis. Patients with more severe steatonecrosis present with all the symptoms characteristic of alcoholic hepatitis. With discontinuance of the offending agent, most of these patients heal with only moderate cirrhosis.

Phospholipidosis is similar to steatonecrosis except that it is the accumulation of phospholipids rather than fatty acids. The phospholipids usually engorge the lysosomal bodies of the hepatocyte.[37] Amiodarone has been documented to cause this reaction. Amiodarone and its major metabolite *N*-desethylamiodarone remain in the liver for several months, even after therapy is discontinued. Usually the phospholipidosis develops in patients who have been treated for more than a year. The patient can present with either elevated transaminases or hepatomegaly; jaundice is rare.[38–40]

### *Toxic Hepatitis*

Drug-induced or toxic hepatitis resembles acute viral hepatitis. The onset of symptoms is usually delayed as much as a week or more. Bioactivation is often important for toxic hepatitis to develop, but may not be the immediate cause of damage. Many of the drugs associated with toxic hepatitis produce metabolites that are not inherently toxic to the liver. They may, however, act as haptens, binding to specific cell proteins and inducing an autoimmune reaction.[41,42] Halothane produces centrolobular necrosis in some patients as described earlier and toxic hepatitis in others. Eosinophilia

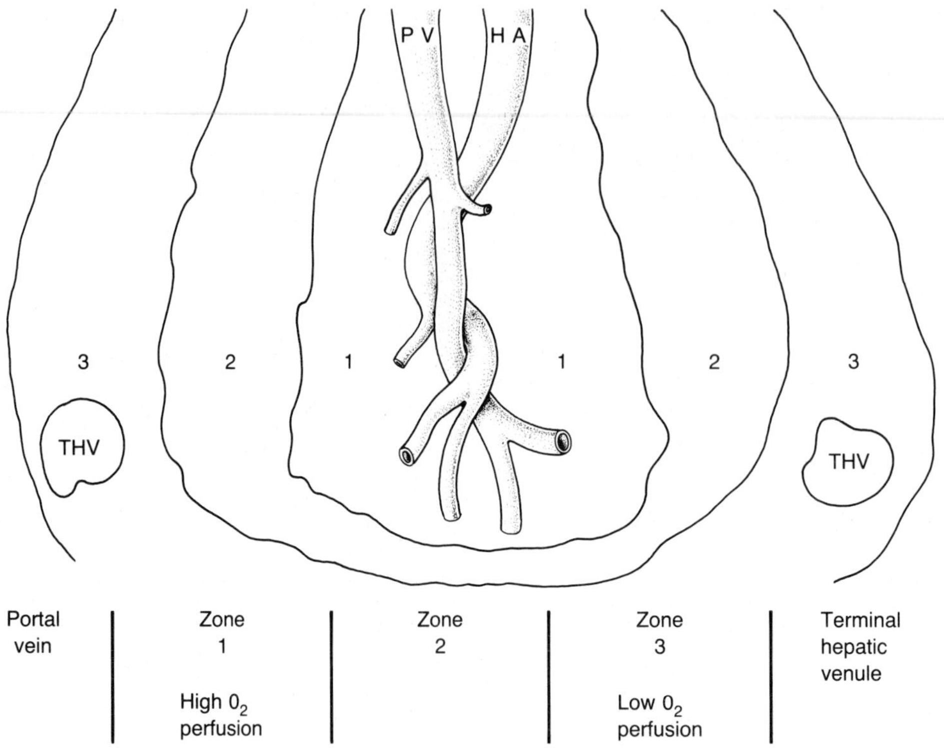


**Figure 32.4** Acinar zones. These zones develop because of the relative oxygenation of the hepatocyte. They are useful in that the location histologically of a hepatotoxic lesion gives a clue to the underlying mechanism of toxicity.

and fever are common in these patients.[43,44] Methyldopa has also been shown to cause toxic hepatitis through the production of a methyldopa–antigen complex.[41] Methyldopa can also induce a lupuslike autoimmune reaction that develops into chronic active hepatitis.[41] These anti-organelle antibodies have now been identified for many drugs associated with toxic hepatitis, including nitrofurantoin.[42]

Isoniazid produces a pattern of hepatocellular necrosis in affected patients that is almost identical to viral hepatitis.[10,45] The long-term administration of isoniazid can lead to some type of hepatic dysfunction in 10% to 20% of those receiving the drug. Severe toxic hepatitis, however, usually develops in only 1% or less of this population.[46–49] Although the exact mechanism is still controversial, patients who are rapid acetylators are believed to have a greater susceptibility. Isoniazid is metabolized by several pathways, acetylation being the major pathway. It is acetylated to acetylisoniazid, which is in turn hydrolyzed to acetylhydrazine. The acetylhydrazine and, to a lesser extent, the acetylisoniazid are directly toxic to the cellular proteins in the hepatocyte.[47,48] The role of acetylator phenotype is even more complex, as studies have shown that rapid acetylators also detoxify acetylhydrazine very rapidly, converting it to diacetylhydrazine.[48] It may be that the relative rates of reaction and affinities of the various pathways actually determine susceptibility to hepatotoxicity.

Acetylator phenotype can be determined prior to the initiation of therapy, but this is seldom done in clinical practice because of the amount of time required and the costs involved. Most methods require the administration of a small dose of another acetylated compound and the determination of serial blood levels. Sulfadimidine is given in doses of 1 g; urine is then collected over an 8-hour period. This method was first introduced in 1939 and is still used in studies of acetylator phenotype today.[50,51] Another method involves the administration of dapsone 5 mg/kg to fasting subjects; blood samples are then drawn at 0, 2, 3, 4, and 5 hours and a half-life is calculated from the data. Rapid acetylators tend to have a half-life less than 2 hours.[52] Alternatively, a blood sample taken 3 hours after a dose of 100 mg dapsone can be assayed for the content of both dapsone and monoacetyldapsone in the blood. Rapid acetylators should have a calculated ratio of monoacetylated dapsone to dapsone greater than or equal to 70%; slow acetylators have values less than or equal to 26%.[53] These methods are contraindicated in persons with hypersensitivity to sulfonamides or sulfones.

**Table 32.2** Types of Cirrhosis[a]

| |
|---|
| Micronodular cirrhosis |
| Macronodular cirrhosis |
| Congestive cirrhosis |
| Biliary cirrhosis |

[a] Cirrhosis, although always a result of the deposition of fibrous tissue, can be subdivided based on the results of a liver biopsy.

Acetylsalicylic acid has also been reported to cause toxic hepatitis in patients taking high doses of the drug. The incidence of this reaction in patients taking more than 2 g of aspirin on a daily basis is high.[54–56] Elevated transaminases are noted in between 20% and 60% of patients in this group. Severe hepatotoxicity is rarer and may have some relationship to serum concentrations greater than 25 mg/dL.[55,56] These patients may go on to develop chronic active hepatitis after the initial insult.

Ketoconazole produces toxic hepatitis or milder forms of hepatic dysfunction in 1% to 2% of patients treated for fungal infections.[57,58] This reaction has been reported to be fatal in many patients. The onset is usually early in therapy, although it can be delayed until several months into therapy. As the relative risk associated with most fungal infections is quite low, the hepatotoxic potential of ketoconazole has relegated it to the level of secondary therapy in most cases.

Chronic active hepatitis is a sequela to the development of toxic hepatitis.[59] It is a progressive necroinflammatory disease that carries a very high mortality rate if not aggressively treated. Methyldopa, isoniazid, nitrofurantoin, and dantrolene have all been associated with its development.[59–61] It is more common in females than males and is characterized by high levels of autoimmune antibodies.[59] Treatment includes the use of such immunosuppressants as prednisone and azathioprine usually in low doses for several months.[59,61]

### *Hypersensitivity Reactions*

Allergic reactions in the liver may manifest as either hepatocellular or cholestatic patterns of injury. Additionally, patients may present with a mixed pattern of both cholestatic and hepatocellular lesions. The sulfonamides, including trimethoprim–sulfamethoxazole, induced in a small number of patients a reaction typical of hepatic hypersensitivity.[62–64] The reaction usually develops within 4 weeks of the start of therapy. It is marked by fever rash, eosinophilia, arthritis, and hemolytic anemia. Formation of granulomas within the liver is often observed on biopsy.[65] The reaction reverses with discontinuation of therapy and reappears upon rechallenge. Many of the other anti-infectives—penicillin, cloxacillin, oxacillin, nitrofurantoin, and erythromycin base—have been associated with this type of reaction.[65–69] The incidence of an allergic liver reaction is low, but fatal in some cases.[65]

Erythromycin and troleandomycin are associated with a classic idiosyncratic hypersensitivity reaction marked by a diffuse rash, pruritus, abdominal pain, and eosinophilia.[69] Granulomas are often seen on biopsy. The incidence of this reaction has been estimated to be 1% to 2% of patients treated with erythromycin.[70] The two macrolide antibiotics produce nitrosoalkanes when metabolized by cytochrome $P_{450}$. Nitrosoalkanes react readily with sulfhydryl groups within the hepatocyte. It is theorized that when enough hepatocytes are damaged by this reaction, there is a release of hepatic intracellular protein that stimulates an allergic reaction within the liver.[70]

Allopurinol has also been associated with a number of reports of hypersensitivity reactions which are classified by the area of the bile canalicular or ductal system that is impaired.[71–73] Canalicular cholestasis is very often associated with long-term estrogen therapy. A significant decrease in bile flow without secondary inflammation is usually seen.[74,75] The actual incidence is very low and decreases as the proportion of estrogen in oral contraceptives decreases. Clinically, these patients present with mild to moderate elevations of serum bilirubin which is often asymptomatic. Androgens are also at times associated with canalicular cholestasis.

α-Tocopherol acetate, an intravenous form of vitamin E, has been noted to cause cholestatic jaundice, involving primarily the canaliculi, in premature infants. The children were being treated with the drug to avoid hemolytic anemia secondary to the vitamin E deficiency often seen in premature infants.[76,77] The incidence of this reaction in this group was very high (greater than 10%) and the mortality, even higher (greater than 50%). The drug was withdrawn from the market because of this problem.

Hepatocellular cholestasis is a much more serious form of cholestatic jaundice in which both parenchyma and bile canalicular cells are involved. Chlorpromazine is the most frequently cited cause of hepatocellular cholestatic jaundice. The reaction occurs in about 1% of all patients treated with the drug.[78] Chlorpromazine has been shown to precipitate bile salts and to decrease total bile flow.[79,80] The reaction typically begins in the first 4 weeks of therapy, but may be delayed several months.[78] The administration of total parenteral nutrition induces cholestatic changes and nonspecific enzyme elevations in as many as 80% of all patients treated, although the exact incidence is probably only around 25%.[81] Patients with low serum albumin concentrations may be at a greater risk than patients with normal serum albumin concentrations.[82] It has also been suggested that aluminum deposition may play a role.[83] This reaction has also been reported to occur rarely with sulfonamides, sulfonylureas, erythromycin estolate and ethyl succinate, captopril, and other phenothiazines.[84–89]

Ductular cholestasis is the least often reported form of cholestatic jaundice. This reaction is similar to canalicular cholestasis in that no inflammation is usually seen. The bile ducts and, to a lesser degree, the canaliculi become plugged with very dense bile casts. The anti-inflammatory agent benoxaprofen is associated with the development of ductular cholestasis. Concurrent renal failure was seen in all cases.[90] Because of this reaction benoxaprofen was withdrawn from the market soon after its introduction.

### *Liver Vascular Disorders*

Focal lesions in hepatic venules, sinusoids, and portal veins have been observed in response to various drugs. The most commonly associated drugs are the cytotoxic agents used to treat cancer, the pyrrolizidine alkaloids, and the sex hormones.[91–95] Veno-occlusive disease is a phlebitis of the central veins in the liver. A centralized necrosis often follows and can result in cirrhosis, usually with a significant amount of concurrent congestion.[92,96] Azathioprine and herbal teas that contain comfrey (a source of pyrrolizidine alkaloids) have been associated with the development of veno-occlusive disease.[93,94] The exact incidence is rare and may, in the case of the pyrrolizidine alkaloids, be dose related.[94]

Peliosis hepatitis is an unusual type of hepatic lesion that can be seen as both an acute and a chronic disease. The liver develops large, blood-filled lacunae within the paren-

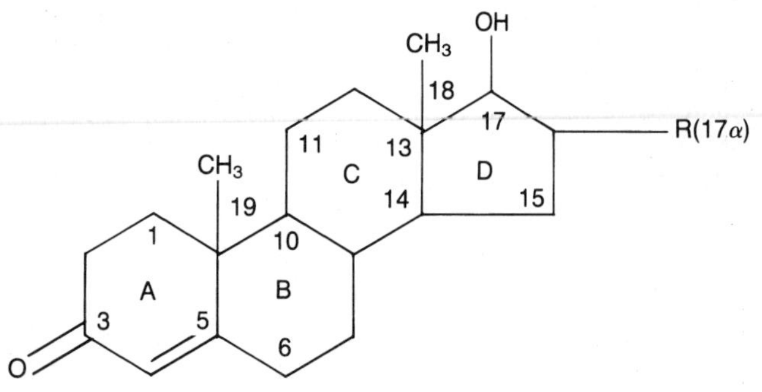


**Figure 32.5** 17α-Testosterone is the most frequently reported cause of the vascular disorder peliosis hepatitis.

chyma.[95,97] Rupture of these lacunae can lead to severe peritoneal hemorrhage. Peliosis hepatitis has been associated with exposure of the liver to androgens, estrogens, tamoxifen, azathioprine, and danazol.[93,98–100] Androgens with a 17α-testosterone structure (Fig. 32.5) are the agents most frequently reported to cause peliosis hepatitis, usually after at least 6 months of therapy. The actual incidence of this reaction is rare; fewer than 25 cases have been reported in the literature in the last 40 years.[101]

### *Cirrhosis*

The deposition of fibrotic tissue and the secondary development of cirrhosis are usually sequelae to a primarily necrotic or cholestatic lesion, but sometimes can be the dominant presenting features of a hepatotoxic reaction. Methotrexate causes periportal fibrosis in a significant number of patients. The lesion results from the action of a bioactivated metabolite produced by cytochrome $P_{450}$.[102,103] This process has most commonly been noted in patients being treated for psoriasis.[102–105] The extent of damage can be reduced or controlled by increasing the dosage interval to a week.[104,105] The addition of leucovorin to the regimen also decreases the rate of fibrosis.[105] Leucovorin is a completely reduced form of folic acid. It is able to act in metabolic reactions without being first reduced by dihydroreductase, the enzyme inhibited by methotrexate. Cells treated with leucovorin may be more resistant to the deteriorating effect of methotrexate. Vitamin A is normally stored in the space of Disse, specifically in Ito cells, and can cause significant hypertrophy and fibrosis when high doses are taken for long periods. Hepatomegaly is a common finding along with other signs of advanced liver disease including ascites and portal hypertension. In patients with vitamin A toxicity, gingivitis and dry skin are also very common.[106] Tragically, patients who develop this hepatotoxic reaction are often extremely interested in their own health and have taken megavitamins to become healthier.

### *Neoplastic Disease*

A large portion of the current literature on adverse reactions and the liver addresses the development of neoplasms after drug therapy. Both carcinoma- and sarcoma-like lesions have been identified. Fortunately, hepatic tumors associated with drug therapy are usually benign and remit when drug therapy is discontinued. Except in rare instances, these lesions are associated with long-term exposure to the offending agent.[5,101]

## Monitoring for Hepatoxicity

Often, no good clinical test is available to determine exactly the type of hepatic lesion, short of biopsy; however, certain patterns of enzyme elevation have been identified and can be helpful (Table 32.3).[107] These enzymes are also useful in monitoring patients on certain potentially hepatotoxic drugs. The specificity of any serum enzyme depends on the distribution of that enzyme in the body. Alkaline phosphatase is usually found in the bile duct epithelium, but it is also found in bone, intestinal, and kidney cells. Alkaline phosphatase, therefore, although indicative of cholestatic disease is not absolutely specific for cholestatic disease.[108] 5′-Nucleotidase is more specific for hepatic disease than alkaline phosphatase, as most of the body's 5′-nucleotidase is stored in the liver. This rule of specificity also holds true within the liver. Glutamate dehydrogenase is a very good indicator of centrolobular necrosis, as it is found primarily in centrolobularly located mitochondria. The sensitivity of serum enzymes as indicators of organ damage depends on the relative concentration and rate of production of the enzyme within the cell. Most hepatic cells have extremely high concentrations of transaminases. Aspartate transaminase (AST or SGOT) and alanine transaminase (ALT or SGPT) are commonly measured. Because of their high concentrations and easy liberation from the hepatocyte cytoplasm, AST and ALT are very sensitive indicators of necrotic lesions within the liver. Once an acute hepatic lesion has begun to develop, it may take weeks to months for these tests to return to normal. An abrupt fall in concentration may indicate the total destruction of the hepatic parenchyma.

Thus, except for serum bilirubin, liver enzymes commonly available to the clinician often have little prognostic value. The serum bilirubin concentration, although nondiscriminatory between types of hepatic dysfunction, can have prognostic value in some disease states.[108] For example, patients with halothane hepatitis have an increased mortality rate when the serum bilirubin concentration is greater than 10 mg/dL.[107,108] The breakdown product of porphyrin, myoglobin, and various cytochromes, bilirubin is actively taken into the hepatic cells, conjugated with glucuronic acid, and excreted into the bile. In the intestine bilirubin is converted to several compounds through the action of bacteria. These urobilinogens are then reabsorbed and excreted via the kidney. When the hepatic production of conjugated bilirubin decreases there is a proportional decrease in the amount of urobilinogen excreted in the urine. Antibiotics, however, can also cause a decrease in urine urobilinogen.[108]

The relative amounts of conjugated (direct) versus unconjugated (indirect) bilirubin are at times useful in differentiating a cholestatic hepatic lesion from an extrahepatic disease or a parenchymal hepatic lesion (Table 32.4). The direct (conjugated) bilirubin would be expected to increase whenever there was a decrease in bile flow. The total bilirubin

**Table 32.3** Patterns of Hepatic Enzyme Elevation Versus Types of Hepatic Lesion[a]

| | Type of lesion | | |
|---|---|---|---|
| *Enzyme* | **Cholestatic** | **Necrotic** | **Chronic** |
| Alkaline phosphatase | XX[b] | X | X |
| 5′-Nucleotidase | XX | X | X |
| γ-Glutamyltransferase (GGTP) | XX | X | X |
| Leucine aminopeptidase | XX | X | X |
| Aspartate transaminase (AST or SGOT) | X | XX | X |
| Alanine transaminase (ALT or SGPT) | X | XX | X |
| Glutamate–oxalate transferase | X | XX | X |
| Malate dehydrogenase | X | XX | X |
| Lactose dehydrogenase (LDH) | X | XX | X |
| Cholinesterase | 0 | −0 | −0 |

[a] Elevations of certain enzymes are characteristic of certain types of liver damage. Transaminases and dehydrogenases, which are cytoplasmic enzymes in the hepatocyte, are much more sensitive to acute parenchymal cell damage. Alkaline phosphatase and the others are found in the canalicular cells and are more sensitive to cholestatic disease. As either disease progresses to a chronic state, however, these differences in sensitivity are less important.

[b] 0, no change; −0, a decrease from the normal range; X, an increase from the normal range; XX, an increase of two or more times the normal range.

would be expected to increase whenever there was a large decrease in the ability of the liver to process bilirubin.

Bilirubin concentrations and serum enzyme elevations give a static picture of the liver's condition; they do not indicate hepatic function. The most widely available tests that indicate hepatic function are the serum proteins and the prothrombin time. As hepatic parenchymal function decreases, serum protein concentrations in the body decrease at a rate determined by each protein's elimination rate. Overhydration and starvation, however, also decrease serum protein concentrations. Additionally, serum protein concentrations give only a rough estimate of the degree of hepatic dysfunction. The prothrombin time increases in a fashion similar to the decrease in serum proteins. The response of the prothrombin time to the administration of 10 mg vitamin K parenterally is often used to differentiate between hepatocellular and cholestatic disease.

Recently, however, the use of radiolabeled aminopyrine has begun to gain in popularity. The breath test uses $^{14}C$-labeled aminopyrine to measure the capacity of the mixed-function oxidase system via the production of $^{14}CO_2$. Because this test requires fairly sophisticated radiation detection equipment it has not become a widely available clinical test for mixed function oxidase activity.[109] The more traditional tests of hepatic function, such as sulfobromophthalein (BSP) excretion or indocyanine green excretion, measure less exact quantities of hepatic clearance. BSP is injected intravenously, absorbed by parenchymal cells, conjugated to glutathione, and then excreted in the bile. A blood sample is taken 45 minutes after the injection, and the result is reported as percentage of dye retained in the blood. BSP is very irritating at the injection site and has rarely been associated with anaphylactic reactions. Indocyanine green follows a similar pathway with the exception of conjugation and is also expressed as percentage of dye retained. Indocyanine green clearance is used in comparative studies of highly extractable, hepatically cleared drugs to measure changes in hepatic blood flow.[110] Hepatobiliary scanning using technetium-99*m*–labeled carriers can also be useful in quantifying the location and extent of obstruction or damage.[108] The use of more sensitive assays such as glutathione-*S*-transferase has also been advocated in particular cases when sensitive early markers of intrinsic damage are needed.[25] In cases of idiosyncratic hypersensitivity reactions a macrophage inhibition test can be useful in predicting which drug may have caused the reaction in question.[111]

In deciding which tests to use in monitoring a patient placed on a hepatotoxic drug, it is important to distinguish the predictable hepatotoxic reaction from the idiosyncratic reaction. Predictable reactions have a high incidence of occurrence and are usually dose related. Reactions to methotrexate and chlorpromazine are examples of predictable hepatotoxic reactions with relatively high incidences of occurrence. Methotrexate, a drug that induces acute parenchymal damage and fibrosis, is best monitored by using

**Table 32.4** Patterns of Bilirubin Elevation[a]

| *Disease* | *Direct bilirubin* | *Indirect bilirubin* | *Urine bilirubin* | *Stool pigments* |
|---|---|---|---|---|
| Hepatocellular | X[b] | X | X | −0 |
| Cholestatic | XX | X | 0 | −0 |
| Hemolysis | 0 | X | 0 | 0 |

[a] The most important use of bilirubin concentration is the differentiation between hepatic disease and extrahepatic disease (usually hemolysis). Extremely high bilirubin concentrations are indicative of a very poor prognosis.

[b] 0, no change from the normal range; −0, a decrease from the normal range; X, an increase from the normal range; XX, an increase of 1.5–2 times the normal range.

measures of acute hepatocellular damage (Table 32.3). The serum transaminases, AST and ALT (SGOT and SGPT), are the measures most commonly used in the clinical setting. Concentrations of these enzymes should be obtained every 2 to 4 weeks depending on the reported characteristics of the reaction in question. Methotrexate, if given weekly to avoid the development of the fibrosis, could be monitored every 4 weeks, as toxicity usually develops over a period of several weeks to months.[104,105] Additionally, some authors recommend that BSP or indocyanine green excretion studies be performed on a regular basis and that patients treated for very long periods of time have a liver biopsy performed every 12 months.[105]

Chlorpromazine, which produces cholestatic lesions, is best monitored with a serum bilirubin concentration and regular determinations of the serum enzymes usually found in high concentrations in the canalicular system (Table 31.3). As the onset of action reported for this reaction occurs in the first 4 weeks of therapy, bilirubin, alkaline phosphatase, and $\gamma$-glutamyltransferase determinations should be obtained every 2 weeks for the first month of therapy and then every month for the next 5 months to pick up the few cases that may be delayed.[78,79]

If a person is in a group at higher risk for the development of a particular reaction the intervals between serum enzyme determinations should be shortened. Isoniazid, for example, carries a greater risk for patients older than 35.[48] Young patients under 14 may also need more intensive monitoring.[49] Isoniazid-induced hepatotoxicity is not a predictable reaction and would not be routinely monitored on a monthly basis, except in these populations. Patients with preexisting liver or kidney disease, in whom even a mild hepatotoxic reaction would have profound negative consequences, should also be more intensely monitored. In patients who are not in high-risk groups or have no preexisting disease, the routine monitoring for idiosyncratic reactions is of little value.

## References


1. Anonymous. Annual survey of births, deaths, marriages and divorces: United States, 1981 Monthly Vital Statistics Report. Washington DC, U.S. Department of Health and Human Services, vol 30, December 1982.
2. Rapport AM. Anatomic considerations, in Schiff L (ed): Diseases of the Liver. Philadelphia, J.B. Lippincott, 1975; pp 1–43.
3. Rowland M, Benet LZ, Graham GG. Clearance concepts of pharmacokinetics. J Pharmacokinet Biopharm 1973;1:123–136.
4. Weibal ER, Staubel W, Enagi HR, et al. Correlated morphometric and biochemical studies on the liver cell. Parts I–II. J Cell Biol 1969;42:68–91.
5. Zimmerman HJ. General considerations, in Zimmerman HJ (ed): Hepatotoxicity, the Adverse Effects of Drugs and Other Chemicals on the Liver. New York, Appleton-Century-Croft, 1978; pp 3–164.
6. Rettie AE, Rettenmeier AW, Howald WN, et al. Cytochrome P-450–catalyzed formation of delta 4-VPA: A toxic metabolite of valproic acid. Science 1987;235:890–893.
7. Recknagel RO, Glende EA Jr. Carbon tetrachloride hepatoxicity: An example of lethal cleavage. CRC Critical Review Toxicol 1973;2:263–297.
8. Forker EL. Mechanisms of hepatic bile formation. Annu Rev Physiol 1977;39:323–347.
9. Kelsey WM, Scharyj M. Fatal hepatitis probably due to indomethacin. JAMA 1967;199:154–155
10. Mitchell JR, Zimmerman HJ, Ishak KG, et al. NIH Conference—Isoniazid liver injury: Clinical spectrum, pathology, and possible pathogenesis. Ann Intern Med 1976;84:181–192.
11. Goldfrank LR, Kristein R, Weisman RS. Acetaminophen, in Goldfrank LR (ed): Toxicologic Emergencies. New York, Appleton-Century-Croft, 1982; pp 49–58.
12. Miller J, Rutherford A. Discussion on atrophy of the liver. Br Med J 1920;2:581–586.
13. Comfort MW, Weir JF. Toxic cirrhosis caused by cincophen. Arch Intern Med 1933;52:685–724.
14. Maddrey WC, Boitnott JK. Drug-induced chronic liver disease. Gastroenterology 1977;72:1348–1353.
15. James OFW. Gastrointestinal and liver function in old age. Clin Gastroenterol 1983;12:671–691.
16. Farah F, Taylor W, Rawlins MD, et al. Hepatic drug acetylation and oxidation—effects of ageing in man. Br Med J 1977;2: 155–156.
17. James OFW. Drugs and the aging liver. J Hepatol 1985;1:431–435.
18. Boyer TD, Rouff SL. Acetaminophen-induced hepatic necrosis and renal failure. JAMA 1971;218:440–441.
19. Trowell J, Peto R, Smith AC. Controlled trial of repeated halothane anaesthetics in patients with carcinoma of the uterine cervix treated with radium. Lancet 1975;2:821–824.
20. Mitchell JR, Thorgiersson SS, Potter WR, et al. Acetaminophen induced hepatic injury: Protective role of glutathione in man and rationale for therapy. Clin Pharmacol Ther 1974;16: 676–684.
21. Black M. Acetaminophen hepatoxicity. Gastroenterology 1980;78:382–392.
22. Seeff LB, Cuccherini BA, Zimmerman HJ, et al. Acetaminophen hepatotoxicity in alcoholics, a therapeutic misadventure. Ann Intern Med 1986;104:399–404.
23. Black M, Raucy J. Acetaminophen, alcohol and cytochrome P-450. Ann Intern Med 1986;104:427–429.
24. Perucca E, Richens A. Paracetamol disposition in normal subjects and in patients treated with antiepileptic drugs. Br J Clin Pharmacol 1979;7:201–206.
25. Beckett GJ, Chapman BJ, Dyson EH, et al. Plasma glutathione-*S*-transferase measurements after paracetamol overdose: Evidence for early hepatocellular damage. Gut 1985;26: 26–31.
26. Timbrell JA. Drug hepatotoxicity. Br J Clin Pharmacol 1983;15:3–14.
27. Maiorino RM, Sipes IG, Gandolf AJ, et al. Quantitative analysis of volatile halothane metabolites in biological tissues by gas chromatography. J Chromatogr 1979;164:63–72.
28. DeGroot H, Noll TL. Halothane hepatotoxicity: Relation between metabolic activation, hypoxia, covalent binding, lipid peroxidation and liver cell damage. Hepatology 1983;3:601–606.
29. Rubin E, Cederbaum AT. Organelle pathology of alcohol-induced hepatic injury, in Fischer MM, Rankin JG (eds): Alcohol and the Liver. New York, Plenum, 1977; pp 167–193.

30. Galambos JT. Alcoholic hepatitis, in Schaffner F, Sherlock S, Leevy CM (eds): The Liver and Its Diseases. New York, Intercontinental Medical Book, 1974; pp 225–267.
31. Zuckerman AJ, Baker SF, Dunkley LJ. The effect of tetracycline on human liver cells in culture. Br J Exp Pathol 1968;49: 20–23.
32. Schultz JC, Adamson JS, Workman WW, et al. Fatal liver disease after intravenous administration of tetracycline in high dosage. N Engl J Med 1963;269:999–1004.
33. Breen KJ, Schenker S, Heimberg M. Fatty liver induced by tetracycline in the rat: Dose–response relationship and effect of sex. Gastroenterology 1975;69:714–723.
34. Bhagwat AG, Warren RE. Hepatic reaction to nitrofurantoin. Lancet 1969;2:1369.
35. Itoh S, Yamaba Y, Matuso S, et al. Sodium valproate-induced liver injury. Am J Gastroenterol 1982;77:875–879.
36. Zimmerman HJ, Ishak KG. Valproate-induced hepatic injury: Analysis of 3 fatal cases. Hepatology 1982;2:591–597.
37. Lullman H, Lullman R, Wasserman O. Drug-induced phospholipidosis. II. Tissue distribution of the amphiphilic drug chlorphentermine. CRC Crit Drug Rev Toxicol 1975;4:185–218.
38. Tordjman K, Klatz I, Bursztyn M, et al. Amiodarone and the liver. Ann Intern Med 1985;98:411–412.
39. Rigas B, Rosenfield LE, Barwick KW, et al. Amiodarone hepatotoxicity. A clinicopathologic study of five patients. Ann Intern Med 1986;104:348–351.
40. Pourcell S, Ireton J, Valencia-Mayoral P, et al. Amiodarone-associated phospholipidosis of the liver: Light, immunohistochemical and electron microscopic studies. Gastroenterology 1984;86:926–936.
41. Neuberger J, Kenna JG, NouriAria K, et al. Antibody mediated hepatocyte injury in methyldopa-induced hepatotoxicity. Gut 1985;26:1233–1239.
42. MacKay IR. Induction by drugs of hepatitis and autoantibodies to cell organelles: Significance and interpretation. Hepatology 1985;5:904–906.
43. Brown BR Jr. Halothane hepatitis revisited. N Engl J Med 1985;313:1347–1348.
44. Zarday Z, Rosenthal WS, Wolff FW. Severe liver toxicity after methyldopa. NY State J Med 1967;67:1897–1899.
45. Black M, Mitchell JR, Zimmerman HJ. Drug-induced chronic liver disease. Gastroenterology 1977;72:1348–1353.
46. Black M, Mitchell JR, Zimmerman HJ, et al. Isoniazid associated hepatitis in 114 patients. Gastroenterology 1975;69:289–302.
47. Maddrey WC. Isoniazid-induced liver disease. Semin Liver Dis 1981;1:129–131.
48. Mitchell JR, Zimmerman HJ, Ishak KG, et al. Isoniazid liver injury clinical spectrum, pathology and probable pathogenesis. Ann Intern Med 1976;84:181–192.
49. Tsagaropolou-Stinga H, Mataki-Emmanou I, et al. Hepatotoxic reactions in children with severe tuberculosis treated with isoniazid–rifampin. Pediatr Infect Dis 1985;4:270–273.
50. Bratton AC, Marshall EK Jr. A new coupling component for sulfadimidine determination. J Biol Chem 1939;128:537–550.
51. Ylitalo P, Rousteenoja R, LesKinen O, et al. Significance of acetylator phenotype in pharmacokinetics and adverse effects of procainamide. Eur J Clin Pharmacol 1983;25:791–795.
52. Kergueris MF, Bourin M, Larousse C. Pharmacokinetics of isoniazid: Influence of age. Eur J Clin Pharmacol 1986;30:335–340.
53. Reidenberg MM, Drayer DE, Levy M, et al. Polymorphic acetylation of procainamide in man. Clin Pharmacol Ther 1975;17:722–730.
54. O'Gorman T, Koff RS. Salicylate hepatitis. Gastroenterology 1977;72:726–731.
55. Miller JJ, Weissman DB. Correlations between transaminase concentrations and serum salicylate concentrations in juvenile rheumatoid arthritis. Arthritis Rheumatol 1976;19:115–118.
56. Zimmerman HJ. Effects of aspirin and acetaminophen on the liver. Arch Intern Med 1981;141:333–342.
57. Heiberg JK, Svejgaard E. Toxic hepatitis during ketoconazole treatment. Br Med J 1981;283:825–826.
58. Lewis JH, Zimmerman HJ, Benson GD, et al. Hepatic injury associated with ketoconazole therapy: Analysis of 33 cases. Gastroenterology 1984;86:503–513.
59. Zimmerman HJ. Drug-induced chronic active hepatic disease. Med Clin North Am 1979;63:567–582.
60. Reynolds TB, Peters RL, Yamada S. Chronic active and lipoid hepatitis caused by a laxative, oxphenisatin. N Engl J Med 1971;285:813–820.
61. Maddrey WC, Boitwott JK. Drug-induced chronic liver disease. Gastroenterology 1977;72:1348–1353.
62. Nair SS, Kaplan JM, Levine LH, et al. Trimethoprim–sulfamethoxazole-induced intrahepatic cholestasis. Ann Intern Med 1980;92:511–512.
63. Dujovne CA, Chan CH, Zimmerman HJ. Sulfonamide hepatic injury. N Engl J Med 1967;277:785–788.
64. Ransohoff DF, Jacobs G. Terminal hepatic failure following a small dose of sulfamethoxazole–trimethoprim. Gastroenterology 1981;80:816–819.
65. Sippel PJ, Agger WA. Nitrofurantoin-induced granulomatous hepatitis. Urology 1981;18:177–178.
66. Valdiva-Barriga V, Feldman A, Orellana J. Generalized hypersensitivity with hepatitis and jaundice after the use of penicillin and streptomycin. Gastroenterology 1963;45:114–117.
67. Reynolds ES, Schlant RC, Gonick HC, et al. Fatal massive necrosis of the liver as a manifestation of hypersensitivity to probenicid. N Engl J Med 1957;256;592–596.
68. Keeffe EB, Reis TC, Berland JE. Hepatotoxicity to both erythromycin estolate and erythromycin ethylsuccinate. Dig Dis Sci 1982;27:701–704.
69. Zafrani ES, Ishak KG, Rudzki C. Cholestatic and hepatocellular injury associated with erythromycin esters: Report of nine cases. Dig Dis Sci 1979;24:385–396.
70. Pessayre D, Larrey D, Funck-Bretano A, et al. Drug interactions and hepatitis produced by some macrolide antibiotics. J Antimicrob Chemother 1985;16:181–192.
71. Simmons F, Feldman B, Gerety D. Granulomatous hepatitis in a patient receiving allopurinol. Gastroenterology 1972;62:101–103.
72. Vanderstigel M, Zafrani ES, Deyone JL, et al. Allopurinol hypersensitivity syndrome as a cause of hepatic fibrin ring granulomas. Gastroenterology 1986;90:188–190.
73. Al-Kawas FH, Seeff LB, Berendson RA, et al. Allopurinol hepatotoxicity. Report of two cases and review of the literature. Ann Intern Med 1981;95:588–590.
74. Kern F, Erfling W, Simon FR, et al. Effect of estrogens on the liver. Gastroenterology 1978;75:512–522.
75. Boelsterli UA, Rakhit G, Balazas T. Modulation of *S*-adenosyl-L-methionate, hepatic $Na^+$,$K^+$-ATPase, membrane fluidity and bile flow in rats with ethinyl estradiol–induced cholestasis. Hepatology 1983;3:12–17.
76. Finer NM, Peters KL, Hayek Z, et al. Vitamin E and necrotizing enterocolitis. Pediatrics 1984;73:387–392.
77. Lorch V, Murphy D, Hoersten L, et al. Unusual syndrome among premature infants associated with a new intravenous vitamin E product. Pediatrics 1985;75:598–601.
78. Ishak KG, Irey NS. Hepatic injury associated with the pheno-

thiazines. Clinicopathological follow-up study of 36 patients. Arch Pathol 1972;93:283–304.
**79.** Carey MC, Hiram PC, Small DM. A study of physiochemical interactions between biliary lipids and chlorpromazine-HCl. Biochem J 1976;153:519–531.
**80.** Walker CO, Combes B. Biliary cirrhosis induced by chlorpromazine. Gastroenterology 1966;51:631–640.
**81.** Bowyer BA, Fleming CR, Ludwig J, et al. Does long term home parenteral nutrition in adult patients cause chronic liver disease? J Parenter Enter Nutr 1985;9:11.
**82.** Nanji AA, Anderson FH. Relationship between serum albumin and parenteral nutrition–associated cholestasis. J Parenter Enter Nutr 1984;8:438.
**83.** Klein GL, Berquist WE, Ament ME, et al. Hepatic aluminum accumulation in children on total parenteral nutrition. J Pediatr Gastroenterol Nutr 1984;3:740.
**84.** Reichel J, Goldberg SB, Ellenberg M, et al. Intrahepatic cholestasis following administration of chlorpropamide. Report of a case with electron microscopic observations. Am J Med 1960;28:654–660.
**85.** Gilbert FI. Cholestatic hepatitis caused by esters of erythromycin and oleandomycin. JAMA 1962;182:1048–1050.
**86.** Bachman BA, Boyd WP, Brady PG. Erythromycin ethylsuccinate–induced cholestasis. Am J Gastroenterol 1982;77:397–400.
**87.** Johnson DF, Hall WH. Allergic hepatitis caused by the propionyl erythromycin ester of lauryl sulfate. N Engl J Med 1961;265:1200–1202.
**88.** Rahmat J, Gelfand RL, Gelfand MC, et al. Captopril-associated cholestatic jaundice. Ann Intern Med 1985;102:56–58.
**89.** Reichel J, Goldberg SB, Ellenberg M, et al. Intrahepatic cholestasis following administration of chlorpropamide. Am J Med 1960;28:654–660.
**90.** Taggart HMA, Alderdice JM. Fatal cholestatic jaundice in elderly patients taking benoxaprofen. Br Med J 1982;284:1372.
**91.** Krivoy N, Raz R, Carter A, et al. Reversible hepatic veno-occlusive disease and 6-thioguanine. Ann Intern Med 1982;96:788.
**92.** Zafrani ES, Pinandeau Y, Dhumeaux D. Drug-induced vascular lesions of the liver. Arch Intern Med 1983;143:495–502.
**93.** Gerlag PGG, Lobatto S, Drissen WMM, et al. Hepatic sinusoidal dilatation with portal hypertension during azathioprine treatment after kidney transplantation. Hepatology 1985;1:339–348.
**94.** Kumara CR, Ng M, Lin JH, et al. Herbal tea induced hepatic veno-occlusive disease: Quantification of toxic alkaloid exposure in adults. Case report. Gut 1985;26:101–104.
**95.** Bagheri SA, Boyer JL. Peliosis hepatitis associated with androgenic anabolic steroid therapy. Ann Intern Med 1974;81:610–618.
**96.** Fajard OLF, Colby JV. Pathogenesis of veno-occlusive liver disease. Arch Pathol Lab Med 1980;104:584–588.
**97.** Schomberg LA. Peliosis hepatitis and oral contraceptives. J Reprod Med 1982;27:753–756.
**98.** Degott C, Rueff B, Kreis H, et al. Peliosis hepatitis in recipients of renal transplants. Gut 1978;19:748–753.
**99.** Nescher G, Dollberg L, Ziman A, et al. Hepatosplenic peliosis after danazol and glucocorticoids for ITP. N Engl J Med 1985;312:242.
**100.** Loomus GN, Aneja P, Bota RA, et al. A case of peliosis hepatitis in association with tamoxifen therapy. Am J Clin Pathol 1983;80:881–883.
**101.** Haupt HA, Rovere GD. Anabolic steroids: A review of the literature. Am J Sports Med 1984;12:469–479.
**102.** Podurgiel BJ, McGill DB, Ludwig J, et al. Liver injury associated with methotrexate therapy for psoriasis. Mayo Clin Proc 1973;48:787–792.
**103.** Hersch EM, Wong VG, Henderson ES, et al. Hepatotoxic effects of methotrexate. Cancer 1966;19:600–606.
**104.** Zachariae H, Bjerring P. Methotrexate in psoriasis with and without leucovorin: Effect of different dosage schedules on acute liver toxicity. Acta Derm Venereol (Stockh) 1982;62:446–448.
**105.** Roenigk HH Jr, Auerbach R, Maibach HI, et al. Methotrexate guidelines—revised. J Am Acad Dermatol 1982;6:145–155.
**106.** Russell RM, Boyer JL, Bagheri SA, et al. Hepatic injury from chronic hypervitaminosis A, resulting in portal hypertension and ascites. N Engl J Med 1974;291:435–440.
**107.** Zimmerman HJ. Chemical hepatic injury and its detection, in Plaa GG, Hewitt WR (eds): Toxicology of the Liver, Target Organ Series. Philadelphia, Raven, 1981, pp 1–46.
**108.** Choppa S, Griffin PH. Laboratory tests and diagnostic procedures in evaluation of liver disease. Am J Med 1985;79:221–230.
**109.** Gallizi J, Long RG, Billing BH, et al. Assessment of the $^{14}C$-aminopyrine breath test in liver disease. Gut 1978;19:40–45.
**110.** Caesar J, Shaldon S, Chiandussi L, et al. The use of indocyanine green in the measurement of hepatic blood flow and as a test of hepatic function. Clin Sci 1961;21:43–57.
**111.** Enat R, Pollack S, Ben-Arieh Y, et al. Cholestatic jaundice caused by cloxacillin: Macrophage inhibition factor test in preventing rechallenge with hepatic drugs. Br Med J 1980;280:982–983.

# Chapter 33 / Pancreatitis and Cholelithiasis

Rosemary R. Berardi, PharmD

## Pancreatitis

Inflammatory disease of the pancreas may be described as either acute or chronic. Although there is no universally accepted classification, acute pancreatitis is usually characterized by a discrete episode of symptoms with restoration of normal exocrine and endocrine function.[1] The acute form of the disease may occur as a single event or recurrent attacks (acute relapsing pancreatitis).

Chronic pancreatitis is differentiated from acute pancreatitis in that it produces irreversible functional and morphologic damage to the pancreas even when the causative factor is eliminated.[1] The term *chronic relapsing pancreatitis* is sometimes used to describe the disease when symptoms (especially pain) are intermittent rather than constant. Symptomatic episodes of chronic pancreatitis may be clinically indistinguishable from acute pancreatitis.

Pancreatic exocrine insufficiency associated with cystic fibrosis and diseases of the endocrine pancreas are discussed in Chapters 56 and 54, respectively.

The prevalence of pancreatitis varies in different geographic areas and depends primarily on etiologic factors. The incidence of acute pancreatitis in the United States is less than 1%, while the number of patients with chronic pancreatitis is largely undefined.[2] The overall male-to-female ratio appears to be nearly 1; however, there is an increased incidence of alcoholic pancreatitis in younger men and of gallstone-related disease in older women.[2]

## Physiology of Exocrine Pancreatic Secretion

The pancreas possesses both endocrine and exocrine functions. The endocrine pancreas secretes insulin, glucagon, and other polypeptide hormones. The exocrine pancreas secretes an average of 2,500 mL of an alkaline pancreatic juice daily. The juice is secreted into the main pancreatic duct (of Wirsung), which enters the duodenum at the ampulla of Vater after joining the common bile duct.[3,4] The final common channel, as well as the bile and pancreatic ducts separately, is encased by the muscular sphincter of Oddi. Pancreatic secretions contain water, electrolytes, and enzymes necessary for the digestive functions of the gastrointestinal tract.

### Composition of Pancreatic Juice

***Water and Electrolytes*** The acinar cells of the pancreas secrete an isotonic fluid that contains sodium, potassium, chloride, calcium, and traces of magnesium, zinc, phosphate, and sulfate. Bicarbonate is secreted primarily by the ductular cells and is the principal ion of physiologic importance. At maximum flow rates, the concentration of bicarbonate may reach 150 mEq/L and the pH of the juice is about 8.3.[3] Water enters the juice passively along osmotic gradients established by active secretion of the electrolytes.[3] The relatively alkaline pancreatic juice neutralizes gastric acid in the duodenum and provides an appropriate pH for maintaining the activity of pancreatic enzymes.

***Enzymes*** Pancreatic juice is protein-rich; more than 90% of the proteins are enzymes or proenzymes secreted by pancreatic acinar cells.[3,4] The proteolytic enzymes are secreted as inactive proenzymes that are activated in the lumen of the duodenum. Enterokinase, an enzyme secreted by the duodenal mucosa, converts trypsinogen to trypsin, which then activates all other proteolytic proenzymes (including chymotrypsin and elastase) in a cascade fashion. Pancreatic juice also contains lipase, amylase, and ribonuclease which are secreted in their active form. Colipase, another constituent of pancreatic secretion, binds to lipase and enhances lipase activity by several different mechanisms.[3,4]

### Regulation of Pancreatic Secretion

Exocrine pancreatic secretions are regulated by both hormonal and neuronal mechanisms, the most important being hormonal control. Two hormones, secretin and cholecystokinin (CCK), augment each other's activity: secretin stimulates ductular cells to increase water and bicarbonate; CCK stimulates acinar cells to secrete a juice that is low in volume and bicarbonate, but rich in protein (enzymes). Secretin's release from the intestinal mucosa is pH dependent and occurs when the duodenal pH is approximately 4.5. The release of CCK from the small intestine is dependent largely on the presence of fatty acids and amino acids in the duodenum.[3,4] Vasoactive intestinal polypeptide (VIP) is structurally similar to secretin and exhibits weak secretin-like effects on exocrine pancreatic secretion.

There are four phases of normal pancreatic exocrine secretion (Table 33.1). A basal rate of secretion is apparently intrinsic to the pancreas. The cephalic phase is stimulated by the sight and smell of food and is thought to be mediated by vagal pathways. Gastric distension and the rate of gastric emptying appear to stimulate an increase in enzyme-rich pancreatic fluid. In the intestinal phase, chyme and acid stimulate pancreatic secretion, largely through the release of secretin and CCK. The pancreas normally secretes more enzymes than are actually needed for digestion. Maldigestion or malabsorption does not usually occur until post-

**Table 33.1** Phases of Pancreatic Secretion

| *Phase* | *Volume* | *Bicarbonate output* | *Enzyme output* |
|---|---|---|---|
| Basal | Low | 2% of maximal | 15% of maximal |
| Cephalic | Moderate | Low | High |
| Gastric | Moderate | Low | High |
| Intestinal | High | pH-dependent increase | 70% of maximal |

Adapted from Perry RS, Gallagher J: Management of maldigestion associated with pancreatic insufficiency. Clin Pharm 1985;4:162, with permission.

meal secretions fall below 15% of normal.[3,4] A comprehensive discussion of pancreatic physiology and the role of pancreatic enzymes in digestion can be found elsewhere.[3–5]

**Protection From Autodigestion**

A number of barriers protect the pancreas from the potential degradative action of its own digestive enzymes. Two important protective mechanisms include the synthesis of enzymes as inactive precursors (proenzymes) that require extrapancreatic trigger enzymes, and the synthesis of protease inhibitors found within the acinar cells and present in normal plasma.[4,6]

## Acute Pancreatitis

Acute pancreatitis is an acute inflammatory disorder of the pancreas caused by intrapancreatic activation of digestive enzymes. The spectrum of the disease varies from mild pancreatitis, which is usually self-limiting, to necrotizing pancreatitis, in which the severity of the attack correlates with the degree of pancreatic necrosis. Use of such descriptive terms as "edematous" and "hemorrhagic" are not meaningful as the appearance of the pancreas is usually not known and the degree of necrosis, not hemorrhage, determines disease severity.

### *Etiology*

Many of the risk factors associated with acute pancreatitis are presented in Table 33.2. Alcohol abuse and biliary tract disease, together, account for 80% to 90% of all cases.[6,7] The remaining 10% to 20% of patients have the disease in association with a variety of processes or in the absence of any known cause (idiopathic).

Acute pancreatitis is frequently associated with ethanol abuse; however, it is not clear whether the acute episodes represent acute or chronic disease. Because of the great functional reserve of the pancreas and the possible insidious loss of pancreatic function, it is possible that many patients presenting with a first acute attack of ethanol-related pancreatitis do, in fact, have chronic pancreatitis.[7] If this recent recognition is correct, then this leaves biliary tract disease as the condition most often associated with acute pancreatitis. Pregnancy is no longer considered a cause of pancreatitis as most pregnant patients develop pancreatitis as a result of coincident processes, most commonly cholelithiasis.[7]

Many drugs have been reported to cause acute pancreatitis, but a definite association is difficult to confirm.[8] This is due, in part, to the fact that most available data are case reports involving only a few patients. In addition, ethical and practical reasons prevent rechallenge with the suspected agent. Table 33.3 lists those drugs that are generally considered to be capable of causing pancreatitis or in which a probable or possible association exists. There appears to be an equivocal association between corticosteroids and pancreatitis.[9] The evidence that cimetidine can cause pancreatitis is weak.[10] Nevertheless, it is probably wise to withdraw the drug in those patients with pancreatitis in whom no other risk factor can be identified. The methods by which drugs induce pancreatitis are unknown and probably involve both direct and indirect mechanisms.

### *Pathophysiology*

The pathophysiology of acute pancreatitis is thought to be related to autodigestion of the pancreas as a result of inappropriate intrapancreatic activation of proteases.[2,6,7] Activated proteolytic enzymes (especially trypsin) digest cell membranes and activate other pancreatic proenzymes within the pancreas. The immediate effects on the pancreas include inflammation, edema, and ischemia, which combine to produce a local and regional necrosis. When digestive enzymes enter the systemic circulation, widespread necrosis of extraabdominal organs may occur.

**Table 33.2** Etiology of Acute Pancreatitis

| | |
|---|---|
| Ethanol abuse | Hyperparathyroidism (hypercalcemia) |
| Biliary tract disease (gallstones) | Pancreatic tumor |
| Idiopathic | Hyperlipidemia |
| Medication | Postoperative (abdominal surgery) |
| Infection | Miscellaneous—scorpion bite, ischemia |
| Abdominal trauma | |

**Table 33.3** Drug-Induced Pancreatitis

| | |
|---|---|
| Definite association | |
| | Azathioprine |
| | Estrogens |
| | Sulfonamides |
| | Tetracyclines |
| | Hydrochlorothiazide |
| | Furosemide |
| Probable Association | |
| | L-Asparaginase |
| | Chlorthalidone |
| | Ethacrynic acid |
| | Phenformin |
| | Valproic acid |
| Possible association (inadequate or contradictory evidence) | |
| | Corticosteroids |
| | Procainamide |
| | Methyldopa |
| | Nitrofurantoin |
| | Cimetidine |

Adapted from Mallory A, Kern F: Drug-induced pancreatitis: A critical review. Gastroenterology 1980;78:813–820, with permission.

In addition to the proteolytic effects, vasoactive substances (kinins, histamine, prostaglandins) are released from the inflamed pancreas into the circulation, causing vasodilation, increased vascular permeability, and edema.[2,6,7] Release of these substances results in a cascade of events that appear to contribute to the development of local and systemic complications.

### *Clinical Presentation*

The clinical presentation of acute pancreatitis is determined by the severity of the inflammatory process. Mild disease is usually confined to the pancreas, whereas severe inflammation and necrosis may damage contiguous organs and produce systemic effects.

**Table 33.4** Signs and Symptoms in Acute Pancreatitis

| *Sign/symptom* | *Frequency (%)* |
|---|---|
| Abdominal pain | 95–100 |
| Epigastric tenderness | 95–100 |
| Nausea and vomiting | 70–90 |
| Low-grade fever | 70–85 |
| Hypotension | 20–40 |
| Mental aberrations | 20–35 |
| Other—jaundice, fat necrosis, pleural effusions, ARDS[a] | Rare (<1) |

[a] Acute respiratory distress syndrome.

Adapted from Levitt MD, Eckfeldt JH: Diagnosis of acute pancreatitis, in Go VLW, Gardner JD, Brooks FP, et al (Eds): The Exocrine Pancreas: Biology, Pathobiology, and Diseases. New York, Raven, 1986, p 482, with permission.

#### Symptoms/Physical Findings

The signs and symptoms of acute pancreatitis and their approximate frequencies are shown in Table 33.4. The initial clinical presentation of the patient ranges from mild abdominal discomfort to excruciating abdominal pain, shock, and respiratory distress.[2,11,12]

Abdominal pain is the major symptom of nearly all patients. The pain is usually epigastric, often radiating to either of the upper quadrants or the back. Five features are characteristic of abdominal pain in acute pancreatitis: (1) the onset is usually sudden; (2) the intensity is usually devastatingly severe; (3) it tends to be steady and boring in quality; (4) it persists for many hours and usually several days; (5) partial relief can be obtained by repositioning the patient so that the knees are flexed against the chest.[11] Marked epigastric tenderness to deep palpation is frequently observed. Bowel sounds are usually diminished or absent. Nausea and vomiting frequently follow the onset of pain.

#### Diagnostic Tests/Procedures

Table 33.5 identifies a number of tests and procedures that are used in the diagnosis of acute pancreatitis; however, many of them do not provide sufficiently reliable information to be of clinical value.[12,13] The diagnosis of acute pancreatitis is usually established by the presence of an increased serum amylase (two to three times the upper limit of normal) in the presence of abdominal pain. An initially elevated

**Table 33.5** Tests and Procedures for Diagnosis of Acute Pancreatitis

| | |
|---|---|
| Useful tests | |
| | Serum or urinary amylase |
| | Serum lipase |
| | Complete blood count |
| | Blood chemistries |
| | Arterial blood gases |
| | x-ray of abdomen or chest |
| | Computed tomography of pancreas |
| Procedures of value in special circumstances | |
| | Endoscopic retrograde cholangiopancreatography |
| | Angiography |
| | Percutaneous transhepatic cholangiography |
| Tests of limited or no value | |
| | Amylase: creatinine clearance ratio |
| | Isoenzymes of amylase |
| | Contrast studies of gastrointestinal tract |
| | Oral cholecystography |
| | Intravenous cholangiography |
| | Biliary scanning |
| | Serum methemalbumin |
| | Serum trypsin, elastase, etc |
| Tests awaiting evaluation | |
| | Plasma fibrinogen |
| | Serum RNase |
| | Peritoneal tap/lavage |

Adapted from Moossa AR: Diagnostic tests and procedures in acute pancreatitis. N Engl J Med 1984;311:639–642, with permission.

serum amylase that returns to normal with resolution of symptoms provides additional support for the diagnosis.

***Serum Amylase*** The serum amylase level usually rises within 24 hours of the onset of symptoms and returns to normal over the next 3 to 10 days. Persistent elevations suggest extensive pancreatic necrosis and/or related complications. Serum amylase elevations do not correlate with either the etiology or the severity of the disease. Many nonpancreatic diseases may be associated with hyperamylasemia, including salivary, renal, hepatobiliary, metabolic, female reproductive tract, and neoplastic diseases.[12,13] Several serum isoamylase enzymes have been identified and may assist in determining the origin of elevated serum amylase concentrations.

***Serum Lipase*** Serum lipase concentrations are usually elevated in acute pancreatitis and may persist longer than serum amylase elevations. Because serum lipase is specific to the pancreas in origin, it is an important diagnostic test.

***Urinary Amylase/Amylase:Creatinine Clearance Ratio*** Urine amylase is increased in acute pancreatitis and may be elevated for 7 to 10 days after serum values have returned to normal. Urinary amylase concentrations are of little clinical value, however, as they reflect the hydration and renal status of the patient. Although some clinicians believe that the amylase:creatinine clearance ratio is a useful test because it accounts for differences in renal function, others believe it is of limited or no value.[12,13]

***Additional Blood Studies*** Leukocytosis, hyperglycemia, hypoalbuminemia, hyperbilirubinemia, and elevations in liver enzymes may be present in varying combinations. The hemoglobin and hematocrit may be elevated as a result of hemoconcentration. Blood calcium levels are usually normal initially but tend to drop over the subsequent 3 to 4 days. A marked fall is an indication of severe necrosis and a bad prognostic sign. Although lipemic serum is often found in patients with acute pancreatitis, evidence suggests that it is probably associated with events preceding the acute attack.

***Radiologic Studies*** A number of radiologic imaging procedures (Table 33.5) reveal abnormalities during the disease course. None, however, provide a positive diagnosis of acute pancreatitis.[12,13]

## *Disease Course/Prognosis/Complications*

In general, the majority of patients with acute pancreatitis recover uneventfully. Mortality rates appear to be influenced by the etiology of the disease and whether the initial episode represents an acute attack or an exacerbation of chronic pancreatitis. There is evidence to suggest that patients with alcoholism-related acute pancreatitis have decreased mortality rates compared with patients with pancreatitis from other causes.[14] Mortality appears to be greater with the first attack than with recurrent acute pancreatitis.

Mortality is increased when identifiable risk factors (Table 33.6) are present upon admission or during the initial 48 hours of hospitalization.[15] Death during the first few weeks usually results from cardiac, respiratory, or renal failure. When death occurs after this period, it is usually associated with local complications.[6]

**Table 33.6** Prognostic Signs Used to Evaluate the Risk of Death or Major Complications From Acute Pancreatitis

| |
|---|
| At admission or diagnosis |
| Age > 55 |
| White blood cell count > 16,000/mm$^3$ |
| Blood glucose > 200 mg/dL |
| Serum lactic dehydrogenase > 350 IU/L |
| Serum aspartate transaminase > 250 IU/dL |
| During initial 48 h |
| Hematocrit fall > 10 percentage points |
| Blood urea nitrogen rise > 5 mg/dL |
| Serum calcium level < 8 mg/dL |
| Arterial $Po_2$ < 60 mm Hg |
| Base deficit > 4 mEq/L |
| Estimated fluid sequestration > 6,000 mL |

Adapted from Ranson JHC: Acute pancreatitis: Surgical management, in Go VLW, Gardner JD, Brooks FP, et al (Eds): The Exocrine Pancreas: Biology, Pathobiology, and Diseases. New York, Raven, 1986, pp 503–511, with permission.

The local and systemic complications of acute pancreatitis are listed in Table 33.7. Local complications usually occur within 2 to 4 weeks of the initial attack.[6,7] A phlegmon is a mass of inflamed pancreas containing patchy areas of necrosis. Pseudocysts are fluid collections of necrotic debris, blood, and pancreatic enzymes. In contrast to true cysts, they do not have an epithelial lining. Pancreatic abscesses are usually secondary infections of necrotic tissue or pseudocysts. The development of a pseudocyst or pancreatic abscess appears to correlate with the severity of the pancreatitis.

Systemic complications included pulmonary, cardiovascular, hematologic, renal, metabolic, and central nervous system abnormalities.[6,7] Pulmonary complications develop in approximately 10% to 20% of patients. Hypotension results from hypovolemia, hypoalbuminemia, the release of kinins, and sepsis. Renal complications are usually caused by hypovolemia.

## *Treatment*

The overall treatment of acute pancreatitis should be aimed at assessing the severity of the attack, minimizing the development of complications, and preventing subsequent episodes. In most patients, the disease is self-limiting and subsides spontaneously within 2 to 7 days of the initiation of supportive care and the reduction of pancreatic secretions. In 10% to 15% of patients, however, the disease takes a fulminiant course. As acute mild pancreatitis can progress to the severe form, all patients should be treated as if they had severe pancreatitis.

### General Supportive Care

A primary goal of therapy is to replace fluid and electrolyte losses that result from the "chemical burn" induced by the pancreatic exudate. In severe pancreatitis, large quantities of fluid are usually sequestered within the peritoneal and

**Table 33.7** Local and Systemic Complications of Acute Pancreatitis

| *Local* | *Systemic* |
|---|---|
| Fat necrosis | Hypotension (hypovolemia, hypoalbuminemia) |
| Pancreatic phlegmon | Metabolic (hypocalcemia, hyperglycemia) |
| Pancreatic pseudocyst | Pulmonary failure |
| Pancreatic ascites | Cardiovascular failure |
| Pancreatic abscess | Renal failure |
| Involvement of contiguous organs | Hematologic (disseminated intravascular coagulation) |
| | Gastrointestinal bleeding |
| | Central nervous system abnormalities |

retroperitoneal spaces. Vomiting and nasogastric suction may contribute to additional fluid losses. The prognosis of the patient depends, to a great extent, on the rapidity and adequacy of volume restoration. Intravenous colloids may be required to maintain intravascular volume and blood pressure in severe pancreatitis, as fluid losses are rich in protein. A high priority should be placed on the frequent monitoring of physical findings and vital signs (see Chapters 102 and 103).

Analgesics should be administered to reduce the severity of abdominal pain. The administration of narcotics has been associated with mild and transient increases in serum amylase and lipase. Because these effects do not appear to be deleterious to the patient, it is not necessary to delay or curtail their administration. A traditional approach is to begin therapy with parenteral meperidine (50–100 mg), as it is thought to cause less spasm of the sphincter of Oddi than other narcotic medications.[16] Increased pancreatic duct pressure is thought to correlate with the severity of pain; however, studies reporting the superiority of meperidine and pentazocine were not conducted in patients with pancreatitis.[16,17] Additionally, the difference in the degree of spasm produced by meperidine and equipotent doses of morphine is thought to be of questionable clinical significance. Therefore, the primary basis for drug selection should be analgesic efficacy. The use of potent narcotics, such as morphine, may be warranted in patients whose pain is unresponsive to meperidine or pentazocine.

### Reduction of Autodigestion

Specific medical therapy of acute pancreatitis is aimed at either directly or indirectly reducing pancreatic secretions or inhibiting the action of proteolytic enzymes. To achieve these goals, a number of manipulations and medications have been investigated. Of these, fasting is the most important, as feeding activates pancreatic secretions and the inflammatory process. The use of nasogastric aspiration appears to offer no clear advantage in patients with mild acute pancreatitis.[6,18,19] Its use is considered to be most beneficial in patients with profound pain, severe disease, paralytic ileus, and intractable vomiting.

Attempts at reducing pancreatic secretions with pharmacologic agents have met with little success. Table 33.8 lists some of the more widely investigated drugs and their potential mechanisms of action. Other agents undergoing study in humans and animals include prostaglandins, secretin, inhibitors of protein synthesis, scavengers of oxygen-derived free radicals, and stimulants of the reticuloendothelial system.

Anticholinergics are not recommended in treating acute pancreatitis as their efficacy is questionable and their side effects may complicate the clinical status of the patient.[20] The $H_2$-receptor antagonists do not appear to be more effective than nasogastric suction or fasting alone in patients with mild to moderate disease.[6,19] Most clinical trials have failed to confirm the value of aprotinin, a proteolytic enzyme inhibitor. Nevertheless, there is evidence to suggest that early administration of the drug may be important in determining its efficacy.[2,18] There are conflicting reports regarding the value of glucagon and calcitonin.[2,18] In contrast, preliminary results of studies with somatostatin look promising.[21] Additional controlled clinical trials are needed to evaluate the efficacy of these agents in severe acute pancreatitis.

### Antibiotics

The use of prophylactic antibiotics does not offer any therapeutic advantage in patients with mild to moderate ethanol-induced pancreatitis.[6,18] Although controlled trials fail to show the benefit of early antibiotic therapy in severe disease, the empiric use of appropriate antibiotics may be warranted in the following situations: severe necrotizing pancreatitis, biliary or pancreatic duct obstruction, and local complications (pancreatic abscess). The selection of an empiric antibiotic regimen should be based on the premise that enteric aerobic gram-negative bacilli and anaerobic

**Table 33.8** Proposed Pharmacologic Agents for Treating Acute Pancreatitis

| |
|---|
| Inhibitors of gastric acid and exocrine pancreatic secretion |
| Anticholinergics |
| $H_2$-receptor antagonists |
| Calcitonin |
| Glucagon |
| Somatostatin[a] |
| Inhibitors of protease enzymes |
| Aprotinin |

[a] Also interferes with release of secretin, gastrin, and other peptide hormones.

microorganisms are often the cause of pancreatic infections. Adjustments in the antibiotic regimen should be made once the results of culture and sensitivity tests are known.

**Management of Complications**

In addition to the preceding measures, the patient with severe acute pancreatitis requires additional medical therapy. This usually includes the intensive treatment of cardiovascular, respiratory, renal, and metabolic complications. Intravenous calcium and magnesium should be used to correct deficiency states. Insulin may be required to treat persistent hyperglycemia. Consideration should be given to the use of parenteral nutrition in patients with severe, protracted pancreatitis who are unable to tolerate enteral feedings.

The use of peritoneal lavage remains controversial. Although removal of toxic pancreatic exudate from the peritoneal cavity may assist in the treatment of early cardiovascular and respiratory complications, it does not prevent necrosis or late abscess formation.[6,22] Frequently, the local complications of acute pancreatitis resolve as the inflammatory process subsides. In other patients, secondary infection occurs, requiring the use of antibiotics and surgical intervention.[6,22]

**Prevention of Recurrence**

Once a patient has recovered from an episode of acute pancreatitis, every effort should be made to identify the etiologic agent and prevent recurrent attacks. For patients with cholelithiasis, correction of their underlying biliary disease should reduce the risk of recurrent pancreatitis.

**Recommendations**

Treatment for mild acute pancreatitis includes administration of intravenous fluids to maintain intravascular volume, analgesics for pain, and measures to reduce pancreatic secretions. Nasogastric aspiration is indicated if pain is severe and if ileus or intractable vomiting is present. The use of anticholinergics, $H_2$-receptor antagonists, and other antisecretory agents does not appear to be of benefit. Antibiotics should not be used in the absence of signs of infection.

Patients with moderate to severe acute pancreatitis should be treated with nasogastric suction and parenteral nutrition when the disease course is prolonged. Antiulcer agents may be necessary to prevent bleeding from stress-related mucosal lesions. It seems reasonable to use antibiotics early in the course of the disease in patients with cholelithiasis or when pancreatic necrosis is likely. Such drugs as glucagon, calcitonin, aprotinin, or somatostatin may be tried, but their efficacy remains unproven.

## Chronic Pancreatitis

Chronic pancreatitis is defined by progressive functional damage to the pancreas that persists even when the causative factor is withdrawn.[1] Permanent destruction of pancreatic tissue usually results in exocrine and endocrine insufficiency. Cystic fibrosis, an important cause of pancreatic exocrine insufficiency in children, is discussed elsewhere.

### *Etiology*

Prolonged alcohol consumption is the main cause of chronic pancreatitis in the United States, accounting for approximately 75% of all cases. In approximately 10% to 15% of patients, no predisposing cause (idiopathic) can be found.[23] Other causes of pancreatitis occur less frequently and include protein-calorie malnutrition, hypercalcemia, heredity, and trauma. Although cholelithiasis may coexist with chronic pancreatitis, gallstones rarely, if ever, lead to chronic disease. The causes of relapsing chronic pancreatitis are similar to those of acute pancreatitis (Table 33.2).

### *Pathophysiology*

The pathophysiology of chronic alcoholic pancreatitis is presumably related to alcohol-induced changes in the composition of pancreatic secretion that lead to the precipitation of protein within the pancreatic ducts.[23] The precipitates form "protein plugs" that occlude the ducts, causing duct dilation, inflammation, acinar cell atrophy, fibrosis, scarring, and eventual calcification. The end result is varying degrees of pancreatic destruction and insufficiency.

### *Clinical Presentation*

**Symptoms/Physical Findings**

Patients with relapsing chronic pancreatitis usually present with symptoms similar to those seen in acute pancreatitis, but their pain is usually intermittent. The main clinical features of chronic pancreatitis are pain, weight loss, diarrhea from malabsorption, diabetes mellitus, and intraductal calcifications.[24]

***Pain*** Abdominal pain is the most prominent clinical feature of chronic pancreatitis and is classically described by many patients as epigastric and radiating through to the back. Characteristically, the pain is deep-seated, positional, and unresponsive to drug therapy. The intensity of the pain varies from mild to severe and does not correlate directly with the inflammatory process or other physical findings. Severe attacks usually last from several days to several weeks and may be aggravated by eating. Up to 50% of alcoholic patients have chronic pain, while the remainder have intermittent attacks or have painless pancreatitis. Nausea, vomiting, and weight loss may accompany the episodes of pain. Although the pathogenesis of the pain is unclear, recent evidence suggests that it may be related to scarring and increased intraductal pressure secondary to continued pancreatic secretion.[24] Abstinence from ethanol may provide relief from pain but does not prevent the continuous development of exocrine dysfunction. The course of pain in chronic pancreatitis is unpredictable, but usually lessens as pancreatic insufficiency progresses.

***Malabsorption*** Permanent destruction of the pancreas and obstruction of the pancreatic ducts lead to a decrease in the amount of pancreatic enzymes that reach the proximal duodenum. Although the secretion of digestive enzymes decreases early in the course of the disease, protein and fat are not malabsorbed until at least 90% of the secretory capacity of the pancreas is lost.[24] Steatorrhea (excessive loss of fat in the feces) and azotorrhea (excessive loss of protein in the feces) are seen in the majority of patients once significant pancreatic destruction occurs. As lipase secretion decreases more rapidly than the secretion of proteolytic enzymes, steatorrhea is an earlier and more severe problem.[24] Diarrhea may occur secondary to fat malabsorption.

In addition to decreased enzyme secretion, severe chronic pancreatitis may affect other gastrointestinal (GI) functions, such as gastric emptying, intraluminal duodenal pH, and bile acids. Abnormally low duodenal pH values have been reported postprandially in severe pancreatic insufficiency.[24] These alterations in GI function may affect the efficacy of exogenous pancreatic enzymes. At least 50% of patients with advanced pancreatic insufficiency present with malabsorption of cobalamin (vitamin $B_{12}$). Weight loss occurs from malabsorption and from avoidance of food, induced by painful responses to eating.

***Other Features*** Diabetes is usually a late manifestation commonly associated with pancreatic calcification. Neuropathy is common, and may result from the additive effects of alcohol abuse and malnutrition. Prolonged jaundice occurs in about 10% of patients and is usually due to common bile duct compression. Mild fever and tachycardia may be present.

#### Diagnostic Tests/Procedures

Numerous tests for diagnosing chronic pancreatitis have been introduced into clinical practice.[24–26] An excellent comprehensive review of the use and value of these tests and procedures has been published.[25] Unfortunately there are no reliable tests for diagnosing mild chronic pancreatitis. Total serum amylase and the amylase:creatinine clearance ratio are of no value in diagnosing and monitoring the course of chronic pancreatitis.[24] The quantitative fecal fat test can be of value in assessing the efficacy of pancreatic enzyme treatment.

Direct tests of pancreatic exocrine function involve the collection of pancreatic juice after stimulation with exogenous hormones such as secretin or cholecystokinin and serve as the best indicator for detecting chronic pancreatic disease. As they require intubation and special collection techniques, they are performed infrequently.[25] Indirect tests of pancreatic secretory capacity (e.g., bentiromide test, dual-label Schilling test) are not as difficult to perform, but are less sensitive (especially in patients with mild disease) and produce a significant number of false positives.[25] Newer imaging techniques are helpful in detecting other possible causes of pain (ductal obstruction secondary to stones or strictures, pancreatic pseudocyst) and in differentiating chronic pancreatitis from pancreatic cancer.[24,25]

### *Disease Course/Prognosis/Complications*

Patients with chronic alcoholic pancreatitis usually present with an initial acute attack followed by successive attacks that are slower to resolve. Continued alcohol abuse leads to chronic abdominal pain and progressive exocrine and endocrine insufficiency. In half of the patients, however, the pain diminishes about 5 to 10 years after the onset of symptoms.[24] The triad of steatorrhea, calcification, and diabetes may develop after 10 to 20 years of heavy ethanol ingestion.

Most patients with chronic pancreatitis are affected by varying degrees of pain, malnutrition, and glucose intolerance. Many complications may occur as a consequence of ethanol and narcotic drug abuse. A minority of patients develop additional severe complications including pancreatic pseudocyst, ascites, or abscess; common bile duct obstruction leading to cholangitis or secondary biliary cirrhosis; and gastrointestinal bleeding resulting from a variety of sources, inducing gastritis, peptic ulcer, and splenic/portal vein thrombosis. Most deaths are due to hepatic, cardiovascular, or malignant disease and rarely are directly related to pancreatitis or its complications.[24]

### *Treatment*

Patients with relapsing chronic pancreatitis are essentially treated like those with acute relapsing pancreatitis. Treatment for uncomplicated chronic pancreatitis is usually directed at two major problems, chronic pain and malabsorption.

#### Chronic Pain

Abstinence from ethanol is the single most important factor in the prevention of chronic pain. Nonnarcotic analgesics such as aspirin or acetaminophen should be tried initially. If the pain does not subside, then a trial of exogenous pancreatic enzymes should be attempted. The administration of pancreatic enzymes early in the course of the disease may afford pain relief by suppressing pancreatic enzyme secretion through a negative-feedback mechanism involving proteases present in the duodenum.[27,28] Beneficial effects seem to occur primarily in patients with mild to moderate disease (without steatorrhea) and treatment appears to be especially useful in patients with a nonalcoholic etiology. The trypsin content within the pancreatic enzyme preparation appears to be crucial, however.[28,29] Frequently, pain relief necessitates the use of narcotic analgesics, which may lead to addiction.

If systemic drug therapy is unsuccessful, percutaneous injection of alcohol into the celiac ganglion may be attempted. Unfortunately, pain relief obtained by this procedure may last only 3 to 6 months and repeated treatments are usually not as effective. If all medical measures fail and severe pain continues, surgical treatment is indicated.

#### Malabsorption

Malabsorption requires treatment when steatorrhea (>7 g fat in feces per 24 hours on a 100-g fat diet) is documented and persistent weight loss occurs in spite of efforts to correct it. As steatorrhea is often the first sign of malabsorption, treatment efficacy is commonly expressed as a reduction in the degree of steatorrhea. The standard therapy for malabsorption resulting from exocrine pancreatic insufficiency is the use of pancreatic enzyme supplements. The combination of enzyme supplementation and reduction in dietary fat (25 g per meal) usually enhances the patient's nutritional status, reduces (not totally corrects) steatorrhea, and alleviates other troublesome symptoms.

***Principles of Enzyme Replacement*** The success of pancreatic enzyme supplementation requires an understanding of several important physiologic factors. First, lipase is rapidly and irreversibly inactivated at a pH less than 4.0, whereas trypsin is more resistant to acid.[24] Second, a critical amount of enzymes must be delivered to the duodenum in sufficient concentrations for digestion to occur. The concentration of enzyme delivered into the duodenum must be 5% to 10% of normal maximal output. This requires that approximately 30,000 IU of lipase and 10,000 IU of trypsin be delivered during a 4-hour postprandial period.[24] Third, gastric and duodenal pH may vary depending on age, etiology of the disease, and disease severity.[24] These factors help to explain why steatorrhea is not as readily corrected as azotorrhea and why there is such a variable response to pancreatic enzyme therapy.

***Pancreatic Enzyme Supplements*** Oral pancreatic enzyme supplements are available as powders, tablets, capsules, and enteric-coated encapsulated microspheres (ECEMs). These products differ in enzyme content and activity, bioavailability, clinical effectiveness, patient acceptance, and cost.[5,30,31] Of major importance is the relatively low potency and variable nature of the lipase content (Table 33.9). Usually, at least six to eight tablets/capsules of the most potent preparations must be taken per meal to reduce steatorrhea. Although controversy exists over the optimal dosage schedule, the consensus is that tablets/capsules should be taken with meals.[31,32] Increasing the frequency of the dosage regimen (e.g., two before, two with, and two after meals, or hourly administration) may further decrease steatorrhea in certain patients; however, the frequency of the dosage regimen must be weighed against patient compliance. Because of the number of tablets/capsules required per dose, the need to take them with each meal or snack, and the cost, compliance (especially among alcoholics) is often poor. An excellent review of the drug therapy associated with the treatment of pancreatic insufficiency has been published.[5]

Gastric inactivation of pancreatic enzymes and inability to correct steatorrhea have led to the development of ECEMs. The polymer used to coat each granule is pH dependent and dissolves in the more alkaline media of the duodenum where the enzymes are released.[5,31,32] Because of this pH dependence, however, it is possible that intragastric pH's greater than 5.0 may liberate the enzymes in the stomach and later inactivate them when the intragastric pH falls to less than 4.0. Conversely, if low duodenal pH's prevail (less than 4.0 to 5.0), the enteric coating will remain intact and the enzymes will be released in more distal portions of the small intestine. A small number of clinical studies have evaluated the efficacy of ECEMs versus conventional formulations in pancreatic insufficiency and found conflicting results.[5,31–34] Although the ECEMs have been shown to reduce steatorrhea, they have not been shown to be more effective than appropriate doses of conventional pancreatic enzyme preparations.[33,34] Results of clinical studies suggest that enteric-coated tablets are ineffective in treating pancreatic enzyme insufficiency.[30,35]

***Adjuncts to Enzyme Therapy*** The use of antacids and $H_2$ antagonists as an adjunct to pancreatic enzyme supplementation has produced conflicting results.[5,31,32,35–37] Theoretically, the use of these agents in conjunction with oral enzymes should maintain luminal gastric and duodenal pH above 4.0 and thereby enhance lipase activity. In addition, increased duodenal pH prevents bile acid precipitation and thus increases fatty acid solubility. The beneficial effects of $H_2$-receptor antagonists appear to result from both an increase in pH and a decrease in intragastric volume.[35–37] Sodium bicarbonate and aluminum hydroxide are more effective than calcium- and magnesium-containing antacids in reducing steatorrhea and do not have the added disadvantage of causing diarrhea.[32,37] Patients whose steatorrhea is not corrected by enzyme replacement therapy and who remain symptomatic may benefit from the addition of $H_2$-receptor antagonists or antacids. Alternatively, the addition of these agents to an ECEM regimen may cause premature dissolution of the enteric coating in the stomach, leading to inactivation of lipase when the gastric pH falls below 4.0.

***Adverse Effects*** Pancreatic enzymes contain nucleic acids and, when given in high therapeutic doses to children with cystic fibrosis, have been reported to cause hyperuricosuria and occasional hyperuricemia.[5,38] Impaired folic acid absorption by oral pancreatic enzymes may lead to folic acid deficiency.[39] Thus, uric acid and folic acid levels should be monitored in patients prone to developing hyperuricemia or folic acid deficiency. Gastrointestinal side effects appear to

**Table 33.9** Enzyme Content of Commonly Prescribed Pancreatic Enzyme Preparations

| *Product* | *Dosage form* | Content (units)[a] | | |
|---|---|---|---|---|
| | | **Lipase** | **Protease** | **Amylase** |
| Viokase | Tablet | 8,000 | 30,000 | 30,000 |
| Ilozyme | Tablet | 11,000 | 30,000 | 30,000 |
| Festal II | Tablet[b] | 6,000 | 20,000 | 30,000 |
| Cotazym | Capsule | 8,000 | 30,000 | 30,000 |
| Ku-Zyme-HP | Capsule | 8,000 | 30,000 | 30,000 |
| Cotazym-S | ECEM[c] | 5,000 | 20,000 | 20,000 |
| Pancrease | ECEM[c] | 4,000 | 25,000 | 20,000 |

[a] Manufacturer's labeled contents (USP units).
[b] Enteric coated.
[c] Enteric-coated encapsulated microspheres.

be dose related but seem to occur less frequently with the ECEM preparations.[33] A hypersensitivity reaction to the powder has been reported.[5]

**Recommendations**

Abdominal pain is the most prominent and challenging clinical feature in chronic alcoholic pancreatitis and may cease with abstinence. Pain management should begin with simple analgesics (aspirin or acetaminophen). If pain persists, the response to exogenous pancreatic enzymes should be evaluated. If these measures fail, the use of more potent narcotics may be considered; however, their use should be individualized (depending on the etiology of the disease) as chronic use is likely to lead to addiction. In patients with alcoholic pancreatitis, celiac ganglion nerve block or appropriate surgery may be necessary, although both have a significant failure rate for pain management. An algorithm for the evaluation and treatment of pain is shown in Figure 33.1.

Most patients placed on a reduced-fat diet and adequate doses of potent conventional pancreatic enzyme supplements achieve a satisfactory nutritional status and become relatively asymptomatic. The dose should be titrated to a reduction in steatorrhea. In those patients who do not have an adequate response, however, consideration should be given to the use of ECEMs. The ECEMs enjoy greater patient acceptance than the conventional dosage forms, as they usually require fewer dosage units per dose to produce an adequate response and they are associated with fewer GI side effects. When cost is based on the number of tablets/capsules required per day, the ECEMs are usually similar in cost to the conventional products. Addition of an $H_2$ antagonist or an antacid to a conventional pancreatic enzyme tablet/capsule regimen should be reserved for those patients who do not respond to enzyme therapy alone. Adjuncts should not be given in conjunction with ECEMs. If antacids are used, aluminum hydroxide is recommended because of its increased efficiency. An algorithm for the treatment of malabsorption resulting from chronic pancreatitis is presented in Figure 33.2.

**Figure 33.1** Algorithm for evaluation and treatment of pain in chronic pancreatitis. *(From DiMagno EP, Clain JE: Chronic pancreatitis, in Go VLW, Gardner JD, Brooks FP, et al (Eds): The Exocrine Pancreas: Biology, Pathobiology, and Diseases. New York, Raven, 1986, p 548, with permission.)*

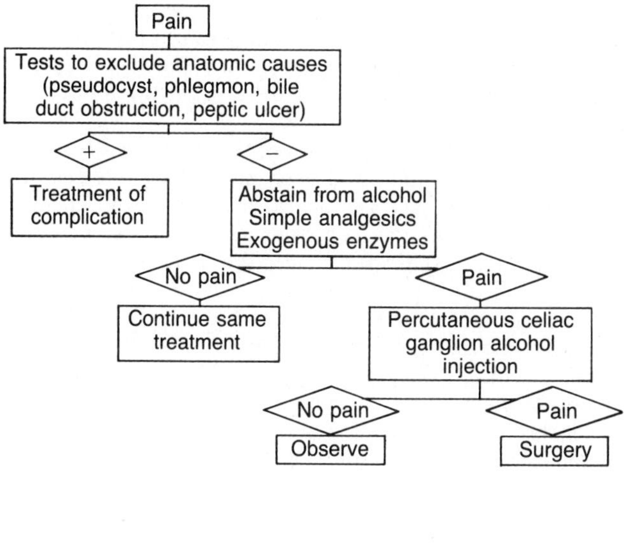


## Nutritional Support in Pancreatic Disease

Nutritional deficits develop rapidly in patients with acute pancreatitis complicated by tissue necrosis, organ failure, and surgery. In addition, a number of factors, including ileus, may preclude oral feeding for prolonged periods of time. Nutritional support should be implemented in patients with acute pancreatitis before protein and calorie depletion becomes advanced. Evidence suggests that as a primary therapeutic modality, parenteral nutrition does not alter the course of acute pancreatitis[40]; however, it should be regarded as a useful adjunct in restoring and maintaining nutritional status.

Parenteral or enteral nutrition (elemental diets) may be necessary for patients with chronic pancreatitis, especially if the patient is chronically debilitated. It appears that the intravenous administration of amino acids and lipids does not significantly stimulate pancreatic secretion.[40,41] When weight loss is refractory to diet and exogenous enzymes, supplementation with medium-chain triglycerides (MCIs) should be considered.

## Surgical Treatment for Pancreatitis

Surgical intervention may be necessary in acute pancreatitis to treat local complications such as pseudocyst or abscess. The surgical correction of biliary disease reduces the risk of recurrent pancreatitis. Peritoneal lavage may be used as an adjunct to treat early cardiovascular or respiratory failure, but has not been shown to decrease overall mortality.[22]

The most common indication for surgery in chronic pancreatitis is abdominal pain refractory to medical therapy. Although the pain may "burn out" as the gland deteriorates, it is unreasonable that a patient wait years for possible spontaneous relief. Surgical procedures that have been shown to alleviate pain include a subtotal or total pancreatectomy, drainage of the pancreatic duct, or interruption of the splanchnic nerves. Complications of chronic pancreatitis including biliary obstruction, pseudocyst, and fistulas may require operative treatment.[42]

## Summary

Despite modern medical knowledge and techniques, much of what we known about the pathophysiologic mechanisms, diagnosis, and treatment of acute and chronic pancreatitis remains incomplete. As time goes on, answers to the many questions surrounding the mysteries of these diseases will become known. Until then, our role as pharmacists is largely supportive, but should include the provision of information to patients and the public regarding the complications and consequences of alcohol-related diseases such as pancreatitis.

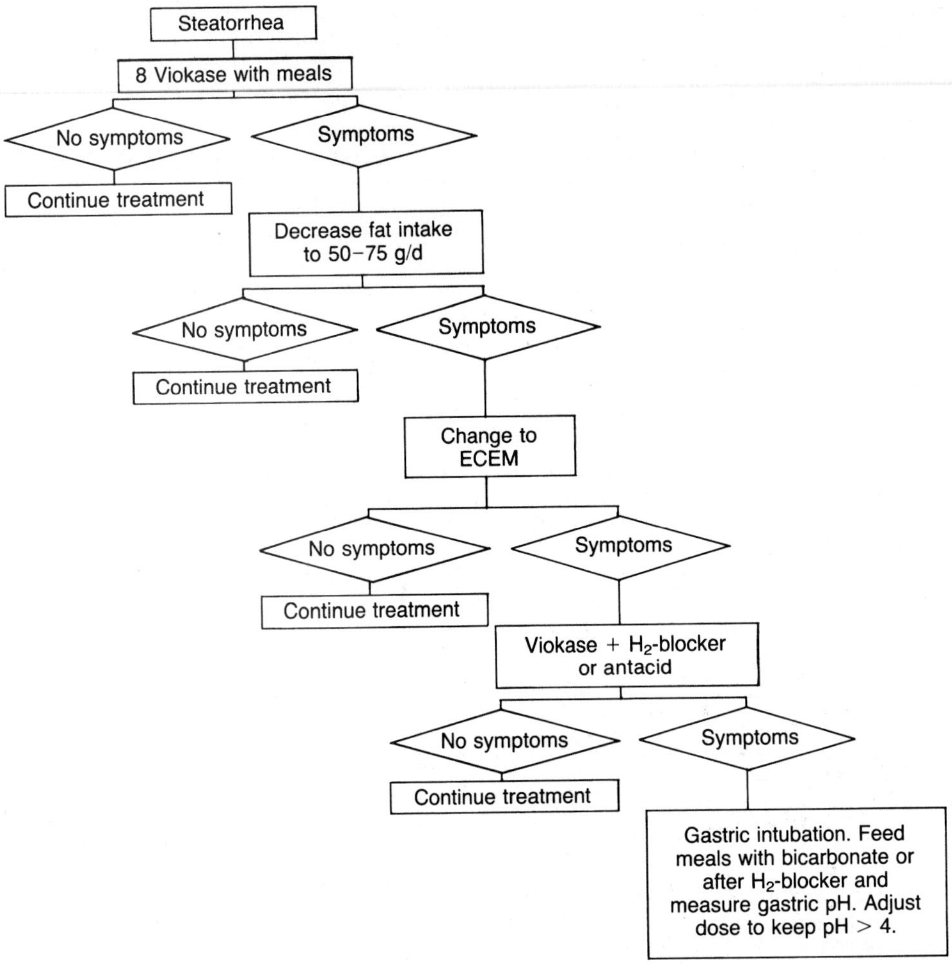


**Figure 33.2** Algorithm for evaluation and treatment of malabsorption resulting from chronic pancreatitis. ECEM, enteric-coated encapsulated microsphere. *(From DiMagno EP, Clain JE: Chronic pancreatitis, in Go VLW, Gardner JD, Brooks FP, et al (eds): The Exocrine Pancreas: Biology, Pathobiology, and Diseases. New York, Raven, 1986, p 556, with permission.)*

## Cholelithiasis

Gallstone formation (cholelithiasis) is the most common biliary tract disease in the United States, occurring in 10% to 20% of the population.[43] Its true prevalence, however, is probably unknown, as many patients with cholelithiasis have asymptomatic (silent) gallstones.[44]

Gallstones are crystalline structures formed by abnormalities in the concentration of bile constituents. They are usually classified according to their chemical composition as either cholesterol or pigment. Cholesterol stones may be composed entirely of cholesterol or may contain large amounts of cholesterol with small amounts of bile salts and unconjugated bilirubin. Pigment stones contain unconjugated bilirubin, bile salts, and only a small amount of cholesterol. Approximately 80% to 85% of patients with cholelithiasis have gallstones consisting primarily of cholesterol, although this percentage varies in different geographic locations and among ethnic groups.[44]

### *Etiology/Pathogenesis*

The formation of cholesterol gallstones requires bile saturated with cholesterol, while the formation of pigment stones requires bile containing excessive amounts of unconjugated bilirubin. As oral therapeutic agents are effective only in treating radiolucent cholesterol stones, pigment stones are not discussed here.

Cholesterol is synthesized within the body and absorbed from the diet. It is eliminated unchanged in the bile and as bile acids. The primary bile acids, cholic acid and chenodeoxycholic acid, are formed from degradation of cholesterol in the liver. These substances are then conjugated in the liver and excreted in the bile, where they undergo enterohepatic circulation or are degraded by intestinal bacteria and converted to deoxycholic acid and lithocholic acid. As cholesterol is insoluble in bile, two detergent-like substances, bile acids and phospholipids (lecithin), help solublize it through the formation of micelles.[45]

Cholesterol supersaturation of the bile is produced by

increased cholesterol secretion, decreased bile salt and lecithin secretion, or a combination of both defects.[45] The most important mechanism is thought to be related to increased biliary secretion of cholesterol. The ultimate cause of cholesterol gallstones is the formation of cholesterol monohydrate crystals and the aggregation of these crystals to produce stones. Several substances (bacteria, mucus, calcium bilirubinate) may serve as nucleating agents, thus requiring less supersaturation of the bile.[45] A comprehensive and detailed description of the complex processes involved in the pathogenesis of gallstones is provided elsewhere.[45]

A number of factors have been associated with cholesterol gallstone formation including increasing age; female gender; obesity; diets high in saturated fats and refined sugars and low in fiber; and drugs such as estrogens and clofibrate.[43,46] Although reports are conflicting, recent studies have not confirmed a direct causal relationship between gallstone formation and oral contraceptives or thiazide diuretics.[43] Cholelithiasis has been associated with such clinical conditions as diabetes, hyperlipidemia, and terminal ileal disease; however, most of the literature suggesting these associations consists of case reports and not controlled studies.[43] The evidence for an association between pregnancy and new gallstone formation is weak.[43]

### *Clinical Presentation*

In approximately 50% of all persons with cholelithiasis, the stones remain in the gallbladder and the patient is asymptomatic.[44] Occasionally, gallstones migrate out of the gallbladder into the cystic or common bile ducts where they cause obstruction of the ducts and increased intraluminal pressure, leading to biliary colic and/or inflammation. Patients may present with mild symptoms, typical chronic cholecystitis, acute cholecystitis, or other complications of biliary disease. The "typical" pain associated with chronic gallstone disease is usually severe and located in the epigastric region or the right upper quadrant, radiating to the right scapula or shoulder. Pain may be precipitated by a large or fatty meal. Nausea or vomiting often accompanies the painful episodes. Fever and chills usually imply an underlying complication.

The diagnosis of cholelithiasis is usually confirmed using oral cholecystography (OCG) or cholecystosonography (ultrasound). Oral cholecystography has traditionally been the best radiologic examination for detecting gallstones. The contrast material used for the test is iopanoic acid (Telepaque), an iodinated lipid-soluble substance that is taken orally in a dose of 3 g the night prior to the procedure. Opacification of the gallbladder occurs about 15 to 20 hours after ingestion of the tablets. While the OCG remains an acceptable diagnostic test, ultrasonography is more rapid and has a lower false-negative rate. Although both the OCG and ultrasound have an overall accuracy of 90% to 98% in detecting cholelithiasis, it appears that ultrasound is replacing the OCG as the primary screening agent for suspected gallstones.[47]

### *Natural History of Gallstones*

Although the natural history of asymptomatic gallstones remains undefined, there is recent evidence to suggest that the risk for developing symptoms or complications requiring surgery is relatively low.[48] In contrast, symptomatic gallstones are more likely to result in such complications as cholecystitis, cholangitis, jaundice, and pancreatitis. The development of acute complications requires hospitalization and appropriate medical and/or surgical therapy. Treatment for these complications is not discussed here because the objective of this chapter is to focus on uncomplicated cholelithiasis and its medical management.

### *Treatment*

#### Surgery

The surgical management of "silent" gallstones remains controversial. The recommendation for a cholecystectomy in a patient with symptomatic gallstones usually depends on several factors including the presence, severity, and frequency of symptoms; the history of a prior complication of gallstone disease; or the presence of an underlying condition that places the patient at an increased risk of developing gallstone complications.[48] For most patients, surgery remains the safest, most effective, and most widely recommended treatment for symptomatic gallstones. The operative mortality associated with a cholecystectomy is less than 1%.[48]

#### Medical Therapy

Until recently, no alternative to the surgical treatment of gallstone disease was available. Development of two oral agents, chenodeoxycholic acid (CDCA) or chenodiol and ursodeoxycholic acid (UDCA), has created a new treatment option for patients unable to undergo surgery either because of increased risk (e.g., increased age, cardiovascular disease) or because they refuse surgery. Oral therapy with CDCA or UDCA is most effective if the gallstones are primarily cholesterol, are radiolucent, are small (diameter < 5 mm), and contain less than 4% calcium.[49] As both CDCA and UDCA must be secreted into the gallbladder to be effective, a functioning gallbladder is necessary.

***Chenodeoxycholic Acid*** The exact mechanism by which exogenous CDCA dissolves cholesterol gallstones is not known; however, it is thought to involve an increase in the percent of CDCA in the bile (from its normal 33% up to 60%–90%) and a reduction in both absolute and relative biliary cholesterol secretion. Although a low gallstone dissolution rate was observed in the National Cooperative Gallstone Study, a number of clinical trials have demonstrated the efficacy of CDCA when administered in a sufficient dose of 13–17 mg/kg/d.[49,50] Obese patients may require a higher dose of 18–20 mg/kg/d. Doses less than 10 mg/kg/d are generally considered to be ineffective. Gallstone dissolution usually requires 6 to 24 months of treatment and should be continued 3 months after apparent dissolution. Complete dissolution rates of 50% to 80% have been reported when optimal doses are used.[49]

A dose-related diarrhea occurs in up to 50% of patients receiving CDCA 15 mg/kg/d. The severity of the diarrhea can be minimized by starting with an initial dose of 250 mg twice daily for several weeks and then gradually increasing the dose by 250 mg/wk until the recommended dose is achieved.

Dose-related increases in serum aspartate and alanine transaminases occur in 30% of patients and may require discontinuation of the drug. Hepatotoxicity has been reported to occur in 3% of patients receiving 750 mg/d. Gallstones recur in up to 50% of patients within 5 years of discontinuation of the drug; however, low-dose prophylactic therapy after dissolution is ineffective and is not recommended.[51] An OCG or ultrasound should be done every 6 to 9 months to document stone dissolution and every several years to detect stone recurrence. A comprehensive review of the medical management of cholesterol gallstones is presented elsewhere.[49]

***Ursodeoxycholic Acid*** Ursodeoxycholic acid is similar in efficacy to adequate doses of CDCA.[49,52] The drug acts by dispersing cholesterol throughout the bile and by decreasing biliary cholesterol secretion. The optimal dose is between 8 and 12 mg/kg/d.[49,52] Unlike CDCA, UDCA therapy is rarely accompanied by diarrhea and hepatotoxicity. There appears to be an increase in efficacy when the entire daily dose is given at bedtime. Combinations of UDCA and CDCA have been reported to result in increased efficacy compared with either drug alone.[49,52]

***Monooctanoin*** Occasionally, gallstones are retained in the biliary tree after a cholecystectomy. A number of stone removal techniques have been employed including endoscopic sphincterotomy and percutaneous extraction through a T-tube tract. When mechanical extraction is not possible, medical therapy of retained cholesterol gallstones can be accomplished by perfusing monooctanoin into a nasobiliary tube or a catheter inserted into the common bile duct. A more in-depth review of this drug and the procedures involved in its administration can be found elsewhere.[53]

## Summary

For most patients with symptomatic cholelithiasis, a cholecystectomy remains the treatment of choice. Factors that influence the decision to treat medically include the patient's symptoms, age, and coexisting diseases. Oral treatment with adequate doses of CDCA is now a therapeutic option for patients with cholesterol gallstones; however, side effects are common, long-term treatment is often required, and the gallstones tend to recur. Low-dose prophylactic therapy does not appear to be effective in preventing gallstone recurrence. Because UDCA is as effective as CDCA and has less potential for causing diarrhea and hepatotoxicity, it may become the drug of choice for the medical treatment of cholesterol gallstones.

## References


1. Sarner M. Pancreatitis: Definitions and classification, in Go VLW, Gardner JD, Brooks FP, et al (eds): The Exocrine Pancreas: Biology, Pathobiology, and Diseases. New York, Raven, 1986, pp 459–464.
2. Hollender LF, Lehnert P, Wanke M. Acute Pancreatitis: An Interdisciplinary Synopsis. Baltimore, Urban & Schwarzenberg, 1983.
3. Meyer JH. Pancreatic physiology, in Sleisenger MH, Fordtran JS (eds): Gastrointestinal Disease: Pathophysiology, Diagnosis, and Management. Philadelphia, W.B. Saunders, 1983, pp 1426–1436.
4. Rinderknecht H. Pancreatic secretory enzymes, in Go VLW, Gardner JD, Brooks FP, et al (eds): The Exocrine Pancreas: Biology, Pathobiology, and Diseases. New York, Raven, 1986, pp 163–183.
5. Perry RS, Gallagher J. Management of maldigestion associated with pancreatic insufficiency. Clin Pharm 1985;4:161–169.
6. Geokas MC, Baltaxe HA, Banks PA, et al. Acute pancreatitis. Ann Intern Med 1985;103:86–100.
7. Steer ML. Etiology and pathophysiology of acute pancreatitis, in Go VLW, Gardner JD, Brooks FP, et al (eds): The Exocrine Pancreas: Biology, Pathobiology, and Diseases. New York, Raven, 1986, pp 465–474.
8. Mallory A, Kern F. Drug-induced pancreatitis: A critical review. Gastroenterology 1980;78:813–820.
9. Steinberg WM, Lewis JH. Steroid-induced pancreatitis: Does it really exist? Gastroenterology 1981;81:799–808.
10. Joffe SN, Lee FK. Acute pancreatitis after cimetidine administration in experimental duodenal ulcers. Lancet 1978;1:383.
11. Banks PA. Acute pancreatitis: Clinical presentation, in Go VLW, Gardner JD, Brooks FP, et al (eds): The Exocrine Pancreas: Biology, Pathobiology, and Diseases. New York, Raven, 1986, pp 475–479.
12. Levitt MD, Eckfeldt JH. Diagnosis of acute pancreatitis, in Go VLW, Gardner JD, Brooks FP, et al (eds): The Exocrine Pancreas: Biology, Pathobiology, and Diseases. New York, Raven, 1986, pp 481–502.
13. Moossa AR. Diagnostic tests and procedures in acute pancreatitis. N Engl J Med 1984;311:639–642.
14. Read G, Braganza J, Howat HT. Pancreatitis: A retrospective study. Gut 1976;17:945–949.
15. Ranson JHC. Etiological and prognostic factors in human acute pancreatitis: A review. Am J Gastroenterol 1982;77:633–638.
16. Gaensler EA, et al. A comparative study of the action of Demerol and opium alkaloids in relation to biliary spasm. Surgery 1948;23:211.
17. Economou G, et al. A cross-over comparison of the effect of morphine, pethidine, pentazocine and phenazocine on biliary pressure. Gut 1971;12:218.
18. DiMagno EP. What is appropriate nonoperative treatment of acute pancreatitis? Dig Dis Sci 1979;24:337–338.
19. Navarro S, Ros E, Aused R, et al. Comparison of fasting, nasogastric suction and cimetidine in the treatment of acute pancreatitis. Digestion 1984;30:224–230.
20. Cameron JL, et al. Evaluation of atropine in acute pancreatitis. Surg Gynecol Obstet 1979;148:206.
21. Usadel KH, Leuschner U, Uberia KK. Treatment of acute pancreatitis with somatostatin: A multicenter double-blind trial. (Letter) N Engl J Med 1980;303:999.
22. Ranson JHC. Acute pancreatitis: Surgical management, in Go VLW, Gardner JD, Brooks FP, et al (eds): The Exocrine Pancreas: Biology, Pathobiology, and Diseases. New York, Raven, 1986, pp 503–511.
23. Sarles H. Chronic pancreatitis: Etiology and pathophysiology, in Go VLW, Gardner JD, Brooks FP, et al (eds): The Exocrine

Pancreas: Biology, Pathobiology, and Diseases. New York, Raven, 1986, pp 527–540.

24. DiMagno EP, Clain JE. Chronic pancreatitis, in Go VLW, Gardner JD, Brooks FP, et al (eds): The Exocrine Pancreas: Biology, Pathobiology, and Diseases. New York, Raven, 1986, pp 541–575.
25. Niederau C, Grendell JH. Diagnosis of chronic pancreatitis. Gastroenterology 1985;88:1973–1995.
26. DiMagno EP, Go VLW, Summerskill WHJ. Relations between pancreatic enzyme outputs and malabsorption in severe pancreatic insufficiency. N Engl J Med 1973;288:813–815.
27. Isaksson G, Ihse I. Pain reduction by an oral pancreatic enzyme preparation in chronic pancreatitis. Dig Dis Sci 1983;28:97–101.
28. Slaff J, Jacobson D, Tillman CR, et al. Protease-specific suppression of pancreatic exocrine secretion. Gastroenterology 1984;87:44–52.
29. Halgreen H, Pedersen NT, Worning H. Symptomatic effect of pancreatic enzyme therapy in patients with chronic pancreatitis. Scand J Gastroenterol 1986;21:104–108.
30. Graham DY. Enzyme replacement therapy of exocrine pancreatic insufficiency in man. N Engl J Med 1977;296:1314–1317.
31. DiMagno EP. Medical treatment of pancreatic insufficiency. Mayo Clin Proc 1979;54:435–442.
32. DiMagno EP. Controversies in the treatment of pancreatic insufficiency. Dig Dis Sci 1982;27:481–484.
33. Graham DY. An enteric-coated pancreatic enzyme preparation that works. Dig Dis Sci 1979;24:9-6-9.
34. Dutta SK, Rubin J, Harvey J. Comparative evaluation of therapeutic efficacy of pH-sensitive enteric coated pancreatic enzyme preparation with conventional pancreatic enzyme therapy in the treatment of exocrine pancreatic insufficiency. Gastroenterology 1983;84:476–482.
35. Regan RT, Malagelada JR, DiMagno EP, et al. Comparative effects of antacids, cimetidine and enteric coating on the therapeutic response to oral enzymes in severe pancreatic insufficiency. N Engl J Med 1977;297:854–858.
36. Regan PT, Malagelada JR, DiMagno EP, et al. Rationale for the use of cimetidine in pancreatic insufficiency. Mayo Clin Proc 1978;53:79–83.
37. Graham DY. Pancreatic enzyme replacement: The effect of antacids or cimetidine. Dig Dis Sci 1982;27:485–490.
38. Stapleton FB, Kennedy J, Nousia-Arvanitakis S, et al. Hyperuricosuria due to high dose pancreatic extract therapy in cystic fibrosis. N Engl J Med 1976;295:246–248.
39. Russell RM, Dutta SK, Oaks EV, et al. Impairment of folic acid absorption by oral pancreatic extracts. Dig Dis Sci 1980;25:369–373.
40. Greenberg GR, Whittaker JS. Role of total parenteral nutrition in pancreatic disease, in Go VLW, Gardner JD, Brooks FP, et al (eds): The Exocrine Pancreas: Biology, Pathobiology, and Diseases. New York, Raven, 1986, pp 611–620.
41. Silberman H, Dixon NP, Eisenberg D. The safety and efficacy of a lipid-based system of parenteral nutrition in acute pancreatitis. Am J Gastroenterol 1982;77:494–497.
42. Adson MA, McIlrath DC. Surgical treatment of chronic pancreatitis, in Go VLW, Gardner JD, Brooks FP, et al (eds): The Exocrine Pancreas: Biology, Pathobiology, and Diseases. New York, Raven, 1986, pp 587–599.
43. Strom BL, West SL. The epidemiology of gallstone disease, in Cohen S, Soloway RD (eds): Contemporary Issues in Gastroenterology: Gallstones. New York, Churchill Livingstone, 1985, pp 1–25.
44. Gracie WA, Ransohoff DF. Natural history and expectant management of gallstone disease, in Cohen S, Soloway RD (eds): Contemporary Issues in Gastroenterology: Gallstones. New York, Churchill Livingstone, 1985, pp 27–43.
45. Holzbach RT, Kibe A. Pathogenesis of cholesterol gallstones, in Cohen S, Soloway RD (eds): Contemporary Issues in Gastroenterology: Gallstones. New York, Churchill Livingstone, 1985, pp 73–100.
46. Bennian LF, Grundy SM. Risk factors for the development of cholelithiasis in man. N Engl J Med 1978;299:1161–1167.
47. Levine MS, Kressel HY, Mintz MC. Radiologic detection of gallstones, in Cohen S, Soloway RD (eds): Contemporary Issues in Gastroenterology: Gallstones. New York, Churchill Livingstone, 1985, pp 129–143.
48. Dempsey DT, Rosato EF. Surgical management of cholelithiasis, in Cohen S, Soloway RD (eds): Contemporary Issues in Gastroenterology: Gallstones. New York, Churchill Livingstone, 1985, pp 191–213.
49. Abate MA. Medical management of cholesterol gallstones. Drug Intell Clin Pharm 1986;20:106–115.
50. Schoenfield LJ, Lachin JM, Baum RA, et al. Chenodiol (chenodeoxycholic acid) for dissolution of gallstones: The National Cooperative Gallstone Study. Ann Intern Med 1981;95:257–282.
51. Marks JW, Lan SP, Baum RA, et al. Low-dose chenodiol to prevent gallstone recurrence after dissolution therapy. Ann Intern Med 1984;100:376–381.
52. Ward A, Brogden RN, Heelk RC, et al. Ursodeoxycholic acid. A review of its pharmacological properties and therapeutic efficacy. Drugs 1984;27:95–131.
53. Abate MA, Moore TI. Monooctanoin use for gallstone dissolution. Drug Intell Clin Pharm 1985;19:708–713.

# Section Four
# Renal Disorders

## *Chapter 34* / Acute Renal Failure

Karen L. Heim-Duthoy, PharmD, Thomas Leither, MS, and Gary R. Matzke, PharmD, FCP, FCCP

Acute renal failure can be defined as an abrupt decrease in renal function or glomerular filtration rate, manifested by an increase in serum creatinine, blood urea nitrogen (BUN), and often diminished urine output. A rise in serum creatinine of 1.0 mg/dL over 2 to 3 days is generally accepted as indicative of acute renal failure[1]; however, some investigators consider smaller increases in serum creatinine indicative of acute renal failure.[2] Regardless of the precise definition, acute renal failure is severe organ failure that is potentially reversible.

The term *acute tubular necrosis* is frequently used interchangeably with acute renal failure, but it is but one of the common types of acute renal failure. Anuric, oliguric, and nonoliguric are other modifiers frequently applied to acute renal failure, and are defined as urine production of less than 50 mL, 50–400 mL, and greater than 400 mL per day, respectively. These classifications have diagnostic and prognostic relevance.

### Epidemiology

Several studies of the frequency of acute renal failure have shown the incidence of severe acute renal failure to range from 20 per million per year in East Germany to as high as 60 per million per year in Britain.[3,4] The clinical course may be rapidly progressive, and multiple dialyses are usually needed. Acute renal failure not requiring dialysis is much more common, being observed in 4% to 5% of patients admitted to general medical/surgical units and in up to 50% of patients who have undergone emergency abdominal aortic aneurysm repair[5,6] (Fig. 34.1).

In developed countries, two thirds to three fourths of patients with acute renal failure have acute tubular necrosis. This often occurs in the hospital setting and is frequently iatrogenic.[5] Acute renal failure is more commonly associated with trauma, infection, snakebites, pregnancy, and poison ingestions in underdeveloped countries.[4]

### Etiology

Acute renal failure may be divided into three broad categories: prerenal, intrinsic renal, and postrenal failure. Prerenal refers to a reduction in glomerular filtration rate that is secondary to diminished renal blood flow. Postrenal causes include obstruction of the flow of urine anywhere from the renal pelvis to the distal urethra. Intrinsic renal causes are those diseases or processes that directly injure the renal parenchyma. This category encompasses a wide variety of systemic and primary renal diseases and includes acute tubular necrosis (Table 34.1).

Acute tubular necrosis and prerenal azotemia each account for 35% to 40% of acute renal failure cases in the general medical/surgical hospital setting,[1] while acute tubular necrosis is the most common cause in many clinical settings (Fig. 34.2).[7,8] Renal disease of glomerular and vascular origin is less common, and accounts for only 10% to 20% of acute renal failure. Obstruction (i.e., postrenal acute renal failure) is important because it is eminently treatable, although it accounts for less than 10% of all cases of acute renal failure.

### Pathophysiology

The pathophysiology of the three most common forms of acute renal failure—prerenal azotemia, acute tubular necrosis, and postrenal obstruction—is of intense interest in experimental research. The pathogenesis of acute renal failure could involve decreased filtration through an altered glomerular membrane, sustained renal hypoperfusion, tubular dysfunction with backleak of filtrate, and intratubular obstruction. The pathophysiology of primary glomerular diseases is discussed in Chapter 38. The pathophysiology of other less common causes of acute renal failure has recently been reviewed and is not elaborated on in this chapter.[9,10]

#### *Decreased Ultrafiltration Coefficient*

Glomerular filtration rate is a function of glomerular transcapillary hydrostatic and oncotic pressure, as well as the filtration coefficient, which is a composite of the surface area and permeability of the glomerular capillary membrane. Consequently, reduction of the filtration coefficient and alterations in glomerular vascular resistance have been proposed as mechanisms for the observed decreases in glomer-

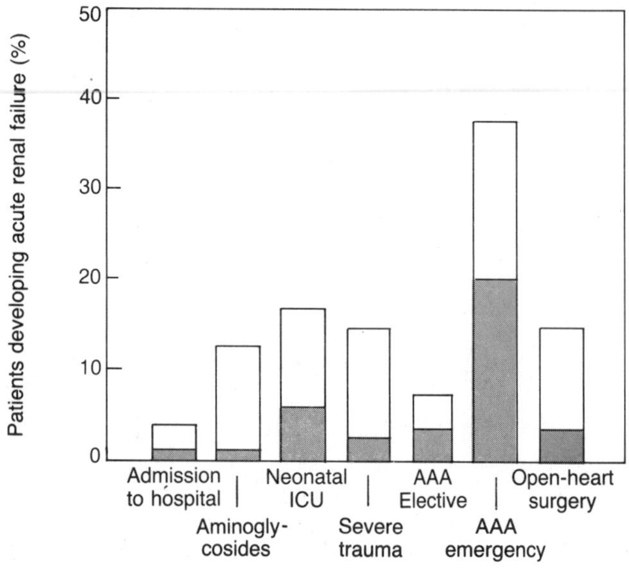


**Figure 34.1** Clinical settings associated with high frequency of acute renal failure. Serum creatinine: 3 mg/dL (nonshaded), 5 mg/dL (shaded). AAA, abdominal aortic aneurysm.

ular filtration rate. There are substantial experimental and human data to support renal vasoconstriction and diminished renal blood flow as a cause of acute tubular necrosis.[11–13] It is important to maintain renal blood flow early in acute tubular necrosis. Volume-expanding agents or vasodilators will not increase glomerular filtration rate in ''established''acute tubular necrosis. A decrease in filtration coefficient could thus be a principal determinant of diminished glomerular filtration rate in ''established'' acute tubular necrosis. This reduction in ultrafiltration coefficient as well as the alterations in glomerular vascular resistances may represent a response to angiotensin II, a vasoactive peptide known to promote an increased vascular resistance and filtration coefficient.[14]

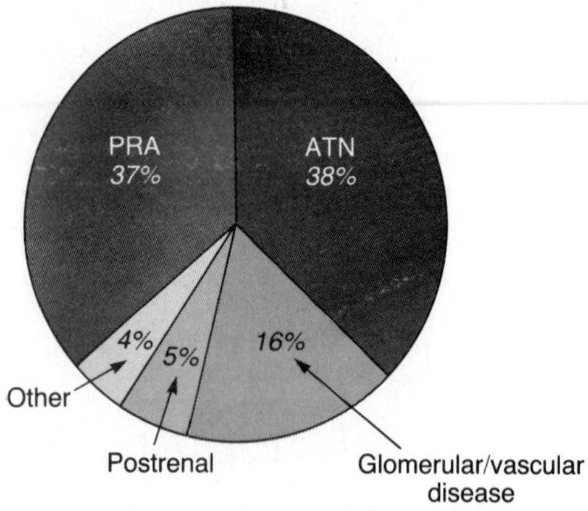


**Figure 34.2** Etiology of acute renal failure in 100 consecutive hospitalized patients. PRA, prerenal azotemia; ATN, acute tubular necrosis. *(Adapted from Rose BD [ed]: Pathophysiology of Renal Disease. New York, McGraw–Hill, 1981, p 55, with permission.)*

### *Renal Hypoperfusion*

Renal blood flow, under normal conditions, is approximately 1 L/min, or 25% of the cardiac output. When the ability of the cardiovascular system to deliver blood to the kidneys is impaired through pump failure or sympathetic discharge (i.e., renal hypoperfusion) prerenal azotemia may result. Heart failure, volume depletion, and shock are the most common causes of prerenal azotemia (Table 34.2).

The kidney is able to maintain glomerular filtration rate and renal blood flow in the presence of moderate reductions in renal perfusion pressure. This is accomplished by intrarenal hemodynamic adjustments collectively called renal autoregulation. Prerenal azotemia results when autoregulation is unable to maintain glomerular filtration rate. During the initial period of decreased renal blood flow, glomerular filtration rate (GFR) may be restored by volume expansion. Prolonged, severe renal hypoperfusion may evolve into an

**Table 34.1** Intrinsic Renal Causes of Acute Renal Failure

| | |
|---|---|
| Glomerular | Vascular |
| Postinfectious glomerulonephritis | Vasculitis |
| Membranoproliferative glomerulonephritis | Polyarteritis nodosa |
| IgA nephropathy | Wegener's granulomatosis |
| Rapidly progressive glomerulonephritis | Cryoglobulinemia |
| Systemic lupus erythematosus | Serum sickness |
| Goodpasture's syndrome | Henoch–Schönlein purpura |
| Vasculitides | Hemolytic–uremic syndrome |
| Idiopathic | Thrombotic thrombocytopenic purpura |
| Tubulointerstitial | Malignant nephrosclerosis |
| Acute tubular necrosis | Arterial thrombosis/embolization |
| Acute interstitial nephritis | Venous occlusion |
| Acute pyelonephritis | Preeclampsia |
| Acute uric acid nephropathy | Cortical necrosis |
| Multiple myeloma | Postpartum renal failure |
| Hypercalcemia | Scleroderma |

**Table 34.2** Causes of Prerenal Acute Renal Failure

| | |
|---|---|
| Decreased cardiac output | Decreased intravascular volume |
| Cardiomyopathy | Hemorrhage |
| Pericardial tamponade | Volume depletion (skin, gastrointestinal, renal losses) |
| Decreased vascular tone | Sequestration (pancreatitis, peritonitis) |
| Bacterial sepsis | |
| Vasodilating drugs | |

established phase of acute renal failure (ARF) where increased renal blood flow does not improve GFR and potentially may result in acute tubular necrosis.[15]

### *Increased Backleak*

Nonselective backleak of filtrate across damaged renal tubules was proposed by Richards in 1929 as the cause of azotemia and oliguria in acute tubular necrosis. Although backleak can be demonstrated in some nephrotoxic and ischemic models, attempts to quantify backleak are not soundly based and have not been conclusive.[15] Although backleak may account in part for the decline in glomerular filtration rate in severe acute renal failure, it cannot explain the total reduction in glomerular filtration rate observed in less severe acute renal failure.

### *Obstruction*

Tubular obstruction was first hypothesized by Minami in 1923 based on the observation of widespread intratubular casts in histologic sections of kidneys from patients with acute tubular necrosis.[15] Although most experimental models support a role for tubular obstruction with cellular casts, this has not been uniformly observed. Evidence supporting obstruction as a role in the course of acute renal failure is the fact that mannitol and/or furosemide increase solute excretion rate and result in an amelioration of acute renal failure; however, these observations have not been consistently reproducible. Thus, the precise role of obstruction in acute renal failure continues to be controversial.

## Clinical Presentation

The history and clinical setting are often helpful in determining the etiology of acute renal failure; for example, acute renal failure after repair of a ruptured abdominal aortic aneurysm likely represents ischemia-induced acute tubular necrosis, whereas the patient with significant volume depletion may have prerenal azotemia; however, the situation is often complex, as many patients with acute renal failure have been exposed to multiple potentially toxic and ischemic insults.[15]

The physical examination often adds invaluable diagnostic information. Prerenal azotemia becomes the likely diagnosis in the presence of signs of decreased effective circulating volume (i.e., decreased blood pressure, increased heart rate with standing). Obstruction of the urinary tract may be accompanied by evidence of prostatic or retroperitoneal disease, while primary or secondary glomerular disease is frequently accompanied by extrarenal pathology.[9,16]

Urine volume may give another clue to the etiology of acute renal failure. Anuria or alternating anuria with polyuria strongly suggests urinary tract obstruction. Oliguria may be seen in prerenal, intrinsic renal, or postrenal failure.

Oliguria has been considered a cardinal feature of acute tubular necrosis, but recent clinical series suggest that the nonoliguric form of acute tubular necrosis is at least as common.[17] Possible explanations for this apparent increased incidence of nonoliguric acute tubular necrosis include earlier and more widespread recognition of renal dysfunction, earlier intervention with diuretics and renal vasculature dilating drugs, or increased use of drugs that generally produce acute tubular necrosis of the nonoliguric type (e.g., aminoglycoside antibiotics).

Examination of the urine sediment is one of the oldest and most frequently used tests to diagnose urinary system disorders. Although the frequency of nonspecific findings on urinalysis has led to a decline in its clinical application by many physicians,[18] the urine should always be examined as part of the initial evaluation of the patient with acute renal failure. Heavy proteinuria ($>3.5$ g/1.73 $m^2$/d) or red blood cell casts are virtually diagnostic of glomerular disease. White blood cell casts with bacteriuria suggest pyelonephritis, while prominent urinary eosinophils suggest allergic interstitial nephritis. The presence of tubular epithelial cells with epithelial and granular casts suggests a tubulointerstitial process, most commonly acute tubular necrosis. Although hyaline casts are commonly observed with dehydration and prerenal azotemia, a paucity of findings on urinalysis is typical in both prerenal and postrenal acute renal failure.

Prerenal azotemia and acute tubular necrosis are often difficult to distinguish because those processes causing prerenal azotemia, if prolonged and severe, may culminate in acute tubular necrosis[15]; however, as aggressive fluid resuscitation (the primary treatment modality for prerenal azotemia) may adversely affect the patient with oliguric acute tubular necrosis, the ability to discriminate between these two disease processes is very important. Invasive hemodynamic monitoring may be helpful in assessing volume states and renal perfusion; however, relatively simple tests of renal tubular function may also be useful in differentiating prerenal azotemia and acute tubular necrosis. These tests assume that the normal physiologic response to decreased effective circulating volume is sodium and water conservation, while in the presence of diffuse tubular injury there is loss of the ability to conserve solute and water (Table 34.3).

Urine osmolality is a measure of the kidney's concentrating ability, and is generally high in patients with prerenal azotemia and near that of serum in patients with acute

**Table 34.3** Diagnostic Parameters for Differentiation of Prerenal Azotemia From Acute Intrinsic Renal Failure

| | *Prerenal* | *Intrinsic* |
|---|---|---|
| Specific gravity | >1.020 | <1.010 |
| Urine osmolality (mOsm) | >500 | <350 |
| Urine/plasma osmolality ratio | >1.3 | <1.1 |
| Urine/plasma urea ratio | >8 | <3 |
| Urine/plasma creatinine ratio | >40 | <20 |
| Creatinine clearance (mL/min) | >20 | <20 |
| BUN/plasma creatinine | >20 | 10 |
| $U_{Na}$ (mEq/L) | <20 | >40 |
| $FE_{Na}$ (%) | <1 | >2 |
| Renal failure index | <1 | >1 |
| $\beta_2$-microglobulin excretion (mg/24 h) | <1 | >50 |

tubular necrosis; however, the frequent finding of indeterminate values limits the usefulness of this test.[19] The concentration of sodium in the urine may also aid in the differential diagnosis. Although a very low value (<10 mEq/L) supports prerenal azotemia, wide overlap among the three most common causes of acute renal failure makes the test very nonspecific.[20] The urine-to-plasma ratios of creatinine, urea, and osmolality may also aid the clinician in making the differential diagnosis. Although a urine-to-plasma osmolality ratio of more than 1.5 strongly suggests prerenal azotemia, considerable interpatient variability makes the creatinine and urea ratios of minimal clinical utility.

The fractional excretion of sodium ($FE_{Na}$), that is, the percentage of filtered sodium excreted in the urine, is normally about 1%. The $FE_{Na}$ is calculated as follows:

$$FE_{Na} = (\text{excreted Na/filtered Na}) \times 100$$

$$= (U_{Vol} \times U_{Na})/(\text{GFR} \times P_{Na}) \times 100$$

where $\text{GFR} = U_{Vol} \times U_{Cr}/P_{Cr} \times \text{time}$. Thus,

$$FE_{Na} = U_{Na} \times P_{Cr} \times 100/U_{Cr} \times P_{Na}$$

$U_{Vol}$ is urine volume, $U_{Na}$ is urine sodium, GFR is glomerular filtration rate, $P_{Na}$ is plasma sodium, $U_{Cr}$ is urine creatinine, and $P_{Cr}$ is plasma creatinine. $FE_{Na}$ appears to have some clinical utility in the differentiation of prerenal azotemia and acute tubular necrosis. $FE_{Na}$ values less than 1% suggest prerenal azotemia; values greater than 2% suggest acute tubular necrosis. As with the other tests described, intermediate results (1%–2%) do not have predictive value. This test, although perhaps the most useful of those available, is not without its problems; there are multiple reports of patients with $FE_{Na}$ values less than 1% who have acute tubular necrosis.[21] This appears to occur primarily in the presence of certain disease states, such as cirrhosis and congestive heart failure. $FE_{Na}$ may be similarly elevated in prerenal azotemia when measured in patients who are receiving diuretics or in those who have chronic renal disease. Therefore, $FE_{Na}$ is often useful but not always conclusive.

Radiologic procedures may also be helpful in differentiating the varying etiologies of acute renal failure. A plain x-ray film of the abdomen showing obstructing calculi in the ureters is suggestive of postrenal obstruction, whereas if renal size is decreased a primary renal cause is likely. Although intravenous urography may provide useful information, the potential of these agents to cause acute renal failure limits their use. Renal ultrasonography and computerized tomography scans are noninvasive tests to examine renal size and shape and, most importantly, to identify hydronephrosis. Although both are reasonably sensitive for the detection of hydronephrosis, occasionally urinary tract obstruction may be present without hydronephrosis. Therefore, when ureteral obstruction is clinically suspected in the setting of acute renal failure, retrograde pyelography should be performed before obstruction is dismissed as an etiology.

In selected cases renal biopsy can influence diagnosis, prognosis, and therapy. It is used when no readily apparent cause of acute renal failure is identifiable or when primary or secondary glomerular disease is suspected.

The diagnostic investigation of acute renal failure should proceed in an organized sequence, with special attention to identifying potentially treatable forms of acute renal failure (i.e., prerenal and postrenal failure). It is not always possible to differentiate prerenal azotemia from acute tubular necrosis, perhaps because of limited understanding of the pathophysiology, progression from prerenal azotemia to acute tubular necrosis, or coexistence of both entities in the same patient. Thus, not infrequently, a careful trial of fluids and diuretics is warranted, as well as serial physical and laboratory examinations.

## Course/Prognosis

The clinical course of acute renal failure varies with the etiology of the renal dysfunction. An excellent outcome is expected for the patient with prerenal or postrenal failure when the underlying disease or process is promptly and effectively treated. The course of acute tubular necrosis has classically been divided into an oliguric phase, a diuretic phase, and a recovery phase. These divisions are now less meaningful with the increased frequency of nonoliguric acute tubular necrosis.

In classic oliguric acute tubular necrosis the average duration of the oliguric phase is 7 to 21 days, with a range of a few hours to 3 to 6 months.[1,15] In some patients this phase may be irreversible.[1,15] When oliguria persists for greater than 1 month the diagnosis of acute tubular necrosis should be reconsidered and other studies pursued to identify an alternative explanation for the acute renal failure. Radionuclide-flow studies may identify renal artery occlusion, while renal biopsy may identify rapidly progressive glomerulonephritis, vasculitis, or acute interstitial nephritis.

During the oliguric phase there is an accumulation of metabolic products secondary to the marked fall in glomerular filtration rate. The rate of accumulation of these substances is determined by the difference between production and excretion. Thus, patients with severe oliguric acute tubular necrosis and hypercatabolic states (e.g., fever, sepsis, severe trauma) will have more marked biochemical rates of change than noncatabolic patients.

The diuretic phase is heralded by a progressive increase in daily urine production. This diuresis is usually an appropri-

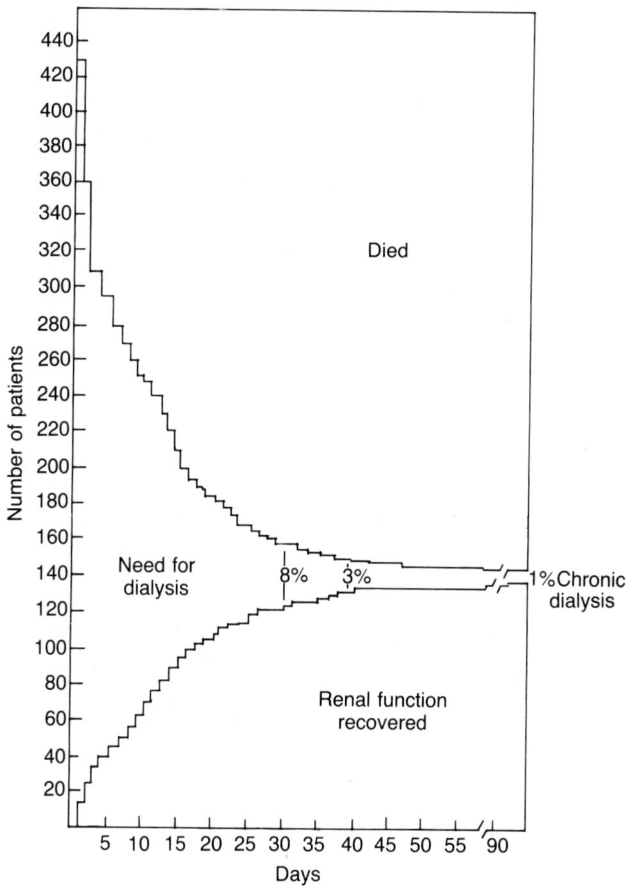


**Figure 34.3** Clinical course of 432 patients with acute tubular necrosis dialyzed at the University of Minnesota 1968–1979. *(From Kjellstrand CM, Pru CE, Jahnke WR, et al: Acute renal failure, in Drukker W, Parsons FM, Maher JF [Eds]: Replacement of Renal Function by Dialysis. Boston, Martinus Nijhoff, 1983, p 559, with permission.)*

ate physiologic response, with the recovering kidneys excreting excess solute and water retained during the oliguric phase. Rarely, the diuresis may be more profound because of the inability of the healing tubules to appropriately conserve salt or water. Serum creatinine and blood urea nitrogen concentrations usually continue to rise during the first few days of the diuretic phase, with descent following as glomerular filtration rate and excretory function increase.

The expected outcome of acute tubular necrosis is recovery of renal function to a degree adequate to sustain life without the need for dialysis in up to 95% of surviving patients.[7] Most improvement in glomerular filtration rate occurs in the first 2 to 4 weeks of the recovery phase, but further improvement may occur during the first 12 months.[15] About 30% to 60% of patients who survive acute tubular necrosis recover full renal function, and only a few (less than 5%) require long-term dialysis therapy (Fig. 34.3). There may be residual tubular defects in addition to impaired glomerular filtration rate. Permanent defects of both urinary concentration and acidification have been described.[22]

Acute renal failure is associated with a high mortality rate.

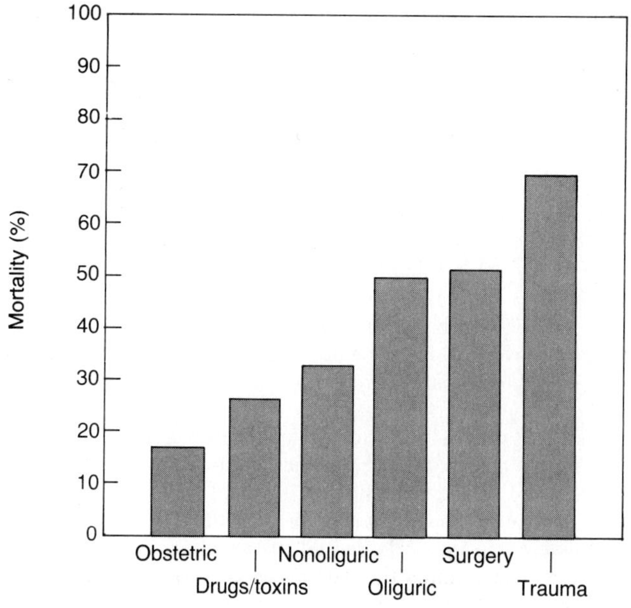


**Figure 34.4** Mortality as a function of the clinical setting and the therapy that patients were receiving. *(Data compiled from References 12 and 23–25.)*

The mortality is highly variable and dependent on the subgroups studied as well as on the definition of acute renal failure (Fig. 34.4). Mortality as low as 25% has been reported. It, however, increases in direct proportion to the observed peak serum creatinine.[5] Patients with nonoliguric acute renal failure have a lower mortality rate than those with oliguric acute renal function (26% versus 50%).[17] Nonoliguric patients have higher renal clearances, lower maximum BUN and serum creatinine values, a decreased duration of azotemia, decreased requirement for dialysis, and a significantly lower incidence of complications.[23]

In patients requiring dialysis the mortality rate is 50% to 70%, and has not significantly changed since dialysis became widely available.[23] This is surprising in light of the important advances in dialysis and care of the critically ill. The lack of improvement in survival may reflect a change in the population being treated for acute renal failure; patients are now older and have more serious underlying medical problems. A major determinant of survival is the underlying condition that precipitated the acute renal failure.[15] Age, oliguria, cardiopulmonary complications, jaundice, and hypercatabolism are associated with a significantly increased risk of mortality.[24] Acute renal failure associated with surgery and trauma has the highest mortality (50%–70%), while obstetrical procedures (15%) and medical etiologies (30%–50%) are associated with a lower mortality rate.[23,25,26]

## Treatment

Mortality remains greater than 70% in most reported series of acute renal failure and has been associated with the underlying disease or initiating event. Therefore, the treatment of acute renal failure is multifactorial and in part directed at ameliorating or removing the insult and its attendant complications.

### *Fluid and Electrolyte Disturbances*

The conversion of oliguria–anuria to nonoliguria has been associated with increased survival and reduced complications in patients with acute tubular necrosis. Therefore, several agents, including mannitol, furosemide, and dopamine, have been extensively evaluated as potential modalities to alter the character and course of acute renal failure. These approaches have yielded controversial results, in part secondary to the uncontrolled design of many of the trials, the small numbers of patients treated, variability in the patient populations, vague and variable diagnostic criteria, and use of markedly different therapeutic regimens.

Mannitol protects the kidney from several types of nephrotoxic insults. The effect may be secondary to enhancement of solute excretion,[27] decreased cell swelling,[28] inhibition of tubular obstruction,[29,30] and/or vasodilation.[31,32] It is difficult to determine whether the effect of mannitol is direct or secondary to the correction of volume status.

The protection effect of furosemide in acute renal failure has been suggested to be the result of decreased tubular obstruction, suppressed tubuloglomerular feedback, or renal vasodilatation.[15] Although the intravenous administration of furosemide to patients with established acute renal failure increases urine flow,[33,34] decreases the time of oliguria–anuria,[35] and reduces the need for dialysis,[35–38] it does not appear to alter the clinical outcome.[33,34]

Despite this evidence that diuretics may have a minimal effect on the prevention of acute renal failure, they are commonly administered in this setting as the benefits are potentially greater than the risks. Mannitol is relatively nontoxic when administered appropriately. Complications of high-dose loop diuretics occur only rarely and include permanent and severe deafness[33,34] and volume depletion. Therefore, mannitol, furosemide, or both may be initially used if blood pressure and volume status are adequate (Table 34.4). Although these treatment modalities may not improve the prognosis of acute renal failure, they increase urine flow and thereby aid in nutritional and fluid management.

Low-dose dopamine has been suggested to protect the kidney in the presence of acute renal failure by decreasing renal vascular resistance and increasing renal blood flow without altering peripheral vascular resistance and systemic arterial pressure.[39] Although low-dose dopamine therapy has been used by several investigators to prevent or treat acute renal failure,[40,42] its therapeutic effect remains controversial.

Conservative therapeutic management of patients with acute renal failure is the primary treatment modality and focuses on the prevention and treatment of complications after the emergent problems have been resolved. The primary objective of conservative treatment is to avoid dialysis and its attendant risks and costs. This may be accomplished by carefully monitoring fluid and electrolyte balance and restricting protein intake.

After normalization of intravascular volume is accomplished, fluid intake should approximate total fluid losses (1 L/d in oliguric patients). If hyponatremia develops and is associated with symptoms, hypertonic saline or dialysis may need to be used.

**Table 34.4** Agents Used in the Treatment of Acute Renal Failure[a]

| *Agent* | *Dosage* | *Special considerations* |
|---|---|---|
| Mannitol (20%) | 25 g IV over 3–5 min, may repeat in 1 h if no response; if urine output follows, 500 mL 20% mannitol with 500–1,000 mg furosemide <20 mL/h for 24 h | Monitor urine output and serum electrolytes to avoid fluid and electrolyte imbalances, particularly fluid overload |
| Furosemide | 100 mg IV; if no response within 1 h, 250 mg IV; if urine output follows, 500–2,000 mg IV per day to maintain urine flow | Monitor for fluid and electrolyte disturbances; rate should not exceed 4 mg/min as hearing loss may result if injected too rapidly |
| Dopamine | 1–5 μg/kg/min | Monitor urinary output |

[a] Agents may exert a beneficial effect when used within 24 h of the onset of oliguria.

Approximately 5% of acute renal failure patients ultimately survive but do not regain normal renal function. In these patients the transition from acute renal failure to chronic renal failure is often difficult to delineate. The treatment of nonemergent electrolyte imbalances is similar in acute renal failure and chronic renal failure patients. Although hyperkalemia is a frequent problem, severe hyperkalemia (serum potassium concentration > 6 mEq/L) may be prevented or avoided with the correction of acidosis and the provision of an adequate supply of carbohydrates. Exogenous potassium administration should obviously be minimized. Potassium-exchange resins (Table 34.5) may be used to treat hyperkalemia in patients with high but stable serum potassium concentrations not associated with severe electrocardiographic changes (i.e., peaked T waves). Sodium polystyrene sulfonate (Kayexalate, Winthrop–Breon) may be given orally or rectally as a retention enema to decrease the serum potassium. Sorbitol suspension is often concomitantly administered with oral Kayexalate to prevent fecal impaction. Kayexalate will remove approximately 1 mEq of potassium per gram when administered orally, or $\frac{1}{2}$ mEq per gram when given as a retention enema. The onset of action is 2 hours after oral administration and even longer after rectal administration. Complications associated with the use of Kayexalate include electrolyte imbalances, fluid overload secondary to the high sodium load (4.1 mEq/g), gastrointestinal upset, and fecal impaction.

**Table 34.5** Agents Used in the Treatment of Hyperkalemia

| *Agent* | *Dosage* | *Onset of action* | *Special considerations* |
|---|---|---|---|
| Kayexalate | 25–50 g PO or rectally as retention enema; sorbitol 20% to be given with Kayexalate PO | 2–3 h | Monitor for fluid, electrolyte, and GI disturbances; concomitant sorbitol to be administered for prevention of fecal impaction |
| Calcium gluconate (10%) | 10–30 mL IV at 1 mL/min | Immediate | Monitor with continuous ECG; calcium and sodium bicarbonate are incompatible |
| Sodium bicarbonate (8.4%) | 50 mL IV over 1–5 min; can be repeated | Minutes | Alkaline load |
| Glucose/insulin | 2–3 g glucose/1 unit Regular insulin; bolus: 50 mL $D_{50}W$ with 10 units Regular insulin; infusion: 1000 mL $D_{10}W$ with 25–50 units Regular insulin IV at 350–500 mL/h | Minutes | Fluid overload and glucose control |

Calcium and phosphorus imbalances are also commonly observed in patients with acute renal failure. Twitching and convulsions may occur as a result of hypocalcemia as well as from other electrolyte or fluid imbalances. Hyperphosphatemia may be prevented or treated by the use of phosphate-binding antacids. These antacids may additionally increase calcium intestinal absorption.

### *Malnutrition*

The caloric and protein requirements for acute renal failure patients are highly variable and dependent on the underlying cause(s) and whether or not dialysis has been initiated. While excessive exogenous protein supplementation may result in the accumulation of uremic waste products, an adequate supply of carbohydrates is required to minimize catabolism.

Although the intake of calories, protein, and fluid may be more liberal for those patients receiving dialysis, there are limits to the removal of these constituents. Excessive hyperalimentation may exacerbate uremia, but exogenous nitrogen is necessary to maintain a positive nitrogen balance and may decrease the hypercatabolic state frequently seen in acute renal failure patients.[43,44] Unfortunately, the optimal amino acid/carbohydrate formula has not emerged from the multiple trials that have been conducted. Blackburn et al[45] observed no significant decrease in BUN or in the rapidity with which BUN decreased in patients receiving an essential amino acid formula compared with those receiving essential amino acids and nonessential amino acids. Proietti et al,[46] however, demonstrated smaller increases in BUN with the administration of balanced amino acid solutions. Although existing data conflict, it appears that balanced solutions of amino acids may be beneficial for patients with acute renal failure and ultimately may improve their prognosis.

### *Complications*

Infection is a common occurrence in patients with acute renal failure and remains the primary cause of death. The urinary tract and pulmonary system are the most common infection sites. These infectious complications of acute renal failure may be secondary to abnormal host-defense mechanisms resulting from impaired leukocyte function and cell-mediated immunity. Uremia, acidosis, malnutrition, and the various invasive procedures may predispose the patients to infection and also increase the severity of infection. The presence of an active infection may also be masked because of impaired immunologic response. Therefore, management of infection is focused primarily on prevention. If infection is suspected, an aggressive therapeutic regimen including multiple bactericidal antibiotics is often required.

Indwelling urinary catheters should not be used for oliguric patients, as they greatly increase the risk of urinary tract infections. If urinary retention is present, straight catheterization may be used on an intermittent basis. Although hemodynamic monitoring with intravascular catheters may be necessary initially, once the patient's cardiovascular status has stabilized, noninvasive methods (i.e., clinical exam, chest x-ray films) may be used for assessment.

Extubation, patient mobilization, and respiratory therapy should be initiated as early as feasible to reduce the risk of pulmonary infection. Fungal infections may result secondary to aggressive prophylactic antibiotic use in these patients. Oral antifungal agents (Mycostatin, Squibb) may be administered concomitantly in uremic patients to prevent *Candida* overgrowth.

Nausea and vomiting are commonly encountered gastrointestinal (GI) problems in these patients and are usually avoided by the early institution of dialysis. GI complications including stress ulceration and GI bleeding are not infrequent in patients with acute renal failure. Antacids may be an effective prophylactic therapy.[47] Cimetidine (Tagamet, Smith, Kline & French) or ranitidine (Zantac, Glaxo and Hoffman–LaRoche) may also be used for the prevention or treatment of GI bleeding. The dose of cimetidine should be reduced in patients with acute renal failure as central nervous system (CNS) side effects may occur with normal doses.[48] These CNS side effects may be difficult to delineate because similar CNS complications may also result from uremia or fluid and electrolyte imbalances. Ranitidine may therefore be the preferred agent, as it appears to lack CNS toxicity. The use of cimetidine is further complicated by drug interactions secondary to inhibition of hepatic enzyme activity.

Cardiovascular complications that may occur with acute renal failure include hypertension, hypotension, cardiac failure, arrhythmias, and pericarditis. Blood pressure elevation may develop secondary to volume overload, especially with prolonged oliguria, and may resolve with the initiation of dialysis. Volume depletion or sepsis may produce hypotension. Cardiac failure and arrhythmias may result from volume overload, electrolyte imbalances, and/or hypertension. Correction of volume and electrolyte imbalances as well as pharmacologic intervention may be necessary in the management of cardiac failure and arrhythmias. Although pericarditis may present as a complication during acute renal failure, it is less frequently symptomatic than during chronic renal failure and may improve with frequent dialysis.

Neurologic manifestations of acute renal failure are variable and may be attributed to disorders of fluid and electrolytes and/or drug toxicity. These abnormalities include lethargy, somnolence, coma, confusion, agitation, neuromuscular irritability, and seizures. These complications usually rapidly improve with dialysis treatment.

The life-threatening complications associated with acute renal failure are especially evident in patients with rapidly progressive courses (Table 34.6). Hyperkalemia, metabolic acidosis, and volume overload are the most frequent of these emergent problems. Prompt treatment of these imbalances is critical if the patient is to survive.

Although serum potassium concentrations may be used to monitor therapy, they do not always correlate with electrocardiographic changes. Electrocardiographic monitoring is useful when peaked T waves are present during hyperkalemia. Therefore, the treatment of hyperkalemia is situationally dependent. If severe and urgent hyperkalemia develops, calcium gluconate can be administered intravenously in conjunction with continuous electrocardiographic monitoring. Calcium gluconate directly antagonizes potassium cardiotoxicity and has an immediate onset of action.

Combination infusions of glucose, insulin, and sodium bicarbonate may also be effective in the treatment of hyperkalemia as the combination shifts potassium intracellularly, while sodium additionally antagonizes the cardiotoxicity of potassium. Sodium bicarbonate should be slowly administered intravenously, as fluid overload may be worsened as a result of the extensive sodium load. Although exchange resins (Kayexalate) may be used for all types of hyperkalemia, their onset of action is slow and not of immediate value in the critical care environment. Dialysis, discussed below, is the most effective means of removing potassium.

Severe metabolic acidosis (pH $< 7.2$ and serum bicarbonate concentrations $< 12$ mEq/L) requires prompt treatment. Although sodium bicarbonate may be administered, dialysis is generally necessary because of the consequences of excessive sodium bicarbonate administration (Chapter 103, Acid-Base Disorders).

The nutritional needs of acute renal failure patients are usually extensive and the delivery of necessary nutrients often requires large volumes, exacerbating volume overload. As a result, oliguric–anuric patients may develop secondary complications. Therefore, aggressive efforts are necessary to prevent volume overload and its attendant complications. Primary management of volume overload consists of fluid restriction. Furosemide (Lasix, Hoechst–Roussell) or mannitol (Osmitrol, Travenol) may be administered to potentially convert an oliguric–anuric to a nonoliguric state. Dialysis, however, is generally indicated in those patients who are oliguric and do not respond to diuretics.

**Table 34.6** Complications of Acute Renal Failure

| | |
|---|---|
| Cardiovascular | Metabolic |
| Arrhythmias | Acidosis |
| Hypertension | Hyperkalemia |
| Myocardial infarction | Hyperphosphatemia |
| Pericarditis | Hyperuricemia |
| Pulmonary edema | Hypocalcemia |
| Gastrointestinal | Hyponatremia |
| Dysgeusia | Neurologic |
| Gastrointestinal bleeding | Asterixis |
| Malnutrition | Coma |
| Nausea | Mental status changes |
| Vomiting | Myoclonus |
| Hematologic | Neuromuscular irritability |
| Anemia | Seizures |
| Hemorrhagic diathesis | Somnolence |
| Infectious | |
| Peritonitis | |
| Pneumonia | |
| Septicemia | |
| Urinary tract infection | |
| Wound infection | |

## *Dialysis*

### Indications

Hyperkalemia, volume overload, severe acidosis, and serious uremic complications such as pericarditis, CNS symptoms, and intractable nausea are the classic indications for

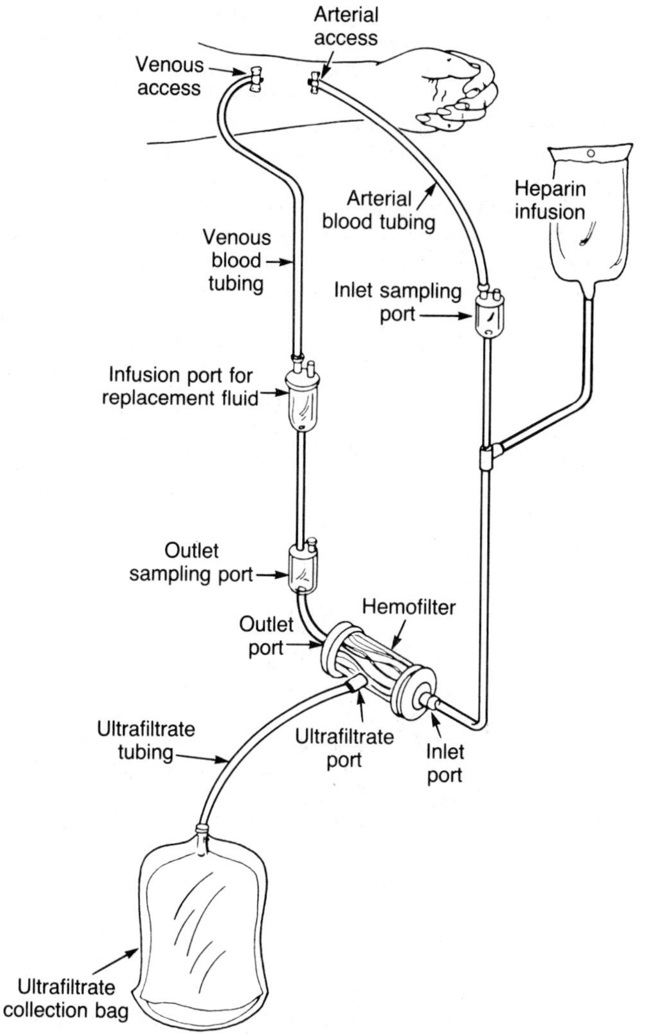


**Figure 34.5** Schematic model of continuous arteriovenous hemofiltration in the patient care setting.

dialysis. In the setting of acute renal failure, dialysis is often begun early or "prophylactically" before these absolute indications are present. This practice is supported by several series showing improved survival and fewer complications when dialysis is initiated to maintain blood urea nitrogen less than 100 mg/dL.[49–51]

## Method

Intermittent hemodialysis and continuous peritoneal dialysis remain the mainstays of dialytic therapy for acute renal failure. Slow continuous hemofiltration is a new technique that employs a small hemofilter and uses the patient's arterial pressure as the driving force for the system.[4] The filter can be hooked to wall suction if ultrafiltration is needed. This system eliminates the need for a sophisticated dialysis delivery system, blood pump, and air detectors (Fig. 34.5). Slow continuous hemodialysis and continuous hemodiafiltration, a combination of hemodialysis and hemofiltration, have recently been described in the treatment of acute renal failure, but their roles are yet to be defined.[4]

Hemodialysis is the most efficient of these methods, being 10 to 20 times more efficient than peritoneal dialysis and slow continuous hemofiltration. It allows prompt correction of life-threatening hyperkalemia and volume overload, as well as short treatment times. Its major disadvantages include a propensity to induce hypotension and arrhythmias.

Peritoneal dialysis offers the advantage of more gentle dialysis, less cardiovascular instability, and no anticoagulation. Its main disadvantages are its relative inefficiency, requiring long or continuous treatment, and the risk of peritoneal infection.

Hemodynamic stability and simplicity make slow continuous hemofiltration attractive, but it too requires continuous treatment and continuous systemic anticoagulation. The ultimate choice of dialysis method for the individual patient depends on the clinical situation and the technical expertise of the treatment center (Table 34.7).

**Table 34.7** Methods of Dialysis for Acute Renal Failure

| *Method* | *Access* | *Advantages* | *Disadvantages* |
|---|---|---|---|
| Intermittent hemodialysis | Scribner shunt<br>Femoral or subclavian venous catheter | Efficient<br>Short treatment time | Cardiovascular instability<br>Anticoagulation |
| Peritoneal dialysis | Peritoneal catheter | Cardiovascular stability<br>No anticoagulation | Inefficient<br>Peritonitis |
| Slow continuous hemofiltration | Scribner shunt | Cardiovascular stability<br>Technically simple | Inefficient<br>Continuous anticoagulation |
| Slow continuous hemodialysis | Scribner shunt<br>Femoral or subclavian venous catheter | Cardiovascular stability | Continuous anticoagulation<br>Technically complicated |
| Continuous hemofiltration | Continuous hemofiltration | Continuous hemofiltration | Continuous hemofiltration |

## Summary

Acute renal failure is a common disease occurring primarily in the hospital setting and frequently iatrogenically. Prerenal azotemia and acute tubular necrosis account for the majority of causes. Prerenal and postrenal failure carry an excellent prognosis when recognized and appropriately treated, while acute tubular necrosis continues to be associated with high mortality. The risk of death correlates most closely with the underlying disease and its complications. Renal function generally returns to a degree obviating the need for dialysis in those patients who survive.

Principles of treatment include prevention by avoidance of iatrogenic renal insults in patients with identified risk, aggressive search for the etiology of renal dysfunction, and early diagnosis. The use of diuretics, dopamine, and amino acids to prevent or modify the course of acute renal failure remains controversial. Nutritional support, an aggressive search for and treatment of infection, and early dialysis may limit complications and improve survival.


## References


1. Rose BD (ed). Pathophysiology of Renal Disease. New York, McGraw-Hill, 1981, pp 55–95.
2. Kahlmeter G, Dahlager JI. Aminoglycoside toxicity—a review of clinical studies published between 1975 and 1982. J Antimicrob Chemother 1984;13(suppl A):9–22.
3. Kjellstrand CM, Pru CE, Jahnke WR, et al. Acute renal failure, in Drukker W, Parsons FM, Maher JF (eds): Replacement of Renal Function by Dialysis. Boston, Martinus Nijhoff, 1983, pp 536–568.
4. Kjellstrand CM, Berkseth RO, Klinkman H. Treatment of acute renal failure, in Schrier RW, Gottschalk CW (eds): Diseases of the Kidney. Boston, Little, Brown and Co., 1987, pp 1501–1540.
5. Hou SH, Bushinsky DA, Wish JB, et al. Hospital-acquired renal insufficiency: A prospective study. Am J Med 1983;74:243–248.
6. Anderson RJ, Schrier RW. Clinical spectrum of oliguric and nonoliguric acute renal failure, in Brenner BM, Stein JH (eds): Contemporary Issues in Nephrology. New York, Churchill Livingstone, 1980, pp 1–16.
7. Kjellstrand CM, Ebben J, Davin T. Time of death, recovery of renal function, development of chronic renal failure and need for chronic hemodialysis in patients with acute tubular necrosis. Trans Am Soc Artif Intern Organs 1981;27:45–50.
8. Balslov JT, Jorgensen HE. A survey of 499 patients with acute anuric renal insufficiency. Am J Med 1963;34:753–764.
9. Suki WN. Renal involvement in systemic disease, in Suki WN, Massry SG (eds): Therapy of Renal Diseases and Related Disorders. Boston, Martinus Nijhoff, 1984, pp 259–382.
10. Arruda JA. Obstructive uropathy, in Brenner BM, Stein JH (eds): Contemporary Issues in Nephrology. New York, Churchill Livingstone, 1983, pp 243–273.
11. Venkatachalam MA, Rennke HG, Sandstrom DJ. The vascular basis for acute renal failure in the rat. Circ Res 1976;38:267–279.
12. Hollenberg NK, Epstein M, Rosen SM, et al. Acute oliguric renal failure in man: Evidence for preferential renal cortical ischemia. Medicine 1968;47:455.
13. Stein JH. The glomerulus in acute renal failure. J Lab Clin Med 1977;90:227–230.
14. Dworkin LD, Ichikawa I, Brenner BM. Hormonal modulation of glomerular function. Am J Physiol 1983;244:F95–F104.
15. Brezis M, Rosen S, Epstein FH. Acute renal failure, in Brenner BM, Rector FC (eds): The Kidney. Philadelphia, W.B. Saunders, 1986, pp 735–799.
16. Glassock RJ, Adler SG, Ward HJ, et al. Primary glomerular diseases, in Brenner BM, Rector FC (eds): The Kidney. Philadelphia, W.B. Saunders, 1986, pp 929–1013.
17. Dixon BS, Anderson RJ. Nonoliguric acute renal failure. Am J Kidney Dis 1985;6:71–80.
18. Schumann GB (ed): Urine Sediment Examination. Baltimore, Williams and Wilkins, 1980, pp 2–9.
19. Miller TR, Anderson RJ, Linas SL, et al. Urinary diagnostic indices in acute renal failure. Ann Intern Med 1978;89:47–50.
20. Pru C, Kjellstrand CM. Urinary indices and chemistries in the differential diagnosis of prerenal failure and acute tubular necrosis. Semin Nephrol 1985;5:224.
21. Diamond JR, Yoburn DC. Nonoliguric acute renal failure associated with a low fractional excretion of sodium. Ann Intern Med 1982;96:597–600.
22. Lewers DT, Mathew TH, Maher JF, et al. Long-term follow-up of renal function and histology after acute tubular necrosis. Ann Intern Med 1970;73:523–529.
23. Finn WF. Recovery from acute renal failure, in Brenner BM, Lazarus JM (eds): Acute Renal Failure. Philadelphia, W.B. Saunders, 1983, pp 753–774.
24. Bullock ML, Umen AJ, Finkelstein M, et al. The assessment of risk factors in 462 patients with acute renal failure. Am J Kidney Dis 1985;5:97–103.
25. Butkus DE. Post-traumatic acute renal failure in combat casualties: A historical review. Milit Med 1984;149:117–124.
26. Kron IL, Joob AW, Van Meter C. Acute renal failure in the cardiovascular surgical patient. Ann Thoracic Surg 1985; 39:590–598.
27. Teshcan PE, Lawson NL. Studies in acute renal failure. Prevention by osmotic diuresis and observations on the effect of plasma and extracellular volume expansion. Nephron 1966;3:1–16.
28. Flores J, DiBona DR, Beck CH, et al. The role of cell swelling in ischemic renal damage and the protective effect of hypertonic solute. J Clin Invest 1972;51:118–126.
29. Burke TJ, Arnold PE, Schrier RW. Prevention of ischemic acute renal failure with impermeant solutes. Am J Physiol 1983;244:F646–F649.
30. Hanley MJ, Davidson K. Prior mannitol and furosemide infusion in a model of ischemic acute renal failure. Am J Physiol 1981;241:F556–F564.
31. Slekurt EE. Changes in renal clearance following complete ischemia of the kidney. Am J Physiol 1945;144:395.
32. Morris CR, Alexander EA, Bruns FJ, et al. Restoration and maintenance of glomerular filtration by mannitol during hypoperfusion of the kidney. J Clin Invest 1972;51:1555–1564.
33. Brown CB, Ogg CS, Cameron JS, et al. High dose furosemide in acute reversible intrinsic renal failure. Scott Med J 1974;19:35.
34. Brown CB, Ogg CS, Cameron JS. High dose frusemide in acute renal failure: A controlled trial. Clin Nephrol 1981;15:90–96.
35. Cantarovich F, Galli C, Benedetti L, et al. High dose frusemide in established acute renal failure. Br Med J 1973;24:449–455.
36. Minuth AN, Terrell JB, Suki WN. Acute renal failure: A study

of the course and prognosis of 104 patients and of the role of furosemide. Am J Med Sci 1976;271:317–324.

37. Fries O, Pozet N, Dubois N, et al. The use of large doses of frusemide in acute renal failure. Postgrad Med J 1971;47:18.
38. Karayannopoulos S. High-dose frusemide in renal failure. Br Med J 1974;2:278–279.
39. Riley AL. Effect of ischemia on renal blood flow in the rat. Nephron 1978;21:107.
40. Talley RC, Forland M, Beller B. Reversal of acute renal failure with a combination of intravenous dopamine and diuretics. Clin Res 1970;18:518.
41. Lindner A. Synergism of dopamine and frusemide in diuretic-resistant, oliguric acute renal failure. Nephron 1983;33:121–126.
42. Davis RF, Lappas DG, Kirklin JK, et al. Acute oliguria after cardiopulmonary bypass: Renal function improvement with low-dose dopamine infusion. Crit Care Med 1982;10:852–856.
43. Giordano C. Use of exogenous and endogenous urea for protein synthesis in normal and uremic patients. J Lab Clin Med 1963;62:231–246.
44. Rose WC. The amino acid requirement of adult man. Nutr Abstr Rev 1957;27:631–647.
45. Blackburn GL, Etter G, Mackenzie T. Criteria for choosing amino acid therapy in acute renal failure. Am J Clin Nutr 1978;31:1841–1853.
46. Proietti R, Pelosi G, Santori R, et al. Nutrition in acute renal failure. Resuscitation 1983;10:159–166.
47. Hastings PR, Skillman JJ, Bushnell LS, et al. Antacid titration in the prevention of acute gastrointestinal bleeding: A controlled, randomized trial in 100 critically ill patients. N Engl J Med 1978;298:1041–1045.
48. Sawyer D, Conner CS, Scalley R. Cimetidine: Adverse reactions and acute toxicity. Am J Hosp Pharm 1981;38:188–197.
49. Conger JD. A controlled evaluation of prophylactic dialysis in post-traumatic acute renal failure. J Trauma 1975;15:1056.
50. Teschan PE, Baxter CR, O'Brien TF, et al. Prophylactic hemodialysis in the treatment of acute renal failure. Ann Intern Med 1960;53:992.
51. Kleinknecht D, Jungers P, Chanard J, et al. Uremic and non-uremic complications of acute renal failure: Evaluation of early and frequent dialysis on prognosis. Kidney Int 1972; 1:190.

# Chapter 35 / Chronic Renal Failure and End-Stage Renal Disease

John A. Opsahl, MD, and David R. P. Guay, PharmD, FCP

The normal human kidneys contain approximately two million functionally integrated glomerulotubular units called nephrons. Under normal conditions these nephrons work in a highly organized fashion to maintain constancy in the internal environment of the body. Although the kidney is most often thought of as an excretory organ, most of the metabolic work of the kidney is directed toward the reclamation of filtered solutes. In addition, the kidney plays an important role in the metabolism of various peptide hormones and is active biosynthetically in the production of renin, ammonia, erythropoietin, and 1,25-dihydroxyvitamin $D_3$.

Renal disease is characterized by disturbances in many of these normal functions. Evidence suggests that even as renal disease develops and adaptations take place, remnant nephrons continue to function in a highly organized fashion. Although whole kidney glomerular filtration rate falls, the glomerular filtration rate of the remnant nephrons rises. This adaptation tends to blunt the drop in whole kidney glomerular filtration rate that would occur in the absence of compensatory changes. For those nephrons with low glomerular filtration rates secondary to the underlying disease, as well as those nephrons with high glomerular filtration rates secondary to compensatory hypertrophy, the fractional excretion of a given solute (amount excreted/amount filtered) is the same. Each nephron, then, contributes to the excretion of solute in a manner proportional to its glomerular filtration rate (the so-called "intact nephron hypothesis").[1,2]

Solute balance is maintained in chronic renal failure by increases in fractional excretion for most solutes such as sodium, potassium, creatinine, blood urea nitrogen, phosphorus, and the solvent water, although the adaptive mechanisms differ in each case. The urinary excretion of any substance is dependent upon the filtered load of that substance plus the net contribution of tubular secretion and tubular reabsorption (Fig. 35.1).

Thus, there are several ways in which remnant nephrons can adapt to maintain solute balance as nephrons are destroyed. Balance for creatinine and blood urea nitrogen, solutes for which tubular secretion or reabsorption is minimal, is achieved through an increase in plasma concentration. This results in an increase in the filtered load presented to each tubule and allows remnant nephrons to increase excretion. Thus, serum creatinine rises in proportion to the decline in glomerular filtration rate and can be used clinically to estimate renal function (Fig. 35.2). As renal tubular reabsorption is the predominant mechanism of regulation of excretion for sodium and phosphorus, balance is achieved in chronic renal failure by a decrease in tubular reabsorption.

$$\text{Excretion} = \text{Filtered load} + \text{Tubular secretion} - \text{Tubular reabsorption}$$

$$\text{Filtered load} = \text{Glomerular filtration rate} \times \text{Plasma concentration}$$

$$\text{Fractional excretion} = \frac{\text{Amount excreted}}{\text{Filtered load}}$$

**Figure 35.1** Determinants of renal solute excretion.

Potassium balance, normally maintained by distal tubular potassium secretion, is maintained via further increases in tubular secretion. Thus, the plasma concentrations of some solutes rise, while the plasma concentrations of others remain relatively constant despite a progressive decline in the number of functioning nephrons. These adaptations, which appear to be solute specific, are discussed in detail later in this chapter.

There may be "trade-offs" to many of these adaptations that actually contribute to the uremic state and its complications.[3,4] Recent evidence suggests that the adaptive mechanisms that maximize whole kidney glomerular filtration rate in the face of loss of functioning nephrons may

**Figure 35.2** Relationship between serum creatinine concentration and creatinine clearance.

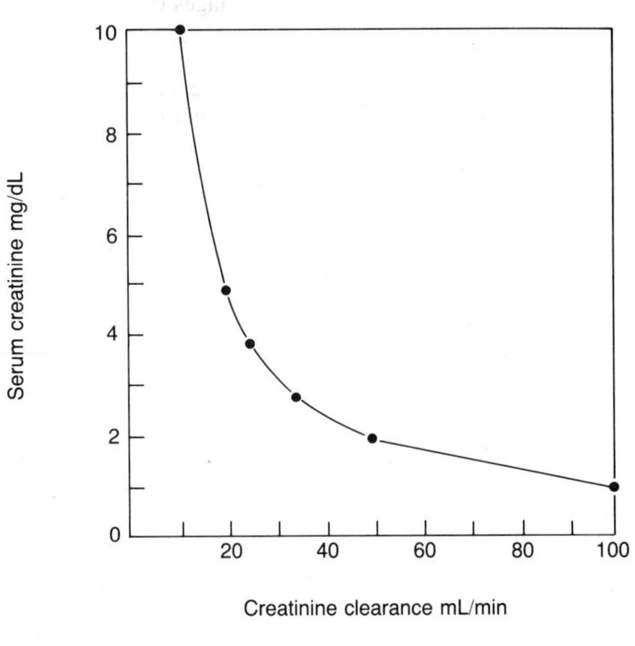

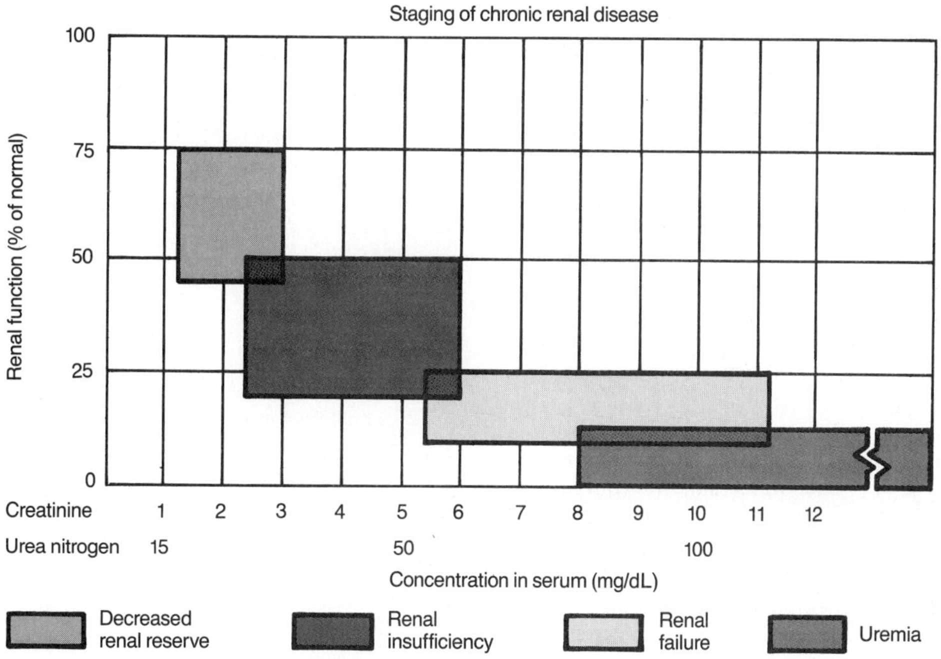


**Figure 35.3** Staging of chronic renal disease. *(Reproduced from Knochel JP: The pathophysiology of uremia. Hosp Practice 1981;16(11):67, with permission. Illustration by Albert Miller.)*

actually be responsible for the inexorable progression of chronic renal failure to end-stage renal disease.[5] An understanding of these renal adaptations is crucial to an understanding of the conservative management of chronic renal failure because many therapeutic interventions follow logically from the disordered physiology.

## Definitions

For practical purposes the clinical course of progressive renal disease is best divided into four stages (Fig. 35.3).[6]

The first of these, *loss of renal reserve*, is clinically silent and patients generally remain asymptomatic. The glomerular filtration rate, as measured by creatinine clearance, may decrease by as much as 50% before the plasma concentrations of urea nitrogen and creatinine rise above the normal range. Patients with this degree of renal functional impairment are often detected as a result of routine laboratory screening.

Further deterioration in renal function results in *renal insufficiency*, which corresponds to a creatinine clearance of 30–50 mL/min. Patients are still asymptomatic for the most part but may develop nocturia secondary to a loss of urinary concentrating ability and/or hypertension secondary to volume expansion from impaired sodium excretion. Laboratory testing reveals a modest elevation in BUN (20–50 mg/dL), increased serum creatinine, and mild anemia. A thorough evaluation to determine the etiology of the renal impairment is especially critical at this point, as the underlying disease process may reverse or stabilize with appropriate treatment.

As the creatinine clearance drops below 30 mL/min, patients develop increasing symptoms from their renal disease and complain of easy fatigability, decreased energy, cold intolerance, abnormal taste sensation, and anorexia. Laboratory abnormalities become more prominent and include progressive azotemia, hyperphosphatemia, hypocalcemia, hyperkalemia, metabolic acidosis, and worsening anemia. This is the stage of *chronic renal failure*.

*Uremia* is a clinical syndrome that develops insidiously with continued decline in renal function. It begins with nonspecific symptoms as seen in chronic renal failure. As the creatinine clearance drops below 10 mL/min, the symptoms become progressively worse. In its severest form, uremia consists of malaise, lack of energy, generalized pruritus, and intractable nausea and vomiting. Manifestations of neuromuscular irritability include leg cramps, myoclonus, asterixis, and clouded sensorium with progression to coma and/or seizures. It is at this stage (preferably before the full syndrome develops) that dialysis is indicated to remove the by-products of protein metabolism thought to be responsible for this symptom complex.

The patient requiring chronic dialysis is said to have *end-stage renal disease* (ESRD).

## Etiology

Many diseases of the kidney, both primary and secondary, can ultimately lead to the total destruction of functioning renal parenchyma. The composition of the chronic dialysis populations at different centers in the United States are remarkably similar and reflect the incidence of those diseases causing chronic renal failure. Our experience with 936 patients who began dialysis in 1980–1984 is detailed in Table 35.1. During 1985 and 1986, the incidence of end-stage renal disease secondary to diabetic nephropathy increased and accounted for roughly 50% of the patients initiating dialysis

**Table 35.1** Etiology of End-Stage Renal Disease

| *Underlying disease* | *Percentage of total patients* |
|---|---|
| Diabetic nephrosclerosis | 34 |
| Chronic glomerulonephritis (all types) | 18 |
| Tubulointerstitial disease (all types) | 13 |
| Hypertensive nephrosclerosis | 12 |
| Polycystic kidney disease | 7 |
| Vascular disease, atheroembolic disease | 4 |
| Unknown and other causes | 12 |

in our center. Other dialysis centers with larger numbers of black patients have a greater percentage of patients with hypertensive nephrosclerosis.

## Pathophysiology

### *Progressive Nature of Renal Disease*

With rare exceptions, chronic renal failure is a progressive disease process that causes total destruction of functioning renal mass. Ultimately, dialysis or renal transplantation is necessary to sustain life. This progression to end-stage renal disease is frequently independent of the activity of the underlying disease process and often occurs when the initiating process is no longer active.[5,7] Clinically there appears to be a critical mass of functioning nephrons below which a predictable steady decline in renal function occurs. This correlates with a serum creatinine concentration of approximately 3 mg/dL and a creatinine clearance of 25–30 mL/min.

The mechanisms responsible for the progressive nature of chronic renal failure have not been completely defined. Based on experimental studies it has been suggested that metabolic factors, such as altered calcium and phosphorus metabolism or hyperlipidemia, as well as adaptive hemodynamic changes participate in progressive nephron destruction.

Disordered calcium and phosphorus metabolism leads to hyperphosphatemia and secondary hyperparathyroidism and may result in the deposition of calcium and phosphorus in the interstitium of the kidney. This in turn incites an inflammatory reaction leading to fibrosis and further destruction of renal parenchyma.[8] Histologic studies in animals and man have indeed demonstrated calcium and phosphorus deposition in the renal interstitium in chronic renal failure.[8,9] Dietary phosphate restriction can ameliorate secondary hyperparathyroidism and has been demonstrated to have a stabilizing effect on renal function in some animal models. Definitive evidence that phosphate restriction alone can slow the rate of decline of renal function in man is lacking.

Recent experimental data suggest that the abnormalities in lipid metabolism that invariably accompany renal disease may also contribute to progressive glomerular injury.[10,11] Additionally, treatment with lipid-lowering agents has a beneficial effect on renal structure and function in experimental models of chronic renal failure.[12,13]

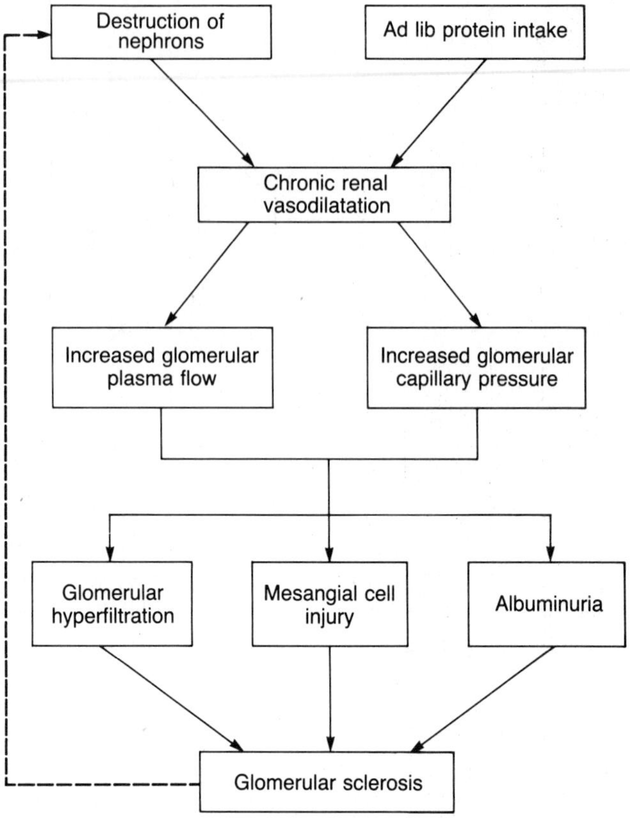


**Figure 35.4** Schematic representation of proposed mechanisms of progressive glomerular sclerosis in chronic renal failure. (*Adapted from Brenner BM, Meyer TW, Hostetter TH: Dietary protein intake and the progressive nature of kidney disease: the role of hemodynamically mediated glomerular injury in the pathogenesis of progressive glomerular sclerosis in aging, renal ablation, and intrinsic renal disease. N Engl J Med 1982;307:657, with permission.*)

Adaptive increments in glomerular plasma flow and glomerular capillary pressure may be important in the progressive nephron destruction seen in chronic renal failure.[14,15] As nephrons are lost to renal disease, residual nephrons increase both in size and in function such that the average plasma flow and glomerular filtration rate of the remaining nephrons rise.[15,16] This adaptation, which tends to maximize total glomerular filtration rate in the residual renal mass, is accomplished in large part by dilatation of the afferent arteriole. Such a reduction in afferent arteriolar resistance results in glomerular hypertension. Increased glomerular capillary pressures and flows, in turn, result in proteinuria as well as increased "trafficking" of plasma proteins through the mesangium.[17] This increased flux of macromolecules could damage mesangial cells and ultimately result in progressive mesangial and glomerular sclerosis (Fig. 35.4).

The exact mechanism that induces afferent arteriolar dilatation and produces the adaptive increases in single-nephron glomerular filtration rates has not been determined. It has been known for some time that a relationship exists between dietary protein intake and glomerular filtration rate.

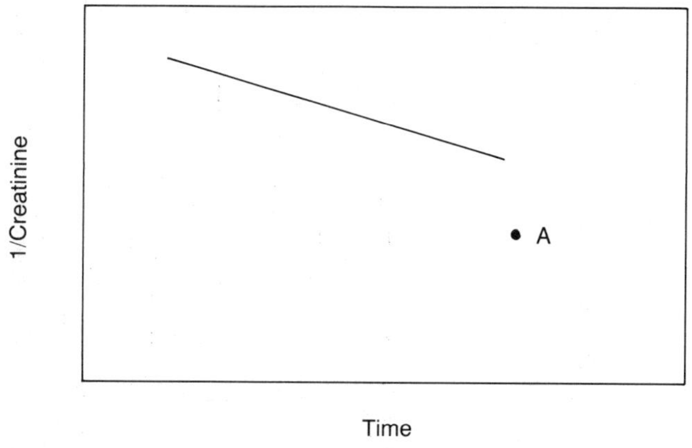


**Figure 35.5** Stylized plot depicting the decline of renal function for a patient with chronic renal failure.

Protein loading induces afferent arteriolar dilatation and increases the whole kidney glomerular filtration rate.[18] This renal vasodilatation is likely hormonally mediated but the exact mechanism is unknown. Evidence is accumulating that a normal dietary protein intake in the face of reduced renal function may result in glomerular capillary hypertension. Additionally, restriction of dietary protein intake in experimental models of chronic renal failure can reduce glomerular capillary hypertension and prevent progressive nephron destruction.[15] Studies of protein restriction in humans with chronic renal failure also suggest that dietary protein restriction can slow the rate of progression of renal disease.[19–23] In a similar manner, pharmacologic intervention with certain antihypertensive agents may specifically reduce both systemic and glomerular capillary pressure, thereby slowing or preventing progressive glomerular injury. Preliminary work in rats with enalapril, an angiotensin-converting enzyme inhibitor, suggests the potential usefulness of this class of medications in the treatment of humans with chronic renal disease.[24,25]

While there is considerable variation in the rate of progression of renal disease from patient to patient and from disease to disease, the rate is relatively constant for any given patient.[26,27] A plot of 1/serum creatinine against time in most patients reveals a predictable rate of loss of renal function (Fig. 35.5). This relationship can be used to predict the time at which the patient is likely to need dialysis (i.e., the point at which the serum creatinine is approximately 10 mg/dL). In addition, such a display of historic data can be very useful in following a patient's course. Whether a change in renal function fits the graph as predicted can be easily determined. If the patient's rate of decline in renal function is greater than predicted, an evaluation for potentially reversible reasons for an accelerated decline in renal function should be initiated.

### *Adaptation to Progressive Nephron Loss*

As nephrons are lost to renal disease many adaptive mechanisms are called into play in an attempt to maintain homeostasis. Many of the adaptive mechanisms have "trade-offs," which at some point can actually become maladaptive by virtue of the problems they create. There do not appear to be any effective adaptive mechanisms to the biosynthetic failure of the kidney which includes decreased ammoniagenesis, decreased production of 1,25-dihydroxyvitamin $D_3$, and decreased erythropoietin production. The adaptive mechanisms to excretory failure appear to be solute specific and are discussed in the following.

#### Sodium Homeostasis

***Normal State*** Sodium balance is maintained with a normal sodium intake of 120–150 mEq/d. The fractional excretion of sodium ($FE_{Na}$) is approximately 1% (see Fig. 35.6).

***Chronic Renal Failure*** Sodium balance is maintained but in a mildly volume expanded state. $FE_{Na}$ increases to as high as 10% to 20%. The exact mechanism whereby $FE_{Na}$ increases is unknown but may be the result of increased levels of "natriuretic hormone." The increased secretion of natriuretic hormone is probably triggered by volume expansion.

***Trade-off*** Volume expansion results in hypertension. Increased levels of natriuretic hormone may interfere with sodium and calcium transport in vascular smooth muscle, resulting in increased resting muscle tone. The resultant

**Figure 35.6** Sodium homeostasis and adaptive mechanisms in chronic renal failure.

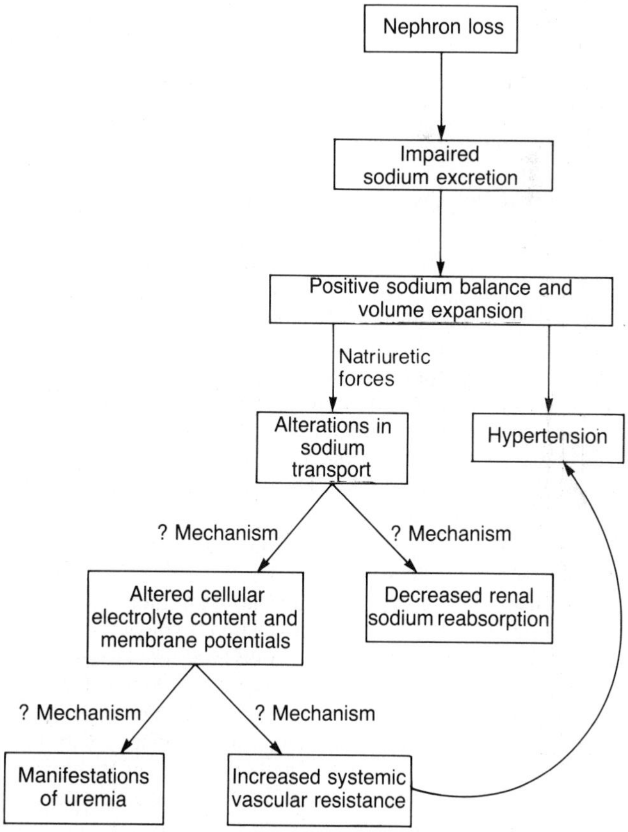

increase in peripheral vascular resistance probably contributes to hypertension. Elevated levels of natriuretic hormone may inhibit sodium and potassium ATPase-dependent pumps in many cells of the body, resulting in altered cellular electrolyte content and membrane potentials that may contribute to the uremic state.

*Clinical Consequences* The ability of the kidney to adjust to abrupt changes in sodium intake is greatly diminished in chronic renal failure. Sodium restriction beyond a no-added-salt diet (80–120 mEq/d) should not be recommended except in the face of hypertension or edema. Although it has been taught that patients with chronic renal failure are frequently "salt wasters" (i.e., develop volume depletion secondary to negative sodium balance when sodium intake is restricted) this is untrue in most cases. In fact, the kidney maintains the ability to lower urinary sodium content to essentially zero, but this can be accomplished only by very gradual sodium restriction over a prolonged time period.[28] In most circumstances, the inappropriate natriuresis and weight loss seen with sodium restriction in patients with chronic renal failure are direct results of the sluggishness of the deadaptation process rather than "salt wasting." Hospitalized patients, therefore, should not routinely be sodium restricted, as they have adapted to their outpatient intake. Negative sodium balance and its resultant volume contraction can result in decreased renal perfusion and subsequent further decline in glomerular filtration rate (GFR). Saline-containing intravenous solutions should be used cautiously in hospitalized patients who are prone to volume overload. Hypertension in chronic renal failure patients is often volume dependent, and diuretics should be used as initial therapy in most cases.

**Potassium Homeostasis**

*Normal State* Potassium balance is maintained with a normal potassium intake of 50–70 mEq/d. Urinary potassium excretion is determined primarily by distal tubular potassium secretion. The fractional excretion of potassium ($FE_K$) is approximately 25% (see Fig. 35.7).

*Chronic Renal Failure* Potassium balance is maintained by an increase in distal tubular potassium secretion in which aldosterone plays an important role. Increased tubular fluid flow rates facilitate distal tubular potassium secretion. $FE_K$ can increase to as high as 125%. The serum potassium concentration is usually maintained in the normal range until advanced renal failure (GFR $<$ 10 mL/min) develops. An increase in aldosterone-mediated potassium secretion by the colon contributes to the maintenance of external balance.

*Clinical Consequences* Although no restriction of dietary intake is usually necessary, patients with chronic renal failure tolerate potassium loads poorly. Potassium-sparing diuretics are relatively contraindicated in chronic renal failure patients because of the high risk of hyperkalemia. $\beta$-Blockers, predominantly via $\beta_2$-antagonistic effects, may interfere with the extrarenal translocation of potassium into cells and result in a further impairment in potassium handling and life-threatening hyperkalemia. Constipation in dialysis patients can interfere with colonic potassium excretion and result in hyperkalemia.

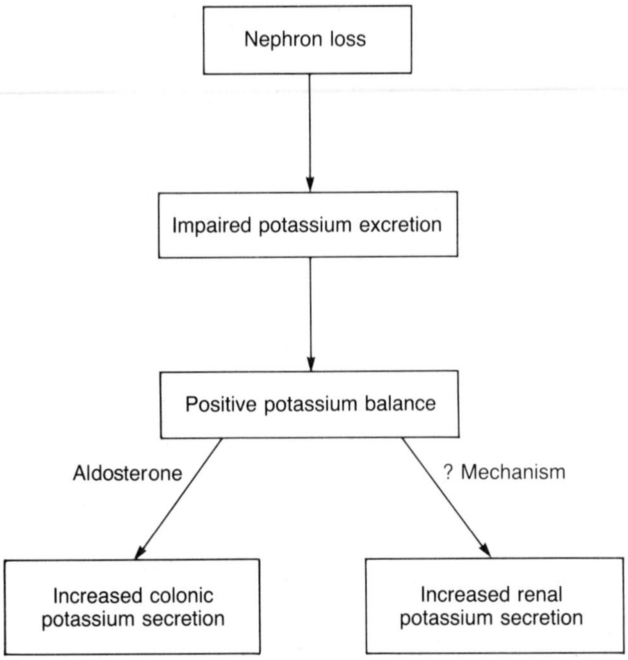


**Figure 35.7** Potassium homeostasis and adaptive mechanisms in chronic renal failure.

**Hydrogen Ion Homeostasis**

*Normal State* Hydrogen ion balance is maintained. Enough hydrogen ion is generated by the kidney to (1) reclaim all filtered bicarbonate and (2) secrete approximately 1 mEq of hydrogen ions per kilogram per day, which are generated from the metabolism of dietary proteins. Renal ammoniagenesis and phosphate excretion provide urinary buffer that facilitates acid excretion (see Fig. 35.8).

*Chronic Renal Failure* All filtered bicarbonate is reclaimed, but the ability of the kidneys to synthesize ammonia is impaired. This decrease in urinary buffer results in decreased net acid excretion and continuous positive hydrogen ion balance. A clinically significant metabolic acidosis is uncommonly seen before the glomerular filtration rate drops below 20 mL/min. The plasma bicarbonate concentration tends to stabilize at 10–20 mEq/L.

*Clinical Consequences* In the presence of metabolic acidosis, bone buffering of hydrogen ions may contribute to renal bone disease. Dietary phosphate restriction or treatment with phosphate binders decreases urinary phosphate excretion and can further impair renal hydrogen ion excretion. The presence of a metabolic acidosis may contribute to the fatigue and decreased exercise tolerance seen in patients with chronic renal failure. Alkali therapy in one form or another is often required.

**Water Homeostasis**

*Normal State* Water balance is maintained. The normal range of urinary osmolality is 50–1,200 mOsm/L.

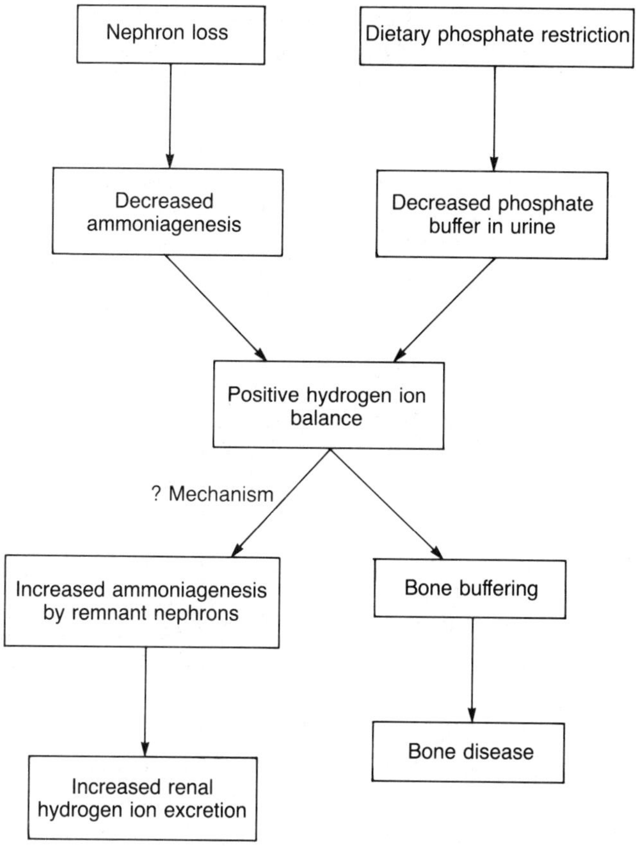


**Figure 35.8** Hydrogen ion homeostasis and adaptive mechanisms in chronic renal failure.

***Chronic Renal Failure*** Water balance is generally maintained but with a limited range of water excretion. As the fractional reabsorption of sodium is decreased secondary to natriuretic hormone, free water generation by the kidney is impaired. An osmotic diuresis caused by a large solute load per remnant nephron results in obligatory water losses. The ability to dilute or concentrate the urine is impaired and urine is isosthenuric (urinary osmolality fixed at that of plasma or approximately 300 mOsm/L).

***Clinical Consequences*** Nocturia is present relatively early in the course of renal disease secondary to the defect in urinary concentrating ability. Fluid restriction is generally not necessary provided sodium intake is controlled, as an intact thirst mechanism maintains total body water and effective plasma osmolality near normal. Because urine volume is relatively fixed at approximately 2 L/day, fluid restriction below this amount should be avoided. Large amounts of free water administered orally or as intravenous fluid may induce hyponatremia and volume overload.

**Phosphorus Homeostasis**

***Normal State*** Phosphate balance is maintained at a normal serum phosphate concentration. The normal tubular reabsorption of phosphate is 80% to 95% (see Fig. 35.9).

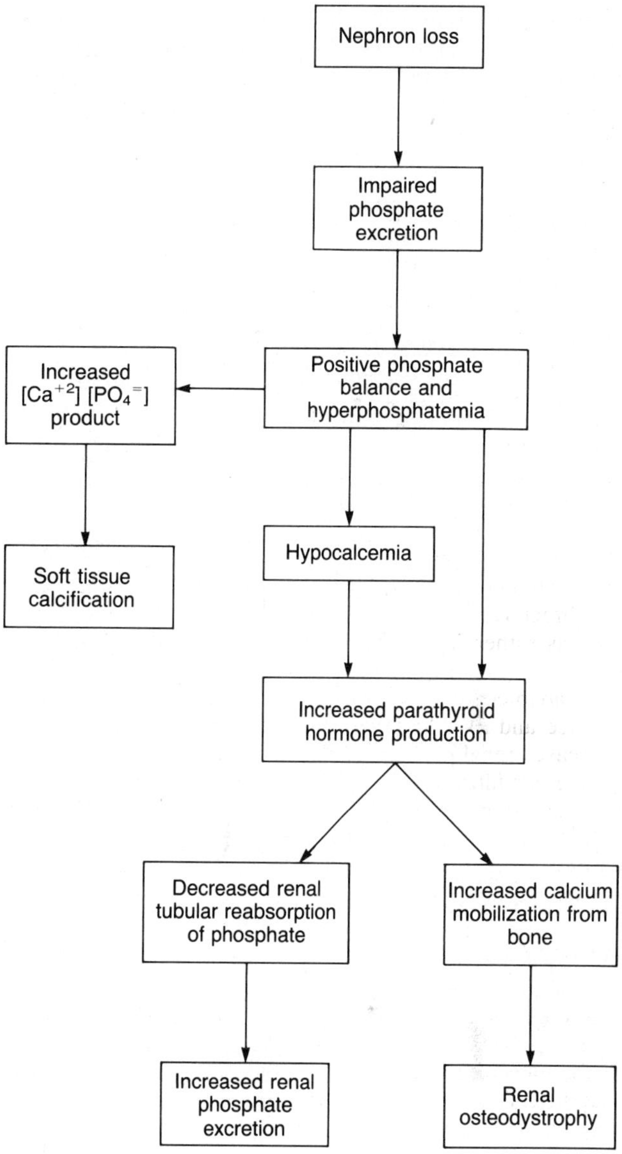


**Figure 35.9** Phosphorus homeostasis and adaptive mechanisms in chronic renal failure.

***Chronic Renal Failure*** Hyperphosphatemia develops and results in hypocalcemia and secondary hyperparathyroidism. Parathyroid hormone decreases proximal tubular phosphate reabsorption and restores phosphate balance. Phosphate balance is maintained with normal serum phosphate concentrations until the glomerular filtration rate falls below 30 mL/min. The tubular reabsorption of phosphate may fall to as low as 15%.

***Trade-off*** Phosphate balance is maintained but hyperparathyroidism induces bone disease. Additionally, parathyroid hormone may itself be a uremic toxin. Hyperparathyroidism and hyperphosphatemia may result in calcification and fibrosis of the renal interstitium and contribute to progression of renal disease.

*Clinical Consequences* The serum phosphate concentration should be controlled with restriction of dairy product intake and use of phosphate binders.

**Calcium Homeostasis**

*Normal State* Calcium balance.

*Chronic Renal Failure* Patients are generally in negative calcium balance. Dietary calcium intake is reduced unavoidably by dietary phosphate restriction. Gastrointestinal absorption of calcium is decreased because of decreased renal synthesis of 1,25-dihydroxyvitamin $D_3$. Renal osteodystrophy results from a combination of vitamin D deficiency and hyperparathyroidism (see Fig. 35.10).

*Clinical Consequences* The initial goal of therapy is to normalize the serum phosphorus concentration with dietary restriction and phosphate binders. Calcium supplementation is indicated for most patients. A vitamin D analogue may be necessary in patients with symptomatic bone disease to suppress parathyroid hormone production, although the use of vitamin D analogues in chronic renal failure patients is thought by some investigators to contribute to deterioration in renal function.[29]

**Protein Homeostasis**

*Normal State* An ad libitum protein intake is maintained. Renal solute excretion keeps pace with solute generation from protein metabolism. Amino acid intake is a determinant of glomerular filtration rate. The kidney maintains a normal BUN and "normal" plasma concentrations of end products of protein metabolism.

*Chronic Renal Failure* The kidneys' ability to excrete the metabolic by-products of protein metabolism is decreased. This results in increased BUN, increased plasma concentrations of organic and inorganic acids, and increased plasma concentrations of many "uremic toxins."

*Trade-off* A normal dietary protein intake in chronic renal failure may result in glomerular injury (glomerulosclerosis) and contribute to the progression of renal failure.

*Clinical Consequences* Dietary protein restriction postpones development of "uremic" symptoms and may retard the progression of renal failure. A high caloric intake should be maintained to avoid calorie-deficiency malnutrition. Dialysis should be initiated when the patient becomes symptomatic from buildup of uremic toxins.

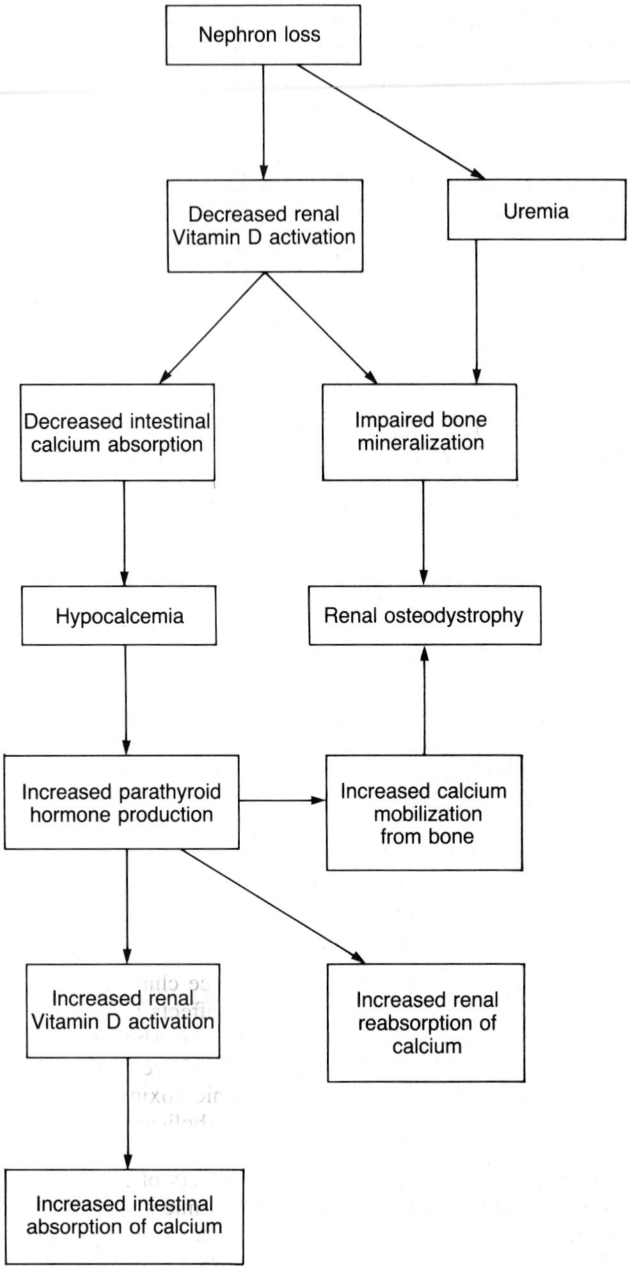


**Figure 35.10** Calcium homeostasis and adaptive mechanisms in chronic renal failure.

### *Uremic State*

Despite multiple investigations, the exact toxin(s) responsible for the manifestations of the uremic syndrome has not been determined. No one toxin is responsible for all of the abnormalities seen in uremia, and the clinical picture likely results from an interplay of multiple factors.

Several mechanisms could contribute to the presence of uremic "toxins" as chronic renal failure progresses. Most likely, the uremic syndrome results from elevations in blood concentrations of various molecules rather than from a depletional syndrome related to prescribed or spontaneous dietary alterations in chronic renal failure. A number of organic compounds are known to accumulate in uremia (Table 35.2). Accumulation could result from several potential mechanisms including the following:

1. Decreased excretion. This would be most typical of the metabolic by-products of protein metabolism that accumulate as the whole kidney glomerular filtration rate falls.
2. Increased secretion of biologically active substances

**Table 35.2** Potential Toxins in Uremia

| | |
|---|---|
| Urea | Lipochromes |
| Cyanate | Insulin |
| Creatinine | Glucagon |
| Methylguanidine | Parathyroid hormone |
| Guanidinosuccinic acid | Natriuretic hormone |
| Other guanidines | Growth hormone |
| Uric acid | Gastrin |
| Cyclic AMP | Renin |
| Pyridine derivatives | Gastric inhibitory peptide |
| Amino acids | Human pancreatic polypeptide |
| Aliphatic amines | Calcitonin |
| Aromatic amines | Prolactin |
| Indoles | $\beta_2$-Microglobulin |
| Phenols | $\beta_1$-Microglobulin |
| Myoinositol | Lysozyme |
| Glucuronic acid | Retinol-binding protein |
| Oxalic acid | $\alpha_2$-Glucoprotein |
| Acetoin | Ribonuclease |
| Middle molecules | |

overproduced as part of the adaptation to the loss of renal mass. The increased secretion of parathyroid hormone and natriuretic hormone noted in chronic renal failure patients may actually contribute to the uremic syndrome.

3. Decreased clearance of endogenous substances normally metabolized by the kidney, including multiple peptide hormones such as parathyroid hormone, gastrin, growth hormone, glucagon, somatostatin, prolactin, calcitonin, and insulin.

The ability of uremic toxins to produce clinical manifestations results in large part from their effects on a cellular level. The uremic syndrome is characterized by prominent alterations in transmembrane transport as well as cellular water and electrolyte content.[30] Uremic toxins may also have direct effects on intermediary metabolism.

It seems most likely that the uremic syndrome results primarily from the retention of by-products of protein metabolism; many manifestations of the uremic syndrome can be improved markedly with protein restriction. The role of other potential toxins has been much more difficult to determine.

## Clinical Presentation

The adaptation to and consequences of renal excretory and biosynthetic failure affect every organ system in the body. Many of these have already been dealt with in the preceding discussions, but a brief review by organ system follows.

### *Cardiovascular System*

Sodium retention and the resultant volume expansion can result in volume overload and pulmonary edema. Hypertension induced by volume expansion and increased systemic vascular resistance increases myocardial work and results in left ventricular hypertrophy. In addition, hypertension represents a major risk factor for cardiovascular disease and the accelerated atherosclerosis seen in these patients. Uremic toxins decrease myocardial contractility. The high cardiac output state induced by anemia may be poorly tolerated in the face of underlying heart disease. Uremic toxins can induce uremic pericarditis, a potentially fatal complication of chronic renal failure.

### *Pulmonary System*

The combination of volume overload and uremic toxin–induced increases in capillary permeability can result in noncardiogenic pulmonary edema.

### *Gastrointestinal Tract*

Anorexia, hiccups, and a metallic taste in the mouth are common in chronic renal failure. In uremia, nausea, vomiting, diarrhea, or abdominal distension may occur. Gastric and colonic mucosal ulcerations with resultant gastrointestinal bleeding are common.

### *Nervous System*

Uremic toxins may increase neuromuscular irritability and result in leg cramps, restless leg syndrome, and reversal of the sleep–wake cycle. Uremic toxins can induce a peripheral neuropathy. The clinical manifestations of uremic encephalopathy include clouded sensorium, coma, seizures, myoclonic jerks, and asterixis. Dialysis dementia can result from aluminum intoxication in chronic dialysis patients.

### *Hematologic System*

A normochromic, normocytic anemia secondary to decreased erythropoietin production and shortened erythrocyte survival is common. A prolongation in the bleeding time and a bleeding diathesis can result from platelet dysfunction and can be corrected by red cell transfusion or administration of cryoglobulin or vasopressin analogues.[31,32]

### *Musculoskeletal System*

Bone disease (renal osteodystrophy) is a common complication of chronic renal failure and end-stage renal disease. Osteomalacia secondary to vitamin D deficiency and osteitis fibrosa secondary to hyperparathyroidism may result in bone pain and bone fractures. Both are characterized by hypocalcemia and increased circulating levels of parathyroid hormone. The long-term use of aluminum-containing antacids or dialysis with water containing aluminum may cause osteomalacia with normal to high serum calcium concentrations and normal to moderately elevated parathyroid hormone concentrations. Calcification of blood vessels or soft tissues may occur secondary to elevation of the calcium–phosphorus product. Parathyroid hormone may induce a myopathy characterized by proximal muscle weakness.

### *Endocrine System*

The hypothalamus is "reset" as seen in other acute illnesses. Most patients are symptomatic as if hypothyroid (i.e., low energy, cold intolerance, constipation) but typically the levothyroxine ($T_4$) concentration is low, and the thyroid-stimulating hormone concentration normal. Hypothermia with decreased heat generation from suppression of cellular sodium transport is common. Hyperglycemia can occur secondary to peripheral resistance to insulin. Diabetic patients with chronic renal failure often present with more frequent hypoglycemic episodes because the kidney is responsible, in large part, for the degradation of insulin. Insulin doses must be adjusted downward as renal failure progresses. Primary hypogonadism as well as hypothalamic abnormalities contribute to sexual dysfunction and sterility.

### *Lipid Abnormalities*

Type IV hyperlipidemia with hypertriglyceridemia and low high-density lipoprotein cholesterol concentrations is very common in chronic renal failure patients secondary to decreased catabolism of lipoproteins. Whether this contributes to the high incidence of cardiovascular disease seen in chronic renal failure and end-stage renal disease patients remains controversial. Similarly, whether treatment directed at the lipid abnormalities benefits these patients is unknown. Administration of clofibrate to patients with reduced renal function is not advisable because of an increased incidence of muscle and liver toxicity secondary to decreased clearance of clofibrinic acid.[33]

### *Dermatologic System*

Dry, flaking skin and generalized pruritus are common manifestations of uremia.

### *Immune System*

An absolute lymphopenia is common in uremic patients. Cell-mediated immunity is impaired secondary to the presence of uremic toxins or protein-calorie malnutrition. A variable mild defect in immunoglobulin production has been described. Defective immune functioning appears to have minor clinical importance.

The exact uremic toxin(s) inducing these effects is unknown. The prevalence of symptoms (and presumably the level of uremic toxins) appears to parallel the rise in blood urea nitrogen in these patients.

## Treatment

The therapeutic management of the patient with chronic renal failure hinges on several important principles. First, those treatments known to slow the rate of progression of renal disease, including protein restriction and aggressive treatment of hypertension, should be applied. Whether therapy with angiotensin-converting enzyme inhibitors would prove particularly beneficial at slowing the rate of decline in renal function in hypertensive or even normotensive patients with chronic renal failure remains unknown. Second, patients must receive dietary instruction to limit protein, potassium, and phosphorus intake and maintain adequate caloric intake. (See Chapter 111.) Phosphate binders and calcium supplements should be used as appropriate. Therapy with alkali should be administered to those patients with a systemic acidosis (serum bicarbonate $< 20$ mEq/L). Third, renal function must be followed closely.

If a patient's renal function is deteriorating more rapidly than predicted (point A, Fig. 35.5), a vigorous search for reversible causes is warranted. Potential reasons for acceleration in the rate of decline of renal function in a patient with chronic renal failure include the following:

1. Volume depletion secondary to inappropriate salt restriction or diuretic therapy
2. Uncontrolled hypertension
3. Relative hypotension (mean arterial blood pressure decreases below the point at which the kidneys are able to maintain renal blood flow by autoregulation)
4. Urinary tract infection
5. Urinary tract obstruction (i.e., papillary necrosis, prostatic hypertrophy)
6. Drug-related effects (see Chapter 36)
   a. Interstitial nephritis
   b. Hemodynamic effects (i.e., nonsteroidal anti-inflammatory drugs)
   c. Direct nephrotoxic effects
7. Congestive heart failure and resultant decrease in renal blood flow

### *Dialysis*

In general, patients are managed conservatively until uremic symptoms become prominent. This uncommonly occurs before the creatinine clearance has dropped to 10 mL/min or less. Criteria for the initiation of dialysis in chronic renal failure (CRF) patients are largely clinical and include nausea and vomiting, uremic encephalopathy (confusion, asterixis, seizures), myoclonus, uremic pericarditis, development of peripheral neuropathy, and development of pruritus. Dialysis is also instituted prophylactically before major surgery.

Once dialysis therapy is initiated, patients need further dietary instruction, as dietary protein intake can be liberalized. (See Chapter 111.) Adequate caloric intake and dietary phosphate restriction remain important goals of dietary management. A no-added-salt diet and fluid restriction to approximately 1,000 mL per day will minimize interdialysis weight gains and hyponatremia. Aggressive antihypertensive therapy remains important, as blood pressure elevation before each dialysis treatment is a strong predictor of future cardiovascular and cerebrovascular mortality.

### *Disordered Calcium and Phosphate Metabolism*

The goal of therapy for disordered calcium and phosphorus metabolism is to normalize the serum concentrations of calcium and phosphate to allow regression of secondary hyperparathyroidism.

#### Phosphate

Initial management hinges upon normalization of hyperphosphatemia because phosphate retention plays a major role in the pathogenesis of secondary hyperparathyroidism and

**Table 35.3** Comparison of Phosphate-Binding Agents Used in the Treatment of Hyperphosphatemia of Renal Failure

| *Agent* | *Trade name* | *Dosage form* | *Sodium content*[a] | *Phosphate-binding capacity* |
|---|---|---|---|---|
| Aluminum carbonate | Basaljel | Capsule | 3.84 | 3+ |
| Aluminum hydroxide | Alternagel | Liquid | 1.15 | 2+ |
| | Amphojel | Liquid | 5.29 | |
| | Nephrox | Liquid | 2.40 | |
| | AluCap | Capsule | 2.30 | |
| | Dialume | Capsule | 2.30 | |
| Aluminum aminoacetate | Robalate | Tablet | <1.00 | 1+ |
| Calcium carbonate | Titralac | Liquid | 11.00 | 4+ |
| | Tums | Tablet | 2.7 | |
| | Os-Cal 500 | Tablet | 4.0 | |
| | Caltrate 600 | Tablet | <1.0 | |

[a] Milligrams per 5 mL liquid or tablet/capsule.

metastatic soft tissue calcification. To achieve normophosphatemia, two modalities may be utilized: (1) modest dietary phosphate restriction 800–1,000 mg/d and (2) phosphate-binding gels that retard phosphate absorption from the gut (Table 35.3). Phosphate-binding gels should be administered with meals to maximize the efficacy of phosphate binding. The dose should be titrated to achieve high normal serum phosphorus concentrations. Hypophosphatemia should be avoided to reduce the risk of osteomalacia. Approximately 5% to 10% of dialysis patients can maintain normophosphatemia without phosphate binders. The safety of aluminum-containing phosphate binders has been questioned because of links between aluminum accumulation and vitamin D–refractory osteomalacia and dialysis dementia.[34,35] High-dose oral calcium carbonate has thus emerged as an alternative to aluminum-containing compounds.[36] Calcium carbonate–containing regimens have the potential advantages of also correcting acidosis and increasing dietary calcium intake; however, hypercalcemia is common at the doses necessary to normalize serum phosphate, limiting application of this modality. Similarly, use of magnesium-containing antacids as phosphate binders is limited by the emergence of life-threatening hypermagnesemia, despite the use of dialysate with very low magnesium concentrations. Currently, the ideal phosphate binder does not exist.

**Calcium**

Once normophosphatemia has been achieved, normocalcemia should be sought using both dietary and pharmacologic means. Serum calcium concentrations at or near the upper limit of normal should be sought to reduce the stimulus for secondary hyperparathyroidism. Low normal serum calcium concentrations in uremia may be insufficient to shut off parathyroid hormone secretion. Dietary calcium intake is often subnormal in renal failure patients because of the reduced intake of phosphate-containing dairy products. Supplementation of dietary intake with elemental calcium 1.0–1.5 g/d has been recommended to produce a neutral or positive calcium balance.[37] This may be achieved by the use of various calcium salts (Table 35.4), although the carbonate salt is often preferred because of its higher elemental calcium content per unit dose and potentially superior bioavailability. In dialysis patients, maintenance of appropriate dialysate calcium concentrations assists in the achievement of normocalcemia. Persistent hypercalcemia may occur if dialysate concentrations exceed 3.6 mEq/L.

In patients who do not achieve normocalcemia with dietary supplementation alone, vitamin D sterol therapy should be added. Although biochemical, radiologic, and histologic improvements in renal osteodystrophy have been noted in patients receiving massive doses of vitamin $D_2$ or $D_3$,[38–40] use of these sterols has been rendered obsolete by the advent of more physiologically active calciferol metabolites with shorter half-lives. Therapy may be initiated with 1,25-dihydroxyvitamin $D_3$ (calcitriol), dihydrotachysterol (DHT), 25-hydroxyvitamin $D_3$ (calcifediol), or 1$\alpha$-hydroxyvitamin $D_3$ (alfacalcidol, not yet available in the United States) (Table 35.5). Hypocalcemia, markedly elevated parathyroid hormone concentrations, increased serum alkaline phosphatase activity, radiologic findings of subperiosteal bone resorption, and bone biopsy findings of osteitis fibrosa generally show equivalent improvement with all these agents.[41–47] Patients who fail to respond to one agent generally do not respond to the others. Patients with aluminum-associated osteomalacia show little or no improvement with vitamin D sterols and generally manifest hypercalcemia early in therapy.

Serum calcium concentrations have been suggested as a sole guide for vitamin D sterol dosage adjustment. Intestinal calcium absorption is substantially augmented in all patients receiving sterol dosages equivalent to 0.5 $\mu$g/d or more of calcitriol. A lack of rise in serum calcium may occur despite increased net accretion of bone. Such patients may then develop hypercalcemia after the serum alkaline phosphatase concentration has declined to normal. Serial serum alkaline phosphatase, calcium, and phosphorus concentrations should be monitored. When serum alkaline phosphatase has normalized, sterol dosage should be decreased.

Whether vitamin D sterols should be used as prophylactic agents in chronic renal failure patients with no evidence of renal osteodystrophy is unclear. Although such therapy may

**Table 35.4** Comparison of Oral Calcium Supplements Used in the Treatment of Hypocalcemia of Renal Failure

| *Salt* | *Trade name* | *Dosage form* | *Calcium content*[a] | *Elemental calcium (%)* | *Dose comparison*[b] |
|---|---|---|---|---|---|
| Glucobionate | Neo Calglucon | Liquid | 115.0 | 6.5 | 44.0 |
| | DorCol Pediatric | Liquid | | | |
| Gluconate | Various | 500-mg tablet | 45.0 | 9.0 | 22.0 |
| | | 650-mg tablet | 58.5 | | 17.0 |
| | | 1,000-mg tablet | 90.0 | | 11.0 |
| Lactate | Various | 325-mg tablet | 42.3 | 13.0 | 24.0 |
| | | 600-mg tablet | 84.5 | | 12.0 |
| Dibasic phosphate | Various | 486-mg tablet | 112.0 | 23.0 | 9.0 |
| Carbonate | Titralac | Liquid | 400.0 | 40.0 | 2.5 |
| | Tums | Tablet | 200.0 | | 5.0 |
| | Os-Cal 500 | Tablet | 500.0 | | 2.0 |
| | Caltrate 600 | Tablet | 600.0 | | 1.7 |

[a] mg/5 mL liquid or tablet.
[b] Number of tablets or milliliters equivalent to 1 g elemental calcium.

retard the development of renal osteodystrophy,[48,49] there is substantial risk because drug-induced hypercalcemia and hyperphosphatemia may accelerate deterioration in renal function.[29,50,51] Most investigators, however, document biochemical and histologic improvement in renal bone disease with no alteration in the rate of decline of renal function provided that hypercalcemia and hyperphosphatemia are avoided.[52–54] We do not routinely use vitamin D supplements until after patients have initiated dialysis.

### Miscellaneous Therapeutic Considerations

Normomagnesemia should be maintained to prevent further perturbations in calcium metabolism.[55] Prevention of hypermagnesemia involves use of appropriate dialysate magnesium concentrations (0.6–1.0 mg/dL) and avoidance of magnesium-containing medications or a diet high in magnesium. Conversely, hypomagnesemia should be avoided as this may decrease parathyroid hormone secretion, reduce responsiveness of bone to parathyroid hormone, and result in hypocalcemia.

Vitamin A increases bone resorption and the increased serum concentrations noted in uremic patients have been thought to contribute to bone disease.[56,57] Thus, vitamin A supplementation is unnecessary and should be avoided.

With appropriate medical therapy, secondary hyperparathyroidism can usually be minimized and osteitis fibrosa usually improved; however, parathyroid surgery may be necessary in selected patients. Criteria for surgery include (1) persistent hypercalcemia (serum calcium > 11.5 mg/dL); (2) a calcium–phosphorus product above 75 to 80 and progressive soft-tissue calcification that persists despite vigorous phosphate restriction and binder use; (3) progressive radiologic lesions of secondary hyperparathyroidism, particularly when associated with severe or debilitating symptoms; (4) intractable pruritus recalcitrant to other therapy; and (5) syndrome of calciphylaxis (a rare syndrome characterized by ischemic necrosis of the skin, muscles, and/or subcutaneous fat caused by vascular calcification).

Total parathyroidectomy is not recommended as the presence of parathyroid hormone appears to be necessary for bone remodeling. Generally, the surgical approach is either

**Table 35.5** Comparison of Vitamin D Analogues Used in the Treatment of Renal Osteodystrophy

| | *Ergocalciferol (vitamin $D_2$)* | *Calcifediol* | *Dihydrotachysterol* | *Alfacalcidol* | *Calcitriol* |
|---|---|---|---|---|---|
| Physiologic dose (μg/d) | 10[a] | 5 | 20 | 1 | 0.5 |
| Pharmacologic dose[b] (μg/d) | 1,200–12,000 | 50–500 | 100–1,000 | 0.25–2.0 | 0.25–2.0 |
| Pharmacologic half-life (d) | Prolonged because of deposition in fat | 16 | 8 | 3–5 | 1–3 |
| Onset of maximal effects (d) | 30–90 | 15 | 7–15 | 5–10 | 2–5 |
| Time for reversal of toxic effects (d) | 17–60 | 7–30 | 3–21 | 3–10 | 1–10 |

[a] 1 μg $D_2$ = 40 IU.
[b] For treatment of renal osteodystrophy.

removal of 3½ to 3¾ of the usual 4 glands or total parathyroidectomy with transplantation of parathyroid tissue to an accessible site such as the forearm[58,59]; however, these implants may spread locally and thereafter be irresectable. Postoperative hypocalcemia, hypophosphatemia, and hypomagnesemia may occur because of a marked increase in bone accretion in relation to bone absorption (''hungry bone syndrome''). The severity of the hypocalcemia depends on the degree of osteitis fibrosa; preoperative treatment with calcitriol may prevent or minimize the risk. Treatment with supplemental calcium and a vitamin D sterol may be necessary for weeks or months. After surgery, efforts to prevent hyperphosphatemia and the recurrence of secondary hyperparathyroidism are necessary.

### *Aluminum Bone Disease*

Aluminum-induced osteomalacia is very often refractory to treatment. Patients with coexisting encephalopathy (dialysis dementia) often die; others have prolonged disability despite institution of treatment. The most important aspect of aluminum intoxication in end-stage renal disease is prevention. Prevention is accomplished by using water purified by deionization or reverse osmosis such that dialysate aluminum concentrations are less than 10 $\mu$g/dL.

Dialysate quality control for aluminum content should be performed at least monthly. Use of dialyzers with a high phosphate clearance and strict compliance with a low-phosphate diet will reduce the dosage of aluminum-containing phosphate binders to the minimum compatible with adequate management of hyperphosphatemia. Effective, safe aluminum-free binders have yet to be developed. Patients at risk for aluminum intoxication may be identified by serial serum aluminum determinations (every 3 months at a minimum) or use of the deferoxamine test to assess tissue load.[60,61] Serum aluminum concentrations greater than 200 $\mu$g/L identify patients at risk for complications of aluminum accumulation.

For patients manifesting aluminum intoxication, institution of dialysis with purified water as discussed before has been documented to reverse hyperaluminemia, although this may take several months.[35] In severe cases, discontinuation of phosphate binders may lead to a rapid decline in serum aluminum concentrations to near-normal values. Chelation therapy with deferoxamine has shown promise in preliminary reports.[62–64] Substantial removal of aluminum during hemodialysis may occur after administration of deferoxamine in contrast to the ineffective removal by hemodialysis alone. Aluminum removal may be further enhanced by hemoperfusion.[65] In severe cases, transplantation may be necessary to treat this disease. The prophylactic use of deferoxamine is an unresolved issue, as not all patients develop aluminum intoxication while taking phosphate binders. Coburn and co-workers have treated aluminum bone disease with a combination of 24,25-dihydroxyvitamin $D_3$ and calcitriol. Addition of the 24,25 metabolite allows the use of higher doses of calcitriol without hypercalcemia. Their results have not been impressive.[66]

### *Anemia in End-Stage Renal Disease Patients*

As in all patients with anemia, treatment is tailored to the etiology of the reduced red cell count. In the small subset of ESRD patients in whom chronic hemolysis develops from hypersplenism with a resultant decrease in red cell survival, splenectomy may be of benefit. Acute hemolysis secondary to exposure to various oxidants,[67–69] excessive formaldehyde in the dialysate, or overheated or hypotonic dialysates will not occur provided proper dialysis monitoring is provided.

Other recognized contributors to the anemia of ESRD include iron and folate deficiencies, osteitis fibrosa associated with hyperparathyroidism, and aluminum intoxication. Iron deficiency, particularly prevalent in the nontransfused hemodialysis patient, can be managed with oral or parenteral iron supplementation.[70–74] Although it has been claimed that iron absorption from the gastrointestinal tract is impaired in patients with chronic renal failure, several studies refute this hypothesis and demonstrate that iron absorption in such patients probably exceeds that seen in the normal population.[75–77] Iron stores should be monitored using ferritin determinations every 4 to 6 months. Caution is advised in the use of parenteral iron as anaphylactic reactions can occur and the indiscriminate use of parenteral iron can lead to iron overload with hemosiderosis. Formulas are available for calculating the total iron–dextran dose necessary to replenish iron stores.[78]

Generally, hemosiderosis does not occur with oral iron, as the intestinal mucosa regulates iron absorption according to the body's iron stores. Iron overload occurs commonly in ESRD patients before the initiation of dialysis because a significant amount of body iron shifts from circulating red blood cells to the reticuloendothelial system as erythropoiesis declines. This overload may be aggravated by blood transfusion. In uncomplicated hemosiderosis, normalization of iron stores can be achieved in regular hemodialysis patients by discontinuation of iron therapy. Dialysis-related blood loss then gradually reduces iron content toward normal.

Only when excessive hemosiderosis is accompanied by clinical or biochemical signs of organ damage (hemochromatosis) are more rigorous measures indicated. Phlebotomy is limited to those hemodialysis patients who have sufficient erythropoiesis with hematocrits above 30% or to patients with significant improvement of anemia after transplantation. In patients who have severe hemosiderosis caused by frequent transfusions and who cannot be transplanted, deferoxamine treatment should be considered. Deferoxamine therapy can be used in conjunction with hemodialysis, hemofiltration, and continuous ambulatory peritoneal dialysis.[79,80] Exact dosing guidelines for deferoxamine use in patients with iron overload have not been reported. Acute side effects such as allergic reactions, bradyarrhythmias and tachyarrhythmias, hypertension and hypotension, headache and rigors, and the rare long-term complication of reversible cataract formation mandate caution in such therapy.[81]

Folate deficiency may develop in hemodialysis patients secondary to reduced dietary intake, use of phenytoin or other anticonvulsants, or loss of the vitamin during dialysis. Oral folic acid or improved dietary intake prevents or corrects folate deficiency megaloblastic anemia.[70]

For the major cause of the anemia of ESRD, erythropoietin deficiency, no truly satisfactory treatment exists at this time. Of the currently available therapies, only androgens have had any impact on this cause of anemia, with parenteral agents such as testosterone enanthate and nandrolone decanoate being the current agents of choice[82]; however, not all patients respond, anemia is rarely corrected, and side effects may be serious. Early clinical trials with recombinant human erythropoietin in dialysis patients have been very promising and this major advance in genetic engineering should have a major impact on the treatment of anemia and iron overload in end-stage renal disease.[83]

Red cell transfusions have been the only sure way to correct the symptoms of tissue hypoxia, but such therapy has only a transient effect and increases the risk of exposure to hepatitis, human T-cell lymphotropic virus type III (HTLV-III), other infectious agents, and iron overload. In addition, transfusion therapy may result in erythroid-marrow suppression, especially if multiple units are infused at once. This is probably because of a negative feedback on residual erythropoietin production. Thus, transfusions should be reserved for those who are clearly symptomatic with anemia or who are active candidates for renal transplantation.

### *Metabolic Acidosis*

The prevention and treatment of severe metabolic acidosis in patients with chronic renal failure may be important for the prevention of the sequelae of the chronic acidotic state, such as bone demineralization, reduced cardiac contractility, increased ventricular irritability, potential for hyperkalemia, and growth retardation in children. Generally, treatment should be instituted when plasma bicarbonate has fallen below 20 mEq/L.

In patients with residual renal function, the use of alkalinizing salts such as sodium bicarbonate or Shohl's solution (a sodium citrate–citric acid mixture, the citrate being metabolized to bicarbonate) may be useful in replenishing depleted body bicarbonate stores.[84] In the adult, therapy is initiated with sodium bicarbonate 20–36 mEq daily or Shohl's solution 30–120 mL daily, both in divided doses four times daily. Doses are subsequently titrated to produce plasma bicarbonate concentrations of 20 mEq/L or greater. Fluid and electrolyte balance should be monitored carefully because of the sodium content of these agents. In addition, excessive doses may cause metabolic alkalosis as well as lethargy or cardiac depression secondary to a decrease in ionized serum calcium concentration. Gastrointestinal distress characterized by gastric distension and flatulence is relatively common with high doses of oral sodium bicarbonate. Patients with renal tubular acidosis (RTA) may require higher doses of these agents. Recommended initial doses of sodium bicarbonate for distal (type 1) and proximal (type 2) RTA of 0.5–2.0 and 4–10 mEq/kg/d, respectively, have been suggested.[84]

Metabolic acidosis in patients undergoing hemodialysis can almost always be managed solely by dialysis. Measures used include dialysis against acetate (a bicarbonate precursor) or bicarbonate baths. This topic is dealt with in greater detail in a recent review.[85]

### *Hypertension in Chronic Renal Failure Patients*

The maintenance of normotension in the hypertensive patient with renal impairment is important not only for the prevention of target organ dysfunction but theoretically also in the slowing of the progression of renal impairment to end-stage renal disease. Such slowing in the rate of decline of renal function has been well documented in diabetic patients.[86,87] As hypertension is dealt with elsewhere in this text (Chapter 10), only those aspects unique to the treatment of hypertension in the patient with renal impairment are discussed here.

It is important to realize that precipitous falls in blood pressure to normotensive levels may be deleterious to renal function in patients with preexisting renal impairment. This may be especially problematic in the patient treated for hypertensive crisis. Target blood pressure should be achieved reasonably slowly to allow adaptation to reduced perfusion pressures. In addition, it is preferable to use antihypertensive agents such as vasodilators that maintain renal blood flow and thus do not contribute to declining renal function.

Diuretics remain the first-line antihypertensive agents in patients with impaired renal function. As creatinine clearance falls below 20–30 mL/min, the thiazide-like diuretics lose their saliuretic action but still maintain a modest antihypertensive effect, possibly because of vasodilation.[88] Saliuresis in these patients can be maintained through the use of potent loop diuretics such as furosemide or bumetanide. However, as creatinine clearance declines further, these agents may become ineffective saliuretics as well. In such patients, a combination of a loop diuretic and a thiazide diuretic or metolazone may acutely prove beneficial, although close clinical and laboratory monitoring should be undertaken to prevent the profound dehydration and metabolic derangement that may ensue.[89] Potassium-sparing diuretics such as spironolactone, triamterene, and amiloride should be used with extreme caution or not at all in patients with renal impairment because of the risk of hyperkalemia. Triamterene should probably be avoided in renally impaired patients also receiving nonsteroidal anti-inflammatory drugs because of the potential risk of precipitating more severe renal impairment.[90]

Although advocated as first- or second-line therapy in the treatment of hypertension, $\beta$-adrenoceptor–blocking agents may reduce renal blood flow and glomerular filtration rate through reduction in cardiac output, thereby placing residual renal function at further risk.[91] Preliminary studies have suggested that nadolol may be an exception in this regard.[92,93] In most patients, however, deterioration in renal function is not seen with $\beta$-blocker therapy.

Similar potential for worsening renal impairment exists with the use of angiotensin-converting enzyme inhibitors in patients with renovascular disease. Acute renal failure has been reported with the use of angiotensin-converting enzyme inhibitors in patients with bilateral renal artery stenosis or renal artery stenosis of a solitary functioning kidney. This probably occurs secondary to loss of renal autoregulation through efferent arteriolar vasodilation. Renal function should be carefully monitored in such patients undergoing angiotensin-converting enzyme inhibitor therapy and such therapy should be withdrawn if renal function deteriorates.[94,95]

The exact role of the calcium channel blockers (nifedipine, diltiazem, verapamil, nitrendipine) as antihypertensive agents in patients with chronic renal failure has not been resolved. Data supporting their efficacy and tolerability have recently been reported.[96,97] Acute renal failure has also been reported with the use of nifedipine in patients with renovascular disease.[98] Although the exact mechanism for this is unknown, it is likely hemodynamic and similar to what has been described with angiotensin-converting enzyme inhibitors.

### *Hypertension in Chronic Dialysis Patients*

The management of hypertension in the chronic dialysis patient is paramount in the prevention of the accelerated atherosclerosis and cardiovascular disease noted in this patient population.[99–101] As hypertension is dealt with in detail in Chapter 10, only those aspects unique to hypertension treatment in the dialysis patient are discussed here.

Of those patients initiating dialysis for end-stage renal disease, 70% to 80% are hypertensive. Dialytic therapy and control of total body sodium through ultrafiltration result in normalization of blood pressure in 50% to 80% of these patients. The percentage of dialysis patients considered to have "dialysis-resistant" hypertension requiring antihypertensive medications varies considerably depending on the approach of the specific dialysis unit or physician, demographic differences, differences in the definition of hypertension in dialysis patients, and the patient's primary disease. In general, antihypertensive medications control elevated blood pressure in the vast majority of these individuals; bilateral nephrectomy is rarely employed today.

The major initial effort in treating hypertension in end-stage renal disease is restriction of salt and water intake, as hypertension is often volume dependent in nature. Massive doses of potent loop diuretics such as furosemide, bumetanide, and ethacrynic acid are generally ineffective in promoting diuresis and expose the patient to the risks of ototoxicity, gastrointestinal upset and bleeding, and hyperglycemia. Although thiazides are ineffective as saliuretics in this patient population, a mild direct antihypertensive effect has been reported.[88]

Patients in whom dietary sodium and water restriction fails to control high blood pressure may benefit from drugs that inhibit the effects of the renin–angiotensin axis, in light of the important role that this hormonal axis may play in the etiology of "dialysis-resistant" hypertension. Inhibition may be accomplished using an angiotensin-converting enzyme inhibitor such as captopril or enalapril, or drugs that interfere with renin release such as the $\beta$-adrenoceptor blockers or the combined $\alpha$-/$\beta$-blocker labetalol.

Bone marrow depression has been noted in up to 10% of renal failure subjects receiving captopril, especially those with autoimmune diseases such as systemic lupus erythematosus (SLE).[102] If captopril therapy is initiated in the dialysis patient, white blood cell counts should be closely monitored and drug doses kept as low as possible. Enalapril, which lacks the sulfhydryl group of captopril, has rarely been associated with bone marrow depression and may become the angiotensin-converting enzyme inhibitor of choice in these patients.[103] The choice of $\beta$-blocker in dialysis subjects should take into account the alterations in drug kinetics with end-stage renal disease and the effect of the dialysis procedure. It would be expected that those agents extensively hepatically metabolized, such as propranolol, timolol, metoprolol, or labetalol, may be easier to dose titrate than those extensively eliminated in unchanged form by the kidney, such as atenolol, nadolol, or acebutolol.

Sympathetic nervous system active agents such as prazosin, methyldopa, clonidine, guanethidine, and reserpine may be required in patients unresponsive to diet plus $\beta$-blocker or diet plus angiotensin-converting enzyme inhibitor therapy. Clonidine appears to be the safest and easiest of these agents to use in the dialysis population. Methyldopa and prazosin should be avoided because of the hypotensive problems that may ensue during the dialysis procedure. In addition, methyldopa can cause significant sedation and postural hypotension and worsen the impotence already noted with increased incidence in this group of patients. Guanethidine should also be avoided because of its propensity to cause severe postural hypotension, severe dialysis hypotension, and impotence. Reserpine is contraindicated because of its frequent side effects and the availability of better tolerated, more effective agents.

Addition of vasodilators such as minoxidil or hydralazine may prove useful in patients resistant to combinations of the previously mentioned agents. In addition, hydralazine is often effective as first-line therapy for hypertension and is generally well tolerated. Monotherapy with this drug is well tolerated in diabetic patients because of the underlying autonomic neuropathy that prevents reflex tachycardia. The incidence of drug-induced SLE does not appear to be increased by the presence of end-stage renal disease. Minoxidil therapy may be associated with a profound reflex tachycardia and most patients should receive a $\beta$-blocker or a central $\alpha_2$ agonist to suppress this. Hirsutism requiring depilatories is an almost universal side effect.[104]

## Summary

Chronic renal failure is a complex disorder characterized by multiple disturbances in renal excretory, biosynthetic, and metabolic function. In the presence of renal disease, the kidney and its component nephrons continue to operate in a highly organized fashion. Many of the adaptations that take place to maintain solute and water homeostasis have "trade-offs" that may contribute to the uremic syndrome. Although thought to be a progressive disease in most patients, recent advances in the understanding of the hemodynamics of chronic renal failure raise the hope that dietary or pharmacologic intervention may postpone or eliminate the need for dialysis for many patients. The treatment of chronic renal failure follows very closely from the disordered physiology and can control or reverse many of the abnormalities. Appropriate pharmacologic intervention can markedly enhance the quality of life of these patients.

## References


1. Bricker NS, Morrin PAF, Kime SW Jr. The pathologic physiology of chronic Bright's disease: An exposition of the "intact nephron hypothesis." Am J Med 1960;28:77.
2. Mazumdar DC, Crosson JT, Lubowitz H. Glomerulotubular relationships in glomerulonephritis. J Lab Clin Med 1975;85: 292–299.
3. Bricker NS. On the pathogenesis of the uremic state: An exposition of the "trade-off hypothesis." N Engl J Med 1972; 286:1093–1099.
4. Bricker NS, Fine LG. The trade-off hypothesis: Current status. Kidney Int 1978;13(suppl 8):S5–S8.
5. Brenner BM, Meyer TW, Hostetter TH. Dietary protein intake and the progressive nature of kidney disease: The role of hemodynamically mediated glomerular injury in the pathogenesis of progressive glomerular sclerosis in aging, renal ablation, and intrinsic renal disease. N Engl J Med 1982;307:652–659.
6. Knochel JP, Seldin DW. The pathophysiology of uremia, in Brenner BM, Rector FC (eds): The Kidney, 2nd ed. Philadelphia, W.B. Saunders, 1981, pp 2137–2183.
7. Brenner BM. Hemodynamically mediated glomerular injury and the progressive nature of kidney disease. Kidney Int 1983;23:647–655.
8. Ibels LS, Alfrey AC, Haut L, et al. Preservation of function in experimental renal disease by dietary restriction of phosphate. N Engl J Med 1978;298:122–126.
9. Alfrey AC, Tomford RC. The case for tubulointerstitial factors, in Narins RG (ed): Controversies in Nephrology and Hypertension. New York, Churchill Livingstone, 1984, pp 557–566.
10. Moorhead JF, Chan MK, El-Nahas M, et al. Lipid nephrotoxicity in chronic progressive glomerular and tubulointerstitial disease. Lancet 1982;2:1309–1311.
11. Fischer GM, Swain ML, Chacko S. Diet and hormone induced lipid deposition in rat kidney: Correlation with systolic blood pressure. Lipids 1982;18:758–759.
12. Kasiske BL, O'Donnell MP, Garvis WJ, et al. Cholesterol synthesis inhibition reduces glomerular injury in the rat 5/6 nephrectomy model of chronic renal failure. (Abstr) Clin Res 1987;35(3):549A.
13. Kasiske BL, O'Donnell MP, Daniels F, et al. The lipid lowering agent clofibric acid ameliorates renal injury in the 5/6 nephrectomy model of chronic renal failure. (Abstr) Clin Res 1985;33(2):488A.
14. Hostetter TH, Rennke HG, Brenner BM. The case for intrarenal hypertension in the initiation and progression of diabetic and other glomerulopathies. Am J Med 1982;72:375–380.
15. Hostetter TH, Olson JL, Rennke HG, et al. Hyperfiltration in remnant nephrons: A potentially adverse response to renal ablation. Am J Physiol 1981;241:F85–F93.
16. Hayslett JP. Functional adaptation to reduction in renal mass. Physiol Rev 1979;59:137–164.
17. Raij L, Keane WF. Glomerular mesangium: Its function and relationship to angiotensin II. Am J Med 1985;79(suppl 36):24–30.
18. Bosch JP, Saccaggi A, Lauer A, et al. Renal functional reserve in humans: Effect of protein intake on glomerular filtration rate. Am J Med 1983;75:943–950.
19. Giovannetti S. Dietary treatment of chronic renal failure: Why is it not used more frequently? Nephron 1985;40:1–12.
20. Rosman JB, Meijer S, Sluiter WJ, et al. Prospective randomized trial of early dietary protein restriction in chronic renal failure. Lancet 1984;2:1291–1296.
21. Oldrizzi L, Rugiu C, Valvo E, et al. Progression of renal failure in patients with renal disease of diverse etiology on protein-restricted diet. Kidney Int 1985;27:553–557.
22. Mitch WE, Walser M, Steinman TI, et al. The effect of a keto acid–amino acid supplement to a restricted diet on the progression of chronic renal failure. N Engl J Med 1984;311:623–629.
23. Giordano C. Early dietary protein restriction protects the failing kidney. Kidney Int 1985;28(suppl 17):S66–S70.
24. Anderson S, Meyer TW, Rennke HG, et al. Control of glomerular hypertension limits glomerular injury in rats with reduced renal mass. J Clin Invest 1985;76:612–619.
25. Raij L, Chiou X, Owens R, et al. Therapeutic implications of hypertension-induced glomerular injury: Comparison of enalapril and a combination of hydralazine, reserpine, and hydrochlorothiazide in an experimental model. Am J Med 1985; 79(suppl 3C):37–41.
26. Rutherford WE, Blondin J, Miller JP, et al. Chronic progressive renal disease: Rate of change of serum creatinine concentration. Kidney Int 1977;11:62–70.
27. Mitch WE, Walser M, Buffington GA, et al. A simple method of estimating progression of chronic renal failure. Lancet 1976;2:1326–1328.
28. Danovitch GM, Bourgoignie J, Bricker NS. Reversibility of the "salt-losing" tendency of chronic renal failure. N Engl J Med 1977;296:14–19.
29. Christiansen C, Rodbro P, Christensen MS, et al. Deterioration of renal function during treatment of chronic renal failure with 1,25-dihydroxycholecalciferol. Lancet 1978;2:700–703.
30. Mitch WE, Wilcox CS. Disorders of body fluids, sodium and potassium in chronic renal failure. Am J Med 1982;72:536–550.
31. Livo M, Marchesi D, Remuzzi G, et al. Uraemic bleeding: Role of anemia and beneficial effect of renal cell transfusion. Lancet 1982;2:1013–1015.
32. Deykin D. Uremic bleeding. Kidney Int 1983;24:698–705.
33. Goldberg AP, Sherrard DJ, Haas LB, et al. Control of clofibrate toxicity in uremic hypertriglyceridemia. Clin Pharmacol Ther 1977;21:317–325.
34. Knoll O, Kellinghaus H, Bertram HP, et al. Gastrointestinal absorption of aluminum in chronic renal insufficiency. Contrib Nephrol 1984;38:24–31.
35. O'Hare JA, Callaghan NH, Murnaghan DJ. Dialysis encephalopathy. Clinical, electroencephalographic and interventional aspects. Medicine 1983;62:129–141.
36. Moriniere PH, Roussel A, Tahiri Y, et al. Substitution of aluminum hydroxide by high doses of calcium carbonate in patients on chronic hemodialysis: Disappearance of hyperaluminaemia and equal control of hyperparathyroidism. Proc Eur Dial Transplant Assoc 1982;19:784–787.
37. Clarkson EM, Durrant C, Phillips ME, et al. The effect of high intake of calcium and phosphate in normal subjects and patients with chronic renal failure. Clin Sci 1970;39:693–704.
38. Verberckmoes R, Bouillon R, Krempian B. Osteodystrophy of dialyzed patients treated with vitamin D. Proc Eur Dial Transplant Assoc 1973;10:217–225.
39. Potter DE, Wilson CJ, Ozonoff MB. Hyperparathyroid bone disease in children undergoing long-term hemodialysis: Treatment with vitamin D. J Pediatr 1974;85:60–66.
40. Eastwood JB, Bordier PJ, Clarkson EM, et al. The contrasting effects on bone histology of vitamin D and of calcium carbonate in the osteomalacia of chronic renal failure. Clin Sci 1974;47:23–42.
41. Frost HM, Griffith DL, Jee WSS, et al. Histomorphometric

changes in trabecular bone of renal failure patients treated with calcifediol. Metab Bone Dis Rel Res 1981;2:285–295.

42. Malluche HH, Goldstein DA, Massry SG. Management of renal osteodystrophy and 1,25-$(OH)_2D_3$. II. Effects on histopathology of bone: Evidence for healing of osteomalacia. Miner Electrolyte Metab 1979;2:48–55.
43. Eastwood JB, Stamp TCB, De Wardener HE, et al. The effect of 25-hydroxyvitamin $D_3$ in the osteomalacia of chronic renal failure. Clin Sci 1977;52:499–508.
44. Kaye M, Chatterjee G, Cohen GF, et al. Arrest of hyperparathyroid bone disease with dihydrotachysterol in patients undergoing chronic hemodialysis. Ann Intern Med 1970;73:225–233.
45. Recker R, Schoenfeld P, Letteri J, et al. The efficacy of calcifediol in renal osteodystrophy. Arch Intern Med 1978;138: 857–863.
46. Massry SG, Goldstein DA, Malluche HH. Current status of the use of 1,25-$(OH)_2D_3$ in the management of renal osteodystrophy. Kidney Int 1980;18:409–418.
47. Sharman VL, Brownjohn AM, Goodwin FJ, et al. Long-term experience of alfacalcidol in renal osteodystrophy. Q J Med 1982;51:271–278.
48. Memmos DE, Eastwood JB, Talner LB, et al. Double-blind trial of oral 1,25-dihyroxy vitamin $D_3$ versus placebo in asymptomatic hyperparathyroidism in patients receiving maintenance hemodialysis. Br Med J 1981;282:1919–1924.
49. Healy MD, Malluche HH, Goldstein DA, et al. Effects of long-term therapy with calcitriol in patients with moderate renal failure. Arch Intern Med 1980;140:1030–1033.
50. Tougard L, Sorensen E, Brochner-Mortensen J, et al. Controlled trial of 1$\alpha$-hydroxycholecalciferol in chronic renal failure. Lancet 1976;1:1044–1047.
51. Chan JCM, Young RB, Alon U, et al. Hypercalcemia in children with disorders of calcium and phosphate metabolism during long-term treatment with 1,25-dihydroxyvitamin $D_3$. Pediatrics 1983;72:225–233.
52. Coen G, Messa F, Massimetti C, et al. 1-Alpha-OH-cholecalciferol (1-alpha-$OHD_3$) and low phosphate diet in predialysis chronic renal failure: Effects on renal function and on secondary hyperparathyroidism. Acta Vitaminol Enzymol 1984;6: 129–135.
53. Mazur AT, Norman ME. Effects of 25-$OHD_3$ on renal function in pediatric patients with chronic renal failure. Miner Electrolyte Metab 1984;10:351–358.
54. Hymes LC, Warshaw BL. Vitamin D replacement therapy and renal function. Am J Dis Child 1984;138:1125–1128.
55. Drueke T. Does magnesium excess play a role in renal osteodystrophy? Contrib Nephrol 1984;38:195–202.
56. Rylance PB, Brown IRF, Howells DW, et al. Relationship between vitamin A and bone disease in chronic renal failure. Nephron 1984;36:131–135.
57. Cundy T, Earnshaw M, Heynen G, et al. Vitamin A and hyperparathyroid bone disease in uremia. Am J Clin Nutr 1983;38:914–920.
58. Diethelm AG, Adams PL, Murad TM, et al. Treatment of secondary hyperparathyroidism in patients with chronic renal failure by total parathyroidectomy and parathyroid autograft. Ann Surg 1981;193:777–793.
59. Mallette LE, Eisenberg KL, Schwaitzberg SD, et al. Total parathyroidectomy and autogenous parathyroid graft replacement for treatment of hyperparathyroidism due to chronic renal failure. Arch Surg 1983;146:727–733.
60. Simon P, Allain P, Aug KS, et al. Prevention and treatment of aluminum intoxication in chronic renal failure. Adv Nephrol 1985;14:439–478.
61. Heaf JG, Nielsen LP. Serum aluminum in haemodialysis patients: Relation to osteodystrophy, encephalopathy, and aluminum hydroxide consumption. Miner Electrolyte Metab 1984;10:345–350.
62. Ackrill P, Day JP, Garstang FM, et al. Treatment of fracturing renal osteodystrophy by deferoxamine. Proc Eur Dial Transplant Assoc 1982;19:203–207.
63. Brown DJ, Dawborn JK, Ham KN, et al. Treatment of dialysis osteomalacia with deferoxamine. Lancet 1982;2:343–345.
64. Malluche HH, Smith AJ, Abreo K, et al. The use of deferoxamine in the management of aluminum accumulation in bone in patients with renal failure. N Engl J Med 1984;311:140–144.
65. Chang TMS, Barre P. Effect of deferoxamine on removal of aluminum and iron by coated charcoal hemoperfusion and hemodialysis. Lancet 1983;2:1051–1053.
66. Coburn JW, Wong EGC, Sherrard DJ, et al. Use of 24,25-$(OH)_2D_3$ in dialysis osteomalacia: Preliminary results. (Abstr) Clin Res 1982;28:532A.
67. Manzler AD, Schreiner AW. Copper-induced acute hemolytic anemia. A new complication of hemodialysis. Ann Intern Med 1970;73:409–412.
68. Neilan BA, Ehlers SM, Kolpin CF, et al. Prevention of chloramine-induced hemolysis in dialyzed patients. Clin Nephrol 1975;10:105–108.
69. Carlson DJ, Shapiro FL. Methemoglobinemia from well water nitrates: A complication of home dialysis. Ann Intern Med 1970;73:757–759.
70. Hutchins L, Lipschitz D. Iron and folate metabolism in renal failure. Semin Nephrol 1985;5:142–146.
71. Parker PA, Izard MW, Maher JF. Therapy of iron deficiency anemia in patients on maintenance dialysis. Nephron 1979;23: 181–186.
72. Strickland ID, Chaput de Saintonge DM, Boulton FE, et al. A trial of oral iron in dialysis patients. Clin Nephrol 1974;2:13–17.
73. Morgan T. The effect of intravenous iron on the haematocrit of patients on maintenance haemodialysis. Med J Aust 1972;1: 852–854.
74. Stewart WK, Fleming LW, Shepherd AMM. Haemoglobin and serum iron responses to periodic intravenous iron–dextran infusions during maintenance haemodialysis. Nephron 1976; 17:121–130.
75. Eschbach JW, Cook JD, Finch CA. Iron absorption in chronic renal disease. Clin Sci 1970;38:191–196.
76. Merrill RH, Tasch R. Iron absorption in hemodialyzed patients. Trans Am Soc Artif Intern Organs 1976;22:69–72.
77. Milman N, Larsen L. Iron absorption in patients with chronic uremia undergoing regular hemodialysis. Acta Med Scand 1976;199:113–119.
78. Hanson DB, Hendeles L. Guide to total dose intravenous iron dextran therapy. Am J Hosp Pharm 1974;31:592–595.
79. Rembold CM, Krumlovsky FA, Roxe DM, et al. Treatment of hemodialysis hemosiderosis with desferrioxamine. Trans Am Soc Artif Intern Organs 1982;28:621–626.
80. Falk RJ, Mattern WD, Lamanna RW, et al. Iron removal during continuous ambulatory peritoneal dialysis using deferoxamine. Kidney Int 1983;24:110–112.
81. Modell B. Advances in the use of iron-chelating agents for the treatment of iron overload. Prog Hematol 1979;11:267–312.
82. Dainiak N. The role of androgens in the treatment of anemia of chronic renal failure. Semin Nephrol 1985;5:147–154.
83. Eschbach JW, Egrie JC, Downing MR, et al. Correction of the anemia of end-stage renal disease with recombinant human erythropoietin. N Engl J Med 1987;316:73–78.
84. American Hospital Formulary Service. Drug Information 86. Bethesda, MD; American Society of Hospital Pharmacists, 1986, pp 1209–1214.

85. Gennari JF. Acid–base balance in dialysis patients. Kidney Int 1985;28:678–688.
86. Parving HH, Andersen AR, Smidt UM, et al. Early aggressive antihypertensive treatment reduces rate of decline in kidney function in diabetic nephropathy. Lancet 1983;1:1175–1179.
87. Mogensen CE. Long-term antihypertensive treatment inhibiting progression of diabetic nephropathy. Br Med J 1982;285: 685–688.
88. Jones B, Nanra RS. Double-blind trial of antihypertensive effect of chlorothiazide in severe renal failure. Lancet 1979;2: 1258–1260.
89. Wollam GL, Tarazi RC, Bravo EL, et al. Diuretic potency of combined hydrochlorothiazide and furosemide therapy in patients with azotemia. Am J Med 1982;72:929–938.
90. Favre L, Glasson P, Vallotton MB. Reversible acute renal failure from combined triamterene and indomethacin: A study in healthy subjects. Ann Intern Med 1982;96:317–320.
91. Wilkinson R. β-Blockers and renal function. Drugs 1982;23: 195–206.
92. Hollenberg NK, Adams DF, McKinstry DN, et al. Beta-adrenoceptor-blocking agents and the kidney: Effect of nadolol and propranolol on the renal circulation. Br J Clin Pharmacol 1979;1(suppl 2):219S–225S.
93. Waal-Manning HJ, Hobson CH. Renal function in patients with essential hypertension receiving nadolol. Br Med J 1980;3:423–424.
94. Hricik DE, Browning PJ, Kopelman R, et al. Captopril-induced functional renal insufficiency in patients with bilateral renal-artery stenoses or renal-artery stenosis in a solitary kidney. N Engl J Med 1983;308:373–376.
95. Chrysant SG, Dunn M, Marples D. Severe reversible azotemia from captopril therapy. Arch Intern Med 1983;143:437–441.
96. Ambroso GC, Como G, Scalamogna A, et al. Treatment of arterial hypertension with nifedipine in patients with chronic renal insufficiency. Clin Nephrol 1985;23:41–45.
97. Moreira J, Barata JD, Olias J. Antihypertensive action of calcium blockade in hypertensive patients with chronic renal disease. Nephron 1985;41:314–319.
98. Diamond JR, Cheung JY, Fang LS. Nifedipine-induced renal dysfunction: Alterations in renal hemodialysis. Am J Med 1984;77:905–909.
99. Lindner A, Charra B, Sherrard DJ, et al. Accelerated atherosclerosis in prolonged maintenance hemodynamics. N Engl J Med 1974;290:697–701.
100. Lowrie EG, Lazarus JM, Hampers CL, et al. Cardiovascular disease in dialysis patients. N Engl J Med 1974;290:737–738.
101. Merrill JP. Cardiovascular problems in patients on long-term hemodialysis, editorial. JAMA 1974;228:1149.
102. Heel RC, Brogden RN, Speight TM, et al. Captopril: A preliminary review of its pharmacological properties and therapeutic efficacy. Drugs 1980;20:409–452.
103. Nicholls MG (ed): Symposium on enalapril. Drugs 1985;30 (suppl 1):1–96.
104. Linas SL, Nies AS. Minoxidil. Ann Intern Med 1981;94:61–65.

# Chapter 36 / Drug-Induced Renal Disease

Paul A. Abraham, MD, and Gary R. Matzke, PharmD, FCP, FCCP

Drugs as well as environmental[1] and occupational[2] agents cause toxic nephropathy. Although such agents as mercury, arsenic, lead, chromium, cadmium, ethylene glycol, and carbon tetrachloride were previously the major nephrotoxins,[3] drugs used for diagnostic and therapeutic purposes now predominate. At present, drug-induced renal structural and functional alterations, including fluid and electrolyte disorders (see Chapters 102 and 103), are significant causes of patient morbidity and mortality.

Recognition of the clinical features of drug nephropathy is necessary for prevention, diagnosis, and treatment of the renal dysfunction that develops during drug therapy. Knowledge of the mechanisms of drug-induced renal disease provides important insights into renal physiology and pathophysiology. Application of these insights has contributed significantly to therapeutic advances. Specifically, recognition of the nephropathy caused by angiotensin-converting enzyme inhibitors helped lead to investigation of their hemodynamic effects and their utilization in preservation of declining renal function.[4]

## Incidence

Drug-induced acute renal failure is a frequent complication of hospital care. During 1979, a prospective study of hospital-acquired acute renal failure identified drug therapy as the etiology for one fifth of cases, with a mortality of 8%.[5] Radiologic-contrast media, aminoglycoside antibiotics, and *cis*-platinum were the agents most commonly implicated. Drugs are also an important cause of acute renal failure in intensive care units. In one analysis, 20.7% of cases were due to pharmacologic agents, particularly radiologic-contrast media.[6] In other studies, an association with aminoglycoside therapy has predominated.[7,8]

Drug nephrotoxicity is also a major reason for acute renal failure requiring specialized care in a nephrology unit. In a multicenter French study, 18.4% of acute renal failure cases admitted for special care were drug induced.[9] Of these cases, 36.9% were due to analgesic and nonsteroidal anti-inflammatory drug use.

While drug-induced acute renal failure is a frequent complication of inpatient care, the incidence in outpatients is unknown; however, it is possible that the incidence may be greater because of the greater over-the-counter availability of potent nonsteroidal anti-inflammatory drugs in the United States.[10–12] In addition, current medical economic incentives for outpatient diagnosis and therapy of more serious medical illnesses could contribute.

Chronic renal failure is another common drug nephropathy. In particular, renal failure resulting from long-term analgesic abuse is a serious worldwide public health concern.[13] Analgesic nephropathy has been reported to cause 36% of end-stage renal disease in areas of Belgium and 20% in areas of Australia.[14] In the United States, analgesic nephropathy is a less common cause of end-stage renal disease; however, in circumscribed geographic regions such as northwest North Carolina, the incidence may be as high as 10%.[15]

## Classification

Drug-induced renal disease is an entity that is heterogeneous with respect to the drugs involved and the lesions produced. No system of classification has been satisfactory. Classification based on mechanisms of toxicity would be preferred, but has been inadequate because of insufficient knowledge. Alternative classifications have included (1) clinical presentations of renal disease (acute and chronic renal failure, hematuria, pyuria, and proteinuria) to emphasize the diagnosis of renal disease, (2) uses of drugs (Table 36.1) to emphasize therapeutics and the multiple nephropathies caused by individual drugs, and (3) renal structural and functional alterations (Table 36.2) to emphasize the diversity of drug nephropathy as well as possible mechanisms of toxicity. The latter approach is used in the present discussion.

## Mechanisms for Renal Susceptibility to Drug Toxicity

The kidneys appear to be more sensitive to drug toxicity than most other body organs. Both immunologic and nonimmunologic mechanisms contribute to this sensitivity. The reasons for renal susceptibility to immune-mediated structural and functional alterations (nephrotic syndrome, glomerulonephritis, and acute allergic interstitial nephritis) are unclear; however, several characteristics of normal renal physiology appear to enhance renal susceptibility to nonimmune mechanisms of drug nephropathy (Fig. 36.1). It is possible that certain of these characteristics could also contribute to immune-mediated mechanisms of drug nephrotoxicity.

### *High Blood Flow and Specialized Hemodynamics*

Although the kidneys constitute only 4.0% of body weight, they receive 20% to 25% of resting cardiac output. Thus, the kidneys have a large exposure to circulating drugs. Within

**Table 36.1** Classification of Nephrotoxic Drugs by Their Therapeutic Use

| | |
|---|---|
| Cardiovascular | Gastrointestinal |
| Thiazide and loop diuretics (I)[a] | Vasopressin (O) |
| Propranolol (H) | Cimetidine (I, P) |
| Triamterene (H, N) | Magnesium antacids (N) |
| Hydralazine (G) | Phosphate enemas (O) |
| Captopril (G, H, I) | Cancer chemotherapy |
| Calcium channel blockers (G, H) | *cis*-Platinum (T) |
| Mannitol (T) | Mitomycin C (V) |
| Low-molecular-weight dextran (O) | Nitrosoureas (methyl CCNU) (I) |
| Antimicrobial | Mithramycin (T) |
| β-lactam antibiotics (I) | Methotrexate (O) |
| Aminoglycosides (T) | Streptozocin (T) |
| Rifampin (I, G) | Immunosuppressive |
| Pentamidine (?) | Cyclosporine (H, I, V) |
| Amphotericin B (T) | Corticosteroids (P) |
| Trimethoprim (P) | Leukocyte A interferon (G, I) |
| Tetracycline (P, T) | Drugs of abuse |
| Acyclovir (O) | Heroin (G, O) |
| Rheumatologic | Amphetamine (V) |
| Gold (G) | Miscellaneous |
| D-Penicillamine (G) | Radiologic-contrast agents (I, T) |
| Nonsteroidal anti-inflammatory drugs (G, H, I, T, PN) | Methoxyflurane anesthesia (T) |
| Acetylsalicylic acid (H) | Ascorbic acid (O) |
| Acetaminophen (T) | Mercurial topical preparations (G) |
| Allopurinol (I, N) | |
| Psychiatric | |
| Lithium (G, I) | |
| Amoxapine (O, T) | |

[a] I, interstitial nephritis; H, hemodynamically mediated; N, nephrolithiasis; G, glomerulopathy; T, tubular necrosis; O, intratubular obstruction; P, pseudo renal failure; V, vasculopathy; PN, papillary necrosis.

the kidney, blood flow is distributed to superficial and deep nephron populations as well as the medulla and papillae. This specialized blood flow is precisely regulated by mechanisms including renal prostaglandins, vasoactive peptides, the sympathetic nervous system, and the renin–angiotensin system. Alterations include total renal blood flow reduction during propranolol therapy[16] and intrarenal blood flow shunting away from superficial nephrons after administration of radiologic-contrast media.[17]

In addition, glomerular blood flow is uniquely specialized to maintain the glomerular filtration rate. Blood pressure within both glomerular afferent and efferent arterioles must be precisely regulated to maintain capillary hydrostatic pressure and glomerular filtration. Alterations of these hemodynamics have been observed when angiotensin-converting enzyme inhibitors,[18] and possibly calcium antagonists,[19] have been administered to patients with ischemic renal vascular disease.

**Table 36.2** Drug-Induced Renal Structural–Functional Alterations

| | |
|---|---|
| Pseudo renal failure | Interstitial nephritis |
| Hemodynamically mediated renal failure | Acute allergic |
| | Chronic |
| Vascular alterations | Papillary necrosis |
| Glomerulopathy | Obstructive nephropathy |
| Nephrotic syndrome | Intratubular |
| Glomerulonephritis | Extrarenal urinary tract |
| Tubular necrosis | Nephrolithiasis |

### *Tubular Epithelial Cell Absorptive and Secretory Functions*

Renal tubular epithelial cells throughout the nephron actively reabsorb filtered solutes from the tubular lumen and absorb other molecules from the contraluminal epithelial membrane for secretion into the luminal fluid. This process is particularly prominent in the proximal tubule, where organic acids and bases are both actively reabsorbed and secreted. Nephrotoxic drugs handled by these organic acid and base transport mechanisms can accumulate within the cell cytoplasm, impair cellular function, and cause tubular necrosis. Cephaloridine, an early first-generation cephalosporin antibiotic that was absorbed from the contraluminal membrane surface, accumulated intracellularly and caused proximal tubular epithelial cell necrosis.[20]

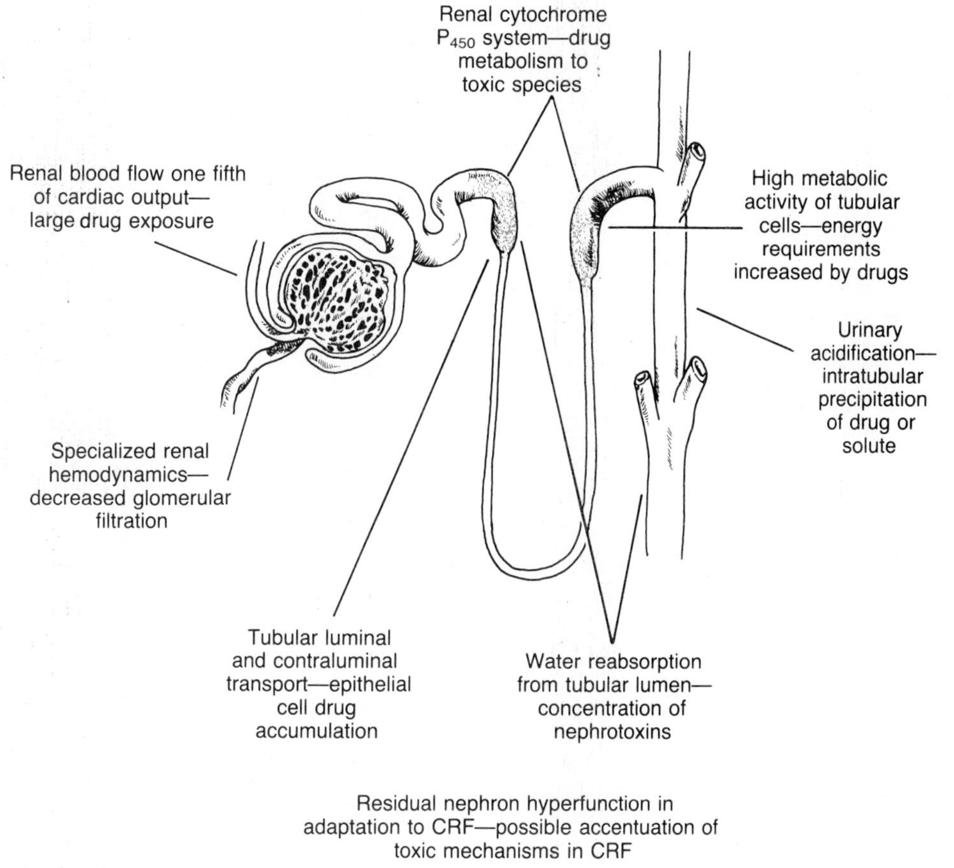


**Figure 36.1** Mechanisms of renal susceptibility to drug toxicity. See text for discussion. CRF, chronic renal failure.

### *Drug Metabolism to Toxic Species*

Renal biochemical pathways inactivate certain toxic molecules, but may also form nephrotoxic drug metabolites. The relative role of renal drug metabolism in the formation of toxic species has been questioned, as whole kidney activity of drug-metabolizing enzymes, including cytochrome $P_{450}$–dependent mixed function oxidases, is lower than liver activity; however, it has now been demonstrated that a cytochrome $P_{450}$–dependent mixed function oxidase system with activity similar to that in the liver is localized in proximal tubule epithelial cells.[21] Other enzymes present in the kidney that contribute to drug metabolism include prostaglandin endoperoxide synthetase, γ-glutamyltranspeptidase, aminopeptidase, *N*-acetyltransferase, sulfotransferase, and uridine diphosphate glucuronyltransferase.[21] Thus, renal biochemical transformation of certain drugs to toxic metabolites may contribute to nephrotoxicity. Oxidation of acetaminophen to a reactive species has been considered a pathogenetic mechanism for analgesic nephropathy.[22]

### *High Energy Requirements*

Renal tubular cells have high energy requirements for active tubular transport and metabolic processes. These normal energy needs appear to be precariously supplied to medullary tubular cells by a specialized blood system that maintains a state of chronic hypoxia.[23] Thus, these cells are sensitive to toxins that increase energy demands or impair energy production or oxygen delivery. Amphotericin B–induced medullary tubular damage appears to result in part from an imbalance between increased cellular energy requirements and inadequate oxygen delivery to this nephron segment.[23]

### *Concentration of Solute in Tubular Lumen*

Ninety-nine percent of the water filtered by the glomerulus is reabsorbed. Normally, 50% to 85% of the reabsorption occurs in the proximal tubule and the remainder in the descending loop of Henle and collecting duct. Systemic volume depletion increases the percentage water reabsorption in the proximal tubule. The consequences of water reabsorption include decreased tubular flow rates and increased luminal concentration of solutes and toxins. During aminoglycoside therapy the occurrence of systemic dehydration and enhancement of water reabsorption appears to increase the risk of toxicity to the tubular epithelium.[24] Increased proximal tubule water reabsorption could facilitate aminoglycoside contact with the tubular epithelium and promote transport into cells.

**Table 36.3** Mechanisms and Principles for Prevention of Drug Nephropathy

| *Mechanism of renal susceptibility* | *Principle for prevention* | *Example* |
|---|---|---|
| A. Large drug exposure resulting from high renal blood flow | 1. Avoid systemic drug administration<br>2. Limit total drug dose | 1. Intraperitoneal administration of cisplatin for intraperitoneal tumor[160]<br>2. Monitor aminoglycoside levels to maintain in therapeutic range[98] |
| B. Specialized renal hemodynamics regulated by vasoactive substances | Avoid drugs that inhibit prostaglandin synthesis | Substitution of nonacetylated salicylates or sulindac for other NSAIDs[40] |
| C. Tubular epithelial cell drug accumulation caused by luminal and contraluminal transport | 1. Inhibit drug absorption from the luminal membrane<br>2. Inhibit drug absorption from the contraluminal membrane | 1. Hydration with chloride anions during cisplatin therapy; calcium supplementation during aminoglycoside therapy[100,111]<br>2. Cilastatin inhibition of imipenem toxicity[161] |
| D. Renal metabolism of drugs to toxic species | Use drugs metabolized by kidney to nontoxic species | Renal metabolism of active sulindac sulfide to inactive sulindac sulfoxide[36] |
| E. Cellular dysfunction resulting from drug-induced increased energy requirements | Decrease cell energy needs by reducing cell membrane transport activity | Furosemide use during amphotericin therapy to reduce ischemia and toxicity to the medullary thick ascending loop of Henle[23] |
| F. Water reabsorption and concentration of nephrotoxins within the tubular lumen promoting increased epithelial cell membrane contact and transport into cells | 1. Prevent dehydration<br>2. Use of osmotic diuresis to increase luminal water concentration and tubular flow rate | 1. NaCl repletion to prevent amphotericin toxicity[119]<br>2. Possible reduction of contrast nephropathy by mannitol diuresis[101] |
| G. Urinary acidification with intratubular precipitation of drug or solute | Alkalinize urine | Urinary alkalinization to prevent uric acid and methotrexate nephropathy[142] |
| H. In chronic renal failure, increased toxin exposure per residual viable nephron as a result of nephron hyperfunction | Avoid drug use or reduce drug dose in renal failure patients | Alternatives to radiologic-contrast agents for renal imaging: ultrasonography, computerized tomography without contrast use, radionuclide studies |

### *Acidification of Urine*

Urine pH can decrease to approximately 4.5 during maximal stimulation of renal tubular hydrogen ion secretion. Certain solutes can precipitate and obstruct the tubular lumen at this acid pH, particularly when urine is concentrated. Urinary acidification contributes to acute uric acid nephropathy as a complication of chemotherapy-induced massive tumor lysis.

### *Increased Function of Individual Nephrons in Adaptation to Chronic Renal Insufficiency*

Each glomerular and tubular unit can be affected to a greater or lesser extent by many diseases that cause chronic renal insufficiency. As a result, certain nephron units can remain relatively uninjured and function at an increased level of activity to compensate for the loss of other nephrons. This hyperfunctioning of remnant nephrons appears to enhance their susceptibility to nephrotoxins, apparently by accentuation of the previously described mechanisms. An example is the greatly increased nephrotoxicity of radiologic-contrast media in patients with chronic renal insufficiency.[25]

## Principles for Prevention of Drug Nephropathy

The basic principle for prevention of drug-induced renal disease is to avoid the use of potentially nephrotoxic diagnostic and therapeutic agents in patients at increased risk for toxicity; however, when exposure to these drugs cannot be avoided, specific techniques may be used to reduce potential nephrotoxicity (Table 36.3). Although many of these approaches remain investigational, others have permitted more aggressive drug administration to maximize efficacy while minimizing toxicity.

## Drug-Induced Renal Structural–Functional Alterations

### *"Pseudo" Renal Failure*

Blood urea nitrogen or creatinine concentrations may increase during drug therapy without a reduction in the glomerular filtration rate. This "pseudo" renal failure is most common during therapy with corticosteroids or tetracyclines, drugs that cause protein catabolism. These drugs increase the concentration of blood urea nitrogen while a normal serum creatinine concentration is maintained. The glomerular filtration rate is accurately indicated by the serum creatinine concentration or creatinine clearance.

Alternatively, pseudo renal failure may be characterized by a rise in the serum creatinine concentration while a normal blood urea nitrogen concentration is maintained. This can occur during therapy with trimethoprim or cimetidine, drugs that competitively inhibit proximal tubular creatinine secretion.[26] This effect is minimal in patients with normal renal function and the serum creatinine concentration usually remains in the normal range.[27] In renal insufficient patients the rise in serum creatinine is greater, as tubular creatinine secretion contributes more to urinary creatinine excretion.[28] Pseudo renal failure also occurs during therapy with cephalosporin antibiotics, particularly cefoxitin, which can increase the serum creatinine concentration by direct interference with creatinine measurement by the Jaffe method.[26] This effect is also most pronounced in renal insufficient patients. During therapy with drugs that can increase the serum creatinine concentration, the glomerular filtration rate can be determined accurately only by inulin clearance or other noncreatinine measures of renal function.

## *Hemodynamically Mediated Renal Failure*

### Reduced Glomerular Capillary Filtration Pressure

Antihypertensive therapy with captopril and enalapril, angiotensin-converting enzyme inhibitors (ACEIs), has resulted in a new syndrome of hemodynamically mediated nephropathy.[18] The glomerular filtration rate of kidneys perfused by stenotic renal arteries can decline rapidly during ACEI therapy and recover upon discontinuation of therapy. The rise in serum creatinine is usually minimal if blood flow to one kidney is normal; however, patients with bilateral renal artery stenosis or a single kidney with renovascular disease may develop severe renal failure. Although the incidence remains to be determined, renal failure has occurred in nine of nine patients with posttransplant renal artery stenosis.[29] The diagnosis can be suspected by the rise in serum creatinine concentration as well as a reversible loss of renal radionuclide imaging by the involved kidney.[30] Renal function of patients with possible renal artery stenosis must be monitored carefully during initiation of ACEI therapy.

The pathogenesis of this nephropathy is a decrease in glomerular capillary hydrostatic pressure sufficient to reduce glomerular ultrafiltration.[31] This occurs in the presence of renal artery stenosis with fixed glomerular afferent arteriole blood flow. In this situation, angiotensin II causes efferent arteriole vasoconstriction to maintain glomerular capillary hydrostatic pressure for ultrafiltration. Therapy with ACEIs reduces angiotensin II production and dilates the efferent arteriole. This reduces glomerular capillary hydrostatic pressure and decreases glomerular ultrafiltration. The pathogenetic principles of this nephropathy are being investigated for application to the diagnosis of renovascular hypertension[32] and prevention of the progressive nature of chronic renal insufficiency.[4]

Calcium channel blockers, like ACEIs, may decrease the glomerular filtration rate in certain patients with arteriosclerotic cardiovascular disease.[19,33] The pathogenesis appears to be hemodynamically mediated, and may involve efferent arteriole vasodilation by inhibition of calcium entry into smooth muscle cells with impairment of vasoconstrictor responsiveness to angiotensin II or norepinephrine.[19] Alternatively, renal insufficiency may have resulted from reduced synthesis of vasodilatory prostaglandins.[19]

### Inhibition of Prostaglandin-Dependent Renal Blood Flow

Nonsteroidal anti-inflammatory drugs (NSAIDs) are commonly prescribed for a variety of disease processes. Their overall safety has resulted in over-the-counter availability of ibuprofen, a potent NSAID; however, these drugs have the potential to cause several nephropathies (Table 36.1), of which hemodynamically mediated acute renal failure is most common.[34]

Patients at greatest risk for this nephropathy generally have medical conditions associated with high plasma renin activity: hepatic disease with ascites, decompensated congestive heart failure, nephrotic syndrome, and glomerulonephritis. Additional risk factors include systemic lupus erythematosus, renal vascular disease, advanced age, hypertension, diabetes mellitus, atherosclerotic cardiovascular disease, diuretic therapy, and volume depletion.[34,35] Reversible oliguric renal failure can occur within days of initiation of NSAID therapy. The creatinine and blood urea nitrogen rise proportionately, the urine sodium concentration is usually low, and the urine sediment is unremarkable.

The pathogenesis of NSAID nephropathy is an imbalance of vasoconstrictive and vasodilatory influences on the kidney. Enhanced activity of renal vasoconstrictors, angiotensin II, norepinephrine, vasopressin, and sympathetic nerve activity is normally counterbalanced by a compensatory increase of renal vasodilator activity to prevent ischemia. This vasodilatory activity includes renal cortical arteriole and glomerular synthesis of prostaglandin $E_2$ and prostacyclin.[36] NSAID therapy inhibits prostaglandin synthesis by preventing cyclooxygenation of arachidonic acid. In high-risk patients, this results in an imbalance of renal vasodilatory and vasoconstrictive influences with subsequent renal ischemia and a decreased glomerular filtration rate.

Vasodilatory prostaglandins are not necessary to maintain renal function in the absence of excess renal vasoconstrictor activity. Thus, NSAID therapy is not considered to have an adverse renal hemodynamic effect in patients without risk factors for this nephropathy; however, a mild reduction in the glomerular filtration rate can occur in normal subjects during prolonged indomethacin therapy.[37] In addition, even aspirin can decrease the glomerular filtration rate of sodium-restricted normal individuals.[38]

These renal hemodynamic effects of NSAIDs have been applied therapeutically to reduce proteinuria in patients with the nephrotic syndrome.[39] The efficacy of various NSAIDs for this purpose is directly proportional to their ability to inhibit renal prostaglandin synthesis.[39]

NSAID-induced acute renal failure is prevented by recognizing high-risk patients and using analgesics with less prostaglandin inhibition: acetaminophen, nonacetylated salicylates, aspirin, and sulindac. When NSAID therapy of high-risk patients is essential, management of predisposing medical problems should be optimized and renal function monitored regularly. The use and pharmacology of sulindac are of particular interest, as it is a potent NSAID that does not inhibit renal prostaglandin synthesis and appears to preserve the renal function of high-risk patients.[40] The mechanism of renal prostaglandin sparing may involve intrarenal metabolism by cytochrome $P_{450}$–dependent mixed-function oxidases of the active drug, sulindac sulfide, to inactive sulindac sulfoxide.[36]

Acute renal failure resulting from NSAID therapy is treated by discontinuation of the NSAID and supportive care. Although renal failure may be severe, recovery is usually rapid without need for dialytic therapy. Occasionally, the hemodynamic insult is sufficiently severe to cause frank tubular necrosis, which can prolong recovery.[41] The differential diagnosis of NSAID hemodynamically mediated acute renal failure must include NSAID-induced acute interstitial nephritis, as steroid therapy may benefit this lesion.[42]

Sulfinpyrazone, a uricosuric congener of phenylbutazone, also appears to cause a hemodynamically mediated acute renal failure.[43,44] Sulfinpyrazone has been used to impair platelet function after myocardial infarction or coronary artery bypass graft surgery. In these settings sulfinpyrazone inhibition of renal prostaglandin synthesis[43] or reduction of renal kallikrein–kinin activity[44] may cause an imbalance in renal hemodynamics and hence renal ischemia. Renal insufficiency may be transient despite continued sulfinpyrazone administration or severe and oliguric with a low urinary sodium concentration.[43,44] Alternative mechanisms of nephrotoxicity include uric acid nephropathy[43] and "pseudo" renal failure, as sulfinpyrazone administration can decrease creatinine clearance without a change in inulin clearance.[45]

### Nonspecific Renal Vasoconstriction

Triamterene is a potassium-sparing diuretic that has been associated with a transient decrease in creatinine clearance in normal subjects[46] and abnormal urinary sediment in hypertensive patients.[47] Triamterene therapy in combination with hydrochlorothiazide has caused reversible acute renal failure in elderly patients,[48] and in combination with indomethacin, it has induced acute renal failure in normal subjects and in a patient at risk for NSAID nephropathy.[49,50] Although acute interstitial nephritis is a potential mechanism,[48] a hemodynamic mechanism is more likely as suggested by the apparent increased risk for nephrotoxicity during combined triamterene/indomethacin therapy.[49] Presumably, triamterene causes renal vasoconstriction that is counterbalanced by increased renal synthesis of vasodilatory prostaglandins.[51] Concomitant NSAID therapy may induce renal ischemia by preventing the compensatory increase in renal prostaglandin synthesis; however, the implications of these observations are unclear, as triamterene and NSAID are frequently used together without apparent nephrotoxicity.

Propranolol, a nonselective $\beta$-adrenergic receptor blocker, causes a 10% to 20% reduction in the renal blood flow of hypertensive patients.[16] The glomerular filtration rate is less consistently reduced.[16] In contrast, nadolol, another nonselective $\beta$-blocker, increases renal blood flow while other $\beta$-blockers do not appear to alter renal hemodynamics.[52] The mechanism of the propranolol-induced decrease in renal blood flow is unknown. As renal function does not decrease with other $\beta$-blockers, the effect is unlikely to result from blockade of $\beta$ receptors or decreased cardiac output. Other postulated mechanisms include renal vasoconstriction resulting from unopposed $\alpha$-adrenergic activity or inhibition of renal vasodilator activity, possibly by the kallikrein–kinin system.[16] The clinical significance of these effects is unknown. At present, however, it appears prudent to avoid propranolol therapy for renal insufficient patients.

Cyclosporine is a potent immunosuppressive agent used since 1976 to prevent rejection of transplanted organs by inhibiting synthesis of and response to interleukin-2.[53] Cyclosporine has dramatically enhanced nonrenal allograft survival and improved renal allograft viability; however, an apparently hemodynamically mediated acute renal failure and a chronic renal failure are major adverse effects of this therapy.[53–55] The pathophysiology has been difficult to assess after renal transplantation because of changes associated with concomitant graft rejection. Renal functional and histopathologic changes have been quantified best in heart and liver transplant patients and during immunosuppression for nonrenal immune diseases such as uveitis and rheumatoid arthritis.[53,55–58]

Overall renal function appears to deteriorate acutely in approximately 80% of patients during the first 6 months of therapy.[53,56] Toxicity is increased by concurrent illnesses, including renal graft rejection, hypotension, and infection, as well as by therapy with other nephrotoxic drugs (aminoglycosides, amphotericin B, and acyclovir).[53] There are no consistent urine sediment abnormalities.[53,57] Additional manifestations of renal dysfunction include hypertension, hyperkalemia, sodium avidity, and hypomagnesemia.[59] Renal biopsy reveals proximal tubular epithelial cell vacuolization and atrophy, thickening of arterioles, mild focal glomerular sclerosis, and interstitial fibrosis.[56,57]

A hemodynamic pathogenesis is suggested by the usually rapid improvement of renal function after cyclosporine dose reduction. Vasoconstriction of preglomerular arterioles may be involved as a consequence of decreased prostacyclin synthesis or stimulation of the sympathetic nervous system.[55,59] Alternatively, direct proximal tubule damage by cyclosporine is possible.[55]

Therapy is limited to dose reduction and treatment of concomitant illness. In most patients, renal function recovers after dose reduction or discontinuation of cyclosporine[58,59]; however, irreversible chronic renal failure can occur with prolonged use.[56,58] Prevention of cyclosporine nephrotoxicity is an important research objective. As toxicity is clearly dose related, clarification of cyclosporine pharmacokinetics and pharmacodynamics relative to immunosuppression and nephrotoxicity is necessary.[59,60]

## *Renal Vascular Alterations*

Systemic polyarteritis nodosa with involvement of small and medium-sized renal arteries has been described after methamphetamine abuse.[61] Patients may have hematuria, proteinuria, renal insufficiency, and hypertension. Renal and visceral vascular aneurysms can be demonstrated by angiography. The pathogenesis may be a toxic reaction to methamphetamine or the result of an associated hepatitis B infection. Penicillin and sulfonamide therapies have also been considered as causes of polyarteritis nodosa, although the associations have been less clear.[61]

Thrombotic microangiopathy (hemolytic–uremic syndrome) involving glomerular afferent arterioles and capillaries has been described during therapy with various drugs, including oral contraceptive agents,[62] cyclosporine,[63] and mitomycin C.[64] The association with mitomycin C is of particular interest because the pathogenesis appears to be a direct toxic effect with a predictable incidence: 1.6% in patients receiving less than 50 mg/m$^2$ and 27.8% in patients receiving more than 70 mg/m$^2$.[65] Nephrotoxicity has occurred after long-term chemotherapy with mitomycin C alone and in combination with 5-fluorouracil, cisplatin, bleomycin, and a vinca alkaloid.[64,66] Microangiopathic hemolytic anemia and thrombocytopenia are usually present. Biopsies of renal, brain, and pulmonary tissue reveal thrombi in small vessels. Renal failure can be severe and irreversible although corticosteroid, vincristine sulfate, plasma exchange, and plasmapheresis therapies have all induced clinical improvement.[67,68]

### *Glomerular Alterations: Nephrotic Syndrome and Glomerulonephritis*

Drug-induced glomerular disease is uncommon, although a variety of agents have been implicated.[69] The mechanism may be immunologic or, less likely, a direct toxic effect. The nephrotic syndrome, defined as proteinuria greater than 3.5 g/d, is the usual manifestation of glomerular damage. Four histopathologic glomerular lesions have been identified: minimal-change, focal segmental glomerulosclerosis, membranous, and membranoproliferative.

Minimal-change nephrotic syndrome is characterized by normal glomeruli under light microscopic examination. When this lesion is drug induced, it is frequently accompanied by an interstitial nephritis. This lesion is most common during NSAID therapy, although ampicillin, rifampin, hydantoin anticonvulsants, and lithium have been implicated.[70] The pathogenesis remains unknown. Nephrotic-range proteinuria resulting from NSAID therapy is frequently associated with an interstitial infiltrate of T lymphocytes, suggesting disordered cell-mediated immunity.[71] These cells may release lymphokines, which increase glomerular capillary permeability to proteins.[42] Proteinuria usually resolves rapidly after discontinuation of the toxic drug, although corticosteroid therapy may be useful in resolving the lesion.[42]

Focal segmental glomerulosclerosis is characterized histopathologically by areas of sclerosis in some glomeruli as well as renal interstitial inflammation and fibrosis. Chronic heroin abuse is the most common cause of this lesion.[72] Blacks may be more susceptible than whites.[72] The pathogenesis is unknown but includes direct toxicity from heroin or contaminants as well as injury from associated bacterial or viral infections. The prognosis is poor; end-stage renal failure develops in most cases. No specific therapy is available although discontinuation of heroin use may prevent progression.[72]

Membranous nephropathy is the most common drug-induced glomerular lesion. It is an immune-mediated disorder characterized by immune complex deposition along glomerular capillary loops. Parenteral gold therapy for rheumatoid arthritis is the most common cause and 0.2% to 5% of patients have been affected.[73] Oral gold therapy appears to be associated with a lesser incidence.[74] The pathogenesis is unclear, but may involve damage to the proximal tubule with subsequent antigen release, antibody formation, and glomerular immune complex deposition.[75] Gold has been identified in proximal tubular cells, but not in the glomerular deposits. Genetic factors appear to be important, as patients with the B-lymphocyte alloantigen HLA-DRW3 or -B8 have increased susceptibility.[76] Mercury found in diuretics, topical skin preparations, and industrial vapors also causes membranous nephropathy.[69,77] The pathogenesis remains unknown, but appears to be immunologically mediated.[69,78] D-Penicillamine[79] and possibly captopril[80] can also cause membranous nephropathy, apparently as an immune response to their sulfhydryl groups.[69]

Membranoproliferative glomerulonephritis is a rare consequence of drug therapy that most commonly occurs with hydralazine-induced systemic lupus erythematosus.[81] Other drug-induced glomerular lesions have only been described in case reports and include rapidly progressive or crescentic glomerulonephritis from D-penicillamine therapy,[79] immune complex glomerulonephritis from nifedipine therapy,[82] and proliferative glomerulonephritis with the nephrotic syndrome from chlorpropamide therapy.[83]

### *Acute Tubular Necrosis*

Acute necrosis of renal tubular epithelium is the most common mechanism of drug-induced renal insufficiency. Proximal tubular cells appear to be the most susceptible. Although multiple drugs have been implicated (see Table 36.4), radiologic-contrast media, aminoglycosides, and cisplatin are the most important.[5]

The initial manifestation of nephrotoxicity by these agents is subclinical proximal tubular proteinuria and enzymuria.[84] Clinical nephrotoxicity becomes apparent later as a rise in the serum creatinine and blood urea nitrogen concentrations, a decline in the creatinine clearance, and disturbances of renal tubular electrolyte and water handling. During repetitive therapy, the cumulative effects of recurrent subclinical toxicity may result in chronic tubulointerstitial disease.[85]

The reason for the reduced glomerular filtration rate in the setting of tubular necrosis remains unclear. The glomerular filtration rate decreases disproportionately more than renal blood flow, suggesting that renal ischemia is not the primary alteration.[86,87] Other possible mechanisms include a shunt of blood away from the glomerulus, reduction of glomerular

**Table 36.4** Drugs That Cause Tubular Necrosis

| *High incidence* | *Low incidence* |
|---|---|
| Radiologic-contrast agents | Mannitol |
| Aminoglycosides | Low-molecular-weight dextran |
| Amphotericin B | Nonsteroidal anti-inflammatory drugs |
| Cisplatin | Methoxyflurane anesthesia |
| Acetaminophen (overdose) | Tetracycline |
| Streptozocin | Amoxapine |
| Cephaloridine | |

capillary filtration pressure, decreased permeability of the glomerular filtration surface, obstruction of tubular lumens by swollen epithelial cells or cellular debris, and backleak of the glomerular ultrafiltrate across damaged tubular epithelia and into the systemic circulation.[86,87] The relative role of each mechanism may depend on the specific nephrotoxic drug.

### Aminoglycoside Nephrotoxicity

The glomerular filtration rate decreases in 5% to 20% of patients treated with aminoglycoside antibiotics, making aminoglycosides the second most common cause of hospital-acquired drug-induced renal disease.[5,88] Pathogenetic mechanisms of this nephropathy have been studied extensively in an attempt to decrease the incidence of toxicity. Furthermore, in this era of cost analysis, individual aminoglycosides have been compared relative to their cost for daily use and additional costs associated with their incidence of nephropathy.[89]

The initial manifestation of aminoglycoside toxicity is increased renal tubular proteinuria ($\beta_2$-microglobulin) during the first 4 days of therapy.[90] After 5 to 7 days of therapy there is a gradual rise in the serum creatinine concentration and decrease in the creatinine clearance. Oliguria (urine volume < 500 mL/d) is uncommon and renal magnesium and potassium wasting can occur. Renal failure is usually mild if aminoglycoside therapy is stopped, although renal replacement therapy with dialysis is occasionally required. Renal dysfunction is usually reversible, even when dialytic therapy is necessary. Atypical presentations of aminoglycoside nephropathy must be evaluated carefully, because not all renal failure that occurs during a course of therapy is aminoglycoside induced. Dehydration, sepsis, and concomitant drug therapy may contribute significantly.

The pathogenesis of aminoglycoside nephrotoxicity is predominantly tubular epithelial cell damage and obstruction of the tubular lumen, although a glomerular mechanism has been considered.[91–93] The tubular toxicity of various aminoglycosides is directly proportional to the number of cationic charges on these molecules: neomycin with six cationic amino groups is more nephrotoxic than streptomycin with three groups, while gentamicin and tobramycin with five amino groups each have intermediate toxicity.[91] These cationic charges facilitate binding of filtered aminoglycosides to renal tubular epithelial cell luminal membranes, which is followed by intracellular transport and concentration in lysozomes.[91] A phospholipidosis results, apparently by aminoglycoside interaction with negatively charged phospholipids (phosphatidylinositol), that inhibits phospholipase activity and causes accumulation of phospholipids. This can be seen histopathologically as abnormal lysozomal structures (myeloid bodies). Membrane function of other cell organelles (e.g., mitochondria) is also affected.[91] Cellular dysfunction and death may result both from release of lysozomal enzymes into the cytosol and from alteration of cellular metabolism caused by reduced activity of membrane-bound enzymes, including Na,K-ATPase.[91] Debris from damaged tubular cells appears to obstruct tubular lumens and decrease the glomerular filtration rate.[92]

Decreased permeability of the glomerular filtration surface may also contribute to reduced renal function. Glomerular structural abnormalities (decreased diameter and density of endothelial fenestrae) can be demonstrated by scanning electron microscopy.[93] The pathogenesis may involve direct toxicity or the effect of an increased angiotensin II concentration stimulated by renal salt wasting and volume depletion.[94,95]

Multiple potential risk factors for aminoglycoside toxicity have been identified and include total cumulative aminoglycoside dose, 1-hour postdose aminoglycoside concentration, trough serum concentration exceeding 2 mg/L, presence of increased or decreased renal function, increased patient age, female gender, associated illness (shock, gram-negative bacteremia, liver disease), dehydration, concomitant drug therapy (cephalosporins, vancomycin, or radiologic-contrast agents), and magnesium deficiency.[96–98] Nomograms to identify patients at risk for aminoglycoside nephrotoxicity have been developed.[99] General guidelines to prevent nephrotoxicity include providing adequate hydration, limiting the total dose administered, avoiding concomitant therapy with other nephrotoxic drugs, maintaining serum aminoglycoside concentrations within the therapeutic range, and monitoring frequently for changes in renal function. By itself, careful maintenance of aminoglycoside concentrations in the therapeutic range has not prevented nephrotoxicity.[88] The specific aminoglycoside used does not appear to significantly affect the risk of nephrotoxicity.[98] Investigational use of calcium supplementation during aminoglycoside therapy has decreased nephrotoxicity, apparently by inhibiting aminoglycoside binding to luminal membranes of renal tubular epithelial cells and preventing uptake into cells.[100]

### Radiologic-Contrast Medium Nephrotoxicity

Administration of radiologic-contrast media is the most common cause of hospital-acquired drug-induced acute renal failure.[5] The spectrum of contrast nephropathy ranges from transient tubular enzymuria to irreversible oliguric renal failure, which requires dialysis therapy.[101] Severe nephrotoxicity is unusual and occurs most frequently in the presence of preexistent severe renal insufficiency. In most cases, toxicity is mild and rapidly reversible. The typical course is an initial transient osmotic diuresis followed by nonspecific glomerular proteinuria and tubular enzymuria. The serum creatinine rises and peaks between 2 and 5 days after exposure, with recovery after 4 to 10 days. Oliguria is present in about 50% of cases. No laboratory test is diagnostic and urinalysis reveals only proteinuria with hyaline and granular casts. The urine sodium concentration and fractional excretion of sodium are frequently low.[102]

The major risk factor for contrast nephropathy is preexistent renal insufficiency.[101] Hospitalized patients with a serum creatinine concentration greater than 1.5 mg/dL have approximately a 30% to 40% incidence, and those with serum creatinine concentrations of 5 mg/dL or greater have approximately a 70% incidence of renal dysfunction after intravenous or intraarterial contrast injection.[101] The increase in serum creatinine observed after contrast administration is not entirely due to direct contrast toxicity, as concomitant medical illnesses and dehydration resulting from fluid restriction, cathartics, and enemas used for study preparation also increase the serum creatinine.[103]

Other risk factors for contrast nephropathy are diabetes

mellitus and conditions associated with decreased renal blood flow including congestive heart failure and dehydration. Large dose, renal arterial site of contrast administration, advanced age, and arteriosclerotic peripheral vascular disease have also been associated with an increased incidence. In addition, multiple myeloma has been considered a relative contraindication for contrast injection; however, it now appears that the toxicity previously associated with multiple myeloma was due to preexistent renal insufficiency. The risk for contrast nephropathy in myeloma patients is minimal if renal function is normal and patients are well hydrated.[101]

The pathogenesis of contrast nephropathy includes both direct tubular toxicity and renal ischemia.[101] The presence of tubular toxicity is indicated by renal tubular enzymuria and biopsy findings of proximal tubular epithelial cell vacuolization and acute tubular necrosis. In addition to the direct toxic effects of contrast media, nonselective proteinuria induced by contrast media may indirectly damage tubular epithelial cells[104]; however, the low urine sodium concentration and fractional excretion of sodium frequently observed with contrast nephropathy indicate good tubular function and suggest that renal ischemia may be a more important mechanism than tubular toxicity. Renal ischemia results from systemic hypotension associated with contrast injection as well as selective renal vasoconstriction. Renal ischemia may also result from dehydration caused by the osmotic diuresis that accompanies use of these hyperosmolar agents (900–1,780 mOsm/kg) and from increased blood viscosity caused by red blood cell crenation and aggregation.[101] A final, less likely mechanism of contrast nephropathy is tubular obstruction caused by intratubular precipitation of uric acid, calcium oxalate, or Tamm–Horsfall glycoprotein.[101]

Contrast nephropathy can be prevented by avoiding contrast use in high-risk patients. If contrast media must be used, prestudy dehydration should be avoided, the smallest adequate dose should be administered, and additional contrast studies should be appropriately delayed to avoid cumulative toxicity. Aggressive hydration and mannitol administration after contrast exposure may also reduce the incidence of nephropathy[101]; however, these measures may not prevent nephropathy in high-risk patients.[105] Dialytic therapy may be necessary to treat established contrast nephropathy. Recovery of renal function is more likely in patients with less severe preexistent renal insufficiency. Use of recently available nonionic contrast media may reduce the risk of toxicity.[106]

### Cisplatin Nephrotoxicity

Cisplatin is an important chemotherapeutic agent with the potential to cause significant renal tubular damage because of the heavy metal, platinum.[107] During early investigations with cisplatin the incidence of nephrotoxicity was 50% to 100%. Subsequently, the incidence of toxicity was decreased to 6% to 13% by limiting the total drug dose and reducing the rate of administration.[108] Concomitant therapy with aminoglycosides can contribute to azotemia, and use with other chemotherapeutic agents can potentiate the characteristic renal magnesium wasting.

Nephrotoxicity is usually reversible and manifests early during therapy as transient proximal renal tubular cell brush border and lysozomal enzymuria.[109] Peak serum creatinine concentrations occur approximately 10 to 12 days after initiation of therapy, with recovery by 21 days. Renal damage, however, can be cumulative, and serum creatinine may continue to rise with subsequent cycles of therapy.[107] Renal magnesium wasting is common and serum magnesium concentrations can decrease progressively with continuing cycles of therapy, even in the absence of azotemia.[107] Hypomagnesemia may be severe and persist long after chemotherapy has ended. Clinical manifestations of magnesium deficiency include seizures, neuromuscular irritability, and personality changes.

The mechanism of cisplatin toxicity involves impairment of cell energy production by binding of platinum to proximal tubular cell sulfhydryl groups, with disruption of cell enzyme activity and uncoupling of oxidative phosphorylation.[108,110] Renal biopsies show sparing of glomeruli, with necrosis of both proximal and distal tubules and collecting ducts.[107] Measures that prevent toxicity include reduction of both dose and frequency of administration. These goals are usually accomplished by administering cisplatin in combination with other chemotherapeutic agents. In addition, vigorous saline hydration is important and furosemide or mannitol diuresis appears to be helpful.[107,108] Investigational techniques that have decreased toxicity are the use of hypertonic saline to reduce tubular cisplatin uptake[111] and the reduction of renal exposure by intraperitoneal administration for peritoneal tumors in conjunction with systemic administration of sodium thiosulfate, a cisplatin neutralizer.[112] Unsuccessful attempts to decrease toxicity have included use of captopril to interrupt cisplatin-induced reflex stimulation of the renin–angiotensin system[113] and use of verapamil to block tubular cell uptake of calcium, a final mediator of cell death.[114]

The pathogenesis of hypomagnesemia includes the renal magnesium wasting resulting from tubular damage and the magnesuric effects of saline hydration and diuretic therapy to prevent tubular toxicity. Anorexia and diarrhea can also contribute.[115] The incidence of hypomagnesemia increases with recurrent cycles of cisplatin and combination chemotherapy.[115] Management requires frequent monitoring of serum magnesium concentrations and repletion with magnesium chloride.[108]

### Amphotericin B Nephrotoxicity

Amphotericin B is an important antifungal agent that causes a dose-dependent reduction in renal function.[116] This decrease is uncommon with a mean total dose of 0.6 g, but occurs in 80% with a dose up to 4 g.[116] Clinical toxicity manifests initially as renal magnesium and potassium wasting. Distal renal tubular acidosis occurs, apparently as a result of backleak of hydrogen ions out of the collecting duct lumen. Nephrogenic diabetes insipidus can occur because of decreased urinary concentrating ability. The glomerular filtration rate ultimately declines.[117]

The renal histopathology includes focal vacuolization of small arterial and arteriolar smooth muscle cells and proximal and distal tubular epithelial cell damage.[118] The pathogenesis appears to involve amphotericin binding to cell membranes with subsequent alterations of membrane permeability, including increased permeability to sodium. Cel-

**Table 36.5** Commonly Used Drugs That Cause Allergic Interstitial Nephritis

| | |
|---|---|
| Penicillins | Allopurinol |
| Cephalosporins | Radiologic-contrast media |
| Aminoglycosides | Sulfinpyrazone |
| Trimethoprim–sulfamethoxazole | Cimetidine |
| | Captopril |
| Rifampin | Clofibrate |
| Erythromycin | Acetazolamide |
| Vancomycin | Amiloride |
| Interferon | Nonsteroidal anti-inflammatory drugs |
| Thiazides | |
| Furosemide | Acetaminophen |
| Triamterene | |

lular damage apparently results in part from oxygen delivery insufficient to meet the energy requirements imposed by alterations of cell membrane permeability.[23] In addition, renal arterial injection of amphotericin B causes intense vasoconstriction and it is probable that vasoconstriction also contributes to renal ischemia.[118]

Amphotericin nephrotoxicity is treated by discontinuation of therapy. Renal tubular dysfunction and glomerular filtration rate can improve, although damage may be irreversible. Salt repletion has decreased the incidence of nephrotoxicity in humans,[119] whereas concomitant mannitol infusion has not been effective.[120]

## *Tubulointerstitial Disease*

### Acute Allergic Interstitial Nephritis

Acute interstitial nephritis is a common drug nephropathy reported to cause 8% of acute renal failures.[121] The clinical experience with methicillin has been most completely documented,[122] although multiple drugs have been implicated (Table 36.5). Signs of nephropathy occur about 17 days (range 2–44 days) after initiation of therapy. These signs (and their approximate incidence)[121–123] include fever (75%), maculopapular rash (25%), eosinophilia (80%), pyuria and hematuria (90%), low-level proteinuria (90%), and oliguria (18%). Eosinophiluria is variably reported to be common or infrequent. Failure to demonstrate eosinophiluria may result from the inadequacy of the staining technique usually used to identify urine eosinophils.[124] Tubular dysfunction, including renal tubular acidosis, hyperkalemia, and salt wasting, occurs occasionally.

Allergic interstitial nephritis resulting from NSAID therapy has a distinctly different clinical presentation.[42] Older patients are affected more frequently, possibly a reflection of the therapeutic indications for these drugs. The onset of nephropathy is delayed a mean of 5.4 months from initiation of therapy. Manifestations of a systemic hypersensitivity response are less frequent, occurring in only 19%. Finally, a concomitant nil lesion nephrotic syndrome is characteristic.

The renal histopathology of allergic interstitial nephritis is a diffuse or focal interstitial infiltrate of lymphocytes, plasma cells, eosinophils and occasional polymorphonuclear neutrophils. Patchy peritubular inflammation with epithelial cell atrophy and necrosis is also present.[121,123] The pathogenesis is an allergic hypersensitivity response.[121–123] In certain cases a humoral, antibody-mediated, mechanism may be involved as indicated by the occasional presence of circulating antibodies to a drug hapten–tubular basement membrane complex, low serum complement levels, and tubular basement membrane deposition of immunoglobulin G and complement. More commonly, a cell-mediated immune mechanism is suggested by the absence of these findings and the presence of a predominantly T-lymphocyte infiltrate with an increased helper: suppressor cell ratio.[125] The pathogenesis of NSAID interstitial nephritis also involves T lymphocytes, possibly in response to altered prostaglandin synthesis.[42]

Prompt and accurate diagnosis of allergic interstitial nephritis is important, as failure to stop the offending drug can result in chronic renal insufficiency. The presence of fever, rash, eosinophilia, or eosinophiluria cannot be used to reliably make the diagnosis, as one or more of these findings are frequently absent. When possible, a renal biopsy is recommended as the most specific and direct method for diagnosis. Alternatively, renal imaging with gallium[67] scintigraphy may be a sensitive, but less specific, noninvasive diagnostic technique.[126] Treatment with corticosteroids appears to be useful in shortening the duration and improving the extent of renal function recovery.[127]

### Chronic Interstitial Nephritis

Lithium and cyclosporine are the most commonly used of the few drugs known to cause this usually progressive and irreversible nephropathy. Semustine (methyl-CCNU), an infrequently used investigational nitrosurea antineoplastic agent, has also predictably caused a chronic tubulointerstitial lesion when the dose has exceeded 1,200 mg/m$^2$.[108,128] Renal function can remain normal during the course of semustine therapy, with a subsequent decrease in renal size and a progressive loss of renal function that ultimately results in end-stage renal failure.

Lithium therapy causes several renal lesions, including chronic interstitial nephritis. The most common of these is nephrogenic diabetes insipidus (polyuria resulting from impaired ability to concentrate the urine), which occurs in 20% to 70% of patients.[129,130] The mechanism is a dose-related collecting duct unresponsiveness to antidiuretic hormone.[131] This appears to result from impaired formation of cellular cAMP in response to antidiuretic hormone and can be ameliorated by amiloride therapy.[130]

Lithium-induced acute renal failure has been observed during episodes of lithium intoxication.[132] The pathogenesis may include dehydration secondary to urinary concentration or direct proximal and distal tubular cell toxicity.[132] Severe renal insufficiency has been reported and is reversible with supportive care, including dialysis to reduce toxic serum lithium concentrations.[132]

Mild renal insufficiency appears to occur in as many as 10% of patients undergoing long-term lithium therapy.[133] Occasional patients have developed end-stage renal failure. The renal lesion includes interstitial fibrosis with focal tubular atrophy and glomerular sclerosis.[134,135] The pathogenesis may involve direct lithium toxicity and a correlation has been observed between the duration of lithium therapy and the decline in the glomerular filtration rate[136]; however, when lithium concentrations have been maintained within the therapeutic range, associated nephrotoxicity has not been convincingly demonstrated. Additional mechanisms of nephrotoxicity include the cumulative effects of acute episodes of lithium toxicity,[134] use of concomitant neuroleptic drugs,[135] and concurrent renal tubulointerstitial disease processes.

Preventive measures include maintenance of lithium concentrations in the therapeutic range, avoidance of dehydration, and close monitoring of renal function. It is unknown whether progression to severe renal failure can be prevented by discontinuing lithium therapy when mild renal insufficiency is first recognized.

Cyclosporine is a potent immunosuppressive drug that has caused interstitial fibrosis and chronic irreversible renal insufficiency. The pathogenesis appears to involve preglomerular arteriole vasoconstriction or direct tubular toxicity, as discussed earlier (Hemodynamically Mediated Renal Failure). Functional and histopathologic changes have been most clearly demonstrated in heart and liver transplant patients and during immunosuppression for nonrenal immune diseases such as uveitis and rheumatoid arthritis.[53,56–58]

**Papillary Necrosis**

Chronic excessive consumption of combination analgesics is a cause of renal tubulointerstitial disease with papillary necrosis. This analgesic or "phenacetin" nephropathy was initially reported from Switzerland in 1953 and has since been recognized as a worldwide public health concern.[13] It has caused as much as 36% of chronic renal failure in certain geographic areas, although the incidence is lower in North America.[14,15] In addition, the incidence of lower urinary tract transitional cell carcinoma is increased in patients with a history of heavy phenacetin use.[137]

Analgesic nephropathy evolves insidiously over years, with clinical expression following a cumulative phenacetin ingestion of 3 kg or more.[138] Women are affected more frequently than men. Upper gastrointestinal irritation with anemia can result from analgesic ingestion. Early renal manifestations include inability to concentrate urine, sterile pyuria, microscopic hematuria, proteinuria, and hypertension. Creatinine clearance declines slowly. The diagnosis is confirmed by intravenous pyelography with the demonstration of papillary necrosis. Frequently, however, urography demonstrates only "chronic pyelonephritis": small kidneys with thin renal cortices and blunted calyces. Renal biopsy reveals nonspecific chronic interstitial inflammation and scarring.

The pathogenesis remains unclear, as evolving analgesic nephropathy is not usually recognized in humans because of the lack of diagnostic markers and as appropriate animal models have been difficult to establish.[139] A combination of analgesics, including phenacetin or acetaminophen and salicylates or nonsteroidal anti-inflammatory drugs, is considered necessary because these agents rarely cause papillary necrosis when used alone.[13] Certain elderly patients, however, may be susceptible to interstitial disease and papillary necrosis when nonsteroidal anti-inflammatory drugs are used alone.[140]

The lesion begins in the papillary tip as a result of accumulation of toxic metabolites, decreased blood flow, and impaired cellular energy production.[138,139] The biochemical mechanisms appear to involve metabolism of phenacetin to acetaminophen, which is then oxidized to toxic free radicals that are concentrated in the papilla during the process of renal water conservation.[138] The ability of the kidney to oxidize acetaminophen has been questioned because of an apparent lack of renal cytochrome $P_{450}$. It now appears that co-oxidation of acetaminophen occurs with renal prostaglandin synthesis.[22] Papillary ischemia results from the ability of both salicylate and acetaminophen to inhibit renal medullary synthesis of vasodilatory prostaglandins. Impaired cellular energy production results from the ability of salicylate to uncouple mitochondrial oxidative phosphorylation.[138]

Public health preventive measures have involved restricted sale of phenacetin and combination analgesics; however, over-the-counter combination analgesics containing aspirin, acetaminophen, and caffeine remain available in the United States.[141] In addition, the substitution of acetaminophen for phenacetin in combination analgesic compounds has not decreased the incidence of analgesic nephropathy.[13] Finally, the extensive use of acetaminophen, aspirin, and nonsteroidal anti-inflammatory drugs, frequently together, constitutes a potential public health problem.

Individuals requiring chronic analgesics may reduce their risk for nephropathy by avoiding combination analgesics and maintaining adequate hydration to prevent renal ischemia and decrease the papillary concentration of toxic substances.[13] Treatment of established nephrotoxicity requires cessation of analgesic consumption, which can prevent progression and may improve renal function.[13] Patients should also be evaluated carefully for associated transitional cell carcinoma of the renal pelvis, calyces, ureters, and bladder.[13] Carcinoma may present years after analgesic nephropathy is diagnosed.

## *Obstructive Nephropathy*

**Renal Tubular Obstruction**

Drug-induced acute renal failure resulting from renal tubular obstruction can be caused by intratubular precipitation of tissue degradation products as well as drugs or their metabolites. Acute uric acid nephropathy after chemotherapy for hematologic malignancies is the most common cause of renal failure resulting from obstruction by tissue degradation products.[142] Acute oliguric or anuric renal failure develops rapidly. The diagnosis is supported by a urine uric acid-to-creatinine ratio greater than 1.[142] Uric acid precipitation can be prevented by pretreatment hydration, urinary alkalinization to pH 7, and administration of allopurinol. Uric acid nephropathy has also been observed at the initiation of therapy with ticrynafen, a novel uricosuric diuretic no longer available in the United States.[61] Patients with hyperuricemia, frequently a result of previous diuretic therapy, were at most risk. Suprofen, a new nonsteroidal anti-inflammatory drug, has recently been associated with acute onset of flank pain and renal insufficiency after the initiation of therapy. Preliminary investigation indicates that this drug is also uricosuric.[143]

Drug-induced muscle necrosis and intratubular precipitation of myoglobin are also a common cause of acute renal failure mediated by tissue degradation products. The pathogenesis may be nontraumatic rhabdomyolysis caused by pressure necrosis in association with stupor and coma resulting from excessive alcohol or heroin.[144] Alternatively, myonecrosis could result from extreme neuromuscular stimulation with phencyclidine[145] or vasoconstriction and ischemia from therapeutic vasopressin infusion.[146]

Precipitation of drugs or their metabolites in a concentrated acid urine was an important cause of acute renal failure with previous generations of sulfonamides.[3] This problem is rare with the currently used more soluble sulfonamides. Methotrexate and a less soluble metabolite, 7-hydroxymethotrexate, have precipitated in acid urine and caused oliguric–anuric renal failure during high-dose chemotherapy.[108,142] Acyclovir therapy for acute herpes zoster has also caused renal insufficiency, possibly by intratubular precipitation of acyclovir in dehydrated oliguric patients.[147] Massive administration of ascorbic acid can result in obstruction of renal tubules with calcium oxalate crystals.[148] Oxalate, a poorly soluble metabolic product of ascorbic acid, can also precipitate and aggravate renal function when administered to patients with acute renal failure or the congenital nephrotic syndrome.[148] Oxalate precipitation may also contribute to methoxyflurane-induced renal failure, although proximal tubular necrosis resulting from fluoride toxicity is the predominant pathogenesis.[149] Low-molecular-weight dextran therapy for volume expansion and rheologic effects has also caused renal failure.[150] As dextran is filtered by the glomerulus, a possible mechanism is intratubular dextran precipitation with obstruction.[150] Renal failure resulting from intratubular precipitation of drugs or their metabolites can be largely prevented by assurance of an adequate urine volume and, in certain cases, urinary alkalinization.

In addition to these drug effects, therapeutic agents not intended for systemic administration can cause renal failure, apparently by tubular obstruction. Severe hyperphosphatemia after administration of a hypertonic phosphate enema has further reduced renal function in a renal insufficient patient, possibly by intratubular precipitation of calcium phosphate.[151] Hypermagnesemia resulting from renacidin irrigation of the renal collecting system has caused end-stage renal failure in a patient with preexistent renal insufficiency.[152] The pathogenesis may have involved renal precipitation of magnesium whitlockite.

**Extrarenal Urinary Tract Obstruction**

Drug therapy is also a cause of renal insufficiency resulting from obstruction of the lower urinary tract. Ureteral obstruction can be caused by renal calculi (see Nephrolithiasis) or retroperitoneal fibrosis resulting from analgesics, methysergide, or radiation therapy.[153] Bladder dysfunction with obstruction can result from anticholinergic therapy, particularly in males with preexisting prostatic hypertrophy. Disopyramide phosphate, an antiarrhythmic agent with anticholinergic effects, has been associated with reversible acute renal failure caused by urinary retention.[154]

### *Nephrolithiasis*

Renal calculus formation, distinct from intratubular precipitation of crystalline material, is presently a rare complication of drug therapy. Historically, calculus formation occurred in 6.1% of patients treated with the poorly soluble sulfonamide sulfadiazine for meningitis and endocarditis.[155] Currently, triamterene therapy appears to be the most frequent cause of calculus formation, with an incidence approximating 1 in 1,500 users of triamterene hydrochlorothiazide.[156] It is unclear, however, whether triamterene or its metabolites actually cause stone formation or are passively absorbed onto the organic matrix of calculi.[157] Other drug-induced calculi include xanthine, hypoxanthine, and oxypurinol stones, which form rarely during allopurinol therapy for conditions in which excess uric acid is produced: Lesch–Nyham syndrome and chemotherapy of lymphosarcoma.[158] Allopurinol inhibits xanthine oxidase and increases the urinary excretion of poorly soluble xanthine, hypoxanthine, and oxypurinol. Finally, massive ingestion of magnesium trisilicate–aluminum hydroxide for gastritis symptoms has been associated with magnesium ammonium phosphate (struvite) stone formation.[159] The pathogenesis could involve hypermagnesuria and increased urinary pH from antacid ingestion.

## Summary

Drug nephrotoxicity is common and includes an expanding spectrum of renal functional and structural alterations. Multiple mechanisms contribute to renal dysfunction and new drugs continue to demonstrate toxicity, frequently by new and unique mechanisms. It is hoped that with increased awareness and knowledge, we can reduce the incidence of this iatrogenic disorder and learn to apply the pathophysiologic principles to therapeutic advantage.

## References

1. Finn WF. Environmental toxins and renal disease. J Clin Pharmacol 1983;23:461–472.
2. Wedeen RP. Occupational renal disease. Am J Kidney Dis 1984;3:241–257.
3. Schreiner GE, Maher JF. Toxic nephropathy. Am J Med 1965;38:409–449.
4. Anderson S, Meyer TW, Rennke HG, et al. Control of glomerular hypertension limits glomerular injury in rats with reduced renal mass. J Clin Invest 1985;76:612–619.
5. Hou SH, Bushinsky DA, Wish JB, et al. Hospital-acquired renal insufficiency: A prospective study. Am J Med 1983;74: 243–248.
6. Werb R, Linton AL. Aetiology, diagnosis, treatment and prognosis of acute renal failure in an intensive care unit. Resuscitation 1979;7:95–100.
7. Kraman S, Khan F, Patel S, et al. Renal failure in the respiratory intensive care unit. Crit Care Med 1979;7:263–266.
8. Wilkins RG, Faragher EB. Acute renal failure in an intensive

care unit: Incidence, prediction and outcome. Anaesthesia 1983;38:628–634.

9. Kleinknecht D, Landais P, Goldfarb B. Analgesic and nonsteroidal anti-inflammatory drug-associated acute renal failure: A prospective collaborative study. Clin Nephrol 1986;25:275–281.
10. Justiniani FR. Over-the-counter ibuprofen and nephrotic syndrome. Ann Intern Med 1986; 105:303.
11. Moss AH, Riley R, Murgo A, et al. Over-the-counter ibuprofen and acute renal failure. Ann Intern Med 1986;105:303.
12. Schneider PD. Nonsteroidal anti-inflammatory drugs and acute cortical necrosis. Ann Intern Med 1986;105:303–304.
13. Consensus conference. Analgesic-associated kidney disease. JAMA 1984;251:3123–3125.
14. Maher JF. Renal failure in America is infrequently due to analgesic abuse. Am J Kidney Dis 1986;7:169–173.
15. Buckalew VM, Schey HM. Analgesic nephropathy: A significant cause of morbidity in the United States. Am J Kidney Dis 1986;7:164–168.
16. Epstein M, Oster JR. Beta blockers and renal functions: A reappraisal. J Clin Hypertens 1985;1:85–99.
17. Lund G, Einzig S, Rysavy J, et al. Role of ischemia in contrast-induced renal damage: An experimental study. Circulation 1984;69:783–789.
18. Hricik DE, Browning PJ, Kopelman R, et al. Captopril-induced functional renal insufficiency in patients with bilateral renal-artery stenoses or renal-artery stenosis in a solitary kidney. N Engl J Med 1983;308:373–376.
19. Diamond JR, Cheung JY, Fang LST. Nifedipine-induced renal dysfunction. Alterations in renal hemodynamics. Am J Med 1984;77:905–909.
20. Tune BM. Effect of organic acid transport inhibitors on renal cortical uptake and proximal tubular toxicity of cephaloridine. J Pharmacol Exp Ther 1972;181:250–256.
21. Hook JB, Smith JH. Biochemical mechanisms of nephrotoxicity. Transplant Proc 1985;17(suppl 1):41–50.
22. Zenser TV, Mattammal MB, Rapp NS, et al. Effect of aspirin on metabolism of acetaminophen and benzidine by renal inner medulla prostaglandin hydroperoxidase. J Lab Clin Med 1983;101:58–65.
23. Epstein FH. Hypoxia of the renal medulla. Q J Med 1985;57:807–810.
24. Whelton A, Solez K. Aminoglycoside nephrotoxicity—a tale of two transports. J Lab Clin Med 1982;99:148–155.
25. D'Elia JA, Gleason RE, Alday M, et al. Nephrotoxicity from angiographic contrast material. A prospective study. Am J Med 1952;72:719–725.
26. Muther RS. Drug interference with renal function tests. Am J Kidney Dis 1983;3:118–120.
27. Collen MJ, Howard JM, McArthur KE, et al. Comparison of ranitidine and cimetidine in the treatment of gastric hypersecretion. Ann Intern Med 1984;100:52–58.
28. Shemesh O, Golbetz H, Kriss JP, et al. Limitations of creatinine as a filtration marker in glomerulopathic patients. Kidney Int 1985;28:830–838.
29. Van der Woude FJ, van Son WJ, Tegzess AM, et al. Effect of captopril on blood pressure and renal function in patients with transplant renal artery stenosis. Nephron 1985;39:184–188.
30. Wenting GJ, Tan-tjiong HL, Derkx FHM, et al. Split renal function after captopril in unilateral renal artery stenosis. Br Med J 1984;288:886–890.
31. Blythe WB. Captopril and renal autoregulation. N Engl J Med 1983;308:390–391.
32. Nally Jr JV, Clarke Jr HS, Grecos GP, et al. Effect of captopril on $^{99}$Tc-diethylenetriaminepentaacetic acid renograms in two-kidney, one clip hypertension. Hypertension 1986;8:685–693.
33. ter Wee PM, Rosman JB, van der Geest S. Acute renal failure due to diltiazem. Lancet 1984;2:1337–1338.
34. Clive DM, Stoff JS. Renal syndromes associated with nonsteroidal antiinflammatory drugs. N Engl J Med 1984;310:563–572.
35. Blackshear JL, Davidman M, Stillman MT. Identification of risk for renal insufficiency from nonsteroidal anti-inflammatory drugs. Arch Intern Med 1983;143:1130–1134.
36. Dibona GF. Prostaglandins and nonsteroidal anti-inflammatory drugs. Effects on renal hemodynamics. Am J Med 1986;80 (suppl 1A:)12–21.
37. Ruilope LM, Robles RG, Paya C, et al. Effects of long-term treatment with indomethacin on renal function. Hypertension 1986;8:677–684.
38. Muther RS, Potter DM, Bennett WM. Aspirin-induced depression of glomerular filtration rate in normal humans: Role of sodium balance. Ann Intern Med 1981;94:317–321.
39. Vriesendorp R, deZeeuw D, deJong PE, et al. Reduction of urinary protein and prostaglandin $E_2$ excretion in the nephrotic syndrome by non-steroidal anti-inflammatory drugs. Clin Nephrol 1986;25:105–110.
40. Ciabattoni G, Cinotti GA, Pierucci A, et al. Effects of sulindac and ibuprofen in patients with chronic glomerular disease. Evidence for the dependence of renal function on prostacyclin. N Engl J Med 1984;310:279–283.
41. Fong HJ, Cohen AH. Ibuprofen-induced acute renal failure with acute tubular necrosis. Am J Nephrol 1982;2:28–31.
42. Abraham PA, Keane WF. Glomerular and interstitial disease induced by nonsteroidal anti-inflammatory drugs. Am J Nephrol 1984;4:1–6.
43. Lijnen P, Boelaert J, van Eeghem P, et al. Decrease in renal function due to sulphinpyrazone treatment early after myocardial infarction. Clin Nephrol 1983;19:143–146.
44. Boelaert J, Lijnen P, Robbens E, et al. Impairment of renal function due to sulphinpyrazone after coronary artery bypass surgery: A prospective double-blind study. J Cardiovasc Pharmacol 1986;8:386–391.
45. Rosenkranz B, Fejes-Toth G, Diener U, et al. Effects of sulfinpyrazone on renal function and prostaglandin formation in man. Nephron 1985;39:237–243.
46. Walker BR, Hoppe RC, Alexander F. Effect of triamterene on the renal clearance of calcium, magnesium, phosphate, and uric acid in man. Clin Pharmacol Ther 1972;13:245–250.
47. Triamterene and the kidney, editorial. Lancet 1986;1:424.
48. Lynn KL, Bailey RR, Swainson CP, et al. Renal failure with potassium-sparing diuretics. NZ Med J 1985;98:629–633.
49. Favre L, Glasson P, Vallotton MB. Reversible acute renal failure from combined triamterene and indomethacin. A study in healthy subjects. Ann Intern Med 1982;96:317–320.
50. Weinberg MS, Quigg RJ, Salant DJ, et al. Anuric renal failure precipitated by indomethacin and triamterene. Nephron 1985;40:216–218.
51. Favre L, Vallotton MB. Relationship of renal prostaglandins to three diuretics. Prostaglandins Leukotrienes Med 1984;14:313–319.
52. Danesh BJZ, Brunton J, Sumner DJ. Comparison between short-term renal haemodynamic effects of propranolol and nadolol in essential hypertension: a cross-over study. Clin Sci 1984;67:243–248.
53. Bennett WM, Pulliam JP. Cyclosporine nephrotoxicity. Ann Intern Med 1983;99:851–854.
54. Curtis JJ, Luke RG, Dubovsky E, et al. Cyclosporine in therapeutic doses increases renal allograft vascular resistance. Lancet 1986;2:477–479.
55. Thiel G. Experimental cyclosporine A nephrotoxicity: A sum-

mary of the International Workshop (Basel, April 24–26, 1985). Clin Nephrol 1986;25(suppl 1):S205–S210.
56. Myers BD, Ross J, Newton L, et al. Cyclosporine-associated chronic nephropathy. N Engl J Med 1984;311:699–705.
57. Palestine AG, Austin III HA, Balow JE, et al. Renal histopathologic alterations in patients treated with cyclosporine for uveitis. N Engl J Med 1986;314:1293–1298.
58. Berg KJ, Forre O, Bjerkhoel F, et al. Side effects of cyclosporine A treatment in patients with rheumatoid arthritis. Kidney Int 1986;29:1180–1187.
59. Bennett WM, Norman DJ. Action and toxicity of cyclosporine. Ann Rev Med 1986;37:215–224.
60. Kahan BD. Individualization of cyclosporine therapy using pharmacokinetic and pharmacodynamic parameters. Transplantation 1985;40:457–476.
61. Porter GA, Bennett WM. Nephrotoxin-induced acute renal failure, in Brenner BM, Stein JH (eds): Contemporary Issues in Nephrology. New York, Churchill Livingstone. 1980, vol 6, pp 123–162.
62. Ridolfi RL, Bell WF. Thrombotic thrombocytopenic purpura. Report of 25 cases and review of the literature. Medicine 1981;60:413–427.
63. Van Buren D, Van Buren CT, Flechner SM, et al. De novo hemolytic uremic syndrome in renal transplant recipients immunosuppressed with cyclosporine. Surgery 1985;98:54–62.
64. Cantrell Jr JE, Phillips TM, Schein PS. Carcinoma-associated hemolytic–uremic syndrome: A complication of mitomycin C chemotherapy. J Clin Oncol 1985;3:723–734.
65. Valavaara R, Nordman E. Renal complications of mitomycin C therapy with special reference to the total dose. Cancer 1985;55:47–50.
66. Jackson AM, Rose BD, Graff LG, et al. Thrombotic microangiography and renal failure associated with antineoplastic chemotherapy. Ann Intern Med 1984;101:41–44.
67. Lyman NW, Michaelson R, Viscuso RL, et al. Mitomycin-induced hemolytic-uremic syndrome. Successful treatment with corticosteroids and intense plasma exchange. Arch Intern Med 1983;143:1617–1618.
68. Grem JL, Merritt JA, Carbone PP. Treatment of mitomycin-associated microangiopathic hemolytic anemia with vincristine. Arch Intern Med 1986;146:566–568.
69. Fillastre J-P, Mery J-P, Druet P. Drug-induced glomerulonephritis, in Solez K, Whelton A (eds): Acute Renal Failure. Correlations Between Morphology and Function. New York, Marcel Dekker, 1984, pp 389–407.
70. Baum M, Piel CF, Goodman JR. Antibiotic-associated interstitial nephritis and nephrotic syndrome. Am J Nephrol 1986;6:149–151.
71. Finkelstein A, Fraley DS, Stachura I, et al. Fenoprofen nephropathy: Lipoid nephrosis and interstitial nephritis. A possible T-lymphocyte disorder. Am J Med 1982;72:81–87.
72. Cunningham EE, Brentjens JR, Zielezny MA, et al. Heroin nephropathy. A clinicopathologic and epidemiologic study. Am J Med 1980;68:47–53.
73. Silverberg DS, Kidd EG, Shnitka TK, et al. Gold nephropathy: A clinical and pathologic study. Arthritis Rheum 1970;13: 812–825.
74. Katz WA, Blodgett Jr RC, Pietrusko RG. Proteinuria in gold-treated rheumatoid arthritis. Ann Intern Med 1984;101: 176–179.
75. Viol GW, Minielly JA, Bistricki T. Gold nephropathy: Tissue analysis by x-ray fluorescent spectroscopy. Arch Pathol Lab Med 1977;101:635–640.
76. Gran JT, Husby G, Thorsby E. HLA DR antigens and gold toxicity. Ann Rheum Dis 1983;42:63–66.
77. Kibukamusoke JW, Davies DR, Hutt MSR. Membranous nephropathy due to skin-lightening cream. Br Med J 1974;2: 646–647.
78. Tubbs RO, Gephardt GN, McMahon JT, et al. Membranous glomerulonephritis associated with industrial mercury exposure. Study of pathogenetic mechanisms. Am J Clin Pathol 1982;77:409–413.
79. Bacon PA, Tribe CR, Mackenzie JC, et al. Penicillamine nephropathy in rheumatoid arthritis: A clinical, pathological and immunological study. Q J Med 1976;45:661–684.
80. Report from the Captopril Collaborative Study Group. Does captopril cause renal damage in hypertensive patients? Lancet 1982;1:988–990.
81. Cush JJ, Goldings EA. Southwestern internal medicine conference: Drug-induced lupus: clinical spectrum and pathogenesis. Am J Med Sci 1985;290:36–44, C3.
82. Hall-Craggs M, Light PD, Peters RW. Development of immune complex nephritis during treatment with the calcium channel-blocking agent nifedipine. Hum Pathol 1984;15:691–694.
83. Appel GB, D'Agati V, Bergman M, et al. Nephrotic syndrome and immune complex glomerulonephritis associated with chlorpropamide therapy. Am J Med 1983;74:337–342.
84. Guarnieri GF, Galli G, Faccini L, et al. Enzymuria ($\alpha$-glucosidase, muramidase, ribonuclease) and proteinuria (total proteins, $\beta_2$-microglobulin, electrophoretic pattern) after cephalosporin and aminoglycoside administration. Contrib Nephrol 1984;42:210–219.
85. Abramowsky CR, Swinehart GL. The nephropathy of cystic fibrosis: A human model of chronic nephrotoxicity. Hum Pathol 1982;13:934–939.
86. Oken DE. Hemodynamic basis for human acute renal failure (vasomotor nephropathy). Am J Med 1984;76:702–710.
87. Myers BD, Moran SM. Hemodynamically mediated acute renal failure. N Engl J Med 1986;314:97–105.
88. Smith CR, Lipsky JJ, Laskin OL, et al. Double-blind comparison of the nephrotoxicity and auditory toxicity of gentamicin and tobramycin. N Engl J Med 1980;302:1106–1109.
89. Holloway JJ, Smith CR, Moore RD, et al. Comparative cost effectiveness of gentamicin and tobramycin. Ann Intern Med 1984;101:764–769.
90. Schentag JJ, Plant ME. Patterns of urinary $\beta_2$-microglobulin excretion by patients treated with aminoglycosides. Kidney Int 1980;17:654–661.
91. Humes HD, Weinberg JM, Krauss TC. Clinical and pathophysiologic aspects of aminoglycoside nephrotoxicity. Am J Kidney Dis 1982;2:5–29.
92. Neugarten J, Aynedjian HS, Bank N. Role of tubular obstruction in acute renal failure due to gentamicin. Kidney Int 1983;24:330–335.
93. Luft FC, Evans PA. Comparative effects of tobramycin and gentamicin on glomerular ultrastructure. J Infect Dis 1980;142: 910–914.
94. Schor N, Ichikawa I, Rennke HG, et al. Pathophysiology of altered glomerular function in aminoglycoside-treated rats. Kidney Int 1981;19:288–296.
95. Luft FC, Aronoff GR, Evans AP, et al. The renin–angiotensin system in aminoglycoside-induced acute renal failure. J Pharmacol Exp Ther 1982;220:433–439.
96. Moore RD, Smith CR, Lipsky JJ, et al. Risk factors for nephrotoxicity in patients treated with aminoglycosides. Ann Intern Med 1984;100:352–357.
97. Zager RA, Prior RB. Gentamicin and gram-negative bacteremia. A synergism for the development of experimental nephrotoxic acute renal failure. J Clin Invest 1986;78:196–204.
98. Meyer RD. Risk factors and comparisons of clinical nephro-

toxicity of aminoglycosides. Am J Med 1986;80(suppl 6B): 119–125.

99. Sawyers CL, Moore RD, Lerner SA, et al. A model for predicting nephrotoxicity in patients treated with aminoglycosides. J Infect Dis 1986;153:1062–1068.

100. Humes HD, Sastrasinh M, Weinberg JM. Calcium is a competitive inhibitor of gentamicin–renal membrane binding interactions and dietary calcium supplementation protects against gentamicin nephrotoxicity. J Clin Invest 1984;73:134–147.

101. Berkseth RO, Kjellstrand CM. Radiologic contrast–induced nephropathy. Med Clin North Am 1984;68:351–370.

102. Fang LST, Sirota RA, Ebert TH, et al. Low fractional excretion of sodium with contrast medium–induced acute renal failure. Arch Intern Med 1980;140:531–533.

103. Teruel JL, Marcen R, Onaindia JM, et al. Renal function impairment caused by intravenous urography. A prospective study. Arch Intern Med 1981;141:1271–1274.

104. Nicot GS, Merk LJ, Charmes JP, et al. Transient glomerular proteinuria, enzymuria, and nephrotoxic reaction induced by radiocontrast media. JAMA 1984;252:2432–2434.

105. Vosnides G, Kalogeropoulos V, Spanos H, et al. Radiocontrast-induced deterioration of renal function in patients with chronic renal failure, in Abstracts of the Eighth International Congress of Nephrology. Athens, University Studio Publishing, 1981, p 306.

106. Albrechtsson U, Hultberg B, Larusdottir H, et al. Nephrotoxicity of ionic and non-ionic contrast media in aorto-femoral angiography. Acta Radiol Diagn 1985;26:615–618.

107. Blachley JD, Hill JB. Renal and electrolyte disturbances associated with cisplatin. Ann Intern Med 1981;95:628–632.

108. Goldberg ID, Garnick MB, Bloomer WD. Urinary tract toxic effects of cancer therapy. J Urol 1984;132:1–6.

109. Coratelli P, Antonelli M, Giangrande MS, et al. *cis*-Platinum nephrotoxicity: Changes in urinary enzyme pattern in patients submitted to two different dosages. Contrib Nephrol 1984;42: 242–247.

110. Weiner MW, Jacobs C. Mechanisms of cisplatin nephrotoxicity. Fed Proc 1983;42:2974–2978.

111. Ozols RF, Corden BJ, Jacob J, et al. High-dose cisplatin in hypertonic saline. Ann Intern Med 1984;100:19–24.

112. Shea M, Koziol JA, Howell SB. Kinetics of sodium thiosulfate, a cisplatin neutralizer. Clin Pharmacol Ther 1984;35: 419–425.

113. Offerman JJG, Mulder NH, Sleijfer DT, et al. Influence of captopril on *cis*-diaminedichloroplatinum–induced renal toxicity. Am J Nephrol 1985;5:433–436.

114. Offerman JJG, Meijer S, Sleijfer DT, et al. The influence of verapamil on renal function in patients treated with cisplatin. Clin Nephrol 1985;5:249–255.

115. Buckley JE, Clarke VL, Meyer TJ, et al. Hypomagnesemia after cisplatin combination chemotherapy. Arch Intern Med 1984;144:2347–2348.

116. Butler WT, Bennett JE, Alling DW, et al. Nephrotoxicity of amphotericin B: Early and late effects in 81 patients. Ann Intern Med 1964;61:175–187.

117. Burgess JL, Birchall R. Nephrotoxicity of amphotericin B, with emphasis on changes in tubular function. Am J Med 1972;53:77–84.

118. Bhathena DB, Bullock WE, Nuttall CE, et al. The effects of amphotericin B therapy on the intrarenal vasculature and renal tubules in man. A study of renal biopsies by light, electron, and immunofluorescence microscopy. Clin Nephrol 1978;9:103–110.

119. Heidemann HTH, Gerkens JF, Spickard WA, et al. Amphotericin B nephrotoxicity in humans decreased by salt repletion. Am J Med 1983;75:476–481.

120. Bullock WE, Luke RG, Nuttall CE, et al. Can mannitol reduce amphotericin B nephrotoxicity? Double-blind study and description of a new vascular lesion in kidneys. Antimicrob Agents Chemother 1976;10:555–563.

121. Linton AL, Clark WF, Driedger AA. et al. Acute interstitial nephritis due to drugs. Review of the literature with a report of nine cases. Ann Intern Med 1980;93:735–741.

122. Ditlove J, Weidmann P, Bernstein M, et al. Methicillin nephritis. Medicine 1977;56:483–491.

123. Kleinknecht D, Vanhille P, Morel-Maroger L, et al. Acute interstitial nephritis due to drug hypersensitivity. An up-to-date review with a report of 19 cases. Adv Nephrol 1983;12: 277–308.

124. Nolan CR, Anger MS, Kelleher SP. Eosinophiluria—a new method of detection and definition of the clinical spectrum. N Engl J Med 1986;315:1516–1519.

125. Cushner HM, Copley JB, Bauman J, et al. Acute interstitial nephritis associated with mezlocillin, nafcillin, and gentamicin treatment for *Pseudomonas* infection. Arch Intern Med 1985;145:1204–1207.

126. Linton AL, Richmond JM, Clark WF, et al. Gallium$^{67}$ scintigraphy in the diagnosis of acute renal disease. Clin Nephrol 1985;24:84–87.

127. Pusey CD, Saltissi D, Bloodworth L, et al. Drug associated acute interstitial nephritis. Clinical and pathological features and the response to high dose steroid therapy. Q J Med 1983;206:194–211.

128. Murray TG. Drug-induced chronic tubulo-interstitial renal disease, in Cotran RS, Brenner BM, Stein JH (eds): Contemporary Issues in Nephrology. New York, Churchill Livingstone, 1983, vol 10, pp 187–209.

129. Baylis PH, Heath DA. Water disturbances in patients treated with lithium carbonate. Ann Intern Med 1978;88:607–609.

130. Batlle DC, von Riotte AB, Gaviria M, et al. Amelioration of polyuria by amiloride in patients receiving long-term lithium therapy. N Engl J Med 1985;312:408–414.

131. Christensen S, Kusano E, Yusufi ANK, et al. Pathogenesis of nephrogenic diabetes insipidus due to chronic administration of lithium in rats. J Clin Invest 1985;75:1869–1879.

132. Fenves AZ, Emmett M, White MG. Lithium intoxication associated with acute renal failure. South Med J 1984;77: 1472–1474.

133. Bendz H. Kidney function in lithium-treated patients. A literature survey. Acta Psychiatr Scand 1983;68:303–324.

134. Hestbech J, Hansen HE, Amdisen A, et al. Chronic renal lesions following long-term treatment with lithium. Kidney Int 1977;12:205–213.

135. Kincaid-Smith P, Burrows GD, Davies BM, et al. Renal-biopsy findings in lithium and prelithium patients. Lancet 1979;2:700–701.

136. Lokkegaard H, Andersen NF, Henriksen E, et al. Renal function in 153 manic–depressive patients treated with lithium for more than five years. Acta Psychiatr Scand 1985;71: 347–355.

137. Piper JM, Tonascia J, Matanoski GM. Heavy phenacetin use and bladder cancer in women aged 20 to 49 years. N Engl J Med 1985;313:292–295.

138. Eknoyan G. Analgesic nephrotoxicity and renal papillary necrosis. Semin Nephrol 1984;4:65–76

139. Bach PH, Hardy TL. Relevance of animal models to analgesic-associated renal papillary necrosis in humans. Kidney Int 1985;28:605–613.

140. Adams DH, Howie AJ, Michael J, et al. Non-steroidal anti-inflammatory drugs and renal failure. Lancet 1986;1:57–60.

141. Physicians Desk Reference for Nonprescription Drugs, 6th ed. Oradell, NJ, Medical Economics Company, 1985.
142. Fer MF, McKinney TD, Richardson RL, et al. Cancer and the kidney: Renal complications of neoplasms. Am J Med 1981;71: 704–718.
143. Abreo K, LaBarre J. Suprofen, acute renal failure, and hematuria. Ann Intern Med 1986;105:799.
144. Cadnapaphornchai P, Taher S, McDonald FD. Acute drug-associated rhabdomyolysis: An examination of its diverse renal manifestations and complications. Am J Med Sci 1980;280:66–72.
145. Patel R, Connor G. A review of thirty cases of rhabdomyolysis-associated acute renal failure among phencyclidine users. Clin Toxicol 1985–86;23:547–556.
146. Affarah HB, Mars RL, Someren A, et al. Myoglobinuria and acute renal failure associated with intravenous vasopressin infusion. South Med J 1984;77:918–921.
147. Bean B, Braun C, Balfour Jr HH. Acyclovir therapy for acute herpes zoster. Lancet 1982;2:118–121.
148. Lawton JM, Conway LT, Crosson JT, et al. Acute oxalate nephropathy after massive ascorbic acid administration. Arch Intern Med 1985;145:950–951.
149. Coggins CH, Fang LS-T. Acute renal failure associated with antibiotics, anesthetic agents, and radiographic contrast agents, in Brenner BM, Lazarus JM (eds): Acute Renal Failure. Philadelphia, W.B. Saunders, 1983, pp 283–320.
150. Feest TG. Low molecular weight dextran: A continuing cause of acute renal failure. Br Med J 1976;2:1300.
151. Biberstein M, Parker BA. Enema-induced hyperphosphatemia. Am J Med 1985;79:645–646.
152. Wilson C, Azmy AF, Beattie TJ, et al. Hypermagnesemia and progression of renal failure associated with renacidin therapy. Clin Nephrol 1986;25:266–267.
153. Critchley JAJH, Smith MF, Prescott LF. Distalgesic abuse and retroperitoneal fibrosis. Br J Urol 1985;57:486–487.
154. Danziger LH, Horn JR. Disopyramide-induced urinary retention: Report of nine cases and review of the literature. Arch Intern Med 1983;143:1683–1686.
155. Dowling HF, Lepper MH. Toxic reactions following therapy with sulfapyridine, sulfathiazole, and sulfadiazine. JAMA 1943;121:1190–1194.
156. Ettinger B, Oldroyd NO, Sorgel F. Triamterene nephrolithiasis. JAMA 1980;244:2443–2445.
157. Werness PG, Bergert JH, Smith LH. Triamterene urolithiasis: Solubility, pK, effect on crystal formation, and matrix binding of triamterene and its metabolites. J Lab Clin Med 1982;99: 254–262.
158. Kranen S, Keough D, Gordon RB, et al. Xanthine-containing calculi during allopurinol therapy. J Urol 1985;133:658–659.
159. Millette CH, Snodgrass GL. Acute renal failure associated with chronic antacid ingestion. Am J Hosp Pharm 1981;38: 1352–1355.
160. Howell SB, Pfeifle CE, Wung WE, et al. Intraperitoneal cisplatin with systemic thiosulfate protection. Ann Intern Med 1982;97:845–851.
161. Birnbaum J, Kahan FM, Kropp H, et al. Carbapenems, a new class of beta-lactam antibiotics. Discovery and development of imipenem/cilastatin. Am J Med 1985;78(suppl 6A):3–21.

# Chapter 37 / Nephrolithiasis

Charles Lee Smith, MD, and David R.P. Guay, PharmD, FCP

Renal stone disease is a common disorder estimated to occur in approximately 12% of the population, with an annual incidence in the United States of 1.6 in 1,000.[1] The recurrence rate is 70% to 81% in males and 47% to 60% in females.[2] For these reasons, an understanding of the pathophysiology and treatment of stone disease is warranted.

## Stone Formation

For clinical stone disease to occur, three conditions must be met. First, a nidus must form. Second, this nidus must be retained within the urinary tract. Third, the nidus must grow to sufficient size to become radiologically apparent or to obstruct the ureter.

### *Nidus Formation*

Three theories have been proposed to explain nidus formation. The first is the matrix theory.[3] All stones, regardless of their crystalline composition, consist of 2% to 3% organic material. The matrix theory proposes that this organic material is the initiating mechanism of calculus formation. A mucoprotein considered unique to stone formers condenses in the urine to serve as a ground substance for mineral precipitation. Studies have conflicted with respect to the uniqueness of this protein to stone formers. Further work has suggested that the mucoprotein found in stones is not essential to the initiation of stone formation but is simply adsorbed to the surface of crystals.[4] Currently most people working in this area do not accept a role for matrix as an initiating event. It may, however, play a role in protecting crystals from dissolution.

The second theory is the inhibitor deficiency theory.[5] The urine is a complex fluid that contains a number of inhibitors of crystallization.[6] Some of these are citrate, sulfate, pyrophosphate, magnesium, glycoaminoglycans, and ribonucleotides. Inhibitors have been shown to inhibit nucleation, crystal growth, and crystal aggregation, all processes considered important to stone formation. The inhibitor deficiency theory proposes a decrease in inhibitor activity in the urine of stone formers that allows precipitation to occur. For the vast majority of stone formers, however, a deficiency of at least recognized inhibitors cannot be demonstrated.

The third theory is the precipitation–crystallization theory. This theory relies on the recognized regions of saturation that exist in an aqueous solution containing minerals.[7] These regions are defined by the solubility product and the formation product. The solubility product is that level of saturation at which the liquid phase is in equilibrium with the solid phase. The formation product is the level of saturation at which spontaneous nucleation occurs. Below the solubility product, the solution is undersaturated. Between the solubility product and the formation product, the solution is supersaturated—a region called metastable. Above the formation product, the solution is oversaturated and spontaneous nucleation occurs. The precipitation–crystallization theory proposes that periods of oversaturation occur that result in precipitation of a crystalline nidus that initiates stone disease. Comparison of levels of saturation between stone formers and non–stone formers has shown the levels in stone formers to be higher; however, extensive overlap between the two groups is present, suggesting that the level of saturation is not a sufficient explanation for stone formation. Nevertheless, the level of saturation is important. Crystallization cannot occur, whether matrix is present or absent and whether inhibitors are present or absent, if a state of supersaturation does not exist.

### *Nidus Retention*

The renal papilla is considered to be the site where actual stone formation occurs. The free particle concept states that crystallization occurs within the nephron and that crystalline mass then attains sufficient size to obstruct the collecting duct.[8] The particle becomes fixed and grows by continuous exposure to a supersaturated urine. Mathematical analysis does not support this free particle concept, as crystalline mass would not be sufficient to obstruct when it reached the tip of the collecting duct.[9]

The fixed particle concept proposes that a site is present within the urinary tract that can serve as a focus for stone formation. Randall plaques are areas of papillary subepithelial calcification and have been proposed as one of these potential sites.[10] Crystals formed within the nephron can adhere to the epithelial lining[11] and studies have suggested a role for the mucin layer of the urinary tract in preventing adherence.[12] Abnormalities in the mucin could result in increased adherence of crystals, thus providing fixed foci for stone formation.

### *Growth of Nidus*

Crystal growth, crystal aggregation, and epitaxy are processes that can increase the crystalline mass. Simple crystal growth can occur. As crystal growth rate is related to the degree of supersaturation of the urine, the higher the level of supersaturation the more rapidly the crystals grow. This is another example of the importance of supersaturation to stone formation. Inhibitors have also been described that prevent or retard crystal growth and could play a role in stone formation by altering the rate of crystal growth. When the formation product is exceeded, many nuclei are formed and these can aggregate to increase the crystalline mass. Inhibitors of crystal aggregation have been described, but their role, if any, in stone formation is not known. Aggregates of crystals tend to be found more in stone formers than in non–stone formers and this has been interpreted as evidence for an abnormality in crystal aggregation.[13] Epitaxy is a process that involves the growth of crystals of one material on the surface of a different material. This process is also poorly understood, although many possible combinations based on the fit of crystal surfaces are possible.[14] Most kidney stones are formed by a combination of all three of these processes.

## Calcium-Containing Stones

Stones that contain calcium are by far the most common type of stone seen. Approximately 90% of all stones analyzed contain calcium.[15] Nine percent of analyzed stones are related to infection, while 81% are composed of predominantly calcium oxalate (73%) and calcium phosphate (8%). Although pure stones of calcium oxalate or calcium phosphate occur, most calcium stones (50%–65%) are a mixture of both types of stone material.[15,16] This section deals with the risk factors for and management of calcium oxalate/calcium phosphate stone disease.

### *Pathogenesis*

The precipitation of calcium oxalate is dependent on the concentrations of calcium and oxalate in the urine and the presence or absence of inhibitors of precipitation. Similarly, the precipitation of calcium phosphate is dependent on the concentrations of calcium and phosphorus in the urine and the presence or absence of inhibitors. In addition, however, calcium phosphate precipitation is pH sensitive; solubility decreases as urine pH increases. Hypercalciuria would predispose to both calcium oxalate and calcium phosphate precipitation, hyperoxaluria would predispose to calcium oxalate precipitation, and increased urine pH would predispose to calcium phosphate precipitation. The main risk factors for calcium stone disease include hypercalciuria, hyperoxaluria, hyperuricosuria, increased urine pH, decreased inhibitors, and low urine volume.[17] Hypercalciuria is the most common risk factor identified in calcium stone formers, being present in 40% to 75% of patients.[18,19] Table 37.1 lists disorders associated with hypercalciuria.

**Table 37.1** Disorders Associated With Hypercalciuria

| | |
|---|---|
| Idiopathic hypercalciuria | Sarcoidosis |
| Dietary calcium excess | Thyrotoxicosis |
| Dietary sodium excess | Hypervitaminosis D |
| Immobilization | Glucocorticoid excess |
| Primary hyperparathyroidism | Paget's disease of bone |
| Renal tubular acidosis | |

### *Idiopathic Hypercalciuria*

Idiopathic hypercalciuria occurs in 40% to 60% of all stone formers.[20,21] This disorder is characterized by urinary calcium excretion in excess of that expected for the level of calcium intake, a normal level of total serum calcium, and the absence of systemic disorders that could lead to excessive calcium excretion.[22] There is controversy surrounding the pathophysiology of this condition. Most agree that there is increased intestinal absorption of calcium.[23,24] The controversy is over whether this is a primary abnormality of intestinal transport or secondary to abnormal vitamin D metabolism or renal handling of calcium or phosphorus.

Intestinal transport of calcium occurs by both active and passive processes. The active transport system is stimulated by vitamin D and occurs primarily in the duodenum whereas passive transport occurs in the jejunum and ileum. The role of vitamin D in these more distal segments is unclear,[25] but studies in humans suggest that this transport system can be stimulated by 1,25-dihydroxyvitamin $D_3$.[26] Increased intestinal transport of calcium in idiopathic hypercalciuria could be achieved through an increase in active transport or the passive process. An increase in jejunal brush border membrane permeability for calcium has been found.[27] Although calcium movement across the brush border membrane is passive, an increase in permeability resulting in increased calcium movement is under the influence of vitamin D,[28] possibly through changes in membrane lipid structure.[29] Thus, abnormal intestinal calcium transport could result from a primary defect in brush border membrane permeability or a change in permeability secondary to an abnormality in vitamin D metabolism.

Balance studies from a number of laboratories have demonstrated that for the same net intestinal absorption of calcium, the calcium excretion is higher in patients with idiopathic hypercalciuria than in normal individuals.[30] This finding is not compatible with a primary abnormality in brush border membrane permeability. To account for the balance data a more widespread abnormality in calcium metabolism would have to exist than simple hyperabsorption of dietary calcium. An abnormality in vitamin D metabolism would be compatible with such a systemic abnormality; however, data are available to suggest that the intestinal hyperabsorption of calcium is not dependent on vitamin D. In normal subjects, vitamin D stimulates calcium absorption in the jejunum and ileum. Magnesium absorption is stimulated in the jejunum but not the ileum.[26] Intestinal perfusion studies in patients with idiopathic hypercalciuria have shown increased jejunal calcium absorption but normal ileal calcium absorption and normal magnesium absorption in both sites.[31] Furthermore, steroids antagonize the action of vitamin D on intestinal absorption of calcium. When administered to patients with idiopathic hypercalciuria, prednisolone led to no change in intestinal calcium absorption.[32] These data suggest that the intestinal hyperabsorption of calcium seen in idiopathic hypercalciuria is independent of vitamin D.

A more direct approach to assessing possible abnormalities in vitamin D metabolism would be to measure circulating levels of the various metabolites. The three major circulating metabolites of vitamin D are 25-hydroxyvitamin D, 1,25-dihydroxyvitamin D, and 24,25-dihydroxyvitamin D.[33] The best measurement of nutritional vitamin D status is assessment of the serum level of 25-hydroxyvitamin D, whereas 1,25-dihydroxyvitamin D is considered the most active metabolite in stimulating intestinal calcium absorption.[33] The last metabolite, 24,25-dihydroxyvitamin D, is probably biologically inactive.[33] Most investigators have found the level of 25-hydroxyvitamin D to be normal in idiopathic hypercalciuria,[34–36] but a few studies have shown elevated levels.[37,38] The mild elevations found in these latter studies would not be expected to stimulate intestinal calcium transport directly, and, in this range, there appears to be no relation between serum concentrations of 25-hydroxyvitamin D and 1,25-dihydroxyvitamin D.[36] A lack of correlation between the serum concentration of 25-hydroxyvitamin D and urinary calcium excretion[37] would further suggest that these mild elevations, if they exist, are not of pathogenetic significance.

The most active metabolite of vitamin D in intestinal calcium absorption is 1,25-dihydroxyvitamin D. Most studies have revealed elevated mean levels of this metabolite in populations of calcium stone formers.[34–36,39,40] There is disagreement as to the cause of the elevated levels of 1,25-dihydroxyvitamin D. The production of 1,25-dihydroxyvitamin D is controlled by parathyroid hormone and phosphorus,[33] and both have been implicated in the pathogenesis of idiopathic hypercalciuria.

Early in the description of idiopathic hypercalciuria, it was proposed that the cause was abnormal calcium handling by the kidney.[23] A fraction of the total serum calcium called ultrafiltrable calcium is filtered at the glomerulus, and approximately 99% of this filtered calcium is reabsorbed by the renal tubule. A primary defect in this tubular reabsorption of calcium could result in an increased excretion of calcium. This defect would lower the serum ionized calcium and stimulate parathyroid hormone secretion, which in turn would increase the production of 1,25-dihydroxyvitamin D; the net result would be an increase in intestinal calcium absorption. This is the mechanism proposed for the renal leak form of idiopathic hypercalciuria.[41] The data in support of this mechanism have been summarized,[42] and a decrease in tubular reabsorption of calcium has been demonstrated.[39,43] Elevated levels of parathyroid hormone have been found by some investigators,[41,44] but others have questioned the existence of the renal leak form of idiopathic hypercalciuria primarily because of an inability to demonstrate elevated levels of parathyroid hormone.[45,46]

Hypophosphatemia results in increased 1,25-dihydroxyvitamin D levels, increased intestinal calcium absorption, and hypercalciuria.[33] Renal tubular phosphate wasting resulting in hypophosphatemia has been proposed as the mechanism for hyperabsorption of dietary calcium.[40] Others have not been able to demonstrate abnormalities in renal phosphorus handling.[39,47,48]

A primary abnormality in vitamin D metabolism with increased production of 1,25-dihydroxyvitamin D has been considered.[31,39] When 1,25-dihydroxyvitamin D is administered to healthy non–stone formers, there is an increase in intestinal calcium absorption, a suppression of parathyroid hormone secretion, a decrease in renal tubular reabsorption of calcium, an increase in the fasting calcium excretion, and hypercalciuria.[49–51] When combined with a low-calcium diet, large doses of 1,25-dihydroxyvitamin D have resulted in a negative calcium balance and evidence of bone resorption.[51] This evidence of bone resorption has not been confirmed by others.[49,50] Although this model in many aspects resembles idiopathic hypercalciuria, the serum phosphorus tends to be higher instead of reduced as is frequently seen in idiopathic hypercalciuria.[51] It may be that an abnormality exists in the proximal tubule that results in both the decrease in serum phosphorus and the increase in 1,25-dihydroxyvitamin D production.

**Table 37.2** Subclassification of Idiopathic Hypercalciuria[a]

| |
|---|
| Absorptive |
| Type I |
| Type II |
| Type III |
| Renal leak |
| Resorptive |

[a] This subclassification is that proposed by Pak.[52]

Currently, we use the subclassification of idiopathic hypercalciuria proposed by Pak[52] and outlined in Table 37.2. Absorptive hypercalciuria is divided into three types. Type I absorptive hypercalciuria is due to intestinal hyperabsorption, but these individuals remain hypercalciuric on a low-calcium diet. Type II absorptive hypercalciuric individuals have normal calcium excretion on a calcium-restricted diet. Type III absorptive hypercalciuria is intestinal hyperabsorption associated with hypophosphatemia. Renal leak hypercalciuria has an elevated fasting calcium:creatinine ratio with evidence of increased parathyroid hormone activity, while resorptive hypercalciuria is due to primary hyperparathyroidism.

The pathogenesis of idiopathic hypercalciuria thus remains unclear. It is very probable that idiopathic hypercalciuria is a heterogeneous disorder and includes some patients with each of the proposed disorders as well as other problems listed in Table 37.1. This then confuses attempts to make them all fit into one pathogenetic pattern. Attempts to study carefully defined populations have just begun[39] but will probably reveal several disorders with different mechanisms.

### *Dietary Causes of Hypercalciuria*

Other etiologies of hypercalciuria are listed in Table 37.1. Excessive dietary calcium is seldom a cause of hypercalciuria. As dietary calcium increases there is a decrease in the fraction absorbed by the intestine.[53] Although net absorption increases as dietary calcium increases, this is moderated by a decrease in fractional absorption and intakes must be in excess of 2,000 mg per day to result in hypercalciuria.[54] Dietary sodium influences urinary calcium excretion. In normal individuals, for each 100 mg/d increase in urinary sodium, there is an approximately 25 mg/d increase in urinary calcium[22]; however, some patients show a remarkable sensitivity to sodium with a hypercalciuria that is virtually unrelated to calcium intake but dependent on a high sodium intake.[55]

### *Immobilization Hypercalciuria*

Immobilization results in an increase in urinary calcium excretion.[56] Bone resorption occurs because of a lack of mechanical stress on bone. This results in a suppression of parathyroid hormone and a fall in the circulating levels of 1,25-dihydroxyvitamin D.[57] The suppression of parathyroid hormone results in a fall in renal tubular calcium reabsorption and a rise in the fasting calcium excretion. There is also a fall in intestinal calcium absorption secondary to decreased levels of 1,25-dihydroxyvitamin D,[58] making dietary therapy of limited usefulness.

### *Primary Hyperparathyroidism*

Around 5% of stone formers seen at referral centers have primary hyperparathyroidism.[21,59] Excessive parathyroid hormone secretion from either a single adenomatous gland or four hyperplastic glands results in increased bone resorption. The high parathyroid hormone concentration also stimulates the production of 1,25-dihydroxyvitamin D and therefore intestinal absorption of calcium. The hypercalciuria thus has an absorptive component as well as a bone resorptive component. Supersaturation of the urine for both calcium oxalate and calcium phosphate occurs with subsequent stone formation.[60]

Approximately 50% of patients with primary hyperparathyroidism form stones.[61] Why 50% of patients form stones and the rest do not has been the subject of study by several investigators. Most patients with this abnormality have hypercalciuria; however, those who form stones have been found by some investigators to have a higher urinary calcium excretion than those who do not form stones.[60,62,63] This has been proposed to be a result of higher levels of 1,25-dihydroxyvitamin D in the stone formers, which leads to an augmented intestinal absorption of calcium.[63] Other investigators have been unable to demonstrate differences between stone formers and non–stone formers in levels of urinary calcium excretion, circulating levels of 1,25-dihydroxyvitamin D, or fractional intestinal calcium absorption.[64] The possibility of differences in inhibitor activity between the stone-forming and non–stone-forming patients with primary hyperparathyroidism has been suggested. Citrate excretion has been found to be the same in the two groups[62,65] or lower in the stone formers,[66] and magnesium excretion is similar in both groups.[62,65,66] Excretion of pyrophosphate is controversial.[66–68] Interestingly, although no difference in the excretion of total acid mucopolysaccharide exists between stone formers and non–stone formers with primary hyperparathyroidism, the potency of these substances in preventing calcium oxalate precipitation is lower in the stone formers.[69]

In summary, most patients with primary hyperparathyroidism have hypercalciuria that is both resorptive and absorptive. This hypercalciuria results in supersaturation of the urine for calcium oxalate and calcium phosphate. Why only 50% of such patients form stones is controversial; it is possible that stone formers have higher circulating levels of 1,25-dihydroxyvitamin D and thus a larger absorptive component to the hypercalciuria. This would make the degree of hypercalciuria diet dependent and introduce variability into the expression of renal stone disease as a manifestation of primary hyperparathyroidism.

### *Renal Tubular Acidosis*

Renal tubular acidosis (RTA) can be defined as an inability, out of proportion to reduction in renal mass, to renally excrete sufficient hydrogen ions to maintain a normal acid–base balance. There are three basic types of RTA: distal (classic, type I, or gradient limited), proximal (bicarbonate wasting or type II), and hyperkalemic renal tubular acidosis (type IV).[70] Renal stone disease associated with hyperkalemic RTA has not been described in the literature. This is surprising as these individuals tend to have persistently acid urine with low urinary ammonia levels[71] reminiscent of idiopathic uric acid stone formers (see Urates and Stones).

Likewise, proximal RTA is generally not considered to result in stone formation.[72] Proximal RTA occurs most often in children and usually with other abnormalities in proximal tubular transport, for example, phosphaturia, glycosuria, uricosuria, and aminoaciduria (known as the Fanconi syndrome).[70] The underlying defect is a decrease in the threshold for proximal tubular reabsorption of bicarbonate. This resetting of the threshold for bicarbonate reabsorption results in a wasting of bicarbonate in the urine (alkaline urine) until the threshold is reached. When the threshold is reached, no more bicarbonate is lost in the urine (acid urine) but hypobicarbonatemia and hyperchloremia are present. Acid–base balance is restored in the presence of a stable metabolic acidosis.[73] The fact that balance is restored is thought to account for the lack of hypercalciuria in this form of RTA. This and the presence of normal to high urinary citrate levels[74] as well as the potential for calcium complexation by amino acids[75,76] may explain the rarity of nephrolithiasis in proximal RTA.

Acetazolamide and dichlorphenamide are carbonic anhydrase inhibitors that produce a tubular abnormality in bicarbonate reabsorption similar to proximal RTA and have been associated with calcium stone formation.[77,78] Unlike isolated proximal RTA or that associated with Fanconi's syndrome, drug-induced proximal tubular bicarbonate wasting is associated with low citrate excretion.[79] A decrease in urinary citrate is seen in virtually all patients on these drugs, but only 4% to 8% develop nephrolithiasis.[80,81] Hypercalciuria may have to exist prior to the administration of a carbonic anhydrase inhibitor, for stone formation to occur.[81]

Distal renal tubular acidosis has been associated with nephrocalcinosis, nephrolithiasis, and metabolic bone disease.[70] This type of RTA is characterized by an inability to generate and/or maintain a steep hydrogen ion gradient across the collecting duct epithelium. More simply, there is an inability to lower the urine pH maximally, even when a systemic acidosis is present and plasma bicarbonate is markedly reduced.[82] Distal RTA can present in the complete form with a depression of plasma bicarbonate and elevation of plasma chloride. It can also present with normal serum electrolytes as the incomplete form.[82] Both forms are associated with nephrocalcinosis and nephrolithiasis; the incomplete form is more common.[83]

The risk factors for stone disease associated with distal RTA are hypercalciuria, persistently alkaline urine, and hypocitraturia.[84] Calcium excretion in patients with distal RTA has varied from normal[85] to markedly elevated.[85,86] It would appear that those with marked hypercalciuria have an associated idiopathic hypercalciuria.[85,87] Indeed, it has been proposed that the hypercalciuria results in tubular damage leading to renal tubular acidosis.[86] In many reported cases of distal RTA, however, hypercalciuria either is not present or is mild.[83,84,88,89]

Several mechanisms for the mild hypercalciuria associated with distal RTA have been proposed. Balance studies in normal individuals with induced metabolic acidosis suggest that there is an ongoing positive net balance of acid.[87] It was proposed that the acid not excreted by the kidneys and not apparently buffered by the bicarbonate buffer system was disposed of by buffers fixed in tissues, namely, bone. This would result in the mobilization of calcium from bone and account for both the hypercalciuria and the osteopenia that had been described. In support of this proposal is the finding that the administration of alkali leads to a reversal of the positive acid balance[90] and to a decrease in urinary calcium excretion.[88] Against this mechanism of hypercalciuria is the finding that parathyroid hormone levels are elevated in metabolic acidosis[91] and specifically in distal RTA.[89] Suppressed levels would be expected if acidosis was mobilizing calcium from bone. Another proposed mechanism is that metabolic acidosis decreases renal tubular reabsorption of calcium, resulting in an increase in urinary calcium excretion.[92,93] This mechanism for hypercalciuria could explain the development of secondary hyperparathyroidism and the reversal of excess parathyroid hormone secretion and hypercalciuria with alkali therapy[89]; however, this mechanism should lead to osteitis fibrosa cystica or hyperparathyroid bone disease. Although osteitis fibrosa cystica has been reported to occur in distal RTA,[94] rickets in children and osteomalacia in adults are the lesions usually present.[95] A defect in the mineralization of bone suggests an abnormality in vitamin D metabolism. Vitamin D must be metabolized before it is metabolically active.[33] The first step in this process takes place in the liver, where it is converted to 25-hydroxyvitamin D. The final step occurs in the kidney, where it is hydroxylated to 1,25-dihydroxyvitamin D, the active metabolite that stimulates intestinal absorption of calcium. This final step has been found to be impaired in metabolic acidosis.[96,97] Thus, metabolic acidosis could lead to low circulating levels of 1,25-dihydroxyvitamin D, resulting in impaired intestinal calcium absorption and bone mineralization.

Hypocitraturia is a common if not universal finding in distal RTA.[98] Citrate is an inhibitor of calcium phosphate precipitation, and deficiency represents a major risk factor for calcium stone disease. Urinary citrate excretion is altered by changes in systemic pH, with acidosis leading to a decrease and alkalosis to an increase in excretion.[99] As citrate excretion is low in both complete and incomplete distal RTA,[100] it has been proposed that in incomplete distal RTA, an intracellular acidosis exists.

Alkaline urine is always found in distal RTA by definition and is also a risk factor. Calcium phosphate is the most common component of stones formed in distal RTA.[101] Alkaline urine pH markedly decreases the solubility of calcium phosphate,[102] thus contributing to the stone formation.

### *Hyperoxaluria*

Hyperoxaluria results in an increase in urinary supersaturation for calcium oxalate. Some of the causes of hyperoxaluria are listed in Table 37.3. Primary hyperoxaluria is a rare disorder of glyoxylate metabolism that occurs primarily in children and leads to renal failure secondary to oxalate deposition, usually before the second decade of life.[103] Two types of this disorder exist as a result of two distinct biochemical abnormalities, but both lead to marked hyperoxaluria and both follow an autosomal recessive mode of inheritance.

Hyperoxaluria has been attributed to a high intake of dietary oxalate. Such foods as rhubarb, spinach, chocolate, tea, nuts, and peanut butter have been found to have a high level of oxalate. Unfortunately, few studies have been done to assess the bioavailability of the oxalate in these foods.[104] Another dietary factor that can increase oxalate excretion is a low dietary calcium intake.[105] Dietary oxalate is felt to be complexed to calcium. Any decrease in available dietary calcium could result in more oxalate being available for absorption. There seems to be greater augmentation of urinary oxalate excretion on a low-calcium diet in those patients with underlying idiopathic hypercalciuria.[106]

Doses of vitamin C in excess of 4 g per day have been reported to increase urinary oxalate[107]; however, a subsequent study in normal individuals failed to show an effect of vitamin C up to 8 g per day on urinary oxalate excretion.[108] The possibility exists that stone formers and non–stone-formers handle ascorbic acid differently. Evidence has been presented suggesting a greater rise in urinary oxalate in stone formers than in non–stone formers after oral ascorbate loading.[109] Although pyridoxine deficiency in experimental animals results in hyperoxaluria,[110] hyperoxaluria of this etiology is rare in humans.

Intestinal disease associated with fat malabsorption has been related to hyperoxaluria.[111] This "enteric" hyperoxaluria occurs when malabsorbed fat binds dietary calcium, thus freeing oxalate for absorption. This has been a major complication of jejunoileal bypass operations for obesity or blood lipid control, but also occurs in any bowel disease resulting in fat malabsorption. The other causes of hyperoxaluria listed in Table 37.3 are associated with acute toxicity and are included for completeness. They have not been associated with recurrent nephrolithiasis.

**Table 37.3** Causes of Hyperoxaluria

| |
|---|
| Primary |
| Type I: Glycolic aciduria |
| Type II: L-Glyceric aciduria |
| Secondary |
| Increased dietary intake |
| Decreased dietary calcium intake |
| Excessive vitamin C intake (?) |
| Enteric |
| Pyridoxine deficiency |
| Ethylene glycol |
| Methoxyflurane |
| Xylitol |

### *Inhibitor Deficiency*

Inhibitor deficiency has been proposed as an etiology for calcium stone disease,[5] but examples of clinical stone disease have been difficult to find. Hypocitraturia associated with distal RTA,[98] acetazolamide therapy,[79] and enteric hyperoxaluria[101] are examples. Idiopathic hypocitraturia has been described[112] but must be confirmed. A role for hyperuricosuria in decreasing inhibitor activity of glycosaminoglycans is discussed under Urates and Stones. Deficiencies of magnesium, pyrophosphate, or glycosaminoglycans have not been convincingly demonstrated.

### *Low Urine Volume*

Low urine volume is a risk factor for calcium stone disease[17] in that it increases the level of supersaturation for both calcium phosphate and calcium oxalate.[113] As urine volumes are an obvious continuum in any population, it is difficult to define "low urine volume." In our experience, urine volumes less than 1,000 mL/d represent a significant independent risk factor.

### *Clinical Characteristics*

Calcium stone disease constitutes 85% to 90% of all stone disease. This stone disease can occur in newborns and the very elderly, but the highest incidence is between 20 and 40 years of age. Noninfection stones in children should suggest inherited disorders such as primary hyperoxaluria or distal RTA, but idiopathic hypercalciuria, even in this age group, is the most common disorder.[114,115] Similarly, in the elderly, primary hyperparathyroidism and drug-induced (i.e., acetazolamide) stone disease should be considered, but idiopathic hypercalciuria is the most common.

Calcium stone disease can be asymptomatic or can present with the severe pain of renal colic. Whether or not a stone passes depends on the size of the stone.[116] Stones less than 4 mm pass spontaneously 93% of the time, stones 4–6 mm pass in 53% of cases, and stones greater than 6 mm rarely pass spontaneously.

Calcium stone disease seldom leads to renal damage even in those patients with frequent stone passage. Exceptions are patients with primary hyperoxaluria, enteric hyperoxaluria, distal RTA, or superimposed infection. These patients need aggressive management to prevent loss of renal function.

Recurrence of calcium stone disease is the rule. Studies that have a follow-up of at least 10 years, with radiologic studies to detect asymptomatic stones and attempts to differentiate new stones from preformed stones, reveal a recurrence rate of 70% to 80% by 20 years.[2] The rate does not appear to decrease with age.[117]

### *Treatment*

Maintenance treatment of calcium stone disease usually depends on reversing the metabolic defect(s) that is/are causing stone formation.[118] As discussed earlier, these defects include hypercalciuria, hyperuricosuria, hyperoxaluria, distal renal tubular acidosis, low urine volume, or any combination. The five elements of this selective approach are that the treatment (1) correct the physicochemical abnormality in urine, (2) overcome physiologic derangements in patients with stones, (3) inhibit stone formation, (4) not cause significant side effects, and (5) prevent extrarenal manifestations of the disease process. Utilization of the selective treatment approach to calcium stone disease has been documented to significantly reduce new stone formation and the need for operative intervention.[119,120]

In general, therapeutic intervention revolves around reducing the urinary concentration of stone-forming materials, increasing the urinary concentrations of inhibitors, or both. Fluid intake is exceedingly important in reducing the urinary concentration of stone-forming substances. A fluid intake sufficient to ensure a urine output of at least 2 L per day is recommended and has been shown to reduce the level of urinary saturation.[113,121]

Hyperabsorption of calcium resulting from absorptive hypercalciuria type I can be treated by means of a low-calcium diet plus an agent that binds calcium in the gut to prevent its absorption. Sodium phytate[122,123] and sodium cellulose phosphate have been used.[124–128] Results with sodium phytate have been disappointing, with little alteration in the natural history of calcium stone disease and a distressing incidence of diarrhea leading to noncompliance with therapy. Sodium cellulose phosphate, an ion-exchange resin used in doses of 2.5–5 g with each meal, has been documented to reduce calcium absorption from the gut. This leads to a decrease in urinary calcium, thus reducing urine brushite saturation and decreasing the propensity for spontaneous nucleation.[124,127,129] Not all investigators have reported successful therapy with cellulose phosphate in absorptive hypercalciuria.[130,131] This treatment does not stimulate parathyroid function or induce bone disease when used in the usual therapeutic doses,[125,129] but may cause hyperoxaluria[128] and reduced magnesium excretion.[124,125,130,131] As magnesium is one of the purported inhibitors of stone formation and hyperoxaluria is a major risk factor,[132,133] it is recommended that oral magnesium supplementation be given separately from cellulose phosphate and that dietary oxalate be moderately restricted.[134] This agent should not be used in patients with renal hypercalciuria or those with low or normal calcium absorption, as secondary hyperparathyroidism may ensue.

Absorptive hypercalciuria type II usually responds to restriction of dietary calcium to 600 mg/d. Orthophosphate is indicated for patients with hypophosphatemic or type III absorptive hypercalciuria. In this disorder, phosphate supplementation is logical as it will suppress 1,25-dihydroxyvitamin D synthesis, thereby reducing calcium absorption and hence excretion.[135,136] It has, however, been used in all patients with idiopathic hypercalciuria and in patients with calcium stone disease of undefined etiology. The urinary saturation of calcium oxalate decreases because of the fall in urinary calcium excretion. The major benefit may be an increase in excretion of pyrophosphate, an inhibitor of both calcium phosphate and calcium oxalate stone formation.[137–139] Orthophosphates are available as acid, neutral, or alkaline salts of sodium or potassium phosphates. All have proven effective in the treatment of recurrent calcium calculi, although the acid preparation may be somewhat inferior to the other preparations. The acid load may result in an increase in urinary calcium and a decrease in urinary citrate.[140] Dosages utilized have ranged from 1,250 to 2,250 mg of elemental phosphorus per day administered in divided doses.

Several studies have documented the efficacy of orthophosphates in preventing calcium-containing calculi.[136,141–143] One double-blind controlled study demonstrated no change in renal stone disease, although this may have resulted from the use of the acid phosphate preparation.[144] Patients with gastrointestinal disorders do not tolerate phosphate therapy, the sodium load may be deleterious in patients with heart failure or hypertension, and diarrhea may limit attainable drug dosage. Dystrophic calcification has been noted by one group of investigators[145] but not verified by others. Phosphate therapy should not be utilized in patients with renal insufficiency and is contraindicated in patients with infection-induced stone disease. The related diphosphonate compounds are exceptionally potent inhibitors of the formation and aggregation of calcium oxalate and calcium phosphate crystals[146,147]; however, the large doses required to modify crystalluria cause bone disease in man; thus, for the present, oral diphosphonates hold little promise of usefulness in stone disease.[148]

Patients with enteric hyperoxaluria have been treated with cholestyramine[149] or diethylaminoethanol-cellulose (DEAE-cellulose),[150] which act as oxalate binders. Cholestyramine, although safely used for many years as a hypolipidemic agent, may be subject to noncompliance because of its physical characteristics and may bind various vitamins, other nutrients, and drugs. DEAE-cellulose, although safe and effective in reducing elevated urinary oxalate excretion, has been used in only a small number of patients and is currently an investigational drug in the United States. Mild hyperoxaluria can be reduced by limiting the intake of such oxalate-rich foods as spinach, rhubarb, strawberries, peppers, parsley, tea, nuts, and chocolate. It is important to counsel patients to avoid coffee, tea, or chocolate beverages as part of their fluid therapy. In addition, the ingestion of megadoses of ascorbic acid should be avoided because of the potential relationship to hyperoxaluria.

Another agent that could potentially reduce the in vivo generation of oxalate is pyridoxine. Pyridoxine is thought to decrease endogenous oxalate production, and hence excretion, by stimulating the conversion of glyoxylic acid to glycine rather than to oxalic acid.[151,152] Pyridoxine therapy has been reported to be successful in some cases of primary hyperoxaluria.[153] Although calcium carbimide can theoretically reduce glyoxalate (and hence oxalate) formation by inhibiting the oxidation of glycolaldehyde via aldehyde dehydrogenase in primary hyperoxaluria,[154] this agent has not been found to decrease urinary oxalate excretion in clinical practice.[155] In addition, succinate is thought to decrease the formation of oxalate by bringing more $C_2$ metabolites into the Krebs cycle. Although succinate has been documented to reduce hyperoxaluria in 74% of patients in one series,[156] poor results were noted in the treatment of hyperoxaluria in another series.[157] Succinate therapy should be regarded as experimental at this time.

Thiazides are thought to represent the "ideal" treatment program for renal leak hypercalciuria as they increase renal tubular reabsorption of calcium,[158–160] restore normal parathyroid function,[161] and reduce serum 1,25-dihydroxyvitamin D concentration[161] and calcium absorption[161,162]; however, many clinicians use these agents for hypercalciuria of any etiology. The fall in urinary calcium leads to a decrease in the level of saturation of brushite and calcium oxalate.[163–165] The mechanism by which renal calcium excretion is reduced by thiazides is unknown although it seems that volume contraction and parathyroid hormone are required.[166,167] Increased tubular reabsorption of calcium induced by thiazides would appear to be the major mechanism. In addition, thiazides have been reported to reduce the urinary excretion of oxalate and increase excretion of zinc and magnesium, two potential stone formation inhibitors.[166,168]

Thiazide-induced potassium depletion may occur, leading to hypocitraturia. This may be deleterious in lieu of the inhibitor effects of citrate, but can be prevented by potassium supplementation with the chloride or citrate salt.[169] Serum calcium may rise but this effect is generally mild.

Although open nonrandomized, noncontrolled or poorly controlled studies have documented the efficacy of thiazides in hypercalciuric stone formers,[119,120,130,166,170] two randomized, well-controlled, recent studies have questioned the value of thiazides in this disorder.[171,172] The methodologic and statistical defects of the noncontrolled trials have been elegantly summarized recently.[173] This controversy will only be answered by further controlled clinical studies utilizing criteria published previously.[173] Thiazides used most commonly in renal stone disorders include hydrochlorothiazide, trichlormethiazide, bendroflumethiazide, chlorthalidone, and chlorothiazide.

Potassium citrate has recently been evaluated for the treatment of all forms of calcium nephrolithiasis, although it is best indicated for the treatment of hypocitraturic calcium stone disease. Citrate excretion has been reported to be decreased in many calcium stone formers.[174–176] Favorable results have been noted in the treatment of calcium nephrolithiasis, especially in hypocitraturic and hyperuricosuric calcium stone formers, in the latter patients because of its effects on both urinary pH and calcium salt crystallization.[177,178] Renal citrate excretion is enhanced by the effect of alkali on the renal handling of citrate. Potassium citrate would seem advantageous over sodium alkali, as it is free of the potential complications of sodium-induced hypercalciuria and sodium urate–induced crystallization of calcium oxalate. As with all potassium-containing preparations, patients should be followed for hyperkalemia and gastrointestinal upset and bleeding.

Administration of oral magnesium to reduce the stone-forming potential in calcium nephrolithiasis has been attempted on the basis of magnesium's crystallization inhibition properties.[132,133] Although a few studies of therapy with magnesium oxide or hydroxide, alone or in combination with pyridoxine, have documented some benefit in calcium stone formers,[179–183] data are too limited to recommend this as a first-line treatment. Investigators have found no significant beneficial effect on urinary formation product or on the rate of crystal growth of calcium oxalate or brushite[184]; however, its use in conjunction with cellulose phosphate therapy may improve the therapeutic response to this calcium-binding agent. Caution should be exercised in its use in patients with renal impairment. Dosage may be limited by the appearance of diarrhea.

## Urates and Stones

Between 5% and 10% of renal stones in the United States are composed of uric acid. A similar percentage applies to most of Europe, but higher figures are reported from Germany, Spain, and Israel[185–187] and lower figures from Sweden.[188] Urates have been proposed to also play a role in calcium stone disease, and both uric acid stone disease and urate involvement in calcium stone disease are discussed.

### *Uric Acid Metabolism*

Uric acid is the end product of purine metabolism. Purines are derived from endogenous sources or the diet and are converted to hypoxanthine and xanthine. Hypoxanthine is oxidized to xanthine and this compound in turn is oxidized to uric acid. Both of these oxidation steps are catalyzed by xanthine oxidase. In many animals uric acid is then oxidized by uricase to allantoin, a water-soluble end product. Man, reptiles, and birds are deficient in uricase activity and cannot convert uric acid to allantoin. Uric acid becomes the end product of purine metabolism and must be excreted; however, uric acid is not as soluble as allantoin in an aqueous medium and thus tends to precipitate.

### *Uric Acid Excretion*

Uric acid is excreted by renal and extrarenal mechanisms. Two thirds of the uric acid excreted per day is cleared through the kidneys and one third, by the intestine. The uric acid lost in the intestine is degraded by uricase-containing bacteria.[189]

Uric acid is handled in the kidney by a four-component system. As protein binding is less than 5%, it is freely filtered at the glomerulus. It is thought that virtually all filtered uric acid is reabsorbed. Tubular secretion of approximately 50% of the original filtered load is followed by further tubular reabsorption. This postsecretory reabsorption amounts to 40% to 45% of the original filtered load. Thus, total excretion of urate is 5% to 10% of the original filtered load, but most if not all of the urate appearing in the urine is derived from that urate secreted by the nephron and escaping postsecretory reabsorption.[190] The site in the nephron of excretion and reabsorption is controversial but is probably in the proximal tubule.[191]

### *Clinical Characteristics*

In addition to renal colic, uric acid gravel is common. This gravel is characteristically reddish in appearance as a result of absorption of urochromes. Passage of gravel is frequently asymptomatic but can be associated with dysuria and hematuria. Occasionally, massive deposition can occur with bilateral ureteral obstruction and acute renal failure.

The age of onset and sex distribution of uric acid stone disease depend on whether or not it is associated with gout. Uric acid stone disease not associated with gout is termed idiopathic and can occur at any age; the male-to-female ratio is 3:1. When associated with gout, this stone disease occurs almost exclusively after the age of 40, with a male-to-female ratio of 12:1.[187,192]

Uric acid stones are radiolucent. Renal colic with no stone seen on a routine flat plate of the abdomen should suggest uric acid stones. They can be seen with an intravenous pyelogram in which they appear as negative filling defects. They are also apparent with computerized tomography and renal ultrasound.

### *Risk Factors*

Inhibitors of uric acid precipitation[193] as well as promoters of precipitation[194] have been proposed; however, studies on uric acid solubility have shown similar levels in non–stone formers and uric acid stone formers,[195] suggesting that the most important factors governing uric acid precipitation are uric acid concentration and pH. Uric acid solubility in the urine is therefore determined by the concentration of undissociated uric acid. Undissociated uric acid concentration is calculated using the equation

$$[A] = [T] \div (1 + 10^{pH - pK}),$$

where [A] is the concentration of undissociated uric acid (in mg/L), [T] is the concentration of total uric acid (in mg/L), pH is the pH of the urine, and $pK = 5.345$.[196] Examination of this formula reveals the marked effect of urine pH below the p$K$ in decreasing the solubility of uric acid.

The risk factors for uric acid stone disease are apparent: hyperuricosuria (increases concentration), low urine volume (increases concentration), and persistently acid urine (decreases solubility).

Hyperuricosuria is not the most common of the three risk factors, being present in only 31% of uric acid stone formers in one large series.[187] It is always a manifestation of the overproduction of uric acid and occurs in the conditions listed in Table 37.4. Of the conditions listed in Table 37.4, gout and high dietary protein intake are the most frequent causes of hyperuricosuria.

Low urine volume secondary to high environmental temperatures may be a contributing factor to the high incidence

**Table 37.4** Classification of Uric Acid Stone Disease

| |
|---|
| Associated with hyperuricosuria |
|   Gout secondary to overproduction of uric acid |
|     Lesch–Nyhan syndrome (hypoxanthine–guanine phosphoribosyl transferase deficiency) |
|     Type I glycogen storage disease (glucose-6-phosphatase deficiency) |
|     Phosphoribosyl pyrophosphate synthetase overactivity |
|     Glutathione reductase overactivity |
| Associated with persistently acid urine |
|   Idiopathic uric acid stone disease |
|   Gout |
|   Gastrointestinal losses of bicarbonate |
|     Chronic diarrhea |
|     Ileostomy |
|     Fistulas |
| Associated with low urine volume |
|   Excessive sweating |
|   Low fluid intake |
|   Gastrointestinal losses |

of uric acid stones in the Middle East.[187] It is also an important risk factor in ileostomy patients and any patient with large gastrointestinal losses of fluids.[197]

The most common risk factor for uric acid stone disease is a persistently acid urine.[198] The urine pH remains below 6 throughout the day.[199] Although there is widespread agreement that the urine is persistently acid, there is controversy as to the mechanism. Early studies proposed that there was an impairment in ammonium excretion by the kidney.[198,200] This could not be confirmed by other investigators,[201,202] who attributed the finding of decreased ammonium excretion to age differences between patients and controls (the patients were older than the controls and ammonium excretion decreases with age) and/or to renal impairment in the patients which is known to decrease ammonium excretion. Subsequent studies again suggested a decreased ammonium excretion but with an elevated titratable acid excretion that was sensitive to changes in dietary protein intake.[203–205] Although there is still controversy, current data suggest that patients with uric acid stones have a persistently acid urine related to an abnormal partitioning of hydrogen ion between ammonium and titratable acid and that this abnormality is more prominent as the level of protein in the diet increases.

### *Urates and Calcium Stone Disease*

Calcium-containing stones occur more commonly among individuals with gout than in the general population.[206] In addition, calcium stone formers with hyperuricosuria or hyperuricemia but with no abnormalities in calcium metabolism have been described.[207] An increased prevalence of hyperuricosuria in calcium stone formers compared with a control group of non–stone formers has been reported.[208] Hyperuricosuria has been identified as a risk factor in 9% to 15% of calcium stone formers.[21,117] Patients with calcium stone disease associated with hyperuricosuria have a more aggressive disease with higher stone formation rates, shorter intervals between stone events,[117] and higher frequency of stones requiring operative management.[117,208] The etiology of the hyperuricosuria has been attributed to a high dietary purine intake, a higher uric acid production for any given purine intake, and alterations in renal handling of uric acid,[205,209,210] although this last mechanism has not been supported by all investigators.[211]

### *Mechanism(s) of Calcium Stone Formation in Hyperuricosuria*

Urates exist in the urine in several forms. In an acid urine, as was discussed in the previous section on uric acid stone disease, urates exist predominantly as undissociated uric acid; however, above pH 6.0, urates associate with monovalent cations, the most abundant being sodium, to form monosodium urate.[212] Potentially, either uric acid or monosodium urate could play a role in calcium stone formation.

Epitaxy is a process by which one crystal form serves as a nidus for a second type of crystal. It has been proposed that either uric acid or monosodium urate could serve as a substrate for calcium oxalate precipitation.[14] In vitro studies showed that monosodium urate readily initiated nucleation of calcium oxalate, whereas uric acid failed to do so.[213] This process was slowed by pyrophosphate, a known inhibitor of calcium oxalate precipitation.[214]

A second proposed mechanism is that urates interfere with the inhibitory action of glycosaminoglycans on calcium oxalate precipitation.[68] Glycosaminoglycans have been shown to be potent inhibitors of the nucleation of calcium oxalate[215] as well as of crystal growth and aggregation.[216] Monosodium urate has been shown to decrease this inhibitory action of glycosaminoglycans.[215] Furthermore, hyperuricosuria leads to supersaturation of the urine for monosodium urate and results in a decrease in the level of supersaturation required for spontaneous precipitation of calcium oxalate.[217]

### *Treatment*

Treatment of uric acid stone disease is dictated by the risk factors present in the individual patient. Treatment is designed to reduce the level of undissociated uric acid to less than 90 mg/L.[196]

Optimal hydration is important in all patients with uric acid stones, not just those found to have low urine volumes. A daily urine output of 2.5 to 3 L per day should be maintained with an emphasis on evening intake to guarantee a high urine flow during the night.[113] The emphasis should be on the volume of urine excreted, not on the volume of fluid consumed.

Allopurinol therapy should be used if hyperuricosuria (>800 mg/d) is present. Allopurinol should be utilized in conjunction with fluid and alkali therapy.[218–221] This drug inhibits xanthine oxidase, thus decreasing the conversion of xanthine and hypoxanthine to uric acid. Although the usual starting dose is 200 to 300 mg once daily, dosage should be adjusted in patients with significant renal dysfunction.[222] Patients should be monitored for the appearance of potentially serious side effects such as precipitation of acute gouty attacks, skin rash (may progress to toxic epidermal necrolysis), vasculitis, blood dyscrasias, and hepatitis. As well, xanthine and oxypurinol stones may develop in patients receiving allopurinol, especially those patients with extremely high purine loads (neoplasia, Lesch–Nyhan syndrome).[223–226]

Alkali therapy is usually required in patients with persistently acid urine. Urine pH should be maintained between 6.5 and 7.0 and not be allowed to drop below 5.5. Also, urine pH should not be allowed to exceed 7.0 to avoid calcium phosphate precipitation. Unless obstruction is complete, systemic alkalinization with intravenous sodium bicarbonate or sodium lactate titrated to produce a urine pH of 6.0–7.0 may be sufficient to result in stone dissolution.[227] Lactate may be the preferred intravenous agent because of its smaller propensity to induce metabolic alkalosis as well as the theoretical advantage of lactate providing the antiketogenic effect of glycogen that may potentiate the acid-neutralizing effect of the sodium ion. Controlled comparative trials are required, however. Intravenous alkalinization may produce total dissolution within only 1 or 2 days of starting therapy. Oral alkalinization may also be adequate for the treatment of incompletely obstructing uric acid stones. Monitoring of therapy with pH strips is recommended. Alkalinization may be achieved with sodium bicarbonate, sodium or potassium citrate, or acetazolamide. Acetazolamide is recommended only if troublesome sodium or fluid retention occurs with sodium salts or if nocturnal pH cannot be raised above 6.0 with conventional therapy.[228] Citrate salts may be preferable to bicarbonate because of better gastrointestinal tolerance. Potassium citrate may be preferable to sodium citrate because of a reduced potential for the development of calcium stones, which may arise from sodium citrate or sodium bicarbonate therapy.[229] Also, monopotassium urate is more soluble than monosodium urate.

Treatment of acute urinary obstruction secondary to uric acid stones requires either open lithotomy or irrigation with or without extraction via percutaneous nephrostomy.[230] Irrigation therapy may be used as primary therapy after nephrostomy tube insertion to decompress the urinary tract. It may also be used as an adjunct to lithotomy or nephrostomy extraction to ensure dissolution of residual stone fragments or stones inaccessible to removal. Irrigation solutions have included 0.1 M sodium bicarbonate (pH 8.4)[231–232] and tromethamine.[233] Bicarbonate is recommended because of greater clinical experience and much lower cost. One to three weeks of therapy has generally been required to effect total stone dissolution.

## Infection Stones

Stones caused by infection are composed of magnesium–ammonium phosphate (struvite) usually combined with carbonate–apatite. Between 9% and 19% of stones analyzed contain struvite.[15,16] Urinary tract infection has been reported in 10% to 12% of stone patients,[234,235] but only 2% to 3% of stone disease is attributed to infection.[21,234,236] One can conclude from these figures that stones caused by infection are probably analyzed more frequently than other stones, that urinary tract infections in stone formers are more common than infection-induced stone formation, and that infection is not a common cause of renal stone disease; however, it is important to recognize this type of stone disease, because it can result in the loss of renal function, can be associated with urosepsis, and has a high rate of recurrence.

### *Pathogenesis*

Infection stones are associated with a highly alkaline urine containing a high concentration of ammonia. Struvite solubility is pH sensitive. It precipitates in an alkaline environment (pH $\geq$ 7.0) and is soluble in an acid solution.[102,237] Carbonate–apatite, a form of calcium phosphate plus carbonate, also is pH sensitive,[107] precipitating in an alkaline solution. Ammonia excretion generally falls in an alkaline urine and, therefore, would not be expected to reach sufficient concentration to precipitate as struvite. Any explanation of the pathogenesis of these stones must account for the high urine pH as well as the increase in the urine concentration of ammonia.

This type of stone disease occurs only in the presence of infection with urease-producing bacteria. Sterile urine from stone formers and non–stone formers has been shown to be undersaturated for struvite.[238] The addition of urease to sterile urine that is undersaturated for struvite results in alkalinization of the urine and supersaturation for struvite.[239] The enzyme urease hydrolyzes urea to form ammonia and carbon dioxide, which on further hydrolysis yield ammonium and bicarbonate plus carbonate. In addition to generation of the ionic species required for stone formation, the hydrolysis of urea also results in alkalinization of the solution. Thus, the requirements for precipitation of struvite and carbonate–apatite (alkaline pH and high ammonia and carbonate concentrations) are met.

Many gram-positive and gram-negative organisms and yeasts as well as T-strain mycoplasma are urease producers.[240] Virtually all *Proteus* sp. are urease producers, whereas *Escherichia coli* seldom, if ever, produces urease. The T-strain mycoplasma *Ureaplasma urealyticum* has been shown to produce urease[241] and has been cultured from struvite stones.[242]

Matrix has been suggested to play a role in infection stones. Ultrastructural studies have demonstrated the production of a bacterial glycocalyx which is proposed to facilitate bacterial adhesion to either uroepithelium or preexisting stone material and to trap mucoproteins (matrix material), struvite, and carbonate–apatite crystals to form the infection stone.[243] Bacteria have been demonstrated to reside within the substance of the stone and not just adhere to the surface.[244] This makes therapy difficult, as antibiotics cannot penetrate the stone to reach the bacteria and any fragment left after surgery constitutes infected material and results in recurrence.

### *Clinical Characteristics*

Infection stone disease is unlike metabolic stone disease in that it is more common in women than men.[245] Also, metabolic stone disease most frequently presents as renal colic. This presentation is uncommon in infection stones which usually present as resistant urinary tract infections or urosepsis. Patients predisposed to urinary tract infection are at risk for this type of stone disease. This group would include anyone with a history of recurrent urinary tract infections with intact anatomy (most commonly women), individuals with bladder dysfunction or obstruction, and those with urinary tract diversions or indwelling bladder catheters. Patients with underlying metabolic stone disease also appear to be at risk. Stones in the urinary tract can serve as foreign bodies, but probably more important, patients with metabolic stone disease are frequently subjected to urologic instrumentation that can introduce bacteria into an otherwise sterile system.[245]

These stones can be either radiolucent or radiopaque depending on the proportion of matrix material. Stones that are predominantly matrix with little or no crystalline material are radiolucent, whereas stones with a great deal of carbonate–apatite are radiodense. These stones are the most common to present as staghorn calculi. Although present in the pelvis of the kidney, these stones send one or more branches into the calyces of the kidney.

Studies have attempted to define the natural history of infection stones if they are left untreated. One study found that in untreated patients with unilateral infection stones, 71% ultimately required a nephrectomy with a mortality rate, primarily from renal failure, of 22%. Bilateral disease appears to fare even less well. Nephrectomy occurred in

44%, with a mortality rate of 80% in those left untreated.[246] A second study found that the mortality rate in bilateral infection stone disease was 25% within 5 years and 40% within 10 years.[247] The severe nature of this stone disease is demonstrated by the fact that 77% of patients requiring nephrectomy for treatment of renal stone disease had infection stones.[248]

### *Treatment*

Treatment of infection (struvite) stones is directed toward (1) surgical removal of all stone material and correction of anatomic abnormalities, (2) eradication and/or long-term suppression of urinary infection, (3) maintenance of an acid urine, and (4) specific treatment of any underlying metabolic disorder.

Surgical removal of stone material is the major therapeutic modality in struvite stone disease. A review of the surgical techniques involved in the removal of struvite calculi is beyond the scope of this chapter, but calculi are commonly removed using standard or extended pyelolithotomy, anatropic nephrolithotomy, pyelonephrolithotomy, and partial nephrectomy.[249–253] The surgical goal is removal of all stone fragments. Numerous adjunctive surgical techniques have been developed to improve surgical success rates. These include regional renal hypothermia, operative radiography, operative nephroscopy, and postoperative irrigations with stone solvents; however, surgical removal is frequently not curative as recurrent stone formation depending on duration of follow-up occurs in 0% to 80% (mean 30% in 6 years) of patients. Surgical removal results in "cure" of infection in only approximately 60% of cases.

Recent reports have stressed the value of postoperative stone solvent irrigations in removing inaccessible macroscopic and microscopic fragments left after surgery.[244,251,253] Suby's G solution[254] and hemiacidrin (Renacidin)[244,251,253,255] have been used successfully, although currently hemiacidrin is the solvent of choice because of better patient tolerance. Both agents contain citric acid and magnesium and are at pH 4. Whether pH is the only important effect or complexes between calcium and citrate and magnesium are additive has not been resolved. Complications in the early years of hemiacidrin use, including death from sepsis and hypermagnesemia,[256] prompted the FDA to withdraw approval for use within the kidney. As a result, informed consent should be obtained prior to this therapy; however, these complications were thought to result from irrigation of an infected urinary tract at high intrarenal pressure. Investigations since 1962 have documented the relative safety of hemiacidrin irrigation provided the urinary tract is kept sterile with systemic antibiotics throughout irrigation therapy, blood magnesium levels are monitored, and intrarenal pressures are kept below 25 cm $H_2O$ to prevent pyelovenous reflux. Hemiacidrin irrigation therapy can result in urothelial irritation and mucosal changes but these are of unknown clinical significance.[257,258]

Irrigation therapy may also be useful as primary therapy for struvite stones, especially in those patients who are high risk or are nonsurgical candidates.[255,257] Although safe and effective, primary dissolution therapy is generally very slow, may not be cost-effective, and risks sepsis and renal damage in patients with large stones unless scrupulous technique is used.

Traditional medical therapy plays an adjunctive role to surgery in the management of infection stones. Antibiotics chosen on the basis of culture and sensitivity results are given pre-, intra-, and postoperatively in an attempt to eradicate the attendant infection. Long-term culture-specific antibiotics are indicated if cessation of therapy results in recrudescence of urinary tract infection. Periodic and routine bacteriologic and radiologic follow-up is necessary.

The Shor regimen (restriction of dietary phosphorus, supplemental aluminum hydroxide to reduce intestinal phosphate absorption) has been successful in preventing recurrence and/or growth of infection stones.[259] Presumably, this treatment works by reducing phosphaturia, which thus reduces urinary saturation with respect to struvite and calcium phosphate; however, this therapy is unacceptable to most patients.

Measures to acidify the urine result in an undersaturated urine with respect to struvite and significantly reduce the level of calcium phosphate saturation. Ammonium chloride appears to be the only effective means of acidifying the urine. Results of urine acidification with ascorbic acid have been quite variable, with some authors citing that 1 to 6 g per day significantly lowers the urine pH[260,261] and other authors denying any significant reduction.[262–264] Also, there is the theoretical risk of precipitating calcium oxalate stone disease by increasing urinary oxalate excretion as a by-product of ascorbic acid metabolism. Even with ammonium chloride, however, it may not be possible to acidify the urine in the presence of urease-producing bacteria.

Hydroxyurea and acetohydroxamic acid, which are structurally similar to urea, act by inhibiting the bacterial enzyme urease.[265] Acetohydroxamic acid forms a stronger, noncompetitive, more slowly reversible bond than hydroxyurea. The reduction in urinary ammonia and pH produced by these agents is said to enhance the effectiveness of concurrent antibiotic therapy, reduce the virulence of bacteria, and permit nonpathologic colonization of the urinary tract (in experimental animal models).[266–268] In vivo confirmation of these findings in humans is lacking.

Although hydroxyurea (in doses of 500–1,000 mg/d) and acetohydroxamic acid (in doses of 250–1,500 mg/d) have been documented to reduce ammonia and urinary alkalinity, convincing evidence of total or even partial stone dissolution in a substantial proportion of patients is lacking.[269–272] In most patients, stone growth ceases during inhibitor therapy. Perhaps the reason for the less-than-convincing results of inhibitor therapy lies in the increase in magnesium and phosphate excretion during short-term therapy. These increases may counteract the effects of the large falls in pH and urinary ammonium excretion on the saturation of struvite and brushite.[273] The clinical importance of these findings await confirmation in long-term studies, however. Of the two agents, acetohydroxamic acid appears to be superior based on a more powerful urease inhibition capacity.[273] Acetohydroxamic acid therapy may be accompanied by side effects in a significant proportion of patients. These include mild headaches, gastrointestinal upset, Coombs-negative hemolytic anemia (dose related, seen more frequently in patients with renal impairment), thrombophlebitis, and psychiatric disturbances (including depression, anxiety, tremulousness). This drug is also teratogenic and should not be used in women of childbearing age without adequate birth control measures. Hydroxyurea therapy has been associated with bone marrow suppression (primarily leukopenia), gastrointestinal upset, skin rashes, and rare central nervous system disturbances such as headache, drowsiness, dizziness, and hallucinations. Use of these agents is not recommended in patients with significant renal impairment (creatinine clearance < 20 mL/min) because of reduced efficacy and increased risk of toxicity.

The role of urease inhibitors is undefined at this time. These agents should always be used in conjunction with antibiotic therapy. Perhaps these agents should be reserved for those patients unable to undergo more definitive operative or irrigation procedures, those patients who have recurrent stones despite optimal management with traditional medical therapy, those patients who are failures of ammonium chloride acidification therapy, and those patients who fail to sterilize their urine despite adequate courses of culture-specific antibiotics.

## Cystine Stones

Cystine stone disease accounts for approximately 1% of stones.[15] It is the result of excess cystine excretion in the urine caused by an inherited abnormality in cystine transport in the kidney. Cystinuria is transmitted as an autosomal recessive gene with an incidence in the population of 1 in 4,000 to 1 in 15,000.

### *Pathophysiology*

Amino acids are freely filtered at the glomerulus and virtually 100% reabsorbed in the proximal tubule. In cystinuria there is a transport defect in the proximal tubule of the kidney for the amino acids cystine, lysine, arginine, and ornithine, and excess excretion of these amino acids occurs. There is also a transport abnormality in the intestine for these same amino acids, leading to a decrease in their intestinal absorption. Even these combined abnormalities of impaired intestinal absorption and renal losses would result in no clinical problems if it were not for the limited solubility of cystine leading to renal stone disease.[274]

Normally, less than 60 mg of cystine is excreted per 24 hours. Homozygotes excrete more than 400 mg per 24 hours; heterozygotes excrete intermediate amounts. Of the amino acids excessively excreted in this disease, cystine is the least soluble. Urine pH has an influence on the solubility of cystine; however, this effect is minimal between pH 5.0 and 7.0; solubility in this pH range is 300–400 mg/L. The solubility rises rapidly above pH 7.0, but these pH values can be attained only with alkali therapy. There is a good correlation between level of saturation of the urine for cystine and crystalluria; thus, inhibitors appear to play no role in the pathophysiology of cystine stone formation.[275]

### *Clinical Characteristics*

The disease presents most frequently in the second to third decade of life; however, it has been reported to present as late as the sixth decade. As there is impairment of intestinal absorption and impaired renal conservation, there has been concern that deficiency of the involved amino acids could lead to other clinical problems. Cystinuria has been reported to occur more frequently in individuals with mental illness or retardation; however, when cystinurics were compared with their normal siblings, no difference in intelligence could be demonstrated and there was no difference from intelligence test norms. Similarly, some investigators have found shorter stature among cystinurics, whereas others have not been able to demonstrate a difference. It would appear that the only significant clinical problem associated with cystinuria is renal stone disease and the consequences of stones. If left untreated, this type of stone disease can result in loss of renal function.

### *Diagnosis*

All stones available should be analyzed; the finding of a cystine stone is diagnostic of cystinuria. Likewise, discovery of cystine crystals, which have a characteristic hexagonal "benzene ring" appearance, on urinalysis is diagnostic of cystinuria. When neither stones nor crystals are present on urinalysis, a qualitative test for cystine is the least expensive way to make a presumptive diagnosis. The cyanide–nitroprusside test is simple to perform and is positive only with excess cystine excretion. When the qualitative test is positive, it should be followed by a quantitative determination. Excess excretion of cystine can also occur in Fanconi's syndrome but in this condition cystine excretion is usually less than 200 mg/d and accompanied by diffuse aminoaciduria, glycosuria, and phosphaturia.

Cystine stones are radiopaque on x-ray as a result of their sulfur content. They have a homogeneous, smooth appearance and are less dense than calcium-containing stones.

### *Risk Factors*

The risk factors for cystine stone formation include excess cystine excretion, acid urine, and low urine volume. Cystine, as noted before, is pH sensitive and an acid pH decreases its solubility. Excess excretion and low urine volume lead to increased levels of saturation at any urine pH.

### *Treatment*

Therapy is aimed at prevention of new stone formation and, when necessary, dissolution of stones. A very low protein diet (0.5 g/kg/d or less), which will reduce the intake of methionine, a precursor of cystine, has been demonstrated to reduce urinary cystine output[276]; however, such protein restriction has proven impractical for most patients. The diet is difficult to prepare and frequently unacceptable. Attempts to reduce the breakdown of methionine to cystine by adding dietary choline have been unsuccessful.[277] Intravenous and oral glutamine has been reported to reduce urinary cystine,[278,279] but this observation has not been confirmed in other studies.[280]

In patients with no stones present in the kidney, treating the risk factors of acid urine and low urine volume may be sufficient. Hydration to ensure a urine output of 3–4 L/d and alkalinization with sodium bicarbonate, sodium citrate, or potassium citrate to achieve a urine pH of 7.0–7.5 usually prevent new stone formation.[281] As the solubility of cystine in relation to pH is predictable, the necessary urine volume can be estimated from the daily cystine excretion rate and urine pH. Urine flow must be maintained at night as well as in the daytime. This usually entails sufficient hydration to cause the patient to arise once nightly to void and to drink fluid.

In patients with cystine stones present in the kidneys the hydration/alkalinization protocol is usually inadequate for medical dissolution and oral D-penicillamine is usually required.[281] D-Penicillamine acts by forming a disulfide complex with cystine that is 50 times more soluble than cystine alone. D-Penicillamine therapy is not tolerated by a substantial proportion of patients because of potentially serious side effects such as systemic lupus erythematosus, proteinuria, nephrotic syndrome, blood dyscrasias, myasthenia gravis, skin rashes, mucositis, and dysgeusia.[282]

Oral $\alpha$-mercaptopropionyl-glycine also forms a disulfide complex with cystine to increase its solubility. It has been effective in stone dissolution and is reported to have a lower incidence of side effects.[283] This agent is currently available only as an investigational drug in the United States. Oral *N*-acetylcystine may reduce the frequency of stone recurrence and possibly promote stone dissolution,[284] but further studies to confirm and extend these observations are necessary before this mode of therapy can be recommended.

While some stones dissolve with treatment, the natural course of cystinuria often involves multiple surgical procedures to alleviate obstruction and colic. Irrigation therapy may be used as primary therapy after nephrostomy tube insertion to decompress the urinary tract. It may also be used as an adjunct to lithotomy or nephrostomy extraction to ensure dissolution of residual stone fragments or of stones inaccessible to removal. Irrigation solutions have included D-penicillamine (pH 8.0),[285] $\alpha$-mercaptopropionyl-glycine,[286] and tromethamine-E.[287] Tromethamine-E appears superior to the other irrigants with regard to decreasing the duration of therapy, but controlled comparative trials are lacking. Primary dissolution therapy has usually required 2 to 13 weeks of treatment time, a definite disadvantage compared with surgical procedures.

## References


1. Sierakowski R, Finlayson B, Landes RR, et al. The frequency of urolithiasis in hospital discharge diagnoses in the United States. Invest Urol 1978;15:438–441.
2. Smith CL. When should the stone patient be evaluated? Early evaluation of single stone formers. Med Clin North Am 1984;68:455–459.
3. Boyce WH. Organic matrix of human urinary concretions. Am J Med 1968;45:673–683.
4. Vermeulen CW, Gill WB. Artificial urinary concretions. Invest Urol 1984;1:370–386.
5. Thomas WC, Howard IE. Studies on the mineralizing propensity of urine from patients with and without renal calculi. Trans Assoc Am Physicians 1959;72:181–187.
6. Fleisch H. Inhibitors and promoters of stone formation. Kidney Int 1978;13:361–371.
7. Pak CYC. Chapter 2, Calcium urolithiasis: Pathogenesis, diagnoses, and management, in: Physical Chemistry of Stone Formation. New York, Plenum, 1978, p 5.
8. Vermeulen CW, Lyon ES, Ellis JE, et al. The renal papilla and calculogenesis. J Urol 1967;97:573–582.
9. Finlayson B, Reid F. The expectation of free and fixed particles in urinary stone disease. Invest Urol 1978;15:442–448.
10. Randall A. The initiating lesions of renal calculus. Surg Gynecol Obstet 1937;64:201–208.
11. Hering F, Lueoend G, Briellman T, et al. Calcification sites in human kidneys: A REM study, in Schwille PO, Smith LH, Robertson WG, et al (eds): Urolithiasis and Related Clinical Research. New York, Plenum, 1985, p 205.
12. Smith C. $^{14}$C-calcium oxalate (CAOX) adherence in the rat bladder, in Schwille PO, Smith LH, Robertson WG, et al (eds): Urolithiasis and Related Clinical Research. New York, Plenum, 1985, p 949.
13. Robertson WG, Peacock M, Nordin BEC. Calcium crystalluria in recurrent renal-stone formers. Lancet 1969;2:21–24.
14. Lonsdale K. Epitaxy as a growth factor in urinary calculi and gallstones. Nature 1968;217:50–58.
15. Herring LC. Observations on the analysis of ten thousand urinary calculi. J Urol 1962;88:545–562.
16. Prien EL, Prien EL Jr. Composition and structure of urinary stone. Am J Med 1968;45:654–672.
17. Robertson WG, Peacock M, Heyburn PJ, et al. Risk factors in calcium stone disease in urinary calculus, in Brockus JG, Finlayson B (eds): International Urinary Stone Conference. Littleton, MA, PSG Publishing, 1981, pp 265–273.
18. Pak CYC. Medical management of nephrolithiasis. J Urol 1982;128:1157–1164.
19. Smith LH, Van Den Berg CJ, Wilson DM. Nutrition and urolithiasis. N Engl J Med 1978;298:87–89.
20. Ljunghall S. Renal stone disease: Studies of epidemiology and calcium metabolism. Scand J Urol Nephrol 1977;S41:4–96.
21. Pak CYC, Britton F, Peterson R, et al. Ambulatory evaluation of nephrolithiasis: Classification, clinical presentation and diagnostic criteria. Am J Med 1980;69:19–30.
22. Lemann J, Adams ND, Gray RW. Urinary calcium excretion in human beings. N Engl J Med 1979;301:535–541.
23. Henneman PH, Benedict PH, Forbes AP, et al. Idiopathic hypercalciuria. N Engl J Med 1958;259:802.
24. Jackson WPU, Dancaster CA. Consideration of the hypercalciuria in sarcoidosis, idiopathic hypercalciuria, and that produced by vitamin D. A new suggestion regarding calcium metabolism. J Clin Endocrinol 1959;19:658–680.
25. Avioli LV. Intestinal absorption of calcium. Arch Intern Med 1972;129:345–355.
26. Krejs GJ, Nicar MJ, Zerwekh JE, et al. Effect of 1,25-dihydroxyvitamin $D_3$ on calcium and magnesium absorption in the healthy human jejunum and ileum. Am J Med 1983;75:973–976.
27. Duncombe VM, Watts RWE, Peters TJ. In-vitro calcium uptake by jejunal biopsy specimens from patients with idiopathic hypercalciuria. Lancet 1980;2:1334–1336.
28. Rasmussen H, Fontaine O, Max EE, et al. The effect of 1,25-dihydroxyvitamin $D_3$ administration on calcium transport in chick intestine brush border membrane vesicles. J Biol Chem 1979;254:2993–2999.
29. Rasmussen H, Matsumoto T, Fontaine O, et al. Role of changes in membrane lipid structure in the action of 1,25-dihydroxyvitamin $D_3$. Fed Proc 1982;41:72–77.

30. Coe FL, Bushinksy DA. Pathophysiology of hypercalciuria. Am J Physiol 1984;247:F1–F13.
31. Brannan PG, Marauski G, Pak CYC, et al. Selective jejunal hyperabsorption of calcium in absorptive hypercalciuria. Am J Med 1979;66:425–428.
32. Zerwekh JE, Pak CYC, Kaplan RA, et al. Pathogenic role of 1-alpha,25-dihydroxyvitamin D in sarcoidosis and absorptive hypercalciuria: Different response to prednisolone therapy. J Clin Endocrinol Metab 1980;51:381–386.
33. DeLuca HF. The transformation of a vitamin into a hormone: The vitamin D story. Harvey Lect 1979–80;75:333–379.
34. Schreiber M, Bichler K-H, Strohmaier WC, et al. Vitamin D metabolism in hypercalciuric patients, in Schwille PO, Smith LH, Robertson WG, et al (eds): Hypercalciuric Patients, Urolithiasis and Related Clinical Research. New York, Plenum, 1985, p 315.
35. Kaplan RA, Haussler MR, Deftos LJ, et al. The role of 1-alpha,25-dihydroxyvitamin D in the mediation of intestinal hyperabsorption of calcium in primary hyperparathyroidism and absorptive hypercalciuria. J Clin Invest 1977;59:756–760.
36. Caldas AE, Gray RW, Lemann J. The simultaneous measurement of vitamin D metabolites in plasma: Studies in healthy adults and in patients with calcium nephrolithiasis. J Lab Clin Med 1978;91:840–849.
37. Berlin T, Bjorkhem I, Collste L, et al. Relation between hypercalciuria and vitamin $D_3$-status in renal stone formers, in Schwille PO, Smith LH, Robertson WG, et al (eds): Urolithiasis and Related Clinical Research. New York, Plenum, 1985, p 253.
38. Elomaa I, Karonen S-L, Kairento A-L, et al. Seasonal variation of urinary calcium and oxalate excretion, serum $25(OH)D_3$ and albumin level in relation to renal stone formation. Scand J Urol Nephrol 1982;16:155–161.
39. Broadus AE, Insogna KL, Lang R, et al. A consideration of the hormonal basis and phosphate leak hypothesis of absorptive hypercalciuria. J Clin Endocrinol Metab 1984;58:161–169.
40. Shen FH, Baylink DJ, Nielsen RL, et al. Increased serum 1,25-dihydroxyvitamin D in idiopathic hypercalciuria. J Lab Clin Med 1977;90:955–962.
41. Pak CYC, Ohata M, Lawrence EC, et al. The hypercalciurias: causes, parathyroid functions and diagnostic criteria. J Clin Invest 1974;54:387–400.
42. Pak CYC. Physiological basis for absorptive and renal hypercalciurias. Am J Physiol 1979;237:F415–F423.
43. Muldowney FO, Freany R, Ryan JG. The pathogenesis of idiopathic hypercalciuria: Evidence for renal tubular calcium leak. Q J Med 1980;49:87–94.
44. Coe FL, Canterbury JM, Firpo JJ, et al. Evidence for secondary hyperparathyroidism in idiopathic hypercalciuria. J Clin Invest 1973;52:134–142.
45. Burckhardt P, Jaeger P. Secondary hyperparathyroidism in idiopathic renal hypercalciuria: Fact or theory? J Clin Endocrinol Metab 1981;53:550–555.
46. Coe FL, Farvus MJ, Crockett T, et al. Effects of low-calcium diet on urine calcium excretion, parathyroid function and serum $1,25(OH)_2D_3$ levels in patients with idiopathic hypercalciuria and in normal subjects. Am J Med 1982;72:25–32.
47. Tzchope W, Ritz E, Schmidt-Gayk H. Is there a renal phosphorus leak in recurrent renal stone formers with absorptive hypercalciuria. Eur J Clin Invest 1980;10:381–386.
48. Barilla DE, Zerwekh JE, Pak CYC. A critical evaluation of the role of phosphate in the pathogenesis of absorptive hypercalciuria. Miner Electrolyte Metab 1979;2:302–309.
49. Adams ND, Gray RW, Lemann J, et al. Effects of calcitriol administration on calcium metabolism in healthy men. Kidney Int 1982;21:90–97.
50. Broadus AE, Erickson SB, Gertner JM, et al. An experimental human model of 1,25-dihydroxyvitamin D–mediated hypercalciuria. J Clin Endocrinol Metab 1984;59:202–206.
51. Maierhofer WH, Gray RW, Cheung HS, et al. Bone resorption stimulated by elevated serum $1,25\text{-}(OH)_2$-vitamin D concentrations in healthy men. Kidney Int 1983;24:555–560.
52. Pak CYC. Chapter 7, Practical guidelines for the diagnosis and management of calcium urolithiasis, in: Calcium Urolithiasis: Pathogenesis, Diagnosis, and Management. New York, Plenum, 1978, p 141.
53. Wilkinson R. Chapter 2, Absorption of calcium, phosphorus and magnesium, in Nordin BEC (ed): Calcium, Phosphate and Magnesium Metabolism. New York, Churchill Livingstone, 1976, p 36.
54. Nordin BEC. Hypercalciuria. Clin Sci Molec Med 1977;52:1–8.
55. Silver J, Friedlaender MM, Rubinger D, et al. Sodium-dependent idiopathic hypercalciuria in renal-stone formers. Lancet 1983;2:484–486.
56. Donaldson CL, Hulley SB, Vogel JM, et al. Effect of prolonged bed rest on bone mineral. Metabolism 1970;19:1071–1084.
57. Stewart AF, Ader M, Byers CM, et al. Calcium homeostasis in immobilization: An example of resorptive hypercalciuria. N Engl J Med 1982;306:1136–1140.
58. Heaney RP. Radiocalcium metabolism in disuse osteoporosis in man. Am J Med 1962;33:188–200.
59. Parks J, Coe F, Favus M. Hyperparathyroidism in nephrolithiasis. Arch Intern Med 1980;149:1479–1481.
60. Peacock M, Marshall RW, Robertson WG, et al. Chapter 35, Renal stone formation in primary hyperparathyroidism and idiopathic stone disease: Diagnosis, etiology and treatment, in Finlayson B, Thomas WC (eds): Colloquium on Renal Lithiasis. Gainesville, University Presses of Florida, 1976, p 339.
61. Parnell DC, Smith LC, Scholz DA, et al. Primary hyperparathyroidism: A prospective clinical study. Am J Med 1971;50: 670–678.
62. Ljunghall S, Danielson BG, Johansson G, et al. Renal stone formation in primary hyperparathyroidism: Role of tubular dysfunction urolithiasis, in Smith LH, Robertson WG, Finlayson B (eds): Clinical and Basic Research. New York, Plenum, 1980, p 89.
63. Broadus AE, Horst RL, Lang R, et al. The importance of circulating 1,25-dihydroxyvitamin D in the pathogenesis of hypercalciuria and renal stone formation in primary hyperparathyroidism. N Engl J Med 1980;302:421–426.
64. Pak CYC, Nicar MI, Peterson R, et al. A lack of unique pathophysiologic background for nephrolithiasis of primary hyperparathyroidism. J Clin Endocrinol Metab 1981;53:536–542.
65. Pak CYC, Holt K. Nucleation and growth of brushite and calcium oxalate in urine of stone-formers. Metabolism 1976;25: 665–673.
66. Smith LH, Van Den Berg CJ, Wilson DM, et al. Urolithiasis in primary hyperparathyroidism. Proc Am Soc Nephrol 1977;9A.
67. Avioli LV, McDonald JE, Signer RA. Excretion of pyrophosphate in disorders of bone metabolism. J Clin Endocrinol Metab 1965;25:912–915.
68. Russell RGG, Hodgkinson A. The urinary excretion of inorganic pyrophosphate in hyperparathyroidism, hyperthyroidism, Paget's disease and other disorders of bone metabolism. Clin Sci 1969;36:435–443.
69. Robertson WG, Knowles F, Peacock M. Urinary acid mucopolysaccharide inhibitors of calcium oxalate crystallization, in Fleisch H, Robertson WG, Smith LH, et al. (eds): Urolithiasis Research. New York, Plenum, 1976, p 331.

**70.** Battle DC, Arruda JAL. Renal tubular acidosis syndromes. Miner Electrolyte Metab 1981;5:83–99.

**71.** Szylman P, Better OS, Chaimowitz C, et al. Role of hyperkalemia in the metabolic acidosis of isolated hypoaldosteronism. N Engl J Med 1976;294:361–365.

**72.** Brenner RJ, Spring DB, Sebatian A, et al. Incidence of radiographically evident bone disease, nephrocalcinosis and nephrolithiasis in various types of renal tubular acidosis. N Engl J Med 1982;307:217–221.

**73.** Leman J, Wilz DR, Brenes LG. Acid, calcium and phosphorus balances in proximal renal tubular acidosis. Kidney Int 1976;10:561.

**74.** de Toni E, Nordio S. The relationship between calcium–phosphorus in metabolism, the "Krebs cycle" and steroid metabolism. Arch Dis Child 1959;34:371–382.

**75.** Milne MD, Stanbury SW, Thomson AE. Observations on the Fanconi syndrome and renal hyperchloremic acidosis in the adult. Q J Med 1952;21:61–82.

**76.** Schwartz WB. Case Records of the Massachusetts General Hospital. N Engl J Med 1958;259:392–400.

**77.** Mackenzie AR. Acetazolamide-induced renal stone. J Urol 1960;84:453–455.

**78.** Wallace MR, MacDiarmid I, Reeder J. Exacerbation of nephrolithiasis by a carbonic anhydrase inhibitor. NZ Med J 1974;79:687–690.

**79.** Harrison HE, Harrison HC. Inhibition of urine citrate excretion and the production of renal calcinosis in the rat by acetazolamide (Diamox) administration. J Clin Invest 1955;34:1662–1670.

**80.** Becker B, Middleton WH. Long-term acetazolamide (Diamox) administration in therapy of glaucoma. AMA Arch Ophthalmol 1955;54:187–192.

**81.** Sutton RAL, Dewar J, Walker VR, et al. Renal calculi and acetazolamide (ACZ) therapy. Proc Am Soc Nephrol 1982;44A.

**82.** Gennari FJ, Cohen JJ. Renal tubular acidosis. Ann Rev Med 1978;29:521–541.

**83.** Cinton-Nadal E, Lespier LE, Roman-Miranda A, et al. Renal acidifying ability in subjects with recurrent stone formation. J Urol 1977;118:704–706.

**84.** Buckalew VM, McCurdy DK, Ludwig GD, et al. Incomplete renal tubular acidosis: Physiologic studies in three patients with a defect in lowering urine pH. Am J Med 1968;45:32–42.

**85.** Buckalew VM, Purvis ML, Shulman MG, et al. Hereditary renal tubular acidosis: Report of a 64 member kindred with variable clinical expression including idiopathic hypercalciuria. Medicine 1974;53:229–254.

**86.** Hamed IA, Czerwinski AW, Coats B, et al. Familial absorptive hypercalciuria and renal tubular acidosis. Am J Med 1979;67:385–391.

**87.** Lemann J, Lennon EJ, Goodman AD, et al. The net balance of acid in subjects given large loads of acid or alkali. J Clin Invest 1965;44:507–517.

**88.** Coe FL, Parks JH. Stone disease in hereditary distal renal tubular acidosis. Ann Intern Med 1980;93:60–61.

**89.** Coe FL, Firpo JJ. Evidence for mild reversible hyperparathyroidism in distal renal tubular acidosis. Arch Intern Med 1975;135:1485–1489.

**90.** Goodman AD, Lemann J, Lennon EJ, et al. Production, excretion and net balance of fixed acid in patients with renal acidosis. J Clin Invest 1965;44:495–506.

**91.** Coe FL, Firpo JJ, Hollandswort DL, et al. Effects of acute and chronic metabolic acidosis on serum immunoreactive parathyroid hormone in man. Kidney Int 1975;8:262–273.

**92.** Lemann J, Litzow JR, Lennon EJ, et al. Studies of the mechanism by which chronic metabolic acidosis augments urinary calcium excretion in man. J Clin Invest 1967;46:1318–1328.

**93.** Sutton RAL, Wong NLM, Dirks JH. Effects of metabolic acidosis and alkalosis on sodium and calcium transport in the dog kidney. Kidney Int 1979;15:520–533.

**94.** Wallach S, Baker RK, Nicastri A. Primary renal tubular acidosis and secondary hyperparathyroidism. Am J Med 1972; 52:809–816.

**95.** Dent CE, Stamp TCB. Chapter 5, Vitamin D, rickets and osteomalacia, in Avioli LV, Krane SM (eds): Metabolic Bone Disease. New York, Academic, 1977, vol 1, pp 237–305.

**96.** Lee SW, Russell J, Avioli LV. 25-Hydroxycholecalciferol to 1,25-dihydroxycholecalciferol: Conversion impaired by systemic metabolic acidosis. Science 1977;195:994–996.

**97.** Langman CB, Bushinsky DA, Farris MI, et al. Ca and P regulation of $1,25(OH)_2D_3$ synthesis of vitamin D–replete rat tubules during acidosis. Am J Physiol 1986;251:F911–F918.

**98.** Dedmon RE, Wrong O. The excretion of organic anion in renal tubular acidosis with particular reference to citrate. Clin Sci 1962;22:19–32.

**99.** Simpson DP. Citrate excretion: A window on renal metabolism. Am J Physiol 1983;244:F223–F234.

**100.** McCurdy DK, Norman ME, Cohn R, et al. Urinary citrate: An alternate to $NH_4Cl$ loading in screening for familial distal (FD) renal tubular acidosis. Proc Am Soc Nephrol 1975;A19.

**101.** Coe FL. Chapter 6, Renal tubular acidosis, in: Nephrolithiasis: Pathogenesis and Treatment. Chicago, Year Book Medical Publishers, 1978, p 116.

**102.** Elliott JS, Quaide WL, Sharp RF, et al. Mineralogical studies of urine: The relationship of apatite, brushite and struvite to urinary pH. J Urol 1958;80:269–271.

**103.** Williams HE. Oxalic acid and the hyperoxaluric syndromes. Kidney Int 1976;13:410–419.

**104.** Brinkley L, McGuire J, Gregory J, et al. Bioavailability of oxalate in foods. Urology 1981;17:534–538.

**105.** Zarembski PM, Hodgkinson A. Some factors influencing the urinary excretion of oxalic acid in man. Clin Chim Acta 1969; 25:1–10.

**106.** Jaegger P, Portman L, Jacquet A-F, et al. Influence of the calcium content of the diet on the incidence of mild hyperoxaluria in idiopathic renal stone formers. Am J Nephrol 1985;5:40–44.

**107.** Lamden MP, Chrystowski GA. Urinary oxalate excretion in man following ascorbic acid ingestion. Proc Soc Exp Biol Med 1954;85:190–192.

**108.** Fituri N, Allavi N, Bently M. Urinary and plasma oxalate during ingestion of pure ascorbic acid: a re-evaluation. Eur Urol 1983;9:312–315.

**109.** Chalmers AH, Cowley DM, Brown JM. A possible etiological role for ascorbate in calculi formulation. Clin Chem 1986;32: 333–336.

**110.** Gershoff SN, Faragalla FF, Nelson DA, et al. Vitamin $B_6$ deficiency and oxalate nephrocalcinosis in the cat. Am J Med 1959;27:72–80.

**111.** Smith CL. Renal complication following jejunoileal bypass surgery, in Linner J (ed): Surgery for Obesity. New York, Springer-Verlag, 1984, pp 42–48.

**112.** Pak CYC, Fuller C. Idiopathic hypocitraturic calcium-oxalate nephrolithiasis successfully treated with potassium citrate. Ann Intern Med 1986;104:33–37.

**113.** Pak CYC, Sakhaee K, Crowther C, et al. Evidence justifying a high fluid intake in treatment of nephrolithiasis. Ann Intern Med 1980;93:36–39.

**114.** Stapleton FB, Roe HN, Roy S, et al. Hypercalciuria in children with urolithiasis. Am J Dis Child 1982;136:675–678.

115. Malek RS, Kelalis PP. Pediatric nephrolithiasis. J Urol 1975; 113:545–551.
116. Sandegaard E. Prognosis of stone in the ureter. Acta Chir Scand 1956;suppl 219;1–67.
117. Coe FL, Keck J, Norton ER. The natural history of calcium urolithiasis. JAMA 1977;239:1519–1523.
118. Pak CYC, Nicar M, Northcutt C. The definition of the mechanism of hypercalciuria is necessary for the treatment of recurrent stone formers. Contrib Nephrol 1982;33:136–151.
119. Pak CYC, Peters P, Hunt G, et al. Is selective therapy of recurrent nephrolithiasis possible? Am J Med 1981;71:615–622.
120. Elomaa I, Ala-Opas M, Porkka L. Five years of experience with selective therapy in recurrent calcium nephrolithiasis. J Urol 1984;132:656–661.
121. Nusiebeh I, Burr RG. The effects of varying water intake and of other measures on the relative saturation of stone-forming salts in the urine of spinal cord patients. Paraplegia 1979–1980; 17:363–370.
122. Boyce WH, Garvey FK, Goven CE. Abnormalities of calcium metabolism in patients with "idiopathic" urinary calculi. Effect of oral administration of sodium phytate. JAMA 1958;166: 1577–1583.
123. Nassim JR, Higgins B. Control of idiopathic hypercalciuria. Br Med J 1965;1:678–681.
124. Pak CYC. Sodium cellulose phosphate: Mechanism of action and effect on mineral metabolism. J Clin Pharmacol 1973;13: 15–27.
125. Pak CYC. Clinical pharmacology of sodium cellulose phosphate. J Clin Pharmacol 1979;19:451–457.
126. Blacklock NJ, MacLeod MA. The effect of cellulose phosphate on intestinal absorption and urinary excretion of calcium. Br J Urol 1974;46:385–392.
127. Pak CYC. Effects of cellulose phosphate and sodium phosphate on formation product and activity product of brushite in urine. Metabolism 1972;21:447–455.
128. Hayashi Y, Kaplan RA, Pak CYC. Effect of sodium cellulose phosphate therapy on crystallization of calcium oxalate in urine. Metabolism 1975;24:1273–1278.
129. Pak CYC, Delea CS, Barther FC. Successful treatment of recurrent nephrolithiasis (calcium stones) with cellulose phosphate. N Engl J Med 1974;290:175–180.
130. Ljunghall S, Backlman U, Danielson BG, et al. Prophylactic treatment of renal calcium stones. Experiences with dietary advice, cellulose phosphate and thiazides. Scand J Urol Nephrol 1980;53:239–248.
131. Backman U, Danielson BG, Johansson G, et al. Treatment of recurrent calcium stone formation with cellulose phosphate. J Urol 1980;123:9–13.
132. Desmars JF, Tawashi R. Dissolution and growth of calcium oxalate monohydrate. I. Effect of magnesium and pH. Biochim Biophys Acta 1973;313:256–267.
133. Bisaz S. Felix R, Neuman WF, et al. Quantitative determination of inhibitors of calcium phosphate precipitation in whole urine. Miner Electrolyte Metab 1978;1:74–83.
134. Pak CYC. A cautious use of sodium cellulose phosphate in the management of calcium nephrolithiasis. Invest Urol 1981;19: 187–190.
135. Van den Berg CJ, Kumar R, Wilson DM, et al. Orthophosphate therapy decreases urinary calcium excretion and serum 1,25-dihydroxyvitamin D concentrations in idiopathic hypercalciuria. J Clin Endocrinol Metab 1980;51:998–1001.
136. Bernstein DS, Newton R. The effect of oral sodium phosphate on the formation of renal calculi and on idiopathic hypercalciuria. Lancet 1966;2:1105–1107.
137. Pak CYC, Hold K, Zerwekh J, et al. Effects of orthophosphate therapy on the crystallization of calcium salt in urine. Miner Electrolyte Metab 1978;1:147–154.
138. Burdette DC, Thomas Jr WC, Finlayson B. Urinary supersaturation with calcium oxalate before and during orthophosphate therapy. J Urol 1976;115:418–422.
139. Fleisch H, Bisaz S, Core AD. Effect of orthophosphate on urinary pyrophosphate excretion and the prevention of urolithiasis. Lancet 1964;1:1065–1067.
140. Lau K, Wolf C, Nussbaum C, et al. Differing effects of acid versus neutral phosphate therapy of hypercalciuria. Kidney Int 1979;16:736–742.
141. Thomas Jr WC. Effectiveness and mode of action of orthophosphates in patients with calcareous renal calculi. Trans Am Clin Climatol Assoc 1971;83:113–124.
142. Edwards NA, Russell RGG, Hodgkinson A. The effect of oral phosphate in patients with recurrent renal calculus. Br J Urol 1965;37:390–398.
143. Oliver I, Weinberger A, Boi-Meir S, et al. Orthophosphate treatment of calcium lithiasis associated with idiopathic hypercalciuria. Urol Int 1974;29:414–420.
144. Ettinger B. Recurrent nephrolithiasis: Natural history and effect of phosphate therapy. Am J Med 1976;61:200–206.
145. Dudley FJ, Blackburn CRB. Extraskeletal calcification complicating oral neutral phosphate therapy. Lancet 1970;2:628–630.
146. Fleisch H, Russell RGG, Bisoy S, et al. The inhibitory effect of phosphonates on the formation of calcium phosphate crystals in vitro and on aortic and kidney calcification in vivo. Eur J Clin Invest 1970;1:12–18.
147. Francis MD, Russell RGG, Fleisch H. Diphosphonates inhibit formation of calcium phosphate crystals in vitro and pathological calcification in vivo. Science 1969;165:1264–1266.
148. Jowsey J, Riggs BL, Kelly PH, et al. The treatment of osteoporosis with disodium ethane-1-hydroxy-1,1-diphosphonate. J Lab Clin Med 1971;78:574–584.
149. Hofmann AF, Poley JR. Role of bile acid malabsorption in pathogenesis of diarrhea and steatorrhea in patients with ileal resection. I. Response to cholestyramine or replacement of dietary long chain triglyceride by medium chain triglyceride. Gastroenterology 1972;62:918–934.
150. Pinto B, Bernshtam J. Diethylaminoethanol-cellulose in the treatment of absorptive hyperoxaluria. J Urol 1978;119:630–632.
151. Gershoff SN, Mayer AL, Kulczycki LL. Effect of pyridoxine administration on the urinary excretion of oxalic acid, pyridoxine, and related compounds in mongoloids and nonmongoloids. Am J Clin Nutr 1959;7:76–79.
152. Balcke P, Schmidt P, Zazgornik J, et al. Pyridoxine therapy in patients with renal calcium oxalate calculi. Proc Eur Dial Transplant Assoc 1983;20:417–421.
153. Will EJ, Bijvoet OLM. Primary oxalosis: Clinical and biochemical response to high-dose pyridoxine therapy. Metabolism 1979;28:542–548.
154. Solomons CC, Goodman SI, Riley CM. Calcium carbimide in the treatment of primary hyperoxaluria. N Engl J Med 1967; 276:207–210.
155. Zarembski PM, Hodgkinson A, Chochran M. Treatment of primary hyperoxaluria with calcium carbimide. N Engl J Med 1967;277:1000–1002.
156. Hautmann R, Hering FJ, Lutzeyer W. Calcium oxalate stone disease: Effects and side effects of cellulose phosphate and succinate in long-term treatment of absorptive hypercalciuria or hyperoxaluria. J Urol 1978;120:712–715.
157. Pinto B, Ruiz-Marcellan FJ, Bernshtam J. Effect of a 5-year treatment program in patients with hyperoxaluric stones. J Urol 1983;130:943–945.

158. Yendt ER, Gagne RJA, Cohanim M. The effects of thiazides in idiopathic hypercalciuria. Am J Med Sci 1966;251:449–460.
159. Harrison AR, Rose GA. The effect of bendrofluazide on urinary and faecal calcium and phosphorus. Clin Sci 1968;34: 343–350.
160. Brickman AS, Massry SG, Coburn JW. Changes in serum and urinary calcium during treatment with hydrochlorothiazide: Studies on mechanisms. J Clin Invest 1972;51:945–954.
161. Zerwekh JE, Pak CYC. Selective effects of thiazide therapy on serum 1,25-dihydroxyvitamin D and intestinal calcium absorption in renal and absorptive hypercalciurias. Metabolism 1980; 29:13–17.
162. Barilla DE, Tolentino R, Kaplan RA, et al. Selective effects of thiazide on intestinal absorption of calcium in absorptive and renal hypercalciurias. Metabolism 1978;27:125–131.
163. Leppla D, Browne R, Hill K, et al. Effect of amiloride with or without hydrochlorothiazide on urinary calcium and saturation of calcium salts. J Clin Endocrinol Metab 1983;57:920–924.
164. Pylypchuk G, Ehrig U, Wilson DR. Effect of hydrochlorothiazide on urine saturation with brushite, in vitro collagen calcification by urine, and urinary inhibitors of collagen calcification. Can Med Assoc J 1978;118:792–797.
165. Pak CYC. Hydrochlorothiazide therapy in nephrolithiasis. Effect on the urinary activity product and formation product of brushite. Clin Pharmacol Ther 1973;14:209–217.
166. Yendt ER, Cohanim M. Prevention of calcium stones with thiazides. Kidney Int 1978;13:397–409.
167. Jorgensen FS. Effect of thiazide diuretics upon calcium metabolism. Dan Med Bull 1976;23:223–230.
168. Pak CYC, Ruskin B, Diller E. Enhancement of renal excretion of zinc by hydrochlorothiazide. Clin Chim Acta 1972;39:511–517.
169. Nicar MJ, Peterson R, Pak CYC. Use of potassium citrate as potassium supplement during thiazide therapy of calcium nephrolithiasis. J Urol 1984;131:430–433.
170. Yendt ER, Guay GF, Garcia DA. The use of thiazides in the prevention of renal calculi. Can Med Assoc J 1970;102:614–624.
171. Brocks P, Dahl C, Wolf H, et al. Do thiazides prevent idiopathic renal calcium stones? Lancet 1981;2:124–125.
172. Scholz D, Schurlle PO, Siegel A. Double-blind study with thiazide in recurrent calcium lithiasis. J Urol 1982;128:903–907.
173. Churchill DN, Taylor DW. Thiazides for patients with recurrent calcium stones: Still an open question. J Urol 1985;133: 749–751.
174. Hodgkinson A. Citric acid excretion in normal adults and in patients with renal calculus. Clin Sci 1962;23:203–212.
175. Nicar MJ, Skula C, Sakhaee K, et al. Low urinary citrate excretion in nephrolithiasis. Urology 1983;21:8–14.
176. Nordin BEC, Smith DA. Citric acid excretion in renal stone disease and in renal tubular acidosis. Br J Urol 1963;35:438–444.
177. Pak CYC, Sakhaee K, Fuller CJ. Physiological and physicochemical correction and prevention of calcium stone formation by potassium citrate therapy. Trans Assoc Am Physicians 1983;96:294–305.
178. Pak CYC, Fuller C, Sakhaee K, et al. Long-term treatment of calcium nephrolithiasis with potassium citrate. J Urol 1985; 134:11–19.
179. Prien Sr EL, Gershoff SF. Magnesium oxide–pyridoxine therapy for recurrent calcium oxalate calculi. J Urol 1974;112:509–512.
180. Gershoff SN, Prien EL. Effect of daily MgO and vitamin $B_6$ administration to patients with recurring calcium oxalate kidney stones. Am J Clin Nutr 1967;20:393–399.
181. Johansson G, Backman U, Danielson BG, et al. Biochemical and clinical effects of the prophylactic treatment of renal calcium stones with magnesium hydroxide. J Urol 1980;124: 770–774.
182. Moore CA, Bunce GE. Reduction in frequency of renal calculus formation by oral magnesium administration. Invest Urol 1964;2:7–13.
183. Melnick I, Landes RR, Hoffman AA, et al. Magnesium therapy for recurring calcium oxalate urinary calculi. J Urol 1971;105: 119–122.
184. Fetner CD, Barilla DE, Townsend J, et al. Effects of magnesium oxide on the crystallization of calcium salts in urine in patients with recurrent nephrolithiasis. J Urol 1978;120:399–401.
185. Scholz D, Schwiller PO, Engelhardt W, et al. Idiopathic uric acid lithiasis—some less known epidemiologic and metabolic findings, in Sperling O, Vahlensieck W (eds): Advances in Urology and Nephrology. Darmstadt, Steinkopff, 1981, vol 16, pp 66–69.
186. Cifuentes-Delatte L, Rapado A, Abehsera A, et al. Uric acid lithiasis and gout, in Cifuentes-Delatte L, Rapado A, Hodgkinson A (eds): Urinary Calculi International Symposium Renal Stone Research. Basel, Karger, 1973, pp 115–118.
187. Frank M, Lazebrik J, DeVries A. Uric acid lithiasis: A study of six hundred and twenty-two patients. Urol Int 1970;25:32–46.
188. Backman U, Danielson BG, Fellstrom B, et al. Kidney stone disease. Experiences from Uppsala, Sweden. Scand J Urol Nephrol 1980;53(suppl):207–211.
189. Sorenson LB. Role of the intestinal tract in the elimination of uric acid. Arthritis Rheum 1965;8:694–703.
190. Steele TH. Renal excretion of uric acid. Arthritis Rheum 1975; 18(suppl):793–804.
191. Weinman EJ, Knight TF. Renal tubular transport of urate. Miner Electrolyte Metab 1978;1:121–128.
192. Melick RA, Henneman PH. Clinical and laboratory studies of 207 consecutive patients in a kidney stone clinic. N Engl J Med 1958;259:307–314.
193. Sperling O, deVries A, Kedem O. Studies on the etiology of uric acid lithiasis. IV. Urinary non-dialyzable substances in idiopathic uric acid lithiasis. J Urol 1965;94:286–292.
194. Pinto B. Isolation and identification of uricine and its effect on uric acid precipitation, in Finlayson B, Thomas WC (eds): Colloquium on Renal Lithiasis. Gainesville, University Presses of Florida, 1976, pp 131–135.
195. Sperling O, deVries A, Studies on the etiology of uric acid lithiasis. Part II. Solubility of uric acid in urine specimens from normal subjects and patients with idiopathic uric acid lithiasis. J Urol 1964;92:331–334.
196. Coe FL, Strauss AL, Tembe V, et al. Uric acid saturation in calcium nephrolithiasis. Kidney Int 1980;17:662–668.
197. Bennett RC, Jepson RP. Uric acid stone formation following ileostomy. Aust NZ J Surg 1966;36:153–158.
198. Henneman PH, Wallach S, Demsey EF. The metabolic defect responsible for uric acid stone formation. J Clin Invest 1962;41: 537–542.
199. Pak Poy RK. Urinary pH in gout. Aust Ann Med 1965;4:35–39.
200. Gutman AB, Yu T. Urinary ammonium excretion in primary gout. J Clin Invest 1965;44:1474–1481.
201. Barzel US, Sperling O, Frank M, et al. Renal ammonium excretion and urinary pH in idiopathic uric acid lithiasis. J Urol 1964;92:1–5.
202. Metcalfe-Gibson A, McCallum FM, Morrison RBI, et al. Urinary excretion of hydrogen ion in patients with uric acid calculi. Clin Sci 1965;28:325–342.
203. Rapoport A, Crassweller PO, Hudson H, et al. The renal

excretion of hydrogen ion in uric acid stone formers. Metabolism 1967;16:176–188.
**204.** Plank GE, Durivage J, Lemieux G. Renal excretion of hydrogen in primary gout. Metabolism 1968;17:377–385.
**205.** Falls WF. Comparison of urinary acidification and ammonium excretion in normal and gouty subjects. Metabolism 1972;21:433–445.
**206.** Yu T-F, Gutman AB. Uric acid nephrolithiasis in gout: Predisposing factors. Ann Intern Med 1967;67:1133–1148.
**207.** Coe FL, Raisen L. Allopurinol treatment of uric-acid disorders in calcium-stone formers. Lancet 1973;1:129–131.
**208.** Fellstrom B, Bachman U, Danielson BG, et al. Urinary excretion of urate in renal calcium stone disease and in renal tubular acidification disturbances. J Urol 1982;127:589–592.
**209.** Coe FL, Kavalach AG. Hypercalciuria and hyperuricosuria in patients with calcium nephrolithiasis. N Engl J Med 1974;291:1344–1350.
**210.** Anton FM, Puig JG, Gaspar G, et al. Renal handling of uric acid in patients with recurrent calcium nephrolithiasis and hyperuricosuria. Nephron 1984;37:123–127.
**211.** Fellstrom B, Backman U, Danielson BG, et al. Renal handling of urate in patients with calcium stone disease. Nephron 1982;31:31–36.
**212.** Pak CYC, Waters O, Arnold L, et al. Mechanism for calcium urolithiasis among patients with hyperuricosuria: Supersaturation of urine with respect to monosodium urate. J Clin Invest 1977;59:426–431.
**213.** Pak CYC, Arnold LH. Heterogenous nucleation of calcium oxalate by seeds of monosodium urate. Proc Soc Exp Biol Med 1975;149:930–932.
**214.** Coe FL, Lawton RL, Goldstein RB, et al. Sodium urate accelerates precipitation of calcium oxalate in vitro. Proc Soc Exp Biol Med 1975;149:926–929.
**215.** Pak CYC, Holt K, Zerwekh JE. Attenuation by monosodium urate of the inhibitory effect of glycosaminoglycans on calcium oxalate nucleation. Invest Urol 1979;17:138–140.
**216.** Bowyer RC, Brockis JG, McCulloch RK. Glycosaminoglycans as inhibitors of calcium oxalate crystal growth and aggregation. Clinica Chim Acta 1979;25:23–28.
**217.** Pak CYC, Barilla DE, Holt K, et al. Effect of oral purine load and allopurinol on the crystallization of calcium salts in urine of patients with hyperuricosuric calcium urolithiasis. Am J Med 1978;65:593–599.
**218.** Cox FL, Raisen L. Allopurinol treatment of uric acid disorders in calcium stone formers. Lancet 1973;1:129–131.
**219.** Smith MJV. Placebo versus allopurinol for renal calculi. J Urol 1977;117:690–692.
**220.** Neto M, Pilloff B, Simon JA. Dissolution of renal uric acid calculus with allopurinol and alkalinization of urine: A case report. J Urol 1976;115:740–741.
**221.** deVries A, Frank M. Prophylaxis of idiopathic and gouty uric acid lithiasis by allopurinol. Urol Int 1967;22:506–516.
**222.** Hande KR, Noone RM, Stone WJ. Severe allopurinol toxicity. Description and guidelines for prevention in patients with renal insufficiency. Am J Med 1984;76:47–56.
**223.** Seegmiller JE. Xanthine stone formation. Am J Med 1968;45: 780–783.
**224.** Greene ML, Fujimoto WY, Seegmiller JE. Urinary xanthine stones—a rare complication of allopurinol therapy. N Engl J Med 1969;280:426–427.
**225.** Landgrebe AR, Nyhan WL, Coleman M. Urinary-tract stones resulting from the excretion of oxypurinol. N Engl J Med 1975;292:626–627.
**226.** Kranen S, Keough D, Gordon RB, et al. Xanthine-containing calculi during allopurinol therapy. J Urol 1985;133:658–659.
**227.** Lewis RW, Roth Jr JK, Polanco EJ, et al. Molar lactate in the management of uric acid renal obstruction. J Urol 1981;125:87–90.
**228.** Freed SZ. Alternating use of an alkalinizing salt and acetazolamide in the management of cystine and uric acid stones. J Urol 1975;113:96–99.
**229.** Sakhaee K, Nicar M, Hill K, et al. Contrasting effects of potassium citrate and sodium citrate therapies on urinary chemistries and crystallization of stone-forming salts. Kidney Int 1983;24:348–352.
**230.** Smith AD, Lee WJ. Percutaneous stone removal procedures including irrigation. Urol Clin North Am 1983;10:719–727.
**231.** Freida FS, Hermady K. Dissolution of uric acid stones. Alternative to surgery. Urology 1976;8:334–335.
**232.** Spataro RF, Linke CA, Basbaric ZL. Use of percutaneous nephrostomy and urinary alkalinization in the dissolution of obstructing uric acid stone. Diagn Radiol 1978;129:629–632.
**233.** Gordon MR, Carrian HM, Politano VA. Dissolution of uric acid calculi with Tham irrigation. Urology 1978;12:395–397.
**234.** Bailey RR, Dann E, Greenslade NF, et al. Renal stones: A prospective study of 350 patients. NZ Med J 1974;79:961–965.
**235.** Modlin M. Renal stone: A study of 520 patients with special reference to the pattern of recurrence. S Afr Med J 1957;312: 824–828.
**236.** Coe FL. Chapter 1, Clinical and laboratory assessment of patients with kidney stones, in: Nephrolithiasis: Pathogenesis and Treatment. Chicago, Year Book Medical Publishers, 1978, p 5.
**237.** Griffith DP, Musker DM. Prevention of infected urinary stones by urease inhibition. Invest Urol 1973;11:228–233.
**238.** Robertson WG, Peacock M, Nordin BEC. Activity products in stone-forming and non–stone–forming urine. Clin Sci 1968;34: 579–594.
**239.** Griffith DP, Musker DM, Itin C. Urease: The primary cause of infection-induced urinary stones. Invest Urol 1976;13:346–350.
**240.** Griffith DP, Bruce RR, Fishbein WN. Chapter 11, Infection (urease)-induced stones, in Coe FL, Brenner M, Stein JH (eds): Contemporary Issues in Nephrology: Nephrolithiasis. New York, Churchill Livingstone, 1980, vol 5, p 230.
**241.** Masover GK, Sawyer JE, Hayflick L. Urea-hydrolyzing activity of a T-strain mycoplasma: *Ureaplasma urealyticum*. J Bacteriol 1976;125:581–587.
**242.** Petterson S, Bronson JE, Grenbaro L, et al. *Ureaplasma urealyticum* in infectious urinary tract stones. Lancet 1983;1: 526–527.
**243.** McLean RJC, Nickel JC, Noakes VC, et al. An in vitro ultrastructural study of infectious kidney stone genesis. Infect Immun 1985;49:805–811.
**244.** Nemoy NJ, Stamey TA. Surgical, bacteriological and biochemical management of "infection stones." JAMA 1971;215: 1470–1476.
**245.** Cox CE. Urinary tract infection and renal lithiasis. Urol Clin North Am 1974;1:279–297.
**246.** Singh M, Chapman R, Tresidder GC, et al. The fate of unoperated staghorn calculus. Br J Urol 1973;45:581–585.
**247.** Wojewski A, Zajaczkowski T. The treatment of bilateral staghorn calculi of the kidneys. Int Urol Nephrol 1974;5:249–260.
**248.** Androulakis P, Frangoulis E, Lefkidis C, et al. Kidney damage in recurrent lithiasis: A survey of 175 cases with clinicopathological observations. Eur Urol 1982;8:261–264.
**249.** Maddern JP. Surgery of the staghorn calculus. Br J Urol 1967;39:237–275.
**250.** Stephenson TP, Bauer S, Hargreave TB, et al. Technique and results of pyelocalycotomy for staghorn calculi. Br J Urol 1975;47:751–758.

251. Bueschen AJ, Zahm MJ, Lloyd LK. Adjuvant surgical techniques in the removal of staghorn calculi. J Urol 1980;123:342–344.
252. Resnick MI, Kursh ED, Cohen AM. Use of computerized tomography in the delineation of uric acid calculi. J Urol 1984;131:9–10.
253. Silverman DE, Stamey TA. Management of infection stones: The Stanford experience. Medicine 1983;62:44–51.
254. Suby HI, Albright F. Dissolution of phosphatic urinary calculi by the retrograde introduction of a citrate solution containing magnesium. N Engl J Med 1943;228:81–91.
255. Dretler SP, Pfister RC, Newhouse JH. Renal-stone dissolution via percutaneous nephrostomy. N Engl J Med 1979;300:341–343.
256. Fostvedt GA, Barnes RW. Complications during lavage therapy for renal calculi. J Urol 1963;89:329–331.
257. Kohler FP. Renacidin and tissue reaction. J Urol 1962;87:102–105.
258. Fam B, Rossier AB, Yalla S, et al. Role of hemiacidrin in the management of renal stones in spinal cord injury patients. J Urol 1976;116:696–698.
259. Lavengood Jr RW, Marshall VF. Prevention of renal phosphatic calculi in the presence of infection by the Shor regimen. J Urol 1972;108:368–371.
260. McDonald DF, Murphy GP. Bacteriostatic and acidifying effects of methiamine, hydrolyzed casein, and ascorbic acid on the urine. N Engl J Med 1959;261:803–805.
261. Murphy FJ, Zelman S, Man W. Ascorbic acid as a urinary acidifying agent: Its adjunctive role in chronic urinary infection. J Urol 1965;94:300–305.
262. Nahata MC, Shimp L, Lampman T. Effect of ascorbic acid on urine pH in man. Am J Hosp Pharm 1977;34:1234–1237.
263. Travis LB, Dodge WF, Minotz AA. Urinary acidification with ascorbic acid. J Pediatr 1965;67:1176–1178.
264. Trang JM, Blanchard J, Conrad KA, et al. Effect of dietary ascorbic acid restriction and supplementation in urine pH in elderly males. JAMA 1984;252:2960–2961.
265. Fishbein WN, Carbone PP. Urease catalysis. II. Inhibition of the enzyme by hydroxyurea, hydroxylamine and acetohydroxamic acid. J Biol Chem 1965;240:2407–2414.
266. Musker DM, Saenz C, Griffith DP. Interaction between acetohydroxamic acid and 12 antibiotics against 14 gram-negative pathogenic bacteria. Antimicrob Agents Chemother 1974;5:106–110.
267. Maclaren DM. Influence of acetohydroxamic acid on experimental proteus pyelonephritis. Invest Urol 1974;12:146–149.
268. Aranson M, Medalia O, Griffel B. Prevention of ascending pyelonephritis in mice by urease inhibitors. Nephron 1974;12:94–104.
269. Smith MJV. Management of infected stone disease with hydroxyurea: A five year follow-up. Proc Eur Dial Transplant Assoc 1983;20:466–468.
270. Griffith DP, Gibson JR, Clinton CW, et al. Acetohydroxamic acid: Clinical studies of a urease inhibitor in patients with staghorn renal calculi. J Urol 1978;119:9–15.
271. Rodman JS, Williams JJ, Peterson CM. Partial dissolution of struvite calculus with oral acetohydroxamic acid. Urology 1983;22:410–412.
272. Williams JJ, Rodman JS, Peterson CM. A randomized, double-blind study of acetohydroxamic acid in struvite nephrolithiasis. N Engl J Med 1984;311:760–764.
273. Burr RG, Naseibeh I. Effect of oral acetohydroxamic acid on urinary saturation in stone-forming spinal cord patients. Br J Urol 1983;55:162–165.
274. Halperin EC, Thier SO. Cystinuria, in Coe FL, Brenner M, Stein JH (eds): Contemporary Issues in Nephrology: Nephrolithiasis. New York, Churchill Livingstone, 1980, vol 5, pp 208–230.
275. Labeeuw C, Gerbaulet C, Pozet C, et al. Cystine crystalluria and urinary saturation in cystine and non-cystine stone formers. Urol Res 1981;9:163–168.
276. Kolb FO, Earll JM, Harper HA. "Disappearance" of cystinuria in a patient treated with prolonged low methionine diet. Metabolism 1967;16:378–381.
277. Zinnser HA. Effect of oral choline in reducing cystine excretion in cystinuria. J Urol 1950;63:929–935.
278. Miyagi K, Nakada F, Oshiro S. Effect of glutamine on cystine excretion in a patient with cystinuria. N Engl J Med 1977;30:196–198.
279. Miyagi K, Nakoda F. Amino acid reabsorption in cystinuria: The effects of monoaminodicarboxylic acids and amido group amino acids with special reference to glutamine. J Jpn Soc Intern Med 1978;67:694–702.
280. Skouby R, Rosenberg LE, Thier SO. No effect of L-glutamine on cystinuria. N Engl J Med 1980;302:236–237.
281. Dahlberg PJ, Van Den Berg CJ, Kurtz SB, et al. Clinical features and management of cystinuria. Mayo Clin Proc 1977;52:533–542.
282. Kean WF, Dwosh IL, Anastassiades TP, et al. Toxicity pattern of D-penicillamine therapy. Arthritis Rheum 1980;23:158–164.
283. Hautmann R, Terhorst B, Stuhlsatz HW, et al. Mercaptopropionyl-glycine: A progress in cystine stone therapy. J Urol 1977;117:628–630.
284. Mulvaney WP, Quilter T, Montera A. Experiences with acetylcysteine in cystinuric patients. J Urol 1975;114:107–108.
285. Stark H, Savir A. Dissolution of cystine calculi by pelviocaliceal irrigation with D-penicillamine. J Urol 1980;124:895–898.
286. Smith AD, Lange PH, Miller RP, et al. Dissolution of cystine calculi by irrigation with acetylcystine through percutaneous nephrostomy. Urology 1979;13:422–423.
287. Tseng CA, Talwalkon YB, Tank EJ, et al. Dissolution of cystine calculi by pelviocaliceal irrigation with tromethamine-E. J Urol 1982;128:1281–1284.

# Chapter 38 / Glomerulonephritis

Charles Halstenson, PharmD, B. L. Kasiske, MD, and William F. Keane, MD

In the first half of the nineteenth century, Richard Bright described the clinical and pathological findings associated with primary glomerular injury; however, not until the middle of the twentieth century were techniques developed that permitted an accurate description of the clinical presentation and natural history of glomerular diseases. Critical to an understanding of human glomerular diseases were the development of immunofluorescence microscopy and the widespread application of percutaneous renal biopsy (1960s).

Knowledge of the pathogenesis of immune-mediated renal disease was significantly advanced by the pioneering studies of serum sickness in rabbits by Dixon et al[1] and Germuth.[2] In these studies the intravenous administration of a foreign antigenic substance, such as bovine serum albumin, led to the formation of antibodies, which then formed antigen–antibody complexes in the circulatory system. It was proposed that the entrapment of these circulating complexes in the glomerulus led to structural injury of the glomerulus.

A much broader understanding of the pathogenesis of immune-mediated renal diseases has developed through rapid advances in the fields of cell biology, immunology, and physiology.[3] In this chapter, the pathogenesis of, clinical presentation of, and therapeutic approaches to frequently encountered glomerular diseases are reviewed.

## Epidemiology

It is difficult to determine the precise incidence of a specific type of renal disease in the general population. Genetic background, as well as host and environmental factors, influences the type and expression of renal disease. The availability of relevant medical care also influences incidence and prevalence data; however, with the development of programs worldwide for the treatment of renal failure, the magnitude of the problem has become evident. Although the precise incidence of chronic renal failure is unknown, approximately 120 people per million develop renal failure each year. In the United States, end-stage renal disease remains the fourth leading cause of death among young adults. Also, in this country alone, there are nearly 80,000 people currently being treated for chronic renal failure by maintenance dialysis or transplantation. About 60% of such patients develop renal failure as a consequence of immunologically mediated glomerular disease.

## Pathophysiology

### *Structure and Function*

An understanding of renal disease requires basic knowledge of the structure and function of the glomerulus. The glomerulus is a unique capillary bed that excludes macromolecules larger than albumin, but allows nonprotein plasma constituents to pass freely. Thus, the glomerular filtration barrier functions as a size-selective barrier that allows water to easily pass while retaining large macromolecules in the circulation. The ultrafiltrate undergoes a series of reabsorptive and secretory processes to form urine. It is through this mechanism that salt and water homeostasis is maintained and the body is rid of a variety of toxic waste materials.

The glomerulus consists of two important components (Fig. 38.1): the filtration barrier and the mesangium. The filtration barrier is composed of three well-defined layers: endothelium, glomerular basement membrane (GBM), and epithelial cells that contain specialized extensions embedded in the outer layer of the GBM.[3] It is across this barrier that fluid flow, which ultimately forms ultrafiltrate, occurs. Under normal conditions, the GBM is believed to function as a compact hydrated gel with a porelike structure. Currently, it is believed that the mesangium not only supports the glomerular capillaries but also modulates flow through these capillaries.

Several studies have demonstrated the presence of fixed, negatively charged sites within glomeruli. These charge sites are detectable in all three layers of the capillary wall: the endothelium, the epithelium, and the GBM. Biochemical and cytochemical studies have shown that the epithelial cell coat is composed of a negatively charged glycoprotein (podocalyxin), made up largely of sialic acid. In addition, the GBM contains an abundance of negatively charged sulfated glycosaminoglycans. These studies have led investigators to conclude that the glomerular filtration barrier functions as both a charge- and a size-selective barrier.[3]

### *Mechanisms of Glomerular Injury*

In its role as a sophisticated ultrafilter, the glomerular capillary is particularly susceptible to immune-mediated injury. Three important mechanisms can induce parenchymal damage (Table 38.1): circulating immune complexes, in situ antigen–antibody interaction, and cell-mediated mechanisms. The first step in the initiation of glomerulonephritis is the production of antibody to an antigen that is recognized as foreign by the host. This antigen may be endogenous or exogenous. For example, endogenous antigens may be intrinsic glomerular antigens or previously sequestered antigens, such as DNA or thyroglobulin. Exogenous antigens are most often viral, bacterial, parasitic, or fungal in origin (Table 38.2). Classically, it has been considered that antigen–antibody complexes are formed in the circulation and then passively entrapped in the glomerulus. Alternatively, recent experimental data have supported the notion that antibodies combine with endogenous glomerular antigens or

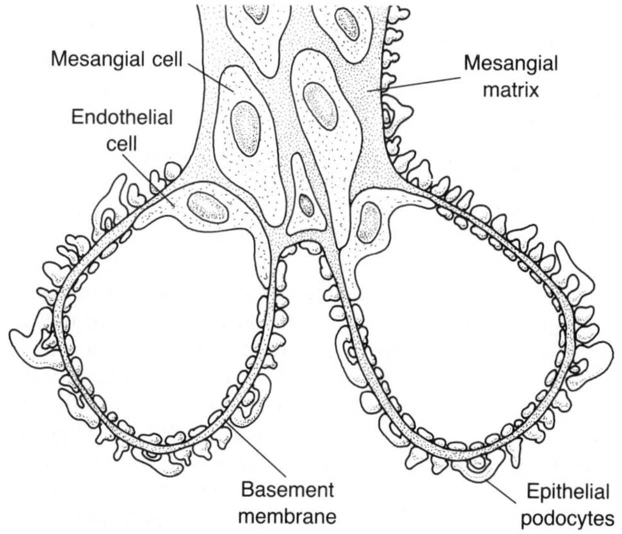


**Figure 38.1** Schematic representation of glomerulus.

**Table 38.2** Antigens Possibly Involved in Immune-Mediated Glomerular Injury

| *Source of antigen* | *Clinical example* |
|---|---|
| **Endogenous Antigens** | |
| Released sequestered cellular antigens | DNA, thyroglobulin |
| Endogenous antigens modified by exogenous source | IgG modified by streptococcal neuroaminidase |
| Tumor antigens | CEA,[a] bronchial and other solid tumors |
| Intrinsic glomerular antigens | Goodpasture's syndrome |
| **Exogenous** | |
| Viral | Hepatitis B |
| Bacterial | Streptococcal organisms |
| Parasitic | Malaria |
| Fungal | *Candida* |

[a] CEA, carcinoembryonic antigen.

exogenous antigens entrapped in the glomerulus and form complexes locally, or in situ.[4] Regardless of the mechanism of formation, these antigen–antibody complexes can be localized along the capillary loop or the mesangium (Fig. 38.1) and are detected by use of immunofluorescence microscopy. Subsequent to antigen–antibody formation, a series of biologic events are triggered that ultimately lead to glomerular injury. This damage is mediated by both humoral and cellular mechanisms. Neutrophils, monocytes, and platelets have been shown to participate in this injury. In addition, the complement and coagulation systems, as well as vasoactive substances, have been proven to participate in immune-mediated injury to the glomerulus.[5] Recently, both macrophages and lymphocytes have been shown to participate in glomerular injury, suggesting an important role for cell-mediated mechanisms.[6,7] This greater understanding of these various pathophysiologic events has allowed therapeutic interventions to be attempted in human renal diseases.

Glomerular injury is often manifested as proteinuria and hematuria. The precise mechanism of hematuria is unknown; however, red blood cells may escape from the capillary lumen into the tubules and urine via gaps in the capillary wall caused by inflammatory injury. The hallmark of glomerular disease is the presence of proteinuria. Recent studies have suggested that abrogation of both the size- and charge-selective properties of the filtration barrier are important pathogenic mechanisms in permitting protein to enter the urine. Indeed, decreases in the fixed negative charge of the filtration barrier, as well as increased size of "pores" in the GBM, may result in proteinuria.

**Table 38.1** Immunologic Mechanisms of Glomerular Injury

| |
|---|
| Circulating immune complexes |
| In situ antigen–antibody interaction |
| Intrinsic glomerular antigen, e.g., GBM antigens |
| Exogenous planted antigens |
| Cell-mediated mechanism |

## Classification/Clinical Presentation

### *Approach to the Patient*

Various classifications of renal disease have been proposed. Some are purely morphologic classifications; others use the manner in which the patient clinically presents. For purposes of this discussion, glomerular disease has been classified according to the manner in which the patient is most likely to present to the physician (Table 38.3). Although not all patients with glomerular disease have proteinuria, most will excrete more than 500 mg per 24 hours. In the initial evaluation of proteinuria and suspected glomerular disease, patients can be divided into two groups: patients with only proteinuria, and patients with significant abnormalities in the urine sediment, for example, red blood cells, white blood cells, or casts (Fig. 38.2). Each group may then be further categorized according to whether or not a patient exhibits clinical evidence of a systemic disease (Fig. 38.2).

### *Determining Presence or Absence of Systemic Disease*

Patients with proteinuria, but few other abnormalities (based on examination of the urine sediment), may present in one of several ways. In fact, the clinical presentation may provide useful diagnostic information (Fig. 38.2). Patients may present with the nephrotic syndrome, that is, urine protein excretion greater than 3 g per 24 hours. Patients with the nephrotic syndrome often have poor appetite, fatigue, weight gain, edema, hypoalbuminemia, and hyperlipidemia. These findings are nonspecific and result from the massive amount of protein lost in the urine. If no other findings suggest a systemic disease as causing the nephrotic syndrome, a renal

**Table 38.3** Clinical Classification of Glomerular Diseases

**Isolated Proteinuria (With or Without Nephrotic Syndrome)**
- Without systemic disease
  - Idiopathic nephrotic syndrome
    - Minimal-change nephropathy
    - Focal glomerulosclerosis
    - Mesangial proliferative nephritis
  - Membranous nephropathy
- With systemic diseases
  - Amyloidosis
  - Diabetes mellitus

**Active Urine Sediment (Red Cells, Red Cell Casts, Proteinuria)**
- Without systemic disease
  - IgA nephropathy
  - Membranoproliferative glomerulonephritis
  - Anti-GBM glomerulonephritis
  - Poststreptococcal glomerulonephritis
- With systemic disease
  - Systemic lupus erythematosus (collagen/vascular disease)
  - Vasculitis syndrome (polyarteritis nodosa, Wegener's granulomatosis)
  - Rapidly progressive glomerulonephritis
  - Thrombotic thrombocytopenic purpura
  - Hemolytic–uremic syndrome
  - Goodpasture's syndrome
  - Infection-related glomerulonephritis (bacterial endocarditis, ventriculoatrial shunt nephritis)

biopsy is likely to disclose either idiopathic nephrotic syndrome or membranous nephropathy (Table 38.3, Fig. 38.2).

Patients with the nephrotic syndrome may also have clinical signs and symptoms that reveal an underlying systemic disease (Table 38.3, Fig. 38.2). For example, diabetes mellitus may cause massive proteinuria with few other urine sediment abnormalities. Patients with diabetes and proteinuria usually have long-standing disease with evidence of other diabetic organ damage. Hypertension, peripheral neuropathy, and diabetic retinopathy are often evident. Systemic amyloidosis is another disease that may cause massive proteinuria with few other urine sediment abnormalities. Amyloidosis may be seen in patients with an underlying chronic disease, such as rheumatoid arthritis, or may occur as a primary disease process. In either case, amyloid infiltration may result in dysfunction of several organ systems.

Patients with proteinuria and an active urine sediment may present with clinical signs and symptoms of a systemic disease (Fig. 38.2). For example, characteristic facial skin rash may suggest systemic lupus erythematosus (SLE). Raised erythematous patches on the skin (palpable purpura) may indicate a small vessel vasculitis, for example, mixed essential cryoglobulinemia or Henoch–Schönlein purpura. Also, the presence of arthritis may suggest an underlying systemic disorder. Collagen vascular diseases, such as SLE or vasculitis, are often associated with signs and symptoms of joint inflammation. Pulmonary symptoms and abnormal chest x-rays may be seen in patients with collagen vascular disease, vasculitis, and Goodpasture's syndrome. Other signs and symptoms of systemic disease may also be helpful to diagnosis. Fever, weight loss, pericarditis, sinusitis, neu-

**Figure 38.2** Glomerulonephritis: clinical presentation. GN, glomerulonephritis; MPGN, membranoproliferative glomerulonephritis; SLE, systemic lupus erythematosus; SBE, subacute bacterial endocarditis; GBM, glomerular basement membrane; TTP, thrombotic thrombocytopenic purpura; HUS, hemolytic–uremic syndrome; AP, anaphylactoid purpura.

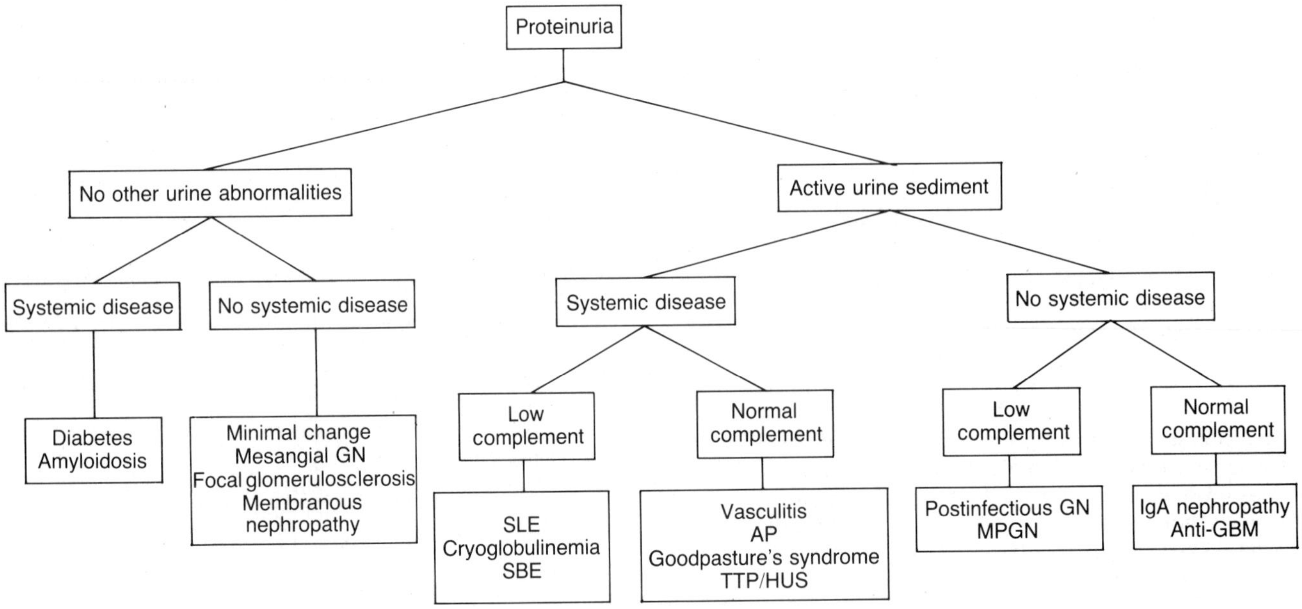

**Table 38.4** Diagnostic Considerations of Renal Diseases Based on Serum Complement Levels

| *Low serum complement level* | *Normal serum complement level* |
|---|---|
| Systemic diseases | Systemic diseases |
| Systemic lupus erythematosus | Vasculitis group |
| Infection-related glomerulonephritis | Polyarteritis nodosa |
| Subacute bacterial endocarditis | Hypersensitivity vasculitis |
| "Shunt" nephritis | Wegener's granulomatosis |
| Cryoglobulinemia | Henoch–Schönlein purpura |
| Primary renal diseases | Goodpasture's syndrome |
| Acute poststreptococcal glomerulonephritis | Primary renal diseases |
| Membranoproliferative glomerulonephritis | IgA nephropathy |
| | Idiopathic rapidly progressive glomerulonephritis |
| | Idiopathic nephrotic syndrome |

rologic abnormalities, and gastrointestinal dysfunction occurring in a patient with proteinuria and an active sediment may all suggest an underlying systemic disorder.

Proteinuria and an active urine sediment may also occur in patients without any of the aforementioned signs and symptoms of systemic disease. Such patients may be asymptomatic or may have a "nephrotic" presentation. Edema, weight gain, decreased urine output, hypertension, and dark-colored urine are often present in these patients.

Measuring serum complement levels is frequently the next step in defining the correct diagnosis. Serum complement levels are characteristically depressed in some glomerular diseases (Table 38.4). In addition, the presence of anti–group B streptococcal antigens, circulating anti-GBM antibodies, or a family history of renal disease may suggest the final diagnosis.

### *Renal Biopsy*

Although diagnosis of the underlying cause of proteinuria and glomerular disease may be possible from the clinical evaluation just described, more often uncertainty persists. In such cases, a percutaneous renal biopsy may provide the definitive diagnosis. The decision to perform a biopsy is based on the risk/benefit ratio. While biopsy may provide information that indicates the most appropriate treatment, some risk is involved. The most common complication of biopsy is hematuria, which may necessitate transfusion in as many as 1.0% of patients biopsied.[8] Though rare, severe hematuria may require treatment with nephrectomy. Mortality from renal biopsy is probably less than 0.1%.[8] Biopsy is contraindicated in patients with a solitary kidney, uncontrolled hypertension, coagulation defects, or poor cooperation. Morphologic diagnosis can usually be made if tissue is examined with light, immunofluorescence, and electron microscopic technique.

### *Course/Prognosis*

The course and prognosis of glomerular disease are extremely variable and depend on the underlying cause. Minimal proteinuria in patients without other urine sediment abnormalities may be relatively benign and require no treatment. The idiopathic nephrotic syndrome (Table 38.3) caused by minimal-change disease often responds to treatment with corticosteroids and has a favorable prognosis, whereas the variant mesangial proliferative disease is somewhat less responsive to treatment, but may also have a favorable outcome. Focal glomerulosclerosis usually does not respond to therapeutic measures and end-stage renal disease is usually the ultimate outcome. Both diabetes and systemic amyloidosis also frequently result in renal failure.

Proteinuria and glomerular diseases associated with a systemic disease may respond favorably to specific therapeutic measures (see later). For example, Goodpasture's syndrome, systemic lupus erythematosus, and systemic vasculitis, all once fatal, may respond favorably to immunosuppressive therapy.

The course and prognosis of glomerulonephritis not associated with systemic disease are extremely variable. Poststreptococcal glomerulonephritis usually has a benign course if complications are carefully managed. Other causes of infection-related glomerulonephritis require specific antibiotic treatment of the underlying infection. In contrast, hereditary nephritis and membranoproliferative glomerulonephritis usually progress to end-stage renal disease. IgA nephropathy is often self-limited, but may lead to renal failure in approximately 15% to 25% of patients.

A unique clinical presentation of glomerular diseases is defined by the syndrome of rapidly progressive glomerulonephritis (RPGN). This presentation usually leads to renal failure in a period of a few months or even a few days. Glomerular diseases associated with RPGN must be treated quickly and aggressively. Although RPGN may be associated with many renal diseases, the most common causes of RPGN include Goodpasture's syndrome, anti-GBM disease, and systemic vasculitis (Table 38.3).

## Treatment

### *Rationale*

The treatment of glomerulonephritis is dependent, in part, on the clinical–histologic category into which it is placed. Careful attention to blood pressure normalization, as well as fluid and electrolyte status, is important in therapy. A variety of therapeutic approaches, including use of corticosteroids and immunosuppressive agents, are commonly used in the treatment of glomerulonephritis; however, it should be recognized that few studies have been performed to define their precise therapeutic efficacy. Plasmapheresis, a relatively new treatment, is a mechanical means of removing substantial volumes from a patient's intravascular fluid compartment and replacing the fluid with a suitable colloid. This technique has been used to remove pathogenic circulating agents such as autoantibodies or immune complexes. Unfortunately, the efficacy of this approach has been clearly demonstrated only in certain clinical syndromes.

The mechanisms of glomerular disease have not been fully explained, although many factors in the immune and inflammatory responses have been identified. These data form the basis for development of different therapeutic regimens. For example, corticosteroids may impact on both immune and inflammatory responses, while many of the cytotoxic drugs influence cellular and humoral immune responses. Various agents that influence coagulation pathways have been used with some success in experimental, as well as human, glomerulonephritis. On the other hand, patients with severe nephrotic syndrome frequently tend to develop vascular thrombosis and embolic disease secondary to a hypercoagulable state. In these patients, anticoagulant agents are required.

Corticosteroids possess both anti-inflammatory and immunosuppressive properties and, therefore, have been employed in a number of inflammatory diseases. The mechanisms by which they produce these effects have not been fully explained. Corticosteroids increase the number of circulating polymorphonuclear leukocytes (PMNs) in the peripheral blood.[9] The increased number results from an accelerated release of cells from the marrow pool and a decreased egress of PMNs from the circulating pool to tissue sites. This delayed egress of PMNs from the circulating pool and subsequent failure to reach an inflammatory site constitute one of the major mechanisms by which corticosteroids prevent inflammatory response. Functional capabilities of the PMNs, such as phagocytosis or bactericidal activity, are relatively unaltered by the standard therapeutic doses of corticosteroids. In contrast to their effect on PMNs, corticosteroids produce a monocytopenia and also inhibit monocyte chemotaxis and bactericidal activity.[9] Secondary tissue damage from the rupture of lysosomes after cellular injury and the accompanying inflammatory response can be modified or eliminated by high concentrations of corticosteroids.[9]

Corticosteroids, in addition to their effect on the inflammatory limb, may inhibit the generation of the immune response in at least three ways: (1) by affecting the processing of the antigen or the release of endogenous antigens, (2) by affecting the function of lymphoid cells and their movement from circulation into the sites where localized cell-mediated immune responses may arise, and (3) by altering the removal and metabolism of immune complexes. The onset of the immunosuppressive effects of corticosteroids is rapid, in contrast to the more delayed onset of the immunosuppressive effects of cytotoxic agents.[9]

Cytotoxic agents were initially developed for use in neoplastic diseases, but because of the observed suppression of the immune system by these agents, they have been employed in the treatment of a number of inflammatory diseases. Several classes of cytotoxic agents are used, including alkylating agents, such as cyclophosphamide and chlorambucil, and antimetabolites, such as azathioprine. The action and the treatment of immunologic renal disease seem to be directed at the cellular limb of the immune response. Azathioprine significantly decreases monocyte function and inhibits sensitization of the lymphocytes.[10] Cyclophosphamide has a more direct effect on lymphocytes, whether they are active or inactive; thus, it is more likely to be effective in treating established autoimmune disease. Cyclophosphamide also alters the circulating pool of mononuclear cells, producing both monocytopenia and lymphocytopenia.[11]

Antiplatelet agents have also been used in the treatment of glomerular disease. It has been shown that platelets are activated in glomerular disease and that platelet factors can cause arteriolar smooth muscle cell proliferation and alter vascular permeability. In addition, increased platelet consumption occurs in various vascular and renal diseases.

Nonsteroidal anti-inflammatory agents are known to decrease prostaglandin production by inhibition of the cyclooxygenase pathway. This decrease in urinary prostaglandin levels may be associated with a decrease in glomerular filtration rate. Nonsteroidal anti-inflammatory agents affect the function of certain prostaglandin-modulated immune responses. Hence, they exert an anti-inflammatory response. Nonsteroidal anti-inflammatory agents may also alter capillary wall permeability, leading to a decrease in protein excretion. This latter effect has prompted their use in patients with severe nephrotic syndrome secondary to focal glomerulosclerosis.

Glomerulonephritis may occur in association with a variety of clinical diseases, but in only a limited number has therapy been of proven benefit. Few studies are available that have adequately controlled for the variability in the clinical expression, as well as the differences in the glomerular histopathology. This lumping together of diseases makes evaluation of their course and treatment difficult to interpret. In addition, many studies of therapeutic trials were short term without long-term follow-up.

### *Complications*

The two most common clinical complications of glomerulonephritis are hypertension and edema. Patients with glomerulonephritis frequently require treatment with antihypertensive and diuretic drugs. Furthermore, in patients with nephrotic syndrome, a hypercoagulable state occurs; therefore, the use of anticoagulants (i.e., warfarin) may be necessary.

Monitoring of therapeutic efficacy in patients with glomerular diseases is based on clinical response and normalization of certain laboratory data. Such parameters as urinary protein excretion, serum albumin, hematuria, renal function, and, in some patients, white blood cell and platelet counts, serum complement levels, and sedimentation rate are routinely followed. These data, coupled with the clinical response to treatment, are used to adjust dosage.

**Table 38.5** Therapeutic Interventions Utilized in Glomerular Diseases[a]

| | *Corticosteroids* | *Cytotoxic agents* | *Other* |
|---|---|---|---|
| **Isolated Proteinuria (With or Without Nephrotic Syndrome)** | | | |
| Without systemic disease | | | |
| Idiopathic nephrotic syndrome | | | |
| Minimal-change nephropathy | + | + | |
| Focal glomerulosclerosis | 0 | ± | |
| Mesangial proliferative nephritis | ± | ± | |
| Membranous nephropathy | ± | ± | |
| With systemic disease | | | |
| Primary amyloidosis | ± | ± | |
| Secondary amyloidosis | 0 | 0 | |
| Diabetes mellitus | 0 | 0 | |
| **Active Sediment** | | | |
| Without systemic disease | | | |
| IgA nephropathy | ± | ± | Phenytoin (?) |
| Membranoproliferative glomerulonephritis | ± | 0 | Anticoagulant, dipyridamole |
| Anti-GBM glomerulonephritis | 0 | ± | Plasmapheresis |
| Poststreptococcal glomerulonephritis | 0 | 0 | PCN/HTN[b] Rx Edema Rx |
| With systemic disease | | | |
| Systemic lupus erythematosus | + | ± | |
| Vasculitis | ± | ± | |
| Rapidly progressive glomerulonephritis | ± | ± | Plasmapheresis |
| Thrombotic thrombocytopenic purpura and hemolytic–uremic syndrome | 0 | 0 | Fresh-frozen plasma |
| Goodpasture's syndrome | ± | ± | Plasma exchange, plasmapheresis, and platelet agents |
| Infection-related glomerulonephritis | 0 | 0 | Antibiotics |

[a] +, proven efficacy; ±, questionable efficacy; 0, no efficacy or not studied.
[b] PCN, penicillin; HTN, hypertension.

### *Isolated Proteinuria With or Without Nephrotic Syndrome*

***Minimal-Change Nephropathy*** Minimal-change nephropathy has been shown to respond more dramatically than any other glomerular disease to corticosteroids or immunosuppressive drug therapy (Table 38.5). Prednisone 1 mg/kg/d (60 mg daily in the adult) in divided doses for approximately 4 weeks results in remission of proteinuria in approximately 95% of the patients[3]; however, nearly 70% relapse within the first year. Prednisone therapy is as beneficial during relapse as during the initial episode. In patients with frequent relapses who show steroid responsiveness, cyclophosphamide and other alkylating agents have been useful in sustaining remission.[3] Conversely, focal segmental glomerulosclerosis is less responsive to corticosteroids. Cytotoxic drug therapy has been used, but experience is limited and the outcome has generally been unfavorable. Corticosteroid nonresponders, frequent relapsers, and steroid-dependent patients have been treated with cyclophosphamide 2 mg/kg/d for not more than 2 to 3 months, with less than a 10% response.[3] Recently, nonsteroidal anti-inflammatory drugs have been used in patients with persistent nephrotic syndrome; generally, the result is decreased proteinuria.[12] Although this effect improves patient management, whether there is a sustained effect on progression of these diseases to renal failure is unknown.

***Mesangial Proliferative Nephritis*** Mesangial proliferative nephrotic syndrome is less responsive to corticosteroids, but experience is limited and the outcome has been generally unfavorable. Most clinicians attempt a course of daily prednisone. Approximately 30% to 50% of the patients treated with prednisone show clinical improvement, and reduction or loss of proteinuria; however, the dramatic therapeutic response seen in minimal-change nephrotic syndrome is not observed in the majority of these patients.[13]

***Membranous Glomerulopathy*** Membranous glomerulopathy is the most common cause of nephrotic syndrome in adults. Both corticosteroids and cytotoxic drugs have been used empirically in this disease, and neither has emerged as the treatment of choice. One controlled trial assessed an alternate-day prednisone treatment regimen in patients with biopsy-proven membranous nephropathy and normal renal function.[14] Although there was initially a significantly greater remission of proteinuria in the corticosteroid therapy group, it was not sustained over the 2-year study interval. At the completion of the study, however, the treatment group appeared to have a significantly greater preservation of renal function. Although results have been considered controversial, current opinion holds that a trial of corticosteroids (120 mg every other day) is indicated in a patient with membranous glomerular disease. Recently, similar beneficial results have been reported in patients treated with methylprednisolone (60 mg daily) for 1 month alternating with daily chlorambucil (2 mg/kg) for 1 month. This alternate-month therapy was used for 6 months. In this study, both sustained remissions and preservation of renal function were significantly greater in the treated group 2 years after treatment.[15]

### *Primary Glomerular Diseases Associated With an Active Urine Sediment*

#### Without Systemic Illness

***IgA Nephropathy*** The majority of patients with IgA nephropathy demonstrate a slowly progressive course, with approximately 10% to 15% eventually contracting end-stage renal disease over 10 to 15 years. Although immunosuppressive therapy has been used in patients with rapidly deteriorating renal function, its benefit has not been clearly defined.[16] Phenytoin, which reduces serum IgA levels, has been clinically studied in IgA nephropathy; however, no demonstrable clinical or pathologic improvement has been noted.[17]

***Membranoproliferative Glomerulonephritis*** There have been two approaches to the treatment of membranoproliferative glomerulonephritis (MPGN). The primary treatment has been alternate-day prednisone for extended periods.[18] McEnery et al evaluated the use of prednisone in an alternate-day regimen over periods of 1.5 to 15 years in 27 children with MPGN. In this uncontrolled trial, they found an 89% survival rate at 15 years after onset, as compared with the 50% survival rate at 6 to 12 years reported by other investigators. Therapy started, on the average, 1.5 years after onset in 23 children with a good response, and 5.2 years after onset in the 4 children with irreversible renal failure. In most, clinical manifestations diminished or disappeared.

The second approach has been long-term treatment with antiplatelet agents and warfarin (Coumadin). Because increased platelet turnover, as well as increased deposition of fibrin/fibrinogen in glomeruli of certain MPGN patients, has been observed, McEnery et al reasoned that antiplatelet agents might provide some beneficial effect. Zimmerman et al evaluated the utilization of warfarin, in doses to response of prothrombin time to 1.5 to 2 times control, and dipyridamole 100 mg four times a day in patients with MPGN in a crossover design.[19] Renal function remained stable over the year-long treatment period in the patients treated with warfarin and dipyridamole. Also, urine protein decreased in the group treated with warfarin and dipyridamole, but was not significantly different from that of the control group.

#### With Systemic Illness

***Systemic Lupus Erythematosus*** Lupus nephritis is a prototype of the autoimmune disease with hyperactive B lymphocytes that produce autoantibodies and high levels of circulating immune complexes. The findings on renal biopsy, taken together with clinical evidence of disease activity, provide a guide for initiation of therapy. Major indications for therapy are the onset of hematuria and proteinuria in the presence of a decline in renal function and the presence of subendothelial deposits. Cellular crescents and necrosis of glomerular tufts are also considered important histologic indicators for initiation of immunosuppressive therapy. Markers that are used to assess therapeutic response include a rise in serum complement, which is decreased in lupus nephritis, disappearance of protein and red blood cells in the urine, and improvement in renal function. Initial treatment of lupus nephritis usually requires high doses of prednisone (1 mg/kg/d) alone or in combination with a cytotoxic agent such as azathioprine or cyclophosphamide.[20] Usually 1 to 3 months of high-dose therapy is required, with subsequent tapering of these agents to low maintenance treatment. In general, the goal of prednisone treatment is to achieve alternate-day dosing to minimize side effects. Cytotoxic agents are frequently continued for 12 to 18 months after resolution of the signs and symptoms of active lupus. Prednisone has been the mainstay of treatment. Combinations of prednisone with cytotoxic agents are frequently utilized in patients with moderate to severe disease, as determined by renal biopsy, decreased complement, red blood cells in the urine, proteinuria, and decreased renal function. Recently, the use of intermittent intravenous cyclophosphamide has been advocated for the treatment of lupus nephritis. It has been shown to be effective and to have a reduced incidence of side effects compared with daily oral cyclophosphamide.[21]

***Systemic Vasculitis*** Vasculitis is a systemic immunologically mediated disease in which glomerulonephritis is a frequent clinical finding. Several forms of vasculitis have been clinically identified. Fauci et al evaluated prospectively 85 patients with Wegener's granulomatosis for 21 years at the National Institutes of Health.[22] Patient treatment followed a protocol calling for use of cyclophosphamide 2 mg/kg body weight per day together with prednisone 1 mg/kg body weight per day, followed by conversion of the prednisone to an alternate-day regimen. Complete remissions were achieved in 79 of the 85 patients (93%). The mean duration of remission was 48.2 ± 3.6 months. Twenty-three patients were off all therapy for a mean duration of 35.3 ± 6.3 months. In addition, long-term remissions can be maintained in a large number of patients by the combination of daily cyclophosphamide and alternate-day prednisone therapy. Similar prospective data in other forms of systemic vasculitis are lacking; however, most clinicians would treat these patients with high-dose corticosteroids. Recently, cyclophosphamide has been used with increasing frequency in patients with systemic vasculitis.

***Rapidly Progressive Glomerulonephritis*** Rapidly progressive glomerulonephritis (RPGN) is a disease with active glomerular inflammation and rapid loss of renal function. Treatment of RPGN frequently utilizes aggressive therapy with "pulse" doses of methylprednisolone. This protocol calls for an intravenous dose of methylprednisolone 15–30 mg/kg daily for 3 days, followed by oral prednisone 2 mg/kg on alternate days. An impressive clinical response has been reported in patients so treated.[23] This therapeutic response to "pulse" prednisone in RPGN has been particularly evident in patients without evidence of glomerular immune reactants. Dramatic responses to a variety of cytotoxic agents, anticoagulants, and plasmapheresis have also been reported. In particular, plasmapheresis, when combined with cytotoxic therapy (cyclophosphamide and prednisone), has been considered the treatment of choice in patients with RPGN secondary to anti-GBM–mediated disease[24]; however, carefully controlled trials have not been performed using these combinations of therapy, and final conclusions regarding their efficacy have not been made.

### *Corticosteroids*

The properties of steroid derivatives are variable (Table 38.6).[9,25] With decreasing equivalences, the sodium-retaining capacity decreases. Elimination half-life increases; also, duration of action increases. Anti-inflammatory activities increase with the newer analogues. Cortisol, the major active glucocorticosteroid produced by the body, is not used as an immunosuppressive drug because of its sodium-retaining characteristics. Prednisolone, an analog of cortisol, is more potent than cortisol on a weight basis and has reduced sodium-retaining activity. Prednisone, another analog, requires bioactivation to prednisolone in the liver. Analogues of intermediate half-life should be used, that is, prednisone/prednisolone, whereas agents such as dexamethasone with prolonged half-life should be avoided in alternate-day drug regimens. Because of the more prolonged biologic effect of longer acting agents on hypothalamic–pituitary–adrenal access, daily dosing results in the axis never being free of suppression. Multiple factors, including selection of the corticosteroid analogue, total dose given, frequency of administration, and duration of therapy, contribute to the overall physiologic effect of the corticosteroid.[9,25] In general, corticosteroid analogues with greater potency per milligram also have a more prolonged biologic effect. Obviously, increasing the amount of drug in a given dose increases the physiologic effect of the steroid. Perhaps less obvious, yet equally important, is the relationship between the frequency of drug administration and the physiologic effect of the steroid. Within a given time period, an increase in the frequency of administration of a given total amount of corticosteroid in divided doses greatly increases the physiologic effect of the steroid. For example, the effect of 10 mg of prednisone given four times daily exceeds that of 40 mg of prednisone given in a single daily dose, and the effect of 40 mg of prednisone as a single daily dose exceeds that of 80 mg of prednisone given on an alternate-day regimen. The total daily average doses of prednisone in these three regimens are identical, but the physiologic effect varies greatly.

The final variable, duration of therapy, is also of major importance. High pharmacologic doses of corticosteroids are well tolerated for brief periods of time, but with prolonged therapy the risk of adverse effects increases and eventually becomes predictable and inevitable.[9,25] Pharmacologic doses of corticosteroids given in daily, or even split, doses are generally well tolerated for approximately 1 or 2 weeks. After this time, such side effects as hypothalamic–pituitary–adrenal access suppression can be observed. This observed pattern is one rationale for "pulse" corticosteroid therapy whenever a short course of high-dose daily steroid is given. Intravenous pulse corticosteroid therapy is considered relatively safe.

When corticosteroids are utilized to suppress immune responses, prednisone therapy is usually initiated with 60–80 mg of the drug per day in three or four divided doses. Although this regimen is extremely powerful in its ability to suppress immune responsiveness, it is just as potent an inducer of adverse corticosteroid effects. Therefore, divided daily doses of prednisone are generally rapidly consolidated into a single daily dose.

Alternate-day steroid therapy provides significant anti-inflammatory and immunosuppressive activity while minimizing undesirable side effects, such as adrenal suppression and increased risk of infection. Only corticosteroid analogues, such as prednisone and prednisolone, should be employed on an alternate-day regimen. Administering dexa-

**Table 38.6** Properties of Steroid Derivatives Used in Pulse Therapy

| *Derivative* | *Equivalent dose (mg)* | *Anti-inflammatory potency* | *Capacity for sodium retention* | *Elimination half-life (min)* | *Duration of action[a] (h)* |
|---|---|---|---|---|---|
| Hydrocortisone | 20 | 1 | 1 | 90 | 8–12 |
| Prednisone | 5 | 3.5 | 0.8 | 60 | 12–36 |
| Prednisolone | 5 | 4 | 0.8 | 200 | 12–36 |
| Methyl prednisolone | 4 | 5 | 0.5 | 180 | 12–36 |
| Dexamethasone | 0.75 | 30 | 0 | 300 | 36–54 |
| Betamethasone | 0.75 | 25 | 0 | 300 | 36–54 |

[a] Duration of hypothalamic–pituitary–adrenal axis suppression after a single dose equivalent to 50 mg of prednisone.

**Table 38.7** Protocol for Conversion to Low-Dose Alternate-Day Prednisone Therapy

| *Prednisone dose (mg/d)* | | |
|---|---|---|
| **Odd day** | **Even day** | **Duration interval (wk)** |
| 15 | 15 | |
| 20 | 10 | 2 |
| 25 | 5 | 2 |
| 30 | None | 2 |
| 25 | None | 4 |
| 20 | None | 4 |
| 15 | None | 4 |
| | | Total duration of conversion $4\frac{1}{2}$ mo |

methazone every other day does not result in a true alternate-day regimen because the prolonged biologic effect of this drug does not allow the adrenal access to escape the effect of steroid on the day the drug is not administered. In addition, the corticosteroid should be administered as a single dose in the morning. Finally, the dose should not exceed 80 mg of prednisone or its equivalent. Higher doses may result in a more prolonged biologic effect, which carries over into the "off" day, thus defeating the intent of the alternate-day regimen. There are many protocols for conversion to alternate-day prednisone dosing; an example is given in Table 38.7. The outlined protocol indicates a gradual dose conversion so that the increased dose is given on the odd day and decreasing doses are given on the even day until all drug is given on the odd day.

The typical steroid withdrawal symptoms are fatigue, weakness, arthralgia, anorexia, nausea, desquamation of the skin, orthostatic dizziness and hypotension, fainting, dyspnea, and hypoglycemia.[26] Recovery of hypothalamus–pituitary axis (HPA) function may take up to 9 months after complete withdrawal from steroids. Canafax et al examined the role of cosyntropin stimulation tests in predicting the adrenal suppression in renal transplant patients being withdrawn from prednisone.[27] Forty-four percent of the patients studied had a suppressed cosyntropin stimulation test, but the suppressed adrenal response could not be predicted consistently by any one factor; however, a history of total prednisone dose greater than 25 g or a duration of steroid therapy greater than 12 months occurred more often among the suppressed patients. Canafax et al concluded that the cosyntropin stimulation tests could be easily performed to identify renal transplant patients at risk of steroid-induced adrenal suppression when rapid steroid tapering is desired.

The adverse effect profile of corticosteroids includes cosmetic complications such as weight gain, changes in facial features and body proportion, acne, and hirsutism. The most devastating complications of long-term corticosteroid therapy are infection, cataracts, atherosclerosis, and avascular necrosis leading to bone collapse; the latter two complications usually are not apparent until after years of treatment. Attempts to minimize the side effects should be made by tapering the drug to an alternate-day regimen or by determining the minimum dose that produces the desired clinical end.

The bioavailability of prednisone may be one potential reason for inadequate clinical response. After prompt absorption, the peak concentration of prednisone has been recorded to occur between 1 and 2 hours. There is extensive first-pass conversion to prednisolone.[28]

There is a relationship among frequency of adverse reactions to prednisone, dose of prednisone utilized, and serum albumin concentration.[29] With an increasing dose and decreased serum albumin (2.5 mg/dL) the incidence of side effects has been shown to increase significantly. This relationship can be explained in part by the dose-dependent plasma protein binding of prednisolone. At low prednisolone concentrations, approximately 90% of prednisolone is plasma protein bound, and at higher concentrations the free fraction of prednisolone increases three- to fourfold. Prednisolone binds primarily to transcortin and also to albumin. Transcortin exists in plasma in limited concentrations and therefore leads to the dose-dependent plasma protein binding of prednisolone.

The bioavailability of prednisone has been recorded to be approximately 80%. After absorption, there is intraconversion of the two steroids, with prednisolone concentration dominating at 4 to 10 times the prednisone concentration after oral or intravenous administration. A small part of the oral dose is excreted in the urine as prednisone (2%–4%) and prednisolone (16%–26%). Prednisolone is oxidated primarily in the liver and renal tissue.

An important facet of prednisone and prednisolone pharmacokinetics is their dose-dependent disposition. There is little change in the half-life with increasing prednisone doses, whereas the dose divided by the area under the serum concentration–time curve (the apparent plasma clearance) and volume of distribution of prednisolone increase with increasing doses.[30]

Plasma clearance may also be an important factor in prednisolone action. Kozower et al[31] demonstrated that patients with a decreased plasma clearance of prednisolone experienced more adverse effects, but did not have a response rate different from that of patients with a higher plasma clearance.

## *Cytotoxic Agents*

### Cyclophosphamide

Cyclophosphamide is generally started at 2 mg/kg orally per day. In a critically ill patient, a dose of 3–4 mg/kg administered intravenously for the first 3 to 4 days of induction may be indicated before conversion to a 2 mg/kg oral dose. Recently, intermittent intravenous cyclophosphamide in a dose of 0.5–1 $mg/mm^2$ has been utilized.[21] This intermittent regimen has potential importance, as certain side effects are dramatically reduced by its use. Doses higher than these levels increase the likelihood of granulocytopenia and the risk of infection without substantially improving the clinically relevant immunosuppressive effect. Generally, pharmacologic daily doses of corticosteroids during the initial induction period with cyclophosphamide or the other cytotoxic agents are used to provide a rapid immunosuppressive effect before the cytotoxic agent has achieved an immunosuppressive effect on its own. During the second week, as the immunosuppressive effect from the cyclophosphamide occurs, expeditious consolidation of the corticosteroid to an alternate-day regimen can be initiated.

After the initial induction, adjustments in the cyclophosphamide dose are made in accordance with circulating peripheral white blood cell counts. In general, the degree of immunosuppression is related to the total circulating white blood cell count; it is modest with a count of 5,000, moderate with a count of 4,000, and substantial at a count of 3,000. Depressing the peripheral white blood cell count below 3,000 by chronic administration of cytotoxic agents usually results in a selective decrease in the granulocyte count without a parallel substantial increase in the degree of immunosuppression. The degree of immunosuppression is also correlated with a total lymphocyte count. A total peripheral lymphocyte count of less than 500 is generally associated with significant immunosuppression. In comparison, the risk of infection is more closely associated with total granulocyte count. By maintaining granulocyte counts greater than 1,000–1,500, the risk of bacterial opportunistic infection is minimized.

Several additional points should be made regarding monitoring of peripheral white blood cell counts in patients undergoing chronic cyclophosphamide therapy. Changes in the peripheral white blood cell count lag behind changes in the cyclophosphamide dose. Consequently, immediate changes in peripheral white blood cell count should not be expected after modification of the cyclophosphamide dose. Frequent white blood cell counts are important during the critical induction period before the individual's chronic cyclophosphamide requirement is established.

Corticosteroids can also affect the response to cytotoxic agents. Steroids do not appear to alter the metabolism of cyclophosphamide, but do affect the response as measured by the white blood cell count. As previously mentioned, steroids produce a circulating granulocytosis and lymphopenia. Patients taking pharmacologic doses of steroids in addition to cyclophosphamide may have relatively less leukopenia. For a given dose of cyclophosphamide, the patient's peripheral white blood cell count is usually higher while on steroids. This factor is particularly important after the induction period with cytotoxic agents, when the steroids administered early in the induction period are being tapered; however, it should be noted that a dose of cyclophosphamide that produces an appropriate therapeutic decrease in the white blood cell count of a patient on daily prednisone may produce profound granulocytopenia when the patient is converted to an alternate-day steroid regimen. With each alteration in steroid dose, the peripheral white blood cell count must be evaluated to determine if a concomitant change is required in the cyclophosphamide dose.

Because steroids produce transient changes in the white blood cell count, additional care is required in evaluating a patient's alternate-day prednisone. In general, blood should be drawn before the steroid is given, and baseline levels for both on and off days should be determined. The count may vary from 2,500 to 4,000 white blood cells, depending upon when the sample is drawn. Appropriate changes in cyclophosphamide dose can be made only if the white blood cell count is interpreted in relation to the steroid dose. After a maintenance dose of cyclophosphamide is established, the white blood cell count remains relatively stable. Periodic checks of white blood cell and platelet counts are required; however, as bone marrow reserve shows a tendency to decline over time with chronic regimens of cytotoxic agents, a gradual reduction in the cyclophosphamide dose may be necessary.

Cyclophosphamide is readily absorbed by oral or parenteral routes and remains inactive until it is biotransformed in the liver. The resultant alkylating metabolites are active and capable of crosslinking DNA.[32] It is probable that certain metabolites are more immunosuppressive and some are more likely to contribute to side effects (e.g., hemorrhagic cystitis) than others.[33]

The metabolism of cyclophosphamide, when used as a chronic daily low-dose immunosuppressive regimen, has not been studied; however, a detailed pharmacologic evaluation after intravenous infusion for neoplastic diseases has been reported.[34] Injected radiolabeled cyclophosphamide rapidly distributed to 64% of body weight. The half-life of plasma cyclophosphamide in patients without prior drug exposure was 6.5 hours, and plasma alkylating activity peaked 2 to 3 hours after infusion. In patients who had received previous doses of cyclophosphamide, the plasma cyclophosphamide half-life was reduced and the peak plasma alkylating activity was higher, suggesting that the liver enzymes required for activation of cyclophosphamide are inducible. The majority of the radiolabeled cyclophosphamide was cleared in the urine (68% in 4 days). Less than 20% of the radiolabeled cyclophosphamide was excreted unmetabolized.

Because there may be delayed clearance of plasma alkylating activity in patients with renal dysfunction treated with cyclophosphamide, the potential for increased drug-related toxicity exists in these individuals.[35] Thus, the safe use of this drug requires additional consideration in patients with altered renal function.

The major adverse effect of the cytotoxic drugs is infection. This is, in part, related to the reduction in circulating granulocytes and monocytes resulting from bone marrow suppression. An increased risk of malignancy has been thought to occur in patients receiving cytotoxic agents over many years. As there is some evidence that autoimmune disease itself carries an increased risk of malignancy, presumably because of altered immune status of the host, the exact contribution of cytotoxic drug therapy to malignancy theory is unclear. Other adverse effects of cyclophosphamide therapy are hemorrhagic cystitis and bladder fibrosis. These localized complications most likely result from active metabolites present in the urine. It is generally believed that bladder complications can be prevented, or at least minimized, by maintenance of adequate hydration with good urinary output. Other side effects include gonadal dysfunction, nausea, vomiting, and hair loss.

Chlorambucil, another alkylating agent, has been used as an immunosuppressive drug. Although the complications and side effects are similar to those of cyclophosphamide, chlorambucil does not induce hemorrhagic cystitis. For this reason, chlorambucil should be considered an alternate agent for patients with hemorrhagic cystitis who require further immunosuppressive therapy.

**Azathioprine**

Azathioprine, along with cyclophosphamide, is frequently used to achieve immunosuppression. Metabolism of azathioprine to 6-mercaptopurine is essential for drug activity. The drug is well absorbed orally and can be used intravenously. Distribution of azathioprine has not been fully characterized, but the drug is rapidly cleared from the blood with a half-life of approximately 1 hour. The metabolites of azathioprine are excreted by the kidneys; only small amounts of azathioprine and 6-mercaptopurine are excreted intact.

Like the alkylating agents, the principal toxic effect of azathioprine is bone marrow depression. Hematologic effects are dose related. Other toxic effects include hepatitis (<3% of patients), alopecia, and stomatitis.

## References


1. Dixon FJ, Feldman JD, Vasquez JJ. Experimental glomerulonephritis: The pathogenesis of a laboratory model resembling the spectrum of human glomerulonephritis. J Exp Med 1961; 113:899–921.
2. Germuth FG. Comparative histologic and immunologic study in rabbits of induced hypersensitivity of serum sickness type. J Exp Med 1953;97:257–283.
3. Keane WF, Michael AF. Renal diseases, in Samter M, Claman HN (eds): Immunological Diseases. Boston, Little, Brown and Co., 1988, p 74.
4. Couser WG, Salant DJ. In-situ immune complex formation and glomerular injury. Kidney Int 1980;17:1–13.
5. Schreiber RD, Mueller-Eberhard HJ. Complement and renal disease, in Zabriskie JB, Fillit H, Villarreal H, et al (eds): Clinical Immunology of the Kidney. New York, John Wiley, 1982, p 77.
6. Cotran RS. Monocytes, proliferation and glomerulonephritis. J Lab Clin Med 1978;92:837–840.
7. Couser WG. Idiopathic rapidly progressive glomerulonephritis. Am J Nephrol 1982;2:57–69.
8. Gault MH, Muehrcke RC. Renal biopsy: Current views and controversies. Nephron 1983;34:1–34.
9. Fauci AS, Dale DC, Balow JE. Glucocorticosteroid therapy: Mechanism of action and clinical considerations. Ann Intern Med 1976;84:304–315.
10. Van Furth R, Gassman AE, Martina MC, et al. The effect of azathioprine (Immuran) on the cell cycle of promonocytes and the production of monocytes in the bone marrow. J Exp Med 1975;141:531–546.
11. Dale DC, Fauci AS, Wolff SM. The effect of cyclophosphamide on leukocyte kinetics and susceptibility to infection in patients with Wegener's granulomatosis. Arthritis Rheum 1973;16:657–664.
12. Torres VE, Velosa JA, Holley KE, et al. Meclofenomate treatment of recurrent idiopathic nephrotic syndrome with focal segmental glomerulosclerosis after renal transplantation. Mayo Clin Proc 1984;59:146–152.
13. Ji-Yun-Y, Melvin T, Sibley R, et al. No evidence for specific role of IgM in mesangial proliferation of idiopathic nephrotic syndrome. Kidney Int 1984;25:100–106.
14. Collaborative study of the adult idiopathic nephrotic syndrome. A controlled study of short term prednisone treatment in adults with membranous nephropathy. N Engl J Med 1979;301:1301–1306.
15. Ponticelli C, Zucchelli P, Imbasciati E, et al. Controlled trial of methylprednisolone and chlorambucil in idiopathic membranous nephropathy. N Engl J Med 1984;310:946–950.
16. Kincaid-Smith P, Nicholls K. Mesangial IgA nephropathy. Am J Kidney Dis 1983;3:90–102.
17. Clarkson AR, Seymour AE, Woodroffe AJ, et al. Control trial of phenytoin therapy in IgA nephropathy. Clin Nephrol 1980;13: 215–218.
18. McEnery PT, McAdams AJ, West CD. Membranoproliferative glomerulonephritis: Improved survival with alternate day prednisone therapy. Clin Nephrol 1980;13:117–124.
19. Zimmerman SW, Moorthy AV, Dreher WH, et al. Prospective trial of warfarin and dipyridamole in patients with membranoproliferative glomerulonephritis. Am J Med 1983;75:920–927.
20. Coggins CH. Overview of treatment of lupus nephropathy. Am J Kidney Dis 1982;2:197–200.
21. Austin HA, Klippel JH, Balow JE, et al. Therapy of lupus nephritis. Controlled trial of prednisone and cytotoxic drugs. N Engl J Med 1986;314:614–619.
22. Fauci AS, Haynes BF, Katz P, et al. Wegener's granulomatosis: Prospective clinical and therapeutic experience with 85 patients for 21 years. Ann Intern Med 1983;98:76–85.
23. Couser WG. Idiopathic rapidly progressive glomerulonephritis. Am J Nephrol 1982;2:57–69.
24. Burns F, Stachura I, Adler S, et al. Effect of early plasmapheresis and immunosuppressive therapy on natural history of anti–glomerular basement membrane glomerulonephritis. Report of a 22 month follow-up. Arch Int Med 1979;139:372–374.
25. Melby JC. Systemic corticosteroid therapy: Pharmacology and endocrinologic considerations. Ann Intern Med 1974;81:505–512.
26. Byyny RL. Withdrawal from glucocorticoid therapy. N Engl J Med 1976;295:30–32.
27. Canafax DM, Mann HJ, Sutherland DER, et al. The use of a cosyntropin stimulation test to predict adrenal suppression in renal transplant patients being withdrawn from prednisone. Transplantation 1983;36:143–146.
28. Gatti G, Perucca E, Frigo GM. Pharmacokinetics of prednisone and its metabolite prednisolone in children with nephrotic syndrome during the active phase and in remission. Br J Clin Pharmacol 1984;17:423–431.
29. Bergrem H. Pharmacokinetics and protein binding of prednisolone in patients with nephrotic syndrome and patients undergoing hemodialysis. Kidney Int 1983;23:876–881.
30. Jusko WJ, Rose JQ. Monitoring prednisone and prednisolone. Ther Drug Monitor 1980;2:169–176.
31. Kozower M, Veatch L, Kaplan MM. Decreased clearance of prednisolone, a factor in the development of corticosteroid side effects. J Clin Endocrinol Metab 1974;38:407–412.
32. Proceedings of the symposium on the metabolism and mechanism of action of cyclophosphamide. Cancer Treat Rep 1976;60: 299.
33. Levy L, Harris R. Effect of *N*-acetyl cysteine on some aspects of cyclophosphamide-induced toxicity and immunosuppression. Biochem Pharmacol 1977;26:1015–1020.
34. Bagley Jr CM, Bostick FW, DeVita Jr VT. Clinical pharmacology of cyclophosphamide. Cancer Res 1973;33:226–233.
35. Mouridsen HT, Jacobsen E. Pharmacokinetics of cyclophosphamide in renal failure. Acta Pharmacol Toxicol 1975;36:409–414.

# Chapter 39 / Drug Dosing in Patients With Impaired Renal Function

Gary R. Matzke, PharmD, FCP, FCCP, and William F. Keane, MD

The treatment of patients with reduced renal function is not limited to the tertiary medical care environment. Many general internists and practicing community nephrologists are now providing primary care for the patient with renal insufficiency. Unfortunately, the information available to these practitioners regarding rational drug use is often outdated, inadequate, or a simplistic presentation of an extremely complex problem. Drug therapy in patients with renal failure is more complex than a simple dose adjustment based on the fractional reduction in glomerular filtration rate. Furthermore, because of the physiologic and biochemical changes associated with uremia, patients with renal insufficiency may respond to a given dose or serum concentration of a drug differently than patients with normal renal function.

Data from the Boston Collaborative Drug Surveillance Program have shown that the incidence of adverse reactions to some drugs (i.e., flurazepam, digoxin, and prednisone) is higher in patients with elevated blood urea nitrogen concentrations.[1] Although this study provides only a "tip of the iceberg" assessment of the relationship between decreased renal function and drug toxicity, it does indicate that adverse drug reactions are more common in patients with reduced renal function. This increased incidence of adverse effects may arise from increased sensitivity of the target organ or altered disposition of the drug compound or both. Increased sensitivity of uremic patients to the central nervous system (CNS)-depressant effects of thiopental was initially reported more than 20 years ago.[2] Recently, Hisaoka and Levy[3] demonstrated that this increased sensitivity may result from the presence of a dialyzable material in uremic blood.

Changes in the disposition of a drug may also lead to an exaggerated pharmacologic response if serum concentrations accumulate excessively. The changes in drug disposition reported in patients with reduced renal function are not caused only by the loss of the renal elimination pathway. There may also be alterations in drug bioavailability, protein binding, volume of distribution, and/or metabolism.[4]

Knowledge of basic pharmacologic/pharmacokinetic principles combined with the drug disposition properties of a particular compound and the degree and type of pathophysiologic alterations associated with renal insufficiency should make it possible for the clinical practitioner to design a therapeutic regimen with a higher degree of safety and efficacy than is possible using empiric means. The objectives of this chapter are to describe the influence of renal failure on drug absorption, distribution, metabolism, and elimination and to provide a practical approach for drug dosage regimen design for dialysis patients and those with reduced renal function.

## Effect of Renal Insufficiency on Drug Disposition

### *Absorption*

There is little quantitative information regarding the influence of impaired renal function on drug absorption and bioavailability.[5] Several factors, such as alterations in gastrointestinal emptying time, gastric pH, and antacid administration, could affect drug bioavailability in this patient population. Edema of the gastrointestinal tract as well as vomiting and diarrhea, frequent complications of renal insufficiency, may also alter drug bioavailability. The assessment of bioavailability in this patient population is further complicated, as most patients with severe renal insufficiency receive multiple medications, many of which cannot be discontinued during the course of a bioavailability study.

Finally, some of the drug absorption (bioavailability) studies in patients with renal failure have not provided an assessment of absolute bioavailability (i.e., they have not included intravenous administration of the drug). Rather, they have documented alterations in the peak concentrations and the time at which peak concentrations were attained or in the fractional amount of drug recovered in the urine. This limited information has been extrapolated to suggest that drug absorption is slowed and/or that the extent of absorption is reduced.[6–8]

The bioavailability of several drug compounds is affected by the extent of their metabolism during the first pass through the gastrointestinal tract and liver. Balant et al[9] have reported an increased bioavailability of three β-blockers, tolamolol, bufuralol, and oxprenolol, in patients with renal failure. These data confirm the observations of increased systemic bioavailability of propranolol,[10] dextropropoxyphene,[11] and dihydrocodeine[12] in patients with renal insufficiency (Fig. 39.1). Although the bioavailability of all these compounds was increased, clinical consequences (development of excessive or unexpected adverse effects) have been demonstrated only with dextropropoxyphene[11] and dihydrocodeine.[13,14] The dissociation between the pharmacokinetic profile and clinical consequences of the β-blockers may be a result of an alteration in the responsiveness of patients with renal disease to these agents, as has been reported with propranolol in the elderly.[15]

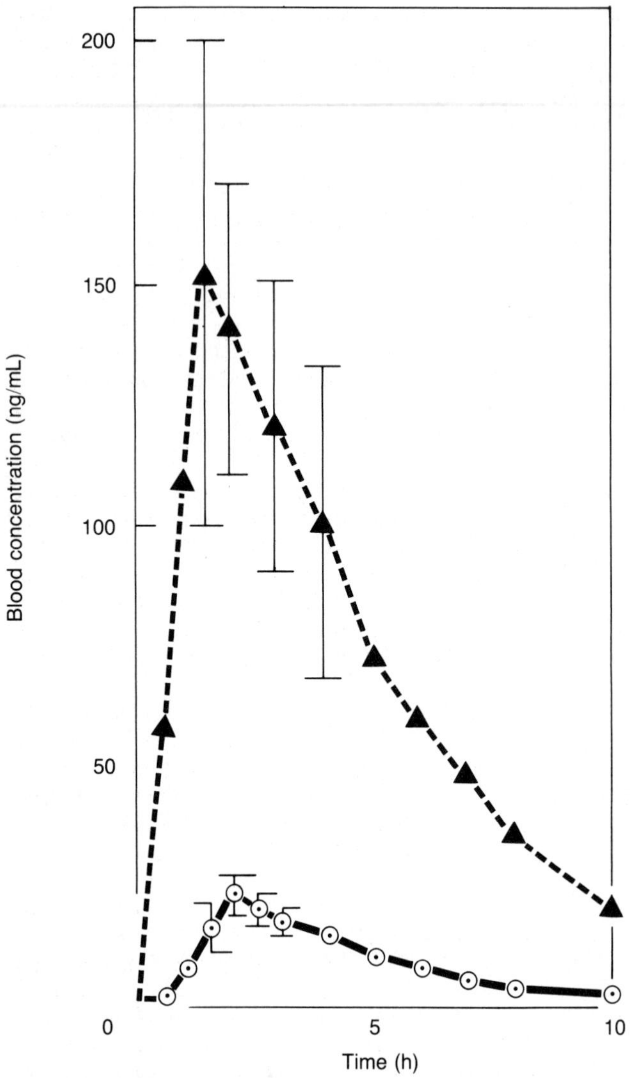


**Figure 39.1** Blood concentrations of propranolol after oral administration of 40 mg to healthy volunteers (○) and patients with chronic renal failure (▲). Values are means ± SEM. Bioavailability (*F*) was 0.19 and 0.62 in volunteers and patients, respectively. *(From Bianchetti G, Graziani G, Brancaccio D, et al: Pharmacokinetics and effects of propranolol in terminal uraemic patients and in patients undergoing regular dialysis treatment. Clin Pharmacokinet 1976;1:373–384, with permission.)*

### *Drug Distribution*

Although most dosage adjustment methods for patients with renal impairment assume that the volume of distribution of a drug is essentially unaltered, recent evidence has indicated that the volume of distribution of many drugs may be significantly increased or decreased.[4,16] Alterations in the distribution volume may result from increased or decreased protein binding, altered tissue binding, or pathophysiologic alterations in body composition, for example, the fractional contribution of total body water to total body weight.

Generally, the plasma protein binding of acidic drugs (warfarin, phenytoin) is decreased in uremia (Table 39.1), whereas the binding of basic drugs (quinidine, lidocaine) is usually normal or only slightly decreased[17] (Table 39.2). The decrease in binding of acidic drugs in uremic plasma has been attributed to qualitative changes in the binding sites, accumulation of endogenous inhibitors of binding, and decreased concentrations of albumin. The first two of these mechanisms appear to account for most of the observed changes in binding.[18] Additionally, the high concentrations of metabolites of some compounds that accumulate in the patient with renal insufficiency may interfere with the protein binding of the parent compound.

**Table 39.1** Protein Binding of Acidic Drugs in Patients With Normal and Impaired Renal Function

| | *Protein bound (%)* | |
|---|---|---|
| ***Drug*** | **Normal** | **IRF**[a] |
| Azlocillin | 35–40 | 25 |
| Cefazolin | 84 | 71 |
| Cefoxitin | 73 | 41 |
| Ceftriaxone | 90 | 80 |
| Clofibrate | 97 | 91 |
| Cloxacillin | 95 | 80 |
| Diazoxide | 94 | 84 |
| Dicloxacillin | 97 | 91 |
| Difunisal | 88 | 56 |
| Doxycycline | 88 | 72 |
| Furosemide | 96 | 94 |
| Metolazone | 95 | 90 |
| Moxalactam | 52 | 36 |
| Naproxen | 99.8 | 99.2 |
| Pentobarbital | 66 | 59 |
| Phenylbutazone | 93–96 | 82–86 |
| Phenytoin | 90 | 74–85 |
| Piretanide | 94 | 88 |
| Salicylate | 92 | 80 |
| Sulfamethoxazole | 66 | 42 |
| Valproic acid | 92 | 77 |
| Warfarin | 99 | 98 |

[a] IRF, impaired renal function.

**Table 39.2** Protein Binding of Basic Drugs in Patients With Normal and Impaired Renal Function

| | *Protein bound (%)* | |
|---|---|---|
| ***Drug*** | **Normal** | **IRF**[a] |
| Amphotericin B | 96.5 | 95.9 |
| Bepridil | 99.7 | 99.85 |
| Chloramphenicol | 55 | 36 |
| Clorazepate | 98 | 95 |
| Diazepam | 98 | 92 |
| Disopyramide | 68 | 72 |
| Ketoconazole | 99 | 98.5 |
| Morphine | 35 | 29 |
| Triamterene | 81 | 57 |

[a] IRF, impaired renal function.

The principal binding protein for several basic drug compounds is $\alpha_1$-acid glycoprotein (AAG), an acute-phase reactant whose concentration is increased in a wide variety of patients, including renal transplant patients and hemodialysis patients.[19] The fraction of those drugs principally bound to AAG, for example, bepridil and disopyramide, may be significantly increased in uremic patients. Thus, patients with renal insufficiency may experience increased or decreased protein binding depending upon the principal binding protein for the drug in question.

Altered tissue binding may also affect the apparent volume of distribution of a drug. The distribution volume of digoxin has been reported to be reduced by 30% to 50% from normal values in patients with renal disease.[4] It has been postulated that this reduction in the distribution volume is secondary to a decrease in tissue binding as a result of competitive inhibition by endogenous or exogenous substances.

Knowledge of protein and tissue binding changes in patients with renal insufficiency is critically important in the interpretation of serum drug concentrations. Numerous investigations have shown that the free concentration of several drugs in plasma correlates more closely with the concentration of drug at the receptor site, and, therefore, with the pharmacologic effect, than does the total concentration of drug in plasma.[20,21] Thus, because an alteration in plasma protein or tissue binding of a drug in an individual patient will likely alter the total drug concentration, the usual expected relationship between total drug concentration and pharmacologic response will be perturbed. For example, the therapeutic range for phenytoin serum concentrations in patients with normal renal function is 10–20 mg/L. As the free fraction is approximately 10% in subjects with normal renal function, the therapeutic free concentration range would then be 1–2 mg/L[21]; however, in patients with end-stage renal disease (ESRD), the free fraction is increased to 15% to 26% (mean ~ 20%), and the total concentration is thus lower as a result of the increased volume of distribution.[18,21] A total serum phenytoin concentration of 7 mg/L in an ESRD patient might therefore be considered subtherapeutic, whereas the free concentration (20% of the total or 1.4 mg/L) is actually in the middle of the therapeutic range.

Thus, in patients with renal insufficiency, particularly those with end-stage renal disease, a "normal" total drug concentration may be associated with either serious adverse reactions secondary to elevated free drug concentrations or subtherapeutic responses because of decreased free drug concentrations. The monitoring of unbound drug concentrations in this patient population is therefore suggested for those drugs that have a narrow therapeutic range and are highly protein bound (free fraction < 30%) and for which marked variability in the free fraction has been reported, for example, phenytoin, disopyramide.[20,21]

### *Metabolism*

Although the role of the kidneys as an excretory organ for drugs and chemicals and their polar metabolites is well described, the kidneys' involvement in the biotransformation of drugs is relatively poorly understood.[22] Recent investigations of drug metabolism in the kidney have suggested that the kidney is very metabolically active and that it may affect the biotransformation of a variety of drugs.[22,23] The renal cytochrome $P_{450}$ system catalyzes the metabolism of a variety of chemicals and drugs with an activity that equals that of the liver on an activity per gram of tissue basis.

Whole kidney homogenate cytochrome $P_{450}$ activity has varied from 14% to 18% of that observed in the liver. Glucuronide, glutathione, and sulfate conjugation activity has also been documented in kidney homogenates. Finally, glucuronyl transferase activity of the kidney in various animal species has been reported to range from 8% to 120% of the liver activity.[22] These limited studies clearly suggest that the kidney possesses considerable drug-metabolizing capability; however, the contribution to the total metabolic activity is generally low, as total kidney weight is far less than liver weight.

Investigations of the effect of chronic renal failure on hepatic enzyme activity in animals have also demonstrated alterations in certain pathways of hepatic drug metabolism.[24,25] Chronic renal failure was associated with a 26% to 71% decrease in hepatic enzyme activity.[24] In each case, the alteration in enzyme activity declined as the extent of renal failure increased.[24] These data suggest that chronic renal impairment may have a detrimental effect not only on drug metabolism in the kidney but also on drug metabolism within the liver.

Recently, Terao and Shen[26] reported that a factor present in the blood of rats with acute renal failure was responsible for the reduced presystemic clearance (first-pass metabolism) of orally administered *l*-propranolol. The metabolism of *l*-propranolol was significantly lower in the livers isolated from rats with acute renal failure compared with livers from normal rats. Moreover, when livers from normal rats were cross-perfused with uremic blood, the extraction of *l*-propranolol was depressed to a level almost identical to that observed in the livers isolated from rats with acute renal failure. When the livers from the renal failure rats were cross-perfused with normal blood, the metabolism of *l*-propranolol was similar to that observed in normal livers perfused with normal blood. These results suggest that the reduction in presystemic hepatic metabolism of *l*-propranolol in this animal model is caused by the presence of an inhibitory factor in uremic blood.

Renal insufficiency, whether acute or chronic in nature, may therefore have a substantial impact on the nonrenal clearance of total (free plus unbound) drug from the systemic circulation (Table 39.3). Thus, the assumption of a constant value for nonrenal clearance or the nonrenal elimination rate constant ($k_{nr}$) in patients with renal insufficiency may need to be seriously reconsidered.

Patients with severe renal insufficiency receiving chronic treatment with some agents may experience accumulation of metabolite(s) as well as parent compound.[27] Although metabolites of several drugs have been reported to have significant pharmacologic and/or toxicologic activity in general, the pharmacokinetics and pharmacology of metabolites are not often fully elucidated in humans. In a sense, the patient with severe renal impairment is being exposed to a "new pharmacologic entity" if the serum concentrations of the metabolite exceed those reported in patients with normal renal function.

The metabolite may have pharmacologic activity similar to that of the parent drug and thus contribute significantly to

**Table 39.3** Effect of End-Stage Renal Disease on Nonrenal (Hepatic) Clearance

| *Increased* | *Unchanged* | *Decreased* |
|---|---|---|
| Antipyrine | Acetaminophen | Acyclovir |
| Bumetanide | Chloramphenicol | Aztreonam |
| Phenytoin | Clonidine | Captopril |
| | Difunisal | Cefmenoxime |
| | Indomethacin | Cefmetazole |
| | Insulin[a] | Cefonicid |
| | Isoniazid[a] | Cefotaxime |
| | Morphine | Cefotiam |
| | Pentobarbital | Cefsulodin |
| | Propranolol | Ceftizoxime |
| | Quinidine | Cilastatin |
| | Tolbutamide | Cimetidine |
| | | Cortisol |
| | | Imipenem |
| | | Metoclopramide |
| | | Moxalactam |
| | | Procainamide |
| | | Procaine |

[a] These drugs may be unchanged or decreased.

clinical response, for example, oxipurinol[27] and desacetyl cefotaxime.[28] Alternatively, the metabolite may have qualitatively dissimilar pharmacologic action, for example, normeperidine, which has a CNS-stimulatory activity that has been reported to produce seizures, while meperidine has CNS-depressant actions.[29,30] Because of the multiplicity of potential interactions of compounds that are primarily metabolized, the practical consequences of metabolite accumulation are difficult to predict and are most often identified in those patients at risk by trial and error (Table 39.4).

### *Renal Elimination*

Measurement of endogenous creatinine clearance is the usual clinical means of determining a patient's renal function.[31,32] This measurement, however, provides only an index of glomerular function. Tubular secretion and tubular reabsorption are also key mechanisms involved in the renal handling of many drug compounds.[32] Alterations in one or more of these three mechanisms secondary to reduction in functional nephron mass may have a dramatic effect on the pharmacokinetics of a drug.

Kamiya et al[33] and Hori et al[34] demonstrated that the type of renal disease may explain in part the differences in pharmacokinetic parameters observed among patients with similar reductions in glomerular filtration rate. The disposition of antibiotic agents extensively secreted by the renal tubules (e.g., ampicillin, cephalexin) was altered to a greater degree in patients with predominantly tubulointerstitial disease compared with those with primary glomerular disease. These data support the earlier observation of this phenomenon with chlorpropamide,[35] and suggest that dosage-adjustment methodologies may need to be developed to take into consideration the impact of altered tubular as well as glomerular function.

Quantitative investigations of renal handling of new drugs will be required to elucidate the relative contribution of tubular and glomerular function to renal drug clearance. The availability of these data should provide a more rational approach to dosage regimen design for those agents that undergo extensive tubular secretion or reabsorption.

In the absence of data delineating the contribution of tubular function to renal elimination, the clinical measurement or estimation of creatinine clearance remains the guiding factor for drug dosage regimen design.[31] The importance of an alteration in renal function on drug elimination thus depends on two factors: the fraction of drug normally

**Table 39.4** Pharmacologic Activity of Metabolites

| *Parent drug* | *Metabolite* | *Pharmacologic activity of metabolites* |
|---|---|---|
| Allopurinol | Oxipurinol | Metabolite primarily responsible for suppression of xanthine oxidase |
| Cefotaxime | Desacetyl cefotaxime | Similar antimicrobial spectrum, but one fourth to one tenth as potent |
| Cephapirin | Desacetyl cephapirin | Similar antimicrobial spectrum, but about one half as potent |
| Chlorpropamide | 2-Hydroxy | Similar in vitro insulin-releasing activity |
| Clofibrate | Chlorophenoxyisobutyric acid | Primarily responsible for hypolipidemic effect and direct muscle toxicity |
| Meperidine | Normeperidine | Less analgesic activity than parent but more CNS-stimulatory effects |
| Procainamide | *N*-Acetyl procainamide | Distinct antiarrhythmic activity, the mechanism of which is different from that of the parent compound |
| Sulfonamides | Acetylated metabolites | Devoid of antibacterial activity, but elevated concentrations are associated with increased toxicity |

**Table 39.5 Methods for Estimation of Creatinine Clearance From Serum Creatinine for Adults[a]**

| *Reference* | *Method* | *Sex* |
|---|---|---|
| Jelliffe[36] | $Cl_{cr} = 100/S_{cr} - 12$ | Male |
| | $Cl_{cr} = 80/S_{cr} - 7$ | Female |
| Jelliffe[37] | $Cl_{cr} = \dfrac{98 - 0.8(\text{age in years} - 20)}{S_{cr}}$ | Male |
| | $Cl_{cr} = Cl_{cr,male} \cdot 0.9$ | Female |
| Mawer[38] | $Cl_{cr} = \text{weight} \cdot \dfrac{[29.3 - (0.203 \cdot \text{age in years})]\,(1 - 0.03S_{cr})}{S_{cr} \cdot 14.4}$ | Male |
| | $Cl_{cr} = \text{weight} \cdot \dfrac{[25.3 - (0.175 \cdot \text{age in years})\,[1 - 0.03S_{cr}]}{S_{cr} \cdot 14.4}$ | Female |
| Cockroft and Graft[39] | $Cl_{cr}\ (\text{mL/min}) = \dfrac{(\text{weight in kg})(140 - \text{age in years})}{72(S_{cr}\ \text{in mg/dL})}$ | Male |
| | $Cl_{cr}\ (\text{mL/min}) = Cl_{cr,male} \cdot 0.85$ | Female |
| Hull et al[40] | $Cl_{cr} = \dfrac{145 - \text{age in years}}{S_{cr}} - 3$ | Male |
| | $Cl_{cr} = Cl_{cr,male} \cdot 0.85$ | Female |
| Wagner[41] | $\text{Log}\ Cl_{cr} = 1.96 - (1.19 \cdot \log S_{cr})$ | Male |
| | $\text{Log}\ Cl_{cr} = 1.85 - (1.18 \cdot \log S_{cr})$ | Female |

[a] $Cl_{cr}$ = creatinine clearance; $S_{cr}$ = serum creatinine.

eliminated by the kidney unchanged and the degree of renal insufficiency.

Measurement of endogenous creatinine clearance requires the collection of total urine output over a defined time period. Because of the time delay involved and problems with completeness of urine collections, measured creatinine clearance values are infrequently used for initial drug dosage regimen design. To facilitate the calculation of initial drug dosage regimens, several methods have been proposed for the estimation of creatinine clearance ($Cl_{cr}$) from such routinely available clinical data as age, sex, height, weight, and serum creatinine[31,36–41] (Table 39.5).

The methodology described by Cockroft and Gault[39] is one of the most frequently utilized. It should be emphasized that this relationship is most accurate for individuals of average muscle mass for their age, weight, and height. In emaciated and obese adult patients incorrect estimates may be obtained. Furthermore, other estimation methods are more applicable for pediatric patients, that is, those less than 12 years of age.[42]

## Drug Dosage Regimen Design for Patients With Renal Insufficiency

Most dosage adjustment guidelines have proposed the use of a fixed dose or interval for patients with broad ranges of renal function.[5,43] For example, moderate renal insufficiency may encompass a creatinine clearance range of 10–50 mL/min, while severe renal insufficiency may be defined as a creatinine clearance of less than 10 mL/min. These categories encompass up to a tenfold range in renal function, and thus the drug regimen may not be optimal for all patients whose renal function lies within the range.

The design of the optimal dosage regimen for patients with renal insufficiency requires an individualized assessment and is dependent on the availability of an accurate characterization of the relationship between the pharmacokinetic parameters of the drug and renal function and an accurate index of the patient's renal function (i.e., creatinine clearance). These relationships may be derived from individual clinical studies or review articles[5,16,43–45] on patients with renal insufficiency, or may be calculated from the kinetic parameters reported in normal volunteers with the method of Welling et al.[46]

Once the kinetic parameters for the patient have been estimated, the best method for dosage regimen adjustment should be selected. Specifically, one must determine if the desired goal is the maintenance of a similar peak, trough, or average steady-state drug concentration. If there is a significant relationship between peak concentration and clinical response (e.g., aminoglycoside)[47] or trough or peak concentration and toxicity (e.g., phenytoin),[21] then attainment of the specific target values is critical. If, however, no specific target values for peak or trough concentrations have been reported (e.g., antihypertensive agents, benzodiazepines), then a regimen goal of attaining the same average steady-state concentration may be appropriate.

Although several methods have been proposed to attain the desired concentration profile, the principal choices are to

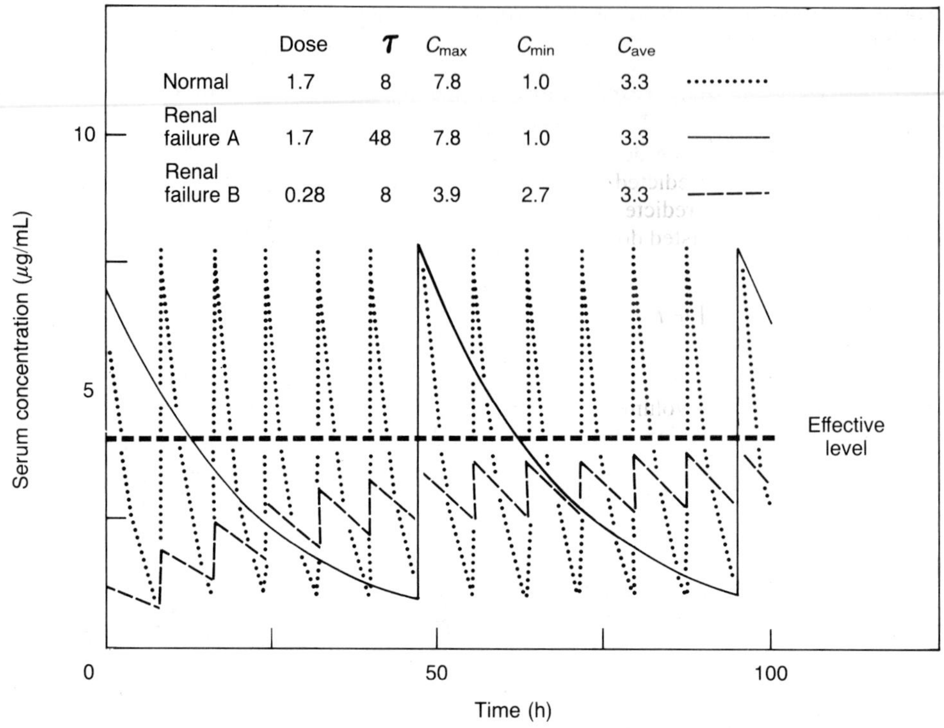


**Figure 39.2** Although the average steady-state concentrations ($C_{ave}$) are identical, the serum concentration–time profile will be markedly different if one changes the dosing interval ($\tau$) and maintains the dose constant versus changing the dose and maintaining the $\tau$ constant.

decrease the dose or prolong the dosing interval. If the size of the dose is reduced while the dosing interval remains unchanged, the desired average steady-state concentration will be similar; however, the peak will be lower and the trough higher (Fig. 39.2). Alternatively, if the dosing interval is decreased and the dose size remains unchanged, the peak and trough concentrations in the patient with reduced renal function will be similar to those in the patient with normal renal function. This dosage adjustment method is generally preferred because it will likely yield significant cost savings as a result of a reduction in nursing and pharmacy time as well as in the supplies associated with frequent drug administration.

Regardless of the approach chosen to adjust the dosage regimen, the first step in the process as previously mentioned is to estimate the drug disposition parameters in the patient with renal insufficiency. The ratio ($Q$) of the estimated elimination rate constant or total body clearance of the patient relative to subjects with normal renal function (creatinine clearance = 120 mL/min) may then be calculated. This parameter may be used to determine the dose or dosing interval alterations necessary for the patient.[48] For example, the following relationship between the elimination rate constant ($k$) and creatinine clearance has been reported for vancomycin[49]:

$$k = 0.0044 + 0.00083(\mathrm{Cl_{cr}})$$

Thus, $k$ for a subject with normal renal function would be calculated as $0.104\ \mathrm{h^{-1}}\ \{0.0044 + [0.00083(120)]\}$, and $k$ for a patient with a creatinine clearance of 10 mL/min would be $0.0127\ \mathrm{h^{-1}}\ \{0.0044 + [0.00083\ (10)]\}$. The ratio of these two values, the quotient or $Q$, for the patient is thus 0.122 (0.0127/0.104).

The maintenance dose ($D_f$) for the patient or the adjusted dosing interval ($\tau_f$) may then be calculated from the following relationships, where $D_N$ is the normal dose and $\tau_N$ is the normal dosing interval:

$$D_f = D_N Q$$

$$\tau_f = \tau_N / Q$$

For this patient situation where $D_N$ = 1,000 mg and $\tau_N$ = 12 hours, the calculated dosage regimen would be either (1) administer 1,000 mg at a prolonged dosing interval of 98 hours ($\tau_f$ = 12 hours/0.122) or (2) maintain the dosing interval of 12 hours and give a reduced dose of 122 mg ($D_f$ = 1,000 mg × 0.122). As the efficacy and toxicity of vancomycin have been associated with the attainment of a peak concentration within a specific range,[50] the optimal regimen for this patient would be to administer 1,000 mg every 98 hours or 4 days.

Application of this dosage adjustment method assumes that the protein binding and volume of distribution of the drug are not altered by renal insufficiency. Thus, this approach cannot be used with accuracy for those drugs with demonstrated differences in these pharmacokinetic parameters. If the elimination half-life, distribution volume, and clearance of the unbound drug are known, even though there may be changes in the "total" drug parameters, this methodology, however, may still be useful.

If the volume of distribution of a drug is significantly altered in patients with renal insufficiency, the estimation of a dosage regimen becomes more complex. If the relationship between volume of distribution and creatinine clearance has been characterized, then the volume of distribution may be estimated. If one assumes the drug can be described by a one-compartment linear model, the predicted volume of distribution may then be used with the predicted elimination rate constant of the drug to yield an adjusted dosing interval and intravenous dose:

$$\tau_f = 1/k\ [\ln(C_{trough}/C_{peak})] + t$$

$$dose_{IV} = kV_D C_{peak}\ [(1 - e^{-k_f\tau_f})/(1 - e^{-k_f t})]$$

$k_f$ = the elimination rate constant, $V_D$ = volume of distribution, $\tau_f$ = dosing interval, and $t$ = infusion duration. For orally administered, rapidly absorbed drugs, the dose can be approximated as

$$dose_{po} = V_D \Delta C$$

where $\Delta C$ = the desired change in plasma concentration. This approach allows for the individualization of a dosage regimen for attainment of specific peak and trough serum concentrations.

Alternately, the predicted volume of distribution and elimination rate constant or the total body clearance may be used to calculate a dosage regimen to maintain a desired average steady-state concentration of the drug ($\overline{C}_{ss}$).

$$dose\ (mg/h) = \overline{C}_{ss}\ (k_f V_D)\ or\ (Cl_f)$$

Depending upon how much variance about the average steady state one desires, the dosing interval may range from hourly to as infrequent as every 48 hours or longer. For example, if the calculated dose were 10 mg/h, the desired average steady-state concentration would be maintained with a dosing interval of 60 mg every 6 hours or 480 mg every 48 hours.

## Drug Dosage Regimen Design for Dialysis Patients

The number of patients with end-stage renal disease who are receiving long-term dialytic therapy has steadily increased since the late 1960s and now is approximately 80,000.[51] Although considerable advances have been made during this time in hemodialysis filter technology[52,53] and the efficiency of the hemodialysis procedure,[54] the effect of hemodialysis on drug disposition once reported has rarely been reevaluated using the newer equipment and technology. Thus, most of the data in the literature probably represent an underestimation of the impact of hemodialysis on drug disposition.

The effect of hemodialysis on drug disposition can be estimated in several ways.[40] The determination of drug concentrations at the start and end of dialysis, with the subsequent calculation of the half-life during dialysis ($t_{1/2,\ HD}$), has frequently been utilized as an index of drug removal by dialysis. Unfortunately, the $t_{1/2,\ HD}$ may not be interpretable because declining plasma drug concentrations during

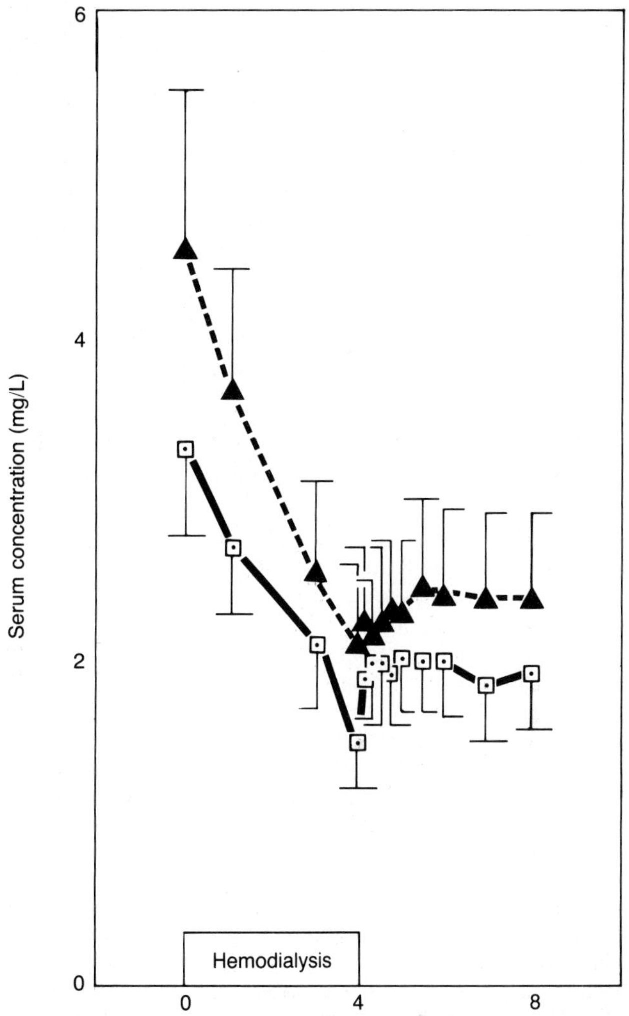


**Figure 39.3** Serum concentration–time profiles of netilmicin (□) and tobramycin (▲) during hemodialysis and in the immediate postdialysis period. Values are means ± SD. The maximum change in serum concentration was 38.3 ± 16.2% with netilmicin and 18.3 ± 3.0% with tobramycin. (*Adapted from Halstenson CE, Berkseth RO, Mann HJ, et al: Aminoglycoside redistribution phenomenon after hemodialysis: Netilmicin and tobramycin. Int J Clin Pharmacol Ther Toxicol 1987;25:50–55, with permission.*)

dialysis represent elimination by the body as well as by dialysis. Furthermore, recent reports of a significant rebound in drug concentrations after dialysis suggest that in some cases the removal of drug by the dialysis procedure may be artificially high or low depending on when after dialysis the concentration is determined[55–57] (Fig. 39.3).

An alternative and more accurate means of assessing the effect of hemodialysis is to calculate the dialyzer clearance ($Cl_D$) of the drug. The dialyzer clearance ($Cl_D$) is calculated as $Cl_D = Q_b\ [(A - V)/A]$, where $Q_b$ is blood flow through the dialyzer, $A$ is the concentration of drug going into the dialyzer filter, and $V$ is the concentration of drug leaving the filter. As drug concentrations are generally determined in plasma, this equation can be modified to $Cl_p = Q_p[(A_p -$

$V_p)/A_p]$ where subscript p represents plasma and $Q_p$ is plasma flow, which equals $Q_b(1 - \text{hematocrit})$. This clearance calculation accurately reflects dialysis drug clearance only if the drug does not penetrate red blood cells or bind to formed blood elements.

Because of potential problems in accurately determining $Q_p$ and the fact that venous plasma concentrations may be concentrated, because water may be removed from the blood at a faster rate than drug when ultrafiltration is performed simultaneously with diffusion during dialysis, the recovery clearance approach has become the benchmark for the determination of dialyzer clearance.[45,57]

Dialyzer clearance can thus be calculated as

$$Cl_D = R/AUC|_0^t$$

where $R$ is the total amount of drug recovered unchanged in the dialysate and $AUC|_0^t$ is the area under the plasma concentration–time curve during hemodialysis. To determine the $AUC|_0^t$ at least two and preferably three to four plasma concentrations should be obtained during dialysis.

Although these techniques for measuring dialyzer clearance in the individual patient may not be feasible or practical in many clinical environments, the following principles may be applied to drug dosage regimen design by using a value of $Cl_D$ calculated by one of the preceding methods that is reported in the literature.[16,43,45]

Because clearance terms are additive, the total clearance during dialysis can be calculated as the sum of total body clearance during the interdialytic period ($Cl_{PT}$) and dialyzer clearance ($Cl_D$):

$$Cl_T = Cl_{PT} + Cl_D$$

The half-life during the period between dialysis treatments and during dialysis can then be calculated from the following relationships using an estimate of the drug's distribution volume ($V_D$), which can be obtained from review articles[16,43,46]:

$$t_{1/2,\,off} = 0.693[V_D/Cl_{PT}]$$

$$t_{1/2,\,on} = 0.693[V_D/(Cl_{PT} + Cl_D)]$$

Once the key pharmacokinetic parameters ($Cl_{PT}$, $Cl_D$, and $V_D$) have been estimated/calculated, they may be used to simulate the plasma concentration–time profile of the drug for the individual patient and ascertain how much to administer and when to administer the next dose of the drug.

For example, AG is a 70-kg male who is estimated to have a drug distribution volume of 19.6 L (0.28 L/kg) and a total body clearance of 0.30 L/h (5 mL/min). Further pertinent data are that the patient undergoes dialysis for 4 hours ($t_D$) with a dialysis filter that has been reported to have a clearance for the current drug ($Cl_D$) of 3.6 L/h (60 mL/min). The patient is to receive 140 mg intravenously of the drug now and be dialyzed in 40 hours. The desired $C_{max}$ after the next dose is given is 7.1 mg/L. What will the plasma concentration be prior to dialysis and after dialysis? What dose should be administered after dialysis (PDD) to achieve the desired $C_{max}$?

$$t_{1/2,\,off\ HD} = 0.693\ [19.6\ L/(0.3\ L/h]$$

$$t_{1/2,\,off\ HD} = 45.3\ hours$$

$$t_{1/2,\,on\ HD} = 0.693\ [19.6\ L/(0.3 + 3.6\ L/h)]$$

$$t_{1/2,\,on\ HD} = 3.5\ hours$$

$$C_{max} = dose/V_D$$

$$C_{max} = 140\ mg/19.6\ L$$

$$C_{max} = 7.1\ mg/L$$

$$C_{preHD} = C_{max}\ [e^{-(Cl_{PT}/V_D)t}]$$

$$C_{preHD} = 7.1\ mg/L\ [e^{-[(0.3\ L/h)/19.6\ L]40}]$$

$$C_{preHD} = 7.1\ mg/L \cdot (0.54)$$

$$C_{preHD} = 3.8\ mg/L$$

$$C_{postHD} = C_{preHD}\ [e^{-\{[(Cl_{PT} + Cl_D)/V_D]\ t_D\}}]$$

$$C_{postHD} = 3.8\ mg/L\ [e^{-\{[(0.3 + 3.6\ L/h)/19.6\ L]\ 4\ h\}}]$$

$$C_{postHD} = 3.8\ mg/L \cdot (0.45)$$

$$C_{postHD} = 1.7\ mg/L$$

$$PDD = V_D\ (C_{max} - C_{postHD})$$

$$PDD = 19.6\ L \cdot (7.1 - 1.7\ mg/L)$$

$$PDD = 106\ mg$$

The time for administration of and the amount of the next dose to be given depend on the desired concentration–time profile and the time after the previous dose when dialysis is initiated. If the desired $C_{max}$ remained 7.1 mg/L and the desired trough concentration prior to administration of the next dose was ≤3.0 mg/L, the variation in the dose that would be required to achieve the desired $C_{max}$ as a function of the time the patient is dialyzed is depicted in Table 39.6.

## Summary

Subtherapeutic or supratherapeutic responses to drugs in uremic patients are often misinterpreted and not recognized as such. The harm done by inappropriate drug use and dosing is not readily quantified but does warrant future

**Table 39.6** Effect of Time of Dialysis on the Simulated Plasma Concentration–Time Profile and Calculated Postdialysis Dose

| | ***Time after dose when dialysis is initiated (h)*** | | | |
|---|---|---|---|---|
| | **4** | **12** | **24** | **48** |
| $C_{preHD}$ (mg/L) | 6.7 | 5.9 | 4.9 | 3.4 |
| $C_{postHD}$ (mg/L) | 3.0 | 2.7 | 2.2 | 1.5 |
| PDD (mg) | 80 | 86 | 96 | 110 |

investigations. Sound pharmacokinetic principles used in concert with reliable population pharmacokinetic estimates should ultimately yield the optimal approach to drug dosage regimen design for patients with impaired renal function. Individualization of therapy should be undertaken whenever clinical therapeutic monitoring tools are available.

## References


1. Jick H. Adverse drug effects in relation to renal function. Am J Med 1977;62:514–517.
2. Dundee JW, Richards RK. Effect of azotemia upon action of intravenous barbiturate anesthesia. Anesthesiology 1954;15: 333–346.
3. Hisaoka M, Levy G. Kinetics of drug action in disease states. XIII. Effect of dialyzable component(s) of uremic blood on phenobarbital concentrations in rats at onset of loss of righting reflex. J Pharmacol Exp Ther 1985;234:180–183.
4. Gambertoglio JG. Effects of renal disease: Altered pharmacokinetics, in Benet LZ, Massoud N, Gambertoglio JG (eds): Pharmacokinetic Basis for Drug Treatment. New York, Raven, 1984, pp 149–171.
5. Bennett WM, Aronoff GR, Morrison G, et al. Drug prescribing in renal failure: Dosing guidelines for adults. Am J Kidney Dis 1983;3:155–195.
6. Tilstone WJ, Dargie H, Dargie EN, et al. Pharmacokinetics of metolazone in normal subjects and in patients with cardiac or renal failure. Clin Pharmacol Ther 1974;16:322–329.
7. Tilstone WJ, Fine A. Furosemide kinetics in renal failure. Clin Pharmacol Ther 1978;23:644–650.
8. Guay DRP, Matzke GR, Bockbrader HN, et al. Comparison of bioavailability and pharmacokinetics of cimetidine in subjects with normal and impaired renal function. Clin Pharm 1983;2: 157–162.
9. Balant LP, Dayer P, Fabre J. Consequences of renal insufficiency on the hepatic clearance of some drugs. Int J Clin Pharmacol Res 1983;3:459–474.
10. Bianchetti G, Graziani G, Brancaccio D, et al. Pharmacokinetics and effects of propranolol in terminal uraemic patients and in patients undergoing regular dialysis treatment. Clin Pharmacokinet 1976;1:373–384.
11. Gibson TP, Giacomini KM, Briggs WA, et al. Propoxyphene and norpropoxyphene plasma concentrations in the anephric patient. Clin Pharmacol Ther 1980;27:665–670.
12. Barnes JN, Williams AJ, Tomson MJF, et al. Dihydrocodeine in renal failure: Further evidence for an important role of the kidney in the handling of opioid drugs. Br Med J 1985;290:740–742.
13. Barnes JN, Goodwin FJ. Dihydrocodeine narcosis in renal failure. Br Med J 1983;286:438.
14. Redfern N. Dihydrocodeine overdose treated with naloxone infusion. Br Med J 1983;287:751–752.
15. Vestal RE, Wood AJJ, Shand DG. Reduced $\beta$ receptor sensitivity in the elderly. Clin Pharmacol Ther 1979;26:181–186.
16. Matzke GR, Keane WF. Use of antibiotics in renal failure, in Peterson PK, Verhoef J (eds): The Antimicrobial Agents Annual. Amsterdam, Elsevier, 1986, pp 472–488.
17. Reidenberg MM, Drayer DE. Alteration of drug–protein binding in renal disease. Clin Pharmacokinet 1984;9(suppl 1):18–26.
18. Liponi DF, Winter ME, Tozer TN. Renal function and therapeutic concentrations of phenytoin. Neurology 1984;34:395–397.
19. Haughey DB, Kraft CJ, Matzke GR, et al. Protein binding of disopyramide and elevated alpha-1-acid glycoprotein concentrations in serum obtained from dialysis patients and renal transplant recipients. Am J Nephrol 1985;5:35–39.
20. Levy RH, Moreland TA. Rationale for monitoring free drug levels. Clin Pharmacokinet 1984;9(suppl 1):1–9.
21. Asconape JJ, Penry JK. Use of antiepileptic drugs in the presence of liver and kidney diseases: A review. Epilepsia 1982;23(suppl 1):S65–S79.
22. Anders MW. Metabolism of drugs by the kidney. Kidney Int 1980;18:636–647.
23. Gibson TP. Renal disease and drug metabolism: An overview. Am J Kidney Dis 1986;8:7–17.
24. Patterson SE, Cohn VH. Hepatic drug metabolism in rats with experimental long-term renal failure. Biochem Pharmacol 1984;35:711–716.
25. Terner UK, Wiebe LI, Noujaim AA, et al. The effects of acute and chronic uremia in rats on their hepatic microsomal enzyme activity. Clin Biochem 1978;4:156–158.
26. Terao N, Shen DD. Reduced extraction of *l*-propranolol by perfused rat liver in the presence of uremic blood. J Pharmacol Exp Ther 1985;233:277–284.
27. Drayer DE. Active drug metabolites and renal failure. Am J Med 1977;62:486–489.
28. Wise R, Willis PJ, Andrews JM, et al. Activity of the cefotaxime (HR756) desacetyl metabolite compared with those of cefotaxime and other cephalosporins. Antimicrob Agents Chemother 1980;17:84–86.
29. Szeto HH, Inturrisi CE, Houde R, et al. Accumulation of normeperidine, an active metabolite of meperidine, in patients with renal failure or cancer. Ann Intern Med 1977;86:738–741.
30. Kaiko RF, Foley KM, Grabinski PY, et al. Central nervous system excitatory effects of meperidine in cancer patients. Ann Neurol 1982;13:180–185.
31. Lott RS, Hayton WL. Estimation of creatinine clearance from serum creatinine concentration—a review. Drug Intell Clin Pharm 1978;12:140–150.
32. Rowland M, Tozer TN (eds): Clinical Pharmacokinetics: Concepts and Applications. Philadelphia, Lea and Febiger, 1980, pp 48–64.
33. Kamiya A, Katsuhiko O, Hori R. Quantitative investigation of renal handling of drugs in dogs with renal insufficiency. J Pharm Sci 1984;74:892–896.
34. Hori R, Okumura K, Kamiya A, et al. Ampicillin and cephalexin in renal insufficiency. Clin Pharmacol Ther 1983;34:792–798.
35. Petitpierre B, Perrin L, Rudhardt M, et al. Behaviour of chlorpropamide in renal insufficiency and under the effect of associated drug therapy. Int J Clin Pharmacol Ther Toxicol 1972;6:120–124.
36. Jelliffe RW. Estimation of creatinine clearance when urine cannot be collected. Lancet 1971;1:975–976.
37. Jelliffe RW. Creatinine clearance: Bedside estimate. Ann Intern Med 1973;79:604–605.
38. Mawer GE, Knowles BR, Lucas SB, et al. Computer-assisted prescribing of kanamycin for patients with renal insufficiency. Lancet 1972;1:12–15.
39. Cockroft DW, Gault MH. Prediction of creatinine clearance from serum creatinine. Nephron 1976;16:31–41.
40. Hull JH, Hak LJ, Koch GG, et al. Influence of range of renal function and liver disease on predictability of creatinine clearance. Clin Pharmacol Ther 1981;29:516–521.

41. Wagner JG. Biopharmaceutics and Relevant Pharmacokinetics. Hamilton, IL, Drug Intelligence Publications, 1971, pp 222–233.
42. Schwartz GJ, Brion LP, Spitzer A. The use of plasma creatinine concentration for estimating glomerular filtration rate in infants, children and adolescents. Pediatr Clin North Am 1987; 34:571–590.
43. Brater DC (ed): Drug Use in Renal Disease. Balgowlah, Australia, ADIS Health Science Press, 1983.
44. Keller F, Offermann G, Lode H. Supplementary dose after hemodialysis. Nephron 1982;30:220–227.
45. Lee CC, Marbury TC. Drug therapy in patients undergoing hemodialysis. Clinical pharmacokinetic considerations. Clin Pharmacokinet 1984;9:42–66.
46. Welling PG, Craig WA, Kunin CM. Prediction of drug dosage in patients with renal failure using data derived from normal subjects. Clin Pharmacol Ther 1975;18:45–52.
47. Moore RD, Lietman PS, Smith CR. Clinical response to aminoglycoside therapy: Importance of the ratio of peak concentration to minimal inhibitory concentration. J Infect Dis 1987; 155:93–99.
48. Rowland M, Tozer TN (eds): Clinical Pharmacokinetics: Concepts and Applications. Philadelphia, Lea and Febiger, 1980, pp 230–246.
49. Matzke GR, McGory R, Halstenson CE, et al. Pharmacokinetics of vancomycin in patients with various degrees of renal function. Antimicrob Agents Chemother 1984;25:433–437.
50. Matzke GR. Vancomycin, in Evans WE, Schentag JJ, Jusko WJ (eds): Applied Pharmacokinetics: Principles of Therapeutic Drug Monitoring, 2nd ed. Spokane, WA, Applied Therapeutics Inc., 1986.
51. Anonymous. The U.S. ESRD program: Selected 1984 statistics. Contemp Dial Nephrol 1985;4:12.
52. Sigdell JE. Technical and functional consideration in choosing a hollow-fiber dialyzer, in Nissenson AR, Fine RN (eds): Dialysis Therapy. Philadelphia, Hanley and Belfus, 1986, pp 51–82.
53. Sigdell JE. Parallel-plate dialyzers, in Nissenson AR, Fine RN (eds): Dialysis Therapy. Philadelphia, Hanley and Belfus, 1986, pp 82–85.
54. Anonymous. Shortened dialysis. Dialysis Transplant 1986;15: 553–563.
55. Keller F, Offerman G, Scholle J. Kinetics of the redistribution phenomenon after extracorporeal elimination. Int J Artif Organs 1984;7:181–188.
56. Halstenson CE, Berkseth RO, Mann HJ, et al. Aminoglycoside redistribution phenomenon after hemodialysis: Netilmicin and tobramycin. Int J Clin Pharmacol Ther Toxicol 1987;25:50–55.
57. Gibson TP. Problems in designing hemodialysis drug studies. Pharmacotherapy 1985;5:23–29.

# Section Five
# Neurologic Disorders

## Chapter 40 / Status Epilepticus

Anthony A. Coniglio, PharmD, and William R. Garnett, PharmD

The term *status epilepticus* (SE) was first used in 1824 by L. F. Calmeil to describe a series of repeated seizures occurring without interruption, where patients did not recover consciousness between attacks and many died.[1] The syndrome most commonly associated with the name SE is tonic–clonic or "convulsive" status, although other types exist. Today, generalized convulsive SE is a neurologic emergency that carries a significant risk of permanent brain damage and death when not promptly and appropriately treated. The longer the generalized convulsive status epilepticus continues, the higher the morbidity and mortality. Despite greater knowledge about the disease process and an improved therapeutic armamentarium, SE still accounts for about one half of the deaths caused by epilepsy.[2]

### Definition/Classification

The current definition and classification of SE, adopted by the International League Against Epilepsy and the World Health Organization (WHO) during the early 1970s, states that "the term status epilepticus is used whenever a seizure persists for a sufficient length of time or is repeated frequently enough to produce a fixed and enduring epileptic condition."[3] The subjective nature of terms such as "sufficient length," "frequently enough," and "fixed and enduring" may create some confusion, although the term is generally applied to continuous seizures lasting at least 30 minutes, even when consciousness is not impaired.

The international classification of SE is provided in Table 40.1, and the terms are compared with traditional terms previously used to describe SE. The broad categories include convulsive status epilepticus, where the patient does not recover to a normal alert state between repeated tonic–clonic attacks, nonconvulsive status epilepticus (e.g., absence status and complex partial status), where the clinical presentation is a prolonged "twilight" state, and continuous partial seizures such as "epilepsia partialis continuans," where consciousness is preserved.[4] Though generalized convulsive SE is considered the most life-threatening, experimental and clinical evidence suggests that focal convulsive SE and nonconvulsive SE also require immediate effective treatment to prevent neuronal damage and neurologic dysfunction.[5]

### Incidence

Between 60,000 and 160,000 Americans have at least one episode of convulsive status epilepticus annually.[6] Accurate prevalence data for nonconvulsive status epilepticus do not exist. The frequency of SE in patients with epilepsy has been reported to be between 2.6% and 6.6%.[7–10] The incidence of SE presenting as the initial ictal event (i.e., prior to a formal diagnosis of epilepsy) may be as low as 12%[11] or as high as 56%[12] in adult patients. In children, frequencies as high as 77% have been reported.[13] The large discrepancy among reported frequency data may be related to the different populations being studied, the inclusion of diverse seizure types and etiologies, and variability in the duration of seizure activity accepted as SE.

### Pathophysiology

#### *Causes*

It is important to distinguish between causes and precipitating factors of SE. The *cause* is the underlying pathologic abnormality that provides the impetus for abnormal electrical activity of the brain. Commonly identified causes of SE in adults and children are listed in Table 40.2; however, the disease is frequently idiopathic and a cause is not identified.

#### *Precipitating Factors*

A *precipitating factor* frequently triggers the manifestation of a SE attack in a patient with an underlying cause for the disease or with preexisting epilepsy. Noncompliance or withdrawal of anticonvulsant therapy is a common precipitating factor in 53% of patients with previous seizures.[14] Concurrent systemic infection is responsible for 5% of all cases of SE, with greater percentages reported for intracranial infection.[7] Additional precipitating factors include emotional stress, alcohol withdrawal, sleep deprivation, electrolyte imbalance, and drug toxicity (e.g., lidocaine,

**Table 40.1** International Classification of Status Epilepticus

| *International* | *Traditional* |
|---|---|
| Generalized SE | |
| Convulsive | |
| Tonic–clonic | Grand mal, epilepticus convulsivus |
| Tonic | |
| Clonic | |
| Myoclonic | |
| Nonconvulsive | |
| Absence | Spike-and-wave stupor, spike and slow-wave or 3/s spike-and-wave SE, petit mal, epileptic fugue, epilepsia minora continua, epileptic twilight state, minor SE |
| Partial SE | |
| Elementary | Focal motor status, focal sensory, epilepsia partialis continuans, adversive SE |
| Somatomotor | |
| Dysphasic | |
| Other types | |
| Complex partial | Epileptic fugue state, prolonged epileptic stupor, prolonged epileptic confusional state, temporal lobe SE, psychomotor SE, continuous epileptic twilight state |
| Unilateral SE | Hemiclonic SE, hemiconvulsion–hemiplegia–epilepsy, hemigrand mal SE, grand mal dimidie |
| Erratic SE (unclassified) | Neonatal status epilepticus |

Compiled from Reference 3.

theophylline, phenothiazines, antihistamines, and street drugs).[2,14] Excessively high plasma concentrations of antiepileptic drugs (AEDs) may also precipitate an episode of SE.

## Clinical Presentation

As stated previously, the definition of SE is applied to clinical or electrical seizures, or both.[5] Electrical seizures must be determined by an electroencephalogram, and may

**Table 40.2** Causes of Status Epilepticus

| |
|---|
| Brain tumors |
| Craniocerebral trauma |
| Cerebrovascular disease |
| Infection |
| Metabolic abnormalities |
| Toxic disorders |
| Encephalopathies |

not always be clinically apparent (i.e., when a patient is comatose). In addition, an accurate identification of the subvariety of SE must be made. This will influence the type and promptness of treatment. Subtypes of convulsive status, for example, have different responses to currently available AEDs.[4] Those patients with primary generalized tonic–clonic SE resulting from a preexisting epileptic condition respond much better to standard therapy than those with secondary generalized tonic–clonic SE caused by acute central nervous system (CNS) impairment.[15]

The diagnosis of SE should not be made until the physician has witnessed at least one generalized tonic–clonic seizure occurring in a patient with a depressed state of consciousness who has a history of repeated seizures without regaining consciousness between episodes.[5] For nonconvulsive or focal motor SE, the diagnosis should not be made until 30 minutes of continuous seizure activity has been observed.[5] If these guidelines for proper diagnosis are followed, the premature administration of large doses of potentially toxic medications may be avoided. Occasionally, a person with intermittent decorticate or decerebrate posturing is mistakenly identified and treated as having SE.[16]

The resulting morbidity and mortality of SE depend on the underlying causes and precipitating factors as well as the response to treatment.[1] Patients often die of seizures, but more frequently they die as a result of the acute illness that precipitated the attack.[17] Mortality rates between 5% and 50% have been reported, although more recent estimates range from 10% to 12%.[4] The reduction in mortality may be a result of the greater understanding of the pathophysiology of SE and improved use of available pharmacologic and supportive modalities.

The morbidity for patients surviving the SE attack is often significant. In a study of 239 children with SE, the prognosis for survivors was poor. Significant sequelae (e.g., epilepsy, mental retardation, or neurologic deficits) occurred in 67% of patients; 50% were normal prior to the episode of SE.[13]

## Physiologic Changes

Certain physiologic changes occur during an episode of SE (Table 40.3). These changes are thought to be related to the violent motor activity of generalized tonic–clonic seizures and to the abnormal neuronal discharges.[5] Neuronal damage after an episode of SE is probably related to excessive metabolic activity of vulnerable neurons in the presence of adequate energy supplies. Another theory ascribes neuronal damage to episodes of transient local hypoxia that occur during seizures caused by a metabolic transition of oxygen sufficiency to insufficiency in the cerebral cortex.[5]

Neuronal damage probably occurs during the late phase of SE (Table 40.3), which suggests that hyperpyrexia, arterial hypotension, hypoxia, and hypoglycemia may be associated with its development.[7] The mean duration of SE in adult patients that do not develop neurologic sequelae is $1\frac{1}{2}$ hours versus 10 hours for those that do and 13 hours for those that die.[4] This relationship emphasizes the importance of prompt, effective treatment of SE to avoid neurologic complications.

Secondary systemic complications may also develop after

**Table 40.3** Physiological Changes in Major Motor Status

| *Transient or early (0–30 min)* | *Late (after 30 min)* |
|---|---|
| Arterial hypertension | Arterial hypotension |
| Cerebral venous pressure raised | Cerebral venous pressure raised or normal |
| $Pa_{O_2}$ low or normal[a] | $Pa_{O_2}$ low or normal |
| $Pa_{CO_2}$ high | $Pa_{CO_2}$ normal |
| $Pcv_{O_2}$ (low or high) | $Pcv_{O_2}$ normal or low |
| $Pcv_{CO_2}$ high | $Pcv_{CO_2}$ normal (or high) |
| Cerebral blood flow increased | Cerebral blood flow increased, normal, or decreased |
| Hyperglycemia | Normoglycemia, hypoglycemia |
| Hyperkalemia | Hyperkalemia |
| Hemoconcentration | Hyperpyrexia (secondary) |
| Lactic acidosis | |

[a] Pa, arterial pressure; Pcv, cerebral venous pressure.

Modified from Treiman DM: General principles of treatment: Responsive and intractable status epilepticus in adults, in Delgado-Escueta AV, Wasterlain CG, Treiman DM, Porter RJ (Eds): Status Epilepticus. New York, Raven, 1983, p 378.

a prolonged SE attack (i.e., greater than 60 minutes) and include autonomic dysfunction (e.g., hyperthermia, excessive sweating, and resulting dehydration). Initial elevations in blood pressure may not be sustained; hypotension and eventually shock may develop. Excessive muscle activity may lead to myolysis (causing elevations in serum enzymes, such as creatinine phosphokinase) and myoglobinuria, leading to renal failure, hyperkalemia, and acute intravascular coagulation. Finally, cardiovascular and respiratory failure may result.[4,5] These conditions have predictive effects on the residual status and functioning of the patient.

Of the various types of SE, generalized tonic–clonic SE clearly causes the most morbidity and mortality; however, other types of SE can also cause residual damage. Both complex partial SE and prolonged focal SE produce neuronal damage and memory loss.[5] It is imperative that focal motor and nonconvulsive status epilepticus be regarded as urgent situations requiring prompt treatment.

## Treatment

### *Convulsive Status Epilepticus*

Convulsive SE may be generalized, or it may be focal in onset and then progress to a generalized condition. In infants, pure clonic SE may occur; pure tonic SE is common in children and adolescents.[7] The most common form of SE in adults is tonic–clonic with bilateral motor activity. This is the most prevalent form of SE and is discussed in detail. Many of the same principles and therapeutic modalities are utilized to treat other, less common forms of convulsive SE (i.e., tonic SE, clonic SE).

The overall goal for treating SE is to stop seizure activity as quickly as possible. The quicker seizure cessation is achieved, the less likely neurologic deficits will develop. Particular attention must be paid to supportive measures, including adequate oxygenation and correction of metabolic anomalies to prevent chronic sequelae.

Table 40.4 outlines the currently recommended management of tonic–clonic SE. This approach is based on historical experience and opinion rather than data generated from comparative trials. The acute nature and severity of the disease and the fact that an effective treatment regimen exists create ethical dilemmas in performing comparative clinical trials on both old and new therapies. The adage "if it's not broken, don't fix it" might be an appropriate analogy to the current treatment recommendations for tonic–clonic SE.

#### Supportive Care

Though the mainstay of therapy in SE consists of administration of AEDs, attention must be paid to the systemic manifestations of prolonged seizure activity (as outlined in the previous section). Specific supportive measures should be instituted simultaneously with AED therapy. Airway management to provide adequate ventilation, oxygenation, and protection from aspiration is essential. The patient should be positioned so that aspiration, suffocation, and physical injury are avoided. A plastic oral airway may be placed if possible. Excessive oral secretions should be suctioned to prevent impairment of airway functioning. The patient should be intubated if airway exchange status is questionable. Unfortunately, these manipulations are often quite difficult to perform on a patient actively seizing.

Blood pressure, pulse rate, and temperature should be carefully monitored. Excessive fluid loss and the subsequent decrease in blood pressure may necessitate increased administration of intravenous fluids. Placing a bladder catheter may also be helpful to monitor the patient's fluid output status. If possible, electrocardiographic (ECG) and electroencephalographic (EEG) monitoring should be used. An indwelling intravenous catheter should be immediately placed an a sample of venous blood obtained for estimates of serum glucose, electrolytes, BUN, calcium, serum AED concentrations (if appropriate), and a toxicology screen (if adequate suspicion exists). Initially, administration of 50 mL of 50% glucose in adults (1–2 mL/kg in children) is recommended. In addition, blood glucose testing (Dextrostix, Visidex, Chemstrip bG) is needed to determine if additional glucose should be administered.

An arterial blood sample for measurement of pH, $Pa_{O_2}$, $Pa_{CO_2}$, and $HCO_3$ should be obtained to assure adequate oxygenation and to determine if the patient is becoming acidotic. An acidotic condition ($pH < 7.35$) is corrected by administration of 50 mEq of sodium bicarbonate ($NaHCO_3$). Repeat blood gas measurements and additional doses of $NaHCO_3$ may be required in patients with compromised respiratory status.

For the patient experiencing a tonic–clonic SE attack outside the hospital environment, every effort should be made to get medical assistance as quickly as possible. In the interim, the patient should be eased to the floor and constrictive clothing should be loosened. Any objects that might harm the patient should be removed. Nothing hard should be

**Table 40.4** Management of Tonic–Clonic Status Epilepticus

| *Time from initiation of observation and treatment (min)* | *Procedure* |
|---|---|
| 0 | Assess cardiorespiratory function as the presence of tonic–clonic status is verified. If unsure of diagnosis, observe one tonic–clonic attack and verify the presence of unconsciousness after the end of the attack. Insert oral airway and administer $O_2$ if necessary. |
| | Insert an indwelling intravenous catheter. Draw venous blood for anticonvulsant levels, glucose, BUN, electrolyte, and CBC stat determinations. Draw arterial blood for stat pH, $Pa_{O_2}$, $Pa_{CO_2}$, and $HCO_3$. Monitor respiration, blood pressure, and ECG. If possible, monitor EEG. |
| 5 | Start IV infusion through indwelling venous catheter with normal saline containing vitamin B complex. Give a bolus injection of 50 mL 50% glucose. |
| 10 | Infuse diazepam IV no faster than 2 mg/min until seizures stop or to total of 20 mg. Also start infusion of phenytoin no faster than 50 mg/min to a total of 18 mg/kg. If hypotension develops, slow infusion rate. (Phenytoin 50 mg/mL in propylene glycol may be placed in a 100-mL volume control set and diluted with normal saline. The rate of infusion should then be watched carefully.) Alternately, phenytoin may be injected slowly by IV push. |
| 30–40 | If seizures persist, two options are available: IV phenobarbital or diazepam IV drip. The two drugs should not be given in the same patient, and an endotracheal tube should be inserted. |
| | IV phenobarbital option: Start infusion of phenobarbital no faster than 100 mg/min until seizures stop or to a loading dose of 20 mg/kg. |
| | Diazepam IV drip option: 100 mg of diazepam is diluted in 500 mL $D_5W$ and run in at 40 mL/h. This should produce serum diazepam levels of 0.2–0.8 $\mu$g/mL. |
| 50–60 | If seizures continue, institute general anesthesia with halothane or pentobarbital and neuromuscular junction blockade. If an anesthesiologist is not immediately available, start infusion of 4% solution of paraldehyde in normal saline; administer at a rate fast enough to stop seizures, or give 50 to 100 mg of lidocaine by IV push. If lidocaine is effective, give 50–100 mg diluted in 250 mL of 5% $D_5W$ IV at a rate of 1–2 mg/min. |
| 80 | If paraldehyde or lidocaine has not terminated seizures within 20 min from start of infusion, institute general anesthesia with halothane and neuromuscular junction blockade. |
| | If status epilepticus reappears when general anesthesia is stopped, consult a neurologist who has expertise in status epilepticus. Seek advice from a regional epilepsy center on the management of intractable status epilepticus. |

Modified from Delgado-Escueta AV, Wasterlain CG, Treiman DM, Porter RJ: Status epilepticus: Summary, in Delgado-Escueta AV, Wasterlain CG, Treiman DM, Porter RJ (Eds): Status Epilepticus. New York, Raven, 1983, p 539.

forced between the patient's teeth as this may cause injury. The patient's head should be turned to the side to prevent aspiration if vomiting occurs. An accurate summary of the details surrounding the onset of the attack and the duration of seizure activity should be recorded and provided to medical personnel as soon as possible.

***Drug Therapy*** The characteristics of an "ideal drug" to treat status epilepticus have been proposed by Treiman[5] (Table 40.5). Although an ideal drug presently does not exist, these properties are useful in determining a rational therapeutic plan for treating SE.

The drug should be available for intravenous administra-

**Table 40.5** Properties of an Ideal Drug for Treatment of Status Epilepticus

| |
|---|
| Rapidly effective against all types of status |
| Available for intravenous administration |
| Potent, so that small volumes can be given rapidly |
| Safe: no cardiorespiratory depression, no depression of consciousness, no systemic side effects |
| Rapidly enters the brain |
| Long distribution half-life |
| Short elimination half-life |
| Useful in oral form as a chronic antiepileptic drug |

Modified from Treiman DM: General principles of treatment: Responsive and intractable status epilepticus in adults, in Delgado-Escueta AV, Wasterlain CG, Treiman DM, Porter RJ (Eds): Status Epilepticus. New York, Raven, 1983, p 381.

tion because of the necessity for rapidly achieving therapeutic plasma concentrations at the effector site (i.e., brain). Intramuscular, nasogastric, and rectal routes are less desirable, as they depend on adequate tissue perfusion for drug absorption and subsequent distribution.[18] The ideal drug should be administered rapidly without concern for adverse effects (e.g., hypotension, cardiac arrhythmias, and respiratory depression). The agent chosen should rapidly enter the brain, and remain for a sufficient duration to prevent further seizure activity.

Table 40.6 describes some pharmacologic and pharmacokinetic parameters of AEDs routinely used in the treatment of SE. The therapeutic plasma concentrations are those specific for generalized convulsive SE and are not based on controlled, prospective dose-ranging studies. Dose–response curves have not been adequately characterized, and many of these recommendations are based only on experience or are extrapolated from studies evaluating drug treatment of chronic epilepsy. The "$t_{1/2}\alpha$" and "$t_{1/2}\beta$" are distribution and elimination half-lives, respectively. The "effective" half-life is an estimation of the length of time a particular agent will exert a therapeutic response after a single dose. This last parameter takes into account relative lipid solubilities, $pK_a$, and distribution characteristics, and can be used when making decisions regarding dosing intervals or the need for continuous infusions.[5,18]

*Diazepam* Intravenous diazepam is the drug of choice for the acute management of generalized tonic–clonic SE.[19] Diazepam stops convulsions within 3 minutes in 33% of patients, and within 5 minutes in 80%.[4] Diazepam has the added benefit of ease of intravenous administration compared with other AEDs. Unfortunately, despite rapid cessation of seizure activity, seizures frequently recur after 15 to 20 minutes. The rapid initial response followed by loss of seizure control is due to the pharmacokinetic characteristics of the drug. Diazepam is extremely lipophilic and rapidly penetrates the brain after intravenous administration. This initial distribution phase is followed by a rapid and extensive redistribution of diazepam into body fat stores, thus decreasing the concentration of drug at the receptor sites.[20] This phenomenon necessitates repeated administration of diazepam or the use of a second drug (e.g., phenytoin) to prevent seizure recurrence.

Intravenous diazepam should be administered at a rate no greater than 2 mg/min until seizures abate (Table 40.4). Although a more aggressive rate of up to 5 mg/min has been suggested, it is not recommended.[18] Complications associated with the intravenous administration of diazepam include respiratory depression, hypotension, and arrhythmias.

**Table 40.6** Pharmacokinetic and Dosing Guidelines for AEDs Commonly Used in SE

| *Drug* | *Usual initial IV dose* | *Administration rate* | *Time to stop SE, $t_{1/2}\alpha$ (min)* | *Mean elimination half-life, $t_{1/2}\beta$ (h)* | *Estimated effective half-life* | *Initial plasma concentration[a] (μg/mL)* |
|---|---|---|---|---|---|---|
| Diazepam | 5–10 mg (0.25–0.4 mg/kg)[b] | 1–2 mg/min (same) | 3–5 | 30–40 | 1.5 min | 0.5–0.8 |
| Phenytoin | 18–20 mg/kg (same) | ≤ 50 mg/min (0.5–1.5 mg/kg/min) | 30 | 22[c] | 22 h | 20–25 |
| Phenobarbital | 300–800 mg (20 mg/kg) | 25–50 mg/min (same) | 20 | 86 | 50–120 h | 20–45 |
| Lorazepam | 4–8 mg (—) | < 2 mg/min (—) | 3 | 15 | 2 h | 0.3–1.0 |
| Paraldehyde[d] | 0.2–0.4 mL/kg[e] (0.1–0.15 mL/kg) | Repeat initial IV dose every 2–4 h prn | — | 7.5 | 6 h | 150–300 |
| Lidocaine | 50–100 mg (0.5–1 mg/kg) | 1–2 mg/min (20–50 μg/kg/min) | 1 | 1.5–2.5 | — | — |

[a] Plasma concentrations have generally not been well established for treatment of SE.
[b] Information in parentheses is for children.
[c] Phenytoin displays nonlinear elimination; this value will change depending on the concentration.
[d] Injectable form is no longer commercially available.
[e] Can also be given IM at a dose of 5–10 mL for adults.

Table compiled from References 5, 16, 19, 20, and 29. Dashes are used for data that could not be extracted from the literature.

Because of the poor solubility of diazepam in water, the commercially available diazepam injection is formulated with 40% propylene glycol and 10% ethyl alcohol. Therefore, rapid infusion may potentiate propylene glycol-induced hypotension and possibly arrhythmias. At an infusion rate of 2 mg/min, no episodes of hypotension occurred in a series of 50 patients with SE.[21] Although an adequate dose–response relationship has not been identified, an administration rate no greater than 2 mg/min is recommended to minimize the hypotensive and arrhythmogenic effects of intravenous diazepam.

A total diazepam dose of 20 mg (Table 40.4) is conservative, and many patients require larger amounts.[20,22,23] Diazepam is a safe drug and can be administered in larger doses with minimal concern for toxicity (provided the rate of administration is appropriate). The significant acute adverse effects include central nervous system (CNS) and respiratory depression. CNS depression may hamper clinical assessment of the patient's response, especially when absence SE is being treated. Both CNS and respiratory depression may be potentiated by the coadministration of other agents, particularly barbiturates; however, as the primary objective in SE is seizure control and as artificial ventilation should be available, diazepam should be administered in doses large enough to induce seizure cessation.

Other possible adverse effects caused by the administration of intravenous diazepam include local complications, such as thrombophlebitis. If proper administration techniques are used and adequate venous access is secured, these complications are negligible.[19] Finally, paradoxical effects have been reported after intravenous diazepam administration. In patients with Lennox–Gastaut syndrome, benzodiazepines and other AEDs have induced brief episodes of tonic SE.[19]

Continuous diazepam infusion is indicated for patients whose seizures are not adequately controlled after appropriate intravenous doses of diazepam and phenytoin (Table 40.4). Despite the paucity of large, controlled clinical trials, intravenous infusion of diazepam appears to be a safe and effective therapy in these treatment-resistant patients.[24]

Stability and compatibility problems with intravenous diazepam infusions have created some confusion and hesitancy in the use of this form of therapy. Contrary to the manufacturer's recommendations, diazepam can be safely diluted and administered as an infusion. The drug is soluble in NaCl 0.9%, Ringer, lactated Ringer, and dextrose solutions. Adsorption of diazepam to the tubing of some infusion sets can be minimized by using glass containers and volume control sets containing cellulose propionate. Plastic containers and infusion sets made of polyvinyl chloride appear to produce the greatest amount of drug absorption.[24] Solutions of diazepam at a concentration of 0.125 mg/mL are stable for 6 to 8 hours in glass containers.[25]

Suggested doses and administration rates for diazepam infusions are provided in Table 40.4. The duration of the diazepam infusion should be determined by the clinical situation, but infusion is usually continued at least 3 hours after seizure cessation.[23] Tolerance may develop with prolonged use. Patients should be continuously monitored clinically and electroencephalographically for seizure activity. If breakthrough seizures occur, an additional bolus dose should be administered and the infusion rate increased.[24] Patients must also be monitored for signs of toxicity, including respiratory depression, hypotension, and arrhythmias.

Although less desirable, rectal delivery of diazepam solution is an alternative to the intravenous route and may be particularly useful in neonates and children. Rectal therapy is effective in the treatment of febrile convulsions and absence SE.[26,27] Intramuscular diazepam is erratically absorbed (especially in adults and those with poor hemoperfusion) and should not be used in the treatment of SE.

Diazepam is cleared from plasma primarily by hepatic (phase I) metabolism. After its redistribution into adipose tissue, diazepam demonstrates a slow elimination half-life of 1 to 2 days. This elimination is age dependent, longer in premature newborns than newborns, and shorter in infants and children than adults. Elderly patients show a longer elimination half-life, caused in part by a change in volume of distribution.[28] The dose of diazepam need not be altered in renal failure, though patients with impaired hepatic metabolism and/or hypoperfusion require close clinical monitoring and possible reduction in infusion rate over time.[18] For a more complete discussion of benzodiazepine pharmacokinetics, the reader is referred to Chapter 51.

Diazepam concentrations between 0.2 and 0.8 mg/L are probably effective in the treatment of SE (Table 40.4), but this therapeutic range has not been rigorously studied.[21] Diazepam assays are not readily available and are impractical to use in the acute clinical setting. Objective measures of response and toxicity exist and should be used in titrating the appropriate diazepam dose in patients with SE.

***Phenytoin*** Phenytoin is an effective agent in the treatment of both partial and generalized convulsive SE, but it is not indicated in the treatment of absence SE.[2] With respect to effectiveness in terminating a convulsive SE episode, intravenous phenytoin is similar to diazepam, although diazepam has a quicker onset of action.[29,30] Because the initial therapeutic effects of diazepam are lost after 15 to 20 minutes (because of the redistribution phenomenon) and seizure activity frequently recurs, the combination of diazepam and phenytoin is recommended (Table 40.4). Brain phenytoin concentrations peak in 15 to 20 minutes, with maintenance of effective brain concentrations and subsequent seizure control for 24 hours or longer after an intravenous loading dose of 18–20 mg/kg (Table 40.6).[29–31]

As with diazepam, adverse effects are associated with the intravenous administration of phenytoin, because the injectable formulation of phenytoin also contains 40% propylene glycol and 10% ethanol. The potential complications of hypotension and cardiac arrhythmias can be minimized by not exceeding an administration rate of 50 mg/min.[32] Elderly patients and those with unstable cardiopulmonary function require an even slower infusion rate.[31] ECG monitoring and frequent blood pressure determinations should be performed during and for 1 hour after the infusion. A phenytoin infusion concentrate that does not contain propylene glycol and alcohol is available in Europe and has been administered rapidly without complications.[33]

Administering phenytoin by rapid intravenous push is impractical. A dose of 18 mg/kg for a 72-kg man would take close to 30 minutes to administer at a rate of 50 mg/min. Intramuscular administration is painful and results in erratic and slow absorption, as phenytoin precipitates at the injection site. Intravenous infusion of phenytoin as a large-volume parenteral also creates difficulties because of its poor solubility with other fluids and the potential formation of a phenytoin acid precipitate.[32]

Phenytoin is soluble in 0.45% and 0.9% sodium chloride and lactated Ringer solution. Admixtures with other drugs or base fluids containing dextrose should be avoided. Sodium chloride 0.9% is an acceptable diluent if the final phenytoin sodium admixture concentration is no less than 100 mg/100 mL and, preferably, 100 mg/25 or 50 mL.[34] In addition to the mixing and administration procedure outlined in Table 40.4, the use of an in-line filter (0.22 or 0.45 $\mu$m) is advocated to prevent minor drug crystals from entering the vein.[31] The solution should be prepared immediately prior to use, and infused within 1 hour.[34]

Local reactions to intravenous phenytoin include painful sensations (burning, aching) and, less frequently, extravasation.[35,36] These effects are thought to be dependent on concentration and rate of administration, and may be minimized by not exceeding a phenytoin concentration of 6.7 mg/mL (in the intravenous admixture fluid) and not administering the drug at a rate greater than 40–50 mg/min.[35] To avoid extravasation, phenytoin should be infused only through a free-flowing, well-positioned intravenous site. Smaller veins (hand, wrist, foot) are best avoided.[35,36]

Patients who have not previously received phenytoin, or those noncompliant patients whose drug concentrations are virtually nonexistent, should be given an intravenous loading dose of 18 mg/kg. This dose should produce initial serum concentrations in the range 20–25 mg/L and 24-hour concentrations greater than 10 mg/L.[37] Phenytoin exhibits an increased volume of distribution in obese subjects.[38] For very obese patients, phenytoin loading doses should be calculated on the basis of ideal body weight (IBW) plus the product of 1.33 times the excess weight over IBW.[38]

For patients with subtherapeutic phenytoin concentrations, the following equation may be used to rapidly estimate an appropriate dose to provide therapeutic serum concentrations:

$$\text{dose (mg)} = (Cp_d - Cp_m)(0.7)(W_{kg})$$

Here $Cp_d$ is the desired serum concentration (generally considered to be between 20 and 25 mg/L for SE), and $Cp_m$ is the measured subtherapeutic serum concentration. The constant 0.7 represents an approximation of the average volume of distribution. $W_{kg}$ is the patient's weight in kilograms. Thus, for a 70-kg patient with a known phenytoin concentration of 4 mg/L who is experiencing an SE attack, a calculated dose of 780 mg should raise the serum concentration to approximately 20 mg/L.

A cautionary note should be emphasized when interpreting serum phenytoin concentrations. Phenytoin is a weak acid and is highly protein bound (approximately 90%) to albumin. In a patient with a normal serum albumin who is not taking other drugs known to displace phenytoin from protein binding sites, a "total" concentration in the range 10–20 mg/L corresponds to a "free" (unbound) concentration of 1–2 mg/L. Although the free phenytoin concentration is responsible for the therapeutic effect, total phenytoin concentrations are generally obtained as they are simpler and less expensive to quantify.[32]

A low total serum phenytoin concentration in the face of a therapeutic free concentration may be caused by decreased serum protein binding or displacement of phenytoin from protein binding sites. Thus, in interpreting phenytoin concentrations, factors altering protein binding (discussed in Chapter 41) should be considered. Measurement of a serum free phenytoin concentration may be indicated in patients with decreased serum albumin or those taking other highly protein-bound drugs. Toxic phenytoin concentrations (i.e., free concentrations > 4.0 mg/L or total concentrations > 40 mg/L) may cause seizure activity and should be avoided.

The decision to initiate chronic phenytoin therapy depends on the clinical situation and the patient's history. For patients with readily correctable causes of their seizures, chronic AED therapy is not warranted. Avoidance of precipitating factors may be all the therapy required. The noncompliant patient should be placed back on phenytoin (or other AEDs) and counseled intensively on compliance. Potential drug interactions should be investigated and doses of phenytoin adjusted accordingly. Any patient presenting with tonic–clonic SE and no identifiable causes should probably be placed on a chronic regimen of phenytoin, at least until a full diagnostic workup is performed. After the initial intravenous loading dose and seizure cessation, a serum phenytoin concentration should be obtained within 12 to 24 hours. Chronic oral administration of phenytoin should be instituted at a dose between 6 and 7 mg/kg/d, 24 hours after the loading dose. The complexities and maintenance dose requirements of phenytoin are reviewed in Chapter 41.

Phenytoin represents an important drug in the treatment of SE. Many patients are successfully treated with phenytoin alone, and diazepam therapy is not always needed.[30] Phenytoin alone is indicated in patients whose seizures follow trauma or other clinical situations where continued evaluation of mental status is important.[2]

***Phenobarbital*** Phenobarbital was among the first effective pharmacologic therapies used in the treatment of SE; it replaced ether and chloroform.[39] Despite the availability of newer agents (e.g., diazepam and phenytoin), phenobarbital is still an important drug in SE, and remains the drug of choice in some institutions.[2,39]

Barbiturates raise the threshold of many neuronal pathways to direct and indirect stimulation, and cause general CNS depression. The ability of phenobarbital to suppress cortical seizure activity at doses that do not cause excessive sedation is an advantage when compared with other barbiturates.[39] Phenobarbital penetrates the CNS at rates similar to those of phenytoin and reaches peak concentrations in 3 to 20 minutes.[40]

An intravenous loading dose of 20 mg/kg (and possibly up to 25 mg/kg) administered at a rate not exceeding 100 mg/min is recommended.[2,4,41] One author suggests a dose of 250–300 mg be given intravenously and, if the patient has not stopped seizing within 20 to 30 minutes, a second dose may be administered. Only occasionally, a third dose is given after an additional 20 minutes.[39] This protocol has produced adequate seizure control with serum concentrations well below the therapeutic range of 25–40 mg/L, without problems of respiratory failure (Table 40.6).[39]

Phenobarbital can be administered rapidly by intravenous push over several minutes. It is soluble in common intravenous fluids and can be mixed without concern of precipitation. A major problem with phenobarbital use is respiratory depression, and ventilatory assistance must be readily available. The coadministration of phenobarbital and diazepam may cause additive respiratory depression. Special precautions should be observed when the two drugs are given concurrently. Also, decreased blood pressure and altered sensorium may occur with phenobarbital administration.

Advantages of using phenobarbital over diazepam are that the depressant effects on respiration, blood pressure, and sensorium are more gradual than those of diazepam and the therapeutic effects of phenobarbital are long-lasting.[2] The main disadvantage is that phenobarbital has a slower onset of action than diazepam. Therefore, the recommendation to use diazepam initially followed by phenytoin in treatment of SE remains appropriate. Although phenobarbital may appear to be a potential alternative to phenytoin, the lack of respiratory and sensorium depression seen with phenytoin outweighs its administration and compatibility problems. For the treatment of neonatal SE, however, phenobarbital is the drug of choice.[7]

***Lorazepam*** None of the three medications discussed so far meet all the desirable characteristics necessary for a single agent in the treatment of SE. Lorazepam may be the drug with properties closest to those described (Table 40.5). The drug has been shown to be effective in both generalized and partial SE, can be rapidly administered by intravenous push, and is relatively safe.[42]

Lorazepam is less lipid soluble than diazepam and is much less extensively tissue bound. This property allows clinically effective CNS concentrations to remain at the receptor site for a longer time after a single dose. Phase II metabolic processes are responsible for the elimination of lorazepam. The elimination half-life of lorazepam is shorter than that of diazepam, and accumulation of lorazepam after repeated administration does not occur.[43]

The efficacy data for lorazepam in SE are largely limited to case reports that suggest the drug is very effective.[42,44] One large, well-controlled, double-blind comparative trial between lorazepam and diazepam found the drugs to be virtually identical in efficacy and adverse effects.[45] Despite the differences in lipophilicity, no statistical differences existed between median times of onset for lorazepam (3 minutes) and diazepam (3–5 minutes). Adverse effects consisted of respiratory depression and respiratory arrest, and occurred in less than 15% in each group. Subjects experiencing adverse effects in the lorazepam group had more underlying medical problems, which possibly predisposed them to adverse drug effects.[45] One shortcoming of this trial was the need to coadminister phenytoin to patients in both groups for ethical reasons. This prevented the assessment of duration of activity for lorazepam when given alone.[45]

The most common adverse effect reported for lorazepam when used to treat SE is sedation.[42] Other effects include confusion, tremor, hallucinations, and respiratory depression.[42,45]

Before intravenous administration, lorazepam must be diluted with an equal volume of compatible diluent, such as sterile water for injection, 0.9% sodium chloride injection, or 5% dextrose injection. Lorazepam injection is available in prefilled syringes that can accommodate diluent directly in the syringe. Once diluted, the solution should be mixed gently, but not shaken vigorously.

Lorazepam may be administered by rapid intravenous push over 2 minutes. Doses for the treatment of SE have ranged from 2 to 10 mg.[42] A common initial dose appears to be 4 mg, which is followed by a second 4-mg dose if seizures have not stopped after 10 minutes.[45]

As a single agent, lorazepam appears to possess those properties necessary for treatment of SE. Whether there is enough evidence to justify a clinical study comparing diazepam and phenytoin with lorazepam alone, poses an ethical and scientific dilemma. Not until this information is available will clinicians feel comfortable using lorazepam as monotherapy in the treatment of SE. The use of lorazepam instead of the combination of diazepam and phenytoin may prove beneficial in certain clinical situations.

***Paraldehyde*** Paraldehyde has been used in the treatment of SE for over 100 years. Poor understanding of its physiochemical properties has led to compatibility problems and adverse effects.[18] The water solubility of paraldehyde decreases with increasing temperature, and the change from room to body temperature may cause precipitation of paraldehyde in the bloodstream, resulting in pulmonary embolization.[46] The drug can be safely administered as a 4% solution in saline.

Paraldehyde is very sensitive to light and air; improper storage leads to decomposition.[46] The revised USP specifications state that paraldehyde must be maintained in well-filled, tight, light-resistant containers not exceeding 30 mL. Any unused portions must be discarded 24 hours after opening.[46]

The pharmacokinetics of paraldehyde make it a desirable agent for SE. After intravenous administration, the drug rapidly distributes to the brain. The drug is 70% to 80% metabolized by the liver and has an elimination half-life between 6 and 7.5 hours.[46]

Paraldehyde can be administered intravenously, intramuscularly, orally, or rectally. Though the latter two routes of administration are frequently impractical during SE, intramuscular paraldehyde provides a reasonable alternative when intravenous administration of drugs is not possible. Near-peak plasma levels occur within 20 minutes.[46] When paraldehyde is administered intramuscularly, caution should be exercised to avoid severe sciatic nerve damage. Also, skin sloughing and sterile abscesses may occur. The drug should be given by injection deep intramuscularly into the buttocks. A glass syringe must be used when injecting paraldehyde (IV or IM) as the drug decomposes plastic syringes and tubing.[46]

For rectal administration, paraldehyde can be diluted 2:1 in oil (olive or cottonseed) or mixed in 200 mL 0.9% NaCl. Absorption from this site is slow, and peak plasma concentrations may not occur for 2 to 4 hours. Slow absorption limits the usefulness of rectal paraldehyde, although it may be the only option in specific clinical situations (e.g., unable to obtain IV access).

Adverse effects reported with paraldehyde include pulmonary hemorrhage, pulmonary edema, metabolic acidosis, hepatitis, and erythematous rash.[40] Oral paraldehyde can cause irritation and ulceration of the mouth and stomach, and often produces foul breath (from exhaled paraldehyde).[46]

Despite the many shortcomings of paraldehyde, it is useful for patients with refractory SE not responding to standard therapy. Situations in which paraldehyde offers particular benefit include the need for initial intramuscular drug administration, SE caused by alcohol withdrawal, and when allergies to safer agents, preclude their use.[46] At this time there are no commercially available sources of injectable paraldehyde.

***Lidocaine*** Lidocaine is recommended as an alternative drug in the treatment of refractory SE (Table 40.4), and may control seizures when diazepam, phenytoin, phenobarbital, and/or paraldehyde have failed. Lidocaine is easy to administer intravenously and has a rapid onset of action, often noted within 20 to 30 seconds. The effectiveness of lidocaine in the treatment of tonic–clonic and simple partial SE was recently confirmed based on review of 148 published cases.[46]

The recommended initial dose is 2–3 mg/kg, but most clinicians administer 50 or 100 mg. Because initial seizure control is lost after 20 minutes, lidocaine infusion at a rate of 1–2 mg/min is recommended, although higher infusion rates (3–10 mg/kg/h) may be necessary.[46] The usually quoted therapeutic range for lidocaine is 2–6 mg/L.[47] This range has been established for the antiarrhythmic effects of the drug; the therapeutic range for SE has not been established. CNS toxicity (e.g., fasiculations, visual disturbances, and tinnitus) may occur at concentrations between 6 and 8 mg/L; seizures and obtundation may develop when concentrations exceed 8 mg/L.[47] Serum lidocaine concentrations should be monitored to avoid drug accumulation and toxicity.

***Valproic Acid*** Although not generally recommended, rectal administration of valproic acid represents an alternative second-line agent in SE. Less experience exists with this form of therapy as compared with paraldehyde or lidocaine. No comparative trials are available assessing valproic acid versus other AEDs in the treatment of SE. A suppository formulation of valproic acid evaluated in a small number of patients was found to be effective when administered with intravenous phenytoin.[48] The slow absorption of valproic acid from the rectal route limits its clinical usefulness in the immediate control of seizure activity. An intravenous dosage form of valproic acid is not currently available but is being investigated.

Until more experience is gained, rectal administration of valproic acid in the acute setting of an SE episode is not generally recommended.

***General Anesthesia*** When first- and second-line SE therapies have failed, the need for an anesthesiologist to induce general anesthesia in the patient becomes paramount. Once the patient has seized for an extended period of time (i.e., ≥60 minutes), general anesthesia may represent the only therapeutic alternative to prevent major metabolic and neurologic sequelae.

As shown in Table 40.4, halothane for inhalation anesthesia[49] or intravenous pentobarbital may be used.[39] As Lederman points out, "few clear and reliable guidelines regarding depth or duration of anesthesia are available, and there are few data regarding the advantages of inhalation versus intravenous agents."[7] The actual method of anesthesia will most likely depend on the individual agents with which the anesthesiologist at each institution is most comfortable and familiar.

## *Nonconvulsive Status Epilepticus*

### Absence Status Epilepticus

Absence SE represents the most frequently observed form of nonconvulsive SE. The clinical manifestations of this disorder include an altered state of consciousness and/or behavior (lethargy, decreased mental function) and manifestation of the classic 3/second spike-and-wave pattern on EEG.[50] Attacks are frequently caused by precipitating factors (similar to tonic–clonic SE) and avoidance of these factors may be the only therapy required. Correction of identifiable causes, such as structural or metabolic aberrations, is paramount.

The acute absence SE attack can be treated by the administration of intravenous diazepam. Seizure cessation may be more difficult in patients with secondary generalized epilepsy than those with primary generalized epilepsy.[51] Chronic therapy to prevent recurrent attacks should be instituted with ethosuximide or valproic acid, as discussed in Chapter 41.

### Complex Partial Status Epilepticus

Complex partial SE occurs when clinical and electroencephalic seizure activity is focal in onset and consciousness is impaired during the attack.[52] Originally thought to be rare,[52] complex partial SE is now believed to be more common.[51] Clinically, the difference between absence SE and complex partial SE is that absence manifests as a prolonged state of one attack, whereas complex partial SE is a continuous series of repeated attacks. Also, patients with complex partial SE experience phases of total unresponsiveness with stereotypical automatisms, whereas patients with absence SE do not.[52]

Treatment recommendations for complex partial SE are similar to those described for absence SE, and include identifying the underlying cause and removing precipitating factors. Few cases of complex partial SE have been reported, making the pharmacologic therapy somewhat empiric. The combination of intravenous diazepam and phenytoin appears to be effective. But in complex partial SE, phenytoin alone may be more beneficial, as it does not produce sedation.[51] This may represent an important advantage when evaluating a disease state with subtle symptoms.

Lorazepam may be a reasonable alternative to the diazepam–phenytoin combination in the treatment of nonconvulsive SE,[53] although sedation limits its usefulness in many instances. Therefore, although intravenous lorazepam is possibly effective, its sedative properties make intravenous phenytoin (as a single agent) a superior choice.

## *Special Populations*

### Neonates

Neonates, infants, and children represent unique patient populations with different etiologies for SE episodes. Neonatal SE is an ominous prognostic indicator. Because of the immature cortical organization of the CNS, seizure activity in the neonate is often subtle and abstruse.[54] Clinical manifestations may be limited to abnormal eye movement, repetitive eye blinking, and repetitive oral buccolingual movements such as sucking or swallowing. The classic tonic and/or clonic movements of the extremities may not be present.[54] Seizure activity must be distinguished from clonus or jitteriness that is not convulsive. The major distinguishing traits of clonus are that it is rhythmic, the alternating movements are of equal amplitudes, it is positional and thus responds to changes in position, it may be ablated by restraining the moving part, and the abnormal eye movements and sucking or swallowing common with seizures do not occur with clonus.[54]

The causes of seizures in neonates are similar to those in adults, but also include amino acid disturbances and drug withdrawal (resulting from addicted mothers).[54] Once correctable causes of seizure activity have been rectified, anticonvulsant therapy should be instituted. AEDs commonly used in the neonate include phenobarbital, phenytoin, diazepam, and paraldehyde.

Phenobarbital, the AED most commonly used in the neonatal period, is given as an intravenous loading dose of 20 mg/kg followed by a maintenance dose of 3.5–5 mg/kg/d.[54] Though a maintenance dose of 5 mg/kg/d might be expected to produce toxic serum phenobarbital concentrations based on the neonate's ability to metabolize the drug, the half-life drops significantly between the first and fourth weeks of life. Serum concentration monitoring and dosage adjustment should be instituted with chronic phenobarbital administration to maintain concentrations between 20 and 40 mg/L.

If phenobarbital alone is ineffective at stopping seizure activity, despite a serum concentration of 40 mg/L, phenytoin should be added. The intravenous route is the most desirable mode of administration, because of unreliable absorption from the oral route and irritation and unpredictable absorption from intramuscular administration.[54] A phenytoin loading dose of 20 mg/kg should be given.

Seizures in the neonatal period are associated with higher mortality and neurologic sequelae (e.g., mental retardation, cerebral palsy, and epilepsy).[55] The best predictors of morbidity and mortality include a 5-minute Apgar score of less than 7, the need for resuscitation during the first 5 minutes after birth, early onset of seizures, seizures lasting longer than 30 minutes, and the number of days on which seizures occurred.[55]

The decision to institute chronic AED therapy in a neonate poses a therapeutic dilemma. The high frequency of neurologic toxicity from long-term AED therapy may outweigh the low risk of subsequent seizure activity.[55] Others recommend phenobarbital prophylaxis for neonates with risk factors such as severe asphyxia, intraventricular hemorrhage, and structural brain abnormalities.[56] Until controlled clinical trials are performed, the decision to institute phenobarbital (or other AEDs) prophylaxis will be based on clinical judgment.

### Infants and Children

The pediatric doses and rates of administration for the AEDs commonly used in the treatment of SE are provided in Table 40.6. The principles of drug administration and monitoring outlined in the previous sections for adults apply to this patient population. Unlike neonates, children tend to have better capacities for metabolic and renal clearance of drugs than adults. Close monitoring of serum concentrations and subsequent dose titration are warranted.

Administration of intravenous phenytoin (9–21 mg/kg) eradicated seizure activity within 3 minutes in 12 out of 13 pediatric patients in SE.[57] This rapid response was produced without concomitant diazepam or phenobarbital administration. The anticipated benefit of lack of sedation was evident and neurologic status was unaltered in all cases. Until these data are replicated in larger clinical trials, the coadministration of intravenous diazepam and phenytoin will remain the treatment of choice in pediatric patients with tonic–clonic SE.

When intravenous access is not readily available, rectal paraldehyde[58] and rectal valproic acid[59] may offer reasonable alternatives as first-line agents in the treatment of SE. Rectal paraldehyde may be given at a dose of 0.3 mL/kg. A second dose should be given within 20 minutes if seizures persist.[58] Valproic acid should be administered rectally at a dose of 20 mg/kg to produce serum concentrations of approximately 50 mg/L.[59] When the rectal route of administration is used to treat SE, careful monitoring of serum AED concentrations is paramount because of the potential for hypoperfusion and poor absorption.

### Elderly

Changes in the pharmacokinetics of AEDs associated with aging should be considered when elderly patients are treated. Decreases in renal clearance and hepatic metabolism of AEDs may occur, resulting in toxic serum AED concentrations. Therefore, close monitoring of serum concentrations is warranted.

Many elderly patients have decreased serum albumin and an increase in the free/total ratio of highly bound AEDs (i.e., phenytoin) should be considered. Monitoring of both free and total serum AED concentrations may be helpful in making therapeutic decisions in this patient population. The free serum concentration should be emphasized over the total serum concentration, as the free (unbound) drug is available for diffusion to the pharmacologic receptors in the brain. Therefore, it is common for the elderly to have "subtherapeutic" total concentrations, yet "therapeutic" free concentrations.

## Summary

Though status epilepticus has been identified for over 150 years, it remains a serious and emergent clinical entity with a high morbidity and mortality. Efforts to more precisely define and classify the various forms of SE have led to greater universal understanding and recognition of the manifestations of the disease. Tonic–clonic SE is the most common and ominous of the various forms of SE and requires immediate treatment. Nonconvulsive SE is now recognized as producing residual morbidity if not appropriately treated. Identification and removal of the causes or precipitating factors of SE are important aspects of therapy. Equal attention must be paid to the systemic physiologic aberrations as well as the seizure activity when treating SE.

Antiepileptic drugs are the mainstay of therapy and intravenous diazepam is frequently the drug of choice because of its rapid onset and ease of administration. Despite these benefits, its short duration of action requires repeated dosing, or the administration of a second intravenous drug such as phenytoin. Alternative agents, and those that may be tried in refractory SE, include phenobarbital, lorazepam, paraldehyde, lidocaine, and valproic acid. For extreme cases, general anesthesia may be required.

The therapy for SE has evolved over time, and is not always supported by data from large, controlled clinical trials. Drugs chosen on a theoretical basis appear to be effective. Formal study is required to determine if other currently available agents, or investigational agents, offer advantages over traditional treatment choices.

## References


1. Calmeil LF. De l'epilepsie etudiae sous le rapport de son siege et de son influence sur la production de l'alientation mentale, thesis, Paris, Didat, 1924.
2. Pellock JM. Status epilepticus, in Pellock JM, Myer EC (eds): Neurologic Emergencies in Infancy and Childhood. Philadelphia, Harper and Row, 1984.
3. Gastaut H. Classification of status epilepticus, in Delgado-Escueta AV, Treiman DM, Porter RJ, Wasterlain CG (eds): Status Epilepticus. New York, Raven Press, 1983, pp. 15–35.
4. Delgado-Escueta AV, Wasterlain CG, Treiman DM, Porter RJ. Status epilepticus: Summary, in Delgado-Escueta AV, Wasterlain CG, Treiman DM, Porter RJ (eds): Status Epilepticus. New York, Raven Press, 1983, pp 537–541.
5. Treiman DM. General principles of treatment: Responsive and intractable status epilepticus in adults, in Delgado-Escueta AV, Wasterlain CG, Treiman DM, Porter RJ (eds): Status Epilepticus. New York, Raven Press, 1983, pp 377–384.
6. Delgado-Escueta AV, Wasterlain CG, Treiman DM, et al. Management of status epilepticus. N Engl J Med 1982; 306(22):1337–1340.
7. Lederman RJ. Status epilepticus. Clev Clin Q 1984; 51:261–266.
8. Oxbury JM, Whitty CWM. Causes and consequences of status epilepticus in adults. A study of 86 cases. Brain 1971;94: 733–744.
9. Janz D. Conditions and causes of status epilepticus. Epilepsia 1961;2:170–177.
10. Celesia GG. Modern concepts of status epilepticus. JAMA 1976;235:1571–1574.
11. Rowan AJ, Scott DF. Major status epilepticus. A series of 42 patients. Acta Neurol Scand 1970; 46:573–584.
12. Roger J, Lob H, Tassmari CA. Status epilepticus, in Vinken RJ, Bruyn GW (eds): Handbook of Clinical Neurology, vol 15. Amsterdam, North-Holland, 1974, pp 145–188.
13. Aicardie J, Chevrie JJ. Convulsive status epilepticus in infants and children. A study of 239 cases. Epilepsia 1970; 11:187–197.
14. Aminoff MJ, Simon RP. Status epilepticus: Causes, clinical features, and consequences in 98 patients. Am J Med 1980; 69:657–666.
15. Cranford RE, Leppik IE, Patrick B, et al. Intravenous phenytoin in acute treatment of seizures. Neurology 1979;29:1474–1479.
16. Leppik IE. Status Epilepticus (State of the science in EEG and Epilepsy—1986). Seattle, WA: American Electroencephalographic Society and American Epilepsy Society, 1986.
17. Hauser WA. Status epilepticus: Frequency, etiology, and neurological sequelae, in Delgado-Escueta AV, Wasterlain CG, Treiman DM, Porter RJ (eds): Status Epilepticus. New York, Raven Press, 1983, pp 3–14.
18. Bleck TP. Therapy for status epilepticus. Clin Neuropharmacol 1983; 6(4):255–269.
19. Tassinari CA, Michelucci DR, Bureau M, et al. Benzodiazepines: Efficacy in status epilepticus, in Delgado-Escueta AV, Wasterlain CG, Treiman DM, Porter RJ (eds): Status Epilepticus. New York, Raven Press, 1983, pp 465–475.
20. Shader RI, Greenblatt DJ. The use of benzodiazepines in clinical practice. Br J Clin Pharmacol 1981;11:55–95.
21. Delgado-Escueta AV, Enrile-Bascal F. Combination therapy for status epilepticus: Intravenous diazepam and phenytoin, in Delgado-Escueta AV, Wasterlain CG, Treiman DM, Porter RJ (eds): Status Epilepticus. New York, Raven Press, 1983, pp 477–485.
22. van der Kleijn E, Baars AM, Vree TB, et al. Clinical pharmacokinetics of drugs used in the treatment of status epilepticus, in Delgado-Escueta AV, Wasterlain CG, Treiman DM, Porter RJ (eds): Status Epilepticus. New York, Raven Press, 1983, pp 421–440.
23. Drugs for epilepsy. Med Letter 1986; 28(723):91–94.
24. Bell HE, Bertino JS. Constant diazepam infusion in the treatment of continuous seizure activity. Drug Intell Clin Pharm 1984; 18:965–970.
25. Mason NA, Cline S, Hyneck ML, et al. Factors affecting diazepam infusion: Solubility, administration-set composition, and flow rate. Am J Hosp Pharm 1981;38:1449–1554.
26. Milligan N, Dhillon S, Richens A, et al. Rectal diazepam in the treatment of absence status: A pharmacodynamic study. J Neurol Neurosurg Psychiatry 1981; 41:914–917.
27. Knudsen FU. Rectal administration of diazepam in solution in the acute treatment of convulsions in infants and children. Arch Dis Childhood 1979;54:855–857.
28. Schmidt D. Benzodiazepines: Diazepam, in Woodbury DM, Penry JK, Pippenger CE (eds): Antiepileptic Drugs. New York, Raven Press, 1982, pp 711–735.
29. Wilder BJ. Efficacy of phenytoin in treatment of status epilepticus, in Delgado-Escueta AV, Wasterlain CG, Treiman DM, Porter RJ (eds): Status Epilepticus. New York, Raven Press, 1983, pp 441–446.
30. Leppik IE, Patrick BK, Cranford RE. Treatment of acute seizures and status epilepticus with intravenous phenytoin, in Delgado-Escueta AV, Wasterlain CG, Treiman DM, Porter RJ (eds): Status Epilepticus. New York, Raven Press, 1983, pp 447–451.
31. Cloyd JC, Gumnit RJ, McLain LW. Status epilepticus: The role of intravenous phenytoin. JAMA 1980; 244(13):1479–1481.
32. Winter ME, Tozer TN. Phenytoin, in Evans WE, Schentag JJ, Jusko WJ (eds): Applied Pharmacokinetics. Spokane, WA, Applied Therapeutics, 1986, pp 493–539.
33. von Albert HH. A new phenytoin infusion concentrate for status epilepticus, in Delgado-Escueta AV, Wasterlain CG, Treiman DM, Porter RJ (eds): Status Epilepticus. New York, Raven Press, 1983, pp 453–456.

34. Carmichael RR, Mahoney DC, Jeffrey LP. Solubility and stability of phenytoin sodium when mixed with intravenous solutions. Am J Hosp Pharm 1980;37:95–98.
35. Earnest MP, Marx JA, Drury LR. Complications of intravenous phenytoin for acute treatment of seizures: Recommendations for usage. JAMA 1983;249(6):762–765.
36. Comer JB. Extravasation from intravenous phenytoin. Amer J IV Ther Clin Nutr 1984; 11(1):23–29.
37. Cranford RE, Leppik IE, Patrick B, et al. Intravenous phenytoin: Clinical and pharmacokinetic aspects. Neurology 1978; 28:874–880.
38. Abernethy DR, Greenblatt DJ. Phenytoin disposition in obesity: Determination of loading dose. Arch Neurol 1985;42:468–471.
39. Goldberg MA, McIntyre HB. Barbiturates in the treatment of status epilepticus, in Delgado-Escueta AV, Wasterlain CG, Treiman DG, Porter RJ (eds): Status Epilepticus. New York, Raven Press, 1983, pp 499–503.
40. Gal P. Phenobarbital and primidone, in Taylor WJ, Diers Caviness MHD (eds): A Textbook for the Clinical Application of Therapeutic Drug Monitoring. Irving, TX, Abbott Laboratories, 1986, pp 237–252.
41. Vining E, Freeman JM. Status epilepticus. Ped Annals 1985;14(1):764–770.
42. Levy RJ, Krall RL. Treatment of status epilepticus with lorazepam. Arch Neurol 1984;41:605–611.
43. Greenblatt DJ, Divoll M. Diazepam versus lorazepam: Relationship of drug distribution to duration of clinical action, in Delgado-Escueta AV, Wasterlain CG, Treiman DM, Porter RJ (eds): Status Epilepticus. New York, Raven Press, 1983, pp 487–491.
44. Homan RW, Walker JE. Clinical studies of lorazepam in status epilepticus, in Delgado-Escueta AV, Wasterlain CG, Treiman DM, Porter RJ (eds): Status Epilepticus. New York, Raven Press, 1983, pp 493–498.
45. Leppick IE, Derivan AT, Homan RW, et al. Double-blind study of lorazepam and diazepam in status epilepticus. JAMA 1983; 249(11):1452–1454.
46. Browne TR. Paraldehyde, chlormethiazole, and lidocaine for treatment of status epilepticus, in Delgado-Escueta AV, Wasterlain CG, Treiman DM, Porter RJ (eds): Status Epilepticus. New York, Raven Press, 1983, pp 509–517.
47. Pieper JA, Rodman JH. Lidocaine, in Evans WE, Schentag JJ, Jusko WJ (eds): Applied Pharmacokinetics. Spokane, WA, Applied Therapeutics, 1986, pp 639–681.
48. Vajda FJ. Valproic acid in the treatment of status epilepticus, in Delgado-Escueta AV, Wasterlain CG, Treiman DM, Porter RJ (eds): Status Epilepticus. New York, Raven Press, 1983, pp 519–529.
49. Opitz A, Marschall M, Degen R, Koch D. General anesthesia in patients with epilepsy and status epilepticus, in Delgado-Escueta AV, Wasterlain CG, Treiman DM, Porter RJ (eds): Status Epilepticus. New York, Raven Press, 1983, pp 531–535.
50. Porter RJ, Penry JK. Petit mal status, in Delgado-Escueta AV, Wasterlain CG, Treiman DM, Porter RJ (eds): Status Epilepticus. New York, Raven Press, 1983, pp 61–67.
51. Thomson T, Svanborg E, Wedlund JE. Nonconvulsive status epilepticus: High incidence of complex partial status. Epilepsia 1986;27(3):276–285.
52. Treiman DM, Delgado-Escueta AV. Complex partial status epilepticus, in Delgado-Escueta AV, Wasterlain CG, Treiman DM, Porter RJ (eds): Status Epilepticus. New York, Raven Press, 1983, pp 69–81.
53. Walker JE, Homan RW, Crawford IL. Lorazapam: A controlled trial in patients with intractable partial complex seizures. Epilepsia 1984;25(4):464–466.
54. Painter MJ. General principles of treatment: Status epilepticus in neonates, in Delgado-Escueta AV, Wasterlain CG, Treiman DM, Porter RJ (eds): Status Epilepticus. New York, Raven Press, 1983, pp 385–393.
55. Gal P. Anticonvulsant therapy after neonatal seizures: How long should it be continued? I. A case for early discontinuation of anticonvulsants. Pharmacotherapy 1985; 5(5):268–273.
56. Hodson A. Anticonvulsant therapy after neonatal seizures: How long should it be continued? II. A case for long-term treatment with anticonvulsants. Pharmacotherapy 1985; 5(5): 274–277.
57. Koren G, Brand N, Halkin H, et al. Kinetics of intravenous phenytoin in children. Ped Pharmacol 1984; 4:31–38.
58. Curless RG, Holzman BH, Ramsay RE. Paraldehyde therapy in childhood status epilepticus. Arch Neurol 1983; 40:477–480.
59. Snead OC, Miles MV. Treatment of status epilepticus in children with rectal sodium valproate. J Peds 1985; 106(2):323–325.

# Chapter 41 / Epilepsy

William R. Garnett, PharmD

Epilepsy has been recognized for at least 2,400 years. In the fifth century BC people with a "falling sickness" were observed. In ancient Rome if a citizen had a seizure it was considered a sign from the gods to adjourn the Senate. Hippocrates was the first to suggest the brain as the origin of the disease but he was long ignored.

Epilepsy is derived from the Greek *epilēpsia* meaning "to come upon, to be grabbed hold of or thrown down, to attack, to seize hold of." Hughlings Jackson stated that "A convulsion is but a symptom and implies only that there is an occasional, excessive, and disorderly discharge of nerve tissue on muscles. This discharge occurs in all degrees. It occurs with all sorts of conditions of ill health, at all ages and under innumerable circumstances." Although this description was written over 100 years ago, it remains a clear, concise description of epilepsy.

Today epilepsy is not considered a simple disease, but is viewed as a symptom of disturbed electrical activity in the brain caused by a wide variety of disorders. Epilepsy is not a single syndrome of similar symptoms, but is a general name given to the wide range of symptoms that reflect the manifold functions of the brain in a pathologically disturbed manner. Epilepsy is a collection of many different types of seizures that vary widely in severity, appearance, cause, consequence, and management. Epilepsy implies a periodic recurrence of seizures with or without convulsions.[1]

A seizure results from an excessive discharge of neurons and is characterized by changes in electrical activity as measured by the electroencephalogram (EEG). In addition, there may be disturbances in consciousness, sensory systems, motor systems, subjective well-being, and objective behavior. A seizure is episodic, is brief, has a beginning and an end, may produce postseizure impairment, and is involuntary. A convulsion implies a violent, involuntary contraction or series of contractions of the voluntary muscles.

Epilepsy is a chronic disorder. In selected patients surgery may offer a cure. Although drug therapy can often control the manifestations of the disease, antiepileptic drugs (AEDs) do not cure epilepsy. The proper treatment of epilepsy begins with a careful classification of the seizure type and selection of the most effective AED. The major determinant of AED selection may be toleration of the drug by the patient. Therefore avoidance of side effects rather than superior efficacy may be the main criterion. Monotherapy is preferred and can control about 80% of all patients with epilepsy. Although epilepsy is a chronic disorder, some patients may be successfully discontinued from AEDs after an extended seizure-free period. The success of AED therapy depends on careful dosage titration based on pharmacokinetic principles, the patient's ability to tolerate side effects, and long-term patient monitoring to ensure compliance, prevent drug interactions, and minimize toxicity.[2,3]

## Epidemiology

At least 8% of the general population have at least one seizure in a lifetime. The incidence of people who develop subsequent chronic seizures (or epilepsy) is harder to define. Some seizures may occur as single events resulting from withdrawal of CNS depressants (e.g., alcohol, barbiturates, and other drugs) or during acute illnesses (e.g., meningoencephalitis) or toxic conditions (e.g., uremia or eclampsia). Also, some people have single seizures for unexplained reasons. These seizures do not represent epilepsy.[4]

The American Epilepsy Foundation estimates that 2% of the general population, or 1 out of every 50 people, has epilepsy. This estimate may be low because of underreporting, improper diagnosis, and failure to seek medical attention.[5] The onset of seizures is greatest during the first year of life. Approximately 80% of patients have their first seizure before age 20. The onset of seizures decreases each decade after the first year until age 60.

## Pathophysiology

### *Mechanism of a Seizure*

Seizure activity is characterized by paroxysmal discharges occurring synchronously in a large population of cortical neurons. This is characterized on the EEG as a sharp wave or "spike." The basic physiology of a seizure episode is traceable to an unstable cell membrane or its surrounding, supportive cells. The seizure originates from the gray matter of any cortical or perhaps subcortical area. Initially, a small number of neurons fire abnormally. This onset propagates by physiologic pathways to involve adjacent or remote areas. The clinical manifestations depend on the site of the focus, on the degree of irritability of the surrounding area of the brain, and on the intensity of the impulse.[1]

The normal firing of neurons is controlled by excitatory and inhibitory neurotransmitters. The development of an action potential in a neuron is similar to that in a cardiac cell. Sodium concentration is high in the extracellular space and low in the intracellular space. The concentrations of potassium are reversed. The major ion species involved in burst activity appears to be calcium. Neurotransmitters (e.g., acetylcholine, norepinephrine, histamine, and corticotropin-releasing factor) enhance the excitability and propagation of neuronal activity, whereas γ-aminobutyric acid (GABA) and dopamine inhibit neuronal activity and propagation. Normal neuronal activity also depends on an adequate supply of glucose, oxygen, sodium, potassium, calcium, and amino acids. Systemic pH is also a factor in precipitating seizures.

Most of what is known about abnormal neuronal activity is derived from in vitro models such as the hippocampal slice model or from animal studies. The generation of epileptogenic discharges appears to depend on the interplay of three major factors. Some neurons must have an inherent ability to elaborate responses leading to paroxysmal bursts. Abnormal neurons recruit normal neurons to propagate the discharge of a seizure. This is augmented by the failure of normal inhibitory activities or by an enhancement of normal excitatory synaptic activities. Thus, a deficiency of inhibitory neurotransmitters such as GABA or an increase in excitatory neurotransmitters would promote abnormal neuronal activity. Interference with normal metabolic processes also promotes seizure activity; however, neither a failure of inhibition nor an enhancement of excitation completely explains the promotion of abnormal propagation. The most recent in vitro experiments suggest that modulation of neuronal activity in favor of the pathologic discharge is also important. This modulation appears to be under cholinergic control. In hippocampal neurons, acetylcholine causes an initial hyperpolarization, followed by a long-lasting depolarization with decreased conductance that leads to prolonged bursting. Differences between acute and chronic foci probably depend more on the degree and intensity of these factors than on fundamentally different mechanisms.[6]

Control of abnormal neuronal activity with AEDs is accomplished by elevating the convulsive threshold of neurons to electrical or chemical stimuli or by limiting the propagation of the seizure discharge from its origin. Raising the threshold most likely involves stabilization of neuronal membranes, whereas limiting the propagation involves depression of synaptic transmission and reduction of nerve conduction.[7]

### *Consequences of a Seizure*

The maintenance of the neuronal membrane action potential requires energy from ATP. Cellular respiration generates ATP and synthesizes neurotransmitters. During a seizure there is a large increase in the demand for brain blood flow to carry off $CO_2$ and to bring substrates for neuronal metabolic activity. The brain has a limited capacity to increase blood flow and during a seizure the brain may use more energy than it can manufacture. The more prolonged the seizure, the more likely the brain is to suffer ischemia that may result in neuronal destruction and brain damage. The developing brain is especially vulnerable and susceptible to damage. Seizure disorders per se do not cause a significant decrease in intelligence.[8]

Seizures beget seizures. There appears to be a positive correlation between the initiation of appropriate AED therapy and the ability to control seizure activity. The failure to control seizures seems to lead to an increase in seizure activity and also to the occurrence of other seizure types.[3] Therefore, appropriate therapy should be initiated early after the diagnosis of epilepsy.

**Table 41.1** Common Causes of Seizures

| | |
|---|---|
| Mechanical | Sudden withdrawal of CNS drugs |
| Trauma | Alcohol |
| Birth injury | Street drugs |
| Neoplasms | Antipsychotics |
| Vascular abnormalities | Antidepressants |
| Metabolic | Antiepileptic drugs |
| Electrolytes | Toxins |
| Water | Fever |
| Glucose | Infection |
| Amino acids | Hereditary |
| Lipids | Idiopathic |
| pH | |

### *Etiology and Precipitation of Seizures*

Seizures occur because small numbers of neurons discharge abnormally. Anything that disrupts the normal homeostasis of the neuronal cell and disturbs its stability may trigger abnormal activity and seizures. As shown in Table 41.1, these disruptions include mechanical disturbances, metabolic disturbances, sudden withdrawal of central nervous system (CNS) drugs, and toxins. A hereditary predisposition to seizures has been suggested. In some cases if an etiology can be found, it can be corrected and the patient will not require chronic AEDs; however, most patients who present with seizures do not have an identifiable cause and have idiopathic epilepsy.[1]

Many factors have been shown to precipitate seizures in susceptible individuals.[5] Hyperventilation may precipitate absence seizures. Sleep, sleep deprivation, sensory stimuli, and emotional stress may initiate seizures. Hormonal changes occurring around the time of menses, puberty, or pregnancy have been associated with the onset of, or an increase in, seizure activity. Birth control pills should be administered with caution to patients with epilepsy. Other precipitating factors include fever, trauma, lack of food, and drugs. A careful history for theophylline, alcohol, phenothiazines, antidepressants (especially maprotiline), and street drug use should be obtained from patients presenting with seizures. Also, AEDs in excessive concentrations may cause seizures.

## Clinical Presentation

### *Diagnosis of Seizures*

The diagnosis of seizures begins with a careful and accurate patient history.[9] The best evaluation of a seizure occurs if the patient has an episode in the presence of a trained observer; however, the frequency may be such that this is impossible. Therefore, the patient and the patient's family should be interviewed carefully to obtain a description of the seizure.

Information that should be obtained includes (1) frequency and duration of episodes, (2) precipitating factors, (3) times at which episodes occur, (4) presence of an aura, (5) ictal activity, and (6) postictal state. Patients may use terms to describe seizures that have no real meaning in seizure classifications. For example, patients may refer to "the little ones" or to "petit mal seizures" that are partial seizures and not absence. The patient's own terms need to be translated into the appropriate seizure classification. Also, the patient may be having more than one seizure type. Patients may not recognize some events as seizures, especially if there are no convulsions or loss of consciousness.

The physical, neurologic, and laboratory evaluations may help identify an underlying etiology. The physical and neurologic examinations may reveal head trauma or signs of other diseases that manifest as seizures. Laboratory tests (e.g., SMA-20, CBC, urinalysis, and special blood chemistries) may identify a metabolic etiology for the seizures (e.g., hypoglycemia, electrolyte abnormalities, or amino acid disturbances). The suspicion of systemic diseases (e.g., lead ingestion, sickle cell anemia, and infections) may be confirmed by laboratory evaluation. A lumbar puncture may be required if the patient has seizures and a fever. In many patients with idiopathic epilepsy, the physical, neurologic, and laboratory evaluations will be normal.

An EEG should be done as soon after the seizure as possible. The EEG is essential in properly classifying seizure types. For example, differentiation between generalized absence seizures and complex partial seizures with loss of consciousness only may be best accomplished by the EEG. The best time to obtain an EEG is while the patient is having a seizure. The EEG may be done under normal conditions, in a sleep-induced state, or in a sleep-deprived state. Clinicians should remember that a patient may have a normal EEG between seizures, while other patients have an abnormal EEG without having epilepsy. EEG results should be combined with the clinical description to classify the seizure type. To facilitate seizure classification, it may be necessary to hospitalize some patients and place them on simultaneous EEG and video monitoring.

Additional tests used in seizure evaluation include computer-assisted tomography (CAT), positron emission tomography (PET), and magnetic resonance imaging (MRI). A psychologic evaluation may be required if the patient is thought to have pseudoseizures or hysterical epilepsy.[10]

### *Classification of Seizures*

The International League Against Epilepsy has developed a classification system that combines clinical description with EEG findings (Table 41.2). Over 90% of seizure patients may be classified using this system.[11,12] This classification has helped identify that all seizures should not be treated the same.[13] The therapeutic range of the AEDs may differ depending on the seizure classification.[14] Therefore, proper seizure classification is essential to therapeutic drug monitoring. Further refinements in seizure classification may result in better drug and dosing selection.

Using the international classification scheme, seizures may be divided into partial, generalized, or unclassified. Partial seizures begin in one hemisphere of the brain and, unless they become secondarily generalized, result in an asymmetric seizure. Partial seizures may be described as focal or unilateral seizures and may be subdivided into simple and complex. Partial seizures manifest as alterations in motor functions, sensory or somatosensory symptoms, or autonomic symptoms. If there is no impairment of consciousness, the seizures are classified as simple partial. If there is impairment of consciousness, the seizures are de-

**Table 41.2** International Classification of Seizures

| *Traditional terminology* | *New nomenclature* |
|---|---|
| Focal motor; Jacksonian seizures | **I. Partial Seizures (seizures begin locally)** |
| | A. Simple (without impairment of consciousness) |
| | 1. With motor symptoms |
| | 2. With special sensory or somatosensory symptoms |
| | 3. With autonomic symptoms |
| | 4. With psychic symptoms |
| Temporal lobe or psychomotor seizures | B. Complex (with impairment of consciousness) |
| | 1. Simple partial onset followed by impairment of consciousness—with or without automatisms |
| | 2. Impaired consciousness at onset—with or without automatisms |
| | C. Secondarily generalized (partial onset evolving to generalized tonic–clonic seizures) |
| | **II. Generalized Seizures (bilaterally symmetrical and without local onset)** |
| Petit mal | A. Absence |
| Minor motor | B. Myoclonic |
| Limited grand mal | C. Clonic<br>D. Tonic |
| Grand mal | E. Tonic–clonic |
| Drop attacks | F. Atonic |
| | G. Infantile spasms |
| | **III. Unclassified Seizures** |
| | **IV. Status Epilepticus (prolonged partial or generalized seizures without recovery between attacks)** |

Compiled from Reference 11.

scribed as complex partial. With complex partial seizures, aberrations of behavior (automatisms) may occur. Complex partial seizures are more likely to progress to a generalized seizure.[15]

Generalized seizures have clinical manifestations that indicate involvement of both hemispheres. Motor manifestations are bilateral. Generalized seizures may be further subdivided by EEG and clinical manifestations.[16]

Absence seizures are manifested by a sudden onset, interruption of ongoing activities, a blank stare, and possibly a brief upward rotation of the eyes. The EEG during the seizure has a characteristic 2–4 cycle/s spike and slow-wave complex.[17]

Tonic–clonic seizures, formerly known as grand mal, are what many people think of as epilepsy. Although they may be preceded by premonitory symptoms known as an aura, the majority of patients lose consciousness without warning. The seizure results in a sudden sharp tonic contraction of muscles followed by a period of rigidity. During this period the patient may fall and be injured. During the seizure the patient may cry or moan, lose sphincter control, bite his(her) tongue, or develop cyanosis. After the seizure the patient may be unconscious for a variable period of time, and frequently goes into a deep sleep. Tonic and clonic seizures may occur separately.[5]

Brief shocklike muscular contractions of the face, trunk, and extremities are known as myoclonic jerks. They may be isolated events or rapidly repetitive.

A sudden loss of muscle tone is known as an atonic seizure. This may be described as a head drop, the dropping of a limb, or a slumping to the ground.[5] These patients often wear protective headware to prevent trauma.

Unclassified seizures include all seizures that cannot be classified because of inadequate or incomplete data.

## Treatment

### *Goals*

Seizures are abnormal events that often result in significant physical and neurologic impairment. The first treatment goal is to control or reduce the frequency of seizures, allowing the patient to live an essentially normal life. Ideally, seizure frequency should be reduced to zero; however, all AEDs have some side effects and the complete suppression of seizures must be balanced against side effects. As therapy is extended for many years, often a lifetime, chronic side effects must be considered. If the patient is overly sedated or develops other significant side effects, some seizure control may have to be sacrificed to improve functioning.

The second treatment goal is to prevent the occurrence of emotional and behavioral aberrations. Despite public awareness programs there are still many misconceptions about epilepsy. These misconceptions often liken epilepsy to mental retardation, to possession by demons, or to punishment by God. Clinicians must work with patients and their families to ensure that these misconceptions are dispelled. Patients may be encouraged to join the Epilepsy Foundation of America or other support groups that encourage patients with epilepsy to lead normal lives. As some AEDs may cause behavioral and cognitive abnormalities, these side effects should be considered in selecting a drug of choice.

**Table 41.3** Principles of Therapy

| |
|---|
| Establish diagnosis and exclude remedial causes |
| Select primary drug most appropriate for seizure type |
| Titrate dose to achieve desired blood concentration (monotherapy is preferred) |
| Consider ''free'' AED concentrations |
| Provide patient education |
| Consider discontinuing AEDs |

### *Principles*[18–22]

***Establish Diagnosis and Exclude Remedial Causes*** Some seizures result from correctable etiologies, for example, metabolic disturbances. Therefore, while AEDs may be used acutely, they would not be indicated for chronic use if the etiology could be identified and corrected. (See Table 41.3.)

***Select Primary Drug Most Appropriate for Seizure Type*** Classification of seizure types and epilepsy syndromes has improved the ability of clinicians to select drugs of choice for specific seizures (Table 41.4). Absence seizures are pharmacologically different from other seizure types. Phenytoin, phenobarbital, and carbamazepine, although effective in generalized and partial seizures, are ineffective in treating absence seizures and in some cases may precipitate an increase in seizure activity. Absence seizures are best treated with ethosuximide or valproic acid. Ethosuximide is effective only in absence seizures and is ineffective against other generalized and partial seizures. If the patient has a combination of absence and other generalized or partial seizures, valproic acid is the preferred first choice because it is the only AED effective against absence and other seizure types. If valproic acid is ineffective in treating a mixed seizure disorder that includes absence, ethosuximide should be used in combination with another AED.

Carbamazepine is recognized as the AED of first choice for partial seizures. Alternatives to carbamazepine are phenytoin, phenobarbital, and valproic acid.

The traditional treatment of tonic–clonic seizures is phenytoin or phenobarbital; however, the use of carbamazepine and valproic acid is increasing because these AEDs have a lower incidence of side effects and equal efficacy.

Recent data suggest that the therapeutic range for AEDs may be different for different seizure types. Blood concentrations may need to be higher to control complex partial seizures than to control tonic–clonic seizures.[14] If initial therapy fails to control seizures, alternative AEDs or a combination of AEDs should be tried to accomplish seizure control.

***Titrate Dose to Achieve Adequate Blood Concentrations of AEDs*** All AEDs are associated with depressed CNS function early in the course of treatment. CNS depression (e.g., drowsiness, lethargy, tiredness) usually lasts only 7 to 10

**Table 41.4** Drugs of Choice for Specific Seizure Disorders

| *New international* | *Commonly used major drugs* | *Commonly used alternative drugs* |
|---|---|---|
| Simple partial | Carbamazepine<br>Phenytoin<br>Phenobarbital | Primidone<br>Valproic acid |
| Complex partial | Carbamazepine<br>Phenytoin<br>Phenobarbital | Primidone<br>Valproic acid |
| Tonic–clonic | Phenytoin<br>Valproic acid<br>Carbamazepine | Primidone |
| Absence | Ethosuximide<br>Valproic acid | Clonazepam<br>Acetazolamide<br>Trimethadione[a] |
| Mixed seizures | Phenytoin<br>Phenobarbital + ethosuximide or valproic acid | Primidone<br>Carbamazepine + clonazepam<br>Acetazolamide |
| Bilateral massive epileptic myoclonus, atonic, infantile spasms[b] | Clonazepam | Phenytoin |
| | ACTH | Phenobarbital<br>Benzodiazepines<br>Acetazolamide |

[a] Previously used; not in common use today.
[b] Difficult group to treat; combinations are the rule.

days. Therefore, except in life-threatening situations (e.g., status epilepticus), AEDs should be started in low doses and gradually increased until seizure control is achieved, intolerable side effects occur, or the maximum therapeutic range has been achieved. A general rule is to initiate therapy with one fourth to one third of the anticipated maintenance dose and increase the dose to maintenance over 3 to 4 weeks.

Although doses of AEDs are frequently cited in milligrams per kilogram, the blood concentration is a more definitive therapeutic endpoint. A therapeutic range has been described for the major AEDs, but there is a large interpatient variability in pharmacokinetic parameters. Therefore, there is a large variation in the milligram-per-kilogram dose required. In compliant patients with low plasma concentrations who are receiving a normal milligram-per-kilogram dose, the dosage may need to be increased.

The blood concentration is a target that should be correlated with clinical outcome. Seizure control may occur before the "minimum" of the range is achieved and side effects may appear before the "maximum" of the range is achieved. Some patients may need and tolerate concentrations beyond the "maximum."

It was once common to start patients with seizures on combination AEDs (e.g., phenytoin and phenobarbital). Numerous studies have demonstrated that many patients can be effectively managed on one AED alone. The reduction in polypharmacy is correlated with a subsequent decrease in side effects. Therefore, the initial treatment of seizures should begin with the most potentially effective single drug.

The initial agent should be titrated until maximum benefit is achieved (i.e., seizure control is achieved or intolerable side effects occur). Patient compliance must be assessed to evaluate the usefulness of the initial agent. Efficacy may be assessed by seizure count.

A second medication may be added if the patient is having continued seizure activity despite good plasma concentrations. The second AED may replace or be added to the initial therapy. If the initial AED is replaced, it should be gradually tapered after the second drug has been titrated to the desired dose.

***Consider "Free" Concentrations of AEDs*** Many AEDs are highly bound to plasma proteins. The unbound or "free" concentration is the active drug capable of penetrating the blood–brain barrier and interacting at the receptor site. Equilibrium dialysis was the only method available to determine free drug concentration. This technique is still the standard used in research, but is too time consuming to be clinically useful.

Several companies have recently marketed ultrafiltration systems that are capable of more rapid separation of free from protein-bound drug. The availability of these systems makes free drug concentrations potentially clinically useful. Despite the ease of using ultrafiltration devices, free level monitoring is not indicated for routine use in all patients.[23] In patients who are not responding or having side effects at "therapeutic" concentrations of total drug, a free concentration may explain the unusual response. For populations known to have altered plasma protein binding (Table 41.5), free rather than total drug concentrations should be measured.

**Table 41.5** Conditions Altering Antiepileptic Drug[a]–Protein Binding

| |
|---|
| Chronic renal failure |
| Liver disease |
| Hypoalbuminemia |
| Burns |
| Pregnancy |
| Malnutrition |
| Displacing drugs |
| Age—neonates and elderly |

[a] Phenytoin and valproic acid are highly protein bound; carbamazepine has variable binding; phenobarbital and primidone are minimally bound; and ethosuximide is not bound to plasma proteins.

***Provide Patient Education*** To promote compliance, to assess safety and efficacy, and to prevent behavioral aberrations, the patient must understand the disease and prescribed medications. This requires patient education. Noncompliance is not influenced by age, sex, psychomotor development, seizure type, or seizure frequency.[24] Compliant patients achieve better seizure control.[25] Patient education should be continuous and compliance stressed at each clinic visit.

***Consider Discontinuing AEDs*** AEDs may not need to be given for a lifetime. Polypharmacy may be reduced and some patients can discontinue AEDs altogether. In reducing polypharmacy, the drug considered less appropriate for the seizure type should be discontinued first and the possibility of drug interactions considered. Reduction of polypharmacy has resulted in a decrease in side effects and an increase in cognitive abilities.[22]

Factors promoting complete withdrawal of AEDs include a seizure-free period of 2 to 4 years, complete seizure control within 1 year of onset, an onset of seizures after age 2 but before age 35, a normal EEG, and use of AEDs for inappropriate reasons. Factors associated with a poor prognosis in discontinuing AEDs despite a seizure-free interval include a history of a high frequency of seizures, repeated episodes of status, combination of seizure types, and development of abnormal mental functioning. A 2-year seizure-free period is suggested for absence and rolandic epilepsy, while a 4-year seizure-free period is suggested for simple partial, complex partial, and absence associated with tonic–clonic convulsions. Withdrawal is generally not suggested for patients with juvenile myoclonic, absence with clonic–tonic–clonic seizures, or clonic–tonic–clonic seizures.[26]

The withdrawal of AEDs should be gradual. Seizure relapses occur most often within the first several months of drug removal. Seizure relapse may be more common if the AEDs are withdrawn over 1 to 3 months compared with 6 months.[27] Sudden withdrawal is to be avoided.

The patient should agree to any plan to reduce or withdraw AED therapy. Some patients may be reluctant to stop medications because of fear of a seizure. Withdrawal may need to be scheduled at the convenience of the patient (e.g., during a summer vacation). A follow-up of 5 years is suggested for any patient successfully withdrawn from AED therapy.

### *Specific Antiepileptic Drugs*

The control of most seizure disorders can usually be accomplished by the careful selection and monitoring of the major AEDs. Reasons for treatment failure are outlined in Table 41.6. (See Tables 41.7, 41.8, and 41.9.) In compliant refractory patients second-line and adjunctive therapy may be tried.

#### Phenytoin

***Therapeutics*** Phenytoin may be used in any generalized seizure type except absence, where it may worsen the condition. Phenytoin is a drug of choice for tonic–clonic seizures. Partial seizures may also be treated with phenytoin.[22]

Phenytoin blocks posttetanic potentiation by influencing synaptic transmission. Proposed mechanisms include altering ion fluxes associated with depolarization, repolarization and membrane stability, altering calcium uptake in presynaptic terminals, influencing calcium-dependent synaptic protein phosphorylation and transmitter release, altering the sodium–potassium ATP-dependent ionic membrane pump, and preventing cyclic nucleotide buildup and cerebellar stimulation.[28]

***Pharmacokinetics*** (See Table 41.7.) Phenytoin is absorbed primarily from the duodenum; little absorption occurs in the stomach or ileum. Absorption is almost complete, with dissolution being the rate-limiting step. Absorption may be prolonged and secondary peaks may be seen. The absorption of phenytoin may be saturable. Enterohepatic cycling of phenytoin occurs, but there is no first-pass metabolism.[29]

The absorption of orally administered phenytoin is affected by the particle size of the administered formulation. Therefore, some brands may be absorbed faster than others. Preparations intended for single daily dosing are indicated as extended-release preparations. The brand of phenytoin that a patient receives should not be switched without careful monitoring.[30] The intramuscular administration of phenytoin is problematic and best avoided, as explained in Chapter 40.

Phenytoin enters the brain quickly, where it is redistributed to other body tissues including saliva and breast milk. It crosses the placenta to reach an equilibrium with mother and fetus. Phenytoin distributes to serum and tissue proteins. Obesity may increase the volume of distribution.[31]

In the blood, phenytoin is highly (~90%) protein bound primarily to albumin. For most patients this binding is predictable and is linear throughout the therapeutic range; however, special populations have altered protein binding (Table 41.5).

**Table 41.6** Reasons for Treatment Failure

| |
|---|
| Inappropriate drug selection |
| Ubiquitous use of phenytoin and phenobarbital for all seizure types |
| Failure to recognize antiepileptic drug of choice |
| Inappropriate dose |
| Failure to evaluate serum drug concentration |
| Failure to maximize serum drug concentration |
| Poor compliance |
| Refractory patients |
| Some patients do not respond despite maximal therapy |

**Table 41.7** Antiepileptic Drug Pharmacokinetic Data

| *AED* | *$t_{1/2}$ (h)* | *Time to steady state (d)* | *% Un-changed* | *$V_D$ (L/kg)* | *% Bioavail-ability* | *Clinically important metabolite* | *% Removed by dialysis* | *% Protein binding* |
|---|---|---|---|---|---|---|---|---|
| Phenytoin | A[a] 10–34<br>C 5–14 | 7–28 | <5 | 0.6–8.0 | 90–95 | No | 4% (H)[b] | 90 |
| Phenobarbital | A 46–136<br>C 37–73 | 14-21 | 20–40 | 0.6 | 90–100 | No | 30% (H)[b] | 50 |
| Primidone | A 3.3–19<br>C 4.5–11 | 1-4 | 40 | 0.43–1.1 | 90–100 | PB[b]<br>PEMA | 30% (H)[b] | 80 |
| Carbamazepine | 12 h if monotherapy; 5–14 h if combination; chronic dosing undergoes autoinduction | 21–28 for completion of autoinduction | <1 | 1–2 | >75 | 10,11-epoxide | <20 | 40–90 |
| Valproic acid | A 8–20<br>C 7–14 | 1–3 | <5 | 0.1–0.5 | 100 | May contribute to toxicity | — | 90–95, binding saturates |
| Ethosuximide | A 60<br>C 30 | 6–12 | 10–20 | 0.67 | Assumed 100 | No | ~50 | 0 |

[a] A, adult; C, child.
[b] H, hemodialysis.
[c] PB, phenobarbital, PEMA, phenylethylmalonamide.

Phenytoin is metabolized in the liver primarily by parahydroxylation to 5-(*p*-hydroxyphenyl)-5-phenylhydantoin (HPPH). HPPH is conjugated and excreted in the urine as a glucuronide. About 80% of an oral dose of phenytoin appears in the urine as HPPH. Abnormally low percentages of HPPH in the urine would indicate a problem with absorption. Phenytoin is a low-extraction drug and its metabolism is not greatly influenced by changes in liver blood flow; however, as the major route of metabolism is hydroxylation, the clearance may be influenced by drugs that stimulate or inhibit liver microsomal enzymes.

Phenytoin displays Michaelis–Menten elimination (i.e., the metabolism changes from first order to zero order) because the enzyme system is saturable. Therefore, after a certain serum concentration, no additional drug can be metabolized. Thus, any change in dosage produces significantly disproportional changes in serum concentrations. The process may be described by the equation

$$D = \frac{V_{max} C_p}{K_m + C_p}$$

where $D$ is the dose (in mg/day), $V_{max}$ is the maximum rate of metabolism, $K_m$ is the serum concentration at which rate of metabolism is half-maximal, and $C_p$ is the serum concentration.

Because $V_{max}$ and $K_m$ are both highly and independently variable, the metabolism of phenytoin may saturate at any concentration and may occur within the therapeutic range. $V_{max}$ has been shown to decline with age and the $K_m$ may be affected by concurrent drug therapy. It is very difficult to predict the resulting outcome of a dosage increase of phenytoin. Also, serum concentrations do not decline by a constant percentage upon discontinuation. Therefore, any dosage change should be followed with careful patient monitoring and serum concentration determinations.

Because of the saturable metabolism, the clinically useful concept of half-life may be inappropriate for phenytoin. Half-life assumes concentration-independent elimination. A better term for phenytoin is the time required to eliminate 50% ($t_{50\%}$). The average $t_{50\%}$ for phenytoin is 22 hours, but may range from 7 to 42 hours. Because of saturation, the $t_{50\%}$ increases with increasing serum concentrations and the time to reach steady-state may be prolonged.

Less than 5% of a dose of phenytoin is excreted unchanged. Renal impairment does not affect the excretion of HPPH. While an inhibitory effect of HPPH on phenytoin metabolism has been suggested, it has not been documented in humans. Neither hemodialysis nor peritoneal dialysis affects the clearance of phenytoin. Clinically insignificant amounts of phenytoin are removed by plasmapheresis.[32]

***Therapeutic Range/Dosing*** The accepted therapeutic range of phenytoin is 10–20 μg/mL in otherwise healthy patients receiving no other medications.[33] This range has evolved from observations that patient response is enhanced as concentrations increase, with 50% of patients showing a decrease in seizures at concentrations greater than 10 μg/mL

**Table 41.8** Summary of Antiepileptic Drug Pharmacologic Data

| *AED* | *Initial dose (mg/kg/d)* | *Therapeutic range (μL/mL total)* | *Side effects* Dose related | *Side effects* Not dose related | *Manufacturer* |
|---|---|---|---|---|---|
| Phenytoin | Loading dose; 20 in status | 10–20 | Nystagmus, ataxia, cognitive impairment, lethargy | Gingival hyperplasia, increase in body hair, coarsening of facial features, acne, folate deficiency, skin rash | Parke–Davis and others |
| Phenobarbital | Loading dose; 20 in status | 15–40 | Sedation, mental dullness, cognitive impairment, hyperactivity, ataxia | Hyperactivity, change in sleep problems, skin rashes | Multiple |
| Primidone | 50–125 mg initial dose; no loading dose required | 5–20 | | | Ayerst |
| Carbamazepine | 2–8 mg; no loading dose required | 4–12 | Double vision, blurred vision, lethargy | Fluid retention, leukopenia, bone marrow suppression, skin rash, GI distress | Ciba–Geigy and others |
| Valproic acid | 7.5–15; no loading dose required | 50–150(?) | GI upset, lethargy | Weight gain, nausea, alopecia, hepatitis | Abbott and others |
| Ethosuximide | 5–7; no loading dose required | 40–100 | GI distress, nausea, drowsiness, hiccups | Headache | Parke–Davis |

and 86% at concentrations greater than 15 μg/mL. The incidence of side effects begins to increase as the phenytoin concentration exceeds 20 μg/mL. At this range the free fraction is 10% of total drug concentration in most patients. Therefore, the therapeutic range of free drug is 1–2 μg/mL. Serum concentrations should be interpreted in concert with clinical response.

Because of the intervariability in the nonlinear elimination of phenytoin, serum concentration is a much better endpoint than total daily dose. The common practice of placing everyone on phenytoin 300 mg/d results in plasma concentrations above and below the desired therapeutic range. The dose of phenytoin must be individually titrated. Loading doses are needed only in status epilepticus. In nonacute

**Table 41.9** CNS Effects of Antiepileptic Drugs

| | *Behavioral/motor* | *Cognitive* |
|---|---|---|
| Phenytoin | Tiredness, ataxia, involuntary movements, alteration of emotional state | Impaired cognitive functioning, decreased attention, decreased problem solving and visuomotor tasks |
| Phenobarbital | Hyperactivity, lethargy, irritability, fussiness, disobedience, altered sleep | Impaired cognitive functioning, impaired short-term memory, decreased memory concentration |
| Carbamazepine | Irritability, difficulty sleeping, agitation, emotional liability | Minimal |
| Valproic acid | Drowsiness | Minimal |

situations, phenytoin may be initiated in doses of 1–3 mg/kg/d and titrated upward.

Because of the saturable metabolism, dose prediction of phenytoin is difficult. There have been several attempts to estimate phenytoin dosing. Bayesian regression-analysis computer programs seem promising in predicting non–steady-state and steady-state dosing[34]; however, this method requires sophisticated computer support. Other forecasting methods require one or two doses with resulting steady-state concentrations. The one-point methods fix either $V_{max}$ or $K_m$ and estimate the other. Population clearance and nomograms methods are clinically useful if used judiciously.[35] Because they fix one independent variable, all one-point methods have the potential for estimating the wrong dose. The reliability of dosage prediction can be enhanced if two different doses and the resulting steady-state values are known. The two values allow for calculation of both $V_{max}$ and $K_m$. Empirically, doses of phenytoin may be increased by 100 mg/d if concentrations are less than 8 μg/mL and by 50 mg/d if concentrations are greater than 9 μg/mL. Any dosage forecasting should be accompanied by careful clinical monitoring.

Based on an average "half-life" of 22 hours, once-a-day dosing has been postulated for phenytoin. A single daily dose should be easier to schedule and could be taken at night if central nervous system (CNS) depression accompanies the dose. Most adult patients can be maintained on a single daily dose of phenytoin; however, children may have more rapid elimination requiring more frequent administration. Adults also have variable elimination rates so everyone cannot be adequately controlled on once-a-day dosing. The larger the dose the more likely split dosing will be required.

***Dosage Forms*** There are three dosage forms for oral administration of phenytoin. The tablet and suspension contain phenytoin acid, while the capsule contains phenytoin sodium. Phenytoin sodium is 92% phenytoin. The parenteral solution is phenytoin sodium. The salt content should be considered in dosage form changes.

If given in equal amounts of phenytoin acid, the tablets, capsules, and suspension have the same bioavailability. Phenytoin capsules are designated as immediate-release or extended-release. Only the extended-release should be used in once-a-day dosing. A single-dose study indicated that phenytoin suspension has the potential for once-a-day dosing.[36] Particle size rather than formulation may determine the rate of absorption.

Phenytoin suspension will settle, producing unequal concentration distribution. A recent study indicated that resuspension could be accomplished without overzealous agitation.[37] Clinicians should remember that there are two different strengths of phenytoin suspension.

If oral administration is not feasible, intravenous administration of phenytoin is preferred over intramuscular administration.

***Adverse Effects*** The side effects of phenytoin may be described as acute, concentration dependent, and chronic. When phenytoin is initiated, the CNS-depressant effects may result in lethargy, fatigue, incoordination, visual blurring, higher cortical dysfunction, and drowsiness. These effects are usually transient and may be minimized by slow dosage titration (Tables 41.8 and 41.9).

When serum concentrations exceed 20 μg/mL, a significant number of patients exhibit nystagmus at a 45° lateral gaze. Ataxia frequently occurs at concentrations above 30 μg/mL. Phenytoin levels greater than 30 μg/mL may induce seizures.[38] At concentrations above 40 μg/mL, mental status changes including coma occur.

It is difficult to determine whether the chronic side effects of phenytoin are concentration or duration dependent. One of the more common chronic side effects is gingival hyperplasia, which occurs in up to 50% of the patients. Suppression of cognitive abilities is also a concern. Other chronic effects include vitamin D deficiency, osteomalacia, folic acid deficiency, carbohydrate intolerance, immunologic disturbances, hypothyroidism, and peripheral neuropathy. Phenytoin is associated with rare hypersensitivity or idiosyncratic reactions resulting in skin rashes, Stevens–Johnson syndrome, pseudolymphoma, bone marrow suppression, lupus-like reactions, and hepatitis.

***Drug Interactions*** Phenytoin is prone to many drug interactions (Table 41.9) and has been extensively reviewed.[39,40] The effects of phenytoin may be enhanced or reduced by drugs that affect its pharmacokinetic parameters. Phenytoin is highly protein bound and may be displaced by other highly protein bound drugs. A decrease in binding results in an increase in free phenytoin. The initial increase in free phenytoin is followed by an increase in clearance, a fall in total phenytoin concentrations, and the reestablishment of normal free phenytoin concentrations. Usually no dosage adjustment is necessary. Problems arise when clinicians react to the lower total phenytoin concentration without considering the free concentration. If protein binding interactions are suspected, free rather than total phenytoin concentrations are a better therapeutic guideline. Drug interactions affecting absorption, metabolism or excretion are potentially more chronically significant because total and free concentrations are affected concurrently. The metabolism of phenytoin can be inhibited (e.g., cimetidine) as well as increased (e.g., phenobarbital).

Phenytoin may interfere with other drugs, altering their pharmacokinetics. The AEDs frequently interact with each other in complex mechanisms. Caution should be used when they are added to or withdrawn from a patient's drug regimen.

Nutritional factors may also interfere with phenytoin. The rate of absorption of phenytoin may be decreased if it is given simultaneously with food. The bioavailability of phenytoin suspension was recently reported to be decreased in patients receiving continuous enteral nutrient tube feedings. A single-dose study of simultaneous administration found no difference in phenytoin bioavailability, indicating that the mechanism was something other than physical contact.[41] A complex interaction of phenytoin with folic acid has also been described, making vitamin ingestion an important part of the drug history. Phenytoin reportedly decreases folic acid absorption, but folic acid enhances the clearance of phenytoin.[42] Replacement of folic acid can reduce phenytoin concentrations and result in loss of efficacy.

*Therapeutic Monitoring* The dose of phenytoin should be individualized using serum concentrations of total or free drug in relationship to the patient's clinical response. A trough level is preferred for evaluation, but because of the usually long $t_{50\%}$, minimal peak-to-trough fluctuation is expected. For a patient experiencing side effects, a peak may be indicated. The initial peak of phenytoin is usually seen in 3 to 12 hours. A secondary peak may also be observed.

Because of the long $t_{50\%}$, the time to reach steady state with phenytoin is prolonged and variable. There usually is no need to obtain serum concentrations on hospitalized patients any more often than every 3 to 4 days, except in critical situations where loading and supplemental doses are given. Outpatients can be monitored every 2 to 4 weeks after a judicious dosage increase. If patients experience signs of toxicity (e.g., nystagmus, ataxia) serum concentrations should be evaluated.

*Other Hydantoins* Mephytoin, ethotoin, and phenacemide are hydantoin derivatives. In general, they are less useful than phenytoin because they are more toxic with the same degree of efficacy; however, for an occasional refractory patient unable to tolerate other AEDs, these hydantoin derivatives may be tried.[43]

**Phenobarbital/Primidone**

*Therapeutics* These AEDs may be considered together because primidone is metabolized to phenobarbital. Primidone is an active AED and has a second metabolite that may be active—phenylethylmalonamide (PEMA). In general because of costs and dosing frequency, phenobarbital should be tried first and primidone reserved for refractory patients. In some patients, primidone will be effective where phenobarbital has failed because of additional AED activity.

Phenobarbital is the drug of choice for febrile seizures and neonatal seizures. It is also useful in generalized seizures (except absence) and may be useful in patients with partial seizures. Primidone shares the same indications but is less useful in partial seizures.[22]

These agents are CNS depressants. They elevate seizure threshold by decreasing postsynaptic excitation, possibly by stimulating postsynaptic GABA-ergic inhibitor responses.[44]

*Pharmacokinetics* Phenobarbital is rapidly and completely absorbed regardless of whether it is given orally, intramuscularly, or rectally.[45,46] The rate of absorption appears to be independent of dose, with peak concentrations being reached 0.5 to 4.0 hours after a dose. The bioavailability of primidone is approximately 90% to 100% (Table 41.7).

Phenobarbital has a biphasic distribution. Initially, phenobarbital penetrates highly perfused organs including the brain. Phenobarbital penetrates the brain at a rate comparable to that of phenytoin, and peak concentrations are achieved 3 to 20 minutes after an intravenous dose.[47] Phenobarbital then distributes evenly to all body tissues including fat. Decreasing the systemic pH drives phenobarbital into body tissues.

Drugs affecting liver enzymes may alter phenobarbital metabolism, but phenobarbital clearance is not affected by liver blood flow. Despite the fact that phenobarbital is a potent enzyme inducer, there is no evidence in humans that it is an autoinducer. The elimination of phenobarbital is linear.[48] Neonates have a longer half-life than adults and children have a shorter half-life. About 20% to 40% of a dose of phenobarbital is excreted in the urine unchanged. Because tubular reabsorption of phenobarbital is pH dependent, the amount excreted renally can be increased by giving diuretics and urinary alkalinizers.

Primidone is metabolized to phenobarbital (3%–5%) and PEMA (30%–45%). The primidone/phenobarbital ratio is highly variable. A significant portion of primidone is excreted unchanged. The half-life of primidone may become shorter after chronic therapy because the phenobarbital metabolite may induce its metabolism.

*Therapeutic Range/Dosing* The therapeutic range of phenobarbital for the treatment of seizures is between 15 and 40 μg/mL. Occasionally, patients respond at lower or higher plasma concentrations. Because of the low plasma protein binding, free concentrations are seldom necessary (Table 41.8).

The accepted therapeutic range of primidone is 5–20 μg/mL. At this concentration, most patients have a phenobarbital concentration that is in the therapeutic range. It is rare that a patient on primidone needs supplemental doses of phenobarbital. PEMA concentrations are not routinely monitored.[49]

In emergency situations phenobarbital may be given by intravenous loading doses (as discussed in Chapter 40). In nonacute situations, phenobarbital should be started in low doses and titrated upward. The dose–concentration effect is linear and maintenance doses can be estimated from the first dose and resulting steady-state concentration.[48] Phenobarbital meets the criteria for predicting maintenance dose with a single serum concentration obtained after the first dose. Because the half-life of phenobarbital is so long the dose can be given as a single-daily dose.[50] Giving the drug at bedtime sometimes minimizes the consequences of CNS depression. Because of its long half-life, phenobarbital takes 3 to 4 weeks to reach steady state. Therefore, rapid dosage adjustments should be avoided in a nonacute situation.

Primidone is not administered as a loading dose. An initial dose of 50–125 mg may be increased every 2 to 4 days until the desired concentration is reached. Because of the short half-lives of primidone and PEMA, the drug should be given in divided doses.

*Adverse Effects* CNS side effects are the primary factors limiting use of phenobarbital. Tolerance usually develops to initial complaints of fatigue, drowsiness, sedation, and depression.[51] In children, paradoxically, the primary side effect is hyperactivity. Phenobarbital impairs higher cortical function. In susceptible patients phenobarbital may precipitate porphyria. Other rare side effects include skin rashes, osteomalacia, and hypotension (Tables 41.8 and 41.9).

The side effects of primidone and phenobarbital are similar and may be difficult to separate. The initial side effects of sedation, nystagmus, and ataxia may be minimized by starting at a low dose and gradually titrating the dose.[52]

*Drug Interactions* Phenobarbital is a potent enzyme inducer and will increase the elimination of any drug metabolized by phase I oxidative processes.[53] Other drugs may alter the concentrations of phenobarbital by altering its metabolism. Valproic acid, phenytoin, cimetidine, and chloramphenicol inhibit phenobarbital metabolism, necessitating a decrease in dose. Ethanol increases the metabolism of phenobarbital. The interactions of primidone are similar.

*Therapeutic Monitoring* Because of its long half-life, there are minimal peak-to-trough fluctuations with phenobarbital. Trough levels are preferred unless patients complain of side effects. Except after loading doses, there is no need to obtain a phenobarbital concentration until steady state has been reached 3 to 4 weeks after initiating therapy or side effects occur. The guidelines for primidone are similar.

**Carbamazepine**

*Therapeutics* This drug was originally approved for the treatment of trigeminal neuralgia; however, clinical trials have shown it to be a safe and effective AED.[54] Carbamazepine's relative lack of side effects as compared with phenytoin and phenobarbital has caused its increased use in a variety of seizure disorders. It may also be useful in selected psychiatric disorders, as discussed in Chapter 49. Carbamazepine is considered the AED of first choice for partial seizures, especially complex partial seizures. It is also useful for generalized seizures other than absence.[22,55]

Animal studies indicate that carbamazepine depresses transmission in the nucleus ventralis anterior of the thalamus. This area has been associated with the generalization and spread of seizure discharge. There is some depression of posttetanic potentiation (PTP) by carbamazepine, but it is of a lesser magnitude than occurs with phenytoin. The exact mechanism by which carbamazepine suppresses seizure spread is obscure. It affects ionic conductance only at concentrations far above those normally produced in man. It may inhibit an increase in cyclic AMP. Other biochemical effects are unknown.

*Pharmacokinetics* Based on bioavailability studies using a reference solution, the absorption of carbamazepine tablets is greater than 75%. The absorption of carbamazepine is slow and erratic because of its low water solubility. Absorption is dissolution rate dependent. Therefore, there may be dose-dependent absorption resulting in less bioavailability at higher doses. The variable absorption results in times to peak of 2 to 24 hours (average 6 hours). There is no first-pass metabolism. Food may enhance the bioavailability of carbamazepine. The suspension dosage form is absorbed faster than the tablets.[56]

Carbamazepine is a neutral and highly lipophilic drug that results in high body tissue binding. Carbamazepine binds to albumin and, to a lesser extent, to $\alpha_1$-acid glycoprotein.[57] The percentage bound may decrease at higher concentrations within the therapeutic range. The usefulness of free carbamazepine concentrations remains to be defined.

Most (98%–99%) of an administered dose of carbamazepine is metabolized by the liver. Although 33 metabolites have been identified for carbamazepine, the major metabolite is 10,11-epoxide carbamazepine.[58] This metabolite has significant anticonvulsant activity in animals, but the exact contribution to seizure suppression in humans is unknown. The formation of 10,11-epoxide carbamazepine is influenced by the presence of other enzyme-inducing drugs.[59]

Carbamazepine has the unique ability to induce its own metabolism. The half-life after a single dose is much longer than the half-life after chronic therapy. The presence of enzyme-inducing drugs reduces the half-life even more. The enzyme induction effect begins within 3 to 5 days after the initiation of therapy and takes 21 to 28 days to complete.[60] Therefore, it is possible to achieve initial concentrations that are within the therapeutic range but have concentrations fall despite continued therapy with good compliance. Some patients who respond well to initial therapy may be labeled refractory or noncompliant if the autoinduction phenomenon is not considered.

*Therapeutic Range/Dosing* Clinical trials indicate that the therapeutic range of carbamazepine is between 4 and 12 μg/mL.[55] Concentrations above 12 μg/mL are associated with an increase in the incidence of CNS-related side effects. The variable contributions of the 10,11-epoxide metabolite and free carbamazepine concentrations have restricted a precise definition of the therapeutic range.

Loading doses of carbamazepine are not clinically indicated. There are significant CNS-depressant effects and gastrointestinal complaints (e.g., nausea and vomiting) associated with large initial doses, but these may be minimized by slow, gradual dosage adjustment. During dosage titration, it should be remembered that carbamazepine clearance increases with time.

Doses may be started at one fourth to one third of the anticipated maintenance dose and increased every 2 to 3 weeks. The ranges for maintenance doses are 7–15 mg/kg/d for adults and 11–40 mg/kg/d for children less than 15 years of age (Table 41.8).

Because of the auto- and heteroinduction of carbamazepine metabolism, it is necessary to administer the drug two to four times per day. While some patients, especially those on monotherapy, can be maintained on twice-a-day therapy, others may require more frequent dosage administration. Children are likely to need more frequent administration. The occurrence of annoying CNS side effects (e.g., such as transient drowsiness, fatigue, lethargy, diplopia) and gastrointestinal complaints (e.g., nausea) may be minimized by giving larger doses at bedtime.

*Dosage Forms* Generic dosage forms of carbamazepine were approved by the FDA in the summer of 1986. The effect of switching brands is undetermined. Based on experience with other AEDs (e.g., phenytoin) this should be done cautiously, if at all, with careful monitoring of efficacy and drug concentrations. It may be necessary to administer the suspension dosage form more frequently than the tablet to prevent excessive peak-to-trough fluctuations.

*Adverse Effects* Side effects (Tables 41.8 and 41.9) of carbamazepine may fluctuate daily, paralleling the rise and decline of serum concentrations.[61]

Neurosensory side effects (e.g., diplopia, blurred vision, nystagmus, ataxia, unsteadiness, dizziness, and headache) are the most common, occurring in 35% to 50% of the patients. They are more common during initiation of therapy and may dissipate with continued treatment. The patient may become tolerant to these effects or they may abate with a reduction in dose. They may also be minimized by giving larger bedtime doses. Dosage manipulation should be tried before the patient is considered to be intolerant of carbamazepine.

Carbamazepine may induce a hyponatremic hyposmolar condition that is similar to the syndrome of inappropriate antidiuretic hormone secretion.[62] The incidence may increase with age. Periodic determinations of serum sodium is recommended. Gastrointestinal discomfort is also frequently reported with carbamazepine.

Until recently, the concern over carbamazepine-induced bone marrow suppression was reinforced by a "black box" warning in the package insert requiring frequent complete blood cell count monitoring. As indicated in several recent reviews, this concern is unfounded.[63,64] Only a few cases of aplastic anemia, the most serious complication, have been reported since 1964. In many cases there were confounding factors that precluded a definite cause-and-effect relationship. Thrombocytopenia and anemia have an incidence of less than 5% and usually respond to a cessation of drug therapy. Leukopenia is the most common hematologic side effect of carbamazepine. An incidence as high as 10% has been reported. In most patients the leukopenia is transient even when the drug is continued. In about 2%, the leukopenia is persistent but even patients with white blood cell counts of 3,000/mL do not seem to have an increase in infection.

Skin rashes are the most frequent hypersensitivity response. These are usually mildly eczematous but may progress to a Stevens–Johnson syndrome. Other rare side effects reported with carbamazepine include hepatitis, osteomalacia, cardiac conduction defects, and lupuslike reactions. Carbamazepine appears to have no or minimal effects on cognitive functioning.[65]

***Drug Interactions*** Because of concentration-dependent efficacy and side effects, drug interactions with carbamazepine are clinically very significant.[66] Drugs may interact with carbamazepine by enzyme induction (e.g., phenytoin, phenobarbital, primidone) or enzyme inhibition (e.g., valproic acid, erythromycin, cimetidine, propoxyphene, and isoniazid). Valproic acid appears to reduce the formation of the 10,11-epoxide metabolite without affecting the concentration of carbamazepine. Because of the empiric use of erythromycin, the interaction of erythromycin with carbamazepine is particularly significant. Carbamazepine may interact with other drugs by inducing their metabolism; for example, carbamazepine increases the metabolism of valproic acid, theophylline, warfarin, and ethosuximide (Tables 41.11 and 41.12).

***Therapeutic Monitoring*** Therapeutic monitoring of carbamazepine should reflect the autoinduction and time to reach steady state. Trough levels are preferred. Samples may be collected at the time of reported side effects. The relationship between time of last dose and sample collection should be noted.

**Valproic Acid**

***Therapeutics*** Valproic acid is a branched-chain carboxylic acid first synthesized in 1881. Until 1963, it was used primarily as an organic solvent, but has since shown efficacy against a variety of seizure disorders. Its relative lack of toxicity as compared with phenytoin and phenobarbital has contributed to its expanded use.[67]

Valproic acid is the only available AED that is effective against absence and other types of generalized seizure types. It is also used in the treatment of partial seizures. Valproic acid is the drug of choice for a patient with absence seizures and another seizure type.[22] It is a second-line agent for patients with febrile seizures who cannot tolerate phenobarbital.[68]

Initially it was felt that valproic acid increased GABA by inhibiting its degradation or by activating its synthesis. While this may explain some of valproic acid effects, the time course for the increase in GABA compared with anticonvulsant effects of valproic acid indicates that inhibition of GABA synthesis does not fully explain how valproic acid prevents seizures. More recently, it was proposed that valproic acid may potentiate postsynaptic GABA responses, may have a direct membrane-stabilizing effect, and may affect the potassium channel.[69]

***Pharmacokinetics*** Valproic acid appears to be completely absorbed from available oral dosage forms when administered on an empty stomach.[70] Peak concentrations occur in ½ to 1 hour with the syrup, 1 to 3 hours with the capsule, and 2 to 6 hours with the enteric-coated tablet.[71] Food delays, but does not decrease, the amount of valproic acid absorbed.

Valproic acid distributes widely throughout the body. It is 90% to 95% protein bound primarily to albumin. The binding sites for valproic acid are saturable and the free fraction may increase as the total concentration increases. The saturable binding may indicate that the free concentration is a better monitoring parameter than the total valproic acid concentration, especially at higher concentrations.[72]

Valproic acid is metabolized primarily by the liver. There is no first-pass metabolism and the clearance is independent of hepatic blood flow. As with other highly protein-bound drugs, an increase in free drug results in an increase in clearance. Thus, the clearance of valproic acid changes at higher concentrations.

The primary route of valproic acid metabolism is $\beta$-oxidation, although up to 40% of a dose may be excreted as the glucuronide. At least ten metabolites of valproic acid have been identified. Some of these may have weak anticonvulsant activity and at least one metabolite may be responsible for the hepatotoxicity reported for valproic acid. One of the lesser oxidative metabolites, 4-*en*-valproic acid, causes significant hepatotoxicity in rats.[73] The formation of this metabolite is increased when valproic acid is given with enzyme-inducing drugs like phenobarbital.[74]

***Therapeutic Range/Dosing*** The minimal effective concentration of valproic acid is 50 $\mu$g/mL; however, there is disagreement on the upper end of the therapeutic range.[75] While 100 $\mu$g/mL is widely quoted as the upper end of the therapeutic range, recent experience indicates that a significant number of patient have improved seizure control when the concentration is increased. Although some reports have linked drowsiness, stupor, and decreases in fibrinogen to concentrations greater than 80–100 μg/mL, there are very few clearly defined concentration-dependent side effects of valproic acid. In refractory or partially responding patients, the concentration of valproic acid may cautiously be titrated upward, provided the patient is closely monitored. As the concentration is pushed upward, the saturable protein binding of valproic acid may become significant and free concentration monitoring may be helpful.

In normal circumstances loading doses of valproic acid are not indicated. Doses of 15–20 mg/kg usually produce concentrations of 75–100 μg/mL. The more common dosing procedure is to start patients on 7.5–15 mg/kg/d in divided doses and increase the dose in 2 to 3 days. Some patients may experience gastrointestinal distress or CNS depression if the initial dose is too high or increased too quickly.

While some patients may have a half-life sufficiently long to permit once-a-day dosing with valproic acid, more frequent dosing is the norm. Based on half-life data, twice-a-day dosing is feasible with any valproic acid dosage form[76]; however, children and other patients taking enzyme inducers may require dosing three to four times per day.

The serum concentration–dose relationship is curvilinear (i.e., the concentration–dose ratio decreases with increasing dose), probably because of increasing free concentrations and a resulting increase in clearance.[77]

***Dosage Forms*** Valproic acid is available as a soft gelatin capsule, an enteric-coated tablet, and a syrup. The soft gelatin capsule is available in several generic forms. The syrup is absorbed more rapidly than either solid. The enteric-coated tablet is not a sustained-release dosage form. The tablet consists of sodium divalproex, which must be metabolized in the gut to valproic acid, and is enteric coated to reduce the incidence of gastrointestinal distress. The enteric coating does cause delayed absorption, though once the enteric coating dissolves, sodium divalproex has absorption, metabolism, and elimination rates similar to those for other dosage forms of valproic acid.

***Adverse Effects*** The most common side effects may cause mild patient discomfort, but are not life-threatening.[78] The most frequently reported side effects are gastrointestinal complaints (up to 20%) including nausea, vomiting, anorexia, and weight gain. Pancreatitis is very rare. The gastrointestinal complaints may be minimized but not totally alleviated with the enteric-coated formulation or by giving the drug with food. Other frequently reported side effects are drowsiness (10%), ataxia (15%), and tremor (10%). These may respond to a modification of dose (Tables 41.8 and 41.9).

The most serious side effect reported with valproic acid is hepatotoxicity. Hyperammonemia is common (50%) but does not necessarily imply liver damage; however, at least 67 fatalities have been attributed to valproic acid hepatotoxicity. Patients dying with valproic acid–associated hepatotoxicity share certain features. Most deaths have occurred in patients who were less than 2 years of age, retarded, and receiving multiple therapy. The hepatotoxicity occurred early in the course of therapy.[79] The multiple therapy may have altered the normal metabolism, leading to increased formation of the potentially liver-toxic 4-*en*-valproic acid.

Thrombocytopenia occurs in 6% to 40% of the patients receiving valproic acid, but is responsive to a decrease in dose. Other hematologic side effects are rare. Alopecia and hair changes occur but are temporary.

Valproic acid causes minimal cognitive impairment.

***Drug Interactions*** Drugs that affect liver enzymes may alter valproic acid kinetics by increasing or decreasing clearance; for example, phenytoin, phenobarbital, primidone, and carbamazepine all increase valproic acid clearance. Because it is highly protein bound, other highly protein-bound drugs may displace valproic acid. Free fatty acids, aspirin and phenytoin may alter valproic acid binding.

Valproic acid is an enzyme inhibitor. The most significant reported interaction is with phenobarbital. The addition of valproic acid to patients taking phenobarbital results in a 30% to 50% decrease in the clearance of phenobarbital and toxicity if the dose of phenobarbital is not reduced.[80]

***Therapeutic Monitoring*** Valproic acid displays diurnal variations in serum concentrations. Therefore, the serum samples should be collected at the same time of day; trough levels are preferred.[81] Because the enteric coating on the sodium divalproex tablets delays absorption, the trough with this formulation may not occur for 2 to 4 hours after a dose. At higher concentrations, the curvilinear serum concentration–dose relationship and saturable protein binding should be considered.

**Ethosuximide**

***Therapeutics*** This is the most effective, least toxic representative of the succimide class of AEDs. It was developed from a systematic search for a more effective treatment of absence seizures.

The only indication for the use of ethosuximide is the treatment of absence seizures[82] for which it is the treatment of choice. It may be used in combination with valproic acid for difficult-to-control absence patients.[83]

The exact mechanism of action of ethosuximide remains elusive. Ethosuximide may inhibit the sodium–potassium ATPase system. Ethosuximide also inhibits NADPH-linked aldehyde reductase, which is necessary for the formation of γ-hydroxybutyrate, which has been associated with the induction of absence seizures. Ethosuximide is not believed to have a direct membrane effect or to affect brain metabolism.[84]

***Pharmacokinetics*** The absorption of ethosuximide is essentially complete. The syrup and the capsule forms are equally bioavailable, but the rate of absorption of the syrup is faster. The time to peak ranges between 3 and 7 hours. There is little first-pass metabolism.[85] Ethosuximide is not bound to plasma proteins or tissues. Only 10% to 20% of a dose of ethosuximide is excreted unchanged in the urine. Metabolism occurs in the liver by hydroxylation. The metabolites are believed to be inactive. There is some evidence of a nonlinear metabolic process.[86]

***Therapeutic Range/Dosing*** The therapeutic range of ethosuximide was defined in a relatively small number of patients by Brown et al.[87] Many unresponsive patients became responders when their drug concentrations were raised to equal those of the responsive patients. The accepted therapeutic range is 40–100 μg/mL, although higher concentrations are occasionally needed.

A loading dose of ethosuximide is not required. The most common dosing procedure is to start patients on 5–7 mg/kg/d in divided doses and increase the dose in 1 to 2 weeks. Doses of 20 mg/kg/d usually result in concentrations of approximately 50 μg/mL. Doses can then be titrated to individual response. Data suggest that patients can be successfully managed on once-a-day therapy; however, gastrointestinal distress appears to be dose related and the total daily dose is usually divided into two equal doses.

*Adverse Effects* Ethosuximide is a relatively benign anticonvulsant. The most frequently reported side effects are nausea and vomiting (up to 40%) and these symptoms may be minimized by administration of smaller doses. Other common side effects include drowsiness, fatigue, lethargy, dizziness, hiccups, and headaches. Rarely, idiosyncratic reactions such as skin rashes, lupus, and blood dyscrasias are reported.[88]

*Drug Interactions* Because ethosuximide is not protein bound, displacement interactions cannot occur. The metabolism of ethosuximide may be induced by carbamazepine. A complex interaction between valproic acid and ethosuximide has been reported. Valproic acid may inhibit the metabolism of ethosuximide, but only if the metabolism of ethosuximide is near saturation.[89]

*Therapeutic Monitoring* Because efficacy is dependent on concentrations greater than 50 μg/mL, trough levels are preferred. Because of the long half-life, minimal peak-to-trough fluctuations are expected.

## *Miscellaneous Antiepileptic Drugs*

### Benzodiazepines

Some benzodiazepines (e.g., diazepam and lorazepam) are used in the acute treatment of status epilepticus (discussed in Chapter 40). On a chronic basis other benzodiazepines such as clonazepam, nitrazepam (not available in the United States), and clobazam (not available in the United States) are more useful, especially in the treatment of seizure types that occur primarily in children.[90]

The exact mechanism of action of these drugs is unknown. They produce several CNS effects and the anticonvulsant effect has been difficult to identify.

Diazepam is the drug of first choice in status epilepticus because it can be administered rapidly. Although diazepam has not been used extensively, it may be of some use in the chronic treatment of infantile spasms.

Clonazepam is an effective adjunctive agent in the treatment of myoclonic seizures, atonic seizures, atypical absence seizures, and infantile spasms. Although clonazepam is effective in the treatment of absence seizures, its use is limited because it has a higher incidence of side effects than conventional AEDs. Clonazepam may also be effective in the treatment of partial seizures. Despite initial response, tolerance to the anticonvulsant effects of clonazepam may occur. CNS side effects have limited the use of clonazepam. Drowsiness, ataxia, and changes in behavior are common, although some tolerance may develop.

The correlation between therapeutic effect and serum clonazepam concentration is undefined. Dosing begins with 0.01–0.03 mg/kg/d given in two to three doses and is increased until the desired response or side effects occur.

### Acetazolamide

The exact role of carbonic anhydrase inhibitors in decreasing brain excitability is not completely defined. The effect may be secondary to the induction of a systemic metabolic acidosis similar to the ketogenic diet. Although acetazolamide is effective in patients with absence seizures, tolerance quickly develops. Therefore, the intermittent use of acetazolamide is more effective. It may be particularly useful in treating the increase in seizures present during menses.[91]

### Bromides

Bromides were the first effective AED; however, their use is limited by significant side effects including skin eruptions, sedation, and psychosis. Bromide use is reserved for patients with myoclonic seizures who are refractory to or intolerant of other AEDs.[92]

### ACTH[93]

This drug is the standard treatment for infantile spasms. Dosages used range between 5 and 180 units, administered in variable dosing regimens. Clinical and EEG improvement is usually evidenced within 3 weeks in 70% to 90% of the patients but relapses are common. The duration of therapy has ranged from 2 weeks to 18 months. ACTH has not been shown to be superior to oral steroids. ACTH can induce Cushing's syndrome.[93]

### Trimethadione

Trimethadione is the most effective, safest representative of the oxazolidinedione class of AEDs; however, it has been replaced by safer more effective therapy (e.g., ethosuximide and valproic acid). It may be used for the treatment of absence seizures in patients refractory to these agents.[94]

## *Chronic Side Effects of Antiepileptic Drugs*

The selection of an anticonvulsant depends on the side effects as well as efficacy. The use of serum concentration monitoring has significantly reduced anticonvulsant toxicity; however, chronic side effects can occur despite serum concentrations within the therapeutic range.[95] The incidence of chronic side effects is greatest with phenytoin (33%), phenobarbital (23%), carbamazepine (15%), and valproic acid (12%). Side effects are lowest in patients on monotherapy and increase with the addition of each additional drug.[96] The risk of side effects must always be balanced with the benefit of preventing seizure activity.

### Cognitive Impairment

The occurrence of nonfebrile seizures has not been associated with a significant change in full-scale IQ. High concentrations of all anticonvulsants affect mental functioning.

Therefore, concern over impairment of cognitive or intellectual abilities by chronic use of AEDs, especially in children, must be considered (Table 41.9).[97]

The comparative effects on cognition have been difficult to interpret because of differences in study design. Phenytoin and phenobarbital cause the most deficits on neuropsychologic tests.[98] Carbamazepine and valproic acid cause less or no impairment in cognition, and cognition improves when patients are switched from phenytoin or phenobarbital to these agents.[99] The apparent absence of cognitive impairment with carbamazepine and valproic acid needs to be confirmed by additional studies.

Patients reduced from polytherapy to monotherapy also demonstrate improvement in cognition.[100] Higher serum concentrations of AEDs are associated with greater degrees of cognitive impairment.[98]

**Behavioral Effects**

The most significant, non–concentration-dependent behavioral abnormality is phenobarbital-induced hyperactivity.[101] Tolerance, dosage titration, and serum concentration monitoring reduce the sleepiness, lethargy, and tiredness reported with AEDs. Reports of beneficial effects of carbamazepine on mood and behavior in seizure patients remain to be confirmed[102] (Table 41.9).

**Teratogenicity**

Children of epileptic mothers have a rate of malformations two to three times that of the general population. It has been difficult, however, to separate the effects of seizures and the general health of the mother from the adverse effect of the drugs.[103] Trimethadione and paramethadione are clearly associated with major malformations. About 30% of infants exposed in utero to phenytoin develop minor craniofacial and digital abnormalities. A smaller percentage develop the fetal hydantoin syndrome characterized by cleft lip and palate and subsequent delays in growth and cognitive development.[104] Valproic acid is associated with a 1% risk of spina bifida. Data on other AEDs are inadequate to assess teratogenicity.

**Osteomalacia[95]**

Phenytoin and phenobarbital have been associated with increased excretion of vitamin D and decreased absorption of calcium,[95] accompanied by hypocalcemia, elevated alkaline phosphatase, reduced bone density, and decreased phosphate; however, overt osteomalacia is rare and seems to require the presence of additional risk factors. Osteomalacia is more common in institutionalized patients with severe disease being treated with multiple therapy. Additional risk factors include decreased exposure to sunlight, inadequate nutrition, malabsorption, and physical inactivity.

**Hepatic Injury**

AEDs may cause acute hepatitis, usually within the first 10 weeks of therapy. Hepatitis associated with valproic acid appears to occur in special populations and may involve the formation of a toxic metabolite. The relation of AEDs to chronic hepatitis has not been well documented.[95]

The more common hepatic occurrence associated with chronic therapy is an increase in liver enzyme concentrations without clinical relevance. This may reflect an adaptive mechanism of the liver that does not reflect toxicity. Therefore, while the increase in liver enzyme concentrations may warrant an evaluation of hepatic damage, a reduction or withdrawal of the AED without definitive evidence of hepatotoxicity is not necessary.

**Blood Disorders**

The incidence of bone marrow suppression secondary to AEDs is rare and appears to occur as a hypersensitivity reaction.[95] Patients often tolerate a leukopenia with carbamazepine that does not require the discontinuation of the drug. Low folic acid levels have been reported in 10% to 91% of epileptic patients. The low folate concentration is not associated with a significant increase in megaloblastic anemia. Therefore, low folate levels are not an a priori reason to give folate supplements. The administration of folate has resulted in an increased clearance of phenytoin and phenobarbital.

**Exacerbation of Seizures**

An often overlooked toxic effect of AEDs is the potential for AED-induced seizures (Table 41.10). EEG telemetry combined with an enhanced knowledge of pharmacokinetics has increased understanding of this adverse effect.

## Special Problems in Epilepsy

### *Drug Interactions*

AEDs have narrow therapeutic ranges, are given chronically, and are frequently given in combination or with other drugs. Drug interactions may occur by a variety of mechanisms that include displacement from protein binding, induc-

**Table 41.10** Exacerbation of Seizures by Anticonvulsants

| |
|---|
| Acute or chronic toxicity |
| High concentrations of phenytoin or carbamazepine |
| Use of AED in a seizure type for which it is not indicated |
| Phenytoin exacerbates absence |
| Phenobarbital exacerbates atonic, myoclonic, and absence |
| Carbamazepine may precipitate generalized convulsive, atonic, and myoclonic seizures when used in children with atypical absence seizures |
| Unmasking one seizure type when another is controlled |
| Attributed to ethosuximide |
| Drug-induced somnolence |
| Phenobarbital and benzodiazepines |
| Sudden withdrawal |
| All anticonvulsants |
| Indirect effects |
| Carbamazepine-induced water intoxication and hyponatremia secondary to inappropriate ADH secretion |

**Table 41.11** Interactions Between Antiepileptic Drugs

| *AED* | *Added drug* | *Effect* |
|---|---|---|
| Phenytoin | Carbamazepine | ↓ Concentration |
| | Methsuximide | ↑ Concentration |
| | Valproic acid | ↓ Total |
| Phenobarbital | Phenytoin | ↑ Concentration |
| | Valproic acid | ↑ Concentration |
| Primidone | Carbamazepine | ↑ Phenobarbital |
| | Phenytoin | ↑ Phenobarbital |
| Carbamazepine | Phenobarbital | ↓ Concentration |
| | Phenytoin | ↓ Concentration |
| | Primidone | ↓ Concentration |
| Valproic acid | Carbamazepine | ↓ Concentration |
| | Phenobarbital | ↓ Concentration |
| | Primidone | ↓ Concentration |
| | Phenytoin | ↓ Concentration |

tion or inhibition of metabolism, self-induction or self-inhibition of metabolism, and altered elimination or altered absorption. Drug interactions are frequent and significant. Some of the interactions between AEDs are summarized in Table 41.11; the interactions between AEDs and other drugs are summarized in Table 41.12. (For more detail the reader should consult Chapter 7.) Screening for drug interactions is a vital part of monitoring patients who are receiving AEDs.

### *Febrile Convulsions*

Febrile convulsions are epileptic events occurring during a febrile illness.[106] Febrile convulsions are divided into simple febrile convulsions (SFCs) and convulsions with fever. SFCs occur in about 4% of children between 6 months and 6 years of age. Approximately 25% to 50% have recurrent episodes within 24 months after the initial seizure. SFCs are not associated with any encephalopathic event and the patient is normal by physical examination and EEG before and after the time of seizure. The seizure is generalized, usually lasts less than 10 minutes, and may be precipitated by a fever greater than 102°F. SFCs do not usually lead to future epilepsy.

There is a smaller subset of patients that have convulsions with fever. These patients are at increased risk of developing future epilepsy. The risk factors that identify this population include abnormal neurologic or developmental status before the febrile convulsion, a family history of febrile seizures, and a complicated seizure history. The seizure is usually focal, lasts longer than 15 minutes, and occurs more than once in 24 hours.

Phenobarbital is effective in preventing febrile convulsions at the usual therapeutic concentration; however, this must be balanced against the known effects of phenobarbital on cognitive abilities. Therefore, the Consensus Development Conference on Febrile Seizures recommended using continuous therapy only in patients at high risk of subsequent epilepsy. The long half-life of phenobarbital prevents its intermittent use. Valproic acid may be an alternative to phenobarbital. Phenytoin and carbamazepine are not effective.

Patients with a history of febrile convulsions should have ready access to an antipyretic when their temperature is greater than 101°F.

### *Neonatal Seizures*

Neonatal seizures are seizures that occur during the newborn period. The incidence of neonatal seizures is 1.5 to 15 per 1,000 live births, but in the neonatal intensive care unit, this increases to 25%.

The diagnosis of neonatal seizures is complex. Abnormal body movement may be difficult to recognize, especially if the brain has been severely damaged; therefore, an EEG

**Table 41.12** Interactions of Antiepileptic Drugs With Other Drugs

| *AED* | *Altered by* | *Result* | *Alters* | *Result* |
|---|---|---|---|---|
| Phenytoin | Antacids | ↓ Absorption | Oral contraceptives | ↓ Efficacy |
| | Disulfiram | ↑ Concentration | Bishydroxycoumarin | ↓ Anticoagulation |
| | Isoniazid | ↑ Concentration | Quinidine | ↓ Concentration |
| | Chloramphenicol | ↑ Concentration | Vitamin D | ↓ Concentration |
| | Propoxyphene | ↑ Concentration | Folic acid | ↓ Concentration |
| | Cimetidine | ↑ Concentration | | |
| | Ethanol | ↓ Concentration | | |
| Phenobarbital | | | Oral contraceptives | ↓ Efficacy |
| Primidone | | | Quinidine | ↑ Metabolism |
| | | | Tricyclics | ↑ Metabolism |
| | | | Corticosteroids | ↑ Metabolism |
| | | | Chlorpromazine | ↑ Metabolism |
| | | | Furosemide | ↓ Renal sensitivity |
| Carbamazepine | Propoxyphene | ↑ Concentration | Warfarin | ↓ Concentration |
| | Cimetidine | ↑ Concentration | Theophylline | ↓ Concentration |
| | Isoniazid | ↑ Concentration | Doxycycline | ↓ Concentration |
| | Erythromycin | ↑ Concentration | | |
| Valproic acid | Salicylates | ↑ Free concentration | | |

may greatly aid in the diagnosis. Neonatal seizures may be caused by a variety of disorders that include trauma and anoxia, congenital abnormalities, metabolic disorders, infections, drug withdrawal, pyridoxine dependency, amino acid disturbances, kernicterus, toxins, and familial seizures.

Treatment of neonatal seizures requires identifying and correcting the precipitating cause if possible. Phenobarbital is the most commonly used antiepileptic drug. Other AEDs include phenytoin, diazepam, paraldehyde, and primidone.

There is significant controversy over the duration of therapy for neonatal seizures. Chronic AED therapy, primarily phenobarbital, is often continued for at least 1 year in the hope of preventing afebrile seizures[107]; however, this is empiric therapy and is not supported by data from controlled clinical trials.[108] In the absence of high risk factors phenobarbital may be discontinued after initial seizure control because of its effects on cognitive functioning.

### *Alcohol and Epilepsy Versus Alcohol Withdrawal Seizures*

On the basis of limited data the prevalence of epilepsy in alcoholics is three times that of the general population, and alcoholism appears to be more prevalent in epileptics than in the general population. There is general agreement that alcohol abuse increases seizure frequency; however, the exact incidence of alcohol-provoked seizures is unknown. The mechanism of alcohol-provoked seizures is also undetermined. Small amounts of alcohol do not appear to induce seizures and may have transient anticonvulsant effects. Alcohol may stimulate liver enzymes and alter AED clearance. In alcoholics with liver disease, protein synthesis may be decreased, altering the binding of AEDs.[109]

The sudden withdrawal of any CNS drug may induce seizures. The clinician must differentiate alcohol withdrawal seizures from epilepsy. Alcohol withdrawal seizures usually occur within the first 24 hours of cessation of drinking. The seizures are generally tonic–clonic and are frequently accompanied by signs of tremulousness, anorexia, gastrointestinal disturbances, insomnia, weakness, and hallucinations. Epileptics usually do not have these symptoms.

Epileptics suffering from alcoholism require AEDs; however, alcohol withdrawal seizures are not epilepsy. The most appropriate time to begin AEDs to prevent alcohol withdrawal seizures is while the patient is still intoxicated; however, most alcohol withdrawal seizures occur before admission. The liberal use of benzodiazepines in alcoholics to prevent delerium tremens may decrease the incidence of alcohol withdrawal seizures. On a chronic basis there are no data to suggest that AEDs prevent alcohol withdrawal seizures. AED therapy for alcohol withdrawal seizures in nonepileptics has recently been shown to possibly enhance seizures because of erratic compliance and sudden cessation of the AEDs.[110]

### *Pregnancy/Sex Hormones/Contraception*

Pregnancy and sex hormones complicate the treatment of epilepsy. The possibility of teratogenic effects of the AEDs has been discussed. About 50% of epileptic women have no change in seizure activity during pregnancy, 40% have an increase, and about 10% have fewer seizures. Seizure activity fluctuates during the menstrual cycle.[103] Seizures decrease during the luteal phase and increase when progesterone levels decline.

Increased seizure activity during pregnancy may result from either a direct effect on seizure threshold or a reduction in AED concentration. During the third trimester the levels of AEDs decrease. For phenytoin, carbamazepine, phenobarbital, ethosuximide, and clorazepate, the decreased levels are attributed to an increase in clearance. The postulated mechanisms for the increased clearance include enhanced metabolic clearance and altered protein binding. The serum concentrations of AEDs should be monitored closely during pregnancy, especially in the third trimester, and the concentrations should be maintained within the therapeutic range. Immediately postpartum the drug clearance returns to normal and the dosages should be decreased.[111] Oral contraceptives may also increase the clearance of AEDs.

AEDs affect sex hormones. The enzyme-inducing AEDs shorten hormone half-life, increase levels of sex hormone–binding globulin, and lower free hormone concentrations. Although decreased libido, potency, and fertility and altered menstrual cycles have been attributed to AEDs, a direct cause-and-effect relationship has not been shown.[112]

The enzyme-inducing AEDs may cause treatment failures in females taking oral contraceptives. Valproic acid and benzodiazepines are not enzyme inducers and have not been associated with this effect. The degree of increased metabolism of estrogen and progesterone is highly variable and unpredictable. Women taking AEDs may require higher doses of oral contraceptives for adequate contraceptive effect. A supplemental form of birth control in addition to oral contraceptives is advised.[113]

### *Head Trauma*

Head trauma may be associated with seizures that develop immediately or have a latent period. Seizures occurring immediately (e.g., within the first week) differ in character and carry a different prognosis. Late seizures, those that begin more than 1 week after injury, require time to develop. It may be 2 to 4 years after the injury before some patients develop seizures.[114]

The incidence rate appears to be higher in trauma associated with combat than in civilian head trauma. The incidence in civilians appears to be about 5% to 11% of patients admitted to neurosurgical units with head trauma. The risk of late epilepsy appears to be increased by complications that include depressed fractures, intracranial bleeding, or early epilepsy. Some of the uncertainty in the assessment of the incidence of epilepsy secondary to head trauma has resulted from a lack of uniformity in the grading of the severity of the head trauma. Rating scales are now recommended and may bring uniformity.

The efficacy of prophylactic AEDs after head trauma is controversial, because of problems with study design.[115] Based on the low incidence of seizure activity secondary to head trauma and the relative toxicity of the AEDs, especially phenytoin, many clinicians would not institute prophylaxis for every head trauma patient who has not experienced a seizure. Other clinicians would elect for prophylaxis. The answer is difficult to obtain because of the large population that would need to be studied for long periods of time to detect differences.[116]

### *Epileptic Syndromes*

Epileptic syndromes are defined on the basis of clinical observation of seizure type, age of onset, EEG characteristics, and prognosis. These syndromes have more or less specific treatment.[5]

Infantile spasms occur in babies and infants and comprise short flexion spans, retarded development, and a characteristic EEG pattern known as hypsarrhythmia. The onset is between the third week and third year of life, and spasms disappear in 2 to 4 years. The treatment of choice for infantile spasms is ACTH.

Lennox–Gastaut syndrome occurs between the ninth month and the ninth year, with the peak around the fourth year of life. The syndrome is characterized by generalized seizures, mental retardation, and slow variants of the spike–wave pattern in the EEG. The generalized seizures are a combination of astatic, tonic–clonic, absence, and myoclonic. Children with Lennox–Gastaut syndrome do not respond to ACTH, but may respond to valproic acid or clonazepam.

Rolandic epilepsy may manifest itself from 9 months to 12 years, with a predilection for ages 7 to 10. This is a focal, not generalized, epilepsy. The seizures are described as short, unilateral, simple brachiofacial focal seizures with paresthesia and/or jerks, tonic hemifacial seizures with hypersalivation and speech arrest, and masticatory seizures.

Hemi-tonic–clonic seizures and tonic–clonic seizures with focal onset may occur, particularly during sleep. Usually only a few seizures occur but there are reports of patients with several seizures per day. Seizures and foci disappear completely at puberty.

Pyknolepsy (frequent absences) has the typical age distribution and EEG characteristics of absence; however, seizures may recur several times per day and can become very frequent, hence pyknoleptic. They may accumulate to a series or to an absence status that may last for hours or days.

### *Special Populations*

While all patients on AEDs require monitoring, some populations require special monitoring because of particular variability in pharmacokinetic properties and hence their response to AEDs. Neonates may metabolize drugs more slowly but eliminate unchanged drug more rapidly. Infants and children may also metabolize drug rapidly. The volume of distribution changes as children grow. The ability to metabolize drugs decreases with age and lower doses of AEDs are required.

Disease states may alter the pharmacokinetics of AEDs. Liver disease may decrease drug metabolism. In addition, if synthesis of albumin decreases, the protein binding of highly bound AEDs will decrease. Patients with chronic renal failure may have decreased elimination of unchanged drug as well as altered protein binding.

### *Surgery for Epilepsy*

Although surgery for epilepsy is rare, it has been done safely for over 30 years.[117] This procedure is usually reserved for patients with complex partial seizures who fail to respond to AED therapy. Patients should have an IQ of at least 70 and no evidence of schizophrenia. Success rates of approximately 80% are reported.

## Summary

Uncontrolled seizures can be a socially devastating disease resulting in impaired progress in school or loss of work. If the seizures are repetitive and prolonged, there is the possibility of brain injury or death.

The treatment of epilepsy begins with a careful identification of the seizure type and selection of the most appropriate anticonvulsant. Therapy should be initiated slowly, except in life-threatening situations, to avoid acute toxicity. The pharmacokinetics and therapeutic plasma range of the AED should be integrated into the clinical monitoring of seizure control to identify the appropriate dose. Patients should be chronically monitored for seizure control, social adjustment, drug interactions, compliance, dosage adjustments, and toxicity. While most patients can be successfully managed on monotherapy, some patients are uncontrollable despite use of multiple AEDs. There is a need for new antiepileptic drugs and continued research in this area.

## References


1. Pellock JM. Seizures and epilepsy, in Kelley VC (ed): Practice of Pediatrics. Philadelphia, Harper and Row, 1986.
2. Delgado-Escueta AV, Treiman DM, Walsh GO. The treatable epilepsies (part 1). N Engl J Med 1983;308:1508–1514.
3. Delgado-Escueta AV, Treiman DM, Walsh GO. The treatable epilepsies (part 2). N Engl J Med 1983;308:1576–1584.
4. Annegers JF, Shirts SB, Hauser WA, et al. Risk of recurrence after an initial unprovoked seizure. Epilepsia 1986;27:43–50.
5. Janz D. Epilepsy: Seizures and syndromes, in Freg HH, Janz D (eds): Antiepileptic Drugs. New York, Springer-Verlag, 1985, pp 3–34.
6. Benardo LS, Pedley TA. Basic mechanisms of epileptic seizures. Cleve Clin Q 1984;51:195–203.
7. Bruni J, Albright PS. The clinical pharmacology of antiepileptic drugs. Clin Neuropharmacol 1984;7:1–34.
8. Ellenberg JH, Hirtz PG, Nelson KB. Do seizures in children cause intellectual deterioration? N Engl J Med 1986;314:1085–1088.
9. Rothner AD. Evaluation of the child with seizures. Cleve Clin Q 1984;51:267–272.
10. Desai BT, Porter RJ, Penry JK. Psychogenic seizures. A study of 42 attacks in six patients with intensive monitoring. Arch Neurol 1982;39:202–209.

11. Commission on Classification and Terminology of the International League Against Epilepsy. Proposal for revised clinical and electroencephalographic classification of epileptic seizures. Epilepsia 1981;22:489–501.
12. Commission on Classification and Terminology of the International League Against Epilepsy. Proposal for classification of epilepsies and epileptic syndromes. Epilepsia 1985;26:268–278.
13. Mattson RH, Cramer JA, Collins JF, et al. Comparison of carbamazepine, phenobarbital, phenytoin and primidone in partial and secondary generalized tonic–clonic seizures. N Engl J Med 1985;313:145–151.
14. Schmidt D, Einicke I, Haenel F. The influence of seizure type on the efficacy of plasma concentrations of phenytoin, phenobarbital and carbamazepine. Arch Neurol 1986;43:263–265.
15. Schomer DL. Partial epilepsy. N Engl J Med 1983;309:536–539.
16. Luders H, Lesser RP, Dinner DS, et al. Generalized epilepsies: A review. Cleve Clin Q 1984;51:205–226.
17. Penry JK. Diagnosis and treatment of absence seizures. Cleve Clin Q 1984;51:283–286.
18. Troupin AS. The measurement of anticonvulsant agent levels. Ann Intern Med 1984;100:854–858.
19. Eadie MJ. Anticonvulsant drugs: An update. Drugs 1984; 27:328–363.
20. Taylor PC, McKinlay I. When not to treat epilepsy with drugs. Dev Med Child Neurol 1984;26:822–827.
21. Beghi E, DiMascio R, Tognoni G. Drug treatment of epilepsy: Outlines, criticism and perspectives. Drugs 1986;31:249–265.
22. Penry JK. Epilepsy: Diagnosis, Management, Quality of Life. New York, Raven, 1986.
23. Levy RH, Schmidt D. Utility of free level monitoring of antiepileptic drugs. Epilepsia 1985;26:199–205.
24. Takaki S, Kurokawa T, Aoyama T. Monitoring drug noncompliance in epileptic patients: Assessing phenobarbital plasma levels. Ther Drug Monit 1985;7:87–91.
25. Peterson GM, McLean S, Millinger KS. A randomized trial of strategies to improve patient compliance with anticonvulsant therapy. Epilepsia 1984;25:412–417.
26. Garnett WR. Discontinuing anticonvulsant medications. Clin Pharm 1984;3:456–457.
27. Todt H. The late prognosis of epilepsy in childhood: Result of a prospective follow-up study. Epilepsia 1984;25:137–144.
28. Yaari Y, Selzer ME, Pincus JH. Phenytoin: Mechanisms of its anticonvulsant action. Ann Neurol 1986;20:171–184.
29. Winter ME, Tozer TN. Phenytoin, in Evans WE, Schentag JJ, Jusko WJ (eds): Applied Pharmacokinetics, 2nd ed. Spokane, WA, Applied Therapeutics, Inc., 1986, pp 493–539.
30. Neuvonen PJ. Bioavailability of phenytoin: Clinical pharmacokinetics and therapeutic implications. Clin Pharmacokinet 1979;4:91–103.
31. Abernathy DR, Greenblatt DJ. Phenytoin disposition in obesity. Arch Neurol 1985;42:468.
32. White RJ, Garnett WR, Sharpe D, et al. Phenytoin removal during plasma exchange. J Clin Apheresis 1987;3:147–150.
33. Kutt H. Phenytoin: Relation of plasma concentration to seizure control, in Woodbury DM, Penry JK, Pippinger CE (eds.): Antiepileptic Drugs. New York, Raven, 1982, pp 241–246.
34. Ludden TM, Beal SL, Peck CC, et al. Evaluation of a Bayesian regression-analysis computer program for predicting phenytoin concentration. Clin Pharm 1986;5:580–585.
35. Welty TE, Robinson FC, Mayer PR. A comparison of phenytoin dosing methods in private practice seizure patients. Epilepsia 1986;27:76–80.
36. Fitzsimmons WE, Garnett WR, Comstock TJ, et al. Single dose comparison of the relative bioavailability of phenytoin suspension and extended capsules. Epilepsia 1986;27:464–468.
37. Sarkar MA, Karnes HT, Garnett WR. Effects of storage and shaking on the settling properties of phenytoin suspension. Neurology 1987;37(suppl 1):93.
38. Stilman N, Masdeu JC. Incidence of seizures with phenytoin toxicity. Neurology 1985;35:1769–1772.
39. Perucca E, Richens A. Drug interactions with phenytoin. Drugs 1981;21:120–137.
40. Cacek AT. Review of alterations in oral phenytoin bioavailability associated with formulation, antacids and food. Ther Drug Monitor 1986;8:166–171.
41. Krueger KA, Garnett WR, Comstock TJ. Effect of two administration schedules of an enteral nutrient formula on phenytoin bioavailability. Epilepsia 1987;28:706–712.
42. Rivey MP, Schottelius DP, Berg MJ. Phenytoin–folic acid: A review. Drug Intell Clin Pharm 1984;18:292–301.
43. Kupferberg HJ. Other hydantoins: Mephenytoin and ethotoin, in Woodbury DM, Penry JK, Pippinger CE (eds): Antiepileptic Drugs, 2nd ed. New York, Raven, 1982, pp 283–296.
44. Prichard JW. Phenobarbital: Mechanism of action, in Woodbury DM, Penry JK, Pippinger CE (eds): Antiepileptic Drugs. New York, Raven, 1982, pp 365–376.
45. Gal P. Phenobarbital and primidone, in Taylor WJ, Caviness MHD (eds): A Textbook for the Clinical Application of Therapeutic Drug Monitoring. Irving, TX, Abbott Laboratories, 1986, pp 237–252.
46. Levy RH, Wilensky AJ, Friel PN. Other antiepileptic drugs, in Evans WE, Schentag JJ, Jusko WJ (eds): Applied Pharmacokinetics, 2nd ed. Applied Therapeutics Inc., Spokane, WA, 1986, pp 540–569.
47. Paulson OB, Gyory A, Hertz MM. Blood–brain barrier transfer and cerebral uptake of antiepileptic drugs. Clin Pharmacol Ther 1982;32:466–477.
48. Browne TR, Evans JE, Szabo GK, et al. Studies with stable isotopes. II: Phenobarbital pharmacokinetics during monotherapy. J Clin Pharmacol 1985;25:51–58.
49. Streete JM, Berry DJ, Pettit LI, et al. Phenylethylmalonamide serum levels in patients treated with primidone and the effects of other antiepileptic drugs. Ther Drug Monit 1986;8:161–165.
50. Wroblewski BA, Garvin WH. Once-daily administration of phenobarbital in adults. Arch Neurol 1985;42:699–700.
51. Mattson RH, Cramer JA. Phenobarbital: Toxicity, in Woodbury DM, Penry JK, Pippinger CE (eds): Antiepileptic Drugs, 2nd ed. New York, Raven, 1982, pp 351–364.
52. Leppik IE, Cloyd JC, Miller K. Development of tolerance to the side effects of primidone. Ther Drug Monit 1984;6:189–191.
53. Kutt H, Paris-Kutt H. Phenobarbital: Interactions with other drugs, in Woodbury DM, Penry JK, Pippinger CE (eds): Antiepileptic Drugs, 2nd ed. New York, Raven, 1982, pp 329–340.
54. Ramsey EG, Wilder BJ, Berger JR, et al. A double-blind study comparing carbamazepine with phenytoin as initial seizure therapy in adults. Neurology 1983;33:904–910.
55. MacKichan JJ. Carbamazepine, in Taylor WJ, Caviness MHD (eds): A Textbook for the Clinical Application of Therapeutic Drug Monitoring. Irving, TX, Abbott Laboratories, 1986, pp 211–224.
56. Graves NM, Kriel RL, Jones-Saete C, et al. Relative bioavailability of rectally administered carbamazepine suspension in humans. Epilepsia 1985;26:429–433.
57. MacKichan J, Zola E. Determinants of carbamazepine and carbamazepine 10,11-epoxide to serum protein, albumin and $\alpha$-1-acid glycoprotein. Br J Clin Pharmacol 1984;18:487–493.
58. Bertilsson L, Tomson T. Clinical pharmacokinetics and pharmacological effects of carbamazepine and carbamazepine 10,11-epoxide. Clin Pharmacokinet 1986;11:177–178.
59. Riva R, Contin M, Albani F, et al. Free concentration of

carbamazepine and carbamazepine 10,11-epoxide in children and adults. Influence of age and phenobarbitone co-medication. Clin Pharmacokinet 1985;10:524–531.
60. Eichelbaum M, Kothe KW, Hoffman F, et al. Use of stable labeled carbamazepine to study its kinetics during chronic carbamazepine treatment. Eur J Clin Pharmacol 1982;23:241–244.
61. Tomson T. Interdosage fluctuations in plasma carbamazepine concentration determine intermittent side effects. Arch Neurol 1984;41:830–834.
62. Sorensen PS, Hammer M. Effects of long-term carbamazepine treatment on water metabolism and plasma vasopressin concentration. Eur J Clin Pharmacol 1984;26:719–722.
63. Hart RG, Easton JD. Carbamazepine and hematological monitoring. Ann Neurol 1982;11:309–312.
64. Pisciotta AV. Carbamazepine: Hematological toxicity, in Woodbury DM, Penry JK, Pippinger CE (eds): Antiepileptic Drugs, 2nd ed. New York, Raven, 1982, pp 533–542.
65. Andrews DG, Bullen JG, Tomlinson L, et al. A comparative study of the cognitive effects of phenytoin and carbamazepine in new referrals with epilepsy. Epilepsia 1986;27:128–134.
66. Baciewicz AM. Carbamazepine drug interactions. Ther Drug Monitor 1986;8:305–317.
67. Rimmer EM, Richens A. An update on valproic acid. Pharmacotherapy 1985;5:171–184.
68. Herranz JL, Armijo JA, Arteaga R. Effectiveness and toxicity of phenobarbital, primidone, and sodium valproate in the prevention of febrile convulsions, controlled by plasma levels. Epilepsia 1984;25:89–95.
69. Johnston P. Valproic acid: Update on its mechanism of action. Epilepsia 1984;25(suppl 1):S1–S4.
70. Cloyd JC, Brundage RC. Valproic acid, in Taylor WJ, Caviness MHD (eds): A Textbook for the Clinical Application of Therapeutic Drug Monitoring. Irving, TX, Abbott Laboratories, 1986, pp 269–280.
71. Albright PS, Bruni J, Suria D. Pharmacokinetics of enteric coated valproic acid. Ther Drug Monit 1984;6:21–23.
72. Hall K, Otten N, Johnston B, et al. A multivariable analysis of factors governing the steady-state pharmacokinetics of valproic acid in 52 young epileptics. J Clin Pharmacol 1985;25:261–268.
73. Nau H, Loscher W. Valproic acid and metabolites: Pharmacological and toxicological studies. Epilepsia 1984;25(suppl 1):S14–S22.
74. Cloyd JC, Kriel RL, Fischer JH. Valproic acid pharmacokinetics in children. II. Discontinuation of concomitant antiepileptic drug therapy. Neurology 1985;35:1623–1627.
75. Chadwick DW. Concentration–effect relationships of valproic acid. Clin Pharmacokinet 1985;10:155–163.
76. Wilder BJ, Karas BJ, Hammond EJ, et al. Twice-daily dosing of valproate with divalproex. Clin Pharmacol Ther 1983;34:501–504.
77. May T, Rambeck B. Serum concentrations of valproic acid: Influence of dose and comedication. Ther Drug Monit 1985;7:387–390.
78. Schmidt D. Adverse effects of valproate. Epilepsia 1984;25(suppl 1):S44–S49.
79. Dreifuss FE, Santilli N. Valproic acid hepatic fatalities: A retrospective review. Neurology 1987;37:379–385.
80. Levy RH, Koch KM. Drug interactions with VPA. Drugs 1982;24:543–556.
81. Bauer LA, Davis R, Wilensky A, et al. Valproic acid clearance: Unbound fraction and diurnal variation in young and elderly adults. Clin Pharmacol Ther 1985;37:697–700.
82. Callaghan N, O'Hare J, O'Driscoll D, et al. Comparative study of ethosuximide and sodium valproate in the treatment of typical absence seizures/petit mal. Develop Med Child Neurol 1982;24:830–836.
83. Rowan AJ, Meiger JWA, deBeer-Pawlikowski N, et al. Valproate–ethosuximide combination therapy for refractory absence seizures. Arch Neurol 1983;40:797–802.
84. Ferrendelli JA, Klank WE. Ethosuximide—mechanisms of action, in Woodbury DM, Penry JK, Pippinger CE (eds): Antiepileptic Drugs, 2nd ed. New York, Raven, 1982, pp 655–661.
85. Garnett WR. Ethosuximide, in Taylor WJ, Caviness MHD (eds): A Textbook for the Clinical Application of Therapeutic Drug Monitoring. Irving, TX, Abbott Laboratories, 1986, pp 225–236.
86. Bauer LA, Harris C, Wilensky AJ, et al. Ethosuximide kinetics: Possible interaction with valproic acid. Clin Pharmacol Ther 1982;31:741–745.
87. Brown TR, Dreifuss FE, Dyken PR, et al. Ethosuximide in the treatment of absence (petit mal) seizures. Neurology 1975;25:515–524.
88. Driefuss FE, Ethosuximide: Toxicity, in Woodbury DM, Penry KJ, Pippinger CE (eds): Antiepileptic Drugs, 2nd ed. New York, Raven, 1982, pp 647–654.
89. Mattson RH, Cramer JA. Valproic acid and ethosuximide interaction. Ann Neurol 1980;7:583–584.
90. Farrell KO. Benzodiazepines in the treatment of children with epilepsy. Epilepsia 1986;27(suppl 1):S45–S51.
91. Woodbury DM, Kemp JW. Sulfonamides and derivatives: Acetazolamide, in Woodbury PM, Penry KJ, Pippinger CE (eds): Antiepileptic Drugs. New York, Raven, 1982, pp 771–790.
92. Woodbury DM, Pippinger CE. Bromides, in Woodbury DM, Penry KJ, Pippinger CE (eds): Antiepileptic Drugs, 2nd ed. New York, Raven, 1982, pp 791–802.
93. Snead CO, Benton JW, Myers GJ. ACTH and prednisone in childhood seizure disorders. Neurology 1983;33:966–970.
94. Booker HE. Trimethadione: Toxicity, in Woodbury DM, Penry JK, Pippinger CE (eds): Antiepileptic Drugs, 2nd ed. New York, Raven, 1982, pp 701–704.
95. Schmidt D. Adverse Effects of Antiepileptic Drugs. New York, Raven, 1982.
96. Collaborative Group for Epidemiology of Epilepsy. Adverse reactions to antiepileptic drugs: A multicenter survey of clinical practice. Epilepsia 1986;27:323–330.
97. Committee on Drugs. Behavioral and cognitive effects of anticonvulsant therapy. Pediatrics 1985;76:644–647.
98. Trimble MR, Thompson PJ. Anticonvulsant drugs, cognitive function, and behavior. Epilepsia 1983;24(suppl 1):S55–S63.
99. Albright P, Bruni J. Reduction of polypharmacy in epileptic patients. Arch Neurol 1985;42:797–799.
100. Ludgate J, Keating J, O'Dwyer R, et al. An improvement in cognitive function following polypharmacy reduction in a group of epileptic patients. Acta Neurol Scand 1985;71:448–452.
101. Reynolds EH, Trimble MR. Adverse neuropsychiatric effects of anticonvulsant drugs. Drugs 1985;29:570–581.
102. Rivinus TM. Psychiatric effects of the anticonvulsant regimens. J Clin Psychopharmacol 1982;2:165–192.
103. Dalessio DJ. Seizure disorders and pregnancy. N Engl J Med 1985;312:359–363.
104. Kelly TE. Teratogenicity of anticonvulsant drugs. Am J Med Genet 1984;19:413–434.
105. Lerman P. Seizures induced or aggravated by anticonvulsants. Epilepsia 1986;27:706–710.
106. Erenberg G. Febrile convulsions: A new look at an old problem. Cleve Clin Q 1984;51:279–282.

107. Gal P. Anticonvulsant therapy after neonatal seizures. How long should it be continued? I. A case for early discontinuation of anticonvulsants. Pharmacotherapy 1985;5:268–273.

108. Hodson A. Anticonvulsant therapy after neonatal seizures. How long should it be continued? II. A case for long term treatment with anticonvulsants. Pharmacotherapy 1985;5:274–277.

109. Chan AWK. Alcoholism and epilepsy. Epilepsia 1985;26: 323–325.

110. Hillbom ME, Hjelm-Jager M. Should alcohol withdrawal seizures be treated with antiepileptic drugs? Acta Neurol Scand 1984;69:39–42.

111. Levy RH, Yerby MS. Effects of pregnancy on antiepileptic drug utilization. Epilepsia 1985;26(suppl 1):S52–S57.

112. Mattson RH, Cramer JA. Epilepsy, sex hormones, and antiepileptic drugs. Epilepsia 1985;26(suppl 1):S40–S51.

113. Mattson RH, Cramer JA, Darney PD, et al. Use of oral contraceptives by women with epilepsy. JAMA 1986;256:238–240.

114. Weiss G, Salazar AM, Vance SC, et al. Predicting posttraumatic epilepsy in penetrating head injury. Arch Neurol 1986;43:771–772.

115. Blackwood DHR, McQueen JK. Anticonvulsant prophylaxis after head injury, in Shorum SD, Birdwood GFB (eds): Rational Approaches to Anticonvulsant Therapy. Berne, Hans Huber Publishers, 1984, pp 65–73.

116. McQueen JK, Blackwood DHR, Harris P, et al. Low risk of late posttraumatic seizures following severe head injury: Implications for clinical trials of prophylaxis. J Neurol Neurosurg Psychiatry 1983;46:899–904.

117. Cahan LD, Sutherling W, McCullough MA, et al. Review of the 20-year UCLA experience with surgery for epilepsy. Cleve Clin Q 1984;51:313–318.

# Chapter 42 / Parkinson's Disease

W. Gary Erwin, PharmD, and Thomas F. Turco, PharmD

The tremor, muscular difficulties, and postural abnormalities that characterize Parkinson's disease, or paralysis agitans, were first described in 1817. These clinical symptoms are representative of the parkinsonism syndrome and result from the degeneration or destruction of dopaminergic neurons, or depletion of the neurotransmitter dopamine within the extrapyramidal system. Idiopathic Parkinson's disease occurs most frequently; other causes of parkinsonian-like syndromes include neurotoxins, trauma, progressive supranuclear palsy, Shy–Drager syndrome, and drugs. A postencephalitic etiology was once common but is no longer considered important.

Parkinson's disease is a disorder of the middle-aged and elderly. The prevalence of the disease is 90 to 100 cases per 100,000 people[1] and the incidence is 20 cases per 100,000 people.[2] It is a progressive, degenerative neurologic motor disorder that most probably results from pathologic aging of neurons within specific areas of the central nervous system (CNS).

## Pathophysiology

### *Etiology*

The etiology of idiopathic Parkinson's disease is unknown. Genetic factors do not appear to play a significant role in disease development. Several endogenous and environmental factors are being investigated. Proposed endogenous causes include a deficiency of nutrient sources (e.g., oxygen) or a lack of "neurotropic" factors, which are proteins necessary for nerve cell function. The deficiency of these substances could potentially decrease dopaminergic neuron survival. Proposed environmental factors include toxic substances, infectious agents, and ischemia. The accumulation of these environmental factors over time may cause cumulative damage. This damage could compound age-related dopamine breakdown and melanin accumulation within cells of the substantia nigra and produce Parkinson's disease. A model neurotoxin is 1-methyl-4-phenyl-1,2,3,6-tetrahydropyridine (MPTP), a meperidine analogue capable of inducing parkinsonism[3]; however, no widespread environmental neurotoxins have been identified. The etiology of Parkinson's disease may include both environmental and endogenous causes.

### *Anatomy/Physiology*

Parkinson's disease occurs as a result of pathologic alterations within the extrapyramidal system, a complex functional unit of the CNS that is involved in control of motor activities. The extrapyramidal system is composed of the basal ganglia, which are symmetrical, subcortical masses of gray matter embedded in the lower portions of the cerebral hemisphere. The components of the basal ganglia (Fig. 42.1) include the caudate nucleus, putamen, medial and lateral globus pallidus, claustrium, amygdala, and related structures in the brain stem including the subthalamic nucleus, substantia nigra (Fig. 42.2), and red nucleus. The putamen and caudate nucleus form the corpus striatum.

Numerous functional relationships and anatomical connections exist between components of the extrapyramidal system and between the extrapyramidal system and the cerebral cortex, cerebellum, thalamus, and reticular formation. A complex circuitry of afferent and efferent neurotransmitter pathways connect parts of the basal ganglia with each other and with other areas of the brain.

Several neurotransmitters are responsible for neuronal transmission within the extrapyramidal system; however, the most important neurotransmitter is dopamine. Approximately 80% of total brain dopamine is located in the corpus striatum.[4] The major dopaminergic neuron system is the nigrostriatal tract that originates in the substantia nigra. Other dopaminergic pathways also exist within the CNS, all originating in the upper brain stem near the substantia nigra.

The widespread distribution of these dopaminergic neurons suggests the possibility that extrapyramidal diseases may be systemwide disorders rather than the result of localized lesions.[1] Stimulation and destruction of these areas result in abnormalities of movement. This suggests that dopamine may exert both an excitatory and/or an inhibitory effect that results in a more generalized modulating influence on nigrostriatal neurons rather than precise control of neuronal discharge.[5] Although the interaction of dopamine with other neurotransmitters (e.g., norepinephrine, serotonin, acetylcholine, and $\gamma$-aminobutyric acid) is poorly understood, acetylcholine is thought to balance the actions of dopamine within the extrapyramidal system.

The metabolic pathway of dopamine is presented in Figure 42.3. Tyrosine, a metabolic precursor of dopamine, is hydrolyzed to dopa by the enzyme tyrosine hydroxylase. Dopa, in turn, is decarboxylated to dopamine by the enzyme dopa decarboxylase. The amount of dopa decarboxylase present in the brain is proportional to the amount of dopamine present.[1] A significant reduction in the brain content and activity of both these enzymes occurs with increasing age,[6] the sharpest drop occurs from ages 15 to 20.[1] Dopamine may be further metabolized to norepinephrine or homovanillic acid (HVA), whose distribution in brain tissue is similar to that of dopamine.[7]

The complex circuitry of the extrapyramidal system is chiefly responsible for maintenance of posture and coordination of body movement which is executed by the motor cortex

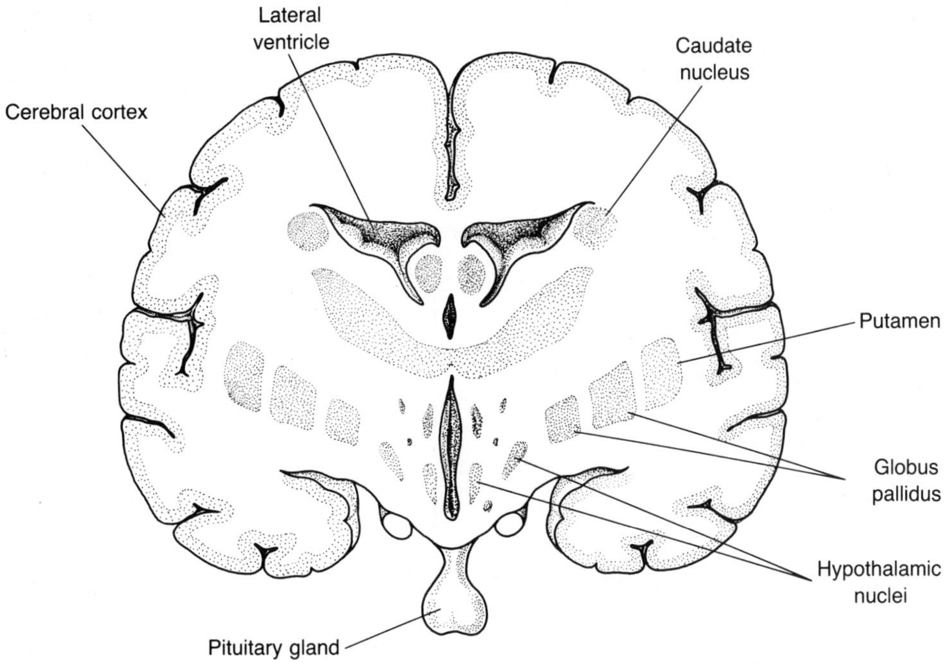


**Figure 42.1** The basal ganglia as viewed from a frontal section of the cerebral hemispheres.

and monitored by the cerebellum. Imbalances of neurotransmitters (e.g., dopamine and acetylcholine) within this complex circuitry lead to a variety of movement disorders.

### *Pathology*

The major site of pathologic involvement in Parkinson's disease is the substantia nigra; the hallmark finding is loss of melanin-containing neuronal cells.[8] The remaining nerve cells have decreased nucleolar volume and melanin content.[9] The most prominent cell loss occurs in the zona compacta of the substantia nigra, but losses also occur in other pigmented nuclei (e.g., the locus ceruleus and dorsal vagus nucleus). The severity of parkinsonism generally correlates with the degree of neuronal loss in the substantia nigra.[10] Parkinson's disease is considered to be an acceleration of normal age-related neuronal cell loss.[11]

**Figure 42.2** Anatomic relationship of substantia nigra to basal ganglia.

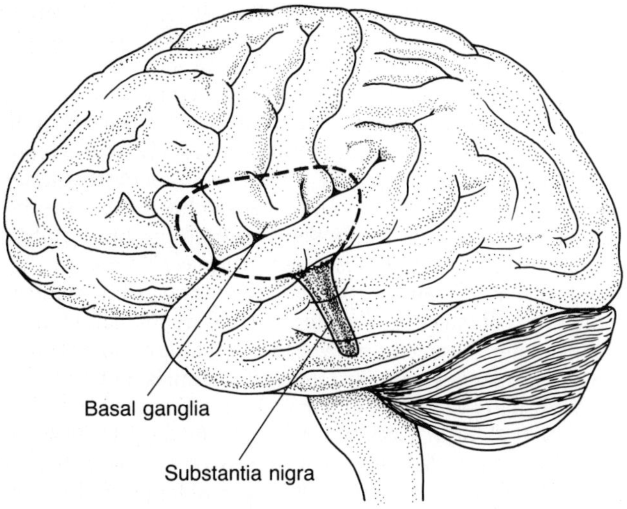


The neuronal degeneration in Parkinson's disease correlates with a decrease in dopaminergic neurotransmission. On autopsy, patients with Parkinson's disease had approximately 10% of the dopamine concentration normally found in the basal ganglia.[7] In addition, levels of dopamine metabolites such as HVA and enzymes such as dopa decarboxylase are reduced in brains of Parkinson's disease patients.[1] The loss of dopamine results in an absolute deficiency of dopamine relative to other neurotransmitters, especially acetylcholine.

A characteristic finding in the remaining neurons of patients with idiopathic Parkinson's disease is Lewy bodies. These are translucent masses of cytoplasmic protein consisting of a dense core surrounded by a filamentous halo. The importance of Lewy bodies is unclear; however, they are not considered a pathologic cause of neuronal destruction.[12,13]

Parkinson's disease is associated with dementia of the Alzheimer type (DAT). Cortical changes indicative of DAT (e.g., neurofibrillary tangles) may be present in significant numbers in Parkinson's disease. Neuronal loss in the nucleus basalis of Meynert has been linked to the pathophysiology of Alzheimer's disease and Parkinson's disease[14,15]; however, involvement of this area may differ in these two disease processes because of differences in the neuropathology present and the extent of neuronal loss. Neuronal loss in this area may contribute to symptoms of Parkinson's disease, Alzheimer's disease, or both.

Parkinson's disease may not be restricted to the substantia nigra, but may be a more generalized brain disorder. Neu-

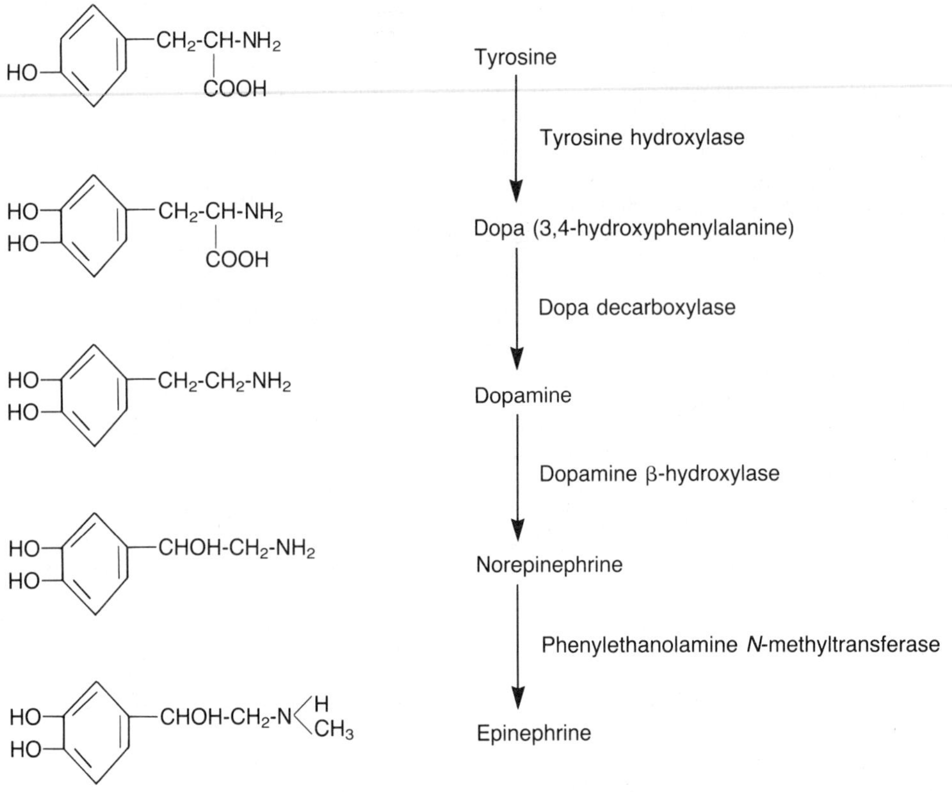


**Figure 42.3** Metabolic pathway for the biosynthesis of catecholamines.

ronal degeneration has been noted in the locus ceruleus, the dorsal motor nucleus of the vagus, and the ventral tegmental area.[16] Lewy bodies have been identified in the hypothalamus of some patients with Parkinson's disease. The significance of these findings in relationship to the movement and mentation difficulties is not thoroughly understood but suggests a nonnigral component. A possible correlation exists between these pathologic findings and the autonomic and endocrine abnormalities observed in these patients.[17,18] Deficiencies of noradrenergic and serotonergic pathways within the spinal cords of Parkinson's disease patients are another possible mechanism for autonomic and sensory disturbances.[19] Cerebrospinal fluid levels of $\beta$-endorphins, which are synthesized in the hypothalamus, are decreased in Parkinson's disease patients.[20]

A decrease in cerebral blood flow has been demonstrated in patients with Parkinson's disease.[21,22] This decrease, however, was not correlated with the severity of dementia symptoms[21] or duration of parkinsonism.[22] Both studies suggest that the decrease in blood flow may be caused by a decrease in metabolic demand because of dopamine deficiency and neuronal loss.

## Clinical Presentation

### *Clinical Features*

Parkinson's disease develops insidiously and progresses slowly in most patients. It is often difficult for a patient to state exactly when the disease began. Initial complaints include aching pains, parasthesias, numbness, and coldness. As the disease progresses the patient displays one or more of the classic clinical features: tremor, rigidity, akinesia or bradykinesia, and postural difficulties.[23]

The tremor is a rhythmic oscillary movement occurring in a relaxed and supported limb, usually the hands. It frequently appears as a "pill-rolling" type movement between the thumb and index finger. Although this resting tremor usually begins unilaterally, it eventually becomes bilateral. Stress worsens the tremor; however, purposeful movement or complete relaxation such as sleep improves it. The tremor may also occur in the feet or perioral region or may not occur at all, as in akinetic Parkinson's disease. A tremor often signifies to the patient the presence of a disease and will often be the patient's presenting medical complaint.

Rigidity is an increased resistance to passive movement in all directions caused by contraction of both the agonist and antagonist of a muscle pair. For example, concurrent contraction of extensor and flexor muscles in the upper extremities of a patient with Parkinson's disease produces "cogwheel" rigidity, a rachetlike, catch–release phenomena.

Akinesia is a complete lack of the ability to initiate or implement voluntary movement, whereas hypokinesia refers to a reduction in such ability and bradykinesia refers to a slowness of movement. The etiology of akinesia and bradykinesia is autonomic dysfunction. An early sign of bradykinesia in Parkinson's disease is masked facies, a lack of emotional reflection that presents as a stare with a relentless, unblinking look. The patient may have difficulty rising and sitting and will often sit with legs uncrossed. Once walking has been initiated, the patient may "freeze" and be totally immobile. There may be a continual decrease in size of handwriting toward the end of a line (micrographia), with a sudden stop. The autonomic dysfunction is also responsible for drooling, excessive sweating, swallowing difficulties, constipation, and postural hypotension.

Bradykinesia combines with rigidity to produce gait abnormalities. Forward flexion of the head and neck, upper extremities, and knees, and adduction of the arms and thighs lead to the characteristic simian posture. Once walking, the patient may fall forward, increase speed disproportionately, and begin to run involuntarily (festination). Stopping may be difficult. The patient's walk is further characterized by a lack of associated walking movements such as normal arm swing.

Postural difficulties involve a loss of reflexes necessary for postural equilibrium and righting reactions. The patient appears unable to make necessary adjustments to maintain posture and center of gravity and frequently falls backward or forward. The falls are usually associated with specific functions (e.g., standing, backing up, turning in tight places, or bending forward).

Initially, Parkinson's disease impairs functional status but not intellectual deterioration; however, there appears to be an association between Parkinson's disease and dementia, and some patients may have significant intellectual deterioration as the disease progresses. Depression is very common although there is controversy over whether it is reactive because the patient is capable of understanding the disability, or endogenous and related to neurotransmitter abnormalities.

### *Diagnosis*

Parkinson's disease is a clinical diagnosis based upon the recognition of abnormal motor symptoms and the exclusion of other causes. This differential diagnosis may be difficult without a clear history of exposure to a neurotoxin or current use of a drug that blocks postsynaptic dopaminergic receptors in the corpus striatum (e.g., phenothiazine and butyrophenone antipsychotics, metoclopramide, and meperidine). (The reader should refer to Chapter 48 for a discussion of drug-induced parkinsonism and its treatment.) Laboratory values in the otherwise healthy Parkinson's disease patient are usually within normal limits; therefore, this information is of secondary importance. As observation of clinical symptoms is the key to diagnosis, the clinician should instruct the patient to perform tasks that would result in a clear display of tremor, rigidity, bradykinesia, or postural difficulties. These include a gentle application of force to the standing patient's chest, while making sure that the patient does not fall; asking the patient to sit and rise from a chair; or asking the patient to support a relaxed arm on a chair. Early manifestations of the disease include the slight loss of motor activity or dexterity. A thorough neurologic examination may uncover these findings and thus signal the clinician to monitor for more diagnostic features of the disease.

## Treatment

### *Overview*

The management of Parkinson's disease is determined by the severity of the disease and includes both supportive care and drug therapy. The classification system developed by Hoehn and Yahr is used most frequently to stage disease severity (Table 42.1).[24] Supportive care, including a planned regimen of rest, exercise, and activities, is the treatment of choice for mild Parkinson's disease (Hoehn and Yahr stages I and II) and is a necessary adjunct to drug therapy in later stages. As the early stages of Parkinson's disease are not accompanied by intellectual deterioration, psychologic support is important to provide an understanding of the disease and encouragement to maintain optimal function.

**Table 42.1** Staging of Severity of Parkinson's Disease

| | |
|---|---|
| Stage I | Unilateral involvement |
| Stage II | Bilateral involvement but no postural abnormalities |
| Stage III | Bilateral involvement with mild postural imbalance; patient leads independent life |
| Stage IV | Bilateral involvement with postural instability; patient requires substantial help |
| Stage V | Severe, fully developed disease; patient restricted to bed or chair |

Compiled from Reference 24.

Drug therapy for Parkinson's disease involves the enhancement of dopaminergic function within the CNS by (1) decreasing cholinergic function (anticholinergics); (2) enhancing endogenous dopamine activity (amantadine); (3) replacing dopamine (levodopa); and (4) stimulating dopamine receptors (dopamine agonists). Although this therapy can substantially improve a patient's functional status (the degree of proficiency in accomplishing activities of daily living) by ameliorating the clinical symptoms of the disease, no medication has been introduced that retards or reverses the disease progression.

### *Initial Drug Therapy*

Initial drug therapy of Parkinson's disease consists of anticholinergic drugs or amantadine (Symmetrel, DuPont). The anticholinergic drugs (Table 42.2) are thought to exert their antiparkinsonism action by antagonizing the effect of acetylcholine. This decreases the absolute excess of acetylcholine present in relation to the amount of dopamine present, thereby correcting the neurotransmitter imbalance. Their effectiveness is limited, with improvement in only 20% to 25% of patients. Anticholinergic drugs are more effective in tremor and ridigity than in bradykinesia. Minor adverse effects of these drugs include dry mouth, blurred vision, constipation, and urinary retention. More serious adverse central effects are delirium, disorientation, anxiety, agitation, hallucinations, and decreased memory function. Patients with preexisting confusion and advanced age are at greater risk of the central effects. To avoid rebound deterioration, anticholinergic drugs should not be abruptly discontinued. Besides initial therapy, anticholinergics are effective adjuncts to levodopa therapy.[25]

Amantadine exerts its antiparkinsonism action by increasing concentrations of dopamine at postsynaptic receptor sites via decreased presynaptic reuptake and enhanced dopamine synthesis and release.[26,27] Amantadine is effective in

**Table 42.2** Anticholinergic Drugs Used in Parkinson's Disease

| *Generic name* | *Trade name* | *Manufacturer* | *Dosage range (mg/d)* |
|---|---|---|---|
| Benztropine | Cogentin | Merck Sharp & Dohme | 1–6 |
| | Generic brands | Various | |
| Biperiden | Akineton | Knoll | 2–8 |
| Diphenhydramine | Benadryl | Parke–Davis | 25–100 |
| | Generic brands | Various | |
| Ethopropazine | Parsidol | Parke–Davis | 100–600 |
| Orphinadrine | Disipal | Riker | 50–250 |
| Procyclidine | Kemadrin | Burroughs–Wellcome | 6–20 |
| Trihexyphenidyl | Artane | Lederle | 2–15 |
| | Tremin | Schering | |
| | Generic brands | Various | |

approximately 50% of patients with Parkinson's disease.[28] The usual initial dose of the drug is 100 mg twice daily. The onset of action of the drug is rapid; however, tolerance to its effects often develops within 6 to 12 weeks after initiation. Adverse CNS effects occur most commonly and include depression, hallucinations, anxiety, dizziness, psychosis, and confusion. Congestive heart failure and seizures are more serious effects but occur rarely. Less serious side effects such as nausea, constipation, and dry mouth occur infrequently. A frequent adverse effect of amantadine is livido reticularis, a diffuse rose color mottling of the skin which is reversible upon drug discontinuation.[28]

### *Levodopa*

Levodopa (Larodopa, Roche; Dopar, Norwich–Eaton) remains the most effective drug in the management of Parkinson's disease. Rigidity, bradykinesia, and tremor are improved in 50% to 60% of patients.[29,30] Unfortunately, a loss of therapeutic efficacy and the appearance of severe adverse effects associated with long-term levodopa use limit the effective treatment period.

Levodopa, a dopamine precursor, is used for treatment because it crosses the blood–brain barrier, whereas dopamine does not. The conversion of levodopa to dopamine within the CNS by the enzyme dopa decarboxylase results in elevated CNS levels of dopamine. This serves to correct the underlying neurotransmitter imbalance. Peripheral conversion of levodopa to dopamine also occurs and causes adverse effects including nausea, vomiting, cardiac arrhythmias, and postural hypotension. By combining levodopa with carbidopa (Sinemet, Merck Sharp & Dohme), a peripheral dopa decarboxylase inhibitor, peripheral conversion of levodopa to dopamine is decreased and increased amounts of levodopa penetrate the blood–brain barrier.[31,32] Therefore, the decreased peripheral dopamine production decreases the frequency of peripheral adverse effects. The combination also provides a levodopa-sparing effect, allowing as much as a 75% reduction in levodopa dose.[1] The usual starting dose of levodopa alone is 100 mg three times daily with a therapeutic range of 2.0 to 8.0 g daily. The dose must be individualized and escalated slowly to the minimum effective dose over several months to prevent gastrointestinal adverse effects. If levodopa is used alone, dietary intake of pyridoxine should be restricted.

The carbidopa/levodopa preparation is available in ratios of 1:4 and 1:10. Carbidopa has a maximum effective daily dose of 100 to 125 mg beyond which there is no greater dopa decarboxylase inhibitory effect.[33] A standard initial dose is one 25/100 tablet twice daily. The dosage is escalated based upon clinical response with the 25/100 tablet until a maximum of eight tablets daily is achieved. If further levodopa is required, one tablet at a time of the 1:4 ratio should be substituted with the 10/100 or 25/250 tablet. Dosage adjustment with the combination product can be more rapid because gastrointestinal effects are minimized. The appropriate dose of levodopa alone or in combination is the minimum amount necessary to accomplish the desired therapeutic effect.

The major long-term complications of levodopa therapy are loss of efficacy and development of adverse effects.[34,35] The loss of efficacy is characterized by the "on–off" phenomenon that occurs in as many as two thirds of patients after 5 years. These response variations may occur in a greater percentage of patients treated with the carbidopa/levodopa combination than with levodopa alone.[36] The "on–off" phenomenon appears as wide fluctuations in functional status ranging from a hyperkinetic to a hypokinetic state, potentially occurring several times a day. The hyperkinetic state is characterized by dyskinesias and good functional status; the hypokinetic state is characterized by akinesia, "freezing" episodes, and painful dystonic spasms. The "on–off" fluctuations are associated primarily with the CNS availability of levodopa at postsynaptic dopamine receptors. Dyskinesias have been correlated with peak dopamine concentrations, but the relationship between therapeutic response and drug concentration is less clear.

In addition to this "on–off" effect, the loss of efficacy may occur as a decreased time of responsiveness to doses of levodopa[34] (e.g., a therapeutic response of 1 hour rather than 4 hours leading to end-of-dose akinesias), a delay in the induction of beneficial effects to a given dose of levodopa,[37] and episodic total unresponsiveness to single doses of levodopa.[38] The loss of efficacy may result from the combination of fluctuating levodopa concentrations in the serum and at postsynaptic dopamine receptors, and disease progression.[39,40]

Long-term adverse effects involving the central nervous system occur frequently and include depression, delirium, agitation, paranoia, delusions, and hallucinations. These occur even more frequently in older patients and in those with underlying confusion. Dementia occurs three times more frequently in Parkinson's disease patients than in aged-matched controls.[41] New cases of dementia also occur more frequently in patients treated with levodopa than in controls. At the present time it is unclear whether levodopa causes dementia and what, if any, relationship exists between the pathophysiologic processes of dementia and Parkinson's disease.

Problems associated with loss of efficacy and long-term adverse effects have led to numerous interventions aimed at prolonging the effective treatment period of levodopa. These interventions attempt to (1) stabilize fluctuating serum concentrations of levodopa, (2) alter the function of postsynaptic dopamine receptors potentially desensitized by chronic drug administration, or (3) prevent desensitization of postsynaptic dopamine receptors by delaying the exposure of the receptor to dopamine.

Stabilization of fluctuating serum dopamine concentrations is important because the greatest contributing factor to the "on–off" phenomenon is the erratic absorption and distribution of levodopa in patients critically dependent upon its delivery.[42] The usual approach to this problem is administration of frequent, small doses. Recent attempts at providing constant dopamine concentrations include administration of intravenous levodopa infusions,[43] supplemental[44] or irreversible[45] dopa decarboxylase inhibitors, controlled-release preparations,[46,47] and continuous duodenal infusions.[48] The benefits of these interventions have been limited because of their lack of therapeutic effectiveness, inability to provide a constant supply of drug, or unrealistic chronic administration procedures.

Attempts to alter the function of potentially desensitized receptors include the use of drug holidays. The holiday consists of tapering levodopa with discontinuation of the drug for 7 to 14 days. During the holiday period there is a dramatic worsening of functional status necessitating hospitalization. After the holiday, therapy is reinstituted at one third to one half of the preholiday dose. The drug holiday is reported to be of long-term benefit for up to 6 months in approximately 60% of patients, with sustained improvement for up to 24 months in approximately 50% of patients.[49] The effectiveness of drug holidays is limited by rapid deterioration of postholiday functional status and questionable benefit in preventing the long-term complications of levodopa.[50] The availability of other drug treatments (e.g., dopamine agonists) has greatly reduced the frequency with which drug holidays are used. Drug holidays are recommended for patients when the addition of other drugs does not improve the progressive deterioration of functional status.

Attempts to prevent desensitization of receptors include use of low-dose rather than high-dose regimens and delay of initiation of therapy. The reported benefits of these two approaches are controversial. Low-dose therapy is reported to provide benefit comparable to that provided by high-dose, daily therapy, with decreased frequency of fluctuations in functional status.[51] Also reported, however, are less initial improvement and similar decline in efficacy.[52] The appropriate time to initiate therapy with levodopa is controversial because of disagreements as to whether the worsening of patient status over time reflects disease progression or long-term exposure to levodopa. Delaying initiation until more severe disabilities in functional status exist may allow the patient to function at higher levels for a longer time.[53] On the other hand, early initiation of therapy could allow patients to remain active longer and maximize quality of life.[39] In general, the proper time to initiate levodopa therapy is when the disease interferes with the patient's daily functioning, when anticholinergic drugs or amantadine are ineffective, or when the patient makes a rational decision to begin therapy after considering all risks and benefits. Arbitrary dosage limits should not be set and levodopa dosage should be individualized.

The pharmacokinetics of levodopa contribute greatly to the problems associated with its availability at CNS receptor sites. There is a poor correlation between levodopa dose and peak plasma concentrations. There is also great interpatient and intrapatient variability in peak plasma concentrations. The elimination half-life of levodopa alone is approximately 1 hour and, when combined with carbidopa, approximately 2 hours. Factors that influence levodopa transport from the proximal small intestine where it is absorbed to its CNS site of action (e.g., concurrent food or drugs, gastric emptying, bioavailability, competition with other dietary amino acids, and enzymatic barriers) may be major determinants of clinical response.

Levodopa should be administered cautiously with monoamine oxidase inhibitors (possible hypertensive crisis), antihypertensive agents (possible additive hypotensive effect), phenytoin (possible reversal of antiparkinson effect), and antipsychotic agents (possible antagonism of levodopa effect).

Despite problems associated with levodopa, it remains the standard of therapy for patients with Parkinson's disease. The carbidopa/levodopa combination is preferable because peripheral adverse effects occur less frequently and less drug is necessary to provide beneficial results. Although there is some evidence that the central adverse effects occur sooner with the combination than with levodopa alone, judicious use of the combination can prolong the effective treatment period. In short, the benefits of using combination therapy versus levodopa alone clearly outweigh the risks.

### *Dopamine Agonists*

The use of dopamine agonists as adjuncts to levodopa therapy is very beneficial in prolonging the effective treatment period. These agents exert their antiparkinsonism effect by direct stimulation of postsynaptic dopamine receptors.[54,55] The only dopamine agonist currently available in the United States is bromocriptine (Parlodel, Sandoz).

Bromocriptine is a beneficial adjunct to levodopa therapy in patients with deteriorating response to levodopa,[56,57] in patients who are experiencing fluctuations in response to levodopa,[58,59] and in patients with limited clinical response to levodopa secondary to inability to tolerate higher doses.[56,58] Bromocriptine is also effective in previously untreated Parkinson's disease patients[60,61]; however, such therapy is not routinely recommended because fewer patients are able to tolerate the adverse effects of bromocriptine compared with levodopa.

**Table 42.3** Investigational and Commercially Available Drugs Used Alone or in Combination With Levodopa in the Treatment of Parkinson's Disease

| *Beneficial results reported* | *Lack of beneficial results reported* |
|---|---|
| Nadolol[73] (Corgard, Squibb) | Naloxone[86] (Narcan, Du Pont) |
| Propranolol[74,75] (Inderal, Ayerst; generic brands, various manufacturers) | Naltrexone[87] (Trexan, Du Pont) |
| Domperidone[76,a] | Buspirone[88] (BuSpar, Bristol–Myers) |
| Lithium[77] (Eskalith, Smith Kline & French; generic brands, various manufacturers) | |
| Benserazide[78,79] | |
| Iron[80,a] | |
| Bupropion[81] (Wellbutrin, Burroughs–Wellcome)[b] | |
| Selegiline[82,83,a] | |
| L-*threo*-3,4-Dihydrophenylserine[84,a] | |
| Mazindol[85,a] | |

[a] Investigational.
[b] Removed from market by manufacturer.

A recommended initial dose of bromocriptine is 1.25 mg once or twice daily. Low-dose regimens (less than 30 mg daily) are as effective as higher dose regimens (greater than 30 mg daily).[62,63] A recent study suggests that average daily doses as low as 12 to 16 mg are effective for a period up to 2 years.[61] The dose of bromocriptine should be escalated slowly by 1.25 mg daily every week and maintained at the minimum amount necessary to accomplish the desired therapeutic effect.

The limiting factor to bromocriptine therapy is adverse effects. These occur in 30% to 50% of patients and are more frequent at higher doses and with rapid escalation of dose. Nausea is the most frequently reported gastrointestinal effect occurring in greater than 50% of patients taking the drug; vomiting rarely occurs. Cardiovascular effects occur infrequently, with the exception of postural hypotension, which is common. CNS effects are most commonly dose limiting and occur in as many as one third of patients taking bromocriptine. These include confusion, hallucinations, and sedation.[58,62,63] The addition of bromocriptine to levodopa therapy will increase the frequency and severity of dyskinesias during periods of good functional status.

Several investigational dopamine agonists have undergone extensive clinical trials in patients with Parkinson's disease. Although these agents are effective in improving functional status in patients with fluctuating responses to levodopa, their usefulness is limited by severe adverse effects. Lergotrile was removed from clinical trials because it caused hepatotoxicity[64]; mesulergine was removed because it produced an increased prevalence of testicular cancer in study animals.[65] Pergolide and lisuride are effective adjuncts to levodopa therapy in some patients; however, both also cause frequent gastrointestinal and central nervous system adverse effects.[66–69] Pergolide, in addition to its arrhythmogenic effect, has a reported bradycardiac effect.[70] The clinical significance of these cardiovascular effects in Parkinson's disease patients without underlying cardiac disease is considered insignificant. Neither agent has demonstrated superiority to bromocriptine.[71,72]

Dopamine agonists should be used in patients who are experiencing deterioration in functional status at maximumly tolerated levodopa doses. Their primary benefit is to allow reductions in levodopa dose while improving functional status. This decreases the frequency and severity of "on–off" fluctuations and prolongs the period in which patients receive benefit from drug therapy. A further consideration with bromocriptine is cost, as the marketed drug product is expensive.

### *Other Drugs*

A wide variety of commercially available and investigational agents have been utilized alone or in combination with levodopa in the treatment of Parkinson's disease (Table 42.3). Results of trials with these agents must be viewed with caution because of the small numbers of patients studied, potential problems with study design, and lack of availability of drug or dosage form in the United States. One investigational agent, selegiline (or deprenyl), a monoamine oxidase B inhibitor, deserves mention. Selegiline has been reported to improve functional status when used as an adjunct to levodopa and to provide a levodopa-sparing effect. The utility of monoamine oxidase B inhibitors in the treatment of Parkinson's disease is undergoing close scrutiny based upon the finding that these agents can prevent the neurotoxicity of MPTP by blocking its oxidation.

### *Surgical Transplantation*

The transplantation of autologous adrenal medullary tissue into the brains of patients with Parkinson's disease offers a new approach to disease management. One report of two patients with severe disease noted minor improvements in rigidity and movement.[89] A more recent report in two patients with severe disease demonstrated significant improvement in rigidity, akinesia, and tremor.[90] The validity, reproducibility, applicability, and long-term benefits of this procedure are unknown.

## Summary

The cause of Parkinson's disease remains a mystery; however, sufficient information regarding its pathophysiology is available to direct treatment measures. Replacement of dopamine can significantly improve a patient's functional status and prolong meaningful life. New drug treatments have yet to be successful in completely eliminating the loss of efficacy and adverse effects associated with levodopa. The goal of management remains maintaining acceptable functional control with the minimum amount of antiparkinson drug necessary.

## Glossary

**Dyskinesias.** Abnormal involuntary movements. In patients with Parkinson's disease these are correlated to peak serum dopamine concentrations and occur during periods of good functional control. Examples include lip smacking, grimacing, and involuntary, rhythmic jerking movements.

**Progressive supranuclear palsy.** Steele–Richardson–Oszewski syndrome. A syndrome with parkinsonian features secondary to reduction of dopamine and loss of dopaminergic receptors. Symptoms appear in the sixth decade and include supranuclear palsy, visual disturbances, axial rigidity, bradykinesia, and disturbances of balance and gait. Tremor is uncommon. This syndrome is characterized pathologically by neuronal loss, granulovacuolar degeneration, gliosis, and neurofibrillary tangles (ultrastructurally different from those in dementia of the Alzheimer type) in the basal ganglia, brain stem, and cerebellar nuclei.

**Shy–Drager syndrome.** Clinical syndrome consisting of parkinsonism symptoms, orthostatic hypotension, and autonomic nervous system dysfunction. Pathologically it is characterized by degeneration in the caudate nucleus, substantia nigra, locus ceruleus, vagal nuclei, and ventral and lateral horns of the spinal cord.

## References


1. McDowell FH, Lee JE, Sweet RD. Extrapyramidal disease, in Baker AB, Baker LH (eds): Clinical Neurology. Philadelphia, Harper and Row, 1986, p 12.
2. Rajput AH, Offord KP, Beard CM, et al. Epidemiology of parkinsonism: Incidence, classification and mortality. Ann Neurol 1984;16(3):278–282.
3. Ballard PA, Tetrud JW, Langston JW. Permanent human parkinsonism due to 1-methyl-4-phenyl-1,2,3,6-tetrahydropyridine (MPTP): Seven cases. Neurology 1985;35(7):949–956.
4. Bentler A, Rosengren E. Occurrence and distribution of catecholamines in brain. Acta Physiol Scand 1959;47:350–361.
5. Teravainen H, Calne D. Motor system in normal aging and Parkinson's disease, in Katzman R, Terry R (eds): The Neurology of Aging. Philadelphia, F.A. Davis Co, 1983, pp 85–107.
6. Carlsson A, Winblad B. Influence of age and time interval between death and autopsy on dopamine and 3-methyltyramine levels in human basal ganglia. J Neural Transm 1976;38(3–4): 271–276.
7. Hornykiewicz O. Metabolism of brain dopamine in human parkinsonism: Neurochemical and clinical aspects, in Coste E, Cote LJ, Yahr MD (eds): Biochemistry and Pharmacology of the Basal Ganglia. Hewlett, NY, Raven, 1966, pp 171–181.
8. Greenfield JG, Bosanquet FD. The brainstem lesions in parkinsonism. J Neurol Neurosurg Psychiatry 1953;16:213–226.
9. Mann DM. Pathogenesis of Parkinson's disease. Arch Neurol 1982;39(9):545–549.
10. Alvord ED, Forno LS, Kusske JA, et al. The pathology of parkinsonism. Adv Neurol 1974;5:175–193.
11. Carlsson A. Some aspects of dopamine in the basal ganglia. Res Publ Assoc Res Nerv Ment Dis 1976;55:181–189.
12. Goldman JE, Yen SH, Chiu FC, et al. Lewy bodies of Parkinson's disease contain neurofilament antigens. Science 1983; 221(4615):1082–1084.
13. Hirsch E, Ruberg M, Dardenne M, et al. Monoclonal antibodies raised against Lewy bodies in brains from subjects with Parkinson's disease. Brain Res 1985;345(2):374–378.
14. Tagliavini F, Pilleri G, Bouras C, et al. The basal nucleus of Meynert in idiopathic Parkinson's disease. Acta Neurol Scand 1984;70(1):20–28.
15. Candy JM, Perry RH, Perry EK, et al. Pathological changes in the nucleus of Meynert in Alzheimer's and Parkinson's disease. J Neurol Sci 1983;59(2):277–289.
16. Uhl GR, Hedreen JC, Price DL. Parkinson's disease: Loss of neurons from the ventral tegmental area contralateral to therapeutic surgical lesions. Neurology 1985;35(8):1215–1218.
17. Langston JW, Forno LS. The hypothalamus in Parkinson's disease. Ann Neurol 1978;3(2):129–133.
18. Goetz CG, Lutge W, Tanner CM. Autonomic dysfunction in Parkinson's disease. Neurology 1986;36(1):73–75.
19. Scatton B, Dennis T, L'Heureux R, et al. Degeneration of noradrenergic and serotonergic but not dopaminergic neurons in the lumbar spinal cord of parkinsonian patients. Brain Res 1986;380(1):181–185.
20. Nappi G, Petraglia F, Martignoni E, et al. $\beta$-endorphin cerebrospinal fluid decrease in untreated parkinsonian patients. Neurology 1985;39(9):1371–1374.
21. Globus M, Mildword B, Melamed E. Cerebral blood flow and cognitive impairment in Parkinson's disease. Neurology 1985; 35(8):1135–1139.
22. Lavy S, Melamed E, Cooper G, et al. Regional cerebral blood flow in patients with Parkinson's disease. Arch Neurol 1979; 36(6):344–348.
23. Klawans HL, Barr A. The extrapyramidal system: A review of function. Clin Neuropharmacol 1983;6(suppl 1):53–58.
24. Hoehn MH, Yahr MD. Parkinsonism: Onset, progression and mortality. Neurology 1967;17(5):427–442.
25. Clough CG, Bergmann KJ, Yahr MD. Cholinergic and dopaminergic mechanisms in Parkinson's disease after long-term l-dopa administration, in Hassler RG, Christ JF (eds): Advances in Neurology, vol 40. New York, Raven Press, 1984, pp 131–140.
26. Stromberg U, Svensson TH. Further studies on the mode of

action of amantadine. Acta Pharmacol Toxicol 1971:30(3–4): 161–171.

27. VonVoightlander PF, Moore KE. Dopamine: Release from the brain in vivo by amantadine. Science 1971;174(4007):408–410.
28. Timberlake WH, Vance MA. Four years treatment of patients with parkinsonism using amantadine alone or with levodopa. Ann Neurol 1978;3(2):119–128.
29. Cotzias GC, Van Woert MH, Schiffer LM. Aromatic amino acids and modification of parkinsonism. N Engl J Med 1967; 276(7):374–379.
30. Yahr MD, Duvoisin RC, Schear MJ, et al. Treatment of parkinsonism with levodopa. Arch Neurol 1969;21(4):343–354.
31. Pletscher A, Bartholini G. Selective rise in brain dopamine by inhibition of extracerebral levodopa decarboxylation. Clin Pharmacol Ther 1971;12(2):344–352.
32. Papavasiliou PS, Cotzias GC, Duby SE, et al. Levodopa in parkinsonism: Potentiation of central effects with a peripheral inhibitor. N Engl J Med 1972;286(1):8–14.
33. Ward CD, Trombley LK, Calne DB, et al. L-dopa decarboxylation in chronically treated patients. Neurology 1984;34 (2):198–201.
34. Marsden CD, Parkes JD. "On–off" effects in patients with Parkinson's disease on chronic levodopa therapy. Lancet 1976; 1(7954):292–296.
35. Marsden CD, Parkes JD. Success and problems of long-term levodopa therapy in Parkinson's disease. Lancet 1977;1 (8007):345–349.
36. deJong GJ, Meerwaldt JD. Response variations in the treatment of Parkinson's disease. Neurology 1984;34(11):1507–1509.
37. Melamed E, Bitton V, Zelig O. Delayed onset of responses to single doses of L-dopa in parkinsonian fluctuators on long-term L-dopa therapy. Clin Neuropharmacol 1986;9(2):182–188.
38. Melamed E, Bitton V, Zelig O. Episodic unresponsiveness to single doses of l-dopa in parkinsonian fluctuations. Neurology 1986;36(1):100–103.
39. Markham CH, Diamond SG. Long-term follow-up of early dopa treatment in Parkinson's disease. Ann Neurol 1986;19 (4):365–372.
40. Leenders KL, Palmer AJ, Quinn N, et al. Brain dopamine metabolism in patients with Parkinson's disease measured by PET. J Neurol Neurosurg Psychiatry 1986;49(8):853–860.
41. Rajput AH, Offord K, Beard CM, et al. Epidemiological survey of dementia in parkinsonism and control population, in Hassler RG, Christ JF (eds): Advances in Neurology, vol 40. New York, Raven Press, 1984, pp 229–234.
42. Nutt JG, Woodward WR. Levodopa pharmacokinetics and pharmacodynamics in fluctuating parkinsonism patients. Neurology 1986;36(6):739–744.
43. Marion MH, Stocchi F, Quinn NP, et al. Repeated levodopa infusions in fluctuating Parkinson's disease: Clinical and pharmacokinetic data. Clin Neuropharmacol 1986;9(2):165–181.
44. Cedarbaum JM, Kutt H, Dhar AK, et al. Effect of supplemental carbidopa on bioavailability of L-dopa. Clin Neuropharmacol 1986;9(2):153–159.
45. Wajsport J, Youdin MBH. A new selective suicide inhibitor of peripheral dopa decarboxylase, in Hassler RG, Christ JF (eds): Advances in Neurology, vol 40. New York, Raven Press, 1984, pp 251–258.
46. Cedarbaum JM, Breck L, Kutt H, et al. Controlled-release levodopa/carbidopa. 1. Sinemet cr3 treatment of response fluctuations in Parkinson's disease. Neurology 1987;37(2):233–241.
47. Nutt JG, Woodward WR, Carter JH. Clinical and biochemical studies with controlled-release levodopa/carbidopa. Neurology 1986;36(9):1206–1211.
48. Kurlan R, Rubin AJ, Miller C, et al. Duodenal delivery of levodopa for on–off fluctuations in parkinsonism: Preliminary observations. Ann Neurol 1986;20(2):262–265.
49. Feldman RG, Kaye JA, Lannon MC. Parkinson's disease: Follow up after drug holiday. J Clin Pharm 1986;26(8):662–667.
50. Mayeau R, Stern Y, Mulvey K, et al. Reappraisal of temporary levodopa withdrawal ("drug holiday") in Parkinson's disease. N Engl J Med 1985;313(12):724–728.
51. Rajput AH, Stern W, Laverty WH. Chronic low-dose levodopa therapy in Parkinson's disease: An argument for delaying levodopa therapy. Neurology 1984;34(8):991–996.
52. Poewe WH, Lees AJ, Stern GM. Low-dose L-dopa therapy in Parkinson's disease: A 6-year follow-up study. Neurology 1986; 36(11):1528–1530.
53. Lesser RP, Fahn S, Snider SR, et al. Analysis of the clinical problems in parkinsonism and the complications of long-term levodopa therapy. Neurology 1979;29(9):1253–1260.
54. Seeman P. Brain dopamine receptors. Pharmacol Rev 1980; 32(3):229–313.
55. Johnson AM, Loew PM, Vigouret JM. Stimulant properties of bromocriptine on central dopamine receptors in comparison to apomorphine, (+)-amphetamine and L-dopa. Br J Pharmacol 1976;56(1):59–68.
56. Jansen ENH. Bromocriptine in levodopa response-losing parkinsonism—a double blind study. Eur Neurol 1978;17(2):92–99.
57. Lieberman A, Kupersmith M, Estey E. Treatment of Parkinson's disease with bromocriptine. N Engl J Med 1976;295 (25):1400–1404.
58. Fahn S, Cote LJ, Snider SR, et al. The role of bromocriptine in the treatment of parkinsonism. Neurology 1979;29(8): 1077–1083.
59. Lieberman AN, Kupersmith M, Gopinathan G, et al. Bromocriptine in Parkinson's disease: Further studies. Neurology 1979;29(3):363–369.
60. Lees AJ, Stern GM. Sustained bromocriptine therapy in previously untreated patients with Parkinson's disease. J Neurol Neurosurg Psychiatry 1981;44(11):1020–1023.
61. Teychenne PF, Bergsrud D, Elton RL, et al. Bromocriptine: Long-term low-dose therapy in Parkinson's disease. Clin Neuropharmacol 1986;9(2):138–145.
62. Teychenne PF, Bergsrud D, Racy A, et al. Bromocriptine: Low-dose therapy in Parkinson's disease. Neurology 1982; 32(6):577–583.
63. Hoehm MM, Elton RL. Low dosages of bromocriptine added to levodopa in Parkinson's disease. Neurology 1985;35(2):199–206.
64. Teychenne PF, Jones EA, Ishak KG, et al. Hepatocellular injury with distinctive mitochondrial changes induced by lergotrile mesylate: A dopaminergic ergot derivative. Gastroenterology 1979;76(3):575–583.
65. Roscol A, Montastruc JL, Roscol O, et al. Mesulergine (cu-32085) in the treatment of Parkinson's disease. Clin Neuropharmacol 1986;9(2):146–152.
66. Jankovic J. Long-term study of pergolide in Parkinson's disease. Neurology 1985;35(3):296–299.
67. Lang AE, Quinn N, Brincat S, et al. Pergolide in late-stage Parkinson disease. Ann Neurol 1982;12(3):243–247.
68. Gopinathan G, Teravainen H, Dambrosia JM, et al. Lisuride in parkinsonism. Neurology 1981;31(4):371–376.
69. Lieberman AN, Goldstein M, Leibowitz M, et al. Lisuride combined with levodopa in advanced Parkinson's disease. Neurology 1981;31(11):1466–1469.
70. Kurlan R, Miller C, Knapp R, et al. Double-blind assessment of potential pergolide-induced cardiotoxicity. Neurology 1986;36 (7):993–995.
71. LeWitt PA, Ward CD, Larsen TA, et al. Comparison of

pergolide and bromocriptine therapy in parkinsonism. Neurology 1983;33(8):1009–1014.

72. LeWitt PA, Gopinathan G, Ward CD, et al. Lisuride versus bromocriptine treatment in Parkinson's disease: A double-blind study. Neurology 1982;32(1):69–72.
73. Foster NL, Newman RP, LeWitt PA, et al. Peripheral beta-adrenergic blockade treatment of parkinsonian tremor. Ann Neurol 1984;16(4):505–508.
74. Owen DAL, Marsden CD. Effect of adrenergic B-blockade on parkinsonian tremor. Lancet 1965;2(7425):1259–1262.
75. Kissel P, Tridon P, Andre JM. Levodopa–propranolol therapy in parkinsonian tremor. Lancet 1974;1(7854):403–404.
76. Langdon N, Malcolm PN, Parkes JD. Comparison of levodopa with carbidopa and levodopa with domperidone in Parkinson's disease. Clin Neuropharmacol 1986;9(5):440–447.
77. Coffey CE, Ross DR, Ferren EL, et al. Treatment of the "on–off" phenomena in parkinsonism with lithium carbonate. Ann Neurol 1982;12(4):375–379.
78. Diamond SG, Markham CH, Treciokas LJ. A double blind comparison of levodopa, madopa and sinemet in Parkinson's disease. Ann Neurol 1978;3(3):267–272.
79. Rinne UK, Molsa P. Levodopa with benserazide or carbidopa in Parkinson's disease. Neurology 1979;29(12):1584–1589.
80. Birkmayer W, Kirkmayer JGD. Iron, a new aid in the treatment of Parkinson's patients. J Neural Transm 1986;67(3–4):287–292.
81. Goetz CG, Tanner CM, Klawans HL. Bupropion in Parkinson's disease. Neurology 1984;34(8):1092–1094.
82. Birkmayer W, Riederer P. Deprenyl prolongs the therapeutic efficacy of combined L-dopa in Parkinson's disease, in Hassler RG, Christ JF (eds): Advances in Neurology, vol 40. New York, Raven Press, 1984, pp 475–481.
83. Heikkila RE, Manzino L, Cabbat FS, et al. Protection against the dopaminergic neurotoxicity of 1-methyl-4-phenyl-1,2,3,6-tetrahydropyridine by monoamine oxidase inhibitors. Nature 1984;311(5985):467–468.
84. Narabayashi H, Kondo T, Nagatsu T, et al. DL-threo-3,4-dihydroxyphenylserine for freezing symptoms in parkinsonism, in Hassler RG, Christ JF (eds): Advances in Neurology, vol 40. New York, Raven Press, 1984, pp 497–502.
85. Delwaide PJ, Mortinella P, Schoenem J. Mazindol in the treatment of Parkinson's disease. Arch Neurol 1983;40(13):788–790.
86. Trabucchi M, Bassi S, Frattola L. Effect of naloxone on the "on–off" syndrome in patients receiving long-term levodopa therapy. Arch Neurol 1982;39(2):120–121.
87. Nutt JG, Rosin AJ, Eisler T, et al. Effect of an opiate antagonist on movement disorders. Arch Neurol 1978;35(12):810–811.
88. Ludwig CL, Weinberger DR, Bruno G, et al. Buspirone, Parkinson's disease, and the locus ceruleus. Clin Neuropharmacol 1986;9(4):373–378.
89. Backlund EO, Granberg PO, Hamberger B, et al. Transplantation of adrenal medullary tissue to striatum parkinsonism. First clinical trials. J Neurosurg 1985;62(2):169–173.
90. Madrazo I, Drucker-Colin R, Diaz V, et al. Open microsurgical autograft of adrenal medulla to the right caudate nucleus in two patients with intractable Parkinson's disease. N Engl J Med 1987;316(14):831–834.

# Chapter 43 / Pain Management

Terry J. Baumann, PharmD, and Mark E. Lehman, PharmD

Humans have always known and sought relief from pain. In fact, the act of relieving pain is as old as the medical profession itself. Today, pain's impact on society is still great, and indeed, pain complaints are the number one reason patients seek medical advice. Approximately one third of all Americans experience pain that requires medical attention.[1] Almost 50 million people are partially or totally disabled because of pain. This costs the American society an estimated $90 billion annually.[1,2]

Unfortunately, pain is often undertreated and pain management greatly misunderstood.[3–8] Marks and Sacher[3] studied hospitalized medical patients receiving narcotic analgesia, and found 73% in severe or moderate distress despite their analgesic regimen. Caregivers' misconceptions regarding narcotic doses, duration of analgesic effect, and fear of addiction were reportedly responsible for this undertreatment.[3] Cohen[4] demonstrated that despite narcotic analgesics, 75% of postsurgical patients were in moderate or marked distress and 45% "cried out" in pain. Fear of addiction and inadequate knowledge of pharmacologic agents were again considered major factors contributing to pain mismanagement.[4] Similar problems are reported in ambulatory patients.[8]

Regrettably, many health care providers do not receive adequate training in this area and new information is not widely disseminated and/or understood. Clearly, pain management is enhanced when a multidisciplinary approach is applied. Thus, understanding the pathophysiology and concepts of pain therapy management and maintaining a working knowledge of individual pain regimens are important to pharmacists and are key factors in reversing the problem of inadequate pain control.

## Definition

An acceptable definition of pain remains an enigma. Originally it was thought to be a punishment from the gods. In fact, the word is derived from the Latin *peone* and the Greek *poine*, meaning "penalty" or "punishment."[8] This punishment theory was advanced by Aristotle, who considered pain a feeling and classified it as a passion of the soul. Two thousand years later Descartes, Galen, and Vaselius postulated that pain was a sensation in which the brain played an important role. In the nineteenth century, Mueller, Van Frey, and Goldscheider hypothesized the concepts of neuroreceptors, nociceptors, and sensory input.[8] These theories developed into this century's definition of pain; a multifactorial phenomenon consisting of the painful stimulus and the interpretation of and reaction to that stimulus.[9]

## Pathophysiology

The pathophysiology of pain is a complex series of afferent and efferent neuronal connections that have not been fully elucidated; however, research over the last 15 years has greatly advanced our understanding of pain transmission.

### *Afferent Pain Transmission*

#### Peripheral Stimulation

The first step leading to the sensation of pain is the stimulation of receptors known as nociceptors. These free nerve endings are found in skin, blood vessels, subcutaneous tissues, muscle fascia, periosteum, viscera, joints, and other structures. They may be specific—responding only to mechanical, thermal, chemical, and ischemic processes alone—or polymodal—responding to one or more of these processes. The exact mechanism that underlies the stimulation of nociceptors is poorly understood; however, bradykinins, prostaglandins, leukotrienes, histamine, and serotonin sensitize these receptors. Receptor activation leads to action potentials that are transmitted along afferent nerve fibers to the spinal cord.[10–15]

In recent years, somatostatin, cholecystokinin, and substance P have been identified as possible neurotransmitters in afferent nociceptive neurons.[16,17] In addition, substance P may play a role in releasing chemicals (histamine and bradykinin) that potentiate nociceptive nerve ending stimulation, possibly causing pain.[10,18,19] In fact, when substance P is blocked by the neurotoxin capsaicin, pain transmission can be significantly reduced, making substance P antagonists a potential future class of analgesics.[20,21]

Afferent fibers are classified as A, B, or C. Large, fast, myelinated A fibers are further divided into alpha, beta, gamma, and delta subfibers. In comparison, C fibers are small, slow, and myelinated and are not subgrouped. Nociceptive transmission takes place only in the A-delta or C fibers.[16] Stimulation of A-delta fibers evokes bright, piercing, well-localized pain, while stimulation of C fibers produces dull, poorly localized, and persistent pain.[15]

#### Gate Control Theory

These afferent, nociceptive, pain fibers synapse in the dorsal horn of the spinal cord along with many other non–pain-transmitting or nonnociceptive neurons (Fig. 43.1). Synapses are made directly onto pain transmission neurons (PTNs) or onto interconnecting neurons (ICNs) that excite PTNs. In addition, large nonnociceptive fibers originating

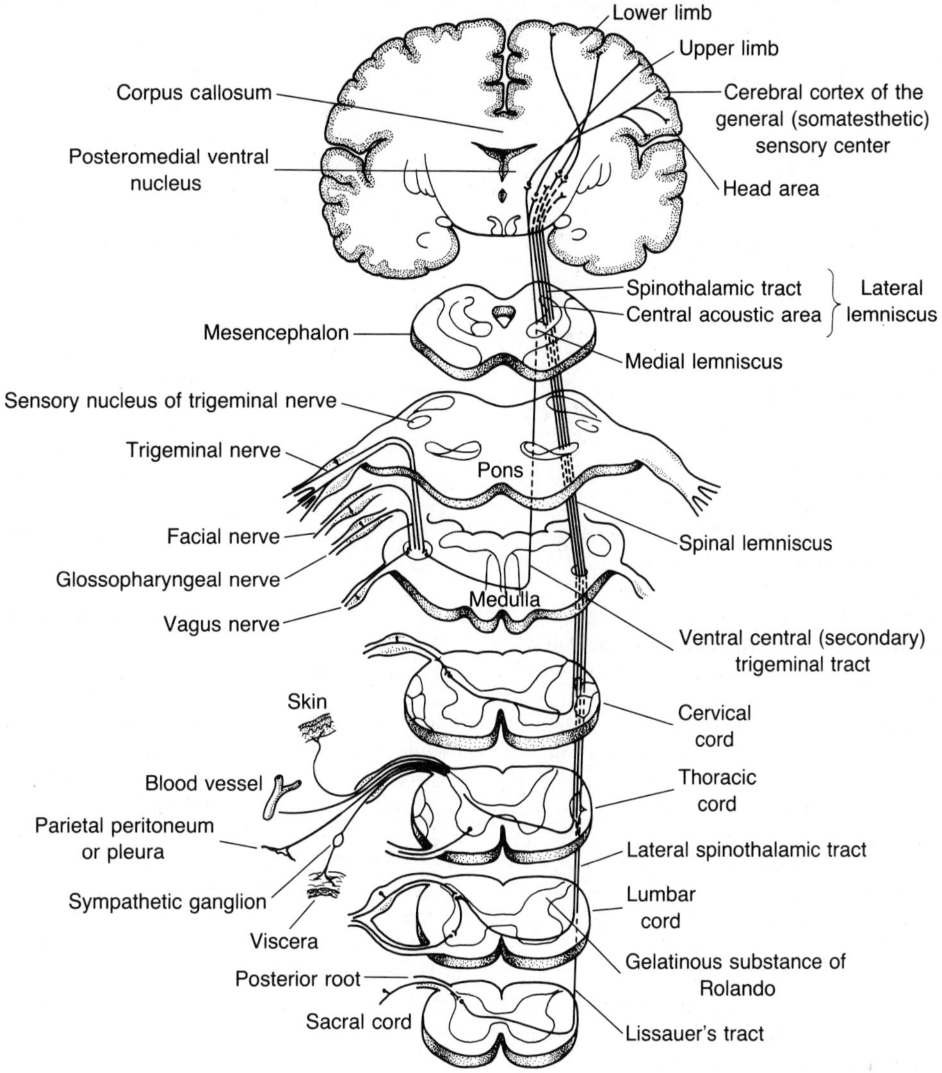


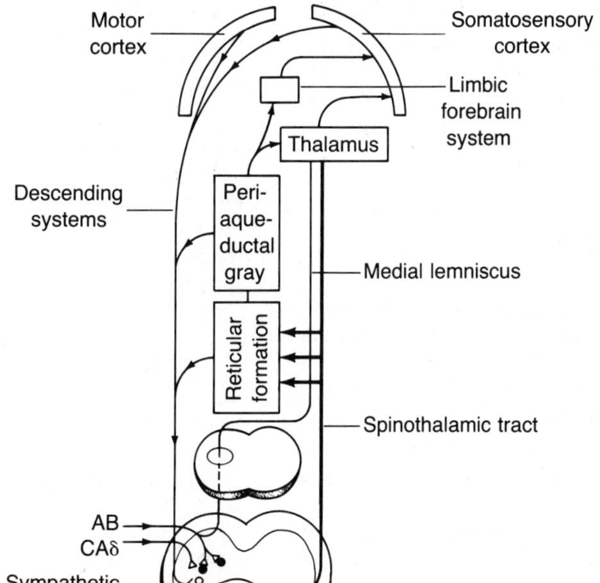


**Figure 43.1** Afferent and efferent pain conduction pathways. *(Top figure adapted from Hospital Practice. Special Reports in the Management of Acute Pain Considerations. New York, H.P. Publishing, January 1977, p 5, with permission. Bottom figure adapted from Stimmel B: Pain, Analgesia and Addiction: The Pharmacology of Pain. New York, Raven, 1983, p 13, with permission.)*

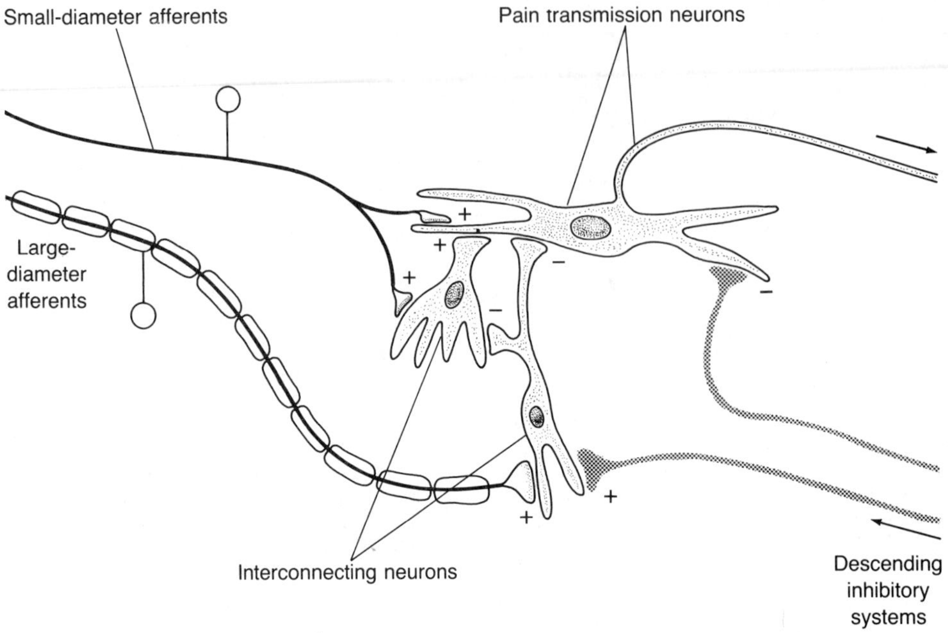


**Figure 43.2** Schematic representation of dorsal horn nociceptive modulation. (+) excitatory connection, (−) inhibitory connection. *(Adapted from Fields HL, Levins JD: Pain mechanisms and management. West J Med 1984;141:349, with permission.)*

either in the periphery or in neurons descending from the spinal cord may inhibit both PTNs and ICNs in the dorsal horn. When large myelinated fibers are stimulated they have an inhibitory affect on pain transmission. Therefore, perception of pain is a complex summation of nonnociceptive and nociceptive neuronal stimulation (Fig. 43.2).[10,22]

Functionally, the importance of the interplay between these different fibers is evident in the analgesic response produced by treatments that stimulate large nonnociceptive neurons, for example, topical irritants, acupuncture, or transcutaneous electrical nerve stimulation (TENS). Although modified, this theory was first explained by Melzack and Wall[23] and is referred to as the ''gate control'' theory of pain transmission.

#### Spinal Cord Transmission

These pain-initiated processes reach the brain through a complex array of ascending spinal cord pathways. In addition, information other than pain impulses is carried along these pathways. Thus, pain is influenced by many factors supplemental to nociception and precludes simple schematic representation; however, one major ascending pathway, the spinothalamic tract, is known to have a major influence on pain transmission and is classically divided into lateral and ventral pathways. The lateral pathway is associated with sharp localized pain and is responsible for the spatial and temporal discriminative aspects of nociception.[8] The ventral pathway makes possible the perception of aching, dull, nonlocalized pain and the reflexes responsible for aversion motivation.[8] Both pathways eventually merge in the thalamus and connect with the cortex.

### *Pain Modulation*

The brain modulates pain through a system that is just beginning to be understood. First evidence of this system was the analgesia produced by selected electrical stimulation of animal brains,[24,25] with subsequent similar results in patients with intractable clinical pain.[26] Almost simultaneously, other investigators discovered opiate receptors within the central nervous system (CNS).[27–29] Dense clusters of opiate receptors are found in the ascending and descending pain pathways and in portions of the brain believed to be essential to the pain modulating system.[8] In 1975, researchers[30,31] identified two pentapeptides (Met-enkephalin and Leu-enkephalin) whose actions were similar to morphine. These enkephalins interact with opiate receptors to form, in part, what is known as the endogenous opiate system.[8] To date, 16 such opioids have been identified[32] and are generically referred to as endorphins. They are often classified as $\beta$-endorphin-like or enkephalin-like.[32] Although both are important in the endogenous opiate system, they originate from different precursors and have different physiologic properties.[32] As the knowledge of endorphins has expanded so has the understanding of opiate receptors. Five such receptors, mu (sometimes split into two subpopulations mu-1 and mu-2), delta, sigma, kappa, and epsilon, have been recognized. These receptors display similar chemical properties but have varying affinities and functions (Table 43.1).[8]

The development of narcotic antagonists (substances that block endogenous opiate receptors) led to the discovery of a highly integrated network associating pain, opiate receptors, and endorphins. Although the endogenous opioid relationship is still not completely defined it may moderate pain through a positive and negative feedback system. Thus, a given nociceptive stimulus activates both peripheral pain transmission pathways (causing pain and termed *positive*

**Table 43.1** Opiate Receptors and Function

| *Opiate receptor* | *Function* |
|---|---|
| $Mu^{-1}$ | Analgesia |
| $Mu^{-2}$ | Respiratory depression |
| | Euphoria |
| | Physical dependence |
| | Constipation |
| Delta | Analgesia |
| Sigma | Autonomic stimulation |
| | Dysphoria |
| | Hallucinations |
| Kappa | Analgesia |
| | Sedation |
| | Miosis |
| Epsilon | Analgesia |

Modified from Stimmel B: Pain, Analgesia and Addiction: The Pharmacology of Pain. New York, Raven, 1983, pp 22 and 96.

*feedback*) and the brain's modulatory network (inhibiting pain and termed *negative feedback*), making the sensation of pain a partial summation of these two processes.[10] Other neurotransmitter substances known to play a role in pain regulation include acetylcholine,[33] dopamine,[34] norepinephrine,[35] and serotonin.[36]

### *Efferent Pain Transmission*

The CNS also contains a highly organized descending system for control of pain transmission. This system influences synaptic transmission of sensory fibers at the dorsal horn level of the spinal cord and is dependent on the biogenic amine neurotransmitters and other networks previously mentioned (Fig. 43.1).[8]

In summary, although progress has occurred in unraveling the pain transmission mystery, understanding of this complex pathway is still limited. Pain without nociception (algodynia) and phantom limb pain (pain in a limb that has been amputated) are very real phenomena, but defy explanation using our present knowledge of neurophysiology.[8] Additional research is needed to clarify the roles of neuromodulaters and neurotransmitters. Although the current pain model is not incorrect, it is certainly incomplete.[2]

## Pain Assessment

Pain is a complex concept,[37] and a proper pain assessment and an accurate diagnosis of the underlying cause are often major obstacles in effective treatment. A patient-oriented approach is essential, and evaluation methods should not differ from those used in other medical conditions.[8] Therefore, a comprehensive history and physical examination are imperative to thoroughly evaluate underlying diseases and possible contributing factors.[8] A baseline description of pain can be obtained by assessing PQRST characteristics (Table 43.2).[38] Attention must also be given to mental factors that alter the pain threshold. Anxiety, depression, fatigue, anger, and fear are particularly noted to lower this threshold, whereas rest, mood elevation, sympathy, diversion, and understanding raise the pain threshold.[38]

**Table 43.2** PQRST Characteristics of Pain

| | | |
|---|---|---|
| P | Palliative factors | What makes the pain better? |
| | Provocative factors | What makes the pain worse? |
| Q | Quality | Describe the pain. |
| R | Radiation | Where is your pain? |
| S | Severity | How does this pain compare with other pain you have experienced? |
| T | Temporal factors | Does the intensity of the pain change with time? |

Modified from Twycross RG: Pain and analgesics. Curr Med Res Opinion 1975; 5:499.

Clinicians must evaluate all components of the pain experience, for example, behavioral (much of our reaction to pain is learned),[39] cognitive (thinking processes alter pain experiences),[15] social (pain expression differs in accordance with social environments),[40] and cultural (cultural background may influence pain tolerance).[40] In addition, separating pain with a known organic cause from that with no known cause (so-called "psychogenic pain") allows for improved treatment regimens.[8] Physical pain is often localized, well described, and relieved with proper analgesic therapy, whereas psychogenic pain, though real, is nonlocalized, ill defined, and not easily treated with conventional analgesics.[8] Proper patient assessment must also include an evaluation of pain management. This includes alleviation of pain symptoms, and an assessment of medication side effects, patient activity, and quality of life.

## Acute and Chronic Pain

Acute pain may be a useful physiologic process warning individuals of disease states and potentially harmful situations. Unfortunately, severe, unremitting, undertreated, acute pain, when it outlives its biologic usefulness, produces many deleterious effects such as extension of myocardial ischemia after myocardial infarction. When pain is not effectively treated, the stress and concurrent reflex reactions often cause hypoxia, hypercapnia, hypotension, excessive cardiac activity, and permanent emotional difficulties. The problems associated with these reactions range from a prolonged recovery time to death.[2]

Under normal conditions, acute pain quickly subsides as the healing process decreases the pain-producing stimuli; however, in some instances pain may persist for months to years, leading to a chronic pain state with features quite different from those of acute pain (Table 43.3). Typically, chronic pain is divided into four subtypes: pain that persists beyond the normal healing time for an acute injury, pain related to a chronic disease, pain without identifiable organic cause, and pain that involves both the chronic and acute pain associated with cancer.[41] Patients in chronic pain often develop severe psychologic problems caused by fear and memory of past pain. In addition chronic pain patients may

**Table 43.3** Characteristics of Acute and Chronic Pain

| *Characteristic* | *Acute pain* | *Chronic pain* |
|---|---|---|
| Relief of pain | Highly desirable | Highly desirable |
| Dependence and tolerance to medication | Unusual | Common |
| Psychologic component | Usually not present | Often a major problem |
| Organic cause | Common | Often not present |
| Environmental contributions and family involvement | Small | Significant |
| Insomnia | Unusual | Common component |
| Treatment goal | Cure | Rehabilitation not a cure |

Modified from Stimmel B: Pain, Analgesia and Addiction: The Pharmacology of Pain. New York, Raven, 1983, p 256.

develop dependence and tolerance to analgesics, have trouble sleeping, and more readily react to environmental changes that can intensify the pain response. Distinguishing between chronic and acute pain states is very important because of drastically different management techniques.[42]

## Acute Pain Management

The obvious way to relieve pain is to eliminate the underlying cause. This is often not possible, however, and symptomatic relief is usually indicated. Therapeutic interventions include pharmacologic treatment, stimulation therapies, and psychologic therapies.

### *Pharmacologic Treatment*

Although pharmacologic agents to effectively treat acute pain are available, they are not always appropriately used. Misunderstanding of the acute pain cycle (Fig. 43.3), inadequate dose titration, fear of analgesic side effects, varying analgesic requirements, inadequate application of current available therapies, and nonappreciation of the complications of untreated pain contribute to ineffective and inappropriate pain management. Adherence to the basic principles of the pharmacologic treatment of pain (Table 43.4) will promote rational pain control decisions. Analgesic agents should be given an adequate trial and often require individual dosage titration. Even in acute pain, administering analgesics as needed (prn) may promote anxiety and contribute to future drug dependence. These drugs should be administered on a regular dosing schedule and not on an as-needed schedule. Side effects should be well understood and excessive sedation avoided. Finally, placebo therapy should never be used to diagnose psychogenic pain and the route of administration should always be geared to the analgesic needs of the patient.

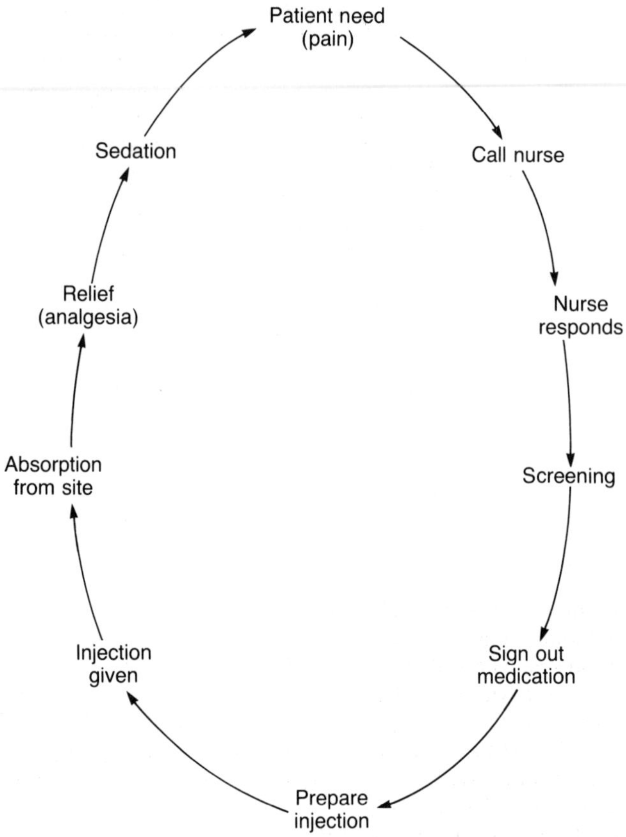


**Figure 43.3** Acute pain cycle. *(Adapted from Graves DA, Foster TS, Batenhorst RL, et al: The evolution of patient-controlled analgesia: A review. Ann Intern Med 1983;99:361, with permission.)*

#### Nonnarcotic Agents

Analgesia should be initiated with the weakest effective analgesic agent having the fewest side effects. Peripherally acting agents, for example, acetaminophen, acetylsalicylic acid (aspirin), and nonsteroidal anti-inflammatory drugs (NSAIDs), are often preferred over centrally acting narcotic agents in the treatment of acute, mild to moderate pain (Tables 43.5 and 43.6). These drugs affect the prostaglandins

**Table 43.4** Pharmacologic Treatment of Pain

| |
|---|
| Identify the source of pain |
| Use the least potent analgesic with the fewest side effects |
| Properly titrate the dose and administer for an adequate duration |
| Do not use analgesics on an as-needed basis |
| Recognize side effects of analgesics |
| Avoid excessive sedation |
| Adjust the route of administration to the needs of the patient |
| Use equianalgesic doses |
| Do not use placebo therapy to diagnose psychogenic pain |

Modified from Stimmel B: Pain, Analgesia and Addiction: The Pharmacology of Pain. New York, Raven, 1983, p 245.

**Table 43.5** Pharmacokinetics of FDA-Approved Nonnarcotic Analgesics

| *Agent* | *Time to peak concentration (h)* | *Elimination half-life (h)* | *Analgesic onset (h)* | *Analgesic duration (h)* |
|---|---|---|---|---|
| Aspirin | 0.25–2 | 0.25–0.33 | 0.5 | 3–6 |
| Diflunisal | 2–3 | 8–12 | 1 | 2–3 |
| Acetaminophen | 0.5–2 | 1–4 | 0.5–1 | 3–6 |
| Mefenamic acid | 2–4 | 2–4 | —[a] | —[a] |
| Ibuprofen | 1–2 | 1–2.5 | 0.5 | 4–6 |
| Fenoprofen | 1–2 | 2–3 | —[a] | —[a] |
| Naproxen | 2–4 | 12–15 | 1 | Up to 7 |
| Naproxen sodium | 1–2 | 12–15 | 1 | Up to 7 |
| Suprofen[b] | 0.5–2 | 2–4 | 1–2 | 4–6 |

[a] Data not available.
[b] Removed from the market July 1987.

Compiled from References 43, 91, 96, and 97.

produced by the arachidonic acid cascade in response to noxious stimuli,[43] thereby decreasing the number of pain impulses received by the CNS. Patient response to mild analgesics varies, with the best results evident in low-grade, somatic-type pain (e.g., headache, myalgia, neuralgia, and dysmenorrhea).[44] Results are poor in intense or sharp visceral pain present after surgery or with headaches of vascular origin.[44] Therapeutic outcomes are also less than desired in those who do not expect "mild" analgesics to relieve pain. Studies comparing the efficacy of these agents have been inconsistent because of problems in presentation, perception, and reproducibility of pain.[44] Therefore, the choice of a particular agent often depends upon availability, cost, pharmacokinetic and pharmacologic characteristics (Tables 43.5, 43.6), and the side effect profile (Table 43.7).

Aspirin or aspirin-like compounds are the most widely used peripherally acting analgesics in the world.[43] This may be because they impart antipyretic and anti-inflammatory action, as well as analgesic effects; however, problems with platelet aggregation defects and direct gastrointestinal irrita-

**Table 43.6** FDA-Approved Nonnarcotic Analgesics

| *Class and generic name* | *Trade name* | *Manufacturer* | *Usual dosage range (mg/d)* | *Maximal dosage (mg/d)* |
|---|---|---|---|---|
| Salicylates | | | | |
| Acetylsalicylic acid (aspirin)[a] | Aspirin | | 325–650 every 4 h | 3,600 |
| | Generic | Various | | |
| Diflunisal | Dolobid | Merck | 250–750 every 8–12 h | 1,500 |
| *para*-Aminophenol | | | | |
| Acetaminophen[a] | Tylenol | McNeil | 325–1,000 every 4–6 h | 4,000 |
| Fenamates | | | | |
| Mefenamic acid | Ponstel | Parke–Davis | 250–500 every 6 h | 1,000 |
| Propionic acids | | | | |
| Ibuprofen[b] | Motrin | Upjohn | 200–400 every 4–6 h | 2,400 |
| | Generic | Various | | |
| Fenoprofen | Nalfon | Dista | 200 every 4–6 h | 3,200 |
| Naproxen | Naprosyn | Syntex | 250–500 every 6–12 h | 1,250 |
| Naproxen sodium[b] | Anaprox | Syntex | 275–550 every 6–12 h | 1,375 |
| Suprofen[c] | Suprol | McNeil | 200 every 4–6 h | 800 |

[a] Available as an over-the-counter preparation.
[b] Available both as an over-the-counter preparation and as a prescription drug.
[c] Removed from the market July 1987.

Compiled from References 43 and 91.

**Table 43.7** Relative Side Effects of FDA-Approved Nonnarcotic Analgesics

| *Agent* | *GI irritation* | *CNS effects* | *Tinnitus* | *Hepatic toxicity* | *Renal toxicity* |
|---|---|---|---|---|---|
| Aspirin | ++++++ | + | +++ | ++ | ++ |
| Diflunisal | +++ | ++ | + | + | + |
| Acetaminophen | + | + | − | ++ | + |
| Mefenamic acid | ++ | + | − | + | ++ |
| Ibuprofen | ++ | ++ | + | + | ++ |
| Fenoprofen | ++ | ++ | + | + | ++ |
| Naproxen | ++ | ++ | + | + | ++ |
| Suprofen[a] | ++ | ++ | − | + | ++ |

[a] Removed from market July 1987.

Compiled from References 43 and 92.

tion leading to nausea, dyspepsia, and epigastric burning have limited their use.[43] Other problems connected with the use of aspirin include a strong association with gastric ulcers (dose related), gastrointestinal bleeding (even with normal doses), tinnitus (dose related), hypersensitivity reactions in patients with asthma, and, when used in doses exceeding 6 g per day, hypoprothrombinemia.[44] These agents should not be used concurrently with other peripherally acting NSAIDs because they may reduce efficacy and increase the potential for side effects.[43]

NSAIDs have effective analgesic and anti-inflammatory properties, but generally cause fewer gastrointestinal problems than aspirin. Particular attention must be given to the effects that NSAIDs have on renal function. Prostaglandins play an important role in counteracting the deleterious effects that release of renin–angiotensin, catecholamines, and vasopressin has on the kidney. When prostaglandin synthesis is inhibited by NSAIDs in patients with poor renal function this control mechanism is lost and severe renal damage may result.[45] Patients suspected of minimal renal function (creatinine clearances below 50 mL/min) who receive NSAIDs must be carefully monitored for further kidney damage. These drugs can also cause rash, tinnitus, nausea, vomiting, a burning sensation in the esophagus and stomach, diarrhea, constipation, and vertigo.[43] There appears to be a great deal of variability from one patient to another in the therapeutic response seen with the NSAIDs. After an adequate drug trial of any of these agents, it is considered rational therapy to switch to another member of this drug group for an additional trial period.

The *para*-aminophenols (acetaminophen and phenacetin) inhibit prostaglandin synthesis in the CNS and manifest both analgesic and antipyretic activity with little anti-inflammatory action.[43] Acetaminophen exhibits a linear dose–response curve, with doses larger than 1,000 mg showing greater efficacy than doses of 650 mg.[43] Phenacetin therapy was linked to renal papillary necrosis and has been removed from the worldwide market.[43] Acetaminophen is relatively free from side effects, although in overdose situations it is highly liver toxic. It can also be used in cases of aspirin allergy.

**Narcotic Agents**

Most clinicians consider the use of narcotic analgesics to be the next logical step in the management of acute pain. The classification of these agents and their equianalgesic doses are outlined in Table 43.8.

The pharmacologic activity of narcotics depends on their affinity for opiate receptors (Table 43.9).[46] Therapeutic activities and side effects range from those exhibited by the pure opiate agonists or stimulators (e.g., morphine), to those seen with the pure opiate antagonists or blockers (e.g., naloxone) (Tables 43.1, 43.9, and 43.10). Partial agonists and antagonists (e.g., pentazocine) compete with agonists for opiate receptor sites and, depending on the inherent ability to either stimulate or block these sites, exhibit mixed agonist–antagonist activity. Mixed agonist–antagonist agents with analgesic activity appear to exhibit selectivity for analgesic receptor sites (Table 43.1).[8] This may result in analgesia with fewer undesirable side effects.

In usual doses, narcotic analgesics do not eliminate pain; instead, they decrease its unpleasantness. Patients report that although their pain is still present, it no longer bothers them. The effects of the analgesics are also relatively selective, and at normal therapeutic concentrations, these agents do not decrease sensitivity to touch, sight, or hearing, or impair intellectual functioning[8]; however, as the dosage increases, so do the undesirable side effects (Table 43.9).

Narcotic analgesics share related pharmacologic attributes and exert their most profound effects on the CNS and gastrointestinal tract.[47] Mood changes, sedation, respiratory depression, nausea, vomiting, decreased gastrointestinal motility, dependence, and tolerance are evident in varying degrees with all agents. Consideration of efficacy and side effect profile assists in the selection of the most appropriate agent.

The route of administration depends on individual patient needs. Oral codeine, oxycodone, meperidine, propoxyphene, and pentazocine are usually used in mild to moderate pain. In addition, the narcotics differ greatly in equianalgesic dose (Table 43.8). Table 43.8 should be used only as a guide because the nature of pain makes it necessary to individualize pain regimens.

In acute pain, analgesics should be given around the clock.

**Table 43.8** Narcotic Analgesics

| *Class and generic name* | *Trade name* | *Manufacturer* | *Route* | *Equianalgesic dose (mg)*[a] |
|---|---|---|---|---|
| **Morphine-like agonists** | | | | |
| Morphine | Generic | Various | IM | 10 |
| | | | PO | 30–60 |
| Hydromorphone | Dilaudid | Knoll | IM | 1.5 |
| | Generic | Various | PO | 7.5 |
| Oxymorphone | Numorphan | Du Pont | IM | 1.0 |
| | | | PO | —[b] |
| Levorphanol | Levo-Dromoran | Roche | SC | 2.0 |
| | | | PO | 4.0 |
| Codeine | Generic | Various | IM | 130[c] |
| | | | PO | |
| Hydrocodone | Generic | Various | IM | —[b] |
| | | | PO | —[b] |
| Oxycodone | Generic | Roxane | IM | —[b] |
| | | Various | PO | 30[c] |
| **Meperidine-like agonists** | | | | |
| Meperidine | Demerol | Winthrop-Breon | IM | 100 |
| | Generic | Various | PO | 300[c] |
| Fentanyl | Sublimaze | Janssen | IM | 0.1 |
| | Generic | Various | PO | —[b] |
| Sufentanil | Sufenta | Janssen | IM | 0.02 |
| | | | PO | —[b] |
| Alfentanil | Alfenta | Janssen | IM | 0.4–0.8 |
| | | | PO | —[b] |
| **Methadone-like agonists** | | | | |
| Methadone | Dolophine | Lilly | IM | 10 |
| | Generic | Various | PO | 10–20 |
| Propoxyphene | Darvon | Lilly | IM | —[b] |
| | Generic | Various | PO | 130–250[d] |
| **Mixed Agonist–Antagonists** | | | | |
| Pentazocine | Talwin | Winthrop–Breon | IM | 30–60 |
| | | | PO | 120–180[d] |
| Butorphanol | Stadol | Bristol | IM | 2.0 |
| | | | PO | —[b] |
| Nalbuphine | Nubain | Du Pont | IM | 10 |
| | | | PO | —[b] |
| Buprenorphine | Buprenex | Norwich–Eaton | IM | 0.3–0.6 |
| | | | Sublingual | 0.4–0.8 |
| Meptazinold[e] | | Wyeth | IM, PO | —[b] |
| Propiram[e] | | Schering | IM, PO | —[b] |
| Ciramadol[e] | | Wyeth | IM, PO | —[b] |
| Profadol[e] | | Parke–Davis | IM, PO | —[b] |
| Dezocine[e] | | Wyeth | IM, PO | —[b] |
| **Antagonists** | | | | |
| Naloxone | Narcan | Du Pont | IV | 0.4–1.2[f] |
| | | | PO | —[b] |
| Levallorphan | Lorfan | Roche | IV | 1.0–2.0[f] |
| | | | PO | —[b] |
| Naltrexone | Trexan | Du Pont | IM | —[b] |
| | | | PO | 50[g] |

[a] Recommended starting doses.
[b] Data not available.
[c] Starting doses lower (codeine—30 mg; oxycodone—5 mg; meperidine—50 mg).
[d] Starting doses lower (propoxyphene—65–130 mg; pentazocine—50 mg).
[e] Currently not marketed in the United States.
[f] Starting doses to be used in cases of opioid overdose.
[g] Starting dose to be used in abstaining opioid-dependent patient.

Compiled from References 47, 91, 93, 94, and 95.

**Table 43.9** Major Adverse Effects of the Narcotic Analgesics

| *Effect* | *Manifestation* |
|---|---|
| Mood changes | Dysphoria, euphoria |
| Somnolence | Lethargy, drowsiness, apathy, inability to concentrate |
| Stimulation of chemoreceptor trigger zone | Nausea, vomiting |
| Respiratory depression | Decreased respiratory rate |
| Interference with hypothalamic function (mostly morphine) | Increase in ADH; decrease in CRF, GnRF, TSH, GH, LRF, and FSH; disordered temperature regulation |
| Decreased gastrointestinal motility | Constipation |
| Increase in sphincter tone (mostly morphine) | Biliary spasm, urinary retention |
| Histamine release (mostly morphine) | Urticaria, pruritus, rarely exacerbation of asthma |
| Tolerance | Larger doses for same effect |
| Dependence | Withdrawal symptoms upon abrupt discontinuation |

Compiled from References 8 and 52.

As-needed schedules often produce wide swings in analgesic plasma concentrations that create wide swings in pain and sedation. This may initiate a vicious cycle where increasing amounts of pain medications are needed for relief.[48] Continuous intravenous methods of narcotic infusion are effective in some postoperative pain,[49] but the probability of unwanted side effects is high. An alternative method that has recently gained prominence is patient-controlled analgesia. With this technique, patients can self-administer preset amounts of intravenous narcotics via a syringe pump electronically interfaced with a timing device. Using this procedure, patients balance pain control with sedation. Additional proposed advantages of this approach over conventional intramuscular dosing are listed in Table 43.11.

Recently, administration of narcotics directly into the CNS (epidural and intrathecal) has shown considerable promise in the control of acute pain (Table 43.12)[50]; however, these methods of analgesia require careful monitoring and are best employed by experienced practitioners only. In addition, reports of marked sedation, convulsions, hallucinations, opioid withdrawal, pruritis, nausea, vomiting, urinary retention, and hypotension have limited widespread use of this technique.[51] Respiratory depression is of concern and can occur within the first 2 hours of opioid administration or manifest as late as 24 hours after single doses of spinal analgesia.[51] Naloxone is used to antagonize this effect but repeated doses may be required.[51] Analgesia as well as side effects is evident at lower doses when the opioids are administered intrathecally instead of epidurally. Intrathecally, single morphine doses of 0.25 to 1 mg are common, whereas epidurally 5- to 10-mg doses are the norm. All opioids administered directly into the CNS should be preservative free.

**Table 43.10** Summary of Narcotic Actions at Opioid Receptors

| *Agent* | Receptor type[a] **Mu-1,-2** | **Kappa** | **Sigma** |
|---|---|---|---|
| Morphine | AG | AG | — |
| Naloxone | ANT | ANT | ANT |
| Pentazocine | ANT | AG | AG |
| Butorphanol | ANT | AG | AG |
| Nalbuphine | ANT | AG | AG |
| Buprenorphine | pAG | ? | — |

[a] AG, agonist; ANT, antagonist; pAg, partial agonist; —, no activity; ?, unknown activity.

Compiled from References 47 and 56.

***Morphine and Congeners*** Despite several newer agents, morphine remains the prototype narcotic analgesic. As new narcotic and nonnarcotic compounds are developed their efficacy and side effect profiles are compared, with morphine as the standard. Many clinicians consider morphine the first-line agent when treating moderate to severe pain. Morphine can be given parenterally, orally, or rectally.

Morphine's CNS effects are numerous. Through direct

**Table 43.11** Advantage of Patient-Controlled Analgesia Over Conventional Intramuscular Therapy

| |
|---|
| Superior pain relief with less sedation |
| Less sedation during daytime hours |
| Decrease delays between request for analgesia and relief |
| Improved pulmonary function tests |
| Fewer postoperative complications |
| Lower potential for overdose |
| Improved sleep patterns |
| More spontaneous daytime activity |

Modified from Graves DA, Foster TS, Batenhorst RL, et al: The evolution of patient-controlled analgesia: A review. Ann Intern Med 1983;99:363.

**Table 43.12** Epidural Opioids

| *Agent* | *Dose (mg)* | *Onset of pain relief (min)* | *Duration of pain relief (h)* |
|---|---|---|---|
| Morphine | 5–10 | 24 | 20 |
| Meperidine | 30–100 | 5–10 | 6 |
| Methadone | 5 | 13 | 7–9 |
| Hydromorphone | 1 | 13 | 12 |
| Fentanyl | 0.1 | 4–10 | 2.5–6 |

Modified from Cousins MJ, Mather LE: Intrathecal and epidural administration of opioids. Anesthesiology 1984;61:299.

stimulation of the chemoreceptor trigger zone, morphine causes nausea and vomiting. This is observed more often in ambulatory patients, often subsides after the initial dose, and may be counteracted by drugs that block postsynaptic dopamine action (e.g., phenothiazine derivatives).[52] Although euphoria and dysphoria have been reported, morphine's unpleasant effects are more frequent when administered to those not experiencing pain.[47] As doses of morphine are increased, the respiratory center becomes less responsive to carbon dioxide, resulting in progressive respiratory depression. This effect is less pronounced in those being treated for severe pain. Respiratory depression is most often manifested as a decrease in respiratory rate, and is further compounded because the cough reflex is also depressed. Morphine-induced respiratory depression can be reversed by pure narcotic antagonists.[52] In patients with emphysema, kyphoscoliosis, and cor pulmonale, extreme caution must be employed when using morphine or any related opioid. Although these patients may be functioning normally, they are already using compensatory breathing mechanisms and are at risk for further respiratory compromise.[52] Precaution is also urged when using narcotic analgesics with alcohol or other CNS depressants. This combination amplifies CNS depression and is potentially quite harmful and possibly lethal.

Therapeutic doses of morphine have minimal effects on blood pressure, cardiac rate, or cardiac rhythm when patients are supine; however, morphine does produce venous and arteriolar vessel dilation, and orthostatic hypotension may result. Hypovolemic patients, those whose blood pressure is being maintained by sympathetic outflow, and patients with acute myocardial infarction are more susceptible to morphine-induced cardiovascular changes (e.g., decreases in blood pressure).[52] As morphine prompts a decrease in myocardial oxygen demand in ischemic cardiac patients, it is often considered the narcotic of choice when using opioids to treat pain associated with myocardial infarction.

Morphine decreases the motility of the entire gastrointestinal tract, in turn reducing biliary and pancreatic secretions. The end result, especially when administered over extended time periods, is constipation. Although not well documented, morphine-induced spasms of the sphincter of Oddi have been observed. Atropine and nitroglycerin can partially reduce these spasms, but the clinical significance of such an occurrence should be assessed on an individual basis.[52] Although morphine's effect on the urinary bladder varies, urinary retention can become a problem in patients with prostate disease.[8] Morphine-induced histamine release often manifests as urticaria and pruritus and, although not seen often, may even exacerbate bronchospasm in patients with a history of asthma.[8] Special attention must be given to patients with increased intracranial pressure and those with head injury secondary to trauma. In these patients morphine can markedly exaggerate this pressure and more readily produce respiratory depression[52] while clouding the neurologic examination results.

Hydromorphone is more potent, has better oral absorption characteristics, and is more soluble than morphine; however, its overall pharmacologic profile parallels that of morphine. Oxymorphone can be administered rectally and by injection. Although it is more potent than morphine, it offers no real pharmacologic advantages. Although levorphanol has an extended half-life and may cause less nausea and vomiting, its overall therapeutic effects are similar to those of morphine.

Codeine is an analgesic that is very effective in mild to moderate pain. It is often combined with other analgesic products and enjoys a popularity that makes it the standard for other oral narcotics. Unfortunately, codeine has the same propensity to produce tolerance and dependence as morphine. Hydrocodone, a derivative of codeine, is also most often seen in combination products and has pharmacologic properties similar to those of morphine. Oxycodone is equal in potency to morphine and is an excellent oral analgesic for moderate to severe pain. This is especially true when the product is used in combination with a peripherally acting nonnarcotic agent; however, its predilection for causing tolerance and dependence, along with its basic opioid characteristics, likens it to morphine.

***Meperidine and Congeners (Phenylpiperidines)*** The prototype phenylpiperidine, meperidine, has a pharmacologic profile comparable to that of morphine; however, it is not as potent and has a shorter half-life. This necessitates larger doses that must be administered more frequently; however, several studies have shown that this is often not done.[3,4] Although meperidine is effective orally, larger doses must be administered to achieve the same effect as obtained with the parenteral form (Table 43.8). With high doses or in patients with renal failure, the metabolite normeperidine accumulates, causing CNS excitability manifested as tremor, muscle twitching, and possibly seizures. Meperidine's effects on the cardiovascular system, gastrointestinal tract, and smooth muscle are less severe than those of morphine, causing considerably less biliary spasm and urinary retention. The combination of monoamine oxidase inhibitors and meperidine should not be used because this mixture can produce an excitation syndrome, hyperpyrexia, and convulsions. In most clinical settings meperidine offers no real advantage over morphine.[47]

Fentanyl, sufentanil, and alfentanil are synthetic opioids structurally related to meperidine. They are most often used in anesthesiology for induction of anesthesia in an attempt to provide cardiovascular stability and limit autonomic response. They are progressively more potent and shorter acting than meperidine (Tables 43.8 and 43.13) and at high doses can produce marked muscle rigidity.

**Table 43.13** Narcotic Analgesic Pharmacokinetics[a]

| *Agent* | *Time to peak (h)* | *Half-life (h)* | *Analgesic onset (min)* | *Analgesic duration (h)* |
|---|---|---|---|---|
| Morphine | 0.5–1 | 2–4 | 15–60 | 3–6 |
| Hydromorphone | 0.5–1 | 2–4 | 15–30 | 4–6 |
| Oxymorphone | 0.5–1 | —[b] | 5–15 | 3–6 |
| Levorphanol | 0.5–1 | 12–16 | 30–90 | 4–8 |
| Hydrocodone | —[b] | 3.3–4.4 | —[b] | 4–6 |
| Codeine | 0.5–1 | 3–4 | 15–30 | 4–6 |
| Oxycodone (PO) | 0.5–1 | 3–4 | 15–30 | 4–6 |
| Meperidine | 0.5–1 | 3–4 | 10–45 | 2–4 |
| Fentanyl | —[b] | 1.5–6.0 | 7–8 | 1–2 |
| Sufentanil (IV) | —[b] | 2.5–3.0 | 1.3–3 | —[b] |
| Alfentanil (IV) | —[b] | 1–2 | —[b] | —[b] |
| Methadone | 0.5–1 | 15–30 | 30–60 | 4–6 (acute) >8 (chronic) |
| Propoxyphene (PO) | 2.0–2.5 | 3.5–15 | 30–60 | 4–6 |
| Pentazocine | 0.25–1 | 2–3 | 15–20 | 3–4 |
| Butorphanol | 0.5–1 | 2.5–3.5 | < 10 | 3–5 |
| Nalbuphine | 1 | 5 | < 15 | 3–6 |
| Buprenorphine | 1 | 2–3 | 15 | 4–8 |
| Naloxone[c] | 0.5–2 | 0.5–1.5 | 2–5 | 0.5–1 |

[a] Based on intramuscular data unless otherwise indicated.
[b] Data not available.
[c] Narcotic antagonist.

Compiled from References 47 and 91–95.

***Methadone and Congeners*** Methadone was synthesized by the Germans during World War II and gained considerable popularity because of its oral efficacy, extended duration of action, and ability to suppress withdrawal symptoms in heroin addicts. With repeated doses the analgesic duration of action is prolonged, but because of metabolite accumulation excessive sedation may also result. Although methadone is quite effective in acute pain,[53] it is usually used to treat the chronic pain of malignancy. The pharmacologic profile resembles that of morphine.

Propoxyphene is one half as potent as codeine, and is more effective than placebo when 65–100 mg is ingested.[54] It is usually used in combination with aspirin or acetaminophen in the treatment of mild to moderate pain. The toxicity profile of propoxyphene is similar to that of codeine.

***Mixed Narcotic Agonist–Antagonists*** Analgesic agents that stimulate the analgesic portion (mu-1, delta, kappa, epsilon) of opioid receptors while blocking the toxicity portion (mu-2, sigma) would be considered ideal (Table 43.1). The mixed agonist–antagonist agents were developed with this ideal in mind. This analgesic class is effective in the treatment of moderate to severe pain and has a ceiling effect on respiratory depression (e.g., after a dose of 30 mg in adults progressively higher doses of nalbuphine do not affect respiratory rate).[55] They have a low abuse potential, cause decreased constipation, and show less biliary spasmotic effects than other narcotic agents; however, psychotomimetic responses (e.g., hallucinations and vivid dreams), reduced analgesic efficacy, a propensity to cause pain and initiate withdrawal in narcotic-dependent populations, and an unfavorable hemodynamic profile have diminished their widespread clinical use.

Pentazocine, the first agonist–antagonist clinically available, is a good oral and parenteral analgesic in moderate to severe pain but causes the most psychotomimetic effects. The oral form has been melted down and used illicitly in combination with tripelennamine; however, the addition of small amounts of naloxone has countered this illegitimate use by blocking the euphoric but not the analgesic effects.

Although decreased in intensity, butorphanol shares pentazocine's penchant to produce hallucinations and increase cardiac workload. Both must be used with caution in patients with myocardial ischemia. Nalbuphine acts similarly to pentazocine and butorphanol but causes a reduced myocardial oxygen demand in patients after myocardial infarction, compared with pentazocine and butorphanol. As nalbuphine blocks the mu receptor and produces analgesia by stimulating the kappa receptor, nalbuphine has also been used postoperatively to simultaneously treat opioid-induced respiratory depression and pain.[56]

Buprenorphine acts as a partial opioid receptor agonist (Table 43.10) and may offer a longer duration of analgesic effect (7 hours) with less respiratory depression than previously mentioned agents.[55] It binds quite strongly to opioid

**Table 43.14** Local Anesthetics

| *Agent* | *Trade name* | *Manufacturer* | *Onset (min)* | *Duration (h)* | *Equivalent concentration (%)* |
|---|---|---|---|---|---|
| **Esters** | | | | | |
| Procaine | Novocain | Winthrop–Breon, | 2–5 | 0.25–0.50 | 2 |
| | Generic | Various | | | |
| Chloroprocaine | Nesacaine | Pennwalt | 6–12 | 0.25–0.50 | 2 |
| Tetracaine | Pontocaine | Winthrop–Breon | 15 | 2–3 | 0.25 |
| **Amides** | | | | | |
| Mepivacaine | Carbocaine, Isocaine | Winthrop–Breon | 3–5 | 0.75–1.5 | 1 |
| | Novocol | Cooke Waite | | | |
| Bupivacaine | Generic | Various | 5 | 2–4 | 0.25 |
| Lidocaine | Generic | Various | 0.5–1 | 0.5–1 | 1 |
| Prilocaine | Citanest | Astra | 1–2 | 0.5–1.5 | 1 |
| Etidocaine | Duranest | Astra | 3–5 | 2–3 | 0.5 |
| Dibucaine | Nupercaine | Ciba–Geigy | 15 | 3–4 | 0.25 |

Compiled from References 66 and 91.

receptors and very large doses of narcotic receptor antagonists (e.g., naloxone) may be needed to reverse the agonist activities.[55] Unlike the previously mentioned narcotics, butorphanol and nalbuphine are not controlled substances.[56] Considering the high cost of storing, recording, and dispensing scheduled drugs, these agents may offer hidden potential economic benefits.

*Narcotic Antagonists* The pure opioid antagonists (e.g., naloxone, levallorphan, and naltrexone) combine competitively to opioid receptors but do not produce an analgesic response. Therefore, they are most often used to reverse the toxic effects of agonist and mixed agonist–antagonist narcotics or in the long-term prevention of opioid abuse.

**Combination Therapy**

The combination of narcotic and nonnarcotic oral analgesics often results in analgesia superior to that produced by either agent alone.[57] Attacking pain on two fronts (peripherally and centrally) enhances pain relief and facilitates the use of lower doses of each agent. This frequently produces a more favorable side effect profile and is the reason hundreds of aspirin and/or acetaminophen–narcotic analgesic combination products are marketed. The clinician should not be limited by the availability of commercially established fixed-ratio combinations. For example, the administration of around-the-clock acetaminophen, aspirin, or other NSAIDs in combination with scheduled narcotic regimens is often very effective in the treatment of pain resulting from bone metastases in advanced cancer.

Not all analgesic combinations are clearly effective. Caffeine in combination with aspirin may offer a slight analgesic advantage over aspirin alone in treating moderate pain[58,59]; however, caffeine's additive analgesic effects are controversial and the benefits of caffeine in combination with aspirin or acetaminophen remain unclear.[60]

Agents shown to potentiate the analgesic efficacy of parenteral narcotics include hydroxyzine and dextroamphetamine.[61,62] Phenothiazines, once thought to possess this potentiating property, apparently offer no inherent analgesic or potentiating characteristics when combined with narcotics, although unwanted sedation may be greatly increased.[8,63]

**Regional Analgesia**

Regional analgesia with properly administered local anesthetics can provide complete relief of pain and block acute pain reflex responses often deleterious in acute pain (Table 43.14).[64] These agents have also been applied directly onto surgical wounds and substantially decreased postoperative narcotic requirements.[65] Regional analgesics relieve pain by blocking nociceptive transmission, interrupting sympathetic reflexes, and preventing increased skeletal muscle activity.[2] Their lipid solubility, protein-binding characteristics, $pK_a$, and vasodilator behavior determine the mechanism of action.[66] Although safe, they readily cross the blood–brain barrier, causing signs of CNS excitation and depression, including dizziness, tinnitus, drowsiness, disorientation, muscle twitching, seizures, and respiratory arrest.[66] Cardiovascular effects include increased PR interval, increased QRS duration, decreased cardiac output, decreased blood pressure, and asystole, with toxic lidocaine levels. Disadvantages of such methods incorporate the need for skillful technical application, the need of frequent administration, and highly specialized follow-up procedures.

### *Stimulation Therapy*

Transcutaneous electrical nerve stimulation (TENS) and electroacupuncture have shown moderate success in managing postoperative pain.[67,68] Although narcotic-like side effects are certainly prevented, a lack of well-controlled studies has prevented this technique from gaining wide acceptance.

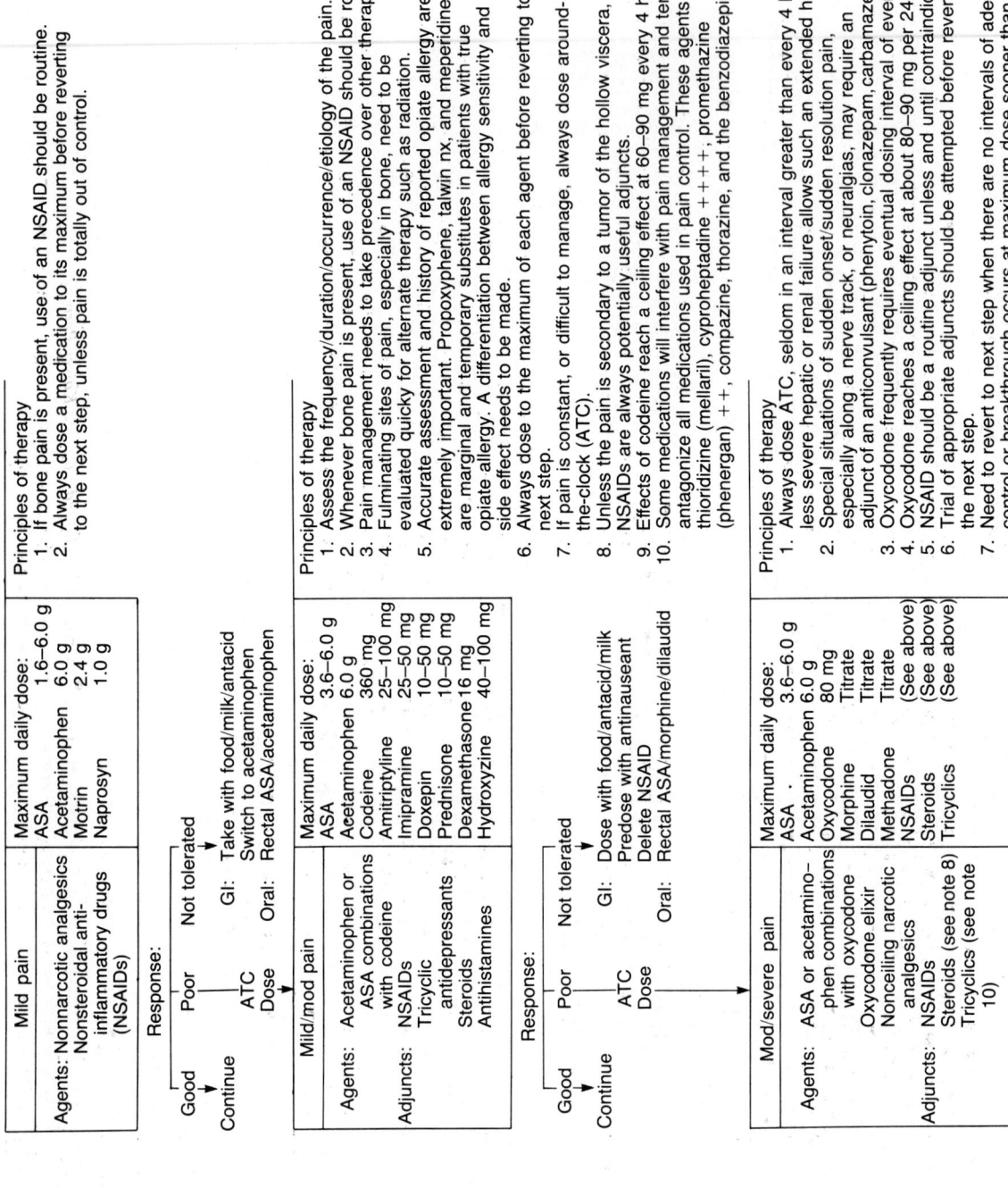

| Mild pain | Maximum daily dose: | |
|---|---|---|
| Agents: Nonnarcotic analgesics | ASA | 1.6–6.0 g |
| Nonsteroidal anti-inflammatory drugs (NSAIDs) | Acetaminophen | 6.0 g |
| | Motrin | 2.4 g |
| | Naprosyn | 1.0 g |

Principles of therapy

1. If bone pain is present, use of an NSAID should be routine.
2. Always dose a medication to its maximum before reverting to the next step, unless pain is totally out of control.

Response:

- Good → Continue
- Poor → ATC Dose ↓
- Not tolerated →
  - GI: Take with food/milk/antacid; Switch to acetaminophen
  - Oral: Rectal ASA/acetaminophen

| Mild/mod pain | Maximum daily dose: | |
|---|---|---|
| Agents: Acetaminophen or ASA combinations with codeine | ASA | 3.6–6.0 g |
| Adjuncts: NSAIDs | Acetaminophen | 6.0 g |
| Tricyclic antidepressants | Codeine | 360 mg |
| Steroids | Amitriptyline | 25–100 mg |
| Antihistamines | Imipramine | 25–50 mg |
| | Doxepin | 10–50 mg |
| | Prednisone | 10–50 mg |
| | Dexamethasone | 16 mg |
| | Hydroxyzine | 40–100 mg |

Principles of therapy

1. Assess the frequency/duration/occurrence/etiology of the pain.
2. Whenever bone pain is present, use of an NSAID should be routine.
3. Pain management needs to take precedence over other therapies.
4. Fulminating sites of pain, especially in bone, need to be evaluated quicky for alternate therapy such as radiation.
5. Accurate assessment and history of reported opiate allergy are extremely important. Propoxyphene, talwin nx, and meperidine are marginal and temporary substitutes in patients with true opiate allergy. A differentiation between allergy sensitivity and side effect needs to be made.
6. Always dose to the maximum of each agent before reverting to the next step.
7. If pain is constant, or difficult to manage, always dose around-the-clock (ATC).
8. Unless the pain is secondary to a tumor of the hollow viscera, NSAIDs are always potentially useful adjuncts.
9. Effects of codeine reach a ceiling effect at 60–90 mg every 4 h.
10. Some medications will interfere with pain management and tend to antagonize all medications used in pain control. These agents are: thioridizine (mellaril), cyproheptadine ++++, promethazine (phenergan) ++, compazine, thorazine, and the benzodiazepines +.

Response:

- Good → Continue
- Poor → ATC Dose ↓
- Not tolerated →
  - GI: Dose with food/antacid/milk; Predose with antinauseant; Delete NSAID
  - Oral: Rectal ASA/morphine/dilaudid

| Mod/severe pain | Maximum daily dose: | |
|---|---|---|
| Agents: ASA or acetaminophen combinations with oxycodone | ASA | 3.6–6.0 g |
| Oxycodone elixir | Acetaminophen | 6.0 g |
| Nonceiling narcotic analgesics | Oxycodone | 80 mg |
| Adjuncts: NSAIDs | Morphine | Titrate |
| Steroids (see note 8) | Dilaudid | Titrate |
| Tricyclics (see note 10) | Methadone | Titrate |
| | NSAIDs | (See above) |
| | Steroids | (See above) |
| | Tricyclics | (See above) |

Principles of therapy

1. Always dose ATC, seldom in an interval greater than every 4 h, unless severe hepatic or renal failure allows such an extended half-life.
2. Special situations of sudden onset/sudden resolution pain, especially along a nerve track, or neuralgias, may require an adjunct of an anticonvulsant (phenytoin, clonazepam, carbamazepine).
3. Oxycodone frequently requires eventual dosing interval of every 3 h.
4. Oxycodone reaches a ceiling effect at about 80–90 mg per 24 h.
5. NSAID should be a routine adjunct unless and until contraindicated.
6. Trial of appropriate adjuncts should be attempted before reverting to the next step.
7. Need to revert to next step when there are no intervals of adequate control or breakthrough occurs at maximum dose sooner than 3 h.

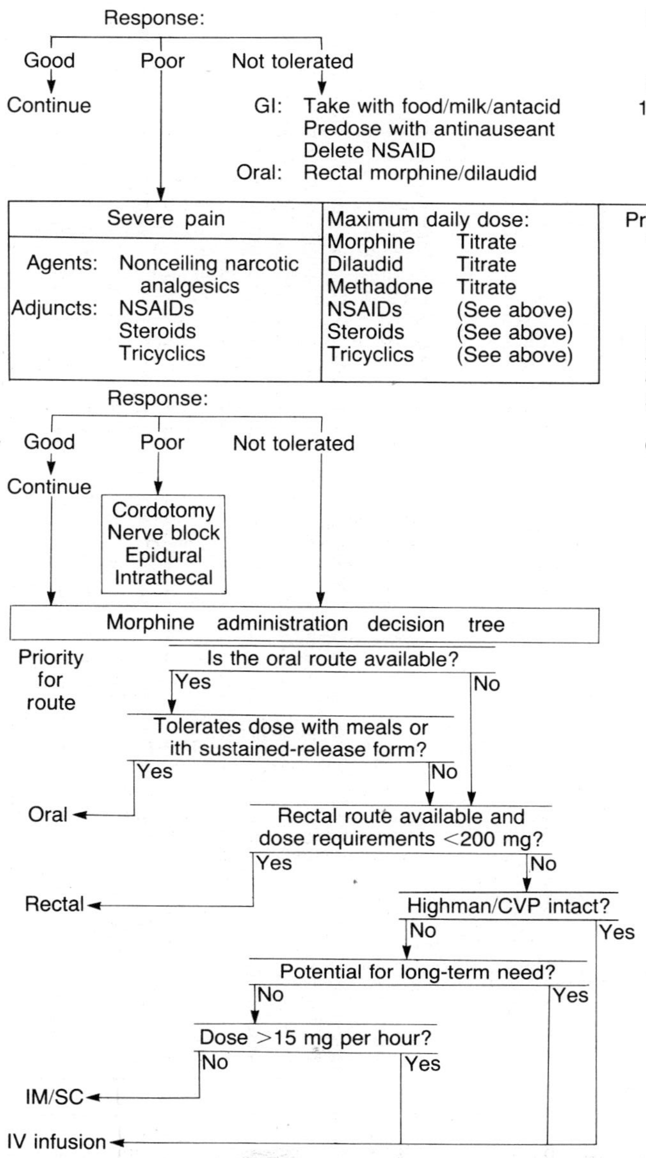


8. Pain resulting from inflammation of neural tissue in CNS (nerve-root compression or CNS metastasis) may require dexamethasone in high dose, 16 mg or more per 24 h. Other steroids do not reach the CNS.
9. Dosing intervals are different for each nonceiling narcotic analgesic.
10. Any time nonpharmacologic options of radiation, chemotherapy, surgical debulking, neurological interventions are used, a total reevaluation of all drug treatment needs to be made.

Principles of therapy

1. Morphine is the drug of choice in this category: (1) multiple products available; (2) multiple route of administration options, such as oral, rectal, IM, SC, IV, epidural, and intrathecal; and (3) a known equipotency between these routes that allows a much easier transition.
2. No real practical dosage limits; can be titrated to patient response.
3. Management should be ATC dosing only.
4. Utilize all possible adjuncts to minimize increases in dose.
5. Initial control may require doses higher than those needed in maintenance.
6. Sustained-release morphine is available when necessary.

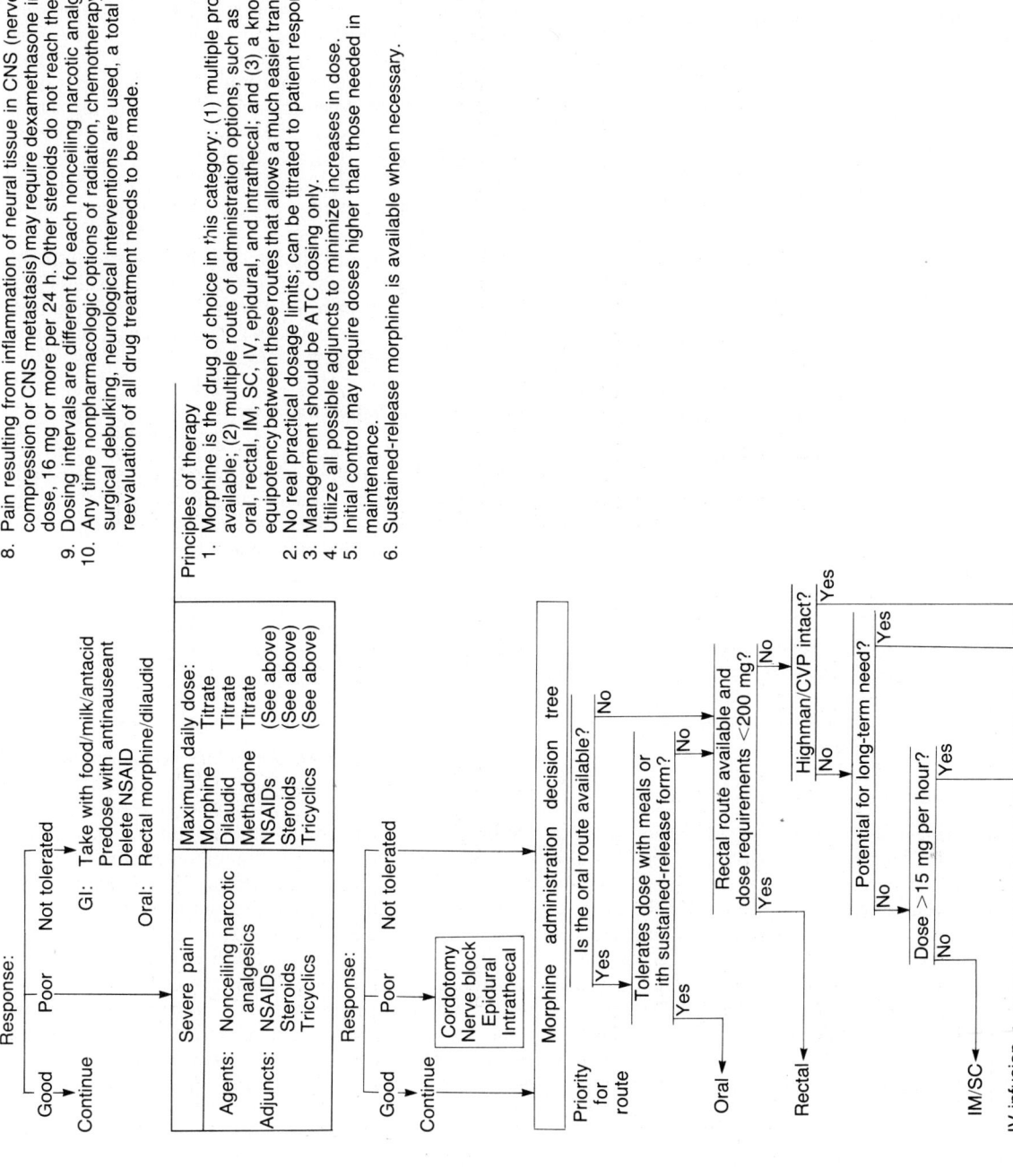

**Figure 43.4** Algorithm for pain management in oncology patients. *(Adapted from the Kaiser Permanente Algorithm for Pain Management in Patients with Advanced Malignant Disease, with permission.)*

### *Psychologic Intervention*

Even though the cognitive, behavioral, and social aspects of pain are well established, psychologic techniques for the treatment of acute pain are not widely employed. Simple interventions (e.g., introductory information about sensations to expect after certain procedures) reduce patient distress and greatly reduce postprocedure suffering.[69] Other successful psychologic techniques include relaxation training, controlled mental imagery, controlled attention or distraction, reinforcement of appropriate actions, hypnosis, and biofeedback.[2]

## Chronic Pain Management

### *Cancer Pain*

Managing the pain of malignant diseases encompasses both acute and chronic management techniques. Thus, pharmacologic treatment and psychologic therapies already mentioned are best combined with neurosurgical methods, anesthetic procedures, and supportive care measures in a multidisciplinary approach to pain relief.[68] The goal is to provide patients with enough pain amelioration to tolerate diagnostic and therapeutic manipulation and permit them to function at a level that will allow freedom of movement and choice.[68] Unfortunately, 25% of patients with cancer die without significant relief of severe pain.[68] Assessment and management techniques described in Tables 43.2 and 43.4 apply to these patients. Special attention must be given to continual reassessment of the painful state and individualization of therapy is always required.[69]

#### Pharmacologic Treatment

Pharmacologic management is the mainstay of therapy and a typical progression of analgesic use is outlined in Figure 43.4. The objective is to prevent the patient from experiencing constant fluctuation between severe pain and pain relief. This is best accomplished by around-the-clock administration schedules which inhibit serum analgesic concentrations from falling below the point at which a patient experiences the suffering of pain. As needed (i.e., prn) schedules are to be employed in conjunction with around-the-clock regimens and are used only when patients experience breakthrough pain. Again, nonnarcotic agents are used as first-line agents, with NSAIDs being especially effective in treating bone pain.[70,71] The choice of narcotic agent remains controversial, but should be based on patient acceptance, analgesic effectiveness, and pharmacokinetic, pharmacodynamic, and side effect profiles. Many clinicians have found morphine both safe and effective when administered by the oral (sustained-release, liquid, and fast-release), subcutaneous, rectal, continual intravenous infusion, patient-controlled intravenous, epidural, or intrathecal route.[51,72–77] Although heroin has shown analgesic and side effect characteristics equal to those of morphine it has no proven superiority.[78] Meperidine is usually not recommended for long-term use because of its relatively short half-life and the CNS hyperirritability of normeperidine, one of its main metabolites.[79] Anticonvulsant drugs,[68] tricyclic antidepressants,[80] levodopa,[81] antihistamines, amphetamines, and steroids[82] are often used as adjuvant pain medications; however, they have enjoyed only limited success as pain relievers, with anecdotal data or retrospective surveys providing most of the rationale for their use.[68]

Anesthetic and neurosurgical approaches have proven successful in alleviating pain but require special expertise and are usually reserved for patients who are refractory to conventional analgesics. They most commonly involve either the sectioning or stimulation of the spinal cord, brain stem, peripheral nerves, or thalamus. These techniques block nociceptive pathways, and subsequently alleviate pain.[68] Cordotomy, the most common procedure, involves interruption of the anterior lateral spinothalamic tract in the cervical or thoracic region. Initially, 90% of patients experience satisfactory pain relief, but this figure drops to 60% after one year and patients often experience intractable pain in previously unrecognized areas.[68]

#### Psychologic and Supportive Care

Previously mentioned psychologic techniques (e.g., relaxation training, controlled mental imagery) are very helpful in relieving pain experienced in malignant disease[2,68] and prove especially useful in conjunction with pharmacologic therapy.

Supportive care, in and outside the hospital, using programs such as the hospice, is one of the cancer patient's greatest allies not only in coping with pain, but in accepting the disease.[83] The positive effect this has on the patient cannot be overstated.

### *Nonmalignant Chronic Pain*

The numerous etiologies that produce nonmalignant chronic pain make treatment complex and management assume multidisciplinary aspects. As pain becomes gradually more chronic, it loses many of the autonomic characteristics evident in the acute stage, and additional symptoms such as depression, sleep disturbances, anxiety, irritability, work problems, and family instability tend to dominate.[8] Patients should not be told that the pain they are feeling is "psychosomatic" or in their head. In most cases, etiology is not as important as symptomatic relief. Objectives in evaluation include establishing an accurate diagnosis, identifying iatrogenic factors, obtaining a comprehensive psychiatric and psychosocial assessment, paying special attention to family and social problems, and obtaining a description of factors that alleviate or exacerbate pain.[8]

Pharmacologic approaches to patient care do not differ from those described previously; however, chronic pain patients most often have received a complete pharmacologic regimen. Adding another "pill" to their therapy will promote dependence and not improve pain control.[8] Other noninvasive or psychologic techniques may prove more successful. An integrated, systematic approach often provided by pain clinics, with a strong emphasis on patient–clinician relationships, is essential. The goal is to improve or maintain the patient's level of functioning, decrease the rate of physical deterioration, decrease pain perception, improve the patient's sense of well-being, improve family and social relationships, and decrease dependency on drug therapy.[8] Patients and clinicians must realize that maximum effective treatment may take months or even years.

## Drug Misuse, Abuse, Tolerance, and Dependence

The tendency of narcotic analgesics to be abused and the problems of tolerance, dependence, and withdrawal have left clinicians with an understandable but often unfounded fear regarding the appropriate use of these agents. Porter and Jick[84] studied 12,000 patients who had received narcotic analgesics for acute pain and found only 4 cases of medically induced dependence. Cohen[4] investigated 109 acute pain patients in five different hospitals and reported that house officers consistently underdosed narcotics and nursing staffs interpreted prn orders to mean "as little as possible." Their overwhelming concern was the fear of "addiction."

The problem associated with dependence and withdrawal is real but often overstated, especially with short-term use. An improper fear of addiction, therefore, promotes inappropriate pain management. "Addiction" is not a medical term but a social one referring to individuals with drug-seeking behaviors. The term should not be used in the patient care setting. With a better understanding of rational analgesic therapy these problems will certainly be minimized.

## Special Pain Populations

### *Elderly*

Aging causes degeneration of neurons in the dorsal column accompanied by diminished sensory awareness, which may change pain perception[85]; however, study results are inconclusive and no age differences have been noted in peripheral nociception.[86] In general the elderly are more sensitive to the effects of analgesics, and individualization of treatment to ensure efficacy and monitoring for adverse effects become even more important than in younger individuals.[8]

### *Children*

For years it was assumed that younger children are less likely to experience pain because their CNS is less advanced.[87] Recent work disputes this theory.[88] Children react to painful stimuli based on their cognitive, social, and emotional development.[87] In acute pain, older children may display discomfort more readily than younger ones, as they have experienced previous pain and the present suffering reminds them of former discomforts and their unpleasant consequences.[89] Children of all ages respond to chronic pain by withdrawal and regression to an earlier stage of development.[87] Pain in children should be treated vigorously with the pharmacologic and nonpharmacologic methods and procedures previously mentioned. Special attention should be given to the anxiety suffered because of separation from parents and to the developmental level of the child reacting to painful stimuli.

### *Narcotic-Dependent Patients*

Patients dependent on street narcotics, those taking methadone to prevent narcotic withdrawal, and medically dependent patients should be treated for acute or chronic pain with the same pharmacologic concepts used for other populations. Traditionally, these patients are among those least favored by clinicians[8] and are often the cause of patient–caregiver conflict and hostility. Rather than using punishment techniques and withholding narcotics, caregivers should treat this group with aggressive pharmacologic methods because of probable tolerance and withdrawal problems not seen in other populations. Care must be taken to adequately meet the individual's immediate need for pain relief. The chronic narcotic problems can be dealt with later, realizing that often, even with good patient–caregiver relations, long-term therapy may not be successful.

## Summary

The importance of proper pain management has been examined by several reviewers and received national prominence by a consensus panel assembled to study the problem by the National Institutes of Health in May 1986. Many of the deficiencies noted were attributed to poor training of health care practitioners in pain assessment and management, improper patient education, and inadequate communication among health care professionals. The panel suggested an integrated approach, utilizing the expertise of many disciplines, as well as individualized pharmacologic and nonpharmacologic strategies as a way of better addressing the problem. Pain relief assessment as part of a quality assurance program was also suggested as a means of ensuring proper therapy.[90] Indeed it is the responsibility of the pharmacist and all health care professionals who deal with pain to communicate therapies and assure proper management in an effort to relieve treatable pain and the suffering that accompanies it.

## References


1. Bonica JJ. Pain research and therapy: Past and current status and future needs, in Ng LKY, Bonica JJ (eds): Pain, Discomfort and Humanitarian Care. New York, Elsevier, 1980, pp 1–46.
2. Chapman CR, Bonica JJ. Acute pain. Current Concepts. Kalamazoo, MI, Scope Publications, 1983.
3. Marks RM, Sacher EJ. Undertreatment of medical inpatient pain with narcotic analgesics. Ann Intern Med 1973;78:173–81.
4. Cohen FL. Postsurgical pain relief: Patients' status and nurses' medication choices. Pain 1980;9:265–274.
5. Perry SW. The undertreatment of pain. Psychiatr Ann 1984;14:808–811.
6. Weis OF, Sriwatanakul K, Alloza JL, et al. Attitudes of patients, housestaff, and nurses toward postoperative analgesic care. Anesth Analg 1983;62:70–74.
7. Angell M. The quality of mercy. N Engl J Med 1982;306:98–99.
8. Stimmel B. Pain, Analgesia and Addiction: The Pharmacology of Pain. New York, Raven, 1983.
9. McLeod DC. Perspectives on Pain and Analgesic Therapy. Chapel Hill, NC, Health Science Consortium, 1980, p 4.

10. Field HL, Levins JD. Pain—mechanisms and management. West J Med 1984;141:347–357.
11. Gilfoil TM, Klavins I. 5-Hydroxytryptamine, bradykinin and histamine as mediators of inflammatory hyperesthesia. Am J Physiol 1965;204:867–876.
12. Ignelzi RJ, Atkinson JH. Pain and its modulation. Part 1. Afferent mechanisms. Neurosurgery 1980;6:577–583.
13. Bessou P, Burgess PR, Perl ER, et al. Dynamic properties of mechanoreceptors with unmyelinated (C) fibers. J Neurophysiol 1971;34:116–131.
14. Bessou P, Perl ER. Response of cutaneous sensory units with unmyelinated fibers to noxious stimuli. J Neurophysiol 1969;32:1025–1043.
15. Chapman CR. New directions in the understanding and management of pain. Soc Sci Med 1984;19:1261–1277.
16. Hokfelt T, Johansson O, Ljungdahl A, et al. Peptidergic neurones. Nature 1980;284:515–521.
17. Hunt SP, Kelly JS, Emson PC, et al. An immunohistochemical study of neuronal populations containing neuropeptides or aminobutyrate within the superficial layers of the rat dorsal horn. Neurosciences 1981;6:1883–1898.
18. Brimijoin S, Lundberg JM, Brodin E, et al. Axonal transport of substance P in the vagus and sciatic nerves of the guinea pig. Brain Res 1980;191:443–457.
19. Gamse R, Holzer P, Lembech F. Decrease of substance P in primary afferent neurones and impairment of neurogenic plasma extravasation by capsaicin. Br J Pharmacol 1980;88:207–218.
20. Yaksh TL, Farb DH, Leeman SE, et al. Intrathecal capsaicin depletes substance P in the rat spinal cord and produces prolonged thermal analgesia. Science 1979;206:481–488.
21. Rosell S, Olgart L, Gazelius B, et al. Inhibition of antidromic and substance P induced vasodilation by a substance P antagonist. Acta Physiol Scand 1981;111:381–382.
22. Cervero F, Iffo A. The substantia gelatinosa of the spinal cord—a critical review. Brain 1980;103:717–772.
23. Melzack R, Wall PD. Pain mechanisms: A new theory. Science 1965;150:971–979.
24. Mayer DJ, Leibeskind JC. Pain reduction by focal electrical stimulation of the brain: an anatomical and behavioral analysis. Brain Res 1974;68:73–93.
25. Mayer DJ, Wolfe TL, Akil H, et al. Analgesia from electrical stimulation in the brain stem of the rat. Science 1971;174:1351–1354.
26. Basbaum AL, Fields HL. Endogenous pain control mechanisms: Review and hypothesis. Ann Neurol 1978;4:451–462.
27. Goldstein A, Lowney LL, Pal BK. Stereospecific and nonspecific interactions of morphine narcotic congener levorphanol in subcellular fractions of mouse brain. Proc Natl Acad Sci USA 1971;68:1742–1747.
28. Pert CB, Pasternak G, Snyder SH. Opiate agonists and antagonists discriminated by receptor binding in brain. Science 1973;182:1359–1361.
29. Simon EJ, Hiller JM, Edelman I. Stereospecific binding of the potent narcotic analgesic (3-H) etorphine to rat-brain homogenate. Proc Natl Acad Sci USA 1973;38:377–384.
30. Hughes F, Smith TW, Kosterlitz HW, et al. Identification of two related pentapeptides from the brain with potent opiate agonist activity. Nature 1975;258:577–580.
31. LI CH, Chung D. Isolation and structure of an untriakontapeptide with opiate activity from camel pituitary glands. Proc Natl Acad Sci USA 1976;73:1145–1148.
32. Copolov DL, Helme RD. Enkephalins and endorphins. Drugs 1983;26:503–519.
33. Armstrong D, Dry RML, Keele CA, et al. Observations on chemical excitants of cutaneous pain in man. J Physiol 1953;120:326–351.
34. Starke K, Taube HD, Borowski E. Presynaptic receptor systems in catecholaminergic transmission. Biochem Pharmacol 1977;26:259–268.
35. Pepeu G. Involvement of central transmitters in narcotic analgesia, in Bonica JJ, Albe-Fessard D (eds): Advances in Pain Research and Therapy. New York, Raven, 1976, vol 1, pp 595–600.
36. Tenen SS. Antagonism of the analgesic effect of morphine and other drugs by *p*-chlorophenylalanine, a serotonin depleter. Psychopharmacology (Berlin) 1968;12:31–50.
37. Turk DC, Kerns RD. Conceptual issues in the assessment of clinical pain. Int J Psychiatry Med 1983–84;13:57–68.
38. Twycross RG. Pain and analgesics. Curr Med Res Opin 1978;5:497–505.
39. Fordyce WE. Learning processes in pain, in Sternbach RA (ed): The Psychology of Pain. New York, Raven, 1978, pp 49–72.
40. Craig KD. Social modelling influences on pain, in Sternbach RA (ed): The Psychology of Pain. New York, Raven, 1978, pp 73–109.
41. Chapman CR, Bonica JJ. Chronic pain. Current Concepts. Kalamazoo, MI, Scope Publications, 1985.
42. American Pain Society. Principles of analgesic use in the treatment of acute pain or chronic cancer pain. Clin Pharm 1987;6:523–532.
43. Amadio P. Peripherally acting analgesics. Am J Med 1984;77:17–26.
44. Pittman AW, Rudd GD. Analgesic Therapy. Carrboro, NC, Health Sciences Consortium, 1984.
45. Zarro V. Nonsteroidal anti-inflammatory drugs: A review. Clin Pharmacol 1984;30:243–246.
46. Pert CB, Snyder SH. Opiate receptor binding of agonists and antagonists affected differentially by sodium. Mol Pharmacol 1974;10:868–879.
47. Hare BD. The opioid analgesics: Rational selection of agents for acute and chronic pain. Hosp Form 1987;22:64–86.
48. Graves DA, Foster TS, Batenhorst RL, et al. The evolution of patient-controlled analgesia: A review. Ann Intern Med 1983;99:360–366.
49. Stapleton JV, Austin KL, Mather LE. A pharmacokinetic approach to postoperative pain: Continuous infusion. Anaesth Intern Care 1979;7:25–32.
50. Lanz E, Theiss D, Riess W, et al. Epidural morphine for postoperative analgesia: A double blind study. Anesth Analg 1982;61:236–240.
51. Cousins MJ, Mather LE. Intrathecal and epidural administration of opioids. Anesthesiology 1984;61:276–310.
52. Jaffe JH, Martin WR. Opioid analgesics and antagonists, in Gilman AG, Goodman LS, Rall TW, et al. (eds): The Pharmacological Basis of Therapeutics. New York, Macmillan, 1985, pp 491–531.
53. Gourlay GK, Wllis RJ, Wilson PR. Postoperative pain control with methadone: Influences of supplementary methadone doses and blood concentration–response relationships. Anesthesiology 1984;61:19–26.
54. Beaver WT. Mild analgesics: A review of their clinical pharmacology (part II). Am J Med Sci 1966;251:576–599.
55. Zola EM, McLeod DC. Comparative effects and analgesic efficacy of the agonist–antagonist opioids. Drug Intell Clin Pharm 1983;17:411–417.
56. Magruder MR, Delaney RD, Difazio CA. Reversal of narcotic-induced respiratory depression with nalbuphine hydrochloride. Anesth Rev 1982;9:34–37.

57. Beaver WT. Combination analgesics. Am J Med 1984;77(3a): 38–53.
58. DeKornfeld TJ, Lasagna L, Frazier TM. A comparative study of five proprietary analgesic compounds. JAMA 1962;182: 1315–1318.
59. Laska EM, Sunshine A, Mueller F, et al. Caffeine as an analgesic adjuvant. JAMA 1984;251:1711–1718.
60. Beaver WT. Caffeine revisted. JAMA 1984;251:1732–1733.
61. Beaver WT, Feise G. Comparison of the analgesic effects of morphine, hydroxyzine and their combinations in patients with postoperative pain, in Bonica JJ, Albe-Fessard D (eds): Advances in Pain Research and Therapy. New York, Raven, 1976; pp 553–565.
62. Forrest WH, Brown BW, Brown CR, et al. Dextroamphetamine with morphine for the treatment of postoperative pain. N Engl J Med 1977;296:712–715.
63. Moore J, Dundee JW. Alterations in response to somatic pain associated with anaesthesia. VII: The effects of nine phenothiazine derivatives. Br J Anaesth 1961;33:422–431.
64. Moore DC. Intercostal nerve block for postoperative somatic pain following surgery of thorax and upper abdomen. Br J Anaesth 1975;47:284–286.
65. Patel JM, Lanzafave RJ, Williams JS, et al. The effect of incisional infiltration of bupivacaine hydrochloride upon pulmonary functions, atelectasis and narcotic need following elective cholecystectomy. Surg Gynecol Obstet 1983;157:338–340.
66. Covino BG. Pharmacology of local anesthetics. Resident Staff Phys 1982;28:60–70.
67. Tyler E, Caldwell C, Ghia JN. Transcutaneous electrical nerve stimulation: An alternative approach to the management of postoperative pain. Anesth Analg 1982;61:449–456.
68. Foley KM. The treatment of cancer pain. N Engl J Med 1985;313:84–95.
69. Johnson JE, Rice VH, Fuller SS, et al. Sensory information instructions in a coping strategy and recovery from surgery. Res Nurs Health 1978;1:4–17.
70. Brodie GN. Indomethacin and bone pain. Lancet 1974;2:1160.
71. Kantor TG. Nonsteroidal anti-inflammatory analgesic agents in management of cancer pain, in: Symposium on the Management of Cancer Pain. Hosp Pract 1984;summer:30–34.
72. Citron ML, Johnston-Early A, Fossieck BE, et al. Safety and efficacy of continuous intravenous morphine for severe cancer pain. Am J Med 1984;77:199–204.
73. Sawe J, Dahlstrom B, Rane A. Steady state kinetics and analgesic effect of oral morphine in cancer patients. Eur J Clin Pharmacol 1983;24:537–542.
74. Meed SD, Kleinman PM, Kantor TG, et al. Management of cancer pain with oral controlled-release morphine sulfate. J Clin Pharmacol 1987;27:155–161.
75. Baumann TJ, Batenhorst RL, Graves DA, et al. Patient-controlled analgesia in the terminally ill cancer patient. Drug Intell Clin Pharm 1986;20:297–301.
76. Nahata MC, Miser AW, Miser JS, et al. Analgesic plasma concentrations of morphine in children with terminal malignancy receiving a continuous subcutaneous infusion of morphine to control severe pain. Pain 1984;18:109–114.
77. Ellison NM, Lewis GO. Plasma concentrations following single oral doses of morphine sulfate in oral solution and rectal suppository. Clin Pharm 1984;3:614–617.
78. Health and Public Policy Committee, American College of Physicians. Drug therapy for severe chronic pain in terminal illness. Ann Intern Med 1983;99:870–873.
79. Kaiko RF, Foley KM, Grabinski PY, et al. Central nervous system excitatory effects of meperidine in cancer patients. Ann Neurol 1983;13:180–185.
80. Walsh TD. Antidepressants in chronic pain. Clin Neuropharmacol 1983;6:271–295.
81. Minton JP. The response of breast cancer patients with bone pain to L-dopa. Cancer 1974;33:358–363.
82. Schell HW. The risk of adrenal corticosteroid therapy with far advanced cancer. Am J Med Sci 1966;252:641–649.
83. Kane RL, Bernstein L, Wales J, et al. Hospice effectiveness in controlling pain. JAMA 1985;253:2683–2686.
84. Porter J, Jick H. Addiction is rare in patients treated with narcotics. (Lett) N Engl J Med 1980;302:123.
85. Procacci P, Bozza G, Buzelli G, et al. The cutaneous pricking pain threshold in old age. Gerontol Clin 1970;12:213–218.
86. Kwentus JA, Harkins SW, Lignon N, et al. Current concepts of geriatric pain and its treatment. Geriatrics 1985;40:48–57.
87. Schechter NL. Symposium on recurrent pains in children: An overview and an approach. Pediatr Clin North Am 1984;31: 949–968.
88. Mather L, Mackie J. The incidence of postoperative pain in children. Pain 1983;15:271–282.
89. Beales JG, Kean JH, Lennox-Holt PJ. The child's perception of the disease and the experience of pain in juvenile chronic arthritis. J Rheumatol 1983;10:61–65.
90. News: Panel cites need for improved pain management. Clin Pharm 1986;5:777–778.
91. Facts and Comparisons. Philadelphia, J.B. Lippincott, 1986.
92. American Hospital Formulary Service. McEvoy GH, McQuarrie GM (eds): Drug Information 87. Bethesda, MD, American Society of Hospital Pharmacists, 1987.
93. Inturrisi CE. Role of opioid analgesics. Am J Med 1984;77(3a): 27–37.
94. Gourlay GK, Cousins MJ. Strong analgesics in severe pain. Drugs 1984;28:79–91.
95. Larijani GE, Goldberg ME. Alfentanil hydrochloride: A new short-acting narcotic analgesic for surgical procedures. Clin Pharm 1987;6:275–282.
96. Hopkinson JH, Smith MT, Bare WW, et al. Acetaminophen (500 mg) versus acetaminophen (325 mg) for relief of pain in episiotomy patients. Curr Ther Res 1974;16:194–200.
97. Levy G. Comparative pharmacokinetics of aspirin and acetaminophen. Arch Intern Med 1981;141:279–281.

# *Chapter 44* / Primary Headache Disorders

Jerry W. Taylor, PharmD, and John D. Cleary, PharmD

Pain is undoubtedly the most significant, if not the most common, reason patients seek medical attention. Foremost among pain problems is headache. Although headaches may occur as a symptom of an underlying medical disease, the majority of headaches are benign. In the broadest sense, headache refers to any kind of pain in or about the head; however, the definition of headache is usually limited to pain in or about the cranium. Headaches are classified into three major categories: primary, psychogenic, and secondary (Table 44.1). This chapter focuses on the characteristics, pathophysiology, management, and prevention of primary headache disorders.

The evaluation of patients with headache includes a careful history to characterize the headache profile (Table 44.2). The use of pertinent laboratory data, diagnostic tests, and physical examination should rule out any underlying organic cause (Table 44.3). Most individuals, however, are viewed as having a "primary headache disorder" because the headache is not secondary to an organic disease. Therefore, the headache profile or clinical history of the headache becomes important in establishing the proper diagnosis. Once the headache type has been recognized, an appropriate treatment program can be initiated.

## Etiology/Pathophysiology

The etiology and pathophysiology of primary headache disorders are poorly understood. Research examining potential etiologic factors and mechanisms contributing to the development of primary headache disorders has produced contradictory findings. The proposed pathophysiologic and etiologic factors discussed are not uniformly accepted. Additional research is needed to clarify this issue.

**Table 44.1** Classification of Headache

- **I. Primary Headache Disorders**
  - A. Muscle contraction headaches
  - B. Vascular headaches
    - 1. Migraine
      - a. Classic migraine
      - b. Common migraine
      - c. Complicated migraine
    - 2. Cluster
      - a. Episodic
      - b. Chronic
        - i. Primary
        - ii. Secondary
      - c. Chronic paroxysmal hemicrania
- **II. Psychogenic Headache Disorders**
- **III. Secondary Headache Disorders**

**Table 44.2** The Headache Profile

| | |
|---|---|
| Time (of day) when attacks tend to occur | Location of pain |
| | Precipitating factors |
| Duration of attack | Factors that relieve or improve headache |
| Intensity of pain | |
| Evolution of the syndrome | Concomitant phenomena |
| Quality of pain | Significance to the patient |

### *Muscle Contraction Headaches*

Muscle contraction (tension) headaches are defined as pain arising in facial, masticular, and occipital muscle groups of the cranium, secondary to fatigue or emotional strain. Muscle contraction headaches may result from psychologic (anxiety, depression, fatigue) or environmental stress.[1] When an individual reacts to stress by prolonged contraction of the head and neck muscles, pain may result from direct mechanical stimulation of pain receptors or tissue ischemia secondary to cranial artery compression. A definite relationship between stress and increased muscle tension or between extent of muscle tension and severity of headache has not been established; however, muscle activity and headache are occasionally linked. A patient's perception of stress may be accompanied by an elevation in muscle tension and may facilitate the development of headache.[2] Whether muscle contraction is the etiologic event, a concomitant occurrence, or a by-product of muscle contraction headache requires further investigation.

**Table 44.3** Evaluation of Patients With Headache

- Obtain a history of the headache or illness.
- Perform a neurologic examination to identify evidence of neurologic abnormalities.
- Obtain a computed tomography (CT) scan of the head if tumor, abscess, or hemorrhage is suspected.
- Perform a lumbar puncture (usually CT scan is done first) if infection is suspected.
- Identify any metabolic abnormalities, electrolyte disturbances, drug effects, and withdrawal symptoms.
- Identify any severe emotional disturbances.
- Suspect temporal arteritis in elderly patients with new-onset headache and obtain sedimentation rate and temporal artery biopsy, if indicated.

## *Vascular Headaches*

### Migraine

Migraine headaches are usually temporal and unilateral in distribution. Migraine headaches have traditionally been accepted as a progression of vascular events. There appears to be an initial period of arterial vasoconstriction, possibly producing an ischemic area in the brain. This neurologic ischemia may correspond to the prodrome of classical migraines. The area of ischemia may dictate the type and quality of the prodrome. Cerebral vasodilation and inflammation usually follow any ischemic event, resulting in pain. The hypothesized mechanisms explaining this cascade of events occurring during a migraine include defective humoral control, abnormal platelet function, and altered calcium homeostasis.[1]

The speculated humoral control defect and abnormal

**Figure 44.1** Physiologic mechanism for migraine.

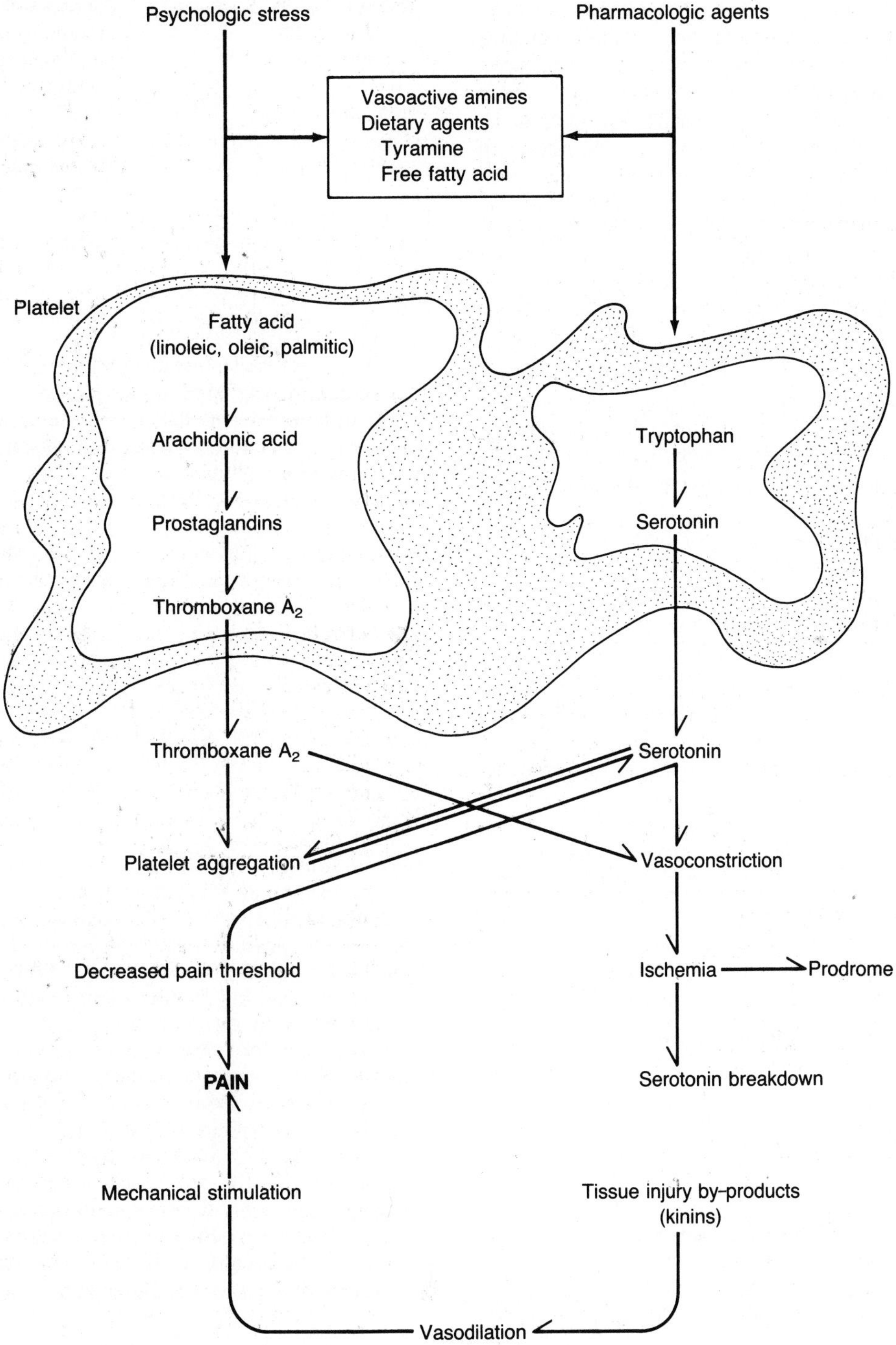

platelet function (biochemical pathway) are displayed (Fig. 44.1). The initial vasospasm in migraine may be mediated by release of the vasoactive amines: serotonin (5-hydroxytryptamine, 5-HT), tyramine, norepinephrine, and epinephrine. Decreased vasoactive amine degradation by platelet monoamine oxidase, increased platelet sensitivity, and increased platelet release of 5-HT and prostaglandins have been suggested as potential mechanisms for the observed vasospasm. Platelet aggregation and 5-HT degradation are, however, clearly abnormal in migrainous compared with nonmigrainous patients.[3–5] Serotonin appears to be the most important vasoactive amine mediating vascular headaches.

Numerous areas have been investigated as etiologic agents in migraine[1,6–9] (Table 44.4). An abnormality in vasoactive amine secretion or response can be identified as a common denominator when these factors are evaluated. For example, psychologic factors or stressors and diet may be involved in elevating catecholamines (i.e., epinephrine and norepinephrine). These catecholamines indirectly cause the release of platelet vasoactive amines which can mediate migranous headaches. Dietary (tyramine and $\beta$-phenylethylamine) products reported to induce migraine include red wine, caffeinated beverages, and chocolate.[10–11] Genetic autosomal trait defects in the ability to conjugate tyramine could also be a cause. Iatrogenic agents[12–15] associated with an increased migraine incidence and possible mechanisms are presented in Table 44.5. These agents probably induce a transient increase in serotonin, initiating a vasoconstrictive reaction; however, the mechanism for causing vascular headaches is unknown. Dietary, psychologic, and pharmacologic causes may also disrupt platelet homeostasis in some patients.[12]

The mechanism producing the physiologic events after the vasoconstrictive phase is not well established. Local increases in monoamine oxidase enzyme release and vascular permeability are believed to result in lowered concentrations of vasoactive amines, primarily serotonin. Without vasoactive amine stimulus, cerebral vasculature passively vasodilates, producing pain.[16] The pattern of vasodilation differs, however, for migraine and cluster headaches. Both migraine and cluster headaches similarly dilate extracranial arterial-vessels at the height of an attack. Migraine additionally dilates intracranial vessels (carotid artery), while the unique vascular phenomenon recognized in cluster headache is the dilation of the ophthalmic artery.[1] Because of different clinical and biochemical properties of these disorders, most clinicians do not accept cluster headache as a migraine variant. The pathophysiology of the vasodilation is probably similar for both migraine and cluster attacks.

**Table 44.4** Migraine-Associated Factors

| |
|---|
| Psychologic factors |
| Stress |
| Personality |
| Enviromental factors |
| Physiologic factors |
| Autonomic nervous system dysfunction |
| Atherosclerosis |
| Epilepsy |
| Autosomal tract defect |
| Immunologic response |
| Hypersensitivity reaction |
| Allergy |
| Metabolic/hormonal abnormality |
| Dietary factors |
| Iatrogenic factors |

**Table 44.5** Migraine-Associated Pharmacologic Agents

| *Mechanism* | *Agent* |
|---|---|
| Serotonin precursor | Tryptophan (various) |
| Inhibitor of granular reuptake and storage of 5-HT | Reserpine (various) |
| | Fenfluramine (Pondimin, Robins) |
| A specific 5-HT reuptake blocker | Fluoxetine (Prozac, Lilly) |
| Platelet aggregator | Ethinyl estradiol (various) |
| | Mestranol (various) |
| Other | Viloxazine (Vivalan, Stuart) |
| | Nicotine (various) |
| | Histamine (Histamine, Lilly) |
| | Cimetidine (Tagamet, Smith Kline & French) |
| | Indomethacin (Indocin, Merck Sharp & Dohme) |

### Cluster Headache

Cluster headache (migrainous neuralgias) is defined as a migraine variant with short severe, episodic, clustering, and unilateral pain over an orbit and the forehead. Factors contributing to the development of cluster headache include stress or emotion, prolonged strain, and pharmacologic vasodilators.[17]

The pathophysiologic explanation of the symptomatology observed during a cluster headache is similar to that for a migraine. An initial vasoconstriction phase has been identified with angiography and radionuclide brain scans that demonstrates significant internal carotid artery narrowing. Thermograms used to localize blood flow show decreased unilateral circulation in supraorbital and frontal arteries prior to the event, with subsequent increased blood flow in the same areas during the attack. Elevated histamine, 5-HT, or bradykinin release and increased $\alpha$-adrenergic and parasympathetic activity are possible causes.[1] Abnormal excitatory parasympathetic impulses transmitted through the nervus intermedius may also be the focal point of the cluster headache.[18]

The pain sensation experienced during migraine and cluster headaches is probably directly related to stimulus of pain nerve fibers, secondary to cranial artery vasodilation, 5-HT depression of the pain threshold or inflammation, and release of prostaglandins.[1,12] Extracranial carotid artery vasodilation distending against pain-sensitive structures surrounding these arteries can result in pain. Edema around the dilated arteries helps intensify the severity of the headache. Sustained dilation of the arterial walls render them less responsive to treatment.[19,20] Later in the attack, the walls of the affected cranial arteries become thickened, and muscular constriction of head and neck muscles follows vascular pain.

The role of altered calcium homeostasis in the constriction of vascular smooth muscle during migraine has recently been investigated. Blockade of calcium channels may prevent the vasomotor effects of vasoactive amines.[21]

## Clinical Presentation/Treatment

### *Muscle Contraction Headaches*

Most patients with muscle contraction (tension) headaches do not seek physician assistance unless the pain is unrelieved by self-medication or the headache becomes severe and/or chronic in nature. An estimated 80% of the adult population will experience tension headaches in their lifetime. The implication that women experience these headaches three times more frequently than males is currently debated.

A headache can occur at any time and is often related to a specific stressful situation. The attack may last for several hours to weeks, with varying intensity. Pain is characterized by a mild, dull ache that is steady and nonthrobbing. The location of discomfort can be unilateral or bilateral, involving temporal, occipital, parietal, or frontal areas. The scalp is usually tender and there may be spasm or tightness of the neck and shoulder muscles.

Success rates in treatment of muscle contraction headaches vary and generally are inversely related to the duration of the illness. Treatment consists of psychotherapy, physical therapy, and pharmacotherapy.

The psychotherapy of tension headaches is directed at unmasking psychologic factors and reducing environmental stress. Education and reassurance that the problem is not serious and can be successfully treated are critical to successful management.

Physical therapy may include application of heat to the head and neck and massage. Manual stretching of neck and occipital muscles, relaxation, and biofeedback training assisted with electromyographic recording from involved muscle groups may also prove beneficial.

Drug therapy may be helpful but is rarely of permanent benefit. Simple analgesics[22] (e.g., aspirin and acetaminophen) are the pharmacotherapy of choice. Nonsteroidal anti-inflammatory agents (NSAIDs) and combination analgesics are equally effective as simple analgesics, but at a greater expense.

In the patient with severe, chronic muscular contraction headaches, it may be necessary to use a mild sedative, anxiolytic, or antidepressive agent.[23] Benzodiazepines are effective for anxiety-related symptoms; long-term use is not recommended. Although many patients are depressed, the effectiveness of the tricyclic antidepressant drugs is probably independent of their antidepressant effects. For a more complete review of side effects and dosing with tricyclic antidepressant drugs, refer to Chapter 50.

### *Vascular Headaches*

**Migraine**

Common migraines occur in approximately 85% of patients who experience migraines; classic migraines occur in approximately 10%. The incidence of migrainous headaches in the general population appears higher for females (29%) than males (19%) and may be higher for individuals with a family history or multiple risk factors. The risk factors include the presence of previously discussed psychologic factors or stressors, dietary agents, genetic traits, or use of associated iatrogenic agents. There appears to be an increased incidence during female menstruation, and about 60% to 80% of migrainous females have improved symptoms during pregnancy.[1,12] Migraine headaches may have an onset in childhood or adolescence. The headache is periodic and lifelong, but tends to lessen in late adult years.[24]

In "classic migraine" the patient experiences a prodrome 15–30 minutes before the headache. The prodrome may be conspicuous sensory, motor, and mood disturbances (i.e., visual scotomata, visual-field defects or scintillations, hemisensory disturbances, or aphasia). When prodromal symptoms persist into or beyond the dilatation or headache phase, the headache is classified as "complicated migraine." In a "common" migraine the patient either fails to recognize or does not experience a prodromal phase.

Migraine headaches usually occur in the early morning hours and rapidly reach a peak intensity within an hour. Duration can vary from a few hours to several days, and may occur daily or only once in several months. Pain is described as a severe pounding and throbbing that may evolve into a milder muscle contraction–type headache lasting days. Migraine headaches are usually temporal and unilateral in distribution. Pain is usually generalized but may be unilateral in and about the eye. Patients commonly report gastrointestinal complaints (e.g., anorexia, nausea, vomiting) and increased sensitivity to light and sound. Patients are incapacitated during attacks and seek a dark quiet place to sleep as this offers relief. Postheadache is characterized by exhaustion, scalp tenderness, and recurrence of headache or sudden head movement.

Migraine patients' conditions can be managed either by treating symptoms once an attack is underway (symptomatic therapy) or by preventing the attack altogether (prophylactic therapy).

In the treatment of migraine, it is essential to educate the patient to begin therapy quickly. Abortive agents are most effective in relieving migraine attacks when taken at the onset of attacks, probably because they act to interrupt the mechanism of the disorder (i.e., defective humoral control, abnormal platelet function, and/or altered calcium homeostasis). Once the migraine headache's vasodilation phase (pain) is established, abortive agents are less effective.

In the patient with infrequent migrainous attacks, management should concentrate on the treatment of each individual attack. Simple analgesics[22,25] may be sufficient for mild forms of migraine, if taken at the onset. Aspirin, 650–975 mg four times a day, is probably the analgesic of choice; acetaminophen (650–975 mg) is an alternative when aspirin cannot be used. Many NSAIDs are similar in efficacy to aspirin, but they exhibit considerable potential for adverse effects at greater expense.

In acute migraine attacks metoclopramide (Reglan)[26,27] can be used to reduce nausea and vomiting and enhance the absorption of other antimigraine products by reducing gastric stasis. Metoclopramide, 10–20 mg by parenteral injection or orally, should be taken at the onset of symptoms and the analgesic 15–30 minutes later. Metoclopramide can be repeated in 4 to 6 hours if necessary. Extrapyramidal symptoms (e.g., tremor, shakiness, and nervousness) may occur, but acute dystonic reactions rarely occur when metoclopramide is used intermittently for acute attacks. The gastric emptying effect of metoclopramide is antagonized by anticholinergic drugs and narcotics.

Ergotamine,[28] an $\alpha$-adrenergic blocking agent and serotonin agonist, is a direct vasoconstrictor of smooth muscle in cranial blood vessels. Its action depends on the tone of the vessels at the time of administration. Ergotamine is widely accepted as the drug of choice for acute migraine management. Ergotamine tartrate is available in oral tablets, sublingual tablets, and suppositories; dihydroergotamine mesylate (DHE-45) is available in parenteral form for injection. Oral ergotamine has a very poor bioavailability with a high "first-pass" effect.[29] Sublingual ergotamine also is probably not absorbed to a useful extent.[30] Suppositories are useful for patients who develop nausea and vomiting early in attacks. Inhaled ergotamine (Medihaler Ergotamine) provides efficient therapy when patients are properly instructed regarding their use. Ergotamine dosage should be limited to no more than 6 mg orally, sublingually, or by rectal suppository in a single attack. The weekly amount should not exceed 10 mg. Dihydroergotamine mesylate,[31,32] 0.25–0.5 mg subcutaneously or intramuscularly, may be given and repeated if needed at 1 to 2 hours. The ergotamine inhaler delivers 0.36 mg per depression and is given at 5-minute intervals with recommendations not to exceed six inhalations per 24 hours. Ergotamine dosage requirements should be titrated for each patient until the appropriate dose is determined for subsequent attacks. Repeated dosing over an extended time interval may be less efficacious by allowing establishment of vasodilation (pain). Total dose requirements can then be given early as a single dose at the onset of headache to abort attacks.[19,20] Major side effects involve the gastrointestinal system, and increased amounts carry the risk of ergotism.[28,33] Ergotism may manifest as nausea, diarrhea, thirst, pruritis, vertigo, muscle cramps, paresthesias, cold skin, or decreased pulses. Overuse of the medication may cause habituation to ergotamine and may lead to severe withdrawal headaches which can last for several days when treatment is stopped.[33] Contraindications include prolonged prodromes, peripheral vascular disease, hypertension, coronary disease, liver and kidney disease, and pregnancy. Caffeine is commonly used in combination with ergotamine to enhance the absorption and action.[28] Other drugs used in combination with ergotamine include antispasmotics, antiemetics, sedatives, analgesics, and other CNS stimulants.

Midrin, a combination of isometheptene mucate 65 mg (a sympathomimetic amine that acts as a vasoconstrictor of cranial arterioles), dichloralphenazone 100 mg (a mild sedative), and acetaminophen 325 mg can be used as an alternative for patients who do not tolerate ergotamine preparation or those who find it ineffective.[34] In comparison with ergotamine, this combination product has fewer side effects, but is also less effective. The recommended dose is one or two capsules at the beginning of an attack, followed by one capsule every 1 to 2 hours as needed up to a maximum of five capsules in 12 hours. The most frequent side effects are dizziness, insomnia, nausea, vomiting, and transient numbness.

The phenothiazine antipsychotic chlorpromazine[23,35,36] has been found effective in severe migraine unresponsive to ergotamine. The drug has several pharmacologic effects, making it difficult to determine its mode of action. The drug is also effective in prophylaxis against vascular headache. Chlorpromazine orally or by intramuscular injection in doses of 50 to 100 mg per day is generally effective, but some patients may require more than 1,000 mg orally in 24 hours. Side effects include sedation, extrapyramidal effects, and orthostatic hypotension. Although tardive dyskinesia can occur after long-term use, it is unusual in younger patients at the lower doses.

Once the patient is in the midst of a severe attack, the pharmacologic measures previously considered are unlikely to help. The use of parenterally administered narcotic analgesics may provide relief as the patient is able to sleep through the attack. This form of therapy should be avoided because of the possible hazards of addiction,[37,38] particularly in patients with recurrent severe headaches. Future management of patients with a history of recurrent attacks should include the use of nonaddicting prophylactic agents and reduction of trigger factors associated with the headache.

Corticosteroids[39] may also be used to bring prolonged migraine attacks under control and lessen the need for narcotics. Therapy is usually limited to a short, decreasing dosage schedule because of long-term side effects. Relief of pain is seen within 8 to 12 hours. Steroids probably act to restore vascular reactivity through their effect on prostaglandin synthesis.

In the later stages of the headache, muscular tension and spasm may predominate. At this point, measures to relax neck muscles (e.g., heat and massage) and antianxiety agents (e.g., benzodiazepines) may afford additional relief.

Prophylactic medication is warranted when a headache of moderate or great severity occurs with a frequency of two or more attacks per month, or when a patient demonstrates a lack of response or is intolerant to ergot alkaloids. Patients with medical problems unable to take abortive therapy and patients with a predictable pattern or regularity of attacks are also candidates for prophylactic therapy. Preventive drugs should decrease the number of headaches and reduce their severity.

Propranolol is widely accepted as the drug of choice for migraine prophylaxis. Propranolol[40] has been used with good results in reducing the frequency and severity of migraine, but this property is not shared by all $\beta$-blockers. Atenolol (Tenormin),[41] metoprolol (Lopressor), and nadolol (Corgard) are effective; timolol (Blocadren), acebutolol (Sectral), and practolol are modestly effective; and oxprenolol, alprenolol, and pindolol (Visken) are completely ineffective. The mechanism by which β-blockers interrupt the frequency of headache is still not fully understood. Effective β-blockers share the property of lack of intrinsic sympathomimetic activity. Other properties that may be important include blockage of vasodilator receptors, membrane stabilization, decreased platelet adhesiveness, and shifting of the oxygen dissociation curve to enhance oxygen release to tissues. The effective dose of propranolol ranges from 80 to 320 mg/d. A trial of at least 2 to 3 months should be given before β-blockers are considered ineffective. Daily doses of other β-blockers are approximately 80–320 mg for nadolol, 50–100 mg for atenolol, and 100–200 mg for metoprolol. β-Blockers have a relatively low index of toxicity. Side effects of the β-blockers include fatigue, dizziness, gastrointestinal symptoms, and sleep disturbances. β-Blockers are relatively contraindicated in patients who have a known history of asthma, diabetes, or heart failure.

Tricyclic antidepressants[42,43] have a beneficial effect in preventing migraine headache independent of their antidepressant action. These agents are often used as an alternative drug choice when β-blockers cannot be used. Tertiary amines, which inhibit the reuptake of serotonin and maintain vasoactive amine stimulus (e.g., amitriptyline and imipramine), are more effective than secondary amines with less serotonergic activity (e.g., protriptyline, nortriptyline, and desipramine). Amitriptyline is more effective than imipramine as it is more slowly metabolized to the less active secondary amine. Initial administration of 25 mg amitriptyline nightly with gradual increases to 100 mg daily as a single or divided dose is usually effective. A 4-week trial period should be used before the drug is considered ineffective. Major initial side effects include anticholinergic activity, sedation, and, with prolonged therapy, weight gain. Drowsiness is better tolerated when the patient takes the medication at night and usually subsides after 1 or 2 weeks.

Methysergide,[44] an ergot alkaloid, is ineffective for the management of an attack in progress, but is one of the most efficacious medications for prophylactic treatment. Methysergide (Sansert) is a potent peripheral antiserotonin agent of complex pharmacologic action. Methysergide additionally inhibits the release of histamine from mast cells, potentiates norepinephrine to produce vasoconstriction, stabilizes platelets against release of serotonin, and appears to manifest central serotonin agonist activity. The dosage is 4–8 mg/d in divided doses with meals to minimize gastrointestinal discomfort. "Drug holidays" of 2 weeks every 3 months, or a minimum of 1 month every 6 months, are required to prevent complications. The medication should be slowly tapered rather than abruptly discontinued to minimize rebound headache. The toxic manifestations and contraindications of methysergide are similar to those of the ergot alkaloids already discussed. Noninterrupted use of methysergide can cause retroperitoneal, pleuropericardial, and subendocardial fibrosis, but these rarely occur until after 7 months. Patients should be counseled to report any flank pain, dysuria, and angina to help in the early detection of early fibrotic changes. Tissue damage can occur but early recognition and discontinuation of therapy may reverse these changes. This medication has serious complications and should be reserved for refractory severe migraine in patients under constant supervision.

Phenelzine (Nardil),[44] a monoamine oxidase inhibitor, is useful in the treatment of resistant causes of migraine not responsive to less toxic prophylactic agents. Phenelzine acts by reducing serotonin metabolism, thus increasing brain serotonin. The patient must be instructed to avoid foods high in tyramine and sympathomimetic medications because of the risk of hypertensive crisis. Phenelzine is usually given in doses of 15 mg two to four times per day. The most common side effects are postural hypotension and symptoms of excessive central stimulation. For a more complete review of side effects and dietary restrictions with phenelzine, refer to Chapter 50.

Clonidine,[45,46] a central sympatholytic antihypertensive agent, has been tried for prevention of migraine, but is no better than placebo in the majority of patients. Clonidine is postulated to act by stabilization of the vasculature that occurs after stimulation of α- and β-adrenergic receptors. Some authorities, however, consider it useful in "dietary" migraine and for patients who have hypertension as well as migraine. The most common side effects are drowsiness and dryness of the mouth. Abrupt discontinuance may produce a rebound headache. The usual adult dose of clonidine is 0.1 to 0.2 mg twice daily.

Cyproheptadine,[44] an antihistamine with serotonin agonist activity, can be used in migraine prophylaxis. Antiplatelet aggregation properties may also contribute to its effectiveness. The usual dose is cyproheptadine 4–20 mg/d, as tolerated. Administration of a larger dose at bedtime and a smaller dose in the morning may be preferred to minimize drowsiness. The major side effects are sedation and weight gain. Response with this agent is often unpredictable and often less than satisfactory.

Analgesics taken regularly can decrease the frequency and intensity of migraine headaches.[47–49] Aspirin and other NSAIDs inhibit prostaglandin activity and synthesis. Additionally, these agents inhibit platelet aggregation and lessen serotonin release, an event thought to be involved in the early stages of migraine attacks. Aspirin 650 mg twice daily and naproxen 250 to 500 mg twice daily are two agents shown to be effective when taken regularly as prophylactic therapy. Some patients benefit from intermittent use for regular and predictable headache. Long-term therapy should be continued at the lowest effective dose. The anti-inflammatory agents may be administered 1 week before menses until the end of the period for relief of menstrual migraine. Usefulness of the agents is limited to renal and gastrointestinal complications.

Calcium channel blockers[50,51] (verapamil, nifedipine, and diltiazem) have recently been shown to be effective in the prophylactic treatment of migraine. Nimodipine, the most efficacious agent, is not available in the United States. Calcium channel blockers are capable of inhibiting the initial vasoconstrictive phase of migraine, whether induced by serotonin, bradykinin, prostaglandin, or other vasoconstrictive agents. In addition to their vasodilatory effects, calcium channel blockers also inhibit platelet aggregation and serotonin release. Divided dosages of nifedipine (30–60 mg/d), verapamil (up to 240 mg/d), or diltiazem (90 mg/d) can significantly reduce the frequency of migraine attacks after approximately 2 weeks of continuous therapy. These agents are generally well tolerated. Most common side effects include flushing, vasodilatory headaches, tachycardia, gastrointestinal disturbances, fluid retention, and rash.

Analgesics and ergot alkaloids are still the drugs of choice for treatment of migraine. Patients may also respond to a period of rest in a darkened room. In an established severe headache, narcotic analgesics are most often helpful, but best avoided. $\beta$-Blockers or other prophylactic measures should be considered in the patient who has frequent headaches or is intolerant to abortive agents. Therapy must be reevaluated at intervals to assess its effectiveness; in the headache-free individual therapy can often be reduced or discontinued after a few months to see if the patient can manage without medication.

Biofeedback adds a new dimension or adjunct in carefully selected patients.[52] The basis of biofeedback comes from Eastern societies that teach self-awareness through the act of physiologic self-discipline. Biofeedback teaches one to control unused or involuntarily controlled functions of the body such as muscle tone and temperature regulation.

Electric devices are used to monitor a particular physiologic function in an individual and then feed the information back to them as visual or auditory signals. The patient learns how to control selected autonomic functions through the use of mind–body training and the repetition of a series of phrases that relax.

Muscle contraction headache patients may benefit from electromyographic (EMG) feedback training, which allows the patient to hear an audible signal or tone proportional to the muscle contractility. Relaxation training leads to a decrease in the audible signals and often a reduction in headache frequency.

Migraine patients are taught to raise the temperature of their hands. The increased peripheral temperature is directly related to local blood flow, enabling the patient to abort migraine attacks. Migraine patients also receive EMG feedback training because muscle relaxation may have prophylactic value.

### Cluster Headache

Cluster headaches are severe headaches that occur in closely packed groups and are followed by periods of remission. Cluster headaches occur in less than 0.001% of the population, with an incidence approximately six times higher in males. The average age of onset is between 10 and 40 years.[1,53] Patients do not have a family history of migraine headache or cluster headaches.

Cluster headaches have a rapid onset without a prodrome. Each headache lasts from a few minutes to several hours, most often 30 to 45 minutes. The periodic clustering of headaches (episodic cluster) usually lasts 6 to 8 weeks, with headache-free periods of months to years. Most often, the attacks occur at night, and more frequently in the spring and fall. Almost 10% of cluster headaches are chronic without remission for periods of greater than 12 months. Chronic cluster headaches may occur without a preceding episodic history or may follow a history of past episodic attacks. A rare subgroup of chronic cluster headaches, chronic paroxysmal hemicrania, has been identified through a unique therapeutic response to NSAIDs (e.g., indomethacin).[54,55]

The location of pain is always unilateral and most often described behind or around the eye. The same side of the head is affected in each bout, although an attack may change sides in different bouts. The pain is excruciating and the patient will often pace, beat the head against objects, and may attempt suicide. During a cluster attack, the patient may demonstrate signs of ipsilateral (affecting the same side) autonomic hyperactivity with rhinorrhea, ptosis, miosis, and tearing. Flushing of the face and ophthalmic region is also very common. Patients with a history of cluster headache may also have an increased incidence of peptic ulcer disease. This may result from hypersensitivity to the histamine released during attacks.[1]

The management of cluster headache is centered around two aspects, the acute attack and the interval of treatment, as an attempt to reduce the frequency and severity of the episodes. Daily administration of a prophylactic medication is warranted when headaches of moderate or great severity recur several times per month. It is of particular urgency in the case of cluster headache in which excruciating pain may strike several times per day.

Individual cluster attacks are difficult to treat as prodromal symptoms are frequently lacking. Pain may awaken the patient from sleep, rapidly attains its maximum intensity, and is short-lived.

The ergot preparations are effective for aborting cluster headache attacks.[54] Aerosol ergot preparations[56] may be effective when used properly. Dihydroergotamine can terminate cluster attack, but effectiveness may be limited by side effects and/or excessive use.

Oral ergot alkaloids are often inadequate in acute attacks, but are often effective if taken an hour before the anticipated time of the attack. If the patient is awakened at night with headache, ergotamine either orally or by suppository at bedtime remains an alternative. Because of the self-limiting nature of cluster attacks in most patients, long-term continuous therapy is not recommended and often unnecessary.

Oxygen,[54,57] a potent cerebral vasoconstrictor, has also been effective in the symptomatic treatment of cluster headache. Inhalation of 100% oxygen through a facial mask at a rate of 6 to 8 L per minute for no longer than 15 minutes is a safe and effective alternative to ergotamine therapy.

Since Ekbom[58] first reported that lithium carbonate was effective in treating chronic cluster headache, others[54,59,60] have reported success in the treatment of episodic and chronic cluster headache attacks. Currently, the mechanism of action in cluster headache is unknown, but effects on platelets as well as on the central nervous system have been postulated.

Lithium is initiated in a dose of 300 to 600 mg/d, and increased to 600–1,200 mg/d as necessary. Prophylaxis is usually started when the attacks begin, and a favorably clinical response often occurs during the first week of therapy.

Plasma lithium concentrations should be monitored as symptoms of toxicity correlate with plasma level. A lithium level between 0.6 and 1.2 mEq/L measured at steady state, 12 hours after the last dose, is usually desired. Optimal plasma levels of lithium for prevention of cluster headache have not been established.

Initial side effects are mild and include tremor, lethargy, nausea, diarrhea, and abdominal discomfort. In cluster headache patients treated with lithium, headaches[59] easily distinguishable from the cluster headache may be observed as a side effect of therapy. These lithium headaches are episodes of moderately severe, throbbing occipital pain lasting 6 to 12 hours. They disappear when lithium is withdrawn. Lithium should be administered with caution to patients with significant renal or cardiovascular disease, dehydration, pregnancy, or concomitant diuretic use.

In patients unresponsive to lithium, methysergide 2 mg three or four times a day is usually effective in shortening the course of cluster headaches.[54,60] Response to treatment usually occurs within 1 week of initiation of the drug. Duration of therapy is limited to no longer than 6 months of continuous use because of the potential complications of long-term use. Doses may be tapered after 2 to 3 weeks of freedom from headaches.

Corticosteroids[54,60–62] have proved effective for cluster headaches not responsive to either lithium or methysergide. High doses of steroids begin to ease pain in 8 to 12 hours, with maximum effectiveness in 2 to 3 days. Prednisone is often given in an initial dosage of 40 to 60 mg orally, administered in divided doses, and rapidly tapered over a 2-week to 1-month period. Steroids seem to suppress and not eliminate the factors producing the headaches; therefore, their usefulness is limited to short-lasting cluster attacks. Long-term use is not recommended to avoid steroid-induced complications.

Other prophylactic measures[54] that have been advocated in the management of cluster headache include β-blockers, tricyclic antidepressants, histamine blockers, nonprescription analgesics, and cyproheptadine, but well-designed, controlled studies are lacking. Calcium channel blockers and chlorpromazine also have been advocated in the management of cluster headache, but further study is needed to establish effectiveness.

Chronic paroxysmal hemicrania may resemble cluster headaches. Some aspects that differentiate the headache types include sex (with women affected more than men), high number of attacks daily without nocturnal preponderance or remission, shorter duration of attacks (15–30 minutes), precipitation by flexion or rotation of the head, and therapeutic response to indomethacin.[55,63,64]

Aspirin is often observed to be partially effective in decreasing the severity of pain in chronic paroxysmal hemicrania patients.[55,64] Many agents used in the management of cluster headache are ineffective. Patients with otherwise typical cluster headaches who do not respond to usual therapy should be given a trial of indomethacin. Indomethacin in doses of 50–150 mg daily, in divided doses, may provide pain relief. Indomethacin should be given after meals and perhaps with antacids to those patients with a higher incidence of peptic ulcer disease.

**Table 44.6** Primary Headache Therapy

- **I. Muscle Contraction Headache**
  - A. Through diagnostic evaluation
  - B. Simple analgesics
  - C. Benzodiazepines (anxiety)
  - D. Antidepressants (depression)
  - E. "Biofeedback"
- **II. Migraine**
  - A. Treatment of individual acute headache episode
    1. Simple analgesics and metoclopramide
    2. Ergotamines
    3. Midrin
    4. Chlorpromazine
  - B. Prophylactic treatment of frequent attacks
    1. β-Blockers
    2. Tricyclic antidepressants
    3. Aspirin or NSAIDs
    4. Calcium channel blockers
    5. Ergotamine preparations
    6. Methysergide
    7. Cyproheptadine, clonidine, or steroids
- **III. Cluster Headaches**
  - A. Treatment of individual acute headache episodes
    1. Migraine regimen (e.g., ergotamines, chlorpromazine)
    2. Oxygen
  - B. Prophylactic treatment of cluster bout
    1. Lithium
    2. Calcium channel blockers
    3. Ergotamines
    4. Methysergide
    5. β-Blockers
    6. Steroids
    7. Indomethacin (chronic paroxysmal hemicrania)
    8. Chlorpromazine

## Summary

Headache pain has many causes but is generally attributed to one of three mechanisms: (1) primary, (2) psychogenic, or (3) secondary to intracranial or systemic illness. A careful patient workup, including patient history, physical examination, and appropriate tests, identifies most headache patients with major life-threatening disease. Appropriate therapy for secondary headaches is directed at correcting the underlying condition.

A variety of strategies can be helpful for primary headache syndromes (Table 44.6). For headaches of muscle contraction origin, treatment includes psychotherapy, physical therapy, and pharmacotherapy. The most effective management of vascular headaches is medication to suppress the acute attack and prevent recurrences.

The wide range of available symptomatic and prophylactic treatment options in the management of vascular headaches indicates that none are wholly effective. Prophylactic medication is warranted when headache of moderate or greater severity recurs with a frequency of two or more attacks per month. Treatment failures may result when patients receive an insufficient dosage of the drug or an inadequate drug trial. Therapy should be continued for 6 to 8 weeks before an agent is considered to be ineffective.

Continuing research into the problem of primary headache disorders will better define pathophysiologic mechanisms and aid the search for less toxic and more efficacious pharmacologic agents.

## References


1. Repschlaeger BJ, McPherson MA. Classification, mechanisms and management of headache. Clin Pharm 1984;3:139–152.
2. Pikoff H. Is the muscular model of headache still viable? A review of conflicting data. Headache 1984;24:186–198.
3. Hanington E. The platelet and migraine. Headache 1986;26: 411–415.
4. Hanington E, Jones RJ, Amess JAL, et al. Migraine: A platelet disorder. Lancet 1981;2:720–723.
5. Coppen A, Swade C, Wood K, et al. Platelet 5-hydroxytryptamine accumulation in migraine. Lancet 1979;2:914.
6. Lance JW. What is migraine? Adv Neurol 1982;33:21–26.
7. Friedman AP. Migraine. Med Clin North Am 1978;62:481–494.
8. Masland WS. Electroencephalography and electromyography in the diagnosis of headache. Med Clin North Am 1978;62: 571–583.
9. Munro J, Brostoff J, Carini C, et al. Food allergy in migraine. Study of dietary exclusion and RAST. Lancet 1980;2:1–4.
10. Kohlenberg RJ. Tyramine sensitivity in dietary migraine: A critical review. Headache 1982;22:30–34.
11. Clover V, Littlewood J, Sandler M, et al. Biochemical predisposition to dietary migraine: the role of phenolsulfotransferase. Headache 1983;23:53–58.
12. Nightingale S. A review of the treatment of migraine. J Clin Hosp Pharm 1984;9:271–282.
13. Krabbe AA, Olesen J. Headache provocation by continuous intravenous infusion of histamine: Clinical results and receptor mechanisms. Pain 1980;8:253–259.
14. Watts DT. The effect of nicotine and smoking on the secretion of catecholamines. Ann NY Acad Sci 1960;90:74.
15. Mann RD. Drug induced disorders of central nervous function, in D'Arcy PF, Griffen JP (ed): Iatrogenic Diseases. Oxford, Oxford University Press, 1986, pp 586–650.
16. Lance JW. Headache. Ann Neurol 1981;10:1–10.
17. Drummond PD. Predisposing, precipitating and relieving factors in different categories of headache. Headache 1985;25:16–22.
18. Anthony M. Plasma free fatty acids and prostaglandin $E_1$ changes in migraine and stress. Headache 1976;16:58.
19. Bradfield JM. A new look at the use of ergotamine. Drugs 1976;12:449–453.
20. Eadie MJ. The management of migraine. Med J Aust 1975;1: 752–754.
21. Peroutka SJ. The pharmacology of calcium channel antagonists: A novel class of anti-migraine agents? Headache 1983;23: 278–283.
22. Peters BH, Fraim CJ, Masel BE. Comparison of 650 mg aspirin and 1000 mg acetaminophen with each other, and with placebo in moderately severe headache. Am J Med 1983;75:36–42.
23. Caviness Jr VS, Phil D, O'Brien P. Headache. N Engl J Med 1980;302:446–450.
24. Diamond S, Dalessio DJ. The practicing physician's approach to headache, in Migraine Headache. Baltimore, Williams and Wilkins, 1978, pp 51–66.
25. Volans GN. The effect of metoclopramide on the absorption of effervescent aspirin in migraine. Br J Clin Pharmacol 1975;2: 57–63.
26. Tokola RA, Neuvonen PJ. Effects of migraine attack and metaclopromide on the absorption of tolfeuamic acid. Brit J Clin Pharmacol 1984;17:67–75.
27. Ross-Lee L, Heazlewood V, Tyrer JH, et al. Aspirin treatment of migraine attacks: Plasma drug level data. Cephalalgia 1982;2: 9–14.
28. Perrin VL. Clinical pharmacokinetics of ergotamine in migraine and cluster headache. Clin Pharmacokinet 1985;10:334–352.
29. Ibraheem JJ, Paalzow L, Tfelt-Hansen P. Low bioavailability of ergotamine tartrate after oral and rectal administration in migraine sufferers. Br J Clin Pharmacol 1983;16:695–699.
30. Tfelt-Hansen P, Paalzow L, Ibraheem JJ. Bioavailability of sublingual ergotamine. Br J Clin Pharmacol 1982;13:239–240.
31. Raskin NH. Repetitive intravenous dihydroergotamine as therapy for intractable migraine. Neurology 1986;36:995–997.
32. Callaham M, Raskin N. A controlled study of dihydroergotamine in the treatment of acute migraine headache. Headache 1986;26:168–171.
33. Horton BT, Peters GA. Clinical manifestations of excessive use of ergotamine preparations and management of withdrawal effect: Report of 52 cases. Headache 1963;4:214–227.
34. Diamond S. Treatment of migraine with isometheptene, acetaminophen and dichloralphenazone combination: A double-blind, crossover trial. Headache 1976;15:282–287.
35. Iserson KV. Parenteral chlorpromazine treatment of migraine. Ann Emerg Med 1983;12:756–758.
36. Lane PL, Ross R. Intravenous chlorpromazine—preliminary results in acute migraine. Headache 1985;25:302–304.
37. Mendelson G, Little TF. Narcotic analgesics in headache. Med J Aust 1981;2:518.
38. Langemark M, Olesen J. Drug abuse in migraine patients. Pain 1984;19:81–86.
39. Kunkel RS. Pharmacologic management of migraine—1985. Cleve Clin Q 1985;52:95–101.
40. Rosen JA. Observations on the efficacy of propranolol for the prophylaxis of migraine. Ann Neurol 1983;13:92–93.
41. Turner P. Beta-blocking drugs in migraine. Postgrad Med J 1984;60(suppl 2):51–55.
42. Couch JR, Hassanein RS. Amitriptyline in migraine prophylaxis. Arch Neurol 1979;36:695–699.
43. Tsuji M, Iida H. Treatment of headache with antidepressant. Folia Psychiatr Neurol Jpn 1984;38:143–150.
44. Scheife RT, Hills JR. Migraine headaches: Signs and symptoms, biochemistry, and current therapy, Am J Hosp Pharm 1980;37: 365–374.
45. Eadie MF. Clonidine in migraine prophylaxis. Aust Prescriber 1979;1:35–37.
46. Kallanranta T, Hakkarainen H, Hokkanen E, et al. Clonidine in migraine prophylaxis. Headache 1977;17:169–172.
47. Welch KMA, Ellis DJ, Keenan PA. Successful migraine prophylaxis with naproxen sodium. Neurology 1985;35:1304–1310.
48. O'Neill BP, Mann JD. Aspirin prophylaxis in migraine. Lancet 1978;2:1179–1181.
49. Ziegler DK, Ellis DJ. Naproxen in prophylaxis of migraine. Arch Neurol 1985;42:582–584.
50. Greenberg DA. Calcium channel antagonists and the treatment of migraine. Clin Neuropharmacol 1986;9:311–328.
51. Solomon GD. Comparative efficacy of calcium antagonist drugs in the prophylaxis of migraine. Headache 1985;25:368–371.
52. Health and Public Policy Committee, American College of Physicians. Biofeedback for headaches. Ann Intern Med 1985;102:128–131.
53. Hannington E, Harper AM. The role of tyramine in the aetiology of migraine and related studies on the cerebral and extracerebral circulation. Headache 1968;8:84–97.
54. Sholar PW. Cluster headache. Johns Hopkins Med J 1982;150: 246–250.

**55.** Hochman MS. Chronic paroxysmal hemicrania: A new type of treatable headache. Am J Med 1981;71:169–170.
**56.** Waldenlind E, Ekbom K, Krabbe A. Ergotamine for cluster headache. A pharmacokinetic study. Acta Neurol Scand 1982; 65(suppl 90):83–84.
**57.** Fogan L. Treatment of cluster headache: A double-blind comparison of oxygen vs. air inhalation. Arch Neurol 1985;42:362–363.
**58.** Ekbom K. Lithium vid kroniska sympton av cluster headache. Opuse Med 1974;19:148–156.
**59.** Mathew NT. Clinical subtypes of cluster headache and response to lithium therapy. Headache 1978;18:26–30.
**60.** Kudrow L. Comparative results of prednisone, methysergide, and lithium therapy in cluster headache, in Green R (ed): Current Concepts in Migraine Research. New York, Raven, 1978, pp 159–163.
**61.** Couch Jr JR, Ziegler DK. Prednisone therapy for cluster headache. Headache 1978;18:219–221.
**62.** Jammes JL. The treatment of cluster headaches with prednisone. Dis Nerv Syst 1978;36:375–376.
**63.** Petty RG, Rose FC. Chronic paroxysmal hemicrania: First reported British case. Br Med J 1983;286:438.
**64.** Kilpatrick CJ, King J. Chronic paroxysmal hemicrania. Med J Aust 1982;1:49–50.

# Section Six
# **Psychiatric Disorders**

# *Chapter 45* / Disorders of Infancy and Childhood

Glen L. Stimmel, PharmD

During the last decade, a substantial scientific base has been established for psychopharmacology of adult patients. Precision in diagnosis has recently been facilitated by the American Psychiatric Association's *Diagnostic and Statistical Manual for Mental Disorders, Third Edition, Revised* (DSM-III-R). This increasing confidence and data regarding psychotropic drugs have also increased attention to child and adolescent psychopharmacology. This review summarizes both the new diagnostic categories of child and adolescent psychiatric disorders and their treatment with medication. Only those disorders treatable with drugs are included.

While the drugs are often the same as those used for adult psychiatric disorders, treatment of children and adolescents typically requires a very different approach. Most adults given psychotropic drugs have major psychiatric disorders—schizophrenia, bipolar illness, and major depression. Most children, however, are given psychotropic drugs to control a symptom or behavior. Another major difference is that with very few exceptions, drug treatment is adjunctive rather than the primary treatment modality for child and adolescent disorders. As will be repeatedly emphasized, drug treatment is often used only after nondrug treatment approaches fail.

## Disruptive Behavioral Disorders: Attention-Deficit Hyperactivity Disorder

### Clinical Presentation

The three essential features are signs of developmentally inappropriate inattention, impulsivity, and hyperactivity. Inattention typically involves the child failing to finish tasks, not seeming to listen, being easily distracted, having difficulty concentrating on schoolwork, and having difficulty sticking to a play activity. Impulsivity is manifest as often acting before thinking, shifting excessively from one activity to another, difficulty in organizing work, needing much supervision, frequently calling out in class, and difficulty awaiting a turn in games or group situations. Hyperactivity typically includes excessive running about or climbing on things, difficulty sitting still or staying seated, excessive moving about during sleep, and acting as "driven by a motor." Symptom presence and severity are variable with the situation and time. It is unusual for a child to display signs of the disorder in all settings or even in the same setting at all times.[1]

Onset is typically by the age of 3 and must be by age 7, though the disorder may not require professional attention until the child enters school. Prevalence is 2% to 3% of prepubertal children in the United States; it is 10 times more common in boys than in girls.[1,2] A 6-month duration of symptoms is necessary for diagnosis.

### Treatment

Severity of symptoms is the primary factor affecting a decision to initiate drug treatment. Drug treatment is reserved for moderate to severe symptom intensity; milder cases can often be successfully treated with environmental manipulation alone. The classes of drugs used for attention-deficit disorder (ADD) with hyperactivity include stimulants, antipsychotic drugs, and the tricyclic antidepressants. Most clinical research has focused on children of average intelligence attending regular schools, so results are not necessarily applicable to inpatients or children with mental retardation or psychosis. Although drug treatment can often successfully ameliorate symptoms, educational, social, and family consequences of the disorder must often be addressed by nondrug treatment approaches.

***Stimulants*** Amphetamines, methylphenidate (Ritalin, Ciba), and pemoline (Cylert, Abbott) represent the most effective drug treatment options for this disorder. Efficacy is optimal when the diagnosis is clear-cut, classic target symptoms are severe and predominant, and the child is of school age rather than preschool.[3] These well-established clinical observations must be viewed cautiously; more severe symptomatology may yield better efficacy only because drug effect is more discernible.[4]

In addition to behavioral effects, stimulants may improve cognitive performance. No study suggests that stimulants impair cognitive performance; rather, reading, memory, and arithmetic performance is often significantly improved. Improved cognitive performance is believed to result from the stimulant drug increasing attention and concentration, not to an effect on a specific cognitive skill.[3,5] The observation that cognitive skills may improve secondary to increased attention and concentration suggests that stimulants are indicated for the target behaviors and are not indicated for primary learning disorders.

Amphetamines were the first drugs to be used for this disorder. Dextroamphetamine is preferred over racemic amphetamine and levoamphetamine because of its greater efficacy and earlier onset of effect.[6,7] Dextroamphetamine improves symptoms in a majority of patients and is significantly more effective than placebo.[3] Methylphenidate is the second stimulant drug found effective for ADD with hyperactivity. Efficacy studies report a 70% to 90% response rate as well as clear superiority over placebo.[8,9] Pemoline is the most recently introduced effective drug and has been shown to be more effective than placebo and either slightly less effective than or equal in efficacy to dextroamphetamine and methylphenidate.[3,9,10]

Two other stimulant drugs have been tried but found inferior in efficacy to the three drugs just described. Deanol looked promising in open clinical trials, but subsequent controlled studies found its efficacy usually only slightly greater than that of placebo.[11] Caffeine also showed early promise, but the majority of controlled studies show no efficacy for ADD with hyperactivity.[12,13]

Of the three effective stimulant drugs, none is favored as the drug of choice. Most efficacy studies find no significant difference between dextroamphetamine and methylphenidate, while pemoline is slightly less effective.[3,12] Pemoline also differs in that its onset of effect requires 2 weeks, with full effect evident at 6 to 8 weeks.[9,10] This disadvantage of slow onset is balanced somewhat by its longer duration of action, which allows once-daily dosing, and lower appetite suppression.[3] Dextroamphetamine appears to cause more growth suppression than methylphenidate, and pemoline has not been reported to have this effect.[3,14] Long-term use of pemoline has been reported to elevate serum concentrations of liver enzymes, indicating possible hepatic damage. From these differences, dextroamphetamine and methylphenidate emerge as first-choice drugs, with pemoline reserved for children who cannot tolerate multiple daily dosing of the first-choice drug because of insomnia or loss of evening appetite.

While initiation and dosage titration procedures vary among clinicians, the following scheme is based upon published recommendations of experienced clinicians.[3,15] The initial dose is dextroamphetamine 2.5 mg or methylphenidate 5 mg. Drug effect is evident in 15 to 30 minutes and lasts 2 to 6 hours. Future dosing increments should be 2.5 and 5 mg, respectively. The dosing schedule can be determined by observing when the loss of positive drug effect occurs during the 2 to 6 hours after an oral dose. Most patients require a two- or three-times-daily dosing schedule. The dose should be raised until no further improvement is seen. Unless side effects become troublesome, the dose should continue to be increased even if moderate but incomplete efficacy is noted. Maximum benefit typically is seen at 40 mg daily of dextroamphetamine or 60 mg daily of methylphenidate. Occasionally, doses need to be raised beyond these amounts. If pemoline must be used, 18.75 mg is the initial dose and amount of dosing increment, with 125 mg daily the typical maximum dose. All drugs should be given after meals to minimize stomachaches and appetite suppression. Both dose and schedule usually require individualization. Insomnia is best treated by giving the last dose earlier or by decreasing the afternoon dose. If loss of efficacy is seen in the evening or early morning, the schedule should be adjusted accordingly. Varying doses and schedules are the hallmark of appropriate prescribing.

A more controversial aspect of stimulant use concerns drug holidays and duration of treatment. Because family members may be more tolerant and less demanding than school personnel, many children can discontinue their drug or take only the morning dose on weekends. Similarly, many children can discontinue drug treatment during vacations and summers. The longest course of treatment should be one school year of continuous use. All children should be given a trial off drugs every year. One very convenient method is to discontinue the drug for summer vacation and not restart for the first 2 weeks of school. If the drug must be restarted, often it can be restarted and adjusted at a lower dose. Drug dosage often varies from year to year, while the schedule usually remains the same.

Gittleman and co-workers[3] identified six examples of mismanagement that concisely portray important clinical management concerns: (1) small doses are given and the child is infrequently seen by the physician, (2) no systematic attempt is made to obtain information from teachers at school regarding response, (3) no "off" periods are used during the school year, (4) parents are put in charge of dosage, (5) deterioration of effectiveness leads to assumption of nonresponse rather than need for dosage increases, and (6) the child is not followed after the drug is discontinued.

Adverse effects of stimulants in children are frequent but usually mild. A 1-month predrug baseline of complaints can help in identifying true drug-induced effects. Anorexia and insomnia occur in about 50% of children given moderate to high doses of stimulants. With proper scheduling of doses, however, both effects can be minimized. While many children will have no appetite for breakfast, lunch and dinner can be minimally affected with the morning dose given after breakfast and the last dose given near midday. Insomnia is specifically a delay in onset of sleep, and can be minimized by adjusting bedtime and/or dosing schedule. Occasionally, dosage reduction is necessary. Headache and abdominal pain occur in 10% of children, particularly in the first few weeks of drug treatment. About 10% of children on higher doses become lethargic and listless. Rare effects include hallucinosis (visual or tactile) and development or reemergence of tics. Heart rate and blood pressure are increased with stimulants, but the magnitude is rarely of clinical importance.[16]

Growth suppression from stimulants represents the side effect of most concern.[17] Although not a consistent finding, growth suppression is more often seen with dextroamphetamine than methylphenidate, and with higher doses than lower doses; taller children seem to be more vulnerable to reduced growth velocity.[14,18] More recent information suggests some tolerance may develop after 1 year,[19] and growth catches up if treatment is interrupted.[20] An early concern with stimulant use in children was an increased likelihood of drug abuse in adolescence, but no evidence has been found to suggest that stimulant abuse is higher in children with a history of stimulant use for ADD with hyperactivity.[21]

*Tricyclic Antidepressants* Imipramine (Tofranil, Geigy) is the most studied antidepressant and it shows limited efficacy for ADD with hyperactivity. Antidepressants are more effective than placebo but inferior to stimulants. Antidepressants are most effective for symptoms of hyperactivity and aggressiveness and much less effective for cognitive dysfunction. Interestingly, therapeutic effect is seen almost immediately, certainly within 4 days, and some tolerance develops.[22] This finding suggests a mechanism very different from the antidepressant action of these drugs. Imipramine should be started at 25–50 mg daily, with a maximum of 5 mg/kg/d.[3] Antidepressants represent backup drugs to the stimulants for treatment of ADD with hyperactivity.

*Antipsychotic Drugs* While stimulant drugs seem to have a more specific beneficial effect on the symptoms of ADD with hyperactivity, antipsychotic drugs decrease hyperactivity but do not improve attention and concentration.[23] Usual doses of chlorpromazine (Thorazine, Smith Kline & French) or thioridazine (Mellaril, Sandoz) range from 50 to 300 mg daily. Major concerns with the use of neuroleptic drugs are the deleterious effects on learning and cognitive functioning and the potential for tardive dyskinesia with long-term use. For most children, the disadvantages far outweigh the advantages of using antipsychotic drugs. Their role should be last-resort agents when stimulants or antidepressants cannot be used, or as temporary adjuncts for marked hyperactivity uncontrolled by stimulants.

*Defined Diets* In 1973 Feingold reported significant reduction of hyperactivity with use of a diet free of salicylates and food additives and published a book containing his clinical observations.[24] This book came at a time of increasing public concern about environmental pollution, a desire for full knowledge of all additives found in prepared food, a heightened aversion to habitual use of medication, and the frustration encountered by parents and physicians in managing childhood hyperactivity. These trends led to widespread experimentation with the Feingold regimen and other defined diets. Controlled studies indicate these diets are only occasionally efficacious, which directly contrasts with parental reports of dramatic improvements.[25,26] An NIH Consensus Development Conference on Defined Diets and Childhood Hyperactivity concluded in 1982 that defined diets should be described to parents as an option, although scientific evidence supports efficacy only in a small proportion of children.[27]

At this time the best approach to treatment of attention-deficit hyperactivity disorder is either dextroamphetamine or methylphenidate for patients with moderate to severe symptomatology. Pemoline remains a secondary treatment option for patients who cannot tolerate multiple daily dosing of first-line drugs because of insomnia or loss of evening appetite.

## Functional Enuresis

### Clinical Presentation

The essential feature is repeated involuntary or intentional voiding of urine by day or at night not caused by any physical disorder. Diagnostic criteria have been somewhat arbitrarily set as involuntary voiding of urine at least twice a month for children between 5 and 6 years old, and once per month for older children. Primary functional enuresis refers to children who have experienced a 1-year period of continence. Nocturnal enuresis is most common (during sleeptime only), but diurnal enuresis (during waking hours) or both can occur. Urination is not associated with a particular sleep stage; it typically occurs in the deeper stages of non–rapid eye movement (non-REM) sleep, but can also occur during the REM stage of sleep.[28] Prevalence at age 5 is 7% for boys and 3% for girls; at age 10 it is 3% for boys and 2% for girls; at age 18 it is 1% for boys and almost nonexistent for girls.[1,3,29]

### Treatment

Most of the studies of drug treatment for functional enuresis were completed in the late 1960s and early 1970s, and relatively little new information has been added in the last 10 to 15 years. Thus, the information in older reviews[30,31] remains valid with the few exceptions to be noted.

Drug treatment for functional enuresis is of short-term benefit, but drug effect does not extend beyond its administration. Nondrug treatments, such as conditioning techniques, have more long-term value, and thus should be given first consideration. Drug treatment is also reliably effective when used intermittently, such as for camping trips or overnight trips away from home.

Tricyclic antidepressant drugs are the only drugs effective for treating enuresis. Dextroamphetamine, monoamine oxidase inhibitors, and anticholinergic drugs are ineffective.[3] The exact mechanism of action is unknown, and previous theories of elimination of stage 4 sleep and peripheral anticholinergic effect of tricyclics have been ruled out as explanations.[3,28] Imipramine has been most studied, although other tricyclics have also been found to be effective. The initial dose of imipramine should be 25 mg at bedtime, with weekly increases of 25 mg if necessary. A nightly dose greater than 75 mg is rarely necessary. Effect is often immediate and is certainly seen within 7 days. Plasma concentrations of imipramine and desipramine do correlate with clinical response, and true nonresponders exist in spite of adequate plasma concentrations.[32] Imipramine efficacy is about 85%; one half of patients have total elimination of bed-wetting and the other half, a significant decrease in the number of episodes. An initially effective dose often becomes ineffective in 2 to 6 weeks, but increasing the dose usually reestablishes control. One week is needed to evaluate the efficacy of a new dose. If drug treatment needs to be given longer than several weeks, attempts to discontinue the drug every 3 to 6 months are advisable, as enuresis may remit spontaneously.[3,32] Before drug treatment begins, an accurate baseline record of bed-wetting frequency must be recorded.

## Developmental Disorders: Mental Retardation

### Clinical Presentation

The essential features of developmental disorders are a significantly subaverage general intellectual functioning (IQ of 70 or below), deficits or impairment in adaptive behavior, and onset before age 18. A discussion of etiologic factors would go far beyond the scope of this chapter, but involves, singly or in combination, genetic factors, environmental biologic factors, and early child-rearing experiences. At any one time, approximately 1% of the population meets the criteria for mental retardation, which is nearly twice as common in males as females. Subtypes of mental retardation are (1) mild (IQ 50–70), representing 85% of cases; (2) moderate (IQ 35–49), 10% of cases; (3) severe (IQ 20–34), 3% to 4% of cases; and (4) profound (IQ below 20), 1% to 2% of cases. The diagnosis of mental retardation is made regardless of whether or not there is a coexisting mental or physical disorder.[1] Behavioral manifestations of mental retardation requiring drug treatment consist primarily of aggressive, assaultive, or self-destructive behavior. Additionally, the prevalence of seizure disorder is high (50%) in the severely retarded and 25% to 30% in the mildly retarded by the age of 22.[33]

#### Treatment

Although there is no drug treatment for mental retardation, antipsychotic drugs are frequently used as treatment for the assaultive, aggressive, or self-destructive behavior seen in some patients. Such a nonspecific indication suggests that these drugs are not being used for their antipsychotic activity but for their ability to decrease the severity or frequency of intolerable behavior.

Most surveys of psychotropic drug use in mental retardation facilities suggest that antipsychotic drugs are usually used too often, in excessive dosage, or for too long. One survey of 2,238 residents in such a facility found that 42% were on antipsychotic drugs; the therapeutic response was generally poor, and in more than 50% of patients, the use of drugs was judged as excessive.[34] The negative component of this issue is that in mentally retarded individuals, antipsychotic drugs often do not reduce inappropriate behaviors and they interfere with the response to reinforcement and performance of workshop tasks.[35] Other studies suggest that only one third of institutionalized mentally retarded individuals receiving antipsychotic drugs actually need them, and that doses can often be reduced by 50% to 67% in those who benefit from drug use.[36] Absence of effective behavioral programs may cause an additional 25% of patients to be continued on antipsychotic drugs.

## Eating Disorders

### *Anorexia Nervosa*

#### Clinical Presentation

This disorder, predominantly found in young women between 10 and 25 years of age, is characterized by weight loss of at least 15% of original body weight (or original plus expected growth in weight) as a result of a disturbance in body image and ultimately unfounded fears of becoming obese even when underweight, and absence of at least three consecutive menstrual cycles.[1] Investigations of abnormal dexamethasone suppression tests (DSTs) and urinary 3-methoxy-4-hydroxyphenylglycol (MHPG) levels have been conducted with positive findings. Abnormalities in both tests were not related to mood of the patients and so probably reflect an intrinsic feature of anorexia nervosa and not a concomitant mood state. All patients less than 75% ideal weight had an abnormal DST, and MHPG was low in most patients.[37] Anorexia is not the result of physical illness and the patient refuses to maintain minimally normal body weight levels if weight is somehow restored.

#### Treatment

Anorexia nervosa is relatively uncommon, but its mortality rate makes effective treatment quite desirable. Outcome studies show mortality rates of 6% to as high as 22%. A follow-up of treated cases showed that 50% continued to have eating difficulties and almost 50% had other signs of psychiatric impairment.[38,39] Various pharmacotherapies have been proposed and attempted, but there are few controlled studies of sufficient populations of anorectics that show both short- and long-term efficacy. Promising results have been found only with cyproheptadine (Periactin, Merck Sharp & Dohme) and amitriptyline (Elavil, Merk Sharp & Dohme).[40,41]

Cyproheptadine has been shown to be effective in terms of weight gain in a group of nonbulimic anorectic patients, but it interferes with treatment for bulimic patients. The drug was used at initial doses of 12 mg per day, given as a liquid concentrate, and these doses were increased by 4 mg every 5 days if a weight gain of 0.5 kg was not achieved, to a maximum dose of 32 mg. This dosage regimen was well tolerated.[41] Although cyproheptadine may not be useful in all patients with anorexia nervosa, its low incidence of side effects and reports of its effectiveness in some patients would suggest that it is a reasonable drug with which to initially attempt weight gain; other drug therapies can be used if the cyproheptadine fails.

Another area of interest in the treatment of anorexia nervosa is in the use of total parenteral nutrition. Two studies[42,43] have shown that total parenteral nutrition can be used safely and effectively in severely ill anorectics; however, the clinician needs to be aware of the potential for wide shifts in electrolyte and fluid balance in these patients during parenteral nutrition (especially in the first days of treatment) which require very close patient monitoring.

### *Bulimia Nervosa*

#### Clinical Presentation

Bulimia nervosa is defined as recurrent episodes of binge eating in which there is rapid consumption of a large amount of food in a defined period of time; for example, over 5,000 calories of easily digested food will be eaten in a binge, which often is terminated by abdominal pain, self-induced vomiting, or sleep. A minimum average of two binge-eating episodes per week for at least 3 months, as well as persistent overconcern with body shape and weight, is necessary for the diagnosis. There are typically repeated attempts to lose weight by severely restrictive diets, self-induced vomiting, laxative abuse, and diuretic abuse. Bulimic patients are aware that this eating pattern is abnormal, and there is fear of not being able to stop eating voluntarily. Depressed mood and self-deprecating thoughts follow the eating binges. A survey of college freshmen indicated that 4.5% of females and 0.4% of males had a history of bulimia.[1,44] Anorexia nervosa and bulimia frequently are found together in a patient; however, they are distinct diagnostic entities. While eating disorders and depressive disorders are related, the nature of the relationship is unclear and not direct.[45] There are many medical complications of eating disorders. Common findings include bradycardia and hypotension secondary to volume depletion, constipation and abdominal bloating, electrolyte disturbance and increased blood urea nitrogen secondary to dehydration, anemia, and mild hypothyroidism.[46]

### Treatment

The occurrence of depressed mood after binge eating has led to the suggestion that bulimia may be a variant of depressive illness and potentially responsive to antidepressant drugs. In addition to a number of uncontrolled studies, several placebo-controlled studies of antidepressant drugs have been completed.[47] Imipramine has been found to significantly reduce the frequency of binge eating. Follow-up on an open basis in one study for up to 8 months found moderate to marked reduction of binge eating in 90% of subjects on antidepressant drug therapy. Desipramine (Norpramin, Merrell Dow) has also been shown to be effective in significantly reducing binge frequency versus placebo.[48] Desipramine dosage ranges from 50 to 200 mg daily and is most effective when the plasma desipramine concentration is 125–275 ng/mL.

Pharmacotherapy and nutritional support should not be viewed as the main focus of treatment, as these approaches serve only as adjuncts to behavior modification and other forms of psychologic intervention. Because of the risk of mortality if extreme weight loss is allowed to continue, a trial of drug treatment or parenteral nutritional support seems quite appropriate.

## Gilles de la Tourette's Syndrome

### Clinical Presentation

This rare disorder of the central nervous system is a syndrome of recurrent, involuntary, repetitive, rapid, and purposeless motor movements of multiple muscle groups, generally accompanied by involuntary vocalizations (throat clearings, coughing, hissing, barking-like noises, snorting, echolalia, and obscenities), any or all of which can be voluntarily suppressed from minutes to hours. The median age of onset is 7 years, with the majority having an onset before age 14. Tourette's syndrome is three times more common in males. The disorder (and its symptoms) waxes and wanes over weeks or months and may spontaneously remit. The disorder must be present for 1 year for a conclusive diagnosis to be made.[1]

An understanding of the various proposed etiologies of this disorder is necessary to allow for understanding of the variety of treatment approaches that have been supported over time. Psychopharmacologic treatment was attempted after 1954 in view of the extensive history of failure of other treatment methods, and 1961 marked the first effective use of haloperidol (Haldol, McNeil) by Seignot in France, followed rapidly by other successful reports, leading researchers to believe that the syndrome was a disorder of dopaminergic activity in the corpus striatum based on the knowledge of the pharmacology of antipsychotics. The frequent exacerbation of illness in a patient previously well controlled by haloperidol, however, led researchers to attempt other forms of chemotherapy, and successes with other treatment methods led to revision of this simplistic dopamine hypothesis.

Currently, the accepted theory is that Tourette's syndrome is a genetically based disorder of central neurotransmitter activity; 47% of females and 28% males have a positive family history.[49] This disorder involves an imbalance in the interaction of dopaminergic, serotonergic, and noradrenergic systems, and it is this multiple-system etiology that best explains the success of a variety of treatment approaches.[50]

### Treatment

Tourette's syndrome is the only disorder discussed in which pharmacotherapy is the primary mode of treatment, although other treatment approaches (e.g., psychotherapy and behavior-management counseling) are frequently useful adjuncts. The emphasis on pharmacologic intervention is the result of satisfyingly high response rates (up to 90% in some studies) when drug treatment is used. For these reasons drug therapy should be initiated whenever symptoms are severe enough to impair the child's ability to function or whenever symptoms are particularly troublesome to the child.[51]

***Haloperidol*** Haloperidol remains the treatment of choice for this disorder, as it is generally quite effective in reducing target symptoms and usually well tolerated by the child, although antiparkinsonian medication may be required to treat or prevent extrapyramidal symptoms. Symptoms may regress within 24 to 48 hours after therapy is initiated and may disappear with proper dosage adjustments.[52]

Therapy with haloperidol should be initiated at low, even ineffective doses (0.025–0.05 mg/kg body weight per day), and increased gradually to avoid extrapyramidal side effects and excessive drowsiness. The daily amount is divided into two or three doses and increased by small increments over a 2- to 3-week period until symptoms are controlled. The dosage should then be readjusted to the lowest level that will provide symptom control with the least amount of troubling side effects.[52] Many patients are maintained on daily doses smaller than 10 mg of haloperidol for long periods of time, but the dosage required may vary between 6 and 180 mg/d (median daily dosage of 9 mg). Such treatment generally results in improvement in about 90% of patients.[53]

Common side effects include drowsiness and extrapyramidal effects of dyskinesias, dystonias, akathisia, akinesia, and pseudoparkinsonism. These side effects have been reported to occur in almost all patients once haloperidol doses of 2 mg/d or greater are used.[53] Because these side effects can mimic symptoms of Tourette's syndrome and cause problems in the child's ability to function (as well as obvious discomfort), frequent attempts at lowering the dose of haloperidol are warranted. If the dose cannot be lowered, then an antiparkinsonian agent such as benztropine (at a starting dose of 0.5 mg PO twice daily) or diphenhydramine will generally reverse side effects. Discontinuation of these additional medications should be attempted in about 4 weeks. Haloperidol-induced phobic disorder has also been reported in 15 patients with Tourette's syndrome.[54]

Chronic, long-term management with haloperidol may be required, but as this disorder may spontaneously remit, attempts to discontinue haloperidol should be made every 6 months. One month per year drug holidays should be instituted, if discontinuation is not possible, to avoid long-term side effects such as tardive dyskinesia.

***Clonidine*** This medication has been used with success in patients who did not respond to or could not tolerate haloperidol, and as such represents a secondary approach to treatment. Clonidine (Catapres, Boehringer Ingelheim) is an imidazoline derivative generally used in the treatment of hypertension, but as an $\alpha$-adrenergic agonist that produces central noradrenergic inhibition, trials in the treatment of Tourette's syndrome were quite rational.

Clonidine has been shown to be generally well tolerated as long as treatment is initiated with a single test dose (generally around 0.15 mg) given in the morning and blood pressure is carefully monitored. If the test dose is tolerated, treatment is begun with a 0.05 mg daily dose, titrated upward every 4 to 7 days to the maintenance dose of 0.15 mg. This dose may be further increased (again, observing for blood pressure changes) over several weeks to control symptoms, and as tolerated by the patients. This treatment approach has been shown to be effective, with a gradual onset of action, in the majority of patients in whom it is used. Furthermore, most patients tolerate the drug well and report increased feelings of calm and well-being with its use.[55,56]

***Pimozide*** Approved for marketing in the United States in 1984 as an orphan drug, pimozide (Orap, McNeil) represents an alternative to haloperidol for Tourette's syndrome.[57] Pimozide differs structurally from phenothiazines and butyrophenones, and possesses selective central dopamine receptor blockade with no effect on noradrenergic receptors. Its elimination half-life is approximately 53 hours, and metabolites are thought to be inactive. Most efficacy studies show pimozide to be equal to haloperidol. It was hoped that pimozide would offer an alternative to haloperidol with fewer adverse effects, but this has not been demonstrated. Extrapyramidal effects are the most frequent adverse reaction and are treatable with anticholinergic drugs such as trihexyphenidyl or benztropine. Pimozide also commonly causes anticholinergic effects. Initial dosing is 1 to 2 mg daily in a divided schedule, increasing every other day to a maximum of 20 mg daily. Most patients need a daily dosage of 10 mg or less. Its long half-life allows once-daily dosing.

At this time the best approach to treatment of Tourette's syndrome is haloperidol at the lowest doses possible, with clonidine or pimozide as secondary agents in those patients in whom haloperidol is ineffective or intolerable.

## Conclusion

Improved precision in the diagnosis of childhood and adolescent psychiatric disorders has led to increased interest in appropriate pharmacotherapy. For several of the disorders discussed, drug treatment is no longer viewed as merely adjunctive, nonspecific, and symptomatic. It is expected that considerable attention will be focused on attempts to gain an understanding of the underlying pathophysiology of some of these disorders, resulting in novel and improved pharmacotherapy in the near future. Eating disorders, in particular, have become a focus of public attention. The use of medication to modify behavior in children remains controversial, and the concerns regarding long-term use and adverse effects are substantial. All pharmacists must maintain an awareness of these issues and the rapid advances in this area to adequately serve the needs of our patients.

## References

1. American Psychiatric Association. Diagnostic and Statistical Manual of Mental Disorders 3rd ed, revised (DSM-III-R). Washington DC, American Psychiatric Association, 1987, pp 27–95.
2. Earls F. Application of DSM-III in an epidemiological study of preschool children. Am J Psychiatry 1982;139:242–243.
3. Klein DF, Gittleman R, Quitkin F, Rifkin A. Diagnosis and Drug Treatment of Psychiatric Disorders: Adults and Children, 2nd ed. Baltimore, William and Wilkins, 1980, pp 590–775.
4. Loney J, Prinz RJ, Mishalow J, et al. Hyperkinetic/aggressive boys in treatment: Predictors of clinical response to methylphenidate. Am J Psychiatry 1978;135:1487–1491.
5. Gittleman R. A controlled study of methylphenidate in combination with academic instruction. Psychopharmacol Bull 1982; 18:112–113.
6. Gross MD. A comparison of dextroamphetamine and racemic amphetamine in treatment of the hyperkinetic syndrome or minimal brain dysfunction. Dis Nerv Syst 1976;37:14–16.
7. Arnold LE, Huestis RD, Smeltzer DJ, et al. Levoamphetamine vs. dextroamphetamine in minimal brain dysfunction. Arch Gen Psychiatry 1976;33:292–301.
8. Lerer RJ, Lerer MP. The effects of methylphenidate on the soft neurological signs of hyperactive children. Pediatrics 1976;57: 521–525.
9. Conners CK, Taylor E. Pemoline, methylphenidate, and placebo in children with minimal brain dysfunction. Arch Gen Psychiatry 1980;37:922–930.
10. Conners CK, Taylor E, Meo G, et al. Magnesium pemoline and dextroamphetamine: A controlled study in children with minimal brain dysfunction. Psychopharmacology 1972;26:321–336.
11. Lewis JA, Lewis BJ. Deanol in minimal brain dysfunction. Dis Nerv Syst 1977;38:21–24.
12. Arnold LE, Christopher J, Huestis R, et al. Methylphenidate vs. dextroamphetamine vs. caffeine in minimal brain dysfunction. Arch Gen Psychiatry 1978;35:473–478.
13. Firestone P, Davey J, Goodman JT, et al. The effects of caffeine and methylphenidate on hyperactive children. J Am Acad Child Psychiatry 1978;17:445–456.
14. Safer D, Allen RP. Side effects from long term use of stimulants in children. Int J Ment Health 1975;4:105–118.

15. Katz S, Saraf K, Gittleman-Klein R, et al. Clinical pharmacological management of hyperactive children. Int J Ment Health 1975;4:157–181.
16. Boileau RA, Ballard JE, Sprague RL, et al. Effect of methyl phenidate on cardiorespiratory responses in hyperactive children. Res Quart 1976;47:590–596.
17. Roche AF, Lipman RS, Overall JE, et al. The effects of stimulant medication on the growth of hyperkinetic children. Pediatrics 1979;63:847–850.
18. Gross MD. Growth of hyperkinetic children taking methylphenidate, dextroamphetamine, or imipramine/desipramine. Pediatrics 1976;58:423–431.
19. Satterfield JH, Cantwell DP, Schell A, et al. Growth of hyperactive children treated with methylphenidate. Arch Gen Psychiatry 1979;36:212–217.
20. Safer DJ, Allen RP, Barr E. Growth rebound after termination of stimulant drugs. J Pediatr 1975;86:113–116.
21. Weiss G, Hechtman L, Perlman T, et al. Hyperactives as young adults: A controlled prospective ten year follow-up of 75 children. Arch Gen Psychiatry 1979;36:675–681.
22. Rapoport J. Antidepressants in childhood attention deficit disorder and obsessive–compulsive disorder. Psychosomatics 1986;27(suppl):30–36.
23. Rapoport J, Abramson A, Alexander D, et al. Playroom observations of hyperactive children on medication. J Am Acad Child Psychiatry 1971;10:524–534.
24. Feingold BF. Why Your Child is Hyperactive. New York, Random House, 1975.
25. Conner CK, Goyette CH, Southwick DA, et al. Food additives and hyperkinesis. A controlled double-blind experiment. Pediatrics 1976;58:154–166.
26. Mattes JA, Gittleman R. Effects of artificial food colorings in children with hyperactive symptoms. Arch Gen Psychiatry 1981;38:714–718.
27. National Institutes of Health Consensus Development Conference, Volume 4, No. 3. Defined Diets and Childhood Hyperactivity. Bethesda, MD, National Institutes of Health, 1982.
28. Mikkelsen EJ, Rapoport JL, Nee L, et al. Childhood enuresis. I. Sleep patterns and psychopathology. Arch Gen Psychiatry 1980;37:1139–1144.
29. Simonds JF, Parraga H. Prevalence of sleep disorders and sleep behaviors in children and adolescents. J Am Acad Child Psychiatry 1982;4:383–388.
30. Blackwell B, Currah J. The psychopharmacology of nocturnal enuresis, in Kolvin I, MacKeith R, Meadow SR (eds): Bladder Control and Enuresis, Clinics in Developmental Medicine. London, Heinemann, 1973.
31. Shaffer D. Enuresis, in Rutter M (ed): Child Psychiatry: Modern Approaches. London, Blackwell Scientific, 1977.
32. Rapoport JL, Mikkelsen EJ, Zavadil A, et al. Childhood enuresis II. Psychopathology, tricyclic concentration in plasma, and antienuretic effect. Arch Gen Psychiatry 1980;37:1146–1152.
33. Roberts JKA. Neuropsychiatric complications of mental retardation. Psychiatr Clin North Am 1986;9:647–657.
34. Tu JB. A survey of psychotropic medication in mental retardation facilities. J Clin Psychiatry 1979;40:125–128.
35. Ferguson DG. Effects of neuroleptic drugs on the intellectual and habilitative behaviors of mentally retarded persons. Psychopharmacol Bull 1982;18:54–56.
36. Zimmerman RL, Heistad GT. Studies of the long-term efficacy of antipsychotic drug in controlling the behavior of institutionalized retardates. J Am Acad Child Psychiatry 1982;21:136–143.
37. Gerner RH, Gwirtsman HE. Abnormalities of dexamethasone suppression test and urinary MHPG in anorexia nervosa. Am J Psychiatry 1981;138:650–653.
38. Hsu LKG. Outcome of anorexia nervosa. Arch Gen Psychiatry 1980;37:1041–1046.
39. Schwartz DM, Thompson MG. Do anorectics get well? Amer J Psychiatry 1981;138:319–323.
40. Herzog DB. Antidepressant use in eating disorders. Psychosomatics 1986;27(suppl):17–23.
41. Halmi KA, Eckert E, LaDu TJ. Anorexia nervosa: Treatment efficacy of cyproheptadine and amitriptyline. Arch Gen Psychiatry 1986;43:177–181.
42. Maloney MJ, Farrell MK. Treatment of severe weight loss in anorexia nervosa with hyperalimentation and psychotherapy. Am J Psychiatry 1980;137:310–314.
43. Pertschuk MJ, Forster J, Buzby G, et al. The treatment of anorexia nervosa with total parenteral nutrition. Biol Psychiatry 1981;16:539–550.
44. Herzog DB, Copeland PM. Eating disorders. N Engl J Med 1985;313:295–303.
45. Swift WJ, Andrews D, Barklage NE. The relationship between affective disorder and eating disorders: A review of the literature. Am J Psychiatry 1986;143:290–299.
46. Brotman AW, Rigotti N, Herzog DB. Medical complications of eating disorders: Outpatient evaluation and treatment. Compr Psychiatry 1985;26:258–272.
47. Pope HG Jr, Hudson JI. Antidepressant drug therapy for bulimia: Current status. J Clin Psychiatry 1986;47:339–345.
48. Hughes PL, Wells LA, Cunningham CJ, et al. Treating bulimia with desipramine. Arch Gen Psychiatry 1986;43:182–186.
49. Kidd KK, Prusoff BA, Cohen DJ. Familial pattern of Gilles de la Tourette's syndrome. Arch Gen Psychiatry 1980;37:1336–1339.
50. O'Quinn AN, Thompson RJ. Tourette's syndrome: An expanded view. Pediatrics 1980;66:420–424.
51. Golden GS. Tourette's syndrome: The pediatric perspective. Am J Dis Child 1977;131:531–534.
52. Serrano AC. Haloperidol—its use in children. J Clin Psychiatry 1981;42:154–156.
53. Woodrow KM. Gilles de la Tourette's disease—a review. Am J Psychiatry 1974;131:1000–1003.
54. Mikkelsen EJ, Detlor J, Cohen DJ. School avoidance and social phobia triggered by haloperidol in patients with Tourette's disorder. Am J Psychiatry 1981;138:1572–1576.
55. Cohen DJ, Detlor J, Young JG, et al. Clonidine ameliorates Gilles de la Tourette's syndrome. Arch Gen Psychiatry 1980;37:1350–1357.
56. Ferre RC. Tourette's disorder and the use of clonidine. J Am Acad Child Psychiatry 1982;21,3:294–297.
57. Colvin CL, Tankanow RM. Pimozide: Use in Tourette's disorder. Drug Intell Clin Pharm 1985;19:421–424.

# Chapter 46 / Organic Brain Syndromes, Alzheimer Type

Larry Ereshefsky, PharmD, Raylene Rospond, PharmD, and Michael Jann, PharmD

The age distribution of the population of the Western nations is increasing. It is estimated that senile dementia, Alzheimer type, has afflicted two to three million individuals in the United States alone. In addition, many elderly people suffer from mild cognitive loss caused by senescence or organic diseases. This "quiet epidemic" can lead to loss of humanity and death. Although the moderate or severely demented patient is readily diagnosed, mild symptoms can be easily overlooked.[1]

Dementia of all etiologies is one of the most commonly encountered organic mental syndromes. The American Psychiatric Association's *Diagnostic and Statistical Manual for Mental Disorders, Third Edition* (DSM-III), has recently been revised (DSM-III-R) with regard to the classification and diagnoses of Organic Brain Syndromes, now classified as Organic Mental Syndromes and Disorders.[2] Organic Mental Syndromes include delirium and dementia of specific etiologies. Organic disturbances associated with intoxication or withdrawal of a drug are now classified as Psychoactive Substance Use Disorders and are discussed in Chapter 47. Organic mental syndromes are neuropsychiatric diseases with a presumptive etiology judged to be related to the disturbance. Organic mental disorders (OMDs) define particular clusters of behavior and physical and neurologic findings where the etiology is either not known (primary degenerative dementia, PDD) or due to cardiovascular disease (multi-infarct dementia). Alzheimer's disease is included in the diagnosis primary degenerative dementia, senile onset (age ≥ 65) or presenile onset (age ≤ 65).

This chapter focuses primarily on the presentation and treatment of dementias. Delirium is usually not treated with medications, except for nonspecific control of behavioral manifestations; however, the features distinguishing between delirium and dementia are reviewed so that patients with reversible forms of organic mental syndromes are identified. Patients with reversible delirium should have the cause for their disturbance treated before the use of psychoactive medication.

## Epidemiology

Dementia's prevalence has been reported to be as high as 10% in persons over 65 and increases to 20% in those over 80.[3] A recent epidemiologic survey reports a prevalence rate for PDD between 1.9 and 5.8 cases per 100 persons over 65.[4] PDD in DSM-III-R is divided into presenile-onset and senile-onset forms, but separation by age is not consistently supported by epidemiologic data[5]; however, recent neuropharmacologic findings indicate that age-specific changes occur in PDD. In postmortem studies of elderly patients, PDD alone or in combination with vascular diseases accounted for approximately 70% of the cases of dementia.[3,4] Alzheimer's disease was first introduced in 1907, and constitutes the most common diagnostic subtype of PDD. As PDD is a diagnosis obtained by excluding other specific etiologies, and Alzheimer's dementia is confirmed only on autopsy, diagnostic heterogeneity is unavoidable. In this chapter, PDD and the term *Alzheimer's disease* (or dementia of the Alzheimer type) are used interchangeably. Alzheimer's disease, however, is a specific type of dementia, with a characteristic pattern of inheritability and central nervous system (CNS) structural abnormality.

## Pathophysiology

### *Structural Changes*

PDD selectively affects neurons in the basal forebrain, amygdala, hippocampus, and cerebral cortex.[6] The major morphologic CNS alterations that occur in PDD include cortical atrophy, neuronal loss, presence of neurofibrillary tangles, and neuritic plaques.[4] Deterioration in neuronal cytoskeletal structures can also occur. These structures are important for supporting neuronal metabolism, surface membrane components, and cellular transport of neurotransmitters and their precursors. These changes can disturb neurotransmission, resulting in alterations in receptor function in specific brain regions.

Neurofibrillary tangles are abnormal neurons in which the cytoplasm is filled with submicroscopic filamentous structures. Neuritic plaques are clusters of degenerating nerve terminals that contain extracellular arrays of linear polypeptide fibrils in a $\beta$-pleated sheet configuration. Other neuropathologic features include neuronal degeneration (particularly in the temporal cortex), dendritic abnormalities, granulovascuolar degeneration, and Hirano bodies present in the hippocampus.[6,7]

In PDD postmortem specimens, a high density of neurofibrillary tangles and neuritic plaques were observed in the cortex and hippocampus, distributed in a pattern matching the regions with significant cell loss (Fig. 46.1). These degenerative changes are progressive and parallel behavioral dysfunction.[9] The hippocampus, entorhinal cortex (temporal lobe area), and amygdala are areas required for normal memory function. Emotional disturbances can result from lesions in the limbic area, amygdala, hippocampus, and prefrontal lobes. As illness progresses, these neurons cease to function and die. In the final stages of PDD, the cortex has lost the majority of its lamination and becomes shrunken.[9]

The hippocampus and entorhinal cortex relay and process

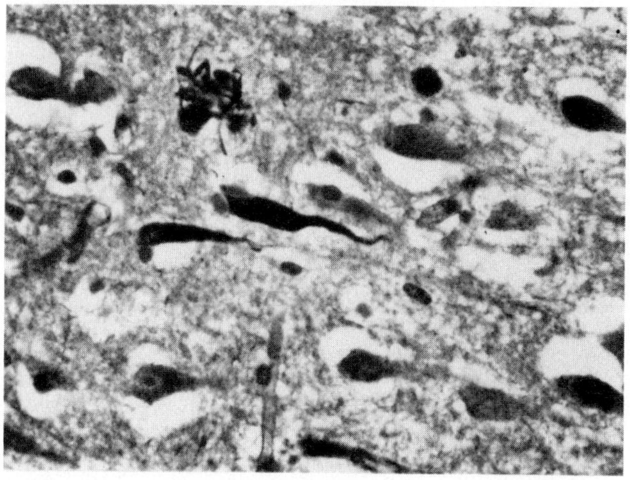

**Figure 46.1** Postmortem human cortex specimen depicting neurofibrillary tangles, neuritic plaques, granulovacuolar changes in cytosol, and inclusion bodies.

neurotransmissions from other CNS control areas. Damage to relatively few cells in the hippocampus can lead to clinically significant dysfunction. In postmortem brains of PDD patients, axonal sprouting of the remaining neurons was demonstrated in the hippocampus.[10] Axonal sprouting, or the generation of new neuronal projections to surrounding tissue, in PDD is preceded by the loss of cholinergic input into the hippocampus. Compensatory growth of the hippocampal neuronal circuitry during PDD is an illustration of CNS plasticity representing homeostatic mechanisms. This process in animal models, and possibly in man, can subsequently affect other CNS areas (e.g., entorhinal cells) and even facilitate cell death.[10]

Various reports have demonstrated a reduced cerebral blood flow (CBF) in PDD and in multi-infarct dementia.[11] In PDD, reduced CBF correlated closely with the severity of dementia and disease duration but not with age. This suggests that PDD is not related to the aging process. Rather, cognitive functions decreased as CBF declined regardless of age. CBF reductions are most likely a result of neuronal atrophy and decreased neuronal metabolism.[11]

### *Role of Aluminum and Silicon*

Various investigators have suggested that brain aluminum and silicon concentrations increase during aging.[4] A Canadian study found increases in brain aluminum concentrations in PDD patients versus normals; however, this was not corroborated by others. Apparently, aluminum is used in processing water in Canada which would explain the elevated concentrations. There are no reports of increased risk of PDD from the chronic use of antacids or antiperspirants containing aluminum and silicon. Correlations between elevated aluminum concentrations and neuropathology in PDD remain to be substantiated.[12]

### *Neuropharmacologic Alterations*

The changes in neuronal structure and function in PDD are paralleled by alterations in CNS neurochemistry and receptor function. Abnormalities in the cholinergic, serotonergic, and noradrenergic neurotransmitter systems are summarized in Table 46.1.[7] Neurotransmitter systems and their receptors have only recently been investigated in the "living brain." Positron emission tomography (PET) scanning techniques, using newly developed ligands such as *para*-iododexetimide $^{123}$I and 3-*N*-methylspiperone $^{11}$C demonstrate that neurochemical changes in PDD involve the cholinergic and serotonergic receptor systems.[13]

**Table 46.1** Neurotransmitter System Changes in Primary Degenerative Dementia, Alzheimer Type

| *System* | *CNS area* | *Activity of area* | *Receptor* | *Binding* |
|---|---|---|---|---|
| Acetylcholine | Subcortical nuclei | Decreased | $M_1$, $M_2$ | Decreased |
| | Other areas? | | Nicotinic | Decreased |
| Noradrenergic | Locus ceruleus | Decreased | $\alpha_1$, $\alpha_2$ | Normal |
| | | | $\beta$ | Normal |
| Serotonin | Raphe nucleus | Decreased | $S_1$, $S_2$ | Decreased |
| | Other areas? | | | |
| GABA/BZ[a] | Diffuse | Normal? | BZ | Normal |
| Enkephalinergic | Diffuse, periaqueductal gray | Normal | $\mu$ | Normal |
| Histamine | Putative system | Normal? | $H_1$, $H_2$ | Unknown |
| | Subcortical nuclei? | | | |
| Dopamine | A-10 subcortical | Normal? | $D_2$ | Decreased?[b] |

[a] GABA, $\gamma$-aminobutyric acid; BZ, benzodiazepine.
[b] Antipsychotic-treated patients demonstrate slight increase in receptor density.

Compiled from Reference 12.

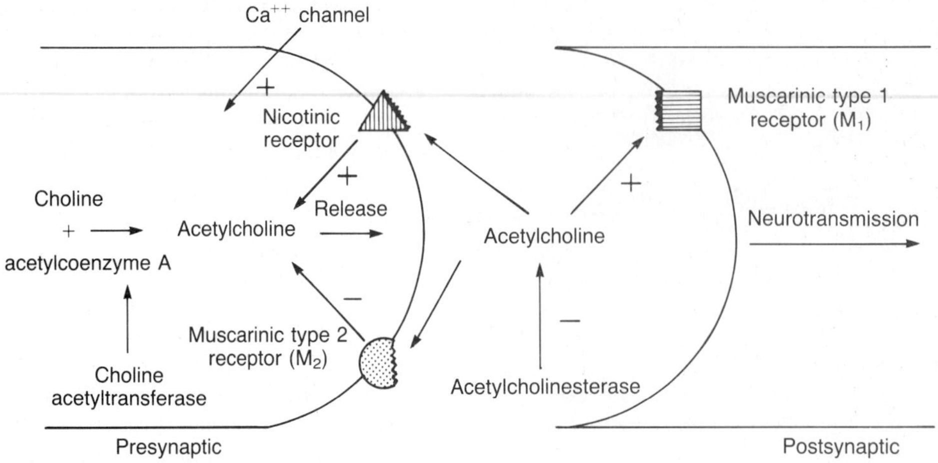


**Figure 46.2** Cholinergic neuronal regulation is modulated by numerous receptor and cellular processes. The muscarinic type 2 receptor, when stimulated, inhibits the release and synthesis of acetylcholine. The nicotinic receptor, when stimulated, facilitates the release of neurotransmitter. Other potential sites of drug action in the treatment of primary degenerative dementia are modulation of enzyme activity, precursor loading, and augmentation of the $Ca^{2+}$ channel.

### *Cholinergic System*

The neuropharmacologic alterations that occur in dementia include a non–age-related decline in the activity of the enzyme choline acetyltransferase and a strong correlation of low choline acetyltransferase activity with profound dementia; however, dementia is not attributed solely to a cholinergic deficiency.[14] Although the etiology of PDD remains to be elucidated, it appears to consistently affect the cholinergic neurons in the cerebral cortex, hippocampus, and amygdala.[6,8,14] Approximately a 40% to 90% decrease in choline acetyltransferase occurs in these brain areas.[4] Studies in animals and humans have implicated cholinergic dysfunction as a common finding in memory and cognitive deficits.[11]

The study of the cholinergic deficit in PDD has focused primarily on the presynaptic neuron and its muscarinic receptor ($M_2$). Figure 46.2 is a diagram of the cholinergic neuron and its synaptic regulation; however, both subtypes of muscarinic receptors ($M_1$ and $M_2$), as measured by autoradiographic techniques, are significantly decreased.[15] A problem in the identification of muscarinic receptors is the limited development and availability of specific ligands for each receptor subtype. Perhaps, utilizing PET scanning methods and *para*-iododexetimide $^{123}I$, $M_1$ and $M_2$ receptor populations in CNS may be further identified.[16]

Recently, Whitehouse et al[8] reported that the density of presynaptic nicotinic cholinergic receptors were decreased in PDD patients postmortem. Nicotine stimulates the release of acetylcholine in the cerebral cortex. The nucleus basilis is the principal source of extrinsic cholinergic innervation of the cortex and has the highest reported concentration of nicotinic binding sites. Thus, degeneration of this nucleus in PDD can result in the reduction of cholinergic transmission to the cortex and to other neuronal systems. The loss of presynaptic $M_2$ and nicotinic receptors, as well as to a lesser degree $M_1$ receptors, can result in a severely dysregulated system.

### *Serotonergic System*

The serotonergic nuclei in the raphe system demonstrate degeneration with numerous neurofibrillary tangles (>50%) present.[7] A decline in the density of serotonin type 2 ($S_2$) receptors in various CNS regions measured by PET correlated with age. Postmortem PDD samples ($N = 12$) demonstrated a significantly increased loss of serotonin receptors ($S_1$ and $S_2$) in the cortex, hippocampus, and amygdala compared with age-matched controls ($N = 13$).[17] Additionally, the loss of $S_1$ receptors was progressive and significantly age related in PDD. Significant dysfunction resulting from $S_1$ receptor depletion might not occur until later stages of PDD. In contrast, $S_2$ receptor losses were 35% greater in the temporal cortex as compared with $S_1$ and not age related. Therefore, the reduction of $S_2$ receptors in PDD may represent a relatively early specific change in the disease process. Rossor et al[18] also measured serotonergic activity in PDD patients (N = 49) postmortem versus control patients ($N = 54$). In contrast with the older, later-onset patients, significant reductions in $S_2$ receptors of "younger" patients was observed.[19] Loss of $S_2$ receptors might indicate the presence of a more severe form of PDD.

These findings are significant when the role of the indoleamine system in CNS function is examined. Stimulation of $S_1$ receptors causes inhibition of neurotransmitter release and contraction of arterial systems.[20] $S_2$ functions include regulation of microcirculation, permeability, and inflammatory processes. Vasoconstriction in superficial, coronary, splanchnic and cerebral blood vessels in man and in other species may be mediated by $S_2$ receptors.[21]

### *Noradrenergic System*

Adrenergic nuclei in the locus ceruleus play a major role in information processing, including adjustment of signal-to-noise ratio, amplification, and intensification of afferent inputs, and alter stress and anxiety tolerance. Noradrenergic nuclei in the locus ceruleus may demonstrate significant neuronal loss in PDD but neurofibrillary tangles rarely appear.[7] Hence, pharmacotherapy to augment the serotonergic or adrenergic systems might enhance function despite the deterioration in the cholinergic system.

### *Other Systems*

Somatostatin (ST), a neuropeptide transmitter, is found in the cerebral cortex and hippocampus. In PDD and Down's syndrome patients, ST concentrations and receptors are decreased to a similar extent as choline acetyltransferase.[4,6,22] The loss of ST receptors appears to correlate with the loss of $S_2$ receptors. Although causality cannot be determined, these two receptor systems demonstrate early changes in the disease.[17,18]

Decreases in observed dopamine type 2 receptor density by PET scan in PDD might be caused either by nonspecific age-related changes or by neuronal atrophy secondary to reduced cholinergic outflow.[13] The interrelationships between serotonergic and dopaminergic systems also form an area of ongoing research.

Investigators have recently focused on the interrelationship of trophic factors such as nerve growth factor (NGF) and choline acetyltransferase activity.[23] Initial evidence, in animals, suggests that hippocampal extracts with high concentrations of NGF augment the cholinergic system. A potential for brain grafting (limited transplantation of nuclei) in humans has also been suggested.

The interrelationships and the roles of nicotinic, muscarinic ($M_1$ and $M_2$), serotonergic ($S_1$ and $S_2$), dopaminergic ($D_2$), and somatostatin transmitter systems in specific CNS areas (i.e., hippocampus, entorhinal cortex) require further research. The combination of pharmacologic challenge techniques and neuroimaging can provide clues into the process of PDD. PDD cholinergic dysfunction and the role of acetylcholine in memory and cognitive functions in humans suggest a useful model for drug development; however, the validity of extrapolating pharmacologic studies in animals, normal persons, or the elderly to patients with PDD is not substantiated. The specific changes in brain pathophysiology, and the resultant neuropharmacologic and receptor alterations, in patients with PDD provide clues to their rational treatment. Many investigational therapies attempt to restore normal brain activity by augmenting function of damaged CNS nuclei or neurotransmitter systems.

## Clinical Presentation

### *Dementia*

Target symptoms commonly observed in dementia and definitions of terminology are listed in Table 46.2.[2] The initial clinical presentation of PDD is subtle and insidious in onset. Often, the first symptoms of an insidious dementia, noticed by others, are the behavioral reactions caused by the patient's awareness of their deterioration. With disease progression, clear-cut changes in orientation (to time and place) and short-term memory become apparent. Occasional forgetfulness can evolve into a complete inability to care for one's self (e.g., not turning off stove, not eating or performing simple hygiene). The patient might begin to demonstrate increased irritability and sensitivity to psychosocial and environmental stress. Mood and affective expression can become extremely labile, rapidly changing from moment to moment. Typical reactive psychologic responses such as denial, anger, anxiety, and depression are likely to occur. With continued deterioration, the patient becomes totally dependent upon the environment for orienting cues. PDD patients typically demonstrate "sundowner's syndrome," meaning that their symptoms worsen at night because of decreased sensory input and orienting stimulation.

**Table 46.2** Target Symptoms of Dementia

| | |
|---|---|
| **Primary Features: "JOMAC"** | |
| Poor Judgment | |
| DisOrientation to time and place | |
| Immediate and short-term Memory impairment | |
| Affective or personality changes | |
| Cognitive impairment including: | |
| Decreased abstraction (inability to understand nonliteral meanings) | Aphasia (impairment in speech) |
| Apraxia (impairment in motor function) | Agnosia/anomia (impairment in recognition and naming) |
| | Perceptual–spatial difficulties |
| **Additional Features and Secondary Responses** | |
| Poor self-care skills | |
| Insomnia | Anxiety |
| Agitation | Psychosis |
| Hypochondriasis | Confusion |
| Depression | Distractability |

Cognitive or intellectual processes gradually deteriorate. Problem-solving skills, memory, abstracting ability, insight, and judgment are reduced. Initially, only immediate recall and short-term memory are affected. Patients confabulate to compensate for memory lapses, for example, claim to have met someone previously and "know" their name. Memory disturbances can also lead to management problems; for example, 1 hour after breakfast, the patient claims not to have eaten. Over time, disease progression can cause severe long-term memory disturbances illustrated by the patient's inability to recognize family members or friends. The presentation can be extremely difficult to monitor objectively. Fluctuations over time and the subjective nature of the findings suggest that systematic assessment tools designed to quantitate the measurement of cognitive and behavioral function can be clinically useful. See Table 46.3 and Figure 46.3 for a list of psychopathometric assessment tools and a list of frequently used questions. Disturbances occur in motor performance and expression including aphasia, anomia, and apraxia. Visual–spatial perceptions, hand–eye coordination, balance, communication skills, and cognitive functions begin to deteriorate while insight is preserved.

**Table 46.3** Neuropsychiatric Rating Scales for Assessment of PPD

| |
|---|
| Dementia Rating Scale |
| Mental Status Check List |
| Mental Test Score (MTS) |
| Plutchik Geriatric Rating Scale (Plut) |
| Stockton Geriatric Rating Scale (SGRS) |
| Geriatric Mental State Schedule (GMS) |
| Short Portable Mental Status Questionnaire |
| Sandoz Clinical Assessment—Geriatric (SCAG) |
| Multidimensional Assessment of Dementia (MAD) |
| Crichton Geriatric Behaviour Rating Scale (CGBRS) |
| Comprehensive Assessment and Referral Evaluation (CARE) |
| Mattis Organic Mental Syndrome Screening Examination (MOMSSE) |

### *Delirium*

In contrast to dementia, delirium presents as an acute change in cognitive function usually as the result of a medical or toxicologic process.[2] The reactive psychologic response to the impaired functional capabilities of the individual are absent. Perceptual disturbances are common and the individual cannot maintain a coherent stream of thought. Sleep disturbance (insomnia or hypersomnolence) and altered psychomotor activity are evident. Patients are disoriented, confused, or incoherent and can be extremely labile in their behavior and mood. Memory, speech, concentration, attention span, and complex cognitive processes (abstraction, mathematics, judgment) are impaired. Agitation, anxiety, tension, and combativeness occur secondary to the disorientation and confusion.

A fluctuating course for the clinical presentation parallels the etiologic disturbance. Dramatic and rapid resolution of the delirium occur once the underlying cause is resolved. Chronic illness with periodic exacerbations such as endocrine disturbances or episodic alcohol intoxication can lead to repeated episodes of delirium with spontaneous mental clearing.

## Diagnosis

Primary degenerative dementia is a diagnosis of exclusion.[1] Dementia and delirium of specific etiology have many possible causes (Table 46.4); however, most cases

**Figure 46.3** Mini-mental state exam.

| Maximum Score | Score | |
|---|---|---|
| | | **Orientation** |
| 5 | ( ) | What is the (year) (season) (date) (day) (month)? |
| 5 | ( ) | Where are we: (state) (country) (town) (hospital) (floor) (or street) (or address) |
| | | **Registration** |
| 3 | ( ) | Name three objects: 1 second to say each. Then ask the patient all three after you have said them. Give 1 point for each correct answer. Then repeat them until the patient learns all three. Count trials and record. |
| | | Number of trials________ |
| | | **Attention and Calculation** |
| 5 | ( ) | Serial 7s. (1 point for each correct) Stop after five answers. Alternatively, spell "world" backward. |
| | | **Recall** |
| 3 | ( ) | Ask for the three objects repeated above. Give 1 point for each correct answer. |
| | | **Language** |
| 9 | ( ) | Name, a pencil, and watch. (2 points) Repeat the following: "No ifs, ands, or buts." (1 point) |
| | | Follow a three stage command: "Take a paper in your right hand, fold it in half, and put it on the floor." (3 points) Read and obey the following: |
| | | Close your eyes (1 point) |
| | | Write a sentence (1 point) |
| | | Copy design (1 point) |
| 30 | ____ | Total score |
| | | Assess level of consciousness along a continuum |
| | | Alert — Drowsy — Stupor — Coma |

**Table 46.4** Causes of Dementia and Delirium With Specific Etiologies[a]

| | |
|---|---|
| Degenerative brain diseases | Medications |
| Pick's disease | Antihypertensives |
| Huntington's disease | β-Blockers |
| Parkinson's disease | Methyldopa |
| Multiple sclerosis | Guanethidine |
| | Reserpine |
| Infections | Antiparkinsonian agents |
| Acute/chronic encephalitis | L-Dopa |
| Herpes simplex encephalitis | Anticholinergics |
| Syphilis (paralysie generale) | Digitalis glycosides |
| Creutzfeldt–Jakob disease | Psychotropics |
| Acquired immune deficiency[b] | Antidepressants |
| | Antipsychotics |
| Exogenous toxins | Lithium |
| Alcoholic dementia | Sedative–hypnotics |
| Wernicke–Korsakoff syndrome | |
| Organic solvents | Metabolic/nutritional |
| CNS anticholinergic syndrome | Uremia, dialysis |
| Wilson's disease | Hepatic failure |
| Alcohol intoxication | Secondary to carcinoma debilitation |
| | $B_{12}$ deficiency |
| Increased intraventricular pressure–hydrocephalus | Hyperlipidemia |
| Hydrocephalic dementia (NPH) | Malnutrition |
| | |
| | Head injury |
| Anoxia | Epilepsy |
| | Trauma |
| Cerebrovascular disorders | |
| Binswanger's disease | Down's syndrome |
| Hypertensive vascular encephalopathy | |
| Systemic lupus erythematosus | |

[a] Excludes PDD or Alzheimer's disease and multi-infarct dementia.
[b] AIDS may become a common source of dementia based upon recent findings.

are linked to central nervous system degenerative diseases such as Alzheimer's or cardiovascular disease.[3] Recently, acquired immune deficiency syndrome (AIDS) has also been reported to be a source of dementia, with approximately 60% of AIDS patients eventually developing dementia.[24,25]

### *Dementia*

Degenerative dementia occurs in approximately 30% of Down's syndrome patients. These patients (almost 100%) develop the neuropathologic changes of PDD by their third decade.[12,14] Therefore, an increased risk for Down's syndrome is suggested in families with a high incidence of PDD. Because of overlapping neuropathologic and neurochemical findings in PDD and Down's syndrome, Down's syndrome can provide a useful model for studying PDD disease processes and has led to the identification of a genetic marker.[14]

Although autopsy has demonstrated the presence of neurofibrillary tangles and neuritic plaques in the cerebral cortex, no peripheral biochemical laboratory test for PDD has been developed.[4] Therefore, a definitive diagnosis is made only upon histological tests obtained from autopsy. The capability of correctly diagnosing PDD has greatly improved from a 10% to 50% error rate to an approximate 90% specificity.[4,5,12,26] A complete evaluation for dementia should include both medical and neuropsychologic assessments (Tables 46.3 and 46.5). This can assist in identifying treatable diseases as well as facilitating an accurate identification of patients with PDD.[7] Improved neuroimaging techniques such as PET and magnetic resonance imaging (MRI) can provide an earlier diagnostic assessment. MRI can detect CNS morphologic lesions with greater resolution than computerized axial tomography (CAT) scans, while PET can quantitate changes in receptor density.

PDD may represent several different biologically distinct diseases.[27] Chui et al[27] compared the age of onset, presence of aphasia, and family history in 146 individuals with PDD. Early onset was significantly associated with more severe language impairment. A positive family history of dementia was found for 45% of the population. The duration of illness and presence of myoclonus and noniatrogenic extrapyramidal disorders were associated with a greater severity of symptoms. Advanced age of the mother at birth and history of head injury were also possible risk factors.[5] Further research of the epidemiologic, genetic, and biochemical parameters is needed to improve the clinician's ability to diagnose PDD.

### *Delirium*

The diagnostic criteria for delirium include clouding of consciousness with reduced capacity to shift, focus, and sustain attention to environmental stimuli.[2] Disorientation

**Table 46.5** Evaluations and Assessments for a Dementia/Delirium Workup[a]

Complete patient history (including family)
Physical examination and vital signs
Neuropsychologic assessment
Chest and skull x-rays, if indicated
Laboratory tests, including serum folate, $B_{12}$, electrolytes, thyroid including TSH, hepatic enzymes, creatinine, glucose, complete blood count, urinalysis
Heavy metal urine screen; if positive, follow-up with blood analysis
Toxicity drug screen including sedatives and bromides
Neuroimaging techniques (i.e., PET, CAT, or MRI), if indicated
Blood, urine, or CSF cultures, if indicated
VDRL, HIV (AIDS screen)
Electroencephalograph, if indicated

[a] TSH, thyroid-stimulating hormone; PET, positron emission tomography; CAT, computerized axial tomography; MRI, magnetic resonance imaging; CSF, cerebrospinal fluid.

and memory disturbances are prominent. Clinical features develop over a short period of time, usually hours to days, and fluctuate over the course of a day. Evidence from history, physical examination, and laboratory tests for a specific etiology related to the disturbance should be found. Behavioral manifestations include perceptual disturbance including misinterpretations, illusion, or hallucinations; incoherent speech; disturbance in sleep–wake cycle; and changes in psychomotor activity level from baseline.

### *Differential Diagnosis*

The differential diagnosis of PDD from other psychiatric, neurologic, and medical causes is essential. The prognosis of PDD is poor and the course of illness is usually downhill with progressive loss of mental capacity and function. Table 46.4 lists possible causes for dementia and delirium with specific etiologies that must be identified or excluded prior to the diagnosis of PDD. Table 46.5 lists the minimum workup usually employed to rule out frequent causes of dementia and delirium. Although beyond the scope of this chapter, the DSM-III-R divides organic mental syndromes and disorders into four groups: delirium, dementia, organic syndromes, and amnestic syndrome.[2]

In contrast to delirium or to other reversible organic mental syndromes, neuroanatomic destruction of CNS nuclei projecting to the cortex occur in PDD. Imaging techniques play an important role in the differential diagnosis of the organic brain disorders. Thorough medical and drug histories, including detailed information regarding the course and progression of the organic disturbance, are essential to the differential diagnostic process. Finally, a complete family history should be obtained, checking for the presence of Down's syndrome or Alzheimer's disease.[14]

In assessing nonspecific behavioral and cognitive target symptoms in patients, a careful differential diagnosis of PDD, delirium, and depressive illness is essential. Depressed individuals can manifest cognitive disturbances that appear to be indistinguishable from "true" dementias. Table 46.6 lists the differences in clinical presentation among dementia, delirium, and depression. A therapeutic trial of an antidepressant or lithium in the depressed patient with "pseudodementia" may reverse the symptoms of the illness and restore the individual's functional capacity. As PDD is a diagnosis of exclusion, a trial of antidepressants is indicated in those patients demonstrating target symptoms consistent with depression, or in those with a positive family or personal history for mood (affective) disorders. Patients with PDD who have locus ceruleus atrophy might also benefit from antidepressant therapy because of its adrenergic augmentation.

## Treatment

The changes in brain pathophysiology, and the resultant neuropharmacologic and receptor alterations, provide clues to the rational treatment of the patient with PDD. Many

**Table 46.6** Differentiating Dementia, Delirium, and Depression

| *Feature* | *Dementia* | *Depression* | *Delirium* |
|---|---|---|---|
| Onset | Unclear, insidious | Clear, recent, often follows a loss | Clear, within hours to days |
| Progression | Relatively stable | Uneven, often no progression | Fluctuation |
| Duration | Long-term; years | Intermediate; months | Short; 1 week |
| Aware of deficits | Often, early on | Usually | Rarely |
| Distressed by deficits | Occasionally | Often | Rarely |
| Affect | Bland, with lability | Appropriate to mood or "masked" | Marked disturbance, lability |
| Test performance | | | |
| Cooperation | Good | Poor | Poor |
| Effort | Good | Poor | Poor |
| Achievement | Deteriorates over time | Variable | Poor |
| Test anxiety | Little | Considerable | Little |
| Responses | Near misses | "Don't know" | Inattention |
| Short-term memory | Often impaired | Selectively impaired | Globally impaired |
| Long-term memory | Unimpaired early in disease | Selectively impaired | Impaired |

investigational therapies attempt to restore normal brain activity by augmenting function of damaged CNS nuclei or neurotransmitter systems. Disease heterogeneity confounds both pathophysiologic and therapeutic research. Whitehouse[23] indicated that the ratio of neuritic plaques to neurofibrillary tangles, as well as the involvement (or not) of the locus ceruleus, can be viable methods of subtyping PDD. The effects of "nonspecific" aging on cognitive functions and memory versus the degenerative changes in PDD are not well defined, thus limiting drug development.

The neuropharmacologic alterations in PDD are the result of a complex interplay of changes in multiple neurochemical systems and their associated receptors. Hence, pharmacotherapy directed toward a single deficit might be only partially effective. Once morphologic changes and atrophy of neurons and cytoskeletal structures occur, pharmacotherapy might be ineffective because of the loss of function within the system affected by the drug.

Pharmacologic therapy for PDD continues to be for the most part empiric. Many drug therapies for PDD currently employed, as well as those in various stages of preclinical and phase I–III evaluation, are based on the evolving understanding of the pathogenesis and neurochemical consequences of this disease. Drug treatment aimed at reversing or retarding the progression of PDD has been disappointing. Table 46.3 lists standardized assessment tools used to quantitate memory, attention span, visual–spatial perceptions, cognition, and abstraction capabilities. These rating scales are essential instruments in evaluating drug therapy. The patient with PDD will have a variable presentation over time and these assessments can help to ensure reproducible findings during the course of longitudinal drug therapy.

### *Behavioral Intervention*

Generally, nonpharmacologic interventions are used initially to treat demented patients. These include environmental manipulations that provide stability, decrease confusion, and minimize change in daily routines, to allow the patient to use remaining skills.[28,29] Because of the progressive nature of this disease, environmental manipulation eventually becomes inadequate and drug therapy is usually needed for symptomatic control. In the mildly to moderately impaired patient, simple reminders such as written notes pasted to medicine cabinets or refrigerator doors serve to increase the individual's function. An orienting environment, without excessive stimulation or activity, should be provided for the patient. A calendar with the current date identified, availability of a radio and television, as well as pictures of family members can help maintain orientation and function. Valuables should not be available to the patient if he or she misplaces items or gives them away; however, personal belongings and items of symbolic importance should be kept in the patient's bedroom and daytime environment. At night, sensory information (e.g., visualization of their surroundings, calendar, pictures, presence of other people) is diminished. If the patient demonstrates clear-cut worsening of behavior at night, then a night lamp should be provided, a radio should be allowed to be kept on at low volume, and a night stand with a light and personal objects of the patient should be within easy reach. This "sundowner's syndrome" can lead to sufficient disorientation that the patient will wander throughout the house or onto the streets. Outside doors should be locked, and safety gates placed to prevent the patient from inadvertently falling down stairs. Repeated verbal reminders should be provided regarding the dangers of wandering at night. If doors need to be locked, than a family member or caretaker should be present in case of emergency or fire.

As the illness progresses, environmental cues will not be sufficient to maintain normal behavior and self-care skills. If the patient remains at home, a caretaker may be needed. Supervision in the kitchen or bathroom may become necessary. Family members must be prepared for the inappropriate behavior of the PDD patient. Lability with intermittent hostility, anger, tearfulness, and dysphoria are seen. The patient's condition can deteriorate, leading to frustration for all involved. Simple short directions must be provided to the patient. Family expectations must be realigned as the patient's functional status diminishes. Eventually, motor and cognitive functions deteriorate, leading to the need for supplemental nursing care.

Prior to placement of the patient into a skilled nursing facility, community-based support services should be pursued. Support groups for the immediate family members can facilitate a better understanding of the available home care–oriented alternatives to the "nursing home." These groups also provide the family with needed psychosocial support. Home day-care services are also often times available for the demented patient who cannot be cared for by a family member. For the mildly to moderately impaired patient, community day-care centers that provide transportation to and from the home are another valuable alternative to the skilled nursing facility.

### *Specific Pharmacotherapy*

Many pharmacologically diverse agents have been studied in the treatment of PDD and memory dysfunction including anabolic steroids, anticoagulants, ergot alkaloids, CNS stimulants and depressants, and vasodilators (Table 46.7).[30] Four classes of pharmacologic agents (cholinomimetic agents, neuropeptides, nootropics, opioid antagonists) have shown the most promise and are discussed here. An overview of nonspecific adjunctive drug therapies is also provided.

#### **Cholinergic Enhancement**

PDD is characterized by a deficiency in the enzyme choline acetyltransferase.[31] Therefore, a major emphasis in the treatment of PDD is enhancement of cholinergic function. Three types of pharmacologic agents have been used to stimulate cholinergic activity: (1) agents that increase acetylcholine (ACH) production in the presynaptic neuron (ACH precursors), (2) agents that inhibit the breakdown of ACH (cholinesterase inhibitors), and (3) agents that directly stimulate cholinergic receptors (cholinomimetic agents). See Figure 46.2 for the potential sites of action for cholinergic agents.[32] The effectiveness of these cholinergic agents is determined largely by drug, dose, age of patient, type of memory function assessed, and degree of cholinergic receptor degeneration.[30,33] Table 46.8 lists cholinergic facilitating agents and their known pharmacokinetic and pharmacodynamic characteristics.

**Table 46.7** Drugs Used for the Treatment of PPD and Memory Dysfunction

| | | |
|---|---|---|
| Cholinergic drugs | Psychotropics[a] | Neuromodulators/$Ca^{2+}$ transport |
| Physostigmine | Antipsychotics | Guanidine |
| Arecoline | Antidepressants | 4-Aminopyridine |
| Oxotremorine | Anxiolytics | 3,4-Diaminopyridine |
| Tetrahydroaminoacridine | Sedative–hypnotics | |
| Bethanechol | | Neuropeptides |
| Acetylcholine precursors | Nootropics | ACTH |
| Choline | Piracetam | Vasopressin |
| Lecithin | Oxiracetam | Desmopressin |
| Deanol | Pramiracetam | RNA |
| | Vincamine | |
| Vasodilators | Meclofenoxate | CNS stimulants |
| Hyperbaric oxygen | Pyrithioxine | Amphetamines |
| Papaverine | | Methylphenidate |
| Isoxsuprine | Opioid Antagonists | Magnesium pemoline |
| Nicotinic acid | Naloxone | Pentylenetetrazol |
| Carbon dioxide | Naltrexone | |
| Cyclandelate | | |
| Nylidrine | | |
| Naftidrofuryl or nafronyl | | |
| Ergoloid mesylates | | |
| Anticoagulants | | |

[a] Nonspecific therapies.

### Acetylcholine Precursors

Choline and lecithin are naturally occurring dietary amino acids, available as food supplements without a prescription, that are precursors for the synthesis of ACH. Phosphatidylcholine is the principal ingredient in lecithin and is metabolized into choline. Deanol (2-dimethylaminoethanol), no longer marketed in the United States, is another acetylcholine precursor that is methylated in the liver to choline.[29] Large amounts of these precursors can, under some conditions, increase brain ACH concentrations[32]; however, large doses are required (e.g., choline >16 g/d, lecithin 20–100 g/d, deanol 300–1,800 mg/d). Doses of this size are often difficult for patients to tolerate; therefore low initial doses (choline 4 g/d, lecithin 10 g/d, and deanol 300 mg/d) followed by slow titration on a weekly basis are recommended. More palatable sources of choline and lecithin (e.g., as chicken noodle soup with high lecithin-content noodles and milk shakes of lecithin solubilized in ethanol) should be considered to improve patient acceptability. Pharmaceutical-grade lecithin containing 90% or greater phosphatidylcholine should be

**Table 46.8** Pharmacodynamics and Kinetics of Cholinergic Facilitating Agents

| *Drug* | *Oral absorption rate*[a] | *CNS penetration* | *Elimination half-life (min)* | *Lipophilic* | *Muscarinic* | *Nicotinic* | *Ganglionic* |
|---|---|---|---|---|---|---|---|
| Choline | ++ | Moderate | | Yes | Yes[b] | Yes[b] | Yes[b] |
| Lecithin | + | Moderate | | Yes | Yes[b] | Yes[b] | Yes[b] |
| Deanol | + | Low to moderate | | Yes | Yes[b] | Yes[b] | Yes[b] |
| Physostigmine | +++[c] | High | 15–40 | Yes | Yes[b] | Yes[b] | Yes[b] |
| Tetrahydroaminoacridine | ++ | High | [d] | Yes | Yes[b] | Yes[b] | Yes[b] |
| Arecoline | ++ | High | 30 | | ++ | | |
| Oxotremorine | | High | 13–43[e] | | ++++ | 0/+ | +[f] |
| Bethanechol | ++ | Poor | | No | ++ | | |

[a] +, Slow absorption; ++, moderate absorption; +++, rapid absorption.
[b] Nonspecific augmentation of all cholinergic transmission.
[c] Absorption variable.
[d] Longer duration of action than physostigmine.
[e] Longer duration of action than arecoline.
[f] High doses.

utilized to minimize calorie load and to increase reproducibility of results. Oral choline is metabolized by intestinal bacteria to trimethylamine, a highly volatile amine excreted in urine, breath, and sweat that produces a fishy odor. Lecithin is preferred, as it does not produce this characteristic odor and yields a more sustained level of free choline in the serum.[34]

The results of most studies show little or no benefit in memory enhancement (Table 46.9). Possible explanations for these negative results are listed in Table 46.10 along with observed adverse reactions to cholinergic agents.[29]

The brain processes and transmits information between nuclei by synaptic transmission. A neuronal "message or signal" comprises both the action potential and the release of discrete quanta of neurotransmitter into the synaptic cleft. The rate of firing of the neuron, as well as the amplitude of the signal, conveys stimulus-specific information. Conduction of an action potential leading to neuronal firing is a prerequisite for successful precursor loading therapy. Assuming that precursor is appropriately utilized by the presynaptic neuron, synthesis to neurotransmitter can only intensify the signal strength resulting from neuronal firing. Precursor therapy does not reverse defects in neuronal responsiveness, activity, or firing rates.

Additionally, the degree to which the synthesis of ACH is

**Table 46.9** Preliminary Reports of Cholinergic Treatment in Patients With PDD, Alzheimer Type

| *Reference* | *Number of patients* | *Age* | *Severity of Alzheimer's* | *Treatment* | *Results* |
|---|---|---|---|---|---|
| Lancet 1977;1:711 | 7 | 70–80 | Severe | Choline PO (5–10 g/d) | Less irritable |
| Lancet 1978;1:508 | 3 | 76–88 | Severe | Choline PO (10 g/d) | No benefit |
| Lancet 1978;2:318 | 10 | 77[a] | — | Choline PO (9 g/d) | No benefit |
| Lancet 1978;2:837 | 8 | 59–78 | Mild | Choline PO (9 g/d) | Slightly improved memory |
| Lancet 1979;1:42 | 1 | 42 | Moderate | Physostigmine IV (1 mg) | Decreased intrusion errors |
| Choline and Lecithin in Brain Disorders, New York, Raven, 1979 | 7 | 42–81 | Moderate | Lecithin PO (25–100 g/d) | Improved associate learning |
| Choline and Lecithin in Brain Disorders, New York, Raven, 1979 | 10 | <65 | Mild to severe | Choline PO (5 g/day) and lecithin (28–100 g/d) | No improvement; deterioration possibly slowed |
| N Engl J Med 1979;31:330 | 18 | 73.2 | — | Choline PO (15 g/d) | No change |
| Science 1979;205:1039 | 14 | — | Mild to moderate | Choline PO (12–20 g/d) | No change |
| Br J Psychiatry 1981;138:46–50 | 11 | — | Mild to moderate | Physostigmine IV (0.25–1 mg) | Slight improvement in picture recognition in 9; clear-cut improvement in 2 |
| Br J Psychiatry 1981;138:46–50 | 7 | — | Mild to moderate | Arecoline PO (4 mg) | Slight improvement in picture recognition |
| J Am Geriatr Soc 1977;25:241 | 14 | 62–80 | Mild to severe | Deanol PO (1.8 g/d) | No change in memory; behaviorally improved |
| Am J Psychiatry 1979;136:1275 | 8 | 64–86 | Mild to moderate | Choline PO (16 g/d) | No change in memory |
| J Gerontol 1982;37:4–9 | 10 | 54–73 | Mild to moderate | Lecithin 53% PO (35 g/d) | No benefit |
| Psychopharm Bull 1983;19:454 | 12 | — | "Early" | Lecithin PO (10.8 g/d) and physostigmine IV (12–15 mg/d) | Improved recall and retrieval; decreased intrusions |
| N Engl J Med 1981;304:1490 | 10 | — | Mild to moderate | Choline PO (9 g/d) and piracetam PO (4.8 g/d) | Marked cognitive improvement in 3 |
| Psychopharm Bull 1984;20:542 | 11 | 67.1[a] | — | Lecithin PO (35 g/d) and piracetam PO (4.8 g/d) | Marked improvement in total recall (73%) |

[a] Average age.

**Table 46.10** Limitations of Cholinergic Precursor Augmentation

| | | |
|---|---|---|
| I. | Cholinergic adverse effects limit dosage[29] | |
| | Muscarinic | Nicotinic |
| | Bronchoconstriction | Muscular fasciculations followed by weakness |
| | Excessive respiratory tract secretions | |
| | Sweating | |
| | Salivation | CNS |
| | Lacrimation | Restlessness |
| | Miosis with spasm of accommodation | Anxiety |
| | Bradycardia | Insomnia |
| | Hypotension | Tremors |
| | Urinary incontinence | Convulsions |
| | Gastrointestinal spasms | Respiratory depression |
| | | Circulatory collapse |
| II. | Receptor desensitization with extended therapy[29] | |
| III. | Loss of ACH neurons capable of producing neurotransmitter[29] | |
| IV. | Inability to facilitate physiologic release of ACH into synapse[29] | |
| V. | Peripherally administered precursors may not enhance central activity[29] | |
| VI. | Increase in brain ACH content does not restore normal central cholinergic activity[35] | |
| VII. | Precursors might increase ACH in selected nuclei, for example, corpus striatum, and not in ACH nuclei modulating memory and cognition[35] | |
| VIII. | Marked reductions in choline acetyltransferase activity are observed, preventing precursor loading from being effective[31] | |

facilitated by precursor loading depends upon the firing rate of the cholinergic neuron. ACH synthesis in cholinergic nerve terminals appears to be directly linked to choline uptake via a sodium-dependent high-affinity transport system that is almost completely saturated under normal conditions. Because under normal conditions the system is completely saturated, this high-affinity uptake process is the rate-limiting step in synthesis of ACH. It requires an increase in neuronal activity to stimulate a secondary low-affinity uptake system to transport the additional choline necessary for ACH synthesis. Choline pretreatment facilitates ACH synthesis only when there is a normal or increased firing rate of the neuron.

Precursor therapy has no effect on firing rate; however, piracetam has generated interest as a potential enhancer of neuronal metabolic activity including firing rate.[32] While the precise mechanism of its effect is unclear, the combination of choline and piracetam has demonstrated significant improvement in some patients (Table 46.10).[35] This improvement appears to be dependent on high intracellular choline concentrations.[36] The combination of lecithin plus piracetam has also resulted in increased therapeutic effect; 73% (8/11) of the PDD patients improved in total recall compared with patients administered placebo in a double-blind, crossover study.[37]

Guanidine (a nucleic acid derivative), 4-aminopyridine, and 3,4-diaminopyridine also have potential for facilitating neuronal utilization of exogenously administered precursors. These investigational compounds stimulate the presynaptic release of ACH and its synthesis. Their mechanism of action is thought to be the facilitation of calcium influx which increases the amount of transmitter released per nerve impulse. Combination of these facilitators of neuronal calcium uptake with precursor might be useful.[32]

**Cholinesterase Inhibitors**

The treatment of PDD with ACH precursors alone or in conjunction with neuronal enhancers is dependent on presynaptic mechanisms. Although ACH esterase inhibitors do not require the presence of an intact presynaptic neuron to augment the synaptic concentrations of ACH, the decline in viable cholinergic neurons is still a major limiting factor. Cholinesterase inhibitors, such as physostigmine (Antilirum) or tetrahydroaminoacridine and diisofluorophosphate (two investigational agents), enhance the cholinergic system by blocking the degradation of ACH in the synapse.

Physostigmine, a tertiary amine with good blood–brain barrier penetration, produces a reversible cholinesterase inhibition. Studies utilizing physostigmine have produced controversial results. Those that demonstrate benefit often produce transient, modest improvement of questionable significance (Tables 46.9 and 46.11). Interpretation of studies utilizing physostigmine is made difficult by many factors. First, all cholinesterase inhibitors are most effective in early stages of PDD, when cholinergic neurons are intact. Second, this early phase of the disease is diagnostically the least precise, occurring when identifying patients for clinical evaluation is the greatest. Third, variability in study design and testing measures further hinder comparative analysis between studies. Last, the required physostigmine dosage varies widely between individuals.[29] There appears to be a biphasic dose–response relationship (i.e., low doses of physostigmine may improve some aspects of memory while higher doses can impair all aspects of memory).[30] Therefore, the best designed studies incorporate a two-phase trial (DF/R = dose finding and ranging) in which the determination of the optimum therapeutic dose precedes the evaluation of patient performance on that drug (Tables 46.9 and

**Table 46.11** Oral Physostigmine Studies

| *Reference* | *Study design*[a] | *Number of patients* | *Age* | *Dose (mg/d)* | *Severity of Alzheimer's* | *Results* |
|---|---|---|---|---|---|---|
| Psychopharmacol Bull 1983;19:451–453 | WO, R, DB, DF/R, PC | 13 | 54–65 | 1.75–14.0 | Not supplied | Memory improvement in 3/4 with AD,[b] 6/8 without AD (?significance) |
| Psychopharmacology 1985;87:147–151 | DB, CO, R, PC | 8 | 58–83 | 3.5–14.0 | Moderate to severe | Improvement in short-term memory $P = 0.001$ at 14 mg/d |
| Psychopharmacol Bull 1986;22:101–105 | DF/R, PC | 12 | — | 3.5–14.0 | Not supplied | Memory improved 7/12 initially; 4/12 clinically consistent improvement |
| Int J Neurosci 1983;18:143–148 | R | 8 | — | $X^c$=3.75 mg per dose $X^c$=0.75 mg per dose | Not supplied | Slight behavior modification; memory nonsignificant change |
| N Engl J Med 1983;308:720 | DB, CO, PC, DF/R | 8 | — | 6.0–15.0 + lecithin 10.8 g/d | "Early" | 8/8 improvement in total recall and retrieval, $P<0.01$ |

[a] PC, placebo-controlled; CO, crossover; DB, double-blind; R, randomized; WO, washout, DF/R, two-step dose ranging.
[b] AD, Alzheimer's disease.
[c] *X*, mean dose.

46.11). Other methodologic difficulties include physostigmine's short duration of action (<1 hour), requiring multiple daily doses, and its high incidence of peripheral cholinergic side effects (nausea, vomiting, and diaphoresis), necessitating simultaneous administration of a quaternary anticholinergic agent.[29]

An alternative to physostigmine is tetrahydroaminoacridine (THA). THA is an investigational centrally acting anticholinesterase available in parenteral and oral preparations. It has a longer duration of action and fewer peripheral side effects than oral physostigmine. Summers and colleagues[38] administered intravenous THA (0.25–1.5 mg/kg) to 12 patients with a mean age of 72.25 years (range 42–85) with moderate to severe PDD. Moderately demented but not severely demented patients demonstrated improvement on orientation questions and global rating scales. Improved performance on memory tasks has also been seen in aged monkeys.

**Cholinomimetic Agents**

ACH precursors and acetylcholinesterase inhibitors share a common limitation: they are dependent on an intact presynaptic neuron to provide a substrate for their activity. This limited efficacy of presynaptic-dependent agents might be circumvented by administering cholinergic agonists (e.g., arecoline, pilocarpine, and oxotremorine) that work directly at postsynaptic receptor sites (investigational for systemic use). Postsynaptic receptor sites may be less severely affected by the disease process (Fig. 46.1). Although arecoline has enhanced learning in young adults and improved cognition in a small number of Alzheimer's patients, its rapid enzymatic hydrolysis results in a half-life too short for effective clinical application.[30,32] Systemic administration produces a high incidence of peripheral side effects.[29] Oxotremorine, a longer acting muscarinic agent, has produced consistent improvement in memory in aged monkeys.[39]

Bethanechol chloride (Urecholine), a pure muscarinic agonist in doses of 0.05–0.7 mg, has been administered intracranially via an implantable continuous infusion pump directly into the ventricular system, bypassing bioavailability problems. The pharmacologic properties of this agent (polar, water soluble) make it suitable for this route of administration, as it does not cross the blood–brain barrier into the periphery when infused into the ventricular system. Preliminary results indicate decreased confusion, increased initiative, and improvement in activities of daily living, without subjective or objective improvement in short-term memory. Complications in 40 patients have included infection ($n = 1$), hemorrhage ($n = 2$), and reversible neurotoxicity ($n = 2$).[40]

Despite the substantial data supporting cholinergic deficits in the pathophysiology of memory dysfunction and PDD, the inconsistent treatment results for cholinomimetics are not surprising if underlying assumptions are considered. One implicit assumption is that the function of muscarinic ($M_1$ and $M_2$) and nicotinic receptors remains normal in PDD. $M_1$ receptors are postsynaptic, and facilitate cellular excitation. $M_2$ receptors are presynaptic on the cholinergic neuronal projection and regulate ACH release.[41,42] $M_2$ receptors are thought to provide negative feedback inhibition of ACH synthesis and release by attenuation of adenylate cyclase activation (Fig. 46.2). These agents might first stimulate neurotransmission by activation of $M_1$ and nicotinic receptors (improve cognitive function) and then inhibit release by activating presynaptic $M_2$ receptors (impair cognitive function). This suggests that specific postsynaptic acting $M_1$ agonists would be rational alternative therapy; however, the number or function of $M_1$ receptors (not on the cholinergic neuron) also appears to be reduced, as evidenced by minimal improvement with investigational $M_1$ agonists in Alzheimer's patients.[43,44] Second, a limitation of any direct-acting cholinomimetic agent is that the drug stimulates receptors based on its pharmacokinetics and CNS penetration. Therefore, a nonphysiologic pattern of receptor activation is produced by drug administration. These abnormal patterns may "flood" the receptor with the agonist compound, resulting in a blockage of "true signal" via neuronal transmission.[31]

To summarize, explanations for the limited efficacy of cholinergic interventions include the following: (1) ACH synthesis and release are dependent on normal neuronal firing activity; (2) cholinesterase inhibitors may be limited by inadequate ACH production from decreasing numbers of intact presynaptic neurons and by their nonspecific augmentation of the neurotransmitter system; (3) muscarinic agonists display a narrow therapeutic window because of receptor interactions; (4) other neurotransmitter or neuropeptide deficits might contribute to the pathophysiology of cognitive dysfunction in PDD.

Similar to the dysregulation hypothesis for depression, PDD might be the result of dysregulation of the cholinergic system relative to other neuronal systems.[45] Hence, augmentation of a single neurotransmitter system (up or down) may not be sufficient to exert therapeutic effects. The pathophysiology should be interpreted within the same context, suggesting that the interdependence of other neurotransmitter systems with the cholinergic system limits the usefulness of present therapies once damage to multiple systems has occurred.

#### Neuropeptides/Nucleic Acids

Neuropeptides function as either neurotransmitters or modulators of neurotransmitters. Neuromodulators cause a longer lasting neurochemical change than do transmitters, reflected as more sustained subsequent behavior.[39] Adrenocorticotropic hormone (ACTH) and vasopressin (antidiuretic hormone, ADH) may modulate the processes of attention, memory, and cognitive deficits of aging. Desmopressin (DDAVP), an analog of vasopressin, and RNA have been studied in the treatment of PPD.[30] By activation of neural pathways that augment attention and concentration, these peptides can partially offset the deficits induced by the decline in cholinergic, serotonergic, and adrenergic function. Peptide therapy might increase the response to a neurologic or weak physiologic stimulus, by amplification of the transmission process in the damaged nuclei.

Investigational peptide derivatives of ACTH, such as the 4- to 10-amino-acid fragment ($ACTH_{4-10}$), and ACTH/MSH, the 7-amino-acid sequence shared by both ACTH and $\alpha$-melanocyte–stimulating hormone (MSH), stimulate neuronal processes through receptor-coupled secondary messenger systems (cAMP, cGMP, phosphoinositol, calmodulin). The second messenger then modulates protein kinase activity which controls the production and degradation of phosphoproteins. Alterations in cellular processes include changes in neurotransmitter release and cellular metabolism that can lead to more normal neuronal function. Other possible mechanisms of neuropeptide action that might lead to positive behavioral and cognitive effects are alteration of the enzymatic activity of the blood–brain barrier or changes in CNS permeability through special transport systems in the pituitary portal system.[46] These peptide fragments or analogs share behavioral properties with ACTH but lack the ability to stimulate corticosteroid release from the adrenal cortex. ACTH peptides seem to affect primarily "secondary" or extrinsic memory-modulating processes, including arousal, attention, and motivation, or to improve mood. ACTH peptides have been found to decrease the strength of stimuli necessary to provoke arousal from relevant environmental triggers, enhance selective attention, and improve "reversal" learning (dependent on ability to attend to changed stimuli and ignore previous memory traces) in studies in animals. These peptides do not modify intrinsic or primary memory mechanisms.

Inconsistent effects on memory task performance were found when single-dose or short-term administration schedules of $ACTH_{4-10}$ (parenteral or insufflation) and ORG 2766 (oral) were used in young normal adults or patients with various memory deficits.[46–48] The lack of persistent effect in humans might indicate a need for higher dosages or longer periods of administration.

ADH appears to facilitate the learning and memorization process at the time of initial acquisition, during consolidation, and during retention[49]; however, ADH's nonspecific CNS stimulation, producing secondary changes in arousal, mood, attention, and memory-modulating processes, is the most likely clinical effect observed. The results of vasopressin administration in PDD patients have been discouraging. Contrary to the positive preclinical data in animals,[39] most carefully controlled trials with severely impaired PDD patients have produced negative results. These findings may result, in part, from the decrease in ADH and its carrier protein, neurohypophysin II, with age.[46]

Another vasopressin analog, 1-desamino-8-D-arginine vasopressin, when administered to college students with varying degrees of mental disorder, produced an enhancement of learning and memory. Cognitive changes appeared to be related to an increased accessibility to knowledge structures necessary for effective and complete encoding of recallable information.[50] Side effects secondary to administration of vasopressin peptides include hypertension, antidiuretic, and corticotrophic effects.[46]

Ribonucleic acid (RNA) theories, in the 1950s and early 1960s, postulated an association among RNA, learning, and memory. Only one study using RNA intravenously resulted in positive effects on memory.[51]

In general, neuropeptides are only partially effective in improving performance on tasks involving recent memory in subjects with mild cognitive impairment caused by aging, dementia, and other trauma.[39] Clinically significant changes in cognitive function are not observed. Future research may clarify these controversial results by employing larger peptide doses for longer periods of time with more appropriately selected patients.

**Table 46.12** Suggested Mechanism or Levels of Action of ''Cerebroactive'' Drugs

| *Drug* | *Vasodilatation* | *Metabolic activation* | *Platelet aggregation* | *CNS neuro-transmitters* | *Hemorrheologic*[a] | *Phospholipid synthesis* |
|---|---|---|---|---|---|---|
| Bamethan[b] | + | | | | | |
| Bencyclane[b] | + | + | + | | | |
| Betahistine[b] | + | | | | | |
| Cyclandelate (Cyclospasmol) | + | + | | | | |
| Cinnarizine[b] | + | | | | | |
| Citilcoline[b] | | | | + | + | + |
| Co-dergocrine[b] | + | + | | + | | |
| Dihydroergocristine (Hydergine) | + | + | + | + | | |
| Eburnamonine[b] | | + | | | | |
| Flunarizine[b] | + | | | | | |
| Isoxsuprine (Vasodilan) | + | | | | | |
| Naftidrofuryl[b] | + | + | | | + | |
| Nicergoline[b] | + | + | + | | | |
| Nicotinic acid derivatives | + | + | | | | |
| Nylidrin (Arlidin) | + | | | | | |
| Pentoxifylline (Trental) | | | + | | + | |
| Papaverine (Pavabid) | + | | | | | |
| Piracetam[b] | + | + | | | | |
| Piribedil[b] | + | | + | | | |
| Raubasine[b] | + | | | | | |
| Suloctidil[b] | | + | + | | | |
| Vincamine[b] | | + | | | + | |

[a] Decreases blood viscosity; increases red blood cell flexibility, microcirculation, and tissue oxygen concentrations.
[b] Investigational agent.

Compiled from Reference 34.

**Metabolic Enhancers**

Studies of cerebral blood flow, oxygen uptake, and glucose utilization indicated that brain carbohydrate metabolism is impaired in a variety of dementias (including PDD). The degree of metabolic reduction has correlated with the severity of the dementia. The impairment of brain carbohydrate metabolism also results in a proportional decrease in the synthesis of ACH. Therefore, enhancement of cerebral metabolic processes would appear to be a rational approach to therapy for PDD patients. A wide variety of agents have been utilized in the search for ''cerebroactive'' drugs (Table 46.12). The majority of these agents were first used for their ''vasodilator'' effects; however, most vasodilating agents have not demonstrated significant efficacy, and only dihydroergotoxin is discussed.

Dihydroergotoxin (DHE, Hydergine) consists of four ergopeptine derivatives, dihydroergocornine, dihydroergocristine, dihydro-$\alpha$-ergocryptine, and dihydro-$\beta$-ergocryptine, in a ratio of 3:3:2:1. Dihydroergotoxin is reported to improve intracellular metabolism of impaired neuronal cells. Clinical trials utilizing dihydroergotoxin have produced controversial results. In two reviews,[52,53] DHE (3.0–4.5 mg/d) produced statistically significant ($P < 0.05$) improvement in several symptoms associated with dementia; however, the small magnitude of improvement and the possible lack of long-term benefit make the clinical significance of the improvement questionable for the moderately to severely ill patient. The cognitive improvement in these studies was attributed to the possible antidepressant effects of DHE. Other studies, however, have indicated that improvement in cognitive function was independent of improvement in affect or mood.[54] DHE produces clinical improvement in most patients with mild senile dementia,[55] but many of the studies did not utilize objective tests of cognitive function, did not determine an optimal dose, or did not analyze the data for a subgroup population in which DHE would be indicated.[56] A therapeutic trial of 6 months' duration utilizing an oral dose of 6 mg/d is sufficient to ascertain the potential benefits of DHE therapy. If a clinically significant response is not observed, DHE should be discontinued.[28]

Clinical study of the combined use of tricyclic antidepressants and DHE is under way (Sandoz Inc., personal communications). It is hoped that the neuromodulating effects resulting from adrenergic receptor activation might be additive to the modest benefits obtained with DHE alone.

**Nootropics**

It is believed that by augmentation of cerebral metabolism, particularly in the cholingeric system, complex brain function such as thinking and memory is improved. These mental processes involve the complex integration of a variety of neurotransmitter and modulating systems. Increased activity in the cholinergic system may facilitate these complex brain mechanisms. Piracetam, 2-oxo-1-pyrrolidine acetamide, belongs to a new class of drugs called nootropic agents ("toward the mind" or "mind-acting"). These agents are thought to enhance cerebral metabolism via an increase in ATP formation and protein synthesis, thereby improving integrative brain mechanisms associated with mental performance.[39,55,57]

By enhancement of cerebral energy metabolism and by augmentation of cerebral electrical activity, these drugs are thought to cause an increase in alertness without the side effects of the CNS stimulants. Drugs in this category include the $\gamma$-aminobutyric acid (GABA) derivatives (piracetam, oxiracetam, pramiracetam), vincamine, pyrithioxine, and centrophenoxine. These drugs are, as yet, investigational in the United States.

Piracetam, currently marketed in Europe, is a cyclic derivative of GABA. Evidence for piracetam's unique mechanism of action includes its lack of direct effect at any presently identified neurotransmitter system, no observed change in regional cerebral blood blow, and its protective effects in reducing cognitive loss secondary to CNS hypoxia or electroconvulsive therapy.[55,56,58] Effects of piracetam may include enhanced learning and memory acquisition and facilitation of interhemispheric transfer of information.[34]

Early studies of piracetam appeared to demonstrate improvement in a mixed population of senile dementia patients. Patients with lower IQs appeared to achieve the most benefit[57,59–61] and lower doses appeared more effective for long-term treatment (2.4 g/d versus 4.8 g/d).[56] In three other double-blind studies, piracetam was found to be superior to placebo for remission of "psychoorganic syndromes"; however, these studies had design and statistical errors including poor matching of piracetam-treated ($n$ = 112) versus placebo-treated ($n$ = 70) patients, reducing the validity of their findings.[34] Other studies indicated no evidence of improvement in cognitive or behavioral symptoms.[58,62] Therefore, the evidence suggesting that piracetam is beneficial in the treatment of the cognitive and behavioral symptoms of PDD is inconsistent.[55]

Despite poor results in humans, memory research in monkeys indicates that piracetam is among the most potent compounds for reversal of short-term memory deficits, although responses are variable.[55,57] Emphasis has been placed on the development of piracetam analogs. Two such analogs, oxiracetam and pramiracetam, have undergone clinical trials. Both agents are considered more potent and efficacious than piracetam and to have greater potential for clinical use.[30]

Nafronyl (naftidrofuryl; Praxilene) is a direct-acting vasodilator that also increases brain utilization of glucose and accelerates aerobic brain metabolism in rats, mice, and humans.[55] This compound may activate succinate dehydrogenase (Kreb's cycle), causing an increase in ATP stores with resultant increases in metabolism.[56] Nafronyl is related to the psychostimulants and there may be a nonspecific effect confounding the efficacy trials. To date, marginal efficacy has been demonstrated for nafronyl.[55]

**Opioid Antagonists**

Several studies have suggested involvement of the endogenous opioid systems (endorphins, enkephalins) in various cerebral functions, including modulation of memory storage, physiologic amnesia, dopamine neuronal activity in the limbic and pituitary systems, and modulation of cortical outflow involved in polymodal information processing (integrative functions) and limbic functions.[63,64] Opioid antagonists might facilitate brain function by these possible mechanisms of action: (1) increased activity of dopaminergic and $\beta$-adrenergic systems that are normally under endogenous opioid inhibition, (2) increased cholinergic and GABAergic system activity, and (3) blockade of enkephalin-induced hippocampal pyramidal cell excitation that might cause impairment of learning.[30,63]

Naloxone hydrochloride (Narcan) in humans without dementia has produced minimal or inconsistent behavioral and cognitive effects at low doses (1–10 mg intravenously).[64,65] Recently, two preliminary reports noted clinical and cognitive improvement of patients with PPD after low intravenous doses of naloxone[66,67]; however, additional clinical trials did not confirm these initial findings.[68–71] Two double-blind trials, using low to high doses of naloxone in patients with PDD, noted no cognitive improvement.[65,69] Tariot et al[70] confirmed these negative results in a recent randomized, double-blind, placebo-controlled trial in 12 patients with PDD. Several studies reported nonspecific behavioral activation as a consequence of naloxone therapy, possibly explaining the beneficial results (Table 46.13).[64–72] Limitations of these trials include their use of a very short acting compound and widely differing dosages. Naltrexone, an opioid antagonist available as an oral preparation, is more potent and longer acting than naloxone (24-hour duration after an oral dose). Naltrexone (Trexan) appears to have negligible toxicity and therefore may be ideal for chronic use.[29]

Similar to the neuropeptides, opioid antagonists may be acting on secondary processes that might potentially offset the primary degenerative damage in the cholinergic system. The modulating effects of naloxone might be too weak to reverse the PDD deficits, explaining the disappointing results to date.

**Other Agents**

In addition to the opioid antagonists, several other compounds are being researched for their possible roles in the treatment of PDD. Destruction of the cholinergic projections from the nucleus basalis of Meynert to the limbic system causes dysfunction in mood, memory, and thought processes. Alzheimer's disease can manifest as a hippocampal dementia with disturbances in mood, memory, and information processing.[73] Therefore, agents that normalize limbic

**Table 46.13** Human Studies With Opioid Antagonists

| *Reference* | *Study design*[a] | *Number of patients* | *Drug and dose* | *Results* |
|---|---|---|---|---|
| Arch Gen Psychiatry 1986;43:727–732 | R, DB, PC | 12 | Naloxone (0.005, 0.1, 2.0 mg/kg) | No improvement in cognitive function; low dose produced behavioral activation |
| N Engl J Med 1983; 308:721–722 | DB, MD, PC | 7 | Naloxone (1, 5, 10 mg) | Significant improvement ($P<0.01$) in clinical test and psychometric tests ($P<0.05$) |
| N Engl J Med 1983;309:556 | Open | 35 | Naloxone (1, 1.2, 2, 5 mg) | No significant improvement documented |
| J Am Geriatr Soc 1985;33:155 | DB | — | Naloxone ("low-dose") | No cognitive change |
| Psychopharm Bull 1983;19:45–47 | Open | 5 | Naloxone (1 mg) | Clinical improvement in 3/5; psychometric improvement in 5/5 |
| Psychopharm Bull 1985;21:680–682 | DB, PC, RD | 12 | Naloxone (0.005, 0.1, 2 mg/kg) | No cognitive improvement; increased irrelevant associations after low dose; behavioral activation occurred |

[a] DB, double-blind; PC, placebo-controlled; RD, random-dosed; R, randomized; MD, multidose.

function, such as sodium valproate (Depakene), carbamazepine (Tegretol), alaproclate (an investigational neuronal serotonin reuptake inhibitor), lithium (lithium carbonate), and the investigational dopaminergic agonist memantine, all show possible promise and deserve further study.[28,29,63,74] The effectiveness of carbamazepine and lithium is associated primarily with the reduction in secondary maniclike target symptoms observed in patients with dementias.[75–77] Lithium therapy must be carefully monitored to reduce the likelihood of neurotoxicity with resultant cognitive and memory disturbances.[78,79] Alaproclate has demonstrated positive effects on the target symptoms of aggressiveness, irritability, and stress incontinence in PDD subjects.[80] Recently, clonidine (Catapres), an $\alpha_2$ agonist capable of modulating noradrenergic outflow by autoreceptor stimulation, has been tried as well.[39]

### *Nonspecific Pharmacotherapy*

Elderly patients with PDD occasionally require adjunctive psychotropic drug therapy to assist in behavioral management. All psychotropics have potential adverse effects on the central nervous, autonomic, or cardiovascular system. Moreover, the pathophysiology of PDD suggests that pharmacologic agents that antagonize muscarinic, adrenergic, or serotonergic function might worsen the cognitive impairments. The nonspecific effects of aging on brain function further compound the PDD patient's sensitivity to psychotropic agents.

In selected patients, psychotropic drugs can improve the quality of the patient's life by ameliorating the secondary affective, psychotic, and anxiety disorders associated with aging and PDD. Calming the agitated and aggressive patient can also be necessary. Nondrug interventions, previously discussed, should be attempted first.

Anticholinergic (antimuscarinic) effects are associated with most psychotropic compounds. Recent work with anticholinergic agents used to treat extrapyramidal symptoms strongly suggests that decrements in learning and memory occur in elderly patients, schizophrenics, and normal persons given therapeutic doses of these agents. Moreover, the detriment in memory functions appears related to the serum concentrations of the anticholinergics.[81–84] Whenever possible, a psychotropic agent with minimal anticholinergic effects should be selected, even though the deleterious effects of antimuscarinic activity with antidepressants and antipsychotics are less clear.

#### Antidepressants

As PDD and major depression may be difficult to distinguish, antidepressant therapy should be considered in the patient with a family or personal history of affective illness (Table 46.6). Patients with symptoms consistent with depression should be evaluated for antidepressant therapy. Additionally, enhancement of biogenic amine activity (norepinephrine and serotonin) might counteract the decreased excitatory influences of the atrophied cholinergic axons in the locus ceruleus and raphe magnus. Trazodone (Desyrel), followed by desipramine (Norpramin), has the least anticholinergic effects of the standard antidepressants. Trazodone's sedative properties make it a good selection for the anxious or insomniac patient; however, orthostatic hypotension is encountered with the same frequency as most tricyclic antidepressants. Nortriptyline (Pamelor) has the least effect on orthostatic blood pressure homeostatic reflexes.[84] Patients sensitive to this adverse effect can usually tolerate nortriptyline. Adjunctive plasma concentration monitoring for nortriptyline is suggested.

For a more complete discussion, refer to Chapter 50.

### Antipsychotic Agents

Antipsychotic agents can, if necessary, be used to treat severe agitation, combativeness, or psychosis in the demented patient. A biphasic response in the elderly, with regard to cognition, is noted with antipsychotic agents. At very low dosages, for example, 1–3 mg/d for haloperidol (Haldol), slight improvements in cognition are noted. At higher doses, negative effects on cognition can occur.[85] Increased sensitivity to adverse effects necessitates cautious dosage titration. Although some studies have suggested superiority of one antipsychotic over another, most controlled trials suggest that these agents are all equally efficacious. Selection of an antipsychotic agent is usually empiric but should include assessment of target symptoms to ascertain the need for sedation and tailoring of the adverse effect profile to the patient's medication and medical history.

The clinical studies to date suggest that low dosages of antipsychotics, for example, thioridazine (Mellaril) 25–50 mg/d initially or its equivalent, can be clinically useful for the management of suspiciousness, hallucinations, insomnia, excitement, hostility, belligerence, and emotional lability; however, these agents do not ameliorate the dementia-specific symptoms of impaired memory, unsociability, poor self-care, or indifference to surroundings. Moreover, in most controlled trials improvements are not dramatic, and 5% to 20% of patients are worsened by therapy.[76] High-potency neuroleptics, for example, fluphenazine (Prolixin), haloperidol (Haldol), or thiothixene (Navane), are safer in patients with cardiovascular disease (see Chapter 48).

### Anxiolytics and Sedative–Hypnotics

Anxiety and insomnia are among the most common complaints of the elderly with organic mental syndromes or disorders. Treatment is not specific, and is aimed at symptom reduction. The stresses of aging, cognitive deterioration, and physical disabilities cause an anxiety reaction in many elderly patients. Adjustment disorders with anxiety from the PDD patient's realization that cognitive function is diminishing are common. The judicious adjunctive use of benzodiazepines can be necessary on occasion to help restore normal sleep patterns or to manage exacerbations of anxiety; however, disinhibition is more likely in brain-damaged individuals, causing paradoxical excitation. Nondrug interventions, including good sleep, hygiene, and relaxation techniques, should be employed first.

Very low dosages should be used initially, preferably as prn regimens. For most individuals, prn doses of diazepam 2 mg for anxiety or triazolam 0.125 mg for insomnia are sufficient. If subchronic therapy is needed, attention to the insidious behavioral deterioration secondary to accumulation of long-acting benzodiazepine drugs and their metabolites is essential. Alternately, withdrawal can precipitate anxiety, insomnia, delirium, panic, psychosis, autonomic nervous system overactivity, and seizures. Buspirone, a nonbenzodiazepine anxiolytic, appears to cause a lesser degree of motor incoordination or dependence/withdrawal. Although the efficacy of buspirone in dementia has not been studied,[86] its pharmacologic profile suggests that deleterious effects on short–term memory and task performance are unlikely.

### Other Drugs

CNS stimulants may nonspecifically counteract age-related problems of fatigue, inattention, amotivation, depression, and motor dysfunction by their euphoric, mood-lifting, or general energizing effects. These nonspecific effects have been postulated to improve function in the PDD patient; however, the majority of data on humans suggests that catecholamine-like agents do not improve, and might often impair, memory. Normal catecholamine function and CNS response to stimulants appear to be dependent upon an intact cholinergic system.[39] The effects of catecholamine facilitators observed in PDD are dependent upon the task variables and dosage. Methylphenidate (Ritalin) in 10- and 30-mg doses failed to produce significant differences in cognitive scores, but did reduce fatigue compared with placebo in a double-blind crossover study.[63] Pemoline magnesium (Cylert), though effective as a stimulant in children, has no effect on general alertness and interest in geriatric patients.[30] Caffeine, and pentylenetetrazole with niacin, also did not significantly improve memory in monkey models.[39] Studies in humans with pentylenetetrazole and pipradol did not improve memory, but changes in mood were observed.[63]

Cardiovascular adverse effects (tachycardia, hypertension, increased myocardial oxygen consumption) and tremulousness can occur frequently in the elderly.[63] Irritability, insomnia, and paranoia result from excessive doses or administration too close to the evening. Chronic use may result in a paranoid psychosis indistinguishable from schizophrenia. Interestingly, amphetamines are reported to be beneficial on performance tests in young healthy subjects and are used by pilots in military and spacecraft. Larger doses (30 mg/d), however, induced agitation and decreased performance. No controlled geriatric trials have been reported.[63]

## Summary

PDD is one of the most common organic brain syndromes of the dementia type. Its etiology and pathophysiology are not completely understood and vigorous research activity is ongoing. Most specific drug therapies are investigational and unfortunately only partially effective. PDD is a syndrome with many possible subtypes, further confounding treatment evaluations. PDD is a progressive disorder, and drug therapy works best on those individuals least impaired. Nondrug therapy, for the most part, should be the primary initial intervention in demented elderly patients. The psychotropic agents are palliative therapies without specificity and with adverse effects to which the elderly are particularly sensitive. Of the currently marketed therapies for PDD in the United States, only DHE (Hydergine) possesses any specificity or effect on core cognitive features; however, the limited magnitude of improvement possible with this drug result in only small gains in cognition in the PDD patient with moderate or severe illness.[87] The role of combination therapies, targeting on the multiple neuronal systems involved, appears logical. Use of piracetam with cholinergic facilitating agents or the combination of DHE with an antidepressant illustrates this approach. Additional controlled studies are sorely needed to validate new therapeutic strategies. The neurochemistry and neurophysiology of this disorder are reviewed in detail, as many of the compounds likely to be marketed are best understood from this framework.

## References


1. Editorial. Dementia—the quiet epidemic. Br Med J 1978;1:1–2.
2. American Psychiatric Association. Diagnostic and Statistical Manual of Mental Disorders, 3rd ed, revised (DSM-III-R). Washington DC, American Psychiatric Association, 1987.
3. Rossor MN. Dementia. Lancet 1982;2:1200–1204.
4. Katzman R: Alzheimer's disease. N Engl J Med 1986;314:964–973.
5. Rocca WA, Amaduccia LA, Schoenberg BS. Epidemiology and clinically diagnosed Alzheimer's disease. Ann Neurol 1986;19: 415–424.
6. Price DL. New perspectives on Alzheimer's disease. Ann Rev Neurosci 1986;9:489–512.
7. Perry EK, Perry RH. A review of neuropathological and neurochemical correlates of Alzheimer's disease. Dan Med Bull 1985;32S:27–34.
8. Whitehouse PJ, Martino AM, Antuono PG, et al. Nicotinic acetylcholine binding sites in Alzheimer's disease. Brain Res 1986;371:146–151.
9. Brun A. The structural development of Alzheimer's disease. Dan Med Bull 1985;32S:25–27.
10. Geddes JW, Monaghan DT, Cotman CW, et al. Plasticity of hippocampal circuitry in Alzheimer's disease. Science 1985;230: 1179–1181.
11. Tachibana H, Meyer JS, Kitagawa Y, et al. Effects of aging on cerebral blood flow in dementia. J Amer Geriatr Soc 1984;32: 114–120.
12. Khachaturian ZS. Diagnosis of Alzheimer's disease. Arch Neurol 1985;42:1097–1105.
13. Wong DF, Wagner HN, Dannals RF, et al. Effects of age on dopamine and serotonin receptors measured by positron tomography in the living brain. Science 1984;226:1393–1396.
14. St. George-Hyslop PH, Tnaz RE, Polinsky RJ, et al. The genetic defect causing familial Alzheimer's disease maps on chromosome 21. Science 1987;235:885–2890.
15. Whitehouse PJ. Receptor autoradiography: Applications in neuropathology. Tren NeuroSci 1985;8:434–437.
16. Frost JJ. Imaging muscarinic cholinergic receptors using I-123 paraiododexetimide and emission computed tomography. Neuroreceptor Conference. Johns Hopkins University, April 18–19, 1986.
17. Cross AJ, Crow TJ, Ferrier IN, et al. Serotonin receptor changes in dementia of the Alzheimer type. J Neurochem 1984;43:1574–1581.
18. Rossor MN, Iversen LL, Reynolds GP, et al. Neurochemical characteristics of early and late onset types of Alzheimer's disease. Br Med J 1984;288:961–964.
19. Crow TJ, Cross AJ, Cooper SJ, et al. Neurotransmitter receptors and monoamine metabolites in the brains of patients with Alzheimer-type dementia and depression, and suicides. Neuropharmacology 1984;23:1561–1569.
20. Peroutka SJ. 5-$HT_1$ receptor sites and functional correlates. Neuropharmacology 1984;23:1487–1492.
21. Leysen JE, De Chaffoy DeCourcelles D, DeClerck F, et al. Serotonin-$S_2$ receptor binding sites and functional correlates. Neuropharmacology 1984;23:1493–1501.
22. Pierotti AR, Harmar AJ, Simpson J, Yates CM. High-molecular weight forms of somatostatin are reduced in Alzheimer's disease and Down's syndrome. Neurosci Lett 1986;63:141–146.
23. Whitehouse PJ. New Clinical Drug Evaluation Unit Annual Meeting, Key Biscayne, FL, May 30, 1986.
24. Hoffman RS. Neuropsychiatric complications of AIDS. Psychosomatics 1984;25:393–400.
25. Barnes DH. AIDS-related brain damage unexplained. Science 1986;232:1091–1093.
26. Cummins JL, Bensen F. Dementia of the Alzheimer type. J Amer Geriatr Soc 1986;34:12–19.
27. Chui HC, Teng EL, Henderson VW, et al. Clinical subtypes of dementia of the Alzheimer type. Neurology 1985;35:1544–1550.
28. Erwin G. Senile dementia of the Alzheimer type. Clinical Pharmacy 1984;3:497–504.
29. Rathmann KL, Conner CS. PDD: Clinical features, pathogenesis, and treatment. Drug Intell Clin Pharm 1984;18:684–691.
30. Galizia VJ. Pharmacotherapy of memory loss in the geriatric patient. Drug Intell Clin Pharm 1984;18:784–791.
31. Lauter H. What do we know about PDD today? Dan Med Bull 1985;32:1–21.
32. Johns CA, Greenwald BS, Mohs RC, et al. The cholinergic treatment strategy in aging and senile dementia. Psychopharmacol Bull 1983;19:185–197.
33. Jarvik ME, Gritz ER, Schneider NG. Drugs and memory disorders in human aging. Behav Biol 1972;7:643–668.
34. Spagnoli A, Tognoni G. Cerebroactive drugs: Clinical pharmacology and therapeutic role in cerebrovascular disorders. Drugs 1983;26:44–69.
35. Mohs RC, Davis KL, Tinklenberg JR, et al. Choline chloride treatment of memory deficits in the elderly. Am J Psychiatry 1979;136:1275–1277.
36. Friedman E, Sherman KA, Ferris SH, et al. Clinical response to choline plus piracetam in senile dementia: Relation to red-cell choline levels. New Engl J Med 1981;304:1490–1491.
37. Smith RC, Vroulis G, Johnson R, et al. Comparison of therapeutic response to long-term treatment with lecithin versus piracetam plus lecithin in patients with PDD. Psychopharmacol Bull 1984;20:542–545.
38. Summers WK, Viesselman JO, Marsh GM, et al. Use of THA in treatment of Alzheimer-like dementia: Pilot study in twelve patients. Biol Psychiatry 1981;16:145–153.
39. Bartus RT, Dean RL, Beer B. An evaluation of drugs for improving memory in aged monkeys: Implications for clinical trials in humans. Psychopharmacol Bull 1983;19:168–184.
40. Harbaugh RE. Intracranial drug administration in PDD. Psychopharmacol Bull 1986;22:106–109.
41. Fine A. Peptides and Alzheimer's disease. Nature 1986;319: 537–538.
42. Mash DC, Flynn DD, Potter LT. Loss of M2 muscarine receptors in the cerebral cortex in PDD and experimental cholinergic denervation. Science 1985;228:1115.
43. Pomara N, Stanley M. The cholinergic hypothesis of memory dysfunction in PDD—revisited. Psychopharmacol Bull 1986;22: 110–118.

44. Weetstein A, Spiegel R. Clinical trials with the cholinergic drug RS86 in PDD and senile dementia of the Alzheimer's type. Psychopharmacology 1984;84:572–573.
45. Siever LJ, Davis KL. Towards a dysregulation hypothesis for depression. Am J Psychiatry 1985;142:1017–1031.
46. Tinklenberg JR, Thornton JE. Neuropeptides in geriatric psychopharmacology. Psychopharmacol Bull 1983;19:198–211.
47. Abuzzahab FS, Will JC, Zimmerman RL. Effects of single dose ACTH 4–10 versus placebo on the memory of symptomatic geriatric volunteers. J Clin Psychopharmacol 1982;2:65–69.
48. Dowson JH. Pharmacological treatment of chronic cognitive deficit: A review. Compr Psychiatry 1982;23:85–98.
49. Kent S. Can drugs halt memory loss? Geriatrics 1981;36:34–41.
50. Weingartner H, Gold P, Ballenger JC, et al. Effects of vasopressin on human memory functions. Science 1981;211:601–603.
51. Cameron DE, Sved S, Solyom L, et al. Effects of ribonucleic acid on memory defect in the aged. Am J Psychiatry 1964;120: 320–325.
52. Hughes Jr, Williams JG. An ergot alkaloid preparation (Hydergine) in the treatment of dementia: Critical review of the clinical literature. J Am Geriatr Soc 1976;24:490–497.
53. Yesavage JA, Westphal J, Rush L. Senile dementia: Combined pharmacologic and psychologic treatment. J Am Geriatr Soc 1981;29:164–170.
54. Gaitz CM, Varner RV, Overall JF. Pharmacotherapy for organic brain syndrome in late life. Arch Gen Psychiatry 1977;34: 839–845.
55. Branconnier RJ. The efficacy of the cerebral metabolic enhancers in the treatment of senile dementia. Psychopharmacol Bull 1983;19:212–219.
56. Reisberg B, Ferris SH, Gershon S. An overview of pharmacologic treatment of cognitive decline in the aged. Am J Psychiatry 1981;138:593–600.
57. Chouinard G, Annable L, Ross-Chouinard A, et al. A double-blind, placebo-controlled study of piracetam in elderly psychiatric patients. Psychopharmacol Bull 1981;17:129.
58. Gustafson L, Reisberg J, Johanson M, et al. Effects of piracetam on regional cerebral blood flow and mental functions in patients with organic dementia. Psychopharmacology 1978;56: 115–117.
59. Stegink AJ. The clinical use of piracetam, a new nootropic drug. Arzneimittelforschung 1972;22:975–977.
60. Diamond SJ, Brouwers EYM. Increase in the power of human memory in normal man through the use of drugs. Psychopharmacology 1976;49:307–309.
61. Mindus P, Cronholm B, Levander SE, et al. Piracetam-induced improvement of mental performance. Acta Psychiatr Scand 1976;54:150–160.
62. Lloyd-Evans S, Brocklehurst JC, Palmer MK. Piracetam in chronic brain failure. Curr Med Res Opin 1979;6:351–357.
63. Reisberg B, London E, Ferris SH, et al. Novel pharmacologic approaches to the treatment of senile dementia of the Alzheimer's type. Psychopharmacol Bull 1983;19:220–225.
64. Tariot PN, Sunderland T, Weingartner H, et al. Naloxone and Alzheimer's disease. Arch Gen Psychiatry 1986;43:727–732.
65. Cohen RM, Cohen MR. Weingartner H, et al. High-dose naloxone affects task performance in normal subjects. Psychiatry Res 1983;8:127–136.
66. Reisberg B, Ferris SH, Anand R, et al. Naloxone effects on primary degenerative dementia. Psychopharmacol Bull 1983;19: 45–47.
67. Reisberg B, Ferris SH, Anand R, et al. Effects of naloxone in senile dementia: A double-blind trial. N Engl J Med 1983;308: 721–722.
68. Blass JP, Reding MJ, Drachman D, et al. Letter to the editor. N Engl J Med 1983;309:556.
69. Steiger WA, Mendelson M, Jenkins T, et al. Effects of naloxone in treatment of senile dementia. J Am Geriatr Soc 1985;33:155.
70. Tariot PN, Sunderland T, Weingartner H, et al. Low- and high-dose naloxone in dementia of the Alzheimer type. Psychopharmacol Bull 1985;21:680–682.
71. Messing RB, Jensen RA, Martinez JL, et al. Naloxone enhancement of memory. Behav Neural Biol 1979;27:266–275.
72. Gallagher M. Naloxone enhancement of memory processes: Effects of other opiate antagonists. Behav Neural Biol 1982;35: 375–382.
73. Ball MJ, Hachinski V, Fox A, et al. A new definition of Alzheimer's disease: A hippocampal dementia. Lancet 1985;1: 14–16.
74. Fleischhacker WW, Buchgeher A, Schubert H. Memantine in the treatment of senile dementia of the Alzheimer type. Prog Neuropsychopharmacol Biol Psychiatry 1986;10:87–93.
75. Essa M. Carbamazepine in dementia. J Clin Psychopharmacol 1986;6:234–236.
76. Rosenbaum AH, Barry MJ. Positive therapeutic response to lithium in hypomania secondary to organic brain syndrome. Am J Psychiatry 1975;132:1072.
77. Risse SC, Barnes R. Pharmacologic treatment of agitation associated with dementia. J Am Geriatr Soc 1986;34:368–376.
78. Christodoulou GN, Kokkevi A, Lykouras EP, et al. Effects of lithium on memory. Am J Psychiatry 1981;138:847–848.
79. Zerbi F, Clemente E, Bezzi G, et al. Memory performances in depressed patients during prophylactic treatment with lithium salts. Bibl Psychiatry 1981;161:190–196.
80. Bergman I, Brane G, Gottfries CG. Alaproclate: A pharmacokinetic and biochemical study in patients with dementia of Alzheimer's type. Psychopharmacology 1983;80:279–283.
81. Tune LE, Strauss ME, Lew MF, et al. Serum levels of anticholinergic drugs and impaired recent memory in chronic schizophrenic patients. Am J Psychiatry 1982;139:1460–1462.
82. Sadeh M, Braham J, Modan M. Effects of anticholinergic drugs on memory in Parkinson's disease. Arch Neurol 1982;39:666–667.
83. Syndulko K, Gilden ER, Hansch EC, et al. Decreased verbal memory associated with anticholinergic treatment in Parkinson's disease patients. Intern J Neurosci 1981;14:61–66.
84. Potamianos G, Kellet JM. Anticholinergic drugs and memory: the effects of benzhexol on memory in a group of geriatric patients. Br J Psychiatry 1982;140:470–472.
85. Aman MG. Psychotropic drugs and learning problems—A selective review. J Learn Diabil 1980;13:87–96.
86. Erwin CW, Linnoila M, Hartwell J, et al. Effects of buspirone and diazepam, alone and in combination with alcohol, on skilled performance and evoked potentials. J Clin Psychopharmacology 1986;6:199–209.
87. Kwentus JA, Hart R, Lingon N, et al. Alzheimer's disease. Am J Med 1986;81:91–96.

# Chapter 47 / Substance Use Disorders

Brian L. Crabtree, PharmD

Drug abuse and drug dependence are among the most common of medical problems. Approximately 40% of all hospitalizations and over 50% of highway fatalities are directly or indirectly related to alcohol or other drugs.[1] Health care costs and lost productivity related to drug use run into the billions. Approximately 70% of youths 12 to 17 years old have tried alcohol and about 30% have tried marijuana. Approximately 8% of the adult population is considered alcohol dependent.[1,2] Although problems associated with drug use are virtually ubiquitous, there is perhaps no other area of medicine that is more variably practiced, understood, and misunderstood. Curricula of schools of the health care professions often provide little formal attention to problems of alcoholism and other drug dependencies.

## Historical Perspective

A discussion of the history of drug abuse and drug dependence is difficult. Although the 1960s brought an explosion of new patterns of drug use, recreational drugs have been used for centuries. Alcohol and opium have been used for their mood-altering effects for hundreds of years. Cocaine was an extraordinarily popular and available drug in the early part of this century. Gasoline sniffing has been a common drug use pattern for many years. Peyote cactus containing mescaline and mushrooms containing psilocybin have been used for centuries. Clearly, however, there are new trends in drug use, and society is continually faced with an increasing diversity of recreational drugs. The so-called "lookalike" and "designer" drugs, as well as the increasing availability of cocaine base, or "crack," are examples.

## Terminology

An important step in understanding substance use disorders and their treatment is the establishment of a standardized working vocabulary. A consensus agreement among scientists and the treatment community with regard to definitions of terms has been difficult. Until recently, there have been no standardized credentials for individuals wishing to offer treatment. As a result, progress in treatment and understanding has been slow, and interpretation of scientific literature difficult. Below is a list of important terms relative to substance use disorders. Although there are no universally accepted definitions, these are widely used and accepted by clinicians.

*Drug abuse.* Use of a drug with the intent of altering mood or feeling state up to, but not beyond, the point of social, family, physical, or occupational dysfunction.

*Drug misuse.* Inappropriate use of a drug intended for therapeutic purposes (e.g., inappropriate prescribing, use of a prescription drug not under the supervision of a physician, self-medication with a nonprescription drug inconsistent with label information).

*Addiction or drug dependence.* Behavioral pattern of compulsive drug use in which obtaining and using a drug constitute the principal focus of the user's life. There is continued use of a drug to alter feelings or prevent withdrawal effects despite medical, social, or occupational contraindications. Although drug dependence is a type of drug abuse (i.e., use of a drug with the intent of altering mood or feeling state), it is possible to be a drug abuser without being drug dependent.

*Physical dependence.* State of physiologic adaptation to chronic use of a drug such that abrupt dosage reduction or discontinuation results in a characteristic abstinence syndrome.

*Tolerance.* State of physiologic adaptation to a drug such that higher-than-usual dosages are required to achieve the usual effect.

*Withdrawal or abstinence syndrome.* Characteristic physical and emotional signs and symptoms precipitated by the abrupt reduction or discontinuation of a drug on which a subject is physically dependent.

*Cross-tolerance and cross-dependence.* Ability of one drug to suppress the manifestations of physical withdrawal produced by another drug and to maintain the physically dependent state.

## Chemically Impaired Health Care Professionals

Health care professionals, including pharmacists, are among the highest risk occupational categories for the development of drug dependency. Recent data from studies of the epidemiology of controlled substance use among pharmacists and physicians indicate that 46% of pharmacists and 62% of pharmacy students have used a controlled substance without a prescription, with the pharmacy students using controlled substances more often for recreational purposes than for self-treatment.[3] Of practicing pharmacists, 19% are occasional or regular users of controlled substances without a prescription, and of pharmacy students, 41% are occasional or regular users (i.e., at least once per month). Physicians and medical students show similar patterns of drug use, with 59% of physicians and 77% of medical students having tried a controlled substance for recreational or self-treatment purposes.[4]

Almost 33% of physicians and 44% of medical students are occasional or regular users of controlled substances. Approximately 38% of medical students are recreational drug users, most commonly using marijuana and cocaine.

Pharmacists and physicians are not well sensitized to their increased risk for the development of drug dependence. Prevalence of drug dependence among health care professionals, including pharmacists, is between 10% and 15%,[5] clearly higher than the lay public, owing to stressful professional responsibilities, ready accessibility to alcohol and other drugs, and a false feeling of invincibility associated with an increased knowledge of drug effects. While health care professionals are often quite knowledgeable about therapeutics, they often know little about drug dependence.

## Substance Use Disorders in the Elderly

Drug abuse has generally been associated with adolescents and young adults. Drug abuse in the elderly has been poorly studied, and it is widely believed that the elderly do not abuse drugs. Although the elderly use a large number of drugs, they are thought to use them in a licit, prescribed fashion. When recognized, inappropriate drug use is often felt to represent drug misuse without considering the possibility of drug abuse, and drug abuse is difficult to detect because of the lifestyle of many elderly. Only a small percentage of the population over the age of 65 have ever tried illegal drugs, although the percentage will rise as the population ages. The exact extent of abuse of legal drugs is unknown. Compared with younger adults, a greater percentage of elderly drug abusers use drugs as coping mechanisms for dealing with depression and stress. As many as 34% of older adults have taken a sedative drug within the last month (a figure significantly higher than in younger adults), and the prevalence of alcohol abuse, frequently in combination with other drugs, is higher than expected, although precise prevalence rates are not known.[6] It is clear that drug abuse among the elderly is more common than previously thought, and that the prevalence of drug abuse will increase with the aging of the population. The elderly may be at greater risk for complications related to drug abuse because of concomitant physical disease and use of multiple drugs.

## Patterns of Use/Clinical Presentation/Pharmacology/Diagnosis

There are many diagnostic classifications of disorders of drug abuse and drug dependence. The system presented here is that of the American Psychiatric Association's *Diagnostic and Statistical Manual of Mental Disorders, Third Edition, Revised* (DSM-III-R).[7] Substance use disorders are divided into two broad categories: psychoactive substance use disorders and psychoactive substance dependence disorders.

The psychoactive substance use disorders include the psychoactive substance–induced organic mental disorders particular to each drug or drug group. *Intoxication* refers to the development of a substance-specific syndrome after recent ingestion and presence in the body of a psychoactive substance and is associated with maladaptive behavior during the waking state caused by the effect of the substance on the central nervous system (CNS). *Withdrawal*, as defined previously, is the development of a substance-specific syndrome after cessation of or reduction in intake of a psychoactive substance that was regularly used by the individual to induce a state of intoxication.

An *organic flashback syndrome* is the reexperiencing of one or more of the perceptual symptoms that had been experienced while intoxicated with a psychoactive substance (e.g., visual or auditory hallucinations or derealization). An organic residual syndrome is characterized by at least 3 months' duration of at least one of the following that is judged to be a consequence of prolonged heavy use of a psychoactive substance:

1. Generalized reduction in goal-directed behavior (e.g., going to school, work, hobbies, often associated with depression, anxiety or irritability)
2. Deficits in cognitive functioning (e.g., difficulty concentrating)

The criteria for substance dependence are the same for each of the psychoactive drugs or drug classes, varying only to fit the unique pharmacologic properties of each drug. To meet criteria for the diagnosis of substance dependence, at least three of the following must be present:

1. Frequent preoccupation with seeking or taking the substance
2. Often takes the substance in larger amounts or over a longer period than intended
3. Tolerance
4. Characteristic withdrawal syndrome
5. Often takes the substance to relieve or avoid withdrawal symptoms
6. Persistent desire or repeated efforts to decrease or control substance use
7. Often intoxicated or impaired by substance use when expected to fulfill social or occupational obligations, or when substance use is hazardous (e.g., does not go to work because hung over or high, goes to work high, drives when drunk)
8. Has given up some important social, occupational, or recreational activity to seek or take the substance
9. Continues to use substance despite a significant social, occupational, or legal problem or a physical disorder that the individual knows is exacerbated by use of the substance

As with most illnesses, the course and prognosis of the disorders of substance use and dependence are variable. Acute intoxication associated with many drugs, especially opiates and cocaine, is potentially fatal. Untreated physical withdrawal from the CNS depressants is potentially life-threatening; however, withdrawal can almost always be successfully managed with proper medical care. Getting patients who are drug dependent to stop using drugs is very difficult, and many patients return to drug use even after treatment. As many as 75% of treated substance-dependent patients relapse at least once. Many patients are, however, able to obtain recovery with treatment and continued care in programs such as Alcoholics Anonymous. Substance dependence, or addiction, can be viewed as a chronic illness that

**Table 47.1** Alcohol Organic Mental Disorders

| |
|---|
| Alcohol intoxication |
| Alcohol idiosyncratic intoxication |
| Alcohol withdrawal |
| Alcohol withdrawal delirium |
| Alcohol hallucinosis |
| Alcohol amnestic disorder |
| Dementia associated with alcoholism |

Compiled from Reference 6.

can be successfully controlled with treatment, but cannot be cured and is associated with a high relapse rate. Without treatment, the course can progress to life-threatening severity, resulting from the effects of the drug, drug contaminants, or medical complications of its use.

## *Central Nervous System Depressants*

### Alcohol

In Western culture, alcohol is the only drug with which obvious self-induced intoxication is socially acceptable in certain circumstances. In the United States, 95% of the adult population has voluntarily consumed alcohol recreationally,[2] and approximately 70% are at least monthly users of alcohol. Approximately 8% of the adult population, around 13 million people, are thought to be alcoholic, described in DSM-III-R as alcohol dependence. Medical complications of alcoholism are common and varied, with virtually all organ systems affected. Common examples of medical complications are liver disease (e.g., cirrhosis, fatty liver), cardiomyopathy, pancreatitis, gastrointestinal disease (e.g., ulcer, varices), anemia, CNS disturbances, and fetal alcohol syndrome.[8]

Alcohol organic mental disorders including alcohol intoxication and withdrawal are listed in Table 47.1. Alcohol organic mental disorders are groups of psychologic or behavioral signs and symptoms caused by ingestion of alcohol. Signs and symptoms of alcohol intoxication and alcohol withdrawal are summarized in Table 47.2. Physical symptoms of alcohol intoxication include slurred speech, ataxia, nystagmus, sedation, and flushed face. Psychologic symptoms include mood change, irritability, loquacity, and impaired attention.[9]

**Table 47.2** Signs and Symptoms of Alcohol Intoxication and Withdrawal

| *Intoxication* | *Withdrawal* |
|---|---|
| Slurred speech | Tremor |
| Ataxia | Tachycardia |
| Nystagmus | Diaphoresis |
| Sedation | Labile blood pressure |
| Flushed face | Anxiety |
| Mood change | Nausea and vomiting |
| Irritability | Hallucinations |
| Euphoria | Seizures |
| Loquacity | Hyperthermia |
| Impaired attention | Delirium |

Alcohol is always a nonspecific CNS depressant drug that does not appear to act by any receptor mechanism.[9] Inhibitory functions of the brain (e.g., impulse control) are depressed at lower alcohol concentrations than excitatory functions (e.g., consciousness and respiration). Although individuals with mild alcohol intoxication may appear stimulated, an effect known as a "disinhibition effect," this behavior is a CNS depressant effect. Alcohol idiosyncratic intoxication is associated with a marked behavioral change, such as aggressive or assaultive behavior, within minutes of the ingestion of alcohol in an amount insufficient to cause intoxication in most people.[8]

Alcohol withdrawal is a cumulative phasic process; that is, symptoms of the initial phases do not diminish as withdrawal progresses to advanced phases. The extent of phasic progression is determined by the amount of alcohol consumed, the abruptness of discontinuation, and overall physical health. Although alcoholics do not uniformly fit the stereotype of the "skid row" individual, patients who are nutritionally deficient, are dehydrated, or have compromised organ system status or other debilitating factors are at risk for more severe withdrawal.

Phase I acute alcohol withdrawal begins within hours of cessation of drinking, lasts 3 to 5 days, and consists of tremor, autonomic hyperactivity including tachycardia, diaphoresis, labile blood pressure, anxiety, and nausea and vomiting. Phase II withdrawal includes perceptual disturbances, which are most commonly auditory or visual, but may be of any type. Phase III includes seizures, usually the generalized clonic–tonic type, lasting 30 seconds to 4 minutes and progressing to status epilepticus in approximately 3% of cases. Between 10% and 15% of untreated alcohol withdrawal patients experience withdrawal seizures. Phase IV is called delirium tremens, a syndrome of acute autonomic hyperactivity and delirium, including severe hyperthermia. The mortality rate for patients who progress to phase IV is approximately 20%. Deaths are frequently related to stroke or cardiovascular collapse. Most alcohol withdrawal patients do not progress beyond phase II, even when they are untreated.[10]

Other alcohol organic mental disorders include alcohol amnestic disorder and dementia associated with alcoholism. Alcohol amnestic disorder is an impairment of both short-term and long-term memory in the presence of an otherwise clear consciousness after prolonged heavy ingestion of alcohol. Alcohol amnestic disorder is frequently also called alcohol "blackouts," a loss of recall for events that occurred under the influence of alcohol. Dementia associated with alcoholism is a loss of intellectual functioning and memory impairment after prolonged heavy ingestion of alcohol that persists at least 3 weeks after discontinuation of alcohol consumption. Interestingly, this is the only instance in which the DSM-III-R criteria mention "alcoholism." What much of the medical community refers to as alcoholism is classified in DSM-III-R as alcohol dependence.

### Barbiturates, Benzodiazepines, and Other Sedative–Hypnotics

Incidence and prevalence of use of sedative–hypnotic drugs are difficult to pinpoint, but recent trends suggest a gradually declining rate of use. Of special interest is the fact that the source of most sedative–hypnotic abuse is prescriptions. Approximately 19% of adults have tried a sedative drug for nonmedical use, with 2.6% having used a sedative in the past month.[2] Shorter acting barbiturates (e.g., pentobarbital, secobarbital) are generally preferred over longer acting drugs (e.g., phenobarbital). A combination of secobarbital and amobarbital, an intermediate-acting barbiturate, is popular among barbiturate users. Shorter acting nonbarbiturate sedative–hypnotics including meprobamate, methyprylon, ethchlorvynol, and glutethimide are also commonly abused. Among the benzodiazepines, faster onset drugs, especially diazepam which has the highest lipophilicity among the benzodiazepines, are often preferred[11]; however, all benzodiazepines have abuse and dependence liability and patients generally cannot be switched from one benzodiazepine drug to another in hopes of decreasing a pattern of drug abuse or dependence behavior.

Barbiturate and similarly acting sedative or hypnotic organic mental disorders include diagnoses analogous to the alcohol organic mental disorders (intoxication, withdrawal, amnestic disorder, etc.), and as barbiturate and barbiturate-like drugs are similar to alcohol pharmacologically (i.e., they are both CNS depressants), their clinical presentations are also similar. An important difference between the barbiturate-like drugs and benzodiazepines is the potential for toxicity at very high doses. Benzodiazepines do not generally cause significant respiratory depression as do the barbiturate-like drugs.[12] Although the clinical presentation of alcohol withdrawal is similar in many respects to that of sedative–hypnotic withdrawal, the time courses may be quite different. Some barbiturates (e.g., phenobarbital, amobarbital) and some benzodiazepines (e.g., diazepam, flurazepam, chlordiazepoxide, clorazepate) have elimination half-lives or active metabolites with elimination half-lives of 24 to greater than 100 hours.[13] As a result, the onset of withdrawal symptoms may be delayed for several days after discontinuation of the drug. Dependence on sedative–hypnotics and benzodiazepines is summarized in Table 47.3.

Long-term use of even therapeutic doses of benzodiazepines may cause physical dependence and withdrawal symptoms after abrupt discontinuation.[14] Patients who have taken benzodiazepines for the treatment of anxiety often experience a rebound increase in anxiety after discontinuation of the antianxiety drug. The heightened autonomic activity of severe anxiety can be easily mistaken for drug withdrawal. A combination of withdrawal and increased anxiety may also occur, and each may intensify the other. Occurrence of hallucinations or seizures would indicate severe physical withdrawal.

### Opiates

Intravenous injection of an opiate causes a warm flushing of the skin and a lower abdominal sensation often described as similar to sexual orgasm. Tolerance may develop rapidly, possibly after the first dose, as many users say they are never able to achieve the same experience again, although a heightened sense of anticipation may also explain the perceived decrease in effect. After the initial "rush," there is a period of apathetic detachment for a few hours before the effect of the drug wears off.[15]

Incidence and prevalence of opiate use are widely variable depending on the drug. Heroin, which gained widespread notoriety during the 1960s and 1970s and which remains the single most commonly used illicit opiate, has been tried by about 1% of the adult population, with less than 0.5% having used it in the last month.[2] The number of heroin-dependent individuals nationally is estimated at around half a million, a number that pales somewhat in comparison with the approximately 13 million alcohol-dependent individuals.

Collectively, use of opiates other than heroin is far more common. Approximately 12% of adults have tried an opiate or opiate-like analgesic for nonmedical use, with around 1% having used an analgesic within 1 month.[2] With the decreased availability of Asian heroin and a subsequent decline in purity of street heroin (frequently to less than 1% pure), new trends in street drug use have emerged since the mid-1970s. Hydromorphone has become widely used among the opiate-using population, with single 4-mg tablets selling for as much as $65. Hydromorphone has a pharmaceutical profile very similar to that of heroin, with the advantage of purity. Drug combinations involving opiates are quite popular. Pentazocine combined with tripelennamine, an antihistamine (so-called "T's and blues"), is an example, although use of the combination has declined with the addition of naloxone, an opiate receptor antagonist, to pentazocine tablets. Opiates are commonly combined with stimulant drugs, especially cocaine, a combination known as a "speedball," although any sedative combined with any stimulant is often referred to as a speedball. Opiate users frequently also drink alcohol, especially when their use of opiate drugs declines because of lack of availability or sometimes after treatment.

Many of the complications of opiate use, especially intravenous use, are related not only to the drug itself, but also to varying purity, contaminants, and techniques of administration such as dirty equipment and use of shared needles. Overdoses, anaphylactic reactions to impurities, nephrotic syndrome, septicemia, endocarditis, and acquired immune deficiency syndrome (AIDS) are examples.[15]

Not all opiate use is street drug use. Some opiate-dependent individuals first obtained their drug during medical treatment and progressed to compulsive drug use and an inability to tolerate the drug-free state, although the number of these individuals may be very small. The prevalence of opiate-dependent health care professionals is extremely high relative to other groups of comparable educational and socioeconomic status. Most impaired health care professionals initially use the drug to relieve depression or fatigue and not generally to achieve an intense euphoria. There are many opiate-dependent individuals who initially used street drugs but now obtain methadone as part of their treatment.

Opioid organic mental disorders include opioid intoxication, withdrawal, and opioid residual disorder. Signs and symptoms of opioid intoxication and withdrawal are summarized in Table 47.4. Physical signs of opioid intoxication include pupillary constriction, sedation, slurred speech, and impaired attention or memory. Psychologic signs include euphoria or dysphoria, apathy, and motor retardation.[15]

Signs and symptoms of opioid withdrawal include lacrimation, rhinorrhea, pupillary dilation, piloerection ("goose pimple flesh"), diaphoresis, diarrhea, yawning, fever and muscle aching, and insomnia.[15] Onset of the acute phase of

**Table 47.3** Dependence on Sedative–Hypnotics[a]

| *Generic name* | *Common trade names [manufacturer]* | *Common street name* | *Oral sedating dose (mg)* | *Physical dependence dose and time needed to produce dependence* | *Time before onset of withdrawal (h)* | *Peak withdrawal symptoms (d)* |
|---|---|---|---|---|---|---|
| **A. Barbiturates** | | | | | | |
| Secobarbital | Seconal, Seco-8 [Lilly] | Reds, Red Devils, Seccies, F-40's, Mexican Reds | 100 | 800–2,200 mg × 35–37 d | 6–12 | 2–3 |
| Pentobarbital | Nembutal [Abbott] | Yellows, Yellow Jackets, Yellow Bullets, Nebbies | 100 | Same | 6–12 | 2–3 |
| Equal parts of seco- and amobarbital | Tuinal [Lilly] | Rainbows, Tuies, Double Trouble | 100 | Same | 6–12 | 2–3 |
| Amobarbital | Amytal [Lilly] | Blue Heavens, Blue Dolls, Blues | 65–100 | Same | 8–12 | 2–5 |
| **B. Nonbarbiturate Sedative-Hypnotics** | | | | | | |
| Glutethimide | Doriden [USV] | Goof Balls, Goofers | 125 | 1.5–3 g × 30 d | 6–12 | 2–3 |
| Ethchlorvynol | Placidyl [Abbott] | | 200 | 1–1.5 g × 30 d | 6–12 | 2–3 |
| Chloral hydrate | Noctec, Somnos, Kessodrate [various] | Jelly Beans, Miki's, Knock-out Drops | 250 | Exact dose unknown; 12 g/d chronically has led to delirium upon sudden withdrawal | | |
| Methyprylon | Noludar [Roche] | Noodlelars | 100 | 30 g × 30 d (est.) | 6–12 | 2–3 |
| Meprobamate | Equanil, Miltown, Meprotabs [various] | — | 400 | 1.6–3.2 g × 270 d | 8–12 | 3–8 |
| **C. Benzodiazepines** | | | | | | |
| Diazepam | Valium [Roche] | Vals | 5–10 | 40–120 mg × 42–120 d | 12–24 | 5–8 |
| Chlordiazepoxide | Librium, Libritabs [Roche] | Libs | 10–25 | 75–600 mg × 42–120 d | 12–24 | 5–8 |
| Flurazepam | Dalmane [Roche] | — | 15–30 | 60–150 mg × 42–120 d (est.) | 8–24 | 3–8 |
| Clorazepate | Tranxene [Abbott] | — | 7.5–15 | 45–180 mg × 42–120 d (est.) | 12–24 | 5–8 |
| Oxazepam | Serax [Wyeth] | — | 15–30 | 90–150 mg × 42–120 d | 8–24 | 2–3 |
| Alprazolam | Xanax [Upjohn] | — | 0.25–8 | 8–16 mg × 42 d (est.) | 8–24 | 2–3 |

[a] Common withdrawal symptoms are tremor, tachycardia, diaphoresis, nausea, vomiting, blood pressure lability, delirium, seizures, and hallucinations.

withdrawal varies with the drug consumed, but ranges from a few hours after stopping the drug with heroin to 3 to 5 days with methadone. The time course of withdrawal ranges from 3 to 14 days. Opioid withdrawal is significantly different from withdrawal from alcohol or other sedative–hypnotics. Of greatest importance is that opioid withdrawal is not fatal unless there is a concurrent medical problem of major concern. This has significant treatment implications, especially where drug therapy is concerned. Although patients in opioid withdrawal may be in great discomfort and incapacitated, they are not delirious. The presence of delirium should raise the question of concurrent withdrawal from another drug, such as alcohol, or another cause of delirium possibly secondary to drug use.

**Table 47.4** Signs and Symptoms of Opioid Intoxication and Withdrawal

| *Intoxication* | *Withdrawal* |
|---|---|
| Euphoria | Lacrimation |
| Dysphoria | Rhinorrhea |
| Apathy | Mydriasis |
| Motor retardation | Piloerection |
| Sedation | Diaphoresis |
| Slurred speech | Diarrhea |
| Attention impairment | Yawning |
| Miosis | Fever |
| | Insomnia |
| | Muscle aching |

## *Central Nervous System Stimulants*

### Cocaine

Cocaine is perhaps the most behaviorally reinforcing of all recreational drugs. That is not to say that dependence on other drugs (e.g., alcohol) is any less "powerful" than that on cocaine, but the pharmacology, pharmacokinetics, and route of administration of cocaine cause intense drug-seeking behavior. The most characteristic systemic effect of cocaine is stimulation of the CNS.[16] In the CNS, cocaine appears to mediate its effects primarily by blocking reuptake of catecholamine neurotransmitters, norepinephrine and dopamine. The most common clinical manifestations of cocaine stimulation of the CNS are intense euphoria, decreased fatigue, and increased alertness. Common slang terms for cocaine are "coke," "snow," "girl," and "nose candy."

Cocaine is rapidly absorbed from virtually all sites of application. Traditionally, cocaine has been administered as the hydrochloride salt form, usually by inhalation, but also by injection. In recent years as the purity of cocaine hydrochloride obtained on the street has declined, many users have converted the cocaine hydrochloride salt to cocaine base, frequently referred to as "freebase."[17] Converting cocaine hydrochloride to cocaine base is accomplished by creating an alkaline environment, such as with the addition of ether or sodium bicarbonate and heat. Combined with sodium bicarbonate, the cocaine base clumps together into rocklike formations commonly referred to as "crack." Cocaine base is stable to heat and can be smoked, and because nonbasic impurities have been eliminated, it is a purer form of the drug. The "rocks" of cocaine base are melted and the vapors inhaled. This form of administration of the drug leads to almost instant absorption and intense euphoria. Peak plasma concentrations greater than 900 ng/mL have been achieved after inhalation of cocaine base vapors. Peak concentrations of 150–200 ng/mL have been achieved after inhalation of 96 mg of pure cocaine hydrochloride powder.[18]

Cocaine is rapidly metabolized and eliminated. The elimination half-life of cocaine is approximately 1 hour and the duration of effect is very short.[16] Coupled with the compensatory CNS depression commonly experienced when the effect of the drug is diminished, the short duration of effect provides a powerful incentive for repeated use of the drug. Many users experience intense drug use cycling, sometimes lasting days, characterized by rapidly repeating doses of cocaine until their supply is exhausted. Monkeys, given a choice between food and cocaine around the clock for 8 days, consistently choose cocaine.[19]

Complications of cocaine use frequently involve cardiovascular system events.[20] Even in small doses, cocaine slows the heart through a vagal stimulation. At higher doses, it increases heart rate because of an overall systemic increase in sympathetic tone. At toxic doses, cocaine causes cardiac failure because of a direct effect on myocardial contractility. Cocaine is also pyrogenic, and hyperthermia is frequently observed in cocaine poisoning. Death is usually related to arrhythmias, shock, or convulsions.

Cocaine is a psychotomimetic drug, sometimes even at systemically nontoxic doses. A kindling phenomenon has been described with cocaine in which neuronal function becomes altered with each dose of the drug. This causes a type of reverse tolerance with increased receptor sensitivity to cocaine, and psychosis may be caused by doses that formerly did not cause psychosis. A toxic psychosis caused by cocaine is characterized by auditory, visual, and frequently tactile hallucinations, paranoid thinking, and looseness of associations. The psychosis is qualitatively very similar to a paranoid schizophrenic psychosis.[21]

Incidence and prevalence of cocaine use increased significantly in the early 1980s. In the mid-1980s, the advent of "crack" at low prices, sometimes \$5 to \$10 for a single dose, has increased use among lower socioeconomic groups. Clearly, cocaine is no longer a drug used primarily by affluent users; 28% of adults have tried cocaine, with approximately 7% having used it in the past month.[2] While use of some drugs seems to be declining slightly, use of cocaine has remained steady.

Cocaine organic mental disorders include cocaine intoxication, withdrawal, delirium, delusional disorder, flashback disorder, and residual disorder. Signs and symptoms of cocaine intoxication are summarized in Table 47.5. Although there is some controversy as to whether cocaine is associated with physical withdrawal upon abrupt discontinuation, most clinicians feel that there is a characteristic syndrome of withdrawal effects although not life-threatening.[15] Cocaine

**Table 47.5** Signs and Symptoms of Cocaine Intoxication and Withdrawal

| *Intoxication* | *Withdrawal* |
|---|---|
| Motor agitation | Fatigue |
| Elation/euphoria | Sleep disturbance |
| Grandiosity | Nightmares |
| Loquacity | Depression |
| Hypervigilance | |
| Tachycardia | |
| Mydriasis | |
| Elevated blood pressure | |
| Sweating or chills | |
| Nausea and vomiting | |

withdrawal consists primarily of fatigue, sleep disturbance, nightmares, and depression, begins within hours of discontinuation of the drug, and lasts up to several days.

**Amphetamines and Other Stimulants**

The physiologic and psychologic effects of amphetamines and other stimulants are qualitatively the same as those of cocaine (i.e., they diminish fatigue, increase alertness, suppress appetite, etc). Amphetamines are psychotomimetic and amphetamine-induced psychosis is a principal experimental model for schizophrenia. Pharmacologically, amphetamines increase the activity of catecholamine neurotransmitters (e.g., norepinephrine, dopamine) by blocking reuptake, increasing release of neurotransmitters, and inhibiting the degradative enzyme monoamine oxidase. The primary differences between cocaine and amphetamines are pharmacokinetic. The onset and duration of effect of amphetamines are not as abrupt as those of cocaine.[15]

The incidence and prevalence of stimulant use (other than cocaine) may be decreasing. Approximately 18% of adults have tried stimulants other than cocaine at least once, with approximately 5% having used them in the past month.[2] In addition to use of stimulants for their euphoric effects, amphetamines and similar drugs are sometimes used by long-distance drivers and students to maintain alertness. When used intravenously, methamphetamine and amphetamine are known as "speed." An increased awareness by state and federal regulatory authorities of diversion of stimulants via so-called weight control clinics has led to renewed efforts to control distribution of these drugs, and prescription of amphetamines may be decreasing. Many states now prohibit prescription of class II stimulants for obesity.

The stimulants include many of the so-called "designer" and "lookalike" drugs. A common example is 3,4-methylenedioxymethamphetamine (MDMA), usually called "ecstasy."[22] Nonprescription stimulant drugs such as caffeine and phenylpropanolamine are frequently packaged in dosage forms designed to resemble more potent amphetamine stimulant drugs.[23] Designer drugs are the result of efforts of amateur organic chemists to manipulate the chemical structure of controlled substances to create drugs with similar effects, but which are not subject to legal prescription controls, although measures have been introduced to allow the U.S. Food and Drug Administration (FDA) to rapidly classify these substances as class I drugs (i.e., no approved medical use and subject to regulatory authority).

### *Phencyclidine*

Phencyclidine was first used as a veterinary anesthetic and briefly as an anesthetic in humans. Phencyclidine is a member of the arylcyclohexylamines. Another member compound, ketamine, is still used clinically as an anesthetic and has many of the same effects as phencyclidine.[15] Phencyclidine, commonly referred to as PCP, angel dust, and crystal, was popular in the 1970s, but as its adverse effects became better known, use declined. Phencyclidine is a frequent substitute or contaminant of other drugs, and its most common pattern of use may now be unintentional. The actual extent of its use is unclear. It is often misrepresented as LSD or THC (tetrahydrocannabinol). THC is virtually unavailable on the street as it is highly unstable when isolated from the marijuana plant. When used intentionally, PCP is commonly smoked with marijuana, referred to as a "crystal joint," but may also be taken orally or intravenously.[24]

**Table 47.6** Signs and Symptoms of Phencyclidine Intoxication

| | |
|---|---|
| Nystagmus | Euphoria |
| Increased blood pressure | Motor agitation |
| Tachycardia | Anxiety and emotional lability |
| Paresthesias | Hostility |
| Ataxia | Delusions |
| Slurred speech | Hallucinations |
| Muscle rigidity | |

Phencyclidine has widely varied actions including CNS stimulation, depression, and hallucinogenic properties. Pharmacologically, it is known to block reuptake of serotonin, dopamine, and norepinephrine, but neurotransmitter antagonists do not effectively block its effects. Phencyclidine may also bind at an opiate receptor associated with psychotomimetic properties, the sigma receptor. In low doses, phencyclidine causes sedation, ataxia, nystagmus, slurred speech, and paresthesias. At higher doses users experience an increase in heart rate, blood pressure, and temperature, diaphoresis, and muscle rigidity. At acutely toxic doses, coma and seizures are known to occur.[25]

Behavioral effects of phencyclidine range from sleep to catatonic detachment to paranoid psychosis to violent hostility. Users are sometimes amnestic for events that occur under the influence of the drug. Psychoses sometimes last weeks. Users with a previous history of schizophrenia are especially susceptible to the psychotomimetic effects of the drug. The only truly characteristic behavioral effect of phencyclidine use is its high unpredictability. The signs and symptoms of phencyclidine intoxication are summarized in Table 47.6.

### *Hallucinogens*

The drugs commonly thought of as being within this category are LSD (lysergic acid diethylamide), psilocybin, DMT (dimethyltryptamine), mescaline, and other related compounds. The incidence and prevalence of hallucinogen use may be decreasing; however, approximately 21% of adults have tried the drugs, with about 2% having used them within a month. These figures may be somewhat misleading, as reporting of use of these drugs generally also includes phencyclidine. Hallucinogenic activity is certainly not unique to these drugs, as discussed for cocaine, amphetamine, phencyclidine, and marijuana. If there is a characteristic effect of the hallucinogens, it is the so-called psychedelic effect, a heightened awareness of sensation with a diminished ability to differentiate boundaries of objects or the self from the environment. Pharmacologically, LSD and related drugs stimulate both presynaptic ($5HT_{1A}$, $5HT_{1B}$, $5HT_{1C}$) and postsynaptic ($5HT_2$) serotonin recognition sites. Hallucinogens, other than LSD, have more potent activity at the $5HT_2$ site.[26] Precisely how the hallucinogens exert their

**Table 47.7** Signs and Symptoms of Hallucinogen Intoxication

| *Psychologic* | *Physical* |
|---|---|
| Perceptual intensification | Mydriasis |
| Depersonalization | Tachycardia |
| Derealization | Diaphoresis |
| Illusions | Palpitations |
| Hallucinations | Blurred vision |
| Synesthesias | Tremor |
| | Incoordination |
| | Dizziness |
| | Weakness |
| | Drowsiness |
| | Paresthesias |

effects remains unclear. LSD, often referred to as "acid," is an extraordinarily potent compound, producing observable CNS effects at doses as low as 25 $\mu$g.[27]

Signs and symptoms of hallucinogen intoxication are summarized in Table 47.7. Physical signs of hallucinogen intoxication include mydriasis, tachycardia, diaphoresis, palpitations, blurred vision, tremor, and incoordination. These symptoms suggest a sympathomimetic effect. Other physical symptoms include dizziness, weakness, drowsiness, nausea, and paresthesias. Psychologic symptoms of intoxication include a subjective intensification of perceptions, depersonalization, illusions, hallucinations, and synesthesias, the overflow of one sensory modality to another (i.e., colors are heard and sounds are seen). Among the hallucinogenic drugs, LSD is the most potent and long acting; it is hundreds of times more potent than both psilocybin and mescaline. DMT is inactive when ingested orally, but can be smoked, inhaled, or injected. There is cross-tolerance among LSD, psilocybin, and mescaline. There is not an observable physical withdrawal syndrome after abrupt discontinuation of hallucinogenic drugs.[27]

Complications from hallucinogen use are primarily psychologic. Users sometimes experience prolonged episodes of panic, the so-called "bad trip." Hallucinogen drug flashbacks are common, occurring in approximately 15% of users, and occur episodically up to several years after the last exposure to the drug. Flashbacks may occur spontaneously, but are also triggered by other drugs, including marijuana, and by anxiety-provoking stimuli. Physical effects of hallucinogen use are relatively nontoxic. Deaths are generally accidents related to intoxication but not to direct effects of the drug. There is no evidence that hallucinogen use causes chromosome damage or genetic defects.[15,27]

### *Marijuana*

Marijuana, referred to as reefer, pot, grass, or weed, is the most commonly used illicit drug. Approximately 64% of adults have tried the drug, with 27% having used it within the last month.[2] Among youths 12–17, 27% have tried marijuana, with 12% having used it within a month. *Cannabis sativa*, the marijuana plant, has been produced in the United States and elsewhere in recent years with increasingly sophisticated growing techniques. Content of $\Delta^9$-tetrahydrocannabinol (THC), the principal psychoactive component, has reached as high as 11%. Hashish, the dried resin of the top of the plant, is much more potent than the plant itself. The pharmacologic mechanism of THC is unknown.[15]

**Table 47.8** Signs and Symptoms of Marijuana Intoxication

| | |
|---|---|
| Tachycardia | Euphoria |
| Conjunctival congestion | Sensory intensification |
| Increased appetite | Apathy |
| Dry mouth | Hallucinations |

Marijuana has been widely used and is believed by many to be a relatively harmless, nonaddictive intoxicant. Chronic exposure to marijuana is not associated with significant physical withdrawal upon abrupt discontinuation, but many chronic users exhibit compulsive drug-seeking and drug use behavior characteristic of addiction or dependence. As experience with the drug is gained, it is clear that marijuana is far from harmless. Acutely, marijuana has many of the effects of alcohol—sedation, a decrease in reactivity and ability to perform complex tasks, and disinhibition. Marijuana also causes hallucinations. Chronic use is associated with all of the risks of tobacco smoking, although marijuana smokers are commonly also tobacco smokers and thus differentiation of effects is often difficult. Endocrine effects including amenorrhea, decreased testosterone production, and inhibition of spermatogenesis have been demonstrated. Marijuana causes an organic residual disorder commonly known as marijuana "amotivational" syndrome, characterized by a behavioral pattern of apathy, dullness, impaired judgment, decreased concentration and memory, loss of interest in personal hygiene, and a general reduction of goal-directed behavior.[28]

The signs and symptoms of marijuana intoxication are summarized in Table 47.8. Cardiovascular effects and reddened conjunctivae are the most prominent physical effects with acute use (e.g., tachycardia, increased blood pressure with large orthostatic changes). Although the duration of effect of marijuana may be only several hours, THC is detectable upon toxicologic screening for up to 4 or 5 weeks, especially in chronic users.[15]

### *Inhalants*

Inhalation of organic solvents including gasoline, glue, aerosols, amyl nitrite, and nitrous oxide remains relatively common and may be increasing in prevalence. Precise determination of incidence and prevalence is difficult because surveys frequently do not include these drugs. Approximately 17% of adults and high school seniors have tried inhalant drugs.[29]

Toluene is a common solvent component. The most recent trend in inhalants is the use of typewriter correction fluid, referred to as "whiting out," which contains trichloroethane and trichloroethylene. Several sudden death reactions related to inhalation of fumes of typewriter correction fluid have been reported.[30–32]

Inhalants are CNS depressants and symptoms of intoxication are similar to those of alcohol. Intoxication is often accompanied by headache and nausea and users may experience hallucinations and delusions. The most serious physical risk of acute use is sudden death, usually from cardiac arrhythmias. Some users die from suffocation by plastic bags that contain the solvent. With chronic use, the drugs are toxic to virtually all organ systems. Psychologic impairment, impaired pulmonary, renal, and hepatic function, neuropathies, encephalopathy, and brain damage have all been observed.[29]

### *Tobacco*

Tobacco is the second most commonly used recreational drug in the United States behind alcohol. Approximately 77% of the adult population have tried tobacco; 40% use tobacco regularly.[2] The health consequences of tobacco use are enormous and well known. A characteristic withdrawal syndrome associated with nicotine, the principal psychoactive component of tobacco, has been observed. Nicotine withdrawal consists of headache, increased appetite, gastrointestinal disturbance, anxiety, irritability, difficulty concentrating, and restlessness. Withdrawal begins within 24 hours of last exposure to nicotine, with some symptoms, such as increased appetite, lasting weeks.[15]

### *Caffeine*

Caffeine is widely consumed in coffee, tea, soft drinks, chocolate, and many analgesic preparations. Health consequences remain controversial. Many soft drinks are now marketed in a caffeine-free form. Caffeinism secondary to excessive intake of caffeine has been well documented but is treated clinically only by discontinuation of the drug. Caffeinism may be observed after the ingestion of as little as 300 mg (equivalent to about two to three cups of coffee) in sensitive individuals, but is more often associated with doses near 1 g. Caffeine intoxication is characterized by restlessness, anxiety, insomnia, flushed face, diuresis, gastrointestinal complaints, muscle twitching, palpitations, and motor agitation.[33]

Physical dependence may occur when daily intake exceeds approximately 500 mg of the drug, about five cups of coffee. It is estimated that approximately 25% of the adult population consume this much caffeine per day. Physical withdrawal from caffeine, beginning around 24 hours after last exposure and lasting several days, consists primarily of headache, anxiety, and restlessness.[33]

### *Anticholinergic Drugs*

Scopolamine, trihexyphenidyl, benztropine, and other anticholinergic drugs have potentially intoxicating effects. Symptoms of an anticholinergic drug–induced toxic psychosis include euphoria, disorientation, hallucinations, and paranoid ideation. Physical symptoms include mydriasis, warm dry skin, tachycardia, dry mouth, ataxia, and constipation with absence of bowel sounds. Users of anticholinergic drugs describe a "buzz" associated with the drugs, and there are reports of individuals presenting to emergency rooms asking for the drugs by name or feigning extrapyramidal symptoms to obtain them.[34,35]

## Pathophysiology

### *Mechanisms of Tolerance, Dependence, and Withdrawal*

Many factors influence the development of drug dependence. As with any disease, a susceptible host must be combined with favorable conditions. Western society is unquestionably drug oriented. Advertising encourages the reward of good behavior and productivity by the use of alcohol, tobacco, and caffeine. Use of drugs, especially alcohol, is often depicted in the context of boisterous camaraderie and good times after a hard day's work or play.

Drug dependence depends on the reinforcing properties of the drug being used (i.e., the drug satisfies a need that demands repetition). Drug dependence most likely evolves in a phasic manner. The euphoriant or other pleasant properties of a drug act initially as reinforcers of drug-seeking behavior; but as tolerance develops, the pleasant effects of the drug are reduced, and higher doses are required to produce the same desirable feelings. Also, the user becomes aware of the need to avoid the pain and discomfort associated with the abstinence syndrome, or drug withdrawal. Many drug-dependent individuals state that their principal motivation for drug use turns relatively quickly from seeking of pleasurable effects to avoidance of unpleasant effects.[36]

Mechanisms of physical dependence involve homeostasis. Drugs disturb biochemical and physiologic systems, and systems therefore adapt to reduce those effects. Such compensatory adaptation leads to the development of tolerance. Therefore, when the drug is withdrawn, the compensatory changes dominate and the user experiences withdrawal symptoms. The clinical manifestations of withdrawal syndromes are generally opposite those of the drugs that produced them. In many cases, the disturbance in homeostatic mechanisms may be long-lasting. Withdrawal may consist of an acute, relatively short phase lasting several days, followed by a more subacute, protracted withdrawal syndrome. Opiate dependence, for example, is associated with a "conditioned abstinence syndrome" lasting several months or longer after cessation of intake and may be precipitated by environmental stimuli previously associated with drug use.[36] Opiate-dependent individuals have reported the onset of physical withdrawal symptoms after merely coming into contact with their previous environment (e.g., the user's neighborhood, the sight of heroin, or the observation of other individuals who are using drugs). Conditioned abstinence may be described as a heightened sensitivity to stimuli, abnormal autonomic responses, dysphoria, and intense craving for the effects of the drug.

There are two types of physiologic tolerance to drugs.[37] The first, dispositional tolerance, also called metabolic or pharmacokinetic tolerance, results from changes in the pharmacokinetics of drugs. Usually, the tolerance is related to increased metabolism. Examples of drugs associated with dispositional tolerance are barbiturates and alcohol. The second type of tolerance is pharmacodynamic tolerance, also known as cellular or functional tolerance. Pharmacodynamic tolerance results from adaptive changes at the site of action of drugs, such as changes in receptor system binding sensitivity. Examples of drugs that exhibit pharmacodynamic tolerance are alcohol and opiates.

### *CNS Depressants*

Alcohol tolerance develops through both dispositional and pharmacodynamic mechanisms.[38] Alcohol is an inducer of liver enzymes and enhances its own metabolism, but the principal mechanism of tolerance appears to be pharmacodynamic. Acute effects of alcohol are mediated by the fluid permeability of cell membranes and alcohol appears to fluidize the cell membrane. When the effect of alcohol is diminished, the structural integrity of the membrane appears to return to levels greater than those present before exposure to alcohol. Greater concentrations of alcohol are then required to refluidize the membrane. Alcohol has a depressing, disordering effect on cell function, and cells compensate by increasing sympathetic activity. In the abrupt absence of alcohol, sympathetic nervous system overactivity appears to cause withdrawal.

The principal mechanism of barbiturate tolerance appears to be dispositional.[39] All barbiturates are potent inducers of liver enzymes and induce their own metabolism. Tolerance to benzodiazepines appears to be primarily pharmacodynamic.[40] The precise cellular mechanism of tolerance to benzodiazepines is not clear, but may be a decrease in the number or sensitivity of benzodiazepine receptors.

Tolerance to opiates appears to be pharmacodynamic.[15] The primary center of the brain for both opiate- and noradrenergic-mediated neurons appears to be the locus ceruleus in the midbrain. Neurons from the locus ceruleus project throughout the cerebral cortex. Although there are multiple subtypes of opiate receptors, the opiate receptor appears to be primarily a presynaptic receptor and has an inhibitory effect on the noradrenergic nerve terminal (i.e., stimulation of the presynaptic opiate receptor inhibits neuronal release of norepinephrine). The endogenous ligand for the opiate receptor is enkephalin. Another presynaptic receptor that serves as an inhibitory receptor for noradrenergic activity is the $\alpha_2$-adrenergic receptor.[41] The presynaptic $\alpha_2$ receptor is a norepinephrine autoreceptor.

Chronic use of exogenous opiates such as heroin, hydromorphone, and methadone causes a decrease in production of the endogenous substance enkephalin, just as administration of exogenous corticosteroids causes a decrease in endogenous production of cortisol. Greater than normal activity at the receptor is associated with a compensatory decrease in the binding sensitivity of the opiate receptor system, also known as downregulation. As the opiate receptor is inhibitory to noradrenergic activity, a downregulation effect would diminish the effect of opiates; thus larger doses would be required to achieve the same degree of inhibition of noradrenergic activity. Abrupt discontinuation of exogenous opiates produces a downregulated inhibitory opiate receptor system and diminished levels of the endogenous ligand, enkephalin. Therefore, opiate withdrawal is a syndrome of noradrenergic hyperactivity.[42]

### *CNS Stimulants*

Tolerance to the stimulants, including cocaine, is pharmacodynamic in nature,[15] but the precise cellular mechanism is unclear; however, tolerance to different pharmacologic effects of stimulants develops at different rates. Tolerance to appetite suppression, for example, develops within days to weeks, whereas tolerance to the euphoric effects and increased alertness develops more slowly. A type of reverse pharmacodynamic tolerance, kindling, was described earlier and has been observed with both cocaine and amphetamines. The neuropharmacology of cocaine and amphetamine withdrawal is not well understood; however, such withdrawal effects as depression, fatigue, and increased sleep and appetite are the opposite of the usual effects of the drug, as is the case with most drugs. Chronic cocaine use may cause catecholamine depletion in the brain.

Tolerance develops to phencyclidine and the LSD-type hallucinogens, although the mechanisms are not clearly understood. Phencyclidine may be associated with a dispositional tolerance. Tolerance to LSD and other hallucinogens that decrease serotonin activity may be related to a compensatory increase in serotonin activity, a type of pharmacodynamic tolerance.[15] Tolerance to marijuana is known, but the mechanism is unclear. Data regarding dispositional tolerance are conflicting and a mechanism of pharmacodynamic tolerance has not been elucidated. The mechanism of tolerance to inhalants is not understood.

### *Disease Concept of Addiction*

Individuals who are drug dependent are frequently regarded as constitutionally weak people who have brought their problems upon themselves and deserve the consequences of their behavior. Even when the lay public and health care professionals acknowledge addiction as a disease process, it is often felt to be self-induced. The disease concept of addiction, using alcoholism as a model, states that addiction is a disease and that individuals who suffer from the disease do not choose to contract the disease any more than someone who suffers from heart disease or diabetes mellitus chooses to contract that illness. A *disease* is defined as "a definite morbid process having a characteristic train of symptoms. It may affect the whole body or any of its parts, and its etiology, pathology, and prognosis may be known or unknown."[43] Alcoholism meets all of the definition criteria.

Discussions of the disease of alcoholism usually focus on three points. The first point involves interindividual differences in response to alcohol, based on the animal model. When a community of rats is offered two sources of water, one a solution of glucose, the other of alcohol, approximately 90% of the animals selectively choose glucose–water after testing both supplies. The remainder prefer alcohol. If the alcohol-preferring rats are separated from the remainder of the population, their offspring are significantly more likely to be alcohol preferring.[44] Data suggest that there is significant interindividual variation in how animals prefer and respond to alcohol and that these differences can be selectively inbred.

The experience of the animal studies led researchers to examine family trends in alcoholism and the possibility that alcoholism can be genetically transmitted. The prevalence of alcoholism among the first-degree relatives of alcoholics (i.e., parents, siblings, children) is approximately 25%, versus 8% in the adult population. Concordance for alcoholism among fraternal twins is approximately 31%, but among identical twins concordance is approximately 54%,[45] although there are conflicting data on this point. When children of alcoholic parents are separated at birth and placed in nonalcoholic homes, they remain two to three times more likely to become alcoholic than adoptees whose biological parents are not alcoholic.[46–48] The difference in concordance between fraternal and identical twins and the greater likelihood of developing alcoholism among adoptees whose biological parents are alcoholic argue for what some clinicians have called a genetic "predisposition." A genetically predisposed individual will not necessarily manifest alcoholic drinking behavior. As stated previously, a susceptible host and favorable conditions must combine for a disease process to occur.

The third point regarding the disease of alcoholism regards possible biochemical abnormalities. Early studies of alcohol-preferring rats showed the presence of a compound called tetrahydropapaveroline (THP), a biosynthetic precursor of morphine. THP is formed as a result of interference of the normal metabolism of biogenic amines by acetaldehyde, a metabolite of alcohol. When THP is administered experimentally to alcohol-avoiding rats, they become alcohol preferring and remain alcohol preferring. Further, they seek alcohol to the point of intoxication and experience withdrawal.[49] Production of THP may occur only when certain concentrations of acetaldehyde are available. The critical acetaldehyde concentration may vary significantly from individual to individual and may be genetically determined. An individual who is genetically predisposed to the development of alcoholism may not manifest the aberrant drinking behavior as long as drinking is done at a level that does not reach the critical acetaldehyde concentration, sometimes called the alcoholism "threshold." In response to environmental factors such as psychosocial stressors, drinking may increase, acetaldehyde levels may increase, and production of THP may occur. The individual may then exhibit the compulsive drug-seeking and drug-using behavior and loss of control over drinking characteristic of addiction. The belief that addiction is a self-induced disease or a constitutional weakness has been dismissed by most clinicians in the addiction treatment field. Willpower and self-discipline cannot control genetics and possible biochemical abnormalities. Given that 95% of the population will try alcohol and that roughly two thirds drink alcohol regularly, the determination of who becomes alcoholic is based on more factors than environmental precipitants. It is highly likely that most "susceptible hosts" will at some time find themselves in favorable circumstances for the development of the disease.

## Treatment

### *Intoxication*

Treatment of drug intoxication, summarized in Table 47.9, is primarily supportive, and vital functions are maintained while waiting for the drug to be eliminated. When absolutely necessary, physical restraint may be required temporarily while a diagnostic evaluation is initiated to rule out other causes for the behavior (e.g., metabolic or fluid and electrolyte disturbances). Whenever possible, drug therapy should be avoided, as psychotropic drug therapy has the potential for worsening a toxic reaction of another psychoactive agent; however, when patients are agitated, combative or assaultive, hallucinatory, or delusional, drug therapy may be required. Drug therapy may also be indicated in the treatment of an acute, potentially fatal overdose, and to speed elimination of the intoxicating substance to hasten recovery. Toxicology screens are useful in the evaluation and treatment process, but many drugs, including cocaine and heroin, are eliminated so rapidly that drug screens may become negative in a matter of hours. When toxicology screens are desired, blood or urine should be collected immediately upon the patient's arrival.

For alcohol, barbiturate, and benzodiazepine intoxication, supportive treatment is the rule. In the case of opiate intoxication, if the patient is unconscious and respiration is depressed, the opiate antagonist naloxone (Narcan, Du Pont) can be used to revive the patient. The usual dosage for naloxone in acute opiate toxicity is 0.4–2.0 mg intravenously, given approximately every 3 minutes as necessary.[50] While naloxone is effective in reversing opiate overdose, it may also precipitate physical withdrawal in physically dependent patients. Patients who fail to respond to a total dosage of 10 mg of naloxone may not have taken an opiate.

Intoxication with stimulants including cocaine, is treated pharmacologically only if the patient is overtly psychotic and agitated. Antipsychotic drugs can be used on a short-term basis, and usually at relatively low doses, for example, haloperidol (Haldol, McNeil) 2–5 mg intramuscularly every 30 minutes to 6 hours as necessary, followed by 5–15 mg orally per day in single or divided doses if the patient is still

**Table 47.9** Treatment of Substance Intoxication

| *Drug class* | *Pharmacologic therapy* | *Nonpharmacologic therapy* |
|---|---|---|
| Alcohol, barbiturates, benzodiazepines, and sedative–hypnotics | None | Support vital functions |
| Opiates | Naloxone 0.4–2.0 mg IV every 3 min | Support vital functions |
| Cocaine and other CNS stimulants | Haloperidol 2–5 mg (or other antipsychotic agent) IM every 30 min to 6 h prn psychotic behavior | Monitor cardiac function |
| Hallucinogens, marijuana, and inhalants | Haloperidol as above | Reassurance; "talk down therapy"; support vital functions |
| Phencyclidine | Haloperidol as above<br>Ascorbic acid or ammonium chloride 2–3 g PO every 6 h and furosemide 40 mg PO daily | Minimize sensory input<br>Cranberry juice ad libitum |

**Table 47.10** Ion Trapping Technique for Increasing Phencyclidine Elimination

| | |
|---|---|
| 1. | Administer ascorbic acid or ammonium chloride 8–12 g/d |
| 2. | Institute hydration with cranberry, plum, or prune juice |
| 3. | When urine pH is below 5.0, force diuresis with oral furosemide 20–40 mg; repeat daily and monitor for adequate hydration |

psychotic after initial treatment.[15] Cardiovascular complications are treated symptomatically with antiarrhythmic agents or other interventions as necessary.

Hallucinogen intoxication is treated in a manner similar to stimulant intoxication. Drug therapy can often be avoided, as patients may respond to careful reassurance, or so-called "talk down" therapy. When necessary, short-term antipsychotic drug therapy can be used as described previously. The same approach applies to marijuana and inhalant intoxication.

Phencyclidine intoxication is more unpredictable and difficult to treat than intoxication with other psychosis-producing drugs. Most clinicians suggest that sensory input be minimized to the extent possible; thus, "talk down" therapy is not recommended and may in fact make the patient worse. If phencyclidine intoxication is suspected, patients should be left alone in a quiet, somewhat darkened room. If behavior is uncontrollable, antipsychotic drug therapy may be necessary. Drug therapy in phencyclidine intoxication is directed primarily at increasing the clearance of phencyclidine through a technique known as ion trapping[51] (Table 47.10). Phencyclidine is a weakly alkaline compound; thus, acidification of the urine ionizes the drug, traps it in the renal tubules, and prevents reabsorption. Phencyclidine base is readily absorbed across the tubular membrane. Ion trapping is accomplished by lowering the urinary pH below 5.0. Ascorbic acid or ammonium chloride at an initial dosage of 2 g every 6 hours can be used and increased within 1 or 2 days to a total of 12 g per day if necessary. Urine pH should be checked daily. Urinary acidification can be enhanced by encouraging the patient to drink plenty of acidic fruit juice (e.g., cranberry juice). Citrus juices do not effectively lower urine pH. When urine pH is successfully lowered below 5.0, excretion of phencyclidine can be enhanced through forced diuresis with furosemide. Treatment with ion trapping should continue until the toxicology screen is negative for phencyclidine for at least 3 days.

### *Withdrawal*

Treatment of drug withdrawal is the primary indication for drug therapy in substance use disorders. Goals of drug therapy include prevention of progression of withdrawal to life-threatening severity, enabling the patient to be sufficiently comfortable and functional to participate in a behavioral treatment program, and supportive drug therapy. The clinician should remember that withdrawal is usually part of a substance dependence disorder. Patients with drug dependence generally cope with almost any stress through the use of a drug. In drug therapy for withdrawal, it is important to avoid reinforcing the patient's drug-seeking and drug-using behavior to the extent possible. Drug withdrawal in the best of circumstances is uncomfortable. Patients must be educated to deal with the stress of withdrawal without seeking drugs. The use of drugs as needed for anxiety or insomnia should be avoided. Treatment of drug withdrawal is summarized in Table 47.11.

### *CNS Depressant Withdrawal*

#### Alcohol

Supportive drug therapy for alcohol withdrawal consists of treatment such as replacement of B vitamins, especially thiamine, to treat or prevent Wernicke's encephalopathy, and fluid and electrolyte replacement to correct dehydration and electrolyte disturbances. Thiamine 100 mg intramuscularly is frequently administered, followed by thiamine 100 mg orally once daily. A multivitamin supplement is also often given. Electrolyte replacement often includes an injection of magnesium sulfate 1 g intramuscularly (2 mL of a 50% solution) for 1 to 3 days. Hypomagnesemia is associated with a lowered seizure threshold.[52]

*Detoxification*, the treatment of acute withdrawal from alcohol, can be accomplished with any drug that is cross-tolerant to alcohol. All of the sedative–hypnotic drugs are cross-tolerant to alcohol, and most have been used to treat alcohol withdrawal. The anticonvulsant carbamazepine has been used in the treatment of alcohol withdrawal in Europe.[53] Most clinicians now agree that the benzodiazepines are the drugs of choice in the treatment of alcohol withdrawal.[52] Compared with the barbiturates and other sedative–hypnotics, benzodiazepines are safer at high doses and have fewer adverse effects on the liver and other organ systems. The choice of benzodiazepine drug is much less clear, as all are effective. Many clinicians use long-acting drugs (e.g., chlordiazepoxide, diazepam) that effectively control withdrawal with few rebound effects after discontinuation. Short- to intermediate-acting drugs (e.g., oxazepam, lorazepam) can also be used and have the advantages of having no active metabolites, being less affected by liver impairment, and having few residual sedative effects after discontinuation. Once a drug is selected, the patient is begun on a dose adequate to control the major symptoms of withdrawal, then gradually tapered over 5 to 7 days. Representative detoxification regimens using benzodiazepines for treatment of alcohol withdrawal are described in Table 47.12. Patients with more severe withdrawal symptoms may require higher doses and longer tapering periods. Monitoring parameters should include the patient's vital signs, presence of tremor, sweating, and other signs and symptoms of withdrawal.

When withdrawal hallucinations are present, short-term antipsychotic drug therapy is indicated. Although any antipsychotic drug would be a correct choice, a high-potency agent with low anticholinergic activity and minimal effect on an already lowered seizure threshold would be most preferable (e.g., haloperidol, fluphenazine, trifluoperazine). Antipsychotic drugs are not indicated in the routine treatment of alcohol withdrawal unless hallucinations or other psychotic symptoms are present.[54]

Alcohol withdrawal seizures do not require treatment with an anticonvulsant drug unless the patient progresses to status epilepticus, as seizures generally end before diaze-

**Table 47.11** Treatment of Withdrawal From Common Drugs of Abuse

| *Drug or drug class* | *Pharmacologic therapy* |
|---|---|
| Alcohol | |
| Detoxification | Chlordiazepoxide 50 mg TID–QID[a] or oxazepam 30 mg TID–QID; taper over 5–7 days |
| Withdrawal hallucinations | Haloperidol 2–5 mg daily × 2–3 d if hallucinations or other symptoms of psychosis persist |
| Withdrawal seizures | Supportive treatment only during seizure unless condition progresses to status; lorazepam 2 mg IM after seizure ends; use higher detoxification dosage and slower taper |
| Supportive drug therapy | Thiamine 100 mg IM, then 100 mg PO daily; multivitamin, one daily; magnesium sulfate 1 g IM × 1–3 d |
| Benzodiazepines | |
| Short- to intermediate-acting | Chlordiazepoxide 50 mg TID–QID or oxazepam 30 mg TID–QID; taper over 5–7 d |
| Long-acting | Chlordiazepoxide 50 mg TID–QID or oxazepam 30 mg TID–QID × 5 d, then taper over additional 5–7 d |
| Barbiturates and other sedative–hypnotics | Pentobarbital tolerance test (Table 48.13); initial detoxification at upper limit of tolerance test; decrease dosage by 100 mg every 2–3 d |
| Opiates | Methadone 20–80 mg PO daily; taper by 5–10 mg daily |
| Mixed-substance withdrawal | |
| Drugs are cross-tolerant | Detoxify according to treatment for longer acting drug used |
| Drugs are not cross-tolerant | Detoxify from one drug while maintaining second drug (or cross-tolerant drug), then detoxify from second drug |
| CNS stimulants | Supportive treatment only; pharmacotherapy generally not used |

[a] TID, three times daily; QID, four times daily.

pam or another drug can be administered.[55] Phenytoin, which is not cross-tolerant to alcohol, does not prevent nor treat withdrawal seizures, and without an intravenous loading dose, therapeutic blood levels of phenytoin are not reached until acute withdrawal is complete.[56] Patients experiencing seizures should be treated supportively. An increase in the dosage and tapering schedule of the benzodiazepine used in detoxification or a single injection of a benzodiazepine may be necessary to prevent further seizure activity. When a benzodiazepine is given by intramuscular injection, lorazepam should be used.[57] Diazepam and chlordiazepoxide are both erratically and poorly absorbed when given intramuscularly.[58] Patients with a history of withdrawal seizures can be predicted to experience an especially severe withdrawal syndrome. In such patients, a higher initial dosage of a benzodiazepine drug and a slower tapering period of 7 to 10 days are advisable.

**Table 47.12** Alcohol Detoxification

| | |
|---|---|
| Chlordiazepoxide | |
| 50 mg TID × 1 d[a] | |
| 50 mg BID × 1 d | |
| 25 mg TID × 1 d | |
| 25 mg BID × 1 d | |
| 25 mg daily × 1 d, then discontinue | |
| Oxazepam | |
| 30 mg TID × 2 d | |
| 30 mg BID × 2 d | |
| 30 mg daily × 1 d, then discontinue | |

[a] TID, three times daily; BID, two times daily.

Compiled from Reference 51.

### Benzodiazepines

Treatment of benzodiazepine withdrawal is very similar to the treatment of alcohol withdrawal, and the same drugs and dosages may be used.[40] The major difference in management is the length of treatment. The onset of withdrawal symptoms in patients physically dependent on the long-acting benzodiazepines may be delayed up to 7 days after discontinuation of the drug. A common approach in detoxification of such patients is to initiate treatment at usual dosages (e.g., chlordiazepoxide 50 mg three times daily, oxazepam 30 mg three times daily) and to maintain the initial dosage for 5 days, with gradual tapering over an additional 5 days. Detoxification in patients physically dependent on shorter acting benzodiazepines is similar to treatment of alcohol withdrawal. Among the benzodiazepines, alprazolam has been suggested to be more difficult to taper and discontinue than the other benzodiazepines.[59] Whether the difficulty is related to a different patient population commonly treated with alprazolam (e.g., panic disorder) or intrinsic differences between alprazolam and other benzodiazepines is not clear.

### Barbiturates and Other Sedative–Hypnotics

Because of the unpredictability and frequently greater severity of withdrawal from barbiturates and other sedative–hypnotic drugs, it is useful to attempt to determine the patient's level of tolerance prior to initiating detoxification. Tolerance

**Table 47.13** Pentobarbital Tolerance Test

| | |
|---|---|
| 1. | Administer pentobarbital 200 mg PO every 2–3 h until intolerance is observed (sedation, slurred speech, nystagmus, ataxia) |
| 2. | Begin detoxification at cumulative dosage required to observe intolerance |
| 3. | Taper daily dosage by 100 mg every 2–3 d |

Compiled from Reference 14.

testing is most often done with pentobarbital (Nembutal, Abbott).[15] The patient is given 200 mg of pentobarbital orally and observed for 2 to 3 hours for signs of a mild intoxication, including sedation, slurred speech, ataxia, and nystagmus. The procedure is repeated until one or more signs of intoxication are observed. The total dosage of pentobarbital required to reach the lower levels of the patient's limit of tolerance can be used as an approximate initial starting dosage for detoxification. The daily dosage can be reduced in decrements of 100 mg every third day at first, then every other day if the patient tolerates initial dosage reductions without difficulty. The pentobarbital tolerance test is summarized in Table 47.13. Monitoring parameters for barbiturate detoxication are the same as for alcohol and benzodiazepine detoxication.

**Opiates**

As mentioned previously, opiate withdrawal is unlike alcohol and sedative–hypnotic drug withdrawal with respect to potential lethality. Opiate withdrawal is not life-threatening unless there is a concurrent life-threatening medical condition. In addition, many patients who are addicted to opiates (i.e., compulsive drug seekers and drug users) are not physically dependent. The purity of street drugs, especially heroin, is often very low. The average volume of usage of street drugs may be insufficient to maintain physical dependence in many patients. Although most patients complain of symptoms of withdrawal such as cramping or insomnia, these symptoms are tolerable and initiation of drug therapy may be avoided. As opiate withdrawal is not life-threatening, observable signs of withdrawal such as mydriasis, pilomotor erection, diaphoresis, or diarrhea should be noted prior to initiation of drug therapy. Unnecessary detoxification with drugs, especially methadone, should be avoided if possible.

The conventional drug therapy for opiate withdrawal has been methadone, a synthetic opiate. Usual starting dosages have been 20–80 mg per day orally; but treatment of withdrawal from heroin usually requires no more than 20 mg of methadone, owing to the low purity of street heroin. The dosage of methadone can be tapered in decrements of 5–10 mg per day until discontinued. Most patients in withdrawal continue to complain of mild symptoms after detoxification is completed. Some patients who are unable to completely discontinue methadone or habitually return to drug use whenever methadone is discontinued are placed in methadone maintenance treatment programs and receive methadone chronically.[15]

Another method of opiate detoxification is the use of clonidine (Catapres, Boerhinger Ingelheim), a centrally acting $\alpha_2$-adrenergic receptor agonist. Use of clonidine can attenuate the noradrenergic hyperactivity of opiate withdrawal without interfering significantly with activity at the opiate receptors. Production of enkephalin and return of receptors to normal levels of sensitivity can occur as rapidly as possible. Advantages of detoxification with clonidine include a more rapid detoxification and an absence of the euphoria sometimes observed with methadone.[60]

Clonidine is generally given in an initial dosage of 6 $\mu$g/kg/d, in three divided doses. Dosage can be increased if necessary to as much as 17 $\mu$g/kg/d. The patient is maintained on the same dosage for 7 days; then, the drug is tapered and discontinued over the next 3 days. A common clonidine side effect is orthostatic hypotension, and the patient's blood pressure should be monitored in the supine and standing positions at least daily. If blood pressure drops to an unacceptably low level (e.g., lying systolic blood pressure less than 90 mm Hg), the dose should be held. If blood pressure has risen in time for the next dose, clonidine can be resumed.[60]

### *Withdrawal From Other Substances*

Withdrawal from other drugs, including cocaine and other stimulants, is primarily supportive. Pharmacotherapy has, however, recently assumed a greater role in treating cocaine withdrawal and dependence. Bromocriptine (Parlodel, Sandoz), a dopamine agonist usually used in the treatment of parkinsonism and hyperprolactinemia, has been used to treat cocaine withdrawal symptoms and to reduce craving for cocaine.[61] Use of bromocriptine is based on the hypothesis that chronic use of cocaine causes dopamine depletion. Use should generally be short term. The precise role of bromocriptine in treating cocaine withdrawal has not been fully elucidated and research into its use continues.

### *Mixed-Substance Withdrawal*

Many drug users practice polypharmacy and it is common for a patient to experience withdrawal from more than one drug. Treatment of withdrawal depends on the individual drug combination. If the drugs are cross-tolerant (e.g., alcohol and diazepam), treatment for withdrawal from diazepam, the longer acting of the two drugs, will also concurrently treat alcohol withdrawal. If the drugs are not cross-tolerant (e.g., alcohol and heroin), withdrawal from each drug must be treated separately. Withdrawal from both drugs can be treated concurrently in a young, otherwise healthy patient, but a more conservative approach is to treat withdrawal from each drug consecutively. While detoxification for one drug is under way, treatment with the second drug (or a drug that is cross-tolerant to the second drug) must be maintained. When detoxification from the first drug is complete, the second drug can be tapered and discontinued according to usual procedures.

### *Substance Dependence*

The treatment of drug dependence, or addiction, is primarily behavioral. The patient must be taught that complete abstinence is the only possible alternative to a life of uncontrollable drug use that will ultimately end in death. There is no intermediate, controllable level of drinking or use of another drug. The prospect of life without alcohol or other drugs is incomprehensible to many patients. Early treatment is directed at penetrating the denial of a problem which is always present. The patient must be educated as to the disease concept of addiction, the effects of drugs, and the permanence of the condition. Although treatment may help patients to reorganize their lives in the absence of the drug, they will never be able to control their drug use. Families must be involved in treatment, not only for the good of the drug-using family member, but for themselves. The course of the patient's illness often has a devastating effect on other family members. Severely depleted self-esteem, denial of the family member's addiction, feelings of responsibility for the family member's drug use, and other behaviors that parallel the addiction process itself are often present. Treatment must be a lifelong process. Aftercare, or what is now being called continued care, should include regular and frequent treatment in some form. Most drug dependence treatment programs embrace a treatment approach based on Alcoholics Anonymous (AA). AA is one of the most successful of all self-help groups. Associated groups include Alanon, a group for family members of alcoholics, and Fellowships Anonymous and Narcotics Anonymous, self-help groups based on the AA concept for users of other drugs.

### Drug Therapy

As previously stated, drug therapy for drug-dependent patients should be minimized to the extent possible. There are, however, several pharmacologic approaches that may be useful in drug dependency.

Disulfiram (Antabuse, Ayerst) is an inhibitor of the enzyme aldehyde dehydrogenase.[15] In the absence of alcohol, disulfiram has minimal effects. In the presence of alcohol, however, the metabolism of acetaldehyde produced by dehydrogenation of alcohol is inhibited, thus causing an acute increase in acetaldehyde levels. Acetaldehyde causes a characteristic reaction consisting of flushing, nausea, vomiting, headache, palpitations, sweating, fever, and hypotension. The patient is made aware of the likelihood of the disulfiram reaction when treatment with disulfiram is initiated, thus providing a pharmacologic disincentive to drink alcohol. If the alcoholic drinks, the experience of the reaction is intended to serve as aversive conditioning to discourage further alcohol consumption. Inhibition of aldehyde dehydrogenase continues as long as 2 weeks after discontinuation of disulfiram.

Patients taking disulfiram should be educated regarding the risk of unsuspected alcohol consumption. Many nonprescription products, including cough syrups and elixirs, contain alcohol. Disulfiram reactions have also been associated with the use of alcohol-containing mouthwashes and even the topical application of alcohol-containing aftershaves. The usual dosage of disulfiram is 250–500 mg per day. The likelihood of a disulfiram reaction is a function of the dose of both disulfiram and alcohol. The most common side effects of disulfiram include rash, headache, lethargy, a metallic taste, and impotency, although impotency from alcohol is far more common than impotency from disulfiram.[62]

Disulfiram is not a cure for alcoholism. It is not intended to be the sole treatment modality for alcoholism, but is intended to serve as an adjunct to behavioral treatment. Although some clinicians have felt disulfiram to be a "crutch" for alcoholics, anything that may help an alcoholic refrain from drinking alcohol, especially in the first several months after initial treatment when relapse is most likely, may be useful.

Naltrexone (Trexan, Du Pont) is an opiate receptor antagonist that blocks the euphoric effects of heroin and other opiates.[63] Although it causes no aversive reaction, blockade of the effects of opiates can interrupt the reinforcement process that leads to further drug use. This can be especially useful during the conditioned abstinence syndrome associated with the first several months after initial withdrawal from opiates, when return to drug use is most likely. Naltrexone is orally active and long acting. The usual dosage is 50 mg daily or 350 mg per week in three divided doses. Patients should be started on naltrexone after detoxification to avoid unintentional precipitation of withdrawal, which would provide a powerful incentive for opiate use. Alternatively, it may be possible to begin naltrexone early in treatment and treat concomitantly with clonidine to attenuate possible withdrawal effects. Research to conclusively document the efficacy and safety of this practice has not been completed. The most common side effects of naltrexone are gastrointestinal disturbance and a naltrexone-precipitated opiate withdrawal syndrome. As with disulfiram, naltrexone is not a cure for opiate dependence and should be used as an adjunct to behavioral treatment.

Tricyclic antidepressants, primarily desipramine (Norpramin, Merrell Dow), have been used in the last several years to decrease cocaine craving.[61] In addition to treating the depression associated with cocaine withdrawal, desipramine may block cocaine-induced euphoria, although data on this question are conflicting. Both desipramine and cocaine block reuptake of brain catecholamines. Competition for common receptor binding sites may decrease the euphoric effect of cocaine. With chronic use, desipramine and cocaine have opposite effects on brain neurotransmitter levels and receptor binding sensitivity, thus possibly relieving the craving for cocaine.

#### Drug Therapy for Dependence Secondary to Other Psychiatric Disorders

The overwhelming majority of drug dependence is primary. A small minority, perhaps 10% or less, appears to be secondary to other psychiatric disorders (e.g., depression, panic disorder, schizophrenia). Depression is a common complaint of many alcoholics, and many are treated with antidepressant drugs. Because the depression is highly likely to be related to drug dependence, patients should be free of alcohol and other drugs for a minimum of 2 weeks before assessment of a primary depressive disorder is made. If a careful diagnostic evaluation reveals a functional psychiatric disorder, however, the appropriate psychotropic drug therapy should be considered.

## Summary

Substance use disorders are one of the great public health issues of contemporary society. Dependence on drugs is a powerful emotional and political issue. As we live in a chemically oriented society, everyone is affected in some way by drug abuse and drug dependence. Health care professionals must be vigilant for problems associated with drug use, not only for our patients, but also for ourselves.

## References


1. Alcoholism, Alcohol Abuse, and Related Problems: Opportunities for Research. Washington DC, National Academy Press, 1980.
2. Miller JD, Cisin IH, Gardner-Keaton H, et al. National Survey on Drug Abuse: Main Findings 1982. Washington DC, US Government Printing Office, 1983.
3. McAuliffe WE, Santangelo SL, Gingras J, et al. Use and abuse of controlled substances by pharmacists and pharmacy students. Am J Hosp Pharm 1987;44:311–317.
4. McAuliffe WE, Rohman M, Santangelo S, et al. Psychoactive drug use among practicing physicians and medical students. N Engl J Med 1986;315:805–810.
5. Farley WJ, Talbott GD. Anesthesiology and addiction. Anesth Analg 1983;62:465–466.
6. Glantz MD. Drugs and elderly adult: An overview, in Glantz MD, Petersen DM, Whittington FJ (eds): Drugs and the Elderly Adult. Washington DC, US Government Printing Office, 1983, pp 1–3.
7. Diagnostic and Statistical Manual of Mental Disorders, 3rd ed, revised (DSM-III-R). Washington DC, American Psychiatric Press, 1987.
8. Victor M, Adams RD. Alcohol, in Petersdorf RG, Adams RD, Braunwald E, et al (eds): Harrison's Principles of Internal Medicine, 10th ed. New York, McGraw-Hill, 1983, pp 1285–1295.
9. Berry MS, Pentreath VW. The neurophysiology of alcohol, in Sandler M (ed): Psychopharmacology of Alcohol. New York, Raven, 1980, pp 43–72.
10. Feuerlein W. Alcohol withdrawal syndromes, in Sandler M (ed): Psychopharmacology of Alcohol. New York, Raven, 1980, pp 215–228.
11. Norman TR, Burrows GD. Benzodiazepine plasma concentrations and anxiolytic response, in Burrows GD, Norman TR, Davies B (eds): Antianxiety Agents: Drugs in Psychiatry, vol 2. Amsterdam, Elsevier, 1984, pp 93–105.
12. Baldessarini RJ. Chemotherapy in Psychiatry: Principles and Practice, 2nd ed. Cambridge MA, Harvard University Press, 1985.
13. Greenblatt DJ, Divoll M, Abernethy DR, et al. Benzodiazepine pharmacokinetics: An overview, in Burrows GD, Norman TR, Davies B (eds): Antianxiety Agents: Drugs in Psychiatry, vol 2. Amsterdam, Elsevier, 1984, pp 79–92.
14. Busto U, Sellers EM, Naranjo CA, et al. Withdrawal reaction after long-term use of benzodiazepines. N Engl J Med 1986;315: 854–859.
15. Jaffe JH. Drug addiction and drug abuse, in Gilman AG, Goodman LS, Rall TW, Murad F (eds): The Pharmacological Basis of Therapeutics, 7th ed. New York, Macmillan, 1985, pp 532–581.
16. Jones RT. The pharmacology of cocaine. Natl Inst Drug Abuse Res Monogr Ser 1984;50:34–53.
17. Washton AM, Gold MS, Pottash AC. "Crack." Early report on a new drug epidemic. Postgrad Med 1986;80:52–58.
18. Fischman MW. The behavioral pharmacology of cocaine in humans. Natl Inst Drug Abuse Res Monogr Ser 1984;50:72–91.
19. Aigner TG, Balster RL. Choice behavior in rhesus monkeys: Cocaine versus food. Science 1978;201:534–535.
20. Duke M. Cocaine, myocardial infarction and arrhythmias—A review. Conn Med 1986;50:440–442.
21. Post RM, Kopanda RT. Cocaine, kindling, and psychosis. Am J Psychiatry 1976;133:627–634.
22. Greer G, Strassman RJ. Information on "ecstasy." Am J Psychiatry 1985;142:1391.
23. Cohen S. The Substance Abuse Problems, vol 2, New Issues for the 1980s. New York, Haworth Press, 1985.
24. Crider R. Phencyclidine: Changing abuse patterns. Natl Inst Drug Abuse Res Monogr Ser 1986;64:163–173.
25. Marwah J, Pitts DK. Psychopharmacology of phencyclidine. Natl Inst Drug Abuse Res Monogr Ser 1986;64:127–133.
26. Titelar M, Lyon RA, Glenum RA. Radioligand binding evidence implicates the brain $5HT_2$ receptor as a site of action for LSD and phenylisopropylamine hallucinogens. Psychopharmacology 1988;94:213–216.
27. Cohen S. The hallucinogens and the inhalants. Psychiatr Clin North Am 1984;7:681–688.
28. Maykut MO. Health consequences of acute and chronic marihuana use. Prog Neuropsychopharmacol Biol Psychiatry 1985; 9:209–238.
29. Nicholi AM. The inhalants: An overview. Psychosomatics 1983; 24:914–921.
30. King GS, Smialek JE, Troutman WG. Sudden death in adolescents resulting from the inhalation of typewriter correction fluid. JAMA 1985;253:1604–1606.
31. Greer JE. Adolescent abuse of typewriter correction fluid. South Med J 1984;77:297–301.
32. Anderson HR, MacNair RS, Ramsey JD. Deaths from abuse of volatile substances: A national epidemiological study. Br Med J 1985;290:304–307.
33. Greden JF. Caffeinism and caffeine withdrawal, in Lowinson JH, Ruiz P (eds): Substance Abuse: Clinical Problems and Perspectives. Baltimore, Williams and Wilkins, 1981, pp 274–286.
34. Rubinstein JS. Abuse of antiparkinsonism drugs: Feigning of extrapyramidal symptoms to obtain trihexyphenidyl. JAMA 1978;239:2365–2366.
35. Smith JM. Abuse of the antiparkinson drugs: A review of the literature. J Clin Psychiatry 1980;41:351–354.
36. Wikler A. Conditioning factors in opiate addiction and release, in Wilner DI, Kossebaum GG (eds): Narcotics. New York, McGraw-Hill, 1965, pp 85–100.
37. Abood LG. Mechanisms of tolerance and dependence: An overview. Natl Inst Drug Abuse Res Monogr Ser 1984;54:4–11.
38. Littleton J. Development of membrane tolerance to ethanol may limit intoxication and influence dependence liability, in Sandler M (ed): Psychopharmacology of Alcohol. New York, Raven, 1980, pp 121–127.
39. Okamoto M. Barbiturate tolerance and physical dependence: Contribution of pharmacological factors. Natl Inst Drug Abuse Res Monogr Ser 1984;54:333–347.
40. Lader M, Petursson H. Tolerance, dependence and abuse in relation to antianxiety drugs, in Burrows GD, Norman TR, Davies B (eds): Antianxiety Agents: Drugs in Psychiatry, vol 2. Amsterdam, Elsevier, 1984, pp 127–141.
41. Guyton AC. Textbook of Medical Physiology, 7th ed. Philadelphia, WB Saunders Co, 1986.
42. Gold MS, Redmond DE, Kleber HD. Noradrenergic hyperactivity in opiate withdrawal supported by clonidine reversal of opiate withdrawal. Am J Psychiatry 1979;136:100–102.
43. Dorland's Illustrated Medical Dictionary, 25th ed. Philadelphia, WB Saunders Co, 1974.
44. Li TK, Lumeng L, McBride WJ, Waller MB. Progress toward a voluntary oral consumption model of alcoholism. Drug Alcohol Depend 1979;4:45–60.
45. Kaij L. Alcoholism in Twins. Stockholm, Almqvist and Wiksell, 1960.

46. Cadoret RJ, Cain CA, Grove WM. Development of alcoholism in adoptees raised apart from alcoholic biologic relatives. Arch Gen Psychiatry 1980;37:561–563.
47. Cloninger CR, Bohman M, Sigvardsson S. Inheritance of alcohol abuse: Cross-fostering analysis of adopted men. Arch Gen Psychiatry 1981;38:861–868.
48. Bohman M, Sigvardsson S, Cloninger CR. Maternal inheritance of alcohol abuse: Cross-fostering analysis of adopted women. Arch Gen Psychiatry 1981;38:965–969.
49. Myers RD, Melchior CL. Alcohol drinking: Abnormal intake caused by tetrahydropapaveroline in brain. Science 1977;196:554–556.
50. Jaffe JH, Martin WR. Opioid analgesics and antagonists, in Gilman AG, Goodman LS, Rall TW, Murad F (eds): The Pharmacological Basis of Therapeutics, 7th ed. New York, Macmillan, 1985, pp 491–531.
51. Done AK, Aronow R, Miceli JN, Lin DCK. Pharmacokinetic observations in the treatment of phencyclidine poisoning. A preliminary report, in Rumack BH, Temple AR (eds): Management of the Poisoned Patient. Princeton, NJ, Science Press, 1977, pp 79–102.
52. Holloway HC, Hales RE, Watanabe HK. Recognition and treatment of acute alcohol withdrawal syndromes. Psychiatr Clin North Am 1984;7:729–743.
53. Sternebring B, Holm R, Wadstein J. Reduction in early alcohol abstinence fits by administration of carbamazepine syrup instead of tablets. Eur J Clin Pharmacol 1983;24:611–613.
54. Mason AS, Granacher RP. Clinical Handbook of Antipsychotic Drug Therapy. New York, Brunner/Mazel, 1980.
55. Hillbom ME, Hjelm-Jager M. Should alcohol withdrawal seizures be treated with anti-epileptic drugs? Acta Neurol Scand 1984;69:39–42.
56. Winter ME, Tozer TN. Phenytoin, in Evans WE, Schentag JJ, Jusko WJ (eds): Applied Pharmacokinetics: Principles of Therapeutic Drug Monitoring, 2nd ed. Spokane, WA, Applied Therapeutics, 1986, pp 493–539.
57. Greenblatt DJ. Clinical pharmacokinetics of oxazepam and lorazepam. Clin Pharmacokinet 1981;6:89–105.
58. Hillestad L, Hansen T, Melsom H, Drivenes A. Diazepam metabolism in normal man. I. Serum concentrations and clinical effects after intravenous, intramuscular, and oral administration. Clin Pharmacol Ther 1974;16:479–484.
59. Browne JL, Hauge KJ. A review of alprazolam withdrawal. Drug Intell Clin Pharm 1986;20:837–841.
60. Gold MS, Pottash ALC, Extein I, et al. Clinical utility of clonidine in opiate withdrawal. Natl Inst Drug Abuse Res Monogr Ser 1981;34:95–100.
61. Kleber HD, Gawin FH. Pharmacological treatments of cocaine abuse, in Washton AM, Gold MS (eds): Cocaine: A Clinician's Handbook. New York, Guilford Press, 1987, pp 118–134.
62. Peachey JE, Naranjo CA. The role of drugs in the treatment of alcoholism. Drugs 1984;27:171–182.
63. Crabtree BL. Review of naltrexone, a long-acting opiate antagonist. Clin Pharm 1984;3:273–280.

# Chapter 48 / Schizophrenic Disorders

Sharyn R. Batey, PharmD

Schizophrenia is a heterogeneous group of related disorders rather than a single disease entity. These illnesses are characterized by disorganized and often bizarre thinking, withdrawn or bizarre behavior, blunted emotional tone or inappropriate affect, delusions, hallucinations, and poor interpersonal skills.

Until the late 1800s, no significant attempt had been made to separate schizophrenia from other psychotic illnesses. In 1896, Emil Kraepelin distinguished dementia praecox (chronic schizophrenia) from manic–depressive (bipolar disorder) psychosis.

In 1911, Eugen Bleuler introduced the concept of symptoms frequently associated with schizophrenia known as the four A's: disturbance in affect, ambivalence, looseness of associations, and autism. This classification and description of the clinical symptoms were generally accepted as standard for diagnosing schizophrenia until the third edition of the *Diagnostic and Statistical Manual of Mental Disorders* (DSM-III) was published in 1980.

## Epidemiology

It is now estimated that 0.5% to 1.5% of the worldwide population will experience a schizophrenic disorder at some point in life.[1] Schizophrenia accounts for 7% to 20% of all psychiatric hospital admissions (between 500,000 and 1,000,000 admissions per year in the United States). Schizophrenia usually begins in adolescence and early adulthood and rarely occurs before adolescence or after 40 years of age. Schizophrenic symptoms usually become pronounced around age 20. Although schizophrenia affects males and females equally, males tend to have an earlier age of onset of the illness. Males are hospitalized for the first time between 15 and 24 years, whereas females usually are first admitted between 25 and 34 years.[2]

Results from twin and adoptee studies indicate a genetic contribution to some forms of schizophrenia. The risk for developing schizophrenia is approximately 0.5% to 1.5% for the general population; however, the risk for persons with a first-degree relative (parent or sibling) with the illness is between 5% and 10%.[1] For children of two schizophrenic parents, the risk is 40%. Twin studies have shown that for the dizygotic twin sibling of a diagnosed schizophrenic, the risk factor is 14%; for the monozygotic twin sibling, the risk factor is 47%.[3]

## Pathophysiology

### *Biochemical Theories*

The most widely accepted and well-supported biochemical etiology explaining schizophrenia is the dopamine theory. This theory states that excessive amounts of the neurotransmitter dopamine may play a profound and unique role in inducing psychotic/schizophrenic symptoms. Pharmacologic evidence supporting this theory includes reports that drugs that increase dopamine (i.e., levodopa, amphetamine, apomorphine) may exacerbate psychotic symptoms.[4–6]

Table 48.1 presents the four areas of the brain where dopamine functions[7] and the effects of antipsychotics on psychosis related to these four areas. While no reliable diagnostic laboratory test for schizophrenia exists, researchers are now working in this area. Plasma homovanillic acid (the major circulating metabolite of dopamine) levels have been associated with psychosis.[8]

### *Neuropeptides*

Another advance related to the pathogenesis of schizophrenia is exploration of the role of endogenous opioids and nonopioid neuropeptides as modulators of dopaminergic brain activity in schizophrenic patients. The antipsychotic efficacy of opioids in patients with schizophrenia may result from an interaction of opioids with the dopaminergic system.[9]

Two nonopioid neuropeptides that have attracted interest in schizophrenic research are neurotensin (NT) and cholecystokinin (CCK). The action of NT in different brain areas implies that it may be possible to modify dopaminergic activity specifically in the mesolimbic system but not in the nigrostriatal areas, thereby potentially avoiding adverse neurologic effects such as extrapyramidal effects and tardive dyskinesia.[10]

CCK is a rapid and powerful excitant of cerebral cortical cells. It coexists with dopamine in neurons that project from the brain stem to the limbic lobe, but not in the nigrostriatal system. CCK may inhibit or inactivate dopamine release in the nucleus accumbens.[11]

### *Psychologic Theories*

Several psychodynamic theories have been proposed to help explain schizophrenic disorders. Schizophrenia may result from disturbances that occur early in personality development and that complicate the maturation process. These disturbances may include the absence of parent–child bonding, ambiguous communication during personality development (i.e., receiving mixed messages), or the "double bind," when two messages are conveyed to the patient at once—one often being nonverbal.[12]

### *Sociologic Theories*

Although schizophrenia is not restricted to certain cultures, environments, or social classes, the disease is most prevalent in impoverished and disadvantaged families and communities. Faris and Dunham proposed a "downward drift"

**Table 48.1** Dopamine Tracks and Effects of Antipsychotics

| *Dopamine track* | *Origin* | *Innervation* | *Function* | *Antipsychotic effect* |
|---|---|---|---|---|
| Mesolimbic | Midbrain ventral tegmental | Limbic structure and nucleus accumbens | Emotional and intellectual | ↓ Hallucinations, delusions, disordered cognition |
| Mesocortical | Ventral tegmental | Frontal cortex | Emotional and intellectual | ↓ Delusions, hallucinations, disordered cognition |
| Nigrostriatal | Substantia nigra | Basal ganglia | Extrapyramidal system-movement | ↑ Motor symptomatology |
| Tuberoinfundibular | Hypothalamus | Pituitary gland | Regulates endocrine functions | ↑ Plasma prolactin levels |

Compiled from References 7 and 26.

hypothesis after observing that patients with schizophrenia tend to move into poverty areas and down the socioeconomic scale.[12]

### *Structural Changes*

Several visual imaging techniques are used in schizophrenia research to explore the nature and pattern of brain deficits and to examine the possibility of localization.[13] While these techniques have not yet had a profound effect on the clinical practice of psychiatry they show promise for expanding our understanding of schizophrenia.[14]

Computerized tomography (CT) scans have suggested that structural changes in the brain, especially ventricular enlargement, occur in a subgroup of chronic schizophrenic patients. Furthermore, there is a correlation between increased ventricular size and the negative symptoms of schizophrenia.[14]

Positron emission tomography (PET) scanning is a noninvasive tool that allows scientists to quantitatively measure physiologic and biochemical functions occurring in live tissue.[14]

Brain electrical activity mapping (BEAM) uses computer analysis to topographically display EEG rhythms and evoked response data on a color video screen, similar to PET scans. This technique has shown slower activity in the frontal lobes of schizophrenic patients consistent with the hypofrontality observed in decreased cerebral blood flow in PET studies.

Using cerebral blood flow (CBF) techniques, investigators have been able to establish a significant correlation between cognitive dysfunction and mean hemispherical cerebral blood flow. In all schizophrenic patients, a reduction in blood flow to the frontal lobe has been noted.[14]

Nuclear magnetic resonance (NMR) is a new imaging technique that obtains cross-sectional pictures of the entire body without exposing the patient to ionizing radiation. NMR yields anatomic pictures comparable to CT scans and allows more careful discrimination between healthy and diseased tissue, thus providing metabolic and biochemical information on organs.[14]

## Differential Diagnosis

The diagnosis of schizophrenia is assigned on the basis of the descriptive presentation of the illness, with care taken to distinguish schizophrenia from different but similar disorders.[15] The differential diagnosis is summarized in Table 48.2.

## Clinical Presentation

Psychiatrists rely on descriptive criteria for diagnosing schizophrenia. The *Diagnostic and Statistical Manual, Third Edition, Revised* (DSM-III-R) criteria for diagnosing schizophrenia are listed in Table 48.3.[15] For a diagnosis of schizophrenia to be assigned, the person must have florid psychotic features with no affective components, and the symptoms must have been present for at least 6 months.[13]

**Table 48.2** Differential Diagnosis of Schizophrenia

- Organic mental disorders
  - Organic delusional syndrome (amphetamine or phencyclidine)
- Mood disorder
  - Bipolar disorder
  - Depressive disorder with psychotic features
- Schizoaffective disorder
- Schizophreniform disorder
- Acute psychotic episode
- Delusional disorder
- Autistic disorders
- Obsessive–compulsive disorder
- Hypochondriasis
- Personality disorders
  - Schizoptypal
  - Borderline
  - Schizoid
  - Paranoid
- Mental retardation
- Medical illnesses
  - Hyperthyroidism
  - Electrolyte imbalance
  - Brain tumor
  - Infections of the central nervous system

Modified from American Psychiatric Association: Diagnostic and Statistical Manual of Mental Disorders, 3rd ed, revised (DSM-III-R). Washington DC, American Psychiatric Association, 1987, pp 192–193.

**Table 48.3** DSM-III-R Diagnostic Criteria for Schizophrenia

A. Either 1, 2, or 3 for at least 2 wk
   1. Two of the following:
      a. Delusions
      b. Prominent hallucinations
      c. Incoherence or marked loosening of associations
      d. Catatonic behavior
      e. Flat or grossly inappropriate affect
   2. Bizarre delusions
   3. Prominent auditory hallucinations
B. During the course of the illness, functioning in such areas as work, social relations, and self-care is significantly below the highest level achieved before the illness
C. Schizoaffective disorder and mood disorders with psychotic features have been ruled out
D. Continuous signs of the illness for at least 6 mo
E. Not resulting from any organic mental disorder

Modified from American Psychiatric Association: Diagnostic and Statistical Manual of Mental Disorders, 3rd ed, revised (DSM-III-R). Washington DC, American Psychiatric Association, 1987, pp 194–195.

The reader is referred to the Glossary at the end of this chapter for definitions. Although the DSM-III-R criteria are the standard diagnostic criteria for schizophrenia, other criteria have been developed to assist in the diagnosis of the illness.[16]

Kurt Schneider developed the Schneiderian First Rank Symptoms of Schizophrenia. A diagnosis of schizophrenia, according to these criteria, is possible only if one of the symptoms listed in Table 48.4 is present in a patient with a clear sensorium.[17] Schneiderian First Rank Symptoms do not occur exclusively in schizophrenic disorders, but when present, they indicate a poor prognosis.

Table 48.5 lists the positive and negative symptoms of schizophrenia. The positive symptoms are associated with abnormal or excess function. The negative symptoms are associated with a deficit of function.[18]

The schizophrenics are divided into two major groups, type I (good prognosis) and type II (poor prognosis), the characteristics of which are listed in Table 48.6.[18]

Schizophrenia is divided into five subtypes based on the predominant group of symptoms present at any one time. For this reason, the subgroup classification for any given patient may change over time depending on the particular symptoms. The diagnostic criteria for the five subtypes of schizophrenia according to DSM III-R[15] are listed in Table 48.7.

The five subtypes of schizophrenia have distinguishing symptoms. The catatonic subtype, which is rarely diagnosed, is characterized by psychomotor symptoms. The disorganized subtype accounts for approximately two thirds of patients diagnosed with schizophrenia. For this diagnosis to be assigned, patients cannot have systematized delusions but they may have a prominent thought disorder. The paranoid subtype accounts for approximately one third of patients diagnosed with schizophrenia[19] and requires that systematized delusions or frequent auditory hallucinations be primary features. The undifferentiated subtype of schizophrenia is assigned when patients have active symptoms of schizophrenia but fail to meet the criteria for either catatonic, paranoid, or disorganized. The residual subtype is used for patients who continue to display the residual symptoms of schizophrenia but no longer have active psychotic symptoms.[20]

**Table 48.4** Schneider's First-Rank Symptoms of Schizophrenia

| |
|---|
| Audible thoughts |
| Voices arguing |
| Voices commenting on one's behavior |
| Somatic passivity |
| Thought withdrawal |
| Thought insertion |
| Thought broadcasting |
| Experiences feelings not his/her own |
| Experiences powerful influence not his/her own but actual performance of the act is his/hers |
| Experiences actions under control of external influence |
| Delusional perception |

**Table 48.5** Positive and Negative Symptoms of Schizophrenia

| *Positive symptoms* | *Negative symptoms* |
|---|---|
| Delusions | Poverty of speech |
| Hallucinations | Blunted affect |
| Formal thought disorder | Withdrawal |
| Bizarre behavior | Anhedonia |
| Disorganized thinking | Apathy |

**Table 48.6** Characteristics of Type I and Type II Schizophrenia

| *Disease characteristic* | *Type I* | *Type II* |
|---|---|---|
| Symptoms[a] | Positive | Negative |
| Onset | Acute | Insidious |
| Precipitating events | Frequent | Rare |
| Prepsychotic history | Good | Poor |
| Course of illness | Exacerbations/remissions | Chronic and deteriorating |
| Social functioning | Intact during remissions | Poor |
| Cognitive functioning | Normal | Impaired |
| Structural brain abnormalities | No evidence | Present |
| Area of brain | Temporolimbic | Prefrontal |
| Antipsychotic response | Good response | Poor response |

[a]Refers to positive and negative symptoms listed in Table 48.5.

**Table 48.7** DSM-III-R Diagnostic Criteria for Subtypes of Schizophrenia

**Catatonic Type**
The clinical picture is dominated by any of the following:
1. Catatonic stupor
2. Catatonic negativism
3. Catatonic rigidity
4. Catatonic excitement
5. Catatonic posturing

**Disorganized Type**
Symptoms include all of the following:
1. Incoherence, marked loosening of associations, or grossly disorganized behavior
2. Flat or inappropriate affect

**Paranoid Type**
Symptoms include all of the following:
1. Preoccupation with one or more systematized delusions or with extensive auditory hallucinations related to a single theme
2. None of the following: incoherence, marked loosening of associations, flat or grossly inappropriate affect, catatonic symptoms, grossly disorganized behavior

**Undifferentiated Type**
Symptoms include all of the following:
1. Prominent delusions, hallucinations, incoherence, or grossly disorganzied behavior

**Residual Type**
A. Absence of prominent delusions, hallucinations, incoherence or grossly disorganized behavior
B. Continuing evidence of the illness, as indicated by two or more of the following:
1. Marked social isolation or withdrawal
2. Marked impairment in role functioning
3. Markedly peculiar behavior
4. Marked impairment in personal hygiene
5. Blunted, flat, or inappropriate affect
6. Digressive, vague, overelaborate, or circumstantial speech, or poverty of speech or content of speech
7. Odd or bizarre ideation, or magical thinking
8. Unusual perceptual experiences
9. Apathy or lack of initiative

Modified from American Psychiatric Association: Diagnostic and Statistical Manual of Mental Disorders, 3rd ed, revised (DSM-III-R). Washington DC, American Psychiatric Association, 1987, pp 196–198.

## Prognosis/Complications

Maintenance antipsychotic medication may prevent relapse of schizophrenia. The primary reason patients are readmitted to psychiatric hospitals is because of noncompliance with antipsychotic medications. Approximately 10% of unmedicated schizophrenic patients relapse each month.[21] Of 3,609 patients studied over several months, 20% relapsed on antipsychotics and 53% relapsed on placebo.[22]

The psychotic symptoms of schizophrenia significantly interfere with social relationship, work, and self-care skills. Antipsychotic agents decrease outward symptoms of schizophrenia; they do little to enable the person to become productive or independent.[23] Failure in academic endeavors, diminished work performance, social isolation, and impairment of interpersonal relationships are other complications of the illness.[24]

## Antipsychotic Agents

Antipsychotics, also called neuroleptics, are used to treat many psychotic conditions in addition to schizophrenia. The antipsychotics are not specific for schizophrenia.[25] Table 48.8 lists the most frequently prescribed antipsychotics by generic and trade name, subdivided into chemical classes. Equivalent dose refers to the dose of each agent that is equivalent to 100 mg of chlorpromazine. The remaining columns list the individual daily dosage ranges for acute and chronic treatment and the available dosage forms.

### *Mechanism of Action*

The antipsychotic activity of these agents results from the central nervous system blockade of the postsynaptic receptors in dopamine-mediated pathways from the midbrain to the limbic system and to the temporal and frontal lobes of the cerebral cortex (Table 48.1). The antipsychotic agents also block dopamine receptors in the substantia nigra, in the midbrain to the caudate nucleus, and in the basal ganglia.[7] The blockade of dopamine receptors in the nigrostriatal system produces extrapyramidal side effects. The blockade of dopamine receptors in the tuberoinfundibular system results in increased release of prolactin from the pituitary.[26] Antipsychotics are also believed to decrease presynaptic dopamine activity.[8]

Two types of brain dopamine receptors have been identified: D-1 and D-2. D-1 receptors increase adenyl cyclase activity whereas D-2 receptors decrease adenyl cyclase. Although most antipsychotics block both D-1 and D-2 receptors, haloperidol blocks only the D-2 receptor. Antipsychotic efficacy is correlated with the ability to block D-2 receptors; however, the clinical effects of D-1 blockade are unknown. Based on a drug's binding affinity for the D-2 receptor, it may be referred to as a high-potency antipsychotic (e.g., haloperidol, thiothixene, etc.) or a low-potency antipsychotic (e.g., chlorpromazine, thioridazine, etc.).[7]

### *Pharmacokinetics*

Even though the pharmacokinetics of antipsychotic medications has not been as thoroughly studied as that of other psychotropic medications, pharmacokinetics should be considered in selection of an agent, dose, and route of administration. Intramuscular injections produce more reliable and higher blood concentrations (4 to 10 times) at a faster rate than oral forms because of variable absorption.[26] The antipsychotics are highly protein bound (most greater than 90%) and very lipophilic.[27] They cross the placenta and are excreted in the maternal milk supply.[26] The antipsychotics are metabolized by microsomal oxidation and by conjugation in the liver.[27] Metabolites are excreted primarily in the urine

**Table 48.8** Antipsychotic Agents

| *Generic name* | *Trade name* | *Manufacturer* | *Approximate equivalent dose (mg)* | *Usual oral dosage range (mg/d)*[a] Acute | Chronic | *Dosage form available*[b] |
|---|---|---|---|---|---|---|
| Aliphatic phenothiazines | | | | | | |
| Chlorpromazine | Thorazine | Smith Kline & French | 100 | 200–2,000 | 200–1,200 | T,L,I,S |
| | Generic brands | Various | | | | |
| Piperidine phenothiazines | | | | | | |
| Thioridazine | Mellaril | Sandoz | 100 | 200–800 | 150–800 | T,L |
| | Generic brands | Various | | | | |
| Mesoridazine | Serentil | Boehringer Ingelheim | 50 | 100–400 | 100–400 | T,L,I |
| Piperazine phenothiazines | | | | | | |
| Trifluoperazine | Stelazine | Smith Kline & French | 5 | 10–60 | 5–40 | T,L,I |
| | Generic brands | Various | | | | |
| Fluphenazine | Prolixin | Princeton Products | 2 | 5–60 | 5–40 | T,L,I,D |
| | Permitil | Schering | | | | |
| Perphenazine | Trilafon | Schering | 10 | 16–64 | 8–64 | T,L,I |
| Thioxanthenes | | | | | | |
| Thiothixene | Navane | Roerig | 2–5 | 10–80 | 10–30 | T,L,I |
| | Generic brands | Various | | | | |
| Chlorprothixene | Taractan | Roche | 100 | 100–600 | 100–400 | T,L,I |
| Butyrophenone | | | | | | |
| Haloperidol | Haldol | McNeil | 2 | 10–100 | 5–40 | T,L,I,D |
| | Generic brands | Various | | | | |
| Dibenzoxazepine | | | | | | |
| Loxapine | Loxitane | Lederle | 10 | 20–250 | 10–100 | T,L,I |
| Dihydroindolone | | | | | | |
| Molindone | Moban | Du Pont | 10 | 20–225 | 10–100 | T,L |

[a] Elderly patients are usually treated with approximately one half of the dose listed.
[b] Dosage forms available: T, tablet/capsule; L, liquid; I, injection (short acting); D, injection (long acting); S, suppository.

and to a lesser extent in the bile.[26] Metabolism and excretion of antipsychotic agents are faster in children and adults than in the fetus, the infant, or the elderly.[27]

The half-lives of most antipsychotics vary from 10 to 20 hours. After chronic administration, adipose tissues become saturated. Pharmacologic effects may persist for months after drug discontinuation, because of leaching of drug from adipose tissue.[25,26]

The use of plasma drug concentrations to monitor therapeutic response is controversial, and plasma level monitoring is not routinely done.[27] Steady-state concentrations achieved by administering a standard dosage of an antipsychotic vary widely among individuals[28]; variations may range from 10- to 100-fold.[27] More work needs to be done in this area before routine blood level monitoring is recommended. Patients who do not respond to standard doses of antipsychotics or those who have excessive side effects are candidates for blood level monitoring.[29]

### *General Prescribing Guidelines*

***Selection of Medication*** Unlike medical conditions there are no objective laboratory tests, biologic markers, or brain imaging techniques to indicate which medication will be most efficacious in treating patients with schizophrenia. The first step is to confirm the diagnosis. A psychotic patient does not necessarily have schizophrenia. Other illnesses in the differential diagnosis must be ruled out to be certain that the patient has schizophrenia and not some other psychotic condition.

***Safety/Efficacy*** All antipsychotics are relatively safe. Concurrent medical problems, however, must be considered in the initial selection and dosing. All currently available antipsychotic agents are efficacious when administered in equivalent dosages, and each agent has its individual profile of side effects[30]; however, there is a wide interpatient variation in response to a given antipsychotic agent. No specific class or subclass of antipsychotics has been shown to be effective for a specific type of psychotic patient or for a patient with a specific diagnosis or cluster of symptoms.[31]

If the patient has a close biologic relative who has been treated successfully with antipsychotic medications, it is likely that the patient would respond in a similar fashion in terms of symptom control, side effects, and perhaps dosage requirements.[26]

***Familiarity With and Availability of Agents*** Hollister[25] suggests that chlorpromazine, thioridazine, fluphenazine, thiothixene, haloperidol, loxapine, and molindone can be successfully used to treat the majority of schizophrenic patients, taking advantage of the full range of potencies and spectrum of side effects. The patient who does not respond to one of the traditional agents is likely to be the exception rather than the rule.

### *Initiation of Therapy*

Factors that influence the initial treatment with antipsychotics include patient's and relatives' previous history of antipsychotic response, age and size of the patient, potential side effects, concurrent medical problems, concomitant medications, and severity of psychotic symptoms.[32]

If a patient has required or tolerated a certain type and dose of medication in the past, that type and dose can be used as a starting point and adjusted on the basis of other considerations.[26] The patient's nonprescription and illicit drug history should also be evaluated. Alcohol, caffeine, and tobacco intake may cause potential drug interactions or misinterpretation of adverse effects of antipsychotic drug therapy. Some recreational drugs (i.e., amphetamine, cocaine, phencyclidine, marijuana) can induce or exacerbate psychotic symptoms.

Patients who are healthy, young adults not on concomitant medications can be dosed more aggressively. Others should be dosed more conservatively. Severity of symptoms will dictate how aggressive dosing and titration must be.[32] The dose of antipsychotic needed to control symptoms in the acute episode is often two to four times the amount needed to maintain control once stabilization has occurred.

Generally, dosing with antipsychotics should be started at the low end of the therapeutic range and administered using a divided schedule.[27] The patient should be observed closely during the first few days on medication and monitored for side effects and for evidence of improvement. If intolerable side effects occur, the dose should be reduced. If side effects are tolerable and there is no improvement in target symptoms, the dose should be increased incrementally every few days until the patient responds or until undesirable side effects occur.[32]

Some clinicians advocate the use of *rapid neuroleptization*, that is, the administration of repeated doses of a high-potency parenteral antipsychotic agent every 30 minutes to an hour over a period of 4 to 6 hours or for shorter periods if sedation is produced.[27] Efficacy with rapid neuroleptization may represent sedation rather than a true antipsychotic effect. The medications produce antipsychotic effects within days rather than hours. Use of an intramuscular benzodiazepine, particularly lorazepam, in doses of 2 mg has been shown to produce immediate behavioral effects similar to the effects of 5 mg of haloperidol intramuscularly.[33]

### *Stabilization of Medication*

In the first few days of antipsychotic treatment, the goal is "medicated cooperation" (i.e., decreasing symptoms of hyperarousal).[34] These symptoms include anxiety, agitation, insomnia, aggressive and assaultive behavior, and positive symptoms such as hallucinations and delusions. Elimination of the thought disorder, increased socialization, and elimination of other negative symptoms of schizophrenia may require weeks to several months of antipsychotic treatment.[32]

The expected pattern of response to antipsychotic medications is gradual over a period of several weeks, with continued improvement from 6 weeks to several months after the optimum dose has been achieved. The antipsychotic should not be switched every few days.[26] An adequate trial of one antipsychotic agent should be a minimum of 4 to 6 weeks after the dosage has been titrated to the maximum dose the patient can tolerate comfortably.[30]

Once the optimum dose is established within the expected range for the acute episode, the patient should be maintained on this dose as long as symptoms are improving.

### *Long-Term Therapy*

As the natural course of schizophrenia fluctuates over time, a patient should not be prescribed a fixed dose of an antipsychotic indefinitely. The patient should be frequently reevaluated for symptom control and potential side effects throughout treatment, and the dosage of medication should be altered as the clinical picture changes.[26]

There is no time limit for the duration of therapy with antipsychotics. Every effort should be undertaken to treat patients with the lowest possible dose of antipsychotic medication.[30]

### *Depot Antipsychotics*

Two antipsychotics are available in long-acting or depot forms. Fluphenazine is available in the enanthate and decanoate salts and haloperidol is available as the decanoate salt. The long-acting forms are beneficial for patients who are unreliable in taking oral medication on a daily basis. Psychotic symptoms should be stabilized on the oral agents before the patient is switched to the depot form of the agents.

### *Adverse Effects*

Table 48.9 presents a classification of various side effects of antipsychotic medications. The side effects of the antipsychotics are discussed with respect to the organ system affected.

#### **Autonomic Nervous System**

Patients receiving antipsychotics frequently experience anticholinergic side effects (e.g., dry mouth, constipation, nasal dryness, dry skin, urinary hesitancy/retention, tachycardia, blurred vision, and inhibition of ejaculation). The low-potency antipsychotics have higher anticholinergic properties than the high-potency agents. The elderly are especially sensitive to anticholinergic effects.[26]

The first four effects are discussed now; the others are discussed later in this chapter. Dry mouth can be relieved by increasing intake of liquids, chewing gum, or sucking on hard candy or ice chips. Anticholinergic agents slow peristaltic movement and decrease the amount of fluid in the intestines which causes the feces to be hard and dry. Patients should be encouraged to increase their exercise level, eat foods with high fiber content, and increase their intake of liquids. Drying of the nasal passages may be mistaken as nasal congestion. The dryness is usually more severe upon

**Table 48.9** Classification of Side Effects of Antipsychotic Medications

| *Generic name* | *Anticholinergic effects* | *Sedation* | *Orthostatic hypotension* | *Acute extrapyramidal effects* |
|---|---|---|---|---|
| Chlorpromazine | +++[a] | +++ | +++ | ++ |
| Thioridazine | ++++ | +++ | +++ | + |
| Mesoridazine | ++++ | +++ | ++ | + |
| Trifluoperazine | ++ | ++ | ++ | +++ |
| Fluphenazine | ++ | ++ | ++ | ++++ |
| Perphenazine | ++ | ++ | ++ | +++ |
| Thiothixene | ++ | ++ | ++ | +++ |
| Chlorprothixene | +++ | +++ | +++ | ++ |
| Haloperidol | + | + | + | ++++ |
| Loxapine | ++ | ++ | ++ | +++ |
| Molindone | ++ | ++ | ++ | +++ |

[a] Severity: +, low; ++, moderate; +++, high; ++++, extremely high.

awakening in the morning, as the patient has been recumbent and breathing through the nasal passages while asleep. Dry skin can be treated by using lotions and decreasing exposure to wind and sun.[26,27]

**Extrapyramidal System**

Several types of extrapyramidal side effects are frequently evident in patients treated with antipsychotics. Table 48.10 lists the early occurring neurologic side effects of the antipsychotic medications. Tardive dyskinesia is a late occurring chronic extrapyramidal effect.

***Acute Dystonia*** Acute dystonia or acute dyskinesia occurs within the first several days of treatment with antipsychotic medication. The reaction can occur after a single dose and usually occurs within 72 hours after initiation of antipsychotic treatment.[35] Dystonic reactions occur most frequently in patients receiving more potent antipsychotics. The symptoms of a dystonic reaction generally affect the head and neck areas of the body. These symptoms may include oculogyric crisis (i.e., the eyes may roll back in the head), trismus (i.e., the face may twist to one side, the tongue may protrude from the mouth in a fixed position), and opisthotonus (i.e., the neck may arch and draw the head backward).[35]

Early reports suggested an incidence of 5%,[26] but more recent studies have found an incidence of as high as 50%.[36] This may reflect increasing use of the high-potency antipsychotics. Patients who do experience these reactions are usually frightened by the involuntary muscle spasms. These reactions most frequently occur in young males, but other patients (older males or females) also have these reactions. Although the acute dystonic reactions are rarely dangerous, in rare cases the respiratory system of the patient is involved. Children experience more severe signs of dystonic reactions than adults, and may have more generalized signs of involvement of the trunk and extremities.[26]

The usual treatment for an acute dystonic reaction is administration of an anticholinergic agent such as benztropine (Cogentin), trihexyphenidyl (Artane),* or diphenhy-

**Table 48.10** Acute Neurologic Side Effects of Antipsychotic Medications

| *Reaction* | *Clinical features* | *Onset (d)* | *Treatment* |
|---|---|---|---|
| Acute dystonia | Spasm of tongue, throat, face, eyes, neck, or back muscles | 1–5 | Use injectable diphenhydramine or benztropine followed by oral anticholinergic agents or benzodiazepines |
| Akathisia | Motor restlessness, inability to stay still | 6–60 | Reduce dose or change antipsychotic; add anticholinergics, benzodiazepines, or β-blockers |
| Pseudo-parkinsonism | Bradykinesia, rigidity, action tremor, rabbit syndrome | 5–90 | Add anticholinergics or amantadine |

* No injectable form available.

dramine (Benadryl). Diazepam (Valium) has also been used. The injectable form is preferred for severe reactions as it provides faster symptom relief. Milder forms of dystonia may be treated safely with oral agents.[35] After the acute dystonic reaction has resolved, the patient may need to be treated with oral medication to prevent recurrence. After several weeks of treatment the dose of the anticholinergic agent can usually be decreased and discontinued without reappearance of the dystonic reaction. Patients who have previously experienced dystonic reactions and who have discontinued antipsychotics are at a high risk of developing the reaction when medications are reintroduced.[37]

***Akathisia*** Akathisia is characterized by an internal motor restlessness. Patients feel as if they are "wound up like a top." Patients may appear restless and have difficulty sitting or lying still, their legs and arms may constantly move, and they frequently walk to decrease the restlessness.[35] Akathisia can occur either early in treatment or after several months. Although the higher potency antipsychotics are frequently associated with akathisia all antipsychotics cause akathisia. The mechanism of action of drug-induced akathisia is vague, but it may be related to postsynaptic dopamine receptor blockade in nonstriatal brain regions. Approximately 20% of patients treated with antipsychotics develop akathisia.[35] Patients between the ages of 30 and 60 are especially prone to akathisia.[27]

Treatment of akathisia is difficult, and anticholinergic medications are frequently ineffective. Benzodiazepines, propranolol (Inderal), and clonidine (Catapres) have been used to treat akathisia with varying degrees of success.[35,38]

***Drug-Induced Parkinsonism*** Parkinsonism involves a triad of signs and symptoms: akinesia, rigidity, and tremor. The antipsychotic-induced parkinsonism resembles Parkinson's disease and is frequently called pseudo-parkinsonism. (See Chapter 42 for a more complete description of Parkinson's disease.)

The mechanism of action for pseudo-parkinsonism is a decrease in dopamine from the substantia nigra in the midbrain to the head of the caudate nucleus in the basal ganglia. Pseudo-parkinsonism usually occurs within 1 month of initiation of drug therapy. Elderly females are more at risk of developing pseudo-parkinsonism than other patient populations.[36]

The treatment of pseudo-parkinsonism includes decreasing the antipsychotic dose, changing to a more anticholinergic antipsychotic, adding an anticholinergic agent (e.g., benztropine or trihexyphenidyl), or increasing dopamine transmission with amantadine (Symmetrel).[35]

***Tardive Dyskinesia*** Tardive dyskinesia is a syndrome of abnormal involuntary muscle movements that usually appears in patients who have received antipsychotics for many years; however, the syndrome may appear in patients treated with antipsychotics for only 3 to 6 months. The syndrome is characterized by gross hyperkinetic activity of the oro-bucco-lingual region and choreoathetoid movements of the arms, hands, feet, and legs. The oro-bucco-lingual movements include smacking, puckering, and sucking lip movement, jaw movements, protrusion of the tongue (fly-catcher tongue), and difficulty swallowing.[35]

Tardive dyskinesia is usually present in the elderly, with a higher prevalence in females. Patients with histories of extended exposure to high doses of antipsychotics, electroconvulsive therapy, organic brain syndrome, and alcohol or drug abuse are at a higher risk of developing tardive dyskinesia. The reported prevalence of tardive dyskinesia in psychiatric patients is between 2% and 50%; however, clinically significant cases are seen in 10% to 20% of all patients exposed to antipsychotics for greater than 1 year.[35]

Drug-induced tardive dyskinesia is believed to be caused by hypersensitive postsynaptic dopamine receptors in the caudate nucleus. Long-term administration of antipsychotics leads to chronic receptor blockade in the basal ganglia and causes the receptors to become hypoactive. Hypoactivity produces dopaminergic receptor supersensitivity and an increase in the actual number of receptors. Thus, tardive dyskinesia may reflect dopaminergic overactivity and cholinergic underactivity.[35]

No marketed antipsychotic appears to have more or less propensity to cause tardive dyskinesia.[39] Patients may show signs of tardive dyskinesia when they are receiving a constant dose of an antipsychotic, when the daily dose is decreased, or when the antipsychotic is discontinued. Increasing the antipsychotic dose temporarily masks the signs of tardive dyskinesia; however, because this unnecessarily exposes patients to more antipsychotic than required and because tardive dyskinesia will reappear and be more severe, this practice is discouraged.

If antipsychotics are abruptly discontinued, patients may initially exhibit signs of transient dyskinesia that often disappear within several days to weeks of discontinuation of drug therapy. This phenomenon is called "withdrawal dyskinesia" and may indicate a predisposition to the subsequent development of tardive dyskinesia if drug therapy is reinstituted.[35]

As there is no known effective treatment for tardive dyskinesia, the best strategy is prevention. Antipsychotics should be used only in patients who actually need the agents, in the lowest possible dose, and for the shortest length of time. Patients should be evaluated periodically for early signs and symptoms of tardive dyskinesia. The Abnormal Involuntary Movement Scale (AIMS) is frequently used for evaluating symptoms of tardive dyskinesia in patients receiving antipsychotics.[35]

For patients who develop tardive dyskinesia, it may be appropriate to discontinue the antipsychotic; however, the benefit-to-risk ratio must be determined for each case. Chronic schizophrenic patients with tardive dyskinesia who cannot function without the antipsychotic should be continued on the lowest effective dose. Lowering the dose of the antipsychotic may initially worsen the movement disorder, but this may be only temporary.[35]

Although no standard effective treatment for tardive dyskinesia is available, many treatments have been tried with varying degrees of success. Benzodiazepines often provide some relief by relaxing muscles, increasing sedation, and increasing $\gamma$-aminobutyric acid (GABA) levels. Agents that decrease dopamine have also been tried (e.g., reserpine, tetrabenazine, and antipsychotics). Cholinergic agents, including deanol,† choline chloride, and lecithin, have been

† No longer marketed in the United States.

used with varying degrees of success. Baclofen (Lioresal), a GABA agonist, and propranolol have also been used.[35]

Drug holidays (defined as regularly scheduled times without psychotropic medication) are a controversial topic. It was once believed that drug holidays might reduce the possibility of development of tardive dyskinesia. More recent evidence has suggested that drug holidays may contribute to the development of tardive dyskinesia.[40]

### Sedation

All antipsychotics can cause some degree of sedation depending upon the level of histaminic properties. The less potent antipsychotics (i.e., chlorpromazine, thioridazine) cause more sedation than the more potent antipsychotics.[26] Administration of the majority of the daily dose at bedtime should eliminate the need for a hypnotic and also decrease the amount of daytime sedation. Sedative effects are usually worse when the patient first begins treatment but often dissipate (but may never be totally eliminated) after several weeks of continued treatment.

### Seizures

Antipsychotics can lower the seizure threshold. The low-potency antipsychotics decrease the seizure threshold more than the piperazine phenothiazines, haloperidol, or molindone.[27] In most patients, antipsychotics do not cause seizures even though most antipsychotics produce epileptic potentials in the EEG. Seizures may occur after sudden changes of dosage at the beginning or discontinuation of antipsychotic treatment.[41]

### Cardiovascular System

Although all antipsychotics can cause cardiovascular effects, the low-potency agents cause more cardiovascular effects than the high-potency agents. These effects include tachycardia, caused by the anticholinergic effects, and orthostatic or persistent hypotension, which is secondary to the $\alpha$-adrenergic blocking effects of the antipsychotics. Mild orthostatic hypotension frequently occurs with initiation of low-potency antipsychotic therapy; however, in most patients this effect quickly dissipates.[27]

Patients who develop severe hypotension must be treated vigorously. A pure-$\alpha$-adrenergic pressor agent such as norepinephrine (Levophed) or phenylephrine (Neo-Synephrine) should be used. Epinephrine (Adrenalin) should not be used to treat severe hypotension in a person receiving antipsychotics. Because epinephrine is both an $\alpha$- and a $\beta$-adrenergic stimulant, the unopposed $\beta$-adrenergic stimulating effects would cause a paradoxical lowering of the person's blood pressure. Also, use of a $\beta$-adrenergic stimulating agent such as isoproterenol (Isuprel) should be avoided.

The antipsychotics have both antiarrhythmic and arrhythmogenic effects. Antipsychotics produce quinidine-like effects on the myocardium and cardiac conduction system. These agents antagonize sympathetic nervous system activity in the hypothalamus and possess local anesthetic properties that serve to stabilize cardiac tissue. The arrhythmogenic effects occur more frequently with low-potency antipsychotics, especially thioridazine. Electrocardiogram changes include increased heart rate, prolonged QT and PR intervals, depressed T waves, and depression of the ST segment.[26] The ECG changes are not usually clinically significant; however, patients with preexisting cardiac abnormalities receiving antipsychotics should be monitored cautiously and a baseline ECG should be obtained.[36]

### Eye

***Blurred Vision*** Blurred vision is usually only a temporary, bothersome anticholinergic side effect of the antipsychotics and usually dissipates after a few weeks of treatment. Anticholinergic medications interfere with visual accommodation and can cause patients to be photosensitive because more light gets into their eyes as a result of mydriasis.[26] Pilocarpine eye drops can help severe refractory cases, and ophthalmic wetting agents can be used for treatment of dry eyes.

***Glaucoma*** Patients with narrow-angle (angle closure) glaucoma should be treated cautiously with antipsychotics and always in conjunction with an ophthalmologist.[27] Antipsychotics can increase intraocular pressure and produce attacks of glaucoma in susceptible patients.

***Pigmentary Retinopathy*** Pigmentary retinopathy results in visual impairment, and possibly blindness. Although very rarely encountered, the retinopathy is most frequently associated with doses of thioridazine greater than 800 mg per day.[34] Pigmentary retinopathy may be caused by melanin deposits in the cornea. Because of this irreversible side effect, thioridazine and its metabolite, mesoridazine, are the only antipsychotics with absolute ceiling daily doses.

### Liver

Although all antipsychotics are metabolized by the liver, hepatic complications are most frequently reported with chlorpromazine. These problems were more commonly observed when the drug was first released, almost 35 years ago. Improved manufacturing techniques have resulted in a decline in chlorpromazine-induced hepatic adverse effects.[27]

Intrahepatic obstructive-type jaundice rarely occurs with antipsychotic treatment, although symptoms may be evident during the first 4 weeks of treatment.[27] The occurrence and severity of the jaundice appear to be idiopathic and not dose related. In patients with jaundice, the antipsychotic should be discontinued and liver function tests monitored until they normalize.[26]

### Urinary Tract

Urinary hesitancy is commonly reported with the low-potency antipsychotics. The anticholinergic effects of these agents cause smooth muscle slowing and paralyze the detrusor muscle of the bladder that is responsible for allowing micturation. Older males with prostatic hypertrophy are especially prone to this effect.[27] Urinary retention is much less frequently encountered than urinary hesitancy and can be treated with bethanechol (Urecholine).

### Blood

Leukopenia and agranulocytosis are rarely reported with antipsychotic medications. A transient decrease in the white blood cell (WBC) count is frequently evident in patients during initial treatment with antipsychotics, although most patients readily compensate for the lowered WBC count.[26] Leukopenia is treated by discontinuing therapy and monitoring the WBC count, which should return to within the normal range. After the WBC count has normalized, patients who require further antipsychotic therapy should be treated with a medication from a different chemical class, and the WBC count carefully monitored.

The low-potency antipsychotics, especially chlorpromazine, are most frequently associated with this rare (incidence less than 0.01%), but potentially toxic adverse effect.[26]

### Skin

***Allergic Reactions*** Allergic reactions usually occur after 2 to 10 weeks of therapy and manifest themselves as maculopapular, erythematous, itchy rashes that are usually evident on the face, neck, extremities, and trunk of the body. The reactions usually disappear after the offending medication has been discontinued. If needed, topical steroids may be used to treat antipsychotic-induced allergic reactions.[26]

***Contact Dermatitis*** Contact dermatitis may occur in people hypersensitive to an antipsychotic.[26] Mixing the concentrate in a sufficient quantity of a nonacidic liquid and having patients quickly swallow the mixture decrease the possibility of contact dermatitis. Patients should not dissolve the tablets in their mouths, and medical personnel who are allergic to antipsychotics should not allow the drug to come into contact with their skin.

***Photosensitivity*** Some patients receiving antipsychotics, especially the low-potency agents such as chlorpromazine, may have photosensitivity reactions after 15–30 minutes of exposure to direct sunlight. Patients who are photosensitive should wear protective clothing and apply a sunscreen to uncovered areas before sun exposure.[34]

Patients receiving high-dose, low-potency antipsychotics, primarily chlorpromazine, for extended periods may develop a blue-gray discoloration of the skin (purple person syndrome). This rare reaction is caused by the interaction of melanin with sunlight.[34]

### Hormonal and Endocrine Systems

Because dopamine regulates prolactin secretion, lowering dopamine will consequently increase serum prolactin levels. Therefore, antipsychotics increase serum prolactin levels via dopamine blockade and hyperprolactinemia is possible.[26] Hyperprolactinemia can cause decreased libido in both males and females as well as gynecomastia and galactorrhea. Amenorrhea and false-positive pregnancy tests have been reported.[27]

Antipsychotics can lower circulating testosterone levels. Lower testosterone levels, coupled with increased serum prolactin levels, can exacerbate the decreased libido in males treated with antipsychotics. The anticholinergic properties of the low-potency agents (especially thioridazine) frequently interfere with ejaculation, often manifested as either delayed or retrograde ejaculation.[26]

***Glucose Metabolism*** Antipsychotic therapy may affect glucose metabolism. This factor should be considered when treating diabetic or prediabetic patients, as glucose levels can be increased.[26]

***Thermoregulation*** The antipsychotics, especially the aliphatic and piperidine phenothiazines, affect the hypothalamus' ability to regulate body temperature. Although mild temperature changes are not usually problematic, patients, especially the elderly, should use extreme caution in high or low temperatures because their ability to conserve or remove body heat has been altered.[26]

***Weight Gain*** The antipsychotics, especially the low-potency agents, often cause weight gain. Patients receiving molindone do not generally report weight gain and may report weight loss. Weight gain may be secondary to the medication's antihistaminic properties which may increase the patient's appetite.[26]

### Neuroleptic Malignant Syndrome

Neuroleptic malignant syndrome (NMS) occurs in 0.5% to 1% of patients receiving antipsychotics.[42] It has been most frequently reported with high-potency antipsychotics given intramuscularly. There is no time course for onset; NMS may appear soon after therapy is initiated or after months of treatment.[43]

Mechanisms proposed for NMS include disruption of the central thermoregulatory mechanism, excess production of heat because of muscle contractions related to dopamine blockade, or the direct effects of antipsychotics on muscle contraction.[43] Males less than 40 who are debilitated and unresponsive to the usual doses of antipsychotics appear to be at a greater risk of developing NMS.[44]

Signs and symptoms of NMS are hyperpyrexia; change in consciousness; dyskinesia; increase muscle tone; dysarthria; autonomic changes of tachycardia, tachypnea, labile blood pressure, diaphoresis, and incontinency; laboratory changes including increases in white blood cells, creatinine phosphokinase, and liver function tests and presence of urinary myoglobin.[42]

Treatment is limited to anecdotal reports as no clinical studies have been done on the syndrome. Discontinuation of the antipsychotic and supportive treatment may be sufficient. Some patients have responded to anticholinergic medications. Bromocriptine (Parlodel), a dopamine agonist, has been used successfully to treat NMS. Dantroline (Dantrium) and benzodiazepines have been used as muscle relaxants in the treatment of NMS.[42]

It is essential that treatment be initiated immediately when NMS is suspected. Approximately 20% to 30% of patients diagnosed as having NMS do not survive.[42] Respiratory and cardiovascular failures are the main causes of death in NMS patients.

## *Toxicity*

The range between therapeutic and toxic doses of antipsychotics is very wide and overdoses are uncommon.[27] In cases where overdoses do occur, gastric lavage should be instituted and activated charcoal can be used to absorb additional quantities of the antipsychotic from the stomach. The anticholinergic properties of the antipsychotic greatly delay gastric emptying times. Emesis is not beneficial as all antipsychotics (except the piperidine phenothiazines) are potent antiemetics and block the chemoreceptor trigger zone.[27] Hypotension after an overdose should be treated with a pure $\alpha$-stimulating agent. Cardiac arrhythmias should not be treated with quinidine or other type 1 antiarrhythmic agents. The central anticholinergic toxic effects can be treated cautiously with physostigmine (Antilirium),[27] as this medication may worsen arrhythmias and decrease the seizure threshold.

#### *Abuse/Withdrawal*

The antipsychotics are rarely used for their recreational effect. Addiction, tolerance, and habituation are not believed to occur with antipsychotics.[26] Tolerance to many anticholinergic side effects develops, and when antipsychotics are discontinued, rebound may occur. The patient may experience insomnia, nightmares, and excessive cholinergic effects such as increased salivation, sweating, abdominal cramps, and diarrhea. The psychosis may reappear as may a transient withdrawal dyskinesia.[26]

#### *Pregnancy/Lactation*

Antipsychotic agents cross the placenta, but their direct teratogenic effect on the developing fetus has not been well established.[30] Antipsychotics can cause withdrawal extrapyramidal symptoms and sedation in newborns exposed to these agents in utero.[27]

Antipsychotics are secreted in the mother's milk. The milk antipsychotic concentration is similar to the corresponding maternal blood antipsychotic concentration.[45] Breastfeeding is discouraged.

#### *Drug Interactions*

Drug–drug interactions[46–48] associated with the antipsychotic agents are summarized in Table 48.11.

## Additional Medications

Several additional medications are used to treat schizophrenia.

#### *Lithium*

The use of lithium in the treatment of schizophrenic patients is controversial. Lithium is not a first-line treatment; however, it may be beneficial in treating chronic schizophrenics who do not respond to antipsychotics.[49,50] Refer to Chapter 49 for a complete review of lithium.

#### *β-Blockers*

Treating schizophrenia with propranolol has resulted in mixed findings. The drug is probably more effective in treating aggression and combative behavior than the actual thought disorder itself.[51] Propranolol combined with antipsychotics increases the plasma concentration of the antipsychotics by decreasing hepatic blood flow and enzyme inhibition; this may be the primary beneficial effect of the agent on schizophrenia.[52]

#### *Benzodiazepines*

The benzodiazepines facilitate GABA (an inhibitory neurotransmitter) transmission. GABA modulates dopamine activity; therefore, benzodiazepines may indirectly decrease dopamine activity. Use of benzodiazepines, especially diazepam, in the treatment of schizophrenia is believed to be due to the agent's modification of both dopaminergic (decrease dopamine release) and GABA-ergic (increase GABA release) transmission.[53] The benzodiazepines have been reported to reduce both positive and negative symptoms of schizophrenia at a faster rate than antipsychotics.[54] The use of benzodiazepines in combination with antipsychotics seems to be justified if the dose of the antipsychotic can be lowered. Refer to Chapter 51 for a complete review of the benzodiazepines.

#### *Carbamazepine*

Carbamazepine (Tegretol) may be useful in treatment of schizophrenic patients unresponsive to antipsychotic medications. This agent has been shown to decrease aggression in schizophrenic patients.[55] Refer to Chapters 41 and 49 for a complete review of carbamazepine.

#### *Clozapine (Investigational Agent)*

Clozapine (Clozaril) has been investigated for more than a decade. Its action on dopamine receptors and dopaminergic functions makes it a unique antipsychotic. This low-potency sedating agent, which is believed to act selectively on the limbic dopamine receptors,[56] does not cause acute extrapyramidal side effects but has extremely high anticholinergic properties. It has been reported not to cause tardive dyskinesia and, therefore, to be of potential benefit in the treatment of psychotic patients with tardive dyskinesia.

Agranulocytosis was reported in Europe at a rate of 1 in 215 patients and at a lethal rate of 1 in 350 patients. In the United States, clinical trials were discontinued in the mid-1970s in response to the high incidence of agranulocytosis. Investigation of clozapine has resumed for patients who have not responded to traditional antipsychotic medications,[57] and is expected to be marketed in 1989.

## Nonpharmacologic Management

As schizophrenia is heterogeneous, there is no single treatment for all patients and treatment must be individualized.[12] The biopsychosocial model of treatment is generally used to treat schizophrenic patients because it incorporates medication and various psychosocial elements.

The foremost treatment for schizophrenic patients is antipsychotic drug therapy. Other types of therapy employed without drug treatment are less effective than drug treatment alone. Before psychotherapy can be effective the more severe symptoms of schizophrenia must be controlled with

**Table 48.11** Drug Interactions Involving Antipsychotic Drugs

| *Interacting compound* | *Mechanism* | *Clinical outcome* |
|---|---|---|
| Antacids | Decrease in gastrointestinal absorption | May decrease antipsychotic efficacy |
| Oral anticoagulants | Antipsychotic may inhibit hepatic microsomal enzymes | May increase anticoagulant activity |
| Antidepressants | Antipsychotic may inhibit hepatic microsomal enzymes | May increase plasma levels of antidepressants and antipsychotics |
| Anticholinergics | Unknown | May decrease plasma levels and decrease efficacy of antipsychotics |
| Barbiturates | Induction of hepatic microsomal enzymes | May decrease plasma levels of antipsychotics |
| Alcohol (and other CNS depressants) | Additive CNS depressant effect | May increase sedation |
| Amphetamine | Antagonism of dopamine blockade | May decrease efficacy of antipsychotics |
| Levodopa | Antagonism of dopamine blockade | May decrease efficacy of antipsychotics |
| Anticonvulsants | Antipsychotic may lower seizure threshold | May decrease efficacy of anticonvulsant |
| β-Blockers | Additive antihypertensive interaction | May exaggerate antihypertensive effects |
| Phenytoin | Decrease in metabolism of phenytoin | May increase anticonvulsant level |
| Oral hypoglycemics, insulin | Antipsychotic may increase blood glucose levels | Alteration in dosage of insulin or oral hypoglycemics may be needed |
| Rifampin, griseofulvin, phenylbutazone, carbamazepine | Possible increase in antipsychotic metabolism | May decrease antipsychotic activity |
| Disulfiram, oral contraceptives | Possible decrease in antipsychotic metabolism | May increase antipsychotic activity |

Modified from Csernansky JG, Whiteford HA: Clinically significant psychoactive drug interactions, in Frances AJ, Hales RE (eds): Psychiatry Update: American Psychiatric Association Annual Review. Washington DC, American Psychiatric Press, 1987, vol 5, p 810.

antipsychotic medication.[22] The nonpharmacologic interventions most frequently used to treat schizophrenia are listed in Table 48.12.

Individual psychotherapy, which offers supportive therapy to the schizophrenic patient, usually produces better results than insight-oriented psychotherapy. Patients with schizophrenia may, in fact, become worse with insight-oriented psychotherapy because it may increase the disorganization of their internal world. Supportive therapy, which allows patients to develop a relationship with one consistent person, can serve to add order to their disorganized internal world.[58]

Group therapy can play a role in the treatment of schizophrenic patients. Again, supportive therapy is better than insight-oriented therapy. Group participation can also serve to increase social interaction and feelings of belonging.[2]

Family therapy can be beneficial to the treatment of schizophrenics. Schizophrenic illness can cause extreme problems in families. Families can learn to deal more effectively with the illness through family therapy.[12]

Behavioral therapy has been used successfully in the treatment of many schizophrenic patients. The structure and limit-setting techniques of this type of therapy can be used to modify or reduce the frequency of bizarre and disturbing behaviors of the schizophrenic patient.[2]

Electroconvulsive therapy is no longer considered a first-line treatment for schizophrenia as it was before the discovery of antipsychotics.[59] It is used to treat schizophrenic patients who do not respond to antipsychotics or other less standard forms of treatment. It is sometimes used in combination with antipsychotics in refractory schizophrenic patients.[59] Electroconvulsive therapy should be considered as a treatment for schizophrenic patients with tardive dyskinesia.[23]

**Table 48.12** Nonpharmacologic Management of Schizophrenia

| |
|---|
| Psychotherapy or supportive therapy |
| Individual |
| Group |
| Family |
| Behavioral therapy |
| Electroconvulsive therapy |

## Summary

As schizophrenia is a heterogeneous illness, the treatment is diverse and frequently less than ideal. Treatment of schizophrenia has changed little over the last 20 years; antipsychotics continue to be the primary treatment. Only after researchers discover the etiology of the disease and are able to subclassify the disease can more successful treatment be targeted at homogeneous subgroups.

## Glossary

**Attention.** Ability to focus on one task in a sustained manner.

**Catatonic behavior.** Marked motor irregularities, usually limited to disturbances associated with a diagnosis of a nonorganic psychotic disorder.

- **Catatonic excitement.** Increased motor activity with no evident purpose and no external stimulatory influence.
- **Catatonic negativism.** Resistance to all instructions or efforts to be moved, for no apparent reason.
- **Catatonic posturing.** Voluntary assumption of an unsuitable or strange position usually maintained for long periods of time.
- **Catatonic rigidity.** Holding a rigid posture against all attempts to be moved.
- **Catatonic stupor.** Decreased responsiveness to surroundings and reduction in spontaneous movements, occasionally to the extreme of appearing unaware of one's environment.
- **Catatonic waxy flexibility.** Extremities can be arranged into any position, which will be held.

**Circumstantial speech.** Speech that is roundabout and delayed in reaching the point.

**Delusion.** False personal belief that cannot be changed with reason; belief is not generally accepted by other members of the culture.

- **Delusion, bizarre.** False belief involving an event that other members of the culture would find completely unbelievable.
- **Delusion of being controlled.** Feelings, thoughts, impulses, or actions experienced as not being one's own.
- **Delusion of persecution.** Belief that one or a group is being cheated, persecuted, conspired against, attacked, or harassed.
- **Delusion of reference.** False belief that events, objects, or other people in one's immediate surroundings have a specific and strange importance, usually of a negative nature.
- **Delusion, somatic.** Pertaining primarily to the functioning of one's body.
- **Delusion, systematized.** Single delusion with multiple elaborations or several delusions that one relates by a single event or idea.

**Depersonalization.** Temporary loss of the feeling of one's own reality because of a change in the perception of self.

**Distractibility.** Frequent drawing of attention to unimportant or irrelevant external stimuli.

**Formal thought disorder.** Disturbance in the form of thought distinct from the content.

**Hallucination.** False sensory perception or sensory perception not caused by external stimuli.

- **Auditory.** Hallucination of sound, most frequently of voices but could be clicks, taps, music, etc.
- **Gustatory.** Taste, most commonly unpleasant.
- **Olfactory.** Smell.
- **Somatic.** Physical experience localized within the body.
- **Tactile.** Touch, on or under the skin.
- **Visual.** Sight, may consist of formed or unformed images.

**Idea of reference.** Idea held less firmly than a delusion of reference.

**Illogical thinking.** Thinking that contains obvious internal contradictions or in which conclusions are reached that are clearly erroneous given the initial starting information.

**Illusion.** Misperception of a real stimulus.

**Incoherence.** Speech that is not understandable because of a lack of logical connections, excessive use of incomplete sentences, irrelevancies, or abrupt changes in subject. Idiosyncratic word usage or distorted grammar.

**Loose association.** Thinking characterized by speech in which ideas switch from one to another completely unrelated topic.

**Magical thinking.** Belief that thoughts, words, or actions cause or prevent specific events.

**Paranoid ideation.** Suspiciousness or belief that one is being harassed, persecuted, or unfairly treated. Less delusional proportion than paranoid delusions.

**Poverty of content of speech.** Speech that is adequate in amount but provides little information because of vagueness and empty repetition.

**Poverty of speech.** Restriction of the amount of speech. Lack of spontaneous speech. Brief replies to direct questions.

**Prodromal.** Early manifestations or symptoms of a disorder.

**Psychomotor agitation.** Excessive, nonproductive, and repetitious motor activity associated with (a feeling of) inner tension.

**Psychosis.** Gross impairment in reality testing and the creation of a new reality.

**Residual.** Stage of illness that occurs after abatement of the full syndrome.

## References


1. Kendler KS. Genetics of schizophrenia, in Francis AJ, Hales RE (eds): Psychiatry Update: American Psychiatric Association Annual Review. Washington DC, American Psychiatric Press, 1986, vol 5, pp 25–47.
2. Strauss JS, Carpenter WT. Schizophrenia. New York; Plenum, 1981.
3. Murray RM, Reveley AM, McGuffin P. Genetic vulnerability to schizophrenia. Psychiatr Clin North Am 1986;9:3–16.
4. Meltzer HY, Stahl SM. The dopamine hypothesis of schizophrenia: A review. Schizophr Bull 1976;2:19–76.
5. Snyder SH. The dopamine hypothesis of schizophrenia: Focus on the dopamine receptor. Am J Psychiatry 1976;133:197–202.
6. Bowers MB. Biochemical process in schizophrenia: An update. Schizophr Bull 1980;6:393–403.
7. Martin MB, Owen CM, Morishia JM. An overview of neurotransmitters and neuroreceptors, in Hales RE, Yudofsky SC (eds): Textbook of Neuropsychiatry. Washington, DC, American Psychiatric Press, 1987, pp 55–86.
8. Pickar D, Labarca R, Doran AR, et al. Longitudinal measure-

ments of plasma homovanillic acid levels in schizophrenic patients. Arch Gen Psychiatry 1986;43:669–676.
9. Schmauss C, Hinderk ME. Dopamine and the action of opiates: A reevaluation of the dopamine hypothesis of schizophrenia with special consideration of the role of endogenous opioids in the pathogenesis of schizophrenia. Biol Psychiatry 1985;20: 1211–1231.
10. Shelly RK, Walsh N. The biochemistry of schizophrenia: A review. Ir Med J 1985;78:139–143.
11. Boza RA, Rotondo DJ. Is cholecystokinin therapeutic in chronic schizophrenia? J Clin Psychiatry 1985;46:485–486.
12. McGlashan TH. Schizophrenia: Psychosocial treatments and the role of psychosocial factors in its etiology and pathogenesis, in Frances AJ, Hales RE (eds): Psychiatry Update: American Psychiatric Association Annual Review. Washington, DC, American Psychiatric Press, 1986, vol 5, pp 96–111.
13. Andreasen NC. Afterword, in Francis AJ, Hales RE (eds): Psychiatry Update: American Psychiatric Association Annual Review. Washington, DC, American Psychiatric Press, 1986, vol 5, pp 112–114.
14. Brown RP, Kneeland B. Visual imaging in psychiatry. Hosp Community Psychiatry 1985;36:489–496.
15. American Psychiatric Association, Diagnostic and Statistical Manual of Mental Disorders, 3rd ed, revised (DSM-III-R). Washington, DC, American Psychiatric Press, 1987.
16. Fenton WS, Mosher LR, Matthews SM. Diagnosis of schizophrenia: A critical review of current diagnostic systems. Schizophr Bull 1981;7:452–472.
17. Mellor CS. First rank symptoms of schizophrenia. Br J Psychiatry 1970;117:15–23.
18. Andreasen NC, Olsen S. Negative v positive schizophrenia: Definition and validation. Arch Gen Psychiatry 1982;39:789–794.
19. Kendler KS, Tsuang MT. Nosology of paranoid schizophrenia and other paranoid psychoses. Schizophr Bull 1981;7:594–610.
20. Pfohl B, Andreasen NC. Schizophrenia: Diagnosis and classification, in Francis AF, Hales RE (eds): Psychiatry Update: American Psychiatric Association Annual Review. Washington, DC, American Psychiatric Press, 1986, vol 5, pp 7–24.
21. Davis JM. Maintenance therapy and the natural course of schizophrenia. J Clin Psychiatry 1985;45:18–21.
22. Davis JM, Gieri B. Pharmacological treatment in the care of schizophrenic patients, in Bellack AS (ed): Schizophrenia. Orlando, FL, Grune and Stratton, 1984, pp 133–173.
23. Van Valkenburg C, Clayton PJ. Electroconvulsive therapy and schizophrenia. Biol Psychiatry 1985;20:699–700.
24. Johnson DAW. Treatment of chronic schizophrenia. Drugs 1977;14:291–299.
25. Hollister LE. Psychopharmacology: Drug side effects and interactions, in Hales RE, Francis AJ (eds): Psychiatry Update: American Psychiatric Association Annual Review. Washington, DC, American Psychiatric Press, 1987, vol 6, pp 698–703.
26. Gelenberg AJ. Psychoses, in Bassuk EL, Schoonover SC, Gelenberg AJ (eds): The Practitioner's Guide to Psychoactive Drugs, 2nd ed. New York, Plenum, 1983, pp 115–165.
27. Baldessarini RJ. Chemotherapy in Psychiatry: Principles to Practice. Cambridge, MA, Harvard University Press, 1985.
28. Boyer WF, Friedel RO. Antidepressant and antipsychotic plasma levels. Psychiatr Clin North Am 1984;7:601–610.
29. Yesavage JA. Psychotropic blood levels: A guide to clinical response. J Clin Psychiatry 1986;47(suppl):16–19.
30. Kessler KA, Waletzky JP. Clinical use of the antipsychotics. Am J Psychiatry 1981;138:202–209.
31. Kane JM. Somatic therapy, in Francis AJ, Hales RE (eds): Psychiatry Update: American Psychiatric Association Annual Review. Washington DC, American Psychiatric Press, 1986, vol 5, pp 78–95.
32. Appleton WS, Davis JM. Practical Clinical Psychopharmacology, 2nd ed. Baltimore, Williams and Wilkins, 1980.
33. Campbell R, Simpson GM. Alternative approaches in the treatment of psychotic agitation. Psychosomatics 1986;27(suppl): 23–26.
34. Lehmann HE. Psychopharmacological treatment of schizophrenia. Schizophr Bull 1970;8:27–45.
35. Tarsey D. Movement disorders with neuroleptic drug treatment. Psychiatr Clin North Am 1984;7:453–471.
36. Levinson DF, Simpson GM. Antipsychotic drug side effects, in Hales RE, Francis AJ (eds): Psychiatry Update: American Psychiatry Association Annual Review. Washington, DC, American Psychiatric Press, 1987, vol 6, pp 704–723.
37. Davis JM, Janicak R, Chang S, et al. Recent advances in the pharmacologic treatment of the schizophrenic disorders, in Grinspoon L (ed): Psychiatry Update. Washington, DC, American Psychiatric Press, 1982, vol 1, pp 178–228.
38. Donlon PT. The therapeutic use of diazepam for akathisia. Psychosomatics 1973;14:222–225.
39. Kane JM, Smith JM. Tardive dyskinesia: Prevalence and risk factors, 1959–1979. Arch Gen Psychiatry 1982;39:473–481.
40. Jeste DV, Potkin SG, Sinha S, et al. Tardive dyskinesia—reversible and persistent. Arch Gen Psychiatry 1979;36:583–590.
41. Itil TM. Use of electroencephalography in the practice of psychiatry. Psychosomatics 1982;23:799–813.
42. Guze BH, Baxter LR. Neuroleptic malignant syndrome. N Engl J Med 1985;313:163–166.
43. Sternberg DE. Neuroleptic malignant syndrome: The pendulum swings. Am J Psychiatry 1986;143:1273–1275.
44. Mueller PS. Neuroleptic malignant syndrome. Psychosomatics 1985;26:654–662.
45. Gelenberg AJ. Pregnancy, psychotropic drugs, and psychiatric disorders. Psychosomatics 1986;27:216–217.
46. Csernansky JG, Whiteford HA. Clinical significant psychoactive drug interactions, in Hales RE, Frances AJ (eds): Psychiatry Update: American Psychiatric Association Annual Review. Washington, DC, American Psychiatric Press, 1987, vol 6, pp 802–815.
47. Hollister LE. Psychopharmacology: Drug side effects and interactions, in Hales RE, Francis AJ (eds): Psychiatry Update: American Psychiatric Association Annual Review. Washington, DC, American Psychiatric Press, 1987, vol 6, pp 698–703.
48. Glassman R, Salzman C. Interactions between psychotropic and other drugs: An update. Hosp Community Psychiatry 1987; 38:236–242.
49. Donaldson SR, Gelenberg AJ, Baldessarini RJ. The pharmacologic treatment of schizophrenia: A progress report. Schizophr Bull 1983;9:504–527.
50. Delva NJ, Letemendia FJ. Lithium treatment in schizophrenic and schizoaffective disorders. Br J Psychiatry 1986;141:387–400.
51. Silver JM, Yudofsky S. Propranolol for aggression: Literature review and clinical guidelines. Int Drug Ther Newslett 1985;20: 9–12.
52. Dominguez RH, Goldstein BJ. Beta-blockers in psychiatry. Hosp Community Psychiatry 1984;35:565,566,568.
53. Greenblatt DJ, Raskin A. Benzodiazepines: New indications. Psychopharmacol Bull 1986;22:77–87.
54. Nestoros JN, Suranyi-Cadotte BE, Spees RC, et al. Diazepam

in high doses is effective in schizophrenia. Neuro-Psychopharmacol Biol Psychiatry 1982;6:513–516.

55. Birkheimer LJ, Curtis JL, Jann MW. Use of carbamazepine in psychiatric disorders. Clin Pharm 1985;4:425–434.

56. Kane JM, Cooper TB, Sachar EJ, et al. Clozapine: Plasma level and prolactin response. Psychopharmacology 1981;73:184–187.

57. Small JG, Milstein V, Marhemke JD, et al. Treatment outcome with clozapine in tardive dyskinesia, neuroleptic sensitivity, and treatment of resistant psychosis. J Clin Psychiatry 1987;48:263–267.

58. Heinrichs DW, Carpenter WT. The psychotherapy of schizophrenic disorders, in Grinspoon L (ed): Psychiatry Update. Washington, DC, American Psychiatric Press, 1982, vol 1, pp 154–166.

59. Major LF. Electroconvulsive therapy in the 1980s. Psychiatr Clin North Am 1984;7:611–623.

# Chapter 49 / Bipolar Disorder

Janet L. Kinney-Parker, PharmD, and Martha P. Fankhauser, MS

For as long as history has been recorded, mood (affective) disorders have been recognized and described. Descriptions of depression are found in ancient Egyptian writings, the Old Testament, and classical Greek literature. Hippocrates was the first to introduce the terms *mania* and *melancholia* and his clinical descriptions are as valid today as they were then. A Roman physician, Areteus, first argued that depression and mania often coexisted in the same individual. He described a group of patients who would "laugh, play, dance night and day, and sometimes go openly to the market crowned, as if victors in some contest of skill" only later to appear "torpid, dull, and sorrowful." Jean Pierre Fabret in 1854 was the first to identify and describe circular insanity (*la folie circulaire*) as a clinically coherent and nosologically distinct entity.

The American Psychiatric Association's *Diagnostic and Statistical Manual of Mental Disorders, Third Edition, Revised* (DSM-III-R), represents our present understanding of bipolar disorder.[1] Bipolar disorder is one of several mood disorders described in the DSM-III-R. The essential feature of the disorder is a disturbance of mood not caused by any other physical or mental disorder.[2] Mood generally involves elation or depression and is the pervasive emotion felt and expressed by an individual. Bipolar disorder (or manic–depressive illness) characterizes individuals who experience extreme mood swings that are outside the range of normal mood changes. Bipolar patients must experience periods of mood elevation (mania or hypomania) that alternate with normal mood states. To be diagnosed as bipolar does not require a history of depression, but most patients experience episodes of depression in their lifetime.

## Epidemiology

Epidemiologic studies of bipolar disorder indicate a prevalence rate of 0.4% to 1.2% of the adult population. The incidence is equally common in men and women.[1] Although mania is rare before puberty, its prevalence increases during adolescence and into adulthood.[3] The onset of bipolar disorder is usually in late adolescence or early twenties, but it may appear after the age of 50.[1,2]

Researchers have utilized family, twin, and adoption studies to examine the genetic influence on bipolar disorder. Bipolar disorder has a higher risk of familial transmission than unipolar depression.[4] Pooled data from family studies indicate that the morbidity risk for developing bipolar disorder is 22.3% for parents, 24.7% for siblings, and 38.9% for children of the bipolar patient. Eighty to ninety percent of bipolar patients have a parent, sibling, or child with an affective disorder. Pooled data from twin studies show a 74.7% concordance in monozygotic twins and a 19.8% concordance in dizygotic twins. Adoption studies have found that 38% of adopted children of parents with bipolar disorder have an affective disorder, whereas only 7% of control adopted children develop an affective disorder.[5]

## Pathophysiology

### *Neurotransmitter Theories*

There are several biologic theories about bipolar disorder.[6] The most prominent and oldest hypotheses regarding mood disorders are those proposing an altered function of monoamine neurotransmitter concentrations in the central nervous system (CNS). In the simplest form, these hypotheses suggest a functional deficit of neurotransmitters (primarily norepinephrine and/or serotonin) in depression (as explained in Chapter 50) and an excess of catecholamines (primarily norepinephrine) in mania. Data supporting these hypotheses are meager and inconsistent. Major support for these theories comes from the proposed mechanisms of action of effective antidepressant and antimanic drugs. Antidepressants increase CNS norepinephrine and serotonin concentrations and antimanic drugs were thought to decrease these concentrations; however, challenging manic patients with monoamine neurotransmitter agonists has not consistently worsened mania.[7]

An increase in brain dopamine concentrations may play a role in causing mania. Drugs that decrease dopamine activity (e.g., lithium and antipsychotic agents) are effective in treating acute mania. Drugs that increase dopamine synthesis (levodopa), stimulate dopamine release (dextroamphetamine), or directly activate dopamine receptors (bromocriptine) may induce mania; however, this is contradictory, as evidence also exists that bromocriptine may be an effective antimanic drug.[8]

Recently, a supersensitivity of neurotransmitter receptors has been proposed as a cause of bipolar illness.[9] Support for this theory arises from the actions of lithium. Lithium prevents the development of dopaminergic supersensitivity, blocks $\beta$-adrenergic supersensitivity (but not the subsensitivity induced by imipramine), and has inconsistent effects on $\alpha$-adrenergic receptor sensitivity. Lithium has no effect on serotonin receptor sensitivity. This theory is appealing, as it fits well with the current theories of depression (see Chapter 50).

### *Neuroendocrine Theories*

Endocrine abnormalities may be related to overactivity of the mesolimbic dopamine pathways along with changes in serotonergic, noradrenergic, cholinergic, and $\gamma$-aminobutyric acid (GABA)-ergic neurotransmitter systems.

Circulating cortisol and cerebrospinal fluid (CSF) cortisol concentrations are elevated in both unipolar and bipolar depressed patients, but less frequently in manic patients.[10] Patients with elevated circulating cortisol (e.g., those with Cushing's syndrome or patients treated with high-dose corticosteroids) often have maniclike states. The mechanism by which elevated cortisol affects mood is not clear but may be related to increased dopamine receptor number and activity.

Although elevated thyroid hormones or thyrotoxicosis can precipitate a maniclike state in patients, circulating thyroid hormone (thyroxine and triiodothyronine) concentrations appear to be normal in manic patients.[10] Thyroid hormones are thought to increase the number and activity of central $\beta$-adrenergic receptors. The overactivity of norepinephrine pathways secondary to thyroid hormones may precipitate mania in predisposed patients. There is some evidence that lithium-induced hypothyroidism may play a role in the pathophysiology of rapid cycling.[6] Patients with rapid manic–depressive cycling (more than four episodes a year) have been shown to have higher thyroid-stimulating hormone (TSH) concentrations than nonrapidly cycling patients on lithium.

Bipolar patients may have altered neurohormonal responses to light and heat from altered noradrenergic activity.[11] Melatonin is secreted from the pineal gland at night and is stimulated by $\beta$-adrenergic pathways. Reports indicate that melatonin is reduced in depression and elevated in mania.[10] The seasonal variation in light and heat may explain the increased incidence of manic episodes during the summer months and of depressive episodes during the winter months. There is some evidence that altering the sleep–wake or light–dark cycle may alter the course of bipolar disorder.[12]

### *Calcium Theories*

Calcium may play a role in the etiology of affective disorders.[13] High serum and CSF calcium concentrations have been found in patients with depression, whereas extracellular calcium concentrations may be low in manic patients.[14] Depression may be associated with an increase, and mania with a decrease, in intracellular calcium-dependent functions. Changes in extracellular and intracellular calcium concentrations can affect the excitability of neuronal firing and may be directly related to the emotional variations seen in affective disorders. The antipsychotics, which are effective for the treatment of mania, have direct calcium channel antagonist effects. Acute lithium treatment decreases calcium transport into cells and may also interfere with the calcium–sodium active transport system. Chronic lithium-treated bipolar patients have increased calmodulin-activated calcium ATPase activity in comparison with controls.[13]

### *Environmental Theories*

Although unclear, the contribution of the environment cannot be denied. Studies have examined the number of independent life events occurring prior to a manic episode. There is an increased frequency of stressful life events, especially difficulty at work and interpersonal conflict, in the period preceding an episode. Approximately two thirds of patients in one study reported that a significant life event preceded the onset of the first manic episode.[15]

### *Dysregulation Hypothesis*

The dysregulation theory proposes that mania and depression are not due simply to increased or decreased activity of certain neurotransmitter or neurohormonal systems but, rather, are due to a failure of regulation or buffering of these systems, as discussed in Chapter 50. Many drugs used to treat affective disorders, including lithium and antidepressants, are thought to correct this abnormality by correcting the "signal-to-noise ratio."[16]

## Clinical Presentation

According to the DSM-III-R, the diagnosis of bipolar disorder cannot be made until an individual has had one or more manic episodes.[1] Bipolar disorder is separated into three subcategories to differentiate the current or most recent episode: manic, depressed, or mixed. The mixed diagnosis is used when individuals have both manic and depressive features, either intermixed or alternating rapidly every few days. Patients with two or more complete cycles (a manic and a depressive episode that succeed each other without a period of normal mood state) have been called "rapid cyclers." Individuals with mixed or rapid cycling episodes have a more chronic course and may be more difficult to treat with medication.

Cyclothymia is another diagnostic classification that requires at least 2 years (1 year for children and adolescents) of numerous hypomanic episodes and numerous depressive periods that do not meet the criteria for a major depressive episode.[1] A residual category is called Bipolar Disorder Not Otherwise Specified, which is used when patients have manic or hypomanic features but do not meet the criteria for any specific bipolar disorder. Included here are bipolar II patients. In another classification of bipolar disorder, bipolar I patients have episodes of depression and mania, whereas bipolar II patients have hypomanic episodes along with episodes of major depression.[2]

An episode of mania is often followed by multiple recurrent episodes of either depression, mania, or hypomania alternating with a normal mood state.[2] Usually there is a period of normal functioning between episodes but approximately 25% to 30% of patients may not fully recover and continue to demonstrate significant impairment in both social and occupational functioning. The length and severity of an episode and the interval between episodes vary from patient to patient. The recurrences may become more frequent as the illness progresses.[2] Untreated episodes may last up to 4 months. A few individuals have episodes that recur regularly at the same time or season of the year. Approxi-

**Table 49.1** DSM-III-R Diagnostic Criteria for a Manic Episode[a]

A. One or more distinct periods when mood was abnormally and persistently elevated, expansive, or irritable
B. During the period of mood disturbance, at least three of the following symptoms persisted (four if the mood was only irritable) and were present to a significant degree
   1. Inflated self-esteem (grandiosity, which may be delusional)
   2. Decreased need for sleep
   3. More talkative than usual or pressure to keep talking
   4. Flight of ideas or subjective experience that thoughts are racing
   5. Distractibility, that is, attention too easily drawn to unimportant or irrelevant external stimuli
   6. Increase in activity (either socially, at work, or sexually) or psychomotor agitation
   7. Excessive involvement in pleasurable activities that have a high potential for painful consequences that is not recognized, for example, buying sprees, sexual indiscretions, foolish business investments, reckless driving
C. Episode of mood disturbance sufficiently severe to cause marked impairment in social or occupational functioning, or hospitalization was necessary
D. At no time during the illness were delusions or hallucinations present at least 2 weeks in the absence of prominent mood symptoms, that is, before the mood symptoms developed or after they remitted
E. Not superimposed on either schizophrenia, schizophreniform disorder, or a delusional disorder
F. Not sustained by a specific organic factor or substance (although there may be an organic precipitant)

[a] A manic episode is defined as meeting criteria A, B, and C. A hypomanic episode meets only criteria A and B (no marked impairment).

Modified from American Psychiatric Association: Diagnostic and Statistical Manual of Mental Disorders, 3rd ed, revised (DSM-III-R). Washington DC, American Psychiatric Association, 1987, p 217.

mately 4% to 6% of patients first diagnosed as having unipolar or major depression will later have an episode of mania. In children, the clinical presentation is usually one of rapid mood swings with short periods of mania and depression. At pubescence, the length and frequency of episodes increase and the disorder is more easily diagnosed.[3]

The DSM-III-R diagnostic criteria for a manic episode are listed in Table 49.1. The clinical presentation and diagnostic criteria for a major depressive episode are the same as those for Bipolar Disorder, Depressed and are discussed in Chapter 50. Bipolar depressed patients tend to have increased sleep (hypersomnia), low energy, carbohydrate craving, and weight gain in comparison with unipolar depressed patients.

Hypomania describes the early stages of mania in which the patient's mood may be elevated, expansive, or irritable and there are associated symptoms such as increased psychomotor activity and flight of ideas[1]; however, the patient does not fit the DSM-III-R criteria for a manic episode because there is no marked impairment in social or occupational functioning. In fact, some patients may actually function better and be more productive and creative during a hypomanic state.

A manic episode usually begins abruptly and symptoms escalate over several days. Target symptoms of mania are listed in Table 49.2. The classic triad of manic symptoms consists of euphoria, psychomotor excitement, and flight of ideas. Manic patients are often considered "high" and are outgoing, overly alert, extravagant, and overly self-confident. They may be playful—punning, joking, laughing, and teasing—and their dress may be flamboyant and their makeup "excessive." The euphoria often leads to disinhibition, grandiosity, and impaired judgment. Frequently they become involved in foolish business adventures, illegal activities, or buying sprees that can cause financial ruin. They tend to lose social inhibitions, have increased sexual and aggressive behavior, make poor decisions, and often take risks that can endanger themselves or others. Grandiose delusions or hallucinations that are consistent with the predominent mood (mood congruent) are present in 15% to 20% of patients.

Although the mood in a manic episode is usually elevated, individuals may become labile, angry, or irritable when people do not go along with their ideas.[17] Overactive manic patients can be garrulous, loud, irritating, intrusive, and often leave everything in disarray. Manic patients may have so much energy and are involved in so many activities that they have no time for sleep. Not sleeping leaves them more time to engage in pleasurable activities, so they rarely complain of this symptom. The decreased need for sleep is often the first clue to a manic episode. The manic patient's attention span is very short and he or she may find it impossible to concentrate. Anything in the environment may elicit a response leading to flight of ideas in which the patient flits rapidly from one topic to another. Yet with close listening, a superficial association can be understood.[17]

The later stages of a manic episode may resemble paranoid schizophrenia with symptoms of bizarre behavior, hallucina-

**Table 49.2** Target Symptoms of Mania

| | | |
|---|---|---|
| Mood | Irritable<br>Expansive<br>Labile | Elated<br>Euphoric |
| Thought content | Flight of ideas<br>Paranoia<br>Hallucinations | Ideas of reference<br>Grandiose delusions |
| Speech | Rapid, pressured<br>Circumstantiality | |
| Behavior | Hyperactive<br>Demanding<br>Distractible<br>Neglect of food<br>Insomnia<br>Decreased inhibitions | Manipulative<br>Assaultive<br>Self-confident<br>Weight loss<br>Decreased need for sleep |

tions, and grandiose delusions. These symptoms are difficult to differentiate and patients may be misdiagnosed as having schizophrenia, schizophreniform disorder, or a paranoid disorder. Blacks and hispanics are at a higher risk for misdiagnosis, as they frequently are not brought in for treatment until the illness has progressed to a more severe state.[18]

Manic patients may need protection, as their lack of judgment and insight can lead to considerable trouble. They are often the last to realize that anything is wrong with their thinking or behavior. Hypomania or mild depressive episodes are usually treated on an outpatient basis. Manic patients may resist treatment, become irritated when help is suggested, and may threaten litigation. As acutely manic patients rarely see the need for hospitalization, involuntary commitment or support and collaboration with the patient's family may be required for treatment.

Inadequately treated bipolar illness can put significant strain on interpersonal relationships. Because a bipolar disorder is usually evident by the midtwenties, education may be interrupted and some patients may have difficulty keeping a job. Bipolar patients tend to become dependent on others for financial support if they are not stabilized on medication. Fortunately, most bipolar patients are adequately controlled on medication and function well in society. The majority of patients who relapse do so because of medication noncompliance. Alcoholism and substance abuse are common in bipolar patients because they try to self-medicate during episodes.[1]

### *Laboratory Tests/Diagnostic Procedures*

Unlike medical illnesses, there are no specific, sensitive diagnostic tests available to assist in the diagnosis of bipolar disorder; however, several potential biologic markers are being investigated. The majority of bipolar depressed patients are dexamethasone suppression test (DST) nonsuppressors, but there is disagreement regarding the manic phase.[7,19] A blunted TSH response to the thyrotropin-releasing hormone (TRH) stimulation test has been reported in manic but not schizophrenic patients.[20] If confirmed, the TRH stimulation test may prove useful in differentiating mania from other psychotic states.

### *Secondary Mania*

Certain medical illnesses, drugs, and drug withdrawal syndromes can induce or present as mania (Table 49.3).[2] Clues to an organic manic episode include a first episode after 40 years of age, history of head trauma, seizures, incontinence, and an abrupt change in behavior and cognition. The diagnostic workup should include a thorough medical, drug, and alcohol history, a complete physical examination, and appropriate laboratory tests.

**Table 49.3** Medical Conditions, Drugs, and Drug Withdrawal Syndromes Reported to Cause Mania

| | |
|---|---|
| **Medical Conditions** | |
| Addison's disease | After electroconvulsive therapy |
| Carcinoid tumors | After closed head trauma |
| Cushing's disease | Subarachnoid hemorrhage |
| Epilepsy | Surgical trauma with subsequent epileptic focus |
| Hyperthyroidism | |
| Infection (postviral encephalitis, influenza) | |
| Multiple sclerosis | |
| **Drugs** | |
| Alcohol | Hallucinogens (marijuana, LSD, mescaline) |
| Amphetamine | Indomethacin |
| Anticholinergics | Isoniazid |
| Antidepressants | L-Dopa |
| Baclofen | Monoamine oxidase inhibitors |
| Benzodiazepines (alprazolam) | Methylphenidate |
| Bromides | Metoclopramide |
| Caffeine | Niridazole |
| Captopril | Phenylpropranolamine |
| Cimetidine | Procainamide |
| Cocaine | Procarbazine |
| Corticosteroids | Quinacrine |
| Diltiazem | Tolmetin |
| Disulfiram | Vitamin $B_{12}$ deficiency |
| Ephedrine | Yohimbine |
| **Drug Withdrawal Syndromes** | |
| Baclofen | Tricyclic antidepressants |
| Clonidine | |

## Treatment

### *Lithium*

Lithium was first used for the treatment of mania in the second century AD by a Greek physician, Seranus Ephesios, who wrote "use should also be made of natural waters, such as alkaline springs."[21] Sir Alfred Garrod, in 1859, used lithium for the cure of gout, rheumatic gout, and urinary calculi. In the late 1800s and early 1900s, lithium was advocated as a mild tonic, a sedative, an anticonvulsant, and a diuretic. In the early 1940s, lithium chloride was introduced as an unmonitored salt substitute for cardiac and hypertensive patients. After numerous reports of severe toxicity and several deaths, lithium was withdrawn from the U.S. market.

In 1949, Cade reintroduced lithium for the treatment of mania after noting that guinea pigs became extremely lethargic and unresponsive to stimuli after intraperitoneal injection of lithium urate.[21] Little progress was made until Shou, in 1954, reported the first controlled study of lithium's antimanic effects. In 1970, the Food and Drug Administration approved the reintroduction of lithium in the United States for the treatment of mania.

Extensive clinical experience and well-controlled studies have shown that lithium is effective in the treatment of acute mania. Lithium is generally 60% to 80% effective in aborting an acute manic or hypomanic episode within 7 to 14 days after starting therapy. Prophylactic lithium therapy is approximately 80% effective in preventing or attenuating recurrences of mania, hypomania, and depression in unipolar and bipolar patients.[22] In bipolar patients, lithium is more effective at preventing the signs and symptoms of mania than those of depression. Lithium appears to be an effective antidepressant in some acutely depressed patients. The complete antidepressant effect of lithium may require up to 3 to 4 weeks, which is similar to standard antidepressant agents.

In April 1984, the National Institutes of Health, in conjunction with the National Institute of Mental Health, convened the Consensus Development Conference on Mood Disorders: Pharmacologic Prevention of Recurrences.[23] The panel concluded that any patient who has a manic episode should be considered for preventative lithium therapy. Patients who have had a depressive episode and a hypomanic episode are also at high risk for recurrence. Other factors increasing the need for medication prophylaxis include the number and frequency of past episodes of depression, family history of bipolar disorder, past suicide attempts or psychotic episodes, past functional incapacity with episodes, and level of social functioning between episodes.[23]

Lithium carbonate (usually combined with other psychotropic agents) is useful in the treatment of various psychiatric disorders, such as schizophrenia, schizoaffective, and impulsive–aggressive behavior. Lithium has been used in the treatment of alcoholism, drug addiction, and premenstrual syndrome with varying degrees of effectiveness. Nonpsychiatric uses of lithium include the treatment of granulocytopenia, syndrome of inappropriate secretion of antidiuretic hormone (SIADH), hyperthyroidism, and migraine and cluster headaches.

**Proposed Mechanism of Action**

Despite numerous investigations into the biologic and clinical properties of lithium, there is no unified theory of lithium's mechanism of action. Lithium is a monovalent cation and belongs to the group of alkali metals. It competes with other monovalent and divalent cations such as calcium, magnesium, potassium, and sodium in body tissues and at binding sites. Lithium has been shown to affect the synthesis, storage, release, and reuptake of central monoamine neurotransmitters including norepinephrine (NE), serotonin (5-hydroxytryptamine, 5-HT), dopamine (DA), acetylcholine (ACH), and $\gamma$-aminobutyric acid (GABA). Initially, lithium increases NE turnover but does not affect the rate of NE synthesis. Chronic lithium administration produces an increased uptake of NE but only insignificant changes in NE turnover.[24] Conflicting results have been reported as to lithium's effects on adrenergic receptors. Lithium is reported to induce a $\beta$-adrenergic receptor subsensitivity, to decrease or have no effect on receptors, or to increase the number of $\beta$-adrenergic receptors. It may also decrease $\alpha_2$-adrenergic receptor sensitivity and increase $\alpha$-receptor density and receptor activation.

Serotonin may play a role in the pathogenesis of depressive episodes but the results with 5-HT in mania are conflicting. Lithium has been shown to have no effect or to increase or to decrease both central and platelet 5-HT.[24] Short-term administration of lithium increases the neuronal uptake of tryptophan which leads to an increased 5-HT synthesis; however, with continued administration, increased uptake of tryptophan, but not increased synthesis of 5-HT, is maintained.

Lithium is reported to reduce dopamine synthesis, increase dopamine striatal turnover, and block dopamine receptor supersensitivity.[24] Lithium has a number of properties similar to those of calcium channel blocking agents. In fact, lithium's known effects on calcium function may explain its therapeutic properties.[13] Increased GABA concentrations are also reported with lithium administration.[25]

Until the etiology of bipolar illness is elucidated, it is only speculative as to which (if any) of the proposed pharmacologic actions accounts for lithium's effectiveness.

**Pharmacokinetics**

***Absorption*** Lithium is readily absorbed from the gastrointestinal tract. The rate and extent of absorption vary depending on the dosage formulation and whether the dose is taken on an empty or full stomach.[26] Conventional lithium carbonate tablets or capsules are 95% to 100% absorbed. Peak plasma concentrations occur within 1 to 3 hours after an oral dose and absorption is usually complete within 6 to 8 hours.[27] Slow-release or controlled-release tablets in the United States are 80% to 97% absorbed. They have a slower absorption with more gradual and delayed peak plasma concentrations that occur within 2 to 6 hours.[26] Absorption is usually complete 6 to 10 hours after oral administration of a sustained-release preparation. Some of the sustained-release lithium preparations available in Europe may be incompletely absorbed. Oral solutions of lithium citrate are rapidly and completely absorbed. Peak concentrations usually occur within 15 to 60 minutes. Patients who ingest lithium on an empty stomach absorb lithium rapidly and may have high peak plasma concentrations. Administering lithium with meals or using a sustained-release product significantly delays absorption, but has no effect on the total amount of lithium absorbed or the area under the time-versus-concentration curve. Concurrent administration of antacids and lithium carbonate does not affect lithium plasma concentrations.[28]

***Distribution*** Lithium is widely distributed into most body tissues and fluids. The distribution phase of lithium follows a biphasic or two-compartment model. The initial distribution phase has a central compartment of 25% to 40% of body weight, and the final distribution space is approximately 50% to 100% of body weight.[27] The volume of distribution of lithium ranges from 0.5 to 1.2 L/kg. Elderly patients have a smaller volume of distribution of about 90% of body weight compared with 120% for younger patients. Distribution is usually complete 6 to 10 hours after oral administration of conventional tablets or capsules. It may take up to 25 to 30 hours for complete distribution of the sustained-release preparations.[26]

Lithium is unevenly distributed into tissues and fluids throughout the body and is not bound to plasma proteins. The plasma concentration equals that found in muscle, heart, lung, and kidney. Concentrations more than twice the plasma concentration are found in the thyroid gland, bone, and some areas of the brain, whereas liver, spinal fluid, and erythrocyte concentrations are 50% or less of the plasma concentration. It takes approximately 3 to 10 days for lithium to equilibrate intracellularly which may account for the delay in therapeutic response.[27]

***Elimination*** Lithium is excreted primarily by the kidney and is not metabolized. Less than 5% of a lithium dose is excreted through the feces, sweat, and saliva.[27] In patients with normal renal function, about 30% to 70% of a single dose is excreted in urine within 6 to 12 hours and 50% to 80% within 24 hours. Lithium has biphasic elimination with an alpha half-life of 0.8 to 1.2 hours and a beta half-life of 20 to 27 hours. The average half-life is approximately 24 hours in adults and 36 hours in geriatric patients. Patients with impaired renal function may have plasma half-lives of 40 to 50 hours.[26]

Lithium clearance is directly proportional to glomerular filtration rate and renal blood flow. Approximately 80% of the lithium filtered through the glomeruli is reabsorbed in the proximal renal tubules.[27] Renal lithium clearance is about 20% of the glomerular filtration rate (GFR) or about 25 mL/min (range, 10–40 mL/min). Because GFR decreases with age, renal clearance of lithium is reduced in the elderly.

Reabsorption of lithium at the proximal tubule is in direct competition with sodium. Any increase in sodium excretion or decrease in plasma sodium proportionately increases lithium reabsorption, resulting in higher lithium plasma concentrations. Dehydration, fever, vomiting, diarrhea, low-sodium diets, sodium-depleting diuretics that act at the proximal tubules, and medications that decrease renal blood flow by inhibiting prostaglandin synthesis can increase plasma lithium concentrations. Sodium loading may increase lithium clearance by reducing the reabsorption of sodium and lithium at the proximal tubule. Postural changes and diurnal variations in renal clearance may also affect lithium clearance.[26,27]

***Therapeutic Blood Concentrations*** Lithium has a narrow therapeutic index in comparison with other psychotropic medications which necessitates close monitoring of plasma concentrations. The usual therapeutic range of lithium is 0.6 to 1.2 mEq/L measured 12 hours after the last dose.[29] Acutely manic patients may require plasma concentrations of 1.0 to 1.5 mEq/L to achieve a therapeutic effect. In general, plasma lithium concentrations higher than the concentrations needed for maintenance therapy should be used to treat acute mania. Onset of the acute antimanic effect of lithium usually occurs within 5 to 7 days; the full therapeutic effect may require 10 to 21 days. When the mania begins to respond to lithium, the dose should be adjusted downward to decrease the risk of lithium toxicity. Recommended plasma concentrations for maintenance therapy are not well defined. One study reported that a minimum of 0.8 mEq/L was required to prevent relapse,[30] but others have reported concentrations as low as 0.4 to 0.6 mEq/L.[31] Maintenance concentrations should be individualized and the patient maintained on the lowest possible dose to prevent relapse. Breakthrough episodes of hypomania or depression during maintenance therapy should be treated by increasing the dose of lithium to achieve plasma concentrations of 1.0 to 1.5 mEq/L until the episode is resolved.

### Initiation of Therapy

***Baseline Assessment*** Before beginning lithium therapy, the patient's medical and drug history should be assessed, looking particularly for evidence of renal, thyroid, cardiovascular, or neurologic disease, for potentially significant drug interactions, and for pregnancy. The recommended guidelines for baseline laboratory testing are listed in Table 49.4.

**Table 49.4** Recommendations for Baseline and Routine Laboratory Testing for Lithium Therapy

| | *Baseline* | *12 months* |
|---|---|---|
| Cardiac | | |
| ECG[a] | * | |
| Pulse | * | |
| Hematologic | | |
| CBC with differential | * | * |
| Metabolic/endocrine | | |
| Weight | * | * |
| Serum electrolytes (sodium, potassium, calcium, phosphate) | * | * |
| $T_3$, $T_4$, and $T_7$ | * | * |
| TSH[b] | * | |
| Renal function | | |
| Serum creatinine[c] | * | * |
| 24-h creatinine clearance[d] | | |
| Urinalysis/osmolality | * | * |
| Specific gravity | * | * |

[a] Those older than 40 or those with preexisting cardiovascular disease.
[b] Thyroid-stimulating hormone is a better indicator of hypothyroidism and should be obtained during maintenance therapy if thyroid function tests change or if the patient exhibits any signs of hypothyroidism.
[c] Measure every 3 months for patients with impaired renal functioning.
[d] Indicated for patients with a history of renal disease or abnormally high serum creatinine or significant increases in serum creatinine.

Laboratory evaluation should include serum creatinine, urinalysis, and electrolytes including calcium and magnesium. A 24-hour creatinine clearance is indicated if the patient has a history of renal disease or if the serum creatinine is abnormal. Thyroid function tests including TSH should be measured and the thyroid palpitated to determine if a goiter is present. A baseline ECG is indicated for all patients over 40 years of age and for those with preexisting cardiovascular disease. A baseline CBC with differential should be obtained to facilitate the monitoring of hematologic changes.

### Initial Dosing

Lithium therapy should be initiated with low doses, 900–1,200 mg per day for prophylaxis and 1,200–1,800 mg per day for acute mania, using a divided dosing regimen. The dose should be gradually increased according to the plasma steady-state concentration drawn 12 hours after the last dose. Approximately 300 mg of lithium carbonate (or 560 mg of lithium citrate) will raise the plasma concentration by 0.2 to 0.4 mEq/L.[32] Lower initial doses should be prescribed in the elderly or in clinical situations that impair lithium excretion (e.g., concomitant diuretic therapy, low-salt diet, renal disease, or decreased cardiac output). Because of poorer compliance with multiple dose regimens, the frequency of dosing should be minimized. Once-a-day dosing at bedtime should be used only in those patients on sustained-release preparations and if they can tolerate the peak concentration side effects.

An alternative method of initiating lithium therapy is to use one of the dose prediction methods. Cooper et al in 1973 developed the first single-point prediction method and this model is the one most commonly used.[33] It is based on a single lithium concentration drawn 24 hours after administering a 600-mg test dose of lithium. The dosage regimen needed to achieve a 12-hour postlithium concentration between 0.6 and 1.2 mEq/L at steady state is obtained from a table. At least five other pharmacokinetic methods for estimating the maintenance dosage requirements of lithium have been proposed (i.e., a modified Cooper method using a 900-mg test dose, a single- and multiple-point method by Perry, and the Zetin and Pepin method that does not utilize lithium concentrations).[34,35] Loading lithium, as is done with other drugs with long half-lives, has also been proposed,[36] but is not commonly utilized or recommended.

Although lithium is not approved by the FDA for children under 12 years of age, it has been used to treat children with mania or aggressive behavior. When therapy is initiated in children, the dose should be low, preferably 300 mg per day in divided doses, with gradual increases after laboratory monitoring. As children normally have a higher renal clearance of lithium, doses relatively higher than those used in adults may be needed to achieve therapeutic concentrations.[37]

***Duration of Treatment*** Although the majority of bipolar patients eventually have recurrences in their lifetime, not all patients should automatically be placed on long-term maintenance lithium therapy after their first manic episode. Patients who have responded to lithium and are tolerating the side effects should be continued on lithium for 9 to 12 months. At this time, a decision must be made about maintenance treatment. Lifetime prophylactic lithium therapy should be given to any patient with two or three previous episodes, with frequent episodes (greater than one per year), or with rapid onset of manic episodes.

***Therapeutic Blood Monitoring*** When monitoring lithium therapy, it is important to draw the blood sample consistently at the same time and interval so that plasma concentrations are comparable. The standardized "therapeutic" lithium concentration requires that the patient receive the same daily dosage for at least 4 to 5 days preceding the blood test (until steady state is reached), the patient should be on a multiple-dose regimen, and the blood sample should be drawn after the absorption and distribution phase. Lithium concentrations should be drawn 12 hours (plus or minus 30 minutes) after the last dose in the evening.[26] Blood samples drawn before or after the 12-hour postdose time can be significantly higher or lower than the reference range and thus be inaccurate. Currently, there is no therapeutic reference range for once-daily dosing with lithium.

When patients are first started on lithium, a plasma concentration should be obtained every 2 to 3 days to minimize the risk of toxicity. A non–steady-state concentration is helpful in patients who may be prone to toxicity. When the desired plasma lithium concentration has been achieved, lithium concentrations should be checked weekly for 3 to 4 weeks. During maintenance therapy, lithium concentrations should be obtained every 1 to 3 months depending on the individual and the frequency of bipolar episodes. Individuals who are prone to lithium toxicity or who have intercurrent illnesses should be carefully supervised by monitoring lithium concentrations at least monthly. In addition, lithium concentrations should be obtained whenever there is suspected toxicity, a possible drug interaction, or a major change in diet.[27]

**Table 49.5** Factors That Can Affect the Accuracy and Reliability of Plasma Lithium Concentrations

| | |
|---|---|
| Compliance before the blood test | Changes in sodium intake or excretion |
| Timing of blood sampling after last dose | Caffeine and alcohol intake |
| Inadequate time to reach steady state | Concomitant drugs that alter lithium clearance |
| Product formulation and bioequivalency differences | Medical illnesses (renal disease, dehydration, etc) |
| Accuracy and reliability of the laboratory | Alterations in diet or physical activity |

Numerous variables influence the accuracy of plasma lithium concentrations (Table 49.5). The most common cause of variation is patient noncompliance or error in the sampling time (obtaining a concentration before or after the 12-hour standardized time). Other possible causes include laboratory error, bioequivalence differences between lithium products, changes in sodium intake, drug interactions, and medical illnesses. If no reason is found for an unusually high lithium concentration and there are no signs of toxicity, a second lithium concentration should be ordered rather than adjusting the dose based on one abnormal result.

***Alternative Monitoring Methods*** The red blood cell (RBC) lithium-to-plasma lithium ratio has been investigated as a method to measure lithium transport across cell membranes and to better understand the mechanism of action of lithium. Lithium distributes into erythrocytes against an electrochemical potential gradient. The carrier-mediated $Na^+$–$Li^+$ countertransport system and the passive "leak" diffusion of lithium across the RBC membrane account for the major transport of lithium. Some studies have shown a decreased activity of the RBC $Na^+$–$Li^+$ countertransport system in bipolar patients as compared with controls.[6] This may result in a higher RBC lithium concentration in bipolar patients. Steady-state lithium concentrations in erythrocytes range from 30% to 90% of concurrent plasma concentrations but are usually 50% or less. The ratio of lithium concentration in erythrocytes to plasma shows wide interindividual variation but minimal intraindividual variation. The relationship of the RBC/plasma lithium ratio to clinical response is not well established.

The RBC/plasma ratio may be used as an indicator of compliance, as patients who have not been taking lithium

**Table 49.6** Lithium Preparations Available in the United States

| *Product* | *Manufacturer* |
|---|---|
| Regular-release capsules (150 mg lithium carbonate, 4.06 mEq) | |
| Lithium carbonate | Roxane |
| Regular-release capsules (300 mg lithium carbonate, 8.12 mEq) | |
| Eskalith[a] | Smith Kline & French |
| Lithonate[a] | Reid–Rowell |
| Lithium carbonate | Roxane |
| Regular-release capsules (600 mg lithium carbonate, 16.24 mEq) | |
| Lithium carbonate | Roxane; generic brands, various |
| Regular-release tablets (300 mg lithium carbonate, 8.12 mEq) | |
| Eskalith (scored)[a] | Smith Kline & French |
| Lithane (scored, contains tartrazine)[a] | Miles |
| Lithium carbonate (scored) | Roxane; generic brands, various |
| Lithotabs (film-coated)[a] | Reid–Rowell |
| Syrup (8 mEq lithium/5 mL as lithium citrate) | |
| Cibalith-S (sugar-free)[a] | Ciba |
| Lithium citrate (sugar-free) | Roxane; generic brands, various |
| Slow-release tablets (300 mg lithium carbonate, 8.12 mEq) | |
| Lithobid (film-coated)[a] | Ciba |
| Controlled-release tablets (450 mg lithium carbonate, 12.18 mEq) | |
| Eskalith CR (scored)[a] | Smith Kline & French |

[a] Trade name.

regularly should have a lower ratio.[38] The primary clinical use of the RBC lithium concentration is to identify patients with RBC concentrations greater than 0.6 mEq/L or a RBC/plasma ratio greater than 0.5, as these individuals may be at higher risk for developing neurotoxic effects.[27] Despite great interest in RBC lithium concentrations, further studies are needed to determine if the ratio is related to diagnosis, response, compliance, side effects, or toxicity.

Because the monitoring of plasma lithium concentrations requires multiple venipunctures, alternative methods, such as saliva lithium concentrations, have been investigated.[27] Lithium is concentrated in saliva and the ratio of saliva to plasma lithium is approximately 2:1 to 3:1. There is wide interpatient variation in the ratio of saliva to plasma but minimal intraindividual variation. The test requires that each patient first have their own saliva/plasma ratio determined; thereafter, saliva concentrations may be used to monitor lithium therapy. Further studies are needed to standardize the test before saliva concentrations can be recommended for routine clinical practice.

Lithium has been measured in urine, cerebrospinal fluid, tears, sweat, muscle tissue, cultured human skin fibroblasts, semen, and breast milk, but these methods have no utility in monitoring lithium therapy at this time.

***Choosing a Product Formulation*** Lithium is available in several salt forms but only the citrate and carbonate salts are marketed in the United States (Table 49.6). Lithium citrate is available only as a syrup (5 mL is equivalent to 8 mEq of lithium, the amount of lithium in a 300-mg lithium carbonate tablet). Lithium carbonate is available in regular-release tablets (300 mg) and capsules (150, 300, and 600 mg), as a slow-release tablet (300 mg), and as a controlled-release tablet (450 mg). Selection of a product is based on patient preference, tolerance of side effects, and cost. Many patients prefer capsules because they cannot tolerate the taste of the tablets or have difficulty swallowing them. The syrup is used primarily for patients who refuse to take medication or who have difficulty swallowing tablets or capsules. Because of increased cost, the slow- and controlled-release products are usually reserved for patients who are experiencing side effects such as nausea or hand tremor with the regular-release products.

### Adverse Effects

Side effects of lithium are divided into those that occur early in therapy but are generally innocuous and transient, and those that occur with long-term therapy and are usually non–dose related. Table 49.7 lists the side effects observed early in therapy.[39,40] Gastrointestinal disturbances such as nausea, diarrhea, anorexia, abdominal pain, and bloating occur commonly but are usually transient. If nausea is significant, patients should take lithium after a meal or snack. Other approaches to alleviate nausea include giving a smaller dose more frequently (e.g., 300 mg QID rather than

**Table 49.7** Early-Onset Benign Side Effects of Lithium

| | |
|---|---|
| Gastrointestinal disturbances | 30% |
| Polyuria | 50% |
| Polydipsia | 50% |
| Muscle weakness | 33% |
| Tremor | 47% |

600 mg BID) or switching to a sustained-release product.[29] Although muscle weakness and lethargy are reported in about 30% of patients, the symptoms are usually transient, and no intervention is generally necessary. As many as 40% of patients receiving lithium initially complain of headache, memory impairment, mental confusion, and a decreased ability to concentrate. Polyuria and polydipsia occur in about 30% to 50% of lithium-treated patients early in therapy and may persist longer than 1 year in up to 23% of patients. Although bothersome, the polyuria and polydipsia are usually innocuous and reversible with discontinuation of lithium. Many patients respond to polydipsia with weight gain, probably because of increased consumption of high-calorie fluids or fluid retention.

Table 49.8 lists the persistent, non–dose-related adverse effects. A fine, rapid intention hand tremor similar to essential tremor may be observed, especially in the fingers. Patients often complain that they are unable to write or to perform fine motor skills. The tremor is worsened by tension, concomitant use of antidepressants or antipsychotics, caffeine, fatigue, and impending toxicity. The tremors are usually noticeable early in therapy and may persist in up to 4% of patients. Although the tremor is usually non–dose related, it may be treated by lowering the dose, by decreasing the peak lithium plasma concentration by dividing doses or switching to a sustained-release product, or by adding a $\beta$-blocker. Propranolol in doses of 10–80 mg daily is most commonly used in the treatment of lithium-induced tremor.[41] Propranolol's effect is usually evident in 30 minutes and the antitremor action may last up to 4 to 6 hours. Other $\beta$-blockers such as nadolol, metoprolol, pindolol, practolol, and oxprenolol have also been used to reduce the lithium-induced tremor. The tremor is not responsive to anticholinergic or antiparkinsonian drugs.

Lithium causes alterations in renal functioning and often produces a mild nephrogenic diabetes insipidus (NDI) manifested as polyuria. Lithium-induced NDI is not related to the classic disease with posterior pituitary dysfunction or vasopressin unavailability. Rather, it is vasopressin unresponsive and may be related to inhibition of the adenylate cyclase system or to blocking of the antidiuretic hormone (ADH) aldosterone.[42] It is characterized by low urine specific gravity, low-osmolality polyuria, and an inability to concentrate urine. Urine volumes of 5 to 6 L per day are not uncommon. Although lithium-induced NDI is not dose related, reduction of the lithium dose or discontinuation of therapy may alleviate the problem. Occasionally the syndrome persists even after lithium is discontinued.[42] Lithium-induced NDI has been treated with loop diuretics, thiazide diuretics, or triamterene. Amiloride, a potassium-sparing diuretic, has been used to treat lithium-induced polyuria and appears to be relatively safe with minimal effects on lithium clearance.[43] Drugs that augment the excretion of ADH are not helpful.

**Table 49.8** Long-Term Non–Dose-Related Side Effects of Lithium

| | |
|---|---|
| **Neurologic** | |
| Tremor | 4% |
| Decreased concentration | |
| Impaired memory | |
| Cogwheel rigidity | |
| **Renal** | |
| Nephrogenic diabetes insipidus | 12% |
| Nephrotoxicity | Uncommon |
| **Cardiovascular** | |
| Nonspecific T-wave changes | 20%–30% |
| Increased premature ventricular contractions | Rare |
| **Thyroid** | |
| Hypothyroidism | 3%–30% |
| Increased TSH | 15% |
| **Hematologic** | |
| Leukocytosis | 30%–45% |
| **Dermatologic** | Uncommon |
| Acne | |
| Psoriasis | |
| Alopecia | |
| Rash | |
| **Weight Gain** | 25% |

The first report that renal damage may occur from chronic lithium therapy was in 1977.[44] Although numerous subsequent studies have examined this issue, no consensus has been reached.[42] Nonspecific nephron atrophy characterized by glomerular sclerosis, tubular atrophy, interstitial fibrosis, and urinary casts has been reported in patients treated with lithium. Tubulointerstitial nephritis clearly exists in some lithium-treated patients; however, lithium may not be the cause, as the age of the patient correlates with renal changes.[45] Patients with affective disorders that have never been treated with lithium also show chronic interstitial nephropathy. A study of renal function in patients receiving lithium for 5 to 17 years found no significant changes in plasma creatinine or renal concentrating capacity, but a moderate decrease in GFR.[46] Thus, it does appear that changes in GFR may occur in some patients after long-term (but not short-term) treatment. Further studies are needed to determine the effect of lithium concentrations, other psychotropic drugs, and affective illness on renal function.

It was previously assumed that renal damage was more common in patients exposed to toxic or high peak concentrations of lithium. Thus, clinicians attempted to maintain relatively constant plasma concentrations by giving the drug in divided daily doses. Recent data suggest that lithium trough concentrations may be of greater importance than peak concentrations. Although still controversial, some investigators report that once-daily dosing results in lower trough lithium concentrations which allows for renal regenerative processes and less polyuria or renal damage.[47]

Lithium has various effects on the thyroid gland, but primarily blocks the release of thyroxine ($T_4$) and triiodothyronine ($T_3$) mediated by thyrotropin. Approximately 15% of patients on maintenance lithium therapy develop transiently elevated TSH concentrations and 5% of patients develop a goiter and/or hypothyroidism. Lithium-induced hypothyroidism is not dose related, is observed ten times more frequently in women, and usually occurs after at least 18 months of therapy.[48] Proposed mechanisms include lithium's interference with thyroid hormone synthesis by increasing iodine uptake or by decreasing iodine release and lithium's inhibition of the TSH-induced thyroid response by interfering with adenylate cyclase activity. Recently, it was proposed that lithium may exacerbate a preexisting autoimmune thyroiditis.[49] Often, symptoms of hypothyroidism (e.g., weight gain, tiredness, low energy, and slowed mental functioning) go unrecognized and are confused with other lithium side effects or symptoms of a depressive episode. Hypothyroidism does not require discontinuation of lithium, as supplemental exogenous thyroid, usually levothyroxine, can be added to the lithium regimen. When lithium is discontinued, the hypothyroidism is almost always reversible.

Lithium may cause a variety of benign and reversible cardiac effects, particularly T-wave flattening or inversion. The cardiac effects of lithium may be secondary to potassium displacement from intracellular myocardial sites. Although rare, lithium may cause myocarditis, sinus node dysfunction, and sinoatrial block and may aggravate ventricular arrhythmias.[50] During lithium intoxication, the ST segment may be depressed and/or the QT interval prolonged. If a patient has significant preexisting cardiac disease, consultation with a cardiologist is recommended before initiation of lithium therapy.

Other long-term side effects include benign reversible leukocytosis, weight gain (25% of patients gain more than 10 pounds), and a variety of dermatologic effects (e.g., acne, alopecia, psoriasis, puritic dermatitis, and ulceration). Dry mouth, alterations in taste, increased glucose tolerance, hypercalcemia, and hyperparathyroidism have been reported.[40,51] Severe disturbances of neuromuscular functioning such as myasthenia gravis and extrapyramidal symptoms are occasionally observed. Cogwheel rigidity often unresponsive to antiparkinsonian medications has been reported after long-term administration.[52] Although rare, a few patients develop lithium-induced neurotoxicity. Muscular hyperirritability (including fasciculations, twitching, clonic movements of limbs), and hyperactive deep tendon reflexes occur in less than 15% of patients receiving lithium. Permanent neurologic sequelae, including cerebellar ataxia, choreoathetoid movements, disturbances in gait and speech, or death, may occur.[52] Patients at risk include the elderly, the physically ill, and those with renal impairment.

### Routine Laboratory Monitoring

During maintenance therapy with lithium, it is important to monitor several laboratory indices to minimize potential long-term side effects. The recommended guidelines for laboratory tests and monitoring are listed in Table 49.4.

The most common indicator of renal function is serum creatinine ($Cr_s$) which can be used to estimate creatinine clearance ($Cl_{Cr}$) using the Cockcroft and Gault equation[53]:

$$Cl_{Cr} = \frac{140 - \text{age (yr)} \times \text{weight (kg)}}{72 \times Cr_s} \times (0.85 \text{ for females})$$

Serum creatinine concentrations should be measured every 6 to 12 months in all patients and every 3 months in patients with impaired renal functioning. Significant changes in the absolute value of the serum creatinine concentration, even if still within the normal range, or a lowering of the estimated creatinine clearance warrant a 24-hour urine collection to determine creatinine clearance. A more sensitive indicator of glomerular filtration rate may be serum $\beta_2$-microglobulin, as it correlates significantly with creatinine clearance. Renal concentrating ability can be determined by urine osmolality or urine specific gravity after a 12-hour overnight fast.[54] A urine osmolality less than 600 mOsm/kg is an indicator of possible tubular dysfunction. Urine osmolality should be evaluated every 12 months or whenever patients complain of increased polydipsia and polyuria.

Thyroid function tests should be performed every 6 to 12 months. The most sensitive test is serum TSH but may not be routinely used because of the expense. A thyroid profile ($T_3$ resin uptake and $T_4$ concentration) plus clinical observation usually serves as a screen for detecting hypothyroidism.

### Toxicity

Lithium is an extremely toxic drug if accidentally or intentionally taken in overdose. Table 49.9 lists the most common signs and symptoms of lithium toxicity. Initial signs of mild toxicity (1.2–1.5 mEq/L) include fine hand tremor, gastrointestinal upset, muscle weakness, and fatigue. An organic brain syndrome manifested by confusion, memory impairment, agitation, EEG changes, and extrapyramidal symptoms (cogwheel rigidity) may be present at therapeutic concentrations, especially in the elderly.[52] Moderate to severe toxic side effects are usually observed at concentrations greater than 1.5 mEq/L. These include agitation, confusion, lethargy, ataxia, dysarthria, aphasia, speech impediments, nystagmus, headache, emesis, increased deep tendon reflexes, coarse tremors, involuntary choreiform movements, muscle fasiculations, clonic–tonic twitching, seizures, respiratory complications, coma, and death.

There are several situations that predispose patients to the risk of elevated lithium concentrations and potential toxicity (Table 49.10). Physically ill patients often become dehydrated or have electrolyte imbalances secondary to poor fluid intake, vomiting, and diarrhea. Concomitant medications that interfere with lithium clearance may lead to lithium toxicity. High-risk patients (e.g., the elderly and those with renal impairment) should be monitored closely for signs of toxicity.

If severe lithium intoxication (concentrations higher than 2.5 mEq/L 12 hours after the last dose) is confirmed by clinical presentation, drug history, or plasma lithium concentrations, then lithium therapy should be discontinued. Treatment of lithium toxicity depends on the severity of the poisoning but should include supportive care with monitoring of vital signs; cardiac, pulmonary and neurologic status; electrolytes; and plasma lithium concentrations. The primary goal of treatment should be to correct any fluid or electrolyte imbalance and to lower lithium concentrations. Alkalinization of the urine along with diuretics (e.g., aceta-

**Table 49.9** Signs of Lithium Toxicity and Treatment

| *Adverse effect* | *Treatment* |
|---|---|
| **Early Signs of Toxicity ([Li] > 1.5 mEq/L)** | |
| Difficulty concentrating, sluggishness, drowsiness, coarse tremor, muscle twitches, dysarthria, loss of appetite, nausea, vomiting, diarrhea, lethargy, confusion, ataxia | 1. Discontinue lithium<br>2. Order lithium concentration stat, then every 1–2 d as required<br>3. Monitor for severe toxicity<br>4. Restart lithium at lower dose when concentrations are again within the therapeutic range |
| **Severe Signs of Toxicity ([Li] > 2.5 mEq/L)** | |
| CNS irritability, muscle twitching, fasciculations, clonic contractions, rigidity, hyperreflexia, nystagmus, convulsions, cardiovascular collapse, permanent neurologic sequelae; level of consciousness may progress from delirium, stupor, and coma to death | 1. Discontinue lithium; gastric lavage for acute ingestion<br>2. Correct fluid and electrolyte imbalance<br>3. Monitor vital signs, cardiac and pulmonary status, and lithium concentrations<br>4. Prevent seizures<br>5. Start hemodialysis if lithium concentration is above 3.0 mEq/L |

zolamide, mannitol and aminophylline) is not recommended except in cases of severe overdose when dialysis is not available. Sodium loading without evidence of sodium depletion may cause hyperosmolality and is not recommended as a method to enhance lithium elimination.

If the lithium concentration is above 3.0 mEq/L, hemodialysis should be started and continued until the concentration is below 1.0 mEq/L. Peritoneal dialysis may be used if hemodialysis facilities are not available. Hemodialysis can increase lithium clearance by 50–90 mL/min and peritoneal dialysis by 15 mL/min.[40] Because of slow equilibrium between intracellular and extracellular compartments, rebound increases in plasma lithium concentrations may occur 5 to 8 hours after dialysis.

Generally, signs of toxicity disappear slowly within 6 to 7 days of lithium poisoning. Several reports of irreversible neurologic deficits with dementia, ataxia, and kidney damage with reduced GFR and concentrating ability have been reported with lithium intoxication.[55]

### Pregnancy and Lactation

In 1970, a Lithium Baby Register was established in Denmark to monitor the incidence of lithium teratogenesis. As of 1980, of 225 cases 25 (11%) were born with congenital malformations. Eighteen of these included Epstein's anomaly and other cardiac abnormalities, seven were stillborn, two had Down's syndrome, and one had intracerebral toxoplasmosis.[56] The high incidence of cardiovascular anomalies suggests that lithium is a teratogen, primarily to the cardiovascular system. Lithium should be discontinued prior to pregnancy and during the first trimester, if not throughout the entire pregnancy.

**Table 49.10** Situations That May Increase Plasma Lithium Concentrations

| | |
|---|---|
| Errors in dosing | Low-sodium diets |
| Salt deficiency | Water deficiency (dehydration) |
| Drug interactions | Physical illness |
| Postpartum changes | Excessive sweating |
| Diuretics | Protracted diarrhea |
| Slimming diets | |
| Renal disease that impairs lithium excretion | |

When lithium is continued during pregnancy or is restarted for the latter part of pregnancy, several precautions are necessary. During pregnancy, GFR increases by 30% to 50%, plasma volume increases by 50%, and there is a cumulative retention of sodium. Renal lithium clearance increases parallel to the increase in GFR; therefore, lithium concentrations decrease as the pregnancy progresses despite unchanged dose. Thus, an increased dose may be necessary to maintain therapeutic plasma concentrations. After delivery, lithium concentrations quickly rise as GFR and plasma volume return to normal.[57] For bipolar patients who can be maintained during pregnancy on no medication, it may be necessary to resume lithium therapy a few weeks before the delivery is expected, to decrease the risk of postpartum mania and/or depression. Guidelines for the use of lithium in pregnant women are outlined in Table 49.11.

Lithium freely crosses the placenta and is found in equal concentrations in maternal and fetal blood.[57] The clinical features of neonatal lithium toxicity include "floppiness," hypotonia, bradycardia, cyanosis, and low Apgar scores. Lithium may impair thyroid function in the fetus, and goiters have been reported.

Lithium passes easily into breast milk. Concentrations in the milk range from 30% to 100% of the mother's plasma concentration, and plasma concentrations in the infant are 10% to 50% of the mother's.[57] For these reasons, breastfeeding is discouraged.

### Drug Combinations

Patients with bipolar disorder receiving lithium frequently require the addition of other medications. Several drug–drug interactions have been reported and are summarized in Table 49.12.[58]

**Table 49.11** Guidelines for Lithium Use in Pregnancy

1. Women in childbearing years should be given lithium only for clear indications.
2. Women should be informed of the teratogenic potential and encouraged to use contraception. Therapeutic abortion is not generally indicated.
3. If a woman desires to get pregnant, lithium should be withdrawn prior to pregnancy if possible and at least for the first trimester. She may be treated with alternative agents if necessary.
4. If lithium is to be continued during pregnancy:
    a. Maternal plasma concentrations should be kept as low as possible.
    b. Plasma concentrations should be closely monitored, at least once a month and weekly during the end of pregnancy.
    c. Fluctuations in plasma concentrations are to be avoided. Divided doses or a sustained-release product should be used.
5. Situations that increase the risk of lithium toxicity should be avoided.
6. Lithium should be discontinued a few days before the date of delivery. It may be restarted after postdelivery stabilization at the same doses used prior to pregnancy.
7. In general, breast-feeding is not recommended.

***With Antidepressants*** Patients with bipolar illness frequently require antidepressants (tricyclic, heterocyclic, or monoamine oxidase inhibitor) along with lithium to treat episodes of acute depression. As psychomotor retardation is more common in bipolar depression, a less sedating antidepressant such as desipramine, nortriptyline, or a monoamine oxidase (MAO) inhibitor may be appropriate. Once the depressive episode has resolved, antidepressants should be gradually withdrawn and discontinued and lithium maintained as the sole prophylactic agent. Increased cycling or induction of mania has occurred when bipolar patients are treated with antidepressants alone or in combination with lithium,[59] but this has not been substantiated by all studies.[60] Thus, patients at high risk for mania or who have frequent cycling should be treated cautiously with long-term antidepressant therapy. There appears to be no long-term prophylactic value in combining lithium and antidepressants.[61] The few controlled studies in bipolar patients using either lithium and a placebo or lithium and imipramine have shown no advantage of the combination maintenance therapy over lithium alone.

Lithium carbonate has been used to potentiate an antidepressant agent in unipolar depressed patients who are initially unresponsive to the antidepressant alone. The addition of lithium to the antidepressant treatment may result in a rapid improvement within days.[62] The rapid onset of antidepressant potentiation suggests that lithium may act by a mechanism different from that usually seen when either lithium or a tricyclic antidepressant is used alone. Tricyclic antidepressants have been found to either not affect or to increase the RBC/plasma lithium ratio (in vitro).[60] The combination of tricyclic antidepressants and lithium may increase lithium-induced tremors, have additive antithyroid effect, or cause extrapyramidal symptoms and seizures.[60]

***With Antipsychotics*** An acute manic episode is generally treated with a combination of an antipsychotic agent (e.g., chlorpromazine, haloperidol) and lithium. In general, mild manic symptoms (or hypomania) respond well to lithium therapy alone. The treatment of acute mania may require doses of antipsychotics higher than those usually given to treat schizophrenia. Antipsychotics (and possibly carbamazepine) appear to have a more rapid onset of action than lithium to control the psychotic symptoms and increased psychomotor activity of acute mania. Once the acute manic episode has been controlled (usually within 7–14 days), the antipsychotic agent should be gradually tapered and discontinued to avoid the possibility of neurotoxicity or extrapyramidal side effects. Lithium should be continued to control disturbances of mood.

Severe adverse effects such as confusion, hyperthermia, severe rigidity, mutism, incontinence of urine, tremor, and irreversible tardive dyskinesia have been reported with the combined use of lithium and haloperidol.[63] Other studies, however, have not shown an increased incidence of these effects.[64,65] The neurotoxic effects may be more closely related to lithium toxicity or to neuroleptic malignant syndrome than to the combination therapy. Other antipsychotics such as chlorpromazine, thioridazine, fluphenazine, and perphenazine in combination with lithium have also been associated with neurotoxicity.

The lithium–antipsychotic neurotoxic syndrome occurs between 24 hours and 3 months after starting the combination therapy. Symptoms usually disappear if the antipsychotic or both drugs are discontinued and the lithium is reinstituted at lower doses. Lithium and antipsychotics may be safely administered together if lower doses of antipsychotics are used and the lithium plasma concentration is maintained below 1.2 mEq/L.

The exact mechanism for increased neurotoxicity with lithium–antipsychotic combination therapy is not known but may be related to increased intracellular lithium concentrations. Patients receiving both lithium and phenothiazines have a higher RBC/plasma lithium ratio than patients not receiving a phenothiazine.[66] Additionally, haloperidol has been reported to increase plasma lithium concentrations.[67]

A recent review of lithium–antipsychotic neurotoxicity suggests that factors that increase the risk of neurotoxicity include large doses of one or both drugs; the presence of acute mania; failure to discontinue drugs when adverse effects occur; preexisting brain damage; a history of extrapyramidal symptoms with antipsychotic therapy alone; the concurrent use of antiparkinsonian drugs; and the presence of other physiologic disturbances such as infection, dehydration, or fever.[68]

An alternative to antipsychotic therapy in acutely manic patients is the use of lorazepam, a short-acting benzodiazepine. Lorazepam (in doses of 2–4 mg orally or 2 mg parenterally every 2 hours as needed to achieve sedation) has been used to control manic agitation during the first 5 to 10 days of lithium therapy.[69] Other benzodiazepines may also prove efficacious in treating the agitation of acute mania and offer the advantage of causing fewer adverse effects.

**Table 49.12** Drug Interactions With Lithium

| *Class/generic name* | *Effect on plasma lithium concentration* | *Significance* |
|---|---|---|
| Antibiotics | | |
| Tetracycline | Possible increase | Case reports; possibly from nephrotoxic effect of antibiotics; tetracycline may be safe |
| Spectinomycin | Possible increase | |
| Tricyclic antidepressants | Unknown | May cause switch to mania; increase in tremors |
| Anti-inflammatory agents | | |
| Ibuprofen | Increase | Case reports of piroxicam and diclofenac sodium increasing lithium concentrations; sulindac may have minimal effect |
| Indomethacin | Increase | |
| Naproxen | Increase | |
| Phenylbutazone | Increase | |
| Antipsychotics | | |
| Chlorpromazine | Possibly increase RBC lithium | All antipsychotics may increase lithium's neurotoxicity |
| Fluphenazine | Possibly increase RBC lithium | |
| Haloperidol | Possibly increase plasma lithium | |
| Perphenazine | Possibly increase RBC lithium | |
| Thioridazine | Possibly increase RBC lithium | |
| Cardiovascular drugs | | |
| Digoxin | Unknown | Case report of CNS confusion and bradycardia |
| Methyldopa | Unknown | Case reports of neurologic toxicity |
| Diuretics | | |
| Carbonic anhydrase inhibitors | | |
| Acetazolamide | Decrease | Increase lithium excretion |
| Loop diuretics | | |
| Furosemide | Unclear | May increase lithium concentrations |
| Ethacrynic acid | Unclear | |
| Distal tubule diuretics | | |
| Thiazides | Increase | Well-documented interaction with increase in lithium concentrations |
| Metolazone | Increase | |
| Chlorthalidone | Increase | |
| Osmotic diuretics | | |
| Mannitol | Decrease | Increase lithium excretion |
| Urea | Decrease | |
| Potassium-sparing diuretics | | |
| Triamterene | Increase | May increase lithium concentrations |
| Spironolactone | Increase | |
| Amiloride | Unclear | May be used to treat lithium-induced polyuria |
| Xanthines | | |
| Theophylline | Decrease | Increase lithium excretion |
| Caffeine | Decrease | |
| Neuromuscular blocking drugs | | |
| Succinylcholine | Unknown | May prolong neuromuscular blockade |
| Pancuronium bromide | Unknown | |
| Miscellaneous | | |
| Sodium chloride | Decrease | Increase lithium excretion |
| Sodium bicarbonate | Decrease | Alkalinization of urine increases lithium excretion |
| Metoclopramide | Unknown | Case report of extrapyramidal symptoms |
| Carbamazepine | Unknown | May have synergistic effect in treating mania and depression; case reports of neurotoxicity |
| Alcohol | Unknown | Increased lithium toxicity in animals; acute alcohol ingestion may increase peak lithium concentration |
| Phenytoin | Possible increase | Case reports of lithium toxicity and changes in phenytoin concentrations |

Compiled from Reference 58.

*With Diuretics* Because approximately 80% of lithium is reabsorbed at the proximal tubule, any drug that affects proximal sodium resorption can significantly alter lithium clearance. Thiazide diuretics decrease tubular readsorption of sodium and indirectly increase lithium reabsorption at the proximal tubule. Thiazide diuretics decrease lithium renal clearance by 24% and increase plasma lithium concentrations by one third.[70] Diuretics and lithium may be given concomitantly as long as lithium doses are lowered and plasma concentrations and electrolytes are monitored closely. Before a patient is started on a thiazide diuretic, the plasma lithium concentration should be within the therapeutic range (0.6–1.2 mEq/L). The dose of lithium should be reduced by about 50%.[71] Plasma lithium concentrations should be ordered biweekly until the concentration restabilizes.

Loop diuretics have less effect on lithium clearance and may not significantly alter lithium concentrations.[72] The effect of potassium-sparing diuretics on lithium clearance has not been sufficiently studied so patients should be closely monitored. Amiloride, a potassium-sparing diuretic, has been used concomitantly with lithium in several patients to reduce lithium-induced polyuria secondary to lithium-induced diabetes insipidus.[43] Osmotic and xanthine diuretics have been shown to increase lithium clearance.[72]

*With Nonsteroidal Anti-inflammatory Agents* Pharmacokinetic studies have found a significant decrease in lithium clearance and a clinically important increase in steady-state plasma lithium concentrations when lithium is combined with nonsteroidal anti-inflammatory agents (NSAIAs) (e.g., indomethacin, 30%–60% increase; phenylbutazone, 20% increase; naproxen, up to 40% increase; and ibuprofen, 12%–66% increase).[73–75] The NSAIAs reduce renal prostaglandin synthesis and thus decrease the urinary excretion of prostaglandins and sodium. Recently, sulindac, a NSAIA with no effect on the renal prostaglandin system in therapeutic doses, was shown not to increase lithium concentrations.[74] Sulindac may offer an advantage over other NSAIAs if further clinical studies confirm that it has a minimal drug interaction with lithium. Aspirin does not appear to affect steady-state plasma concentrations of lithium and is considered the drug of choice for patients who require an anti-inflammatory agent.[76]

### Sodium Intake

Low-sodium diets or restriction of sodium intake significantly increases plasma lithium concentrations.[77] Therefore, patients should notify their physician before reducing their sodium intake. Heavy exercise, sauna baths, hot weather, high humidity, and fever may promote sodium loss. Patients should be cautioned to maintain adequate sodium and fluid intake. Increases in sodium consumption via high-sodium diets may increase lithium clearance. When drugs with a high sodium content are used concomitantly with lithium, plasma lithium concentrations should be monitored.

### Electroconvulsive Therapy

Electroconvulsive therapy (ECT) is an alternative to lithium therapy in treating acute mania or severe depression in patients who refuse medication, have medical contraindications to medication, or are unresponsive to medication. Acute neurotoxicity and delirium have been reported in patients receiving lithium and ECT. Lithium should be withdrawn and discontinued at least 2 days before ECT and should not be resumed until 2 to 3 days after the last ECT.[78]

### Patient Education

Lithium, perhaps even more so than other psychotropic drugs, requires special patient instructions. The Lithium Information Center at the University of Wisconsin publishes a booklet (*Lithium and Manic Depression: A Guide*) that is helpful in educating patients and family members about lithium and bipolar disorder.[79] Because most patients take lithium for many years, the clinician must address the psychologic implications of long-term drug therapy. Patients should be informed about the need to take medication regularly and the importance of accurate plasma lithium concentrations. Because lithium has a narrow therapeutic range, it is essential that patients and family members know the initial symptoms of toxicity as well as the side effects. Patients should be instructed on how to minimize side effects and on what to do if they experience symptoms of toxicity.

The need for ample fluid and sodium intake should be discussed, as dehydration and low-sodium diets may precipitate toxicity. Patients should be told to drink at least two to three quarts of fluid each day and to avoid excessive use of coffee, tea, cola, and other caffeine-containing beverages. Patients should be warned that alcohol intake may increase the potential for toxicity. Women of childbearing age should be educated about the teratogenic effects of lithium and advised of appropriate birth control methods. Because of lithium's numerous drug interactions, patients should be instructed to inform all health care professionals that they are taking lithium.

## *Carbamazepine*

Although lithium is the drug of choice for bipolar disorder, there remains a need for alternative drugs. Approximately 20% of bipolar patients have an inadequate response to lithium despite therapeutic blood concentrations. Many patients cannot take lithium because of age, pregnancy, renal or cardiac disease, or intolerance to the side effects. Carbamazepine is the first drug that has been extensively studied as an alternative treatment for bipolar disorder. Studies indicate that carbamazepine has antimanic, antidepressant, and prophylactic effects in bipolar disorder. Approximately 70% of acute manics respond to carbamazepine, 48% of patients show good to moderate antidepressant response, and effective prophylaxis is provided in approximately 60% to 75% of patients.[80] In most studies, approximately 60% of manic subjects who were first unresponsive to lithium responded to carbamazepine within the first several days of treatment. Therefore, carbamazepine is particularly useful in patients who have failed on lithium therapy or are rapid cyclers. Although less is known about carbamazepine's acute antidepressant effect, one study reported a typical lag time of 2 to 4 weeks for the onset of antidepressant effect.[81]

### Proposed Mechanism of Action

The precise mechanism of action of carbamazepine in affective disorders remains to be elucidated. Like lithium, it has a multiplicity of biochemical effects. Carbamazepine, which

**Table 49.13** Routine Laboratory Monitoring for Carbamazepine

| *Laboratory test* | *Pretreatment* | *2 wk* | *4 wk* | *6 wk* | *8 wk* | *Quarterly* | *Yearly* |
|---|---|---|---|---|---|---|---|
| CBC[a] | Yes | × | × | × | × | × | |
| Platelet count[a] | Yes | × | × | × | × | × | |
| Liver function | Yes | | | | | | × |
| Renal function | Yes | | | | | | × |
| Electrolytes | Yes | × | × | × | × | × | |
| Plasma carbamazepine concentration | | × | × | × | × | × | |

[a] If leukopenia develops, CBC and platelets should be monitored at 2-week intervals until the concentrations return to baseline; if possible, dose should be decreased until values return to normal.

is structurally similar to imipramine, was initially synthesized for its possible antidepressant effect. Carbamazepine blocks the reuptake of NE, decreases GABA turnover, and blocks accumulation of cyclic AMP. It has complex effects on dopaminergic function, but neither these effects nor its serotonergic effects are thought to contribute to its efficacy in bipolar disorder.[80]

In animal models, carbamazepine is effective in inhibiting amygdala and limbic kindling. Because of its stabilizing effect on limbic kindling, carbamazepine may help to stabilize dysregulated limbic system neural activity, a theory that correlates well with the dysregulation hypothesis of affective disorders.[82]

### Initiation of Therapy

***Baseline Assessment*** Carbamazepine has been associated with serious side effects and drug interactions. Therefore, the same conditions and monitoring procedures used in seizure disorders should be used when treating psychiatric disorders. Before therapy is initiated, baseline laboratory testing should include a complete blood count with differential and platelet count, liver enzymes, serum electrolytes, blood urea nitrogen, urine specific gravity, serum creatinine, neurologic assessment, and ECG if the patient is over 40 years old or has preexisting cardiac disease.[80]

***Dosing*** Carbamazepine doses should not be increased rapidly to a mean dose or plasma concentration range because moderate to severe side effects may occur with rapid titration. During an acute manic episode, carbamazepine should be started at 200 mg daily for the first 2 days, followed by 200 mg twice daily for the next 2 days, then 200 mg three times daily.[83] If 600 mg daily is not enough to provide an adequate response (improvement is usually seen in 4 to 10 days), the dosage can be gradually increased by 200 mg per day until optimal response is observed. Doses less than 2200 mg per day are generally effective.

Carbamazepine therapy can be initiated during the symptom-free period with an initial dose of 200 mg daily for the first 7 days, followed by 200 mg twice daily for the next week, and then increased to 200 mg three times daily for maintenance therapy. Doses as low as 200 to 400 mg daily are effective in some patients and may be tried if adverse reactions occur at 600 mg per day.[83]

***Plasma Concentrations*** There appears to be no direct relationship between dose of carbamazepine and plasma concentration, nor is there any significant correlation between plasma concentration and degree of antimanic or antidepressant response.[83] Despite the poor correlation between plasma concentration and clinical response, most clinicians attempt to maintain plasma concentrations of carbamazepine between 4 and 12 μg/mL. One study reported that the concentration of the 10,11-epoxide metabolite was correlated with antidepressant efficacy, but further studies are needed to determine its clinical usefulness.[84] Steady-state concentrations should be obtained twice a month during the first 2 months of treatment. Plasma concentrations may drop initially because of carbamazepine's autoinduction of its own metabolism, and appropriate increases in dosage must be made to maintain therapeutic concentrations. Once steady-state concentrations are stabilized, plasma carbamazepine concentrations can be monitored every 2 to 3 months.

### Routine Laboratory Monitoring

The recommended routine laboratory tests for carbamazepine are listed in Table 49.13. Although hematologic toxicity is rare with carbamazepine, the manufacturer recommends that laboratory testing be done regularly throughout maintenance therapy. Complete blood counts should be obtained every 2 weeks during the first 2 months of therapy and every 3 to 6 months thereafter.[85] A transient leukopenia can occur in approximately 10% (range 2%–60%) of patients during the first few months of treatment and does not require discontinuation of the drug. If symptoms of bone marrow suppression occur, a complete blood count with differential, platelet count, and liver enzymes should be done to rule out aplastic anemia, leukopenia, or thrombocytopenia. According to the (Tegretol) package insert, carbamazepine should be discontinued if severe leukopenia occurs (fewer than 4,000 WBC/$mm^3$ or fewer than 1,500 neutrophils/$mm^3$), if the platelet count is lower than 100,000/$mm^3$, if hematocrit is less than 32%, if hemoglobin is less than 11 mg/dL, if erythrocytes are fewer than $4.0 \times 10^6/mm^3$, if the reticulocyte count is below 0.3% (20,000/$mm^3$), or if serum iron is greater than 150 μg/dL.[86]

Carbamazepine may cause hyponatremia or water intoxication secondary to its antidiuretic activity. Patients who have low baseline serum sodium concentrations or who complain of fatigue, irritability, or decreased concentration should be evaluated for hyponatremia. Electrolyte monitoring is recommended every 2 weeks during the first 2 months of treatment and every 4 months thereafter.[80]

A mild transient elevation of liver enzymes is commonly seen during initial carbamazepine treatment but does not necessitate drug discontinuation. A fairly rare and potentially fatal hepatic reaction (granulomatous hepatitis) has been reported with carbamazepine, so yearly monitoring of liver function tests is recommended.

### Adverse Effects

There are several dose-related neurologic side effects of carbamazepine, including drowsiness, dizziness, fatigue, clumsiness, ataxia, diplopia, and blurred vision. These side effects usually occur during the first few weeks of therapy and may be minimized by initiating therapy with low doses and gradually increasing the dose to achieve the desired therapeutic response. Side effects may also be alleviated rapidly by dose reduction. Neurologic toxicity can occur in up to 60% of patients receiving carbamazepine and may be the most bothersome adverse effect.[87]

Gastrointestinal side effects occur in up to 15% of patients and include nausea, vomiting, and diarrhea.[88] The gastrointestinal side effects may be minimized by administering the drug with food. Approximately 8% of patients may develop dermatologic reactions including erythema multiforme, urticaria, Stevens–Johnson syndrome, lichenoid or eczematous rashs, bullous eruptions, exfoliative dermatitis, and toxic epidermal necrolysis.

Idiosyncratic hematologic effects reported with carbamazepine include aplastic anemia, agranulocytosis, megaloblastic anemia, thrombocytopenia, leukopenia, eosinophilia, and hemolytic anemia.[85] Although the hematologic toxicity of carbamazepine has been well publicized, serious or fatal toxicity is fairly uncommon. As of 1982, twenty-two cases of aplastic anemia had been reported; this is a prevalence rate of fewer than one in 50,000 patients. A more thorough discussion of carbamazepine's adverse effects can be found in Chapter 41.

### Pregnancy and Lactation

No definitive answers are available as to the absolute risk of teratogenicity with carbamazepine. Most studies have been in patients with epilepsy which itself increases the incidence of teratogenesis. Minor malformations (face, fingers, and

**Table 49.14** Drug Interactions With Carbamazepine

| *Drug* | *Effect* |
|---|---|
| Antipsychotics | Possible neurotoxicity; decreased haloperidol concentrations |
| Cimetidine | Increased carbamazepine concentrations caused by enzyme inhibition |
| Clonazepam | May cause no interaction or may decrease effectiveness of clonazepam |
| Corticosteroids | Decreased steroid effect caused by enzyme induction |
| Digoxin | One report of bradycardia, causal relationship not established |
| Doxycycline | Decreased effectiveness of doxycycline caused by enhanced metabolism |
| Erythromycin | Increased concentrations of carbamazepine |
| Ethosuximide | Decreased ethosuximide concentrations caused by enzyme induction |
| Isoniazid | Increased concentrations of carbamazepine |
| Lithium | Possible neurotoxicity |
| Monoamine oxidase inhibitors | Because of its structural similarity to tricyclic antidepressants, carbamazepine may cause toxicity |
| Oral contraceptives | Breakthrough bleeding caused by enhanced metabolism |
| Phenobarbital | Decreased phenobarbital and/or carbamazepine concentrations caused by enzyme induction |
| Phenytoin | Decreased phenytoin and/or carbamazepine concentrations caused by enhanced metabolism |
| Primidone | Decreased primidone and/or carbamazepine concentrations caused by enhanced metabolism |
| Propoxyphene | Increased concentrations of carbamazepine caused by enzyme inhibition |
| Sodium valproate | Variable effects; decreased concentrations of valproic acid caused by enhanced metabolism |
| Theophylline | Decreased concentrations of theophylline caused by enhanced metabolism |
| Verapamil | Increased concentrations of carbamazepine caused by enzyme inhibition |
| Warfarin | Decreased effect of warfarin caused by enhanced metabolism |

toes) and microcephaly have been reported with most of the anticonvulsants including carbamazepine.[89] Whether these result from drug therapy or from the epilepsy remains unknown. Carbamazepine, when administered alone, is rarely associated with fetal abnormalities and, therefore, may be an alternative to lithium during the first trimester.

If carbamazepine is ingested during pregnancy, the clinician should expect plasma concentrations to decrease as the pregnancy progresses. Carbamazepine concentrations must be carefully monitored and adjustments in dosage made as needed.[89] Maternal plasma concentrations and umbilical cord concentrations of carbamazepine are identical. Concentrations of carbamazepine in breast milk are about 60% of the mother's plasma concentration[90]; however, breast-feeding is not discouraged unless the infant is somnolent and sucks poorly.[89]

### Drug Combinations

Carbamazepine is known to interact with numerous drugs.[91] Table 49.14 lists the well-known drug interactions and the effect of each drug combination. Lithium and carbamazepine may be synergistic in the treatment of refractory bipolar patients.[92] Usually, carbamazepine is added to lithium therapy for nonresponsive or poorly controlled patients. Lithium has also been used to rapidly potentiate the antidepressant response of carbamazepine nonresponders.[92] Although there were no problems with toxicity or drug interactions in early studies, neurotoxicity has recently been observed when plasma concentrations of both drugs were within the accepted therapeutic ranges.[93] Clinical symptoms included confusion, drowsiness, generalized weakness, lethargy, coarse tremor, hyperreflexia, and cerebellar signs. The neurotoxic syndrome resolved quickly when one or both agents were discontinued.

In the majority of clinical trials, carbamazepine has been combined with antipsychotics or antidepressants. Recently, two cases were reported in which patients receiving a combination of carbamazepine and haloperidol developed lethargy, confusion, slurred speech, and disorientation.[94] Symptoms cleared quickly with discontinuation of the drugs.

## *Investigational Therapies*

Numerous drugs have been tried for the treatment of bipolar affective disorder (Table 49.15), some on the basis of empirical clinical experience and some on the basis of the proposed hypotheses for bipolar disorder.[95,96] To date, reports of efficacy are based on case reports and open or double-blind studies with small numbers of subjects.

**Table 49.15** Possible Alternatives to Lithium

| | |
|---|---|
| Adrenergic agents | Serotonergic agents |
| α-Methyl-paratyrosine | Fenfluramine |
| Clonidine | L-Trytophan |
| Propranolol | Miscellaneous |
| Anticonvulsants | Aldosterone |
| Acetazolamide | Ascorbic acid |
| Clonazepam | Bupropion |
| Phenytoin | Clorgyline |
| Sodium valproate | Demeclocycline |
| Cholinergic agents | Levothyroxine |
| Diisopropylfluorophosphate | Naloxone |
| Lecithin | Reserpine |
| Physostigmine | Spironolactone |
| Dopaminergic agents | Verapamil |
| Bromocriptine | |
| D-Amphetamine | |
| Piribedil | |

Drugs that reduce the availability of NE have been suggested for use in bipolar disorder. Both clonidine and propranolol have been utilized in a few patients with some success. A major drawback of these drugs is their ability to induce depression. Drugs that increase cholinergic activity have also been tried. Physostigmine is effective but has little practical applicability. Lecithin appears to have some promise but reports of its efficacy need to be confirmed. Because of the effects of antipsychotics and lithium on dopamine, other drugs that increase available dopamine (i.e., bromocriptine, piribedil, and D-amphetamine) have been tried experimentally, with inconsistent results. Anticonvulsants such as valproic acid, clonazepam, and phenytoin have shown antimanic effects comparable to those of lithium in open and controlled studies.

The permissive hypothesis of affective disorders suggests that drugs that increase serotonin might be effective. L-Tryptophan in doses of 1.5 to 3 g was found to be effective in the treatment of acute mania in two out of three double-blind, placebo-controlled, crossover studies. In each study, L-tryptophan was given concurrently with pyridoxine and ascorbic acid to obtain appropriate concentrations in the CNS.

If the calcium hypothesis of bipolar disorder is correct, then calcium channel blockers such as verapamil, which act by lowering calcium influx intracellularly, should be effective. Preliminary data suggest that verapamil significantly improves manic symptoms.[97]

Further studies are needed to confirm the effectiveness of all the proposed alternatives to lithium and carbamazepine in the treatment of bipolar disorder.

## References

1. Mood disorders, in Diagnostic and Statistical Manual of Mental Disorders, 3rd ed, revised (DSM-III-R). Washington DC, American Psychiatric Press, 1987, pp 213–233.
2. Keller MB. Differential diagnosis, natural course, and epidemiology of bipolar disorders, in Hales RE, Frances AJ (eds): American Psychiatric Association Annual Review. Washington DC, American Psychiatric Press, 1987, vol 6, pp 10–31.
3. Puig-Antich J. Affective disorders in childhood: A review and perspective. Psychiatr Clin North Am 1980;3:403–424.

4. Rice J, Reich T, Andredson NC, et al. The familial transmission of bipolar illness. Arch Gen Psychiatry 1987;44:441–447.
5. Schlesser MA, Altshuler KZ. The genetics of affective disorder: data, theory and clinical applications. Hosp Community Psychiatry 1983;34:415–422.
6. Potter WZ, Rudorfer MV, Goodwin FK. Biological findings in bipolar disorders, in Hales RE, Frances AJ (eds): American Psychiatric Association Annual Review. Washington DC, American Psychiatric Press, 1987, vol 6, pp 32–60.
7. Baldessarini RJ. A summary of biomedical aspects of mood disorders. McLean Hosp J 1981;6:1–34.
8. Silverstone T. Dopamine in manic depressive illness: A pharmacological synthesis. J Affective Disord 1985;8:225–231.
9. Wood K. The neurochemistry of mania. The effect of lithium on catecholamines, indoleamines and calcium mobilization. J Affective Disord 1985;8:215–223.
10. Cookson JC. The neuroendocrinology of mania. J Affective Disord 1985;8:233–241.
11. Lewy AJ, Nurnberger JI, Wehr TA, et al. Supersensitivity to light: Possible trait marker for manic–depressive illness. Am J Psychiatry 1985;142:725–727.
12. Wehr TA, Sack DA, Rosenthal NE, et al. Sleep and biological rhythms in bipolar illness, in Hales RE, Frances AJ (eds): American Psychiatric Association Annual Review. Washington DC, American Psychiatric Press, 1987, vol 6, pp 61–80.
13. Meltzer HL. Lithium mechanisms in bipolar illness and altered intracellular calcium functions. Biol Psychiatry 1986;21:492–510.
14. Dubovsky SL, Franks RD. Intracellular calcium ions in affective disorders: A review and an hypothesis. Biol Psychiatry 1983;18:781–797.
15. Ambelas A. Life events and mania. A special relationship. Br J Psychiatry 1987;150:235–240.
16. Siever LJ, Davis KL. Overview: Toward a dysregulation hypothesis of depression. Am J Psychiatry 1985;149:1017–1031.
17. Lehmann HE. Affective disorders: Clinical features, in Kaplan HI, Sadock BJ (eds): Comprehensive Textbook of Psychiatry, 4th ed. Baltimore, Williams and Wilkins, 1985, pp 786–807.
18. Mukherjee S, Shukla S, Woodle J, et al. Misdiagnosis of schizophrenia in bipolar patients: A multiethnic comparison. Am J Psychiatry 1983;140:1571–1574.
19. Graham PM, Booth J, Boranga G, et al. The dexamethasone suppression test in mania. J Affective Disord 1982;4:201–211.
20. Extein I, Pottash ALC, Gold MS, et al. Using the protirelin test to distinguish mania from schizophrenia. Arch Gen Psychiatry 1982;39:77–81.
21. Georgotas A, Gershon S. Historical perspectives and current highlights on lithium treatment in manic–depressive illness. J Clin Psychopharmacol 1981;1:27–31.
22. Page C, Benaim S, Lappin F. A long-term retrospective follow-up study of patients treated with prophylactic lithium carbonate. Br J Psychiatry 1987;150:175–179.
23. Consensus Development Panel. Mood disorders: Pharmacologic prevention of recurrence. Am J Psychiatry 1985;142:469–476.
24. Jefferson JW, Greist JH, Ackerman DL, et al. Mechanism of action, in Jefferson JW, Greist JH, Ackerman DL, et al (eds): Lithium Encyclopedia for Clinical Practice, 2nd ed. Washington DC, American Psychiatric Press, 1987, pp 436–441.
25. Berrettini WH, Nurnberger JI, Theodore AH, et al. Reduced plasma and CSF beta-aminobutyric acid in affective illness: Effect of lithium carbonate. Biol Psychiatry 1983;18:185–194.
26. Amdisen A, Carson SW. Lithium, in Evans WE, Schentag JJ, Jusko WJ (eds): Applied Pharmacokinetics: Principles of Therapeutic Drug Monitoring, 2nd ed. San Francisco, Applied Therapeutics, 1986, pp 979–1008.
27. Ereshefsky L, Jann MW. Lithium, in Mungall D (ed): Applied Clinical Pharmacokinetics, 2nd ed. New York, Raven, 1983:245–270.
28. Goode DL, Newton DW, Ueda CT, et al. Effect of antacid on the bioavailability of lithium carbonate. Clin Pharm 1984;3:284–287.
29. Ereshefsky L, Gilderman AM, Jewett CM. Lithium therapy of manic depressive illness. Part II: Monitoring. Drug Intell Clin Pharm 1979;13:492–497.
30. Prien RF, Caffey EM. Relationship between dosage and response to lithium prophylaxis in recurrent depression. Am J Psychiatry 1976;133:567–570.
31. Hullin RP. Minimum serum lithium concentrations for effective prophylaxis, in Johnson FN (ed): Handbook of Lithium Therapy. Baltimore, University Park Press, 1980, pp 243–247.
32. Ereshefsky L, Gilderman AM, Jewett CM. Lithium therapy of manic depressive illness. Part I: Target symptoms, pharmacology and kinetics. Drug Intell Clin Pharm 1979;13:403–408.
33. Cooper TB, Bergner PE, Simpson GM. The 24-hour serum lithium concentration as a prognosticator of dosage requirements. Am J Psychiatry 1973;130:601–603.
34. Rosenberg JG, Binder RL, Berlant J. Prediction of therapeutic lithium dose: Comparison and improvement of current methods. J Clin Psychiatry 1987;48:284–286.
35. Browne JL, Patel RA, Huffman CS, et al. Comparison of pharmacokinetic procedures for dosing lithium based on analysis of predictive error. Drug Intell Clin Pharm 1988;22:227–231.
36. Kook KA, Stimmel GL, Wilkins JN, et al. Accuracy and safety of a priori lithium loading. J Clin Psychiatry 1985;46:49–51.
37. Campbell M, Perry R, Green WH. Use of lithium in children and adolescents. Psychosomatics 1984;25:95–106.
38. Ayd FJ. Checking for compliance with lithium therapy. Int Drug Ther Newsl 1981;16:33–34.
39. Vestergaard P. Clinically important side effects of long-term lithium treatment: A review. Acta Psychiatr Scand 1983;67 (suppl 305):11–33.
40. Reisberg B, Gershon S. Side effects associated with lithium therapy. Arch Gen Psychiatry 1979;36:879–887.
41. North DS, Roerig JL. Ineffectiveness of metoprolol in controlling lithium-induced tremor. Clin Pharm 1982;1:264–266.
42. Lippmann S. Is lithium bad for the kidneys? J Clin Psychiatry 1982;43:220–224.
43. Ayd FA. Amiloride therapy for lithium-induced polyuria. Int Drug Ther Newsl 1985;20:18–19.
44. Hestbech J, Hansen HE, Amidsen A, et al. Chronic renal lesions following long-term treatment with lithium. Kidney Int 1977;12:205–213.
45. Walker RG, Bennett WM, Davis BM, et al. Structural and functional effects of long-term lithium therapy. Kidney Int 1982;21(suppl 2):513–519.
46. Lokkegaard H, Anderson NF, Henriksen E, et al. Renal function in 153 manic–depressive patients treated with lithium for more than five years. Acta Psychiatr Scand 1985;71:347–355.
47. Plenge P, Mellerup ET, Bolwig TG, et al. Lithium treatment: Does the kidney prefer one daily dose instead of two? Acta Psychiatr Scand 1982;66:121–128.
48. Jefferson JW, Griest JH, Ackerman DL, et al. Hypothyroidism and nontoxic goiter, in Jefferson JW, Griest JH, Ackerman DL (eds): Lithium Encyclopedia for Clinical Practice, 2nd ed. Washington DC, American Psychiatric Press, 1987, pp 356–360.
49. Calabrese JR, Gulledge AD, Hahn, et al. Autoimmune thyroiditis in manic–depressive patients treated with lithium. Am J Psychiatry 1985;142:1318–1321.

50. Mitchell JE, Mackenzie TB. Cardiac effects of lithium therapy in man: A review. J Clin Psychiatry 1982;43:47–51.
51. Mallette LE, Eichhorn E. Effects of lithium carbonate on human calcium metabolism. Arch Intern Med 1986;146:770–776.
52. Ghadirian AM, Lehman HE. Neurological side effects of lithium: Organic brain syndrome, seizures, extrapyramidal side effects and EEG changes. Compr Psychiatry 1980;21:327–335.
53. Gelenberg AJ, Wojcik JD, Coggins CH, et al. Renal function monitoring in patients receiving lithium carbonate. J Clin Psychiatry 1981;442:428–431.
54. Rifkin A, Quitkin F, Klein DF. Organic brain syndrome during lithium carbonate treatment. Compr Psychiatry 1973;14:251–254.
55. Schou M. The recognition and management of lithium intoxication, in Johnson FN (ed): Handbook of Lithium Therapy. Baltimore, University Press, 1980, pp 394–402.
56. Jefferson JW, Griest JH, Ackerman DL, et al. Teratogenesis, in Jefferson JW, Griest JH, Ackerman DL et al (eds): Lithium Encyclopedia for Clinical Practice 2nd ed. Washington DC, American Psychiatric Press, 1987, pp 640–645.
57. Weinstein MR. Lithium treatment of women during pregnancy and in the postdelivery period, in Johnson FN (ed): Handbook of Lithium Therapy. Baltimore, University Press, 1980, pp 421–429.
58. Salem R. A pharmacist's guide to monitoring lithium drug–drug interactions. Drug Intell Clin Pharm 1982;16:745–747.
59. Wehr TA, Goodwin FK. Rapid cycling in manic–depressives induced by tricyclic antidepressants. Arch Gen Psychiatry 1979;36:555–559.
60. Jefferson JW, Ayde FJ. Combining lithium and antidepressants. J Clin Psychopharmacol 1983;3:303–307.
61. Prien RF, Kupfer DJ, Mansky PA, et al. Drug therapy in the prevention of recurrences in unipolar and bipolar affective disorders. Report of the NIMH Collaborative Study Group comparing lithium carbonate, imipramine, and a lithium carbonate–imipramine combination. Arch Gen Psychiatry 1984;41: 1096–1104.
62. Louie AK, Meltzer HY. Lithium potentiation of antidepressant treatment. J Clin Psychopharmacol 1984;4:316–321.
63. Ayd FJ. Combined lithium–neuroleptic therapy. Psychiatr Ann 1984;14:294–295.
64. Goldney RD, Spence ND. Safety of the combination of lithium and neuroleptic drugs. Am J Psychiatry 1986;143:882–884.
65. Tupin JP, Schuller AB. Lithium and haloperidol incompatibility reviewed. Psychiatric J Univ Ottawa 1978;3:245–251.
66. Von Knorring L, Smigan L, Perris C, et al. Lithium and neuroleptic drugs in combination: Effect on lithium RBC/plasma ratio. Int Pharmacopsychiat 1982;17:287–292.
67. Schaffer CB, Batra K, Garvey MJ, et al. The effect of haloperidol on serum concentrations of lithium in adult manic patients. Biol Psychiatry 1984;19:1495–1499.
68. Hansten PD. Lithium and neuroleptic agents. Drug Interaction Newsl 1982;2:17–19.
69. Modall JG, Lenox RH, Weiner S. Inpatient clinical trial of lorazepam for the management of manic agitation. J Clin Psychopharmacol 1985;5:109–113.
70. Lippmann S, Wagermaker H, Tucker D. A practical approach to management of lithium concurrent with hyponatremia, diuretic therapy and/or chronic renal failure. J Clin Psychiatry 1981;42:304–306.
71. Ayd FA. Drug–drug interactions that matter: Lithium/diuretics. Int Drug Ther Newsl 1984;19:32.
72. Jefferson JW, Greist JH, Baudhuin M. Lithium: Interactions with other drugs. J Clin Psychopharmacol 1981;1:124–134.
73. Kristoff CA, Hayes PE, Barr WH, et al. Effect of ibuprofen on lithium plasma and red blood cell concentrations. Clin Pharm 1986;5:51–55.
74. Ragheb MA, Powell AL. Lithium interaction with sulindac and naproxen. J Clin Psychopharmacol 1986;6:150–154.
75. Ragheb M. Ibuprofen can increase serum lithium level in lithium-treated patients. J Clin Psychiatry 1987;48:161–163.
76. Reiman JW, Diener U, Frolich J. Indomethacin but not aspirin increases plasma lithium ion concentrations. Arch Gen Psychiatry 1983;40:283–286.
77. Hansen HH, Amdisen A. Lithium intoxication (report of 23 cases and review of 100 cases from the literature). Q J Med 1978;47:123–144.
78. Ayd FA. Lithium–ECT induced cerebral toxicity. Int Drug Ther Newsl 1981;16:21–23.
79. Bohn J, Jefferson JW. Lithium and Manic Depression: A Guide. Madison, University of Wisconsin, Lithium Information Center, 1987 rev ed.
80. Birkhimer LJ, Curtis JL, Jann MW. Use of carbamazepine in psychiatric disorders. Clin Pharm 1985;4:425–434.
81. Post RM, Uhde TW, Roy-Burne PP, et al. Antidepressant effects of carbamazepine. Am J Psychiatry 1986;143:29–43.
82. Post RM, Uhde TW. Are the psychotropic effects of carbamazepine in manic–depressive illness mediated through the limbic system? Psychiatr J Univ Ottawa 1985;10:205–219.
83. Okuma T. Therapeutic and prophylactic effects of carbamazepine in bipolar disorders. Psychiatr Clin North Am 1983;6:157–174.
84. Post RM, Uhde TW, Ballenger JC, et al. Carbamazepine and its 10,11-epoxide metabolite in plasma and CSF. Relationship to antidepressant response. Arch Gen Psychiatry 1983;40:673–676.
85. Hart RG, Easton JD. Carbamazepine and hematological monitoring. Ann Neurol 1982;11:309–312.
86. Geigy Pharmaceuticals. Tegretol package insert. Ardsley, NY, 1985, August.
87. Reynolds EH. Neurotoxicity of carbamazepine, in Penry JK, Dalby DD (eds): Advances in Neurology. New York, Raven, 1975, pp 343–353.
88. Suria A, Killam EK. Antiepileptic drugs: Carbamazepine, in Glaser GH, Penry JK, Woodbury DM (eds): Antiepileptic Drugs: Mechanisms of Action. New York, Raven, 1980, pp 563–575.
89. Dalessio DJ. Seizure disorders and pregnancy. N Engl J Med 1985;312:559–563.
90. Anderson PO. Drugs and breast feeding: A review. Drug Intell Clin Pharm 1977;11:208–223.
91. Baciewicz AM. Carbamazepine drug interactions. Ther Drug Monit 1986;8:305–317.
92. Post RM, Kramlinger RG, Uhde TW. Carbamazepine–lithium combination: Clinical efficacy and side effects. Int Drug Ther Newsl 1987;22:5–8.
93. Shukla S, Godwin CD, Long LEB, et al. Lithium–carbamazepine neurotoxicity and risk factors. Am J Psychiatry 1984;141: 1604–1606.
94. Yerevanian BI, Hodgman CH. A haloperidol–carbamazepine interaction in a patient with rapid-cycling bipolar disorder. Am J Psychiatry 1985;142:785–786.
95. Jann MW, Garrelts JC, Ereshefsky L, et al. Alternative drug therapies for mania: A literature review. Drug Intell Clin Pharm 1984;18:577–589.
96. Post RM, Uhde TW. Clinical approaches to treatment-resistant bipolar illness, in Hales RE, Frances AJ (eds): American Psychiatric Association Annual Review. Washington DC, American Psychiatric Press, 1987, vol 6, pp 125–150.
97. Dubovsky SL, Franks RD, Allen S, et al. Calcium antagonists in mania: A double-blind study of verapamil. Psychiatry Res 1986;18:309–320.

# Chapter 50 / Depressive Illness

Barbara G. Wells, PharmD, and Peggy E. Hayes, PharmD

Mood disorders (affective disorders) are among the most common mental disorders encountered in clinical practice and are divided into bipolar disorders and depressive disorders. The essential feature of mood disorders is a major disturbance of mood. Mood is defined as a pervasive and sustained emotion that, in the extreme, markedly affects the person's perception of the world. A mood disorder occurs when a mood disturbance is combined with certain associated symptoms for a minimal duration of time. Bipolar disorders (discussed in Chapter 49) refer to patients who have episodes of mania and/or hypomania alternating with episodes of depression.[1]

Depressive disorder includes patients who have one or more episodes of depression without a history of mania or hypomania. Various names (or classifications) used to describe depression have included reactive, unipolar, psychotic and neurotic, exogenous and endogenous, agitated and retarded, primary and secondary, and involutional melancholia.[2] Clinicians are currently using the classification (Table 50.1) and diagnostic criteria for depressive disorders listed in the *Diagnostic and Statistical Manual of Mental Disorders, Third Edition, Revised* (DSM-III-R), published by the American Psychiatric Association in 1987.[1] Two types of depressive disorders are listed in the DSM-III-R: major depression and dysthymia. This chapter focuses on the diagnosis and treatment of major depression. The use of standardized criteria (Table 50.2) has greatly improved clinicians' ability to correctly diagnose and appropriately treat major depression.

Patients with major psychiatric illness have an increased mortality risk (death expectancy), largely from suicides, medical illness, and accidents.[3] The most frequent complication of depression is suicide. Approximately 15% of patients with unrecognized or inadequately treated depression commit suicide; this is approximately 30 times the rate of occurrence in nondepressed patients.[3] Although adequate treatment may reduce the risk of suicide, depressive illness is underdiagnosed and many patients do not receive adequate treatment.[3,4]

Recently, several significant advances have been made in the recognition and treatment of depressive illness. Depression is no longer viewed as a disease that can be cured by "pulling oneself up by the boot straps." Although supportive counseling and psychotherapy are important treatments for social and interpersonal problems, antidepressant drugs are the primary treatment modality for major depression.

## Epidemiology

The true prevalence of depressive illness in the United States is unknown. Depressive symptoms may occur in 13% to 20% of the population. The lifetime prevalence for depression is about 15% (10% in males and 20% in females).[5] A recently completed National Institute of Mental Health Epidemiological Catchment Area (ECA) study provides the most up-to-date, comprehensive epidemiologic data of psychiatric disorders,[6,7] In this extensive community survey, 6-month prevalence rates for affective disorders (mood disorders) were 6%, while only 32% sought treatment.[6] Major depression was the most common of the mood disorders studied.[7]

All studies have reported that depression is twice as frequent in females as males.[1,5–8] Although depression can occur at any age, the average age of onset for women was once believed to be 35 to 45 years of age, and that for men reportedly peaked after age 55[2]; however, the ECA study reported that the highest rates of major depression occurred in adults 25–44 years old; therefore, our understanding of age of onset and course of the illness may require revision.[7] The DSM-III-R reports that the age of onset for major depression is the late twenties.[1] Depressive disorders are quite common during adolescence.[7] As many as 20% to 35% of elderly patients with concurrent medical illness are reported to be depressed.[8]

A genetic factor has been identified as a predisposing factor in the development of depressive illness. Depressive illness tends to cluster in families, and relatives of patients with depressive illness are two to three times more likely to develop depressive illness than controls. Approximately 17% of patients with major depressive illness have at least one first-degree relative (father, mother, brother, or sister) with a history of depressive illness compared with 5.6% of the first-degree relatives of a normal control group.[9] Patients with delusional depression have a somewhat higher rate of major depression among first-degree relatives (28.2%).[10] The children of depressed patients have an increased risk for depression. Published twin studies of depressive illness estimate the concordance rate for monozygotic (identical) twins to be 43% and the rate for dizygotic (fraternal) twins to be 19%.[5]

## Pathophysiology

The etiology of depressive illness is too complex to be totally explained by a single social, developmental, or biologic theory. A variety of factors appear to work together to cause or precipitate depressive illness. Patients with depressive illness have symptoms that may reflect changes in brain monoamine neurotransmitters, for example, norepinephrine (NE) or serotonin (5-HT).[11,12]

Although life is filled with events that cause pain (e.g., death of a loved one, loss of a job, major illness, loss of

**Table 50.1** Classification of Depressive Disorders

| |
|---|
| Major depression[a,b] |
| Single episode |
| Recurrent[c] |
| Dysthymia[d,e] |

[a] Further subclassified by current state as unspecified, in full remission, in partial remission, mild, moderate, severe (without psychotic features), or with psychotic features.
[b] For major depressive episodes specify if chronic and if melancholic type.
[c] Specify if seasonal pattern.
[d] Specify primary or secondary type.
[e] Specify early or late onset.

Modified from American Psychiatric Association. Diagnostic and Statistical Manual of Mental Disorders, 3rd ed, revised (DSM-III-R). Washington DC, American Psychiatric Association, 1987, pp 218–224.

functioning through advancing age), not everyone becomes depressed. Most individuals adjust to life's challenges and suffer only mild, transient dysphoric feelings; however, some individuals exposed to these psychosocial stressors or unfortunate life events become "stuck" in their depressed mood. Biologic factors (genetics, medical illness, and monoamine-depleting drugs) may place certain individuals at high risk for developing a depressive illness.[12]

The biogenic amine theory of depressive illness states that depression is caused by a reduction (or deficiency) or neurotransmitters (e.g., NE or 5-HT) at postsynaptic adrenergic receptor sites. According to the catecholamine theory the deficiency is of NE; in the indoleamine theory the deficiency is of 5-HT. A neurotransmitter deficiency results in a faulty transmission of impulses within the central nervous system (CNS).[13] In depression, this biochemical deficiency may be located in the limbic system, including the diencephalon, and may explain the large number of physical symptoms present in depressed patients. The diencephalon regulates a significant number of important physiologic functions (e.g., sleep, appetite, energy, psychomotor function). Furthermore, monoamine-depleting drugs (e.g., reserpine) produce depressive conditions in some patients taking these agents.[10]

Antidepressants enhance the availability of NE or 5-HT at the postsynaptic receptor site and therefore alleviate a hypothesized neurotransmitter deficiency in depressed patients.[11]

The biogenic amine theory, however, does not totally explain the etiology of depression and/or the therapeutic effects of the antidepressants. The receptor sensitivity theory of depression attempts to explain the occurrence of depression in terms of enhanced sensitivity of receptors. The long-term administration of antidepressants (3 weeks) effects a downregulation of presynaptic and postsynaptic receptors. A downregulated postsynaptic receptor may be associated with diminished function, whereas downregulation of presynaptic receptors may enhance function. The $\beta$-adrenergic receptor (postsynaptic receptor) is downregulated after long-term treatment with all known effective chemical treatments of depression, as well as electroconvulsive therapy. Therefore, supersensitive $\beta$-adrenergic receptors may play a role in the etiology of depression. The serotonergic type 2 receptor, a postsynaptic receptor, is also downregulated, while the serotonin type 1 receptor, a presynaptic receptor, is unaffected by antidepressant treatment.[11,13]

The dysregulation hypothesis emphasizes a failure to regulate brain neurotransmission rather than a simple increase or decrease in activity of one neurotransmitter as underlying the etiology of depression.[14]

A deficiency of serotonergic activity may be highly correlated with suicide completed by violent methods. Postmortem levels of 5-HT and 5-hydroxyindoleacetic acid (the major metabolite of 5-HT) in brain tissue, or cerebrospinal fluid are generally found to be reduced in patients who commit suicide or make violent suicide attempts. Furthermore, an increase in the number of serotonin type 2 receptors (or upregulation) has been reported in suicide patients.[15]

For several years investigators have searched for biologic markers to assist in the diagnosis and treatment of depressed patients. Approximately 45% to 60% of patients with major depressive disorders have a neuroendocrine abnormality, including hypersecretion of cortisol, lack of cortisol suppression after dexamethasone administration, or abnormal or diminished thyroid-stimulating hormone (TSH) response to thyrotropin-releasing hormone (TRH).[5,11,16] Neuroendocrine abnormalities involving the hypothalamic–pituitary–adrenal (HPA) axis are the most extensively reported. Cortisol hypersecretion is most evident in depressed patients with biologic symptoms. The dexamethasone suppression

**Table 50.2** DSM-III-R Diagnostic Criteria for Major Depressive Illness

A. At least five of the following symptoms have been present during the same 2-week period and represent a change from previous functioning; at least one of the symptoms is either (1) depressed mood or (2) loss of interest or pleasure.
   1. Depressed mood
   2. Markedly diminished interest or pleasure in all, or almost all, activities
   3. Significant weight loss (not dieting) or weight gain, or decrease or increase in appetite
   4. Insomnia or hypersomnia
   5. Psychomotor agitation or retardation (objective)
   6. Fatigue or loss of energy
   7. Feelings of worthlessness or excessive or inappropriate guilt (may be delusional)
   8. Diminished ability to think or concentrate, or indecisiveness
   9. Recurrent thoughts of death, recurrent suicidal ideation, or a suicide attempt or a specific suicide plan

B. The mood disturbance is not due to an organic factor or is not a normal reaction to the death of a loved one.
C. The patient does not have delusions or hallucinations without prominent mood symptoms.
D. The patient does not have schizophrenia, schizophreniform, or a delusional disorder.

Modified from American Psychiatric Association: Diagnostic and Statistical Manual of Mental Disorders, 3rd ed, revised (DSM-III-R). Washington DC, American Psychiatric Association, 1987, pp 222–223.

test (DST) is the most specific measure of HPA axis overactivity. Dexamethasone administration suppresses endogenous ACTH and adrenal corticosteroid production in normal subjects for 24 hours by artificially elevating plasma cortisol levels; this elevation activates the negative-feedback loop and reduces cortisol production. Failure of dexamethasone to suppress plasma cortisol concentrations indicates overactivity or dysregulation of the HPA axis.[11,16]

An abnormal response to dexamethasone has been associated with major depressive illness. The standardized procedure for the overnight DST involves administering dexamethasone 1 mg orally at 11 PM and then obtaining blood samples for serum cortisol the following day at 4 and 11 PM. The DST results are considered abnormal (e.g., positive or nonsuppressed) if either of the postdexamethasone plasma cortisol samples measures greater than 5 $\mu$g/dL. Several medical and psychiatric conditions as well as drugs may interfere with the accurate interpretation of DST results and should be considered when interpreting DST findings.[16] Psychotropic drug withdrawal may be an underrecognized confounding variable in abnormal DST results.[17] Although the DST is a promising research strategy, it is not recommended as a routine screening test; it is reserved for patients whose diagnosis is in doubt, and then only to confirm clinical impressions.[16,18]

Another abnormal endocrine response seen in some depressed patients is a deficient or blunted TSH response to TRH. A baseline TSH is obtained; then 500 $\mu$g of TRH is infused over 30 seconds. Serial TSH measurements are obtained 15, 30, and 45 minutes after infusion. An increase in plasma TSH of 10–20 $\mu$U/mL above baseline is considered a normal response. An increase of less than 7 $\mu$U/mL is considered a blunted response and occurs in 25% to 35% of patients with major depression. This test, especially in conjunction with the DST, may be useful in diagnosing depressive illness.[11,19]

Abnormalities in all-night EEG sleep recording have been reported in some depressed patients. Studies have shown that the onset of rapid eye movement (REM) sleep occurs sooner than in the normal population (REM latency). There may also be a decrease in slow-wave sleep and a shift of REM sleep activity to the first half of the night.[5,11]

## Clinical Presentation

### *Diagnosis*

When a patient presents with depressive symptoms, it is necessary to investigate the possibility of medical, psychiatric, and drug-induced causes (Table 50.3).[2,5] Depressive symptoms may be present in several medical illnesses and are often evident during the initial clinical workup. Also, the knowledge that one has a physical illness can trigger a secondary depressive illness. Because depressive illness is frequently missed in patients with medical disorders, the cause of depressive symptoms in the medically ill should be carefully assessed. It is important to diagnose depressive illness in this group, because the illness will frequently respond to antidepressive therapy.

Clinicians should also be alert for depressive illness, as the primary disease, in some patients with alcoholism. Alcohol may worsen depressive illness. Although depressive symptoms may be present in patients with Alzheimer's disease, depression is commonly the primary illness in the elderly who manifest intellectual difficulties.

The differential diagnosis of clinical depression and normal grief caused by the death of a loved one (bereavement) is often difficult, because of overlapping symptoms. Grief is characterized as a self-limited reaction to loss that requires no intensive medical intervention. The DSM-III-R suggests that uncomplicated bereavement be designated major depression when the symptoms are prolonged (duration varies among different cultural groups) and are severe.[1] Suicidal thoughts, psychomotor retardation, and feelings of worthlessness usually are uncommon in a grief reaction, and when

**Table 50.3** Common Medical Illnesses, Psychiatric Illnesses, and Drug Therapy Associated With Depression

| | | |
|---|---|---|
| **A. Medical Illnesses** | | **B. Psychiatric Illnesses** |
| Endocrine diseases | Metabolic disorders | Alcoholism |
| Hyperthyroidism | Electrolyte imbalance | Generalized anxiety disorder |
| Hypothyroidism | Hypokalemia | Panic disorder |
| Addison's disease | Hyponatremia | Eating disorder |
| Cushing's disease | Hepatic encephalopathy | Schizophrenia |
| Deficiency states | Cardiovascular disease | **C. Drug Therapy** |
| Pernicious anemia | Cerebral arteriosclerosis | Alcohol |
| Wernicke's encephalopathy | Congestive heart failure | Antihypertensives |
| Severe anemia | Myocardial infarction | Reserpine |
| Infections | Neurologic disorders | Methyldopa |
| Encephalitis | Alzheimer's disease | Propranolol hydrochloride |
| Influenza | Huntington's disease | Guanethidine sulfate |
| Mononucleosis | Multiple sclerosis | Hydralazine hydrochloride |
| Tuberculosis | Parkinson's disease | Clonidine hydrochloride |
| AIDS | Poststroke | Diuretics—hypokalemia or hyponatremia |
| Collagen disorders | Malignant disease | Oral contraceptives |
| Systemic lupus erythematosus | | Steroids/ACTH |

Compiled from References 2, 7, and 12.

present, suggest that bereavement is complicated by major depression.[1,5]

All depressed patients, especially the elderly, should have a complete physical examination, mental status examination, and basic laboratory workup, including a complete blood count with differential, thyroid function tests, and electrolyte determinations to identify any potential medical problems. Patients who are placed on antidepressants should have a baseline ECG, especially if they are over 40 years of age.[5]

### *Clinical Features*

According to DSM-III-R diagnostic criteria (Table 50.2), the cardinal symptom of major depression is a depressed (or dysphoric) mood (may be an irritable mood in children or adolescents) or loss of interest or pleasure.[1] This feeling is excessive and accompanied by other emotional, physical, and intellectual symptoms that must have been present nearly every day for at least 2 weeks. Therefore, the clinician must consider presenting symptoms, as well as the duration of the illness, and the patient's current level of social and/or occupational functioning. The presence or absence of a precipitating life event may have little diagnostic value. Significant stressors or life events may trigger depressive illness in some but not others, possibly because of genetic or other biological factors.[1,5]

***Emotional Symptoms*** Major depression is characterized by a persistent, diminished ability to experience pleasure. A loss of interest and pleasure in usual activities, hobbies, or work is common. Patients appear sad or depressed, and a change in personality may be noted. They are often pessimistic and believe that nothing will help them feel better. Patients often weep or report crying spells. The presence of intense hopelessness and complete or near total loss of interest and pleasure in usual activities may identify patients at risk for suicide after discharge.[4] Anxiety symptoms are present in almost 90% of depressed outpatients.

Patients often feel they have let others down. These guilt feelings are unrealistic and may reach delusional proportions. Patients may feel they are responsible for the sins of the world and that they deserve punishment; they may view their present illness as a punishment. A depressed patient may hear voices (auditory hallucinations) telling him that he is a bad person and that he should kill himself. Depression with psychotic features usually requires hospitalization, especially if the patient becomes a danger to self or others.

***Physical Symptoms*** These symptoms often motivate the patient, especially the elderly, to seek medical attention. The elderly are more likely to complain of physical symptoms than emotional ones. Patients may request nonprescription drugs for their complaints.

Chronic fatigue is a common complaint, and patients complain of loss of energy and feeling tired with a decreased ability to perform normal, daily tasks. Fatigue often seems worse in the morning and does not improve with rest. Complaints of pain, especially headache, often accompany fatigue.

Sleep disturbances generally present as frequent early morning awakening (terminal insomnia), with difficulty returning to sleep. This may coexist with difficulty falling asleep (initial insomnia) and frequent nighttime awakening. Other patients complain of increased sleep or hypersomnia, although they experience daytime exhaustion or fatigue.

Appetite disturbances, including complaints of decreased appetite, often result in substantial weight loss. Some patients lose two or more pounds per week without dieting, and a few severely depressed patients literally starve themselves to death. Others overeat and gain weight, although they may not actually enjoy eating.

Some patients exhibit gastrointestinal complaints, others cardiovascular complaints, especially heart palpitations. Patients frequently present with a loss of sexual interest or libido.

***Intellectual or Cognitive Symptoms*** These symptoms include a decreased ability to concentrate, slowed thinking, and a poor memory for recent events. Patients may appear confused and indecisive. Depression should be considered when these symptoms are present in the elderly.

***Psychomotor Disturbances*** Patients may appear noticeably slowed or retarded in physical movements, thought processes, and speech (psychomotor retardation). Conversely, depression may be accompanied by psychomotor agitation manifesting as purposeless, restless motion (e.g., pacing, wringing of hands, and outbursts of shouting).

### *Suicide Risk Evaluation and Management*

Suicide is one of the leading causes of death for all ages and the leading cause of death in adolescents and young adults under 25. The suicide rate among adolescents has actually tripled within the last several years; however, the elderly remain the age group at greatest risk for suicide. Although the elderly account for only 11% of the population, they commit approximately 25% of all suicides.[8] Depressive illness accounts for two thirds of all suicides; most of the remaining suicides are due to alcoholism.[4]

Patients should be assessed for the presence of suicidal thoughts whenever depressive symptoms are present. Widely held myths regarding suicide include the belief that people are more likely to commit suicide if they are asked about it; that people who attempt or talk about suicide are just looking for attention and are not serious; that suicidal people are crazy; and that most suicides are caused by a sudden traumatic event.

Factors that increase the risk for suicide include increasing age, being widowed, being unmarried, unemployment, living alone, a history of a previous psychiatric admission, and depression.[3] The presence of a very detailed plan with the intention and ability to carry it out indicates strong intent and a high risk of suicide. Although women attempt suicide two to three times more often than men, men succeed about three times more frequently. Additional factors that increase suicide risk are prior attempts, family history of suicide, anniversary of a loss, presence of a serious medical problem, lack of a social support system, and refusal to seek help.

In assessing the severity of suicidal thoughts, the clinician must be sensitive to hints of suicidal ideation including a change in personality, a sudden decision to make a will or give away possessions, and recent purchase of a gun or obtaining (or hoarding) of a large supply of medications including antidepressants or other potentially toxic substances.

When suicidal intent is suspected, it is important to ask, "Are you thinking about hurting or killing yourself?" If the risk is determined to be significant, the patient must be referred to the appropriate health care professional and a family member must be contacted.

### *Classification/Prognosis*

Depressive disorders are divided into major depression and dysthymia. Single or recurrent episodes of major depression are subclassified in the DSM-III-R (Table 50.1) according to severity (mild, moderate, or severe). A severe depression may present with or without psychotic symptoms. Psychotic symptoms include delusions (a false fixed belief) and hallucinations that are entirely consistent with the depressed mood (mood-congruent).[1] Furthermore, a depressive episode may be further classified as chronic (the current episode has lasted 2 years without a period of 2 months or longer in remission of depressive symptoms), melancholic or seasonal. Melancholic type is a severe form of depression believed to be particularly responsive to drug therapy. Melancholia has distinct physical symptoms, including diurnal mood swings (symptoms are worse in the morning), early morning awakening, and significant weight loss.[1] In seasonal depression there is a regular temporal relationship between depression and a particular 60-day period of the year.[1] The seasonal type of depression has recently been identified and was not included in previous editions of the DSM.

The course of depressive illness is variable. Although 20% of patients have only a single episode, relapse occurs in about 80%. The average number of depressive episodes per lifetime is five or six.[5] Most treated episodes last approximately 3 months, while untreated episodes last about 6 to 13 months.[1,5] Although most individuals usually function well between episodes, in about 20% to 35% of the patients, the disease is chronic with considerable residual symptoms and social impairment.

Dysthymia is a chronic disturbance of mood involving either depressed mood or loss of interest in most activities, but not of sufficient severity or duration of symptoms to meet the criteria for major depression. There is a history of a depressed mood more days than not for at least 2 years. Patients with dysthymia may have superimposed major depression that may be the reason they seek treatment. The differential diagnosis of dysthymia and major depression is difficult, as both disorders share symptoms and differ only in duration and severity.[1]

### *Depression in the Elderly*

Although major depression is common and may occur for the first time in the elderly, it is often overlooked or misdiagnosed. Depressive symptoms may be atypical in the elderly; they may complain of multiple somatic or hypochondriacal symptoms and not sadness or loss of interest. Complaints of memory disturbances may be mistaken as dementia, thus the term "pseudodementia." The role of drugs and medical problems should be carefully assessed.[8]

## Treatment

Several drug classes play a role in the pharmacotherapy of major depression. Historically, the tricyclic antidepressants (TCAs) have been the mainstay of clinical management. Fortunately, the number of marketed antidepressant compounds is gradually expanding. The major marketing claim for the new agents has been less frequent side effects, especially cardiovascular and anticholinergic; none, however, claim to be more effective than the traditional TCAs. Plans for the marketing of bupropion (Wellbutrin, Burroughs-Wellcome) in the United States were suspended in February 1985 because the risk of seizures was found to increase almost 10-fold between doses of 450 and 600 mg daily. Studies to further assess bupropion's seizure potential are ongoing. Nomifensine was withdrawn from worldwide markets in 1986, five months after it was introduced in the United States, because of reports of serious hypersensitivity reactions.[20]

Currently marketed antidepressant agents and suggested therapeutic plasma concentration ranges and dosages are listed in Table 50.4.[21] All antidepressants except the monoamine oxidase inhibitors (MAOIs) are considered to have equal therapeutic efficacy in groups of depressed patients, although an individual patient may respond better to one compound than another. Approximately 65% to 70% of patients with varying types of depression improve with drug therapy compared with 30% to 40% who improve with placebo.[22] The number of responders may increase to approximately 80% to 90% when plasma drug monitoring is used.[23] Major depression with psychotic symptoms responds less well to antidepressant medications alone than depression without psychotic symptoms. Either electroconvulsive therapy (ECT) or antidepressants in combination with antipsychotics are considered appropriate choices for the treatment of psychotic depression.[24]

There are no simple algorithms for initial drug selection. Drug selection is often based on a patient's prior history of positive response to a particular agent or differences in adverse effect profiles. Thus, an adequate medication history is exquisitely important in drug selection decisions.

Historically the MAOIs were considered less effective and more toxic than the TCAs and were used only as second- or third-choice agents. Additional research suggests that the MAOIs may be more effective than the TCAs for depressive illness with atypical symptoms (e.g., hysterical, phobic, or obsessive–compulsive features).[25] In addition, MAOIs (as well as TCAs) are effective in patients with panic disorder with agoraphobia (discussed in Chapter 51).

### *Antidepressants*

#### Mechanism of Action

Traditionally, the therapeutic effects of TCAs were believed to be mediated by their ability to block the reuptake of NE and 5-HT at the presynaptic monoaminergic neuron.[26] Table 50.5 depicts the relative potencies of the various antidepressants in antagonism of reuptake of these neurotransmitters. Study of the neuropharmacologic effects of the antidepres-

**Table 50.4** Adult Dosages for Currently Available Antidepressant Medications

| *Generic name* | *Trade name* | *Manufacturer* | *Suggested therapeutic plasma concentration range (ng/mL)* | *Initial dose[a] (mg/d)* | *Usual dosage range[a] (mg/d)* |
|---|---|---|---|---|---|
| Tricyclic antidepressants | | | | | |
| Tertiary amines | | | | | |
| Amitriptyline | Elavil | Merck Sharp & Dohme | 120–250[b] | 50–75 | 50–300 |
| | Endep | Roche Products | | | |
| | Generic | Various | | | |
| Doxepin | Adapin | Pennwalt | 110–250[b] | 50–75 | 50–300 |
| | Sinequan | Roerig | | | |
| | Generic | Various | | | |
| Imipramine | SK-pramine | Smith Kline & French | 200–300[b] | 50–75 | 50–300 |
| | Tofranil | Geigy | | | |
| | Generic | Various | | | |
| Trimipramine | Surmontil | Ives | | 50–75 | 50–300 |
| Secondary amines | | | | | |
| Desipramine | Norpramin | Merrell Dow | 125–300 | 50–75 | 50–300 |
| | Pertofrane | USV Pharmaceuticals | | | |
| | Generic | Various | | | |
| Nortriptyline | Aventyl | Lilly | 50–150 | 25–50 | 50–150 |
| | Pamelor | Sandoz Pharmaceutical Division | | | |
| Protriptyline | Vivactil | Merck Sharp & Dohme | 70–240 | 10–20 | 15–60 |
| Dibenzoxazepine | | | | | |
| Amoxapine | Asendin | Lederle | 200–400[c] | 50–150 | 50–600 |
| Tetracyclic | | | | | |
| Maprotiline | Ludiomil | Ciba | 200–300[b] | 50–75 | 50–225 |
| Bicyclic | | | | | |
| Fluoxethine | Prozac | Dista Products | | 20 | 20–80 |
| Triazolopyridine | | | | | |
| Trazodone | Desyrel | Mead Johnson | | 50–150 | 50–600 |
| | Generic | Various | | | |
| Monoamine oxidase inhibitors | | | | | |
| Phenelzine | Nardil | Parke–Davis | | 45 | 60–90 |
| Tranylcypromine | Parnate | Smith Kline & French | | 20 | 20–40 |
| Isocarboxazide | Marplan | Roche | | 20 | 20–60 |

[a] Doses listed are total daily doses; elderly patients are usually treated with approximately one half of the dose listed.
[b] Parent drug plus demethylated metabolite.
[c] Parent drug plus hydroxymetabolite.

Modified from Wells BG: Tricyclic antidepressants, in Taylor WJ, Caviness MHD (Eds): A Textbook for the Clinical Application of Therapeutic Drug Monitoring. Irving, TX, Abbott Laboratories, 1986, p 451.

sants, iprindole and mianserin (unavailable in the United States), has generated renewed interest in the mechanisms of action of these drugs because these compounds have minimal ability to block the reuptake of NE or 5-HT. Thus, these older theories are giving way, and newer ones being advanced.

Changes in the sensitivity of amine receptor systems have been proposed as a component of the mechanism underlying the efficacy of antidepressant drugs. Long-term treatment with antidepressants reduces (downregulates) postsynaptic $\beta$-adrenergic sensitivity.[27,28] Changes in sensitivity of the presynaptic $\alpha_2$-adrenergic receptors may be less important, because these effects are more variable and more short term.[29] The serotonin type 2 receptor, a postsynaptic receptor, is also downregulated, while the serotonin type 1 receptor, a presynaptic receptor, is unaffected.[11,13] The dysregulation hypothesis as a biologic theory of depression emphasizes a failure of regulation of neurotransmitter sys-

**Table 50.5** Relative Potencies of Norepinephrine and Serotonin Reuptake Blockade and Side Effect Profile of Antidepressant Drugs

| | *Reuptake antagonism* | | | | | | |
|---|---|---|---|---|---|---|---|
| | **Norepinephrine** | **Serotonin** | ***Anticholinergic effects*** | ***Sedation*** | ***Orthostatic hypotension*** | ***Seizures*** | ***Conduction abnormalities*** |
| Tertiary amines | | | | | | | |
| Amitriptyline | ++[a] | ++++ | ++++ | ++++ | +++ | +++ | ++++ |
| Doxepin | ++ | ++ | +++ | ++++ | ++ | +++ | ++ |
| Imipramine | +++ | +++ | +++ | +++ | ++++ | +++ | ++++ |
| Trimipramine | + | + | ++++ | ++++ | +++ | +++ | ++++ |
| Secondary amines | | | | | | | |
| Desipramine | ++++ | + | ++ | ++ | +++ | ++ | +++ |
| Nortriptyline | +++ | ++ | +++ | +++ | + | ++ | +++ |
| Protriptyline | +++ | ++ | +++ | + | ++ | ++ | ++++ |
| Dibenzoxazepine | | | | | | | |
| Amoxapine[b] | +++ | ++ | +++ | ++ | + | +++ | ++ |
| Tetracyclic | | | | | | | |
| Maprotiline | +++ | + | +++ | +++ | ++ | ++++ | +++ |
| Triazolopyridine | | | | | | | |
| Trazodone | 0 | ++ | 0 | +++ | +++ | ++ | + |

[a] ++++, high; +++, moderate; ++, low; +, very low; 0, none.
[b] Also blocks dopamine receptors.

Modified from Bryant SG, Brown CS: Current concepts in clinical therapeutics: Major affective disorders, Part 1. Clin Pharm 1986;5:310.

tems. In accordance with this hypothesis antidepressants may pre- and postsynaptically reequilibrate the noradrenergic neurotransmitter system, thus correcting the dysregulation underlying the depression.[14]

MAOIs are known to increase concentrations of NE, 5-HT, and dopamine as a result of inhibition of monoamine oxidase, the intracellular enzyme that degrades these substances. Chronic treatment with MAOIs is associated with changes in receptor sensitivities similar to those demonstrated with long-term TCA treatment.[30]

### Side Effects

***Tricyclic Antidepressants*** Before treatment begins patients should be given a thorough explanation of common side effects and should be encouraged to continue in treatment until an antidepressant response occurs or an adequate trial has been completed. For an in-depth review of the management of antidepressant-induced side effects, the reader is referred to the review by Pollack and Rosenbaum.[31] Therapeutic failure is often caused by inadequate dose or inadequate duration of therapy, and may be associated with patient noncompliance.

The most frequently occurring side effects associated with TCAs are anticholinergic, sedation, and orthostatic hypotension (Table 50.5). The secondary amine TCAs and amoxapine are less likely to cause these side effects than the tertiary amine TCAs; however, trazodone, a nontricyclic agent is almost devoid of anticholinergic properties. Patients often develop some tolerance to these side effects during the first few weeks of treatment.

Anticholinergic side effects include dry mouth, constipation, blurred vision, exacerbation of narrow-angle glaucoma, urinary retention, poor concentration, memory dysfunction, and decreased sweating.[32] Constipation is a potentially serious complaint and may lead to impaction or paralytic ileus; stool softeners or bulk laxatives are considered the treatment of choice. Patients receiving TCAs with potent anticholinergic effects are more likely to experience confusion and delirium, especially elderly patients with preexisting organic mental disorder. The TCAs, like other anticholinergic drugs, may worsen choreas such as tardive dyskinesia.[33]

Drowsiness or sedation is attributed primarily to antihistaminic ($H_1$) effects. This may be a beneficial effect in some depressed patients who have insomnia. The tertiary amine TCAs and trazodone are more likely to cause sedation than the secondary amine TCAs.

Antidepressants may produce several undesirable cardiovascular side effects. Side effects vary with the drug employed (Table 50.5). ECG changes[34,35] and orthostatic blood pressure changes[36] do not correlate well with steady-state plasma concentrations within the therapeutic range; however, it is apparent that TCA overdose causes serious cardiac arrhythmias. TCAs are usually considered to produce cardiotoxicity at plasma concentrations above 1,000 ng/mL and almost certain death at 3,000 ng/mL.[37]

The most common serious cardiovascular complication of the antidepressants at therapeutic concentrations is orthostatic hypotension, which may occur as a result of $\alpha_1$-adrenergic blockade. Greater than 20% of patients taking imipramine experience a postural blood pressure drop of over 35 mm Hg systolic.[38] This orthostatic drop is maximal well below therapeutic levels, and there is little tendency to accommodate to this effect[36]; however, the orthostatic effect of nortriptyline in healthy depressed patients was not clinically important.[39] Nortriptyline caused negligible orthostatic problems compared with imipramine, even in patients with conduction disease. Preexisting impairment of ventricular function increases the likelihood of developing orthostatic hypotension.[40]

TCAs may modestly increase heart rate, especially early in treatment. Except for patients with coronary artery disease, this may not be clinically important.[38]

In patients without heart disease, TCAs at therapeutic plasma concentrations frequently prolong the PR and QRS intervals, but rarely cause symptomatic conduction disturbance.[40] At plasma concentrations only slightly above the therapeutic range, nortriptyline frequently delays intraventricular conduction, and plasma concentrations above 200 ng/mL have been associated with conduction defects.[41]

Patients with bundle branch block are at risk of developing high-degree atrioventricular block when treated with TCAs. If TCAs are prescribed for patients with bundle branch block, measures of cardiac conduction (ECGs, 24-hour continuous ECG recordings), blood pressure measurements, and TCA plasma concentrations should be monitored. ECT could be an alternative treatment for these patients.[40]

TCAs may worsen agitation and psychosis in patients with depression with psychotic symptoms or schizophrenia. Approximately 20% to 30% of patients who receive antidepressants experience behavioral disturbances, sometimes manifested as a "switch" from depression to hypomania or mania. This effect usually occurs during the first 4 weeks of treatment, and is more likely to occur in bipolar patients than in patients with major depression.[42]

Abrupt withdrawal of antidepressants has been associated with symptoms suggestive of cholinergic rebound (e.g., dizziness, nausea, diarrhea, malaise, anxiety, insomnia, and restlessness) especially if the dose exceeds 300 mg.[43]

Allergic reactions associated with TCAs include rash, urticaria, photosensitization, and drug fever. Cross-sensitivity between various drugs in this class has been reported. Agranulocytosis and allergic–obstructive jaundice have also been reported rarely.

TCAs lower the seizure threshold, and cause seizures in 0.001% to 4% of nonepileptic patients.[44] Desipramine, trazodone, and MAOIs are appropriate choices for depressed patients with a history of seizure disorder.[45]

***New Antidepressants*** For a comprehensive review of the side effects of new antidepressants, the reader is referred to the review by Hayes and Kristoff.[20]

Maprotiline blocks reuptake of NE with little effect on 5-HT. It has intermediate sedative and anticholinergic effects and may cause less orthostatic hypotension than imipramine; however, an exanthemous rash occurs in approximately 4% of patients.[46] It is more seizurogenic than the standard TCAs. Maprotiline is contraindicated in patients with abnormal EEGs or those with a history of seizure disorder. In hospitalized depressed patients maprotiline treatment was associated with seizures in 15.6% of patients, while TCA therapy was associated with seizures in 2.2%.[47] Therefore, maprotiline should be initiated at 75 mg daily and as low as 25 mg daily in elderly patients. Dosage should be gradually increased, and for most outpatients total daily dosage should not exceed 150 mg daily. In hospitalized depressed patients, dosage may be gradually increased to a maximum of 225 mg daily. In overdose, symptoms of toxicity are similar to those of the TCAs. Maprotiline has one of the poorest morbidity rates.[2]

Amoxapine, the demethylated metabolite of loxapine, has intermediate sedative and anticholinergic potency.[48] Because of postsynaptic dopamine-blocking effects, its use is associated with a risk of neuroleptic malignant syndrome, tardive dyskinesia and other extrapyramidal side effects including akinesia, rigidity, tremor, akathisia, and dystonia.[49] Although associated with less cardiotoxicity than other TCAs, amoxapine is possibly more toxic in overdose.[50] It has been associated with a disproportionate number of seizures and deaths.[2] It offers no advantage over standard TCAs or other new antidepressants.

Trazodone, a triazolopyridine with 5-HT potentiating effects, has few anticholinergic side effects but has considerable sedative effects. It is a potent $\alpha$-adrenergic blocker and therefore has considerable potential for causing orthostasis.[51] Initially, trazodone was felt to be a good choice for depressed patients with cardiac conduction disease for whom standard TCAs pose a serious risk; however, it may increase cardiac irritability in some patients as evidenced by anecdotal reports of ventricular ectopy.[52] It is notable that although drowsiness, ataxia, nausea, and vomiting may be observed after acute trazodone overdose, serious cardiovascular or neurologic toxic effects are rarely reported.[20]

A rare but potentially serious side effect of trazodone therapy is priapism, which is reported to occur between 1 in 1,000 and 1 in 10,000 male patients.[53] Some cases have required surgical intervention (1 in 23,000), and permanent impotence may result.[54]

Trazodone's low incidence of anticholinergic adverse effects and relative safety in overdose make it a good choice for some depressed patients, especially the elderly and those with suicidal risk.

Fluoxetine, marketed in February 1988, is discussed later under investigational agents.

***Monoamine Oxidase Inhibitors*** The most common side effect of MAOIs is postural hypotension[55]; this is more significant with phenelzine than tranylcypromine. Anticholinergic side effects, especially dry mouth and constipation, are common, but are mild compared with those associated with imipramine or amitriptyline.

Phenelzine, the most frequently prescribed MAOI, has mild to moderate sedating effects. Tranylcypromine is structurally similar to the amphetamines and may exert a stimulant effect. Insomnia may be a problem for some patients treated with tranylcypromine, especially if the last dose is administered late in the afternoon.[32]

Dose-related impotence in males[56] and orgasmic inhibition in females[57] have been reported. In addition, fever[58] and brisk deep tendon reflexes[55] may occur.

The hydrazine MAOIs, phenelzine and especially isocarboxazide, are associated with hepatocellular damage. Tranylcypromine and pargyline are nonhydrazine MAOIs and should be selected over the hydrazine derivatives for patients with a history of liver disease.[55] Isocarboxazide is more hepatotoxic than phenelzine and is rarely prescribed.

Hypertensive crisis, a potentially fatal but rare adverse reaction, occurs only when MAOIs are taken concurrently with certain foods or drugs, especially those high in tyramine (Tables 50.6 and 50.7). Ten milligrams of tyramine can cause

**Table 50.6** Dietary Restrictions for Patients Taking Monoamine Oxidase Inhibitors

| | |
|---|---|
| Aged cheeses[a] | Fermented foods |
| Sour cream[b] | Canned figs |
| Yogurt[b] | Raisins |
| Cottage cheese[b] | Pods of broad beans[a] |
| American cheese[b] | Yeast extract[a] |
| Mild Swiss cheese[b] | Meat extract (Marmite, Bovril) |
| Wine[c] (especially chianti and sherry) | Soy sauce |
| Beer | Chocolate[d] |
| Herring (pickled, salted dry)[a] | Coffee[e] |
| | Liqueurs |
| Sardines | Ripe avocado |
| Anchovies | Canned, aged, or processed meats |
| Liver | |

[a] Clearly warrants absolute prohibition.
[b] Up to 2 oz daily is acceptable; other cheeses or cheese products should be avoided.
[c] 3 oz white wine or a single cocktail is acceptable for reliable patients.
[d] Up to 2 oz daily is acceptable.
[e] Up to 2 cups daily is acceptable; larger amounts of decaffeinated coffee are acceptable.

Compiled from References 48 and 60.

a marked pressor effect and 25 mg can result in serious hypertensive crisis.[60] These incidents may culminate in cerebrovascular accident and death.[55] Symptoms of hypertensive crisis include occipital headache, stiff neck, nausea, vomiting, sweating, and sharply elevated blood pressure. Phentolamine, an $\alpha$ blocker, is considered a specific treatment for hypertensive crisis.

Education of patients taking MAOIs regarding dietary and medication restrictions is extremely important. Printed and verbal patient instructions should be provided. Patients unable to read and those with difficulty understanding or remembering medication instructions should not be prescribed MAOIs unless they have a supportive network. Patients should be instructed regarding the necessity of consulting a health professional prior to taking other prescribed or over-the-counter medications. Patients should be informed of the symptoms of hypertensive crisis and advised to go immediately to the emergency room if symptoms occur.

### Pharmacokinetics

The pharmacokinetic properties of the antidepressants are summarized in Table 50.8. With the exception of protriptyline, TCAs are rapidly absorbed after oral administration, and plasma concentrations peak within 2 to 6 hours. Although absorption appears to be complete, bioavailability is low (30%–70% for most TCAs). This is accounted for by the first-pass effect, the degree of which shows great interindividual variation.[21]

TCAs have a large volume of distribution. Imipramine has a combined absorption/distribution phase of 2 to 6 hours after oral administration. These drugs concentrate in brain and cardiac tissue, and there is a strong correlation between plasma and brain concentrations at steady state in laboratory animals.[61] Substantial amounts of TCAs pass into breast milk, and breast-feeding is, therefore, inadvisable.[21]

The TCAs, in particular the tertiary amines, are strongly bound to plasma albumin. In addition, they bind to erythrocytes, $\alpha_1$-acid glycoprotein, and lipoprotein. Small changes in the degree of protein binding can markedly change the volume of distribution and other pharmacokinetic parameters. Disease states may dramatically alter the extent of binding, and this may affect interpretation of plasma concentrations.

TCAs are cleared primarily by hepatic metabolism to biologically active metabolites (Table 50.8). Major metabolic pathways are demethylation, aromatic and aliphatic hydroxylation, and glucuronide conjugation. Enterohepatic circulation has been described.[22] Although the metabolism of TCAs appears to be linear within the usual dosage range,[62] saturation of metabolic pathways may occur in the overdosed patient.

The elimination half-lives of the TCAs vary greatly among individual patients. Similar doses of the same drug may produce a 30-fold interindividual difference in plasma concentration, and this may be genetically determined.[21]

***Altered Pharmacokinetics*** Factors reported to influence TCA plasma concentrations include disease states, genetics, age, cigarette smoking, and concurrent drug administration.

Hepatic disease may reduce metabolic clearance of TCAs and increase plasma concentrations.[63] Chronic renal failure does not alter nortriptyline metabolism.[64] In renal failure, however, the 10-hydroxy metabolite (believed to be active) may accumulate and protein binding may be diminished,[65] with resultant enhanced sensitivity to drug.

The data on the effect of age on steady-state plasma concentrations of TCAs are often conflicting. Clinicians should be alert to the possibility of higher-than-expected plasma concentrations of some TCAs in the elderly population. An age-related increase in steady-state plasma concentrations was reported with imipramine and amitriptyline, but not with desipramine or nortriptyline.[66] Dose-related kinetics cannot be ruled out in the elderly; therefore, plasma level monitoring may be more difficult.

**Table 50.7** Medication Restrictions for Patients Taking Monoamine Oxidase Inhibitors

| | |
|---|---|
| Amphetamines | Epinephrine |
| Appetite suppressants | Guanethidine |
| Asthma inhalants | Levodopa |
| Buspirone | Local anesthetics containing sympathomimetic vasoconstrictors |
| Carbamazepine | |
| Cocaine | |
| Cyclobenzaprine | Meperidine |
| Decongestants (topical and systemic, including phenylephrine, phenylpropanolamine, pseudoephredine) | Methyldopa |
| | Methylphenidate |
| | Other antidepressants |
| | Other monoamine oxidase inhibitors |
| Dextromethorphan | Reserpine |
| Dopamine | Sympathomimetics |
| Ephedrine | Tryptophan |

Compiled from References 22 and 48.

**Table 50.8** Pharmacokinetic Properties of Antidepressants

| *Generic name* | *Elimination half-life (h)*[a] | *Time of peak plasma concentration (h)* | *Plasma protein binding(%)* | *% Bioavailable* | *Clinically important metabolites* |
|---|---|---|---|---|---|
| Tricyclic antidepressants | | | | | |
| Tertiary amines | | | | | |
| Amitriptyline | 9–46 | 1–5 | 90–97 | 30–60 | Nortriptyline<br>10-Hydroxynortriptyline |
| Doxepin | 8–36 | 1–4 | 68–82 | 13–45 | Desmethyldoxepin |
| Imipramine | 6–34 | 1.5–3 | 63–96 | 22–77 | 2-Hydroxyimipramine<br>Desipramine<br>2-Hydroxydesipramine |
| Trimipramine | 7–40 | 3 | 94–96 | 18–63 | None |
| Secondary amines | | | | | |
| Desipramine | 11–46 | 3–6 | 73–92 | 33–51 | 2-Hydroxydesipramine |
| Nortriptyline | 16–88 | 3–12 | 87–95 | 46–70 | 10-Hydroxynortriptyline |
| Protriptyline | 54–198 | 6–12 | 90–94 | 75–90 | None |
| Dibenzoxazepine | | | | | |
| Amoxapine | 8–30[b] | 1–2 | 90 | —[c] | 8-Hydroxyamoxapine |
| Tetracyclic | | | | | |
| Maprotiline | 28–105 | 4–24 | 88 | 79–87 | Desmethylmaprotiline |
| Bicyclic | | | | | |
| Fluoxetine | 48–72[d] | 6–8 | 95 | —[c] | Norfluoxetine |
| Triazolopyridine | | | | | |
| Trazodone | 6–11 | 1–2 | 92 | —[c] | *meta*-Chlorophenyl-piperazine |

[a] Biologic half-life in slowest phase of elimination.
[b] Amoxapine, 8 h; 8-hydroxyamoxapine, 30 h.
[c] No data available.
[d] Metabolism may not be proportional to dose; half-life of norfluoxetine is 7–9 days.

Modified from Wells BG: Tricyclic antidepressants, in Taylor MJ, Caviness MHD (Eds): A Textbook for the Clinical Application of Therapeutic Drug Monitoring. Irving, TX, Abbott Laboratories, 1986, p 454.

Controversy surrounds the issue of cigarette smoking and plasma concentrations of TCAs. Lower levels of imipramine, desipramine, amitriptyline, and nortriptyline have been reported in smokers than nonsmokers; however, two studies found no difference in amitriptyline or nortriptyline concentrations between smokers and nonsmokers.[21]

***Plasma Concentrations and Clinical Response*** Studies in acutely depressed patients have demonstrated a correlation between antidepressant effect and plasma concentrations for some TCAs. The relationship between maintenance plasma concentrations and prevention of relapse is inconclusive. For other depressive conditions (e.g., dysthymia) the relationship between plasma concentrations and clinical effect is not clear. Although the prognosis for dysthymia is usually good, antidepressant treatment is more effective for major depression than dysthymia.

The patient's clinical response, not plasma concentration, dictates dosage adjustments. Some patients with plasma concentrations outside the therapeutic range respond, while others are unresponsive regardless of their plasma concentrations.

For nortriptyline and imipramine there is adequate evidence to allow recommendation of optimal plasma concentrations with confidence. For the other TCAs evidence is less consistent and more sparse. Minimal information is available with the new agents. Current suggested therapeutic plasma concentration ranges are shown in Table 50.4.

Research suggests a linear or sigmoid relationship between plasma concentrations of imipramine (plus desipramine) and antidepressant response in patients taking imipramine.[23,67] The therapeutic range is, therefore, defined by a lower concentration for efficacy and a higher concentration associated with more side effects, but with minimal change in therapeutic response.

Six studies have demonstrated a curvilinear (or therapeutic window) relationship between nortriptyline plasma concentrations with antidepressant response.[21] The reason for poorer response at higher plasma concentrations is unclear. Because cardiotoxicity may be associated with nortriptyline plasma concentrations above 200 ng/mL, this level is considered the upper limit.[68]

For other antidepressants the relationship between plasma concentration and clinical response is inadequately studied, and evidence is conflicting and difficult to evaluate. For additional information, the reader is referred to the American Psychiatric Association Task Force report on blood level measurement of TCAs and clinical outcome.[69]

Many TCAs have hydroxylated metabolites that are phar-

**Table 50.9** Potential Indications for Determination of Plasma Concentrations of Tricyclic Antidepressants

| | |
|---|---|
| Inadequate response | Physical illness |
| Relapse | Overdose or suspected toxicity |
| Serious or persistent side effects | Suspected drug interactions |
| Higher-than-standard doses | Suspected noncompliance |
| Elderly patients | Changing brands |
| Cardiac disease | |

Modified from Wells BG: Tricyclic antidepressants, in Taylor WJ, Caviness MHD (Eds): A Textbook for the Clinical Application of Therapeutic Drug Monitoring. Irving, TX, Abbott Laboratories, 1986, p 458.

macologically active and also cardiotoxic.[70] The need to measure plasma concentrations of these metabolites is unclear, but this practice may be meaningful for amitriptyline and nortriptyline because the steady-state concentrations of the 10-hydroxy metabolite (not available through most clinical laboratories) often exceed those of the parent compound.

***Monitoring*** Because of interindividual variations in plasma concentrations achieved by a given dose, approximately 40% of patients given standard doses may not obtain plasma concentrations within the desired therapeutic range.[71] In addition, the TCAs have a narrow therapeutic index and a therapeutic window exists for nortriptyline. Although plasma level monitoring of TCAs may be useful in maximizing therapy, routine measurements are not necessary for effective therapy.

The usual indications for plasma level monitoring are shown in Table 50.9. A patient who fails to respond to a TCA with a linear dose–response relationship (e.g., imipramine) may respond to a dosage increase without the necessity of a plasma level determination, provided side effects and noncompliance are not problematic; however, failure to respond to a TCA with a curvilinear dose–response relationship (nortriptyline) would necessitate a plasma concentration determination. In nonresponding patients plasma concentration determinations suggest whether dosage adjustment or alternate therapy is indicated.

**Table 50.10** Pharmacokinetic Drug Interactions Involving Tricyclic Antidepressants

| |
|---|
| Elevates plasma concentrations of TCAs |
| Cimetidine |
| Ethanol, acute ingestion |
| Haloperidol |
| Methylphenidate |
| Phenothiazines |
| Propoxyphene |
| Lowers plasma concentrations of TCAs |
| Barbiturates |
| Charcoal |
| Ethanol, chronic ingestion |
| Elevates plasma concentrations of interacting drug |
| Hydantoins |
| Oral anticoagulants |

Compiled from Reference 73.

**Table 50.11** Pharmacodynamic Drug Interactions of Tricyclic Antidepressants

| *Interacting drug* | *Effect* |
|---|---|
| Androgens | Delusions, hostility |
| Clonidine | Decreased antihypertensive efficacy |
| Disulfiram | Acute organic brain syndrome |
| Estrogens | Increased or decreased antidepressant response; increased toxicity |
| Guanethidine | Decreased antihypertensive efficacy |
| Methyldopa | Decreased antihypertensive efficacy; tachycardia; CNS stimulation |
| Monoamine oxidase inhibitors | Increased therapeutic and possible toxic effects of both drugs; hypertensive crisis; delirium; seizures; hyperpyrexia |
| Sympathomimetics | Increased pharmacologic effects of direct-acting sympathomimetics; decreased effects of indirect-acting sympathomimetics |
| Thyroid hormones | Increased therapeutic and possible toxic effects of both drugs; CNS stimulation; tachycardia |

Compiled from Reference 73.

Plasma concentrations should be obtained at steady state. Except for protriptyline, steady state is achieved after a minimum of 1 week at constant dosage. Protriptyline may continue to accumulate for 3 to 4 weeks or longer. Sampling should be done during the elimination phase, usually in the morning, 12 hours after the last dose. Samples collected in this manner are comparable for patients on once-daily, twice-daily, or three-times-daily regimens.[72] Samples are generally collected in glass syringes or Venoject tubes (Kimble-Terumo, Inc.).

When interpreting plasma concentration data, the clinician must consider other factors that may influence plasma levels, including drug factors (Tables 50.10 and 50.11)[73] and nondrug factors (Table 50.12).

**Table 50.12** Nondrug Factors That Influence Plasma Concentrations of Tricyclic Antidepressants

| |
|---|
| Elevates plasma concentrations |
| Acute inflammatory illness |
| Aging |
| Basic urine |
| Hepatic disease |
| Weight loss |
| Lowers plasma concentrations |
| Cigarette smoking |
| Acid urine |

*Individualized Dosage Regimens* A nonresponding patient with a steady-state plasma concentration ($Cp_{ss}$) below the therapeutic range should have an upward dosage adjustment. The new daily dose may be calculated according to the following formula:

$$\text{New dose} = \text{desired } Cp_{ss} \frac{\text{present dose}}{\text{present } Cp_{ss}}$$

This assumes that metabolism remains linear within the dosage range employed, systemic availability remains constant, and neither enzyme inhibition nor stimulation occurs during dosage adjustment. Because these assumptions cannot be absolutely assured, a cautious approach is advised, with a gradual titration to the calculated dose, especially if side effects are already evident.

There are several methods of predicting oral doses necessary to achieve steady-state plasma concentrations within the desired therapeutic range.[21] These methods may be particularly useful when treating patients especially susceptible to TCA adverse effects. The published reports should be consulted for proper application of these methods.

**Drug Interactions**

Minimal information is available regarding drug interactions associated with the new antidepressants. Tables 50.10 and 50.11 summarize drug interactions associated with the TCAs.

Barbiturates induce hepatic microsomal enzymes (cytochrome $P_{450}$ system) to increase metabolism of TCAs, resulting in lower TCA plasma concentrations. Not unexpectedly, drugs that inhibit microsomal enzymes (e.g., oral contraceptives, cimetidine, and methylphenidate) cause increased TCA concentrations.[74]

TCAs may reverse the hypotensive effects of certain sympatholytic antihypertensives (e.g., guanethidine, methyldopa, and clonidine) because of inhibition of presynaptic uptake of the antihypertensive or desensitization at the $\alpha_2$-presynaptic receptor. Similarly, because of inhibition of presynaptic uptake, TCAs may increase the vasopressor response to direct-acting sympathomimetics such as phenylephrine, epinephrine, and NE. The vasopressor response to indirect-acting sympathomimetics such as ephedrine is decreased.[74]

Administration of TCAs concurrently with warfarin may result in prolonged prothrombin times and potential bleeding in some cases. Coadministration of TCAs and thyroid hormone may result in increases in the therapeutic and toxic effects of both drugs because of enhanced receptor sensitivity.[74]

Although MAOIs and TCAs may be safely coadministered in many patients with apparent increased efficacy compared with monotherapy, severe reactions and fatalities have occurred with their concomitant administration. These reactions include hypertensive crises, hyperpyrexia, excitation, and convulsions, and usually occur when TCAs are added to established MAOI therapy.[74]

In addition, side effects of any antidepressant drug would be additive with those of other drugs with similar pharmacologic effects (e.g., anticholinergic, sedative, or hypotensive effects).

**Special Populations**

*Elderly Patients* Depression is commonly overlooked in the elderly. It is particularly important to screen for medical conditions that may underlie depressive illness. Before initiating antidepressive treatment, the elderly patient should undergo a complete physical examination including the cardiovascular, cerebrovascular, ophthalmologic, gastrointestinal and urinary systems.

Both drug metabolism and tolerance to side effects are often decreased in the aged.[22] Organic mental disorders, postural hypotension, and anticholinergic effects can be particularly problematic.

Antidepressants with weak anticholinergic and sedative potencies are usually preferred in this population. Desipramine and nortriptyline are often selected because of weak anticholinergic effects and the low likelihood of inducing postural hypotension, respectively. Trazodone may also be useful because of weak anticholinergic effects, but may be excessively sedating. MAOIs are not routinely recommended, as they have not been adequately evaluated in this age group for safety or efficacy. In addition, they may produce potentially dangerous hypotension and may interact with other medications commonly given to elderly patients.

High-potency antipsychotics (e.g., fluphenazine, trifluoperazine, and haloperidol) are sometimes prescribed for elderly depressed patients with agitation or paranoid delusions. Low-potency antipsychotics (e.g., chlorpromazine and thioridazine) are usually avoided because of their hypotensive, anticholinergic, and sedative effects.

Dosage is usually begun at approximately one half those listed in Table 50.4. An initial daily dose of 10 mg of desipramine or its equivalent may be appropriate for an elderly infirm patient. Divided daily doses are usually preferable to single daily doses, to minimize anticholinergic and cardiotoxic actions.

Determination of steady-state plasma concentration is considered desirable in the elderly. These patients, as well as those with cardiovascular or hepatic disease, should have their plasma concentration monitored and ideally maintained at the lower end of the suggested therapeutic range. In addition, regular ECGs are an important part of monitoring elderly patients, patients with cardiovascular disease, and those receiving higher-than-standard doses of TCAs.

*Pediatric Patients* Depression in children and adolescents is more commonly recognized today than a decade ago. In addition to the classic symptoms of depression, children may also present with guilt, aggression, conduct disorders, learning disorders, or phobias. The only FDA-approved antidepressant for children over 6 years of age is imipramine for the treatment of enuresis. Antidepressants should be initiated in this patient population at a dosage somewhat lower than that used in adults; however, adolescents usually require adult doses and 6 to 8 weeks may be required before an antidepressant response occurs.

Because children have smaller adipose compartments than adults, antidepressants are less extensively distributed to inactive storage sites. Imipramine has been reported to be 26% free (unbound) in the neonate compared with 14% free in the adult. Differences in protein binding might account for the greater susceptibility of children to side effects[75]; however, children demethylate imipramine to a greater extent than adults.[76] Increased cardiotoxicity of imipramine in children has been suggested by reports of prolonged PR and QR intervals and first-degree atrioventricular block at doses of 5 mg/kg.[77]

The relationship between TCA plasma concentrations and antidepressant response has not been studied as well in the pediatric population as in adults. In prepubertal depression, optimal response correlated with total plasma concentrations of imipramine plus desipramine greater than 220 ng/mL.[78] Prepubertal depressions have been treated with imipramine 1.5–5 mg/kg/d,[79] although the manufacturer recommends a dose not to exceed 2.5 mg/kg/d in children.

***Pregnant/Lactating Patients*** Although TCAs have been administered during the first trimester of pregnancy without harmful effects to the fetus, they should be avoided if possible. Irritability, hyperhidrosis, tachycardia, tachypnea, and cyanosis have been reported in neonates with a history of maternal ingestion of TCAs; however, severely depressed or potentially suicidal pregnant patients may receive a trial of TCAs if potential benefits are felt to outweigh risks. Because the safety of MAOIs has not been established during pregnancy, they, too, should be used only when potential benefits justify possible risks to the fetus.[80]

Nursing women should be cautioned about breast-feeding while taking antidepressants. Although it is not known if MAOIs are distributed into human milk, TCAs are excreted in small amounts into breast milk. The clinical effects of such exposure are unknown.[80]

### Toxicity

About 3% of patients have potentially toxic TCA plasma concentrations from usual therapeutic doses.[63] Fourteen percent of those receiving usual doses of amitriptyline had steady-state plasma amitriptyline (plus nortriptyline) concentrations greater than 300 ng/mL (308–912 ng/mL).[81] Although some patients have plasma imipramine (plus desipramine) concentrations of 600–900 ng/mL without side effects, because these levels have not been associated with increased efficacy, it is considered advisable to lower the plasma concentrations to within the presumed therapeutic range.[79]

Manifestations of TCA overdose include coma, acute brain syndrome (delirium), liver damage, respiratory depression, paralytic ileus, cardiac rhythm and conduction disturbances, and seizures. Generally, ingestion of 1.5 g of amitriptyline (or its equivalent) is considered a serious toxicity. In amoxapine and maprotiline overdose, seizures are a particularly complicating feature, and toxicity with these drugs appears more serious than overdoses with other antidepressants.[82,83]

TCAs often produce cardiotoxic effects at plasma concentrations above 1,000 ng/mL and almost certain death at 3,000 ng/mL.[37] Significant ECG effects associated with toxicity include bundle branch block, heart block, and arrhythmias.

Because TCAs possess toxic potential and prolonged elimination, repeated assessment of plasma concentrations and liver function is recommended.[84] TCA plasma concentrations are unlikely to be a factor in the initial assessment of an overdose attempt because they are rarely available on a stat basis.

All patients with a history suggesting TCA toxicity should have a baseline ECG and should be monitored for at least 6 hours. Patients may be discharged if they are symptom free and without anticholinergic signs. The toxicology literature should be consulted for details of treatment of TCA overdose, including management of seizures, conduction defects, arrhythmias, and hypotension. Lidocaine and phenytoin have been used successfully for management of cardiac problems, but quinidine and procainamide are contraindicated.[2] Cardiac monitoring may be discontinued when the ECG has been normal for 2 days or when the plasma concentration falls below 500 ng/mL.[85] Seizures may be treated with phenytoin or diazepam.[2] The reader is referred to Chapter 9 for usual supportive management of overdose.

### Clinical Application

***Dosing*** Usually, dosage is initiated conservatively in divided doses to minimize side effects. Adults may be started at 50–75 mg daily of most antidepressants, and the dose may be increased by 25–50 mg every third day. Recommended initial doses and dosage ranges are shown in Table 50.4.

Caution is urged when discontinuing one antidepressant and initiating another. The same patient may show different levels of tolerance to side effects and different metabolic capabilities for different drugs.

Although sleep, appetite, and energy levels usually improve within 1 week, an antidepressant (mood-elevating) response may not be observed for 2 to 3 weeks.[86] A 4-week trial at a maximum dosage or therapeutic plasma concentration at the upper therapeutic range is considered adequate. Patients should be informed about the expected lag time before the onset of clinical response.

An antidepressant response with a MAOI may require 2 to 4 weeks (6 weeks in some patients). Response may correlate with 60% to 80% platelet MAO inhibition.[87] This degree of platelet MAO inhibition usually requires 60 mg daily of phenelzine.

To minimize postural hypotension, phenelzine is usually dosed three or four times daily. Tranylcypromine may produce a faster antidepressant response than other MAOIs, with some patients responding within 3 to 5 days.[88] A dose from 10 mg two to three times daily to 20 mg twice daily may be used, with the last dose given no later than 4 PM to lessen the likelihood of insomnia.

After an antidepressant response is achieved, drug therapy is usually continued for an additional 6 to 12 months. This may reduce the risk of relapse by 20% to 50%.[89] Antidepressants should be gradually tapered and discontinued over several weeks. Patients who suffer from recurrent episodes of depression may require long-term drug maintenance[48]; however, TCAs should be used prophylactically only in patients with a history of frequent relapse or history of severe relapses with suicide attempts.

After the patient has developed some tolerance to side effects, it may be possible to give the entire dose at bedtime. This may improve compliance and enhance sleep; however, it is preferable to maintain divided daily doses in the elderly, patients with preexisting cardiac compromise, and those taking large doses.

***Monitoring*** Several monitoring parameters, in addition to plasma concentrations, are useful in managing patients with TCAs. Patients must be monitored for side effects and remission of previously documented target symptoms. The presence of side effects does not indicate adequate dosage.[90] Because antidepressant therapy has been associated with bone marrow suppression, leukocyte and differential counts should be performed on those who develop fever or sore throat during the first year of TCA therapy. When TCAs are given concurrently with adrenergic neuronal blocking antihypertensives (e.g., guanethidine, methyldopa, clonidine), blood pressure should be regularly monitored.

***Refractory Patients*** A patient who has failed to respond to an antidepressant with preferential NE reuptake–inhibiting effects should generally be given a trial with a drug having preferential 5-HT reuptake–inhibiting properties (Table 50.5). Patients who have failed to respond to adequate trials of both 5-HT and NE potentiating antidepressants may be candidates for MAOI therapy. Some patients who failed to respond to TCAs will respond favorably when a low-dose antipsychotic is added to the regimen.[91] Others respond favorably when 25 mg of L-triiodothyronine is added.[92] This may be a therapeutic alternative even in refractory patients with normal thyroid function measurements. The combination of lithium and antidepressant in refractory patients may also improve therapeutic response.[91]

Another therapeutic alternative in treating refractory patients is a trial of a combination of a TCA and a MAOI.[93] This treatment should be reserved for healthy refractory patients whose lives are significantly impaired by depression. Although this combination is not approved by the FDA, data suggest the safety of concurrent use of these drugs. The reader is referred to other sources for guidelines governing the use of this combination,[48,93,94]

Significant differences in TCA plasma concentrations have been reported when switching from one brand to another.[95] An initial favorable response may be lost and differences in side effects have been reported.[48] When brands are changed, patients should be monitored for altered response or side effects.

### *Investigational Agents*

Several investigational antidepressants are under clinical study in the United States. Clomipramine is a TCA that exerts a relatively selective effect on 5-HT metabolism and may have specific activity against phobic symptoms and obsessive–compulsive disorder.[96]

Mianserin is a tetracyclic compound with minimal anticholinergic effects, probably less cardiotoxicity than the TCAs, and few psychotropic drug interactions. Side effects include weight gain and drowsiness.[97]

Fluoxetine (Prozac, Dista Products), a bicyclic antidepressant, is a selective 5-HT presynaptic reuptake inhibitor with little affinity for muscarinic, histaminic ($H_1$), or noradrenergic receptors.[98] Fluoxetine's efficacy in major depression is comparable with the TCAs and it has a similar onset of action. Fluoxetine appears to have an advantageous side-effect profile compared with available antidepressants. It has a low frequency of sedation, lacks orthostatic hypotensive properties and cardiovascular conduction effects, and has a potential to cause weight loss and not weight gain. Side effects reported more frequently with fluoxetine than with TCAs include nausea, nervousness, and insomnia.[99] Although few reported cases of overdose with fluoxetine have been reported, it appears to be a relatively safe drug. Postmarketing experience with this drug will clarify its clinical usefulness and better define its side-effect profile.[100]

### *Electroconvulsive Therapy*

In the acute treatment of severe depression, no treatment modality has been shown superior to electroconvulsive therapy (ECT).[101] A rapid therapeutic response (7–14 days) has been reported. Unfortunately, a negative social stigma surrounds the use of ECT. Relapse rates during the year following ECT are high unless maintenance antidepressant medications are prescribed. Factors to be considered in determining the appropriateness of ECT include severity of depression (suicide risk), medical indications and contraindications, and nonresponsiveness to other treatments.[102] An absolute contraindication to ECT is increased intracranial pressure, and relative contraindications include brain tumor, recent myocardial infarction, and large aneurysms.[101] Although bilateral ECT may be more effective in certain patients or conditions, unilateral ECT (to the nondominant hemisphere) may cause less memory disturbance and confusion. The use of an anesthetic (e.g., methohexital) and a neuromuscular blocking agent (e.g., succinylcholine) has decreased the morbidity associated with ECT.[103] The Consensus Conference on ECT summarizes the efficacy, risks, adverse effects, and general guidelines for administration.[101]

### *Psychotherapy*

The comparative value of psychotherapy and pharmacotherapy in treatment of depression has not been adequately studied. Weissman et al[104] reported that for acute depressive episodes in ambulatory patients, once-weekly interpersonal psychotherapy can be equal to TCAs, and that the combination is superior to either treatment alone. For maintenance treatment psychotherapy is reported to improve social functioning.[105] Supportive, behavioral or cognitive psychotherapy is usually chosen for treatment of major depression.

## Conclusion

Although depressive disorders are among the most common illnesses occurring in clinical practice, they are often undiagnosed and untreated. Pharmacologic treatments remain the mainstay of management of major depression. Antidepressant medications are known to influence a variety of receptors both peripherally and in the CNS, and are associated with many side effects. Safe and effective use of antidepressants requires a thorough understanding of their pharmacology and principles of monitoring for efficacy and adverse effects. Although plasma concentration monitoring is unnecessary in most patients, it is recommended in certain populations.

The search for more effective antidepressants with more favorable adverse effect profiles must be continued. Pharmacokinetic applications become more important as the relationship between plasma concentrations and response and adverse effects become further elaborated and as practical methods of dosage prediction are better defined.

## References


1. American Psychiatric Association. Diagnostic and Statistical Manual of Mental Disorders, 3rd ed, revised (DSM-III-R). Washington, DC, American Psychiatric Association, 1987.
2. Bryant SG, Brown CS. Current concepts in clinical therapeutics: major affective disorders, part 1. Clin Pharm 1986;5:304–318.
3. Tsuang MT, Simpson JC. Mortality studies in psychiatry. Arch Gen Psychiatry 1985;42:98–103.
4. Fawcett J, Scheftner W, Clark D, et al. Clinical predictors of suicide in patients with major affective disorders: A controlled prospective study. Am J Psychiatry 1987;144:35–40.
5. Winokur G. Unipolar depression, in Winokur G, Clayton P(eds): Medical Basis of Psychiatry. Philadelphia, W.B. Saunders Co, 1986, pp 60–79.
6. Myers JK, Weissman MM, Tischler GL, et al. Six month prevalence of psychiatric disorders in three communities. Arch Gen Psychiatry 1984;41:959–967.
7. Regier DA, Burke JD. Psychiatric disorders in the community: Epidemiologic catchment area study, in Frances AJ, Hales RE (eds): American Psychiatric Association, Annual Review. Washington, DC, American Psychiatric Press, 1987, vol 6, pp 610–624.
8. Jenike MA. Affective illness, in Jenike MA (ed): Handbook of Geriatric Psychopharmacology. Littleton, MA, PSG Publishing Co, 1985, pp 39–96.
9. Weissman MM, Gershon ES, Kidd KK, et al. Psychiatric disorders in the relatives of probands with affective disorder. Arch Gen Psychiatry 1984;41:13–21.
10. Leckman JF, Weissman MM, Prusoff BA, et al. Subtypes of depression. Arch Gen Psychiatry 1984;41:833–838.
11. Baldessarini RJ. Biology of depressive disorder, in Baldessarini RJ (ed): Biomedical Aspects of Depression and Its Treatment. Washington, DC, American Psychiatric Press, 1983, pp 7–84.
12. Akiskal HS. Toward a psychobiological integration: Affective illness as a final common path to adaptive failure, in Whybrow PC, Akiskal HS, McKinney WT (eds): Mood Disorders Toward a New Psychobiology. New York, Plenum, 1984, pp 173–199.
13. Charney DS, Menkes DB, Heninger GR. Receptor sensitivity and the mechanism of action of antidepressant treatment. Arch Gen Psychiatry 1981;38:1160–1180.
14. Siever LJ, Davis KL. Overview: Toward a dysregulation hypothesis of depression. Am J Psychiatry 1985;142:1017–1031.
15. Mann JJ, Stanley M, McBride PA, et al. Increased serotonin 2 and $\beta$-adrenergic receptor binding in the frontal cortices of suicide victims. Arch Gen Psychiatry 1986;43:954–959.
16. Hayes PE, Ettigi PG. Dexamethasone suppression test in diagnosis of depressive illness. Clin Pharm 1983;2:538–545.
17. Kraus RP, Hux M, Grof P. Psychotropic drug withdrawal and the dexamethasone suppression test. Am J Psychiatry 1987; 144:82–85.
18. Arana GW, Baldessarini RJ, Ornsteen M. The dexamethasone suppression test for diagnosis and prognosis in psychiatry. Arch Gen Psychiatry 1985;42:1193–1204.
19. Extein I. Gold MS. Psychiatric applications of thyroid tests. J Clin Psychiatry 1986;47:13–16(S).
20. Hayes PE, Kristoff CA. Adverse reactions to five new antidepressants. Clin Pharm 1986;5:471–480.
21. Wells BG. Tricyclic antidepressants, in Taylor WJ, Caviness MHD (eds): A Textbook for the Clinical Application of Therapeutic Drug Monitoring. Irving, TX, Abbott Laboratories, 1986, pp 449–465.
22. Baldessarini RJ. Antidepressant agents, in Chemotherapy in Psychiatry: Principles and Practice. Cambridge, MA, Harvard University Press, 1985 pp 130–234.
23. Glassman A, Perel J, Shostak M, et al. Clinical implication of imipramine plasma levels for depressive illness. Arch Gen Psychiatry 1977;34:197–204.
24. Minter RE, Mandel MR. A prospective study of the treatment of psychotic depression. Am J Psychiatry 1979;136:1470–1472.
25. Davison JRT, Miller RD, Turnbull CD, et al. Atypical depression. Arch Gen Psychiatry 1982;39:527–534.
26. Rehavi M, Skolnick P, Hulihan B, et al. High affinity binding of $^3$H-desipramine to rat cerebral cortex: Relationships to tricyclic antidepressant–induced inhibition of norepinephrine uptake. Eur J Pharmacol 1981;70:597–599.
27. Banerjee S, Kung L, Riggi S, et al. Development of $\beta$-adrenergic receptor subsensitivity by antidepressants. Nature 1977;268:455–456.
28. Sulser F. New perspectives on mode of action of antidepressant drugs. Trends Pharmacol Sci 1979;1:92–94.
29. Charney DS, Heninger GR, Sternberg DE, et al. Presynaptic adrenergic receptor sensitivity in depression. Arch Gen Psychiatry 1981;38:1334–1340.
30. Cohen RM, Ebstien RP, Daly JW, et al. Chronic effects of a monoamine oxidase–inhibiting antidepressant: Decreases in functional $\alpha$-adrenergic autoreceptors precede the decrease in norepinephrine-stimulated cyclic adenosine 3′:5′-monophosphate systems in rat brain. J Neurosci 1982;2:1588–1595.
31. Pollack MH, Rosenbaum JF. Management of antidepressant-induced side effects: A practical guide for the clinician. J Clin Psychiatry 1987;48:3–8.
32. Blackwell B. Side effects of antidepressant drugs, in American Psychiatric Association Update. Washington, DC, American Psychiatric Press, 1987, vol 6, pp 724–745.
33. Richardson J, Richelson E. Antidepressants: Clinical update for medical practitioners. Mayo Clin Proc 1984;59:330–337.
34. Vieth R, Bloom V, Bielkski R, et al. ECG effects of comparable plasma concentrations of desipramine and amitriptyline. J Clin Pharmacol 1982;2:394–398.
35. Spiker D, Weiss A, Chang S, et al. Tricyclic antidepressant overdose: Clinical presentation and plasma levels. Clin Pharmacol Ther 1975;18:539–546.
36. Glassman A, Bigger J, Giardina E, et al. Clinical characteristics of imipramine-induced orthostatic hypotension. Lancet 1979;1:468–472.
37. Petit J, Spiker D, Ruwitch J, et al. Tricyclic antidepressant plasma levels and adverse effects after overdose. Clin Pharmacol Ther 1977;21:47–51.
38. Glassman A. Cardiovascular effects of tricyclic antidepressants. Ann Rev Med 1984;35:503–511.
39. Roose S, Glassman A, Siris S, et al. Comparison of imipramine- and nortriptyline-induced orthostatic hypotension: A meaningful difference. J Clin Psychopharmacol 1981;1:316–319.
40. Roose SP, Glassman AH, Giardina EGV, et al. Tricyclic antidepressants in depressed patients with cardiac conduction disease. Arch Gen Psychiatry 1987;44:273–275.
41. Vohra J, Burrows G, Hunt D, et al. The effect of toxic and therapeutic doses of tricyclic antidepressant drugs on intracardiac conduction. Eur J Cardiol 1975;3:219–227.
42. Picklar D, Cowdry RW, Lis AP, et al. Mania and hypomania

during antidepressant pharmacotherapy: Clinical and research implications, in Post RM, Ballenger JC (eds): Neurobiology of Mood Disorders. Baltimore, Williams and Wilkins, 1984, pp 836–845.

43. Dilsaver SC, Feinberg M, Greden JF. Antidepressant withdrawal symptoms treated with anticholinergic agents. Am J Psychiatry 1983;140:249–251.
44. Peck AW, Stern WC, Watkinson C. Incidence of seizures with tricyclic antidepressant drugs and bupropion. J Clin Psychiatry 1983;44(5,sec 2):197–201.
45. Itil T, Soldatos C. Epileptic side effects of psychotropic drugs: Practical recommendations. JAMA 1980;244:1460–1463.
46. Wells BG, Gelenberg AJ. Chemistry, pharmacology, pharmacokinetics, adverse effects, and efficacy of the antidepressant maprotiline hydrochloride. Pharmacotherapy 1981;1:121–139.
47. Bryan GE, Marsh EE, Jabbari B, et al. Incidence of seizures in patients receiving tricyclic and tetracyclic antidepressants. Ann Neurol 1983;14:153–154.
48. Bernstein JG. Handbook of Drug Therapy in Psychiatry. Boston, John Wright PSG, 1983, pp 74–76.
49. Ayd F. Amoxapine side effects: An update. Int Drug Therapy Newsl 1984;19:21–23.
50. Holden JM, Kerry RJ, Orme JE, et al. Amoxapine in depressive illness. Curr Med Res Opin 1979;6:338–341.
51. Bryant SG, Ereshefsky L. Trazodone: Review and evaluation of its antidepressant properties. Clin Pharm 1982;1:406–417.
52. Janowsky D, Curtis G, Zisook S, et al. Ventricular arrhythmias possibly aggravated by trazodone. Am J Psychiatry 1983;140:796–797.
53. Mead Johnson Pharmaceutical Division. Desyrel package insert. Evansville, IN, 1985.
54. Aronoff GM. Trazodone associated with priapism. Lancet 1984;1:856.
55. Klein DF, Gittelman R, Quitkin F, et al. Diagnosis and Drug Treatment of Psychiatric Disorders: Adults and Children, 2nd ed. Baltimore, Williams and Wilkins, 1980.
56. Rapp MS. Two cases of ejaculatory impairment related to phenelzine. Am J Psychiatry 1979;136:1200–1201.
57. Barton JL. Orgasmic inhibition by phenelzine. Am J Psychiatry 1979;136:1616–1617.
58. Atkinson R, Ditman K. Tranylcypromine: A review. Clin Pharmacol Ther 1965;6:631–655.
59. Brown CS, Bryant SG. Monoamine oxidase inhibitors: Safety and efficacy issues. Drug Intell Clin Pharm 1988;22:232–235.
60. Neil JF, Licata SM, May SJ, et al. Dietary noncompliance during treatment with tranylcypromine. J Clin Psychiatry 1979; 40:33–37.
61. Glotzbach R, Preskorn S. Brain concentration of tricyclic antidepressants: Single-dose kinetics, and relationship to plasma concentrations in chronically dosed rats. Psychopharmacology 1982;78:25–27.
62. Montgomery S, McAuley R, Montgomery D, et al. Dosage adjustment from simple nortriptyline spot level predictor tests in depressed patients. Clin Pharmacokinet 1979;4:129–136.
63. DeVane L, Wolin R, Rovere R, et al. Excessive plasma concentrations of tricyclic antidepressants resulting from usual doses: A report of six cases. J Clin Psychiatry 1981;42:143–147.
64. Dawling S, Crome P, Heyer E, et al. Nortriptyline therapy in elderly patients: Dosage prediction from plasma concentration at 24 hours after a single 50 mg dose. Br J Psychiatry 1981;139: 413–416.
65. Reidenberg M. The binding of drug to plasma proteins and the interpretation of measurements of plasma concentrations of drugs in patients with poor renal function. Am J Med 1977; 62:466–470.
66. Nies A, Robinson D, Friedman M, et al. Relationship between age and tricyclic antidepressant plasma levels. Am J Psychiatry 1977;134:790–793.
67. Gram L, Reisby N, Ibsen I, et al. Plasma levels and antidepressant effect of imipramine. Clin Pharmacol Ther 1976;19: 318–324.
68. Burrows G, Vohra J, Dumovic P, et al. Tricyclic antidepressant drugs and cardiac conduction. Prog Neuropsychopharmacol 1977;1:329–334.
69. Anonymous. Tricyclic antidepressants—Blood level measurements and clinical outcome: An APA task force report. Am J Psychiatry 1985;142:155–162.
70. Potter WZ, Calil HM, Sutfin TA, et al. Active metabolites of imipramine and desipramine in man. Clin Pharmacol Ther 1982;31:393–401.
71. Glassman A, Perel J. Tricyclic blood levels and clinical outcome, a review of the art, in Lipton M, DiMascio A, Killam K (eds): Psychopharmacology: A Generation of Progress. New York, Raven, 1978, pp 917–922.
72. Ziegler V, Biggs J, Rosen S, et al. Imipramine and desipramine plasma level: Relationship to dosage schedule and sampling time. J Clin Psychiatry 1978;39:660–663.
73. Mangini R. Drug Information Facts. St. Louis, Facts and Comparisons Division, J. B. Lippincott Co, 1984.
74. Hansten PD. Drug interactions, 5th ed. Philadelphia, Lea and Febiger, 1985.
75. Winsberg B, Perel J, Hurwic M, et al. Imipramine protein binding and pharmacokinetics in children, in Forrest I, Carr J, Usdin E (eds): The Phenothiazines and Structurally Related Drugs. New York, Raven, 1974.
76. Perel J, Irani F, Hurwic M, et al. Tricyclic antidepressants: Relationships among pharmacokinetics, metabolism, and clinical outcome, in Garattini S (ed): Depressive Disorders. Stuttgart/New York, Schattaur Verlag, 1978.
77. Saraf K, Klein D, Gittleman-Klein R, et al. EKG effects of imipramine treatment in children. J Am Acad Child Psychiatry 1978;17:60–69.
78. Puig-Antich J, Perel J, Luptaken W. Plasma levels of imipramine and desmethylimipramine and clinical response in prepubertal major depressive disorder. J Am Acad Child Psychiatry 1979;18:616–627.
79. DeVane CL. Tricyclic antidepressants, in Evans W, Schentag J, Jusko W (eds): Applied Pharmacokinetics. San Francisco, Applied Therapeutics, 1980, pp 549–585.
80. Bryant SG, Brown CS. Current concepts in clinical therapeutics: Major affective disorders, part 2. Clin Pharm 1986;5:385–395.
81. Preskorn S, Simpson S. Tricyclic-antidepressant–induced delirium and plasma drug concentrations. Am J Psychiatry 1982; 139:822–823.
82. Koval G, VanNuis C, Davis T. Seizures associated with amoxapine. Am J Psychiatry 1982;139:845.
83. Knudsen K, Heath A. Effects of self-poisoning with maprotiline. Br Med J 1984;288:601–603.
84. Kuhn W, Jones D, Lippmann S, et al. Clinical and pharmacological considerations in elimination of tricyclic antidepressants and metabolites after overdose. J Clin Psychopharmacol 1984;4:158–160.
85. Preskorn SH, Irwin HA. Toxicity of tricyclic antidepressants—Kinetics, mechanisms, intervention: A review. J Clin Psychiatry 1982;43:151–156.
86. Hollister LE. Treatment of depression with drugs. Ann Intern Med 1978;89:78.
87. Stern SL, Rush AJ, Mendels J. Toward a rational pharmacotherapy of depression. Am J Psychiatry 1980;137:545–552.

**88.** Quitkin F, Rifkin A, Klein DF. Monoamine oxidase inhibitors: Review of effectiveness. Arch Gen Psychiatry 1979;36:749–760.

**89.** Quitkin FM, Rifkin A, Klein DF. Prophylaxis of affective disorders: Current status of knowledge. Arch Gen Psychiatry 1976;33:337–341.

**90.** Preskorn S, Weller E, Weller R, et al. Plasma levels of imipramine and adverse effects in children. Am J Psychiatry 1983;140:1332–1335.

**91.** Stern SI, Mendels J. Drug combinations in the treatment of refractory depression: A review. J Clin Psychiatry 1981;42: 368–373.

**92.** Goodwin FK, Prange AJ Jr, Post RM, et al. Potentiation of antidepressant effects by L-triiodothyronine in tricyclic nonresponders. Am J Psychiatry 1982;139:34–38.

**93.** Spiker DG, Pugh DD. Combining tricyclic and monoamine oxidase inhibitor antidepressants. Arch Gen Psychiatry 1976; 33:828–830.

**94.** White K, Pistole T, Boyd JL. Combined monoamine oxidase inhibitor–tricyclic antidepressant treatment: A pilot study. Am J Psychiatry 1980;137:1442–1445.

**95.** Ostroff R, Docherty J. Tricyclics, bioequivalency, and clinical response. Am J Psychiatry 1978;135:1560–1561.

**96.** Shopsin B, Cassano GB, Conti L. An overview of new "second generation" antidepressant compounds: Research and treatment implications, in Enna SJ, Malick JB, Richelson E (eds): Antidepressants. New York, Raven, 1981.

**97.** Conti L, Cassano GB, Sarteschi P. Clinical experience with mianserin, in Drykonigen G, Rees WL, Ogara RC (eds): Mianserin HCl. Progress in Pharmacotherapy of Depression. Amsterdam, Excerpta Medica, 1979.

**98.** Stark P, Fuller RW, Wong DT. The pharmacologic profile of fluoxetine. J Clin Psychiatry 1985;46(3,sec 2):7–13.

**99.** Wernicke JF. The side effect profile and safety of fluoxetine. J Clin Psychiatry 1985;46(3,sec 2):59–67.

**100.** Sommi RW, Crismon ML, Bowden CL. Fluoxetine: A serotonin-specific, second-generation antidepressant. Pharmacotherapy 1987;7:1–15.

**101.** Anonymous. Consensus: Electroconvulsive Therapy. JAMA 1985;254:2103–2108.

**102.** Greenblatt M. Efficacy of ECT in affective and schizophrenic illness. Am J Psychiatry 1977;134:1001–1005.

**103.** Allen RE, Pitts FN, Summers WK. Drug modification of ECT: Methohexital and diazepam. Biol Psychiatry 1980;15:257–264.

**104.** Weissman MM, Prusoff BA, DiMascio A, et al. The efficacy of drugs and psychotherapy in the treatment of acute depressive episodes. Am J Psychiatry 1979;136:555–558.

**105.** DiMascio A, Weissman MM, Prusoff BA, et al. Differential symptom reduction by drugs and psychotherapy in acute depression. Arch Gen Psychiatry 1979;36:1450–1456.

# Chapter 51 / Anxiety Disorders

Peggy E. Hayes, PharmD, and Cynthia Kristoff Kirkwood, PharmD

Anxiety is a universal feeling state and is part of the fabric of everyday life. Anxiety is often an unpleasant emotion, involving a feeling of apprehension and nervousness, caused by the perception of actual or potential (anticipatory) danger that threatens the security of the individual.

Everyone experiences a certain degree of anxiety when faced with a stressful situation. Usually the response is reasonable and adaptive, enabling individuals to "rise to the occasion," and contains a built-in control mechanism to return to a normal physiologic state. For some, the reaction to fear or stress is frequently abnormal (or maladaptive), irrational, and excessive, and severely impairs normal daily functioning. The distinction between normal (adaptive) and pathologic (maladaptive) anxiety is not always clear. Anxiety may be a consequence of psychosocial or medical stress, a symptom of a mental or physical illness, secondary to certain drugs, or a psychiatric illness (i.e., an anxiety disorder).

Anxiety disorders are among the most frequent mental disorders encountered in clinical practice, and may have replaced depressive illness as the most common psychiatric illness. The lifetime prevalence rate for anxiety disorders was recently estimated at 16%, with more illness in women than men.[1] Unfortunately, only 25% of anxious patients seek treatment and some do not receive the most appropriate treatment. Furthermore, even when an appropriate therapy is administered, treatment failures are common.[2]

The health consequences of persons with untreated or inadequately treated anxiety disorders are not well researched. Untreated anxious patients tend to be high utilizers of health care facilities for nonpsychiatric reasons.[2] An increased rate of hospitalization and an increased incidence of peptic ulcer disease, hypertension, heart disease, and cardiovascular mortality (men) in anxious individuals has been reported.[3] Therefore, anxiety may have pronounced health consequences in patients with certain medical illnesses.

## Differential Diagnosis

The differential diagnosis of anxiety disorders includes several medical and psychiatric illnesses, as well as prescription and nonprescription drugs. Evaluation of the anxious patient requires a complete physical and mental status examination, appropriate laboratory tests, and a thorough knowledge of the patient's medical, psychiatric, and drug history.[3–5]

To appropriately treat anxiety, the clinician must determine the underlying cause. Situational anxiety, probably more accurately termed "worry" or "apprehension," is a normal response to a stressful situation (e.g., problems at work, interpersonal conflict, or financial problems). Although the symptoms are severe, they are temporary and usually last no more than 2 or 3 weeks. Situational anxiety is not classified as an anxiety disorder. Although short-term, "as-needed" treatment with an anxiolytic agent such as a benzodiazepine is very common and may provide some symptomatic relief, prolonged drug therapy is unnecessary.[4,5]

### *Medical Diseases Associated With Anxiety*

Anxiety symptoms are part of the initial clinical presentation in several medical illnesses, thus complicating the distinction between anxiety and medical disorders.[3–5] Also, the knowledge that one has a physical illness may trigger anxious feelings and further complicate therapy and interfere with rehabilitation. Physical disorders most closely associated with anxiety involve the cardiovascular, respiratory, digestive, and endocrine systems (Table 51.1).[3–5]

Physical symptoms of anxiety frequently present in cardiovascular and respiratory disorders include palpitations, tachycardia, chest pain or tightness, shortness of breath, dyspnea, and hyperventilation. Anxiety is frequently a complication in the postmyocardial infarction (MI) patient that may have a direct physiologic effect upon survival. Anxiety occurs in most MI patients, and may be moderate to severe in half of them.[6] After hospital discharge, anxiety and depression may interfere with patients' recovery and subsequent return to work. Thus, patients often require follow-up care for these symptoms. The recognition and treatment of anxiety are important goals in the management of the MI patient.[4,5,7]

Endocrine disorders (e.g., hyperthyroidism, hypoglycemia, and pheochromocytoma) are commonly considered in the differential diagnosis of anxiety. Symptoms of increased adrenergic activity (i.e., palpitations, sweating, insomnia, and shortness of breath) overlap with physical symptoms present in anxiety disorders.[7]

"Functional" gastrointestinal disorders (e.g., irritable bowel syndrome) account for 50% to 60% of the gastrointestinal complaints seen by physicians. The majority of these patients have a psychiatric illness such as an anxiety disorder.[7]

### *Psychiatric Diseases Associated With Anxiety*

Anxiety may be a concomitant symptom of several major psychiatric illnesses. For example, anxiety symptoms are common in patients with mood disorders (e.g., depression

**Table 51.1** Common Medical Disorders Associated With Anxiety Symptoms

| |
|---|
| **Cardiovascular/Respiratory System** |
| Arrhythmias, angina, chronic obstructive lung disease, hypertension, hyperventilation, mitral valve prolapse, myocardial infarction, pulmonary embolus |
| **Endocrine System** |
| Cushing's disease, hyperthyroidism, hypothyroidism, hypoglycemia, pheochromocytoma |
| **Gastrointestinal System** |
| Colitis, irritable bowel syndrome, peptic ulcer |
| **Miscellaneous** |
| Epilepsy, migraine, pain, pernicious anemia |

Compiled from References 3 and 5.

and mania), schizophrenia, organic mental syndromes (e.g., delirium and dementia), and substance use disorders (e.g., alcohol and drug intoxication and withdrawal).[4,5]

### *Drug-Induced Anxiety*

The two major classes of pharmacologic agents that produce anxiety symptoms are the central nervous system (CNS) stimulants and depressants. CNS stimulants include nicotine, caffeine, cocaine, sympathomimetic amines, amphetamines, and other anorexic agents including nonprescription products containing phenylpropanolamine (Table 51.2).[3] Anxiety occurs during the use of these drugs in a dose-dependent manner, but ingestion of minimal amounts may result in marked anxiety in susceptible individuals.[3,5] Patients with a history of panic attacks may be hypersensitive to even small doses of caffeine.[5] Caffeine and nonprescription drugs are of special importance as possible inducers of anxiety symptoms in the elderly. Anxiety occasionally occurs during the use of CNS depressants (e.g., ethanol, barbiturates, meprobamate, and the benzodiazepines), especially in children and the elderly; however, anxiety complaints are far more common as complications of drug withdrawal after the abrupt discontinuation of chronic administration of these agents.[5] Pharmacists should include these drugs in the medication history of all patients, especially those complaining of nervousness, the elderly, and those with a history of anxiety.

**Table 51.2** Drugs Associated With Anxiety Symptoms

| |
|---|
| **CNS Depressants** |
| Anxiolytics/sedatives, ethanol, narcotic agonists (withdrawal) |
| **CNS Stimulants** |
| Prescription products |
| Albuterol (Proventil, Ventolin), amphetamines (Dexadrine), cocaine, diethylpropion (Tenuate), fenfluramine (Pondimin), isoproterenol (Isuprel, Medihaler Iso), methylphenidate (Ritalin) |
| Nonprescription products |
| Caffeine (Nodoz, Vivarin), ephedrine (Efedron Nasal), naphazoline (Privine, Allerest Eye Drops), oxymetazoline (Afrin, Dristan), phenylephrine (Neo-Synephrine, Allerest Nasal, Sinex), phenylpropanolamine (Dexatrim, Acutrim), pseudoephedrine (Sudafed, Novafed) |
| **Miscellaneous** |
| Anticholinergic toxicity, baclofen (Lioresal), digitalis toxicity, dapsone (Arlosulfon), cycloserine (Seromycin), quinacrine (Atabrine) |

## Epidemiology

Epidemiologic studies conducted in the United States estimate the prevalence rate for anxiety disorders to be 4% to 8% of the adult population.[1] The recently completed National Institute of Mental Health (NIMH) Epidemiological Catchment Area (ECA) Study provides the most up-to-date, comprehensive data. In this extensive community survey, 6-month prevalence rates for anxiety disorders exceeded those for depressive illness and averaged 8.3%; phobias were the most common anxiety disorder reported. The lifetime prevalence rate for anxiety disorders was 16%.[1,2]

In general, anxiety disorders constitute a group of heterogeneous illnesses that develop before age 30, and are more common in women and in those with a family history of anxiety and depression. Patients with an anxiety disorder are at risk for developing another anxiety disorder or a major depression.[2] Anxiety disorders are generally chronic in nature, and although symptoms wax and wane over time, patients are rarely completely symptom free.[3,8]

## Classification/Clinical Presentation

*The Diagnostic and Statistical Manual*, third edition, (DSM-III) of the American Psychiatric Association (APA),[9] published in 1980, classified anxiety disorders into four main categories (Table 51.3); however, the revised edition (DSM-III-R), published in 1987, includes several major changes in categorization (Table 51.3).[10] Anxiety disorders are classified together because anxiety and avoidance behavior are the characteristic features of these illnesses.

### *Generalized Anxiety Disorder*

The DSM-III-R diagnostic criteria for generalized anxiety disorder (GAD) are presented in Table 51.4.[10] These criteria extend the time frame for the presence of symptoms to 6 months (instead of 1 month as in the DSM-III) and the number of required symptoms to six (instead of three as in the DSM-III).[9,10] Stricter criteria should assist in defining a more homogeneous population of patients with GAD.

The essential feature of GAD is unrealistic or excessive anxiety and worry about two or more life circumstances (e.g., finances, illness, misfortune), without panic or phobic symptoms. In children and adolescents this may be worry about academic, athletic, and social performance. Symptoms of GAD are both psychologic (tension, fear, difficulty in concentrating, and apprehension) and somatic or physical

**Table 51.3** DSM-III and DSM-III-R Classifications of Anxiety Disorders

| *DSM-III* | *DSM-III-R* |
|---|---|
| A. Phobic disorders | A. Phobic disorders |
| Agoraphobia | Social phobia |
| Agoraphobia with panic attacks | Simple phobia |
| Social phobia | B. Panic disorder |
| Simple phobia | With agoraphobia |
| B. Anxiety states | Without agoraphobia |
| Panic disorder | C. Agoraphobia without a history of panic disorder |
| Generalized anxiety disorder | D. Generalized anxiety disorder |
| Obsessive–compulsive disorder | E. Obsessive–compulsive disorder |
| C. Posttraumatic stress disorder | F. Posttraumatic stress disorder |
| D. Atypical anxiety disorder | G. Atypical anxiety disorder |

Compiled from References 9 and 10.

**Table 51.4** DSM-III-R Diagnostic Criteria for Generalized Anxiety Disorder

A. Unrealistic or excessive anxiety and worry about two or more life circumstances for a period of 6 months or longer; in children and adolescents, anxiety and worry may include academic, athletic, and social performance
B. At least 6 of the following 18 symptoms are often present when anxious (do not include symptoms present only during panic attacks)
   Motor tension
   1. Trembling, twitching, or feeling shaky
   2. Muscle tension, aches, or soreness
   3. Restlessness
   4. Easy fatigability
   Autonomic hyperactivity
   5. Shortness of breath or smothering sensation
   6. Palpitations or tachycardia
   7. Sweating or cold clammy hands
   8. Dry mouth
   9. Dizziness or lightheadedness
   10. Nausea, diarrhea, or other abdominal distress
   11. Hot or cold flashes or chills
   12. Frequent urination
   13. Trouble swallowing or "lump in the throat"
   Vigilance and scanning
   14. Feeling keyed up or on edge
   15. Startling easily
   16. Difficulty concentrating or "mind going blank" because of anxiety
   17. Trouble falling or staying asleep
   18. Irritability
C. It cannot be established that an organic factor initiated and maintained the disturbance (e.g., hyperthyroidism, caffeine)

Modified from American Psychiatric Association: Diagnostic and Statistical Manual of Mental Disorders, 3rd ed, revised (DSM-III-R). Washington DC, American Psychiatric Association, 1987, pp 252–253.

(tachycardia, palpitations, tremor, sweating, and gastrointestinal upset).[10] Many symptoms of GAD overlap with those of depressive illness making the differential diagnosis often difficult.[8]

Generalized anxiety disorder has a gradual onset, usually in the early twenties, but may be precipitated in later life by severe psychologic stressors. This disease generally follows a chronic fluctuating course of spontaneous exacerbations and remissions and is often complicated by secondary depression.[8] Unlike most anxiety disorders, a genetic component does not appear to play a role in the development of the illness and both sexes are equally affected.[2]

### *Phobic Disorders*

The essential feature of a phobic disorder is an irrational fear of a specific object, activity, or situation. Fear is a disturbing feeling that danger is close at hand. Unlike most anxiety disorders, the object of this fearful feeling is clearly recognized. Although the individual recognizes the fear as unreasonable considering the actual danger involved, it persists, resulting in avoidance of the feared situation.[10]

Two types of phobic disorders are listed in the DSM-III-R: social phobia and simple phobia. Patients with either phobia are usually not severely impaired in terms of daily functioning and seldom seek psychiatric treatment.

Social phobia is characterized by a persistent, irrational fear of behaving in an embarrassing or humiliating manner in public, when the individual is the focus of others' attention. The common basis of the fear is exposure to public scrutiny. Specific social activities such as public speaking, eating in a restaurant, or using a public restroom are avoided, or endured with intense discomfort, by patients with social phobia.[10]

Simple phobia is an irrational fear of a specific object or situation such as thunderstorms, snakes, insects, or heights. Apart from contact with the feared object or situation, the simple phobic is usually free of symptoms. Most persons simply avoid the feared object and adjust to certain restrictions of their activities.[10] Simple phobia is the most common anxiety disorder in the general population; however, very few persons seek treatment.

## *Panic Disorder*

Beginning in 1980, the DSM-III classified panic disorder as a diagnostic illness separate from generalized anxiety disorder. Before this, patients with excessive anxiety over prolonged periods of time were diagnosed as having anxiety neurosis (later renamed generalized anxiety disorder); patients with panic attacks (panic anxiety) were simply considered to have a more severe form of anxiety neurosis.

Two major events occurred in the 1960s that caused clinicians to consider panic disorder as a separate illness: (1) the discovery that monoamine oxidase inhibitors and tricyclic antidepressants blocked spontaneous panic attacks,[11] and (2) the finding that an infusion of sodium lactate administered to patients with a history of panic attacks usually triggered a panic attack, although panic attacks were not precipitated in control subjects or in anxious patients.[12]

Panic disorder begins as a series of acute or unprovoked (spontaneous) anxiety attacks, involving an intense, terrifying fear, similar to that caused by life-threatening danger. Patients often describe an overwhelming sense of doom, a fear of dying or losing control, and numerous physical symptoms (Table 51.5).[10] Although the panic attacks may seem interminable to the patient, they usually last no more than 20 to 30 minutes, with the peak intensity of symptoms within the first 10 minutes. Often patients seek help at a nearby physician's office or emergency room, only to have their symptoms resolve upon arrival. Consequently, multiple referrals and misdiagnoses are common.[13] Approximately 40% of patients with panic attacks have mitral valve prolapse, as compared with 9.5% of the population.[14]

The disease is often progressive and many patients develop anticipatory (chronic) anxiety. Between attacks, patients are frequently worried, anxious, fearful, restless, cannot relax, and wear out easily. Most patients eventually develop symptoms of avoidance behavior or agoraphobia, leading to the diagnosis of panic disorder with agoraphobia. Agoraphobia is the fear of being in places or situations where escape might be difficult (or embarrassing) or where help might not be available in the event of a panic attack.[10] As a result, patients often avoid specific situations (e.g., crowded places, stores, bridges, and travel away from home) where they fear a panic attack may occur. In the majority of patients with agoraphobia, panic attacks are the initial event causing the subsequent development of avoidance behavior; however, because not all reported cases of agoraphobia are preceded by panic attacks, agoraphobia (without panic attacks) is a separate diagnosis in the DSM-III-R.[10]

Panic disorder with agoraphobia is more common in women than men (2:1 to 4:1), with the onset of symptoms first evident in young adulthood. Patients frequently report a history of childhood separation anxiety and childhood phobias. Panic disorder is frequently a chronic, relapsing illness that often requires lifetime treatment. It is a familial illness with approximately 25% to 30% of patients having at least one first-degree relative (father, mother, brother, or sister) with a similar condition, compared with only 2% among relatives of healthy controls. Complications of this disorder include depression, suicide, and alcohol dependence.[3,5]

**Table 51.5** DSM-III-R Diagnostic Criteria for Panic Disorder

A. One or more panic attacks (discrete periods of intense fear or discomfort) have occurred that were unexpected and were not triggered by situations in which the person was the focus of others' attention
B. At least four attacks have occurred within a 4-week period. One or more attacks have been followed by at least a 1-month period of persistent fear of having another attack
C. At least four of the following symptoms developed during at least one of the attacks
   1. Dyspnea (shortness of breath) or smothering sensations
   2. Dizziness, unsteadiness, or faintness
   3. Palpitations or accelerated heart rate (tachycardia)
   4. Trembling or shaking
   5. Sweating
   6. Choking
   7. Nausea or abdominal distress
   8. Feelings of unreality (depersonalization)
   9. Numbness or tingling sensations (paresthesias)
   10. Hot and/or cold flashes
   11. Chest pain or discomfort
   12. Fear of dying
   13. Fear of going crazy or doing something uncontrolled

   *Note:* Attacks involving fewer than four symptoms are limited-symptom attacks.

D. At least four of the C symptoms developed suddenly and increased in intensity within 10 min of the beginning of the first symptom
E. Not caused by a known organic factor (e.g., amphetamines, caffeine, thyrotoxicosis), or other psychiatric disorders (e.g., depression, substance abuse)

   *Note:* Mitral valve prolapse may be an associated condition but does not preclude a diagnosis.

Modified from American Psychiatric Association: Diagnostic and Statistical Manual of Mental Disorders, 3rd ed, revised (DSM-III-R), Washington DC, American Psychiatric Association, 1987, pp 237–238.

## *Obsessive–Compulsive Disorder*

This disorder is characterized by obsessions (recurrent ideas or thoughts that are persistent and unwanted and cannot be eliminated by logic or reasoning) and compulsions (a repetitive and unwanted urge to perform an act often contrary to one's wishes or standards). These behaviors seem purposeful such as handwashing, bathing, or cleaning, but because of their repetitive nature, are actually senseless. Anxiety occurs when the individual attempts to resist the obsessions or compulsions.[10]

Although obsessive–compulsive disorder was once considered rare (with an estimated prevalence of 0.05%),[15] the NIMH community survey reported a prevalence rate that ranged from 1.3% to 2.0%, suggesting that this illness may be more common than previously believed.[1] This anxiety disorder usually begins before the age of 25 and is often chronic; the most common complication is depression. Unlike most anxiety disorders, obsessive–compulsive disorder is profoundly disabling and prolonged hospitalizations are common.[15]

### *Posttraumatic Stress Disorder*

Posttraumatic stress disorder is a pathologic reaction to a psychologically traumatic experience that is outside the range of usual human experience, such as a serious accident, natural disaster, combat, or torture. Symptoms may be acute or delayed and are characterized by reexperiencing the traumatic event through nightmares and flashbacks. There is persistent avoidance of situations that are reminders of the trauma. Other symptoms include emotional detachment or numbing, autonomic hyperactivity with hypervigilance, difficulty sleeping, irritability, and outbursts of anger.[10] This disorder is frequently seen among Vietnam War veterans. The prevalence of posttraumatic stress disorder has not been well studied, but additional data from the NIMH community survey should be helpful. Depression and alcohol dependence are serious complications of this disorder.[5]

### *Atypical Anxiety Disorder*

This diagnosis is given when a patient presents with prominent anxiety or phobic avoidance but fails to meet criteria for a specific anxiety disorder.[10]

## Pathophysiology

Although the pathophysiology of the anxiety disorders is unknown, scientists have proposed theories regarding the neurobiology of anxiety disorders by studying the biochemical activity of anxiolytic and anxiogenic agents. The norepinephrine and the benzodiazepine receptor models of anxiety are theories that have attracted the most interest.

### *Noradrenergic Model*

The basic premise of the noradrenergic theory is that the autonomic nervous system of anxious patients (especially those with panic attacks) overreacts to various stimuli. Patients clearly display symptoms of peripheral autonomic hyperactivity (e.g., hyperventilation, palpitations, and tremulousness) and thus appear to have increased noradrenergic activity.[5]

The locus cerulus (LC), a small brain stem nucleus, may play a major role in regulating anxiety. The LC contains 70% of the brain's noradrenergic neurons and has widespread projections to the limbic system as well as the cerebral and cerebellar cortices. The LC serves as an alarm center associated with increased adrenergic activity in response to fearful or anxiety-producing stimuli.[16]

Drugs with anxiolytic or antipanic effects (e.g., the benzodiazepines and antidepressants) inhibit LC activity or firing. (The exception is buspirone, a new nonbenzodiazepine anxiolytic, that increases LC neuronal transmission.[17]) Drugs that stimulate LC activity (e.g., yohimbine, isoproterenol, and caffeine) are usually anxiogenic or produce anxious symptoms. Patients with anxiety disorders, especially those with panic disorder, are more susceptible to the effects of anxiogenic agents.[18] Furthermore, administration of drugs that inhibit LC activity (e.g., imipramine and alprazolam) diminish or block the anxiogenic effects.[19] Altered noradrenergic function or receptor sensitivity may underlie the origin of certain anxiety disorders, especially panic disorder.[18,19]

### *Benzodiazepine Receptor Model*

Studies to determine the mechanism of action of the benzodiazepines led to the discovery, in 1977, of the benzodiazepine binding sites in rat brain tissue.[20] Since then, similar receptors have been identified on the nerve cells of human brain. The receptors are functionally and perhaps structurally linked to the neurotransmitter, $\gamma$-aminobutyric acid (GABA).[21] GABA is the most important inhibitory neurotransmitter in the CNS and is involved in nerve transmission in nearly one third of brain impulses. The benzodiazepines are believed to decrease anxiety by enhancing GABA-mediated inhibition at presynaptic and postsynaptic sites throughout the CNS. The benzodiazepine receptor may be important in the regulation of generalized anxiety disorder symptoms.[21,22]

There is also increasing evidence for involvement of the neurotransmitter serotonin in the etiology and regulation of anxiety symptoms. At least one serotonin type 1A agonist drug (buspirone) has been marketed as an antianxiety agent; several other drugs are currently being investigated. Additional research will clarify the exact role of serotonin in anxiety disorders.

## Treatment

### *Generalized Anxiety Disorder*

Treatment of generalized anxiety disorder usually consists of both psychologic and pharmacotherapeutic interventions. Once generalized anxiety disorder is diagnosed, an individualized treatment approach must be determined. Selection of a therapeutic plan depends upon the patient's age, medication history, medical status, personality, and degree of incapacitation. Psychotherapy is often the least invasive and safest treatment modality. For patients experiencing anxiety symptoms severe enough to produce dysfunction or discomfort, however, temporary use of an antianxiety medication is indicated.[8]

The benzodiazepines are the most efficacious and widely prescribed agents for the amelioration of anxiety symptoms. Although barbiturates and meprobamate are occasionally prescribed, they account for only 7% of all anxiolytic prescriptions. Barbiturate use is limited by the rapid development of tolerance, high potential for abuse, lethality in overdosage, excessive sedation, and significant drug interactions.[23] These agents should be avoided in the management of generalized anxiety disorder.[8] Buspirone, autonomic blocking agents, and antihistamines are additional anxiolytic options (Table 51.6).

**Table 51.6** Nonbenzodiazepine Antianxiety Agents

| *Class/generic name* | *Brand name* | *Manufacturer* | *Approved for anxiety* | *Usual dosage range[a] (mg/d)* |
|---|---|---|---|---|
| Diphenylmethanes | | | | |
| Diphenhydramine | Benadryl | Parke–Davis | No | 25–200 |
| | Generics | Various | | |
| Hydroxyzine | Vistaril | Pfizer | Yes | 50–400 |
| | Atarax | Roerig | | |
| | Generics | Various | | |
| Propanediols | | | | |
| Meprobamate | Equanil | Wyeth | Yes | 400–1,600 |
| | Miltown | Wallace | | |
| | Generics | Various | | |
| β-Blockers | | | | |
| Propranolol | Inderal | Ayerst | No | 80–160 |
| | Generics | Various | | |
| Azaspirodecanadiones | | | | |
| Buspirone | BuSpar | Mead Johnson | Yes | 15–60[b] |

[a] Elderly patients are usually treated with approximately one half of the dose listed.
[b] The dosage range in elderly patients appears to be the same, but is not established.

### Nonpharmacologic Therapy

Most patients require psychologic therapy, alone or in combination with medication, to overcome fears and learn to improve coping abilities.[8] Consideration of the patient's clinical symptoms, personality, and life problems aids in the choice of psychologic therapy. Supportive psychotherapy provides explanations and encouragement, and allows formulation of strategies to effectively manage anxiety-provoking situations. Dynamic psychotherapy, used in patients with personality disorders, examines the causes of anxiety, relating past experiences to the patient's present reactions. Behavioral therapy is indicated in patients with avoidance behavior. Patients with anxiety secondary to impaired interpersonal relations may benefit from group therapy. Relaxation therapy (biofeedback, relaxation exercises, meditation) may aid in the relief of tension in some patients,[8] but is usually inadequate treatment when used alone in patients with severe anxiety.

### Benzodiazepine Therapy

The benzodiazepines are the drugs of choice in the management of generalized anxiety disorder. Discovered in the 1930s, these agents were not marketed in the United States until 1960. Benzodiazepine use peaked approximately 10 years ago. Currently, these agents account for 5% of all prescriptions dispensed by community pharmacies.[24]

***Indications*** All benzodiazepines possess anxiolytic properties, but only 8 of the 13 marketed in the United States have FDA-approved labeling indications for the treatment of generalized anxiety disorder (Table 51.7). Flurazepam, temazepam, and triazolam are marketed as sedative–hypnotic agents, while clonazepam is indicated for use as an anticonvulsant.[22] Alprazolam has proven efficacy in panic disorder with agoraphobia and possibly depressive illness; however, alprazolam is not, as yet, FDA approved for these indications. Differences in marketed clinical indications often represent the manufacturers' marketing strategies rather than any major inherent differences in pharmacologic properties.[24]

***Mechanism of Action*** The benzodiazepine receptor model of anxiety (described under Pathophysiology) theorizes that benzodiazepines ameliorate anxiety through potentiation of the inhibitory activity of GABA.[21,22] Benzodiazepine binding sites are present in highest density in the cortical and limbic-forebrain areas of the CNS.[22] The benzodiazepine receptor is functionally (and perhaps physically) coupled to the GABA receptor and the associated chloride (Cl) ion channel in the postsynaptic nerve cell membrane. When the benzodiazepine receptor is activated in the presence of GABA, the chloride ion channels open and allow an influx of chloride ions into the cell. This results in a negatively charged, hyperpolarized membrane that prevents further depolarization by excitatory neurotransmitters.[24] This benzodiazepine-GABA-Cl interaction may also enhance or trigger activity of other neurotransmitters.[25]

***Pharmacokinetics*** Although benzodiazepines have similar pharmacologic activity, differences in their pharmacokinetic properties may assist the clinician in choosing an appropriate anxiolytic (Table 51.8). After a single dose, the onset, intensity, and duration of pharmacologic effects are important factors to consider when using benzodiazepines for the short-term, intermittent, or as needed (prn) treatment of anxiety.

The primary determinant of a drug's onset of effect after a single oral dose is the rate of drug absorption. Because of high lipophilicity, diazepam and clorazepate are rapidly absorbed and quickly distributed into the CNS. Therefore, the onset of anxiolytic effect occurs within 30 to 60 minutes

**Table 51.7** Benzodiazepine Antianxiety Agents

| *Generic name* | *Brand name* | *Manufacturer* | *Approved indications* | *Approved dosage range*[a] *(mg/d)* | *Approximate equivalent dose (mg)* |
|---|---|---|---|---|---|
| Alprazolam | Xanax | Upjohn | Anxiety | 0.75–4 | 0.5 |
| | | | Anxiety–depression | | |
| Chlordiazepoxide | Librium | Roche | Anxiety | 25–200 | 10 |
| | Generics | Various | Alcohol withdrawal | | |
| | | | Preop sedation | | |
| Clorazepate | Tranxene | Abbott | Anxiety | 7.5–90 | 7.5 |
| | | | Seizure disorders | | |
| Diazepam | Valium | Roche | Anxiety | 2–40 | 5 |
| | Generics | Various | Alcohol withdrawal | | |
| | | | Muscle spasm | | |
| | | | Preop sedation | | |
| | | | Status epilepticus | | |
| Halazepam | Paxipam | Schering | Anxiety | 20–160 | 20 |
| Lorazepam | Ativan | Wyeth | Anxiety | 0.5–10 | 1 |
| | Generics | Various | Preop sedation | | |
| Oxazepam | Serax | Wyeth | Anxiety | 30–120 | 15 |
| | | | Anxiety–depression | | |
| | | | Alcohol withdrawal | | |
| Prazepam | Centrax | Parke–Davis | Anxiety | 20–60 | 10 |

[a] Elderly patients are usually treated with approximately one half of the dose listed.

and produces a rapid and intense relief of anxiety. High lipophilicity increases the extent of drug distribution into the periphery, particularly adipose tissue, resulting in a shorter duration of effect after a single dose.[22] Clinically, patients perceive a rapid onset of action, but some may experience an unpleasant feeling of drowsiness, relaxation, or loss of control.[22] This "rush" may be euphoric and may increase abuse potential.[26] Chlordiazepoxide's onset of effect is much slower, because of decreased lipophilicity, slower absorption, and passage into the CNS.

Lorazepam, oxazepam, and prazepam are also less lipophilic than diazepam and have a slower onset of effect. Oxazepam absorption is slow and peak levels are not obtained until 2 to 4 hours after a single dose; however, like lorazepam, oxazepam's anxiolytic effects are long-lasting because extensive distribution does not occur.[23] Prazepam, a prodrug, is very slowly absorbed and requires hepatic dealkylation to *N*-desmethyldiazepam (*N*-DMDZ), with peak levels delayed until 6 hours after a single dose. Drugs with slow absorption rates are not recommended for the immediate (acute) relief of anxiety.

Parenteral administration through the intramuscular route

**Table 51.8** Pharmacokinetics of Benzodiazepine Antianxiety Agents

| *Generic name* | *Peak plasma level (h)* | *Elimination half-life, parent (h)* | *Metabolic pathway* | *Clinically significant metabolites* | *Protein binding (%)* |
|---|---|---|---|---|---|
| Alprazolam | 1–2 | 12–15 | Oxidation | None | 80 |
| Chlordiazepoxide | 1–4 | 5–30 | *N*-Dealkylation | Desmethylchlor-diazepoxide | 96 |
| | | | Oxidation | Demoxepam | |
| | | | | *N*-DMDZ[a] | |
| Clorazepate | 1–2 | Prodrug | Oxidation | *N*-DMDZ | 97 |
| Diazepam | 0.5–2 | 20–80 | Oxidation | *N*-DMDZ | 98 |
| Halazepam | 1–3 | 14 | Oxidation | *N*-DMDZ | 97 |
| Lorazepam | 2–4 | 10–20 | Conjugation | None | 85 |
| Oxazepam | 2–4 | 5–20 | Conjugation | None | 97 |
| Prazepam | 6 | Prodrug | Oxidation | *N*-DMDZ | 97 |

[a] *N*-Desmethyldiazepam, half-life 36–200 h.

Compiled from References 22 and 24.

should be avoided with diazepam and chlordiazepoxide secondary to variability in the rate and extent of drug absorption. Intramuscular lorazepam provides rapid, reliable, and complete absorption, but the preparation must be refrigerated.[22]

After chronic dosing, the rate and extent of drug accumulation are functions of the drug's elimination half-life, clearance, and formation of active metabolites. Differences in clinical effects that occur during and after repeated dosage with the benzodiazepines are related in part to variability in metabolism and metabolite accumulation.

The benzodiazepines undergo two primary metabolic processes, hepatic microsomal oxidation (N-dealkylation or aliphatic hydroxylation) and glucuronide conjugation. With the exception of lorazepam and oxazepam (which are conjugated only), all benzodiazepines are oxidated first, then conjugated, and excreted renally. Oxidation may be impaired in such clinical situations as liver disease, in the elderly, and with the simultaneous use of drugs that inhibit oxidation. Impaired oxidation results in higher levels of the parent drug and/or an active metabolite.[22] Benzodiazepine conjugation is not affected by these factors.

Many benzodiazepines are converted (through N-demethylation) to *N*-DMDZ, an active metabolite with a long elimination half-life of 36 to 200 hours (Table 51.8).[24] *N*-DMDZ is further oxidated to oxazepam, then conjugated, and excreted. After multiple dosing, accumulation of *N*-DMDZ is slow and extensive, providing a long-lasting antianxiety effect. If oxidation of *N*-DMDZ is impaired, the half-life is prolonged and complications of drug accumulation (e.g., drowsiness, sedation) may result.[22] Although diazepam and halazepam possess anxiolytic activity, their primary metabolite is *N*-DMDZ. Chlordiazepoxide is also active and is converted into a number of active metabolites.

Clorazepate and prazepam are considered prodrugs because *N*-DMDZ is primarily responsible for their anxiolytic effects. Before absorption, clorazepate is rapidly metabolized in the stomach through a pH-dependent process.[27] Alterations of stomach pH (e.g., administration of antacids) may decrease the rate of *N*-DMDZ formation. Prazepam requires first-pass liver transformation before *N*-DMDZ is formed.

Benzodiazepines with short half-lives (e.g., alprazolam, lorazepam, oxazepam) reach steady-state plasma concentrations rapidly and drug accumulation after repeated dosing is minimal. Alprazolam is oxidized to $\alpha$-hydroxyalprazolam, which accounts for approximately 17% of the total dose. This metabolite probably contributes little to clinical effects, however.[28] Neither oxazepam nor lorazepam is converted into active metabolites.[22]

Benzodiazepine protein binding is extensive, especially in benzodiazepines with long elimination half-lives. Patients with hypoalbuminemia may have increased sensitivity to clinical effects and benzodiazepines with lower protein binding (e.g., oxazepam, alprazolam) should be used.

***Clinical Use*** Knowledge of benzodiazepine pharmacokinetics may assist the clinician in selecting an agent for a particular clinical situation. After multiple dosing, drugs with long elimination half-lives may take 1 to 2 weeks to reach steady state and thus full therapeutic effect. In the elderly, secondary to a decreased capacity for oxidation and alterations in the volume of distribution, drug accumulation may result. Patients with hepatic diseases are also at risk for drug accumulation and subsequent complications. Therefore, intermediate- or shorter acting benzodiazepines are preferred for chronic use in the elderly and those with liver disorders because of minimal accumulation and achievement of steady state within 1 to 3 days.

Benzodiazepines with long elimination half-lives may be dosed once a day at bedtime and may provide both hypnotic and daytime anxiolytic activity. Agents with shorter elimination half-lives should be administered in divided daily doses.

***Drug Interactions*** Drugs interacting with the benzodiazepines generally fall into two categories—CNS depressants and drugs that interfere with benzodiazepine metabolism (Table 51.9). Simultaneous use of alcohol and a benzodiazepine results in additive sedative effects and lowers the therapeutic index of the benzodiazepine.[29] In addition, concurrent ingestion of any drug with CNS depressant properties (e.g., phenothiazines, antihistamines, narcotics, barbiturates, anticonvulsants, antidepressants) may potentiate the sedative action of the benzodiazepines. When ingested alone in an overdose attempt, benzodiazepines are rarely life-threatening; however, the combination of benzodiazepines with alcohol or other CNS depressant agents (e.g., antidepressants) is potentially fatal.

Cimetidine, an $H_2$ receptor antagonist, competitively inhibits the metabolism of drugs that require oxidation through the hepatic microsomal $P_{450}$ enzyme system.[30] A prolonged elimination half-life and decreased plasma clearance of single doses of diazepam, chlordiazepoxide, and alprazolam were reported after treatment with cimetidine [31–33]; how-

**Table 51.9** Drug Interactions With the Benzodiazepines

| *Drug* | *Effect* |
|---|---|
| Alcohol | Decreases clearance of chlordiazepoxide and diazepam; additive psychomotor impairment |
| Disulfiram | Decreases clearance of chlordiazepoxide and diazepam by 40%–50% |
| Cimetidine | Increases elimination half-life and decreases clearance of alprazolam, diazepam, and chlordiazepoxide |
| Isoniazid | Decreases metabolism of diazepam |
| Rifampin | Induces metabolism of diazepam |
| Antacids | Decreases rate and extent of clorazepate absorption<br>Decreases rate, but not extent, of diazepam and chlordiazepoxide absorption |
| Oral contraceptives | Increases the free concentration of chlordiazepoxide and slightly decreases clearance; decreases clearance and increases half-life of diazepam after low-dose estrogen oral contraceptives |

Compiled from References 22 and 30–35.

ever, cimetidine failed to inhibit metabolism of oxazepam and lorazepam because these agents are conjugated.[34] Greenblatt and associates[35] failed to demonstrate adverse psychomotor effects when cimetidine was added to diazepam therapy, despite mean increases in diazepam and *N*-DMDZ plasma concentrations of 62% and 54%, respectively. Thus, the clinical importance of this interaction is minimal in healthy patients on chronic benzodiazepine therapy; however, when chronic therapy is indicated in the elderly or debilitated patients receiving cimetidine, oxazepam or lorazepam is the benzodiazepine of choice. Ranitidine (Zantac), a $H_2$ receptor antagonist that does not inhibit oxidative metabolism, has no clinically important effects on the pharmacokinetics of diazepam or lorazepam.[36]

Antacids may decrease the rate and extent of clorazepate absorption. The rate but not extent of diazepam and chlordiazepoxide absorption is decreased by concurrent antacid ingestion.[24] Other agents that may impair benzodiazepine metabolism include disulfiram, isoniazid, and low-dose estrogens.

***Adverse Drug Reactions*** The most common adverse effects associated with benzodiazepine therapy involve CNS depression. This is clinically manifested as drowsiness, sedation, blurred vision, psychomotor impairment, and ataxia.[24] A transient mild drowsiness is commonly experienced by patients during the first few days of treatment; however, a tolerance to this effect soon develops. Disorientation, confusion, aggression, and excitement have been reported, particularly in the elderly.[24]

Impairment of memory and recall may occur during benzodiazepine treatment. The memory loss induced by the benzodiazepines and barbiturates typically is limited to events occurring after drug ingestion (or anterograde amnesia).[37] The anterograde amnesia is secondary to disordered consolidation processes that store information and is not an impairment in the perception or retrieval of information.[38] The extent of benzodiazepine-induced memory impairment is unknown because it may go unrecognized by the clinician and the patient. Complaints of forgetfulness in patients receiving benzodiazepines, especially the elderly, should be explored for drug-induced amnesia.

***Abuse, Dependence, Withdrawal, and Tolerance*** The widespread use of benzodiazepines has generated public concern about the occurrence, severity, and extent of benzodiazepine abuse. The long-term use of benzodiazepines has caused increased interest regarding the development of dependence.[39]

Abuse is defined by the World Health Organization as the persistence of sporadic, excessive drug use inconsistent with or unrelated to acceptable medical practice. Benzodiazepine abuse is rare in the general population of users; however, individuals with a history of multiple drug abuse (e.g., alcohol, sedatives) are at the greatest risk of becoming benzodiazepine abusers.[39]

Benzodiazepine dependence as demonstrated by the appearance of withdrawal symptoms upon discontinuation of therapy is well documented. Although first reported in patients taking excessive doses of benzodiazepines, it has recently been recognized that a mild withdrawal syndrome occurs in up to 44% of patients ingesting therapeutic doses of benzodiazepines for as little as 4 to 6 weeks.[40,41] The symptoms of mild benzodiazepine withdrawal include anxiety, insomnia, malaise, anorexia, diaphoresis, and perceptual changes. In more severe cases of withdrawal, tremor, orthostasis, nausea, vomiting, seizures, and psychosis may occur.[42] The onset of withdrawal symptoms in patients ingesting agents with short elimination half-lives occurs much earlier than in those taking agents with long elimination half-lives where symptoms begin 3 to 8 days later.[43] Other factors associated with an increased incidence or severity of benzodiazepine withdrawal include a long duration of therapy and high dosages. Abrupt discontinuation and the use of short elimination half-life benzodiazepines (e.g., lorazepam, oxazepam, and alprazolam) may produce a more severe withdrawal, including seizures as early as 24 hours after discontinuation.[42,43] A rapid drop in the drug's plasma concentration may unmask the hypersensitive benzodiazepine receptors responsible for symptoms of withdrawal.[24]

Recent reports of severe withdrawal symptoms and lack of cross-tolerance with diazepam have caused concern regarding long-term alprazolam therapy. Alprazolam is often used to treat panic disorder and depression in high doses for prolonged periods of time. In certain patients, alprazolam may have to be withdrawn with greater individualization and more cautiously (0.5 mg/week) than recommended by the package insert (0.5-mg decrease every 3 days).[44]

Brief interrupted courses of benzodiazepine therapy at the lowest effective dose may minimize or prevent benzodiazepine withdrawal syndrome. Chronic benzodiazepine administration should be avoided whenever possible. If benzodiazepine therapy exceeds 6 weeks, a slow dosage taper over several weeks is recommended.[24] A benzodiazepine with a long elimination half-life (e.g., diazepam) may be substituted for agents with short elimination half-lives (e.g., lorazepam, oxazepam, alprazolam) and patients should receive these drugs for a few weeks before gradual drug discontinuation. In patients receiving alprazolam, carbamazepine may be a useful alternative to diazepam.[45]

Although tolerance develops to the sedative, muscle relaxant, and anticonvulsant activities, the benzodiazepines do not appear to lose anxiolytic efficacy.[8,24] The efficacy of benzodiazepines in long-term clinical trials (i.e., greater than 4 months of chronic use) has not been reported; however, many patients obtain beneficial anxiolytic effects from chronic ingestion of these agents.

***General Prescribing Guidelines*** The goals of benzodiazepine therapy in generalized anxiety disorder are to relieve symptoms of anxiety and to improve the patient's overall functioning. All benzodiazepines are equally effective anxiolytics and consideration of pharmacokinetic properties and the clinical situation of the patient may aid in selection of the most appropriate agent.

Diazepam and clorazepate are preferable in situations where a rapid onset of effect is necessary. Agents with short elimination half-lives are recommended for the elderly, for patients with hepatic disorders, and for those receiving drugs that impair oxidative metabolism. Drug and metabolite accumulation and toxicity may result if long elimination half-life benzodiazepines are used in these situations, but can be minimized by lowering the dosage or decreasing the frequency of drug administration.

Benzodiazepine dosage requirements vary widely among patients and must be individualized and carefully titrated to avoid adverse effects. In the adult patient, start with low doses (e.g., diazepam 2 mg TID or its equivalent) and titrate the dose to relief of anxiety symptoms and appearance of adverse effects (diazepam, maximum 40 mg daily). After initial response is achieved, the agents with long-elimination half-lives may be dosed at bedtime and dosage adjustments should be made on a weekly basis. Side effects such as drowsiness and sedation can be managed by a decrease in dosage or an increase in dosage frequency.[24]

In most patients, the duration of therapy will be limited. For chronic anxiety, benzodiazepine usage should be limited to brief treatment of episodes (not longer than 6 weeks). Problems with drug withdrawal are infrequently encountered in patients receiving usual therapeutic doses for less than 4 months, when the benzodiazepine is tapered. The overall incidence of benzodiazepine abuse is rare, but may occur in patients with alcohol or sedative–hypnotic dependence.

The elderly patient requires additional monitoring when benzodiazepines are used. They are more sensitive to the CNS depressant effects, additive CNS depression with other agents, and problems associated with accumulation of the long-elimination half-life benzodiazepines. The elderly may be susceptible to benzodiazepine-induced sedation, impaired daytime functioning, and memory problems that may be enhanced by other drugs with CNS depressant effects.

Patient education should include the anticipated length of drug therapy, potential side effects, and consequences of the ingestion of alcohol and other CNS depressants. Patients should understand that medications provide symptomatic relief, but do not solve any underlying psychologic problems. Patients should be told not to decrease or discontinue benzodiazepine usage without contacting their physician.

**Buspirone Therapy**

Marketed as an anxiolytic in the United States in 1986, buspirone is a member of a unique chemical class called the azaspirodecanediones. Buspirone is structurally and pharmacologically unlike benzodiazepines, barbiturates, and meprobamate. Buspirone lacks the anticonvulsant, muscle relaxant, and hypnotic properties characteristic of the benzodiazepines.[46] Cross-tolerance between buspirone and the benzodiazepines has not been demonstrated, and buspirone was unsuccessful in the management of benzodiazepine withdrawal.[47,48]

***Indications*** Buspirone is indicated in the treatment of generalized anxiety disorder. Double-blind, placebo-controlled clinical trials[49,50–53] found buspirone to be superior to placebo and as efficacious as diazepam at the end of 4 weeks when given in equipotent doses (mg per mg). In double-blind, 4-week comparisons in patients with generalized anxiety disorder, buspirone was equivalent in efficacy to diazepam,[54] clorazepate,[49,55] and alprazolam and lorazepam[56]; however, other investigators[57,58] report that buspirone is unsatisfactory compared with lorazepam and diazepam, especially in patients with severe anxiety.

***Mechanism of Action*** Buspirone's anxiolytic mechanism of action is unknown; however, it does not appear to act directly through the benzodiazepine–GABA-Cl receptor complex nor to decrease noradrenergic neuron firing in the locus ceruleus. Evidence suggests buspirone possesses activity as a serotonin agonist and binds to serotonin type 1a receptors to produce anxiolysis.[59]

Buspirone also possesses both dopamine agonist and indirect dopamine antagonist properties.[60] Dopaminergic effects are probably not responsible for buspirone's therapeutic efficacy, but may be of concern in the potential development of side effects associated with postdopamine receptor blockade.

***Pharmacokinetics*** After an oral dose, buspirone is rapidly and completely absorbed, and undergoes extensive first-pass metabolism. The mean systemic bioavailability is approximately 4%.[61] Food does not alter buspirone's absorption, but decreases the degree of first-pass metabolism which increases buspirone's bioavailability; the clinical significance of this finding is unknown.[61] The mean elimination half-life of buspirone is reported to be 2.1 to 2.7 hours.[62,63] Buspirone is 95% protein bound to both albumin and $\alpha_1$-acid glycoprotein.[61]

Buspirone is eliminated primarily by oxidative metabolism and is converted into active and inactive metabolites. One pharmacologically active metabolite, 1-pyrimidinylpiperazine, possesses approximately one fifth the anxiolytic activity of buspirone as measured by the Vogel anticonflict paradigm in animals. This metabolite probably contributes little to the compound's anxiolytic activity.[61] Buspirone's metabolites lack postsynaptic dopamine receptor binding properties; thus, metabolism may play a major role in minimizing adverse effects associated with postsynaptic dopaminergic blockade.[64] Although unaffected by age, buspirone's clearance is markedly decreased in patients with cirrhosis and to a lesser extent in patients with renal impairment.[61]

***Adverse Drug Reactions*** A major advantage of buspirone over other antianxiety agents is the claim that it lacks sedative effects. Five of nine clinical trials reported a significantly higher incidence of sedation and drowsiness in the diazepam,[51,54] clorazepate,[49,55] and alprazolam and lorazepam[56] groups as compared with the buspirone group. The remaining four trials[49,50,52,53] reported sedative effects more frequently in the benzodiazepine patients; however, the incidence of drowsiness after single 10- or 20-mg doses of buspirone in normal persons was reported to be comparable with that for the benzodiazepines (diazepam 10 mg or lorazepam 2.5 mg) and significantly greater than that for placebo.[24] Although drowsiness does occur in normal persons when daily doses of buspirone exceed 20 mg, the incidence of sedation appears to be less than with benzodiazepines at equipotent doses.[65]

Other side effects reported during buspirone therapy include dizziness, nausea, headaches, nervousness, and dysphoria (especially with large single doses of 20–40 mg).[66] Potential problems secondary to postsynaptic dopaminergic blockade (e.g., gynecomastia, galactorrhea, extrapyramidal symptoms) were observed in fewer than 0.57% of patients in clinical trials.[67] The long-term safety of buspirone has not been published.

*Drug Interactions* Few data are available on drug interactions with buspirone. Buspirone was reported to increase the area under the concentration-versus-time curve (AUC) of haloperidol. Although the clinical significance of this interaction is not known,[24] the manufacturer recommends avoidance of this combination of drugs.[67] In comparative trials with benzodiazepines, buspirone (but not the benzodiazepines) lacked a pharmacokinetic interaction with alcohol and failed to potentiate the performance impairment of alcohol.[24] Four occurrences of elevated blood pressure were reported in patients taking a monoamine oxidase inhibitor and buspirone concurrently. Therefore, concomitant use of buspirone and a monoamine oxidase inhibitor is not recommended.[68] In vitro experiments suggest that buspirone may displace weakly protein bound drugs such as digoxin; the clinical relevance of this finding is not known.[67]

*Abuse, Dependence, and Withdrawal* Physical dependence and withdrawal symptoms have not been reported in studies in animals or humans.[69,70] The results of human trials indicate that buspirone has a low potential for abuse.[71,72] To date, postmarketing experience supports a lack of patient abuse and dependence for buspirone.

*General Prescribing Guidelines* The recommended initial dose of buspirone is 5 mg three times a day with dosage increments of 5 mg per day every 2 to 3 days as needed.[67] The usual therapeutic dose of buspirone is 20–30 mg/d,[49–56] with a maximum dose of 60 mg daily.[67] The onset of anxiolysis is not immediate, requiring a week or more before clinical effects occur; maximum effects may not be evident for 4 to 6 weeks.[69]

Buspirone possesses specific characteristics that distinguish it from other anxiolytic agents. Thus different guidelines must be used for successful therapy with buspirone. Buspirone has minimal sedating properties and is not useful in clinical situations requiring immediate anxiolytic effects or for patients who take anxiolytics as needed. Therefore, buspirone is an alternative for patients who are unable to tolerate the sedative effects and psychomotor impairment of benzodiazepines, especially the elderly.

Buspirone is not cross-tolerant with the benzodiazepines and thus will not prevent or treat symptoms of benzodiazepine withdrawal. When a patient is switched from a benzodiazepine to buspirone, the benzodiazepine should be tapered slowly before buspirone is initiated.

Patients who will potentially have the most beneficial response to buspirone are newly diagnosed anxious patients who have not received previous benzodiazepine therapy. Prior benzodiazepine use may predict a less favorable therapeutic outcome with buspirone. Benzodiazepine exposure may lead to certain expectations of anxiolytic drug effects (immediate response and sedation) that buspirone typically does not demonstrate.[43] Therefore, patients who have received benzodiazepines should be advised of the differences between effects of previous drugs and buspirone, particularly at the outset of therapy. Buspirone may become the anxiolytic of choice in patients with a history of alcohol or drug abuse because of the low potential for dependency and abuse. Additional clinical experience with buspirone will better define guidelines for appropriate clinical use and adverse drug reactions.

### Adrenergic Blocking Agents

Propranolol, a $\beta$-adrenergic blocking drug, was first used in the treatment of generalized anxiety disorder in 1966. Additional clinical trials reported that propranolol and other $\beta$-blocking agents were especially useful in patients with prominent cardiovascular symptoms of anxiety (e.g., palpitations, tremors); however, other studies reported conflicting results.[73] Most studies were limited by a small sample size, an inadequate drug dosage and duration of treatment, and a crossover study design.[73,74]

$\beta$-Blocking drugs are less effective anxiolytics than benzodiazepines[73] and their usefulness may be entirely restricted to those anxiety patients whose physical symptoms, especially cardiovascular complaints, have not adequately responded to benzodiazepine therapy. Additive effects have been reported, with the combination of diazepam and propranolol, but additional study is required.[74]

Propranolol therapy is usually well tolerated with few adverse effects, provided a complete medical examination is performed. Patients with bradycardia, heart block, or cardiac failure should not receive $\beta$-blocking agents. Propranolol should also not be used in patients with asthma, bronchospasm, or Raynaud's disease.[23] Side effects reported with propranolol use in anxious patients are similar to those reported during antihypertensive therapy and include fatigue, lightheadedness, bradycardia, nausea, and insomnia.[23] Most adverse effects may be eliminated by reducing the dose or administering the dose early in the day to avoid insomnia.

Doses of propranolol ranging from 40 to 360 mg/d are used in the management of generalized anxiety disorder.[73] Although propranolol has a short elimination half-life (2–6 hours), $\beta$-blockade usually lasts 8 to 12 hours after a single dose. Propranolol should be dosed at least twice a day.[23,73] Propranolol 10 mg twice a day should be used initially and gradually titrated to anxiolytic response. The usual duration of therapy is not well defined, but may parallel the benzodiazepines. Upon discontinuation of therapy, propranolol dosage should be tapered to avoid rebound anxiety and cardiovascular effects.[23,73]

Propranolol may be a useful alternative to the benzodiazepines in patients with generalized anxiety disorder who may be at risk for dependence or those who experience intellectual impairment.

### Antihistamines

Hydroxyzine is commonly used in the treatment of anxiety and tension associated with psychiatric and physical diseases, and diphenhydramine is used for its sedative and calming effects.[23] Although the antihistamines are less effective anxiolytics than the benzodiazepines, they lack potential for dependence.[8]

The usual dose of hydroxyzine is 50 to 100 mg four times daily.[23] The antihistamines have anticholinergic effects that may be problematic, especially in the elderly. Additive CNS

**Table 51.10** Drugs Used in the Treatment of Panic Disorder With Agoraphobia

| *Class/generic name* | *Brand name* | *Manufacturer* | *Antipanic dosage range[a] (mg/d)* | *Comments* |
|---|---|---|---|---|
| Tricyclic antidepressants | | | | |
| Imipramine | Tofranil<br>Generics | Geigy<br>Various | 150–300 | Effective<br>Problems: lag time, side effects |
| Monoamine oxidase inhibitors | | | | |
| Phenalzine | Nardil | Parke–Davis | 45–90 | Effective<br>Problems: patient acceptance, dietary restrictions, side effects |
| Benzodiazepines | | | | |
| Alprazolam | Xanax | Upjohn | 4–10 | Effective in high doses<br>Problems: long-term therapy needs further study |
| Diazepam | Valium<br>Generics | Roche<br>Various | 30–40 | Possibly effective, needs more study |
| Clonazepam | Klonopin | Roche | 3–6 | Possibly effective, needs more study |
| Miscellaneous agents | | | | |
| Propranolol | Inderal<br>Generics | Ayerst<br>Various | 240 | Questionable efficacy |
| Clonidine | Catapres<br>Generics | Boehringer Ingelheim<br>Various | 0.5 | Tolerance develops to antipanic effects |

[a] Dosage used in clinical trials but not FDA approved.

depressant effects may result when antihistamines are combined with alcohol, narcotic analgesics, tricyclic antidepressants, and other CNS depressants.

### *Panic Disorder With Agoraphobia*

For several years, panic disorder has been effectively treated with either the tricyclic antidepressant, imipramine or the monoamine oxidase inhibitor, phenelzine. Presently, several additional agents including the benzodiazepines are undergoing extensive study for the treatment of panic disorder (Table 51.10). Most clinicians combine antipanic medications with behavioral therapy, and approximately 85% of the patients report moderate to marked global improvement.[75–77] Antipanic medications enhance behavioral therapy, which is most effective in patients whose panic disorder is under pharmacologic control.[75–77]

#### Nonpharmacologic Therapy

Most patients require behavioral therapy to alleviate their phobic-avoidance behavior. The antiphobic but not the antipanic properties of behavioral therapy are well researched.[75–77] Patients often acknowledge that although their panic attacks no longer occur, their fears and avoidance (or agoraphobia) of situations remain firm.

Behavioral therapy requires patients to confront the phobic situations gradually, starting with the least feared situation and working up.[78] Once the panic attacks are controlled with medications, patients learn they can reenter phobic situations without having a panic attack.

Although approximately one third of the panic patients with agoraphobia show clinically noticeable improvement with behavioral therapy alone,[75–77] most clinicians believe a combination of antipanic drugs and behavioral therapy is the most effective treatment approach. If the patient is not on medication, panic attacks may be experienced during desensitization (physical exposure), further reinforcing avoidance behavior. For patients who cannot or will not take medication, behavioral treatment alone is certainly indicated.

#### Tricyclic Antidepressants

Several double-blind, placebo-controlled studies have demonstrated the efficacy of imipramine in blocking panic attacks.[75–77,79,80] All studies used concomitant behavioral therapy to assist in the management of the phobic-avoidance behavior.

In 1978, Zitrin and associates[75] reported that imipramine effectively blocked panic attacks within 3 to 5 weeks, in patients with panic disorder with agoraphobia. But maximal improvement (including antiphobic response) did not become evident until 6 to 10 weeks. In the absence of panic attacks, the anticipatory anxiety level diminished, followed by decreased phobic avoidance. Approximately 18% of the imipramine-treated patients experienced stimulatory (amphetamine-like) side effects that prevented a medication increase and interfered with overall treatment outcome.

Reducing the dose often eliminated the unpleasant effects. Approximately 30% of the imipramine-treated agoraphobic patients (versus 9% in the placebo group) dropped out of the study. During the 12-month follow-up, 30% of the imipramine-treated agoraphobic patients relapsed versus 14% of those receiving placebo.

Although imipramine is the only tricyclic antidepressant studied using controlled conditions, all agents in this class may be effective; however, trazodone and amoxapine may be less effective than the other antidepressants.[81]

### Monoamine Oxidase Inhibitors

The majority of studies assessing the efficacy of the monoamine oxidase inhibitors in the treatment of panic disorder were poorly designed and lacked sufficient dosage and duration of treatment, sufficient sample size, and valid ratings of panic attacks.[24] Sheehan et al[13] conducted the most definitive trial comparing phenelzine (45 mg/d) and imipramine (150 mg/d) with placebo. Both drugs were found effective and superior to placebo on a variety of measures (phobic anxiety, fears, general anxiety, agoraphobic avoidance, work and social disability), with a slight edge for phenelzine on several scales. As with imipramine, the initial response to phenelzine was often delayed and did not become maximal for 6 to 10 weeks.

### Alprazolam and Other Benzodiazepines

Until recently benzodiazepines did not appear effective in blocking panic attacks or preventing phobic-avoidance behaviors, although they decreased anticipatory anxiety. This assumption was based on the clinical observation that patients receiving benzodiazepines continued to have panic attacks that subsequently cleared, after imipramine treatment; however, recent preliminary trials suggest that alprazolam, diazepam, and clonazepam are possibly effective in treating panic disorder with agoraphobia when taken in sufficiently high doses (Table 51.10).[82–86] Presently, alprazolam is the best researched and most widely used benzodiazepine for the treatment of panic disorder.[82–84]

Sheehan and associates[82] reported results of a single-blind, 8-week study comparing alprazolam and ibuprofen. Patients receiving alprazolam (mean daily dose 5.4 mg) significantly improved, but those on ibuprofen did not. Depression as a symptom did not respond. Alprazolam's antipanic response was rapid (some responded within the first week) and appeared dose related. The most frequently reported side effect was drowsiness.

Preliminary results from a large multicenter, double-blind, placebo-controlled trial of alprazolam (mean dose 5.6 mg/d) in 560 patients with panic disorder and agoraphobia with panic attacks have been reported.[83] Significantly greater reductions in panic attacks, phobia, anxiety, and work and social disability were reported in the alprazolam group compared with the placebo group. Alprazolam was well tolerated, with less than a 5% dropout rate secondary to side effects. Sedation was the principal side effect reported, but improved over time.

Several reports of the efficacy of clonazepam in treating panic disorder with agoraphobia have been published.[85,86] Study results appear promising with doses of 3–6 mg/d. The most frequently reported side effects were depression and initial nausea. Tolerance to the therapeutic effects did not develop over the study period of 12 months. No serious adverse consequences were encountered. Because of its long half-life (20–40 hours), clonazepam can be administered in a twice-daily dosage schedule with less risk of rebound anxiety and withdrawal symptomatology than other short-acting benzodiazepines.[86] Controlled studies are needed to assess more accurately the use of clonazepam in the treatment of panic and agoraphobic patients.

### Clinical Guidelines

Effective therapeutic agents in the treatment of panic disorder with agoraphobia include the tricyclic antidepressant imipramine, the monoamine oxidase inhibitor phenelzine, and the benzodiazepine alprazolam.

***Selection of Initial Drug Therapy*** All three drugs (imipramine, phenelzine, alprazolam) appear equally effective, although controlled trials comparing them are needed. (The FDA has not approved product labeling for any drug for the treatment of panic disorder.) Clinicians generally select the initial drug using the following clinical indicators: onset of therapeutic effect, acute and chronic side effects, problems with drug withdrawal, certain individual characteristics (e.g., presence of depression, age, previous drug history), and drug costs.

A clear disadvantage of phenelzine is patient acceptance. Patients fear side effects and are apprehensive about the dietary restrictions associated with the monoamine oxidase inhibitors.[81,87] Therefore imipramine or alprazolam is frequently the first drug selected. Problems with imipramine are well documented and include stimulatory or amphetamine-like side effects with symptom worsening, a lag time of 3 to 5 weeks before an antipanic response occurs, a lag time of up to 12 weeks before an antiphobic effect is maximal, and toxicity when taken in an overdose. For patients who cannot tolerate the anticholinergic side effects of imipramine, a switch to desipramine may be helpful.[88] Imipramine is available as a generic product and is the least expensive antipanic drug marketed.

Problems associated with the use of alprazolam are not as clearly defined as those with the antidepressants. Patient acceptance of alprazolam is not usually a problem and, except for sedation, side effects are rarely reported.[81] Significant antipanic response has been observed within the first week or two of therapy.[82–84] Alprazolam should be used cautiously in patients whose illness is complicated by depression.[81,82] Antidepressants are probably superior to alprazolam and other benzodiazepines in managing concurrent depression. Antidepressants should be selected first for patients who are clinically depressed or have a family history of depression. A recent report[89] noted that 33% of patients with panic disorder treated with alprazolam 3–10 mg/d developed symptoms consistent with DSM-III criteria for major depression despite symptom remission. No patient met criteria for major depression at the beginning of the study. Therefore, all panic patients receiving alprazolam should be monitored for symptoms of depression. Continued research on potential withdrawal complications after long-term use will further define alprazolam's role in treating these patients. Alprazolam is not available as a generic drug and is the most expensive antipanic drug to use.

*Initiation of Therapy* The guiding principle for using imipramine and phenelzine in panic disorder is to start low, push high, and treat for an appropriate period of time.[81] Side effects often interfere seriously with the buildup of optimal dosage, compromising treatment response and contributing to patient noncompliance.[75–77]

With imipramine, treatment can be initiated with 10–25 mg/d at bedtime and slowly increased as tolerated to 100–200 mg/d over a 2- to 4-week period.[81] Although an occasional patient will respond to 50 mg/d or less, most require at least 150 mg/d,[80] or a plasma concentration of 100–150 ng/mL.[90] If this dose is not effective, a higher dose (up to 300 mg/d) should be used.[90,91] When stimulatory side effects occur, the dose should be decreased until the symptoms subside; then slow medication increase can be resumed. Many of these symptoms resolve if treatment continues longer than 2 to 3 weeks. The principal side effects are anticholinergic (e.g., dry mouth, blurred vision, and tachycardia).[81]

The starting dose of phenelzine is 15 mg/d, increased by 15 mg/d every 3 to 4 days until 60 mg/d is reached. A dose of less than 45 mg/d is rarely effective. Dosages may be increased (up to 90 mg/d) if improvement is not achieved after 8 to 12 weeks.[81,87] If a patient has previously been receiving a tricyclic agent, 1 to 2 weeks should lapse before phenelzine is started to prevent any potential drug interaction between the tricyclic agent and phenelzine. Anticholinergic side effects are less severe than with the tricyclic agents, but postural hypotension and insomnia are often more of a problem. After 3 weeks, most of the unpleasant side effects subside.[81]

Hypertensive crisis after the ingestion of tyramine-containing foods or sympathomimetic drugs is the most serious, potentially life-threatening event encountered with phenelzine. Symptoms include a severe headache, usually accompanied by throbbing, flushing, and a heavy thumping of the heart. Patients should be instructed that if symptoms occur, they must go immediately to the nearest emergency room. They must never lie down, as this only increases intracranial pressure. (Refer to Chapter 50 for a complete list of the food and drug restrictions and a more complete discussion of side effects.) Patients should be counseled and given a printed list of these restrictions. Patients should observe the food, drink, and drug restrictions for at least 24 hours before starting the first dose of phenelzine, and for 2 weeks after stopping therapy.

The starting dose of alprazolam is 0.25 or 0.50 mg/d in two or three divided doses, which is slowly increased over several weeks. During the initial weeks of therapy, patients may pass through two or three dosage plateaus followed by some tolerance to side effects and some loss of benefit before reaching a final ideal dose. Patients have been responsive to doses as low as 1.5–2.0 mg/d.[81] Most patients require 3–6 mg/d, although others may need doses of 6–10 mg/d to maximize response.[82,83] Patients appear to tolerate the initial side effects of alprazolam (e.g., sedation) much better than those of imipramine and phenelzine. If the dose becomes too high, a mild intoxication (incoordination, slurred speech, disinhibition) may be encountered.[91]

*Termination of Therapy* Optimal length of therapy is unknown, and most patients continue to improve for 6 to 10 months, then slow medication taper may be initiated over a 1- to 3-month period. The most frequently encountered problem is relapse or reemergence of panic attacks in approximately 30%.[81] Reinstitution of medication usually results in renewed clinical response. After 3 months, medication taper may be attempted again. Many patients may be successfully tapered off medication during the second year of therapy.[81,90]

Withdrawal symptoms (as discussed under Benzodiazepines) may be observed with alprazolam if this medication is suddenly discontinued or tapered too rapidly. The tapering of alprazolam dosage should be individualized; some panic patients are able to tolerate decreases of only 0.25 mg or less per week.

*Patient Education* Many patients are reluctant to take medications for fear that drugs will worsen their illness or that they will become addicted. Side effects are often perceived as a worsening of the illness and may contribute to noncompliance and prevent necessary medication increases. Patients should be informed regarding the lag time before a therapeutic response is evident. Patients taking phenelzine should be instructed about possible food and drug interactions. Patients who receive alprazolam or another benzodiazepine should be told not to decrease or discontinue therapy unless authorized by their physician.

### Summary

Many advances have been made in the treatment of panic disorder with agoraphobia. Panic disorder is classified as a separate disease state and not simply a more severe form of generalized anxiety disorder. The efficacy of imipramine and phenelzine in treating panic attacks has been known since the early 1960s; however, the clinical use and important aspects of patient education are just now being fully appreciated. Although the benzodiazepine alprazolam appears to be an effective antipanic agent, problems with drug withdrawal may limit its long-term use in some patients.

## *Other Anxiety Disorders*

### Simple and Social Phobias

Simple phobic patients are not responsive to drugs, although they are highly responsive to behavioral therapy.[75,77,91] The use of antidepressant medications may be detrimental in patients with simple phobia.

Although there is no established treatment for social phobia, some patients may respond to monoamine oxidase inhibitors or $\beta$-blocking agents,[91,92] while benzodiazepines and tricyclic antidepressants are believed to have limited value.[92] Evidence to support the use of $\beta$-blocking drugs in treating social phobia comes from reports of their positive effect on performance anxiety.[91] Propranolol 40 mg 1 hour before the performance may be quite helpful, as physical symptoms of anxiety frequently add to the patient's distress. Three types of behavioral treatment (desensitization or exposure, social skills training, cognitive restructuring) have been found useful in controlled studies. No comparisons of various behavior therapies or pharmacologic treatments have been conducted.[26]

### Obsessive–Compulsive Disorder

Obsessive–compulsive disorder is the most difficult anxiety disorder to treat. This disorder is profoundly disabling and refractory to most traditional psychologic treatments; however, psychotherapy is still the treatment of choice in obsessive–compulsive disorder uncomplicated by depression. When depression is a feature, antidepressants should be added as adjunctive therapy.[15] Other psychotropic agents (e.g., antipsychotic agents and benzodiazepines) should be avoided.[15]

Clomipramine, an antidepressant, marketed as Anafranil (Ciba) in several foreign countries, may have unique effects in the treatment of obsessive–compulsive disorder and is presently in Phase III clinical trials in the United States for this disorder. Clomipramine may have an antiobsessive effect that is at least partially independent of its antidepressant effect.[93] A response rate of about 50% for clomipramine in carefully controlled studies is typical; the placebo response rate is less than 10%.[94]

### Posttraumatic Stress Disorder

The treatment of posttraumatic stress disorder is quite difficult. Behavioral therapy is often used in conjunction with drug treatment. Antipsychotic agents, benzodiazepines, propranolol, and lithium have been tried, usually with limited success.[95] Antidepressants may be the treatment of choice because of posttraumatic stress disorder's shared symptomatology with panic disorder and depression.[95] Additional controlled trials in patients with posttraumatic stress disorder are warranted.

## Summary

Theories about anxiety disorders have undergone major revisions over the past several years. Anxiety disorders are quite common, occurring in approximately 4% to 8% of the population. The proper management of anxiety disorders begins with the correct diagnosis; not all patients should receive antianxiety agents. Nonpharmacologic interventions are often effective alone or when combined with drug therapy.

The current classification for anxiety disorders includes several subtypes. The diagnosis determines the type of drug and nonpharmacologic intervention selected. While benzodiazepines remain the drugs of choice for generalized anxiety disorder and situational anxiety, other agents may be preferable for other types of anxiety. The new anxiolytic agent buspirone may prove useful for patients who need chronic therapy for generalized anxiety disorder or who cannot tolerate benzodiazepines. Antidepressants (imipramine and phenelzine) are extensively used in patients with panic disorder with agoraphobia. The benzodiazepine alprazolam has recently been shown to be effective in this illness. The pharmacologic treatment of other anxiety disorder types (i.e., phobic disorders, obsessive–compulsive disorder, and posttraumatic stress disorder) is not as well studied and further research is needed to better define the most appropriate treatment.

## References

1. Robins LN, Helzer JE, Weissman MM, et al. Lifetime prevalence of specific psychiatric disorders in three sites. Arch Gen Psychiatry 1984;41:949–958.
2. Weissman MM. The epidemiology of anxiety disorders: rates, risks, and familial patterns, in Tuma AH, Maser JD (eds): Anxiety and the Anxiety Disorders. Hillsdale, NJ, Lawrence Erlbaum Associates, 1985, pp 275–296.
3. Cameron OG. The differential diagnosis of anxiety: Psychiatric and medical disorders. Psychiatr Clin North Am 1985;8:3–23.
4. Schuckit MA. Anxiety related to medical disease. J Clin Psychiatry 1983;44:31–36.
5. Hayes PE, Dommisse CS. Current concepts in clinical therapeutics: Anxiety disorders, part I. Clin Pharm 1987;6:140–147.
6. Cassem NH, Hackett TP. Psychological aspects of myocardial infarction. Med Clin North Am 1977;61:711–721.
7. Weiner, H. The psychobiology and pathophysiology of anxiety and fear, in Tuma AH, Maser JD (eds): Anxiety and the Anxiety Disorders. Hillsdale, NJ, Lawrence Erlbaum Associates, 1985, pp 333–354.
8. Hoehn-Saric R, McLeod DR. Generalized anxiety disorder. Psychiatr Clin North Am 1985;8:73–88.
9. American Psychiatric Association. Diagnostic and Statistical Manual of Mental Disorders, 3rd ed (DSM-III). Washington DC, American Psychiatric Association, 1980.
10. American Psychiatric Association. Diagnostic and Statistical Manual of Mental Disorders, 3rd ed, revised (DSM-III-R). Washington DC; American Psychiatric Association, 1987.
11. Klein DF, Fink M. Psychiatric reaction patterns to imipramine. Am J Psychiatry 1962;119:432–438.
12. Pitts FN, McClure JN. Lactate metabolism in anxiety neurosis. New Engl J Med 1967;277:1329–1336.
13. Sheehan DV, Ballenger JC, Jacobsen G. Treatment of endogenous anxiety with phobic, hysterical and hypochondriacal symptoms. Arch Gen Psychiatry 1980;37:51–59.
14. Agras WS. Stress, panic, and the cardiovascular system, in Tuma AH, Maser JD (eds): Anxiety and the Anxiety Disorders. Hillsdale, NJ, Lawrence Erlbaum Associates, 1985, pp 1363–1368.
15. Lelliott PT, Monteiro WO. Drug treatment of obsessive–compulsive disorder. Drugs 1986;31:75–80.
16. Redmond DE, Huang YH. New evidence for a locus coeruleus–norepinephrine connection with anxiety. Life Sci 1979;25:2149–2162.
17. Sanghera MK, McMillan BA, German CD. Buspirone, a non-benzodiazepine anxiolytic, increases locus coeruleus noradrenergic neuronal activity. Eur J Pharmacol 1983;86:107–110.
18. Charney DS, Heninger GR, Breier A. Noradrenergic function in panic anxiety. Arch Gen Psychiatry 1984;41:751–763.
19. Charney DS, Heninger GR. Noradrenergic function and the mechanism of action of antianxiety treatment. I. The effect of

long-term alprazolam treatment. Arch Gen Psychiatry 1985;42: 458–467.

20. Moehler H, Okada T. Benzodiazepine receptor: Demonstration in the central nervous system. Science 1977;198:849–851.
21. Skolnick P, Paul SM. Benzodiazepine receptors in the central nervous system. Int Rev Neurobiol 1982;23:103–140.
22. Greenblatt DJ, Shader RI, Abernathy DR. Current status of benzodiazepines, part I. N Engl J Med 1983;309:354–358.
23. Schatzberg AF, Cole JO (eds): Antianxiety agents, in Manual of Clinical Psychopharmacology. Washington DC, American Psychiatric Press, 1986, pp 139–171.
24. Dommisse CS, Hayes PE. Current concepts in clinical therapeutics: Anxiety disorders, part II. Clin Pharm 1987;6:196–215.
25. File SE. Neurochemistry of anxiety, in Burrows GD, Norman TR, Davies B (eds): Drugs in Psychiatry, vol II, Antianxiety Agents. Amsterdam, Elsevier, 1984, pp 13–32.
26. Griffiths RR, McLeod DR, Bigelow GE, et al. Comparison of diazepam and oxazepam: Preference, liking and extent of abuse. J Pharmacol Exp Ther 1984;229:501–508.
27. Saleto B. Early clinical pharmacology of tranquilizers, in Hippius H, Winokur G (eds): Clinical Psychopharmacology, part II. Amsterdam, Excerpta Medica, 1983, pp 97–122.
28. Dawson GW, Jue SG, Brogden RN. Alprazolam: A review of its pharmacodynamic properties and efficacy in the treatment of anxiety and depression. Drugs 1984;27:132–147.
29. Greenblatt DJ, Shader RI, Abernathy DR. Current status of benzodiazepines, part II. New Engl J Med 1983;309:410–416.
30. Sedman AJ. Cimetidine drug interactions. Am J Med 1984;76: 109–114.
31. Klotz U, Antilla VJ, Reimann I. Cimetidine/diazepam interactions. Lancet 1979;2:699.
32. Desmond PV, Patwardhan RV, Schenker S, et al. Cimetidine impairs the elimination of chlordiazepoxide in man. Ann Intern Med 1980;93:266–268.
33. Abernathy DR, Greenblatt DJ, Divoll M, et al. Interaction of cimetidine with the triazolobenzodiazepines alprazolam and triazolam. Psychopharmacology 1983;80:275–278.
34. Greenblatt DJ, Abernathy DR, Koepke HH, et al. Interaction of cimetidine with oxazepam, lorazepam, and flurazepam. J Clin Pharmacol 1984;24:187–193.
35. Greenblatt DJ, Abernathy DR, Morse DS, et al. Clinical importance of the interaction of diazepam and cimetidine. N Engl J Med 1984;310:1639–1643.
36. Abernathy DR, Greenblatt DJ, Eshelman FN, et al. Ranitidine does not impair oxidative or conjugative metabolism: Noninteraction with antipyrine, diazepam and lorazepam. Clin Pharmacol Ther 1984;35:188–192.
37. Roth T, Hartse KM, Saab PG, et al. The effects of flurazepam, lorazepam and triazolam on sleep and memory. Psychopharmacology 1980;70:231–237.
38. Scharf MB, Khosla N, Lysaght R, et al. Anterograde amnesia with oral lorazepam. J Clin Psychiatry 1983;44:362–364.
39. Busto U, Sellers EM, Naranjo CA, et al. Patterns of benzodiazepine abuse and dependence. Br J Addict 1986;81:87–94.
40. Fontaine R, Chouinard G, Annable L. Rebound anxiety in anxious patients after abrupt withdrawal of benzodiazepine treatment. Am J Psychiatry 1984;141:848–852.
41. Power KG, Jerrom DWA, Simpson RJ, et al. Controlled study of withdrawal symptoms and rebound anxiety after six week course of diazepam for generalized anxiety. Br Med J 1985;290: 1246–1248.
42. Higgit AC, Lader MH, Fonagy P. Clinical management of benzodiazepine dependence. Br Med J 1985;291:688–690.
43. Busto U, Sellers EM, Naranjo CA, et al. Withdrawal reaction after long-term therapeutic use of benzodiazepines. New Engl J Med 1986;315:854–859.
44. Upjohn Company. Xava package insert. Kalamazoo, MI, 1987, Jan.
45. Klein E, Udhe TW, Post RM. Preliminary evidence for the utility of carbamazepine in alprazolam withdrawal. Am J Psychiatry 1986;143:235–236.
46. Goa KL, Ward A. Buspirone: A preliminary review of its pharmacological properties and therapeutic efficacy as an anxiolytic. Drugs 1986;32:114–129.
47. Schweiser E, Rickels K. Failure of buspirone to manage benzodiazepine withdrawal. Am J Psychiatry 1986;143:1590–1592.
48. Lader M, Olajide D. A comparison of buspirone and placebo in relieving benzodiazepine withdrawal symptoms. J Clin Psychopharmacol 1987;7:11–15.
49. Goldberg HL, Finnerty R. Comparison of buspirone in two separate studies. J Clin Psychiatry 1982;43:87–91.
50. Jacobson AF, Dominguez RA, Goldstein BJ, et al. Comparison of buspirone and diazepam in generalized anxiety disorder. Pharmacotherapy 1985;5(5):290–296.
51. Rickels K, Weisman K, Norstad N, et al. Buspirone and diazepam in anxiety: A controlled study. J Clin Psychiatry 1981;43:81–86.
52. Pecknold JC, Familamiri P, Chang H, et al. Buspirone: anxiolytic? Prog Neuropsychopharmacol Biol Psychiatry 1985;9:639–642.
53. Wheatley D. Buspirone: Multicenter efficacy study. J Clin Psychiatry 1982;43:92–94.
54. Feighner JP, Merideth CH, Hendrickson GA. A double-blind comparison of buspirone and diazepam in outpatients with generalized anxiety disorder. J Clin Psychiatry 1982;43:103–107.
55. Cohn JB, Bowden CL, Fisher JG, et al. Double-blind comparison of buspirone and clorazepate in anxious outpatients. Am J Med 1986;10S–16S.
56. Cohn JB, Wilcox CS. Low-sedation potential of buspirone compared with alprazolam and lorazepam in the treatment of anxious patients: A double-blind study. J Clin Psychiatry 1986; 47:409–412.
57. Olajide D, Lader M. A double-blind comparison of buspirone and diazepam in outpatients with chronic anxiety. Proceedings of the 14th CINP, Florence, Italy, June 19–23, 1984.
58. Scheibe G, Buchheim P, Bender W, et al. Busiprone versus lorazepam: A double-blind study in outpatients with anxiety syndromes. Proceedings of the 14th CINP, Florence, Italy, June 19–23, 1984.
59. VanderMaelen CP, Matheson GK, Wilderman RC, et al. Inhibition of serotonergic dorsal raphe neurons by systemic and iontophoretic administration of buspirone, a non-benzodiazepine anxiolytic drug. Eur J Clin Pharmacol 1986;129:123–130.
60. Cimino M, Ponzio F, Achilli G, et al. Dopaminergic effects of buspirone, a novel anxiolytic agent. Biochem Pharmacol 1983; 32:1069–1074.
61. Gammans RE, Mayol RF, Labudde JA. Metabolism and disposition of buspirone. Am J Med 1986;80:41S–51S.
62. Mayol RF, Adamson DS, Gammans RE, et al. Pharmacokinetics and disposition of $^{14}$C-buspirone HCl after intravenous and oral dosing in man. Clin Pharmacol Ther 1985;37:210.
63. Gammans RE, Mayol RF, Mackenthun AV, et al. The relationship between buspirone bioavailability and dose in healthy subjects. Biopharm Drug Dispos 1985;6:139–145.
64. Temple DL, Yevich JP, New JS. Buspirone: Chemical profile of a new class of anxioselective agents. J Clin Psychiatry 1982; 43:4S–9S.
65. Bond A, Lader M, Shrotriya R. Comparative effects of a repeated dose regime of diazepam and buspirone on subjective ratings, psychological tests and the EEG. Eur J Clin Pharmacol 1983;24:463–467.

66. Newton RE, Marunycz JD, Alderdice MT, et al. Review of the side effect profile of buspirone. Am J Med 1986;80:17S–21S.
67. Mead Johnson Pharmaceutical Division/Bristol Myers. BuSpar package insert. Evansville, IN, 1986, Oct.
68. Mead Johnson Pharmaceutical Division/Bristol Myers. Monoamine oxidase inhibitor interaction information. Evansville, IN, 1987, March letter.
69. Tyrer P, Murphy S, Owen RT. The risk of pharmacological dependence with buspirone. Br J Clin Pract 1985;39:91–93.
70. Leonard BE. Neuropharmacological profile of buspirone: A non-benzodiazepine anxiolytic with specific mid-brain modulating properties. Br J Clin Pract 1985;39:74–81.
71. Cole JO, Orzack MH, Beake B, et al. Assessment of the abuse liability of buspirone in recreational sedative users. J Clin Psychiatry 1982;43:69–74.
72. Griffith JD, Josinski DR, Casten GP, et al. Assessment of the abuse liability of buspirone in alcohol-dependent patients. Am J Med 1986;80:30S–35S.
73. Noyes R. Beta-adrenergic blocking drugs in anxiety and stress. Psychiatric Clin North Am 1985;8:119–132.
74. Hayes PE, Schulz SC. Beta-blockers in anxiety disorders. J Affective Disorders 1987;13:119–130.
75. Zitrin CM, Klein DF, Woemer MG. Behavior therapy, supportive psychotherapy, imipramine and phobias. Arch Gen Psychiatry 1978;35:307–316.
76. Zitrin CM, Klein DF, Woemer MG. Treatment of agoraphobia with group exposure in vivo and imipramine. Arch Gen Psychiatry 1980;37:63–72.
77. Zitrin CM, Klein DF, Woemer MG, et al. Treatment of phobias: I. Comparison of imipramine and placebo. Arch Gen Psychiatry 1983;40:125–138.
78. Mavissakalian M. Exposure treatment of agoraphobia, in Grinspoon L (ed): American Psychiatric Association, Annual review, vol 3. Washington DC, American Psychiatric Press, 1983, pp 448–460.
79. Klein DF, Zitrin CM, Woerner MG, et al. Treatment of phobias: II. Behavior therapy and supportive therapy: Are there any specific ingredients? Arch Gen Psychiatry 1983;40:139–145.
80. Mavissakalian M, Perel JM. Imipramine in the treatment of agoraphobia: Dose–response relationships. Am J Psychiatry 1985;142:1032–1036.
81. Ballenger JC. Pharmacotherapy of the panic disorders. J Clin Psychiatry 1986;47:27S–32S.
82. Sheehan DV, Coleman JH, Greenblatt DJ, et al. Some biological correlates of panic attacks with agoraphobia and their response to a new treatment. J Clin Psychopharmacol 1984;4:66–75.
83. Ballenger JC, Rubin R, DuPont R, et al. Treatment of agoraphobia/panic disorder with alprazolam: Preliminary results from a large multicenter placebo-controlled trial. Presented to the Annual NCDEU Meeting, Key Biscayne, Florida, April, 1985.
84. Dunner DL, Ishiki D, Avery DH, et al. Effect of alprazolam on anxiety and panic attacks in panic disorder: A controlled study. J Clin Psychiatry 1986;47:458–460.
85. Spier S, Tesar G, Rosenbaum JF, et al. Clonazepam in the treatment of panic disorder and agoraphobia. J Clin Psychiatry 1986;47:238–242.
86. Pollack MH, Tesar GE, Rosenbaum JF, et al. Clonazepam in the treatment of panic disorder and agoraphobia: A one-year follow-up. J Clin Psychopharmacol 1986;6:302–304.
87. Sheehan DV, Claycomb JB, Kouretas N. Monoamine oxidase inhibitors: Prescription and patient management. Int J Psychiatry Med 1980–1981;10:99–121.
88. Muskin PR, Fyer AJ. Treatment of panic disorder. J Clin Psychopharmacol 1981;1:81–90.
89. Lydiard RD, Laraia MT, Ballenger JC, et al. Emergence of depressive symptoms in patients receiving alprazolam for panic disorder. Am J Psychiatry 1987;144:664–665.
90. Ballenger JC, Peterson GA, Laraia MT, et al. A study of plasma catecholamines in agoraphobia and the relationship of serum tricyclic levels to treatment response, in Ballenger JC (ed): Biology of Agoraphobia. Washington DC, American Psychiatric Press, 1984, pp 27–64.
91. Noyes R, Chaudry DR, Domingo DV. Pharmacologic treatment of phobic disorder. J Clin Psychiatry 1986;47:445–452.
92. Liebowitz MR, Fyer AB, Gorman JM, et al. Phenelzine in social phobia. J Clin Psychopharmacol 1986;6:93–97.
93. Mavissakalian M, Turner SM, Michelson L, et al. Tricyclic antidepressants in obsessive–compulsive disorder: antiobsessional or antidepressant agents? Am J Psychiatry 1985;142:572–576.
94. Insel PR, Mueller EA, Gillin JC, et al. Tricyclic response in obsessive–compulsive disorder. Prog Neuropsychopharmacol Biol Psychiatry 1985;9:25–31.
95. vanderKolk BA. Psychopharmacological issues in posttraumatic stress disorder. Hospital and Community Psychiatry 1983;34:683–691.

# Chapter 52 / Sleep Disorders

Michael Z. Wincor, PharmD

## Sleep Physiology

Although we spend about one third of our lives sleeping, most of us take this psychophysiologic phenomenon for granted. This chapter will briefly review the nature of normal sleep and describe the epidemiology, classification, pathophysiology, clinical features, and management of a number of major sleep disorders. Before describing sleep, it should be noted that we definitely require sleep, although we do not know why, and that exact sleep needs vary greatly among individuals.

Sleep has been studied in various ways. Behaviorally, one can observe changes in an organism with respect to body position, responsiveness to external stimuli, and eyelid closure. Anatomically, sleep-regulating centers in the brain stem have been identified. Neurochemically, various neurotransmitters are involved in sleep mechanisms (e.g., norepinephrine appears to be involved in wakefulness and dreaming sleep, while serotonin appears to be involved in nondreaming sleep). In addition, there is evidence of an interaction between the cholinergic system and the noradrenergic system as well as contributions by various other neurotransmitters, including several endogenous peptides.[1]

### Electrophysiology and Sleep Stages

Currently, the standard method for observing and measuring sleep is electrophysiologic in nature. In the laboratory, sleep is recorded polygraphically, with electroencephalograms (EEGs), electrooculograms (EOGs) from both eyes, and electromyograms (EMGs) generally of the mentalis and submentalis muscles.[2] Two EOGs, one EEG, and one EMG would be the minimal recordings utilized in scoring sleep stages. In addition, several other physiologic measures may be necessary, as will be discussed.

Wakefulness is characterized by an EEG of low voltage, fast activity, random eye movements and blinks, and relatively high muscle tone. The EEG of stage 1 sleep is described as low voltage, mixed frequency (relatively slower than that found in wakefulness). Slow-rolling eye movements and a muscle tone lower than that of wakefulness are observed. The subjective experience of stage 1 sleep varies widely among individuals; some experience it as wakefulness, others as drowsiness, and yet others as sleep. Stage 2 sleep is characterized by an EEG that continues to be relatively low voltage, mixed frequency but with two particular waveforms known as "spindles" and "K complexes"; muscle tone is somewhat lower than that of stage 1.

Stages 3 and 4 continue with low muscle tone and are characterized by high-amplitude, slow activity in the EEG known as delta waves; hence, these two stages together are often referred to as delta sleep. A major difference between the two stages is simply the percentage of delta waves per unit of recording. Stages 1–4 are collectively known as non–rapid eye movement (NREM) sleep, distinguishing them from rapid eye movement (REM) sleep.

REM sleep is characterized by a low-voltage, mixed-frequency EEG (similar in many respects to that of stage 1), very low muscle tone (as low as or lower than that seen in any other stage of sleep), and bursts of bilaterally conjugate rapid eye movements (as though the sleeper is watching a movie or actively observing some activity). Classical dreaming occurs during REM sleep and dream reports can be obtained 80% to 90% of the time when subjects are awakened during or at the end of REM periods.

### Sleep Cycle

The architecture of sleep in the normal young adult is cyclic. From wakefulness, the sleeper quickly passes through stages 1 and 2, spending a moderate block of time in delta sleep. Some 90 minutes after sleep onset, the sleeper enters the first REM period of the night, which may last only 5 to 7 minutes. The cycle is repeated four to five times each night, with relatively predictable variations. As the night progresses, less time is spent in delta sleep; most delta sleep occurs in the first half of the night. REM periods become longer and more intense, both physiologically and psychologically, as the night progresses. The final REM period of the night may last 30 to 60 minutes. In general, one spends approximately 75% of the night in NREM sleep and the remaining 25% in REM sleep.

In the elderly, however, the typical sleep architecture just described may be quite different, with a considerable decrease in delta sleep, an increase in light sleep, an increase in awakenings, and a generally more disrupted night of sleep.[3] There may be a slight decrease in total sleep time during the night compared with young adults. The contribution of daytime napping and specific sleep pathology (e.g., sleep apnea and nocturnal myoclonus) to this apparent decrease in sleep is unclear. In randomly selected, noncomplaining, elderly individuals, the incidence of sleep apnea and nocturnal myoclonus may be as high as 40%.[4]

Those parameters that can be measured objectively in the sleep laboratory and are of particular relevance to sleep disorders and drug effects on sleep are listed in Table 52.1.

Latency to sleep onset is defined as the amount of time taken to fall asleep after going to bed. The number of awakenings and number of stage shifts during the night indicate how disrupted sleep has been. REM intensity, or the frequency of bursts of rapid eye movements, may at times be a more subtle indicator of changes in REM sleep than simply

**Table 52.1** Sleep Parameters

| |
|---|
| Latency to sleep onset |
| Total sleep time |
| Sleep stage duration |
| Sleep stage percentage of total sleep time |
| Number of awakenings during the night |
| Number of stage shifts during the night |
| REM intensity |
| Other physiologic measurements |

the total number of minutes spent in REM sleep during the night. Finally, other physiologic measurements may include electrocardiogram, respiration, oxygen saturation, and activity of the anterior tibialis muscles.

### *Classification of Sleep Disorders*

In the 1970s, a group of clinically oriented sleep researchers organized the Association of Sleep Disorders Centers. This group developed a complete scheme for classifying sleep disorders.[5] Only a basic outline is given in Table 52.2. A modified outline can be found in Appendix E of the *Diagnostic and Statistical Manual of Mental Disorders, Third Edition* (DSM-III) published in 1980 by the American Psychiatric Association; however, this outline is not included in the revised edition (DSM-III-R). Sleep disorder clinicians have had the opportunity to work with the current classification for several years, and there is an international effort under way for revision and modification. The revised classification scheme is expected to be finalized no earlier than 1988.

Disorders of initiating and maintaining sleep (DIMS) are equivalent to insomnia, whereas disorders of excessive somnolence (DOES) are equivalent to excessive daytime sleepiness. Disorders of the sleep–wake schedule involve disturbances of biologic rhythms, and the parasomnias include a number of miscellaneous disorders. There is a considerable amount of overlap with respect to possible etiologies among the major categories of disorders, with the exception of the parasomnias. The determining factor in defining a patient's sleep problem is often the nature of the subjective complaint (i.e., "Doctor, I'm not sleeping well at night" versus "Doctor, I'm always sleepy").

## Parasomnias

Although a number of miscellaneous sleep disorders have been identified (Table 52.3), only three—somnambulism, night terrors, and nightmares[6]—are discussed here. For a discussion of enuresis, refer to Chapter 45.

**Table 52.2** Classification of Sleep and Arousal Disorders

| |
|---|
| Disorders of initiating and maintaining sleep (DIMS) |
| Disorders of excessive somnolence (DOES) |
| Disorders of the sleep–wake schedule |
| Disorders associated with sleep, sleep stages, or partial arousals (parasomnias) |

Compiled from Reference 5.

**Table 52.3** Parasomnias

| |
|---|
| Sleepwalking (somnambulism) |
| Sleep terror (pavor nocturnus) |
| Sleep-related enuresis |
| Nightmares |
| Sleep-related bruxism |
| Sleep-related headbanging |

### *Somnambulism*

Somnambulism (sleepwalking) is generally a delta sleep phenomenon. About 15% of children are reported to have had at least one sleepwalking episode, compared with 2% to 5% of the general adult population. Although the individual appears to be navigating fairly well, there is significant impairment of critical skills and reactivity. Fortunately, the disorder is usually "outgrown." Treatment consists primarily of protecting the individual from injury. Theoretically, sleepwalking may be prevented by suppressing delta sleep. Although most benzodiazepines suppress delta sleep, the benefit of treatment over simple protection from injury is questionable because of the unknown risks of long-term, continuous exposure of a developing child to delta sleep suppressants.[6]

### *Night Terrors*

Pavor nocturnus (sleep terrors or night terrors) is reported to be a problem in 1% to 3% of children. It generally occurs in delta sleep and is characterized by extreme vocalizations, motility, and autonomic changes. Fortunately for the sleeper, recall of frightening content is minimal or absent. Usually, the parents of a child with night terrors are considerably more disturbed by the events than the sleeper. Although the sleeper may awaken with tachycardia and be moist from perspiration, the absence of frightening content results in nothing psychologic with which to associate the event. Again, treatment consists primarily of waiting until the disorder is "outgrown." Reservations regarding the use of delta sleep suppressants also apply for this disorder.[6]

### *Nightmares*

Nightmares ("bad dreams") are a current problem for 5% of the general population. Nightmares, unlike night terrors, are a REM phenomenon and are associated with frequent and elaborate recall of "frightening dream" content. There is actually less motility and less variability in autonomic parameters in nightmares than in night terrors. Once REM suppressant drug withdrawal is ruled out as a causative factor, the usual treatment consists of psychologic intervention. This may be as simple as a parent providing comfort and reassurance to a child with an occasional nightmare or as complex as intensive psychotherapy for an adult with frequent, highly disturbing nightmares.[6]

## Sleep Apnea

### *Definition/Overview*

Generally, sleep apnea has an onset in adulthood, usually over the age of 30, and is more prevalent in men.[7] In addition, approximately 40% of the elderly may have sleep apnea.[8] Many persons with sleep apnea, especially the elderly, are asymptomatic (i.e., they have no complaints that would have brought this condition to the attention of a physician or sleep disorder specialist).

Sleep apnea is a condition characterized by repeated episodes of cessation of breathing.[7] After each apneic episode, there is a very brief arousal during which breathing resumes. These arousals are often called "mini-arousals," as the patient may be unaware of them even though the EEG clearly indicates activation. In severe cases, there may be as many as several hundred "mini-arousals" during a single night. Symptoms may include morning headache, irritability, and general difficulty with daytime functioning. Often, the bed partner reports that the patient snored very loudly, stopped breathing, and then gasped for air. There often is a history of recent weight gain associated with the onset of symptoms. Common complications of sleep apnea include arrhythmias, systolic or diastolic hypertension, and signs of pulmonary arterial hypertension and right ventricular failure.

There are three types of sleep apnea: obstructive, central, and mixed. Obstructive sleep apnea is caused by something obstructing the airway. The problem may be as simple as the tongue falling back across the airway or enlarged tonsils. Electrophysiologic recording of both nasal/oral airflow and thoracic respiratory effort demonstrates that airflow stops while respiratory effort continues. In central sleep apnea, the problem may reside in the respiratory centers of the brain stem in that respiratory effort ceases and, as a result, nasal/oral airflow stops as well. In mixed sleep apnea, typically central respiratory effort stops, the airway becomes obstructed, and then even when respiratory effort resumes, there is no airflow. In any of these cases, as oxygen saturation falls (which can be measured by means of an earlobe oximeter), the brain automatically produces a "mini-arousal" that results in resumption of breathing. The complaint by the patient, insomnia versus excessive daytime sleepiness, is quite subjective; however, obstructive sleep apnea appears to be more highly associated with complaints of excessive daytime sleepiness, whereas central apnea appears to be more closely associated with complaints of insomnia.[7]

### *Treatment*

Treatment differs with the type of sleep apnea under consideration. For the obstructive type, sometimes simple weight loss is sufficient to eliminate the problem. Unfortunately, weight reduction may result in only limited improvement.[7] Removal of enlarged tonsils may be the necessary intervention. When life-threatening complications of repeated episodes of hypoxemia (e.g., arrhythmias, pulmonary hypertension, right ventricular failure) are of concern, a tracheostomy may be the intervention of choice. Patients may go about their daily activities with the opening plugged and then remove the plug during sleep. Immediately after tracheostomy, some individuals describe a phenomenal change in how they feel. A more complicated surgical procedure, uvulopalatopharyngoplasty (UPPP), has been performed successfully in about 50% of patients; it involves surgical enlargement of the pharyngeal airspace. Unfortunately, in many cases, long-term follow-up has been lacking. A more recent, and very promising, approach is the use of nasal continuous positive airway pressure (nasal CPAP) throughout the night, but only a small number of patients have been successfully treated for long periods of time.[7]

The single most important pharmacologic intervention in the treatment of sleep apnea is the avoidance of all central nervous system (CNS) depressants (e.g., alcohol, anxiolytics, hypnotics, narcotics). Any agent that interferes with the brain's ability to produce an apnea-terminating "mini-arousal" is potentially lethal. Even drugs that show little or no effect on respiratory function during wakefulness could potentially interfere with the "mini-arousals." Active pharmacologic intervention has met with mixed and unpredictable results. Tricyclic antidepressants, particularly protriptyline (Vivactil) in a dose of 10 mg, have been used in the treatment of both obstructive and central sleep apnea.[9] This drug may act by decreasing REM sleep or by increasing the tonus of the musculature of the oropharynx. Respiratory stimulants, such as medroxyprogesterone[10] and acetazolamide,[11] have also been tried. These medications have only limited efficacy, and no studies have shown their long-term effectiveness.[7]

## Narcolepsy

### *Definition/Overview*

Narcolepsy typically begins before the age of 25 and continues for the remainder of life. The incidence of narcolepsy in the adult population is about 0.1%, with men and women being equally affected.[7]

Narcolepsy, in its classic form, has four cardinal features, which are listed in Table 52.4.[7,12] Narcoleptics fall asleep at some of the most inopportune times throughout the day and also have highly disturbed nighttime sleep. They are extremely sleepy most of the time, feel lethargic, have impaired performance, and generally feel miserable.

Cataplexy, present in about 70% to 80% of narcoleptics, is characterized by brief episodes of muscle weakness and/or paralysis that may cause the person to collapse, while remaining conscious. These episodes may last seconds to minutes. They are often precipitated by emotionally charged stimuli (e.g., laughter, anger, excitement).

Sleep paralysis and hypnagogic hallucinations occur in

**Table 52.4** Narcolepsy Tetrad

| |
|---|
| Excessive daytime sleepiness |
| Cataplexy |
| Sleep paralysis |
| Hypnagogic hallucinations |

about 25% to 50% of patients. These phenomena occur during the transition between wakefulness and sleep, and are very short (1 minute or less). Sleep paralysis is particularly frightening to the patient because the musculature is inhibited while the patient is still awake and, therefore, aware of the paralysis. Hypnagogic hallucinations are brief dreamlike experiences, but more fragmented and perhaps more bizarre than a typical dream.

Sleep laboratory evaluation of the narcoleptic confirms the existence of excessive sleepiness (with an ability to fall asleep very quickly at any time) and generally disturbed nighttime sleep, as well as sleep-onset REM periods. Although normal sleepers take an average of at least 90 minutes after sleep onset to reach the first REM period, narcoleptics can enter a REM period immediately after falling asleep. The occurrence of sleep paralysis, cataplexy, and sleep-onset REM periods has led to the conclusion that narcolepsy represents an abnormality in the regulatory mechanisms of REM sleep. It is clear that the etiology is not psychologic or epileptic. There appears to be a genetic predetermination manifested at puberty, perhaps by the action of a single gene.[7]

### *Treatment*

Treatment consists of both pharmacologic and nonpharmacologic interventions. Counseling the patient and significant others is a necessity. Often, the family, and even the patient, begin to think that the patient is a lazy, nonproductive member of society; they fail to recognize the crippling effects of narcolepsy. Long-term support groups exist locally and nationally for narcoleptics. Good sleep habits must be encouraged. If the patient's daily schedule allows, several daytime naps can be of immense benefit. After a 15- or 20-minute nap, the patient may feel relatively refreshed for several hours.

Pharmacologic treatment consists of two separate approaches—one directed toward the excessive daytime sleepiness and the other directed toward cataplexy.[13] For daytime sleepiness, CNS stimulants are employed. Most commonly, methylphenidate (Ritalin) is used at a starting dose of 2.5 mg twice daily; less often, pemoline (Cylert) may be prescribed in a dose of 18.75 mg/d. Amphetamines are generally avoided because of the higher risk of abuse, habituation, and tolerance. For the cataplexy, imipramine (Tofranil) had been used in the past, but currently protriptyline (Vivactil) at an initial dose of 5 mg/d is favored. The efficacy may, to some extent, be based on the anticholinergic activity of the agent. Although other tricyclic antidepressants are more anticholinergic than protriptyline, they are also more sedating. The rationale is to avoid further sedation of an already extemely sleepy individual. Finally, there has been interest in $\gamma$-hydroxybutyrate as a treatment for narcolepsy and further investigations are currently under way.

General principles of drug therapy include using the lowest effective dose possible, employing gradual titration and careful monitoring for therapeutic and adverse effects, and temporarily withdrawing the stimulant when tolerance has developed (perhaps timing the withdrawal to coincide with a vacation period so that the patient is not severely affected by the resulting increase in symptomatology). In addition, cataplexy may be treated on an as-needed basis in some patients. If the patient, for instance, recognizes that the cataplexy is associated with a specific stimulus and its occurrence is predictable, then protriptyline may be taken for only a day or two before and during the expected occurrence.

## Insomnia

### *Definition/Overview*

Insomnia is the most commonly encountered sleep disorder and occurs more frequently among females and the elderly. Reports from various surveys indicate that for a majority of the population over the age of 16, sleeping can be a problem. Approximately 38% of the population admit that insomnia is a current problem.[6,14]

In defining insomnia, two factors must be considered. First, there must be a relative lack of sleep; however, no particular number of hours of sleep defines insomnia. An individual who requires only 5 hours of sleep per night and sleeps 5 hours does not suffer from insomnia. On the other hand, an individual who sleeps 7 hours but requires 8 hours per night for peak daytime performance may indeed have insomnia. Second, there must be a subjective complaint. The patient must say that he is not sleeping as well as he thinks he should and that it is interfering with his daytime performance. In many respects, an insomniac's sleep is not that dramatically different from that of a good sleeper; however, the insomniac perceives it as poor sleep.[6,15] As yet, there is no definitive way of measuring the quality of sleep electrophysiologically in the sleep laboratory.

Insomnia can be assessed (viewed) from various perspectives. For example, the degree of severity (i.e., from mild to severe) clearly has implications with respect to treatment decisions. Whether the insomnia is transient or chronic is important in both diagnosis and treatment. Finally, the pattern of a typical night's sleep (i.e., difficulty falling asleep, difficulty staying asleep [numerous awakenings during the night], early morning awakening [waking up 3 to 4 hours earlier than expected with an inability to return to sleep], or some combination of these problems) is also important in diagnosing the sleep disorder and planning subsequent treatment.

There are numerous causes for insomnia (Table 52.5). Medical causes may include pain (e.g., arthritis, pruritus, duodenal ulcer). Pain not only interferes with the ability to fall asleep, but also may lead to increased nocturnal arousals and a generally "lighter" sleep. Nocturia, as part of a medical disorder or the result of too late a dose of a diuretic, may cause fragmentation of sleep. Psychologic or psychiatric causes include worry, excitement, and anxiety. Almost everyone is familiar with an occasional bout of insomnia associated with emotional arousal. In addition, some type of sleep disturbance almost always accompanies an acute episode of any of the major psychiatric disorders and is often one of the diagnostic criteria. Other miscellaneous causes of a sleep disturbance may include disruption of circadian rhythms (e.g., jet lag), sleep apnea (more often central type), nocturnal myoclonus, and drug effects.

**Table 52.5** Common Medical Causes, Psychologic/Psychiatric Causes, and Miscellaneous Causes Associated With Insomnia

| | |
|---|---|
| **A. Medical Causes** | |
| Pain | |
| Nocturia | |
| Thyrotoxicosis | |
| **B. Psychologic/Psychiatric Causes** | |
| Worry | Schizophrenia |
| Excitement | Depression |
| Anxiety | Mania |
| **C. Miscellaneous Causes** | |
| Disruption of circadian rhythms | |
| Sleep apnea | |
| Nocturnal myoclonus | |
| New sleeping environment | |
| Stressful life events | |
| Drugs—stimulants, diuretics, alcohol | |
| Drug dependency/withdrawal | |

### *Treatment*

An initial consideration in treating insomnia must be whether the problem is transient or persistent. In general, use of hypnotics is most appropriate for transient or short-term insomnia. Transient insomnia may be associated with work shift change, jet lag, or situational factors (e.g., exciting or disturbing circumstances, anxiety, acute pain). Although a brief trial of a hypnotic may be acceptable in treating some persistent insomnias, for many such an approach would be either inappropriate and/or unsafe.

There are a number of common examples of persistent insomnia. If insomnia is secondary to a treatable medical problem or is drug induced, the primary problem should be identified and treated. If the sleep disturbance is one symptom of a major psychiatric disorder, selection and titration of a psychotropic agent could be the most appropriate treatment. For disruptions of circadian rhythm, it is possible to readjust the internal clock. An example would be delayed sleep phase syndrome, where the patient's ability to sleep simply does not coincide with the time period set aside for sleep. By means of chronotherapy, the patient's internal clock is reset by 2 to 3 hours each night for a number of consecutive nights until ultimately the body is sleepy at the same time the patient wants to be sleeping.[16] Other examples of persistent insomnia include sleep apnea syndrome (discussed earlier) and nocturnal myoclonus.

Nocturnal myoclonus (periodic leg movement) is characterized by periodic (every 20–40 seconds), stereotypic, myoclonic movements of the anterior tibialis muscles during sleep, resulting in arousals. Like the arousals of sleep apnea, the patient may experience several hundred per night and yet not be aware of them the following day. This condition is age related, showing a marked increase in incidence in individuals over 40. Nocturnal myoclonus has been treated with the benzodiazepine clonazepam (Klonopin), starting at a dose of 0.5 mg at bedtime and titrating up if necessary.[17] Benzodiazepines do not necessarily decrease the number of movements, but patients report subjective improvement in sleep. Tricyclic antidepressants and levodopa reportedly exacerbate nocturnal myoclonus.

Although not a sleep disorder, restless legs syndrome is a related condition that can certainly affect the ability to fall asleep. This is characterized by uncomfortable sensations in the legs at rest that can be relieved by movement. Codeine and related compounds (e.g., oxycodone) and carbamazepine (Tegretol), given at bedtime, have helped some patients.[18]

For both persistent and transient or short-term insomnia, several nonpharmacologic interventions are available to assist in promoting sleep. Often, hypnosis or relaxation techniques are helpful; this is particularly true if a patient simply needs to relax to allow sleep to occur. Some patients need to develop improved sleep habits. These may involve a carefully designed ritual of going to bed or setting the bedroom aside as an environment only for sleep (as opposed to reading, paying bills, or watching television). Greater attention must be paid to regularity with respect to time to go to bed and time to get up. The patient may need to be reminded to omit alcohol and caffeine in the evening. Others may benefit from psychotherapy. Timing of meals and exercise may need modification. A heavy meal too close to bedtime in a patient with gastroesophageal reflux will likely lead to more disturbed sleep. Excessive exercise just before bedtime may actually worsen sleep as compared with exercise in the afternoon. Finally, the sleeper should ideally have a comfortable bed in secure surroundings. Still, there are times, as mentioned before, when hypnotic drugs are indicated.

## Hypnotics

### *The Ideal Hypnotic*

Although the ideal hypnotic does not exist, it might be useful to describe such an agent. A hypnotic should rapidly induce sleep and have a duration of action sufficiently long to maintain sleep throughout the night, but not so long that there is impaired daytime functioning the next morning. Repeated use on consecutive nights should not result in dependence or tolerance; and abrupt discontinuation should not lead to drug-withdrawal insomnia or rebound insomnia. The drug should have a high therapeutic index and should normalize disturbed sleep without disturbing the sleep of a normal sleeper.

### *Classification and Pharmacology of Selected Agents*

A number of the more commonly used agents are presented in Table 52.6. The barbiturates include pentobarbital, secobarbital, and amobarbital. These agents are capable of suppressing REM sleep as well as delta sleep. Upon abrupt withdrawal, there is a REM rebound. Other disadvantages of the barbiturates include induction of liver enzymes causing a number of drug interactions, toxicity in overdose because of a narrow therapeutic index, and loss of effectiveness in inducing and maintaining sleep within 14 consecutive nights of use at a consistent dose.[19]

The nonbarbiturate nonbenzodiazepines, originally touted as superior to the barbiturates, have (with the exception of

**Table 52.6** Hypnotics—Classification and Dosage

| *Drug class/generic name* | *Trade name* | *Manufacturer* | *Dosage range (mg)* |
|---|---|---|---|
| Barbiturates | | | |
| Pentobarbital | Nembutal | Abbott | 100–200 |
| | Generic | Various | |
| Secobarbital | Seconal | Lilly | 100–200 |
| | Generic | Various | |
| Amobarbital | Amytal | Lilly | 100–200 |
| | Generic | Various | |
| Nonbarbiturate nonbenzodiazepines | | | |
| Ethchlorvynol | Placidyl | Abbott | 500–1,000 |
| Glutethimide | Doriden | USV | 500–1,000 |
| | Generic | Various | |
| Methyprylon | Noludar | Roche | 200–400 |
| Chloral hydrate | Noctec | Squibb | 500–2,000 |
| | Generic | Various | |
| Antihistamines | | | |
| Diphenhydramine | Benadryl | Parke–Davis | 25–100 |
| | Generic | Various | |
| Doxylamine | Unisom | Leeming | 25–100 |
| Pyrilamine | Nervine | Miles | 25–100 |
| | Generic | Various | |
| Benzodiazepines | | | |
| Flurazepam | Dalmane | Roche | 15–30 |
| | Generic | Various | |
| Temazepam | Restoril | Sandoz | 15–30 |
| | Generic | Various | |
| Triazolam | Halcion | Upjohn | 0.125–0.50 |
| Amino acids | | | |
| L-Tryptophan[a] | Trofan | Upsher–Smith | 1,000–4,000 |
| | Generic | Various | |

[a] Not FDA approved as a drug; available as a nutritional supplement.

chloral hydrate) most of the disadvantages of the barbiturates plus some additional ones. For example, they have a higher abuse potential, and overdoses are more difficult to manage. In the case of glutethimide overdose, the clinician is dealing with a CNS depressant overdose as well as anticholinergic toxicity. In several European countries these agents are not available; however, despite controversy over their availability for more than a decade, they remain on the market in the United States.

Although chloral hydrate lacks some of the disadvantages just mentioned, it does interact with other drugs that are highly protein bound and may cause gastrointestinal irritation. In addition, chloral hydrate has been found to lose its effectiveness in inducing and maintaining sleep, similar to the barbiturates.[20]

Antihistamines are available as nonprescription sleep aids and are used in an attempt to take advantage of their sedative side effects. Diphenhydramine and doxylamine are more sedating than pyrilamine, while pyrilamine causes more gastrointestinal side effects. By subjective report, diphenhydramine 50 mg has a soporific effect equivalent to that of pentobarbital 60 mg,[21] but increasing dosages do not necessarily produce a linear increase in therapeutic response. Even at therapeutic doses the antihistamines may cause considerable anticholinergic activity, which can be particularly bothersome in elderly patients. These effects include dry mouth, constipation, blurred near vision, urinary retention, and central anticholinergic effects (e.g., confusion, disorientation, impairment of short-term memory, and perhaps even visual and tactile hallucinations). Unfortunately, few objective (i.e., sleep laboratory) data are available regarding the hypnotic efficacy of antihistamines.

The amino acid L-tryptophan, a serotonin precursor, became popular as a natural hypnotic. Serotonin appears to be a major neurotransmitter involved in NREM sleep. Unfortunately, the overall efficacy of this agent is unclear. Although some insomniacs respond well, others do not. Also, the factors that predict response to L-tryptophan have yet to be identified.[22] Probably the major side effect of L-tryptophan is gastrointestinal upset, which has been likened by previously pregnant women to morning sickness. It should be noted that this agent does not have an FDA-approved labeling indication for the treatment of insomnia.

The benzodiazepines come closest to the ideal hypnotic. Indeed, the conclusion of a Consensus Development Conference on Drugs and Insomnia at the National Institute of Mental Health was that when pharmacotherapy is indicated, benzodiazepines are preferable.[23] Extensive reviews of these agents can be found elsewhere[24–27]; hence, only a brief discussion follows. Flurazepam was the first benzodiazepine marketed as a hypnotic. Its favorable profile includes a wide margin of safety and few drug interactions. In addition, flurazepam produces little or no REM suppression at lower doses; even at higher doses REM suppression is not followed by REM rebound upon abrupt discontinuation of the drug (probably because of the slow elimination of its long-acting active metabolite, desalkylflurazepam, with a half-life of 47–100 hours). Whether flurazepam lacks a withdrawal phenomenon has yet to be established. Sleep patterns may need to be followed for several weeks beyond discontinuation of the drug to clarify this issue. Flurazepam had the additional advantage of remaining effective at a consistent dose for at least 28 consecutive nights of use. It does suppress delta sleep and the long-acting metabolite, desalkylflurazepam, accumulates over time. This could prove to be problematic with respect to impaired daytime functioning, especially in the elderly.

Temazepam has the advantage of a short to intermediate elimination half-life (average half-life, 14.7 hours). It shares many of the properties of flurazepam with respect to effects on sleep. The major question concerns its ability to induce sleep (i.e., the drug could take 1 to 2 hours to work). This is a formulation issue that is being addressed by the manufacturer.

Triazolam is unique in that it is ultrashort to short acting, with a half-life of 3 hours and a rapid onset of less than 30 minutes. While it may suppress REM sleep in the first half of the night, there appears to be compensation for this in the second half of the night. Triazolam seems to have little effect on delta sleep. It is the least likely of the benzodiazepines to produce morning hangover. Like flurazepam and temazepam, it increases the general quality of sleep, decreases nocturnal awakenings, and increases total sleep time. There has been speculation among clinicians, but only limited data, that triazolam has greater potential to produce psychomotor impairment and anterograde amnesia than other benzodiazepines; whether this is a function of dose and potency or a unique risk of triazolam is as yet unclear.[28]

### *Drug-Withdrawal Insomnia and Rebound Insomnia*

Drug-withdrawal insomnia was described in association with abrupt discontinuation of the older hypnotics.[29] After the drug suppressed REM sleep with chronic use, its removal would result in a dramatic increase in REM sleep to as much as 40% of total sleep time. The REM sleep could be extremely intense with frightening dreams or nightmares. Sleep would be so disrupted that without proper counseling, the patient would think that the hypnotic was definitely needed and would immediately resume use. This led to a standard treatment plan of very gradual tapering of a hypnotic, especially when the dose had exceeded the usual dosage range and had been administered for prolonged treatment periods. Patient counseling regarding the natural psychophysiologic changes to be expected after drug withdrawal was recommended.

Rebound insomnia, after abrupt discontinuation of a drug, is a phenomenon described recently by Kales.[30] Rebound insomnia is described as a worsening of sleep, even beyond what it was like before drug treatment was initiated. Kales claims that this phenomenon is a characteristic of the shorter acting benzodiazepines; however, studies have produced mixed results on this matter and the predictability of rebound insomnia remains controversial.

### *Problems/Controversies*

Two important issues with respect to insomnia and hypnotics are that no one drug is ideal for every insomniac and that not all insomniacs should be treated with hypnotics. Hypnotics are to be used almost exclusively in the treatment of transient or short-term insomnia.[23] The implication is that a thorough assessment is made of every patient with a complaint of insomnia. Although hypnotic-induced sleep may be unnatural in some respects, the ultimate measure of efficacy is improved or optimal daytime performance.

The problem of delayed psychomotor impairment with flurazepam, especially in the elderly, can be avoided by using a shorter acting agent such as temazepam or triazolam. The possible problem of delayed onset of activity with temazepam can be avoided by using a more rapidly acting agent such as triazolam or flurazepam. The possible problem of psychomotor impairment and anterograde amnesia with triazolam may be avoided by careful titration from a low starting dose. In general, the choice of drug depends upon the pharmacokinetic and side effect profile as well as the expected therapeutic outcome.

There may be some concern that because patients can develop dependence, hypnotics should be totally avoided; however, if hypnotics are used appropriately—for brief periods and at low doses—this risk is low. Also, drug dependence insomnia, in which sleep worsens with long-term use of hypnotics even while the patient continues to take the drug,[29] should not be a problem.

The issue of hypnotic use in chronic insomnia is more difficult. Few data are available regarding the efficacy and safety of hypnotics when taken for more than 1 to 2 months. If a thorough sleep evaluation has been made, a hypnotic trial may be initiated in some chronic insomniacs (e.g., the patient with nocturnal myoclonus); however, longer use increases the risks of dependence, tolerance with resulting escalation of dose, and difficult withdrawal. If such a trial is undertaken in a chronic insomniac, the prescriber must carefully and frequently evaluate the patient for significant improvement in sleep and daytime performance, as well as the persistence of the therapeutic effect at a constant dose.

### *General Principles of Clinical Use*

A careful diagnosis of the sleep problem must be made to avoid the use of hypnotics in patients with sleep apnea, patients who use alcohol or other CNS depressants, pregnant patients, and individuals in whom alert nighttime performance is mandatory (e.g., firemen, pilots). Although the benzodiazepines are extremely safe, caution should be used when prescribing them to a patient with a high suicidal risk. Most overdoses involve alcohol in combination with other drugs and such a hypnotic–alcohol combination could be fatal.

The benefit that the patient is seeking must be determined. Ideally, the patient is seeking both improved sleep and improved daytime functioning. Simply increasing the number of hours of sleep is generally not a sufficient reason for prescribing a hypnotic. Once the hypnotic is chosen, the lowest effective dose to achieve a clear-cut benefit should be used. This requires following the patient regularly, assessing therapeutic effect, and educating the patient regarding the need to begin with a low dose and give it an adequate trial. Especially in elderly patients, daytime sequelae must be monitored as well. Hypnotics should typically be used for short-term treatment. This usually means several days to several weeks. The longer the treatment, the more important it is to have the patient try a night or two without the drug after several nights of good sleep. This may decrease the risk of tolerance and may also indicate to the patient that the drug need not be taken every night. Finally, when the drug is discontinued, the patient must be informed of possible temporary withdrawal effects.

## Summary

A fascinating psychophysiologic phenomenon, sleep, has been described as a cyclic activity that can be observed and measured electrophysiologically. Considering that the association between the REM period and dreaming was discovered little more than three decades ago[31] and that sleep disorder medicine is considerably younger than that, it is amazing how much is known about sleep and its disorders. Still, much remains to be clarified. Disorders have been described that manifest as excessive daytime sleepiness (obstructive sleep apnea and narcolepsy), insomnia (transient as well as persistent types), and unusual behaviors and mental activity during sleep (sleepwalking, night terrors, and nightmares).

Not all complaints of patients regarding sleep should be treated with hypnotics; indeed, some sleep disorders may be worsened by hypnotics or other drugs. With careful diagnosis and treatment tailored to the individual and the particular problem, more people will not only sleep better, but will also perform considerably better while awake.

## References

1. Monnier M, Gaillard JM. Biochemical regulation of sleep. Experientia 1980;36:21–4.
2. Rechtschaffen A, Kales A (eds). A manual of standardized terminology, techniques and scoring system for sleep stages of human subjects. Washington, DC: US Government Printing Office, Public Health Service Publications, 1968, publication 204.
3. Carskadon MA, Van den Hoed J, Dement WC. Sleep and daytime sleepiness in the elderly. J Geriatr Psychiatry 1980;13: 135–151.
4. Ancoli-Israel S, Kripke DF, Mason WJ, et al. Sleep apnea and PMS in a randomly selected elderly population: Final prevalence results. Sleep Res 1986;15:101.
5. Sleep Disorders Classification Committee, Association of Sleep Disorders Centers. Diagnostic classification of sleep and arousal disorders. Sleep 1979;2:1–137.
6. Kales A, Soldatos CR, Kales JD. Sleep disorders: Insomnia, sleepwalking, night terrors, nightmares, and enuresis. Ann Intern Med 1987;106:582–592.
7. Kales A, Vela-Bueno A, Kales JD. Sleep disorders: Sleep apnea and narcolepsy. Ann Intern Med 1987;106:434–443.
8. Ancoli-Israel S, Kripke DF, Mason W, et al. Sleep apnea and periodic leg movements in an aging sample. J Gerontol 1985;40: 419–425.
9. Conway WA, Zorick F, Piccione P, et al. Protriptyline in the treatment of sleep apnea. Thorax 1982;37:49–53.
10. Strohl KP, Hensley MJ, Saunders NA, et al. Progesterone administration and progressive sleep apneas. JAMA 1981;245: 1230–1232.
11. White DP, Zwillich CW, Pickett CK, et al. Central sleep apnea: Improvement with acetazolamide therapy. Arch Intern Med 1982;142:1816.
12. Dement WC, Carskadon MA, Guilleminault C, et al. Narcolepsy: Diagnosis and treatment. Primary Care 1976;3:609–623.
13. Campbell RK. The treatment of narcolepsy and cataplexy. Drug Intell Clin Pharm 1981;15:257–262.
14. Bixler EO, Kales A, Soldatos CR, et al. Prevalence of sleep disorders in the Los Angeles metropolitan area. Am J Psychiatry 1979;136:1257–1262.
15. Carskadon MA, Dement WC, Mitler MM, et al. Self reports versus sleep laboratory findings in 122 drug-free subjects with complaints of chronic insomnia. Am J Psychiatry 1976;133: 1382–1388.
16. Weitzman ED, Czeisler CA, Coleman RM, et al. Delayed sleep phase syndrome. Arch Gen Psychiatry 1981;38:737–746.
17. Channa N, Peled R, Rubin AH, et al. Periodic leg movements in sleep: Effect of clonazepam treatment. Neurology 1985;35:408–411.
18. Telstad W, Sorensen O, Larsen S, et al. Treatment of restless legs syndrome with carbamazepine: A double blind study. Br Med J 1984;288:444.
19. Kales AK, Bixler EO, Kales JD, et al. Comparative effectiveness of nine hypnotic drugs: Sleep laboratory studies. J Clin Pharmacol 1977;17:207–213.
20. Kales A, Allen C, Scharf MB, et al. Hypnotic drugs and their effectiveness: All night EEG studies of insomniac subjects. Arch Gen Psychiatry 1970;23:226–232.
21. Teutach G, Mahler DL, Brown CR, et al. Hypnotic efficacy of diphenhydramine, methapyrilene, and pentobarbital for nighttime sedation. Clin Pharmacol Ther 1975;17:195–201.
22. Schneider-Helmert D, Spinweber CL. Evaluation of L-tryptophan for treatment of insomnia: A review. Psychopharmacology 1986;89:1–7.
23. National Institute of Mental Health, Consensus Development Conference. Drugs and insomnia: The use of medications to promote sleep. JAMA 1984;251:2410–2414.
24. Dement WC. Rational basis for the use of sleeping pills. Pharmacology 1983;27(suppl 2):3–38.
25. Wincor MZ. Insomnia and the new benzodiazepines. Clin Pharm 1982;1:425–432.
26. Kales A, Kales JD. Sleep laboratory studies of hypnotic drugs: Efficacy and withdrawal effects. J Clin Psychopharmacol 1983; 3:140–150.
27. Rickels K. Clinical trials of hypnotics. J Clin Psychopharmacol 1983;3:133–139.
28. Griffiths RR, Lamb RL, Ator NA, et al. Relative abuse liability of triazolam: Experimental assessment in animals and humans. Neurosci Biobehav Rev 1985;9:133–151.
29. Kales A, Bixler E, Tan T, et al. Chronic hypnotic-drug use: Ineffectiveness, drug-withdrawal insomnia, and dependence. JAMA 1974;227:513–517.
30. Kales A, Scharf M, Kales J. Rebound insomnia: A new clinical syndrome. Science 1978;201:1039–1041.
31. Aserinsky E, Kleitman N. Regularly occurring periods of eye motility and concomitant phenomena during sleep. Science 1953;118:273–274.

# Section Seven
# Endocrine and Exocrine Disorders

## Chapter 53 / Thyroid Disorders

Marie A. Smith, PharmD

The syndromes associated with excessive production (hyperthyroidism) and deficiency (hypothyroidism) of thyroid hormones are the most common disorders of the thyroid gland. Although symptoms and signs are systemic and generalized, they are quite characteristic, ranging from subclinical to life-threatening. An understanding of the normal physiology of the thyroid provides a basis for the pharmacologic approach to treatment. In addition, several measurements of thyroid hormone function or responsiveness are quite useful in both the diagnosis and the monitoring of treatment.

### Hyperthyroidism

Hyperthyroidism, or thyrotoxicosis, is a disorder with multiple etiologies (Table 53.1). The most common cause of hyperthyroidism is Graves' disease (toxic diffuse goiter or Basedow's disease). Although the diagnosis of Graves' disease is straightforward, the clinical features and diagnosis of the less common forms of hyperthyroidism are more subtle and often misleading.

#### *Epidemiology*

Graves' disease is a relatively common thyroid disorder that affects predominantly females (7:1 ratio), with a peak onset in the third and fourth decades of life. A distinct familial predisposition has been observed in patients with Graves' disease and has been associated with certain HLA types.[1] Among family members of Graves' disease patients, patterns of clinical and immunologic overlap exist with Hashimoto's disease, pernicious anemia, and other autoimmune diseases.[2]

#### *Etiology and Pathogenesis*

Although the exact cause of Graves' disease is unknown, the remarkable familial patterns, resemblance to Hashimoto's thyroiditis, and associated disturbances of the autoimmune system provide definite clues. An underlying autoimmune disorder as a possible etiology of Graves' disease has been seriously considered since the discovery of long-acting thyroid stimulator (LATS) as an IgG immunoglobulin with thyroid-stimulating properties. In addition, there is a general hypertrophy of lymphoid tissue in the disease and focal collections of lymphocytes are found in hyperplastic thyroid tissue. Circulating antimicrosomal thyroid antibodies (anti-MAb) are detected in approximately 86% and antithyroglobulin antibodies (Anti-TGAb) in about 50% of patients with Graves' disease.[2]

The pathogenesis of Graves' disease also appears to be related to an autoimmune phenomenon involving genetic dysfunction of immunologic control because of suppressor-T-lymphocyte abnormalities. In the normal immunologic system, B lymphocytes interact with helper T lymphocytes to stimulate the production of immunoglobulins. Suppressor T lymphocytes maintain immunologic control of the system by preventing B lymphocytes from producing inappropriate immunoglobulins. In Graves' disease, an aberration of suppressor T-lymphocytes may be responsible for the production of abnormal thyroid-stimulating and antithyroid immunoglobulins.[3] The presence of glandular lymphocytic infiltrates, IgG immunoglobulins, and antithyroid antibodies provides support for an autoimmune etiology in Graves' disease.

#### *Clinical Presentation*

The classic clinical presentation of Graves' disease includes thyrotoxicosis, diffuse goiter, infiltrative ophthalmopathy, and pretibial myxedema. Clinical manifestations vary according to severity, age, and underlying diseases. Despite the interpatient differences in clinical presentation, usual signs and symptoms reflect an increased metabolism of all body systems and adrenergic stimulation of the cardiac and neurologic systems (Table 53.2).

The patient with Graves' disease usually appears restless, wasted, and emotionally labile and has rapid speech. Often, the hyperthyroid patient complains of heat intolerance and perspiring at rest as well as during periods of anxiety or exertion. The skin has a smooth, velvety texture and localized nonpitting myxedema of the shins, forearms, or exten-

**Table 53.1** Etiology and Frequency of Hyperthyroidism

| *Etiology* | *Relative frequency (%)* |
|---|---|
| Graves' disease | 70–85 |
| Toxic multinodular goiter | 5–15 |
| Solitary toxic nodule | 3–30 |
| Thyroiditis (including hashitoxicosis) | 4–23 |
| Drug-induced thyrotoxicosis | Rare |
| Pituitary or trophoblastic tumors | Rare |
| Ectopic (struma ovarii) | Very rare |

sor surfaces of the fingers, a hallmark of Graves' disease. These lesions are often raised, slightly hyperpigmented, pruritic, and thickened. The nail beds may be softened, resulting in nail detachment (onycholysis) and a characteristic reverse half-moon appearance.

The most characteristic ocular features of hyperthyroidism are staring, infrequent blinking, lid lag, and lid retraction. Specific findings of infiltrative ophthalmopathy are useful in establishing Graves' disease and include proptosis, periorbital edema, chemosis, and conjunctival injection. Exophthalmos (eyeball protrusion) may be unilateral in the early stages of disease, with progression to symmetric involvement.

The thyroid gland is usually but not always enlarged. The gland is usually symmetrically enlarged and slightly tender, and has a palpable thrill in Graves' disease. Graves' goiters are usually two to four times the normal gland size.

Thyroid hormone excess has multiple effects on the cardiovascular system, including increased cardiac output and blood volume, tachycardia, widened pulse pressure, palpitations, arrhythmias (especially atrial fibrillation), and systolic murmurs. More than 75% of elderly hyperthyroid patients present with abnormal cardiovascular signs. Palpitations and congestive heart failure may be indicative of not only the direct stimulation of the myocardium by excess thyroid hormones but also the diminished cardiovascular reserve common in the elderly. The incidence of atrial fibrillation is 15% to 40% in elderly hyperthyroid patients; this may often be the presenting feature, while new or exacerbated angina is noted in approximately 25% of patients.[4]

Despite hyperphagic episodes, most hyperthyroid patients lose weight. Common effects on the gastrointestinal system include increased motility, gastric emptying, and frequency of bowel movements. Hyperdefecation, anorexia, nausea, and vomiting occur occasionally. Polydypsia and polyuria

**Table 53.2** Systemic Signs and Symptoms of Thyroid Disorders

| *Organ system* | *Hyperthyroidism* | *Hypothyroidism* |
|---|---|---|
| General | Heat tolerance, weight loss with increased appetite, increased sweating, hyperkinetic speech and behavior | Cold intolerance, weight gain with anorexia, hoarseness, fatigue, decreased sweating, mental slowing |
| Head | Thinning of hair, fine texture | Puffy facies, large tongue, dry/brittle hair, thinning eyebrows |
| Eyes | Exophthalmos, lid lag, lid retraction, stare, blurred vision | Ptosis, edematous lids |
| Neck | Goiter with or without bruits/thrills | Goiter in primary hypothyroidism |
| Cardiac | Palpitations, high-output failure, increased pulse and systolic pressure, murmurs, angina | Cardiomegaly, low-output failure, dyspnea |
| Gastrointestinal | Loose stools, hyperdefecation | Constipation |
| Genitourinary | Polyuria, amenorrhea or decreased duration of menses | Dysmenorrhea, menorrhagia |
| Neuromuscular | Fatigue, weakness, tremor, quick deep tendon reflexes | Delayed deep tendon reflexes, muscle weakness |
| Extremities | Pretibial myxedema, warm/moist skin | Pretibial myxedema, cool/dry skin, brittle nails, yellow tint |
| Emotional | Nervousness, irritability, lability, insomnia | Depression, apathy, lethargy |

are frequent complaints, yet normal electrolyte balance is maintained.

A fine tremor of the fingers is often observed as a sign of hyperthyroidism. Other neuromuscular effects include hyperactivity, muscle weakness and fatigue, emotional lability, anxiety, distractability, and hyperactive deep tendon reflexes. Nervous symptoms predominate in younger individuals, whereas cardiovascular and myopathy are seen more commonly in older hyperthyroid patients.

Occasionally, a thyrotoxic patient may present with atypical findings or an absence of the common clinical manifestations previously mentioned. Often seen in elderly patients, this is known as "apathetic" or "masked" hyperthyroidism. Presenting symptoms may be fatigue, listlessness, mental dullness, delayed speech, apathetic affect, congestive heart failure, and low-grade fever, which may obscure an accurate diagnosis.[5]

### *Diagnosis*

Graves' disease can often be diagnosed on the basis of clinical manifestations, but should be confirmed by laboratory assessment. When diffuse thyroid enlargement (accompanied by a bruit) is associated with ophthalmopathy, Graves' disease presents a classic clinical picture. In florid thyrotoxicosis, laboratory tests reveal increased levothyroxine ($T_4$) and triiodothyronine ($T_3$), radioactive $T_3$ uptake ($RT_3U$), free $T_3$ or $T_4$ index ($FT_3I$ or $FT_4I$), and radioactive iodine ($^{131}I$) uptake (RAIU). If laboratory tests reveal a normal serum $T_4$, $RT_3U$, and RAIU, there may be increased serum $T_3$ and $FT_3I$, as seen in $T_3$ thyrotoxicosis. Thyroid scanning has a minor role in the diagnosis of thyrotoxicosis, except in patients with nodules. As thyroid-stimulating hormone (TSH) concentrations are uniformly normal or low in patients with Graves' disease, this assay is not useful in the diagnosis. Determination of antibody titers may provide supportive evidence for Graves' disease. Positive anti-MAb and TgAb assays establish only that autoimmunity is present and do not indicate thyrotoxicosis.

Hyperthyroidism can also affect the synthesis and degradation of a number of substances in the blood. An increase may be noted in total and ionized calcium, sex steroid binding globulin, angiotensin-converting enzyme, alkaline phosphatase, ferritin, and factor VIII; cholesterol levels may be decreased.[6] Although these are nonspecific indicators, they may be supportive evidence of hyperthyroidism.

### *Clinical Course*

In classic Graves' disease, symptoms of thyrotoxicosis, thyroid enlargement, and proptosis gradually develop over a period of weeks or months. The onset of the disease has occurred after emotional trauma and weight reduction, but whether this bears a causal relationship in the development of Graves' disease is controversial. Presently, the natural course of the thyrotoxic process is commonly altered with pharmacologic or definitive therapy. Before the availability of treatment, hyperthyroidism would exhibit periods of exacerbation and remission. Patients with mild symptomatology often experience spontaneous remission to a euthyroid state in 1 year or more.

If left untreated, thyrotoxicosis can be a fatal disease, with mortality estimates of 11%. Deaths are usually attributed to cardiovascular complications (congestive heart failure or myocardial infarction) or infections associated with muscle weakness and debilitation.[2]

### *Other Hyperthyroid States*

#### Toxic Nodular Goiter

Toxic multinodular goiter is most frequently seen in elderly patients with a long history of simple goiter and accounts for about 10% of hyperthyroidism cases. The incidence increases with age, with an onset often in the fifth or sixth decade of life and a predilection for women. The onset of hyperthyroidism is often subtle and results from one or more autonomous thyroid nodules growing within the multinodular goiter. Clinical manifestations usually do not occur until the autonomous nodular tissue is greater than 4 cm and has supraphysiologic secretions that suppress the nonautonomous tissue.[7]

The degree of thyrotoxicosis is typically less than that seen with Graves' disease; however, the physiologic effect on specific organ systems, especially the cardiovascular system, may be significant. Arrhythmias or congestive heart failure may be precipitated or exacerbated with thyrotoxicosis while other clinical findings are absent or subtle. Ophthalmopathy is rare and may signal the development of Graves' disease. The patient may experience dysphagia, cough, and hoarseness.

An observed or palpable nodular goiter establishes a diagnosis of thyroid disease. Conventional laboratory tests may be indicative of borderline thyrotoxicity. A serum $T_3$ concentration in the normal range for a young adult may actually indicate thyrotoxicosis in an elderly patient, as $T_3$ concentrations usually decline with age. The $FT_4I$ and 24-hour RAIU are normal in most cases. Scanning after administration of $^{131}I$ or $^{99m}Tc$ may delineate nodular areas that are not visible or palpable. The advantages of using $^{99m}Tc$ over $^{131}I$ include smaller radiation dose and shorter test duration. Although the $T_3$ suppression test is often useful in defining autonomous hyperfunctioning in multinodular goiter, it can subject the elderly patient to cardiac difficulties. Today, most clinicians confirm the diagnosis with a therapeutic trial of propylthiouracil or methimazole.

#### Subacute Thyroiditis

Subacute thyroiditis, known as granulomatous, giant cell, or deQuervain's thyroiditis, is a spontaneous, remitting inflammatory thyroid condition that appears to have a viral etiology. Clinical manifestations usually include fever, malaise, difficulty swallowing, and local or referred pain. Only 50% of patients exhibit symptoms of hyperthyroidism. Two laboratory tests, hallmarks of the disease, are a markedly increased erythrocyte sedimentation rate and depressed or undetectable RAIU. Other thyroid laboratory test results vary according to the stage of the disease. In early stages, serum $T_4$ concentration is high and protein-bound iodine (PBI) is elevated secondary to leakage of iodoproteins. Later, the laboratory results may mimic hypothyroidism with low $T_4$ and elevated TSH concentrations as glandular hormone is depleted. Spontaneous recovery of thyroid function commonly occurs and treatment is primarily symptomatic (heat, rest, analgesics). Propranolol may be used to control hyperthyroid symptoms and is withdrawn once the RAIU returns to normal values.[8]

### $T_3$ Thyrotoxicosis

Although hyperthyroidism usually involves excessive $T_4$ concentrations, $T_3$ thyrotoxicosis with preferential $T_3$ secretion and a normal or low $T_4$ concentration has been reported in association with Graves' disease, toxic goiters, and hyperfunctioning adenomas. The diagnosis should be suspected in a patient with hyperthyroid symptoms and laboratory findings of a normal or low $T_4$ concentration and $FT_4I$ combined with a normal or increased RAIU. Elevated $T_3$ concentrations may precede the onset of $T_4$ thyrotoxicosis and can be useful as a harbinger of relapse after a course of antithyroid medication.[9]

### Drug-Induced Thyrotoxicosis

Hyperthyroidism can be transiently associated with excessive ingestion of thyroxine (factitious thyrotoxicosis). Thyroid medications may be taken by healthy, euthyroid patients who desire an increased metabolism for weight reduction. This etiology should be considered in patients with a low RAIU concentration, even if the patient denies taking thyroid medication. If the patient is taking $T_3$, the serum $T_4$ concentrations should be low or borderline normal. Serum thyroglobulin concentrations are usually low in patients with factitious hyperthyroidism.[10]

Iodine-induced hyperthyroidism (Jod–Basedow disease) is not common as an etiology for drug-induced hyperthyroidism. Most cases appear in patients with underlying multinodular goiters or autonomous nodules triggered by an excessive iodine intake. Some patients may have subclinical Graves' disease that is expressed with the ingestion of iodine.[11] Thyrotoxicosis has also been reported after the use of radiocontrast dyes containing iodine.[12]

Lithium is known to interfere with the release of preformed thyroid hormones. Thyrotoxicosis has been reported after lithium withdrawal,[13] probably as a result of unmasking of an underlying hyperthyroidism. The iodine-rich antiarrhythmic drug amiodarone can elevate serum $T_4$ concentrations for several months. Its association with hyperthyroidism is caused by excess iodine release from the drug and is considered rare.[14]

### Hyperthyroidism and Drug Effects

Hyperthyroidism alters the kinetics of digitalis; there is an increased volume of distribution and possible increase in the renal clearance of digitalis. As hyperthyroid patients seem to be "resistant" to the digitalis effect, increased doses may be required for a therapeutic effect. Hyperthyroid patients may also be more sensitive to catecholamines and should use sympathomimetic drugs (e.g., asthma, cold, and allergy preparations) cautiously to avoid thyrotoxic and cardiac symptoms. There seems to be increased renal clearance and metabolism of insulin, so patients may require more insulin to maintain blood glucose control. In thyrotoxicosis, synthesis and catabolism of vitamin K–dependent clotting factors are increased, while the half-life is decreased. Thus, hyperthyroid patients usually require less warfarin for anticoagulation.

## *Treatment*

Three common treatment modalities are used in the management of hyperthyroidism: antithyroid medications, radioactive iodine, and surgery (Table 53.3). The overall therapeutic objectives are to eliminate the excess thyroid hormone and minimize the associated symptoms of hyperthyroidism. Therapy must be individualized, as the decision is dependent on type and severity of hyperthyroidism, patient's age and sex, existence of nonthyroidal conditions, and response to previous antithyroid therapy.

### Thiourea Drugs

The only two drugs approved for the treatment of hyperthyroidism in the United States are classified as thioureylenes, which incorporate a

$$\begin{array}{c} S \\ \| \\ N{-}C{-}N \end{array}$$

group into their ring structures.

***Mechanism of Action*** The two antithyroid compounds used clinically are propylthiouracil (PTU) and methimazole. Although it was once thought that they interfered with the thyroid's ability to trap inorganic iodide or release stored hormone into circulation, it is now clear that the main mechanism of PTU and methimazole is interference with the biosynthesis of thyroid hormone.[15] The exact mechanism of action is not completely known, but these compounds inhibit primarily (1) the "organification" process of iodide binding to thyroglobulin to form monoiodotyrosine and diiodotyrosine, and (2) the coupling reaction of monoiodotyrosine and diiodotyrosine to form $T_3$ and $T_4$.

In addition to the major thyroidal action, PTU and methimazole have significant extrathyroidal effects. PTU, but not methimazole, inhibits peripheral conversion of $T_4$ to $T_3$.[16] This effect is acutely dose related and occurs within hours of PTU administration. The antithyroid drugs may have direct immunologic action distinct from any thyroidal effects, which has therapeutic implications for autoimmune thyroid conditions such as Graves' disease. In patients with Graves' disease, antithyroid drug treatment has been associated with lower thyroid-stimulating antibody titers and restoration of normal suppressor-T-cell function.[17]

***Pharmacokinetics*** Both antithyroid drugs are well absorbed from the gastrointestinal tract, with peak serum concentrations about 1 hour after ingestion. The drugs are actively concentrated in the thyroid gland. The serum half-lives of PTU and methimazole are approximately 1 and 5 hours, respectively, and are not appreciably affected by thyroid status. Serum clearance is slowed in patients with renal or severe hepatic failure, but the clinical implications are not well known. PTU is approximately 60% to 80% protein bound to albumin, while methimazole is not. Methimazole freely crosses the placental barrier and appears in

**Table 53.3** Pharmacologic Agents Used in the Management of Hyperthyroidism

| *Agent* | *Mechanism of action* | *Dose* | *Toxicity* | *Comments* |
|---|---|---|---|---|
| Thioamides | | | | |
| Propylthiouracil (PTU) | Blocks organification of hormone synthesis and peripheral conversion of $T_4$ to $T_3$; possibly immunosuppressive | Initially: 400–800 mg/d (max 1,200 mg/d)<br>Maintenance: 50–300 mg/d | Skin rash, arthralgias, hypoprothrombinemia, hepatitis, gastrointestinal upset, transient leukopenia, agranulocytosis | Used in children, young adults, and pregnant patients; onset in 2–4 wk; cross-sensitivity incidence about 50% |
| Methimazole (Tapazole, Lilly) | Same as PTU, but no interference with $T_4$ to $T_3$ peripherally | Initially: 40–80 mg/d<br>Maintenance: 10–30 mg/d | Similar to PTU, cholestatic jaundice, nephrotic syndrome, ageusia | Freely crosses placenta and appears in breast milk |
| Iodides | | | | |
| Lugol's solution (8 mg iodide/drop)<br>Saturated solution of potassium iodide (SSKI) (40 mg iodide/drop) | Blocks release of thyroid hormones; decreases vascularity of the gland | 6 mg iodide/d is an effective dose; for surgery preparation, 5–10 drops TID for 10–14 d before surgery | Hypersensitivity reactions: skin rash, rhinorrhea, metallic taste, parotid swelling | Used as preoperative preparation, and for patients with mild disease or thyroid storm |
| Adrenergic blockers | | | | |
| Propranolol (Inderal, Ayerst) | Blocks peripheral action of thyroid hormone; blocks peripheral conversion of $T_4$ to $T_3$ | 10–40 mg PO every 6 h; 0.5–1.0 mg IV slowly | Symptoms of $\beta$ blockade: bradycardia, congestive heart failure; inhibits sympathetic response to hypoglycemia; exacerbates asthma | Used for symptomatic relief while awaiting onset of thioamides, RAI, or surgery; thyroid storm |
| Reserpine | Catecholamine depletion | 1–3 mg IV every 8 h | Symptoms of sympathetic blockade; nasal stuffiness, hypotension, CNS effects | Used in thyroid storm, but propranolol is the drug of choice |
| Radioactive iodine (RAI) | Destruction of thyroid gland | 80–100 $\mu$Ci/g of thyroid tissue | Hypothyroidism; potential genetic damage, leukemias | Used in adults, elderly cardiac patients, or those who are poor surgical risks; slow onset of 2–4 wk; full effect 3–6 mo |
| Surgery | Subtotal or total thyroidectomy | | Hypothyroidism, hypoparathyroidism, vocal cord damage, surgical risks | Used in pregnancy in second trimester, patients with contraindications to RAI or thioamides or a malignancy; higher incidence of complications with second operation |

breast milk, whereas PTU crosses the placental membranes only one tenth as well.[18]

***Dosing/Monitoring*** PTU is available as 50-mg tablets, and methimazole as 5- and 10-mg tablets. Methimazole is approximately 10 times potent than PTU. Initial therapy with PTU ranges from 400 to 800 mg daily usually in four divided doses. Methimazole is given in three divided doses totaling 40 to 80 mg/d. These starting doses are dependent on the severity of thyrotoxicosis and should be gradually reduced on a monthly basis to a maintenance daily dose of 50 to 300 mg for PTU or its equivalent. Clinical improvement is related to the magnitude of the intrathyroidal hormone pool (colloid stores) and its rate of release. Once the pool is reduced, clinical improvement should occur if the dose is sufficient to block new hormonal biosynthesis. Usually within 4 to 8 weeks of initiating therapy, clinical symptoms are diminished and circulating thyroid hormone concentrations are normalized. At this time the tapering regimen can be started. If clinical improvement is not observed, the following factors should be considered: (1) noncompliance, (2) insufficient dosage to block hormone synthesis, or (3) inadequate dosing interval (especially if using a single-daily dose).

Baseline laboratory evaluations of $T_4$ (radioimmunoassay), $RT_3U$, and $FT_4I$, and a white blood cell (WBC) count with a differential should be performed before antithyroid drug therapy is initiated. The decline in serum $T_4$ concentrations along with symptom improvement should signal the clinician to taper the dose to its lowest point to maintain a normal serum $T_4$ concentration. This euthyroid dose should be maintained for 12 to 24 months. One month after therapy starts or the regimen changes, the therapeutic response should be monitored with repeat $T_4$, $RT_3U$, and $FT_4I$ assays. In addition to laboratory determinations, clinical signs may be useful in monitoring the response to antithyroid drug therapy (Table 53.4). The WBC count can be useful as an indicator of the development of agranulocytosis as an adverse effect of therapy.

**Table 53.4** Monitoring of Antithyroid Drug Therapy Response

| *Response* | *Signs* |
|---|---|
| Continuing Graves' disease or relapse | Recurrence of hyperthyroid symptoms<br>Blunted response of TSH to TRH test<br>Abnormal thyroid suppressibility<br>Sustained elevation of serum thyroid-binding globulin concentration<br>Positive test for thyroid-stimulating antibodies |
| Remission | Decrease in thyroid gland size<br>Lower maintenance dose required<br>Decrease in RAIU<br>Normal thyroid suppressibility<br>Normal TSH response to TRH test |

***Adverse Effects*** Adverse reactions to PTU and methimazole have an overall incidence of 3% to 12% depending on the dose and the drug. Pruritic maculopapular rashes, arthralgias, and fevers occur in up to 5% of patients and may occur at greater frequency with higher doses and in children. Rashes often disappear spontaneously but if persistent may be managed with antihistamines.

Perhaps one of the most common side effects is a benign transient leukopenia characterized by a WBC count of less than 4,000/mm$^3$. This condition occurs in up to 12% of adults and 25% of children and sometimes can be confused with the mild leukopenia seen in Graves' disease. This mild leukopenia is not a harbinger of the more serious adverse effect of agranulocytosis, so therapy can usually be continued. If a *minor* adverse reaction occurs with one antithyroid drug, the alternate thiourea may be tried, but cross-sensitivity occurs in about 50% of patients.[15]

Agranulocytosis is the most serious adverse effect of thiourea drug therapy and is characterized by fever, malaise, gingivitis, oropharyngeal infection, and a granulocyte count less than 250/mm$^3$. This toxic reaction has occurred with both thioureas; the incidence varies from 0.5% to 6%. It is higher in patients over age 40 receiving a methimazole dose greater than 40 mg/d or the equivalent dose of PTU. Agranulocytosis almost always develops in the first 3 months of therapy with a sudden onset, often undetectable by routine monitoring. Once antithyroid drugs are discontinued, clinical improvement is seen over several days to weeks. Patients should be counseled to discontinue therapy and contact their physician if flulike symptoms such as fever, malaise, sore throat, or bacterial infection develop.[19]

Another serious toxic reaction seen with PTU is a drug-related hepatotoxicity that can be severe and fatal. Methimazole has been associated with cholestatic jaundice, nephrotic syndrome, and ageusia. Vasculitis, a lupuslike syndrome, and hypoprothrombinemia have also been reported more frequently with PTU. Patients who have experienced a *major* adverse reaction to one thiourea drug should not be converted to the alternate drug, as significant cross-sensitivity exists.[15]

***Prognosis*** Antithyroid drug therapy induces permanent remission rates of 30% to 50%. Other patients relapse once therapy is discontinued. Patients who relapse after the initial course of therapy are less likely to have a remission with subsequent courses of therapy. Patient characteristics for a favorable outcome include a small goiter (less than 50 g), short duration of disease (less than 6 months), no previous history of relapse with antithyroid drugs, and low maintenance dosage requirements.[20] Relapse usually occurs within the first few months after discontinuing antithyroid therapy. As there are no specific and reliable predictors of relapse, it is important that patients be followed every 6 to 12 months after remission occurs. If a relapse occurs, alternate therapy with radioiodine may be tried rather than a second course of antithyroid drugs.

***Clinical Controversies*** One of the clinical controversies surrounding the use of the thiourea drugs is whether drug dosage or duration of therapy affects the remission rate with antithyroid drugs. Romaldini et al[21] compared remission rates in a prospective study of patients receiving high doses of PTU (mean dose of 693 mg/d) or methimazole (60 mg/d) for 1 to 2 years. Findings revealed that the high-dose group had a nearly twofold higher remission rate (75.4% versus 41.6%) after a mean follow-up period of 42 months; however, this high-dose group also had a higher incidence of side effects, especially hepatotoxicity. Thus, the high-dose regimen has not received widespread clinical use.

Another study has focused on the duration of therapy and remission rates. Greer et al[22] reported remission rates of 30% to 40% (standard success rates) whether the thiourea drugs were given only until a euthyroid state was obtained (2 to 6 months) or for the conventional 1 to 2 years. Therefore, most clinicians administer antithyroid medications for at least 12 months.

Some thyroidologists have advocated a single daily dose of PTU or methimazole for a dosage frequency. Although a once-a-day regimen for the entire treatment period may be effective for patients with mild disease, most clinicians initiate therapy with a three- or four-times-daily schedule until the patient is euthyroid and then consider a single-dose schedule. As methimazole has a longer half-life (5 hours) and biologic effect (40 hours), it seems to be the preferred thiourea for once-daily dosing.[22] The potassium perchlorate discharge test has been used to predict with high accuracy which patients can be effectively managed with a single-dose regimen.[23]

Although it is not recommended, some clinicians use thyroxine concomitantly with full-dose antithyroid therapy to suppress hypothyroidism and goiter formation resulting from PTU or methimazole therapy. Despite this potential advantage, the combination of antithyroid drugs with thyroid hormone has several major limitations. These undesirable aspects include taking multiple drugs, a higher dosage requirement of the antithyroid drug (associated with a greater incidence of adverse effects), and difficulty in assessing the onset of spontaneous remission.[20]

**Iodides**

Iodide was the first form of drug therapy for Graves' disease. Its mechanism of action is to acutely block thyroid hormone release, inhibit thyroid hormone biosynthesis by interfering with intrathyroidal iodide utilization (the Wolff–Chaikoff effect), and decrease the size and vascularity of the gland. This early inhibitory effect provides symptom improvement within 2 to 7 days of initiating therapy. The iodides' effects are transient and limited because of the thyroid gland's ability to "escape" from the inhibitory effects. Therefore, iodides are limited mainly to use as adjunctive therapy to prepare a patient with Graves' disease for surgery, restore a euthyroid state in a patient treated with RAI or surgery who has a recurrence of hyperthyroidism, or shorten the time to a euthyroid state after RAI therapy.[15]

Potassium iodide is available either as a saturated solution (SSKI), which contains 40 mg of iodide per drop, or as Lugol's solution, which contains 8 mg of iodide per drop. A typical starting dose of SSKI is 3–10 drops daily (120–400 mg) in water or juice. When used to prepare a patient for surgery, it should be administered 7 to 14 days preoperatively. As an adjunct to RAI, SSKI should not be used before, but rather 1 week after, RAI treatment so that the radioactive iodide can concentrate in the thyroid. After 1 month, the dose can be titrated to the minimal dose required to control the condition. Potassium iodide therapy can usually be discontinued 3 to 6 months after RAI. The most frequent toxic effect with iodide therapy is hypersensitivity reactions (skin rashes, drug fever, rhinitis, conjunctivitis).

**Adrenergic Blockers**

As many of the manifestations of hyperthyroidism are mediated by $\beta$-adrenergic receptors, $\beta$-blockers (especially propranolol) have been used widely to ameliorate hyperthyroid symptoms such as palpitations, anxiety, tremor, and heat intolerance. The effects of other $\beta$-blockers have not been widely studied. Both propranolol and nadolol block the peripheral conversion of $T_4$ to $T_3$; however, the contribution of this effect to the overall therapeutic effect is probably small.

$\beta$-Blockers are usually used as adjunctive therapy with antithyroid drugs, RAI, or iodides; for Graves' disease or toxic nodules; in preparation for surgery; or in thyroid storm. The only conditions for which $\beta$-blockers are primary therapy for hyperthyroidism are thyroiditis and iodine-induced hyperthyroidism. Propranolol 20 to 40 mg four times daily is effective in ameliorating most hyperthyroid symptoms and maintaining a pulse of 80 beats per minute. Younger or more severely toxic patients may require as much as 240–480 mg/d, as there seems to be an increased clearance rate in these patients.[15] Caution should be taken in using any $\beta$-blocker in patients with congestive heart failure (except that solely caused by high output such as in hyperthyroidism), asthma, chronic obstructive pulmonary disease, or diabetes mellitus.

**Radioactive Iodine**

Radioactive iodine is administered as a colorless and tasteless liquid that is well absorbed and concentrates in the thyroid. Initially, RAI disrupts hormone synthesis by incorporating into thyroid hormones and thyroglobulin. $^{131}I$ has a half-life of 8 days and delivers $\beta$ radiation to a maximal depth of 2 mm. Over a period of weeks, follicular cells exposed to the radiation are damaged and the hyperthyroid state is attenuated. The goal of therapy is to destroy overactive thyroid cells, which usually requires a single dose of 4,000–8,000 rads. Benefits from RAI are seen within 1 month of treatment, but 3 to 6 months are required for nearly 60% of patients to attain a euthyroid state after a single nonablative RAI dose. The remaining 40% become euthyroid within a year, requiring two or more doses. It is advisable that a second RAI dose be given 6 to 12 months after the first RAI treatment and the major effects of the first dose have been noted.

The slow onset of effect with RAI does warrant symptomatic control with adjunctive therapy. Iodides should be administered 1 to 14 days *after* RAI to prevent interference with the uptake of RAI in the thyroid gland. Thioamides can be given before RAI to attain a euthyroid state; however, they should be suspended from 1 week before to 1 week after RAI administration to allow maximum $^{131}I$ uptake and concentration in the gland. $\beta$-Adrenergic blockers may be administered anytime without compromising RAI therapy, accounting for their role as a mainstay of adjunctive therapy to RAI treatment.[15]

The acute, short-term side effects of $^{131}I$ therapy are minimal and include mild thyroidal pain and tenderness, dysphagia, and some transient thinning of the hair. A secondary consequence of RAI is the development of primary hypothyroidism. Nearly 50% of patients are clinically hypothyroid 10 years after RAI treatment and approximately 80% at 20 years. If hypothyroidism persists longer than 2 months, it will most likely be permanent. The often feared long-term complications of radiation-induced carcinogenesis or teratogenesis have not been documented in long-term follow-up studies.[24,25]

**Surgery**

Surgical removal of the thyroid gland is the most definitive treatment of hyperthyroidism. Traditional preparation of the patient for thyroid surgery includes administration of PTU or methimazole until the patient is biochemically euthyroid (6 to 8 weeks usually) and then adding iodides (500 mg/d) for 10 to 14 days before surgery to decrease the vascularity of the gland. Propranolol has also been used for several weeks in the preoperative period in doses sufficient to maintain the resting pulse at a maximum 80 beats per minute. As $T_3$ and $T_4$ concentrations remain elevated postoperatively, propranolol therapy should be continued 7 to 10 days after thyroid surgery. A combined pretreatment with propranolol and 10 to 14 days of potassium iodide has been advocated.[26]

Surgery appears to be as safe as nonsurgical treatment for hyperthyroidism if performed by an experienced surgeon. Complications of thyroid surgery include hypothyroidism (less frequently than with RAI), hypoparathyroidism, and vocal cord paralysis.

**Clinical Considerations**

There is no optimal treatment for hyperthyroidism; treatment is individualized on the basis of the patient's age and health condition. Often the treatment decision is empiric. The thioamides are the preferred treatment for children, young adults, and pregnant women. Thyrotoxicosis is usually a self-limiting disease and the risk of hypothyroidism secondary to RAI or surgery makes thioamides a reasonable treatment alternative. Patients with a large gland, diffuse goiter, and long duration of disease may not have a good prognosis with thioamides. Noncompliant patients and those with swallowing difficulty may require another form of therapy. RAI is the preferred treatment for debilitated, cardiac, and elderly patients and patients who have had a failure or toxic reaction on drug therapy. RAI is also used in patients who relapse after surgery. Thyroidectomy is considered the treatment of choice for carcinoma, extremely large goiters (over 80 g), and patients with contraindications to thioamides (i.e., allergy or adverse effects) or RAI (i.e., pregnancy).

***Graves' Disease*** In the treatment of Graves' disease in children and adolescents, most clinicians use the thiourea drugs as initial therapy. RAI therapy is avoided to obviate the eventual hypothyroidism requiring lifetime thyroid supplementation and the potential long-term carcinogenic or genetic effects of RAI. Two therapy alternatives, RAI and thioureas, are used in young adults 18 to 30 years old. In adults over 30, RAI is the treatment of choice. Pharmacologic induction of euthyroidism with iodides or thioureas usually expedites clinical recovery and reduces the risk of radiation-induced thyroiditis. $\beta$-Adrenergic blockage, if not contraindicated, may prevent symptoms associated with excessive thyroid hormones. As RAI takes effect after several weeks, pharmacologic therapy should be tapered and monitored to maintain euthyroidism.

Approximately 0.2% of pregnancies are complicated by Graves' disease. As RAI is contraindicated in pregnancy, antithyroid drug therapy is usually the treatment of choice. PTU is the preferred agent because it does not cross the placental membranes as well as methimazole and does not enter breast milk. To prevent goiter and suppression of fetal thyroid function, PTU is usually prescribed in daily doses of 300 mg or less and tapered to 50–150 mg daily after 4 to 6 weeks. Concomitant thyroid hormone has been advocated to prevent fetal goiter, but thyroxine does not cross the placenta well. Long-term administration of iodides (even vaginal povidone–iodine) may lead to iodine crossing the placental membrane and causing fetal goiter. Also, long-term use of propranolol should be avoided because of its association with fetal respiratory depression, small placenta, intrauterine growth retardation, and postnatal bradycardia and hypoglycemia. If acute symptoms occur or preoperative preparation is required, propranolol or iodides may be used cautiously for less than 7 days. Surgery should only be performed during the second trimester to avoid spontaneous abortion.[27]

Serum TSH and $T_4$ concentrations should be monitored closely in pregnant patients treated with antithyroid drug therapy. $T_4$ concentrations should be maintained in the normal range for pregnancy, which is usually 12–17 $\mu$g/dL (somewhat higher than the usual 4–12 $\mu$g/dL) because of high thyroid-binding globulin concentrations. As Graves' disease spontaneously improves in the third trimester, antithyroid drug therapy may be discontinued. Postpartum follow-up is crucial because relapse often occurs after delivery.

***Toxic Nodules*** The preferred therapy for patients with toxic nodules is surgery or RAI, except that surgery is usually selected for young patients. Toxic multinodular goiter and a solitary toxic nodule are well suited to RAI, as nonautonomous areas are suppressed and fail to incorporate radioactive iodine. Therefore, the normal thyroid tissue is selectively protected from the destruction of RAI. Elderly or cardiac patients with toxic multinodular goiter require pretreatment with antithyroidal drugs to deplete intrathyroidal stores before RAI is administered so that a release of thyroid hormones does not exacerbate an underlying condition.

***Thyroid Storm*** Thyroid storm is a life-threatening medical emergency characterized by severe thyrotoxicosis, high fever (often greater than 103°F), tachycardia, tachypnea, dehydration, delirium, coma, nausea, vomiting, and diarrhea. Its pathogenesis is not well known, but it typically follows surgery or infection. An increased quantity of thyroid hormones in conjunction with a heightened sympathetic and adrenal output contributes to the multiple systemic manifestations of thyroid storm. Thyroid storm may occur at any age and has an average duration of 72 hours, although symptoms may persist for up to 8 days if treatment is not aggressive. The aims of pharmacotherapy include four major

**Table 53.5** Drug Dosages Used in the Management of Thyroid Storm

| *Drug* | *Regimen* |
|---|---|
| Propylthiouracil | 900–1,200 mg/d PO in four or six divided doses |
| Methimazole | 90–120 mg/d PO in four or six divided doses |
| Sodium iodide | Up to 2 g/d IV in single or divided doses |
| Lugol's solution | 5–10 drops TID in water or juice |
| Saturated solution of potassium iodide | 1–2 drops TID in water or juice |
| Propranolol | 40–80 mg every 6 h |
| Reserpine | 0.25 mg PO every 8 h |
| | 2.5–5.0 mg IV or IM every 8 h |
| Guanethidine | 10–50 mg PO every 8 h |
| Lithium | 600–1,500 mg/d PO in three or four divided doses |
| Dexamethasone | 5–20 mg/d PO or IV in divided doses |
| Prednisone | 25–100 mg/d PO in divided doses |
| Methylprednisolone | 20–80 mg/d IV in divided doses |
| Hydrocortisone | 100–400 mg/d IV in divided doses |

areas: (1) inhibition of the synthesis and release of thyroid hormones, (2) reversal of the peripheral effects of hormones and catecholamines, (3) supportive treatment of vital systems, and (4) elimination of the precipitating cause. Specific agents used in thyroid storm are outlined in Table 53.5. PTU is the preferred thioamide because it interferes with the production of thyroid hormones and blocks the peripheral conversion of $T_4$ to $T_3$. Iodides, which rapidly block the release of preformed thyroid hormones, should be administered after PTU is initiated to inhibit iodide utilization by the overactive gland.

The use of lithium in thyroid storm is controversial, but it shares iodide's inhibition properties on the thyroid gland. Depleting agents such as reserpine and guanethidine are classic therapy in decreasing tachycardia, agitation, and nervousness; however, propranolol is quite effective in antagonizing the catecholamine-mediated autonomic hyperactivity and is advantageous over classic agents (reserpine and guanethidine) with rapid onset, short duration of action, and fewer gastrointestinal and psychogenic side effects. Supportive treatment can include adrenocorticosteroids to prevent hypoadrenalism, antipyretics, fluid and electrolyte replacement, sedatives, digitalis, antiarrhythmics, insulin, and antibiotics. Mortality rates in thyroid storm range from 7% to 10% and are significantly reduced by accurate, continuous, and aggressive treatment, especially when adrenergic blocking agents are employed.[28]

## Hypothyroidism

Hypothyroidism is characterized by a progressive slowing of systemic functions because of insufficient thyroid hormone synthesis. Cretinism refers to a developmental abnormality related to thyroid deficiency from birth; myxedema is a severe form of hypothyroidism with an accumulation of hydrophilic mucopolysaccharides that infiltrate the dermal layers. The prevalence of hypothyroidism is about 1% in women and 0.1% in men; it seems greater in psychiatric or depressed patients with depressing illness. The prevalence rises to nearly 6% or 7% in women after age 60.[29]

### *Epidemiology/Etiology*

Hypothyroidism can be classified as primary (thyroprivic), secondary (pituitary), or tertiary (hypothalamic) as outlined in Table 53.6. Goiter formation results from excessive TSH stimulation in response to low circulating concentrations of $T_3$ and $T_4$. Nongoitrous forms can be primary or thyroidal in nature (i.e., congenital, idiopathic, or iatrogenic) or secondary, which involves the suprathyroidal structures (i.e., Sheehan's postpartum pituitary hemorrhage, head injury, tumors, or idiopathic atrophy of the hypophysis). Iatrogenic hypothyroidism is most commonly caused by RAI or surgery; idiopathic atrophy of the thyroid may be the end stage of autoimmune destruction with Hashimoto's thyroiditis; congenital hypothyroidism is cretinism. Goitrous forms of the disease include Hashimoto's thyroiditis, iodine deficiency, drug-induced disease, and inherited biosynthetic defects.

Hashimoto's thyroiditis (chronic or lymphocytic thyroiditis) is the most common cause of goitrous hypothyroidism, with an incidence similar to that of Graves' disease (3 to 6 per 10,000 annually). It has a high predilection for women (15:1), with peak occurrence in middle age. Similar to Graves' disease, there is a strong genetic predisposition. Hashimoto's thyroiditis is characterized by diffuse enlargement and lymphocytic infiltration of the gland, an autoimmune disturbance, and hypothyroidism.

Multinodular goiters are a common disorder that affect predominantly women and occur in nearly 4% of adults over age 30. The etiology appears to be the presence of longstanding TSH stimulation, which may be exacerbated by iodide deficiency, dietary goitrogens (i.e., rutabagas, turnips, cabbage), or enzymatic defects. Clinically, the patient may be euthyroid and develop hypothyroidism or hyperthyroidism with time.

**Table 53.6** Etiology of Hypothyroidism

| *Origin of deficiency* | *Etiology* |
|---|---|
| Thyroidal | |
| Thyroprivic | Congenital development defect (cretinism) |
| | Primary idiopathic |
| | Postablation (RAI or surgery) |
| Goitrous | Hereditary biosynthetic defects |
| | Iodine deficiency (not in North America) |
| | Drug-induced thyrotoxicosis (iodides, lithium, PTU, methimazole) |
| | Chronic autoimmune thyroiditis (Hashimoto's) |
| | Goitrogens (dietary) |
| Suprathyroidal | Pituitary or hypothalamic disease |

**Table 53.7** Thyroid Hormone Synthesis and Secretion Inhibitors

| *Mechanism of action* | *Substance* |
|---|---|
| Blocks iodide transport into thyroid | Bromine<br>Fluorine<br>Lithium |
| Impairs organification and coupling of thyroid hormones | Thioamides<br>Sulfonylureas<br>Sulfonamides?<br>Salicylamides?<br>Antipyrone? |
| Inhibits thyroid hormone secretion | Iodide (large doses)<br>Lithium |

Drug-induced hypothyroidism can result from any substance that interferes with the biosynthesis, release, or peripheral conversion of thyroid hormones (Table 53.7). The thioamides and iodides, used therapeutically in hyperthyroidism, may be goitrogenic if excessive doses are employed. Lithium has been associated with goiter and hypothyroidism. Lithium acts similarly to the iodides by inhibiting the release of thyroid hormone. The onset of diffuse goiter with or without hypothyroidism appears within 5 months to 2 years of treatment and usually occurs in patients with a strong family history of or prior thyroid abnormalities. Goiters usually subside with discontinuation of lithium or administration of thyroxine.[30] Large doses of chlorpropamide (3–7 g) and tolbutamide depress $^{131}I$ uptake by interfering with iodide binding; however, this effect is uncommon at usual sulfonylurea dose ranges.[31]

Iatrogenic hypothyroidism is most commonly a result of RAI treatment in Graves' disease. Hypothyroidism may not be manifest until several years after RAI administration, but virtually all patients eventually become hypothyroid. The incidence of hypothyroidism at 5 years after RAI treatment varies from 10% to 50%. Another significant cause of hypothyroidism is surgical removal of the gland. The incidence is reported at 5% to 40% of patients undergoing thyroidectomy but is highly dependent on surgical technique, follow-up, and function of the thyroid remnant.[2]

### *Pathogenesis*

As antibodies to thyroglobulin or colloid or microsomal components are often present, pathogenesis may involve an autoimmune process related to defects in the suppressor T lymphocytes. In addition, cell-mediated immunity against thyroid antigens has been found. Hashimoto's thyroiditis often coexists with other autoimmune disorders such as rheumatoid arthritis, collagen vascular diseases, and Graves' disease. It is postulated that Hashimoto's and Graves' diseases may actually be variant manifestations of the same autoimmune process, as mild thyrotoxicosis may precede the onset of hypothyroidism.

### *Clinical Presentation*

The manifestations of cretinism are present at birth or, more commonly, are evident within the first several months. The neonate is persistently jaundiced, constipated, and somnolent, and has a hoarse cry and feeding problems. Normal childhood development is markedly delayed and typical physical features of short stature, broad flat nose, protruding tongue, sparse hair, wide set eyes, dry skin, and protruding abdomen become evident. Mental development is also retarded and intellectual attainment depends on the rapidity of hormonal replacement.

In the adult, hypothyroidism ranges from subclinical, with no overt symptoms, to the classic presentation of large tongue, husky voice, brittle nails and hair, fatigue, cold intolerance, constipation, cool and dry skin, slow reflexes, apathy, and weight gain. Cardiac findings include decreased pulse, stroke volume, and cardiac output, as well as cardiomegaly, edema, and effusions. There is an obvious metabolic slowdown as the disease progresses to myxedema with symptoms of coarse voice, slurred speech, memory impairment, and puffy facies. If left untreated, myxedema can progress to a potentially life-threatening condition often labeled "myxedema coma," marked by hypothermia, hypoventilation, respiratory acidosis, hyponatremia, hypotension, and a comatose state.

There is a paucity of symptoms in the extremes of age. Both the hypothyroid neonate and elderly patient typically have very few or no symptoms. In the elderly, many of the clinical signs and symptoms of hypothyroidism may inadvertently be attributed to old age. In many elderly patients hypothyroidism is not recognized until late in the course of the disease.[4]

#### Diagnosis

As many patients may not present with overt symptoms, the signs and symptoms are not an absolute means of diagnosis but a guide to laboratory tests that can confirm a clinical suspicion. Decreased serum $T_4$ concentrations and $FT_4I$ are common to all types of hypothyroidism. The serum TSH concentration is invariably increased in thyroprivic (primary) and goitrous varieties of hypothyroidism, yet may be normal or undetectable in pituitary or hypothalamic types. An elevated serum TSH concentration is highly specific for and diagnostic of primary hypothyroidism.

Other manifestations of hypothyroidism include increased serum cholesterol, triglyceride, and low-density lipoprotein concentrations in primary disease; elevations of serum creatine phosphokinase, lactic dehydrogenase, and serum glutamic–oxaloacetic transaminase concentrations; and abnormally slow deep tendon reflexes. Electrocardiographic changes may include bradycardia, low amplitude, and flat T waves. The x-ray films show cardiomegaly or pericardial effusion. Thyroglobulin antibodies are present in 80% of Hashimoto's patients, whereas antimicrosomal antibodies are present in 97%.[2]

#### Course

Naturally occurring hypothyroidism has an insidious onset and often is not noticed by the patient. Symptoms are often general in nature (i.e., fatigue, constipation, weight gain,

**Table 53.8** Thyroid Preparations Used in the Treatment of Hypothyroidism

| *Drug/dosage form* | *Content* | *Relative equivalency* | *Comments* |
|---|---|---|---|
| Thyroid, USP<br>Armour Thyroid, USV<br>¼, ½, 1, 1½, 2, 3, 4, and 5 grain tablets | Desiccated hog, beef, or sheep thyroid gland | 1 grain (equivalent to 60 $\mu g$ of $T_4$) | Unpredictable hormonal content; poor stability; inexpensive; generic brands may not be bioequivalent |
| Thyroglobulin<br>Proloid, Parke–Davis<br>½, 1, 1½, 2, and 3 grain tablets | Partially purified hog thyroglobulin | 1 grain | Standardized biologically to give $T_4$:$T_3$ ratio of 2.5:1; more expensive than thyroid extract; no clinical advantage |
| L-Thyroxine<br>Synthroid, Flint; Levothyroid, USV<br>25, 50, 100, 150, 175, 200, and 300 $\mu g$ tablets; 500 $\mu g$ tablet | Synthetic $T_4$ | 100 $\mu g$ | Stable; predictable potency; generics may not be bioequivalent; when switching from natural thyroid to L-thyroxine, lower dose by ½ gr; variable absorption between products; $t_{1/2}$ = 7 d, so daily dosing |
| Liothyronine<br>Cytomel, Smith Kline and French<br>5 and 25 $\mu g$ tablets | Synthetic $T_3$ | 25 $\mu g$ | Uniform absorption; rapid onset; $t_{1/2}$ = 1.5 d, multiple daily dosing; monitor response with TSH assays |
| Liotrix<br>Euthyroid, Parke–Davis; Thyrolar, USV<br>¼, ½, 1, 2, and 3 strength tablets | Synthetic $T_4$:$T_3$ in 4:1 ratio | | Stable, predictable, expensive; lacks therapeutic rationale because $T_4$ is converted to $T_3$ peripherally |

drowsiness) and especially in the elderly may be attributed to advancing age. Patients may not present until the disease is quite advanced with myxedematous signs. Postablative hypothyroidism (i.e., after RAI or surgery) occurs more suddenly with symptoms recognized by the patient. Hashimoto's thyroiditis begins with a gradual enlargement of the thyroid, which may remain unchanged for several years. Signs and symptoms of mild hypothyroidism may occur in 20% of patients when first discovered.[2]

### *Treatment*

The goal of therapy is to restore thyroid hormone in tissues to provide symptomatic relief and reverse the biochemical abnormalities of hypothyroidism. Any of the commercially available thyroid preparations accomplishes this goal (Table 53.8). When $T_4$ is administered, $T_3$ is formed by tissue deiodinases so that adequate serum concentrations of both hormones are maintained. The thyroid preparations are either natural (i.e., desiccated thyroid, thyroglobulin) or synthetic (levothyroxine, liothyronine, liotrix) in origin.

#### Natural Thyroid Hormones

Desiccated thyroid is derived from hog, beef, or sheep thyroid gland. The *United States Pharmacopeia* requires that the preparation contain 0.17% to 0.23% organic iodine by weight. With these requirements, there is a variable potency in the quantities and proportions of $T_4$ and $T_3$. Only the Armour brand is biologically standardized, making it preferable to generic preparations that may not be bioequivalent. In addition, the animal protein source may be antigenic in allergic or sensitive patients. Even though desiccated thyroid is inexpensive, its limitations do not render it a drug of choice for hypothyroid patients. Thyroglobulin is a purified hog gland extract biologically standardized to yield a $T_4$:$T_3$ ratio of 2.5:1. It has no clinical advantages and is not widely used.

#### Synthetic Thyroid Hormones

Levothyroxine ($T_4$) is one of the more common thyroid preparations because it is chemically stable, is relatively inexpensive, is free of antigenicity, and has uniform potency. L-Thyroxine has a half-life of 7 days, affording once-daily dosing. Absorption of L-thyroxine varies from 35% to 78%, with most patients absorbing 60% to 65%. Generic preparations may not be bioequivalent with brand name products and have resulted in inadequate thyroid replacement. Therefore, substitution of multisource thyroid preparations should not be encouraged.[32]

Liothyronine ($T_3$) is chemically pure with a known potency and has a shorter half-life of 1.5 days; it requires multiple daily dosing. Although it is widely used diagnostically in the $T_3$ suppression test, $T_3$ has some major clinical disadvantages, including a higher incidence of cardiac adverse effects, higher cost, and difficulty in monitoring with conventional laboratory tests.

Liotrix is a combination of synthetic $T_4$ and $T_3$ in a 4:1 ratio that attempts to mimic the natural hormonal secretion.

It is chemically stable and pure and has a predictable potency. The major limitations to this product are high cost and lack of therapeutic rationale, as about 35% of $T_4$ is peripherally converted to $T_3$.

***Dosing/Monitoring*** The average thyroid replacement dose is between 100 and 200 mg of thyroxine daily; however, there is a wide range of replacement doses, necessitating individualized therapy. The initial $T_4$ dose is highly dependent on patient's age, severity of deficiency, and duration of disease.

In young, healthy adult patients with recent onset of disease, a thyroxine dose of 100–200 μg daily will maintain a euthyroid state in nearly 90% of hypothyroid patients.[33] Further dosage adjustments should be made at monthly intervals until the patient is euthyroid. In young patients with long-standing disease and patients over 45 without known cardiac disease, therapy should be initiated with 50 μg of $T_4$ daily and the dose increased to 100 μg/d after 1 month. The recommended initial daily dosage for older patients or those with known cardiac disease is only 25 μg of $T_4$. Patients should be followed closely, with the dosage titrated upward in 12.5- or 25-μg increments at monthly intervals to prevent the elderly patient's cardiovascular system from being overstressed. Some patients may experience an exacerbation of angina with higher doses of thyroid hormone.

In congenital hypothyroidism, full maintenance therapy should be instituted early to improve the prognosis for mental and physical development. The average maintenance dose of $T_4$ in neonates and children is 3.5 μg/kg/d, or approximately 100 μg/m $^2$ of body surface area.

Patients with subclinical hypothyroidism (many times seen in the elderly) have no signs or symptoms, normal serum $T_4$ and $T_3$ concentrations, and an elevated basal TSH concentration. Treatment in this case is quite controversial, but most clinicians supplement with thyroid hormone provided such treatment does not pose significant risk.

Once euthyroidism is attained, patients are usually maintained on that stable daily dose of $T_4$ for their lifetime. The ability to measure serum TSH concentrations has improved the accuracy with which thyroid hormone replacement can be monitored. Plasma TSH concentrations begin to fall within hours and may be normalized in 2 weeks. The primary indices used to monitor thyroid hormone replacement are serum $T_4$ and TSH concentrations, which should be checked monthly until a euthyroid state is achieved. Serum $T_4$ concentrations can be useful when noncompliance, malabsorption, overtreatment, or change in $T_4$ preparation bioequivalence is suspected. The expected range of serum $T_4$ concentrations in patients receiving replacement therapy is higher than that of normal persons. This may occur because the biologic effect of $T_3$ is absent and must be supplemented by a higher thyroxine dose. The usual serum range in treated patients is 6–17 μg/dL compared with a normal range of 5–12 μg/dL.[33] An elevated TSH concentration indicates insufficient replacement. The appropriate dose maintains the TSH concentration in the normal range. If biochemical or clinical signs of hypothyroidism persist despite suppression of TSH concentrations to normal, the response to thyrotropin-releasing hormone (TRH) should be evaluated. If TSH is still elevated, the dose of thyroid hormone should be increased. If the response to TRH is low or normal, there may be a peripheral, rather than pituitary, resistance to thyroid hormone.

***Adverse Effects*** Serious untoward effects are unusual if dosing is appropriate and the patient is carefully monitored during initial treatment. Patients with an underlying or past history of bipolar affective disorders may exhibit manic behavior on thyroid hormone supplementation. Gross overtreatment may be fatal secondary to cardiac causes.[34] Allergic or idiosyncratic reactions can occur with the natural animal derivate products such as desiccated thyroid and thyroglobulin, but these are extremely rare with the synthetic products used today.

Hypothyroidism with coexisting cardiovascular disease can result in complications with thyroid hormone replacement. If replacement doses are too high or titrated too aggressively, cardiac patients may have more frequent angina episodes, arrhythmias, congestive heart failure, or myocardial infarction. In such patients, partial correction of hypothyroidism often provides a balance between cardiovascular disease and thyroid deficiency.

***Prognosis*** A patient with uncomplicated myxedema receiving a typical dose of $T_4$ of 150 μg/d will have an increase in metabolic activity and be out of the myxedematous zone within a week of initiating therapy. Plasma TSH concentrations begin to drop within hours and may be in the normal range after 2 weeks.[35] An impressive diuresis usually occurs within 2 or 3 days, with an improvement in the puffy facial appearance and weight loss. Speech, skin temperature, mental alertness, and physical activity show improvement within 72 hours.

In children with hypothyroidism developing beyond 2 to 3 years of age, normal central nervous system (CNS) and physiologic development are expected with thyroid replacement therapy; however, in congenital or neonatal hypothyroidism, CNS development is dependent on the severity of the disease and the time at which therapy is begun. Retrospective studies have shown that the earlier the treatment begins, the better the prognosis for mental development. Three months of age seems to be a critical time after which treatment may not normalize intellectual development.[36]

Myxedema coma is the end stage of long-standing uncorrected hypothyroidism. Clinical features include hypothermia, advanced stages of hypothyroid symptoms, and altered sensorium ranging from delirium to coma. Mortality rates of 60% to 70% necessitate immediate and aggressive therapy with intravenous thyroxine 500 μg to saturate the thyroxine-binding globulins. If cardiac disease is present, the initial dose should be 200 μg intravenously. Consciousness, lowered TSH concentrations, and normal vital signs are expected within 24 hours. Maintenance doses are guided by clinical response. Supportive therapy must be instituted to maintain adequate ventilation, euglycemia, blood pressure, and body temperature.

### Clinical Considerations

Myxedema during pregnancy has been associated with congenital hypothyroidism, spontaneous abortions, and mental retardation; however, normal infants have been born to hypothyroid women. Congenital hypothyroidism may result from maternal–fetal transfer of destructive antibodies in women with Hashimoto's thyroiditis. As thyroid hormone does not cross the placental membranes, thyroid replacement does not affect the fetus. Typical doses of $T_4$ can be initiated in the absence of cardiac abnormalities and should be monitored with $T_4$ (radioimmunoassay) and $FT_4I$ assays monthly in the first trimester to ensure adequate replacement. TSH assays should not be used because of human chorionic gonadotropin interference.

Hypothyroidism may affect the metabolism and clinical efficacy of several medications. Digitalis preparations have a decreased volume of distribution in the hypothyroid state, resulting in increased sensitivity to the digitalis effect. Therefore, many hypothyroid patients achieve a therapeutic effect at lower digitalis doses. Insulin degradation may be delayed in hypothyroidism, thereby requiring a lower insulin dose. The anticoagulant response to warfarin is delayed because of increased half-life of clotting factors. Therefore, the hypothyroid patient may achieve anticoagulation on a lower warfarin dose. Respiratory depressants such as barbiturates, phenothiazines, and narcotic analgesics should be avoided, as there is an increased sensitivity that may increase carbon dioxide retention and precipitate myxedema coma.

## Summary

Although the exact etiology of thyroid disorders is unknown, recent research indicates that the two most common disorders, Graves' disease and Hashimoto's thyroiditis, involve the autoimmune system. Regardless of the etiology, the treatment objectives are to normalize the production of thyroid hormone and minimize the associated systemic symptoms of hypothyroidism and hyperthyroidism. While many patients present with "textbook" clinical manifestations, thyroid disorders are often nonspecific or subclinical in the neonate and elderly. The diagnosis must be based on biochemical findings in addition to the clinical presentation. Effective treatment must be individualized and take into consideration the patient's age, sex, health status, and severity of thyroid disease.

## References

1. Freidman JM, Fialkow PJ. The genetics of Graves' disease. Clin Endocrinol Metab 1978;7:47–65.
2. DeGroot LJ, Larsen PR, Refetoff S, et al. The Thyroid and Its Diseases, 5th ed. New York, John Wiley and Sons, 1984.
3. Okita N, Row VV, Volpe R. Suppressor T-lymphocyte deficiency in Graves' disease and Hashimoto's thyroiditis. J Clin Endocrinol Metab 1981;52:528–533.
4. Gambert SR. Atypical presentation of thyroid disease in the elderly. Geriatrics 1985;40:63–69.
5. Blum M. Thyroid function and disease in the elderly. Hosp Pract 1981;16:105–108, 110, 113.
6. Ladenson PW. Diseases of the thyroid gland. Clin Endocrinol Metab 1985;14:145–173.
7. Spaulding SW, Lippes H. Hyperthyroidism: Causes, clinical features, and diagnosis. Med Clin North Am 1985; 69:937–951.
8. Volpe R. Subacute (de Quervain's) thyroiditis. Clin Endocrinol Metab 1979;8:81–95.
9. Hollander CS, Shenkman L, Mitsuma T, et al. Hypertriiodothyroninemia as a premonitory manifestation of thyrotoxicosis. Lancet 1971;2:731–733.
10. Mariotti S, Martino E, Cupini C, et al. Low serum thyroglobulin as a clue to the diagnosis of thyrotoxicosis factitia. N Engl J Med 1982;307:410–412.
11. Fradkin JE, Wolff J. Iodine-induced thyrotoxicosis. Medicine 1983;62:1–20.
12. Silas AM, White AG. Hyperthyroidism after use of contrast medium. Br Med J 1975;4:162.
13. Rosser R. Thyrotoxicosis and lithium. Br J Psychiatry 1976;128: 61–66.
14. Melmed S, Nademane K, Reed AW, et al. Hyperthyroxinemia with bradycardia and normal thyrotropin secretion after chronic amiodarone administration. J Clin Endocrinol Metab 1981;53: 997–1001.
15. Cooper DS, Ridgway EC. Clinical management of patients with hyper-thyroidism. Med Clin North Am 1985;953–971.
16. Chopra IJ. A study of extrathyroidal conversion of thyroxine ($T_4$) to 3′, 3′, 5-triiodothyronine ($T_3$) in vitro. Endocrinology 1977;101:453–463.
17. McGregor AM, Petersen MM, McLachlan SM, et al. Carbimazole and the autoimmune response in Graves' disease. N Engl J Med 1980;303:302–307.
18. Cooper DS, Bode HH, Nath B, et al. Methimazole pharmacology in man: Studies using a newly developed radioimmunoassay for methimazole. J Clin Endocrinol Metab 1984;58:473–479.
19. Cooper DS, Goldminz D, Levin AA, et al. Agranulocytosis associated with antithyroid drugs. Ann Intern Med 1983;98:26–29.
20. Wartofsky L. Guidelines for the treatment of hyperthyroidism. Am Fam Phys 1984;30:199–210.
21. Romaldini JH, Bromberg N, Werner RS, et al. Comparison of effects of high and low dosage regimens of antithyroid drugs in the management of Graves' hyperthyroidism. J Clin Endocrinol Metab 1983;57:563–570.
22. Greer MA, Kammer H, Bouma DJ. Short-term antithyroid drug therapy for the thyrotoxicosis of Graves' disease. N Engl J Med 1977;297:173–176.
23. Barnes HV, Bledsoe T. A simple test to select the thioamide schedule in thyrotoxicosis. J Clin Endocrinol Metab 1972;35: 250–255.
24. Holm LE, Dahlqvist I, Engs M, et al. Malignant thyroid tumors after iodine-131 therapy: A retrospective cohort study. N Engl J Med 1980;303:188–219.
25. Robertson JS, Gorman CA. Gonadal radiation dose and its genetic significance in radioiodine therapy of hyperthyroidism. J Nucl Med 1976;17:826–835.
26. Feek CM, Sawers JS, Irvine CW, et al. Combination of potassium iodide and propranolol in preparation of patients with Graves' disease for thyroid surgery. N Engl J Med 1980;302: 883–885.
27. Burrow GN. The management of thyrotoxicosis in pregnancy. N Engl J Med 1985;313:562–565.
28. Raber J. The pharmacotherapy of thyroid storm. Drug Intell Clin Pharm 1980;14:344–352.

29. Sawin CT, Chopra D, Azizi F, et al. The aging thyroid: Increased prevalence of elevated serum thyrotropin in the elderly. JAMA 1979;242:247–250.
30. Shopsin B. Effect of lithium on thyroid function. Dis Nerv Syst 1970;31:237–244.
31. Nikkila EA, Jakobson T, Josipii SG, et al. Thyroid function in diabetic patients under long-term sulfonylurea treatment. Acta Endocrinol 1960;33:623.
32. Ingbar JC, Braverman LE, Ingbar SH. Equivalence of thyroid preparations. JAMA 1980;244:1095.
33. Stock JM, Surks MI, Oppenheimer JH. Replacement dosage of L-thyroxine in hypothyroidism. N Engl J Med 1974;290:529–533.
34. Bhasin S, Wallace W, Lawrence JB, et al. Sudden death associated with thyroid hormone abuse. Am J Med 1981;71:887–890.
35. Ridgway EC, McCammon JA, Benotti J, et al. Acute metabolic responses in myxedema to large doses of intravenous L-thyroxine. Ann Intern Med 1972;77:549-555.
36. Klein AH, Meltzer S, Kenny FH. Improved prognosis in congenital hypothyroidism treated before three months. J Pediatr 1972;89:912–915.

# Chapter 54 / Diabetes Mellitus

George E. Francisco, Jr, PharmD

Diabetes mellitus is a term that describes a series of complex and chronic metabolic disorders characterized by symptomatic glucose intolerance. Because diabetes appears to be a heterogeneous group of disorders, there is no commonality in regard to the age of onset, genetic predisposition, or development of complications. It is known, however, that all diabetics eventually show abnormalities of insulin secretion and complications of the disease, such as vascular abnormalities; most manifest some degree of cellular resistance to insulin.

Currently there are more than 10 million diabetics in the United States, and estimates reveal that this number will double by the year 2000. Over 600,000 new cases of diabetes are diagnosed each year. If left untreated, the disease can directly or indirectly affect virtually every organ in the body. Although technological advances can correct many of the ocular changes associated with this disease, diabetes is still the leading cause of blindness in the United States.

## Pathogenesis/Classification

Until recently diabetes was classified primarily by age of onset. Such terms as juvenile onset, adult onset, brittle, chemical, overt, and latent often made the understanding of diabetes difficult. The National Diabetes Data Group has reclassified diabetes, and this new classification has been adopted by the American Diabetes Association.[1] The two main types of diabetics include insulin-dependent diabetes mellitus (IDDM or type I) and non–insulin-dependent diabetes mellitus (NIDDM or type II). A much smaller group includes diabetes secondary to various drugs and diseases, impaired glucose tolerance (IGT), and gestational diabetes mellitus (GDM). See Table 54.1 for a more complete classification.

### *Type I*

This type of diabetes usually occurs in childhood or early adulthood and accounts for only 5% to 10% of all diabetics. These patients are often thin, have an absolute lack of insulin, and are prone to develop ketoacidosis if insulin is withheld. This is probably a heterogeneous disorder; heredity, viruses, and autoimmune syndromes have been linked to its development.

### *Type II*

Type II diabetes usually manifests in adulthood around age 40 or later. More than 90% of diabetics are of the type II or non–insulin-dependent type. Type II diabetes also appears to be a heterogeneous mix, although it is more genetically linked than is type I diabetes.[2] About 90% of patients with NIDDM are obese and may not display the classic symptoms of diabetes. They may initially be hyposecretors, normal secretors, or hypersecretors of insulin; however, the insulin does not appear to be useful in the transport of glucose into cells because of hidden receptors, desensitized receptors, or low quality of insulin. Type II diabetics do not usually progress to ketoacidosis (except during periods of stress); therefore, insulin replacement is not an absolute necessity for initial therapy. (See Table 54.2 for a more thorough differentiation between type I and II diabetes.)

### *Other Types*

Other diabetics may have preexisting pancreatic disease or some type of hormone excess (e.g., ACTH, cortisol) resulting from endocrine disease or hormone treatment. Diabetes may also result from the use of certain medications (e.g., thiazide diuretics) or from insulin receptor abnormalities. These patients have either known or very likely causes for their diabetes.

Gestational diabetes mellitus (GDM) refers to onset of glucose intolerance during pregnancy, usually in the second or third trimester. These patients almost always require insulin therapy during pregnancy, but may be asymptomatic postdelivery. Patients with GDM should be tested and reclassified accordingly after delivery.

### *Impaired Glucose Tolerance*

Impaired glucose tolerance (IGT) is the term given to patients who have higher-than-normal plasma glucose levels but are not diagnostic for diabetes. (Remember that the definition of diabetes is based on *symptomatic* glucose intolerance.) Although about 25% of these patients go on to develop diabetes mellitus, it is important not to label these patients as diabetic until a definite diagnosis has been made as there are often insurance and job limitations placed on diabetics. Medications are many times implicated as the cause of IGT (see Table 54.3).

## Metabolism and Utilization of Carbohydrates, Proteins, and Fats

### *Insulin*

Before understanding the etiology, manifestations, or complications of diabetes, one must first be familiar with normal carbohydrate, protein, and fat metabolism. Carbohydrates

**Table 54.1** Classification of Diabetes Mellitus and Impaired Glucose Tolerance

1. Diabetes mellitus
   a. Type I: insulin-dependent diabetes mellitus (IDDM)
   b. Type II: non–insulin-dependent diabetes mellitus (NIDDM)
2. Secondary causes of diabetes mellitus
   a. Pancreatic disease and endocrinopathies
      i. Chronic pancreatitis, cystic fibrosis, pancreatectomy, hemochromatosis
      ii. Acromegaly, Cushing's disease, glucagonoma, pheochromocytoma, primary aldosteronism
   b. Drugs: catecholamines, glucocorticoids, oral contraceptives, thiazide and loop diuretics
   c. Genetic syndromes: Huntington's chorea, hyperlipidemia, muscular dystrophy
3. Impaired glucose tolerance (IGT)—causes
   a. Pre–diabetes mellitus
   b. Secondary to pancreatic disease, drugs, and genetic syndromes (see secondary causes of diabetes mellitus above)
   c. Gestational glucose intolerance

are broken down in the body to glucose. The glucose is absorbed from the gastrointestinal tract into the bloodstream; it is then oxidized in skeletal muscle to produce energy. Glucose is also stored in the liver in the form of glycogen and is converted in adipose tissue to fats and triglycerides. Insulin, which is produced in, stored in, and released from the $\beta$ cells of the pancreas, facilitates these processes. It increases uptake of glucose by the tissues, increases liver glycogen levels, decreases glycogen breakdown (glycogenolysis) by the liver, increases synthesis of fatty acids, decreases breakdown of fatty acids into ketone bodies, and promotes incorporation of amino acids into proteins.[3]

Insulin is normally released from the pancreas at a rate of 0.5–1 U/h. Additional insulin is also released when the blood sugar is in excess of 100 mg/dL. The average adult pancreas secretes 25–50 units of insulin per day. Insulin is cleared metabolically by the liver, peripheral tissues, and kidneys. Hence, it is not unusual for patients with renal disease to require less insulin simply because insulin is not being metabolized.

Glucose can actively diffuse into the brain without the aid of insulin, but muscle and fat require the presence of insulin to utilize glucose for energy. If glucose is not available to muscle and adipose tissue, these tissues will convert amino acids to carbohydrate (called gluconeogenesis). If these tissues are further deprived of glucose, they will eventually metabolize stored fats, resulting in the production of free fatty acids that are eventually oxidized to ketone bodies.[3]

The body normally maintains plasma glucose concentrations between 40 and 160 mg%. A plasma glucose concentration of at least 40 mg% is necessary for normal brain function. In addition, glucose is the primary source of nutrition for cells. Therefore, a high plasma concentration implies that glucose is not being transported into cells for energy production. Plasma concentrations in excess of 180 mg%, however, may exceed the kidney's filtering threshold; consequently glucose, which is not necessarily present in the urine, spills into the urine; higher concentrations may actually cause an osmotic diuresis. Of course, as these plasma values are only averages, there may be significant interpatient variation.

**Table 54.2** General Characteristics of Type I and Type II Diabetics

| *Characteristic* | *Type I diabetes* | *Type II diabetes* |
|---|---|---|
| Age of onset | Usually during childhood or adolescence | Usually age 40 or older |
| Rapidness of onset | Usually abrupt | Usually gradual |
| Family history | Usually little family history of diabetes | Positive history for diabetes is common |
| Etiology | Unknown; postulated causes include heredity, autoimmune diseases, and viral infections | Unknown, but heredity is highly associated with occurrence |
| Body weight | Usually thin and undernourished | Obesity is common |
| Insulin | Secretion is markedly diminished early in the disease and may be totally absent later in the disease; insulin therapy is mandatory | Levels may be low (indicating deficiency), normal, or high (indicating insulin resistance); insulin therapy may not be required |
| Ketosis | Common, especially with proper insulin control | Uncommon; if present, usually associated with severe stress or infection |
| Symptoms | Polyuria, polydipsia, polyphagia, weight loss | May be asymptomatic; polyuria and/or polydipsia may be present |

**Table 54.3** Drugs Causing Significant Elevations in Plasma Glucose Concentrations[a]

| *Drug* | *Proposed mechanism* |
|---|---|
| α-Adrenergic agonists/sympathomimetics | Increased glycogenolysis, gluconeogenesis |
| β-Adrenergic blockers | Decreased insulin release (NIDDM only) |
| Diazoxide | Decreased insulin secretion and utilization |
| Glucocorticoids | Increased gluconeogenesis |
| Oral contraceptives | Mechanism unknown—glucose appears to be affected by both estrogen and progestin components |
| Phenytoin | Decreased insulin secretion |
| Thiazide and loop diuretics | Mechanism unclear |

[a] Other drugs have been reported to elevate plasma glucose concentrations; however, they have not been included in this table, as the significance of their hyperglycemic effects is debatable.

### *Other Substances*

In addition to insulin, other substances in the body aid in the regulation of blood glucose.[3]

***Glucagon*** The alpha cells of the endocrine pancreas produce glucagon, which has an effect opposite that of insulin. Glucagon secretion is stimulated during fasting to prevent blood glucose values from dropping too low. Glucagon increases blood glucose by increasing glycogenolysis and gluconeogenesis in the liver.

***Growth Hormone*** Secreted from the anterior pituitary, growth hormone also opposes the action of insulin by interfering with the body's ability to utilize glucose. One stimulus for growth hormone secretion is hypoglycemia.

***Somatostatin*** Somatostatin is produced in the gamma cells of the pancreas. It inhibits both insulin and glucagon secretion and suppresses growth hormone. This results in a fall in blood glucose levels because of the suppression of glucagon. In addition, somatostatin inhibits absorption of glucose from the gastrointestinal tract.

***Epinephrine*** Epinephrine, secreted by the adrenal medulla, acts to increase blood glucose levels by stimulating the conversion of glycogen to glucose in the liver. Similarly, drugs, such as ephedrine and phenylpropanolamine, which stimulate the release of epinephrine and other catecholamines, can also produce an elevation in plasma glucose levels via the same mechanism.

***Glucocorticoids*** Compounds with glucocorticoid activity elevate plasma glucose by stimulating gluconeogenesis, thereby causing a marked increase in liver glycogen. They do not, however, increase glycogen in any other body cells. In fact, glucocorticoids decrease glycogen stores in all other cells because they decrease glucose uptake and utilization by these cells.

***Thyroid Hormone*** Thyroid hormone elevates blood glucose by increasing the rate of absorption of glucose from the gastrointestinal tract. Moreover, thyroid hormone increases liver gluconeogenesis and glycogenolysis.

## Clinical Presentation

The classic symptoms of diabetes include polyuria (excessive urination), polydipsia (thirst), and polyphagia (increased appetite with increased calorie intake). As plasma glucose levels increase to about 180 mg/dL, the reabsorptive capacity of the kidneys (i.e., the "renal threshold") for glucose is exceeded, resulting in spillage of glucose into the urine. Higher urine glucose levels then result in an osmotic diuresis. This diuresis produces the symptom of polyuria, which can lead to dehydration with accompanying polydipsia. As glucose cannot be adequately transported into cells, the "hunger sensation" is triggered, resulting in polyphagia. Type I diabetics often experience these symptoms along with weight loss, weakness, and dry skin. The onset of these symptoms is rapid, and secondary ketoacidosis is common.[4]

Type II diabetes, on the other hand, has a gradual onset and may be present without symptoms. As the type II diabetic is usually obese (except for the elderly who are usually of normal weight), weight loss and/or polyphagia may be absent or go unnoticed. Polyuria may be a presenting complaint, but most type II diabetics are discovered because of an abnormal blood or urine glucose on routine physical examination.

Blurred vision (resulting from glucose-induced changes in the lens), itchy skin, slow-healing skin lesions, recurrent vaginal infections caused by *Candida*, and a history of complications during pregnancy (e.g., stillbirths or a baby whose birthweight is over 9 pounds) are other possible signs of diabetes that warrant further investigation.[1]

A definitive diagnosis of diabetes is made by a combination of symptoms, screening tests, and/or diagnostic tests. The symptoms of diabetes, as described in the previous section, are more evident in the type I diabetic.

### *Screening Tests*

It has been estimated that about 2.5% of the U.S. population may have diabetes that will go undetected unless screened. Persons who should be screened for diabetes include those with a strong family history of diabetes mellitus, persons who are markedly obese, women with a morbid obstetrical history or a history of babies of over 9 pounds at birth, and all women between 24 and 28 weeks of pregnancy.[1,5]

**Table 54.4** Diagnostic Criteria for Diabetes Mellitus

Nonpregnant adults—must display ONE
  a. Random plasma glucose ≥ 200 mg/dL **plus** classic signs and symptoms (polyuria, polydipsia, polyphagia, weight loss)
  b. Fasting plasma glucose level ≥ 140 mg/dL on at least two occasions
  c. Fasting plasma glucose < 140 mg/dL **plus** at least two sustained glucose levels during the OGTT (one 0- to 2-h glucose level and the 2-h level should be ≥200 mg/dL)

Children—must display ONE
  a. Random plasma glucose ≥ 200 mg/dL **plus** classic signs and symptoms (polyuria, polydipsia, ketonuria, weight loss)
  b. Fasting plasma glucose ≥ 140 mg/dL on at least two occasions **plus** at least two sustained glucose levels during the OGTT (one 0- to 2-h glucose level and the 2-h level should be ≥200 mg/dL)

Pregnant women—diagnosis of gestational diabetes is made if two plasma glucose values equal or exceed the following

| | |
|---|---|
| Fasting | 105 mg/dL |
| 1 h | 190 mg/dL |
| 2 h | 165 mg/dL |
| 3 h | 145 mg/dL |

The recommended screening test for nonpregnant adults and children is a fasting plasma glucose level. The patient should fast 10 to 14 hours prior to the test and should have discontinued any medications that may lower or raise plasma glucose 3 days before testing if at all possible. Other screening tests have included urine glucose determinations, 2-hour postprandial plasma glucose determinations, or random plasma glucose levels. In pregnant women a 50-g oral glucose load is recommended for screening.[5]

### *Diagnostic Tests*

Most patients can be diagnosed as diabetic on the basis of classic signs and symptoms plus a positive screening test (see the following criteria); however, those patients who have only *one* of the following should undergo diagnostic testing with an oral glucose tolerance test (OGTT):

1. Positive screening test
2. Presence of obvious signs and symptoms of diabetes such as polydipsia, polyuria, polyphagia, or weight loss
3. Incomplete clinical picture (such as glucosuria)
4. Equivocal findings of a random plasma glucose level

For a meaningful glucose tolerance test, the patient should have fasted for the past 10 to 14 hours and should have discontinued glucose-altering medications 3 days before the test day. The patient should be instructed not to smoke or drink coffee just before and during the test, as false elevations in plasma glucose may occur. A fasting plasma glucose is then drawn. The patient is administered a standard glucose-containing solution (75 g for nonpregnant adults, 100 g for pregnant women, and 1.75 g/kg ideal body weight up to 75 g for children). In nonpregnant adults and children, blood samples are drawn every 30 minutes for 2 hours. In pregnant women, blood samples are drawn every hour for 3 hours. Plasma glucose values should peak in about 1 hour, remain under 200 mg% throughout the test, and return to fasting values by the 2-hour interval. [1,5] See Table 54.4 for specific diagnostic criteria. Those patients who have abnormal test results and cannot be diagnosed as diabetic are classified as having impaired glucose tolerance. Criteria for the diagnosis of IGT are listed in Table 54.5.

**Table 54.5** Criteria for Impaired Glucose Tolerance

Children—must display BOTH
  a. Fasting plasma glucose < 140 mg/dL
  b. 2-h OGTT plasma level > 140 mg/dL

Nonpregnant adults—must display ALL
  a. Fasting plasma glucose < 140 mg/dL
  b. 2-h OGTT level between 140 and 200 mg/dL
  c. 0- to 2-h OGTT level ≥ 200 mg/dL

Once the diagnosis of diabetes has been made, it is important to classify the patient as having either type I or type II diabetes. Usually the classification can be made on the basis of age, suddenness of onset, and physical characteristics of the patient. C-peptides have also been used to distinguish between type I and II diabetics. Proinsulin is cleaved in the pancreas to form insulin and C-peptide molecules. Therefore, patients with no insulin production have little, if any, production of C-peptides.[6] Regardless of the criteria used to classify the diabetic, it is important to remember that the type I diabetic has an absolute lack of insulin and must be given exogenous insulin to sustain life and prevent ketoacidosis. Therapy for type II diabetes, on the other hand, can often be started without oral medication or insulin.

## Treatment

The treatment of diabetes varies considerably between type I and type II diabetes. Type I diabetics have an absolute lack of insulin, so that diet, exercise, and insulin are necessary for proper management. The therapy for type II diabetes also consists of diet and exercise; however, oral medications or insulin may or may not be required. The goals of diet for the two types of diabetics are also quite different. The goal of therapy, however, is consistent: to maintain the plasma glucose in an acceptable range throughout the day so that the patient remains nonsymptomatic. Desirable plasma glucose concentrations are listed in Table 54.6.

### *Patient Education*

Successful treatment of diabetes often involves some lifestyle change (e.g., diet, exercise, or taking medication) for the patient. The patient, therefore, must be involved in the decision-making process. Consequently he or she must understand as much as possible about diabetes. The patient must understand why the symptoms of diabetes are occurring and how a controlled blood glucose concentration will alleviate the symptoms. The long-term complications of diabetes must be explained to the patient, stressing that newer evidence indicates that many of these complications can be curtailed or prevented with a tightly controlled blood glucose concentration. Finally, the patient must understand that medications alone will not control the disease or its complications—that a sensible regimen of diet, exercise, and "awareness" is as important as any diabetic medication.

### *Diet*

The cornerstone of therapy in the diabetic is diet; however, the goals of diet for type I and type II diabetics are different. Type I diabetics are usually thin, possibly even below ideal body weight. Hence, the goal of diet is not to lose weight but to provide the proper number of calories needed for the patient and to provide the proper composition of these calories. In the past, diabetics were taught to avoid carbohydrates, but it is now accepted that 55% to 60% of the calories in a diabetic's diet should consist of carbohydrates, 15% of protein, and no more than 30% of total calories should be derived from fat (primarily from polyunsaturated fats). The carbohydrates should be of the complex type (starches, oligosaccharides, and "fiber-containing" carbohydrates) as opposed to simple sugars.[7]

Calories should be spread as evenly as possible throughout the major daily meals. In general, meals taken 4 to 5 hours apart allow adequate time for the postprandial glucose concentration to return to preprandial levels.[8] Patients with diabetes have greater-than-normal incidence of hyperlipidemia, atherosclerosis, and hypertension (reasons for which are discussed later). Dietary recommendations related to these conditions should be observed.

The goal of diet for the type II diabetic may be slightly different. Although it is accepted that the type I diabetic cannot be treated with diet alone, often proper diet and exercise can control the plasma glucose concentration in many type II diabetics. The type II patient still needs to have the proper distribution of calories and usually needs to lose weight, as it is the weight reduction that actually makes insulin receptors more accessible and aids in the transport of glucose into cells. Those type II diabetics who are initially diet controlled usually fail at using diet to control their diabetes as a long-term goal. While conscientious at first, these patients usually slip into old eating habits and ultimately lose control of the disease.[9]

**Table 54.6** Goals of Therapy

| *Parameter* | *Normal* | *Acceptable* | *Fair* | *Poor* |
|---|---|---|---|---|
| Fasting plasma glucose (mg/dL) | 115 | 140 | 200 | >200 |
| Postprandial plasma glucose (mg/dL) | 140 | 175 | 235 | >235 |
| Glycosylated hemoglobin[a] (%) | 6 | 8 | 10 | >10 |

[a] Increase limits 10% for elderly patients.

Another reason for diet failure in the diabetic is the "exchange" program. Patients are often given complicated diets, often they cannot follow the diets, or they cannot afford the exchange foods, or the diet is too complicated to fit into the rest of the family's diet. Therefore, it is important for a dietician or other knowledgeable health professional to work with the patient in adapting the patient's usual diet and eating habits to the new diabetic diet.[9]

It is becoming increasingly evident that all diabetics (type I and type II) should begin monitoring either urine or blood glucose concentration at home to see which foods adversely affect the control of their blood glucose (see Monitoring). Unless the patient has some way of monitoring progress, diet usually fails as a means of controlling diabetes.

### *Exercise*

Unless contraindicated, appropriate physical activity should be recommended to improve insulin sensitivity and possibly improve glucose tolerance. Exercise can also help to promote weight loss and maintain ideal body weight when combined with restricted caloric intake.[10] Exercise, however, is not recommended if the patient has poorly controlled, labile blood glucose levels or is at increased risk from diabetic complications (discussed later). Strenuous exercise is usually not wise in the patient prone to developing hypoglycemia unless the patient is well educated about the symptoms and consequences of hypoglycemia and has taken proper measures to anticipate and treat this condition.[11]

### *Oral Hypoglycemics*

For the type II diabetic who has successfully lost weight and who has maintained proper caloric distribution but has still failed to control blood glucose adequately, the clinician is faced with initiating drug therapy. The dilemma now arises as whether to choose an oral hypoglycemic agent or to begin the patient on insulin. In the late 1960s the University Group Diabetes Program (UGDP) study examined diet alone versus diet plus oral hypoglycemia (tolbutamide) versus diet plus insulin in controlling short- and long-term diabetes.[12] One of the findings of the study was that prolonged use of an oral hypoglycemic agent greatly increased cardiovascular mor-

**Table 54.7** Oral Hypoglycemic Agents

| *Generic (Trade)* | *Onset (h)* | *Half-life (h)* | *Duration (h)* | *Recommended starting dose* Nonelderly | Elderly | *Maximum dose per day* | *Metabolism/ elimination* |
|---|---|---|---|---|---|---|---|
| **First-Generation Agents** | | | | | | | |
| Tolbutamide (Orinase) | 1 | 5.6 | 6–12 | 1–2 g/d | 500 mg/d to 500 mg twice daily | 2–3 g | Metabolized in liver to inactive metabolites that are excreted renally |
| Acetohexamide (Dymelor) | 1 | 5 | 10–14 | 250 mg–1.5 g/d | 125–250 mg/d | 1.5 g | Metabolized in liver; metabolite's potency is equal to or greater than that of parent compound; renally eliminated |
| Tolazamide (Tolinase) | 4–6 | 7 | 10–14 | 100–250 mg/d | 100 mg/d | 750 mg–1 g | Metabolized in liver; metabolite less active than parent compound; renally eliminated |
| Chlorpropamide (Diabinese) | 1 | 35 | 72 | 250 mg/d | 100 mg/d | 500 mg | Metabolized in liver; also excreted unchanged in the urine |
| **Second-Generation Agents** | | | | | | | |
| Glyburide (Diaβeta, Micronase) | 1.5 | 10 | 24 | 2.5 mg/d | 1.25–2.5 mg/d | 20 mg | Metabolized in liver; 50% of metabolites eliminated in urine, 50% in feces |
| Glipizide (Glucotrol) | 1 | 3–7 | 10–24 | 5 mg/d | 2.5–5 mg/d | 40 mg | Metabolized in liver to inactive metabolites; renally eliminated |

tality. Physicians were advised against using oral hypoglycemics in most patients, especially in younger type II diabetics. Since that time, however, numerous flaws in the statistical design of the study have been uncovered, and patients on oral hypoglycemics are not believed to have a greater cardiovascular risk because of the medication.

Although controversy regarding the overall safety and long-term efficacy of oral hypoglycemic agents still exists, this form of therapy is preferred by most physicians and type II diabetics, especially since it does not involve daily injections. There are still many who advocate starting younger type II diabetics on insulin, whereas elderly patients, patients with poor eyesight, patients living alone, or patients who cannot otherwise draw up and administer insulin may be started on an oral hypoglycemic agent.

Oral agents exert their initial effect by increasing beta cell insulin secretion. After several months, insulin levels return to pretreatment values while glucose levels remain improved. This suggests that oral agents exert extrapancreatic as well as pancreatic effects on glucose metabolism.[13] Approximately 60% to 70% of all patients with type II diabetes have an initial response to sulfonylurea therapy. About 5% to 20% of patients experience secondary failure because of the patient's reluctance to follow a prescribed dietary plan, because of progression of the disease, or because of the occurrence of an underlying stressful condition or disease.[5]

The older oral hypoglycemics include tolbutamide, chlorpropamide, tolazamide, and acetohexamide (see Table 54.7). Tolbutamide is a short-acting sulfonylurea, initially prescribed once a day but usually requiring two or three doses per day to adequately control plasma glucose. It is metabolized by the liver to inactive metabolites that are excreted in the urine. On a weight basis, tolbutamide is the least potent of the first-generation hypoglycemics. Many clinicians consider this drug safer than other agents, particularly in patients with renal impairment or in the elderly.[14,15]

Tolazamide (Tolinase) is an intermediate-acting sulfonylurea that is metabolized by the liver. The metabolites of this drug are excreted renally and demonstrate weak hypoglycemic and diuretic activity. Tolazamide is usually administered once or twice a day.[14,15]

Acetohexamide (Dymelor) is also an intermediate-acting sulfonylurea and is usually administered once or twice a day. It is metabolized in the liver to an active metabolite which has more than twice the potency of the original drug. In addition, acetohexamide has diuretic activity and is a potent uricosuric agent.

Chlorpropamide is partially metabolized by the liver to

active metabolites and partially excreted unchanged in the urine. This drug has the longest duration of action of the oral hypoglycemic agents (about 60 hours) and is usually prescribed once per day. There is rarely sufficient reason to administer chlorpropamide more than once per day. Chlorpropamide can cause significant water retention and hyponatremia, primarily by promoting the release of antidiuretic hormone. In addition, a disulfiram-like reaction is experienced most commonly with this hypoglycemia agent when alcohol is ingested.

Second-generation sulfonylureas are so named because they are more potent than the older agents, have a quicker onset of action, and exhibit a longer duration of action. Currently the two agents marketed in the United States include glyburide (Diaβeta, Micronase) and glipizide (Glucotrol). These agents are metabolized by the liver and have a duration of action of up to 24 hours. These drugs appear to lower glucose by increasing the binding of insulin to receptors and by increasing the efficacy of endogenous insulin by decreasing peripheral resistance to the insulin.[15,16] It has been argued that these agents promote a greater release of insulin after the noon and evening meals than do the first-generation drugs. Moreover, except for hypoglycemia, the second-generation oral hypoglycemics appear to produce fewer side effects than do the older drugs.

The absorption of glipizide is impaired by meals; hence, it should be taken on an empty stomach; however, because of glipizide's rapid onset of action, patients should be instructed to eat within 30 minutes after ingesting the drug. Glipizide has three active metabolites that are excreted primarily renally. Although the maximum daily dose is 40 mg, the manufacturer recommends dividing doses that exceed 15 mg to avoid hypoglycemic reactions.

Glyburide appears to have a biphasic half-life, the first of which is 5 hours, the second 10 hours. The drug has no active metabolites and is eliminated equally by renal and hepatic mechanisms. The duration of action may be longer than that of glipizide, theoretically allowing for once-a-day dosing in most patients.[16] Glyburide can produce a mild diuresis with an increase in free water clearance.

Hypoglycemia is the major complication of all sulfonylurea drugs. It is particularly troublesome with chlorpropamide because of its long duration of action. Elderly patients are more susceptible to the hypoglycemia, especially when they skip meals or when there is some degree of renal or liver impairment. Other side effects of sulfonylureas include hematologic reactions such as leukopenia, thrombocytopenia, and hemolytic anemia; skin reactions, particularly rashes, purpura, and pruritus; antithyroid activity; and diffuse pulmonary reactions. Renal side effects of these drugs include mild diuresis, seen especially with tolazamide and acetohexamide, as well as significant fluid retention and hyponatremia occurring with chlorpropamide.[5,15] Gastrointestinal side effects include nausea, vomiting, and cholestasis (with or without jaundice). Cholestatic jaundice has been identified more often with chlorpropamide than with any other oral agent. If jaundice results from any of these drugs, it is recommended that the patient be switched to insulin therapy rather than to another oral agent.[5]

Those patients who are at least 40 years of age at the onset of NIDDM, have been diabetic for less than 5 years prior to the initiation of sulfonylurea therapy, and have a fasting plasma glucose concentration of less than 300 mg/dL appear to be the best candidates for sulfonylurea therapy.[5,17] The dosage of these agents should be increased every 1 to 2 weeks until satisfactory control has been achieved or until the maximum dose has been reached. It the maximum dose of the drug does not provide adequate control, then it is common practice to try another oral agent. If control has not been achieved after two agents, the patient is then a candidate for insulin therapy. No benefit has been demonstrated using two sulfonylurea drugs simultaneously.

Primary failure with an oral hypoglycemic medication occurs when a patient does not respond initially to the drug; however, when initial glycemic control has been achieved with an oral agent and then lost, the patient is considered to be a secondary drug failure. Secondary failure occurs in 5% to 10% of patients per year.[5] Some reasons include failure to follow prescribed diet, progression of the disease, or underlying stressful conditions such as infection, pregnancy, or cardiovascular disease. In these situations the patient should be temporarily switched to insulin therapy. After recovery from an intercurrent disease or condition, reinstatement of oral hypoglycemic therapy may be successful.

### *Insulin*

#### Characteristics

Insulins may be categorized according to their strength, onset and duration of action, species source, and purity. Each of these factors plays a role in determining the type and dose of insulin that is best suited to an individual patient.

***Strength*** Prior to 1980, three strengths of insulin were available: U-40, U-80, and U-100. (The numeral following the "U" indicates the number of units of insulin per milliliter.) In an attempt to purify and standardize the various insulin products, U-80 is no longer produced. Although the vast number of diabetics today use U-100 insulin, U-40 and U-500 insulins are available. U-40 syringes are color-coded "red"; U-100 products are color-coded "orange with black lettering." Some pediatric patients may require other strengths of insulin (e.g., U-10). Special diluents and empty sterile vials are available from the manufacturer to prepare such dilutions.

***Onset/Duration*** Table 54.8 compares the onset, peak, and duration of various insulin preparations. Regular insulin is a clear, colorless solution. Until the advent of the insulin infusion pump, regular insulin was rarely used by itself for maintenance therapy because of its short duration of action. It was found that the addition of acetate buffers, protamine, or zinc to regular insulin could greatly prolong its effect. Consequently, the addition of protamine and zinc led to the NPH and Protamine Zinc & Iletin (PZI) lines of insulin, while the addition of acetate buffers and zinc led to the Lente series. As regular insulin is a solution, it can be administered by the intravenous, intramuscular, or subcutaneous route. All other types of insulin, however, are suspensions and can be administered subcutaneously only.[18]

NPH and Lente insulins are considered "intermediate-acting" insulins. Because their duration of action usually lies between 18 and 24 hours, a single injection of either NPH or

**Table 54.8** Onset, Peak, and Duration of Various Insulin Preparations

| *Type of insulin* | *Onset (h)* | *Peak (h)* | *Duration (h)* |
|---|---|---|---|
| Short-acting | | | |
| Regular | 0.5–1 | 2–4 | 5–7 |
| Semilente | 1–2 | 4–6 | 12–16 |
| Intermediate-acting | | | |
| NPH | 1–2 | 6–14 | 18–24 |
| Lente | 1–2 | 6–14 | 18–24 |
| Long-acting | | | |
| PZI | 6–8 | 18–24 | 36 |
| Ultralente | 4–6 | 18–26 | 36+ |

Lente is usually the first step in chronic maintenance of the insulin-dependent diabetic. NPH is produced by combining zinc, protamine, and Regular insulins. Protamine is a foreign protein and can produce high antibody titers and symptoms of allergy in a small number of patients. Lente insulin is produced by adding acetate buffers and zinc to regular insulin. The resultant product may produce local allergic manifestations in patients with metal allergies.[19]

Although NPH and Lente are essentially identical in their onset, peak, duration of action, and cost, they differ in their ability to be combined with other types of insulin. Any product in the Lente series can be mixed with another product in the same series; the combination is stable for 1 month at room temperature or for 3 months under refrigeration; however, as Lente is made with an excess of zinc, a mixture of Regular and Lente insulins tends to interact 15 minutes to 24 hours after the two have been combined. This ultimately alters the intended ratio of Regular to Lente. Once the reaction has occurred, the new product is stable for 1 month at room temperature or for 3 months under refrigeration.[20] When NPH and Regular insulins are combined, a reaction between the protamine and Regular insulin occurs within 15 minutes after mixing. The resultant product is again stable for 1 month at room temperature or for 3 months in the refrigerator; hence, to avoid this reaction, the dose must be administered immediately after it is drawn up.[20] These interactions may be especially important to the homebound patient who must have someone draw up dosages for several days at one time.

***Species Source*** All insulins currently marketed are one of four types: beef, pork, beef-pork mixture, or "semisynthetic." Beef insulin differs from human insulin by three amino acids, thus theoretically being the most antigenic of the insulins. Pork insulin differs from human insulin by only one amino acid. Semisynthetic insulins are also known as "Human" insulins because their amino acid structure is identical in composition to human insulin and consequently is less antigenic than either beef or pork insulins. The semisynthetic insulins are produced either by recombinant DNA technology or by modification of beef insulin.[21]

Eli Lilly & Company manufactures a beef–pork combination in their Iletin I series and single-species insulin in the Iletin II series. Squibb–Novo markets only single-species insulin (either pork or beef). Lilly's "Human" insulin is produced from *Escherichia coli* by recombinant DNA technology. Squibb–Novo's "Human" insulin is prepared by modifying beef insulin. A more detailed listing of these insulins has been included in Table 54.9.

***Purity*** "Purity" refers to the amount of proinsulin and other impurities present in a given insulin product. Theoretically, the less proinsulin a patient receives, the fewer insulin antibodies the patient produces. All insulins produced in the United States contain less than 25 ppm of proinsulin. The term "improved single peak" refers to most Lilly insulins whose concentration of proinsulin is less than 20 ppm. "Purified" insulins are even less antigenic, containing less than 10 ppm of proinsulin.[15,22] Similarly, the human insulin products, containing virtually no proinsulin, are classified as "purified" insulins. The term "standard" insulin in Table 54.9 refers to any product containing 10–25 ppm of proinsulin.

**Dosing**

There are a number of methods for dosing insulin. For the hospitalized patient, many clinicians prefer a "sliding scale" approach. Blood glucose concentrations are ordered several times a day (e.g., every 4 hours, every 6 hours, or at specified times—7 AM, 11 AM, 4 PM, and midnight) such that fasting values and values before meals are obtained. Subcutaneously administered Regular insulin is then ordered in an amount that increases with the increase in blood glucose. For example, a typical order may be to give no insulin for a blood glucose less than 200 mg/dL, 4 units for a blood glucose of 200–249 mg/dL, 6 units for a blood glucose of 250–299 mg/dL, and 8 units for a value of 300 mg/dL or greater. Of course, any reasonable scale and/or dose can be utilized, depending on the patient's sensitivity to insulin, the severity of the hyperglycemia, and other factors. When the patient's insulin requirement has stabilized over 2 to 3 days, the number of units required during the last 24 hours is totaled. The patient can then be given a single injection of an intermediate-acting insulin; the beginning dose is two thirds to three fourths of the 24-hour Regular insulin dose and is given 30 minutes before breakfast. The dose can then be "fine-tuned" over the next several days.

In an attempt to avoid long hospitalizations to stabilize a patient on Regular insulin and then convert to NPH or Lente, some clinicians initially prescribe 0.5–1.2 U/kg of an intermediate-acting insulin or a combination of Regular and an intermediate-acting insulin[5,17]; either regimen is administered subcutaneously 30 minutes before breakfast. The dose is then adjusted on an outpatient basis through continued blood glucose monitoring.

It is important to note that type I diabetics often go through a "honeymoon phase" after the initial diagnosis of diabetes. During this period, insulin requirements diminish so that the patient is taking a very low dose of insulin. Regardless of how low the dose may become, patients should be encouraged to remain on insulin during this period to decrease the likelihood of producing antibodies to the insulin and becoming insulin resistant.[23]

As the type II diabetic is usually not prone to ketoacidosis, there is less urgency to initiate aggressive therapy. This individual can be started on a single injection of 15–20 U/day

**Table 54.9** Insulins

| *Brand name* | *Manufacturer* | *Origin* | *Concentration* |
|---|---|---|---|
| **Short-Acting Insulins** | | | |
| Standard insulin | | | |
| Regular Iletin I | Lilly | Beef, pork | U-40, U-100 |
| Regular insulin | Squibb–Novo | Pork | U-100 |
| Semilente Iletin I | Lilly | Beef, pork | U-40, U-100 |
| Semilente insulin | Squibb–Novo | Beef | U-100 |
| Purified | | | |
| Beef Regular Iletin II | Lilly | Beef | U-100 |
| Pork Regular Iletin II | Lilly | Pork | U-100, U-500 |
| Regular purified pork insulin | Squibb–Novo | Pork | U-100 |
| Velosulin | Nordisk–USA | Pork | U-100 |
| Semilente purified pork | Squibb–Novo | Pork | U-100 |
| Human (Purified) | | | |
| Humulin R | Lilly | Human (recombinant DNA) | U-100 |
| Novolin R | Squibb–Novo | Semisynthetic | U-100 |
| **Intermediate-Acting Insulins** | | | |
| NPH (Standard) | | | |
| NPH Iletin I | Lilly | Beef, pork | U-40, U-100 |
| NPH insulin | Squibb–Novo | Beef | U-100 |
| NPH (Purified) | | | |
| Beef NPH Iletin II | Lilly | Beef | U-100 |
| Pork NPH Iletin II | Lilly | Pork | U-100 |
| NPH purified pork | Squibb–Novo | Pork | U-100 |
| Insulatard NPH | Nordisk-USA | Pork | U-100 |
| NPH (Human) | | | |
| Humulin N | Lilly | Human (recombinant DNA) | U-100 |
| Novolin N | Squibb–Novo | Semisynthetic | U-100 |
| Lente (Standard) | | | |
| Lente Iletin I | Lilly | Beef, pork | U-40, U-100 |
| Lente insulin | Squibb–Novo | Beef | U-100 |
| Lente (Purified) | | | |
| Lente Iletin II | Lilly | Beef | U-100 |
| Lente Iletin II | Lilly | Pork | U-100 |
| Lente purified pork | Squibb–Novo | Pork | U-100 |
| Lente (Human) | | | |
| Novolin L | Squibb–Novo | Semisynthetic | U-100 |
| Humulin L | Lilly | (recombinant DNA) | U-100 |
| NPH–Regular combination (Purified) | | | |
| Mixtard (70% NPH, 30% Regular) | Nordisk-USA | Pork | U-100 |
| NPH-Regular combination (Human) | | | |
| Novolin 70/30 | Squibb-Novo | Semisynthetic | U-100 |
| **Long-Acting Insulins** | | | |
| PZI and Ultralente (Standard) | | | |
| Protamine Zinc & Iletin I | Lilly | Beef, pork | U-40, U-100 |
| Ultralente Iletin I | Lilly | Beef, pork | U-40, U-100 |
| Ultralente insulin | Squibb–Novo | Beef | U-100 |
| Purified | | | |
| Protamine Zinc & Iletin II | Lilly | Beef | U-100 |
| Protamine Zinc & Iletin II | Lilly | Pork | U-100 |
| Ultralente purified beef | Squibb–Novo | Beef | U-100 |

of an intermediate-acting insulin. Blood glucose levels can then be followed and the insulin adjusted accordingly. Recent studies have shown that almost 90% of type II diabetics can be initially controlled on less than 20 units of insulin per day.[5,24]

The American Diabetes Association suggests that when a patient's insulin dosage exceeds 30 units per day, the dose may be split into two injections and may contain both Regular and an intermediate-acting insulin. The first injection, consisting of an intermediate-to-Regular ratio of 2:1, is given 30 minutes before breakfast. The second injection is given 30 minutes before the evening meal; the ratio of intermediate-acting to Regular insulin is 1:1. These regimens are known as "intensive dose" regimens.[17,25]

**Storage, Preparation, and Administration**

Patients should be taught proper storage, dosage preparation, and administration techniques for their insulin. These guidelines are presented in Table 54.10.

### *Monitoring Therapy*

Regardless of whether the patient's therapy consists of diet and exercise, diet and exercise plus a sulfonylurea, or diet and exercise plus insulin, the success of the therapy must be closely monitored. Such monitoring instruments as urine testing, blood or plasma glucose testing, glycosylated hemoglobins, and C-peptides have all been employed in patients with varying degrees of success. The choice of method depends upon the severity of the diabetes, the progression of the disease, economic factors, and the patient's willingness and ability to monitor therapy.

In the home setting, urine glucose concentrations have been the mainstay of assessing diabetic control until recently when many have advocated the use of whole blood glucose concentration as a means of monitoring diabetic control. Initially and for any patient who has been relatively difficult to control, urine glucose determinations are usually made several times a day (e.g., a fasting level, before the noontime meal, in the afternoon, and at bedtime). When the patient has been consistently controlled for several weeks, the frequency of this testing may be reduced to once or twice a day.

Urine testing is the least expensive monitoring device, but the results are not always easily interpretable. The tests, listed in Table 54.11, utilize either the glucose oxidase or the copper reduction method to detect glucose in the urine. The glucose oxidase method is a qualitative test, which is specific for glucose and yields few false-positive results. The copper reduction method is a better quantitative test, but will react with any reducing substance, thereby producing false-positive results. With either test the presence of glucose results in a color change which can then be correlated with a relative urine glucose concentration.

Urine tests, although inexpensive and relatively easy to perform, have several limitations. First, a randomly collected urine specimen may correspond to a blood glucose concentration several hours previously. One tries to overcome this obstacle by using a "double-voided" specimen, whereby the patient urinates, drinks a full glass of water, and in approximately 30 minutes recollects and tests a second urine specimen. Another drawback of urine testing rests with the lack of correlation between urine and blood glucose values.

Although we state that the average person begins to spill glucose into the urine when the serum glucose approaches 180 mg/dL, this figure actually fluctuates greatly among patients. In addition, there can even be intrapatient variation depending on the progression of the disease and day-to-day stress factors. The values themselves can be difficult to interpret. For example, a negative urine glucose cannot discern among the adequately controlled patient, the person who is hypoglycemic, and the patient who is hyperglycemic but whose blood glucose value has not exceeded the renal threshold for spilling into the urine.

Clinitest is the only commercially available test that utilizes the copper reduction method. The tablets are available as "5-drop" and "2-drop" methods, the former testing for low to intermediate values and the latter, for higher values of urinary glucose. In this respect, Clinitest is superior to the glucose oxidase tests, which detect primarily low glucose concentrations; however, besides being influenced by a large number of drugs (Table 54.12), Clinitest requires a test tube and a dropper for accurate results. Moreover, the tablets themselves are corrosive and can cause serious chemical burns if ingested.

For patients in the hospital or office setting, blood glucose determination has become the standard for diabetes monitoring. In the laboratory usually serum or plasma is utilized for glucose determinations. These values may be slightly higher than those obtained on whole blood although in almost all cases, the differences have no clinical significance. More recent advances in blood glucose monitoring have allowed patients and health professionals to monitor glucose levels using chemically impregnated strips or hand-held electronic glucose monitoring machines that utilize many of these strips. These strips or machines are designed to be able to monitor whole blood glucose from several drops of blood obtained by a fingerstick.[26,27]

There are several differences in the various commercially available strips. The strip itself cannot monitor a true blood glucose concentration but measures a range within which the patient's value lies. Many of these strips, however, can be inserted into a machine which can then measure and display an accurate blood glucose value (see Table 54.13). When used without the machine, the patient's blood interacts with the chemicals on the strip to produce a color change that corresponds to a range of blood glucose values. Some strips maintain this color for several hours or days while other strips begin to fade after a few minutes. Two drawbacks to the use of either strips or glucose monitoring machines include the relative expense, especially if the patient has to monitor blood values several times a day, and the educational level required of the patient, as the machines must be calibrated and the test properly performed to obtain accurate results.

The glycosylated hemoglobin (hemoglobin $A_{1c}$) may be useful for monitoring long-term control of diabetes. Glucose can react in a concentration-dependent manner with amino groups of amino acids to produce glycosylated products.[28] For example, chronic elevation of blood glucose results in an increase in the presence of glycosylated hemoglobins, of which hemoglobin $A_{1c}$ is a major component. Hemoglobin

**Table 54.10** Patient Information on the Storage and Administration of Insulin

1. Unopened vials of insulin should be stored in the refrigerator but should not be placed in a part of the refrigerator where the insulin might freeze. Freezing may alter the desired effect of the insulin. An opened vial of insulin that is being used daily should be stored at room temperature, away from windows, lamps, or any other places in which temperature could be altered. Insulin stored at room temperature causes less pain and fewer local reactions upon injection than does refrigerated insulin. Insulin that is refrigerated is usable until the expiration date stamped on the vial. Insulin stored at room temperature expires after 3 months.
2. All supplies for administering an insulin dosage should be close at hand. These include insulin syringes, cotton balls and 70% isopropyl alcohol or alcohol swabs, and the insulin. The alcohol should be clear in appearance and should not contain any soaps or perfumes that might cause a local irritation resembling an insulin allergy. U-100 syringes are available as standard or Lo-Dose. The Lo-Dose syringes can accurately measure single units of insulin and the numbers on the barrel of the syringe are easy to read; these syringes are useful for patients who are administered less than 50 units of insulin per injection. Syringes can be capped after use, stored in the refrigerator, and reused until the needle starts to dull.
3. All insulins except "Regular" are cloudy in appearance and need to be gently agitated before a dosage is drawn. The vial should not be shaken vigorously but should be gently agitated or rolled between the palms of the hands.
4. The plunger on the syringe should be pulled back to the appropriate number of units desired.
5. The insulin vial should be inverted and the needle should be inserted into the rubber stopper in the vial. The plunger should be pressed all the way into the barrel of the syringe; the plunger should then be pulled back, allowing the correct number of units of insulin to enter the barrel of the syringe.
   *Note*: If you are drawing up two different kinds of insulin (Regular and NPH, for example), the technique is slightly different. Calculate the TOTAL number of units to be withdrawn from the two vials, and pull the plunger back to this point. Insert the needle into the Regular insulin vial (ALWAYS draw up the Regular insulin first); inject into the vial an amount of air equal to the number of units of Regular insulin you will be withdrawing. Then withdraw the correct number of Regular units. Remove the needle from the vial and insert it into the NPH vial. Inject the remaining air into the NPH vial, being careful not to inject any Regular insulin into this vial. Pull back on the plunger, allowing the correct number of units of NPH insulin to enter the barrel of the syringe. Remove any air bubbles from the syringe as outlined below.
6. Air bubbles should be tapped toward the needle and gently expelled from the syringe. Injecting an air bubble subcutaneously is not harmful; however, air in the syringe indicates that the full dose of insulin has not been properly drawn up. Therefore, every attempt should be made to ensure that air bubbles have been expelled from the syringe, leaving the correct number of units of insulin in the syringe for injection.
7. A subcutaneous injection is made into fat (not merely "under the skin" as many people think). The most popular places for injecting insulin are the backs of the arms (triceps area), the abdomen, and the inner thigh areas. Patients who administer their own injections usually prefer the abdomen or thighs. Absorption is usually fastest from the abdomen, slowest from the thigh; therefore, it is important NOT to rotate injection sites from abdomen to thigh to arm but rather to rotate sites of injection within a general area. Not rotating sites with each injection may lead to a "calloused" area, affecting the actual subcutaneous tissue and altering insulin's absorption from that area.
8. After the site for injection is chosen, the area should be cleaned with alcohol. This should be done in a circular fashion, beginning in the center of the circle working outward about 2 in. Allow a few seconds for the alcohol to evaporate.
9. If you are right-handed, pinch up the fat at the site of injection with your left hand, being careful not to touch the area where the needle will enter the skin. Hold the syringe in your right hand as you would a pencil. The needle should be aimed perpendicular (90°) to the skin unless the patient is very thin and has too little subcutaneous tissue (in which case the needle should be inserted at a 45° angle). Using a slight wrist action, quickly insert the needle through the skin into the subcutaneous tissue. The entire length of the needle should be below the skin surface.
10. While the needle is still in the subcutaneous tissue, gently pull back on the plunger about 2 units—this is called "aspirating." (If you are right-handed, this can be done by using the thumb of your right hand or by letting go of the pinched up area with your left hand and using your left hand to aspirate.) If any blood comes back into the syringe, you may have inserted the needle into a vein—DO NOT INJECT! If no blood appears in the syringe after aspirating, you can assume it is okay to inject.
    *Note*: Many health professionals are no longer teaching the technique of aspiration, as they claim it is rare for the needle to be inserted into a large vein.
11. Slowly push the plunger in all the way until it stops. Gently pull out the needle. You may use a cotton ball to GENTLY wipe the inection area after pulling out the needle, but do NOT massage the area of injection as this will alter the rate of insulin absorption.

**Table 54.11** Tests for Urine Glucose Determination

| *Product* | *Detection method* | *Range detected (%)* |
|---|---|---|
| Chemstrip uG | Glucose oxidase | 0, ¼, ½, 1, 2, 3, 5 |
| Clinitest (5-drop) | Copper reduction | 0, ¼, ½, ¾, 1, ≥2 |
| Clinitest (2-drop) | Copper reduction | 0, ≤½, ½, 1, 2, 3, 5 |
| Diastix | Glucose oxidase | 0, 1/10, ¼, ½, 1, ≥2 |
| TesTape | Glucose oxidase | 0, 1/10, ¼, ½, ≥2 |

$A_{1c}$ usually constitutes 4% to 8% of the total hemoglobin, but may constitute up to 15% of the total with chronic hyperglycemia. As the life span of an average red blood cell is 120 days, bringing the blood glucose under control for 4 to 6 weeks will result in a fall in the percentage of hemoglobin $A_{1c}$. On the other hand, a patient must have experienced hyperglycemia for 1 to 4 weeks before the hemoglobin $A_{1c}$ concentration rises substantially.[28,29] Methods for measuring glycosylated hemoglobins have not been standardized, however. Some tests that measure other glycosylated derivatives may be affected by short periods of hyperglycemia. Other conditions, such as sickle cell anemia, bleeding, or hemolysis that affect the average life span of the red blood cell can also yield misleading results with glycosylated hemoglobin monitoring.

Most patients show an interest in monitoring their urine or blood glucose initially but seem to lose interest after a short time. Factors contributing to this loss of interest include expense and lack of knowledge as to what to do with the results of these tests. Therefore, patients must be educated as to the short- and long-term benefits of day-to-day monitoring of glucose. Daily monitoring of glucose allows the patient to fine-tune dietary constraints. For example, some patients can eat peanuts but find that peanut butter substantially raises their blood glucose concentration. Other patients find that they can eat certain types of bread but must avoid others. Still other patients find that small amounts of sucrose do not significantly affect their blood or urine glucose concentrations. Thus, patients become more involved in their own therapy.

Exercise also affects daily blood glucose concentrations. Monitoring daily urine or blood glucose values allows the patient to define how much and what kind of exercise is appropriate. For the insulin-dependent diabetic, the amount and type of exercise may dictate which parts of the body are best for insulin injections. Running may increase the absorption of insulin that has been injected into the thighs, resulting in hypoglycemia or shorter duration of action of the insulin.[30]

**Table 54.12** Drugs That Cause False-Positive Results With Copper Reduction Tests for Glucosuria

| | |
|---|---|
| *para*-Aminosalicylic acid | Methyldopa |
| Ascorbic acid | Nalidixic acid |
| Cephalosporins | Penicillins (large doses) |
| Chloral hydrate | Probenecid |
| Isoniazid | Salicylates |
| Levodopa | Streptomycin |
| Metaxalone | |

Certain prescription and nonprescription drugs can alter blood glucose concentrations (listed in Table 54.3). Daily monitoring of glucose allows the patient to determine if taking one or more of these drugs causes individual loss of diabetic control. Additionally, other short-term factors affect daily insulin requirements. Factors that increase insulin requirements include infection, trauma, stress, and the second and third trimesters of pregnancy.[17] Conversely, exercise and early pregnancy decrease insulin requirements in most individuals. Consequently, daily monitoring of urine or blood glucose not only can detect these factors but can also help to define to what extent these factors affect an individual patient.

Self-monitoring of urine or blood glucose, therefore, is essential in helping the patient and physician to detect acute and chronic factors that affect the patient's overall control of diabetes. Moreover, daily monitoring involves the patient in his/her own therapy, which is essential to the overall success of any therapeutic regimen.

## *Adjusting Therapy*

### Recognizing, Treating, and Preventing Hypoglycemia

Hypoglycemia is the most common side effect from sulfonylurea or insulin therapy. During the waking hours, the usual symptoms of hypoglycemia include sweating, tachycardia, palpitations, and tremor. Especially when the blood glucose level falls below 40 mg/dL, central nervous system signs such as headache, confusion, visual disturbances, irritability or other personality changes, seizures, or unconsciousness may occur. Hypoglycemia may occur during the night or early morning hours while the patient is asleep, producing such symptoms as nightmares, night sweats, and headache.[31]

In some diabetics (especially the elderly diabetic) and nondiabetic individuals, a mildly depressed blood glucose level (50–70 mg/dL) can produce epinephrine release with resulting symptoms. It is often hard in these cases to document the hypoglycemia; consequently, the patient may experience these episodes for months or years before a definitive diagnosis is made.

Although there are several causes of hypoglycemia, by far the most frequent cause in the insulin-dependent diabetic is not eating at the proper times. Despite frequent warnings, many diabetics let their lifestyle dictate their eating habits. It is not uncommon for someone to skip breakfast because he or she is late for work. Working through lunch or making a late dinner engagement are other common causes. Unfortunately, insulin's onset, peak, and duration of action are not as flexible! A significant increase in exercise or taking too much antidiabetic medication also produces hypoglycemia. Another cause of hypoglycemia, especially in the insulin-dependent diabetic, is a defect in glucagon secretion.[32] Other counterregulatory mechanisms may also be adversely affected, such as the impairment of epinephrine's action

**Table 54.13** Reflectance Photometers for Home Glucose Monitoring

| *Meter* | *Manufacturer* | *Blood glucose range (mg/dL)* | *Strip used* | *Comments* |
|---|---|---|---|---|
| Glucometer II | Ames | 40–400 | Glucostix | Strip can be read manually |
| Memory Glucometer | Ames | 20–450 | Glucostix | Strip can be read manually |
| Accu-Chek II | Boehringer, Mannheim | 20–500 | Chemstrip bG | Strip can be read manually; little or no color fading after several hours |
| Glucoscan 2000 | Lifescan | 25–450 | Glucoscan | Strip cannot be read manually |
| Glucoscan 3000 | Lifescan | 25–450 | Glucoscan | Strip cannot be read manually |
| Diascan | Home Diagnostics | 10–600 | Diascan | Strip can be read manually |

resulting from the administration of a $\beta$-adrenergic blocking drug.

Hypoglycemia occurring in the early morning hours can produce a rebound hyperglycemia because of the release of counterregulatory hormones (glucagon, cortisol, or growth hormone). This rebound hyperglycemia, often accompanied by glucosuria and possibly ketonuria, is known as the Somogyi phenomenon.[33] Although often hard to diagnose, this phenomenon must be distinguished from the "dawn phenomenon," a relative resistance to insulin's effect during the early morning hours. The dawn phenomenon also results in hyperglycemia and is thought to result from excessive action of growth hormone.[34]

The immediate treatment of hypoglycemia in a conscious patient involves the administration of food, preferably sugar. A candy bar, five or six Lifesavers, 4 to 6 oz of a sugar-containing soft drink, a piece of fruit, or a tablespoonful of sugar dissolved in fruit juice usually reverses the symptoms in 10 to 20 minutes. In the unconscious patient, 1 mg of glucagon injected subcutaneously should provide relief within 10 to 15 minutes. Once the patient regains consciousness, oral sugar should then be administered. In the hospitalized hypoglycemic patient 50 mL of $D_{50}W$ provides rapid reversal of symptoms.

The long-term prevention of hypoglycemia involves altering the patient's dietary habits, exercise patterns, or medication dosage. If insulin has been implicated as the cause of hypoglycemia, the dosage may have to be reduced, split into two or more injections, or both. Hypoglycemia (ultimately leading to hyperglycemia) resulting from the Somogyi phenomenon can be corrected by decreasing the insulin dose by 10% in the insulin-dependent patient and by 30% to 40% in the non–insulin-dependent diabetic.[17]

### Treating Hyperglycemia With Oral Hypoglycemics

Many patients taking sulfonylureas mistakenly assume that the drug by itself will adequately control their diabetes. Therefore, any patient taking an oral agent who has been controlled but who is now hyperglycemic should be asked the following questions:

Have you been taking your medication as prescribed?
Have you run out of your medication during the past several days?
Have you continued to follow the same diet and exercise plan during the past month? Have you experienced a weight gain during this period?
Have you experienced any recent "stresses" (infection, trauma, altered lifestyle, increased pressures)?
Have you been measuring urine or blood glucose values during the past month? Is this hyperglycemia a new phenomenon or has it evolved over the past few weeks?
Have you experienced any symptoms of hypoglycemia (i.e., increased heart rate, irritability, night sweats, nightmares) recently?
Have you experienced any symptoms of hyperglycemia (i.e., increased urination, increased thirst) recently?
Have you taken any new medications—prescription or nonprescription—during the past month?

Correctable factors should first be determined. For example, if the patient has deviated from the standardized diet and exercise plans, every attempt should be made to reinstitute these programs. If increased work or family pressures have triggered the hyperglycemia, whether these pressures are acute or will continue to exist for an indefinite period of time must be ascertained. If there is evidence of infection or other "stress," many times the patient will not respond to an oral agent. In such cases, the patient must be started on short-term insulin therapy (preferably "Human" insulin to minimize production of antibodies)[35] until the problem subsides, at which time the patient can be restarted on an oral sulfonylurea.

If there is no apparent reason for the existing hyperglycemia, it must be assumed that the diabetes has worsened. At this point, urine or blood glucose determinations performed three or four times per day will be beneficial in deciding if the dose needs to be increased and/or administered more than once a day, if the patient needs a trial with a more potent oral agent, or if the patient must be converted to insulin therapy.

Although there are no definitive guidelines for beginning sulfonylurea therapy, the patient's age and fasting blood glucose level may narrow the choice of agents. Tolbutamide is the shortest acting of the sulfonylureas, and often once-a-day therapy is not sufficient for the younger patient with an elevated fasting blood glucose. Therefore, another first-generation agent or one of the second-generation agents may be used. Conversely, tolbutamide may be an excellent choice in the newly diagnosed elderly diabetic, as a hypoglycemic episode may be more dangerous in this patient. Moreover, chlorpropamide, while beneficial for many patients, should be considered as a second- or third-choice agent in the elderly because of its long duration of action.

Usually if the patient's blood glucose is not adequately controlled with maximum doses of one oral agent, a more potent oral agent is indicated; however, if the second oral drug proves unsuccessful, the patient should be considered a candidate for insulin therapy.[5]

**Adjusting Hyperglycemia With Insulin**

It is not uncommon for patients who have begun insulin therapy, whether they be type I or type II diabetics, to reject the notion of daily insulin injections, much less multiple daily injections. Thus, noncompliance resulting from anger, denial, or fear may be more widespread than is expected. It is also more common for patients receiving insulin therapy to experience the Somogyi or dawn phenomenon. Therefore, in the patient who is no longer controlled on his or her current insulin regimen, an attempt should be made to find answers to the following questions:

Is the patient administering the correct number of units of the correct insulin(s) at the correct time(s) per day?
Has the insulin been stored under appropriate conditions?
If the patient is using an insulin suspension, is the bottle being properly agitated to promote proper resuspension?
Is the patient drawing up the insulin correctly (especially if using two different kinds of insulin)?
Is the patient rotating injection sites but still staying in the same general anatomic area (e.g., abdomen, thighs)?
Is the patient injecting the insulin correctly?
Has the patient experienced any itching, redness at the site of injection, or any other evidence of insulin allergy?
Have there been any recent dietary modifications (time of meals, type of food consumed, amount of food consumed)?
Has the patient continued to follow the same exercise plan during the past month?
Has the patient gained or lost any weight during the past month?
Has the patient experienced any daytime or nocturnal symptoms of hypoglycemia recently?
Has the patient experienced any recent "stresses" (infection, trauma, altered lifestyle, increased pressures, etc.)?
Has the patient tested urine or blood consistently during the past month? Is the hyperglycemia a new phenomenon or has it evolved over several weeks?
Has the patient experienced any recent symptoms of hyperglycemia?
Has the patient taken any new medications—prescription or nonprescription—during the past month?

Assuming that there have been no errors in diet, in exercise, or in the storage, dose preparation, or administration of the insulin, the patient's dosage will need adjustment. The patient's weight, symptoms of hypo- or hyperglycemia, evidence of the Somogyi effect, and times during the day in which the patient is hypoglycemic offer invaluable clues as to how to adjust the insulin dosage.

***Weight*** A weight gain may indicate that the patient's insulin dosage is too large. Excess insulin promotes fat storage and hypoglycemia, which results in rebound hyperglycemia, thus seeming to require extra insulin to reduce the high blood glucose.[17,36] This effect may snowball, ultimately resulting in the patient remaining hyperglycemic while simultaneously gaining weight. Symptoms of hypo- and hyperglycemia may verify this suspicion. In this case, the insulin dosage must actually be adjusted downward.

***Somogyi Effect*** Hyperglycemia occurring during the early morning hours may be caused by a shorter-than-anticipated duration of action of the insulin or by nocturnal hypoglycemia resulting in rebound hyperglycemia (Somogyi effect). Blood glucose levels measured at midnight and during the early morning hours may be of help in determining the cause of the hyperglycemia. Questioning the patient about symptoms of nocturnal hypoglycemia (nightmares, night sweats) may also help to differentiate between the two causes of the problem. If the Somogyi effect is suspected, a decrease in insulin dose will alleviate the problem.

***Times of Hyperglycemia*** This is by far the most important factor in determining how to adjust insulin therapy. Blood glucose levels collected at various times throughout the day can pinpoint the times at which the patient consistently loses control. For patients who have a high midmorning blood glucose but who are otherwise normoglycemic throughout the day, addition of Regular insulin to the current dose of intermediate-acting insulin will help to correct the problem. If a patient experiences hyperglycemia during the night and/or has a high fasting value, splitting the dose of intermediate-acting insulin such that the patient receives two thirds of the total dose before breakfast and one third before supper will help achieve tighter control. If the patient resists the concept of two injections per day, another possible solution to the problem may be to convert the patient to a long-acting insulin (Ultralente). A patient who exhibits hyperglycemia during the evening hours may benefit from a dose of Regular insulin just before supper.

## Complications

As diabetes progresses, it affects the vasculature throughout the body. Larger blood vessels such as coronary, cerebral, and peripheral vessels may be more prone to occlusion. These macrovascular complications can ultimately lead to coronary heart disease, stroke, or peripheral vascular disease (intermittent claudication). Likewise, the microvascular circulation may be damaged, ultimately producing such complications as nephropathy, retinopathy, and peripheral neuropathy.

### *Macrovascular*

Although seen in both type I and type I diabetics, macrovascular complications are much more prevalent in type II than in type I diabetics. In fact, 60% of deaths in non–insulin-dependent diabetics have been attributed to macrovascular complications, whereas there is only a 30% macrovascular-related mortality rate in insulin-dependent diabetics.[37,38] The mechanism by which these changes occur is unclear, but has been most often attributed to an altered metabolism of low-density lipoprotein (LDL) cholesterol or to a direct effect of diabetes on arterial wall cells. The most important factors that can be addressed to reverse these complications include lowering of cholesterol levels, adequate treatment of hypertension, and cessation of smoking. There is a clear association between poor blood glucose control and elevated cholesterol levels. Moreover, tight metabolic control in type I and type II diabetics has been found to decrease very low density lipoprotein (VLDL), LDL, and total cholesterol levels. Conversely, high-density lipoprotein (HDL) levels have not been found to be affected significantly by tight glycemic or metabolic control.[39–41]

### *Microvascular*

These complications occur almost exclusively in the type I diabetic. Although the mechanism of diabetic nephropathy, retinopathy, and neuropathy has not been fully elucidated, these complications have been linked to increased sorbitol levels resulting from glucose metabolism via a polyol pathway.[5,38] This ultimately produces increased capillary basement membrane thickening, altered lipid metabolism, and increased platelet adhesiveness.

The renal complications of diabetes may occur independently or in conjunction with hypertension. Proteinuria, azotemia, and increased serum creatinine are indicative of the nephropathy and impending renal impairment. Dialysis or renal transplant is indicated if the nephropathy progresses to complete renal failure.

Diabetes is the leading cause of new blindness in the United States. Diabetes-associated retinopathy may be of the nonproliferative or proliferative type. Nonproliferative retinopathies may be asymptomatic with little vision impairment. Proliferative retinopathy, on the other hand, can produce greatly diminished vision or sudden blindness.[38] Fortunately, many diabetics with retinopathy can be treated with laser photocoagulation, thus preserving much of their eyesight.

Associated with increased sorbitol levels, neuropathy is a painful diabetic complication and is difficult to manage. Symptoms may begin as tingling or burning sensations, particularly in the calves, ankles, and feet with a definite loss in vibratory sensation. Later the patient may lose all sensation in a particular area, thus not being able to detect hot, cold, or pain. Circulation may be impaired to these areas because of atherosclerosis, and it is not uncommon for diabetics to undergo amputation of toes, feet, or legs. Phenytoin, perphenazine–amitriptyline, clonidine, and other drugs have been used with anecdotal success to treat the pain associated with diabetic neuropathy.[42–44] New therapy protocols with aldose reductase inhibitors such as tolrestat and sorbinil have shown promise in reducing the painful symptoms and possibly restoring some of the electrophysiologic conductance.[45]

Autonomic neuropathies involving the gastrointestinal, genitourinary, and cardiovascular systems are also complications of diabetes. Gastric paresis produces symptoms of anorexia, bloating, and vomiting from delayed gastric emptying. Metoclopramide has been successfully used to manage this condition.[46] Genitourinary problems include neurogenic bladder, impotence in males, and *Candida* vaginitis in females.

Once one of the microvascular complications has developed, the process is irreversible. Consequently, preventing the complication, retarding its onset, and limiting its progression are current areas of diabetic research. Animal studies demonstrate that poor metabolic control accelerates the occurrence and progression of microvascular complications. Data in humans correlating tight glycemic control with a reduced incidence of microvascular complications look promising but are still not definitive.[47–49]

## Special Problems Associated With Therapy

### *Ketoacidosis*

***Pathophysiology*** Ketoacidosis presents much more often in the type I diabetic and is considered a medical emergency. As there is a lack of circulating insulin, hyperglycemia is always present, resulting in hyperosmolar serum and a subsequent osmotic diuresis. The body relies on fatty acid metabolism and gluconeogenesis as a means of energy production. With an absence of insulin, fat metabolism is impaired, and fatty acid intermediates are converted to highly acidic, two- and four-carbon ketones.[50] These ketones are initially excreted in the urine as sodium and potassium salts. As the osmotic diuresis continues, however, hypovolemia and prerenal azotemia develop, leading to a decrease in the glomerular filtration rate.

The acidosis causes potassium to move from intracellular to extracellular spaces. With a relative decrease in glomerular filtration rate, an apparent hyperkalemia develops (although the patient is actually in a negative potassium balance because of initial renal excretion of potassium). Acidosis is also a potent respiratory stimulant, and hyperventilation is common. Although hyperventilation lowers $Paco_2$, total body hydrogen ion concentrations are relatively unaffected.

***Clinical Presentation*** Patients with ketoacidosis often complain of thirst, weakness, fatigue, nausea, and vomiting. Abdominal pain and "not being able to get enough air" are also common complaints. "Fruity" breath caused by ketone accumulation may be detectable, and the patient may be drowsy or inattentive; coma is possible but is not a classic finding. The patient usually feels warm and dry, although the body temperature may actually be subnormal. Laboratory findings include hyperglycemia, ketonemia, azotemia, glucosuria, and ketonuria. Serum potassium may be normal or elevated because of the intracellular to extracellular shift.

***Treatment*** Intravenous fluids and low-dose Regular insulin constitute the current treatment of diabetic ketoacidosis. Initially 1–2 L of normal saline (NS) are administered at a rate of 200 mL/h or faster to replete sodium; the intravenous fluid can then be changed to half-normal saline ($\frac{1}{2}$NS). Regular insulin (10–20 units) is given as a bolus into the intravenous line. A second intravenous site is then usually established, and a continuous insulin drip is subsequently prepared by adding 100 units of Regular insulin to a liter of NS or $\frac{1}{2}$NS. The administration rate is approximately 0.1 unit of insulin per kilogram per hour.[51] The first intravenous is used to adjust fluid and electrolyte therapy, while the second is used to adjust insulin therapy. Care should be taken not to drop the blood glucose too quickly (usually 100 mg/dL/h is desirable to avoid possible cerebral edema). When the blood glucose has dropped to approximately 250 mg/dL, the intravenous fluid is changed to $D_5\frac{1}{2}NS$. The insulin drip should be continued until serum ketones are no longer detected.

Careful attention should be given to serum potassium, phosphate, and bicarbonate concentrations. As the hyperglycemia is brought under control, hypokalemia may develop. Potassium may be added to the intravenous as either potassium chloride or potassium phosphate. Phosphate buffers may have been depleted with the acidosis; however, potassium should not be administered as the phosphate salt unless hypophosphatemia is present. Although serum bicarbonate is initially low, levels usually return to normal with correction of the acidosis, and bicarbonate replacement is rarely indicated.

### *Insulin Requirements of the Surgical Patient*

Diabetics scheduled for surgery usually do not receive breakfast on the day of surgery, and administration of insulin might lead to profound hypoglycemia; however, the "stress" of surgery has a tremendous hyperglycemic effect such that withholding insulin can lead to dehydration, an impaired inflammatory response, and possible ketoacidosis (in the type I diabetic). Therefore, plasma glucose values should ideally be less than 300 mg%.

The diet-controlled diabetic usually needs no exogenous insulin but should at least be covered by a sliding scale order should the need for insulin arise. "Human" insulin should be utilized to minimize the formation of insulin antibodies. The patient controlled with oral hypoglycemics should have the medication held on the day of surgery and needs to have an order for a sliding scale. The insulin-dependent diabetic should receive one-half of his or her usual dose of an intermediate-acting insulin and should likewise have an order for sliding scale insulin after surgery.[52]

### *"Sick-Day" Guidelines for Insulin-Dependent Diabetics*

When a patient feels too ill to eat, the question often arises as to how much (if any) insulin is needed. Although insulin requirements on "sick days" vary among individuals, most would agree that insulin should not be discontinued, as infection, stress, and other factors significantly increase plasma glucose. Extra fluids (up to 12 glasses) should be consumed, especially if the patient has a fever. Patients should be instructed to record the amount of fluid they consume as well as the number of times they urinate, vomit, or have loose stools. Urine should be tested with each urination; if it contains ketones or more than 2% glucose, the patient's physician should be contacted. Similarly, any patient having difficulty breathing or breathing over 24 times per minute (symptoms of respiratory alkalosis) should seek medical attention. Although it is normal to feel tired or sleepy when sick, any patient who feels very sleepy or cannot pay attention should have someone seek medical help immediately.

## References


1. National Diabetes Group. Classification and diagnosis of diabetes mellitus and other categories of glucose tolerance. Diabetes 1979;28:1039–1057.
2. Rotter JI, Rimoin DL. The genetics of the glucose intolerance disorders. Am J Med 1981;70:116–126.
3. Cahill GF. Disorders of carbohydrate metabolism: Diabetes mellitus, in Wyngaarden JB, Smith LH (eds): Cecil Textbook of Medicine. Philadelphia, W.B. Saunders, 1982, pp 1054–1056.
4. Gerich JE. Insulin-dependent diabetes mellitus: Pathophysiology. Mayo Clin Proc 1986;61:787–791.
5. American Diabetes Association. The Physician's Guide to Type II Diabetes (NIDDM): Diagnosis and Treatment. New York, American Diabetes Association, 1984, pp 1–112.
6. Hoekstra JBL, van Rijn HJM, Erkelens DW, et al. Review: C-peptide. Diabetes Care 1982;5:438–446.
7. Arky R, Wylie-Rosett J, El-Beheri B. Examination of current dietary recommendations for individuals with diabetes mellitus. Diabetes Care 1982;5:59–63.
8. Crapo PA. Nutrition update. Clin Diabetes 1983;1:12–14.
9. Ary DV, Toobert D, Wilson W, et al. Patient perspective on factors pertaining to nonadherence to diabetes regimen. Diabetes Care 1986;9:168–172.
10. Bogardus C, Ravussin E, Robbins DC, et al. Effects of physical training and diet therapy on carbohydrate metabolism in patients with glucose intolerance and non–insulin dependent diabetes mellitus. Diabetes 1984;33:311–318.
11. Zimman B. Exercise in diabetes treatment. Clin Diabetes 1983;1:18–22.
12. The University Group Diabetes Program. A study of the effects of hypoglycemic agents on vascular complications in patients with adult onset diabetes. Diabetes 1970;19:(suppl 2):1–26.
13. Skillman TG, Feldman JM. The pharmacology of sulfonylureas. Am J Med 1981;70:361–372.
14. Lebovitz HE, Feinglos MN. The oral hypoglycemic agents, in Ellenberg M, Rifkin H (eds): Diabetes Mellitus: Theory and Practice. New Hyde Park, NY, Medical Examination Publishing Co., 1983, pp 591–610.
15. Antidiabetic agents, in American Hospital Formulary Service Drug Information 86. Bethesda, American Society of Hospital Pharmacists, 1984, pp 1562–1594.
16. Gavin JR. Dual actions of sulfonylureas and glyburide: Receptor and post-receptor effects. Am J Med 1985;79(suppl 3B): 34–43.
17. Gregerman RI. Diabetes mellitus, in Barker LR, Burton JR, Zieve PD (eds): Principles of Ambulatory Medicine. Baltimore, Williams and Wilkins, 1986, pp 951–986.
18. Home PD, Alberti KGMM. The new insulins: Their characteristics and clinical indications. Drugs 1982;24:401–413.
19. Deckert T. Intermediate-acting insulin preparations: NPH and lente. Diabetes Care 1980;3:623–626.
20. Personal communication, Dr. SM Chernish, Clinical Investigation Division, Lilly Research Laboratories, Jan 21, 1983.
21. Ahrens ER, Gossain VV, Rovner DR. Human insulin: Its development and clinical use. Postgrad Med 1986;80:181–187.
22. Galloway JA. Insulin treatment for the early 80's: Facts and questions about old and new insulins and their usage. Diabetes Care 1980;3:615–622.
23. Cahill GF, McDevitt HO. Insulin-dependent diabetes mellitus: The initial lesion. N Engl J Med 1981:304:1454–1465.
24. Wilson RM, Clarke P, Barkes H, et al. Starting insulin treatment as an outpatient: Report of 100 consecutive patients followed up for at least one year. JAMA 1986;256:877–880.

25. Cryer PE, Gerich JE. Glucose counterregulation, hypoglycemia and intensive insulin therapy in diabetes mellitus. N Engl J Med 1985;313:232–241.
26. Bergman M, Felig P. Self-monitoring of blood glucose levels in diabetics: Principles and practice. Arch Intern Med 1984; 144:2029–2034.
27. Geffner ME, Kaplan SA, Lippe BM, et al. Self monitoring of blood glucose levels and intensified insulin therapy. JAMA 1983;249:2913–2916.
28. Goldstein DE, Parker KM, England JD, et al. Clinical application of glycosylated hemoglobin measurements. Diabetes 1982; 31(suppl 3):70–78.
29. Bunn HF. Evaluation of glycosylated hemoglobin in diabetic patients. Diabetes 1981;30:613–617.
30. Ruderman NV, Schneider S. Exercise and the insulin-dependent diabetic. Hosp Pract 1986;21(suppl 5A):41–51.
31. Galloway JA. The complications of insulin therapy, in Bressler R, Johnson DG (eds): Management of diabetes mellitus. Boston, John Wright–PSG, 1982, pp 91–114.
32. Gossain VV, Rovner DR. Pancreatic glucagon: Possible implications of the hyperglycemic hormone in diabetes control. Postgrad Med 1982;72:87–96.
33. Prout TE. Diabetes mellitus, in Harvey AG, Johns RJ, McKusick VA, et al (eds): The Principles and Practice of Medicine. New York, Appleton-Century-Crofts, 1980, pp 795–815.
34. Bolli GB, Gerich JE. The dawn phenomenon—a common occurrence in both non–insulin-dependent and insulin-dependent diabetes mellitus. N Engl J Med 1984;310:746–750.
35. Deckert T. The immunogenicity of new insulins. Diabetes 1985;34(suppl 2):94–96.
36. Wilson DE. Excessive insulin therapy: Biochemical effects and clinical repercussions. Ann Intern Med 1983;98:219–227.
37. Ganda OP. Pathogenesis of macrovascular disease in the human diabetic. Diabetes 1980;29:931–942.
38. Feingold KR. Preventing the Vascular Complications of Diabetes. New York, HP Publishing, 1987, pp 2–16.
39. Dunn FL. Lipids and diabetes: Guidelines for treatment. Clin Diabetes 1986;4:34–41.
40. Feingold KR, Siperstein MD. Diabetic vascular disease. Adv Intern Med 1985;31:309–340.
41. Colwell JA, Winocour PD, Lopes-Virella M, et al. New concepts about the pathogenesis of artherosclerosis in diabetes mellitus. Am J Med 1983;75(suppl 5B):67–80.
42. Ellenberg M. Diabetic neuropathy: Clinical aspects. Metabolism 1976;25:1627–1655.
43. Spritz N. Nerve disease in diabetes mellitus. Med Clin North Am 1978;62:787–798.
44. Joseifek LF, Bleeker ML. Peripheral neuropathy, in Barker LR, Burton JR, Ziere PD (eds): Principles of Ambulatory Medicine. Baltimore, Williams and Wilkins, 1986, pp 1200–1215.
45. Kador PF, Kinoshita JH, Sharples NE. Aldose reductase inhibitors: A potential new class of agents for the pharmacological control of certain diabetic complications. J Med Chem 1985;28:841–849.
46. Clements RS, Bell DS. Diabetic neuropathy: Peripheral and autonomic syndromes. Postgrad Med 1982;71:50–67.
47. Camerini-Davalos RA, Velasco C, Glasser M, et al. Drug-induced reversal of early diabetic microangiopathy. N Engl J Med 1983;309:1551–1556.
48. Dahl-Jorgensen K, Brinchman-Hansen O, Hanssen KF, et al. Rapid tightening of blood glucose leads to transient deterioration of retinopathy in insulin dependent diabetes mellitus: The Oslo study. Br Med J 1985;290:811–815.
49. Dahl-Jorgensen K, Brinchman-Hansen O, Hanssen KF, et al. Effect of near normoglycaemia for two years on progression of early diabetic retinopathy, nephropathy, and neuropathy: The Oslo study. Br Med J 1986;293:1195–1199.
50. McGarry JD, Foster DW. Ketogenesis and its regulation. Am J Med 1976;61:9–13.
51. Levine SN, Lowenstein JE. Treatment of diabetic ketoacidosis. Arch Intern Med 1981;141:713–715.
52. Byyny RL. Management of diabetes during surgery. Postgrad Med 1980;68:191–202.

# *Chapter 55* / Disorders of the Adrenal Gland

John G. Gums, PharmD

The adrenal glands were first characterized by Eustachius in 1563 (Table 55.1). After Addison identified a case of adrenal insufficiency in man, adrenal anatomy and physiology flourished. Most of the work done in the early and mid-1900s centered on the glucocorticoid cortisol. But with the discovery of aldosterone by Simpson and Tait in 1952, adrenal pharmacology turned toward the mineralocorticoid. Conn followed with his classical description of primary aldosteronism in 1955,[1] and numerous clinicians and investigators have continued the discovery of the variety of disease processes promoted through the adrenal gland.

## Physiology/Anatomy/Biochemistry

There are two adrenal glands located extraperitoneally to the upper poles of each kidney (Fig. 55.1). The right gland tends to be higher than the left. On average, each adrenal gland weighs 4 g and is 2–3 cm in width and 4–6 cm in length. The gland is fed by small arteries from the abdominal aorta and renal and phrenic arteries. Drainage of the adrenal gland occurs via the renal vein on the left and the inferior vena cava on the right.

The adrenal cortex occupies 90% of the total gland. The adrenal medulla accounts for the remaining 10% and is responsible for the secretion of catecholamines. The adrenal cortex comprises[2] three separate zones. The zona glomerulosa, 15% of the total adrenal cortex, is responsible for aldosterone production. The zona reticularis, the innermost zone, making up 60% of the cortex, is responsible for basal cortisol production. The zona fasciculata occupies 25% of the adrenal cortex, is highly cholesterol bound, and is responsible for all androgen production.

The adrenal cortex is responsible for the secretion of three types of hormones (Fig. 55.2). The first of these is the glucocorticoids. Cortisol, the end metabolite, is responsible for the regulation of fat, carbohydrate, and protein metabolism. The second group is the mineralocorticoids, of which aldosterone is the principle end product. Aldosterone maintains electrolyte and volume homeostasis by altering potassium secretion and renal tubular sodium reabsorption. The androgens, testosterone and estradiol, are the major end products of the third type. Androgens have influence within the reproductive system as well as affecting primary and secondary sex characteristics.

### *Hormone Production and Metabolism*

Cortisol production is accomplished via two successive hydroxylations, the first at the 21-position by 21-hydroxylase, yielding 11-deoxycortisol, and the second at the 11-position by 11-hydroxylase, yielding cortisol or hydrocortisone.

Aldosterone is a by-product of the 21-hydroxylation of pregnenolone to form deoxycorticosterone. The oxidation of 18-hydroxycorticosterone to aldosterone is a unique feature of the zona glomerulosa, explaining why aldosterone is not affected during disease processes limited to the zonae fasciculata and/or reticularis.

Androgens have a 19-carbon nucleus and serve as precursors to more potent analogs produced in the periphery. The adrenal gland can synthesize estradiol and estrone from testosterone and androstenedione, respectively; however, the quantities are extremely small. The relative rates of production for the various steroids produced by the adrenal gland are listed in Table 55.2.

Glomerular filtration is responsible primarily for the elimination of endogenously produced glucocorticoids. The half-life of cortisol is 70 to 120 minutes; with aldosterone, the half-life is only 15 minutes because of an extremely high first-pass effect.

Metabolism and conversion of the various steroids can be altered by a variety of disease states and medicinal compounds. Metabolism is reduced in chronic liver disease, hypothyroidism, infancy, the elderly, anorexia nervosa, and protein-calorie malnutrition. Drugs such as mitotane, phenytoin, rifampin, aminoglutethimide, and barbiturates are all capable of affecting steroid metabolism and/or production.

### *Regulation of Hormone Secretion*

The regulation of glucocorticoid secretion is accomplished by the pituitary hormone, adrenocorticotropic hormone (ACTH). Under normal conditions, ACTH is released from the anterior pituitary in response to corticotropin-releasing factor (CRF), which is secreted by the median eminence of the hypothalamus (Fig. 55.3). After release ACTH stimulates the adrenal gland to release cortisol and to a lesser extent aldosterone and androgens. The rising cortisol concentration inhibits the secretion of CRF and ACTH through a negative-feedback mechanism.

Regulation of adrenal androgens is accomplished in a manner similar to cortisol regulation. Therefore, when plasma androgen reaches sufficient concentrations, production is terminated via a negative-feedback loop. Androgen release is increased during puberty and affected by certain disease states and drugs.

Regulation of aldosterone secretion is considerably more complex. The renin–angiotensin system has the ability to respond to electrolyte and volume changes to increase or decrease aldosterone secretion. Renin production and sub-

**Table 55.1** Landmarks in Adrenal Cortical History

| *Date* | *Discovery* | *Investigator* |
|---|---|---|
| 1563 | Adrenal described | Eustachius |
| 1855 | Adrenal insufficiency in man | Addison |
| 1856 | Adrenalectomy fatal in dog | Brown |
| 1895–1904 | Discovery of epinephrine | Oliver |
| 1910 | Hypoglycemia of Addison's disease | Porges |
| 1927 | First active adrenal cortical extract | Hartman |
| 1932 | Life of patient with Addison's disease prolonged with salt | Loeb |
| 1936 | The "alarm reaction" | Selye |
| 1938 | Synthesis of desoxycorticosterone | Reichstein |
| 1948 | Partial synthesis of cortisone | Sarrett |
| 1949 | First anti-inflammatory use of cortisone | Hench/Kendall |
| 1952 | Discovery of aldosterone | Simpson/Tait |
| 1955 | Discovery of primary aldosteronism | Conn |

sequent aldosterone secretion are stimulated by blood pressure lowering, erect posture, salt depletion, $\beta$-adrenergic stimulation, and central nervous system excitation. These processes are inhibited by salt loading, angiotensin II, vasopressin, potassium, calcium, blood pressure increases, and a variety of drugs. The conversion of renin substrate to angiotensin I and subsequently to angiotensin II is the initial stimulus for aldosterone synthesis. Angiotensin II is acted upon by aminopeptidase and converted to angiotensin III. Angiotensin II and III are both capable of stimulating the zona glomerulosa to secrete aldosterone. After aldosterone secretion, increases in sodium, water, and blood pressure are seen, thereby turning off the stimulus for renin release.

## Hyperfunction of the Adrenal Gland

### *Cushing's Disease*

In 1932, Cushing first described a syndrome of pituitary basophilism that attracted national attention. It was not until this time that patients with unexplained central obesity, cutaneous striae, osteoporosis, weakness, hypertension, diabetes mellitus, and congestion had a definite diagnosis. Cushing emphasized that the disease was of pituitary origin. Ten years later, Albright focused his attention on the sugar hormone he believed was originating from the adrenal cortex.[3]

**Figure 55.1** Anatomy of the adrenal gland. A, artery; V, vein.

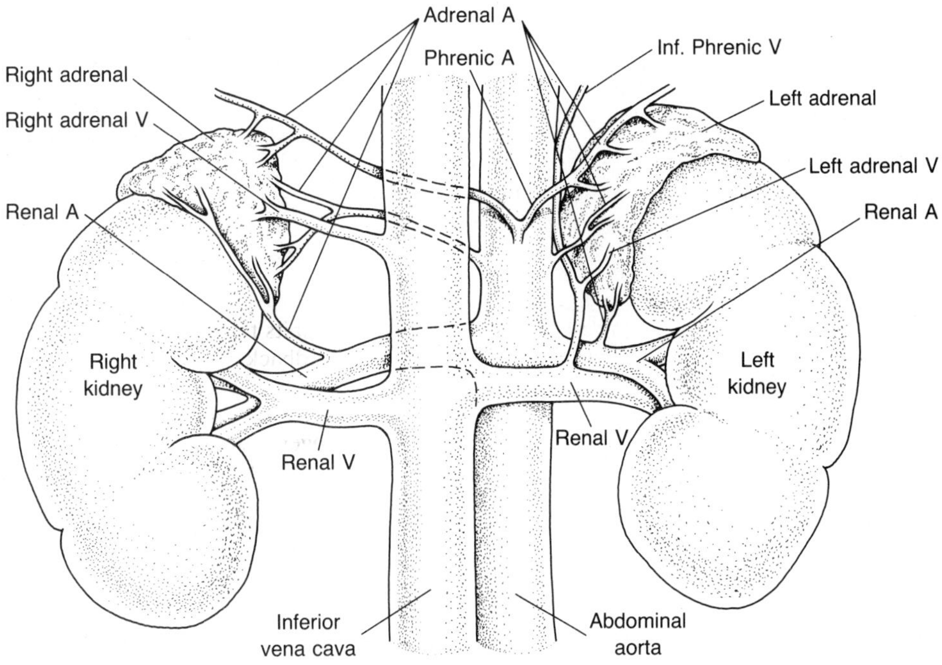

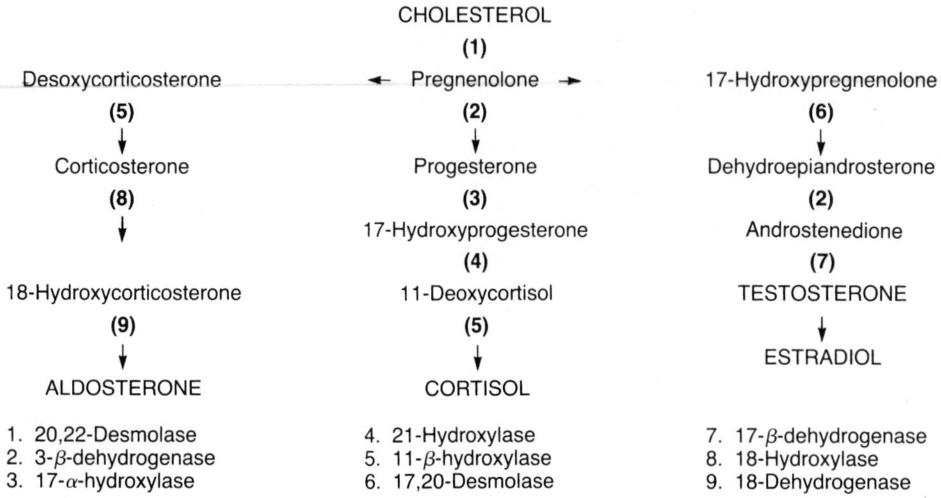


**Figure 55.2** The cholesterol pathway with major enzymes and endpoints. *(From Grodsky GM: Chemistry and functions of the hormones: Adrenal and gonads, in Martin DW, Mayes PA, Rodwell VW (Eds): Harper's Review of Biochemistry. Los Altos, CA, Lange Medical Publications, 1983, pp 494–510.)*

After development of the method for measuring urinary steroids, Daughaday discovered elevated steroids in the urine of Cushing's disease patients. Finally, the end product was identified and Cushing's disease was correctly explained as an excess of cortisol in the plasma (hypercortisolism).

### Etiology

The etiology of Cushing's disease is varied. Pituitary-dependent disease accounts for 60% to 70% of the Cushing's cases. The remaining 30% to 40% are approximately equally divided between adrenal adenomas,[4] adrenal carcinomas,[5] and ectopic ACTH-secreting tumors. The most common form arises from ACTH oversecretion from the pituitary, with the net result of chronic stimulation of the adrenal gland leading to bilateral adrenal hyperplasia (BAH). The majority of these disorders can be traced to a pituitary-dependent tumor. In selected patients, an abnormal CRF secretion from the hypothalamus may exacerbate the disorders or serve as a separate etiology.

**Table 55.2** Rate of Production and Plasma Concentrations of Various Steroids

| *Steroid* | *24-h secretion (mg)* | *Plasma concentration (ng/mL)* |
|---|---|---|
| Aldosterone | 0.15 | 0.16 |
| Androstenedione | 2.40 | 1.50 |
| Corticosterone | 2.50 | 3.00 |
| Cortisol | 16.0 | 100.00 |
| 11-Deoxycorticosterone | 0.60 | 0.16 |
| 11-Deoxycortisol | 0.40 | 1.70 |
| Progesterone | 0.0 | 0.20 (male)<br>12.0 (female) |
| Testosterone | 0.20 | 5.60 (male)<br>0.50 (female) |

The majority of adrenal cortex tumors are benign adenomas. Adrenal carcinoma is found more often in children than adults with Cushing's disease. Ectopic ACTH syndrome refers to excessive ACTH production resulting from a nonendocrine tumor, usually of the pancreas, thymus, or lung. To distinguish between the various etiologies, a careful history and some pertinent laboratory work are required (Table 55.3).

### Clinical Presentation

The clinical symptoms most commonly seen with Cushing's disease are listed in Table 55.4.[6] The most common of these findings include central obesity and facial rounding. Patients are often described as having moon facies with a buffalo hump. Fat accumulation is often noted at the supraclavicular and dorsocervical areas as well.

**Figure 55.3** Regulation of cortisol secretion under normal conditions.

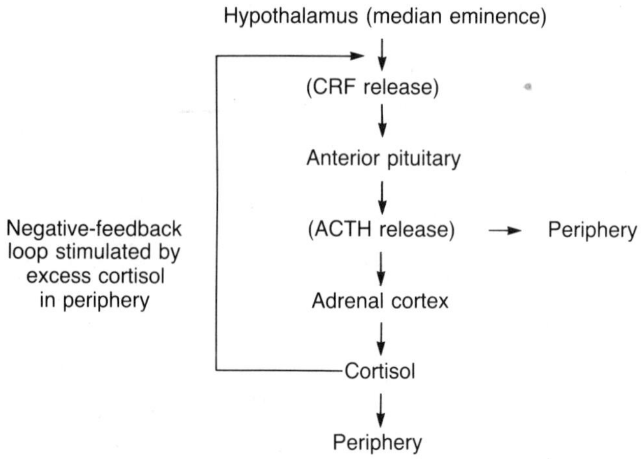

**Table 55.3** Various Etiologies of Cushing's Disease and Their Respective Differences

| | *Pituitary dependent* | *Adrenal adenoma* | *Adrenal carcinoma* | *Ectopic ACTH syndrome* |
|---|---|---|---|---|
| Course | Slow | Slow | Rapid | Rapid |
| Symptoms | Mild to moderate | Mild to moderate | Severe | Atypical |
| Dominant sex/age | Female/male | None noted | Children | Male/female |
| Virilization | + | + | +++ | + |
| Abdominal mass | 0 | 0 | ++ | 0 |
| Plasma ACTH concentration | Slightly elevated | 0 | 0 | 0 |
| Dexamethasone suppression test | 50% suppression or greater | No suppression | No suppression | No suppression |
| Iodocholesterol scan | Bilateral uptake | Unilateral uptake | No uptake | Bilateral uptake |

About 50% of patients exhibit some peripheral obesity and fat accumulation. Facial plethora is caused by an underlying atrophy of the skin and connective tissue. Striae take on a red to purple color and are usually present along the lower abdomen. Excess androgen secretion is responsible for the 80% of female patients who present with hirsutism.

Diagnosis of Cushing's is relatively easy, but the differentiation between etiologies can be difficult.[7,8] Tests used to diagnose Cushing's include measurement of 24-hour urine for free cortisol, 1-mg overnight dexamethasone suppression test, plasma ACTH assay, eight-dose dexamethasone suppression test, adrenal vein catheterization, or iodocholesterol nuclear scan.[7]

Patients with Cushing's disease have an abnormal urinary free cortisol content. Elevated urinary free cortisol concentrations are highly suggestive of Cushing's disease. Normal reference values for urinary free cortisol are 20–90 $\mu$g per 24-hour period. It is not unusual to detect a two- or threefold increase in urine cortisol in the patient with hyperfunction of the adrenal gland. Starvation, topical steroid application, and hydration from water loading are all capable of falsely elevating the urine cortisol concentrations. As other pathologic conditions can increase the amount of free cortisol, additional tests should be performed to confirm the diagnosis.

In the overnight dexamethasone suppression test, 1 mg of dexamethasone is administered at 11:00 PM. The next morning, at 8:00 AM, plasma cortisol is obtained for analysis. The Cushing's patient will not exhibit a suppressed cortisol concentration via the negative-feedback loop, and the morning cortisol concentration will be elevated (greater than 5 $\mu$g/100 mL).[9]

**Table 55.4** Clinical Features in Patients With Hypercortisolism

| *Feature* | *% Patients* |
|---|---|
| Obesity | 90 |
| Hypertension | 85 |
| Facial plethora | 84 |
| Glucose intolerance | 80 |
| Menstrual dysfunction | 76 |
| Hirsutism | 72 |
| Striae | 67 |
| Myopathy | 65 |
| Muscular weakness | 58 |
| Osteoporosis | 55 |
| Psychiatric change | 55 |

Urinary examination of steroids can be used in the diagnosis of Cushing's. Greater than 10 mg of 17-hydroxycorticosteroid per gram of creatinine is indicative of hypercortisolism.

The normal circadian rhythm of cortisol demonstrates a 60% to 80% decline between 8:00 AM and 11:00 PM. This rhythm is lost in the Cushing's disease patient.

Additionally, plasma ACTH concentrations can be measured. Patients with adrenal tumors and ectopic ACTH syndrome present with suppressed plasma ACTH concentrations.[10] Hypothalamic or pituitary-dependent patients have a plasma ACTH excess. While the plasma ACTH concentration is specific for certain etiologies, the assay lacks the sensitivity needed to differentiate between a low ACTH concentration and a high to normal measurement.

The high-dose dexamethasone suppression test operates under the same principle as the low-dose test.[11] The main difference is in total dose (16 mg) and the time to test the patient (48 hours). The high-dose test has its main application in differentiating the adrenal hyperplasia patient from the patient with another form of hypercortisolism. The adrenal hyperplasia patient generally demonstrates a 50% reduction in urinary steroids over baseline, whereas the others generally do not suppress.

The two newer techniques for substantiating the diagnosis and differentiating an etiology in Cushing's disease are adrenal catheterization and nuclear scan. Selective adrenal vein catheterization can distinguish adrenal adenoma from adrenal hyperplasia. The procedure is an invasive one and requires skill and quality equipment. Intraadrenal hemorrhage follows this procedure in as many as 10% of patients. Nuclear scanning uses a cholesterol compound, iodocholesterol, which is taken up by the adrenal gland. Once in the gland the iodinated cholesterol can be scanned and read for uptake percentage. After the nuclear scan, a differential diagnosis can be made between hyperplasia and tumor-producing Cushing's disease.

**Table 55.5** Summary of Tests Used to Diagnose Cushing's Syndrome[a]

| *Test* | *Normal* | *Hyperplasia* | *Adenoma* | *Carcinoma* | *Ectopic ACTH* |
|---|---|---|---|---|---|
| Plasma | | | | | |
| Cortisol (μg/100 mL, AM/PM) | 17/8 | 30/25 | 35/35 | 50/50 | 35/35 |
| ACTH (pg/mL) | 150 | 50–500 | 50 | 10 | 500–1,000 |
| Urine: 17-hydroxycorticosteroid (mg/d) | | | | | |
| Basal | 2–10 | 15 | 30 | 50 | 30 |
| After ACTH | 2–5× ↑ | 3–5× ↑ | ↕ | ↕ | 2× ↑ |
| Dexamethasone 2 mg/d | 3 | 4 | 30 | 50 | 30 |
| Dexamethasone 8 mg/d | 3 | 3 | 30 | 50 | 30 |
| Nuclear: Iodocholesterol uptake pattern | B | B | U | N | B |

[a] ↑, increase; ↕, no change; B, bilateral; U, unilateral; N, no uptake.

**Differential Diagnosis**

While the diagnosis of Cushing's disease is not a difficult one, at times the clinician needs to differentiate it from other syndromes that mimic Cushing's signs and symptoms. Pseudo-Cushing's syndrome is the name given to a group of diseases that can mimic Cushing's disease. Patients with obesity, chronic alcoholism, depression, and acute illness of any type can cloud the diagnosis of Cushing's. Depressed patients while mimicking the urinary steroid abnormalities of Cushing's disease do not resemble a Cushing's patient in appearance. In chronic alcoholics, the laboratory panel returns to baseline after cessation of drinking. The obese patient often has normal cortisol concentrations on both serum and urinary screening.

Iatrogenic Cushing's syndrome, induced by administration of glucocorticoids, can often be indistinguishable from Cushing's disease. A careful history and serum determination in a basal state can aid the clinician in making the diagnosis.

Several additional procedures have been used to diagnose Cushing's disease. These include ACTH loading, metyrapone testing, and insulin-induced hypoglycemia. The reliability of these tests is questionable, but they may help to confirm the diagnosis when previous tests are inconclusive.[9] Table 55.5 summarizes the tests used to diagnose Cushing's disease.

**Treatment**

The treatment of Cushing's disease is dependent on the etiology of the hypercortisolism.[12] If left untreated, Cushing's syndrome is associated with a high percentage of morbidity and mortality. Associated disorders such as diabetes mellitus, cardiovascular disease, and electrolyte disorders limit the survival of the Cushing's patient to 4 to 5 years after initial diagnosis if left untreated. Many treatment plans are available depending on the etiology of the disease (see Table 55.6).

*Adrenal Adenoma* The treatment of choice for adrenal adenoma is surgical removal. Surgical removal is associated with relatively few side effects and a high cure rate. The contralateral gland in the patient with adrenal adenoma is usually atrophic. Therefore, steroid replacement is needed both perioperatively and postoperatively. Table 55.7 outlines an approach to steroid replacement for three separate routes of hydrocortisone. Therapy should be continued 2 to 3 months after surgery. In time, an alternate-day dosing scheme can be used, with discontinuation of therapy 4 to 6 months postoperatively.

*Adrenal Carcinoma* The treatment of adrenal carcinoma is surgical removal[5]; however, unlike the adenoma patient, patients with adrenal carcinoma have an unpredictable outcome. Often, the complete tumor cannot be excised, leaving the patients with some degree of symptomatology and extraadrenal involvement. Irradiation can be used if metastases are discovered. In the patient with adrenal carcinoma who is not a surgical candidate, the focus of treatment is on pharmacologic intervention (e.g., mitotane).

The adrenolytic agent 1-chloro-2-[2,2-dichloro-1-(4-chlorophenyl)ethyl]benzene (mitotane, Lysodren, Bristol–Myers) is a cytotoxic drug that structurally resembles the insecticide chlorophenothane (DDT). Mitotane appears to

**Table 55.6** Possible Treatment Plans in Cushing's Disease Based on Etiology

| *Etiology* | *Treatment* |
|---|---|
| Adrenal adenoma | Surgery plus postoperative replacement therapy |
| Adrenal carcinoma | Surgery<br>Mitotane |
| Ectopic ACTH syndrome | Surgery<br>Chemotherapy<br>Irradiation<br>Adrenal inhibitors (metyrapone, aminoglutethimide, trilostane) |
| Pituitary-dependent | Surgery<br>Irradiation<br>Cyproheptadine, metyrapone, trilostane, or mitotane |

**Table 55.7** Steroid Replacement in the Adrenal Adenoma Patient

| | *Hydrocortisone dose* | | |
|---|---|---|---|
| | **IV** | **IM** | **PO** |
| Operation day | 300 mg | 50 mg before surgery | |
| Postoperative day | | | |
| 1 | 200 mg | 50 mg every 12 h | |
| 2 | 150 mg | 50 mg every 12 h | |
| 3 | 100 mg | 50 mg every 12 h | |
| 4 | | 50 mg every 12 h | 25 mg every 6 h |
| 5 | | 25 mg every 12 h | 25 mg every 6 h[a] |
| 7 | | | 25 mg every 6 h |
| 8–10 | | | 25 mg every 8 h |
| 11–20 | | | 25 mg every 12 h |
| 21 or more | | | 20 mg at 8 AM<br>10 mg at 4 PM |

[a] Add fludrocortisone 0.05–0.2 mg PO daily.

selectively inhibit adrenocortical function without causing cellular destruction.[13] Regeneration of cells within the zonae fasciculata and reticularis occurs with resultant atrophy of the adrenal cortex. The zona glomerulosa is minimally affected during acute therapy but can become damaged after long-term treatment. Mitotane decreases cortisol secretion rate, plasma cortisol concentrations, urinary free cortisol, and plasma concentrations of the 17-substituted steroids. Mitotane inhibits the 11$\beta$-hydroxylation of 11-desoxycortisol and 11-desoxycorticosterone in the cortex. The net result is reduced synthesis of cortisol and corticosterone.

Mitotane appears to be the drug of choice in inoperable functional and nonfunctional adrenal carcinoma. Tumor regression is seen in approximately 50% of the patients, with most regressions occurring between the second and fourth month of therapy. Seventy-five percent of patients exhibit a 30% fall in urinary steroids, with 50% of patients showing an improved clinical response after 5 months of treatment. Patient survival appears prolonged, although no adequate clinical trials are available to support this assumption. Approximately 80% of mitotane-induced side effects are restricted to the gastrointestinal tract: nausea, vomiting, diarrhea, and anorexia.

Before initiation of therapy the patient should be hospitalized. The recommended dose of mitotane is 9–10 g daily, divided into three or four doses. If a higher dose is tolerated dosage increases should be attempted every 3 to 7 days. The maximum daily dose is approximately 16 g. Pediatric dosing of mitotane is accomplished by using 0.1–0.5 mg/kg/d in divided doses. Mitotane should be continued as long as clinical benefits occur. Cortisol secretion rate, plasma cortisol concentration, urinary free cortisol, and urinary steroid production should be monitored to assess mitotane response.

***Ectopic ACTH Syndrome*** In the treatment of ectopic ACTH syndrome, surgical removal of the responsible tumor is the treatment of choice. As multiple sources of tumors exist, location of the ectopic site is essential. Approximately 10% of patients are cured after surgery; the remaining 90% receive postoperative medication.

In the pharmacologically managed patient, metyrapone (Metopirone, Ciba) was shown to be effective and remains the agent of choice.[14] In the ectopic ACTH syndrome patient, metyrapone inhibits 11$\beta$-hydroxylase activity, resulting in inhibition of cortisol synthesis. Initially, patients may demonstrate an increase in plasma ACTH concentrations because of a sudden drop in cortisol. Metyrapone is biologically active after oral administration. Nausea, vomiting, vertigo, headache, dizziness, abdominal discomfort, and allergic rash have been reported after administration.[15]

Two days before the test, patients must be medication free. Adults are given 750 mg orally every 4 hours for six doses. Urine samples are obtained for 17-hydroxyketosteroids, and plasma ACTH concentrations are measured. In the patient with adrenal hypercortisolism, the steroid production in the urine will be depressed after metyrapone administration. Patients with ectopic-producing ACTH syndrome maintain elevated concentrations of cortisol in the urine even after inhibition within the adrenal gland.

A second agent used in the treatment of ectopic ACTH syndrome is aminoglutethimide.[16,17] Initially, aminoglutethimide (Cytadren, Ciba) was used to treat refractory forms of epilepsy, but it was later discovered to be a potent inhibitor of cortisol synthesis. Aminoglutethimide inhibits the conversion of cholesterol to pregnenolone early in the cortisol pathway. Plasma cortisol concentrations are reduced by up to 50% after aminoglutethimide therapy. Side effects include severe sedation, nausea, ataxia, and skin rashes. Most of the reactions are dose dependent, and they limit its use in most patients. Alone, aminoglutethimide is indicated for short-term use in inoperable Cushing's disease with ectopic ACTH syndrome as the suspected underlying etiology. Aminoglutethimide is available as 250-mg tablets.

Aminoglutethimide may be used in combination with metyrapone. Smaller doses of both drugs can be used, therefore minimizing the toxicity associated with either agent. The combination therapy appears effective for various etiologies of Cushing's disease and is useful in the inoperable patient.

A third alternative agent in the treatment of Cushing's disease caused by a disturbance in the hypothalamic–pituitary axis is trilostane.[18] Trilostane (Modrastane, Winthrop) is a synthetic steroid that blocks the adrenal cortical enzymes responsible for cortisol synthesis. The most common adverse reactions include diarrhea, stomach upset, bloating, belching, mucosal burning, and headache. Initial therapy should be started at 30 mg four times a day, with dosage titration every 3 to 4 days with urinary steroid and electrolyte measurements. Dosages above 480 mg/d are not recommended. Trilostane is available as 30- and 60-mg capsules.

Mitotane has been tried in the past in patients with ectopic ACTH syndrome; however, its side effect profile generally limits its use.

Spironolactone has been used for its competitive antagonism of aldosterone in the treatment of Cushing's disease. Spironolactone can provide symptomatic relief of the hypertension and hypokalemia often seen in Cushing's disease.

### *Pituitary-Dependent Cushing's Syndrome*

The etiology of Cushing's disease of pituitary origin is unknown. Autopsy reports of pituitary-dependent Cushing's patients reveal that 50% to 80% have some form of pituitary tumor, usually basophilic adenoma.[19] Other studies using radiologic exams reported the incidence of tumors to be 10% to 30%.[20] Another proposed etiology is an abnormal hypothalamic control of ACTH secretion. Because the pituitary-dependent Cushing's patient exhibits abnormal levels of cortisol, prolactin, and growth hormone, some investigators feel that excess ACTH is the primary etiology.[19] Currently, the optimal form of therapy utilizes the hypothalamus, pituitary, and adrenal glands as avenues for intervention.

Bilateral surgery had been the mainstay of therapy for years[21]; however, 10% of patients developed Nelson's syndrome. Nelson's syndrome, which involves sella turcica enlargement and hyperpigmentation, is caused by postoperative hypothalamic stimulation. Therefore, adrenalectomy should be accompanied by some form of hypothalamic inhibition.

A relatively new approach involves transsphenoidal resection of the pituitary microadenoma.[4,12] The advantages of this procedure include preservation of pituitary function, low complication rate, and high clinical improvement rate.

Irradiation (4,000–5,000 rads) of the pituitary has provided clinical improvement in approximately 70% of patients.[19] Improvement is usually not seen until 6 months after therapy and can create pituitary-dependent hormone deficiencies. Most clinicians reserve pituitary irradiation for the patient with a mild case of Cushing's disease or as an adjunct to another therapy.

Other forms of therapy used in the past include monoamine neurotransmitters, acetylcholine, and the serotonin blocker cyproheptadine. Cyproheptadine (Periactin, Merck Sharp & Dohme) can decrease ACTH secretion, especially in the Cushing's patient who presents in a state of hypersecretion. The initial dose should be 4 mg, given twice daily. Morning plasma cortisol concentrations, as well as 24-hour urinary cortisol (free) concentrations, should be monitored. Side effects are minor and include sedation and hyperphagia.

The focal point in the management of Cushing's disease is proper diagnosis of the underlying etiology. Figure 55.4 provides an algorithm for the proper diagnosis of the disease and accurate identification of the correct etiology.

**Figure 55.4** Algorithm for diagnosing Cushing's disease.

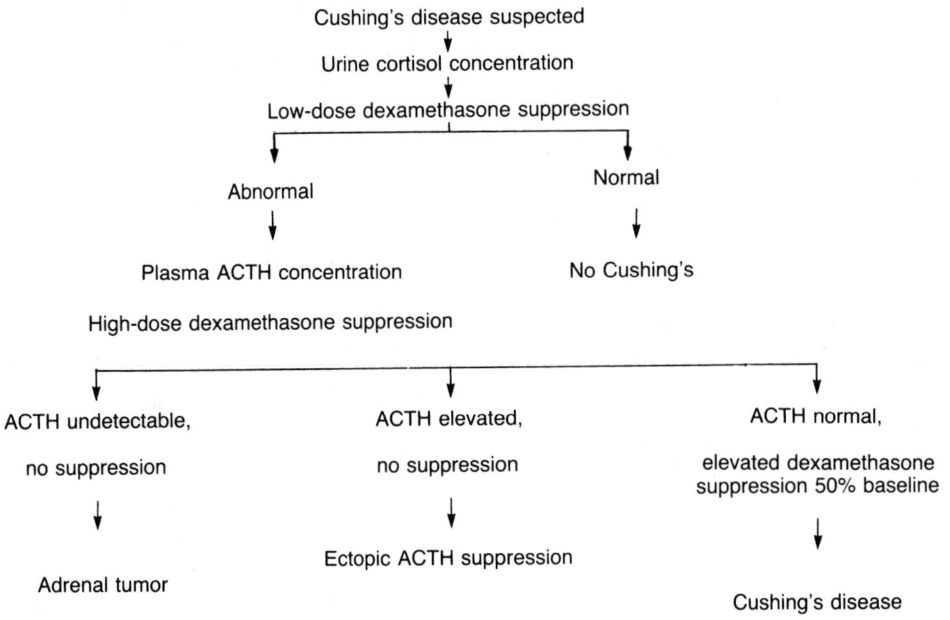

**Table 55.8** Syndromes of Mineralocorticoid Excess

A. Primary aldosteronism
   1. Aldosterone-producing adenoma (APA)
   2. Bilateral adrenal hyperplasia (BAH)—idiopathic
   3. Adrenal carcinoma
   4. Glucocorticoid-remediable hyperaldosteronism
B. Secondary aldosteronism
   1. Nonhypertensive
      a. Sodium depletion
      b. Hemorrhage
      c. Pregnancy
      d. Edema
      e. Bartter's syndrome
      f. Diuretic therapy
   2. Hypertensive
      a. Accelerated and renal vascular hypertension
      b. Renin-secreting tumors
      c. Necrotizing vasculitis
      d. Estrogen therapy

### *Hyperaldosteronism: Primary Aldosteronism*

Excess aldosterone is categorized as either primary or secondary aldosteronism (Table 55.8).[22–24]

#### Etiology

Primary aldosteronism implies that the physiologic abnormality is within the adrenal cortex. Etiologies include a solitary adrenal adenoma, multiple adenomas, hyperplastic tissue, or adrenal cortex carcinoma.[22] Of the possible etiologies responsible for primary aldosteronism, 75% to 85% are adrenal adenomas, 14% to 24% bilateral hyperplasia, and the remaining 1% carcinoma.

#### Clinical Presentation

The incidence of primary aldosteronism is relatively uncommon, occurring in approximately 1% of all hypertensive patients. The disease is more common in women aged 20 to 50 years. Signs and symptoms include arterial hypertension, muscle weakness, fatigue, nocturnal polyuria, polydipsia, reduced glucose tolerance, metabolic alkalosis, and headache.[22] Hypokalemia, suppressed renin activity, elevated plasma aldosterone concentrations, hypernatremia, hypomagnesemia, and a suppressed bicarbonate concentration are all characteristic of laboratory findings in primary aldosteronism.[23]

The absolute diagnosis is relatively easy to make based on clinical findings and pertinent laboratory findings[25–28]; however, as in Cushing's disease, the discovery of the underlying etiology is mandatory to assure proper treatment. Table 55.9 lists the various abnormalities that must be ruled out when suspicion of hyperaldosteronism is high.

A serum potassium concentration below 3.5 mEq/L with a concurrent urinary potassium content greater than 30 mEq/24 h is indicative of primary aldosteronism.

Differentiation between aldosterone-producing adenoma (APA) and bilateral adrenal hyperplasia (BAH) is imperative in formulation of a proper treatment plan. On a clinical and biochemical basis there exists little evidence to distinguish APA from BAH.[23] A majority of the adenomas are singular and small, less than 1 cm. The left adrenal gland is affected at a higher rate than the right. The tumors are usually avascular and under partial physiologic control. The APA patient responds well to ACTH, implying tumor regulation, but response is poor to angiotensin.[10] Circadian rhythm is maintained, with the rhythm becoming blocked after dexamethasone suppression.

The underlying abnormality in BAH remains a mystery, but some investigators feel a hormone factor stimulates the zona glomerulosa, resulting in increased sensitivity to angiotensin II.[29] In contrast to APA patients, patients with BAH are able to maintain control of the renin–angiotensin system with little effect from ACTH loading.

To distinguish APA from BAH, numerous methods have been tried, but the most satisfactory method appears to be adrenal localization. The two methods used to localize the adrenal are adrenal vein catheterization and adrenal imaging.[22] As adrenal vein catheterization is invasive and has a significant morbidity, clinicians are using this procedure less often. Adrenal imaging involves the cholesterol derivative, $^{131}$I-19-iodocholesterol.[22,24] Iodocholesterol is taken up by the adrenal gland similar to cholesterol. After uptake, the adrenals can be visualized for "hot" areas of

**Table 55.9** Differential Diagnosis of Primary Aldosteronism

| *Disease* | *Plasma renin concentration* | *Plasma aldosterone concentration* | *Blood pressure* | *Serum potassium concentration* |
|---|---|---|---|---|
| Primary aldosteronism | Low | High | High | Low |
| Edematous disorders | High | High | Normal | Low |
| Malignant hypertension | High | High | High | Low |
| Congenital adrenal hyperplasia | Low | Low | High | Low |
| Cushing's syndrome | Low to normal | Low to normal | High | Low |
| Liddle's syndrome | Low | Low | High | Low |
| Bartter's syndrome | High | High | Low to normal | Low |
| Licorice ingestion | Low | Low | High | Low |
| Low-renin essential hypertension | Low | Low to normal | High | Normal |

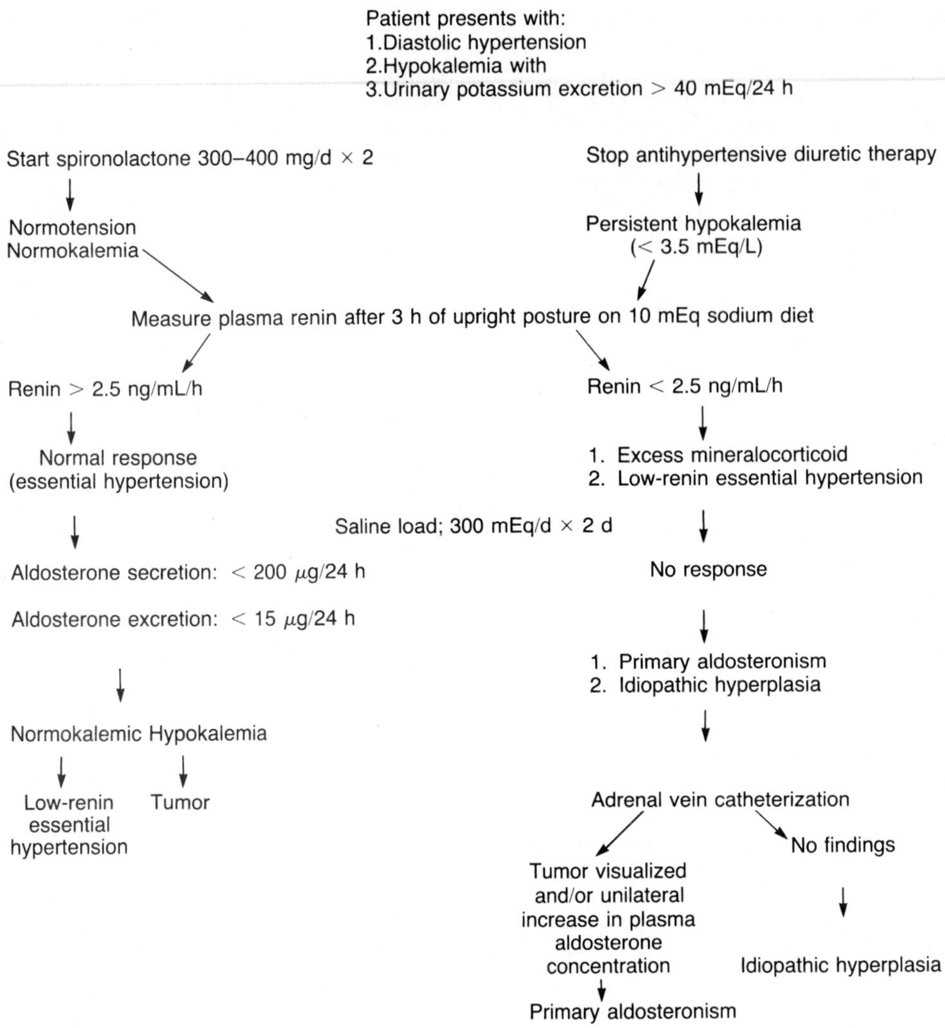


**Figure 55.5** Flow chart for the diagnosis of primary aldosteronism.

increased or sustained uptake. Patients with APA normally have unilateral visualization compared with the bilateral visualization seen with patients who have BAH.[29]

Why is the differentiation between APA and BAH so important if both are producing excess aldosterone? The answer is treatment.[30] Surgical removal of the adenoma is generally the treatment of choice. In patients with BAH, pharmacologic intervention is useful in controlling or limiting the symptoms.

### Treatment

***BAH-Dependent Hyperaldosteronism*** Spironolactone, a competitive inhibitor of aldosterone, is the drug of choice in BAH-dependent hyperaldosteronism.[30] Spironolactone (Aldactone, Searle) has the capability of inhibiting aldosterone biosynthesis within the adrenal gland, making it extremely useful in overstimulated BAH patients.[22] Spironolactone is orally available, with most patients responding to doses in the range 200–400 mg per day. The clinician should wait between 4 and 6 weeks before reassessing the patient for urinary electrolytes and blood pressure control.

***APA-Dependent Hyperaldosteronism*** The treatment of choice for APA-dependent aldosteronism remains surgical removal of the adenoma. If no primary lesion is found, resection of one and one half of the adrenal glands can be attempted with supplemental spironolactone therapy.

In summary, the diagnosis of primary aldosteronism is made through the observation of elevated blood pressure, low serum potassium, high urinary potassium, and elevated serum aldosterone (Fig. 55.5). Differentiating between the various etiologies can be difficult, but patients who present with adrenal adenomas can be distinguished from patients with hyperplasia using one method of adrenal localization. Treatment depends on the etiology, with surgical resection well accepted as the treatment of choice in adenomas, and spironolactone in patients with hyperplasia.

## *Hyperaldosteronism: Secondary Aldosteronism*

Secondary aldosteronism results from stimulation of the zona glomerulosa by an extraadrenal factor, usually the renin–angiotensin system. Excessive potassium intake can create a physiologic increase in aldosterone, as can oral contraceptive use, pregnancy (10 times normal by third trimester), and menses. Congestive heart failure, cirrhosis, renal artery stenosis, and Bartter's syndrome can also lead to elevated aldosterone concentrations.

Treatment of secondary aldosteronism is dictated by the etiology. Removal of the extraadrenal source of the excess aldosterone should resolve the disorder. Medical therapy with spironolactone is the mainstay of treatment until an exact etiology can be diagnosed.

### *Miscellaneous Hyperadrenal Disorders*

#### Adrenal Virilism

Virilism, excessive secretion of androgens from the adrenal gland,[31] is more commonly seen in females, with hirsutism being the dominant feature.[31] Women who present with hirsutism may also have voice deepening, increased muscle mass, menstrual abnormalities, or clitoral enlargement.[32] While virilism may be easy to diagnose based on clinical symptoms, diagnosis on a biochemical basis is difficult. The most common etiology of virilism involves one of many possible congenital enzyme defects. Depending on the enzyme deficiency, accumulation of a variety of androgens, notably testosterone, can develop.

Treatment of virilism centers around suppression of the pituitary–adrenal axis with exogenous glucocorticoids. Choice of steroids is variable, with the focus of treatment being the establishment of an alternate-day therapy.

#### Hirsutism

Hirsutism (hypertrichosis) is defined as more hair than is cosmetically acceptable. The majority of cases occur in women with no underlying endocrine abnormality. Some cases of hypertrichosis are related to a wide variation in hairiness as well as hereditary factors. In general, people who are dark-haired, pigmented whites of either sex from the Mediterranean and southern Europe stock are more prone to genetic hypertrichosis. If virilism and/or defeminization are concurrently present, the chances of the hirsutism arising from an endocrine abnormality increase.[33]

Endocrinopathies without masculinization can predispose to hirsutism in patients with documented pituitary tumors, Cushing's disease, or excessive use of steroids/androgens.[33] Hirsutisms related to certain drugs, namely phenytoin and diazoxide, have been documented. In the patient with hirsutism, congenital adrenal hyperplasia, adrenal tumors, and ovarian tumors must be ruled out.[33]

Idiopathic hirsutism accounts for approximately 50% of cases. Evaluation of patients with hirsutism should include historical data, severity, areas of the body involved, and cosmetic measures that have been tried in the past. Menstrual status, fertility, and drug use (oral contraceptives, hormones) must be evaluated in the initial workup.

In patients whose etiology suggests ovarian or adrenal tumor, a laboratory examination should consist of urinary 17-ketosteroids. To exclude ovarian tumor, blood testosterone and androstenedione concentrations should be measured. To exclude Cushing's disease, a routine Cushing's workup should be performed (see Cushing's Disease).

Cosmetic measures should be attempted as first-line therapy in hirsutism. Electrolysis is helpful for small, isolated facial hairs and modest mustache and beard formations. Depilatory creams and bleaching can be used by some patients for larger areas of the body. Only when cosmetic surgery is ineffective should suppressive therapy be used. Glucocorticoids, such as dexamethasone, can be used, but may induce cushingoid symptoms even in doses of 0.5 mg per day. Oral contraceptives can be used in patients who require contraception concurrently. If oral contraceptives are used, a progestin with low androgen activity (norethynodrel or ethynodiol diacetate) should be employed.

## Hypofunction of the Adrenal Gland

Primary adrenal insufficiency, or Addison's disease, involves the destruction of all regions of the adrenal cortex.[34] Deficiencies arise in cortisol, aldosterone, and the various androgens. Secondary insufficiency usually results from a hypothalamic–pituitary deficiency of ACTH, producing low concentrations of androgen and cortisol. Secondary disease classically presents with normal concentrations of mineralocorticoids.

Approximately 90% of the adrenal cortex must be destroyed before adrenal insufficiency symptoms demonstrate themselves clinically.[34] Specific etiologies for both primary and secondary insufficiency are listed in Table 55.10. The most common reason for secondary insufficiency is the overuse of exogenous glucocorticoids. Symptoms common to both subsets of insufficiency include weakness (100%), weight loss (100%), increased pigmentation (95%), hypotension (90%), and vitiligo (20%).

### *Addison's Disease*

Distinguishing Addison's disease from secondary insufficiency is difficult; however, the following guidelines may be helpful:

1. Hyperpigmentation is usually not seen in secondary adrenal insufficiency because of low amounts of melanocyte-stimulating hormone (MSH).
2. Aldosterone secretion is usually preserved in secondary insufficiency.
3. Weight loss, dehydration, and electrolyte abnormalities are generally not as common and less severe in secondary insufficiency.

**Table 55.10** Etiologies of Primary and Secondary Adrenal Insufficiency

| *Primary insufficiency* | *Secondary insufficiency* |
|---|---|
| Tuberculosis | Tumors of the third ventricle |
| Amyloidosis | Craniopharyngioma |
| Hemochromatosis | Hypopituitarism |
| Adrenal vein thrombosis | Corticosteroid administration |
| Bilateral adrenalectomy | |
| Autoimmune adrenalitis | |

**Table 55.11** Relative Potencies of Glucocorticoids

| *Glucocorticoid* | *Anti-inflammatory potency* | *Equivalent potency (mg)* | *Sodium-retaining potency* |
|---|---|---|---|
| Hydrocortisone | 1.0 | 20.0 | 2.0 |
| Prednisolone | 4.0 | 5.0 | 1.0 |
| Prednisone | 3.5 | 5.0 | 1.0 |
| Cortisone | 0.8 | 25.0 | 2.0 |
| Triamcinolone | 5.0 | 4.0 | 0.0 |
| Methylprednisolone | 5.0 | 4.0 | 0.0 |
| Betamethasone | 25.0 | 0.60 | 0.0 |
| Dexamethasone | 30.0 | 0.75 | 0.0 |

Treatment of Addison's disease must include adequate patient education, so that the patient is aware of treatment complications, expected outcome, missed doses, and drug side effects. The agents of choice are prednisone, hydrocortisone, and cortisone, with the treatment objective being the establishment of the lowest effective dose while still mimicking the normal diurnal adrenal rhythm[34] (Table 55.11). Usually, a twice-daily dosing schedule is adequate, with the dose used dependent on the steroid chosen. A morning dose of cortisol (25 mg), hydrocortisone (20 mg), or prednisone (5 mg) followed by an evening dose of the same agent at 50% of the morning dose is usually sufficient. To replace the mineralocorticoid loss, 9$\alpha$-fluohydrocortisone can be used. A dose of 0.1–0.2 mg by mouth once a day is adequate. If parenteral therapy is needed, 2–5 mg of deoxycorticosterone trimethylacetate in oil intramuscularly every 3 to 4 weeks can be used.

Adverse effects must be monitored closely. Symptoms include gastric upset, edema, hypertension, hypokalemia, insomnia, excitability, and diabetes mellitus. In addition, weight, blood pressure, and electrocardiogram should be monitored regularly.

The endpoint of therapy is difficult to assess in most patients, but a reduction in the excess pigmentation is a good clinical marker. The treatment of secondary adrenal insufficiency is identical to treatment of primary disease, except that mineralocorticoid replacement is usually not necessary. Patient education should still be stressed, with emphasis placed on establishing an alternate-day regimen.

### Advantages of Alternate-Day Therapy Regimen

The dilemma of prolonged steroid administration is sometimes lessened by the use of an alternate-day therapy (ADT) regimen.[35] ADT minimizes the hypothalamic–pituitary suppression as well as some of the adverse effects seen with once-daily therapy. This can be especially important in the treatment of the child and young adult, in whom growth suppression is a major concern. ADT is not recommended for initial management, but rather in the management of the stabilized patient who needs long-term therapy.[21] The transfer of a patient from a once-daily steroid to an alternate-day steroid is a gradual process. The patient is exposed to "on" and "off" days; the "on"-day dose is gradually increased as the "off"-day dose is reduced, over a period of 14 days. By the 14th day, the patient is consuming medication only on the "on" day.

### Acute Adrenal Insufficiency

Adrenal crisis, or Addisonian crisis, is characterized by an acute adrenocortical insufficiency. In cases of adrenal crisis, the body's need for corticosteroids exceeds the currently available supply. Adrenal crisis represents a true endocrine emergency. Events that can precipitate an adrenal crisis include anything that increases the requirements dramatically. Stressful situations, surgery, infection, and trauma are all potential triggering events, especially in the patient with some underlying adrenal or pituitary insufficiency. The most common cause of adrenal crisis is adrenal insufficiency brought on by chronic use of glucocorticoids.

Early symptoms of acute adrenal insufficiency include myalgias, malaise, anorexia, weakness, and weight loss. As the situation continues, vomiting, fever, hypotension, and shock develop. Hyponatremia, hypoglycemia, and hypercalcemia may also be present.

Treatment of adrenal crisis involves the administration of parenteral glucocorticoids. Hydrocortisone (Solu-cortef, Upjohn) is the agent of choice because of its mineralocorticoid activity as well as its glucocorticoid effects. Hydrocortisone is started at 100 mg intravenously through rapid infusion and is followed by a continuous infusion of 100 mg over an 8-hour interval. Intravenous administration is continued for 48 hours, at which time oral hydrocortisone may be started at a dose of 50 mg every 8 hours for another 48 hours. After oral maintenance therapy, a hydrocortisone taper is initiated until the dosage is 30–50 mg per day in divided doses. Fluid replacement is often required and may be accomplished with 5% dextrose and isotonic (normal) saline ($D_5NS$) at a rate of ½–1 L/h for several hours. Electrolytes should be monitored and repeated as needed. If hyperkalemia is present after the hydrocortisone maintenance phase, additional mineralocorticoid is usually required. Fludrocortisone acetate (Florinef, Squibb) in a dose of 0.1 mg by mouth daily is the agent of choice. Adrenal hemorrhage can result from multiple etiologies, but septicemia is the most common.[35] Symptoms include shaking chills, headache, vertigo, vomiting, rash, and death in 6–48 hours if not treated. Treatment includes steroids, norepinephrine, and intravenous antibiotics. *Pneumococcus*, *Staphylococcus*, and *Hemophilus influenzae* are the most common organisms found on autopsy. The use of steroids should be as in adrenal crisis. Norepinephrine is used to improve vascular tone, as circulatory collapse can quickly occur.

### Hypoaldosteronism

Hypoaldosteronism is rare and usually associated with low renin status, complete heart block, or severe postural hypotension, or it may occur postoperatively after tumor removal.[2]

Laboratory analysis reveals low serum sodium and high serum potassium concentrations. As the deficiency lies in the mineralocorticoid, replacement with 9α-fluohydrocortisone in a dose of 0.1–0.3 mg is usually effective. Patients should be followed for blood pressure response as well as electrolyte status.

### Limited ACTH Reserve

Limited ACTH reserve is a disease process caused by some form of pituitary dysfunction. In patients with hypopituitarism, there is enough ACTH to maintain adrenal response but inadequate amounts to respond to stress or stimulus. A variety of endocrine disorders can include a limited pituitary reserve.

## Congenital Adrenal Hyperplasia

Because many enzyme systems are needed to complete the complex cholesterol-to-cortisol pathway, enzyme deficiencies may lead to disruptions of the normal cascade of events (Fig. 55.2). This group of enzyme disorders is known as congenital adrenal hyperplasia, mainly because of the resultant chronic adrenal gland stimulation that occurs after the enzyme deficiency.[36] Any enzyme deficiency is capable of affecting any one or all three of the steroid pathways.[37] Therefore, treatment should be focused on replacement of the deficient hormone as well as turning off of the chronic stimulation causing the hyperplasia. Six of the most common enzyme deficiencies are briefly discussed.

### 20-Hydroxylase (Cholesterol Desmolase) Deficiency

A deficiency of 20-hydroxylase leads to an enlarged adrenal gland that is almost always full of cholesterol. Infants with this disorder generally present with female genitalia and have a poor prognosis. Blood and urine concentrations of all steroids are low, with elevated ACTH concentrations.

### 3β-Hydroxysteroid Dehydrogenase Deficiency

Patients with this disorder present with both cortisol and aldosterone deficiencies. Increased concentrations of pregnenolone and cholesterol are commonly seen.

### 17α-Hydroxylase Deficiency

After progesterone synthesis, one major pathway for the production of cortisol and estradiol is dependent on 17α-hydroxylase. As the aldosterone pathway is not affected, replacement of the mineralocorticoid is not necessary. Patients with this disorder are generally hypertensive, with low concentrations of cortisol and estrogens.

### 21-Hydroxylase Deficiency

This most common form of congenital adrenal hyperplasia results in excessive concentrations of progesterone and 17α-hydroxyprogesterone and low concentrations of cortisol and aldosterone. Patients who exhibit this disorder may not be diagnosed until later in life, when the salt-wasting becomes clinically evident. In milder forms of this disorder, children may go undiagnosed for 2 to 10 years when acne, early appearance of pubic hair, voice lowering, or increased muscularity becomes bothersome. Once replacement therapy begins, most children mature normally.

### 11β-Hydroxylase Deficiency

This enzyme marks the final step in the biosynthesis of cortisol and corticosterone. The enzyme is found only in the adrenal cortex. Patients with this disorder exhibit low plasma cortisol and aldosterone concentrations. In addition, high ACTH and melanocyte-stimulating hormone concentrations are present. Patients classically present with hypertension in secondary aldosterone excess, and virilism from androgen excess. Often this disorder is mistaken for Cushing's disease, but no glucose intolerance, often seen with Cushing's disease, occurs.

### 18-Hydroxysteroid Dehydrogenase Deficiency

This enzyme disorder is restricted to the zona glomerulosa and results in a sole defect in aldosterone synthesis. The deficiency results in sodium depletion, potassium retention, hypotension, and increased plasma renin activity. Therapy should be identical to that for Addison's disease, with mineralocorticoid replacement but no glucocorticoid replacement.

## Long-Term Therapy With Glucocorticoids

While the use of glucocorticoids is essential in some patients, the chronic administration of steroids can cause problems in and of itself. Hypothalamic–pituitary–adrenal (HPA) suppression occurs in all patients exposed to chronic glucocorticoids. Symptoms of HPA suppression mimic those seen in the Addisonian patient, with the exception of hyperpigmentation. Classically, these patients exhibit low blood cortisol and ACTH concentrations, low baseline steroid excretion, and abnormal ACTH and metyrapone tests. Upon discontinuation of glucocorticoid administration, most patients recover normal HPA axis function; however, full recovery may not be seen for months. As suppression of the HPA axis can occur at any dose and at any time, prudent use of long-term steroids, with adequate follow-up, is advisable in all patients.

## References

1. Conn JW. Primary aldosteronism, a new clinical syndrome. J Lab Clin Med 1955;45:6–17.
2. Liddle GW. The adrenals, in Williams RH (ed): Textbook of Endocrinology. Philadelphia, W.B. Saunders, 1981, pp 249–290.

3. Albright F. Cushing syndrome. Harvey Lect 1942–43;38:123–186.
4. Scott HW, Foster JH, et al. Cushing's syndrome due to adrenocortical tumor. Ann Surg 1965;162:505–516.
5. Hutter AM, Kayhoe DE. Adrenal cortical carcinoma. Am J Med 1966;41:581–592.
6. Vagnucci AH, Evans E. Cushing's disease with intermittent hypertension. Am J Med 1986;80:83–88.
7. Gold EM. The Cushing syndromes: Changing views of diagnosis and treatment. Ann Intern Med 1979;90:829–844.
8. Anon DC, Tyrrell JB, Fitzgerald PA, et al. Cushing's syndrome: Problems in diagnosis. Medicine 1981;60:25–35.
9. Weiss ER, Rayyis SS, Nelson DH, et al. Evaluation of stimulation and suppression tests in the etiological diagnosis of Cushing's syndrome. Ann Intern Med 1969;71:941–949.
10. May ME, Carey RM. Rapid adrenocorticotropic hormone test in practice: Retrospective review. Am J Med 1985;79:679–684.
11. Tyrrell JB, Findling JW, Arno DC, et al. An overnight high-dose dexamethasone suppression test for rapid differential diagnosis of Cushing's syndrome. Ann Intern Med 1986;104:180–186.
12. Orth DN, Liddle GW. Results of treatment in 108 patients with Cushing's syndrome. N Engl J Med 1971;285:243–247.
13. Temple TE, Jones DJ, et al. Use of o,p'DDD to correct hypercortisolism without inducing aldosterone deficiency in the treatment of Cushing's disease. N Engl J Med 1969;281:801–805.
14. Dickstein G, Lahar M, Shen-Orr, et al. Primary therapy for Cushing's disease with metyrapone. JAMA 1986;255:1167–1169.
15. Spiger M, Jubiz W, Meikle AW, et al. Single-dose metyrapone test: Review of a four-year experience. Arch Intern Med 1975; 135:698–700.
16. Anonymous. Aminoglutethimide. Med Lett Drugs Ther 1981; 23:71–72.
17. Anonymous. Aminoglutethimide. Med Lett Drugs Ther 1985; 27:87–88.
18. Anonymous. Trilostane. Med Lett Drugs Ther 1985;27:87–88.
19. Bondy PK. Disorders of the adrenal gland, in Wilson JD, Foster DW (eds): Williams Textbook of Endocrinology, Philadelphia, W.B. Saunders Company, 1985, p 816.
20. Burns TW. Endocrinology, in Sodeman WA, Sodeman TM (eds): Pathologic Physiology: Mechanisms of Disease. Philadelphia, W.B. Saunders, 1979, pp 1023–1031.
21. Federman DD. The adrenal, in Ribensten E, Federman DD (eds): Medicine. New York, Scientific American, 1986, pp 3(IV) 1–3(IV)14.
22. Weinberger MM, Grim CE, Mollified JW, et al. Primary aldosteronism: Diagnosis, localization, and treatment. Ann Intern Med 1979;90:386–395.
23. Ferriss H, Beevers G, Brown J. Clinical, biochemical and pathological features of low-renin ("primary") hyperaldosteronism. Am Heart J 1978;95:375–388.
24. Ganguly A, Donohue JP. Primary aldosteronism: Pathophysiology, diagnosis and treatment. J Urol 1983;129:241–247.
25. Lyons DF, Kern DC, Brown RD, et al. Single dose captopril as a diagnostic test for primary aldosteronism. J Clin Endocrinol Metab 1983;57:892–896.
26. Stokes GS, Monaghan JC, Menme BA. Use of an intravenous sodium load in screening for primary hyperaldosteronism. Aust NZ J Med 1984;14:201–207.
27. Arteaga E, Klein R, Biglieri EG. Use of the saline infusion test to diagnose the cause of primary aldosteronism. Am J Med 1985;79:722–728.
28. Gordon RD. The diagnosis of primary hyperaldosteronism. Aust NZ J Med 1984;14:195–196.
29. Banks WA, Kastin AJ, Biglieri EG, et al. Primary adrenal hyperplasia: A new subset of primary hyperaldosteronism. J Clin Endocrinol Metab 1984;58:783–785.
30. Siragy H, Carey RM. Management of primary aldosteronism. Drug Ther 1986;16:89–103.
31. Kenney FM, Hashida Y, Askari AH, et al. Virilizing tumors of the adrenal cortex. Am J Dis Child 1968;115:445–458.
32. Thorn GW. The adrenal cortex. Johns Hopkins Med J 1968;123: 49–77.
33. Kuttenn F, Couillin P, Girard F, et al. Late-onset adrenal hyperplasia in hirsutism. N Engl J Med 1985;313:224–231.
34. Nerup J. Addison's disease—clinical studies. A report of 108 cases. Acta Endocrinol 1974;76:127–141.
35. Claman HN. Glucocorticoids II: The clinical responses. Hosp Pract 1983;18:143–151.
36. Bongiovanni AM, Root AW. The adrenogenital syndrome. N Engl J Med 1963;268:1283–1289, 1342–1351, 1391–1399.
37. Finkelstein M, Shaefer JM. Inborn errors of steroid biosynthesis. Physiol Rev 1979;59:353–406.

# Chapter 56 / Cystic Fibrosis

John A. Bosso, PharmD

Cystic fibrosis is the most common lethal, genetically inherited disease affecting the white population. It is a disease involving mainly the exocrine glands and thus affects a number of organs or organ systems (Table 56.1). The more common manifestations of the disease involve the gastrointestinal and pulmonary systems, with most of the observed morbidity and mortality associated with the latter. Gastrointestinal manifestations include maldigestion and malabsorption secondary to pancreatic enzyme deficiency. Pulmonary pathology is due to production of viscous secretions and comprises chronic obstructive pulmonary disease and pneumonia. Although considered a pediatric disease since it was first described by Anderson in 1938,[1] early diagnosis and more effective therapy now enable many patients to survive into adulthood. Care of these patients should be multidisciplinary and involve a wide variety of therapeutic interventions. This chapter concentrates on the pathophysiology and pharmacotherapeutics of cystic fibrosis.

## Epidemiology

Cystic fibrosis is inherited through an autosomal (Mendelian) recessive genetic mode. This implies that each parent must be at least a carrier (heterozygous) for the trait and with such a couple, each child would have a one-in-four chance of having the disease, a one-in-two chance of being a carrier, and a one-in-four chance of being normal (having neither the disease nor the trait). The incidence of cystic fibrosis is greatest in the white population, with a rate of 1 in 2,000 live births in the United States.[2] The incidence of the trait (carrier state) in this group is about 5%. The frequency of the disease is considerably less in other races, occurring in 1 in 17,000 blacks and about 1 in 90,000 Orientals.[3] Why the incidence of this disease, with its high morbidity and altered fertility, is not decreasing is unknown. It has been speculated that the high cystic fibrosis gene frequency may result from such factors as heterozygote advantage, multiple loci, or genetic drift.[4]

## Pathophysiology

### *Gastrointestinal Tract*

Involvement of the gastrointestinal tract in cystic fibrosis is due to both the increased viscosity of mucous secretions and a relative deficiency of pancreatic digestive enzymes. In 7% to 10% of cystic fibrosis patients, the first gastrointestinal manifestation of the disease is an intestinal obstruction that occurs shortly after birth and is known as meconium ileus. This complication is caused by an inability to evacuate the abnormally viscid meconium in these patients. A similar condition, known as meconium ileus equivalent or distal intestinal obstruction syndrome, occurs in older cystic fibrosis patients; it is also thought to result from abnormally viscous gastrointestinal secretions and fecal impaction. This condition can be confused with constipation secondary to failure to take sufficient pancreatic enzymes with ingested food.

A deficiency of pancreatic digestive enzymes, also known as pancreatic achylia, is present in 85% of cystic fibrosis patients. Pancreatic lesions include fibrosis, fatty replacement, and cyst formation and are thought to be secondary to obstruction of small pancreatic ducts by secretions and cellular debris.[5] These secretions are predominantly acid mucopolysaccharide in nature. Inspissated eosinophilic material is also present in acini and ductules. As a result, pancreatic secretions (as reflected by duodenal aspirates) are viscous and low in volume and in concentrations of pancreatic enzymes and bicarbonate. Affected enzyme levels include trypsin, chymotrypsin, carboxypeptidase, amylase, and lipase. The degree of deficiency of any of these enzymes varies from one patient to the next. This leads to a maldigestion of ingested nutrients including fats and protein.

Because of the lipase deficiency, fat-soluble vitamin (A, D, E, and K) deficiencies sometimes occur. Whether lipase is involved in fat-soluble vitamin absorption directly (e.g., micelle formation) or indirectly, with continuing steatorrhea resulting in abnormally high losses of these nutrients in the feces, is unclear. While pancreatic involvement is predominantly exocrine in nature, insulin deficiency has been described in many older cystic fibrosis patients. This complication involves an increase in the number of insulin receptors on peripheral blood monocytes with decreased affinity for insulin.[6] Despite a concomitantly increased tissue affinity for insulin, 8% of cystic fibrosis children over 12 years of age require insulin therapy.[7]

The liver is sometimes involved in cystic fibrosis. While biliary cirrhosis secondary to bile duct obstruction occurs, fatty infiltration may be more common, occurring in about 30% of patients in a pattern unrelated to nutritional status. Bile duct obstruction occurs with inspissated eosinophilic material and may be focal or multilobular.[8] Such hepatic involvement is rarely clinically evident, but can lead to portal hypertension and thus bleeding esophageal varices and hypersplenism.[9] Hepatic changes may be present at any age.

**Table 56.1** Organ Involvement in Cystic Fibrosis

| *Organ system/organ* | *Abnormality* | *Consequence* |
|---|---|---|
| Gastrointestinal tract | | |
| Pancreas | Digestive enzyme deficiency | Maldigestion |
| | | Malnutrition |
| | Insulin deficiency | Glucose intolerance |
| Intestines | Viscous secretions | Obstruction |
| Liver | Biliary cirrhosis/fatty infiltration | Portal hypertension/ esophageal varices |
| Pulmonary system | Viscous secretions | Chronic obstructive disease |
| | | Hypoxia |
| | | Cor pulmonale |
| | Infection | Pneumonia/sinusitis |
| Sweat glands | Failure to reabsorb NaCl | Hyponatremia |
| Reproductive system | Obstruction of epididymis, vas deferens, and seminal vesicles | Aspermia (sterility) |
| | Viscous cervical mucus | Decreased fertility |
| Hematologic system | Chronic disease? | Anemia |
| Joints | Unknown | Arthritis |

### *Pulmonary System*

Involvement of the respiratory tract accounts for the vast majority of morbidity and mortality associated with cystic fibrosis. Manifestations within this organ system result from the accumulation of viscous mucus in the small airways. The presence of such abnormal mucus would present a clearance challenge to normal lungs, but cystic fibrosis patients also have a defect in mucociliary clearance.[10] There are two important consequences of this pulmonary condition: obstruction and infection.

Obstruction of both small and large airways by thick mucus results in air trapping, bronchiectasis, and atelectasis, leading to a chronic obstructive pulmonary disease phenomenon not unlike emphysema in presentation (although little alveolar septal destruction occurs). Hyperinflation or dilation of the airspaces is the common lesion.[11] Further, the persistence of this same mucus makes it an excellent growth medium for microorganisms, and pulmonary infections are commonplace despite normal host defense mechanisms.[12]

While bacterial infection is thought to be the major factor in this portion of the respiratory disease, viruses and other nonbacterial pathogens probably play an important role as well.[13] The three most common bacterial pathogens isolated from the respiratory secretions (sputum) of cystic fibrosis patients are *Staphylococcus aureus*, *Pseudomonas aeruginosa*, and *Hemophilus influenzae*. *Proteus* and *Klebsiella* species are observed much less frequently. The mucoid strains of *Pseudomonas aeruginosa* commonly observed in cystic fibrosis may be particularly resistant to antibiotics.[14] Recently, the isolation of *Pseudomonas cepacia* from the sputum of cystic fibrosis patients has become more common.[15] The significance of the presence of this organism is unclear at this time, and whether it is directly responsible for some of the morbidity of end-stage cystic fibrosis or is merely an incidental finding remains to be clarified. The presence of these bacteria is believed to be responsible for some of the destructive changes in the lungs of cystic fibrosis patients; these changes result from direct damage by bacterial toxins and from the body's immune reaction to the presence of the bacteria. For example, it has been shown that *P. aeruginosa* elaborates a number of extracellular toxins that may be responsible for direct or indirect pulmonary damage, increases mucin production in respiratory epithelium, and stimulates the production of immune complexes which may also contribute to local damage.[16] The occasional presence of *Aspergillus fumigatus* in the sputum of these patients may also contribute to the pulmonary pathology.

The major consequence of these pulmonary processes is a decrease in gas exchange by the lungs. The challenge of moving air into and out of such congested airways often requires the use of accessory muscles, resulting in an increased anterior–posterior chest diameter (also referred to as "barrel chest"), a flattened diaphragm, and pulmonary hypertension. Pneumothorax has also been reported.[17] Right ventricular failure (cor pulmonale) can occur secondary to the pulmonary hypertension. While seldom overt clinically, findings such as right ventricular hypertrophy, increased heart weight, and right atrial and right ventricular chamber dilation are usually present at autopsy.[18] It is unclear whether digital clubbing, a common finding in cystic fibrosis as well as other chronic pulmonary conditions, is due to chronic hypoxia.

The upper respiratory tract is also involved; sinusitis and nasal polyposis occur in 90% and 10%–25% of patients, respectively.[19,20] Sinusitis is chronic in character and acute symptoms are unusual. While its etiology is not entirely clear, sinusitis may result from obstruction of the sinus ducts, preventing drainage, and is apparently not related to the underlying lung disease.[21] The bacteria generally isolated in these cases of sinusitis include *P. aeruginosa*, *H. influenzae*, streptococci, and anaerobes. It is not clear whether the presence of these bacteria represents true infection or merely colonization. The need for antimicrobial therapy has not been established.

Nasal polyps result from distension of submucous glands with ductular dilatation secondary to the accumulation of inspissated eosinophilic material. Polyps are often multiple and bilateral and can cause partial or complete nasal obstruction.

### *Sweat Glands*

The abnormally high concentrations of both sodium and chloride in the sweat of cystic fibrosis patients can result in the need for supplementary dietary intake of these electrolytes and form the basis for the diagnosis of the disease. The sodium and chloride are not excreted in abnormally high concentrations by the sweat glands. Instead, there is a failure of the sweat ducts to reabsorb these electrolytes in a normal fashion,[22] apparently because of a chloride impermeability in the sweat ducts.[23] Similar abnormalities are seen in the excretions of the salivary glands.

### *Reproductive System*

Of males with cystic fibrosis, 95% are sterile because of abnormal development or obstruction of the epididymis, vas deferens, and seminal vesicles, with resulting aspermia. Females also have less than normal fertility because of the production of abnormal cervical mucus. There is late maturation of the reproductive system in both sexes.[24] Nonetheless, because of greater life expectancy in these patients, we are seeing increasing numbers of cystic fibrosis mothers. The course of pregnancy in these individuals is related to pregravid nutritional and pulmonary status.[25]

### *Hematologic System*

Anemia is observed in some cystic fibrosis patients despite chronic hypoxia.[26] This anemia is characterized by decreased hematocrit, serum ferritin, and vitamin E and by increased carboxyhemoglobin and is often responsive to treatment with iron and vitamin E.[27]

### *Joints*

Arthritis has been reported in a small number of cystic fibrosis patients. This arthritis may be either mono- or polyarticular and is usually nondestructive. The etiology of arthritis in this population is unknown and the usual causes of the disease in the general pediatric population can normally be ruled out. Theoretical mechanisms of arthritis in cystic fibrosis include hypertrophic pulmonary osteoarthropathy secondary to chronic pulmonary disease and polycythemia with resultant hyperuricemia. This condition usually occurs in patients 15 years of age or older,[28–30] but has been reported in younger children.[31]

## Diagnosis

Cystic fibrosis is normally diagnosed on the basis of an abnormal sweat test. In such a test, a sample of sweat is collected (often with the use of pilocarpine iontophoresis) and the concentration of chloride is determined.[32] A chloride concentration of 60 mEq/L or greater is considered diagnostic; 98% of cystic fibrosis patients have a sweat chloride concentration in this range. The remaining 2% have sweat chloride concentrations between 50 and 60 mEq/L. Nonetheless, the results of a sweat test are not necessarily proof-positive of the presence or absence of cystic fibrosis. The presence of chronic obstructive pulmonary disease, exocrine pancreatic insufficiency, and/or a positive family history of the disease helps to confirm the diagnosis.

## Clinical Presentation

The clinical signs and symptoms of cystic fibrosis occur as direct consequences of the pathophysiologic processes described before. Thus, the clinical findings can be conveniently subdivided by organ system.

### *Gastrointestinal Tract*

Intestinal symptomatology is secondary to obstruction and maldigestion of nutrients. Obstruction manifested as meconium ileus or meconium ileus equivalent causes symptoms such as vomiting of bile-stained material, abdominal distension, and pain. Pain may be an especially prominent feature when obstruction results in intussusception.

The more frequent gastrointestinal clinical presentation is steatorrhea and malnutrition, resulting from maldigestion of ingested food. Stools are characterized by their foul smell, bulky, greasy nature, and abnormally high number per day and may precipitate rectal prolapse. The stool's high fat content results from the relative lipase deficiency. Perhaps the most significant consequence of maldigestion is malnutrition. Cystic fibrosis children characteristically fall below age-related norms for both weight and height.

### *Pulmonary System*

The respiratory symptoms of cystic fibrosis are those of obstructive disease and pneumonia. Hypoxia with resultant cyanosis and digital clubbing are common. Likewise, labored breathing with retractions and resultant increased anterior–posterior chest diameter, flattened diaphragm, and overaeration observed on chest roentgenogram are frequent findings.

Acutely, a patient's respiratory status follows a cyclical pattern, from a state of relative well-being to one of acute pulmonary deterioration theoretically paralleling the course of the infectious process. Marked declines in pulmonary status (secondary to infection) are referred to as acute respiratory exacerbations and are generally associated with symptoms of acute bacterial pneumonia. Thus, fever, increased cough, increased sputum production, change in sputum character (e.g., from yellow to green with increased viscosity), increased respiratory rate, dyspnea on exertion, increased oxygen requirements, and decreased exercise tolerance are commonly described.

Concomitantly, laboratory tests reveal an increased white blood cell count with increased polymorphonuclear leukocytes and immature forms. Tests of pulmonary function often demonstrate decreased forced vital capacity and forced expiratory volume, increased residual volume, hypoxia, and hypercapnia.

### *Other Symptoms*

The relative insulin deficiency observed in older cystic fibrosis patients is often asymptomatic and only detected on laboratory analysis of serum performed for other reasons. Symptomatic patients present as untreated cases of diabetes mellitus type II. Cases of cor pulmonale are not usually clinically evident until signs of left ventricular failure ensue. An enlargement of the heart is often noted on routine chest roentgenogram prior to that time, however. Signs and symptoms of anemia and arthritis with cystic fibrosis patients do not differ from those in other patients.

While the abnormal loss of sodium and chloride in the sweat of cystic fibrosis patients seldom results in profound symptoms such as those of heat prostration, this phenomenon has formed the basis of some large-scale public awareness/screening programs because of the resultant "salty" taste on the skin of affected patients.

### *Course of Disease*

Cystic fibrosis is a heterogeneous disease in terms of initial presentation, organ involvement, and clinical course. Most patients are not diagnosed at birth (only 7%–10% have meconium ileus) but are diagnosed later in life, based on a history of recurrent respiratory infections, steatorrhea, and/or failure to thrive.

The course of the disease after diagnosis varies markedly from one patient to the next. Some patients have a rapid downhill course based on pulmonary involvement; others suffer only from gastrointestinal complaints for many years.

While the expected life span of cystic fibrosis patients has doubled in the last 15 to 20 years, some patients still die early in life secondary to a fulminant pulmonary process. Some, on the other hand, because of minimal involvement and a mild course, are not diagnosed until their second or third decade of life.

## Treatment

### *Gastrointestinal Tract*

#### Pancreatic Enzyme Supplementation

The backbone of gastrointestinal therapy in cystic fibrosis is pancreatic enzyme replacement. The preferred products are microencapsulated (Cotazym S, Organon, and Pancrease, McNeil). These products protect the contained enzymes from destruction by gastric acid and may be given in much lower doses than their predecessors, which were susceptible to acid breakdown.

Before the introduction of microencapsulated enzyme products, various maneuvers were utilized to circumvent or overcome the problem of acid breakdown. The most obvious of these was to administer large quantities of enzyme. Enteric coated products met with limited success and histamine $H_2$ receptor antagonists were sometimes used to reduce the pancreatic enzyme dose. While there has been much controversy in the past regarding the relative amounts of various enzymes in the many pancreatic enzyme products available, such discussions pale in significance when considering the proven superiority of the microencapsulated products.[33] The comparative contents of commercially available enzyme preparations may be found elsewhere.[34]

For patients who are unable to swallow these capsules, the contents may be emptied into applesauce, jelly, or some other vehicle provided that the patient does not chew the microencapsulated beads. Bulk powder is available for infants and other children unable to use capsules.

Side effects of pancreatic enzyme products are unusual. Perianal irritation resembling diaper rash may occur in infants fed excess quantities of pancreatic enzyme powders. Hyperuricosuria has also been reported to occur secondary to pancreatic enzyme use.

#### Vitamin Supplementation

While clinically evident fat-soluble vitamin deficiencies are unusual in those patients taking adequate pancreatic enzymes and receiving a balanced diet, obvious vitamin K deficiency has been reported, manifested as bleeding diathesis.[35–37] Demineralization of bone has also been described.[38] Further, appropriate laboratory tests (serum carotene, vitamin E, and cholecalciferol concentrations) document other deficiencies, leading to recommendations for additional supplementation of these vitamins.[39–41] Water-miscible vitamin A 4,000 IU/d, vitamin E 50 mg/d, and vitamin K 5 mg orally twice a week have been recommended.

#### Meconium Ileus

Treatment of meconium ileus or meconium ileus equivalent can sometimes be limited to the use of enemas with contrast materials such as Gastrografin (Squibb) or Hypaque (Winthrop–Breon).[42] Unfortunately, surgery is more often necessary to treat this condition and prevent its complications.

### *Cardiovascular System*

Various modalities have been used in attempts to treat the pulmonary hypertension and secondary cor pulmonale of cystic fibrosis. These treatments, which include the pulmonary vasodilator, tolazoline (Priscoline, CIBA), inotropic agents such as digoxin (Lanoxin, Burroughs–Wellcome) and isoproterenol (Isuprel, Winthrop–Breon), and diuretics, have all resulted in limited and transient effects.[43–45] This is most likely due to the fact that none of these modes of therapy addresses the underlying cause of the cor pulmonale, hypoxia.

### *Pulmonary System*

Management of the pulmonary component of cystic fibrosis can be broken down into two areas: respiratory therapy and antibiotic therapy.

**Respiratory Therapy**

The cornerstone of pulmonary therapy is percussion and postural drainage, which aid in the clearance of pulmonary mucus and are performed as often as five times a day or more during an acute exacerbation. It should be noted that the benefits of percussion and postural drainage are acute in nature,[46,47] that data demonstrating long-term benefit are scant,[47] and that exercise alone may be just as effective in helping to clear mucus.[48] Percussion is often preceded by nebulizer therapy during which nebulized sterile water or 0.9% sodium chloride is breathed to liquefy pulmonary secretions. Bronchodilators and/or mucolytic agents (e.g., *N*-acetylcysteine) may be added to the nebulizer solution to prevent bronchospasm and further liquefy pulmonary secretions, respectively. While the effects of bronchodilators administered by inhalation are readily demonstrated with pulmonary function tests, those of mucolytic agents are not as obvious and a number of attempts to demonstrate the effects of inhaled *N*-acetylcysteine (Mucomyst, Mead Johnson) have been unsuccessful.[49–51] Many patients prefer not to use *N*-acetylcysteine because of its unpleasant taste and odor and because it often induces bronchospasm.

As some cystic fibrosis patients have a reactive airway component to their pulmonary disease, systemic bronchodilators such as theophylline may be of benefit. Responsiveness to such agents should be documented, however, before a contracted course is begun. Normal antiasthmatic doses of most bronchodilators should be appropriate for cystic fibrosis patients; however, theophylline clearance may be different in cystic fibrosis patients,[52–54] and bioavailability of some products may be decreased[54] (sometimes necessitating the use of higher-than-usual doses). The determination of a theophylline dose in a specific cystic fibrosis patient should be based upon that individual's dose–serum concentration relationship (i.e., individual pharmacokinetic values). As cystic fibrosis patients are at high risk of developing the complications of influenza, influenza vaccine should be administered to them on a yearly basis.

**Antibiotic Therapy**

The use of antibiotics in cystic fibrosis patients is both controversial and fraught with difficulty. Controversy exists because of the observation that during treatment for an acute pulmonary exacerbation, clinical improvement occurs despite failure to eradicate bacterial pathogens from the sputum, suggesting that the bacteria present are colonizers rather than pathogens which argues against the use of antibiotics in these patients.

Further, there is a paucity of controlled trials documenting a therapeutic benefit from antibiotics. Beaudry and colleagues studied 22 patients given either cloxacillin or gentamicin and carbenicillin for acute pulmonary exacerbations.[55] No difference in response was noted. On the other hand, Hyatt and co-workers reported a comparative trial in which 15 patients received a combination of oxacillin, sisomicin, and carbenicillin and 9 patients received oxacillin alone.[56] In terms of failure rate, the results favored the combination therapy. Wientzen and colleagues conducted a trial in 20 patients who received either tobramycin or placebo; the results tended to support tobramycin use although the placebo group may have included more severely affected patients.[57] Additionally, there is a considerable body of both direct and indirect evidence pointing to the pathogenicity of such bacteria as *Pseudomonas aeruginosa*, which when considered in light of the few favorable controlled clinical trials leads one to realize the need for antibiotic therapy. Despite the ongoing nature of this controversy, most clinicians caring for cystic fibrosis patients do prescribe antibiotic treatment.[58]

Once one is committed to antibiotic therapy, a number of other unresolved issues emerge:

Should antibiotics be prescribed only during an acute exacerbation?

Should antibiotics be used on a "prophylactic" basis to suppress bacterial growth and perhaps decrease the incidence of hospitalization?

Should hospitalization and intensive antibiotic therapy be performed on a regularly scheduled basis regardless of acute clinical condition as recommended by some European experts?[59]

Should antibiotics be selected based on specific culture and susceptibility results or based on potential pathogens and susceptibility patterns?

Is there an ideal length of treatment for intravenous antibiotics or should length of therapy be governed by clinical or laboratory endpoints?

Can some of the newer β-lactam antibiotics with enhanced activity against gram-negative bacteria be used alone in these patients to take advantage of attractive safety profiles or would such a practice lead only to the rapid emergence of resistance as has been demonstrated with cefoperazone[60] (Cefobid, Roerig) and azlocillin (Azlin, Miles)?[61,62]

Unfortunately, the answers to these and other questions regarding antibiotic use in cystic fibrosis remain unanswered.

As mentioned before, most clinicians do treat pulmonary exacerbations with antibiotics. Specific therapy is directed at proven or likely pathogens such as *Pseudomonas aeruginosa* and *Staphylococcus aureus*, and usually includes an aminoglycoside and an extended-spectrum penicillin. While growing, the evidence supporting the clinical superiority of such combinations over single-agent therapy is not totally convincing[61–66]; however, the fact that they are synergistic in vitro[67] and the possibility that they may act to suppress or delay the emergence of resistance[68,69] provide an attractive argument for their use. Further, in vitro synergism has been reported to persist even in the face of resistance to one of the single agents.[70] It should be noted, however, that early experience with the newer β-lactams ceftazidime (Fortaz, Glaxo and others)[71] and aztreonam (Azactam, Squibb),[72] when used alone in this condition, has been impressive. Whether rapid and/or extensive emergence of resistance to these agents occurs with their continued use as single-antibiotic therapy remains to be seen. Unlike other cases of pneumonia, organism-specific drug treatment may be based on results from sputum cultures in cystic fibrosis patients, as good agreement between sputum and thoracotomy cultures has been demonstrated.[73] Typically, such results lead to prescription of aminoglycoside/β-lactam combinations. While complete eradication of *S. aureus* and *H. influenzae* is a practical goal or endpoint of this type of antibiotic therapy,

**Table 56.2** Antibiotics With Altered Pharmacokinetics in Cystic Fibrosis Patients

| | |
|---|---|
| Gentamicin | Cloxacillin |
| Tobramycin | Dicloxacillin |
| Amikacin | Azlocillin |
| Netilmicin | Piperacillin |
| Trimethoprim–Sulfamethoxazole | Ceftazidime |
| Methicillin | Ceftriaxone |

the total eradication of *Pseudomonas* species is infrequent and transient.

One other problem with antibiotic use in cystic fibrosis emerges at this point, specifically, altered pharmacokinetic disposition of some antibiotics in most cystic fibrosis patients (Table 56.2). As is true for theophylline, many cystic fibrosis patients have increased total body clearance for many antibiotics including the aminoglycosides, some of the β-lactams, and trimethoprim–sulfamethoxazole. Thus, higher doses of these agents may be necessary to produce therapeutic concentrations. Unfortunately, these alterations in pharmacokinetics are neither consistent nor predictable.

Increased total body clearance along with variable changes in elimination rate (and serum half-life) and apparent volume of distribution has been reported for the aminoglycosides gentamicin,[74] tobramycin,[75] amikacin,[76] and netilmicin.[77] Interestingly, a concomitant increase in renal clearance has not been demonstrated for these agents, leading some to speculate about extrarenal pathways (such as accumulation in pulmonary secretions) for aminoglycoside elimination in cystic fibrosis patients,[78,79] Similarly, altered pharmacokinetic disposition has been reported for some β-lactam antibiotics including methicillin,[80] cloxacillin,[81] dicloxacillin,[82] azlocillin,[83] piperacillin,[84] ceftazidime,[85] and ceftriaxone.[86] In these cases, increased total body clearance could be accounted for by increased renal clearance. Of note is the observation that other β-lactams that do not undergo significant renal tubular secretion, such as imipenem and cefsulodin, have not been found to exhibit increased total body clearance in cystic fibrosis patients.[87,88] It should also be pointed out that renal function (as reflected by glomerular filtration rate and renal blood flow) is not different in cystic fibrosis patients as compared with non–cystic fibrosis controls.[89] A study of the disposition of trimethoprim–sulfamethoxazole conducted by Reed and colleagues revealed a decreased half-life and increased clearance of this combination in cystic fibrosis patients.[90]

The mechanism accounting for these changes is unknown. These alterations in antibiotic pharmacokinetics necessitate increased dosage in many, but not all cystic fibrosis patients. For example, experience with netilmicin revealed a dosage requirement range of 7 to 17 mg/kg/d to achieve peak concentrations (one-half hour after the end of a drug infusion) of 8 μg/mL.[91] The mean dosage requirement was approximately 12 mg/kg/d. Peak concentrations of this magnitude are felt to be necessary to adequately treat pneumonia caused by gram-negative organisms.[92,93]

While the pharmacokinetics of antibiotics may correlate with the severity of pulmonary disease,[94,95] it is not possible to predict changes in antibiotic pharmacokinetics in cystic fibrosis patients based upon markers of clinical status or disease progression. Attempts to correlate antibiotic pharmacokinetics with Schwachman scores, a gross method for quantitation of disease status,[96] have been unsuccessful.[81,97] Attempts to guide aminoglycoside dosing are often based on serum concentrations measured during a course of therapy. This method may also meet with limited success because of the changing pharmacokinetic disposition of aminoglycosides during an acute pulmonary exacerbation.[91]

An additional method of antibiotic administration that is intuitively attractive in patients with pneumonia is inhalation of aerosolized solutions. Such a route of administration should, theoretically, deliver the drug to the actual site of infection and perhaps avoid systemic toxicity. While many classes of antibiotics have been administered to cystic fibrosis patients in this fashion, often in conjunction with systemic antibiotics, no clear effect or advantage can be consistently demonstrated.[98–102] Why this form of therapy does not yield positive results is unclear but probably is due to failure of aerosolized particles to reach the small airways. This mode of antibiotic therapy cannot, therefore, be recommended on a routine basis.

Despite these inherent difficulties, a number of recommendations regarding the use of systemic antibiotics in cystic fibrosis can be made. The selection of antibiotics should be based on specific culture and sensitivity results. While the goal of bacterial eradication is desirable, other attainable endpoints may be more reasonable. A return to the preexacerbation clinical status or pulmonary function status is a practical endpoint for antibiotic therapy. Aminoglycosides should be initially dosed at the upper end of the normal dose range (6–7.5 mg/kg/d for tobramycin) and serum concentrations should be determined frequently so that dosage can be appropriately adjusted to achieve peak concentrations of at least 8 but not exceeding 12 μg/mL. It should be kept in mind that aminoglycoside serum half-lives may lengthen during the course of treatment so that a constant relationship between dose and serum concentrations may not exist. Upward adjustments in dosage should therefore be made with some degree of caution and should be followed with further determination of serum concentrations. β-Lactam antibiotics such as extended-spectrum penicillins should be prescribed with aminoglycosides to take advantage of their frequent synergy and prevent the emergence of resistance. These agents should be prescribed in large doses to delay stepwise resistance. Ticarcillin, azlocillin, and piperacillin should be prescribed in a dosage of at least 350 mg/kg/d divided into four to six doses. Selection among these agents should be based upon local susceptibility patterns and cost considerations. The possible increased incidence of fever and exanthema with the newer penicillins[103] should be kept in mind.

Oral antibiotics should be prescribed in outpatients with susceptible pathogens in their sputum. This form of therapy should also be limited in length, with specific endpoints identified as treatment commences. Agents with activity against common pathogens such as *S. aureus* and *H. influenzae* are useful in this setting. These typically include such antibiotics as first-generation cephalosporins, trimethoprim–sulfamethoxazole, and amoxicillin–clavulanic acid. The use of such agents on a "prophylactic" basis is discouraged as the presently available data suggest that a beneficial effect[104] does not outweigh the risk of development of resistance among the common bacterial pathogens of cystic fibrosis. Newer oral antibiotics are currently being introduced. One of these, the quinolone ciprofloxacin, has been evaluated in adults with cystic fibrosis and appears to be as efficacious as standard intravenous antibiotic therapy.[105] This type of agent may decrease the need for frequent hospitalization in some patients but must be used prudently.[106]

## Summary

The prognosis for cystic fibrosis patients has improved substantially in the last few decades because of early diagnosis, aggressive management, and improved antibiotic therapy. Nonetheless the average life span for these patients has risen only into the third decade of life. Presumably because of the heterogeneous nature of the clinical presentation and course of the disease, there are still early deaths and substantial morbidity throughout life.

Pharmacotherapeutic intervention plays an important role in the management of these patients but is complex. The clinician is, as yet, faced with many unresolved issues in attempting to apply sound therapeutic principles in this population. Although close attention should be paid to pharmacologic treatment, the approach to these patients should be multifaceted and multidisciplinary in character. In addition to the involvement of such pediatric subspecialties as gastroenterology, pulmonology, pharmacology, and infectious disease, contributions from such areas as nutrition and social work should be a regular and ongoing part of the management effort.

## References


1. Anderson DH. Cystic fibrosis of the pancreas and its relation to celiac disease. Am J Dis Child 1938;56:344–399.
2. Steinberg AG, Brown DC. On the incidence of cystic fibrosis of the pancreas. Am J Hum Genet 1960;12:416–424.
3. Wright SE, Morton NE. Genetic studies on cystic fibrosis in Hawaii. Am J Hum Genet 1968;20:157–169.
4. Klinger KW. Genetics of cystic fibrosis. Semin Respir Med 1985;6:243–251.
5. Park RW, Grand RJ. Gastrointestinal manifestations of cystic fibrosis: A review. Gastroenterology 1981;81:1143–1161.
6. Lippe BM, Kaplan SA, Neufeld ND, et al. Insulin receptors in cystic fibrosis: Increased number and altered affinity. Pediatrics 1980;65:1018–1022.
7. Matthews LW, Drotar D. Cystic fibrosis—A challenging long-term disease. Pediatr Clin North Am 1984;31:133–52.
8. di Sant'Agnese P, Blanc W. A distinctive type of biliary cirrhosis of the liver associated with cystic fibrosis of the pancreas. Pediatrics 1956;18:387–409.
9. Stern RC, Stevens DP, Boat RF, et al. Symptomatic hepatic disease in cystic fibrosis: Incidence, course and outcome of portal systemic shunting. Gastroenterology 1976;70:645–649.
10. Sanchis J, Dolovich M, Rossman C, et al. Pulmonary mucociliary clearance in cystic fibrosis. N Engl J Med 1973;288:651–654.
11. Davis PB. Pathophysiology of pulmonary disease in cystic fibrosis. Semin Respir Med 1985;6:261–270.
12. Schiøtz PO. Systemic and mucosal immunity and non-specific defense mechanisms in cystic fibrosis patients. Acta Paediatr Scand 1982;suppl 301:55–62.
13. Petersen NT, Høiby N, Mordhorst CH, et al. Respiratory infections in cystic fibrosis patients caused by virus, chlamydia, and mycoplasma. Possible synergism with *Pseudomonas aeruginosa*. Acta Paediatr Scand 1981;70:623–628.
14. Marks MI. The pathogenesis and treatment of pulmonary infections in patients with cystic fibrosis. J Pediatr 1981;98:173–179.
15. Isles A, Maclusky I, Corey M, et al. *Pseudomonas cepacia* infection in cystic fibrosis: An emerging problem. J Pediatr 1984;104:206–210.
16. Vasil ML. *Pseudomonas aeruginosa*: Biology, mechanisms of virulence, epidemiology. J Pediatr 1986;108:800–805.
17. McLaughlin FJ, Matthews WJ, Strieder DJ, et al. Pneumothorax in cystic fibrosis: Management and outcome. J Pediatr 1982;100:863–869.
18. Royce SW. Cor pulmonale in infancy and early childhood: Report on 34 patients with special reference to the occurrence of pulmonary disease in cystic fibrosis of the pancreas. Pediatrics 1951;8:255–274.
19. Gharib R, Allen RP, Joos HA, et al. Paranasal sinuses in cystic fibrosis. Am J Dis Child 1964;108:499–502.
20. Shwachman H, Kulczycki LL, Mueller HL, et al. Nasal polyposis in patients with cystic fibrosis. Pediatrics 1962;30:389–401.
21. Ledesma-Medina J, Osman MZ, Girdany BR. Abnormal paranasal sinuses in patients with cystic fibrosis of the pancreas. Pediatr Radiol 1980;9:61–64.
22. Schulz IJ. Micropuncture studies of the sweat formation in cystic fibrosis patients. J Clin Invest 1969;48:1470–1477.
23. Quinton PM. Chloride impermeability in cystic fibrosis. Nature 1983;301:421–422.
24. Reiter EO, Stern RC, Root AW. The reproductive endocrine system in cystic fibrosis: I. Basal gonadotropin and sex steroid levels. Am J Dis Child 1981;135:422–426.
25. Palmer J, Dillon-Baker C, Tecklin JS, et al. Pregnancy in patients with cystic fibrosis. Ann Intern Med 1983;99:596–600.
26. Vichinsky EP, Pennathur-Das R, Nickerson B, et al. Inadequate erythroid response to hypoxia in cystic fibrosis. J Pediatr 1984;105:15–21.
27. Ater JL, Herbst JJ, Landaw SA, et al. Relative anemia and iron deficiency in cystic fibrosis. Pediatrics 1983;71:810–814.
28. Athreya BH, Borns P, Rosenlund ML. Cystic fibrosis and hypertrophic osteoarthropathy in children. Am J Dis Child 1975;129:634–637.
29. Matthay MA, Matthay RA, Mills DM, et al. Hypertrophic osteoarthropathy in adults with cystic fibrosis. Thorax 1976;31:572–575.
30. Grossman H, Denning CF, Baker DH. Hypertrophic osteoarthropathy in cystic fibrosis. Am J Dis Child 1964;107:1–6.
31. McGuire S, Monaghan H, Tempany E. Arthritis in childhood cystic fibrosis. Ir J Med Sci 1982;151:253–254.
32. Gibson LE, Cooke RE. A test for concentrations of electrolytes in sweat in cystic fibrosis of the pancreas using pilocarpine by iontophoresis. Pediatrics 1959;23:545–549.
33. Cho YW, Aviado DM. Pancreatic enzyme preparations, with

special reference to enterically coated microspheres of pancrelipase. J Clin Pharmacol 1981;21:224–237.

34. Bosso JA, Herbst JJ. Pancreatic enzymes, in: Guide to Drug Therapy in Cystic Fibrosis. Atlanta, National Cystic Fibrosis Research Foundation, in press.
35. Torstenson OL, Humphrey GB, Edson JR, et al. Cystic fibrosis presenting with severe hemorrhage due to vitamin K deficiency. Pediatrics 1970;45:857–861.
36. Dolan TF, Gibson LE. Possibility of cystic fibrosis in infants with vitamin K deficiency. J Pediatr 1970;77:515.
37. Walters TR, Koch HF. Hemorrhagic diathesis and cystic fibrosis in infancy. Am J Dis Child 1972;124:641–642.
38. Mischler EH, Chesney J, Chesney RW, et al. Dimineralization in cystic fibrosis. Am J Dis Child 1979;133:632–635.
39. Congden PJ, Bruce G, Rothburn MM, et al. Vitamin status in treated patients with cystic fibrosis. Arch Dis Child 1981;56: 708–714.
40. Solomons NW, Wagonfeld JB, Rieger C, et al. Some biochemical indices of nutrition in treated cystic fibrosis patients. Am J Clin Nutr 1981;34:462–474.
41. Harrigs JT, Mullen DPR. Absorption of different doses of fat soluble and water miscible preparations of vitamin E in children with cystic fibrosis. Arch Dis Child 1971;46:341–344.
42. Wagget J, Johnson DG, Borns P, et al. The nonoperative treatment of meconium ileus by Gastrografin enema. J Pediatr 1970;77:407–411.
43. Stern RC, Borkat G, Hirschfeld SS, et al. Heart failure in cystic fibrosis: Treatment and prognosis of cor pulmonale with failure of the right side of the heart. Am J Dis Child 1980;134:267–272.
44. Moss AJ. The cardiovascular system in cystic fibrosis. Pediatrics 1982;70:728–741.
45. Whitman V, Stern RC, Bellet P, et al. Studies on cor pulmonale in cystic fibrosis: I. Effects of diuresis. Pediatrics 1975;55:83–85.
46. Feldman J, Traver GA, Taussig LM. Maximal expiratory flows after postural drainage. Am Rev Respir Dis 1979;119:239–245.
47. Desmond KJ, Schwenk WF, Thomas E, et al. Immediate and long-term effects of chest physiotherapy in patients with cystic fibrosis. J Pediatr 1983;103:538–542.
48. Zach MS, Purrer B, Oberwaldner B. Effect of swimming on forced expiration and sputum clearance in cystic fibrosis. Lancet 1981;2:1201–1203.
49. Wanner A, Rao A. Clinical indications for and effects of bland, mucolytic and antimicrobial aerosols. Am Rev Respir Dis 1980;122:79–103.
50. Waring WN. Current management of cystic fibrosis. Adv Pediatr 1976;23:401–438.
51. Rao S, Wilson DB, Brooks RC, et al. Acute effects of nebulization of *N*-acetylcysteine on pulmonary mechanics and gas exchange. Am Rev Respir Dis 1970;102:17–22.
52. Larsen GL, Barron RJ, Landay RA, et al. Intravenous aminophylline in patients with cystic fibrosis. Pharmacokinetics and effect on pulmonary function. Am J Dis Child 1980;134:1143–1148.
53. Isles A, Spino M, Tabachnik E, et al. Theophylline disposition in cystic fibrosis. Am Rev Respir Dis 1983;127:417–421.
54. Valet SB, Schwartz RH, Brooks JG. Pharmacokinetics of theophylline and bioavailability of sustained release theophylline preparation in patients with cystic fibrosis. Ann Allergy 1983;50:161–165.
55. Beaudry PH, Marks MI, McDougall D, et al. Is anti-*Pseudomonas* therapy warranted in acute respiratory exacerbations in children with cystic fibrosis? J Pediatr 1980;97:144–147.
56. Hyatt AC, Chipps BE, Kumor KM, et al. A double-blind controlled trial of anti-pseudomonas chemotherapy of acute respiratory exacerbations in patients with cystic fibrosis. J Pediatr 1981;99:307–311.
57. Wientzen R, Prestidge CB, Kramer RI, et al. Acute pulmonary exacerbations in cystic fibrosis. A double-blind trial of tobramycin and placebo therapy. Am J Dis Child 1980;134:1134–1138.
58. Nelson JD. Management of acute pulmonary exacerbations in cystic fibrosis: A critical appraisal. J Pediatr 1985;106:1030–1034.
59. Szaff M, Høiby N, Flensborg EW, et al. Frequent antibiotic therapy improves survival of cystic fibrosis patients with chronic *Pseudomonas aeruginosa* infection. Acta Pediatr Scand 1983;72:651–657.
60. Jewett CV, Ledbetter J, Lyrene RK, et al. Comparison of cefoperazone sodium vs methicillin, ticarcillin, and tobramycin in treatment of pulmonary exacerbations in patients with cystic fibrosis. J Pediatr 1985;106:669–672.
61. McLaughlin FJ, Matthews WJ, Strieder DJ, et al. Clinical and bacteriological responses to three antibiotic regimens for acute exacerbations of cystic fibrosis: Ticarcillin–tobramycin, azlocillin–tobramycin, and azlocillin–placebo. J Infect Dis 1983;147:559–567.
62. Michalsen H, Bergan T. Azlocillin with and without an aminoglycoside against respiratory tract infections in children with cystic fibrosis. Scand J Infect Dis 1981;29(suppl):92–97.
63. Parry MF, Neu HC, Merlino M, et al. Treatment of pulmonary infections in patients with cystic fibrosis: A comparative study of ticarcillin and gentamicin. J Pediatr 1977;90:144–148.
64. Møller NE, Høiby N. Antibiotic treatment of chronic *Pseudomonas aeruginosa* infection in cystic fibrosis patients. Scand J Infect Dis 1981;24(suppl):87–91.
65. Friis B. Chemotherapy of chronic infections with mucoid *Pseudomonas aeruginosa* in lower airways of patients with cystic fibrosis. Scand J Infect Dis 1979;11:211–217.
66. Krause PJ, Young LS, Cherry JD, et al. The treatment of exacerbations of pulmonary disease in cystic fibrosis: Netilmicin compared with netilmicin and carbenicillin. Curr Ther Res 1979;25:609–617.
67. Scribner RK, Marks MI, Weber AH, et al. Activities of various $\beta$-lactams and aminoglycosides, alone and in combination, against isolates of *Pseudomonas aeruginosa* from patients with cystic fibrosis. Antimicrob Agents Chemother 1982;21:939–943.
68. Gerber AU, Vastola AP, Brandel J, et al. Selection of aminoglycoside-resistant variants of *Pseudomonas aeruginosa* in an in vivo model. J Infect Dis 1982;146:691–697.
69. Gerber AU, Craig WA. Aminoglycoside-selected subpopulations of *Pseudomonas aeruginosa*. J Lab Clin Med 1982;100: 671–681.
70. Aronof SC, Klinger JD. In vitro activities of aztreonam, piperacillin and ticarcillin combined with amikacin against amikacin-resistant *Pseudomonas aeruginosa* and *P. cepacia* isolates from children with cystic fibrosis. Antimicrob Agents Chemother 1984;25:279–280.
71. Blumer JL, Stern RC, Yamashita TS, et al. Cephalosporin therapeutics in cystic fibrosis. J Pediatr 1986;108:854–860.
72. Bosso JA, Black PG, Matsen JM. Efficacy of aztreonam in pulmonary exacerbations of cystic fibrosis. Pediatr Infect Dis J 1987;6:393–397.
73. Thomassen MJ, Klinger JD, Badger SJ, et al. Cultures of thoracotomy specimens confirm usefulness of sputum cultures in cystic fibrosis. J Pediatr 1984;104:352–356.
74. Kearns GL, Hilman BA, Wilson JT. Dosing implications of

altered gentamicin disposition in patients with cystic fibrosis. J Pediatr 1982;100:312–318.

**75.** Kelly HB, Menendez R, Fan L, et al. Pharmacokinetics of tobramycin in cystic fibrosis. J Pediatr 1982;100:318–321.

**76.** Finkelstein E, Hall K. Aminoglycoside clearance in patients with cystic fibrosis. J Pediatr 1979;94:163–164.

**77.** Bosso JA, Townsend PL, Herbst JJ, et al. Pharmacokinetics and dosage requirements of netilmicin in cystic fibrosis patients. Antimicrob Agents Chemother 1985;28:829–831.

**78.** Levy J, Smith AL, Koup JR, et al. Disposition of tobramycin in patients with cystic fibrosis: A prospective controlled study. J Pediatr 1984;105:117–124.

**79.** Mendelman PM, Smith AL, Levy J, et al. Aminoglycoside penetration, inactivation, and efficacy in cystic fibrosis sputum. Am Rev Respir Dis 1985;132:761–765.

**80.** Yaffe SJ, Gerbracht LM, Mosovich LL, et al. Pharmacokinetics of methicillin in patients with cystic fibrosis. J Infect Dis 1977;135:828–831.

**81.** Spino M, Chai RP, Isles AF, et al. Cloxacillin absorption and disposition in cystic fibrosis. J Pediatr 1984;105:829–835.

**82.** Jusko WJ, Mosovich LL, Gerbracht LM, et al. Enhanced renal excretion of dicloxacillin in patients with cystic fibrosis. Pediatrics 1975;56:1038–1044.

**83.** Bosso JA, Saxon BA, Herbst JJ, et al. Azlocillin pharmacokinetics in patients with cystic fibrosis. Antimicrob Agents Chemother 1984;25:630–632.

**84.** Prince AS, Neu HC. Use of piperacillin, a semisynthetic penicillin, in the therapy of acute exacerbations of pulmonary disease in patients with cystic fibrosis. J Pediatr 1980;97: 148–151.

**85.** Padoan R, Brienza A, Crossignani RM, et al. Ceftazidime in treatment of acute pulmonary exacerbations in patients with cystic fibrosis. J Pediatr 1983;103:320–324.

**86.** Michalsen H, Bergan T. Pharmacokinetics of antibiotics in children with cystic fibrosis with particular reference to netilmicin. Acta Paediatr Scand 1982;suppl 301:101–105.

**87.** Reed MD, Stern RC, O'Brien CA, et al. Pharmacokinetics of imipenem and cilastatin in patients with cystic fibrosis. Antimicrob Agents Chemother 1985;27:583–588.

**88.** Reed MD, Stern RC, Yamashita TS, et al. Single-dose pharmacokinetics of cefsulodin in patients with cystic fibrosis. Antimicrob Agents Chemother 1984;25:579–581.

**89.** Spino M, Chai RP, Isles AF, et al. Assessment of glomerular filtration rate and effective renal plasma flow in cystic fibrosis. J Pediatr 1985;107:64–70.

**90.** Reed MD, Stern RC, Bertino JS, et al. Dosing implications of rapid elimination of trimethoprim–sulfamethoxazole in patients with cystic fibrosis. J Pediatr 1984;104:303–307.

**91.** Bosso JA, Relling MV, Townsend PL, et al. Intrapatient variations in aminoglycoside disposition in cystic fibrosis. Clin Pharm 1987;6:54–58.

**92.** Moore RD, Smith CR, Lietman PS. Association of aminoglycoside plasma levels with therapeutic outcome in gram-negative pneumonia. Am J Med 1984;77:657–662.

**93.** Noone P, Parsons MC, Pattison JR, et al. Experience in monitoring gentamicin therapy during treatment of serious gram negative sepsis. Br J Med 1974;1:477–481.

**94.** MacDonald NE, Anas NG, Peterson RG, et al. Renal clearance of gentamicin in cystic fibrosis. J Pediatr 1983;103: 985–990.

**95.** Nahata MC, Lubin AH, Visconti JA. Cephalexin pharmacokinetics in patients with cystic fibrosis. Dev Pharmacol Ther 1984;7:221–228.

**96.** Shwachman H, Kulczycki LL. Long-term study of 105 patients with cystic fibrosis: Studies made over 5- to 14-year period. Am J Dis Child 1958;96:6–15.

**97.** Jacobs RF, Trang JM, Kearns GL, et al. Ticarcillin/clavulanic acid pharmacokinetics in children and young adults with cystic fibrosis. J Pediatr 1985;106:1001–1007.

**98.** Pines A, Raafat H, Plucinski K. Gentamicin and colistin in chronic purulent bronchial infections. Br Med J 1967;2:543–545.

**99.** Pines A, Raafat H, Siddigin GM, et al. Treatment of severe *Pseudomonas* infections of the bronchi. Br Med J 1970;1: 663–665.

**100.** Stephens D, Garey N, Isles A, et al. Efficacy of inhaled tobramycin in the treatment of pulmonary exacerbations in children with cystic fibrosis. Pediatr Infect Dis 1983;2:209–211.

**101.** Huang HN, Hiller GT, Macni CM, et al. Carbenicillin in patients with cystic fibrosis: Clinical pharmacology and therapeutic evaluation. J Pediatr 1971;78:338–345.

**102.** Nolan G, McIvor P, Levison H, et al. Antibiotic prophylaxis in cystic fibrosis: Inhaled cephaloridine as an adjunct to oral cloxacillin. J Pediatr 1982;101:626–630.

**103.** Møller NE, Eriksen KR, Feddersen C, et al. Chemotherapy against *Pseudomonas aeruginosa* in cystic fibrosis. A study of carbenicillin, azlocillin or piperacillin in combination with tobramycin. Eur J Respir Dis 1982;63:130–139.

**104.** Loening-Bauke VA, Mischler E, Myers M. A placebo-controlled trial of cephalexin therapy in the ambulatory management of patients with cystic fibrosis. J Pediatr 1979;95:630–637.

**105.** Bosso JA, Black PG, Matsen JM. Ciprofloxacin versus tobramycin plus azlocillin in pulmonary exacerbations in adult patients. Am J Med 1987;82(suppl 4A):180–184.

**106.** Stutman HR. Summary of a workshop on ciprofloxacin use in patients with cystic fibrosis. Pediatr Infect Dis J 1987;6: 932–935.

# Section Eight
# Immunologic Disorders

## Chapter 57 / Immunodeficiency Diseases

Jeffrey C. Delafuente, MS

Immunodeficiencies are a diverse group of diseases with varying pathogenesis, genetic inheritance, etiology, and clinical presentation. The first human immunodeficiency disease was reported in 1952.[1] Since that time more than 20 different forms of immunodeficiency have been recognized. The World Health Organization has classified the immunodeficiencies into four major categories: predominantly antibody defects, common variable immunodeficiency, predominantly cell-mediated immunity defects, and immunodeficiencies associated with other major defects (Tables 57.1–57.4).[2] Although the functional and cellular abnormalities of the various immunodeficiency diseases have been characterized, the pathogenesis for most of these diseases remains unknown. None of these diseases has been associated with any human leukocyte antigen (HLA)–linked immune response gene; however, many of these disorders are caused by genetic defects associated with the X chromosome.[3]

An exact incidence for the various immunodeficiency diseases is not available. Fortunately, these serious and often fatal diseases are rare. A few of the more common immunodeficiency diseases are discussed in this chapter, but even these diseases are quite rare in the population. A succinct review of the human immune system precedes the discussion of these diseases. Methods frequently used to evaluate immune responses are also discussed.

### The Immune System

The immune system is a highly complicated and regulated system. It is categorized into two major components: the cellular immune system and the humoral immune system.

#### *Cellular Immunity*

Cellular immunity is that specific immune response to antigens mediated primarily by lymphocytes and macrophages, with minor participation by other cell types. The cellular immune system is responsible for functions such as organ transplant rejection, killing of tumor or virus-infected cells, and delayed cutaneous hypersensitivity.

Lymphocytes are divided into two major categories, T and B cells. T lymphocytes are responsible for both regulation and mediation of cellular immunity. B lymphocytes are responsible primarily for antibody production. Lymphocytes that are neither T nor B cells are referred to as null cells. Null cells may be progenitors of the natural killer cells responsible for killing virus-infected cells and tumor cells in the body. Macrophages and monocytes process and present foreign antigens to lymphocytes, initiating the immune response. Macrophages and monocytes also secrete soluble substances that serve as regulatory signals for lymphocytes.

Figure 57.1 illustrates the complexity of the cellular interactions within the immune system. Uncommitted bone marrow stem cells differentiate into mature T lymphocytes within the thymus gland. B-lymphocyte maturation probably takes place within the bone marrow or fetal liver. Subpopulations exist within each lymphoid cell type. For example, T lymphocytes contain subpopulations of regulatory cells, which include helper and suppressor T lymphocytes. A delicate balance between these two cell types maintains a homeostatic functioning immune system.

Many of the regulatory and effector functions of T lymphocytes are mediated through the production and secretion of soluble mediators, known as lymphokines. In addition to soluble mediators, cell-to-cell contact may also be required for certain immune responses.

#### *Humoral Immunity*

The humoral immune system involves plasma cell production of immunoglobulins (antibodies). Plasma cells are derived from mature B lymphocytes. The five classes of immunoglobulins in humans are found in serum, secretions, and other biologic fluids and tissues. Immunoglobulin class–specific functions and characteristics are summarized in Table 57.5. Other humoral constituents include complement proteins, kinins, and prostaglandins. As shown in Figure 57.1, immunoglobulin production is regulated by helper and suppressor T lymphocytes.

**Table 57.1** Predominantly Antibody Defects

| | Usual phenotypic expression | | | | | | |
|---|---|---|---|---|---|---|---|
| *Designation* | **Serum Ig** | **Serum antibodies** | **Circulating B cells** | **Circulating T cells** | **CMI** | *Presumed pathogenesis/ differentiation defect* | *Inheritance* |
| X-linked agammaglobulinemia | All isotypes decreased | Decreased | Usually absent | Normal | Normal | Intrinsic defect in pre-B- to B-cell differentiation | X-linked |
| X-linked hypogammaglobulinemia with growth hormone deficiency | All isotypes decreased | Decreased | Absent or very low | Normal | Normal | Unknown; probably defect in pre-B- to B-cell differentiation | X-linked |
| Autosomal recessive agammaglobulinemia | All isotypes decreased | Decreased | Decreased | Normal | Normal | ? Intrinsic defect in pre-B- to B-cell differentiation | AR |
| Ig deficiency with increased IgM (and IgD) | IgM and IgD increased | IgM increased, other isotypes decreased | Normal IgM- and IgD-bearing cells | Normal | Normal | Intrinsic isotype switch defect; failure of $IgM^+$, $IgD^+$ B-cell maturation to $IgG^+$, $IgA^+$, $IgE^+$, B cells | X-linked or AR or AD |
| | IgG and IgA decreased | IgG and IgA decreased | No IgG- or IgA-bearing cells | Normal | Normal | | Unknown |
| IgA deficiency | $IgA_1$ or $IgA_2$ decreased | IgA decreased | Immature sIgA B cells | Usually normal | Usually normal | Defective IgA (± IgG subclass) B-cell maturation: intrinsic? extrinsic (T-cell)? | Unknown: some AR, some AD (frequent in families with common variable ID) |
| | $IgA_1$, $IgA_2$, and $IgG_2$ decrease with or without $IgG_4$ decrease | IgA and IgG decreased | Immature sIgA B cells | Normal | Normal | | |
| | $IgA_1$ or $IgA_2$ decreased | $IgA_1$ or $IgA_2$ decreased | Immature sIgA B cells | Normal | Normal | | |

| | | | | | | | |
|---|---|---|---|---|---|---|---|
| Selective deficiency of other Ig isotypes | Decreased IgM, $IgG_1$, $IgG_2$, $IgG_3$, or $IgG_4$ | Decrease of the deficient isotype | ? Normal | Normal | Normal | Differentiation defect of IgM B cell to isotype-specific plasma cell | Unknown |
| Kappa chain deficiency | Ig (kappa) decreased | Decreased | Normal or decreased kappa $B^+$ cells | Normal | Normal | Unknown | Unknown |
| Antibody deficiency with normal or hypergamma-globulinemia | Normal | Decreased | Near normal | Normal | Variable | B-cell differentiation defect; defective T-cell help | Unknown |
| ID with thymoma | All isotypes decreased | Decreased | Absent or very low | Variable | Variably decreased | Unknown defect in HSC to pre-B-cell maturation (? excessive T-suppressor activity) | None |
| Transient hypogam-maglobulinemia of infancy | IgG and IgA decreased | Decreased | Normal | Decreased T help | Variable | IgG/IgA B-cell to IgG/IgA plasma cell differentiation defect: delayed maturation of T help; ? other | Unknown |

AR, autosomal recessive; AD, autosomal dominant; Ig, immunoglobulin; CMI, cellular-mediated immunity; ID, immunodeficiency; sIg, surface immunoglobulin; HSC, hematopoietic stem cell.

**Table 57.2** Common Variable Immunodeficiency

| | *Usual phenotypic expression* | | | | | | |
|---|---|---|---|---|---|---|---|
| *Designation* | Serum Ig | Serum antibodies | Circulating B cells | Circulating T cells | CMI | *Presumed nature of basic defect* | *Inheritance* |
| Common variable immunodeficiency with predominant B-cell defect | | | | | | | |
| Near-normal B-cell number with primarily $IgG^+$ and $IgM^+$ cells | Decreased | Decreased | Near-normal numbers but abnormal proportions of subtypes | Variable | Variable | Intrinsic defect in cell differentiation of immature to mature B cells | Unknown, AR, AD |
| Very low B-cell number | Decreased | Decreased | Decreased | Variable | Variable | Intrinsic defect in pre-B- to B-cell maturation | Unknown, AR, AD |
| "Nonsecretory" B cells with plasma cells | Decreased | Decreased | Normal numbers but abnormal proportions of subtypes | Normal | Normal | Intrinsic defect in B-cell maturation at plasma cell level | Unknown |
| Normal or increased B-cell number | Decreased | Decreased | Normal or increased | Variable | Variable | Intrinsic defect in B-cell to plasma cell maturation | Unknown |
| Common variable immunodeficiency with predominant immunoregulatory T-cell disorder | | | | | | | |
| Deficiency of T helper cells | Decreased | Decreased | Normal | Variable | Variable | Immunoregulatory T-cell disorder: defect in thymocyte to helper-T-cell differentiation | Unknown |
| Presence of activated T suppressor cells | Decreased | Decreased | Normal | Variable | Variable | Immunoregulatory helper-T-cell disorder | Unknown |
| Common variable immunodeficiency with autoantibodies to B or T cells | Decreased | Decreased | Decreased | Decreased | Variable | Variable; no differentiation defect known | Unknown |

AR, autosomal recessive; AD, autosomal dominant; Ig, immunoglobulin; CMI, cellular-mediated immunity.

**Table 57.3** Predominantly Cell-Mediated Immunity Defects

| *Designation* | Usual phenotypic expression: Serum Ig | Serum antibodies | Circulating B cells | Circulating T cells | CMI | *Presumed nature of basic defect* | *Inheritance* |
|---|---|---|---|---|---|---|---|
| Combined immunodeficiency with T-cell defect | Near-normal or progressive decrease | Decreased | Normal | Decreased | Decreased | Unknown: defect involves T-cell differentiation | Unknown, AR |
| Purine nucleoside phosphorylase deficiency | Normal | Normal | Normal | Progressive decrease | Progressive decrease | T-cell defect from toxic metabolites resulting from enzyme deficiency | AR |
| Severe combined immunodeficiency with adenosine deaminase deficiency | Decreased | Decreased | Decreased | Decreased | Decreased | T- and B-cell defects from toxic metabolites resulting from enzyme deficiency | AR |
| Severe combined immunodeficiency | | | | | | | |
| Reticular dysgenesis | Decreased | Decreased | Decreased | Decreased | Decreased | Defective differentiation of T and B cells; lymphomyeloid maturation defect | AR |
| Low T and B cells | Decreased | Decreased | Decreased | Decreased | Decreased | Lymphoid maturation defect of both T and B cells | AR or X-linked |
| Low T cells, normal B cells (Swiss) | Decreased | Decreased | Normal | Decreased | Decreased | Lymphoid maturation defect of both T and B cells | AR or X-linked |
| "Bare lymphocyte syndrome" | Decreased | Decreased | Decreased | Decreased | Decreased | Differentiation defect with lack of HLA determinants on T and B cells | AR |
| ID with unusual response to EBV | Decreased after EBV infection in some | Decreased after EBV infection in some | Decreased after EBV infection in most | Normal | Normal | Unknown | X-linked or AR |

AR, autosomal recessive; AD, autosomal dominant; Ig, immunoglobulin; CMI, cellular-mediated immunity; ID, immunodeficiency; EBV, Epstein–Barr virus.

**Table 57.4** Immunodeficiencies Associated With Other Major Defects

| | *Usual phenotypic expression* | | | | | | |
|---|---|---|---|---|---|---|---|
| ***Designation*** | **Serum Ig** | **Serum antibodies** | **Circulating B cells** | **Circulating T cells** | **CMI** | ***Presumed nature of basic defect*** | ***Inheritance*** |
| Transcobalamin deficiency | All isotypes decreased | Decreased | Normal | Normal | Normal | Defect in $B_{12}$ transport resulting in defective cell proliferation; defect in B-cell to plasma cell differentiation | AR |
| Wiskott–Aldrich syndrome | Increased IgA, IgE; decreased IgM | Decreased | Normal | Progressive decrease | Progressive decrease | Cell membrane defect affecting all hematopoietic stem cell derivatives | X-linked |
| Ataxia telangiectasia | Often decreased IgA, IgE, IgG; increased IgM (monomers) | Variably decreased | Normal | Decreased | Decreased | Unknown: defective T-cell maturation | AR |
| Third- and fourth-pouch/arch syndrome (DiGeorge) | Normal (?) | Decreased | Normal | Decreased | Decreased | Embryopathy: abnormal thymus with resultant T-cell defects | None |

AR, autosomal recessive; AD, autosomal dominant; Ig, immunoglobulin; CMI, cellular-mediated immunity.

**Table 57.5** Characteristics of Human Immunoglobulins

| *Antibody class* | *Biological activity* | *Number of subclasses* | *Serum half-life (d)* | *Serum concentration (mg/dL)* |
|---|---|---|---|---|
| IgG | Toxin neutralizing<br>Opsonization<br>Bacteriolytic<br>Complement activation | 4 | 23 | 550–1,900 |
| IgM | Toxin neutralizing<br>Bacteriolytic<br>Complement activation | 2 | 5 | 45–145 |
| IgA | Toxin neutralizing<br>Secretory antibody | 2 | 6 | 60–330 |
| IgD | Antigen receptor on B cells | 0 | 3 | 2–5 |
| IgE | Mediates allergic reactions<br>Binds to mast cells | 0 | 3 | ~ 0.02 |

## Evaluation of Immune Function

### *Cellular Immunity*

Cellular immunity can be evaluated both in vivo and in vitro. Delayed cutaneous hypersensitivity testing is used in the clinical setting to evaluate cellular immune function. When certain antigens are injected intradermally into an immunologically competent person, a delayed-type hypersensitivity reaction occurs. Antigens often used include mumps, purified protein derivative (PPD), trichophyton, and *Candida albicans*. Erythema and induration are usually measured after 48 hours. Delayed cutaneous hypersensitivity is often depressed in congenital and acquired immunodeficiencies, as well as in many other disease states.

Lymphocytes and lymphocyte subpopulations can be enumerated using a variety of different methods. Although quantification of lymphocyte numbers may be helpful for diagnosis,

**Figure 57.1** Overview of the human immune system. Pluripotent stem cells differentiate in primary lymphoid organs into mature T or B lymphocytes. T lymphocytes have regulatory and effector functions; B cells are responsible for antibody production. Soluble substances secreted by immunocompetent cells such as macrophage interleukin-1 and T-cell interleukin-2 enhance immune responses, whereas other substances such as prostaglandins suppress immune responses. $T_E$, effector T cells; $T_S$, suppressor T cells; $T_H$, helper T cells; M, macrophages; B, B cells; P, plasma cells.

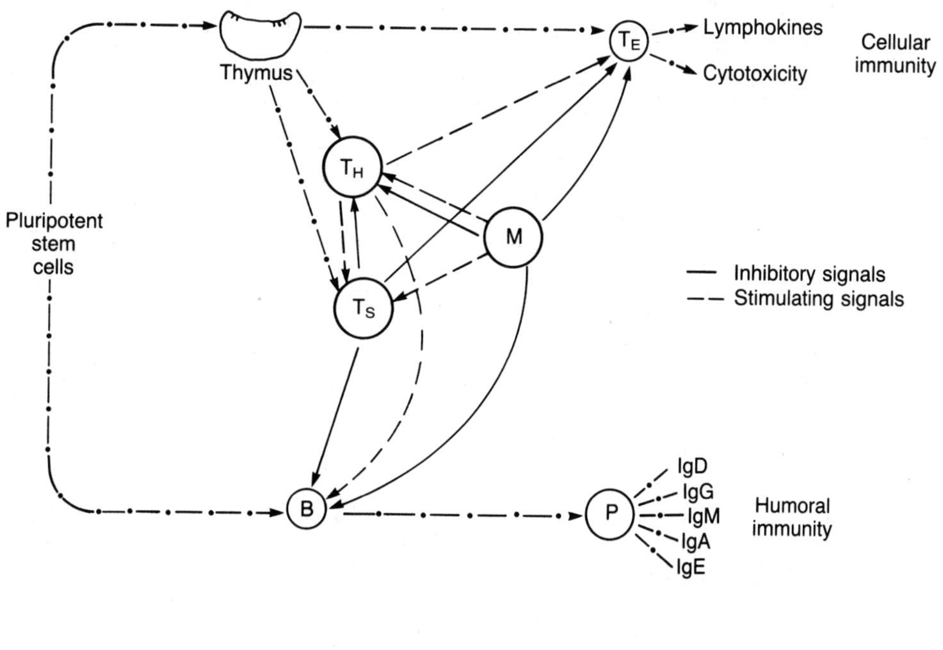

assessment of lymphocyte function may be more meaningful. A useful tool to assess lymphocyte function is measurement of in vitro lymphocyte proliferation in response to various stimuli, such as nonspecific mitogens, specific antigens, or allogeneic cells. Failure of lymphocytes to proliferate in vitro is evidence suggestive of cellular defects. Decreased in vitro lymphocyte proliferation is seen not only in certain immunodeficiency diseases, but also in a number of other diseases.

### *Humoral Immunity*

Serum immunoglobulin concentrations can be measured by a number of different methods to screen for antibody deficiency. In some immunodeficiency disease states, total immunoglobulin concentrations may be normal; however, antigen-specific antibodies may not be present. Various in vitro assays are available to measure concentrations of antigen-specific antibodies in serum and other biologic fluids. Lymphocytes may also be cultured in vitro to assess their ability to produce antibodies. Complement deficiencies are detected by measuring individual complement components or complement lytic activity in serum.

## Antibody Deficiency Diseases

Antibody deficiency disorders may occur as congenital or acquired diseases, with deficiencies of all immunoglobulin classes or of only one class or subclass of immunoglobulin. The inability to form an antibody against a specific antigen, or the absence of an immunoglobulin subclass, may be seen in patients with normal total serum immunoglobulin concentrations. Therefore, routine screening for total immunoglobulin concentrations can be misleading. The general clinical features of antibody deficiency diseases are shown in Table 57.6. Clinical characteristics may range from asymptomatic, as seen in selective IgA deficiency, to severe recurrent pyogenic bacterial infections, as seen in X-linked agammaglobulinemia.

### *X-Linked Agammaglobulinemia*

This disease is also known as congenital, infantile, or sex-linked agammaglobulinemia or as Bruton's disease. The term agammaglobulinemia is a misnomer, as small amounts of serum immunoglobulin may be present.[4] The majority of patients do well during the first 6 to 9 months of life because of the presence of maternal antibody. As maternal antibody concentrations decrease, recurrent pyogenic infections begin to appear during infancy and early childhood. Common infectious organisms include pneumococci, streptococci, and *Hemophilus*.[3,4] Common types of infection include sinusitis, pneumonia, otitis, furunculosis, meningitis, and septicemia. Chronic fungal and viral infections are not usually a common problem because T-lymphocyte function remains intact.[4] These patients are at risk of developing vaccine-associated poliomyelitis and infections from certain enteric pathogens, such as echoviruses and *Giardia lamblia*.[5] Patients may present with chronic diarrhea or spruelike symptoms and protein-losing enteropathies.

This disease occurs only in boys. Currently, there are no markers to identify to heterozygotes. The diagnosis is suspected if serum IgA, IgG, and IgM concentrations fall below the 95% confidence limits for age- and race-matched controls.[4] The pathogenetic defect appears to be a block in the maturation of pre-B-cell to B-cell differentiation.[5] There are few B cells in peripheral circulation, but the normal number of pre-B cells in bone marrow.[4] Normal or increased numbers of T cells are found in the circulation and cellular immunity is normal. X-linked agammaglobulinemia is associated with other disease states, such as rheumatoid arthritis, leukemia, and other lymphoreticular malignancies.[4] Prognosis is reasonably good if immunoglobulin replacement (discussed later in this chapter) is initiated early.

**Table 57.6** Common Clinical Features of Antibody Deficiencies

| |
|---|
| Recurrent pyogenic infections with encapsulated bacteria |
| Chronic sinopulmonary problems |
| Enteroviral infections |
| Low or absent antibodies in serum and secretions |
| B cells may be present in circulation |

### *Common Variable Agammaglobulinemia*

This deficiency is also known as agammaglobulinemia with immunoglobulin-bearing B lymphocytes, idiopathic late-onset immunoglobulin deficiency, and common variable immunodeficiency. Unlike X-linked agammaglobulinemia, this immunodeficiency can occur at any age with a similar incidence in males and females.[5] Its clinical presentation may be similar to that of X-linked agammaglobulinemia. In common variable immunodeficiency there is a high incidence of gastrointestinal abnormalities with a spruelike syndrome, often caused by *Giardia lamblia*, and a high incidence of gastrointestinal tumors. One third of these patients develop pernicious anemia.[5] Other complications include bronchiectasis and lymphoreticular malignancies.

Patients with common variable agammaglobulinemia usually have a normal number of circulating B lymphocytes, although some patients have been described with decreased numbers of B cells. As implied in the name of the disease, variable pathogenetic mechanisms are responsible for this immunodeficiency. The major defect is in the differentiation of mature B lymphocytes into antibody-secreting plasma cells.[3] Abnormal function of regulatory T lymphocytes may be a factor in some patients, with either an abnormality in helper T cells or overactive suppressor cells.[5–7] Autoantibodies to lymphocytes may also be involved.[5]

### *Selective IgA Deficiency*

The most common immunodeficiency in man is selective IgA deficiency, with a frequency of approximately 1 in 700 people.[5] Many individuals are unaware that they have abnormally low serum IgA concentrations, as many of these people never exhibit any signs or symptoms of this disorder. IgA is the major immunoglobulin in secretions providing mucosal immunity, and as would be expected, infections of the respiratory, gastrointestinal, and genitourinary tracts predominate in symptomatic patients. IgA may prevent bacteria from attaching to mucosal surfaces. Usually, encapsulated bacteria are responsible for recurrent infections and there is no evidence for increased susceptibility to viral pathogens. IgA deficiency may be associated with certain autoimmune diseases, such as rheumatoid arthritis, systemic lupus erythematosus, pernicious anemia, and thyroiditis.[8] It is not understood why some patients with this deficiency remain healthy while others become seriously ill.

Decreased serum IgA concentrations have been reported to occur with phenytoin and penicillamine therapy.[4,9] Apparently, phenytoin can induce suppressor cells, causing hypogammaglobulinemia.[9] This drug-induced problem resolves when the drugs are discontinued. It is possible to have normal serum IgA concentrations with an absence of IgA in secretions because of a deficiency of secretory component, necessary for IgA transport across mucosal surfaces into secretions.[10]

There is no specific therapy for IgA deficiency other than appropriate antibiotics for specific infections. Replacement of serum IgA is not useful, as it will not be transported into secretions. Secretory IgA must be produced locally in the mucosa to enter secretions. Many of these patients have antibodies directed against IgA.[11]

### *Treatment*

The treatment for most antibody-deficiency diseases is replacement therapy with γ-globulin. γ-Globulin can be administered by either intramuscular or intravenous route. A large multicenter crossover study showed that there are no differences between intramuscular and intravenous therapy in preventing acute and chronic infections.[12]

Many problems are associated with intramuscular therapy, including (1) acute pain at the injection site, (2) prolonged pain (several days) caused by prolonged distribution of the bolus from the injection site, (3) limitation of dose by small muscle mass in infants and children, (4) degradation of the γ-globulin by proteolytic enzymes at the injection site before absorption, (5) low serum IgG concentrations, and (6) delayed (1–2 weeks) time to peak serum concentrations.

Intravenous γ-globulin has eliminated many of the problems of intramuscular therapy and is now the preferred route for most patients. The recommended minimum dose of intravenous γ-globulin for antibody deficiency is usually 100–200 mg/kg every 4 weeks. This dose increases the serum IgG concentration approximately 250 to 300 mg/dL over baseline.[13] Higher doses may be given, but there are no data showing better efficacy with larger doses. There is large interpatient variability, but little intrapatient variability, in the pharmacokinetics of intravenous γ-globulin. It is therefore necessary to establish a time–dose relationship for each patient. Sequential serum IgG concentrations should be obtained every 7 days throughout two cycles of therapy.[13] The goal of treatment is to maintain trough serum IgG concentrations above 350 mg/dL. Optimal doses for intravenous γ-globulin have not been established.[13]

Selective IgA deficiency patients should never receive any γ-globulin preparation containing IgA because of the risk of life-threatening anaphylaxis. Also, patients with common variable hypogammaglobulinemia with undetectable IgA concentrations can develop IgE anti-IgA antibodies and have anaphylactic reactions to γ-globulin treatment.[14]

## Cellular Immunodeficiency Diseases

### *Combined Immunodeficiency With Predominant T-Cell Defect*

This immunodeficiency, also known as Nezelof's syndrome, is characterized by lymphopenia. Patients have normal serum immunoglobulin concentrations, although they often fail to make specific antibody in response to a foreign antigen. The general clinical features of cellular immunodeficiencies are shown in Table 57.7. Patients with Nezelof's syndrome often present with recurrent or chronic infections of the lung, skin, genitourinary tract, and blood and failure to thrive.[3] Delayed cutaneous hypersensitivity testing is negative and lymphocytes fail to proliferate in vitro to mitogenic stimulation. Long-term prognosis in these patients is poor.

### *Severe Combined Immunodeficiency Disease*

This disorder presents as a heterogeneous clinical entity and is the most severe form of immunodeficiency. The most common clinical symptoms are failure to thrive and severe illness in the first few months of life.[15] Persistent oral and perianal candidiasis is frequent. Intractable diarrhea and malabsorption, often secondary to enteric viral infections, are common.[15] Pneumonia from *Pneumocystis carinii* is often seen.[5]

This disease is inherited as an autosomal recessive or X-linked recessive trait, with about 75% of cases occurring in males.[5,15] Both cellular immunity and humoral immunity are affected. Patients exhibit delayed cutaneous hypersensitivity anergy, impaired in vitro lymphocyte proliferation, and inability to reject transplants. Specific antibody formation in response to vaccinations does not occur. Variants of this disease are listed in Table 57.3.

The pathogenesis of this disease is very heterogeneous. In some patients there is a total absence of B lymphocytes, while in others markedly elevated numbers of circulating B lymphocytes are found.[16] Lymphocyte dysfunction is the result of defects in differentiation occurring at one or more sites.[17] In addition, increased suppressor-T-cell activity or decreased helper-T-cell function may have a role in the pathogenesis of this disease.[16] Evidence also suggests that in some patients B-lymphocyte dysfunction is secondary to abnormal T-lymphocyte function[18,19] and that partial B-cell function can be restored when exposed to normal T-cell helper factors.[16,17]

**Table 57.7** Common Clinical Features of Cellular Immunodeficiencies

| |
|---|
| Recurrent infections with opportunistic organisms such as fungi, viruses, and *Pneumocystis carinii* |
| Lack of delayed cutaneous hypersensitivity |
| High incidence of malignancy |
| Major developmental defects |

### *Treatment*

The cellular immunodeficiency diseases are not easily treated. The only useful treatment is immunologic reconstitution. Advances in bone marrow transplantation have made it possible to restore both cellular and humoral abnormalities in severe combined immunodeficiency.[20,21] If immunocompetent-tissue transplantation is unsuccessful, death is almost a certainty within the first year of life. The only other therapeutic alternative is to keep these patients in a totally sterile environment.[3]

## Immunodeficiency Associated With Other Major Defects

### *Wiskott–Aldrich Syndrome*

This syndrome is characterized by severe eczema, thrombocytopenia, and opportunistic infections. There is abnormal cellular immunity and a decreased ability to make antigen-specific antibody. In addition, these patients have decreased platelet survival and platelet function. Patients usually die from overwhelming viral or bacterial infections, hemorrhagic episodes, or tumors within the first decade of life.[22,23] Complete remission of this disease from bone marrow transplantation has been reported.[4]

### *Third- and Fourth-Pouch Syndrome*

This disorder, also known as DiGeorge syndrome, results from dysmorphogenesis of the third and fourth pharyngeal pouches during embryogenesis.[4] This causes either hypoplasia or aplasia of the thymus and parathyroid glands. Other embryologic abnormalities include right-sided aortic arch, aberrant origin of the left subclavian artery, low-set ears, midline facial clefts, and hypertelorism.[24] Cardiac defects are often responsible for deaths in these patients. The diagnosis is usually suspected because of hypocalcemia and tetany during the neonatal period.[4] Abnormal cellular immunity is present and infections are frequent during infancy. Thymus gland or thymic epithelial cell transplants have been successful in controlling the immunologic abnormalities, but reconstitution may last only a few years.[24]

## Effects of Aging on Immune Responses

Aging is associated with a partial failure of the immune system. This abnormality, referred to as immunosenescence, may contribute to the high incidence of neoplastic, infectious, and autoimmune diseases in the elderly.[25] Both cellular and humoral immunity may be affected. Many studies show a decrease in the total number of mature T lymphocytes in peripheral blood of elderly subjects, although this is not a consistent finding.[26–28] Elderly individuals may exhibit delayed cutaneous hypersensitivity anergy and decreased lymphocyte proliferation in vitro to various stimuli.

Although the absolute number of circulating B lymphocytes does not change with aging, senescent B cells lose their ability to function and respond normally.[29,30] Abnormal regulation of antibody production is a common finding in the elderly. This is evident in the high incidence of autoantibody production, decreased ability to produce antibodies to foreign antigens, and occurrence of benign monoclonal gammopathies. Abnormal antibody production in the elderly is a result of both altered B-lymphocyte function and impaired immunoregulatory T lymphocytes.[25]

There is no specific treatment available to reverse immunosenescence. It is important that all elderly persons receive appropriate vaccinations to enhance their immunity to common infectious pathogens. Because of the increasing geriatric population and because their associated chronic diseases are risk factors for severe pneumococcal and influenza illnesses, the future mortality from these diseases is likely to increase unless steps are taken to provide immunization to all elderly individuals. All elderly persons should be routinely immunized against pneumococcus, influenza, and tetanus.

Pneumococcal vaccine and influenza vaccine can be given together at the same time at different sites without increased side effects.[31] Influenza vaccine is given annually, but pneumococcal vaccine is given only once. All elderly persons should be given a detailed immunization record to ensure that additional doses of pneumococcal vaccine are not given.[31]

## References


1. Bruton OC. Agammaglobulinemia. Pediatrics 1952;9:722–727.
2. Meeting report. Primary immunodeficiency diseases. Report prepared for the WHO by a scientific group on immunodeficiency. Clin Immunol Immunopathol 1983;28:450–475.
3. Buckley RH. Immunodeficiency. J Allergy Clin Immunol 1983; 72:627–641.
4. Cooper MD, Buckley RH. Developmental immunology and the immunodeficiency diseases. JAMA 1982;248:2658–2669.
5. Rosen FS, Cooper MD, Wedgwood RJP. The primary immunodeficiencies, parts 1 and 2. N Engl J Med 1984;311:235–242, 300–310.
6. Geha RS, Schneeberger E, Merler E, et al. Heterogeneity of "acquired" or common variable agammaglobulinemia. N Engl J Med 1974;291:1–6.
7. Waldmann TA. Disorders of suppressor cells with common variable hypogammaglobulinemia and selective IgA deficiency, in Waldmann TA (moderator): Disorders of suppressor immunoregulatory cells in the pathogenesis of immunodeficiency and autoimmunity. Ann Intern Med 1978;88:226–238.
8. Ammann AJ, Hong R. Selective IgA deficiency: Presentation of 30 cases and a review of the literature. Medicine 1971;50:223–236.
9. Dosch HM, Jason J, Gelfand EW. Transient antibody deficiency and abnormal T suppressor cells induced by phenytoin. N Engl J Med 1982;306:406–409.
10. Strober W, Krakauer R, Klaeveman HL, et al. Secretory component deficiency: A disorder of the IgA immune system. N Engl J Med 1976;294:351–356.

11. Koistinen J, Heikkila M, Leikola J. Gammaglobulin treatment and anti-IgA antibodies in IgA-deficient patients. Br Med J 1978;2:923–924.
12. Ammann AJ, Ashman RF, Buckley RH, et al. Use of intravenous gamma globulin in antibody immunodeficiency: Results of a multicenter controlled trial. Clin Immunol Immunopathol 1982;22:60–67.
13. Pirofsky B. Intravenous immune globulin therapy in hypogammaglobulinemia. Am J Med 1984;76(3A):53–60.
14. Burks AW, Sampson HA, Buckley RH. Anaphylactic reactions after gamma globulin administration in patients with hypogammaglobulinemia. Detection of IgE antibodies to IgA. N Engl J Med 1986;314:560–564.
15. Gelfand EW, Dosch HM. Diagnosis and classification of severe combined immunodeficiency disease. Birth Defects 1983;19:65–72.
16. Pahwa SG, Pahwa RN, Good RA. Heterogeneity of B lymphocyte differentiation in severe combined immunodeficiency disease. J Clin Invest 1980;66:543–550.
17. Pahwa RN, Pahwa SG, Good RA. T-lymphocyte differentiation in vitro in severe combined immunodeficiency. J Clin Invest 1979;64:1632–1641.
18. Seeger RC, Robins RA, Stevens RH, et al. Severe combined immunodeficiency with B lymphocytes: In vitro correction of defective immunoglobulin production by addition of normal T lymphocytes. Clin Exp Immunol 1976;26:1–10.
19. Dosch HM, Lee JWW, Gelfand EW, et al. Severe combined immunodeficiency disease: A model of T cell dysfunction. Clin Exp Immunol 1978;34:260–267.
20. Reinherz EL, Geha R, Rappeport JM, et al. Reconstitution after transplantation with T-lymphocyte–depleted HLA haplotype–mismatched bone marrow for severe combined immunodeficiency. Proc Natl Acad Sci USA 1982;79:6047–6051.
21. Reisner Y, Kapoor N, Kirkpatrick D, et al. Transplantation for severe combined immunodeficiency with HLA-A, B, C, D, DR incompatible parental marrow cells fractionated by soybean agglutinin and sheep red blood cells. Blood 1983;61:341–348.
22. Parkman R, Rappeport J, Geha R, et al. Complete correction of the Wiskott–Aldrich syndrome by allogeneic bone-marrow transplantation. N Engl J Med 1978;298:921–927.
23. Perry GS, Spector BD, Schuman LM, et al. The Wiskott–Aldrich syndrome in the United States and Canada (1892–1979). J Pediatr 1980;97:72–78.
24. Thong YH, Robertson EF, Rischbieth HG, et al. Successful restoration of immunity in the DiGeorge syndrome with fetal thymic epithelial transplant. Arch Dis Child 1978;53:580–584.
25. Delafuente JC. Immunosenescence. Clinical and pharmacologic considerations. Med Clin North Am 1985;69:475–586.
26. Hallgren HM, Jackola DR, O'Leary JJ. Unusual pattern of surface marker expression on peripheral lymphocytes from aged humans suggestive of a population of less differentiated cells. J Immunol 1983;131:191–194.
27. Nagel JE, Chrest FJ, Pyle RS, et al. Monoclonal antibody analysis of T-lymphocyte subsets in young and aged adults. Immunol Commun 1983;12:223–237.
28. Barrett DJ, Stenmark S, Wara DW, et al. Immunoregulation in aged humans. Clin Immunol Immunopathol 1980;17:203–211.
29. Ceuppens JL, Goodwin JS. Regulation of immunoglobulin production in pokeweed mitogen–stimulated cultures of lymphocytes from young and old adults. J Immunol 1982;128:2429–2434.
30. Ennist DL, Jones KH, St. Pierre RL, et al. Functional analysis of the immunosenescence of the human B cell system: Dissociation of normal activation and proliferation from impaired terminal differentiation into IgM immunoglobulin-secreting cells. J Immunol 1986;136:99–105.
31. Centers for Disease Control. Prevention and control of influenza: Recommendation of the Immunization Practices Advisory Committee. Ann Intern Med 1985;103:560–565.

# Chapter 58 / Systemic Lupus Erythematosus

Mark B. Burlingame, PharmD, and Jeffrey C. Delafuente, MS

Systemic lupus erythematosus (SLE) is a fluctuating, multisystem disease with a diversity of clinical presentations. Because of this variability, other diseases are often considered and subsequently "ruled out" before a diagnosis is made. Abnormal immunologic function and formation of antibodies against "self" antigens underlie the pathogenesis of this disease.

*Lupus* is the Latin word for "wolf" and was first used to describe erosive skin lesions that looked as though a wolf had eaten away the flesh.[1] The term *lupus erythematosus* was first used in 1851 by Cazenave, a Frenchman who described an illness in a patient with manifestations occurring only in the skin.[1,2] It is not surprising that SLE was first recognized as a skin disorder, as cutaneous manifestations constitute one of the most common clinical features of the disease. Further descriptions by Kaposi in 1872 and Osler in 1895 led to the concept of a multisystem disease, as it became recognized that patients developed other complications such as fever, pneumonia, and anemia as well as involvement of the joints, heart, kidneys, and other organ systems.[1,2]

Autoantibodies in this disease became apparent with the development of the lupus erythematosus (LE) cell test in 1948 and the fluorescent antinuclear antibody (ANA) test in 1957.[1,2] Recognition of SLE as an autoimmune disease of multisystemic nature led the American Rheumatism Association (ARA) to develop criteria for identifying lupus patients (Table 58.1). These criteria were originally developed in 1971 and revised in 1982 and are used primarily for determining SLE patients for clinical studies.[3] To classify a patient as having SLE, 4 or more of the 11 criteria must be present. Although these criteria may be helpful, diagnosis requires additional serologic and immunopathologic evaluations.

## Epidemiology

The incidence of SLE has been reported as 1.0 to 7.6 per 100,000 population per year, with a prevalence of 5.8 to 51.0 per 100,000 population.[4] The disease occurs predominantly in women, with a reported female:male ratio approaching 10:1.[5] This predominance is most visible during reproductive years which has led to the suggestion that SLE development may be related to hormonal factors. The incidence in blacks and some other races appears higher than in whites.[5,6] An earlier age of disease onset has also been reported in blacks compared with whites.[6,7] Although the most typical SLE patient is a young adult female, the disease can occur in people of any age, race, and sex.

## Pathophysiology

### *Autoantibodies*

A major event in the development of SLE is excessive and abnormal autoantibody production. Many of these antibodies are directed against nuclear constituents of the cell and are called collectively antinuclear antibodies. An SLE patient often has many antinuclear antibodies in serum and tissue. These are antibodies against such nuclear constituents as double-stranded or native DNA (dsDNA), single-stranded or denatured DNA (ssDNA), RNA, nuclear ribonuclear protein (nRNP), nucleohistone, and an acidic nuclear protein called Sm antigen.[8,9] Patients with SLE also have antibody to cytoplasmic constituents such as ribosome, a glycoprotein named Ro, and a soluble tissue protein referred to as the lupus anticoagulant (La).[8,10] Antibodies may also be directed against circulating cells such as lymphocytes, red cells, granulocytes, and platelets as well as against clotting factors (lupus anticoagulant).[11–14] Sometimes antibodies may be directed against cardiolipin, which produces a false-positive serologic test for syphilis.[8] Antineuronal antibodies have also been observed and may correlate with neuropsychiatric SLE.[15]

The abnormal and excessive production of these autoantibodies may be related to a defect in lymphocyte regulation. Although the absolute number of lymphocytes is decreased in SLE, there is an increase in B-cell activity and subsequently an increase in antibody production.[12] There is some evidence that the increase in B-cell activity may be related to a loss of suppressor T-cell function, with a resultant reduction in autoregulation of B-cell activity.[11,12]

The mechanism of tissue injury in SLE is not completely understood but is thought to be related to immune complex formation, primarily DNA–anti-DNA immune complexes.[16] The model states that immune complexes are not completely removed by the reticuloendothelial system and deposit in the kidney and other tissues, resulting in cell damage, complement fixation, and inflammation.

The etiology of abnormal autoantibody production and development of SLE is still unknown. Many factors have been implicated as having a role in the expression of the disease and some of these factors are discussed here.

### *Environment*

It has been suggested that SLE is caused by an infectious virus or some other transmissible agent. Findings that suggest this include the observation of tubuloreticular structures in the kidneys, increased levels of antiviral antibodies in SLE patients, presence of lymphocytotoxic antibodies in

**Table 58.1** The 1982 Revised Criteria for Classification of Systemic Lupus Erythematosus[a]

| *Criterion* | *Definition* |
|---|---|
| Malar rash | Fixed erythema, flat or raised, over the malar eminences, tending to spare the nasolabial folds |
| Discoid rash | Erythematous raised patches with adherent keratotic scaling and follicular plugging; atrophic scarring may occur in older lesions |
| Photosensitivity | Skin rash as a result of unusual reaction to sunlight, by patient history or physician observation |
| Oral ulcers | Oral or nasopharyngeal ulceration, usually painless, observed by a physician |
| Arthritis | Nonerosive arthritis involving two or more peripheral joints, characterized by tenderness, swelling, or effusion |
| Serositis | Pleuritis—convincing history of pleuritic pain or rub heard by a physician or evidence of pleural effusion<br>*or*<br>Pericarditis—documented by ECG or rub or evidence of pericardial effusion |
| Renal disorder | Persistent proteinuria greater than 0.5 g/d or greater than 3+ if quantitation not performed<br>*or*<br>Cellular casts—may be red cell, hemoglobin, granular, tubular, or mixed |
| Neurologic disorder | Seizures—in the absence of offending drugs or known metabolic derangements, e.g., uremia, ketoacidosis, or electrolyte imbalance<br>*or*<br>Psychosis—in the absence of offending drugs or known metabolic derangements, e.g., uremia, ketoacidosis, or electrolyte imbalance |
| Hematologic disorder | Hemolytic anemia—with reticulocytosis<br>*or*<br>Leukopenia—fewer than 4,000/$mm^3$ total on two or more occasions<br>*or*<br>Lymphopenia—fewer than 1,500/$mm^3$ on two or more occasions<br>*or*<br>Thrombocytopenia—fewer than 100,000/$mm^3$ in the absence of offending drugs |
| Immunologic disorder | Positive LE cell preparation<br>*or*<br>Anti-DNA; antibody to native DNA in abnormal titer<br>*or*<br>Anti-Sm; presence of antibody to Sm nuclear antigen<br>*or*<br>False-positive serologic test for syphilis known to be positive for at least 6 months and confirmed by *Treponema pallidum* immobilization or fluorescent treponemal antibody absorption test |
| Antinuclear antibody | An abnormal titer of antinuclear antibody by immunofluorescence or an equivalent assay at any point in time and in the absence of drugs known to be associated with "drug-induced lupus" syndrome |

[a] The proposed classification is based on 11 criteria. For the purpose of identifying patients in clinical studies, a person shall be said to have systemic lupus erythematosus if any 4 or more of the 11 criteria are present, serially or simultaneously, during any interval of observation.

From Tan EM, Cohen AS, Fries JF, et al: The 1982 revised criteria for the classification of systemic lupus erythematosus. Arthritis Rheum 1982;25:1271–1277.

household contacts of SLE patients, and occurrence of antibodies to denatured DNA in laboratory workers who have been exposed to SLE sera.[5] These findings have been inconsistent and attempts to isolate a virus have been unsuccessful. It has also been suggested that a viral or bacterial antigen may trigger the disease by stimulating an abnormal immune response in genetically predisposed individuals.[16]

### *Hormones*

The higher incidence of SLE in women of reproductive age has led to the belief that the disease may be under hormonal control. Studies in mice suggest that estrogen enhances, and androgen inhibits, the expression of autoimmunity.[16]

### *Genetics*

There is good evidence for the existence of genetic predisposition in the development of SLE. Seven to twelve percent of SLE patients have a first- or second-degree relative with the disease.[17] A 69% concordance of disease has been reported in monozygotic twins; however, the risk in dizygotic twins is the same as that in first-degree relatives.[16] Much attention has been focused on the major histocompatibility complex of man, HLA, and its association with SLE. Antigens encoded by the HLA-D region, specifically, the D-related (DR) antigens HLA-DR2 and HLA-DR3, have been associated with the disease.[16,17] Other HLA-associated antigens, MT1 and MT2, have also been linked to SLE.[17] Hereditary deficiencies of various components of the complement system have been associated with autoimmune diseases, although this is probably not a major factor predisposing to SLE. Deficiencies of C2 and C4 appear to correlate best with development of a lupuslike illness.[16,17]

## Clinical Presentation

As previously mentioned, SLE is a multisystemic disease. Table 58.2 lists many of the signs and symptoms that may present in a patient with SLE. While certain of these may be more common than others, each patient presents differently and the course of the disease is highly unpredictable. Furthermore, lupus is not static, and most patients have fluctuations or "flare-ups" during the course of the disease.

Such signs and symptoms as fatigue, fever, anorexia, and weight loss are referred to as constitutional manifestations and are frequently seen in patients with active disease.[18] Musculoskeletal involvement (e.g., arthralgia, myalgia, arthritis) is very common in SLE. Approximately 90% of patients develop this type of manifestation at some time during the course of the disease.[18] Joint involvement tends to be symmetrical and may affect multiple sites. Objective evidence of musculoskeletal disease is often missing, although a few patients may present with deforming arthritis or rheumatoid nodules.[18]

**Table 58.2** Clinical Signs and Symptoms of Systemic Lupus Erythematosus

| *Common features* | *Uncommon features* |
|---|---|
| Arthritis | Hepatomegaly |
| Arthralgias | Splenomegaly |
| Fever and constitutional symptoms | Retinopathy |
| Mucocutaneous involvement | Myalgias |
| Nephritis | Raynaud's phenomenon |
| Pleuritis | Abdominal pain |
| Pericarditis | |
| Libman–Sacks disease | |
| Lymphadenopathy | |
| Neuropsychiatric disease | |
| Anemia | |
| Leukopenia | |

Cutaneous manifestations are seen in approximately 85% of patients.[18] The most well known of these is the butterfly rash, which occurs over the bridge of the nose and the malar eminences and is often observed after sun exposure. The classic butterfly rash is generally seen in fewer than 50% of patients; however, one series reported a malar rash in 61% of 150 patients with SLE.[6] Another common skin manifestation is an erythematous, maculopapular rash which often resembles a cutaneous drug reaction.[18] This rash may also be produced by sun exposure. In fact, photosensitivity is common to many SLE patients who present with cutaneous manifestations. Patients should use sunscreens when outdoors for prolonged periods. Skin lesions characteristic of discoid lupus occur in 15% to 20% of patients.[18] Discoid lupus may be considered a chronic cutaneous form of SLE without other organ involvement. Other cutaneous manifestations include vasculitis (which may be ulcerative), livedo reticularis, erythema around the base of the nails, and alopecia.[18] Certain individuals are said to develop subacute cutaneous lupus erythematosus. These people develop a widespread rash in association with mild systemic disease and are thought to represent a subset of SLE, somewhere between discoid lupus erythematosus and severe SLE.[18]

After musculoskeletal and skin, the next most common manifestation of SLE involves the serous membranes.[6] Pleurisy may present as pleuritic pain, a pleural rub, or a pleural effusion. As many as 40% of patients may have a pleural effusion, which is usually exudative in nature.[19] Pericarditis is the most common cardiac manifestation of SLE. Pericarditis presents clinically in 20% to 30% of patients but may be evident echocardiographically in up to 75% of patients.[20]

Pulmonary involvement in SLE is not restricted to the pleura. Lupus pneumonitis may present acutely with fever, dyspnea, tachypnea, cough, rales, and patchy infiltrates or chronically with interstitial fibrosis.[21] Other pulmonary manifestations include atelectasis and diaphragmatic elevation and dysfunction.

In addition to pericarditis, other cardiovascular effects of SLE include myocarditis and endocarditis (Libman-Sacks disease), either of which may be accompanied by cardiac rhythm disturbances.[20] Atherosclerotic heart disease is occurring with increasing frequency in lupus patients as treatment modalities improve and patients live longer.[22] It is thought that corticosteroid therapy may contribute significantly to the development of heart disease in these patients.

Clinical evidence of kidney involvement is observed in approximately 50% of SLE patients and has been recognized as a significant factor associated with mortality,[23] although different types of lupus nephritis may be prognostically quite different.[24,25] A discussion of lupus nephritis is presented later.

Neuropsychiatric manifestations of SLE may present in a diversity of ways, from psychosis to seizure to peripheral neuropathy. This aspect of lupus is seen in 25% to 40% of patients and may be an important factor contributing to morbidity and mortality.[22,26]

The effects of SLE on the gastrointestinal tract are usually related to serositis or vasculitis and commonly present as

**Table 58.3** Antinuclear Antibody: Patterns, Antigens, and Specificities

| *Pattern* | *Antigen* | *Disease* |
|---|---|---|
| Peripheral | Double-stranded DNA | SLE |
| Speckled | Acidic nuclear protein | Rheumatoid arthritis |
| | Ribonucleoprotein | SLE |
| | Extractable nuclear antigen | Scleroderma |
| | | Mixed connective tissue disease |
| Homogeneous | Deoxyribonucleoprotein | Rheumatoid arthritis |
| | Histone | SLE |
| Nucleolar | Nucleolar RNA | Progressive systemic sclerosis |

abdominal pain. Hepatomegaly may present in some patients although liver dysfunction does not appear to be characteristic of lupus. Pancreatitis may also be present in an occasional patient.[19]

The clinical workup of an SLE patient may reveal nonspecific findings such as splenomegaly or lymph node enlargement. Ocular involvement sometimes occurs and may consist of lesions in the fundus called "cytoid bodies" or conjunctivitis like that seen in Sjögren's syndrome.[19]

### *Hematologic Manifestations*

Anemia is found in many cases of SLE. It is usually an anemia of chronic disease, with a mild normochromic, normocytic smear and low serum iron but adequate iron stores. Some patients may develop a hemolytic anemia with a positive Coombs' test.[12]

Leukopenia is present in nearly half of SLE patients. The leukopenia is generally not severe, as the total white blood cell count rarely falls below 2,000/mm$^3$.[27] Both granulocytes and lymphocytes may be affected but there is usually a much larger decrease in the amount of circulating granulocytes.[12] The absolute number of both T lymphocytes and B lymphocytes decreases.[12]

Thrombocytopenia is less common than anemia or leukopenia in SLE. Many patients have a shortened platelet survival time, with the bone marrow compensating by increasing the production of thrombocytes.[12] Another interesting finding in less than half of patients is the presence of an autoantibody referred to as the lupus anticoagulant (LA).[13,14] The presence of LA inhibits the prothrombinase complex and often results in prolongation of the activated partial thromboplastin time and, less commonly, prolongation of the prothrombin and thrombin times. Bleeding is rare and occurs only in conjunction with thrombocytopenia or a clotting factor deficiency. In fact, the presence of LA has been associated with an increased risk of thrombosis.[14] LA has also been associated with a biologic false-positive VDRL.[13]

Other laboratory abnormalities seen in SLE include an increase in the erythrocyte sedimentation rate, a decrease in serum albumin, and an increase in $\gamma$-globulins although patients with nephrotic syndrome may have decreased $\gamma$-globulins.[28] Serologic abnormalities are discussed further under Diagnosis.

### *Lupus Nephritis*

Clinical evidence of renal involvement, such as a rising serum creatinine or proteinuria, is generally associated with a poorer outcome than in patients without renal involvement[23]; however, the extent and course of renal disease are quite variable and many lupus nephritis patients do very well. The World Health Organization (WHO) has classified lupus nephritis on the basis of histologic characteristics. This system identifies lupus nephritis as mesangial, focal proliferative, diffuse proliferative, membranoproliferative, or membranous glomerulonephritis.[24] Many patients progress from one form of nephritis to another during the course of the disease. For example, a common progression is focal proliferative to diffuse proliferative glomerulonephritis. There is some evidence that the proliferative form of lupus nephritis, especially diffuse proliferative glomerulonephritis, is associated with a poorer outcome compared with other forms[24,25]; however, the prognostic value of the WHO histologic classification system is uncertain. It has been suggested that a chronicity index based on renal biopsy information would be a much better prognostic indicator.[24]

### *Diagnosis*

As mentioned earlier, the 1982 ARA criteria should not be the primary means for diagnosing SLE, although many of the criteria may be valuable in the diagnostic process. Epidemiologic characteristics, clinical signs and symptoms, and common laboratory abnormalities are all used in diagnosing SLE.

Once the disease is highly suspected, serologic tests may be useful in making the final diagnosis. The LE cell test recognizes phagocytic cells that engulf whole nuclear protein. This test lacks sensitivity and specificity and has been supplanted by other tests.[27] A serologic test extensively used to diagnose suspected SLE is the fluorescent antinuclear antibody (ANA) test. This test is very sensitive but not very specific for SLE.[3] That is, nearly all SLE patients are ANA positive, but other disease states may also be associated with a positive test (Table 58.3); however, in other diseases many of the positive ANA tests are of a lower titer.[28] The pattern of immunofluorescence of the ANA test may also be of diagnostic value (Table 58.3). A homogeneous pattern is not specific for SLE, whereas a peripheral pattern is very specific and confirms the diagnosis of lupus.[29]

**Table 58.4** Drug Treatment of Systemic Lupus Erythematosus

| *Drug class* | *Drug* | *Dose* | *Indication* |
|---|---|---|---|
| NSAID | Various agents | Anti-inflammatory dose | Mild disease: fever, arthritis, skin rash, serositis |
| Antimalarial | Hydroxychloroquine | 200–400 mg PO daily | Mild disease: arthritis, skin rash, serositis |
| | Chloroquine | 250–500 mg PO daily | |
| Corticosteroid | Prednisone | 1–2 mg/kg/d PO (or equivalent) | Initial control of severe disease |
| | | <1 mg/kg/d (or equivalent) | Control of mild disease or maintenance after disease suppression with higher doses |
| | Methylprednisolone | 1 g IV daily × 3 d | Life-threatening disease |
| Cytotoxic | Azathioprine | Up to 4 mg/kg/d PO | Most commonly used in severe lupus nephritis |
| | Cyclophosphamide | Up to 4 mg/kg/d PO | |
| | Cyclophosphamide | 0.5–1.0 g/m$^2$ IV every 3 mo | |

Assays for detecting antibodies to specific nuclear constituents may also be diagnostically useful. Antibodies to native DNA (dsDNA) and to Sm antigen are quite specific for SLE.[30]

### *Prognosis*

In earlier years, SLE was associated with a poor prognosis. For example, one report of cases diagnosed between 1949 and 1953 showed a 4-year survival rate of 51%.[31] Today, probably as a result of improved treatment and improved diagnostic techniques that allow earlier diagnosis, the 10-year survival rate has been reported at approximately 90%.[32]

The most important prognostic sign is that of lupus nephritis. A 10-year survival rate of 87% in patients without evidence of nephritis compared with 65% in patients with nephritis has been reported.[23] Central nervous system (CNS) involvement may also be associated with a poorer prognosis,[22,26] although this is probably not as significant as nephritis. Death from SLE is usually a result of kidney involvement, CNS disease, or infection[22,23]; however, cardiovascular disease as a cause of death is prominent in patients with disease of longer duration.[22]

Pregnancy in SLE patients has been associated with exacerbation of disease during pregnancy, exacerbation of disease during early postpartum, and a greater incidence of spontaneous abortion.[33,34] Once born, however, the infants appear to do as well as the general population.[34] Modification of drug therapy for SLE is usually not required during pregnancy. During labor and postpartum, an increase in corticosteroid dosage may decrease postpartum exacerbations of the disease.[34] The risks of pregnancy should be discussed with the patient but should not be an absolute contraindication to pregnancy.

## Treatment

### *Drugs*

Therapeutic management of SLE is not optimal because the disease process is not completely understood. Drug therapy consists of agents that suppress the immune response or inflammation.[16] Table 58.4 lists common agents that have been used in the United States to control SLE. In general, the choice of drug therapy depends on the extent and severity of disease.

#### Nonsteroidal Anti-inflammatory Drugs

As discussed earlier, such signs and symptoms as fever, arthritis, skin rash, and serositis are among the most common in patients with active disease. Therefore, in many patients with mild disease, initial treatment with a nonsteroidal anti-inflammatory drug (NSAID) is the most logical choice.

The choice of a NSAID in SLE is empiric. There is no evidence of superiority of one drug to another. The choice of drug may depend on such factors as response of the patient, tolerance to gastrointestinal irritation, development of adverse reactions, and cost of medication (aspirin being the least expensive). The dose used should be adequate to provide anti-inflammatory effects. For example, it has been stated that SLE patients using aspirin often improve with daily doses of 2.4–3.0 g. The effectiveness of a NSAID should be evaluated after an adequate trial of 2 to 4 weeks.[35]

SLE patients taking NSAIDs may develop changes in renal function because of drug effects and not the underlying disease. These changes may be manifested as increases in serum creatinine and BUN and a decrease in creatinine clearance. It has been suggested that high urinary prostaglandin excretion may be a characteristic of patients with SLE and make them more susceptible to the renal sequelae from prostaglandin inhibition.[36] Awareness of this effect is important, as declining renal function might be mistakenly attributed to progression of lupus nephritis. There also exist reports of an association between aseptic meningitis in SLE patients and the use of ibuprofen, tolmetin, and sulindac.[35,37]

#### Antimalarial Drugs

Antimalarial agents such as chloroquine and hydroxychloroquine have been used successfully in the management of discoid lupus and SLE.[38] In general, the manifestations of SLE that respond best to antimalarials are cutaneous manifestations, arthralgia, pleuritis, and mild pericardial inflammation.[38] Malaise and lethargy may also respond. Because these drugs are not effective immediately, they are best used in long-term management. Response occurs in 1 to 2 months in most patients.[39]

It is not known how these drugs work in lupus. It is believed that the 4-aminoquinolone moiety of the antimalarial may be necessary to be effective.[38] For example, pyrimethamine is an effective antimalarial drug, but differs in chemical structure and is ineffective in treating SLE. Several theories exist for the mechanism of action of antimalarials including reduced sensitivity to ultraviolet light, inhibitory effects on antibodies, anti-inflammatory activity, binding to nucleoprotein, and inhibition of the LE cell reaction.[38]

Dosage and duration of therapy depend upon patient response, tolerance to side effects, and development of retinal toxicity, which is a potentially irreversible adverse reaction associated with long-term therapy.[38] Current recommended doses for antimalarials in SLE are hydroxychloroquine 200–400 mg daily and chloroquine 250–500 mg daily.[37] Side effects of these drugs include malaise, dizziness, irritability, gastrointestinal disturbance (e.g., nausea), dermatitis, pigmentary changes of the skin and hair, and reversible cycloplegia resulting from deposition of the drug in the cornea.[38,40] The frequency of side effects reported in the literature is probably much higher than in present practice because of the higher dosages used previously.[40]

Retinal toxicity is rare when the currently recommended doses are used and may be least common with hydroxychloroquine[37,39,40]; however, because of the possibility of permanent damage associated with the retinopathy, an ophthalmologic evaluation should be done every 4 to 6 months.[38,39] If retinal abnormalities are noted, antimalarial therapy should be discontinued.

### Corticosteroids

Corticosteroid therapy is commonplace in therapeutic regimens for SLE. Although evidence for improved survival with corticosteroid therapy in SLE is inadequate, these agents are known to be effective in suppressing the clinical expression of disease and are considered by many to be a major factor in the improved prognosis of recent years.[37,41]

A patient with the diagnosis of SLE does not automatically require corticosteroid therapy. Mild disease with such manifestations as fever, arthralgia, pleuritis, or skin manifestations may respond adequately to NSAIDs or antimalarials; however, a patient with clinical manifestations that are more serious or unresponsive to other drugs may be an appropriate candidate for corticosteroids.

The goal of treatment when using corticosteroids in SLE is to suppress and maintain suppression of active disease with the lowest dose possible. In patients with mild disease, low-dose therapy (e.g., 15–20 mg prednisone daily) is adequate; however, in patients with more severe disease (e.g., severe hemolytic anemia or cardiac involvement) higher doses, such as prednisone 1–2 mg/kg daily, may be required.[37] Once adequate suppression of disease is achieved, the dose should be reduced to the minimum amount required for continued disease suppression. Because there may be a poorer prognosis associated with CNS disease in SLE, corticosteroid therapy has been examined with reference to this specific indication.[37] Corticosteroids in CNS lupus may be more difficult to evaluate because of the potential for steroid-induced CNS manifestations, which may be difficult to distinguish from disease exacerbation. It appears that high-dose corticosteroids may be beneficial in the treatment of neuropsychiatric manifestations of lupus; however, controlled clinical trials are needed.[26]

Because of the increased morbidity and mortality associated with lupus nephritis, there exists an ongoing examination of various therapeutic regimens to determine optimal drug therapy. The role of corticosteroids in lupus nephritis is not entirely clear. Patients with mesangial or membranous lupus nephritis tend to do well irrespective of treatment[25]; however, patients with proliferative lupus nephritis, the diffuse type in particular, tend to fare much worse.[24,25] It is thought that high-dose prednisone (i.e., >1 mg/kg daily) increases the survival of patients with diffuse proliferative glomerulonephritis,[25] although it is not yet known if prednisone alone represents optimal treatment of lupus nephritis. Prednisone in combination with other agents may be of greater benefit and is discussed under Cytotoxic Drugs. The decision to begin tapering should be accompanied by monitoring of disease activity with serologic studies (e.g., anti-dsDNA antibody and serum complement levels) and renal function studies, as well as consideration of nonrenal exacerbation of disease and complications of prolonged high-dose corticosteroids.[28,41]

Steroid pulse therapy is the administration of short-term, high-dose, intravenous corticosteroids with the goal of inducing remission in SLE patients with serious, life-threatening disease, such as diffuse proliferative glomerulonephritis, CNS involvement, or hemolytic disease, although it has also been used in patients without life-threatening disease.[42] A standard pulse regimen consists of intravenous methylprednisolone 1 g daily for three consecutive days. Several reports have shown disease suppression in patients with renal and nonrenal disease, although not all patients respond.[42–45] Many of those who do respond eventually relapse and may require additional courses of pulse therapy. Methylprednisolone pulse therapy is not without adverse effects, including infection, gastrointestinal and taste disturbances, hyperglycemia, palpitations, facial flushing, hypertension, and CNS effects.[46] Sudden death has also been reported with this form of therapy.[46] Thus, pulse therapy represents an alternative and possibly effective mode of treatment for patients with life-threatening disease and/or disease unresponsive to other therapeutic trials.

### Cytotoxic Drugs

Perhaps the most controversial issue concerning drug therapy for SLE is the role of cytotoxic (or immunosuppressive) drugs. Included in this category are the alkylating agent cyclophosphamide and the antimetabolite azathioprine.[47] These agents have been the mainstays of immunosuppressive therapy in the United States. Both are known to suppress and stabilize extrarenal disease activity; however, evaluation has focused almost exclusively on lupus nephritis, the major factor associated with morbidity and mortality in SLE. Furthermore, most study patients had diffuse proliferative glomerulonephritis, as patients with other histologic types of nephritis tend to do better regardless of the type of treatment. Both cyclophosphamide and azathioprine have been shown to delay the onset of nephritis and prolong survival in the New Zealand mouse, the animal model of SLE.[37] Results in human trials, however, have been inconclusive and contradictory, probably because of the variable presentation and variable course of disease and because trials were short and included few patients.[48] More recent clinical trials of these agents define the endpoint "mortality" as the number of patient deaths plus the number of patients progressing to end-stage renal disease. This is done to allow for comparison with earlier trials when chronic dialysis and renal transplantation were not readily available.[47,48] Also, in many clinical trials, patients receiving cytotoxic drugs also continue to use low-dose prednisone for control of nonrenal manifestations.

Azathioprine has not been shown to be clearly more effective than prednisone alone. Although some studies have shown azathioprine to be associated with improved survival and a steroid-sparing effect, other studies indicate no significant advantage.[49,50] Azathioprine is given orally in doses up to 4 mg/kg per day. Azathioprine is generally less toxic than cyclophosphamide, but adverse reactions may be serious and include infection, herpes zoster, cancer, sterility, and hepatotoxicity.[49,51] Thus, it is not clear whether possible benefits outweigh risks to justify its role in the therapeutic management of SLE.

The case for cyclophosphamide is only slightly more convincing. Although most reports have been inconclusive, there may be a slight advantage associated with cyclophosphamide in the high-risk patient. Treatment with cyclophosphamide plus prednisone versus prednisone alone in patients with diffuse proliferative glomerulonephritis has been studied.[52] Treatment was for 6 months and the follow-up was reported at 4 years. The cyclophosphamide group had a lower incidence and lower average rate of clinical recurrence of nephritis as indicated by creatinine clearance and/or proteinuria; however, there was no difference in the percentage of patients alive with stable or improved renal function. This would seem to indicate that standard measures of renal function may not be sufficient predictors of outcome.

A report on clinical trials in lupus nephritis at the National Institutes of Health (NIH) suggested that cytotoxic drug regimens comprising either oral azathioprine plus oral cyclophosphamide or intravenous cyclophosphamide alone were more effective in controlling disease activity than prednisone alone.[53] The mean observation period was 3.5 years; however, the difference in renal function status between treatment groups was not significant. This report stated that because of the low frequency and late appearance of complete renal failure in lupus nephritis patients, standard measures of renal function are weak indicators of outcome in short-term trials, thus making it difficult to detect a significant difference among treatment regimens. It appears that longer clinical trials or better indicators of outcome in SLE patients with life-threatening nephritis are required to indicate if significant advantages exist for a particular cytotoxic agent.

Longer NIH trials have been reported that utilize a chronicity index based on renal biopsy information as a predictor of renal functional outcome.[51,54] One report indicated a marginal advantage of oral cyclophosphamide over oral prednisone alone after a mean follow-up of 85 months.[54] Another NIH report indicated a statistically significant advantage of intermittent (every 3 months), intravenous cyclophosphamide (0.5–1.0 g/m$^2$ of body surface area) plus low-dose prednisone over prednisone alone in patients with active lupus glomerulonephritis after a mean follow-up of 7 years.[51] The most significant benefit was observed in high-risk patients who were identified as having chronic histologic change based on the chronicity index.

Of course, cyclophosphamide therapy is not without risk. Serious toxic effects include infection, herpes zoster, bladder complications (hemorrhagic cystitis and cancer), and sterility, although intermittent, intravenous cyclophosphamide accompanied by adequate hydration may minimize bladder complications.[51]

At this time, evidence supporting the usefulness of cytotoxic drugs in the management of SLE is minimal; however, there may be a role for such drugs as cyclophosphamide in management of the lupus nephritis patient with serious disease.

### *Plasmapheresis*

Another potential treatment for severe cases of SLE is removal of autoantibodies and immune complexes from serum using plasmapheresis, a process whereby 3–4 L of plasma is exchanged per week, with the cells of the patient being returned in a plasma substitute or in plasma from healthy donors.[37] In addition to removal of cytotoxic constituents from serum, plasmapheresis may also affect immunologic responses by improving reticuloendothelial phagocytic cell function and increasing antibody production.[55] Because of the potential for enhancing antibody production, it has been suggested that plasmapheresis be accompanied by corticosteroid and/or cytotoxic drug therapy.[55]

Clinical improvement after plasmapheresis has been reported in uncontrolled observations[55]; however, one trial showed no difference in improvement between "sham pheresis" and a plasma exchange group.[56] Plasmapheresis is of questionable benefit and should be reserved for patients with disease refractory to conventional drug therapy.

## Drug-Induced Systemic Lupus Erythematosus

A drug-induced SLE-like syndrome was first described in 1945 and was associated with the use of sulfadiazine.[57] Today, it is recognized that procainamide and hydralazine are by far the most common SLE-inducing drugs, although numerous other drugs have been implicated.[57]

Although many drugs have been associated with an SLE-like syndrome, not all of these reported cases satisfy the 1982 revised ARA criteria for identification of SLE patients. Furthermore, many drugs produce a positive ANA test (Table 58.5) without clinical disease.[57]

The epidemiologic characteristics of drug-induced SLE are different from those of idiopathic SLE. The average ages of onset of procainamide- and hydralazine-induced SLE are 62 and 53 years, respectively.[57] This is much later in life compared with idiopathic SLE, probably because the majority of people who use these drugs are older. Other observations include a greater percentage of white patients and an

**Table 58.5** Drugs Associated With Developing Antinuclear Antibodies

| | |
|---|---|
| Hydralazine | Quinidine |
| Procainamide | Sulfasalazine |
| Phenothiazines | Methyldopa |
| Phenytoin | Levodopa |
| Ethosuximide | Lithium |
| β-Blockers | |

absence of female predominance when compared with idiopathic SLE.[57] Risk factors for development of drug-induced SLE include high daily dosage (hydralazine), slow acetylator phenotype, family history of autoimmune disease, and HLA-DRw4 phenotype.[57]

Musculoskeletal symptoms are the most common clinical manifestations, while renal and CNS involvement is rare or absent in both procainamide- and hydralazine-induced SLE.[57] Renal involvement may not occur because of a lack of complement deposition in the kidney.[57]

A positive ANA test is found in all cases of procainamide-induced SLE and nearly all hydralazine-induced cases.[57] These antibodies are primarily against ssDNA and not dsDNA as in idiopathic SLE. Other laboratory manifestations that may be seen in drug-induced SLE include the presence of LE cells, an elevated erythrocyte sedimentation rate, a positive VDRL test, a positive rheumatoid factor (procainamide), normochromic and normocytic anemia, mild leukopenia, and occasionally mild thrombocytopenia. Immunoglobulin levels may be elevated; complement levels are usually normal.[57]

There is some evidence that the presence of antihistone antibodies correlates with symptomatic drug-induced lupus, although one clinical trial noted the presence of antihistone antibodies in 32% of asymptomatic patients who had drug-induced antinuclear antibodies.[58] Another study in patients with procainamide-induced SLE suggested that IgG antiguanosine antibody levels may be a better indicator of symptomatic drug-induced lupus.[59]

If signs and symptoms of SLE appear in a patient and are thought to be drug related, the drug should be discontinued.[57] If the lupus is drug induced, the clinical manifestations should disappear in days to weeks.[57] A NSAID might be useful in treating musculoskeletal manifestations. Other, more aggressive drugs should not be necessary unless manifestations are deemed more serious.

## Summary

SLE is a disease that affects multiple organ systems and consists of abnormal immunologic function and the development of autoantibodies. The disease is quite variable in clinical presentation and progression. The cause of lupus is unknown although several factors (e.g., environment, hormones, genetics) may predispose an individual to development of the disease. Although SLE was once thought to be rapidly fatal, today 90% of patients survive 10 years.

Drug therapy is nonspecific and is aimed at suppressing the inflammation and abnormal immune response associated with active disease. Clinical trials with various agents have often been inadequate and contradictory and the therapeutic management of lupus is not optimal. Nevertheless, drug therapy of recent years probably has contributed significantly to the improved survival of these patients. As the understanding of SLE progresses, we can expect to see the development of more specific and optimal treatment.

## References


1. Blotzer JW. Systemic lupus erythematosus. I. Historical aspects. Md State Med J 1983;32:439–441.
2. Schur PH. Historical perspective and changing history, in Schur PH (ed): The Clinical Management of Systemic Lupus Erythematosus. Orlando, Grune and Stratton, 1983, pp 1–8.
3. Tan EM, Cohen AS, Fries JF, et al. The 1982 revised criteria for the classification of systemic lupus erythematosus. Arthritis Rheum 1982;25:1271–1277.
4. Michet CJ, McKenna CH, Elveback LR, et al. Epidemiology of systemic lupus erythematosus and other connective tissue diseases in Rochester, Minnesota, 1950 through 1979. Mayo Clin Proc 1985;60:105–113.
5. Hochberg MC, Arnett FC. Systemic lupus erythematosus: Epidemiology and genetics. Md State Med J 1983;32:524–528.
6. Hochberg MC, Boyd RE, Ahearn JM, et al. Systemic lupus erythematosus: A review of clinico-laboratory features and immunogenetic markers in 150 patients with emphasis on demographic subsets. Medicine 1985;64:285–295.
7. Hochberg MC. The incidence of systemic lupus erythematosus in Baltimore, Maryland, 1970–1977. Arthritis Rheum 1985;28: 80–86.
8. Lafer EM, Rauch J, Andrzejewski C, et al. Polyspecific monoclonal autoantibodies reactive with both polynucleotides and phospholipids. J Exp Med 1981;153:897–909.
9. Notman DD, Kurata N, Tan EM. Profiles of antinuclear antibodies in systemic rheumatic diseases. Ann Intern Med 1975;83: 464–469.
10. Bell DA, Maddison PJ. Serologic subsets in systemic lupus erythematosus. An examination of autoantibodies in relationship to clinical features of disease and HLA antigens. Arthritis Rheum 1980;23:1268–1273.
11. Decker JL, Steinberg AD, Reinertsen JL, et al. Systemic lupus erythematosus: Evolving concepts. Ann Intern Med 1979;91: 587–604.
12. Budman DR, Steinberg AD. Hematologic aspects of systemic lupus erythematosus. Current concepts. Ann Intern Med 1977;86:220–229.
13. Colaco CB, Elkon KB. The lupus anticoagulant. A disease marker in antinuclear antibody negative lupus that is cross-reactive with autoantibodies to double-stranded DNA. Arthritis Rheum 1985;28:67–74.
14. Gastineau DA, Kazmier FJ, Nichols WL, et al. Lupus anticoagulant: An analysis of the clinical and laboratory features of 219 cases. Am J Hematol 1985;19:265–275.

15. How A, Dent PB, Liao SK, et al. Antineural antibodies in neuropsychiatric systemic lupus erythematosus. Arthritis Rheum 1985;28:789–795.
16. Steinberg AD, Raveche ES, Laskin CA. Systemic lupus erythematosus: Insights from animal models. Ann Intern Med 1984;100:714–727.
17. Arnett FC, Reveille JD, Wilson RW, et al. Systemic lupus erythematosus: Current state of the genetic hypothesis. Semin Arthritis Rheum 1984;14:24–35.
18. Ziminski CM. Systemic lupus erythematosus. III: Nonrenal manifestations I. Md State Med J 1983;32:699–701.
19. Ziminski CM. Systemic lupus erythematosus. IV: Nonrenal manifestations II. Md State Med J 1983;32:774–776.
20. Ansari A, Larson PH, Bates HD. Cardiovascular manifestations of systemic lupus erythematosus: Current perspective. Prog Cardiovasc Dis 1985;27:421–434.
21. Segal AM, Calabrese LH, Ahmad M, et al. The pulmonary manifestations of systemic lupus erythematosus. Semin Arthritis Rheum 1985;14:202–224.
22. Rubin LA, Urowitz MB, Gladman DD. Mortality in systemic lupus erythematosus: The bimodal pattern revisited. Q J Med 1985;55:87–98.
23. Wallace DJ, Podell T, Weiner J, et al. Systemic lupus erythematosus—survival patterns. Experience with 609 patients. JAMA 1981;245:934–938.
24. Austin HA, Muenz LR, Joyce KM, et al. Prognostic factors in lupus nephritis. Contribution of renal histologic data. Am J Med 1983;75:382–391.
25. Pollack VE, Dosekun AK. Evaluation of treatment in lupus nephritis: Effects of prednisone. Am J Kidney Dis 1982;2(suppl 1):170–177.
26. Abel T, Gladman DD, Urowitz MB. Neuropsychiatric lupus. J Rheumatol 1980;7:325–333.
27. Meyerhoff J. Systemic lupus erythematosus. VI: Hematologic and serologic abnormalities. Md State Med J 1983;32:935–939.
28. Systemic lupus erythematosus, in Rodnan GP, Schumacher HR, Zvaifler NJ (eds): Primer on the Rheumatic Diseases. Atlanta, Arthritis Foundation, 1983, pp 49–58.
29. Burnham TK. Antinuclear antibodies (ANA). How useful is the ANA test today? Int J Dermatol 1985;24:41–44.
30. D'Amelio R. Clinical diagnosis of systemic lupus erythematosus. Contrib Nephrol 1985;45:181–184.
31. Merrell M, Shulman LE. Determination of prognosis in chronic disease, illustrated by systemic lupus erythematosus. J Chron Dis 1955;1:12–32.
32. Hochberg MC, Carole AD, Feinglass EJ, et al. Survivorship in systemic lupus erythematosus. Effect of antibody to extractable nuclear antigen. Arthritis Rheum 1981;24:54–59.
33. Gimovsky ML, Montoro M, Paul RH. Pregnancy outcome in women with systemic lupus erythematosus. Obstet Gynecol 1984;63:686–692.
34. Fine LG, Barnett EV, Gabriel MD, et al. Systemic lupus erythematosus in pregnancy. Ann Intern Med 1981;94:667–677.
35. Schmidt MC. Systemic lupus erythematosus. IX: Nonsteroidal anti-inflammatory drugs and antimalarial agents. Md State Med J 1984;33:296–298.
36. Kimberly RP, Gill JR, Bowden RE, et al. Elevated urinary prostaglandins and the effects of aspirin on renal function in lupus erythematosus. Ann Intern Med 1978;89:336–341.
37. Stevens MB, Hahn BH. Management of systemic lupus erythematosus. Bull Rheum Dis 1982;32:35–42.
38. Dubois EL. Antimalarials in the management of discoid and systemic lupus erythematosus. Semin Arthritis Rheum 1978; 8:33–51.
39. Decker JL. Management, in Schur PH (ed): The Clinical Management of Systemic Lupus Erythematosus. Orlando, Grune and Stratton, 1983, pp 259–276.
40. Lanham JG, Hughes GRV. Antimalarial therapy in SLE. Clin Rheum Dis 1982;8:279–298.
41. Urman JD, Rothfield NF. Corticosteroid treatment in systemic lupus erythematosus. Survival studies. JAMA 1977;238:2272–2276.
42. Isenberg DA, Morrow WJW, Snaith ML. Methylprednisolone pulse therapy in the treatment of systemic lupus erythematosus. Ann Rheum Dis 1982;41:347–351.
43. Ponticelli C, Zucchelli P, Banfi G, et al. Treatment of diffuse proliferative lupus nephritis by intravenous high-dose methylprednisolone. Q J Med 1982;51:16–24.
44. Kimberly RP, Lockshin MD, Sherman RL, et al. High-dose intravenous methylprednisolone pulse therapy in systemic lupus erythematosus. Am J Med 1981;70:817–824.
45. Eyanson S, Passo MH, Aldo-Benson MA, et al. Methylprednisolone pulse therapy for nonrenal lupus erythematosus. Ann Rheum Dis 1980;39:377–380.
46. Elenbaas J. Steroid pulse therapy in systemic lupus erythematosus. Drug Intell Clin Pharm 1983;17:342–343.
47. Donadio JV, Holley KE, Ilstrup DM. Cytotoxic drug treatment of lupus nephritis. Am J Kidney Dis 1982;2(suppl 1):178–181.
48. Donadio JV. Chemotherapy of lupus nephropathy. Contrib Nephrol 1985;45:200–202.
49. Hahn BH, Kantor OS, Osterland CK. Azathioprine plus prednisone compared with prednisone alone in the treatment of systemic lupus erythematosus. Report of a prospective controlled trial in 24 patients. Ann Intern Med 1975;83:597–605.
50. Decker JL, Klippel JH, Plotz PH, et al. Cyclophosphamide or azathioprine in lupus glomerulonephritis. A controlled trial: Results at 28 months. Ann Intern Med 1975;83:606–615.
51. Austin HA, Klippel JH, Balow JE, et al. Therapy of lupus nephritis. Controlled trial of prednisone and cytotoxic drugs. N Engl J Med 1986;314:614–619.
52. Donadio JV, Holley KE, Ferguson RH, et al. Treatment of diffuse proliferative lupus nephritis with prednisone and combined prednisone and cyclophosphamide. N Engl J Med 1978;299:1151–1155.
53. Dinant HJ, Decker JL, Klippel JH, et al. Alternative modes of cyclophosphamide and azathioprine therapy in lupus nephritis. Ann Intern Med 1982;96:728–736.
54. Carette S, Klippel JH, Decker JL, et al. Controlled studies of oral immunosuppressive drugs in lupus nephritis. A long-term follow-up. Ann Intern Med 1983;99:1–8.
55. Lewis EJ. Phasmapheresis for the treatment of severe lupus nephritis: Uncontrolled observations. Am J Kidney Dis 1982;2 (suppl 1):182–187.
56. Wei N, Huston DP, Lawley TJ, et al. Randomised trial of plasma exchange in mild systemic lupus erythematosus. Lancet 1983;1:17–22.
57. Stratton MA. Drug-induced systemic lupus erythematosus. Clin Pharm 1985;4:657–663.
58. Epstein A, Barland P. The diagnostic value of antihistone antibodies in drug-induced lupus erythematosus. Arthritis Rheum 1985;28:158–162.
59. Weisbart RH, Yee WS, Colburn KK, et al. Antiguanosine antibodies: A new marker for procainamide-induced systemic lupus erythematosus. Ann Intern Med 1986;104:310–313.

# Section Nine
# Bone and Joint Disorders

## Chapter 59 / Osteomalacia and Osteoporosis

Steven F. Bauwens, PharmD

Osteomalacia and osteoporosis are members of a larger group of diseases known as metabolic bone diseases. Metabolic bone disease is commonly defined as a reduction of measurable bone mineral content of varying etiology; it is also called *osteopenia*. Although the two diseases are related in that they affect the quality of bone present, their specific effects on bone are quite different. Consequently, each disease process is discussed separately. Although osteomalacia and osteoporosis are different disease states, they do share the commonality of affecting the formation and resorption of bone. To appreciate fully this difference, it is necessary to understand the dynamic process associated with bone as a tissue. This chapter will discuss bone metabolism in general and the means of evaluating the metabolic bone disease present. Osteomalacia and osteoporosis are then discussed individually.

### Bone Structure, Composition, and Mineralization

The skeleton has two basic functions, structural support and depot for calcium, phosphorus, basic hydroxyl groups, and magnesium. Bone mineral crystals consist of hydroxyapatite containing primarily calcium and phosphorus. In addition, there is a close relationship between parathyroid hormone (PTH) and vitamin D, which together act to maintain serum calcium concentrations the moment any fluctuation occurs. Table 59.1 describes the relationship of these agents to serum calcium.[1] It is important to remember that the maintenance of serum extracellular calcium concentrations always takes precedence over the structural function of bone. Consequently, any deficiency of calcium will be balanced by drawing from bone mineral stores.[2]

The vitamin D system has recently been described in detail.[3] This compound, which is both a vitamin and a hormone, is activated by a complex series of events, as shown in Figure 59.1.[4] The primary function of vitamin D is to increase the serum calcium concentration. It accomplishes this by increasing intestinal absorption of calcium and phosphorus, increasing resorption of bone mineral, and probably increasing renal retention. When calcium is not available via the intestine, vitamin D resorbs calcium from bone.[3]

Calcitonin, another major calcium-regulating hormone in man, is secreted by the parafollicular cells of the thyroid in response to postprandial elevations in serum calcium. It acts to increase mineral stores in bone and increase urinary calcium loss.[2]

These factors contribute to the close control of calcium and also have an effect on the process that maintains bone integrity, called *bone turnover*, or *remodeling*. This renewal of old bone occurs on bone surfaces in discrete packages called bone multicellular units (BMUs),[5] by several cells specific for bone remodeling, as shown in Tables 59.2 and 59.3.[6] Several bone cells and a number of noncollagenous proteins are involved in the remodeling process, which relies on the intricate interaction of these various factors.

The bone surfaces involved in the remodeling process may be seen in Figure 59.2. The series of events constituting bone remodeling are illustrated in Figure 59.3. Under resting conditions, bone surfaces are lined by flat, relatively inactive cells.[7] A remodeling signal, believed to be induced by PTH or 1,25-dihydroxyvitamin D (1,25-$(OH)_2D$), stimulates maturation of the osteoclasts that reside over a focal area of bone surface.[2] Within 3 weeks of maturation, the osteoclasts remove 0.1 $mm^3$ of bone, after which the osteoclasts are replaced by osteoblasts. These cells synthesize osteoid, a collagenous substance.

Mineralization occurs about 10 days after the nonmineralized matrix is laid down. The time from resorption to completion of mineralization is 90 to 100 days. As resorption is more rapid than formation, an empty volume of bone, called the remodeling space, exists temporarily; it constitutes about 0.5% to 1.0% of the skeleton at any given time. The balance between bone resorption and formation is called the *remodeling balance*. Any alteration in the remodeling activation frequency results in an immediate dysequilibrium between the resorption and formation phases. Although this sequence of events for remodeling is the same for all bone,

**Table 59.1** Hormonal Regulation of Calcium and Phosphorus Metabolism

| *Hormonal regulation and activity* | *Parathyroid hormone* | *Calcitriol* | *Calcitonin* |
|---|---|---|---|
| Hormone source | Chief cells of parathyroid glands | Proximal tubule of kidney | Parafollicular cells of thyroid gland |
| Factors that stimulate hormone release | Decreased serum calcium concentration | Increased parathyroid hormone<br>Decreased serum calcium concentration<br>Decreased serum phosphate concentration | Increased serum calcium concentration |
| Factors that inhibit hormone release | Increased serum calcium concentration<br>Increased calcitriol concentration | Decreased parathyroid hormone<br>Increased calcium concentration<br>Increased serum phosphate concentration | Decreased serum calcium concentration |
| End-organ effects | | | |
| Intestine | No direct effect<br>Indirect action on bowel by stimulation of calcitriol in kidney | Stimulation of intestinal absorption of calcium and phosphate ions | Unknown |
| Kidney | Conversion of calcifediol to calcitriol by stimulation of hydroxylase<br>Increase in fractional reabsorption of filtered calcium<br>Promotion in fractional reabsorption of filtered calcium<br>Promotion of urinary excretion of phosphate | Unknown | Unknown |
| Bone | Stimulation of osteoclasts (resorption)<br>Stimulation of aggregation of osteoclast precursors | Potent stimulation of osteoclastic resorption | Inhibition of osteoclastic resorption |
| Net effect on serum concentration of calcium and phosphate | Increased serum calcium concentration<br>Decreased phosphate concentration | Increased calcium concentration<br>Increased phosphate concentration | Decreased serum calcium concentration (transient) |

Adapted from Kaplan FS: Osteoporosis. Clin Symp 1983;35:1–32, with permission.

differences in bone composition likely result in different remodeling rates.[7] Specifically, trabecular bone remodels (turns over) faster than cortical bone. This concept is important, as different bone sites, seen in Table 59.4,[8] have quite different quantities of cortical and trabecular bone.

It is also important to understand the differences between cortical and trabecular bone. Cortical bone, also called compact bone, makes up 80% of the skeleton and the dense outer layer of bone predominating in the shaft of long bones such as the radius. Trabecular bone, also called spongiosa, has a honeycomb configuration that provides a much greater surface area per unit volume than does cortical bone. Consequently, trabecular bone turns over more rapidly than does cortical bone. Because of these kinetic differences, quantitative changes in the two bone types do not necessarily correlate well in a given individual.[9]

## Quantification of Bone Mineral Content

### *Noninvasive Techniques*

Bone can be quantified using several noninvasive techniques, including radiography, photon absorptiometry, computerized tomography scan, and neutron activation. Table 59.5 compares the noninvasive quantifying techniques. At present, single-photon absorptiometry is recommended for measurement of the forearm (primarily cortical bone), and dual-photon absorptiometry for the spine and hip (primarily trabecular bone and combination of trabecular and cortical bone, respectively).

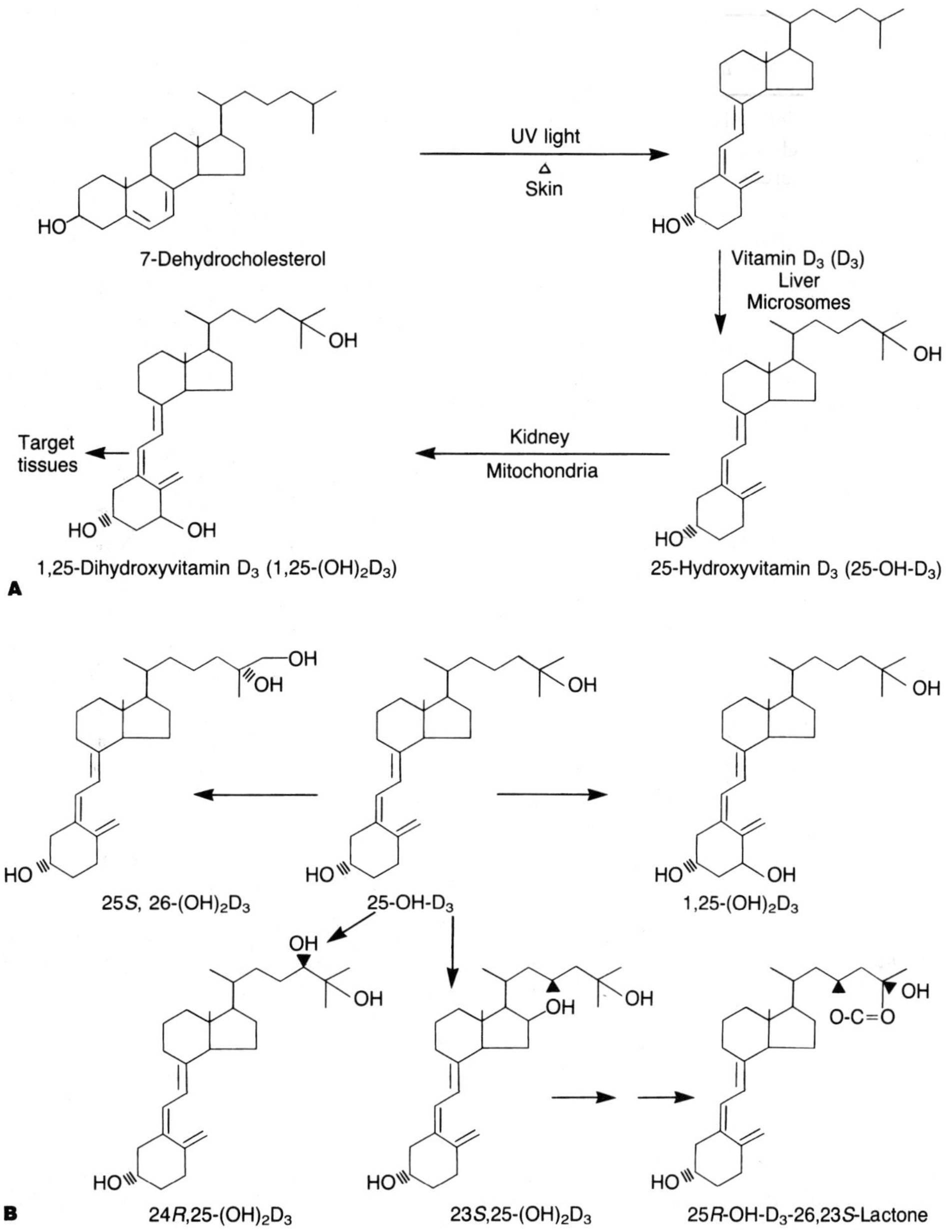


**Figure 59.1** Formation and metabolism of vitamin D (A) and some of its metabolites (B). (*Adapted from Bauwens SF, Drinka PJ, Boh LB: Primary osteoporosis: Pathogenesis and management strategies. Clin Pharm 1986;5:641, with permission.*)

### *Iliac Crest Biopsy*

The quality and quantity of bone, as well as the rate of turnover, can be studied by obtaining an intact core of cortical and trabecular bone from the iliac crest. From this sample, the specific bone tissue volumes (osteoid, mineralized bone, and marrow space) are quantified, as are surface bone cell types (osteoclast, osteoblast, and inactive lining cells). Tetracycline is frequently given before the biopsy, because it is incorporated into newly mineralized bone.[10] A tetracycline agent is administered for 3 days and discontinued for 11 days; then, a second tetracycline is given for another 3 days. The specific tetracycline used does not appear to make any difference. A commonly employed regimen consists of demeclocycline (Declomycin, Lederle) 300 mg twice daily initially, followed by doxycycline (various manufacturers) 100 mg twice daily as the second tetracycline. The bone biopsy is performed 3 days after the last dose of tetracycline. Histologic examination of the bone under normal conditions shows two distinct bands of tetracycline under a fluorescent microscope. The distance between the two bands provides the basis for measuring the

**Table 59.2** Bone Cells and Related Functions

| *Bone cell* | *Function* |
|---|---|
| Osteoprogenitors | Give rise to the bone-forming cells found on endosteal and periosteal surfaces of bone |
| Osteoblasts | Responsible for bone matrix synthesis, appear on surfaces of bone undergoing growth and development |
| | Synthesize bone collagen and several noncollagenous bone proteins |
| Osteocytes | Derived from osteoblasts |
| | Buried within mineralized bone matrix; connected to one another and to surface osteoblasts by projections |
| | Thought to provide nutrition to bone |
| Osteoclasts | Rich in lysosomal enzymes |
| | When in contact with bone surface, easily penetrate it forming the BMU |

Adapted from Boskey AL, Posner AS: Bone structure, composition, and mineralization. Orthop Clin North Am 1984;15:597–612, with permission.

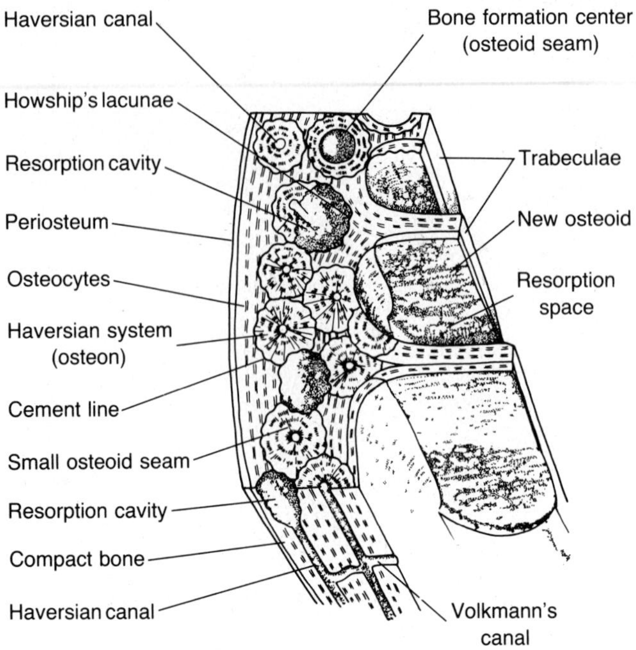


**Figure 59.2** Cross and longitudinal section of bone showing the remodeling units in cortical bone and on endosteal surfaces. *(Adapted from Parfitt AM, Duncan H: Metabolic bone disease affecting the spine, in Rothman R, Simeone F [Eds]: The spine, 2nd ed. Philadelphia, W.B. Saunders, 1982, p 777, with permission.)*

rate of mineralization. From these data, patients may be categorized into fast mineralizers (high turnover) and slow mineralizers (slow turnover). At present the bone biopsy is useful for differentiating osteomalacia from osteoporosis, but, especially in the case of osteoporosis, knowledge of the rate of mineralization has not been of particular benefit in selection of a particular form of therapy. It may in the future. It should be noted that iliac crest biopsy without tetracycline labeling is widely available but offers limited information, whereas histomorphometry of tetracycline-labeled samples is available at only a limited number of medical centers in the United States.

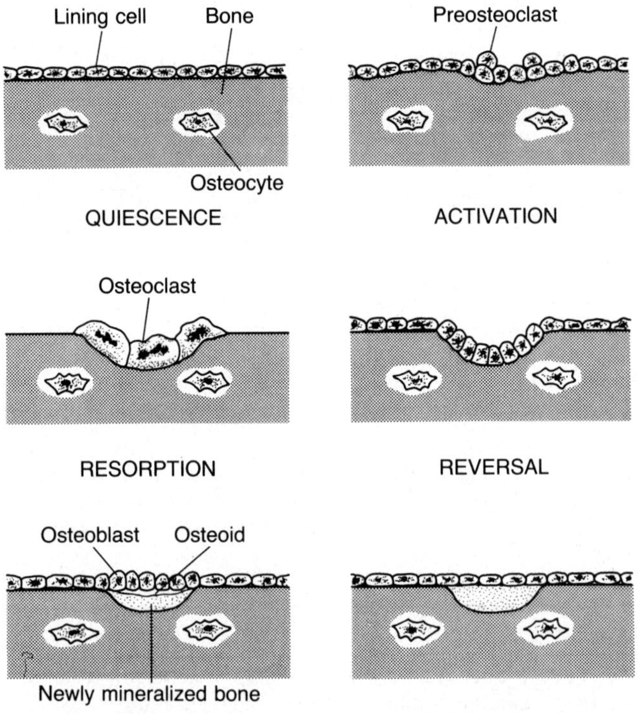


**Figure 59.3** The remodeling process for both cortical and trabecular bone. After activation, osteoclasts are mobilized on the bone surface. The osteoclasts resorb a pocket of bone called the Howship lacuna. Osteoblasts lay down new bone until the pocket is filled. *(From Bauwens SF, Drinka PJ, Boh LB: Primary osteoporosis: Pathogenesis and management strategies. Clin Pharm 1986;5:642, with permission.)*

**Table 59.3** Noncollagenous Bone Proteins With Functions

| *Protein* | *Function* |
|---|---|
| Osteocalcin | Triggers resorption |
| | Regulates mineral deposition |
| Osteonectin | Coordinates binding of mineral to collagen |
| | Regulates rate of mineral growth |
| Phosphoproteins | Regulates/promotes mineral deposition |
| Sialoprotein | Unknown |
| Proteoglycan | Regulates/promotes mineral deposition and growth |
| Proteolipid | Promotes mineral deposition |

Adapted from Boskey AL, Posner AS: Bone structure, composition, and mineralization. Orthop Clin North Am 1984;15:597–612, with permission.

**Table 59.4** Proportions of Cortical and Trabecular Bone According to Site

| *Site* | *% Cortical bone* | *% Trabecular bone* |
|---|---|---|
| Hip | | |
| Trochanteric region | 50 | 50 |
| Neck | 75 | 25 |
| Vertebrae | <33 | >66 |
| Forearm | | |
| Distal | 30–50 | 50–70 |
| Middle | 95 | 5 |

Adapted from Cummings SR, Kelsey JL, Nevitt MC, et al: Epidemiology of osteoporosis and osteoporotic fractures. Epidemiol Rev 1985;7:178–208, with permission.

## Laboratory Evaluation

Recently available advanced biochemical tests have somewhat improved the ability to diagnose specific types of metabolic bone disease; however, the pathogenesis of some diseases, such as osteoporosis, is multifactorial and as such is not well described by chemical abnormalities. Further, some of the newer tests are expensive, of variable reliability, and not widely available. With this in mind, basic biochemical testing should be used to classify the metabolic bone disease into broad categories, after which the appropriate advanced testing can be selected. Table 59.6 lists the chemical abnormalities found in the various types of osteomalacia and osteoporosis.[11] Basic and advanced biochemical tests are discussed in greater detail under each disease process.

## Osteomalacia

The term *osteomalacia* refers to a group of disorders that have in common a delay in the initiation of mineralization of new bone matrix as it is laid down, resulting in skeletal deformities. Rickets is the equivalent form of osteomalacia in children and adolescents, the difference being that in rickets the growth plate is affected primarily by a defect in the calcification of the epiphyseal cartilage. Even though the skeleton of the individual stops growing, bone turnover continues throughout life. Consequently, unmineralized matrix accumulates in every part of the skeleton in patients with osteomalacia.

A detailed description of the clinical syndrome was first made in 1645. The disease state was discovered during the industrialization of Northern Europe, where sweatshops and densely crowded cities reduced the amount of sunlight exposure and the thick smoke reduced the amount of ultraviolet light. It was not until 1822, however, that the suggestion was made that the disease might be caused by lack of sunlight exposure. Between 1909 and 1937, seasonal variations were observed in the incidence of the disease, cod liver oil was noted to prevent the disease, and the antirachitic factor (i.e., vitamin D) was identified as a fat-soluble

**Table 59.5** Noninvasive Measurements of Bone Mineral Density

| *Technique* | *Bone type* | *Measurement location* | *Radiation dose[a] (mrem)* | *Advantages* | *Disadvantages* |
|---|---|---|---|---|---|
| Radiography (measures cortical thickness) | Cortical | Metacarpals | <5 | Simple, widely available, inexpensive | Difficulty determining cortical borders; poor correlation with other cortical bone measurements |
| Single-photon absorptiometry | Primarily cortical | Forearm | <5 | Good precision, widely available, inexpensive | Does not correlate well with trabecular bone, especially in disease state |
| Dual-photon absorptiometry | Primarily trabecular | Vertebra, hip | 5–15 | Good precision, widely available, moderately expensive | Lacks three-dimensional localization; values include calcification of superimposed aorta and facet joints |
| Single-energy computerized tomography | Trabecular | Vertebra | 200 | Three-dimensional localization | Does not distinguish calcified tissue from soft tissue; high radiation exposure; expensive |
| Dual-energy computerized tomography | Trabecular | Vertebra | 400 | Three-dimensional localization; distinguishes calcified from soft tissue | Very high radiation exposure; very expensive; may have limited availability |

[a] Radiation exposure of chest roentgenogram = approximately 20 mrem.

**Table 59.6** Biochemical Indices of Selected Types of Osteoporosis and Osteomalacia

| | *SCa* | *SPh* | *Alk Ph* | *PTH* | *25-OH-D* | *1,25-(OH)$_2$D* | *U Ca* | *U Hypro* |
|---|---|---|---|---|---|---|---|---|
| Osteoporosis | | | | | | | | |
| Postmeno-pausal | WNL | WNL | WNL | WNL | WNL | WNL | WNL, ↓ | WNL |
| Senile | WNL | WNL | WNL | WNL | WNL | WNL | WNL, ↓ | WNL |
| Osteomalacia | | | | | | | | |
| Vitamin D dependent | ↓ | ↓ | ↑ | ↑ | ↓ | WNL, ↑, ↓ | ↓ | WNL |
| Vitamin D resistant | WNL, ↓ | ↓ | ↑ | ↑ | ↓ | WNL, ↑, ↓ | ↓ | WNL |

SCa, serum calcium; SPh, serum phosphate; Alk Ph, alkaline phosphatase; PTH, parathyroid hormone; U Ca, urinary calcium; U Hypro, urinary hydroxyproline; WNL, within normal limits.

Adapted from Frost HM: Tetracycline based histological analysis of bone remodeling. Calcif Tiss Res 1969;3:211–237, with permission.

sterol.[12] Although this information should have made osteomalacia extinct, it is still present today in varying degrees.

### *Epidemiology*

The exact incidence of osteomalacia is not really known. In the United States, the specific incidence has not really been well studied because it is believed, perhaps erroneously, to be of little clinical importance. Dietary and environmental sources of vitamin D in this country should be adequate[12]; however, a recent study in the United States showed that 22% of patients with hip fractures had abnormally low 25-hydroxyvitamin D (25-OH-D) concentrations and 30%, hyperosteoidosis.[13] This study demonstrates part of the confusion with the criteria defining osteomalacia. The incidence is lower when only chemical and radiographic criteria (hypocalcemia, hypophosphatemia, elevated alkaline phosphatase, and pseudofractures) are used than when such criteria as blood 25-OH-D concentrations and bone biopsy are used. Many believe that the actual incidence is much higher than commonly reported.

### *Pathophysiology*

Osteomalacia results when histologic normal bone matrix is produced by osteoblasts but mineralization of the matrix is delayed or does not occur. This defect in mineralization of the matrix of mature bone leads to the accumulation of nonmineralized or poorly mineralized osteoid in both cortical and trabecular bone. Therefore, there is less mineral than normal in a given volume of bone.[13,14] There are numerous causes of osteomalacia as seen in Table 59.7; however, there are some universal findings.

The pathogenesis of osteomalacia may be explained in two ways: as an abnormality in osteoblast function and as defective cellular function.[7] Osteoblast dysfunction is responsible for the increased thickness observed at the osteoid seams. Matrix synthesis continues at a normal rate while maturation and mineralization are defective. Though many different types of osteomalacia exist, a deficiency of one or more active metabolites of vitamin D, along with a deficiency of phosphorus, is responsible for the decreased osteoblast function. Further, hypophosphatemia may be responsible for the osteoblast's abnormal function. The vitamin D deficiency seen in osteomalacia, although partly responsible for the hypophosphatemia, probably impairs the osteoblast at a cellular level, reducing its capacity to retain phosphate.[15]

### *Clinical Presentation*

Bone pain, especially of the spine, ribs, pelvis, and lower extremities, invariably accompanies osteomalacia. Muscle strain, weight bearing, or pressure worsens the pain; pain also may be worse at night. Skeletal pain is often vague and ill defined, and many patients with long-standing osteomala-

**Table 59.7** Etiology of Osteomalacia

| *Type of osteomalacia* | *Specific contributory diseases* |
|---|---|
| Vitamin D deficiency | |
| Vitamin D malabsorption | Gastric surgery<br>Bile salt deficiency<br>Pancreatic disease<br>Intestinal mucosal disease |
| Impaired 25-OH-D formation | Liver disease |
| Impaired 25-OH-D catabolism | Anticonvulsants |
| Impaired renal excretion | Nephrotic syndrome |
| Impaired 1,25-(OH)$_2$D formation | Vitamin D dependency<br>Chronic renal failure |
| 1,25-(OH)$_2$D resistance | |
| Phosphate depletion | Nutrition<br>Chronic antacids<br>Hemodialysis |
| Primary hypophosphatemia | Familial<br>Sporadic |
| Renal tubular acidosis | |
| Mineralization inhibitor | Fluoride (as single agent)<br>Diphosphonates<br>Chronic renal failure<br>Aluminum |

cia have been misdiagnosed as having muscular rheumatism, arthritis, and herniated lumbar disks.[16]

Skeletal deformities are caused by softening of the bone and include bowing, gibbus, and pigeon chest. The spinal manifestations may lead to scoliosis, kyphosis, and shortening of the spine. Of importance is that, in general, abrupt changes in height caused by vertebral collapse are not seen unless osteoporosis is also present. In fact vertebral collapse may be protective because the osteomalacia produces increased elasticity that dissipates acute stress more easily.[16]

Muscle weakness is frequently seen, and proximal weakness in the lower extremities may lead to a waddling gait similar to that seen with muscular dystrophy.[16] Unwillingness to tense muscles because of increased pain may appear as muscle weakness. Hypocalcemia may be present to such an extent that paresthesias, muscle cramps, and frank tetany occur.

#### Biochemical Changes

Commonly seen in osteomalacia are low serum calcium and phosphate and increased alkaline phosphatase concentrations[12]; however, in mild cases, which perhaps are the most frequently encountered, these parameters are normal even though the histologic evidence suggests osteomalacia. Urinary excretion of less than 100 mg of calcium over 24 hours is suggestive of osteomalacia and should warrant a workup. In more severe cases, numerous laboratory changes may be seen depending on the etiology of the osteomalacia.

#### Roentgenographic Changes

Skeletal x-ray films show a generalized picture of osteopenia in both cortical and trabecular bone. Vertebral biconcavity usually affects adjacent vertebra and the upper and lower borders of the same vertebra. Osteosclerosis, especially of the spine, may occur. The most distinctive feature, however, is the occurrence of pseudofractures, also called Milkman's fractures (after the physician who first described them) or Looser's zones. These represent stress fractures in which the normal process of healing is impaired by the mineralization defect of osteomalacia and appear on roentgenograms as symmetric radiolucent bands. They most commonly appear adjacent and perpendicular to the periosteal surface in ribs, in pubic rami, in the outer borders of the scapulae, and near the ends of long bones.[7] Pseudofractures may progress to complete fractures, or complete fractures without pseudofractures may occur with minimum trauma, particularly in the ribs.[16] Fractures and pseudofractures associated with osteomalacia also usually show increased uptake of bone-seeking isotopes with external scanning, sometimes misinterpreted as a primary malignancy with metastases to bone.[17]

### *Etiology*

Once the diagnosis of osteomalacia is made, the difficult search for the specific cause is undertaken. On the basis of concentrations of vitamin D and its metabolites, five broad categories of osteomalacia emerge: dietary (deficiency/malabsorption), liver (disease/enzyme induction), renal failure, dependency, and resistance. Other factors that may be involved include hypophosphatemia and local tissue factors. Bone cell abnormalities and mineralization defects may be different in different forms of osteomalacia, but it is not possible at this time to ascribe a specific histologic feature or bone remodeling defect to a specific etiologic factor in osteomalacia.

### *Treatment*

#### General

Treatment of the patient with osteomalacia is generally quite rewarding. Persons who have been debilitated by the disease can become asymptomatic within 2 to 3 months; however, it must be remembered that when osteoporosis occurs concurrently with the osteomalacia, recovery is incomplete and the patient is still at risk of sustaining a fracture. In all cases, management of the underlying disease states is undertaken whenever feasible.

Regardless of the type of osteomalacia, the primary form of therapy is vitamin D or one of its metabolites; the dose and duration differ markedly according to the specific etiology. In cases where phosphorus is depleted, supplemental phosphorus may be given, oftentimes alone.

Treatment of osteomalacia may be divided into two phases.[7] The first phase ranges from the beginning of treatment to renewal of normal mineralization. During this time optimal concentrations of vitamin D metabolites are established, and normal osteoblastic function is restored, allowing mineralization to resume. In vitamin D depletion, this phase lasts a few days, but in patients requiring pharmacologic doses, it may last weeks to months. The second phase, a reparative process in which vitamin D stores are repleted, lasts until normal bone structure is restored, which may take weeks to months, depending on the severity of the osseous changes.

#### Specific

When vitamin D is used to correct the deficiency, larger doses are used initially until healing begins; then the dose is reduced to a maintenance dose. The overall risk of toxicity is small. There is some controversy, however, as to whether use of the higher dose is required to initiate healing or simply begins the healing more quickly.[15] During the first phase, body stores of vitamin D and metabolites are repleted; however, the amount needed to replete the stores varies between disease states, between patients, and even within the same patient at various times. It is, therefore, most rational to begin with a dose of vitamin D that is below the expected dose required to manage the specific type of osteomalacia (Table 59.8). At a constant dose, steady-state equilibrium is reached in 4 to 6 weeks. It takes at least 4 additional weeks for the clinical, biochemical, and radiologic effects to be seen. Consequently, once a steady-state concentration is obtained, further increments in dose should not be made for at least 8 weeks.

**Table 59.8** Usual Range of Vitamin D Doses for Types of Osteomalacia Classified by Mechanism

| *Disease* | *Vitamin D dose*[a] *(mg/d)* |
|---|---|
| Vitamin D deficiency | 0.025–0.1 |
| Vitamin D malabsorption | 0.1–10.0[b] |
| Liver disease (impaired 25-OH-D formation) | 0.25–1.0 |
| Anticonvulsants (increased 25-OH-D metabolism) | 0.1–0.5 |
| Impaired formation of 1,25-$(OH)_2D$ (vitamin D dependent, CRF[c]) | 1.0–5.0[b] |
| Vitamin D resistance | Varies |

[a] Use of either ergocalciferol ($D_2$) or cholecalciferol ($D_3$).
[b] Exact dose depends on specific cause.
[c] Chronic renal failure.

Compiled from References 7 and 15.

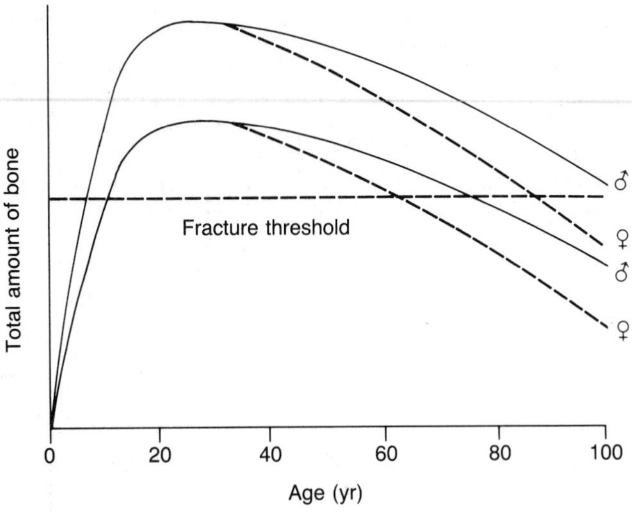


**Figure 59.4** Representation of bone gain and loss throughout life in relation to fracture threshold. This threshold is reached at an earlier age in women than in men, and is reached earlier in both men and women whose peak bone mass is lower (dashed lines) than in those who gained more mass (solid lines). (*Adapted from Parfitt AM, Duncan H: Metabolic bone disease affecting the spine, in Rothman R, Simeone F [Eds]: The Spine, 2nd ed. Philadelphia, W.B. Saunders, 1982, p 824, with permission.*)

The dose needed to produce healing may be monitored by following serum alkaline phosphatase; as this concentration starts to fall, the dose of vitamin D should be reduced until the lowest possible dose is found. In most circumstances, the final maintenance dose is slightly lower than the dose needed to produce healing.

The various vitamin D metabolites are now under intensive study to determine their indications in osteomalacia. When 25-OH-D (ergocalciferol [$D_2$], various manufacturers; cholecalciferol [$D_3$], various manufacturers) is used, the previously described principles should be followed with respect to dosing. If 1,25-$(OH)_2D_3$ (calcitriol, Rocaltrol, Roche) is used, it may be initiated at a dose higher than the expected maintenance dose, because its half-life is shorter than that of other vitamin D preparations.

## Osteoporosis

Osteoporosis is a disease that is frequently defined as a universal, gradual reduction in bone mass to a point where the skeleton is compromised, resulting in fractures with minimal trauma. Estimates of the annual incidence of hip fractures alone range from approximately 147,000 to 200,000 in the United States, with approximately 80% resulting from minor trauma.[18] In 1980 alone, the cost for hip fractures was $1 billion; an estimated 50,000 women die each year from complications of fractures and an additional 40,000 require institutionalization as a result of disability caused by the hip fracture.

### *Epidemiology*

Maximal bone mineral content of cortical bone occurs in men and women in the fourth decade of life, and thereafter slowly declines (Figure 59.4). In women, cortical bone loss proceeds at a rate of 3% per decade until menopause, at which time it accelerates to about 9% per decade until age 75, when it returns to normal.[9] Men begin cortical bone loss with 30% more bone mass than do women, and lose it at 3% to 4% per decade throughout life. Age-related hip fractures increase exponentially with age.[19] By age 90, 33% of women and 17% of men have sustained a hip fracture; 17% to 67% of these patients die within a year of the fracture.[18]

Measurements of trabecular bone mineral content are more variable than measurements of cortical bone. Dual-photon absorptiometry of the lumbar spine has demonstrated a 6% per decade loss in women and a 2% per decade loss in men throughout life.[20] A more recent series found an 8% per year decrease in vertebra centra bone mineral loss when measured longitudinally in oophorectomized women.[21] This discrepancy in rates of loss may result from the methods used for measurement, patient selection criteria, and type of study.

Cortical and trabecular bone loss varies widely from site to site, resulting in a poor correlation between axial and peripheral sites. Therefore, bone mineral density should be measured at all available scanning sites to determine the variance in bone loss in an individual's entire skeleton.

### *Pathophysiology*

Osteoporosis is not a single disease entity with a single cause, but rather a very heterogeneous disease process involving a number of contributing etiologic factors.

#### Age-Related Changes in Bone

The peak bone mass attained at skeletal maturity differs among individuals; it is possibly the single most important factor regarding future bone status. When less bone is present at skeletal maturity, the individual is closer to the critical level at which fractures occur (Fig. 59.4). If, however, sufficient bone has accumulated during growth, this fracture threshold may never be reached.

A biphasic pattern of bone loss has been described: a protracted slow phase that occurs in both sexes and a transient accelerated phase that occurs in women after menopause.[22] For cortical bone, the loss begins at around age 40 for both sexes, at a rate of about 0.3% to 0.5% annually, and increases with age until the ninth decade where it slows or ceases.[9,22] Over a lifetime, women lose about 35% of their cortical bone, men about 23%. In women, a superimposed pattern of 2% to 3% per year immediately follows menopause for 8 to 10 years.[9]

Trabecular bone loss is less well defined. Most densitometry studies suggest an early onset of bone loss, perhaps at age 30–35, with a linear decline in bone mass.[9] Cross-sectional densitometry data show that women have a decrease of 2.4% per year, while men have a 1.2% loss per year.[23,24] Only two studies have found an accelerated loss after natural menopause.[22]

### Other Age-Related Contributory Factors

Four basic factors appear to contribute to the onset of age-related bone loss, specifically decreased osteoblast function, decreased calcium absorption, biochemical imbalances, and, in women, menopause. After age 40, less bone is formed than is resorbed at any given BMU.[22] This imbalance in the coupled remodeling process appears to increase with age. It is not the result of osteoblast senescence, as fracture repair in the elderly does not appear to be delayed. Therefore, the impairment in the regulation of the osteoblast may be the result of abnormalities of systemic or local factors, such as skeletal growth factor, bone-derived growth factor, or macrophage-derived growth factor.

Calcium absorption decreases with age in both sexes, especially after the age of 70.[25,26] Concurrent with this decrease in calcium absorption is a 50% decrease in 1,25-OH-D seen in aging, probably the cause of the diminished calcium absorption.[26] Impairment of 1$\alpha$-hydroxylase, which is responsible for activation of 1,25-$(OH)_2D$, has been shown to occur in elderly patients with vertebral or hip fractures.[27]

Other factors are an increase in parathyroid hormone (PTH), proposed to be due to the decreased calcium absorption,[28] and increased PTH activity stemming from increases in urinary cAMP and nephrogenous cAMP excretion (both measures of the biologic action of PTH).[22] An increase in PTH would lead to increased bone turnover by increasing the number of BMUs and, when uncoupling occurred, would lead to increased bone loss.[29] Calcitonin, a potent antiresorptive compound, may cause age-related bone loss, as patients with decreased calcitonin concentrations also have lower bone mineral density (BMD) than normal persons.

Lastly, menopause in women has consistently been implicated as contributing to bone loss. Interestingly, the relationship between estrogen deficiency and accelerated bone loss is best shown in oophorectomized women, and proof of this relationship in natural menopause is more difficult secondary to gradual ovarian failure.[30,31] Attempts to find an estrogen receptor in bone have failed. Menopause, therefore, appears to be only one of several possible causes of bone loss.

The contribution of hormones to male bone loss is less well defined, as men do not go through a process equivalent to menopause. Gonadal function does decrease in men, and overt male hypogonadism is associated with vertebral fractures.[22]

### Clinical Heterogeneity

Riggs and Melton[32] postulated that at least two types of involutional osteoporosis exist. Type I, most often referred to as postmenopausal osteoporosis, affects primarily trabecular bone in women within 15 to 20 years of their menopause. The rate of trabecular bone loss is three times normal, while the rate of cortical loss is only slightly above normal. Consequently, vertebral and distal forearm fractures are the main type of fractures seen. Type II or senile osteoporosis affects men and women over the age of 70. Cortical and trabecular bone density values show a proportionate loss, the rate of loss of both being only slightly higher than in age-matched controls. The clinical manifestations of type II osteoporosis are multiple wedge and hip fractures. Table 59.9 compares some characteristics of types I and II.

### Biochemical Changes

Unlike osteomalacia, frank abnormalities of serum calcium, phosphate, or alkaline phosphatase concentrations are unusual. Alkaline phosphatase may be slightly increased if

**Table 59.9** Two Proposed Types of Involutional Osteoporosis

| | *Type I* | *Type II* |
|---|---|---|
| Age (yr) | 51–75 | >70 |
| Sex ratio (F:M) | 6:1 | 2:1 |
| Type of bone loss | Mainly trabecular | Trabecular and cortical |
| Rate of bone loss | Accelerated | Slightly increased |
| Fracture sites | Vertebrae and distal radius | Vertebrae and hip |
| Parathyroid function | Decreased | Increased |
| Calcium absorption | Decreased | Decreased |
| Metabolism of 25-OH-D to 1,25-$(OH)_2D$ | Secondary decrease | Primary decrease |
| Primary causes | Factors related to menopause | Factors related to aging |

Adapted from Riggs BL, Melton LJ: Involutional osteoporosis. N Engl J Med 1986;314:1676–1686, with permission.

measured after a fracture. Other laboratory values include PTH, serum 1,25-$(OH)_2D$, and serum calcitonin. Serum PTH has not been found to be consistently changed, having been shown to be both increased and decreased in postmenopausal osteoporotic women.[10] A decrease in 1,25-$(OH)_2D$ of about 30% has been shown in postmenopausal women, correlating well with the changes seen in intestinal calcium absorption. Abnormalities in serum calcitonin, although reported, have not been found consistently.

### *Clinical Presentation*

Although osteoporosis is a disease of the entire skeleton, its major clinical manifestations involve the axial skeleton. The usual finding is fracture, most commonly of the vertebra, hip, or forearm, but any bony site may be fractured if sufficient bone mass is lost. These fractures frequently occur after apparently minor trauma, such as bending over, lifting, jumping, and falling from the standing position. Recurrent fractures are common, and the course is not predictable in that there may be several months or several years between fractures.

The most frequent type of fracture is of vertebral bodies, which result in back pain and spinal deformity. Pain resulting from collapse of a vertebra varies enormously. Some patients may have a fracture with no clinical presentation; the fracture is found on routine x-ray film or may be manifest simply as a reduction in stature. Alternatively, acute pain may occur after the fracture, followed by complete resolution in 2 to 3 months until the next fracture, or chronic back pain may be manifested as a nagging, deep, dull pain localized to the general area of the fracture. Multiple fractures with or without pain may lead to dorsal kyphosis and exaggerated cervical lordosis, frequently referred to as dowager's or widow's hump. It should be noted that vertebral collapse only very rarely leads to spinal cord compression, and although osteoporosis may involve the entire skeleton, generalized skeletal pain is not seen.

Although very long lists of the secondary causes of osteoporosis may be compiled, the scientific nature of these etiologies is not well founded.[7] Many of them were proposed before age-related bone loss was well understood and present techniques to measure bone mineral density were available. Further, because of differences before and after skeletal maturity, an etiologic factor of secondary osteoporosis occurring in an adult will not be true in a child unless actually documented. Table 59.10 provides a list of reasonably well-documented causes of secondary osteoporosis.

**Table 59.10** Documented Causes of Secondary Osteoporosis Known to Affect Adults

| | |
|---|---|
| Genetic | Osteogenesis imperfecta |
| | Homocystinuria |
| Endocrine | Hypogonadism |
| | Hyperadrenocorticism |
| | Hyperthyroidism |
| | Hyperparathyroidism |
| | Growth hormone deficiency |
| Nutritional | Calcium deficiency |
| | Protein deficiency |
| | Ascorbic acid deficiency |
| | Intestinal malabsorption |
| Drug-induced | Heparin |
| | Anticonvulsants |
| | Methotrexate |
| | Ethanol |
| Miscellaneous | Metabolic acidosis |
| | Rheumatoid arthritis |
| | Trauma |
| | Disease |

Adapted from Parfitt AM, Duncan H: Metabolic bone disease affecting the spine, in Rothman R, Simeone F (Eds): The Spine, 2nd ed. Philadelphia, W. B. Saunders, 1982, pp 775–905, with permission.

### *Treatment*

Many difficulties prevent evaluations of possible therapeutic interventions for osteoporosis. Not only are symptoms episodic and unrelated to the severity of the disease state, but, even when fractures have occurred, further fractures may continue though reduction of bone mass may be stopped or significantly slowed. Consequently, the only way to show true effectiveness of a given treatment is to demonstrate a significant decrease in the fracture rate, which requires many years of follow-up. To date, no controlled prospective trial for any form of therapy has used this approach. A more realistic approach is to show that an increase in the amount of bone has occurred or to significantly reduce the rate of loss. It seems reasonable that if this can be shown, the risk of fracture would also be reduced.

There are two approaches to management of this disease state: prevent the loss of enough bone such that fractures do not occur, or, in an individual who has already suffered an osteoporotic fracture, prevent further fractures. Table 59.11 shows the various agents used to manage bone loss and their effects on bone tissue.

**Table 59.11** Various Therapeutic Agents and Proposed Effects on Bone Remodeling

| |
|---|
| Preventative therapy |
| Decrease remodeling sequence |
| Estrogen |
| Vigorous exercise |
| Decrease bone turnover |
| Estrogens |
| Calcium |
| Androgens and anabolic steroids |
| Calcitonin |
| Increase bone mass |
| Bypass remodeling sequence |
| Sodium fluoride |
| Exploit remodeling sequence |
| ADFR regimen |

Adapted from Parfitt AM, Duncan H: Metabolic bone disease affecting the spine, in Rothman R, Simeone F (Eds): The Spine, 2nd ed. Philadelphia, W. B. Saunders, 1982, pp 775–905, with permission.

## Calcium

The association between calcium intake and bone loss became apparent when it was learned that intestinal calcium absorption decreases with age in both sexes. The importance of calcium intake, however, is somewhat controversial in that some areas with both low and high daily calcium intake appear not to have significant differences in the incidence of fracture.[33] Although seemingly contradictory, this might stem from the ethnic differences of the groups studied and the measurement techniques used.

Administration of calcium has been shown to have several effects on bone metabolism: an increase in net calcium absorption, a decrease in serum PTH concentrations, a decrease in 1,25-$(OH)_2D$ concentrations (though not below that necessary for increased calcium absorption), and a transient decrease in bone turnover.[34]

***Effect on Calcium Balance*** Some early studies used calcium balance as a criterion for assessing the effect of a specific calcium intake, as techniques were not available to measure small changes in bone mass.[35] Those patients maintained on high doses of calcium (about 2,500 mg/d) showed improvement in both absorption and balance for periods of 3 months to 3 years. More recent studies, however, have shown improvement in absorption and balance for up to 6 months, at which time these effects are significantly diminished or lost.[36] The apparent benefit seen in the former studies probably resulted from calcium-induced suppression of bone resorption, followed by a decrease in formation caused by the close coupling of the two processes.[1]

***Effect on Bone Mass and Fracture Rates*** The effect of calcium on bone loss has only recently been elucidated. The specific calcium dose, duration of follow-up, patient selection, and outcome vary greatly. These studies have concentrated on cortical bone. Currently there are no data from controlled trials documenting the effects of calcium on trabecular bone. Studies have included follow-up of 3 years or less; conclusions cannot be made concerning the long-term effects of calcium. The literature seems to support a daily elemental calcium intake of 1,000–1,500 mg to prevent bone loss, and at least 1,500 mg daily in those who have already lost substantial quantities of bone or who have sustained a fracture. Two recent studies, however, did not find any correlation between calcium intake and densitometry.[4] Because of such data, controversy exists as to what role calcium does or should have in the management of osteoporosis. Nevertheless, there is no disagreement that all patients, regardless of age, should meet the basic daily nutritional requirements for calcium. Further, use of calcium in combination with other types of therapy, such as exercise or estrogens, has not been adequately studied.

***Supplementation*** In the United States more than two thirds of all women between the ages of 18 and 30 ingest less than the recommended daily allowance (RDA) for calcium, which is 800 mg elemental calcium daily. More than 75% of women older than 35 have calcium intakes less than the RDA. Between 60% and 70% of men between the ages of 15 and 35, on the other hand, maintain intakes above the RDA, and 75% of men maintain intakes above 500 mg daily for most of their adult lives.[36]

**Table 59.12** Calcium Content of Various Foods

| *Food* | *Serving size* | *Calcium content (mg)* |
|---|---|---|
| Milk (skim) | 1 qt | 1,212 |
| Milk (whole) | 1 qt | 1,152 |
| Sardines | 8 medium | 354 |
| Yogurt (low-fat) | 1 cup | 345 |
| Swiss cheese | 1 oz | 250 |
| Red salmon | $\frac{1}{2}$ cup | 250 |
| Turnip greens, cooked | $\frac{1}{2}$ cup | 245 |
| Creamed cottage cheese | 1 cup | 211 |
| Cheddar cheese | 1 oz | 211 |
| Ice cream | 1 cup | 200 |
| American processed cheese | 1 oz | 150 |
| Spinach (frozen, chopped, cooked) | $\frac{1}{2}$ cup | 113 |
| Chocolate fudge | $3\frac{1}{2}$ oz | 100 |

Considerable controversy surrounds calcium requirements for the elderly, primarily because the current RDA was established for all adults older than 51 years. Calcium may be ingested either in food or by oral supplementation. Table 59.12 lists select foods with high calcium content, primarily dairy products. Based on the recommendation of 800 mg daily, three servings of foods are required given normal serving sizes. Although some studies have found dietary calcium to be the most absorbable form of calcium, intake of sufficient quantities of foods may be prohibitive, particularly if the individual does not like or cannot ingest dairy products.[4]

When dietary intake is inadequate, oral calcium supplements are a convenient means of ensuring adequate intake. The various preparations on the market provide varying amounts of calcium, depending on the particular product chosen. Calcium carbonate contains more elemental calcium by weight (40%) than the gluconate (9%) or lactate (13%) salts, dibasic calcium phosphate (31%), or chelated calcium (20%). Table 59.13 lists some common forms of calcium and their calcium content.

Calcium carbonate is the most commonly recommended form of calcium because of its high calcium content and low cost. This salt, however, requires an acidic medium for adequate absorption. Although it has been estimated that by age 60 about 20% of the elderly may be achlorhydric, recent data show that if calcium carbonate is administered with meals, adequate absorption occurs even in the presence of documented achlorhydria.

Another consideration regarding product selection is which carbonate salt should be recommended. Virtually no bioavailability data exist on calcium supplements; however,

**Table 59.13** Oral Calcium Supplementation Products

| Preparation | Tablet size: mg | Tablet size: mg elemental calcium/tablet | To supply one g elemental calcium (tablets/d) |
|---|---|---|---|
| Calcium carbonate (40% elemental calcium) | | | |
| Generic | 650 | 260 | 4 |
| Cal-Sup (Riker Laboratories, Inc.) | 750 | 300 | 4 |
| Caltrate (Lederle Laboratories) | 1,500 | 600 | 2 |
| Os-Cal 500 (Marion Laboratories) | 1,250 | 500 | 2 |
| Tums (Norcliff–Thayer, Inc.) | 500 | 200 | 5 |
| Titralac (3M Company) | 420 | 168 | 6 |
| Generic calcium gluconate (9% elemental calcium) | 650 | 58.5 | 17 |
| Generic calcium lactate (13% elemental calcium) | 650 | 84.5 | 12 |
| Generic dibasic calcium phosphate (23% elemental calcium) | 500 | 115 | 9 |

recent data have shown that many preparations have unacceptable dissolution rates, while others virtually do not dissolve at all. Incomplete or unacceptable dissolution rates are indicative of poor bioavailability.

*Effect of Thiazides on Calcium Metabolism* Thiazide diuretics promote a decrease in renal calcium excretion. While several investigators have attempted to use this effect to improve calcium balance and thus bone mineral content, to date no prospective controlled data have shown this to be a beneficial therapy, either alone or in combination with other therapy.[37]

### Vitamin D and Metabolites

The recommended daily allowance for vitamin D has not been well studied but was recently decreased from 400 IU daily to 200 IU daily for adults. Interestingly, of the data that do exist, it has been shown in a group of housebound elderly that 400 IU daily was necessary to maintain serum calcifediol concentrations at more than 10 ng/mL, the acceptable low to normal serum concentration. Vitamin D stimulates an active calcium transport system that increases calcium absorption in the small intestine and also acts on bone mineralization by maintaining calcium and phosphorus serum concentrations via a trophic effect on bone.[2]

*Vitamin D* Although pharmacologic doses of vitamin D are considered standard therapy for management of osteoporosis by some clinicians, no data demonstrate benefits from vitamin D administration. Any improvement in osteoporotic patients treated with vitamin D may well be the result of treating unrecognized subclinical osteomalacia.[38] Furthermore, one study showed that 2 of 63 elderly patients became hypercalcemic after taking a daily dose of 2,000 IU.[39] Studies have failed to show beneficial effects of vitamin D in doses of 2,000–5,000 IU daily, with or without calcium supplementation.[4] With these doses, hypercalcemia and hypercalciuria were commonly produced. Further, a recent study was unable to demonstrate any difference between 400 IU vitamin D daily with calcium and 5,000 IU weekly with supplemental calcium.[40] Consequently, current data suggest that no more than 400–800 IU of vitamin D be given daily. If supplemental calcium is given, the two compounds should not be in the same dosage form, as some data suggest that calcium in the same preparation as vitamin D promotes inactivation of the vitamin D.[14]

*Vitamin D Metabolites* The more potent forms of vitamin D, calcitriol and 1$\alpha$-hydroxyvitamin D, increase intestinal absorption of calcium; however, this beneficial effect is also accompanied by hypercalcemia and hypercalciuria, both of which require a decrease in dose or dietary calcium restriction. Furthermore, the long-term effects of these agents on calcium balance, bone mass, and fracture rates have not been studied. Little information on the use of other vitamin D metabolites, calcifediol and 24,25-$(OH)_2D$, is available at this time.

### Hormonal Therapy

The association between estrogen deficiency and osteoporosis has been known for almost half a century. Despite the widespread use of estrogens in the management of osteoporosis, the specific mechanism by which they are effective remains unclear. No estrogen receptor has been found in bone, but they decrease bone resorption, increase calcitriol concentrations, and increase intestinal calcium absorption and retention. Postmenopausal women given estrogens have a more positive calcium balance than untreated women.[33] These data further suggest that women receiving estrogen therapy require a total calcium intake of 900–1,000 mg of calcium, while untreated women required 1,500 mg of elemental calcium daily to maintain a zero-calcium balance. Unfortunately, the relationship among estrogen dose, daily calcium intake, and calcium balance has not been investigated in long-term studies.

***Effect of Estrogens on Bone Mass and Fracture Rates*** A number of studies have shown that estrogens preserve both cortical and trabecular bone when given in a variety of doses and types. A substantial increase in bone mass occurs early after estrogen therapy has been initiated (within 3 years) and is followed by a stabilizing effect on the bone mass. This transient increase in bone mass may result from depression of bone resorption after estrogen therapy, resulting in a depressed remodeling space and consequently a one-time increase in bone mass.[33,41]

Numerous case-control studies have shown that various types and doses of estrogens are effective in decreasing the incidence of fractures, primarily of the distal radius and forearm.[30,42]

***Dosage and Duration of Estrogen Therapy*** The effects of treating women with estrogens and then removing the estrogen have been well described.[43] A group of women treated with estrogens for 4 years, followed by 4 years of no estrogen, showed the same degree of bone loss as a control group followed for 8 years; all the bone loss in the former group occurred during the nondrug phase of the study. Thus, once initiated, estrogens may be indicated for life. Studies on the use of estrogen during the period of menopausal bone loss (i.e., ~ 10 years) have not been undertaken. It may be possible to discontinue or substitute the estrogen therapy.

A dose–response relationship exists between bone mass and conjugated estrogen (Premarin, Ayerst, various generics) doses of 0.3–2.5 mg.[4] Further, bone loss is inconsistently maintained at doses less than 0.6 mg of conjugated estrogens, while doses above 0.6 mg appear to be no more effective than 0.6 mg. Consequently, current data and the majority of opinion suggest that 0.625 mg conjugated estrogens or its equivalent is optimal for preservation of bone mass.

Recent data have shown use of 0.3 mg conjugated estrogens with 1 g elemental calcium to maintain bone mass in postmenopausal women. These results are very significant as they suggest that a lower dose of estrogen may be used when combined with another agent, potentially reducing the risk of higher dose (0.625 mg), long-term therapy.

***Effect of Progesterones on Bone Mass*** Progesterones also retard bone loss, and the mechanism probably differs from that of estrogen.[4] Three studies have shown that addition of progesterone to estrogen actually promotes new bone formation, though not all progestational agents appear to have beneficial effects on bone. Additional data are needed in this area.

***Risks of Long-Term Hormonal Therapy*** The association between estrogen use and breast and endometrial cancer, both estrogen-sensitive tissues, has long been appreciated and continues to be of major concern. Studies in the mid-1970s linked an increase in the incidence of endometrial cancer to the use of estrogens, whose use was in vogue at the time.[4] These studies indicated an increased risk 1.7 to 8.0 times that of the normal population; this risk increased with prolonged exposure and high-dose therapy. A 3- to 6-year latency period is required between the first exposure to estrogen and the onset of increased risk of cancer.

The addition of a progestogen to an estrogen regimen reverses the hyperplasia and facilitates complete sloughing of the endometrium.[44] In fact, it has been suggested that progesterones actually protect against endometrial cancer. The major disadvantage of adding progesterone to an estrogen is the return of light-to-moderate withdrawal bleeding. Bleeding at any other time of the administration cycle should be considered abnormal, and an endometrial biopsy performed. A frequently used regimen is medroxyprogesterone (Provera) 5–10 mg for the last 13 days of estrogen administration.

Data on the risk of breast cancer with estrogen use suggest a 0.5 to 3.3 risk, depending on the particular study involved. This type of information is vital, as the risk of developing breast cancer is higher than that of endometrial cancer, and the outcome is less favorable.

Other effects long-term estrogens may have on postmenopausal women include possible beneficial effect on coronary artery disease, changes in blood lipids (increased high-density lipoproteins [HDLs] and decreased low-density lipoproteins [LDLs] and very-low-density lipoproteins [VLDLs]), increase in coagulation problems (though not well substantiated), increased incidence of gallbladder disease, and increased incidence of thromboembolic disease. Most of these data are derived from younger women using oral contraceptives and have not been documented in elderly postmenopausal women.

**Fluoride**

Fluoride (sodium fluoride, various manufacturers) is the first agent discussed so far that has the potential to increase bone mass. The predominant effect on bone is to increase bone formation.[45] The fluoride ion substitutes for hydroxy radicals in the hydroxyapatite crystals to form fluorapatite, resulting in increased bone crystallinity and a decrease in solubility. The net effect is a more stable mineral system more resistant to resorption. Fluoride produces a positive uncoupling favoring formation over resorption, resulting in increased bone mass.[40] The increased quantity of mineralized bone appears to make the newly formed bone more resistant to compressive forces, but torsional strain results in hip fractures more easily.[46]

Trabecular bone, particularly of the axial skeleton, is responsive to fluoride therapy.[40] While a twofold increase has been demonstrated in trabecular bone mass in about 50% of patients receiving fluoride for 2 years, about 40% of patients show no response to fluoride. Further, not only is it not known why this occurs, but with our current evaluation techniques, it is not possible to predict who will be a responder.[40] Loss of vertebral bone mass, number of vertebral fractures before treatment, and bioavailability of the fluoride product are not responsible for this apparent variability of response. The effect of fluoride on cortical bone is less well studied, but available data suggest no change or a decrease in cortical bone density. The effect of fluoride on fracture rates has not been systematically studied in patients with osteoporosis.

***Dose*** The dose of fluoride used is 40–50 mg daily supplemented with at least 1,000 mg of elemental calcium. Fluoride is available as sodium fluoride 2.2 mg, containing 1.1 mg elemental fluoride. Calcium and fluoride should be given individually to prevent chemical binding, as about 25% less fluoride is absorbed when fluoride and calcium are administered concurrently.[40] A commercial preparation of sodium fluoride 8.3 mg and calcium carbonate 364 mg per tablet (Florical) is available, but data on the bioavailability of calcium in this product are lacking.

*Adverse Effects* The adverse effects are primarily gastrointestinal and rheumatic and are seen in up to 50% of patients. Gastrointestinal symptoms include nausea, vomiting, diarrhea, abdominal pain, and occasional gastrointestinal bleeding. Rheumatic symptoms include plantar facial pain, periarticular pain, synovitis, and arthritis. Symptoms disappear within 1 to 3 weeks after discontinuation of the fluoride and reappear if it is reinstituted, even at a lower dose.

Many questions presently surround the use of fluoride in patients with osteoporosis. Two large, prospective, randomized studies are presently under way in the United States to evaluate the crucial issues concerning fluoride: its relative effects on cortical versus trabecular bone and its effect on fracture rates of different bone types. Until these data become available, fluoride should be considered an investigational agent.

**Calcitonin**

The Food and Drug Administration has approved calcitonin for prevention of progressive bone loss in postmenopausal osteoporosis. Despite this approval, the exact role calcitonin should play in overall management is not well defined. Studies have shown calcitonin (salmon calcitonin, Calcimar, USV; Miacalcin, Sandoz) to decrease resorption, probably by decreasing activation of the BMU.[7] When administered in daily doses of 100 IU subcutaneously with 500 mg elemental calcium, a significant increase in total body calcium was observed[4]; however, there were no significant differences between fractures in treated and control patients. Other studies have shown 50 and 100 IU to produce similar effects. Interestingly, a recent study showed that only 50% of patients responded at all to a given dose of calcitonin. As was the case with fluoride, it was impossible to predict who would respond.

Overall, the combination of calcium and calcitonin preserves bone mass in some patients, but it is unclear what the optimal dose should be. Apparently without adverse effects, the drug is quite expensive (about $6.50 per 100 IU) and available only in parenteral form. Additional studies are needed to determine the optimal dose, its effectiveness compared with other regimens, and its effect on fracture rates.

**Other Agents**

Several other agents have been used in the management of osteoporosis. Parathyroid hormone (PTH) stimulates bone turnover, differentiation of new bone and remodeling units, and renal tubular reabsorption of calcium. Although these are theoretical benefits, the few studies reported do not show any significant benefit.

Limited data are available on the use of androgens and anabolic steroids. Oxandrolone (Anavar, Searle) has not been shown to have a beneficial effect on bone mass. Methandrostenolone (various generic preparations) increases total body calcium in postmenopausal women, but a demonstrable effect, at least on cortical bone, was not seen. Stanozolol (Winstrol, Winthrop), in combination with calcium, increased total body calcium and decreased numbers of vertebral fractures in postmenopausal osteoporotic women, though statistical significance was not achieved.

Diphosphonates are known to be potent inhibitors of crystal growth and dissolution that slow bone turnover and inhibit bone resorption. Ethane-1-hydroxy-1,1-diphosphonate (EHDP, etidronate, Didronel, Norwich–Eaton) is currently the only diphosphonate available in the United States. In clinical trials for osteoporosis, however, diphosphonates have not been shown to have beneficial effects.

**Activation–Depression–Free–Repeat Regimen**

Perhaps the most exciting approach to management of osteoporosis is the theoretical model first described by Frost and now referred to as the activation–depression–free–repeat (ADFR) regimen.[47] This model exploits the normal remodeling sequence as it is now understood. The first phase requires use of an agent that increases the activation of new BMUs; this could be achieved by administration of PTH, thyroid hormone, 1,25-$(OH)_2D$, or growth hormone. The second phase would shift the bone balance within the particular BMU with such agents as calcitonin and diphosphonates, which would inhibit the activation of newly generated osteoblasts but not osteoclasts. The net result would be an overfilling of the BMUs with osteoblasts because of the absence of inhibiting factors; thus, bone mass would increase. This approach to therapy is currently under study.

**Exercise**

The role of exercise in the management of osteoporosis continues to be studied. Exercise can increase bone mass proportional to the amount of stress placed on a particular extremity.[48] Occupations that require moderate to heavy physical exertion show similar results: the greater the physical activity, the higher the skeletal mass.[48]

Because prevention of bone loss should begin early in life, there is some concern over vigorous exercise by women. Amenorrhea occurs in 25% to 40% of highly trained endurance women athletes and is caused by low gonadotropin concentrations. These amenorrheic runners have lower lumbar mineral densities and normal radial densities, and experience running-related fractures more frequently, compared with controls.[49] There is a great deal of concern that osteoporosis may occur earlier in these amenorrheic athletes.

Physical exercise is apparently beneficial in the maintenance of skeletal bone mass. Currently unknown is how much or what type of weight-bearing exercise produces optimal results. This information is especially vital because many debilitated elderly may not be capable of enduring extensive weight-bearing activities. Current recommendations suggest regular exercise, for at least 45 minutes three times a week, particularly during skeletal development, to help maximize peak bone mineral content. Immobilization should be minimized to the extent possible, and an appropriate vigorous exercise program initiated as soon as the mobilization period has ended.

## Summary

Osteomalacia and osteoporosis comprise several metabolic bone diseases. Osteomalacia is a disease of decreased bone mineralization with multiple etiologies, all which have in common an impairment in vitamin D homeostasis. Depending on the specific etiology involved, therapy almost exclusively revolves around vitamin D in some form.

Osteoporosis, a disease of decreased bone mass, clinically manifests as a fracture. Like osteomalacia, osteoporosis has a number of etiologies, but unlike osteomalacia, it is unclear how identification of the etiology should affect implementation of a specific therapeutic regimen. Prevention of age-related bone loss produces the most desirable outcome. Treatment of established osteoporosis is much less satisfactory; however, as our understanding of the natural history of the disease state increases and more controlled studies are completed, better treatment regimens will become available. In the interim, a good understanding of the bone remodeling process will enable the clinician to realize the therapeutic implications of various treatment regimens.


## References


1. Kaplan FS. Osteoporosis. Clin Symp 1983;35:1–32.
2. Parfitt AM, Gallagher JC, Heaney RP, et al. Vitamin D and bone health in the elderly. Am J Clin Nutr 1982;36:1014–1031.
3. DeLuca HF. The metabolism and function of vitamin D, in Makin HLJ (ed): Biochemistry of Steroid Hormones, 2nd ed. Oxford, Blackwell Scientific, 1975, pp 71–82.
4. Bauwens SF, Drinka PJ, Boh LB. Primary osteoporosis: Pathogenesis and management strategies. Clin Pharm 1986;5:639–659.
5. Frost HM. Bone remodelling and its relationship to metabolic bone disease. Springfield, IL, Charles C. Thomas, 1973.
6. Boskey AL, Posner AS. Bone structure, composition, and mineralization. Orthop Clin North Am 1984;15:597–612.
7. Parfitt AM, Duncan H. Metabolic bone disease affecting the spine, in Rothman R, Simeone F (eds): The Spine, 2nd ed. Philadelphia, W.B. Saunders, 1982, pp 775–905.
8. Cummings SR, Kelsey JL, Nevitt MC, et al. Epidemiology of osteoporosis and osteoporotic fractures. Epidemiol Rev 1985;7: 178–208.
9. Mazess RB. On aging bone loss. Clin Orthop 1982;165:239–252.
10. Frost HM. Tetracycline based histological analysis of bone remodeling. Calcif Tiss Res 1969;3:211–237.
11. Burtis WJ, Lang R. Chemical abnormalities. Orthop Clin North Am 1984;15:653–669.
12. Doppelt SH. Vitamin D, rickets, and osteomalacia. Orthop Clin North Am 1984;15:671–686.
13. Doppelt SH, Neer RM, Daly M, et al. Vitamin D deficiency and osteomalacia in patients with hip fractures—an unrecognized epidemic, in Frame B, Potts JT Jr (eds): Clinical Disorders of Bone and Mineral Metabolism. Amsterdam, Excerpta Medica, 1983, p 491.
14. Schenk RK, Olah AJ. What is osteomalacia? Adv Exp Med Biol 1985;128:549–562.
15. Parfitt AM, Kleerekoper M. Clinical disorders of calcium, phosphorus and magnesium metabolism, in Maxwell M, Kleeman CR (eds): Clinical Disorders of Fluid and Electrolyte Metabolism, 3rd ed. New York, McGraw-Hill, 1979, pp 947–1152.
16. Frame B, Parfitt AM. Osteomalacia: Current concepts. Ann Intern Med 1978;89:966–982.
17. McFarlane JD, Lutkin JE, Burwood MA. The demonstration by scintigraphy of fractures in osteomalacia. Br J Radiol 1977;50: 369–371.
18. Nickens HW. A review of factors affecting the occurrence and outcome of hip fractures with special reference to psychosocial issues. J Am Geriatr Soc 1983;31:166–170.
19. Melton LJ, Riggs BL. Epidemiology of age-related fractures, in Avioli LV (ed): The Osteoporotic Syndrome—Detection, Prevention, Treatment. New York, Grune and Stratton, 1983, pp 45–72.
20. Riggs BL, Wahner HW, Dunn WL, et al. Differential changes in bone mineral density of the appendicular and axial skeleton with aging. J Clin Invest 1981;67:328–335.
21. Genant HK, Cann CE, Ettinger B. Quantitative computed tomography of vertebral spongiosa: A sensitive method for detecting early bone loss after oophorectomy. Ann Intern Med 1982;97:699–705.
22. Riggs BL, Melton LJ. Involutional osteoporosis. N Engl J Med 1986;314:1676–1686.
23. Meier DE, Orwoll ES, Jones JM. Marked disparity between trabecular and cortical bone loss with age in healthy men: Measurement by vertebral computed tomography and radial photon absorptiometry. Ann Intern Med 1984;101:605–612.
24. Meunier P, Coupron P, Edouard C, et al. Physiological senile involution and pathological rarefaction of bone: Quantitative and comparative histological data. Clin Endocrinol Metab 1973; 2:239–256.
25. Bullamore JR, Gallagher JC, Wilkinson R. Effect of age on calcium absorption. Lancet 1970;2:535–537.
26. Gallagher JC, Riggs BL, Eisman J, et al. Intestinal calcium absorption and serum vitamin D metabolites in normal subjects and osteoporotic patients: Effect of age and dietary calcium. J Clin Invest 1979;64:729–736.
27. Slovik DM, Adams JS, Neer RM, et al. Deficient production of 1,25-dihydroxyvitamin D in elderly osteoporotic patients. N Engl J Med 1981;305:372–374.
28. Gallagher JC, Riggs BL, Jerpbak CM, et al. The effect of age on serum immunoreactive parathyroid hormone in normal and osteoporotic women. J Lab Clin Med 1980;95:373–385.
29. Delmas PD, Stenner D, Wahner KG, et al. Increase in serum $\gamma$-carboxyglutamic acid protein with aging in women: Implications for the mechanism of age-related bone loss. J Clin Invest 1983;71:1316–1321.
30. Lindsay R, Hart DM, Forrest C, et al. Prevention of spinal osteoporosis in oophorectomized women. Lancet 1980;2:1151–1154.
31. Genant HK, Cann CE, Ettinger B, et al. Quantitative computed tomography for spinal mineral assessment, in Christiansen C (ed): Osteoporosis: An International Symposium. Copenhagen, Aolborg-Sitz-Bogtrykkeri, 1984, pp 65–72.
32. Riggs BL, Melton LJ. Evidence for two distinct syndromes of involutional osteoporosis. Am J Med 1983;75:899–901.
33. Heaney RP, Recker RR, Saville PD. Menopausal changes in calcium balance performance. J Lab Clin Med 1978;92:953–963.
34. Recker RR, Saville PD, Heaney RP. Effect of estrogens and calcium carbonate on bone loss in postmenopausal women. Ann Intern Med 1977;87:649–655.

35. Harrison M, Fraser R, Mullan B. Calcium metabolism in osteoporosis: Acute and long-term responses to increased calcium intake. Lancet 1961;1:1015–1019.
36. Heaney RP, Gallagher JC, Johnston CC, et al. Calcium nutrition and bone health in the elderly. Am J Clin Nutr 1982;36:986–1013.
37. Christiansen C, Christiansen MS, McNair P, et al. Prevention of early postmenopausal bone loss: Controlled two year study in 315 normal females. Eur J Clin Invest 1980;10:273–279.
38. Slovik DM. The vitamin D endocrine system, calcium metabolism and osteoporosis. Spec Top Endocrinol Metab 1983;5:83–148.
39. Johnson KR, Jobber J, Stonawski BJ. Prophylactic vitamin D in the elderly. Age Aging 1980;9:121–127.
40. Riggs BL. Treatment of osteoporosis with sodium fluoride: An appraisal. Bone Mineral Res 1984;2:366–393.
41. Parfitt AM. The morphologic basis of bone mineral measurements: Transient and steady state effects of treatment in osteoporosis. Miner Electrolyte Metab 1980;4:273–287.
42. Johnson RE, Specht EE. The risk of hip fracture in postmenopausal females with and without estrogen drug exposure. Am J Public Health 1981;71:138–144.
43. Lindsay R, Aitken JM, Anderson JB, et al. Long-term prevention of postmenopausal osteoporosis by estrogen. Lancet 1976; 2:1038–1041.
44. Hulka BS, Fowler WC, Kaufman DG, et al. Estrogen and endometrial cancer: Cases and two control groups from North Carolina. Am J Obstet Gynecol 1980;137:92–96.
45. Baylink DJ, Bernstein DS. The effects of fluoride therapy on metabolic bone disease: A histologic study. Clin Orthop 1967; 55:51–85.
46. Inkovaara J, Heikinheimo R, Jarvinen V, et al. Prophylactic fluoride treatment and aged bone. Br Med J 1975;3:73–74.
47. Frost HM. Treatment of osteoporosis by manipulation of coherent bone cell populations. Clin Orthop 1979;143:227–244.
48. Riggs BL, Hodgson SF, Hoffman DL, et al. Treatment of primary osteoporosis with fluoride and calcium. Clinical tolerance and fracture occurrence. JAMA 1980;243:446–449.
49. Drinkwater BL, Nilsson K, Chesnut GH, et al. Bone mineral content of amenorrheic and eumenorrheic athletes. N Engl J Med 1984;311:277–281.

# *Chapter 60* / Rheumatoid Arthritis and the Seronegative Spondyloarthropathies

Arthur A. Schuna, MS, and Beth D. Vejraska, PharmD

## Rheumatoid Arthritis

Rheumatoid arthritis is the most common systemic inflammatory disease characterized by symmetrical joint involvement. Extra-articular involvement including rheumatoid nodules, vasculitis, scleritis, neurologic dysfunction, pericarditis, lymphadenopathy, splenomegaly, and chronic lung disease are manifestations of the disease. Although the usual disease course is chronic, resulting in progressive destruction of the involved joints, some patients spontaneously enter a remission.

### *Epidemiology*

Rheumatoid arthritis is estimated to have an incidence of 2% to 3% and does not have any racial predilections. The disease is three times more common in women. In people aged 15–45, women predominate by a ratio of 6:1; the sex ratio is approximately equal among patients in the first decade of life and in those over 60.

The factors that initiate the inflammatory process are unknown. Epidemiologic data suggest that a genetic predisposition and exposure to unknown environmental factors may be necessary for expression of the disease.[1,2] It has been observed that HLA-DRw4 (HLA = human leukocyte antigen, an antigen characterized in histocompatibility typing) is found in 70% of patients with rheumatoid arthritis but in only 28% of normal controls. Rheumatoid arthritis is six times more common among dizygotic twins and nontwin children of parents with rheumatoid factor–positive, erosive rheumatoid arthritis than in children whose parents do not have the disease. If one of a pair of monozygotic twins is affected, the other twin has a 30 times greater risk of developing the disease.

### *Pathophysiology*

Chronic inflammation of the synovial tissue lining the joint capsule results in the proliferation of this tissue. The inflamed, proliferating synovium characteristic of rheumatoid arthritis is called pannus (Fig. 60.1). This pannus invades the cartilage and eventually the bone surface, producing erosions that lead to destruction of the joint.

Infectious agents have been postulated as a cause of rheumatoid arthritis. Supporting evidence includes the similarity between rheumatoid arthritis and acute inflammatory arthritides associated with known infectious agents (e.g., rheumatic fever following streptococcal infection, Lyme arthritis, postviral arthritis) and experimentally induced synovitis resembling rheumatoid arthritis produced by the injection of bacterial cell wall fragments in rats. No specific infectious agent has been isolated from the joints of patients suffering from rheumatoid arthritis.

The immune system is a very complex network of checks and balances designed to discriminate self from nonself (foreign) tissues. It helps rid the body of infectious agents, tumor cells, and products associated with the breakdown of cells. In rheumatoid arthritis, this system attacks the synovial tissue and other connective tissues.

The immune system has both humoral and cellular immune functions. The humoral component is necessary for the formation of antibodies. These antibodies are produced by B lymphocytes. Most patients with rheumatoid arthritis form antibodies called rheumatoid factors. These rheumatoid factors are a heterogeneous group of antibodies consisting of IgM, IgG, and IgA. Of patients with rheumatoid arthritis, 70% have IgM rheumatoid factors in their serum (these patients are characterized as seropositive or rheumatoid factor positive). Most tests for rheumatoid factor measure IgM rheumatoid factor. Patients who are seronegative may have rheumatoid factors in the other immunoglobulin classes.

Rheumatoid factors have not been identified as pathogenic. The quantity of these circulating antibodies does not always correlate with disease activity. Seropositive patients tend to have a more aggressive course of illness than seronegative patients. Immunoglobulins can activate the complement system. The complement system amplifies the immune response by encouraging chemotaxis (directing inflammatory cells to the site of inflammation), phagocytosis (engulfing cells or debris by inflammatory cells), and the release of lymphokines by mononuclear cells.

The cellular component of the inflammatory process consists of polymorphonuclear cells and lymphocytes (see Fig. 60.2). Damage to synovial tissues is caused by lysosomal enzymes and other cytotoxic substances (i.e., collagenases, other enzymes, free oxygen radicals) released from these inflammatory cells. Lymphocytes may be either B cells (derived from bone marrow) or T cells (derived from thymus tissue). T cells may be either helper or suppressor T cells, which modulate the inflammatory response. The majority of lymphocytes isolated from rheumatoid synovial tissue are T cells. It has been observed that patients with rheumatoid arthritis have an abnormal ratio of helper to suppressor T cells compared with normal controls.

Vasoactive substances may also play a role in the inflammatory process. Histamine, kinins, and prostaglandins are

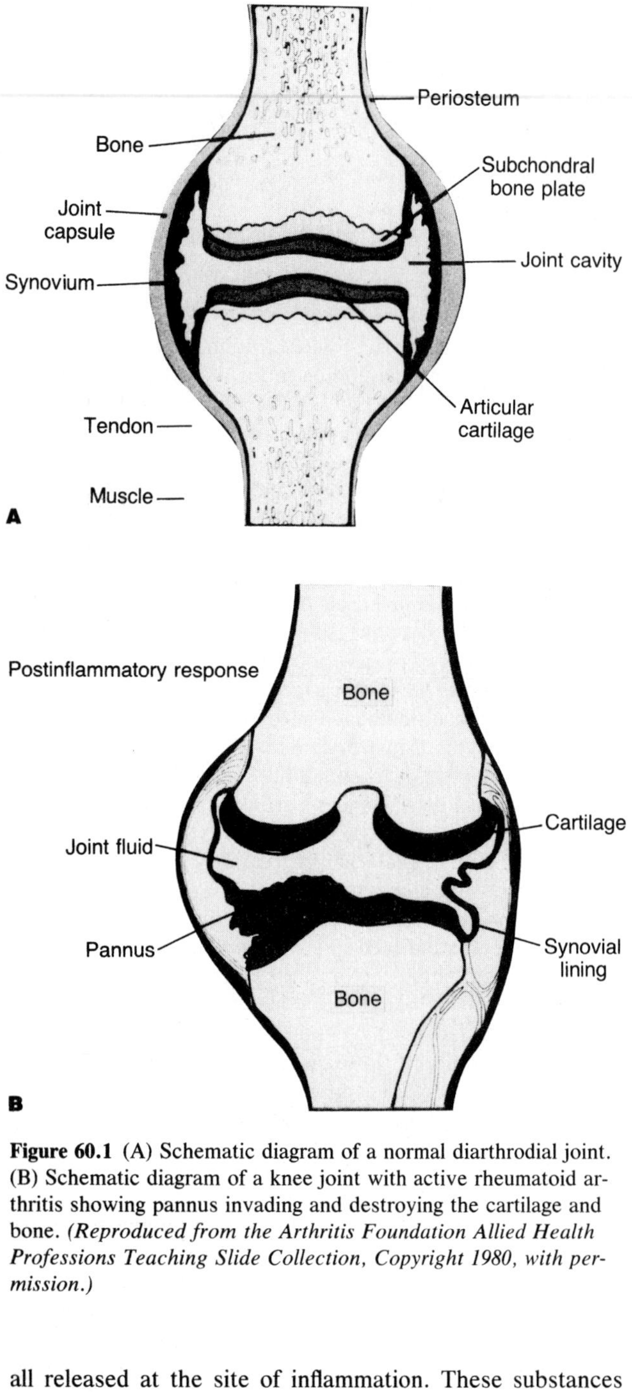


**Figure 60.1** (A) Schematic diagram of a normal diarthrodial joint. (B) Schematic diagram of a knee joint with active rheumatoid arthritis showing pannus invading and destroying the cartilage and bone. *(Reproduced from the Arthritis Foundation Allied Health Professions Teaching Slide Collection, Copyright 1980, with permission.)*

all released at the site of inflammation. These substances increase both blood flow to the site of inflammation and permeability of blood vessels. These substances cause the edema, warmth, erythema, and pain associated with inflamed joints and also make it easier for granulocytes to pass from blood vessels to the site of inflammation.

The end results of the chronic inflammatory changes are variable. Loss of cartilage may result in a loss of joint space. The formation of chronic granulation or scar tissue can lead to loss of joint motion or bony fusion (called ankylosis). Laxity of tendon structures can result in a loss of support to the affected joint, leading to instability or subluxation. Tendon contractures may also occur, leading to chronic deformity.[3–6]

**Table 60.1** American Rheumatism Association Criteria for the Diagnosis of Rheumatoid Arthritis[a]

1. Morning stiffness
2. Pain on motion or tenderness of at least one joint
3. Swelling of one joint (soft tissue or fluid)
4. Swelling of at least one other joint with a symptom-free interval no longer than 3 mo
5. Symmetric swelling of joints
6. Subcutaneous nodules over bony prominences or extensor surfaces or near joints
7. Typical radiographic changes, including periarticular osteoporosis
8. Positive serum test for rheumatoid factor
9. Synovial fluid with poor mucin clot upon addition of a weak acetic acid solution
10. Synovial histopathology compatible with rheumatoid arthritis
    a. Marked villous hypertrophy
    b. Proliferation of synovial cells
    c. Lymphocyte/plasma cell infiltration of subsynovium
    d. Fibrin deposition within or upon microvilli
11. Characteristic histopathology of rheumatoid nodules biopsied at any site

| *Degree of certainty of diagnosis* | *Number of criteria needed* |
|---|---|
| Classical rheumatoid arthritis | 7 |
| Definite rheumatoid arthritis | 5 |
| Probable rheumatoid arthritis | 3 |

[a] These symptoms must be present for 6 weeks.

### *Clinical Presentation*

The symptoms of rheumatoid arthritis usually develop insidiously over the course of several weeks to months (Table 60.1). Prodromal symptoms include fatigue, weakness, loss of appetite, and joint pain. Stiffness and muscle aches (myalgias) may precede the development of joint swelling (synovitis). Fatigue tends to be more of a problem in the afternoon. The fatigue begins earlier in the day during disease flares and subsides as disease activity lessens. Most commonly, joint involvement tends to be symmetrical; however, early in the disease some patients present with an asymmetrical pattern involving one or a few joints, which eventually develops into the more classic presentation. About 20% of patients develop an abrupt onset of their illness with fevers, polyarthritis, and constitutional symptoms (depression, anxiety, fatigue, anorexia, and weight loss).[1,2] Patients may be classified according to the interference of the condition in the activities of daily living (see Table 60.2).

#### Joint Involvement

The joints most frequently affected by rheumatoid arthritis are the small joints of the hands, wrists, and feet (see Fig. 60.3). In addition, elbows, shoulders, hips, knees, and ankles may be involved. Patients usually experience joint stiffness, typically worse in the morning. The duration of

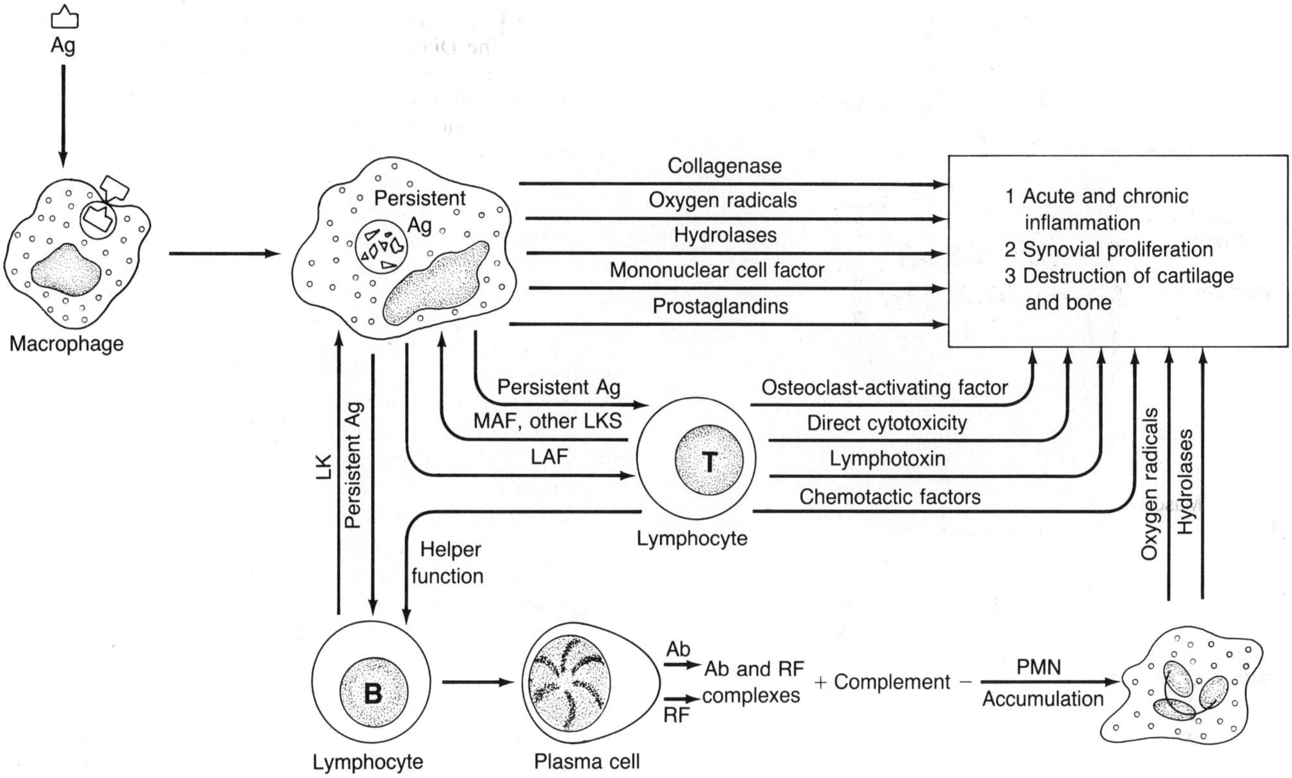


**Figure 60.2** Pathogenesis of the inflammatory response. Ag, antigen; Ab, antibody; LAF, lymphocyte-activating factor; LK, lymphokines; MAF, macrophage-activating factor; RF, rheumatoid factor. *(From Snyderman R: Mechanisms of inflammation and tissue destruction in the rheumatic diseases, in Wyngaarden JB, Smith LH [Eds]: Cecil Textbook of Medicine, 17th ed. Philadelphia, W. B. Saunders, 1985, with permission.)*

stiffness tends to be directly correlated with disease activity. The duration of stiffness reported usually exceeds 30 minutes and may persist all day. Chronic inflammation with lack of an adequate exercise program results in loss of range of motion, atrophy of muscles, weakness, and deformity.

On examination, the swelling of the joints may be visible or may be apparent only by palpation. The swelling feels soft and spongy, as it is caused by proliferation of soft tissues or fluid accumulation within the joint capsule. The swollen joint may appear erythematous and feel warmer than nearby skin surfaces, especially early in the course of the disease. In contrast, the swelling associated with osteoarthritis is usually bony (caused by osteophytes) and is infrequently associated with signs of inflammation.

**Table 60.2** Functional Classification of Rheumatoid Arthritis

| | |
|---|---|
| Class I | Capable of all activities without handicap |
| Class II | Able to conduct normal activities despite handicap of discomfort or limited mobility of one or more joints |
| Class III | Functional capacity adequate to perform only a few of the normal duties of usual occupation |
| Class IV | Confined to bed or wheelchair, capable of little or no self-care |

Hand involvement is manifest by pain, swelling, tenderness, and grip weakness during the acute phase and subluxation, instability, ulnar deviation, and muscle atrophy in the chronic phase of the disease. Functional difficulties with clasp, grasp, and pinch alter both strength and fine motor movement. This affects the activities of daily living (ADL) necessary for self-care. Tenosynovitis involving the flexor tendons of the hands often results in restriction of motion or locking of digits in a flexed position. Tenosynovitis of the extensor tendons of the hand may result in pain, swelling, and spontaneous rupture with loss of function.

Deformity of the hand may be seen with chronic inflammation. Subluxations of the wrists and metacarpophalangeal (MCP) joints may be observed. The thumbs may develop flexion at the MCP joint and hyperextension of the interphalangeal (IP) joint, which may make pinch grip difficult. Involvement of tendons in the hands can result in either hyperextension at the proximal interphalangeal (PIP) joint and flexion of the distal interphalangeal (DIP) joint (called a swan-neck deformity; see Fig. 60.4) or flexion at the PIP joint with hyperextension of the DIP joint (called a boutonniere deformity; see Fig. 60.5). Ulnar deviation of the fingers may also occur as a result of tendon abnormalities associated with rheumatoid arthritis (see Fig. 60.6).

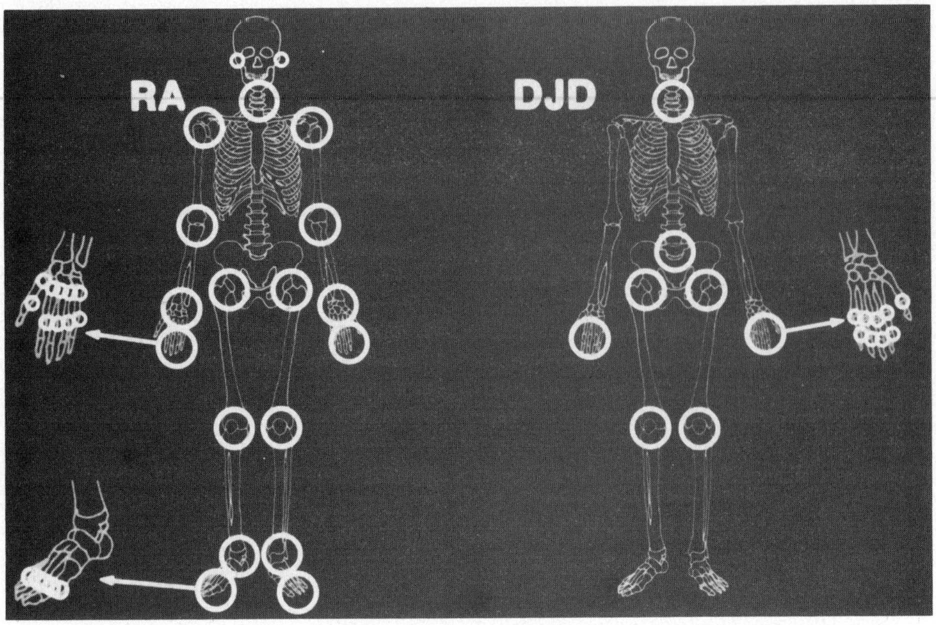


**Figure 60.3** Patterns of joint involvement in rheumatoid arthritis (RA) and degenerative joint disease (DJD). *(Reproduced from the Arthritis Foundation Allied Health Professions Teaching Slide Collection, Copyright 1980, with permission.)*

Wrist involvement results in joint space narrowing, collapse, and subluxation, leading to grip weakness. Destruction of the cartilage at the radioulnar joint results in pain on pronation (rotation of the forearm with the palm downward) and supination (rotation of the forearm with the palm upward) of the hand and limits its use in twisting, wringing, or percussive activities. Carpal tunnel syndrome, caused by entrapment of the median nerve by inflamed synovium, results in pain and tingling in the fingers and grip weakness.

Swelling at the elbow is most evident at the radial–humeral joint. Shoulder pain may result from involvement of the joint itself or from tendon inflammation (tendinitis) or inflammation of the bursa (bursitis) near the deltoid muscle.

The knee can also be involved, with loss of cartilage, instability, and joint pain. Synovitis of the knee may cause a cyst to form behind the knee (called a popliteal cyst or Baker's cyst). These cysts may become painful as they become tense or rupture, producing a clinical picture much like that seen with thrombophlebitis secondary to the release of inflammatory components into the calf muscle area. Chronic joint pain leads to muscle atrophy, which can result in a laxity of the ligamentous structures that support the knee, causing instability. Maintenance of an adequate range of motion of the knee is essential to normal gait.

Involvement of the ankle may result in a soft spongy swelling, either anterior or posterior to the malleoli. Involvement of the subtalar joint, which controls inversion and eversion of the foot, may result in difficulty walking on uneven ground. The metatarsophalangeal (MTP) joints are commonly involved in rheumatoid arthritis, making walking difficult. Subluxation of the metatarsal heads leads to "cock-up" toe deformities. Subluxation may also cause a flexion

**Figure 60.4** Swan-neck deformity in rheumatoid arthritis. *(Reproduced from the Arthritis Foundation Allied Health Professions Teaching Slide Collection, Copyright 1980, with permission.)*

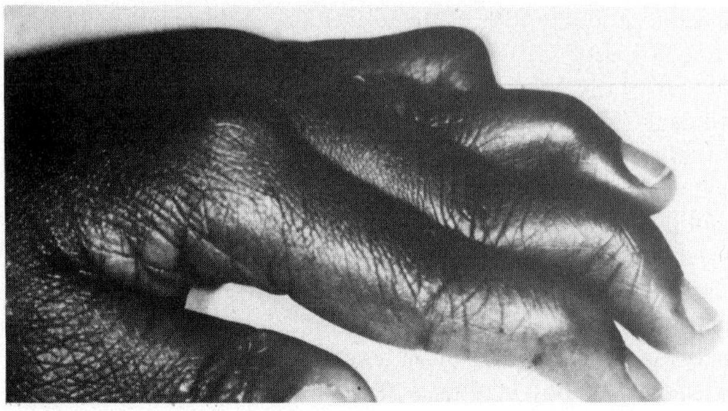

**Figure 60.5** Boutonniere deformity in rheumatoid arthritis.

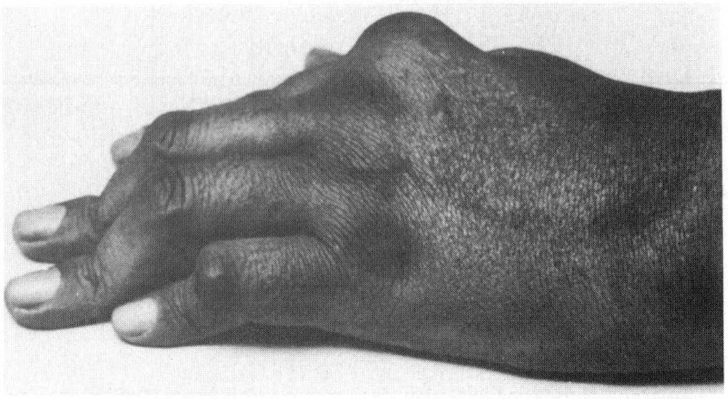

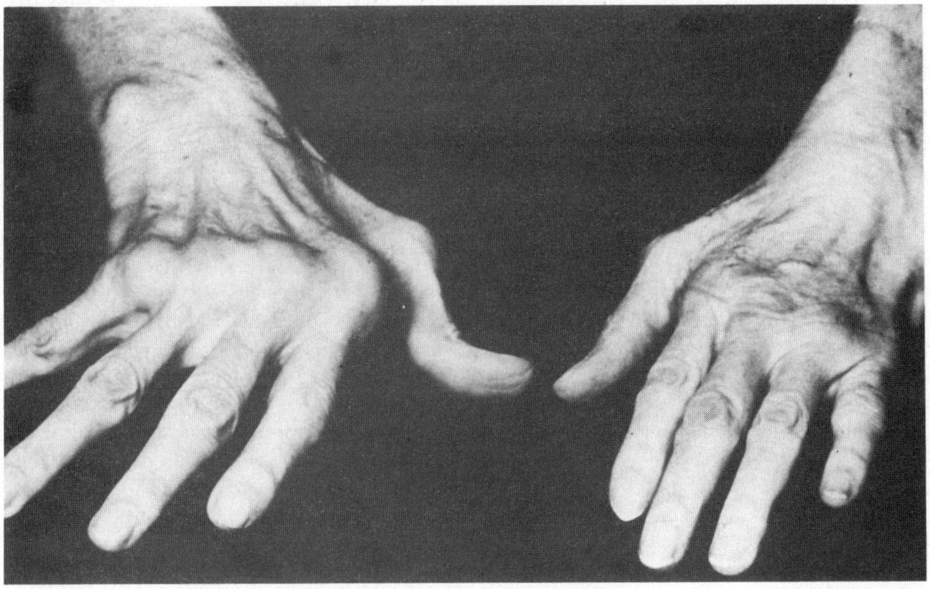

**Figure 60.6** Ulnar deviation of the fingers of the right hand. *(Reproduced from the Arthritis Foundation Allied Health Professions Teaching Slide Collection, Copyright 1980, with permission.)*

deformity at the proximal interphalangeal joint of the toe, leading to pressure necrosis of the joint secondary to irritation caused by shoes. Hallux valgus (lateral deviation of the digit) and bunion or callus formation may occur at the great toe (see Fig. 60.7). A widening of the foot commonly occurs with long-standing disease.

Involvement of the spine usually occurs in the cervical vertebrae; lumbar vertebral involvement is rare. Involvement of the first ($C_1$) and second ($C_2$) cervical vertebrae can lead to instability of this joint. Patients with this problem are at a greater risk for spinal cord compression, although this complication is rare.

**Figure 60.7** Foot involvement of rheumatoid arthritis with hallux valgus deformity of the first digit and hammer toe deformity of the second through fifth digits bilaterally. *(Reproduced from the Arthritis Foundation Allied Health Professions Teaching Slide Collection, Copyright 1980, with permission.)*

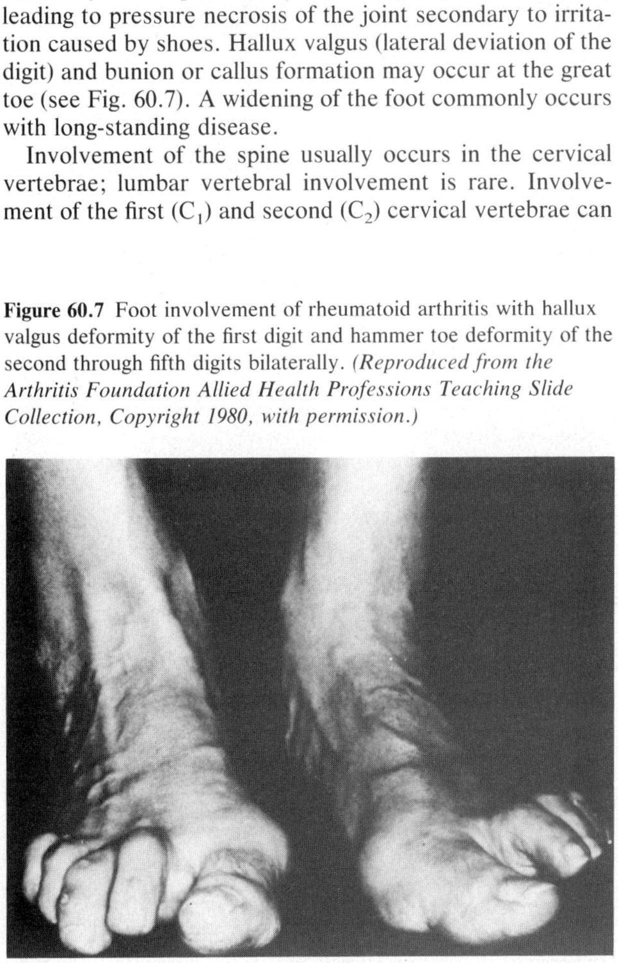

The temporomandibular joint (jaw) can be affected, resulting in malocclusion and difficulty in chewing food. Inflammation of the cartilage in the chest can lead to chest wall pain. Hip pain may occur as a result of destructive changes in the hip joint, soft tissue inflammation (e.g., bursitis), or referred pain from nerve entrapment at the lumbar vertebrae.

### Extra-articular Involvement

***Rheumatoid Nodules*** Rheumatoid nodules occur in 20% of patients with rheumatoid arthritis. These nodules are most commonly seen on the extensor surfaces of the elbows, forearms, and hands but may also be seen on the feet and at pressure points elsewhere on the body. They may also develop on the pleural lining of the lung and rarely in the meninges. Rheumatoid nodules are asymptomatic and do not require any special intervention. Nodules are more commonly observed in patients with erosive, destructive disease.[7]

***Vasculitis*** Vasculitis may result in a wide variety of clinical presentations. Invasion of blood vessel walls by inflammatory cells results in obliteration of the vessel, producing infarction of tissue distal to the area of involvement. Most commonly, small-vessel vasculitis produces infarcts near the ends of the fingers or toes, especially around the nail beds. These infarcts are usually of little consequence. Vasculitis may also cause the breakdown of skin, especially in the lower extremities, producing ulcers that may be indistinguishable in appearance from stasis ulcers. However, these ulcers do not heal with the usual modes of treatment used for stasis ulcers. Involvement of larger vessels with vasculitis can result in life-threatening complications. Infarction of vessels supplying blood to nerves can cause irreversible motor deficit. Involvement of vessels supplying other organ systems can lead to visceral involvement and a polyarteritis nodosa–like illness. Fortunately, the more serious vasculitic picture is rarely seen.

***Pulmonary Complications*** Rheumatoid arthritis may involve the pleura of the lung, which is often asymptomatic. Pleural fluid obtained from patients with effusions characteristically has a low glucose concentration (frequently 10–50 mg/dL). Pulmonary fibrosis may also develop as a result of rheumatoid involvement; smoking appears to increase the risk of this complication. Rheumatoid nodules may develop in lung tissue and may be difficult to distinguish from neoplasms. Interstitial pneumonitis and arteritis are rare, potentially life-threatening complications of rheumatoid arthritis.

***Ocular Manifestations*** These include keratoconjunctivitis sicca and inflammation of the sclera, episclera, and cornea. Atrophy of the lacrimal duct may result in a decrease in tear formation, causing dry and itchy eyes, termed *keratoconjunctivitis sicca*. When this is observed in association with rheumatoid arthritis, it is referred to as Sjögren's syndrome. Artificial tears may be used to relieve symptoms. Inflammation of the superficial layers of the sclera (episcleritis) is generally self-limiting. Involvement of deeper tissues (scleritis) usually results in a more serious, painful, and chronic inflammation. Nodules may develop on the sclera.

***Cardiac Involvement*** This occurs in rheumatoid arthritis but is rarely symptomatic. Pericarditis may occur, resulting in the accumulation of fluid. Although many patients show evidence of previous pericarditis at autopsy, the development of clinically evident pericarditis with tamponade is a rare complication. Cardiac conduction abnormalities and aortic valve incompetence, caused by aortic root dilatation, may occur. Myocarditis is a rare complication of rheumatoid arthritis.

***Other Complications*** Lymphadenopathy may occur in patients with rheumatoid arthritis, particularly in nodes proximal to more actively involved joints. Renal involvement is rare but can be associated with treatment including nonsteroidal anti-inflammatory drugs (NSAIDs), gold salts, and penicillamine. Amyloidosis is a rare complication of long-standing rheumatoid arthritis. It appears to be more common in Europe than in this country.

Rheumatoid arthritis in association with splenomegaly and neutropenia is known as *Felty's syndrome*. Leukopenic patients are more susceptible to infection. The decrease in granulocytes appears to be mediated by the immune system, as splenectomy does not result in improvement of the patient.[8]

### *Laboratory Findings*

Hematologic tests often reveal a mild to moderate anemia with normocytic, normochromic indices. The hematocrit may fall as low as 30%. The anemia is usually inversely related to inflammatory disease activity and is referred to as an anemia of chronic disease. This type of anemia does not respond to iron therapy and can present a diagnostic dilemma, as NSAIDs may induce gastritis and chronic blood loss leading to iron deficiency anemia. Laboratory tests useful in differentiating these anemias include stool guaiac (or other stool tests for occult blood), serum iron/iron binding capacity ratio (decreased in iron deficiency), and mean corpuscular volume (more likely to be decreased in iron deficiency). Other causes of anemia must also be considered in the differential diagnosis (see Chapter 69).

Thrombocytosis is another common hematologic finding with active rheumatoid arthritis. Platelet counts rise and fall in direct correlation with disease activity. Thrombocytopenia may result from the toxicity of gold salts, penicillamine, or immunosuppressive therapy. Thrombocytopenia may also be observed in Felty's syndrome or vasculitis.

Although leukopenia is associated with Felty's syndrome, it may be associated with the toxicity of gold, penicillamine, and immunosuppressive drugs. Leukocytosis is commonly seen as a result of corticosteroid treatment.

The erythrocyte sedimentation rate (ESR) is usually elevated in patients with rheumatoid arthritis and other inflammatory diseases. This test is very nonspecific, and although the ESR usually falls as patients respond to therapy, there is a large variability among patients in response to treatment.

Rheumatoid factor is present in 60% to 70% of patients with rheumatoid arthritis. The usual laboratory test for rheumatoid factor is an antibody specific for IgM rheumatoid factor. Patients with rheumatoid arthritis and a negative test for rheumatoid factor may have IgG or IgA rheumatoid factors, but tests for these are not routinely available. Rheumatoid factor tests are usually reported positive at a specific serum dilution. Serum is diluted to a standard series of dilutions; the greatest dilution that yields a positive test result is reported (e.g., rheumatoid factor positive at 1:640). Higher dilutional titers of rheumatoid factors usually indicate a more severe disease, but like the ESR, the large interpatient variability makes this test difficult to use as a means of assessing patient progress. Rheumatoid factor may be positive in patients without rheumatoid arthritis (Table 60.3).

**Table 60.3** Diseases Associated With a Positive Rheumatoid Factor

| |
|---|
| Rheumatic diseases |
| Rheumatoid arthritis |
| Sjögren's syndrome (with or without arthritis) |
| Systemic lupus erythematosus |
| Progressive systemic sclerosis |
| Polymyositis/dermatomyositis |
| Infectious diseases |
| Bacterial endocarditis |
| Tuberculosis |
| Syphilis |
| Infectious mononucleosis |
| Infectious hepatitis |
| Leprosy |
| Other causes |
| Aging |
| Interstitial pulmonary fibrosis |
| Cirrhosis of the liver |
| Chronic active hepatitis |
| Sarcoidosis |

Antinuclear antibodies (ANAs) are detected in 25% of patients with rheumatoid arthritis. These antibodies usually have a diffuse pattern of immunofluorescence. Tests for antibodies to double-stranded DNA (usually positive in systemic lupus erythematosus, SLE) are negative. Serum complement is usually normal, although complement concentrations of joint fluid are often depressed from consumption secondary to the inflammatory process. In patients with vasculitis, serum complement concentrations may be low.

Synovial fluid usually is turbid because of the large number of leukocytes in inflammatory fluid. White cell counts of 5,000 to 50,000/$mm^3$ are not uncommon in inflamed joints. The fluid is usually less viscous than that in normal joints or in fluid associated with osteoarthritis. Glucose concentrations of joint fluid are normal or low compared with those in serum drawn at the same time as synovial aspirates. The decrease is not as profound as the decrease associated with joint infection or SLE.

Radiologic manifestations of rheumatoid arthritis include soft tissue swelling and osteoporosis near the joint (periarticular osteoporosis). Erosions tend to occur later in the course of the disease and are usually seen first in the MCP and PIP joints of the hands and the MTP joints of the feet. Erosions are usually first seen at the margin of the joint near the interface of the head of the bone with the synovial tissue (see Fig. 60.8).

### *Treatment*

The goals of treatment in patients with rheumatoid arthritis are to relieve pain, to preserve joint function, and to prevent further disease progression. These goals may not be achievable in all patients even with an optimal treatment program. Although drugs play a very important role, nondrug therapy should always be used in conjunction with pharmacologic approaches to management.

#### Nondrug Therapy

Nondrug therapy consists of rest, physical therapy, occupational therapy, social services, and surgical intervention. The goals of physical therapy are to preserve and maintain range of motion and prevent muscle atrophy. Chronic joint pain and inflammation can lead to decreased activity. This decrease in use can result in a loss in range of motion, atrophy, and weakness of the affected limb or joint.

An exercise program designed to move joints through their full range of motion is helpful in preventing these complications. It is useful in maintaining muscle tone, decreasing the likelihood of joint instability. Initially the exercises are done without weights or added resistance. Gradually, resistance is added to improve strength and endurance. In addition to exercise, adequate rest must also be provided. Overuse of joints from excessive physical activity can aggravate ar-

**Figure 60.8** Radiograph of normal hand (right) and hand affected by rheumatoid arthritis (left) with joint space narrowing, periarticular osteoporosis, and erosions (see arrows). *(Reproduced from the Arthritis Foundation Allied Health Professions Teaching Slide Collection, Copyright 1980, with permission.)*

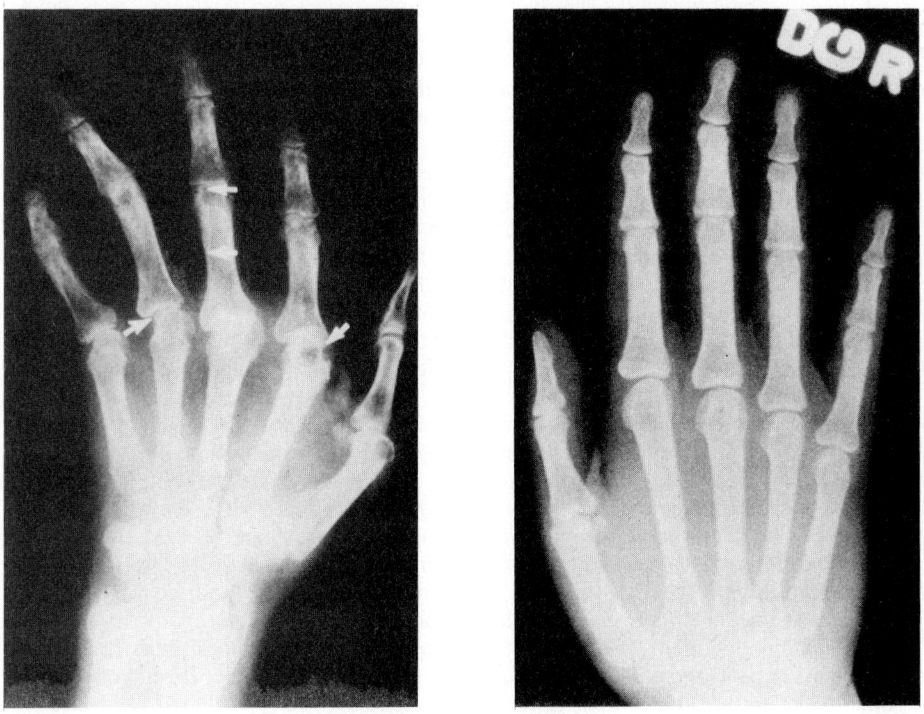

thritic symptoms. Joint protection and work-simplification measures may be necessary to assist the patient in maintaining self-care.

Prosthetic devices may be of benefit in selected patients. Canes and crutches can be used to unload major symptomatic weight-bearing joints and to provide additional support for unstable joints. Cervical collars, wrist splints, and knee braces may restrict motion of painful joints. Resting and supporting symptomatic joints will diminish pain in many patients with rheumatoid arthritis.

Surgical procedures are necessary in some patients with rheumatoid arthritis. Removal of the synovium (synovectomy) can relieve pain and swelling in isolated, active joints. The synovium does regrow and the procedure does not routinely provide permanent relief of symptoms. Joint replacement may be necessary when severe destructive changes have occurred in major weight-bearing joints. Procedures to improve the functional capabilities of hand and foot joints may be necessary in some patients.[9]

**Drug Therapy**

Figure 60.9 provides an algorithm for the treatment of rheumatoid arthritis. The initial pharmacologic treatment of choice for most patients is salicylates or NSAIDs. These drugs are analgesic at lower doses and require regular scheduled dosing at higher dosage levels to achieve an anti-inflammatory effect.

In general, the newer NSAIDs have similar toxic effects, are no more effective in clinical trials, and are more costly compared with aspirin. Therapeutic effect varies among patients receiving these agents, and most clinicians recommend a trial of several of these agents before progressing to more costly and toxic therapeutic alternatives.

NSAIDs work by a different mechanism than do other therapies for inflammatory arthritis. The combination of an NSAID with other treatment is additive. NSAIDs block some of the manifestations of the inflammatory response but do not appear to alter the progression of the disease.

Patients who fail to get adequate relief of their inflammation or who show evidence of disease progression while taking NSAIDs are candidates for more aggressive treatment. The slow-acting antirheumatic drugs (SAARDs), such as gold, hydroxychloroquine, and penicillamine, are usually added to an NSAID. These drugs characteristically have a 2- to 6-month delay between initiation of treatment and onset of action. They are also more toxic and require frequent monitoring to avoid serious complications. Patients who fail to respond to a 6-month trial of therapy or who have serious toxic effects from one agent may be switched to another SAARD.

Methotrexate, azathioprine, and cyclophosphamide are antineoplastic drugs with proven activity in the management of rheumatoid arthritis. Azathioprine is the only drug in this class that has FDA approval for the treatment of rheumatoid arthritis. These agents are generally reserved for patients who have failed to respond to the SAARDs or for patients with life-threatening complications.

Corticosteroids are reserved for short-term management of patients with severe limitation of their daily activities while waiting for a therapeutic response to a SAARD, or for patients who fail all other treatments. The dosage is usually limited to the smallest dose that provides a therapeutic effect. Intra-articular injections of long-acting corticosteroids may be useful in patients with monoarthritis. Injections of corticosteroids may be of benefit in the management of soft tissue inflammations (e.g., tendonitis, bursitis). See Table 60.4 for laboratory monitoring parameters for antirheumatic drugs.

***Salicylates*** Many clinicians choose aspirin for the initial treatment of rheumatoid arthritis. Administered on a regular basis in divided doses, plain aspirin tablets are the least expensive and a good initial choice.[10] Alternative formulations are available for use in patients with aspirin intolerance. The simple analgesic and antipyretic actions of aspirin may be achieved at relatively low doses. When used to reduce the inflammation associated with rheumatoid arthritis, higher dosages are required.[11] An adequate anti-inflammatory dosage of 0.9 g four times a day, preferably with meals, is the usual initial regimen. The dose is gradually increased by one or two tablets a week until therapeutic benefit or toxic effects develop.

The optimal dosage at which a patient should be maintained is slightly less than that which causes tinnitus. Tinnitus may be an unreliable indicator of toxicity in children and older patients in whom more serious, if not fatal, metabolic disturbances may occur before tinnitus is observed. Serum salicylate concentration monitoring is necessary in the young, the elderly, and those with preexisting or undetected hearing loss. Patients with high-tone hearing loss before salicylate therapy often do not experience tinnitus, even with very high salicylate concentrations. A serum salicylate concentration between 15 and 30 mg/dL is considered therapeutic. A decrease in dosage generally reverses most toxic effects, although some patients require drug cessation. Blood salicylate concentrations may also be useful in assessing patient compliance.

Low doses of salicylate are eliminated via first-order kinetic processes; however, as salicylate dosage is increased, most metabolic pathways of the drug become saturated, prolonging the serum half-life. Analgesic doses of salicylate have a plasma elimination half-life of 2.5 hours; anti-inflammatory doses result in an elimination half-life of 16 to 18 hours. Plasma protein binding site saturation also occurs at higher dosages, creating a decrease in the apparent volume of distribution. These factors cause large increases in serum salicylate concentrations with even small incremental dosage increases. These effects may be offset by shifts in salicylate metabolism and excretion toward nonsaturable pathways. Total clearance for a given salicylate dose eventually stabilizes and remains constant. Because of the complexity of salicylate pharmacokinetics, 5 to 7 days is required to reach a new steady-state blood concentration after a change in dosage. Incremental changes greater than 650 mg/d are not recommended.

Salicylate and its metabolites are excreted primarily in the urine and should be used with caution in patients with impaired renal function. Because of its inhibitory effect on renal prostaglandin synthesis, aspirin may further reduce glomerular filtration and renal blood flow. It has also been shown to blunt the diuretic effects of furosemide and spironolactone and may block the uricosuric action of probenecid and sulfinpyrazone. Hepatic abnormalities have been seen in association with high blood salicylate concentrations, and close monitoring is advisable, particularly in patients with

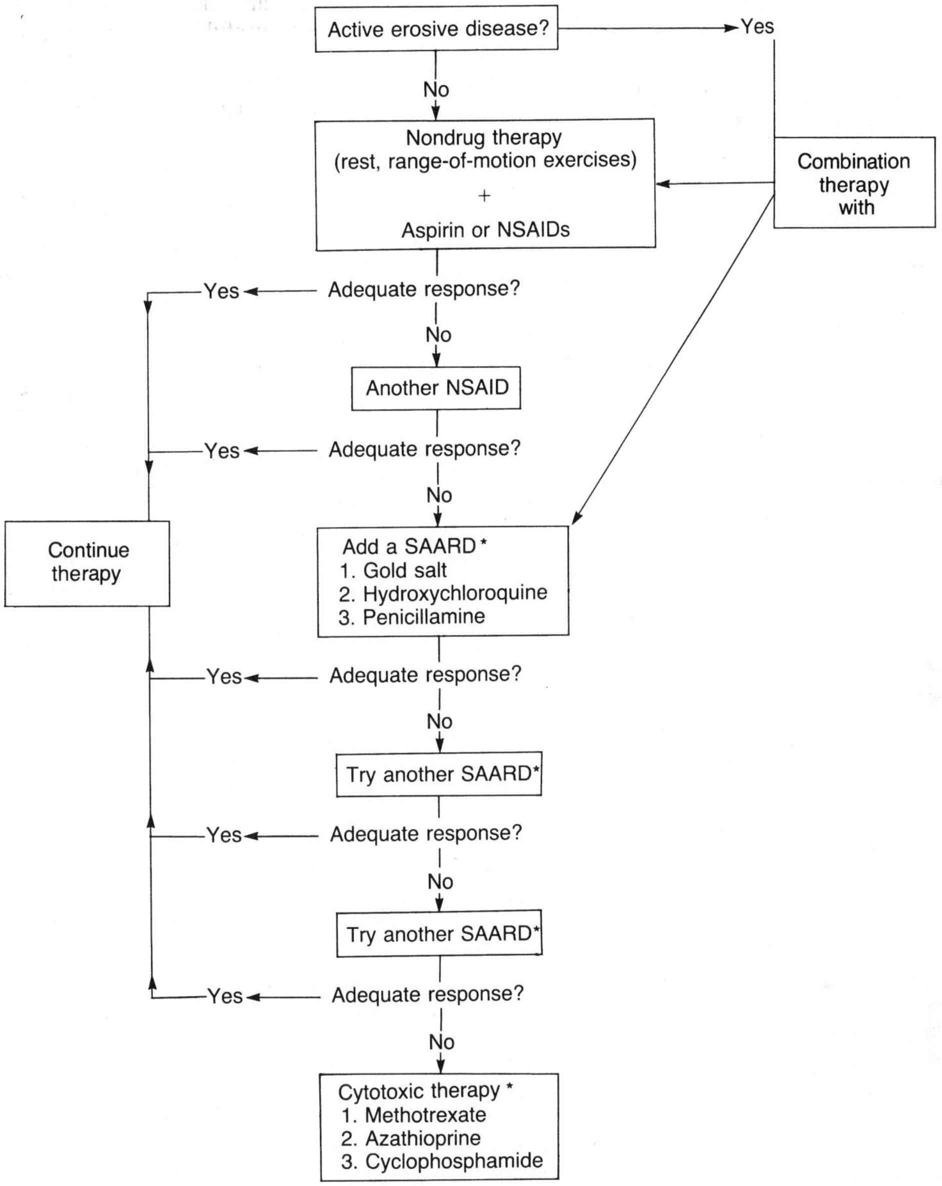


**Figure 60.9** Algorithm for treatment of rheumatoid arthritis. *Corticosteroids may be necessary for patients with severe inflammatory disease, in any of these phases, to enable the patient to be more functional while awaiting the beneficial effects of therapy or treatment failure.

systemic lupus erythematosus, juvenile rheumatoid arthritis, or adult-onset Still's disease. Salicylate usage has been implicated in the development of Reye's syndrome in children, but the liver pathology of that disease is quite different from that found in aspirin-induced hepatotoxicity.

While many salicylate preparations commonly cause gastrointestinal blood loss, this is usually minimal and may not require a change in therapy.[12] Inhibition of gastric prostaglandin synthesis is presumably responsible for some gastric damage, as prostaglandins stimulate production of gastric mucus that protects against autodigestion. Direct contact of aspirin particles with the mucosa causes superficial gastric erosions and bleeding, but severe gastrointestinal hemorrhage is uncommon. Although salicylates may aggravate peptic ulcer disease, there is no evidence relating dyspepsia after aspirin ingestion to the occurrence of severe bleeding. Gastrointestinal upset may be alleviated by giving the drug with meals or antacids. Regular use of therapeutic doses of antacids may, however, produce an increase in urinary pH and a resulting increase in salicylate excretion, as the renal excretion of salicylate is highly pH dependent. Use of urine acidifiers could, likewise, theoretically increase serum salicylate concentrations.

If gastrointestinal intolerance occurs in the presence of a desired therapeutic response, a buffered or enteric-coated preparation may be initiated. These preparations are usually better tolerated and less irritating than regular aspirin and generally provide reliable absorption. A number of salts of

**Table 60.4** Laboratory Monitoring Parameters for Antirheumatic Drugs

| *Drug* | *Trade name* | *Monitoring parameter* |
|---|---|---|
| Salicylates | | Serum assays (salicylates) |
| NSAIDs | | Complete blood counts |
| | | Renal function tests |
| Gold salts | | Complete blood counts |
| Aurothioglucose | Solganol | Platelet counts |
| Gold sodium thiomalate | Myochrysine | Urinalysis |
| Auranofin | Ridaura | |
| Antimalarials | | Ophthalmologic examination |
| Hydroxychloroquine | Plaquenil | (with red light peripheral |
| Chloroquine | Aralen | visual field testing) |
| Penicillamine | Cuprimine | Complete blood counts |
| | Depen | Platelet counts |
| | | Urinalysis |
| Azathioprine | Imuran | Complete blood counts |
| | | Platelet counts |
| | | AST or ALT serum assays[a] |
| Cyclophosphamide | Cytoxan | Complete blood counts |
| | | Platelet counts |
| | | Urinalysis |
| Methotrexate | | Complete blood counts |
| | | Platelet counts |
| | | AST or ALT serum assays |

[a] AST, aspartate aminotransferase (formerly SGOT); ALT, alanine aminotransferase (formerly SGPT).

salicylic acid are also available as alternatives to aspirin. Sodium salicylate, magnesium salicylate, choline salicylate, choline magnesium trisalicylate, and salicyl salicylate may produce fewer adverse gastrointestinal effects, but may also be pharmacologically inferior to aspirin.

The only absolute contraindications to the use of aspirin are a history of severe gastrointestinal bleeding, coagulopathies, or a history of aspirin hypersensitivity. Nasal polyps and asthma are associated with aspirin hypersensitivity. In these patients aspirin challenge may result in bronchospasm, rhinorrhea, or anaphylaxis. Patients intolerant of aspirin might also display a cross-sensitivity to other nonsteroidal drugs. A cautious trial with an alternative nonacetyl salicylate preparation may be used in patients who describe a previous allergy to aspirin.

Of the many potential interactions between salicylates and other drugs, few are clinically important. Concurrent use of salicylates with other NSAIDs should be discouraged, as salicylates decrease serum concentrations of many of these drugs, usually via protein displacement. No data indicate that salicylate/NSAID combinations have a synergistic effect, and there may be additive toxicity. Salicylates may potentiate the hypoglycemic effects of sulfonylurea drugs, necessitating a reduction in dosage.

Corticosteroids may cause a decrease in serum salicylate concentrations. Aspirin may also increase the bone marrow–depressing effects of high-dose methotrexate; the importance of this interaction with the small doses of methotrexate used in rheumatoid arthritis patients is not known. Aspirin displaces warfarin-type anticoagulants from protein binding sites, and an increased tendency for bleeding exists when these drugs are used simultaneously. Aspirin irreversibly inhibits platelet aggregation. Several days are necessary for reversal of this effect, as new platelets must be released into circulation before bleeding time normalizes. Nonacetylated salicylates have less effect on platelet aggregation. Patients undergoing elective surgery should be advised to discontinue aspirin 7 to 10 days before a procedure.

*Nonsteroidal Anti-inflammatory Drugs* If patients do not tolerate or respond inadequately to salicylates, NSAIDs should be used. The efficacy and toxicity of these drugs are comparable to those of salicylates. Like aspirin, the NSAIDs are anti-inflammatory, analgesic, and antipyretic. The mechanism of action is prostaglandin synthesis inhibition; however, it is unlikely that all NSAIDs act only on prostaglandins and by only one mechanism.[13]

Clinical trials have not shown superiority of any of these agents over the others for the management of rheumatoid arthritis. There may be a large intersubject variability in response to these drugs.[14] Inadequate response or loss of response to one NSAID does not imply inefficacy of other NSAIDs. Treatment with an alternative NSAID is appropriate in these instances before considering the addition of more expensive and more toxic agents. Attempts to correlate free and total serum/synovial drug concentrations with clinical response have met with limited success in most studies. As a result, pharmacokinetic monitoring is not used.

All currently marketed NSAIDs are rapidly and reliably absorbed. They are best administered with food to decrease gastric irritation. Food may delay absorption of ibuprofen and ketoprofen and impair absorption of fenoprofen; how-

**Table 60.5** Dosage Regimens for Nonsteroidal Anti-inflammatory Drugs

| *Drug* | *Trade name* | *Clearance half-life (h)* | *Recommended anti-inflammatory daily dosage* | | *Dosing schedule* |
|---|---|---|---|---|---|
| | | | **Adult** | **Children** | |
| Fenoprofen | Nalfon | 2-3 | 2.4–3.0 g | — | QID |
| Ibuprofen | Motrin<br>Rufen | 1-3 | 1.2–2.4 g | 10 mg/kg | TID to QID |
| Indomethacin | Indocin | 1.5-2 | 75–200 mg | 2.5 mg/kg | QID |
| Ketoprofen | Orudis | 2-4 | 150–300 mg | — | TID to QID |
| Meclofenamate | Meclomen | 2-4 | 300–400 mg | — | QID |
| Naproxen | Naprosyn | 12-15 | 0.5–1 g | 10 mg/kg | BID |
| Piroxicam | Feldene | 24-36 | 20 mg | — | QD |
| Sulindac | Clinoril | 18 | 200–400 mg | 6 mg/kg | BID |
| Tolmetin[a] | Tolectin | 1 | 0.6–2 g | 25 mg/kg | QID |

[a] FDA approved for juvenile arthritis.

ever, these effects are minimal. Some NSAIDs, such as sulindac and fenbufen, are inactive prodrugs, metabolized in the liver to their active forms. All the drugs are highly plasma protein bound, primarily to albumin. With regular dosing, it will take four to five half-lives to reach steady-state plasma concentrations. As a result, short-acting drugs reach plateau concentrations within 24 to 48 hours. NSAIDs with longer half-lives may require days to weeks to achieve maximum plasma concentration.[15] Sufficient time must be allowed for an adequate clinical trial with one agent before its use is considered a treatment failure. Normally, a trial period of 2 to 3 weeks is required before treatment is defined as a failure or success. See Table 60.5 for recommended anti-inflammatory dosages of NSAIDs and serum half-lives.

NSAIDs are extensively metabolized by the liver, but with little first-pass effect (except for aspirin deacetylation). Most metabolites are excreted by the kidneys, with little clearance of unchanged drug. Most of the NSAIDs inhibit the renal prostaglandin synthesis necessary for maintenance of intrarenal blood flow, especially in cases of mild to moderate renal function impairment. This leads to a rise in BUN and serum creatinine, in addition to salt and water retention with consequent edema and weight gain. Decreases in plasma renin concentrations have been observed. NSAIDs may block the action of diuretics, resulting in sodium and fluid retention and possibly increased blood pressure. Rarely, NSAIDs have been reported to cause interstitial nephritis.

Gastrointestinal irritation is the most commonly encountered side effect of the NSAIDs. This toxic effect results largely from inhibition of prostaglandins' protective effect on gastric mucosa and direct irritation of mucosal tissues. These effects may be minimized by administration of the drug with food or antacids. Concurrent cimetidine or ranitidine may be indicated for use in selected patients. Possible CNS toxic effects include fatigue, headache, dizziness, nightmares, depression, anxiety, and tinnitus.

Other side effects occasionally observed with NSAIDs include visual blurring, morbilliform rashes, and rare reports of Stevens–Johnson syndrome and anaphylactic reactions. Clinicians should be aware of the possibility of renal or hepatic toxicity, especially with long-term use. Clinically important drug interactions exist between most NSAIDs and other highly protein-bound drugs, such as the oral anticoagulants and hypoglycemics. Patients receiving these drugs in combination should be monitored for enhanced therapeutic effects. Displacement from protein by other drugs, such as aspirin, results in decreased plasma concentrations and increased clearance of NSAIDs. Concurrent use of two NSAIDs should be discouraged, as the combination may lead to additive or synergistic toxicity rather than increased efficacy.[16] Future research may disclose that agents indeed have slightly different mechanisms of action that lead to added efficacy. This theory, however, requires further investigation.

*Gold* Rheumatoid arthritis was first treated with gold salts in the early 1930s, because of the success of their use in treating tuberculosis, a disease theorized at the time to be of a common etiology. The relatively high incidence of toxic effects from the regimens used at that time limited the use of gold compounds. Studies confirming gold's clinical efficacy and safety in rheumatoid arthritis were not published until the early 1960s. Today it is the most common initial choice among rheumatologists for remission-inducing therapy. Studies have shown gold to be most effective in early, nonerosive rheumatoid arthritis, but it also has demonstrated efficacy in long-standing disease with active synovitis.

The mechanisms of action for gold remain unclear. It has been shown to affect processes of inflammation, the immune system, and cellular biochemistry.

The two intramuscular gold salts used are gold sodium thiomalate (Myochrysine, Merck Sharp & Dohme), prepared as an aqueous solution, and aurothioglucose (Solganol, Schering), a suspension in oil. Both compounds are water soluble and contain 50% gold by weight, attached to a sulfhydryl moiety. The drugs are approximately equal in efficacy. Some studies suggest that aurothioglucose may be less toxic.[17] After injection, most gold is bound to albumin and reaches peak serum concentrations (700 $\mu$g/dL) in a few hours. Aurothioglucose has somewhat lower peak serum concentrations because of a slower absorption rate. The serum half-life ranges from 14 to 168 days with chronic dosing, and steady-state concentrations (approximately 50%

of the initial peak) are achieved in 6 to 8 weeks. Serum concentrations directly reflect the administered dose but show little correlation with efficacy or toxicity. Gold is widely distributed throughout body tissues and fluids. Amounts of gold ranging from 30% to 45% are retained in the body, depending on dose and frequency of administration. Approximately 40% of an administered dose is eliminated, 70% in the urine and 30% fecally. After termination of therapy, gold may be detectable in the serum for up to 1 year.

The standard regimen of parenteral gold for adults with RA consists of a test dose of 10 mg intramuscularly, followed by 25–50 mg given at weekly intervals. The beneficial effects of gold therapy usually are not observed before 400–500 mg is given. Patients failing to achieve benefits after a 1,000-mg cumulative dose of gold are usually considered treatment failures. After a favorable response, injection intervals may be progressively lengthened to 2 to 4 weeks. The usual maintenance dosage is 25–50 mg monthly. Barring signs of toxicity, maintenance therapy may be continued indefinitely or gold may be ceased after several years of remission.

Auranofin, a triethylphosphine gold compound containing 29% gold by weight, is administered orally and has been shown to be nearly as effective as the parenteral gold salts in treating RA. Auranofin differs from the injectable forms of gold in pharmacokinetics.[18] Auranofin is rapidly but incompletely (25%) absorbed via the oral route. Peak plasma concentrations (80 $\mu$g/dL) are significantly lower with oral gold, and steady-state plasma concentrations are attained after approximately 12 weeks. Total body retention of auranofin is less than that of parenteral gold. Elimination of auranofin is dose dependent, with the majority (95%) eliminated via the fecal route.

The usual dosage of auranofin for adults with rheumatoid arthritis is 3 mg twice daily; lower doses are less effective and higher doses are associated with more gastrointestinal toxicity. As with parenteral gold, onset of response to auranofin may be delayed by 3 to 12 months.

Cutaneous reactions are the most common toxic manifestations of gold therapy, ranging from a transient, nonspecific dermatitis to rare, life-threatening exfoliative dermatitis.[19] The character of the rash is variable, but it is often pruritic. Stomatitis occurs less frequently and may accompany dermatitis or appear independently. Most clinicians recommend discontinuance of gold therapy if mucocutaneous reactions occur. Patients may be rechallenged with gold when the rash clears (1–4 months) if the previous reaction was not severe. Renal toxicity is manifested by mild to moderate proteinuria or hematuria, usually requiring cessation of therapy. Hematologic complications include reversible thrombocytopenia, anemia, leukopenia, and severe bone marrow aplasia. Vasomotor (nitritoid) reaction, characterized by weakness, dizziness, nausea, vomiting, diaphoresis, and facial flushing, may follow administration of the parenteral gold salts. Substitution of another parenteral gold salt may be advantageous for these patients. Some patients may experience a flare in their rheumatoid arthritis after an injection of gold. These reactions typically resolve a few days after the injection and recur with the next injection. This reaction is often resolved with use of a different gold salt. Other rare but serious complications of gold therapy include hepatitis, colitis, and pneumonitis.

Many side effects observed with auranofin are similar to those seen with injectable gold compounds. In addition, mild and transient diarrhea and abdominal cramps are commonly observed. Symptoms are generally seen early in therapy, may improve with time or dosage reduction, and rarely require discontinuance of drug. The toxic effects observed with parenteral gold compounds occur less commonly with auranofin; rates of withdrawal from gold therapy because of drug intolerance are lower with oral gold.

In view of the potential serious toxicity of gold, laboratory parameters must be monitored (see Table 60.4). The patient should also be interviewed and examined for evidence of skin or mouth lesions and other symptoms of gold toxicity. If serious rash, proteinuria, or hematologic complications appear, gold administration should be discontinued. Patients previously treated with gold may be rechallenged after the toxic effect(s) subsides if the reaction observed is not severe or life-threatening; however, patients in remission after initial treatment with gold salts are less likely to develop remission after a second course of gold.[20]

Long-term outcome of gold therapy would suggest that only 15% to 20% of patients continue treatment after 3 to 5 years.

***Antimalarials*** Use of antimalarial agents in the treatment of rheumatoid arthritis began in the early 1950s, after the fortuitous discovery of improvement in two patients' rheumatoid arthritis while they were being treated with quinacrine for systemic lupus erythematosus and discoid lupus. Chloroquine and hydroxychloroquine, developed later, are used today as remission-inducing agents for rheumatoid arthritis. Because of previous problems with dose-related ocular toxicity associated with chloroquine, hydroxychloroquine is preferred by most rheumatologists.

The mechanism by which antimalarials work in rheumatoid arthritis is not fully understood. These agents affect several physiologic processes that regulate inflammatory and immune response, including sulfhydryl–disulfide interchange, enzymatic reactions, and nucleoprotein interaction.

Chloroquine and hydroxychloroquine differ chemically by only one hydroxyl substitution on an aliphatic side chain, which renders hydroxychloroquine less potent but also less toxic on a milligram-per-milligram basis. Pharmacokinetic parameters of the two drugs are similar. Chloroquine and hydroxychloroquine are rapidly and well absorbed from the gastrointestinal tract, with peak plasma concentrations attained within 1 to 2 hours. Serum concentrations are variable and dose dependent; steady-state concentrations are reached after several weeks of therapy. Approximately 50% of the drug is protein bound. Plasma elimination half-life ranges from 70 to 120 hours and is more prolonged with higher doses. Chloroquine and hydroxychloroquine are widely distributed in body tissue, especially in the eyes and skin, where concentrations greatly exceed those found in the plasma.

Because antimalarial agents bind to melanin, affinity for pigmented tissue is high. The drugs are 30% to 50% metabolized by the liver. Excretion of unchanged drug and metabolites is via the kidneys and may be increased by urinary acidification. Small amounts of drug may be present in the urine for months to years after cessation of therapy. Attention to renal and hepatic function is necessary, with appropriate dosage adjustment to avoid potential toxicity. A 50% dosage reduction is suggested with glomerular filtration rates less than 10 mL/min.

The recommended dosages are 3.5–4.0 mg/kg/d for chloroquine and 6.0–6.5 mg/kg/d for hydroxychloroquine, based on lean body weight, or a maximum dosage of 250 mg chloroquine or 400 mg hydroxychloroquine daily.[21] Several weeks to months may lapse before clinical improvement is observed; a minimum trial of 6 months is recommended before considering alternative therapy.

The major complication limiting the use of antimalarial agents in rheumatoid arthritis is ocular toxicity. Mild defects in accommodation or convergence and corneal deposits are most common. Visual problems associated with accommodation defects are reversible with discontinuation of the drug; corneal deposits are asymptomatic. A more serious complication is retinal toxicity, which may lead to loss of vision. Antimalarials concentrate in the pigmented tissues of the eye, in the uveal tract and retinal epithelium. The degree of binding is dependent on the plasma concentration of drug, with higher concentrations producing the greatest potential for toxicity. As these drugs are retained in body tissues, retinopathy may persist indefinitely after treatment cessation. Daily dosage and duration of treatment are the most important risk factors related to development of retinal toxicity.[22] Symptoms of retinopathy include blurred vision, night blindness, and scotomas. Classic chloroquine retinopathy shows macular pigmentary mottling or clumping, progressing to a "bull's-eye" lesion. The less severe findings of mild pigmentary abnormalities or visual field defects found only with red test objects are generally reversible and are often termed *premaculopathy*. Severe pigmentary changes and visual field loss to a white test object are characteristic of "true retinopathy" and often progress to severe loss of vision, even after medication is discontinued. Patients should receive an ophthalmologic examination with red light testing of peripheral visual fields at initiation of antimalarial therapy and every 6 months thereafter. If a pigmentary abnormality or visual field defect is found, medication should be discontinued.

Gastrointestinal effects, nausea, and vomiting are common with antimalarials. Rashes (variable in appearance) and exacerbation of psoriatic skin lesions may occur. Reversible changes in skin pigmentation have been noted, in addition to bleaching of hair and rare alopecia. Mild and reversible neurologic complications include headache, vertigo, insomnia, depression, agitation, and muscle weakness.

Studies have shown the antimalarial compounds to be of moderate efficacy in the treatment of rheumatoid arthritis. Complete remission is achieved in approximately 15% of patients; partial remission is observed in 50% to 55%. Antimalarials enjoy the lowest dropout rate (3%–7%) secondary to toxic and side effects but have a treatment failure rate of about 30%. Early disease may be most responsive to antimalarial therapy, but this does not preclude a good response in patients with disease of long duration who have active synovitis.[23]

***Penicillamine*** Penicillamine, found to be effective as a disease-suppressive agent in rheumatoid arthritis, was originally used as a chelating agent for removal of excess tissue copper in patients with Wilson's disease. Since its approval for use in rheumatoid arthritis in 1978, penicillamine has become established as one of the major second-line drugs used in the United States. It is usually considered after a trial of gold therapy has been abandoned. There appears to be a higher incidence of toxic effects with penicillamine in patients who have a history of toxic responses to gold treatment, but this does not contraindicate its use.[24] Rheumatoid arthritis patients with HLA-DRw3 histocompatibility antigen may be at greater risk of developing adverse reactions to penicillamine. A history of allergy to penicillin is not a contraindication to the use of penicillamine.

As with most remission-inducing drugs, the mechanism of action of penicillamine in the treatment of rheumatoid arthritis is poorly understood. It is neither cytotoxic nor anti-inflammatory, but evidence suggests it may act via an immunoregulatory mechanism.[25] Other proposed mechanisms include its copper chelating properties, oxidation–reduction reactions with sulfhydryl groups on proteins, a direct effect on collagen, and vitamin $B_6$ antagonism.

Penicillamine is well absorbed from the gastrointestinal tract, with peak serum concentrations occurring within 2 to 3 hours. The drug is approximately 80% protein bound. Steady-state serum concentrations rise gradually with prolonged therapy and likewise decline slowly upon termination of treatment, suggesting accumulation of drug in body tissues.[26] The drug is extensively metabolized, with little free penicillamine recovered in the urine. A biphasic elimination process has been observed, with a rapid elimination half-life of 1 to 5 hours and a slow elimination half-life of 4 to 8 days.

Because of a high incidence of toxic and adverse reactions to the drug, penicillamine administration must be individualized and generally cannot follow a fixed protocol. A latency period of 8 to 12 weeks may be required before a full therapeutic effect is observed. The drug is introduced gradually, with slow incremental changes until a clinical response is achieved. Penicillamine therapy is typically initiated with a single daily dose of 125–250 mg. Incremental changes are generally made at 8-week intervals by 125–250 mg/d as needed and tolerated. The drug is best absorbed when taken approximately 90 minutes before a meal and apart from any other medications.[27] Simultaneous administration of iron preparations in particular has been shown to inhibit penicillamine absorption. Most patients benefiting from the drug show clinical improvement within 6 months. Doses greater than 750 mg daily increase toxicity and are not more efficacious.

Although penicillamine is considered equal in efficacy to other remission-inducing drugs, toxic and adverse effects have limited its clinical usefulness. Most serious reactions develop during the initial 18 months of therapy. Hematologic toxicity, including leukopenia, thrombocytopenia, and aplastic anemia, has been observed. Thrombocytopenia may precede impending bone marrow aplasia. Proteinuria and microscopic hematuria may indicate renal toxicity. Protein excretion exceeding 2 g per 24 hours or evidence of nephrotic syndrome or gross hematuria warrants cessation of therapy. See Table 60.4 for recommended laboratory monitoring.

Induction of autoimmune syndromes has been observed with penicillamine. These include Goodpasture's syndrome, myasthenia gravis, polymyositis, pemphigus, systemic lupus erythematosus, and Sjögren's syndrome. Discontinuance of drug is indicated if any of these conditions occurs. Concern for these toxic effects has caused most rheumatologists to consider the drug only after gold or hydroxychloroquine treatment failure.

Skin rashes are commonly encountered with the use of penicillamine. Rashes observed early in treatment are often mild but pruritic and usually respond to dosage reduction. Rashes of later onset are generally more severe and may require discontinuance of the drug. Hypogeusia (blunting of taste perception) is commonly seen early and gradually clears even with continued therapy. Other frequently encountered side effects include nausea, dyspepsia, diarrhea, and stomatitis.

About 20% to 30% of patients tolerate long-term treatment with penicillamine. Treatment complications occur in 50% to 80% of patients but require discontinuation in only 30% to 40%.[28] Another 20% to 30% of patients discontinue penicillamine secondary to treatment failure.

***Immunosuppressive Drugs*** Although the use of antineoplastic drugs in rheumatoid arthritis dates back to the early 1950s, the clinical availability and efficacy of corticosteroids caused a decline in the use of antineoplastic drugs until the mid-1960s. The immunosuppressive drugs used most commonly today are azathioprine, cyclophosphamide, and methotrexate. Because of their potential for serious long-term side effects, their role in therapy is limited to cases of severe erosive rheumatoid arthritis refractory to other conventional remission-inducing agents.

Immunosuppressive drugs presumably modify immunopathogenic and inflammatory mechanisms important in the pathology of rheumatoid arthritis, but their precise actions remain unknown. Although each drug has unique adverse effects, all carry the potential risk of serious problems such as mutagenesis or teratogenesis, sterility, neoplasia, infection, and bone marrow suppression.[29] Continuous monitoring of blood counts is necessary, with appropriate dosage modification to maintain the leukocyte count above 3,000–3,500 cells/mm$^3$.

Azathioprine is the sole immunosuppressive agent approved in the United States for treatment of rheumatoid arthritis. A purine analog, it is quickly converted in vivo to 6-mercaptopurine (6-MP), which is responsible for most of the pharmacologic effects. It is well absorbed, with peak plasma concentrations occurring at about 2 hours. It is 30% protein bound and has a plasma elimination half-life of 60 to 90 minutes. It is hepatically metabolized by xanthine oxidase to its major metabolite, 6-thiouric acid, which is excreted in the urine. Azathioprine doses should be reduced by two thirds in patients taking concurrent allopurinol.[17] Dosage should be reduced by 25% in patients with renal failure (glomerular filtration rate $<$ 10 mL/min).[30] Azathioprine is generally administered in doses of 1.5–3.0 mg/kg/d, with further adjustment according to the degree of resulting myelosuppression or therapeutic response. Clinical effects are usually seen within 3 to 4 weeks of initiation of therapy.

The major toxic effect of azathioprine is bone marrow suppression, manifested by leukopenia, thrombocytopenia, or anemia. These suppressive effects are reversible with dosage adjustment. Gastrointestinal intolerance, nausea, and vomiting are commonly observed. Hepatotoxicity occurs infrequently but may be severe. Hepatic fibrosis has been reported in patients without changes in liver function enzymes. Azathioprine has been associated with an increased incidence of infection and oncogenesis.

Cyclophosphamide is thought to be more effective than or equal to azathioprine for the treatment of rheumatoid arthritis, and both are considered approximately equal in efficacy to gold or penicillamine.[31] Cyclophosphamide has been shown to be of particular value in treating rheumatoid vasculitis. It is, however, significantly more toxic than other immunosuppressive agents. Cyclophosphamide is a nitrogen mustard alkylating agent, well absorbed orally and metabolized to its active form by the liver. The drug itself is not significantly protein bound, although several of its metabolites are. Its plasma half-life is about 6.5 hours and may be significantly prolonged with concurrent administration of xanthine oxidase inhibitors. As roughly 70% of a dose is ultimately found in the urine, renal failure may result in impaired excretion of the drug's active metabolites and increased risk of toxicity. A 25% to 50% dosage reduction is recommended with glomerular filtration rates less than 10 mL/min.[30] The usual initial dosage of cyclophosphamide in rheumatoid arthritis patients is 1.5–3.0 mg/kg/d. Clinical efficacy may be observed within 2 to 4 weeks.

Adverse effects of cyclophosphamide are frequent and serious. It inhibits rapidly dividing cell populations, such as those in the bone marrow, hair follicles, and gastrointestinal tract.[32] Although suppression of all marrow elements is seen, neutropenia is the most serious. Changes in leukocyte count often lag 10 to 14 days behind a given cyclophosphamide dose. This necessitates close monitoring and strict avoidance of dosage increases more frequent than every 30 days. The risk of bone marrow toxicity increases with duration of treatment.

Alopecia is common but is generally not total or irreversible. Gastrointestinal intolerance, nausea, and vomiting have been observed. Cystitis is a frequent (15%–30% incidence), potentially serious problem, apparently related to the direct alkylating effects of the drug and its metabolites on bladder mucosa. Although cystitis is usually reversible, bladder fibrosis, hemorrhage, and bladder carcinoma may occur. Onset of hemorrhagic cystitis is an absolute indication for discontinuation of drug. Cyclophosphamide has also been shown to cause pneumonitis and pulmonary fibrosis, an increased incidence of infections, sterility, chromosomal abnormalities, teratogenesis, and oncogenesis.

Methotrexate, a folic acid antagonist, is effective in rheumatoid arthritis because of its immunosuppressive and anti-inflammatory properties. It is equal in efficacy to other immunosuppressive agents in the treatment of rheumatoid arthritis and is associated with fewer side effects. Methotrexate is readily absorbed from the gastrointestinal tract and produces peak serum concentrations at approximately 1 to 2 hours with a half-life of 2.0 to 4.5 hours. It is 50% to 60% protein bound and may be displaced by certain drugs such as sulfonamides, salicylates, tetracycline, and chloramphenicol, increasing the risk of toxicity. Up to 80% to 90% of an administered dose is excreted unchanged in the urine within 24 hours. It is cleared by filtration and active secretion. Active secretion may be inhibited by weak organic acids, such as salicylates and NSAIDs. Impaired renal function has been noted to be an important factor in the development of the pancytopenia associated with methotrexate.[33] Patients with creatinine clearance less than 50 mL/min will require substantial (50%) dosage reduction.

Methotrexate may be administered orally or parenterally with equal efficacy; the oral route is used more often for patient convenience.[34] The usual dosage range is 5–20 mg, commonly given in divided doses over 24 to 36 hours at weekly intervals. Use of pulse therapy and lower doses is thought to decrease toxicity and is comparable in efficacy to daily treatment.[35]

The most common adverse effects seen with methotrexate involve the gastrointestinal tract, including nausea, vomiting, anorexia, diarrhea, and stomatitis. Bone marrow suppression, primarily leukopenia and thrombocytopenia, may be seen and is reversible with dosage modification, as are most gastrointestinal effects. Pulmonary fibrosis or pneumonitis may occur in 4% to 5% of patients (see Chapter 24). Patients present with a dry cough, malaise, fever, and dyspnea. The diagnosis of methotrexate pulmonary toxicity is one of exclusion; discontinuation of methotrexate usually results in a reversal of pulmonary symptoms. Sterility and teratogenesis have also been seen. Unlike other immunosuppressive agents, methotrexate engenders a low risk of oncogenesis.

Methotrexate therapy has been associated with both acute hepatitis and hepatic fibrosis.[36] Low-dose methotrexate commonly results in elevated liver function enzymes, but these do not predict the presence of hepatic fibrosis. Serum aspartate aminotransferase and alanine aminotransferase assays should be performed monthly. Persistent elevations of greater than twice normal values are an indication for decreasing the methotrexate dose. Baseline liver biopsies should be obtained in patients at risk for hepatotoxicity, including the aged, the obese, diabetic patients, previous alcohol users, or patients with previous hepatic disease. Routine liver biopsies are recommended after every 1.5-g cumulative dose increment. Cirrhosis or moderate to severe fatty changes warrant cessation of therapy. The incidence of hepatic fibrosis in patients taking methotrexate for rheumatoid arthritis may be less than that observed in psoriatic patients receiving methotrexate.

***Corticosteroids*** Corticosteroids are effective for rheumatoid arthritis because of a combination of anti-inflammatory and immunosuppressive effects; there is little evidence indicating any effect on the underlying disease process. The use of systemic steroids in patients with rheumatoid arthritis is indicated for symptomatic relief during exacerbations of disease activity, during the interim period before therapeutic effects of SAARDs are observed, and in refractory cases of rheumatoid arthritis as a "last resort." It has been suggested that they might be used during stages of active inflammation, in low dose, as an adjunctive therapy.[37,38] In any case, the challenge and goal in the clinical use of corticosteroids are to achieve maximal therapeutic efficacy with minimal adverse effects.

Corticosteroids inhibit leukocyte migration to the inflammatory site and alter other cellular processes. Corticosteroids are also potent inhibitors of prostaglandin synthesis, albeit through a mechanism slightly different from that of the NSAIDs. The magnitude of effects produced is directly related to the duration of action of the drug, the dose, and the interval between doses.[39] Ideally one could maintain adequate disease suppression if high doses were used for long periods of time. This approach is impractical and unacceptable owing to the drugs' serious side effects.

The corticosteroids used most commonly for oral administration are methylprednisolone and prednisone. In patients with severe, progressive, active disease, daily administration of prednisone may be appropriate for symptomatic control while awaiting a therapeutic response from remission-inducing drugs. The drug is best given as a single morning dose, as this most closely simulates the normal diurnal cortisol cycle and minimizes potential hypothalamic–pituitary–adrenal (HPA) axis suppression. Patients with very active inflammatory disease may require divided doses for initial treatment. Once the disease is adequately controlled, continual attempts should be made to reduce the dose or convert to alternate-day dosage regimens.[40] Unfortunately, the latter form of therapy is often not adequate for control of RA symptoms. Patients treated with steroids for extended periods of time may experience withdrawal syndromes or flares of disease, even with small dosage decrements.[41]

Adverse effects from steroids are many and diverse. These include the manifestations of Cushing's syndrome and HPA suppression (see Chapter 55). Musculoskeletal effects, including osteoporosis, compression fractures, aseptic bone necrosis, and myopathy, are frequently seen with long-term use. Steroids may aggravate peptic ulcer disease and can induce diabetes mellitus and hypertension. Effects on immune response are manifested by suppression of delayed hypersensitivity and increased susceptibility to infections.

Metabolism of steroids is enhanced by drugs that induce hepatic microsomal enzymes, such as phenytoin, barbiturates, and rifampin. Steroids may decrease serum salicylate concentrations by induction of hepatic enzymes or increased renal excretion. They may also increase requirements for insulin or oral hypoglycemics, antihypertensives, and glaucoma medications.

Intrasynovial steroid injections are useful for patients with one or two acutely inflamed joints whose arthritis is otherwise satisfactorily controlled.[42] Long-acting corticosteroid agents such as triamcinolone hexacetonide or methylprednisolone acetate are used for this purpose. The onset of action is 24 to 72 hours after administration. Duration of benefit in the injected joint is variable, with some patients experiencing relief for several months and others only a few days. Most patients note some systemic effect from a local injection. The number of injections of a single joint, bursa, or tendon sheath should, however, be limited to no more than two or three per year because of the risk of accelerated degenerative arthritis, decreased tensile strength of tendons, and avascular necrosis. Patients receiving intraarticular steroid injections should be advised to reduce the activity of an injected joint for 1 to 2 weeks after injection. An exacerbation of inflammation in the injected joint may be seen in 5% of patients because of an inflammatory response to the steroid crystals.

## Seronegative Spondyloarthropathies

The seronegative spondyloarthropathies are a group of rheumatic diseases characterized by spinal involvement and negative rheumatoid factors. Peripheral joint involvement, when it exists, tends to be asymmetrical and often involves fewer joints than does rheumatoid arthritis. Psoriatic arthritis, ankylosing spondylitis, Reiter's syndrome, and arthropathy associated with inflammatory bowel disease are some of these disorders. The long-term outcome of patients with these diseases is usually a lesser degree of functional disability compared with rheumatoid arthritis patients. The clinical presentation of these diseases, especially early in their course, may be difficult to distinguish from that of seronegative rheumatoid arthritis. The distinction is important because of the differences in the approach to treatment and clinical outcomes.[2,43]

There is a genetic predisposition for these diseases. HLA-B27 histocompatibility antigen is positive in a much higher proportion of patients with these disorders than in the general population. Environmental factors play a role in some of these disorders. Reiter's syndrome has occurred in epidemics following outbreaks of *Salmonella* and *Shigella* gastroenteritis and may also be associated with venereal infections.

### *Psoriatic Arthritis*

Psoriatic arthritis occurs in 7% of patients with psoriasis. There are four major patterns of joint involvement: (1) the classical presentation involving predominantly the distal interphalangeal joints of the hands; (2) arthritis mutilans, in which severe destructive changes, with resorption of bone, result in "telescoping" (shortening) of digits; (3) the oligoarticular pattern, in which a few joints are involved; and (4) symmetric polyarthropathy, which mimics seronegative rheumatoid arthritis. There is no relationship between the clinical course of the skin disease and the course of the joint activity. There is a relationship among psoriatic nail changes, pitting and onycholysis (lifting of the distal portion of the nail from the nail bed), and joint involvement. Digits often develop a characteristic "sausagelike" appearance with diffuse swelling of the finger, as opposed to the articular swelling observed in rheumatoid arthritis. Inflammation of tendon insertion sites is commonly seen and results in pain. Involvement of the sacroiliac joints is seen in 20% of patients. There are no specific laboratory tests to help identify this disorder.

Most patients respond well to NSAIDs. Indomethacin is believed by most clinicians to be particularly effective. Gold salts have been effective in psoriatic arthritis. Hydroxychloroquine may also be useful, but exacerbations of the patient's skin disease can occur. Methotrexate is an effective treatment for the arthritis and skin disease; however, precautions must be taken to avoid hepatotoxicity. Prednisone may be useful in treating both skin and joint disease; however, the complications of long-term treatment with corticosteroids make their use in chronic management less desirable.

### *Ankylosing Spondylitis*

This disease involves primarily the axial skeleton. Inflammation of the spinal column and sacroiliac joints leads to eventual fusion of these joints with a resultant loss of motion. The disease is more often diagnosed in males. HLA-B27 is positive in 90% of patients with ankylosing spondylitis (compared with 6%–8% of the normal population). Enthesopathy (inflammation of tendinous attachments to bone) is the predominant pathologic finding in patients with ankylosing spondylitis. Asymmetric peripheral arthritis may be seen in one third of the patients. Involvement of the lower extremities is more common than upper-extremity arthritis. Inflammation of rib articulations can result in bony fusion and a decrease in the ability to expand the chest with breathing. Inflammation of the eye (iritis) occurs in 25% of patients. Topical corticosteroids may be required to relieve the inflammation. Involvement of the aortic root can lead to cardiac murmurs and rarely to serious cardiac disease. Involvement of the cardiac conduction system can lead to electrocardiographic abnormalities and arrhythmias.

Patients usually present with back pain and stiffness that typically improves with activity. NSAIDs are the primary mode of treatment. Indomethacin is particularly effective for most patients. Although these drugs provide temporary relief, nothing appears to alter the clinical course of the disease. In severe cases, the end result of the chronic inflammation is bony fusion of the spine (radiographically giving the spine the classic bamboo appearance). Physical therapy is essential to help prevent flexion deformities.

### *Reiter's Syndrome*

Reiter's syndrome is an inflammatory disease with the classic triad of symptoms of arthritis, urethritis, and conjunctivitis. Some patients do not demonstrate all three symptoms seen in the classic presentation.

The arthritis is typically asymmetrical in distribution. Enthesopathy is a common feature in Reiter's syndrome; heel pain and calcification of the plantar fascial insertion (calcaneal spur) are also common. Urethritis may occur episodically during the course of the disease. Conjunctivitis may be asymptomatic; other serious inflammatory eye diseases have also been reported. Characteristic skin rashes associated with Reiter's syndrome include circinate balanitis (a scaly erythematous rash surrounding the head of the penis) and keratoderma blennorrhagicum (a dry scaly rash on the soles of the feet and the palmar surface of the hands, accompanied by vesicles). Painless ulcers of mucous membranes of the mouth and genitalia may occur. The usual course of Reiter's disease is characterized by acute exacerbations and asymptomatic intervals, although chronic arthritis may also be seen. Some patients may have a single episode of illness lasting weeks to months. There is a strong association between Reiter's syndrome and bacterial dysentery or venereal infections.

Treatment is symptomatic, with NSAIDs being the primary form of therapy. Injections of corticosteroids into inflamed tendon insertion sites may be of value in isolated inflamed tendonitis. The value of gold, penicillamine, hydroxychloroquine, and immunosuppressive agents has not been evaluated in controlled studies.

### *Arthritis Associated With Inflammatory Bowel Disease*

This has been observed in 11% of patients with ulcerative colitis and 21% of patients with Crohn's disease. Joint distribution is usually asymmetrical and often involves only a few joints. An ankylosing spondylitis–like picture may be seen. The synovitis usually is not chronic in nature and does not result in deformity. Colectomy usually results in resolution of the arthritis associated with ulcerative colitis. Analgesics and NSAIDs may be used for symptomatic treatment.

## Controversies in Therapy

The choice of initial treatment in rheumatoid arthritis is controversial. Aspirin has been the standard with which all nonsteroidal agents have been compared and remains the initial treatment of many clinicians. Studies comparing newer nonsteroidal agents with aspirin show them to be equally effective. Although most of the newer nonsteroidal agents produce fewer gastrointestinal symptoms than aspirin, the incidence of peptic ulcer disease has not been proven to be more frequent with aspirin therapy. These studies routinely use plain aspirin tablets and not the buffered or enteric-coated formulations that may have less gastrointestinal toxicity. Aspirin is less expensive than other nonsteroidal agents. Education is necessary to convince the patient to take appropriate anti-inflammatory doses, which exceed dosages commonly used for analgesic purposes.

Another controversy in treatment is the appropriate time to institute SAARD therapy. Traditionally, SAARDs are considered in patients who have failed to achieve adequate symptomatic relief or who have developed erosive disease. SAARDs appear to be more effective when begun in early disease. The arguments against early use of SAARDs are increased patient cost and toxic effects.

The relative efficacy of the SAARDs and the order of preference are controversial. Most rheumatologists would use gold as their initial choice; however, a good case could be made for hydroxychloroquine, as the cost of monitoring therapy is less and initial response rates are comparable. Most clinicians are concerned about the autoimmune toxicity of penicillamine and would relegate it to last choice within this group of drugs.

The ability of these drugs to prevent erosions remains an issue. Some studies suggest a decrease in the formation of new erosions when the SAARDs are used. The difficulty with this assessment includes the lack of information about the natural course of untreated rheumatoid arthritis. Such a study would be unethical at this time. Another problem in assessing erosive disease is the relative insensitivity and lack of standardization of radiologic technique. Although radiologic assessment is used clinically to determine the efficacy of the patient's treatment regimen, it cannot be assured that changing a patient's therapy will alter the course of the disease.

The role of lymphopheresis and total lymphoid irradiation in the management of rheumatoid arthritis has not been ascertained. Lymphopheresis, a technique that removes lymphocytes from the patient's blood, and irradiation of lymph nodes have been demonstrated to result in clinical improvement in rheumatoid arthritis. These procedures are expensive, produce a short-term benefit, and have risks of toxicity.

## Summary

Rheumatoid arthritis is the most common inflammatory arthritis, affecting approximately 3% of the population. The disease is characterized by symmetrical swelling and stiffness of the involved joints. The stiffness is usually more prominent in the morning. Extra-articular features of rheumatoid arthritis include rheumatoid nodules, vasculitis, and ocular, cardiac, and pulmonary complications. The course of the disease is highly variable. Treatment is aimed at relieving pain and inflammation and maintaining and preserving joint function. The initial drug treatment is either aspirin or NSAIDs; several of these agents should be tried before progressing to other agents. Nondrug therapy, including exercise and adequate rest periods, should be used early in the course of treatment. One of the slow-acting antirheumatic drugs—gold, hydroxychloroquine, or penicillamine—may be added to NSAID therapy in patients who have had an inadequate response to initial treatment or who have developed destructive disease. Methotrexate, azathioprine, and cyclophosphamide may be effective in patients failing to respond to or having serious toxic effects from the SAARDs. Their use must be weighed against the potential for long-term toxicity. Corticosteroids are a useful adjunct for treatment, but because of adverse effects should be used in the lowest possible dose for the shortest possible treatment interval.

The seronegative spondyloarthropathies are a cluster of inflammatory rheumatic diseases that include psoriatic arthritis, ankylosing spondylitis, Reiter's syndrome, and the arthropathy associated with inflammatory bowel disease. These diseases have many of the features of rheumatoid arthritis but are distinctly different, with a greater tendency for asymmetrical peripheral joint inflammation and involvement of the axial spine. Psoriatic arthritis may be treated in much the same way as rheumatoid arthritis. The efficacy of SAARDs in the management of the other seronegative diseases has not been proven.

## References


1. Harris ED. Rheumatoid arthritis: The clinical spectrum, in Kelly WN, Harris ED, Ruddy S, et al (eds): Textbook of Rheumatology, 2nd ed. Philadelphia, W. B. Saunders, 1985.
2. Rodnan GP, Schumacher HR (eds). Primer of the Rheumatic Diseases, 8th ed. Atlanta, Arthritis Foundation, 1983.
3. Graziano FM, Bell CL. The normal immune response and what can go wrong. Med Clin North Am 1985;69:439–452.
4. Harris ED. Pathogenesis of rheumatoid arthritis, in Kelley WN, Harris ED, Ruddy S, et al (eds): Textbook of Rheumatology, 2nd ed. Philadelphia, W. B. Saunders, 1985.
5. Amstutz HC, Bluestone R, Cracchiolo A, et al. Diagnosis and treatment of rheumatoid arthritis and other forms of joint destruction. Ann Intern Med 1975;82:241–256.
6. Snyderman R. Mechanisms of inflammation and leukocyte chemotaxis in the rheumatic diseases. Med Clin North Am 1986; 70:217–235.

7. Moore CP, Wilkens RF. The subcutaneous nodule: Its significance in the diagnosis of rheumatoid arthritis. Semin Arthritis Rheum 1977;7:63–79.
8. Hard ER. Extraarticular manifestations of rheumatoid arthritis. Semin Arthritis Rheum 1979;8:151–176.
9. St. Clair EW, Polisson RP. Therapeutic approaches to the treatment of rheumatoid arthritis. Med Clin North Am 1986;70: 285–304.
10. Ruddy S. The management of rheumatoid arthritis, in Kelley WN, Harris ED, Ruddy S, et al (eds): Textbook of Rheumatology, 2nd ed. Philadelphia, W. B. Saunders, 1985;pp 979–992.
11. Plotz PH. Aspirin and salicylate, in Kelley WN, Harris ED, Ruddy S, et al (eds): Textbook of Rheumatology, 2nd ed. Philadelphia, W. B. Saunders, 1985; pp 725–752.
12. Hadler NH. The argument for aspirin as the NSAID of choice in the management of rheumatoid arthritis. Drug Intell Clin Pharm 1984;18:34–38.
13. Ehrlich GE. Other NSAIDs of choice for rheumatoid arthritis. Drug Intell Clin Pharm 1984;18:39–41.
14. Hart FD, Huskisson EC. Nonsteroidal anti-inflammatory drugs: Current status and rational therapeutic use. Drugs 1984;27:232–255.
15. Bollet AJ. Nonsteroidal anti-inflammatory drugs, in Kelley WN, Harris ED, Ruddy S, et al (eds): Textbook of Rheumatology, 2nd ed. Philadelphia, W. B. Saunders, 1985; pp 752–773.
16. Porter RS. Factors determining efficacy of NSAIDs. Drug Intell Clin Pharm 1984;18:42–51.
17. Bunch TW, O'Duffy JD. Disease-modifying drugs for progressive rheumatoid arthritis. Mayo Clin Proc 1980;55:161–179.
18. Furst DE. Mechanism of action, pharmacology, clinical efficacy and side effects of auranofin. Pharmacotherapy 1983;3:284–296.
19. Gibbons RB. Complications of chrysotherapy. Arch Intern Med 1979;139:343–346.
20. Evers AE, Sundstrom WR. Second course gold therapy in the treatment of rheumatoid arthritis. Arthritis Rheum 1983;26: 1071–1075.
21. Mackenzie AH. Antimalarial drugs for rheumatoid arthritis. Am J Med 1983;75(suppl)Dec:48–58.
22. Rynes RI. Ophthalmologic safety of long-term hydroxychloroquine sulfate treatment. Am J Med 1983;75(suppl)July:35–39.
23. Bell CL. Hydroxychloroquine sulfate in rheumatoid arthritis: Long-term response rate and predictive parameters. Am J Med 1983;75(suppl)July:46–50.
24. Stein HB, Ruedy J, Atkins CJ, et al. Penicillamine and other remittive agents in rheumatoid arthritis: Comparisons and interaction. Clin Invest Med 1984;7:59–63.
25. Jaffe IA. Penicillamine: An anti-rheumatoid drug. Am J Med 1983;75(suppl)Dec:63–67.
26. Muijsers AO, Van de Stadt RJ, Henrichs AMA, et al. D-Penicillamine in patients with rheumatoid arthritis. Arthritis Rheum 1984;27:1362–1368.
27. Schuna AA, Osman MA, Patel RB, et al. Influence of food on the bioavailability of penicillamine. J Rheumatol 1983;10:95–97.
28. Weiss AS, Markenson JA, Weiss MS, et al. Toxicity of D-penicillamine in rheumatoid arthritis. Am J Med 1978;64:114–120.
29. Steinberg AD, Plotz PH, Wolff SM, et al. Cytotoxic drugs in treatment of nonmalignant diseases. Ann Intern Med 1972;76: 619–642.
30. Bennett WM, Aronoff GR, Morrison G, et al. Drug prescribing in renal failure: Dosing guidelines for adults. Am J Kidney Dis 1983;3:155–193.
31. Decker JL. Azathioprine and cyclophosphamide as slow-acting drugs for rheumatoid arthritis. Am J Med 1983;75(suppl)Dec: 74–78.
32. Kovarsky J. Clinical pharmacology and toxicology of cyclophosphamide: Emphasis on use in rheumatic diseases. Semin Arthritis Rheum 1983;12:359–371.
33. MacKinnon SK, Starkebaum G, Willkens RF. Pancytopenia associated with low dose pulse methotrexate in the treatment of rheumatoid arthritis. Semin Arthritis Rheum 1985;15:119–126.
34. Letendre PW, DeJong DJ, Miller DR. The use of methotrexate in rheumatoid arthritis. Drug Intell Clin Pharm 1985;19:349–358.
35. Hoffmeister RT. Methotrexate therapy in rheumatoid arthritis: 15 years experience. Am J Med 1983;75(suppl)Dec:69–73.
36. Groff GD, Shenberger KN, Wilke WS, et al. Low dose oral methotrexate in rheumatoid arthritis: An uncontrolled trial and review of the literature. Semin Arthritis Rheum 1983;12:333–347.
37. Myles A. Corticosteroid treatment in rheumatoid arthritis. Br J Rheumatol 1985;24:125–127.
38. Masi AT. Low dose glucocorticoid therapy in rheumatoid arthritis: Transitional or selected add-on therapy? J Rheumatol 1983;10:675–683.
39. Fauci AS, Dale DC, Balow JE. Glucocorticosteroid therapy: Mechanisms of action and clinical considerations. Ann Intern Med 1976;84:304–314.
40. Fauci AS. Alternate-day corticosteroid therapy. Am J Med 1978;64:729–731.
41. Dixon RB, Christy NP. On the various forms of corticosteroid withdrawal syndrome. Am J Med 1980;68:224–229.
42. Fitzgerald RH. Intrasynovial injection of steroids. Mayo Clin Proc 1976;51:655–659.
43. Calin A. Seronegative spondyloarthritides. Med Clin North Am 1986;70:323–336.

# Chapter 61 / Osteoarthritis

Larry E. Boh, MS, RPh

Osteoarthritis (OA) is a very common, slowly progressive disorder not clinically apparent until later in life. It affects primarily the weight-bearing joints of the peripheral and axial skeleton, causing pain, limitation of motion, deformity, and progressive disability. Terms such as osteoarthrosis, degenerative joint disease (DJD), or hypertrophic arthritis are used to describe this disease, though none of these terms is satisfactory. Osteoarthrosis implies a lack of inflammation and excess materials in the joint. Degenerative joint disease suggests a wearing out, deterioration, or breakdown of the joint. Hypertrophic arthritis, the earliest historic designation, describes only one aspect of the disease, the overgrowth of bone and cartilage. As articular cartilage is a very anabolic, synthetic, and reparative tissue[1–3] and because inflammation is present, [4–7] the best designation is osteoarthritis.

## Historical Perspective

An interesting phylogenetic observation is that OA occurs in most mammals surviving the evolutionary process and was present in prehistoric mammals.[6] OA has been observed in all vertebrates with bony skeletons, from modern animals, reptiles, birds, and mammals to the giant dinosaurs.[8] Interestingly, OA has not been observed in animals with cartilaginous skeletons such as sharks.[6] Of further intrigue is the observation of OA in whales, dolphins, and fish. These findings are contrary to the "wear-and-tear" theory because these species are constantly supported by water.[8]

OA was not identified as a separate clinical entity until 1907 by Garrod, despite numerous clinical and pathologic descriptions in the late eighteenth and early nineteenth centuries.[6] Between 1907 and 1910 the differentiation between rheumatoid arthritis (RA) and OA was made in terms of clinical and pathologic presentation. Presently, a variety of distinct clinical syndromes of OA are recognized. These range from primary generalized osteoarthritis to secondary localized osteoarthritis, which are at times difficult to distinguish.[9]

## Epidemiology

Osteoarthritis is the most prevalent of the rheumatic diseases and a common cause of decreased productivity and disability.[8] Numerous epidemiologic surveys have reported on the incidence and clinical characteristics of osteoarthritis. Review of these studies requires close attention to the variations in analytical techniques used and the populations studied.[10] In the United States an estimated 40.5 million adults have some evidence of osteoarthritis based on roentgenograms of the hands and feet.[11] Symptoms or disability occurs in only about 5 million. Autopsy studies have demonstrated that degenerative joint changes begin to occur by the second decade and that by age 40, despite being asymptomatic clinically, 90% of all patients have some degree of joint changes.[6]

### *Age, Sex, and Race*

Most strongly associated with the development of osteoarthritis is the aging process. A survey conducted from 1960 through 1962 reported that incidence and overall disease severity increased with age for persons with OA of the hands and feet. Incidence ranged from 4% for persons 18 to 24 years old to 85% for those 75 to 79. It is interesting that OA had a higher incidence in men under 45 and in women over 55 (Table 61.1).[11,12]

Incidence of OA of the knee and hip as reported in the HANES study was similar (Table 61.2).[12,13] The overall rates of Grade II findings were 0.2% and 8.6% in persons 25–34 and 65–74 years old, respectively. The rate of incidence of moderate to severe OA of the hips increases from 0.2% among men 25–34 years old to 2.3% among men 65–74 years old. For women 65–74 years old, it is about 1.2%. The study also demonstrated that 1% to 2% of the population between the ages of 25 and 74 reported limitation of some type of activity and required assistance.

In summary, comparison of all age groups shows that in the United States men and women are equally affected by OA. In Great Britain, similar findings were obtained; the number of joints affected and the severity of involvement are similar in men and women until age 54 but are more severe and generalized in women over 55.[14]

OA is less prevalent in blacks than in whites.[8,12] Among the black population of South Africa the incidence of OA of the hands, feet, and hips and of the presence of Heberden's nodes (bony enlargements of distal interphalangeal joints) is low. This difference is postulated to be related to differences in life styles or occupations. Osteoarthritis appears to be more prevalent in American Indians as compared with the overall U.S. population.[11]

### *Obesity*

The relationship between obesity and OA remains controversial.[12,15] Excess body weight appears to be associated with more severe OA of the knee but not the hip.[12] An increased incidence of OA in non–weight-bearing joints has also been reported; however, other authors suggest that obesity itself is not a factor in the induction or aggravation of degenerative joint disease.[15] Instead, obesity may be secondary to the limitation brought on by the joint pain.

**Table 61.1** Prevalence of Osteoarthritis of the Hands and Feet by Age, Gender, and Severity: U.S. Health Examination Survey, 1960–1962

| | *Men (%)* | | *Women (%)* | |
|---|---|---|---|---|
| *Age* | **Grade II** | **Grades III, IV** | **Grade II** | **Grades III, IV** |
| 18–24 | 7.2 | 0.0 | 1.6 | 0.0 |
| 25–34 | 13.5 | 0.1 | 6.2 | 0.0 |
| 35–44 | 29.2 | 1.0 | 18.1 | 1.5 |
| 45–54 | 43.9 | 3.1 | 39.3 | 7.0 |
| 55–64 | 48.4 | 14.8 | 49.9 | 25.3 |
| 65–74 | 51.0 | 24.8 | 47.0 | 37.7 |
| 75–79 | 47.7 | 33.2 | 35.9 | 53.9 |

Compiled from References 11 and 12.

### *Occupation*

Osteoarthritis related to occupation and leisure activity has been reported,[16–18] but also remains controversial. The mechanism for development of OA was related to repetitive trauma to the joints. Dock workers have a higher incidence of OA of the fingers, elbows, and knees than age-matched controls.[17] Observation of women working in a hand-weaving factory demonstrated that the pattern of OA hand involvement was related to the type of work.[16] Other studies have failed to demonstrate an association between OA and trauma.[12,18] In athletic runners, evaluation of knee and hip joints supported the relative absence of OA.[12,18,19]

## Pathophysiology

Osteoarthritis is primarily a disease of cartilage. The pathologic changes involve two major processes that ultimately lead to joint failure:

1. A progressive structural breakdown of articular cartilage that lines the joint surface in weight-bearing areas
2. Dense, smooth-surfaced bone formation (eburnation) at the base of the cartilage lesion and formation of osteophytes at the joint margins

The etiopathogenesis suggests that the process comprises more than the ''wear and tear'' that occurs with aging. No single factor causes OA; instead, several factors appear to contribute to the breakdown of joint cartilage, including biochemical abnormalities, inflammation, and crystal deposition.[6–9,20–30]

Before these factors are discussed, it is useful to clinically classify OA into primary and secondary forms (Table 61.3). *Primary* or idiopathic OA describes failure of the cartilage in the absence of any known underlying predisposing factor. If OA is affected by an identifiable underlying local or systemic pathogenetic factor such as infection, nutrition, or trauma, it is classified as *secondary* OA. (For a more detailed discussion of secondary OA, see Reference 8.)

**Table 61.2** Prevalence of Osteoarthritis of the Knee and Hip by Age, Gender, and Severity: U.S. Health and Nutrition Examination Survey, 1971–1975

| | *Men (%)* | | *Women (%)* | |
|---|---|---|---|---|
| *Age* | **Grade II** | **Grades III, IV** | **Grade II** | **Grades III, IV** |
| **Knee** | | | | |
| 25–34 | 0.0 | 0.0 | 0.1 | 0.0 |
| 35–44 | 1.6 | 0.1 | 1.0 | 0.5 |
| 45–54 | 2.1 | 0.2 | 3.1 | 0.9 |
| 55–64 | 3.1 | 1.0 | 10.4 | 0.9 |
| 65–74 | 6.3 | 2.0 | 11.4 | 6.6 |
| 25–74 | 2.1 | 0.5 | 3.6 | 1.3 |
| **Hip** | | | | |
| 25–34 | 0.2 | 0.5 | — | — |
| 35–44 | 0.1 | 0.0 | — | — |
| 45–54 | 0.6 | 0.1 | — | — |
| 55–64 | 1.9 | 0.7 | 1.2 | 1.6 |
| 65–74 | 2.3 | 2.3 | 1.5 | 1.2 |
| 55–74 | 2.1 | 1.4 | 1.4 | 1.4 |

Compiled from References 11 and 12.

**Table 61.3** Classification of Osteoarthritis

| *Primary* | *Secondary* |
|---|---|
| Idiopathic | Trauma—acute/chronic |
| Generalized | Underlying joint disorder |
| | Local (fracture/infection) |
| | Diffuse (rheumatoid arthritis) |
| Erosive | Systemic metabolic or endocrine disorders |
| | Wilson's disease |
| | Acromegaly |
| | Hyperparathyroidism |
| | Hemochromatosis |
| | Paget's disease |
| | Diabetes mellitus |
| | Obesity |
| | Crystal deposition disease |
| | Basic calcium phosphate crystal disease |
| | Calcium pyrophosphate dihydrate |
| | Hydroxyapatite |
| | Other calcium-containing crystals |
| | Monosodium urate monohydrate |
| | Neuropathic disorders |
| | Intra-articular corticosteroid overuse |
| | Avascular necrosis |
| | Bone dysplasia |

Compiled from References 8 and 15.

The two most common concepts held by the lay public and many health practitioners are that OA (1) is a wear-and-tear disease and (2) is related to the aging process. The wear-and-tear theory suggests that repeated use of a joint leads to abrasion of the cartilage from continuous motion and degeneration from impact loading.[7] Joint lubrication is provided by the fluid squeezed out of the cartilage. This lubrication keeps the joint surfaces apart and hence prevents damage from shear forces. Presently, there is no evidence of a difference in joint fluid between OA-affected and normal persons.[7] In contrast, impact loading such as occurs during repetitive tasks seen in arms of baseball pitchers, knees of basketball players, or ankles of ballet dancers causes changes in the cartilage. With excessive loads, the subchondral bone can develop microfractures that heal by callus formation and remodeling, thereby forming stiffer less compliant bone that leads to cartilage degeneration.[7]

Aging has been implicated as an etiologic factor, as the disease commonly occurs in the elderly. This would suggest that cartilage composition changes as an individual ages. Articular cartilage demonstrates a constant biochemical composition throughout life, unlike nonarticular cartilage. In addition, changes in cartilage have not been observed in aged humans with or without OA.[30]

Other etiologic factors include heredity, obesity, inflammatory joint disease, and genetic and metabolic factors.[7,21,25,28]

To help the reader understand the relationships and changes associated with osteoarthritis, the normal cartilage function and biochemistry and the mechanics of a diarthrodial joint are reviewed. More detailed reviews of cartilage biochemistry can be found elsewhere.[1,3,5,6,21,26]

## *Normal Cartilage*

### Function

In the free-moving diarthrodial joint (Figure 61.1) cartilage functions to cover the ends of the opposed bone. (Two to five millimeters thick, this avascular, aneural, and alymphatic tissue has a calcified base covering a thin layer of cortical bone known as the subchondral plate.) Because of its frictionless surface, cartilage provides a smooth gliding surface during movement of the joint and serves as a shock absorber or load support. Upon compression from weight loading, it is easily deformed; up to 40% of its height can be compressed. As a result, when a load is applied, cartilage can provide a large contact area and disperse this force more uniformly to the underlying bone.

### Biochemistry

Histologically, cartilage is a gel composed of a hypocellular (<5% chondrocytes) matrix containing 75% to 80% water by weight. The remainder (20%–25%) of the cartilage matrix consists of two types of macromolecules: type II collagen and large aggregates of proteoglycans (PGs). Chondrocytes control the synthesis and degradation of this matrix. Because of the avascular nature of adult cartilage, chondrocytes receive their nutrition from the synovial fluid. The cyclic movement and loading of joints increase the flow of nutrients to the cartilage, while immobilization reduces the supply.

Type II collagen contributes to the structure, tensile strength, and shape of the cartilage. In the superficial layers of cartilage, the collagen fibers are parallel to the

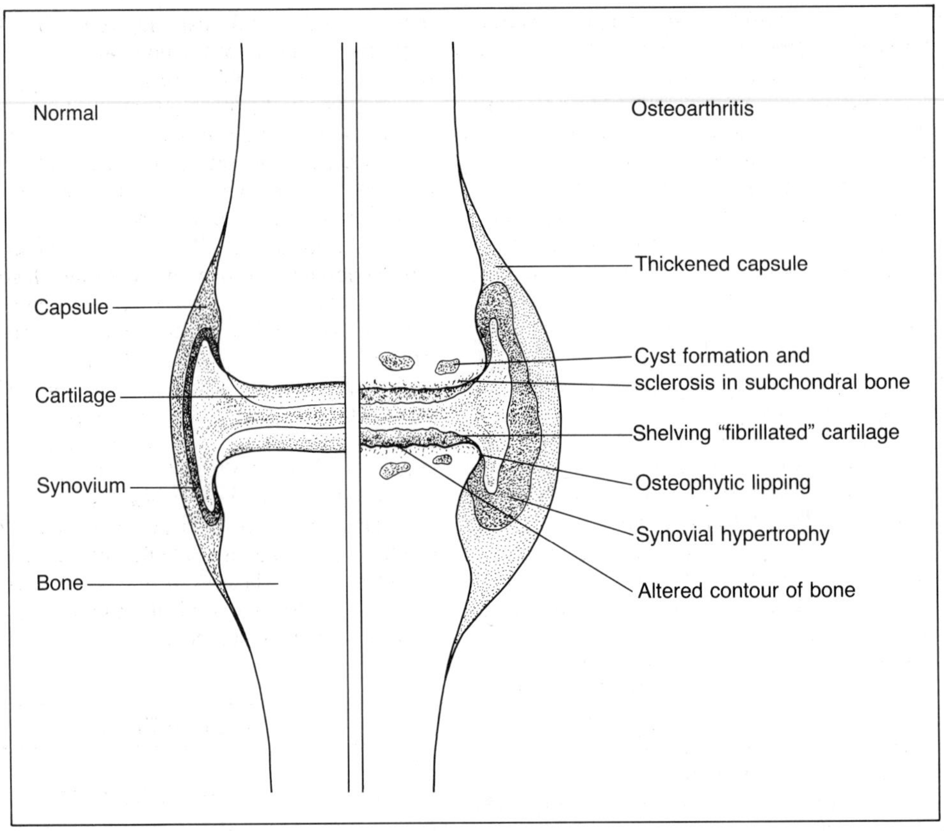


**Figure 61.1** Diagrammatic cross section of a normal joint and a joint affected by osteoarthritis. (*Reproduced from Dieppe PA, Bacon PA, Banji AN, et al: Osteoarthritis: Slide Atlas of Rheumatology. London, Gower Medical Publishing, with permission.*)

surface, thereby protecting the cartilage surface from the abrasive forces generated during motion. In contrast, the collagen fibers in the deeper layers are perpendicular to the cartilage surface. They penetrate the layer of calcified cartilage at the base, thereby anchoring to the subchondral bone.

The large aggregates of PGs provide the ''stuffing material'' for the matrix. Each aggregate consists of a linear protein linked to repeating chains of disaccharides called glycosaminoglycans (GAG). The GAG include chondroitin 6-sulfate, chondroitin 4-sulfate, and keratin sulfate. By covalently binding to the protein core, these molecules form a proteoglycan subunit. The subunits then combine with long hyaluronate molecules to form aggregates. The aggregates retain and maintain the water content of the cartilage because of their highly hydrophilic and anionic properties. These characteristics give cartilage its resilience and load-bearing properties. Under pressure, these compounds release water and enhance solute flux and chondrocyte nutrition; then, on removal of pressure, the compounds regain their water content. Interestingly, it is also this property that renders the PG molecular structure vulnerable to degradation by proteolytic enzymes; cleavage of only one or two peptide bonds can totally alter the properties of this molecule.[7] When protease degradation of its proteoglycans has been experimentally induced, cartilage has maintained its shape but lost its elastic properties.[7]

## *Osteoarthritic Cartilage*

### Biochemical Changes

Several changes have been reported in the composition of osteoarthritic cartilage (Table 61.4). These biochemical changes are thought to be important in explaining cartilage degradation in osteoarthritis. The initial change appears to be an increase in the water content of the cartilage matrix despite the reduction in proteoglycans, which are very hydrophilic. The reason for this change is unknown, but the increase implies a failure on the part of the collagen network to restrain the PGs, thereby allowing them to increase hydration and expand.[7] The decrease in proteoglycan content appears to correlate with the severity of the disease.[29] Increased synthesis of smaller, less mature proteoglycans

**Table 61.4** Changes in Osteoarthritic Cartilage

| |
|---|
| Decrease in tissue content of proteoglycans |
| Decrease in proteoglycan aggregation |
| Decrease in chondroitin sulfate chain length |
| Change in glycosaminoglycan composition |
| Increase in water content |
| Increase in collagen and proteoglycan synthesis |
| Increase in cellular activity of articular chondrocytes |

has also been reported.[28] Soon after these changes in water content occur, the GAG composition changes, reflecting a reduction in keratin sulfate compared with chondroitin sulfate. Further, the ratio of chondroitin 6-sulfate to chondroitin 4-sulfate decreases. These changes may result in decreased PG–collagen interaction in the cartilage. The collagen content does not appear to change until severe disease is present. Increases in collagen synthesis and in the distribution and diameter of the fibers have been noted.

Originally, researchers believed that cartilage passively eroded away. In fact, however, cellular activity increases, suggesting that the articular cartilage is responding with a reparative process.[9,20] This increase in activity appears to continue only until the disease is advanced, suggesting a possible failure of the chondrocytes.[27]

Despite the increase in matrix synthesis controlled by the chondrocytes, there continues to be loss of proteoglycan and increase in water content, implying that degradation is proceeding faster than synthesis. Further increases in enzymes such as the lysosomal enzymes of the chondrocytes (cathepsins B and D), neutral proteoglycanase, proteases and sulfatases (which can degrade GAGs), and collagenase are reported in osteoarthritic tissue.[3,9,30]

In summary, the slow progressive changes in osteoarthritis consist of an increase in water content, loss of PG, and reduction of PG aggregates of cartilage and appear to be related to mechanical as well as enzymatic alterations. The net result is the failure of cartilage to repair itself. The series of pathologic changes that occur result in loss of cartilage, eburnation of bone, and severe clinical symptoms.

#### Pathologic Changes

Coexistent with the biochemical changes are a series of pathologic changes in the cartilage and bone (Fig. 61.1). The early pathologic changes are not well defined, but the intermediate and late-stage changes in osteoarthritis are well described. The changes are similar for weight-bearing and non–weight-bearing joints and for idiopathic OA and secondary osteoarthritis.[29] The following changes are observed in cartilage:

1. Fibrillation, a splitting of the noncalcified cartilage believed to be related to the biochemical changes described earlier
2. Horizontal splitting of cartilage between the calcified and uncalcified layers secondary to shearing damage
3. Cartilage thinning and erosions progressing to focal exposure of the calcified cartilage and underlying bone as a result of grinding damage or abrasive wear

As destruction of the cartilage progresses, pathologic changes in subchondral bone occur. The appearance varies considerably depending on the site of cartilage loss; areas lacking the protective layer of cartilage demonstrate the most changes. The superficial portion of subchondral bone contains necrotic osteocytes. Increased osteoblastic and osteoclastic activity with osteolytic foci or cysts is observed below the superficial layer. The exposed area of bone may contain fibrous or chondroid tissue, presumably reflecting reactive bone resorption and vascular changes. With continued progression, the cartilaginous layer is completely eroded, leaving denuded subchondral bone that becomes dense, smooth, and glistening (eburnation). This alters the physical properties of the bone and results in a brittle, stiffer bone that is less able to resist the stress of bearing weight. The subchondral bone can then develop sclerosis and microfractures. Microfractures result in the production of callus and increased amounts of osteoid. New bone formation at the joint margins, away from the area of cartilage destruction, is referred to as osteophytes. An interesting observation is that osteophytes can occur in the absence of cartilage destruction and, conversely, cartilage destruction can occur in the absence of osteophytes. Osteophytes may be an attempt to stabilize joints and may not be part of the destructive aspects of osteoarthritis.

The joint capsule and synovium also show a variety of pathologic changes secondary to OA. Inflammation, such as synovitis, is seen and may result from the release of inflammatory mediators initiated by cartilage breakdown.

Figure 61.2 summarizes graphically the cellular and metabolic changes of osteoarthritic cartilage. In response to an insult by an unknown etiologic factor, the cartilage increases chondrocyte synthesis and release of degradative enzymes, resulting in the biochemical changes described earlier and altered cartilage resilience.

## Clinical Presentation

### *Signs/Symptoms*

The clinical presentation depends on the duration of disease, the joints affected, and the severity of joint involvement (Table 61.5). The predominant symptom is a localized deep, aching pain associated with the affected joint. If more than one joint is involved or if systemic symptoms are present, another form of arthritis or connective tissue disease should be considered.

Early in the course of the disease, pain occurs when the joint is first used and is relieved by rest or removal of weight from the affected joint. Later, the pain occurs with minimal motion or activity and may be present even during rest. The pain that occurs is not related to the destruction of cartilage, because cartilage is aneural. Rather, the pain arises from other intraarticular or periarticular structures. Weather or changes in the barometric pressure also seem to aggravate the pain.[8]

The joints most commonly affected in primary OA are the distal and proximal interphalangeal (DIP and PIP) joints of the hand, the first carpometacarpal joint, knees, hips, cervical and lumbar spine, and the first metatarsophalangeal (MTP) joint of the toe. In addition to pain in the affected joint, limitation of motion, stiffness, crepitus, and deformities may be present. The limitation of motion that develops as the disease progresses is related to the loss of articular surfaces, muscle spasms, capsular contracture, and mechanical blockage secondary to osteophytosis. The stiffness observed with OA is typically confined to the involved joint and lasts less than 30 minutes. When generalized stiffness is present, other inflammatory rheumatic disorders should be considered. Crepitation, or the crackling–grating sound heard as the joint moves, is related to irregularity of the joint surface and loss of cartilage. Joint enlargement is typically related to bony proliferation or in some cases thickening of

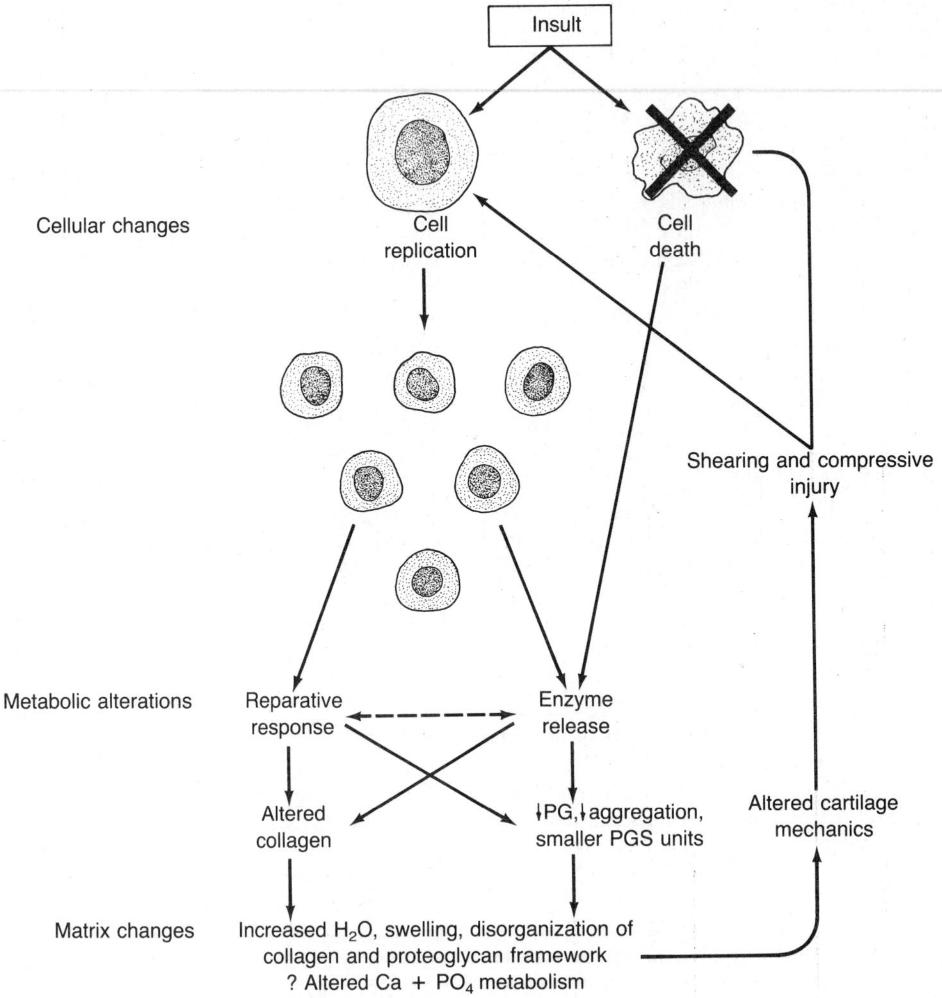


**Figure 61.2** Pathogenesis of cartilage change in osteoarthritis based on cellular metabolic and matrix changes. (*Reproduced from Primer on the Rheumatic Diseases, 8th ed. Atlanta, GA, Arthritis Foundation, 1983, p 105, with permission.*)

the synovium and joint capsule. The presence of a warm, red, tender joint may suggest an inflammatory type of synovitis.

Finally, joint deformity may be present in the later stages of OA and is the result of subluxation, collapse of subchondral bone, formation of bone cysts, or bony overgrowths.

### Physical Examination

Physical examination of the affected joint or joints reveals pain, tenderness, crepitus, and possible joint enlargement. The specific findings reported on physical examination of the commonly affected joints are discussed here.

***Hands*** Heberden's and Bouchard's nodes are bony enlargements (osteophytes) of the DIP and PIP joints, respectively. Heberden's nodes usually develop slowly, are nonpainful, occur on both lateral and medial aspects of the joint, and are approximately 10 times more common in women than men.[8] Occasionally, these nodes become red, warm, swollen, and painful, usually as a result of trauma or use. A strong female hereditary predominance is demonstrated upon questioning of the patient.

In patients with first carpometacarpal joint involvement, pain and tenderness are common. The increase in osteophytosis gives the radial aspect of the hand the characteristic square appearance termed the *shelf sign*.

***Knees*** The knee is one of the most commonly affected joints. It is important to localize the symptoms because the joint has three separate articulations: the patellofemoral and the medial and lateral compartments. Pain related to climbing stairs is typically associated with patellofemoral joint involvement. Presentation with a bowlegged deformity (genu varum) is caused by medial compartment involvement; knock-knee deformity (genu valgum) results from lateral compartment involvement. The symptoms include pain, tenderness, crepitation, limited extension with passive or active motion, and joint instability. These symptoms may cause the patient to limit the use of this joint, thereby

**Table 61.5** Clinical Presentation of Osteoarthritis

| |
|---|
| Age |
| Usually elderly |
| Sex |
| Age <45 more common in men; |
| >45 more common in women (hands) |
| **Symptoms** |
| Pain |
| Deep, aching |
| Pain on motion |
| Early in disease—pain with use |
| Late in disease—pain at rest |
| Stiffness |
| Rarely exceeds 15 min; related to weather |
| Localized to involved joints |
| Limited joint motion |
| Instability of weight-bearing joints |
| Crepitus, crackling |
| **Signs/Physical Examination** |
| Monoarticular or oligoarticular; asymmetrical involvement |
| Joints frequently involved |
| Hands—DIP, PIP, first carpometacarpal joint |
| Foot—first metatarsophalangeal |
| Hips, knees, cervical spine, lumbar spine |
| Observations on joint examination |
| Bony proliferation or occasional synovitis |
| Local tenderness |
| Crepitus |
| Muscle atrophy |
| Limited motion with passive/active movement |
| Effusions |
| Characteristics of synovial fluid |
| High viscosity |
| Mild leukocytosis (<2,000 WBC/$mm^3$) |
| **Laboratory Values** |
| No specific test |
| ESR, hematologic survey, chemistry survey are normal |
| No systemic manifestations |

Compiled from References 8, 15, 30, and 31.

causing muscle atrophy. Transient joint effusions may also occur. The synovial fluid is typically noninflammatory (white blood cell count < 2,000/$mm^3$ with normal protein).

***Hips*** The symptoms of OA of the hip frequently appear in older individuals, especially in men.[15] Hip osteoarthritis is associated with buttock or groin pain that is exacerbated when the patient is bearing weight, standing up, or walking. Pain located on the outside of the hip is typically bursitis, and should not be confused with hip disease. Stiffness is common, especially after inactivity, and joint motion may be limited.

***Spine*** Degenerative changes result from involvement of the intervertebral disks, vertebral bodies, or posterior apophyseal articulations. In the lumbar spine area L3–4 involvement is most common. The resulting nerve root compression can cause pain, paresthesias, loss of reflexes, and muscle weakness in the distribution of the affected nerve root.

***Feet*** The involvement in the feet is limited primarily to the first metatarsophalangeal joint. Pain, tenderness, and stiffness are the predominant symptoms.

Other joints not commonly involved include the shoulder, elbow, acromioclavicular, sternoclavicular, and temporomandibular joint. (For a more detailed discussion, see Reference 15.)

### *Laboratory Findings*

No specific clinical laboratory abnormalities occur in primary OA. Erythrocyte sedimentation rate (ESR), routine chemistry studies, complete hematologic surveys, and urinalysis are generally normal. The rheumatoid factor test is negative. Analysis of the synovial fluid reveals fluid with high viscosity. This fluid demonstrates a mild leukocytosis (< 2,000 WBC/$mm^3$), with predominantly mononuclear cells. In the case of secondary osteoarthritis associated with an underlying metabolic disorder or endocrinopathy, specific laboratory tests are indicated to identify the cause.

### *Radiologic Evaluation*

Radiologic evaluation is an absolute necessity in the diagnosis of OA. In early, mild OA, radiographic changes may be normal. With the progression of degenerative changes in cartilage, the joint space may begin to narrow, subchondral bony sclerosis occurs, and marginal osteophyte and cyst formation may develop. Late in the disease process, subluxation and deformity sometimes occur. In general, osteoporosis and joint erosions are not seen, but they do occur in a subset of patients with erosive OA. Radiologic criteria for the diagnosis of osteoarthritis are listed in Table 61.6.[8] Specifically, weight-bearing radiographs at the knee provide better definition of the joint space.

**Table 61.6** Criteria for Radiologic Diagnosis of Osteoarthritis[a]

| |
|---|
| Formation of osteophytes in the joint margins or at ligamentous attachments (e.g., tibial spine) |
| Periarticular ossicles, mainly distal and proximal interphalangeal joints |
| Narrowing of joint space associated with sclerosis of subchondral bone |
| Cystic areas with sclerotic walls situated in the subchondral bone |
| Altered shape of bone end (e.g., head of femur) |

[a] The following five-step grading system is used according to the number of criteria present: 0 = no OA, 1 = doubtful OA, 2 = minimal OA, 3 = moderate OA, 4 = severe OA.

Adapted from Brandt KD: Osteoarthritis: Clinical patterns and pathology. In Kelly WN (Ed): Textbook of Rheumatology, 2nd ed. Philadelphia, W.B. Saunders, 1985, p 1435, with permission.

### *Diagnosis*

The diagnosis of osteoarthritis depends on clinical evaluation of the patient history, affected joint(s), and radiologic findings. Not until all these components are evaluated can an accurate diagnosis be made.

### *Prognosis*

The prognosis for patients with primary OA is variable and depends on the joint involved. If a weight-bearing joint or the spine is involved, there is the potential for considerable morbidity and significant disability. In the case of secondary OA, the prognosis depends on the underlying cause of osteoarthritis. Treatment of the cause may prevent further progression but does not reverse joint changes already present.

## Treatment

Successful therapeutic management of the patient with OA depends on accurate diagnosis of the degree and extent of joint involvement. As many patients are commonly asymptomatic, radiologic diagnosis and clinical examination and history are paramount. Further, the optimal treatment approach must be individualized to include, as appropriate, physical therapy, occupational therapy, dietary considerations, drug therapy, surgery, and patient education. The major goals are to relieve pain, preserve or improve function, and minimize the disability.

### *Nondrug Therapy*

An effective management plan requires more than drug therapy. The first step is to educate the patient about the extent, degree of involvement, prognosis, and management approach. At the same time, the patient should be warned about various arthritis quackery schemes. Several excellent sources of patient information on osteoarthritis are available from the local or national Arthritis Foundation. Specifically, the Arthritis Foundation provides literature about the disease and information about clinics and other local agencies offering physical and economic assistance.

#### Diet

For the overweight patient, dietary counseling is an important recommendation. It is not only the excess weight that can contribute to the progression of the disease but also the contraction of the muscles that span and stabilize the joint.[32] Further, obese patients scheduled to undergo total joint replacement of the hips or knees generally have a poorer surgical outcome and postoperative prognosis than patients of normal weight.[33] Weight reduction requires a motivated patient and participation in a supervised program.

#### Physical/Occupational Therapy

Physical therapy—with heat or cold treatments and an exercise program—helps to maintain and regain joint range of motion, relieve pain, and reduce muscle spasms. Such simple measures as a warm bath or warm water soaks may be effective in reducing pain and diminishing stiffness. With heat application, patients should be cautioned to avoid lying on the heat source for longer than 30 minutes to minimize the risk of burns. Other heat application techniques consist of diathermy or ultrasound to the affected joints (but not in patients with artificial metal joints as the potential for deep thermal burns exists). These techniques are reserved primarily for deep-seated joints (hips/spine) and are more costly than simpler forms of heat application.[33] Transcutaneous electrical nerve stimulation (TENS), the transmission of an electrical current from the skin to a peripheral nerve, may provide some pain relief.[9]

Exercise programs using isometric techniques are designed to strengthen the muscles and improve joint function and motion. The program should favor isometric over isotonic exercises, as the latter can aggravate the affected joint. Typical exercises consist of quadriceps-setting exercises and straight leg raises designed to strengthen knee and leg muscles. Each exercise should be taught and then observed before the patient is allowed to exercise at home. The exercises should be performed three to four times daily. If severe pain develops during exercise, the patient should be instructed to decrease the number of exercises. If necessary, various assistive devices, including splints, canes, walkers, and braces, can be used during exercise or daily activities.

#### Surgery

Surgical procedures are indicated for patients with severe disease or those individuals with intractable pain or impaired function. For patients with mild disease of the knee, an osteotomy will correct the malalignment seen with genu varum or genu valgum. Joint debridement may also be indicated to remove free cartilage fragments, eliminate locking, and reduce pain. If osteophytes are large, removal may be attempted to increase joint range of motion. For severe, advanced disease a partial or total arthroplasty is performed primarily to relieve pain, although improvement of motion is also possible. The increased motion more commonly occurs with hip than with knee joint replacements. An arthrodesis or joint fusion can also be performed to reduce the pain associated with degenerative changes but it will restrict motion of that joint.

### *Drug Therapy*

Drug therapy in OA is directed at the symptomatic relief of pain and inflammation when present. Currently, no medication has been shown to be effective in preventing the progression of OA.[34,35] The regimen of choice requires an individualized approach. Some patients with mild symptoms may require only analgesics; those with signs of active inflammation may benefit from the use of an anti-inflammatory medication.

#### Analgesics

The pain that occurs in OA is not related to the degenerating cartilage as cartilage is aneural. Rather, a variety of factors—microfractures in subchondral bone, irritation of periosteal nerve endings, ligamentous stress secondary to bone deformity, and venous congestion caused by remodeling of subchondral bone—contribute to the pain.[36]

**Table 61.7** Nonsteroidal Anti-inflammatory Drugs

| *Chemical classification* | *Generic* | *Brand* | *Manufacturer* |
|---|---|---|---|
| Salicylates | Acetylated | | |
| | Aspirin | Various | Various |
| | Aspirin, buffered | Various | Various |
| | Enteric coated | Various | Various |
| | Sustained release | Various | Various |
| | Nonacetylated | | |
| | Choline salicylate | Arthropan | Purdue Frederick |
| | Choline magnesium trisalicylate | Trilisate | Purdue Frederick |
| | Diflunisal | Dolobid | Merck Sharp & Dohme |
| | Salsalate | Disalcid | Riker |
| | | Various | Various |
| | Magnesium salicylate | Various | Various |
| | Sodium salicylate | Various | Various |
| Fenamates | Meclofenamic acid | Meclomen | Parke–Davis |
| | Mefenamic acid | Ponstel | Parke–Davis |
| Acetic acids | Diclofenac[a] | Voltaren | Ciba–Geigy |
| | Etodolac[a] | Ultradol | Ayerst |
| | Indomethacin | Indocin | Merck Sharp & Dohme |
| | | Various | Various |
| | Sulindac | Clinoril | Merck Sharp & Dohme |
| | Tolmetin | Tolectin | McNeil |
| Propionic acids | Carprofen[a] | Rimadyl | Roche |
| | Fenbufen[a] | Cinopal | Lederle |
| | Fenoprofen | Nalfon | Dista |
| | Flurbiprofen[a] | Ansaid | Upjohn |
| | Ibuprofen | Motrin | Upjohn |
| | | Rufen | Boots |
| | | Various | Various |
| | Ketoprofen | Orudis | Wyeth |
| | Naproxen | Naprosyn | Syntex |
| | | Anaprox | |
| Pyrazolones | Phenylbutazone | Azolid | USV |
| | | Butazolidin | Geigy |
| | | Various | Various |
| Oxicam | Piroxicam | Feldene | Pfizer |

[a] Soon to be released.

The major analgesics of choice are aspirin and acetaminophen in doses of 325–650 mg four times daily. To achieve anti-inflammatory activity, aspirin in doses greater than 3.6 g/d is necessary. The zero-order kinetics of anti-inflammatory doses of aspirin has been well described[37,38]; monitoring of serum salicylate concentrations for efficacy or toxicity is required. The serum half-life of salicylates ranges from 2 hours for analgesic doses to more than 20 hours for anti-inflammatory doses. Serum concentrations should be measured after five half-lives. The relationship of serum salicylate concentrations to clinical response or toxicity has been described.[37,38] Therapeutic levels are between 15 and 30 mg/dL. Plasma concentrations greater than 30 mg/dL generally correlate with the onset of tinnitus, except in children or in the elderly patient who has preexisting hearing loss.

Aspirin is also highly protein bound; increasing doses result in an increase in the apparent volume of distribution as protein binding site saturation occurs. Low albumin concentrations, increasing age, and highly protein bound drugs can increase the toxic effects from salicylates.[37,38] Urinary pH changes can affect the excretion of salicylates severalfold, as an alkaline urine increases the excretion of salicylates. In the choice of a particular aspirin product, several factors related to toxicity should be considered; a large variety of acetylated and nonacetylated salicylate products exist (Table 61.7).

First, salicylates can cause adverse gastrointestinal effects ranging from mild discomfort to gastric ulcers. To minimize these effects, the salicylates should be taken with food or milk. Also, enteric-coated products cause less gastric mucosal injury compared with buffered or plain aspirin.[39] The nonacetylated salicylate products also produce less gastrointestinal irritation and bleeding than plain aspirin.[39] Second, the decreased platelet aggregation observed with aspirin is

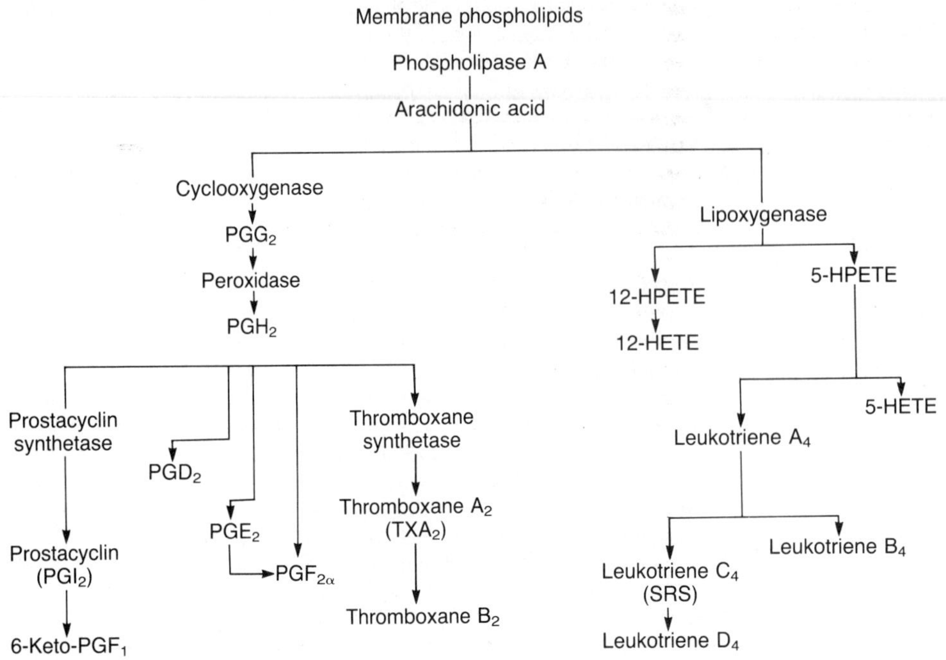


**Figure 61.3** Outline of arachidonic acid metabolism. HPETE, hydroperoxyeicosatetraenoic acid; HETE, hydroxyeicosatetraenoic acid; $PGE_2$, prostaglandin $E_2$; $PGF_{2\alpha}$, prostaglandin $F_{2\alpha}$. *(Compiled from References 47 and 48.)*

not seen with the nonacetylated salicylate products.[39] These nonacetylated salicylates are a safer alternative in the patient with a bleeding disorder or in those patients scheduled to undergo a surgical procedure. Third, a clinically important syndrome of aspirin intolerance exists in some patients. Administration of aspirin can result in two kinds of reactions: type A—bronchoconstriction, vasomotor rhinitis, and nasal polyps or laryngeal edema; type B—urticaria and angioedema. Type A occurs in 2% to 4% of asthmatics with cross-sensitivity to other nonsteroidal anti-inflammatory agents (although a nonacetylated salicylate may be tolerated). This reaction appears to be related to inhibition of prostaglandin synthesis.[40] Type B reactions generally occur with other salicylates.[40–43] Other toxic responses to aspirin products include impaired renal function and increases in serum transaminases. The last factor to consider in selection of a product is cost. Nonacetylated products are considerably more expensive than plain aspirin.

For patients who need only analgesic therapy, acetaminophen 650 mg four times daily provides analgesia comparable to that provided by aspirin 650 mg four times daily. The lack of anti-inflammatory properties precludes its usefulness in patients with evidence of inflammation. Generally, acetaminophen is well tolerated by patients, but when taken in excess or by patients with liver disease it may cause toxic hepatitis.[43,44]

Narcotics such as codeine should be used only rarely because of the potential for drug dependence. Patients should be instructed to use the narcotics for severe pain and for the shortest duration possible. Ideally, prescriptions should be written for a limited quantity with only one or two refills.

**Anti-inflammatory Drugs**

Nonsteroidal anti-inflammatory drugs (NSAIDs) provide analgesic effects at lower doses and anti-inflammatory activity at higher doses. Several NSAIDs from a variety of chemical classes are available (Table 61.7); more products are in various phases of clinical testing in Europe and the United States.[45]

As a class of compounds, the NSAIDs are all comparably effective in reducing pain and modifying or diminishing the inflammatory process. Though the exact mechanism of action is unknown, a major component of the activity of all NSAIDs is believed to be related to the inhibition of prostaglandin biosynthesis[46,47] by inhibition of the enzyme cyclooxygenase (Fig. 61.3).

The choice of a particular NSAID is frequently a matter of prescriber preference based on past treatment, cost, patient preference, toxic effects, and compliance. In general, the NSAIDs are indicated after simple analgesics have failed to relieve pain, toxic effects have developed, or inflammation is present. All NSAIDs appear to be as effective as aspirin in terms of analgesia or anti-inflammatory properties and cause fewer gastrointestinal complaints than aspirin.[45,47–52] These characteristics have encouraged many physicians to select the NSAIDs before aspirin; however, the NSAIDs are considerably more expensive.

The pharmacokinetics of the individual NSAIDs are similar.[45,48,49] All are well absorbed after oral administration, are highly protein bound (> 90%), and have a low volume of distribution (< 0.2 L/kg). Elimination is dependent on hepatic biotransformation to inactive metabolites (except sulindac, which is metabolized to an active form), with renal excretion of less than 5% of the unchanged drug. Total body clearance is low (for most NSAIDs, < 200 mL/min). They readily penetrate the joint fluid in concentrations generally half those found in blood.[51] Therapeutic monitoring of serum and synovial drug concentrations has not been successfully applied.[49] The anti-inflammatory effect generally peaks after 2 to 3 weeks, irrespective of the half-life. Analgesic effectiveness usually occurs 1 to 2 hours after taking the NSAID and lasts up to 24 hours. The most variable property appears to be the serum half-life, which ranges from 1 hour for tolmetin to 60 to 90 hours for phenylbutazone.

Patient response to the NSAIDs is typically variable and highly individual.[51] A patient may respond well to one drug in a particular chemical class but have little or no benefit from another NSAID in the same class. Therefore, it is reasonable to try other NSAIDs, in a selective manner, after an adequate trial (2–3 weeks) at an adequate dose (either anti-inflammatory or analgesic). Patients should always be instructed that a trial with more than one product may be necessary and compliance with the scheduled regimen is important in evaluating effectiveness. Combination of nonsteroidal anti-inflammatory agents with other NSAIDs or aspirin increases toxic effects while providing no added benefit.[46]

Gastrointestinal complaints are the most common toxic effects observed with the NSAIDs and account for many treatment failures. To minimize toxic effects, administration with food or milk should be encouraged, except for the enteric-coated products, as milk or antacids may destroy the enteric coating and cause increased gastrointestinal symptoms. Diarrhea can occur but is more commonly observed with meclofenamate than the other NSAIDs. Gastrointestinal bleeding and ulceration can occur without subjective complaints, necessitating close monitoring of stools for change of color (and hematology profiles if gastrointestinal bleeding is suspected). Additionally, guaiac-positive stools do not always indicate toxic responses to NSAIDs and other pathologic processes causing gastrointestinal bleeding should be considered.[53] All NSAIDs have the potential to cause gastrointestinal bleeding through a variety of mechanisms, including interference with the cytoprotective barrier produced by the prostaglandins.[46,47]

NSAIDs have also been shown to cause a variety of renal complications, including peripheral edema, transient acute renal insufficiency, tubulointerstitial nephropathy, hyperkalemia, and renal papillary necrosis.[54,55] Many of these complications may be mediated by inhibition of prostaglandins, which have an important role in the regulation of intrarenal blood flow in vasoconstricted states.[54,55] Highly prone to developing renal insufficiency are patients with congestive heart failure, cirrhosis/ascites, or volume contraction (from any cause) and the elderly. Clinical findings associated with NSAID-induced renal syndromes include an increased serum creatinine, BUN, serum potassium, and peripheral edema and a weight gain. Prostaglandin-mediated renal effects are reversible upon discontinuance of therapy. Recent data suggest that sulindac and possibly the nonacetylated salicylates are less likely to cause renal insufficiency.[54,55] Nevertheless, close monitoring for this complication is required.

Other toxic effects include hypersensitivity reactions, rash, hepatitis, or central nervous system complaints such as drowsiness, dizziness, headaches, depression, confusion, and tinnitus.[42,47,56] Additionally, all the agents that inhibit cyclooxygenase affect platelet function to some extent. Aspirin inhibition is irreversible and 5 to 7 days is required before platelet function returns to normal, whereas the other NSAIDs cause a reversible inhibition that allows platelet function to return to normal sooner (1–3 days) after discontinuance. In either case, the nonacetylated salicylate products may be preferable for the patient with a bleeding disorder or as a temporary treatment before elective surgical procedures.

Significant drug interactions with the NSAIDs are frequently related to the ability of the highly protein bound NSAID to displace other highly protein bound drugs, such as oral anticoagulants, oral hypoglycemics, and anticonvulsants. In the case of oral anticoagulants, the NSAIDs have the potential to cause gastrointestinal bleeding, inhibit platelet aggregation, displace oral anticoagulants, and compete for metabolism, all resulting in increased toxicity. Many other interactions are of theoretical concern but nevertheless require careful monitoring for enhanced effectiveness. NSAIDs may also antagonize the effects of diuretics and other antihypertensives.[57]

A major controversy in the treatment of OA with NSAIDs is whether these agents actually help or hinder the progression of osteoarthritis.[58,59] Experimental data in animals have demonstrated the ability of salicylates and some NSAIDs to suppress proteoglycan biosynthesis in articular cartilage.[58,59] The effect of suppression appears to be greater in osteoarthritic cartilage than in normal cartilage. Additionally, a retrospective radiographic study reported that indomethacin administration may be associated with joint destruction greater than that seen in control subjects.[60] Further experimental and clinical data in humans are necessary to confirm the finding and the subsequent implications of not using or limiting the use of the NSAIDs in the treatment of OA.

### Corticosteroids

Systemic corticosteroid therapy is not recommended in the treatment of osteoarthritis.[36] The side effects associated with prolonged use outweigh any potential benefits of therapy. The use of intra-articular corticosteroids (IAC) is a more controversial issue. Significant relief of pain has been reported with the injection of IAC into the knee. The pain relief has usually been temporary and, in some studies, comparable to that obtained with injection of saline solutions or procaine.[36] Concern over increased damage from overuse after the amelioration of pain and studies of cartilage degeneration following IAC injections in animals have resulted in recommendations for avoiding frequent injections.[36] If used, IAC should be administered infrequently at intervals of 4 to 6 months for any given joint. If no improvement occurs from one or two injections, then further treatment is not likely to succeed.[36] After injection, the patient should be instructed to minimize joint activity or stress loading for several days. Injection of corticosteroids into the ligaments or pericapsular areas can be beneficial and is associated with reduced risks relative to IAC administration.[8,36]

## Summary

Osteoarthritis is a very common, slowly progressive disorder that affects diarthrodial joints. It is characterized by a progressive deterioration of articular cartilage that results in loss of articular cartilage and osteophyte formation. Clinically, the manifestations occur later in life and consist of gradual onset of joint pain, stiffness, and limitation of motion. The treatment goal is reduce pain, maintain function, and prevent further destruction. An individualized approach consisting of nondrug and drug therapy can be successful in attaining these goals, with analgesics and NSAIDs playing an important role.

## References


1. Mankin HJ. The reaction of articular cartilage to injury and osteoarthritis. N Engl J Med 1974;291:1285–1292, 1335–1340.
2. Mankin HJ, Johnson ME, Lippiello LO. Biochemical and metabolic abnormalities in articular cartilage from osteoarthritic human hips. J Bone Joint Surg 1981;63A:131–139.
3. Hammerman D, Klagsbrun M. Osteoarthritis: Emerging evidence for cell interactions in the breakdown and remodeling of cartilage. Am J Med 1985;78:495–499.
4. Ehrlich GE. Osteoarthritis beginning with inflammation. JAMA 1975;232:157–159.
5. Peyron J. Inflammation in osteoarthritis (OA): A review of its role in clinical picture, disease progress, subsets and pathophysiology. Semin Arthritis Rheum 1981;11:115S–116S.
6. Bland JH, Cooper SM. Osteoarthritis: A review of the cell biology involved and evidence for reversibility. Management rationally related to known genesis and pathophysiology. Semin Arthritis Rheum 1984;14:106–133.
7. Brandt KD. Pathogenesis of osteoarthritis, in Kelley WN (ed): Textbook of Rheumatology, 2nd ed. Philadelphia, W.B. Saunders, 1985.
8. Brandt KD. Osteoarthritis: Clinical patterns and pathology, in Kelley WN (ed): Textbook of Rheumatology, 2nd ed. Philadelphia, W.B. Saunders, 1985.
9. Anonymous. Osteoarthritis, in Primer of Rheumatic Diseases, 8th ed. Atlanta, Arthritis Foundation, 1983.
10. Peyron JG. Epidemiologic and etiologic approach of osteoarthritis. Semin Arthritis Rheum 1979;8:288–306.
11. National Center for Health Statistics. Prevalence of osteoarthritis in adults by age, sex, race, and geographic area, United States, 1960–1962. Vital and Health Statistics, series 11, no. 15. Washington DC, US Government Printing Office, 1966.
12. Scott JC. Osteoarthritis. I: Epidemiology. Md State Med J 1984; 33:712–716.
13. National Center for Health Statistics. Basic data on arthritis: Knee, hip, and sacroiliac joints in adults ages 25–74 years, United States, 1971–1975. Vital and Health Statistics, Series 11, No. 213, Washington DC, US Government Printing Office, 1979.
14. Kellgren JH, Lawrence JS, Bier F. Genetic factors in generalized osteoarthrosis. Ann Rheum Dis 1963;22:237–255.
15. Moskowitz RW. Clinical and laboratory findings in osteoarthritis, in McCarty DJ (ed): Arthritis and Allied Conditions, 10th ed. Philadelphia, Lea and Febiger, 1985.
16. Halder NM, Gillings DB, Imbus HR, et al. Hand structure and function in an industrial setting. Arthritis Rheum 1978;21:210–220.
17. Partridge RH, Duthie JR. Rheumatism in dockers and civil servants: A comparison of heavy manual and sedentary workers. Ann Rheum Dis 1968;27:559–568.
18. Macys JR, Bullough PG, Wilson PD. Coxarthrosis: A study of the natural history based on a correlation of clinical, radiographic, and pathologic findings. Semin Arthritis Rheum 1980; 10:66–80.
19. Panush RS, Schmidt C, Caldwell JR, et al. Is running associated with degenerative joint disease? JAMA 1986;255:1152–1154.
20. Bland JH. The reversibility of osteoarthritis: A review. Am J Med 1983;5:16–26.
21. Lee P, Rooney PJ, Sturrock RD, et al. The etiology and pathogenesis of osteoarthrosis: A review. Semin Arthritis Rheum 1974;3:189–219.
22. Cooke TDV. Pathogenetic mechanisms in polyarticular osteoarthritis. Clin Rheum Dis 1985;11:203–238.
23. Troyer H. Experimental models of osteoarthritis: A review. Semin Arthritis Rheum 1982;11:362–374.
24. Radin EL. The physiology and degeneration of joints. Semin Arthritis Rheum 1972–1973;2:245–257.
25. Howell DS, Sapolsky AI, Pita JC, et al. The pathogenesis of osteoarthritis. Semin Arthritis Rheum 1976;5:365–383.
26. Nimni ME. Collagen: Its structure and function in normal and pathological connective tissues. Semin Arthritis Rheum 1974;4: 95–150.
27. Mankin HJ, Dorfman H, Lippiello L, et al. Biochemical and metabolic abnormalities in articular cartilage from osteoarthritic hips. II. Correlation of morphology with biochemical and metabolic data. J Bone Joint Surg 1971;53A:523–537.
28. Gardner DL. The nature and causes of osteoarthrosis. Br Med J 1983; 286:418–424.
29. Ettinger WH. Osteoarthritis. II: Pathology and pathogenesis. Md State Med J 1984;33:811–814.
30. Mankin HJ. Normal articular cartilage and the alterations in osteoarthritis, in Lombardino JG (ed): Nonsteroidal Antiinflammatory Drugs. New York, Wiley-Interscience, 1985.
31. Blotzer JW. Osteoarthritis. III: Clinical features. Md State Med J 1984;33:907–910.
32. Brandt KD. Management of osteoarthritis, in Kelley WN (ed): Textbook of Rheumatology. Philadelphia, W.B. Saunders, 1985.
33. Hochberg MC. Osteoarthritis: Pathophysiology, clinical features, management. Hosp Pract 1984;12:41–53.
34. Huskisson EC, Doyle DV, Lanham JG. Drug treatment of osteoarthritis. Clin Rheum Dis 1985;11:421–431.
35. Doyle DV, Lanham JG. Routine drug treatment of osteoarthritis. Clin Rheum Dis 1984;10:277–291.
36. Lemperg RK. Arnoldi CC. The significance of intraosseous pressure in normal and diseased states with special reference to the intraosseous engorgement-pain syndrome. Clin Orthop 1978;136:143–156.
37. Dromgoole SH, Furst DE. Salicylates, in Evans WE (ed): Applied Pharmacokinetics. San Francisco, Applied Therapeutics, 1980.
38. Dromgoole SH, Furst DE, Paulus HE. Rational approaches to the use of salicylates in the treatment of rheumatoid arthritis. Semin Arthritis Rheum 1981;11:257–283.
39. Graham DY, Smith JL. Aspirin and the stomach. Ann Intern Med 1986;104:390–398.
40. Szczeklik A, Gryglewski RJ, Czerniawska-Mysik G. Clinical

patterns of hypersensitivity to nonsteroidal antiinflammatory drugs and their pathogenesis. J Allergy Clin Immunol 1977;60: 276–284.
41. Moore-Robinson M, Warin RP. Effect of salicylates in urticaria. Br Med J 1967;1:262–264.
42. Abrishami MA, Thomas J. Aspirin intolerance—a review. Ann Allergy 1977;39:28–37.
43. Barker JD, de Carle DJ, Anuras S. Chronic excessive acetaminophen use and liver damage. Ann Intern Med 1977:87:299–301.
44. Black M, Raucy J. Acetaminophen, alcohol and cytochrome P-450, editorial. Ann Intern Med 1986;104:427–429.
45. Marsh CC, Schuna AA, Sundstrom WR. A review of selected investigational nonsteroidal antiinflammatory drugs of the 1980s. Pharmacotherapy 1986;6:10–25.
46. Simon LS. Nonsteroidal antiinflammatory drugs. N Engl J Med 1980;302:1179–1185, 302:1237–1243.
47. Craig GL, Buchanan WW. Antirheumatic drugs: Clinical pharmacology and therapeutic use. Drugs 1980;20:453–484.
48. Verbeeck RK, Blackburn JL, Loewen GR. Clinical pharmacokinetics of nonsteroidal anti-inflammatory drugs. Clin Pharmacokinet 1983;8:297–331.
49. Porter RS. Factors determining efficacy of NSAIDs. Drug Intell Clin Pharm 1984;18:42–51.
50. Wallis WJ, Simkin PA. Antirheumatic drug concentrations in human synovial fluid and synovial tissue. Clin Pharmacokinet 1983;8:496–522.
51. Hadler NM. The argument for aspirin as the NSAID of choice in the management of rheumatoid arthritis. Drug Intell Clin Pharm 1984;18:34–38.
52. Scott DL, Roden S, Marshal T, et al. Variations in responses to nonsteroidal antiinflammatory drugs. Br J Clin Pharmacol 1982; 14:691–694.
53. Bahrt KM, Korman LY, Nashel DJ. Significance of a positive test for occult blood in stools of patients taking anti-inflammatory drugs. Arch Intern Med 1984;144:2165–2166.
54. Clive DM, Stoff JS. Renal syndromes associated with nonsteroidal antiinflammatory drugs. N Engl J Med 1984;310:563–572.
55. Garella S, Matarese RA. Renal effects of prostaglandins and clinical adverse effects of nonsteroidal antiinflammatory agents. Medicine 1984;63:165–181.
56. Lewis JH. Hepatic toxicity of nonsteroidal anti-inflammatory drugs. Clin Pharm 1984;3:128–138.
57. Webster J. Interactions of NSAIDs with diuretics and $\beta$-blockers: Mechanisms and clinical implications. Drugs 1985;30: 32–41.
58. Palmoski MJ, Brandt KD. Effects of salicylate and indomethacin on glycosaminoglycan and prostaglandin $E_2$ synthesis in intact canine knee cartilage ex vivo. Arthritis Rheum 1984;27: 398–403.
59. Palmoski MJ, Brandt KD. Effects of some nonsteroidal antiinflammatory drugs on proteoglycan metabolism and organization in canine articular cartilage. Arthritis Rheum 1980;23: 1010–1020.
60. Ronningen H, Langeland N. Indomethacin treatment in osteoarthritis of the hip joint. Does the treatment interfere with the natural course of the disease? Acta Orthop Scand 1979;50:169–174.

# *Chapter 62* / Gout and Hyperuricemia

David W. Hawkins, PharmD

Hyperuricemia and gout occur in individuals who have some abnormality in either the production or the elimination of uric acid, or both. Men are affected 10 times more often than women, and the mean age of onset of gout is 47 years.

Hyperuricemia may be an asymptomatic condition, with an increased serum uric acid as the only apparent abnormality. Statistically, hyperuricemia is defined as a serum urate concentration greater than two standard deviations above the population mean. At 37°C, the serum is saturated with urate at a concentration of 7 mg/dL; hyperuricemia may be defined biochemically as a serum urate concentration of 7.1 mg/dL or higher.

Gout is a disease evoked by the deposition of sodium urate crystals in and about the joints and cartilage and in the kidneys and by the precipitation of urinary uric acid stones.[1] These pathologic events are more likely to occur when hyperuricemia is present, but they sometimes develop in people with serum urate concentrations below the saturation point.

## Pathophysiology

In humans, uric acid is the end product of the degradation of purines. It serves no known physiologic purpose and therefore is regarded as a waste product. In lower animals, the enzyme uricase breaks down uric acid to the more soluble allantoin, and thus uric acid does not accumulate. Conversely, in humans, a miscible pool of uric acid exists. Under normal conditions, the amount of cumulated uric acid is about 1,200 mg. The size of the urate pool may increase to 18,000 to 31,000 mg in individuals with gout.

### *Overproduction of Uric Acid*

The purines from which uric acid is produced originate from three sources: dietary purine, conversion of tissue nucleic acid to purine nucleotides, and de novo synthesis of purine bases. The purines derived from these three sources enter a common metabolic pathway, leading to the production of either nucleic acid or uric acid. When purine metabolism is normal, the average human produces about 600 to 800 mg of uric acid each day.

Along the pathway are several enzyme systems regulating the direction of purine metabolism. An abnormality in any of these regulatory systems could result in overproduction of uric acid. Excessive uric acid may also occur as a consequence of increased breakdown of tissue nucleic acids associated with myeloproliferative and lymphoproliferative disorders. Dietary purines play an insignificant role in the generation of hyperuricemia in the absence of some derangement in purine metabolism or elimination.

To date only two enzyme defects of purine metabolism are known to cause an overproduction of uric acid, namely, phosphoribosyl pyrophosphate (PRPP) synthetase and hypoxanthine–guanine phosphoribosyl transferase (HGPRT) (Fig. 62.1). The defect associated with PRPP synthetase results in an increased intracellular concentration of PRPP. The buildup of PRPP accelerates the rate of purine biosynthesis de novo and, consequently, the production of uric acid.

HGPRT is responsible for the conversion of guanine to guanylic acid and hypoxanthine to inosinic acid. These two conversions require PRPP as the cosubstrate and are important reutilization reactions involved in the synthesis of nucleic acids. A deficiency in the HGPRT enzyme would lead to an increased metabolism of guanine and hypoxanthine to uric acid and more PRPP to interact with glutamine in the first step of the purine pathway.[2] Complete absence of HGPRT results in the childhood Lesch–Nyhan syndrome, characterized by choreoathetosis, spasticity, mental retardation, and markedly excessive production of uric acid. A partial deficiency of the enzyme may be responsible for marked hyperuricemia in otherwise normal healthy individuals.

### *Underexcretion of Uric Acid*

Hyperuricemia does not occur as long as a balance exists between uric acid production and elimination. Uric acid is eliminated in two ways. Most of the uric acid produced each day is excreted in the urine. About 200 mg is eliminated through the gastrointestinal tract, after enzymatic degradation by colonic bacteria. In the presence of renal failure, the elimination of uric acid through the gastrointestinal tract increases several times.

A decline in the urinary excretion of uric acid leads to hyperuricemia and an increased miscible pool of sodium urate. This situation may arise if any component involved in the renal handling of uric acid is altered. Almost all the urate in plasma is freely filtered across the glomerulus; therefore, any reduction in the glomerular filtration rate will be associated with a proportionate increase in serum urate concentration. After glomerular filtration, urate undergoes passive tubular reabsorption, active tubular secretion, and then passive tubular reabsorption again. In the initial part of the proximal tubule, 98% to 100% of the filtered urate is reabsorbed back into the bloodstream. Therefore, the final concentration of uric acid in the urine is largely dependent upon postsecretory reabsorption. If there is some specific defect in tubular secretion of urate or some other substance is

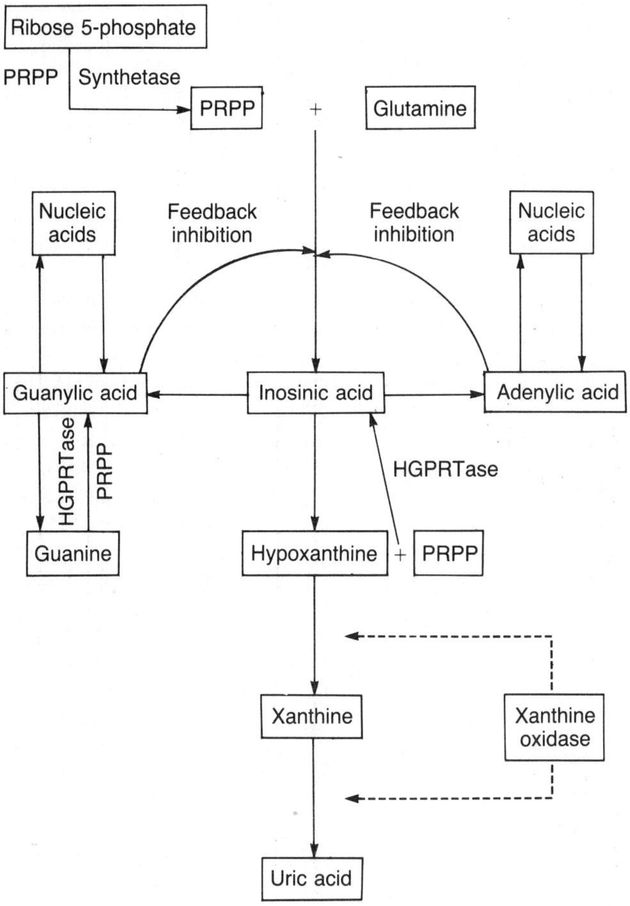


**Figure 62.1** Purine biosynthesis and degradation. PRPP, phosphoribosyl pyrophosphate; HGPRTase, hypoxanthine–guanine phosphoribosyl transferase.

competing with urate for tubular secretory sites, then the amount of uric acid excreted decreases and hyperuricemia ensues. Likewise, an increase in the postsecretory reabsorption of urate, as may occur secondary to plasma volume contraction, would lead to a decrease in urate excretion, and thus a rise in the serum urate concentration.

A variety of conditions are associated with hyperuricemia (Tables 62.1 and 62.2). On the basis of the previous discussion, these conditions must either increase the production of uric acid or decrease its excretion. Some of these conditions are known to affect both production and elimination of uric acid (e.g., glycogen storage disease type 1). The pathophysiologic approach to the treatment of hyperuricemia requires determining whether the patient is overproducing or underexcreting uric acid. This can be accomplished by placing the patient on a purine-free diet for several days and then measuring the amount of uric acid excreted in 24 hours. Patients who are overproducing uric acid excrete more than 600 mg of uric acid per day. Hyperuricemic individuals who excrete less than 600 mg of uric acid per 24 hours may be defined as relative underexcretors of uric acid. Individuals who excrete more than 1,000 mg of uric acid per 24 hours on a regular diet are also judged to be overproducers of uric acid.

**Table 62.1** Conditions Associated With Hyperuricemia

| | |
|---|---|
| Primary gout | Diabetic ketoacidosis |
| Myeloproliferative disorders | Lactic acidosis |
| Lymphoproliferative disorders | Starvation |
| Chronic hemolytic anemia | Toxemia of pregnancy |
| Pernicious anemia | Glycogen storage disease type 1 |
| Psoriasis | Obesity |
| Sarcoidosis | Congestive heart failure |
| Renal dysfunction | Down's syndrome |
| Lead toxicity | Hyperparathyroidism |
| Acute alcoholism | Hypoparathyroidism |
| Acromegaly | Hypothyroidism |

## Clinical Characteristics of Gout

Gout is a disease manifested by acute attacks of arthritis, nephrolithiasis, gouty nephropathy, and aggregated deposits of sodium urate (tophi) in cartilage, tendons, synovial membranes, and elsewhere.[3]

### *Acute Gouty Arthritis*

Acute attacks of gouty arthritis are characterized by rapid onset of excrutiating pain, swelling, and inflammation. The attack is typically monoarticular at first, most often affecting the first metatarsophalangeal joint and then, in order of frequency, the insteps, ankles, heels, knees, wrists, fingers, and elbows.

The predilection of acute gout for peripheral joints is probably related to the low temperature of the joint and the high intraarticular urate concentration, brought about by synovial effusions during the day and a twofold increase in water reabsorption over urate from the joint during sleep.

The development of crystal-induced inflammation involves a number of chemical mediators causing vasodilation, increased vascular permeability, and chemotactic activity for polymorphonuclear leukocytes. Phagocytosis of urate crystals by the leukocytes results in rapid lysis of cells and a discharge of proteolytic enzymes into the cytoplasm. The inflammatory reaction that ensues may last from 3 to 14 days, if left untreated.

Although acute attacks of gouty arthritis may occur without apparent provocation, a number of conditions in the right circumstances may precipitate an attack. These include stress, trauma, surgery, rapid lowering of serum uric acid by ingestion of uric acid–lowering agents, and ingestion of certain drugs known to elevate serum acid acid concentrations.

**Table 62.2** Drugs Capable of Inducing Hyperuricemia and Gout

| | |
|---|---|
| Diuretics | Nicotinic acid |
| Salicylates (<2 g/d) | Ethanol |
| Pyrazinamide | L-Dopa |
| Ethambutol | Cytotoxic drugs |

### *Uric Acid Nephrolithiasis*

Nephrolithiasis occurs in 10% to 25% of patients with gout and in hyperuricemic patients with no history of gout.[4] Factors that predispose individuals to uric acid nephrolithiasis include excessive urinary excretion of uric acid, an acidic urine, and a highly concentrated urine. The stones may be of three types: pure uric acid stones, mixed uric-acid–calcium oxalate stones, and calcium oxalate stones.

Uric acid has a $pK_a$ of 5.5. Therefore, when the urine is acidic, uric acid exists primarily in the un-ionized, less soluble form. At a urine pH of 5.0, for example, only 6–8 mg of uric acid is soluble in 100 mL of urine. When the urine pH is 7.0, the solubility of uric acid is increased to 124–160 mg per 100 mL of urine. In patients with uric acid nephrolithiasis, urinary pH is typically less than 6.0 and frequently less than 5.5. When an acidic urine is saturated with uric acid, spontaneous precipitation of stones may occur.

### *Gouty Nephropathy*

There are two types of gouty nephropathy.[5] The formation of uric acid crystals in the collecting tubules or ureter is related to acute hyperuricaciduria and is a well-recognized complication in patients with myeloproliferative or lymphoproliferative disorders. The blockade of urine flow leads to acute renal failure.

The other type is caused by the chronic deposition of urate crystals in the renal parenchyma. Microtophi may form, with a surrounding giant cell inflammatory reaction. A decrease in the kidney's ability to concentrate urine and the presence of proteinuria may be the earliest pathophysiologic disturbances. Hypertension and nephrosclerosis are common complications and chronic renal insufficiency could ultimately develop. Long-standing hyperuricemia by itself does not appear to be a predisposing factor, as chronic gouty nephropathy is very rare in the absence of gouty arthritis.

### *Tophaceous Gout*

Tophi (urate deposits) are uncommon in the general population of gouty subjects and are a late complication of hyperuricemia. The most common site of tophaceous deposits in patients with recurrent acute gouty arthritis is the base of the great toe; however, visible tophi may also occur in the ear lobes, olecranon bursa, ankles, heels, knees, wrists, and hands. Eventually even the hips, shoulders, and spine may be affected. In addition to causing obvious deformities, tophi may damage surrounding soft tissue, cause joint destruction and pain, and even lead to nerve compression syndromes including carpal tunnel syndrome.

## Treatment

This discussion on the management of gout and hyperuricemia includes a review of the treatment options available for acute attacks of gouty arthritis and uric acid nephrolithiasis and some general recommendations regarding prophylactic treatment programs as well as the management of asymptomatic hyperuricemia.

### *Acute Gouty Arthritis*

The treatment of acute attacks of gouty arthritis is accomplished with colchicine or nonsteroidal anti-inflammatory agents.[6] Colchicine can be given orally or parenterally. The usual oral dose is 0.5 or 0.6 mg at hourly intervals until the joint symptoms subside; the patient develops nausea, vomiting, or diarrhea; or the patient has taken a maximum of 12 tablets. About 75% to 95% of patients with acute gouty arthritis respond favorably to colchicine when ingestion of the drug is begun within 12 to 24 hours of the onset of joint symptoms. If the ingestion of colchicine is delayed longer than 24 hours after the onset of acute symptoms, the probability of success with the drug diminishes significantly.[7]

The major problem associated with the use of oral colchicine is development of gastrointestinal toxicity before relief from gout occurs, in 50% to 80% of patients. The elderly patient is likely to become severely dehydrated and may incur serious electrolyte losses.

When given intravenously, the initial dose of colchicine is 2–3 mg. If relief is not obtained after 6 hours, an additional dose may be given. The colchicine should be diluted with 20 mL of normal saline before administration to minimize sclerosis of the vein. The intravenous administration of colchicine eliminates most of the gastrointestinal symptoms associated with the oral dose but subjects the patient to the risk of local extravasation with inflammation and necrosis of the surrounding tissue. Very small difficult-to-inject veins and renal impairment represent relative contraindications to intravenous colchicine therapy.

Both phenylbutazone and indomethacin have proved to be as effective as colchicine in the treatment of acute gouty arthritis.[8] As gastrointestinal toxicity occurs far less frequently with these two drugs than with colchicine, they are preferred. Patients with acute gouty arthritis and borderline cardiac reserve or overt congestive heart failure should be treated with indomethacin rather than phenylbutazone. Side effects unique to indomethacin include headache and dizziness. Both drugs have been implicated in the cause of peptic ulceration and bleeding, but with short-term therapy this is not likely to occur. Also, the hematologic toxic effects associated occasionally with phenylbutazone therapy would be unusually rare in instances where the drug use is limited to several days.

When indomethacin or phenylbutazone is used in the treatment of acute gouty arthritis, it is customary to start with a relatively large dose for the first 24 to 48 hours and then to taper the therapy over 3 to 4 days to minimize the risk of recurrent attacks. For example, 75 mg of indomethacin should be given initially, followed by 50 mg every 6 hours for 2 days, then 50 mg every 8 hours for 1 or 2 days. With phenylbutazone, 300–400 mg should be given initially, then 200 mg four times a day for 2 days and 100 mg four times a day for 2 additional days before discontinuing the drug.

A number of other nonsteroidal anti-inflammatory agents (e.g., naproxen, fenoprofen, and ibuprofen) also appear to be effective in relieving the inflammation of acute gout. If further testing and clinical experience indicate a lower incidence of adverse reactions to these agents, then it is likely that they will become the drugs of choice in the treatment of gouty arthritis.

Adrenocorticotropic hormone (ACTH) and corticosteroids may be used to treat acute attacks of gouty arthritis, but they are reserved primarily for resistant cases. Doses of 40–80 USP units of ACTH gel are given intramuscularly every 6 to 8 hours for 2 to 3 days and then the doses are reduced in stepwise fashion and discontinued. Intraarticular administration of hydrocortisone in a dose of 25–50 mg may be useful in treating acute gout limited to a single joint; oral administration of prednisone in doses of 40–60 mg daily may be used in patients with multiple-joint involvement. As rebound attacks may occur upon steroid withdrawal, 0.6 mg of colchicine should be given two or three times daily during and several days after steroid therapy.

### *Nephrolithiasis*

The medical management of uric acid nephrolithiasis includes adequate hydration, control of urine hyperacidity, avoidance of purine-rich foods, moderation of protein intake, and prevention of recurrent uric acid stones.[9]

Maintenance of a 24-hour urine volume of 2–3 L with an adequate intake of fluids is desirable for all gouty patients, but especially for those with excessive (>1.0 g/d) uric acid excretion. Hydration should be accompanied by the use of alkalinizing agents, with the objective of making the urine less acid, but not alkaline. Urine pH should be maintained at 6.0–6.5. In this pH range, up to 85% of uric acid will be in the form of the soluble urate ion.

Reduction of urine acidity can be accomplished by the administration of sodium bicarbonate or Shohl's solution (40 g citric acid and 98 g sodium citrate per liter). With the former, 2–6 g/d is given in equally divided doses at 6- to 8-hour intervals. A dose of 20–60 mL of Shohl's solution per day, given in three or four divided doses, provides an equivalent amount of alkali. If use of a sodium salt is contraindicated, potassium citrate may be used instead. One must keep in mind that the older patient with uric acid kidney stones may also have hypertension, congestive heart failure, or renal insufficiency and obviously should not be exposed to overload with alkalinizing sodium salts or unlimited fluid intake. Acetazolamide, a carbonic anhydrase inhibitor, produces rapid and effective urinary alkalinization and is sometimes used in conjunction with alkali therapy. When a 250-mg dose of acetazolamide is given at bedtime, the excretion of an acidic urine in the early morning hours is avoided. The usual tachyphylaxis (rapid tolerance) to this drug is obviated by the daily repletion dose of bicarbonate.

Since the advent of allopurinol, a low-purine, low-protein diet in the patient with uric acid lithiasis is no longer as critical as it once was; however, it is still advisable to instruct the patient to avoid foods rich in purine and to limit the protein to not more than 90 g/d. Such a diet is still palatable and reduces appreciably the amount of uric acid in the urine.

The drug of choice in recurrent uric acid lithiasis is allopurinol. It is effective in reducing both serum and urinary uric acid levels, thus preventing the formation of calculi. It is also recommended as prophylactic treatment in the patient who is going to receive cytotoxic agents for the treatment of lymphoma or leukemia. The marked increase in uric acid production associated with cytolysis of a neoplasm predisposes a patient to the development of uric acid nephrolithiasis.

### *Prophylactic Therapy*

After the first attack of acute gouty arthritis or after the passage of the first renal stone, a decision to institute prophylactic therapy must be entertained. If the first episode was mild and responded promptly to treatment, and if the patient's serum urate concentration was only minimally elevated or the 24-hour urinary uric acid excretion was not excessive (<700 mg/24 h), then prophylactic treatment can be withheld. Some patients never have a second attack or a second stone. Others may not experience a second gouty episode for 5 to 10 years. A wait-and-see attitude, therefore, seems justified in patients who meet the conditions described.

On the other hand, if the patient had a severe attack of gouty arthritis or a complicated course of uric acid lithiasis, or if the patient's serum uric acid was substantially elevated (>10.0 mg/dL) or the 24-hour urinary excretion of uric acid was excessive, then prophylactic treatment should be instituted immediately after resolution of the acute episode. Therapeutic intervention would also be appropriate for patients with frequent (i.e., more than two or three per year) attacks of gouty arthritis even if the serum uric acid concentration is normal or only minimally elevated.

Recurrences of acute gouty arthritis may be prevented with continuous colchicine therapy, a uricosuric agent, allopurinol, or combination therapy consisting of colchicine plus a uricosuric agent or allopurinol. The choice of treatment depends on the serum urate concentration, the amount of uric acid excreted in a 24-hour period, and the renal function status of the patient.[10]

Prophylactic therapy with low-dose oral colchicine, 0.5–0.6 mg twice daily, may be effective in preventing recurrent arthritis in patients with no evidence of visible tophi and a normal to slightly elevated serum urate concentration. Patients do not become tolerant of daily colchicine, and, if they sense the beginning of an acute attack, they should increase the dose to 1 mg every 2 hours; in most instances the attack will abort after 1 or 2 mg of colchicine. If the serum urate concentration is within the normal range, and the patient has been symptom free for a period of a year, maintenance colchicine may be discontinued. The patient should be advised, however, that discontinuation of the treatment program may be followed by an exacerbation of acute gouty arthritis.

Patients with a history of acute gouty arthritis and a significantly elevated serum uric acid concentration are probably best managed with antihyperuricemic therapy. Colchicine at a dose of 0.5 mg twice daily should be administered during the first 6 to 12 months of antihyperuricemic therapy to minimize the risk of acute attacks that may occur during reequilibration of serum to tissue urate concentration. The therapeutic objective of antihyperuricemic therapy is to reduce the serum urate concentration below 6 mg/dL, well below the saturation point.

Reduction of the serum urate concentration can be accomplished pharmacologically by increasing the renal excretion of uric acid or by decreasing its synthesis. The drugs most widely used to increase uric acid excretion are probenecid and sulfinpyrazone. Several other uricosuric drugs are being used in Europe, but they have not been approved for use in the United States.

### Uricosuric Drugs

Uricosuric drugs increase the renal clearance of uric acid by inhibiting the renal tubular reabsorption of uric acid. Therapy with uricosuric drugs should be started at a low dose to avoid marked uricosuria and possible stone formation. The maintenance of adequate urine flow and alkalinization of the urine with sodium bicarbonate or Shohl's solution during the first several days of uricosuric therapy further diminish the possibility of uric acid stone formation. Probenecid is given initially at a dose of 250 mg twice a day for 1 to 2 weeks, then 500 mg twice a day for 2 weeks. Thereafter, the daily dose is increased by 500-mg increments every 1 to 2 weeks until satisfactory control is achieved or a maximum dose of 3.0 g is reached. The initial dose of sulfinpyrazone is 50 mg twice a day for 3 to 4 days, then 100 mg twice a day, increasing the daily dose by 100-mg increments each week until the serum urate concentration is in the desired range.

The major side effects associated with uricosuric therapy are gastrointestinal irritation, rash and hypersensitivity, precipitation of acute gouty arthritis, and stone formation. These drugs are contraindicated in patients who are allergic to uricosuric agents and in patients with impaired renal function (i.e., creatinine clearance below 50 mL/min).

### Xanthine Oxidase Inhibitor

Currently, allopurinol is the only approved drug used for inhibiting uric acid synthesis.[11] Both allopurinol and its major metabolite, oxypurinol, are xanthine oxidase inhibitors, and thus impair the conversion of hypoxanthine to xanthine and xanthine to uric acid. Allopurinol also lowers the intracellular concentration of PRPP. Because of the long half-life of its metabolite, allopurinol can be given once daily. An oral daily dose of 300 mg is usually sufficient. Occasionally, as much as 600–800 mg/d may be necessary.

Allopurinol is the antihyperuricemic drug of choice in patients with a history of urinary stones or impaired renal function, in patients who have lymphoproliferative or myeloproliferative disorders and need pretreatment with a xanthine oxidase inhibitor before initiation of cytotoxic agents, and in patients who are overproducers of uric acid. The major side effects of allopourinol are skin rash, leukopenia, occasional gastrointestinal toxicity, and increased frequency of acute gouty attacks with the initiation of therapy.

### *Asymptomatic Hyperuricemia*

The management of asymptomatic hyperuricemia is controversial.[12] The purported benefits from treatment include prevention of acute gouty arthritis, tophi, nephrolithiasis, and gouty nephropathy. The first three complications are easily controlled should they develop; therefore, it is reasonable to withhold antihyperuricemic therapy in patients with only minimal degrees of hyperuricemia. Urate nephropathy, however, is an irreversible process even with appropriate therapy. Available data indicate that gouty nephropathy is extremely rare in the absence of articular gout, and evidence that elevation of uric acid by itself may cause renal disease is weak and inconclusive.[13]

As the risk of gouty arthritis or nephrolithiasis rises with increasing serum urate and urinary acid concentrations, antihyperuricemic therapy is appropriate at some point. The argument lies at what degree of hyperuricemia or urinary excretion of uric acid treatment should be instituted. Even though the answer is somewhat arbitrary, epidemiologic data show that patients with serum urate concentrations greater than 10 mg/dL have a greater than 50% chance of developing gouty arthritis, if this persists. This risk runs even higher in elderly patients. Moreover, it has been shown that the risk of nephrolithiasis is about 20% when urinary uric acid excretion is less than 700 mg/d, but 50% when the value exceeds 1,100 mg/d.

## Summary

Hyperuricemia may lead to acute arthritis, chronic gout, or kidney stones or remain asymptomatic. Asymptomatic hyperuricemia need not be treated, especially if the serum urate concentration remains below 10 mg/dL.

Acute gouty arthritis requires either colchicine or a nonsteroidal anti-inflammatory drug to treat the underlying inflammatory condition. The management of uric acid kidney stones includes hydration and alkalinization of the urine. Prevention of recurrent gouty arthritis or recurrent nephrolithiasis and treatment of chronic gout all require hypouricemic therapy with either a uricosuric drug or allopurinol. Allopurinol is the hypouricemic drug of choice in patients with a history of uric acid stones or renal insufficiency and in patients known to be overproducers of uric acid.

## References

1. Wyngaarden JB, Kelley WN. Gout and Hyperuricemia. New York, Grune and Stratton, 1976.
2. Wilson JM, Young AB, Kelley WN. Hypoxanthine–guanine phosphoribosyltransferase deficiency. N Engl J Med 1983;309:900–910.
3. Boss GR, Seegmiller JE. Hyperuricemia and gout: Classification, complications, and management. N Engl J Med 1979;300:1459–1468.
4. Yu T. Nephrolithiasis in patients with gout. Postgrad Med 1978;63:164–170.
5. Klineberg JR. Role of the kidneys in the pathogenesis of gout. Postgrad Med 1978;63:45–150.

6. Mangini RJ. Drug therapy reviews: Pathogenesis and clinical management of hyperuricemia and gout. Am J Hosp Pharm 1979;36:497–504.
7. Wisner DE, Simkin PA. Management of gout and hyperuricemia. Primary Care 1984;11:283–294.
8. Simkin PA. Management of gout. Ann Intern Med 1979;90: 812–816.
9. German DC, Holmes EW. Hyperuricemia and gout. Med Clin North Am 1986;70:419–436.
10. Edwards NL. The diagnosis and management of gouty arthritis. Compr Ther 1983;9(9):14–19.
11. Rundles RW. The development of allopurinol. Arch Intern Med 1985;145:1492–1503.
12. Liang MH, Fries JF. Asymptomatic hyperuricemia: The case for conservative management. Ann Intern Med 1978;88: 666–670.
13. Fessel WJ. Renal outcomes of gout and hyperuricemia. Am J Med 1979;67:74–82.

# Section Ten

# Disorders of the Eyes, Ears, Nose, and Throat

## Chapter 63 / Drug-Induced Ear and Eye Toxicity

Timothy S. Lesar, PharmD

A large number of medications have been identified as toxic to the ears or eyes. These adverse reactions vary from minor, reversible effects to serious, permanent impairment of hearing, vestibular function, or vision. Knowledge of the potential toxic effects of drugs and of methods limiting toxicity will minimize these adverse effects. The major drugs associated with ocular or ototoxic effects as well as characteristics of the toxic effects, risk factors, monitoring parameters, and management of adverse effects are reviewed in this chapter.

### Drug-Induced Ototoxicity

Toxic effects on the structures of the inner ear include temporary or permanent ototoxicity resulting from adverse effects on the cochlea, producing hearing loss, and/or the vestibular apparatus, producing vertigo, ataxia, lightheadedness, and other symptoms. The overall incidence of drug-induced ototoxicity is unknown; however, drug-induced deafness has been estimated to occur in 3 per 1,000 medical patients.[1]

#### *Manifestations and Risk Factors*

The primary symptoms of drug-induced ototoxicity are the cochlear signs of tinnitus and hearing loss and the vestibular signs of lightheadedness, nystagmus, ataxia, vertigo, and nausea and vomiting. Tinnitus is a subjective ringing, buzzing, ticking, clicking, screaming, or roaring noise. It may be quite distressing to patients, and in some cases may mask concomitant hearing loss. Drug-induced tinnitus may precede or occur concomitantly with hearing impairment, although several drugs produce tinnitus without hearing loss. Patients with drug-induced hearing impairment may notice muffling of speech, fullness of the ear, and hearing loss affecting selected or all frequencies depending on the responsible agent or severity of toxicity. Raising of the patient's voice may alert the clinician to possible hearing loss. Hearing ability is measured by audiometry. In pure-tone audiometry, the "threshold" of hearing pure tones at frequencies as low as 250 Hz is measured. The threshold is defined as the minimum effective sound pressure capable of evoking a hearing sensation 50% of the time. Hearing thresholds are measured in decibels (dB) with the level 0 dB defined as the normal hearing level in healthy young adults. A decrease of 10–20 dB in hearing is considered mild, 21–40 dB moderate, and more than 40 dB severe hearing loss. Hearing loss at frequencies of 500 to 3,000 Hz (speech range) will produce the most clinically noticeable deafness. Most patients do not detect or complain of hearing loss unless impairment exceeds 30 dB at frequencies less than 3,000–4,000 Hz; however, most humans can hear frequencies up to 20,000 Hz. Evaluation of drugs for ototoxicity typically involves audiograms performed at 250–8,000 Hz, with *ototoxicity* defined as an increase in auditory threshold of 15–20 dB. Drug-induced hearing loss at high frequencies may not be detected, thereby underestimating the true incidence of ototoxicity. It is important to detect subclinical hearing loss at high frequencies (>4,000 Hz) and less than 30 dB. Early, minor hearing loss may be reversible with dosage reduction or drug discontinuation, whereas more severe toxic effects may be irreversible. Minor degrees of impairment are caused by degeneration of sensory hair cells, and the subsequent use of ototoxic drugs may result in a similar minor degree of toxicity; however, because of the preexisting damage, the additional hearing loss may be clinically important. Clinicians should be aware of the ototoxic potential of medications and watch for hearing loss. Recommendations for audiometric monitoring of patients receiving ototoxic drugs involve the selection of high-risk patients, establishment of baseline hearing levels, serial audiometry during therapy, and audiometry tests after drug discontinuation. The clinical usefulness of audiometric monitoring is limited by the need for patient cooperation, the inability to perform sensitive testing, and the need to continue lifesaving medications despite toxic effects. The decision to alter drug therapy if a patient is experiencing ototoxicity should be based on careful assessment of the risk-to-benefit ratio.

When damage to the vestibular apparatus occurs, the patient may complain of lightheadedness, headache, giddiness, whirling sensations, a bouncing, spinning, or lurching of the room or objects, inability to focus or fixate on ocular images, nausea, vomiting, and cold sweats. These symptoms occur primarily when the patient is in motion. The patient may display nystagmus, ataxia, and unsteady gait and posture. The symptoms of vestibular toxicity tend to improve gradually with time because of increased reliance upon visual and proprioceptive inputs and central compensatory mechanisms for equilibrium. If these abilities are impaired, compensation does not occur and vestibular toxicity may severely disrupt the patient's ability to function.

Risk factors associated with an increased incidence of drug-induced ototoxicity include increased drug concentrations and/or prolonged exposure of the inner ear to the drug, concomitant use of more than one ototoxic drug, dehydration, fever, noise exposure, preexisting hearing loss, bacteremia, heredity, prior exposure to ototoxic agents, and possibly old age.[2–4]

Organ-specific drug toxicity such as ototoxicity may result from a unique susceptibility of the injured tissue to the drug, accumulation of the drug within the organ, or a combination of both factors. Inner ear injury may result from reversible inhibition of normal physiologic functions, such as endolymph formation, which if inhibited for prolonged periods of time results in degeneration of tissue dependent upon the particular physiologic function. Direct toxic effects on the sensory end organs (i.e., hair cells) also play a role in drug-induced toxicity.

## *Antimicrobial Agents*

### Aminoglycoside Antibiotics

Because of the frequency, severity, irreversibility, and cumulative effects of their toxicity, these drugs are among the most ototoxic of all drugs. All aminoglycosides are thought to produce ototoxicity, although the individual agents differ in severity, frequency, and site (cochlear versus vestibular) of damage. Aminoglycoside ototoxicity may occur after parenteral administration, aerosolization, oral use, topical use, wound or cavity irrigation, or possibly topical otic administration. Auditory toxicity (cochlear damage) usually occurs after 2 to 5 days or more of therapy, and may regress or progress after drug discontinuation. Tinnitus frequently precedes or coincides with the development of ototoxicity. The tinnitus is usually high pitched or ringing, possibly intermittent initially and subsequently becoming constant. Tinnitus may continue for several days to 2 weeks after discontinuation of therapy.[3,5–16] Hearing loss is typically bilateral and symmetric but may occur unilaterally, particularly with amikacin, kanamycin, and netilmicin.[3,5] Some reversible decrease in hearing may occur after single doses. High-frequency (>3,000–4,000 Hz) hearing loss is evident first, and loss may progress to all frequencies. Clinically, the patient may initially notice loss of sound discrimination ("muffled voices") rather than decreased sensitivity and complain of fullness of the ears.

The degree of hearing impairment ranges from minor loss of sensitivity or discrimination at high frequencies to complete deafness. Damage to the cochlea by aminoglycosides is thought to be irreversible; however, up to 50% of patients show partial or complete recovery of hearing within 2 weeks of drug discontinuation.[3,5]

Aminoglycoside-induced vestibular toxicity may occur with or without concomitant hearing loss, but is more likely to occur alone or concurrent with hearing loss during gentamicin, streptomycin, and tobramycin therapy (i.e., these are more vestibulotoxic) than with netilmicin, kanamycin, or amikacin therapy. Vestibular toxicity may initially present as headache, nausea and vomiting, trouble with ocular fixation or focus, giddiness, or lightheadedness. These symptoms may coexist with more severe vestibular symptoms such as vertigo, nystagmus, ataxia, and gait instability. Symptoms are minimal or absent when the patient is bedridden and are exacerbated upon sitting, standing, or eye closure. The vestibular symptoms may persist for 1 to 2 weeks, followed by 2 weeks to 2 months of adaption. During this period symptoms decrease, and may be present only when the patient ambulates, makes quick movements, or closes the eyelids. The compensation period may be lengthened or less complete in patients with visual impairment or proprioceptive deficits. After adaption to vestibular damage, symptoms usually occur only during eyelid closure.

The reported incidence of aminoglycoside ototoxicity ranges from 0.6% to 30% for auditory toxicity (usually defined as a loss of 15–20 dB at 250–8,000 Hz) and 0% to 75% for vestibular toxicity. The frequency reported depends on the drug, as well as study design and definition of ototoxicity. Neomycin is thought to be the most auditory (cochlear) toxic aminoglycoside and for this reason, as well as nephrotoxicity, is never administered parenterally; however, neomycin-induced ototoxicity has been reported after topical, aerosolized, intrawound, intracavitary, and oral administration. Vestibular toxicity from neomycin occurs less frequently. Streptomycin is the most vestibular toxic aminoglycoside, producing this adverse effect in 20% to 75% of patients depending on dose. Streptomycin is associated with a 4% to 15% incidence of hearing impairment. Of the commonly used parenteral aminoglycosides (kanamycin, gentamicin, tobramycin, amikacin, and netilmicin), clinical differences in ototoxic potential are less clearly defined. Gentamicin is more vestibulotoxic than cochleotoxic, whereas kanamycin, amikacin, and netilmicin are more cochleotoxic than vestibulotoxic; tobramycin is equally cochleotoxic and vestibulotoxic. Significant differences in ototoxic potential of aminoglycosides have been demonstrated in studies in animals; however, clinical studies demonstrate a similar incidence of auditory toxicity with gentamicin, amikacin, and tobramycin, whereas netilmicin has been reported to have similar or less auditory toxicity than the other aminoglycosides. The ranges of reported incidence of auditory toxicity for individual agents are 10% to 60% for kanamycin,[4] 2% to 24% for gentamicin, 0.4% to 22% for tobramycin, 3% to 24% for amikacin, and 0.5% to 10% for netilmicin. Most studies report an overall incidence of 3% to 10% for aminoglycoside toxicity; however, the risk for an individual patient depends on the presence of risk factors.[3,5,6,9]

Vestibular toxicity occurs most frequently with gentamicin (up to 15%), then tobramycin (up to 4.6%), and less commonly with amikacin and netilmicin (1.3%). Because of the lack of comparative trials, the true relative frequency of vestibular toxicity has not been well established.

The mechanism for the ototoxicity produced by aminoglycosides is most likely a combination of the drug accumulation in the perilymph and endolymph and the unique sensitivity of various cells within the inner ear to the toxic effects

**Table 63.1** Risk Factors Associated With Aminoglycoside Ototoxicity

| | |
|---|---|
| Total dose | Exposure to high-intensity noise |
| Total daily dose | Advanced age |
| Impaired renal function | Intrinsic ototoxic potential of drug |
| Multiorgan failure | Bacteremia |
| Concomitant ototoxic drug | Fever |
| Elevated serum concentrations | Dehydration |
| Prior aminoglycoside therapy | Advanced age ? |
| Hereditary susceptibility | Concomitant ear infection |

Complied from References 3, 4, 6, 8, 10, 11, 13, 14, 27, 46, and 47.

of these antibiotics. Aminoglycosides enter and leave the inner ear fluids slowly, resulting in accumulation of drug upon continued administration and prolonged persistence of drug upon discontinuation. The elimination half-life of aminoglycoside from perilymph is three to five times (10–15 hours) the serum elimination half-life in experimental animals. The pathologic findings in animals demonstrate that the earliest sign of aminoglycoside toxicity is degeneration of the outer hair cells of the organ of Corti at the basal turn of the cochlea. The site specificity of the damage at the basal turn corresponds with the clinical finding of early high-frequency hearing loss. With continued exposure to aminoglycosides, hair cell death progresses toward the apex of the cochlea (to affect lower frequency hearing). Eventually, inner hair cells, other organ of Corti cells, the stria vascularis, and Reissner's membrane may degenerate. After death of the hair cells, retrograde degeneration of the auditory nerve occurs. Vestibular toxicity is characterized by damage to hair cells of the crest of the crista in the ampulla of semicircular canals. The exact mechanism by which sensory hair cell damage occurs remains controversial, but may involve alteration of endolymph electrolyte composition, direct toxicity to the hair cells, or both. The site specificity of ototoxicity (cochlear versus vestibular) may result from differences in endolymph production mechanisms or in hair cell membrane lipid characteristics between the two sites.[3]

A large number of risk factors have been associated with the development of aminoglycoside ototoxicity (Table 63.1). Controlling serum concentrations of the aminoglycosides may minimize the incidence of ototoxicity, although the relationship between serum concentration and ototoxicity has not been well established. Serum concentrations should be monitored and dosage adjustments made to maintain "peak" (gentamicin, tobramycin, netilmicin $< 10–12\ \mu g/mL$; karamycin, amikacin $< 32\ \mu g/mL$) and "trough" (gentamicin, tobramycin, netilmicin $< 2\ \mu g/mL$; kanamycin, amikacin $< 10\ \mu g/mL$) concentrations within recommended ranges. Many patients exhibit ototoxicity despite appropriate serum concentrations because of the presence of the additional risk factors listed in Table 67.1.

The concurrent use of other ototoxic drugs, particularly loop diuretics, has been associated with increased ototoxicity. Ethacrynic acid appears to result in clinically significant increases in ototoxicity, whereas the increase in incidence is much less with furosemide and bumetanide[17]; however, diuretic-induced dehydration may potentiate aminoglycoside toxicity. High noise levels produce ototoxic lesions similar to those produced by aminoglycosides, and studies in animals suggest an additive effect. Previous aminoglycoside or other ototoxic drug therapy may produce subclinical toxicity, with subsequent courses of aminoglycoside producing clinically significant toxicity.[5]

The potential for ototoxicity should be considered in all patients receiving aminoglycosides. An assessment for the presence of risk factors should be performed. Serum concentrations should be monitored early in therapy and doses adjusted appropriately. Additional ototoxic agents should be avoided or used sparingly if possible. Symptoms indicating ototoxicity should be noted and follow-up audiometry or vestibular function tests used if appropriate. Fluid status should be monitored and dehydration avoided. Noise exposure should be kept to a minimum. If ototoxicity occurs, the drug should be discontinued, if possible, and replaced with a nonototoxic agent.

### Erythromycin

Cases of reversible erythromycin ototoxicity after oral, intravenous and intraperitoneal administration have been reported.[18] Both base and salt forms of erythromycin have been associated with ototoxicity, suggesting that any form of the drug may produce toxicity. Ototoxicity is characterized by a bilateral, sensorineural impairment (caused by nerve damage) of hearing at high frequencies. Tinnitus may be present and has been described as "blowing." Signs of vestibular toxicity may be present in some patients. Erythromycin ototoxicity is associated with the administration of large doses ($\geq 4$ g/d); however, smaller ($\geq 2$ g/d) daily doses may produce toxic effects in patients with impaired hepatic or renal function. Doses less than 2 g/d are not associated with toxic effects except when administered intraperitoneally to peritoneal dialysis patients. Ototoxicity usually occurs within 4 to 8 days of starting the ototoxic dose, and may occur as little as 12 hours to as long as 32 days after initiation of therapy. Onset of recovery from hearing loss may begin within 24 hours to 3 days, and complete recovery occurs 2 to 30 days after dose reduction or discontinuation. Risk factors include high dose ($\geq$ 2–4 g) combined with renal impairment, hepatic failure, intravenous administration, increased age, and possibly female sex. The mechanism of erythromycin ototoxicity is unknown. Cochlear hair cell damage has been demonstrated after instillation of erythromycin into the middle ear. The risk for erythromycin ototoxicity may be minimized by limiting doses to $\leq 2$ g/d in patients with renal or hepatic failure and those of extreme age.

**Vancomycin**

Auditory toxicity is the most important adverse neurotoxic effect of vancomycin.[19–22] Ototoxicity is characterized by initial high-frequency hearing loss and tinnitus, progressing to permanent impairment of hearing at all frequencies. Hearing loss may continue after drug discontinuation; however, hearing improvement does occur in some patients. Ototoxicity is thought to occur with increased frequency when peak serum concentrations exceed 45–60 $\mu$g/mL, and is rare at peak concentrations less than 30 $\mu$g/mL. The mechanism of vancomycin ototoxicity is unclear, as the drug is nontoxic in animal models, although vancomycin is reported to produce cochlear histologic changes similar to those produced by the aminoglycosides. Use of vancomycin concomitantly with other ototoxic agents or in patients with risk factors may increase the frequency of this adverse effect.

**Minocycline**

The tetracycline antibiotic minocycline is associated with a high frequency of reversible ototoxicity manifested by vestibular symptoms.[23,24] Common symptoms include dizziness, vertigo, ataxia, lightheadness, and a "spaced out" feeling frequently accompanied by nausea, vomiting, and tinnitus. The frequency, onset, and severity of vestibular toxicity appear to be related to dosage regimen and possibly female sex. Minocycline administered as 50 mg orally every 12 hours produces toxic effects in 11% to 14%, 75 mg every 12 hours in 53%, 100 mg every 12 hours in 60% to 77%, and with higher doses in up to 97%. The onset of symptoms occurs earlier (within 24 hours) with loading doses or high-dose regimens. Onset of symptoms occurs between 1 and 3 days in patients receiving 100 mg every 12 hours. Symptoms are often severe enough to require drug discontinuation or greatly impair daily activities in 5% to 52% of patients and appear to be dose related. The risk of developing vestibular side effects is two to three times higher for females than for males given the same dose. This sex difference may be related to the higher serum concentrations found in females compared with males administered the same dose. Patients prescribed minocycline should be informed of the vestibular effects and their impact on ability to perform tasks requiring motor coordination, such as driving. Because of the vestibular toxicity, minocycline is no longer considered the drug of choice for *Neisseria meningitidis* prophylaxis. Vestibular effects abate within 48 hours of discontinuation of minocycline in three fourths of affected patients; however, 15% may have symptoms persisting 72 hours or longer.

### *Antimalarial Agents*

Quinine and chloroquine have been associated with reversible and irreversible ototoxicity.[25] Quinine in small doses frequently produces tinnitus, and in therapeutic doses (>200–300 mg) it produces reversible hearing loss, tinnitus, and dizziness in 20% of patients. Severe sensorineural deafness may occur with prolonged therapy at high doses. Hearing loss typically affects lower frequencies. The mechanism by which quinine produces ototoxicity is unclear; however, cystic degeneration of the stria vascularis, degeneration of cochlear neurons, and loss of hair cells occur. Injury may be caused by spasm of cochlear blood vessels, producing anoxia and subsequent cellular damage. Chloroquine has also been associated with tinnitus, ataxia, and imbalance upon rapid head turning. Severe, irreversible sensorineural deafness has been reported with as little as 1 g. Deafness may develop or progress after drug discontinuation. Chloroquine has been shown to accumulate in the pigmented cells of the stria vascularis, producing cell death and disruption of endolymph production. Similar to quinine, chloroquine may produce cochlear vascular spasm. Hydroxychloroquine and primaquine are associated with tinnitus.

### *Nonsteroidal Anti-inflammatory Agents*

Salicylates and other nonsteroidal anti-inflammatory agents may produce reversible ototoxicity. Aspirin (and other salicylates) produces dose/concentration-related auditory toxicity. Tinnitus is characterized as a high-pitched ringing or hissing noise that frequently precedes and/or occurs concomitantly with hearing loss. Hearing loss may occur equally at all frequencies or predominantly at high frequencies. Deafness is typically bilateral and symmetrical; however, cases of unilateral hearing loss have been reported. Rare cases of vertigo have been reported with aspirin. The ototoxic effects of aspirin occur in 0.3% to 1.7% of patients. The frequency of toxicity is clearly dose/concentration-related, with daily doses above 2.7 g or concentrations above 25–30 mg/dL associated with increased incidence of ototoxicity. Doses above 4 g per day produce tinnitus in approximately 50% and hearing loss in 25% of patients. Ototoxicity has been reported after oral, intravenous, and topical salicylate administration.

Salicylate ototoxicity is reversible, with recovery occurring within 24 to 72 hours regardless of the degree of hearing loss. Rare cases of irreversible hearing loss have been reported with aspirin. The mechanism by which salicylates produce ototoxic symptoms is unclear as no inner ear morphologic changes have been demonstrated in studies in animals. A proposed mechanism is production of vasoconstriction of inner ear blood vessels resulting in tissue ischemia. Vasoconstriction results from inhibition of vasodilating prostaglandins.[26–29] Other nonsteroidal anti-inflammatory drugs (NSAIDs) have been associated with a lower incidence of similar ototoxic symptoms. Ibuprofen, naproxen, fenoprofen, phenylbutazone, sulindac, tolmetin, piroxicam, indomethacin, and diflunisal have been reported to produce ototoxic symptoms in 1% to 3% of patients. Indomethacin produces vertigo and/or dizziness in 3% to 9% of patients.[10]

### *Loop Diuretics*

The potent "loop" diuretics, ethacrynic acid, furosemide, and bumetanide, produce a similar dose-related ototoxicity, but differ in the individual frequency and severity. Ethacrynic acid is associated with significantly greater ototoxicity than furosemide and bumetanide. Ototoxicity usually manifests as a rapid onset of hearing loss (within minutes of a large rapidly administered intravenous dose), occasionally accompanied by tinnitus and symptoms of vestibular toxicity. Toxicity of ethacrynic acid may result from a cysteine adduct metabolite and is related to dose and rate of administration. Doses less than 200 mg/d intravenously and 400 mg/d orally are unlikely to cause ototoxicity. Hearing loss occurs typically at middle and high frequencies, although occasional loss of discrimination at all frequencies may occur. Hearing loss is usually reversible within 1 to 24 hours of drug discontinuation, although a number of cases of permanent hearing loss have been reported.

Furosemide produces similar ototoxic symptoms; however, the frequency and severity of toxicity are less. Like ethacrynic acid, rapid infusions of furosemide produce dramatic, reversible hearing loss. Large doses (>120 mg) administered at rates of 4 mg/min or less are unlikely to produce ototoxicity, whereas rates of 25 mg/min produce toxicity in 50%, and rates of 67 mg/min in 100% of patients.[30–32] The majority of cases of furosemide ototoxicity have occurred with doses greater than 240 mg, although doses as low as 40 mg have been associated with toxicity. Ototoxicity has been reported after oral administration of furosemide 160–800 mg/d. Most patients recover from furosemide ototoxicity within several hours of drug discontinuation; however, permanent hearing impairment does occur.

Bumetanide is five to six times more ototoxic than furosemide on a milligram-to-milligram basis; however, the diuretic potency of bumetanide is 40 times that of furosemide. Data in both animals and humans suggest that bumetanide produces two to seven times less ototoxicity than furosemide. Large clinical studies report that bumetanide produces ototoxicity effects in 1.1% to 1.7% of patients, whereas furosemide produces toxic effects in 3% to 6.5%.[31]

Loop diuretic–induced ototoxicity appears to result from inhibition of enzymes in the stria vascularis. This results in a loss of endocochlear potential because of reduction in the endolymph–perilymph potassium and sodium concentration differences and corresponds to the rapid onset and recovery of hearing loss encountered clinically. Morphologic changes in the organ of Corti and outer sensory hair cells have been demonstrated with ethacrynic acid, and the degeneration of hair cells corresponds to the permanent ototoxicity encountered clinically. Risk factors for development of loop diuretic ototoxicity include rapid infusion rate of large doses, large doses, renal failure, hepatic failure, cardiac failure, the specific diuretic administered, previous ototoxic drugs, and concomitant use of ototoxic agents.[30–32]

### *Antitumor Agents: Cisplatin*

Cisplatin, a potent antineoplastic agent, produces a high incidence of ototoxicity. The primary manifestation of cisplatin ototoxicity is hearing loss,[33] although vestibular toxicity has also been reported. The hearing loss produced by cisplatin occurs in 30% to 70% of patients receiving 50–100 mg/m$^2$. Hearing frequencies above 2,000–3,000 Hz (usually 4,000–8,000) are most commonly affected. Hearing loss is usually bilateral (less commonly unilateral) and symmetrical and caused by degeneration of the outer hair cells of the organ of Corti. Hearing loss tends to occur early in therapy (after one or two treatments) and may occur suddenly. Tinnitus frequently accompanies hearing loss and occurs intermittently, but is not predictive of impending ototoxicity. Ototoxicity may be more frequent in children and older patients and those with preexisting hearing loss. Other chemotherapeutic agents including bleomycin, dactinomycin, mechlorethamine, vincristine, and cytarabine have been reported to cause hearing loss and tinnitus. Methotrexate has been reported to produce tinnitus.

### *Topically Applied Drugs*

Several drugs may be ototoxic when applied to the middle ear (or into the external auditory canal in patients with perforated tympanic membranes).[8,16] Studies in animals have demonstrated the ototoxic effects of topically applied aminoglycosides, chloramphenicol, polymyxin, erythromycin, and tetracycline. Use of these antimicrobials in patients with otitis media with perforated tympanic membrane or during ear surgery may result in ototoxicity. Drugs diffuse readily from the middle ear to the inner ear through the round window membrane. Other ototoxic compounds include lidocaine and the antiseptic chlorhexidine. For these reasons, ototopical medications must be used carefully during ear surgery or in patients with perforated tympanic membranes.

### *Other Medications*

Several other medications are associated with ototoxicity. A complete listing is beyond the scope of this chapter and comprehensive listings are suggested.[34–37] Commonly used medications and associated ototoxic effects are listed in Table 63.2.

## Drug-Induced Oculotoxicity

Drugs administered both systemically and nonsystemically may produce adverse effects on the eye and surrounding tissues. Comprehensive compilations of drugs producing ocular toxicity are available.[38–40] Adverse effects of drugs may involve external ocular functions and structures—oculomotor function, eyelids, lacrimation, conjunctiva, and cornea—or internal structures—trabecular meshwork, ciliary body, iris, lens, retina, and optic nerve. This section reviews the major types of drug-induced ocular toxicity and discusses the medications most commonly associated with specific adverse effects. Nonspecific alterations of visual functions as an extension of pharmacologic effects are not addressed and the reader is referred to comprehensive texts available.

### *External Ocular Structures*

#### Oculomotor Function

Alteration of the control of external ocular muscles produces oculomotor dysfunction and results in nystagmus, oculogyric crisis, strabismus, and ocular weakness and paralysis. The external ocular muscles are innervated by cranial nerves III, IV, and VI and serve to place an object on the fovea rapidly, maintain the object near the fovea, maintain eye position with respect to changes in head and body movement, align visual axis to maintain bifoveal fixation, and maintain eye position with respect to target. The drugs most commonly associated with oculomotor dysfunction are the

**Table 63.2** Ototoxic Drugs

| *Drug* | *Comment* |
|---|---|
| Antimicrobials | |
| Aminoglycoside | See text |
| Antimalarials | See text |
| Ampicillin | Reversible hearing loss |
| Capreomycin | Reversible hearing loss, tinnitus |
| Chloramphenicol | Reversible hearing loss |
| Clindamycin | Tinnitus |
| Colistin | Hearing loss |
| Cotrimoxazole | Reversible hearing loss |
| Doxycycline | Tinnitus |
| Erythromycin | See text |
| Furazolidone | Hearing loss, tinnitus |
| Metronidazole | Tinnitus |
| Minocycline | See text |
| Paromomycin | Auditory/vestibular toxicity |
| Polymyxin B | Reversible hearing loss |
| Rifampin | Reversible hearing loss |
| Sulfonamides | Tinnitus and vertigo |
| Tetracycline | Tinnitus |
| Thiabendazole | Tinnitus |
| Vancomycin | See text |
| Salicylates and NSAIDs | See text |
| Loop diuretics | See text |
| Antitumor agents | See text |
| Miscellaneous | |
| Aminophylline | Tinnitus |
| Antihistamines | Tinnitus |
| Caffeine | Tinnitus |
| Carbamazepine | Tinnitus |
| Contraceptive steroids | Reversible hearing loss |
| Deferoxamine | Permanent hearing loss |
| Diazoxide | Reversible hearing loss |
| Haloperidol | Tinnitus |
| Levodopa | Tinnitus |
| Lidocaine | Tinnitus, ototoxic with topical use |
| Metaproterenol | Tinnitus |
| Molindone | Tinnitus |
| Monoamine oxidase inhibitors | Tinnitus |
| Morphine | Tinnitus |
| Penicillamine | Tinnitus |
| Pentazocine | Tinnitus |
| Propranolol | Tinnitus |
| Propoxyphene | Hearing loss, tinnitus |
| Propylthiouracil | Hearing loss, tinnitus |
| Quinidine | Reversible hearing loss, tinnitus, vertigo |
| Tricyclic antidepressants | Hearing loss, tinnitus |
| Verapamil | Tinnitus |

anticonvulsants (e.g., phenytoin and phenobarbital), which produce broken pursuit movements and nystagmus, and the antipsychotic drugs (phenothiazines and butyrophenones), which produce oculogyric crisis. Nalidixic acid, corticosteroids, ethanol, and vincristine may produce cranial nerve palsies. Complete listings of medications associated with altered oculomotor dysfunction are available[38,39] (see Table 63.3).

**Lacrimation**

The tear film serves a number of purposes in maintaining ocular function. Tears maintain an optically uniform corneal surface, provide a mechanism for flushing debris from the eye, act as lubricants, provide nutrition to the corneal epithelium, and provide an antibacterial function. The tear film consists of three layers: the superficial oily layer, the

**Table 63.3** Drug-Induced Oculotoxic Effects

| *Drug* | *Adverse ocular effects* |
|---|---|
| Anti-inflammatory agents | |
| Corticosteroids | Glaucoma, cataracts, pseudotumor cerebri, exophthalmos, ptosis, chemosis |
| Cyclosporine | Decreased visual acuity |
| Gold salts, auranofin | Conjunctivitis, corneal deposits |
| Ibuprofen | Blurred vision, color vision disturbance, optic neuritis (all rare) |
| Indomethacin | Corneal deposits, retinopathy (both rare) |
| Ketoprofen | Pseudotumor cerebri |
| Phenylbutazone | Conjunctivitis, blurred vision, corneal deposits |
| Piroxicam | Burning eyes, blurred vision |
| Salicylates | Conjunctivitis |
| Antimicrobial agents | |
| Amiodaquine | Corneal deposits, retinopathy |
| Clofazamine | Conjunctival deposits, corneal deposits, pigmentary retinopathy |
| Chloramphenicol | Optic neuritis |
| Chloroquine/hydroxychloroquine | Conjunctival deposits, corneal deposits, pigmentary retinopathy |
| Diethylcarbamazine | Ocular inflammation |
| Ethambutol | Optic neuritis, retinal changes |
| Gentamicin | Pseudotumor cerebri |
| Griseofulvin | Corneal deposits, pseudotumor cerebri |
| Isoniazid | Optic neuritis |
| Minocycline | Conjunctival deposits |
| Nalidixic acid | Altered color vision, visual disturbance, optic neuritis, pseudotumor cerebri |
| Nitrofurantoin | Extraocular muscle paralysis, pseudotumor cerebri |
| Quinine | Retinal ischemia (in overdose) |
| Rifampin | Keratoconjunctivitis |
| Streptomycin | Nystagmus |
| Sulfonamides | Conjunctivitis, optic atrophy |
| Suramin | Keratoconjunctivitis, optic atrophy |
| Tetracycline | Conjunctival pigmentation, pseudotumor cerebri |
| Vaccinations | Optic atrophy |
| Antineoplastic agents | |
| BCNU/CCNU/methyl-CCNU | Optic neuritis, optic atrophy, retinopathy |
| Busulfan | Keratoconjunctivitis sicca, cataracts |
| Carmustine | Retinopathy, retinal infarcts/hemorrhage |
| Chlorambucil | Keratitis, retinal hemorrhage, papilledema, cataracts |
| Cisplatin | Retinopathy, optic neuritis, papilledema |
| Cyclophosphamide | Keratoconjunctivitis sicca, blurred vision |
| Cytosine arabinoside | Corneal opacities, keratoconjunctivitis |
| Doxorubicin | Lacrimation, conjunctivitis |
| 5-Fluorouracil | Lacrimation, keratoconjunctivitis, tear duct fibrosis |
| Methotrexate | Conjunctivitis |
| Mitotane | Cataracts, retinopathy |
| Nitrogen mustard | Uveitis |
| Procarbazine | Nystagmus, diplopia, retinal hemorrhage, papilledema |
| Tamoxifen | Corneal opacity, retinopathy (only at high dose) |
| Vinca alkaloids | Diplopia, optic neuropathy |
| Cardiovascular agents | |
| Amiodarone | Corneal opacities, transient blurred vision with large doses, retinal toxicity |
| Diazoxide | Lacrimation |
| Digitalis glycoside | Blurred vision, halos around objects, color vision disturbance |
| Ergot alkaloids | Central retinal artery occlusion |
| Guanethidine | Conjunctival hyperemia, ptosis |
| Metoprolol | Dry eyes |
| Minoxidil | Optic neuritis |

**Table 63.3** Drug-Induced Oculotoxic Effects (continued)

| *Drug* | *Adverse ocular effects* |
|---|---|
| Nifedipine | Transient retinal ischemia |
| Propranolol | Dry eyes, conjunctivitis, inflammatory pseudotumor |
| Quinidine | Dry eyes, keratopathy, blurred vision, corneal deposits, retinopathy |
| Reserpine | Conjunctival hyperemia |
| Central nervous system | |
| Amantadine | Transient blurred vision |
| Barbiturates | Nystagmus, ptosis |
| Bromocriptine | Myopia |
| Carbamazepine | Nystagmus, cataracts |
| Ethchlorvynol | Optic neuritis |
| Lithium | Blurred vision |
| Narcotic analgesics | Miosis |
| Phenothiazine | Conjunctival deposits, corneal deposits, cataracts, retinopathy, oculogyric crisis |
| Protriptyline | Rare corneal deposits |
| Phenytoin | Nystagmus, cataracts, ptosis |
| Trimethadione | Glare, photophobia, blurred vision, altered color vision |
| Miscellaneous agents | |
| Allopurinol | Cataracts |
| Clomiphene | Blurred vision |
| Contraceptives (oral) | Occlusion of retinal vasculature, retinal edema, optic neuritis, corneal edema |
| Dantrolene | Lacrimation |
| Deferoxamine | Cataracts, optic neuritis, retinopathy |
| Disulfiram | Optic neuritis |
| Isotretinoin | Conjunctivitis, dry eyes, corneal opacities, myopia, optic neuritis |
| Penicillamine | Rare retinopathy, ocular myasthenia gravis |
| Thiazide diuretics | Myopia, decreased tear production |
| Diphenhydramine | Filamentary keratitis, myopia |

aqueous layer, and the mucoid layer. Medications have been associated with both hyposecretion and hypersecretion of tears[35–37] (Table 63.3).

Secretion of tears by the lacrimal gland is under parasympathetic control, and drugs with anticholinergic properties are the most frequent cause of decreased tear secretion. Sedative–hypnotic (e.g., barbiturates) drugs reduce tear production when ingested for a prolonged period.[41,42] Thiazide diuretics may produce decreased tear secretion. Busulfan has been reported to produce a dry-eye syndrome with an extreme decrease in tear production.[43] Drug-induced hypersecretion of tears is most commonly produced by cholinergic drugs or is secondary to external ocular irritation caused by drug secretion into the tears. The increased tear production associated with doxorubicin, methotrexate, and 5-fluorouracil (5-FU) appears to result from ocular irritation.[43–45] Increased tearing is frequently associated with drug-induced conjunctival and corneal inflammation and irritation (see below). After severe inflammation, as might occur in the Stevens–Johnson syndrome, scarring of the conjunctiva may result in a dry eye from damage to tear component–producing cells and glands.

### Conjunctiva and Cornea

The major drug-induced toxic effects involving the conjunctiva and cornea are inflammation of the conjunctiva (conjunctivitis), cornea (keratitis), or both (keratoconjunctivitis) and formation of deposits in the conjunctiva and/or the cornea.

Inflammation of the conjunctiva and/or cornea may be a result of drug hypersensitivity or a direct toxic effect.[46] External ocular inflammation (secondary to drug hypersensitivity) may be a local reaction or part of a systemic hypersensitivity reaction. Severe inflammation of the eyelids, conjunctiva, and cornea, as occurs in the Stevens–Johnson syndrome, may result in symblepharon (adhesions between the bulbar and palpebral conjunctiva) and subsequently corneal scarring.

Commonly used medications associated with allergic conjunctivitis and keratoconjunctivitis include chloral hydrate, sulfa drugs, phenytoin, allopurinol, salicylates and other nonsteroidal anti-inflammatory agents, and quinidine.[38–40,41,46] Nonallergic inflammation of the conjunctiva and/or cornea results from a direct irritant or toxic effect on the involved tissues. Severe conjunctivitis and keratitis may be produced by antineoplastic agents (e.g., doxorubicin, cytarabine, busulfan, cyclophosphamide, 5-fluorouracil, and methotrexate) as a result of the secretion of the antineoplastics into the tears.[44,45–48] Isotretinoin produces or exacerbates preexisting blepharoconjunctivitis in approximately 40% to 50% of patients. The blepharoconjunctivitis is dose related and may be transient, improving without dose reduction.[44,49] Auranofin and injectable gold salts produce conjunctivitis in 3% to 10% of patients and may rarely produce corneal ulcers.[50] Other systemic medications have been associated with external ocular inflammation, although rarely.[38] Almost any topical ophthalmic medication may produce inflammation of either the allergic or the nonallergic type. Systemic and topical medications must be considered as possible etiologies in patients presenting with external ocular inflammation.[39]

Prolonged therapy with certain medications may result in the formation of deposits or opacities within the conjunctiva or cornea. Conjunctival deposits have been reported after prolonged therapy (>10 years) with tetracyclines for acne vulgaris.[50] These deposits are located in conjunctival cysts and range from unpigmented to black in color. Topical epinephrine may produce similar brown to black conjunctival deposits as a result of collections of adrenochrome within the conjunctiva, primarily within the light-exposed palpebral fissure.[38] Long-term, high-dose therapy with a phenothiazine, particularly chlorpromazine, may produce a brownish discoloration of the conjunctiva.[51,52] Such changes may be caused by the photosensitizing actions of chlorpromazine, resulting in protein complexation and denaturization or deposition of chlorpromazine derivatives followed by excess melanin production. Phenothiazine conjunctival discoloration occurs in patients with concomitant marked corneal and lens deposits. Clearing of the conjunctival pigmentation occurs once chlorpromazine is discontinued.

Other medications have been associated with conjunctival deposits or discoloration, including amiodarone, gold salts, iron supplements, quinoline derivatives, and penicillamine.[38,39] The conjunctival deposit/discoloration is usually of minimal clinical significance other than for cosmetic reasons.

Drug-induced corneal deposits are also of minimal clinical importance as the deposits are usually reversible and rarely cause intolerable symptoms. The quinoline antimalarial agents, for example, chloroquine and hydroxychloroquine (less commonly amiodaquine and quinacrine), produce dose-related corneal deposits.[38,39,41,53,54] The deposits, which form a whorllike pattern, are usually gray to golden in color when found in the superficial corneal epithelium and may be more yellowish when found in the stroma. Corneal deposits may appear within weeks to months of initiation of therapy at doses greater than 250 mg per day chloroquine or 400 mg hydroxychloroquine. At these doses, 30% to 70% of patients will develop opacities, whereas the incidence is only 0% to 4% at lower doses unless used for prolonged periods of time.[55] Symptoms produced by corneal deposits include decreased corneal sensation, blurred vision, glare, and photophobia; however, these symptoms are seldom intolerable and infrequently require drug discontinuation. The corneal deposits that develop in response to the quinolines is unrelated to the retinopathy associated with these agents.[53]

Amiodarone causes corneal deposits similar to those produced by chloroquine.[38,56] The development of amiodarone-induced cornea verticillata is dose and duration related. At doses less than 200 mg/d, only minor or no deposits develop. At doses above 400 mg/d over 90% of patients develop deposits. At doses of 400 mg or greater, deposits develop within 10 days in some patients and by 1 to 2 months in almost all patients. The deposits are clinically indistinguishable from those produced by chloroquine. The deposits develop to a point and do not progress despite continued constant administration, and produce symptoms in only 4% to 6% of patients. The major patient complaints are blurred vision, glare, photophobia, and halos around lights. Like chloroquine, corneal deposits result from deposition of drug–phospholipid complexes. The drug apparently reaches the cornea primarily by secretion into the tears. Use of artificial tears has been reported to decrease the incidence/severity of the deposits, probably as a result of drug dilution. The lack of deposits in children is most likely due to the more rapid tear turnover rate in this population. The corneal deposits typically clear 3 to 12 months after drug discontinuation, disappearing slowly at first and then more rapidly. Unlike chloroquine, severe retinopathy appears to rarely occur with amiodarone.

Chlorpromazine produces two types of corneal deposit: (1) cornea verticillata, similar to that produced by chloroquine and amiodarone; and (2) a fine, diffuse, brownish granular deposit. The cornea verticillata occurs only with prolonged use of high doses (>2,000 mg/d) and is similar to that described with chloroquine. The mechanism of chlorpromazine-induced cornea verticillata is assumed to be identical to that for the disease induced by chloroquine and amiodarone. The diffuse granular deposits produced by chlorpromazine are throught to be similar to those found in the conjunctiva, being located primarily within the palpebral fissure. The incidence of corneal deposits has been associated with the total dose of chlorpromazine administered. In patients receiving less than 0.5 kg total dose, deposits are rare, whereas patients receiving greater than 1–2.5 kg demonstrate higher frequencies of corneal deposits. Others have suggested that daily dosage rate rather than total dose is important, with doses less than 300 mg/d rarely producing deposits. Corneal deposits are rarely seen in patients without chlorpromazine-induced lens deposits (see below). Corneal deposits occur in 20% to 50% of patients with lens deposits. The corneal deposits rarely cause clinical symptoms and are frequently reversible upon drug discontinuation. Other antipsychotics (e.g., loxapine, dibenzoxazepine, trifluoperazine, fluphenazine, prochlorperazine, chlorprothixine, perphenazine, thiothixene, and possibly thioridazine) have occasionally been associated with corneal deposits.[57,58]

Other medications associated with the development of corneal opacities include indomethacin, gold salts, iron salts, vitamin D, cytarabine, isotretinoin, phenylbutazone, protriptyline, tamoxifen, silver protein (argyrol), vinblastine, and quinidine.[38,39,49,59,60]

### *Internal Ocular Structures*

Medications may alter the function of or be toxic to internal structures of the eye, resulting in drug-induced glaucoma (see Chapter 64), cataracts, retinopathy, and optic neuritis. Unlike the adverse effects on the external ocular structures, adverse effects on internal structures may produce significant irreversible impairment of vision.

#### Lens

Other than reversible changes in accommodation caused by ciliary body constriction/relaxation, the major adverse drug effects on the lens are cataracts (lens opacities) and myopia. Commonly used medications that produce cataracts with significant frequency include the phenothiazines, corticosteroids, and topical parasympathomimetic agents used in the treatment of glaucoma.

Cataracts caused by phenothiazines, like the conjunctival and corneal deposits, are most common with chlorpromazine. The mechanism of phenothiazine-induced cataracts is thought to be a photosensitivity reaction similar to that which produces the conjunctival and corneal deposits. The incidence of chlorpromazine-induced cataracts is greater than that of corneal or conjunctival deposits and is dose and duration related. Fifty percent of patients given a total dose of 0.5 kg and 90% of patients given a total dose of 2.5 kg demonstrate deposits. Deposits are rare with doses less than 0.5 kg. Dosage rate also appears to play an important role, with higher rates (>2 g/d) producing deposits within months of initiation of therapy and rates less than 300 mg/d infrequently producing cataracts unless therapy is prolonged. Lenticular opacities almost universally appear prior to corneal and conjunctival deposits. Phenothiazine-induced cataracts rarely produce symptoms and are typically slowly reversible upon drug discontinuation or switching to an alternative antipsychotic.

Corticosteroids administered systemically or topically to the eye have been identified as cataractogenic.[61–64] Cataracts have not been clearly demonstrated after topical skin application, but considering the systemic absorption from the skin, such patients should be considered at risk.

The cataracts are usually bilateral and symmetric, although 10% of patients may demonstrate asymmetric opacities. The reported incidence of cataracts in patients receiving corticosteroid therapy ranges from 5% to 96%. Dose and duration were previously thought to be closely related to incidence of cataracts, but there appears now to be no relation between dosage rate, total dose, duration of therapy, or age of patient and cataracts, and development of cataracts appears to be a function of individual susceptibility. Corticosteroid-induced cataracts rarely produce symptoms; however, cataracts requiring removal have been reported in up to 9%. Alterations of lens capsule permeability, decreased lens ATPase, altered lens electrolyte concentrations, decreased aqueous humor potassium and ascorbic acid, and increased aqueous humor pH are possible etiologies of corticosteroid cataracts. Lens opacities produced by corticosteroids are thought to be largely irreversible; however, cases of progression after discontinuation and regression (primarily in children) during therapy and after discontinuation have been reported. Other commonly used medications associated with cataracts are listed in Table 63.3.

Myopia has been reported to occur during therapy with a number of medications.[38,39] The primary mechanisms include ciliary muscle contraction, producing accommodation, and hydration of the lens, increasing the refractive power. Parasympathomimetics and narcotics produce myopia because of ciliary muscle contraction. Drugs that produce myopia as a result of lens hydration include corticosteroids; tetracyclines; bromocriptine; sulfonamide antibiotics; sulfa derivatives such as thiazide diuretics, spironolactone, and acetazolamide; and antihistamines. Myopia is typically transient, disappearing with discontinuation or, in many cases, with continued dosing.

**Retina and Optic Nerve**

Toxic effects on the sensory retina and optic nerve are the most important organ-specific adverse effects of drugs on the eye. These effects may impair vision significantly and occasionally are irreversible. Monitoring for drug-induced retinal and optic nerve toxicity is essential for early recognition. Commonly used medications producing significant retinal toxicity include the phenothiazines, quinoline antimalarials, antineoplastic agents, and deferoxamine.

The phenothiazine antipsychotic thioridazine produces a toxic pigmentary retinopathy. The development of retinopathy is clearly dose dependent, with doses above 800–1,200 mg/d associated with a high frequency of retinopathy.[38,40,65,66] Doses less than 800 mg/d are generally considered safe; however, cases of retinopathy have occurred with doses less than 800 mg/d. Symptoms of toxic retinopathy often occur within 2 weeks to 3 months of initiation of high-dose thioridazine. Patients may complain of blurred vision, brown-colored vision, or other abnormalities of color vision, decreased night vision, and scotomas (blind spots) around the area of central vision. Some patients may retain normal central visual acuity. These early symptoms may be associated with retinal edema or optic disk hyperemia, or the fundus may appear normal. Within weeks to months, funduscopic evaluation may detect diffuse, fine, deep retinal pigment deposits in the pole posterior to the equator of the globe. The macula may be spared in some cases. With continued therapy, the pigment granules begin to coalesce and may form plaques of pigment. Eventually, multiple large areas of depigmentation appear associated with atrophy of the retinal pigment epithelium, choriocapillaris, and retina. Retinal arteriole attenuation may occur. Vision testing will demonstrate normal to decreased central acuity, constricted visual field and paracentral scotomas, and altered color vision. Thioridazine produces retinopathy after binding to the melanin of the retinal pigmented epithelium (RPE) and choroid, inhibiting oxidative phosphorylation within the retina and producing outer rod segment degeneration. Cellular debris from rod degeneration accumulates, producing the characteristic pigmentary changes in the retina. Upon discontinuation of thioridazine, visual acuity, night vision, and color vision generally improve; however, some patients show no improvement in vision and even progression of retinopathy. Early pigmentary changes generally clear with discontinuation; however, later changes may be permanent. All patients starting on high-dose, long-term thioridazine therapy should have an ophthalmologic exam and be routinely examined for vision and funduscopic changes. Patients complaining of blurred vision, altered color vision, decreased night vision, or blind spots must be carefully examined. If retinopathy occurs, thioridazine should be discontinued and an alternative drug chosen. Chlorpromazine has been rarely associated with the development of retinal pigmentation. Doses of 800–2,400 mg/d for approximately 2 years are required to produce retinopathy. The chlorpromazine-induced retinopathy is less severe than that produced by thioridazine and is reversible upon drug discontinuation.

The quinoline antimalarial agents, chloroquine and hydroxychloroquine, produce a dose-dependent toxic retinopathy.[67,68] Although most cases of toxicity have been reported with chloroquine, hydroxychloroquine is thought to be equally toxic. Daily doses less than 250 mg chloroquine or 400 mg hydroxychloroquine are only rarely (<5%) associated with the development of retinal damage. Larger doses produce retinopathy in up to 15% of patients continuing therapy for more than 1 year and may be more toxic in patients with systemic lupus erythematosus. Older studies suggested that total dosage consumption was important; however, recent data suggest that the dosage rate is the most important determinant of risk, with daily doses of chloroquine less than 4.5 mg/kg and of hydroxychloroquine less than 6.5 mg/kg only rarely associated with toxicity.[68] Retinopathy produced by quinoline derivatives is unrelated to the development of corneal deposits. Early changes are similar to retinal changes seen with age and are difficult to identify without a baseline evaluation. Symptoms are frequently absent at this stage, or the patient may complain of blurred vision. With continued chloroquine use, the classic retinal findings of increased macula granular pigmentation surrounded by alternating concentric rings of hypo- and hyperpigmented retinal epithelium (''bull's-eye retinopathy'') develop. At this stage, symptoms of blurred vision, reading difficulties with missing words or letters (caused by paracentral scotomas), photophobia, decreased night vision, flashes or streaks of light, large visual field defects, and altered color vision are present. Symptoms do not always parallel the retinal findings. Advanced retinopathy is characterized by a generalized retinopathy; disruption of the retinal pigmented epithelium, attenuated retinal arterioles, optic disk pallor, and severe visual impairment may occur. Retinopathy is thought to occur as a result of the binding of chloroquine to the melanin of the retinal pigmented epithelium and the choroid, decreasing retinal protection from toxic free radicals and resulting in injury and death of inner retinal cell layers (rods and cones).

Early retinal toxicity with absent or minimal symptoms is usually reversible with drug discontinuation; however, when the bull's-eye lesion and significant symptoms are present, retinopathy remains stable when the drug is stopped, although some improvement in vision may occur. Occasionally, retinopathy may progress despite drug discontinuation; such ''progressive'' retinopathy is more likely to occur when more severe retinal damage has occurred during therapy. Rare cases of retinopathy appearing and progressing after drug discontinuation have been reported. Because of the irreversible nature of all but early retinopathy, close monitoring for ocular toxicity is required during chloroquine therapy. A baseline exam is mandatory, with follow-up monitoring every 4 to 6 months during therapy. Useful monitoring parameters include ophthalmoscopic exam, visual fields with white and red targets, visual acuity, and retinal electrophysiologic studies. Chloroquine and hydroxychloroquine retinopathy may be limited by administering doses less than 4.5 mg/kg/d (chloroquine) or 6.5 mg/kg/d (hydroxychloroquine), a careful, conscientious monitoring program, and discontinuation at first signs of retinopathy. Drug holidays during the summer months and use of dark sunglasses to decrease sun exposure may be of value in limiting toxic effects. Infrequent cases of retinal abnormalities after therapy with amiodaquine, quinine, mepacrine, and quinacrine have also been reported.[53–55]

Retinal toxicity occurs with the use of a number of other medications. Long-term use of oral contraceptives has been rarely associated with retinal abnormalities including retinal vein occlusion, retinal arteriole occlusion, retinal hemorrhage, altered macula function, abnormal color vision, and possible accelerated progression of retinitis pigmentosa.[69] Deferoxamine therapy for hemosiderosis has been associated with the development of pigmentary retinopathy after administration of 12–96 g of deferoxamine over 4 to 17 days. Symptoms of blurred vision and color vision abnormalities occurred concomitantly with the bilateral retinopathy. After drug discontinuation, some regression of retinopathy occurred; however, baseline vision was not regained.[70] Prolonged high-dose (>240 mg/d) tamoxifen therapy has been reported to produce a retinopathy characterized by fine, white refractile retinal opacities, cystoid macular edema, and occasional depigmentation of retinal pigmented epithelium.[71] The calcium channel blocker nifedipine may produce transient retinal ischemia, purportedly because of a ''steal'' phenomenon with resultant transient decreased acuity and visual field defects.[72] Cardiac glycoside toxicity frequently produces disturbance of vision (particularly color vision) because of inhibition of Na–K ATPase in the sensory retina cells. Prolonged cardiac glycoside therapy may rarely produce irreversible retinopathy.[73] Other medications associated with retinopathy are listed in Table 63.3.

### Optic Nerve and Visual Tracts

Adverse effects of drugs on the optic nerve and visual tracts include optic neuropathy, optic atrophy, and papilledema. Optic neuropathy, an inflammation of the optic nerve, produces symptoms including blurred vision, scotomas, constricted visual fields, altered color vision, and occasionally edema or hyperemia of the optic disk. Ethambutol produces a dose-dependent optic neuropathy (either axial or periaxial) after 1 to 3 months of therapy.[38,39,41,74,75] Axial (or central) neuropathy is more common than periaxial neuropathy and is characterized by decreased visual acuity, central scotomata, and disturbance of red–green color vision. Subtle swelling of the optic disk and splinter hemorrhages may be present when symptoms occur suddenly. Periaxial optic neuropathy is characterized by the presence of paracentral scotomata without significant decreases in visual function or color vision disturbance. The incidence of optic neuropathy is rare (0.8%–1.7%) at doses of 15 mg/kg/d or less; however, doses greater than 25 and 50 mg/kg/d produce optic neuritis in 5% and 10%, respectively. Optic neuropathy may be preceded by peripheral neuropathy. The mechanism of toxicity is thought to be an ethambutol metabolite–induced chelation and subsequent decrease in zinc content of the retina and optic nerve. Ethambutol-induced optic neuropathy is generally reversible within 3 months of drug discontinuation; more severely affected patients recover more slowly. Some experts recommend administration of 100–250 mg zinc sulfate three times daily in patients with optic neuropathy. Patients failing to recover after drug discontinuation may show regression of visual loss when given high-dose hydroxycobalamin (40 mg/d). Continued therapy with ethambutol in patients with optic neuropathy may produce optic atrophy and irreversible visual loss. All patients receiving ethambutol should undergo baseline visual exam, including visual acuity, visual field, and color vision tests. Patients should be warned of possible ocular toxicity and should be counseled to immediately report decreased visual acuity, trouble in reading, blind spots, and abnormal color vision. Patients receiving doses greater than 15 mg/kg/d should undergo visual examinations monthly.

Isoniazid also produces optic neuropathy, particularly in malnourished patients, and presents with symptoms similar to those seen with ethambutol. The optic neuropathy usually responds to therapy with pyridoxine. Deferoxamine produces a bilateral optic neuropathy with symptoms similar to those observed with ethambutol. The mechanism of toxic optic neuropathy may be similar to that of ethambutol-induced disease, with chelation and a subsequent decrease in retinal zinc and/or copper.[74] Deferoxamine-induced optic neuropathy may occur within 4 days to 3 months. Long-term or high-dose therapy with chloramphenicol is associated with optic neuropathy when total doses exceed 75–100 g.[76] Optic neuropathy with chloramphenicol is characterized by sudden decrease in visual acuity, halos around objects, scotomata, altered color vision, and orbital pain with onset of neuropathy. A funduscopic exam may demonstrate papilledema, disk hyperemia, flame hemorrhage, and exudates. Discontinuation of chloramphenicol produces total regression of symptoms. Continuation of therapy may result in optic nerve atrophy. Other agents reported to produce optic neuropathy or optic atrophy include minoxidil, propoxyphene (in overdose), carmustine, vincristine, cisplatin, ethchlorvynol, sulfonylurea hypoglycemics and other sulfa derivatives, barbiturates, and possibly oral contraceptives and isotretinoin. Optic neuropathy has also been reported after vaccination for measles/mumps/rubella, influenza, and swine flu.

Papilledema, or swelling of the optic disk secondary to a benign increase in intracranial pressure (pseudotumor cerebri), may be produced by a number of medications. The primary symptoms are headache and enlarged blind spot, with swelling of the optic disk upon funduscopy. Drugs associated with papilledema include corticosteroids (also corticosteroid withdrawal), tetracyclines, oral contraceptives, isotretinoin, aminoglycosides, and nalidixic acid. Drug discontinuation commonly results in regression of all symptoms; however, total or partial visual loss may occur in some patients.

## Summary

Adverse drug reactions involving the ears and eyes are relatively uncommon; however, because of the delicate and complicated structure and function of these organs, significant irreversible damage may be produced when toxicity occurs. Awareness of potential ototoxic and oculotoxic drugs as well as of factors increasing the risk of toxicity allows the clinician to minimize the frequency and consequences of toxicity.

## References


1. The Boston Collaborative Surveillance Program. Drug-induced deafness. JAMA 1973;224:515–516.
2. Brown RD, Feldman AM. Pharmacology of hearing and ototoxicity. Annu Rev Pharmacol Toxicol 1978;18:233–252.
3. Bendush CL. Ototoxicity: Clinical considerations and comparative information, in Whelton A, Neu HC (eds): The Aminoglycosides. Microbiology, Clinical Use and Toxicology. New York, Marcel Dekker, 1982.
4. Bergstrom L, Thompson PL. Ototoxicity, in Northern JL (ed): Hearing Disorders, 2nd ed. Boston, Little Brown, 1984, pp 253–266.
5. Moore RD, Smith CR, Lietman PS. Risk factors for the development of auditory toxicity in patients receiving aminoglycosides. J Infect Dis 1984;149:23–30.
6. Fee WE. Aminoglycoside ototoxicity in the human. Laryngoscope 1980;90(suppl 24):1–9.
7. Garrison L, Dutro M. Ototoxicity from topical neomycin. (Lett) Clin Pharm 1982;1:301.
8. Mittelman H. Ototoxicity of "ototopical" antibiotics: Past, present and future. Trans Am Acad Ophthalmol Otol 1972;76: 1432–1441.
9. Matz GJ, Lerner SA. Prospective studies of aminoglycoside ototoxicity in adults, in Lerner SA, Matz GJ, Hawkins JE (eds): Aminoglycoside Ototoxicity. Boston, Little Brown, 1981.
10. Brummett RE. Drug induced ototoxicity. Drugs 1980;19:412–428.
11. Marlow FI. Ototoxic agents. Otolaryngol Clin North Am 1978; 11:791–800.
12. Hybels RL. Drug toxicity of the inner ear. Med Clin North Am 1979;63:309–319.
13. Snavely SR, Hodges GR. The neurotoxicity of antibacterial agents. Ann Intern Med 1984;101:92–104.
14. Quick CA. Chemical and drug effects on the inner ear, in Parella MM, Shumrick DA (eds): Otolaryngology, 2nd ed. Philadelphia, W.B. Saunders, 1980, vol 2.
15. Wersall J. Recent otological evaluation of aminoglycoside antibiotics. J Antimicrob Chemother 1984;13(suppl A):31–36.
16. Stupp H, Kupper K, Lagler F, et al. Inner ear concentrations and ototoxicity of different antibiotics in local and systemic administration. Audiology 1973;12:350–363.
17. Smith CR, Leitman PS. Effect of furosemide on aminoglycoside-induced nephrotoxicity and auditory toxicity in humans. Antimicrob Agents Chemother 1983;23:133–137.
18. Haydon RC, Thelin JW, Davis WE. Erythromycin ototoxicity: Analysis and conclusions based on 22 case reports. Otolaryngol Head Neck Surg 1984;92:678–684.
19. Traber PG, Levine DP. Vancomycin ototoxicity in a patient with normal renal function. Ann Intern Med 1981;95:458–460.
20. McHenry MC, Gavan TL. Vancomycin. Pediatr Clin North Am 1983;30:31–47.
21. Farber BF, Moellering RC. Retrospective study of the preparations of vancomycin from 1974 to 1981. Antimicrob Agents Chemother 1984;23:138–141.
22. Ajodhia JM, Dix MR. Drug induced deafness and its treatment. Practitioner 1976;216:561–570.
23. Gump DW, Ashikaga T, Fink T, et al. Side effects of minocycline: Different dosage regimens. Antimicrob Agents Chemother 1977;12:642–646.
24. Drew TM, Altman R, Black K, et al. Minocycline for prophy

laxis of infection in *Neisseria meningitidis*: High rate of side effects in recipients. J Infect Dis 1976;133:194–198.

25. Dwivedi GS, Mehra YN. Ototoxicity of chloroquine phosphate. A case report. J Laryngol Otol 1978;92:701–703.
26. Shinn AF. Drugs and ototoxicity. US Pharmacist 1978;May: 54–64.
27. Porter J, Jick H. Drug induced anaphylaxis, convulsions, deafness and extrapyramidal symptoms. Lancet 1977;1:587–588.
28. Miller RR, Jick H. Acute toxicity of aspirin in hospitalized medical patients. Am J Med Sci 1977;274:271–279.
29. Miller RR. Deafness due to plain and long acting aspirin tablets. J Clin Pharmacol 1978;18:468–471.
30. Gallhager KL, Jones JR. Furosemide induced ototoxicity. Ann Intern Med 1979;91:744–745.
31. Tuzel IH. Comparison of adverse reactions to bumetanide and furosemide. J Clin Pharmacol 1981;21:615–619.
32. Brummett RE, Bendrick T, Himes D. Comparative ototoxicity of bumetanide and furosemide when used in combination with kanamycin. J Clin Pharmacol 1981;21:628–636.
33. Morosu MJ, Blair R. A review of cisplatin ototoxicity. J Otolaryngol 1983;12:365–369.
34. Davies DM. Drug induced deafness. Adv Drug React Bull 1978;69:244–277.
35. Worthington EL, Lunin LF, Heath M, et al. Index-Handbook of Ototoxic Agents, 1966–1971. Baltimore, Johns Hopkins University, 1973.
36. Drucker T. Drugs that can cause tinnitus. ATA Newslett 1979; 4:3–5.
37. Miller JJ. Handbook of Ototoxicity. Boca Raton, FL, CRC Press, 1980.
38. Fraunfelder FT, Meyer SM. Drug Induced Ocular Side Effects and Drug Interactions, 2nd ed. Philadelphia, Lea and Febiger, 1982.
39. Grant WM. Toxicity of the eye, 3rd ed. Springfield IL, Charles C Thomas, 1986.
40. Anonymous. Adverse ocular effects of systemic drugs. Med Let 1976;18:63–64.
41. Spiteri MA, James DG. Adverse ocular reactions to drugs. Postgrad Med J 1983;59:343–349.
42. Miller D. Systemic medications. Int Ophthalmol Clin 1981; 21:177–183.
43. Fraunfelder FT, Meyer M. Ocular toxicity of antineoplastic agents. Ophthalmology 1983;90:1–3.
44. Sugar J. Ocular side effects of systemic therapy of cutaneous diseases. Int Ophthalmol Clin 1985;21:173–183.
45. Vizel M, Oster MW. Ocular side effects of cancer chemotherapy. Cancer 1982;49:1999–2002.
46. Perry HD. Drugs and toxins. Int Ophthalmol Clin 1982; 18:97–108.
47. Griffen JD, Garnick MB. Eye toxicity of cancer chemotherapy: A review of the literature. Cancer 1981;48:1539–1549.
48. Ritch PS, Hansen RM, Hever OK. Ocular toxicity from high dose cytosine arabinoside. Cancer 1983;51:430–432.
49. Fraunfelder FT, LaBraico JM, Meyer SM. Adverse ocular reactions possibly associated with isotretinoin. Am J Ophthalmol 1985;100:534–537.
50. Messmer E, Font RL, Sheldon G, et al. Pigmented conjunctival cysts following tetracycline/minocycline therapy. Ophthalmology 1983;90:1462–1468.
51. Gowdey CW, Coleman LM, Crawford EM. Ocular changes and phenothiazine derivatives in long-term residents of a mental retardation center. Psych J Univ Ottawa 1985;10:248–253.
52. Bond WS, Yee GC. Ocular and cutaneous effects of chronic phenothiazine therapy. Am J Hosp Pharm 1980;37:74–78.
53. Portnoy JZ, Callen JP. Ophthalmologic aspects of chloroquine and hydroxy-chloroquine therapy. Int J Dermatol 1983;22: 273–278.
54. Zeuhlke RL, Lillis PJ, Tice A. Antimalarial therapy for lupus erythematosus: An apparent advantage of quinacrine. Int J Dermatol 1981;20:57–61.
55. Tobin DR, Kruhel GB, Rynes RI. Hydroxychloroquine. Seven-year experience. Arch Ophthalmol 1982;100:81–83.
56. Ingram DV, Jaggarao NSV, Chamberlain DA. Ocular changes resulting from therapy with amiodarone. Br J Ophthalmol 1982;66:676–679.
57. Gaultieri T, Lefler H, Guimond et al. Corneal and lenticular opacities in mentally retarded young adults treated with thioridazine and chlorpromazine. Am J Psychiatry 1982;139:1178–1180.
58. Rasmussen K, Kirk L, Faurby A. Deposits in the lens and cornea of the eye during long term chlorpromazine medication. Acta Psychiatr Scand 1980;53:1–4.
59. Bron AJ, McLendon BF, Camp AV. Epithelial deposition of gold in the cornea in patients receiving systemic therapy. Am J Ophthalmol 1979;88:354–360.
60. Beck M, Mills PV. Ocular assessment of patients treated with tamoxifen. Cancer Treat Rep 1979;63:1833–1834.
61. Lien EJ, Koda RT. Structure–side effect sorting of drugs: V. Glaucoma and cataracts associated with drugs. Drug Intell Clin Pharm 1981;15:434–439.
62. Havener WH. Ocular Pharmacology, 5th ed. St. Louis, C.V. Mosby, 1983.
63. Santamaria J. Steroidal agents: Their systemic and ocular complications. Ocular Inflammation Ther 1983;1:19–26.
64. Sammartino JP. Ocular toxicity of systemic drugs. Am Fam Physician 1985;31:226–229.
65. Fishman GA. Toxic retinopathies. Contemp Ophthalmol 1980;1:1–5.
66. Ball WA, Caroff SN. Retinopathy, tardive dyskinesia, and low dose thioridazine. Am J Psychiatry 1986;143:256–257.
67. Olansky AJ. Antimalarials and ophthalmologic safety. Am Acad Dermatol 1982;6:19–23.
68. Marks JS. Chloroquine retinopathy: Is there a safe daily dose? Ann Rheum Dis 1982;41:52–58.
69. Petursson GS, Fraunfelder FT, Meyer M. Oral contraceptives. Ophthalmology 1981;88:368–371.
70. Lakhanpal V, Shocket SS, Jiji R. Deferoxamine (Desferal) induced toxic retinal pigmentary degeneration and presumed optic neuropathy. Ophthalmology 1984;91:443–451.
71. Kaiser-Kupfer M, Kupfer C. Rodrigues MM. Tamoxifen retinopathy. A clinicopathologic report. Ophthalmology 1981;88: 89–93.
72. Pitlik S, Manor R, Lipshitz I, et al. Transient retinal ischemia induced by nifedipine. Br Med J 1983;287:1845–1846.
73. Weleber RG, Shults WT. Digoxin retinal toxicity. Clinical and electrophysiologic evaluation of cone dysfunction syndrome. Arch Ophthalmol 1981;99:1568–1572.
74. Dukes MNG (ed): Meyler's Side Effects of Drugs, 10th ed. New York, Elsevier, 1984.
75. Karmon G, Savir H, Zevin D, et al. Bilateral optic neuropathy due to combined ethambutol and isoniazid therapy. Ann Ophthalmol 1979;11:1013–1017.
76. Godel V, Nemet P, Lazar M. Chloramphenicol optic neuropathy. Arch Ophthalmol 1980;98:1417–1421.

# Chapter 64 / Glaucoma

Timothy S. Lesar, PharmD

Glaucoma is a group of ocular diseases characterized by increased intraocular pressure (IOP), optic nerve atrophy, optic disk changes, and loss of visual field. Two major types of glaucoma have been identified: open angle and closed angle. Either type may be a primary, inherited disorder; secondary to disease, trauma, or drugs; or congenital. Glaucoma occurs in 0.5% to 1.5% of the population over the age of 40 and is responsible for 12% to 15% of the blindness in the United States. In this chapter, the pathophysiology, clinical findings, and drug therapy of glaucoma are reviewed.

See Figure 64.1 for a diagram of the eye.

In glaucoma, the optic disk changes and retinal nerve fiber damage result from the increased IOP. Susceptibility to visual loss at a given IOP varies considerably; some patients do not demonstrate damage at high IOPs, whereas other patients have progressive visual field loss despite an IOP in the "normal" range. Although IOP poorly predicts which patients will have visual field loss, an IOP greater than 21 mm Hg is considered "suspicious." The mean "normal" IOP as measured by applanation tonometry is $15.5 \pm 2.5$ mm Hg,[1] with a non-Gaussian frequency distribution with skewness to higher IOPs. Intraocular pressures consistently greater than 21 mm Hg are found in 5% to 7% of the general population. The incidence increases with age such that abnormal IOP is found in 15% of those 70 to 75 years old. Intermittently very high IOP is found in patients with angle-closure glaucoma.

Glaucoma is classified as primary, secondary, or congenital (Table 64.1). Primary glaucomas are genetically determined disorders and may be open angle or closed angle. Secondary glaucomas are also either open angle or closed angle but result from trauma, disease (both ocular and systemic), or pharmacologic agents. Both primary and secondary glaucomas may be caused by a combination of open-angle and closed-angle mechanisms.

## Aqueous Humor and Intraocular Pressure

Constant inflow of aqueous humor from the ciliary body (Fig. 64.2) and resistance to outflow result in an intraocular pressure great enough to produce an outflow rate equal to the inflow rate. Despite considerable research, the physiologic and pharmacologic controls of aqueous inflow and outflow and, therefore, of IOP have not been completely defined. Aqueous humor is formed in the ciliary body through both ultrafiltration and secretion. Fluid pressure gradients produce an ultrafiltrate of the blood in the stroma of the ciliary process. Because ultrafiltration depends upon pressure gradients, blood pressure and IOP changes influence aqueous formation. Osmotic gradients produced by active secretion of sodium and bicarbonate, and possibly other solutes such as ascorbate, into the aqueous humor result in movement of water from the pool of stromal ultrafiltrate into the posterior chamber, forming the aqueous humor. Carbonic anhydrase appears to be involved in the secretion of such solutes, explaining the IOP-lowering effects of carbonic anhydrase inhibitors such as acetazolamide.[1–5] Receptor systems controlling aqueous outflow have not been fully elucidated but pharmacologic studies suggest that β-adrenergic agents increase inflow[6] whereas α-adrenergic,[7,8] α-adrenergic blocking,[7] β-adrenergic blocking,[3,6] dopamine blocking,[9] and adenylate cyclase stimulating[10] agents decrease aqueous inflow. Aqueous humor produced by the ciliary body is secreted into the posterior chamber at a rate of approximately 2 μL/min.[4] The pressure in the posterior chamber produced by the constant inflow pushes the aqueous humor between the iris and lens and through the pupil into the anterior chamber of the eye (Fig. 64.3).

Aqueous humor in the anterior chamber leaves the eye by two routes: (1) filtration through the trabecular meshwork to Schlemm's canal and (2) traversal of the anterior face of the iris and absorption into iris blood vessels (uveoscleral outflow). Outflow via the trabecular meshwork accounts for drainage from the eye of 1.5–1.8 μL aqueous humor per minute. Uveoscleral outflow occurs at a rate of 0.2–0.5 μL/min. Cholinergic agents such as pilocarpine increase outflow by physically pulling open the meshwork pores through ciliary muscle contraction. The outflow of aqueous is increased by β-adrenergic agonists such as epinephrine and albuterol.[11] The net effect of β-adrenergic agents is a decrease in IOP. Cholinergic agents such as pilocarpine may decrease uveoscleral outflow[12]; however, the net effect of cholinergic agents is a decrease in IOP. The increased IOP in open-angle glaucoma results from the decreased facility for aqueous outflow through the trabecular meshwork.

The balance between the inflow and outflow of aqueous humor in the eye determines the intraocular pressure (Fig. 64.3). The intraocular pressure is measured by tonometry—either indentation tonometry, applanation tonometry, or a noncontact method using an air pulse. The noncontact applanation tonometer measures the pressure required to flatten the cornea with a steadily increasing stream of air. These methods may result in slightly different pressure readings. The average intraocular pressure measured in large populations is $15.5 + 2.5$ mm Hg; however, the distribution of pressures around the mean is skewed to the right (toward higher readings).[13] Intraocular pressure is not constant and changes with pulse, blood pressure, forced expiration or coughing, neck compression, and posture. Intraocular pressure demonstrates considerable circadian variation, primar-

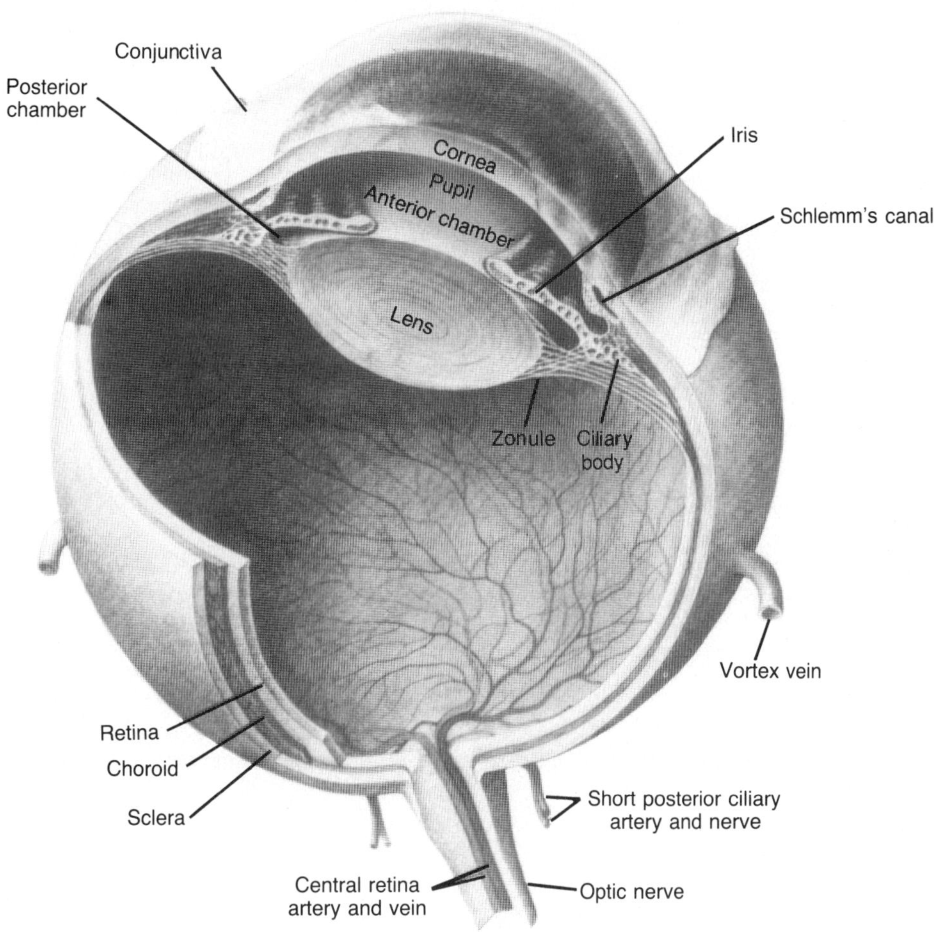


**Figure 64.1** The human eye. *(From Newel FW. Ophthalmology: Principles and Concepts, 5th ed. St. Louis, C.V. Mosby, 1982, with permission.)*

ily because of changes in the rate of aqueous formation.[13] This circadian variation results in a minimum IOP at approximately 6 PM and a maximum IOP at awakening. The circadian IOP variation is usually less than 3–4 mm Hg; however, it may be greater in patients with glaucoma.[1] This circadian variation makes single measurements of IOP by tonometry a poor screening test for glaucoma.[14]

**Table 64.1** Classification of Glaucoma

I. Primary glaucoma
   A. Open angle
   B. Angle closure
      1. With pupillary block
      2. Without pupillary block
II. Secondary glaucoma
   A. Open angle
      1. Pretrabecular
      2. Trabecular
      3. Posttrabecular
   B. Angle closure
      1. With pupillary block
      2. Without pupillary block
III. Congenital glaucoma

Approximately 0.5% to 1% per year of individuals with IOP between 21 and 30 mm Hg develop optic disk changes and visual field loss (i.e., glaucoma) over 5 to 15 years.[15] Recent data suggest that more subtle retinal damage, such as alteration of color vision, decreased contrast sensitivity, and peripheral acuity, occurs in a higher percentage of patients with IOP greater than 21 mm Hg.[16] The incidence of visual field defects increases to as high as 28% in individuals with IOP above 30 mm Hg.[17] For a given abnormal IOP, the incidence of glaucoma increases with age.[18] In patients with preexisting optic nerve damage, the worse the existing damage, the more sensitive the eye is to a given IOP.[19] About 25% to 30% of patients with glaucomatous visual field loss have an IOP less than 21 mm Hg.[20] Thus, the IOP is a poor predictor of optic nerve damage.

Additional clinical findings in glaucoma include optic nerve damage (reflected in changes of the optic disk) and loss of visual field. The *optic disk* is the portion of the optic nerve ophthalmoscopically visible as it leaves the eye. The small

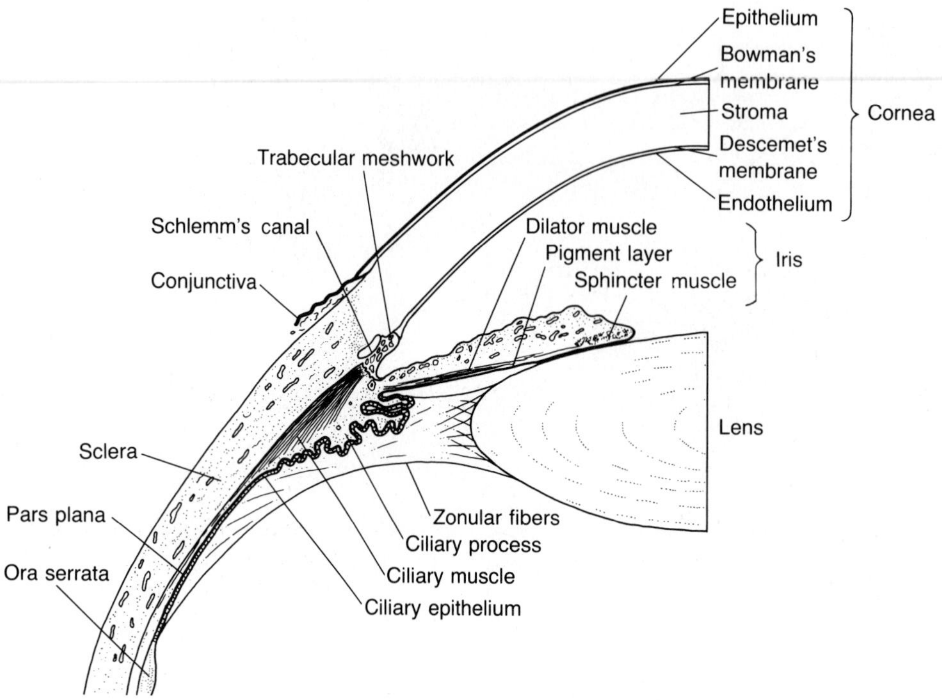


**Figure 64.2** The anterior chamber angle and surrounding structures. *(From Vaughn D, Asbury T. General Ophthalmology, 10th ed. Los Altos, CA, Lange Medical Publications, 1983, with permission.)*

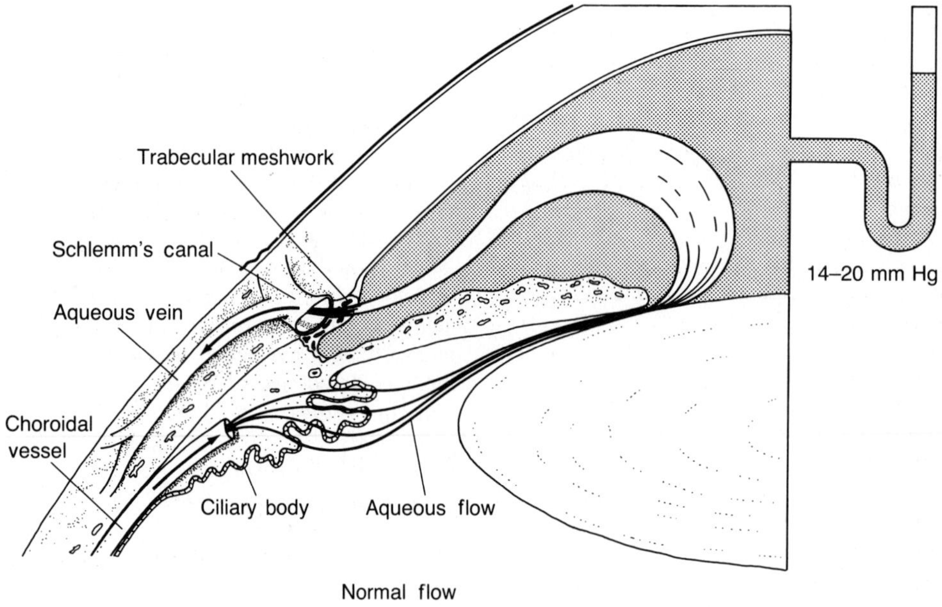


**Figure 64.3** Cross section of anterior segment of the eye, demonstrating aqueous humor formation and flow and outflow pathways. *(From Kolker A, Hetherington S. Becker-Shaffer's Diagnosis and Therapy of the Glaucomas, 5th ed. St. Louis, C.V. Mosby, 1983, with permission.)*

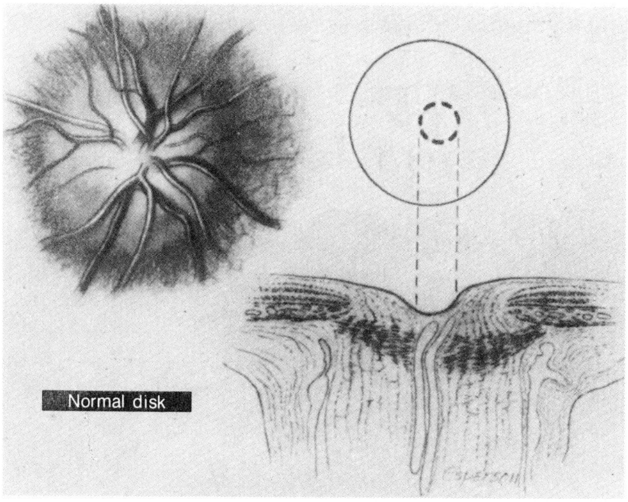


**Figure 64.4** The normal optic disk and cup. *(From Kolker A, Hetherington S. Becker-Shaffer's Diagnosis and Therapy of the Glaucomas, 5th ed. St. Louis, C.V. Mosby, 1983, with permission.)*

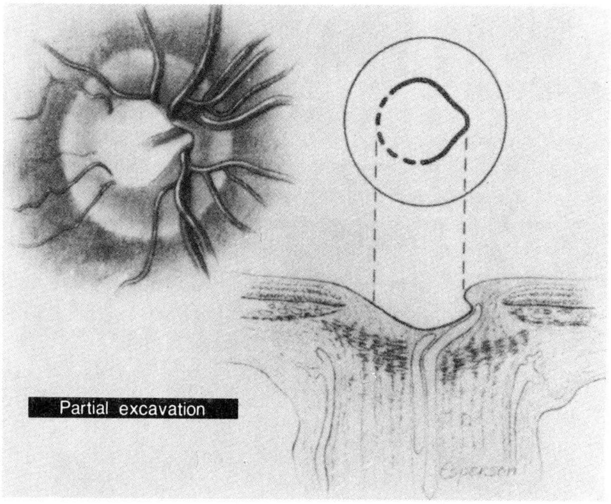


**Figure 64.5** Early optic disk and cup changes in glaucoma. *(From Kolker A, Hetherington S. Becker-Shaffer's Diagnosis and Therapy of the Glaucomas, 5th ed. St. Louis, C.V. Mosby, 1983, with permission.)*

depression within the disk is termed the *cup* (Fig. 64.4). A normal physiologic cup does not extend below the retinal surface and has a diameter less than one third that of the disk (cup:disk ratio less than 0.33). The common alterations of the optic disk found in glaucoma are listed in Table 64.2 (Fig. 64.5). These disk changes result from optic nerve degeneration and increased IOP on the disk structures.[1–3]

Determination of visual field allows assessment of optic nerve damage and is a primary monitoring parameter in treatment. The peripheral visual field is measured using a perimeter. Characteristic visual field loss occurs in glaucoma (Table 64.3), but loss of central visual acuity does not occur until late in the disease. Therefore, IOP, optic disk changes, and perimetry are the primary diagnostic and monitoring parameters.[1,2,18]

**Table 64.2** Optic and Visual Field Findings in Glaucoma

| |
|---|
| Optic disk findings |
| Cup:disk ratio greater than 0.5 |
| Progressive increase in cup size |
| Cup:disk ratio asymmetry greater than 0.2 |
| Vertical elongation of the cup |
| Excavation of the cup |
| Deepening of the cup |
| Increased exposure of lamina cribrosa |
| Pallor of the cup |
| Splinter hemorrhages |
| Cupping to edge of disk |
| Notching of the cup (usually superior or inferior) |
| Visual field defects in glaucoma |
| General peripheral visual field constriction |
| Isolated scotomas (blind spots) |
| Nasal visual field depression (nasal step) |
| Enlargement of the blind spot |
| Large arclike scotomas |

The mechanism by which increased IOP produces optic nerve damage remains controversial.[18,21,22] The vasogenic theory suggests that optic nerve damage results from insufficient blood flow to the retina secondary to the high perfusion pressure required in the eye with high IOP. The insufficient blood flow produces degeneration of axonal (axoplasmal) fibers of the retina. A second theory suggests that the increased IOP may disrupt axoplasmal flow directly or by "arching" of the lamina cribrosa. Both mech-

**Table 64.3** Considerations in Treating Ocular Hypertension

| |
|---|
| Risk factors |
| IOP over 30 mm Hg |
| Suspicious optic disk findings |
| Family history of glaucoma |
| Systemic vascular disease |
| Increased age (over 65–70) |
| Asymmetric cups |
| High myopia |
| Optic disk hemorrhages |
| Increasing IOP over time |
| Retinal nerve fiber defects |
| Diabetes mellitus |
| Black patients |
| Patient characteristics |
| One-eyed patients |
| Young patients (longer exposure to high IOP) |
| Unreliable patients |
| Unreliable visual fields |
| Optic disk not visualized |
| Patient desires treatment |
| Patient with retinal vascular occlusion |

anisms could be operative in producing the optic nerve damage observed in glaucoma. The classic disk enlargement of glaucoma results from axon degeneration.

## Primary Open-Angle Glaucoma

Primary open-angle glaucoma (POAG) is a bilateral, genetically determined disorder constituting 60% to 70% of all glaucomas and 90% to 95% of primary glaucomas.[2,18] POAG manifests as an increased IOP that results in optic nerve degeneration characterized by disk changes and visual field loss (Table 64.2). POAG is a chronic, slowly progressive disease found primarily in individuals older than 50, although it may occur earlier.[18] Symptoms do not present until significant visual field constriction occurs. Central visual acuity is typically maintained, even in the late stages of the disease.[1] POAG is a bilateral disease; however, one eye may have higher IOP and greater progression of disease than the other. Detection and diagnosis involves measurement of the IOP, measurement of facility of outflow, evaluation of the optic disk, and assessment of the visual fields. Elevated IOP (greater than 21 mm Hg) without disk changes or visual field loss with increased IOP is observed in 5% to 7% of individuals and is known as ocular hypertension or "glaucoma suspect." The presence of disk changes or field loss with increased IOP confirms the diagnosis of glaucoma. Typical disk changes and field loss may be found at an IOP less than 21 mm Hg (i.e., "low-tension" glaucoma).

The basic, underlying disorder of POAG is a decreased outflow facility, resulting in an imbalance between aqueous production and aqueous outflow. The flow of aqueous from the posterior chamber to the trabecular meshwork is normal; however, histologic changes in the meshwork or Schlemm's canal in glaucomatous eyes appear to produce an increase in resistance to aqueous outflow.

Secondary open-angle glaucoma has many causes including systemic diseases, trauma, surgery, rubeosis, lens changes, ocular inflammatory diseases, and medications. A system for classifying secondary glaucomas into pretrabecular, trabecular, and posttrabecular forms has been proposed.[23] This classification allows drug therapy to be chosen on the basis of the pathogenic mechanism involved. In pretrabecular forms, a membrane overlies the meshwork and does not allow aqueous to flow out. The membrane may be fibrovascular, such as neovascular growth in diabetics, fibrous ingrowth, or the result of inflammation. Trabecular forms of secondary glaucoma result from either an alteration of meshwork or an accumulation of material in the intertrabecular spaces. This type of glaucoma may result from accumulation of cells, pigment or protein in the trabeculum, or alteration of the meshwork secondary to trauma, corticosteroids, edema, inflammation, and trauma. The posttrabecular forms result primarily from disorders causing increased episcleral venous blood pressure. Examples of such conditions include Sturge–Weber syndrome, retrobulbar tumors, and carotid-cavernous fistulas.

### *Treatment*

All patients with increased IOP demonstrating optic disk changes or visual field defects (i.e., glaucoma by definition) should be treated. Treatment of the patient with ocular hypertension remains controversial, as only 0.5% to 1% per year develop visual field loss. Treatment of ocular hypertension in these patients is based on the presence or absence of risk factors known to increase the chance of developing visual field loss and on the presence of certain individual traits (Table 64.3). Persons with ocular hypertension with additional risk factors usually require a topical agent such as pilocarpine, carbachol, epinephrine, dipivefrin, or a β-blocker.[24] Therapy is initiated in one eye to assess efficacy and tolerance. The frequent side effects of anticholinesterase inhibitors and carbonic anhydrase inhibitors result in an unfavorable risk:benefit ratio in the ocular hypertension patient and are rarely indicated.[16,18,25,26] The goal of therapy is to lower the IOP to a level associated with a decreased risk of optic nerve damage. Drug therapy should be monitored by regular measurement of IOP, examination of the optic disk, assessment of the visual fields, and evaluation of the patient for drug side effects. Patients who are unresponsive to or intolerant of a drug should be switched to an alternative agent rather than given an additional drug. Patients failing to respond adequately to simple topical therapy may require multiple drugs, cholinesterase inhibitors, or carbonic anhydrase inhibitors; however, many authorities prefer to discontinue all medication in such patients and closely monitor for development of disk changes or visual field loss.[25,26]

The goal of drug therapy in the glaucoma patient is reduction of the IOP to a level at which no further optic nerve damage occurs. Effectiveness is determined by monitoring IOP and assessing the optic disk and visual fields for disease progression. Drug therapy is initiated in a stepwise manner, starting with lower concentrations of a well-tolerated topical agent (e.g., pilocarpine 1%–2%), a β-blocker (timolol, betaxolol, or levobunolol), or epinephrine. The choice of initial drug depends on individual patient characteristics and concurrent disease states.

Pilocarpine, the parasympathomimetic agent of choice in POAG, is available as an ophthalmic solution, an ocular insert, and a hydrophilic polymer gel (Table 64.4).[27,28] Pilocarpine in POAG or ocular hypertension is initiated as 0.5% to 1% solution, one drop three to four times daily. Both drug concentration and frequency may be increased if IOP reduction is inadequate. Patients with darkly pigmented eyes frequently require higher concentrations of pilocarpine than patients with lightly pigmented eyes. Concentrations of pilocarpine above 4% are rarely required in patients other than those with darkly pigmented eyes. Increasing the concentration of pilocarpine may not result in a greater IOP reduction but may increase the duration of action.[18] Administration more often than every 3 to 4 hours is inconvenient and exposes the patient to a higher risk of side effects. Instead, such patients should be switched to an alternative form of pilocarpine or to an alternative agent.

The pilocarpine ocusert is a solid, elliptical, sustained-release device designed for placement in the conjunctival sac and delivery of pilocarpine over a 7-day period. The ocusert should be placed in the eye at bedtime so early side effects occur during sleep. The advantages of the ocusert are

**Table 64.4** Topical Agents Used in the Treatment of Glaucoma

| *Drug* | *Form* | *Strength (%)* | *Brand name* | *Dose frequency*[a] | *IOP reduction (h)* Onset | Peak | Duration | *Mechanism* |
|---|---|---|---|---|---|---|---|---|
| Parasympathomimetics | | | | | | | | |
| Pilocarpine | Solution | 0.25–10 | Numerous | Q 8 h–Q 4 h | 0.75–1 | 1.25 | 4–14 | Increased trabecular outflow facility |
| | Gel | 4 | Pilocarpine HS | Q 24 h at HS | 1 | 3–12 | 18–24 | |
| | Ocusert | 20, 40 μg/h | Ocusert Pilo | Weekly at HS | 1 | 1.5–2 | 7 d | |
| Carbachol | Solution | 0.75–3 | Isopto-Carbachol | Q 12 h–Q 6 h | 1 | 2–4 | 6–8 | |
| Physostigmine | Solution | 0.25, 0.5 | Isopto-Eserine | Q 12 h– Q 8 h | — | 2–4 | 12–36 | |
| | Ointment | 0.25 | Eserine | Q 24 h– Q 8 h | — | 2–6 | 12–36 | |
| Demecarium | Solution | 0.125, 0.25 | Humorsol | Q 24 h–Q 12 h | — | 12–24 | 7–28 d | |
| Echothiophate | Solution | 0.03–0.25 | Phospholine Iodide | Q 24 h–Q 12 h | 4–8 | 12–24 | 7–28 d | |
| Isoflurophate | Ointment | 0.025 | Floropryl | Q 3 d–Q 8 h | — | 12–24 | 7 d | |
| Adrenergic agents | | | | | | | | |
| Epinephrine HCl | Solution | 0.25–2 | Glaucon | Q 12 h | 0.5–1 | 4–8 | 12 | Increased outflow facility |
| Bitartrate | Solution | 2[b] | Epitrate | | | | | |
| Borate | Solution | 0.5–2 | Epinal | | | | | |
| Dipivefrin | Solution | 0.1 | Propine | Q 12 h | 0.5–1 | 4–8 | 12 | |
| β-Adrenergic blocking agents | | | | | | | | |
| Timolol | Solution | 0.25, 0.5 | Timoptic | Q 24 h–Q 12 h | 0.25–0.5 | 1–2 | 12–24 | Decreased aqueous inflow |
| Betaxolol | Solution | 0.5 | Betoptic | Q 12 h | 0.25–0.5 | 1–2 | 12–24 | |
| Levobunolol | Solution | 0.5 | Betagan | Q 24 h–Q 12 h | 0.25–0.5 | 1–2 | 12–24 | |

[a] Q *x* h, every *x* h; HS, at bedtime.
[b] Equivalent to 1.1% epinephrine base.

convenience of weekly placement, possibly improved control of diurnal IOP increases, and decreased frequency of side effects. The disadvantages include increased cost, discomfort, undetected loss of the device, and increased dexterity required for unit placement.[27–29] Pilocarpine gel (Pilocarpine HS) is a product containing 4% pilocarpine in a hydrophilic polymer gel. The slow dissolution of the gel and increased ocular contact time, which improve ocular absorption, result in control of IOP for a 24-hour period. Treatment with pilocarpine gel 4% is equivalent to treatment with pilocarpine solution 4% four times daily or timolol 0.5% twice daily.

Ocular side effects of pilocarpine include miosis, which decreases night vision and vision in patients with central cataracts and constriction of the visual field. Pilocarpine ciliary muscle contraction produces accommodative spasm, particularly in younger patients still able to accommodate (pre-presbyopic). Pilocarpine also may produce frontal headache, browache, periorbital pain, eyelid twitching, and conjunctival irritation or injection early in therapy, which tends to decrease in severity over 3 to 5 weeks of continued therapy. Systemic cholinergic side effects of pilocarpine are rare, but may be seen in patients using high concentrations (6%–8%) or with overzealous use in treatment of acute angle closure. Other side effects associated with direct-acting miotics include retinal detachment, allergic reaction, exacerbation of inflammatory disorders, permanent miosis, cataracts, precipitation of angle-closure glaucoma, and, rarely, miotic cysts of the pupillary margin.

Carbachol is a potent, direct-acting miotic agent; its duration of action is longer than that of pilocarpine (8–10 hours) because of resistance to hydrolysis by cholinesterases. Patients with an inadequate response to or intolerance of pilocarpine as a result of ocular irritation or allergy frequently do well on carbachol. The ocular and systemic side effects of carbachol are similar but more frequent, constant, and severe than those of pilocarpine.

The $\beta$-blocking agents produce ocular hypotensive effects by decreasing the production of aqueous by the ciliary body, without producing significant effects on aqueous outflow facility. The mechanism by which $\beta$-blockers decrease aqueous inflow remains controversial, but is most frequently attributed to $\beta_2$-adrenergic receptor blockade in the ciliary body.[29,30]

Three ophthalmic $\beta$-blockers are presently available: timolol, levobunolol, and betaxolol. Timolol and levobunolol are both nonspecific $\beta$-blocking agents, whereas betaxolol is a $\beta_1$-adrenergic selective agent. The three agents reduce IOP to a similar degree. Because of $\beta_1$ specificity, betaxolol is less likely to produce the systemic side effects caused by $\beta_2$-adrenergic blockade, such as bronchospasm. Because of their systemic side effects, ophthalmic $\beta$-blockers should be used with caution in patients with pulmonary diseases, sinus bradycardia, second- or third-degree heart block, congestive heart failure, diabetes, and myasthenia gravis and in patients receiving oral $\beta$-blocker therapy.[30,31]

Epinephrine is a first-line agent in the treatment of glaucoma and, when combined with other antiglaucoma medications, may be useful in refractory patients.[32,33] Dipivefrin is a prodrug of epinephrine formed by addition of two pivaloyl groups to the epinephrine molecule. The mechanism of action by which epinephrine lowers IOP has not been fully elucidated; however, recent data suggest that epinephrine produces an increase in outflow facility. Compared with $\beta$-blockers or miotics, epinephrine reduces IOP less.[18] For this reason epinephrine is used as initial therapy in patients with mild to moderate increases in IOP or in combination with other agents. Epinephrine is available as epinephrine hydrochloride, epinephrine bitartrate, and epinephryl borate solutions. Epinephryl borate and epinephrine hydrochloride are labeled as the concentration of epinephrine base; however, epinephrine bitartrate 2% is equivalent to epinephrine base 1.1%. The various salts of epinephrine produce equivalent IOP-lowering effects and adverse reactions. Patients with minor ocular irritation may occasionally benefit from use of the less acidic epinephryl borate salt.[18]

A factor limiting the usefulness of epinephrine is the high frequency of local ocular side effects. Tearing, burning, ocular discomfort, browache, conjunctival hyperemia, punctate keratopathy, allergic blepharoconjunctivitis, rare loss of eyelashes, stenosis of the nasolacrimal duct, and blurred vision may occur. Prolonged use (over 1 year) may result in deposition of pigment (adrenochrome) in the conjunctiva and cornea. Pigment may also deposit in soft contact lenses, turning them black.[18] These side effects may occur less frequently with dipivefrin. Epinephrine may produce mydriasis (particularly when combined with a $\beta$-blocker) and may precipitate acute angle-closure glaucoma in patients with narrow anterior chambers. A relative contraindication to the use of epinephrine is aphakia (i.e., after cataract removal) because of the development of degeneration of the macular portion of the retina. Macular edema occurs in 20% to 30% of aphakic eyes treated with epinephrine.[3,18,32] Systemic side effects of epinephrine include headache, faintness, increased blood pressure, tachycardia, arrhythmias, tremor, pallor, anxiety, and increased perspiration.[18,32–34] Epinephrine should be used with caution in patients with cardiovascular diseases, cerebrovascular diseases, aphakia, angle-closure glaucoma, hyperthyroidism, and diabetes mellitus and in patients undergoing anesthesia with halogenated hydrocarbon anesthetics.[3,18,34]

Therapy is started in one eye (except in patients with very high IOP or advanced field loss) to evaluate drug efficacy and tolerance.[18] Monitoring of therapy should be individualized: IOP should be measured every 1 to 3 months; the disk should be visualized and the visual field measured every 6 to 12 months or after any change in drug therapy. In patients who fail therapy, the drug concentration and/or frequency should be increased (do not use more than one drop per dose). Patients responding to but intolerant of initial therapy may be switched to another drug or an alternative dosage form of the same medication. For patients failing to respond to high concentrations of the initial drug, either a switch should be made to an alternative agent after 1 day of concurrent therapy or another topical drug may be added and used in combination. The need to use combination therapy should be documented by therapeutic trial. Patients prescribed combinations that include timolol or epinephrine should be instructed to instill these agents first as they improve ocular absorption of subsequently instilled agents.[35] Because of the frequency of side effects, topical cholinesterase inhibitors and carbonic anhydrase inhibitors are considered second-line agents to be used in patients who fail less toxic therapy.

The cholinesterase inhibitors used in the treatment of POAG include the reversible inhibitor physostigmine and the irreversible inhibitors echothiophate, demecarium, and isoflurophate (Table 64.4); however, because of the significant ocular and systemic toxic effects of these agents, the cholinesterase inhibitors are reserved primarily for patients not responding to or intolerant of other therapy. The ocular and periocular parasympathomimetic side effects are more common and severe than with pilocarpine or carbachol. In addition to the parasympathomimetic effects, the cholinesterase inhibitors may produce severe fibrinous iritis (particularly with the irreversible inhibitors), synechiae, iritic cysts, conjunctival thickening, and occlusion of the nasolacrimal ducts. Cataracts occur at high frequency with the use of cholinesterase inhibitors, particularly echothiophate. The incidence of cataracts appears to increase with increasing concentration, with up to 60% of patients developing cataracts at higher concentrations.[3] The inhibition of systemic pseudocholinesterase by these agents decreases the rate of succinylcholine hydrolysis, resulting in prolonged muscle paralysis.[3,18]

The role of cholinesterase inhibitors in glaucoma is limited by the frequency and potential toxicity of these agents. In phakic patients, cholinesterase inhibitors should be administered only if intolerance or failure results from use of other antiglaucomatous medications.

The cholinesterase inhibitors should be used with caution in patients with asthma, retinal detachments, narrow angles, bradycardia, hypotension, heart failure, Down's syndrome, epilepsy, parkinsonism, peptic ulcer, and ocular inflammation and in those receiving cholinesterase inhibitor therapy for myasthenia gravis or exposure to carbamate or organophosphate insecticides and pesticides. Nasolacrimal occlusion should always be used when cholinesterase inhibitors are administered.

**Table 64.5** Carbonic Anhydrase Inhibitors

| Drug | Form | Strength (mg) | Brand name | Dose | IOP reduction (h) Onset | Peak | Duration |
|---|---|---|---|---|---|---|---|
| Acetazolamide | Injection | 500 | Diamox | 500 mg IV or IM | 2 min | 0.25–0.5 | 2–5 |
| | Tablets | 125, 250 | Diamox | 125–250 mg BID–QID | 1–1.5 | 2–4 | 8–12 |
| | Capsules | 500 | Diamox Sequels[a] | 500 mg BID | 2 | 8–12 | 12–24 |
| Dichlorphenamide | Tablets | 50 | Daranide | 25–50 mg BID–QID | 0.5–1 | 2–4 | 6–12 |
| Ethoxzolamide | Tablets | 125 | Cardrase | 62.5–125 mg BID–QID | 1–2 | 2–4 | 6–12 |
| Methazolamide | Tablets | 50 | Neptazane | 25–100 mg BID–TID | 2–4 | 6–8 | 10–12 |

[a] Sustained-release capsule.

Carbonic anhydrase inhibitors are indicated in patients failing to respond to or tolerate maximum topical therapy. Carbonic anhydrase inhibitors (CAIs) reduce IOP by decreasing ciliary body aqueous humor secretion by 40% to 60%.[3,18] The exact mechanism by which CAIs inhibit aqueous production is not known, as the role carbonic anhydrase plays in aqueous production is undefined. The available CAIs (Table 64.5) produce equivalent IOP reduction but differ in potency, side effects, dosage forms, and duration of action.

Despite their excellent effects on elevated IOP of any etiology, the CAIs frequently produce intolerable side effects. As a result, CAIs are considered second- or third-line agents in the treatment of POAG. On average, only 30% to 60% of patients are able to tolerate CAI therapy for prolonged periods.[3] Intolerance to CAI therapy most commonly results from a symptom complex that may include malaise, fatigue, anorexia, nausea, weight loss, altered taste, depression, and decreased libido.[3,18,36] Elderly patients tolerate CAIs less frequently than younger patients.[37] The four available CAIs produce the same spectrum of side effects; however, the drugs differ in the frequency and severity of the side effects listed.[3,18,35] Acetazolamide sustained-release capsules (Diamox Sequels) and methazolamide (Neptazane) are commonly considered the best-tolerated CAIs.[3,18,35,36] Carbonic anhydrase inhibitors should be used with caution in patients with sulfa allergies, respiratory acidosis, pulmonary disorders, renal calculi, electrolyte imbalance, hepatic disease, renal disease, diabetes mellitus, or Addison's disease. Concurrent use of a CAI and a diuretic may rapidly produce hypokalemia. High-dose salicylate therapy may increase the acidosis produced by CAIs, while the acidosis produced by CAIs may increase the toxicity of salicylates.[3,18,36–39]

A number of drugs or drug combinations may need to be tried before an effective and well-tolerated regimen is identified. A suggested stepwise approach to therapy is shown in Figure 64.6.

Medications may fail to control progression of visual field loss despite attainment of an IOP less than 20 mm Hg. Such patients may be particularly sensitive to even "normal" IOP, are frequently found to have advanced field loss, and may require IOP in the midteens.[18] Large circadian fluctuations may also contribute to progressive nerve damage in the face of normal IOP. When drug therapy fails, surgical procedures may be required to improve aqueous outflow.

Treatment of secondary glaucomas is similar to that of POAG; however, the choice of drug should be based more on the underlying cause of the IOP. Miotics are effective if the drugs improve aqueous outflow through the meshwork; however, if most of the meshwork is covered, blocked, or damaged so that the action of miotics to open the trabecular meshwork has limited effect, the drug will be ineffective. In addition, patients with inflammation should not be treated with miotics, as increased pain and possible inflammation may result. Depending on the effect of the underlying disease on the outflow routes, epinephrine may or may not be useful. Such drugs as β-blockers and carbonic anhydrase inhibitors may be the most useful agents in the treatment of secondary open-angle glaucoma, as these drugs decrease aqueous production and do not rely on improving damaged outflow pathways. β-Blockers and carbonic anhydrase inhibitors are also the primary agents used in the prevention and treatment of increased IOP in the postoperative period.[24]

### *Patient Education*

The other important consideration in patients failing to respond to drug therapy is compliance. A large percentage of patients fail to use topical ophthalmic drugs correctly.[40] The patient should be taught the following procedure: Wash and dry the hands. With a forefinger, pull down the outer portion of the lower lid to form a "pocket" to receive the drop. Grasp the dropper bottle between the thumb and fingers with the hand braced against the cheek or nose with the head upward. Place the dropper over the eye while looking at the tip of the bottle; then, look up and place a single drop in the eye. The lids should be closed but not squeezed or rubbed for 1 to 3 minutes after instillation. This increases the ocular availability of the drug. Alternatively, nasolacrimal occlusion may be used to improve ocular bioavailability. The patient induces nasolacrimal occlusion for 1 minute by placing the index finger over the nasolacrimal drainage system in the corner of the eye.[41] This maneuver as well as

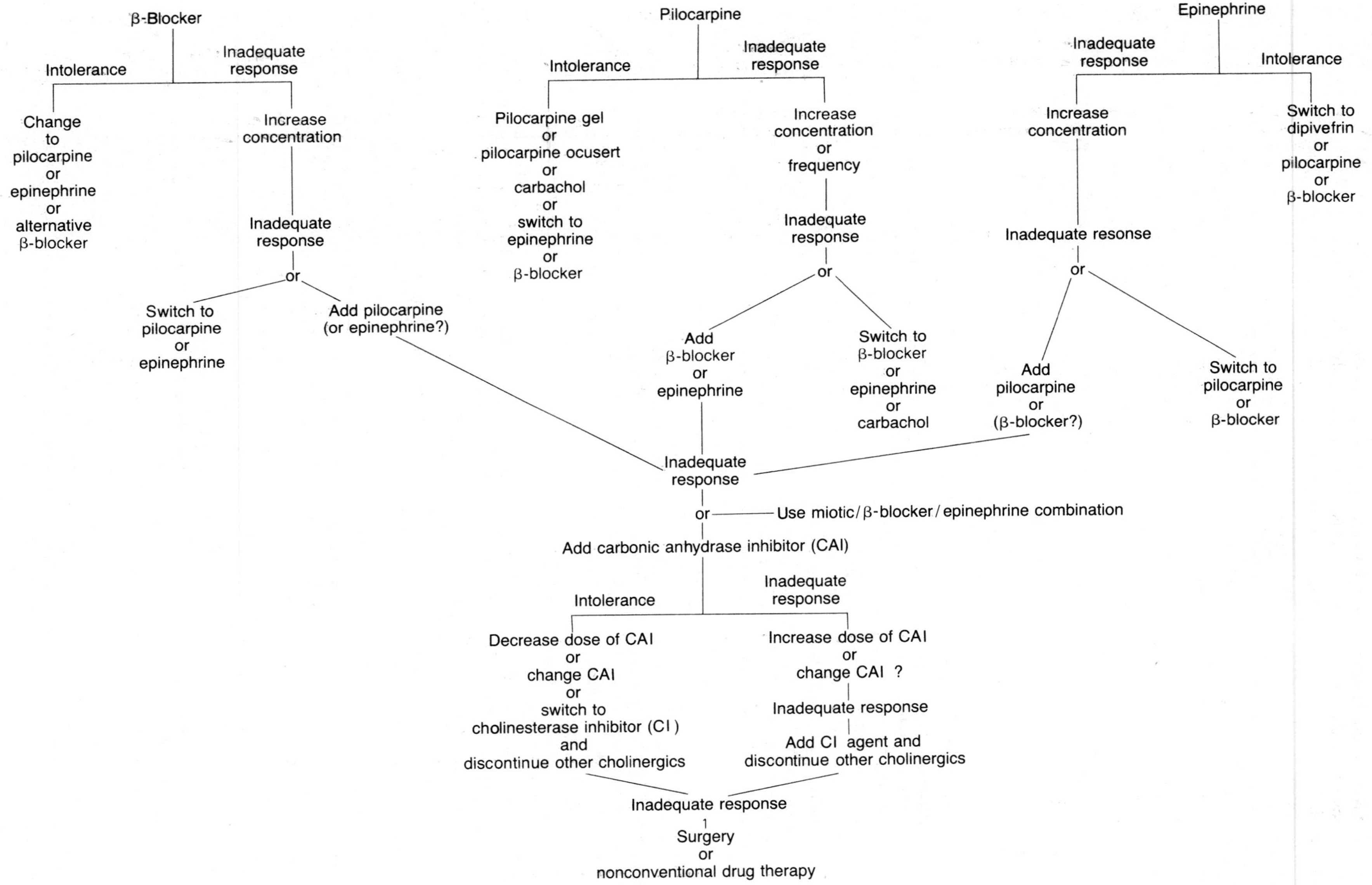


**Figure 64.6** Suggested stepwise approach to the drug treatment of glaucoma. Start with β-blocker, pilocarpine, or epinephrine; initial drug choice depends upon patient characteristics (see text). Choice of alternative drug therapy (alter dosage form or change drug) in intolerant patient depends upon type of adverse reaction encountered. Need for combination drug therapy should be documented through therapeutic trial.

eyelid closure decreases punctal drainage of drug, thereby decreasing the amount of drug available for systemic absorption from the nasopharyngeal mucosa. Use of more than one drop per dose does not significantly improve response but may increase side effects. When two drugs are to be administered, instillations should be separated by at least 3 to 5 minutes to prevent the drug administered first from being washed out. The patient should be taught not to touch the dropper bottle tip with eye, hands, or any surface. The patient should be fully informed of the expectations of therapy and the need to continue therapy despite a lack of symptoms. Possible side effects of the medication and ways of reducing them should be discussed. Compliance will be improved by finding well-tolerated and convenient drug regimens. For example, the use of once-a-day pilocarpine gel or a weekly pilocarpine ocusert may greatly improve compliance over the use of pilocarpine solution four times daily.

### *Prognosis*

In most cases of POAG the prognosis is excellent. Progression to blindness is rare when POAG is discovered early and adequately treated. Patients with advanced visual field loss rarely have continued field loss if the IOP is maintained at less than 18 mm Hg; however, of patients with IOP greater than 22 mm Hg, 30% have loss of vision.[18] Thus, the keys to treatment of POAG are an effective, well-tolerated drug regimen, close monitoring of therapy, and compliance.

## Angle-Closure Glaucoma

Primary angle-closure glaucoma accounts for only 5% or less of primary glaucomas; however, when acute angle-closure occurs, it must be treated as an emergency to avoid visual loss. Angle-closure glaucoma results from mechanical blockage of the trabecular meshwork by the iris. Blockage of the meshwork occurs intermittently, resulting in extremely high IOP and symptoms of acute angle-closure glaucoma. Between attacks of angle-closure glaucoma, the IOP is normal unless the patient has concomitant POAG. Primary angle-closure glaucoma occurs in patients with inherited shallow anterior chambers, which produce a narrow angle between the cornea and iris or tight contact between the iris and lens ("pupillary block") (Figs. 64.7 and 64.8). Secondary angle-closure glaucoma results from any cause (i.e., synechiae) of trabecular meshwork blockade by the iris. The presence of a narrow angle is determined by visualization of the angle by gonioscopy.

Other tests for angle-closure glaucoma involve provocation of angle closure–induced IOP increase. These tests attempt to produce angle closure through mydriasis (dark room test, mydriasis test) or by gravity (prone test) and measure any increase in IOP resulting from the provocative test.[1,2,18]

Two major types of primary angle-closure glaucoma have been described: angle closure with pupillary block and angle closure without pupillary block. Angle closure with pupillary block (Figure 64.7) results when the iris is in firm contact with the lens. This produces a relative block of aqueous flow through the pupil to the anterior chamber, resulting in a

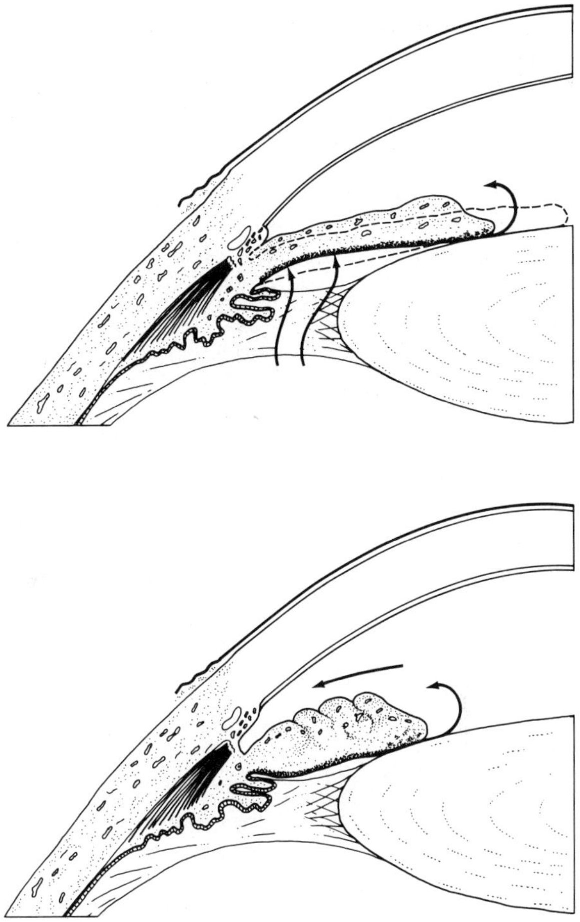

**Figure 64.7** In the narrow-angle eye, the lens is displaced anteriorly in relation to the ciliary body and the iris root. When the eye is miotic (dotted line), the iris lies firmly against the lens, producing pupillary block, but the iris root is pulled away from the trabecular meshwork. In middilation, pupillary block is present but the lax iris bows forward to block the meshwork. With further dilation, pupillary block is broken and the iris does not bow forward, allowing aqueous to flow to the meshwork. *(From Kolker A, Hetherington S. Becker-Shaffer's Diagnosis and Therapy of the Glaucomas, 5th ed. St. Louis, C.V. Mosby, 1983, with permission.)*

bowing forward of the iris which blocks the trabecular meshwork. Angle closure with pupillary block (Figure 64.8) most commonly occurs when the pupil is in middilation. In this position the combination of pupillary block and relaxed iris allows the greatest bowing of the iris; however, angle closure may occur during miosis or mydriasis.

Angle-closure glaucoma without pupillary block occurs in patients with an abnormality called a *plateau iris*. The iris root of these patients is inserted anteriorly, very close to the trabecular meshwork. Mydriasis causes the peripheral iris to bunch up and block the meshwork. The mydriasis produced by anticholinergic drugs or any other drug results in precipitation of both types of angle-closure glaucoma, whereas drug-induced miosis may produce pupillary block.[1,2,18]

Patients with untreated angle-closure glaucoma typically

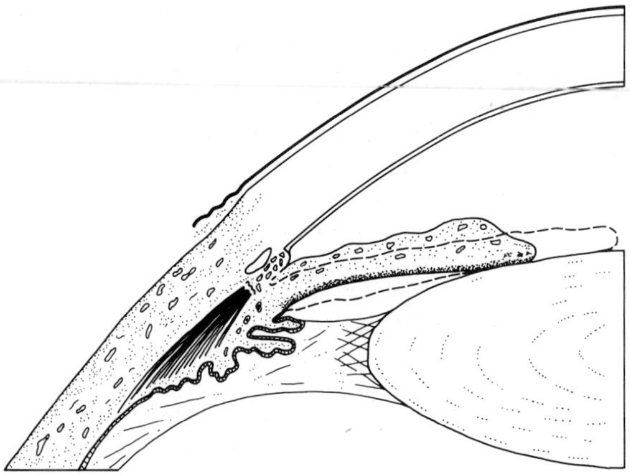

**Figure 64.8** In an eye with plateau iris, the iris is attached anteriorly on the ciliary body. In miosis (dotted line), the root of the iris is pulled away from the meshwork and pupillary block is minimal. In mydriasis, the root of the iris bunches up, blocking the meshwork and producing angle closure. *(From Kolker A, Hetherington S. Becker-Shaffer's Diagnosis and Therapy of the Glaucomas, 5th ed. St. Louis, C.V. Mosby, 1983, with permission.)*

experience intermittent prodromal symptoms brought on by precipitating events. The symptoms include blurred or hazy vision with halos around lights, caused by a hazy, edematous cornea, and occasionally headache.

Intraocular pressure increase during such prodromal episodes is not great enough or long enough to produce the other symptoms of a full-blown attack. Such prodromal attacks last 1 to 2 hours, at which time pupillary block is broken by further mydriasis or miosis, or miosis occurs in patients with plateau iris. Acute angle closure produces the symptoms associated with an edematous cornea: ocular pain or discomfort, nausea, vomiting, abdominal pain, and diaphoresis. On examination, the patient is found to have a closed angle, narrow anterior chamber, hyperemic conjunctiva, and an edematous and hyperemic optic disk. The rate at which IOP increases may be a determinant of when full-blown symptoms occur. Visual fields demonstrate generalized constriction. In prolonged attacks, total loss of vision may occur if the IOP is high enough. Tonometry reveals IOPs as high as 40–90 mm Hg.[1–3,18]

The goal of initial therapy for angle-closure glaucoma is rapid reduction of the IOP to preserve vision and to avoid surgical or laser iridectomy on a hypertensive, congested eye. Iridectomy is the definitive treatment of angle-closure glaucoma; it produces a hole in the iris that allows aqueous to flow directly from the posterior chamber to the anterior chamber. Drug therapy involves administration of pilocarpine, hyperosmotic agents, and a secretory inhibitor (carbonic anhydrase inhibitor or β-blocker). With miosis produced by pilocarpine, the peripheral iris is pulled away from the meshwork. Pilocarpine 1%–2% is instilled every 5 minutes for three doses, then every 15 to 30 minutes until the angle opens. Higher concentrations may be used when lower concentrations fail to open the angle. The unaffected contralateral eye should be treated with the miotic every 6 hours to prevent development of angle closure. Miotics may worsen angle closure by increasing pupillary block and producing anterior movement of the lens because of drug-induced accommodation. At IOPs greater than 60 mm Hg, the iris may be ischemic and unresponsive to miotics; as the pressure drops and the iris responds, miosis occurs. During this period of time, the tendency to use excessive amounts of pilocarpine must be avoided. Nasolacrimal occlusion should be induced to prevent systemic toxicity from the large amounts of pilocarpine administered.

An osmotic agent should be administered in all cases as these drugs produce the most rapid decrease in IOP (Table 64.6). Oral glycerin or isosorbide can be used if an oral agent is tolerated; if not, intravenous mannitol should be used. Aqueous humor production can be decreased during an acute attack by application of a topical β-blocking agent in combination with miotic and hyperosmotic agents. Acetazolamide orally or parenterally may lower IOP in patients with inadequate response to other therapy.[42,43] Once the IOP is

**Table 64.6** Osmotic Agents Used in Glaucoma

| *Drug* | *MW*[a] | *Strength (%)* | *Dose* | *Route* | *Distribution*[b] | *Ocular penetration*[c] | *IOP reduction (h)* Onset | Peak | Duration |
|---|---|---|---|---|---|---|---|---|---|
| Mannitol | 182 | 5, 10, 15, 20, 25 | 1–2 g/kg | IV | Extra-cellular | Poor | 0.25 | 0.5–1 | 6–9 |
| Urea | 60 | 30 | 1–1.5 g/kg | IV | Total | Good | 0.25 | 1–2 | 5–6 |
| Sodium ascorbate | 198 | 20 | 0.5–1 g/kg | IV | Total | Good | 0.5 | 1–2 | 8–12 |
| Glycerin | 92 | 50, 75 | 1–1.5 g/kg | PO | Extra-cellular | Moderate | 0.25 | 0.5–1.5 | 4–6 |
| Isosorbide | 146 | 45 | 1–2 g/kg | PO | Total | Good | 0.25 | 0.5–1.5 | 4–6 |
| Ethanol | 46 | 40–50 | 2–3 mL/kg | PO | Total | Good | 0.5 | 1–2 | 8 |

[a] MW, molecular weight.
[b] Distribution in body water.
[c] Prefer poor intraocular penetration for IOP reduction.

**Table 64.7** Drugs That May Induce or Potentiate Glaucoma

| *Open-angle glaucoma* | *Angle-closure glaucoma* |
|---|---|
| Corticosteroids (high risk) | Topical anticholinergics (high risk) |
| Topical anticholinergics | Topical sympathomimetics (high risk) |
| Systemic anticholinergics (low risk) | Antihistamines |
| Heterocyclic antidepressants (low risk) | Systemic anticholinergics |
| Phenothiazines (low risk) | Heterocyclic antidepressants |
| Vasodilators (low risk) | Antihistamines |
| Cimetidine ?? (low risk) | Phenothiazines |
| | Benzodiazepines (low risk) |
| | Theophylline (low risk) |
| | Vasodilators (low risk) |
| | Systemic sympathomimetics (low risk) |
| | CNS stimulants (low risk) |
| | Tetracyclines (low risk) |
| | Carbonic anhydrase inhibitors (low risk) |
| | Monoamine oxidase inhibitors (low risk) |
| | Topical cholinergics (low risk) |

controlled, pilocarpine should be given every 6 hours until iridectomy is performed.

Patients failing all other medical therapies may respond to retrobulbar anesthesia. Retrobulbar anesthesia blocks ciliary body aqueous production and ocular congestion as well as relieves pain.[3,18] Because peripheral iridectomy essentially "cures" primary angle-closure glaucoma, long-term drug therapy is not used.

## Medications of Potential Hazard in Glaucoma

A number of medications have been associated with increased IOP or carry labeling that cautions use of the medication in glaucoma patients. The potential for a medication to produce or worsen glaucoma depends on the type of glaucoma and whether or not the patient is adequately treated.

Patients with treated, controlled POAG are at minimal risk of induction of an increase in IOP by systemic medications with anticholinergic properties or vasodilators; however, in the untreated glaucoma suspect or uncontrolled POAG patient, the potential of these medications to increase IOP should be considered. Topical anticholinergic agents used to produce mydriasis may result in an increase in IOP. Potent anticholinergic agents such as atropine or homatropine are most likely to increase the IOP. Weaker anticholinergics such as tropicamide that produce less cycloplegia are less likely to increase the IOP and are favored, along with phenylephrine, when mydriasis is desired in the POAG patient. Topical or systemic glucocorticoids may produce increased IOP in both normal individuals and patients with POAG. Patients with POAG appear to be particularly susceptible to glucocorticoid-induced increases in IOP. Glucocorticoids reduce the facility of aqueous outflow through the trabecular meshwork. The decreased facility of outflow appears to result from the accumulation of extracellular material blocking the trabecular channels. The potential of a glucocorticoid to increase IOP is related to its anti-inflammatory potency and intraocular penetration. The increase in IOP induced by glucocorticoids appears to be an inherited trait. Within the general population, 66.2% have an IOP increase of 1.6 mm Hg after 4 weeks of 0.1% dexamethasone, 28.8% have an increase of 10 mm Hg, and 5% have an increase of 16 mm Hg or more.[18] Thus, patients should be treated with the lowest potency and dose and for the shortest time possible when steroids are indicated.[44]

In patients predisposed to angle-closure glaucoma (i.e., narrow anterior chambers), angle closure may be produced by any drug that produces mydriasis. The topical use of anticholinergics or sympathomimetic agents is most likely to result in angle closure. Systemic anticholinergic and sympathomimetic agents must also be used with caution in such patients. The patient should be instructed to avoid the use of such over-the-counter agents as cold remedies, appetite suppressants, and anti–motion sickness and sleep aids, which contain anticholinergic or sympathomimetic ingredients. As previously discussed, potent miotic agents such as echothiophate may produce angle closure by increasing pupillary block. Drugs associated with potentiation of glaucoma are listed in Table 64.7.[45]

## Summary

Glaucoma is a group of primary and secondary diseases, management of which presents a considerable challenge. Successful therapy requires rational use of antiglaucoma medications by the clinician and patient compliance with the selected regimen, combined with conscientious monitoring for side effects and disease progression. The reward for successful therapy is considerable, the maintenance of vision. The overview of the clinical findings, pathology, and drug therapy presented in this chapter provides the clinician with the fundamentals necessary to understand and treat glaucoma.

## References


1. Newell FW. Ophthalmology: Principals and Concepts, 5th ed. St. Louis, C.V. Mosby, 1982.
2. Vaughn D, Asbury T. General Ophthalmology, 10th ed. Los Altos, CA, Lange Medical Publications, 1983.
3. Havener WH. Ocular Pharmacology, 5th ed. St. Louis, C.V. Mosby, 1983.
4. Sears M. The aqueous, in Moses RA (ed): Adler's Physiology of the Eye: Clinical Applications, 7th ed. St. Louis, C.V. Mosby, 1981.
5. Green K. Physiology and pharmacology of aqueous humor inflow. Surv Ophthalmol 1984;28:208–214.
6. Araie M, Takase M. Effects of various drugs on aqueous humor dynamics in man. Jpn J Ophthalmol 1981;25:91–111.
7. Mittag T. Ocular effects of selective alpha-adrenergic agents: A new drug paradox? Ann Ophthalmol 1983;15:201–202.
8. Hodapp E, Kolker E, Kass M, et al. The effect of topical clonidine on intraocular pressure. Arch Ophthalmol 1981;99: 1208–1211.
9. Chiou GCY. Ocular hypotensive actions of haloperidol, a dopaminergic antagonist. Arch Ophthalmol 1984;102:143–145.
10. Sears ML. Regulation of aqueous flow by the adenylate cyclase receptor complex in the ciliary epithelium. Am J Ophthalmol 1985;100:194–198.
11. Yablonski ME. Mechanism of action of topical epinephrine. Ann Ophthalmol 1984;16:307–308.
12. Bleiman BS, Schwartz AL. Paradoxical intraocular pressure response to pilocarpine. Arch Ophthalmol 1979;97:1305–1306.
13. Moses RA. Intraocular pressure, in Moses RA (ed): Adler's Physiology of the Eye: Clinical Applications, 7th ed. St. Louis, C.V. Mosby, 1981.
14. Smith J. Diurnal intraocular pressure: correlation to automated perimetry. Ophthalmology 1985;92:858–861.
15. Kass MA. When to treat ocular hypertension. Surv Ophthalmol 1983;28:229–232.
16. Drance SM. The early structural and functional disturbances of chronic open-angle glaucoma. Ophthalmology 1985;92:853–857.
17. Armaly MF. Interpretation of tonometry and ophthalmoscopy. Invest Ophthalmol 1971;11:75–80.
18. Kolker A, Hetherington J. Becker–Shaffer's Diagnosis and Therapy of the Glaucomas, 5th ed. St. Louis, C.V. Mosby, 1983.
19. Grant MW, Burke JF. Why do some people go blind from glaucoma. Ophthalmology 1982;89:991–998.
20. Drance SM. Low tension glaucoma. Enigma and opportunity. Arch Ophthalmol 1985;103:1131–1133.
21. Maumenee AE. Causes of optic nerve damage in glaucoma. Ophthalmology 1983;90:741–752.
22. Krakau CET, Bengtsson B, Holmin C. The glaucoma theory updated. Acta Ophthalmol 1983;61:737–741.
23. Ritch R, Shields MB. The secondary glaucomas. St. Louis, C.V. Mosby, 1982.
24. Shields MB, Braverman SD. Timolol in the management of secondary glaucomas. Surv Ophthalmol 1983;28(suppl):266–271.
25. Shields MB. A revisit: Ocular hypertension, glaucoma suspect, pre-glaucoma or glaucoma? Ann Ophthalmol 1985;17:456.
26. Phelps CD. In response to Johnson and Zimmerman. Ann Ophthalmol 1985;17:598–600.
27. Zimmerman TJ. Pilocarpine. Ophthalmology 1981;88:85–88.
28. Zimmerman TJ, Wheeler TM. Miotics, side effects and ways to avoid them. Ophthalmology 1982;89:76–80.
29. Remis LL, Epstein DL. Treatment of glaucoma. Ann Rev Med 1984;35:195–205.
30. Neufeld AH, Bartels SP, Liu JH. Laboratory and clinical studies on the mechanism of action of timolol. Ophthalmology 1983;28:286–290.
31. Lesar T. Comparison of ophthalmic beta-blocking agents. Clin Pharm 1987;6:461–463.
32. Podos SM. Epinephrine. Ophthalmology 1980;87:721–723.
33. Podos SM, Ritch R. Epinephrine as initial therapy in selected cases of ocular hypertension. Surv Ophthalmol 1980;25:188–194.
34. Selvin BL. Systemic effects of topical ophthalmic medications. South Med J 1983;76:349–356.
35. Kooner KS, Zimmerman T. Pearls in glaucoma management. Ann Ophthalmol 1985;16:507–508.
36. Lichter PR, Newman LP, Wheeler NC, et al. Patient tolerance to carbonic anhydrase inhibitors. Am J Ophthalmol 1978;85: 495–502.
37. Shrader CE, Thomas JV, Simmons RJ. Relationship of patient age and tolerance to carbonic anhydrase inhibitors. Am J Ophthalmol 1983;96:730–733.
38. Fraunfelder FT, Meyer SM, Bagby GC, et al. Hematologic reactions to carbonic anhydrase inhibitors. Am J Ophthalmol 1985;100:79–81.
39. Anderson CJ, Kaufman PL, Sturm RJ. Toxicity of combined therapy with carbonic anhydrase inhibitors and aspirin. Am J Ophthalmol 1978;86:516–519.
40. Zimmerman TJ, Zalta A. Facilitating compliance in glaucoma therapy. Surv Ophthalmol 1983;28(suppl):252–257.
41. Zimmerman TJ. Improving the therapeutic index of topically applied drugs. Arch Ophthalmol 1984;102:551–553.
42. Kramer P, Ritch R. The treatment of acute angle closure glaucoma revisited. Ann Ophthalmol 1984;16:1101–1103.
43. Airaksinen PJ, Saari KM, Tiainen TJ, et al. Management of acute closed-angle glaucoma with miotics and timolol. Br J Ophthalmol 1979;63:822–825.
44. Francois J. Corticosteroid glaucoma. Ophthalmologica 1984; 188:76–81.
45. Abel SR. Drug induced potentiation of glaucoma. US Pharmacist 1981;December:76–81.

# Chapter 65 / Allergic Rhinitis

J. Russell May, PharmD

Rhinitis is inflammation of the nasal mucous membrane. Allergic rhinitis is caused by mucous membrane exposure to inhaled allergenic materials that elicit a specific immunologic response. It is characterized by sneezing, nasal discharge, and conjunctival itching.

There are two types of allergic rhinitis. Seasonal rhinitis, commonly known as hay fever, occurs in response to specific allergens that are present seasonally, in the spring or fall. These allergens include pollen from trees, grasses, and weeds. Perennial rhinitis is a year-round disease caused by nonseasonal allergens such as house dust, animal hair, and house mites. Unfortunately, some patients have a combination of these two types of allergic rhinitis, suffering all year with seasonal exacerbations.

## Magnitude of Problem

Allergic rhinitis is one of the most common medical disorders found in humans. It affects 10% to 20% of adults and children.[1,2] Allergic rhinitis should be treated because of its potential interference with normal daily functions and because it may lead to some potentially serious complications, such as otitis media, sinusitis, facial and dental abnormalities, hearing loss, poor speech development, and recurrent upper respiratory tract infections.

## Epidemiology

### *Predisposing Factors*

Family history is one of the primary factors predisposing to development of allergic rhinitis. Although the details of genetic control are questionable, some have postulated that it is a function of several genetic factors that have antigen-specific and nonspecific effects. Regulatory genes (ones that regulate other genes but do not produce functional enzymes) may control antigen-specific responses, while structural genes may control the amount of immunoglobulin E (IgE) produced by an individual in response to any antigen.[3] The risk of developing allergic rhinitis is approximately 30% for children with unilateral family history (one parent with allergies) and slightly higher for children with bilateral family history (both parents with allergies).[4] Symptoms of seasonal allergic rhinitis usually begin by the time a person reaches 20 years of age. Patients with perennial rhinitis develop the disease later. About 80% develop perennial rhinitis by age 40, with the majority of these being women.[5]

Allergen exposure is another predisposing factor. For allergic rhinitis to occur, an individual must be exposed to an allergen that elicits the allergic response in that individual. Many potential sufferers never develop symptoms because they never come into contact with the appropriate allergen.

Higher rates of positive skin tests have been observed in people in higher socioeconomic classes and in people who live in suburban areas compared with those living in more polluted intercity areas.[4,6] Further epidemiologic studies are needed to confirm and rationalize these findings.

### *Allergens*

Allergens that produce seasonal allergic rhinitis are the protein components of airborne pollen grains from a variety of trees, grasses, and weeds. Ragweed and grass pollen are the most common offenders in the United States; however, this changes with the geographic region. In general, tree pollens cause symptoms in the spring, grass pollens cause symptoms in the early to middle summer, and weed pollens are the culprit in the late summer to early fall. Patients who are hypersensitive to all three may have overlapping problem periods that can lead to a misdiagnosis of perennial rhinitis.

To complicate matters further, the antigenic components of many grasses are similar, resulting in cross-allergenicity. These include fescue, Kentucky bluegrass, orchard, redtop, and timothy. Fortunately, the trees that produce many of the offending airborne pollens produce pollens that are antigenically distinct. These trees include ash, beech, birch, cedar, hickory, maple, oak, poplar, and sycamore.

Mold spores may also act as allergens. Spores are present year-round; however, there are seasonal increases because of mold growth on decaying vegetation.

The list of allergens that can produce perennial rhinitis is extensive and includes house dust, animal hair, fungus spores, house mites, animal dander, feathers, jute, kapok, newspaper, tobacco, and wood dust. Whether or not foods produce allergic rhinitis is controversial. Food allergies are commonly characterized by urticaria and angioedema.

## Pathophysiology

### *Nasal Physiology*

Knowledge of nasal physiology aids in the understanding of allergic rhinitis. The nose performs three air-conditioning functions to prepare the air for the lungs. During the fraction of a second air is in the nose, it is heated, humidified, and cleaned. The cleaning process plays a role in the development of allergic rhinitis. As the air passes through the nose, the turbulence throws particulate matter against a mucous blanket. The rhythmic movements of the nasal cilia cause the mucous blanket to move posteriorly at approximately 9 mm/min, where it is eventually shallowed[7]; therefore, foreign particles are removed via the gastrointestinal tract and do not reach the lungs.

The vascular tissue in the nose is erectile. Stimulation of sympathetic fibers causes vasoconstriction, reduction in erectile tissue size, and airway widening. Parasympathetic stimulation causes vasodilation, increase in erectile tissue size, and airway narrowing.

Located in the nasal mucosa are the mast cells, which act as local regulators of blood flow by releasing mediators such as histamine.[8] Histamine has a direct effect on $H_1$ vascular receptors, causing increased airway resistance. Histamine increases epithelial permeability, which may allow allergens to penetrate the submucosa, where the mast cell density is greater.[9]

### *The Immune Response*

Although the local immunology of the nose is complex and not completely understood, it is known that IgE is the immunoglobulin of most importance in allergic rhinitis. IgE possesses a high affinity for specific receptors found on the surface of mast cells in the nasal mucosa. When an antigen combines with IgE molecules, mast cell mediators are released. Patients with allergic rhinitis have a high IgE titer and may be easily sensitized to inhaled allergens.

## Clinical Presentation

### *Symptoms*

The IgE-mediated release of chemical mediators from mast cells produces characteristic symptoms including nasal vasodilation and edema (stuffy nose), stimulation of the itch receptor (itchy nose), and increased mucous secretion (runny nose). The parasympathetic response is also triggered, adding to vascular dilatation and production of nasal secretions. Similar mechanisms are responsible for the ocular symptoms that usually accompany allergic rhinitis (conjunctival erythema, pruritus, and tearing).

For seasonal sufferers, symptoms worsen as the season progresses because of a "priming" effect, where the amount of pollen necessary to produce the same level of symptoms decreases.[10,11] A ragweed-sensitive patient, when exposed to pollen out of season, responds with modest symptoms. During ragweed season, when the nasal mucosa is already irritated, exposure to pollen elicits a more severe response.

### *Complications*

As previously mentioned, allergic rhinitis should be treated because of some potential complications. Chronic malaise and fatigue may develop in addition to the nasal symptoms, leading to absenteeism from school or work. Loss of smell or taste and chronic coughing and clearing of the throat are also common.

The role of allergic rhinitis in the development of otitis media with effusion remains controversial, with estimates of allergy as a predisposing factor ranging from 0% to 80%.[12] Negative middle ear pressure is associated with otitis media in children.[13,14]

Certain facial and dental abnormalities may result from allergic rhinitis.[8] Constant nose rubbing can cause a transverse nasal crease across the lower nose and dark circles under the eyes known as *allergic shiners*. Because of blocked nasal passages, patients with rhinitis become mouth breathers, and in children, this can lead to dental malocclusion and orthodontic problems.

Adults with chronic allergic rhinitis frequently have thickening of the sinus membranes, known as hyperplastic sinusitis, and polyps of the nose or sinuses.[5] At one time it was postulated that patients with chronic allergic rhinitis actually had chronic bacterial infections of nasal membranes and sinuses and developed allergic reactions to the bacteria[15]; however, this remains unproven. Other potential complications of chronic allergic rhinitis include hearing loss secondary to otitis media, epistaxis in children, poor speech development, and recurrent upper respiratory infections.

### *Diagnosis*

Three methods have been employed to aid in the diagnosis of allergic rhinitis: history, skin testing, and IgE measurements. A thorough history, including time, place, and circumstances associated with the onset of symptoms, is helpful in diagnosis. Identification of specific causative allergens is extremely difficult. For example, a reaction induced by mowing the yard may not be caused by grass pollens, but by the disturbance of various weeds, molds, or other plants in the lawn. A patient history is of limited utility in diagnosing perennial rhinitis if its cause is house dust or mites because the pattern and presentation of symptoms are not as clear.

Skin testing is a valuable tool when correlated with patient history. Two different methods are available. The intradermal test is performed by injecting 0.01 to 0.05 mL of diluted allergen between the layers of skin. The epicutaneous test, also known as the scratch test or prick test, is performed by making a superficial wound in the outermost layer of skin. A drop of antigen is placed on the wound and allowed to diffuse into the underlying skin. With both procedures, a positive test produces a wheal and flare within 15 to 30 minutes. Of these tests, the epicutaneous appears to be preferable because it is more specific and sensitive.[16,17]

Several problems with skin testing have been identified.[18] The use of antigen extracts has been criticized because of variability in potency and stability. The test results may vary depending on the anatomic site at which the test is performed. Also, the concurrent use of antihistamines or sympathomimetics may alter the test response. Selection of allergens for testing is controversial. The allergen extracts available are numerous and include extracts of tree, grass, weed pollens, molds, foods, and other miscellaneous inhalants. Selection should be based on patient history.

The radioallergosorbent test (RAST) is an in vitro assay of specific IgE. Its use is rarely justified in clinical practice because it is more expensive and less specific than skin tests[19]; however, elevated total serum IgE in the presence of a positive history may be a useful screening test in certain

**Table 65.1** Relative Sedative Effects of Antihistamines

| | |
|---|---|
| High | Low |
| Diphenhydramine hydrochloride | Chlorpheniramine maleate |
| Promethazine hydrochloride | Dexchlorpheniramine maleate |
| | Brompheniramine maleate |
| | Triprolidine hydrochloride |
| Moderate | Cyproheptadine |
| Azatadine | |
| Tripelennamine hydrochloride | Low to none |
| Carbinoxamine maleate | Terfenadine |
| Trimeprazine | |

situations.[20] These IgE measurements may be useful when specific allergen extracts are not available, when negative controls produce a wheal reaction, or when antihistamine therapy cannot be discontinued.[16]

## Treatment

### *Avoidance*

Avoidance of the offending allergens is a simple and direct method of preventing allergic rhinitis: unfortunately, this is often difficult. Patients who are allergic to animal hair and dander may benefit from removal of pets from the house. Covering mattresses and pillows with plastic covers is one method of reducing exposure to dust mites. Filter masks can also be worn while gardening or mowing the lawn.

Careful housecleaning aids in reducing house dust, but it may only benefit patients with a low-grade sensitivity, as dust is difficult to eliminate completely. A change of residence is a fairly drastic step but it may considerably alter exposure to household molds and dust mites. Central air-filtration systems for houses are expensive and minimally effective.[21,22]

Patients with seasonal allergic rhinitis may elect to take vacations to pollen-free areas or remain indoors during pollen season. When avoidance is impractical, or not possible, or produces partial response, several pharmacologic approaches can be used to treat allergic rhinitis.

### *Treatment/Prevention of Symptoms*

Common therapeutic modalities for treating allergic rhinitis are directed at relief of symptoms. This group includes antihistamines, decongestants (both oral and topical), topical corticosteroids, and topical cromolyn sodium.

#### Antihistamines

Histamine $H_1$ receptor antagonists are antihistamines that prevent the binding of histamine from the receptor sites. This prevents the histamine response (increased airway resistance) in sensory nerve endings and blood vessels. It is likely, although still unproven, that the histamine-induced increase in epithelial permeability is inhibited.[9]

Antihistamines are more effective at preventing the actions of histamines from occurring than in reversing these actions once they have taken place. Reversal of symptoms is, at least in part, caused by the anticholinergic properties of these drugs. This activity is responsible for the drying effect of antihistamines, which reduces the problem of nasal, salivary, and lacrimal gland hypersecretion. Antihistamines antagonize capillary permeability, wheal-and-flare formation, and itching.

Histamine $H_2$ receptor antagonists, such as cimetidine and ranitidine, may have some effect on histamine-induced nasal blockage but not on sensory nerves.[9] These agents do not currently have a role in treating allergic rhinitis.

In general, the antihistamines are well absorbed, have a large volume of distribution, and are metabolized by the liver. There appears to be considerable interpatient variation in mean serum half-life.[23] Also, the therapeutic effects of these agents are more prolonged than might be predicted by their half-lives.

Sustained-release products have been available for several years. Although published data to support their use are lacking, many patients claim they are beneficial. In some patients, the duration of action is similar to that of the traditional tablet forms.[24]

Drowsiness is usually the chief complaint of patients who take antihistamines. Drowsiness can interfere with a patient's ability to drive a car or operate machinery and may interfere with a patient's ability to function adequately at the workplace. The sedative effects of antihistamines vary from class to class. Table 65.1 lists common antihistamines in order from the most to the least sedating.

The sedative effects of antihistamines can be useful in patients who suffer from sleeplessness caused by the symptoms of allergic rhinitis. In these patients, a bedtime dose may prove beneficial. Tolerance occurs within 24 hours of the first dose.[25] The mechanism for sedation is not well understood, but its central effect depends on the drug's ability to cross the blood–brain barrier.[26] Most antihistamines are lipid soluble and cross this barrier easily.

A major advance in antihistamine therapy occurred with the release of the first peripherally acting agent, terfenadine. Studies have confirmed terfenadine's lack of sedation compared with other antihistamines and placebo.[27]

Anticholinergic (drying) effects lend to the agents' therapeutic efficacy. Dry mouth, difficulty in voiding urine, constipation, and potential cardiovascular effects may be troublesome. Table 65.2 lists common antihistamines in order from those with the most anticholinergic effects to those with the least effects. Keep in mind that the differences may be small. Patients with a predisposition to urinary retention

**Table 65.2** Relative Anticholinergic Effects of Antihistamines

| | | |
|---|---|---|
| High | | |
| | Ethanolamine class | |
| | | Diphenhydramine hydrochloride |
| | | Carbinoxamine maleate |
| | | Clemastine fumarate |
| | Phenothiazine class | |
| | | Promethazine hydrochloride |
| | | Trimeprazine |
| Moderate | | |
| | Alkylamines | |
| | | Chlorpheniramine maleate |
| | | Dexbrompheniramine maleate |
| | | Triprolidine hydrochloride |
| | Piperadines | |
| | | Cyproheptadine |
| | | Azatadine |
| Low | | |
| | Butyrophenone | |
| | | Terfenadine |

(e.g., elderly males, those on concurrent anticholinergic therapy) should use antihistamines with caution. Caution should also be used in patients with increased intraocular pressure, hyperthyroidism, and cardiovascular disease.

Other side effects of antihistamines include loss of appetite, nausea, vomiting, epigastric distress, constipation, and diarrhea.

Antihistamines are more effective when taken approximately 1 to 2 hours before the anticipated exposure to the offending allergen. If tolerance develops to the therapeutic effect, change to an agent in a different chemical class may be effective.[28]

Patients should be counseled about the proper use of antihistamines. Side effects, especially drowsiness, should be emphasized. Patients should be warned against taking other central nervous system depressants, including alcohol. Patients should be told not to take a double dose when a dose is missed. Taking the antihistamine with meals or at least a full glass of water will help prevent the gastrointestinal side effects (nausea, vomiting, and epigastric distress). Patients should check with their pharmacist and read labels before taking over-the-counter medications. Many cold products and sleep aids contain antihistamines. Patients should be instructed not to use more than one antihistamine at a time. Table 65.3 lists the recommended dosages of the commonly used agents.

**Table 65.3** Oral Dosages of Common Antihistamines and Decongestants

| *Drug* | *Dosage and interval* |
|---|---|
| Antihistamines | |
| Diphenhydramine hydrochloride | |
| Adults | 25–50 mg every 6–8 h |
| Children | 5 mg/kg/d divided every 6 h (up to 25 mg per dose) |
| Chlorpheniramine maleate | |
| Adults | 4 mg every 6 h |
| Children | 0.35 mg/kg/d divided every 6 h (up to 2 mg per dose) |
| Promethazine hydrochloride | |
| Adults | 25 mg at bedtime |
| Children | 0.5 mg/kg/d at bedtime (up to 25 mg per dose) |
| Terfenadine | |
| Adults | 60 mg every 12 h |
| Decongestants | |
| Pseudoephedrine hydrochloride | |
| Adults | 60 mg every 4–6 h<br>120 mg every 12 h[a] |
| Children 6–12 yr | 30 mg every 4–6 h |
| 2–5 yr | 15 mg every 4–6 h |
| Ephedrine | |
| Adults | 25–50 mg every 4 h |
| Children | 2–3 mg/kg/d divided every 4 h (up to 25 mg every 4 h) |
| Phenylpropanolamine | |
| Adults | 25 mg every 4 h or 50 mg every 8 h[a] |
| Children 6–12 yr | 12.5 mg every 4 h |
| 2–5 yr | 6.25 mg every 4 h |

[a] Dosage for sustained-release products.

**Table 65.4** Duration of Action of Topical Decongestants

| *Drug* | *Duration (h)* |
|---|---|
| Short-acting | Up to 4 |
| Phenylephrine hydrochloride | |
| Intermediate-acting | 4–6 |
| Naphazoline hydrochloride | |
| Tetrahydralazine hydrochloride | |
| Long-acting | Up to 12 |
| Oxymetazoline hydrochloride | |
| Xylometazoline hydrochloride | |

### Decongestants

Topical and systemic decongestants are sympathomimetic agents that act on adrenergic receptors in the nasal mucosa, producing vasoconstriction. Decongestants shrink swollen mucosa and improve ventilation.

***Topical Decongestants*** Topical decongestants are applied directly to swollen nasal mucosa via drops or sprays. Table 65.4 lists some of the common topical decongestants and their duration of action. The use of these agents results in little or no systemic absorption.

Because these agents are extremely effective and available to patients over-the-counter, they are widely used. Prolonged use of these agents results in a condition known as rhinitis medicamentosa or "status asthmaticus of the nose." This condition is thought to be caused by severe nasal edema and reduced receptor sensitivity.[16] Patients who develop this condition use more spray more often with less response. While the methods used to treat this "addiction" have not been formally studied, several are commonly used. Abrupt cessation works, but it is difficult because of rebound congestion which may leave the patient congested for several days or weeks. Sleeping may become difficult. Nasal steroids have been used successfully, but they take several days to work. Weaning the patient off topical decongestants can be accomplished by decreasing the dosing interval or the concentration over several weeks. Combining the weaning process with nasal steroids may prove useful.

Other side effects of topical decongestants include burning, stinging, sneezing, and dryness of the nasal mucosa.

Patients should be counseled on the use of topical decongestants to prevent rhinitis medicamentosa. Patients should be instructed to use as small a dose as possible as infrequently as possible and only when absolutely necessary (e.g., at bedtime to aid in falling asleep). Duration of therapy should always be limited to 3 to 5 days.

***Systemic Decongestants*** Oral decongestants are not as effective on an immediate basis as the topical agents but they may last longer and cause less local irritation. Also, rhinitis medicamentosa is not a problem. The most commonly used agents are pseudoephedrine, phenylpropanolamine, and ephedrine.

The pharmacokinetic variables for pseudoephedrine, phenylpropanolamine, and ephedrine are summarized in Table 65.5.

The therapeutic index for phenylpropanolamine is very low. It can produce severe or life-threatening hypertension at less than three times the usual over-the-counter dose of 37.5 mg.[29,30] The therapeutic index for ephedrine is also low; doses exceeding two to three times the therapeutic dose can cause clinically important hypertension.[29]

Pseudoephedrine appears to be the safest of the three. Doses of 180 mg have been shown to produce no measurable change in blood pressure or heart rate.[31] In higher doses (210–240 mg), pseudoephedrine has raised both blood pressure and heart rate.[32] All three systemic decongestants can cause mild central nervous system stimulation, even at therapeutic doses.

Table 65.3 lists the usual doses for pseudoephedrine, phenylpropanolamine, and ephedrine. Because most of the studies on the effect of decongestants on blood pressure were performed in normotensives, hypertensive patients should, unless absolutely necessary, avoid these drugs, especially phenylpropanolamine and ephedrine. Severe antihypertensive reactions can occur with any of these agents when given with monoamine oxidase inhibitors.[33]

As with antihistamines, patients should be encouraged to read product labels to avoid therapeutic duplications. As most over-the-counter appetite suppressants contain phenylpropanolamine, they should not be taken in combination with decongestants.

### Combination Products

Numerous products combining an antihistamine with a decongestant are available. The combination seems rational because of the different mechanisms of action. Two well-controlled studies have documented the efficacy of pseudoephedrine in combination with triprolidine.[34,35] On the basis of these two studies, the Food and Drug Administration upgraded this product's designation to "effective." As pre-

**Table 65.5** Pharmacokinetic Variables of Systemic Decongestants

| *Drug* | *Half-life (h)* | *Mechanism of metabolism or elimination* |
|---|---|---|
| Pseudoephedrine | 3–8[a] | Partially metabolized; majority excreted unchanged in urine |
| Ephedrine | 3–6[a] | Majority excreted unchanged in urine |
| Phenylpropanolamine | 3–4 | Majority excreted unchanged in urine |

[a] Dependent on urinary pH.

viously mentioned, patients should read labels to avoid therapeutic duplication. Specific symptoms should be treated with a single drug when possible.

### Topical Steroids

The desired benefits of corticosteroids must be weighed against the potential risks. While corticosteroids are universally accepted to be effective in allergic rhinitis, concern over side effects has limited their systemic use. Topical steroids appear to be effective with minimal side effects.

Recent in vivo studies have shown several effects of topical steroids on the nasal mucosa: a decrease in the number of epithelial mediator cells,[10] reduction in epithelial permeability,[36] reduction of the secretory response to stimulation of nasal cholinergic receptors,[37] and partial inhibition of the immediate allergen-induced nasal symptoms.[38] The effects of nasal steroids appear to be local rather than systemic. After nasal administration of steroids, nasal symptoms improve; however, eye symptoms remain.[39]

Topical steroids produce only minor side effects, the most common being sneezing, stinging, and epistaxis. Suppression of the hypothalmic–pituitary–adrenal axis has not been a problem with therapeutic doses.[40] Local infections with *Candida albicans* have occurred rarely.

Beclomethasone dipropionate and flunisolide are the most commonly used agents. In adults, 42 $\mu$g (one inhalation) of beclomethasone dipropionate is inhaled into each nostril every 6 to 12 hours. With flunisolide, 50 $\mu$g (two inhalations) is inhaled into each nostril every 8 to 12 hours in adults and every 12 hours in children (6–14 years). These agents appear to be equally effective.

The therapeutic benefits of topical steroids are not immediate. Patients need to understand this to ensure cooperation and continuation of therapy. Some patients notice improvement in a few days, but peak responses may not be observed for 2 to 3 weeks. Blocked nasal passages should be cleared with a decongestant before administration to ensure adequate penetration of the spray. Topical steroids should not be used in patients with nasal septum ulcers or recent nasal surgery or trauma.

### Cromolyn Sodium

Cromolyn sodium is a mast cell stabilizer. This is a local effect seen in lung mucosa, nasal mucosa, and eyes. A nasal solution is used for the symptomatic prevention and treatment of allergic rhinitis.

Cromolyn sodium has the unique property of preventing antigen-triggered mast cell degranulation and release of the mediators of allergic reactions, including histamine.[41] One hypothesis on the mechanism is that the drug interferes with calcium transport across the mast cell membrane. Cromolyn sodium has no direct antihistaminic, anticholinergic, or anti-inflammatory properties.

Like topical steroids, the most common side effects result from local irritation—sneezing and nasal stinging.

The dose in adults and children over 6 is one spray in each nostril three to four times a day at regular intervals.

For seasonal rhinitis, treatment should be initiated just before the usual start of the offending allergen's season. Treatment should continue throughout this season. In perennial rhinitis, the effects may not be seen for 2 to 4 weeks; therefore, antihistamines or decongestants may be needed during this initial phase of therapy. As the cromolyn sodium begins to work, the need for these medications should decrease.

Cromolyn sodium must come into contact with the entire nasal lining; therefore, patients should be instructed to clear nasal passages before administration. Inhaling through the nose during administration aids in this process. One author has theorized that if 90% of the nasal lining is reached by the spray, allergic reactions in the remaining 10% can evoke symptoms in the entire mucous membrane.[9]

### Future Drug Therapy

Several new agents will soon be available for the treatment of allergic rhinitis. How these agents compare with those just described remains to be seen.

***Ipratropium*** Ipratropium is a topical anticholinergic shown to reduce the watery discharge in allergic and nonallergic rhinitis.[42] This agent blocks the glandular but not the vascular cholinergic receptors.

***Fenterol*** This $\beta_2$ adrenoreceptor agonist is in the same pharmacologic class as the antiasthmatic agents albuterol and metaproterenol. Topical nasal application has provided some protection against allergen-induced sneezing, nasal discharge, and blockage.[43]

***Astemizole and Mequitazine*** These peripherally acting, nonsedating antihistamines are similar to terfenadine.

***Budesonide and Fluocortin Butyl*** Budesonide is a topical corticosteroid that has been compared with flunisolide in patients with seasonal allergic rhinitis.[44] Both were effective; however, there were more complaints of nasal irritation in the flunisolide-treated group. Fluocortin butyl, another new topical corticosteroid, may have a higher ratio of local anti-inflammatory activity to systemic activity compared with other topically applied steroids.[45]

***Ketotifen and Oxatomide*** These are interesting agents that have mast cell–stabilizing effects similar to those of cromolyn but are effective orally.[46,47] They are also potent antihistamines.

Other agents that may be used are the calcium channel blockers. Topical verapamil may have a slight effect on mediator cells in the nose[9]; the mechanism is not clear. Further studies need to be performed to determine if this class of drugs has a role in the treatment of allergic rhinitis.

## *Immunotherapy*

### History

The first report of the use of grass pollen extract injections to treat allergic rhinitis successfully was published in 1911 by Noon.[48] The therapy was first called desensitization; however, this did not seem appropriate because skin reactivity remained. The name was changed to hyposensitization.

While the term *hyposensitization* is still used today, immunotherapy has become the most accepted terminology.

Immunotherapy was widely used for many years without the benefit of controlled clinical trials. In 1954, Frankland and Augustin reported 80% improvement in patients receiving grass pollen extract compared with 33% improvement in a placebo group.[49] Numerous studies are available today documenting the effectiveness of immunotherapy. Opponents have argued that most of the benefit is caused by placebo effect and patient bias. The use of immunotherapy remains somewhat controversial today, even in light of the increase in documentation of benefits.

### Mechanism of Action

The immunologic mechanism explaining the improvement from immunotherapy remains unclear. Numerous immunologic changes have been documented, including suppression of seasonal rises of IgE antibodies[50]; decreased basophil reactivity and sensitivity to allergens[51]; and generation of antigen-specific suppressor cells.[52]

### Adverse Reactions

Adverse reactions that can occur with immunotherapy are substantial. Among the most common are mild local reactions consisting of induration and swelling at the site of injection. Other more serious reactions, such as hives, asthma, laryngeal spasm, and anaphylactic shock, have occurred but are rare. Severe reactions are treated with epinephrine and antihistamines. Immunotherapy with bee and wasp venoms is associated with a higher risk of anaphylactic reactions. Immunotherapy with inhalant allergen extracts conducted by experienced personnel appears to be safe. Recent studies have failed to demonstrate any consequences of long-term administration of allergen extracts such as induction of circulating immune complexes or immune complex–like disorders.[53]

### Therapeutic Use

Certain patients are most likely to benefit from immunotherapy. Patients who are uncontrolled by medication and are unable to avoid the offending allergen are candidates for immunotherapy. Patients with intolerable side effects (e.g., drowsiness, nervousness, urinary retention) or those who become resistant to medication should consider immunotherapy. Patients with coexisting disease states that limit the use of medication (e.g., hypertension, diabetes) may also consider immunotherapy.

The selection of antigens should be based on patient history and skin test results. Numerous regimens for administration of selected allergens have been suggested. In general, very dilute solutions (1:100,000 to 1:1,000,000,000) are given one to two times per week. The concentration is increased until the maximum tolerated dose is achieved. This maintenance dose is continued every 2 to 6 weeks, depending on clinical response. Best results are usually obtained when injections are given year-round rather than on a seasonal basis.[54]

### Future Developments

***Allergoids*** Treatment of allergens with formaldehyde has resulted in products with substantially less allergenicity but only slightly less immunogenicity. This means a higher therapeutic-to-toxic ratio. Thus, maintenance doses are achieved much faster and patients may need booster shots only every 3 months.

***Polymerized Extracts*** These extracts have advantages similar to those of allergoids. The pollen allergen extracts are treated with glutaraldehyde.

***Other Routes of Administration*** Immunotherapy with grass pollen extracts administered locally in the nose has been shown to reduce symptoms.[55] In an effort to decrease side effects from this treatment, a lower dose was studied, but was shown not to be effective.[56] Oral administration of grass pollen extract has been tried unsuccessfully.[57] More work is needed in these areas.

## Summary

Allergic rhinitis is one of the most common diseases in man. Treatment is justified in most cases because of the potential for complications. Therapeutic modalities include avoidance and pharmacologic management with antihistamines, topical and systemic decongestants, topical steroids, cromolyn sodium, and immunotherapy. Future developments in these treatment modalities look promising.

## References

1. Mullarkey MF. A clinical approach to rhinitis. Med Clin North Am 1981;65:977–986.
2. Settipane GA. Rhinitis: An introduction, in Settipane GA (ed): Rhinitis. Providence, RI, New England and Regional Allergy Proceedings, 1982, pp 1–10.
3. Kantor FS. Allergic rhinitis, in Wyngaarden JB, Smith LH (eds): Cecil Textbook of Medicine. Philadelphia, W.B. Saunders, 1982, pp 1800–1803.
4. Smith JM. The epidemiology of allergic rhinitis, in Settipane GA (ed): Rhinitis. Providence, RI, New England and Regional Allergy Proceedings, 1982, pp 86–91.
5. Winkenwerder WL, Gay LN. Perennial allergic rhinitis: An analysis of 198 cases. Bull Johns Hopkins Hosp 1937;61:90–100.
6. Barbee RA, Lebowitz MD, Thompson HC, et al. Immediate skin test reactivity in a general population sample. Ann Intern Med 1976;84:129–133.
7. Connell JT. Nasal disease: Mechanisms and classifications. Ann Allergy 1983;50:227–235.
8. Ballow M. Allergic rhinitis and conjunctivitis. Postgrad Med 1984;76:197–206.
9. Mygind N. Mediators of nasal allergy. J Allergy Clin Immunol 1982;70:149–159.
10. Holmes TH, Treuting T, Wolff HG. Life situations, emotions,

and nasal disease. Evidence on summative effects inhibited in patients with hay fever. Psychosom Med 1951;13:71–82.
11. Connell JT. Quantitative intranasal pollen challenge. II. Effect of daily pollen challenge, environmental pollen exposure, and placebo challenge on the nasal membrane. J Allergy 1968;41: 123–139.
12. Bernstein JM. Otitis media with effusion: An allergic disease? Compr Ther 1980;6:15–21.
13. O'Conner RD, Ort H, Leong AB, et al. Tympanometric changes following nasal challenge in children with allergic rhinitis. Ann Allergy 1984;53:468–471.
14. Bluestone CD, Beery QC, Andrus WS. Mechanics of the eustachian tube as it influences susceptibility to and persistence of middle ear effusions in children. Ann Otol Rhinol Laryngol 1974;83(suppl 11):27–34.
15. Grove RC, Cook RA. Etiology and nature of chronic hyperplastic sinusitis. Arch Otolaryngol 1933;18:622–629.
16. Mygind N. Clinical investigations of allergic rhinitis and allied conditions. Allergy 1979;34:195–208.
17. Brown WG, Halonen MJ, Kalterborn WT, et al. The relationship of the respiratory allergy, skin test reactivity, and serum IgE in a community population sample. J Clin Immunol 1979;63: 328–335.
18. Norman PS. Allergic rhinitis. J Allergy Clin Immunol 1985;75: 531–545.
19. Adkinson NF. The radioallergosorbent test: Uses and abuses. J Allergy Clin Immunol 1980;65:1–4.
20. Hayes J, Mullarkey MF, Hill JS, et al. Simple and significant discriminators of allergic rhinitis. J Allergy Clin Immunol 1979; 63:201.
21. Hirsch D. Effect of central air conditioning and meteorologic factors on indoor spore counts. J Allergy Clin Immunol 1978;62: 22–26.
22. Kooistra JB, Pasch R, Reed CE. The effects of air cleaners on hay fever symptoms in air conditioned homes. J Allergy Clin Immunol 1978;61:315–319.
23. Simons FER, Simon KJ. $H_1$ receptor antagonists. Clinical pharmacology and use in allergic disease. Pediatr Clin North Am 1983;30:899–914.
24. Fowle ASE, Hughes DTD, Knight GJ. The evaluation of histamine antagonists in man. Eur J Clin Pharmacol 1971;3:215–220.
25. Bye CE, Claridge R, Peck AW, et al. Evidence for tolerance to central nervous effects of the histamine antagonist, triprolidine, in man. Eur J Clin Pharmacol 1977;12:181–186.
26. Douglas WD. Histamine and 5-hydroxytryptamine (serotonin) and their antagonists, in Gilman AG, Goodman LS, Rall TW, et al (eds): The Pharmacological Basis of Therapeutics, 7th ed. New York, Macmillan, 1985, pp 605–638.
27. Kemp JP, Buckley CE, Gershwin ME, et al. Multicenter, double-blind trial of terfenadine in seasonal allergic rhinitis and conjunctivitis. Ann Allergy 1985;54:502–509.
28. Cooper JW. Antihistamines and decongestants in the treatment of chronic rhinitis, in Settipane GA (ed): Rhinitis. Providence, RI, New England and Regional Allergy Proceedings, 1982, pp 103–107.
29. Pentel P. Toxicity of over-the-counter stimulants. JAMA 1984; 252:1898–1903.
30. Horowitz JD, Lang WJ, Howes LG, et al. Hypertensive response induced by phenylpropanolamine in anorectic and decongestant preparations. Lancet 1980;1:60–61.
31. Empey DW, Young GA, Letley E, et al. Dose response study of the nasal decongestant and cardiovascular effects of pseudoephedrine. Br J Clin Pharmacol 1980;9:351–358.
32. Drew CDM, Knight GT, Hughes DTD, et al. Comparison of the effects of D-(−)-ephedrine and L-(+)-pseudoephedrine on the cardiovascular and respiratory systems in man. Br J Clin Pharmacol 1978;6:221–225.
33. Hansten PD. Monoamine oxidase inhibitor interactions, in Drug Interactions, 5th ed. Philadelphia, Lea and Febiger, 1985.
34. Diamond L, Gerson K, Cato A, et al. An evaluation of triprolidine and pseudoephedrine in the treatment of allergic rhinitis. Ann Allergy 1981;47:87–91.
35. Connell JT, Williams BO, Allen S, et al. A double blind controlled evaluation of Actifed and its individual constituents in allergic rhinitis. J Intern Med Res 1982;10:341–347.
36. Sorenson H, Mygind N, Pedersen CB, et al. Long term treatment of nasal polyps with beclomethasone dipropionate aerosol. III. Morphological studies and conclusions. Acta Otolaryngol 1976;82:260–263.
37. Molm L, Wihl JA, Lamm CJ, et al. Reduction of metacholine-induced nasal secretion by treatment with a new topical steroid in perennial non-allergic rhinitis. Allergy 1981;36:209–214.
38. Okuda M, Senba O. Effects of beclomethasone dipropionate spray on subjective and objective findings in perennial allergic rhinitis. Clin Otolaryngol 1980;5:315–321.
39. Mygind N. Local effects of intranasal betamethasone dipropionate aerosol in hay fever. Br Med J 1973;4:464–466.
40. Small P, Black M, Frenkiel S, et al. Beclomethasone dipropionate in the management of rhinitis—a review. Ann Allergy 1982;49:127–130.
41. Foreman JC, Garland LG. Cromoglycate and other antiallergic drugs: A possible mode of action. Br Med J 1976;1:820–821.
42. Borum P, Larsen FS, Mygind N. Nasal metacholine provocation and ipratropium therapy of perennial rhinitis. Acta Otolaryngol 1979;360(suppl):35–39.
43. Borum P, Mygind N. Inhibition of the immediate allergic reaction in the nose by beta-2 adrenostimulant fenterol. J Allergy Clin Immunol 1980;66:25–32.
44. Pipkorn U, Geterud A. A comparative trial testing budesonide and flunisolide nasal sprays in patients with seasonal allergic rhinitis. Ann Allergy 1984;52:183–186.
45. Hartley TF, Lieberman PL, Meltzer EO, et al. Efficacy and tolerance of fluocortin butyl administered twice daily in adult patients with perennial rhinitis. J Allergy Clin Immunol 1985;75: 501–507.
46. Craps LP. Immunologic and therapeutic aspects of ketotifen. J Allergy Clin Immunol 1985;76:389–393.
47. Richards DM, Brogden RN, Heel RC, et al. Oxatomide. Drugs 1984;27:210–231.
48. Noon L. Prophylactic inoculation against hay fever. Lancet 1911;1:1572–1573.
49. Frankland AW, Augustin R. Prophylaxis of summer hay fever and asthma: Controlled trial comparing crude grass pollen extracts and isolated main protein component. Lancet 1954;1: 1055–1057.
50. Lichtenstein LM, Ishizaka K, Norman PS, et al. IgE antibody measurements in ragweed hay fever: Relationship to clinical severity and the results of immunotherapy. J Clin Invest 1973; 52:472–482.
51. Pruzansky JJ, Patterson R. Histamine release from leucocytes of hypersensitive patients. II. Reduced sensitivity of leucocytes after injection therapy. J Allergy 1967;39:44–50.
52. Rocklin RE, Sheffer AL, Greindar DK, et al. Generation of antigen specific suppressor cells during allergy desensitization. N Engl J Med 1980;302:1213–1219.
53. Levinson AI, Summers RJ, Lawley TJ, et al. Evaluation of adverse effects of long term hyposensitization. J Allergy Clin Immunol 1979;62:109–114.
54. Rocklin RE. Clinical and immunologic aspects of allergen

specific immunotherapy in patients with seasonal allergic rhinitis and/or allergic asthma. J Allergy Clin Immunol 1983;72: 323–334.

55. Georgitis JW, Clayton WF, Wypych JI, et al. Further evaluation of local intranasal immunotherapy with aqueous and allergoid grass extracts. J Allergy Clin Immunol 1984;74:694–700.

56. Georgitis JW, Nickelson JA, Wypych JI, et al. Local nasal immunotherapy: Efficacy of low dose aqueous ragweed extract. J Allergy Clin Immunol 1985;75:496–500.

57. Cooper PJ, Darbyshire J, Nunn AJ, et al. A controlled trial of oral hyposensitization in pollen and asthma rhinitis in children. Clin Allergy 1984;14:541–550.

# Section Eleven
# Dermatologic Disorders

## *Chapter 66* / Common Skin Disorders: Acne and Psoriasis

Jean A. Rumsfield, PharmD, and Dennis P. West, MS, FCCP

There are nearly 2,000 skin disorders readily visible and brought to the attention of health care practitioners. Skin rash is a frequent reason for visits to physicians.[1] The pharmacist's role in dermatology can be quite varied, and depends upon the particular cutaneous abnormality. The pharmacist may screen patients to identify dermatologic disorders, identify drug-induced causes of dermatoses, initiate drug therapy (considering vehicle and active ingredients), and monitor for therapeutic effect, adverse reactions, and patient compliance.

The clinician's approach to solving dermatologic problems involves analysis, assessment, establishment, and initiation of a treatment plan followed by careful drug monitoring (Table 66.1). This algorithm is similar to problem-solving approaches in other disease states, but major differences include the development of an objective data base by physical examination of the integument and lesions as well as description of the dermatoses in specific, brief, concise, and uniform terminology.

Important aspects of the physical examination of the skin, a definition of lesion types, and a review of the basic structure and physiology of skin are presented. This review is designed to assist the pharmacist in understanding normal and abnormal skin pathophysiology and in identifying common dermatologic disorders and appropriate treatment regimens. Examination of the skin should include notations on color and consistency of lesions, distribution over body surface, configuration, size, border, and other superficial characteristics.

### Lesion Morphology

#### *Color*

Lesion color, attributed to a variety of causes, is of major diagnostic importance. Hyperpigmentation is usually related to increased deposition of melanin in the skin. Pregnancy, sunlight, and oral contraceptives are only a few causes of hyperpigmentation. Cyanosis or blue skin color can be caused by an increased amount of reduced hemoglobin secondary to hypoxia. A reddish-blue hue may denote capillary stasis or increase in red blood cell numbers.

Erythema (redness) is a hallmark of many dermatologic disorders (e.g., sunburn, and inflammation) and may be caused by dilation of blood vessels, increased number of vessels, or increased blood flow. A yellow hue may be caused by increased bilirubin or carotenoid levels. Light or white skin is defined as hypopigmentation and may be secondary to decreased amounts of melanin. A purple-red or violaceous hue may result from aging of a lesion that was formerly erythematous (red) when it was new (such as a bruise). The consistency of color should also be noted. Some lesions have consistent color throughout, while others may vary in color from the border to an area of central clearing.

#### *Distribution*

The distribution of lesions may be helpful in determining a diagnosis (Figs. 66.1 and 66.2). Lesions may be localized to an anatomic area or generalized over the surface of the body. Lesions involving only exposed areas or body-fold areas (intertriginous) should be differentiated.

#### *Configuration*

Configuration is also essential to diagnosis and may be defined as the relationship of one lesion to another or how lesions are grouped together. Lesions are often described as clustered (a group of lesions close together), linear (in a straight line), annular (circular), polycyclic (two or more rings touching), serpiginous (snakelike with wavy borders), or geographic (large and maplike). Lesion size can be approximated; borders should be categorized as well demarcated (sharply circumscribed), scalloped, or diffuse (ill-defined).

Superficial characteristics such as elevations or depressions in skin, changes in texture, firmness, and presence of moisture or dried exudate should also be noted. Usually, the characteristics of a lesion are communicated in a few singular terms describing the morphologic "type" of lesion. Description of lesion "type," along with color, distribution, and configuration, is the most accepted method of communicating what is noted by physical assessment. Use of

**Table 66.1** An Approach to Solving the Dermatologic Problems of Patients[a]

| *Knowledge base* | | *Patient data base* |
|---|---|---|
| Dermatologic manifestations | Analyze the problem | Subjective data<br>Objective data |
| Therapeutic endpoints<br>Risk *v* benefit | Assess the problem<br>Establish "optimum" treatment plan for the patient | |
| Pharmaceutic and pharmacokinetic considerations<br>Drug/disease/lab interactions<br>Monitoring parameters | Monitor the patient<br>Therapeutic effect<br>Adverse affects<br>Compliance | |
| No resolution | | Resolution of the problem |

[a] The approach to any dermatologic problem is basically the same; however, the distribution of responsibilities between physician and pharmacist varies, depending upon the diagnosis and whom the patient approaches first.

uniform terminology aids in diagnosis and allows others to visualize the lesions. The glossary at the end of the chapter defines the most common lesion types.

## Acne

Acne is a common, self-limiting, multifactorial disease involving the sebaceous follicles of the face and upper trunk. Acne affects 80% of the population between the ages of 12 and 25.[2] In the United States, at least 350,000 patients have acne severe enough to require treatment at any time. Although acne is generally self-limiting and non–life-threatening, the psychologic effect on patients is profound. This is reflected in the amount of money spent on acne therapy in the United States each year. Sales of nonprescription acne medications exceed $100 million; an equivalent amount is spent on antiacne prescription drugs.[2] The pharmacist plays a major role in educating patients on causes of acne, recommending treatment regimens, and counseling on proper drug use.

### *Pathophysiology*

The causes of acne are multifactorial and not completely understood (Fig. 66.3). Etiologic theories of acne include the role of androgens, *Propionibacterium acnes*, sebum production, and follicle growth.

Sebaceous follicles, which normally produce substances to "moisturize" the skin, are found on the face, chest, back, and shoulders. A cross-sectional view of the sebaceous follicle (Fig. 66.4) illustrates the opening to the skin (orifice or "pore") and a long narrow canal extending into the dermis. Sebaceous glands develop at puberty in response to androgen stimulation and are attached to the follicle canal by sebaceous ducts. Sebum produced in sebaceous glands is transported through ducts to the canal and onto the surface of the skin. The follicular canal may also contain fine vellus hair, keratinous material (similar to skin surface cells), and bacteria (usually *P. acnes*). Acne is believed to be caused by a derangement in the structure or function of the normal sebaceous follicle.

Formation of the primary lesion, the comedo (or comedone), may be simplistically thought of as plugging of the sebaceous follicle. Histologically, a widening of the follicular canal along with an increase in cell production is seen.[3] Sebaceous glands atrophy and sebum mixes with excess loose cells in the follicular canal to form a keratinous plug. This lesion clinically appears as a "blackhead" or open comedo. Trauma or inflammatory changes in the primary lesion may lead to formation of a "whitehead" or closed comedo. If the follicular wall is damaged or ruptured by trauma or irritation, the contents of the follicle may extrude into dermis and initiate an inflammatory reaction clinically seen as a pustule or cyst. Factors that induce or transform acne lesions are unknown.

#### Androgens

Androgens stimulate growth of sebaceous follicles and enhance production of sebum. During the second decade, sebum production closely parallels both androgen production and the presence of acne. Although testosterone is the most potent androgen, its metabolites and weaker androgens (e.g., androstenedione, dehydroepiandrosterone, and dehydroepiandrosterone sulfate) are increased in acne patients and may stimulate sebaceous gland activity.[4] Skin, hair follicles, and sebaceous glands can metabolize androgens to active dihydrotestosterone and acne-prone skin may demonstrate increased metabolic activity.[4] These abnormalities are not, however, found in all acne patients and more specific diagnostic tools are being developed to assess endocrine abnormalities in acne.

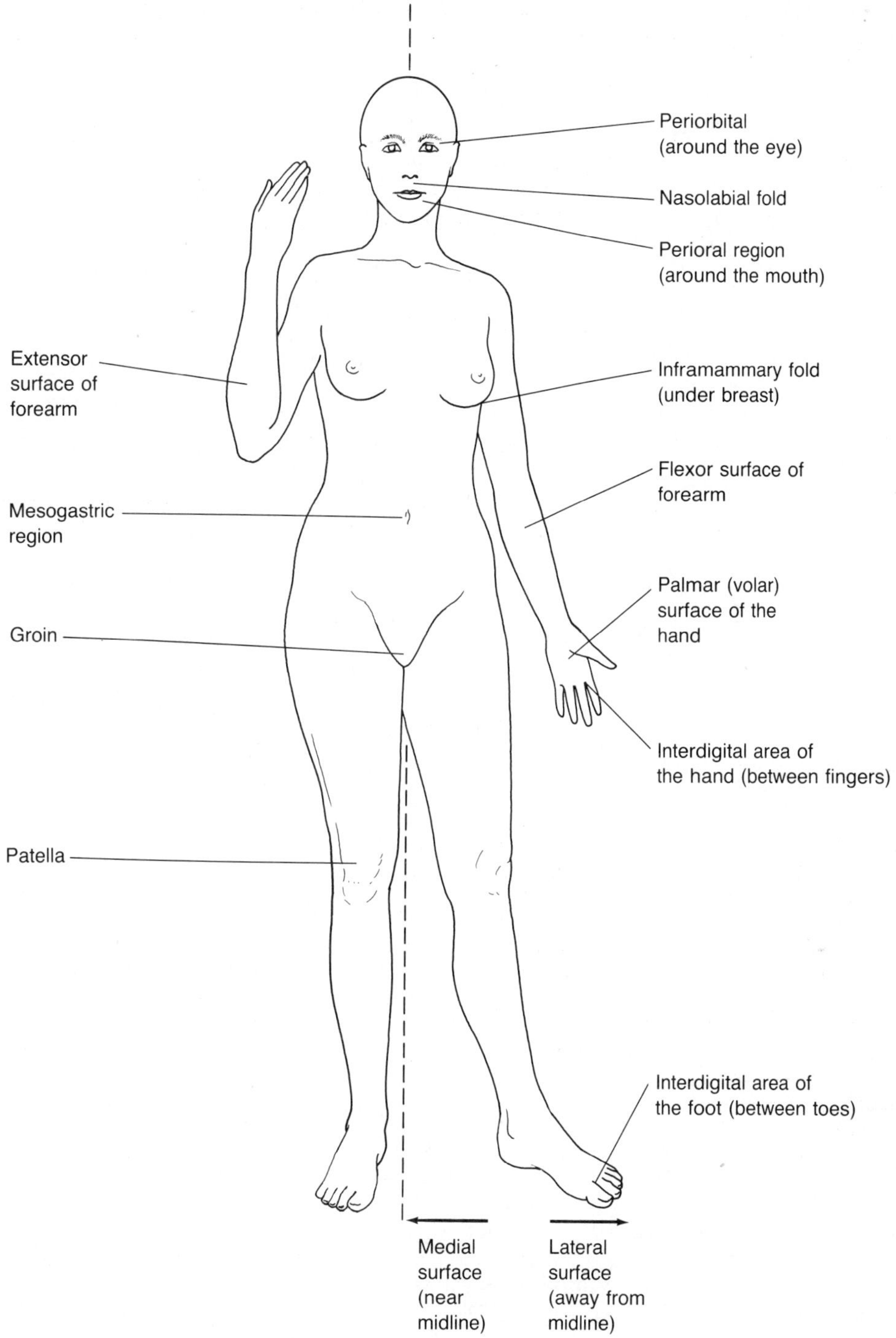


**Figure 66.1** Anterior (ventral) surfaces of the body.

### Sebum Production

Sebum is produced in the sebaceous glands and consists of glycerides, wax esters, squalene, and cholesterol. At times, a relationship between increased sebum secretion and severity of acne is present.[5] The glyceride component of sebum is converted to free fatty acids and glycerol by lipases, products of *P. acnes*.[3] Free fatty acids may irritate the follicular wall and cause increased cell turnover and inflammation.[5] More recently this has been considered an oversimplification; glycerol has been identified as a "substrate" for *P. acnes*, while free fatty acids may function as a measure of *P. acnes* activity and viability.

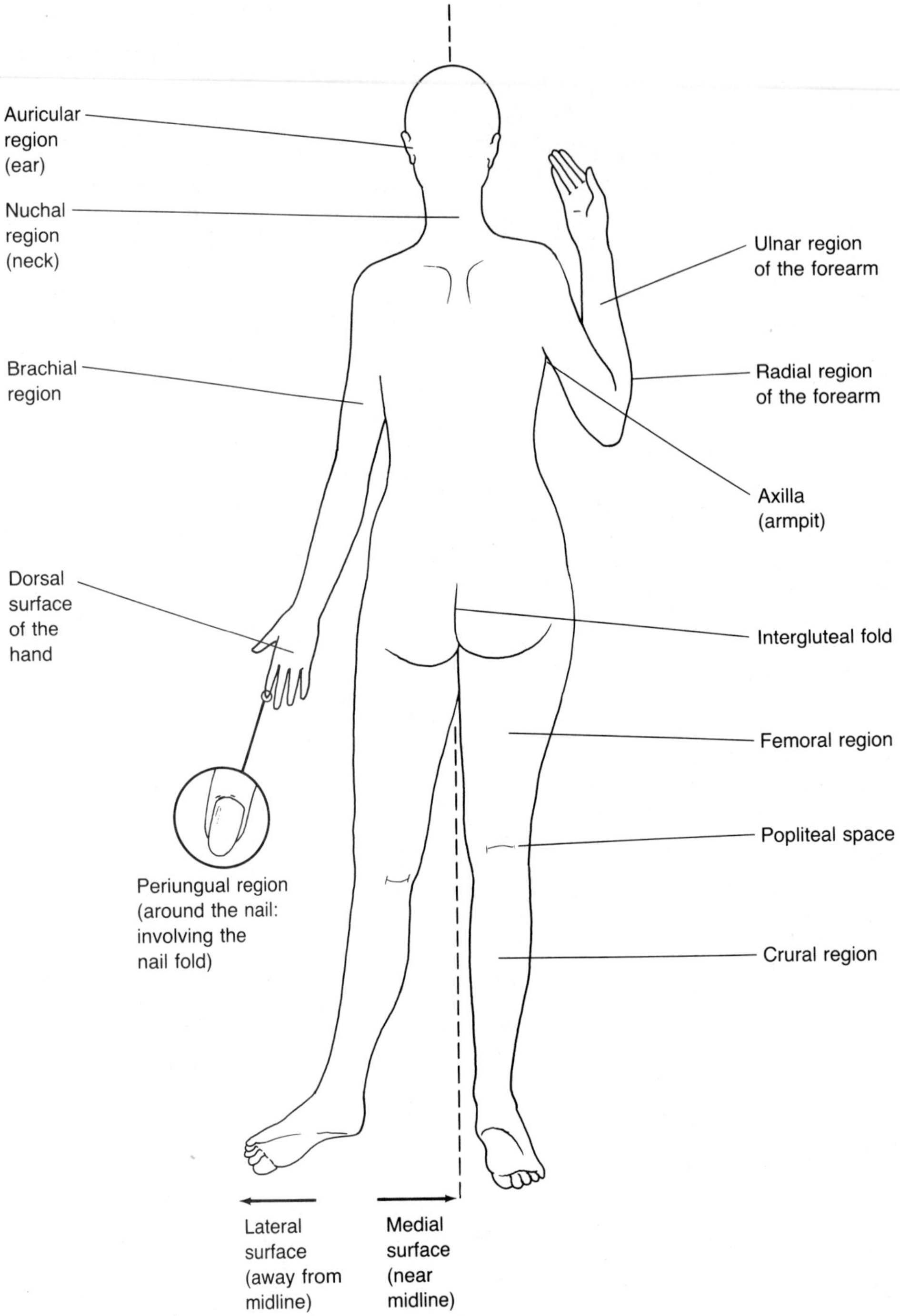


**Figure 66.2** Posterior (dorsal) surfaces of the body.

### Follicle Growth

Abnormal alterations in the follicle wall and its cell growth (keratinization) have been noted histologically in association with acne.[5] The increased production of loosely adherent keratin cells has been correlated with obstruction of the follicles seen in comedo formation. Whether this abnormality is inherent or secondary to irritation or other factors is uncertain.

### Bacteria

*P. acnes* is part of the normal flora in the sebaceous follicle and plays an important role in the initial development and maintenance of the inflammatory response present in acne. Although *P. acnes* counts are typically higher in patients with acne and antibiotic therapy reduces these counts, the pathogenic role of *P. acnes* is not that of simple infection. *P. acnes* may be considered antigenic and capable of causing

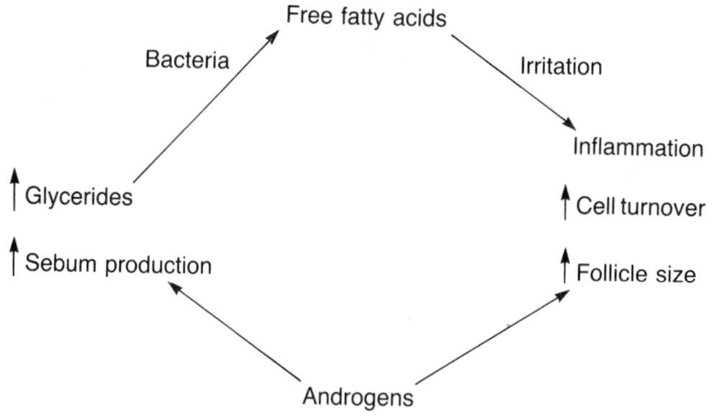


**Figure 66.3** Acne pathogenesis.

increased antibody formation (IgG, IgM), leading to an inflammatory response.[3] Immune complex–mediated complement activation as a result of *P. acnes* may lead to vascular leakage, mast cell degranulation, and leukocyte chemotaxis.[3] Levels of antibodies to *P. acnes* are higher in patients with severe forms of acne than in normal controls. *P. acnes* may activate the complement cascade via both classic and alternate pathways and produce direct tissue damage.[3] Also, there is evidence that chemotactic factors may be secreted by *P. acnes*, diffuse through the follicle wall, and activate neutrophil chemotaxis and complement.[2] Hydrolytic enzymes released by complement activation may damage the follicle wall and lead to more severe, inflammatory acne. Neutrophils are an important factor in inflammatory acne and patients with nodulocystic acne may demonstrate neutrophil defects of either very high or low chemotaxis as well as impaired phagocytosis. *P. acnes* may also evoke a cell-mediated immune response, but this is yet to be clarified.[3] Although the exact cause of acne is unclear, its pathogenesis involves many factors that are interrelated (Figs. 66.3 and 66.4).

### *Clinical Presentation/Treatment*

Clinically, acne ranges from mild (few open comedones) to severe (multiple inflamed cysts, nodules, and pustules). Acne lesions may take as long as a month to develop and 3 to 6 weeks to heal completely. Fibrosis associated with healing may lead to permanent scarring. Most forms of adolescent acne are self-limiting, but more severe forms may be persistent and require more advanced treatment. There is no "cure" for inflammatory acne, but aggressive therapy may modify or inhibit involvement. An important goal of therapy is to prevent or minimize scarring, and the treatment of choice depends on severity and individual patient tolerance. As acne is a multifactorial process, multiple treatment approaches may be required for control. Various medications may be grouped according to their action on the pathogenesis of acne (Table 66.2).

Achievement of clinical effectiveness by any given therapeutic regimen may require 6 to 8 weeks. Patients may also notice an "exacerbation" of acne after initiation of therapy. Inflammatory acne lesions may take approximately 4 weeks to "surface"; therefore, new follicular plugging should be well controlled after 2 months of effective therapy. For topical agents, all acne-prone areas should be treated, as the purpose of therapy is to prevent new lesions.[6]

#### Benzoyl Peroxide

Benzoyl peroxide is an accepted, effective treatment for mild and moderately severe acne. The mechanism of action is uncertain, although benzoyl peroxide is decomposed on the skin by cysteine, liberating free oxygen radicals that oxidize bacterial proteins.[7] Daily application of 10% benzoyl peroxide for 2 weeks can reduce free fatty acid levels by 50% and *P. acnes* levels by 98%.[7] Benzoyl peroxide is also a primary irritant that increases the sloughing rate of epithelial cells, loosens the follicular plug structure, and thus is comedolytic.[7] Dryness and irritation from benzoyl peroxide may limit therapy in some patients and contact dermatitis may occur in 1% to 3%.[8] To limit irritation and increase patient tolerance

**Figure 66.4** Cross-sectional view of the sebaceous follicle.

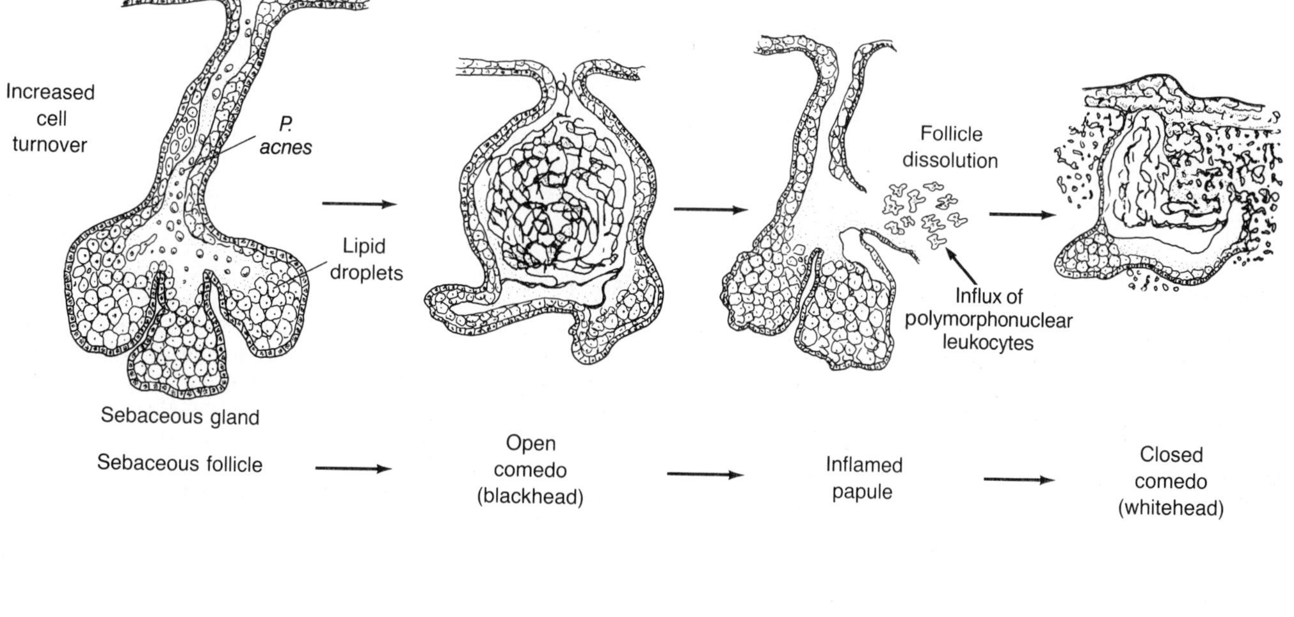

**Table 66.2** Agents That Decrease Pathogenic Mechanisms in Acne

| *Cell turnover* | *P. acnes* | *Inflammation* | *Sebum production/secretion* |
|---|---|---|---|
| Benzoyl peroxide | Benzoyl peroxide | Sulfur | Corticosteroids |
| Tretinoin | Tetracycline | Resorcinol | Estrogens |
| Salicylic acid | Erythromycin | Nonsteroidal anti-inflammatory drugs | Isotretinoin |
| Abrasives | Clindamycin | Isotretinoin | |
| Isotretinoin | Trimethoprim–sulfamethoxazole | | |
| | Minocycline | | |
| | Isotretinoin | | |

to benzoyl peroxide one may initiate therapy with a low potency (2.5%) and increase strength (5% to 10%) or slowly increase application frequency (every other day, each day, then twice a day). Benzoyl peroxide is available in soaps, lotions, creams, and gels. Gel formulations are usually most potent, while the lotions and soaps are of weaker potency. Gels are usually alcohol, propylene glycol, or water based; the alcohol-based preparations generally cause more dryness and irritation. Fair or moist skin is usually more sensitive to irritation from benzoyl peroxide; thus, patients should be advised to apply medication to dry skin (at least 30 minutes after washing) to decrease irritation. The oxidizing capability of benzoyl peroxide may bleach colored fabrics (e.g., washcloths, pillow cases).

### Tretinoin

Tretinoin (topical vitamin A acid) is unique in its effect on the follicular epithelium. Tretinoin increases cell turnover in the follicular wall and decreases cohesiveness of cells, leading to extrusion of existing comedones and inhibition of the formation of new comedones.[9] Tretinoin also decreases the number of cell layers in the stratum corneum from 14 to 5.[7] A "flare" of acne may suddenly appear after 3 to 6 weeks of treatment followed by clinical clearing by 8 to 12 weeks.[9] Irritation, erythema, and peeling often limit successful therapy and allergic contact dermatitis has been reported in a few cases,[9] although not as frequently as with benzoyl peroxide. Tolerance to irritation may be managed by titrating strength and frequency of application. Tretinoin is currently available in 0.05% solution (most potent), 0.01% and 0.025% gel, and 0.05% and 0.1% cream (least potent). Treatment initiation with 0.05% cream is usually recommended for mild acne in people with fair complexions, 0.01% gel for moderate acne in fair skin with oily complexion, and 0.025% gel for severe acne with oily skin.[9]

Patients should be advised to apply the medication to dry skin approximately 30 minutes after washing to minimize erythema and irritation. Slowly increasing application frequency from every other day to daily, then twice daily over a few weeks to months may increase tolerance to tretinoin. Increased sensitivity to sun exposure, wind, cold, and other irritants has also been evident in patients using tretinoin. A combination of benzoyl peroxide each morning and tretinoin at bedtime may enhance efficacy and be less irritating than either agent used alone.[10]

### Sulfur/Resorcinol/Salicylic Acid

These topical agents are keratolytic and mildly antibacterial. The term *keratolytic* refers to the effect of solubilization of the intracellular cement of keratin cells in the stratum corneum. Although evidence for efficacy in treatment of acne is conflicting, each agent has been classified as effective by an advisory review panel of the Food and Drug Administration. Combinations of these agents are often considered synergistic (e.g., sulfur and resorcinol, salicylic acid, and benzoyl peroxide). These products may be less irritating than benzoyl peroxide and tretinoin; however, they are not considered effective comedolytic agents as are benzoyl peroxide and tretinoin. Disadvantages of these agents include the odor created by hydrogen sulfide upon reaction of sulfur with the skin, the brown scale from use of resorcinol, and salicylism from long-term use of high concentrations of salicylic acid on permeable (inflamed and/or abraded) skin.

### Topical Antibiotics

Topical antibiotics (e.g., clindamycin, erythromycin, and tetracycline) have been used effectively to treat acne by concentrating medication to the affected area and subsequently decreasing the risk of systemic toxicity. Clinical trials that compare the efficacy of topical with systemic antibiotics are difficult to evaluate as early formulations often were extemporaneously prepared or different vehicles were used.[11,12]

Clindamycin is considered the most effective topical antibiotic for acne although there are no well-controlled trials. In one study, in vivo topical clindamycin significantly reduced the numbers of *P. acnes*, while topical erythromycin and tetracycline did not[13]; however, reduction of the percentage of free fatty acids in sebum has been noted with the use of topical tetracycline and erythromycin.[13]

Disadvantages of topical antibiotic dosage forms include occasional irritation and stinging upon application. Although tetracycline is the most frequently prescribed oral antibiotic for acne, it is the least frequently prescribed topical antibiotic. On the skin, tetracycline photooxidizes to produce a visible yellow tinting with a relative lack of efficacy.[13] Diarrhea and pseudomembranous colitis may occur from the use of topical clindamycin.[14,15] Antimicrobial resistance from widespread use of topical antibiotics for acne has been postulated but not substantiated as a clinical problem.[13]

**Oral Antibiotics**

There are few well-controlled, double-blind studies of the efficacy of oral antibiotics in acne. Nevertheless, oral antibiotics are considered effective and relatively safe for inflammatory types of acne.[13,16] Tetracycline (and derivatives), erythromycin, clindamycin, and trimethoprim–sulfamethoxazole can significantly decrease the percentage of free fatty acids in skin surface lipids as well as decrease numbers of *P. acnes*.[13] Tetracycline exhibits additional activity by reducing the amount of keratin in sebaceous follicles and by inhibiting chemotaxis, phagocytosis, complement activation (by the alternate pathway), and cell-mediated immunity.[13] Tetracycline also appears to have a greater affinity for inflammatory cells and bacteria, resulting in higher drug concentrations in areas of inflamed skin.[13] Drawbacks to the use of tetracycline include a drug–food interaction with dairy products, photosensitivity, gastrointestinal disturbances, and predisposition to suprainfections (i.e., vaginal candidiasis).

Clindamycin use for acne is limited by diarrhea and risk of pseudomembranous colitis. Erythromycin may have a safer adverse effect profile compared with tetracycline, with a similar efficacy profile.[13,17] In refractory cases, minocycline or doxycycline may be effective because of greater lipid solubility and enhanced penetration into tissue and sebaceous follicles.[7,18] Disadvantages of minocycline include a high incidence of vestibular toxicity and discoloration of skin and teeth.[18] Although trimethoprim–sulfamethoxazole may be effective in tetracycline-resistant acne, it should perhaps be reserved for refractory cases to minimize the risk of resistance.[13,19]

Another consideration in the use of oral antibiotics for acne is a potential interaction with oral contraceptives. Ampicillin and tetracycline apparently decrease the intestinal flora needed to hydrolyze conjugated ethinyl estradiol excreted into the bile; thus, enterohepatic recirculation is interrupted and the amount of active estrogen is reduced.[20] The clinical importance of this interaction is not well established, but several pregnancies have been reported with concurrent use of ampicillin or tetracycline and oral contraceptives.[20] Women taking oral contraceptives (especially agents containing less than 50 μg estrogen) should be informed of the potential for this interaction, especially before initiation of long-term oral antibiotics.

**Isotretinoin**

Isotretinoin is indicated for patients with severe recalcitrant cystic acne unresponsive to conventional therapies. It has multiple actions against cystic acne, including (1) decreased sebum production and change in sebum composition, (2) inhibition of *P. acnes* growth within follicles, (3) inhibition of inflammation, and (4) altered patterns of keratinization within follicles (decreased size and increased differentiation).[21] After a 16-week course of therapy, isotretinoin produces a greater than 70% success rate followed by a prolonged remission of more than 20 months.[22]

Adverse effects from isotretinoin are numerous, frequent, and often dose related. At least 90% of patients receiving isotretinoin experience dry lips, and 30% may show dryness and desquamation of the face. Hypertriglyceridemia may be found in more than 25% of patients. Conjunctivitis and eye irritation may be noted by patients, especially those using contact lenses. Muscle and joint pain, including complaints of backache, are common and may be attributed to catabolic effects on mesenchymal tissues of cartilage, connective tissue, and bone. Skeletal hyperostosis was first noted in patients taking high-dose, long-term isotretinoin for disorders of keratinization, but more recently asymptomatic hyperostosis has occurred in patients on short-course regimens for acne. The relative risk and clinical significance of these skeletal changes are undetermined.

An increase in creatinine phosphokinase and blood glucose, as well as photosensitivity, pseudotumor cerebri, and excess granulation tissue, has occurred during use of isotretinoin.[22] The incidence of teratogenicity in babies of mothers exposed to isotretinoin is high and well documented. Of 16 case reports of adverse pregnancy outcomes in women exposed to isotretinoin, 9 were spontaneous abortions and 7 were babies with major birth defects (e.g., hydrocephalus, small or partially occluded external auditory canals, and cardiac abnormalities).[23] In addition, five normal pregnancies were reported, but timing of exposure to isotretinoin was uncertain.[23]

Other oral agents investigated for the treatment of acne include ibuprofen, zinc, spironolactone, prednisone, dexamethasone, and oral contraceptives.

Acne is a common self-limiting disease with several effective therapeutic modalities. Recognition of the pathogenic factors causing acne, selection of an appropriate treatment regimen, and monitoring for adverse effects can often lead to a successful outcome. The pharmacist should convey concepts of therapy to the patient and emphasize the importance of compliance.

## Psoriasis

Psoriasis is a common chronic disease characterized by recurrent exacerbations and remissions of thickened, erythematous, and scaling lesions. Statistics indicate that approximately 1% of the U.S. population has psoriasis.[24] There is no known "cure" for psoriasis and the annual cost of chronic care is estimated to be at least 5% of the individual U.S. median income.[24]

This debilitating disease occurs in all racial groups and has equal distribution between men and women.[3,25] The mean age of onset is 27 years, with approximately 35% of cases occurring before age 20[26]; however, the age of onset is widely variable from infancy to old age.

### *Pathophysiology*

The cause of psoriasis is unknown and the lack of an adequate animal model has impeded research. There are several hypotheses regarding the pathophysiology of psoriasis. Factors to consider include genetics, various trigger factors (i.e., stress, infection, trauma, drugs), defects in skin cell cycle, and disruption in arachidonic acid metabolism.

The search for an inherent skin defect as a pathogenic mechanism for psoriasis has provided much information and numerous hypotheses. Psoriatic epidermal cells proliferate at a rate sevenfold faster than normal epidermal cells.[27,28] The germinative cell population increases in psoriatic skin, and duration of the cell cycle is calculated at 37.5 hours (versus 300 hours in normal skin).[28] Lesion-free skin in psoriatic patients is generally considered to be involved, as epidermal proliferation is elevated in apparently normal skin.[29]

Other abnormalities found in psoriatic skin include evidence of increased metabolic activity and increased cGMP, DNA, RNA, IgG, and C3.[28,29] In psoriatic lesions, arachidonic acid levels are 30 times normal, 12-L-hydroxy-5,8,10, 14-eicosatetraenoic acid (HETE) levels are 80 times normal, and prostaglandin $E_2$ levels are 50% higher than normal. Glucocorticoids normalize levels of arachidonic acid and HETE by inhibition of phospholipase A and may be partly responsible for regression of psoriatic lesions.[28] Although the exact cause of psoriasis is unknown, treatment approaches are reliable and offer good control of the disorder.

### Genetics

There is a significant genetic component in psoriasis, but the exact mode of inheritance is uncertain. Approximately 36% of patients with psoriasis have at least one immediate relative with the disorder.[26] Monozygotic twins have a higher concordance for psoriasis than dizygotic twins.[26] Studies of histocompatibility antigens in psoriatics indicate statistically significant associations on the B, C, and D loci, more specifically, HLA-B13, HLA-B17, and HLA-B37.[25,30] The most significant risk is with HLA-CW6, where the relative likelihood for developing psoriasis is 9 to 15 times normal.[7] In addition, the B13 and B17 loci appear to be linked with the gene that expresses CW6.[29]

### Exogenous Trigger Factors

Factors such as climate, stress, infection, trauma, and drugs may aggravate psoriasis. Warm seasons and sunlight reportedly improved psoriasis in 80% of patients, while 90% reported worsening in cold weather. Also, stress worsened psoriasis in 30% to 40% of patients. The exact role stress plays in exacerbation of psoriasis is uncertain.

Infection has retrospectively been identified as a common precipitating factor in psoriasis. A review of 245 cases of psoriatic children indicates that 25% had initial onset of the disease after clinically documented infections, while 54% had exacerbation during a 2- to 3-week interval after an upper respiratory infection.[31] Another study indicates that exacerbation of psoriasis 1 to 2 weeks after acute streptococcal infection is common.[32]

Psoriasis may also occur at the site of injury to normal-appearing skin (Koebner response). The incidence is variable, ranging up to 76% in retrospective studies and 51% in prospective studies.[29] The Koebner response may be induced by a variety of causes including rubbing, venipuncture, bites, surgery, and pressure. The mechanism for development of the Koebner response is unknown and is not unique to psoriasis. The length of time between injury and lesion development, although variable, is usually a few days to weeks. Lithium carbonate and β-adrenergic-blocking agents are the drugs most commonly noted to exacerbate psoriasis.[33,34]

## *Clinical Presentation*

The clinical appearance of psoriatic lesions, although not scarring, may almost be categorized as disfiguring, especially for patients with severe disease in cosmetic areas.

In general, psoriatic lesions are characterized by sharply demarcated, erythematous papules and plaques often covered with silver-white fine scales. Initial lesions are usually small papules that enlarge over time and coalesce into large plaques, sometimes as serpiginous or geographic forms. If the fine scale is removed, a salmon-pink lesion is exposed, perhaps with punctate bleeding from prominent dermal capillaries (Auspitz sign).

The appearance of psoriatic lesions also varies depending on the area of the body affected and the type of psoriasis. Scalp psoriasis ranges from diffuse scaling on an erythematous scalp to thickened plaques with exudation, microabscesses, and fissures. Trunk, back, arm, and leg lesions may be generalized, scattered, discrete, droplike lesions (guttate) or large plaques. Palms, soles, face, and genitalia may be involved as well. Affected nails are often pitted with collections of subungual keratotic material. Yellow spots under the nail plate may also be seen.

Patients with pustular psoriasis have lesions with a mixture of brown and white noninfected pustules associated with erythema and scaling. Usually, pustular psoriasis affects the palms and soles symmetrically, but infrequently more severe forms of generalized pustular psoriasis (von Zumbusch variety) may occur with erythroderma, "lakes" of coalescent pustules, fever, malaise, and leukocytosis.

Psoriatic arthritis is a distinct clinical entity in which both psoriatic lesions and inflammatory "arthritis" occur. Classically, distal interphalangeal joints and adjacent nails are involved, but knees, elbows, wrists, and ankles may also be involved. Skin lesions usually precede joint involvement, although the reverse may occur, or skin lesions and joint disease may occur simultaneously. The clinical appearance of psoriasis may sometimes be confused with numerous other dermatologic diseases; thus, the differential diagnosis is extensive and histopathology may be helpful.

## *Treatment*

As psoriasis is often a lifelong relapsing and remitting disease, modes of therapy should be selected with long-term consequences in mind. Major factors of consideration include the extent and site of disease involvement and the age of the patient. The goal of therapy is to achieve complete clearing of lesions, but partial clearing is acceptable at times using regimens with decreased toxicity and increased patient acceptability. Drug treatments for psoriasis are listed in Table 66.3.

**Table 66.3** Drug Treatments for Psoriasis

| *Topical* | *Systemic* |
|---|---|
| Emollients and keratolytics | Ultraviolet A light and oral psoralens |
| Coal tar | Methotrexate |
| Anthralin | Retinoids |
| Corticosteroids | |

### Emollients/Keratolytics

Moisturizers or emollients hydrate the stratum corneum (after application of an occlusive oily film) and minimize evaporation of water from the stratum corneum.[35] Hydration causes the stratum corneum to swell and flatten the surface contour. Moisturizers may decrease the binding forces within the horny layer, enhance desquamation, and eliminate scaling.[35] Moisturizers may also increase pliability of the skin, have antipruritic activity, and possess mild vasoconstrictor activity. Moisturizers often need to be applied three times a day to achieve a beneficial response. Adverse effects include folliculitis or allergic contact dermatitis.

Keratolytics are used to remove scale, smooth the skin, and decrease hyperkeratosis.[35] Salicylic acid, the most frequently used keratolytic agent, is generally applied in concentrations of 2% to 10% or higher. A possible mechanism of salicylic acid keratolysis is that it causes a decrease in corneocyte-to-corneocyte cohesion in the abnormal horny layer of psoriatic skin. Lower concentrations of salicylic acid exhibit a keratin-dispersing effect, while concentrations of 5% or higher have a corneolytic (exfoliative) action.[36] Although salicylic acid may enhance percutaneous penetration of some drugs it also produces local irritation.[35] Application of salicylic acid to large areas of skin may induce salicylism with symptoms of nausea, vomiting, tinnitus, or hyperventilation.[37]

### Coal Tar

Although tar derivatives have been used to treat skin diseases for two millennia, relatively little is known about their composition or mechanism of action.[38] Tars are derived from wood such as pine or juniper, shale (ichthammol), and bituminous coal (coal tar). In recent years, wood and shale tars have fallen out of use because they possess relatively less efficacy than coal tar.[39] Coal tar contains thousands of hydrocarbon compounds formed from distillation of bituminous coal.[38] When applied to normal skin, coal tar causes predominantly transient epidermal hyperplasia during the first 2 weeks of therapy followed by a cytostatic effect with epidermal thinning.[40] There is additional evidence that coal tar can crosslink with DNA, and in combination with ultraviolet light, may increase prostaglandin synthesis in the skin. Suppression of DNA synthesis in the epidermis may be measured via the hairless mouse model used to predict antipsoriatic effectiveness of coal tar derivatives.[41]

Coal tar is an effective treatment for psoriasis; however, its disadvantages include unpleasant odor, ability to stain skin and clothing, ability to reversibly darken or alter light hair colors, and ability to tarnish silver in jewelry. Coal tar is usually applied topically to lesions (often at bedtime), but may also be used in bath water and as a shampoo.

Concern with the long-term use of coal tar is risk of carcinogenicity. Crude coal tar contains many polynuclear aromatic hydrocarbons that are known carcinogens. Retrospective studies of psoriatic patients treated with crude coal tar have not indicated any increase in cancer cases compared with controls[38]; however, there are cases indicating a higher rate of cutaneous carcinoma in patients exposed to tar and ultraviolet light. Controlled studies are needed to determine the carcinogenicity risk associated with the clinical use of crude and refined coal tars.

### Anthralin

Anthralin, an anthrone derivative of chrysarobin (from the South American araroba tree), is used topically to treat psoriasis.[42] Although anthralin (under the name dithranol) has been used for 70 years in Great Britain, it has only recently been extensively used in the United States. Anthralin appears to inhibit DNA synthesis by intercalation between DNA strands.[43] Another possible mechanism is that anthralin may decrease epidermal proliferation by mitochondrial inhibition. Irritation and inflammation are common with anthralin therapy and, to a point, correlate with clinical efficacy.[42,44] Other hypotheses support the role of anthralin-generated free radicals in producing both antipsoriatic effects and irritation.[45]

Inflammation, irritation, and staining of skin and clothing (via oxidation and binding to keratins) are often therapy-limiting effects. Fortunately, anthralin exerts its clinical effects at low cellular concentrations; therefore, short-contact therapy regimens (application for 20 minutes) have been found effective with decreased side effects.[46] Titrating the strength of anthralin slowly from a low concentration (0.1%–0.25%) to a higher concentration (0.5%–1%) may minimize irritation.

Anthralin was traditionally formulated in stiff paste bases to provide adherence to plaques. More recently, cream formulations have been developed that are more cosmetically appealing and appear as clinically effective. The patient must apply anthralin products only to affected areas of skin, as contact with uninvolved skin may result in excessive and unwanted irritation and staining, which usually disappears within 1 to 2 weeks of discontinuation. Staining of affected plaques is a sign of resolution, however, as cell turnover has been slowed enough to take up the stain.[43] Despite the demonstrated efficacy of anthralin, some patients will not tolerate local irritation and staining.

### Topical Corticosteroids

Topical corticosteroids may play an important adjunctive role in the treatment of psoriasis by decreasing erythema, pruritus, and scaling. The mechanism of topical steroids' efficacy in psoriasis is uncertain. Steroid receptors have been identified in the skin, and synthesis and mitosis of DNA in epidermal cells have been halted by topical steroids in hairless mice.[47] Topical corticosteroids appear to inhibit phospholipase A, lowering the amounts of arachidonic acid, prostaglandins, and leukotrienes in the skin.[48]

A wide variety of topical steroids are available in different potencies and vehicles. The choice of steroid and vehicle depends on the severity and extent of involvement, the area of the body to be treated, and the anticipated duration of treatment. Topical steroids are available in ointments, creams, lotions, gels, and sprays.

Ointments are considered the most clinically effective in psoriasis because of their hydrating effect and ability to enhance penetration of the steroid into the skin by lipophilicity.[49] Ointments are not suited for use in areas such as the axilla, groin, or other intertriginous areas where maceration and folliculitis may develop secondary to the occlusive effect. Creams are often preferred by patients and may be used in intertriginous areas even though their water content

**Table 66.4** Topical Corticosteroid Vasoconstrictive (Anti-inflammatory) Potency[a]

| |
|---|
| **Group 1** |
| Betamethasone dipropionate 0.05% in optimized vehicle (Diprolene) |
| **Group 2** |
| Amcinonide 0.1% ointment (Cyclocort) |
| Betamethasone dipropionate 0.05% ointment (Diprosone) |
| Diflorasone diacetate 0.05% ointment (Florone, Maxiflor) |
| Fluocinonide 0.05% cream, ointment, gel (Lidex) |
| Halcinonide 0.1% cream (Halog) |
| **Group 3** |
| Betamethasone valerate 0.1% ointment (Valisone) |
| Betamethasone dipropionate 0.05% cream (Diprosone) |
| Triamcinolone acetonide 0.5% cream (Aristocort, Kenalog) |
| Diflorasone diacetate 0.05% cream (Maxiflor, Florone) |
| **Group 4** |
| Fluocinolone acetonide 0.025% ointment (Synalar) |
| Triamcinolone acetonide 0.1% ointment (Aristocort, Kenalog) |
| Flurandrenolide 0.05% ointment (Cordran) |
| **Group 5** |
| Betamethasone valerate 0.1% cream (Valisone) |
| Triamcinolone acetonide 0.1% cream (Aristocort, Kenalog) |
| Hydrocortisone valerate 0.2% cream (Westcort) |
| **Group 6** |
| Desonide 0.05% cream (Tridesilon) |
| **Group 7** |
| Dexamethasone 0.1% cream (Decadron) |
| Hydrocortisone 2.5% cream (Hytone) |
| Hydrocortisone 1% cream (Hytone) |

[a] Ranked according to vasoconstrictive potency category.

Modified from Cornell RC, Stoughton RB: Correlation of the vasoconstriction assay and clinical activity in psoriasis. Arch Dermatol 1985;121:66, with permission.

makes them more drying than ointments. Table 66.4 lists some commonly available topical corticosteroids.

In severe, acute forms of psoriasis, and other inflammatory dermatoses, a patient may be instructed to apply a high-potency topical steroid every 2 hours for 24 to 48 hours, followed by application three or four times a day. For maintenance, application two to four times a day is adequate. Adverse reactions are of several types and common. Local tissue atrophy, degeneration, and striae are manifestations of steroid effect on collagen synthesis and fibroblast growth. If detected early, atrophy and striae may be reversible upon drug discontinuation, but in many cases of prolonged therapy with high-potency agents these changes may be permanent. Thinning of the epidermis may result in visible distended capillaries (telangiectasias) and purpura. Acneform eruptions and masking of symptoms of bacterial or fungal skin infections have been reported.

Systemic consequences of topical corticosteroid use include risk of suppression of the hypothalamic–pituitary–adrenal axis, hyperglycemia, and development of cushingoid features. Avoidance of prolonged therapy with high-potency agents minimizes the risk of these side effects. Tachyphylaxis and rebound flare of psoriasis after abrupt cessation of topical corticosteroid therapy can also occur. With proper monitoring, topical corticosteroids are a safe and effective adjunct to psoriasis treatment.

### Systemic Therapy–Photochemotherapy: Oral Psoralen and Long-Wave Ultraviolet A Light

The use of psoralens with ultraviolet A light (PUVA) has been studied since the early 1970s and was approved by FDA in 1982. Efficacy studies indicated that control of psoriasis occurred in nearly 90% of patients.[50]

Psoralens react with nucleic acids and intercalate between base pairs. When DNA is irradiated with long-wave ultraviolet light (320–400 nm, UVA), the psoralens covalently bind to pyrimidine bases forming a crosslink.[51] PUVA may also affect immune responses in the skin and circulating lymphocytes, as demonstrated by decreased ability to mount delayed hypersensitivity responses to contact sensitizers and increased risk of cutaneous cancer in treated patients.[52,53]

Candidates for PUVA therapy usually have severe incapacitating psoriasis unresponsive to topical therapies without history of photosensitivity, skin cancers, cataracts, or x-ray therapy of the skin. Methoxsalen (8-methoxypsoralen) is usually dosed at 0.6–0.8 mg/kg and is given 2 hours before exposure to UVA. Serum methoxsalen concentrations usually peak within 0.5 to 2 hours of ingestion; however, there is a large interindividual and intraindividual variation in absorption that may complicate titration of effective therapy.[54] Dosing of UVA is determined by patient skin type and history of previous response to ultraviolet radiation.

### Methotrexate

Methotrexate is indicated in the treatment of severe forms of psoriasis (e.g., psoriatic arthritis, erythrodermic psoriasis, pustular psoriasis, and extensive psoriasis) refractory to other therapy.[55] Methotrexate appears to act directly on the proliferating epidermal cells of psoriasis.[56] Through inhibition of the synthesis of thymidylate, one of the precursors to the DNA base pairs, cell division is halted. Biochemical inhibition by methotrexate is somewhat specific for cells in the S phase of the cell cycle; thus, its action is targeted against the majority of psoriatic cells found in this phase (six times normal).[56] Psoriatic cells may be more dependent on the thymidylate pathway and may further target the action of methotrexate to diseased skin.

Several dosage and administration regimens for methotrexate have been used in the treatment of psoriasis, but the "triple-dose" regimen is probably the most common.[56] This regimen involves oral methotrexate administration at 12-hour intervals for three doses to provide inhibition for the 36-hour cell cycle period in psoriasis. After a test dose of 2.5–5 mg, the patient is usually given 2.5 mg every 12 hours for three doses per week. This dose is increased by 2.5 mg per week to maximum effect and minimum toxicity.

As therapy is often prolonged, a baseline liver biopsy is recommended before treatment and at intervals of 1.0–1.5 g cumulative dose of methotrexate.[55] Leukocyte and platelet counts should be monitored every 4 weeks with hemoglobin, serum creatinine, aspartate and alanine transaminases, alkaline phosphatase, and urinalysis performed every 3 to 4 months.[55] A yearly chest x-ray film is also recommended.

Careful patient selection to exclude those with significant risk factors allows highly effective treatment of psoriasis with relatively low risk of toxicity.

### Etretinate

Etretinate is a derivative of vitamin A (retinol) that is effective in treating severe pustular and erythrodermic forms of psoriasis. Summaries of preliminary testing in the United States indicate that of 642 psoriatic patients treated with etretinate, 15% had clearing, 37% had greater than 75% clearing, 31% had 50% to 75% clearing, and 17% had unsatisfactory response.[57]

The mechanism of etretinate's effect on psoriasis is unknown. An antikeratinizing effect and an alteration of cell proliferation have been noted with decreased levels of polyamines.[58] Phosphorylation of proteins within erythrocyte membranes is altered in psoriatic patients and normalized with etretinate therapy. Doses of 1 mg/kg/d are used and are titrated to the lowest effective dose. Although the half-life of etretinate is approximately 12 hours, it appears to be stored in adipose tissue and may be detected in serum for a year after discontinuation.[58] The predominant active metabolite of etretinate, acitretin (etretin, Ro 10-1670), is minimally stored in fat and, therefore, much more rapidly excreted; however, it has a side effect profile similar to that of the parent compound.[59]

Peeling of palms and soles, softening of the nails, diffuse hair loss, and dryness of mucous membranes occur in patients taking etretinate. As with isotretinoin, etretinate therapy often results in an increase in serum triglycerides and cholesterol, with a lowering of high-density lipoprotein. Transient increases in aspartate and alanine transaminases and lactate dehydrogenase have been reported from etretinate therapy along with a few documented cases of hepatitis.[60,61] Careful patient selection and monitoring are essential for optimum results with etretinate therapy.

## Summary

Rational dermatologic therapy must be principled in the pathogenesis of the disorder. Major advances in recent years have allowed a better understanding of disease mechanisms and have produced a high level of interest in the field of dermatopharmacology.

Common skin disorders such as acne and psoriasis are excellent clinical models for demonstrating broad areas of potential pharmacologic intervention and therapeutic benefit. There are obviously many other common dermatologic disorders where these same principles apply.

## Glossary: Skin Lesion Types

**Atrophy.** Usually denotes decrease in thickness of the skin or a depression (hypotrophic), or a nodular-like scarring reaction (hypertrophic). Repeated insulin injections may cause lipoatrophy.

**Bulla.** An elevated fluid-filled lesion greater than 1 cm. These "large blisters" may be tense or flaccid to palpation.

**Crust.** Dried exudate on top of a lesion. Exudate may be thin or thick and red, yellow, or brown in color.

**Cyst.** Similar to a tumor or nodule but saclike, containing either fluid or solid material. A cyst is usually not transparent as is a vesicle or bulla. Cysts are common lesions in severe acne.

**Erosion.** A superficial denuded area of skin (small ulcer). Unlike an ulcer, an erosion usually damages the epidermis only.

**Excoriation.** An abrasion of the skin caused by mechanical means. Excoriations may be caused by trauma from fingernails and may result in exudate and crusting.

**Fissure.** A linear break in the skin through the epidermis to the dermis.

**Lichenification.** A raised flat lesion, often with transverse ridges and leatherlike texture from long-term rubbing or scratching. Lichenification is a common sign in several forms of dermatitis.

**Macule.** A flat lesion (in the plane of the skin) denoted by a change in normal skin color. Usually well circumscribed with distinct outline and no elevation or depression of skin (e.g., a "freckle" is a macule).

**Nodule.** Usually an elevated, rounded lesion like a papule but larger than 1 cm in diameter.

**Papule.** An elevated solid lesion less than 1 cm in diameter (pea-sized). Like a pea, the surface may be smooth or rough, soft or firm. Papules may consist of superficial skin "debris" and may range in color from red and yellow to black.

**Patch.** May also be a macule but usually implies an area larger than 1 cm.

**Plaque.** An elevated patch but usually larger than 1 cm in diameter and "flat"-topped. Plaques may sometimes consist of many papules grouped together.

**Purpura.** Extravasation of blood through vessel walls (e.g., bruise). Purpuric lesions the size of pinpoints are known as petechiae. Lesions greater than 2 cm in diameter are called ecchymoses.

**Pustule.** An elevated, round, well-circumscribed lesion filled with pus. It may be used to describe an inflamed papule. Pustules contain cellular debris of yellow, green, or white color and may occur around follicles.

**Scale.** Overaccumulation of loose epidermal cells. Scale may be white, yellow, or brown, shiny or dull, and dry or greasy.

**Telangiectasia.** A permanent enlargement in the caliber (and usually an increase in the number) of capillaries near the surface of the skin. Telangiectasias appear as outlines of vessels through the skin and usually blanche (turn white) when pressure is applied.

**Tumor.** A description used to define size and not malignancy. A tumor is usually an elevated round lesion greater than 2–3 cm in diameter.

**Ulcer.** Destruction of the skin down to the dermis. Ulcers may be any size or shape, but depth is an important criterion.

**Vesicle.** An elevated lesion that is less than 1 cm in diameter, filled with clear, red, or yellow fluid, and well circumscribed. An example of a vesicle is a blister formed via the cleavage between layers of skin.

**Wheal.** Similar to a plaque (elevated, round, or flat topped, red or pink) but edematous and pruritic. Urticaria (hives) are examples of wheals that persist about 24 hours.

## References


1. Johnson M-L, Johnson KG, Engel A. Prevalence, morbidity, and cost of dermatologic diseases. J Am Acad Dermatol 1984; 11:930–936.
2. Shalita AR, Freinkel RK. Acne. J Am Acad Dermatol 1984;11: 957–959.
3. Solomon JA, Pochi PE. Acne vulgaris, in Stone J (ed): Dermatologic Immunology and Allergy 1985. St. Louis, C.V. Mosby, pp 649–660.
4. Pochi PE. Hormonal therapy of acne. Dermatol Clin 1983; 1:377–384.
5. Shalita AR. Acne vulgaris: Current concepts in pathogenesis and treatment. Int J Dermatol 1976;15:182–187.
6. Melski JW, Arndt KA. Topical therapy for acne. N Engl J Med 1980;302:503–506.
7. Arndt KA. Acne, in Manual of Dermatologic Therapeutics, 3rd ed. Boston, Little Brown and Company, 1983.
8. Eaglstein WH. Allergic contact dermatitis to benzoyl peroxide. Arch Dermatol 1968;97:527.
9. Thomas JR III, Doya JA. The therapeutic uses of topical vitamin A acid. J Am Acad Dermatol 1981;4:505–513.
10. Hurwitz S. The combined effect of vitamin A acid and benzoyl peroxide in the treatment of acne. Cutis 1976;17:585–590.
11. Franz TJ. On the bioavailability of topical formulations of clindamycin hydrochloride. J Am Acad Dermatol 1983;9:66–73.
12. Eady EA, Holland KT, Cunliffe NJ. Should topical antibiotics be used for the treatment of acne vulgaris? Br J Dermatol 1982; 107:235–246.
13. Eady EA, Holland KT, Cunliffe WJ. The use of antibiotics in acne therapy: Oral or topical administration? J Antimicrob Chemother 1982;10:89–115.
14. Becker LE, Bergstresser PR, Whiting DA, et al. Topical clindamycin therapy for acne vulgaris. Arch Dermatol 1981;117: 482–485.
15. Parry MF, Rha CK. Pseudomembranous colitis caused by topical clindamycin phosphate. Arch Dermatol 1986;122:583–594.
16. Ad Hoc Committee on the Use of Antibiotics in Dermatology. Systemic antibiotics for treatment of acne vulgaris, efficacy and safety. Arch Dermatol 1975;111:1630–1636.
17. Gammon WR, Meyer C, Lantis S, et al. Comparative efficacy of oral erythromycin versus oral tetracycline in the treatment of acne vulgaris. J Am Acad Dermatol 1986;14:183–186.
18. Jonas M, Cunha BA. Minocycline. Ther Drug Monit 1982;4: 137–145.
19. Nordin K, Hallander H, Fredriksson T, et al. A clinical and bacteriological evaluation of the effect of sulphamethoxazole–trimethoprim in acne vulgaris, resistant to prior therapy with tetracyclines. Dermatologica 1978;157:245–253.
20. Hansten PD, Horn JR. Inhibition of oral contraceptive efficacy. Drug Interactions Newslett 1985;5(2):7–10.
21. Rumsfield JA, West DP, Tse CST, et al. Isotretinoin in severe, recalcitrant cystic acne: A review. Drug Intell Clin Pharm 1983; 17:329–333.
22. Shalita AR, Cunningham WJ, Leyden JJ, et al. Isotretinoin treatment of acne and related disorders: An update. J Am Acad Dermatol 1983;9:629–638.
23. Anonymous. Adverse effects with isotretinoin. FDA Drug Bull 1983;13:21–23.
24. Krueger GG, Bergstresser PR, Lowe NJ, et al. Psoriasis. J Am Acad Dermatol 1984;11:937–947.
25. Watson W. Psoriasis: Epidemiology and genetics. Dermatol Clin 1984;2:363–371.
26. Farber EM, Nail ML. The natural history of psoriasis in 5,600 patients. Dermatologica 1974;148:1–18.
27. Weinstein GD, McCullough JL, Ross PA. Cell kinetic basis of pathophysiology of psoriasis. J Invest Dermatol 1985;85:579–583.
28. Baden HP. Biology of the epidermis and pathophysiology of psoriasis and certain ichthyosiform dermatoses, in Soter NA, Baden HP (eds): Pathophysiology of dermatologic diseases. New York, McGraw-Hill, 1984, pp 101–126.
29. Krueger GG. Psoriasis: Current concepts of its etiology and pathogenesis, in Dobson RL, Thiers BH (eds): Yearbook of Dermatology. Chicago, Yearbook Medical Publishers, 1981.
30. Russell TJ, Schultes LM, Kuban DJ. Histocompatibility (HL-A) antigens associated with psoriasis. N Engl J Med 1972;287:738–740.
31. Nyfors A, Lemholt K. Psoriasis in children: A short review and a survey of 245 cases. Br J Dermatol 1975;92:437–442.
32. Whyte HJ, Baughman RD. Acute guttate psoriasis and streptococcal infection. Arch Dermatol 1964;89:350–356.
33. Skoven I, Thormann J. Lithium compound treatment and psoriasis. Arch Dermatol 1979;115:1185–1187.
34. Neumann HAM, van Joost T. Adverse reactions of the skin to metoprolol and other beta-adrenoreceptor-blocking agents. Dermatologica 1981;162:330–335.
35. Marks R. Topical therapy for psoriasis: General principles. Dermatol Clin 1984;2:383–388.
36. Weirich EG. Dermatopharmacology of salicylic acid. I: Range of dermatotherapeutic effects of salicylic acid. Dermatologica 1975;151:268–273.
37. Davies MG, Briffa DV, Greaves MW. Systemic toxicity from topically applied salicylic acid. Br Med J 1979;1:661.
38. Lin AN, Moses K. Tar revisited. Int J Dermatol 1985;24:216–218.
39. Polano MK. Topical skin therapeutics. London, Churchill Livingstone, 1984, p 95.
40. Lavker RM, Grove GL, Kligman AM. The atrophogenic effect of crude coal tar on human epidermis. Br J Dermatol 1981;105: 77–82.
41. Lowe NJ, Breeding J, Wortzman MS. The pharmacological variability of crude coal tar. Br J Dermatol 1982;107:475–479.
42. Ashton RE, Andre P, Lowe NJ, et al. Anthralin: Historical and current perspectives. J Am Acad Dermatol 1983;9:173–192.
43. Swanbeck G, Thyresson N. Interaction between dithranol and nucleic acids. Acta Derm Venereol (Stockh) 1965;45:344–348.
44. Barr RM, Misch KJ, Hensby CN, et al. Arachidonic acid and prostaglandin levels in dithranol erythema: Time course study. Br J Clin Pharmacol 1983;16:715–717.
45. Finnen MJ, Lawrence CM, Shuster S. Inhibition of dithranol inflammation by free-radical scavengers. Lancet 1984;2:1129–1130.
46. Gorsulowsky DC, Voorhees JJ, Ellis CN. Anthralin therapy for

psoriasis: A new look at an old compound. Arch Dermatol 1985; 121:1509–1511.

47. Cornell RC, Stoughton RB. The use of topical steroids in psoriasis. Dermatol Clin 1984;2:397–409.
48. Hammarstrom S, Hamberg M, Duell EA, et al. Glucocorticoid in inflammatory proliferative skin disease reduces arachidonic and hydroxyeicosatetraenoic acids. Science 1977;197:994–996.
49. Burdick KH, Haleblian JK, Poulsen BJ, et al. Corticosteroid ointments: Comparison by two human bioassays. Curr Ther Res 1973;15:233–242.
50. Bickers DR. Position paper—PUVA therapy. J Am Acad Dermatol 1983;8:265–270.
51. Cole RS. Light-induced crosslinking of DNA in the presence of a furocoumarin (psoralen). Biochem Biophys Acta 1970;217:30–39.
52. Thorvaldsen J, Volden G. PUVA-induced diminution of contact allergic and irritant skin reactions. Clin Exp Dermatol 1980;5:43–46.
53. Elmets CA, Bergstresser PR. Ultraviolet radiation effects on immune processes. Photochem Photobiol 1982;36:715–719.
54. Goldstein DP, Carter DM, Ljunggren B, et al. Minimal phototoxic doses and 8-MOP plasma levels in PUVA patients. Invest Dermatol 1982;78:429–433.
55. Roenigk HH, Auerbauch R, Maibach HI, et al. Methotrexate guidelines revised. J Am Acad Dermatol 1982;6:145–155.
56. Weinstein GD. Chemotherapy for psoriasis. Dermatol Clin 1984;2:431–438.
57. Dicken CH. Retinoids: A review. J Am Acad Dermatol 1984;11:541–552.
58. Ellis CN, Grekin RC, Kragtalle K, et al. Retinoids, in Stone J (ed): Dermatologic Immunology and Allergy. St. Louis, C.V. Mosby, 1985, pp 851–876.
59. Kingston TP, Matt LH, Lowe NJ. Etretin therapy for severe psoriasis. Arch Dermatol 1987;123:55–58.
60. Weiss VC, Layden T, Spinowitz A, et al. Chronic active hepatitis associated with etretinate therapy. Br J Dermatol 1985;112:591–597.
61. Weiss VC, West DP, Ackerman R, et al. Hepatotoxic reactions in a patient treated with etretinate. Arch Dermatol 1984;120:104–106.

# Chapter 67 / Drug-Induced Skin Diseases

Jean A. Rumsfield, PharmD, and Dennis P. West, MS, FCCP

Skin reactions to medications occur in approximately 2% to 3% of medical inpatients.[1] Skin rash is a frequent reason for patient visits to physicians.[2] Establishment of a relationship between medication use and subsequent development of cutaneous reactions, however, is often difficult. Unfortunately, mechanisms underlying adverse drug reactions are poorly understood and few diagnostic tests are available to properly establish cause and effect. Patients with cutaneous reactions are often taking more than one drug, making detection of the causative agent difficult. The picture is further complicated because small doses of a drug may evoke severe reactions even if that agent was previously well tolerated.[3]

## Drug History

A thorough and organized approach is essential to proper diagnosis of a drug-induced skin reaction. Patient evaluation should include (1) a comprehensive drug history, (2) awareness of the various clinical manifestations of drug allergy and cutaneous reactions, (3) awareness of the factors that favor the development of allergic reactions to drugs, and (4) awareness of the immunologic and nonimmunologic mechanisms involved in cutaneous reactions to drugs.[4,5]

Although several in vitro and in vivo tests have been used to diagnose drug allergy, the availability and reliability of these tests are limited. Patch testing, useful in determining contact dermatitis, has limited applications in drug allergy, particularly in delayed hypersensitivity reactions, fixed-drug eruptions, and toxic epidermal necrolysis.[6] Scratch or prick testing with drugs and/or metabolites may be useful in type I reactions (i.e., penicillin allergy) although there are practical limitations to this method. The in vitro radioallergosorbent test (RAST) may be used to detect IgE or IgG antibodies and has produced the most reliable results in detecting penicillin allergy.[6] The modified Coombs test and bacteriophage inhibition test have even higher sensitivity for detecting IgG and IgE antibodies, although more elaborate laboratory resources are required.[6]

The lymphocyte transformation test is considered the most reliable in vitro test for diagnosis of both immediate and delayed drug reactions, but results appear to depend on the type of drug or type of skin eruption.[6] Dechallenge/rechallenge continues to be regarded as the most definitive method in ascertaining drug-induced reactions. It is often not an option if a patient has experienced a potentially life-threatening reaction or if the suspected agent cannot be discontinued. In some cases, rechallenge may not result in the same reaction and further clouds the picture.

A patient may experience a skin reaction while on multiple drugs. Most authorities advise that the first drug(s) to consider is that initiated within the week preceding the reaction. This short temporal relationship does not hold for all drugs (e.g., onset perhaps 2 weeks after discontinuation of semisynthetic penicillins, onset perhaps 6 months for $\beta$-blocker–induced psoriasiform eruptions, onset of 2 months to perhaps 5 years for drug-induced systemic lupus erythematosus).[7] Each drug should be individually considered as a potential cause.

*A Guide to Drug Eruptions*[8] is updated at 4-year intervals and is a useful source of information on drug-induced skin reactions. The tables in this chapter are not all-inclusive, and consultation of additional, more recently updated resources is encouraged. With an increased number of drugs undergoing shorter premarketing phases, a greater number of skin reactions are expected to occur during postmarketing surveillance. The pharmacist plays an important role in identifying possible drug-induced skin reactions and in monitoring or preventing recurrence.

## Clinical Presentation

It is important to recognize the clinical manifestations of a drug allergy. Symptoms of an allergic drug reaction usually have an acute onset, may last several minutes to months, or may occur periodically throughout an exposure period. An accurate description of the characteristics of a cutaneous drug reaction should be obtained. Although drug hypersensitivity is impossible to predict, certain drug and host factors increase the likelihood of a reaction.

Drug allergy is more frequent in older individuals[9] and may be related to the development of the immune response and to increased exposure to drugs.

Individual genetic factors may also predispose an individual to drug allergy: differences in drug metabolism, differences in immune response, differences in tissue receptor sites, differences in elaboration of immunologic mediators.[10]

In addition, a previous history of allergic reactions may increase the risk of development of an allergic reaction. Hepatic and renal disorders may alter drug metabolism and provoke an allergic response.[11]

To induce an immune response (i.e., hypersensitivity reaction), the drug or its metabolite must act as, or form, a complete antigen. For example, proteins contained in sera, vaccines, biologicals, and allergens may act as complete antigens; however, most drugs are small molecules and must bind with larger molecules to create a complete antigen. Haptens are drugs capable of this. Once a complete antigen is formed, the immune system reacts to neutralize, destroy, or eliminate it from the host.

The route of administration may influence drug allergy. For example, topical application of drugs has the greatest propensity to induce allergy, followed by the intravenous route and the oral route. Although not strictly dose related, such factors as the number of drugs, the dose of drug, and the duration of therapy may influence the likelihood of developing a hypersensitivity reaction.[10]

The host's ability to react to antigenic material is the basis for specific immune reactions. The ultimate physiologic role of the immune system is to differentiate "self" from "nonself" and eliminate foreign materials from the body. The type of immunologic mediation of hypersensitivity determines the category of reaction and thus the clinical presentation of drug-induced skin disorders.

## Classification of Hypersensitivity Reactions

Allergy is defined as altered immunologic reactivity to an antigen that results in pathologic reactivity. Potential antigens (e.g., foreign materials, haptens, or altered host material) induce immune reactivity manifested by production of reactive antibodies or sensitized lymphocytes capable of reacting with the antigen. Hypersensitivity reactions were originally classified by Gell and Coombs[12] into four main clinical types: type I — anaphylactic, type II — cytotoxic, type III — immune complex mediated, and type IV — cell mediated. A fifth type is described by Roitt[13] as an antibody-mediated stimulation injury. The most frequently occurring are types I and IV.

### *Type I*

A type I reaction is an immediate hypersensitivity. It occurs when a specific antibody (IgE) to an antigen is formed and attaches to a mast cell or basophil. On reexposure, an interaction between the attached antibody and antigen occurs, resulting in degranulation of the mast cell or basophil and release of pharmacologically active mediators. Table 67.1 lists drugs frequently implicated in type I reactions.

These mediators (e.g., histamine, serotonin, slow-reacting substance A [SRS-A], and vasoactive amines) cause increased capillary dilatation and permeability, bronchospasm, and vasoconstriction. The clotting mechanism may be activated by consumption of several components (including fibrinolysins).

Tissue and organs with high concentrations of mast cells (e.g., skin, mucous membranes of the gastrointestinal tract and respiratory system, and bronchial smooth muscle) are more frequently involved. Anaphylactic shock, the more severe form of type I reaction, involves several organs.

Clinical manifestations of type I reactions relate to local mediator effects and the exposed area. For example, upper respiratory tract symptoms may include sinus headache, itching of eyes, tearing, sneezing, watery nasal discharge, itching of nose, and throat irritation. These symptoms may occur within minutes of oral administration or inhalation of drug particles. Symptoms are often diagnosed as allergic rhinitis or conjunctivitis. Lung involvement may include the asthmalike symptoms of wheezing, dyspnea, dry cough, and tightness in the chest.

**Table 67.1** Drugs Frequently Implicated in Type I Hypersensitivity Reactions

| |
|---|
| Adrenocorticotropic hormone |
| Aminopyrine |
| Bromsulphalein |
| Cephalosporins |
| Chymotrypsin |
| Heparin |
| Insulin |
| Meprobamate |
| Penicillins |
| Penicillinase |
| Procaine |
| Salicylates |
| Streptomycin |
| Sulfonamides |
| Tetracyclines |

Compiled from References 14–18.

Oral use of a drug may lead to symptoms affecting primarily the gastrointestinal tract, including glossitis, cardiospasm, nausea, vomiting, irritable bowel, diarrhea, steatorrhea, and possible hemorrhage. The causative agent may be the drug or the additives used to maintain drug stability or provide color.

Skin involvement is one of the most common manifestations of a type I hypersensitivity reaction. Clinical symptoms may include urticaria, pruritus, angioedema, weeping, erythema, and vesicopapular lesions. If these symptoms occur shortly after drug administration, a type I hypersensitivity reaction should be suspected.

Treatment should be individualized according to the particular drug involved, route of administration, organ system or tissue involved, severity of reaction, and clinical signs and symptoms. Treatment may require drugs that block mediator effects (e.g., antihistamines), drugs that reverse or counteract mediator effects (e.g., adrenergic agents), and drugs that inhibit mediator secretion (e.g., theophylline and corticosteroids). Another approach is to prevent the reaction by inducing hyposensitization. Using this mechanism, the immune system develops blocking antibodies (IgG) that bind allergen and thus prevent binding to mast cells. This technique has been used in patients allergic to penicillin.

### *Type II*

Type II reactions are cytotoxic and include such clinical conditions as hemolytic anemia, agranulocytosis, thrombocytopenia, and vascular endothelium disorders.

Antigen or hapten attaches to some component of the target cell; for example, in the vascular system, the target may be an erythrocyte, a leukocyte, a thrombocyte, or endothelium of the vessel wall. Specific antibodies (IgG or IgM) then react to antigenic constituents of the cell or to an antigen that is bound to the cell, causing activation of complement. Activated complement, a complex group of serum proteins, increases capillary permeability, causes chemotaxis, and promotes phagocytosis by polymorphonuclear leukocytes (PMNs), resulting in the release of cellular enzymes causing cytotoxic or cytolytic injury to the cell.

**Table 67.2** Drugs Frequently Implicated in Type II Hypersensitivity Reactions (Vascular Endothelium)

| | |
|---|---|
| Chlorpromazine | Phenytoin |
| Iodides | Propylthiouracil |
| Penicillins | Quinidine |
| Phenylbutazone | Sulfonamides |

Compiled from References 4, 17, and 19.

Clinical manifestations depend upon the target cells involved and the severity of the reaction depends on the degree of immunologic destruction of target cells. For example, whether erythrocytes, leukocytes, thrombocytes, or vascular endothelium is involved, the cytotoxic/cytolytic effects are similar and result in hemolytic anemia, agranulocytosis, thrombocytopenic purpura, or vascular purpura, respectively. Although cytotoxic mechanisms have not been clearly established for cutaneous drug reactions, the drugs most frequently implicated in purpura and other hemorrhagic lesions are listed in Table 67.2. Treatment includes discontinuation of the offending agent and management of clinical manifestations.

### *Type III*

Type III reactions are known to be immune complex mediated (e.g., Arthus reaction and serum sickness). Table 67.3 lists drugs that cause type III reactions.

Immune complexes are formed when antigen binds to antibody (usually IgM or IgG). Rather than being cleared from the circulation by phagocytosis, these complexes deposit on target tissues and in vascular endothelium. Complement is activated, leading to chemotaxis of neutrophils; protein-digesting enzymes (lysozymes) are released, causing tissue injury. The type and severity of reaction depend on quantity of immunoreactive complexes, location, and presence of vasoactive amines.

The Arthus reaction occurs as a local reaction, with hemorrhagic necrosis often occurring at the site of injection within 12 to 24 hours. This reaction usually involves large amounts of antigen in the target tissue and circulating antibodies that interact to cause complement activation resulting in localized tissue damage.

A serum sickness reaction is caused by circulating antigen–antibody complexes that penetrate the walls of blood vessels and deposit in the basement membrane. Complement is then fixed and activated. The result is a systemic reaction that involves highly vascular target organs (e.g., kidney). Penicillin is the most common cause of serum sickness, although the frequency of serum sickness is relatively rare.

Clinical features include pruritus, arthralgias with periarticular edema, angioedema, low-grade fever, enlarged lymph nodes, and urticarial or maculopapular rash. The onset of symptoms may be a few hours (for the accelerated type) to 3 weeks after drug exposure. Laboratory determinations are generally not diagnostic. Hypergammaglobulinemia and elevated erythrocyte sedimentation rate are commonly noted.

Treatment is generally accomplished with antihistamines and analgesics to control the symptomatic complaints of pruritus and pain. If the reaction is severe, short-term oral corticosteroid therapy may be beneficial.

**Table 67.3** Drugs Frequently Implicated in Type III Hypersensitivity Reactions

| |
|---|
| Adrenocorticotropic hormone |
| Arsenicals |
| Azathioprine |
| Barbiturates |
| Bismuth |
| Dextran–iron complex |
| Digitalis |
| Erythromycin |
| Griseofulvin |
| Heparin |
| Insulin |
| Iodides |
| Iodinated-radiocontrast media |
| Isoniazid |
| Nitrofurantoin |
| Penicillins |
| Phenolphthalein |
| Phenylbutazone |
| Phenytoin |
| Probenecid |
| Procainamide |
| Propylthiouracil |
| Quinidine |
| Quinine |
| Salicylates |
| Streptomycin |
| Sulfonamides |
| Tripelennamine |
| Vaccines |
| Viomycin |

Compiled from References 14, 16, and 19.

### *Type IV*

Type IV reactions are commonly known as cell-mediated reactions. The pathogenesis for allergic contact dermatitis has been established, but the mechanism of generalized cell-mediated reactions (''delayed'' hypersensitivity) has not been determined.

In classical allergic contact dermatitis, a complete antigen is produced by binding haptens to various proteins in skin. Amino and sulfhydryl groups of cystine and cysteine are known binding sites for haptens. The same allergen may conjugate with more than one type of protein. Thus, a clinical reaction may actually represent combined responses to simultaneous binding of multiple haptens and multiple proteins.

When T lymphocytes are exposed to allergen, there is blast transformation and proliferation of the clone of ''sensitized'' cells, as well as ''elicitation'' or release of lymphokines. Drugs frequently implicated in type IV hypersensitivity reactions are listed in Table 67.4.

Clinical features of type IV reactions include eczematous dermatitis. Symptoms of acute contact dermatitis include papulovesiculation, erythema, and edema. Chronically, the skin may show scaling, erythema, lichenification, and hypopigmentation or hyperpigmentation.

**Table 67.4** Drugs Frequently Implicated in Type IV Hypersensitivity Reactions

| |
|---|
| Benzyl alcohol |
| Chromate compounds |
| Ethylenediamine compounds |
| Formaldehyde |
| Lanolin |
| Mercury derivatives (merthiolate, mercurochrome, thimerosal) |
| Neomycin |
| Nickel |
| *para*-Aminobenzoic acid compounds (local anesthetics such as benzocaine) |
| Parabens |
| Peru balsam |
| Phenylenediamine compounds |

Compiled from References 14, 16, 17, and 20.

Treatment, as well as prevention, includes avoidance of the allergen. Topical corticosteroids, compresses, and antipruritic systemic and/or topical agents are commonly used.

### *Nonimmunologic Drug Reactions*

Nonimmunologic cutaneous reactions to drugs may be more common than immunologic allergic reactions.[21] Mechanisms of nonimmunologic cutaneous reactions include direct activation of effector pathways, cumulative toxicity or overdose, secondary side effects, drug interactions, metabolic changes, and exacerbation of preexisting dermatologic conditions. Drugs may cause release of mast cell contents by direct contact, resulting in clinical symptoms such as urticaria. Agents that cause physical degranulation of mast cells (without IgE antibody production) include opiates, polymyxin B, hydralazine, and iodinated-radiocontrast media. Drugs may also activate complement in the absence of antibody.[21] This may be a common mechanism in urticaria induced by iodinated-radiocontrast media.[21]

Anaphylaxis from aspirin and nonsteroidal anti-inflammatory agents may be caused by inhibition of cyclooxygenase and alteration of arachidonic acid metabolism.[21] Cumulative toxicity may result from deposition of drugs or metabolites in the skin. Pigmentation changes from prolonged use of silver, mercury, gold, or chlorpromazine are examples of cumulative toxicity. Reversible hair loss after administration of chemotherapeutic agents is an example of a secondary side effect of a drug. Alteration in normal flora permitting overgrowth of an organism (i.e., candidiasis during administration of a broad-spectrum antibiotic) is an example of an ecologic disturbance mechanism. Drugs may also exacerbate a preexisting dermatologic disease, as when $\beta$-blocking agents induce psoriasiform dermatitis.

## Patterns of Cutaneous Reactions

As any drug may induce cutaneous reactivity, a complete review of drug-induced skin reactions is not possible; however, an in-depth description of common cutaneous drug reactions, clinical course, possible mechanisms, etiologies, and management is presented. Maculopapular reactions and urticaria are the most common types.

### *Maculopapular Eruptions*

Macular or maculopapular skin reactions are common drug-induced skin eruptions. Morbilliform, exanthematous, scarlatiniform, or rubellaform are common morphologic descriptions of maculopapular eruptions. Such reactions often start on the trunk or in areas of pressure or trauma and are frequently symmetrical. Flat or raised, reddened lesions, varying from a few millimeters to confluent large areas, are characteristic, but vesicles may be present. Involvement of mucous membranes or palms and soles is variable and infrequent; mild fever may also accompany the reaction.[21]

The course of a maculopapular eruption is variable and may be classified as an "early" or "late" reaction.[8] In an early reaction, the eruption appears within 2 to 3 days of drug administration in previously sensitized patients. Sensitization may occur without symptoms or rash because drug fever (or elevated temperature), for example, often goes unnoticed. Also, fever may be a symptom of the disease for which the drug is being prescribed.[8] The "late" reaction appears approximately 9 days after drug exposure, although with previous sensitization the onset may be quicker. Because of individual patient differences, reactions may occur any time from the first day of exposure to 2 weeks after therapy. A maculopapular rash usually fades a few days after discontinuation of the causative agent. Occasionally, eruptions decrease or disappear even with continued medication use and may not always recur with drug rechallenge.[21]

The variable and unpredictable course of maculopapular eruptions makes identification of the mechanism or pathogenesis difficult. A hypersensitivity reaction, possibly secondary to cell-mediated allergy, has been suggested by skin testing, lymphocyte transformation, and macrophage-migration inhibition tests.[6] The fact that these tests are positive in a small portion of patients with maculopapular eruptions suggests the likelihood of a different mechanism. Immune complex reactions have also been suggested.[6] Although definitive cause-and-effect relationships have been established for the penicillins, many other drugs have been associated with maculopapular eruptions (see Table 67.5).

Serologic tests rarely establish a diagnosis of drug-induced delayed hypersensitivity; thus, patient history may often be the only diagnostic clue. Maculopapular rashes generally do not persist for prolonged periods, although recurrence may present as more serious and extensive exfoliative skin reactions.[6]

### *Urticaria*

Urticarial lesions consist of raised, pruritic erythematous wheals (hives) ranging in size from a few millimeters to "geographic" lesions extending over the chest or trunk. The raised edematous and plaquelike features of these lesions may result from localized vasodilation and transudation of fluid from small cutaneous blood vessels. This edematous response is induced by degranulation of mast cells in the dermis, causing release of histamine and other mediators of inflammation. The causes of mast cell degranulation are

**Table 67.5** Drugs Commonly Associated With Maculopapular Eruptions

| |
|---|
| Allopurinol |
| Barbiturates |
| Benzodiazepines |
| Carbamazepine |
| Chloramphenicol |
| Erythromycin |
| Ethionamide |
| Gold salts |
| Hydantoin derivatives |
| Ibuprofen |
| Indomethacin |
| Isoniazid |
| Nitrofurantoin |
| Penicillins |
| Penicillamine |
| Phenothiazines |
| Phenylbutazone |
| Piroxicam |
| Pyrazolon derivatives |
| Rifampin |
| Streptomycin |
| Sulfonamides (including sulfonylureas and thiazide diuretics) |
| Sulindac |
| Tetracyclines |
| Tolmetin |

Compiled from Reference 8.

numerous and not limited to drugs (foods, allergens, infection, heat, and cold are examples). Drugs frequently associated with urticaria are listed in Table 67.6.

Drug-induced urticaria may be caused by IgE-dependent, circulating immune complexes or by nonimmunologic activation of effector pathways.[21] In IgE-dependent reactions the drug (antigen) forms a bridge between the IgE molecule and the surface of the mast cell, resulting in degranulation and liberation of histamine. Clinically, urticarial lesions may appear within minutes to hours of drug exposure in a sensitized patient; this is termed an *immediate reaction*. Reactions that occur within 12 to 36 hours of drug exposure are called *accelerated reactions*. In some cases, urticarial lesions may be the first manifestation of anaphylaxis; thus, close monitoring is indicated.

Hypersensitivity that is established during administration of the drug with symptoms not appearing until 8 to 21 days after exposure is termed a *late reaction*. Other symptoms that may accompany urticaria in late reactions include fever, lymphadenopathy, joint swelling, and arthralgias.

Some drugs do not require an allergic mechanism to induce urticaria. Certain amines may displace histamine from intracellular storage sites, while other drugs directly degranulate mast cells through complement or arachidonic acid–dependent pathways.[8,21] Examples include acetylsalicylic acid, atropine, opiates, quinine, thiamine, pilocarpine, iodinated-radiocontrast dyes, and nonsteroidal anti-inflammatory agents. Drug concentrations may play a role in the appearance of these reactions.

The course of acute urticaria is variable, but the condition usually resolves within 1 to 3 days. Chronic urticaria has a more prolonged, sometimes indefinite course. For example, it may be stimulated from penicillin found in dairy products or by molds within the environment.[6] Identification of the causative agent in urticaria may be difficult when multiple drugs and exposures to foodstuffs and environmental allergens are considered. Appropriate management depends on the severity of symptoms and the ability to identify and remove the offending agent. Recent reports indicate that the tricyclic antidepressant doxepin may block $H_1$ and $H_2$ receptors and may be effective in patients with chronic urticaria.[23] Topical agents other than mild antipruritic agents are not necessary and topical antihistamines (used for local anesthetic effect) are best avoided because of their high incidence of contact sensitization.[24]

**Table 67.6** Drugs Frequently Associated With Urticaria

| | |
|---|---|
| Acetylsalicylic acid | Opiates |
| Gold | Penicillins |
| Heparin | Sulfonamides |
| Ibuprofen | Sulindac |
| Indomethacin | Tartrazine |
| Iodinated-radiocontrast media | Tolmetin |
| Naproxen | |

Compiled from References 8 and 22.

### *Fixed-Drug Eruptions*

The fixed-drug eruption is the only cutaneous reaction for which drugs or chemicals are considered the sole cause (see Table 67.7). A fixed-drug eruption consists of an erythematous round or oval lesion ranging from a few millimeters to 20 cm in diameter.[8] Initially, one lesion appears; other lesions may subsequently occur. With time the color turns to a dusky-red or violaceous hue. The lesion may also be edematous with formation of vesicles or bullae. The patient may complain of itching in the affected area, but sensations of warmth or burning are more common without additional systemic symptoms. Lesions may appear on any part of the skin or mucous membranes, although the lips and genitalia are more commonly affected.[25] Healing occurs over 7 to 10 days after discontinuation of the offending agent and often leaves a dark hyperpigmented patch. Reexposure to the offending drug results in recurrence of the eruption (within 30 minutes to 8 hours) in the exact location as the previous reaction.[25] The recurrence after rechallenge in the same site led to the label "fixed-drug eruption."

The pathogenesis of fixed-drug eruption is not well understood. In some cases, topical application of the drug to the affected area will reexacerbate the reaction.[25]

Usually, a single drug is responsible for a fixed-drug eruption, although some patients react to multiple agents (especially when the compounds are chemically related).[25] Diagnosis may be established by biopsy. The drug should not be readministered as extensive bullous lesions may occur.[8] The use of systemic corticosteroids or antihistamines has no apparent effect on the course of fixed-drug eruptions.[25]

**Table 67.7** Drugs That Frequently Produce Fixed-Drug Eruptions

| | |
|---|---|
| Barbiturates | Ibuprofen |
| Dapsone | Ipecac |
| Digitalis compounds | Metronidazole |
| Diphenhydramine | Phenolphthalein |
| Disulfiram | Phenothiazines |
| Epinephrine | Phenylbutazone |
| Erythromycin | Quinidine |
| Gold | Sulfonamides |
| Griseofulvin | Sulindac |
| Hydralazine | Tetracyclines |
| Hydroxyurea | Trimethoprim |

Compiled from References 8, 22, and 25.

**Table 67.8** Drugs That Frequently Produce Photosensitivity Reactions

| | |
|---|---|
| Amiodarone | Piroxicam |
| Carbamazepine | Protriptyline |
| Dacarbazine | Quinidine |
| Furosemide | Sulfonamides |
| Ketoprofen | Sulfonylureas |
| Naproxen | Sulindac |
| Oral contraceptives | Tetracyclines |
| Phenothiazines/chlorpromazine | Thiazides |
| Phenylbutazone | |

Compiled from References 6, 8, 22, and 27.

### *Photosensitivity*

Sun- and drug-induced cutaneous reactions are increasingly more common, not only because of increased use of tanning booths and emphasis on tanning, but also because of the increased number of photosensitizing chemicals in cosmetics and drugs. Clinically, photosensitivity reactions appear very similar to a sunburn and may include erythema; edema; papules; and plaquelike and, perhaps, urticarial lesions, sometimes with vesicle formation. The hallmark of photosensitivity eruptions is their appearance on areas of skin receiving the greatest exposure to sunlight (e.g., the tops of the ears, nose, cheeks, lateral and lower posterior surfaces of the neck, extensor surfaces of the forearms, and dorsa of the hands).[8] In some cases, the eruption may extend to non–sun-exposed areas and generalize over the body.[26] Chronically, reactions may become hyperpigmented or hypopigmented, perhaps atrophic and with yellowish papules as well as telangiectasias.

Phototoxic and photoallergic reactions are two different types of photosensitivity conditions that are often difficult to differentiate. Phototoxic reactions are the most common and depend on the dose of drug and the amount of sunlight. A phototoxic reaction occurs in 100% of those exposed to adequate amounts of drug and sunlight on first exposure to such stimuli. The drug or metabolite is thought to act as a chromophore, absorbing ultraviolet light (usually longwave). The ultraviolet light activates the drug or metabolite to emit energy that may damage adjacent tissue. The wavelength of light needed to produce a reaction is dependent on the absorption spectrum of the drug.[8] The resulting damage appears as an intensified sunburn with desquamation and peeling.

A photoallergic reaction is less common and, by definition, dependent on an antigen–antibody or cell-mediated hypersensitivity phenomenon.[26] Photoallergic reactions do not generally occur upon first exposure and require a sensitization period to the drug or metabolite. It is postulated that ultraviolet light reacts with the drug or metabolite in the skin to produce a hapten. The hapten combines with a tissue antigen to form a complete antigen that elicits an allergic response on subsequent exposure. Once sensitization is achieved, minimal amounts of drug are usually needed to produce a reaction.[8] Topically applied drugs or chemicals and airborne allergens may also produce photosensitivity reactions at their point of contact with the skin. Ingredients found in perfumes, deodorants, and after-shave lotions are examples of photocontactants. See Table 67.8 for drugs that frequently produce photosensitivity reactions.

Diagnosis of photosensitivity reactions is usually based on history and clinical presentation, although histology or patch testing may be helpful.[26] Discontinuation of the offending agent should result in slow regression of the eruption, although 10% to 20% of patients may have a persistent photosensitivity for prolonged periods.[6,28] Management for acute reactions includes avoidance of sunlight, topical remedies (e.g., cool wet dressings, soothing shake-lotions, corticosteroids), and topical or systemic antipruritic agents.[26]

Identification and removal of the inciting agent are ideal. In cases where this is not possible, sunscreens, or psoralen–ultraviolet light treatment (PUVA), have been used.[28] The use of sunscreens to prevent photosensitive reactions may be problematic. Most sunscreens do not block the entire spectrum of ultraviolet light that may be responsible for mediating many photoreactions. Paradoxically, sunscreens may also produce a photocontact eruption in sensitized patients.[6,8,27] *para*-Aminobenzoic acid, a common ultraviolet–$\beta$-blocking ingredient in sunscreens, is chemically similar to thiazides, sulfonylureas, furosemide, and carbonic anhydrase inhibitors. Patients allergic to such agents should use alternative sunscreens containing oxybenzone or cinoxate to avoid cross-reactivity.

### *Alopecia*

Many drugs have been associated with partial or total hair loss, either as an extension of their pharmacologic effect or as an adverse reaction with an unknown mechanism[29] (see Table 67.9).

**Table 67.9** Drugs Associated With Alopecia

| | |
|---|---|
| Carbamazepine | Hydantoin derivatives |
| Clofibrate | Propranolol |
| Colchicine | Valproate sodium |
| Ethionamide | Vitamin A (overdose) |

Compiled from References 8, 22, and 29.

**Antimitotics/Cytostatics**

Hair loss from cytostatic agents is well recognized and occurs because of a direct effect of the drug on the hair follicle. The incidence of alopecia in patients receiving high-dose cyclophosphamide has ranged from 21% to 48%.[30]

Cyclophosphamide inhibits mitosis of actively growing hair follicles, resulting in a thinned and weakened hair shaft susceptible to damage with minor trauma.[30] The extent of alopecia appears to be dose dependent and may often occur within 4 to 6 days of the first dose.[31] Regrowth usually occurs after discontinuation of drug, although shedding of normal mature hairs may continue for a prolonged period.[31]

**Anticoagulants**

Heparin and warfarin may sometimes induce alopecia 2 to 3 months after initiation of therapy.[31] The exact mechanism is unknown, although it is postulated that actively growing hairs are prematurely entered into the telogen (resting phase) and shed.[8] Higher doses (and not duration of exposure) are thought to influence primarily the degree of hair loss, which may be diffuse and/or extensive. Regrowth occurs after discontinuation of the drug.[31]

**Thioamides**

Agents used to treat hyperthyroidism may not only cause a dose-dependent hair loss, but may change the texture of the remaining hair to dry, brittle, and lusterless.[8] This may be an extension of thioamide pharmacologic effect, as hypothyroidism presents with a similar picture.

**Oral Contraceptives**

Two types of alopecia are associated with oral contraceptive use. First, a diffuse hair loss sometimes occurs within 1 to 4 months of discontinuation of oral contraceptives.[31] This is analogous to postpartum alopecia, as pregnancy slows the conversion of actively growing hair to mature hair. Second, during oral contraceptive therapy, a more diffuse alopecia, similar to the male pattern, may occur.[32] Progesterone stimulation via the androgenic effects of oral contraceptives may cause this type of alopecia.

## *Vasculitis*

Vasculitis is characterized by inflammation and damage of blood vessels that may affect various organ systems. It commonly appears on the lower extremities or pressure-dependent areas of the skin as red or purple (purpuric) lesions. These lesions range in size from a pinpoint to several centimeters. Early lesions are often macular, although they are commonly raised (palpable) and may have hemorrhagic bullae.[33] Lesions may persist 1 to 4 weeks or longer and in some cases become yellow to brown upon healing.[33] Systemic symptoms such as burning, stinging, malaise, arthralgias, and fever may be present. Other organ systems, including the liver, kidney, brain, and joints, may also be affected. Table 67.10 lists drugs that frequently cause vasculitis.

It is often difficult to distinguish between various types of vasculitis and to identify a cause. Although skin tests or in vitro testing assists in the diagnosis, identification of a causative source is difficult. Management includes removal of the offending or suspected agent.[33] Bedrest and compression of lesions may promote healing. Although their efficacy is not well documented, oral corticosteroids have been used by some clinicians to inhibit cell-mediated immunity, decrease inflammation, and suppress immunoglobulin synthesis.[33] Cyclophosphamide, plasmapheresis, indomethacin, sulfones, colchicine, and aspirin have been tried with variable success.[33] Interestingly, some therapeutic modalities are listed as causative agents, suggesting that further research is needed to identify the pathogenic processes involved in vasculitis.

**Table 67.10** Drugs That Cause Vasculitis

| | |
|---|---|
| Allopurinol | Phenylbutazone |
| Anticoagulants | Phenytoin |
| Cimetidine | Piroxicam |
| Hydralazine | Propylthiouracil |
| Ibuprofen | Quinine |
| Indomethacin | Sulfonamides |
| Penicillins | Thiazides |

Compiled from References 6, 8, 21, and 22.

## Hyperpigmentation

Drugs may produce color changes in the skin by a variety of mechanisms including deposition of melanin in the dermis and stimulation of melanin formation. Appearance, location, mechanism, and course of hyperpigmentation induced by commonly used drugs vary by pharmacologic grouping. Drugs known to induce pigmentary changes include hydantoins, metals (see Table 67.11), antimalarials, phenothiazines, oral contraceptives, tetracyclines, chemotherapeutic agents (see Table 67.12), and amiodarone.

**Hydantoin Derivatives**

Approximately 10% of patients taking phenytoin or related agents develop a brown patchy hyperpigmentation on light-exposed areas.[8] Although the hyperpigmentation deepens with light exposure, it usually does not disappear during winter months.[35] Hydantoin derivatives appear to cause an increase in melanin of the basal layer and induce dispersion of melanin granules in an animal model.[35] Women appear to be affected more than men, suggesting a hormonal origin with light as a triggering factor.[35]

**Antimalarial Agents**

Approximately 25% of patients taking antimalarials for more than 3 or 4 months develop pigmentation changes.[34] The pigmentation patterns vary and include patchy, irregular blue-black or gray lesions on pretibial areas or diffuse facial hyperpigmentation. A transverse band in the middle of the nail has also been reported.[8,34] The onset of pigmentation changes has ranged from 4 to 20 months, with discontinuation of therapy resulting in lightening but persistence of lesions.[34] Quinacrine causes a diffuse lemon-yellow skin

**Table 67.11** Heavy Metal–Induced Hyperpigmentation

| *Agent* | *Color* | *Region involved* | *Special feature* |
|---|---|---|---|
| Mercury | Gray brown<br>Slate green | Skin folds (topical)<br>Gingival pigmentation (systemic) | Caused by deposition of metallic granules and increased melanin production; formerly used in bleaching agents |
| Silver | Slate gray<br>Blue gray | Sun-exposed areas, mucosa sclerae, nails | Silver granule deposition that activates melanin production; occurs months to years after ingestion |
| Bismuth | Blue gray | Skin, conjunctiva, oral and vaginal mucosa; black line along gingival margin | Deposition of metallic granules or interaction with bacteria in mouth; more common with parenteral use |
| Arsenic | Brown<br>Bronze | Trunk, "raindrop"-shaped hyperkeratotic papulonodular lesions; palms, soles | Activates enzymes that form melanin and deposit in skin; used systemically for psoriasis and as a health tonic; pigmentation appears 1–20 yr after exposure |
| Gold | Blue gray | Periorbital, generalized chrysiasis, sun-exposed areas | Caused by deposition of metallic particles in epidermis, occurs months to years after exposure and is permanent |

Compiled from References 8 and 34.

discoloration that gives the patient a jaundiced appearance. Scleral coloration is slight and pigmentation returns to normal 1 to 4 months after therapy.[34]

### Phenothiazines

Pigmentation changes induced by phenothiazines (e.g., chlorpromazine, thioridazine) range from a bronze color in sun-exposed areas to a violet, purplish gray with long-term exposure.[34] Forehead, cheeks, nose, hands, and upper extremities are most commonly affected. An increased deposition of melanin occurs in the dermis and phenothiazine–melanin complexes are believed responsible for color changes. Pigmentation is not usually totally reversible but may fade slowly in winter months or upon discontinuation of therapy.[8,34]

### Oral Contraceptives

Melasma, characterized by irregular brown macules on the cheeks, forehead, or upper lip, is a frequent cutaneous reaction to oral contraceptives.[32] Estrogen, progesterone, or sun exposure may be responsible for the increased melanin deposition in the dermis and epidermis.[34] Onset usually occurs within 1 to 20 months, but hyperpigmentation may persist after discontinuation.[32] Sunscreens may be helpful in minimizing the extent of hyperpigmentation.

### Tetracyclines

Bluish pigmentation of previously inflamed skin may result from tetracycline deposition after prolonged high-dose therapy.[8,34] Several types of pigmentation changes have been reported with the use of minocycline. Blue-black coloration in areas of active scarring, generalized blue-gray pigmentation on sun-exposed areas, generalized muddy hue, and discoloration of teeth have been noted.[34] Coloration commonly fades after cessation of therapy.[36]

### Amiodarone

A gray-blue coloration in sun-exposed areas has been reported in up to 10% of patients receiving amiodarone.[37] The discoloration may be caused by the incorporation of amio-

**Table 67.12** Chemotherapeutic Agents Associated With Hyperpigmentation

| *Agent* | *Color* | *Region involved* | *Special feature* |
|---|---|---|---|
| Busulfan | Brown | Face, forearms, chest, trunk, hands | Accelerates melanin formation by enzymes; incidence more frequent in dark-skinned patients; resolves on discontinuation |
| Bleomycin | Brown | Linear bands on chest, back | Incidence 8%–20%; reversible on discontinuation |
| Doxorubicin | Black-brown | Tongue, palms, soles, nails | Increased incidence in dark-skinned patients; reversible on discontinuation |
| Mechlorethamine (topical) | Brown | Areas of contact | Toxic effect on keratinocytes; increased melanocytes; some aggregation |

Compiled from Reference 34.

darone into lysosomes, causing an accumulation of polar lipids.[37] Symptom onset has ranged from 6 to 39 months after initiation of therapy and discontinuation may cause slow fading of the lesion.[34]

## Erythema Multiforme/Stevens–Johnson Syndrome

Erythema multiforme is a cutaneous reaction of variable morphology that evolves and changes over time. Initially, a round, 1- to 10-cm, erythematous macule may appear, which becomes edematous and papular over time.[38] These lesions may enlarge into plaques or form concentric rings of erythema and clearing with a central vesicular or necrotic area. Lesions with zones of concentric color change are termed "iris" or "target" lesions and may enlarge and coalesce into polycyclic configurations. Hands, feet, limbs, mucous membranes, and face are the sites most commonly affected, with an acute onset often preceded by mild upper respiratory symptoms. Lesions begin to resolve in 4 to 5 days, with complete healing in 2 to 4 weeks, although new lesions can appear during this period.[38] Postinflammatory hyperpigmentation may occur after healing.

Stevens–Johnson Syndrome (SJS) is considered a severe variant of erythema multiforme with extensive mucosal and conjunctival edema, erosions, high fever, myalgias, vomiting, diarrhea, and arthralgias. Skin lesions may be severe with large bullae and areas of denudation. The onset of these lesions is variable, but healing usually occurs within 6 weeks. Complications include keratitis, conjunctival scarring, blindness, pneumonia, dehydration, and esophagitis.[38]

The pathogenesis of erythema multiforme and SJS is not completely elucidated. Evidence indicates that both an immune complex mechanism and cell-mediated immune reactivity may be involved.[6] Identification of the etiologic factor is also difficult, as erythema multiforme may be precipitated by totally unconnected factors. Drugs are frequently implicated (see Table 67.13), but viruses, bacteria, fungi, vaccines, and other diseases have been associated with erythema multiforme.[38]

Diagnosis of erythema multiforme is based largely on history, clinical appearance, and histology. Often, prodromal symptoms are treated with antibiotics; thus, etiology (e.g., virus, bacteria, or drug) is difficult to clarify. As mild forms of erythema multiforme are self-limiting, usually only symptomatic treatment is instituted, for example, tap water compresses for blisters and necrosis, antihistamines for pruritus, and one-half-strength hydrogen peroxide gargle for oral lesions. Patients should be carefully monitored for progression to more severe forms or development of complications. The efficacy of using systemic corticosteroids for severe erythema multiforme and SJS is not clearly defined. A decision to use systemic corticosteroids should be made on an individual basis.

**Table 67.13** Drugs Associated With Erythema Multiforme

| | |
|---|---|
| Barbiturates | Propranolol |
| Carbamazepine | Quinine |
| Diflunisal | Salicylates |
| Hydantoins | Sulfonamides |
| Ibuprofen | Sulfonylureas |
| Penicillins | Sulindac |
| Phenolphthalein | Thiazides |
| Phenylbutazone | |

Compiled from References 6, 8, 22, and 38.

## Toxic Epidermal Necrolysis

Although toxic epidermal necrolysis (TEN) is considered common, its true incidence may not be correctly estimated because of misdiagnosis and confusion with similar severe skin reactions. In many cases, there is a prodromal state of malaise, sore throat, pyrexia, headache, and myalgias, followed by an acute onset of cutaneous manifestations within hours or days.[6,8,39] The eruption may present in various forms, often as a macular lesion with a burning sensation that enlarges over the body. The lesions may form large flaccid bullae within the erythema or directly progress to massive detachment of the epidermis. At this point, the epidermis is easily rubbed off by light pressure with outer coverings of ruptured bullae clinging to underlying tissue. Because lesions may appear on any area of skin (e.g., palms, soles, mouth, throat, nose, trachea, eyelids, conjunctiva, cornea, and vagina), the picture may be similar to a second-degree burn or scald. Hairy areas are less commonly involved.

Complications are numerous and include fluid and electrolyte imbalance from loss of epidermis; septicemia; erosion of the mucous membranes of the mouth, nose, urethra, vagina, or rectum; corneal ulceration; and conjunctivitis. Internal organs may also be involved in severe cases, with possible manifestation of pneumonia, hepatocellular damage, gastrointestinal ulceration, nephritis, and myocardial damage.[6]

The pathogenic mechanisms responsible for TEN are unknown. The onset of TEN after drug exposure suggests a hypersensitivity–immunologic reaction, although there is little supporting evidence.[40] A TEN-like eruption has occurred in patients with a graft-versus-host reaction after bone marrow transplant or blood transfusion.[41]

Normocytic anemia, leukopenia, granulocytopenia, and neutropenia are commonly present in TEN with no readily accountable cause.[40,41] Drugs are often implicated as precipitating factors, but this is also difficult to verify because many patients receive multiple drugs (see Table 67.14). Other factors associated with TEN include vaccinations; viral, bacterial, and fungal infections; and neoplasia.[39]

**Table 67.14** Drugs Associated With Toxic Epidermal Necrolysis

| | |
|---|---|
| Allopurinol | Penicillins |
| Barbiturates | Phenylbutazone |
| Chloramphenicol | Quinine |
| Hydantoin derivatives | Sulfonamides |
| Ibuprofen | Sulindac |
| Indomethacin | Tolmetin |

Compiled from References 8 and 22.

The prognosis for TEN depends on the patient's age, extent of skin involvement, concurrent diseases, and complications.[6] Mortality is about 3% within the first 3 or 4 days of the acute episode.[6,8] After the acute episode, the epidermis may regenerate within 2 to 3 weeks, with complete healing in 6 weeks.[8] Management includes identification and withdrawal of the inciting factor, fluid and electrolyte maintenance, treatment or prevention of bacterial involvement, and prevention of ocular complications. Management should be tailored to the individual case; some clinicians prefer referral to a burn unit.

Although the empiric use of systemic corticosteroid therapy is well documented, it is controversial because of a lack of well-controlled studies. Some clinicians advocate corticosteroid use only within the first 48 to 72 hours of onset to prevent progression of complications[39]; others attribute delayed morbidity to systemic steroid use.[40] Without a definitive cause or known pathogenesis, supportive care is necessary to minimize mortality from TEN.

## Summary

Unfortunately, there are currently no methods to determine unequivocally if a medication is the cause of a particular skin eruption. Diagnosis is based largely on clinical appearance and morphology of lesions, history, and in some cases in vitro tests or rechallenge. A thorough history of drug and chemical exposure must be obtained, including the use of nonprescription medications and topical medications that may alter the morphologic appearance of the original lesion. The clinician should also consider the possibility of reaction to excipients or dyes contained in the drug formulation.

## References


1. Shapiro S, Slone D, Siskind V, et al. Drug rash with ampicillin and other penicillins. Lancet 1969;2:969–972.
2. Johnson M, Johnson KG, Engel A. Prevalence, morbidity, and cost of dermatologic diseases. J Am Acad Dermatol 1984;11: 930–936.
3. Baer RL, Witten VM. Drug eruptions, in: Yearbook of Dermatology 1960–1961 Series. Chicago, Yearbook Medical Publishers, 1961, pp 9–37.
4. Witte K, West DP. Immunology of adverse reactions to drugs. Pharmacotherapy 1982;2:54–65.
5. Witte KW, West DP. Immunology of adverse reactions to antimicrobial agents, in Jeljaszewicz J, Pulverer G (eds): Antimicrobial Agents and Immunity. London, Academic, 1986:217–249.
6. Schulz KH. Cutaneous manifestations of drug allergy, in De Weck AL, Bundgaard H (eds): Allergic Reactions to Drugs. Berlin, Springer-Verlag, 1983, pp 135–162.
7. Bruinsma W. Drug monitoring in dermatology. Int J Dermatol 1986;25:166–168.
8. Bruinsma W. A Guide to Drug Eruptions. Oosthuizen, the Netherlands, De Zwaluw, 1982.
9. Nelson HS. Allergic reactions to drugs. Adv Asthma Allergy 1976;3:18–35.
10. Bellanti JA. Immunology III. Philadelphia; W. B. Saunders, 1985;379–390.
11. Sell S. Immunology, Immunopathology, and Immunity, 3rd ed. Hagerstown, Harper and Row, 1980.
12. Gell PGH, Coombs RRA. Clinical Aspects of Immunology, 2nd ed. Oxford, Blackwell, 1968.
13. Roitt IM. Clinical manifestations, in Essential Immunology. Oxford, Blackwell, 1984, pp 262–263.
14. Parker CW. Drug allergy (parts 1, 2, and 3). N Engl J Med 1975;292:511–514, 732–736, 957–960.
15. DeSwarte RD, Smith BC. Allergic reactions to drugs, in Lockey RF (ed): Allergy and Clinical Immunology. Garden City, Medical Examination Publishing Co, 1979, pp 861–893.
16. Cluff LE, Caranasos GJ, Stewart RB. Clinical manifestations, in Clinical Problems With Drugs. Philadelphia, W. B. Saunders, 1975, vol 5, pp 80–96.
17. Van Arsdel P. Adverse drug reactions, in Middleton E, Reed C, Ellis EF (eds): Allergy: Principles and Practice. St. Louis, C. V. Mosby, 1978.
18. Avery GS (ed): Drug Treatment, 2nd ed. Sidney, ADIS Press, 1979.
19. Symmers WSC. The occurrence of gingivitis and of other generalized diseases of connective tissues as a consequence of the administration of drugs. Proc R Soc Med 1962;55:20–28.
20. Baer RL, Gigli I. Allergic eczematous contact dermatitis, in Fitzpatrick TB, Eisen AZ, Wolff K (eds): Dermatology in General Medicine. New York, McGraw-Hill, 1979, pp 512–519.
21. Wintroub BU, Stern R. Cutaneous drug reactions: Pathogenesis and clinical classification. J Am Acad Dermatol 1985;13:167–179.
22. Bigby M, Stern R. Cutaneous reactions to nonsteroidal anti-inflammatory drugs. J Am Acad Dermatol 1985;12:866–876.
23. Greene SL, Reed CE, Schroeter AL. Double-blind crossover study comparing doxepin with diphenhydramine for the treatment of chronic urticaria. J Am Acad Dermatol 1985;12:669–675.
24. Yaffe SJ, Bierman CW, Cann HM, et al. Antihistamines in topical preparations. Pediatrics 1973;51:299–301.
25. Korkij W, Soltani K. Fixed drug eruption. Arch Dermatol 1984;120:520–524.
26. Epstein JH, Wintroub BU. Photosensitivity due to drugs. Drugs 1985;30:42–57.
27. Drugs that cause photosensitivity. Med Lett 1986;28:51–52.
28. Robinson HN, Morison WL, Hood AF. Thiazide diuretic therapy and chronic photosensitivity. Arch Dermatol 1985;121: 522–524.
29. Brodin MB. Drug-related alopecia. Dermatol Clin 1987;5:571–579.
30. Hood AF. Cutaneous complications of immunosuppressive agents. Dermatol Clin 1983;1:591–606.
31. Rook A, Wilkinson DS, Ebling FJG (eds): Alopecia of chemical origin, in Textbook of Dermatology. Oxford, Blackwell, 1979, pp 1773–1774.
32. Jelinek JE. Cutaneous side effects of oral contraceptives. Arch Dermatol 1970;101:181–186.
33. Mackel SE. Treatment of vasculitis. Med Clin North Am 1982;66:941–954.
34. Granstein RD, Sober AJ. Drug and heavy metal–induced hyperpigmentation. J Am Acad Dermatol 1981;5:1–18.
35. Moller H. Pigmentary disturbances due to drugs. Acta Derm Venereol (Stockh) 1966;46:423–431.

36. Basler RSW. Minocycline-related hyperpigmentation. Arch Dermatol 1985;121:606–608.
37. Trimble JW, Mendelson DS, Fetter BF, et al. Cutaneous pigmentation secondary to amiodarone therapy. Arch Dermatol 1983;119:914–918.
38. Huff JC, Weston WL, Tonnesen MG. Erythema multiforme: A critical review of characteristics, diagnostic criteria, and causes. J Am Acad Dermatol 1983;8:763–775.
39. Parsons JM. Management of toxic epidermal necrolysis. Cutis 1985;36:305–311.
40. Westly ED, Wechsler HL. Toxic epidermal necrolysis. Arch Dermatol 1984;120:721–726.
41. Goeens J, Song M, Fondu P. Haematological disturbances and immune mechanisms in toxic epidermal necrolysis. Br J Dermatol 1986;114:255–259.

# Chapter 68 / Burns

Dianne M. Brundage, PharmD, and Dabney Yarbrough III, MD

Successful management of burn patients requires a multidisciplinary approach, and is based upon a solid knowledge base of the epidemiology, pathophysiology, and therapy available. This chapter focuses on the aforementioned topics and the appropriate fluid and nutritional management of the burn patient as well as management of wounds and infective processes. The pharmacodynamic and pharmacokinetic drug studies that have been done in thermally injured patients and animals are also discussed.

## Epidemiology

Although the exact rate of occurrence of burns is not known, it has been estimated that about 1% of the population of the United States (over 2 million people) are burned or scalded each year. Of these, 500,000 seek medical attention. Another 500,000 of those burned require confinement to bed for some period of time. Approximately 100,000 individuals are admitted to hospitals for treatment of acute burns, and about 6,000 people die from burn injuries every year. Children and elderly individuals constitute more than half of the deaths reported in some series of burn patients.[1–3]

## Classification

There are four major categories of burns: thermal (includes flame and scald burns), electrical (contact and flash), chemical, and radiation (extremely rare).

The quickest and most easily remembered method for estimating the area of burn is the rule of nines. According to the rule of nines, the total body surface area (BSA) of skin is divided into areas equal to 9% (or multiples thereof). The head is equal to 9% of BSA; the arms are 9% each; the legs are 18% each; the anterior trunk is 18%; the posterior trunk is 18%; and the perineum is 1% of BSA. This method is relatively inaccurate in children and adults with small body surface area; therefore, another method, the Lund and Browder chart (Fig. 68.1), may be used. The area and the depth of involvement of burn injury should be recorded on an accurate diagram.

The depth of burns is estimated from clinical observation of the appearance and sensitivity of the wound.[4] First-degree burns, or superficial burns, may include sunburns. A first-degree burn involves the epidermis only. Generally there is no blistering; however, redness, skin warmth, and mild edema are present. First-degree burns may be painful because sensitive nerve endings remain intact. These burns usually heal uneventfully in 3 to 10 days. Treatment of first-degree burns generally requires no care other than avoidance of reinjury and relief of pain and fever. This type of burn is not included in the calculation for fluid resuscitation.

Second-degree burns (often referred to as superficial second-degree, superficial dermal, or partial-thickness burns) involve the entire epidermis and may extend into the dermis layer. Second-degree burns may be superficial or deep. In superficial second-degree burns, most of the dermal layer is spared and healing is more rapid. Second-degree burns may blister, are moist, and are painful because injured nerve endings are irritated. These burns generally heal spontaneously within 3 weeks, with minimal scarring. Deep second-degree burns involve the epidermis and most of the dermis, sparing only the base of hair follicles and glands. These burns may require 3 to 6 weeks to heal. Deep second-degree burns may cause very severe scarring. Skin grafts may be advisable in areas where integrity of the skin or cosmetic appearance is important.

Third-degree (or full-thickness) burns destroy all of the skin elements, including the epidermis and the dermis. They may extend into subcutaneous fat, muscle, and bone. They are usually pearly white or charred in appearance. The eschar, the coagulated tissue protein, lacks sensation and is hard and parchmentlike. If third-degree wounds are extensive (if the diameter exceeds 3–4 cm), grafting is required to achieve wound closure.

Flame burns are usually a mixture of partial- and full-thickness burns and have irregular margins. Scald burns are often seen in children and may be partial- or full-thickness injuries. Superheated steam may cause full-thickness burns and severe respiratory tract injury. Flash burns are usually a uniform partial-thickness injury of exposed areas. Electrical burns may cause severe necrosis of underlying muscles, tendons, nerves, and bone with minimal involvement of the skin surface.

## Initial Assessment and Care

Stopping the burning process is the initial step in treatment of the burn victim. In patients with chemical burns, it is imperative that clothing be removed as quickly as possible to stop the continuing injury from the chemical agent. Chemical burns should be thoroughly irrigated with water.

Another important aspect of management of a burn patient is to make sure that an adequate airway is present. Victims of burns sustained in a closed space may suffer inhalation injury. Mechanical airway problems may be immediately apparent but in most instances do not develop for 30 minutes to 1 hour after the burn injury. Airway compromise resulting

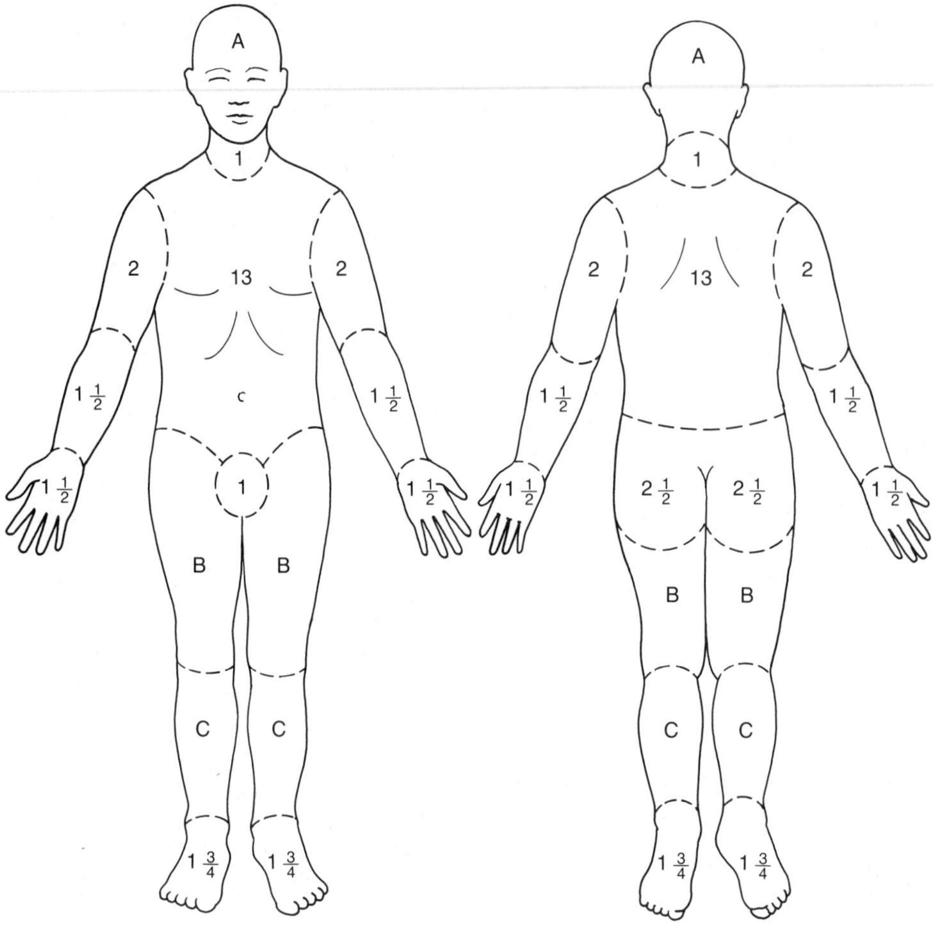


| Relative percentage of areas affected by growth | Age (years) | | | | | |
|---|---|---|---|---|---|---|
| | 0 | 1 | 5 | 10 | 15 | Adult |
| A. One half of head | $9\frac{1}{2}$ | $8\frac{1}{2}$ | $6\frac{1}{2}$ | $5\frac{1}{2}$ | $4\frac{1}{2}$ | $3\frac{1}{2}$ |
| B. One half of one thigh | $2\frac{3}{4}$ | $3\frac{1}{4}$ | 4 | $4\frac{1}{4}$ | $4\frac{1}{2}$ | $4\frac{3}{4}$ |
| C. One half of one leg | $2\frac{1}{2}$ | $2\frac{1}{2}$ | $2\frac{3}{4}$ | 3 | $3\frac{1}{4}$ | $3\frac{1}{2}$ |

Total percent burned ______ 2° + ______ 3° = ______

**Figure 68.1** Lund and Browder chart for estimating percentage burn and for plotting burned areas.

from burn injury is usually due to accumulation of edema fluid in the soft tissues of the airway. The onset may be very rapid after the institution of intravenous fluid resuscitation. The clinical signs of facial burns, singed eyebrows or nasal hair, carbon deposits on the mucosa, acute inflammatory changes in the mucosa and pharynx, carbonaceous sputum, and/or hoarseness may be predictors of inhalation injury. Intubation should be performed as soon as the need for airway access is established. A patent airway should be maintained until upper airway edema resolves, usually 2 to 5 days.

Victims who upon physical exam have singed nasal hairs, mucosal burns of the mouth and pharynx, and hoarseness and stridor are at risk for developing progressive upper airway obstruction. In these victims the mouth, throat, and larnyx should be examined for damage. Most airway obstruction occurs within 24 to 48 hours of the burn. Patients with inhalation injury may need chest x-rays several times during the first 48 hours because chest x-rays may remain normal up to 48 hours after burn injury.[4] Fiber-optic bronchoscopy may be done to show upper airway and laryngeal injury. Xenon scans or ventilation perfusion scans may determine regional lung abnormalities before x-ray changes become evident. Pulmonary function tests can also be used to evaluate lower respiratory tract injury.[5] Therapy for inhalation injury in patients with normal blood gases consists of administration of warm humidified oxygen, use of bronchodilators, postural drainage, percussion, spirometry, intermittent positive-pressure breathing, mucolytic agents, and fiber-optic bronchoscopy to remove soot and exudate. Constricting burn eschars of the chest may require escharotomy for relief of mechanical restriction of thoracic expansion. Steroids[6–8] and prophylactic antibiotics[6,9] have not been found to be of benefit. Tracheostomy or cricothyroidotomy through burned, contaminated tissues should be only a last resort because of the greatly increased incidence of pulmonary infection.

Early respiratory problems usually are the result of smoke inhalation. Inhalation of noxious products of combustion results in bronchospasm, chemical necrosis of tracheal and bronchial epithelium, chemical pneumonia, and pulmonary edema. Rarely is there true heat injury of the lower airway; therefore, the terms *pulmonary burn* and *respiratory burn* are misnomers.

Initial fluid and electrolyte resuscitation is necessary when burns cover greater than 15% to 20% of the total body surface area in adults, or greater than 10% to 15% of the total body surface in children (see Fluid Resuscitation). The massive fluid losses in the burn patient are caused by the increased capillary permeability induced by the burn. The result is massive third-space fluid losses, decreased plasma and blood volumes, decreased cardiac output, and hypovolemic shock with increased peripheral vascular resistance and inadequate peripheral tissue perfusion. The treatment is replacement of the fluid losses.

Immediate wound care of the burn patient involves, first, removal of the patient's clothing. Peripheral circulation should be maintained in patients who have extremity burns. Rings, bracelets, and other constricting items of clothing should be removed. After initial debridement of all tissue, the burn should be reclassified according to the appearance of the wound. Application of antibiotic creams or ointments should be delayed until all wounds are properly cleaned and classified. After this has been accomplished, initial dressings can be applied.

Additional treatment of the burn patient should include a history of illness and/or surgery that may complicate care. A careful physical examination should be performed. Particular attention should be paid to the external auditory canal and eardrum, eyes, nares, neck, and abdomen. Careful examination of the extremities distal to circumferential burns for evidence of impaired circulation is necessary. The collection of edema fluid beneath a tight, unyielding circumferential burn eschar of the extremities results in increasing tissue pressure as edema fluid accumulates. This may obstruct lymphatic, venous, and arterial circulation, causing impaired distal tissue perfusion and tissue necrosis. The eschar should be incised in the midlateral and/or midmedial lines of the extremities or the anterior axillary lines of the chest.

A nasogastric tube should be inserted and attached to suction if the patient has greater than 25% total body surface area burn. Virtually all patients with major burns exhibit paralytic ileus for 3 to 4 days after the injury. Nasogastric suction is necessary during this period of time to prevent vomiting and aspiration.

A bladder catheter should be inserted to measure hourly urine output and to assess the level of hemoglobinuria present. Extensive erythrocyte hemolysis and/or muscle injury may produce a grossly visible pigmenturia. A combination of fluid and an osmotic diuretic, such as mannitol, may be administered to clear the pigment load rapidly and minimize the incidence of renal failure caused by pigment deposition in the renal tubules. Accurate measurement of urine output during the fluid resuscitation phase is crucial to proper monitoring and fluid assessment in burn patients.

All burns require tetanus prophylaxis. If a victim has had a tetanus booster in the last 5 years, a booster should be administered intramuscularly. Tetanus immunoglobulin is recommended if the victim has not had a booster in more than 5 years, the wound is heavily contaminated, or previous immunization is uncertain.

A thorough history of the immediate injury should be obtained as part of the initial assessment. The history should include the burning agent, if possible, the circumstances in which the injury occurred, whether or not toxic substances were released from surrounding combustible material, the nature of the accident, any loss of consciousness for brief periods, and any other aspects of injury that may have been noted.

Analgesics may be administered as necessary to burn patients to accomplish the necessary procedures. All medications should be given by the intravenous route because absorption may be altered in those patients with greater than 20% to 25% body surface area burn.[10] Medications given via the intramuscular or subcutaneous route may be absorbed erratically, or perhaps not at all, because of underperfused tissue sites. Once perfusion is restored to these areas, the intramuscularly or subcutaneously administered analgesic may be absorbed too quickly, which may result in a respiratory depression.

The American Burn Association has established criteria for transfer of patients to a burn center:

1. Third-degree burns involving more than 10% BSA
2. Second-degree burns involving more than 20% BSA
3. Significant burns involving the hands, face, feet, or perineum
4. Burns with associated injuries (i.e., fractures)
5. High-voltage electrical injuries
6. Burn patients with significant smoke inhalation

## Fluid Resuscitation

When the extent of burn exceeds 15% to 20% of body surface area, a significant amount of plasma leaks from the intravascular fluid space into damaged tissues, producing edema, hypovolemia, and ultimately inadequate tissue perfusion and perhaps shock. The most common serious side effects or complications of inadequate or delayed fluid resuscitation in burn patients are metabolic acidosis and acute renal failure.[10] The increase in capillary permeability is due to the loss of vascular integrity during the burn/thermal injury process. Fluid shifts from the intravascular compartment to the vascular cellular space occur, and plasma proteins, principally albumin, are also lost into the injured tissue. With the loss of intravascular volume, cardiac output also decreases. Hematocrit may often rise as the intravascular volume contracts, with the net loss of plasma. The continued loss of intravascular plasma volume results in hypotension, with further depression of cardiac output.

Decreased cardiac output results in decreased perfusion and tissue acidosis and, ultimately, in hypovolemic burn shock. The shift of fluid from the intracellular spaces is inadequate to maintain intravascular fluid volume; therefore, rapid replacement of fluid is necessary within the first 8 hours of acute thermal injury. During the period of decreased cardiac output, the kidney pertusion is decreased. Cardiac output begins to rise and return to normal with adequate fluid resuscitation in the first 24 hours. After 48 hours, cardiac output starts to increase to higher-than-normal values, reflecting the onset of a postburn hypermetabolic phase. Thus, once adequate fluid resuscitation is achieved, renal blood flow returns to normal as manifested by urine output. This reinforces the importance of having a patient catheterized to monitor this parameter more carefully.

Several formulas have been developed to approximate the fluid requirements for burn shock resuscitation. A balanced electrolyte solution is used for several formulas because it approximates the intravascular fluid that is lost into the injured tissue areas. Glucose-free Ringer's lactate solution is the most commonly used balanced electrolyte solution.[11] Most formulas for fluid resuscitation estimate volumes to be used at 2 to 4 mL/kg of body weight per percent of total body surface burn (Table 68.1). For example, according to the Parkland formula, a 70-kg man with a 40% BSA burn would require $4 \times 70 \times 40$ or 11,200 mL of Ringer's lactate solution in the first 24 hours. Ringer's lactate contains 130 mEq of sodium per liter and also lactate, which is metabolized to bicarbonate and helps to correct the metabolic acidosis that may accompany the major thermal injury. Half of the estimated fluid requirements are administered within the first 8 hours of thermal injury. The 8-hour period begins with the time of injury. If arrival at the hospital is delayed 4 hours, one half of the fluid calculated must be replaced during the next 4 hours to maintain adequate perfusion. The remainder of fluid administered during the next 16 hours is determined by the clinical criteria used in evaluating the patient, such as urine output, mental status, pulse rate, blood pressure, and other clinical signs. Colloids may also be a part of fluid resuscitation. Theoretically, during this initial phase there is such marked permeability that the colloids administered could leak into the wound, thereby increasing interstitial oncotic pressure and prolonging the duration of wound edema or adversely affecting outcome. Experimentally, it has been found that restoration and maintenance of plasma protein content are not effective until 8 hours after a burn, when adequate levels can be maintained by infusion.[12] Another factor to be considered in colloid therapy is the expense. For the past 20 years, the trend in the United States has been away from the use of colloids during the first 24 hours. After this initial 24- to 36-hour period, colloids may be administered to patients. Whether early colloid administration is of benefit has not yet been demonstrated.[13]

Hypertonic crystalloid solutions have been used in resuscitation of burn patients.[12,14,15] These solutions, which contain 250 mEq of sodium per liter, are used to reduce the volume of fluid infused and, therefore, decrease the possibility of edema; however, because these solutions are hypertonic, hypernatremia may result. Serum sodium concentrations exceeding 160 mEq/L are associated with numerous side effects. If hypertonic crystalloid solutions are used, it is recommended that serum sodium level and osmolality be closely monitored during therapy to prevent hypernatremia. While the main advantage of this method is the use of less fluid, the biggest concern is inadequate fluid resuscitation. In the elderly, where congestive heart failure is a major concern, the large volumes administered have not been shown to cause congestive heart failure in the acute phase of thermal injury; however, congestive heart failure may become evident later, three to seven days after injury.

**Table 68.1** Formulas for Estimating Fluid Requirements for Adults for the First 24 Hours Postburn

| *Name of formula* | *Fluid used* | *Formula* |
|---|---|---|
| Evans | Normal saline | 1 mL/kg/% burn |
| | Colloid | 1 mL/kg/% burn |
| | 5% Dextrose in water | 2,000 mL |
| Parkland | Ringer's lactate | 4 mL/kg/% burn |
| Brooke | Colloid | 0.5 mL/kg/% burn |
| | Ringer's lactate | 1.5 mL/kg/% burn |
| | 5% Dextrose in water | 2,000 mL |
| Modified Brooke | Ringer's lactate | 2 mL/kg/% burn |
| Hypertonic | Sodium 250 mEq/L | Titrate to urine output 0.5–1.0 mL/kg/h |

A large-bore intravenous catheter (14 or 16 gauge) should be inserted into a peripheral vein in an unburned area for fluid administration. A careful scrub is necessary and aseptic techniques should be used for each intravenous line inserted.

Once fluid therapy is initiated, the formulas (see Table 68.1) are only guidelines. Therapy should be modified according to the clinical response of the patient. Parameters that should be monitored are urine output, heart rate, blood pressure, peripheral signs of perfusion, mental status, and, if central lines have been placed, hemodynamic parameters. Clinically, the burn patient should be assessed for hydration status. In the patient without head trauma or excessive drug sedation, confusion or alterations in mental status may indicate hypovolemia, and additional volume replacement may be warranted. The goal of urine output is 30 to 60 mL/h for adults and 1 mL/kg/h for children below 30 kg in body weight. Inadequate urine output may be a sign of hypovolemia, which should be treated with additional volume loading before treatment with diuretics is started. Goals for heart rate in burn patients should be 100 to 120 beats per minute. Heart rates exceeding 140 beats per minute may indicate an intravascular volume deficit. Patients that may require invasive monitoring of hemodynamic response to fluid resuscitation include those patients that have had an inadequate response to fluid administration to 6 mL/kg of body weight per percent of burn area, patients with other major trauma, and patients with a history of coronary artery or valvular heart disease, cerebral injury, or edema.

During the second day of therapy for fluid resuscitation,

crystalloids and colloids can be administered as needed to maintain clinical goals. During this first 48-hour period, there can be a weight gain of as much as 15% to 20% of normal weight because of fluid therapy. Fluids should be administered to maintain adequate urine output and should be followed by vital signs, levels of serum sodium and other electrolytes, and osmolalities.

Dextrose-containing solutions can be used after the first day.[15] These solutions can aid in the excretion of the large sodium doses received during resuscitation and can also help prevent water loss by evaporation. Between 2 and 3 mL/kg of body weight per percent burn area is lost in terms of evaporation each day. Fluid replacement should be guided by daily body weight determinations, assessment of appropriate insensible losses, and monitoring of urine output. Preburn weight should be reached by days 7 to 10 postburn as an ultimate goal of fluid management.

## Burn Wounds

### *Pathophysiology*

The mechanism of tissue injury common to thermal burns, electrical burns, and some chemical burns is thermal denaturation of protein with destruction of critical intracellular enzyme systems. The degree of destruction of skin by heat is determined by several factors:

1. Temperature of the burning agent
2. Duration of exposure to the burning agent
3. Thickness of the skin
4. Efficiency of heat transfer mechanisms (chiefly the cooling effect of cutaneous blood flow)
5. Presence of insulating materials such as hair and skin oils

Histologic examination of the burn wound reveals three distinct zones: a central zone of coagulation, a surrounding zone of stasis (of blood flow), and an outer zone of hyperemia.[16]

### *Treatment*

Once the patient is stabilized and the admission evaluation is completed, the burn wound should be gently debrided. Loose bullae should be excised and hair removed from all burned areas. In cases where a burn may be near hair, the hair should be shaved at least 2–3 cm beyond the area of burn and the rest of the hair controlled in such a manner that it does not contaminate the burn surface. Once debridement is completed, the burn wound should be bathed with a mild antibacterial soap and covered with a topical antimicrobial agent. Analgesics may be administered during this time to allow these procedures to occur relatively pain free.

The use of effective topical antimicrobial agents has been associated with an approximately 50% reduction in mortality in burn patients.[17] Three agents used today are mafenide acetate (Sulfamylon), silver sulfadiazine (Silvadene), and silver nitrate. Mafenide acetate is an 8.5% formulation in a water-miscible base. It is an excellent bacteriostatic agent and is particularly effective in suppressing clostridia. It is uniquely active against *Pseudomonas* species and penetrates the eschar. The disadvantages of mafenide include pain upon application, cutaneous hypersensitivity, and carbonic anhydrase inhibition with bicarbonate diuresis. Some patients may develop a rash, which responds to antihistamines.

Silver sulfadiazine is a 1.0% cream that is similar in its bacteriostatic spectrum to mafenide. It is painless on application and hypersensitivity is rare. Silver sulfadiazine has been associated with transient leukopenia. This agent does not penetrate the eschar well, and if bacterial density in the burn wound increases, this agent should be discontinued and mafenide substituted.

Silver nitrate, a 0.5% aqueous solution, is useful in those burn patients who have a hypersensitivity to sulfonamide drugs. Profound electrolyte imbalances may occur, with the loss of sodium, chloride, calcium, and potassium into the dressings that are needed for this particular agent. It is active only at the burn wound surface, and is inactive against clostridia.

Topical antimicrobial agents may fail to control bacterial infection in the burn wound and these organisms can go on to cause bacteremias and generalized sepsis. The systemic signs of infection that must be monitored include ileus, hypothermia or hyperthermia, glucose intolerance, tachycardia, and hypotension. Prophylactic antibiotics, such as penicillin, have not been shown to be effective in preventing infections in burn patients.[18,19] Therefore, routine use of penicillin or other prophylactic antibiotics during the initial phase of thermal injury is not recommended.

Burn wound infections can occur despite adequate topical antimicrobial agent therapy. Signs of burn wound infections include conversion of a partial-thickness burn to a full-thickness burn, hemorrhagic discoloration of subeschar tissue, blistering in the healing partial-thickness burns (herpes infection), discoloration of unburned skin marginal to the burn wound, hemorrhagic lesions with a central necrosis in unburned skin (ecthyma gangrenosum), and an accelerated eschar separation.[19] The most accurate method of monitoring the burn wound is biopsy. Biopsy material should be examined for demonstration of organisms within tissue, and the number of organisms per gram of tissue reported.

## Curling's Ulcer

Curling's ulcer is an acute stress ulceration of the stomach or duodenum that occurs in burned patients. The ulcerations may be single or multiple, gastric or duodenal. Acute erosions may appear within 72 hours of burn injury; incidence peaks 7 to 14 days postburn. They usually manifest as relatively asymptomatic upper gastrointestinal bleeding. Possible causes include energy-deficient mucosal cells, back-diffusion of acid, and gastric acid hypersecretion. Antacid administration may be used to maintain gastric pH above 5. If necessary, $H_2$-receptor antagonists can be added to obtain desired gastric acid pH control; however, higher dosages and increased frequency of administration may be necessary for adequate control (see Pharmacokinetics/Pharmacodynamics in Burn Patients). Surgery may be required for massive bleeding or perforation.

## Nutritional Support

Cuthbertson[20] originally described the metabolic response to major trauma as a biphasic response. The ebb phase begins immediately after the injury and is characterized by hypotension, decreased total body blood flow, and poor tissue perfusion. Correlated with this is a general hypometabolic state, with a decrease in total body oxygen consumption below normal levels. The flow phase begins after successful resuscitation in the burn patient. During this phase, cardiac output is restored to normal and may rise to two to two and one-half times normal somewhere between days 5 and 10 postburn. During this period, there is a concomitant hypermetabolic response in the burn patient. The magnitude of the hypermetabolic response is proportional to the size of the thermal injury and increases in a linear relationship with the size of burn to a burn size of approximately 50% to 60% of the total body surface.[21,22] For burns greater than 60% of total body surface area, the metabolic rate remains essentially constant.[22] The hypermetabolic state continues until the burn wound either heals or is closed by skin grafting, or is fully mature and blanched. Therefore, nutritional support plays a vital role in the treatment of burn patients. The metabolic rate of the patient is also proportional to the amount of nitrogen excreted in the urine. While 80% to 90% of nitrogen appears in the urine as urea, 20% to 25% of total daily nitrogen losses can be through the skin.[22] Alanine and glutamine are found in increased quantities in the circulation after severe burns.[22] Increased urinary excretion of creatinine and 3-methylhistidine result from muscle proteolysis.[22] Decreased lean body mass and weight loss occur in burn patients who receive no nutritional support. In patients with burns exceeding 40% of body surface area, weight losses can be 30% of the preinjury weight if nutritional support is not provided.[22]

What causes this hypermetabolic response in burn patients? Catecholamines may be the major mediators in this response in the thermally injured patient. Blockade of $\beta$ receptors diminishes the postburn hypermetabolic rate, respiratory rate, minute ventilation, and concentrations of free fatty acids; however, full $\beta$-blockade decreases only a portion of the hypermetabolism in the thermally injured patient which suggests that other hormonal mediators may be involved.[22]

The goals of nutritional support in the thermally injured patient should be to provide calories adequate to match the injury demands and nitrogen adequate to replace body protein stores. An ileus may develop in patients with burns greater than 30% of body surface area soon after injury; therefore, the gastrointestinal tract initially cannot be used for nutrition. The gastrointestinal tract may return to functional status within 24 to 72 hours of burn injury. The elderly or patients who have inhalation injury or complicating diseases may experience a prolonged period of ileus after thermal injury, and bowel activity may not return for a longer period. Once evidence of gut function is present (passage of stool or flatus) enteral feedings can be instituted.

Direct and indirect measurements of metabolic rate and caloric and protein requirements may be made chemically, by calorimetry and by oxygen consumption and carbon dioxide production. Ideal daily caloric intake for adult burn patients is calculated with the following formula: 25 kcal per kilogram body weight plus 40 kcal per percent body surface area burn.[23] Another approach is to provide twice the basal energy expenditure, as calculated by the Harris–Benedict equation.[21] There are no definitive guidelines for protein requirements in burn patients. Severely burned patients may lose over 200 g of protein per day during the first weeks of injury.[21] Suggested formulas for estimation of protein requirements include 94 g/m$^2$/d for burns greater than 40% BSA; 2.5 g/kg/d for an adult (3–5 g/kg/d for a child) for any percent BSA burn; and 1 g/kg plus 3 g per percent BSA burn for adults (3 g/kg plus 1 g per percent BSA burn for a child).[21] It is important to realize that these formulas can only guide therapy. Individualized therapy is the key to successful management of the burn patient. The principles and monitoring parameters for nutritional support should be followed (see Chapters 104–110).

## Infection and Immunology

The leading cause of mortality from severe thermal burns is infection.[24] The body's first line of defense against bacterial invasion, the skin, is destroyed during thermal injury, and the eschar provides an excellent growth medium for microorganisms. The eschar, which is avascular, prevents the body's defenses from inhibiting the growth of these microorganisms. The thermal injury also causes severe immunosuppression, which alters the host's ability to fight infection. Therefore, it is advisable to begin antibiotic therapy even before definitive microbiologic information becomes available. Aggressive antibiotic therapy needs to begin early because systemic sepsis can occur within 48 hours.[24] Many institutions begin therapy with an aminoglycoside and a penicillinase-resistant penicillin together until appropriate cultures are available and more appropriate therapy can be determined. It is recommended that serum concentrations of aminoglycosides be determined in burn patients because of the rapid elimination of these drugs in thermally injured patients.

Staphylococcal infections in a burn patient must be considered serious and appropriate antibiotic therapy must be started immediately. It is important for the clinician to be aware of any problems with methicillin-resistant *Staphylococcus aureus*. If this pathogen is a problem in the unit, it is advisable to begin systemic vancomycin therapy immediately.

The signs and symptoms that must be monitored during an infective process include white cell counts and differentials, temperatures, chest x-rays, and appropriate tests that monitor organ function (e.g., creatinine clearance). Also, cultures of infected areas should be repeated every few days.

Host defenses play an important role in the resolution of the infective process. White blood cell chemotactic activity that occurs in response to inflammatory stimuli is impaired after burn injury.[24,25] Both phagocytic and bacterial activities of white cells are depressed after thermal injury. Serum complement levels, serum immunoglobulin levels, and the ability to produce specific antibodies either in vivo or in vitro are also decreased. Studies of T cells have shown that cell function is dramatically affected in all patients with burns exceeding 20% body surface area.[24] This is important because immune function depends upon T cells. Helper T cells aid in amplifying the immune response to infection, while suppressor T cells inhibit or regulate the magnitude and duration of a response. In burn patients, there is increased suppressor cell activity and decreased helper cell activity. This is an important consideration when dealing with antibiotic therapy in burn patients.

## Pharmacokinetics/Pharmacodynamics in Burn Patients

Thermal injuries cause a number of physiologic alterations that involve the cardiovascular, hepatic, renal, and dermatologic systems. The degree of burn and the complications resulting from thermal injury may produce changes in the pharmacokinetics and pharmacodynamics of drugs.

Changes in cardiac output can alter the pharmacokinetics of some drugs by changing the characteristics of absorption, distribution, and elimination. Variations in plasma volume and red blood cell mass may also alter these same factors. The plasma protein concentration is important for those drugs that are highly protein bound since the activity of these drugs is likely to depend more on the unbound than the total drug concentration. Studies have shown significant postburn alterations in the concentrations of the important drug-binding proteins, albumin and $\alpha_1$-acid glycoprotein (AAG).[26,27] Investigations have shown that on day 1 after thermal injury, AAG concentrations were 36 to 99 mg/dL, well within normal limits. Five to twenty-five days after injury, AAG concentrations had risen to 221 to 268 mg/dL. Concentrations peaked as early as 9 days after injury in some and remained elevated at 17 and 25 days in others. Martyn et al[27] found that AAG concentrations correlated well ($r$ = 0.70) with imipramine free (unbound) fraction; as AAG concentrations increased, free imipramine levels decreased. It was concluded that basic drugs that are highly bound to AAG may show progressive, increased binding after thermal injury. Such binding changes can alter the interpretation of total serum or plasma drug concentrations. Bloedow and co-workers[26] reported similar AAG levels in burn patients. They examined the free fraction for other drugs bound primarily to AAG. They found decreased free fractions (increased protein binding) of imipramine, lidocaine, meperidine, and propranolol. Albumin concentrations have been shown to decrease in burn patients[28] and tend to remain in the range 1.0–3.0 g/dL for several weeks. This is consistent with the fact that the skin contains the largest fraction of exchangeable albumin[29] and thermal destruction of skin results in significant loss of albumin. A generalized increase in capillary permeability further depletes plasma albumin levels, particularly in the early phase of burn injury.[30] Additional fluctuations in albumin may be attributed to an increase in catabolism, transfusion of albumin-containing fluid, and massive fluid resuscitation.[31] Bloedow and co-workers[26] found increased free fractions of diazepam, phenytoin, and salicylate in burn patients as compared with controls. This confirms the same observation made by Bowdle and co-workers,[32] who found a two- to threefold increase in the free fraction of plasma phenytoin in burn-injured patients who had serum albumin concentrations approximately 50% of normal. They also noted a fivefold increase in the free fraction of valproic acid in the presence of a 50% decrease in albumin. Similar findings have been made for diazepam.[27] For highly protein bound drugs, monitoring of free drug and serum protein concentrations may be more appropriate than monitoring of total serum drug concentrations, in burn-injured patients.

Renal dysfunction of varying degree may occur secondary to burn trauma. The renal clearance of a drug after a burn injury may be affected by tubular necrosis, altered renal blood flow, and altered protein binding.[28] Glomerular filtration rate is a function of four parameters: the mean transcapillary hydraulic pressure, the ultrafiltration coefficient, the renal blood flow rate, and the protein concentration rate in afferent plasma.[33] Renal blood flow may increase as a result of several factors. An increase in cardiac output related to the burn surface area may increase renal blood flow. Fever caused by bacterial endotoxins may increase cardiac output and renal blood flow. Hypervolemia resulting from extracellular overhydration may contribute to an increase in renal blood flow. Some investigators have observed decreased creatinine clearances in patients with greater than 15% burn. Although maximum reductions occurred 2 to 4 days after injury, clearances usually normalized within 2 to 3 weeks. Other investigators have observed elevated glomerular filtration rates within the first 2 weeks of burn trauma.[33] Values were found to be 200% of those found in normal subjects. Drugs eliminated primarily by the kidney that have been studied in burn patients are tobramycin,[33] vancomycin,[34,35] gentamicin,[36,37] ceftazidime,[38] piperacillin,[39] cimetidine,[40–42] and amikacin.[43]

For drugs that are renally eliminated, correlation between drug clearance and creatinine clearance (estimated and measured) is inconsistent. Vancomycin clearance has been shown to exhibit both modest[34] and good[35] correlation with creatinine clearance. It is not clear why the results differ. The method of determining creatinine clearance may account for part of the difference. Investigators have found that three methods of estimating creatinine clearance provide reasonably accurate predictions of measured creatinine clearance[44]; however, wide variability between measured and predicted creatinine clearance was observed, and all methods tended to overestimate creatinine clearance when measured creatinine clearances were less than 60 mL/min per 1.73 $m^2$. Because of the wide variability between measured and predicted creatinine clearances, and between measured and predicted drug clearances, serum concentrations should be monitored for those drugs with narrow therapeutic ranges to maximize efficacy and prevent toxicity.[45,46]

Little work has been done on the effects of thermal injury on hepatic clearance of drugs in humans. The effects of thermal injury on hepatic clearance have been studied in the rat model[47] for phenytoin,[32] pentobarbital,[48,49] quinidine,[48] lidocaine,[48] and theophylline.[48] The volume of distribution and total body clearance of phenytoin in rats increase as a result of decreased protein binding and lower albumin concentrations. While the effects of thermal injury on phenytoin clearance and volume of distribution have not been studied in humans, plasma samples from burn patients have shown a two- to threefold increase in the free fraction of phenytoin and low serum albumin concentrations.[32] Thermally injured rats had prolonged clearance and elimination half-life for pentobarbital, increased volume of distribution and decreased clearance for quinidine, and increased volume of distribution for lidocaine.[48] There were no changes in pharmacokinetic parameters for theophylline in the thermally injured rat model.[48] Diazepam kinetics have been studied in patients with severe burns.[50] Volume of distribution, elimination half-life, and free fraction of diazepam were increased over values obtained from control patients. These patients were on cimetidine, which has been reported to inhibit the clearance of diazepam.[51] Because of the limited information on hepatic clearance of drugs in burn patients, more pharmacokinetic information is needed before any definitive recommendations can be made.

## Summary

The care of the hospitalized burn patient requires a multidisciplinary approach by a number of specially trained people. The physician is responsible for coordinating the available expertise and institutional capabilities that are important in patient care and is responsible for the coordination of all medical services provided in the appropriate management of the burn patient. Occupational and physical therapists play an important part in the rehabilitation of the burn patient. Their activities need to begin in the critical care period, which later is extended into step-down units and often into discharge from the burn facility. The social worker, the clinical psychologist, and/or the psychiatrist play an important part in the psychologic support of the burn patient.

The critical care, or primary burn, nurse is key to the care of the patient and must maintain accurate records and pay particular attention to the monitoring devices (arterial lines, Swan–Ganz catheters, intravenous lines, urinary catheters, infusion devices). The nurse needs to be aware of the signs and symptoms of infection and the goals of medical, physical, and psychologic therapy.

The burn team may also include an infectious disease specialist, a pulmonary medicine specialist, a respiratory therapist, a dietician, a nutritionist, a pharmacist, and burn technicians. Orchestration of this multidisciplinary team by the physician is essential to the successful outcome of the seriously burned patient.

## References


1. US Department of Health and Human Services. Detailed diagnoses and surgical procedures for patients from short-stay hospitals: United States, 1979. DHHS Publication No. (PHS) 82-1274-1, 1985.
2. Herndon DN, Curreri PW, Abston S, et al. Treatment of burns. Curr Probl Surg 1987;24:341–397.
3. Wachtel TL. Epidemiology, classification, initial care, and administrative considerations for critically burned patients. Crit Care Clin 1985;1:3–26.
4. Moncrief JA. Burns. I. Assessment. JAMA 1979;242:72–74.
5. Herndon DN, Langner F, Thompson P, et al. Pulmonary injury in burned patients. Surg Clin North Am 1987;67:31–46.
6. Stone HH, Rhame DW, Corbitt JD, et al. Respiratory burns: A correlation of clinical and laboratory results. Ann Surg 1967;165:157–168.
7. Wroblewski DA, Bower GC. The significance of facial burns in acute smoke inhalation. Crit Care Med 1979;7:335–338.
8. Moylan JA, Chan CK. Inhalation injury—an increasing problem. Surgery 1978;180:34–37.
9. Moylan JA, Alexander Jr G. Diagnosis and treatment of inhalation injury. World J Surg 1978;2:185–191.
10. Moncrief JA. Burns. II. Initial treatment. JAMA 1979;242: 179–182.
11. Demling RH. Fluid resuscitation after major burns. JAMA 1983;250:1438–1440.
12. Demling RH. Fluid replacement in burned patients. Surg Clin North Am 1987;67:15–30.
13. Demling RH. Burns. N Engl J Med 1985;313:1389–1398.
14. Bowser-Wallace BH, Cone JB, Caldwell Jr FT. Hypertonic lactated saline resuscitation of severely burned patients over 60 years of age. J Trauma 1985;25:22–26.
15. Demling RH. Fluid and electrolyte management. Crit Care Clin 1985;1:27–45.
16. Achauer BM, Martinez SE. Burn wound pathophysiology and care. Crit Care Clin 1985;1:47–58.
17. Monafo WW, Freedman B. Topical therapy for burns. Surg Clin North Am 1987;67:133–145.
18. Durtschi MB, Orgain C, Counts GW, et al. A prospective study of penicillin in acutely burned hospitalized patients. J Trauma 1982;22:11.
19. Luterman A, Dacso CC, Curreri PW. Infections in burn patients. Am J Med 1986;81(suppl 1A):45–52.
20. Cuthbertson DP. The metabolic response to injury and its nutritional implications: Retrospect and prospect. JPEN 1979;3:108–129.
21. Pasulka PS, Wachtel TL. Nutritional considerations for the burned patient. Surg Clin North Am 1987;67:109–131.
22. Goodwin CW. Metabolism and nutrition in the thermally injured patient. Crit Care Clin 1985;1:97–117.
23. Curreri PW, Richmond D, Marvin J, et al. Dietary requirements of patients with major burns. J Am Diet Assoc 1974;65:415–417.
24. Munster AM, Winchurch RA. Infection and immunology. Crit Care Clin 1985;1:119–127.
25. Hansbrough JF, Zapata-Sirvent RL, Peterson VM. Immunomodulation following burn injury. Surg Clin North Am 1987;67: 69–92.
26. Bloedow DC, Hardin TC, Simmons MA, et al. Serum drug binding in burn patients. Clin Pharmacol Ther 1982;31:204.
27. Martyn JA, Abernathy DR, Greenblatt DJ. Plasma protein binding of drugs after severe burn injury. Clin Pharmacol Ther 1984;35:535–539.
28. Sawchuk RJ. Drug absorption and disposition in burn patients, in Benet LZ, Massoud N, Gambertoglio JG (eds): Pharmacokinetics Basis for Drug Treatment. New York, Raven, 1984, pp 333–348.
29. Rothschild MA, Ovaty M, Schrieber SS. Albumin metabolism. Gastroenterology 1973;64:324–327.
30. Martyn JA, Greenblatt DJ, Quinby WC. Diazepam kinetics in patients with severe burns. Anesth Analg 1983;62:293–297.

31. Sawchuk RJ, Rector TS. Drug kinetics in burn patients. Clin Pharmacokinet 1980;5:548–556.
32. Bowdle TA, Neal GD, Levy RH, et al. Phenytoin pharmacokinetics in burned rats and plasma protein binding of phenytoin in burned patients. J Pharmacol Exp Ther 1980;213:97–99.
33. Loirat P, Rohan J, Baillet A, et al. Increased glomerular filtration rate in patients with major burns and its effect on the pharmacokinetics of tobramycin. N Engl J Med 1978;299:915–919.
34. Rotschafer JC, Crossley K, Zaske DE, et al. Pharmacokinetics of vancomycin: Observations in 28 patients and dosage recommendations. Antimicrob Agents Chemother 1982;22:391–394.
35. Brater DC, Bawdon RE, Anderson SA, et al. Vancomycin elimination in patients with burn injury. Clin Pharmacol Ther 1986;39:631–634.
36. Glew RH, Moellering RC, Burke JF. Gentamicin dosage in children with extensive burns. J Trauma 1976;16:819–823.
37. Zaske DE, Sawchuk RJ, Gerding DN, et al. Increased dosage requirements of gentamicin in burn patients. J Trauma 1976;16:824–828.
38. Farringer JA, Krinsky DL, Dimick AR. Single-dose pharmacokinetics of ceftazidime in burn patients. Drug Intell Clin Pharm 1986;20:468.
39. Shikuma LR, Ackerman BH, Solem LD, et al. Altered piperacillin disposition in burn and surgical patients. Drug Intell Clin Pharm 1986;20:461.
40. Martyn JA, Greenblatt DJ, Abernethy DR. Increased cimetidine clearance in burn patients. JAMA 1985;253:1288–1291.
41. Ziemniak JA, Watson WA, Saffle JR, et al. Cimetidine kinetics during resuscitation from burn shock. Clin Pharmacol Ther 1984;36:228–233.
42. Martyn JA. Clinical pharmacology and drug therapy in the burned patient. Anesthesiology 1986;65:67–75.
43. Zaske DE, Sawchuk RJ, Strate RG. The necessity of increased doses of amikacin in burn patients. Surgery 1978;84:603–608.
44. Lott RS, Uden DL, Wargin WA, et al. Correlation of predicted versus measured creatinine clearance values in burn patients. Am J Hosp Pharm 1978;35:717–720.
45. Zaske DE, Bootman JL, Solem LB, et al. Increased burn patient survival with individualized dosages of gentamicin. Surgery 1982;92:142–149.
46. Solem LD, Zaske DE, Strate RG. Ecthyma gangrenosum: Survival with individualized antibiotic therapy. Arch Surg 1979;114:580–583.
47. Durlofsky L, Fruncillo RJ. Impaired drug-metabolizing ability in the burned rat. J Trauma 1982;22:950–953.
48. Fruncillo RJ, DiGregorio GJ. Pharmacokinetics of pentobarbital, quinidine, lidocaine, and theophylline in the thermally injured rat. J Pharm Sci 1984;73:1117–1121.
49. Fruncillo RJ, DiGregorio GJ. The effect of thermal injury on drug metabolism in the rat. J Trauma 1983;23:523–529.
50. Martyn JA, Greenblatt DJ, Quinby WC. Diazepam kinetics in patients with severe burns. Anesth Analg 1983;62:293–297.
51. Klotz U, Riemann I. Delayed clearance of diazepam due to cimetidine. N Engl J Med 1980;302:1012–1014.

# Section Twelve
# Hematologic Disorders

## Chapter 69 / Anemias

William J. Spruill, PharmD, and William E. Wade, PharmD

Anemias are a group of diseases characterized by a decrease in circulation of either hemoglobin or red blood cells (RBCs), resulting in a decrease in the oxygen-carrying capacity of blood. Anemia can be caused by reduction of the number of RBCs, the size of RBCs, or the hemoglobin content of the RBCs. Anemia, often a sign of an underlying disease, is characterized in laboratory terms as a decrease in the oxygen-carrying pigment hemoglobin, or as a hematocrit below the specified "normal" values. Classically, anemias are conditions in which the red cell mass is less than normal; practically, anemias are diagnosed indirectly by measurement of the hemoglobin concentration and hematocrit.

Our study of anemias begins with a review of the classification systems, definitions, pathophysiology, and laboratory tests and procedures used in describing and diagnosing anemias. Then, some specific anemias are described in detail.

Anemias are classified by several, often confusing methods. Table 69.1 shows three commonly used methods and gives some examples.

Iron deficiency anemia, anemia of chronic disease, and anemias associated with acute bleeding each account for roughly 25% of all anemias.[1] The remaining 25% are anemias resulting from such conditions as bone marrow damage, decreased erythropoiesis, and hemolysis.

### Maturation and Development

In the normal adult, RBCs are formed in the marrow of the vertebra, ribs, sternum, clavical, pelvic (iliac) crest, and proximal epiphyses of the long bones, such as the upper ends of the femur and humerus. In a child, most bone marrow space is hematopoietically active because of high RBC requirements. With increasing age, available bone space exceeds blood cell production requirements and much marrow space is filled with inactive fatty reserve marrow. This reserve space can be reactivated if other hematopoietic marrow fails or RBC life span decreases.

Like all blood cells, RBCs originate from undifferentiated mesenchymal "stem" cells in the bone marrow. Upon specific stimulation by the hormone erythropoietin, the stem cell differentiates into a committed stem cell that then undergoes mitosis; one cell remains in the stem cell pool and the other committed stem cell serves as the initial precursor for erythrocyte formation. In this manner, all blood cells can develop from a similar stem cell population, which is normally self-sustaining. Stem cells contain the DNA necessary for mitosis and the RNA necessary for protein synthesis.

In normal RBC formation (normoblastic erythropoiesis), the committed stem cell undergoes a dynamic maturation process involving multiple mitotic divisions, with folate- and vitamin $B_{12}$-dependent synthesis and splitting of RNA and DNA. This process is accompanied by the ongoing incorporation of hemoglobin and iron into the gradually maturing RBC, which is then released from the marrow into the circulating blood as a reticulocyte. This maturation process takes about 1 week. Over the next several days the reticulocyte loses its nucleus, shrinks slightly, and develops into a mature enucleated RBC called an erythrocyte. Normally, less than 2% of all circulating RBCs are reticulocytes; thus, the reticulocyte count or percentage is a good indicator of increased RBC formation. All blood cells, including RBCs, go through this gradual maturation process, first forming a primitive blast cell precursor, then progressing to a pro. . .cyte form, a . . .cyte form, a meta. . .cyte form, and eventually a mature cell. Each stage results in changes in cytoplasm, nucleus, and cell size. The cytoplasm of immature cells is predominantly blue and contains large amounts of RNA which has an affinity for basic or blue dye (methylene blue); hence, immature cells are called diffusely basophilic erythrocytes, polychromatophilic macrocytes, or reticulocytes. As the cell matures the cytoplasm becomes less blue and more red. Because the earlier forms of each cell line (eosinophil, neutrophil, basophil, monocyte, thrombocyte, erythrocyte, and lymphocyte) appear similar morphologically, it is often difficult to distinguish the various immature forms of blood cells; these immature forms are usually reported on CBC reports without differentiation as to their eventual mature cell form. Immature cells are simply reported as "blast," "pro," "meta," and so on. Table 69.2 outlines the terminology used for the immature erythrocyte

**Table 69.1** Classification Systems for Anemias

**Morphology**

Classifies anemias on the basis of red blood cell size (microcytic, normocytic, macrocytic) and hemoglobin content (hypochromic, normochromic, hyperchromic)

- Macrocytic
  - Megaloblastic anemias
    - Vitamin $B_{12}$ deficiency
    - Folic acid deficiency anemia
- Hypochromic microcytic
  - Iron deficiency anemia
  - Genetic anomaly
    - Sickle cell anemia
    - Thalassemia
    - Other hemoglobinopathies (abnormal hemoglobins)
- Normocytic
  - Recent blood loss
  - Hemolysis
  - Bone marrow failure
  - Anemias of chronic disease
  - Renal failure
  - Endocrine disorders
  - Myeloplastic anemias

**Etiology**

Classifies anemias on the basis of three fundamental mechanisms

- Deficiency
  - Iron
  - Vitamin $B_{12}$
  - Folic acid
  - Pyridoxine
- Central—Caused by impaired bone marrow function
  - Anemia of chronic disease
  - Anemia of senescence
  - Malignant bone marrow disorders
- Peripheral
  - Bleeding (hemorrhage)
  - Hemolysis (hemolytic anemias)

**Pathophysiology**

Classifies anemias on the basis of evaluation of pathophysiologic etiology

- Excessive blood loss
  - Recent hemorrhage
    - Trauma
    - Peptic ulcer
    - Gastritis
    - Hemorrhoids
  - Chronic hemorrhage
    - Vaginal bleeding
    - Peptic ulcer
    - Intestinal parasites
    - Aspirin and other nonsteroidal anti-inflammatory agents
- Excessive red cell destruction
  - Extracorpuscular (i.e., outside the cell) factors
    - RBC antibodies
    - Drugs
    - Physical trauma to RBCs (artificial valves)
    - Excessive sequestration in the spleen

**Table 69.1** (continued)

  - Intracorpuscular factors
    - Heredity
    - Disorders of hemoglobin synthesis
- Inadequate production of mature RBCs
  - Deficiency of nutrients ($B_{12}$, folic acid, iron, protein)
  - Deficiency of erythroblasts
    - Aplastic anemia
    - Isolated (often transient) erythroblastopenia
    - Folic acid antagonists
    - Antibodies
  - Conditions in which bone marrow is infiltrated
    - Lymphoma
    - Leukemia
    - Myelofibrosis
    - Carcinoma
  - Endocrine abnormalities
    - Hypothyroid
    - Adrenal insufficiency
    - Pituitary insufficiency
  - Chronic renal disease
  - Chronic inflammatory disease
    - Granulomatous diseases
    - Collagen vascular diseases
  - Hepatic disease

precursors in normoblastic erythropoiesis. Immature cells are large and progressively decrease in size as they mature.

Two abnormal forms of erythropoiesis, microcytic and megaloblastic, result in mature microcytes and macrocytes, respectively. Megaloblasts are larger nucleated precursors that proceed through stages of development similar to those of normoblastic erythropoiesis (yet abnormal). Megaloblasts are typically seen with $B_{12}$ and folic acid deficiency anemias.

### *Stimulation of Erythropoiesis*

Production of RBCs is initiated by the hormone erythropoietin, which is produced mainly (90%) by the kidneys in response to a decrease in tissue oxygen caused by a decreased hemoglobin. This decreased tissue oxygen signals the kidneys to increase production and release into the plasma of erythropoietin, which (1) stimulates stem cells to differentiate into rubriblasts, (2) increases the rate of mitosis, (3) increases the release of reticulocytes from the marrow, and (4) induces hemoglobin formation. When hemoglobin synthesis is accelerated, the critical hemoglobin concentration necessary for maturity is reached more rapidly and a

**Table 69.2** Erythrocyte Maturation Sequence

| | |
|---|---|
| Least mature form | Rubriblast (pronormoblast) |
| Second cell formed | Prorubricyte |
| Third cell formed | Rubricyte (last mitotic stage) |
| Fourth cell formed | Metarubricyte |
| Fifth cell formed | Reticulocyte (basophilic erythrocyte) |
| Most mature form | Erythrocyte (nonnucleated) |

feedback mechanism stops further RBC nucleic acid synthesis so that the last mitotic division is skipped, causing an earlier release of reticulocytes. The appearance of these cells is another indication that RBC production is being stimulated.

### *Synthesis of Hemoglobin*

Hemoglobin is composed of two identical half molecules and its synthesis within the RBCs is under genetic control. Hemoglobin is a tetrahedron, that is, a four-sided crystal geometric molecule containing a protein (globin) component composed of two $\alpha$ and two $\beta$ chains; each chain is linked to a heme group consisting of a porphyrin ring structure with an iron atom chelated at its center that is capable of binding oxygen. The globin portion of hemoglobin consists of two pairs of polypeptide chains containing 141 to 146 amino acids, depending on the type of hemoglobin (i.e., Hb A, Hb $A_2$, Hb F, Hb S, etc). These polypeptide chains are attached to and folded around each heme structure, giving hemoglobin its unique tetrahedron shape.

The initial step in the synthesis of heme from succinyl coenzyme A and glycine requires the presence of pyridoxine phosphate (vitamin $B_6$) as a catalyst. After it is synthesized in the cytoplastic mitochondria of RBCs, heme diffuses into the extramitochondrial space to combine with the completed $\alpha$ and $\beta$ chains and form hemoglobin.

A defect or block in hemoglobin synthesis can lead to abnormally appearing, usually hypochromic, RBCs, reflecting a lack of hemoglobinization. Because the cell remains in the marrow longer, waiting for proper hemoglobin synthesis to occur, an increased number of cell divisions may occur, resulting in a final mature erythrocyte that is smaller than normal—a microcyte.

A defect in hemoglobin synthesis as well as certain acquired defects in erythropoietic precursor cell metabolism may cause changes in iron incorporation, producing a cell with an excess of nonheme iron within the cytoplasm. These cells, called sideroblasts, cause sideroblastic anemia which is usually macrocytic. Other hereditary defects in heme synthesis can lead to overproduction of heme precursors, causing the disease porphyria.

Lastly, genetic expression of an abnormal amino acid substitution in either the $\alpha$- or $\beta$-globin chains can lead to a variety of hemoglobinopathies causing such hemolytic diseases as sickle cell anemia and thalassemia. Hundreds of these abnormal hemoglobin diseases exist, and are best diagnosed by hemoglobin electrophoresis.

Under normal conditions, the body produces approximately 6.25 g of hemoglobin per day. The maximal output of hemoglobin in the event of a hemolytic disease has been calculated to be 40 g per day. Consequently, the normal RBC survival time of 120 days can decrease to 18 to 20 days before an anemia occurs, if the bone marrow functions at maximal capacity. When the hemolytic destruction of RBCs exceeds marrow production capacity, anemia develops, causing the hemoglobin value to decrease to a "steady-state" level at which production is equal to destruction. Hemoglobin values in these hemolytic anemias, such as sickle cell anemia, remain stable unless other factors further shorten RBC life span.

### *Incorporation of Iron Into Heme*

Iron is delivered to the bone marrow for incorporation into the RBC's hemoglobin molecule by a specific plasma transport protein (globulin) called transferrin. Each molecule of transferrin can bind two molecules of iron. Transferrin then attaches itself to the RBC and iron passes through the membrane into the RBC.

Circulating transferrin is normally only about 30% saturated with iron. The remaining transferrin (approximately 70%) is not bound to iron and represents the total iron-binding capacity (TIBC). Transferrin also delivers extra iron to other body storage sites such as the liver, marrow, and spleen for later use. This iron is stored as ferritin or hemosiderin. Ferritin consists of a ferric hydroxyphosphate core surrounded by a protein shell called apoferritin. Hemosiderin can be described as compacted ferritin molecules with an even greater iron-to-protein-shell ratio; physiologically it is a more stable but less available form of storage iron.

### *Absorption of Iron*

The average daily diet contains approximately 12 to 15 mg of iron, in mainly the ferric ($Fe^{3+}$), nonabsorbed form. This is first ionized by stomach acid and then reduced to the ferrous state ($Fe^{2+}$) and absorbed primarily in the duodenum and, to a lesser extent, in the jejunum. Iron overload is prevented by a mechanism described as "the intelligent behavior of the small intestine," whereby only the amount of iron lost per day is absorbed. This represents about 10% (1 mg) of daily dietary intake. Up to 8–12 mg per day can be absorbed if iron requirements increase. A hereditary gastrointestinal disease, hemochromatosis, results from the loss of regulation of iron absorption; the resultant iron deposition in various tissues causes multiple-organ-system failure.

### *Normal Destruction of Red Blood Cells*

Older blood cells are destroyed in the marrow by phagocytic breakdown (Fig. 69.1). The amino acids from the globin chains return to an amino acid pool; the porphyrin heme structure splits, forming biliverdin and releasing its iron. Iron returns to the iron pool for reuse, while biliverdin is further enzymatically reduced to bilirubin. This bilirubin is released from the marrow into the plasma, where it binds to albumin and is transported to the liver for glucuronide conjugation and excretion via the bile. Should the liver be unable to carry out this conjugation in the normal manner, as seen with intrinsic liver disease or oversaturation of conjugation enzymes by excessive cell hemolysis, the result would be an elevated indirect (unconjugated) bilirubin laboratory value. Should there be an obstruction in the excretion pathway of the conjugated bilirubin, an elevated direct bilirubin would result. Comparison of direct and indirect bilirubin values helps determine if the defect in bilirubin clearance occurs before or after blood enters the liver.

The hemoglobin in red blood cells destroyed by intravascular hemolysis attaches to a haptoglobin and is carried back to the marrow for processing in the normal manner.

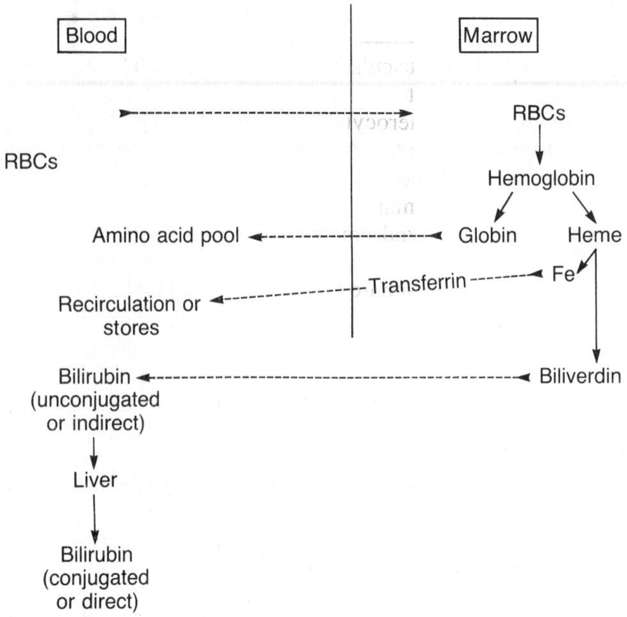


**Figure 69.1** Destruction of red blood cells (RBCs).

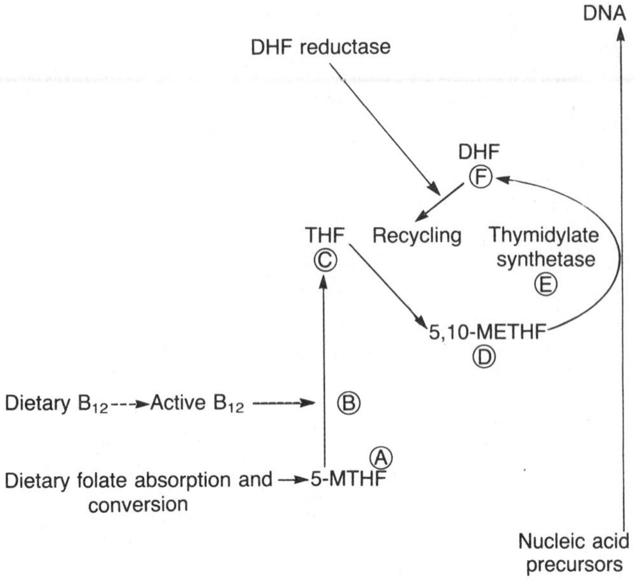


**Figure 69.2** Drug-induced megaloblastosis. DHF, dihydrofolate; THF, tetrahydrofolate; 5-MTHF, 5-methyl THF; 5,10-METHF, 5,10-methylene THF.

## Pathophysiology

The pathologic processes responsible for development of various anemias are described in this section. Specific details are given under Clinical Presentation and Treatment.

### *Iron Deficiency Anemia*

In iron deficiency anemia (IDA), the iron stores are depleted prior to development of anemia; therefore, the earliest change observed is a decrease in serum ferritin relative to baseline. Unfortunately IDA is not usually detected at this level. With continuing iron depletion, the hemoglobin drops slightly and serum ferritin falls below 12. TIBC increases and serum iron concentration decreases. The hemoglobin, hematocrit, and RBC indices usually remain normal. In the later stages of IDA, the hemoglobin and hematocrit fall below normal values and a microcytic, hypochromic anemia develops. Microcytosis may precede hypochromia, as erythropoiesis is programmed to maintain normal hemoglobin concentration in deference to cell size. As a consequence, even slightly abnormal hemoglobin and hematocrit values may indicate significant depletion of iron stores and should not be ignored. Conversely, with treatment of IDA, these monitoring parameters return to normal in reverse order of their occurrence.

### *Megaloblastic Anemias*

Megaloblastosis results from interference in folic acid and vitamin $B_{12}$-interdependent nucleic acid synthesis in the immature erythrocyte. Because DNA and RNA synthesis is retarded, one or more mitotic cell divisions are skipped, resulting in an abnormally large cell. Synthesis of the RNA and DNA necessary for cell division depends upon a series of reactions catalyzed by vitamin $B_{12}$ and folic acid (Fig. 69.2). In this process dietary folates are absorbed and converted (*A*) to 5-methyl tetrahydrofolate (5-MTHF), which is then converted via a $B_{12}$-dependent (*B*) reaction to tetrahydrofolate (THF) (*C*). After gaining a carbon, this THF is converted to a folate cofactor (*D*), 5,10-methylene tetrahydrofolate (5,10-METHF), used by thymidylate synthetase (*E*) in the biosynthesis of nucleic acids. The 5,10-METHF cofactor is converted to dihydrofolate (DHF) (*F*) during biosynthesis. Normally, dihydrofolate reductase enzyme (*F*) reduces DHF back to tetrahydrofolate (*C*), which can again pick up a carbon and be recycled to produce more 5,10-METHF (*D*). Several drugs (Table 69.3) have been reported to cause a folic acid deficiency megaloblastic anemia by either interfering with folate absorption or inhibiting the dihydrofolate reductase necessary for conversion of dihydrofolate to its active tetrahydrofolate form. Recent information[2] indicates that although phenytoin may induce a megaloblastic anemia, folic acid supplementation in these patients may decrease phenytoin's anticonvulsant activity. Routine supplementation is therefore not recommended; however, close monitoring for this potential interaction is advised.

### *Anemia of Chronic Disease*

Anemia of chronic disease (ACD) is a hypoproliferative anemia that accompanies infectious, inflammatory, or neoplastic diseases lasting more than 1 or 2 months. ACD is caused primarily by a block in the release of iron from the reticuloendothelial cells of the marrow, along with a decreased RBC life span, the mechanism for which is not yet understood. Examination of bone marrow reveals an abundance of iron, so it appears that the mechanism for release of this iron is the central defect. Additionally, certain diseases such as chronic renal failure also decrease erythropoietin

**Table 69.3** Drug-Induced Megaloblastosis[a]

| |
|---|
| Impaired absorption or folate inactivation |
| Phenytoin[3–5] |
| Phenobarbital[5,6] |
| Primidone[5,6] |
| Alcohol[7,8] |
| Oral contraceptives[9–13] |
| Sulfasalazine[14,15] |
| Inhibition of dihydrofolate reductase necessary for conversion of DHF to THF, the metabolically active folate cofactor for nucleic acid synthesis |
| Methotrexate[16] |
| Trimethoprim[17–20] |
| Triamterene[21,22] |
| Inadequate or inactive vitamin $B_{12}$ |
| Neomycin[23,24] |
| Colchicine[25] |

[a] Only phenytoin, phenobarbital, primidone, and methotrexate are associated with a frequent incidence of reported megaloblastosis.

production, further exacerbating anemia of chronic disease. Although these anemias are usually mild, they often alert the physician to an underlying, as yet undiagnosed chronic disease. Table 69.4 lists diseases commonly associated with ACD.

### *Anemia of Senescence*

Many factors predispose elderly patients to development of anemia: iron, $B_{12}$, or folic acid deficiency; anemia of chronic disease; or a combination. Anemia of senescence is used to describe anemias in the elderly that are not due to commonly recognized causes. This type of anemia is characterized by an overall reduction in hematopoietic capability and reserve, and is analogous to the "wearing out" of the hematopoietic system.[26]

**Table 69.4** Causes of Anemia of Chronic Disease

| |
|---|
| Chronic infections |
| Tuberculosis |
| Other chronic lung infections |
| Subacute bacterial endocarditis |
| Osteomyelitis |
| Chronic urinary tract infections |
| Chronic inflammation |
| Rheumatoid arthritis |
| Systemic lupus erythematosus |
| Other rheumatoid (collagen vascular) diseases |
| Inflammatory osteoarthritis |
| Gout |
| Chronic inflammatory liver diseases |
| Malignancies |
| Carcinoma |
| Hodgkin's disease |
| Leukemia |
| Multiple myeloma |

**Table 69.5** Common Classes of Hemolytic Anemias

| |
|---|
| Intrinsic (intracorpuscular)—usually genetically inherited |
| Membrane defect |
| Hereditary spherocytosis |
| Hereditary elliptocytosis |
| Hemoglobin defect |
| Sickle cell anemia |
| Thalassemia syndrome |
| Metabolic defect |
| Glucose-6-phosphate dehydrogenase (G6PD) deficiency |
| Many other enzyme deficiencies |
| Extrinsic |
| Membrane defect—autoimmune hemolytic anemia associated with |
| Lymphoproliferative cancers |
| Systemic lupus erythematosus and other autoimmune disorders |
| Mononucleosis and other viral infections |
| Mycoplasma infections |
| Drugs (methyldopa, penicillin) |
| Hemoglobin defect |
| Oxidants that may cause unstable hemoglobin to clump |
| Metabolic defects |
| Oxidants that may cause G6PD-deficient cells to hemolyze |

### *Hemolytic Anemia*

The normal 120-day life span of a red blood cell derives from its inherent flexibility in passage through the microvasculature and spleen without disruption of the cell membrane or sequestration and phagocytosis by reticuloendothelial cells. Hemolysis, as defined by a RBC life span less than 120 days, results from one of three primary defects: alteration in cell shape or deformability, loss of membrane integrity, and changes in adherence properties of the cell membrane. Defects in one of the three main components of the RBC can cause a decreased life span leading to a hemolytic anemia: (1) membrane defects, leading to spherocytes or even cell fragments, changes in membrane permeability causing swollen or shrunken cells, and modifications of the membrane surface; (2) alterations in the solubility or stability of hemoglobin; and (3) alterations in cell metabolism (enzymopathies) responsible for maintaining cell dimensions and hemoglobin solubility. These changes in membrane integrity, hemoglobin stability, and cell metabolism originate intrinsically or extrinsically. Table 69.5 lists examples of the different classes of hemolytic anemias.

#### Laboratory Evaluations of Anemias

Several laboratory tests are used to evaluate anemias.

1. *Hemoglobin* (normally 12–16 g/dL in females and 14–18 g/dL in males). The higher values in males result from stimulation of RBC production by androgenic steroids. Hemoglobin can decrease as a result of a decrease in the quantity of RBCs or a decrease in the number of RBCs.
2. *Hematocrit* (normally 35%–40% in females and 42%–52% in males) is the actual volume of RBCs in a

unit volume expressed as a percentage. A low hematocrit indicates a reduction in either number or size of RBCs or an increased plasma volume.

3. *Red blood cell count* (normally 4.5–6.0 million/$mm^3$ for men and 4.0–5.5 million/$mm^3$ for women) is an indirect estimate of the hemoglobin content of the blood.
4. *RBC indices* (Wintrobe indices) were introduced in 1934 by Maxwell Wintrobe to describe certain morphologic characteristics of the RBC.
   a. *Mean corpuscular volume* (MCV) (normally 80–100 fL or $\mu m^3$ in adults) indicates macrocytic, normocytic, or microcytic morphology, as it represents the average volume, measured with a Coulter counter, of the RBC. It is based on the relationship of average RBC size to hematocrit. For example, if the average size of the RBC is increased, then the same number of RBCs will have a slightly larger total cell mass and an increased hematocrit, whereas if the average size is decreased, the hematocrit will be decreased. Folic acid and vitamin $B_{12}$ deficiency anemias are macrocytic.
   b. *Mean corpuscular hemoglobin* (MCH) (normally 27–31 pg in adults) is the average weight of hemoglobin in a RBC. Two morphologic changes, microcytosis and hypochromia, can reduce MCH. A microcytic cell contains less hemoglobin because it is a smaller cell, whereas a hypochromic cell has a low MCH because of the decreased amount of hemoglobin present in a normocytic cell. Cells commonly are both microcytic and hypochromic. MCH alone cannot distinguish between microcytosis and hypochromia. The most common cause of an elevated MCH is macrocytosis.
   c. *Mean corpuscular hemoglobin concentration* (MCHC) is the weight of hemoglobin per volume of cells (that is, concentration). MCHC is independent of cell size and therefore is more useful than MCH in distinguishing between microcytosis and hypochromia. A low MCHC always indicates hypochromia, as a microcyte with a normal hemoglobin concentration will have a low MCH but a normal MCHC.
5. *Total reticulocyte count* (normally 0.5%–1.5% of total red blood cells in adults). Occasionally, a patient's hematocrit decreases while the absolute number of reticulocytes remains the same. This results in a falsely elevated reticulocyte percentage. For example, if a patient's hematocrit decreases by 50% (from 50% to 25%) the corresponding reticulocyte percentage doubles. This problem is corrected by expressing the reticulocyte count as an absolute number; to do this, the percentage reticulocytes (expressed as a decimal) is multiplied by the total red blood cell count. A corrected percentage reticulocytes can also be calculated by multiplying it by the patient's hematocrit and then dividing the product by an average normal hematocrit (for men or women).

   Corrected reticulocyte count (%) =

$$\text{observed \%} \times \frac{\text{patient's Hct}}{\text{normal Hct}}$$

6. *Serum iron* (normally approximately 65–185 $\mu$g/dL) is the concentration of iron bound to transferrin. Normally, transferrin is about one-third bound (saturated) to iron. Unfortunately, the serum iron level of many patients with iron deficiency anemia remains within the lower limits of normal, giving a false-negative test. There is also a 20% to 30% diurnal variation in serum iron levels (it is best to draw blood in the morning) and a 20% to 25% day-to-day variation among individuals. Consequently, as a diagnostic tool, serum iron levels are best interpreted in conjunction with the total iron-binding capacity. Serum iron is decreased with iron deficiency anemia and anemias of chronic disease and is increased with hemolytic anemias and iron overload.
7. *Total iron-binding capacity* (TIBC) (normally 250–440 $\mu$g/dL) is an indirect measurement of serum transferrin, determined by adding an excess of iron to plasma to saturate all transferrin with iron. The excess (unbound) iron is then removed and the serum iron concentration is determined. Unlike the serum iron level, the TIBC is remarkably constant. The finding of a low serum iron and a high TIBC indicates IDA.
8. *Serum ferritin* (normally 12–300 ng/mL). The concentration of ferritin (storage iron) in the serum is proportional to total iron stores and, consequently, is a reliable indicator of body iron stores. Low serum ferritin levels are virtually diagnostic of IDA as they are decreased only in IDA, whereas serum iron may be decreased in IDA and anemia of chronic disease.
9. *Folic acid level* (normal values vary depending on assay method used). Decreased levels indicate a folate deficiency megaloblastic anemia that may coexist with a vitamin $B_{12}$ deficiency anemia.
10. *Vitamin $B_{12}$ level* (normal values vary depending on assay method used). Low levels indicate vitamin $B_{12}$ deficiency "pernicious" anemia.
11. *The Schilling test* is used to diagnose vitamin $B_{12}$ deficiency anemia caused by a $B_{12}$ absorption defect resulting from lack of an intrinsic factor (pernicious anemia). An oral dose of cobalt-labeled vitamin $B_{12}$ is administered. If sufficient intrinsic factor is being produced gastrointestinally, the $B_{12}$ will be absorbed. Concomitantly, a large intramuscular dose of nonlabeled vitamin $B_{12}$ is given to saturate tissue binding sites and flush the radiolabeled $B_{12}$ into the urine. Normally, approximately 33% of the absorbed radiolabeled $B_{12}$ appears in the urine over 24 hours. Patients with pernicious anemia excrete less than 8% of the original oral radiolabeled dose. After several days, this test is repeated, except that the oral radiolabeled $B_{12}$ is administered with a sufficient amount of intrinsic factor. Results within the normal range indicate that the defect is in intrinsic factor production as opposed to dietary lack of vitamin $B_{12}$.

Table 69.6 lists laboratory changes commonly seen with various anemias.

## Clinical Presentation and Treatment

### *Iron Deficiency Anemia*

As previously stated, IDA is usually microcytic and hypochromic. It is believed to occur in approximately 25% of patients with anemia. The most commonly cited causes of

**Table 69.6** Laboratory Changes in Anemias

| | Parameter[a] | |
|---|---|---|
| | **Increased** | **Decreased** |
| Iron deficiency anemia | TIBC<br>Free erythrocyte<br>Protoporphyrin | Hemoglobin<br>Hematocrit<br>MCV<br>MCHC<br>Ferritin<br>Iron |
| Vitamin $B_{12}$ deficiency | MCV<br>Unconjugated bilirubin<br>Lactate dehydrogenase<br>Transferrin saturation | $B_{12}$ (but may be normal)<br>Reticulocyte count |
| Folic acid deficiency | MCV<br>Unconjugated bilirubin<br>Lactate dehydrogenase<br>Transferrin saturation | Folate<br>Reticulocyte count |
| Anemia of chronic disease | Transferrin saturation<br>Bilirubin<br>Protoporphyrin<br>Marrow sideroblast iron | Hemoglobin<br>MCV<br>MCHC<br>Iron (may be normal)<br>TIBC |
| Hemolytic anemia | Reticulocyte count<br>Unconjugated bilirubin<br>Urinary urobilinogen<br>Fecal urobilinogen<br>Spherocyte count<br>Urinary hemosiderin | |

[a] MCV, mean corpuscular volume; MCHC, mean corpuscular hemoglobin concentration; TIBC, total iron-binding capacity.

Compiled from References 26, 27, 31, and 32.

IDA include inadequate dietary intake, inadequate absorption from the gastrointestinal tract, increased iron demands, blood loss, and certain diseases.[28] Dietary deficiencies most frequently result from reduced consumption of animal protein and ascorbic acid[29] as a consequence of chronic alcoholism, food faddism, prolonged illness with anorexia, or poor nutrition. Inadequate absorption from the gastrointestinal tract is usually a sequel to such disorders as malabsorption syndromes, postgastrectomy states, the presence of certain foods or drugs, or unrelenting diarrhea. Demands for iron may increase during infancy, pregnancy, adolescence, or old age. Blood loss may occur as a result of many disorders, including trauma, hemorrhoids, peptic ulcers, gastritis, gastrointestinal carcinoma, diverticular disease, copious menstrual flow, nose bleeds, or postpartum bleeding.[30] Diseases contributing to the development of iron deficiency anemia include rheumatoid arthritis (with chronic aspirin ingestion), various carcinomas, and renal disease. With iron deficiency anemia, the possibility of a multifactorial etiology must always be kept in mind.

***Signs and Symptoms*** Presenting symptoms of IDA are listed in Table 69.7.[31] These symptoms usually do not appear until the hemoglobin concentration falls below 8 or 9 g/100 mL. These symptoms differ based on the speed of onset of development of the anemia.

***Laboratory Findings*** Hemoglobin concentrations below 11 g/100 mL and hematocrits less than 38% usually indicate a decrease in red blood cell mass that may be caused by iron deficiency. Low concentrations of ferritin (less than 10–12 $\mu$g/L) are indicative of iron deficiency. In patients with inflammatory disorders, however, these values may be within normal limits despite the presence of iron deficiency. Liver disease causes an elevation in serum ferritin; thus, ferritin should not be used for diagnostic purposes in patients with even mild hepatic pathology. Transferrin saturation is calculated by dividing the serum iron concentration by the total iron-binding capacity and multiplying by 100. One major disadvantage of this test is the large biologic variation in serum iron levels. Iron concentrations are highest in the morning and lowest at night. Therefore, it is generally

**Table 69.7** Signs and Symptoms of Anemias

| |
|---|
| All anemias |
| Fatigue |
| Pallor |
| Jaundice |
| Hepatosplenomegaly |
| Tachycardia |
| Wide pulse pressure |
| Pale mucous membranes |
| Cardiac decompensation |
| Shortness of breath |
| Edema |
| Dizziness |
| Lightheadedness |
| Weakness |
| Vitamin $B_{12}$ deficiency |
| Dysphagia |
| Anorexia |
| Weight loss |
| Beefy red tongue |
| Psychosis |
| Forgetfulness |
| Paresthesia of hands and toes |
| Ataxia |
| Positive Romberg sign |
| Positive Babinski sign |
| Impaired vibratory sense |
| Impaired position sense |
| Impaired urinary function |
| Hemolytic anemia |
| Painful crises |
| Abdominal pain |
| Hemoglobinuria |
| Cholelithiasis |
| Leg ulcers |
| Fever (rare) |
| Jaundice (rare) |
| Lymphadenopathy (rare) |
| Angina (rare) |
| Syncope (rare) |
| Congestive heart failure (rare) |
| Iron deficiency anemia |
| Koilonychia (spooning of nails) |
| Angular stomatitis |
| Glossitis |
| Achlorhydria |
| Craving for substances low in iron (clay, ice, cornstarch) |
| Folic acid deficiency |
| Dysphagia |
| Anorexia |
| Weight loss |
| Beefy red tongue |
| Personality changes |
| Generalized malnutrition |
| Ecchymosis |
| Purpura |
| Loss of skin elasticity |
| Early graying of hair |

Compiled from References 27, 32, and 38.

recommended that blood for transferrin saturation testing be drawn in the morning or early afternoon hours. Low values (below 15%) at these times will likely indicate iron deficiency anemia; however, as mentioned before, low serum transferrin saturation values may also be present in inflammatory disorders. Fortunately, the TIBC usually helps to differentiate the diagnosis in these patients; a TIBC greater than 400 μg% suggests IDA, whereas values below 200 μg% usually represent inflammatory disease.

Free erythrocyte protoporphyrin can also be used in the diagnosis of IDA. Iron normally binds with protoporphyrin to form heme. When iron levels are low, the serum concentration of protoporphyrin not bound to iron is elevated. This test is very helpful in distinguishing between iron deficiency and thalassemia minor, as values are normal in the latter and elevated in the former. Unfortunately, free erythrocyte protoporphyrin is also elevated in inflammatory disorders and lead poisoning and, thus, is less effective in distinguishing iron deficiency in patients in whom these other two conditions are also present.

***Diet*** Food plays a significant role in the prevention as well as treatment of IDA. It is now well known that iron absorption varies greatly with different foods. Iron is poorly absorbed from vegetables, grain products, dairy products, and eggs, while it is best absorbed from meat, fish, and poultry. Substitution of meat for eggs, milk, or cheese in a mixed meal has been shown to quadruple the absorption of iron from the entire meal.[33] Beverages have also been shown to affect iron absorption. For example, orange juice doubles the absorption of iron from an entire meal, whereas tea and milk reduce absorption to less than one half.[34,35] It is thus recommended that meat, orange juice, and other ascorbic acid–rich foods be included in meals and that if milk and tea are used, they be consumed in moderation between meals.

***Therapeutic Iron Preparations*** In most cases of IDA, oral iron therapy with soluble ferrous iron salts is the recommended treatment. The dose depends upon the patient's ability to tolerate the administered iron. In patients with iron deficiency, it is generally recommended that approximately 200 mg elemental iron be administered each day.[36] The percentage of iron absorbed progressively decreases as the dose increases, but the absolute amount absorbed increases.[29] Food interferes with the absorption of iron; therefore, iron should preferably be administered one or more hours before meals. Previous studies have shown that addition of ascorbic acid does not enhance absorption from oral iron preparations when given on an empty stomach.[29] Ferrous sulfate, ferrous gluconate, and ferrous fumarate are the most frequently prescribed oral iron preparations. Approximately 60–65 mg elemental iron is provided per 300- to 325-mg sulfate salt tablet, approximately 37–39 mg elemental iron per 300- to 325-mg gluconate tablet, and 33 mg elemental iron per 100-mg fumarate tablet. Administration of 40–75 mg elemental iron three times a day before meals is effective therapy for most IDA patients.

Adverse reactions at this dose are primarily gastrointestinal in nature and consist of discoloration of feces (dark), constipation or diarrhea, nausea, and vomiting. Failure to develop at least some of these symptoms, even mildly, may indicate noncompliance. Should these side effects be intolerable, the dose may be taken with meals or the total daily dose may be reduced to 110–120 mg elemental iron. Administration of iron with meals, however, reduces the amount of iron absorbed by more than one half.

Therapeutic doses of iron raise the hemoglobin value by 1–2 g% per week. As the hemoglobin level approaches normal, the rate of increase slows progressively. A hemoglobin response of less than 2 g/100 mL over a 3-week period is unacceptable and should be further evaluated. Additionally, reticulocytosis occurs 7 to 10 days after initiation of iron therapy. If the patient does not develop reticulocytosis, the diagnosis needs to be reevaluated.

Iron therapy should continue for a period sufficient to completely restore the serum level and also to replenish some iron stores. The time required to accomplish this goal varies from patient to patient, but in general, 3 to 6 months of therapy is necessary.[37] Patients with negative iron balances caused by bleeding may require iron replacement therapy for only a month after correction of the underlying lesion, whereas patients with recurrent negative balances may require long-term treatment. This latter group may require as little as 30–60 mg of elemental iron daily.

Failure to respond to the preceding treatment regimen necessitates reevaluation of the situation. Common causes of treatment failures include noncompliance with therapy, misdiagnosis (e.g., inflammation), malabsorption, and blood loss equal to the rate of production. Malabsorption can be ruled out by the iron test in which plasma iron levels are determined at half-hour intervals for 2 hours following the administration of 50 mg elemental iron as liquid ferrous sulfate. If plasma iron levels increase by more than 50 ng% during this time, absorption is satisfactory.

Parenteral iron therapy may be necessary when there is evidence of iron malabsorption, when intolerance of orally administered iron exists, and when noncompliance is a problem. Iron dextran may be given intramuscularly (Z-tract administration) or intravenously in these situations. Equations for calculating the dose in patients with IDA and anemia secondary to blood loss are given in Table 69.8. When administered intravenously, the dose should not exceed 50 mg iron per minute (1 mL/min). The manufacturer suggests that no more than 100 mg of iron dextran be administered daily; however, there are numerous reports that describe how the total dose of iron dextran needed was administered as a single dose either by intravenous infusion or direct intravenous administration. If the total dose required to correct the anemia is given in a single dose, one must be aware of the increased possibility of such adverse reactions as arthralgia, myalgia, and fever. Other adverse reactions to iron dextran include staining of the skin, pain at the injection site, allergic reactions, and anaphylaxis (rare).

**Table 69.8** Equations for Calculating the Dose of Iron Dextran for Patients With Iron Deficiency Anemia and Anemia Secondary to Blood Loss

**Iron Deficiency Anemia**

$$\text{mg of iron} = W \times (100 - \%\text{Hb}) \times 0.3$$

where $W$ is the patient's weight in pounds and %Hb is the patient's observed hemoglobin expressed as a percentage of the normal hemoglobin concentration (assuming that 14.8 g of hemoglobin per 100 mL is equivalent to 100% concentration)

If the patient weighs 13.6 kg (30 pounds) or less, the dose is 80% of the calculated amount.

**Anemia Secondary to Blood Loss (hemorrhagic diathesis or long-term dialysis)**

$$\text{mg of iron} = \text{blood loss} \times \text{hematocrit}$$

where blood loss is in milliliters and hematocrit is expressed as a decimal fraction

### *Megaloblastic Anemias*

#### Vitamin $B_{12}$ Deficiency

Vitamin $B_{12}$ is a water-soluble vitamin that humans obtain by ingestion of animal foodstuffs containing $B_{12}$, primarily meat and dairy products. Body stores of vitamin $B_{12}$ range from 2 to 3 mg, with the daily requirement being approximately 2 $\mu$g. Thus, a person would have to be deprived of $B_{12}$ for 3 to 4 years before developing $B_{12}$ deficiency. As previously stated, vitamin $B_{12}$ is necessary for DNA synthesis; it is also important in metabolic reactions involving folic acid and in maintaining the integrity of the neurologic system.

The three major causes of vitamin $B_{12}$ deficiency are inadequate intake, decreased absorption, and inadequate utilization.

Inadequate dietary consumption of vitamin $B_{12}$ is rare. It is usually seen only in patients who are strict vegetarians, as body stores are large and meats and vegetables are a readily available source.

Decreased absorption of vitamin $B_{12}$ occurs in patients with a deficiency of an intrinsic factor. A decrease in the production of the intrinsic factor results in acquired pernicious anemia, while dysfunction of the intrinsic factor causes congenital pernicious anemia. $B_{12}$ deficiency may also result from overgrowth in the bowel of bacteria that utilize $B_{12}$ or from injury or removal of ileal receptor sites where vitamin $B_{12}$ and intrinsic factor complex. Blind loop syndrome, fish tapeworm infestations, intestinal resections, tropical sprue, regional enteritis, and Crohn's disease may all contribute to the development of vitamin $B_{12}$ deficiency.

In the portal blood, vitamin $B_{12}$ is bound to a transport protein, transcobalamin II, which rapidly delivers the vitamin to sites of utilization and storage. In persons with a transcobalamin II deficiency, $B_{12}$ cannot be transported from the blood to utilization and storage sites. Consequently, the patient has a normal $B_{12}$ level but evidence of frank $B_{12}$ deficiency.

***Signs and Symptoms*** As is true in most forms of anemia, certain symptoms are cardiovascular in origin and result when the body can no longer tolerate the increased cardiac output stimulated by the anemia. These symptoms are listed in Table 69.7. Other manifestations of $B_{12}$ deficiency are glossitis, pallor, icterus, dysphagia, hepatosplenomegaly, anorexia, weight loss, and certain neurologic manifestations. Subacute degeneration of the nervous system as a consequence of demyelination progressing to axonal degeneration and eventual neuronal death may occur. The earliest neurologic symptom suggesting $B_{12}$ deficiency is paresthesias of the hands and toes. Forgetfulness, irritability, psychosis, weakness, depression, dementia, loss of intellectual function, ataxia, impaired vibratory and position sense, impaired urinary bladder function, and positive Romberg and Babinski signs may be present.[38]

***Laboratory Findings*** Once anemia has been confirmed with a low red blood cell count and low hemoglobin/hematocrit, the red cell indices must be examined. In macrocytic anemias, mean corpuscular volume is usually elevated above 100 $\mu m^3$. Leukopenia and thrombocytopenia may be present. The peripheral blood smear demonstrates macrocytosis accompanied by hypersegmented polymorphonuclear leukocytes (one of the earliest and most specific indications of this disease) and oval macrocytes. Serum lactate dehydrogenase, bilirubin, iron, and transferrin saturation are elevated, while the reticulocyte count is low. Serum $B_{12}$ levels are usually low.[39]

***Therapy*** Reports in the literature conflict as to the most appropriate therapy for vitamin $B_{12}$ deficiency. All patients with pure $B_{12}$ deficiencies probably demonstrate some hematologic response to treatment with either folic acid or vitamin $B_{12}$; however, conversion of the bone marrow to normoblastic morphology would probably not be completed with the administration of folic acid alone. Some authorities think that the treatment of pure vitamin $B_{12}$ deficiency is daily administration of 100 $\mu$g of $B_{12}$ for 3 to 5 days, followed by monthly injections for life.[32] Others, however, support the use of small doses of $B_{12}$ to prevent the too rapid conversion of bone marrow to normoblastic morphology.[38] These individuals administer 2 to 5 $\mu$g $B_{12}$ for 2 days and then 100 $\mu$g monthly. This dosage regimen promotes the maximum rate of increase of hemoglobin.

Vitamin $B_{12}$ deficiency is usually treated with 100 $\mu$g intramuscularly on a monthly basis. There is no evidence that larger doses produce a better state of health. In patients diagnosed with $B_{12}$ deficiency secondary to a lack of intrinsic factor, the treatment of choice is administration of exogenous vitamin $B_{12}$ intramuscularly. The recommended dose is 30 $\mu$g daily for 5 to 10 days, followed by a monthly maintenance dose of 100–200 $\mu$g. Oral therapy with vitamin $B_{12}$ is inferior to parenteral therapy and should be used only in patients who have a history of dietary $B_{12}$ deficiency with normal gastrointestinal absorption and no evidence of intrinsic factor deficiency.[40] Major side effects of vitamin $B_{12}$ therapy include sodium retention and hypokalemia. These adverse effects are more likely to occur in the patient with compromised cardiovascular status, because of an expansion of the intravascular volume secondary to the sudden increase in production of red blood cells.

In patients with chronic anemia, cardiac failure may result from a reflex increase in cardiac output and sodium retention in response to reduced vascular volume and accumulation of fluid. If dyspnea, anginal pain, or evidence of cerebral hypooxygenation is present, administration of packed cells is in order. Usually, administration of one unit of packed red blood cells is the treatment of choice. Care must be exercised to prevent cardiac overload. Small doses of diuretics may also be beneficial in these situations.

**Folic Acid Deficiency**

Folic acid is a heat-labile vitamin that is necessary for the production of nucleic acids, proteins, amino acids, purines, thymine, and hence DNA and RNA. As humans are unable to synthesize the total daily folate requirement, they must depend on a dietary source of this vitamin. Major dietary sources of folate include fresh vegetables and fruits, such animal organs as liver and kidney, yeast, and mushrooms. Even though body demands for folate are high (because of high red blood cell synthesis and turnover), the minimum daily requirement is 50–100 $\mu$g. The body stores approximately 10–20 mg folate; thus, cessation of dietary folate intake would result in depletion of all body stores within a few months. Folic acid deficiency results in the development of large functionally inmature erythrocytes termed megaloblasts.

The major causes of folic acid deficiency include inadequate intake, decreased absorption, hyperutilization, and inadequate utilization. Folic acid deficiency is associated with poor eating habits seen in elderly patients, alcoholics, food faddists, the poor, and the chronically ill or demented. Decreased absorption of folic acid may occur in patients with malabsorption syndromes, such as nontropical and tropical sprue, and after the administration of certain drugs.

Hyperutilization of folic acid may occur in states in which the rate of cellular division is increased. Examples include pregnancy, hemolytic anemia, and the growth spurts seen in adolescence and infancy. This is primarily of importance when the daily intake of folate is borderline, resulting in inadequate replacement of folate stores.

***Signs and Symptoms*** Table 69.7 lists signs and symptoms commonly observed in patients with folate deficiency. For the most part, these symptoms have an insidious onset, which often precludes early identification of the etiology. As can be seen in Table 69.7, the symptoms associated with folate deficiency are similar to those seen in patients with $B_{12}$ deficiency. The major difference between these two disease entities is the relative absence of neurologic manifestations in folate-deficient megaloblastic anemia.

Table 69.6 lists laboratory changes commonly associated with folate deficiency megaloblastic anemia. These findings are similar to those seen in vitamin $B_{12}$ deficiency anemia with the exception of decreased serum and red cell folate levels.

***Therapy*** Folic acid deficiency is treated by administration of exogenous folic acid. It is recommended that therapy be initiated with 50 $\mu$g/d orally for 2 days, followed by 2 mg orally twice a week or 0.5 mg daily. It is also recommended that patients with a folic acid deficiency be placed on diets containing foods high in folates. For patients with cardiovascular problems, the approach is the same as that for $B_{12}$ deficiency anemia.

Pyridoxine deficiency produces a severe hypochromic microcytic anemia characterized by splenomegaly, hepatomegaly, and elevation of serum iron level with saturation of the iron-binding capacity because iron cannot be incorporated into the heme structure.

### *Anemia of Senescence*

One of the most common clinical problems observed in the elderly is anemia.[26] As many as 7.5% of men and 20% of women over the age of 65 years suffer from this disorder. Fortunately, most of these cases can be treated.

There are several causes of anemia in the elderly. It is thought that approximately 45% of elderly anemic patients suffer from iron deficiency. Another 10% have megaloblastic anemia resulting from a deficiency of either vitamin $B_{12}$ or folic acid. In the remaining 45%, the more common cause is anemia of chronic disease; less common and often refractory causes include anemia associated with malignancy or a premalignant condition.[41]

#### Hypochromic Microcytic Anemia

Hypochromic microcytic anemia is the most commonly observed anemia in the elderly and generally results from iron deficiency; other causes include thalassemia (especially thalassemia minor) and heavy metal poisoning (mostly lead). Patients with hypochromic microcytic anemia and a normal or elevated serum iron level must be evaluated for the presence of heavy metal poisoning; hemoglobin electrophoresis may be necessary for diagnosing thalassemia.

Elderly patients with hypochromic microcytic anemia may present with a history of recurrent epistaxis, bleeding hemorrhoids, or bleeding from the genitourinary tract. Most cases are caused by occult gastrointestinal blood loss associated with the presence of gastrointestinal malignancy, ulcer disease, or the ingestion of medications that contribute to gastrointestinal bleeding.

Treatment of hypochromic microcytic anemia consists of oral iron supplementation. These products are well absorbed when administered on an empty stomach; however, elderly patients frequently show poor tolerance. In such cases, it may be necessary to take the supplement with meals. A pediatric elixir is available for those who have difficulty swallowing tablets; however, the iron content of these elixirs is low and they may stain teeth and dentures.

Hypochromic anemia may also be seen in patients with anemia of chronic disease. These patients frequently have a low serum iron concentration and low iron-binding capacity, which results in a low or normal iron saturation. In these patients, the problem is iron utilization rather than iron availability. These anemias are usually associated with an inflammatory process such as rheumatoid arthritis, chronic infection (tuberculosis, bacterial endocarditis, abscesses, etc.), and malignant disorders. These patients do not respond to hematinics, but treatment of the underlying disease generally resolves the anemia.

#### Macrocytic Anemia

The second most common form of anemia found in the elderly is macrocytic anemia. It generally results from a deficiency of vitamin $B_{12}$ or folic acid or from the use of drugs that compete with these vitamins or interfere with nuclear maturation and DNA synthesis.

Folic acid deficiency may occur as a result of dietary deprivation, malabsorption from the gastrointestinal tract, or competition with drugs for absorption or metabolism (estrogens and phenytoin). It is treated by oral administration of 1 mg folic acid daily.

Vitamin $B_{12}$ deficiency resulting from dietary deprivation is rare. Gastrointestinal malabsorption is a much more frequent cause of this deficiency in the elderly. As discussed under Megaloblastic Anemias, the Schilling test is an excellent means of determining whether malabsorption is the problem. The $B_{12}$ deficiency is treated by exogenous administration of crystalline vitamin $B_{12}$ intramuscularly.

#### Normochromic Normocytic Anemia

The least common anemia seen in elderly patients is normochromic normocytic anemia. Patients with this form of anemia are divided into two categories: those with elevated reticulocyte counts and those with low or normal reticulocyte counts. The reticulocyte count is extremely useful in that it is the number of new red blood cells in the circulation and indicates to the clinician whether the bone marrow is responding normally (elevated reticulocyte count) or abnormally (low or normal reticulocyte count).

Anemia in the geriatric patient with an elevated reticulocyte count most commonly occurs as a result of acute or recent blood loss. If the patient demonstrates sustained anemia with an elevated reticulocyte count and no bleeding can be documented, the patient most likely has a hemolytic anemia (inappropriately rapid destruction of red blood cells). Elderly patients with hemolytic anemia usually develop this disease process because of a defect in the red cell environment (enlargement or increased activity of the spleen). Acquired hemolytic anemia not associated with splenomegaly is usually immune in nature and can be detected with the Coombs test. Drugs are an important cause of immune hemolytic anemia in the elderly, with methyldopa and cephalosporin antibiotics the major offenders.

Normochromic normocytic anemia with a low or normal reticulocyte count implies that the bone marrow is unable to respond normally to the anemia. This form of anemia is often associated with a systemic disease or hematologic disorder that can be diagnosed only upon examination of the bone marrow; however, the most common form of this anemia, anemia of chronic disease, is more easily diagnosed by examining the serum iron concentration and total iron-binding capacity along with serum transferrin saturation. In these patients, iron is readily available; however, it is poorly utilized in erythropoiesis. As previously stated, this form of anemia is almost always associated with a systemic inflammatory disease (rheumatoid arthritis; chronic renal failure; chronic infection, i.e., tuberculosis; mycotic infections; suppurative infections) or cancer. These forms of anemia respond only to suppression or cure of the underlying disease.

### *Anemia of Chronic Disease*

All cases of anemia of chronic disease are characterized by the presence of inflammation. The anemia is usually hypoproliferative (that is, the expected rise in erythrocyte production does not occur in response to the anemia). Inflammation increases destruction of erythrocytes (decreases the life span by one half to two thirds) and blocks the release of iron by the reticuloendothelium, resulting in an increase in serum ferritin levels.[42] Inflammation is not always apparent, and its presence may have to be inferred from an elevated erythrocyte sedimentation rate. The degree of anemia is generally proportional to the severity of inflammation.[43]

Disease states that may contribute to anemia include rheumatoid arthritis, systemic lupus erythematosus, renal failure, and regional enteritis. Anemia of chronic disease is most frequently seen in systemic lupus erythematosus, although it is also seen in renal failure when the blood urea nitrogen exceeds 50 mg%.

Table 69.6 lists laboratory changes found in anemias of chronic disease. The anemia found in these patients is usually normochromic and normocytic.[44] There is a lack of erythroid hyperplasia and an increase in reticuloendothelial iron in the bone marrow. Apparently, in response to chronic disease, the marrow becomes less active and erythrocyte production slows down. Even though serum iron levels may be within normal limits, the bone marrow cannot generate red blood cells because of the limited iron available for erythropoiesis.

The treatment of anemia of chronic disease is somewhat less specific than treatment of other anemias. Usually, recovery from the anemia occurs with recovery from the inflammatory process. During inflammation, iron therapy is ineffective by either the oral or the parenteral route. Cobalt and especially corticosteroids have been effective in the treatment of rheumatoid arthritis and its anemia. Red cell transfusions should be limited to situations in which oxygen transport is inadequate because of other medical problems.

## *Hemolytic Anemia*

Hemolytic anemia is one of the least common forms of anemia encountered in clinical practice. Although hemolysis in itself is uncommon, the mechanisms responsible for decreasing the survival time of red blood cells are numerous. The severity of hemolytic anemia varies with the mechanism. Hemolysis may be mild, chronic, compensated, and lifelong or acute, severe, and life-threatening.

Hemolysis is defined as reduction of the survival time of erythrocytes in the circulation to less than 120 days. Anemia occurs when the rate of destruction exceeds the capacity of the bone marrow to compensate by increasing erythropoiesis. Normal bone marrow has the ability to increase the production of erythrocytes eightfold; however, this response is not immediate. Therefore, anemia is more pronounced when the onset of hemolysis is acute and severe or when the rate of erythropoiesis is reduced.[45] Changes in cell membrane, hemoglobin stability or solubility, and cell metabolism are major factors that lead to decreased erythrocyte survival time. These changes may be caused by intrinsic or extrinsic mechanisms. Intrinsic defects are intracorpuscular changes and are often genetically determined; extrinsic defects, or extracorpuscular changes, are usually the cause of acquired hemolytic anemia. Acquired disorders result mainly from a direct effect upon the membrane and less often from alterations in hemoglobin or metabolism.

### Hemolytic Anemias Secondary to Membrane Defects

Hereditary spherocytosis is the most common inherited disorder of the red cell membrane. Other forms are rare and are not discussed in this chapter. In this disorder, red blood cells lose their flexible biconcave characteristics and become tight spheres. These altered cells can still deliver oxygen to body cells; however, when these rigid cells enter the splenic microcirculation, they cannot pass through the pores lining the sinusoids of the spleen and consequently become trapped in the splenic pulp and eventually destroyed by the reticuloendothelial cells. These patients are at risk of developing cholelithiasis or cholecystitis, pigment bile stones, mild jaundice, and splenomegaly. The treatment of choice for hereditary spherocytosis is splenectomy. Although the spherocytosis persists, the hemolysis is no longer a problem once the spleen has been removed.

Paroxysmal nocturnal hemoglobinuria, although rare, is a condition characterized by increased intravascular lysis of red blood cells by the patient's endogenous complement. This condition appears to be exacerbated by the presence of the mild acidosis that accompanies sleep. As a consequence of the hemolysis, a hypochromic microcytic iron deficiency anemia can also develop. Neutropenia, thrombocytopenia, an increased predisposition to repeated venous thromboses, and terminal evolution into an acute leukemia are other complications. There is no satisfactory therapy for paroxysmal nocturnal hemoglobinuria, although repeated transfusions with red blood cells washed in normal saline may be necessary. Some investigators have reported the use of corticosteroids and androgens as effective in selected cases.[46]

Acanthocytosis, or "spur cell anemia," is a more common form of acquired membrane defect and is frequently a complication of severe hepatocellular disease in which abnormal lipid metabolism results in an imbalance in the cholesterol and phospholipid accumulated on the red blood cell membrane. Consequently, hemolysis occurs.

Extrinsic hemolytic anemias occur most commonly as a result of the premature destruction of red cells affected by antibodies to red cell antigens. Such immune-related hemolysis is usually associated with warm-reacting antibodies of the IgG type or cold antibodies of the IgM type. Warm-antibody hemolytic anemias are frequently associated with malignancies of the lymphoproliferative system, collagen vascular diseases, and infectious diseases (particularly viral). In this form of anemia, antibodies and complement coat the surface of the red blood cell. These antibody-coated red blood cells attach to reticuloendothelial cells, which then phagocytose fragments of the red cell membrane (but not hemoglobin). These phagocytosed red cells may detach from the reticuloendothelial cells and function in the same manner as spherocytes in hereditary spherocytosis. Any damaged red cells that reattach to reticuloendothelial cells may eventually be completely phagocytosed. It must be kept in mind that a relatively large proportion of cases of warm-antibody immune hemolysis have no demonstrable cause and are therefore termed idiopathic acquired immune hemolytic anemia.

Laboratory changes suggestive of warm-antibody immune anemia can be detected with the direct Coombs or antiglobulin test. In this test, the patient's red cells react with anti–human globulin antiserum from rabbits, revealing the IgG antibody or complement or both on the surface of the red cell.

Treatment consists of therapy for the primary underlying disorder. If initial therapy is unsuccessful or if the anemia is idiopathic, specific therapy for the anemia is necessary. Corticosteroids have been shown to be effective by interfering with the "recognition" of the antibody-coated red cells by the reticuloendothelial cells. These agents are successful in 60% to 80% of cases.[47] Response is usually seen within 7 days of the initiation of therapy with 60–100 mg prednisone daily. The steroid should then be tapered gradually over 3 to 6 months. In approximately 60% to 70% of patients, remission is achieved or the condition is controlled with low-dose maintenance corticosteroids. If steroid therapy is unsuccessful after 3 weeks of treatment, splenectomy may be necessary. Splenectomy is beneficial in approximately 50% to 60% of cases, with resolution of hemolysis or a reduction in maintenance steroid therapy.[48] Unfortunately, splenectomy is not uniformly successful, as antibody-coated red blood cells can be destroyed by reticuloendothelial cells in other areas of the body, especially the liver. If hemolysis persists after corticosteroid therapy and/or splenectomy, the use of immunosuppressive or cytotoxic drugs may be necessary. Azathioprine and cyclophosphamide produce a clinical response in 50% to 60% of these resistant cases. Patients usually respond 1 to 3 months after initiation of therapy; generally therapy is continued 6 to 12 months.[49]

Cold-reacting immune hemolysis is less common than the warm antibody disease. It too can be found in patients with collagen disease, lymphoid malignant disorders, or mycoplasma pneumonia.

Cold-agglutinin syndrome is caused by an IgM complement–fixing antibody that binds to red blood cells at low temperatures. With rising temperatures, this antibody leaves the red blood cell. In patients developing this syndrome, these antibodies are present in titers greater than 1:1,000 and have increased thermal amplitude so that the antibody activity is demonstrated at high temperatures. Patients with this condition typically present in northern climates generally during winter months. Symptoms similar to those found in Raynaud's phenomenon may occur upon exposure to cold. Additionally, a small number of patients develop dramatic intravascular hemolysis and hemoglobinuria upon exposure to cold. The cold-agglutinin titer is generally high and the direct Coombs test is positive for complement components on the red blood cells and negative for immunoglobulin.

Therapy for cold-reacting immune hemolysis is primarily supportive. Corticosteroids and splenectomy have not been shown to be beneficial. Protection from cold is the primary means of treatment and thus it may be necessary for patients to move to warmer climates. Chronic folic acid administration and transfusions may be needed. Blood or other products must be prewarmed to body temperature before intravenous infusion to prevent life-threatening agglutination and hemolysis. Some patients may respond to azathioprine or cyclophosphamide therapy.

#### Metabolic Disorders

The two major metabolic pathways necessary for normal red blood cell metabolism are the hexose monophosphate shunt, with its associated enzyme systems, and the Embden–Myerhof pathway of anaerobic glycolysis. The former is responsible primarily for maintaining hemoglobin in the reduced state and thus preventing the formation of methemoglobin; the latter metabolizes glucose to lactic acid which leads to ATP formation.

The most common metabolic abnormality resulting in a hemolytic syndrome is glucose-6-phosphate dehydrogenase deficiency in the hexose monophosphate shunt pathway. Hemoglobin is oxidized to methemoglobin and then to sulfhemoglobin. Heinz bodies of denatured hemoglobin form, resulting in damage to the red cell membrane. Hemolysis results from the action of the spleen and reticuloendothelial system on these damaged cells. The disease more typically presents in whites of Mediterranean descent upon exposure to oxidant drugs and chemicals or with infection.

Therapy for this condition consists of avoidance of oxidant medications and chemicals. Currently, there is no specific therapy that compensates for the enzyme deficiency.

### References


1. Bergin JJ. Evaluation of anemia. Postgrad Med J 1985;77:253–269.
2. MacCosbe PE, Toomey K. Interaction of phenytoin and folic acid. Clin Pharm 1983;2:362–369.
3. Blair JA, Matty AJ, Acid microclimate in intestinal absorption. Clin Gastroenterol 1974;3:183–197.
4. Hoffbrand A, Necheles TF. Mechanisms of folate deficiency in patients receiving phenytoin. Lancet 1968;2:528.
5. Wickramasinghe SN, Williams G, Saunders J, et al. Megaloblastic erythropoiesis and macrocytosis in patients on anticonvulsants. Br Med J 1975;4:136–137.
6. Klipstein FA. Subnormal serum folate and macrocytosis associated with anticonvulsant drug therapy. Blood 1964;23:68–86.
7. Eichner ER. The hematologic disorders of alcoholism. Am J Med 1973;54:621–630.
8. Wu A, Chanarin I, Slavin G, et al. Folate deficiency in the alcoholic—its relationship to clinical and hematological abnormalities, liver disease and folate stores. Br J Haematol 1975;29:469–478.
9. Necheles TF, Snyder LM. Malabsorption of folate polyglutamates associated with oral contraceptive therapy. N Engl J Med 1970;282:858–859.
10. Paton A. Oral contraceptives and folate deficiency. Lancet 1969;1:418.
11. Shojania AM, Hornady G, Barnes PH. Oral contraceptives and serum folate levels. Lancet 1968;1:1376–1377.
12. Shojania AM, Hornady G, Barnes PH. Oral contraceptives and folate metabolism. Lancet 1969;1:886.
13. Streiff RR. Folate deficiency and oral contraceptives. JAMA 1970;214:105.
14. Halsted CH, Gandhi G, Tamerra T. Sulfasalazine inhibits the absorption of folates. N Engl J Med 1981;305:1513–1517.
15. Franklin JL, Rosenberg IH. Impaired folic acid absorption in inflammatory bowel disease: Effects of salicylazosulfapyridine (Azulfidine). Gastroenterology 1973;64:517–525.
16. Douglas IDC, Price LA. Bone marrow toxicity of methotrexate: A reassessment. Br J Haematol 1973;24:625–631.
17. Chanarin I, England JM. Toxicity of trimethoprim–sulphamethoxazole in patients with megaloblastic haemopoiesis. Br J Med 1972;1:651–653.
18. Tamtamy SE. Co-trimoxazole and the blood. Lancet 1974;1:929–930.
19. Jewkes RF, Edwards MS, Grant BJG. Haematological changes

in a patient on long term treatment with trimethoprim–sulphonamide combination. Postgrad Med J 1970;46:723–726.
20. Kahn SB, Fein SA, Brodsky T. Effects of trimethoprim on folate metabolism in man. Clin Pharmacol Ther 1968;9:550–560.
21. Lieberman FL, Bateman JR. Megaloblastic anemia possibly induced by triamterene in patients with alcoholic cirrhosis: Two case reports. Ann Intern Med 1968;68:168–173.
22. Corcino J, Waxman S, Herbert V. Mechanism of triamterene induced megaloblastosis. Ann Intern Med 1970;73:419–424.
23. Dobbins WO, Herrero BA, Mansbach CM. Morphological alterations associated with neomycin induced malabsorption. Am J Med Sci 1968;255:63–77.
24. Jacobson E. An experimental malabsorption syndrome induced by neomycin. Am J Med 1960;28:524–533.
25. Webb DI, Chodos RB, Mahar CQ, et al. Mechanism of vitamin B-12 malabsorption in patients receiving colchicine. N Engl J Med 1968;279:845–850.
26. Lipschitz DA, Mitchell CO, Thompson C. The anemia of senescence. Am J Hematol 1981;11:47–54.
27. Hobbs J, Rodriguez AR. Megaloblastic anemias. Am Fam Physician 1980;22:128–136.
28. Gerbino PP. Treatment of the common anemias. Am Druggist 1979;179(4):39–43.
29. English EC, Finch CA. Iron deficiency: A systematic approach. Drug Ther 1984;14(4):19–20, 25–27.
30. Stucky WJ. Common anemias: A practical guide to diagnosis and management. Geriatrics 1983;38:42–48.
31. Oski FA. The nonhematologic manifestations of iron deficiency. Am J Dis Child 1979;133:315–321.
32. Freedman ML. Common hematologic problems: Diagnosis and treatment. Geriatrics 1983;38:119–123, 127–130, 134.
33. Cok JD. Food iron absorption in human subjects. III. Comparison of the effect of animal proteins on non-heme iron absorption. Am J Clin Nutr 1976;29:859–867.
34. Dallman PR, Siimes MA, Stekel A. Iron deficiency in infancy and childhood. Am J Clin Nutr 1980;June:86–118.
35. Monsen ER, Hallberg L, Layrisse M, et al. Estimation of available dietary iron. Am J Clin Nutr 1978;31:134–141.
36. Beutler E. Iron preparations: New and old. Blood 1960;15:65–89.
37. Dallman PR. Iron deficiency: Diagnosis and treatment. West J Med 1981;134:496–503.
38. Cooper BA. Megaloblastic anemia: When to suspect it, how to treat it. Drug Ther Hosp 1984;9:55–57, 61–62, 67–69.
39. Christensen DJ. Diagnosis of anemia: Clues to greater precision. Postgrad Med J 1983;73:293–297, 300.
40. McEvoy GK. American Hospital Formulary Service Drug Information 86, 28th ed. Bethesda, MD, American Society of Hospital Pharmacists, 1986, pp 1855–1859.
41. Howe RB. Anemia in the elderly: Common causes and suggested diagnostic approach. Postgrad Med J 1983:73:153–160.
42. Bonnet JD. Normocytic, normochromic anemia. Postgrad Med J 1977;61:139–142.
43. Finch CA. Anemia of chronic disease. Postgrad Med J 1978; 64:107–109, 112–113.
44. Ward PC. Investigation of nonpoikilocytic normochromic normocytic anemia. Postgrad Med J 1979;65:232, 234–235, 238, 241–243.
45. Brain MC. Hemolytic anemia: A systematic approach to management. Postgrad Med J 1978;64:127–133.
46. Forget BG. Hemolytic anemias: Congenital and acquired. Hosp Pract 1980;15:67–78.
47. Murphy S, LoBuglio AF. Drug therapy of autoimmune hemolytic anemia. Semin Hematol 1976;13:323–334.
48. Bowdker AJ. The role of the spleen and splenectomy in autoimmune hemolytic disease. Semin Hematol 1976;13:335–348.
49. Axeksib JA, LoBuglio AF. Immune hemolytic anemia. Med Clin North Am 1980;64:597–606.

# Chapter 70 / Coagulation Disorders

Keith A. Rodvold, PharmD, and William R. Friedenberg, MD

This chapter describes a pathophysiologic approach to the diagnosis and management of patients with common coagulation disorders. The chapter is divided into two sections. Fundamental concepts of hemostasis and thrombosis are presented first. Next, the clinical application of these fundamentals with regard to hemostatic disorders and thrombotic disorders is discussed. The general categories of disorders contrast congenital bleeding illnesses with acquired disorders of coagulation. Treatment of each coagulation disorder is discussed.

## Regulation of Hemostasis

Hemostasis is the spontaneous arrest of bleeding from damaged blood vessels. Thrombogenesis and hemostasis are similar processes; an intravascular thrombus results from a pathologic disturbance of hemostasis. Hemostasis and thrombosis are regulated by a multifactorial balance between procoagulant and anticoagulant molecular events.[1,2] The factors that determine the exact balance between clot formation (coagulation) and dissolution (fibrinolysis) are not completely understood; however, they involve the dynamic interaction of four major components: (1) the vessel wall, (2) platelets, (3) the coagulation cascade, and (4) the fibrinolytic system. The following is a brief description of our current understanding of the main components of the hemostatic system and their physiologic interactions and regulation.

### *Vessel Wall and Platelets*

Primary hemostasis is dependent on a blood vessel and circulating platelets. The vessel wall plays key roles in vasoconstriction, formation of platelet plugs and regulation of coagulation and fibrinolysis (Fig. 70.1). Platelets are essential for normal hemostasis and perform four distinct functions in response to vascular damage: (1) continual maintenance of vascular integrity by sealing over minor deficiencies of the endothelium, (2) initial arrest of bleeding through the formation of platelet plugs, (3) stabilization of the hemostatic plug by contributing procoagulant activity to the coagulation system to form fibrin, and (4) promotion of vascular healing by stimulating endothelial cell migration and medial smooth muscle cell migration and proliferation. The formation of a platelet plug proceeds through the sequence of platelet adhesion to exposed subendothelial connective tissue structures; platelet aggregation by adenosine diphosphate (ADP), thromboxane $A_2$ and thrombin recruitment; contribution of platelet coagulant activity to the coagulation process which stabilizes the plug with a fibrin mesh; and retraction of the platelet mass to provide a dense thrombus.

### *Coagulation System*

The coagulation system generates and stabilizes the fibrin clot, whereas the fibrinolytic system dissolves the polymerized fibrin clot. These two systems serve two interrelated and opposing functions. Fibrinogen is cleaved by thrombin to form fibrin, the substance of clot. Thrombin occupies a central position in the hemostatic system (Fig. 70.1); it is involved in platelet aggregation, fibrin formation, and the modulation of fibrinolysis.

Currently, 12 plasma proteins have been recognized as coagulation factors (Table 70.1). In addition, tissue factor (a lipoprotein) and calcium are sometimes designated as factors III and IV, respectively. It is convenient to divide the coagulation factors into three groups on the basis of biochemical properties. These groups include vitamin K–dependent factors (II, VII, IX, and X), contact activation factors (XI and XII, prekallikrein, high-molecular-weight kininogen), and thrombin-sensitive factors (V, VIII, XIII, and fibrinogen).

Coagulation factors as well as key enzymes in the fibrinolytic system generally circulate as inactive forms (zymogens). Coagulation of blood entails a cascading series of proteolytic reactions. At each step a clotting factor undergoes limited proteolysis and becomes an active protease (designated by a lowercase "a", as in Xa). This clotting factor enzyme activates the next clotting factor until ultimately an insoluble fibrin clot is formed. This ability to generate large quantities of fibrin rapidly necessitates mechanisms that localize clot formation to the specific site of vascular injury and maintain blood fluidity.

Clotting is initiated by either an intrinsic or an extrinsic pathway, with subsequent factor interactions that converge upon a final, common pathway (Fig. 70.2). Both pathways are activated when normal components of the vascular endothelium come into contact with blood. Tissue factor is the cofactor that catalyzes the activation of factor VII. Because tissue factor is not found in the blood (found in many organs including the brain, lungs, kidneys, liver) it is said to be "extrinsic" to blood and therefore initiates the extrinsic clotting pathway. In the extrinsic system, factor VII undergoes proteolytic activation by factor XIIa, factor XIa, and kallikrein. Factor VIIa, calcium, tissue thromboplastin, and factor X form a lipoprotein complex that results in activation of factor X. From this step onward, the extrinsic system is identical to the intrinsic system.

In the intrinsic pathway, all the protein factors necessary

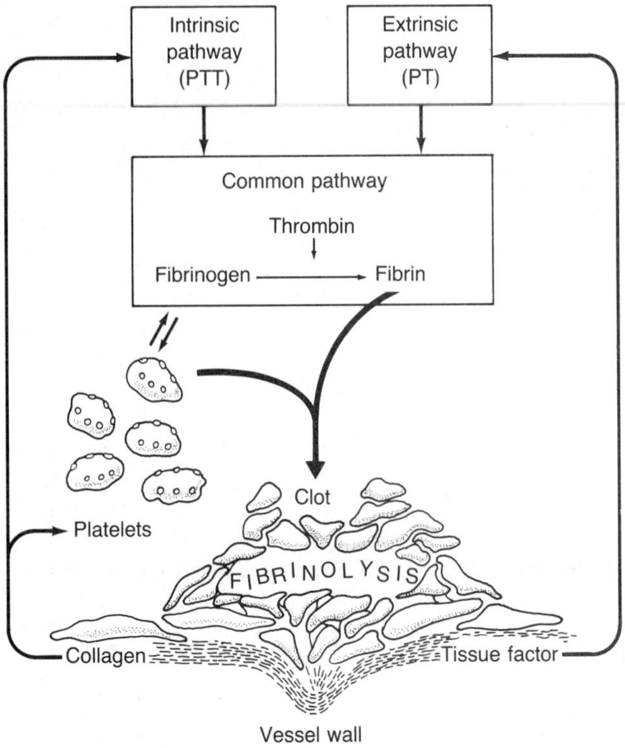


**Figure 70.1** Simplified scheme of the hemostatic system, showing interaction of vessel wall platelets, coagulation pathways, and fibrinolytic system. Not shown are regulatory and inhibitory mechanisms. (*From Stead RE: Regulation of Hemostasis, in Goldhaber SZ (Ed): Pulmonary Embolism and Deep Vein Thrombosis. Philadelphia, W.B. Saunders, 1985, p 28, with permission.*)

for coagulation are present in the circulating blood. The intrinsic pathway is initiated by the contact activation phase, when circulating factor XII comes into contact with subendothelial collagen or basement membrane. Other contact activation factors, high-molecular-weight kininogen and prekallikrein, also participate in the contact activation phase. Factor XI is activated by factor XIIa, with high-molecular-weight kininogen participating as a cofactor. Once formed, factor XIa activates factor IX to factor IXa. Factor VIII, factor IXa, calcium, and platelet phospholipid form a lipoprotein complex with prothrombin and activate it to thrombin.

The intrinsic and extrinsic pathways converge in the common pathway to generate thrombin, which in turn cleaves fibrinogen to form a fibrin gel. The fibrin monomer can then be polymerized and stabilized into an insoluble clot.

### *Fibrinolysis*

The fibrinolytic system is part of the repair of the damaged endothelium. Once the fibrin polymer has been formed, it is very resistant to disruption and must be enzymatically digested by the serine protease plasmin. Plasminogen, the circulating precursor, is also trapped within the fibrin meshwork but can be converted to active plasmin by plasma and vascular plasminogen activators. Once formed, plasmin enzymatically digests fibrin to release a number of fibrin degradation products (fibrin split products). These products are themselves potent anticoagulants that inhibit fibrin generation and polymerization.

As seen in Figure 70.2, the activation of thrombin is absolutely central in the coagulation system. Thrombin itself is important in fibrin formation, fibrin stabilization, induction of platelet aggregation, activation of factors V and VII, and activation of protein C with its anticoagulant and profibrinolytic effects. Given this powerful and multifocal activation of the hemostatic system, it is not surprising that the generation of thrombin is the focus of important regulatory controls. Regulation involves naturally occurring circulating protease inhibitors; the major ones inactivate the proteases involved in hemostasis. Antithrombin III is the major inhibitor of thrombin and is present in excess amounts in plasma. Antithrombin III complexes with and inactivates not only thrombin but also the other serine proteases (XIIa, XIa, IXa, Xa). Patients with a hereditary or acquired deficiency of antithrombin III have a high incidence of recurrent thromboembolic disease. Protein C, a vitamin K–dependent protein, has recently been recognized as an important inhibitor of coagulation and stimulator of fibrinolysis. Whereas antithrombin III specifically neutralizes the activated serine proteases, protein C inactivates two other cofactors in the coagulation cascade, Va and VIIIc.

Thus, thrombin potentially may initiate both positive- and negative-feedback loops, which regulate further thrombin generation. The delicate balance between clot formation and dissolution may be readily perturbed, in either direction, by a number of pathologic and pharmacologic mechanisms.

### *Simple Tests*

Laboratory support in the diagnosis of coagulation disorders and monitoring of therapy is designed to provide rapid, relatively nonspecific information.[3–5] Detailed, specific analysis of individual coagulation factors may be more time consuming and is undertaken usually only after abnormalities are identified by generalized screening tests. Moreover, laboratory results within the normal range do not necessarily confirm that hemostasis is normal. Thus, a convincing personal or family history of abnormal bleeding is as important as an abnormal laboratory value. The following is a brief review of simple tests that are available in most hospital or clinic settings. These tests are summarized in Table 70.2.

***Bleeding Time*** In conjunction with the platelet count, determination of the bleeding time allows the examiner to make fundamental decisions regarding abnormalities of primary hemostasis. Patients with an abnormal bleeding time but a normal platelet count are arbitrarily designated as having qualitative abnormalities of platelet function. Such patients include those with von Willebrand's disease, those who have recently ingested various antiplatelet drugs (i.e., aspirin), and those with uremia.

***Prothrombin Time*** The prothrombin time (PT) assesses the function of the extrinsic system and common pathway of the coagulation system. In particular, the test measures the

**Table 70.1** Blood Coagulation Factors

| *Factor*[a] | *Synonym* | *Role* |
|---|---|---|
| I | Fibrinogen | Terminal substrate of the coagulation system, polymerizes into fibrin fibers upon proteolysis by thrombin |
| II | Prothrombin | Vitamin K–dependent zymogen of the serine protease thrombin |
| V | Proaccelerin Labile factor | Nonenzymatic procofactor for factor Xa in the prothrombinase complex |
| VII | Proconvertin | Vitamin K–dependent zymogen of factor VIIa that activates factor X via the extrinsic pathway and factor IX via the alternate pathway |
| VIII | Antihemophilic factor A | Nonenzymatic pro-cofactor of factor IXa in the factor X activation complex |
| IX | Antihemophilic factor B, Christmas factor | Vitamin K–dependent zymogen of factor IXa that activates factor X |
| X | Stuart–Prower factor | Vitamin K–dependent zymogen of factor Xa, the protease of the prothrombinase complex |
| XI | Plasma thromboplastin antecedent | Zymogen of protease factor XIa that converts factor IX to factor IXa |
| XII | Hageman factor | Zymogen of factor XIIa that activates factor XI and prekallikrein |
| XIII | Fibrin–stabilizing factor | Zymogen of a transglutaminase that covalently crosslinks fibrin monomers with each other |
| Prekallikrein | Fletcher's factor | Zymogen of kallikrein that activates factor XII and cleaves high-molecular-weight kininogen to liberate bradykinin |
| High-molecular weight kininogen | Flaujeac's, Fitzgerald's, or Williams' factor | Nonenzymatic contact activation cofactor of factor XIIa and kallikrein |

[a] Coagulation factors are numbered with Roman numerals in order of their discovery. The most frequent synonyms are listed. Factor III (tissue factor) and factor IV (calcium ions) have been omitted from the table.

From Rugger: ZM (Ed): Clinics in Haematology. New York, W.B. Saunders, p 282, with permission.

activity of the vitamin K–dependent factor, factor VII. PT reflects the time required for fibrin strands to appear after the addition of tissue thromboplastin and calcium to a patient's plasma. Thus, the PT yields evidence about the current synthetic capacity of the liver, the adequacy of vitamin K absorption, and the inhibition of clotting factor synthesis by warfarin.

***Activated Partial Thromboplastin Time*** The activated partial thromboplastin time (APTT) measures the activity of the intrinsic system and common pathway. APTT reflects the time required for a fibrin clot to form after calcium and an activating agent are added to the patient's plasma. The APTT is widely used for monitoring heparin therapy.

***Thrombin Time*** The thrombin time (TT) assesses the clotting of plasma by thrombin and is affected by quantitative and qualitative abnormalities of fibrinogen. The TT measures the time required for the formation and the appearance of the fibrin clot. The test bypasses all earlier steps of the coagulation pathway. It is commonly used to monitor the effect of systemic fibrinolytic therapy and can be modified for monitoring heparin therapy.

## Congenital Disorders

### *Hemophilia*

The inherited plasma coagulation disorders result from rare defects in single coagulation proteins. The two X-linked disorders, hemophilia A (factor VIII deficiency) and hemophilia B (factor IX deficiency), account for almost all known congenital coagulation defects.

Hemophilia A is also called classic hemophilia and is the oldest known congenital coagulopathy.[6] The writers of the Talmud decreed that boys whose older brothers or cousins had bled to death after circumcision need not undergo the procedure. In general, only males are affected by the disease, but females are carriers. The incidence of hemophilia A in the overall population is approximately 1 per 10,000, or

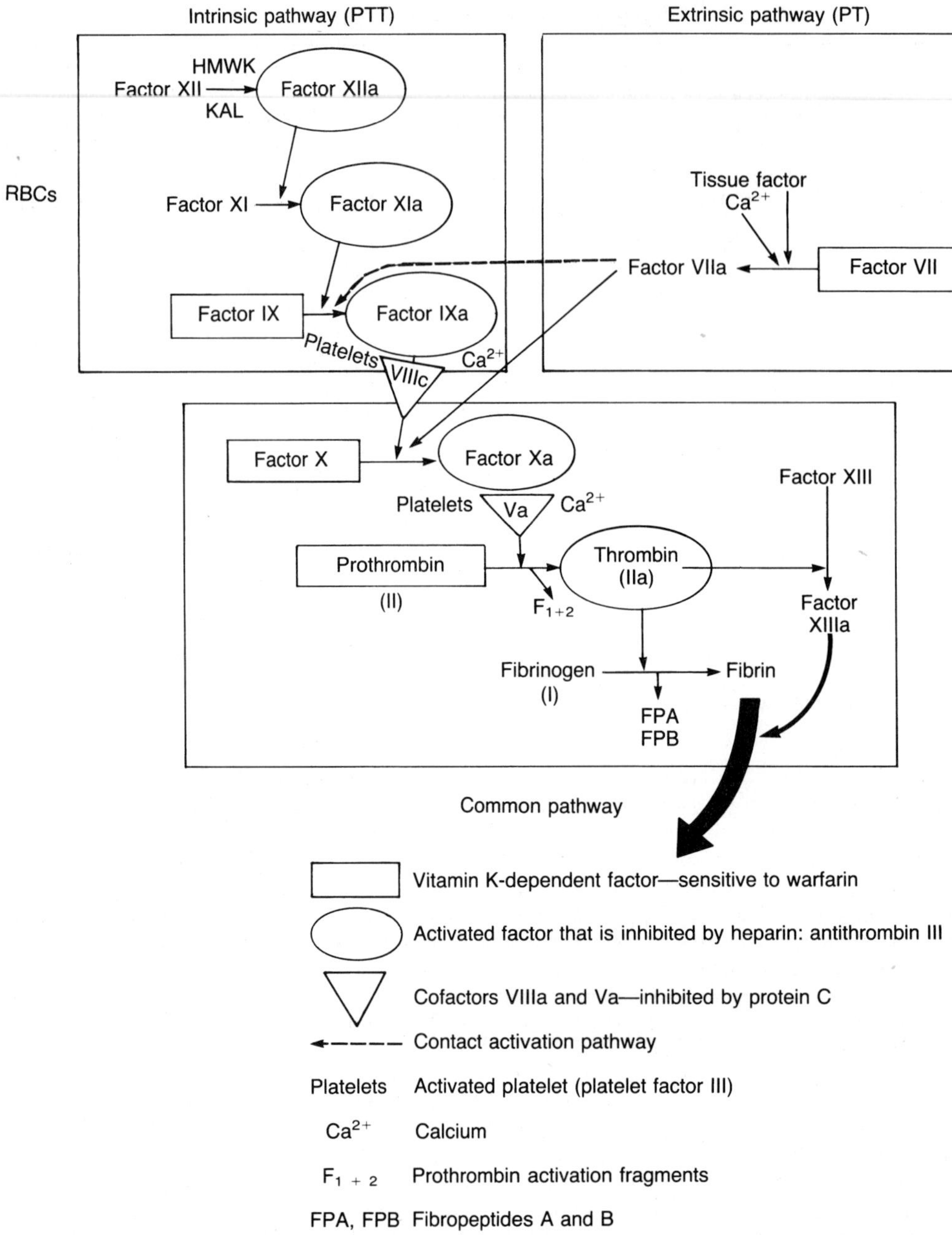


**Figure 70.2** The coagulation pathways. Important features include the contact activation phase, vitamin K–dependent factors (affected by warfarin), the activated serine proteases that are inhibited by heparin: antithrombin III, and the role of platelets and calcium. Factors VIIIc and Va are nonenzymatic cofactors that are inactivated by protein C. The protime (PT) measures the function of the extrinsic and common pathways; the partial thromboplastin time (PTT) measures the function of the intrinsic and common pathways. HMWK, high-molecular-weight kininogen; KAL, kallikrein. *(From Stead RB: Regulation of hemostasis, in SZ Goldhaber (Ed): Pulmonary Embolism and Deep Vein Thrombosis. Philadelphia, W.B. Saunders, 1985;pp 27–40.)*

2 per 10,000 males.[7] The National Heart and Lung Institute estimates the frequency to be 25 per 100,000 males in the United States of which approximately 85% have hemophilia A (factor VIII deficiency) and the remaining have hemophilia B (factor IX deficiency). Both hemophilia A and hemophilia B are recessive sex-linked diseases; the defective gene is located on the X chromosome. Affected males have no normal allele on their X chromosome and no gene on their Y chromosome; thus, their sons would be normal and their daughters would be obligatory carriers. Female children of hemophiliacs have one normal allele (the normal X chromosome from the mother) and, therefore, do not have a hemorrhagic tendency. Sons of a female carrier and a normal male have a 50% chance of being hemophiliacs, whereas

**Table 70.2** Laboratory Procedures

| *Procedure* | *Reagent content* | *Normal range* | *System tested* | *Disease detected* |
|---|---|---|---|---|
| Template bleeding time | None | 1–8 min | Platelets and capillaries | Thrombocytopathy, von Willebrand's disease |
| Activated partial thromboplastin time (APTT) | Phospholipid contact activator | 42 s | Intrinsic | Mild (40%–50%) deficiencies of factors VIII, IX, and XI (hemophilias); deficiency of factor XII; von Willebrand's disease; disseminated intravascular coagulation; heparin therapy |
| Prothrombin time (PT) | Tissue thromboplastin | 10–12 s | Extrinsic | Factor VII deficiency (acquired or hereditary), vitamin K deficiency |
| Thrombin time (TT) | Thrombin | 20–24 s | Conversion of fibrinogen to fibrin | Hypofibrinogenemia and dysfibrinogenemia, fibrin split products, and presence of heparin |

Modified from Triplett DA: Hemostasis: A Case Oriented Approach. New York, Igaku-Shoin, 1985, p 66, with permission.

daughters have a 50% chance of being carriers. This mode of inheritance with a ''skipped generation''—the female carriers being children of the hemophiliacs do not express the disease but pass it on to the next male generation—was first described accurately early in the nineteenth century. The most celebrated carrier was Queen Victoria. One of her sons was a hemophiliac and at least two of her daughters were carriers. Victoria's daughters spread hemophilia throughout the royal families of Europe.

Hemophilia has been observed in few females.[7] This can occur if a hemophiliac marries a female carrier or if the ''normal'' X chromosome in the carrier female undergoes extreme lyonization. *Lyonization* is the process by which one of the X chromosomes in a female degenerates and does not produce effective gene products. There have been extremely rare cases where patients have had either one X chromosome or an autosomal dominant mode of transmission. In the older literature many of these cases of female hemophilia were thought to have been von Willebrand's disease.

Before 1947, it was thought that all patients with sex-linked, hereditary bleeding disorders had classic hemophilia resulting from factor VIII (antihemophiliac factor) deficiency.[8] In 1947, blood from one patient with presumed classic hemophilia was found to correct the clotting abnormality in another patient. Subsequent investigators showed that both of these disorders were inherited as sex-linked recessive disorders with identical means of inheritance, but one was due to a deficiency of factor IX (plasma thromboplastin component or Christmas factor).

Modern techniques of molecular biology have been successful in cloning the gene for factor VIII production.[6] The gene is 186,000 bases long. The coagulant material originates from liver cells, although other tissues such as the kidney, spleen, and lymph glands have also been found to be sources of the coagulant material (factor VIII:C). This protein cofactor is missing in hemophilia A. The entire factor VII molecule consists of this factor VIII coagulant material, along with a larger molecule, von Willebrand's factor (vWF), which is the protein that mediates adhesion of platelets to the subendothelium.[7,9,10] This part of the molecule is absent, decreased or defective in von Willebrand's disease. Von Willebrand's factor circulates as a complex with factor VIII:C in normal plasma and appears to stabilize the latter. Antibodies have been produced to both the factor VIII coagulant material and the von Willebrand's factor and are called factor VIII:C antigen and von Willebrand's factor antigen, respectively (Table 70.3).

At least 200 hemophiliac factor genes have been examined and at least seven different mutations have been pinpointed.[6] Four of the changes have been single base changes leading to a truncated factor VIII and severe hemophilia. One mutation was the substitution of an incorrect amino acid, resulting in a relatively mild form of the disease. The other three mutations are deletions of several thousand nucleotides and cause severe hemophilia. Classic hemophilia A is caused by a deficiency of factor VIII coagulant material, with the degree of deficiency depending upon the degree of genetic defect. Von Willebrand's factor appears to be synthesized in endothelial cells. In patients with classic hemophilia, there is a deficiency of factor VIII coagulant material but not of von Willebrand's factor.

All patients with hemophilia B have decreased factor IX clotting activity.[8] The molecular basis for this decrease varies; some patients have decreased synthesis of a normal molecule, whereas others appear to have normal amounts of factor IX antigen with markedly decreased coagulant activity and thus are thought to have an abnormal protein with

**Table 70.3** Nomenclature for Factor VIII

| | |
|---|---|
| Factor VIII coagulant protein (VIII:C) | Protein that activates factor X with other factors and is missing in hemophilia A |
| VIII:C:Ag | Antigenic expression of VIII:C |
| Von Willebrand's factor (vWF) | Protein that mediates adhesion of platelets and is abnormal in quality or quantity in von Willebrand's disease; it circulates complexed to VIII:C, stabilizing the latter |
| vWF:Ag | Antigenic expression of vWF |
| VIII:C–WF | Complex of VIII:C and vWF that circulates in plasma |

From Ruggeri ZM (Ed): Clinics in Haematology. Philadelphia, W.B. Saunders, 1987 p 344, with permission.

retained antigenic characteristics. There are several variants of factor IX deficiency, one of which is hemophilia $B_m$.[8,11] This disorder is characterized by a prolonged PT, as in most patients with hemophilia B this test is normal. The subscript "m" refers to the family name of the original patient. These patients have been shown to have the factor IX molecule by the presence of cross-reactive material (CRM positive). The specific protein abnormality has been identified in several different types of these variants. It is this abnormal protein that is felt to interfere with a factor VII–tissue factor activation of factor X, thereby prolonging the PT. The mechanism of this interference is unknown. About 5% of hemophilia B patients are hemophilia $B_m$ variants. There are several other variants of hemophilia B, but they all have similar clinical manifestations.

The complete amino acid sequence for the circulating factor IX molecule has been delineated and the gene for factor IX has been cloned. The entire gene is 35,000 nucleotides long.[11]

Molecular biologists use various techniques to detect carriers of either hemophilia A or B. In addition, prenatal diagnosis can be carried out if sufficient fetal DNA is obtained by cell culture of amniotic fluid or by biopsy of the chorionic villi.[6,11]

It should be possible to cure hemophiliacs by introducing the appropriate gene into their cells. Gene therapy for many diseases is not yet possible but should be in the future.[6,11]

### Clinical Presentation

***Hemophilia A*** Clinical bleeding is usually correlated with the degree of deficiency of factor VIII:C. Patients with less than 1% factor VIII:C are classified as severe hemophiliacs, those with 1% to 5% are moderate hemophiliacs, and those with greater than 5% are mild hemophiliacs.[7,12] Most bleeding episodes are characterized by joint and muscle hemorrhage, with prolonged bleeding after trauma or surgery. Minor trauma and abrasions, which are frequently controlled with platelet plugs, do not pose clinical problems in patients with hemophilia.

Joint hemorrhages frequently involve the large joints, especially the weight-bearing ones. These episodes are frequently spontaneous, begin in childhood, and can lead to disabling arthropathies.

Muscle hematomas, especially psoas hematomas, can lead to false diagnoses, including appendicitis, and can also compress nerves leading to weakness or paralysis. Bleeding into vital organs can cause significant dysfunction: retroperitoneal bleeding can obstruct one or both kidneys or bleeding into the oral cavity can obstruct the airway. Occasionally, bleeding into the subperiosteum after trauma can cause pseudotumors with bone necrosis.

Although mucous membrane bleeding is more common in disorders affecting platelet function, genitourinary, gastrointestinal, and intracranial bleeding may occur.

***Hemophilia B*** Hemophilia B (Factor IX:C Deficiency) is similar in all of its clinical manifestations to hemophilia A, with the severity of the disorder paralleling the degree of factor deficiency.[8]

### Diagnosis

Patients who have spontaneous bleeding or bleeding out of proportion to what is expected clinically from an injury or surgical procedure may have a coagulopathy. Screening tests to detect coagulopathies include platelet count, bleeding time, PT, and APTT (Table 70.4).[5,13] A TT can provide rapid information on the later stages of the coagulation mechanism and may also be useful. Depending on the results of these tests, other tests including specific factor assays may be utilized to establish the correct diagnosis.

The APTT is an excellent test for screening deficiencies in the pathways of coagulation and has been reported to detect 99% to 100% of hemophilia A patients.[5,13] The sensitivity of the test is therefore excellent. If clinically normal patients are screened, there is an approximately 2% false-positive rate; this rate is approximately 11% for patients being evaluated for abnormal bleeding. Normal APTT and PT essentially rule out a significant plasma coagulation defect. Preoperative screening for coagulation disorders with the APTT shows that the incidence of clinically inapparent coagulopathies is so low that false-positive results greatly outnumber true-positive results and make screening pointless. The most critical piece of information is an adequate clinical assessment, including a medical history related to any prior history of bleeding problems. In patients for whom a clinical assessment is not possible, patients who have clinical evidence to suggest a bleeding disorder, such as liver disease and malabsorption, or patients undergoing procedures that may interrupt normal coagulation, such as extracorporeal circulation, screening tests are recommended.

Ideally, the APTT is sensitive to factor deficiency states of less than 30% activity. Patients with a normal PT but an abnormal APPT typically have deficiencies of factors that are unique to the intrinsic system (i.e., factors VIII, IX, XII, and XI). The specific factor assay for factor VIII or IX will reveal the appropriate defect. The exception to this is the

**Table 70.4** Tests in Patients With Hemophilia A, Hemophilia B, and Von Willebrand's Disease

| | *Hemophilia*[a] | | *Von Willebrand's disease* | | | | | |
|---|---|---|---|---|---|---|---|---|
| | **A** | **B** | **I** | **II-A** | **II-B** | **II-C** | **IID** | **III** |
| PTT | A | A | A | A/N | A/N | A/N | A/N | A |
| PT | N | N/A[b] | N | N | N | N | N | N |
| Factor VIII:C | A | N | A | A/N | A/N | A/N | A/N | A |
| vWF:Ag | N | N | A | A/N | A/N | A/N | A | A |
| vWF:R | N | N | A/N | A | A | A | A | A |
| RIPA | N | N | A/N | A | A[c] | A | A | A |
| vWF multimers | | | | | | | | |
| In plasma | N | N | Reduced, absent | Largest absent | Largest absent | Largest absent | Largest absent | None |
| In platelets | N | N | N | Largest absent | All present | Abnormal triplet | Aberrant bands | None |
| Factor IX:C | N | A | N | N | N | N | N | N |
| TT | N | N | N | N | N | N | N | N |
| Bleeding time | N | N | A | A | A | A | A | A |
| Platelet adhesion | N | N | A | A | A | A | A | A |
| Other factors | N | N | N | N | N | N | N | N |

[a] A, abnormal, N, Normal.
[b] Prothrombin time is abnormal in hemophilia $B_m$.
[c] Platelet aggregation with ristocetin is increased.

deficiency of factor IX in hemophilia $B_m$ in which case the PT as well as the APTT is prolonged.

In addition, any patient with factor VIII deficiency should undergo the laboratory tests necessary to define von Willebrand's disease to be sure that the patient does not have this disorder or a variant thereof (see later) (Table 70.4).

#### Treatment

The total care of hemophilia requires a multitude of medical and paramedical personnel.[12] In the United States and the United Kingdom, the treatment of hemophilia has become centralized because of federally funded regional comprehensive hemophilia programs. In addition to centralizing the treatment, the federal government has supported the high cost of hemophilia treatment, thus decreasing the difficulty of providing care to both the institution and the patient. These patients frequently require primary care physicians, hematologists, orthopedic surgeons, nurses, physical medicine specialists, dentists, genetic counselors, psychologists, social workers, and vocational counselors along with pharmaceutical services and inpatient and outpatient treatment facilities associated with adequate coagulation testing.

In addition to some of the previously mentioned preventive medicine aspects necessary from birth, children need to be educated in some degree of physical protection during usual play. Passenger restraints in automobiles are especially important to children with hemophilia. Physical exercise is encouraged along with a daily program to improve muscle and joint function.

Newborn male infants who may be hemophiliacs should not be circumcised until the diagnosis is excluded. Blood should be obtained from a peripheral vein and not from a femoral or jugular vein puncture because of the danger of hematoma formation. Babies with hemophilia should receive routine immunizations, including immunization against hepatitis B. These small-gauge needles do not usually cause hematomas.

Genetic counseling with a neutral attitude should be offered and female relatives who may be carriers should be tested. Female relatives who are carriers may have a mild to moderate bleeding diathesis and can be forewarned of any difficulty with either trauma or surgery.

As children grow they may be taught to administer their own factor concentrate so that they may achieve independence. Concurrent illnesses can complicate hemophilia. Minor infections are frequently associated with bleeding into the site of inflammation and need to be followed closely.

As all hemophiliacs are exposed to blood products, they are at high risk of acquiring bloodborne infections, including hepatitis and AIDS. Newly diagnosed hemophiliacs can be protected against hepatitis B with a specific vaccine, but they still are at high risk of non-A,non-B hepatitis. With multiple exposures to either cryoprecipitate or factor concentrate, the incidence of non-A,non-B hepatitis approaches 100%. There is a very high incidence of liver enzyme elevation in patients with hemophilia, but its significance is unclear. Very few patients become symptomatic and the liver disease rarely progresses to end-stage cirrhosis.

Prior to the development of an antibody test for AIDS, many blood products were contaminated with the virus and therefore almost all frequently transfused hemophiliacs have acquired human immunodeficiency virus (HIV) seropositivity.[14,15] Once HIV antibody tests became available, all blood products were screened for HIV. In addition, heating of factor concentrate appears to markedly decrease the chances of infectivity. Future hemophiliacs may have a markedly decreased chance of becoming infected with HIV. The likelihood of developing AIDS after seroconversion to a positive antibody test is unknown and there appears to be a fairly constant yearly rate (5%–8%) of conversion of hemophiliacs who become HIV positive. Hemophiliacs should therefore be watched closely for signs and symptoms of opportunistic infections so that they may be treated with the appropriate medication.

***Hemophilia A*** Patients with severe factor VIII:C deficiency may be treated with either cryoprecipitate or commercial factor VIII concentrate.[7,12] The factor is quantitated in units, where 1 unit of factor VIII is the amount found in 1 mL of pooled plasma. Cryoprecipitate, in general, contains approximately 70 to 100 units per 10- to 20-mL bag. The usual half-life of factor VIII is 8 to 12 hours and must be individualized. One way of calculating the appropriate initial dose is based upon the observation that each unit of factor VIII infused per kilogram of body weight yields a 2% rise in plasma factor VIII levels. The general goal is to achieve a factor VIII level of 25% to 30% to maintain hemostasis. To achieve this in 8 to 12 hours, it is necessary to have twice this level immediately after the infusion to allow for the decay with time. This level of factor is satisfactory for joint or muscle hemorrhage, but with severe bleeding or major surgical procedures the level should be raised to and maintained at 50% to 80% for up to a week.

Mild factor VIII:C deficiency may be treated with 1-desamino-8-D-arginine vasopressin (desmopressin acetate, DDAVP), which transiently increases the factor VIII level.[16] If the patient has a mild bleeding episode, such as a hemarthrosis, DDAVP 0.3–0.4 μg/kg over 15 to 30 minutes may be given and factor levels obtained to ensure that an adequate increment has been achieved. If successful, future episodes can be treated without monitoring factor levels. The injection can be repeated in 12 to 24 hours, but the factor increments become attenuated with frequent dosages. Use of DDAVP reduces exposure to non-A,non-B hepatitis virus and HIV.

Kinetic studies can be done to predict the factor VIII level and half-life in the individual patient. Changes in volume and clinical status such as a new infection may change the half-life considerably.

Inhibitors (antibodies) can develop in approximately 5% to 10% of patients with hemophilia for unknown reasons.[17] These inhibitors are usually IgG immunoglobulins, which do not precipitate human factor VIII and do not fix complement. They are directed against the factor VIII:C coagulant portion of the complex. These antibodies may be recognized when a calculated dose of factor VIII does not produce the expected plasma level. A 1:1 mixture of the patient's plasma and normal plasma will still have markedly prolonged APTT, whereas in the usual deficiency state the APTT returns to the normal range. This is standard procedure in most laboratories, with the level of the inhibitor in Bethesda Units. Patients with coagulant factor antibodies require specialized care. To overcome the inhibitor, high doses of factor VIII, cytotoxic chemotherapy (i.e., cyclophosphamide), porcine factor VIII, a prothrombin complex concentrate (such as Konyne and Proplex), and anti-inhibitor–coagulant complexes (such as Autoplex and FEIBA) have been used.[17–19]

The risk of hepatitis is less likely with single-donor plasma or cryoprecipitate than with products made from pooled plasma (factor VIII concentrate).[12] Reduction in donor exposure can best be achieved in patients who require infrequent or low-dose treatment with plasma products (e.g., single-donor plasma), such as patients with mild hemophilia or small children with hemophilia. Patients requiring frequent high-dose factor replacement eventually are exposed to a great many donors, even if single-donor plasma or cryprecipitate is used.

Lyophilized concentrates of factor VIII are prepared by various techniques that do not provide a good source of functionally active von Willebrand's factor. Most concentrate is made from plasma pooled without regard to blood type, so isoagglutinins to red cell antigens A and B are present and can cause hemolysis.

Porcine factor VIII concentrate is intended primarily for use in patients who have developed inhibitors against factor VIII:C. The neutralizing activity of these inhibitors is usually weaker against nonhuman as opposed to human factor VIII coagulant. The occasional allergic reactions are usually managed with antihistamines and corticosteroids. Some patients have developed inhibitors to porcine as well as human factor VIII, but others have no anamnestic response.

***Hemophilia B*** Factor IX deficiency can be treated with either plasma or prothrombin complex concentrate (PCC).[8,12] The latter is prepared by fractionation of pools of plasma from hundreds to thousands of donors and contains factors IX and X with variable amounts of factors VII and II. Activated forms of factors VII, IX, and X may be present. A vial of lyophilized material contains approximately 500–1,000 units of factor IX in 20–30 mL when reconstituted. About 40% of the factor IX measured in vitro can be recovered in the patient. When large quantities of factor IX have to be administered, PCC is preferable to plasma. It is stable at refrigerator temperatures and rarely causes allergic reaction, so it may easily be self-administered. Because it is made from pooled plasma, viruses, especially non-A,non-B hepatitis, may be transmitted. Also, because of the presence of activated coagulation factors there exists the possibility of thromboembolic phenomenon which has been reported in a few patients, especially postoperative or liver disease patients. Five to ten units of heparin per milliliter of reconstituted PCC has been recommended to counteract the excessive thrombotic tendency. Although PCC is the mainstay of therapy for severe hemophilia B, plasma may be used to treat the mild disorder. In addition, PCC is widely used without heparin to treat hemorrhage in patients with inhibitors of factor VIII.

The half-life of factor IX:C is approximately 24 hours, with normal hemostasis being achieved when plasma levels are approximately 10% to 25%. Each unit of factor IX infused per kilogram body weight yields a 1% rise in the level of factor IX. As with factor VIII, the success of infusion and achievement of appropriate levels should be monitored with factor IX assays. Although hemostasis is usually achieved between 10% and 25%, plasma levels of 40% have been recommended for severe muscle and joint bleeding, with factors of 60% recommended for major surgery. With major surgery, replacement therapy should be continued for at least a week.

The incidence of factor IX antibodies, perhaps 2% to 3% of the population, is less than that of factor VIII antibodies;

however, in patients with severe hemophilia B the incidence is as high as 12%.

Anti-inhibitor–coagulant complexes (AICCs) such as Autoplex and FEIBA are deliberately activated PCCs developed for the treatment of hemorrhage in patients with coagulant inhibitors.[17] Each brand has its own unit system related to in vitro inhibitor-neutralizing capacity. Several controlled studies on the use of single doses of PCC or AICC in joint hemorrhages in patients with inhibitors have been published. With 75 units per kilogram of either Konyne or Proplex (both nonactivated PCCs), 50% of hemarthroses were halted, as opposed to 29% by an albumin placebo. Similar studies have shown equivalent results with Autoplex 50 U/kg. Individual reports have documented control of critical hemorrhage with AICC. If one dose does not work, higher or repeated doses may sometimes be effective.

## *Von Willebrand's Disease*

Von Willebrand's disease is probably the most common inheritable coagulopathy.[7,9,10] The first clinical description of the disease was made by von Willebrand in 1926. Von Willebrand's disease is caused by a deficiency, quantitative or qualitative, of von Willebrand's factor and results both in abnormal platelet function and in defective blood coagulation clotting. Von Willebrand's factor (vWF) is a glycoprotein that can be found in classic hemophiliac plasma and in normal plasma. At first, it was called factor VIII–related antigen or protein, as antibodies had been raised against protein fractions containing factor VIII coagulant activity. It is now known that factor VIII:C is distinct from vWF, but forms a dissociable complex with it: the factor VIII complex (Table 70.3).[20] Von Willebrand's factor can normally be detected not only in plasma but in vessel walls and platelets. Almost all of the vWF in platelets is located in the alpha granules. Within endothelial cells, vWF has been located on the plasma membrane and in the endoplasmic reticulum of the cytoplasm, as well as in cell-specific organelles.

Von Willebrand's factor has a dual role in hemostasis, facilitating platelet adhesion to injured vessel walls and binding the antihemophiliac factor (factor VIII:C) in a complex, thus serving as a carrier of factor VIII:C in plasma.

The basic subunit of vWF is a protein chain with a molecular weight of approximately 230,000. The subunits are held together in a very complex way by disulfide bonds, forming proteins that vary widely in molecular weight. Von Willebrand's factor consists of a series of multimers ranging from 800,000 to 14,000,000 in molecular weight. The large multimers are thought to be the most hemostatically efficient, with a greater potential for interaction with platelets and binding to the subendothelium. Von Willebrand's factor must join the platelets with the subendothelium to cause effective platelet function.

In 1973 Howard[21] showed that the antibiotic ristocetin causes platelet aggregation dependent upon vWF. Platelet aggregation with ristocetin became a model system in the study of platelet–vWF interactions. Von Willebrand's factor activity was measured on the basis of platelet aggregation and expressed as ristocetin cofactor activity. As ristocetin and vWF agglutinate platelets fixed with paraformaldehyde or formalin, formalin-fixed platelets are now used to measure this activity.

High-molecular-weight forms of vWF seem to have the highest ristocetin cofactor activity and appear to be the most efficient in promoting adhesion in these systems. Some commercial factor VIII concentrates contain only low-molecular-weight multimers of vWF and are less efficient in promoting platelet adhesion.

Von Willebrand's factor appears to be the carrier protein for factor VIII:C as it circulates in normal blood. Although the site of factor VIII:C has not been established, factor VIII:C antigen has been demonstrated in the endothelial cells lining liver sinusoids, but not in other types of endothelium. Von Willebrand's factor also seems to be a stimulator of factor VIII:C production, because when vWF is given to a patient with von Willebrand's disease who lacks the complete complex, the factor VIII:C activity in the patient's blood increases more than can be explained by the factor VIII:C activity in the infused material.

### Clinical Presentation

Von Willebrand's disease is usually inherited in the heterozygous form as an autosomal dominant disorder.[7,9,10] Genetic variants are defined according to the qualitative and quantitative abnormalities of vWF, which run true in affected kindreds. One affected person may be markedly different from another within a kindred with respect to the amount of factor deficiency but not the type of deficiency. Types I, II-A, II-B, and II-D are inherited as autosomal dominant characteristics, whereas types II-C and III are inherited as autosomal recessive disorders. These genetic variants are described under Diagnosis.

Patients with von Willebrand's disease frequently present with mucosal bleeding such as epistaxis, gingival bleeding, easy bruising, menorrhagia, and postsurgical bleeding, especially after operations on mucosal surfaces such as tonsillectomy, vaginal surgery, and dental surgery. In the most severe forms of the disease the bleeding starts in early childhood and tends to decrease with age or with pregnancy. In milder forms the disease may not be discovered until an episode of trauma or surgery when the patient is an adult. The bleeding into joints and muscles characteristic of hemophilia is rare in von Willebrand's disease.

### Diagnosis

Von Willebrand's disease and its variants are defined by the type of abnormality in vWF—quantitative, qualitative, or both (Table 70.4).[7,9,10] Von Willebrand's factor activity is measured as the bleeding time and by the ristocetin cofactor test. The bleeding time has been shown to be reasonably reproducible and accurate when obtained by the template technique. The ristocetin cofactor test measures the ability of the patient's plasma to agglutinate normal washed, fresh or formalin-fixed platelets in the presence of ristocetin. Ristocetin-induced platelet aggregation (RIPA) is measured on platelet-rich plasma with an aggregometer.

Von Willebrand's factor is also measured by quantitation of von Willebrand's antigen, usually by electrophoresis with precipitating antibody to von Willebrand's factor or by radioimmunoassay.

The multimeric structure of von Willebrand's factor is demonstrated by electrophoresis in sodium dodecyl sulfate–agarose or acrylamide gels. The multimers are then identified with radiolabeled antibody to vWF and autoradiography. The bands separate on the basis of their molecular size, and the relative proportions of large and small multimers can be demonstrated. Genetic variants are defined by the results of these tests. Factor VIII:C coagulant activity is usually low and commensurate with the degree of vWF deficiency. In some patients, however, factor VIII:C levels may approach normal. In the following, each type of von Willebrand's disease is described with respect to the preceding tests and the pattern of inheritance (Table 70.4).[7,9,10]

***Type I*** The most common form of von Willebrand's disease is inherited as an autosomal dominant disorder and expressed as a decrease in von Willebrand's antigen and vWF; multimers of all sizes are found in plasma and platelets. Although the amount of vWF is usually proportional to the level of von Willebrand's antigen, the amount of factor VIII:C may be higher. RIPA is normal or decreased. The bleeding time is usually prolonged. Type I von Willebrand's disease appears to result from production of decreased amounts of structurally normal vWF.

***Type II*** Type II von Willebrand's disease was originally described as a normal concentration of von Willebrand's antigen with a qualitative defect in von Willebrand's protein. Ristocetin cofactor activity (vWF) is low compared with the concentration of von Willebrand's antigen. The differentiation of types A–D is based upon the multimeric pattern of vWF in plasma and platelets. The response of platelets to ristocetin is also an important characteristic.

Type II-A von Willebrand's disease is inherited as an autosomal dominant disorder and is characterized by the absence from plasma of large and medium-sized von Willebrand's multimers and the absence from platelets of large multimers. There is marked reduction in ristocetin cofactor and in the response to ristocetin of platelet aggregation. Factor VIII antigen and coagulant material may be decreased or normal. DDAVP increases the numbers of small multimers in plasma but does not increase large multimers. This disease is probably a defect in the ability to make large multimers of vWF.

Type II-B is inherited as an autosomal dominant disorder and is characterized by the absence from plasma of large multimers. They are present in platelets. Plasma levels of von Willebrand's antigen, factor VIII coagulant material, and vWF may be decreased or normal. Aggregation of platelets in response to ristocetin is increased, with strong agglutination in the presence of ristocetin too weak to agglutinate normal platelets. DDAVP may cause a sudden release of large multimers, causing widespread platelet aggregation with marked thrombocytopenia. This disorder appears to result from a qualitative defect in the formation of large multimers, causing enhanced affinity of cellular binding sites.

Type II-C is a rare variant that is characterized by the absence of large multimers from both plasma and platelets and an increase in the smallest multimer. It is inherited as an autosomal recessive disorder. Von Willebrand's factor and RIPA are undetectable; the level of factor VIII:C is very low.

Type II-D is an autosomal dominant disorder characterized by an abnormal multimeric pattern: patients lack the large multimers, and the smallest multimers do not have the normal triplet pattern.

***Type III*** A few patients have been found to have a severe plasma deficiency of vWF, with essentially no protein being found in either plasma or platelets. Factor VIII:C activity is low in proportion to the markedly reduced vWF and von Willebrand's antigen. Type III is inherited as an autosomal recessive disorder; heterozygotes appear normal. The bleeding time is severely prolonged.

***Pseudo von Willebrand's Disease*** This is also known as platelet-type von Willebrand's disease because it results from an abnormality in the platelet instead of in vWF. It is inherited as an autosomal dominant disorder; the platelets bind normal vWF at concentrations of ristocetin lower than those needed for normal platelets to bind. RIPA is enhanced. Von Willebrand's factor alone without ristocetin may aggregate platelets. Multimeric analysis may show depletion of the large multimers of vWF and may resemble type II-B disease. Some patients have chronic thrombocytopenia. DDAVP and cryoprecipitate may result in platelet aggregation and worsen the thrombocytopenia.

***Acquired von Willebrand's Disease*** Patients with altered immune status have been reported to develop a disorder resembling von Willebrand's disease, with prolonged bleeding times and reduced levels of factor VIII–related activities.[22,23] Patients with systemic lupus erythematosus and other collagen diseases, monoclonal gammopathies, lymphoproliferative disease, and Wilms' tumor have been reported to have this disease. In some cases, inhibitors (antibodies) have been detected in the plasma that are capable of binding to factor VIII–von Willebrand factor complex, removing it at an accelerated rate.

### Treatment

In addition to improving the factor VIII:C level it is important to improve the bleeding time in patients with von Willebrand's disease.[7,9,10] The highly concentrated commercial concentrates used for hemophilia A are not suitable because they may lack high-molecular-weight multimers and therefore fail to correct the bleeding time. Although use of fresh-frozen plasma is possible, it is frequently limited by the large volume necessary to correct the deficiency. When the type of von Willebrand's disease is unclear prior to multimeric analysis, the defect is severe, or the trauma is serious, thus requiring correction with a high degree of certainty, cryoprecipitate is the treatment of choice. Despite adequate correction of the factor VIII:C level with appropriate amounts of cryoprecipitate calculated to achieve a factor VIII level appropriate for the clinical conditions, the bleeding time frequently is corrected for only 6 to 12 hours. There is usually a discrepancy between vWF activity and factor VIII:C level 24 hours after the infusion if more cryoprecipitate is not given. Therefore, bleeding time should guide treatment and cryoprecipate usually needs to be given every 12 hours.

In mild von Willebrand's disease, DDAVP may be used because any plasma product carries the risk of transmitting hepatitis.[16,24] Intravenous DDAVP, at 0.3–0.4 $\mu$g/kg over 15 to 30 minutes, usually induces a dose-dependent increase in all factor VIII–related activities, with both factor VIII:C and vWF increasing two- to threefold. This usually lasts 4 to 8 hours and is effective in mild or moderate type I disease and in type II-A disease. The dose may be repeated in 8 to 12 hours but the response diminishes with continued treatment, and laboratory monitoring should be initiated if treatment is extended. DDAVP also stimulates the release of plasminogen activator and some investigators prophylactically administer fibrinolytic inhibitors (i.e., aminocaproic acid, Amicar).

Side effects of DDAVP are minimal and consist of occasional facial flushing, headache, and palpitations. Water retention can occur and hypertension is exaggerated.

Patients with mild hemophilia A may also be treated with DDAVP, but both patients with severe type I von Willebrand's disease and severe hemophiliacs do not respond well. In Type II-A, DDAVP increases plasma vWF, but the qualitative abnormality is not corrected and the bleeding time may be shortened but not normalized.[24] DDAVP should not be used before the type of von Willebrand's disease is defined by multimeric analysis, because in type II-B, in vivo platelet aggregation and severe thrombocytopenia may occur. DDAVP is also not beneficial in types II-C and II-D.

Menorrhagia is a frequent problem in women with von Willebrand's disease. Oral contraceptives may be very effective in controlling this symptom. Inhibitors of the fibrinolytic system may be of special value in those tissues rich in fibrinolytic activity such as the ear, nose, and throat region and especially with tooth extractions. Patients with von Willebrand's disease should be encouraged to avoid aspirin and nonsteroidal anti-inflammatory drugs because of their effects on platelet function which may possibly increase the risk of serious bleeding.

### *Other Congenital Factor Deficiencies*

In addition to deficiencies in factors VIII and IX, congenital deficiencies in fibrinogen, in factors II, V, VII, X, XI, XII, and XIII, in contact factors, and in combinations of other factors have been reported to form multiple defects.[25] Contact factor abnormalities including deficiencies in factor XII (the Hageman factor), high-molecular-weight kininogen (the Fitzgerald factor), and prekallikrein (Fletcher factor) all prolong the APTT but do not lead to any bleeding diathesis. The only contact factor deficiency that causes bleeding diathesis is factor XI deficiency. As most of these other deficiencies are inherited as autosomal recessive disorders, they are rare. Some patients with abnormal molecules, such as fibrinogen, may have increased tendency for thromboembolic phenomenon. The usual treatment for these deficiencies is fresh-frozen plasma, although there may be instances in which prothrombin complex concentrate is necessary to treat factor II, VII, or X deficiency. Cryoprecipitate may be used to treat a fibrinogen deficiency.

## Acquired Coagulation Disorders

### *Disseminated Intravascular Coagulation*

Disseminated intravascular coagulation (DIC) may be an acute or chronic process.[17,26,27] Acute DIC is usually an overwhelming clinical syndrome characterized by depletion of coagulation factors and platelets and evidence of excessive fibrinolysis, which presumably is an attempt to compensate for microvascular clotting. Normally, a constant, balanced dynamic process of clotting and fibrinolysis operates to prevent organ dysfunction, bleeding, or clotting. In acute DIC, this process is disrupted by some sort of injury that causes excessive intravascular coagulation, overcoming normal inhibitory processes. In subacute or chronic DIC, the balance between depletion and synthesis of coagulation factors in the circulation may make diagnosis difficult. Some of the known clinical settings in which acute and chronic DIC occurs are listed in Table 70.5.

Acute DIC is usually an overwhelming clinical syndrome that becomes obvious when the patient begins bleeding from multiple sites.[17,26,27] The patient is frequently hypotensive and there is associated organ dysfunction, resulting in azotemia and oliguria. Because of the depletion of coagulation factors in the plasma there is usually a deficiency of fibrinogen, factors V, VIII, and XIII, and antithrombin III. Thrombocytopenia is present and excessive fibrinolysis is frequent, with low plasminogen and increased fibrin split products. Factors released from platelets, such as platelet factor III, platelet factor IV, and $\beta$-thromboglobulin, are frequently elevated because of the consumption of platelets during the process. Active fibrinolysis occurs, as shown by the increase in concentration of split products of fibrin and fibrinogen; blood plasminogen concentrations may decrease.

DIC can be better understood by reconsidering the Shwartzman phenomenon, which consists of DIC, bilateral renal cortical necrosis, and death from central nervous system bleeding. The Shwartzman reaction characteristically follows two spaced intravenous injections of bacterial endotoxin into experimental animals and, in part, is believed to be mediated by one or more episodes of DIC. The first injection has little effect; the second injection, given 6 to 72 hours after the first, produces dramatic effects, resulting in agglutination of platelets and while cells in many organs associated with fibrin thrombi in small blood vessels. The generation of thrombi is felt to be the mechanism by which the Shwartzman reaction occurs.

By studying the sequence of changes in the blood during the Shwartzman reaction, we can better understand why certain clinical situations such as infection, pregnancy, and malignancy may predispose patients to DIC. Early in these settings, fibrinogen, acting as an "acute-phase reactant," can be elevated. Likewise, in the Shwartzman reaction, after the first exposure to endotoxin, there is progressive elevation in fibrinogen levels for 48 hours. After the second injection there is an abrupt decrease in fibrinogen associated with thrombocytopenia and the other hemostatic abnormalities common to acute DIC. It is felt that whatever underlying disease state predisposes to DIC, it generates thromboplastin, which converts prothrombin to thrombin leading to all the subsequent events in the coagulation cascade.

#### Clinical Presentation

Acute DIC occurs secondary to many clinical conditions as listed in Table 70.5.[17,26,27] Sepsis is one of the more common causes and, although more frequently linked to gram-negative bacteria, it may occur with gram-positive organisms, fungi, and viruses as well. As mentioned before, acute DIC

**Table 70.5** Etiology and Clinical Settings of Disseminated Intravascular Coagulation

| *Acute disseminated intravascular coagulation* | *Chronic disseminated intravascular coagulation* |
|---|---|
| Obstetrics | Malignant neoplasia |
| Septic and saline-induced abortion | Solid tumors |
| Abruptio placentae and placenta previa | Leukemia (especially |
| Prolonged retention of a dead fetus | promyelocytic leukemia) |
| Amniotic fluid embolism | Vascular disorders |
| Infections | Giant hemangioma |
| Gram-negative sepsis (for example, meningococcemia) | Aortic aneurysms |
| Gram-positive sepsis (less common) | Valvular heart disease |
| Rickettsial (Rocky Mountain spotted fever) | Liver disease |
| Protozoal (malaria) | |
| Viral (congenital rubella) | |
| Shock | |
| Hypovolemic | |
| Hypoperfusion | |
| Tissue injury | |
| Prolonged surgery | |
| Trauma | |
| Burns | |
| Heat stroke | |
| Anaphylaxis | |

From Fruchtman S, Aledort LM: Etiology and clinical settings of disseminated intravascular coagulation. J Am Coll Cardiol 1986;8(suppl B):159B–167B, with permission.

may be seen in late pregnancy either associated with abruptio placentae and placenta previa or associated with a dead fetus or amniotic fluid embolism. Patients who have severe hypotension, who require prolonged surgery, or who suffer tissue injury such as burns or heat stroke may experience DIC.

Subacute and chronic DIC is more commonly associated with malignancies, especially solid tumors. Mucin-producing adenocarcinomas, especially those originating in the gastrointestinal tract or the prostate and sometimes in other organs such as the lung or breast, may be associated with smoldering DIC. Promyelocytic leukemia is almost always associated with DIC to the point that prophylactic treatment has been recommended. In addition, vascular disorders (such as giant hemangiomas) and chronic liver disease have been associated with smoldering DIC.

**Diagnosis**

Disseminated intravascular coagulation should be suspected on clinical grounds in any of the previously mentioned clinical situations. It should also be considered if the patient develops bleeding from many sites, including oozing from intravenous lines or from invasive procedure. Disseminated intravascular coagulation should be suspected with multiple-organ-system failure. Massive bleeding from the gastrointestinal tract or genitourinary system, peripheral cyanosis of the extremities, renal failure, or purpura fulminans may dominate the clinical picture.

The laboratory diagnosis of DIC is based upon a complete battery of laboratory tests.[17,26,27] A single laboratory abnormality is insufficient for a diagnosis of DIC. The relative importance of any particular laboratory test is controversial. Routine tests of blood coagulation including PT, APTT, and TT should be done. The PT is usually prolonged, while the APTT is more variable and frequently normal. Occasionally, both tests may be decreased, rather than increased. The TT is usually prolonged, because of the absolute decrease in fibrinogen as well as the presence of fibrin split products, which inhibit the reaction of thrombin on fibrinogen. As liver disease frequently causes abnormalities in these tests, it can be difficult to separate patients who have decreased synthesis of coagulation factors secondary to liver disease from those with DIC. Fibrinogen levels below 150 mg/dL and platelet counts below $150{,}000/mm^3$ are seen in 95% of all DIC patients. In addition, 75% of patients have schistocytes (red blood cell fragments). Unfortunately, these findings may also be observed in severe liver disease and hypersplenism. Depressed antithrombin III levels are seen in most patients. Fibrin split products are not usually greater than 100 $\mu$g/dL in chronic liver disease but are quite elevated in patients with DIC; thus, this finding is more specific. Mild elevations in fibrin split products may be seen in many other inflammatory diseases and in association with hematomas and deep vein thrombosis, but these are usually less than 40 $\mu$g/dL. Paracoagulation tests, such as the ethanol gelation or the protamine sulfate precipitation test, measure fibrin monomers and should be specific for DIC but are of low specificity in most clinical series. Factor VIII and V levels should be decreased in DIC; however, these tests may be quite variable. The most specific findings are a low platelet count associated with elevated fibrin split products and depressed antithrombin III and fibrinogen levels. As the generation of thrombin is the sine qua non of DIC, it would be useful to measure thrombin in plasma. A radioimmunoassay has been developed for measuring thrombin, but clinical studies have not yet been done. Thrombin cleaves fibrinopeptides A and B from fibrinogen; thus, fibrinopeptides A and B should be elevated in patients with DIC. Initial studies of fibrinopeptide A in patients suspected of having DIC have shown a good correlation, but other inflammatory conditions such as systemic lupus erythematosus, infections, and thrombosis may also result in elevated levels, thus decreasing the specificity of this test.

**Treatment**

Most important in the treatment of DIC is treatment of the underlying disease.[17,26,27] In patients in whom the disease is self-limited, such as a pregnant woman with abruptio placentae or retained placenta, delivery of the fetus with the products of conception usually returns hemostasis to normal. In those patients who have overwhelming sepsis or shock, antibiotics and treatment of hypotension are the mainstays of treatment. In patients who are receiving maximum treatment for the underlying condition, but in whom the process is worsening or in whom bleeding develops, either replacement of deficient factors or the use of anticoagulants has been tried. Fresh-frozen plasma provides volume to expand the intravascular space and replaces clotting factors including fibrinogen. If hypofibrinogenemia is severe, cryoprecipitate may be useful, because in addition to the factor VIII in each unit there is a significant amount of fibrinogen. Although it has been argued that replacement of coagulation factors "adds fuel to the fire," in practice this does not appear to make the situation worse and frequently hemostasis is improved. Antithrombin III (which should remove thrombin from the circulation) is present in fresh-frozen plasma and may be beneficial. Purified antithrombin III has been used, but there are no controlled trials to demonstrate its efficacy.

Anticoagulation is controversial in patients with DIC and specific guidelines are not available.[17,26,27] Anecdotal reports of improvement in individual patients abound, but controlled clinical studies are lacking. Heparin has not been shown to reduce morbidity or mortality in uncontrolled series. Heparin rarely restores the coagulopathy to normal, although both the deficiency of coagulation factors and the thrombocytopenia may improve. If the patient does not respond to the replacement of coagulation factor alone, heparin followed by factor replacement may improve the coagulopathy. If the patient has an underlying condition that can be brought under control, improvement of the coagulopathy may provide sufficient time for the DIC to abate. Heparin may be given either as an intravenous bolus (every 4 hours) or as a continuous intravenous infusion via pump. In those patients who have progressive organ dysfunction, such as azotemia with or without ischemia of the extremities, heparin may provide improvement.

Heparin with replacement of coagulation factors, including fresh-frozen plasma, cryoprecipitate, and platelets, has been recommended routinely for patients with acute promyelocytic leukemia. In those patients with metastatic carcinoma of the prostate, in whom hormonal therapy may be very efficacious, prophylactic anticoagulation prior to institution of chemotherapy may be life-saving if the patient has DIC.

Antifibrinolytics (i.e., aminocaproic acid, Amicar) have been used in patients in whom the dominant clinical picture is one of excessive fibrinolysis. Most clinicians prefer to use aminocaproic acid only in conjunction with heparin, unless the patient has recently had cardiopulmonary bypass surgery or has carcinoma of the prostate, the two clinical conditions in which isolated fibrinolysis without generation of thrombin has been well documented. In patients with chronic liver disease who manifest dominant fibrinolysis, inhibition of the fibrinolytic system has been attempted but is generally unsuccessful.

## *Vitamin K Deficiency*

Vitamin $K_1$ is necessary for carboxylation of factors II, VII, IX, and X to make complete $\gamma$-carboxyglutamic acid molecules from glutamic acid residues.[17] When vitamin K deficiency occurs, the inactive precursors of these coagulation factors, which do not bind calcium, accumulate in the plasma and act as vitamin K antagonists. These have been called protein induced by vitamin K antagonists (PIVKA). Vitamin K is also necessary for the active form of protein C, which inhibits the activated factor V and VIII molecules. In most clinical situations, vitamin K deficiency causes a bleeding diathesis as a result of the marked deficiency of factors II, VII, IX, and X.

Vitamin K is found in green vegetables and is synthesized by bacteria in the large intestine. Naturally occurring vitamin $K_1$ is fat soluble, but the synthetic analogues are water soluble so that they may be administered parenterally.

***Hemorrhagic Disease of the Newborn*** Infants may become deficient in vitamin K because of the absence of this vitamin in human milk and because their gut has not had sufficient time to be colonized by bacteria. In addition, some infants may have immature ability to synthesize vitamin K–dependent clotting factors from the liver. These infants usually bleed from the umbilical cord, from the gastrointestinal tract, or occasionally into the brain after birth.

Although the normal neonate has a mild deficiency of coagulation factors, if vitamin K deficiency exists, the vitamin K–dependent factors are usually less than 25% of normal. In this situation the PT and APTT are prolonged, but TT, fibrinogen, and platelet count are normal. Levels of vitamin K–dependent factors will substantiate the diagnosis.

Infants usually respond to 1 mg of vitamin $K_1$ parenterally on the first day, which can be repeated every 8 hours until the clotting tests have returned to normal. If there is life-threatening hemorrhage, fresh-frozen plasma should correct the defect immediately. Prophylactic vitamin $K_1$ is given on some obstetrical units routinely, although it may not be necessary. Premature or low-birth-weight neonates should probably receive vitamin $K_1$.

***Malabsorption*** Patients may become vitamin K deficient because of poor nutrition or malabsorption.[17] A careful dietary history is important in this regard. Patients with a poor diet may have other manifestations of malabsorption, such as vitamin deficiencies and anemia. Broad-spectrum antibiotics may sterilize the large intestine postoperatively, and if vitamin $K_1$ is not administered, the patient may become vitamin K deficient even more quickly than from simply the lack of parenteral vitamin K.

Malabsorption resulting from diseases of the small intestine such as celiac disease, amyloidosis, Whipple's disease, and short-bowel syndrome may cause abnormal development in children, weight loss, muscle wasting, steatorrhea, as well as other manifestations of malnutrition such as vitamin deficiencies and anemia. Significant malabsorption can occur even without symptoms of diarrhea or steatorrhea, requiring quantitation of fat excretion to confirm the presence of malabsorption.

Severe vitamin K deficiency is also seen in obstructive jaundice where bile salts do not reach the small intestine and therefore vitamin K cannot be absorbed. Patients with malabsorption from small-bowel disease or obstructive jaundice require parenteral administration of vitamin K. Vitamin $K_1$ 10 mg weekly is usually sufficient.

## *Liver Disease*

### Clinical Presentation

Severe hepatocellular disease may cause a significant coagulopathy as a result of the lack of synthesis of coagulation factors.[17,28] The liver synthesizes the majority of blood coagulation factors including fibrinogen (factor I) and factors II, VII, IX, X, XI, XII, XIII, and V. In addition, plasminogen, antithrombin III, and $\alpha_2$-antiplasmin are synthesized by the liver. The factor VIII–von Willebrand factor complex is usually elevated rather than reduced in liver disease. Factor VIII:C is felt to be synthesized by many organs in addition to the liver. In chronic liver disease, plasminogen activator derived from endothelial cells is not cleared by the reticuloendothelial system, leading to a fibrinolytic state. In addition to the defect in synthesis of these coagulation factors, DIC may occur. If hepatocellular disease is so severe that a coagulation defect occurs, patients have a poor prognosis.

PT, APTT, and TT are useful in screening for a deficiency of liver-dependent factors. The PT is sensitive to deficiencies in the vitamin K–dependent factors (factors II, VII, IX, and X). The APTT helps to determine deficiencies in factor IX as well as some other factors. The TT is helpful in detecting hypofibrinogenemia and dysfibrinogenemia as well as the presence of fibrin degradation products that interfere with fibrin polymerization. Another test that is sometimes useful in hepatic disease is the measurement of clotting time using snake venom, which is not affected by heparin and removes fibrinopeptide A from fibrinogen. This test indicates the degree of dysfibrinogenemia. As defects in polymerization may occur before severe hypofibrinogemia, this may be an indication of the degree of liver dysfunction.

Factor V is synthesized by hepatic cells but is not dependent upon vitamin K. Therefore, it may be useful in distinguishing vitamin K deficiency from liver disease. The deficiency of antithrombin III occurs with severe hepatocellular disease and may contribute to the development of DIC. Tests of the lytic system, such as an euglobulin clot lysis time, may show increased activity, either because of decreased clearance of fibrinolytic factors or because of DIC. In acute hepatic failure, plasminogen may be low, reflecting both decreased synthesis and increased catabolism associated with DIC.

### Treatment

Patients with liver disease should be evaluated with a PT, APTT, TT, and platelet count.[17,28] Although patients can have severe abnormalities in these tests, bleeding may not occur. Patients who are not bleeding should not be treated. Conversely, major bleeding may occur with normal tests secondary to esophageal varices or peptic ulcer disease. To be sure there is no vitamin K deficiency contributing to the abnormalities, most clinicians administer 10 to 25 mg of vitamin $K_1$ for one or several days to be sure that the liver is synthesizing to its capacity. When a patient bleeds in association with a coagulopathy, replacement therapy may correct or improve the bleeding tendency. Fresh-frozen plasma supplies all the missing coagulation factors, but fluid overload may be a serious problem. Usually one to two units (250–500 mL) of fresh-frozen plasma is necessary every 6 hours in a seriously ill patient. If the patient has ascites, the half-life of many of these factors is decreased, and it is difficult to correct the coagulopathy. Prothrombin complex concentrates can be given, but there is an increased risk of precipitating intravascular coagulation and causing DIC if it is not already present. In general, the use of these concentrates is not recommended. Only when the administration of fresh-frozen plasma does not correct the coagulopathy and the patient continues to have serious bleeding should PCCs be considered.

The use of heparin and antifibrinolytic drugs (aminocaproic acid) is controversial. Aminocaproic acid has been tried and may be successful, especially with mucosal bleeding from the genitourinary tract; however, acute renal failure may occur. Heparin has not been demonstrated to improve survival and may exacerbate the underlying coagulopathy even if DIC is present. In the few clinical studies that have been done, both controlled and uncontrolled trials have not shown any definite benefit with heparin in severe acute hepatic necrosis. Platelet transfusions may also be necessary if thrombocytopenia occurs secondary to hepatocellular disease and/or hypersplenism.

## References

1. Ratnoff OD. The role of haemostatic mechanisms. Clin Haematol 1981;10:261–281.
2. Lammle B, Griffin JH. Formation of the fibrin clot: The balance of procoagulant and inhibitory factors. Clin Haematol 1985;14:281–342.
3. Lowe GDO. Laboratory evaluation of hypercoagulability. Clin Haematol 1981;10:407–442.
4. Giddings JC, Peake IR. Laboratory support in the diagnosis of coagulation disorders. Clin Haematol 1985;14:571–595.
5. Suchman AL, Griner PF. Diagnostic uses of the activated

partial thromboplastin time and prothrombin time. Ann Intern Med 1986;104:810–816.
6. Lawn RM, Vehar GA. The molecular genetics of hemophilia. Sci Am 1986;254:48–54.
7. Mammen EF. Congenital coagulation disorders. Semin Thromb Hemost 1983;9:22–28.
8. Mammen EF. Congenital coagulation disorders. Semin Thromb Hemost 1983;9:28–30.
9. Zimmerman TS, Ruggeri ZM, Folcher CA. Factor VIII/von Willebrand factor. Prog Hematol 1983;13:279–309.
10. Homberg L, Nilsson IM. Von Willebrand disease. Clin Haematol 1985;14:461–488.
11. Thompson AR. Structure, function, and molecular defects of factor IX. Blood 1986;67:565–572.
12. Kasper CK, Dietrich SL. Comprehensive management of haemophilia. Clin Haematol 1985;14:489–512.
13. Bowie EJ, Owen CA. The significance of abnormal preoperative hemostatic tests. Prog Hemost Thromb 1980;5:179–209.
14. Gallo RC. The AIDS virus. Sci Am 1987;256:46–56.
15. Kim HC, Nahum K, Raska K, et al. Natural history of acquired immunodeficiency syndrome in hemophiliac patients. Am J Hematol 1987;24:169–176.
16. de la Fuente B, Kasper CK, Rickles FR, et al. Response of patients with mild and moderate hemophilia A and von Willebrand's disease to treatment with desmopressin. Ann Intern Med 1985;103:6–14.
17. Prentice CRM. Acquired coagulation disorders. Clin Haematol 1985;14:413–442.
18. Tengborn L, Hedner V. Management of haemophilia A with antibodies: The effect of combined treatment with factor VIII, hydrocortisone and cyclophosphamide. Thromb Haemost 1985; 54:776–779.
19. Bona RD, Pasquale DH, Kalish RI, et al. Porcine factor VIII and plasmapheresis in the management of hemophiliac patients with inhibitors. Am J Hematol 1986;21:201–207.
20. Marder VJ, Mannucci PM, Firkin BG, et al. Standard nomenclature for factor VIII and von Willebrand factor: A recommendation by the International Committee on Thrombosis and Haemostasis. Thromb Haemost 1985;54:871–872.
21. Howard MA, Sawers RJ, Firkin BG. Ristocetin: A means of differentiating von Willebrand's disease into two groups. Blood 1973;41:687–690.
22. Joist JH, Cowan JF, Zimmerman TS. Acquired von Willebrand's disease. N Engl J Med 1978;298:988–991.
23. Lazarchick J, Pappas AA, Kizer J, et al. Acquired von Willebrand syndrome due to an inhibitor specific for von Willebrand factor antigens. Am J Hematol 1986;21:305–314.
24. Gralnick HR, Williams SB, McKeown LP, et al. DDAVP in type IIa von Willebrand's disease. Blood 1986;67:465–468.
25. Mammen EF. Congenital coagulation disorders. Semin Thromb Hemost 1983;9:1–73.
26. Roseman B. Disseminated intravascular coagulation: A review. Oral Surg 1985;59:551–556.
27. Fruchtman S, Aledort LM. Disseminated intravascular coagulation. J Am Coll Cardiol 1986;8:159B–167B.
28. O'Grady JG, Langley PG, Isola LM, et al. Coagulopathy of fulminant hepatic failure. Semin Liver Dis 1986;6:159–163.

# Chapter 71 / Sickle Cell Anemia

Clarence E. Curry, Jr, PharmD, and Eula D. Beasley, PharmD

Though Herrick[1] has generally been credited with the discovery of sickle cell anemia (SCA), Konotey-Ahulu[2] has presented evidence that the problem had been recognized in Africa by Ghanians long before the earliest description offered in the medical literature after the turn of this century. Such information suggests that SCA is not as distinctly modern a problem as we may have thought.

After Herrick's case report of a 20-year-old black male West Indian student observed in 1904, but unreported until 1910, many investigators became interested in this disorder and subsequently made contributions to the literature. In 1917, Emmel[3] offered pertinent information regarding the familial nature of the disease. He also suggested that sickling of red blood cells might occur because of a decreased oxygen supply. Huck later showed that the sickling characteristic was contained in the red cell as opposed to the plasma.[4] He also suggested that the sickling process was reversible. The reversibility of the sickle shape was subsequently demonstrated by Hahn and Gillespie,[5] who showed that the process depended on the degree of oxygenation of plasma hemoglobin. A state of reduced oxygen tension results in the sickle form. In 1930, Scriver and Waugh confirmed in vivo the reversibility of the sickling process.[6] In 1940, Ham and Castle discussed the pathogenesis of in vivo sickling.[7] They suggested that sickling results in increased blood viscosity, which causes decreased blood circulation resulting in increased deoxygenation leading to greater sickling.

Neel and Beet, working independently, provided evidence that sickle cell anemia and sickle cell trait were inheritable.[8,9] In a 1948 paper, Watson et al speculated that the sickling that occurred in adult patients was due to a different type of adult hemoglobin.[10] Their speculation was based on observations of infants who did not show sickling until they were about 4 months old. In 1949, Nobel Laureate Linus Pauling and his co-workers, using moving boundary electrophoresis, reported that hemoglobin from a patient with SCA had a mobility different from that of hemoglobin from a normal adult.[11] As a result, the hemoglobin of sickle cell anemia patients was referred to as sickle hemoglobin or hemoglobin S (Hb-S) and the hemoglobin of normal individuals, hemoglobin A (Hb-A).

## Etiology

The biochemical defect that leads to the development of hemoglobin S involves the substitution of valine for glutamic acid as the sixth amino acid in the $\beta$ polypeptide chain. Hemoglobin C, another abnormal hemoglobin commonly included in the sickle cell disease group, is produced by the substitution of lysine for glutamic acid as the sixth amino acid in the $\beta$ chain (see Figure 71.1). The $\alpha$ chains of Hb-S and Hb-A are structurally identical. Therefore, sickling and the related sequelae have to be explained on the basis of the chemical difference in the $\beta$ chain. When deoxygenated, both Hb-S and Hb-A have similar physical properties in dilute solutions; however, in concentrated solutions, deoxygenated Hb-S is insoluble and forms a gel, whereas deoxygenated Hb-A remains soluble and in solution. The solubility difference represents the physiochemical basis for sickling.[12]

## Incidence

Hemoglobin S is commonly thought to be found only in Africa, but it occurs in areas around the Mediterranean, such as in certain parts of Greece and Italy; it also occurs in parts of India, Iran, and Turkey. It is the most commonly found sickle gene.

Sickle cell trait appears to offer a considerable degree of protection against malaria. Abnormal sickled RBCs are less easily parasitized by *Plasmodium falciparum* than are normal RBCs. As a result, those persons who are heterozygous for the sickle gene (trait) have a selective advantage in regions (tropical areas) where malaria is hyperendemic[13]; however, Thompson found that adults with the trait, unlike children, were sick more often from this infection than adults with Hb-C or normal homozygotes.[14]

Hemoglobin S is also the most frequently found sickle gene among the black population in the United States, where the frequency of sickle cell trait is about 8%.[15]

Hemoglobin C is found chiefly in West and Northern Africa or in descendents of people from this area, with the highest frequency in northern Ghana.[16] Hb-C has a frequency in the U.S. population of about 3%. Other abnormal hemoglobins seen in various areas are hemoglobin E (Asian subcontinent) and hemoglobin D (India, Pakistan, Afghanistan, and Iran).

Figure 71.2 illustrates the genetic profiles possible for offspring of parents with normal hemoglobin, sickle cell trait, and sickle cell anemia. A person with entirely normal hemoglobin is designated AA. A person with the sickle cell trait is designated AS. Sickle cell anemia is represented as SS.

When one parent has normal hemoglobin and the other carries the sickle cell trait (example 1), the children may have either normal hemoglobin or sickle cell trait. No child from this union would have sickle cell anemia.

When both parents carry the trait (example 2), there is a 50% chance a child will carry sickle cell trait, a 25% chance a child will have sickle cell anemia, and a 25% chance the child will be normal.

(*a*) Hb-A

| Position | 1 | 2 | 3 | 4 | 5 | 6* | 7 |
|---|---|---|---|---|---|---|---|
| β Chain | Valine– | Histidine– | Leucine– | Threonine– | Proline– | Glutamate– | Glutamate |

(*b*) Hb-S

| Position | 1 | 2 | 3 | 4 | 5 | 6* | 7 |
|---|---|---|---|---|---|---|---|
| β Chain | Valine– | Histidine– | Leucine– | Threonine– | Proline– | Valine– | Glutamate |

(*c*) Hb-C

| Position | 1 | 2 | 3 | 4 | 5 | 6* | 7 |
|---|---|---|---|---|---|---|---|
| β Chain | Valine– | Histidine– | Leucine– | Threonine– | Proline– | Lysine– | Glutamate |

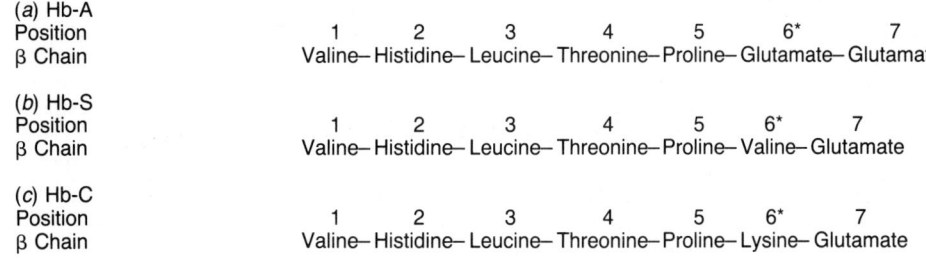

**Figure 71.1** The sixth-position (*) amino acid in the $\beta$ chain differentiates (*a*) Hb-A from (*b*) Hb-S and (*c*) Hb-C.

If one parent has sickle cell anemia and the other parent has normal hemoglobin (example 3), all children will carry the trait.

Offspring from the union of one parent with sickle cell anemia and the other with sickle cell trait have a 50% chance of having sickle cell anemia and a 50% chance of carrying sickle cell trait (example 4).

The union of two persons with sickle cell anemia, if able to produce offspring, would produce only children with sickle cell anemia.[17]

## Pathophysiology

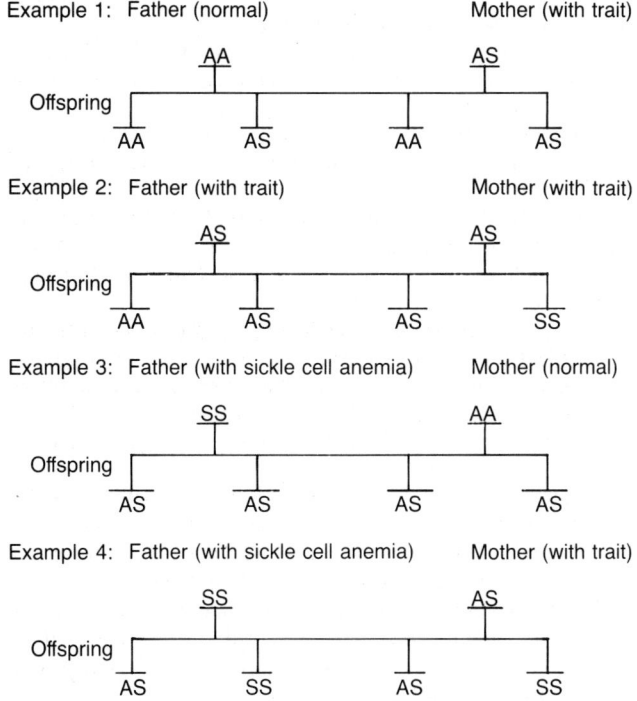

In the pathogenesis of sickle cell disease, three known problems appear to constitute the basis of the various clinical manifestations: impaired circulation, destruction of red blood cells, and stasis of blood flow. These three problems probably relate directly to two major disturbances involving red blood cells. The first involves damage to the membrane of RBCs containing hemoglobin S. These cells may lose potassium and water, leading to a dehydrated state which enhances the formation of sickled forms. After continually repeating this process, the RBC membrane probably retains greater quantities of calcium and develops a more rigid form, that of an irreversibly sickled cell.

**Figure 71.2** Inheritance scheme for the sickle gene. A, hemoglobin A (normal); S, hemoglobin S (sickle hemoglobin).

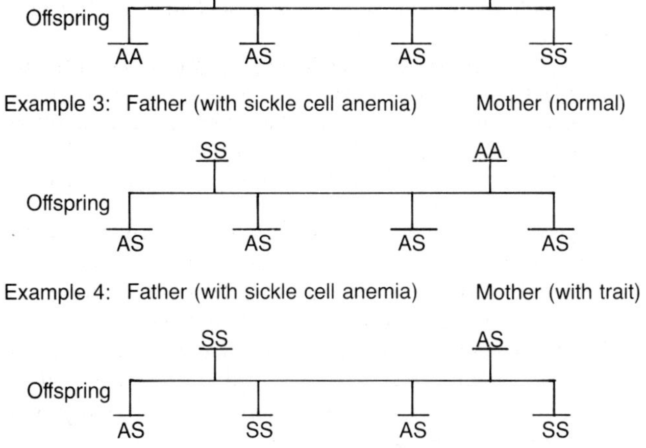


When the blood of patients with sickle cell disease is deoxygenated, blood viscosity increases. This second disturbance has been related to an alteration of the flow properties of red cells containing polymerized hemoglobin S. These cells have more difficulty deforming themselves than normal cells and, as a result, remain more rigid, retarding their flow, particularly through the microcirculation. Recent evidence suggests that significant amounts of intracellular polymerized hemoglobin S, enough to bring about a change in normal erythrocyte flow, may exist at oxygen saturation levels as high as 80% to 90%[18]; however, such a finding has yet to be specifically related to the actual clinical events in the SCA patient. The presence of sickled RBCs increases blood viscosity and encourages sludging in the capillaries and small venous vessels. Such obstructive events lead to local tissue hypoxia which tends to accentuate the pathologic process. Other events such as the elevation of fibrinogen or globulin level, or both, also increase blood viscosity and, thus, would aggravate the hematologic environs in the sickle cell patient (for example, during infections).[19] Jensen et al have shown that the cycle of sickling and unsickling that occurs in response to variations in oxygen tension results in loss of the cell membrane containing hemoglobin. This sickle–unsickle cycle leads to loss of the membrane and to production of the irreversibly sickled cell (ISC). Membranes of ISCs are permanently deformed regardless of the oxygenation state of the hemoglobin within the cell.[20]

Intravascular destruction of sickle cells may occur at an accelerated rate in this disease. In view of the various stresses of circulation, including rigid deoxygenated cells and repetitive sickle–unsickle cycles, cell fragmentation is a likely result.[21]

That some cells of patients with sickle cell disease contain increased amounts of hemoglobin F has been known for some years. It has also been noted that hemoglobin F does not appear to participate in the gelling of deoxygenated Hb-S. Irreversibly sickled cells are smaller than the other red cells of patients with SCA. ISCs also exhibit a higher mean corpuscular hemoglobin concentration (MCHC) and a lower concentration of hemoglobin F. Hemoglobin F appears to be distributed heterogenously among the RBCs in SCA. Nevertheless, increased levels of fetal hemoglobin moderate or even ameliorate the disease in some patients, thereby producing more benign forms of SCA.[22–25]

The pathogenesis of a number of clinical manifestations associated with sickle cell disease is not easily attributed directly to the sickling phenomenon. Other factors may be responsible. For example, alterations in reticuloendothelial function in SCA may be noted early in the sickle cell disease patient when splenic phagocytotic action decreases. This defect may be related to the increased susceptibility of many of these patients to infection (particularly pneumococcal disease) and to disseminated intravascular coagulation (DIC).[19] Several reports[26–29] suggested that patients with SCA have a deficient pneumococcal opsonization, although the exact nature of the defect is debatable.[30,31]

## Clinical Presentation

The term *sickle cell disease* (SCD) does not exclusively imply that the patient is homozygous for hemoglobin S (Hb-SS). Sickle cell anemia is a form of SCD in which both abnormal genes code for formation of hemoglobin S; however, varying degrees of anemia may be present in other variants of SCD.

As previously noted, a person who carries sickle cell trait has one normal gene (A) and one abnormal gene (S, C, D, etc). Such a person would not belong in the SCD group. A person with a genotype of AS is often referred to as a heterozygote; however, caution must be exercised because other heterozygous states can be pathologic (e.g., SC, S Thal).[3]

Hemoglobin disorders can be screened by hemoglobin electrophoresis on cellulose acetate, followed by solubility testing for sickling in all blood samples showing anything other than the usual hemoglobin A. If such tests suggest the presence of abnormal hemoglobin patterns, confirmation should be sought using such methods as citrate agar electrophoresis, quantitation of hemoglobin fractions, alkali denaturation, and family studies.[32]

Persons with sickle cell trait are usually asymptomatic. Some clinical signs and symptoms have occasionally been associated with sickle cell trait. An impairment of renal function, which probably arises from the sickling of red cells, tends to promote a more dilute urine. Such patients may be at some risk of dehydration during periods in which the body normally conserves water, such as hot and dry weather. Hematuria has also been noted and probably also relates to sickling within the kidney.

Castro and Scott[33] have recently shown that a group of persons with sickle cell trait had a small but statistically significant decrease in red cell size and in MCHC; however, the decreases did not affect the blood hemoglobin or hematocrit levels. The cause is unknown. Though some persons with sickle cell trait may experience abnormalities under certain conditions, these instances are not routine and trait carriers are not considered to have clinical disease.

The usual clinical signs and symptoms associated with Hb-SS disease include chronic anemia, fever and pallor, arthralgia, scleral icterus, abdominal pain, weakness, anorexia, fatigue, enlargement of spleen, liver, and heart, and hematuria. Contrast this with the picture of Hb-SC disease, which is characterized primarily by mild anemia (hemoglobin levels above 9 g/100 mL), infrequent episodes of pain, persistence of splenomegaly into adult life, and excessive target cells in the peripheral blood smear.[34]

These patients usually appear asthenic, with rather long extremities and tapered fingers. The abdomen is protuberant with exaggerated lumbar lordosis. The chest is frequently barrel-shaped. Both height and weight are usually below average. Such a patient displays a tendency to delayed sexual maturity and a reduced level of fertility. Female patients show some menstrual abnormalities more often than normal women.[35]

**Table 71.1** Manifestations of Sickle Cell Disease: Crises and Complications

| *Crisis* | *Characteristic* |
|---|---|
| Vaso-occlusive | Infarction/pain |
| Hemolytic | Massive hemolysis |
| Splenic sequestration | Sequestration of red blood cells |
| Aplastic | Bone marrow failure |

| *Organ system* | *Complication* |
|---|---|
| Pulmonary | Acute chest syndrome |
| Neurologic | Various, including cerebrovascular accident |
| Dermatologic | Chronic ulcers |
| Cardiovascular | Hypertrophy |
| Genitourinary | Priapism, hematuria, hyposthenuria |
| Skeletal | Aseptic necrosis, osteomyelitis |
| Ocular | Retinal problems |
| Hepatic | Cholelithiasis |

### *Sickle Cell Crisis*

Chronic hemolytic anemia in the SCD patient is periodically interrupted by crises. Crises are more common in childhood than in adulthood for the average patient. Patients with Hb-SS disease experience crises more often on average than patients with Hb-SC or some other variants. Crises are often precipitated by fever, infections, dehydration, hypoxia, acidosis, and sudden temperature alterations. Often, multiple factors are at work in bringing about a crisis. The time between crises is called the steady-state period, and patients not in crisis are said to be in the steady state.[2] Clinically, four types of crisis are generally described (Table 71.1).[36–38]

*Aplastic (Hypoplastic) Crisis* The bone marrow becomes hypoplastic. There may be associated pain. There is a definite drop in reticulocytes accompanied by a rapidly developing severe anemia.

***Hemolytic Crisis*** The patient affected shows a rate of hemolysis even greater than that usually present. Hemoglobin and red blood cell levels fall, often without a change in reticulocytes and with a hyperplastic bone marrow. This crisis may be accompanied by pain and fever. An increase in the icteric state is usually observed.

***Splenic Sequestration Crisis*** This crisis is described as sudden massive enlargement of the spleen and liver resulting from the sequestration by these organs of blood from the reticuloendothelial system. There is a dramatic fall in hematocrit and hemoglobin concentration, with no evidence of marrow failure and accelerated hemolysis. The condition is most often seen in infants and children because they have intact spleens that have not undergone multiple infarctions and fibrosis. Because repeated infarctions lead to autosplenectomy as the disease progresses, the incidence of this type of crisis declines as adolescence approaches. It is rarely seen in adult Hb-SS patients but may be seen in adult Hb-SC or sickle cell thalassemia patients.

***Vaso-occlusive (Infarctive) Crisis*** This most common type of crisis has a number of clinical manifestations. Pain usually occurs over the involved areas, but there may be no change in hemoglobin or other laboratory values. Laboratory changes that may be seen include leukocytosis, increased serum fibrinogen, and decreased serum pH and bicarbonate. The following are the usually observed manifestations:

*Sickle cell dactylitis (hand–foot syndrome).* A condition reported to occur in infancy and early childhood. The dorsal aspects of the hands and feet, as well as the fingers and toes, swell. The episodes are painful and accompanied by erythema. There usually is no permanent damage.

*Involvement of joints and extremities.* This form of crisis may be caused by areas of infarction over long bones or of periarticular tissues of the larger joints. Often, the pain mimics that of rheumatic fever. Pain may migrate from one site to another. Mild temperature elevations may be noted.

*Abdominal involvement.* These crises may simulate an acute abdominal process suggesting surgical intervention. The episodes are usually due to areas of infarction in abdominal structures. The pain may be severe and episodic in nature. Though the usual duration is about 3 or 4 days, protracted courses are occasionally encountered. Low-grade fever is often present.

*Hepatic involvement.* This type of crisis is characterized by a rise in the serum bilirubin level well beyond the steady-state value, as some degree of hyperbilirubinemia is common in sickle cell disease. It is associated with right upper quadrant pain. Widespread intrahepatic sickling may occur, leading to hepatocellular necrosis and swelling. Such an extensive occurrence could be fatal. These severe obstructive jaundice processes, as well as episodes of cholelithiasis, must be distinguished early in affected patients. Hepatic crises are seen more often in the older sickle cell patient.

*Pulmonary involvement.* Lung infarctions occur in both children and adults. Children seem to have pulmonary episodes most often as a result of infection. It may sometimes be very difficult to distinguish between infection and infarction and, indeed, both may be present. Infection is usually due to the pneumococcus; infarction is often related to embolization from sickled RBCs or pieces of necrotic bone marrow tissue.

### *Complications*

Acute chest syndrome is the pulmonary illness that occurs in sickle cell disease patients and is characterized by cough, dyspnea, chest pain, fever, pulmonary infiltration, and an equivocal response to antibiotic therapy.[39] Pulmonary infarcts seem more often to involve the lower lobes of the lungs and are a frequent cause of pleural effusions. Pneumonia appears to occur most often in the middle and upper lobes. These pulmonary manifestations can and do occur in the absence of bone, joint, or abdominal pain. There is some degree of disagreement over the predominant cause of acute chest syndrome. Oppenheimer and Esterly reviewed autopsy findings on 36 patients with sickle cell anemia; intimal proliferation and pulmonary infarcts had occurred in more than one fifth of the cases.[40] Sprinkle and associates recently reviewed 100 cases in children and found little evidence of bacterial infection to support the clinical picture seen.[39] These data contrast dramatically with those of Barrett-Conner, who showed pulmonary infarction in only 5% of 66 cases.[41] Furthermore, it is possible that intravascular fluid overload with pulmonary edema can occasionally simulate sickle cell lung disease in the sickle cell patient hospitalized for other causes.[42] Sudden death may occur after the occlusion of large vessels in the absence of infarction. Pulmonary edema has been a common finding in patients who have died suddenly, the pulmonary capillaries of such patients being overly distended from packed sickled cells.[43]

Neurologic abnormalities can occur in both adults and children. These manifestations are uncommon except for cerebral vascular accidents and their associated sequelae. Vaso-occlusive processes occasionally lead to cerebral vascular occlusion in which patients show signs and symptoms similar to those of stroke. These include drowsiness, paralysis, transitory or permanent blindness, aphasia, visual disturbances, spinal cord infarction, and convulsions. The onset is sudden, but occasionally may be gradual. Milder symptoms may occur as a result of vascular stasis. Some patients recover rapidly and completely. Others are left with permanent neurologic deficits.

Chronic leg ulcers are a difficult problem and a common finding in many young adults with Hb-SS disease. The inner aspect of the lower leg just above the ankle seems to be the site most often affected. Ulcers are often seen after trauma or infection. They are usually slow to heal (several weeks to a year).

Cholelithiasis is another disorder frequently observed in sickle cell patients. Both children and adults can be affected.

As with any anemia, cardiovascular abnormalities, including cardiac enlargement and various murmurs, occur. Patients complain of various degrees of exertional dyspnea, tachycardia, and palpitation owing to the decreased oxygen-carrying capacity of the system. Effects are most prominent in Hb-SS disease.

Priapism is a very painful complication that develops in certain male patients. It is caused by sickling in the sinusoids of the penis. This produces a sustained painful erection that might last several hours or several days. A patient might become impotent after repeated episodes.

Destructive bone and joint problems are frequently seen. Aseptic necrosis, particularly of the femoral or humeral heads, causes permanent damage and disability. This problem is seen both in patients with Hb-SS disease and in heterozygous patients. Patients are also susceptible to an increased incidence of osteomyelitis. The organism most often responsible is *Salmonella*.

Ocular problems occur in the form of transient monocular blindness, visual field defects from retinal hemorrhage, retinal detachment, or vitreous hemorrhage, venous microaneurysms, and neovascularization in the adult. Patients with Hb-SC disease are most likely to suffer from these disorders.

Renal complications include unilateral hematuria and hyposthenuria. Death from renal disease is unusual except in long-term survivors.

## Treatment

### *Painful Crises*

#### Hydration and Analgesia

Hydration and analgesia are the mainstays of treatment for painful crises; however, there is no consensus on specific guidelines for their use. In hospitalized patients, infusion of 4 L or more of fluid per day in adults and 2,500 mL/m$^2$ in children has been recommended.[44] Glucose-in-saline solutions (for example, 5% glucose in one-half normal saline[45] or 5% glucose in one-quarter normal saline[46]) are appropriate in this setting. The superiority of a given intravenous fluid has not been established. Outpatients may be managed through oral consumption of 2 to 3 L of fluid per day.[44] Overhydration should be avoided, however, because vigorous intravenous fluid therapy has been associated with the development of pulmonary edema in some hospitalized patients.[39]

Despite the common and frequent use of analgesics in sickle cell patients, controlled studies to determine the optimal regimen are lacking. For hospitalized patients, intramuscular meperidine is often prescribed at dosages ranging from 75 to 125 mg every 3 to 4 hours.[44] The use of meperidine and other narcotics is often limited by the fear of promoting addiction or inducing tolerance to the drugs. Additionally, concern regarding meperidine-induced seizures has prompted some clinicians to limit the use of this agent; however, prudent use can minimize this side effect. Seizures are a concern when high doses of meperidine are used. They probably result from the accumulation of normeperidine, a meperidine metabolite. Factors that may predispose a patient to development of seizures include doses greater than 100 mg every 2 hours for more than 24 hours, renal failure, alkaline urine, concurrent use of enzyme inducers, and coadministration of phenothiazines. Shimomura et al consider parenteral morphine the drug of choice for pain associated with sickle cell crisis. Morphine has been noted to have the advantage of a longer duration of action than meperidine. Hydromorphone is also a good alternative analgesic. During a crisis, analgesics may be more effective if given on a schedule rather than as needed. This allows maintenance of a desired level of analgesia.[47]

Intravenous infusions, even more so, produce steady levels of analgesia. Cole et al[48] reported their 5 years of experience with intravenous narcotic therapy in pediatric patients in severe sickle cell pain crisis. Intravenous infusions of morphine or meperidine were found to be effective in controlling pain. Patients who during earlier episodes had received only bolus narcotic injections preferred the continuous infusions. Side effects, including nausea, vomiting, lethargy, and abdominal distention, occurred more frequently with the continuous infusion than with bolus administration. This was probably due to the use of higher doses, as infusions were reserved for patients with more severe pain. Accurate dosing and close monitoring are needed to minimize the risk of complications with continuous narcotic infusions.

There is some concern that the course of acute sickle cell chest syndrome may be prolonged by administration of narcotics.[39]

Agents that may be used in the outpatient management of painful crises include, but are not limited to, acetaminophen combined with codeine, propoxyphene, or oxycodone.[44]

#### Oxygen

Although oxygen is still utilized in the treatment of sickle cell crisis, controlled clinical trials of this intervention are lacking. Oxygen administration is, of course, widely recommended for events that produce hypoxemia.[49]

In an attempt to elucidate the effects of oxygen on erythropoiesis and sickled erythrocytes, Embury et al[49] administered oxygen continuously for 5 days to patients who were not in crisis. Arterial oxygen tensions, which initially ranged from 72 to 83 mm Hg, increased to 146 to 175 mm Hg within the first 3 hours. Oxygen inhalation resulted in a decrease in the number of irreversibly sickled cells; however, there was a decline in erythropoietin levels and number of reticulocytes. The decline was a delayed effect, occurring after the first 2 days of therapy. After oxygen inhalation was discontinued, erythropoietin and reticulocyte levels increased, as did levels of irreversibly sickled cells, reaching levels higher than those before oxygen therapy in two of the three patients. Acute painful episodes occurred in these patients. It is suggested that when indicated, oxygen inhalation be administered on an intermittent rather than a continuous basis. Solanski[50] reported one case in which overzealous use of oxygen resulted in an excessive partial pressure and is believed to have caused an acute suppression of erythropoiesis.

#### Dextran

Dextran decreases erythrocyte aggregation and blood viscosity and thus improves microcirculation. These actions prompted the study of dextran use in sickle cell populations. Although dextran use in sickle cell crisis is still sometimes advocated, its benefit has not been established in controlled trials, despite early positive results in a limited number of patients.[51–53]

### Alkali

Alkali administration has been evaluated in sickle cell disease, as it has been demonstrated that sickling is enhanced at lower pH. In contrast to early reports, controlled studies have failed to show a benefit from this therapy.[51,54]

### Splenectomy

Early therapy for sickle cell disease included splenectomy. This was based on the belief that anemia in these patients was due to hypersplenism. Results with this intervention have varied greatly. Thus, splenectomy should be used cautiously, except in splenic sequestration crisis.[51]

### Miscellaneous Agents

Other agents that have been suggested for use in sickle cell crisis include carbonic anhydrase inhibitors, glucose-6-phosphate dehydrogenase inhibitors, papaverine hydrochloride, vasodilators, antithyroid drugs, blood coagulation inhibitors, fibrinogenolytic agents, steroids, pyridoxine hydrochloride, and DDAVP (an antidiuretic hormone derivative).[51,55] These agents, however, are not widely used.

A newer agent, pentoxifylline, is being studied for the treatment of painful crises. Pentoxifylline is a synthetic xanthine derivative approved for the treatment of peripheral vascular disease. Intravenous pentoxifylline was administered to 20 patients with homozygous sickle cell anemia who were experiencing vaso-occlusive crises. All patients showed a measurable improvement in duration and intensity of pain compared with previous crises.[56] Oral pentoxifylline was administered to an 18-year-old patient who had been experiencing weekly painful crises since childhood. A decrease in viscosity was noted. The patient did not experience subsequent painful crises, although hemolysis continued to occur once a month. The patient no longer required analgesics at any time, although she had previously required continuous analgesic medication.[57]

Pentoxifylline may prevent vaso-occlusive complications because of its ability to decrease blood viscosity and improve microcirculation during hemolytic crises.[57] It has been demonstrated in vitro that the deformability of red blood cells from patients with homozygous sickle cell anemia is improved by the addition of pentoxifylline.[58]

## *General Management*

### Folic Acid

Folic acid demands are increased in sickle cell patients because of accelerated erythropoiesis. Low serum folate levels are common and megaloblastic changes have been reported.[55,59,60] The incidence of megaloblastic anemia in association with sickle cell disease, however, is unknown. Although folic acid supplementation has become standard, it is not clear whether it is necessary for all patients with sickle cell anemia. Patients who are at increased risk of folate deficiency include infants, pregnant women, and adolescents.[61]

Despite the common use of folate, controlled studies assessing therapy are lacking. A double-blind controlled study of folate supplementation in 117 Jamaican children aged 6 months to 4 years did not support the need for routine folate supplementation. Folic acid 5 mg/d did not result in significant improvement in hemoglobin levels, growth characteristics, occurrence of infections, or painful episodes; however, the mean corpuscular volume was significantly lower in the folate-treated group, suggesting the existence of a marginal folate deficiency in patients receiving placebo. The authors caution that the results of this study may not be applicable elsewhere because of dietary differences.[61] Although 5 mg/d was administered in this study, 1 mg/d is more than adequate for supplementation.[55,60,62] There exists at least a theoretical argument for prescribing folate supplementation in all sickle cell patients. Additionally, patients may benefit clinically from a placebo effect.

### Zinc

Selected sickle cell patients have benefited from zinc supplementation. In two experiments involving young male patients, administration of zinc 15 mg orally twice daily produced an increase in testosterone levels, height, and weight.[63] An earlier study showed similar positive effects with the administration of zinc (as the acetate) 15 mg orally three times daily.[64] As a result of these findings, it is recommended that sickle cell patients be screened for zinc deficiency and, if found deficient, supplemented.

### Transfusions

Transfusion therapy may be the most effective means of treating sickle cell disease; however, its use is usually restricted to life-threatening complications.[65] Transfusions have yielded favorable results in several clinical settings, including prophylactic therapy prior to surgery, after central nervous system infarction, and before childbirth.[51]

Blood transfusion after a stroke is a common practice today. Chronic transfusion in these patients has been shown to decrease the chance of further strokes and halt clinical progression. Although it is not certain whether transfusion therapy improves the arteriogram, it does prevent the recurrence of cerebrovascular accidents.[66]

Sarnaik et al[67] described a prophylactic transfusion program in 27 children who had experienced at least one episode of central nervous system infarction. Transfusions were given on an outpatient basis initially at 3-week intervals. The frequency was later adjusted to maintain a hemoglobin level of 10–12 g/dL, a hemoglobin S quantitation of 25% or less, and a peripheral smear with little or no sickling. Twenty-five patients had no recurrences of CNS events. The other two patients had only transient recurrences. Twelve of the twenty-seven completely recovered neurologic function and an additional twelve showed definite improvement. Although the remaining three patients showed no improvement, they had nonprogressive neurologic deficits. A decrease in hospitalizations for sickle cell–related complications was also noted. In this study the duration of therapy ranged from 1 to 9 years.

When transfusion therapy is used in stroke victims, the questions whether and when transfusions may be safely stopped remain unresolved, because strokes have occurred after cessation of therapy.[44] It has been suggested that transfusion regimens be maintained for more than 2 years.[66]

In light of the beneficial effects of transfusions, it has been suggested that chronic transfusions be considered in patients diagnosed as having sickle cell disease. Chronic transfusions reduce the proportion of circulating sickle cells. This approach may, at the least, prevent many serious complications and improve the quality of life.[66] One case report of a patient with severe sickle cell disease who received continuous transfusions over a 13-year period records eradication of the symptoms of the disease.[65]

Risks associated with the use of transfusion therapy include iron overload, transfusion-related infection such as hepatitis or AIDS, and sensitization to the blood received. A chelation process or the use of young red blood cells (neocytes), which allows the frequency of transfusions to be reduced, may combat the problem of iron overload. Although the hepatitis vaccine reduces the risk of hepatitis B it offers no protection against non-A, non-B hepatitis. Routine blood screening offers protection against exposure to the AIDS virus. Lastly, the use of compatible donor blood decreases the risk of sensitization.[44,66]

### Gelation Inhibitors

Many therapeutic approaches are aimed at inhibiting the gelation of deoxyhemoglobin S. This inhibition can be effected by alteration of the sickle hemoglobin.[68] Additionally, as gelation is concentration dependent, decreasing sickle hemoglobin concentration (for example, by increasing the concentration of fetal hemoglobin) markedly delays gelation.[69] Agents that have been used in the past include cyanate and urea. In addition, hydroxyurea and azacytidine are being evaluated, as is cetiedil, an agent that is not presently commercially available in the United States.[70]

Cyanates have been shown to block intracellular polymerization.[71] Some therapeutic benefit has been suggested; however, not all studies have been supportive of cyanate use.[72] Toxicity, especially polyneuropathy, has limited its usefulness[73]; however, toxicity has not been reported with extracorporeal treatment. Consequently, only extracorporeal administration of cyanate salts should be considered for clinical use.[51,69] Extracorporeal therapy should be used only in patients with severe, debilitating manifestations of sickle cell disease.[73]

Urea is another agent that initially was considered for therapy in sickle cell disease; later, its use was limited because it was feared that toxic effects would be produced at the doses necessary to derive therapeutic benefit.[45,54]

Several small studies have shown beneficial effects after hydroxyurea administration. Platt[74] found that 5-day courses of hydroxyurea 50 mg/kg/d orally in three divided doses result in increases in fetal reticulocytes and fetal hemoglobin. Reticulocytes increased within 48 to 72 hours, peaked in 7 to 11 days, and decreased by 18 to 21 days. Veith et al[75] also reported increases in fetal hemoglobin after short courses of hydroxyurea. Long-term therapy has yielded significant improvement in one study.[76] In contrast, minimal therapeutic benefit was seen in a study in which treated patients experienced marrow toxicity.[77] Hydroxyurea is believed to cause stimulation of fetal hemoglobin as a result of the erythroid regeneration that follows cytoreduction.

Zidovudine, an agent recently approved for treatment of patients with AIDS, has also been shown to cause significant increases in fetal hemoglobin and a decrease in irreversibly sickled cells. Hemolysis is also decreased with azacytidine therapy. The effect of azacytidine on fetal hemoglobin synthesis, however, is transient. Repeated courses would be needed unless methods of prolonging the effect are found. Minimal side effects have been noted during treatment. The most common side effects have been gastrointestinal. There is also a potential for development of bone marrow toxicity. Thus far, marrow toxicity has not been a common problem in studies involving sickle cell patients, although it has occurred. This effect was accompanied by a slowed response to azacytidine therapy.[78–80]

Cytarabine also stimulates fetal reticulocyte production. The increase in fetal reticulocytes is preceded by a marked decrease in absolute reticulocyte count.[76]

Cetiedil citrate, an agent not presently available commercially in the United States, is the prototype of agents that affect primarily red blood cell membranes.[69] An iminoester developed from 3-thienyl acid,[70] this vasodilator is used in Europe to treat intermittent claudication and other vascular disease.

In a double-blind randomized study, cetiedil was superior to placebo in decreasing the duration of crises and reducing the number of painful sites. Cetiedil use, however, did not reduce parenteral analgesic requirements. No serious adverse effects occurred. The most common side effects were nausea, vomiting, headache, and dry mouth. The incidence of these side effects was similar to that in the group receiving placebo. The exact mechanism of action is not known; however, the beneficial effects may result from its ability to produce peripheral vasodilation, reduce plasma fibrinogen concentration and blood viscosity, inhibit platelet aggregation, and inhibit calmodulin.[70] Calmodulin is a protein important in the activation of calcium-dependent enzymes in red blood cell membranes. In vitro, cetiedil alters ion transport across the red blood cell membrane. This increases sodium concentration, as well as water content, inside the cell. The result is an increase in cell size and a decrease in concentration of sickle hemoglobin.[68]

Other agents that are being evaluated for their potential to inhibit gelation include aromatic amino acids, oligopeptides containing hydrophobic groups, bis(3,5-dibromosalicyl)-fumarate and related compounds, butylurea, disodium carbamyl phosphate, cystamine, pyridoxal HCl, methylacetimidate HCl, dimethyladipimidate, glyceraldehyde, dibromoacetylsalicylic acid, and nitrogen mustard.[71]

### Bone Marrow Transplantation

A report by Johnson et al[81] prompts consideration of a possible role for bone marrow transplantation in the treatment of sickle cell anemia in selected patients. While being treated for leukemia, an 8-year-old girl with sickle cell anemia received a bone marrow transplant. Subsequently, the hemoglobin A and S levels assumed those of the donor who only carried the trait. The patient, however, experienced graft-versus-host disease. This potential adverse reaction is one of the major limitations of this treatment approach.

### Prophylaxis of Pneumococcal Infections

In early trials the pneumococcal vaccine was found to be effective in preventing infection in sickle cell patients. Later studies yielded less impressive results, with some deaths from infection.[82] John et al[83] reported the occurrence of pneumococcal infections despite immunization with the 14-valent pneumococcal vaccine in a study of pediatric patients with Hb-SS disease. Almost all infections (10 of 11) were due to serotypes present in the vaccine, with type 23 accounting for one half of the cases. Type 23 is known to be poorly antigenic. Types 6 and 19 are also known to cause little antibody formation. Anglin et al[84] evaluated the effects of immunization of nasopharyngeal colonization. Despite prior administration of the pneumococcal vaccine, 64% of the nasopharyngeal isolates in patients with sickle cell anemia were serotypes contained in the vaccine.

Until late 1983 the available pneumococcal vaccine was a 14-valent product. It now contains 23 capsular polysaccharide types. Whether studies that utilize only the 23-valent product yield more impressive results is yet to be seen.

Prophylactic penicillin has also been used in an effort to decrease the occurrence of pneumococcal infections. In a study involving 242 pediatric patients with homozygous sickle cell anemia, the use of benzathine penicillin 600,000 units per month intramuscularly was evaluated. Although seven pneumococcal infections occurred in patients assigned to receive penicillin therapy, no pneumococcal infections occurred while the patients were still receiving the drug; however, infections occurred within 11 months of cessation of penicillin therapy. This prompted the researchers to recommend that penicillin be continued beyond the age of 3.[83] Other investigators have also expressed concern for the high risk of infection after the discontinuation of antibiotic therapy.[82]

Oral administration of penicillin has also been evaluated. In a study of oral penicillin (125 mg twice a day in children less than 15 kg in weight and 250 mg twice a day in children greater than 15 kg in weight), a reduction in the occurrence of pneumococcal colonization was reported.[84] In a multicenter randomized, double-blind, placebo-controlled clinical trial conducted by the Prophylactic Penicillin Study Group (PROPS), oral penicillin was found to decrease significantly the incidence of pneumococcal septicemia. The dose of penicillin V potassium used in this study was 125 mg twice a day. The risk of septicemia caused by *Streptococcus pneumoniae* was decreased by 84% in the patients who received penicillin. Additionally, no deaths were reported in the penicillin-treated group in contrast to three deaths in the placebo group. PROPS researchers recommend neonatal detection of sickle cell anemia, with prophylactic penicillin therapy beginning not later than 4 months after birth.[85]

Potential noncompliance is a concern with long-term oral penicillin use. The occurrence of pneumococcal septicemia with some subsequent deaths has been reported in patients who were prescribed penicillin, but were noncompliant. A 66% compliance rate to oral penicillin regimens was reported in one study. The use of an intensive educational program is believed to have contributed to this high compliance rate.[86]

Researchers have not noted the emergence of penicillin-resistant strains as a result of prophylactic penicillin use.[82–84]

Some clinicians recommend the use of *Hemophilus* type b vaccine in addition to pneumococcal vaccine in children with sickle cell disease.[87]

### Aseptic Necrosis of the Bone

When this condition presents at early stages of the disease, bed rest alone may be adequate. It gives the diseased bone an opportunity to repair itself. Analgesic therapy may also be required. More advanced disease may necessitate surgery, such as replacement of a joint with a prosthesis.[44]

### Idiopathic Unilateral Renal Hematuria

In cases of idiopathic unilateral renal hematuria, a high fluid intake should be maintained to prevent clotting and urethral colic. If blood loss continues, iron therapy may be needed. Nephrectomy should be reserved for cases involving extensive blood loss.[55]

### Priapism

Most therapeutic approaches may be ineffective in treating priapism in sickle cell patients. Therapy has included hot baths, ice packs, alkalinization, transfusions, anticoagulants, and estrogens.[55,88] Successful use of pentoxifylline has also been reported.[89] More invasive approaches to the treatment of priapism include aspiration of the corpora cavernosa[55,90] and more extensive surgery.[91]

## References


1. Herrick JB. Peculiar elongated and sickle-shaped red blood corpuscles in case of severe anemia. Arch Intern Med 1910;6: 517–521.
2. Konotey-Ahulu FID. The sickle cell diseases: Clinical manifestations including the "sickle crisis." Arch Intern Med 1974;133: 611–619.
3. Emmel VE. A study of the erythrocytes in a case of severe anemia with elongated and sickle-shaped red blood corpuscles. Arch Intern Med 1917;20:586–598.
4. Huck JG. Sickle cell anemia. Bull Johns Hopkins Hosp 1923; 34:335–344.
5. Hahn EV, Gillespie EB. Sickle cell anemia: Report of case greatly improved by splenectomy; experimental study of sickle cell formation. Arch Intern Med 1927;39:233.
6. Scriver JB, Waugh TR. Studies on a case of sickle-cell anemia. Can Med Assoc J 1930;23:375–380.
7. Ham TH, Castle WB. Relation of increased hypotonic fragility and of erythrostasis to the mechanism of hemolysis in certain anemias. Trans Assoc Physicians 1940;55:127–132.
8. Neel JV. The inheritance of sickle cell anemia. Science 1949; 110:64–66.
9. Beet EA. The genetics of the sickle cell trait in a Bantu tribe. Ann Eugenics 1949;14:279–284.
10. Watson J, Stahman AW, Bilello FP. Significance of the paucity of sickle cells in newborn Negro infants. Am J Med Sci 1948; 215:419–423.
11. Pauling L, Itano HA, Singer SJ, et al. Sickle cell anemia, a molecular disease. Science 1949;110:543–548.

12. Knox-Macaulay HHM. Molecular biology and inheritance, in Fleming AF (ed): Sickle-Cell Disease: A Handbook for the General Clinician. New York, Churchill Livingstone, 1982, pp 1–21.
13. Allison AC. Protection afforded by sickle cell trait against subtertian malarial infections. Br Med J 1954;1:290.
14. Thompson GR. Significance of hemoglobins S and C in Ghana. Br Med J 1962;1:682.
15. Headings VE, Scott RB. Current and potential options for preventing hemoglobinopathies. South Med J 1975;68:1129–1432.
16. Cerami A, Washington E. Sickle Cell Anemia. New York, Third Press, 1974.
17. Ferguson AD, Carrington HT, Scott RB. Studies in sickle cell anemia—a clinical review. Med Ann DC 1955;24:517–532.
18. Rodgers GP, Noguchi CT, Schechter AN. Noninvasive techniques to evaluate the vaso-occlusive manifestations of sickle cell disease. Am J Pediatr Hematol Oncol 1985;7:245–253.
19. Rickles F, O'Leary DS. Role of coagulation system in pathophysiology of sickle cell disease. Arch Intern Med 1974;133: 635–641.
20. Jensen WM, Bromberg PA, Bessis MC. Microincision of sickled erythrocytes by a laser beam. Science 1967;155:704–707.
21. Bensinger TA, Gillete PN. Hemolysis in sickle cell disease. Arch Intern Med 1974;133:624–631.
22. Charache S, Conley G. Rate of sickling of red cells during deoxygenation of blood from persons with various sickling disorders. Blood 1964;24:25–48.
23. Ali S. Milder variation of sickle cell disease in Arabs in Kuwait associated with unusually high level of fetal hemoglobin. Br J Hematol 1970;19:613–619.
24. Edington G, Lehamann H. Expression of the sickle cell gene in Africa. Br Med J 1955;2:1328.
25. Perrine BP, Brown MJ, Clegg JB, et al. Benign sickle-cell anemia. Lancet 1972;2:1163–1167.
26. Bjornson AB, Gaston MH, Zellner CL. Decreased opsonization for *Streptococcus pneumoniae* in sickle cell disease: Studies on selected complement components and immunoglobulins. J Pediatr 1977;91:371.
27. Winkelstein JA, Drachman RH. Deficiency of pneumococcal serum opsonizing activity in sickle cell disease. N Engl J Med 1968;279:459.
28. Johnston RB, Newman SL, Struth AG. An abnormality of the alternate pathway of complement activation in sickle cell disease. N Engl J Med 1973;288:803.
29. Chudwin DS, Wara DW, Matthay KK, et al. Increased serum opsonic activity and antibody concentration in patients with sickle cell disease after pneumococcal polysaccharide immunization. J Pediatr 1983;102:51–54.
30. Winkelstein JA. Pneumococcal infections in sickle cell disease. J Pediatr 1977;91:521.
31. Winkelstein JA. The role of complement in the host's defense against *Streptococcus pneumoniae*. Rev Infect Dis 1981;3:289.
32. Scott RB, Castro O. Sickle cell thalassemia: Interpretation of test results. JAMA 1981;246:81.
33. Castro O, Scott RB. Red blood cell counts and indices in sickle cell trait in a black American population. Hemoglobin 1985;9: 65–67.
34. Rucknagel DL. The genetics of sickle cell anemia and related syndromes. Arch Intern Med 1974;133:595–606.
35. Samuels-Reid J, Scott RB. Characteristics of menstruation in sickle cell disease. Fertil Steril 1985;43:139–141.
36. Diggs LW, Anatomic lesions, in Abramson H, Bertles JF, Wethers DL (eds): Sickle Cell Disease: Diagnosis, Management, Education and Research. St. Louis, C.V. Mosby, 1973; p 189.
37. Pearson HA, Diamond LK. The critically ill child: Sickle cell disease crises and their management. Pediatrics 1971;48:629–635.
38. Rosenthal CJ, Lever RD. Current therapy of sickle cell disease. Drug Ther 1978;3:12–26.
39. Sprinkle RH, Cole T, Smith S, et al. Acute chest syndrome in children with sickle cell disease. Am J Pediatr Hematol Oncol 1986;8:105–110.
40. Oppenheimer EH, Esterly J. Pulmonary changes in sickle disease. Am Rev Respir Dis 1971;103:853–859.
41. Barrett-Conner E. Acute pulmonary disease in sickle cell anemia. Am Rev Respir Dis 1971;104:159–165.
42. Young RC, Castro O, Baxter RP, et al. The lung in sickle cell disease: A clinical overview of common vascular, infectious and other problems. J Natl Med Assoc 1981;73:19–26.
43. Bromberg PH. Pulmonary aspects of sickle cell disease. Arch Intern Med 1974;133:652–657.
44. Smith JA. Management of sickle cell disease: Progress during the past 10 years. Am J Pediatr Hematol Oncol 1983;5:360–366.
45. Cooperative Urea Trials Group. Clinical trials of therapy for sickle cell vaso-occlusive crises. JAMA 1974;228:1120–1124.
46. Cooperative Urea Trials Group. Therapy for sickle cell vaso-occlusive crises: Controlled clinical trials and cooperative study of intravenously administered alkali. JAMA 1974;228:1129–1131.
47. Shimomura SK, Harris S. Pain management of patients with sickle cell anemia. Hosp Pharm 1979;14:332–336.
48. Cole TB, Sprinkle RH, Smith SJ, et al. Intravenous narcotic therapy for children with severe sickle cell pain crisis. Am J Dis Child 1986;140:1255–1259.
49. Embury SH, Garcia JF, Mohandas N, et al. Effects of oxygen inhalation on endogenous erythropoietin kinetics, erythropoiesis and properties of blood cells in sickle cell anemia. N Engl J Med 1984;311:291–295.
50. Solanski DL. Sickle cell anemia, oxygen treatment and anaemic crisis. Br Med J 1983;287:725–726.
51. Alluoch JR. The treatment of sickle cell disease: A historical and chronological literature review of the therapies applied since 1910. Trop Geogr Med 1984;36(suppl):S1–S26.
52. Oski FA, Viner ED, Purugganan H, et al. Low molecular weight dextran in sickle cell crisis. JAMA 1965;191:43.
53. Watson-Williams, EJ. Sickle cell crisis treated with rheomacrodex. Lancet 1963;1:1053.
54. Cooperative Urea Trials Group. Treatment of sickle cell crisis with urea in invert sugar. JAMA 1974;228:1125–1128.
55. Charache S. The treatment of sickle cell anemia. Arch Intern Med 1974;133:698–705.
56. Khosla AA, Chintu C. A pilot study: An open clinical trial of pentoxifylline in patients with painful sickle cell crises. East Afr Med J 1984;61:829–837.
57. Keller F, Leonhardt H. Amelioration of blood viscosity in sickle cell anemia by pentoxifylline: A case report. J Med 1979;10:429–433.
58. Ambrus JL, Ambrus CM, Bannerman R, et al. Studies on the management and prevention of vaso-occlusive crises in sickle cell disease. J Med 1984;15:385–407.
59. MacIver JE, Went NL. Sickle cell anemia complicated by megaloblastic anemia of infancy. Br Med J 1960;1:775–779.
60. Lindenbaum J, Klipstein FA. Folic acid deficiency in sickle-cell anemia. N Engl J Med 1963;269:875–882.
61. Rabb LM, Grandison Y, Mason K, et al. A trial of folate supplementation in children with homozygous sickle cell disease. Br J Haematol 1983;54:589–594.

62. Alperin JB. Folic acid deficiency complicating sickle cell anemia. Arch Intern Med 1967;120:298–306.
63. Prasad AS, Abbasi AA, Rabbani P, et al. Effect of zinc supplementation on serum testosterone level in adult male sickle cell anemia subjects. Am J Hematol 1981;10:119–127.
64. Prasad A, Zafrallah C. Zinc supplementation and growth in sickle cell disease. Ann Intern Med 1984;100:367–371.
65. Finch C, Lee MY, Leonard JM. Continuous RBC transfusions in a patient with sickle cell disease. Arch Intern Med 1982;142: 279–282.
66. Piomelli S. Chronic transfusions in patients with sickle cell disease. Am J Pediatr Hematol Oncol 1985;7:51–55.
67. Sarnaik S, Soorya D, Kim, et al. Periodic transfusions for sickle cell anemia and CNS infarction. Am J Dis Child 1979;133:1254–1257.
68. Weinraub M, Standish R. Cetiedil: A vasodilator with interesting therapeutic possibilities. Hosp Formulary 1986;21:1095–1101.
69. Luskey K, Schechter AN, Hercules JI. New approaches to the therapy of sickle cell diseases. Texas Rep Biol Med 1980–81;40: 305–312.
70. Benjamin LJ, Berkowitz LR, Orunjir E, et al. A collaborative double-blind randomized study of cetiedil citrate in sickle cell crisis. Blood 1986;67:1442–1447.
71. Chang H, Ewert SM, Bookchin RM, et al. Comparative evaluation of fifteen anti-sickling agents. Blood 1983;61:693–704.
72. Peterson CM, Tsairis P, Ohnishc A, et al. Sodium cyanate induced polyneuropathy in patients with sickle cell disease. Ann Intern Med 1974;81:152–158.
73. Diederich D, Curran M, Odenbaugh A, et al. Extracorporeal treatment of erythrocytes in sickle cell anemia: Hemoglobin carbamylation. Texas Rep Biol Med 1980–81;40:313–322.
74. Platt OS, Orkin SH, Dorer G. Hydroxyurea enhances fetal hemoglobin production in sickle cell anemia. J Clin Invest 1984;74:652–656.
75. Veith R, Galanello R, Papayannopoulou T, et al. Stimulation of F-cell production in patients with sickle cell anemia treated with cytarabine or hydroxyurea. N Engl J Med 1985;313:1571–1575.
76. Charache S, Dover GJ, Moyer MA, et al. Hydroxyurea-induced augmentation of fetal hemoglobin production in patients with sickle cell anemia. Blood 1987;69:109–116.
77. Dover GJ, Humphries RK, Moore TG. Hydroxyurea induction of hemoglobin F production in sickle cell disease: Relationship between cytotoxicity and F cell production. Blood 1986;67:735–738.
78. Ley TJ, DeSimone J, Noguchi CT, et al. 5-Azacytidine increases gamma-globulin synthesis and reduces the portion of dense cells in patients with sickle cell anemia. Blood 1983;62: 370–380.
79. Dover GJ, Charache S, Boyer SH, et al. 5-Azacytidine increases HbF production and reduces anemia in sickle cell disease: Dose–response analysis of subcutaneous and oral dosage regimens. Blood 1985;66:527–532.
80. Humphries RK, Dover G, Young NS, et al. 5-Azacytidine acts directly on both erythroid precusors and progenitors to increase production of fetal hemoglobin. J Clin Invest 1985;75:547–557.
81. Johnson FL, Look AT, Gockerman T, et al. Bone-marrow transplantation in a patient with sickle-cell anemia. N Engl J Med 1984;311:780–783.
82. Buchanan GR, Smith SJ. Pneumococcal septicemia despite pneumococcal vaccine and prescription of penicillin prophylaxis in children with sickle cell anemia. Am J Dis Child 1986;140:428–432.
83. John AB, Ramlal A, Jackson H, et al. Prevention of pneumococcal infection in children with homozygous sickle cell disease. Br Med J 1984;288:1567–1570.
84. Anglin DL, Siegel JD, Pacini DL, et al. Effect of penicillin prophylaxis on nasopharyngeal colonization with *Streptococcus pneumoniae* in children with sickle cell anemia. J Pediatr 1984;104:18–22.
85. Gaston MH, Vertu JI, Woods G, et al. Prophylaxis with oral penicillin in children with sickle cell anemia. N Engl J Med 1986;314:1593–1599.
86. Buchanan GR, Siegel JD, Smith SJ, et al. Oral penicillin prophylaxis in children with impaired splenic function: A study of compliance. Pediatrics 1982;70:926–930.
87. Scott RB. Advances in the treatment of sickle cell disease in children. Am J Dis Child 1985;139:1219–1222.
88. Serjeant GR, DeCeular K, Maude GH. Stilboestrol and stuttering priapism in homozygous sickle-cell disease. Lancet 1985;2: 1274–1276.
89. Rardin KB, Washington TG, Beasley EB. Use of pentoxifylline in treating priapism in two patients with sickle cell anemia. Paper presented to 21st Annual ASHP Midyear Clinical Meeting. Las Vegas, NV, Dec 9, 1986.
90. Sousa CM, Catoe BL, Scott RB. Studies in sickle cell anemia: Priapism as a complication in children. J Pediatr 1962;60:52–54.
91. Pantaleo-Gandais O, Chacon RC, Plaza N. Priapism: Evaluation and treatment. Urology 1984;24:345–346.

# Chapter 72 / Drug-Induced Hematologic Disorders

Michael D. Parr, PharmD, and Michael Doukas, MD

Drug-induced hematologic disorders (DIHDs) are an expected complication of therapy in most patients who are treated with antineoplastic agents; however, in patients receiving other types of drug therapy, DIHDs are an uncommon side effect. The development of DIHDs in patients receiving medications is often an idiosyncratic reaction that may be life-threatening. The incidence of DIHDs depends on a number of factors including the cell line affected, the specific drug, the dose of drug, and possibly genetic predisposition. The exact incidence of DIHDs is difficult to predict, but studies on drug-induced agranulocytosis in Sweden demonstrated an incidence of approximately 0.01% in the general population.[1–3] Mortality from DIHDs has decreased in recent years but still ranges from 11% to 48%.[1–3] The Swedish studies demonstrated a higher incidence of agranulocytosis in the elderly population and a greater risk in females as opposed to males.

Diagnosis of DIHDs is often difficult, as a number of different disease states may cause symptoms and laboratory abnormalities similar to those of aplastic anemia, agranulocytosis, and other disorders. In addition, patients may be taking a number of different medications at the time the blood disorder first appears. Therefore a process of elimination must be used to determine which drug is the culprit. Before a drug can be implicated it must be determined that the patient was actually taking it. Next, a temporal relationship between initiation of drug therapy and onset of symptoms must be established.

Depending on the results of the investigation, a drug can be placed into one of five categories.[4]

1. *Causative reaction*. The drug in question is regarded as the actual cause of the DIHD because it meets the criteria described in the preceding paragraph and because the reaction has been previously reported in the literature.
2. *Probable reaction*. Drugs in this category are related temporally to the DIHD. In addition, there exist reports in the literature that the drug causes blood abnormalities; however, the data are not reproducible.
3. *Possible reaction*. The medications that fall into this class are primarily new drugs, for which there are insufficient data in the literature documenting this reaction; however, a temporal relationship exists.
4. *Coincident reaction*. Drug exposure occurred, but another cause is found (i.e., a disease).
5. *Negative relationship*. No temporal relationship exists.

Because of the severity of these disorders, rechallenging the patient with the suspected drug is in most cases unethical. In vitro testing to determine if the suspected drug is the actual culprit would therefore be advantageous. Unfortunately, in vitro testing is expensive and frequently does not yield conclusive results, because DIHDs arise by a variety of mechanisms. Clinicians often never find the exact cause of the blood disorder in a given patient.

The mechanisms by which drugs induce blood disorders differ because of the wide variety of chemical structures involved. In addition, a particular drug may cause a DIHD by several different mechanisms (i.e., quinidine). DIHDs can be classified into four types:

1. Abnormal sensitivity of a stem cell population to the drug or a metabolite
2. Genetic predisposition (i.e., oxidative hemolytic anemia)
3. Abnormal metabolism of the drug, causing formation of a toxic metabolite
4. Immune-mediated effect on a mature cellular component of the blood or on the stem cell population

Investigators have also hypothesized that certain drugs may cause changes in the microenvironment of the bone marrow, resulting in DIHDs.[5] Combination of viral infection with drug exposure may have an additive effect speculated to cause DIHDs affecting T lymphocytes and stem cells.[6] Presently, however, neither changes in the microenvironment nor concomitant viral infections have been documented as causes of DIHDs.

To better understand the mechanisms just discussed, a basic knowledge of hematopoiesis and immunology is needed. Hematopoiesis is a process of cell differentiation which is controlled by hematopoietic hormones and the microenvironment (lymphocytes, macrophages, and stroma). Theoretically, all blood cells originate from a pool of pluripotent stem cells[7] (see Fig. 72.1). A *stem cell* is a primitive cell capable of self-renewal and differentiation. Pluripotent stem cells begin to differentiate into colony-forming units (CFUs) dedicated to specific cell lines. Cells from one CFU develop into mature blood cells. Figure 72.2 shows the differentiation of a neutrophil from a stem cell; the arrows indicate several possible sites where drugs can induce agranulocytosis. Some investigators feel that the earlier a DIHD occurs in the differentiation process, the more severe the disorder will become.[8] A thorough discussion of the immune system is beyond the scope of this chapter; therefore, the reader is encouraged to review the article by Tami et al[9] to gain a better understanding of the immune system.

Any cell lines can be affected in DIHDs including white blood cells (WBCs), red blood cells (RBCs), and platelets. A drug-induced decrease in all three cell lines accompanied by a hypoplastic bone marrow is called drug-induced aplastic anemia. A drug-induced decrease in white blood cells alone

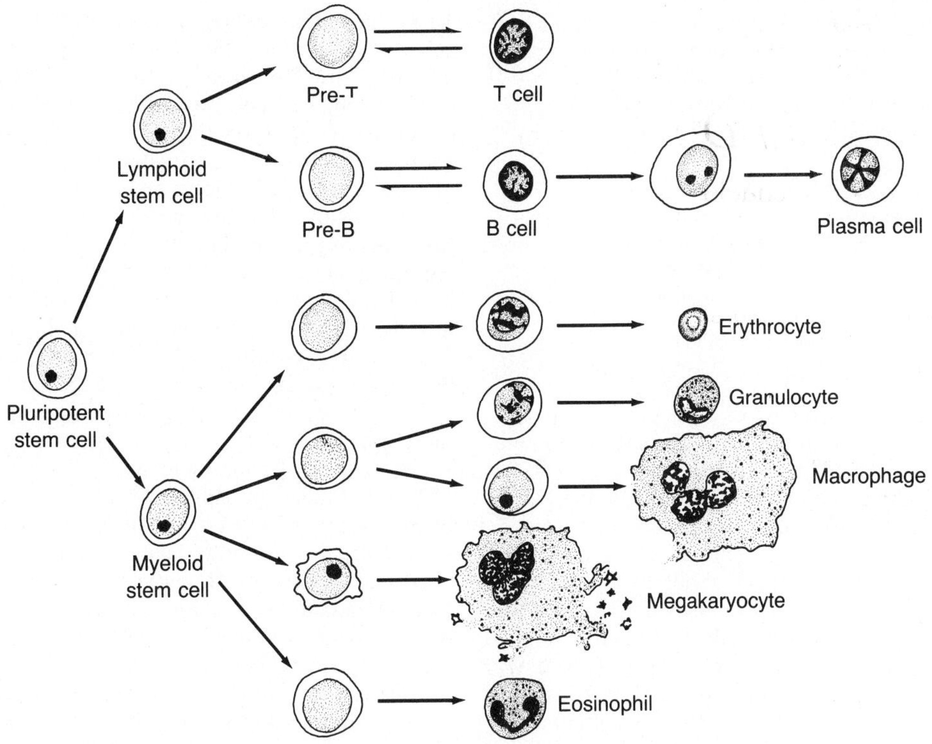


**Figure 72.1** The process of maturation of blood cellular components from pluripotent stem cells to mature granulocytes, erythrocytes, and other cells. *(From Cline MJ, Golde DW: Controlling the production of blood cells. Blood 1979;53:159, with permission.)*

is termed drug-induced agranulocytosis. Drugs can affect RBCs by causing a number of different anemias, including drug-induced immune hemolytic anemia, drug-induced oxidative hemolytic anemia, or drug-induced megaloblastic anemia. A medication-induced decrease in platelets is called drug-induced thrombocytopenia.

## Drug-Induced Aplastic Anemia

Drug-induced aplastic anemia (DIAA) can be defined as a *pancytopenia* (a decrease in all the cellular components of peripheral blood) with a hypocellular bone marrow (a bone

**Figure 72.2** Differentiation of the stem cell to the mature neutrophil. The arrows indicate possible sites of drug-induced agranulocytosis. *(From Young GAR, Vincent PC: Drug-induced agranulocytosis. Clin Haematol 1980;9:483–504, with permission.)*

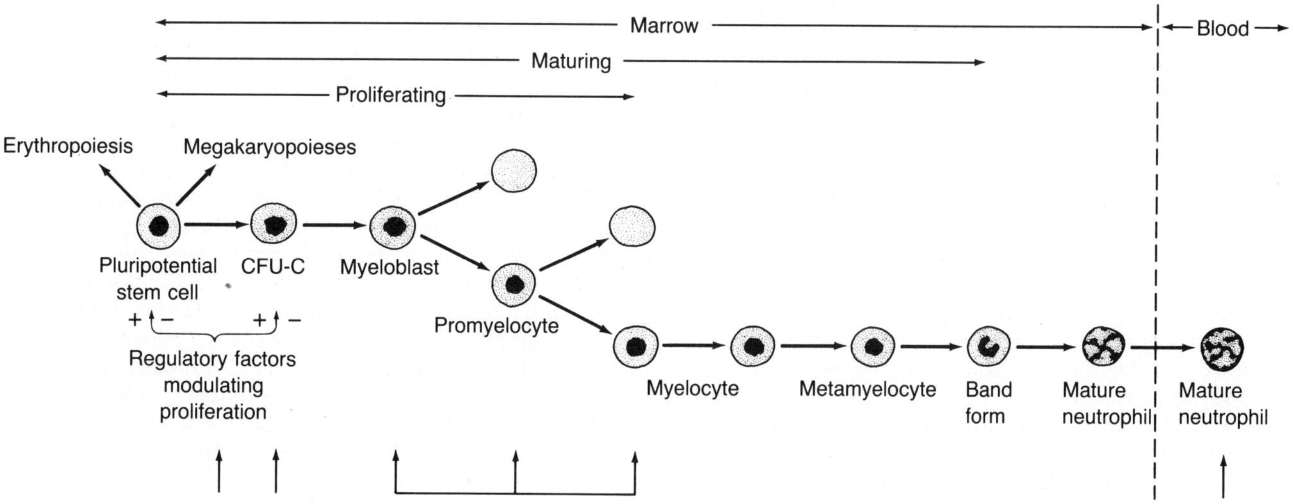

**Table 72.1** Drugs Associated With Aplastic Anemia

| | |
|---|---|
| Acetazolamide | Oral antidiabetics |
| Antihistamines | Oxyphenbutazone |
| Carbamazepine | Penicillamine |
| Chloramphenicol | Phenobarbital |
| Chloroquine | Phenothiazines |
| Chlorothiazide | Phenytoin |
| Gold salts | Propylthiouracil |
| Indomethacin | Quinidine |
| Methimazole | Sulfonamides |

marrow demonstrating a decreased production of blood cells); no gross evidence of increased peripheral blood cell destruction should be observed. The bone marrow must be free of neoplastic infiltration or significant myelofibrosis.[10] There also must be no history of exposure to antineoplastic agents or to intensive radiation. The onset of DIAA is insidious; symptoms usually appear about $6\frac{1}{2}$ weeks after initiation of the offending agent.[11] The disease often appears after the drug has been discontinued. Symptoms include fatigue, weakness, stomatitis, easy bruisability, petechiae, and purpura. Less common manifestations are infection and bleeding, which are seen later. Table 72.1 lists a number of drugs associated with DIAA.

The etiology of DIAA is felt to be damage to the hematopoietic stem cell. The earlier the stem cell is affected in the maturation process, the greater the likelihood that the DIAA will be long term.[8] There is no evidence that DIAA occurs as a result of destruction of the microenvironment of the bone marrow.[10] Three mechanisms have been proposed as causes of damage to the stem cell line.[11] First, there may be a dose-dependent toxic effect on hematopoiesis. The second mechanism is idiosyncratic, implying abnormal pharmacokinetics of the suspected drug or hypersensitivity of the stem cells to the bone marrow–destructive effects of the drug. The third mechanism is a drug- or metabolite-induced immune reaction specific to the stem cell population.

The dose-dependent mechanism for development of aplastic anemia can best be illustrated by the antineoplastic agents. This type of toxicity can be beneficial in particular situations, such as bone marrow transplantation. In bone marrow transplantation, large doses of chemotherapeutic drugs are given to prepare patients for infusion of the donor marrow.

Patients who develop DIAA at doses that are tolerated by the large majority of patients receiving the drug fall into the idiosyncratic category. Drugs causing DIAA in a minority of patients can imply abnormal pharmacokinetics of a drug. An excellent example is chloramphenicol-induced aplastic anemia. Investigators have hypothesized that this cause of DIAA is the result of abnormal metabolism of chloramphenicol. The nitrobenzene ring present on chloramphenicol is thought to be reduced to form a nitroso group on the chloramphenicol molecule.[12] The nitroso group could then interact with DNA in the stem cell, causing chromosomal damage and eventually cell death. A second type of chloramphenicol-induced bone marrow depression can also be seen. This reaction is dose dependent and reversible. In this reaction the chloramphenicol affects primarily the erythroid cell line as a result of injury to the mitochondria.[12] Other drugs thought to induce aplastic anemia include phenytoin and carbamazepine. Metabolites of phenytoin and carbamazepine are theorized to bind covalently to macromolecules in the cell and then either cause cell death through direct toxic effects on the stem cell or cause the death of lymphocytes involved in regulating hematopoieis.[13]

Phenylbutazone-induced aplastic anemia is thought by some to result from low phenylbutazone clearance.[10,11] It has been suggested that the drug accumulates to a toxic concentration and kills the stem cell population. Researchers have demonstrated a decreased clearance of phenylbutazone in some patients with phenylbutazone-induced aplastic anemia[10,11]; however, the medication has never been shown to be toxic to stem cells in high concentration. The exact mechanism of phenylbutazone-induced aplastic anemia is therefore still unclear.

Genetic predisposition may also influence the development of DIAA. Studies in animals and a case report of chloramphenicol-induced aplastic anemia in identical twins suggest a genetic predisposition to development of DIAA.[10,12]

DIAA has also been hypothesized to result from development of an immune reaction. The mechanism may be similar to that in drug-induced immune agranulocytosis or drug-induced immune hemolytic anemia (discussed later). Appearance of antibodies to chloroquine and subsequent bone marrow suppression support this hypothesis.[11] Drugs could also affect the function of suppressor T cells, which in turn could initiate the inhibition of stem cell production.[11] The clinical success of anti-thymocyte globulin in the treatment of possible DIAA may also indicate a drug effect on suppressor-T-cell function in DIAA.[14]

The 2-year survival rate for a patient who develops DIAA is approximately 62%.[11] As with all DIHDs, the suspected offending agent must be removed. Early withdrawal of the agent may allow reversal of the aplastic anemia.[11] Patients with DIAA need to be treated symptomatically for infection and bleeding. Anti-thymocyte globulin has been employed to reverse the aplastic anemia (in doses of 20 mg/kg body weight per day by intravenous infusion for 8 consecutive days).[15] Corticosteroids have been used in DIAA but their efficacy is questionable.[11] If bone marrow suppression continues after anti-thymocyte globulin and corticosteroid therapy, the only viable option at present is bone marrow transplantation.

## Drug-Induced Agranulocytosis

Drug-induced agranulocytosis (DIA) can be defined as a drug-mediated reduction in the mature myeloid cells in the blood (granulocytes and immature granulocytes [bands]) to a total count of 2,000 cells/mm$^3$ or less. Symptoms of agranulocytosis include sore throat, fever, malaise, weakness, and chills. The symptoms can appear rapidly, within 7 to 14 days after initiation of the offending agent, or, as in the case of phenothiazine-induced agranulocytosis, patients can be asymptomatic at the time of diagnosis. In the large majority of cases, the DIA resolves over time.[4] Table 72.2 lists medications that have been reported to cause DIA.

DIA may develop by a number of different mechanisms. Initially, it was thought that drugs affected only mature granulocytes. In recent years, however, studies have dem-

**Table 72.2** Drugs Associated With Agranulocytosis

| | |
|---|---|
| Acetaminophen | Levodopa |
| Acetazolamide | Levamisole |
| Acetylsalicylic acid | Lincomycin |
| Allopurinol | Meprobamate |
| *para*-Aminosalicylic acid | Methazolamide |
| $\beta$-Lactam antibiotics | Methimazole |
| Benzodiazepines | Methyldopa |
| Brompheniramine | Metronidazole |
| Carbamazepine | Nitrofurantoin |
| Captopril | Oxyphenbutazone |
| Chloramphenicol | Penicillamine |
| Chlorpropamide | Pentazocine |
| Cimetidine | Phenothiazines |
| Clindamycin | Phenylbutazone |
| Clomipramine | Phenytoin |
| Dapsone | Primidone |
| Desipramine | Procainamide |
| Doxycycline | Propranolol |
| Ethacrynic acid | Propylthiouracil |
| Ethosuximide | Pyrimethamine |
| Fenoprofen | Quinine |
| Flucytosine | Rifampin |
| Gentamicin | Streptomycin |
| Gold salts | Sulfa antibiotics |
| Griseofulvin | Thiazide diuretics |
| Hydralazine | Tocainide |
| Hydroxychloroquine | Tolbutamide |
| Ibuprofen | Vancomycin |
| Imipramine | |
| Indomethacin | |
| Isoniazid | |

onstrated a possible toxic effect of drugs on the myeloid colony-forming unit in bone marrow.[16,17] DIA can be classified into three types.[18] The type I reaction is immune mediated and involves the drug or drug metabolite, antibodies, and neutrophils. A type II reaction is associated with accumulated drug toxicity in hypersensitive individuals. The final type, type III, represents other etiologies induced by a combination of both immune and toxic mechanisms.

Drug-induced immune agranulocytosis (type I) has been theorized to develop by one of four different mechanisms.[19] The first mechanism involves drug absorption on the membrane of the neutrophil. The drug membrane complex then acts as a hapten to stimulate antibody formation. The antibodies produced attach to the drug–membrane complex, causing destruction of WBCs through complement activation and removal of the reticuloendothelial system (RE system) (Fig. 72.3). This hapten-type reaction is often seen when drugs are given in large doses. Penicillin derivatives are frequently associated with this type of agranulocytosis. The dose at which this immune-mediated reaction occurs is usually above 150 mg/kg/d for the majority of penicillin derivatives, but the reaction has also occurred at lower doses.[17,20,21]

The second mechanism behind immune-mediated agranulocytosis is called the "innocent bystander phenomenon." In this reaction the drug combines with a drug-specific antibody. The complex is nonspecifically absorbed to the

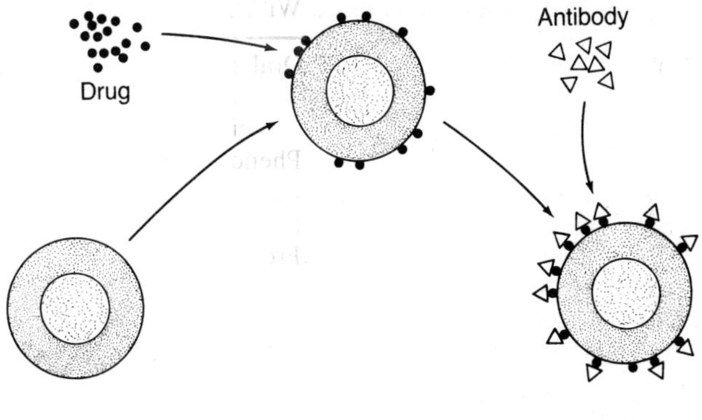


**Figure 72.3** Drug absorption mechanism. The drug binds to the membrane of the blood cell. Antibodies are formed to the drug–membrane complex (a hapten). The antibodies then attach to the complex and cell toxicity occurs. *(From Petz LD, Garratty G: Acquired Immune Hemolytic Anemias. New York, Churchill Livingston, 1980, pp 267–304, with permission.)*

neutrophil membrane and complement is activated. The cell is then cleared by the RE system (Fig. 72.4). Quinidine has been associated with this type of reaction.

A similar type of immune response involves a protein carrier that combines with the drug and then attaches to the cell membrane. This in turn causes antibody formation. The antibodies attach to the drug protein carrier–membrane complex and activate complement. The cell is then cleared by the RE system (Fig. 72.5).

The final mechanism for an immune-mediated reaction is the production of autoantibodies to a membrane "spoiled" by the offending drug. The drug produces an alteration in the neutrophil membrane that induces the formation of autoantibodies (antibodies that attach directly to the neutrophil). These antibodies attach to the neutrophil, causing cellular destruction (Fig. 72.6).

The onset of symptoms in disorders that arise by immune-mediated mechanisms is rapid (7–15 days). In the case of penicillin-induced agranulocytosis, the patient can often be

**Figure 72.4** "Innocent bystander" mechanism. The drug induces antibody formation. The antibodies and drug form a complex in the serum and the complex nonspecifically binds to the cell membrane. Complement is activated. *(From Petz LD, Garratty G: Acquired Immune Hemolytic Anemias. New York, Churchill Livingstone, 1980, pp 267–304, with permission.)*

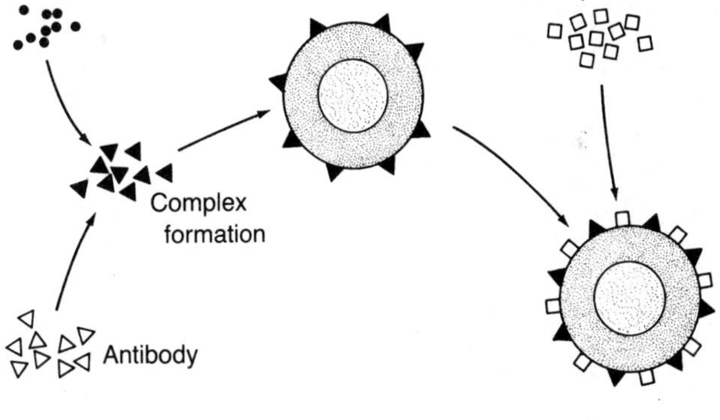

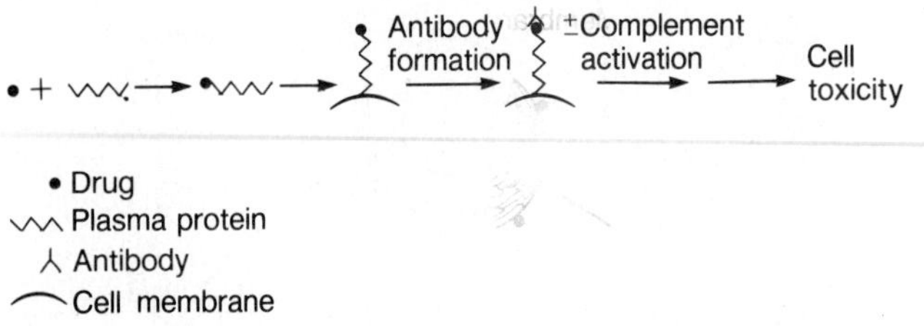


**Figure 72.5** Protein carrier mechanism. The drug combines with a plasma protein. The complex then attaches to the cell membrane, and antibody formation is stimulated. Antibodies later attach to the complex and activate complement. *(From Young GAR, Vincent PC: Drug-induced agranulocytosis. Clin Haematol 1980;9:483–504, with permission.)*

restarted on a lower dose of penicillin after the neutropenia has resolved without any relapse of DIA.[20,21] Because of the rapid onset of symptoms and the dose-related phenomenon, a second mechanism could be involved with penicillin-induced agranulocytosis. This mechanism involves accumulation of the drug to a toxic concentration in hypersensitive individuals (type II reaction). Researchers have shown in in vitro cell cultures that penicillin derivatives in high concentration inhibit growth of myeloid colony-forming units in patients recovering from DIA.[22,23] Penicillin derivatives may therefore exert WBC suppression by several mechanisms.

Antithyroid medications such as propylthiouracil and methimazole produce agranulocytosis in about 0.3% to 0.6% of patients.[24] The mechanism by which antithyroid agents cause agranulocytosis is unknown but antibodies to granulocytes have been demonstrated.[25] In a study by Cooper et al[24] agranulocytosis occurred more frequently in older patients (>40 years) within 2 months of initiation of therapy. The investigators also reported a possible dose–response relationship with methimazole. In patients receiving less than 30 mg a day of methimazole, no agranulocytosis occurred, but in patients receiving higher doses, neutropenia was observed. There appeared to be no dose–response relationship with conventional doses of propylthiouracil.

Another group of drugs known to cause a type II DIA is the phenothiazines. The onset of phenothiazine-induced agranulocytosis is approximately 2 to 15 weeks after initiation of therapy.[19] Short-term toxicity is not usually observed in patients taking phenothiazines chronically; however, there is one report of acute agranulocytosis in a child who accidentally ingested a large quantity of chlorpromazine.[16] Usually, patients ingest 10 to 20 g of a phenothiazine chronically before the onset of neutropenia. Phenothiazine-induced agranulocytosis occurs most frequently in females over the age of 50. The mechanism by which phenothiazines cause the DIA has been studied primarily with chlorpromazine.[4] Chlorpromazine is thought to affect cells that are in the phase of the cell cycle in which the enzymes needed for DNA synthesis are manufactured ($G_1$ phase) or the phase in which cells are resting and not committed to cell division ($G_0$ phase).[4] The antipsychotic agents are known to precipitate proteins and may coprecipitate polynucleotides, so they can no longer participate in nucleic acid synthesis. Chlorpromazine also increases the loss of macromolecules from the intracellular pools that are essential for cellular replication.[4] When bone marrow from a patient with phenothiazine-induced agranulocytosis is examined it initially appears to have no cellularity (aplastic), but over time it becomes highly hyperplastic. It is felt that the toxic effects of the phenothiazines are not observed in all patients taking the medications because the majority of patients have enough bone marrow reserve to overcome the toxic effects.[4]

The primary treatment for DIA is removal of the offending drug. After discontinuation of the drug, most cases of neutropenia resolve over time and only symptomatic treatment (i.e., antimicrobials for infections) is necessary.

**Figure 72.6** Autoantibody mechanism. A drug induces an alteration in the cell membrane. Autoantibodies are formed to the altered cell membrane and cell toxicity occurs. *(From Young GAR, Vincent PC. Drug-induced agranulocytosis. Clin Haematol 1980;9:483–504, with permission.)*

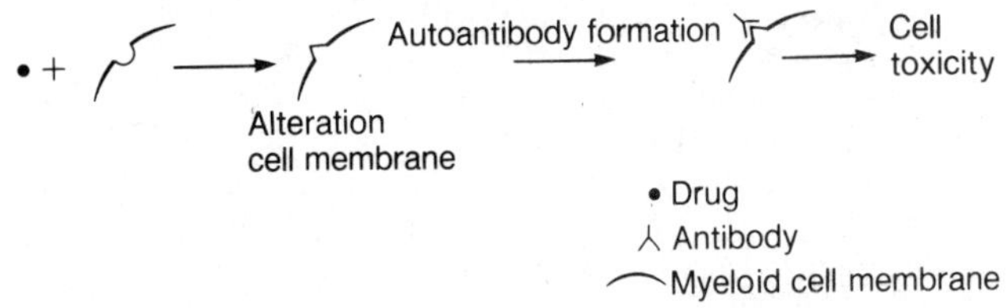


## Drug-Induced Hemolytic Anemia

Drug-induced hemolytic anemia (DIHA) is a disorder in which RBCs are damaged or destroyed (hemolyzed). The mechanisms by which DIHA arises can be divided into two categories: immune and metabolic. The immune mechanism may be similar to that in immune-regulated agranulocytosis or it may involve suppression of regulator cells, which allows production of autoantibodies. The second type of mechanism involves the induction of hemolysis by metabolic abnormalities in the RBCs. Patients with DIHA can present with signs of intravascular or extravascular hemolysis. The onset of DIHA is variable and depends upon the drug and mechanism of hemolysis. Table 72.3 lists drugs that have been associated with DIHA.

**Table 72.3** Drugs Associated With Hemolytic Anemia

| | |
|---|---|
| Acetaminophen | Methysergide |
| *para*-Aminosalicylic acid | Nomifensine |
| Cephalosporins | Penicillins |
| Chlorpromazine | Probenecid |
| Chlorpropamide | Procainamide |
| Hydralazine | Quinidine |
| Hydrochlorothiazide | Quinine |
| Ibuprofen | Rifampin |
| Isoniazid | Sulfonamides |
| Levodopa | Streptomycin |
| Mefenamic acid | Tetracycline |
| Melphalan | Tolbutamide |
| Methadone | Triamterene |
| Methyldopa | |

## Drug-Induced Immune Hemolytic Anemia

As stated earlier the proposed mechanisms by which drug-induced immune hemolytic anemia (DIIHA) arises are similar to the mechanisms by which DIA evolves. The first mechanism is absorption of the drug to the RBC membrane to form a hapten and subsequent antibody formation. A study by Yust et al[26] demonstrated that once the RBCs are coated with the antibodies, the cells are destroyed either by phagocytosis or by cell-mediated cytotoxicity. The effector cells in both processes are mononuclear phagocytes.[26] Mainly penicillin and cephalosporin derivatives, in high doses, are associated with this type of immune reaction.[27] Other drugs that have been reported to cause DIIHA by this process include tetracycline[28] and certain antineoplastic agents (i.e., cyclophosphamide, cisplatin, and melphalan).[29]

DIIHA has also been reported to occur as a result of the "innocent bystander phenomenon." Quinidine and phenacetin are the prototype drugs in this reaction. Drugs that induce this reaction form complexes with drug-specific antibodies that adhere to the RBC membrane. Complement then lyses the RBC membrane.[27] This type of mechanism is associated with acute intravascular hemolysis. A metabolite of nomifensine (an antidepressant agent removed from the market by the manufacturer) has also been shown to cause DIIHA by this mechanism.[30]

A third type of immune-mediated mechanism has been observed with cephalosporin derivatives. The cephalosporins combine with nonspecific proteins, including albumin, IgG, IgA, and fibrinogen, and adhere to the RBC. The binding is not immunologic in origin and hemolytic anemia has not been associated with this reaction (Fig. 72.7). The reaction can, however, cause difficulties in cross-matching patients for blood transfusions, because of the nonspecific binding of antibodies to the RBC membrane.[27]

Typically, patients in whom the direct Coombs test (also called direct antiglobulin test) is positive because of systemic disease have antibodies attached to their RBC membranes. These antibody-coated cells are then removed by the reticuloendothelial system, which in turn causes an extravascular hemolysis. Methyldopa has long been known to produce a Coombs-positive hemolytic anemia, but the clinical course does not follow the typical presentation of an immune hemolytic anemia. First, the majority of patients who have a positive direct Coombs test for reasons other than methyldopa develop extravascular hemolysis; however, of the 15% to 20% of patients who have a positive direct Coombs test after taking methyldopa, only 0.8% develop hemolysis. Second, the time between development of a hemolytic anemia and a positive direct Coombs test is usually short. Patients with methyldopa-induced hemolytic anemia present 18 months to 4 years after initiation of the drug, but most patients have a positive direct Coombs test much earlier (3–6 months). Another differentiating factor in the development of methyldopa-induced hemolysis is that although hemolysis may subside promptly after discontinuation of the drug, the Coombs test may remain positive for 7 to 20 months.[27] Patients who are Coombs test positive but are not hemolyzing can receive blood transfusions without any adverse effects.[28]

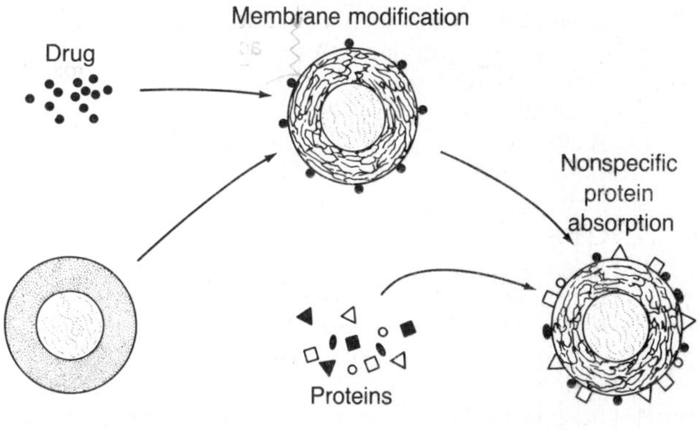


**Figure 72.7** Nonspecific binding of protein mechanism. The drug combines with the cell membrane, which in turn causes a nonspecific binding of serum protein. This reaction is seen primarily with the cephalosporins; no cell lysis or toxicity occurs. *(From Petz LD, Garratty G: Acquired Immune Hemolytic Anemias. New York, Churchill Livingstone, 1980, pp 267–304, with permission.)*

Because of the many contradictions in methyldopa-induced hemolytic anemia and our past misunderstanding of the immune system, a number of mechanisms by which this disorder may arise have been proposed over the years. The most plausible mechanism is inhibition by methyldopa of the proliferation of nonspecific suppressor T cells.[31] This inhibition of suppressor T cells allows unregulated production of autoantibodies by plasma cells. The increase in autoantibodies causes the Coombs test to turn positive, but this study still does not explain why only a small number of patients with a positive direct Coombs test develop hemolytic anemia. Recently, however, Kelton et al[32] demonstrated that methyldopa also impairs reticuloendothelial cell function. The patients involved in the study were receiving methyldopa and were Coombs test positive with or without hemolysis. The patients with an impairment of the reticuloendothelial system could not clear the RBCs coated with autoantibodies from their bloodstream; therefore, hemolysis did not occur. In patients presenting with hemolysis, no impairment of the reticuloendothelial system was demonstrated. Procainamide has also been reported to cause a positive direct Coombs test and hemolytic anemia. The hemolysis may resolve rapidly after discontinuation of the drug, but the direct Coombs test can remain positive for many months.[33] Other drugs that have been reported to cause an autoimmune hemolytic anemia include levodopa, mefenamic acid, and cimetidine.[27]

Treatment for DIIHA comprises removal of the offending agent and supportive care.

## Drug-Induced Oxidative Hemolytic Anemia

Drug-induced oxidative hemolytic anemia (DIOHA) is a hereditary condition that is most often associated with a glucose-6-phosphate dehydrogenase (G6PD) deficiency, but can also occur as a result of other enzyme defects (i.e., NADH methemoglobin reductase, GSH peroxidase). The concentration of G6PD is decreased in 13% of American black males, in 3% of American black females, and in some

**Table 72.4** Drugs Associated With Oxidative Hemolytic Anemia

| | |
|---|---|
| Ascorbic acid | Menadiol |
| Aspirin | Methylene blue |
| Benzocaine | Nitrofurantoin |
| Chloramphenicol | Nitrofurazone |
| Chloroquine | Phenazopyridine |
| Dapsone | Salazosulfapyridine |
| Diazoxide | |

other ethnic groups (e.g., Greeks, Sardinians, and Sephardic Jews).[34] DIOHA occurs when the following conditions exist[35]:

1. Abnormal increases in oxidative stress exceed the normal sources of reducing power.
2. Structural abnormalities of the RBC hemoglobin molecule render the cells more susceptible to oxidant stress despite normal reducing sources.
3. There is a deficiency of reducing power in the RBC; therefore, the cell cannot react appropriately to normal increases in oxidative stress.

The excessive oxidative stress can cause denaturation of the hemoglobin molecule and increase RBC membrane rigidity which causes cell lysis. The degree of hemolysis depends on the severity of the enzyme deficiency and the oxidative stress; however, the dose required for hemolysis to occur is often below prescribed quantities of the suspected agent.[35] Any drug that places oxidative stress on the RBC will cause DIOHA, but severe hemolysis is rare.[35] An interesting case of DIOHA occurred in a child when dapsone (an oxidizing agent) was transferred through the breast milk of the mother taking the drug.[36] For a list of agents that can cause DIOHA refer to Table 72.4.

The treatment for DIOHA is removal of the drug. No other therapy is usually necessary, as most cases of DIOHA are mild. Patients should be advised to avoid medication capable of inducing the hemolysis.

## Drug-Induced Megaloblastic Anemia

Drug-induced megaloblastic anemia (DIMA) is the result of abnormal development of RBC precursors called megaloblasts in the bone marrow. Examination of peripheral blood will show a rise in the mean corpuscular hemoglobin. These megaloblastic changes are due to direct or indirect effects of the drug on DNA synthesis. The abnormality can be seen in any portion of the replication process including DNA assembly, base precursor metabolism, and RNA synthesis.[37] The antineoplastic agents most frequently cause DIMA because of their pharmacologic action on DNA replication, but other drugs such as co-trimoxazole, phenytoin, and the barbiturates have also been implicated. Co-trimoxazole has been reported to cause DIMA at both low and high doses.[38,39] The DIMA produced by co-trimoxazole is thought to occur most frequently in patients with a partial $B_{12}$ or folate deficiency.[37] Patients with adequate stores of these vitamins are probably at low risk of developing DIMA, because drug

**Table 72.5** Drugs Associated With Megaloblastic Anemia

| | |
|---|---|
| *para*-Aminosalicylic acid | Neomycin |
| Azathioprine | Nitrofurantoin |
| Chloramphenicol | Oral contraceptives |
| Colchicine | Phenobarbital |
| Cyclophosphamide | Phenytoin |
| Cytarabine | Primidone |
| 5-Fluorodeoxyuridine | Pyrimethamine |
| 5-Fluorouracil | Sulfasalazine |
| Hydroxyurea | Triamterene |
| 6-Mercaptopurine | Trimethoprim |
| Methotrexate | Vinblastine |

affinity for human dihydrofolate reductase is low. Phenytoin, primidone, and phenobarbital have been postulated to cause DIMA either by inhibiting folate absorption or by increasing the catabolism of folate. In both instances, a relative deficiency of folate is produced. Table 72.5 lists drugs that have been suggested to produce DIMA.

When DIMA is related to chemotherapy, no real therapeutic option is available and DIMA is an accepted side effect of therapy. If DIMA occurs as a result of co-trimoxazole, a trial course of folinic acid 5–10 mg up to four times a day may correct the anemia.[38,39] Folic acid supplementation (1 mg daily) often corrects the DIMA produced by phenytoin or phenobarbital, but some clinicians have suggested that folic acid supplementation decreases the effectiveness of the anti-epileptic medications.

## Drug-Induced Thrombocytopenia

The mechanisms by which drugs induce thrombocytopenia (DIT) are similar to those for DIA and DIHA, that is, toxic and immune-mediated reactions. If the toxic effect of the drug is direct, there will be a decrease in megakaryocytes in the bone marrow. This differs from an immune reaction in which there is increased peripheral destruction of platelets and an increased number of megakaryocytes. Early symptoms of DIT include increased bruising, petechiae, ecchymosis, and epistaxis. Bleeding from mucous membranes and severe purpura can appear later in the disorder. Patients who develop DIT must be transfused when their platelet count drops below 20,000/mm$^3$ and they are actively bleeding.

Drugs that induce thrombocytopenia by their toxic effects are primarily cancer chemotherapy agents; however, organic solvents, pesticides, and amrinone have also been implicated. Amrinone has been shown to cause thrombocytopenia in up to 18.6% of the patients taking the drug.[40] The thrombocytopenia is mild and occurs 24 hours to 2 weeks after initiation of the drug orally. Although the investigators demonstrated an amrinone-dependent antibody, they felt that because of the rapid onset, the dose-related response, and the absence of anamnestic effect, the disorder was indicative not of an immune-mediated reaction, but probably of a toxic reaction.[40] Amphotericin B has also been implicated in a case of thrombocytopenia. The mechanism proposed was a toxic effect on the bone marrow, as no peripheral destruction of the patient's platelets occurred.[41]

**Table 72.6** Drugs Associated With Thrombocytopenia

| | |
|---|---|
| Acetazolamide | Hydrochlorothiazide |
| Acetylsalicylic acid | Hydroxychloroquine |
| Allopurinol | Isoniazid |
| Aminoglutethimide | Meclofenamate |
| *para*-Aminosalicylic acid | Morphine |
| Amrinone | Penicillin |
| Cephalothin | Phenylbutazone |
| Chlorothiazide | Phenytoin |
| Cimetidine | Procainamide |
| Desipramine | Quinidine |
| Diazepam | Quinine |
| Digitoxin | Rifampin |
| Furosemide | Sulfisoxazole |
| Gold heparin | Trimethoprim |

In the majority of patients, DIT is caused by an immune reaction. The mechanisms are similar to those described earlier in the chapter. Formation of a hapten between the drug and a molecule on the platelet membrane is observed with penicillin derivatives, trimethoprim, and heparin. A complete list of medications known to cause DIT is provided in Table 72.6. The thrombocytopenia seen with this type of immune reaction occurs 7 to 15 days after initiation of the drug and patients are frequently receiving large doses of the medication (i.e., penicillin derivatives > 150 mg/kg).[42,43] The recovery period is often short.[44]

Heparin can cause at least two types of thrombocytopenia.[45] The first is mild and occurs 2 to 4 days after initiation of therapy. The platelet count slowly returns to normal after the initial drop. The patients develop no major sequelae from the thrombocytopenia. The mechanism for this type of reaction may be sequestration of platelets.[45] The second type of heparin-induced thrombocytopenia is the severe form and may be associated with thrombosis.[45,46] The platelet count generally begins to drop 6 to 12 days after starting heparin therapy. In addition, patients may develop thrombocytopenia and thrombosis even on low-dose heparin.[45,47] The reaction is mediated by the formation of antibodies to the platelet–heparin complex. The antibodies attach to the complex and fix complement, allowing activation of arachidonic acid and endoperoxide by the platelets.[48] The platelets subsequently aggregate and form a thrombus. The incidence of heparin-induced thrombocytopenia with thrombosis has been reported to be three to four times higher with bovine sources of heparin than with porcine sources,[49,50] but Green et al[51] demonstrated no differences between animal sources of heparin. In addition, in one patient, switching from a bovine source to a porcine source in the face of active thrombocytopenia and thrombosis did not eliminate the disorder.[52]

The thrombocytopenia induced by gold salts is also related to formation of antibodies to platelets.[53,54] The incidence of gold-induced thrombocytopenia is 1% to 3%, and the onset is often abrupt and severe.[53] The autoantibody formed to the platelet appears to be associated with human leukocyte antigens (HLAs), which are located on the platelet membrane and on a number of other different cells in the body.[53,54] HLAs are specific antigens that allow the body to differentiate between antigens (i.e., tissue, platelets, etc.) that are part of a particular individual genetic makeup (self antigens) and genetically dissimilar antigens (non-self antigens). Recognition of HLAs controls the immunologic response of an individual to a particular antigenic stimulus. In some types of autoimmune disease, HLAs are associated with development of the disease. The recognition of these HLAs in combination with antigenic determinants causes the patient's immune system to attack the body. A similar reaction occurs in gold-induced thrombocytopenia. The gold salts and the HLAs interact, causing the platelets to be recognized as non-self and thus inducing destruction of the platelets. The HLA most commonly associated with induction of autoantibodies is DR-3, but DR-4 may also interact with the antibodies.[53–55] The exact mechanism by which gold causes the formation of autoantibody-regulated DR-3 and DR-4 antigens has not been elucidated.

The third mechanism described for DIT is the "innocent bystander" immune response. The most commonly implicated drug is quinidine and the DIT is frequently related to high doses.[56] Quinidine may also form a hapten with the platelet membrane to produce thrombocytopenia.[57]

The primary treatment for DIT is removal of the offending drug and symptomatic treatment of the patient. In the case of heparin-induced thrombocytopenia with thrombosis, some clinicians recommend the administration of antiplatelet drugs. At the present time, however, there have been no studies that demonstrate the efficacy of antiplatelet agents. In addition, it appears that large doses of steroids have no effect.[58] In gold salt–induced thrombocytopenia, however, some investigators feel that prednisone 60 mg daily is beneficial in correcting the thrombocytopenia.[53]

## Summary

The occurrence of a drug-induced blood disorder is rare. The mechanisms often involve either an immune or a toxic effect on the affected blood cell line. The primary treatment is removal of the drug and symptomatic support of the patient.

## References


1. Arneborn P, Palmblad J. Drug-induced neutropenia—a survey for Stockholm 1973–1978. Acta Med Scand 1982;212:289–292.
2. Arneborn P, Palmblad J. Drug-induced neutropenia in the Stockholm region 1973–1975; frequency and causes. Acta Med Scand 1978;204:283–286.
3. Arneborn P, Palmblad J. Drug-induced neutropenias in the Stockholm region 1976–1977. Acta Med Scand 1979;206:241–243.
4. Pisciotta V. Drug-induced agranulocytosis. Drugs 1978;15:132–143.

5. Haak HL. Experimental drug-induced aplastic anemia. Clin Haematol 1980;9:621–639.
6. Levy M. The combined effect of viruses and drugs in drug-induced diseases. Med Hypotheses 1984;14:293–296.
7. Cline MJ, Golde DW. Controlling the production of blood cells. Blood 1979;53:156–165.
8. Niewg HO. Aplastic anemia (panmyelopathy), in Girdwood RH (ed): Blood Disorders Due to Drugs and Other Agents. Amsterdam, Excerpta Medica, 1974.
9. Tami JA, Parr MD, Thompson JS. The immune system. Am J Hosp Pharm 1986;43:2483–2493.
10. Vincent PC. In vitro evidence of drug action in aplastic anemia. Blut 1984;49:3–12.
11. Heimpel H, Heit W. Drug-induced aplastic anaemia: Clinical aspects. Clin Haematol 1980;9:641–662.
12. Yunis AA, Miller AM, Salem Z, et al. Chloramphenicol toxicity: Pathogenetic mechanisms and the role of the p-$NO_2$ in aplastic anemia. Clin Toxicol 1980;17:359–373.
13. Gerson WT, Fine DG, Spielberg SP, et al. Anticonvulsant-induced aplastic anemia: Increased susceptibility to toxic drug metabolites in vitro. Blood 1983;61:889–893.
14. Thomas ED, Storb R. Acquired severe aplastic anemia: Progress and perplexity. Blood 1984;64:325–328.
15. Champlin R, Ho W, Gale RP. Antithymocyte globulin treatment in patients with aplastic anemia. N Engl J Med 1983;308:113–118.
16. Burckart GJ, Snidow J, Bruce W. Neutropenia following acute chlorpromazine ingestion. Clin Toxicol 1981;18:797–801.
17. Neftel KA, Muller MR, Hauser SD, et al. More on penicillin-induced leukopenia. N Engl J Med 1983;308:901.
18. Heit WF. Hematologic effects of antipyretic analgesics: Drug-induced agranulocytosis. Am J Med 1983;75:65–68.
19. Young GA, Vincent PC. Drug-induced agranulocytosis. Clin Haematol 1980;9:483–504.
20. Kirkwood CF, Smith LL, Rustagi PK, et al. Neutropenia associated with $\beta$-lactam antibiotics. Clin Pharm 1983;2:569–578.
21. Homayouni H, Gross PA, Setia V, et al. Leukopenia due to penicillin and cephalosporin homologues. Arch Intern Med 1979;139:827–828.
22. Irvine AE, Morris TC, Kelly GJ, et al. Ticarcillin-induced neutropenia corroborated by in vitro CFU-C toxicity. Acta Haematol 1983;70:364–368.
23. Neftel KA, Hauser SP, Muller MR. Inhibition of granulopoiesis in vivo and in vitro by $\beta$-lactam antibiotics. J Infect Dis 1985; 152:90–98.
24. Cooper DS, Goldmiriz D, Lewin AA, et al. Agranulocytosis associated with antithyroid drug. Ann Intern Med 1983;98:26–29.
25. McIntyre PA, Laleli YR, Hodkinson BA, et al. Evidence for antileukocyte antibodies as a mechanism for drug-induced agranulocytosis. Trans Assoc Am Physicians 1971;84:217–225.
26. Yust I, Frisch B, Goldsher N. Simultaneous detection of two mechanisms of immune destruction of penicillin-treated human red blood cells. Am J Hematol 1982;13:53–62.
27. Petz LD. Drug-induced immune haemolytic anaemia. Clin Haematol 1980;91:455–482.
28. Simpson MB, Pryzbylik J, Innis B, et al. Hemolytic anemia after tetracycline therapy. N Engl J Med 1985;312:840–842.
29. Doll DC, Weiss RB. Hemolytic anemia associated with antineoplastic agents. Cancer Treat Rep 1985;69:777–782.
30. Salama A, Mueler-Eckhardt C. The role of metabolite-specific antibodies in nomifensine-dependent immune hemolytic anemia. N Engl J Med 1985;313:469–474.
31. Kirtland HH, Mohler DN, Horwitz DA. Methyldopa inhibition of suppressor-lymphocyte function. A proposed cause of auto immune hemolytic anemia. N Engl J Med 1980;302:825–832.
32. Kelton JG. Impaired reticuloendothelial function in patients treated with methyldopa. N Engl J Med 1985;313:596–600.
33. Kleinman S, Nelson R, Smith L, et al. Positive direct antiglobulin tests and immune hemolytic anemia in patients receiving procainamide. N Engl J Med 1984;311:B809–B812.
34. Wallach J (ed.): Interpretation of Diagnostic Tests: A Handbook Synopsis of Laboratory Medicine, 3rd ed. Boston, Little, Brown, 1978.
35. Gordan-Smith EC. Drug-induced oxidative haemolysis. Clin Haematol 1980;9:557–586.
36. Sanders SW, Zone JJ, Foltz RL, et al. Hemolytic anemia induced by dapsone transmitted through breast milk. Ann Intern Med 1982;96:465–466.
37. Scott JM, Weir DG. Drug-induced megaloblastic change. Clin Haematol 1980;9:587–605.
38. Magee F, O'Sullivan H, McCann SR. Megaloblastosis and low-dose trimethoprim–sulfamethoxazole. Ann Intern Med 1981;95:657.
39. Kobrinsky NL, Ramsay NK. Acute megaloblastic anemia induced by high-dose trimethoprim–sulfamethoxazole. Ann Intern Med 1981;94:780–781.
40. Ansell J, Tiarks C, McCue J, et al. Amrinone-induced thrombocytopenia. Arch Intern Med 1984;144:949–952.
41. Chan CP, Tuazon CU, Lessin LS. Amphotericin-B–induced thromobocytopenia. Ann Intern Med 1982;96:332–333.
42. Murphy MF, Riordant T, Minchinton RM, et al. Demonstration of an immune-mediated mechanism of penicillin-induced neutropenia and thrombocytopenia. Br J Haematol 1983;55:155–160.
43. Salamon DJ, Nusbacher J, Stroupe T, et al. Red cell and platelet-bound IgG penicillin antibodies in a patient with thrombocytopenia. Transfusion 1984;24:395–398.
44. Miescher PA, Graf J. Drug-induced thrombocytopenia. Clin Haematol 1980;9:505–519.
45. Johnson RA, Lazarus KH, Henry DH. Heparin-induced thrombocytopenia: A prospective study. Am J Hematol 1984;17:349–353.
46. Cines DB, Kaywin P, Bina M, et al. Heparin-associated thrombocytopenia. N Engl J Med 1980;303:788–795.
47. Cheng TC. Thrombocytopenia associated with minidose heparin therapy. Postgrad Med 1981;70:73–78.
48. Arthur CK, Isbister JP, Aspery EM. The heparin induced thrombosis–thrombocytopenia syndrome (H.I.T.T.S.): A review. Pathology 1985;17:82–86.
49. King DJ, Kelton JG. Heparin-associated thrombocytopenia. Ann Intern Med 1984;100:535–540.
50. Bell WR, Royall RM. Heparin-associated thrombocytopenia: A comparison of three heparin preparations. N Engl J Med 1980;303:902–907.
51. Green D, Martin GJ, Shoichet SH, et al. Thrombocytopenia in a prospective, randomized, double-blind trial of bovine and porcine heparin. Am J Med Sci 1984;288:60–64.
52. Guay DR, Richard A. Heparin-induced thrombocytopenia—association with a platelet aggregating factor and cross-sensitivity to bovine and porcine heparin. Drug Intell Clin Pharm 1984;18:398–401.
53. Armstrong RD, Faith A, Panayi GS, et al. Gold-induced thrombocytopenia: Detection of anti-platelet antibody. Clin Rheumatol 1983;2:183–188.
54. Adachi JD, Bensen WG, Singal DP, et al. Gold induced thrombocytopenia: Platelet associated IgG and HLA typing in three patients. J Rheumatol 1984;11:355–357.
55. Coblyn JS, Weinblatt M, Holdsworth D, et al. Gold-induced

thrombocytopenia. A clinical and immunogenetic study of twenty-three patients. Ann Intern Med 1981;95:178–181.

56. Kelton JG, Meltzer D, Moore J, et al. Drug-induced thrombocytopenia is associated with increased binding of IgG to platelets both in vivo and in vitro. Blood 1981;58:524–529.

57. Chong BH, Berndt MC, Koutts J, et al. Quinidine-induced thrombocytopenia and leukopenia: Demonstration and characterization of distinct antiplatelets and antileukocyte antibodies. Blood 1983;62:1218–1223.

58. Rector TS, Cipolle RJ, Seifert RD, et al. Characteristics of heparin-associated thrombocytopenia. Am J Hosp Pharm 1979; 36:1561–1565.

# 3 Diseases of Infectious Origin

# Chapter 73 / Use of Laboratory Tests in Infectious Diseases

Michael N. Dudley, PharmD

The treatment of infectious diseases provides a unique opportunity for the clinician to individualize drug therapy. No other group of diseases is more amenable to ex vivo study of drug effects—one can indeed study the etiology of a disease in the absence of a host. This possibility has resulted in the development and utilization of many in vitro tests of antimicrobial activity; however, although clinicians have an impressive array of tests to guide them in the selection of antimicrobials, there remains considerable controversy regarding the usefulness of even some of the most fundamental measures of antimicrobial activity.[1] This chapter reviews the basic principles of tests available in the clinical laboratory that are useful in the diagnosis and treatment of infectious diseases.

## Laboratory Tests Confirming the Presence of Infection

### *Colonization Versus Infection*

One of the most difficult tasks confronting the clinician is the differentiation between infection and colonization with potential pathogens in certain body sites. *Colonization* may be defined as invasiveness of an organism *without* disease in a host. *Infection* implies the presence of an organism within tissues that results in a *response* of the host's immune defenses. Table 73.1 lists some common colonizing organisms and the associated body sites; however, it should be stressed that while in many instances the organisms recovered from these sites are regarded as "normal flora," many of these same organisms are capable of initiating infection when introduced into certain body tissues or fluids. These same organisms may also become invasive in the absence of adequate host defenses.

### *Nonspecific Tests*

#### White Blood Cell Count and Differential

Moderate to high elevation of the total white blood cell count often indicates the presence of systemic infection. In bacterial infections, the total white blood cell count usually rises above the normal range (5–10,000/mm$^3$). The leukocytosis may be mild, particularly in elderly patients or in less serious infections, or it may exceed 50,000 cells/mm$^3$ in overwhelming sepsis; however, the absolute white blood cell count remains a nonspecific test as elevations may be observed in noninfectious diseases (e.g., leukemia, rheumatoid arthritis) or during drug therapy (e.g., corticosteroids, lithium).

The differential count may be of further use in defining the cause of the leukocytosis and occasionally the etiology of infection. Table 73.2 displays the normal differential of the white blood cell count for an adult. Bacterial infections generally result in an increase in neutrophils (polymorphonucleur leukocytes, PMNs, "segs"), the principal cell type involved in cell-mediated host response to bacterial infection. Microscopic examination of a peripheral blood smear may disclose morphological changes in the cytoplasm of these cells (e.g., toxic granulations, vacuolization) that are suggestive of bacterial infection. Immature cells ("bands," "stabs") are often released from the bone marrow into the peripheral circulation during acute infection. This so-called "shift-to-the-left" (so named because of the location of these cells in diagrams depicting neutrophil maturation in basic immunology texts) may exceed 10% to 20% of the total number of white blood cells.

Leukocytosis secondary to bacterial infection does not occur in all hosts. For example, bacterial infections are frequently a complication of neutropenia of cancer chemotherapy; these patients are incapable of developing a leukocytosis in response to bacterial infection. Indeed, the outcome of infection in these patients is highly dependent on a rise in white blood cell count. In the elderly, leukocytosis is frequently absent during an acute bacterial infection.

Lymphocytosis is most frequently associated with viral infection. For example, acute Epstein–Barr virus infection (mononucleosis) produces an absolute leukocytosis with a lymphocytic predominance. These lymphocytes are frequently described as being "atypical" because of their morphological appearance on microscopic examination.

Monocytosis is less frequently associated with acute bacterial infection, although its presence has been associated with the response of certain infections (e.g., tuberculosis) to chemotherapy.

#### Other Tests

Table 73.3 lists other nonspecific laboratory tests that may be useful in diagnosing infection. Large elevations of the erythrocyte sedimentation rate (ESR, "sed" rate) are associated with acute or chronic infection, particularly endocarditis, chronic osteomyelitis, and intraabdominal infection.[2] Unfortunately, a normal ESR does not exclude the possibility of infection. Serum complement concentrations, particularly the C3 component, are often reduced in serious infections because of consumption during the host defense process. Other acute phase reactants such as C-reactive proteins may be elevated in acute infection and may support a clinical diagnosis of infection. The nitroblue tetrazolium

**Table 73.1** Organisms Frequently Regarded as Normal, Colonizing Flora

| | |
|---|---|
| Skin | Upper Respiratory Tract |
| Diphtheroids (e.g., *Corynebacterium* sp.) | *Bacteroides* sp. |
| Propionibacteriaceae | *Hemophilus* sp. |
| Staphylococci | *Neisseria* sp. |
| Streptococci | Streptococci |
| Gastrointestinal tract | Genital Tract |
| *Bacteroides* sp. | *Corynebacterium* sp. |
| *Clostridium* sp. | Enterobacteriaceae |
| Diphtheroids | *Lactobacillus* sp. |
| Enterobacteriaceae (e.g., *Escherichia coli, Klebsiella* sp.) | *Mycoplasma* sp. |
| *Fusobacterium* sp. | Staphylococci |
| Streptococci (anaerobic) | Streptococci |

(NBT) reduction test detects changes in white blood cell membrane enzyme production and utilization. This test has been utilized for differentiation of bacterial versus nonbacterial causes of leukocytosis; however, the actual usefulness of this test has recently been questioned and appears to be limited.[3]

## Laboratory Identification of Pathogens

### *Direct Examination*

One of the most rapid and readily available methods for the laboratory diagnosis and identification of pathogens is direct examination of body fluids or tissues believed to be infected. Gram stain characteristics (positive, negative, or variable) and morphological appearance (e.g., coccus or bacillus) provide rapid, preliminary identification of bacteria and may be of great usefulness in selecting empiric lifesaving antimicrobial therapy in critically ill patients. Table 73.4 lists some common infecting pathogens grouped according to Gram stain and other characteristics. Certain other bacterial (e.g., mycobacteria) and fungal pathogens may be best identified microscopically using special reagents or stains. Other pathogens may be identified through special stains, "wet" mounts, "fixed" slides, or specimens treated with fluorescent antibody specific for an antigen associated with a pathogen.

**Table 73.2** Normal White Blood Cell Differential in an Adult

| | |
|---|---|
| Neutrophils (PMNs[a]) | 50–70% |
| Immature neutrophils (bands, stabs) | 3–5% |
| Metamyelocytes | 0–1% |
| Lymphocytes | 20–40% |
| Monocytes | 0–7% |
| Eosinophils | 0–5% |
| Basophils | 0–1% |

[a] Polymorphonuclear leukocytes.

**Table 73.3** Some Nonspecific Laboratory Tests Utilized in the Diagnosis of Infectious Disease

| |
|---|
| White blood cell count |
| Erythrocyte sedimentation rate (ESR, "sed rate") |
| Serum complement |
| "Acute phase" reactants (e.g., haptoglobin, C-reactive protein, $\alpha_1$-antitrypsin, fibrinogen) |
| Nitroblue tetrazolium (NBT) test for neutrophils |

### *Cultures*

Growth and subsequent identification of etiologic agents from body fluids or tissues believed to be infected remain the most frequently utilized method of determining the etiology of infection. Most clinical laboratories are now capable of cultivating aerobic and anaerobic gram-positive and gram-negative bacteria and certain fungi. Culture of more fastidious bacteria, which may require special media or conditions (e.g., mycobacteria, chlamydia, *Legionella* sp.), and viral cultures are often only performed in larger hospitals or reference laboratories because of the expense of equipment and time involved in processing samples.

Assurance of proper collection and handling of specimens greatly enhances the correct interpretation and usefulness of culture of infected material. Careful collection of certain specimens (e.g., urine, sputum) to avoid contamination with commensal organisms is necessary to obtain meaningful results. When more fastidious organisms are suspected to be present in a sample, rapid transport of the specimen in appropriate media or containers to the microbiology laboratory for processing is necessary to ensure recovery of the pathogen. For example, anaerobic bacteria from an abscess are best recovered when fluid for culture is collected by aspiration rather than on an easily obtained cotton swab.

Once growth of a pathogen is established, bacteria are identified by fermentation properties, morphology, and growth characteristics on selective media. Biochemical profiling has become increasingly important in the rapid identification of bacteria. For example, *Pseudomonas aeruginosa* can be readily differentiated from certain other hospital-acquired gram-negative aerobic bacilli by the oxidase test, which takes only a few minutes to perform. This information may be of great value in the selection or adjustment of empiric antibiotic therapy in a patient infected with this pathogen.

Recent technological advances have enabled the rapid detection of growth of bacteria present in certain specimens. One automated blood culturing system (Bactec) employs bottles of growth media containing $^{14}C$-labeled carbohydrates and amino acids. Patient blood samples for culture are inoculated into these bottles and incubated. Early growth of bacteria is detected through determination of radiolabeled $CO_2$ produced by bacteria growing in bottles. Another system (Septacheck) utilizes a slide containing different growth media which is "rinsed" with inoculated blood culture media through periodic inversion of the bottles. Growth is detected by visual inspection of the slides. Both systems have been shown to detect the presence of certain bacteria in blood cultures significantly sooner than conventional methods, which involve visual inspection of bottles for

**Table 73.4** Examples of Important Bacterial Pathogens Classified According to Staining Characteristics, Morphology, and Other Salient Features

- **Gram-Positive Cocci**
- Staphylococci
  - Coagulase-positive
    - *Staphylococcus aureus*
  - Coagulase-negative
    - *Staphylococcus epidermidis*
- Streptococci
  - Anaerobes
    - Peptostreptoccus
    - *Streptococcus pneumoniae* (diplococcus, pneumococcus)
  - Group A, β-hemolytic
    - *Streptococcus pyogenes*
  - Group B
    - *Streptococcus agalactiae*
  - Group D
    - Enterococcal species
      - *Enterococcus faecalis*
      - *Enterococcus durans*
      - *Enterococcus faecium*
    - Nonenterococcal species
      - *Streptococcus bovis*
      - *Streptococcus equinus*
    - Viridans group
      - *Streptococcus sanguis*
      - *Streptococcus mitior*
      - *Streptococcus mutans*
      - *Streptococcus milleri*
- **Gram-Positive Bacilli**
- *Bacillus* sp.
  - *Bacillus cereus*
- *Clostridium* sp.
  - *Clostridium difficile*
  - *Clostridium perfringens*
  - *Clostridium tetani*
- Diphtheroids
  - *Corynebacterium diphtheriae*
  - *Corynebacterium* JK strain
- *Listeria monocytogenes*
- **Gram-Negative Bacilli**
- Anaerobes
  - *Bacteroides fragilis*
- *Campylobacter* sp.
- Enterobacteriaceae
  - *Citrobacter* sp.
  - *Enterobacter* sp.
  - *Escherichia coli*
  - *Klebsiella* sp.
  - *Serratia* sp.
  - *Morganella* sp.
  - *Proteus*
    - Indole-negative—*P. mirabilis*
    - Indole-positive—*P. vulgaris*
  - *Providencia* sp.
- *Pseudomonas* sp.
  - *Pseudomonas aeruginosa*
  - *Pseudomonas cepacia*
  - *Pseudomonas maltophilia*
- **Gram-Negative Cocci**
  - *Branhamella (Neisseria) catarrhalis*
  - *Neisseria gonorrhoeae*
  - *Neisseria meningitidis*
- **Mycobacteria (acid-fast bacilli)**
  - *Mycobacterium avium–intracellulare*
  - *Mycobacterium fortuitum*
  - *Mycobacterium tuberculosis*
- **Fungi**
- Yeasts
  - *Torulopsis glabrata*
  - *Candida* sp.
  - *Cryptococcus neoformans*
- *Aspergillus* sp.
  - *Aspergillus fumigatus*

turbidity or "blind" subculturing from bottles onto solid media.[4]

Rapid identification of bacteria may be accomplished by analysis of the fermentation properties of an organism with commercially available biochemical testing panels. A suspension of the organism is inoculated into several small chambers containing various sugars or other reagents. After an appropriate period of incubation, the results are noted and reduced to a code number which is then used to identify the bacteria in a reference manual.

An increasing number of laboratories are capable of isolation of viral pathogens. Appropriately collected specimens are inoculated into tissue culture, and the virus type is identified by characteristic changes in culture cell morphology.

***Effects of Antimicrobial Therapy on Culture Results*** Growth of organisms in specimens collected from patients receiving antimicrobial therapy may be slowed or inhibited by antibiotic present in the specimen; this is particularly true in blood cultures where more fastidious organisms are present. This problem is partially remedied by the presence of sodium polyanetholesulfonate (SPS), a polyanionic compound added to most blood culture media for its anticoagulant properties. In addition, SPS appears to be capable of inactivating the aminoglycoside and polymyxin classes of antibiotics.[5,6] Many β-lactam antibiotics are inactivated by β-lactamase, which some laboratories add routinely to all blood culture bottles. Thiol broth (Difco Laboratories, Detroit, MI) has also been reported to inactivate some penicillins and gentamicin.[7]

Two commercially available methods of inactivating antimicrobials "carried over" into blood culture media have become available for clinical use. The Antibiotic Removal Device (ARD, Marion Scientific) consists of a bottle containing resin beads that are capable of binding (and thus inactivating) many frequently used antibiotics (Table 73.5).

**Table 73.5** Methods Reported to Inactivate Various Antimicrobials in Vitro[5–15]

| *Drug* | *β-Lactamase* | *SPS[a]* | *ARD[b]* | *Bactec 16B* | *Thiol Broth* |
|---|---|---|---|---|---|
| Aminoglycosides | | | | | |
| amikacin, gentamicin, kanamycin, tobramycin | | X | X | X | X[c] |
| Amphotericin B | | | X | X | |
| Cephalosporins | | | | | |
| cefazolin, cephalexin, cephalothin, cefoxitin, cefotaxime | X | | X | X | |
| Cefamandole | X | | | X | |
| Moxalactam | | | | X | |
| Clindamycin | | | X | X | |
| Erythromycin | | | X | X | |
| Ketoconazole | | | X | | |
| Metronidazole | | | X | | |
| Penicillins | | | | | |
| ampicillin, cloxacillin, carbenicillin, methicillin, nafcillin, oxacillin | X | | X | X | X[d] |
| Azlocillin | X | | | X | |
| Mezlocillin | X | | | X | |
| Ticarcillin | X | | X | X | |
| Tetracycline | | | X | X | |
| Trimethoprim–sulfamethoxazole | | | X | X | |
| Vancomycin | | | X | X | |

[a] Sodium polyanetholesulfonate.
[b] Antibiotic Removal Device (Marion Scientific).
[c] Gentamicin only tested.
[d] Carbenicillin, oxacillin, and nafcillin only tested.

Use of this device involves injection of a blood sample for culture into a bead-containing bottle; this bottle is then rotated for approximately 45 minutes to ensure contact of the sample with the beads. Blood is then removed from this bottle and inoculated into blood culture media for processing as usual.[8] Alternatively, commercial sources of bottled blood culture media containing antibiotic-binding resins (e.g., Bactec 16B) are now available, thus eliminating the extra handling required by the ARD. Table 73.5 depicts the antibiotics reportedly "inactivated" by these methods.[9] Data on the Bactec 16B system have been largely extrapolated from studies where parallel processing of blood cultures from patients receiving antibiotics demonstrated recovery of organisms only from aliquots treated with the ARD or resin beads; thus, complete inactivation of antibiotics was "'assumed" in many cases.[10] Studies evaluating the efficiency of both of these systems in the removal of known amounts of certain antibiotics reveal that not all of the antibiotic present is bound[11]; this appears to be the case for some of the newer, more potent β-lactam components (e.g., imipenem). Most studies, however, have shown both methods to be highly effective in detecting bacteremia in patients receiving antimicrobial therapy as compared with conventional methods.[12–14] These systems may be most useful for recovery of organisms from patients who are receiving antibiotics and are suspected of having bacteremia of unknown etiology; however, the role of these devices in monitoring therapy in patients with bacterial infections of established etiology (e.g., *Staphylococcus aureus* endocarditis) is not known.[15]

### *Immunodiagnosis of Infection*

For many bacterial, fungal, and viral infections, routine culture of an etiologic agent is neither feasible nor possible. For many infections, immunologic methods that detect the presence of antibody directed against a pathogen are used in the definitive diagnosis of infection. Antibodies may be detected by immunodiffusion, immunofluorescence, and immunoassay (e.g., enzyme-linked immunosorbent assay, ELISA).

Similar principles are also utilized in detection of bacterial, fungal, and viral antigens in clinical specimens. The methods include agglutination, immunoelectrophoresis, and immunoassay. These methods have the advantages of usually being rapid and of having acceptable sensitivity (i.e, the ability to detect a true positive test) and specificity (i.e., the ability of a test to give a negative result in the absence of disease). Many tests (e.g., latex agglutination test for identification of the group A streptococcus) can be performed in a physician's office in less than an hour.[16]

## Evaluation of the Pharmacodynamic Properties of Antimicrobials

### *In Vitro Susceptibility Testing*

Assessment of antimicrobial activity against a specific pathogen is an important guide for selection of appropriate antimicrobial therapy. Despite widespread acceptance of many methods, there yet remain numerous controversies surrounding the performance and interpretation of these tests.[1,17] Nevertheless, in vitro antibiotic susceptibility testing remains an important means of individualizing patient pharmacotherapy of certain infectious diseases.

#### Minimum Inhibitory Concentration

The "time-tested" method of evaluating antimicrobial activity against bacteria has utilized liquid media to determine the minimum inhibitory concentration (MIC). Varying concentrations of an antimicrobial are prepared in liquid growth medium (i.e., broth), usually in serial twofold dilutions (Fig. 77.1). A standard number of bacteria (inoculum) are added to each tube and the mixture is incubated at a standard temperature (usually 37°C) for 18–24 hours. After incubation, tubes are examined for growth (i.e., clarity versus turbidity); the minimum inhibitory concentration is defined as the tube containing the lowest concentration of antibiotic that prevented visible growth (Fig. 73.1).

The MIC may also be determined on solid medium using an agar-dilution method. In fact, susceptibility testing of certain more fastidious bacteria (e.g., *Mycobacterium tuberculosis*) may be accomplished only on solid medium. As with the tube-dilution method, the agent to be tested is diluted in molten agar to make known concentrations of drug. Molten agar is then transformed into petri dishes and allowed to harden. After the agar has hardened, bacterial inocula are applied to the surface of the agar in drops or with calibrated multitip prongs (Steers replicator). Plates are then incubated and inspected for growth. As with the tube-dilution method, the MIC is the plate with the lowest drug concentration on which no growth of the organism is observed.

***Interpretation*** Although the MIC serves as a quantitative measure of a drug's activity against bacteria, clinical use of the MIC value is facilitated through interpretative guidelines of categories familiar to most clinicians. On the basis of the MIC (or its correlates), an organism may be designated as "susceptible," "moderately susceptible," "conditionally susceptible," or "resistant" to the agent tested.

Organisms termed susceptible to an antibiotic would have the lowest MICs and thus would be the organisms most likely eradicated during therapy of human infection using usual doses of an antimicrobial. Resistant organisms are those bacteria with higher MICs, suggesting that less than optimal clinical results might be anticipated if the tested drug was utilized in the treatment of an infection resulting from these organisms. Moderately susceptible organisms constitute a middle range of bacteria that might be less likely to be effectively treated than those in the susceptible range; therefore, the drug should be used at maximum doses. For some bacteria, the number of strains with MICs in this range is small and thus organisms with a certain MIC may be termed "indeterminant," meaning that organisms may be either susceptible or resistant. Both the "moderately susceptible" and "indeterminant" classifications serve as a "buffer zone" to avoid major changes in the interpretation of the MIC value (i.e., susceptible versus resistant) which will inherently vary plus-or-minus one twofold dilution step (see later). Finally, organisms may be termed "conditionally susceptible" to a drug. This classification is usually applied in those instances in which organisms are inhibited by high drug concentrations achievable only in certain body fluids

**Figure 73.1** Tube-dilution MIC determination for gentamicin against a strain of *Pseudomonas aeruginosa*. The gentamicin concentrations in each tube (from left to right) are 0 (C), 0.5, 1, 2, 4, 8, and 16 μg/mL, respectively. Tubes are shown following a 20-hour incubation at 37°C. Turbidity is seen in the tubes containing no drug (C) and 0.5, 1, and 2 μg/mL gentamicin; the tubes containing 4, 8, and 16 μg/mL gentamicin are clear. The MIC of this organism for gentamicin is 4 μg/mL.

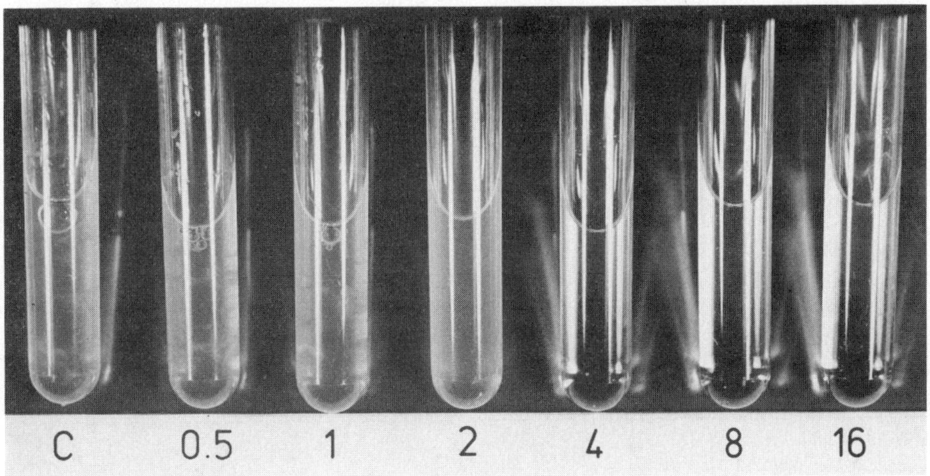

(e.g., urine); however, this classification has been deleted from recently approved standards for susceptibility testing although some laboratories may continue to use it.[18]

The MIC should not be regarded as an "all-or-none" phenomenon, as numerous effects of subinhibitory concentrations of an antibiotic on bacteria have been described.[17] Moreover, subpopulations of bacteria within an inoculum may be inhibited by drug concentrations below the MIC, while others may require concentrations much higher than the measured MIC. These subpopulations may be important determinants of clinical response to antimicrobial therapy.

It is emphasized that while these interpretative classes are of great value in selecting antimicrobial therapy, they are not accurate predictors of success or failure of drug therapy.[17] Drug therapy of infectious diseases caused by organisms susceptible to the agent used is not an assurance of a clinical cure, as numerous other factors may be important in achieving a good clinical result. For example, *Salmonella typhi* may be susceptible in vitro to the aminoglycosides, tetracyclines, and cephalosporins; however, only ampicillin, chloramphenicol, and folate antagonists have been shown to be effective therapy of enteric fever. The results of drug susceptibility testing must be applied in the context of the site of infection, the pharmacodynamic and pharmacokinetic properties of the drug, and the clinical status of the patient.

Table 73.6 lists interpretative categories and their respective MIC "breakpoints" for susceptible, moderately susceptible, and resistant classifications for some frequently used antimicrobials. Breakpoint concentrations are selected on three criteria.[21] First, the pharmacokinetic properties of the

**Table 73.6** Interpretive Breakpoints (μg/mL) for Broth-Dilution MIC Testing

| *Drug* | *Susceptible* | *Moderately susceptible* | *Resistant* |
|---|---|---|---|
| Aminoglycosides | | | |
| Amikacin, kanamycin | ≤ 16 | 32 | ≥ 64 |
| Gentamicin, tobramycin | ≤ 4 | 8 | ≥ 16 |
| Netilmicin | ≤ 4 | 8–16 | ≥ 32 |
| Aztreonam | ≤ 8 | 16 | ≥ 32 |
| Cephalosporins | | | |
| Cefazolin, cephalothin, cefamandole, ceforanide, cefonicid, cefuroxime, ceftazidime | ≤ 8 | 16 | ≥ 32 |
| Cefotaxime, ceftizoxime, ceftriaxone, moxalactam | ≤ 8 | 16–32 | ≥ 64 |
| Cefoperazone | ≤ 16 | 32 | ≥ 64 |
| Clindamycin | ≤ 0.5 | 1–4 | ≥ 8 |
| Erythromycin | ≤ 0.5 | 1–4 | ≥ 8 |
| Imipenem | ≤ 4 | 8 | ≥ 16 |
| Penicillins | | | |
| Amoxicillin/clavulanate | | | |
| *Hemophilus* sp. | ≤ 4/2 | — | ≥ 8/4 |
| Others | ≤ 8/4 | 16/8 | ≥32/16 |
| Ampicillin | | | |
| *Hemophilus* sp. | ≤ 2 | — | ≥ 4 |
| Enterobacteriaceae | ≤ 8 | 16 | ≥ 32 |
| Azlocillin (for *Pseudomonas aeruginosa*) | ≤ 64 | — | ≥ 128 |
| Mezlocillin, piperacillin, ticarcillin with or without clavulanate | ≤ 16 | 32–64 | ≥ 128 |
| Nafcillin, oxacillin | ≤ 2 | — | ≥ 4 |
| Penicillin G | | | |
| *Neisseria gonorrhoeae*, nonenterococcal streptococci | ≤ 0.12 | 0.25–2 | ≥ 4 |
| Enterococci | — | ≤ 8 | ≥ 16 |
| Quinolones | | | |
| Ciprofloxacin | ≤ 1 | 1<MIC≤ 2 | > 2 |
| Enoxacin[a] | ≤ 2 | 4 | > 4 |
| Norfloxacin | ≤ 4 | — | > 4 |
| Tetracyclines | 4 | 8 | 16 |
| Trimethoprim–sulfamethoxazole | 2/38 | — | 4/76 |
| Vancomycin | 4 | 8–16 | 32 |

[a] Tentative

Compiled from References 18–20.

drug in man are of obvious importance. Serum and tissue concentrations following usual doses should normally exceed the MIC of an organism; however, the magnitude and duration of time that these concentrations should exceed the MIC are controversial and appear to vary according to the drug class and bacterial species. Second, the population distribution of MICs of a group of bacteria for a drug is considered. Figure 73.2 depicts the distribution of MICs for cefotetan, a cephalosporin antibiotic.[22] Breakpoints set in the areas of a peak are less desirable, as a large number of organisms would be affected by changes resulting from the usual twofold dilution variability of the test; that is, many organisms would fluctuate between different interpretative categories. Third, the clinical efficacy of an agent against bacteria with a given MIC is considered in clinical trials. Although the clinical response of patients cannot always be correlated with the MIC of an infecting pathogen, observations on the response of a large number of patients with infections resulting from organisms with MICs in a borderline range may be useful in selecting final breakpoints.

***Limitations*** The MIC is regarded as the most standardized quantitative measure of antimicrobial activity; however, it is not without some limitations. Preparation of several serial twofold drug dilutions and inoculation with bacteria are both time consuming and expensive, and thus not feasible in most clinical laboratories. This disadvantage has been largely bypassed by the development of techniques using smaller volumes of liquid medium and automation (see later). Bacterial growth medium and cation content can significantly affect the activity of many drugs. For example, aminoglycoside[23] and quinolone[24] antibiotics are less active against *Pseudomonas aeruginosa* in medium supplemented with physiological concentrations of magnesium and calcium cations than in medium without these additions. The MICs of many antibiotics that are highly bound to plasma proteins are significantly higher in medium containing human serum than in unsupplemented medium.[25] The inoculum size (the amount of bacteria tested) significantly affects the MIC of some drugs against certain organisms. This is particularly true for most $\beta$-lactam antibiotics and gram-negative bacilli, where a 100-fold increase in the size of the inoculum increases the MIC to an extent that organisms might be considered susceptible at a lower inoculum, but resistant at a larger one. Fortunately, a series of guidelines for standardization of these variables and other factors for performance of these tests has recently been published and has been largely adopted by most clinical and research laboratories.[18]

#### Disk Diffusion Assay

In view of the impracticality of performing MIC testing on a large number of organisms against numerous drugs in a clinical hospital laboratory, Kirby and Bauer developed a rapid, convenient method of determining the susceptibility of bacteria to several antibiotics in the 1950s.[26] Paper disks impregnated with a fixed amount of antibiotic are placed onto an agar surface with a "lawn" of the bacteria to be tested. Drug diffuses from the disk into the medium, with drug concentrations in the agar decreasing proportionally to the distance from the disk. The plate is incubated and bacteria grow on the surface of the agar, except in areas

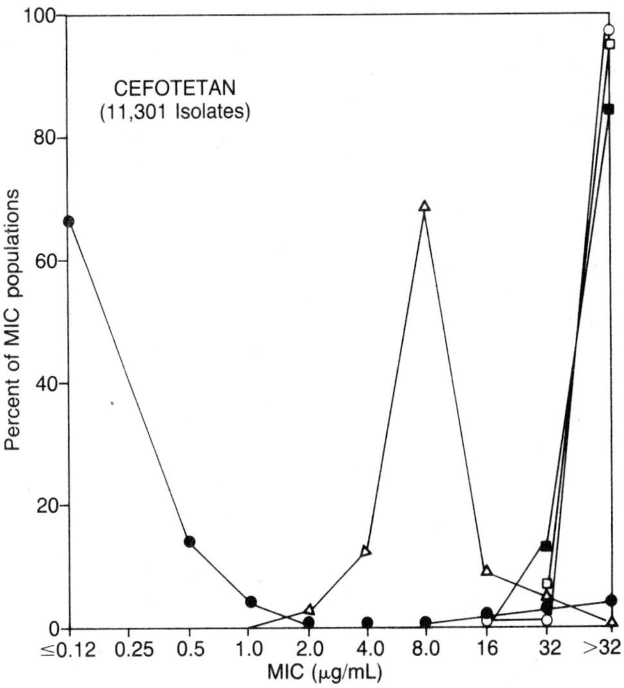


**Figure 73.2** Distribution of MICs of *Pseudomonas aeruginosa* (■), *Acinetobacter* sp (□), *Enterobacteriaceae* (●), *Staphylococcus aureus* (△), and enterococci (○) for cefotetan. *(From Ayers LW, Jones RN, Barry AL, et al: Cefotetan, a new cephamycin: comparison of in vitro antimicrobial activity with other cephems, beta-lactamase stability, and preliminary recommendations for disk diffusion testing. Antimicrob Agents Chemother 1982;22:875, with permission.)*

where the drug concentration in the agar exceeds the MIC. Thus, "zones of inhibition" are produced and their diameters are measured using calipers or other devices.

Interpretation of the zone size is facilitated by the log–linear relationship between the MIC and the zone of inhibition produced by a disk containing a fixed amount of drug. As shown in Figure 73.3, the zone sizes of organisms with higher MICs tend to be small while more susceptible organisms tend to have large zones. "Scattergrams" are constructed using the MICs and zones of inhibitions measured on agar from studies of a large number of bacteria (Fig. 73.3). Using MIC breakpoints (i.e., susceptible, resistant), the corresponding zone breakpoints are constructed. As shown in Figure 73.3, this relationship is not perfect in that some organisms with higher MICs occasionally have large zones, and vice versa. Boundaries for zone breakpoints are usually constructed to avoid the most unsatisfactory "major" error of classifying an organism susceptible by the diffusion test (i.e., large zone) when it is resistant according to the more quantitative MIC test.

The disk diffusion method has proved extremely useful in the assessment of the activity of many antibiotics against large numbers of bacteria routinely isolated in a clinical laboratory. Like the MIC test, numerous factors may influence the size of the zones of inhibition; thus, standardization of techniques, drug content in disks, and other factors has been necessary. With the availability of newer automated

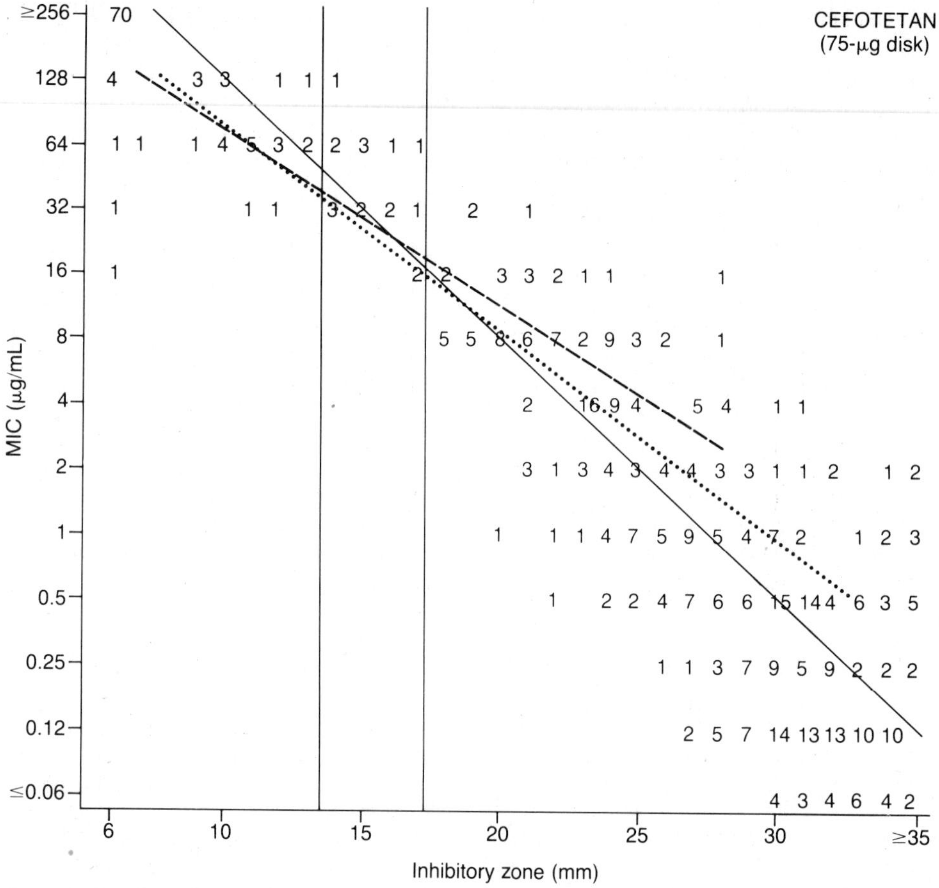


**Figure 73.3** Scattergram showing the relationship between MIC and zone of inhibition for cefotetan. Numbers represent numbers of isolates with a given MIC and zone of inhibition. Regression lines for MICs from 0.01 to 256 (—), 0.5 to 256 (···), and 2 to 256 (- - -) mg/L are drawn for comparison. Vertical lines indicate corresponding breakpoints for resistant (MIC > 64 mg/mL, zone size < 15 mm) and susceptible (MIC ≤ 16 mg/L; zone size > 18 mm). *(From Ayers LW, Jones RN, Barry AL, et al: Cefotetan, a new cephamycin: comparison of in vitro antimicrobial activity with other cephems, beta-lactamase stability, and preliminary recommendations for disk diffusion testing. Antimicrob Agents Chemother 1982;22:875, with permission.)*

susceptibility systems using broth media and the increasing emphasis on determination of the MIC of clinical isolates, this technique is slowly being phased out in many clinical laboratories.

### *Automated Antimicrobial Susceptibility Testing*

The availability of many new antimicrobials as well as the greater demand for rapid quantitative susceptibility testing of clinical isolates has led to the development of several automated systems for determining antimicrobial susceptibility. Most of these systems test drugs and bacteria in very small volumes of broth as is done with the tube-dilution method. Transmission or scattering of light through cuvettes or microdilution wells containing drug and bacteria is periodically or continuously monitored and recorded in a computer. In many systems, incubation for as little as 3 hours is all that is required to obtain results. Studies comparing many of these newer systems with standard techniques of broth or agar dilution have documented good agreement between methods.[27]

## Special in Vitro Tests of Antimicrobial Activity

### *Minimum Bactericidal Concentration*

While the MIC is useful in determining the lowest concentration of drug capable of inhibiting an organism's growth, it may also be of value in determining if an antimicrobial will kill the organism (i.e., if it is bactericidal). The ability of an antibiotic to exert a bactericidal effect at clinically achievable drug concentrations may be assessed by determination of the minimum bactericidal concentration (MBC). The test is performed using the results from broth-dilution MIC testing. An aliquot of broth from each dilution without evidence of bacterial growth (i.e., "clear" to tubes) is inoculated onto antibiotic-free agar and incubated for 24 hours. The MBC is defined as the lowest concentration of drug that results in a 99.9% reduction in the initial bacterial density (3 log drop). For example, if $1 \times 10^5$ CFU of bacteria per milliliter was originally inoculated into broth medium, then only $10^2$ CFU of bacteria per milliliter must remain after exposure in liquid medium to meet the criteria for bactericidal activity.

Bactericidal activity of an antimicrobial agent alone (or in combination) may be crucial in the area of certain infections, such as bacterial endocarditis. Some strains of bacteria normally "killed" by certain antibiotics are sometimes only inhibited by them; these strains are often termed "tolerant." The existence of antimicrobial tolerance has been defined as the situation where the MBC:MIC ratio is greater than or equal to 32.[28] Tolerance has been described primarily with β-lactam antibiotics and includes many strains of bacteria, particularly *Staphylococcus* sp. and *Streptococcus* sp. The clinical significance of tolerance in many of these strains, particularly with *Staphylococcus aureus*, is controversial.[29]

### *Timed-Kill Curve*

Although the MBC test yields information on the net reduction in bacteria over a 24-hour period, it may be desirable to characterize the *rate* of killing of bacteria during exposure to antimicrobials alone or in combination. Figure 73.4 depicts an example of a timed-kill curve for varying concentrations of ciprofloxacin, a fluoroquinolone antibiotic, against *Pseudomonas aeruginosa*. As shown in this example, the rate of bacterial killing and the selection of resistant bacteria are concentration dependent. The timed-kill curve analysis appears to be most useful in research studies evaluating antimicrobial activity alone or in combination, and perhaps in some selected instances in the clinical setting for selection and assessment of antibiotic therapy of serious infections resulting from certain bacteria.

### *Testing of Antimicrobial Combinations*

It is occasionally desirable to assess the effect of various combinations of antibiotics against a bacterial pathogen. Generally, *antimicrobial synergism* is defined as an interaction between two or more agents that results in an effect greater than that expected from the sum of their independent effects. Alternatively, combinations may be considered *antagonistic* if a combination of antimicrobials exerts an effect less than that observed when each agent is considered independently. Combinations of antimicrobials not synergistic or antagonistic may be termed *indifferent* if the agents appear to work similarly alone or in combination, or *additive* if the effects of a combination simply reflect addition of each of their respective activities.[30]

**Figure 73.4** Timed-kill curve showing the effect of 4 mg/L (□), 2 mg/L (+), and 0.4 mg/L (◇) ciprofloxacin on a strain of *Pseudomonas aeruginosa* (△ = control). *(From M. N. Dudley, unpublished observations.)*

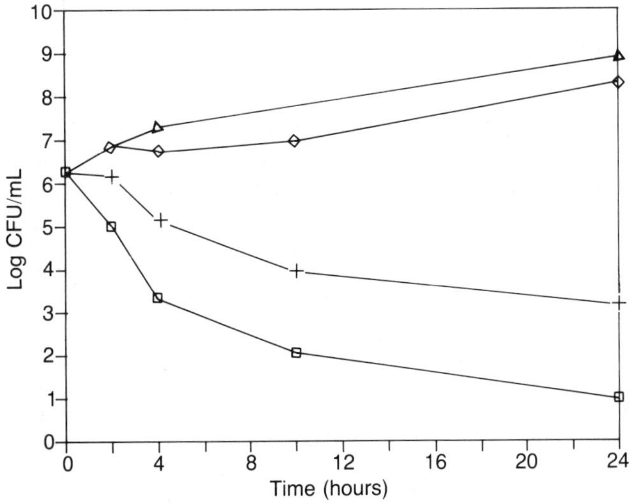


The clinical significance of antimicrobial synergism and antagonism has been the subject of several reviews.[30,31] Older as well as more recent studies suggest that the presence of antimicrobial synergism may enhance the clinical response in neutropenic patients with infection; this appears to be particularly true in bacteremia or infections resulting from *P. aeruginosa*.[31] Other studies in enterococcal endocarditis, particularly in animal models, have stressed the importance of antimicrobial combinations resulting in a synergistic effect for optimal cure of valve infection.[32]

In vivo antagonism between antimicrobials and correlation with in vitro observations have been observed less frequently. The most often cited example of in vivo antagonism is from the study of Lepper and Dowling.[33] They demonstrated a higher fatality rate in adults with pneumococcal meningitis treated with penicillin plus a tetracycline (an antagonistic combination in vitro) than in those treated with penicillin alone.[33] Sande et al also demonstrated in vitro and in vivo antagonism between chloramphenicol and gentamicin in rabbits in which meningitis had been experimentally induced with *Listeria monocytogenes*.[34]

Table 73.7 lists several examples of drug combinations frequently associated with synergism or antagonism in vitro.

While the definitions just introduced appear straightforward in description, the most appropriate methodology for use in the clinical laboratory to detect these interactions is unsettled.[35] Some methods are capable of describing interactions of antimicrobials only on the basis of inhibitory properties, while others utilize bactericidal endpoints. The methodologies frequently employed in research as well in clinical laboratories are briefly described below.

#### **Checkerboard/Isobologram**

This method is most frequently utilized in testing antimicrobial combinations because of its versatility and simplicity.[36] Concentrations of one antimicrobial are prepared in the range four to five dilutions below and one to two dilutions above the MIC. A similar scheme is used for the second antimicrobial so that a "checkerboard" of all possible combinations (in twofold dilutions of the MIC) of each drug exists. This test may be performed using liquid medium (and thus inhibitory or bactericidal endpoints may be used) or by the agar-dilution method. Bacteria are then added and the results (i.e., inhibition or bactericidal activity) are recorded as with MIC or MBC testing. The lowest concentration of drug within each respective row or column that inhibits growth (or is bactericidal) is plotted on $x$ and $y$ axes to form an isobologram (Fig. 73.5). The line connecting the respective MICs for each drug is the line of additivity. An inward

**Table 73.7** Examples of Drug Combinations Frequently Synergistic or Antagonistic in Vitro Against Bacteria and Fungi

| *Drug combinations* | *Example* |
|---|---|
| Synergistic | |
| Aminoglycosides | |
| + A broad-spectrum penicillin[a] | Gram-negative bacilli |
| + A cephalosporin | Gram-negative bacilli |
| + Ampicillin or penicillin G | Enterococci |
| + Antistaphylococcal penicillin | Staphylococci |
| Penicillins | |
| Nafcillin or oxacillin + rifampin | Staphylococci |
| Broad-spectrum penicillin[a] + a third-generation cephalosporin | Gram-negative bacilli |
| Antifungals | |
| Amphotericin B + flucytosine | *Cryptococcus neoformans* |
| Antagonistic | |
| Broad-spectrum penicillin | |
| + A cephalosporin | *Enterobacter cloacae*, *Pseudomonas aeruginosa*, *Citrobacter* sp. |
| + Chloramphenicol | *Streptococcus pneumoniae* |
| Aminoglycoside + chloramphenicol | Enterobacteriaceae |

[a] Mezlocillin, piperacillin, ticarcillin, or azlocillin

bowing of the plotted line indicates an additivity or synergism; an outward bowing denotes antagonism.

Alternatively, an isobologram may be expressed mathematically by calculation of the fractional inhibitory concentration index (FIC index).[36] The FIC index is calculated as

$$\text{FIC} = \frac{A}{\text{MIC}_A} + \frac{B}{\text{MIC}_B}$$

where $A$ or $B$ is the lowest concentration of drug that is inhibitory in the presence of the second drug, and the MIC is the minimum inhibitory concentration of the drug when tested alone. With this method, synergy is defined as an FIC index less than or equal to 0.5, additivity is an FIC index equal to 1, and antagonism corresponds to an FIC index greater than or equal to 2. As described previously, bactericidal endpoints (i.e., MBCs) may alternatively be used in this equation.

### Timed-Kill Curves

Combinations of two antimicrobials may increase or decrease the rate of killing relative to that observed with either antibiotic alone. To detect this interaction, the timed kill is performed as described earlier, except that two antibiotics at fixed concentrations are incubated with bacteria over a given period of time (Fig. 73.6). Synergism with this method is defined as a greater than or equal to 100-fold increase in killing of bacteria with the combination as compared with either drug alone when tested at the same concentration (Fig. 73.5).[36]

### Other Methods

Other less frequently utilized qualitative methods of evaluating antimicrobials include the double-disk diffusion test. This test is performed by placing two disks containing one of each of the antibiotics to be tested on solid medium in such proximity that their zones of inhibition would not be expected to overlap. A synergistic or additive interaction is observed when there is an extension of these zones of inhibition between the two drugs.

Other more elaborate methods of evaluating antimicrobial combinations include spectrophotometric analysis[37] and the use of in vitro kinetic models.[38] With the spectrophotometric method, growth rate constants of bacteria as a function of drug concentration alone or in combination are compared with those observed in unexposed organisms. In vitro kinetic models expose bacteria to changing concentrations of two drugs as would occur in vivo. The number of viable organisms surviving exposure to both drugs as a function of time with the combination regimen is compared with the results of single-drug experiments. Both techniques have been limited to use in the research laboratory.

### Interpretation and Use

Considerable controversy exists regarding the clinical significance of in vitro synergy (see Chapter 78). Moreover, it still remains unclear as to which of these methods best predicts in vivo synergy, as there often is a discrepancy between the conclusions obtained using different tests. For example, one study found significant disagreements in the conclusions of checkerboard and killing curve techniques which varied depending on the criteria used for defining synergism as well as other technical factors.[39] In some cases, synergism between two drugs against an organism reflects increased killing of bacteria; in others, a synergistic effect may simply reflect the prevention by the second drug of the growth (and thus "emergence") of resistant subpopulations of bacteria that would normally grow to detectable numbers during a 24-hour incubation with a single drug.[35]

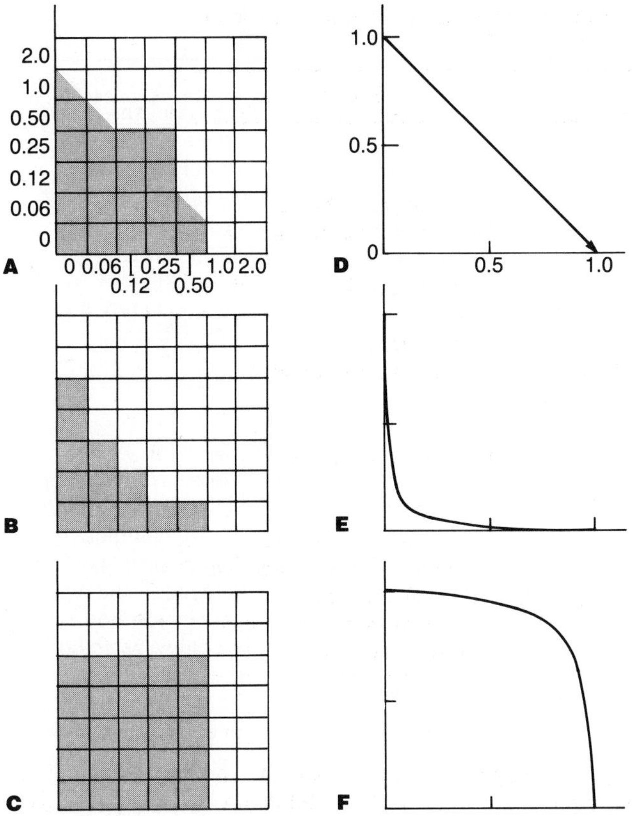


**Figure 73.5** (A–C) Assessment of antimicrobial combinations using the "checkerboard" dilution technique. Increasing concentrations of each drug are found as one moves from the lower left corner upward (first drug) and to the right (second drug). Shaded areas depict areas of visible growth after incubation. (D–F) Corresponding isobolograms from the results, plotted as fractions of the MIC of each drug. Panels A/D, B/E, and C/F depict additivity, synergy, and antagonism, respectively. *(Adapted from Krogstad DJ, Moellering RC, Jr: Antimicrobial combinations, in Lorian V (Ed): Antibiotics in Laboratory Medicine, 2nd ed. Baltimore, Williams and Wilkins, 1986, p 548, with permission.)*

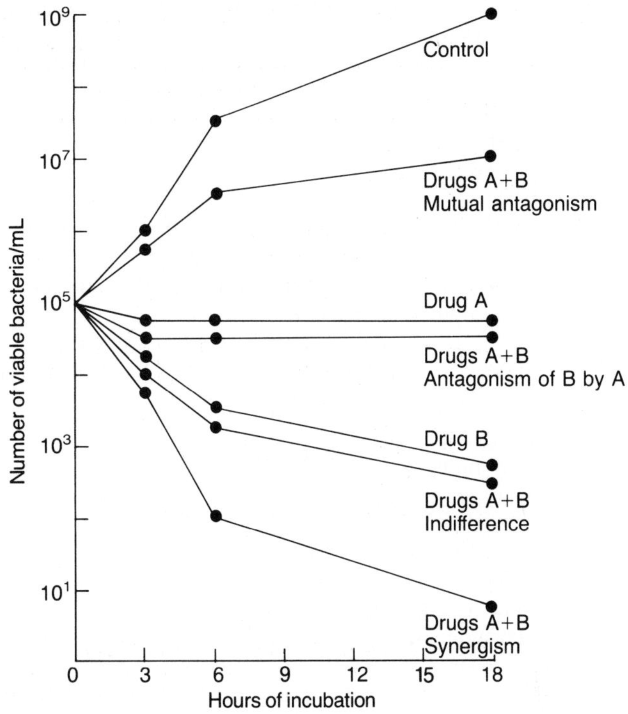


**Figure 73.6** Timed-kill curve illustrating synergistic, antagonistic, and indifferent effects of two antibiotics at fixed concentrations at various intervals during incubation. *(From Rahal JJ: Antibiotic combinations: the clinical relevance of synergy and antagonism. Medicine 1978;57:181, with permission.)*

Testing of antimicrobial combinations in the clinical laboratory appears to be useful in certain situations. It is often necessary to assess the activity of certain antibiotic combinations against antibiotic-resistant bacteria isolated from a patient (e.g., gram-negative bacilli). In this setting, it is hoped that the strain that is resistant to one or both of the single drugs might become "susceptible" to the combination through a synergistic interaction. In other cases, a synergistic combination may be desired when either of the drugs alone is only bacteriostatic against an organism. For example, most enterococci (e.g., *Enterococcus faecalis*) are inhibited but not killed by clinically achievable concentrations of penicillin derivatives. In certain enterococcal infections (e.g., bacterial endocarditis), the bacteriostatic activity of ampicillin or penicillin alone is inadequate treatment; thus, a combination of penicillin or ampicillin with an aminoglycoside is used for a synergistic bactericidal effect. In vitro synergy testing may be performed to guide the selection of optimal antibiotic combinations in this setting.

## Laboratory Monitoring of Antimicrobial Therapy

The pharmacokinetic properties of antimicrobials are of great interest because of the importance of delivery of adequate drug concentrations to the site of infection. Unlike other drugs for which the site of action is relatively constant, antimicrobials must attain inhibitory concentrations in a variety of body tissues and fluids. With better understanding of the pharmacokinetic properties of newer as well as older antimicrobial agents, the pharmacokinetic determinants of both efficacy and toxicity have been more completely defined.

### *Serum Bactericidal Titer*

Determination of the bactericidal titer of a serum sample from a patient receiving antimicrobial therapy is frequently used clinically to monitor antimicrobial activity in vivo. The test is similar to the determination of the MIC and MBC. The greatest dilution of a patient's serum sample that kills a standard inoculum of the infecting pathogen is determined. The test is performed by dilution of a serum sample collected from a patient receiving antimicrobial therapy (usually a "peak" or "trough" sample). The sample is diluted (usually in twofold increments) and a standard inoculum of bacteria is added to each dilution. Samples are incubated for 18–24 hours at a standard temperature; the serum inhibitory (or bacteriostatic) titer is read as the greatest dilution of serum that prevents visible growth. The serum bactericidal titer is determined by subculture of dilutions showing no growth on antibiotic-free agar. Bactericidal endpoints (i.e., 99.9% reduction in the initial inoculum) are determined as for the MBC test; the greatest dilution of serum that meets the criteria for bactericidal activity is termed the *serum bactericidal titer*.

Although the test has been most often applied to serum samples, it has also been modified for measurement of bactericidal activity in other tissues, such as synovial and cerebrospinal fluid, sputum, and urine.[40]

### Interpretation

The SBT is theoretically useful for monitoring antibiotic therapy because it integrates information regarding the antibiotic susceptibility of the infecting pathogen and the in vivo pharmacology of the antibiotic in a given patient. Indeed, the serum bactericidal titer may be mathematically derived by dividing the serum drug concentration by the MBC.[41]

As described previously, some bacteria may be considered tolerant to certain antimicrobials. Because the MBC is seldom determined in clinical laboratories, tolerant strains of bacteria may be detected by comparison of the serum inhibitory and bactericidal titers. For example, a serum inhibitory titer of 1:64 with a bactericidal titer of 1:2 would be indicative of a tolerant organism.

The SBT is probably most useful in assessing the activity of antimicrobial combinations against a pathogen. Several studies have noted enhancement of the serum bactericidal activity observed with a single drug by addition of a second agent. The serum bactericidal assay has been utilized as a means of investigating synergism between drugs in vivo.[42]

### Limitations

The same technical factors that influence the results of MIC and MBC tests are applicable to the serum bacteriostatic and bactericidal assays. In particular, the use of serum versus broth for making dilutions of the sample may be important, particularly for highly protein-bound drugs. Binding of drugs to serum proteins may be decreased when the sample is diluted in growth medium rather than serum because of dilution of proteins in the original sample. Thus, large dilutions would result in a greater free fraction of bioactive drug. These and other issues surrounding the performance and interpretation of the SBT necessitate standardization to make the test of greater clinical value.[41]

### Use

The serum bactericidal assay has been utilized in the management of patients with bacterial endocarditis, osteomyelitis, pneumonia, bacteremia, urinary tract infections, septic arthritis, and meningitis.[40,41] Despite widespread use of the test, there are no definitive data defining the optimal titer associated with cure of these infections. On the basis of studies on endocarditis, infection in the immunocompromised host, and osteomyelitis, most studies suggest that dosage regimens should achieve a peak bactericidal titer of 1:8 or greater.[40]

The SBT has also been used as a guide for changing from parenteral to oral antibiotic therapy of endocarditis or bone and joint infections.[40] Use of the test in this setting provides confirmation of adequate oral absorption of antibiotics to allow for prolonged therapy in the outpatient setting.

More recently, the SBT has been employed in the evaluation of new antimicrobial agents. In many cases, however, most of the information obtained in these analyses could be gained simply through comparison of the serum drug level and the MIC or MBC of a pathogen. The test appears to be most useful in studying the combined effects of combination antimicrobial regimens,[43] or of drugs with active metabolites.[44]

In view of the uncertainty regarding the clinical significance of the titer, its unstandardized nature, and the laboratory cost for its performance, recommendations for its clinical use are provided in Table 73.8.

**Table 73.8** Suggested Clinical Use of the Serum Bactericidal Titer

| |
|---|
| Infective Endocarditis |
| May be helpful in infections caused by organisms known to be only moderately susceptible to each of the antibiotics alone, and a combination is employed for synergism (e.g., enterococcal endocarditis) |
| Titer may be helpful in the assessment of patients responding poorly to antibiotic therapy |
| Oral Antibiotic Therapy |
| May be helpful in individual patients for adjusting doses of oral agents to achieve activity similar to that observed during parenteral therapy |

## *Tissue Versus Serum Concentrations of Antibiotics*

While extravascular distribution (or so-called "tissue penetration") of antibiotics is regarded as important for effective therapy of certain infections, the clinical usefulness of antibiotic concentration data in homogenates of excised tissue samples is not known. This is due to the artifactual (and occasionally misleading) data arising from dilution of drug present in the interstitial (and the most likely to be infected) space by intracellular water released upon homogenation of an excised tissue sample. Moreover, drug bound to extravascular proteins, or present in blood circulating to the tissue, further complicates the interpretation of drug concentrations measured in these studies. Perhaps not surprisingly, there is little clinical correlation of "tissue" levels with clinical efficacy. Therefore, measurement and attempted application of antibiotic concentration data derived from homogenates of tissue samples in the clinical setting should be discouraged.

In contrast, measurement of antibiotic concentrations in certain extravascular fluids may be useful and correlate well with efficacy. Determination of the antibiotic concentration in peritoneal and cerebrospinal fluid may be of use in the individualization of drug dosage and may optimize therapy of infections in these fluids. Difficulty in obtaining certain specimens (e.g., CSF), however, may limit the degree of monitoring of drug pharmacokinetics in these fluids.

In view of these problems, monitoring of serum concen-

**Table 73.9** "Therapeutic" Serum Concentrations for Selected Antimicrobial Agents

| *Drug* | *Time of collection* | *Target concentrations (mg/L)* | *Comments* |
|---|---|---|---|
| Aminoglycosides[46–60] Gentamicin Tobramycin | Peak (1 h after the start of a 15- to 45-min infusion) | <5 | Urinary tract infections |
| | | >5 | Bacteremia |
| | | >6 | Bacterial pneumonia |
| | | >12 | Endocarditis caused by *Pseudomonas aeruginosa* |
| | Trough | <2–3 | High trough concentrations are most likely a *result* and not a *cause* of nephrotoxicity |
| Amikacin | Peak | <15 | Urinary tract infections |
| | | >20 | Bacteremia |
| | | >24 | Bacterial pneumonia, other serious infections |
| | Trough | <9–10 | See comments regarding trough gentamicin/tobramycin concentrations |
| Flucytosine[67–70] | Peak (2 hours postdose) | <100 | Levels consistently exceeding this concentration are associated with hematological toxicity |
| | | | 5-Fluorouracil concentrations associated with toxicity have been detected in some patients receiving flucytosine |
| Vancomycin[71–75] | Peak (1–2 h after a 30- to 60-min infusion) | 20–35 | Recommendations should be considered tentative, as definitive data correlating these concentrations with efficacy and toxicity are not available |
| | Trough | <10 | |
| Chloramphenicol[62–65] | Peak (0.5–1.5 h after 0.5-h IV infusion of succinate salt, or 1.5–3.0 h after oral dose of palmitate) | 10–25 | Serum concentrations exceeding 25 may be, but are not always, associated with toxicity |

trations of antibiotics remains the most convenient and reproducible method for individualization of therapy. For most drugs the therapeutic window (toxic versus antimicrobial concentration) is large; moreover, both toxic and efficacious concentrations in vivo are not defined for many agents, particularly $\beta$-lactam antibiotics. Therefore, serum concentration monitoring is not warranted for most agents in the clinical setting because of unproven clinical value; however, serum concentration determinations (with appropriate interpretation and dosage adjustment) may be useful for the agents listed in Table 73.9.

### *Serum Antibiotic Assay*

A relationship between serum antibiotic concentrations and clinical response has been suggested in a few settings. Anderson et al[45] demonstrated that of 42 cases of "breakthrough" bacteria (recurrence of bacteremia in patients receiving appropriate antibiotic therapy for at least 24 hours), more than half of the plasma antibiotic concentrations were below the MIC of the infecting organism. This was particularly the case in patients with early breakthrough bacteremia (between 24 and 72 hours after the start of therapy). This study concluded that the failure to maintain inhibitory concentrations of both $\beta$-lactam and aminoglycoside antimicrobials may have been responsible for some of the observed relapses.

As with all drugs, possible correlations between toxicity and serum concentrations have been the subject of great interest. Unfortunately, it is usually difficult to directly relate a blood level with toxicity. Differences in pharmacologic response between patients, effects of drug toxicity on the pharmacokinetics of the agents potentially responsible, and dissociation between serum and receptor drug concentrations may all play a role in obscuring these issues. As with all drugs, toxicity should always be suspected on the basis of clinical presentation and not solely on the basis of measured drug concentration.

#### Assay Methodology

***Microbiological Assay*** Bioassay of antimicrobial agents is performed by several methods. The most commonly employed method is a modification of the disk diffusion technique used for determining antibiotic susceptibility. Paper disks are placed onto, or wells are punched into the surface of, agar containing bacteria known to be highly susceptible to the agent to be assayed. A fixed volume (usually 10 $\mu$L) of known concentration (standards) of the drug to be assayed or sample is placed on the disks or in the wells. The measured zone of inhibition and the logarithm of drug concentration are plotted; the drug concentration in unknown samples is determined from measurement of the zone site surrounding disks spotted with unknown concentrations of drug and the plotted standards.

Advantages of this method include its relative ease of

performance and low cost for equipment. Disadvantages include possible interference by other antibiotics present in this sample, lack of precision, and slow turnaround time.

***Enzyme Multiple Immunoassay Technique*** This technique (EMIT) involves measurement of the activity of an enzyme in the presence of the drug. The unknown sample or standard is mixed with an enzyme. This mixture is subsequently mixed with antibodies directed against the drug. Antibodies bind to the drug–enzyme complex, thus inactivating it. Some of the enzyme, however, remains unbound and is active; the residual activity is related to the drug concentration. Advantages of the EMIT involve rapid turnaround time, good precision, and relatively short sample preparation and run time. Disadvantages include some problems with cross-reactivity (e.g., amikacin and gentamicin) and relatively moderate cost for equipment and reagents.

***Fluorescence Polarization Immunoassay*** This technique (FPIA) involves application of the principles of fluorescence when molecules are exposed to light. Fluorescein-labeled drug and antibody directed against the drug are added in constant amounts to samples or standards. The antibody–fluorescein-labeled drug complex results in a change in the fluorescence polarization. Changes in fluorescence polarization occur because of competition for antibody between drug present in the sample and fluorescein-labeled drug added to the sample; therefore, high drug concentrations in the sample reduce the extent of binding of fluorescein-labeled drug to antibody and, thus, the extent of reduction in fluorescence polarization.

Advantages of this technique include automation through the use of the TDX system (Abbott laboratories, North Chicago, IL). Disadvantages include the expense for reagents and capital purchase of the automated system.

***Radioimmunoassay*** This technique (RIA) involves the interaction among radiolabeled drug, unlabeled antibiotic, and antibody directed against the drug. Equilibrium between antibody and the sources of antigen-radiolabeled drug and drug sample is allowed to occur and the amount of bound or free radiolabeled drug is determined using standard radiometric methods of detection. Advantages of the system include good precision; disadvantages include the expense of the disposal of radioactive wastes.

***High-Pressure Liquid Chromatography*** In this technique (HPLC) the principles of separation of different molecular species are used by passing a mobile solvent phase over a stationary phase. Drugs with a polarity similar to that of the stationary phase will be retained for a time on the column and then released. These temporarily retained substances are detected using ultraviolet, fluorescence, electrochemical, or radiometric methods. The detector response is proportional to the amount of molecules ''seen''; standard curves containing known drug concentrations are related to the detector response, usually recorded as peak area or peak height. Advantages include rapid turnaround time, precision, and ability to detect metabolites. Disadvantages include the cost of instruments and the expertise required to perform certain assays.

**Timing of Collection of Serum Samples**

Generally, peak and trough samples are collected to assess maximum and minimum antimicrobial concentrations. Some authorities have recommended collection of an additional sample toward the middle of the dosing interval to more accurately describe the terminal elimination phase, or to obtain measurable drug concentrations when trough levels are expected to be low or perhaps undetectable.

Samples for determination of the trough drug concentration should be collected just prior to the next dose. Timing the collection of samples to obtain meaningful peak concentration data appears to be critical. Generally, it is desirable to allow for the distribution phase of the drug to have been completed to more closely characterize extravascular concentrations. Moreover, most pharmacokinetic interpretive methods use the more simplified one-compartment body model. Therefore, samples for determining the peak concentration are generally collected 1 hour after the start of a 15- to 45-minute intravenous infusion, but there are some exceptions (see Table 73.9). Serum concentrations of orally administered drugs also tend to peak 1 hour after the dose. Clinicians should ensure that the proper dosing history and sample collection times be recorded to facilitate proper interpretation of serum concentration data.

It is often recommended that one should wait for ''steady-state'' pharmacokinetic conditions (approximately four half-lives) before determining serum antibiotic levels. Although this approach simplifies pharmacokinetic interpretation and adjustment of drug doses to some extent, it may be clinically unsound in the treatment of certain infectious disease. For many infections, achievement of therapeutic serum concentrations early during the course of antibiotic therapy may be an important determinant of survival from an infection (see later). One should ensure that adequate serum concentrations of certain agents have been achieved in critically ill patients and *not* delay collection of samples simply because ''steady-state'' pharmacokinetic conditions do not exist. Indeed, one can apply appropriate methods for the analysis of drug concentration data at non–steady-state conditions to aid in pharmacokinetic parameter estimation and dosage adjustment.

**Aminoglycosides**

***Assay Methods*** Gentamicin, tobramycin, and amikacin are the most frequently used and thus assayed aminoglycosides in the United States. Analytical methods include RIA, bioassay, EMIT, HPLC, fluorescence immunoassay (FIA), and FPIA.[46] Studies comparing the sensitivity, accuracy, and reproducibility of these methods have noted excellent agreement among these methods. At present, FPIA and EMIT appear to be the preferred methods in most laboratories.

***Serum Concentrations and Efficacy*** Numerous studies have attempted to correlate serum concentrations with clinical response. Early studies by Noone et al[47] and Jackson and Riff[48] concluded that peak serum tobramycin or gentamicin concentrations greater than 4–5 mg/L are associated with a higher therapeutic response in gram-negative sepsis, while peaks exceeding 8 mg/L appear to be necessary in patients with gram-negative pneumonia. Although these studies are frequently cited as evidence supporting the monitoring and adjustment of aminoglycoside concentrations, they were limited with respect to the small number of patients studied, differences in underlying disease, and use of other antimicrobials.

More recent studies have examined the influence of serum levels on the response of gram-negative bacteremia and pneumonia to aminoglycoside therapy. Septicemic patients with 1-hour postinfusion peak gentamicin or tobramycin concentrations exceeding 5 mg/mL, or amikacin concentrations exceeding 20 mg/mL, during the first 48 hours had a greater survival rate than those with peak levels below these concentrations. Similarly, survival was lowest in those patients with peak concentrations below these concentrations ($P < 0.05$).[49] No correlation between trough aminoglycoside concentrations and survival was found. A similar relationship between peak plasma levels (greater than 6 mg/L for tobramycin or gentamicin or 24 mg/L for amikacin) and successful outcome was demonstrated in patients with gram-negative pneumonia.[50] Other recent studies have also confirmed the importance of high peak aminoglycoside plasma concentrations in successful therapy of infection.[51,52]

In summary, available data for several studies support the attainment of high peak aminoglycoside concentrations, particularly in the early stages of therapy. Trough aminoglycoside concentrations appear to be less important predictors of clinical efficacy.

***Serum Concentrations and Toxicity*** Controversy surrounding the influence of serum aminoglycoside concentrations on the development of nephrotoxicity and ototoxicity has existed for several years. Several studies have suggested that trough concentrations exceeding 2 mg/L[53–55] or 4 mg/L[56] for gentamicin and tobramycin and 10 mg/L for amikacin[57] predispose patients to nephrotoxicity. More recent analysis of several variables concluded that the initial peak[58,59] aminoglycoside concentration is highly correlated with the development of nephrotoxicity; however, many of these studies simply demonstrated that high concentrations were most likely the *result*, not the *cause*, of the reduction in glomerular filtration rate.

Several studies have attempted to correlate serum aminoglycoside concentrations with the development of ototoxicity (vestibular and cochlear); however, as with evaluations of studies of nephrotoxicity, absolute peak and trough levels have been difficult to correlate with toxicity and it is likely that alleged relationships have simply reflected higher average concentrations resulting from excessive doses. Indeed, a recent study concluded that only total dose and duration of aminoglycoside therapy were the most significant drug factors predisposing patients to ototoxicity.[60]

Correlation of peak or trough aminoglycoside concentrations with therapeutic or toxic outcome has been difficult. Indeed, controversy regarding the appropriate time for collection of "peak" levels still exists; thus, the results of published studies might be expected to be inconsistent.[46,61] Nevertheless, it appears that sufficient data exist to support the monitoring of peak aminoglycoside concentrations for efficacy. Trough aminoglycoside levels are useful for detecting accumulation of drug caused by nephrotoxicity and may precede changes in other correlates of renal function (e.g., serum creatinine). Trough levels are also of use in pharmacokinetic analyses to facilitate dose adjustment.

**Chloramphenicol**

***Assay Methods*** Chloramphenicol is assayed using biological, radioenzymatic, and HPLC methods.[62] HPLC appears to be the most sensitive, accurate, and precise method; it is also capable of measuring chloramphenicol succinate, the prodrug of chloramphenicol used for intravenous injection. Analysis of the serum concentrations of the unhydrolyzed succinate salt of chloramphenicol may be of value in determining the systemic bioavailability of chloramphenicol in certain patient populations.

***Collection of Samples*** Peak serum chloramphenicol concentrations occur between 1.5 and 3 hours after oral administration of the palmitate salt. Peak concentrations after intravenous administration are more variable because of differences in the rate of hydrolysis from the succinate salt, but generally occur between 0.5 and 1.5 hours after a 30-minute infusion.[62]

***Serum Concentrations and Efficacy*** There are no data correlating serum chloramphenicol concentrations with efficacy; however, peak concentrations between 10 and 25 mg/L are generally recommended.[62–64]

***Serum Concentrations and Toxicity*** Dose-related toxic conditions associated with chloramphenicol are reversible bone marrow suppression and the "gray baby" syndrome. Both conditions have been associated with doses exceeding 100 mg/kg/d.[62] A recent study demonstrated that peak and trough serum chloramphenicol concentrations exceeding 25 and 15 mg/L, respectively, occurred in nine patients with signs and symptoms of toxicity[65]; however, an additional 27 neonates in this series tolerated serum chloramphenicol concentrations exceeding 25 mg/L without symptoms of toxicity. Therefore, it does not appear that serum concentrations are valuable in identifying patients in a "toxic" condition.

**Flucytosine**

***Assay Methods*** Flucytosine is assayed by bioassay, nonspecific fluorometric detection, gas–liquid chromatography, and HPLC.[66] Presently, most laboratories utilize a bioassay or HPLC for analysis of clinical samples.

***Serum Concentrations and Efficacy*** There are no data correlating serum concentrations and efficacy.

***Serum Concentrations and Toxicity*** Toxic conditions arising during flucytosine therapy include leukopenia and thrombocytopenia.[67] Serum level data obtained from patients receiving doses associated with hematologic side effects suggest that sustained "peak" concentrations exceeding 100–125 mg/L may be associated with toxicity.[67–69] Other studies have detected low concentrations of 5-fluorouracil in patients receiving flucytosine; half of the serum samples in one series contained 5-fluorouracil concentrations known to be hematotoxic.[70] While correlation between serum flucytosine and 5-fluorouracil concentrations has been observed,[70] 5-fluorouracil concentrations were not predictive of toxicity in one large series.[69]

### Vancomycin

***Assay Methods*** Vancomycin is usually assayed by bioassay, HPLC, RIA, FIA, and FPIA. All of these methods give accurate results, with FPIA the most precise and perhaps the most convenient because of automation.[71]

***Serum Concentrations and Efficacy*** There are no definitive data correlating peak or trough serum concentrations with efficacy; however, most dosage regimens used in clinical studies and dosing nomograms provide peak concentrations between 25 and 40 mg/L and trough concentrations less than 10 mg/L.[72]

***Serum Concentrations and Toxicity*** Intravenous administration of vancomycin has been associated with the development of ototoxicity and nephrotoxicity in some patients; however, reformulated preparations of vancomycin appear to be infrequently associated with nephrotoxicity. Ototoxicity (transient or permanent) appears to be related to serum levels exceeding 40 mg/L,[72] although toxicity has been noted at lower concentrations. The "red-man" syndrome, which has been reported after rapid[73] and, more recently, slow[74] infusions of vancomycin, has not been correlated with serum levels, but may occur more frequently with higher doses.[75]

## References


1. Greenwood D. In vitro veritas? Antimicrobial susceptibility tests and their clinical relevance. J Infect Dis 1981;144:380–381.
2. Sox HC, Liang MH. The erythrocyte sedimentation rate: guidelines for rational use. Ann Intern Med 1986;104:515–523.
3. Ravel R. Clinical Laboratory Medicine, 4th ed. Chicago, Yearbook Medical Publishers, 1984, pp 472–473.
4. Weinstein MP, Reller LB, Mirrett S, et al. Clinical comparison of an agar slide, blood culture bottle with tryptic soy broth and a conventional blood culture bottle with supplemented peptone broth. J Clin Microbiol 1985;21:815–818.
5. Edberg SC, Bottenbley CJ, Gam K. Use of sodium polyanethol sulfonate to selectively inhibit aminoglycoside and polymyxin antibiotics in a rapid blood level assay. Antimicrob Agents Chemother 1976;9:414–417.
6. Krogstad DJ, Murray PR, Granich GG, et al. Sodium polyanethol sulfonate inactivation of aminoglycosides. Antimicrob Agents Chemother 1981;20:272–274.
7. Murray PR, Niles AC. Inactivation of penicillins by thiol broth. J Clin Microbiol 1982;16:982–984.
8. Wallis C, Milnick JL, Wende RD, et al. Rapid isolation of bacteria from septicemic patients by use of an antimicrobial agent removal device. J Clin Microbiol 1980;11:462–464.
9. Lindsey NJ, Riely PH. In vitro antibiotic removal and bacterial recovery from blood with an antibiotic removal device. J Clin Microbiol 1981;13:503–507.
10. Peterson LR, Shanholtzer CJ, Mohn ML, et al. Improved recovery of microorganisms from patients receiving antibiotics with the antimicrobial removal device. Am J Clin Pathol 1983;80:692–696.
11. Weinberg E, Shungu DL, Gadebusch HH. Effectiveness of the antimicrobial removal device, BACTEC 16B medium, and thiol broth in neutralizing antibacterial activities of imipenem, norfloxacin, and related agents. J Clin Microbiol 1984;19:207–209.
12. McGuire NM, Kauffman CA, Hertz CS, et al. Evaluation of the BACTEC antimicrobial removal system for detection of bacteremia. J Clin Microbiol 1983;18:449–451.
13. Carlson GC, Tenover FC, Plorde JJ. Increased detection of staphylococcal bacteremia using an anti-microbial removal device. Am J Clin Pathol 1985;84:509–512.
14. Appelbaum PC, Beckwith DG, Dipersio JR, et al. Enhanced detection of bacteremia with a new BACTEC resin blood culture medium. J Clin Microbiol 1983;17:48–51.
15. Wright AJ, Thompson RL, McLimans CA, et al. The antimicrobial removal device. Am J Clin Pathol 1982;78:173–177.
16. Nahata M. Rapid diagnostic tests for streptococcal pharyngitis. Clin Pharm 1986;5:160–161.
17. Washington JA. Discrepancies between in vitro activity of and in vivo responses to antimicrobial agents. Diagn Microbiol Infect Dis 1983;1:25–31.
18. National Committee for Clinical Laboratory Standards. Methods for Dilution Antimicrobial Susceptibility Tests for Bacteria that Grow Aerobically; Approved Standard. NCCLS publication M7-A. Villanova, PA, NCCLS, 1985, pp 579–618.
19. Barry AL, Fass RJ, Anhalt JP, et al. Ciprofloxacin disk susceptibility tests: interpretive zone size standards for 5-$\mu$g disks. J Clin Microbiol 1985;21:880–883.
20. Rudrik JT, Cavalieri SJ, Britt EM. Proposed quality control and interpretive criteria for disk diffusion susceptibility testing and enoxacin. J Clin Microbiol 1985;21:332–334.
21. Acar JF, Goldstein FW. Disk susceptibility test, in Lorian V (ed): Antibiotics in Laboratory Medicine, 2nd ed. Baltimore, Williams and Wilkins, 1986, pp 27–63.
22. Ayers LW, Jones RN, Barry AL, et al. Cefotetan, a new cephamycin: comparison of in vitro antimicrobial activity with other cephems, beta-lactamase stability, and preliminary recommendations for disk diffusion testing. Antimicrob Agents Chemother 1982;22:859–877.
23. Medeiros AA, O'Brien TF, Wacker WEC, Yulug NF. Effect of salt concentration on the apparent in vitro susceptibility of *Pseudomonas* and other gram-negative bacilli to gentamicin. J Infect Dis 1971;124(suppl):S59–S64.
24. Blaser J, Dudley MN, Gilbert D, et al. Influence of medium and method on the in vitro susceptibility of *Pseudomonas aeruginosa* and other bacteria to ciprofloxacin and enoxacin. Antimicrob Agents Chemother 1986;29:927–929.
25. Nightingale CM, Dudley MN. Protein binding and antimicrobials, in Cunha BA, Ristuccia A (eds): Antimicrobial Therapy. New York, Raven Press, 1984, pp 379–387.
26. Bauer AW, Kirby MM, Sherris JC, et al. Antibiotic susceptibility testing by a standardized, single-disk method. Am J Clin Pathol 1966;45:493–496.
27. Thornsberry C. Automation and mechanization in antimicrobial susceptibility testing, in Lorian V (ed): Antibiotics in Laboratory Medicine, 2nd ed. Baltimore, Williams and Wilkins, 1986, pp 151–158.
28. Sabath LD, Wheeler N, Laverdiere M, et al. A new type of penicillin resistance of *Staphylococcus aureus*. Lancet 1977;1: 443–447.

29. Kaye D. The clinical significance of tolerance of *Staphylococcus aureus*, editorial. Ann Intern Med 1980;93:924–926.
30. Rahal JJ. Antibiotic combinations: the clinical relevance of synergy and antagonism. Medicine 1978;57:179–195.
31. Klastersky J, Zinner SH. Synergistic combinations of antibiotics in gram-negative bacillary infections. Rev Infect Dis 1982;4: 294–301.
32. Scheld WM, Mandell GL. Enigmatic enterococcal endocarditis. Ann Intern Med 1984;100:904–905.
33. Lepper MM, Dowling HF. Treatment of pneumococcic meningitis with penicillin compared with penicillin plus aureomycin. Arch Intern Med 1951;88:489–494.
34. Strausbaugh LJ, Sande MA. Factors influencing the therapy of experimental *Proteus mirabilis* meningitis in rabbits. J Infect Dis 1978;137:251–260.
35. Moellering RC. Antimicrobial synergism—an elusive concept. J Infect Dis 1979;140:639–641.
36. Krogstad DJ, Moellering RC, Jr. Antimicrobial combinations, in Lorian V (ed): Antibiotics in Laboratory Medicine, 2nd ed. Baltimore, Williams and Wilkins, 1986, pp 532–595.
37. King TC, Krogstad DJ. Spectrophotometric assessment of dose–response curves for single antimicrobial agents and antimicrobial combinations. J Infect Dis 1983;147:758–764.
38. Zinner SH, Dudley MN, Blaser J. In vitro models for the study of combination antibiotic therapy in neutropenic patients. Am J Med 1986;80(Suppl 6B):156–159.
39. Norden CW, Wentzel H, Keleti E. Comparison of techniques for measurement of in vitro antibiotic synergism. J Infect Dis 1979;140:629–633.
40. Wolfson JS, Swartz MN. Serum bactericidal activity as a monitor of antibiotic therapy. N Engl J Med 1985;312:968–975.
41. Reller LB. The serum bactericidal test. Rev Infect Dis 1986;8: 803–808.
42. Barriere SL, Kapusnik JE, Ely E, et al. Analysis of a new method for assessing activity of combinations of antimicrobials. Area under the bactericidal activity curve. J Antimicrob Chemother 1985;16:49–59.
43. Tod JK, Folliver P. Subtraction serum bactericidal assay: a method for estimating in vivo effects of antibiotic combinations. J Infect Dis 1979;140:807–810.
44. Reller LB. Interaction of cefotaxime and desacetylcefotaxime against pathogenic bacteria. Diagn Microbiol Infect Dis 1984;2: 55S–61S.
45. Anderson ET, Young LW, Hewitt WL. Simultaneous antibiotic levels in "breakthrough" gram-negative rod bacteremia. Am J Med 1986;61:493–497.
46. Zaske D. Aminoglycosides, in Evans WE, Schentag JJ, Jusko WJ (eds): Applied Pharmacokinetics, 2nd ed. San Francisco, Applied Therapeutics, 1986, pp 331–381.
47. Noone P, Parsons TMC, Pattison JR, et al. Experience in monitoring gentamicin therapy during treatment of serious gram-negative sepsis. Br Med J 1974;1:477–481.
48. Jackson GG, Riff LJ. Pseudomonas bacteremia: pharmacologic and other bases for failure of treatment with gentamicin. J Infect Dis 1971;124(suppl):S185–S191.
49. Moore RD, Smith CR, Lietman PS. The association of aminoglycoside plasma levels with mortality in patients with gram-negative bacteremia. J Infect Dis 1984;149:443–448.
50. Moore RD, Smith CR, Lietman PS. Association of aminoglycoside plasma levels with therapeutic outcome in gram-negative pneumonia. Am J Med 1984;77:657–662.
51. Deziel-Evans LM, Murphy JE, Martin LJ. Correlation of pharmacokinetic indices with therapeutic outcome in patients receiving aminoglycosides. Clin Pharm 1986;5:319–324.
52. Moore RD, Lietman PS, Smith CR. Clinical response to aminoglycoside therapy: importance of the ratio of peak concentration to minimum inhibitory concentration. J Infect Dis 1987;155:93–99.
53. Dahlgren JG, Anderson ET, Hewitt WL. Gentamicin blood levels: A guide to nephrotoxicity. Antimicrob Agents Chemother 1975;8:58–62.
54. Lerner SA, Seligsohn R, Matz GJ. Comparative clinical studies of ototoxicity and nephrotoxicity of amikacin and gentamicin. Am J Med 1977;62:915–923.
55. Lau WK, Young LS, Black RE, et al. Comparative efficacy and toxicity of amikacin/carbenicillin vs. gentamicin/carbenicillin in leukopenic patients. Am J Med 1977;62:959–966.
56. Goodman EL, Van Gelder J, Holmes R, et al. Prospective comparative study of variable dosage and variable frequency regimens for administration of gentamicin. Antimicrob Agents Chemother 1975;8:434–438.
57. Smith CR, Maxwell RR, Edwards CQ, et al. Nephrotoxicity induced by gentamicin and amikacin. Johns Hopkins Med J 1978;142;85–90.
58. Moore RD, Smith CR, Lipsky JJ. Risk factors of nephrotoxicity in patients treated with aminoglycosides. Ann Intern Med 1984;100:352–357.
59. Sawyers CL, Moore RD, Lerner SA, et al. A model for predicting nephrotoxicity in patients treated with aminoglycosides. J Infect Dis 1986;153:1062–1068.
60. Moore RD, Smith CR, Lietman PS. Risk factors for the development of auditory toxicity in patients receiving aminoglycosides. J Infect Dis 1984;149:23–30.
61. Blaser J, Simnen HP, Gonzenbrach HR, et al. Aminoglycoside monitoring: timing of "peak" levels is critical. Ther Drug Monit 1985;7:303–307.
62. Nahata MC. Chloramphenicol, in Evans WE, Schentag JJ, Jusko WJ (eds): Applied Pharmacokinetics, 2nd ed. San Francisco, Applied Therapeutics, 1986, pp 437–462.
63. Ambrose P. Clinical pharmacokinetics of chloramphenicol and chloramphenicol succinate. Clin Pharmacokin 1984;9:222–228.
64. Ekblad H, Ruuskanen O, Lindbert R, et al. The monitoring of serum chloramphenicol levels in children with severe infections. J Antimicrob Chemother 1985;15:489–494.
65. Mulhall A, deLouvois J, Hurley R. Chloramphenicol toxicity in neonates: its incidence and prevention. Br Med J 1983;287: 1424–1427.
66. Warnock DW, Richardson MD, Turner A. High performance liquid chromatographic (HPLC) and other non-biological methods for quantitation of antifungal drugs. J Antimicrob Chemother 1982;10:467–478.
67. Kauffman CA, Frame PT. Bone marrow toxicity associated with 5-fluorocytosine therapy. Antimicrob Agents Chemother 1977;11:244–247.
68. Bennett JE, Dismukes WE, Duma RJ, et al. A comparison of amphotericin B alone and combined with flucytosine in the treatment of cryptococcal meningitis. N Engl J Med 1979;301: 126–131.
69. Stamm AM, Diasio RB, Dismukes WE, et al. Toxicity of amphotericin B plus flucytosine in 194 patients with cryptococcal meningitis. Am J Med 1987;83:236–242.
70. Diasio RB, Lakings DE, Bennet JE. Evidence for conversion of 5-fluorocytosine to 5-fluorouracil in humans: Possible factor in 5-flucytosine clinical toxicity. Antimicrob Agents Chemother 1978;14:903–908.
71. Pfaller MA, Krogstad DJ, Granich GG, et al. Laboratory evaluation of five assay methods for vancomycin: bioassay,

high-pressure liquid chromatography, fluorescence polarization immunoassay, radioimmunoassay, and fluorescence immunoassay. J Clin Microbiol 1984;20:311–316.

72. Moellering RC. Pharmacokinetics of vancomycin. Antimicrob Chemother 1984;14(suppl D):43–52.

73. Newfield P, Roizen MF. Hazards of rapid administration of vancomycin. Ann Intern Med 1979;91:581.

74. Davis RL, Smith AL, Koup JR. The "red man's syndrome" and slow infusion of vancomycin. Ann Intern Med 1986;104:285–286.

75. Polk RE, Healy D. Garson M, et al. Vancomycin and the "red man's" syndrome. Presented at the 26th Interscience Conference on Antimicrobial Agents and Chemotherapy, New Orleans, LA, 1986 (Abstract 32).

# Chapter 74 / Selection of Antimicrobial Regimens

Steven L. Barriere, PharmD

Choosing an antimicrobial agent to treat or prevent an infection is far more complicated than simply matching a drug to a known or suspected pathogen. Although many may feel, and perhaps rightfully so, that antimicrobial therapy is more art than science, there is a generally accepted systematic approach to the selection and evaluation of an antimicrobial regimen (Table 74.1). Unfortunately, all too often we are tempted to ignore the systematic approach to designing an optimum regimen in favor of broad-spectrum therapy that will "cover everything." This approach is not only unsystematic, but it is expensive, and potentially more toxic, and will lead to widespread resistance and difficult-to-treat superinfections.

Another abuse of antimicrobial agents is their application when, in fact, they are not needed. The best example of this is the well-recognized and widespread practice of prescribing antibacterials for self-limited, clinical conditions that are most likely viral in origin.

Initial selection of antimicrobial therapy is nearly always "empiric." That is, therapy begins before the offending organism is identified. Infectious diseases are generally acute and delay in beginning antimicrobial therapy may result in serious morbidity or even mortality. An example is the rapidly lethal nature of various forms of meningitis. Thus, antimicrobial therapy selection is based upon the information gathered from the patient's history and physical examination and from the results of Gram stains or rapidly performed serologic tests. This information coupled with knowledge of the most likely offending organism(s) and an institution's local susceptibility patterns allows for a rational selection of drugs to treat the patient.

This chapter outlines, in some detail, the systematic approach to selection of antimicrobial therapeutic regimens. The principles for selection of antimicrobial prophylactic regimens are discussed in Chapter 89.

## Confirming the Presence of Infection

### *Fever*

The presence of a temperature greater than the expected 98.6°F (37°C) "normal" body temperature is considered a hallmark of infectious diseases. Generally, body temperature, measured by the oral route, of greater than 99.5–100.5°F (37.5–38.0°C) is considered to be significant. Normal diurnal variations may raise body temperature to 99.5°F (37.5°C). Many other, noninfectious causes of fever exist and must be ruled out before searching further for infection.[1,2] These noninfectious etiologies of fever may be referred to as "false-positives." Although these certainly may confuse the clinician, even more troublesome are "false negatives": the absence of fever in a patient with signs and symptoms consistent with an infectious disease. Several types of infection do not produce fever (e.g., uncomplicated cystitis), but more important are true false-negatives induced by antipyretics, undetected antimicrobial therapy, or overwhelming infection. The patient or family should be carefully questioned to assess the ingestion of any medication that can mask fever. These include aspirin, acetaminophen, nonsteroidal anti-inflammatory agents, and corticosteroids. Similarly, treatment of a disease state with only partially effective therapy may also temporarily reduce fever and other signs of infection. A good example is the use of bacteriostatic drugs in a patient with infective endocarditis.

Additionally, the use of antipyretics should be discouraged during the treatment of infection unless absolutely necessary. The common practice of administering an antipyretic during the treatment of infection may mask a poor therapeutic response. Moreover, elevated body temperature, unless very high (>105°F), is not harmful, and may be beneficial.[3] Artificial means of reducing elevated body temperature (e.g., cooling blankets) are generally unnecessary, and may even be dangerous. Fever patterns are felt by many to be helpful in establishing the etiology of the increased temperature. For example, high spiking fevers are felt to be more consistent with an infectious process, whereas sustained fevers are associated with collagen vascular disease or malignancy. Although these guidelines may be generally true, there are reports of drug-induced fever which was high and spiking. Additionally, many subacute infectious processes such as mycobacterial and fungal infections may produce relatively modest but sustained elevations in temperature. Overall, characterization of the fever pattern offers little in the general assessment of the patient.

### *Signs and Symptoms*

Most infections result in elevated white blood cell counts (leukocytosis) because of the mobilization of granulocytes and/or lymphocytes to ingest and destroy invading microbes. The generally accepted range of "normal" values for white blood cell counts is between 4,000 and 10,000/mm$^3$. Values above or below this hold important prognostic and diagnostic value.

Classically, bacterial infections are associated with elevated granulocyte counts (neutrophils, basophils), often with immature forms (band neutrophils) seen in peripheral blood smears ("left shift"). The presence of immature forms is an indication of increased bone marrow response to the infection. With infection, peripheral leukocyte counts may be

**Table 74.1** Systematic Approach to Selection of Antimicrobials

A. Confirmation of the presence of infection
  1. Fever
  2. Signs and symptoms
  3. Predisposing factors
B. Identification of the pathogen (Chapter 73)
  1. Collection of infected material
  2. Stains
  3. Serologies
  4. Culture
C. Selection of presumptive therapy
  1. Host factors
  2. Drug factors
D. Monitoring of therapeutic response
  1. Clinical assessment
  2. Laboratory tests
  3. Assessment of therapeutic failure

**Table 74.2** Factors Predisposing to Infection

Alterations in normal flora of the host
Disruption of natural barriers
  Skin/mucous membranes
  Cilia of respiratory tract
  pH and motility of bowel
  Flow of urine and tears
Immunosuppression secondary to
  Malnutrition
  Underlying disease (hereditary or acquired)
  Hormones (e.g., pregnancy, corticosteroids)
  Drugs (e.g., cytotoxic agents)
Age

very high, but are generally never higher than 30,000 to 40,000/mm.[3] Since leukocytosis indicates the normal host response to infection, low leukocyte counts after the onset of infection indicate an abnormal response and are generally associated with a poor prognosis of bacterial infection.[4] Relative lymphocytosis, even with normal or slightly elevated total white cell counts, is generally associated with viral or fungal infections. Many types of infections, however, may be accompanied by a completely normal white blood cell count and differential.

The classic signs of pain and inflammation may be manifested by swelling, erythema, tenderness, and purulent drainage. Unfortunately, these are only visibly apparent if the infection is superficial or in a bone or joint. The manifestations of inflammation in deep-seated infections such as meningitis, pneumonia, endocarditis, and urinary tract infection must be ascertained by examining tissues or fluids. For example, the presence of polymorphonuclear leukocytes (neutrophils) in spinal fluid, lung secretions (sputum), and urine is highly suggestive of bacterial infection.

Symptoms referable to an organ system must be carefully sought out, for they not only help in establishing the presence of infection, but also aid in narrowing the list of potential pathogens. For example, a febrile patient with complaints of flank pain and dysuria may well have pyelonephritis. In this situation, enteric gram-negative bacilli, especially *Escherichia coli*, are the predominant pathogens; however, if a febrile patient has no symptoms referable to an organ system, but only constitutional complaints, the list of possible infectious diseases is quite long.[1] A febrile individual with cough and sputum production probably has a pulmonary infection. What is not so evident, however, is the etiologic organism in this situation, as it may be bacteria, mycobacteria, viruses, or mycoplasmas.[5] In this situation attention to the patient's history and background disease states is important. Even more important is careful examination of infected material (in this case sputum) to try and ascertain the identity of the pathogen (see later).

### *Predisposing Factors*

Table 74.2 lists factors that predispose patients to infection. Generally, immunosuppressive disease states lead to a wide variety of infections (e.g., acquired immune deficiency syndrome), while other diseases may predispose the patient to a certain type of infectious disease (e.g., recurrent meningococcal infection with complement deficiency). Information from the patient's history regarding underlying disease is vitally important, as the presence of an underlying condition not only may predispose patients to infection, but may modify the likely offending pathogen. For example, purulent meningitis in an otherwise healthy adult is almost invariably caused by meningococci or pneumococci, whereas this same infection in a patient with a lymphoma may be caused by *Listeria monocytogenes*, which will infect a normal adult only very rarely.[6]

Many factors predisposing to infection are related to disruption of the host's integumentary barriers. For example, trauma, burns, and iatrogenic wounds induced in surgery all may lead to a substantial risk of infection depending upon the severity and location of the injury or disruption.

Controversy remains over the exact role that certain risk factors play. For example, the more frequent incidence of urinary tract infections in diabetic patients may simply be the result of manipulation of the urinary tract (catheterizations) during frequent hospitalizations, rather than a predisposition to the disease itself. Additionally, there is some doubt over the immunosuppressive role of pregnancy in dissemination of chronic granulomatous diseases such as tuberculosis.

## Identifying the Pathogen

Infected body materials must be sampled before institution of any antimicrobial therapy for two reasons. First, Gram stain of the material may rapidly reveal bacteria or fungi, or acid-fast stain may detect mycobacteria or actinomycetes. Second, delay in obtaining infected fluids or tissues until after therapy is started may result in false-negative culture results. This is particularly true in patients with urinary tract infections, meningitis, and septic arthritis.[7]

In addition to the potentially infected materials being

brought forth by the patient (sputum, urine, stool, wound or sinus drainage), samples of other less accessible fluids or tissues must be obtained based on localizing signs or symptoms (e.g., spinal fluid in meningitis, joint fluid in arthritis). Abscesses and cellulitic areas should also be aspirated. Finally, blood cultures should nearly always be performed in the febrile patient. Blood culture collection is usually timed to sharp elevations in temperature, indicating pyrogen release by the microorganisms in the bloodstream; however, in selected diseases, especially endocarditis, the bacteremia is qualitatively continuous, so cultures may be obtained at any time.[8]

Gram staining techniques, culture methods, and serologic identification, as well as susceptibility testing, are covered in detail in Chapter 73. Emphasis must be placed on the proper collection and handling of specimens, and careful assessment of Gram stain or other rapid serologic test results, in guiding the clinician toward appropriate selection of initial antimicrobial therapy.

## Selecting the Presumptive Therapy

In the selection of rational antimicrobial therapy for a given clinical situation, a variety of factors must be considered. These include the severity and acuity of the disease, host factors, factors related to the drugs used, and the necessity for use of multiple agents. Additionally, there are generally accepted "drugs of choice" for the treatment of most pathogens (see the Appendix).

The severity and/or acuity of the infectious process dictates the necessity for use of so-called "empiric" antimicrobial therapy. In most cases, therapy is started before results of culture and susceptibility testing are available, because a delay of 24–48 hours would be incurred. This delay would, obviously, compromise the health of the patient if the infection were rapidly progressive. Moreover, a great deal of antibiotic use occurs in ambulatory patients, who are unlikely to return for treatment after having been seen by a physician. Thus, therapy is often begun "empirically" or without knowledge of the exact infecting organism(s). Empiric therapies are directed at organisms that are known to frequently cause the infection in question. These organisms are discussed in the following chapters.

To define the most likely infecting organisms, a careful history and physical examination (as described above) must be performed. In addition, a variety of host factors should be considered, to help identify the likely etiologic agent as well as to assist in the selection of the best initial or empiric therapy for the patient.

### *Host Factors*

In evaluating a patient for initial or empiric therapy the factors listed in Table 74.3 should be considered. Allergy to the antimicrobial agents being considered for therapy would seem to preclude their use; however, a very careful assessment of allergic histories must be performed, as many patients may confuse common adverse drug effects, such as gastrointestinal disturbance, with true allergic reactions.[9] Among the most commonly cited antimicrobial allergies are those to penicillin and/or related compounds. One can find many authoritative sources that recommend other $\beta$-lactam compounds, especially cephalosporins, in this setting, because of suggestive evidence that no more than 5% to 10% of patients with penicillin allergy will react to a cephalosporin.

**Table 74.3** Host Factors in Selection of Antimicrobial Therapy

| |
|---|
| Allergy of history of adverse drug reactions |
| Age of patient |
| Pregnancy |
| Genetic or metabolic abnormalities |
| Renal and hepatic function |
| Site of the infection |
| Concomitant drug therapy |
| Underlying disease state(s) |

Approximately 8% of patients who give a history of penicillin allergy react to a cephalosporin, whereas 2% who give a negative allergic history react.[10] Only about 10% of patients who give a history of penicillin allergy have a positive skin test to either penicilloyl-polylysine or one of the minor determinants[11]; however, it was recently demonstrated that in over 70 patients who were skin test positive to one or more penicillin determinants, none reacted to subsequent exposure to parenteral cephalosporins.[11] This information supports the older data that cross-reactivity between these two classes of $\beta$-lactams is very low.

In the absence of complete penicillin skin-testing capabilities, a rule of thumb for giving cephalosporins to penicillin-allergic patients is to avoid their use in patients who give a good history for immediate or accelerated reactions (anaphylaxis, laryngospasm) and to use them cautiously in patients with a history of delayed reaction such as rash.

The patient's age is an important factor, both in trying to identify the likely etiologic agent and in assessing the patient's ability to detoxify or eliminate the drug(s) to be used. The best example is bacterial meningitis where the pathogens differ as the patient grows from the neonatal period, to infancy and childhood, and into adulthood.[6] A neonate's hepatic and liver function is not well developed, but becomes extremely efficient during infancy and childhood, and slowly wanes with increasing age. Thus, both drug selection and drug dosage must be adjusted based upon the age of the patient.

Specific patient groups require additional considerations when using antimicrobials. For example, neonates (especially when premature) may develop kernicterus when given sulfonamides. This results from displacement of bilirubin from serum albumin.[12] Chloramphenicol is well established as a cause of the "gray baby" syndrome. This syndrome results from the inability of the newborn's liver to metabolize (and detoxify) the drug, leading to shock and cardiovascular collapse.[13] Thus, serum concentrations of chloramphenicol must be monitored to ensure that concentrations of the drug do not exceed 20–25 $\mu$g/mL.

Although it is generally believed that the elderly are more predisposed to adverse drug effects, there are no clear-cut explanations.[14] Hepatotoxicity from the antimicrobial agent

**Table 74.4** Routes of Antimicrobial Elimination and Dose-Related Toxic Effects

| *Drug* | *Primary route of elimination* | *Degree of accumulation*[a] | *Dose-related toxic effect(s)* |
|---|---|---|---|
| **Penicillins** | | | |
| Ampicillin | Renal | Significant | CNS (seizures, etc.) |
| Azlocillin | Renal/hepatic[b] | Moderate | ? Platelet dysfunction |
| Carbenicillin | Renal | Significant | Platelet dysfunction, CNS toxicity, sodium overload |
| Methicillin | Renal | Moderate | ? Nephritis |
| Mezlocillin | Renal/hepatic[b] | Moderate | ? Platelet dysfunction |
| Nafcillin | Renal/hepatic[b] | Insignificant | ? Neutropenia |
| Oxacillin | Renal/hepatic[b] | Insignificant | ? Neutropenia |
| Penicillin G | Renal | Significant | CNS toxicity, hyperkalemia |
| Piperacillin | Renal/hepatic[b] | Moderate | ? Platelet dysfunction |
| Ticarcillin | Renal | Significant | CNS toxicity, platelet dysfunction |
| **Cephalosporins** | | | |
| Cefamandole | Renal | Significant | Hypoprothrombinemia |
| Cefazolin | Renal | Significant | CNS toxicity |
| Cefonicid | Renal | Significant | None |
| Cefoperazone | Hepatic/renal[b] | Moderate | Hypoprothrombinemia |
| Ceforanide | Renal | Significant | None |
| Cefotaxime | Renal/hepatic[b] | Moderate | None |
| Cefotetan | Renal | Significant | Hypoprothrombinemia |
| Cefoxitin | Renal | Significant | None |
| Ceftazidime | Renal | Significant | None |
| Ceftizoxime | Renal | Significant | None |
| Ceftriaxone | Renal/hepatic[b] | Insignificant | None |
| Cefuroxime | Renal | Significant | None |
| Moxalactam | Renal | Significant | Hypoprothrombinemia, platelet dysfunction |
| **Aminoglycosides** | Renal | Significant | Nephrotoxicity, ototoxicity |
| **Tetracyclines** | Renal (except doxycycline) | Significant | Exacerbation of azotemia, possible hepatotoxicity |

isoniazid has been documented to increase in frequency with age.[15]

During pregnancy, not only is the fetus at risk for drug teratogenicity, but the pharmacokinetic disposition of certain drugs may be altered.[16] Penicillins, cephalosporins, and aminoglycosides are cleared from the peripheral circulation more rapidly during pregnancy. This is probably due to the marked increases in intravascular volume, glomerular filtration rate, and hepatic/metabolic activities, especially during late pregnancy. The net result is that maternal serum antimicrobial concentrations may be as much as 50% lower during this period than in the nonpregnant state. Increased dosages of certain compounds may be necessary to achieve therapeutic levels during late pregnancy.

Inherited or acquired metabolic abnormalities influence the therapy of infectious diseases in a variety of ways. For example, patients with impaired peripheral vascular flow may not absorb drugs given by intramuscular injection. Additionally, certain metabolic states may predispose patients to enhanced drug toxicity. For example, patients who are phenotypically slow acetylators of isoniazid are at greater risk for development of peripheral neuropathy.[17] Patients with severe deficiency of glucose-6-phosphate dehydrogenase (G6PD) may develop significant hemolysis when exposed to drugs such as sulfonamides, nitrofurantoin, nalidixic acid, antimalarials, dapsone, and perhaps chloramphenicol.[18] Although mild deficiencies are found in blacks, the more severe forms of the disease are generally confined to persons of eastern Mediterranean origin.

Patients with diminished renal and/or hepatic function will accumulate drugs unless the dosage is adjusted. Although many antimicrobial reactions are idiosyncratic, there are significant dose-related toxic effects associated with a number of agents. Table 74.4 lists drugs by antimicrobial class and identifies the route of elimination and the dose-related toxic effect to be avoided.

Clear-cut identification of the site of the infection or the likely source of a bacteremia can aid in defining the most likely organisms. For example, the overwhelming majority of urinary tract infections are caused by enteric gram-negative bacilli, especially *E. coli*.[19] In contrast, bone and joint infections in children are nearly always due to *Staphylococcus aureus*.[20] Bacterial pneumonia in an adult, acquired in the community, is very likely caused by *Strepto-*

**Table 74.4** (continued)

| *Drug* | *Primary route of elimination* | *Degree of accumulation*[a] | *Dose-related toxic effect(s)* |
|---|---|---|---|
| **Miscellaneous** | | | |
| Aztreonam | Renal | Moderate | None |
| Chloramphenicol | Hepatic | Moderate | Gray baby syndrome, marrow suppression |
| Clindamycin | Hepatic | Moderate | None |
| Erythromycin | Hepatic | Insignificant | Ototoxicity |
| Imipenem | Renal | Significant | CNS toxicity |
| Metronidazole | Hepatic/renal | Moderate | Encephalopathy, neuropathy |
| Polymyxins | Renal | Significant | Nephrotoxicity, neuropathy, neuromuscular blockade |
| Sulfonamides | Renal/hepatic[b] | Moderate | Kernicterus |
| Trimethoprim | Renal | Moderate | Megaloblastic anemia |
| **Antifungal Agents** | | | |
| Amphotericin B | Unknown | Insignificant | Most adverse effects increase in frequency with cumulative dose, not individual dosage size |
| Flucytosine | Renal | Significant | Marrow suppression, ? hepatotoxicity |
| Miconazole | Hepatic | Insignificant | ? Hepatotoxicity |
| Ketoconazole | Hepatic | Insignificant | None |
| **Antiviral Agents** | | | |
| Acyclovir | Renal | Significant | CNS toxicity, nephrotoxicity |
| Vidarabine | Hepatic/renal[b] | Insignificant | ? CNS toxicity |
| **Antitubercular Agents** | | | |
| Isoniazid | Hepatic | Insignificant | Neuropathy |
| Ethambutol | Renal | Moderate | Optic neuritis |
| Rifampin | Hepatic | Insignificant | ? None |

[a] Accumulation of parent compound and/or active/toxic metabolites in patients with decreased capacity of primary route of elimination.

[b] Accumulation is probably significant in combined hepatic and renal failure, but data are sparse.

*coccus pneumoniae*, whereas this same infection, acquired in the hospital, is more likely due to enteric gram-negative bacilli such as *Klebsiella, Enterobacter,* or *Pseudomonas*. The most common source of bacteremias is the urinary tract, and the majority of the bacteremias from this site are caused by enteric gram-negative bacilli.[19] In contrast, bacteremia from an intravenous catheter site is very likely caused by staphylococci.[21]

Any concomitant therapy the patient is receiving may influence selection of drug therapy, dosage, and monitoring. For example, administration of chloramphenicol to a patient who is also receiving phenytoin may result in phenytoin toxicity. This is caused by an inhibition of phenytoin metabolism by chloramphenicol. Additionally, the selected antimicrobial therapy itself may adversely affect the management of another disease. A list of significant drug interactions involving antimicrobials and antimicrobial interference with laboratory tests is provided in Table 74.5.

Concomitant disease states may influence the selection of therapy. Certain diseases predispose patients to a particular infectious disease or alter the type of infecting organism. For example, patients with diabetes mellitus and resulting peripheral vascular disease often develop lower extremity soft tissue infections. Patients with chronic lung disease or cystic fibrosis develop frequent pulmonary infections, which may be caused by microorganisms somewhat different from those found in otherwise normal hosts.

Patients with immunosuppressive diseases such as malignancies or acquired immunologic deficiencies are highly predisposed to infections, and the types of organisms may be vastly different from what would be expected. For example, patients undergoing chemotherapy for acute forms of leukemia are often profoundly granulocytopenic and are predisposed to infections caused by staphylococci, enteric gram-negative bacilli, and fungi. In contrast, patients with the acquired immune deficiency syndrome (AIDS) often become infected with an enormous variety of organisms, such as the protozoans *Pneumocystis carinii, Cryptosporidium, Toxoplasma gondii,* and *Isospora belli*; the viruses cytomegalovirus and herpes simplex; the fungi *Cryptococcus neoformans* and *Histoplasma capsulatum*; and mycobacteria.[22]

**Table 74.5** Antimicrobial Interactions

| *Antimicrobial agent* | *Other agent* | *Results of interaction* |
|---|---|---|
| Aminoglycosides | Neuromuscular blocking drugs | Increased neuromuscular blockade |
| | Other nephrotoxins or ototoxins (e.g. cisplatin, amphotericin B, ethacrynic acid, vancomycin, cyclosporine) | Increased nephrotoxicity or ototoxicity |
| | Penicillins | Inactivation of both drugs (a particular problem in renal failure and when obtaining drug levels) |
| Sulfonamides | Sulfonylureas | Hypoglycemia |
| | Phenytoin | Increased serum concentration of phenytoin leading to toxicity |
| | Oral anticoagulants (warfarin derivatives) | Enhanced hypoprothrombinemia |
| Chloramphenicol | Phenytoin, tolbutamide, ethanol | Increased serum concentration of other agents and enhanced pharmacologic effect or increased toxicity |
| Ciprofloxacin | Theophylline | May increase theophylline concentrations |
| | | $Mg^{2+}$- and $Al^{3+}$-containing antacids inhibit intestinal absorption |
| Metronidazole (also cefamandole, moxalactam, cefoperazone) | Ethanol (including ethanol-containing medications) | Disulfiram-like reaction |
| Erythromycin | Theophylline | Increased serum theophylline concentration |
| | Cyclosporin | Cyclosporin serum concentrations may be increased |
| Rifampin | Coumarin anticoagulants | Decreased anticoagulant effect (increased metabolism of drug) |
| | Quinidine | Decreased effect of quinidine |
| | Digoxin | Decreased effect of digoxin |
| | Methadone | Narcotic withdrawal |
| | Propranolol | Decreased effect of propranolol |
| | Oral contraceptives | Decreased effect (pregnancy) |
| Tetracyclines | Antacids, iron, calcium | Inhibit intestinal absorption of tetracycline |
| Penicillins and cephalosporins | Uricosuric agents (probenecid, high-dose aspirin, etc.) | Block excretion of β-lactams, causing higher serum levels |
| | Copper reduction test for glycosuria (Clinitest tablets) | False-positive test for glycosuria (not seen with glucose oxidase method) |
| Isoniazid | Phenytoin | Increased serum concentrations of both |

## *Drug Factors*

### Pharmacokinetics

In the selection of an antimicrobial agent for empiric therapy, the kinetic disposition of the agent is an important consideration. This is partly because we should be selecting drugs that are best suited for the patient's elimination capacity.

As described previously, chronic renal and hepatic dysfunction predisposes patients to certain types of infections, thereby dictating the type of therapy. Additionally, it would be desirable, whenever possible, to select agents that either will not worsen the underlying dysfunction or will not be dependent upon that organ system for detoxification or removal from the body. This is certainly not always possible and we often must select drugs that will accumulate to a significant extent in renal and/or hepatic failure.

The precision of dosage regimen design depends in part on the dose-related toxic effects of the drug and its therapeutic index (ratio of toxic to therapeutic concentrations). Additionally, we must have knowledge of the extent of elimination/accumulation of the drug. For example, if a drug is only partially eliminated unchanged by the kidneys, then we would expect only modest accumulation, even in patients with end-stage renal disease, and the tendency might be to not adjust the dose; however, if the therapeutic index were very small, then careful dosage adjustment would be imperative. In contrast, relatively ''nontoxic'' compounds such as β-lactam agents, many of which are almost entirely eliminated unchanged, are often given with little regard for the degree of excretory function. This practice should be avoided, however, because certain rare adverse effects such as hemolytic anemia and convulsions may occur, and it has been suggested that colonization and superinfection probably are more frequently encountered with excessively high doses of these drugs.[23]

Finally, in the present era of cost containment, giving unnecessarily large doses of expensive drugs is not cost effective. An excellent example is administration of ''full'' doses of a drug like cefazolin to a patient with poor renal function. Not only is this potentially toxic to the central nervous system, but doses as small as 250–500 mg once daily would be adequate.

The antimicrobial agents that must be most carefully dosed because of potential toxicity include the aminoglycosides, vancomycin, chloramphenicol, and flucytosine. All these drugs have relatively well-described therapeutic ranges that need not and should not be exceeded. This list is not all inclusive and careful attention to the elimination characteristics of antimicrobial agents prescribed for specific patients is necessary to ensure optimal therapy, avoid adverse effects, and contain costs.

**Tissue Penetration**

The relevance of tissue concentrations of antimicrobials has long been disputed. Because methods to measure the concentrations of antimicrobial agents have become widely used as research tools, a great deal of data has been generated in this area. Unfortunately, primarily because of methodologic problems, much of the generated information is flawed and is relatively meaningless, often because healthy tissues were sampled for analysis, when penetration into diseased or infected tissues is more important. Penetration into certain healthy tissue may be relevant for surgical prophylaxis, but even this is questionable. Some of the difficulties with interpreting these data include a lack of correlation with clinical outcome and poor understanding of whether the antimicrobial agents are present in a biologically active form. An example of the former problem is the recognized efficacy of drugs with low biliary concentrations in the treatment of cholecystitis and/or cholangitis, and the absence of enhanced efficacy of drugs whose primary route of elimination is biliary excretion of active drug. An example of the latter difficulty is abscess penetration, where various factors such as acid pH, white cell products, and various enzymes may inactivate even high concentrations of certain drugs.

The central nervous system is one body site where antimicrobial penetration is relatively well defined, and correlations with clinical outcome are established.[24] Cerebrospinal fluid (CSF) concentrations of antimicrobial agents necessary to eradicate bacterial meningitis have been defined, and drugs that do not reach significant concentrations in CSF should be avoided in treating meningitis. Apart from the bloodstream, other body fluids for which drug concentration data are clinically relevant include urine, synovial fluid, and peritoneal fluid.

Caution must be taken in selecting an antimicrobial agent for clinical use on the basis of tissue/fluid penetration. Apart from CNS penetration data, more attention should be paid to clinical efficacy, antimicrobial spectrum, toxicity, and cost than to comparative data on penetration into a given body site.

**Drug Toxicity**

As the Hippocratic oath states "Above all, do no harm," it is incumbent upon health professional to avoid toxic drugs whenever possible. Certainly, if one has the choice of two drugs that are equally efficacious yet one is less toxic, then the decision is clear. The less toxic drug, even if more costly, should be selected. Unfortunately, all too often we are faced with much more difficult decisions, not only whether to select one drug regimen over another but whether or not to use drugs at all in a given clinical situation. In making these choices, we must assess the risk/benefit ratio for the use of each drug.

An example of the application of risk/benefit analysis in the decision to use a drug is the indication for administering isoniazid prophylactically to prevent tuberculosis. Because the hepatotoxicity of isoniazid increases in frequency with age, persons over 35 who are candidates for isoniazid prophylaxis (positive skin test) must have additional risk factors of tuberculosis to balance the potential toxic effects. These include evidence of recent skin test conversion, immunosuppression, or previous gastrectomy. Patients over 35 without additional risk factors are more likely to suffer toxic effects from isoniazid than to derive benefit from its use.[25]

An excellent example of selection of drugs with equivalent efficacy on the basis of toxicity is afforded us in a study that compared chloramphenicol, ticarcillin, and clindamycin, all in combination with gentamicin, in the treatment of intraabdominal infection.[26] This study found that the efficacies of all drug regimens were equivalent. Therefore, the selection of one of these regimens for treatment of a specific patient would be based on toxicity and cost. Among the three drugs compared in the study neither ticarcillin nor clindamycin has been associated with an adverse reaction as uniformly fatal as the aplastic anemia sometimes caused by chloramphenicol. Although this effect is very rare (1 in 40,000), neither of the other two drugs has ever been associated with such a serious toxic effect, so the *routine* use of chloramphenicol for this indication would be precluded. Therefore, either ticarcillin or clindamycin should be used, with one chosen over the other on the basis of cost and other minor factors.

Attention must be paid to the potential adverse effects that would be likely in the individual patient. For example, patients with underlying renal disease or who have received recent prior courses of aminoglycoside therapy may be at increased risk of ototoxicity or nephrotoxicity from additional aminoglycosides.[27] This type of patient should not receive further therapy with this group of drugs if possible.

**Cost**

With the recent introduction of prospective reimbursement, understanding the cost of antimicrobial therapy is more important than ever. The total cost of antimicrobial therapy includes much more than just the acquisition cost of the drugs, more even than the cost of preparation and administration of the products.

The total economic impact of antimicrobial therapy is detailed in Table 74.6. Many ancillary costs affect the true

**Table 74.6** Total Economic Impact of Antimicrobial Therapy

| | |
|---|---|
| Drug acquisition cost | Monitoring |
| Storage/inventory cost | Adverse effects |
| Preparation | Impact on length of stay |
| Distribution | Cost of control systems |
| Administration | |

cost of therapy. These include objective factors such as storage, preparation, and administration, as well as more subjective items such as the costs of adverse effects. Data presently available do not allow us to readily calculate the total economic impact of antimicrobial therapy. Recently, however, Holloway et al[28] performed a cost analysis of the comparative toxicity of two aminoglycosides. They found that despite an increased frequency of toxicity for gentamicin, the extremely low cost of the product more than outweighed the difference in "total" cost resulting from an adverse effect. This type of analysis is necessary for careful assessment of the total cost of therapy.

## Combination Antimicrobial Therapy

In the selection of a drug regimen for a given patient, consideration must be given to the necessity for using more than one drug. Combinations of antimicrobials are generally used for the following reasons: (1) to broaden the spectrum of coverage for empiric therapy, (2) to achieve synergistic activity against the infecting organism, (3) to prevent the emergence of resistance, and (4) to reduce dosage of the drugs or prevent toxic effects. Examples of application of each of these rationales follow.

### Broadening the Spectrum of Coverage

Increasing the "coverage" of antimicrobial therapy is generally necessary in mixed infections where multiple organisms are likely to be present. This is the case in intraabdominal and female pelvic infections in which a variety of aerobic and anaerobic bacteria may produce disease. Traditionally, a combination of a drug active against aerobic gram-negative bacilli, such as an aminoglycoside, and a drug active against anaerobic bacteria, such as metronidazole or clindamycin, is selected. Newer β-lactam compounds, which possess good activity against both of these types of organisms, such as cefoxitin or imipenem, may be adequate to replace the combination and thereby reduce the cost of therapy.

The other clinical situation in which increased spectrum of activity is desirable is in nosocomial infection. Hospital-acquired infections, except as noted previously, are generally caused by only one organism, but many different organisms may be possible. Therefore, broad-spectrum therapy is generally prescribed at least initially. Again, newer β-lactam agents such as the third-generation cephalosporins may be adequate in certain situations to replace aminoglycoside-containing combinations; however, the enhanced gram-negative spectrum of these compounds has been achieved at the expense of gram-positive activity. Thus, most infectious disease consultants would add a drug with good antistaphylococcal activity to the regimen, such as a penicillinase-resistant penicillin or vancomycin. This is especially true in immunosuppressed patients in whom such broad-spectrum coverage is dictated by the likelihood of staphylococci and enteric gram-negative bacilli.

### Synergism

The achievement of synergistic antimicrobial activity is advantageous for infections caused by enteric gram-negative bacilli in immunosuppressed patients. Traditionally, combinations of aminoglycosides and β-lactams have been used, as these drugs together generally act synergistically against a wide variety of bacteria; however, the data supporting the superior efficacy of synergistic over nonsynergistic combinations are weak. At best, it would appear that synergistic combinations produce better results in infections caused by *Pseudomonas aeruginosa* and, perhaps, in patients with persistent neutropenia.[29] The data strongly support the superior efficacy of combinations in which both drugs are active against the infecting pathogen; however, these data were accrued using older drugs less potent than those currently available.[29] Evidence against the necessity for synergistic combinations includes the efficacy in this setting of β-lactam combinations, which are infrequently synergistic, and the efficacy of newer broad-spectrum cephalosporins as single agents.[30,31]

The concept of broad-spectrum coverage in immunosuppressed patients takes on new meaning when pulmonary infection is present. In this setting, especially in patients with lymphoproliferative disorders, the possible organisms include fungi, protozoa (*Pneumocystis carinii*), viruses (cytomegalovirus), and bacteria (*Legionella* spp. and others). Thus, empiric regimens escalate in size beyond antibacterial regimens consisting of two or three agents; regimens in immunocompromised patients may include trimethoprim–sulfamethoxazole, amphotericin B, erythromycin, and possibly acyclovir. Such an approach should be avoided whenever possible, and every attempt should be made to establish the diagnosis by means of bronchoscopy or other minimally invasive procedures.

### Preventing Resistance

The use of combinations to prevent the emergence of resistance is widespread but not often realized. The only circumstance in which this has been clinically useful is in the treatment of tuberculosis. The prevalence of resistance to a first-line drug such as isoniazid or rifampin in a population of organisms may be as high as 1 in $10^6$–$10^8$. As the bacterial load in a patient with active tuberculosis often exceeds this, two drugs are given to reduce the likelihood of encountering resistance to less than 1 in $10^{10}$.[32]

### Reducing Dosages

There are two good examples of dosage reduction by means of combining antimicrobial agents. The goal is to reduce the toxic effects caused by either drug. The classic example is the development of the triple sulfonamide combination. Each agent in the combination is relatively insoluble in aqueous medium but by combination of three separate but similar agents in lower dosage, the solubility problem and the resultant sulfonamide crystalluria were diminished.

A more recent example is a study comparing the efficacy of amphotericin B alone with that of amphotericin B in reduced dosage plus flucytosine in the treatment of cryptococcal meningitis.[33] Although there were some methodologic problems with this investigation, a shorter duration of therapy, and thus a lower total dose of amphotericin B in the combination with flucytosine, was as effective as the drug given alone at a higher dose for a longer period of time. Unfortunately, although nephrotoxicity was less in the groups given the lower dose of amphotericin B, one third of the patients receiving flucytosine suffered bone marrow suppression.

**Disadvantages**

Although the combination of drugs has potentially beneficial effects, potentially serious liabilities also exist, for example, additive nephrotoxicity from drugs such as aminoglycosides, amphotericin, and possibly vancomycin.[34] Inactivation of aminoglycosides by penicillins may be clinically significant when excessive doses of the penicillin are given to a patient in renal failure.[35] Accumulation of the penicillin has resulted in decreased serum concentrations of aminoglycosides in vivo. This same reaction can *falsely* lower aminoglycoside concentrations, even in properly dosed patients, if serum samples containing both drugs are not properly handled (frozen until assay or promptly assayed).

The combination of cephalothin and an aminoglycoside has been demonstrated in several controlled studies to be synergistically nephrotoxic.[36] However, none of the comparison groups in these studies were given an aminoglycoside alone; rather, a penicillin *plus* an aminoglycoside was used. It therefore is not clear that the higher incidence of nephrotoxicity seen in the cephalothin–aminoglycoside groups resulted from an interaction, as penicillins have been shown to *prevent* aminoglycoside toxicity.[37] The higher incidence of nephrotoxicity with cephalothin may result from an *absence* of a protective effect. This has not been demonstrated for any other currently available cephalosporins.

Finally, one must be concerned with the use of potentially antagonistic combinations. Antagonism has been demonstrated experimentally when a bacteriostatic drug (chloramphenicol) diminished the bactericidal and curative effects of gentamicin[38]; however, there are few clinical data that demonstrate this antagonism in humans. The most frequently cited example is the study of the treatment of pneumococcal meningitis in which a group of patients who received chlortetracycline in addition to penicillin G had a higher rate of mortality from the infection.[39] Such combinations should probably be avoided, whenever possible.

Of more current relevance is the increasing use of $\beta$-lactam antimicrobials in combination. A drug such as amdinocillin, which acts at a different receptor site than other $\beta$-lactam agents, may be synergistic with penicillins and cephalosporins; however, cephalosporins or other agents that are capable of inducing $\beta$-lactamase production in bacteria such as *Enterobacter cloacae* and *Pseudomonas aeruginosa* may antagonize the effects of enzyme-labile drugs such as penicillins.[30] This mechanism of antagonism is clearly demonstrable in vitro and in experimental models of infection. Although clinical failures of such combinations have not yet been found to result from this mechanism, the laboratory data are highly supportive of avoiding these combinations except in patients in whom the toxic effects of aminoglycosides are very likely to develop or are developing.

## Monitoring the Therapeutic Response

### *Clinical Assessment*

Once antimicrobial therapy has been instituted, the patient must be monitored carefully for a therapeutic response. Clinical assessment of the patient on a daily basis, or more or less often as needed, is clearly the most effective. Subjective findings in addition to an objective assessment (physical examination) are very valuable. For example, one of the most revealing signs of improving health is when patients begin to be concerned with their physical appearance.

Apart from the basics of the physical examination such as vital signs, the clinical assessment for monitoring purposes should focus on the organ system initially identified as diseased or as the nidus for systemic infection. For example, for a patient with pneumonia, the physical exam involves auscultation and percussion of the chest, listening for improvement in breath sounds. Roentgenograms, various scans, and other noninvasive examinations are very useful for checking the progress of selected diseases. Other procedures such as endoscopy, biopsies, and lumbar punctures are of somewhat more limited use because of their invasiveness.

### *Laboratory Tests*

Laboratory tests that are most useful in monitoring antimicrobial therapy include various serologic techniques for detection of antigens or antibodies, cultures of originally infected fluids or tissues, and testing of the patient's serum for bactericidal activity against the infecting organism. An example of a very useful serologic tool is the detection of antibodies to *Coccidioides immitis*, the cause of coccidioidomycosis. There is a very good correlation between disease activity and antibody levels circulating in serum.[40]

Obviously, one would expect cultures that originally grew the pathogen to become sterile during therapy. The time it takes for this to occur varies widely and ranges from a matter of hours for uncomplicated urinary tract infection to as long as several weeks in the case of tuberculosis.

Serum bactericidal titers are occasionally used in the management of selected infections. Although the data supporting their use are weak, most clinicians test the ability of the patient's serum to kill the infecting organism in bacterial endocarditis.[41] The goal is to achieve levels of activity of $\geq$1:16 dilutions. That is, serum obtained from the patient during antimicrobial therapy can be diluted at least 16-fold and still contain enough of the antimicrobial agent to kill the infecting organism. Another clinical situation in which these titers have been used is osteomyelitis in children, for whom oral antimicrobial therapy may be used for most of the duration of therapy.[42]

Determinations of serum (or other fluid) levels of antimicrobials may be useful in ensuring outcome and/or preventing toxicity (Table 74.7). Achievement of adequate amino-

**Table 74.7** Antimicrobial Agents for Which Serum Concentration Determinations Are Useful

| | |
|---|---|
| Chloramphenicol | Amikacin |
| Flucytosine | Gentamicin |
| Vancomycin | Netilmicin |
| | Tobramycin |

glycoside concentrations within the first few days of therapy of gram-negative infection correlates with better therapeutic outcome.[43] Additionally, ensuring that excessive concentrations of certain drugs such as chloramphenicol and flucytosine are avoided will prevent toxic effects.

Various methods are available to individualize drug dosages. The purpose of individualization is to tailor the dose of the drug administered to the patient's infectious process (e.g., urinary tract infection versus meningitis), as well as to the patient's excretory and metabolic capacity. The rationale has been, in part, discussed previously, but the complete individualization analysis involves more than the simple recognition that a drug dosage should be adjusted. Reliance upon simple formulas or nomograms may be hazardous, as these methods of dosage adjustment seldom, if ever, consider all of the possible factors that may affect kinetic disposition.[44] For example, although several nomograms are available to adjust aminoglycoside dosage, none of the "easier" more popular methods allows for "abnormally" low or high volumes of distribution.

Changes in the distribution volume may have significant impact on the efficacy and/or safety of therapy. An unexpectedly low volume of distribution (as in the dehydrated patient) will result in higher, potentially toxic concentrations, whereas a larger than expected volume (as in patients with edema or ascites) will result in low, potentially subtherapeutic concentrations. There are various methods to individualize dosage regimens for the specific patient at hand. All are reasonably effective as long as careful attention is paid to the factors that have been outlined. The most effective methods use measured serum concentrations of the drugs rather than estimations from renal function tests to assess true drug clearance from the body.[44]

## *Failure of Antimicrobial Therapy*

A variety of factors may be responsible for apparent lack of response to therapy, including those directly related to the host, those related to the pathogen, and, although unlikely, laboratory error in identification and/or susceptibility testing. Factors directly related to the antimicrobial agents being utilized constitute only a small proportion of the possibilities.

## *Failures Caused by Drug Selection*

Factors directly related to drug selection include an inappropriate drug selection or dosage or route of administration. For example, selection of a bacteriostatic drug for endocarditis or administration of a drug by intramuscular injection in a patient with compromised peripheral circulation (e.g., shock) may result in inadequate therapy. Malabsorption of a drug product because of gastrointestinal disease (e.g., short bowel syndrome) or a drug interaction (e.g., complexation of tetracyclines with divalent cations resulting in reduced absorption) will lead to potentially subtherapeutic serum concentrations.

Accelerated drug elimination is also possible. This may occur in patients with cystic fibrosis or during pregnancy, when more rapid clearance or larger volumes of distribution may result in low serum concentrations particularly for aminoglycosides.

Inactivation of antimicrobial agents by other drugs may occur, as in the case of aminoglycoside inactivation by penicillins. Finally, a common cause of failure of therapy is poor penetration into the site of infection. This is especially true for the so-called "privileged" sites, such as the central nervous system, the eye, and the prostate gland.

### Failures Caused by Host Factors

Host defenses must be considered in evaluation of a patient who is not responding to antimicrobial therapy. Patients who are immunosuppressed (e.g., granulocytopenia from chemotherapy, AIDS) may respond poorly to therapy because their own defenses are inadequate to eradicate the infection despite seemingly adequate drug regimens. A good example is the poor response of infection seen in granulocytopenic patients when their white cell counts remain low during therapy. This contrasts with the much better response obtained when granulocyte counts rise during the therapy.[45]

Other host factors are related to the necessity for surgical drainage of abscesses or removal of foreign bodies and/or necrotic tissue. If these situations are not corrected, they result in persistent temperature elevations and, occasionally, bacteremia despite adequate antimicrobial therapy.

### Failures Caused by Microorganisms

Factors related to the pathogen include the development of drug resistance during therapy. For example, the induction of β-lactamase production by newer cephalosporins may result in development of resistance in species of *Enterobacter, Pseudomonas aeruginosa,* and other organisms.[46] Superinfection with resistant organisms occasionally can occur and leads to apparent failure of therapy. Mixed infections caused by aerobic and anaerobic bacteria in which only aerobes are initially identified and treated may result in persistent anaerobic infection (abscess).[47] This is especially true in intraabdominal and pelvic infections and soft tissue infections of the extremities in patients with poor vascular supply.

### Failures Caused by Laboratory Errors

Finally, although this factor should never be encountered, there may be situations where the microbiology laboratory erroneously reports the identification or susceptibility of an organism. For example, failure to identify a group D streptococcus as enterococcus may lead to therapy with penicillin alone, which may well fail because of inadequate bactericidal activity. Another example would be the reporting of cephalosporin susceptibility of methicillin-resistant *Staphy-*

*lococcus aureus* (MRSA). Although some isolates of MRSA may appear susceptible in vitro, treatment of these organisms with a cephalosporin may well fail.[48]

## Non-antimicrobial Therapy

Several modalities are available for management of infectious diseases which are either adjunctive to appropriate antimicrobial therapy or are the only effective means of controlling the infection. These include surgical procedures (discussed before), antipyretics for management of very high temperature, and the correction of various host abnormalities.

Antipyretics (e.g., aspirin, acetaminophen) should be used only to keep temperatures below dangerous levels (≥ 105°F in adults; ≥ 103°F in children). If temperature is below these levels and is not producing any clinical problems, antipyretics should not be used. There is some experimental and limited clinical evidence that elevation of temperature actually is beneficial in eradication and/or control of the infection. If antipyretics must be given, they should be given on a regular basis so as to avoid wide swings in body temperature that may make the patient even more uncomfortable.

Host abnormalities may be responsible for predisposition to or persistence of infection, including cardiac or pulmonary disease, immunosuppressive disorders, and structural abnormalities of various organ systems. (For complete discussions of these factors, the reader is referred to chapters on the individual disease states.) Administration of various adjunctive measures such as granulocyte transfusions, immunoglobulins, antitoxins, and immunostimulatory agents may be beneficial depending upon the circumstances. Obviously, prevention of infection is more desirable than treatment of an established disease. Therefore, active or passive immunization is often used to either prevent or abort many infectious diseases (Table 74.8). Finally, there has been a great deal of interest in recent years in either reconstitution of immunity (e.g., with interferons, interleukins) or immunostimulation (e.g., with granulocyte/macrophage colony stimulating factor). These are not yet widely applied, but a great deal of research is taking place.

The results thus far have shown that interferons are effective in prevention of the common cold and other viral infections, but appear to be ineffective in the treatment of established viral infections (e.g., herpesvirus). Immunostimulatory drugs appear promising in vitro, but limited clinical trials to date have produced mixed results.

**Table 74.8** Agents Used for Active or Passive Immunization

| *Passive* | *Active* |
|---|---|
| Antitoxins | Bacterial vaccines |
| Botulism | Cholera |
| Diphtheria | Diphtheria |
| Tetanus | Hemophilus |
| Immunoglobulins | Meningococci |
| Hepatitis A or B | Pertussis |
| Pertussis | Pneumococci |
| Poliomyelitis | Tetanus |
| Rabies | Tuberculosis (BCG) |
| Rubella | Typhoid |
| Tetanus | Viral vaccines |
| Vaccinia | Hepatitis B |
| Varicella | Influenza |
| | Measles |
| | Mumps |
| | Poliomyelitis |
| | Rabies |
| | Rubella |
| | Smallpox |
| | Yellow fever |

## Summary

The complex interrelationship among a host, a microorganism, and antimicrobial agents makes selection of an antimicrobial regimen to treat an infectious disease more complex than treatment of most other disease states.

The presenting signs and symptoms of infection are often difficult to distinguish from autoimmune or malignant diseases. Various predisposing factors may significantly alter the likelihood of infection and/or the likelihood of a certain type of infection. To judiciously and rationally select appropriate antimicrobial therapy, careful attention must be paid to identification of the pathogen, various host factors that influence drug selection, and factors related to the pharmacologic characteristics of the drugs themselves. Integration of all of these data allows composition of a drug regimen that is effective, minimally toxic and inexpensive, and results in minimal alteration of the host's protective normal flora. Once therapy has been instituted, it can be "tailored," given the results of culture and susceptibility testing as well as the clinical response of the patient.

**Appendix** Drugs of Choice

| | *First choice* | *Alternative* |
|---|---|---|
| **Gram-Positive Cocci** | | |
| *Streptococcus* (groups A, B, C, G, and *S. bovis*) | Penicillin G[a] or V[b] or ampicillin | Erythromycin, FGC,[c,d] vancomycin |
| *Streptococcus pneumoniae* | Penicillin G or V or ampicillin | Erythromycin, FGC,[c,d] cefuroxime,[e] chloramphenicol[e] |
| *Streptococcus*, viridans group | Penicillin G ± gentamicin[f] | Vancomycin |

**Appendix** Drugs of Choice (continued)

| | *First choice* | *Alternative* |
|---|---|---|
| *Enterococcus* | Ampicillin (or penicillin G) + gentamicin[g] (in serious infection) | Vancomycin and gentamicin (nitrofurantoin or tetracycline: urinary tract infection) |
| *Staphylococcus aureus* | | |
| Penicillinase-negative | Penicillin G or V | FGC,[c,d] clindamycin, vancomycin |
| Penicillinase-positive | PRP[h] | FGC,[c,d] vancomycin, clindamycin[i] |
| Methicillin-resistant | Vancomycin ± rifampin or gentamicin | Trimethoprim–sulfamethoxazole ± rifampin |
| **Gram-Negative Cocci** | | |
| *Branhamella catarrhalis* | Trimethoprim–sulfamethoxazole | Amoxicillin–clavulanate, erythromycin |
| *Neisseria gonorrhoeae* | | |
| Uncomplicated infection | Amoxicillin/probenecid or ceftriaxone | Ampicillin, APPG,[j] tetracycline, spectinomycin |
| DGI[k] | Penicillin G or ampicillin | Tetracycline, TGC[l] |
| *Neisseria meningitidis* | Penicillin G | Chloramphenicol, cefuroxime[e] |
| **Gram-Positive Bacilli** | | |
| *Clostridium perfringens* | Penicillin G | Clindamycin, metronidazole |
| *Clostridium tetani* | TIG[m] | Penicillin, tetracycline |
| *Clostridium difficile* | Vancomycin[n] | Metronidazole, bacitracin |
| *Corynebacterium diphtheriae* | Antitoxin + penicillin G | Erythromycin |
| *Corynebacterium* JK | Vancomycin ± gentamicin | |
| *Listeria monocytogenes* | Ampicillin ± gentamicin | Trimethoprim–sulfamethoxazole |
| **Gram-Negative Bacilli** | | |
| *Acinetobacter* spp. | Gentamicin ± ESP[o,p] | Amikacin, ceftizoxime, ceftazidime, imipenem |
| *Aeromonas hydrophila* | Trimethoprim–sulfamethoxazole | Gentamicin |
| *Bacteroides fragilis* (and others) | Metronidazole | Clindamycin, cefoxitin, chloramphenicol, ESP[o], ampicillin/sulbactam, ticarcillin/clavulanate |
| *Bordetella pertussis* | Erythromycin | Trimethoprim–sulfamethoxazole |
| *Campylobacter* sp. | Erythromycin | Tetracycline, chloramphenicol, ciprofloxacin |
| *Enterobacter* sp. | Gentamicin + ESP[o,p] | Amikacin, aztreonam, TGC[l] |
| *Escherichia coli* | Gentamicin ± a penicillin[q] | FGC,[c,d] amikacin, ESP[o] |
| *Gardnerella vaginalis* | Metronidazole | Ampicillin |
| *Hemophilus influenzae* | TGC[l,r] or cefuroxime or ampicillin | Trimethoprim–sulfamethoxazole, chloramphenicol |
| *Klebsiella pneumoniae* | FGC[c,d] or gentamicin ± FGC | TGC,[l,r] trimethoprim–sulfamethoxazole, amikacin |
| *Legionella* sp. | Erythromycin ± rifampin | Ciprofloxacin (?) |
| *Pasteurella multocida* | Penicillin G | Tetracycline |
| *Proteus mirabilis* | Ampicillin | FGC,[c,d] gentamicin, trimethoprim–sulfamethoxazole |
| *Proteus* (indole-positive) (including *Providencia rettgeri, Morganella morganii, Proteus vulgaris*) | Gentamicin ± ESP[o,p] | TGC,[l] amikacin, trimethoprim–sulfamethoxazole |
| *Providencia stuartii* | Amikacin ± ESP[o,p] | TGC,[l] gentamicin, trimethoprim–sulfamethoxazole |
| *Pseudomonas aeruginosa* | Gentamicin or tobramycin + ESP[o,p] | Amikacin, ceftazidime, aztreonam, imipenem, ciprofloxacin |
| *Pseudomonas cepacia* | Trimethoprim–sulfamethoxazole | Chloramphenicol |
| *Salmonella typhi* | Chloramphenicol | Trimethoprim–sulfamethoxazole, ampicillin |
| *Salmonella* (nontyphi) | Ampicillin[s] | Trimethoprim–sulfamethoxazole, chloramphenicol, ciprofloxacin |
| *Serratia marcescens* | Gentamicin or amikacin ± ESP[o,p] | TGC,[l] trimethoprim–sulfamethoxazole |

**Appendix** (continued)

| | *First choice* | *Alternative* |
|---|---|---|
| *Shigella* | Trimethoprim–sulfamethoxazole[s] | Chloramphenicol, ampicillin, ciprofloxacin, norfloxacin |
| **Miscellaneous Organisms** | | |
| *Actinomyces israelii* | Penicillin G | Tetracycline |
| *Nocardia* | Sulfonamide[t] | Trimethoprim–sulfamethoxazole, minocycline, erythromycin |
| *Chlamydia* | Tetracycline or erythromycin | Sulfonamide |
| *Mycoplasma pneumoniae* | Erythromycin | Tetracycline |
| *Rickettsia* | Tetracycline | Chloramphenicol |
| *Treponema pallidum* | Penicillin G | Tetracycline, erythromycin |
| *Borrelia burgdorferi* (Lyme Agent) | Tetracycline | Penicillin, erythromycin, ceftriaxone |
| **Fungi** | | |
| *Aspergillus* sp. | Amphotericin B | |
| *Candida* sp. | Amphotericin B or ketoconazole[u] | Flucytosine[v] |
| *Coccidioides immitis* | Amphotericin B | Ketoconazole, miconazole |
| *Cryptococcus neoformans* | Amphotericin B ± flucytosine[v] | Ketoconazole |
| *Histoplasma capsulatum* | Amphotericin B | Ketoconazole |
| *Mucor* | Amphotericin B | |
| *Sporothrix schenkii* | Iodides[w] | Amphotericin B |
| **Viruses** | | |
| Herpes simplex | Trifluridine[x] or acyclovir[y] | Vidarabine, idoxuridine[x] |
| Influenza A | Amantadine | |
| Varicella zoster | Acyclovir | Vidarabine |
| Cytomegalovirus | Ganciclovir | |
| Epstein–Barr | Acyclovir (?) | |
| Human immunodeficiency virus (HIV) | Zidovudine | |

[a] Either aqueous penicillin G or benzathine penicillin G (pharyngitis only).
[b] Only for soft tissue infections or upper respiratory infections (pharyngitis, otitis media).
[c] First-generation cephalosporins—cephalothin, cephapirin, or cefazolin.
[d] Some penicillin-allergic patients may react to cephalosporins.
[e] For the treatment of meningitis.
[f] Gentamicin should be added if tolerance or "moderately susceptible" (MIC $\geq$ 0.1 $\mu$g/mL) organisms are encountered; streptomycin may be used but is more toxic in the elderly.
[g] Must be added for synergy in cases of endocarditis, meningitis, and perhaps bacteremic pyelonephritis.
[h] Penicillinase-resistant penicillin: nafcillin or oxacillin; methicillin is probably more nephrotoxic.
[i] Not reliably bactericidal, so should not be used for endocarditis.
[j] Aqueous procaine penicillin G.
[k] Disseminated gonococcal infection.
[l] Third-generation cephalosporins—cefotaxime, ceftizoxime, ceftriaxone.
[m] Tetanus immune globulin.
[n] Oral administration only.
[o] Extended-spectrum penicillin—ticarcillin, mezlocillin, or piperacillin.
[p] Combination therapy is probably required only in severely immunosuppressed patients.
[q] Ampicillin, ticarcillin, mezlocillin.
[r] Should be used only in meningitis.
[s] Antibiotics should not be given for gastroenteritis, as the carrier state may be prolonged without significant clinical benefit.
[t] Sulfisoxazole, sulfadiazine (preferred for CNS disease), trisulfapyrimidines.
[u] Mucocutaneous disease only.
[v] May be added to amphotericin for potential synergy, but only if in vitro susceptibility is documented. Resistance develops frequently if used alone. Urinary tract infections caused by *Candida* are amenable to monotherapy.
[w] Lymphocutaneous disease only.
[x] Keratitis only.
[y] Topical form for primary genital disease only; oral form to treat severe genital disease, and to prevent recurrence of genital infections; IV form for severe mucocutaneous, disseminated, or meningoencephalitic disease.

## References


1. Esposito AL, Gleckman RA. A diagnostic approach to the adult with fever of unknown origin. Arch Intern Med 1979;139:575–579.
2. Young EJ, Fainstein V, Musher DM. Drug-induced fever: Cases seen in the evaluation of unexplained fever in a general hospital population. Rev Infect Dis 1982;4:69–77.
3. Atkins E. Fever: The old and the new. J Infect Dis 1984;149: 339–345.
4. McCue JD. Improved mortality in gram-negative bacillary bacteremia. Arch Intern Med 1985;145:1212–1216.
5. Donowitz GR, Mandell GL. Empiric therapy for pneumonia. Rev Infect Dis 1983;5(suppl):S40–S51.
6. Bell WE. Treatment of bacterial infections of the central nervous system. Ann Neurol 1981;9:313–327.
7. Lewin EB. Partially treated meningitis. Am J Dis Child 1974; 128:145–147.
8. Lerner PI, Weinstein L. Infective endocarditis in the antibiotic era. N Engl J Med 1966;274:323–331.
9. Parker CW. Drug allergy. N Engl J Med 1975;292:511–514, 732–735, 957–961.
10. Saxon A. Immediate hypersensitivity reactions to β-lactam antibiotics. Rev Infect Dis 1983;5(suppl 2):S368–S378.
11. Saxon A, Beall GN, Rohr AS, et al. Immediate hypersensitivity reactions to β-lactam antibiotics. Ann Intern Med 1987;107:204–215.
12. Kantor HI, Sutherland DA, Leonard JT, et al. Effect on bilirubin metabolism in the newborn of sulfisoxazole administered to the mother. Obstet Gynecol 1961;17:494–500.
13. Powell DA, Nahata MC. Chloramphenicol: new perspectives on an old drug. Drug Intell Clin Pharm 1982;16:295–300.
14. Gardner ID. The effect of aging on susceptibility to infection. Rev Infect Dis 1980;2:801–810.
15. Kopanoff DE, Snider DE Jr, Caras GJ. Isoniazid-related hepatitis. A US Public Health Cooperative Surveillance Study. Am Rev Respir Dis 1978;117:991–1001.
16. Chow AW, Jewesson PJ. Pharmacokinetics and safety of antimicrobial agents during pregnancy. Rev Infect Dis 1985;7:287–313.
17. Snider DE. Pyridoxine supplementation during isoniazid therapy. Tubercle 1980;61:191–196.
18. Swanson M. Drugs, chemicals, and hemolysis. Drug Intell Clin Pharm 1973;7:6–24.
19. Roberts JA. Urinary tract infections. Am J Kidney Dis 1984;4: 103–117.
20. Waldvogel FA, Vasey H. Osteomyelitis: the past decade. N Engl J Med 1980;303:360–370.
21. Winston DJ, Dudnik DV, Chapin M, et al. Coagulase-negative staphylococcal bacteremia in patients receiving immunosuppressive therapy. Arch Intern Med 1983;143:32–36.
22. Armstrong D, Gold JWM, Dryjanski J, et al. Treatment of infections in patients with the acquired immune deficiency syndrome. Ann Intern Med 1985;103:738–743.
23. Tillotson JR, Finland M. Bacterial colonization and clinical superinfection of the respiratory tract complicating antibiotic treatment of pneumonia. J Infect Dis 1969;119:597–624.
24. Scheld WM. Theoretical and practical considerations of antibiotic therapy for bacterial meningitis. Pediatr Infect Dis 1985;4: 74–83.
25. Bailey WC, Byrd RB, Glassroth JL, et al. Preventive treatment of tuberculosis. Chest 1985;87(suppl):128S–132S.
26. Harding GKM, Buckwold FJ, Ronald AR, et al. Prospective randomized comparative study of clindamyin, chloramphenicol, and ticarcillin, each in combination with gentamicin, in therapy for intraabdominal and female genital tract sepsis. J Infect Dis 1980;142:384–393.
27. Moench TR, Smith CR. Risk factors for aminoglycoside nephrotoxicity, in Whelton A, Neu HC (eds): The Aminoglycosides—Microbiology, Clinical Use and Toxicology. New York, Marcel Dekker, 1982, 401–415.
28. Holloway JJ, Smith CR, Moore RD, et al. Comparative cost effectiveness of gentamicin and tobramycin. Ann Intern Med 1984;101:764–769.
29. Anderson ET, Young LS, Hewitt WL. Antimicrobial synergism in the therapy of gram-negative rod bacteremia. Chemotherapy 1978;24:45–54.
30. Barriere SL. Therapeutic considerations in using combinations of newer β-lactam antibiotics. Clin Pharm 1986;5:24–33.
31. Moellering RC. Can the third generation cephalosporins eliminate the need for antimicrobial combinations? Am J Med 1985;79(suppl 2A):104–109.
32. Snider DE, Cohn DL, Davidson PT, et al. Standard therapy for tuberculosis 1985. Chest 1985;87(suppl):117S–124S.
33. Bennett JE, Dismukes WE, Duma RJ, et al. A comparison of amphotericin B alone and combined with flucytosine in the treatment of cryptococcal meningitis. N Engl J Med 1979;301: 126–131.
34. Farber BF, Moellering RC. Retrospective study of the toxicity of preparations of vancomycin from 1974 to 1981. Antimicrob Agents Chemother 1983;23:138–141.
35. Ervin FR, Bullock WE, Nuttall CE. Inactivation of gentamicin by penicillins in patients with renal failure. Antimicrob Agents Chemother 1976;9:1024–1031.
36. Wade JC, Schimpff SC, Wiernik PH. Antibiotic-combination associated nephrotoxicity in granulocytopenic patients with cancer. Arch Intern Med 1981;141:1789–1793.
37. English J, Gilbert DN, Kohlhepp S, et al. Attenuation of experimental tobramycin nephrotoxicity by ticarcillin. Antimicrob Agents Chemother 1985;27:897–902.
38. Sande MA, Overton JW. In vivo antagonism between gentamicin and chloramphenicol in neutropenic mice. J Infect Dis 1973;128:247–250.
39. Lepper MH, Dowling HF. Treatment of pneumococcic meningitis with penicillin compared with penicillin plus aureomycin. Arch Intern Med 1951;88:489–494.
40. Hardenbrook MH, Barriere SL. Coccidioidomycosis: Evaluation of parameters used to predict outcome with amphotericin B therapy. Mycopathologia 1982;78:65–71.
41. Weinstein MP, Stratton CW, Ackley A, et al. Multicenter collaborative evaluation of a standardized serum bactericidal test as a prognostic indicator in infective endocarditis. Am J Med 1985;78:262–269.
42. Prober CG. Oral antibiotic therapy for bone and joint infections. Pediatr Infect Dis 1982;1:8–10.
43. Moore RD, Smith CR, Lietman PS. Association of aminoglycoside plasma levels with therapeutic outcome in gram-negative pneumonia. Am J Med 1984;77:657–662.
44. Lesar TS, Rotschafer JC, Strand LM, et al. Gentamicin dosing errors with four commonly used nomograms. JAMA 1982;248: 1190–1193.

**45.** Bodey GP. Antibiotics in patients with neutropenia. Arch Intern Med 1984;144:1845–1851.

**46.** Sanders CC, Sanders WE. Microbial resistance to newer generation $\beta$-lactam antibiotics: clinical and laboratory implications. J Infect Dis 1985;151:399–406.

**47.** DiPiro JT, Mansberger JA, Davis JB. Current concepts in clinical therapeutics: intraabdominal infections. Clin Pharm 1986;5:34–50.

**48.** Cafferkey MT, Hone R, Keane CT. Antimicrobial chemotherapy of septicemia due to methicillin-resistant *Staphylococcus aureus*. Antimicrob Agents Chemother 1985;28:819–823.

# Chapter 75 / Central Nervous System Infection

John C. Rotschafer, PharmD, Humphrey Z. Zokufa, PharmD, and Irving Steinberg, PharmD

Central nervous system infections include a wide variety of clinical conditions and etiologies.[1–4] Meningitis, meningoencephalitis, encephalitis, brain and meningeal abscesses, and shunt infections are all included under this heading. These infections may be caused by a variety of bacteria, fungi, viruses, and parasites.[1–4] The ability to rapidly diagnose and institute effective therapy is paramount to patient survival without neurological sequelae. The initial examination of cerebrospinal fluid and possibly a repeat examination 12 hours later can be useful in differentiating bacterial, fungal, and viral infections.

Central nervous system infections are divided into septic and aseptic infections. Septic or bacterial infections are the result of hematogenous spread from a primary point of infection, parameningeal seeding from a localized infection, or trauma or congenital defects in the central nervous system. Aseptic infection is a term broadly used to describe chemical irrigants and viral, fungal, parasitic, tubercular, sarcoid, neoplastic, and syphilitic processes of the central nervous system.

In most cases of bacterial meningitis there are several steps in the sequence of the disease process. First, the organism (usually encapsulated) attaches to the epithelial cells of the nasopharyngeal and/or oropharyngeal mucosa.[1,2] The organisms then penetrate the mucosal barrier, invading the bloodstream.[1,2] If the organisms survive the natural defense mechanisms of the blood and cause bacteremia, the meninges may become seeded with microorganisms causing meningitis.[1,2]

Signs and symptoms of central nervous system infection have clinical features similar to those of a variety of infectious diseases. Fever, peripheral leukocytosis with a left shift, and malaise are often common observations.[1,4] Clinical symptoms in the elderly may be uniquely different, resembling stroke or endocarditis.[3,4] Signs and symptoms in the neonate may be limited to fever and irritability. Usually, the cerebrospinal fluid (CSF) pattern of pleocytosis (an increase in the number of leukocytes, especially lymphocytes, in the CSF), protein concentration, and glucose concentration with respect to time can be used to differentiate viral, fungal, and bacterial etiologies.[1–4]

Several additional factors are important in the diagnosis of central nervous system infections. The clinical setting (hospital, community, or long-term care center) may give some clue as to the etiology of infection. Whether the central nervous system is anatomically intact or has recently been traumatized is of key importance in the proper diagnosis. The age of the patient and the season of the year may also assist in identifying likely pathogens.[1–4] Integration of clinical, demographic, and laboratory data is crucial to the proper diagnosis and the selection of appropriate antimicrobial agents. The purpose of this chapter is to present relevant aspects of the pathogenesis, pathophysiology, and antimicrobial therapy of central nervous system infections.

## Anatomy and Physiology of the Central Nervous System

### *Meninges*[5]

The skull and vertebrae protect the central nervous system from blunt or penetrating trauma (Fig. 75.1). The brain is suspended in these structures by cerebrospinal fluid and is surrounded by the meninges. The meninges are made up of three separate membranes. The dura mater, or pachymeninges, lies directly beneath and is adherent to the skull. The other two membranes are referred to collectively as the leptomeninges. The pia mater lies directly over the brain tissue itself. The arachnoid is the middle layer between the dura mater and pia mater. Between the pia mater and arachnoid is the subarachnoid space, which serves as the conduit for cerebrospinal fluid. By definition, meningitis is an infection of the subarachnoid space.

### *Cerebrospinal Fluid*[5,6]

Approximately 85% of cerebrospinal fluid is produced within the fourth and lateral ventricles by the choroid plexus (Fig. 75.1). Cerebrospinal fluid volume in the central nervous system is related to patient age. Infants have approximately 40 to 60 mL of cerebrospinal fluid, whereas older children have approximately 80 to 100 mL. Adults have approximately 110 to 160 mL of cerebrospinal fluid. Cerebrospinal fluid is produced at the rate of approximately 0.5 mL/min and flows unidirectionally downward through the spinal cord. Cerebrospinal fluid is removed by the arachnoid villi (Fig. 75.1) and vertebral venus plexus located in the spinal cord and does not recommunicate with the point of production.

Cerebrospinal fluid (Table 75.1) is normally clear, has a protein content <50 mg/dL, has a glucose concentration approximately 50% to 66% of the simultaneous peripheral concentration, has a physiologic pH, and usually contains fewer than five white blood cells per cubic millimeter all of which should be mononuclear.

### *Blood–Brain Barrier/Blood–Cerebrospinal Fluid Barrier*[5–7]

The central nervous system has natural barriers to the exchange of drugs and endogenous compounds among the blood, brain, and cerebrospinal fluid. The blood–brain bar-

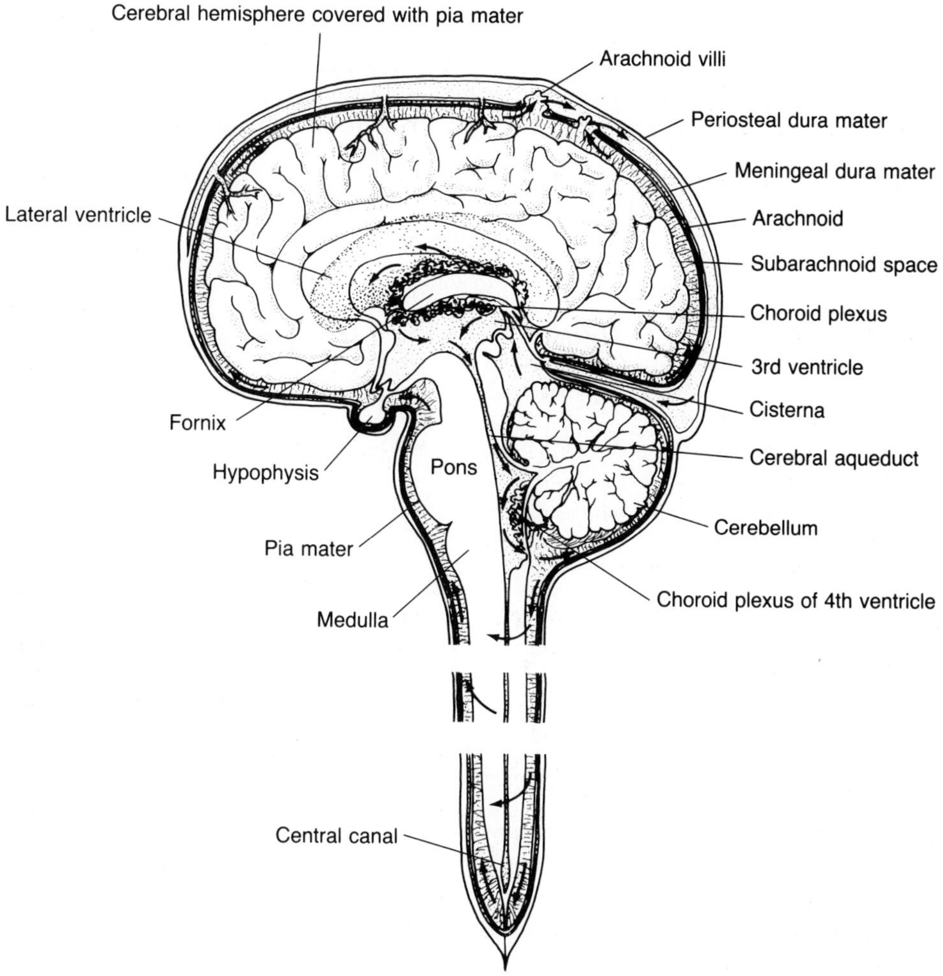


**Figure 75.1.** Diagram of the central nervous system.

rier consists of tightly joined capillary endothelial cells. Drug entry into brain tissue is accomplished by direct passage through the capillary endothelial cell. Having traversed this barrier, the drug must then penetrate the glial cells which envelop the capillary structure.

Passage of chemical substances into the cerebrospinal fluid is controlled by the blood–cerebrospinal fluid barrier. This barrier is created by the ependymal cells of the choroid plexus which function similarly to renal tubular epithelial cells. Like the active transport system in the kidney, the functions of the choroid plexus can be inhibited by the administration of probenecid. The natural functioning of the choroid plexus is also inhibited by the inflammatory process associated with meningitis.

Several factors influence the transfer of antibiotic from capillary blood into the central nervous system. With in-

**Table 75.1** Mean Values of the Components of Normal and Abnormal Cerebrospinal Fluid

| *Component* | *Normal CSF* | *Abnormal CSF* |
|---|---|---|
| Glucose | 30–70 mg/100 mL | <50 mg/100 mL (50%–60% of peripheral serum glucose) |
| Protein | <50 mg/100mL | >150 mg/100 mL |
| White blood cells | <10/mm$^3$ (mononuclear) | >1,200/mm$^3$ (with 95% PMNs for bacterial meningitis) |
| Lactic acid | <14 mg/100 mL | >35 mg/100 mL |
| pH | 7.3 | 7.1 |

**Table 75.2** Penetration of Antimicrobial Agents into the Cerebrospinal Fluid

| | |
|---|---|
| Therapeutic concentration in CSF without inflammation of meninges | Sulfonamides<br>Trimethoprim<br>Chloramphenicol<br>Isoniazid<br>Rifampin |
| Therapeutic concentration in CSF with inflammation | Penicillin G<br>Ampicillin<br>Ticarcillin ± clavulanic acid<br>Carbenicillin<br>Mezlocillin<br>Piperacillin<br>Cefuroxime<br>Ceftizoxime<br>Ceftazidime<br>Imipenem<br>Aztreonam |
| Nontherapeutic concentration with or without inflammation | Amikacin<br>Streptomycin<br>Gentamicin<br>Kanamycin<br>Tobramycin<br>Polymyxin<br>Most quinolones |

creased meningeal inflammation, there will be greater antibiotic penetration (Table 75.2). Antibiotics of smaller molecular weight are more capable of passing biological barriers than are compounds of large molecular weight. Only antibiotics that are un-ionized at the physiologic or pathologic pH are capable of diffusion. Compounds that are highly lipid soluble penetrate more readily than water-soluble compounds. Antibiotics that are not extensively protein bound in the serum provide a larger free fraction of drug capable of passing into the cerebrospinal fluid. Passage of large polar antibiotics into the cerebrospinal fluid must be assisted by a saturable carrier transport system.

Problems of cerebrospinal fluid penetration may also be overcome by direct instillation of antibiotics by intrathecal, intracisternal, or intraventricular administration[8–11] (Table 75.3). The advantages of direct instillation, however, must be weighed against the risks of invasive central nervous system procedures. Intrathecal administration of antibiotics is unlikely to produce therapeutic concentrations in the ventricles because of the unidirectional flow of cerebrospinal fluid.[9] Although intraventricular administration may be preferred over intrathecal administration, the former requires neurosurgical placement of an Ommaya or Rickham reservoir.[8] Another option to maintain antibiotic concentrations within the cerebrospinal fluid is to limit drug clearance by interfering with antibiotic transport out of the central ner-

**Table 75.3** Intraventricular and Intrathecal Antibiotic Dosage Recommendations

| *Antibiotic* | *Dose (mg)* | *Expected CSF concentration*[a] *(mg/L)* | *Reference* |
|---|---|---|---|
| Ampicillin | 10–50 | 60–300 | 58–60 |
| Methicillin | 25–100 | 160–600 | 58–60 |
| Nafcillin | 75 | 500 | 60 |
| Cefazolin | 1–2 mg/kg, 50 mg maximum | 300 | 53 |
| Cephalothin | 25–100 | 160–600 | 58–60 |
| Chloramphenicol | 25–100 | 160–600 | 58, 59, 61 |
| Gentamicin | 1–10 | 6–60 | 58–62 |
| Tobramycin | 1–10 | 6–60 | 62 |
| Amikacin | 5–10 | 60 | 63, 64 |
| Vancomycin | 5 | 30 | 65–67 |

[a] Assumes adult CSF volume = 150 mL.

vous system. With most $\beta$-lactam antibiotics, the use of probenecid will reduce the rate of antibiotic clearance from cerebrospinal fluid.

## Bacterial Meningitis

### *Clinical Presentation*

On initial presentation, differentiation of patients with bacterial, viral, or fungal meningitis is virtually impossible. Patients will present with variable common complaints of fever, stiffness of the neck and/or back, nuchal rigidity, positive Brudzinski's sign (flexion of both legs and thighs upon forcible flexion of the neck), and positive Kernig's sign (inability of patient to extend leg completely when lying on back with thigh flexed at right angles to trunk).[1–3] Later in the course of the disease, the patient may experience seizures, focal neurologic deficits, and hydrocephalus.[1–3] The most likely bacterial pathogens causing meningitis as associated with age are presented in Table 75.4.

The diagnosis of bacterial meningitis is usually made on the basis of examination of cerebrospinal fluid collected soon after the diagnosis is suspected. The presence of 200 to 10,000 white blood cells per cubic millimeter ($\geq$95% polymorphonuclear cells), an elevated cerebrospinal fluid protein concentration >50 mg/dL, and a cerebrospinal fluid glucose concentration below 50% of the simultaneously obtained peripheral value may suggest bacterial meningitis. In some cases of viral meningitis, the initial examination of cerebrospinal fluid may reveal predominantly polymorphonuclear cells.[12] For these reasons, cerebrospinal fluid white blood cell counts, glucose concentration, and protein concentration cannot always be relied on to establish or rule out bacterial meningitis because the ranges for these tests overlap significantly with those for viral, tuberculous, and fungal meningitis.[13]

Several rapid diagnostic methods are available for identifying potential pathogens from cerebrospinal fluid.[14–17] Counterimmunoelectrophoresis (CIE), latex fixation, and coagglutination tests provide for the rapid identification of *Streptococcus pneumoniae*, *Neisseria meningitidis*, and type B *Hemophilus influenzae*.[3,14] All of these tests work on the principle of bringing potential capsular antigens of the pathogen causing meningitis in contact with a specific antibody, causing an antigen–antibody reaction. This capsular antigen–antibody reaction can be observed visually and can be accomplished quickly without waiting for culture results. The sensitivity and specificity of these tests vary with the manufacturer of the antibody, the density of antigen present in the CSF, and the pathogen being tested. Manufactured antisera are not available to all strains of potentially pathogenic bacteria.

In the case of gram-negative meningitis where cerebrospinal fluid may contain endotoxin, the limulus lysate assay may be of value. If endotoxin present in cerebrospinal fluid is brought into contact with amebocyte lysate from *Limulus polyphemus* (horseshoe crab), the specimen gels.[15] Some additional tests of questionable diagnostic value, because they are nonspecific, are determinations of cerebrospinal fluid pH and lactate levels.[16] Not to be overlooked as a valuable diagnostic tool is the Gram stain of cerebrospinal fluid prior to antibiotic therapy which may be positive in >80% of adult patients found to be culture positive.[17]

### *Treatment*

Because of compromised phagocytosis in the cerebrospinal fluid caused by impaired opsonic activity and reduced levels of complement and immunoglobulin,[18] peak cerebrospinal fluid antibiotic concentration should be approximately ten times the minimum bactericidal concentration (MBC) of microorganisms causing bacterial meningitis.[19] The level of antibiotics in the cerebrospinal fluid is a function of the permeability properties of the antibiotic across the blood–

**Table 75.4** Meningitis: Most Likely Infecting Microorganism at Various Ages

| *Age commonly affected* | *Most likely causative microorganism* | *Risk factors for all ages* | *Less likely causative microorganism* |
|---|---|---|---|
| Newborn–1 month | *Escherichia coli*<br>*Klebsiella* spp.<br>*Enterobacter* spp.<br>Group B streptococcus | Respiratory tract infection<br>Otitis media<br>Mastoiditis<br>Head trauma | *Listeria monocytogenes*<br>Herpes simplex type 2 |
| 1 month–4 years | *Hemophilus influenzae*<br>*Neisseria meningitidis*<br>*Streptococcus pneumoniae* | Alcoholism<br>Splenectomy<br>Sickle cell disease<br>High-dose steroids | Viruses |
| 5–9 years | *N. meningitidis*<br>*H. influenzae*<br>*S. pneumoniae* | Immunosuppression<br>Immunoglobulin deficiency | Viruses |
| 10–29 years | *N. meningitidis*<br>*S. pneumoniae*<br>*H. influenzae* | | Viruses |
| 30–70 years | *S. pneumoniae*<br>*N. meningitidis* | | *L. monocytogenes*<br>Viruses |

**Table 75.5** Antimicrobial Agents of First Choice and Alternative Choice in Treatment of Various Types of Meningitis Caused by Gram-Positive Microorganisms

| *Type of meningitis* | *Antibiotic of first choice*[a] | *Alternative choice of antibiotic*[a] |
|---|---|---|
| *Streptococcus pneumoniae* | Penicillin G 200,000–300,000 units/kg/day (4 million units every 4 h IV) | Chloramphenicol 25 mg/kg every 6 h IV<br>Cefuroxime 2–3 g every 6–8 h IV (max 3 g every 8 h)<br>Cefotaxime 2 g every 4 h IV<br>Ceftizoxime 3–4 g every 8 h IV<br>Ceftriaxone 2 g every 12 h IV |
| Group B streptococcus | Penicillin G 200,000–300,000 units/kg/day (4 million units every 4 h IV) | Chloramphenicol 25 mg/kg every 6 h IV<br>Cefuroxime 2–3 g every 6–8 h IV (max 3 g every 8 h)<br>Cefotaxime 2 g every 4 h IV<br>Ceftizoxime 3–4 g every 8 h IV<br>Ceftriaxone 2 g every 12 h IV |
| Staphylococcal | | |
| *S. aureus* (penicillin-resistant) | Nafcillin 2 g every 4 h IV<br>Cefotaxime 2 g every 4 h IV | Vancomycin 30–40 mg/kg/d IV |
| *S. aureus* (methicillin-resistant) | Vancomycin 30–40 mg/kg/d | — |
| *S. epidermidis* (penicillin-resistant) | Nafcillin 2 g every 4 h IV<br>Cefotaxime 2 g every 4 h IV | Vancomycin 30–40 mg/kg/d IV |
| *S. epidermidis* (methicillin-resistant) | Vancomycin 30–40 mg/kg/d | |
| *Listeria monocytogenes* | Ampicillin 2 g every 4 h IV | Trimethoprim 10 mg/kg/d IV<br>Sulfamethoxazole 50 mg/kg/d IV |

[a] Recommended doses for adult patients with normal renal function and/or hepatic function.

CSF barrier. Only lipid-soluble compounds reach the brain readily because they can cross the blood–brain barrier. In the presence of meningeal inflammation some antibiotics (e.g., ampicillin, penicillin G) can achieve adequate levels in CSF; others (e.g., clindamycin and aminoglycosides) do not.

Cultures of cerebrospinal fluid and blood are mandatory in any patient in whom bacterial meningitis is suspected because isolation and identification of the causative agent can assist in selection of the best antimicrobial therapy for the patient (Tables 75.5 and 75.6).

## *Causative Agents*

### *Neisseria meningitidis* (Meningococcus)

*Neisseria meningitidis* meningitis is most commonly found in children and young adults.[1–3] The source of the infection is usually an asymptomatic carrier.[1] Most cases usually occur in the winter or spring at a time when viral meningitis is relatively uncommon.[1–3] Four serogroups of *N. meningitidis* are primarily responsible for this type of meningitis. Serogroups A and C are usually associated with epidemics of meningitis, while serogroup B is the primary cause of isolated cases of meningitis.[1–3,20] Serogroup Y is more frequently associated with pneumonia and is rarely associated with meningitis.[1,3]

Patients are initially colonized and at some point develop a bacteremia, which likely occurs prior to the patient's hospital admission. As a result of the bacteremia, there is metastatic seeding; the meninges are the most common site.[1,3] Following meningitis, there is a unique immune reaction that distinguishes meningococcal meningitis from other bacterial causes.[1,3] Approximately 10 to 14 days after the onset of the disease and despite successful treatment, the patient develops a characteristic immunologic reaction of fever, arthritis (usually involving large joints), and pericarditis.[1,3] At this time, examination of synovial fluid will reveal a large number of polymorphonuclear cells, elevated protein concentration, and normal glucose concentration.[1,3] Cultures of synovial fluid will be sterile.[1,3] The reaction may last a week or longer and no additional antibiotic therapy is required[1,3]; however, the patient may benefit from nonsteroidal anti-inflammatory agents or aspirin therapy.

Approximately 50% of such patients die within the first 24 hours as a result of an acute fulminant course associated with meningococcemia.[1–4] Other patients develop a picture of chronic meningococcemia that is characterized by episodes of fever, arthritis, and a morbilliform rash which reoccurs every 48 to 72 hours and persists for 24 hours.[1–4]

Seizures and coma are uncommon with meningococcal meningitis. Patients may behave aggressively and are often maniacal. Patients may develop 6th, 7th, and 8th cranial

**Table 75.6** Antimicrobial Agents of First Choice and Alternative Choice in Treatment of the Various Types of Meningitis Caused by Gram-Negative Microorganisms

| *Type of meningitis* | *Antibiotic of first choice*[a] | *Alternative choice of antibiotic*[a] |
|---|---|---|
| Meningococcal (*Neisseria meningitidis*) | Penicillin G 200,000–300,000 units/kg/day (4 million units every 4 h IV) | Chloramphenicol 25 mg/kg every 6 h IV<br>Cefuroxime 2–3 g every 6–8 h<br>Cefotaxime 2 g every 4 h IV<br>Ceftizoxime 3–4 g every 8 h IV<br>Ceftriaxone 2 g every 12 h IV |
| *Escherichia coli* | Ampicillin 2 g every 4 h IV | Chloramphenicol 25 mg/kg every 6 h IV<br>Cefuroxime 2–3 g every 6–8 h IV (max 3 g every 8 h)<br>Cefotaxime 2 g every 4 h IV<br>Ceftizoxime 3–4 g every 8 h IV<br>Ceftriaxone 2 g every 12 h IV |
| *Hemophilus influenzae*<br>β-Lactamase-positive<br>β-Lactamase-negative | <br>Chloramphenicol 25 mg/kg every 6 h IV<br>Ampicillin 2 g every 4 h IV | Cefuroxime 2–3 g every 6–8 h IV (max 3 g every 8 h)<br>Cefotaxime 2 g every 4 h IV<br>Ceftizoxime 3–4 g every 8 h IV<br>Ceftriaxone 2 g every 12 h IV |
| Gram-negative bacillary (*Pseudomonas aeruginosa*) | Piperacillin 3 g every 4 h IV and tobramycin 5–7.5 mg/kg/d | Ceftazidime 2 g every 8 h IV<br>Imipenem 1 g every 6 h IV |

[a] Recommended doses for adult patients with normal renal function and/or hepatic function.

nerve dysfunction noted by deafness and transiently impaired ocular movements. Deafness unilaterally, or more commonly bilaterally, may develop early or late in the disease course and is permanent.[21] Aphasia is uncommon with meningococcal meningitis. Fortunately, most neurologic complications are rare.[1–4]

The presence of petechiae may be the primary clue that the underlying pathogen is *N. meningitidis*.[1–4] Approximately 50% of patients with meningococcal meningitis have purpuric lesions, petechiae, or both.[1–4] Patients may have an obvious or subclinical picture of disseminated intravascular coagulation (DIC) which may progress to infarction of the adrenal glands and renal cortex and cause widespread thrombosis.[1–4]

Aggressive early intervention with high-dose intravenous crystalline penicillin G, 50,000 units/kg every 4 hours (or adjusted for renal function), is usually recommended for treatment of *N. meningitidis* meningitis.[1–4] Chloramphenicol is bactericidal for *N. meningitidis* and may be used in place of penicillin G.[1–4] Several third-generation cephalosporins (e.g., cefotaxime) approved for the treatment of meningitis are acceptable alternatives to penicillin G (Table 75.2).

Close contacts of patients contracting *N. meningitidis* meningitis are at an increased risk of developing meningitis. Secondary cases of meningitis can develop within 30 days contact with the index case.[20] Risk factors in these contacts have been estimated at 200 to 1,000 times that of the general population.[20] Young children are at the greatest risk of contracting *N. meningitidis*; however, close contacts of all ages are at risk.

Prophylaxis should be started without delay and without the aid of culture and sensitivity studies, as most secondary cases occur within the first week of index case contact. The delay involved in obtaining cultures and sensitivity studies would put the close contact at high risk of contracting the disease. Adult patients should receive 600 mg of rifampin every 12 hours for four doses. Children 1 month to 12 years should receive 10 mg/kg of rifampin every 12 hours for four doses, and children younger than 1 month should receive 5 mg/kg every 12 hours for four doses.[20] Rifampin, unlike many other antibiotics, can eliminate pharyngeal colonization of meningococci.

Vaccination is of limited value in that sporadic cases of the disease are caused primarily by serogroup B and vaccines are available only for serogroups A, C, Y, and W–135.[20] Patients being vaccinated should also receive rifampin as there may be up to a 2-week delay in achieving protective antibody titers after vaccination.[20] Patients receiving rifampin should be counseled as to the expected red-to-orange color change in urine and other body secretions.

### *Streptococcus pneumoniae* (Pneumococcus or diplococcus)

Pneumococcal meningitis occurs in the very young (1–4 months) and the very old.[3,22] It is the most common cause of meningitis in adults and accounts for 12% of meningitis episodes in children 2 months to 10 years. Approximately 50% of cases are secondary to primary infections involving parameningeal foci such as the ear or paranasal sinuses. Pneumonia, endocarditis, cerebrospinal fluid leak secondary to head trauma, splenectomy, alcoholism, sickle cell disease, and bone marrow transplantation may all predispose the patient to the development of pneumococcal meningitis.[1–4] Failure to develop a pleocytosis in CSF is a poor prognostic sign. Case fatality rates in children are highest with this organism and approach 30%.

Bacteremia tends to be less common with *Streptococcus pneumoniae* than with *Neisseria meningitidis*. Neurologic complications such as coma and seizures are common with pneumococcal meningitis.[3] Traumatic tears of the dura, fracture of the cribriform plate or paranasal sinuses, nasal meningocele, repeated episodes of otitis media, and osteomyelitis of the skull floor are risk factors for recurrent pneumococcal meningitis.[1–5]

Treatment with intravenous crystalline penicillin G 50,000 units/kg every 4 hours in adult patients with normal renal function usually results in a favorable prognosis. There have been limited reports of penicillin-resistant *S. pneumoniae*.[23] Although these resistant strains are not a prevalent problem, their ultimate impact has yet to be defined.

Chloramphenicol represents a useful alternative to penicillin G and is bactericidal for *S. pneumoniae*.[1–5,18] Several third-generation cephalosporins may serve as alternatives to penicillin in the treatment of pneumococcal meningitis; however, third-generation cephalosporins containing a 3-methylthiotetrazole substitution (e.g., cefoperazone and moxalactam) should be avoided as the ratio of achievable antibiotic concentrations in cerebrospinal fluid to minimum bactericidal concentration of the *S. pneumoniae* is too low to be considered curative.[24–32] Such drugs as cefuroxime, cefotaxime, ceftizoxime, and ceftriaxone may prove useful alternatives to penicillin G.[24–32] Outcome may depend on the serotype of the microorganism (especially type 3), whether the infection is primary or secondary, and the number of white blood cells in cerebrospinal fluid.[1]

Chemoprophylaxis and vaccination for close contacts of an index case with *S. pneumoniae* meningitis are not recommended as the risk of acquiring secondary disease in this population is very slight.[20] Pneumococcal vaccine may help prevent future infections in patients with CSF leak and underlying chronic diseases.

### Gram-Negative Meningitis

Over the last 20 years, the incidence of gram-negative meningitis, excluding *Hemophilus influenzae*, has been increasing in both children and adults.[18] Currently, enteric gram-negative organisms are the fourth leading cause of meningitis, with only *Streptococcus pneumoniae*, *Hemophilus influenzae*, and *Neisseria meningitis* having a higher incidence.[18]

There are several predisposing factors to the development of gram-negative meningitis. Congenital defects, accidental cranial trauma, or neurosurgery alter the anatomical defenses and may predispose the patient to this form of meningitis. The use of antimicrobial agents with exclusive gram-positive activity preoperatively in neurosurgery may also predispose the patient to development of a gram-negative infection. Any form of communication between the skin and subarachnoid space, such as a dermal sinus, greatly increases the risk of gram-negative meningitis. Gram-negative bacteremia by itself is an infrequent cause of meningitis without some form of central nervous system trauma. Other risk factors for the development of gram-negative meningitis include diabetes, malignancy, urinary tract infection in neonates, cirrhosis, parameningeal infection, spinal anesthesia, and hospitalization in general.

Elderly debilitated patients may also be at increased risk of gram-negative meningitis but lack classic signs and symptoms of the disease. Nuchal rigidity may be difficult to diagnose because of the presence of cervical arthritis in the elderly. The presence of a low-grade temperature and changes in mental status without other obvious cause should prompt lumbar puncture. The two most common organisms causing gram-negative meningitis in the postneonatal period are *Escherichia coli* and *Klebsiella pneumoniae* which are responsible for 60% to 70% of cases.[18]

The optimal antimicrobial agent(s), route of administration, and duration of therapy for gram-negative bacillary meningitis have yet to be defined.[2]

Cases of *Pseudomonas aeruginosa* meningitis should be treated with an antipseudomonal penicillin plus an aminoglycoside. Because of poor aminoglycoside penetration of the cerebrospinal fluid, intrathecal or intraventricular administration should be considered, especially in situations in which the patient fails to respond to initial management with parenteral antibiotics.[7–11] Preservative-free forms of gentamicin and tobramycin are available for direct administration into the cerebrospinal fluid.

Other gram-negative organisms causing meningitis can likely be treated with a third-generation cephalosporin such as cefotaxime, ceftizoxime, ceftriaxone, ceftazidime, or moxalactam.[24–33] In situations where the offending organism is not initially known, moxalactam and ceftazidime may not reliably produce cerebrospinal fluid antibiotic concentrations >10 times the minimum bactericidal concentration for gram-positive organisms.[19,24–33] Cefoperazone produces unreliable antibiotic concentrations in the cerebrospinal fluid because of its high protein binding and should not be a drug of first choice for gram-negative meningitis.[31] In adults, daily doses of 8 to 12 g per day of these third-generation cephalosporins or 1 g of ceftriaxone should produce cerebrospinal fluid concentrations of 5 to 20 mg/L.

Limitations to the use of third-generation cephalosporins with a 3-methylthiotetrazole substitution, like cefoperazone and moxalactam, in gram-negative meningitis may include such adverse reactions as bleeding disorders, resistance caused by inducible $\beta$-lactamases, and superinfection resulting from the broad spectrum of antimicrobial activity. None of the third-generation cephalosporins are effective for *Listeria monocytogenes* and perhaps only ceftazidime would be effective in treating *P. aeruginosa* meningitis. Although chloramphenicol is a bactericidal antibiotic for *H. influenzae*, *N. meningitidis*, and *S. pneumoniae*, the antibiotic produces only a bacteriostatic effect for most gram-negative organisms.[34]

Trimethoprim–sulfamethoxazole produces cerebrospinal fluid levels of 1.9 to 5.7 mg/L for the former and 20 to 63 mg/L for the latter when given parenterally in doses of 10 mg/kg/d (trimethoprim) and 50 mg/kg/d (sulfamethoxazole).[18,35] In addition to several of the Enterobacteriaceae, trimethoprim–sulfamethoxazole may be useful for *Acinetobacter* sp. and *Serratia* sp. meningitis.[18] One additional advantage of trimethoprim–sulfamethoxazole is that the antibiotic concentrations are not dependent on the extent of meningeal inflammation.

### *Hemophilus influenzae*

*Hemophilus influenzae* is the most common cause of meningitis in children 6 months to 3 years.[1] *H. influenzae* meningitis after age 6 may indicate parameningeal foci of infection, middle ear infection, and cerebrospinal fluid leakage.[1] The disease is often a complication of primary involvement of the middle ear, paranasal sinuses, or lungs. Spread of the organism may then occur either via the veins draining these areas or via bacteremia originating from the local focus of infection.[1]

Coma and seizures commonly occur early in the course of the disease.[1] When seizures occur, they usually begin as a Jacksonian seizure on the left side progressing to generalized seizures. Deafness can develop within 24 to 36 hours after the onset of meningitis.[21] Morbilliform and petechial rashes are very uncommon but may resemble the rash seen with meningococcal infection.[1–5] Sterile subdural effusions are common with *H. influenzae* but not other forms of meningitis.[1] These effusions may provoke fever after initial defervescence, seizures, and vomiting, necessitating repeated subdural paracentesis.

Approximately 10% to 25% of *H. influenzae* are ampicillin resistant.[36] For this reason, initial therapy is usually chloramphenicol and ampicillin. Once bacterial susceptibilities are available, chloramphenicol can be discontinued if the organism is ampicillin sensitive. Regardless of whether ampicillin or chloramphenicol is used alone to manage the meningitis, both drugs are bactericidal for *H. influenzae*.[37,38] As an alternative, certain second- and third-generation cephalosporins (such as cefuroxime and cefotaxime) are very active against $\beta$-lactamase-producing and non–$\beta$-lactamase-producing strains of *H. influenzae* and appear to be very effective in this form of meningitis.[24–32.]

Because cases of *H. influenzae* meningitis occur in clusters, treatment of close contacts of patients is usually recommended.[39] Usually, secondary cases, those resulting from close contact with the index case, occur within 30 days of the onset of disease.[20] As with meningococcal meningitis, close contacts may be at 200 to 1,000 times the risk of the general population for acquiring *H. influenzae* meningitis.[20] A recent study performed in Texas questions whether close day-care contacts actually have a higher incidence of meningitis than a base population and whether rifampin prophylaxis is indicated.[40]

Close contacts are usually defined as household members, individuals sharing sleeping quarters, crowded confined populations, day-care attendees, and nursing home residents.[20] The disease may also be transmitted in the laboratory, sexually, or nosocomially. Without intimate contact with the index patient's respiratory secretions, the risk of acquiring *H. influenzae* meningitis is low.[20]

The goal of prophylaxis is to protect close contacts from the index case by eliminating nasopharyngeal and oropharyngeal carriage of *H. influenzae*. Cultures are of no immediate value and may cause a delay in starting effective prophylaxis. Like meningococcal meningitis, secondary cases of meningitis may occur within 1 week of contact with the index case. Withholding chemoprophylaxis pending the results of the culture and sensitivity tests would put the close contact at risk of acquiring meningitis and is not recommended.

Prophylaxis for *H. influenzae* is recommended when at least one member of the same household as the index case is less than 6 years of age, when persons were in close daily contact (greater than 4 hours) with the index case 1 week prior to the onset of meningitis, for hospital personnel who have intimate contact with respiratory secretions, and for day-care attendees.[20] Prophylaxis is not indicated for persons having casual contact with the index case at work or school, most hospital employees, and now possibly day-care contacts.[20,40] For household contacts, once a decision has been made to provide chemoprophylaxis, the entire family (household) of the identified group should be treated.[20] The index case should also receive chemoprophylaxis prior to discharge from the hospital as there are reports of recolonization even after successful antibiotic therapy.[20]

Adults should receive 600 mg of rifampin daily for 4 days.[20] Children 1 month to 12 years should receive 20 mg/kg (maximum 600 mg) per day for 4 days, and children less than 1 month should receive 10 mg/kg per day for 4 days.[20] Minocycline is an alternative to rifampin chemoprophylaxis; however, there is a high incidence of vestibular reactions. Patients receiving *H. influenzae* prophylaxis should be carefully monitored as failures do occur and patients may go on to develop meningitis.

Children 18 months or older should now be routinely immunized with hemophilus B *conjugate* vaccine (PROHIBIT).[20,41] This vaccine will replace the old *polysaccharide* vaccine (B-CAPA-I). The conjugate vaccine may also prove useful in children younger than 18 months.

### *Listeria monocytogenes*

*L. monocytogenes* is a gram-positive diphtheroid-like organism, and is responsible for 2% of all reported cases of meningitis. The disease affects primarily neonates, immunocompromised adults, and the elderly.[2] In the immunocompromised patient, the cerebrospinal fluid resembles that found in bacterial meningitis.

Usually, the patient's gastrointestinal tract becomes colonized with the organisms, which then penetrate the gut lumen and, if there is not a sufficient cell-mediated response (T-lymphocyte macrophages), bacteremia, meningitis, meningoencephalitis, or cerebritis may develop.[2,42] Infection of the brain may be diffuse or localized, possibly involving the cerebral hemispheres, thalamus, and brain stem. Approximately 75% of *L. monocytogenes* infections in compromised hosts result in central nervous system seeding.[42]

The incidence of *L. monocytogenes* meningitis tends to peak in the summer and early fall.[1] As with gram-negative meningitis, the presentation may be subtle and insidious. Clinical suspicion should prompt lumbar puncture. *L. monocytogenes* produces primarily a mononuclear cerebrospinal fluid response.[2,42] One common laboratory error seen with *L. monocytogenes* is the tendency to misidentify the organism on Gram stain as a diphtheroid or streptococcus.

Treatment of *L. monocytogenes* meningitis with penicillin G or ampicillin may result in only a bacteriostatic effect. Usually the combination of penicillin G or ampicillin with an aminoglycoside results in a bactericidal effect. Patients should be treated for 18 to 21 days to prevent the possibility of relapse.[1,42] Usually combination therapy is employed for at least 10 days and the remaining course of therapy is completed with penicillin G alone. Trimethoprim–sulfamethoxazole may be an effective alternative if the organism is very susceptible, as adequate CSF penetration is achieved with trimethoprim–sulfamethoxazole.

### *Mycobacterium tuberculosis*

*Mycobacterium tuberculosis* var. *hominis* is the primary cause of tubercular meningitis.

The most useful, although often unelicited, diagnostic clue is a history of known contact with an index case of tuberculosis. Usually there is some evidence of pulmonary involvement with hilar adenopathy; however, tubercular meningitis may exist in the absence of disease in the lung or extrapulmonary sites. The tuberculin skin test (purified protein derivative, PPD) is negative in 5% to 50% of cases.[43]

Upon initial examination, cerebrospinal fluid usually contains from 50 to 500 white blood cells/mm$^3$ which may be 75% to 80% polymorphonuclear cells.[1,43] Over time the pattern of white blood cells in the cerebrospinal fluid will shift to lymphocytes and monocytes. Cerebrospinal fluid glucose levels may initially be normal and over time may gradually decrease.[1,43] Protein concentration within the cerebrospinal fluid may be normal to slightly elevated.[1,43]

One potentially useful diagnostic sign unique to tubercular meningitis is paralysis of the sixth cranial nerve which initially may be unilateral and then progress to become bilateral.[1] Acid-fast bacilli on microscopic examination of cerebrospinal fluid are seen in 90% of culture-positive cases. Cultures of cerebrospinal fluid may be positive in 45% to 90% of cases depending upon the quantity of cerebrospinal fluid used in the culture, pathogen density, and the experience of the laboratory in culturing *M. tuberculosis*. Positive culture results may take up to 8 weeks, providing little help with initial diagnosis.

Isoniazid (INH) is the mainstay in virtually any regimen to treat *M. tuberculosis*.[4,43] Isoniazid penetrates cerebrospinal fluid with or without meningeal inflammation. Usually, *M. tuberculosis* has minimum inhibiting concentrations of 0.05 to 0.20 mg/L.[43] Other antitubercular antibiotics capable of penetrating the cerebrospinal fluid without meningeal inflammation are ethionamide and cycloserine which produce cerebrospinal fluid concentrations that approximate those in serum.[43] Pyrazinamide, rifampin, ethambutol, and streptomycin penetrate cerebrospinal fluid only in the presence of meningeal inflammation.[43]

In children the usual dose of isoniazid is 15 to 20 mg/kg/d (maximum 500 mg/d). Adults usually receive 8 to 10 mg/kg/d or a daily dose of 300 to 600 mg/d. Supplemental doses of pyridoxine hydrochloride (vitamin $B_6$) 50 mg/d are usually recommended to prevent the peripheral neuropathy associated with isoniazid administration.[43] Concomitant administration of rifampin is recommended 15 to 20 mg/kg/d (maximum 600 mg/d) for children and 600 mg/d for adults.[43] At present the duration of therapy is not clearly defined. Patients should be treated for a minimum of 9 months or longer with multiple-drug therapy. Some authors have suggested, in addition to the rifampin and isoniazid, daily doses of ethambutol, 25 mg/kg/d for the first 1 to 2 months and then 15 mg/kg/d thereafter, or streptomycin, 1 g/d intramuscularly for adults or 20 to 40 mg/kg/d in children for the first 6 to 8 weeks and then the same dosage twice weekly.[43]

The use of steroids for tubercular meningitis remains controversial. In some cases administration of steroids has resulted in a dramatic clearing of sensorium, remission of cerebrospinal fluid abnormalities, reduction in fever, and elimination of headaches.[43]

With early diagnosis and treatment, tubercular meningitis has a mortality rate of 10% to 20%,[2,43] The most useful prognostic indicator is the level of patient consciousness at the start of therapy. Patients comatose at the start of therapy have a mortality rate of 50% to 70%.[2,43] Other negative prognostic factors include old age, poor nutrition, evidence of miliary disease, initial high CSF protein concentrations, presence of hydrocephalus, and evidence of elevated intracranial pressure.

Ten to thirty percent of patients surviving the disease have physical or mental sequelae.[43]

### *Cryptococcus neoformans*

Cryptococcal infections are acquired by inhalation from the environment. Immunocompetent hosts are able to contain the infection to the lungs and/or hilar nodes. In immunocompromised hosts, the organisms disseminate and seed the meninges, skin, prostate, bone, kidneys, eyes, liver, spleen, adrenals, and lymph nodes.[44] Frequently, these lesions reach sufficient size to be seen macroscopically and are called cryptococcomas or torulomas.

The symptoms, as with several forms of meningitis, are insidious. Fever, history of headaches, altered mentation, and evidence of focal neurologic deficits may be present.[44] Usually, signs of meningeal irritation are not present. The diagnosis is usually based on the presence of a pulmonary disease which may produce only mild symptoms, and the presence of skin lesions. The diagnosis is usually made by culture or by the detection of cryptococcal antigen. Tests for cryptococcal antigen are very sensitive and can also be used as a prognostic indicator. Patients with an initial titer <1:256 usually have an excellent prognosis.[44]

Examination of cerebrospinal fluid usually reveals small numbers of white blood cells (<150/mm$^3$) which are primarily lymphocytes.[44] The organism can be seen microscopically when stained with india ink. Cerebrospinal fluid cultures are positive in >90% of cases.[44,45] In addition to cerebrospinal fluid cultures, urine cultures should be obtained as *C. neoformans* can be recovered in 35% of cases.[44] There is also a latex agglutination test for rapid identification of cryptococcal antigen in cerebrospinal fluid.[44] This test is positive in >90% of culture-positive cases. The test can also be used to follow the patient's prognosis using the level of antigen titer.[44]

Patients with *C. neoformans* infections are usually treated with systemic amphotericin B.[39,44,45] Doses of 1 to 1.5 mg/kg/d (total doses of 2 to 3 g over 6 weeks) are usually given and result in approximately two thirds of patients being cured.[39,44,45] *C. neoformans* meningitis has a mortality rate of approximately 25%; an additional 10% of patients die of other underlying diseases.[44] Flucytosine has been used alone to treat these infections; however, the high incidence of resistance to it usually results in failure.[44] Comparative studies evaluating amphotericin B alone versus the combination of amphotericin B and 5-flucytosine suggest significant differences in outcome favoring combination therapy.[39]

Cerebrospinal fluid should be sampled weekly for determination of the antigen titer to *C. neoformans*. The antigen titer should decrease with treatment. If the patient fails to respond, amphotericin B can be administered intrathecally or intraventricularly into the cerebrospinal fluid. In the past, ketoconazole and miconazole have not been recommended because of poor penetration into cerebrospinal fluid; however, recent studies using high doses of ketoconazole have demonstrated therapeutic antifungal levels of drug in cerebrospinal fluid.[46] Further studies are required to evaluate the role of these agents in treatment of this form of meningitis.

## Viral Meningitis

Viral meningitis is virtually impossible to differentiate from other causes of meningitis without the presence of distinguishing clinical features such as the dermatomal lesions of herpes zoster, the vesicular lesions of genital herpes simplex, or the parotitis of mumps. The most common viral cause of meningitis is the enteroviruses, which are polioviruses, coxsackie viruses, and echoviruses[47]; however, mumps virus, lymphocytic choriomeningitis virus, herpes viruses, varicella, human immunodeficiency virus, and arboviruses can also cause viral meningitis.[47] Enteroviruses are RNA viruses present in the gastrointestinal tract and cause 80% to 90% of cases of viral meningitis where a viral etiology can be identified.[47] These RNA viruses are typically spread by the fecal–oral route and typically affect children less than 14 years old but can affect all age groups. Viral meningitis is usually a seasonal disease peaking in summer and early fall, reflecting the seasonal prevalence of the enteroviruses.[47]

The clinical syndrome seen with viral meningitis may vary depending upon the age of the patient. Common signs and symptoms in adults include headache, fever, nuchal rigidity, malaise, drowsiness, nausea, vomiting, and photophobia. Only fever and irritability may be evident in the infant, and meningitis must be ruled out as a cause of fever when no other localized findings in a child are observed. Examination of cerebrospinal fluid usually reveals a pleocytosis with 10 to 1,000 white blood cells/mm$^3$ which are predominantly lymphocytic; however, 20% to 75% of patients with viral meningitis may have a predominance of polymorphonuclear cells on the initial examination of cerebrospinal fluid.[47] Initial cerebrospinal fluid findings may not differ from those found in bacterial meningitis; however, patients whose cerebrospinal fluid contains more than 2,000 white blood cells/mm$^3$ ($\geq$95% polymorphonuclear cells), a protein concentration greater than 200 mg%, and reduced glucose concentrations probably do not have viral meningitis.[47]

Because of the difficulty in differentiating viral infection from bacterial infection, patients are usually managed with antibiotics until culture results are available. In situations where there is a question of viral illness and the patient is clinically stable, antibiotics can be withheld for 12 hours. Then, a second lumbar puncture can be performed and the cerebrospinal fluid white blood cell count and differential can be compared with those from the initial examination.[48] Ninety percent of patients with viral meningitis initially presenting with a predominance of neutrophils experience a pattern shift to a predominance of monocytes within 8 hours.[48]

The second most common cause of viral meningitis is mumps virus which is responsible for approximately 10% to 20% of cases.[47] The usual presenting symptom is parotitis, which usually precedes symptoms of meningitis by 3 to 10 days, but may follow the onset of these symptoms by 1 or 2 weeks. While parotitis is most commonly associated with mumps, other viruses such as cytomegalovirus, coxsackie virus, Epstein–Barr virus, and lymphocytic choriomeningitis virus can all cause parotitis. Parotitis may not develop in as many as 20% to 50% of cases of mumps-associated meningitis. The disease tends to be a relatively benign and self-limited disease that has its peak occurrence between April and July.

Lymphocytic choriomeningitis virus is also an RNA virus. The disease is typically transmitted to humans through contact with an infected rodent. The disease can occur year round but is more common in the winter. There is usually a prodrome of arthralgias, nausea, lightheadedness, anorexia, hair loss, and pneumonitis. The virus can usually be recovered in blood or cerebrospinal fluid. Diagnosis is usually made on a retrospective basis with the observation of a fourfold increase in acute versus convalescent titers.

Both types 1 and 2 of herpes simplex have been associated with infections of the central nervous system.[47] Herpes simplex type 1 is associated with meningoencephalitis while herpes simplex type 2 is associated predominantly with meningitis. Herpes simplex type 2 infection of the meninges is most likely hematogenously spread from an initial genital site of infection. Young, sexually active adults are the primary group affected. Aseptic meningitis usually occurs during or after an attack of genital or rectal herpes. While herpes simplex type 2 virus can frequently be cultured from cerebrospinal fluid, herpes simplex virus type 1 is not. The diagnosis is usually made by culture or a fourfold rise in complement-fixing antibody to the virus. Recently, a variety of assay methods have been used to detect herpes simplex virus antibody in cerebrospinal fluid. These tests may provide for useful retrospective assessment of cerebrospinal fluid for herpes simplex.[49] It is paramount that diagnosis be established as early as possible as the disease has a high mortality rate and, unlike other viral encephalitides, specific and effective therapy is available. The definitive diagnosis can be established only with a brain biopsy. Although a herpes simplex etiology may be strongly suspected on the basis of local findings after clinical evaluation, in only half of these patients will the clinical diagnosis be confirmed by brain biopsy. Brain biopsy also allows for an alternative diagnosis to be made if herpes simplex is ruled out.

Vidarabine (ARA-A) has been the mainstay of therapy for herpes simplex encephalitis. A placebo-controlled trial has shown a decreased mortality rate when vidarabine was used to treat confirmed herpes simplex encephalitis.[50] Vidarabine is usually used in a dose of 15 mg/kg/d. Because of its poor solubility in water, the drug must be mixed in large volumes of parenteral fluid and infused over a 12-hour period. In addition, patients receiving vidarabine should be monitored for leukopenia, megaloblastic anemia, thrombocytopenia, and a parkinsonian-like neurologic syndrome. Treatment with vidarabine is usually continued for 10 days or until the results of brain biopsy are available.

Acyclovir is currently replacing vidarabine as the drug of choice for herpes simplex encephalitis. Recent studies have shown a significantly (19% versus 50%) lower mortality rate for patients treated with acyclovir as compared with vidarabine.[51] An ongoing study by the National Institute of Allergy and Infectious Diseases has compared acyclovir with vidarabine in 68 biopsy-proven cases. The mortality for the acyclovir group was 31% as compared with 54% for the patients receiving vidarabine.[52] In patients with normal renal function, acyclovir is usually administered as 10 mg/kg every 8 hours.

Thirty to forty percent of patients with uncomplicated herpes zoster infection have a mild pleocytosis and/or a slightly increased cerebrospinal fluid protein but rarely have meningitis. As with several of the other viral agents, herpes zoster tends to be a self-limited disease and does not require treatment.

Although there are over 250 different varieties of arboviruses, only four have been associated with aseptic meningitis or encephalitis. These four include St. Louis encephalitis virus, Eastern equine encephalitis virus, Western equine encephalitis virus, and the California encephalitis group of viruses. These groups of viruses are transmitted primarily by mosquitos. For this reason, outbreaks tend to peak during the summer months.

## Shunt Infections

With hydrocephalus, surgical shunting procedures are used to produce a decompression of the two lateral ventricles by diverting cerebrospinal fluid from the ventricles into another body compartment.[53] The two most popular techniques are ventriculoatrial (VA) and ventriculoperitoneal (VP) shunts. In the VP shunt, fluid is diverted into the peritoneal cavity; the VA shunt diverts cerebrospinal fluid into the right atrium.

Inevitably a surgical procedure leaving a foreign device in place is associated with infection. Shunt infections have a lifetime incidence of 1.5% to 39%, with most studies reporting a rate of 10% to 15%.[53] In the last 15 years, the incidence of shunt infections has decreased by 50%. There appears to be no difference in infectious risk whether the surgical procedure is the initial placement or a revision.

Children requiring shunt placement prior to 3 months of age, elderly patients requiring shunt procedures, lengthy surgical procedures, surgical emergencies, and possibly the type of shunt are all potential risk factors for infection. If a VA shunt is used and the distal catheter tip is at or below T7 in children, the risk of infection seems to increase.[53] Optimal placement of the VA distal catheter tip in adults is between T5 and T7.[53] Children with VA shunts require further revision with growth.

*Staphylococcus epidermidis* is the primary cause of VA and VP shunt infections. *Staphylococcus aureus* is the second leading cause of shunt infection with an estimated incidence of 25%.[53] Collectively, *Klebsiella* sp., *Escherichia coli*, and *Proteus* sp. cause approximately 5% to 10% of shunt infections.[53] *Hemophilus influenzae*, *Streptococcus pneumoniae*, and *Neisseria meningitidis* cause approximately 5% of all shunt infections.[53] Approximately 70% of all shunt infections are clinically apparent within 2 months of the shunting procedure.[53] Eighty percent are evident within 6 months of surgery.[53] A variety of etiologies have been postulated for shunt infections. One obvious possibility is site contamination at the time of surgery. A second possibility is hematogenous spread of organisms that contaminate the shunt. Organisms may migrate in a retrograde fashion from a contaminated distal catheter tip.

Several factors are involved in the infectious process: the magnitude of pathogen contamination, the intrinsic virulence of the offending organism, and the presence or absence of functioning host defense mechanisms. With *S. epidermidis* there may be "slime" production that allows the organism to colonize and adhere to the shunt and protect the organism from phagocytosis.

Tenderness along the path of the catheter across the rib margin is suggestive of a VP infection. Approximately one third of patients with a VP infection will present with abdominal symptoms.[53] Several complications can arise from both VA and VP shunts. Chronic bacteremia, nephritis, hypocomplementemia, and septic pulmonary embolization may result with VA shunts. Complications from VP shunts include infectious peritonitis, bowel obstruction secondary to adhesions, bowel perforation, and peritoneal cysts.

### *Clinical Presentations*

Diagnosis is usually based on clinical suspicion. In patients with shunts every febrile episode should be evaluated as a possible shunt infection. Blood cultures are usually positive in about 95% of patients with VA shunts but in only 20% of patients with VP shunts.[53] Obtaining cerebrospinal fluid percutaneously from the shunt reservoir or tubing is the most useful diagnostic procedure. These cultures are usually positive in more than 95% of patients not receiving antibiotics.[53] While shunt cultures of cerebrospinal fluid may be positive, cerebrospinal fluid obtained by lumbar puncture may be culture negative. As a rule, cerebrospinal fluid is not as reactive in shunt infections as in other central nervous system infections. Cerebrospinal fluid white blood cell counts average $<100/mm^3$.[2,53] Presence of white blood cells in cerebrospinal fluid correlates well with culture results. When more than 100 white blood cells are seen per cubic millimeter of cerebrospinal fluid, the cultures are positive in more than 90% of cases. When cerebrospinal fluid contains fewer than 20 white blood cells/$mm^3$, less than 50% of the cultures are positive.[53] If cultures are negative but cerebrospinal fluid white count remains elevated the patient should be evaluated for an anaerobic or fungal infection. Hypoglycorrhachia (low glucose concentrations in CSF) is usually not severe.

### *Treatment*

Treatment usually involves the use of parenteral antibiotics, intraventricular antibiotic administration, and possibly shunt removal. Systemic antibiotic therapy should be started based on the suspected initial pathogen and the usual antimicrobial patterns of susceptibility. Serious consideration should be given to the possibility of methicillin-resistant strains of both *Staphylococcus aureus* and *Staphylococcus epidermidis*. Depending on the organism, various synergistic combinations of systemic antibiotic therapy may be used. In adults, nafcillin or cefotaxime can be used at doses of 12 g per day. In children, nafcillin 300 mg/kg/d or cefotaxime 200 mg/kg/d can be used initially.[53] When methicillin-resistant strains are suspected, adults with normal renal function should receive vancomycin 2 g/d, gentamicin 5 mg/kg/d, and rifampin 1,200 mg/d.[53] In children, vancomycin 40 mg/kg/d should be used along with gentamicin 5 mg/kg/d and rifampin 20 mg/kg/d. Vancomycin and gentamicin dosages should be adjusted as guided by patient renal function and follow-up serum concentrations.

Both VA and VP shunts have a percutaneous port that allows direct installition of antibiotics into the ventricles. Treatment with parenteral and intraventricular antibiotics will result in 35% to 55% of patients being successfully treated without removal of the shunt.[53] An external ventricular drainage device, established by exteriorizing the infected shunt or by placing a ventricular catheter, is preferred over immediate replacement with a new shunt.

Several factors should be evaluated when direct methods are used for instillation of antibiotics into the central nervous system. Consideration should be given to total cerebrospinal fluid volume, sensitivity of the offending pathogen, desired antibiotic concentration in cerebrospinal fluid, and variability in pharmacokinetics of antibiotics in cerebrospinal fluid. As previously discussed, cerebrospinal fluid volume varies with age. If antibiotic is delivered to one ventricle, or into the intralumbar space, only a fraction of cerebrospinal fluid volume is available for drug distribution. Over the next several hours, the antibiotic begins to distribute. With intrathecal administration, distribution of antibiotic throughout the CSF is unlikely. For these reasons, the initial antibiotic concentration in cerebrospinal fluid at the point of injection may be several thousand micrograms per milliliter. This may be potentially irritating and toxic to sensitive neurologic tissue. The sensitivity of the bacterial pathogen and an estimate of cerebrospinal fluid volume (40–60 mL for infants, 60–100 mL for young children, 1 mL CSF per pound body weight for older children and adults)[3] can be used to arrive at a dose that will produce the desired ratio between the cerebrospinal fluid antibiotic concentration and the sensitivity of the pathogen.

## Brain Abscesses

Brain abscesses are relatively uncommon, with an estimated incidence of 4 per 1,000,000 population.[54–56] Brain abscesses may be caused by a parameningeal focus, extension from a skull fracture, penetrating wound, craniofacial osteomyelitis, dental sepsis, bacterial meningitis, or as a complication of neurosurgery.[54–56] Infections outside the central nervous system having a bacteremic component (e.g., pneumonia) can result in seeding of the brain with microorganisms and abscess formation. Parameningeal infections (e.g., middle ear or sinuses) cause a brain lesion by direct extension or through vascular channels. The two most likely groups of patients are young males in their thirties and children between 4 and 7 years of age (often with a history of congenital heart disease).[54–56]

A prerequisite for the development of a brain abscess is a focal area of ischemia or necrosis. Polycythemic thromboses, hypoxia, or septic emboli can cause ischemia which can create a microaerophilic environment ideal for anaerobic organisms. Abscesses tend to locate in the white matter, which is more poorly vascularized than the gray matter, and the junction between white and gray matter. The inflammation related to the abscess may be associated with cerebral edema increasing intracranial pressure. This further interferes with blood flow to an already ischemic area.

### *Clinical Presentation*

Most patients have a history of symptoms less than 2 weeks. The primary symptom is headache, which occurs in approximately 75% of patients.[54] Approximately 50% of patients complain of nausea and vomiting and one third of patients may have seizures.[54] Fever may or may not be present. Altered states of consciousness with lethargy, confusion, irritability, and coma are not uncommon. An underlying history of congenital heart disease, otitis, sinusitis, or pulmonary infection with this constellation of symptoms should heighten the suspicion of a possible brain abscess.

As the abscess begins to enlarge, symptoms become consistent with those of a space-occupying lesion. Most patients at this stage begin to experience significant neurologic sequelae such as hemiplegia, focal or generalized seizures, papilledema, and nuchal rigidity.[54–56] Attempts to obtain cerebrospinal fluid by lumbar puncture should be approached cautiously, as elevated intracranial pressure may precipitate herniation of the brain stem because of the sudden release in pressure once the needle is inserted into the intrathecal space. Evidence of papilledema may indicate the presence of elevated intracranial pressure; however, computerized tomography has shown evidence of intracranial pressure in patients without evidence of papilledema. Cerebrospinal fluid is also of little diagnostic value for brain abscess. Usually, patients have an elevated opening pressure on lumbar puncture, pleocytosis with several hundred white blood cells (primarily lymphocytes), elevated cerebrospinal fluid protein concentration, and normal cerebrospinal fluid glucose concentration.[54–56] X-rays demonstrate an abnormality in approximately 50% of patients.[54] Perhaps the most useful diagnostic tool is computerized tomography with and without contrast. Radionuclide brain scan and arteriography may also be of some help in making the diagnosis.

Over the past several years, several improvements have been made in the isolation and identification of bacteria responsible for causing brain abscesses. Use of anaerobic transport media and expeditious processing on the part of the microbiology laboratory have greatly improved the yield of bacteria from clinical specimens. In most cases, at least two or more species of bacteria are isolated from a bacterial abscess in the central nervous system. Often these bacteria tend to be a mixture of aerobes and anaerobes.

The most common bacterial cause of abscess is streptococci, most notably *Streptococcus milleri*, *Streptococcus viridans*, nonhemolytic streptococci, enterococcus, $\beta$-hemolytic streptococcus, and *Peptostreptococcus*. *Bacteroides* spp. are found in 25% to 60% of patients.[54–56] The *Entero-*

*bacteriaceae* and *Staphylococcus aureus* are also associated with brain abscesses. Opportunistic organisms should also be considered when dealing with the immunosuppressed patient.

### *Treatment*

Treatment of brain abscesses is usually accomplished with parenteral antibiotics and surgical removal of purulent material. As in meningitis, antibiotic selection should be guided by the likelihood that the antibiotic selected will produce satisfactory antibiotic concentrations at the site of infection. As meningitis may not be present with brain abscess, antibiotic selection should be based on the ability of the antibiotic to enter the central nervous system independent of meningeal inflammation. Some consideration should also be given to the change in environment caused by the abscess. Differences in pH, oxygen tension, presence of white blood cells, and presence of purulent material may affect antibiotic performance, as with aminoglycosides the activity of which is decreased by low pH and oxygen tension. Studies done to date demonstrate that penicillin G, chloramphenicol, and clindamycin produce satisfactory but sometimes inconsistent levels in brain tissue.[54] Ampicillin, nafcillin, and cloxacillin have been shown to produce poor concentrations in brain tissue.[54] Metronidazole has been shown to produce therapeutic concentrations, even after oral administration.[54] Usually initial antibiotic regimens include combinations of penicillin G, chloramphenicol, or metronidazole with cefotaxime. These regimens are aimed at *Streptococcus*, anaerobes including *Bacteroides fragilis*, enteric bacilli, and *Hemophilus* spp. Patients are usually treated for 6 to 8 weeks. Very aggressive antibiotic regimens are used (penicillin G 20–40 million units/d, ampicillin 12–18 g/d, cefotaxime 12 g/d, and metronidazole 30 mg/kg/d, with dosages adjusted for age, renal function, or hepatic function).[54–56]

Once the abscess lesion has been localized and if the lesion is operable, neurosurgery may be indicated if the patient has continuous increases in intracranial pressure, continued reduced levels of consciousness, or an increase in neurologic deficits. Aspiration, marsupialization, and excision of the abscess represent standard alternatives. Patients who are at increased surgical risk because of underlying medical conditions, multiple abscesses, inoperable lesions, concomitant meningitis/ependymitis, or concomitant hydrocephalus may not be candidates for neurosurgery. Bartlett has shown that with relatively small abscesses, parenteral antibiotics by themselves may effect reduction and elimination of the abscess.[57]

Approximately 50% of patients with brain abscesses recover without neurologic sequelae.[54] Of the remaining patients, 25% have sequelae but likely can lead a normal life. The other 25% have substantial sequelae that compromise their quality of life.[54] Approximately 10% of patients are severely retarded or cannot be cared for at home.[54] The condition of the patient at the time of presentation to the hospital is a major determining factor in clinical outcome. Patients who are herniating or rupturing or who have substantial underlying diseases are unlikely to have a favorable clinical prognosis.

## Summary

Paramount to successful intervention in treating central nervous system infections are prompt diagnosis and aggressive treatment to prevent serious sequelae. The availability of rapid diagnostic methods for meningitis caused by certain bacteria, *Cryptococcus neoformans*, and herpes simplex is helpful.

Treatment of central nervous system infections is adequately achieved if bactericidal cerebrospinal fluid concentrations of antimicrobial agent are present. Some third-generation cephalosporins (e.g., cefotaxime) achieve these concentrations when meningeal inflammation is present and when given at high doses. Adequate cerebrospinal fluid concentrations are achieved by amphotericin B for cryptococcal meningitis and by acyclovir for viral meningitis caused by herpes simplex.

Prophylaxis for patients who are at a high risk for central nervous system infections or who are in close contact with patients having bacterial meningitis has, or will have, a significant impact in reducing morbidity and mortality from these infections.

## References


1. Weinstein L. Bacterial meningitis, in Molavi A, LeFrock JL (eds): The Medical Clinics of North America. Philadelphia, W.B. Saunders, 1985, pp 219–229.
2. McGee ZA, Kaiser AB. Acute meningitis, in Mandell GL, Douglas RG, Bennett JE (eds): Principles and Practice of Infectious Diseases, 2nd ed. New York, John Wiley and Sons, 1985, pp 560–573.
3. Bolan G, Barza M. Acute bacterial meningitis in children and adults, in Molavi A, Lefrock JL, (eds): The Medical Clinics of North America. Philadelphia, W.B. Saunders, 1985, pp 219–229.
4. Ellner J. Chronic meningitis, in Mandell GL, Douglas RG, Bennett JE (eds): Principles and Practice of Infectious Diseases, 2nd ed. New York, John Wiley and Sons, 1985, pp 573–579.
5. Greenlee JE. Anatomic considerations in central nervous system infections, in Mandell GL, Douglas RG, Bennett JE (eds): Principles and Practice of Infectious Diseases, 2nd ed. New York, John Wiley and Sons, 1985, pp 551–560.
6. Allinson RR, Stach PE. Intrathecal drug therapy. Drug Intell Clin Pharm 1978;12:347–359.
7. Richards ML, Prince RA, Kenaley KA, et al. Antimicrobial penetration into cerebrospinal fluid. Drug Intell Clin Pharm 1981;15:341–368.
8. Ratcheson RA, Ommaya AK. Experience with the subcutaneous cerebrospinal fluid reservoir. N Engl J Med 1968;279:1026–1031.
9. Kaiser AB, McGee ZA. Aminoglycoside therapy of gram-negative bacillary meningitis. N Engl J Med 1975;293:1215–1220.
10. McCracken GH, Mize SG. A controlled study of intrathecal

antibiotic therapy in gram-negative enteric meningitis of infancy. Report of the Neonatal Meningitis Cooperative Study Group. J Pediatr 1976;89:66–72.

11. Wright PF, Kaiser AB, Bowmann CM, et al. The pharmacokinetics and efficacy of an aminoglycoside administered into the cerebral ventricles in neonates: implications for further evaluation of this route of therapy in meningitis. J Infect Dis 1981;143: 141–147.
12. Powers WJ. Cerebrospinal fluid lymphocytosis in acute bacterial meningitis. Am J Med 1985;79:216–220.
13. Ratzan KR. Viral meningitis, in Molavi A, LeFrock JL (eds): The Medical Clinics of North America. Philadelphia, W.B. Saunders, 1985, pp 399–413.
14. Edwards EA, Muehl PM, Peckinpaugh RO. Diagnosis of bacterial meningitis by counterimmunoelectrophoresis. J Lab Clin Med 1972;80:449–454.
15. Case MJ, Ryther SS, Novitsky TJ. Detection of endotoxin in antibiotic solutions with lumulus amoebocyte lysate. Antimicrob Agents Chemother 1983;23:649–652.
16. Rutledge J, Benjamin D, Hood L, et al. Is the CSF lactate measurement useful in the management of children with suspected bacterial meningitis? J Pediatr 1981;98:20–24.
17. Provine H, Gardner P. The Gram-stained smear and its interpretation. Hosp Pract 1974;9:85–91.
18. LeFrock JL, Smith BR, Molavi A. Gram-negative bacillary meningitis, in Molavi A, LeFrock JL (eds): The Medical Clinics of North America. Philadelphia, W.B. Saunders, 1985, pp 243–256.
19. Sande MA. Antibiotic therapy of bacterial meningitis: lessons we've learned. Am J Med 1981;7:507.
20. Shapiro ED. Prophylaxis for bacterial meningitis, in Molavi A, LeFrock JL (eds): The Medical Clinics of North America. Philadelphia, W.B. Saunders, 1985, pp 269–280.
21. Dodge PR, Davis H, Feigin RD, et al. Prospective evaluation of hearing impairment as a sequela of acute bacterial meningitis. N Engl J Med 1984;311:869–874.
22. Griseler PJ, Nelson KE, Levin S, et al. Community-acquired purulent meningitis: a review of 1,316 cases during the antibiotic era 1954–1976. Rev Infect Dis 1980;2:725–745.
23. Feldman C, Kallenbach JM, Miller SD, et al. Community acquired pneumonia due to penicillin-resistant pneumococci. N Engl J Med 1985;313:615–617.
24. Landesman SH, Corrado ML, Shah PM, et al. Past and current roles for cephalosporin antibiotics in the treatment of meningitis. Am J Med 1981;71:693–703.
25. Nelson JD. Emerging role of cephalosporins in bacterial meningitis. Am J Med 1985;79(suppl):47–51.
26. Perfect JR, Durack DT. Pharmacokinetics of cefoperazone, moxalactam, cefotaxime, trimethoprim, and sulphamethoxazole in experimental meningitis. J Antimicrob Chemother 1981;8:49–58.
27. Schaad UB, McCracken GH, Loock CA, et al. Pharmacokinetic and bacteriologic efficacy of moxalactam, cefotaxime, cefoperazone, and Rocephin in experimental meningitis. J Infect Dis 1981;143:156–163.
28. Overturf GD, Cable DC, Forthal DN, et al. Treatment of bacterial meningitis with ceftizoxime. Antimicrob Agent Chemother, 1984;25:258–262.
29. Schaad UB, Krucko J, Pfenninger J. An extended experience with cefuroxime therapy of childhood bacterial meningitis. Pediatr Infect Dis 1984;3:410–416.
30. Congeni BL. Comparison of ceftriaxone and traditional therapy of bacterial meningitis. Antimicrob Agents Chemother 1984;25: 40–44.
31. Cable D, Overturf G, Edralin G. Concentrations of cefoperazone in cerebrospinal fluid during bacterial meningitis. Antimicrob Agents Chemother 1983;23:688–691.
32. Neu HC. The new beta lactamase stable cephalosporins. Ann Intern Med 1982;97:408–419.
33. Fong IW, Tomkins KB. Review of *Pseudomonas aeruginosa* meningitis with special emphasis on treatment with ceftazidime. Rev Infect Dis 1985;7:604–612.
34. Rahal JJ, Simberboff MS. Bactericidal and bacteriostatic action of chloramphenicol against meningeal pathogens. Antimicrob Agents Chemother 1979;16:13–18.
35. Levitz RE, Quintiliani R. Trimethoprim–sulfamethoxazole for meningitis. Ann Intern Med 1984;100:881–890.
36. Thornsberry C, McDougal LK. Ampicillin resistant *Haemophilus influenzae*. Postgrad Med 1982;71:133–145.
37. Schulking ML, Atemeier WA, Ayoub EM. A comparison of ampicillin and chloramphenicol therapy in *Hemophilus* meningitis. Pediatrics 1971;48:411–416.
38. Girgis NI, Yassin MW, Sandorn WR, et al. Ampicillin compared with penicillin and chloramphenicol combined in the treatment of bacterial meningitis. J Trop Med Hyg 1972;75:154–157.
39. Bennett JE, Dismakes WE, Duma RJ. A comparison of amphotericin B alone and combined with flucytosine in the treatment of cryptococcal meningitis. N Engl J Med 1979;301:126–131.
40. Murphy TV, Clements JF, Breedlove JA, et al. Risk of subsequent disease among day-care contacts of patients with systemic *H. influenzae* type B disease. N Engl J Med 1986;316:5–10.
41. Recommendations of the Immunization Advisory Committee. Update: Prevention of *Haemophilus influenzae* type B disease. MMWR 1988;37:13–16.
42. Rubin RH, Hooper DC. Central nervous system infection in the compromised host, in Molavi A, LeFrock JL (eds): The Medical Clinics of North America. Philadelphia, W.B. Saunders, 1985, pp 281–296.
43. Molavi A, LeFrock JL. Tuberculous meningitis, in Molavi A, LeFrock JL (eds): The Medical Clinics of North America. Philadelphia, W.B. Saunders, 1985, pp 315–331.
44. Sabetta JR, Andriole VT. Cryptococcal infection of the central nervous system, in Molavi A, LeFrock JL (eds): The Medical Clinics of North America. Philadelphia, W.B. Saunders, 1985, pp 333–344.
45. Bell WE. Treatment of fungal infections of the central nervous system. Ann Neurol 1980;9:417–422.
46. Craven PC, Graybill JR, Jorgensen JH, et al. High dose ketoconazole for treatment of fungal infections of the central nervous system. Ann Intern Med 1983;98:160–167.
47. Ratzan KR. Viral meningitis, in Molavi A, LeFrock JL (eds): The Medical Clinics of North America. Philadelphia, W.B. Saunders, 1985, pp 399–413.
48. Feign RD, Shackelford PG. Value of repeat lumbar puncture in the differential diagnosis of meningitis. N Engl J Med 1973;289: 571–574.
49. Kahlon J, Chatterjee S, Lakeman FD, et al. Detection of antibodies to herpes simplex virus in the cerebrospinal fluid of patients with *H. simplex* encephalitis. J Infect Dis 1987;155:38–43.
50. Whitley RJ, Soong SJ, Dolin R, et al. Adenine arabinoside therapy of biopsy-proven herpes simplex encephalitis: National Institute of Allergy and Infectious Diseases Collaborative Antiviral Study. N Engl J Med 1977;297:289–294.
51. Skoldenberg B, Forsgen M, Alestig K, et al. Acyclovir versus vidarabine in herpes simplex encephalitis. Lancet 1984;2:707–711.

52. Ho DD, Hirsch MS. Acute viral encephalitis. Med Clin North Am 1985;69:415–429.
53. Gardner P, Leipzig T, Phillips P. Infections of central nervous system shunts, in Molavi A, LeFrock JL (eds): The Medical Clinics of North America. Philadelphia, W.B. Saunders, 1985, pp 297–314.
54. Kaplan K. Brain abscess, in Molavi A, LeFrock JL (eds): The Medical Clinics of North America. Philadelphia, W.B. Saunders, 1985, pp 345–360.
55. Silverberg AL, DiNubile MJ. Subdural empyema and cranial epidural abscess, in Molavi A, LeFrock JL (eds): The Medical Clinics of North America. Philadelphia, W.B. Saunders, 1985 pp 361–374.
56. Farley E, Musher DM. Spinal epidural abscess, in Molavi A, LeFrock JL (eds): The Medical Clinics of North America. Philadelphia, W.B. Saunders, 1985 pp 375–384.
57. Bartlett JG. Recent developments in the management of anaerobic infections. Rev Infect Dis 1983;5:235–245.
58. Salmon JH. Ventriculitis complicating meningitis. Am J Dis Child 1972;124:35–40.
59. McLaurin RL. Infected cerebrospinal fluid shunts. Surg Neurol 1973;1:191–195.
60. Wald SL, McLaurin RL. Cerebrospinal fluid antibiotic levels during treatment of shunt infections. J Neurosurg 1980;S2:41–46.
61. Sells CJ, Shurtleff DB, Loeser JD. Gram-negative cerebrospinal fluid shunt associated infections. Pediatrics 1977;59:613–619.
62. Kaiser AB, McGee ZA. Aminoglycoside therapy of gram-negative bacillary meningitis. N Engl J Med 1975;293:1215–1220.
63. Sklaver AR, Greenman RL, Hoffman TA. Amikacin therapy of gram-negative bacteremia and meningitis. Arch Intern Med 1978;138:713–716.
64. Wirt TC, McGee ZA, Oldfield EH, Meacham WF. Intraventricular administration of amikacin for complicated gram-negative meningitis and ventriculitis. J Neurosurg 1979;50:95–99.
65. Congeni BL, Tan J, Salstrom SD. Kinetics of vancomycin after intraventricular and intravenous administration. (Abstr) Pediatr Res 1979;13:459–463.
66. Visconti EB, Peter G. Vancomycin and cerebrospinal fluid shunt infections. J Neurosurg 1979;51:245–246.
67. Pau AK, Samego RA, Fisher MA. Intraventricular vancomycin: Observation of tolerance and pharmacokinetics in two infants with ventricular shunt infections. Pediatr Infect Dis 1986;5:93–96.

# Chapter 76 / Lower Respiratory Tract Infections

Michael D. Reed, PharmD, and Madolin K. Witte, MD

The treatment of infections arising within the respiratory tract continues to be a common yet therapeutically challenging clinical concern. Respiratory infections remain the major cause of morbidity from acute illness in the United States[1] and most likely represent the single most common reason patients seek medical attention.[2] These demographic data have far-reaching implications in consideration of the dramatic changes that are occurring in methods of health care reimbursement within our country today. This chapter focuses upon bacterial and viral infections involving the lower respiratory tract, which includes the tracheobronchial tree and lung parenchyma.

## Lung Defenses

A description of lower respiratory tract infections would be incomplete without a discussion of the physiologic mechanisms by which the lungs normally resist infection. The respiratory tract has an elaborate system of host defenses which include humoral mechanisms, cellular mechanisms, and important mechanical mechanisms such as the mucociliary transport system.[3] When functioning properly, the host defenses of the respiratory tract are markedly effective in protecting against pathogen invasion and in removing potentially infectious agents from the lungs. For the most part, infections in the lower respiratory tract occur only when these defense mechanisms are impaired. Examples of impaired defenses would include dysgammaglobulinemia or compromised ciliary function caused by the chronic inflammation that accompanies cigarette smoking. In addition, local defenses may be overwhelmed when a particularly virulent microorganism or excessive inoculum invades lung parenchyma. Most likely, the majority of pulmonary infections follow colonization of the upper respiratory tract with potential pathogens which, after achieving sufficiently high concentrations, gain access to the lung via aspiration of oropharyngeal secretions.[4] In contrast, and less commonly, microbes enter the lung via the blood from an extrapulmonary source or by the inhalation of infected aerosolized particles.[3] The specific type of pulmonary infection caused by an invading microorganism is determined by a variety of host factors, including age, the anatomic features of the airway, and specific characteristics of the infecting agent. The most common infections involving the lower respiratory tract include bronchitis, bronchiolitis, pneumonia, and lung abscess.

## General Approach to Diagnosis

Lower respiratory tract infections in both children and adults are most commonly a result of either viral or bacterial invasion of lung parenchyma. The diagnosis of viral infections rests primarily on the recognition of a characteristic constellation of clinical signs and symptoms or on the results of serologic laboratory tests, and treatment is largely supportive. In contrast, the effective and expedient treatment of bacterial infections in the lower tract depends, in large part, on the isolation of the etiologic agent from lung tissue or secretions. Sputum Gram stain and culture, which are both noninvasive and readily available, are the tests most widely performed for this purpose; however, because many of the bacteria that may constitute normal upper respiratory tract flora are known pathogens in the lung,[5] the isolation of these agents from expectorated sputum contaminated with oropharyngeal secretions can be difficult to interpret.[6] Despite this limitation, properly collected and processed sputum specimens are a valuable diagnostic tool in the majority of patients with uncomplicated lower respiratory tract infections.[7] In patients unable to expectorate sputum, such as obtunded or debilitated patients and most young children, transtracheal aspiration may be performed to obtain specimens for microbiologic studies. Performed properly, transtracheal aspiration is a safe technique for sampling lower respiratory tract secretions and yields bacteriologic results more reliable than those obtained from routine sputum collection.[8] More invasive diagnostic techniques, such as transthoracic needle aspiration, transbronchial lung biopsy, and open lung biopsy, offer a high diagnostic yield but carry a substantial increased risk of morbidity including pneumothorax and bleeding[9]; thus, their routine use in the diagnosis of pulmonary infections is not recommended. Treatment of the patient with uncomplicated lower respiratory tract infection should be based on the results of properly collected sputum cultures interpreted in light of current knowledge of the most common lung pathogens and their antibiotic sensitivity patterns. Invasive diagnostic methods should be reserved for serious infections not responding to empiric therapy and pulmonary infections in the immunocompromised patient.

## Bronchitis

The *bronchiolitides* (i.e., bronchitis and bronchiolitis) refer to an inflammatory condition of the tracheobronchial tree that is usually associated with a generalized respiratory infection. The infectious agents are usually of viral origin, and the inflammatory process does not extend to include the alveoli. The diagnosis of bronchitis or bronchiolitis is based primarily upon clinical considerations. In an attempt to more specifically describe bronchitis, the disease entity is frequently classified as either acute or chronic. Acute bronchitis most commonly occurs in the young and old, whereas bronchiolitis is a disease of infancy. Chronic bronchitis is primarily a disease afflicting adults.

## *Acute Bronchitis*

### Epidemiology

Acute bronchitis most commonly occurs during the winter months, following a pattern very similar to those of other acute respiratory tract infections. Cold, damp climates and/or the presence of high concentrations of irritating substances such as air pollution or cigarette smoke may precipitate attacks.[10]

### Etiology

Respiratory viruses are by far the most common infectious agents associated with acute bronchitis. The common cold viruses, rhinovirus and coronavirus, and lower respiratory tract pathogens, including influenza virus, adenovirus, and respiratory syncytial virus, account for the majority of cases. In children, similar pathogens are observed with the addition of the parainfluenza viruses. While the true incidence remains to be defined, *Mycoplasma pneumoniae* also appears to be a frequent cause of acute bronchitis. Although a variety of bacteria including *Streptococcus pneumoniae*, *Streptococcus* spp., *Staphylococcus* spp., and *Hemophilus* spp. may be isolated from throat or sputum culture, it is probable that these organisms represent contamination by normal flora of the upper respiratory tract rather than true pathogens. While a primary bacterial etiology for acute bronchitis appears rare, secondary bacterial infection may be involved; however, the exact significance of a secondary bacterial infection is not well established.[11]

### Pathogenesis

Because acute bronchitis is primarily a self-limiting illness and rarely a cause of death, limited data are available describing the actual pathology or pathophysiology. In general, infection of the trachea and bronchi yields hyperemic and edematous mucous membranes with an increase in bronchial secretions. Destruction of respiratory epithelium can range from mild to extensive and may affect bronchial mucociliary function.[12,13] In addition, the increase in bronchial secretions, which can become thick and tenacious, further impairs mucociliary activity. The probability of permanent damage to the airways as a result of acute bronchitis remains unclear and a hotly debated issue; however, epidemiologic evaluations support the belief that acute respiratory infections may be associated with the pathogenesis of chronic obstructive lung disease.[10,14]

### Clinical Presentation

The initial manifestations of acute bronchitis are primarily upper respiratory in nature. Depending upon the etiologic agent, symptoms may be predominantly nasal as with the common cold or may also involve the pharynx as in nasopharyngitis. Nonspecific complaints including malaise and headache frequently accompany the coryza and sore throat. Cough is the hallmark of acute bronchitis and occurs early. The onset of cough may be insidious or abrupt and will persist despite the resolution of nasal or nasopharyngeal complaints. Frequently, the cough is initially nonproductive but then progresses, yielding mucopurulent sputum. In older children and adults, the sputum is raised and expectorated; in the young child, sputum is often swallowed resulting in gagging and vomiting. Slight substernal discomfort may result from the coughing. Dyspnea, cyanosis, or signs of airway obstruction are rarely observed unless the patient has serious underlying pulmonary disease (e.g., emphysema, chronic obstructive pulmonary disease). Fever, when present, rarely exceeds 39°C and appears most commonly with adenovirus, influenza virus, and *M. pneumoniae* infections.

Initial physical examination is generally unimpressive, usually revealing a variable degree of rhinitis. Chest examination may reveal rhonchi and coarse, moist rales bilaterally. Chest radiographs, when performed, are usually normal. Bacterial cultures of expectorated sputum are generally of limited utility as a result of inability to avoid normal nasopharyngeal flora by the sampling technique. Routine viral cultures are unnecessary and usually unavailable; however, cultures of respiratory secretions for *M. pneumoniae*, influenza virus, and *Bordetella pertussis* should be obtained when epidemiologic considerations and vaccination history would suggest their involvement. The white blood cell count is usually normal or slightly elevated ($>10{,}000/mm^3$) with a predominance of neutrophils in approximately one third of the cases.

### Treatment

The treatment of acute bronchitis is symptomatic and supportive in nature. Bed rest and mild analgesic–antipyretic therapy are often helpful in relieving the associated lethargy, malaise, and fever. Aspirin or acetaminophen (650 mg in adults or 10 mg/kg per dose in children) should be administered every 4 hours. In children, acetaminophen is the preferred agent because of the possible association between aspirin use and the development of Reye's syndrome.[15]

Patients suffering from acute bronchitis frequently medicate themselves with over-the-counter cough and cold remedies containing various combinations of antihistamines, sympathomimetics, and antitussives despite the lack of definitive evidence supporting their effectiveness. In fact, the tendency of these agents to dehydrate bronchial secretions may aggravate and prolong the recovery process. Patients should be encouraged to drink fluids to prevent overall dehydration and possibly decrease the viscosity of respiratory secretions. Mist therapy and/or the use of a vaporizer may further promote the thinning and loosening of respiratory secretions.[16] Persistent, mild cough, which may be bothersome, may be treated with dextromethorphan; more severe coughs may require codeine or other similar such agents.[17] In severe cases, cough may be persistent enough to disrupt sleep and the use of a mild sedative–hypnotic, concomitantly with a cough suppressant, may be desirable; however, antitussives should be used cautiously when the cough is productive. The primary or supplemental use of expectorants is questionable as their clinical effectiveness has not been well established.[18]

Routine use of antibiotics in the treatment of acute bronchitis should be discouraged; however, in patients who exhibit persistent fever or respiratory symptomatology for more than 4–6 days, the possibility of a concurrent bacterial infection should be suspected. When possible, antibiotic therapy should be directed toward the respiratory pathogen (i.e., *Streptococcus pneumoniae*, *Hemophilus influenzae*) demonstrating a predominate growth upon throat culture. *Mycobacterium pneumoniae*, if suspected by history or positive cold agglutinins (titers $\geq$ 1:32), may be treated with erythromycin. During known epidemics involving the influenza A virus, amantidine or ramantidine may be effective in minimizing associated symptomatology if administered early in the course of the disease.[19] In severe cases occurring in debilitated patients or patients with underlying cardiac or pulmonary disease, aerosolized ribavirin therapy may be beneficial. At present, however, the exact role of ribavirin therapy remains to be defined (see Bronchiolitis).

## *Chronic Bronchitis*

### Epidemiology

Chronic bronchitis is a nonspecific disease that affects primarily adults. Current estimates suggest that between 10% and 25% of the adult population 40 or older suffer from chronic bronchitis. Despite prevailing confusion surrounding the diagnosis and treatment of chronic bronchitis, it is clear from these figures that this disease entity is responsible for substantial health care dollar expenditures and lost wages.[20] Similar to acute bronchitis, cold, damp climates, as well as the presence of elevated airborne concentrations of irritating substances, may favor this disease.[21,22] Chronic bronchitis occurs more commonly in men than in women.

### Etiology

Despite the recognition for decades of chronic bronchitis as a specific disease entity, the exact cause of this disease (or syndrome?) remains unidentified. Current data and experience suggest that chronic bronchitis is a result of several contributing factors; the most prominent of these include cigarette smoking, exposure to occupational dusts, fumes, and environmental pollution, and bacterial (and possibly viral) infection. The influence that each of these factors and others, either alone or in combination, contributes to the etiology and prevalence of chronic bronchitis remains ill defined. Cigarette smoke is a well-known airway irritant and is believed by many to be the predominant factor in the etiology of chronic bronchitis.[22] Studies of lungs from smoking and nonsmoking individuals have clearly demonstrated a substantial increase in the number of alveolar macrophages,[21] as well as the presence of bronchial inflammation, in individuals who smoke cigarettes.[22] Although the majority of patients who suffer from chronic bronchitis have a positive smoking history, no history of smoking can be identified in as many as 10% of cases. These findings suggest that additional airway irritants, either alone or more probably in combination, are responsible for the pathogenesis of chronic bronchitis.

In addition to the preceding, the influence of recurrent respiratory tract infections during childhood or young adult life on the later development of chronic bronchitis remains unclear. The available data suggest that recurrent respiratory infections at a young age do predispose individuals to the development of chronic bronchitis[14,20]; however, it is unclear whether these recurrent respiratory tract infections are a result of unrecognized anatomic abnormalities of the airways or impaired pulmonary defense mechanisms. In any case, either of these physical conditions would appear to predispose an individual to the later development of chronic bronchitis.

### Pathogenesis

As previously discussed, the chronic inhalation of irritating, noxious gases compromises the normal secretory and mucociliary function of bronchial mucosa. In chronic bronchitis, the bronchial wall is thickened and the number of mucus-secreting goblet cells in the surface epithelium of both larger and smaller bronchi is markedly increased.[23] In contrast, goblet cells are generally absent from the smaller bronchi of normal individuals.[24] In addition to the increased number of goblet cells, hypertrophy of the mucus glands and dilatation of the mucus gland ducts are also observed.[23] As a result of these changes, chronic bronchitics have substantially more mucus in their peripheral airways, further impairing normal lung defenses. This increased quantity of tenacious secretions within the bronchial tree frequently causes mucus plugging of the smaller airways. Accompanying these changes are squamous cell metaplasia of the surface epithelium, edema and increased vascularity of the basement membrane of larger airways, and variable chronic inflammatory cell infiltration.[23] Continued progression of this pathology can result in residual scarring of small bronchi, augmenting airway obstruction and the weakening of bronchial walls.

### Clinical Presentation

The hallmark of chronic bronchitis is cough which, depending upon the severity of the disease, may range from a mild "smoker's" cough to severe incessant coughing productive of purulent sputum. Coughing may be precipitated by multiple stimuli including simple, normal conversation. Expectoration of the largest quantity of sputum usually occurs upon arising in the morning, though many patients expectorate sputum throughout the day. The expectorated sputum is usually tenacious and can vary in color from white to yellow-green. As a result, many patients complain of a frequent bad taste in their mouth and halitosis. In the absence of an acute pulmonary exacerbation of chronic bronchitis or another concurrent or underlying illness, most chronic bronchitics remain professionally and socially active.[25]

The diagnosis of chronic bronchitis is based primarily on clinical assessment and history. By definition, any patient who reports the coughing up of sputum on most days for at least 3 consecutive months each year for 2 consecutive years suffers from chronic bronchitis.[26,27] The diagnosis of chronic bronchitis is made only when the possibilities of bronchiectasis, cardiac failure, cystic fibrosis, and lung carcinoma have been effectively excluded. In an attempt to be more specific in the diagnosis, some investigators have added lost wages for 3 or more weeks to the criteria. In addition, many clinicians attempt to subdivide their patients into one of three subgroups: (1) those patients with "simple" chronic bronchitis, (2) those with chronic or recurrent mucopurulent bronchitis (based upon the presence of mucopurulent sputum confirmed by microscopic analysis), and (3) those with chronic obstructive bronchitis (based upon the clinical history and the presence of airway obstruction documented by pulmonary function testing).[20] Much of the confusion and controversy surrounding the diagnosis, clinical assessment, and evaluation of therapeutic intervention in chronic bronchitis results from inconsistencies in the definition and application of diagnostic criteria.

With the exception of pulmonary findings, the physical examination of patients with mild to moderate chronic bronchitis is usually unremarkable. Chest auscultation usually reveals inspiratory and expiratory rales, rhonchi, and mild wheezing with an expiratory phase that is frequently prolonged. Normal vesicular breathing sounds are diminished. Depending upon the severity of the disease, an increase in the anteroposterior (AP) diameter of the thoracic cage (observed as a "barrel chest"), hyperresonance on percussion with obliteration of the area of cardiac dullness, and depressed diaphragms with limited mobility are often observed. In more advanced stages, cyanosis is common and may be accompanied by a compensatory erythrocytosis. Clubbing of the digits is infrequent, but when observed, is usually reflective of advanced disease. In more advanced stages of chronic bronchitis, physical findings associated with cor pulmonale including cardiac enlargement, hepatomegaly, and edema of the lower extremities may be observed. In general, chronic bronchitics tend to maintain at least normal body weight, and are commonly obese. Radiographic studies are of limited value either in the diagnosis or as a means of sequentially following a patient. In advanced disease with chronic pulmonary hypertension, enlargement of the right ventricle may be observed. A decrease in vital capacity and a prolongation of expiratory flow are usually found upon pulmonary function studies.

Although the results may frequently be difficult to interpret, the microscopic and laboratory assessment of sputum is considered an important component in the overall evaluation of patients with chronic bronchitis. When performed, a fresh sputum specimen obtained as an early morning sample is preferred. Comparison of the cellular constituents of chronic bronchitic sputum with those of normal sputum[28] can provide insight into the degree of activity of the disease processes. An increased number of polymorphonuclear granulocytes often suggests continual bronchial irritation, whereas an increased number of eosinophils may suggest an allergic component which should be further investigated. Ciliated epithelial cells may also be identified and appear to correlate with the amount of coughing the patient has undergone to produce the sputum.[25] Gram staining of the sputum often reveals a mixture of both gram-positive and gram-negative bacteria, reflecting normal oropharyngeal flora and tracheal colonization by *Streptococcus pneumoniae* and *Hemophilus influenzae*. The role of sputum culture in the assessment of lung infection in chronic bronchitis remains controversial[20] and is discussed in further detail later.

**Treatment**

From the preceding discussion, it is obvious that the approach to the treatment of chronic bronchitis must be multifactorial. A complete occupational/environmental history for the determination of exposure to noxious, irritating gases, as well as preference toward cigarette smoking must be assessed. Often easier discussed than accomplished, honest yet reasonable attempts should be made with the patient to reduce the number of cigarettes smoked daily or to eliminate their use altogether. In an organized, coordinated cessation program (e.g., counseling, hypnotherapy), the adjunctive use of nicotine substitutes (e.g., nicotine gum) may promote reduction or complete withdrawal from cigarette smoking. Often just as difficult is the modification of exposure to irritating substances within the workplace.

During acute pulmonary exacerbations of the disease, a patient's ability to mobilize and expectorate sputum may be dramatically reduced. In these instances, attempts at postural drainage techniques, with instruction from a respiratory therapist, may assist in promoting clearance of pulmonary secretions. This instruction may require the assistance of a respiratory therapist. In addition, humidification of inspired air may promote the hydration (liquefaction) of tenacious secretions allowing for more productive removal. The use of mucolytic aerosols (e.g., *N*-acetylcysteine) is of questionable therapeutic value, particularly in consideration of their propensity to induce bronchospasm.[29] Similarly, the value of pre- and postpostural drainage bronchodilator aerosols remains to be defined. In contrast, oral or aerosolized bronchodilators may be of benefit to some patients during acute pulmonary exacerbations. For those patients that consistently demonstrate clinical limitation in airflow, a therapeutic challenge of bronchodilators should be considered.

In contrast to the preceding, further treatment recommendations are less clear. Our approach to the treatment is hampered by a lack of uniformity in definition of chronic bronchitis, as well as lack of consensus as to what constitutes an acute pulmonary exacerbation. In the most simple terms, an acute pulmonary exacerbation of chronic bronchitis is characterized by an increased cough, dyspnea, and alterations in appearance and amount of sputum produced. As previously discussed, some clinicians have added to these clinical findings a change in a patient's "normal" quiescent state, as well as lost wages. Substantial confusion relative to treatment guidelines has resulted from these less than critical and oftentimes conflicting opinions in our understanding of what establishes an acute pulmonary exacerbation of chronic bronchitis. Furthermore, this confusion has dramatically limited our understanding of the therapeutic impact of antimicrobial therapy.

A plethora of studies have attempted to describe a beneficial effect of antibiotic administration upon the acute and chronic treatment of chronic bronchitics (see Tables 76.1 and 76.2 for selected citations). Numerous comparative evaluations including placebo-controlled studies have sug-

**Table 76.1** Comparative Studies of Antibiotic Therapy for Acute Exacerbations of Chronic Bronchitis

| *Study* | *Drug regimen* | *Therapeutic outcome* |
|---|---|---|
| P. C. Elmes et al Br Med J 1957;2:1272–1275 | Oxytetracycline versus placebo | Treatment reduced time lost from work |
| D. G. Berry et al Lancet 1960;1:137–139 | Oxytetracycline versus placebo | Treatment group demonstrated more rapid improvement |
| M. A. DeKock et al South Afr Med J 1970;44: 1064–1065 | Tetracycline versus trimethoprim–sulfamethoxazole | No difference |
| A. Pines et al Br J Dis Chest 1972;66:107–115 | Tetracycline versus chloramphenicol versus placebo | ⅔ patients improved with treatment; ½ with placebo |
| British Thoracic Association Br J Dis Chest 1972;66:199–206 | Tetracycline versus trimethoprim–sulfamethoxazole | No difference |
| M. B. Nicotra et al Ann Intern Med 1982;97:18–21 | Tetracycline versus placebo | No difference |

Adapted from Sachs FL, Chronic bronchitis, in Pennington JE (Ed): Respiratory Infections: Diagnosis and Management. New York, Raven, 1983, with permission.

gested definite clinical benefit, whereas other similar studies have not. The antibiotics most frequently selected (e.g., ampicillin, tetracycline, chloramphenicol, trimethoprim–sulfamethoxazole) possess in vitro activity against the common sputum isolates *H. influenzae*, *S. pneumoniae*, and *M. pneumoniae* (tetracycline, erythromycin, chloramphenicol). In general, these conflicting results appear independent of which antibiotic was used or regimen compared. Expanding this further, Nicotra and colleagues[30] were unable to demonstrate any benefit of tetracycline 50 mg four times daily over placebo in chronic bronchitics who required hospitalization for their acute pulmonary exacerbation. Thus, the wide disparity that exists in the results from these studies, combined with the difficulties in recognition and lack of standardized diagnostic criteria noted previously, serves as the basis for the enormous controversy surrounding the use of antibiotics in chronic bronchitis. These issues have been expertly reviewed by Tager and Speizer[31] and Sachs[20] who provide insight into this problem and clinically relevant "consensus" recommendations.

From these reviews and others, it is apparent that it is extremely difficult to assess when an acute pulmonary exacerbation of chronic bronchitis has occurred. Attempts at sequentially following serum antibody titers to a large number of microorganisms (bacteria and viruses), as well as using sputum colony counts as an indicator of an acute exacerbation, have been met with limited success.[20] Furthermore, and just as confusing, is the issue of prophylaxis against acute pulmonary exacerbations by the continuous administration of antimicrobial agents (Table 76.2). Clinical opinion and the currently available data suggest that the decision to use antibiotics for the prevention and/or treatment of an acute exacerbation of chronic bronchitis should be made on an individual patient-specific basis. In those patients whose history suggests recurrent exacerbations of their disease that might be attributable to certain specific events (i.e., seasonal—winter months), a trial of prophylactic antibiotics might be beneficial. If no clinical improvement is noted over an appropriate period (e.g., 2–3 months per year for 2–3 years), one might elect to discontinue further attempts at prophylactic therapy. Similarily, such patient-specific trials could be performed in individuals experiencing acute exacerbations. Although less than desirable, this method of clinical assessment might distinguish those patients who will benefit from antibiotics from those who will not. Needless to say, a substantial amount of study is required to fully describe the role, if any, of antibiotics in the treatment of chronic bronchitis.

## *Bronchiolitis*

### Epidemiology

Bronchiolitis is an acute viral infection of the lower respiratory tract of infants that shows a definite seasonal pattern. The disease most commonly affects infants during the first year of life, with peak attack rates occurring in children between the ages of 2 and 10 months. Infectious bronchiolitis

**Table 76.2** Comparative Studies of Administration of Prophylactic Antibiotics to Patients With Chronic Bronchitis

| *Study* | *Drug regimen* | *Therapeutic outcome* |
|---|---|---|
| J. Buchanan et al<br>Lancet 1958;719–722 | Tetracycline versus control | Fewer exacerbations/ patient/year with therapy |
| J. McC. Murdoch et al<br>Br Med J 1959;2:1277–1285 | Tetracycline versus control | Fewer exacerbations with therapy |
| N. Datta et al<br>Lancet 1960;2:723–727 | Oxytetracycline versus penicillin and sulfa versus control | No significant differences |
| C. M. Fletcher et al<br>Br Med J 1966;1:1317–1322 | Oxytetracycline versus control | Less time lost from work; no difference in exacerbations |

Adapted from Sachs FL: Chronic bronchitis, in Pennington JE (Ed): Respiratory Infections: Diagnosis and Management. New York, Raven, 1983, with permission.

is unusual in children older than 2 years of age. The occurrence of bronchiolitis peaks during the winter months and persists through early spring. This pattern of occurrence reflects that of the primary etiologic agent, respiratory syncytial virus. Bronchiolitis remains one of the major reasons infants under 6 months require hospitalization. Current estimates suggest that the hospitalization rate for infants younger than 6 months for bronchiolitis approximates 6 per 1,000 children per year.[32] The incidence of bronchiolitis appears to be more common in males than females.

### Etiology

Respiratory syncytial virus is the most common cause of bronchiolitis, accounting for 45% to 60% of all cases.[32,33] During epidemic periods, the incidence of respiratory syncytial virus–induced bronchiolitis can exceed 80%. Parainfluenza viruses type 3 (10%–15%), type 1 (5%–10%), and type 2 (1%–5%) are the second most common etiologic pathogens, constituting as a group nearly 25% of cases. Although initially spurring much controversy,[34] current data fail to establish any role of bacterial agents as either primary or secondary pathogens.

### Clinical Presentation

A prodromal period usually lasting from 2 to 7 days precedes the onset of clinical symptoms. These symptoms usually occur after a 4- to 6-day incubation period after exposure to adults or older children with the common cold or other viral respiratory infections. During this prodromal period, infants may be irritable and restless and have a mild fever. The most common clinical signs of bronchiolitis are cough and coryza. As symptoms progress, infants may experience vomiting, diarrhea, noisy breathing, and an increase in respiratory rate. For those infants presenting to a hospital, examination reveals a rapid pulse and a respiratory rate between 40 and 80 breaths per minute. Breathing is labored with retractions of the chest wall, nasal flaring, and grunting. Chest auscultation reveals wheezing and inspiratory rales. Mild conjunctivitis may be observed in up to one third of infants, whereas 5% to 10% may have a concurrent otitis media. As a result of limited oral intake due to coughing combined with vomiting and diarrhea, infants are frequently dehydrated. The increased work of breathing and tachypnea most likely further increases fluid loss. In most cases, this clinical picture persists between 3 and 7 days. Although the hospital course of bronchiolitic children is often variable, substantial clinical improvement is usually observed within the first 2 days, with gradual improvement and resolution over the next 7–21 days.

The diagnosis of bronchiolitis is based primarily on history and clinical findings. It is important for the clinician to attempt to differentiate between bronchiolitis and a host of other clinical entities affecting infants which may produce a similar picture of dyspnea and wheezing. Asthma, pneumonia (anatomic airway abnormalities, cystic fibrosis), foreign bodies, gastroesophageal reflux, and salicylism are the primary disease entities that may present in a fashion similar to bronchiolitis. The ability to identify specific viral pathogens is often limited by the limited availability of special virology laboratories. The recent availability of the enzyme-linked immunosorbent assay (ELISA) and fluorescent antibody staining techniques of nasopharyngeal secretions has increased our ability to identify viral antigens within several hours.[35]

Multiple clinical laboratory determinations have been used to assist in the differential diagnosis of bronchiolitis. Roentgenographic evaluation of the chest in children with bronchiolitis yields variable findings. The peripheral white blood cell count is usually normal or only slightly elevated. In those children requiring hospitalization, abnormalities in blood gas tensions are frequent and appear to relate to disease severity.[36] Hypoxemia is common and acts to increase the respiratory drive, whereas hypercarbia is seen only in the most severe cases. Despite the presence of moderate degrees of hypoxemia, clinical cyanosis is unusual.

**Treatment**

The mainstay of therapy for bronchiolitis is oxygen therapy. Reversal of hypoxemia is usually achieved by the administration of 40% oxygen. Adequate fluids should be provided to prevent or correct dehydration. Clinical assessment combined with blood gas determinations is used to monitor the effectiveness of therapy. Aerosolized $\beta$-adrenergic therapy appears to offer little benefit for the majority of patients,[37,38] though some clinicians suggest the careful use of bronchodilators in selected hospitalized infants.[39] Similarly, controlled trials of corticosteroids have failed to reveal any therapeutic benefit (or harmful effect) when administered to bronchiolitic infants.[40,41] As a result, the routine use of systemically administered corticosteroids is discouraged. Although it has been common practice to place children with bronchiolitis in mist tents, there are no data to document the effectiveness of this practice. As bacteria do not represent primary pathogens in the etiology of bronchiolitis, antibiotics should not be routinely administered. Despite this fact, many clinicians frequently administer antibiotics initially while awaiting culture results, as the clinical and radiographic findings in bronchiolitis are often suggestive of a possible bacterial pneumonia.

The recent availability of the antiviral agent ribavirin expands the clinician's therapeutic armamentarium of clinically effective antiviral drugs, and may offer a new approach to the treatment of bronchiolitis and other lower respiratory tract viral infections. Ribavirin is a synthetic nucleoside that possesses antiviral properties in vitro against a variety of RNA and DNA viruses, including influenza A, influenza B, parainfluenza, and respiratory syncytial virus.[42–44] Use of the drug requires special equipment (small-particle aerosol generator) and specifically trained personnel for administration via oxygen hood or mist tent; special care must be taken to avoid drug particle deposition and the resultant clogging of respiratory tubing in mechanical ventilators. The potential for mechanical ventilator malfunction can be easily prevented by following simple precautionary procedures.[44]

When administered as small particles via aerosol, ribavirin has been shown to ameliorate the clinical course of both influenza A and B infections in adults, as well as to diminish the systemic symptoms, fever, and viral shedding associated with respiratory infections caused by respiratory syncytial virus[42–44]; however, limited data are currently available describing the utility of this form of therapy in many clinical situations. Because of the method available for drug administration, the limited availability of special aerosol devices, and cost, most centers are presently reserving the use of ribavirin for more severely ill patients, including those with underlying cardiac or pulmonary disease.

## Pneumonia

### *Epidemiology*

Prior to the antibiotic era, pneumonia was referred to as "the captain of the men of death" and bore a mortality rate in excess of 50%.[45] While the availability of antimicrobial therapy has significantly improved the outcome in this disease, pneumonia remains the most common infectious cause of death in the United States.[46] Pneumonia occurs throughout the year, with the relative prevalence of disease resulting from different etiologic agents varying with the seasons. It occurs in persons of all ages, though the clinical manifestations are most severe in the very young, the elderly, and the chronically ill.

### *Pathogenesis*

Microorganisms gain access to the lower respiratory tract by three routes. They may be inhaled as aerosolized particles or may enter the lung via the bloodstream from an extrapulmonary site of infection; however, aspiration of oropharyngeal contents, a common occurrence in both healthy and ill persons during sleep, is the major mechanism by which pulmonary pathogens gain access to the normally sterile lower airways and alveoli.[47] When pulmonary defense mechanisms are functioning optimally, aspirated microorganisms are cleared from the region before infection can become established; however, aspiration of potential pathogens from the oropharynx can result in pneumonia if lung defenses are impaired. Factors that promote aspiration, such as altered sensorium and neuromuscular disease, may result in an increase in the size of the inoculum delivered to the lower respiratory tract, thereby overwhelming local defense mechanisms. Lung infections with viruses suppress the antibacterial activity of the lung by impairing alveolar macrophage function and mucociliary clearance, thus setting the stage for secondary bacterial pneumonia.[48] Mucociliary transport is also depressed by ethanol and narcotics and by obstruction of a bronchus by mucus, tumor, or extrinsic compression. All of these factors can severely impair the pulmonary clearance of aspirated bacteria.

In addition to the myriad of factors that promote the development of pneumonia by impairing lung defenses, characteristics of bacterial colonization of the upper airway can influence the development of lower respiratory tract infections. The high carriage rate of *Streptococcus pneumoniae* in the pharynx of normal persons (60% infants, 25% children and their parents) accounts for this organism being the most common cause of acute bacterial pneumonia.[49] The demonstrated resistance of normal respiratory epithelial cells to colonization with aerobic gram-negative rods is reflected in the low incidence of pneumonia caused by this group of bacteria in otherwise healthy adults. In contrast, the high prevalence of oropharyngeal colonization by gram-negative bacilli in elderly and seriously ill patients is associated with in vitro and in vivo evidence of increased attachment and adherence of these organisms to upper airway epithelial cells,[50] and accounts for the high incidence of gram-negative bacillary pneumonia in this patient population. Thus, it is clear that host factors are extremely important in determining whether or not pneumonia will develop after endogenous aspiration. Likewise, the causative agent in most cases of pneumonia is determined by the host factors of age and underlying health status, as well as by the clinical setting in which the infection occurs.

The vast majority of pneumonia cases acquired in the community by otherwise healthy adults are due to one of two organisms: *Streptococcus pneumoniae* (pneumococcus) and *Mycoplasma pneumoniae*. Pneumococcus is the most common cause of bacterial pneumonia in all age groups and accounts for approximately 70% of all acute bacterial pneumonias in the United States.[51] *M. pneumoniae* is believed to account for 10% to 20% of cases.[52] Community-acquired pneumonias caused by *Staphylococcus aureus* and gram-negative rods are observed primarily in the elderly, especially those residing in nursing homes, and in association with alcoholism and other debilitating conditions.[53,54] Gram-negative aerobic bacilli and *Staphylococcus aureus* are also the leading causative agents in hospital-acquired pneumonia.[55] Anaerobic bacteria are the most common etiologic agents in pneumonia that follows the gross aspiration of gastric or oropharyngeal contents. Pneumonia in infants and children is caused by a wider range of microorganisms, and unlike adults, nonbacterial pathogens predominate.[56] Most pneumonias in the pediatric age group are due to viruses, especially respiratory syncytial virus, parainfluenza, and adenovirus. *M. pneumoniae* is an important pathogen in older children, and other nonbacterial pathogens such as *Chlamydia trachomatis*, *Ureaplasma urealyticum*, *Pneumocystis carinii*, and cytomegalovirus are frequent causes of pneumonia during the first 3 months of life. Beyond the neonatal period, the pneumococcus is the major bacterial pathogen in childhood pneumonia followed by *Hemophilus influenzae* type B, group A streptococcus, and *Staphylococcus aureus*.

## *Clinical Presentation*

### Gram-Positive Pneumonias

***Streptococcus pneumoniae (Pneumococcus)*** Pneumococcus is an aerobic, gram-positive coccus which appears as lancet-shaped pairs on Gram stain. It is by far the most frequent cause of acute bacterial pneumonia in the United States, accounting for over 70% of cases. Although it occurs sporadically throughout the year, the overall incidence is highest in the winter months. It occurs most frequently in the elderly, often after a viral respiratory infection, and in children less than 5 years old. Patients with splenic dysfunction, diabetes mellitus, and chronic cardiopulmonary or renal disease are at increased risk. Despite the availability of antibiotics, the disease is associated with a 10% to 20% mortality, especially in the elderly, bacteremic patient.[57] Its onset is classically abrupt, with shaking, chills, fever, severe pleuritic chest pain, and cough productive of rust-colored, purulent sputum developing in up to 90% of patients. On physical examination, the patient is typically dyspneic, with tachypnea, chest wall retractions, and grunting respirations. Decreased respiratory excursion on the affected side (splinting) may also be observed. Early cases may exhibit only localized, fine rales on auscultation. Diminished bronchial breath sounds, dullness to percussion, increased tactile fremitus, whispered pectoriloquy, and egophony accompany lobar consolidation. Pleural friction rubs are common. Sterile pleural effusions occur in approximately 25% and empyema in 1% of cases, and their presence is suggested by the findings of decreased tactile fremitus with diminished breath sounds and dullness to percussion. Nonpulmonary findings include tachycardia, myalgias, nausea and vomiting, and disorientation and confusion.

Laboratory findings in these patients include a peripheral leukocytosis with neutrophilia and an increased percentage of immature granulocytes. Pneumococcus is isolated from blood cultures in approximately 30% of cases.[54] A properly collected and Gram-stained sputum specimen that reveals polymorphonuclear leukocytes and numerous lancet-shaped diplococci is highly suggestive of the diagnosis of pneumococcal pneumonia. Counterimmunoelectrophoresis to detect pneumococcal polysaccharide antigen is positive in approximately one half of patients with both bacteremic and nonbacteremic pneumococcal pneumonia, and may be a useful diagnostic adjunct when an adequate sputum sample is unobtainable. Although the "classic" finding on chest radiographs is dense lobar or segmental consolidation, patchy bronchopneumonia is frequently observed. Thus, an etiologic diagnosis cannot be made solely on the basis of roentgenographic criteria.

***Staphylococcus aureus*** *Staphylococcus aureus* is a gram-positive coccus that grows in pairs and clusters; it is a bacterium that elaborates an array of extracellular toxins. While *S. aureus* is a much less frequent cause of pneumonia in the general population than pneumococcus, accounting for only 2% to 5% of community-acquired cases, it is an important pathogen in certain patient populations. It is the third leading cause of nosocomial pneumonias, accounting for 11% to 14% of cases,[55] and is seen with increased frequency in the settings of antecedent viral respiratory infections (especially influenza A) and prior antibiotic use. In addition, it is the most common aerobic pathogen causing aspiration pneumonia. In pediatric patients, *S. aureus* pneumonia is most commonly seen during the first 3 months of life and in young patients with cystic fibrosis. Although most cases of staphylococcal pneumonia are primary infections, approximately 25% result from hematogenous spread from an extrapulmonary infection. The availability of potent antistaphylococcal antibiotics has reduced the rate of mortality from this infection from 80% to approximately 30%.[54]

The illness is characterized by abrupt onset and rapid progression with fever, chills, dyspnea, productive cough, and pleuritic chest pain. Rales and rhonchi are present on chest auscultation. The elaboration of a multitude of extracellular toxins by the *S. aureus* probably accounts for the extensive tissue destruction that is characteristic of staphylococcal pneumonia, including erosion of bronchial and arterial walls, hemorrhage, thrombosis, and infarction. As a result, frank hemoptysis is not uncommon in this disease, and abscess formation is frequent, developing in up to 25% of cases of staphylococcal pneumonia. Pleural effusions are present in approximately 25% of cases, while the incidence of empyema approaches 10%.

Laboratory findings are largely nonspecific and may include an elevated white blood cell count and arterial hypoxemia. Blood cultures are positive in approximately 20% of cases, and sputum Gram stain reveals gram-positive cocci in clusters and polymorphonuclear leukocytes. Chest radiographs typically reveal bilaterally patchy bronchopneumonia, though in hematogenously acquired cases, multiple round densities may be seen in the lung periphery. The presence of thin-walled air-containing cysts, or pneumatoceles, suggests the diagnosis of staphylococcal pneumonia.

***Group B β-Hemolytic Streptococcus*** Group B β-hemolytic streptococcus (*Streptococcus agalactiae*), a rare cause of pneumonia in adults, is the most common bacterial pathogen causing pneumonia in the early neonatal period. In this age group, the infection causes a clinical picture nearly indistinguishable from hyaline membrane disease (HMD), with respiratory distress and hypoxemia developing within hours of birth. The radiographic findings of reticulogranular ("ground glass") infiltrates and the air bronchogram closely resemble those seen in HMD. This disease follows a fulminant course and has a mortality rate between 60% and 90%.[58]

### Gram-Negative Pneumonias

Aerobic gram-negative bacteria are a common cause of both community-acquired and hospital-acquired pneumonias. Members of the Enterobacteriaceae (*Klebsiella pneumoniae*, *Enterobacter* spp., *Serratia*, *Escherichia coli*, *Proteus* spp.) and *Pseudomonas* spp. account for most nosocomial pneumonias, and probably result from increased upper airway colonization with subsequent endogenous aspiration or inhalation of aerosolized bacteria from contaminated respiratory therapy apparatus.[59] These organisms also cause pneumonia in neonates and in ambulatory patients with chronic illness, especially alcoholism and diabetes mellitus, while the other significant gram-negative respiratory pathogens, *Hemophilus influenzae* and *Legionella pneumophilia*, cause disease in both healthy and chronically ill individuals. Their high incidence and mortality make this group of pathogens of great clinical importance.

***Klebsiella pneumoniae*** *Klebsiella pneumoniae*, a nonmotile encapsulated gram-negative rod, is the most common pathogen causing gram-negative bacillary pneumonia. This infection is seen with increased incidence in middle-aged to elderly men and in the settings of nursing home residence, alcoholism, hospitalization, and prior antibiotic therapy. In this patient population, *K. pneumoniae* pneumonia is associated with a mortality rate that exceeds 50%.[54] Infected individuals typically present acutely ill, with fever, chills, dyspnea, pleuritic chest pain, and productive cough. The sputum is generally thick, tenacious, and brick red in color, though purulent yellow-green sputum has also been associated with infection by this pathogen. Similar to *Staphylococcus aureus*, *K. pneumoniae* has a tendency to produce necrosis of lung tissue and blood vessels, and thus hemoptysis and abscess formation are not uncommon.[59] Blood cultures are positive in approximately 25% of cases, whereas other laboratory findings are usually nonspecific and unhelpful. The diagnosis usually rests on isolation of the organism from culture of lower respiratory tract secretions. Roentgenographic features are variable and include lobar consolidation, especially involving the right upper lobe, or less commonly, bronchopneumonic or perihilar distribution of infiltrates. Abscess formation and effusions are common, and bulging of interlobar fissures is considered a distinctive radiographic finding of this disease.

***Other Enterobacteriaceae*** *Serratia marcescens*, *Escherichia coli*, *Proteus* spp., *Providencia* spp., and *Morganella* spp. are all capable of causing pneumonia. Pulmonary infections caused by these pathogens are seen in settings very similar to that in which *K. pneumoniae* occurs, affecting older individuals with underlying chronic illness and within the hospitalized environment. The infections caused by these organisms also closely mimic *K. pneumoniae* in their clinical manifestations.

*E. coli* ranks after *K. pneumoniae* as the second most common cause of community-acquired gram-negative bacillary pneumonia, and is the third leading cause of nosocomial pneumonias due to this group of bacteria.[55,59] Unlike other gram-negative pneumonias, most cases develop after hematogenous spread from genitourinary or gastrointestinal tract infections, and as such the organism is generally easily identified in culture from one or more sites.

*S. marcescens* causes hospital-acquired infections of the lungs, genitourinary tract, blood, and wounds and outbreaks of *Serratia* pneumonia have been associated with the use of contaminated aerosol nebulizers and fiberoptic bronchoscopes.[60] Certain strains of this organism produce a dark red pigment that stains the sputum and can result in the clinical phenomenon of "pseudohemoptysis."

***Pseudomonas Species*** *Pseudomonas aeruginosa*, the most commonly isolated species of *Pseudomonas*, is an aerobic, motile gram-negative bacillus. It is widely prevalent in the hospital environment and requires no growth factors, utilizing carbon dioxide as its sole carbon source and ammonium as its nitrogen source. It ranks second only to *K. pneumoniae* as a cause of nosocomial pneumonia.[61] Although hematogenous seeding of the lungs may occur in the neutropenic or severely burned patient, endogenous aspiration from a colonized oropharynx is the most common mechanism of infection. While only 5% of healthy adults carry *Pseudomonas* species within their upper airway, this bacterium can be isolated from up to 50% of hospitalized patients, especially those with malignancies.[62] In addition, outbreaks of *Pseudomonas* pneumonia have occurred secondary to exogenous inhalation of the pathogen from contaminated respiratory therapy apparatus.[61] Clinical manifestations are similar to those seen in *K. pneumoniae*. Radiographic findings are diffuse, patchy bronchopneumonic infiltrates, frequently accompanied by pleural effusions. Despite the availability of "antipseudomonal" antibiotics, the mortality from this illness remains within the range 50% to 70%.

A different clinical picture is seen with *Pseudomonas* lung infections in patients with cystic fibrosis. Multiple morphotypes of *P. aeruginosa*, and less commonly *P. cepacia* and *P. maltophilia*, can be isolated from the lower respiratory tract of these individuals. Although some patients may experience asymptomatic colonization, signs and symptoms of chronic infection are seen in the vast majority and recurrent acute pneumonia due to *Pseudomonas* is typical.

***Hemophilus influenzae*** *Hemophilus influenzae* is a gram-negative pleomorphic coccobacillus that exists as both encapsulated and nonencapsulated strains. The encapsulated organisms are responsible for most infectious diseases caused by this organism, with *H. influenzae* type B being most prevalent in children. *H. influenzae* has long been recognized as a leading cause of bacterial pneumonia in children under 10, with a peak incidence in the age group 6 months to 2 years.[63] Recently, this organism has been increasing in importance as an etiologic agent in acute pneumonia in adults, accounting for approximately 8% of cases in this population, with chronic bronchitis, chronic obstructive pulmonary disease, and alcoholism being common predisposing conditions.[64]

In pediatric patients, *H. influenzae* pneumonia is almost always preceded by coryza, with gradually worsening of "cold" symptoms over several days. Cough, fever, decreased appetite, irritability, and tachypnea ensue. While this subacute course is most common, approximately one third of patients experience acute onset of fever, productive cough, and respiratory distress. Bacteremia and extrapulmonary infections, including meningitis and pericarditis, are frequent occurrences in children. Pleural effusions, which develop early in the course of the illness, may be observed in as many as 75% of cases.[63] Typical radiographic findings include segmental or lobar infiltrates, although diffuse bronchopneumonia has also been described.

Laboratory findings include leukocytosis with an increased percentage of mature and immature granulocytes. Blood cultures are positive in over 90% of patients, and the causative organism can be isolated from approximately 50% of pleural fluid specimens. Because of the difficulties in obtaining sputa from pediatric patients and the significant carriage rate of *H. influenzae* in the upper airway of normal children, the bacteriologic diagnosis generally cannot be made solely on the basis of culture of respiratory tract secretions. In addition to isolation of the organism from blood or pleural fluid, identification of *H. influenzae* type B antigens in body fluids by counterimmunoelectrophoresis or latex agglutination may be helpful in establishing the etiologic diagnosis.

Two different clinical presentations of *H. influenzae* pneumonia are seen in adults. The most common by far is the bronchopneumonia form, which develops most frequently in patients with underlying chronic lung disease and is believed to represent, in most patients, an exacerbation of chronic bronchitis. Affected individuals typically develop worsening cough and tachypnea along with low-grade fever and constitutional symptoms. Bacteremia is present in approximately one quarter of cases. Because asymptomatic colonization of the lower respiratory tract with *H. influenzae* occurs in patients with chronic lung disease, culture of sputum or transtracheal aspirates may not be reliable in this population, and the diagnosis rests on antigen detection or isolation of the bacteria from pleural fluid. In the second form of *H. influenzae* pneumonia, which occurs in approximately 15% of patients, segmental or lobar involvement predominates. The course of this illness is more acute, with sudden onset of cough, fever, and pleuritic chest pain. Bacteremia occurs in nearly three quarters of cases, and *H. influenzae* type B is the strain most commonly isolated. In addition to lobar or segmental infiltrates, early pleural reaction is typically seen on chest radiographs.

***Legionella pneumophilia*** Of the several *Legionella* species known to cause pneumonia in humans, *L. pneumophilia* is by far the most important. While this organism gained widespread notoriety after the American Legion outbreak in 1976, retrospective immunologic and bacteriologic analyses have identified it as being the etiologic agent in outbreaks of illness occurring more than 20 years ago.[65] *L. pneumophilia* is a fastidious, poorly staining gram-negative bacillus that elaborates exotoxin and endotoxin. It is a water and soil organism and is most probably transmitted by air, aerosol, or water. Outbreaks of illness caused by *L. pneumophilia* have been linked to excavation sites and contaminated water from air conditioners and showers. Person-to-person transmission has not been demonstrated.[65] In addition to outbreaks of disease, *L. pneumophilia* causes sporadic illness that peaks in summer and fall. Individuals who are male, middle-aged or older, immunocompromised, chronic bronchitics, or cigarette smokers are at increased risk. The incidence of sporadic cases of *L. pneumophilia* pneumonia in children is similar to that in adults, accounting for 1% to 5% of community-acquired pneumonias that require hospitalization.[66]

Legionnaire's disease, caused by *L. pneumophilia*, is characterized by multisystem involvement, including rapidly progressive pneumonia. It has a gradual onset, with prominent constitutional symptoms such as malaise, lethargy, weakness, and anorexia occurring early in the course of the illness. A dry, nonproductive cough is initially present which over several days becomes productive of mucoid or purulent sputum. Fevers exceeding 40°C develop in over half of patients and are typically unremitting and associated with a relative bradycardia. Pleuritic chest pain and progressive dyspnea may be seen, and fine rales are found on lung exam, progressing to signs of frank consolidation later in the course of the illness. Large pleural effusions, empyema, and lung abscess are uncommon in this disease. Extrapulmonary manifestations remain evident throughout the course of the illness and include diarrhea, nausea, vomiting, myalgias, and arthralgias. Substantial changes in a patient's mental status, often out of proportion to the degree of fever, are seen in approximately one fourth of patients. Obtundation, hallucinations, grand mal seizures, and focal neurologic findings have also been associated with this illness. Although abnormalities in hepatic and renal function may be noted on laboratory assessment, these are usually of limited clinical significance. Chest roentgenograms initially reveal patchy alveolar infiltrates which may be bilateral. Progression to lobar or multilobar consolidation is frequent, as are small pleural effusions.

Laboratory findings include leukocytosis with predominance of mature and immature granulocytes in 50% to 75% of patients. Urinalysis may reveal proteinuria, hematuria, and casts; liver function tests (e.g., serum glutamic–oxaloacetic transaminase, serum glutamic–pyruvic transaminase, bilirubin) may be abnormal. Hyponatremia and hypophosphatemia have also been frequently reported. Because *L. pneumophilia* stains poorly with commonly used stains, routine microscopic examination of sputum is of little diagnostic value. While it exhibits slow growth and has highly selective growth requirements, *L. pneumophilia* has been successfully isolated from tissue using specialized medium. In addition to diagnosis by culture, fluorescent antibody testing can be performed to diagnose Legionnaire's disease. Serologic diagnosis using the indirect fluorescent antibody technique is the most widely available, and three quarters of affected individuals demonstrate a fourfold rise in titer; however, as the mean time required for seroconversion is 2 weeks, serology is not diagnostic during the acute phase of the illness. Direct fluorescent antibody examination of respiratory tract secretions, lung tissue, or pleural fluid is the most rapid means of establishing the diagnosis. The sensitivity of this method approaches 70% for sputum and 90% for lung tissue, and diagnostic specificity is high for both.[67] Because this diagnostic test is complex and difficult to perform, it is unavailable in most clinical laboratories. As such, the diagnosis of Legionnaire's disease is often initially presumptive, based on a suggestive clinical presentation.

### Anaerobic Pneumonia

A variety of gram-positive and gram-negative anaerobic bacteria endogenous to the upper airway may cause pneumonitis when large quantities of oropharyngeal secretions are aspirated into the lower airways. The organisms most frequently implicated are *Peptostreptococcus* spp., *Fusobacteria*, *Bacteroides melaninogenicus*, *Bacteroides fragilis*, and *Peptococcus* spp.; polymicrobial infections with anaerobes and aerobes such as *Staphylococcus aureus*, *Streptococcus pneumoniae*, and gram-negative bacilli are common.[2] Anaerobic pneumonitis is most likely to occur in individuals predisposed to aspiration by impaired consciousness, and may be more prevalent in those with periodontal disease or dysphagia. In addition, bronchogenic carcinoma is an associated underlying condition that should be suspected in patients with anaerobic pneumonia who do not appear predisposed to aspiration.[68]

The course of the illness is typically indolent with cough, low-grade fever, and weight loss, although an acute presentation may occur. Rigors are notable for their absence and bacteremia is rare. Putrid sputum, when present, is highly suggestive of the diagnosis. Chest radiographs reveal infiltrates typically located in dependent lung segments, and lung abscesses develop in 20% of patients 1 to 2 weeks into the course of the illness.[68]

### Nonbacterial Pneumonia

Viruses, mycoplasma species, chlamydial species, and parasites are recognized causes of pneumonia syndromes in all age groups. The designation "atypical pneumonia," in distinction to the "typical" bacterial pneumonia most commonly seen in adults, has been used to describe the illness caused by many of these agents.

***Mycoplasma pneumoniae*** *Mycoplasma* species are the smallest of free-living organisms, and share some properties of both viruses and bacteria. These prokaryocytes lack a cell wall, are inhibited by specific antibody, and stain with routine bacteriologic stains. *M. pneumoniae* causes human disease throughout the year, with a slightly increased incidence in fall and early winter. During summer months when other causes of pneumonia are less common, *M. pneumoniae* is responsible for a greater proportion of cases. Both infection and disease from *M. pneumoniae* are common, with two thirds of children age 2–5 and 97% of persons over 17 having detectable serum antibody to the organism.[69] Overall, *M. pneumoniae* is responsible for approximately 20% of pneumonia cases, though in enclosed populations such as military recruits and college dormitory residents it may cause more than 50% of pneumonia cases.[52] Infection is spread by close person-to-person contact, and the incubation period is 2–3 weeks. *M. pneumoniae* infections are unusual in children under 5 years of age and show a peak incidence in older children and young adults. Only 3% to 10% of persons infected with *M. pneumoniae* develop pneumonia, with the majority of respiratory tract involvement being manifested as pharyngitis and tracheobronchitis.[70] Asymptomatic infection is apparently common.

*M. pneumoniae* presents with a gradual onset of fever, headache, and malaise, with the appearance 3–5 days after the onset of illness of a persistent, hacking cough which initially is nonproductive. Sore throat, ear pain, and rhinorrhea are often present. Chills are only occasionally seen, and pleuritic pain is uncommon. Lung findings are generally limited to rales and rhonchi; findings of consolidation are rarely present. Nonpulmonary manifestations are extremely common and include nausea, vomiting, diarrhea, myalgias, arthralgias, polyarticular arthritis, skin rashes, myocarditis and pericarditis, hemolytic anemia, meningoencephalitis, cranial neuropathies, and Guillain–Barré syndrome. Systemic symptoms generally clear in 1 to 2 weeks, while respiratory symptoms may persist up to 4 weeks. Although the course of mycoplasmal pneumonia is usually benign and self-limited, severe respiratory disease may develop in patients with sickle cell disease, agammaglobulinemia, and chronic obstructive lung disease.[70]

Radiographic findings are generally more impressive than the patient's physical findings, and include patchy or interstitial infiltrates which are most commonly seen in the lower lobes. Small unilateral, transient pleural effusions are common but large effusions and empyema are rare. Roentgenographic abnormalities resolve slowly, and 4 to 6 weeks may be required for complete resolution.

Sputum Gram stain may reveal mononuclear or polymorphonuclear leukocytes, with no predominant organism. While *M. pneumoniae* can be cultured from respiratory secretions using specialized medium, its growth is slow and 2–3 weeks may be necessary for culture identification. Indirect evidence of infection by *M. pneumoniae* is the presence of elevated levels of serum cold hemagglutinins. These IgM antibodies develop in approximately half of patients with mycoplasmal pneumonia and can be elevated in other illnesses, especially viral infection.[69] A definitive diagnosis can also be made by demonstrating a fourfold or greater rise in serum antibodies to *M. pneumoniae*; however, as this test also requires 2–4 weeks for results, the diagnosis of mycoplasmal pneumonia during the acute phase of the illness must be based on the characteristic history, the appropriate clinical setting, and typical physical findings.

***Viral Pneumonia*** Viruses are not a common cause of pneumonia in adults except in the immunosuppressed. Influenza virus, usually type A, is the most common cause of pneumonia in the adult civilian population, whereas adenoviruses cause most cases in military trainees.[54] In contrast, viruses are by far the most common agents producing pneumonia in infants and young children, with respiratory syncytial virus, parainfluenza, and adenovirus producing most cases.[56]

All viral respiratory tract infections occur more commonly in the winter, and rapid person-to-person spread through susceptible populations is typical. Underlying cardiac or pulmonary disease predisposes to increased incidence and severity of viral lower respiratory tract infection, especially with influenza virus in adults and respiratory syncytial virus in children. Radiographic findings are nonspecific and in-

**Table 76.3** Empiric Antimicrobial Therapy for Pneumonia in Adults[a]

| *Clinical setting* | *Usual pathogen(s)* | *Presumptive therapy* |
|---|---|---|
| Previously healthy, ambulatory patient | Pneumococcus, *Mycoplasma pneumoniae* | Erythromycin |
| Elderly (nursing home residence)[b] | Pneumococcus, *Klebsiella pneumoniae Staphylococcus aureus, Hemophilus influenzae* | Semisynthetic penicillin[c] plus aminoglycoside; or ticarcillin/clavulanate cephalosporin[d]; imipenem |
| Chronic bronchitis | Pneumococcus, *H. influenzae* | Ampicillin, tetracycline, TMP–SMZ, cefuroxime |
| Alcoholism[b] | Pneumococcus, *K. pneumoniae, S. aureus, H. influenzae* | Semisynthetic penicillin[c] or ticarcillin/clavulanate plus aminoglycoside; cephalosporin[d]; imipenem |
| Recent influenza | Pneumococcus, *S. aureus* | Semisynthetic penicillin[c] or cephalosporin (e.g., cefazolin) |
| Aspiration | | |
| Community | Mouth anaerobes | Penicillin |
| Hospital | Mouth anaerobes, *S. aureus*, gram-negative enterics | Penicillin or clindamycin |
| Nosocomial pneumonia[b] | *K. pneumoniae, Pseudomonas aeruginosa, S. aureus, Escherichia coli* | Ticarcillin, piperacillin, mezlocillin, aztreonam, or imipenem plus aminoglycoside; or ceftazidime |

[a]See Treatment of Bacterial Pneumonia. TMP–SMZ = trimethoprim–sulfamethoxazole.
[b]Ciprofloxacin may prove to be a viable alternative for initial therapy in these patients.
[c]Semisynthetic penicillin (e.g., nafcillin, oxacillin).
[d]Second- or third-generation cephalosporin (e.g., cefuroxime, ceftriaxone, cefotaxime, ceftazidime).

Adapted from Pennington JE: Community-acquired pneumonia and acute bronchitis, in Pennington JE (Ed): Respiratory Infection: Diagnosis and Management. New York, Raven Press, 1983.

clude bronchial wall thickening and perihilar or diffuse interstitial infiltrates. Pleural effusions may be seen, especially in adenovirus and parainfluenza pneumonia.

The clinical pictures produced by respiratory viruses are sufficiently variable and overlap to such a degree that an etiologic diagnosis cannot confidently be made on clinical grounds alone. Although virus isolation in tissue culture is possible, 7 or more days is often required for virus identification; thus, this method usually cannot be relied upon for definitive diagnosis during the acute phase of illness. Serologic tests for virus-specific antibodies are often used in the diagnosis of viral infections. The diagnostic fourfold rise in titer between acute and convalescent phase sera may require 2–3 weeks to develop; however, same-day diagnosis of viral infections is now possible through the use of indirect immunofluorescence tests on exfoliated cells from the respiratory tract. The immunofluorescence technique is adaptable to other respiratory viruses, providing the potential for rapid diagnosis of a wider range of viral infections in the future.

### *Treatment of Bacterial Pneumonia*

The treatment of bacterial pneumonia, like the treatment of most infectious diseases, initially involves broader empiric therapy that should be narrowed so that it is specifically directed once the causative pathogen(s) has been identified. Empiric antibiotic therapy should be instituted that is effective against probable pathogens after appropriate cultures and specimens for laboratory evaluation have been obtained. Multiple factors that help define the potential pathogens involved include patient age, previous and current medication history, underlying disease(s), major organ function, and present clinical status. These factors must be evaluated to properly select an effective empiric antibiotic regimen, as well as the most appropriate route for drug administration (e.g., oral, parenteral).

Numerous antibiotics are available and the majority have been shown to be effective in the treatment of bacterial pneumonia. Superiority of one compound over another when both demonstrate similar in vitro activity and tissue distribution characteristics is difficult to define. Our opinions on viable empiric agents for the treatment of bacterial pneumonias relative to a patient's underlying disease are shown in Table 76.3 for adults and Table 76.4 for children. As mentioned before, once the causative pathogen is identified, the empiric antibiotic regimen should be changed to an effective therapeutic agent with a more narrow antimicrobial spectrum. A complete listing of antimicrobial agents for specifically directed therapy is beyond the scope of this chapter. The *Medical Letter Handbook of Antimicrobial Therapy* is a recommended, authoritative source for the reader to consult.[71]

The plethora of commercially available antimicrobial agents with documented bacterial and clinical effectiveness in the treatment of pneumonia often appears endless. These large numbers of often expensive drugs mandate our critical evaluation of these agents for selection clinically, as well as for inclusion into hospital formularies. Similarities in in vitro

**Table 76.4** Empiric Antimicrobial Therapy for Pneumonia in Pediatric Patients[a]

| *Age* | *Usual pathogen(s)* | *Presumptive therapy* |
|---|---|---|
| <1 month | Group B streptococcus, *Staphylococcus aureus*, *Escherichia coli* | Semisynthetic penicillin[b] plus aminoglycoside or cephalosporin[c]; imipenem |
| | Cytomegalovirus (CMV), respiratory syncytial virus (RSV), adenovirus | Ribavirin for RSV |
| 1–3 months | *Chlamydia, Ureaplasma,* CMV, *Pertussis, Pneumocystis carinii* (afebrile pneumonia syndrome) | Erythromycin, TMP–SMZ |
| | RSV | Ribavirin |
| | Pneumococcus, *S. aureus* | Semisynthetic penicillin[b] or cephalosporin[c] |
| 3 months–6 years | Pneumococcus, *Hemophilus influenzae*, RSV, adenovirus, parainfluenza | Ampicillin or cephalosporin[d] Ribavirin for RSV |
| >6 years | Pneumococcus, *Mycoplasma pneumoniae*, adenovirus | Erythromycin |

[a] TMP–SMZ = trimethoprim–sulfamethoxazole.
[b] Semisynthetic penicillin (e.g., nafcillin, oxacillin).
[c] Third-generation cephalosporin (e.g., ceftriaxone, cefotaxime).
[d] Second-generation cephalosporin (e.g., cefuroxime).

activity, resistance to bacteria-inactivating enzymes, and overall effectiveness often make rational therapeutic decisions difficult and potentially even appear random. For community-acquired pneumonia, the bacteriologic causes remain relatively constant, even within specific geographic areas and patient populations. In contrast, antibiotic selection within the hospital environment may be more difficult because of changes in antibiotic activity in vitro and the development of pathogen resistance. Moreover, the potential of certain β-lactam antibiotics to induce bacterial β-lactamase[72] may impact greatly on our dependence on, and selection of, these agents over the next several years. These facts underscore the importance of sequentially documenting the epidemiology of pathogens and infectious diseases within a specific practice or institution. As a result, an antimicrobial agent for a specific infectious disease favored in one practice site may not be the most desirable selection in another, despite similarities in size and practice. Multiple variables must be considered in selection of the most appropriate antimicrobial agent, particularly in our present cost-conscious environment. (See Chapter 74.)

Numerous investigators have demonstrated that antibiotic concentrations in respiratory secretions in excess of the pathogen minimum inhibitory concentration (MIC) are necessary for successful treatment of pulmonary infections.[73,74] The concept of a blood–bronchus barrier, analogous but dissimilar to the blood–brain barrier, has been used to assess the characteristics of drug penetration into pulmonary secretions.[73] The ability of a drug to penetrate respiratory secretions depends upon multiple physicochemical factors, including molecular size, lipid solubility, and degree of ionization at serum and biologic fluid pH. Studies performed in animals and cystic fibrosis patients suggest that larger molecular size favors the accumulation of drugs in bronchial secretions.[75,76] This finding contrasts with data on drug penetration of other physiologic compartments, such as the cerebrospinal fluid, and may be a result of the trapping of lower molecular weight compounds in mucin pores. The importance of this finding cannot be overemphasized; however, the rate at which a drug may accumulate in certain respiratory secretions would appear to remain an important factor relative to the drug's clinical efficacy in treating pulmonary infections. The un-ionized form of a drug and lipid solubility also appear to favor drug penetration.[73,74] It should be noted that the pH of infected bronchi is often more acidic than that of normal tissue and blood.[77,78] Fewer data are available assessing the influence of drug protein binding on the rate and amount of respiratory secretion penetration. As the degree of protein binding has been shown to influence a drug's ability to traverse membranes, a similar relationship would be expected within the lung.[73,74] Thus, it is prudent to assess the pharmacokinetic–pharmacodynamic correlates of drug binding to serum proteins, tissue distribution, and in vitro potency when selecting an antimicrobial regimen. These concepts relating to overall drug penetration of respiratory secretions, and others, have lead to the clinical practice of administering certain antibiotics (e.g., aminoglycosides) to achieve high peak serum concentrations on the assumption that higher (and possibly more effective) biologic fluid concentrations of the drug will be achieved. Substantial clinical experience supports this practice for treating pulmonary infections with certain antibiotics, though more data are needed to describe the relationships between these variables and clinical response.

Prior to the availability of newer β-lactam antibiotics possessing consistent potent activity against multiple gram-negative pathogens, the administration of antibiotics via aerosol or direct endotracheal instillation was promoted by some investigators.[79,80] This method of drug administration is an attempt to provide increased "topical" concentrations of antibiotics that do not appear to penetrate respiratory secretions effectively while reducing the likelihood of systemic toxicity. In addition, greater local concentrations of antibiotics, particularly for the polymyxins and aminoglycosides, are believed to partially overcome the substantial decrease in antibiotic bioactivity observed when these agents interact with the purulent material present in infectious foci.[81,82] Despite these potential theoretical advantages, the role of antibiotic aerosols or direct endotracheal instillation in clinical practice remains ill defined.

Sputum is frequently assessed as possibly representing the pharmacodynamic interface for pulmonary infections. It should be noted that sputum represents only one of many pulmonary fluids and secretions, though sputum may serve as a reservoir for pathogen growth. These beliefs have led many investigators to assess antibiotic concentrations in sputum, frequently describing sputum drug concentrations as a ratio of serum drug concentrations.[74] Although sputum drug concentrations provide us with some insight into the characteristics of drug penetration of respiratory secretions, caution should be exercised in the interpretation of these data. Current data describing sputum drug concentrations are often difficult to interpret because of differences in analytical techniques, method of sputum sampling, and the random nature of sampling times relative to drug dose. Moreover, representation of sputum drug concentrations as a ratio of serum drug concentration can be misleading and most probably should be described relative to absolute drug concentration or apparent sputum area under the curve. To more accurately describe the distribution characteristics of antimicrobial agents in sputum, research studies should be designed to allow sequential repeated sputum sampling over a dosage interval under both first-dose and steady-state conditions.[83,84]

Prevention of some cases of pneumonia is possible through the use of vaccines against selected infectious agents.[85] Inactivated influenza virus vaccines formulated annually to contain antigens representative of expected prevalent strains are widely available and generally well tolerated. Immunization is recommended for individuals likely to experience serious complications from influenza infection, such as patients with underlying heart or lung disease, chronic renal disease, and the elderly. Although it should not replace active immunization, amantadine may be administered for prevention of influenza A infection, beginning as soon as possible after exposure and continuing for at least 10 days. The recommended dose is 5 mg/kg/d in two to three divided doses not to exceed 150 mg/d in children 1 to 9 years old, and 200 mg/d in two divided doses in patients 9 or older.

Polyvalent polysaccharide vaccines are available for two of the leading causes of bacterial pneumonia, pneumococcus and *Hemophilus influenzae* type B; however, these vaccines are poorly immunogenic in children under 2, and thus are of no benefit in an age group at relatively high risk for pneumonia caused by these pathogens. Specific indications for these vaccines are outlined in Chapter 90. Rifampin prophylaxis may be used to prevent *H. influenzae* type B in young children who have been in close contact with a patient with invasive disease resulting from *H. influenzae*. The drug should be given orally once daily for 4 days in a 20 mg/kg dose (maximum 600 mg/d) to all household contacts in households where there are children other than the index case less than 4 years of age.

The supportive care of the patient with pneumonia includes the use of humidified oxygen for hypoxemia, administration of bronchodilators when bronchospasm is present, and chest physiotherapy with postural drainage if there is evidence of retained secretions. Additional therapeutic adjuncts include adequate hydration, optimal nutritional support, and fever control.

## Lung Abscess

A lung abscess is a localized area of suppuration within pulmonary parenchyma accompanied by necrosis of lung tissue. While a multitude of factors may predispose to the development of lung abscess, the majority are due to aspiration of infected oropharyngeal secretions.[86] Periodontal disease, oropharyngeal infections, depressed sensorium and decreased cough reflex resulting from alcoholism, anesthesia, or neurologic disorders, and esophageal disease causing impaired swallowing all predispose to the development of lung abscess. Endobronchial obstruction caused by foreign body or tumor, septic emboli, and bland or septic pulmonary infarction may also lead to lung abscess formation. Secondary lung abscesses complicating bacterial pneumonia account for approximately 20% of cases, and most commonly follow infections with *Staphylococcus aureus* and *Klebsiella pneumoniae*.[87]

### *Pathogenesis*

The bacteriology of primary lung abscess reflects that of the oropharyngeal flora and, as such, is characteristically anaerobic and polymicrobial. Using transtracheal aspiration to obtain specimens for microbiologic studies, Bartlett et al[86] recovered anaerobic bacteria from 93% of patients with primary lung abscess, with the most common isolates being *Bacteroides melaninogenicus*, *Fusobacterium nucleatum*, and anaerobic or microaerophilic gram-positive cocci. Mixed infections with anaerobes and aerobes were seen in nearly half. *S. aureus* and enteric gram-negative bacilli are more common isolates in patients whose disease developed in the hospital than in community-acquired cases.[88] The microbiology of lung abscess in pediatric patients is similar to that reported for adults.[89]

The most common sites for the development of lung abscess are the portions of the lung that are dependent in the supine position. These include the posterior segments of the upper lobes and the apical segments of the lower lobes, with the right lung being involved far more frequently than the left. The infection begins as a pneumonitis, with alveolar edema and an inflammatory infiltrate, and progresses to necrotizing pneumonia, characterized by multiple small cavitations. If treatment is delayed or inadequate, further progression of the infection and necrosis results in the formation of a single large abscess cavity which becomes bound by fibrosing inflammatory tissue that limits its further extension. The abscess cavity may communicate with a bronchus or with the pleural space.

### *Clinical Presentation*

The course of primary lung abscess is gradually progressive, with most patients having symptoms for several weeks prior to diagnosis.[87] General malaise, low-grade fever, weight loss, night sweats, and pleuritic chest pain are frequent complaints. Patients commonly exhibit a cough productive of copious amounts of sputum, which in approximately half of the cases is putrid.[54] Physical findings may include signs of frank consolidation, localized rales, or, in late cases, cavernous breath sounds.

The chest radiograph is diagnostic of lung abscess and typically reveals a single, thin-walled cavity which may contain an air–fluid level. Etiologic diagnosis depends on bacteriologic studies on lower airway secretions. Because the normal inhabitants of the oropharynx are the leading pathogens in lung abscess, cultures of expectorated sputum specimens are of little value in diagnosis of this disease entity. Transtracheal aspiration is 80%-90% accurate in establishing an etiologic diagnosis in anaerobic and aerobic lung abscess,[90] and is a safe and useful diagnostic adjunct when a specific bacteriologic diagnosis is necessary; however, the consistent microbiology of primary lung abscesses within a given clinical setting makes the likelihood of success of properly chosen "empiric therapy" high.

### *Treatment*

Antimicrobial therapy is the keystone of treatment of lung abscess. Prolonged treatment may be necessary to achieve cure without relapse. Initial treatment with parenteral antibiotics until defervescence and clinical improvement are achieved is generally recommended. Thereafter, oral therapy may be instituted and continued until satisfactory radiographic clearing has occurred, a process that may take several months. The choice of antimicrobial agent(s) should be based on results of bacteriologic studies when available, or on the clinical setting in which the infection occurred. Lung abscesses acquired in the community are almost universally caused by anaerobic organisms, and penicillin G remains the drug of choice for primary lung abscess in this setting. Even those patients from whom *Bacteroides fragilis* or aerobic microbes are recovered generally are cured with this drug alone.[91] Because *S. aureus* and gram-negative bacilli, as well as anaerobes, are often implicated in hospital-acquired lung abscesses, clindamycin may be a superior therapeutic agent in these patients, and is the drug of choice when penicillin treatment is contraindicated.[91,92] Chloramphenicol also exhibits moderately good activity against the common anaerobic pathogens and may be used as an alternative therapy.

The time course of resolution of primary lung abscess treated with appropriate antimicrobial agents depends on the size and location of the abscess cavity. In a review of 60 patients with primary lung abscess, Weiss[93] noted 80% radiographic resolution within 1 month of therapy for cavitations less than 3 cm in diameter, whereas in larger abscesses, resolution occurred in only 30% by 1 month. By 3 months, 70% showed complete radiographic resolution. Abscesses involving the right upper lobe resolved more slowly than those in other locations. Because of the eminent success of properly chosen antimicrobial therapy in the treatment of these infections, surgical drainage of primary lung abscess is rarely indicated. Bronchoscopy may be useful in excluding foreign body and malignancy as predisposing conditions and, if the cavity of the abscess communicates with a bronchus, may aid in drainage. The mortality rate for primary lung abscess is 5% to 10%[86]; however, the prognosis for patients with severe underlying disease, such as a malignancy and immunosuppression, is much more guarded.

## References


1. Wilder CS. Acute respiratory illnesses reported to the US National Health Survey during 1957–1962. Am Rev Resp Dis 1963;88:14–21.
2. George WL, Finegold SM. Bacterial infections of the lung. Chest 1982;81:502–507.
3. Reynolds HY. Normal and defective respiratory host defenses, in Pennington JE (ed): Respiratory Infections: Diagnosis and Management. New York, Raven, 1983, pp 1–23.
4. Johanson WG Jr, Higuchi JH, Chanduri TR, et al. Bacterial adherence to epithelial cells in bacillary colonization of the respiratory tract. Am Rev Resp Dis 1980;121:55–63.
5. Todd JK. Bacteriology and clinical relevance of nasopharyngeal and oropharyngeal cultures. Pediatr Infect Dis 1984;3:159–163.
6. Heinemann HS, Chawla JK, Lofton WM. Misinformation from sputum cultures without microscopic examination. J Clin Microbiol 1977;6:518–527.
7. Davidson M, Tempest B, Palmer DL. Bacteriologic diagnosis of acute pneumonia. Comparison of sputum, transtracheal aspirates and lung aspirates. JAMA 1976;235:158–163.
8. Bartlett JG. Diagnostic accuracy of transtracheal aspiration bacteriologic studies. Am Rev Resp Dis 1977;115:777–782.
9. Matthay RA, Moritz ED. Invasive procedures for diagnosing pulmonary infection. A critical review. Clin Chest Med 1981;2:3–18.
10. Monto AS, Ross HW. The Tecumseh study of respiratory illness. X. Relation of acute infections to smoking, lung function and chronic symptoms. Am J Epidemiol 1978;107:57–64.
11. Mills EL. Viral infections predisposing to bacterial infections. Ann Rev Med 1984;35:469–479.
12. Carson JL, Collier A, Clyde WA Jr. Ciliary membrane alterations occurring in experimental *Mycoplasma pneumoniae* infection. Science 1979; 206:349–350.
13. Reed SE, Bayde A. Organ cultures of respiratory epithelium infected with rhinovirus and parainfluenza virus studied by scanning electron microscope. Infect Immun 1972;6:68–76.
14. Lebowitz MD, Burrows B. The relationship of acute respiratory illness history to the prevalence and incidence of obstructive lung disorders. Am J Epidemiol 1977;105:544–554.
15. Daniels SR, Greenberg RS, Ibrahim MA. Scientific uncertainties in the studies of salicylate use and Reye's syndrome. JAMA 1983;249:1311–1316.
16. Dulfano MJ, Adler K. Wooten O. Physical properties of sputum. IV. Effects of 100 percent humidity and water mist. Am Rev Resp Dis 1973;107:130–132.
17. Committee on Drugs. Use of codeine and dextromethorphan-

containing cough syrups in pediatrics. Pediatrics 1978;62;118–122.

18. Kuhn JJ, Hendley JO, Adams KF, et al. Antitussive effect of guaifenesin in young adults with natural colds. Objective and subjective assessment. Chest 1982;82:713–718.
19. Hayden FG, Monto AS. Oral rimantadine hydrochloride therapy of influenza A virus H3N2 subtype infection in adults. Antimicrob Agents Chemother 1986;29:339–341.
20. Sachs FL. Chronic bronchitis. Clin Chest Med 1981;2:79–89.
21. Reynolds HY, Merrill WW. Airway changes in young smokers that may antedate chronic obstructive lung disease. Med Clin North Am 1981;65:667–689.
22. Niewoehner DE, Kleinerman J, Rice DB. Pathologic changes in the peripheral airways of young cigarette smokers. N Engl J Med 1974;291:755–758.
23. Heard BE, Khatchatourov V, Otto H, et al. The morphology of emphysema, chronic bronchitis and bronchiectasis: definition, nomenclature and classification. J Clin Pathol 1979;32:882–892.
24. Breeze RG, Wheeldon EB. The cells of the pulmonary airways. Am Rev Resp Dis 1977;116:705–777.
25. Reynolds HY. Chronic bronchitis and acute infections exacerbations, in Mandell GL, Douglas RG Jr, Bennett JE (eds): Principles and Practice of Infectious Diseases, 2nd ed. New York, John Wiley and Sons, 1985; pp 387–390.
26. American Thoracic Society. Definitions and classifications of chronic bronchitis, asthma and pulmonary emphysema. Am Rev Resp Dis 1962;85:762–768.
27. Definition and classification of chronic bronchitis for clinical and epidemiologic purposes. A report to the Medical Research Council by their Committee on the Aetiology of Chronic Bronchitis. Lancet 1965;1:775–779.
28. Murray PR. Macroscopic and microscopic evaluation of respiratory specimens. Clin Lab Med 1982;2:259–267.
29. Lourenco RV, Cotromanes E. Clinical aerosols. II. Therapeutic aerosols. Arch Intern Med 1982;142:2299–2308.
30. Nicotra MB, Rivera M, Awe RJ. Antibiotic therapy of acute exacerbations of chronic bronchitis. A controlled study using tetracycline. Ann Intern Med 1982;97:18–21.
31. Tager I, Speizer FE. Role of infection in chronic bronchitis. N Engl J Med 1975;292:563–571.
32. Foy HM, Cooney MK, Maletzky AJ, et al. Incidence and etiology of pneumonia, croup and bronchiolitis in preschool children belonging to a prepaid medical care group over a four year period. Am J Epidemiol 1973;97:80–92.
33. Henderson FW, Clyde Jr WA, Collier AM, et al. The etiologic and epidemiologic spectrum of bronchiolitis in pediatric practice. J Pediatr 1979;95:183–190.
34. Sell SHW. Some observations on acute bronchiolitis in infants. Am J Dis Child 1960;100:31–39.
35. Sarkkinen HK, Halonen PE, Arstila PP, et al. Detection of respiratory syncytial, parainfluenza type 2, and adenovirus antigens by radioimmunoassay and enzyme immunoassay on nasopharyngeal specimens from children with acute respiratory disease. J Clin Microbiol 1981;13:258–265.
36. Hall CB, Hall WJ, Speers DM. Clinical and physiologic manifestations of bronchiolitis and pneumonia. Outcome of respiratory syncytial virus. Am J Dis Child 1979;133:798–802.
37. Phelan PD, Williams HE. Sympathomimetic drugs in acute viral bronchiolitis. Their effect on pulmonary resistance. Pediatrics 1969;44:493–497.
38. Rutter N, Milner AD, Hiller EJ. Effects of bronchodilators in respiratory resistance in infants and young children with bronchiolitis and wheezy bronchitis. Arch Dis Child 1975;50:719–722.
39. Ellis EF. Therapy of acute bronchiolitis. Pediatr Res 1977;11: 263–264.
40. Dabbous IA, Tkachyk JS, Stamm SJ. A double-blind study on the effects of corticosteroids in the treatment of bronchiolitis. Pediatrics 1966;37:477–484.
41. Leer Jr JA, Green JL, Heimlich EM, et al. Corticosteroid treatment in bronchiolitis. A controlled collaborative study in 297 infants and children. Am J Dis Child 1969;117:495–503.
42. McClung HW, Knight V, Gilbert BE, et al. Ribavirin aerosol treatment of influenza B virus infection. JAMA 1983;249: 2671–2674.
43. Hall CB, McBride JR, Walsh EE, et al. Aerosolized ribavirin treatment of infants with respiratory syncytial viral infection. A randomized double-blind study. N Engl J Med 1983;3008: 1443–1447.
44. McBride JT. Ribavirin and RSV: a new approach to an old disease. Pediatr Pulmonol 1985;1:294–295.
45. Osler W. The Principles and Practice of Medicine, 4th ed. New York, Appleton, 1901, p 108.
46. Centers for Disease Control, Annual Summary 1983. MWR 1984;32:121.
47. Huxley EJ, Viroslav J, Gray WR, et al. Pharyngeal aspiration in normal adults and patients with depressed consciousness. Am J Med 1978;64:564–568.
48. Toews GB. Pulmonary clearance of infectious agents, in Pennington JE (ed): Respiratory Infections: Diagnosis and Management. New York, Raven, 1983, p 31–39.
49. Gray BM, Converse GM III, Dillon HC. Epidemiologic studies of *Streptococcus pneumoniae* in infants: acquisition, carriage and infection during the first 24 months of life. J Infect Dis 1980;142:923–933.
50. Johanson WG Jr, Woods DE, Chadhuri TR. Association of respiratory tract colonization with adherence of gram-negative bacilli to epithelial cells. J Infect Dis 1979;139:667–673.
51. Frame PT. Acute infectious pneumonia in the adult. Newsletter, American Thoracic Society, Basics Resp Dis 1982;10:1–8.
52. McHenry MC. The infectious pneumonias. Hosp Pract 1980;15: 41–52.
53. Gleckman RA, Roth RM. Community-acquired bacterial pneumonia in the elderly. Pharmacotherapy 1984;4:81–88.
54. Carden DL, Gibb KA. Pneumonia and lung abscess. Emerg Med Clin North Am 1983;1:345–370.
55. LaForce FM. Hospital-acquired pneumonia: epidemiologic summary and clinical approach, in Pennington JE (ed): Respiratory Infections: Diagnosis and Management. New York, Raven, 1983, pp 135–142.
56. Klein JO. Emerging perspectives in management and prevention of infections of the respiratory tract in infants and children. Am J Med 1985;78:38–44.
57. Briggs DO. Pulmonary infections. Med Clin North Am 1977;61: 1163–1183.
58. Pass MA, Gray BM, Khare S, et al. Prospective studies of group B streptococcal infections in infants. J Pediatr 1979;95:437–443.
59. Pierce AK, Sandord JP. State of the art: aerobic gram-negative bacillary pneumonias. Am Rev Resp Dis 1974;110:647–658.
60. Yu VL. *Serratia marcescens*. Historical perspective and clinical review. N Engl J Med 1979;300:887–893.
61. Crane LR, Lerner AM. Gram-negative bacillary pneumonias, in: Pennington JE (ed): Respiratory Infections: Diagnosis and Management. New York, Raven, 1983, pp 227–250.
62. Schimpff SC, Young VM, Greene WH, et al. Origin of infection in acute nonlymphocytic leukemia: significance of hospital acquisition of potential pathogens. Ann Intern Med 1972;77: 707–714.
63. Ginsburg CM, Howard JB, Nelson JD. Report of 65 cases of *Haemophilus influenzae* B pneumonia. Pediatrics 1979;64: 283–286.

**64.** Norden CW. *Hemophilus influenzae* infections in adults. Med Clin North Am 1980;507–527.

**65.** Meyer RD, Finegold SM. Legionnaire's disease. Ann Rev Med 1980;31:219–232.

**66.** Orenstein WA, Overturf GD, Leedom JM, et al. The frequency of *Legionella* infection prospectively determined in children hospitalized with pneumonia. J Pediatr 1981;99:403–406.

**67.** Edelstein PH, Meyer RD, Finegold SM. Laboratory diagnosis of Legionnaire's disease. Am Rev Resp Dis 1980;121:317–327.

**68.** Bartlett JG. Anaerobic bacterial pneumonitis. Am Rev Resp Dis 1979;119:19–23.

**69.** Broughton RA. Infections due to *Mycoplasma pneumoniae* in childhood. Pediatr Infect Dis 1986;5:71–85.

**70.** Murray HW, Tuazon C. Atypical pneumonias. Med Clin North Am 1980;64:507–527.

**71.** Anonymous. The choice of antimicrobial drugs. Med Lett Drugs Ther 1986;28:33–40.

**72.** Sanders CC. Novel resistance selected by the new expanded-spectrum cephalosporins: a concern. J Infect Dis 1983;147:585–589.

**73.** Pennington JE. Penetration of antibiotics into respiratory secretions. Rev Infect Dis 1981;3:67–73.

**74.** Smith BR, LeFrock JL. Bronchial tree penetration of antibiotics. Chest 1982;83:904–908.

**75.** Saggers BA, Lawson D. Some observations on the penetration of antibiotics through mucus in vitro. J Clin Pathol 1966;19:313–317.

**76.** Saggers BA, Lawson D. In vivo penetration of antibiotics into sputum in cystic fibrosis. Arch Dis Child 1968;43:404–409.

**77.** Matthews LW, Spector S, Lemm J, et al. Studies on pulmonary secretions. I. The over-all chemical composition of pulmonary secretions from patients with cystic fibrosis, bronchiectasis and laryngectomy. Am Rev Resp Dis 1963;88:199–204.

**78.** Bodem CR, Lampton LM, Miller DP, et al. Endobronchial pH. Relevance to aminoglycoside activity in gram-negative bacillary pneumonia. Am Rev Resp Dis 1983;127:39–41.

**79.** Klastersky J, Carpentier-Meunier F, Kahan-Copperis L, et al. Endotracheally administered antibiotics for gram-negative bronchopneumonia. Chest 1979;75:586–591.

**80.** Gough PA, Jordan NS. A review of the therapeutic efficacy of aerosolized and endotracheally instilled antibiotics. Pharmacotherapy 1982;2:367–377.

**81.** Bryant RE, Hammond D. Interaction of purulent material with antibiotics used to treat pseudomonas infections. Antimicrob Agents Chemother 1974;6:702–707.

**82.** Levy J, Smith AL, Kenny MA, et al. Bioactivity of gentamicin in purulent sputum from patients with cystic fibrosis or bronchiectasis: comparison with activity in sputum. J Infect Dis 1983;148:1069–1076.

**83.** Blumer JL, Stern RC, Klinger JD, et al. Ceftazidime therapy in patients with cystic fibrosis and multiply-drug-resistant pseudomonas. Am J Med 1985;79(suppl 2A):37–46.

**84.** Mendelman PM, Smith AL, Levy J, et al. Aminoglycoside penetration, inactivation, and efficacy in cystic fibrosis sputum. Am Rev Resp Dis 1985;132:761–765.

**85.** Report of the Committee on Infectious Diseases: American Academy of Pediatrics, 19th ed. Evanston, IL, 1982.

**86.** Bartlett JG, Gorbach SL, Tally FP. Bacteriology and treatment of primary lung abscess. Am Rev Resp Dis 1974;109:510–518.

**87.** Bartlett JG. Anaerobic infection of the lung and pleural space. Am Rev Resp Dis 1974;110:56–77.

**88.** Bartlett JG, Gorbach SL, Finegold SM. The bacteriology of aspiration pneumonia. Am J Med 1974;56:202–207.

**89.** Brook I, Finegold SM. Bacteriology and therapy of lung abscess in children. J Pediatr 1979;94:10–12.

**90.** Irwin RS, Garrity FL, Erickson AD, et al. Sampling lower respiratory tract secretions in primary lung abscess. Comparison of the accuracy of four methods. Chest 1981;79:559–565.

**91.** Bartlett JB, Gorbach SL. Treatment of aspiration pneumonia and primary lung abscess. JAMA 1975;234:935–937.

**92.** Levison ME, Mangura CT, Lorber B, et al. Clindamycin compared with penicillin for the treatment of anaerobic lung abscess. Ann Intern Med 1983;98:466–471.

**93.** Weiss W. Cavity behavior in acute primary nonspecific lung abscess. Am Rev Resp Dis 1973;198:1273–1275.

# Chapter 77 / Ophthalmic Infections

Richard G. Fiscella, RPh, MPH, Charles A. Biggio, RPh, and Paul R. O'Dea, RPh

The main function of the eye is to convert light signals to nerve impulses which are transmitted to the brain to provide a visual image. The eye is composed of different refractive media that allow light rays to pass to the back of the eye or retina, which in turn converts the light rays to nerve impulses. The cornea, aqueous fluid, lens, and vitreous fluid are important refractive structures. These are lucid in a normal eye and enable uninterrupted light transmission; however, if the eye tissues are abnormal in any way, the light is interrupted, and thus vision is adversely affected.

Vision can be decreased or lost through ocular infections. Bacterial corneal ulcers may cause permanent scarring even if the infectious process is stopped. Endophthalmitis may cause destruction of delicate intraocular structures even though the eye may be "sterilized." Although some ocular infections may be self-limiting, most should be treated appropriately to prevent permanent ocular damage. This chapter will describe infective processes involving periocular and ocular structures. It will also review antimicrobial therapy and present current clinical aspects of ophthalmic treatment.

The eye presents a unique treatment situation unlike any other part of the body. Therapy may vary from the use of topical medication for a bacterial conjunctivitis to topical, periocular, intraocular, and intravenous therapy for the treatment of endophthalmitis. The route of administration used depends on the availability of the drug at the site of infection in inhibitory concentrations. As mentioned earlier, an external ocular infection may be treated with an antimicrobial agent that is applied only topically in ointment or drop form (see Table 77.1). When the infectious processes involve deeper ocular structures, effective treatment modalities must incorporate other routes of administration to achieve adequate tissue levels. In some severe corneal ulcers and in infections in the inner layers of the eye (endophthalmitis), subconjunctival injections are employed. In addition, endophthalmitis usually requires direct injections into the vitreous (intravitreal) to achieve effective tissue levels. Drugs must penetrate in effective concentrations and yet be nontoxic to ocular structures.

## Anatomy

The eyelids are movable folds of tissue that serve to protect the eye (Fig. 77.1). The skin of the lids, the thinnest in the body, is loose and elastic. Elasticity permits extreme swelling and subsequent return to normal shape and size. Four types of glands in the lid are the meibomian glands, the glands of Moll and Zeis, and the accessory lacrimal glands (Krause and Wolfring). The meibomian glands produce a sebaceous substance on the surface of the tear film that prevents rapid evaporation of the normal tear layer. The glands of Zeis are small, modified sebaceous glands connected with the follicles of the eyelashes. The glands of Moll are unbranched simple sinuous tubule sweat glands. The accessory lacrimal glands (Krause and Wolfring) supply most of the needed moisture to the conjunctival sac and cornea. The blood supply to the lids is derived mainly from the ophthalmic, zygomatic, and angular arteries. The lymphatics drain into the preauricular, parotid, and submaxillary lymph glands.

The lacrimal apparatus consists of the lacrimal gland, accessory glands, puncta, canaliculi, tear sac, and nasolacrimal duct (Fig. 77.2). The lacrimal gland is a tear-secreting gland located in the anterior superior temporal portion of the orbit. Several secretory ducts connect this gland to the superior conjunctival fornix. Tears pass over the cornea and the bulbar and palpebral conjunctiva, moistening the surfaces of these structures. They drain into the lacrimal canaliculi through the upper and lower lacrimal puncta. Diverticula may be a part of the normal structure and susceptible to higher bacterial (*Actinomyces*) or fungal infection.

The lacrimal sac is the dilated portion of the lacrimal drainage system that lies in the bony lacrimal fossa. The nasolacrimal duct is the downward continuation of the lacrimal sac. It opens into the inferior meatus lateral to the inferior turbinate.

All passages of the lacrimal drainage system are lined with epithelium. Tears pass into the puncta by capillary attraction. The combined forces of the capillary attraction in the canaliculi, gravity, and the pumping action of the orbicularis oculi muscle on the lacrimal sac aid to continue the flow of tears down the nasolacrimal duct in the nose and nasopharynx.

The conjunctiva is a thin, transparent mucous membrane that covers the posterior surface of the lids (the palpebral conjunctiva), as well as the anterior surface of the sclera (the bulbar conjunctiva). It also connects the skin at the lid margin (a mucocutaneous junction) with the corneal epithelium at the limbus.

The conjunctiva is rich in blood vessels which are derived from the anterior ciliary and palpebral arteries and a few pain fibers which arise from the ophthalmic division of the fifth cranial nerve. The conjunctiva is also rich in lymphatics.

The cornea (see Figure 77.3) is a clear transparent, avascular tissue whose main function is to refract light. The iris is the anterior part of the uveal tract. The uveal tract consists of the iris, choroid, and ciliary body. The iris is a circular membrane that dilates or constricts to control the amount of light entering the eye. The lens is a transparent, avascular

**Table 77.1** Instillation of Ophthalmic Ointments and Drops

**How to Instill Eye Drops**
1. Wash hands
2. Remove cap from plastic bottle
3. Tilt head slightly back
4. Gently pull down lower lid
5. Hold bottle vertically with dropper pointed downward close to front of eye
6. Instill drops into pocket between eye and lid
7. Release eyelid, close eyes, and roll eyes slowly in circular manner
8. Replace and tighten cap

**How to Use Eye Ointment (Salve)**
1. Wash hands
2. Remove cap from tube
3. With one hand, gently pull lower lid down
4. While looking up, squeeze a small amount of ointment (about $\frac{1}{4}$ to $\frac{1}{2}$ in.) inside lower lid; be careful not to touch tip of tube to eye or fingers
5. Close eye gently and, keeping it closed, roll eyeball in all directions; temporary blurriness may occur
6. Replace cap on tube

When opening tube for the first time, squeeze out the first $\frac{1}{4}$ in. and discard, as it may be too dry.

structure located between the iris and the vitreous. The lens is responsible for the focusing or accomodative power of the eye. The vitreous, located behind the lens, occupies approximately four fifths of the total volume of the eyeball and lends support for ocular structures. It is a clear, gellike material that is made up of about 99% water; the rest of the gel consists of hyaluronic acid and collagen fibers. The retina is the thin layer of nervous tissue that consists of the sensory layer and the pigment epithelium. In retinal detachments, the sensory layer is normally separated from the pigment epithelium, which is firmly attached to the choroid.

Alterations of its normal defense systems subject the eye to microbial infection. The major mechanisms of defense are the tears and the repetitive movement of the eyelid. These provide media for the flow of antibacterial substances and a constant mechanical washing of the cornea.[1] Specific antibacterial agents carried by the tears include lysozyme, lactoferrin, $\beta$-lysine, and immunoglobins A and G. The acute inflammatory reaction and development of specific bacterial, fungal, and viral immunity also play an important role in the external defenses of the eye.

### *Infections of the Eyelids*

Lid disorders are among the most common ocular problems. The patient with disorders of the eyelids has varied complaints. There are many pain fibers in the tissues near the lid margins. Consequently, if there is inflammation with stretching of tissues, as in hordeolum, the patient complains of moderately severe pain. In marginal blepharitis, there is no pain but the patient complains of red-rimmed eyes. Because of the proximity of the lid margins to the conjunctiva, frequent attacks of conjunctivitis are a common complaint.

**Figure 77.1** Cross section of the upper lid. *(From Vaughn D, Asbury T: General Ophthalmology, 10th ed. Los Altos, CA, Lange Medical Publications, 1983, p 43, with permission.)*

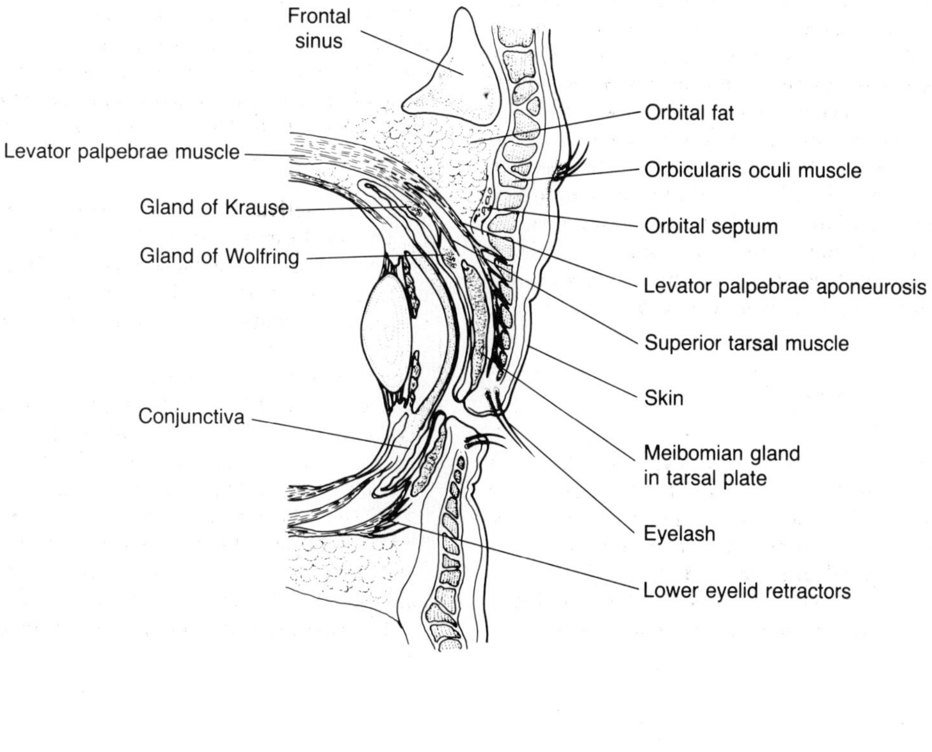

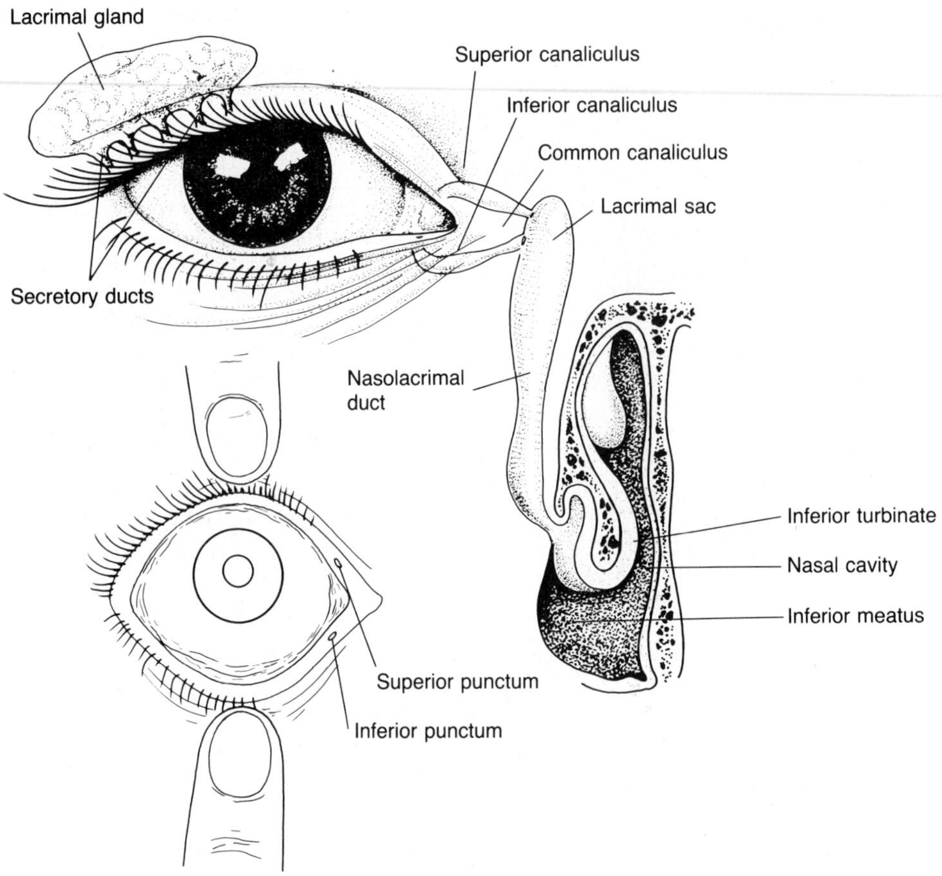


**Figure 77.2** The lacrimal drainage system. *(From Vaughn D, Asbury T: General Ophthalmology, 10th ed. Los Altos, CA, Lange Medical Publications, 1983, p 43, with permission.)*

Bacterial infections of the eyelids range from very mild to quite severe. The most common of these are folliculitis, impetigo, erysipelas, and infectious eczematoid dermatitis.[2,3] Folliculitis is a staphylococcal infection of the hair follicles around the lids and is characterized by an itching and a burning sensation in the affected areas. Impetigo is usually caused by a combined staphylococcal and streptococcal infection manifested by a vesiculopustular eruption. Eyelid involvement in erysipelas varies from mild edema to vesicle formation which may suppurate. The causative organism is $\beta$-hemolytic streptococcus. If the condition goes untreated, gangrene of the eyelids may develop. Systemic effects include malaise, fever, and headaches. Infectious eczematoid dermatitis usually occurs as a toxic and/or allergic reaction to staphylococcal products. The eczema subsides when the infection clears.

In mild bacterial infections treatment consists of topical antibiotic ophthalmic ointment therapy plus hot compresses. For the treatment of infectious eczematoid dermatitis, a local steroid–anti-infective ophthalmic ointment is indicated. Measures to improve lid hygiene, such as scrubbing the lids with a dilute solution of baby shampoo, are often beneficial in recurrent superficial staphylococcal infections.[4]

For the most severe bacterial infections, systemic antibiotics are recommended. Penicillin is used for streptococcal infections and tetracycline or a penicillinase-resistant penicillin, such as dicloxacillin, for other infections. In more severe cases, an attempt should be made to identify the causative organism and initiate appropriate therapy based on culture and sensitivity results.

In staphyloccocal blepharitis the patient typically complains of local irritation and burning. If treated inadequately, staphylococcal blepharitis frequently lasts years, producing chronically red eyelid margins and possible scarring. The longer the disease has been present the more difficult it is to treat effectively.

Staphylococcal or ulcerative blepharitis is best treated with topical antibiotic ophthalmic ointments, such as bacitracin 500 units/g or erythromycin 5 mg/g. In recurrent cases, the utilization of a systemic antibiotic should be considered; dicloxacillin or erythromycin 250–500 mg four times a day may be employed. Although tetracyclines are not very effective against staphylococci, there is evidence that they have a salutary effect upon the ocular components of rosacea[5] and thus could be helpful. The observation that adults with staphylococcal blepharitis often have concomitant rosacea and/or seborrheic blepharitis suggests that there may be an underlying dermatologic disorder.[6] When antibiotic ophthalmic ointment therapy is initiated, the ointment should be applied four times a day for 1 to 2 weeks, then reduced to twice a day. Once the eyelid appears normal, application can be reduced to daily at bedtime. If a sebor-

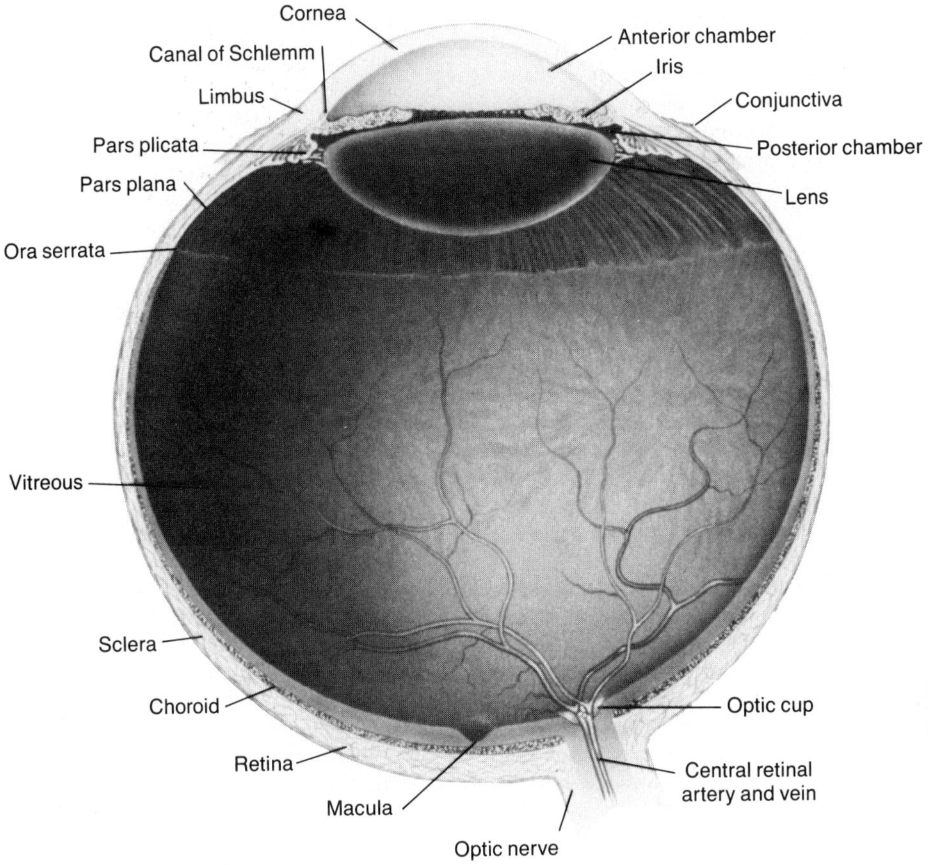


**Figure 77.3** Diagrammatic representation of horizontal (meridional) section through a left human eye.

rheic condition is present, the scalp should be shampooed with an antiseborrheic agent, such as selenium sulfide; however, in refractory cases, mild corticosteroid solutions applied to the scalp or mild corticosteroid cream applied to the forehead may provide relief.

### Hordeolum (Sty)

Hordeolum externum is a staphylococcal infection of the eyelash follicle and Moll's or Zeis' glands. Hordeolum internum is a staphylococcal infection of a meibomian gland.[7] Both types are self-limiting and respond well to the frequent application of hot compresses. Incision and drainage of the purulent material may be necessary if the process does not begin to resolve itself within 48 hours. Topical use of antibacterials is warranted if the hordeolum recurs. In cases of severe internal hordeolum, systemic antistaphylococcal therapy is warranted.

### Chalazion

Chalazion is a sterile granulomatous inflammation of a meibomian gland, of unknown cause, characterized by localized swelling in the upper or lower eyelid. In general, a fully developed chalazion is differentiated from hordeolum by the absence of acute inflammatory signs. They seldom subside spontaneously. If chalazions recur in the same area, a biopsy should be performed to rule out malignancy.[8] If a chalazion is so large that it presses against the cornea, it may distort vision. Therefore, excision may be indicated; however, an injection of 0.05 mL triamcinolone acetonide (diluted 1:1 with normal saline to yield a concentration of 5 mg/mL) may be effective in the elimination of the lesion.[9]

### Impetigo

Impetigo of the eyelids occurs by the spread of the causative bacteria, staphylococcus and/or streptococcus, from other facial areas. Mild cases can be treated with bacitracin or erythromycin ophthalmic ointment. Systemic medication may be required for more severe cases. An isoxazoyl penicillin, such as oxacillin, cloxacillin, or dicloxacillin, or a cephalosporin such as cephalexin in a dose of 250–500 mg orally four times a day can be utilized. If the culture reveals only streptococcus, then penicillin VK 250–500 mg orally four times a day is the appropriate drug.

### Meibomianitis

Meibomianitis is an uncommon, bilateral, and chronic inflammation of the meibomian glands. It occurs during or after the middle years of life and is generally preceded by or associated with blepharitis. The patient complains of chronically red and irritated eyes and a slight but continuous discharge. The meibomian glands are prominent, the lid margins are red, and there is a conjunctival discharge.

Treatment consists of the application of hot, moist compresses, repeated manual expression of the meibomian glands, and topical antibiotic therapy. Systemic tetracyclines often yield significant improvement. The application of 1% silver nitrate ophthalmic solution to the eyelid margins is sometimes effective.

#### Herpes Simplex Blepharitis

The lesions associated with herpes simplex are characterized by small vesicles with surrounding erythema. They are sometimes associated with similar lesions of the lip and must be differentiated from those of herpes zoster or impetigo. Treatment of this condition is nonspecific[10]; however, application of a topical antiviral agent (e.g., trifluridine) may be indicated to prevent corneal involvement. If the lesions are secondarily infected, topical antibiotic ointments may be utilized. Corticosteroids are contraindicated as their use may predispose to corneal involvement.

#### Herpes Zoster Blepharitis

Herpes zoster infection of the eyelids is characterized by vesicular lesions along the superficial branches of the ophthalmic division of the trigeminal nerve. No specific treatment is available for herpes zoster. Periocular pain usually precedes the development of vesicles. The pain associated with herpes zoster may be severe and management with appropriate analgesic therapy may be warranted. The usefulness of such potent corticosteroid topical agents as fluocinolone, betamethasone 17-valerate, flurandrenolide, and flucinonide is questionable for the general treatment of herpes zoster. Certainly none of these agents could be applied to the eyelids, and the use of systemic steroids is controversial. Zoster immune globulin has not been found to be beneficial in the treatment or prevention of the disease.[11]Acyclovir 0.3% ophthalmic ointment (investigational) may be of some benefit, but further clinical studies are necessary to substantiate its effectiveness.

#### Pediculosis (Lice Infestation)

Adult lice thrive in the cilia, and their eggs (nits) cling to the eyelashes. Infestation of the eyelid is extremely rare and is almost always secondary to pubic infestation in the patient or through sexual contact. Mechanical removal of the lice and the nits with forceps under slit-lamp visualization should be attempted. Pediculosis of the cilia can be treated with either 1% yellow mercuric oxide ophthalmic ointment or 1% to 3% ammoniated mercury ophthalmic ointment twice a day for 1 week. Anticholinesterases such as 0.25% physostigmine ophthalmic ointment are effective but cause intense miosis and spasms of accommodation and must be used a minimum of 10 days, as they do not affect the nits, and the treatment must cover the entire life cycle of the lice.[12] $\gamma$-Benzene hexachloride 1% is highly effective against adult lice when applied to the eyelid. Its use is controversial because of potential eye toxicity.[12,13]

### *Infections of the Lacrimal Apparatus*

Patients with disorders of the lacrimal apparatus complain of tearing or dry eyes. In the event of tearing without associated symptoms, the disorder is usually in the lacrimal drainage system or, rarely, the result of hypersecretion. Paradoxic lacrimation (an occasional complication of seventh nerve palsy) is a condition in which salivary gland fibers innervate the lacrimal gland. If the eyes are dry, there is faulty production of tears. The symptoms are investigated by irrigation to test the patency of the canaliculi and the nasolacrimal ducts and by palpation of the nasolacrimal gland. If the complaint is dry eyes, the quantity of tear production should be assessed (Schirmer test) and the appearance of the tear film should be studied with the aid of a slit-lamp.

There are many causes of tearing, for example, conjunctivitis, keratitis, iritis, and foreign bodies; however, if tearing is the only symptom, the cause in the great majority of cases will be found in the lacrimal drainage apparatus.

#### Dacryocystitis

Infection of the lacrimal sac is a common acute or chronic disease. It is most often unilateral and is always secondary to obstruction of the nasolacrimal duct.[14] In acute dacryocystitis the usual infectious agent is *Staphylococcus aureus* or, occasionally, $\beta$-hemolytic streptococcus. In chronic dacryocystitis, *Streptococcus pneumoniae* is the predominant organism. *Hemophilus influenzae* may be the pathogen in children. Cultures are difficult to obtain, and therapy should consist of a systemically administered cephalosporin or a penicillin that is active against penicillinase-producing staphylococci. Obstruction of the nasolacrimal duct is the basic cause of dacryocystitis, and the disease is usually persistent until the obstruction is relieved. As probing is usually unsuccessful in adults, dacryocystorhinostomy is usually necessary if symptoms are severe.

#### Canaliculitis

Canaliculitis is an uncommon, chronic unilateral condition caused by infection with *Actinomyces israelii, Candida albicans*, or *Aspergillus* species.[15] Curettage of the necrotic material in the involved canaliculus followed by forceful irrigation is usually effective.

#### Dacryoadenitis

Acute inflammation of the lacrimal gland is a rare unilateral condition that may be seen in children as a complication of mumps, measles, or influenza, and in adults in association with gonorrhea. It also may develop after injury to the lacrimal gland or as a retrograde infection from a bacterial conjunctivitis. Swelling is most prominent at the upper outer aspect of the eye under the lid. If bacterial infection is present, usually staphylococci, then appropriate systemic antibiotic therapy should be employed. Incision may be necessary if the pus collects in the gland under tension. Chronic dacryoadenitis is sometimes seen bilaterally as a manifestation of sarcoidosis. It usually occurs in blacks and is self-limited. Chronic dacryoadenitis may also occur in lymphosarcoma, tuberculosis, and lymphatic leukemia.

**Table 77.2** Differentiation of the Common Types of Conjunctivitis

| *Feature* | *Bacterial* | *Viral* | *Chlamydial* |
|---|---|---|---|
| Tearing | Moderate | Profuse | Moderate |
| Exudate | Moderate to profuse | Minimal | Minimal in adults, copious in newborns |
| Preauricular adenopathy | Uncommon | Common | Common only in inclusion conjunctivitis |
| Stained scrapings and exudates | Bacteria, PMNs[a] | Monocytes | PMNs, plasma cells, inclusion bodies |
| Associated sore throat and fever | Occasionally | Occasionally | Never |
| Matting of lids on awakening | Yes | No | Absent in adults, present in newborns |
| Follicles (palpebral conjunctiva) | Usually absent | Present | Present in adults, absent in newborns |
| Response to specific antibiotic therapy | Yes | No | Yes |
| Duration | Up to several weeks | Several weeks | Persistent |

[a] PMN, polymorphonuclear cell.

Compiled from References 16 and 17.

## Conjunctivitis

Inflammation of the conjunctiva (conjunctivitis) is the most common eye disease in the western hemisphere. It varies in severity from a mild hyperemia with tearing (hay fever conjunctivitis) to a severe necrotic process (membranous conjunctivitis).

### *Clinical Presentation*

The important symptoms of conjunctivitis are a foreign body sensation, a scratching or burning sensation, a sensation of fullness around the eyes, itching, and, when the cornea is affected, photophobia. (See Table 77.2 for differential diagnosis of conjunctivitis.)

Foreign body sensation and scratching or burning are often associated with the swelling and papillary hypertrophy that normally accompany conjunctival hyperemia. If there is pain, the cornea is probably also affected. Pain that is more severe on waking and improves during the day suggests staphylococcal infection; pain that is severe during the day and better on waking suggests keratoconjunctivitis sicca. Itching, if complained of spontaneously rather than in response to questioning, usually indicates that the patient has an allergic conjunctivitis of the immediate hypersensitivity type.

The important signs of conjunctivitis are hyperemia; tearing; exudation; pseudoptosis; papillary hypertrophy; chemosis; follicles, pseudomembranes, and membranes on the conjunctiva; granulomas; and preauricular adenopathy (Table 77.3).

In the differential diagnosis of conjunctivitis as the cause of a red, painful, or irritated eye, it is important to rule out keratitis, iritis, and acute glaucoma (see Table 77.3). The causal organisms can then be identified by microscopic examination of the stained conjunctival material. Before treatment is started, cultures and antibiotic sensitivity tests should be performed. Acute and chronic bacterial conjunctivitis are common types. The acute types occasionally become chronic but are usually self-limited, lasting a maximum of 2 weeks if untreated.

**Table 77.3** Distinguishing Features of Conjunctivitis, Keratitis, and Iritis

| *Feature* | *Conjunctivitis* | *Keratitis/iritis* |
|---|---|---|
| Vision | Normal | May be reduced |
| Pain | Gritty irritation | True pain |
| Conjunctivitis | Diffuse injection | Ciliary flush |
| Exudate | Minimal to profuse | Usually none |
| Matting of lids | May be present | Absent |
| Photophobia | Absent | Present |
| Lacrimation | Usually absent | Present |
| Pupil | Normal | Usually small |

Compiled from Reference 17.

**Table 77.4** Etiologic Classification of Infectious Conjunctivitis

A. Bacterial
  1. Purulent
    *Neisseria gonorrhoeae*
    *Neisseria meningitidis*
  2. Acute catarrhal (pinkeye)
    Pneumococcus (*Streptococcus pneumoniae)* (temperate climates)
    *Hemophilus aegyptius* (Koch–Weeks bacillus) (tropical climates)
  3. Subacute catarrhal–*Hemophilus influenzae (*temperate climates)
  4. Chronic, including blepharoconjunctivitis
    *Staphylococcus aureus*
    Moraxella lacunata (diplobacillus of Morax–Axenfeld)
  5. Rare types (acute, subacute, chronic)
    *Neisseria (Branhamella) catarrhalis*
    Coliforms
    *Proteus*
    *Corynebacterium diphtheriae*

B. Chlamydial
  1. Trachoma (*Chlamydia trachomatis*)
  2. Inclusion conjunctivitis (*Chlamydia oculogenitalis*)
  3. Lymphogranuloma venereum (LGV) (*Chlamydia lymphogranulomatis*)
  4. Psittacosis (*Chlamydia psittaci*)
  5. Rare types–agents of parakeet psittacosis, feline pneumonitis, and ovine abortion

C. Viral
  1. Acute viral follicular conjunctivitis
    Pharyngoconjunctival fever caused by adenovirus types 3 and 7
    Epidermic keratoconjunctivitis caused by adenovirus types 8 and 19
    Herpes simplex virus
    Newcastle disease
    Acute hemorrhagic conjunctivitis caused by enterovirus type 70; rarely, coxsackievirus type A28
  2. Chronic follicular conjunctivitis
    Molluscum contagiosum virus
  3. Viral blepharoconjunctivitis
    Vaccinia caused by vaccinia–variola viruses
    Varicella and zoster caused by varicella zoster viruses
    Measles virus

D. Rickettsial: nonpurulent conjunctivitis with hyperemia and minimal infiltration, often a feature of rickettsial diseases
    Typhus
    Murine typhus
    Scrub typhus
    Rocky Mountain spotted fever
    Mediterranean fever
    Q fever

E. Fungal (rare)
  1. Catarrhal, complicating blepharitis
    *Candida*
  2. Granulomatous
    *Rhinosporidium seeberi*
    *Coccidioides immitis* (San Joaquin Valley fever)
    *Sporothrix schenckii*

F. Parasitic (rare but important) chronic conjunctivitis and blepharoconjunctivitis caused by
    *Onchocera volvulus* (Central America, Africa)
    *Thelazia californiensis*
    *Loa loa*
    *Ascaris lumbricoides*
    *Trichinella spiralis*
    *Schistosoma hematobium* (bladder fluke)
    *Taenia solium* (cysticercus)
    *Phthirius pubis* (pediculus pubis, pubic louse)
    Fly larvae (*Oestrus ovis*, etc.) (ocular myiasis)
    Caterpillar hair

**Table 77.4** (continued)

G. Secondary to dacryocystitis or canaliculitis
 1. Conjunctivitis secondary to dacryocystitis
  Pneumococci or β-hemolytic streptococci
 2. Conjunctivitis secondary to canaliculitis
  *Actinomyces israelii*, *Candida* sp., *Aspergillus* sp. (rarely)

From Vaughn D, Asbury T: General Ophthalmology, 10th ed. Los Altos, CA, Lange Medical Publications, 1983, p 58, with permission.

### *Etiology/Treatment*

**Bacterial Conjunctivitis**

Most bacterial conjunctival infections are caused by staphylococci, streptococci, pneumococci, *Moraxella* spp., or *Hemophilus* spp. (Table 77.4). Anaerobic organisms have been recovered but their role remains in doubt.[18,19] In most cases of bacterial conjunctivitis the organisms can be identified by the microscopic examination of stained conjunctival scrapings, which reveals numerous polymorphonuclear neutrophils. Direct examination and culture study are recommended for all cases and are mandatory if the disease is purulent, membranous, or pseudomembranous. Antibiotic sensitivity studies are also highly desirable, so that an appropriate drug can be started at once. It is important to culture both eyes even though the patient may exhibit symptoms in only one. In this way the "normal" flora (see Table 77.5) of the uninvolved eye can be differentiated from the flora of the inflamed, involved eye. Hot compresses may provide desirable symptomatic relief in the early stages of the disease. Antibiotics should be continued 4 or 5 days after all symptoms have subsided.

**Table 77.5** Bacterial Flora of the Healthy Eye

| *Organism group* | *% Incidence*[a] |
|---|---|
| Staphylococci | |
| *S. epidermidis* (*S. albus*, coagulase-negative) | 65–80 |
| *S. aureus* (coagulase positive) | 15–35 |
| Diphtheroids (*Corynebacterium* sp.) | 20–50 |
| Streptococci | |
| *S. pneumoniae* (pneumococcus) | 2–8 |
| Other α-hemolytic streptococci | 2–4 |
| β-Hemolytic streptococci | 1 |
| Miscellaneous | |
| *Bacillus* sp. | 2 |
| *Proteus* sp. | |
| Coliforms | |
| *Neisseria* sp. | |
| *Hemophilus* sp. | |
| *Branhamella* (*Neisseria*) *catarrhalis* | |
| No growth | 15–40 |

[a] Total percentage is greater than 100 because more than one organism can be grown from cul de sac, for example, *S. epidermidis* and diphtheroids.

Compiled from Reference 20.

Most organisms exude a purulent or mucopurulent discharge. *Neisseria gonorrhoeae* causes a severe discharge. Pseudomembranes, which rarely accompany bacterial conjunctivitis, suggest an infection with *Streptococcus pyogenes*.[21] True membranes are present with diphtheria. The organisms involved produce bilateral irritation and injection (conjunctival blood vessel congestion), a purulent exudate, as mentioned, with agglutination of the lids on waking, and occasionally lid edema. The infection usually starts in one eye and is spread to the other by the hands. It may spread from one person to another by fomites.

Topical preparations of neomycin, with gramicidin, and polymyxin B sulfate are generally good combinations because of their broad antibacterial spectrum and because they are seldom used systemically; however, neomycin produces allergic reactions in 5% to 10% of patients if therapy is continued for longer than a week. In addition, it may also produce punctate epithelial erosions of the cornea. Sulfacetamide or sulfasoxazole ophthalmic preparations cause fewer side effects but are less effective. Erythromycin as a 0.5% ointment is also a useful ophthalmic preparation against gram-positive cocci, but staphylococci rapidly develop a resistance to this antibiotic. Chloramphenicol 0.5% ophthalmic solution is nonirritating and penetrates the cornea and conjunctiva well, but lacks the wide antibacterial spectrum of neomycin, polymyxin B, and gramicidin. A few cases of aplastic anemia have been reported with the use of chloramphenicol eye drops. Topical gentamicin or tobramycin should be reserved for more serious infections caused by sensitive organisms. Conjunctivitis caused by *Staphylococcus aureus* should be treated with bacitracin ophthalmic ointment 500 units/g, five to six times a day, decreasing the frequency of application as the condition improves. As this organism causes a chronic conjunctivitis, treatment should continue daily at bedtime for 1 month after all signs of the infection have vanished.[22]

Systemic antibiotics are required for the treatment of diphtheritic, gonococcal, tularemic, and granulomatous conjunctivitis. Diphtheritic conjunctivitis may be treated by daily intramuscular injections of procaine penicillin 300,000 to 1 million units. Either diphtheria antitoxin, penicillin, or chloramphenicol may be applied topically to prevent corneal involvement.

Gonorrheal conjunctivitis should be treated vigorously to prevent serious involvement of the cornea. This infection is usually acquired by sexual contact with an infected partner or by autoinoculation. There is usually a marked ocular reaction with a copious amount of thin and serous, then heavy, purulent discharge. The inflammatory reaction may be relatively mild. Recommended therapy is 4.8 million units of procaine penicillin G administered in two intramuscular injections at one visit, together with 1 g of probenecid orally at least 30 minutes before the injections. The value of concomitantly administered penicillin G (100,000 units/mL) eye drops is questionable. In adults, cefoxitin (1 g) or cefotaxime (500 mg) intravenously four times a day for 5 days may be substituted for penicillin. Alternative therapy could consist of spectinomycin (2–4 g) in one intramuscular injection with topical tetracycline as an optimal adjunct. Gonococcal infection caused by penicillinase-producing organisms usually responds to spectinomycin.

### Chlamydial Conjunctivitis

Although sporadic cases occur in the white population in the United States, trachoma, caused by *Chlamydia trachomatis*, is rare here except among the American Indians of the southwestern states, where it is mild and relatively uncomplicated; however, with over 400 million of the world's population afflicted, it is one of the most common of all chronic human diseases. The disease, which eventually produces corneal scarring, is a leading cause of blindness in the world.

The current recommended treatment is a 4- to 6-week course of oral tetracyclines. Topical sulfonamide therapy may be added. In children less than 9 years old or in pregnant women, oral sulfonamides or erthromycin should be substituted because of the side effects caused by tetracyclines on developing teeth. Although trachoma can probably be cured by topical treatment alone, it requires a much longer treatment than therapy with systematically administered antibiotics. Tetracycline 1% ophthalmic ointment applied twice a day, 6 days a week for 10 weeks, is the recommended therapy. Systemic therapy consists of tetracycline 1 to 1.5 g/d orally in four divided doses, or doxycycline 100 mg/d, or erythromycin 1 g/d orally in four divided doses. Several courses are sometimes necessary for an actual cure.[23]

Inclusion conjunctivitis, caused by *Chlamydia oculogenitalis*, usually bilateral, is a common disease, especially in sexually active young people. Characteristically, the chlamydial agent infects the urethra of the male and the cervix of the female. Transmission is generally from the genitourinary tract to the eyes in adults. Indirect transmission can also occur in inadequately chlorinated swimming pools. Chlamydial (inclusion) disease in adults produces a chronic follicular conjunctivitis with minimal redness and irritation. Treatment consists of a 6-week course of oral tetracycline 1–1.5 g/d in four divided doses, or erythromycin 1–1.5 g/d in four divided doses for pregnant women or children less than 9 years old. In addition, topical sulfonamide therapy should be utilized.

### Viral Conjunctivitis

Viral conjunctivitis is the most common type of infectious conjunctivitis and with few exceptions there is no specific treatment. Some viruses produce severe, disabling diseases, others only mild, rapidly self-limited diseases. Therapy should be directed toward prevention of complications, reduction of secondary bacterial infection, and relief of symptoms. Among the viral diseases of the conjunctiva for which there is no specific treatment are Newcastle virus disease, adenovirus infections, echovirus disease, epidemic keratoconjunctivitis, and rubeola.

***Herpes Simplex***[24] Herpes simplex virus conjunctivitis is an uncommon disease of young children. It is characterized by unilateral injection, irritation, mucoid discharge, pain, and mild photophobia. It occurs only in primary attacks of herpes simplex virus infection, and is often associated with herpes simplex keratitis, in which the cornea shows discrete epithelial lesions that usually coalesce to form single or multiple dendrites. As the conjunctivitis is self-limited, therapy usually is not necessary. A topical antiviral agent may be applied to prevent corneal involvement. The use of steroids is contraindicated, as they aggravate herpes simplex disease and convert it from a short, self-limited process to a severe prolonged process.

***Herpes Zoster*** Simple herpes zoster conjunctivitis may be left untreated; more severe forms, especially when keratitis and iridocyclitis occur, are best treated with topical steroids. Acyclovir has been tried in patients with severe intraocular involvement. The use of systemic steroids has been shown to reduce the duration of acute trigeminal pain and the incidence of postinfection trigeminal neuralgia. They are contraindicated when a coexistent malignant disease such as lymphoma is present, as an increase in mortality may occur with the administration of systemic steroids. Herpes zoster must not be confused with herpes simplex in which topical steroids aggravate an existing keratitis.

## Keratitis

Infections of the cornea usually occur after injury such as trauma or contact lens wear or in a compromised cornea as in prolonged steroid use, keratitis sicca, or diabetes. The most frequent causes of bacterial keratitis include *Pseudomonas aeruginosa, Staphylococcus aureus, Streptococcus pneumoniae*, and *Staphylococcus epidermidis*. Less common bacterial agents are *Proteus, Serratia, Escherichia coli*, and *Klebsiella*. Fungal infections normally follow trauma to the cornea caused by vegetative matter; the most common invaders include *Candida, Fusarium*, and *Aspergillus*. Although the incidence of viral keratitis is much lower than that of bacterial or fungal keratitis, recurrence is common because the virus remains dormant in adjacent ganglia, which are shed in response to physical or psychological stress.

The dominance of pathogens changes with geography[25,26]: Gram-positive cocci have the highest incidence among microorganisms responsible for corneal ulceration and are most prevalent in parts of the northern and eastern United States. Gram-negative rods rank second nationwide; fungi are rare in the North but occur in significant numbers in the southern and western portions of the United States.

### *Clinical Presentation*

Microbial infections of the cornea are characterized by epithelial defects surrounded by edema and folds. Stromal involvement is often present as is anterior chamber inflammation. With continued progression, corneal neovascularization, hypopyon, and corneal thinning appear.

Specific bacteria produce distinctive clinical characteristics.[27] Staphylococcal infections are localized and well defined. Pneumococcus ulcers have regular edges with hypopyon. *Pseudomonas* causes rapid necrosis and characteristic mucopurulent discharge.

Filamentous fungi (*Fusarium, Aspergillus*) display as a gray or dirty-white rough, textured surface with elevated margins.[10] Branching lines radiate from the fungal ulcer and satellite lesions may appear. Yeast fungi (*Candida*) appear as oval outlines with a plaquelike surface. Fungal infections are rapidly destructive, with ulceration that may thin the cornea to the point of perforation.

Herpes simplex keratitis is identified by characteristic dendritic figures. The deeper stromal infections display blotchy, cheesy-white infiltrates that may lie under the ulcer.[27]

## *Treatment*

### Antimicrobial Therapy

The field of ophthalmology is divided in its initial methods of treatment of bacterial ulcers. Traditional theory holds that the selection of the initial antibiotic regimen should be based upon the results of a Gram stain and the gross morphology of the bacterium (Table 77.6). Others support a "shotgun" or empiric approach, with selection based upon the prevalence of pathogens known to be producing this disease in the community.[28,29]

**Table 77.6** Therapy of Corneal Infections

**Empiric Therapy**
Cefazolin 100 mg/mL drops and gentamicin 9–18 mg/mL drops every 15 to 60 min
Cefazolin 100 mg and gentamicin 20–40 mg for subconjunctival injections every 12–24 h for 2–4 days
**Traditional Therapy**[28]
Gram-positive cocci
Topical: alternating cefazolin 50–100 mg/mL or bacitracin 100,000 U/mL and gentamicin or tobramycin 9–18 mg/mL every 15–60 min
Subconjunctival: cefazolin 100 mg every 12–24 h (may add gentamicin or tobramycin 20–40 mg)
Gram-negative cocci
Topical: bacitracin 100,000 U/mL
Subconjunctival: aqueous penicillin G 100,000 U (erythromycin lactobionate if penicillin allergic); note: if gonorrheal, treat systemically
Gram-positive rods (uncommon)
Topical: gentamicin 4–18 mg/mL every 15–60 min
Subconjunctival: gentamicin 20–40 mg every 12–24 h
Gram-negative rods
Topical: gentamicin or tobramycin 9–18 mg/mL every 15–60 min (if *Pseudomonas*, add carbenicillin 4 mg/mL)
Subconjunctival: gentamicin or tobramycin 20–40 mg every 12–24 h

Proponents of the traditional treatment cite increased risk of adverse reactions, possible antagonism of antibiotic combinations, and increased risk of superinfection as major risks of the empiric theory. Those that support the empiric theory are quick to point out the unreliability of the Gram stain and the uncertainty of basing an antibiotic regimen upon such. Both schools agree that initial choices of therapy should be changed not solely on the basis of culture and sensitivity results but also on clinical progression of the ulcer. Antibiotic administration should be by topical instillation of concentrated antibiotics and possibly subconjunctival injection. Although, individually, subconjunctivally and topically administered antibiotics are equally effective, choice of route should depend upon compliance, pain of subconjunctival injections, expense of subconjunctival injection, and questionable effectiveness of drops because of tear washout. When used concomitantly, subconjunctival injections yield temporarily high concentrations to supplement the moderate but sustained drug levels provided by topically administered drops.[26,30] Antibiotics should be administered intravenously only when corneal perforation threatens infection of intraocular processes.[31]

Because routine in vitro bacterial susceptibility tests assume attainment of the usual plasma levels of antibiotics, they do not accurately reflect the activity of high concentrations achieved by topical instillation and therefore may not accurately predict clinical response. Initial therapy should not be changed if there is evidence of improvement. Only if the ulcer has failed to respond to initial treatment should therapy be changed as indicated by the culture and sensitivity report.

If corneal scrapings fail to identify specific bacteria, broad-spectrum treatment is indicated. If the ulcer still fails to improve, the clinician should investigate other etiologies (fungal, viral, chemical).

### Special Considerations

Many corneal ulcers are mixed infections. This possibility must be considered in unresponsive conditions. Excessive tearing occurring in children or associated with extemporaneous solutions that are not within a comfortable range of pH or tonicity may result in a washout of the antimicrobial drop. In these cases, subconjunctival injections should become the mainstay of treatment.

Ophthalmic ointments create a physical barrier preventing subsequent antibiotic solutions from contacting the corneal epithelium.[32] After a decrease in purulence and a reduction in ulcer size, the intervals between antimicrobial instillation and/or frequency of instillation should be prolonged to reduce the inhibition of corneal reepithelialization caused by concentrated antimicrobial solutions.[33]

Natamycin is the first-line treatment in fungal infections of the cornea. This drug provides broad-spectrum antifungal action without the pain and corneal irritation caused by the old standard, amphotericin B. Other available alternatives include miconazole and ketaconazole. *Candida* infections refractory to natamycin may respond to nystatin or flucytosine, although natamycin is the only commercially available ophthalmic antifungal agent.

Therapy of viral infections begins with mechanical debridment of the involved rim along with a rim of normal epithelium, followed by topical instillation of vidarabine or idoxuridine 5 times daily for 2 to 3 weeks; or trifluorothymidine may be used every hour while awake and every 2 hours at night for 2 to 3 weeks.[27] Trifluorothymidine penetrates stromal areas well.

### Other Treatments

In addition to antimicrobials, other drug treatment is required for conditions secondary to the ulcer. Anterior chamber reaction is often associated with corneal ulcers. The resultant decreased mobility of the iris allows adhesions to form, usually at pupillary margins. Treatment with atropine or scopolamine will help prevent synechia formation.

Steroid use should be withheld whenever possible for at least 24 hours after antimicrobial testing and successful treatment. Steroid use is indicated especially when the visual axis is involved or when the inflammatory reaction is severe. Once committed to this treatment, its discontinuation must be tapered with topical use just as with other routes of steroid administration. Topical steroid use in epithelial viral keratitis is contraindicated. The use of steroids here and in other persistent corneal infections may aid in preventing corneal melting and resulting perforation.[26,27]

If transient increases of intraocular pressure result from the keratitis, reduction can be achieved with hyperosmotics, carbonic anhydrase inhibitors, or $\beta$ blockers. Miotics should be avoided.

A 1% intravenous solution of potassium iodide has been used concomitantly to minimize the corneal reaction to the infection. By supporting the osmolarity of the cornea and by aiding the glycolytic and phosphorylation processes, much of the damage caused by corneal edema can be prevented. Success has been observed in fungal infections.[32]

If corneal perforation occurs or is imminent despite antimicrobial treatment, penetrating keratoplasty is indicated.

## Sinus Thrombosis, Preseptal and Orbital Cellulitis

These diseases result from infection of preseptal and pretarsal spaces of the eyelids and of orbital spaces. Inoculation may be direct by trauma or surgery or may be secondary to sinusitis, otitis media, or dental abscess. The most common microbial agents are *Staphylococcus aureus* and *Hemophilus influenzae* although traumatic injury may introduce anaerobes.[34,35]

### *Clinical Presentation*

Moderate to severe swelling of the lids, proptosis, and chemosis are symptomatic of *H. influenzae*. Cellulitis is characterized by blue-purple discoloration of the lid. Preseptal cellulitis produces purulent discharge while a displaced globe indicates orbital cellulitis. Progressive loss of consciousness and facial weakness suggest fungal involvement.

### *Treatment*

Initial choice of intravenous antibiotic treatment should be based upon Gram stain findings.[34]

| *Organism in Gram stain* | *IV antibiotics* |
|---|---|
| Gram + cocci | Methicillin and penicillin G |
| Gram + rods | Penicillin G |
| Gram − rods | Gentamicin and penicillin G |
| Gram − cocci | Ampicillin |
| None (posttrauma/postsurgery) | Methicillin, penicillin G and gentamicin |
| None (secondary to paranasal sinusitis) | Under age 5: methicillin and ampicillin<br>Over age 5: methicillin and penicillin G |

Progression of signs and symptoms despite antibiotic therapy suggests abscess formation, which requires surgical drainage. Phycomycosis is treated with amphotericin B.

## Endophthalmitis

Endophthalmitis is a devastating intraocular inflammation and infection involving the inner layers of the eye. Prognosis is guarded and the chance of any useful vision is highly dependent on many factors that will be discussed later. It is a dreaded clinical situation that should be treated as an ocular emergency.

### *Epidemiology/Etiology*

The incidence of endophthalmitis varies depending on multiple factors. The geographic location, the type of surgical procedure performed, the use of preoperative antibiotics, and the type of penetrating injury may all have some bearing on the incidence of endophthalmitis.

For instance, in some countries, the incidence of endophthalmitis after cataract surgery is more than 1%. In the United States, the reported incidence in most studies is less than 0.1%.[36,37]

The type of surgical procedure performed has some influence. Keratoplasty and glaucoma procedures have a very low incidence of endophthalmitis in the immediate postoperative period; however, the infection rate for filtering bleb surgery in glaucoma, for an extended period of time, jumps dramatically. Rates from 1% to 18% have been reported.[38–40]

Although no specific incidence of fungal endophthalmitis has been reported, it is generally believed to be on the increase with the use of broad-spectrum antibiotics, indwelling catheters, hyperalimentation, antineoplastic agents, immunosuppressive therapy, and parenteral drug abuse.[41]

### *Pathophysiology*

Endophthalmitis is an inflammatory process that involves the inner structures of the eye. In many instances, it is commonly of bacterial origin, although as previously noted, fungal endophthalmitis is on the increase. Panophthalmitis is considered an inflammatory process involving all layers of the eye, including external structures. Endophthalmitis can develop from both exogenous and endogenous sources. The microflora that are responsible for endogenous and exogenous endophthalmitis do vary somewhat. Bacterial pathogens isolated most commonly include *Staphylococcus aureus*, *S. epidermidis*, gram-negative bacteria, *Streptococcus viridans, Bacillus cereus,* and *Peptostreptoccus intermedius*.

Endogenous endophthalmitis usually arises from embolic phenomena. The most common sources of emboli include heart valves, metastatic systemic infections, including various cancers, and injection site abscesses or direct introduction of microorganisms into the bloodstream in intravenous drug abusers.[42]

Fungal and bacterial infections are often seen, with *Candida* endophthalmitis being the most common form of endogenous endophthalmitis.[43,45]

Viral endophthalmitis, though more commonly diagnosed as a retinitis, may exhibit many of the signs and symptoms of an endogenous endophthalmitis and therefore may be treated as aggressively. Patients with viral retinitis have had both herpes simplex type I and cytomegalovirus isolated for systemic and ocular aspirates.[46,47] Many viral infections that involve the deeper layers within the eye have been seen in immunocompromised hosts.

Exogenous sources of endophthalmitis include penetrating trauma, postoperative infections, and filtering blebs that become secondarily infected. Depending on the source of infection, the offending organism may vary.

In postoperative endophthalmitis, staphylococcal infections are the largest causative agent. In one series, *Staphylococcus epidermidis* was the cause of 58.8% of cases of endophthalmitis from cataract extraction and 80% of single organisms cases were gram positive.[48]

### *Clinical Presentation*

Most patients with endophthalmitis present with pain in the eye, diminished red reflex (light reflects back in clear media as a red reflection), hypopyon, and decreased visual acuity. Some variation may exist, and case reports of painless endophthalmitis[49] or no hypopyon have been reported. A slight leukocytosis may sometimes be seen. *Bacillus cereus* causes a very virulent form of endophthalmitis with accompanying ocular proptosis and lymphadenopathy.[43]

Occasionally, an acute inflammatory response arises that is indistinguishable from a bacterial or fungal endophthalmitis. Such cases of *sterile endophthalmitis* are treated as bacterial infections, if any doubt exists. Culture information is very important in determining the pathogenicity and prognosis in endophthalmitis. Aqueous fluid aspirations have been reported to be negative in many cases of endophthalmitis, while vitreous cultures have in turn been positive. The recommended procedure is to obtain culture and sensitivities of the site of entry (if applicable) and of the aqueous and vitreous fluids. Samples should be cultured for aerobic, anaerobic, and fungal growth. Gram and Giemsa stains are invaluable for initial treatment information. Endophthalmitis is truly an ophthalmic emergency. Treatment should be aggressive, with empiric wide-spectrum antibacterial coverage, until culture and sensitivity results are known (Table 77.7).

**Table 77.7** Empiric Endophthalmitis Treatment—Adult Doses

| | |
|---|---|
| **Intravenous Antibiotics** | |
| Aminoglycoside (gentamicin) + cefazolin[a] | Dosage individualized using serum concentrations |
| **Topical Therapy** | |
| Gentamicin fortified drops (13.6 mg/mL)[b] + cefazolin drops (100 mg/mL) | Alternate drops every 15–30 min |
| **Intravitreal Injection** | |
| Gentamicin 100 to 200 μg | |
| Clindamycin 450 μg | All per 0.1 mL |
| Dexamethasone 360 μg | |
| **Vitrectomy Solution**[c] | |
| Balanced salt solution | 500 mL |
| Dexamethasone | 8 mg |
| 5% Dextrose in water | 10 mL |
| Sodium bicarbonate 8.4% | 13.1 mL |
| Gentamicin | 8 μg/mL |
| Clindamycin | 9 μg/mL |

[a] In a patient with a true penicillin allergy, clindamycin, 900 mg every 8 h, may be substituted for cefazolin.

[b] These patients should be continuously observed for epithelial toxicity.

[c] Vitrectomy solutions may vary among the various institutions. Antibiotics may vary depending on results of culture and sensitivity tests. Subconjunctival injections (if indicated) are given in Table 77.8.

The main prognostic indicators for good visual acuity seem to be the virulence of the organism causing the infection and the interval of time before treatment. Patients that respond with the best visual acuities are those that seem to have less virulent organisms isolated, prompt and aggressive treatment, and a normal host immune response.[50]

### *Treatment*

In endophthalmitis, the goal of treatment is attainment of adequate and nontoxic vitreal levels of drug. This helps to preserve the delicate retinal and other intraocular tissue function by decreasing inflammation and eradicating the infectious organisms.

The inflammatory and/or infection processes involve most structures of the eye including the vitreous cavity. Penetration through the blood–retina barrier into the vitreous fluid by most routes of administration is poor. Thereapy consists of topical, intravenous, intraocular, and possibly periocular administration of anti-infectives and/or corticosteroids.[51]

Corticosteroids are indicated when an overwhelming inflammatory condition threatens to destroy the sensitive intraocular structures. Corticosteroids are employed in endophthalmitis concomitantly with antimicrobial agents. It is hardly appropriate to sterilize an infected eye if the delicate intraocular contents of the eye have been destroyed by inflammation. Corticosteroids may be given by periocular, subconjunctival, topical, or intraocular route. Intravitreal injections of corticosteroids are given by some clinicians together with antibiotics when a bacterial endophthalmitis is suspected. Dexamethasone phosphate in the dose of 360 μg/0.1 mL has proved to be nontoxic to the retina.[52]

Investigators have recommended the use of dexamethasone 16 μg/mL in the vitrectomy solution or 5 to 10 mg subconjunctivally when these routes are indicated.[45] In some instances, topical prednisolone acetate, to quiet anterior segment inflammation, or oral prednisone in high doses (1–2 mg/kg) is employed for short-term use should posterior inflammation or membrane formation continue or increase. Corticosteroid usage definitely is effective in reducing the inflammatory process, which may be detrimental to the eye. The clinician's judicious use of such potent agents may be of great benefit in a situation that may otherwise be hopeless.

An exhaustive review of prophylactic antibiotics for ophthalmic surgery was made by Starr.[53] His conclusions were that properly selected antibiotics over a 1- to 2-day course were effective in reducing the postoperative incidence of endophthalmitis. Ocular flora were decreased or eradicated; therefore, one of the main sources of endophthalmitis is considerably reduced.

Most ocular pharmacokinetic studies of various antimicrobial agents have been performed in animals, with the majority being studies in rabbits. Although the rabbit is not a perfect model, many of the results exhibit good correlation to the human eye.[54] Studies of the ocular penetration of antimicrobial agents in humans are somewhat limited because of inadequate sampling techniques.

Therefore, antibacterial treatment of endophthalmitis raises some controversy. Investigators have been divided as to the need for antibiotics given by direct intravitreal route versus alternative routes of administration. Responses from systemic, periocular, and topical routes of administration have been poor. This is due to restrictions of the penetration of drugs by the blood–ocular barrier. It is a lipoidal barrier and drug usually crosses in proportion to its lipid solubility. The blood–ocular barrier consists of the blood–aqueous barrier and the blood–retina barrier. The blood–aqueous barrier is composed of tight junctions of the ciliary body epithelium and capillary endothelium, and allows for increased drug penetration when inflamed. Studies have shown that inflamed eyes generally have better penetration of antibiotics into the aqueous fluid.[54]

The blood–retina barrier (BRB) is much harder to traverse than the blood–aqueous barrier. The blood–retina barrier consists of the tight junctions between retinal pigment epithelial cells and endothelial cells of the retinal blood vessels. Antibiotic penetration into the vitreous does not increase significantly during inflammatory states as it does in the anterior chamber. Penicillin or moxalactam[45] penetrates the vitreous fluid in levels high enough to achieve minimum inhibitory concentrations for most organisms. One study indicated that cefazolin (2 g IV) was the only antistaphylococcal agent that consistently gave vitreous levels effective against *S. aureus* and *S. epidermidis*.[55] Therapy is directed at achieving the highest nontoxic concentration of antibiotic in the eye, at the first signs and symptoms of endophthalmitis, to prevent any further destruction of the intraocular structures.

Both the emergence in the late 1900s of different pathogens, especially gram-negative bacilli, and the poor vitreous penetration of most antibiotics contributed to the poor visual prognosis in endophthalmitis. Therefore, intravitreal antibiotics were revived in the 1970s as a means of directly instilling antibiotics into the eye. Since that time many publications have supported the use of intravitreal antibiotics, antifungals, and antivirals for the treatment of endophthalmitis.[56] Nontoxic doses have been determined for many antimicrobials (see Table 77.8.)

Most topical antibiotics penetrate the aqueous fluid and, in a vitrectomized patient, may reach inhibitory concentrations in the eye. Some physicians use fortified eye drops to increase the aqueous levels of antibiotics. Cefazolin (100 mg/mL) and fortified gentamicin (13.6 mg/mL) drops are advocated for empiric treatment of bacterial keratitis.[57] Because higher aqueous levels are achieved, the logical extension of this regimen has been for the treatment of endophthalmitis. No good clinical study has proved these fortified drops to be any more effective in endophthalmitis.

Intravenous antibiotics are of questionable value in endophthalmitis. Studies justifying aggressive intravenous antibiotic treatment in endophthalmitis are not abundant. Drug concentrations in the eye depend on whether the drug crosses the blood–ocular barrier, the drug clearance from the eye, and the concentration of free drug in the blood. As mentioned before, the blood–ocular barrier is the largest obstacle to drug penetrating the eye, especially the vitreous. Organic acids, such as penicillin or cefazolin, may be actively transported out of the vitreous by the ciliary body and retinal pigment epithelium. All compounds are removed to some extent by diffusion into the anterior chamber and out by the normal aqueous outflow mechanism.

Empiric endophthalmitis treatment recommendations are given in Table 77.7. Broad-spectrum coverage with intravenous aminoglycoside (gentamicin) and a cephalosporin (cefazolin is indicated because of its effective intravitreal levels against staphylococcus from intravenous therapy) would be most appropriate. Cefazolin must be used with caution in someone who has a true penicillin allergy; an alternative may be the use of clindamycin and gentamicin. Clindamycin and gentamicin by the intravenous route are indicated if the patient is suspected of having *Bacillus cereus* endophthalmitis because of their reported synergy against that organism. Topical treatment may consist of an alternating dose of gentamicin fortified and cefazolin every 15 minutes to one-half hour for a couple of days, after which the results of culture and sensitivity tests will determine the dose. A change to regular-strength gentamicin drops is recommended when possible to prevent any epithelial toxicity. Intravitreal antibiotics are usually given immediately upon the patient's initial presentation. A normal *intravitreal cocktail* may consist of (per 0.1 mL) 200 μg gentamicin, 450 μg clindamycin, and 360 μg dexamethasone. If vitrectomy is indicated, gentamicin 8 μg/mL, clindamycin 9 μg/mL, and dexamethasone 16 μg/mL may be added to the vitrectomy

**Table 77.8** Antimicrobial Concentrations for Treatment of Ophthalmologic Infections[a]

| | *Topical (%)* | *Subconjunctival injection (mg/0.5 mL)* | *Intravitreal injection (mg/0.1 mL)* | *Vitrectomy solution (μg/mL)* |
|---|---|---|---|---|
| **Penicillins** | | | | |
| Ampicillin | | 100–200 | 5 | |
| Carbenicillin | 10 | 100–150 | 0.5–2 | |
| Methicillin | 5–10 | 100–200 | 2 | 20 |
| Oxacillin | 6.6 | 100 | 0.5 | 10 |
| Penicillin G | 0.1–0.2 MU/mL[b] | 0.3–1 MU | 200–300 U | 80 |
| Piperacillin | 5–10 | 100 | | |
| Ticarcillin | 5–10 | 100 | | |
| **Cephalosporins** | | | | |
| Cefamandole | | 12.5 | | |
| Cefazolin | 5–10 | 100 | 0.5–2 | |
| Cefotaxime | 5–10 | | | |
| Ceftriaxone | | | 2 | |
| Cephalothin | 5 | 50–125 | 2 | |
| Moxalactam | 10 | 100 | 1.25 | |
| **Aminoglycosides** | | | | |
| Gentamicin | 0.3–1.5 | 10–20 | 0.1–0.4 | 8 |
| Amikacin | 0.5–1.5 | 25 | 0.2–0.4 | 10 |
| Tobramycin | 0.3–1.5 | 5–20 | 0.1–0.5 | 10 |
| Netilmicin | | 10–20 | 0.25 | 10 |
| Neomycin | 0.3–3.3 | 250–500 | | |
| **Miscellaneous** | | | | |
| Vancomycin | 5 | 25 | 0.5–1 | |
| Clindamycin | 1–5 | 15–49 | 0.3–1 | 9 |
| Erythromycin | 0.5 (ointment) 1.5 | 50–100 | 0.5 | |
| Choramphenicol | 0.5,1 (ointment) | 50–100 | 2 | 10 |
| Tetracycline | 1 (suspension) (ointment) | | | |
| Chlortetracycline | 1 (ointment) | | | |
| Bacitracin | 100,000 U/mL | 10,000 U | | |
| Polymyxin B | 5–10,000 U/g | 100,000 U | | |
| Sulfacetamide | 10,30,30 (ointment) | | | |
| **Antivirals** | | | | |
| Acyclovir | 3 (ointment) | 0.080 | 20 | |
| Idoxuridine | 0.1<br>0.5 (ointment) | | | |
| Vidaribine | 3 (ointment) | 0.040 | 8 | |
| Trifluridine | 1 | | | |
| **Antifungal** | | | | |
| Amphotericin B | 0.25–1.5 | 0.1–0.2 | 0.005 | |
| Nystatin | 100,000 U/mL (suspension) | | | |
| Flucytosine | 1 | | | |
| Miconazole | 1 | | | |
| Natamycin | 5 (suspension) | | | |

[a] Solution, except where noted.
[b] MU, million units.

solution. Intravenous, vitrectomy, topical, and intravitreal antibiotics may be changed as the results of culture and sensitivity tests become available.

If fungal endophthalmitis is suspected, an intravitreal injection of amphotericin 5 $\mu g$/0.1 mL is recommended. Intravenous amphotericin along with oral 5-fluorocytosine (50–150 mg/kg) may also be indicated. A vitrectomy may be performed with an intravitreal injection of amphotericin B given after the procedure, as amphotericin B is compatible only in $D_5W$ and not a balanced salt solution or normal saline. Subconjunctival administration of miconazole has also been found to be effective in some cases of fungal endophthalmitis. Topical natamycin is of questionable value because penetration is only into the cornea and possibly the anterior chamber, with negligible concentrations in the posterior chamber.

## Glossary

**Blepharitis.** Inflammation of the eyelids.
**Chalazion.** Meibomian gland granulomatous inflammation.
**Chemosis.** Swelling of the conjunctiva.
**Dacryocystitis.** Infection of the lacrimal sac.
**Dendrites.** Branching-like process seen with herpes simplex infections.
**Endophthalmitis.** Extensive intraocular inflammation or infection.
**Filtering bleb surgery.** Surgical procedure that allows aqueous fluid to percolate under the conjunctiva, thereby reducing intraocular pressure.
**Fornix.** Conjunctival cul-de-sac.
**Fortified eye drops.** Compounded drops in a concentration higher than those commercially available.
**Giemsa stain.** Differential staining of blood smears.
**Hordeolum (sty).** Infection of the glands of the eye.
**Hypopyon.** Collection of white blood cells in the anterior chamber.
**Iridocyclitis.** Inflammation of the iris and ciliary body.
**Keratoconjunctivitis sicca.** Dry eye.
**Limbus.** Junction between cornea and sclera.
**Orbital septum.** A fibrous membrane extending from the orbit onto the lids; these are mostly considered the posterior fascia of the musculus orbicularis oculi.
**Proptosis.** Displacement outward of the globe.
**Pseudoptosis.** Condition resembling ptosis.
**Ptosis.** Drooping eyelid.
**Rosacea.** Vascular and follicular dilatation involving the nose and cheeks.
**Seborrheic blepharitis.** Blepharitis related to overactivity of the sebaceous glands.
**Tarsus.** Fibrous plates giving support to the eyelids.
**Tenon's capsule.** Membrane located below the conjunctiva that continues around the eye.

## References


1. Thygeson P. Nonspecific defense mechanisms of the eye. Int Ophthalmol Clin 1984;24:1–11.
2. Duke-Elder S (ed): System of Ophthalmology: Diseases of the Eyelids. St. Louis: C. V. Mosby, 1974, vol 13, part 1.
3. Locatcher-Khorazo D, Segal BC. Microbiology of the Eye. St. Louis, C. V. Mosby, 1972.
4. Wilson LA (ed): External Diseases of the Eye. New York, Harper and Row, 1979.
5. Brown SI, Shahinian L. Diagnosis and treatment of ocular rosacea. Ophthalmology 1978;85:779–786.
6. Lempert SL, Jenkins MS, Brown SI. Chalazia and rosacea. Arch Ophthalmol 1979;97:1652–1655.
7. Bullen CL, Liesegang TJ, McDonald TJ, et al. Ocular complications of Wegener's granulomatosis. Ophthalmology 1983;90: 279–290.
8. Harvey JT, Anderson RL. The management of meibomian gland carcinoma. Ophthalmic Surg 1982;13:56–60.
9. Pizzarello LD, Jakobiec FA, Hofeldt AJ, et al. Intralesional corticosteroid therapy of chalazia. Am J Ophthalmol 1978;85: 818–821.
10. Fitzpatrick TB, Eisen AZ, Wolff K, et al (eds): Dermatology in General Medicine, 2nd ed. New York, McGraw–Hill, 1979.
11. Brunell PA, Gershon AA. Passive immunization against varicella-zoster infections and other modes of therapy. J Infect Dis 1973;127:415–423.
12. Couch JM, Green WR, Hirst LW, et al. Diagnosing and treating Phthirus pubis palpebrarum. Surv Ophthalmol 1982;26:219–225.
13. Awan KJ. Pediculosis and phthiriasis, in Fraunfelder FT, Roy FH (eds): Current Ocular Therapy. Philadelphia, W. B. Saunders, 1980.
14. Jones LT, Wobig JL. Surgery of the Eyelids and Lacrimal System, New York, Aesculapius Publishers, 1976.
15. Richards WW. Actinomycotic lacrimal canaliculitis. Am J Ophthalmol 1973;75:155–157.
16. Vaughn D, Asbury T. General Ophthalmology, 10th ed. Los Altos, CA, 1983.
17. Barza M, Baum J. Ocular infections. Med Clin North Am 1983; 67:131–152.
18. Brook I. Anaerobic and aerobic bacterial flora of acute conjunctivitis in children. Arch Ophthalmol 1980;98:833–835.
19. Perkins RE, Kundsin RB, Pratt MV, et al. Bacteriology of normal and infected conjunctiva. J Clin Microbiol 1975;1:147–149.
20. Bogigian GM. Handbook of External Diseases of the Eye. Fort Worth, TX, Alcon Labs, 1980.
21. Kluever HC. Streptococci in inflammation of the eye: Report of 18 cases. Am J Ophthalmol 1935;18:805–810.
22. Ellis P. Ocular Therapeutics and Pharmacology, 7th ed. St. Louis, C. V. Mosby, 1985.
23. Schachter J, Dawson CR. Human chlamydial infections. Littleton, MA, P.S.G. Publishing, 1978.
24. Ostler HB. Herpes simplex: the primary infection. Surv Ophthalmol 1976;21:91–99.
25. Musch DC, Sugar A, Meyer R. Demographic and predisposing factors in corneal ulceration. Arch Ophthalmol 1983;101:1545–1548.

**26.** Wilhelmus K. Bacterial corneal ulcers. Int Ophthalmol Clin 1984;24(2):1–16.

**27.** Foulks G, Pavan-Lampton D. Cornia and external disease, in Pavan-Lampton D (ed): Manual of Ocular Diagnosis and Therapy, 2nd ed. Boston, Little, Brown, 1985, pp 76–97, 434–347.

**28.** Barza M, Baum J. Ocular infections. Med Clin N Am 1983;67 (1):131–151.

**29.** Baum J. Antibiotic use in ophthalmology, in Duane T (ed): Clinical Ophthalmology. Philadelphia, Harper and Row, 1985, vol 4, pp 1–20.

**30.** Baum J. Treatment of bacterial ulcers of the cornea in the rabbit: a comparison of administration by eye drops and subconjunctival injections. Trans Am Ophthalmol Soc 1982;80:369–390.

**31.** Baum J, Jones D. Initial therapy of suspected microbial corneal ulcers. Surv Ophthalmol 1979;24:97–116.

**32.** Havener W. Ocular Pharmacology. 4th ed. St. Louis, C. V. Mosby, 1978.

**33.** Petroutsos G, Guimaraes R, Girand J, et al. Antibiotics and corneal epithelial wound healing. Arch Opthalmol 1983;101: 1775–1778.

**34.** Jones D. Microbial preseptal and orbital cellulitis, in Duane T (ed): Clinical Ophthalmology. Philadelphia, Harper and Row, 1985, vol 4, pp 1–19.

**35.** Goldenberg R. Lateral sinus thrombosis. Arch Otolaryngol 1985;111:56–58.

**36.** Allen HF, Mangiaracine AB. Bacterial endophthalmitis after cataract extraction: a study of 22 infections in 20,000 operations. Arch Ophthalmol 1964;72:454–462.

**37.** Allen HF, Mangiaracine AB. Bacterial endophthalmitis after cataract extraction: II. Incidence in 36,000 consecutive operations with special reference to preoperative topical antibiotics. Arch Ophthalmol 1974;91:3–7.

**38.** Sugar HS, Zekman T. Late infection of filtering conjunctival scars. Am J Ophthalmol 1958;46:155.

**39.** Christensen L, Robinson PJ. Late infection of filtration blebs. Trans Pacific Coast Ottophthalmol Soc 1963;44:95–101.

**40.** Hattenhauer JM, Lipsich M. Late endophthalmitis after filtering surgery. Am J Ophthalmol 1971;72:1097–1101.

**41.** Peyman GA, Sanders D, Goldberg MF (eds): Principles and Practice of Ophthalmology. Philadelphia, W. B. Saunders, 1980, pp 1654–1656.

**42.** Elliott J, O'Day D, Gutow G, et al. Mycotic endophthalmitis in drug abusers. Am J Ophthalmal 1979;88:66–72.

**43.** O'Day D, Smith R, et al. The problem of *Bacillus* species infection with special emphasis on the virulence of *Bacillus cereus*. Ophthalmology 1981;88:833–838.

**44.** Brinton G, Topping T, et al. Posttraumatic endophthalmitis. Arch Ophthalmol 1984;102:547–550.

**45.** Peyman GA, Schulman J. Intravitreal Surgery: Principles and Practices. Norwalk CT, Appleton-Century-Crofts, 1986.

**46.** Pepose JS, Hilborne LH, Cancilla PA, et al. Concurrent herpes simplex and cytomegalovirus retinitis and encephalitis in the acquired immune deficiency syndrome (AIDS). Ophthalmology 1984;91:1669–1677.

**47.** Pepose JS, Holland G, et al. Acquired immune deficiency syndrome: pathogenic mechanisms of ocular disease. Ophthalmology 1985;92:472–484.

**48.** Pulianto CA, Baker AS, Haat J, et al. Infectious endophthalmitis: review of 36 cases. Ophthalmology 1982;89:921–929.

**49.** Deutsch T, Goldberg MF. Painless endophthalmitis after cataract surgery. Ophthalmic Surg 1984;15:837–840.

**50.** Vastine D, Peyman GA, Guth S. Visual prognosis in bacterial endophthalmitis treated with intravitreal antibiotics. Ophthalmic Surg 1979;10(3):76–83.

**51.** Lemp M. Diagnosis and treatment of tear deficiencies, in Duane T (ed): Clinical Ophthalmology. Philadelphia, Harper and Row, 1985, vol 4, pp 1–10.

**52.** Graham RO, Peyman GA. Intravitreal injection of dexamethasone. Treatment of experimentally induced endophthalmitis. Arch Ophthalmol 1974;92:149–156.

**53.** Starr M. Prophylactic antibiotics for ophthalmic surgery. Surv Ophthalmol 1983;27:353–373.

**54.** Barza M. Treatment of bacterial infections of the eye, in Remington J, Swartz M (eds): Current Clinical Topics in Infectious Disease. New York, McGraw Hill, 1984, vol. 5.

**55.** Axelrod J, Klein R, et al. Human vitreous levels of selected antistaphylococcal antibiotics. Am J Ophthalmol 1985;100:570–575.

**56.** Lesar T, Fiscella R. Antimicrobial drug delivery to the eye. Drug Intell Clin Pharm 1985;19:642–654.

**57.** Jones D. Decision-making in the management of microbial keratitis. Ophthalmology 1981;88:814–820.

# Chapter 78 / Skin and Soft Tissue Infections

Larry H. Danziger, PharmD, and Erkan Hassan, PharmD

Infections of the skin and soft tissues are some of the most common infections seen both in and out of the hospital setting. These infections may involve any/or all layers of the skin, fascia, and muscle. These infections may spread far from the initial site of infection leading to more severe infectious complications such as gram-negative sepsis, or to a glomerulonephritis as a sequela of a streptococcal infection.

The treatment involved in skin and soft tissue infections may at times necessitate both medical and surgical management. This chapter presents details of the pathogenesis and management of some of the more important infections involving the skin and soft tissues.

## Cellulitis

Cellulitis is generally an acute, spreading infectious process that initially affects the epidermis and dermis and may subsequently spread within the superficial fascia. This process is characterized by inflammation, but with little or no necrosis or suppuration of soft tissue. A variety of bacteria are responsible for the several types of cellulitis most commonly encountered (see Table 78.1).

In normal circumstances the skin and subcutaneous tissues are extremely resistant to infection. Even when high concentrations of bacteria are applied topically or injected into the soft tissue a resultant infectious process is rare.[1,2] Various conditions are necessary to produce skin infections, including (1) a high concentration of bacteria (> $10^5$ microorganisms), (2) occlusion of the blood supply to the area in question, (3) availability of proper nutrients, and (4) damage of the corneal layer allowing for bacterial penetration.[3]

### *Pathophysiology/Etiology*

The majority of infectious processes of the skin and soft tissues result from the disruption of normal host defenses such as skin puncture, abrasion, or introduction of some foreign body. The clinical infection seen in this setting depends upon both the type of microorganism present and the site of inoculation. A large percentage of these infections are caused by the normal skin flora (see Table 78.2). The exposed areas of the body (face, neck, etc.) generally have the highest bacterial density and *Staphylococcus epidermidis* is the most frequently found microorganism, whereas the axillary and groin areas (moister areas) are most frequently colonized with gram-negative bacilli.[4] As most bacterial inoculations of skin encounter intact skin or local intact host defense mechanisms, infections are aborted or very limited in nature. Therefore, epidemiologic data on this topic are sparse.

Bacterial infections of the skin can be classified as primary (pyodermas) or secondary. Primary bacterial infections are produced by a single bacterial species of generally normal skin (e.g., impetigo, erysipelas). Secondary infections, however, develop in areas of already damaged skin and very often show a polymicrobic pattern upon culture.

Classical cellulitis is caused by group A $\beta$-hemolytic streptococci or by *Staphylococcus aureus*. Occasionally, other gram-positive cocci, such as *Streptococcus pneumoniae* or group B streptococci, in the newborn, can be the etiologic agent.

### *Clinical Presentation*

The involved area may be extensive and is characterized by erythema and edema of the skin; the lesion is nonelevated and has poorly defined margins. Tender lymphadenopathy associated with lymphatic involvement is common. This is all associated with malaise, fever, and chills. There is usually a history of an antecedent wound from minor trauma, an ulcer, or surgery.

Cellulitis of an incised wound may be caused by any microorganism but the most aggressively spreading lesions are caused by group A streptococcus or *Clostridium perfringens* (the latter type of infection can occur from 6 to 48 hours after surgery).

It is important to note that it is often impossible to differentiate streptococcal and staphylococcal cellulitis. A Gram stain of a smear obtained by injection and aspiration of 0.5 mL of saline (using a small-gauge needle) into the advancing edge of the erythematous lesion may help in making the diagnosis but often yields negative results.[5] Generally, the diagnosis is made on clinical grounds, that is, the appearance of the lesion.

Cellulitis is considered a serious disease because of the propensity of the infection to spread through lymphatic tissue and to the bloodstream. When the lower extremities are involved in older patients it may be complicated by thrombophlebitis.

Erysipelas (Saint Anthony's fire) is a distinct type of superficial cellulitis of the skin with extensive lymphatic involvement. It is almost always due to *Streptococcus pyogenes* (group A streptococci). Other streptococci (in the newborn) and very rarely *Staphylococcus aureus* can cause similar skin lesions.

Erysipelas most commonly occurs in infants, young children, and the elderly, and frequently in patients with nephrotic syndrome.[6] Erysipelas also occurs in areas of preexisting lymphatic obstruction or edema. This infection

**Table 78.1** Bacterial Classification of Types of Cellulitis

| *Lesion* | *Common causative agent* |
|---|---|
| Erysipelas | Group A streptococcus (*Streptococcus pyogenes*) |
| Gangrenous cellulitis | Group A streptococcus, anaerobic streptococci plus some second microorganism (*Staphylococcus aureus* or *Proteus* spp.) |
| Crepitant cellulitis | *Clostridia* sp., *Bacteroides* sp., peptostreptococci |
| Miscellaneous cellulitis | Group A streptococci, *S. aureus*, *Hemophilus influenzae* |

manifests as a warm, painful, edematous, indurated lesion sharply circumscribed by an elevated border. It is most commonly found on the skin of the face in adults (involving the bridge of the nose and cheeks). Fever and leukocytosis are also common.

The causative agent usually cannot be cultured from the surface skin lesion but the streptococci may sometimes be aspirated from the edge of the advancing lesion.[5,7] The microorganism most likely gains access via some small break in the skin (i.e., accidental injury, ulcer, or surgical wound). Approximately one third of patients have had a preceding streptococcal respiratory infection.

Gram-negative cellulitis can be caused by a wide variety of organisms, such as *Escherichia coli*, *Proteus* spp., *Klebsiella* spp., *Enterobacter* spp. and anaerobes (especially *Bacteroides* spp.). These types of infections are often polymicrobic in nature (see Bacterial Diabetic Foot Infection) and involve peptostreptococcus or other anaerobic microorganisms. Acute cellulitis with mixed flora generally occurs in diabetics where the skin is adjacent to some site of trauma, where surgery has been done on the abdomen or perineum, or where host defenses have been compromised (vascular insufficiency or venous insufficiency ulcers). As with other types of cellulitis, warmth, redness, and induration are observed, and there may also be gas formation (crepitus). If the cellulitis progresses it can lead to areas of gangrene. As these infections often occur in poorly controlled diabetics and patients with alterations in host defense mechanisms and/or with poor nutrition, generalized systemic findings such as hypotension, dehydration, and altered mental status are common. Often, needle aspiration of the leading edge of the lesion and subsequent Gram staining and culture are helpful in making a diagnosis. A leukocytosis of greater than 20,000 is not uncommon.

**Table 78.2** Predominant Microorganisms of Normal Skin

| |
|---|
| Yeast (*Pityrosporon ovale*) |
| *Staphylococcus epidermidis* |
| Diphtheroids |
| *Staphylococcus aureus* |
| Streptococcal species |
| Anaerobic micrococci |
| Gram-negative bacilli (*Bacillus* and *Micrococcus*—soil organisms) |

*Hemophilus influenzae* cellulitis occurs most often in young children. Most adults have bactericidal antibody and/or anticapsular antibodies to *H. influenzae* and so are less often infected. Humans are the only known natural hosts for this gram-negative microorganism, which seems to occur most often in children between 1 and 5. *H. influenzae* is carried in the oropharynx and nasopharynx as part of the normal flora. This infection characterically causes a purple-red cellulitis of the face, neck, or upper extremities.[8]

*H. influenzae* cellulitis frequently occurs in close association with an upper respiratory tract infection.[9] In young children the lesion has margins that are indistinct, blue-red to purple-red in color, and surrounded by an area of edema and induration. Regional lymphadenopathy is rarely present. In adults, the blue-red to purple-red discoloration may not be present.

Fever (in the range 39–40°C) and elevated white blood cell count (about 20,000 $cm^3$) are common. Blood cultures are positive for *H. influenzae* in roughly 80% of patients. Aspiration, Gram stain, and culture of the margin of cellulitis are positive in approximately 50% of all cases.[10]

## Treatment

Antimicrobial therapy of bacterial cellulitis depends upon the type of bacteria either suspected or documented to be present, which will generally coincide with the clinical presentation. Local care often aids in the rapid resolution of symptoms. Surgical intervention as a mode of therapy is rarely indicated in the treatment of cellulitis.

As streptococcal cellulitis is indistinguishable clinically from staphylococcal cellulitis, administration of a semisynthetic penicillin (nafcillin or oxacillin 1–2 g IV every 4 hours) is recommended until a definitive diagnosis, by skin or blood cultures, can be made in the treatment of classical cellulitis.[10,11] If documented to be a mild cellulitis secondary to streptococci, then parenteral penicillin should be used. Procaine penicillin G 600,000 units intramuscularly every 8 to 12 hours or penicillin VK 250–500 mg orally four times daily for 10–14 days is adequate. For more severe streptococcal infections aqueous penicillin G 600,000 to 2 million units IV every 4 to 6 hours should be used.[10,11]

In penicillin-allergic patients, erythromycin 500 mg orally and/or parenterally four times daily may be used.[10,11] A first-generation cephalosporin such as cefazolin may also be used for these patients. For mild infections of susceptible strains, 500 mg every 8 hours may be used; for more severe infections, 1–2 g every 6–8 hours can be used depending on the severity of the infection. When erythromycin or cephalosporins cannot be used, because of documentation of a significant allergic reaction to β-lactam antibiotics or isolation of a methicillin-resistant staphylococcal strain, vancomycin 1 g intravenously every 12 hours should be used (in adults with normal renal function).

Local care of cellulitis includes elevation and immobilization of the involved area to decrease local swelling. Cool sterile saline dressings can decrease the local pain and can be followed later with moist heat to aid in localization of the

**Table 78.3** Treatment Regimens for Gram-Negative or Mixed Bacterial Cellulitis[a]

| | |
|---|---|
| Single gram-negative aerobe | Aminoglycoside[b] or cephalosporin (first- or second-generation depending on severity of infection or susceptibility pattern)[10] |
| Polymicrobic infection without gram-positive anaerobes | Aminoglycoside[b] + penicillin G 0.6–1.0 million units every 4–6 h or a semisynthetic penicillin (i.e., nafcillin 1–2 g every 4–6 h depending on isolation of staphylococci or streptococci) |
| Polymicrobic infection with anaerobes | Aminoglycoside[b] + clindamycin 900 mg every 8 h[10,11] or metronidazole 0.5–0.75 g every 8 h<br>or<br>Single-drug therapy with second- or third-generation cephalosporin[112,121,122] (i.e., cefoxitin 1–2 g every 6 h or ceftizoxime 1–2 g every 8 h) |

[a] For penicillin-allergic patients, use vancomycin 0.5–1.0 g every 8–6 hours with dosage adjustments made for renal dysfunction.

[b] Aminoglycoside—2 mg/kg loading dose, then maintenance dose determined by serum concentrations.

cellulitis. In general, incision and drainage are not necessary in the absence of necrosis or suppuration.

When treated promptly with parenteral antibiotics, the majority of patients with cellulitis are cured rapidly. Failure to respond to therapy may be indicative of an underlying local or systemic problem or misdiagnosis.

Mild to moderate cases of erysipelas in adults are treated with procaine penicillin G 600,000 units intramuscularly twice daily or penicillin VK 250–500 mg orally four times daily for 7–10 days.[12] Dramatic improvement is generally expected 24–48 hours after treatment has begun. Penicillin-allergic patients can be treated with erythromycin 250–500 mg orally every 6 hours for 7–10 days. Strains resistant to erythromycin have been documented so some caution is warranted.[12] For more serious infections parenteral aqueous penicillin G 2–8 million units daily should be administered intravenously and the patient should be hospitalized.[10,13]

For cellulitis caused by gram-negative bacilli or a mixture of microorganisms, immediate antimicrobial chemotherapy as determined by Gram stain is essential, along with appropriate surgical excision of necrotic tissue and drainage. If there is no obvious focus for the infection some internal source should be sought (i.e., perforated viscus or rectal tear) and repaired if possible. Specific antibiotic therapy is directed toward not only gram-negative enteric bacilli but also anaerobic gram-negative organisms (e.g., *Bacteroides*) and anaerobic streptococci, as this type of infectious process is often polymicrobic in nature. Many different treatment regimens are possible depending on the bacteriology of the lesion (see Table 78.3).

Because this infection can progress very quickly to very serious tissue invasion, therapeutic intervention should be immediate. If treated early, a quick response can be seen. Unfortunately, as this infection often occurs in patients with compromised immune defense systems, even with therapeutic intervention the disease process may still progress. If the infectious process is secondary to some systemic cause (e.g., diabetes), the treatment course can be prolonged and may be associated with high mortality and morbidity.

In mild *Hemophilus influenzae* infections for children less than 20 kg, either ampicillin 50–100 mg/kg/d in four divided doses or amoxicillin (not recommended for use in infants 4 weeks of age or less) 20–40 mg/kg/d in three divided doses may be used. For adults, ampicillin 250–500 mg every 6 hours or amoxicillin 250–500 mg every 8 hours may be used.

For penicillin-allergic patients, either cephalosporins (cefaclor, cefuroxime) or trimethoprim–sulfamethoxazole may be used. For severe infections in young children it is recommended that chloramphenicol 50–100 mg/kg/d in four divided doses plus ampicillin as described earlier be used until results of culture and sensitivity tests are known because of the increasing documentation of *H. influenzae* strains resistant to ampicillin and chloramphenicol individually.[14]

Dosage adjustments for chloramphenicol should be determined by use of serum concentrations, as the pharmacokinetics of the drug may change in critically ill children and adults when given either intravenously or orally.[15,16] Data are now available that support the concept of dosage alterations in patients with underlying liver, renal, or gastrointestinal dysfunction.[17–19] In general, for severe infections, maintenance of serum concentrations of chloramphenicol in the range 10–20 $\mu$g/mL is usually associated with successful outcome and with a low incidence of toxicity.[20]

## Lymphangitis

Acute lymphangitis refers to an inflammation involving lymphatic subcutaneous channels. This acute process is secondary to a bacterial pathogen, most frequently group A streptococci, but may occasionally be caused by *Staphylococcus aureus* or *Pasteurella multocida*.[1,21,22] Chronic lymphangitis is not generally associated with pain or systemic signs of infection. Chronic lymphangitis is most commonly caused by sporotrichoids (a type of fungus).[22] The remainder of this discussion pertains only to acute lymphangitis.

### *Clinical Presentation*

Acute lymphangitis is not contained locally but spreads along the lymphatic channels. Systemic manifestations of this infection often develop rapidly before any sign of infection at the initial site of inoculation is evident, or even after the initial lesion has subsided. The systemic symptoms are often more profound than would be expected from examination of the cutaneous lesion. Acute lymphangitis is characterized by the rapid development of fine red linear streaks extending proximally from the extremities.

These linear streaks may be a few to several centimeters wide and extend from the initial site of infection toward the regional lymph nodes, which are usually enlarged and tender. Often associated with this is peripheral edema of the involved extremity.[1,22]

Systemic symptoms are often prominent and include fever, chills, malaise, and headache. Generally, an elevation in the peripheral white blood cell count is noted (>10,000/mm$^3$). Cultures of the affected lesions will not yield positive results, as the infection resides within the lymphatic channels; however, the offending pathogen can often be identified by Gram stain of the initial lesion if done early in the course of the disease.

Identification of a peripheral lesion associated with proximal red linear streaks directed toward the regional lymph nodes is diagnostic of acute lymphangitis. At times, thrombophlebitis and acute lymphangitis in the lower extremities may be confused, as both are associated with red linear streaking and tender areas; however, in thrombophlebitis no portal of entry is identifiable.

### *Treatment*

Penicillin is the treatment of choice for acute lymphangitis. For mild cases 600,000 units of intramuscular procaine penicillin G once or twice daily initially; then, over time (24–48 hours) the patient may be converted to oral penicillin VK 250–500 mg four times daily for a total of 10 days.[22] In more severely ill patients with bacteremia, aqueous penicillin G 600,000 to 2 million units is given intravenously every 4 to 6 hours.

If the suspicion is high that *Staphylococcus aureus* is the causative pathogen, a semisynthetic penicillinase-resistant penicillin should be used (i.e., nafcillin 1–2 g every 4–6 hours depending on the severity of the infection). For penicillin-allergic patients, erythromycin 250–500 mg four times daily for 10–14 days may be used.

## Lymphadenitis

Lymphadenitis may refer to acute or chronic inflammation of the lymph nodes. Lymphadenitis occurs when bacteria reach the lymph nodes and elicit an inflammatory response. This process may be restricted to a solitary node or to a certain anatomic region (regional lymphadenitis) or may be a generalized phenomenon.

Lymphadenitis can be caused by a variety of pathogens (see Table 78.4) including bacteria, viruses, fungi, protozoa, helminths, and chlamydia.[21,22] Acute regional lymphadenitis is more common in children than adults. Recently, *Staphylococcus aureus* has become the most frequently isolated pathogen in acute suppurative lymphadenitis.

**Table 78.4** Types and Causes of Regional Lymphadenitis

| | |
|---|---|
| Pyogenic—bacterial | |
| Cervical | *Staphylococcus aureus* or with or without group A streptococci |
| Suppurative | Epitrochlear—group A streptococci plus *S. aureus* |
| Suppurative iliac | Staphylococci or streptococci |
| Nonpyogenic | |
| Tuberculous cervical (scrofula) | *Mycobacterium tuberculosis* *Mycobacterium scrofulaceum* |
| Cat scratch disease | Not identified (viral?) |
| Chlamydial | Lymphogranuloma venereum—*Chlamydia trachomatis* |
| Fungal | |
| Histoplasmosis | *Histoplasura capsulatum* |

### *Clinical Presentation*

Commonly involved sites include the submaxillary and anterior and posterior cervical, inguinal, and axillary lymph nodes. Pharyngitis and tonsillitis are common precursor diseases of cervical lymphadenitis. Suppurative iliac lymphadenitis resulting from infections of the leg, perineum, or abdominal wall can lead to psoas space abscess.

On examination, the area around the node is swollen and the node or nodes are usually tender and greater than 3 cm in diameter. The skin overlying the node is generally erythematous, warm, and edematous. Fever is also commonly present. Often prominent are systemic symptoms, including temperature from 37.7 to 39.0°C, chills, and malaise. The white blood cell count is generally elevated from 12,000 to 15,000/mm$^3$.

### *Treatment*

Early antimicrobial therapy of localized lymphadenitis will lead to rapid resolution of the problem. Because lymphadenitis following skin infections may be caused by either staphylococci or streptococci the drug of choice is a penicillinase-resistant penicillin (same recommendations as for lymphangitis).[22] In cases in which there is lack of improvement, aspiration or surgical drainage is an appropriate consideration.

## Pressure Sores

The terms *decubitus ulcer*, *bed sore*, and *pressure sore* are used interchangeably. In reality, the decubitus ulcer and the bed sore are types of pressure sores. The term decubitus ulcer is derived from the Latin word *decumbere*, meaning "lying down." Pressure sores, however, can develop regardless of what position a patient is in. Pressure sores are most frequently seen in chronically debilitated persons, in the elderly, and in persons with serious spinal cord injury (resulting from deprivation of sensory feedback mechanisms).

Pressure sores and their infectious complications have been known to medical practitioners for centuries, as evidenced by their documented presence on Egyptian mummies.[23] Until the twentieth century the only form of therapy was the application of topical medicinals. In more recent years the combination of antibiotics and surgery has led to decreased morbidity.[24] With advances in resuscitation of patients with spinal cord injuries and the increased number of debilitated geriatric patients, this problem has gained increased attention.

### *Epidemiology*

The absolute incidence of pressure sores has been suggested to be between 61 and 86 per 100,000 population.[25,26] General surveys of hospitalized patients indicate that from 3% to 4.5% develop pressure sores during their hospital stay.[25,27] Generally, those patients who are at risk for pressure sores are elderly or chronically ill young patients who are immobilized either to bed or wheelchair, and may have altered mental status often associated with incontinence.[25–27] Care of this population is estimated to cost between $15,000 and $20,000 more per patient; overall hospitalization is prolonged and nursing time increased by 50% per patient.[28] More recently, it has been estimated that considering the cost of curing the pressure sore and cost associated with patient productivity losses, in the United States alone more than $2 billion dollars is spent annually.

### *Pathophysiology*

Many factors are thought to predispose patients to the formation of pressure sores: paralysis, paresis, immobilization, malnutrition, anemia, infection, and advanced age. Four factors thought to be most critical to their formation are pressure, shearing forces, friction, and moisture; however, there is still debate as to the exact pathophysiology behind pressure sore formation.[29,30]

It is widely believed that pressure is the essential element in the formation of pressure sores. The areas of highest pressure are most often generated over the bony prominences. Pressure measurement studies have been conducted with people sitting in wheelchairs, and the points of greatest pressure were directly under and just lateral to the ischial tuberosities.[31] Studies have shown that when the pressure is relieved intermittently within a 2-hour period, only minimal changes occur in soft tissue and skin structures.[32] Therefore, both the degree of pressure and the length of time that the pressure is applied are of importance.

Shearing forces are caused by the sliding of adjacent parallel surfaces of soft tissues in an unequal fashion. Clinically, this situation can occur when the head of a bed is raised, causing the upper torso to slide downward, transmitting pressure to the sacrum and other areas. This effect results in occlusion or distortion of vessels, leading to compromise of the dermis.[33] At the same time, shearing forces are created by sitting and gravity; the posterior sacral skin area can become fixed secondary to friction with the bed. The effects of friction and shearing forces combine, resulting in transmission of force to the deep portion of the superficial fascia and leading to further damage of soft tissue structures.

Compounding the problems of shearing and friction forces are the macerating effects of excessive moisture in the local environment, resulting from incontinence and/or perspiration. This factor is of critical importance, because when combined with the other forces, it increases the risk of pressure sore formation fivefold.[34]

### *Clinical Presentation*

The persistence of the causative factors as discussed previously often results in pressure sore formation. Without treatment an initial small localized area of ulceration can rapidly progress to 5–6 cm within days. The visible ulcer is just a small portion of the actual wound; up to 70% of the total wound is below the skin. A pressure gradient phenomenon is created by which the wound takes on conical nature; the smallest point is at the skin surface and the largest portion of the defect is at the base of the ulcer (see Fig. 78.1).

Pressure sores can occur anywhere on the body. Over 95% of all pressure sores are located on the lower part of the body (65% in the region of the pelvis and 3.4% on the lower extremities) (see Fig. 78.2). The most common sites on the lower portion of the body are the sacral and coccygeal areas, ischial tuberosities, and greater trochanter.

Clinically, pressure sores vary greatly in their severity, ranging from an abrasion to large lesions that can penetrate

**Figure 78.1** Distribution of forces involved with sore formation in a conical fashion. *(From Reuler JB, Cooney TG: The pressure sore: Pathophysiology and principles of management. Ann Intern Med 1981;94:661–666, with permission.)*

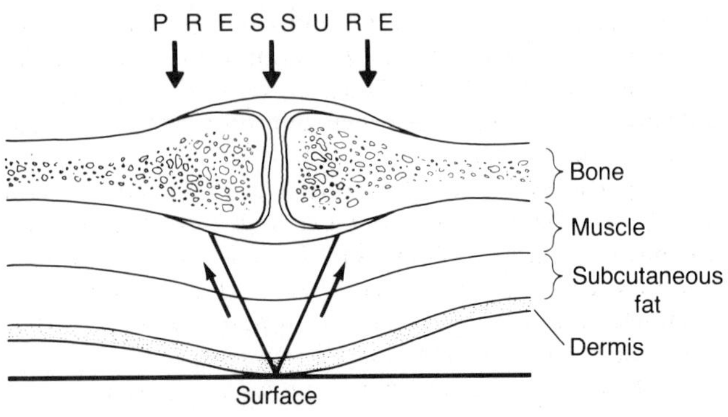

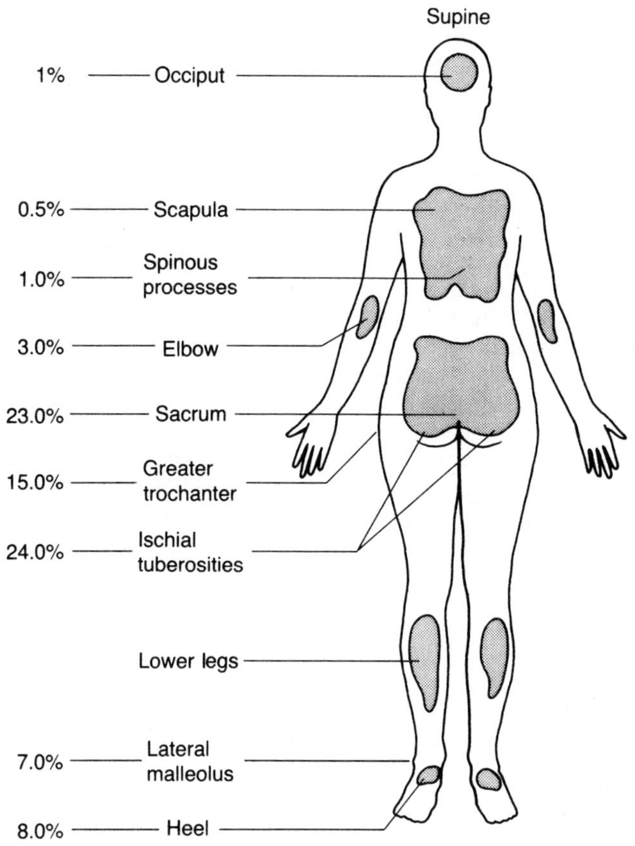


**Figure 78.2** Supine view of areas where pressure sore formation tends to occur. *(Adapted from Reuler JB, Cooney TG: The pressure sore: Pathophysiology and principles of management. Ann Intern Med 1981;94:661–666, with permission.)*

into the deep fascia involving both bone and muscle. Numerous systems for classification of pressure sores have been described, but the most frequently used system was devised by Shea.[35] This system describes the progression of the pressure sore through four stages. A stage 1 pressure sore is generally reversible, is limited to the epidermis, and resembles an abrasion. It is best described as an irregularly shaped area of soft tissue swelling, with induration and heat. A stage 2 sore may also be reversible; it extends through the dermis to the subcutaneous fat along with extensive undermining. A stage 3 sore or ulcer extends further into subcutaneous fat along with extensive undermining. A stage 4 sore or ulcer is characterized by penetration into deep fascia involving both muscle and bone. Stage 3 and 4 lesions are unlikely to resolve on their own and often require surgical intervention.

Complications of pressure sores are not uncommon and may be life-threatening. The most frequently encountered complications are infectious in nature. Pressure sores are routinely colonized by a wide variety of microorganisms; gram-negative aerobes and anaerobes are most often associated with the infections.[36] Systemic infections are not infrequent, with the most common organisms being gram-negative aerobes and anaerobes. Extension to the bone can occur and can lead to osteomyelitis and pyarthroses.[37]

### *Treatment*

#### Prevention

Prevention is the single most important aspect in the management of pressure sores. Prevention is far easier and less costly than the intensive care necessary for the healing and eventual closure of pressure sores. Of primary importance then is the ability to identify those patients who are at high risk so that preventative measures may be instituted.

Friction and shearing forces can be minimized by proper positioning. Skin care and prevention of soilage are important, with the intent being to keep the surface relatively free from moisture. Patients with problems of incontinence should be frequently cleaned, and efforts should be made to keep the involved areas dry. Natural sheepskin is thought to be useful in minimizing the effects of moisture, shearing forces, and friction.[38] Relief of pressure is probably the single most important factor in preventing pressure sore formation. The research done by Dinsdale[39] and Kosiach et al[31] has led to the belief that the patient should never be allowed to remain in one position for up to 2 hours. Relief even for 5 minutes once every 2 hours is felt to give protection against pressure sore formation.[32]

A variety of pressure relief systems are available (both active and passive). Devices are used to prevent pressure sore formation at either some local or a general site. The principal objective is to disperse pressure over a greater surface area or change the location of pressure contact points, preventing pressures from progressing to a critical level. These devices can be divided into three categories[40]: (1) support of specific pressure areas of the body, such as hips, heels, backs, and elbows; (2) aids in moving or turning the patient; (3) devices that attempt to support the entire body surface. Mechanical devices, however, do have certain disadvantages, including mechanical breakdown, technical complexity, and inability to be useful in all settings because of size and weight.

#### Medical Management

The medical approach to the treatment of pressure sores depends upon the stage of the disease. Medical management is generally indicated for lesions that are of moderate size and of relatively shallow depth (stage 1 or 2 lesions) and are not located over a bony prominence. Depending on their location and severity from 30% to 80% of these ulcers will heal without an operation.[41] Generally, medical treatment is not indicated for the management of those ulcers that extend through superficial fascia or into bone (stage 3 and 4). When the disease becomes this severe surgical intervention is almost always necessary.

Management of pressure sores differs little from that of other wounds; the basic principles of wound care still apply. The process of wound healing can be characterized by three phases. First, in response to necrosis and soft tissue destruction, an inflammatory reaction occurs. Second, usually 4–5

**Table 78.5** Chemical Debriding Agents

| |
|---|
| Enzymes |
| Sutilains (Travase) |
| Collagenase (Santyl/Biozyme-C) |
| Fibrinolysis and desoxyribonuclease (Elase) |
| Trypsin (Granulex) |
| Papin (Panafil) |
| Streptokinase/streptodornase (not commercially available) |
| Elements |
| Dextranomer (Debrisan) |
| Hydrogen peroxide |
| Silver nitrate |

days after the injury, cellular proliferation occurs. In this stage granulation tissue forms and collagen is deposited, reducing the effective size of the wound. Third, in the final phase, reepithelialization and contraction of the wound occur. Therefore, wound closure is the result of granulation, contraction, and epithelialization. This reparative process can be retarded by necrotic tissue, local infection, continued pressure on the wound, or various systemic factors (anemia, edema, diabetes mellitus, malnutrition). These concomitant secondary factors should be corrected to allow for maximal healing of the wound, in this case the pressure sore.

The goal of topical therapy is to clean and decontaminate the ulcer, to promote wound healing by permitting the formation of healthy granulation tissue, or to prepare the wound for an operative procedure. The main factors to be considered for successful topical therapy (local care) are (1) relief of pressure, (2) cleaning measures (debridement), (3) disinfection, and (4) stimulation of granulation tissue. Before any topical agents can be employed effectively, good wound care is necessary.

***Debridement*** The goals of debridement and cleansing measures are removal of devitalized tissue and reduction of bacterial contamination, which can slow granulation time and therefore impede healing. Debridement can be accomplished by surgical, mechanical (wet-to-dry dressing changes), or chemical means.

Chemical debridement is time consuming and is an extremely controversial issue (see Table 78.5). None of the currently available debriding agents has been documented to be superior to wet-to-dry dressings.[40,42] Surgical debridement rapidly removes necrotic material from the wound, but the associated risks include destruction of surrounding viable tissue, inadvertent enlargement of the ulcer, and possible extension of any existing infection. Mechanical debridement routinely uses the wet-to-dry dressing technique, which can be very painful and may possibly disrupt newly formed granulation tissue.[44] To avoid these problems wet-to-moist or wet-to-wet dressing changes have been suggested.[45] Another effective mechanical therapy is hydrodebridement—use of the whirlpool (Hubbard tank) to remove necrotic tissue and debris; it is a useful adjunct to both surgical and chemical debridement.

Collagenase is thought by many to be the most effective enzymatic debriding agent.[46,47] Collagenase is able to dissolve undenatured collagen fibers, which anchor necrotic tissue to the surface of the wound, without damaging granulation tissue. Collagenase is effective only within the pH range 6–8, so cleansing of the wound with an acidic solution should be avoided. Collagenase is inhibited by many cleansing agents (e.g., hexachlorophene, benzalkonium chloride) and many heavy metal–containing antiseptics (silver nitrate, thimerosal).[46] Dakin's solution and buffered (pH 7.0–7.5) normal saline solution will not inhibit enzymatic activity. Generally, collagenase need only be applied to a clean wound once daily, unless the wound is extremely soiled. Adverse reactions to collagenase are rare. It may cause irritation and inflammation of normal skin located at the edges of the wound.[28]

In a double-blind randomized study, 28 advanced dermal ulcers were treated with either collagenase or placebo. Significant improvement was observed in 14 of 17 patients in the treatment group. Reported side effects were minimal.[48] Rao and Sane treated 21 patients suffering from chronic decubitus ulcers with collagenase; the ulcers exhibited a significant reduction in odor, pus, inflammation, and necrosis.[49]

Sutilains (Travase) is a proteolytic enzyme that selectively digests necrotic tissue and has minimal activity in digesting collagen. Sutilains functions optimally in the pH range 6.0–6.8.[28,50] A loose wet dressing should be used and kept moist to allow the best environment for release of the enzyme. The entire dressing process should be repeated every 6–8 hours.[46] Sutilains is inactivated by the same agents as is collagenase. Adverse reactions reported with the use of sutilains include burning pain, paresthesias, transient dermatitis at the site of application, and occasional bleeding.[46,49] Sutilains has been documented to improve healing rates in studies in both animals and humans. In one such study, 18 patients with second- and third-degree burns, stasis ulcers of peripheral vascular disease, decubitus ulcers, and traumatic wounds were treated with sutilains three times daily.[50] Although not uniformly successful, sutilains did improve healing of these various wounds.

Other enzymatic debriding agents are also available but not as commonly used. Elase is a combination of two hydrolytic enzymes, fibrinolysin and desoxyribonuclease; the former degrades the fibrin present in a clot or fibrinous exudate, whereas the latter dehydrolyzes the DNA in the denatured protein of devitalized tissue. Adverse reactions are usually rare and include local irritation and hyperemia when high concentrations are used.[51] This product is used in conjunction with dressing changes and applied one to three times daily. Trypsin destroys the bonds between arginine and lysine. This enzyme product is rapidly inactivated by a low-pH environment; therefore, its use on an infected wound may not be appropriate. It should be used with dressing changes two to three times daily.

To date no specific enzymatic preparation has been shown to be more effective than any other product and use depends on user preference. These agents are an aid, not a substitute, in the debridement process.

Dextranomer (Debrisan) is purported to both clean and debride wounds. It consists of beads composed of hydrophilic dextran molecules crosslinked with *O*-glycerylene groups. The material is chemically inert and is believed to work by molecular and capillary absorption of fluid from the wound.[52]

Jacobson et al evaluated 47 patients with matching donor site wounds treated with dextranomer or not treated.[53] Seventy-seven percent of the dextranomer-treated wounds were microscopically less inflamed, softer, and more pliable, without crust coverings, than those left untreated. In one single-blind, randomized study, 51 chronic leg ulcers were treated with either dextranomer or wet saline compresses, twice daily for 7 days.[54] The wounds treated with dextranomer demonstrated a statistically significant increase in tissue granulation, a decrease in pus and debris, and a decrease in wound pain. Lastly, a controlled trial comparing dextranomer, collagenase, and a mixture of sugar and egg white showed a higher incidence of complete healing (43%—dextranomer, 10%—collagenase) and improved healing (86%—dextranomers, 46%—collagenase) for dextranomer-treated patients.[55] No improvement was seen in the ulcers of those patients treated with the egg white–sugar mixture.

Dextranomer appears to be effective in cleansing exudative venous stasis and decubitus ulcers. It also appears to increase tissue granulation, decrease wound inflammation, and decrease pus and debris; however, its cost and application techniques limit its usefulness. Few controlled trials are available with which to accurately gauge this drug's efficacy.

Application of dextranomer should be preceded by cleansing of the wound, with the site left moist. The site is then packed with dry beads to a depth of 1/8 to 1/4 in. and covered with gauze. Two to three times daily the material should be removed and the application repeated. No major adverse reactions have been reported with the use of dextranomer, although application and removal of the beads may cause intermittent pain, bleeding, blistering, and erythema in some patients.

***Disinfection*** A number of agents have been used to disinfect pressure sores (see Table 83.6) as well as other types of open wounds; however, objective clinical trials evaluating their efficacy are lacking. The agents used for disinfection and wound cleansing are classified as soaps, astringents, disinfectants, and topical antibiotics. These agents are used to reduce the bacterial content of open wounds. Most pressure sores are infected with both aerobic and anaerobic microorganisms; however, disinfectants have not been shown to penetrate tissue effectively to completely eradicate these organisms.[56] Therefore, use of these agents does not produce sterile wounds, but may decrease the number of bacteria present to fewer than 100,000 organisms per gram of tissue. This is important since infecting organisms can retard wound healing by depriving cells of oxygen.[56] A number of investigators have documented that bacterial counts greater than 100,000 organisms per gram of tissue can interfere with wound healing.[57,58]

Paradoxically, there is debate as to whether disinfectants help or interfere with wound healing. Branemark and associates reported that many disinfecting agents microscopically cause tissue damage within already existing wounds and therefore may delay wound healing.[59] Studies of the effects of various topical antimicrobials and povidone–iodine upon wound healing have yielded inconsistent results.[60,61]

The role of topical antibiotics (see Table 78.6) is still unclear. These products do not penetrate deeper tissue and

**Table 78.6** Disinfecting Agents

| | |
|---|---|
| Acetic acid | Topical antibiotics |
| Sodium hypochlorite (Dakin's) | Neomycin |
| | Gentamicin |
| Sodium oxychlorosene | Chloramphenicol |
| Hydrogen peroxide | Bacitracin |
| Povidone–iodine | Polymyxin B |
| Hexachlorophene | Metronidazole |

have not been documented to reduce bacterial counts by statistically significant amounts.[28] Problems with resistance, systemic toxicity, and sensitization further cloud any potential benefit.[28,56]

Although disinfectants do not sterilize a wound and may interfere with wound healing, they may be a potential benefit. These agents can be used to help clean the wound (by decreasing the bacterial counts), but should be stopped when the wound is clean and granulation appears to be occurring.

***Granulation/Epithelialization*** After the pressure sore has been adequately debrided and disinfected and pressure, friction, and moisture have been kept to a minimum, granulation and reepithelialization begin. An agent that promotes and hastens this process would obviously be desirable. Many agents (see Table 78.7) have been suggested, but hardly any evidence of a supportive nature exists.

Karaya has been used successfully in the treatment of excoriated skin sites around ostomies. This probably led to its use in the treatment of pressure sores, to hasten granulation[62]; however, the data and number of patients evaluated are too small to draw any conclusion of possible benefit. Some researchers have cautioned against its use because it is a potential irritant and/or it may disrupt the overlying fragile epithelial tissue present on the healing wound.[28]

Sugar—either powdered, granulated, or a paste—has been claimed to be an effective granulating agent for wounds for two reasons.[63–65] First, sugar is thought to work by attracting the bacteria to a growth site more hospitable than the diseased tissue (the new site is then removed with dressing changes).[66] Second, the hypertonicity of the sugar may directly stimulate wound healing.[66] The only randomized study done to date compared a sugar–egg white mixture with collagenase and dextranomer.[55] Although only 17 patients were evaluated, none of the 5 patients randomized to the sugar–egg white protocol responded. Caution should be used if sugar is selected because bacterial contamination (with *Bacillus* spp.) and other excipients present in the commercial product (cornstarch, tricalcium phosphate) may lead to problems.[67]

Some other agents that have been used but found to be effective in only a small number of patients include insulin,[68] Gelfoam,[69] and benzoyl peroxide.[70] The objective evidence available to support the use of these products is poor.

A different approach to decreasing the time needed for wound healing is aimed at wound dressing materials (see Table 78.7). Wound dressing materials should keep the wound moist, allow free exchange of air, act as a physical

**Table 78.7** Agents Used to Promote Granulation and Epithelialization

| | |
|---|---|
| Pharmacologic agents | Occlusive dressings |
| Karaya | Hydrocolloid occlusive dressing (Duoderm) |
| Sugar | |
| Insulin | |
| Powdered gelatin | Polyurethane film dressing (Op-Site) |
| Gelatin sponge (Gelfoam) | |
| Benzoyl peroxide | |
| Dextranomer | Silicone spary |
| Scarlet red | Silicone foam |
| Mercurochrome | |

barrier to bacteria, and prevent physical damage. Two newer agents are of some interest. Hydrocolloid occlusive dressing (Duoderm) is opaque and impermeable to water and oxygen.[56] This dressing absorbs moisture from the wound exudate and forms a gellike covering over the wound. Op-Site is a polyurethane film that is semipermeable, allowing evaporation. One study compared Op-Site, Duoderm, wet-to-dry dressing, and a control in pigs.[44] Significantly faster reepithelialization and greater collagen synthesis were noted in the wounds covered with Op-Site and Duoderm. Both wet-to-dry gauze dressing changes and Duoderm lead to damaged epithelium during removal. At present, only minimal data are available regarding the use of these agents in humans.[71,72] The major appeal of these occlusive-type dressings is that they need be changed only once every several days versus several times daily for the traditional wet-to-dry dressing technique.

Another nonpharmacologic approach to shorten healing time has been the use of oxygen.[73] It has been suggested that oxygen stimulates phagocytosis, granulation tissue growth, and bacterial stasis.[46] The idea is to enclose the wound in some type of chamber and apply hyperbaric oxygen. Various techniques have been used with varying degrees of success but have never been studied in a controlled fashion.[73,74]

Unfortunately, although as previously stated more than 2,000 agents have either been studied or used in the treatment of pressure sores, few controlled trials have been done that show any single agent to be efficacious. Whichever agent is selected, it must be evaluated on its own merits by the clinician, as limited scientific data are available.

### Recommendations

Some broad major guidelines can be recommended for the treatment of pressure sores (stages 1 and 2):

1. Relieve pressure
2. Avoid unnecessary friction and shearing forces
3. Prevent patient from lying in a moist environment
4. Use debridement, either pharmacologic or via minor surgical approach
5. Keep the wound clean by pharmacologic means or through use of a physical barrier
6. Use occlusive dressing (may also lead to increased healing and simplify the nursing care routine) if possible

For stage 3 and 4 pressure sores surgical management is most likely the major approach, with follow-up according to guidelines 1–6.

## Infections in Intravenous Drug Abusers

Infectious complications are the most frequent cause of illness and hospitalization of intravenous drug abusers.[75] Intravenous drug abusers are predisposed to a number of infectious complications including endocarditis, septic arthritis, osteomyelitis, pneumonia, and a variety of skin and soft tissue infections. Abscess formation and cellulitis at the site of injection are the most common infectious complications encountered in this population.[75] These skin and soft tissue infections are most frequently located on the upper extremities.

Soft tissue infections of the intravenous drug abuser are generally polymicrobic in nature, and usually more than two types of bacteria are isolated per patient.[76–78] *Staphylococcus aureus* or streptococcal species are believed to account for the majority of organisms isolated in these patients (range 37.5%–60.6%). The role of anaerobic bacteria in these infections is unclear. Investigators have reported the presence of anaerobic bacteria in 6% to 67% of patients with soft tissue infections.[76–78] Why differences exist among researchers with respect to the bacteriology of these types of infections is unknown. It is possible that the bacteriology of infections in intravenous drug abusers may be different depending upon geographic location.[77]

Data from various researchers support the belief that the source of organisms causing infectious complications in intravenous drug abusers is the patient and not the drug of abuse or drug use paraphernalia[77–79]; however, "street heroin" has been reported to be contaminated by a number of organisms. Organisms causing infection are believed to originate from multiple sources, including the mouth, the crushing of drug prior to injection, saliva (to moisten the cotton used to filter materials prior to injection), the blowing of clots from needles and syringes, or the use of poor injection technique which introduces bacteria into the skin.[77,80]

Generally, those patients with mild infections present with typical signs and symptoms of localized cellulitis and lymphangitis (see Cellulitis and Lymphangitis). The lesion will be erythematous, with swelling, increased skin temperature, and almost always lymphadenitis.[81] Occasionally cellulitis presents as a necrotizing cellulitis which is associated with a high mortality rate. It is characterized by signs of systemic illness, severe pain, swelling, a turbid watery pus, and occasionally soft tissue crepitus.

Nondrug treatment modalities for soft tissue infections in intravenous drug abusers include rest and immobilization of the involved extremity. When indicated, incision and drainage are of extreme importance. All available material should be aspirated and cultured for both aerobes and anaerobes, and examined by Gram stain. Blood cultures should be obtained, as between 25% and 35% of patients may be bacteremic.[77,82]

Very little attention has been focused on the antibiotic regimens for this patient population. A well-localized cutaneous infection in a non–toxic-appearing patient can be treated with local incision and drainage followed by appropriate dressing change techniques with or without an oral antibiotic. In this case, in which gram-positive microorganisms are most frequently involved, a semisynthetic penicillin would be appropriate.[82,83] Also, the clinician should be aware that a growing number of resistant gram-positive stains are being reported and, if isolated, treatment should be modified accordingly.

The more seriously ill appearing patient or a patient with extensive cellulitis or deep-seated infections requires the above nondrug treatment modalities in addition to parenteral antibiotics. In these patients a penicillinase-resistant penicillin (nafcillin 9–12 g/d) and an aminoglycoside (gentamicin 2 mg/kg loading dose followed by a maintenance dose based on renal function) should be initiated. Intravenous drug abusers have been reported to have a more rapid rate of aminoglycoside elimination, and a larger-than-normal volume of distribution; therefore these patients require close monitoring of serum concentrations.[84]

If the patient presents with a soft tissue infection associated with systemic toxicity, and watery, foul-smelling exudate, the suspicion should be high that anaerobes are present. In this case the combination of an aminoglycoside and an antianaerobic agent (clindamycin 900 mg IV every 8 hours or metronidazole 500–750 mg every 8 hours) should be instituted. Use of either clindamycin or metronidazole is warranted considering the increasing trend of *Bacteroides fragilis* and *Bacteroides melaninogenicus* resistance to penicillin.[85]

The antibiotic regimen should be modified on the basis of the final culture results. Many intravenous drug abusers have been documented to self-medicate themselves with antibiotics, which may account for the noted changes in patterns of susceptibility.[77]

## Infected Bite Wounds

One of the common problems seen in emergency rooms in the United States is the bite wound. If left untreated, complications including soft tissue infection or osteomyelitis may occur, possibly requiring extensive debridement or amputation. Approximately 1 to 2 million people in this country are bitten by dogs annually. The incidence of other bites (cats, humans, snakes) remains undetermined. Most of the data presently available derive from anecdotal case reports, making therapeutic decisions often controversial.

### *Dog Bites*

Dog bites account for 80% to 90% of all animal bite wounds requiring medical attention.[86] Dog bites commonly occur in individuals less than 20 years of age (52.2% of reported cases) who are most often male (57.8%). Over 70% of bites are to the extremities.[87] Occasionally, facial bites may occur, seen most often in children under 15, and can be a lethal event via exsanguination.

Health care providers see two distinct groups of patients seeking medical attention for dog bites.[88] The first group of patients presents 8–12 hours after the injury. These patients require general wound care, repair of tear wounds, or rabies and/or tetanus therapy. The second group of patients presents more than 12 hours after the injury has occurred. These patients usually have clinical signs of infection and seek medical attention for infection-related complaints (i.e., pain, purulent discharge, swelling). Those patients at greatest risk of acquiring an infection after a bite have had a puncture wound (usually the hand), have not sought medical attention within 12 hours of the injury, and are older than 50.[89,90]

The infected dog bite is usually characterized by a localized cellulitis and pain at the site of injury. The cellulitis usually spreads proximally from the initial site of injury. If *Pasteurella multocida* is present, a rapidly progressing cellulitis with a gray malodorous discharge may be encountered. Fewer than 20% of patients have a concomitant adenopathy or lymphangitis. Fever is uncommon. Wounds close to bones or joints may lead to infections of these structures.

Infections from dog bite wounds are due predominantly to organisms documented to be from the dog's oral flora.[91] Studies examining the normal flora of the dog frequently isolate *P. multocida*, *Staphylococcus aureus*, coagulase-negative staphylococci, and various unnamed organisms.[92,93] Wound site cultures in both infected and noninfected patients have similar bacteria present, with aerobic organisms (including facultative bacteria) isolated from 74% and anaerobic organisms isolated from 41%. The most frequently isolated organisms from infected and noninfected wounds are *S. aureus*, *P. multocida*, *Bacteroides* sp., and *Fusobacterium* sp.[88] Cultures obtained from noninfected bite wounds unfortunately have not been of value in predicting the subsequent development of infection.

Documentation of the mechanism of injury is important; if possible, an immunization history of the animal should be obtained. It is also important that the patient's tetanus immune status be determined.

Wounds should be thoroughly irrigated with a sterile saline solution. Proper irrigation significantly decreases the rate of subsequent infection.[89] Several management techniques used in the treatment of bite wounds remain controversial; these include the extent and type of debridement,[89] the use of primary closure within 24 hours of the injury,[88,94] and indications for the use of antibiotics.

Data on the role of prophylactic antimicrobial therapy for the early noninfected bite wound are controversial.[95,96] Until recently most suggestions concerning the use of prophylactic antibiotics were based on retrospective studies or upon observations of complicated cases. Callaham[89] demonstrated that patients treated with penicillin VK 40,000 IU/kg four times a day for 5 days had an infection rate of 10% compared with a 25% infection rate for those patients treated with placebo. Although a trend toward benefit with the use of prophylactic antibiotics was noted there was no statistical difference in infection rates between groups. Elenbass et al[97] reported that prophylactic administration of oxacillin 500 mg four times a day for 5 days in a similar number of patients did not improve outcome compared with administration of placebo in adult patients with noninfected full-thickness wounds presenting within 24 hours of injury.

As controlled studies have not definitively showed any benefit to the prophylactic use of antibiotics for noninfected bites, they are not routinely recommended; however, a semisynthetic penicillinase-resistant penicillin orally or a cephalosporin should be used for puncture wounds, wounds to the hands, and wounds in compromised hosts.[98,99] Tetracycline is recommended as an alternative form of therapy for those patients allergic to penicillins. If this is a problem (as in growing children or pregnant women), then erythromycin may be considered (in this case, sensitivities should be obtained, as *P. multocida* isolates will be resistant in up to 50% of cases). Prophylactic therapy should be given for 5 days. In addition to irrigation and antibiotics, when indicated the injured area should be immobilized and elevated.

Infections developing within the first 24 hours of a bite are most often caused by *P. multocida* and should be treated with penicillin (tetracycline is an alternative for penicillin-allergic patients).[98] For severe infections, intravenous penicillin therapy should be started and followed by oral therapy when the signs of cellulitis have subsided. Treatment should be given for 10 to 14 days. Semisynthetic penicillinase-resistant penicillins should be avoided in these cases because of their poor activity against *P. multocida*. For those infections developing more than 24 hours after the bite, therapy includes a penicillinase-resistant penicillin or a cephalosporin and should be given for a full 10 to 14 days.[98] Results of a Gram stain should be used to confirm the appropriateness of therapy.

Tetanus does not commonly occur after dog bites; however, it is a theoretical possibility. If the immunization history of a patient with anything other than a clean minor wound is not known, tetanus/diphtheria toxoids (Td) and tetanus immune globulin (TIG) should be administered. Patients with wounds that do not require immunization with tetanus/diphtheria toxoid are those who have had three or more immunization doses of TIG within the past 5 years. Patients who have received three or more doses of TIG within the last 10 years or patients who received two doses of TIG within the first 24 hours of injury do not require additional TIG therapy.[100]

As the rabies virus can be transmitted via saliva, rabies may be a potential complication of a bite. When the symptoms of rabies develop after a bite the prognosis for survival is poor. Roughly 3% of rabies cases documented in animals were in dogs (the most frequent vectors are skunks, raccoons, and bats).[101]

Once a patient has been exposed to rabies the treatment objectives consist of thorough irrigation of the wound, tetanus prophylaxis, antibiotic prophylaxis if indicated, and immunization. Postexposure prophylaxis immunization consists of BOTH passive antibody administration and vaccine administration. The only exceptions to antibody administration are patients who have been previously immunized with the appropriate degree of documented rabies antibody titers.

### *Cat Bites*

Cats are probably the second most common cause of animal bite wounds in the United States, but unfortunately very few data are available on the incidence and infection rate of these bites.[91] The major problems associated with cat bites are puncture wounds and scratches usually located on the lower extremities. Approximately 40% of cat bites and scratches become infected. These infections are frequently caused by *P. multocida*, which has been isolated in the oropharynx of 50% to 70% of healthy cats.[90] Both tularemia (*Pasteurella tularensis*) and rabies have also been transmitted by cat bites.[96] The management of cat bites is similar to that discussed for dog bites. Antibiotic therapy with penicillin is the mainstay and therapy is as described for dog bites.

### *Human Bites*

Infected human bites can occur as bites from the teeth or from blows to the teeth (clenched-fist injuries). Human bites are generally more serious than animal bites and carry a higher likelihood of infection. Infections can occur in up to 50% of patients with human bites.[102]

Self-inflicted bites most commonly occur on the lips or around the fingernails (from sucking or biting the nail).[103] Bites by others can occur to any part of the body but most often involve the hands. Bites to the hand are most serious and more frequently become infected.[99] The clenched-fist injury is a traumatic laceration caused by one person hitting another in the mouth and is one of the most serious of bite wounds. The areas most commonly affected by this injury are the third and fourth metacarpophalangeal joints.

Patients with infected bites to the hand may develop a painful, throbbing, swollen extremity. The wound often has a purulent discharge and the patient complains of a decreased range of motion. In addition to a cellulitis, other complications such as osteomyelitis, septic arthritis, and tenosynovitis can occur. Loss of a digit or hand has been reported.

Infections caused by these injuries are similar and most often caused by the normal oral flora, which include both aerobic and anaerobic microorganisms. The most frequent aerobic organisms are streptococcal species, *Staphylococcus aureus*, *Hemophilus parainfluenzae*, *Klebsiella pneumoniae*, and *Eikenella corrodens*.[104,105] The most common anaerobic organisms are *Bacteroides* sp., *Fusobacterium* sp., *Peptostreptococcus* sp., and *Peptococcus* sp.[104,105] Anaerobic microorganisms have been isolated in the range of 40% of human bite and 55% of clenched-fist injuries.

Management of bite wounds consists of aggressive irrigation, surgical debridement, and immobilization of the affected area. Primary closure for human bites is not generally recommended. If damage to a bone or joint is suspected, radiographic evaluation should be undertaken. Tetanus toxoid may be indicated and its need evaluated.

Patients with noninfected bite injuries should be given prophylactic antibiotic therapy. The drug of choice is penicillin, but if *S. aureus* is suspected, a penicillinase-resistant penicillin should be used with the penicillin. Prophylactic therapy should be given for 3 to 5 days as for prophylaxis for dog bites. A first-generation cephalosporin is not recommended, as the sensitivity to *E. corrodens* is variable.[106] For infected bite wounds, penicillin and a penicillinase-resistant penicillin should be empirically started and changed pending the culture results. Hospitalization for minor wounds is not necessary if surgical repair of vital structures has not been necessary. Those patients suffering serious injuries should be started on intravenous antibiotics. Duration of therapy for infected bite injuries should be 7 to 14 days.

When indicated, tetanus toxoid and antitoxin therapy should be instituted. Antibiotic therapy should always be used in clenched-fist injuries. Therapy should include penicillin (or ampicillin) plus a penicillinase-resistant penicillin until the final cultures are available. Therapeutic failures have been documented when either first-generation cephalosporins or penicillinase-resistant penicillins have been used alone, most likely because of their poor and variable activity against *E. corrodens*.[107,108] Therapy should be continued from 7 to 14 days.

## Bacterial Diabetic Foot Infection

With the development of insulin (1923) the patterns of morbidity and mortality for diabetic patients changed dramatically. Diabetes mellitus is estimated to affect between 3 and 10 million people in the United States.[109,110] Disorders of the foot are the most common complication of diabetes, requiring hospitalization (roughly 20% of all hospitalizations) at an annual cost of between 100 and 200 million dollars.[111] It has been suggested that up to 25% of diabetic patients give a history of some significant soft tissue infection at some time during the course of their illness.[112] The most common septic problem leading to hospitalization of diabetics is infections of the lower extremities.[113]

Three key factors are involved in the causation of diabetic foot problems: neuropathy, angiopathy, and some immunologic defect. Any of these disorders can occur singly; however, they frequently occur together.

Diabetic involvement of the autonomic nervous system plays an important part in the pathogenesis of foot lesions. Recent experimental work seems to indicate that diabetic neuropathy is caused by nerve swelling resulting from an increased polyalcohol sorbitol accumulation secondary to hyperglycemia.[114] This neuropathy may affect the motor nerve supply of small intrinsic muscles of the foot, may cause diminished sensory perception (absence of pain), or may damage the sympathetic nerve supply, which can result in an absence of sweating. This leads to dry cracked skin which can become secondarily infected.

Atherosclerosis is more common in the diabetic than in the nondiabetic; it appears at a younger age and progresses more rapidly. Also, diabetics and nondiabetics differ in regard to which blood vessels are involved and the extent of the involvement. Diabetics may have problems with small vessels (microangiopathy) and large vessels (macroangiopathy) that can result in varying degrees of ischemia, ultimately leading to infections.

Diabetic patients may have normal humoral immunity, normal levels of immunoglobulins, and a normal antibody response. The defect in host defense mechanisms appears to be at the cellular level.[114] Patients with hyperglycemia have been documented to have impaired phagocytosis and intracellular microbicidal function compared with nondiabetics.[115] The exact defects in the host defense system of diabetics are not completely understood.

Although the bacteriology of the diabetic foot infection has been known to be polymicrobic (an average of 2.5 to 5.8 isolates per culture), it has only been within the last 10 years that the true spectrum of microorganisms present has come to be appreciated. Previously, the emphasis was on the importance of *Staphylococcus aureus*, streptococci, and aerobic gram-negative bacilli in causing infections of the lower extremities of diabetics. Recently, with the advent of more sophisticated culture techniques, obligate anaerobes have been shown to have a significant part in the bacterial flora of these infections.[112,116,117] The most common aerobic isolates are *Proteus mirabilis*, group D streptococcus, *Escherichia coli*, and *Staphylococcus aureus*. The principal anaerobic isolate was *Bacteroides fragilis*, followed by *Peptococcus* and *Peptostreptococcus*.

Superficial culturing of the infected wound is not very reliable. The correlation between superficial culturing techniques and a true deep culture (via biopsy) is poor.[117] Therefore, cultures and sensitivity tests should be done preferably with deep culture materials.

Clinical signs and symptoms of infection of the diabetic foot may not be present secondary to the angiopathy and neuropathy. Often when the infection is noticed it is even more extensive than it appears. Certain lesions are typical of diabetic foot infections; these include paronychia (infection of the soft tissue adjacent to the nail), infections of the middle foot secondary to painless trauma, a toe web space infection, or a mal perforans puncture wound (infection of the sole of the foot over the head of the metatarsals). Diabetic foot infections may be further complicated by necrotizing skin and soft tissue infections and/or osteomyelitis. Osteomyelitis is one of the most serious complications of foot care in diabetic patients. In one review, roughly one third of 247 patients with osteomyelitis were diabetic.[118]

In the treatment of diabetic foot infections the use of intravenous antibiotics alone often is not adequate. In addition to the need for local wound care, immobilization of the extremity in question, control of hyperglycemia (some researchers feel that serum glucose below 200 mg/dL will avoid problems with phagocytosis), drainage, debridement, and amputation are often necessary.

Knowledge of the polymicrobic flora involved in these infections is useful in determining the most appropriate approach to antibiotic therapy. Considering that an average of 2.5 to 5.8 organisms per specimen are present, various antibiotic regimens have been advocated by many researchers. Suggested therapy has included such regimens as gentamicin plus ampicillin,[117] cloxacillin plus kanamycin,[119] gentamicin plus clindamycin,[114] or just one of the penicillinase-resistant penicillins alone.[120] Some of these regimens are inadequate, as they evolved prior to newer culture techniques that demonstrated the importance of anaerobes; others may place the patient at a greater risk for toxicity. When an aminoglycoside is used in these patients, care must be taken to avoid compromising renal function because they may already have an underlying component of diabetic nephropathy.

Recently, data have been presented showing that the use of single broad-spectrum $\beta$-lactam antibiotics[112,114,121,122] along with appropriate medical and/or surgical management is effective. The use of cefoxitin as the antibiotic of choice has been evaluated in three studies,[112,121,122] one of which is the only completed double-blind study[122] concerning this topic. These studies have shown that cefoxitin therapy will result in anywhere from a 60% to 90% microbiologic or clinical cure in treated patients. One study[122] compared ceftizoxime to cefoxitin in 53 patients with either diabetic or peripheral vascular disease lower extremity infections. Although clinical responses were satisfactory in 82% of patients treated with ceftizoxime, compared with 68% for cefoxitin, these differences were not statistically significant.

Initial (empiric) therapy for diabetics requiring hospitalization for lower extremity infections should be cefoxitin 2 g every 6 hours (or ceftizoxime 2 g every 8 hours, as determined by cost), adjusted as necessary for renal dysfunction. As deep wound tissue culture information becomes available and the clinical condition of the patient is assessed, the therapy should be changed accordingly.

## Burn Wound Infections

A number of physiologic alterations are observed in severely burned patients. These changes include dramatic shifts in body fluids and electrolytes because of increased capillary permeability,[123] airway distress from direct thermal injury,[124] increases in metabolic rate,[125] and sepsis.[126] Infection coupled with multiorgan system failure in patients with burns over more than 40% of their total body surface area is the major cause of death. The most reasonable way to prevent the sequelae of the burn wound infection is to prevent the burn wound from becoming infected.

### *Pathophysiology/Etiology*

The burn patient is predisposed to infection for three reasons: (1) breakdown of the skin's protective barrier; (2) formation by the coagulated skin and exudate (eschar) of an excellent growth medium for bacteria; and (3) depression of nonspecific, humoral, and cellular immunologic function.

Phagocytic cells (i.e., polymorphonuclear leukocytes, neutrophils, monocytes) migrate to an injured area to kill invading organisms. The burn patient may have impaired polymorphonuclear leukocyte chemotactic function, resulting in an inability to phagocytose and destroy the opportunistic organism. This impaired function is directly related to burn size and the patient's prognosis.[127] In addition, serum complement levels are diminished, resulting in impaired migration of phagocytic cells to the area of damage.

Thermal injury also impairs the majority of functions within the immune system. Burns covering more than 20% of the body surface dramatically impair T-cell lymphocyte function. T cells are responsible for recognizing antigens (i.e., bacteria) and stimulating B-cell lymphocytes to differentiate and promote antibody formation. Therefore, T cell depression may impair nearly all immune functions. T suppressor cells normally act as a protective mechanism to prevent overzealous immunologic responses. The functioning of these cells is impaired with burn injury. The humoral system of a burn patient is also affected. Decreased amounts of fibronectin and $\gamma$-globulin have been reported.[128]

Most burn wounds are initially free of major contamination from bacteria, as the heat encountered destroys not only the cutaneous elements but also the surface microorganisms. Normally, the burn wound becomes colonized with bacteria within 48 hours of the injury. These burn areas are almost always colonized by organisms from the patient's own gastrointestinal tract. Within the first 48 hours, gram-positive bacteria proliferate and anytime thereafter gram-negative bacteria can be found within the burn wound.

The causative microorganisms in burn wound infections are not constant but continually changing.[129] Prior to the availability of penicillin, gram-positive bacteria were the most frequently isolated microorganism. The majority of burn wound infections are now caused primarily by gram-negative bacteria. Initially, *Pseudomonas aeruginosa* was the most common bacteria identified; however, the use of potent antibiotics has reduced its overall incidence. No single strain is responsible for the majority of burn wound infections. Some other commonly isolated gram-negative bacteria include *Enterobacter cloacae*, *Providencia stuartii*, *Serratia marcescens*, and *Klebsiella* sp.

If the bacterial concentration at the burn site exceeds $10^5$ microorganisms per gram of tissue, then spread to viable tissue and bacteremia usually occur.[129] This process of seeding the systemic circulation with organisms from the burn site is termed *burn wound sepsis*. Burn wound sepsis is characterized by deterioration of the burn wound and, subsequently, signs of systemic sepsis.

### *Treatment*

The full impact of a particular mode of therapy in the burn patient is difficult to determine because of the influence of various treatment modalities on the profoundly altered host defense systems. Nutrition, burn wound excision, debridement, and topical and/or systemic antibiotic therapy may all improve the functioning of the immune system and therefore affect outcome.

One of the major goals of burn wound therapy is to prevent the wound from becoming infected. Therapy includes prompt removal of necrotic tissue from the burn injury and immediate closure of the wound with skin grafts. One of the main methods for controlling burn wound sepsis is prevention of local burn wound infection with the appropriate topical antibiotics. The use of topical antibiotics is aimed at controlling the rate of bacterial proliferation in the burn to allow the injury to heal (form granulation tissue) without leading to systemic sepsis. The use of topical antimicrobial agents has led to a decreased incidence of conversion of partial-thickness to full-thickness wounds by local infection.

Several topical antibiotics have been used effectively in preventing bacterial proliferation within the burn wound. The four most commonly used products are described here.

***Silver sulfadiazine*** One of the most commonly used topical agents, silver sulfadiazine has demonstrated bacteriostatic activity against most gram-positive and gram-negative bacteria.[130] After removal of the serous discharge and as much of the eschar as possible, 3 mm of silver sulfadiazine is applied to the burn area twice daily. The area either may be covered with a light dressing or may be left uncovered (this allows for free range of motion). This agent does not penetrate deep extensive burns. Allergic skin reactions have been reported in approximately 1.3% of patients.[130] Leukopenia may occur early in therapy (approximately 5% incidence); however, it is usually reversible and may not necessitate withdrawal of the drug. Many patients report a soothing effect at the burn site upon application of the drug. Those involved with routine application of this drug should wear protective gloves. Bacterial resistance to silver sulfadiazine has been reported.[131] To avoid this some centers have begun to alternate silver sulfadiazine with other agents such as sodium mafenide (sodium mafenide in the morning and silver sulfadiazine in the evenings). Silver sulfadiazine is most useful as a prophylactic agent, prior to major bacterial colonization of the burn wound site, because of its poor ability to penetrate the eschar.

***Sodium Mafenide*** This agent is effective against most gram-positive and gram-negative microorganisms including anaerobes. At present few reports of resistance have been documented. One of its unique properties is its ability to almost totally penetrate the eschar.[131] After the area is cleaned, this agent should be applied to a depth of 3 mm; the site either may be left uncovered or may be covered with a light dressing (apply twice daily). Mafenide usually causes pain at the wound site when applied, which may last between 30 and 60 minutes. In addition, approximately 5% of patients develop an allergic reaction (a macular papular rash) to this drug.[131] Those applying the cream should wear gloves. Both mafenide and its metabolite (*p*-carboxybenzenesulfonamide, a deaminated metabolite) are carbonic anhydrase inhibitors; therefore, absorption may cause a metabolic acidosis. Postburn hyperventilation may be accentuated by the metabolic acidosis caused by mafenide. Mafenide is used as a topical agent in burn wound therapy when bacteria resistant to silver sulfadiazine have been isolated and when rapid penetration of a thick eschar is necessary.[132] Because of mafenide's ability to penetrate the eschar, it is useful in the presence of a thick eschar (as in electrical burns).

***Silver Nitrate*** A 0.5% concentration of silver nitrate is effective against most gram-positive and gram-negative microorganisms including some *Pseudomonas* strains. This drug should be used early to prevent bacterial growth as well as to delay the separation of dead tissue. Once bacterial growth has occurred, silver nitrate will not be effective for bacterial killing, as it does not penetrate tissues well. Although it is painless and does not cause local allergic reactions, hyponatremia and hypochloremia may occur. Other problems include staining of surrounding skin (as well as sheets and other hospital supplies) and methemoglobinemia. The need for bulky wet dressings and side effects limit silver nitrate's role in the therapy of burn patients.[132]

***Povidone–Iodine and Gentamicin Cream*** These agents have been used in the treatment of burn patients but have limited usefulness. Povidone-iodine does not penetrate the eschar and may cause local pain because of its drying effect. A rise in protein-bound iodine may also occur. Povidone–iodine should not be used if the burn occupies greater than 20% of the total body surface, as the resultant absorption may lead to metabolic acidosis[133] and renal failure. Povidone–iodine's most useful role is in the treatment of small burn areas as an aid in drying out and healing grafts. Gentamicin cream may produce bacterial resistance, especially to *Pseudomonas* strains. Treating large burn areas with gentamicin cream may lead to systemic absorption with the risk of ototoxicity and nephrotoxicity.

***Other Agents*** Use of systemic antibiotics with the intent of avoiding burn wound infection is not recommended. Prophylactic systemic antibiotic administration has been advocated in an attempt to prevent the development of cellulitis. Currently, most data do not support the prophylactic use of antibiotics (penicillin) to prevent cellulitis (caused by group A $\beta$-hemolytic streptococci) because such use may result in superinfections or the emergence of resistant microorganisms.[126–128] Centers that have discontinued the use of prophylactic antibiotics have not witnessed any significant increase in streptococcal cellulitis[126,134,135]; however, one group of researchers has documented delayed wound colonization and decreased incidence of burn wound sepsis after a prophylactic oral antibiotic regimen (neomycin–erythromycin–nystatin). But it must be pointed out that all patients were treated within a laminar-flow environment.

When burn wound infections do occur, they are commonly caused by a single strain of gram-negative bacteria.[136] Biopsy specimens of a suspected infection site producing 100,000 or more bacteria per gram of tissue indicate infection that requires aggressive therapy. In addition to surgical excision to the fascial plane, systemic antibiotic therapy should be instituted. Antibiotic selection should be directed toward the organism isolated by Gram stain of the biopsy specimen or the most likely pathogen for the specific burn unit. The value of administration of local antibiotic directly into burn tissue having minimal or no vascularity is not known. Use of aminoglycosides is the mainstay of therapy but is complicated because of the altered pharmacokinetics in burn patients.[137] Usually, acceptable aminoglycoside doses have been reported to result in low serum concentrations and may potentially lead to suboptimal treatment and clinical failure. The aminoglycoside half-life in the burn patient has been documented to be unusually short, especially in young patients. These patients therefore require aggressive initial therapy, with early serum concentration determinations to individualize therapy.

Burn patients may also encounter difficulty with fungal infections. Wound discoloration to a dark, infected-appearing tissue should raise the suspicion of a fungal infection. Confirmation of a fungal wound infection is best made by biopsy of the tissue. Common organisms causing fungal infections include *Aspergillus, Mucor, Candida,* and *Geotrichum* species. The treatment of choice for a fungal infection is extensive surgical excision and debridement to noninfected tissues. Systemic or topical therapy is directed toward the offending pathogen and plays only a secondary role. If a clinical picture consistent with systemic fungal sepsis is present or blood cultures are positive for fungi, systemic antifungal therapy (usually with amphotericin B) is required.

## References


1. Simmons RL, Ahrenholz DH. Infections of skin and soft tissues, in Simmons RL, Howard RJ (eds): Surgical Infections. New York, Appleton-Century-Crofts, 1982, pp 507–683.
2. Roettinger W, Edgerton MT, Kurtz LD, et al. Role of inoculation site as a determinant of infection in soft tissue wounds. Am J Surg 1973;126:354–358.
3. Ducan WC, McBride ME, Knox JM. Experimental production of infection in humans. J Invest Dermatol 1970;54:319–323.

4. Noble WC, Somerville DA. Microbiology of the Human Skin. Philadelphia, W.B. Saunders, 1974.
5. Hook EW, Hooton TM, Horton C, et al. Microbiologic evaluation of cutaneous cellulitis in adults. Arch Intern Med 1986; 146:295–297.
6. Ferriere P. Acute post-streptococcal glomerulonephritis and its relationship to the epidemiology of streptococcal infections. Minn Med 1975;58:598–602.
7. Uman SJ, Kunin CM. Needle aspiration in the diagnosis of soft tissue infections. Arch Intern Med 1975;135:959–961.
8. Nelson J, Ginsburg C. An hypothesis on the pathogenesis of *Hemophilus influenzae* buccal cellulitis. J Pediatr 1976;88:709–710.
9. Granoff C, Nankerves G. Cellulitis due to HF type B antigemia and antibody responses. Am J Dis Child 1976;130:1211–1214.
10. Swartz MN. Cellulitis and superficial infections, in Mandell GL, Douglas RG, Bennett JE (eds): Principles and Practice of Infectious Diseases, 2nd ed. New York, John Wiley and Sons, 1979, pp 598–609.
11. Magnussen CR. Skin and soft tissue infections, in Reese R, Douglas G (eds): A Practical Approach to Infectious Diseases, 2nd ed. Boston, Little, Brown, 1983, pp 239–265.
12. Peter G, Smith A. Group A streptococcal infections of the skin and pharynx. N Engl J Med 1977;297:311–317.
13. Goepel JR, Richards DG, Harris DM, et al. Fulminant *Streptococcus pyogenes* infection. Br Med J 1980;281:1412.
14. Katz S, Klein J, Yow M, et al. Ampicillin resistant strains of HF type B. Pediatrics 1975;55:145–146.
15. Slaughter R, Pieper J, Cerra F, et al. Chloramphenicol sodium succinate kinetics in the critically ill patient. Clin Pharmacol Ther 1982;28:69–77.
16. Kauffman R, Tirumoosthi M, Buckley J, et al. Relative bioavailability of intravenous chloramphenicol succinate and oral chloramphenicol palmitate in infants and children. J Pediatr 1981;99:963–967.
17. Marks M, LaFerriere C. Chloramphenicol: recent developments and clinical indications. Clin Pharm 1982;1:315–320.
18. Brasfield J, Record K, Griffen W, et al. Chloramphenicol and chloramphenicol succinate concentration in patients with renal impairment. Clin Pharm 1983;2:355–358.
19. Azzollini F, Gazzanega A, Lodola E, et al. Elimination of chloramphenicol and thiamphenicol in subjects with cirrhosis of the liver. Int J Clin Pharmacol 1976;6:130–143.
20. Feder HM, Osier C, Madefazo EG. Chloramphenicol: a review of its use in clinical practice. Rev Infect Dis 1981;3:479–491.
21. Swartz M. Lymphadenitis and lymphangitis, in Mandell GL, Douglas RG, Bennett JE (eds): Principles and Practice of Infectious Diseases. New York, John Wiley and Sons, 1985, pp 618–624.
22. Dajani AS, Garcia RE, Wolinski E. Etiology of lymphadenitis in children. N Engl J Med 1963;268:1329–1341.
23. Thompson J. Pathological changes in mummies. Proc R Soc Med 1961;54:409–415.
24. Davis JS. The operative treatment of scars following bed sores. Surgery 1938;3:1–7.
25. Peterson NC, Bittmann B. The epidemiology of pressure sores. Scand J Plast Reconstr Surg 1971;6:62–66.
26. Barbenel JC, Horden MM, Nicol SM, et al. Incidence of pressure sores in the Greater Glasgow Health Board area. Lancet 1977;2:548–550.
27. Manley MT. Incidence, contributory factors and costs of pressure sores. S Afr Med J 1978;53:217–222.
28. Sather MR, Weba CE, George J. Pressure sores and the spinal cord injury patient. Drug Intell Clin Pharm 1977;11:154–169.
29. Parish LC, Witkowski JA. Coping with decubitus ulcers. Drug Ther 1979;9:133–136.
30. Daniel R, Hall E, MacLeod M. Pressure sores—a reappraisal. Ann Plast Surg 1979;3:53–63.
31. Kosiak M, Kubicek WG, Olson M, et al. Evaluation of pressure as a factor in the production of ischial ulcers. Arch Phys Med Rehabil 1958;39:623–629.
32. Kosiak M. Etiology of decubitus ulcers. Arch Phys Med Rehabil 1961;42:19–29.
33. Reichel SM. Shearing force as a factor in decubitus ulcers in paraplegics. JAMA 1958;166:762–763.
34. Reuler JB, Cooney TG. The pressure sore: pathophysiology and principles of management. Ann Intern Med 1981;94:661–666.
35. Shea JD. Pressure sores—classification and management. Clin Orthop 1975;112:89–100.
36. Galpen JE, Chow AW, Bayer AS, et al. Sepsis associated with decubitus ulcers. Am J Med 1976;61:346–350.
37. Sugarmann B, Haives S, Musher D, et al. Osteomyelitis beneath pressure sores. Ann Intern Med 1983;143:683–688.
38. Cooney TG, Reuler JB. Pressure sores. West J Med 1984;140: 622–624.
39. Dinsdale SM. Decubitus ulcers: role of pressure and function in causation. Arch Phys Med Rehabil 1974;55:147–152.
40. Antypas PG. Management of pressure sores. Curr Probl Surg 1980;17:229–244.
41. Morgan JE. Topical therapy of pressure ulcers. Surg Gynecol Obstet 1975;141:945–947.
42. Morgan JE. Topical therapy of pressure sores. Surg Gynecol Obstet 1975;141:945–947.
43. Carpendale M. A comparison of four beds in the prevention of tissue ischemia in paraplegic patients. Paraplegia 1974;12:21–32.
44. Alvarez OM, Mertz AM, Englstein WH. The effect of occlusive dressings on collagen synthesis and re-epithelialization in superficial wounds. J Surg Res 1983;35:142–148.
45. Stuzin J, Engrav L, Buehler P. Care of open wounds. Compr Ther 1982;8:32–34.
46. Nierman MM. Treatment of dermal and decubitus ulcers. Drugs 1978;15:226–230.
47. Varma AO, Burgatch E, German FM. Debridement of dermal ulcers with collagenase. Surg Gynecol Obstet 1973;136:281–282.
48. Lee LK, Ambrus JL. Collagenase therapy for decubitus ulcers. Geriatrics 1975;(May):91–98.
49. Rao DB, Sane P, Georgien EL. Collagenase in the treatment of dermal and decubitus ulcers. J Am Geriatr Soc 1975;23:22–24.
50. Coopwood TB. Evaluation of a topical enzymatic debridement agent—Sutilains ointment. South Med J 1976;69:834.
51. Rodeheaver G, Wheeler C, Reye G, et al. Side effects of topical proteolytic enzyme treatment. Surg Gynecol Obstet 1979;148:562–566.
52. Heel RC, Morton P, Brogden RN, et al. Dextranomer: A review of its general properties and therapeutic efficacy. Drugs 1979;18:89–102.
53. Jacobson S, Rothman V, Arturson G, et al. A new principle for cleaning of infected wounds. Scand J Plast Reconstructr Surg 1976a;10:97–101.
54. Fleden CH, Wilkstrom K. Controlled trial with dextranomer (Debrisan) on venous leg ulcers. Curr Ther Res 1978;24:753–760.
55. Parish LC, Collins E. Decubitus ulcers: a comparative study. Cutis 1979;23:106–110.
56. Longe RL. Current concepts in clinical therapeutics: pressure sores. Clin Pharm 1986;5:669–681.

57. Daltrey DC, Rhodes B, Chattwood JG. Investigation into the microbial flow of healing and non-healing decubitus ulcers. J Clin Pathol 1981;34:701–705.
58. Conolly WB, Hunt TK, Dunphy JE. Management of contaminated surgical wounds. Surg Gynecol Obstet 1969;135:593–601.
59. Branemack PI, Ekholm R, Albrektsaen B, et al. Tissue injury caused by wound disinfectants. J Bone Joint Surg 1967;49A: 46–62.
60. Geronemus R, Mertz P, Eaglstein W. Wound healing. The effects of topical antimicrobial agents. Arch Dermatol 1979; 115:1311–1314.
61. Dennis D, Luterman A, Ramenofsky F, et al. Does PVP–iodine interfere with wound healing? Infect Surg 1983;4:371–374.
62. Wallace G, Hayter J. Karaya for chronic skin ulcers. Am J Nurs 1974;74:1094–1098.
63. Trouillet J, Chastie J, Fagen J, et al. Use of granulated sugar in treatment of open mediastinitis after cardiac surgery. Lancet 1985;2:180–184.
64. Gordon H, Middleton K, Seal D, et al. Sugar and wound healing. (Lett) Lancet 1985;2:663–664.
65. Rostenberg A, Wasserman E, Medansky R. Sugar paste in the treatment of leg ulcers. Arch Dermatol 1985;78:94.
66. Verkonick PJ. A preliminary report of decubitus care. Am J Nurs 1961;61:68–69.
67. Addison MK, Walterspiel J. Sugar and wound healing. (Lett) Lancet 1985;2:665.
68. Gerber RM, Van Ort SR. Topical application of insulin in decubitus ulcers. Nurs Res 1979;28:16–19.
69. Freeman LW, Joyner JF. Adsorbable gelatin sponge in the treatment of decubitus ulcers. JAMA 1963;184–188.
70. Pace WE. Treatment of cutaneous ulcers with benzoylperoxide. Can Med Assoc J 1976;115:1101–1106.
71. Braverman AM, Nasar MA. The treatment of superficial decubitus ulcers. Practitioner 1981;225:1842–1843.
72. Nasar MA. Treating pressure sores. (Lett) Br Med J 1978;1: 1624–1625.
73. Olenjniczaks S, Zrelinski A. Topical oxygen promotes healing of leg ulcers. Resident Staff Physician 1977;23:165–242.
74. Fischer BH. Topical hyperbaric oxygen treatment of pressure sores and skin ulcers. Lancet 1969;2:405–409.
75. White AG. Medical disorders in drug addicts. JAMA 1973;223: 1469–1471.
76. Webb D, Thadepalli H. Skin and soft-tissue polymicrobial infections from intravenous abuse of drugs. West J Med 1979; 130:200–204.
77. Orangio GR, Pitlick SD, Latta PD, et al. Soft-tissue infections in parenteral drug abusers. Ann Surg 1984;199:97–100.
78. Moustoukas N, Nichols R, Smith J, et al. Contaminated street heroin. Relationship to clinical infections. Arch Surg 1983;118: 746–749.
79. Tuazon CV, Hill R, Sheayren JN. Microbiologic study of street heroin and injection paraphernalia. J Infect Dis 1974;1299:327–329.
80. Tuazon CV, Sheagren JN. Increased rate of carriage of *Staphylococcus aureus* among narcotic addicts. J Infect Dis 1974; 129:725–727.
81. Haw T, Kallick C. Surgical infection in drug addicts. World J Surg 1980;4:403–413.
82. Crane L, Levine D, Aervos M, et al. Bacteremia in narcotic addicts at Detroit Medical Center. Microbiology, epidemiology, risk factors, and empiric therapy. Rev Infect Dis 1986;8: 364–373.
83. Markowitz N, Pohlod D, Saravolatz L, et al. In vitro susceptibility patterns of methicillin-resistant and susceptible *Staphylococcus aureus* strains in a population of parenteral drug abusers from 1972 to 1981. Antimicrob Agents Chemother 1983;23:450–457.
84. King CH, Creger RJ, Ellner JJ. Pharmacokinetics of tobramycin and gentamicin in abusers of intravenous drugs. Antimicrob Agents Chemother 1985;27:285–290.
85. Louria D. Surgical infections in drug addicts (invited commentary). World J Surg 1980;4:412–413.
86. Callaham M. Dog bites. JAMA 1980;244:2327–2328.
87. Harris D, Imperato PJ, Oken B. Dog bites—an unrecognized epidemic. Bull NY Acad Med 1974;50:981–1000.
88. Goldstein EJC, Citron DM, Finegold SM. Dog bite wounds and infection: a prospective clinical study. Ann Emerg Med 1980;9:508–512.
89. Callaham ML. Treatment of common dog bites: infection risk factors. JACEP 1978;7:83–87.
90. Rest JG, Goldstein EJC. Management of human and animal bite wounds. Emerg Med Clin North Am 1985;3:117–126.
91. Goldstein EJC, Citron DM, Finegold SM. Role of anaerobic bacteria in bite wound infections. Rev Infect Dis 1984;6(suppl 1):s177–s183.
92. Baile WE, Stowe EC, Schmitt AM. Aerobic bacterial flora of oral and nasal fluids of canines with reference to bacteria associated with bites. J Clin Microbiol 1978;7:223–231.
93. Saphir DA, Carter GR. Gingival flora of the dog with special reference to bacteria associated with bites. J Clin Microbiol 1976;3:344–349.
94. Lee M, Buhr A. Dog bites and local infections with *Pasteurella septica*. Br Med J 1960;1:169–171.
95. Callaham ML. Prophylactic antibiotics in common dog bite wounds: A controlled study. Ann Emerg Med 1980;9:410–414.
96. Goldstein EJC. Bites, in: Mandell GL, Douglas RG, Bennett JE (eds): Principles and Practice of Infectious Diseases. New York, John Wiley and Sons, 1985, 632–635.
97. Elenbass RM, McNaoney WK, Robinson WA. Prophylactic oxacillin in dog bite wounds. Ann Emerg Med 1982;11:248–251.
98. Elliot DL, Tolle SW, Goldberg L, et al. Pet-associated illness. N Engl J Med 1985;313:985–995.
99. Nunley D, Suski T, Atkins A, et al. Hand infections in hospitalized patients. Am J Surg 1980;140:374–376.
100. Centers for Disease Control, Advisory Committee. Diphtheria, tetanus, and pertussis guidelines for vaccine prophylaxis and other preventive measures. Ann Intern Med 1981;95:723–728.
101. Rabies—United States. MMWR 1982;31:379–380.
102. Mann RJ, Hoffeld TA, Farmer CB. Human bites of the hand: Twenty years of experience. J Hand Surg 1977;2:97–99.
103. Brook I. Bacteriologic study of paronychia in children. Am J Surg 1981;141:703–705.
104. Goldstein EJC, Citron DM, Wield B, et al. Bacteriology of human and animal bite wounds. J Clin Microbiol 1978;8:667–672.
105. Peeples E, Boswick JA, Scott FA. Wounds of the hand contaminated by human and animal saliva. J Trauma 1980;20: 383–389.
106. Goldstein E, Gombert M, Agyare E. Susceptibility of *Eikenella corrodens* to newer beta-lactam antibiotics. Antimicrob Agents Chemother 1980;18:832–833.
107. Goldstein E, Miller T, Citron D, et al. Infections following clenched-fist injury: A new perspective. J Hand Surg 1978;3: 455–459.
108. Goldstein E, Barene M, Miller TA. *Eikenella corrodens* in hand infections. J Hand Surg 1983;8:563–566.
109. Dinerstein C, Mason R, Giron F. Lower extremity complications of diabetes mellitus. Surg Rounds 1984;7(7):26–41.

110. Gocke T. Infections complicating diabetes mellitus, in Grieco M (ed): Infections in the Abnormal Host. New York, Yorke Medical Books, 1982, pp 585–600.
111. Levin M, Boniuk I, Anderson C, et al. Prevention and treatment of diabetic complications. Arch Intern Med 1980;140: 691–696.
112. LeFrock J, Blais F, Schell RF, et al. Cefoxitin in the treatment of diabetic patients with lower extremity infections. Infect Surg 1983;2:361–374.
113. Pratt T. Gangrene and infections in the diabetic. Med Clin North Am 1965;49:987–1004.
114. LeFrock JL, Joseph WS. Lower extremity infections in diabetics. Infect Surg 1986;5:135–145.
115. Bagdade JO, Root RK, Bilger RJ. Impaired leukocyte function in patients with poorly controlled diabetes. Diabetes 1974;23: 9–15.
116. Louie JT, Bartlet JG, Tally FP, et al. Aerobic and anaerobic bacteria in diabetic foot ulcers. Ann Intern Med 1976;85:461–463.
117. Sharp CS, Bessman AN, Wagner FW, et al. Microbiology of deep and superficial tissues in infected diabetic gangrene. Surg Gynecol Obstet 1979;149:217–219.
118. Waldvogel FA, McDoff G, Swartz MN. Osteomyelitis: A review of clinical features, therapeutic considerations and unusual aspects. N Engl J Med 1970;282:198–216.
119. Little JR, Kobayski GS. Bacteriology and infection of the diabetic foot, in Levin ME, O'Neal W (eds): The Diabetic Foot, 2nd ed. St. Louis, C.V. Mosby, 1977, pp 97–105.
120. Williams HT, Hutchinson KJ, Brown GD, et al. Gangrene of the foot in diabetics. Arch Surg 1974;108:609–612.
121. Fierer J, Daniel D, Davis C. The fetid foot: lower-extremity infections in patients with diabetes mellitus. Rev Infect Dis 1979;1:210–217.
122. Hughes C, Johnson C, Bamberger D, et al. A randomized double-blind trial of ceftizoxime vs cefoxitin for therapy of lower extremity infections in patients with diabetes mellitus and/or peripheral vascular disease. Proceedings of the 14th International Congress of Chemotherapy, Kyoto, Japan, 1985, pp 2331–2332.
123. Arturson G. Microvascular permeability to macromolecules in thermal injury. Acta Physiol Scand 1979;463(suppl):111–122.
124. Reed GF, Camp HL. Upper airway problems in severely burned patients. Ann Otol 1969;78:741–751.
125. Wilmore DW, Long JC, Mason AD, et al. Catecholamines: mediator of the hypermetabolic response to thermal injury. Ann Surg 1974;180:653–669.
126. Shires G, Dineen P. Sepsis following burns, trauma, and intra-abdominal infections. Arch Intern Med 1982;142:2012–2022.
127. Warden GD, Mason AD, Pruitt BA. Suppression of leukocyte chemotaxis in vitro by chemotherapeutic agents used in the management of thermal injuries. Ann Surg 1975;181:363–369.
128. Lanser ME, Saba TM, Scovill WA. Opsonic glycoprotein (plasma fibronectin) levels after burn injury: Relationship to extent of burn and development of sepsis. Ann Surg 1980;192: 776–782.
129. Lindberg RB, Moncreif JA, Mason AD. Control of experimental and clinical wound sepsis by topical application of sulfamylon compounds. Ann NY Acad Sci 1986;150:950–960.
130. Pegg SP. The role of drugs in the management of burns. Drugs 1982;24:256–260.
131. Pegg SP, Ramsay K, Meldrum L, et al. Clinical comparison of maphenide and silver sulphadiazine. Scand J Plast Reconstr Surg 1979;13:95–101.
132. Yurt R, Shires G. Burns, in Mandel G, Douglas R, Bennett J (eds): Principles and Practice of Infectious Diseases, 2nd ed. New York, John Wiley and Sons, 1985, pp 628–632.
133. Pretsch J, Meakins JL. Complications of providing iodine absorption in topically treated burn patients. Lancet 1976;1: 280–282.
134. Drutschi MB, Orgain C, Counts GW, et al. A prospective study of prophylactic penicillin in acutely burned hospitalized patients. J Trauma 1982;22:11–14.
135. Harburchak DR, Pruitt BA. Use of systemic antibiotics in the burned patient. Surg Clin North Am 1978;58:1119–1132.
136. Aurreri PW. Overview of recent progress in the treatment of burn wound infection. J Trauma 1981;21(suppl):674–676.
137. Zaske DE, Sawchuk RJ, Gerding DN, et al. Increased dosage requirements of gentamicin in burn patients. J Trauma 1976;16:824–828.

# Chapter 79 / Infective Endocarditis

Joseph T. DiPiro, PharmD, and John Fisher, MD

*Endocarditis* refers to inflammation of the endocardium, the membrane lining the chambers of the heart and covering the cusps of the heart valves. The term *infective endocarditis* more specifically refers to the syndrome resulting from colonization or invasion of the endocardium, especially the heart valves themselves, by various types of microorganisms. Other terms such as acute and subacute bacterial endocarditis have been based upon presentation of the disease. Acute bacterial endocarditis is a fulminating endocardial infection associated with high fevers, systemic toxicity, and death within a few days to weeks. This syndrome is most frequently observed with infection of previously normal valves caused by notoriously virulent bacteria such as *Staphylococcus aureus*, *Streptococcus pyogenes* (group A β-hemolytic streptococci), *Streptoccus pneumoniae* (pneumococcus), and *Neisseria gonorrhoeae*. Subacute bacterial endocarditis is considered to be a more indolent infection caused by less invasive organisms such as viridans streptococci, occurring in a setting of prior valvular heart disease. It has become increasingly clear that the clinical presentation is not a reliable indicator of the causative organisms and much overlap exists. In addition, fungal endocarditis has become more common. Therefore, the more encompassing term *infective endocarditis* is preferred.

Endocarditis may be associated with prosthetic heart valves that are placed for native valvular dysfunction. Prosthetic valvular endocarditis may be referred to as "early" if it occurs within 60 days of surgery or "late" if it occurs more than 60 days after surgery.

## Epidemiology and Etiology

Although infective endocarditis is not considered a common problem, it has been reported as a diagnosis in 1 of 1,000 hospital admissions (range: 0.16 to 5.4 per 1,000).[1,2] The disorder is more common in males (1.7:1). The majority (54%) of affected patients are 31 to 60 years old, with 26% and 21% of cases occurring in patients less than 30 years and greater than 60 years, respectively.[3] Endocarditis caused by group D streptococci is generally encountered in individuals 61 to 67 years old. Infective endocarditis is relatively uncommon in children.

Prosthetic valve endocarditis has been reported to occur in 1% to 9.4% (average of 2.6%) of patients who have undergone valve replacement.[4] About two thirds of cases occur as late infections, most frequently involving the aortic (59% of cases) or mitral valve (31%).[4]

Numerous factors predisposing to infective endocarditis have been observed. Any type of structural heart disease increases the risk of endocarditis, particularly where there is turbulence of blood flow. Rheumatic heart disease has been associated with 37% to 67% of cases over the past two decades, and congenital heart disease has been associated with 6% to 24% of cases.[2] Even though valvular heart disease is an important factor, in up to 50% of instances there may be no demonstrable predisposing cardiac condition. Other predispositions to infective endocarditis include arteriovenous fistulae (including access for hemodialysis), intracardiac pacemakers and valvular prostheses, and leutic heart disease. Intravascular devices, such as flow-directed, balloon-tipped, and central venous catheters, are associated with nosocomial endocarditis.[5] Finally, intravenous drug abusers are at greater risk of heart valve infection from the systemic introduction of microorganisms by contaminated needles and syringes.

Endocarditis resulting from streptococci and staphylococci accounts for 80% to 90% of infections involving native valves and two thirds of infections involving prosthetic valves, although the list of causative organisms has become increasingly longer (Table 79.1). Coagulase-negative staphylococcus is the primary pathogen in early prosthetic valve endocarditis. In late infections, non–group D streptococci are the most common isolates (29% of cases).[4]

### Streptococci

These organisms are the major cause of infective endocarditis, particularly in patients with valvular heart disease. Viridans streptococci are isolated most frequently. Because streptococci are found as normal flora in many body sites, including the skin, oral cavity, gastrointestinal tract, and vagina, there are many opportunities for these organisms to enter the bloodstream. Enterococci are a less frequently observed, but often more troublesome, cause of endocarditis. Enterococci generally result in endocarditis with a subacute course, and are a more frequent cause of endocarditis in intravenous drug abusers than other streptococci.

### Staphylococci

With regard to incidence, staphylococci are second only to streptococci as a cause of endocarditis. In certain clinical settings, staphylococci are actually more common causes of the disease. For example, in intravenous drug abusers, *S. aureus* is the most frequent organism encountered in valve infections, and coagulase-negative staphylococci are the most frequently recognized cause of prosthetic valve endocarditis recognized after valve replacement. Unlike streptococci, staphylococci frequently cause endocarditis in patients with no previous heart disease. Moreover, the

**Table 79.1** Etiologic Agents in Infective Endocarditis

| | *Percentage of cases* | |
|---|---|---|
| *Organisms* | **Native valves** | **Prosthetic valves (early plus late)** |
| Streptococci | 60–80 | 26 |
| Viridans streptococci | 30–40 | 18 |
| Enterococci | 5–18 | 7 |
| Other streptococci | 15–25 | 1 |
| Staphylococci | 20–35 | 41 |
| Coagulase-positive | 10–27 | 14 |
| Coagulase-negative | 1–3 | 27 |
| Gram-negative bacilli | 1.5–13 | 14 |
| Fungi | 2–4 | 14 |
| Miscellaneous bacteria | <5 | 8 |
| Mixed infections | 1–2 | — |
| "Culture negative" | <5–24 | 2 |

From Gnann JW, Cobbs CG: Infections of prosthetic valves and intravascular devices, in Mandel GL, Douglas RG, Bennett JE (Eds): Principles and Practice of Infectious Diseases. New York, John Wiley and Sons, 1983, pp 530–539, with permission.

mortality rate from staphylococcal endocarditis is very high (about 40%), with the exception of intravenous drug abusers (where the mortality rate is only a few percent).

### Gram-Negative Bacilli

Endocarditis caused by gram-negative bacilli is relatively uncommon; however the incidence appears to be increasing. Patients at higher risk include intravenous drug abusers and those with prosthetic valves. The organism most commonly associated with gram-negative rod endocarditis is *Pseudomonas aeruginosa*. This has become a relatively common pathogen among intravenous drug abusers in the Detroit area.[6] Other gram-negative bacilli associated with endocarditis include other pseudomonads, *Serratia marcescens*, *Escherichia coli*, *Enterobacter*, *Citrobacter*, *Salmonella*, and *Hemophilus*. Generally, these infections have a poor prognosis with mortality rates as high as 60% to 80%.

### Fungi

Fungi are associated with fewer than 3% of cases of endocarditis. Most patients with fungal heart valve infections have undergone recent cardiovascular surgery, are intravenous drug abusers, have received prolonged treatment with intravenous catheters or antibiotics, or have been immunosuppressed. *Candida*, *Histoplasma*, and *Aspergillus* are the most common genera involved, and the underlying mortality is high for the following reasons: (1) the large, bulky vegetations that often form; (2) the tendency for fungi to invade the myocardium; (3) the systemic septic embolization that often occurs; (4) poor penetration of vegetations by antifungals; (5) low toxic/therapeutic ratio of agents such as amphotericin B; and (6) lack of consistent fungicidal activity of available antifungal agents.[7]

## Pathophysiology

The development of infective endocarditis requires the occurrence of several independent factors. Although many questions remain, major factors in the process have been well identified. The steps in the process are as follows:

1. The endothelial surface must be altered to become a suitable site for the adherence of bacteria. This occurs with turbulent blood flow, as with stenotic or insufficient valves and ventricular septal defects. In addition, trauma or exogenous stresses may alter the endothelial surface. Examples of stresses include infection at other sites, hypersensitivity states, cold exposure, simulated high altitude, hormonal manipulations, and cardiac lymphatic obstruction.[8] Changes in endothelial surface have also been observed with malignancies and chronic diseases.
2. With changes in the endothelial surface, platelet and fibrin deposition occurs and these deposits are referred to as nonbacterial thrombotic endocarditis (NBTE). These deposits are believed to be a prerequisite for bacterial adherence to endothelial surfaces.
3. Given a focus of NBTE, and the occurrence of bacteremia, the endocardial surface may become colonized.[9] Most often, bacteremia is the result of trauma to a mucosal surface having a high concentration of resident bacteria, that is, the gastrointestinal tract or genitourinary tract. Procedures most likely to produce transient bacteremia include dental procedures, gastrointestinal procedures, and urologic examinations or operations.[10]
4. All bacteria do not have the same capability to adhere to NBTE. Those most likely to adhere include staphylococci, certain streptococci and other organisms such as *Pseudomonas aeruginosa*.[11] Specific factors, such as dextran production by oral streptococci, allow them to adhere more avidly to NBTE.[12]
5. After colonization of the endothelial surface begins, fibrin and platelets continue to aggregate and a vegetation forms. The protective cover of fibrin and platelets allows unimpeded bacterial growth to concentrations as high as $10^9$ to $10^{10}$ per gram of tissue.

The vegetations that form may be single or multiple and vary in size from a few millimeters to centimeters. Most appear on the atrial surface of the mitral or tricuspid valve or the ventricular surface of the aortic or pulmonic valve. With the formation of vegetations, destruction of underlying valvular tissue may occur. Even with resolution of the process, fibrosis of tissue with some dysfunction may result. Continuing destruction may lead to perforation of the valve leaflet or rupture of the chordae tendoniae, papillary muscle, or even the interventricular septum. Occasionally, valvular stenosis may occur. Abscesses may develop in the valve ring or in myocardial tissue.

Because of the friability of some vegetations, fragments may be released downstream. These infected particles are referred to as septic emboli. These emboli more commonly affect organs with high blood flow, such as kidneys, spleen, brain, or heart, but may involve any tissue of the body resulting in abscess or infarction. Immune phenomena may result from the continuous antigenic stimulus of bacteremia. Immune complexes consisting of antigen, antibody, and complement circulate and may be deposited in organs such as the kidney, producing local inflammation and damage (glomerulonephritis). Other potential pathologic changes include the development of mycotic aneurysms, cerebral infarction, splenic infarctions and abscesses, pulmonary emboli with right-sided endocarditis, and skin manifestations such as petechiae, Osler's nodes, and Janeway's lesions.

The pathogenesis of prosthetic valvular endocarditis (PVE) differs from endocarditis of native valves. With early PVE it is believed that bacteria are introduced during the surgery itself or the perioperative period. Bacteria may originate from the skin of the patient or operating room personnel, from a contaminated bypass pump,[13] or from intravascular catheters, cannulas, and pacemakers that may be used in these patients. The recently placed, nonendothelialized valve is much more susceptible to bacterial colonization than native valves. With late PVE the mechanism is similar to that which occurs in native valve endocarditis. In a patient who has recovered from valve replacement surgery, transient bacteremia may occur as discussed previously, particularly after dental procedures and urologic and gastrointestinal surgery. The bacteria entering the bloodstream may adhere to and colonize the valvular material. With early or late PVE, valve ring abscess or myocardial abscess may develop. Valve dehiscence and incompetence may then result. Large vegetations may encroach on valvular outflow tracts.

## Clinical Presentation

### *Manifestations*

The presentation of patients with endocarditis is highly variable and any organ system may be involved (Table 79.2). Fever is the most common finding and is often accompanied by other nonspecific symptoms. The fever may be relatively low grade, particularly in subacute cases. Heart murmurs are found in 85% of patients at presentation, with a much lower percentage documented as new or changing murmurs. Other common findings include evidence of embolic phenomena (e.g., splenic or renal infarction) and skin manifestations.

Peripheral manifestations of infective endocarditis are common and include skin manifestations such as Osler's nodes, Janeway's spots, splinter hemorrhages, petechiae, as well as clubbing and Roth spots. A brief description of each is provided here.

*Osler's Nodes* Purplish or erythematous subcutaneous papules or nodules that may appear on the pads of the fingers and toes. These lesions may be 2 to 15 mm in size and are painful and tender. These lesions are not specific for infective endocarditis, and may be the result of embolic or immunologic phenomena. They are uncommon in acute endocarditis.

*Janeway's Lesions* Hemorrhagic, painless plaques that may develop on the palms of the hands or soles of the

**Table 79.2** Occurrence of Symptoms and Physical Findings With Infectious Endocarditis

| *Symptom* | *Percentage of patients* | *Physical finding* | *Percentage of patients* |
|---|---|---|---|
| Fever | 80 | Fever | 90 |
| Chills | 40 | Heart murmur | 85 |
| Weakness | 40 | Changing murmur | 5–10 |
| Dyspnea | 40 | New murmur | 3–5 |
| Sweats | 25 | Embolic phenomenon | >50 |
| Anorexia | 25 | Skin manifestations | 18–50 |
| Weight loss | 25 | Osler's nodes | 10–23 |
| Malaise | 25 | Splinter hemorrhages | 15 |
| Cough | 25 | Petechiae | 20–40 |
| Skin lesions | 20 | Janeway's lesion | <10 |
| Stroke | 20 | Splenomegaly | 20–57 |
| Nausea/vomiting | 20 | Septic complications | 20 |
| Headache | 15 | Mycotic aneurysms | 20 |
| Myalgia–arthralgia | 15 | Clubbing | 12–52 |
| Edema | 15 | Retinal lesion | 2–10 |
| Chest pain | 15 | Signs of renal failure | 10–15 |
| Abdominal pain | 10–15 | | |
| Delirium–coma | 10 | | |
| Hemoptysis | 10 | | |
| Back pain | 10 | | |

Adapted from Scheld WM, Sande MA: Endocarditis and intravascular infections, in Mandell GL, Douglas RG, Bennett JE (Eds): Principles and Practice of Infectious Disease, New York, John Wiley and Sons, 1983, pp 504–530, with permission.

feet. These lesions are also believed to be embolic in origin.

*Splinter Hemorrhages* Thin, linear hemorrhages found under the nail beds of the fingers or toes. These lesions are not specific for infective endocarditis and may be the result of traumatic injuries.

*Petechiae* Small, erythematous, hemorrhagic lesions that are not painful or tender. These lesions may appear anywhere on the skin but are more frequent on the anterior trunk. They are nonblanching and resolve after a few days. The buccal mucosa and palate may also be affected.

*Clubbing of the Fingers* Proliferative change in the soft tissues about the terminal phalanges that may be observed in long-standing bacterial endocarditis.

*Roth Spot* Retinal infarct with central pallor and surrounding hemorrhage.

Arthritis, arthralgias, or myalgias occur relatively commonly in infective endocarditis. Up to 44% of patients may have musculoskeletal symptoms with multiple joint involvement sometimes resembling rheumatic fever.[14]

Embolic phenomena may occur in up to one third of cases and may result in significant complications. Renal artery emboli may cause flank pain with hematuria, splenic artery emboli may cause abdominal pain, pulmonary emboli may cause pleuritic pain with hemoptysis, and cerebral emboli may result in hemiplegia or alteration in mental status. Splenomegaly is also a frequent finding and is more common in patients with endocarditis of prolonged duration.

As stated before, the clinical presentation of endocarditis is highly variable and a diagnosis based on clinical findings is unreliable. In some patients, endocarditis may take a rapid and fulminant course ("acute endocarditis"). This severe form often involves normal valves, and is most frequently caused by pyogenic staphylococci, pneumococci, or gonococci. Fever and chills may be prominent, and numerous petechiae and evidence of embolic phenomena may be observed.

In the majority of patients with endocarditis, the disease begins insidiously and gradually worsens. The patient may present with nonspecific findings such as fatigue, weakness, low-grade fever, weight loss, and anorexia, often with arthralgias. Mucocutaneous lesions, as well as clubbing and splenomegaly, may be observed.

Infections of prosthetic valves are also generally indolent and difficult to diagnose. Examination frequently reveals signs of valvular dysfunction (particularly new or changing murmurs), persistent low-grade fever, or splenomegaly. Embolic phenomena and petechiae may also be observed.

In intravenous drug abusers, microorganisms may be introduced through contaminated needles, but most often the causative bacteria are those found on the skin (particularly *Staphylococcus aureus*). These patients are generally young and there is a male predominance. Fever is the most common finding, and often there are pulmonary manifestations (pleuritic chest pain, hemoptysis, increased sputum production). In addition, an extracardiac focus of infection may be found.

### *Laboratory Findings*

Patients with endocarditis virtually always have some laboratory abnormalities; however, many are not specific for endocarditis. For example, a normocytic, normochromic anemia with a low serum iron and low iron-binding capacity is expected as in the anemia of other chronic diseases. Anemia may not be present, however, in more acute presentations.

Despite a continuous bacteremia, leukocytosis is not a prominent finding except in acute endocarditis. The white blood cell count is usually normal or only slightly elevated, sometimes with a mild left shift.

The erythrocyte sedimentation rate (ESR) is elevated in over 90% of patients, although this is a nonspecific marker of inflammation. An increased ESR may be helpful in supporting a diagnosis of endocarditis when used to confirm clinical suspicions. Rheumatoid factor is positive in about one half of patients with endocarditis.

A number of special studies have been devised to aid in the diagnosis of endocarditis. One such study attempts to detect teichoic acid antibodies in the serum. This substance is present in the cell wall of staphylococci and can be detected in 95% of patients with endocarditis caused by staphylococci.[15] As with other tests, this evaluation may serve only to support other clinical evaluations.

### *Blood Cultures*

The location of infected vegetations explains the continuous presence of causative organisms in the bloodstream. Therefore, the majority of blood cultures will yield the culprit microorganism. Collection of two or three separate samples of venous blood for culture during the first 24 hours has been recommended.[16] This is reasonable provided there is no evidence of cardiac decompensation, in which case several samples should be collected for culture and empiric treatment begun immediately. Well over 90% of patients with endocarditis should have a positive blood culture result with three blood samples. If antimicrobials have been administered, the rate of positive cultures declines significantly. Up to five or six blood samples may need to be collected to maximize detection of bacteria. Also, special growth media that contain resins that bind antimicrobials in serum may be used, thereby allowing low numbers of bacteria that may be present to grow. With any venous sampling for blood cultures, it is important that meticulous skin cleansing and sample preparation technique be adhered to so that contamination of culture media by skin bacteria is minimized. In contrast to bacterial valvular infections, only about one half of patients with fungal endocarditis have positive blood cultures.

### *Other Tests*

Echocardiography is often used in identifying and localizing valvular lesions and is helpful for diagnosing endocarditis when blood cultures are negative or in planning for surgical intervention. This technique, however, is not very sensitive for small vegetations.[17] Cardiac catheterization is sometimes performed to determine the need for surgical intervention.

Electrocardiograms and chest roentgenograms may be performed but they are often normal in patients with endocarditis.

### *Prognosis*

Without the use of appropriate antimicrobial therapy and surgical intervention (if required), recovery from infective endocarditis is rare; however, recovery can be expected in most patients with proper management. Factors that increase the mortality from endocarditis include (1) congestive heart failure, (2) culture-negative endocarditis, (3) endocarditis caused by resistant organisms, (4) endocarditis resulting from *Staphylococcus aureus*, (5) fungal endocarditis, and (6) prosthetic valve endocarditis. Indeed, mortality with PVE can be as high as 74% with early PVE and 43% with late PVE.[4]

## Treatment

### *General Considerations*

The most important treatment approaches for infective endocarditis include antimicrobial therapy and surgical intervention. Parenteral antimicrobials should be begun as soon as possible after the diagnosis of endocarditis is established. The antimicrobial agent used should be selected on the basis of culture and susceptibility results, and should be bactericidal. Studies in animals and humans have determined that a prolonged treatment course is necessary to prevent recurrence. If cardiac failure develops or worsens in the face of aggressive and appropriate medical management, then surgical intervention (usually valve replacement) should be considered. In the course of treatment, coincident problems, such as arrhythmias, should be treated with standard measures. The patient with endocarditis may also have renal or central nervous system dysfunction that necessitates an intensive care environment.

### *Surgery*

Surgery is an important aspect in the treatment of endocarditis, and the importance of early surgical intervention in some patients has become well recognized.[18] In most patients, the surgical procedure performed is valve replacement (usually of the aortic valve), with the objective of removing all infected tissues and restoring proper hemodynamic function. The recognized indications for surgical intervention include the following:

- Congestive heart failure
- Evidence of valvular dysfunction
- Multiple septic embolic episodes
- Endocarditis caused by resistant organisms
- Failure of appropriate medical therapy
- Most cases of endocarditis caused by Enterobacteriaceae, *Pseudomonas*, or fungi
- Local suppurative complications such as a myocardial abscess
- Almost all cases of prosthetic valve endocarditis

Replacement of an infected valve under the conditions listed is recommended even in the presence of active and uncontrolled infection. The timing of surgery is determined by the hemodynamic status and not the status of the infection. The major cause of death in these patients is heart failure or the result of septic embolization and not the infection. In fact, when valve replacement surgery is performed in the face of active infection the frequency of reinfection is surprisingly low.[19] The aggressive use of early surgical intervention is particularly important in prosthetic valve endocarditis.[20] If on the basis of valvular function, surgery is deemed to be inevitable, even in a stable patient, recent evidence suggests that early valve replacement is preferable to waiting for the completion of antimicrobial therapy.

### *Antimicrobial Therapy*

The initiation of prompt bactericidal antimicrobial regimens for endocarditis is of utmost importance. Prior to initiation of antimicrobials, adequate blood samples should be collected for culture. Then, during therapy, blood cultures should be repeated at intervals to ensure that bacteremia has ceased. Parenteral antimicrobials are preferred to provide the greatest chance of achieving bactericidal concentrations. For some types of endocarditis, oral regimens may be instituted after a patient is stabilized on a course of parenteral antimicrobials for at least a few weeks. For many pathogens, the use of synergistic antimicrobial combinations will be important. This is particularly true for enterococci, for which combinations of penicillin or ampicillin and aminoglycosides are used, and for methicillin-resistant *Staphylococcus epidermidis*, for which combinations of vancomycin, gentamicin, and rifampin have been used.

A long duration of therapy is required for adequate treatment of infective endocarditis even for very susceptible pathogens. Microorganisms in the vegetations are enclosed in an area where host defenses are impaired and where organized fibrin deposits protect the microorganisms from phagocytic cells.[7] In addition, the concentrations of bacteria in these vegetations are believed to be very high. Moreover, many bacteria are not actively dividing and thus are limiting the bactericidal action of some agents. For most patients, 4 to 6 weeks of therapy is required. Specific recommendations for treating infective endocarditis caused by various organisms follow.

#### Viridans Streptococci

These organisms are the most common cause of infective endocarditis and antimicrobial regimens have been fairly well established; however, it has been recently recognized that viridans streptococci are actually heterogeneous with regard to their susceptibility to penicillin. Some strains exhibit only intermediate susceptibility while others remain exquisitely susceptible. Although most viridans streptococci are penicillin sensitive (penicillin MIC $< 0.1$ $\mu$g/mL), up to 20% may be resistant (MIC $> 0.1$ $\mu$g/mL) to penicillin.[21,22] Additionally, some isolates may be penicillin "tolerant," where the MBC:MIC ratio is greater than 10:1.[23] Penicillin susceptibility determines the antimicrobial regimen that should be used.[24] Penicillin remains very active against non–group D enterococci and other streptococci such as *Streptococcus pyogenes*. First-generation cephalosporins and vancomycin are acceptable alternatives to penicillin for these gram-positive cocci.[25,26]

For penicillin-susceptible streptococci, the standard regimen is penicillin G intravenously for 4 weeks (Table 79.3).[27] Short courses (e.g., 2 weeks of penicillin alone) often prove ineffective.[28] A first-generation cephalosporin or vancomycin is acceptable in patients who are allergic or intolerant to penicillin.[29–31] Single-drug therapy is likely to be effective in relatively uncomplicated cases in young patients with penicillin-susceptible organisms.

Combination antimicrobial regimens are recommended in some patients. Combinations of cell wall–active agents (penicillins, cephalosporins, or vancomycin) with aminoglycosides are synergistic in vitro and also in vivo.[32–34] Many clinicians have added aminoglycosides, such as streptomycin or gentamicin, to β-lactams or vancomycin even for penicillin-susceptible organisms, citing relatively large series of patients and high cure rates.[27,35] Nevertheless, the need for the addition of aminoglycosides in uncomplicated cases caused by penicillin-susceptible streptococci is not well documented. Others have concluded that the use of aminoglycosides is not necessary.[36,37] Also, the use of penicillin/streptomycin combination may allow shorter regimens. In one report by Wilson,[38] a regimen of penicillin plus streptomycin used for 2 weeks was successful in treating penicillin-susceptible streptococcal endocarditis.

Combination therapy (usually penicillin with streptomycin) has been recommended in patients with more severe disease.[29] Specifically, patients with complicated courses, disease with a duration of greater than 3 months, or prosthetic valve endocarditis should receive penicillin plus streptomycin, where the streptomycin is given for the first 2 weeks of therapy. For tolerant organisms, the approach to therapy is controversial.[31] Some recommendations suggest the use of penicillin with streptomycin or ampicillin with gentamicin. Streptomycin should be avoided in some patients, generally those over 65 (who are more susceptible to ototoxicity) or those with eighth nerve impairment.

#### Enterococci

Enterococci are a common cause of endocarditis with a relatively high mortality.[39] These infections tend to be much more difficult to treat mainly because enterococci are much less susceptible to antimicrobials than other streptococci. MICs for enterococci may be as high as 12 μg/mL for penicillin, 3 μg/mL for ampicillin, 3 μg/mL for vancomycin, 25 μg/mL for cephalosporins, 25 μg/mL for gentamicin, and greater than 2,000 μg/mL for streptomycin.[26] The MBCs of these organisms may be much greater than the MICs. Because of the relative tolerance of these bacteria, most β-lactam antibiotics are not bactericidal at the concentrations usually achieved in serum. Because endocarditis must be treated with a bactericidal regimen, combination antimicrobial therapy is required. Penicillins and aminoglycosides are synergistic in vitro against enterococci.[40–42]

The standard treatment for enterococcal endocarditis is penicillin and an aminoglycoside, where both agents are given for 6 weeks (Table 79.3). Ampicillin and gentamicin have been used increasingly, as these agents have greater in vitro activity and many strains show high-level streptomycin resistance (i.e., MIC > 2,000 μg/mL).[43] Cephalosporins or penicillinase-resistant penicillins should not be used for these infections since their in vitro activity against enterococci is relatively poor. In penicillin-allergic patients, vancomycin may be used in combination with an aminoglycoside.[44,45] The value of this combination is not well documented, and it may pose a greater risk of nephrotoxicity.[46] An alternative to the use of vancomycin in penicillin-allergic patients is penicillin desensitization.

The components of combination therapy for enterococcal endocarditis continue to be debated. Although penicillin has been the β-lactam of first choice, ampicillin is more active against enterococci in vitro.[47] No differences between penicillin and ampicillin have been demonstrated in patients, however. For the aminoglycoside component, streptomycin has traditionally been the agent of first choice, yet 20% to 50% of enterococci may exhibit high-level resistance to streptomycin.[43] Most of the isolates that are resistant to streptomycin are susceptible to gentamicin. Also, the synergistic effect with penicillins is greater with gentamicin than with streptomycin.[41,48–50] In a rabbit model of enterococcal endocarditis, gentamicin was more effective than streptomycin when used with penicillin for streptomycin-sensitive and streptomycin-resistant isolates.[42] Thus, gentamicin is preferred by many infectious disease specialists. It should be pointed out that a clinical benefit of gentamicin has not been demonstrated in patients when streptomycin-susceptible isolates were treated. Furthermore, gentamicin poses a greater risk of nephrotoxicity and cochlear toxicity, while streptomycin has a greater potential for vestibular toxicity but is less nephrotoxic.

#### Staphylococci

Coagulase-negative and coagulase-positive staphylococci are frequent causes of endocarditis. Coagulase-negative staphylococci are prominent causes of prosthetic valve endocarditis, whereas *Staphylococcus aureus* is more common in intravenous drug abusers. Appropriate management of staphylococcal endocarditis requires consideration of several factors: (1) Does the infection involve a native valve or prosthetic valve? (2) Is the patient an intravenous drug abuser? (3) How likely is methicillin resistance? (4) Should combination or oral therapy be considered?

Another factor influencing the selection of antimicrobial therapy for staphylococcal endocarditis is that some staphylococci are "tolerant" to frequently used antimicrobials.[51] These tolerant organisms are less susceptible to antimicrobials, but not through enzymatic degradation of the antimicrobial (e.g., production of β-lactamase). Although the mechanism of staphylococcal tolerance is not well understood it may involve extrachromosomal factors (such as plasmids). In the patient infected with tolerant organisms, either persistent bacteremia or lack of clinical improvement may be observed despite acceptable MICs for the agent chosen. MBCs for these organisms are found to be greater than eight times the MICs. In contrast, for most nontolerant staphylococci, the MIC and MBC are almost the same. When staphylococci are studied after 24 hours in culture, up to 60% appear to be tolerant to penicillins and cephalosporins[52]; however, if they are observed at 48 hours only 4% to

**Table 79.3** Recommended Antimicrobial Regimens for Infective Endocarditis Caused by Gram-Positive Cocci

| *Antimicrobial agent* | *Dosage*[a] | *Duration* | *Comments* |
|---|---|---|---|
| **Streptococci (Penicillin-Susceptible)** | | | |
| 1. Penicillin G | 20 million units IV daily | 4 wk[b] | May be used alone in uncomplicated cases |
| *or* | | | |
| Procaine penicillin | 1.2 million units IM every 6 h | | |
| *with* | | | |
| Streptomycin | 0.5 g IM every 12 h (or 10 mg/kg, whichever is lower) | 2 wk | Add to penicillin for complicated cases; use for 4 wk with tolerant organisms |
| *or* | | | |
| Gentamicin (with normal renal function) | 1–1.5 mg/kg IV every 8 h | | |
| 2. Cephalothin | 2 g IV every 4 h | 4 wk | Penicillin allergy |
| *or* | | | |
| Cefazolin | 1–2 g IV or IM every 6 h | | |
| *with* | | | |
| Streptomycin | 0.5 g IM every 12 h (or 10 mg/kg, whichever is lower) | 2 wk | 1–1.5 mg/kg IV every 8 h |
| *or* | | | |
| Gentamicin (with normal renal function) | | | |
| 3. Vancomycin | 0.5 g IV every 6 h (alone) | 4 wk | Penicillin allergy |
| **Enterococci** | | | |
| 1. Penicillin G | 20 million units IV daily | 6 wk | |
| *or* | | | |
| Ampicillin | 2 g IV every 4 h | | |
| *with* | | | |
| Streptomycin | 1 g IM every 12 h for 2 wk followed by 0.5 g every 12 h for 4 wk | 6 wk | 1 mg/kg IV every 8 h |
| *or* | | | |
| Gentamicin | | | |
| 2. Vancomycin | 0.5 g IV every 6 h | 6 wk | Penicillin allergy |
| *with* | | | |
| Streptomycin or gentamicin | As above | 6 wk | |
| ***Staphylococcus aureus*** **(Methicillin-Susceptible)** | | | |
| 1. Oxacillin or nafcillin | 1.5–2 g IV every 4 h | 4–6 wk | For addicts, 4 wk may be adequate |
| Rifampin | 300 mg PO every 8 h | 4–6 wk | Add if poor response |
| Gentamicin | 1 mg/kg every 8 h | 5 d | Add to $\beta$-lactam for PVE[c] |
| 2. Cephalothin or cefazolin | 1.5–2 g IV every 4 or 6 h, respectively | 4–6 wk | Alternative to penicillins |
| 3. Vancomycin | 500 mg IV every 6 h | 4–6 wk | Alternative to penicillins |
| ***Staphylococcus aureus*** **(Methicillin-Resistant)** | | | |
| Vancomycin | 500 mg IV every 6 h | 4–6 wk | Possibly add aminoglycoside |

**Table 79.3** Recommended Antimicrobial Regimens for Infective Endocarditis Caused by Gram-Positive Cocci (*continued*)

| *Antimicrobial agent* | *Dosage* | *Duration* | *Comments* |
|---|---|---|---|
| ***Staphylococcus epidermidis* (Methicillin-Susceptible)** | | | |
| 1. Oxacillin or nafcillin | 1.5–2 g IV every 4 h | 4–6 wk | Use 6 wk for PVE |
| Rifampin | 300 mg PO every 8 h | 6 wk | Add to above for PVE |
| Gentamicin | 1 mg/kg IV every 8 h | 2 wk | Use for initial 2 wk with PVE |
| 2. Cephalothin or cefazolin | 1.5–2 g every 4 or 6 h, respectively | 4 wk | Alternative for native valves |
| ***Staphylococcus epidermidis* (Methicillin-Resistant)** | | | |
| Vancomycin | 500 mg IV every 6 h | 4–6 wk | Use 6 wk for PVE |
| Rifampin and gentamicin | As above | | Use for PVE |

[a] Assumes average-size adult with normal renal function.
[b] The penicillin portion of this regimen may be used for 2 weeks (with 2 weeks of aminoglycoside) in uncomplicated cases and penicillin-susceptible organisms.
[c] Prosthetic valvular endocarditis.

5% are found to be tolerant.[17] Cross-tolerance of penicillins with cephalosporins or vancomycin has also been reported.[53] The overall implications of tolerance are not clear and controversy continues. When various antimicrobial combinations (e.g., β-lactams with aminoglycosides) are tested against tolerant staphylococci, synergistic activity is observed; however, the benefit of using combination therapy for patients infected with tolerant staphylococci has not yet been demonstrated.

For patients infected with methicillin-sensitive *S. aureus* (MSSA) the recommended therapy would be a penicillinase-resistant penicillin or a first-generation cephalosporin (such as cephalothin or cefazolin) (Table 79.3). Oxacillin or nafcillin should be the penicillin of choice since methicillin is associated with a higher incidence of renal toxicity (interstitial nephritis). If a patient is allergic to penicillins, a cephalosporin may be used unless there is a history of type 1 sensitivity to penicillin. Vancomycin is a second alternative. Generally, the agent should be continued for 4 to 6 weeks. A shorter duration of therapy may be successful in intravenous drug abusers.[54]

The use of cephalosporins (particularly cefazolin) has been somewhat controversial for MSSA endocarditis. In the majority of studies these agents appear effective; however, there are reports of failures with cephalosporins despite in vitro susceptibility.[55–58] Other agents such as clindamycin or rifampin should not be used alone because of the reported high rates of relapse and the rapid development of resistance (particularly with rifampin).[59]

The value of combination therapy for MSSA endocarditis has been assessed in both intravenous drug abusers[52,60,61] and nonaddicts.[61,62] In a trial by Abrams and associates,[60] β-lactams alone or combined with 2 weeks of an aminoglycoside did not produce differing results in intravenous drug abusers. There was no significant difference in the number of days with fever, days until bacteriologic resolution, occurrence of embolic phenomenon, need for surgery, or mortality. In a trial by Korzeniowski and associates,[61] no advantage was found for aminoglycosides in terms of survival or relapse rates; however, the addition of aminoglycoside shortened the time to defervescence and the time to clearance of bacteremia. Trials conducted in nonaddicts have also failed to demonstrate the advantage of adding an aminoglycoside to β-lactam therapy in terms of patient survival.[61,62]

From in vitro studies, combinations of antimicrobials do appear to be of benefit because they are synergistic.[63,64] Also, in animal models of endocarditis (usually in rabbits) combinations of penicillins with aminoglycosides eradicate organisms from vegetations more rapidly than penicillins alone.[65] For these reasons, some clinicians prefer to add an aminoglycoside during the initial 2 weeks of therapy for MSSA endocarditis. In more complicated cases, such as with prosthetic valve endocarditis, the value of aminoglycosides is not documented but combination therapy is often used. Other agents, such as rifampin, may be added in cases where staphylococci are not eradicated by the standard regimens. In some cases, the addition of rifampin may result in dramatic patient improvement.[61]

The need for combination regimens for tolerant organisms is not clear. In clinical studies, the in vitro observation of tolerance occurring with antimicrobial failure has been infrequent[66,67]; however, there are reports of failures with β-lactams or vancomycin used for tolerant staphylococci in which the subsequent addition of gentamicin or rifampin was effective.[67,68]

Over the past few years, greater numbers of *S. aureus* have been found resistant to methicillin and isoxazolyl penicillins. They have been termed methicillin-resistant *S. aureus* (MRSA). Moreover, these organisms can be associated with endocarditis and are as virulent as MSSA. For these organisms, vancomycin should be the agent of first choice. Virtually all MRSA are susceptible to vancomycin. Although cephalosporins may appear to be active in vitro against these organisms, this is artifactual and these agents should not be used for therapy.[69,70]

Coagulase-negative staphylococci (primarily *Staphylococcus epidermidis*) are important causes of endocarditis particularly with prosthetic valves. The prevalence of methicillin-resistant *S. epidermidis* (MRSE) as a cause of endocarditis appears to be increasing, and in one report, 79% of isolates from infected prosthetic valves were resistant to methicillin.[20] At present, all coagulase-negative staphylococci isolated from infected prosthetic valves should be assumed to be methicillin-resistant. As with MSSA, MRSE are virtually all susceptible to vancomycin.[71,72] Most of these isolates are also susceptible to rifampin in vitro; however, resistant mutants routinely emerge when rifampin is used alone.[71] When used in combination with $\beta$-lactams or vancomycin, resistance to rifampin is unusual.

Because of the demonstrated in vitro activity of vancomycin against MRSE, it is the drug of choice in the treatment of endocarditis caused by this organism. If methicillin susceptibility can be demonstrated, then a penicillinase-resistant penicillin, oxacillin or nafcillin, should be used. Of interest is a series of 68 patients with prosthetic valve endocarditis caused by MRSE, in which Karchmer and associates[20] found that vancomycin was more effective than $\beta$-lactams and that the combination of vancomycin with rifampin and/or gentamicin (the latter for the first 2 weeks of therapy only) was more effective than vancomycin alone. On the basis of this study, the current preferred treatment for prosthetic valve endocarditis caused by MRSE is vancomycin with rifampin for 6 weeks (see Table 79.3). The addition of gentamicin is controversial and is the subject of ongoing studies.

The value of combination therapy for methicillin-susceptible *S. epidermidis* has yet to be fully demonstrated but is recommended for the treatment of prosthetic valve endocarditis.[65] For native valve infections the usual therapy should consist of 4 weeks of vancomycin or a penicillinase-resistant penicillin, based on in vitro susceptibility. Cephalothin or cefazolin are suitable alternatives for methicillin-susceptible isolates. In the unusual event that staphylococci causing endocarditis were proven to be susceptible to penicillin G then this agent would be preferred.

### Gram-Negative Bacilli

Gram-negative bacilli are occasional causes of infective endocarditis in intravenous drug abusers, in patients with prosthetic valves, and less frequently as a cause of native valve endocarditis in nonaddicts. Overall, there is very little clinical information on which to base solid recommendations for treatment. In most cases, surgical intervention with valve replacement is a necessary component of therapy.[73] For antimicrobial therapy, the combination of an aminoglycoside and an extended-spectrum $\beta$-lactam agent is generally recommended.

One group of investigators reviewed the therapeutic outcome of patients with *Pseudomonas* endocarditis and compared the benefit of combining varying doses of aminoglycosides with or without valve replacement.[74] When patients were treated with "low doses" of aminoglycosides (<5 mg/kg/d gentamicin) without or with surgery, the survival rates were 25% and 50%, respectively. When "high-dose" aminoglycoside therapy was used (at least 8 mg/kg/d gentamicin), the survival rates improved to 65% and to 86% if high-dose therapy was combined with surgery. Even in the higher dosage regimens the frequency of aminoglycoside toxicity was low.

For the treatment of *Pseudomonas* endocarditis, standard therapy should be an antipseudomonal $\beta$-lactam in combination with an aminoglycoside (e.g., ticarcillin plus tobramycin).[75] In vitro, the most active antipseudomonal $\beta$-lactams are piperacillin, azlocillin, or ceftazidime. As *Pseudomonas* may possess inducible $\beta$-lactamases, these $\beta$-lactams should always be combined with an aminoglycoside. Although most of the commonly used aminoglycosides (gentamicin, tobramycin, amikacin, netilmicin) should be effective, tobramycin and amikacin generally have greater in vitro activity against *Pseudomonas*. In some institutions where resistance to gentamicin is frequent, tobramycin or amikacin may be the aminoglycoside of choice.

The appropriate regimen for the treatment of gram-negative bacillary endocarditis caused by Enterobacteriaceae depends upon the results of in vitro susceptibility testing. For *Escherichia coli* and *Proteus mirabilis*, $\beta$-lactam agents are also often combined with aminoglycosides. Some organisms, such as *Serratia marcescens* and *Klebsiella pneumoniae*, may be particularly refractory to antibiotic therapy. The advent of new cephalosporins, carbapenems, and monobactams may allow greater flexibility in the treatment of gram-negative endocarditis, but data are incomplete at present. It is hoped that long-term use of aminoglycosides might be avoided by employment of these newer agents. Whichever agents are chosen, treatment should generally be continued for 6 weeks. In light of the recalcitrant nature of many valvular gram-negative bacillary infections, consultation with a cardiac surgeon upon confirmation of the diagnosis is mandatory in the opinion of the authors.

### Fungi

These infections occur infrequently and are usually fatal. There are scant clinical data from which solid treatment recommendations may be made. Proper management will be somewhat suggested by the specific type of fungal endocarditis being treated. Amphotericin B, with or without flucytosine, along with valve replacement is recommended for *Candida* and *Aspergillus* endocarditis. For native valve fungal infections caused by *Histoplasma capsulatum*, antifungals alone have been successful except in cases of heart failure, uncontrolled infection, or systemic emboli, although so few instances of this form of endocarditis have occurred that firm recommendations cannot be made.[76] For almost all cases of prosthetic valve endocarditis caused by fungi, combined antifungal and surgical therapy is required.

The antifungal of choice for these infections is amphotericin B. After a test dose of 1 mg, amphotericin B should be administered in a dose of 0.5 to 0.7 mg/kg/d to a total cumulative dose of 1.5 to 3 g. This dose is usually given over 6 to 12 weeks.[77,78] For some organisms (such as *Cryptococcus* and *Candida*) the addition of oral flucytosine (5-fluorocytosine) to amphotericin B may result in synergistic antifungal action.[79] The use of this combination for the treatment of endocarditis, however, is controversial as there is little clinical documentation of benefit. Flucytosine should not be used alone because resistance may develop during therapy.

### Anaerobic Bacteria

Anaerobic bacteria are uncommon causes of infective endocarditis, and these infections are often fatal. The treatment recommendations for anaerobic endocarditis are based upon incomplete data. For most anaerobic infections, except those caused by *Bacteroides fragilis*, penicillin G is effective and should be given intravenously at 20 million units daily divided in six doses.[80] For the treatment of *B. fragilis* endocarditis only one agent is recommended—metronidazole. This compound is bactericidal against a wide array of anaerobic organisms including *B. fragilis*. Less satisfactory alternatives for *B. fragilis* endocarditis, such as carbenicillin, ticarcillin, piperacillin, or cefoxitin, may be considered. The requirement for a bactericidal agent in the treatment of endocarditis precludes the use of static agents such as clindamycin and chloramphenicol.

## *Monitoring*

The evaluation of treatment regimens for endocarditis includes assessment of signs and symptoms, reculture of blood, in vitro microbiologic tests (such as MIC, MBC, or serum bactericidal titer), antimicrobial serum concentration determinations, and other tests that may be necessary in the evaluation of organ function (particularly central nervous system, pulmonary, renal, and cardiac).

### Signs and Symptoms

The most frequent finding with endocarditis is fever, and with successful treatment fever usually declines to about normal within a week of initiating therapy. Persistence of fever may indicate ineffective antimicrobial therapy. Continued low-grade fever may also be caused by emboli, infections of intravascular catheters that have been in place for long periods of time, or even a drug reaction. In some patients, low-grade fever may persist even with appropriate antimicrobial therapy. With defervescence, the patient should begin to feel better and other symptoms, such as lethargy or weakness, should subside. Also, it must be remembered that bacteriostatic or partially effective agents may interrupt bacteremia while they are being administered and result in temporary resolution of symptoms; however, these agents may have little effect on bacteria deep within valvular vegetations, and when the antimicrobial is stopped the clinical signs and symptoms of infection may reappear.

### Blood Cultures and Bacterial Susceptibility

With effective therapy, blood cultures should be negative within a few days. If bacteria continue to be isolated from blood beyond the first few days of therapy, it may indicate that the antimicrobials being used are inactive against the pathogens, or that the doses used are not producing adequate concentrations in serum. After the initiation of therapy, blood cultures should be rechecked, possibly daily, until they are found negative. During the remainder of therapy, frequent blood culturing is not necessary.

For all isolates from blood cultures, MICs and MBCs should be determined if possible. The antimicrobials tested should include those being used and alternatives that may be required. The determination of MBC is particularly important in this situation as MICs will not identify tolerant organisms. The MBC is generally considered to be the lowest concentration of antimicrobial that kills 99.9% of the original innoculum.[16] It should be remembered that many factors can affect the performance of these tests (e.g., the size of the inoculum, the medium used, the duration of incubation).

In some instances it may be useful to determine if synergy exists for the antimicrobials chosen for use in combination. In vitro determinations of synergy are summarized in Chapter 73 and are recommended for patients with endocarditis caused by enterococci or unusual organisms. These tests can be very time consuming and expensive, so they should be performed only in carefully selected individuals.

### Serum Bactericidal Titer

Serum bactericidal titers (SBTs) have been used for many years and in association with a number of infectious diseases.[81,82] The SBT is the greatest dilution of a patient's serum sample, obtained while the patient is receiving antimicrobial treatment, that kills greater than 99.9% of an inoculum of the infecting pathogen in vitro over 18 to 24 hours.

In animal models of endocarditis the majority of studies of SBT conclude a relationship between SBT and outcome from infection.[81] In humans, however, there is a poor correlation with outcome from endocarditis.[83] In two reports that do suggest a relationship, an SBT wih a dilution greater than or equal to 1:8 correlated with a successful outcome.[84,85] For most streptococci causing endocarditis it is usually easy to achieve an SBT greater than or equal to 1:8; however, for many staphylococci or enterococci it may be difficult.

SBTs are affected by several variables that are addressed in greater detail in Chapter 73. Primary variables include method of diluting serum (using broth or serum), bacterial inoculum size, timing of collection of the blood sample (peak or trough), and measurement of the test endpoint. When referring to SBTs most clinicians mean a blood sample drawn when the antimicrobial concentration is likely to be at a peak.

At present, no firm conclusions can be presented about the value of SBTs in the treatment of infective endocarditis.[16,81] Therefore, a clinician could justifiably decide not to use them at all. If SBTs are used, then a target of greater than or equal to 1:8 should be used and attempts made to adjust antimicrobial dosage accordingly. These tests will be most useful when the causative organisms are moderately susceptible to antimicrobials, when less well established regimens are used, or when response to therapy is suboptimal. In addition, SBTs may be helpful in determining that a decrease in antimicrobial dose is acceptable when a patient is at high risk of drug toxicity. If bactericidal dilutions in the SBT are very high, the dosage could theoretically be decreased. As only patients with serious infections require consideration for SBTs and these same individuals are often already receiving the maximum antibiotic doses recommended by the manufacturers, increased dosage based upon satisfactory SBTs may not be warranted. Obviously, there is room for additional study in this area.

#### Serum Drug Concentration

Of the agents commonly used for infective endocarditis, serum concentration determinations are commonly performed for aminoglycosides (except streptomycin) and vancomycin. With any of the agents there are very few clinical data to support the necessity of attaining any specific serum concentrations. In general, most clinicians would agree that the serum concentration of the antimicrobial should exceed the MBC of the organism.

For aminoglycosides, several studies have attempted to correlate clinical outcome with serum concentrations achieved; however, very little of this work involves patients with endocarditis. In one important trial with endocarditis caused by *Pseudomonas aeruginosa*, the investigators noted improved outcome when gentamicin was used in high dosages (8 mg/kg/d) that resulted in peak serum concentrations of 12 to 20 μg/mL.[74,75] These investigators justify the use of these unusually high doses because of the high mortality from *Pseudomonas* endocarditis. When aminoglycosides are given in combination therapies for endocarditis caused by gram-positive cocci, acceptable peak serum concentrations should be in the more traditional ranges (5–8 μg/mL for gentamicin and tobramycin, and 20–35 μg/mL for amikacin).

As with aminoglycosides, there is very little information to suggest what are "appropriate" serum concentrations for vancomycin when treating endocarditis. In general, peak serum concentration should not exceed 40 μg/mL to avoid ototoxicity, although a clear correlation of excessive peak vancomycin concentrations with toxicity has not been fully demonstrated.[86] For staphylococcal and enterococcal endocarditis, optimal vancomycin trough concentrations are greater than 10 μg/mL, as the MBCs of some strains may be as high as 12 to 16 μg/mL and it is desirable to maintain serum concentrations above the MBCs for as much of the dosing interval as possible.

### *Anticoagulation*

For patients with native valve endocarditis, the use of anticoagulants is contraindicated. These patients may experience increased frequency of bleeding complications, possibly from areas of embolic infarction or from mycotic aneurysms. With prosthetic valve endocarditis the use of anticoagulants is controversial; however, it is probably best that patients that require anticoagulants for prosthetic valves be continued on them during endocarditis therapy. In one published report, patients with PVE whose anticoagulants were discontinued experienced an increased frequency of major central nervous system emboli.[87] When warfarin is used in patients with PVE, the prothrombin time-to-control ratio should be maintained at about 1.5 and careful assessment of the patient for bleeding complications should be performed. If the patient is at high risk for bleeding complications, aspirin with dipyridamole may be substituted for warfarin.

## Prevention

Antimicrobials have been used to prevent the development of endocarditis in patients who were believed to be at high risk.[88,89] The use of antimicrobials for this purpose requires consideration of (1) the types of patients who are at high risk for developing endocarditis, (2) the circumstances that increase the risk of endocarditis, and (3) the organisms that are likely to cause endocarditis. The primary objective of prophylaxis is to diminish the likelihood of endocarditis in high-risk individuals who are undergoing procedures significantly associated with bacteremia.

### *Patients at Risk*

Patients with certain underlying cardiac lesions, particularly those with prosthetic heart valves and certain other conditions, are recognized to be at high risk for developing endocarditis (Table 79.4). One problem with the generation of such a list of high-risk patients is that up to one half of patients developing endocarditis are not in a high-risk category. Patients with coronary artery disease, atherosclerotic plaques, atrial septal defects, cardiac pacemakers, or surgically corrected cardiac defects without prosthetic implants as the only risk factor are believed to be at low risk of endocarditis.

### *Procedures Causing Bacteremia*

Bacteremia accompanies many everyday events, such as brushing teeth; however, certain procedures may cause a transient but intense bacteremia. For procedures involving the gums and oral structures, viridans streptococci frequently enter the bloodstream, whereas instrumentation and surgery of the gastrointestinal and genitourinary tracts more often result in enterococcal bacteremia. For some gastrointestinal procedures (particularly endoscopy), the incidence of endocarditis is very low, and those organisms found in infected patients are often not those susceptible to recom-

**Table 79.4** Conditions for Which Endocarditis Prophylaxis Is Recommended

| |
|---|
| Recommended |
| Prosthetic cardiac valves (including biosynthetic valves) |
| Most congenital cardiac malformations |
| Surgically constructed systemic–pulmonary shunts |
| Rheumatic and other acquired valvular dysfunctions |
| Idiopathic hypertrophic subaortic stenosis |
| Previous history of bacterial endocarditis |
| Mitral valve prolapse with insufficiency |
| Not recommended |
| Isolated secundum atrial septal defect |
| Secundum atrial defect repaired without a patch 6 or more months earlier |
| Patent ductus arteriosus ligated and divided 6 or more months earlier |
| After coronary artery bypass graft surgery |

From Kaye D: Prophylaxis for infective endocarditis: An update. Ann Intern Med 1986; 104:419–423, with permission.

**Table 79.5** Procedures for Which Endocarditis Prophylaxis Is Indicated

| | |
|---|---|
| Oral cavity and respiratory tract | |
| | All dental procedures likely to induce gingival bleeding |
| | Tonsillectomy or adenoidectomy |
| | Surgical procedures or biopsy involving respiratory mucosa |
| | Bronchoscopy, especially with rigid bronchoscope |
| | Incision and drainage of infected tissue |
| Genitourinary and gastrointestinal tracts | |
| | Cystoscopy |
| | Prostatic surgery |
| | Urethral catheterization |
| | Urinary tract surgery |
| | Vaginal surgery |
| | Gallbladder surgery |
| | Colonic surgery |
| | Esophageal dilatation |
| | Sclerotherapy for esophageal varices |
| | Colonoscopy |
| | Upper gastrointestinal tract endoscopy with biopsy |
| | Proctosigmoidoscopic biopsy |

From Kaye D: Prophylaxis for infective endocarditis; An update. Ann Intern Med 1986;104:419–423, with permission.

mended prophylactic regimens; however, current recommendations suggest prophylaxis for these procedures in high-risk patients (Table 79.5).[89]

### *Antibiotic Regimens*

Antimicrobials are used in these situations to prevent the development of endocarditis. The most important mechanism by which antimicrobials prevent endocarditis is not known. It is believed that antimicrobials work primarily by decreasing the incidence and intensity of bacteremia after a procedure. In addition, antimicrobials may prevent multiplication of bacteria at the valve site (thereby allowing more time for host defenses to work), or they may even interfere with adherence of bacteria to cardiac lesions.[90] Recommended antimicrobial regimens are based not on controlled clinical trials demonstrating their effectiveness, but on known in vitro activity against organisms commonly causing endocarditis and in consideration of the practicality of administering antimicrobials to mostly ambulatory patients.

The duration of antimicrobial prophylaxis necessary is not precisely known, but is now believed to be relatively short.

**Table 79.6** Recommended Regimens for Prophylaxis of Endocarditis in Adults

| | |
|---|---|
| **Dental or Respiratory Procedures** | |
| Standard regimen | |
| For dental procedures that cause gingival bleeding and for oral or respiratory tract surgery | Penicillin V 2 g PO 1 h before, then 1 g 6 h later; or penicillin G 2 × $10^6$ units IV or IM 0.5–1 h before, then 1 × $10^6$ units 6 h later |
| Special regimens | |
| When maximal protection is desired (e.g., with prosthetic valves) | Ampicillin 1–2 g IV or IM plus gentamicin 1.5 mg/kg 0.5 h before, then 8 h later (or penicillin V 1 g may be given 6 h later) |
| For penicillin allergy | Erythromycin 1 g PO 1 h before, then 0.5 g 6 h later |
| | *or* |
| | Vancomycin 1 g IV over 1 h starting 1 h before the procedure with no repeat dose |
| **Gastrointestinal or Genitourinary Tract Procedures** | |
| Standard regimen | |
| For procedures listed in Table 79.5 | Ampicillin 2 g IM or IV plus gentamicin 1.5 mg/kg 0.5–1 h before, then 8 h later |
| Special regimens | |
| Oral regimens for minor or repetitive procedures in low-risk patients | Amoxicillin 3 g PO 1 h before, then 1.5 g 6 h later |
| Patients allergic to penicillin | Vancomycin 1 g IV over 1 h plus gentamicin 1.5 mg/kg IM or IV 1 h before, then repeated 8–12 h later |

Adapted from Kaye D: Prophylaxis for infective endocarditis: An update. Ann Intern Med 1986;104:419–423, with permission.

From one animal model it was determined that bactericidal activity was necessary for 9 hours after bacterial challenge to prevent endocarditis.[91] Recommended antimicrobial regimens for prophylaxis of endocarditis are presented in Table 79.6.

## References

1. Von Reym CF, Levy BS, Arbeit RD, et al. Infective endocarditis: Analysis based on strict case definitions. Ann Intern Med 1982;94:505–518.
2. Kaye D. Definitions and demographic characteristics, in Kaye D (ed): Infective Endocarditis. Baltimore, University Park Press, 1976, p 1.
3. Watanakunakorn C. Changing epidemiology and newer aspects of infective endocarditis. Adv Intern Med 1977;22:21–47.
4. Gnann JW, Cobbs CG. Infections of prosthetic valves and intravascular devices, in Mandel GL, Douglas RG, Bennett JE (eds): Principles and Practice of Infectious Diseases. New York, John Wiley and Sons, 1983, pp 530–539.
5. Pelletier LL, Petersdorf RG. Infective endocarditis: A review of 125 cases from the University of Washington Hospitals, 1963–1972. Medicine 1977;56:287–313.
6. Cohen PS, Maguire JH, Weinstein L. Infective endocarditis

caused by gram-negative bacteria: A review of the literature, 1945–1977. Prog Cardiovasc Dis 1980;22:205–242.

7. Scheld WM, Sande MA. Endocarditis and intravascular infections, in Mandell GL, Douglas RG, Bennett JE (eds): Principles and Practice of Infectious Diseases. New York, John Wiley and Sons, 1983 pp 504–530.
8. Sande MA. Experimental endocarditis, in Kaye D (ed): Infective Endocarditis. Baltimore, University Park Press, 1976, p 11.
9. Okell CC, Elliott SD. Bacteraemia and oral sepsis. With special reference to the aetiology of subacute endocarditis. Lancet 1935;2:869–872.
10. Everett ED, Hirschman JV. Transient bacteremia and endocarditis prophylaxis: a review. Medicine 1977;56:61–77.
11. Gould K, Ramirez-Ronda CH, Holmes RK, et al. Adherence of bacteria to heart valves in vitro. J Clin Invest 1975;56:1364–1370.
12. Pelletier LL, Coyle M, Petersdorf R. Dextran production as a possible virulence factor in streptococcal endocarditis. Proc Soc Exp Biol Med 1978;158:415–420.
13. Blakemore WS, McGarrity GJ, Thurer RJ, et al. Infection by airborne bacteria with cardiopulmonary bypass. Surgery 1971; 70:830–838.
14. Churchill MA, Geraci JE, Hunder GG. Musculoskeletal manifestations of bacterial endocarditis. Ann Intern Med 1977:87; 754–759.
15. Tuazon CU, Sheagren JW. Teichoic antibodies in the diagnosis of serious infections with *Staphylococcus aureus*. Ann Intern Med 1976;84:543–546.
16. Washington JA. The role of the microbiology laboratory in the diagnosis and antimicrobial treatment of infectious endocarditis. Mayo Clin Proc 1982;57:22–32.
17. Bayer AS. Staphylococcal bacteremia and endocarditis: state of the art. Arch Intern Med 1982;142:1169–1177.
18. Dinubile MJ. Surgery in active endocarditis. Ann Intern Med 1980;96:650–659.
19. Jung JY, Saab SB, Almond CH. The case for early surgical treatment of left-sided primary infective endocarditis. J Thorac Cardiovasc Surg 1975;70:509–518.
20. Karchmer AW, Archer GL, Dismukes WE. *Staphylococcus epidermidis* causing prosthetic valve endocarditis: microbiologic and clinical observations as guides to therapy. Ann Intern Med 1983;98:447–455.
21. Roberts RB, Krieger AG, Schiller NL, et al.Viridans streptococcal endocarditis: the role of various species, including pyridoxal dependent streptococci. Rev Infect Dis 1979;1:955–965.
22. Carey RB, Brause BD, Roberts RB. Antimicrobial therapy of vitamin B6-dependent streptococcal endocarditis. Ann Intern Med 1977;87:150–154.
23. Pulliam L, Inokuchi S, Hadley WK, et al. Penicillin tolerance in experimental streptococcal endocarditis. Lancet 1979;2:957.
24. Hook EW, Guerrant RL. Therapy of infective endocarditis, in Kaye D (ed): Infective Endocarditis. Baltimore, University Park Press, 1976, p 167–184.
25. Bourgault AM, Wilson WR, Washington JA. Antimicrobial susceptibilities of species of viridans streptococci. J Infect Dis 1979;140:316–321.
26. Atkinson BA. Species incidence and trends of susceptibility to antibiotics in the United States and other countries: MIC and MBC, in Lorian V (ed): Antibiotics in Laboratory Medicine. Baltimore, Williams and Wilkins, 1986, pp 995–1152.
27. Wolfe JC, Johnson WD. Penicillin-sensitive streptococcal endocarditis. In vitro clinical observations on penicillin–streptomycin therapy. Ann Intern Med 1974;81:178–181.
28. Tompsett R, Robbins WC, Berntsen C Jr. Short term penicillin and dihydrostreptomycin therapy of streptococcal endocarditis. Results of the treatment of thirty five patients. Am J Med 1958;24:57–67.
29. Sande MA, Scheld WM. Combination antibiotic therapy of bacterial endocarditis. Ann Intern Med 1980;92:390–395.
30. Kaye D. Antibiotic treatment of streptococcal endocarditis. Am J Med 1980;69:650–652.
31. Bisno AL, Dismukes WE, Durack DT, et al. AHA committee report. Treatment of infective endocarditis due to viridans streptococci. Circulation 1981;63:730A–733A.
32. Sande MA, Irvin RG. Penicillin–aminoglycoside synergy in experimental *Streptococcus viridans* endocarditis. J Infect Dis 1974;129:572–576.
33. Watanakunakorn C, Glotzbecker C. Synergism with aminoglycosides of penicillin, ampicillin, and vancomycin against group D streptococci and viridans streptococci. J Med Microbiol 1977; 10:133–138.
34. Drake TA, Sande MA. Studies of chemotherapy of endocarditis: correlation of in vitro, animal model, and clinical studies. Rev Infect Dis 1983;5:S345–S354.
35. Wolfe JC, Johnson WD. Penicillin-sensitive streptococcal endocarditis. In vitro and clinical observations on penicillin–streptomycin therapy. Ann Intern Med 1974;81:178–181.
36. Malacoff RF, Frank E, Andriole VT. Streptococcal endocarditis (nonenterococcal, non-group A). Single vs combination therapy. JAMA 1979;241:1807–1810.
37. Karchmer AW, Moellering RC, Maki DG, et al. Single-antibiotic therapy for streptococcal endocarditis. JAMA 1979;241: 1801–1806.
38. Wilson WR, Thompson RL, Wilkowsky CJ, et al. Short-term therapy for streptococcal infective endocarditis. Combined intramuscular administration. JAMA 1981;245:360–363.
39. Mandeel GL, Kaye D, Levison ME, et al. Enterococcal endocarditis: an analysis of 38 patients observed at New York Hospital–Cornell Medical Center. Arch Intern Med 1970;125: 258–264.
40. Wilson WR, Wilkowske CJ, Wright AJ, et al. Treatment of streptomycin-susceptible and streptomycin-resistant enterococcal endocarditis. Ann Intern Med 1984;100:816–823.
41. Watanakunakorn C. Penicillin combined with gentamicin or streptomycin: synergy against enterococci. J Infect Dis 1971; 124:581–586.
42. Hook EW, Roberts RB, Sande MA. Antimicrobial therapy of experimental enterococcal endocarditis. Antimicrob Agents Chemother 1975;8:564–570.
43. Moellering RC, Wennersten C, Medrek T, et al. Prevalence of high-level resistance to aminoglycosides in clinical isolates of enterococci. Antimicrob Agents Chemother 1970:335–340.
44. Westenfelder GO, Paterson PY, Reisberg BE, et al. Vancomycin–streptomycin synergism in enterococcal endocarditis. JAMA 1973;223:37–40.
45. Watanakunakorn C, Tisone JAC. Synergism between vancomycin and gentamicin or tobramycin for methicillin-susceptible and methicillin-resistant *Staphylococcus aureus*. Antimicrob Agents Chemother 1982;22:903–905.
46. Farber BF, Moellering RC. Retrospective study of the toxicity of preparations of vancomycin from 1974 to 1981. Antimicrob Agents Chemother 1983;23:138–141.
47. Simon HJ. Antimicrobial susceptibility of group D hemolytic streptococci (enterococci). Am J Med Sci 1967;253:259–265.
48. Serra P, Brandimark C, Martino P, et al. Synergistic treatment of enterococcal endocarditis. In vitro and in vivo studies. Arch Intern Med 1977;137:1562–1567.
49. Weinstein AJ, Moellering RC. Penicillin and gentamicin therapy for enterococcal infections. JAMA 1973;223:1030–1032.
50. Moellering RC, Wennersten C, Weinberg AW. Synergy of

penicillin and gentamicin against enterococci. J Infect Dis 1971;124(suppl):207–209.

51. Sabath LD, Wheeler N, Laverdier M, et al. A new type of penicillin resistance of *Staphylococcus aureus*. Lancet 1977;1: 443–447.
52. Rajashekaraiah KR, Rice T, Rao VS, et al. Clinical significance of tolerant strains of *Staphylococcus aureus* in patients with endocarditis. Ann Intern Med 1980;93:769–801.
53. Rahal JJ. Symposium on current problems in staphylococcal infections: staphylococcal bacteremia and endocarditis. Proceedings of the 20th Interscience Conference on Antimicrobial Agents and Chemotherapy. New Orleans, Sept 22–24, 1980. Washington DC, American Society for Microbiology.
54. Parker RH, Fossieck BE. Intravenous followed by oral antimicrobial therapy for staphylococcal endocarditis. Ann Intern Med 1980;93:832–834.
55. Bryant RE, Alford RH. Unsuccessful treatment of staphylococcal endocarditis with cefazolin. JAMA 1977;237:569–570.
56. Quinn EL, Pohlod D, Madhavan T, et al. Clinical experiences with cefazolin and other cephalosporins in endocarditis. J Infect Dis 1973;128:S386–S391.
57. Burgess HA, Evan RJ. Failure of cephaloridine in a case of staphylococcal endocarditis. Br Med J 1966;2:1244.
58. Reinarz JA, Kier CM, Guckian JC. Evaluation of cefazolin in the treatment of bacterial endocarditis and bacteremia. J Infect Dis 1973;128:S392–S396.
59. Watanakunakorn C. Clindamycin therapy of *Staphylococcus aureus* endocarditis. Clinical relapse and development of resistance to clindamycin, lincomycin, and erythromycin. Am J Med 1976;60:419–425.
60. Abrams B, Sklaver A, Hoffman T, et al. Single or combination therapy of staphylococcal endocarditis in intravenous drug abusers. Ann Intern Med 1979;90:789–791.
61. Korzeniowski O, Sande MA. The National Collaborative Endocarditis Study Group. Combination antimicrobial therapy for *Staphylococcus aureus* endocarditis in patients addicted to parenteral drugs and in non-addicts. Ann Intern Med 1982;97: 496–503.
62. Watanakunakorn C, Baird IM. Prognostic factors in *Staphylococcus aureus* endocarditis and results of therapy with penicillin and gentamicin. Am J Med Sci 1977;273:133–139.
63. Richmond AS, Simberkoff MS, Schaeffer S, et al. Resistance of *Staphylococcus aureus* to semisynthetic penicillins and cephalothin. J Infect Dis. 1977;135:108–112.
64. Tuazon CU, Lin MYC, Sheagren JN. In vitro activity of rifampin alone and in combination with nafcillin and vancomycin against pathogenic strains of *Staphylococcus aureus*. Antimicrob Agents Chemother 1978;13:759–761.
65. Karchmer AW. Staphylococcal endocarditis: laboratory and clinical basis for antibiotic therapy. Am J Med 1985;78(suppl B):116–127.
66. Denny AE, Peterson LR, Gerding DN, et al. Serious staphylococcal infections with strains tolerant to bactericidal antibiotics. Arch Intern Med 1970;139:1026–1031.
67. Faville RJ, Zaske DE, Kaplan EL, et al. *Staphylococcus aureus* endocarditis: combined therapy with vancomycin and rifampin. JAMA 1978;240:1963–1965.
68. Gopal V, Bisno AL, Siverblatt FJ. Failure of vancomycin treatment in *Staphylococcus aureus* endocarditis: in vivo and in vitro observations. JAMA 1976;236:1604–1606.
69. Myers JP, Linnemann CC. Bacteremia due to methicillin-resistant *Staphylococcus aureus*. J Infect Dis 1982;145:532–536.
70. Craven DE, Kollisch NR, Hsieh CR, et al. Vancomycin treatment of bacteremia caused by oxacillin-resistant *Staphylococcus aureus*: comparison with beta-lactam antibiotic treatment of bacteremia caused by oxacillin-sensitive *Staphylococcus aureus*. J Infect Dis 1983;147:137–143.
71. Archer GL. Antimicrobial susceptibility and selection of resistance among *Staphylococcus epidermidis* isolates recovered from patients with infections of indwelling foreign devices. Antimicrob Agents Chemother 1978;14:353–359.
72. Sabath LD, Garner C, Wilcox C, et al. Susceptibility of *Staphylococcus aureus* and *Staphylococcus epidermidis* to 65 antibiotics. Antimicrob Agents Chemother 1976;9:962–969.
73. Cooper R, Mills J. *Serratia* endocarditis. A followup report. Arch Intern Med 1980;140:199–202.
74. Reyes MP, Brown WJ, Lerner AM. Treatment of patients with pseudomonas endocarditis with high dose aminoglycoside and carbenicillin therapy. Medicine 1978;57:57–67.
75. Reyes MP, Lerner AM. Current problems in the treatment of infective endocarditis due to *Pseudomonas aeruginosa*. Rev Infec Dis 1983;5:314–321.
76. Leisen JCC, Lang DM, Quinn EL. Fungal organisms, in Magilligan DJ, Quinn EL (eds): Endocarditis, Medical and Surgical Management. New York, Marcel Dekker, 1986, pp 27–35.
77. Cohen J. Antifungal chemotherapy. Lancet 1982;2:532–537.
78. Medoff G, Kobayashi GS. Strategies in the treatment of systemic fungal infections. N Engl J Med 1980;302:145–155.
79. Utz JP, Garriques IL, Sande MA, et al. Therapy of cryptococcosis with a combination of flucytosine and amphotericin B. J Infect Dis 1975;132:368–373.
80. Nastro FL, Sarma RJ. Infective endocarditis due to anaerobic microaerophilic bacteria. West J Med 1982;137:18–23.
81. Wolfson JS, Swartz MN. Serum bactericidal activity as a monitor of antibiotic therapy. N Engl J Med 1985;312:968–975.
82. Reller LB. The serum bactericidal test. Rev Infect Dis 1986;8: 803–808.
83. Coleman DL, Horwitz RI, Andriole VT. Association between serum inhibitory and bactericidal concentrations and therapeutic outcome in bacterial endocarditis. Am J Med 1982;73:260–267.
84. Klastersky J, Daneau D, Swings G, et al. Antibiotic activity in serum and urine as a therapeutic guide in bacterial infections. J Infect Dis 1974;129:187–193.
85. Carrizosa J, Kaye D. Antibiotic concentrations in serum, serum bactericidal activity, and results of therapy of streptococcal endocarditis in rabbits. Antimicrob Agents Chemother 1977;12: 479–483.
86. Cheung RPF, DiPiro JT. Vancomycin: an update. Pharmacotherapy 1986;6:153–169.
87. Wilson WR, Geraci JE, Danielson GK, et al. Anticoagulant therapy and central nervous system complications in patients with prosthetic valve endocarditis. Circulation 1978;57:1004–1007.
88. Kaye D. Prophylaxis for infective endocarditis: An update. Ann Intern Med 1986;104:419–423.
89. Shulman S, Amren DP, Bisno AL, et al. Prevention of bacterial endocarditis: a statement for health professionals by the Committee on Rheumatic Fever and Infective Endocarditis of the Council on Cardiovascular Disease in the Young. Circulation 1984;70:1123A–1127A.
90. Glauser MP, Bernard JP, Moreillon P, et al. Successful single-dose amoxicillin prophylaxis against experimental streptococcal endocarditis. Evidence for two mechanisms of protection. J Infect Dis 1983;147:568–575.
91. Durack DT, Petersdorf RG. Chemotherapy of experimental streptococcal endocarditis: I. Comparison of commonly recommended prophylactic regimens. J Clin Invest 1973;52:592–598.

# *Chapter 80* / Tuberculosis

Steven C. Ebert, PharmD

Throughout history, tuberculosis has assumed a prominent role as a disease that has affected society as well as the practice of medicine. Referred to as the "white plague" and as "phthisis" (indicative of the wasting character of the disease), it has been the cause of countless human deaths dating back to prehistoric man. The term *tubercle* initially referred to the substance found in the lungs of patients with the disease that was felt to be "a degeneration of the natural occupant of the cell, or the epithelial scales."[1] English physicians in the 1800s attributed tuberculosis to "abuse of the body" through physical or moral transgressions, or to "the defective system handed down from father and mother to child—the result of accumulating vices of life, and of injudicious marriages,"[1] which supposedly accounted for the prevalence of the disease within families.

Tuberculosis was a major cause of death in Europe when the Industrial Revolution drew workers formerly dwelling in rural areas into a crowded, unsanitary urban lifestyle. Though a bane to mankind, the disease was paradoxically the impetus for many of the early discoveries in medicine, including the monumental findings of Robert Koch and the discovery of streptomycin. Today, in this era of chemotherapy of infectious diseases, tuberculosis remains a disease that has proven difficult to eliminate. The challenges for today's clinician are to identify patients with atypical as well as classic forms of the disease and to ensure effective monitoring of and compliance with drug therapy.

## Etiology

Human tuberculosis is almost invariably caused by *Mycobacterium tuberculosis*, a nonmotile, slow-growing, nonspore-forming aerobic bacillus that resides primarily in humans. Of the approximately 20 other species of the genus *Mycobacterium*, only *M. bovis* causes tuberculosis in the normal host, whereas a variety of species (*M. kansasii*, *M. fortuitum*, and *M. avium-intracellulare*) may cause disease in immunosuppressed individuals. The term "acid-fast" is often used to describe the genus *Mycobacterium* because of its ability to resist decolorization with acid–alcohol after staining with carbol–fuchsin. The organisms are also tolerant of the acidic environment of the stomach, and it is not unusual to isolate organisms from the gastric contents of patients diagnosed with tuberculosis.

## Epidemiology

In 1985, 22,575 new cases of tuberculosis were reported in the United States, a rate of 9.4 cases per 100,000 persons.[2] For the period 1953 through 1984, the case rate has declined annually by an average of 6.4% per year. From 1984 to the present the case rate has remained stable and perhaps even increased slightly.[2] Before the discovery of streptomycin, approximately 40,000 persons died annually from tuberculosis, compared with 1,807 reported deaths in 1982. Currently, over 10 million people in the United States are infected with *M. tuberculosis* as documented by skin test. The frequency of skin test positivity varies with age from approximately 1% in young children to 10% in adults over age 65.[3]

Based on the average rate of decline of new cases diagnosed annually since 1953, it is possible that tuberculosis could be eliminated within the United States by the year 2100. For this to occur, support from health care agencies in identifying and contacting all persons exposed to infected individuals would be necessary. Factors that make the complete eradication of tuberculosis unlikely include the continued influx of immigrant populations with high infection rates, the presence of disease caused by drug-resistant bacteria, the increasing rate of infection with human immunodeficiency virus, and the apathy expressed by both physicians and patients toward assurance of effective treatment.

The presence or absence of certain factors will influence an individual's likelihood of acquiring tuberculosis. Persons exposed to individuals with active pulmonary tuberculosis constitute the group at highest risk for acquiring the disease. Studies of skin tests performed on close contacts of patients with tuberculosis reveal conversion rates as high as 27%, depending on the infectivity of the patient's sputum.[3] Between 5% and 15% of these converters go on to develop the active form of the disease.

Geographic location also influences the propensity for developing tuberculosis. Individuals from underdeveloped countries are at extremely high risk. In the United States, persons living in metropolitan areas with populations greater than 250,000 are at a risk twice that of the national average. Residents of coastal states (Atlantic, Pacific, or Gulf of Mexico) and Alaska and Hawaii possess case rates higher than average, possibly because of their large immigrant populations.[2]

Age has not generally been considered a risk factor for acquisition of tuberculosis. The higher rates of skin test positivity observed in the elderly are usually attributed to their higher cumulative chance of exposure. Recent studies, however, have documented an increased incidence of newly acquired skin test positivity in elderly patients, particularly those residing in nursing homes. Elderly patients may therefore be at risk for contracting tuberculosis as a nosocomial disease.[4] Others have suggested that children constitute a high-risk group for acquiring the disease. In most instances, children who contract tuberculosis are household contacts of infected individuals. Any increased risk for children is probably due to the larger amount of their time spent in the home compared with adults than to any influence of age.[3]

Other patient factors associated with an increased risk for contracting tuberculosis include low socioeconomic status, non-Caucasian race, and male sex.

Finally, it appears that patients with AIDS or AIDS-related complex appear to be at increased risk for acquiring tuberculosis. Data from the Centers for Disease Control in 1986 suggest that approximately 4% of AIDS patients also have tuberculosis, compared with less than 1% of the general population.[2] The majority of AIDS patients who have tuberculosis also have other risk factors (i.e., immigrants such as Haitians, residence in highly populated areas, low socioeconomic status).[5] However, the diagnosis of tuberculosis should not be excluded in AIDS patients with respiratory tract infections who do not possess these other risk factors.[6]

## Pathophysiology

The host–parasite relationship between man and *M. tuberculosis* is incredibly diverse. The extent of infection may range from a solitary granuloma that is undetectable on chest x-ray to widely disseminated disease involving virtually every organ system in the body.

For all practical purposes, tuberculosis is invariably transmitted from person to person via microsize droplet nuclei which are dispersed by either coughing or sneezing. The classic studies of Riley in the late 1950s[7] demonstrated the ability of air circulated from a hospital ward of patients with tuberculosis to cause disease in guinea pigs. When the air was filtered or exposed to ultraviolet radiation, the animals were not infected.[7]

"Primary infection" is initiated by the alveolar implantation of organisms in droplet nuclei that are small enough (1–5 μm) to escape the ciliary epithelial cells of the upper respiratory tract. The degree of subsequent progression of infection to clinical disease depends on the initial inoculum size as well as the state of the host's cell-mediated immune system.[3] Once implanted, the organisms multiply and are ingested by pulmonary macrophages where they continue to multiply, albeit more slowly. Intracellular organisms then spread to involve regional lymph nodes in the hilar, mediastinal, and retroperitoneal areas. Depending on the concentration of antigen present and the inflammatory response evoked, tissue necrosis and calcification of the originally infected site and regional lymph node may occur, resulting in the formation of a radiodense area referred to as a *Ghon complex*.

After this stage of lymph node involvement, organisms spread via the bloodstream to a variety of organ systems including other lymph nodes, bone and bone marrow, the liver, kidneys, and, most commonly, the posterior apical region of the lungs. Seeding of these particular sites probably occurs because of their relatively high blood flow but limited lymphatic drainage.[3] Nodular infiltrates that may arise in the apices of the lung secondary to this hematogenous spread are referred to as *Simon foci*.

Concurrent with the proliferation of organisms is the development of delayed hypersensitivity via activation and multiplication of T lymphocytes with subsequent enhancement of the mycobactericidal activity of macrophages. When activated lymphocytes reach an adequate number (usually 1–3 months after infection), tissue hypersensitivity results as evidenced by the presence of a positive tuberculin skin test. Activated macrophages may then act to limit the hematogenous spread of organisms. The arrest of mycobacterial proliferation is characterized pathologically by formation of granulomas of two types: *proliferative* granulomas, which are stable and can effectively limit the spread of the organism; and *caseating* granulomas, so named for their cheese-like appearance, which have a necrotic center, are relatively unstable, and permit the limited growth of *M. tuberculosis* within them.[3]

The size of the inoculum of organisms delivered, the integrity of the host's cell-mediated immune system, the rate at which it arrests the proliferation of organisms, and the presence or absence of other underlying factors influence the subsequent clinical course of the disease. Between 85% and 95% of patients who experience primary disease have no further clinical manifestations other than a positive skin test either alone (70%) or in combination with radiographic evidence of stable granulomas (20%).[8] Approximately 1% of patients (usually children or elderly) experience "progressive primary" disease, which occurs before skin test conversion. This form of the disease is characterized by progressive pneumonia originating at the site of the primary infection (usually the lower lobes) and frequently by dissemination leading to meningitis and often to involvement of the upper lobes of the lung as well.

The remaining 4% to 14% of patients develop "reactivation disease," which arises subsequent to the hematogenous spread of the organism.[8] The vast majority of those who experience reactivation do so within 1 year of the primary infection, and nearly all will within 2 years. The apical areas of the lung are the most common site for reactivation (85% of cases). This typically originates as a small lesion which is visualized as an alveolar infiltrate. The resultant inflammatory response produces caseating granulomas which eventually will liquify and cavitate. The aerobic environment of a cavity enhances growth of the organism; bacterial counts within the cavity may be as high as $10^8$ organisms per milliliter of sputum. Fluid within the cavity is easily aerosolized by coughing, which results in the spread of the organism to other areas within the upper and lower respiratory tracts as well as into the surrounding environment. Partial healing may result from fibrosis of cavities and other infected sites, but the potential exists for breakdown of these areas and subsequent reactivation.[3] If left untreated, pulmonary tuberculosis will eventually spread to involve the entire respiratory tract, resulting in hypoxia, respiratory acidosis, and death.

A significant number of patients with the reactivation form of the disease present with infections at extrapulmonary sites. Although the total number of cases of tuberculosis in the United States reported per year has continued to decline, the number of extrapulmonary cases has remained constant, currently accounting for approximately 15% of new cases.[9] Organs and systems most commonly involved include the central nervous system (meningitis and cranial tuberculomas), peritoneum, genitourinary tract, lymphatic system, skeletal system, pericardium, adrenal glands, and liver.[9] Occasionally, a massive inoculum of organisms may be introduced into the bloodstream, causing widely disseminated disease and granuloma formation known as *miliary tuberculosis*. This form of the disease acquired its name from the millet seed–like appearance of the small granulomas viewed on chest x-ray as well as in films of other soft tissues.[8] As with the pulmonary form, extrapulmonary tuberculosis that is left untreated may result in mortality.

Occasionally, patients experience the reactivation form of the disease more than 2 years after primary infection. In the United States, development of tuberculosis in patients with a positive skin test is statistically more likely to be caused by reactivation rather than reinfection. Reinfection is uncommon because of the low rate of exposure in this country and because previously sensitized individuals possess some degree of immunity to reinfection.[10] Risk factors felt to pose an increased risk for reactivation disease, despite a lapse of more than 2 years since primary infection, include x-ray evidence of inactive pulmonary tuberculosis; immunosuppressed states including immunosuppressive drug therapy, chronic renal failure, and hematologic malignancy; pulmonary silicosis; and gastrectomy for peptic ulcer disease.[3]

## Clinical Presentation

The clinical presentation of pulmonary tuberculosis is nonspecific, indicative only of a slowly evolving infectious process. A patient with subclinical or early disease may be completely asymptomatic. When the population of organisms increases to a certain point, however, the patient begins to complain of generalized malaise, anorexia, weight loss, and fatigue as well as intermittent fevers with alternating chills and night sweats. Subsequently, a cough with increasing sputum production develops. Often insidious in onset, the cough is frequently attributed to other causes, such as a viral syndrome or exacerbation of chronic bronchitis. Pleuritic chest pain may or may not be a concurrent complaint. Hemoptysis may also occur, and is usually indicative of advanced disease.

Expectoration and/or swallowing of sputum containing large numbers of organisms may result in extension of disease involving the upper respiratory or gastrointestinal tract. Ulceration of the pharynx, larynx, tongue, and oral mucosa as well as otitis media, gastric ulceration, and perirectal abscess may occur.[3]

Physical exam is again nonspecific, suggestive only of slowly progressive pulmonary disease. Dullness to chest percussion suggests consolidation in involved areas of the lung. Rales and increased vocal fremitus are frequently observed upon auscultation. In patients in whom impaired oxygenation has developed, cyanosis and clubbing of the digits may be seen.

Abnormal laboratory data are usually limited to moderate elevations of white blood cell count with a lymphocyte predominance. Other abnormal values may occasionally be observed, but are too infrequent to be useful diagnostically.[3]

Clinical features associated with extrapulmonary tuberculosis vary depending on the organ system(s) involved, but typically consist of slowly progressive compromise of organ function with low-grade fever and other constitutional symptoms as mentioned previously. Concurrent pulmonary disease may or may not also be present.[9]

Confirmatory diagnosis of a clinical suspicion of tuberculosis must be made via chest x-ray, microbiological examination of sputum or other infected materials, and skin testing. A positive result from one or more of these procedures must be observed to initiate treatment. Whether one or more of these tests is positive depends on the site and extent of infection as well as the underlying physical status of the patient.

A chest x-ray should be routinely ordered in patients suspected of having tuberculosis to assist in the initial diagnosis and to assess the extent of disease in those previously diagnosed. While no pathognomonic pattern exists, a number of radiographic findings occur that are characteristic of tuberculosis. In the reactivation form of the disease, ongoing infection is characterized by patchy infiltrates of the upper segments or apices of the lung.[3] In advanced cases, cavitation is commonly observed. Granulomas in various stages of development are also seen frequently. In quiescent disease, calcification of granulomas often occurs. Thickening of the pleura and apical scarring are also seen in patients with past history of active disease. Early primary tuberculosis is often characterized by a discrete lower lobe lesion with enlarged hilar lymph nodes. Subsequent active disease in the lower lobes of the lung, however, is radiographically indistinct from other bacterial pneumonias.[3]

Examination of sputum is important in providing microbiologic evidence of tuberculosis.[11] Acid-fast bacilli may be detected in the sputa of virtually all patients with active pulmonary tuberculosis. Sputum collected in the morning is considered to have the highest number of organisms per volume and hence the highest yield; however, multiple sputum collections over a 24-hour period are recommended. For patients unable to produce sputum, fiberoptic bronchoscopy may be performed and samples obtained through biopsy or washings.[12] Alternatively, induction of sputum production or aspiration of gastric contents may be attempted. Once obtained, sputum should be sent for acid-fast stain and culture. The slow-growing characteristics of *Mycobacterium* dictate that culture results will not be available for 4–8 weeks. Cultures should nonetheless be performed because they are of higher diagnostic sensitivity than staining techniques in detecting positive sputa.[3] They are also useful in distinguishing *M. tuberculosis* from other mycobacteria as well as for screening for drug-resistant organisms.

The purified protein derivative (PPD) tuberculin skin test is the method most widely used for detecting tuberculous infection.[13] It may be used for identifying patients with subclinical infection as well as active disease. PPD as it exists today was developed in 1941 and consists of proteins derived from a single strain of *M. tuberculosis*. To distinguish it from skin tests for other mycobacteria, it is designated PPD-S, in recognition of its developer, Florence Seibert. One test unit of PPD-S (1 TU) contains 0.00002 mg of protein.[13] Current preparations of PPD-S contain Tween 80 as a stabilizer, which prevents the protein from adhering to the inside of the container or syringe, which would result in loss of potency.[13]

Three test strengths of PPD-S are available: first strength (1 TU), intermediate strength (5 TU), and second strength

(250 TU). The intermediate-strength form is almost invariably used for routine screening and diagnostic purposes. First-strength PPD-S is sometimes used for testing patients in whom a severe reaction may be expected (i.e., patients with a known prior positive test), though few data exist to support this practice.[14] Second-strength PPD-S may be used in testing patients with depressed cell-mediated immunity who have had a negative result with the intermediate-strength test, but appear likely to have tuberculosis on the basis of clinical criteria.

The basis for use of the tuberculin skin test is the fact that the majority of persons infected with *M. tuberculosis* manifest cutaneous hypersensitivity to the PPD antigen because of the recruitment of T lymphocytes that were sensitized during the primary infection. This results in the development of erythema and induration (swelling) at the test site, which are maximal at 48 hours after test administration. Even after effective chemotherapy has been given, cutaneous hypersensitivity persists, albeit to a gradually decreasing extent.[12]

The Mantoux method of PPD administration, which is the most reliable technique, consists of the intradermal injection of 0.1 mL of PPD containing 5 TU into the volar or dorsal surface of the forearm using a 27-gauge needle, keeping the bevel upward. A small wheal should be visible at the site to confirm intradermal disposition of the PPD. The test is read 48–72 hours after injection by measuring the diameter of the zone of induration. It is important that the size of the induration, not erythema, be measured. Although 48 hours is usually considered the best time for reading test results, a positive reaction remains for at least 5 days after the test has been administered.[14]

The definition of a positive tuberculin skin test is subject to a variety of criteria, as is its interpretation. In general, a positive test is defined as the development of an indurated reaction greater than 10 mm in diameter at 48 hours.[13] Studies in patients tested with PPD have shown a direct relationship between the reaction size and the probability of infection with *M. tuberculosis*. In these studies, a bimodal distribution of reaction sizes was observed, with one group having reactions between 0 and 4 mm and the other group with reaction sizes of 10–25 mm. A value of 10 mm was therefore selected as a point to classify the groups as noninfected or infected, respectively.[14]

The cutoff point of 10 mm for skin test reactivity may not be the ideal value for use in all subsets of patients; it may be higher or lower depending on the competency of the patient's immune system and the presence or absence of other factors that influence the size of the reaction. For example, some cross-reactivity toward PPD-S may be demonstrated in individuals who have been infected with nontuberculous mycobacteria.[15] Here, the presence of test reactivity may not imply true tuberculous infection. In such geographic areas as the southeastern United States, where infection from nontuberculous mycobacteria is endemic, many individuals without tuberculosis react to PPD with indurations of 5 to 12 mm. For these individuals, a higher cutoff point (e.g., 15 mm) would appear appropriate.[15] On the other hand, for individuals residing in areas with no nontuberculous mycobacteria (such as Alaska), the risk of a false-positive test result is much less, and a cutoff point lower than 10 mm could be used. For testing individuals who are likely to be recently infected with *M. tuberculosis*, such as the close contacts of an infected patient, a smaller cutoff point would again be indicated because of a higher degree of suspicion that any reaction would represent true infection.

While the tuberculin skin test alone cannot induce cutaneous hypersensitivity de novo, it may sufficiently enhance the low-level reactivity present in some patients so that conversion of a "doubtful" test result (1–9 mm) to a "positive" result (>10 mm) could occur after repeat testing. This "booster effect" occurs in patients with small reactions to PPD resulting either from past tuberculous infection or from infection with nontuberculous mycobacteria, and potentially may be misinterpreted as a true positive test.[16] All individuals identified during routine PPD screening as having a doubtfully positive reaction of less than 10 mm should be retested 1 week later. This should allow sufficient time for boosting to occur. Those whose reaction size increases to greater than 10 mm after the repeat test are identified as boosters and may be presumed to have latent infection which may not require treatment; nonboosters are considered to be without infection, and any subsequent positive skin test should be viewed as indicative of recent infection requiring treatment.[12,16]

As described above, false-positive tuberculin skin test results may occur in some patients. False-negative results also occur and may result from faulty test material, poor administration technique, observer error, or impairment of the host's immune system (Table 80.1).[14] To minimize the incidence of false-negative results, proper storage and administration techniques for tuberculin should be observed. Other skin test controls (mumps, *Candida*, trichophyton) should be applied to test for anergy when a negative skin test result is observed despite a clinical suspicion of tuberculosis.

While conventional diagnostic techniques are successful in identifying the majority of patients with infection from *M. tuberculosis*, diagnosis in others such as those with extrapulmonary disease or individuals who are anergic remains an enigma. Recent advances in in vitro immunologic testing for immune complexes appear promising in improving the diagnostic yield in these patients.[3,12]

## Treatment

Active pulmonary disease in tuberculosis is defined as the presence of clinical and radiographic signs of active respiratory tract infection with demonstration of the presence of *M. tuberculosis* by skin test and preferably also by sputum stain and/or culture. Chemotherapy of tuberculosis is the cornerstone of effective treatment. Three goals of chemotherapy exist: to eliminate as many organisms from the body as possible, thereby limiting the incidence of relapse to less than 5%; to prevent the development of resistance, which could result in treatment failure; and to minimize toxicity and cost of treatment while maximizing patient compliance.[17,18]

Three subpopulations of mycobacteria are postulated to exist within the body, each of which is treated best with certain antituberculous agents.[18,19] Most numerous are the extracellular, rapidly dividing bacteria; these are killed most readily by isoniazid (INH) and streptomycin and to a lesser extent by rifampin. A second group comprises those orga-

**Table 80.1** Reasons for False-Negative Tuberculin Skin Tests

| |
|---|
| Faulty testing material |
| Outdated material |
| Improper storage |
| Bacterial contamination |
| Adsorption onto container (not Tween stabilized) |
| Improper administration |
| Dose too small |
| Injection made too deeply |
| Improper interpretation |
| Delay in interpretation |
| Bias by interpreter |
| Faulty technique |
| Depression of tuberculin sensitivity |
| Noninfectious diseases that impair the immune system |
| Sarcoidosis |
| Amyloidosis |
| Lymphomas |
| Leukemias |
| AIDS |
| Viral infections |
| Rubeola |
| Influenza |
| Epstein–Barr virus |
| Hepatitis A or B |
| Varicella zoster virus |
| Polio |
| Cytomegalovirus |
| Live attenuated viral vaccines |
| Drug therapy |
| Topical or systemic corticosteroids |
| Immunosuppressive or cytotoxic drugs |
| Miscellaneous |
| Elderly (> 60 years) |
| Crohn's disease |
| Solid tumors |
| Radiation therapy |
| Systemic lupus erythematosus |
| Miliary tuberculosis |
| Uremia |

Adapted from Reichman LB: Tuberculin skin testing: the state of the art. Chest 1979;76 (suppl):764–770, with permission.

nisms residing within caseating granulomas; these organisms are usually in a dormant metabolic state but on occasion will increase their activity for short periods of time. Rifampin is unique in its ability to kill these organisms. The final subset are the intracellular mycobacteria present within macrophages. The acidic environment within macrophages inhibits the activity of most agents, but pyrazinamide (PZA) is most active here and readily kills intracellular bacteria. INH and rifampin are also active to a lesser extent.

The regimen of INH and streptomycin that was used in the 1950s had to be continued for 18–24 months to be effective; this regimen killed only extracellular organisms and required that other bacterial populations, or "persisters," migrate to extracellular sites where they would be more susceptible to, or could be destroyed by, the host's immune system.[18] Today, by combining antituberculous agents directed at all populations of bacteria, one can effect eradication of mycobacteria in the lung in a much shorter period of time. Use of shorter courses of therapy allows less time for adverse effects to occur and is less costly as well.

The emergence of resistance during therapy is also minimized with the use of combinations of drugs. It is estimated that $10^{11}$ organisms are present in a patient with cavitary tuberculosis.[19] As approximately 1 in $10^6$ bacteria is resistant to INH, it is very likely that monotherapy with INH for cavitary tuberculosis will fail as a result of the development of resistance. By combining INH with rifampin, to which 1 in $10^7$ organisms is resistant, the frequency of resistance to both antibiotics becomes 1 in $10^{13}$; that is, there is only a 1% chance of resistance developing to both INH and rifampin when given concurrently.

Current practices of chemotherapy for tuberculosis utilize combinations of two classes of agents: those that rapidly eliminate extracellular organisms from the sputum and decrease infectivity ("early bactericidal" drugs such as INH and streptomycin), and those that destroy slowly dividing organisms within granulomas and macrophages ("sterilizing" drugs such as rifampin and PZA).[20–22] As mentioned previously, this allows courses of therapy as short as 6 months to be used while preventing resistance from occurring. Bacteriostatic drugs such as ethambutol are of use in present-day regimens only when resistance to one or more bactericidal agents is suspected.[23]

Two distinct phases of this "short-course" form of chemotherapy are employed. The initial or "induction" phase may be from 2 weeks to 3 months in duration. The goal of this phase is to rapidly destroy extracellular bacteria and thereby render the sputum noninfectious. Daily dosing of drugs is required because of the relatively rapid growth of this target population of bacteria. INH and rifampin constitute the core regimen for this phase. They may be used alone or in combination with streptomycin or ethambutol when resistance is suspected. PZA may be added to the initial regimen if even more rapid killing is desired.

The second or "continuation" phase is of longer duration and is designed to eliminate "persisters" from the body. Combined therapy with INH and rifampin is again used here; addition of other agents appears to offer no benefit.[22] The duration of the continuation phase depends on the combination of agents that is used in the initial phase: if INH and rifampin (with or without ethambutol or streptomycin) were used initially, the continuation phase of treatment would be given until a total of 9 months of therapy is achieved; if INH, rifampin, and PZA were given (with either ethambutol or streptomycin) initially for 2 months, continuation therapy with INH and rifampin need only be given for an additional 4 months to yield 6 months total.[20,21] During the continuation phase INH and rifampin may be dosed twice weekly rather than daily. The organisms remaining at this point reside mainly within macrophages of granulomas and grow more slowly, allowing a longer dosing interval to be used. In addition, because rifampin is most active against organisms with intermittent spurts of growth activity, twice-weekly dosing theoretically may potentiate its action. Twice-weekly dosing is also less expensive and usually results in better patient compliance; however, a missed dose on twice-weekly therapy results in the patient missing 50% of that week's dose.

In summary, two frequently used "short-course" regimens exist. The most common regimen in the United States utilizes INH and rifampin (with or without ethambutol or streptomycin) given daily for 2 weeks to 3 months followed by INH and rifampin given either daily or biweekly to complete a course of 9 months. A shorter course of therapy that has also been shown to be successful involves an initial 2 months of therapy with four agents (INH, rifampin, and PZA with either ethambutol or streptomycin given daily) followed by a continuation phase of INH and rifampin. A variety of other regimens have been tested, but offer no advantage over those described.[22,24]

On occasion, use of INH or rifampin may be precluded because of adverse effect or resistance. Resistance to INH is most commonly acquired in noncompliant patients but may be primary in infected immigrant populations from Asia or Mexico.[25] When INH cannot be used for treatment a regimen of rifampin, PZA, and ethambutol or streptomycin given for 12 months is recommended. Because of its enormous value in treatment of tuberculosis, INH should probably be included in initial therapy for suspected resistance until results of sensitivity testing are known, after which it may be withdrawn if necessary.[24,25]

Limited studies have shown PZA to be an effective alternative to rifampin. When rifampin is contraindicated, a 9-month regimen of INH, PZA, and streptomycin may be used.[20] Alternatively, an 18-month course of INH and ethambutol is also acceptable.

### *Patient Factors*

Certain subsets of patients require special consideration by the clinician when selecting an appropriate chemotherapeutic regimen.

Patients in whom relapse of disease occurs despite adequate treatment usually present within 6 months after completion of therapy. Noncompliance is the major cause of therapeutic failure, and relapse is usually due to organisms that are susceptible to the antituberculous drugs used initially.[18,25] A direct relationship exists between the duration of previous therapy and the likelihood of resistant bacteria on relapse.[25] Patients who require retreatment should be considered to be infected with resistant organisms until proven otherwise. In general, therapy with INH and rifampin should be reinstated along with two additional drugs, usually PZA and streptomycin. This regimen may be altered when the sensitivity pattern becomes known.

Tuberculosis in children may be treated with regimens similar to those used in adults. A regimen of both INH and rifampin 10–20 mg/kg given daily for 1 month followed by rifampin 10–20 mg/kg and INH 20–40 mg/kg twice weekly for 8 months has been shown to be highly effective.[26]

Females with tuberculosis should be cautioned against becoming pregnant, as the disease poses a risk to the fetus as well as to the mother. Treatment regimens for tuberculosis in pregnant patients should involve agents with minimal teratogenic potential. A study that examined the incidence of birth defects resulting from various antituberculous drugs concluded that the risk to infants born to mothers treated with INH or ethambutol was equal to that in normal populations.[27] Rifampin therapy was also associated with a low complication rate, but too few pregnancies were studied to be conclusive. Treatment with streptomycin resulted in a higher-than-normal rate of infant malformations, mainly in the form of ototoxicity.[27] The teratogenic potential of PZA is unknown, and its use should therefore be avoided. Pregnant females with tuberculosis should probably receive INH and ethambutol for a period of 18 months. If a third drug is necessary, rifampin may be added for a total duration of therapy of 9 months. Alternatively, INH and ethambutol may be used during pregnancy and rifampin added after delivery, but whether this would allow a total course of less than 18 months to be given is unknown.

Patients with end-stage renal disease may be at increased risk for active tuberculosis because of an impairment in cell-mediated immune function.[28] Regimens need to be modified to compensate for decreased excretory function. Rifampin can be given at full doses, and the dose of INH need be reduced only in anephric patients who are slow acetylators. The daily dose of ethambutol should be reduced to 5–8 mg/kg daily. Streptomycin should be used with caution in patients with renal failure; a dose of 3–5 mg/kg may be given after each dialysis, with close monitoring of serum concentrations. It is unclear to what extent the dose of PZA should be modified in renal failure.

Extrapulmonary tuberculosis has traditionally been considered to be a more severe form of the disease, and recommendations for treatment usually include three or more drugs given for an extended period of time. From a theoretical standpoint, patients with only extrapulmonary disease probably harbor fewer organisms than do those with pulmonary tuberculosis. Considering the fact that the extravascular penetration of most antituberculous agents is excellent, it would appear that short-course therapy would be adequate for treatment. A recent study has confirmed this theory, demonstrating a 95% success rate for a 9-month treatment regimen of INH and rifampin.[29]

Patients receiving immunosuppressive therapy would appear to be at risk for rapid progression of tuberculosis. In general, however, a 9- to 12-month course of therapy with INH and rifampin appears adequate. Ethambutol should probably be added routinely during the initial phase of treatment. Reductions in the doses of immunosuppressive agents during therapy do not appear to be necessary.[30]

Although most antituberculous agents are dosed on a milligram-per-kilogram basis, the clearance of antituberculous agents does not appear to be influenced by weight.[31] Obese individuals may potentially receive excessive doses and be at risk for drug toxicity. In general, ideal body weight should therefore be used when calculating doses for obese patients.

### *Monitoring*

Patients should be monitored clinically and microbiologically to assess response to therapy. Symptoms such as fever, malaise, anorexia, and cough should decrease markedly within the first 2 weeks of therapy. Occasionally, fever will persist for a longer period of time despite adequate treatment. Sputum should be cultured every 2–4 weeks until two consecutive cultures are negative. In general, patients with a positive sputum culture but negative smear will undergo conversion more rapidly than patients with both a positive culture and smear.[32]

One hundred percent of compliant patients have negative sputum cultures after 6 months of appropriate therapy. In 1985, however, only 75% of patients treated for tuberculosis in the United States had negative sputum cultures documented after 6 months of therapy.[33] Others had no follow-up sputum cultures performed (18%) or were lost to follow-up (3%), which suggests failure of patients and/or their physicians in assuring adequate follow-up. It is important to note that 9-month regimens for tuberculosis assume culture conversion at 3 months, with 6 months of therapy continued after conversion.[22] Patients receiving INH and rifampin should actually be treated for 6 months after sputum conversion or for a total of 9 months, whichever is longer. This rule does not apply to patients treated with 6-month short-course regimens. After completion of treatment, patients should be examined every 3 months for 1 year for signs and symptoms of relapse. Follow-up chest x-rays are not necessary in asymptomatic individuals after treatment.[24]

## *Pharmacology of Antituberculosis Drugs*

### Isoniazid

Because chemotherapy is the most important component of therapy for tuberculosis, a brief discussion of the clinical pharmacology of the drugs used for treatment is indicated. Isoniazid, or isonicotinylhydrazide (INH), was introduced in 1952 as the first orally administered mycobactericidal agent. It is the most widely used agent for treatment of tuberculous infections in the world today.

INH acts by inhibiting synthesis of mycolic acids, which are a major component of the mycobacterial cell wall. It undergoes active transport into the bacterium where it acts to kill actively growing organisms in the extracellular environment and inhibits the growth of dormant organisms present within macrophages and in caseating granulomas. Primary resistance to INH occurs in about 1 in $10^6$ organisms, and is due to decreased active uptake of the drug.[34]

INH is completely absorbed in the gastrointestinal tract after oral administration and is distributed widely throughout the body. Bioavailability may be reduced when the drug is taken with meals and antacids or in patients with intestinal malabsorption syndromes.

Metabolism accounts for 70% to 90% of the elimination of INH. The drug undergoes hydrolysis forming a hydrazine moiety and isonicotinic acid either initially or after acetylation of the hydrazine side chain (Fig. 80.1). Monoacetyl hydrazine may be excreted unchanged in the urine, further acetylated to the diacetyl form, or hydroxylated to an electrophilic intermediate. The latter compound is felt to be responsible for the hepatotoxic effects seen in patients treated with INH.[35] The rates of acetylation of INH and monoacetyl hydrazine are dependent on an individual's phenotypic classification as either a slow or rapid acetylator. Caucasians are equally divided into slow and rapid acetylators (Fig. 80.2), whereas the Eskimos and Japanese are primarily rapid and the Egyptians primarily slow acetylators. The elimination rate of INH is dependent on acetylator phenotype, with half-lives of 1–2 and 2–5 hours observed in rapid and slow acetylators, respectively.[36]

Because of the small amount of INH excreted unchanged via the kidneys, dose adjustment in patients with impaired renal function is necessary only in slow acetylators with a creatinine clearance less than 10 mL/min. A reduction of daily dose by 50% is recommended in patients with severe hepatic disease to prevent drug accumulation and lessen the chance for hepatotoxicity.

Therapy with INH results in development of adverse effects in approximately 5.5% of patients. A transient elevation in serum transaminases occurs in 12% to 15% of patients and usually occurs within the first 8–12 weeks of therapy.[35] Overt hepatotoxicity, however, occurs in only 1% of cases. Destruction of hepatocytes by accumulation of reactive hydrazine metabolites is most frequently cited as the cause. Risk factors for hepatotoxicity include patient age (Table 80.2) and preexisting liver disease. Consumption of alcohol is probably not a risk factor if it has not resulted in preexisting liver disease.

INH also may result in neurotoxicity, most frequently presenting as peripheral neuropathy.[35] Central nervous system effects such as ataxia, mental status changes, or exacerbation of preexisting convulsive disorders are also occasionally observed. INH exerts its neurotoxic effect through enhanced elimination of pyridoxine and/or competitive inhibition with pyridoxine in its action as a cofactor in the synthesis of synaptic neurotransmitters.[35] Patients with pyridoxine deficiency such as alcoholics, children, and the malnourished are at increased risk, as are patients who are slow acetylators of INH and those predisposed to neuropathy such as diabetics. Coadministration of as little as 6 mg of pyridoxine daily will reduce the incidence of these neurotoxic effects from 20% to less than 1%.[34,35]

Other adverse effects occasionally seen with INH therapy include a lupuslike syndrome which may involve rash, fever, vasculitis, arthralgias, and cytopenias.

INH is usually administered as a daily dose of 5 mg/kg (maximum 300 mg) orally with pyridoxine 50 mg given concurrently. For twice-weekly therapy, a dose of 15 mg/kg (maximum 900 mg) is used. Patients should be monitored for signs of hepatitis (malaise, anorexia, nausea, jaundice) and neurotoxicity (paresthesias, tingling, numbness, mental status changes, seizures). Serum glutamic–oxaloacetic and glutamic–pyruvic transaminases may be monitored monthly with the knowledge that any elevations are usually transient and will resolve with continued therapy. INH should be discontinued if transaminase values rise to greater than five times baseline values and/or symptoms of hepatitis develop.

INH has been reported to inhibit the metabolism of phenytoin, carbamazepine, primidone, and warfarin.[36] Patients who are being treated with these agents should be monitored closely and appropriate dose adjustments should be made when necessary.

***Effect of Acetylator Phenotype on Hepatotoxicity*** When the monoacetyl hydrazine metabolite was identified as the cause of INH-induced hepatotoxicity, a number of investigators postulated that patients who were rapid acetylators would constitute a high-risk group for development of liver damage. Rapid acetylators were thought to produce larger amounts of this compound than their slow acetylator counterparts. A few early retrospective studies tended to confirm this theory.[37]

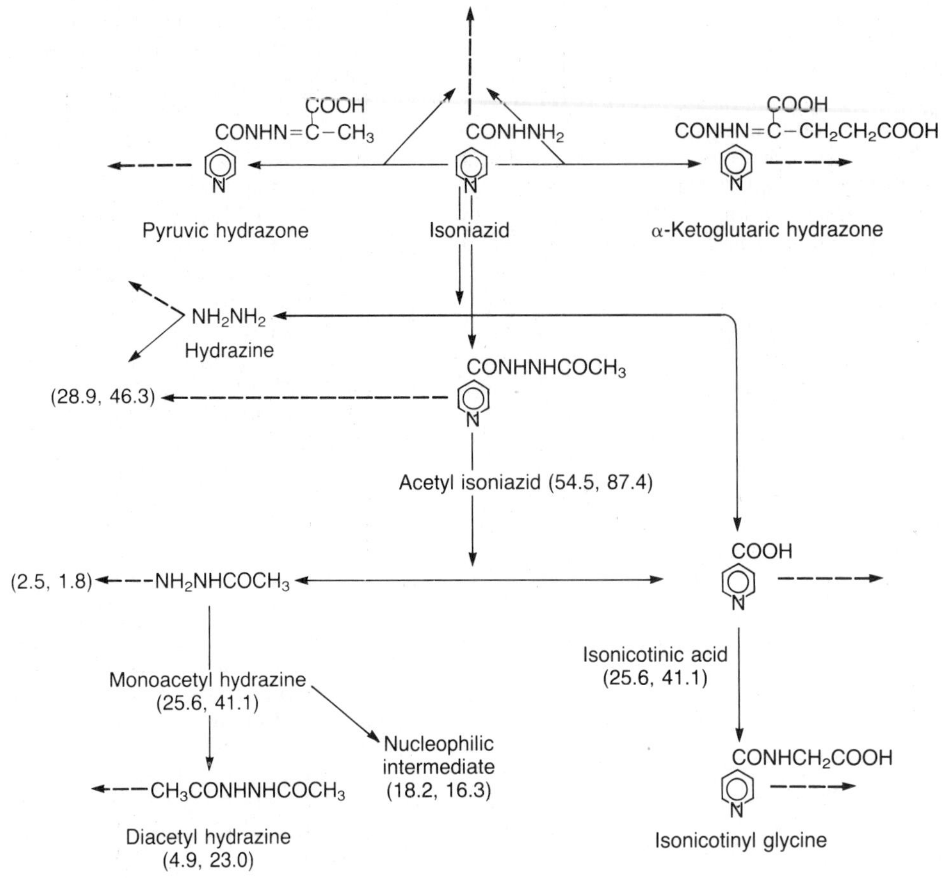


**Figure 80.1** Pathways for the metabolism of isoniazid in man. Numbers in parentheses are percentages of each metabolite formed in slow and rapid acetylators, respectively. ----, renal elimination. *(From Weber WW, Hein DW: Clin Pharmacokinet 1979;4:401–422, with permission.)*

More recent prospective studies using larger subject populations have suggested that rapid acetylators are not at increased risk for hepatitis from INH.[38] Upon review of the metabolic pathways for INH in humans (Fig. 80.1) it becomes apparent that although rapid acetylators may initially generate a higher proportion of monoacetyl hydrazine than do slow acetylators, they also convert the monoacetyl form more readily to the nontoxic diacetyl form. The net amount of monoacetyl hydrazine recovered is the same in both groups. On the basis of this information, prospective testing of an individual's acetylator phenotype for the purpose of lessening the chance for hepatotoxicity appears unnecessary.

**Figure 80.2** Bimodal distribution of isoniazid half-lives as related to acetylation status. Isoniazid 5 mg/kg was administered to patients intravenously. Light bars indicate rapid acetylators; dark bars, slow acetylators. *(From Tiiten H: Isoniazid and ethionamide serum levels and inactivation in Finnish subjects. Scand J Resp Dis 1969;50:110, with permission.)*

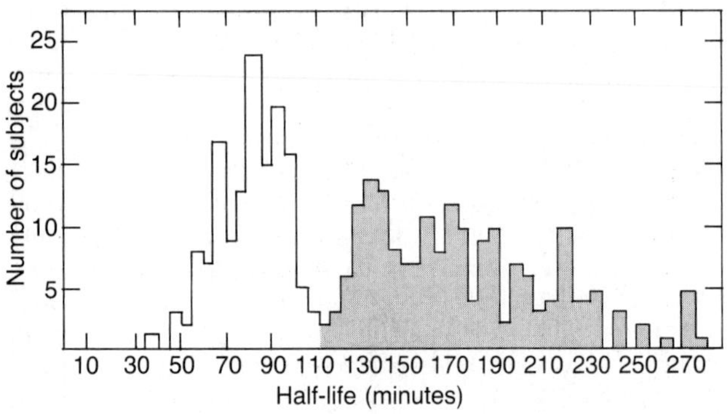


**Table 80.2** Effect of Age on Incidence of Hepatitis From Isoniazid

| *Age* | *Frequency (%)* |
|---|---|
| 0–19 | 0.3–0.6 |
| 20–34 | 0.3–2.2 |
| 35–49 | 1.2–3.2 |
| 50–64 | 2.3–3.4 |
| >65 | 2.3–4.2 |

Adapted from American Thoracic Society,[41] Comstock and Edwards,[44] and Dash et al.[45]

**Rifampin**

The introduction of rifampin in 1967 revolutionized the treatment of tuberculosis by providing successful treatment using shorter courses of therapy. Combined therapy with rifampin and INH results in sterilization of tuberculosis lesions much more rapidly than can be achieved with INH alone.[12,34] Rifampin possesses the ability to kill the slow-growing mycobacteria present within macrophages and in caseating granulomas, thereby acting synergistically with INH which is bactericidal primarily against actively dividing extracellular organisms.[17,34] Approximately 1 of every $10^{7-8}$ mycobacteria is inherently resistant to rifampin, usually because of an altered RNA polymerase. Resistance develops rapidly when rifampin is used as a single agent in therapy. Therefore, it is imperative that it be used only in combination with other antituberculous agents.

Because of its high lipid solubility at physiologic pH, rifampin distributes well into most body tissues, including cerebrospinal fluid.[39] This is evidenced by the fact that body secretions such as sweat, urine, saliva, and tears will be colored orange in a patient receiving rifampin. Patients who wear soft contact lenses should be cautioned that their lenses may be dyed permanently.

Approximately 85% of a dose of rifampin is eventually metabolized. The parent drug is largely excreted in the bile and undergoes enterohepatic circulation as does its primary metabolite, desacetylrifampin, albeit to a lesser extent. A smaller proportion of drug is hydrolyzed to formylrifampin. Rifampin appears to cause proliferation of the smooth endoplasmic reticulum in hepatocytes, resulting in an increase in cytochrome $P_{450}$ oxidase metabolic activity. This can increase the rate of metabolism of a variety of drugs, including rifampin itself.[36]

Dose adjustment of rifampin is unnecessary in patients with impaired renal function because of its extensive metabolism. In patients with hepatic dysfunction, rifampin may accumulate and result in hyperbilirubinemia by competing with bilirubin for uptake by hepatocytes.[35] Dose adjustment in patients with liver disease is therefore indicated to minimize the occurrence of hyperbilirubinemia.

Adverse effects associated with rifampin are infrequent and rarely necessitate withdrawal of drug. Elevations in hepatic enzymes have been attributed to rifampin in 10% to 15% of patients, with overt hepatotoxicity occurring in less than 1%. Rifampin has the potential to augment the hepatotoxicity of INH by increasing microsomal enzyme activity, which is the enzyme system responsible for converting monoacetyl hydrazine into a hepatotoxic intermediate. When INH and rifampin are used together, elevations in serum transaminases occur in 20% to 30% of patients, usually within the first 8 weeks of therapy.[35] In most cases this is transient in nature. More frequent adverse effects of rifampin include rash, fever, and gastrointestinal distress.

Allergic reactions to rifampin have been reported, and occur mainly in patients receiving therapy at twice weekly intervals. Sensitization of the immune system and development of antirifampin antibodies are postulated to occur, with subsequent rechallenge resulting in symptoms.[35] These reactions may take the form of a flulike syndrome, with development of fever, chills, headache, arthralgias, and, rarely, hypotension and shock. Alternatively, hemolytic anemia or acute renal failure may occur.

As mentioned previously, rifampin's induction of hepatic enzymes may enhance elimination of a number of drugs including theophylline, steroids, narcotics, oral hypoglycemics, and warfarin. In addition, an increase in vitamin D metabolism has been reported with rifampin, with development of osteomalacia in some cases.[35]

Rifampin is administered orally at a dose of 10 mg/kg (maximum 600 mg) daily or 15 mg/kg twice to three times weekly. Patients should be monitored for signs of hepatotoxicity as well as skin appearance and renal function. Patients who interrupt therapy should be restarted on the drug cautiously to avoid allergic reactions. Females who use oral contraceptives should be advised to use another form of contraception during therapy. Finally, the discolorizing effects of rifampin on urine, other secretions, and contact lenses should be discussed with the patient.

**Ethambutol**

Ethambutol, or *d*-ethylenediimino-di-1-butanol, was first used in the treatment of tuberculosis in the early 1960s. Its mechanism of action against mycobacteria is probably through inhibition of bacterial RNA synthesis. It is a slow-acting tuberculostatic agent which has a delayed onset of activity in vitro, although studies performed in vivo have shown that ethambutol enhances phagocytic killing of intracellular mycobacteria.[23] Because of its static activity, ethambutol is used only in combination with bactericidal agents. Primary resistance to ethambutol is rare, and resistance during therapy develops infrequently, probably because a series of stepwise mutations are necessary for it to occur.

Approximately 80% of a dose of ethambutol is excreted unchanged in the urine via both glomerular filtration and tubular secretion. The remaining fraction is oxidized to the aldehyde or carboxylic acid form. The serum half-life for ethambutol is normally 3–5 hours but increases to 10 hours in anephric patients.

Dose adjustment of ethambutol in patients with hepatic dysfunction is unnecessary. A 50% reduction in daily dose is indicated in patients with a creatinine clearance between 10 and 30 mL/min, and a 65% reduction of the normal dose in those with a creatinine clearance less than 10 mL/min.[36] During hemodialysis the half-life of ethambutol is reduced to 2 hours, but only a small fraction of the total amount of drug in the body is removed because of its large volume of distribution. Therefore, usually no supplemental dose is required after dialysis.[36]

Retrobulbar neuritis is the major adverse effect noted in patients treated with ethambutol. Incidence is dose related, with occurrence rates of 5% in patients receiving daily doses of 25 mg/kg but less than 1% in those treated with 15 mg/kg daily.[35] Patients usually complain of a change in visual acuity and/or inability to see the color green. Risk factors for toxicity include high (25 mg/kg/d) doses of drug and decreased renal function leading to drug accumulation. Avoidance of ethambutol use in children is recommended because of the difficulty in monitoring visual acuity in this group. Other adverse effects that may be observed include rash, fever, arthralgias, and gastrointestinal irritation.

Ethambutol is administered orally at a daily dose of 15 mg/kg or as a biweekly dose of 50 mg/kg. Patients should have baseline tests of renal function and visual acuity, with follow-up tests of vision every 1–2 months.

### Pyrazinamide

Pyrazinamide is a pyrazine analog of nicotinamide. Originally developed in the 1950s, PZA was used only sparingly after clinicians noted the frequent occurrence of hepatotoxicity with daily doses of 3,000 mg or more. The recent discovery that smaller daily doses are associated with a much lower incidence of adverse effects has prompted a resurgence in the use of PZA as a second-line and, in some cases, first-line agent for treatment of tuberculosis.[17]

PZA is tuberculostatic in vitro using conventional culture media, but is bactericidal toward actively dividing organisms residing in the acidic environment within macrophages. Studies conducted in animal models of tuberculosis have demonstrated the ability of PZA in combination with INH to sterilize tuberculous lesions more rapidly than INH alone.[17] The precise mechanism of action of PZA on mycobacteria is unknown.

PZA undergoes extensive biotransformation in vivo, with 95% to 99% of a dose being excreted in the form of metabolites. It is hydrolyzed primarily to pyrazinoic acid, with subsequent hydroxylation and excretion via the kidney.[36] Pyrazinoic acid has some antituberculous activity, but other metabolites do not. The usual half-life of PZA in serum is 9–10 hours.

Reduction of the daily dose of PZA in patients with impaired renal function is apparently unnecessary. A reduction of dose in patients with hepatic dysfunction is indicated, judging from the dose-dependent hepatotoxicity observed with the drug. No specific guidelines have been established, but a 50% reduction of daily dose in patients with severe hepatic disease would appear appropriate.

As mentioned previously, hepatotoxicity is the major limiting adverse effect seen with PZA therapy. Results of early studies that used doses of 3 g daily reported a 15% incidence of hepatitis.[35] The incidence is much lower when daily doses of 1–2 g are used. Patients at risk are primarily those with preexisting impairment in hepatic function.

PZA's primary metabolite, pyrazinoic acid, may compete with uric acid for elimination via the kidney, resulting in exacerbation of gout in susceptible individuals. PZA also frequently causes gastrointestinal irritation with nausea and vomiting.

PZA is administered orally at a daily dose of 15–30 mg/kg up to a maximum of 2,000 mg. A dose of 50 mg/kg may be given twice weekly. Patients should undergo baseline testing for hepatic function and should be monitored for symptoms of hepatitis.

### Streptomycin

Streptomycin was released in 1947 and was the first antibiotic to be used in treatment of tuberculosis. It is one of three aminoglycoside antibiotics (along with amikacin and kanamycin) that are active against mycobacteria. Although it is bactericidal in vitro, streptomycin diffuses poorly into granulomas and macrophages and lacks activity in the intracellular environment. Therefore, it is active only against extracellular organisms and clinically has only static activity when used alone. Approximately 1 in $10^6$ mycobacteria is inherently resistant to streptomycin.[34]

Renal excretion as unchanged drug accounts for 90% of the elimination of streptomycin. Its serum half-life is 2–3 hours in normal individuals and may approach 100 hours in anuric patients. Hemodialysis reduces serum concentrations by 25% to 30%.[36] Dosage regimens of streptomycin must be altered in patients with impaired renal function. This may be accomplished most easily by lengthening the interval between doses.

Impairment of 8th cranial nerve function is the most important adverse effect of streptomycin. Vestibular function is most frequently affected, but hearing may also be impaired. If treatment with streptomycin continues despite the occurrence of toxicity, damage may not be completely reversible.[35] Pain on injection and sterile abscess formation may also occur during therapy with streptomycin. Streptomycin is the least nephrotoxic of the aminoglycosides, with an estimated incidence of renal toxicity of less than 1%. Neuromuscular blockade has been reported to occur rarely.

For treatment of tuberculosis, streptomycin is administered at a dose of 1,000 mg daily for 2 months followed by biweekly injections when continued for the remainder of treatment. Although the intramuscular route is preferred, intravenous injections may be given over a 1-hour period. Patients should be monitored for signs of ototoxicity including tinnitus, tone deafness, nystagmus, vertigo, nausea, or vomiting. Baseline audiometric testing should be performed and repeated every 1–2 months. In patients with impaired renal function, serum concentrations may be used as a guide for adjustment of dosage regimens. In general, values greater than 60 μg/mL should be avoided.[34,35]

### *para*-Aminosalicylate

*para*-Aminosalicylic acid (PAS) is rarely used in present-day chemotherapeutic regimens for tuberculosis. Originally discovered by Lehman in 1946, its activity against *M. tuberculosis* has been demonstrated to be much less than that of contemporary agents.[34] In addition, the large daily doses required and the high incidence of gastrointestinal irritation make it unsuitable for routine use. It is therefore used only when other more active agents are contraindicated because of resistance, allergy, or adverse effects.

Approximately 45% of a dose of PAS is excreted in the urine as the acetylated metabolite, which possesses antimycobacterial activity. Another 15% is excreted as other metabolites, most notably a glycine conjugate which is also active. The remaining 40% is excreted unchanged in the urine. The usual serum half-life of PAS is 1 hour.[36] A reduction in dose should be made in patients with severe renal disease but is not necessary for those with hepatic impairment.

Adverse effects are frequent and usually gastrointestinal in nature, with anorexia, nausea, abdominal pain, and diarrhea all common. A lupuslike syndrome may also develop with fevers, malaise, joint pain, and hematologic abnormalities. Patients who develop hypersensitivity to PAS reportedly may develop cross-sensitivity to INH or streptomycin.[35]

PAS is administered orally at a dose of 8–12 g daily, usually divided into three or four doses and taken with meals to minimize gastric upset. Patients should receive periodic complete blood counts and be followed closely to ensure compliance. PAS may inhibit the acetylation of INH and therefore increase its serum concentrations. Conversely, PAS has been reported to decrease the bioavailability of rifampin by interfering with its absorption.

### Ethionamide, Cycloserine, and Capreomycin

Ethionamide, cycloserine, and capreomycin are used infrequently because of their lesser activity and higher incidence of adverse effects compared with conventional agents. As with PAS, they are used in substitution for first- and second-line agents only when indicated because of resistance, allergy, or adverse effects. Ethionamide, or $\alpha$-ethyl thioisonicotinamide, is structurally similar to isoniazid. It is less active than INH, however, and is bacteriostatic only. Organisms resistant to INH are also resistant to ethionamide. Its adverse effects are also similar to those of INH but occur more frequently.[3,34]

Cycloserine is a cyclic derivative of the amino acid serine. Another bacteriostatic agent, it acts to inhibit cell wall synthetic processes that require D-alanine. Cycloserine is used infrequently because of its high incidence of adverse effects involving the central nervous system including headaches, tremor, vertigo, nystagmus, confusion, visual disturbances, lethargy, and seizures.[3,34]

Capreomycin is a cyclic polypeptide antibiotic produced by *Streptomyces capreolus*. It is bacteriostatic, acting to inhibit bacterial protein synthesis. It must be administered daily via the intramuscular route to be effective. Frequent adverse effects include pain on injection, eosinophilia, ototoxicity, and nephrotoxicity.[3,34]

### New Agents

The choice of antituberculosis agents has not changed appreciably since the introduction of rifampin in the 1970s. Recently, data have been published demonstrating the impressive in vitro activity of 4-quinolone antibiotics such as ciprofloxacin against *M. tuberculosis* and nontuberculous mycobacteria.[42] Pending confirmatory studies performed in vitro and in vivo, these agents may serve as useful alternatives to current first- and second-line agents when resistance or adverse effect precludes their use in the treatment of tuberculosis.

## *Nondrug Therapy*

Initial respiratory isolation of patients with pulmonary tuberculosis is recommended. Confinement of the patient to a closed hospital room and use of masks by all visitors are generally practiced; however, use of a mask by the patient alone to limit dissemination of organisms is probably just as efficacious. The institution of chemotherapy will rapidly render a patient's sputum noninfectious.[40] Isolation may be discontinued and the patient discharged after 10–14 days of treatment, even if sputum cultures and smears are still positive.[12,41] Respiratory isolation is not necessary for tuberculosis limited to extrapulmonary sites.

Surgical intervention including lobectomy was once a common mode of treatment for tuberculosis. Today, indications for surgery are limited to removal of necrotic tissue or drainage of abscesses and other sites of fluid collection.[12,18]

All close contacts of patients diagnosed with pulmonary tuberculosis should be skin tested, with a repeat test given after 3 months to detect late converters. Those with positive tests should receive prophylactic therapy. Because of their higher risk for progressive primary tuberculosis, children who are close contacts may receive prophylactic therapy immediately upon identification, with discontinuation at 3 months if a skin test at that time is negative.[41]

## *Prophylaxis*

Prophylactic therapy for tuberculosis consists of daily administration of 10–15 mg/kg (maximum 300 mg) of INH for a period of 1 year. The term "prophylaxis" is inaccurate because it implies that therapy is used to prevent infection. Rather, candidates for INH prophylaxis have already been infected, but receive therapy to prevent progression to active disease.[43]

A patient should receive INH prophylaxis if he/she has an appreciable risk for developing active tuberculosis. As therapy with INH may result in adverse effects, notably hepatotoxicity, it should be restricted to those in whom the risk for adverse effects from INH is less than their lifetime risk for developing active tuberculosis.[44,45] Children constitute one such group; as noted before, those who are exposed to an individual with active tuberculosis should be assumed to be infected and receive INH for at least 3 months. If the skin test and/or chest x-ray are positive at 3 months, a total of 12 months of therapy is indicated.

Other individuals who are considered eligible for INH prophylaxis include certain asymptomatic persons with a positive tuberculin skin test. A 1-year course of INH should be given to those who possess risk factors in addition to their skin test positivity. As active tuberculosis occurs most frequently in skin test–positive individuals within 2 years after test conversion,[45] any person who is considered "newly infected" should receive INH prophylaxis. Newly infected patients are defined as those who have converted their skin test to positive (greater than 10 mm) within the last 2 years, or who have a recent history of exposure to an infected individual and a skin test reading of 5 mm or more.[41] The lifetime risk for the development of active disease in these patients without treatment is approximately 5%.[45]

Asymptomatic individuals with a positive tuberculin test of unknown duration also require prophylactic therapy if they possess other factors that could potentially increase their risk of developing active disease. Such risk factors include evidence of parenchymal lesions suggestive of nonprogressive tuberculous infection on chest x-ray; silicosis; diabetes mellitus; prolonged (more than 2 months) therapy with corticosteroids or other immunosuppressive drugs; presence of hematologic or reticuloendothelial diseases such as leukemias, lymphomas, or AIDS; chronic hemodialysis; and patients who are postgastrectomy.[41] To date, only the radiographic presence of nonprogressive infection and postgastrectomy state have been associated with an increased risk of active disease.[43] Nevertheless, tuberculin-positive patients with any of these conditions should receive INH prophylaxis until evidence to the contrary has been presented.

Tuberculin-positive individuals who have received either INH prophylaxis or adequate treatment for tuberculosis in the past and subsequently develop one of the risk factors just listed are probably not candidates for an additional course of INH prophylaxis; however, these patients should be monitored for any signs of recurrence of disease.

The use of INH prophylaxis in patients with a positive tuberculin skin test of unknown duration and no other risk factors is of questionable benefit. As the lifetime risk of active disease is unknown but assumed to be less than that of recently infected individuals, the decision to use INH is more dependent on their likelihood of developing hepatotoxicity. For patients less than 35 years of age, the incidence of INH-induced hepatotoxicity is very low (Table 80.2),[45] and prophylactic treatment may be indicated. For those older than 35, the risk of hepatotoxicity rises appreciably and appears to outweigh the risk of developing active tuberculosis. INH prophylaxis therefore should not be given to patients 35 and older who have a positive tuberculin test of unknown duration as their only risk for tuberculosis. Younger patients, particularly those under 21, should receive prophylaxis. Evidence supporting INH prophylaxis in patients between ages 21 and 35 is less definitive.[46]

Patients in whom INH prophylaxis is considered should have a chest x-ray performed to rule out active disease. Baseline laboratory tests for hepatic function should be performed. INH prophylaxis is contraindicated in patients with hepatic dysfunction because of an increased risk for hepatotoxicity. If infection with INH-resistant organisms is suspected, combined therapy with INH and rifampin should be used; the use of rifampin alone for prophylaxis has not been shown to be reliable.[47]

Screening for active disease through annual chest x-rays has been suggested for all patients and employees who have completed a course of prophylaxis as well as for those who have chosen not to receive INH. This practice appears to be unnecessary, however, as individuals diagnosed with pulmonary tuberculosis caused by reactivation are almost always symptomatic and may be detected from history and clinical presentation.[48]

***Use of BCG Vaccine*** The bacille Calmette–Guérin (BCG) is an attenuated, hybridized strain of *Mycobacterium* that is genetically similar yet distinct from *M. tuberculosis* and *M. bovis*, the two most common human pathogenic species. It was originally developed in 1921 and is used as a prophylactic vaccine against tuberculosis. Administration of BCG vaccine is compulsory in 64 countries and is officially recommended in 118 others.[49]

Vaccination with BCG produces a subclinical infection resulting in sensitization of T lymphocytes and immunity to *M. tuberculosis*, as well as cutaneous hypersensitivity and a positive tuberculin skin test.[49] This invalidates any subsequent use of skin test positivity as a sign of true tuberculous infection as long as the effect of the vaccine persists, usually about 10 years. Because of this interference, BCG vaccination should be used only in geographic areas where tuberculosis infection rates are sufficiently high to preclude the use of the PPD skin test as a screening tool and where health programs are inadequate to detect newly infected individuals. Such areas include underdeveloped countries in Asia, Africa, and South America as well as arguably in certain metropolitan areas within the United States and other developed countries where large immigrant populations exist.

The success of BCG in preventing tuberculosis remains uncertain. While some studies cite protection rates of as high as 80%, others show no or even negative protection rates with BCG.[50] Attempts to explain the wide discrepancy in protection rates invoke differences in study design, in the nutritional status of subjects, in the presence of atypical mycobacterial infection, in the frequency and virulence of *M. tuberculosis*, and in the potency of the vaccine.[49,50] On the basis of these and other data, certain conclusions about the vaccine may be made. Administration of BCG is not effective in reducing the rate of primary infection with *M. tuberculosis*, nor is it effective in preventing reinfection when given to previously tuberculin-positive individuals. BCG is, however, effective in reducing the rate of progression of primary infection to active disease.[51] Therefore, the protective benefits of BCG may be masked in countries with high rates of tuberculosis caused by reinfection rather than reactivation of latent disease. Protective benefits are highest when BCG is given to tuberculin-negative individuals residing in or traveling to areas endemic for tuberculosis.[49–51]

Patients who have received BCG in the past may still be screened using PPD skin testing, although positive results are subject to interpretation. A vaccination scar should be identified or documentation of BCG administration obtained for confirmatory purposes. What reaction size should be considered "significant" depends upon history of exposure to an active case of tuberculosis as well as the time elapsed since vaccination.[52]

## References


1. Smith E. Lectures on certain views on the nature and treatment of phthisis pulmonalis. Br Med J 1857;1:107–111.
2. Centers for Disease Control. Tuberculosis provisional data—United States, 1986. MMWR. 1987;36:254–255.
3. Des Prez RM, Goodwin RA. *Mycobacterium tuberculosis*, in Mandell GL, Douglas RG, Bennett JE (eds): Principles and Practice of Infectious Diseases, 2nd ed. New York, John Wiley and Sons, 1985, p 1383.
4. Stead WW, Te T. The significance of the tuberculin skin test in elderly persons. Ann Intern Med 1987;107:837–842.
5. Sunderam G, McDonald RJ, Maniatis T, et al. Tuberculosis as a manifestation of the acquired immunodeficiency syndrome (AIDS). JAMA 1986;256:362–366.
6. Louie E, Rice LB, Holzman RS. Tuberculosis in non-Haitian patients with acquired immunodeficiency syndrome. Chest 1986;90:542–545.
7. Riley RL, Mills CC, Nyka W, et al. Aerial dissemination of pulmonary tuberculosis: A two-year study of contagion in a tuberculosis ward. Am J Hyg 1959;70:185–196.
8. Geppert EF, Leff A. The pathogenesis of pulmonary and miliary tuberculosis. Arch Intern Med 1979;139:1381–1383.
9. Alvarez S, McCabe WR. Extrapulmonary tuberculosis revis-

ited: a review of experience at Boston City and other hospitals. Medicine 1984;63:25–55.

10. Stead WW. Pathogenesis of a first episode of chronic pulmonary tuberculosis in man: recrudescence of residuals of the primary infection or exogenous reinfection? Am Rev Resp Dis 1967; 95:729–745.
11. Strumpf IJ, Tsang AY, Sayre JW. Reevaluation of sputum staining for the diagnosis of pulmonary tuberculosis. Am Rev Resp Dis 1979;119:599–602.
12. Glassroth J, Robins AG, Snider DE. Tuberculosis in the 1980's. N Engl J Med 1980;302:1441–1450.
13. Snider DE. The tuberculin skin test. Am Rev Resp Dis 1982; 125(suppl):108–118.
14. Reichman LB. Tuberculin skin testing: The state of the art. Chest 1979;76(suppl):764–770.
15. Bass LB, Sanders RV, Kirkpatrick MB. Choosing an appropriate cutting point for conversion in annual tuberculin skin testing. Am Rev Resp Dis 1985;132:379–381.
16. Thompson NJ, Glassroth JL, Snider DE, et al. The booster phenomenon in serial tuberculin testing. Am Rev Resp Dis 1979;119:587–597.
17. Snider DE, Cohn DL, Davidson PT, et al. Standard therapy for tuberculosis 1985. Chest 1985;87(suppl):117S–124S.
18. Alford RH, Manian FA. Current antimicrobial management of tuberculosis, in Remington JS, Schwatz MN (eds): Current Clinical Topics in Infectious Diseases. McGraw-Hill, New York, 1987, pp 204–226.
19. Mitchison DA. Basic mechanisms of chemotherapy. Chest 1979;76(suppl):771–781.
20. Aquinas SM. Short-course therapy for tuberculosis. Drugs 1982;24:118–132.
21. Angel JH. The case for short-course chemotherapy of pulmonary tuberculosis. Drugs 1983;26:1–8.
22. Stratton MA, Reed MD. Short-course drug therapy for tuberculosis. Clin Pharm 1986;5:977–987.
23. Crowle AJ, Sbarbaro JA, Judson FN, et al. The effect of ethambutol on tubercle bacilli within cultured human macrophages. Am Rev Resp Dis 1985;132:742–745.
24. Deresinski SC. A stepwise guide for treating tuberculosis. West J Med 1984;141:546–548.
25. Suwanogool S, Smith SM, Smith LG, et al. Drug resistance encountered in the retreatment of *Mycobacterium tuberculosis* infections. J Chron Dis 1984;37:925–931.
26. Kendig EL. Evolution of short-course antimicrobial treatment of tuberculosis in children, 1951–1984. Pediatrics 1985;75:684–686.
27. Snider DM, Layde PM, Johnson MW, et al. Treatment of tuberculosis during pregnancy. Am J Resp Dis 1980;122:65–79.
28. Andrew OT, Schoenfeld PY, Hopewell PC, et al. Tuberculosis in patients with end-stage renal disease. Am J Med 1980; 68:59–65.
29. Dutt AK, Moers D, Stead WW. Short-course chemotherapy for extrapulmonary tuberculosis: nine years' experience. Ann Intern Med 1986;104:7–12.
30. Dautzenberg B, Grosset J, Fechner J, et al. The management of thirty immunocompromised patients with tuberculosis. Am Rev Resp Dis 1984;129:494–496.
31. Geiseler PJ, Manis RD, Maddux MS. Dosage of antituberculosis drugs in obese patients. Am Rev Resp Dis 1985;131:944–946.
32. Kim TC, Blackman RS, Heatwole KM, et al. Acid-fast bacilli in sputum smears of patients with pulmonary tuberculosis: prevalence and significance of negative smears pretreatment and positive smears post-treatment. Am Rev Resp Dis 1984;129: 264–268.
33. Centers for Disease Control. Bacteriologic conversion of sputum among tuberculosis patients—United States. MMWR 1985; 34:747–750.
34. Mandell GL, Sande MA. Drugs used in the chemotherapy of tuberculosis and leprosy, in Gilman AG, Goodman LS, Gilman A (eds): The Pharmacological Basis of Therapeutics. New York, Macmillan, 1980, p 1200.
35. Girling DJ. Adverse effects of antituberculosis drugs. Drugs 1982;23:56–74.
36. Holdiness MR. Clinical pharmacokinetics of the antituberculosis drugs. Clin Pharmacokinet 1984;9:511–544.
37. Mitchell JR, Thorgeirsson UP, Black M, et al. Increased incidence of isoniazid hepatitis in rapid acetylators: Possible relation in hydrazine metabolites. Clin Pharmacol Ther 1975; 18:70–79.
38. Alexander MR, Louie SG, Guernsey BG. Isoniazid-associated hepatitis. Clin Pharm 1982;1:148–153.
39. Holdiness MR. Cerebrospinal pharmacokinetics of the antituberculosis drugs. Clin Pharmacokinet 1985;10:532–534.
40. Kamat SR, Dawson JJY, Devadatta S, et al. A controlled study of the influence of segregation of tuberculosis patients for one year on the attack rate of tuberculosis in a 5-year period in close family contacts in south India. Bull WHO 1966;34:517–532.
41. American Thoracic Society. Treatment of tuberculosis and tuberculous infection in adults and children. Am Rev Resp Dis 1986;134:355–363.
42. Fenlon CH, Cynamon MH. Comparative in vitro activities of ciprofloxacin and other 4-quinolones against *Mycobacterium tuberculosis* and *Mycobacterium intracellulare*. Antimicrob Agents Chemother 1986;29:386–388.
43. Anonymous. Chemoprophylaxis for tuberculosis. Tubercle 1981;61:69–72.
44. Comstock GW. Prevention of tuberculosis among tuberculin reactors: Maximizing benefits, minimizing risks. JAMA 1986; 256:2729–2730.
45. Dash LA, Comstock GW, Flynn JPG. Isoniazid preventive therapy: retrospect and prospect. Am Rev Resp Dis 1980; 121:1039–1044.
46. Taylor WC, Aronson MD, Delbanco TL. Should young adults with a positive tuberculin test take isoniazid? Ann Intern Med 1981;94:808–813.
47. Livengood JR, Sigler TG, Foster LR, et al. Isoniazid-resistant tuberculosis: A community outbreak and report of a rifampin prophylaxis failure. JAMA 1985;253:2847–2849.
48. Nemcek AA, Forrest JV, Barrett-Connor E. The low yield of routine radiographic screening of tuberculin-positive hospital employees. Am J Infect Control 1985;13:52–56.
49. Grange JM, Gibson J, Osborn TW, et al. What is BCG? Tubercle 1983;64:129–139.
50. Clemens JD, Chuong JJH, Feinstein AR. The BCG controversy: A methodological and statistical reappraisal. JAMA 1983;249:2362–2369.
51. ten Dam HG, Pio A. Pathogenesis of tuberculosis and effectiveness of BCG vaccination. Tubercle 1982;63:225–233.
52. Snider DE. Bacille Calmette–Guérin vaccinations and tuberculin skin tests. JAMA 1985;253:3438–3439.

# Chapter 81 / Gastrointestinal Infections and Enterotoxigenic Poisonings

Tom A. Larson, PharmD

Collectively, gastrointestinal infections are thought to be one of the more common causes of morbidity and mortality around the world. In some developing countries, diarrhea, which is the major manifestation of intestinal infection, is the leading cause of mortality in infants and young children.[1] Frequently, because of the self-limited nature of infectious diarrhea and the potential economic burden of identification, the infectious agents go unidentified; however, protozoans (see Chapter 83), bacteria, and viruses are thought to account for the vast majority. This chapter focuses primarily on bacterial and viral causes of gastrointestinal infections.

## Bacterial Infections

The bacteria most commonly responsible for acute infectious diarrhea in the United States are *Campylobacter*, *Escherichia coli*, *Shigella*, *Salmonella*, *Yersinia*, and enterotoxin-producing *Staphylococcus aureus*. Although not a leading cause of diarrhea in North America, the vibrios most certainly are a leading cause on a global scale.

Bacteria-induced diarrheas are frequently grouped according to the mechanisms by which they produce disease. The two most commonly recognized are mucosal invasion of bacteria and enterotoxin-stimulated hypersecretion. Cholera is the classic type of acute toxin-induced diarrhea. The second major mechanism by which bacteria cause diarrhea is by tissue invasion. Bacteria responsible for the second type, tissue invasion, are *Salmonella*, *Shigella*, *Yersinia*, *Campylobacter*, and enteropathogenic *E. coli*.

## Invasive (Dysentery-like) Diarrhea

### *Bacillary Dysentery*

Bacillary dysentery, a self-limited intestinal infection caused by *Shigella*, is characterized by fever and abdominal pain with small volumes of feces often containing blood and mucus. The shigellae are gram-negative bacilli belonging to the family Enterobacteriaceae. Four species most often associated with disease are *S. dysenteriae*, *S. flexneri*, *S. boydii*, and *S. sonnei*. In a similar fashion, enterotoxic *Escherichia coli* (ETEC) may also cause an intestinal disorder that is difficult to differentiate from shigellosis based on symptoms alone. *E. coli* also belongs to the family Enterobacteriaceae. Of the hundreds of *E. coli* serotypes, only a few cause invasive-type diarrhea.

#### Epidemiology

The shigellae have worldwide distribution, with regional differences in prevalence of subgroups responsible for disease. For example, in the United States the common causes of shigellosis are *S. sonnei* and *S. flexneri* and cases caused by other shigellae are most often acquired on travel to other countries. Epidemics are uncommon in areas of the world where sanitation standards are high. Areas of poor sanitation and personal hygiene and high population density are at risk even in developed countries.

The majority of cases are thought to result from person-to-person transmission which is anal–oral in nature. A few well-documented food- and water-associated outbreaks have been reported. In the tropics, peak incidence of shigellosis correlates well with peak infestation of flies, suggesting that flies may be an important vector of transmission. Peak incidence in the United States is in late summer.

Shigellosis is primarily a disease of children, with the highest incidence between ages 1 and 4. Infection among infants is uncommon and only one third of all cases occur in adults. The reported incidence in the United States ranges from about 15,000 to 20,000 cases per year.[2]

#### Pathogenesis

*Shigella* species are very efficient at causing disease. Ingestion of as few as 200 viable organisms has been shown to cause disease in healthy adults. This probably explains the ease with which the disease is transmitted from person to person. This is contrasted by the comparatively large inoculum of *E. coli* required to initiate infection ($>10^8$). *Shigella* species and enteroinvasive *E. coli* cause dysentery upon penetrating the epithelial cells lining the colon.[3] The bacteria multiply within the submucosa, and rarely extend beyond the mucosa. Penetration of the mucosa results in distortion of the crypts, sloughing of mucosal cells, and submucosal accumulation of inflammatory cells with microabscess formation. These may coalesce, forming larger abscesses. Infection frequently involves the entire colon. Some *Shigella* species have been shown to produce an enterotoxin; however, the role that it plays in pathogenesis of the disease is unclear. Watery diarrhea commonly precedes the dysentery and may be a result of these toxins much like that of *Vibrio cholerae* and enterotoxigenic *E. coli*.

#### Clinical Presentation

Signs and symptoms are initially nonspecific: nausea, fever, abdominal tenderness of the lower quadrants, and hyperactive bowel sounds. Watery diarrhea appears within 48 hours,

**Table 81.1** Comparison of Solutions Used in Oral Maintenance and Rehydration

| | *Electrolytes (mEq/L)* | | | | | | |
|---|---|---|---|---|---|---|---|
| *Product* | $Na^+$ | $K^+$ | $Cl^-$ | Bicarbonate | Other cations | Carbohydrates (g/L) | *Osmolality (mOsm/L)* |
| Lytren (Mead Johnson) | 30 | 20 | 25 | 45 | 17 | 70 | 583 |
| Pedialyte (Ross) | 45 | 20 | 35 | 30 | — | 25 | 388 |
| Pedialyte RS (Ross) | 75 | 20 | 65 | 30 | — | 25 | 314 |
| WHO solution (Unicef) | 90 | 20 | 80 | 30 | — | 20 | 333 |
| Infalyte powder (Penwalt) | 50 | 20 | 40 | 30 | — | 20 | 251 |
| Gatorade | (20–24) | 3 | 17 | 30 | — | (46–58) | 305 |
| Jell-O (1/2 strength) | (6–17) | 0.2 | — | — | — | 80 | 600 |
| Cola | (0–6.5) | (0–4) | — | 13 | — | (100–120) | (390–750) |
| 7-Up | (5–7) | 2 | — | — | — | (74–102) | 535 |
| Kool-Aid | 1 | 1 | — | — | — | — | (250–590) |
| Grape juice | 3 | (31–34) | — | 32 | — | 156 | 1180 |
| Orange juice | 2 | (46–65) | — | 50 | — | 90 | (540–740) |

and is followed by dysentery within a couple of days. Stools are greenish color and often contain mucus and/or blood.[4] Proctoscopic exam reveals hyperemic mucosa, increased mucus secretion, and multiple superficial bleeding ulcers.

Laboratory findings are quite variable. White blood cell counts are inconsistent and range from a leukopenia to a pronounced leukocytosis with a "left shift." Fluid and electrolyte loss may be significant, particularly in infants and elderly patients. Stool culture will establish *Shigella* species as the causative agent. Immunofluorescent labeled antiserum will give rapid and precise diagnosis; however, it is not readily available.

If untreated, bacillary dysentery usually lasts about 1 week (range 1–30 days). Complications are unusual and include severe dehydration, convulsions resulting from fluid and electrolyte loss (primarily in children), septicemia, perforated colon, arthritis, and hemolytic–uremic syndrome. Mortality is rare, but it may be more likely with *S. dysenteriae*.

**Treatment**

Shigellosis is generally a self-limited disease. Patients most often become afebrile and completely recover within 4–7 days. Approximately 10% experience a recurrence. Treatment of bacillary dysentery generally includes correction of fluid and electrolyte disturbances and, sometimes, antimicrobials, especially in the very young and elderly (see Tables 81.1 and 81.2). Fluid and electrolyte losses can generally be replaced with oral therapy, as dysentery is generally not associated with significant fluid loss (Table 81.1). Intravenous replacement is necessary only for those patients with severe illness.

Initial assessment of fluid loss is essential for rehydration. Weight loss is the most reliable means of determining the extent of water loss. If this is not possible, clinical signs can be helpful in determining approximate deficits (Table 81.3). Physical assessment is generally more reliable in young children and infants than in adults. When losses are mild to moderate, oral rehydration therapy (ORT) is often successful. Fluid loss greater than 10% body water is considered severe and parenteral replacement is often indicated.

The most important component of ORT solutions is glucose (Table 80.1). Glucose enhances the absorption of sodium from the intestine and water is passively absorbed along with the sodium. Glucose concentrations of 5% or more may cause an osmotic diarrhea which makes the condition appear worse. Sodium content should be between 50 and 90 mEq/L.[5] Infants may have significant insensible water loss, and often require additional plain water if the solutions with higher sodium concentration are used. Soft drinks that have been decarbonated (by stirring vigorously), liquid gelatin desserts with twice the water content, and fruit juices are all adequate substitutes for ORT solutions. Lactase deficiency may result from diarrheal illness, necessitating withholding milk or lactose-containing formula for at least 24 hours. Lactase deficiency may last up to 10 days. Breast milk is generally well tolerated by infants.

With mild to moderate dehydration, fluid loss should be replaced within 24 hours, with half of the deficit being given in the first 8 hours if possible. It is not recommended that food or other fluids (except breast milk) be given for the first 12–24 hours of rehydration therapy. Initially, easily digested foods (bananas, applesauce, etc.) may be added slowly as tolerated. A normal diet can usually be restarted slowly and lactose-containing foods should be avoided until at least 24 hours after the diarrhea has stopped.

Because shigellosis is usually a self-limited disease and antibiotic resistance is an increasing concern, some clinicians feel antibiotics should be reserved for the severely ill; however, because antibiotic therapy has been shown to both

**Table 81.2** Antibiotic Selection

| *Organism* | *First choice* | *Alternative* |
|---|---|---|
| *Clostridium difficile* | Vancomycin, metronidazole | Bacitracin |
| *Campylobacter* | Erythromycin | Tetracycline, clindamycin, gentamicin, 5-quinolones |
| *Escherichia coli* | Cotrimoxazole | |
| *Salmonella typhi* | Chloramphenicol (if from Mexico, India, or Southeast Asia—amoxicillin or cotrimoxazole) | Ampicillin, cotrimoxazole, 5-quinolones |
| Other *Salmonella* species | Cotrimoxazole | Ampicillin |
| *Shigella* | Cotrimoxazole | Ampicillin, nalidixic acid, 5-quinolones |
| *Vibrio* | Tetracycline | Cotrimoxazole, ampicillin, chloramphenicol, furazolidone |
| *Yersinia enterocolitica* | Aminoglycoside | Cotrimoxazole, chloramphenicol, third-generation cephalosporins |
| *Yersinia pseudotuberculosis* | Ampicillin, streptomycin | Tetracycline |

shorten the period of fecal shedding (usually 1–4 weeks in patients not receiving antimicrobials) and attenuate the clinical illness, many clinicians and patients prefer to treat with antibiotics.[6] Cotrimoxazole and ampicillin have been shown to be equivalent for treatment of shigellosis caused by susceptible strains; however, with an increasing incidence of ampicillin-resistant strains in much of the world, cotrimoxazole has become the treatment of choice.[7] Bicozamycin, a nonabsorbable agent, has been shown to be as effective as cotrimoxazole. This is surprising as the disease is invasive by nature and systemic absorption was thought to be required for therapeutic effect. Apparently, this may not be so.[8] Other antibiotics shown to have activity include sulfamethoxazole, nalidixic acid, the quinolones, and furazolidone. Clinical recovery after furazolidone treatment has been found to be slow and in some cases ineffective for treatment of severe shigellosis in children.[7] Antispasmodics and agents that inhibit intestinal peristalsis should not be used, as they may prolong fever and diarrhea, worsen the dysentery, and possibly contribute to development of toxic megacolon.[9] Vaccines for prevention of shigellosis are currently under investigation. Preliminary results are encouraging, although an ideal vaccine has yet to be developed.[10]

**Table 81.3** Signs of Dehydration

| *% Body weight loss as water* | *Clinical signs* |
|---|---|
| <4 (mild) | Decreasing tearing, dry mucous membranes |
| 4–8 (moderate) | Decreased skin turgor, sunken fontanelles, sunken eyes, increased pulse, reduced urine flow |
| 8–12 (severe) | Decreased blood pressure, muscle cramps, variable alertness |

### *Salmonellosis*

Salmonellae are gram-negative bacilli belonging to the family Enterobacteriaceae. The genus *Salmonella* has three species (*S. typhi*, *S. enteritidis*, and *S. choleraesuis*) of which there are over 1,700 different serotypes. Reports to the Centers for Disease Control show serotype *S. typhimurium* as the most common isolate. Although there are over 1,700 serotypes, the 10 most commonly isolated serotypes accounted for 71% of all isolates. The number of reported isolates increased from 19,659 in 1968 to 38,881 in 1983.[11]

Human disease caused by *Salmonella* generally falls into four categories: acute gastroenteritis, bacteremia, extraintestinal localized infection, and enteric fever (typhoid and paratyphoid fever).

#### Epidemiology

Salmonellosis is a disease primarily of infants, children, and adolescents. One third of all cases reported to the Centers for Disease Control were in persons less than 1 year of age and most cases were children under 10. As with shigellosis, there is a seasonal pattern with greatest frequency in the summer months.[12]

Contaminated food or water has been implicated in the majority of cases. Direct fecal–oral transmission occurs less frequently but is particularly important in children. Foods most often implicated in human salmonellosis are poultry, poultry products, beef, pork, and dairy products. Pets, particularly turtles, have been shown to be a common source of infection.

Most reports of outbreaks occur sporadically within households and institutions. It is quite common for family contacts to acquire infection. Person-to-person contact and use of common fomites are likely responsible for outbreaks in neonatal and pediatric wards.[13] While the incidence of *Salmonella* infection overall has increased over the past decade, that attributed to *S. typhi* has declined.

### Pathophysiology

Salmonellae are much more sensitive to lower gastric pH than shigellae. Therefore, a relatively larger inoculum is required to cause infection ($10^5$ to $10^{12}$ bacteria). Agents that decrease gastric acidity or decrease gastric emptying time may predispose patients to infection. Other predisposing conditions include previous antibiotics, which alter the protective normal flora, lack of previous exposure to salmonellae, and immunodeficient states.

Enterocolitis caused by salmonellae appears to occur secondary to mucosal invasion of microorganisms. The different serotypes have a broad range of invasive potential. Some salmonellae like *S. choleraesuis*, the most invasive, are frequently associated with bacteremia and metastatic localization, whereas others such as *S. anatum* seldom cause disease. Mucosal invasion, however, does not appear to completely explain the extensive fluid loss of some patients. Some investigators have suggested enterotoxin production or local inflammatory exudates as possible mechanisms of pathology; however, these require further study.[14]

Organisms that invade beyond the mucosa enter the mesenteric lymphatics causing a local hyperplasia and monocytic infiltrates. Lymphatic flow then carries bacteria to the general circulation via the thoracic duct. Most circulating bacteria are cleared by the reticuloendothelial system; however, bacteria not cleared may cause metastatic infection in various organs.

Symptoms such as headache, fever, malaise, and abdominal pain, are apparently, at least in part, caused by endotoxins; however, other, as yet unclear, mechanisms may also play a role.

### Clinical Presentation

***Enterocolitis*** Most patients experience symptoms within 24 hours of ingestion. Patients often complain of nausea and vomiting followed by crampy abdominal pain, fever, and diarrhea, although the actual presentation is quite variable. Some patients do not have increased stool frequency, while others have more than one stool per hour. Stools are generally loose, and may be mucoid and/or bloody (dysentery-like). Temperatures usually range between 100 and 102°F, but may be higher. Diarrhea and fever usually spontaneously resolve within 1 to 5 days, but may last 2 weeks. Cases lasting longer should suggest other pathology.[15]

Stool cultures inevitably yield the causative organism if taken early; however, recovery of organisms continues to decrease with time so that by 3 to 4 weeks, only 5% to 15% of adult patients are passing salmonella. Infants and children tend to pass bacteria for longer periods than adults. Some patients may continue to shed salmonella for a year or longer. These "chronic carrier" states are rare for serotypes other than *S. typhi*.

***Bacteremia*** Salmonellae can produce bacteremia without classic enterocolitis or enteric fever. The clinical syndrome is characterized by persistent bacteremia and prolonged intermittent fever with chills. Stool cultures are frequently negative. This is most frequent and highly likely with serotype *S. choleraesuis* infections (50%). Leukocyte counts are often within the normal range.

***Localized Infections*** Extraluminal infection and/or abscess formation can occur at any site; these may follow any of the other syndromes, or may be the primary presentation. Metastatic infections have been reported to involve bone, cysts, heart, kidney, liver, lungs, pericardium, spleen, and tumors. The clinical presentation is usually determined by the organ system(s) involved. Polymorphonuclear leukocyte counts are often elevated.

***Enteric Fever (Typhoid and Paratyphoid)*** Enteric fever caused by *S. typhi* is called typhoid fever. If caused by any other serotype, it is referred to as paratyphoid fever. The clinical presentations of typhoid fever and paratyphoid fever are generally indistinguishable, although, in retrospect, paratyphoid fever tends not to be as severe as typhoid fever. Time to onset of symptoms is inversely related to the inoculum size. The onset of symptoms is gradual; nonspecific symptoms of fever, dull headache, malaise, anorexia, and myalgias are most common. Initially, fever tends to be remittent, but gradually progresses over the first week to temperatures that are often sustained over 104°F. Many patients have vague abdominal discomfort with constipation or diarrhea. Other frequently encountered symptoms include chills, nausea, vomiting, cough, weakness, and sore throat. Symptoms generally slowly subside within 4 weeks; however, without treatment, illness may be prolonged, lasting 2 months or longer.[16]

Physical examination generally reveals an acutely ill patient. An erythematous maculopapular rash known as rose spots appears primarily on the abdomen in 15% to 50% of patients. The abdomen may also be tender, particularly in the lower quadrants. Hepatomegaly and/or splenomegaly may also be present in 50% of the cases, and cervical lymph nodes may be enlarged. Auscultation of the chest will often reveal moist rales. In 5% to 10% of patients an altered state of consciousness is present.[16]

A normochromic anemia may develop rapidly without evidence of gastrointestinal loss; however, intestinal bleeding may be contributory. Leukopenia may be caused by a relative decrease in polymorphonuclear leukocytes. White cell counts, however, may range from 1,200 to 20,000/mm$^3$. As many as one third of the patients have elevated levels of the liver enzymes glutamic–oxaloacetic transaminase and alkaline phosphatase. Transient proteinuria with normal creatinine clearance can occur early.[14–16]

About 80% of patients have positive blood cultures. Bacteremia persists in about one third for several weeks if not treated. Diagnostic tests, other than culture, are unreliable.

Intestinal perforation, thrombophlebitis, toxemia with circulatory collapse, intestinal hemorrhage, and pneumonia all contribute to a fatality rate of 1% to 2%. Without treatment, mortality may be 10%.

### Treatment

***Enterocolitis*** Most patients require no therapeutic intervention. When required, the most important part of therapy for salmonella entercolitis is fluid and electrolyte replacement. The vast majority of patients respond quite nicely to oral replacement (Table 81.1, see section on rehydration); however, if vomiting prevents this or the patient presents with severe hypovolemia, intravenous solutions may be necessary. Antimicrobials are not indicated as part of the therapy of uncomplicated enterocolitis as they have not been shown to shorten the course of this self-limited disorder. In addition, antibiotics may prolong the excretion of organisms in the stool.[17] One reason for prolonged excretion of salmonella with antibiotics may be related to altered intestinal flora. Antibiotic therapy should be considered if there is suspected transition to one of the other salmonella syndromes (bacteremia, localized infection, or enteric fever) or if underlying conditions predispose to systemic spread.

***Bacteremia and Localized Infections*** Chloramphenicol or amoxicillin is most frequently used for the treatment of these syndromes. Cotrimoxazole, which has been shown to be effective in treatment of localized salmonella infections, should be considered when the organism is resistant to both chloramphenicol and amoxicillin. When bactericidal activity is desired, as with endocarditis or other intravascular infections, ampicillin is the preferred agent. The duration of antibiotic therapy should be dictated by the site; for example, osteomyelitis should be treated for 4–6 weeks or longer.

***Enteric Fever (Typhoid and Paratyphoid)*** Chloramphenicol has been the mainstay of therapy in most areas of the world. Although a number of antibiotics have demonstrated activity against salmonella, chloramphenicol has been shown to attenuate the disease course more consistently; however, chloramphenicol resistance is often encountered in Mexico, Southeast Asia, and India because of an R factor, which also transfers resistance to sulfonamides, tetracycline, and streptomycin. Ampicillin, amoxicillin, and cotrimoxazole are also effective, although response is not as predictable as with choramphenicol. These agents should be considered alternatives, and used when chloramphenicol is contraindicated or chloramphenicol resistance is suspected.[18,19] Therapy should be continued for at least 2 weeks. Clinical response to antibiotics is often seen within 2 days; however, temperatures slowly normalize within 3–5 days.

Some clinicians feel that severely ill patients may have a beneficial response to a short course of corticosteroids. One recent study using large doses of dexamethasone given intravenously during the first 48 hours supports this opinion.[20]

Antidiarrheal agents or laxatives should not be used because they may prolong illness or precipitate perforation.

## *Campylobacteriosis*

The *Campylobacter* species are non–spore-forming, gram-negative bacilli. Of the six recognized species *C. jejuni* and *C. coli* are considered the major pathogens for humans.[21] Although recognized for their ability to cause disease in the late 1940s, the routine isolation techniques required for speciation of *Campylobacter* were not readily available until the 1970s.

### Epidemiology

*Campylobacter* species are now thought to be a major cause of diarrhea, comparable to *Salmonella* and *Shigella*. Although occurring in all age groups, about 80% of cases reported to the Centers for Disease Control surveillance program were in persons less than 35 years old.[22,23] Most reported cases occur during the summer months.

Mammals (such as livestock, dogs, and cats) and birds (including poultry) are thought to be the primary reservoirs of *Campylobacter*. Transmission of infection appears to be by the fecal–oral route (direct contact with human or animal feces) or by ingestion of contaminated food or water.

### Pathophysiology

*Campylobacter* is susceptible to acid, much like *Salmonella*, and so a larger inoculum is required to initiate infection. This inoculum is thought to be lower when the bacteria are ingested along with foods, antacids, or histamine ($H_2$)-blocking agents.

Conditions in the upper small intestine are favorable for multiplication. Tissue invasion by bacteria has been demonstrated in the jejunum, ileum, and colon. In addition to the invasive mechanism, extracellular toxins and enterotoxins have been demonstrated; however, the role they play in development of disease is as yet unclear.

### Clinical Presentation

Incubation usually ranges from 1 to 12 days with the average being 2–4 days. The most common symptoms include diarrhea of varying consistency and severity, abdominal pain, nausea, vomiting, headache, myalgias, malaise, and fever. Bowel movements may be numerous and may range from loose to watery (cholera-like), bloody (dysentery-like), foul smelling, and melenic. Cramping and abdominal pain are usually relieved by defecation. Generalized abdominal pain with tenderness and fever may mimic appendicitis.[22]

The disease is self-limiting and signs and symptoms usually resolve in about a week, but may persist longer in 10% to 20% of patients. A reactive arthritis, which usually disappears within 6 months, may be seen in as many as 5% of cases. Complications of campylobacteriosis, including thrombophlebitis, abscess, septicemia, peritonitis, empyema, urinary tract infection, and cholecystitis, are relatively uncommon but occur more frequently in those who are immunocompromised.

### Treatment

As with other acute diarrheal illnesses, fluid and electrolyte support is a mainstay of therapy. The majority of *Campylobacter*-induced fluid loss can be managed with oral rehydration solutions (Table 81.1); however, severe hypovolemia with shock requires intravenous fluid replacement.

Antibiotic therapy is not necessary in the majority of cases.[24] Antibiotics should be considered when the patients have severe bloody diarrhea, continued fever (>102°F), persistence of symptoms beyond 7 days, worsening symptoms, or compromised immune systems or are very old or very young. *Campylobacter* species are susceptible to erythromycin, tetracycline, chloramphenicol, clindamycin, ciprofloxacin, and the aminoglycosides. Currently, erythromycin is felt to be the agent of choice[25]; however, two recent studies have been unable to demonstrate erythromycin therapy as any more likely to alter the clinical course than placebo.[24,26] The self-limited nature of the disease is suggested as a possible explanation. Both studies were able to show that erythromycin hastens the bacteriological cure, which may be of epidemiological benefit. Antimotility drugs may impede the resolution of infection.[24]

### *Yersiniosis*

The genus *Yersinia* includes six species known to cause disease in humans. Of these, *Y. enterocolitica* and *Y. pseudotuberculosis* are more likely to be associated with intestinal infection. There are marked geographic differences in the predominant serotypes causing infection.

#### Epidemiology

*Y. enterocolitica* and *Y. pseudotuberculosis* are important etiologic agents of gastroenteritis. Most cases occur in children and young adults with over 75% of reported cases in persons less than 20 years of age.[27,28] The incidence of cases appears to be on the increase, perhaps reflecting an increased awareness and improved isolation techniques. Peak incidence occurs during the winter months.

The organisms have been isolated from a variety of food sources, and some of these have been associated with outbreaks. *Y. enterocolitica* has also been isolated from a number of mammals; however, the possible transmission of disease from these reservoirs to humans is poorly understood.

#### Pathophysiology

The pathophysiology of yersiniosis in humans is not clearly understood. It appears that the bacteria invade the intestinal mucosa causing local necrotic lesions, and invade local lymph nodes producing a purulent lymphadenitis. With septicemia, localized purulent lesions may be found in various organs.

#### Clinical Presentation

These bacteria cause a wide spectrum of clinical syndromes. The majority of cases present with enterocolitis that is mild and self-limited. Symptoms, generally lasting 1–3 weeks, include abdominal pain, diarrhea, and fever. A clinical syndrome seen in older children and adolescents presenting with fever, right lower quadrant pain, and leukocytosis may be clinically indistinguishable from appendicitis.[27]

As many as one third of adults with *Y. enterocolitica* may have an immunologically mediated polyarthritis within 1 month of the onset of diarrhea. Joints involved frequently include the fingers, wrists, toes, ankles, and knees. Symptoms often resolve spontaneously, but may persist for several months.[29] Other syndromes that frequently occur are erythema nodosum and exudative pharyngitis. Septicemia caused by either *Y. enterocolitica* or *Y. pseudotuberculosis* is uncommon and is most often reported in patients with underlying disease. Signs and symptoms are similar to those seen with other gram-negative bacteremias. Other organ systems may secondarily be infected. The mortality rate of bacteremia may be as high as 50% to 75% despite antibiotic therapy.

#### Treatment

The utility of antimicrobials for treating *Yersinia*-associated enterocolitis and mesenteric adenitis is difficult to evaluate, as these diseases are generally self-limited and are easily managed with oral rehydration solutions (Table 81.1). As a result, controlled trials with cotrimoxazole have failed to demonstrate beneficial effects[28]; however, in severe disease, bacteremia, or localizing forms of the disease, antibiotic treatment is indicated. *Y. enterocolitica* is generally susceptible to third-generation cephalosporins, aminoglycosides, chloramphenicol, tetracycline, and cotrimoxazole. *Y. enterocolitica* is usually resistant to penicillin G and frequently resistant to ampicillin and first-generation cephalosporins. Suggested antibiotics of choice[25] are shown in Table 81.2. *Y. pseudotuberculosis* is generally susceptible to antibiotics active against *Y. enterocolitica*, as well as ampicillin.

## Enterotoxigenic (Cholera-like) Diarrhea

### *Cholera (Vibrio cholerae)*

Vibrios are aerobic, curved, gram-negative bacilli commonly found in surface water. The two species most often causing human illness are *Vibrio cholerae* and *Vibrio parahemolyticus*. Although the disease caused by each species is strikingly different, only *V. cholerae* is discussed because it best characterizes the secretory-type diarrheas. *V. cholerae* is distinguished by serotyping, somatic (O) antigens: Ogawa, Inaba, and Hikojima.

#### Epidemiology

Cholera has been endemic in the Ganges delta, West Bengal, Bangladesh, and southern Asia (including Southeast Asia) since at least 1817. Three different biotypes have been pandemic several times since then: Classic, El Tor, and a new classic variant. Contaminated water sources have been shown to be a primary vector for transmission of disease. During epidemics, contaminated food and direct contact are undoubtedly also vectors. Many individuals will have asymptomatic infections. The ratio of symptomatic to asymptomatic infections is about 1:30 (or less) for the El Tor biotype versus 1:2–4 for the "classic" biotype. There is no evidence for any carrier of the organism other than humans. Excreted bacteria may remain viable for up to a week in water, with El Tor variants surviving slightly longer than classic biotypes. There appears to be an inverse relationship between attack rate and age. After clinical disease about 90% to 100% protection from recurrence is seen for several years.[30–33]

### Pathophysiology

Most pathology of cholera is thought to result from an enterotoxin produced by the bacteria. The toxin has been well characterized. It contains two subunits: A (activating moiety) and B (binding moiety). The subunit B binds to a $GM_1$ monosialosyl ganglioside of the epithelial cell wall, causing the subunit A to enter the cell. This causes increased intracellular adenylate cyclase activity. The resulting increase in cyclic AMP causes secretion of chloride ion into the intestinal lumen. The toxin likely acts along the entire intestinal tract; however, most fluid loss occurs in the duodenum where secretory capacity is greatest. The effects of the toxin persist for many hours.[31]

Cholera toxin does not appear to affect the glucose-facilitated sodium resorptive capacity of the gut. The net effect of cholera toxin is isotonic secretion (primarily in the small intestine), which exceeds the absorptive capacity of the intestinal tract (primarily the colon).

### Clinical Presentation

The incubation period of *V. cholerae* is 6–48 hours. The clinical presentation is characterized by a spectrum from the asymptomatic state to the most severe typical cholera syndrome. In the most severe state this disease can progress to death in a matter of 2–4 hours if not treated. More typically, however, progression from the first watery stool to shock takes two to three times longer, with death delayed up to several days. Some patients may experience a prodrome, a sense of fullness and borborygmus, prior to the first watery stool. Initial stools generally do not have the "rice water" appearance that is classically seen with cholera.

Most signs and symptoms are a direct result of fluid and electrolyte loss. These frequently include poor skin turgor, sunken eyes, cyanosis, shallow or absent pulses, tachycardia, hypotension, and tachypnea. The presentation generally correlates well with the severity of fluid loss from diarrhea. Patients may have ileus, and collection of fluid within the intestines can cause intravascular depletion without diarrhea.

Surprisingly, despite the profound intravascular fluid loss, and even in cases where peripheral pulses are absent, patients are generally easily aroused and give appropriate responses to questioning. In children, however, altered consciousness and even convulsions may be the first sign of hypoglycemia.[34] Hypokalemia is often seen in children, perhaps as a reflection of a potassium loss with diarrhea greater than that of adults. Altered consciousness, muscle weakness and cramping, cardiac arrhythmias, and ileus may be manifestations of electrolyte losses. Other complications include acidosis, renal failure secondary to volume depletion, iatrogenic water intoxication from over rehydration, and aspiration pneumonia.

### Treatment

The mainstay of treatment for cholera consists of replacement of fluid and electrolytes lost from the gastrointestinal tract. Volume loss can be dramatic, with a few patients losing a liter or more of isotonic fluid every hour. The amounts of water and salts given are dictated by those that are lost. Most cases of hypovolemia can be managed with oral rehydration therapy on an outpatient basis with solutions that are easily prepared at home. Several commercially prepared packets are on the market; however, if they are not available, solutions are easily prepared with common household staples for most mild cases. Table 81.1 shows some of the solutions available for oral replacement. An important component of these solutions is glucose or glucose precursors (sucrose). The glucose is necessary to maximize glucose-facilitated sodium absorption. Sucrose (table sugar) and rice powder have been reported to be adequate alternatives to glucose.[35]

Intravenous therapy is usually required only in severe cases, as initial replacement prior to oral therapy, or when patients are unable to take or retain oral replacement solutions. When initial replacement is emergent, solutions should be infused rapidly. Infusion rates of 50–100 mL/min will rehydrate most patients within the first hour. Once initial volume has been replaced, further rates of administration should be directed to match losses. Often, therapy can then be switched to oral replacement as rehydration is accomplished.

Hypoglycemia is a serious complication, particularly in children and infants. Convulsions or altered states of consciousness may be the first sign of hypoglycemia and should be evaluated and treated promptly. Hypokalemia is also more likely to develop in children. If not promptly detected and corrected, hypokalemia may result in cardiac arrest.

Antibiotics have been shown to shorten the duration of diarrhea, decrease the volume of fluid lost, and shorten the duration of the carrier state.[36] The tetracyclines are the drugs selected most often.[25] When the tetracyclines are not available or desirable, as in pregnancy or young children, ampicillin is an appropriate alternative. Other agents such as chloramphenicol, cotrimoxazole, and furazolidone have also been effective.[37] Increasing multiple-antibiotic resistance may dictate regional antibiotic selection. Antibiotics need only be given for 3–5 days in most cases. Lindebaum et al[36] found about 20% relapse with antibiotic therapy of less than 48 hours.

## *Enterotoxigenic Escherichia coli*

*E. coli* is a gram-negative bacillus belonging to the family Enterobacteriaceae. *E. coli* causes three types of diarrheal illness: enterotoxigenic, invasive, and enteropathogenic. The most common of these is the toxin-induced diarrhea, enterotoxigenic, which in many respects is similar to that of *V. cholerae*. Invasive *E. coli* diarrhea, which is briefly discussed with bacillary dysentery, and enteropathogenic *E. coli*, which is problematic in nurseries and young children, are much less common. Although not recognized as a significant cause of diarrhea until the second half of this century, enterotoxigenic *E. coli* (ETEC) is now incriminated as being the most common cause of traveler's diarrhea, the most common cause of diarrhea in children in certain areas of the world, and a common cause of food and/or water–associated outbreaks.[38]

### Pathophysiology

ETEC are capable of producing two plasmid-mediated enterotoxins: heat-labile toxin (HLT) and heat-stable toxin (HST). HLT, a cholera-like toxin, has two subunits (A and B) which have similar antigenic properties and have a similar action on the gut mucosa. The net effect of this toxin on the mucosa is production of a cholera-like secretory diarrhea. HST has a rapid onset of action, is not antigenic, has a low molecular weight, and probably acts only on the small intestine.[39]

### Clinical Presentation

Diarrhea caused by ETEC is often characterized by abrupt onset of watery diarrhea with or without abdominal cramping. Severe cases may be indistinguishable from cholera. Usually, there is no blood or pus in the stool. Signs and symptoms are directly dependent on the extent of fluid loss, which in most cases is subclinical. Most ETEC diarrhea resolves within 24 to 48 hours without complication.

### Treatment

Most patients do not require specific therapy, although some will have sufficient loss of fluid and electrolytes to require replacement therapy. Most cases respond readily to oral rehydration therapy.

Fruit juices or soda (soft drinks) will be adequate replacement for mild cases. Other ORT solutions that are available are listed in Table 81.1. When fluid and electrolyte loss is severe (weight loss > 10%) intravenous therapy may be required.

Because this is a short-lived disease that responds well to ORT, antibiotic therapy is seldom necessary. Antibiotic prophylaxis has, however, been shown to effectively prevent the development of ETEC diarrhea.[40] Effective prophylactic agents include tetracycline, cotrimoxazole, neomycin, and furazolidone.[41] Because multiple-antibiotic resistance among ETEC has developed in many countries, many prescribers prefer to reserve antibiotics for treatment of symptomatic patients.[6,40]

## *Pseudomembranous Colitis (Clostridium difficile)*

Pseudomembranous colitis (PMC) was first reported in 1883 and first associated with antibiotic therapy in 1955. While described in the preantibiotic era, the incidence has increasingly been associated with antibiotic administration. Recent evidence suggests that PMC is the result of toxins produced by *Clostridium difficile*.[42]

### Epidemiology

*C. difficile* is a spore-forming, gram-positive, obligate anaerobic bacillus. The incidence of intestinal colonization is variable, ranging from over 70% in infants to 3% in healthy adults.[43] With antibiotic-altered flora, reports of colonization among adults increase to 20% to 46%. The relation between the colonized state and active disease is poorly understood. Newborn infants may be colonized with toxin-producing strains yet have no clinical disease.

The exact incidence of PMC within the United States is not known. It occurs most often in high-risk groups: the elderly, debilitated patients, cancer patients, surgery patients, or any patient receiving antibiotics. PMC has been associated most often, but not necessarily, with antimicrobials, particularly with clindamycin, ampicillin or cephalosporins. As many as 10% of selected patients receiving clindamycin may acquire PMC.[43]

### Pathophysiology

Pseudomembranous colitis is thought to be caused by toxins produced by strains of *C. difficile*. Two toxins (A and B) have been described.[44] As yet these toxins are not well characterized and there may be other toxins as well. The exact mechanism by which these toxins produce human disease remains to be elucidated. The toxins appear to act on mucosal membranes, causing necrosis, inflammation, increased peristalsis, and loss of fluid and electrolytes.

### Clinical Presentation

Symptoms can occur from several days after the start of antibiotic therapy to several weeks after antibiotics are discontinued. The onset of illness is often abrupt. PMC is characterized by fever, cramping, abdominal pain and tenderness, and profuse greenish diarrhea (watery or mucoid) either during or after antibiotic therapy. Fevers of 103–105°F, marked leukocytosis, and hypoalbuminemia are also common.[44]

Pseudomembranous lesions, which look like whitish-yellow raised plaques, can be found anywhere in the colon. Diagnosis is made by visualization of pseudomembranes. A diagnostic dilemma exists, as some persons will have positive stool cultures and/or positive cytotoxin assays and no demonstrable pseudomembranes. This group of patients has been classified as having *C. difficile*–associated diarrhea. Recent evidence suggests that about 23% of these cases resolve spontaneously within 48 to 72 hours.[45] Because the cytotoxins can be demonstrated within 24 hours of stool collection, some of these patients may receive inappropriate antibiotic therapy. Most pseudomembranous plaques are distal and are easily seen with sigmoidoscopy; however, they may occur anywhere in the colon or rectum. Therefore, when sigmoidoscopy and proctoscopy are negative PMC cannot be ruled out.

### Treatment

As with all types of diarrhea, supportive care is of primary concern. Fluid and electrolyte losses may be significant. If possible, it is ideal to stop the offending antibiotic. In many cases of antibiotic-associated diarrhea, patients respond to supportive care alone after discontinuation of the inducing antibiotic. Teasley et al[45] showed that 23% of patients with *C. difficile*–associated diarrhea had resolution within 72 hours simply by discontinuing the inducing agent. If the patient has not improved within 72 hours, has severe disease, requires continuation of the inducing antibiotic, or is a high-risk patient, such as the elderly and debilitated, antibiotic therapy should be promptly initiated.

*C. difficile* is usually susceptible in vitro to vancomycin, metronidazole, bacitracin, rifampin, ampicillin, and cephalosporins. Clinically, however, resistance to rifampin develops quickly and β-lactamase produced by intestinal flora inactivates ampicillin and cephalosporins making these antibiotics ineffective. Many isolates are resistant to tetracyclines or erythromycin.

Vancomycin 500–2,000 mg/d for 10 days has historically been suggested as the treatment of choice. Vancomycin's efficacy is well documented, very likely a reflection of excellent activity against *C. difficile* and poor absorption from the GI tract. Doses of 125 mg four times daily have been shown to result in fecal concentrations greater than 300 mg/mL, far exceeding the MIC break point of susceptibility.[46] Vancomycin should be given orally because gastrointestinal concentrations after parenteral administration are very low and unpredictable.

Relapse after discontinuation of vancomycin may occur in 12% to 39% of patients. This is thought to be caused by failure to restore normal flora and/or residual spores. Retreatment with vancomycin is often successful.

Although vancomycin has been the drug of choice for several years, some authors now suggest that in many cases metronidazole may be the agent of choice.[25,45] A large prospective study comparing metronidazole (1 g/d) and vancomycin (2 g/d) among 101 veterans with antibiotic-associated diarrhea and stool cultures positive for *C. difficile* showed no statistically significant difference in efficacy, toxicity, or relapse rate.[45] These results are somewhat surprising in light of metronidazole being well absorbed and other reports suggesting metronidazole to be a potential PMC-inducing agent. The number of study patients with PMC was not large and although metronidazole and vancomycin appear to be equally effective more experience is required. Because of its mutagenic and tumorigenic potential in laboratory experiments, metronidazole should not be used indiscriminately in pregnant women.

A second alternative agent for treatment of *C. difficile*–associated diarrhea and colitis is bacitracin. Bacitracin is poorly absorbed from the gastrointestinal tract allowing for high fecal concentrations. Young et al[47] recently reported that bacitracin 80,000 units/d given orally was less effective than vancomycin 500 mg/d in clearing *C. difficile* from stools; however, both were comparable in control of symptoms of colitis. The number of other reported cases is far too few to suggest bacitracin as any more than an alternative agent. Further studies are required.

Anion exchange resins have been used with variable success in mild cases.[44] Tedesco found moderate success with exchange resins.[44] Response was slow and limited to only mild disease. The usual adult dose of cholestyramine is 4 g three to four times daily for 3 to 19 days. Cholestyramine has been shown to bind vancomycin; however, in vitro data suggest that there is no loss of antibiotic activity.[48] Concomitant administration should be avoided or administration of antibiotics and exchange resins should be separated by several hours.

Drugs that inhibit peristalsis such as diphenoxylate are contraindicated. Some patients have become worse after use of these drugs. They may be particularly dangerous to use in infants. Slowing of fecal transit time is thought to result in extended toxin-associated damage.[49]

## Acute Viral Gastroenteritis

Acute viral gastrointestinal disorders have been appreciated only relatively recently. The exact incidence is unknown; however, these disorders are thought to account for a significant percentage of illness classified as "nonbacterial." Two groups of viruses known to cause significant morbidity and even mortality among children and adults are the rotavirus and Norwalk virus groups.[50,51] This section serves as an introduction to the current theories of the epidemiology, pathophysiology, and therapeutics of each group.

### *Rotaviruses*

#### Etiology/Epidemiology

Rotaviruses, also called infantile gastroenteritis virus, reovirus-like or orbivirus-like, are wheel-shaped RNA viruses. Distribution is worldwide. Although rotaviruses have been isolated from a variety of mammals and birds, the exact mechanism of transfer or principal vectors of infection are poorly understood. Water, food, or inspired droplets have been suspected; however, it is generally thought that the primary route is fecal–oral. Although infection is most often seen in children, adults can be infected and may act as a potential reservoir for transmission. Outbreaks are not thought to be common among infants; however, this age group may be more susceptible to complications as evidenced by a higher hospitalization rate.

Rotaviruses have been associated with up to 50% of enteritis in hospitalized children.[50] The incidence of rotavirus infections in the United States peaks in January and February. Incubation and duration of viral shedding are thought to range from 1 to 4 days and 6 to 10 days, respectively.

#### Pathophysiology

The exact mechanism by which the rotaviruses cause diarrhea is not known. Limited human histologic studies show mild intestinal villous shortening, reticular cell enlargement, shortened columnar epithelial cells, mononuclear infiltration of the lamina propria, and decreased microvillae. Rotavirus infection may cause altered sugar absorption.

#### Clinical Presentation

The highest frequency of rotavirus-associated diarrhea appears between ages 6 and 24 months. Clinical manifestations of rotavirus infections vary from asymptomatic (which is common in adults) to severe nausea, vomiting, and diarrhea with dehydration. Symptoms are characterized initially by nausea and vomiting, which causes varying degrees of dehydration. Diarrhea occurs in most patients and lasts from 1 to 9 days, but some patients experience only loose stool with no increase in frequency.[51] Other signs and symptoms include fever, irritability, lethargy, pharyngeal erythema, rhinitis, red tympanic membranes, and palpable cervical lymph nodes.

Dehydration and electrolyte disturbances occur more frequently in children. Severe cases of dehydration may result and precipitate death. Death may occur as soon as 24 hours after initial symptoms. Fortunately this is uncommon, but illustrates that this disease can very quickly result in significant fluid depletion. Reye's syndrome has also been reported following rotavirus infection. Neonates may have asymptomatic rotavirus particles in their stool. Some evidence suggests that institutionalized infants are more susceptible to spread than those taken care of at home.[51]

Exposure may result in immunologic protection for several years. Human milk that contains rotavirus antibodies appears to have a passive protective effect and may be an effective form of treatment among immunodeficient patients.

Laboratory findings reflect the degree of vomiting and/or diarrhea. Dehydration may result in elevated blood urea nitrogen and urine specific gravity. Electron microscopy, fluorescent virus precipitin test, radioimmunoassay, enzyme-linked immunosorbent assay (ELISA), and latex agglutination are reliable ways to detect rotavirus, with the latter three most practical for general use.

#### Treatment

Treatment of rotavirus-associated vomiting and/or diarrhea is directed at prevention or correction of dehydration. Several oral rehydration solutions are suggested for fluid and electrolyte replacement (Table 81.1). In severe cases, parenteral rehydration may be necessary.

Studies are being conducted to explore active and passive immunity as viable means of prevention or treatment. These include administration of human or bovine milk containing rotavirus antibodies, administration of attenuated rotavirus vaccine, and DNA sequencing for either rotavirus vaccines or antibodies.[10]

### *Parvovirus-like Agents*

#### Etiology/Epidemiology

Parvovirus-like agents constitute a group of viruses 25–32 nm in diameter that can cause acute gastroenteritis. The Norwalk agent was the first of these agents to be described. Subsequently, several other agents have been described that are thought to cause a similar syndrome. These are named according to the location of the outbreak of illness or contaminated source: Norwalk, Hawaii, MC, W, Ditchling, Cockle, Parramatta, Snow Mountain, and Marin County.

As with most viruses, epidemiology of the parvovirus-like agents is poorly understood. Only recently with the introduction of new technology have researchers been able to appreciate these agents as widespread and common. The disease is thought to affect all age groups and is nonseasonal. Studies of prevalence of antibody production have shown the incidence to increase from about 10% in 3- to 4-year-olds to more than 50% by age 50. The exact vectors of transmission are not known; however, the fecal–oral route is thought to be important. Several outbreaks have been associated with contaminated food or water.

#### Pathophysiology

The pathology of this disease is similar to that caused by the rotavirus agents. Human volunteer studies have shown histopathologic changes to appear within 24 hours of viral challenge, with clinical manifestations within 48 hours. Brush border enzyme activity may be decreased, but generally returns to preinfection levels within 2 weeks. This may result in lactose intolerance. The exact mechanisms of virus-induced vomiting or diarrhea are unknown.

#### Clinical Presentation/Treatment

This disease is characterized by sudden onset of abdominal cramps plus nausea and/or vomiting. Other frequent complaints are myalgias, headaches, and malaise which are accompanied by fever in about 50% of cases. Signs and symptoms generally last only 48–72 hours. Complications are rare.

The disease is generally self-limited and does not require therapy. On occasion, oral rehydration may be required if fluid loss is severe. Rarely is parenteral hydration necessary.

## Bacterial Food Poisoning

Food poisoning results from the ingestion of food containing pathogenic microorganisms, preformed toxins that were produced by microorganisms, or other toxic compounds. Although a number of bacteria can cause food poisoning (Table 81.4), this discussion is limited to a common cause of bacterial food poisoning, *Staphylococcus aureus*, and the frequently deadly type of bacterial food poisoning, botulism.

### *Staphylococcal Food Poisoning*

Staphylococcal food poisoning results from the ingestion of food contaminated by a preformed enterotoxin produced by certain strains of *S. aureus* growing within the food. The exact incidence of staphylococcal food poisoning is unknown, perhaps a reflection of an illness that is usually mild and of short duration, allowing it to go unrecognized and unreported, but is thought to be quite common.

Toxigenic *S. aureus* is a common component of the normal skin flora of humans. Often the offending organism can be recovered from the person preparing the contaminated food. Common foods reported to be contaminated include salads, custard-filled pastries, ham, sausages, poultry, and dairy products. Enterotoxin production generally results from leaving foods at room temperatures, allowing the staphylococci to grow. At least five heat-stable toxins (A, B, C, D, E) are responsible. These toxins apparently have little or no local effect on the digestive tract. The exact mechanism by which the toxins produce disease is unknown but probably involves central stimulation of the vomiting center in the brain.

Symptoms are rapid in onset, generally occurring within 1 to 6 hours of ingestion of toxin-containing foods. The condition is often characterized by nausea, vomiting, abdominal cramps, and diarrhea that is short in duration usually lasting less than 12 hours. Myalgias, headache, sweating, and chills are sometimes also present. Complications are rare and most often related to dehydration.[52,53]

Treatment is generally required only in severe cases. Oral rehydration therapy is often sufficient (Table 81.1); however, in protracted cases, intravenous rehydration may be required. Antibiotics have not been shown to be beneficial.

### *Botulism*

Foodborne botulism results from the ingestion of food contaminated with preformed toxins produced by *Clostridium botulinum*, an anaerobic, spore-forming, gram-positive ba-

**Table 81.4** Food Poisonings

| *Organism* | *Time to symptoms (h)* | *Principal foods* | *Peak incidence (USA)* | *Principal mechanism of pathophysiology* | *Duration* | *Treatment* |
|---|---|---|---|---|---|---|
| *Staphylococcus aureus* | 1–6 | Salad, pastries, ham, poultry | Summer | Preformed toxins (A–E) (heat stable) | 12 h | Supportive |
| *Bacillus cereus* | 1–6 | Meats, vegetables, fried rice | None | Preformed toxins | 12 h | Supportive |
| | 8–16 | | | Toxin production (in vivo) | 24 h | Supportive |
| *Clostridium perfringens* (type A) | 6–24 | Meats, poultry | Fall, winter, spring | Toxin production (in vivo) | 24 h | Supportive |
| *Vibrio parahemolyticus* | 16–72 | Shellfish | Spring, summer, fall | Toxin production and tissue invasion | 2–7 d | Supportive |
| *Salmonella* spp. | 16–48 | Beef, poultry, water, eggs, dairy products | Summer | Tissue invasion | 2–7 d | Supportive |
| *Shigella* spp. | 16–48 | Salad, water | Summer | Tissue invasion | 2–7 d | Supportive |
| Enteropathogenic *Escherichia coli* | 16–48 | Water | None | Tissue invasion | 2–7 d | Supportive |
| *Campylobacter* | 16–48 | Poultry, dairy products, clams, water | Spring, summer | Tissue invasion | 2–7 d | Supportive |
| Enterotoxigenic *E. coli* | 16–72 | Water | None | Toxin production (in vivo) | 1–7 d | Supportive |
| *Vibrio cholerae* | 16–72 | Water | — | Toxin production (in vivo) | 2–12 d | Supportive, antibiotics |
| *Yersinia enterocolitica* | 16–48 | Dairy products | — | Toxin production and/or tissue invasion | 1–30 d | Supportive |
| *Clostridium botulinum* | 12–72 | Canned fruits, vegetables, meats | None | Preformed toxins A, B, and E (children and adults) Toxin production (in vivo) (infants) | | Supportive (including mechanically assisted ventilation), trivalent antitoxin |

cillus. Clostridia are commonly found in a variety of environmental sources. Although clostridia are strict anaerobes, the spores are resistant to a variety of environmental conditions. Botulism is almost always associated with improper preparation and/or storage of food which allows the spores to germinate.

Eight distinct toxins have been described and specific toxin types appear to be geographically distributed. The toxins, which are produced by the bacteria and released upon lysis, are the most potent biological or chemical toxins known to man. They have been shown to prevent the release of the neurotransmitter acetylcholine at the peripheral cholinergic nerve terminal. Blockade is most evident in cranial nerves and at the neuromuscular junction.[54]

Clinical manifestations are a direct result of the toxin-induced cholinergic blockade. The disease is most often characterized by dysphagia, dry mouth with furrowed tongue, diplopia, dysarthria, fatigue, constipation, dyspnea, and a descending paralysis. Symptoms usually appear within 12–72 hours of ingestion; however, they may be delayed up to several days. Some patients experience nausea, vomiting, or diarrhea prior to the neurologic symptoms. Patients are normally alert, oriented, and without sensory deficit. Descending paralysis often includes ophthalmoplegia, ptosis, facial weakness, and upper and lower muscle weakness. Phrenic nerve blockade may result in diaphragm paralysis. Death is usually a direct result of or is due to complications arising from respiratory failure.[55]

Treatment of botulism consists primarily of respiratory support and use of botulinum antitoxin. Respiratory failure may occur prior to involvement of other upper muscle groups. Patients should be monitored for respiratory failure continuously in an intensive care unit. An endotracheal tube should be placed or tracheostomy performed before severe respiratory dysfunction occurs. If evaluation is performed within several hours of ingestion, gastric lavage or induction of vomiting is suggested. Cathartics and high enemas can also be used to remove residual toxin from the bowel; however, they are contraindicated in cases of ileus.

Although the effectiveness of antitoxin is unknown, patients diagnosed as having botulism should receive botulinum antitoxin. Large, prospective, placebo-controlled studies evaluating the effectiveness of trivalent antitoxin have not been, and are not likely to be, conducted. Limited data comparing pre- and post-antitoxin eras suggest that patients with toxin type E botulism may benefit.[56] A recent retrospective review of 132 cases of type A botulism reported to the Centers for Disease Control between 1973 and 1980 suggested trivalent antitoxin to be beneficial.[57] After controlling for age and incubation period, patients treated with antitoxin were reported to have a lower fatality rate and a shorter clinical course than those who did not receive antitoxin. Interestingly, patients receiving antitoxin within the first 24 hours of onset of symptoms had a shorter clinical course but about the same mortality rate as those receiving antitoxin late.

Botulinum antitoxin is a concentrated preparation of equine globulins obtained from horses immunized with toxins A, B, and E. Each 10-mL vial of trivalent antitoxin contains 7,500 IU of type A, 5,500 IU of type B, and 8,500 IU of type E antitoxin. Data on the pharmacokinetics of the individual antitoxins are limited.[58]

Before receiving botulinum antitoxin, patients should be tested for sensitivity because trivalent antitoxin is equine in origin. Current recommendations for dosing are that after sensitivity testing (outlined in package insert) one vial be given intravenously and one vial be given intramuscularly. After 4 hours, if signs and symptoms worsen, one vial should be given intravenously; another vial may be given intravenously after 12 to 24 hours. Antitoxin may be obtained from the Centers for Disease Control, Atlanta, Georgia.

Other agents used experimentally as adjunctive therapy are guanidine and 4-aminopyridine which have been shown to increase acetylcholine release. Data are limited yet promising.[59]

Prevention should always be stressed. Botulinum toxins are heat labile and readily destroyed by 10 min of boiling. All home-canned foods should be processed according to directions and boiled instead of just warmed prior to eating.

## References


1. Walsh JA, Warren KW. Selective primary health care: An interim strategy for disease control in developing countries. N Engl J Med 1979;301:967–974.
2. Shigellosis—United States, 1983. MMWR 1984;33(43):616.
3. LaBrec E, Schneider H, Magnani T. Epithelial cell penetration as an essential step in the pathogenesis of bacillary dysentery. J Bacteriol 1964;88:1503–1518.
4. DuPont HL, Hornick R, Dawkins A. The response of man to virulent *Shigella flexneri* 2a. J Infect Dis 1969;119:296–299.
5. Santosham M, Daum RS, Dillman L, et al. Oral rehydration therapy of infantile diarrhea. N Engl J Med 1982;306:1070–1076.
6. DuPont HL, Reves RR, Galindo E, et al. Treatment of travelers' diarrhea with trimethoprim/sulfamethoxazole and with trimethoprim alone. N Engl J Med 1982;307:841–844.
7. DuPont HL. Nonfluid therapy and selected chemoprophylaxis of acute diarrhea. Am J Med 1985;78(suppl 6B):81–90.
8. Ericsson CD, DuPont HL, Sullivan P, et al. Bicozamycin, a poorly absorbable antibiotic, effectively treats travelers' diarrhea. Ann Intern Med 1983;98:20–25.
9. DuPont HL, Hornick R. Adverse effects of Lomotil therapy in shigellosis. JAMA 1973;226:1525–1528.
10. Edelman R. Prevention and treatment of infectious diarrhea: speculations on the next ten years. Am J Med 1985;78(suppl 6B):99–106.
11. Anonymous. Human salmonella isolates—United States, 1983. MMWR 1984;33(49):693.
12. Anonymous. Salmonella surveillance summary for 1980. Atlanta, GA, Centers for Disease Control, 1982.
13. Baine WB, Gangarosa EJ, Bennett JV. Institutional salmonellosis. J Infect Dis 1973;128:357–360.
14. Hook EW. *Salmonella* species (including typhoid fever), in Mandell GL, Douglas RG, Bennett JE (eds): Principles and Practice of Infectious Diseases. New York, John Wiley and Sons, 1985, pp 1256–1269.

15. Rubin RH, Weinstein L. Salmonellosis: Microbiologic, Pathologic, and Clinical Features. New York, Stratton Intercontinental Medical Book Corporation, 1977.
16. Hoffman TA, Ruiz CJ, Counts GW, et al. Waterborne typhoid fever in Dade County, Florida: Clinical and therapeutic evaluation of 105 bacteremic patients. Am J Med 1975;59:481–487.
17. Aserkoff B, Bennett JV. Effect of antibiotic therapy in acute salmonellosis on the fecal excretion of salmonellae. N Engl J Med 1969;281:636–640,
18. Butler T, Rumans L, Arnold K. Response of typhoid fever caused by chloramphenicol-susceptible and chloramphenicol-resistant strains of *Salmonella typhi* to treatment with trimethoprim–sulfamethoxazole. Rev Infect Dis 1982;4:551–561.
19. Pillay N, Adams EB, Coombes DN. Comparative trial of amoxicillin and chloramphenicol in treatment of typhoid fever in adults. Lancet 1975;2:333–337.
20. Hoffman SL, Punjab NH, Kumala S, et al. Reduction of mortality in chloramphenicol-treated severe typhoid fever by high-dose dexamethasone. N Engl J Med 1984;310:82–88.
21. Blaser MJ, Taylor DN, Feldman PA. Epidemiology of *Campylobacter jejuni* infections. Epidemiol Rev 1983;5:157–176.
22. Pitkanen T, Ponka A, Pettersson T, et al. Campylobacter enteritis in 188 hospitalized patients. Arch Intern Med 1983;143: 215–219.
23. Finch MJ, Riley LW. Campylobacter infections in the United States—results of an 11-state surveillence. Arch Intern Med 1984;144:1610–1612.
24. Nolan CM, Johnson KE, Coyle MB, et al. *Campylobacter jejuni* enteritis: efficacy of antimicrobial and antimotility drugs. Am J Gastroenterol 1983;78:621–626.
25. Sanford JP. Guide to Antimicrobial Therapy 1985. San Antonio, TX, Antimicrobial Therapeutics, Inc., 1985.
26. Anders BJ, Lauer BA, Paisley JW, et al. Double-blind placebo controlled trial of erythromycin for treatment of campylobacter enteritis. Lancet 1982;1:131–132.
27. Marks MI, Pai C, Lafleur L, et al. *Yersinia enterocolitica* gastroenteritis: a prospective study of clinical bacteriologic and epidemiologic features. J Pediatr 1980;96:26–31.
28. Pai C, Gillis F, Tuomanen E, et al. Clinical and laboratory observations: placebo controlled double-blind evaluation of trimethoprim–sulfamethoxazole treatment of *Yersinia enterocolitica* gastroenteritis. J Pediatr 1984;104:308–311.
29. Winblad S. Arthritis associated with *Yersinia enterocolitica* infections. Scand J Infect Dis 1975;7:191–195.
30. Anonymous. Cholera in a tourist returning from Cancun, Mexico. New Jersey MMWR 1983;32:357.
31. Gill DM. The mechanism of action of cholera toxin. Adv Cyclic Nucleotide Res 1977;8:85.
32. Svennerholm A, Jeriborn M, Gothefors L, et al. Mucosal antitoxin and antibacterial immunity after cholera disease and after immunization with a combined B subunit–whole cell vaccine. J Infect Dis 1984;149:884–893.
33. Hug MI, Sanyal SC, Samadi AR, et al. Comparative behaviour of classical and El Tor biotypes of *Vibrio cholerae* 01 isolated in Bangladesh during 1982. Diar Dis Res 1983;1:5–9.
34. Hirschhorn N, Lindenbaum J, Greenough WC, et al. Hypoglycemia in children with acute diarrhea. Lancet 1966;2:128–132.
35. Molla AM, Sarker SA, Hossain M, et al. Rice-powder electrolyte solution as oral therapy in diarrhea due to *Vibrio cholerae* and *Escherichia coli*. Lancet 1982;1:1317–1319.
36. Lindebaum J, Greenough WB, Islam MR. Antibiotic therapy of cholera in children. Bull WHO 1967;37:529.
37. Karchmer AW, Curlin GT, Hug MJ, et al. Furazolidone in paediatric cholera. Bull WHO 1970;43:373–378.
38. Guerrant RL, Moore RA, Kirschenfeld PM, et al. Role of toxigenic and invasive bacteria in acute diarrhea of childhood. N Engl J Med 1975;293:567–573.
39. Guerrant RL, Hughes JM, Chang B, et al. Activation of intestinal guanylate cyclase by heat stable enterotoxin of *E. coli*: studies of tissue specificity, potential receptors, and intermediates. J Infect Dis 1980;142:220–228.
40. Immunizations and chemoprophylaxis for travelers. Med Lett Drug Ther 1985;27:33–36.
41. Gracey M. Traveler's diarrhea: is drug therapy for prophylaxis and treatment of real benefit? Drugs 1984;27:1–5.
42. Bartlett JG, Chang TW, Gurwith M, et al. Antibiotic-associated pseudomembranous colitis due to toxin-producing clostridia. N Engl J Med 1978;298:531–534.
43. Fekety R, Kim KH, Brown D, et al. Epidemiology of antibiotic-associated colitis. Isolation of *Clostridium difficile* from the hospital environment. Am J Med 1981;70:906–908.
44. Tedesco FJ. Pseudomembranous colitis: pathogenesis and therapy. Med Clin North Am 1982;66:655–663.
45. Teasley DG, Olson MM, Gerding DN, et al. Prospective randomized study of metronidazole versus vancomycin for clostridium-associated diarrhea and colitis. Lancet 1983;2:1043–1046.
46. Bartlett JG. Treatment of antibiotic-associated pseudomembranous colitis. Rev Infect Dis 1984;6(suppl):S235–S241.
47. Young GP, Ward P, McDonald M, et al. Comparison of oral bacitracin with vancomycin in therapy of antibiotic-associated colitis. Gastroenterology 1984;86:1306.
48. King C, Barrier SL. Analysis of in vitro interaction between vancomycin and cholestyramine. Antimicrob Agents Chemother 1981;19:326–329.
49. Novak E, Lee DG, Seckman CE, et al. Unfavorable effect of atropine–diphenoxylate therapy in lincomycin-caused diarrhea. JAMA 1976;235:1451–1454.
50. Brandt CD, Kim HW, Rodriguez WJ, et al. Pediatric viral gastroenteritis during eight years of study. J Clin Microbiol 1983;18:71–78.
51. Hjelt K, Krasilnikoff PA, Gravballe PC, et al. Clinical features in hospitalized children with acute gastroenteritis. Acta Paediatric Scand 1985;74:96–101.
52. Feig M. Staphylococcal food poisoning. A report of two related outbreaks, and a discussion of the data presented. Am J Public Health 1950;40:279.
53. Holmberg SD, Blake PA. Staphylococcal food poisoning in the United States: New facts and old misconceptions. JAMA 1984;251:487–489.
54. Gunderson CB. The effects of botulinum toxin on the synthesis, storage, and release of acetylcholine. Prog Neurobiol 1980;14:99.
55. Hughes JM, Blumenthal JR, Mirson MA, et al. Clinical features of types A and B foodborne botulism. Ann Intern Med 1981;95:442–445.
56. Whittaker RL, Gilbertson RB, Garrutt AS. Botulism, type E: Report of eight simultaneous cases. Ann Intern Med 1964;61:448–454.
57. Tacket CO, Shandera WX, Mann JM, et al. Equine antitoxin use and other factors that predict outcome in type A foodborne botulism. Am J Med 1984;76:794–798.
58. Hatheway CH, Snyder JD, Seals JE, et al. Antitoxin levels in botulism patients treated with trivalent equine botulism antitoxin to toxin types A, B, and E. J Infect Dis 1984;150:407–412.
59. Sellin LC. Botulism—an update. Military Med 1984;149:12–16.

# *Chapter 82* / Intraabdominal Infections

Joseph T. DiPiro, PharmD, and John A. Mansberger, MD

Despite the introduction of many new antimicrobials and advances in diagnostic and surgical techniques the treatment of intraabdominal infection continues to pose many challenges. The nature of these infections varies considerably depending on the site of infection, the underlying disease process, and the status of the patient's own defense mechanisms. Optimal therapeutic management usually requires a combination of surgical procedures, antimicrobials, and other measures to maintain vital organ function.

Intraabdominal infections are those contained within the peritoneum or retroperitoneal space (Fig. 82.1). The peritoneal cavity extends from the undersurface of the diaphragm to the floor of the pelvis and contains the stomach, most of the small bowel, the large bowel (including the sigmoid colon), liver and gallbladder, and spleen. The duodenum, pancreas, kidney, adrenals, great vessels (aorta and vena cava), and most mesenteric vascular structures reside in the posterior retroperitoneum. These infections may be diffuse, spread throughout the peritoneum, or localized. Also, they may be contained within visceral structures such as the liver, spleen, or pancreas, or the female reproductive organs. Two general types of intraabdominal infection are discussed throughout this chapter, peritonitis and abscess. Peritonitis is defined as the acute, inflammatory response of peritoneal lining to microorganisms, chemicals, irradiation, or foreign body injury. This chapter deals only with peritonitis of infectious origin. An abscess is a purulent collection of fluid separated by a more or less well defined wall from surrounding tissue. It usually contains necrotic debris, bacteria, and neutrophils. These processes differ considerably to their presentation and the required approach to treatment.

## Etiology

Peritonitis may be classified as either "primary" or "secondary." With primary peritonitis an intraabdominal focus of disease may not be evident. Bacteria may be transported from the bloodstream to the peritoneal cavity where the inflammatory process begins. In secondary peritonitis a focal disease process is evident within the abdomen. In most cases this involves perforation of a hollow structure of the gastrointestinal tract and subsequent escape of intestinal contents.

Primary peritonitis has been reported to occur infrequently in normal infants and children and sometimes in association with nephrotic syndrome. It occurs in 10% to 20% of patients with cirrhotic ascites, in immunocompromised patients in general, and commonly, in patients undergoing peritoneal dialysis. The overall incidence of primary peritonitis is much less than that of secondary peritonitis. Recent paracentesis, upper gastrointestinal endoscopy, portacaval anastomosis, arterial or umbilical vein catheterization, and barium enema or sigmoidoscopy appear to increase the risk of primary peritonitis.

Table 82.1 summarizes many of the potential causes of secondary peritonitis. These include inflammatory processes of the gastrointestinal tract or abdominal organs, mechanical problems such as bowel obstruction, vascular occlusions that may lead to gangrene of the intestines, and neoplasias that may cause intestinal perforation or obstruction. Other possible causes include those resulting from traumatic injuries or postoperative infections.

Abscesses are the result of chronic inflammation and most often occur without preceding peritonitis. They may be located within one of the spaces of the peritoneal cavity or in one of the visceral organs. These collections often have a fibrinous capsule and may take from a few days to years to form.

The causes of intraabdominal abscess somewhat overlap those of peritonitis. Appendicitis is the most frequent cause followed by pancreatitis and lesions of the genitourinary tract (particularly in women). Other potential causes of intraabdominal abscesses include diverticulitis, lesions of the biliary tract, osteomyelitis of the spine, perforating tumors in the abdomen, trauma, and leaking sutures after intestinal anastomosis. For certain diseases, such as appendicitis and diverticulitis, abscesses occur much more frequently than peritonitis.

**Table 82.1** Causes of Secondary Bacterial Peritonitis

| | |
|---|---|
| Miscellaneous causes | Vascular causes |
| Diverticulitis with perforation | Mesenteric arterial occlusion |
| Appendicitis | Mesenteric ischemia without occlusion |
| Crohn's disease | Mesenteric venous occlusion |
| Salpingitis | Trauma |
| Empyema of the gallbladder | Blunt abdominal trauma and small-bowel rupture |
| Necrotizing pancreatitis | Penetrating abdominal trauma |
| Neoplasms | Iatrogenic intestinal perforation |
| Intestinal obstruction | Intraoperative events |
| Perforation | Peritoneal contamination during abdominal operation |
| Mechanical GI problems | Leakage from gastrointestinal anastomosis |
| Any cause of small-bowel obstruction | |

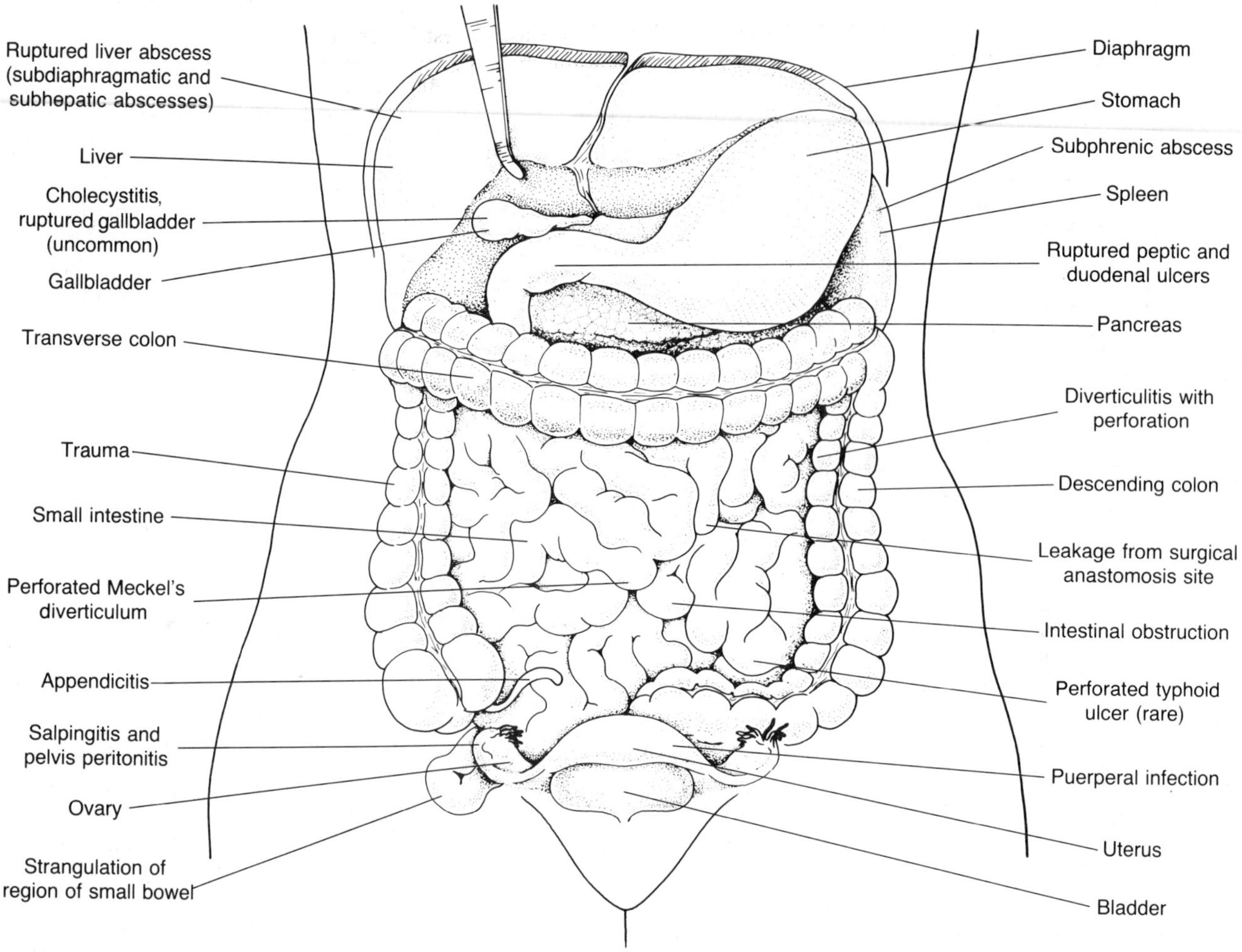


**Figure 82.1** Sites and common causes of peritonitis. (*From Maddux MS, Nishikawa RA: Anaerobic Infections: Considerations for the Hospital Pharmacist, Part 2. Chicago, University of Illinois, 1984, p 10, with permission.*)

## Microflora of Gastrointestinal Tract and Female Genital Tract

A full appreciation of the nature of these processes requires an understanding of the normal microflora within the gastrointestinal tract. There are striking differences in gastrointestinal flora contained within the various segments of the gastrointestinal tract (Table 82.2) and this bacterial environment usually determines the severity of infectious processes in the abdomen.[1] Generally, the low pH of the stomach eradicates bacteria that enter. Perforation of the stomach as a result of peptic ulcer is serious enough to require prompt surgical intervention, but the potential for serious intraabdominal infectious complications is generally not significant, as few bacteria reside in a stomach that has fluid with a very low pH. In fact, the concentration of bacteria in the stomach can be directly related to gastric pH. With achlorhydria bacterial counts may rise to $10^{5-7}$/mL. The normally low bacterial count also changes with gastric outlet obstruction and gastric cancer, in patients that have been on cimetidine, or in the presence of blood.[2] In each of these situations the concentration of bacteria may increase by 1,000- or 10,000-fold.

The biliary tract (gallbladder and bile ducts) is sterile in most healthy individuals but in certain groups it is likely to be colonized by aerobic gram-negative bacilli (particularly *Escherichia coli* and *Klebsiella* spp.) and enterococci.[3] Groups more likely to be colonized include those over the age of 70, or those with acute cholecystitis, jaundice, or common bile duct stones.[4] Because these groups are more frequently colonized they are at greater risk of infection that develops in the biliary tract.

At the distal ileum, particularly just before the ileocecal junction, bacterial counts of aerobes and anaerobes are quite high. In the colon there may be 400 to 500 different types of bacteria, with bacterial concentrations often reaching $10^{11}$/mL, and anaerobic bacteria outnumbering aerobic bacteria by over 1,000 to 1. Fortunately, most colonic bacteria are not pathogens, as they cannot survive in environments outside the colon. The presence of stool has significant implications on colonic flora, as studies have shown that up to 50% of the dry mass of stool is bacteria. Perforation of the

**Table 82.2** Usual Microflora of the Gastrointestinal Tract

| Site | Commonly found bacteria | Approximate concentration (log no. organisms/mL) | |
|---|---|---|---|
| | | Aerobes | Anaerobes |
| Stomach[a] | *Streptococcus, Lactobacillus* | $10^0$–$10^2$ | Rare |
| Biliary tract | Normally sterile (*Escherichia coli* or *Klebsiella* enterococci in some patients) | 0 | 0 |
| Proximal small bowel | *Streptococcus* (including enterococci), *E. coli, Klebsiella, Lactobacillus,* diphtheroids | $10^2$ | Few |
| Distal ileum | *E. coli, Klebsiella, Enterobacter,* enterococci, *Bacteroides fragilis, Clostridium,* peptostreptococci | $10^4$–$10^6$ | $10^5$–$10^7$ |
| Colon | *Bacteroides* spp., peptostreptococci, *Clostridium, E. coli, Klebsiella,* enterococci, *Enterobacter* (and many others) | $10^5$–$10^8$ | $10^9$–$10^{11}$ |

[a] With achlorhydria, H-2 antagonist therapy, gastric cancer, or gastric outlet obstruction, bacterial counts may rise to $10^5$/mL.

colon therefore results in the release of very large numbers of anaerobic and aerobic bacteria into the peritoneum.[5] The colonic flora are generally stable unless broad-spectrum antimicrobials have been in use, where increases in *Candida* or resistant bacteria are noted.

The lower female genital tract is generally colonized by a large number of aerobic and anaerobic bacteria. Anaerobes may number $10^9$/mL and often include lactobacilli, eubacteria, clostridia, anaerobic streptococci, and less frequently, *Bacteroides fragilis*. Aerobic bacteria are most often streptococci and *Staphylococcus epidermidis*, and these may number $10^8$/mL.

## Pathophysiology

Intraabdominal infection results from entry of bacteria into the peritoneal or retroperitoneal spaces. In primary peritonitis the route of bacterial spread is not apparent. Bacteria may enter the abdomen via the bloodstream or the lymphatic system, by transmigration through the bowel wall, or via the fallopian tubes in females. Hematogenous bacterial spread (through the bloodstream) more likely occurs with tubercular peritonitis or peritonitis associated with cirrhotic ascites.[6] With peritonitis resulting from peritoneal dialysis, bacteria are routinely introduced through the peritoneal catheter from skin.[7] In secondary peritonitis, bacteria most often enter the peritoneum or retroperitoneum as a result of disruption of the integrity of the gastrointestinal tract caused by diseases or injuries. Also, peritonitis or abscess may result from contamination of the peritoneum during a surgical procedure, or from lesions of the female genital tract.

The physiologic characteristics of the peritoneal cavity determine the nature of the response to infection or inflammation within it. The peritoneum is lined by a highly permeable, serous membrane of large surface area, approximately that of skin. The normal peritoneal cavity contains about 50 mL of a serous fluid that is normally sterile, is low in protein and leukocytes, and contains no fibrinogen. These conditions change drastically with peritoneal infection or inflammation as will be described later.

After bacteria are introduced into the peritoneal cavity there is an immediate response to contain the insult.[7] Humoral and cellular defenses respond first; then peritoneal and omentum tissues migrate to the affected area. A limited bacterial inoculum is rapidly handled by defense mechanisms. Under certain conditions the bacterial insult is not contained and bacteria disseminate throughout the peritoneal cavity, resulting in peritonitis. This is more likely to occur in the presence of a foreign body or where there is (1) a large bacterial inoculum, (2) continuing bacterial contamination, (3) contamination involving a mixture of organisms that by synergistic action are particularly virulent.

When bacteria become dispersed throughout the peritoneum the inflammatory process involves the majority of the peritoneal lining. There is an outpouring into the peritoneum of serous fluid containing leukocytes, fibrin, and other proteins which form exudates on the inflamed peritoneal surfaces and begin to form adhesions between peritoneal structures. This process, combined with a paralysis of the intestines, may result in confinement of the contamination to one or more locations within the peritoneum. Fluid also begins to collect in the bowel and distension may result. The fluid and protein shift into the abdomen may be so dramatic that there is a decreased circulating blood volume, which causes decreased cardiac output and possibly hypotension. The fluid imbalance may be worsened by accompanying fever, vomiting, or diarrhea. At this point a sympathetic response (sweating, tachycardia, and cutaneous vasoconstriction) may be evident. With an inflamed peritoneum, bacteria and the endotoxins are easily absorbed into the bloodstream and this may result in septic shock. Other foreign substances that may be present in the peritoneal cavity potentiate peritonitis. These adjuvants, notably feces, dead tissues, barium, mucus, bile, and even hemoglobin, have detrimental effects on host defense mechanisms, particularly on bacterial phagocytosis.

Peritonitis often results in mortality because of the effects on multiple organ systems. As mentioned before, fluid shifts and endotoxins may cause hypotension and shock. Fluid loss from the vasculature with generalized peritonitis is similar to that which occurs after a 50% second-degree burn. Hypoalbuminemia may result from protein loss into the peritoneum. Pulmonary function may be compromised because the inflamed peritoneum inhibits proper ventilation. Then, atelectasis and pulmonary shunting of blood may result in hypoxemia. With fluid loss and hypotension, renal perfusion may be compromised and acute renal failure is a potential threat.

If the body is successful in localizing peritoneal contamination but fails to completely eliminate bacteria, an abscess results. This collection of necrotic tissue, bacteria, and white blood cells may be at single or multiple sites and may be within one of the spaces of the peritoneal cavity or in one of the visceral organs. The location of the abscess is often related to the site of primary disease.[8] Abscesses resulting from appendicitis tend to appear in the right lower quadrant or the pelvis; those resulting from diverticulitis tend to appear in the left lower quadrant or pelvis.

An abscess begins by the combined action of neutrophils, bacteria, fibrin, and other inflammatory components. Bacteria may release heparinases which cause local thrombosis and tissue necrosis. Others produce fibrinolysins, collagenases, or other enzymes that allow extension of the process into surrounding tissues. Neutrophils that have gathered in the abscess cavity die in 3 to 5 days, releasing lysosomal enzymes that liquify the core of the abscess. A mature abscess may have a fibrinous capsule that isolates bacteria and the liquid core from opsonins and antimicrobials.

In this environment the oxygen tension is low, anaerobic bacteria thrive, and the size of the abscess may increase. Also, abscesses are hypertonic, resulting in additional influx of fluid. Hypertonicity will then promote the formation of bacterial L forms, which would be resistant to antimicrobial agents that disrupt cell walls. This process may continue and stabilize for long periods of time and not be readily evident to patient or physician. In some instances the abscess may resolve, and infrequently it may erode into adjacent organs or it may rupture and cause diffuse peritonitis. If the abscess ruptures near the skin it may result in a fistulous tract or drain through a surgical wound.

### *Microbiology of Intraabdominal Infections*

Because of the diverse bacteria present in the gastrointestinal tract, secondary intraabdominal infections are often polymicrobial.[9] The mean number of isolates of microorganisms from infected intraabdominal sites has ranged from 2.5 to 5.0, including an average of 1.4 to 2.0 aerobes and 2.4 to 3.0 anaerobes.[5,10] Anaerobic organisms are isolated in most patients. Purely aerobic or anaerobic infections are uncommon, as would be infections caused by fungi. The frequencies with which specific bacteria were isolated in secondary bacterial peritonitis are given in Table 82.3.[11] *E. coli* and *Bacteroides* spp. were most often isolated from the infectious site as well as from blood cultures. This pattern of infecting bacteria is similar to that seen in intraabdominal abscesses. With abscesses, though, anaerobic bacteria are even more frequently isolated.

**Table 82.3** Causative Organisms in Patients With Secondary Bacterial Peritonitis

| *Aerobes* | | *Anaerobes* | |
|---|---|---|---|
| **Organism** | **% Patients** | **Organism** | **% Patients** |
| *Escherichia coli* | 66 | *Bacteroides fragilis* | 47 |
| *Proteus* | 25 | Other *Bacteroides* | 49 |
| *Klebsiella* | 29 | *Peptostreptococcus* | 18 |
| *Pseudomonas* | 9 | *Peptococcus* | 13 |
| *Streptococcus* (including enterococcus) | 30 | *Clostridium* | 23 |
| | | *Fusobacterium* | 11 |
| *Staphylococcus* | 7 | | |

From Wilson SE: Secondary bacterial peritonitis, in Wilson SE, Finegold SM, Williams RA (Eds): Intra-abdominal Infection. New York, McGraw–Hill, 1982, pp. 62–68, with permission.

Primary bacterial peritonitis presents quite a different microbiologic picture, as these infections are often caused by single organisms. Primary peritonitis in children is usually caused by *Streptococcus pneumoniae* or group A streptococcus.[12] When peritonitis occurs in association with cirrhotic ascites, again, single bacteria—most often enteric organisms—are usually responsible.[6] *E. coli* is isolated most frequently, followed by streptococcal species (including pneumococcus), *Klebsiella*, *Bacteroides* spp., *Pseudomonas aeruginosa*, and numerous other organisms. Occasionally, primary peritonitis may be caused by *Mycobacterium tuberculosis*. Peritonitis in patients undergoing peritoneal dialysis is most often caused by common skin organisms: *Staphylococcus epidermidis*, *Staphylococcus aureus*, streptococci, and diphtheroids.[7] Occasionally, aerobic gram-negative bacilli may cause infections, particularly in patients undergoing dialysis during hospitalization.

Some visceral abscesses differ in character from most intraabdominal abscesses. Hepatic abscesses may be polymicrobial (involving *E. coli* and anaerobes) or occasionally may be caused by amoeba. Pancreatic abscesses are also often polymicrobial, involving enteric bacteria that ascend through the biliary system or occasionally staphylococci as a result of hematogenous spread. Splenic abscesses usually result from hematogenous dissemination of bacteria such as *S. aureus*, streptococci, and occasionally *Salmonella* or anaerobic organisms.

### *Bacterial Synergism*

There is much variation in infectious consequences after the introduction of bacteria into the peritoneal cavity. These differences are partially attributed to the competence of patient immune defenses against infection as well as factors related to the infecting bacteria. The size of the bacterial inoculum and the number and types of bacterial species present significantly affect patient outcome. Altemeier[13] noted a direct correlation between peritonitis mortality rates and the number of bacterial species cultivated from peritoneal fluid. The combination of aerobic and anaerobic organisms appears to greatly increase the risk of infection. In animal studies, combinations of aerobic and anaerobic bacteria were much more lethal than infections caused by the aerobes or anaerobes alone.

In intraabdominal infections, facultative bacteria may provide an environment conducive to the growth of anaerobic bacteria.[14] Although many bacteria isolated in mixed infections are nonpathogenic by themselves, their presence may be essential for the pathogenicity of the bacterial mixture. The role of facultative bacteria in mixed infections may include (1) promotion of an appropriate environment for anaerobic growth, (2) production of nutrients necessary for anaerobes, or (3) production of extracellular enzymes that promote tissue invasion by anaerobes.

Animal models of intraabdominal infection have been devised that demonstrate that aerobic and anaerobic bacteria are important participants. In one series of experiments, gelatin capsules containing a mixture of 22 aerobic and anaerobic bacteria were implanted intraperitoneally into rats.[14] After implantation of the capsules, a two-stage disease process was apparent. During the first 5 days, acute generalized peritonitis was observed and the mortality rate was 39%. After 5 days, mortality from intraabdominal infection was not observed; however, almost all surviving animals had intraabdominal abscesses when sacrificed at 2 weeks. During the peritonitis stages, *E. coli* was noted in the bloodstream of most animals, and *E. coli*, *B. fragilis*, and enterococci were isolated from peritoneal exudates. Bacteremia could not be demonstrated during the abscess stage, but abscesses were found to contain predominantly anaerobic bacteria (*B. fragilis* and *Fusobacterium varium*) but also *E. coli* and enterococcus.

In further experiments, defined inocula of *E. coli*, enterococci, and *B. fragilis* were placed in the gelatin capsule implants alone or in varying combinations.[14] *E. coli* was shown to reliably produce peritonitis in a significant percentage of animals whether or not it was introduced in combination with the other bacteria. *B. fragilis* reliably produced abscesses, whether or not it was given in combination with other bacteria. The combination of *E. coli* with *B. fragilis* resulted in a 65% early mortality and abscesses in 100% of survivors. Enterococci or *F. varium* introduced alone did not result in mortality or abscesses.

These experiments support the concept that aerobic enteric bacteria and anaerobic bacteria are pathogens in intraabdominal infection. Aerobic bacteria, particularly *E. coli*, appear responsible for the early mortality from peritonitis, while anaerobic bacteria are major pathogens in abscesses, with *B. fragilis* predominating. The role of enterococci as a pathogen was not clear, as it failed to produce peritonitis or abscesses when given alone, but it may still participate in the infectious process by creating an environment favorable to other pathogens. The extension of this model is relatively limited because it simulates untreated intraabdominal infection after free perforation of the colon.

The role of anaerobic bacteria in intraabdominal infection has been a continuing source of controversy. Anaerobic bacteria and enterococci are present in the gastrointestinal tract, and these bacteria, especially *B. fragilis*, are isolated from many intraabdominal infections; however, Stone et al[15] demonstrated that after traumatic injury to the colon or with a ruptured appendix, even though anaerobic bacteria could be isolated in all cases, those same anaerobic bacteria were isolated in only 10% of patients 1 to 2 hours after the abdomen was opened. They concluded that exposure to atmospheric oxygen was the most important factor in reducing the numbers of anaerobic bacteria and that specific antianaerobic antimicrobials are not always necessary. On the other hand, Nichols[10] obtained quantitative and qualitative cultures at regular intervals intraoperatively, in patients with peritonitis, and found no selective suppression of anaerobes by exposure to air. At this time most clinicians acknowledge the importance of anaerobic bacteria as pathogens in intraabdominal infection and recommend specific therapies directed against these bacteria.

Enterococcus can be isolated from many intraabdominal infections in humans, but its role as a pathogen is not clear.[16] In numerous studies, antimicrobial regimens that are not effective against enterococci in vitro have been successful in treating intraabdominal infections. Although enterococcal bacteremia accompanying intraabdominal infection occurs relatively infrequently, antibiotics ineffective against enterococcus in vitro, such as cephalosporins, have been successfully used alone. Others have noted that enterococcal infection occurs in the presence of factors indicating failure of the host's defenses (e.g., immunocompromised patients).

## Clinical Presentation

Intraabdominal infections have a wide spectrum of manifestations, often depending on the specific disease process, its location, and concurrent host factors. Peritonitis is usually easily recognized but intraabdominal abscesses may often continue for considerable periods of time either unrecognized or attributable to an unrelated disease process.

Generalized bacterial peritonitis usually commands the immediate attention of the physician, as the patient most often presents in acute distress. The patient lies still, usually on his or her back, possibly with hips slightly flexed. Any movement of the patient, including deep breaths, worsens the generalized abdominal pain, so the patient exhibits voluntary guarding of the abdomen and respirations are shallow and frequent. There is generalized abdominal tenderness on examination and after a short period of time the abdominal muscles become rigid, a product of involuntary guarding; this is called a "board abdomen." Bowel sounds are at first faint, then absent; abdominal distension ensues. Sometimes the patient has nausea often accompanied by vomiting. Because of the secretion of serous fluid into the peritoneal cavity the vascular volume may contract. This, as well as the physiologic response to stress, causes a tachycardia. Initially the patient's temperature is normal but increases to 100 to 102°F within the first few hours and up to 103°F within 6 to 8 hours. Because of the fluid loss into the peritoneum and vomiting, the patient may appear dehydrated, and a decreased urine output would be noted.

If peritonitis continues untreated the patient may go into hypovolemic shock from fluid loss into the peritoneum. This may be accompanied by generalized sepsis as the inflamed peritoneum absorbs bacteria and toxins from the suppurative process into the bloodstream. Dehydration with hypovolemic shock is the major factor for mortality in the early stage of peritonitis.

Laboratory evaluations usually demonstrate leukocytosis (15,000–20,000 WBC/mm$^3$), with neutrophils predominating. The hematocrit and the blood urea nitrogen may be elevated because of the dehydration. Early after the insult the patient is usually alkalotic because of hyperventilation and vomiting. As the process progresses the patient may become acidotic from hypovolemia or presence of devitalized tissue. At this stage serum lactic acid will probably be elevated. Abdominal radiographs may be useful, as free air in the abdomen (indicating intestinal perforation) or distension of the small or large bowel is often evident.

The presentation of primary peritonitis can be quite different from that of secondary peritonitis. Primary peritonitis can develop over a period of days to weeks, evident as an acute febrile illness. Usually the patient has nausea, vomiting (sometimes with diarrhea), abdominal tenderness, and hypoactive bowel sounds although the abdominal signs are variable. The patient's temperature or white blood cell count may be only mildly elevated. The cirrhotic patient may have worsening encephalopathy.

Patients on chronic peritoneal dialysis usually have abdominal pain and tenderness, possibly with nausea and vomiting, but fever is not a consistent finding. In these patients a cloudy dialysate drainage is often noted as a first sign of peritonitis.

With primary peritonitis, routine evaluative procedures would be performed (e.g., serum chemistries, complete blood count, abdominal radiographs, blood cultures), but also, if possible, ascitic fluid collected by paracentesis or peritoneal dialysate should be examined. In the presence of peritonitis, ascitic fluid usually contains greater than 300 leukocytes/mm$^3$ and bacteria may be evident on Gram stain of a centrifuged specimen; however, in 60% to 80% of patients with cirrhotic ascites, the Gram stain is negative.

Intraabdominal abscesses pose a more difficult diagnostic challenge as the symptoms are often neither specific nor dramatic. The patient may complain of abdominal pain or discomfort but these symptoms are not reliable. Fever is usually present; often it is low grade, but it can be a high, spiking pattern. The patient may have paralytic ileus and abdominal distension. The abdominal examination is unreliable; tenderness and pain may be present, and a mass can possibly be palpated.

Peritonitis may result from an abscess that ruptures, spreading bacteria and toxins throughout the peritoneum. In other patients, the entry of bacterial toxins into the systemic circulation from the abscess may lead to progressive multisystem organ failure (renal, hepatic, or cardiac).

Laboratory studies are generally not helpful in the diagnosis of intraabdominal abscess although most patients will have leukocytosis. Some patients may have positive blood cultures, while others, particularly diabetics, may have hyperglycemia. The finding of *Bacteroides* or any two enteric bacteria in the bloodstream is often indicative of an intraabdominal infectious process.

At present, there are a number of noninvasive methods for diagnosis of intraabdominal abscesses, but definitive diagnosis often requires exploratory laparotomy. Collections of gas or an air–fluid level in the peritoneum may be evident on plain abdominal radiographs. Gastrointestinal contrast studies may show displacement of abdominal structures. Ultrasound may detect abscess in some cases although it is relatively nonspecific. More recent imaging techniques, computerized tomography and magnetic resonance imaging, are capable of locating many intraabdominal abscesses.

Intraabdominal infection caused by disease processes at specific sites often produces characteristic manifestations that are helpful in diagnosis. For example, a patient with diverticulitis may exhibit stabbing left lower quadrant abdominal pain and constipation. Fever and leukocytosis are often present and a tender mass is sometimes palpable. With appendicitis, the findings are typically inconsistent but many patients have a sudden onset of periumbilical or epigastric pain, which is usually colicky and shifts to the right lower quadrant. The location of pain may vary, as the appendix can be in many locations in the abdomen. A mass may be palpable on abdominal or rectal examination. The patient's temperature is generally mildly elevated early and then increases. Leukocyte counts are usually 12,000–15,000. If perforation and diffuse peritonitis were to occur the manifestations just described would apply. More frequently though, appendiceal perforation results in a local abscess.

Abscesses in specific locations may produce clues to their existence. Pelvic abscesses may be palpable by pelvic examination. A subdiaphragmatic abscess may result in pleural effusion or dyspnea. Retroperitoneal abscesses may cause lumbar or psoas muscle spasm resulting in lower back pain and may cause the patient to flex the legs at the hip.

Intraabdominal infections associated with the biliary tract may coincide with symptoms of acute cholecystitis. These include right upper quadrant abdominal pain and tenderness, sometimes radiating to the back, nausea and vomiting, and often a low-grade fever and leukocytosis. If there are stones present in the common bile duct, the patient is usually jaundiced and serum alkaline phosphatase may be elevated. In the infrequent but serious event of infected bile with common bile duct obstruction (cholangitis), the patient will usually have a high spiking fever, chills, and jaundice.

The presentation and outcome of any intraabdominal infection are significantly influenced by the status of the patient. Those who are malnourished, have undergone multiple traumatic injuries, or are at the extremes of age are more likely to succumb to intraabdominal infection or require an extended period for recovery. In addition to these factors, those with such associated diseases as diabetes mellitus, malignancies, renal failure, and cirrhosis, are recognized to be at greater risk for most infectious processes, including intraabdominal infections. Other risk factors often relating to intraabdominal infection are the use of corticosteroids, particularly in patients with Crohn's disease, and radiation therapy for tumors. Also, use of antimicrobial agents may prevent the prompt diagnosis of abscesses, particularly subphrenic. In some instances acute intraabdominal infectious processes may become chronic with the initiation of antimicrobial agents.

## Treatment

### *General Approach*

The treatment of intraabdominal infection most often requires the coordinated use of a combination of modalities. The three major modalities are (1) prompt surgical intervention, (2) support of vital functions, and (3) appropriate antimicrobial therapy.

The foundation of treatment is either (1) the correction of intraabdominal disease processes or injuries that have caused infection or (2) drainage of collections of purulent material. Antimicrobials are an important adjunct to surgical procedures in the treatment of intraabdominal infections; however, the use of antimicrobial agents without surgical intervention is usually not adequate. For some specific situations (e.g., most cases of primary peritonitis), surgical procedures may not be required, and antimicrobial agents become the mainstay of therapy.

In the early phase of serious intraabdominal infections much attention is paid to maintenance of body organ system functions. With generalized peritonitis, large volumes of intravenous fluids are required to restore vascular volume and improve cardiac function. Adequate hourly urine output should be maintained to ensure proper renal function. This is done by correcting hypovolemia and restoring cardiac output. The use of diuretics to improve urine output once these factors are corrected is controversial since they may worsen fluid deficits. Respiratory function is assisted by the use of nasal oxygen, and ventilatory support in severely ill patients. Often, the critically ill patient with intraabdominal infection will require intensive care monitoring, particularly if there is cardiovascular or respiratory instability. Also, isolation procedures may be required if the infectious process poses a threat to other hospitalized patients.

An additional important component of therapy is parenteral nutrition. Intraabdominal infections often directly involve the gastrointestinal tract or disrupt its function (i.e., paralytic illness). After other therapeutic measures are begun, the return of gastrointestinal function may take a few days to a few weeks and occasionally months. In this interim, parenteral nutrition allows patient recovery and wound healing while maintaining nutritional status.

### *Surgical Management*

The type of surgical procedure performed in treating intraabdominal infections depends on the underlying disease process, the extent or location of the infectious process, and the nature of coexisting injuries or illnesses. The goals of surgical procedures for intraabdominal infection are (1) to stop continuing bacterial contamination and reduce the numbers of bacteria in the peritoneum, (2) to remove foreign material from the abdomen, and (3) to provide drainage of purulent collections. In attempting to reach these goals the surgeon usually performs an exploratory laparotomy to visualize the extent of injury. Any observed defects, such as perforation of the gastrointestinal tract, are corrected, most often by oversewing the perforation or resecting the injured area and leaving either a primary anastomosis of intestine to intestine or an enterostomy. All foreign material, necrotic tissue, feces, blood, or pus should be removed from the operative field and the peritoneum should be copiously irrigated with up to 20 L of sterile 0.9% sodium chloride, to decrease the concentrations of bacteria or other noxious substances.

The most valuable microbiologic information may be obtained at the time of operation or percutaneous abscess drainage. If pus or fluids are found that are believed infected, it is best to aspirate 2–3 mL into a syringe, remove any air, and tightly cap the syringe. The specimen should be brought promptly to the microbiology lab where a Gram stain should be performed immediately and cultures prepared for identification of aerobic bacteria and anaerobic bacteria. If there is no fluid available for collection, culture swab devices may be applied to the infected area. A swab transported under anaerobic conditions is required and it should be analyzed as just described.

### *Fluid Therapy*

Aggressive fluid repletion and management are required for successful treatment of intraabdominal infections. Fluid therapy is instituted for the purposes of achieving or maintaining proper intravascular volumes and adequate urine output and correcting acidosis. Intravascular volume is often decreased in patients with severe intraabdominal infections because fluids accumulate in the abdomen; they collect in a "third space" at the expense of the vasculature. Loss of fluid through vomiting, diarrhea, or a nasogastric suction tube contributes to dehydration. Intravascular volume can be assessed by blood pressure and heart rate but more accurately by measurement of central venous pressure or pulmonary capillary wedge pressure (see Chapter 103). When a contracted vascular volume is accompanied by hemorrhage, the hematocrit initially is about normal, but if there is no hemorrhage the hematocrit is usually elevated as an indication of hemoconcentration. Urine output should be continuously monitored in severely ill patients by use of a transurethral bladder catheter, quantitated hourly, and it should equal or exceed 1 mL/kg body weight per hour.

In patients with peritonitis, hypovolemia is often accompanied by acidosis, so a reasonable intravenous fluid would be lactated Ringer's, which contains the bicarbonate precursor, lactate, as well as sodium, potassium, and calcium. In the initial hour of treatment a large volume of solution may need to be administered to restore intravascular volume. Although this volume may frequently approach 4 L, much more fluid may be required to restore vital functions. For a few hours thereafter fluids may be required at the rate of 1 L/h. Maintenance fluids should be instituted (after intravascular volume is restored) with 0.9% sodium chloride and potassium chloride (20 mEq/L) or 5% dextrose and 0.45% sodium chloride with potassium chloride (20 mEq/L). The administration rate should be based on estimated daily fluid loss through urine and nasogastric suction, including 0.5–1.0 L for insensible fluid loss. Potassium would not routinely be included if the patient is hyperkalemic or has renal failure.

Some clinicians recommend the use of intravenous colloids (5% albumin or 6% hetastarch) for volume repletion, although these agents do not have a demonstrated advantage for this purpose. Their added expense may not be justified. For patients whose hematocrit is decreased because of blood

**Table 82.4** Likely Intraabdominal Pathogens

| *Type of infection* | *Aerobes* | *Anaerobes* |
|---|---|---|
| Primary bacterial peritonitis | | |
| Children (spontaneous) | Pneumococci, group A *Streptococcus* | — |
| Cirrhosis | *Escherichia coli*, *Klebsiella*, pneumococci (many others) | — |
| Peritoneal dialysis | *Staphylococcus*, *Streptococcus* | — |
| Secondary bacterial peritonitis | | |
| Gastroduodenal | *Streptococcus*, *E. coli* | — |
| Biliary tract | *E. coli*, *Klebsiella*, enterococci | *Clostridium* or *Bacteroides* (infrequent) |
| Small or large bowel | *E. coli*, *Klebsiella* spp., *Proteus* spp. | *Bacteroides fragilis* and other *Bacteroides*, *Clostridium* |
| Appendicitis | *E. coli*, *Pseudomonas* | *Bacteroides* spp. |
| Abscesses | *E. coli*, *Klebsiella*, enterococci | *B. fragilis* and other *Bacteroides*, *Clostridium*, anaerobic cocci |
| Liver | *E. coli*, *Klebsiella*, enterococci, staphylococci, amoeba | *Bacteroides* (infrequent) |
| Spleen | *Staphylococcus*, *Streptococcus* | — |

loss, whole blood should be administered. Aggressive fluid therapy must often be maintained in the postoperative period, as the insult initiated by peritonitis continues. For the first few days after operation, fluid may still sequester in the peritoneal cavity, posing a continued risk of hypovolemia.

### *Antimicrobial Therapy*

The approach to antimicrobial therapy of intraabdominal infection—in particular, the choice of antimicrobials used and the route of administration—has been the subject of much debate in recent years. Whatever agents are chosen and by whatever route they are administered, the goals of antimicrobial therapy remain the same: (1) to control bacteremia and the establishment of metastatic foci of infection, (2) to reduce suppurative complications after bacterial contamination, and (3) to prevent local spread of existing infection. Once suppuration has occurred (e.g., an abscess has formed), a cure by antibiotics alone is very difficult to achieve; antimicrobials may serve to improve the results that would have been attained with surgery alone. In a few instances, such as *selected* patients with pyogenic liver abscess, surgical intervention is not always indicated and percutaneous drainage accompanied by antimicrobial therapy may be justified.

Antimicrobial agents should be started as soon as the presence of intraabdominal infection is suspected, so they are usually begun before identification of infecting bacteria is complete. Therapy must be initiated based on what are the likely pathogens. Predominant pathogens, as discussed in the previous section, vary depending on the site of intraabdominal infection and the underlying disease process. Likely pathogens, those against which antimicrobial agents should be directed, are listed in Table 82.4.

The importance of providing antimicrobial coverage for aerobic and anaerobic pathogens was demonstrated with the previously described rat model of intraabdominal contamination.[14] When gentamicin, an agent with excellent activity against aerobic gram-negative bacilli but no activity against anaerobic bacteria, was administered alone to the animals, most of the peritonitis was prevented and the mortality rate was reduced to 4%; however, most surviving animals still had intraabdominal abscesses when sacrificed at 12 days. When clindamycin, an agent with excellent activity against anaerobic bacteria but no activity against aerobic gram-negative bacilli, was administered alone, the frequency of peritonitis and mortality remained about 40% while abscess formation was prevented in most survivors. As expected, when gentamicin and clindamycin were administered concurrently, mortality rates (from peritonitis) and abscess formation were both significantly reduced.

Using this same rat model, selected single-drug therapies, such as carbenicillin, moxalactam, cefoxitin, and cefotaxime, have also resulted in a significant reduction in the frequency of peritonitis *and* intraabdominal abscesses.[17] Antimicrobial agents with good activity against aerobic gram-negative, enteric bacilli successfully reduced mortality rates from peritonitis, while agents active against *Bacteroides fragilis* and other anaerobes reduced the incidence of intraabdominal abscesses.

### Clinical Assessment

Many studies have been conducted evaluating or comparing the effectiveness of antimicrobials for treatment of intraabdominal infections, but, unfortunately, little valuable information has been generated. Substantial differences in patient outcomes from treating intraabdominal infections with a variety of agents have not been demonstrated. Solomkin et al[18] noted that trials of antimicrobial therapy for intraabdominal infection often had serious defects in design, and these defects usually prevented the detection of differences between agents.

The inability to demonstrate differences between antimicrobial regimens in treating intraabdominal infection has been noted by other authors. Thadepalli[19] has observed that before the introduction of sulfonamides, the mortality from intraabdominal trauma was around 48%. "With the introduction of sulfadiazine in 1942 it fell to 8 to 11 percent," Thadepalli noted. "Interestingly, it has remained unchanged since then."[19] Others have noted that despite advances in antimicrobial therapy, generalized peritonitis and subphrenic abscesses continue to result in mortality rates approaching 50% and 30%–40%, respectively.[20,21]

In recent years, single agents (most often second- and third-generation cephalosporins or acylaminopenicillins) have been compared with combination drug regimens containing aminoglycosides. In almost all trials, the single-agent regimen has fared as well as the combination therapy; however, many of these trials included patients at relatively low risk. Often, the definition of intraabdominal infection was extended to include patients with acute intraabdominal bacterial contamination, such as after penetrating traumatic injuries, or "peritonitis" was extended to include patients with cholecystitis and diverticulitis. In fact, many of the reported trials with intraabdominal infections were conducted primarily with patients who had bacterial contamination of the abdomen as a result of traumatic injuries. If most of these patients are treated a few hours after injury, bacterial infection (peritonitis or abscess) is not established and most infectious complications are avoided. In this group, antimicrobial agents are used to prevent infection rather than treat it.

Comparative trials of antimicrobials in patients who have sustained intraperitoneal bacterial contamination from traumatic injuries have most often included a combination of aminoglycoside with clindamycin versus a cephalosporin (cefoxitin, cefamandole, third-generation cephalosporins). In three controlled, comparative trials, cefoxitin was shown to be equivalent to the combination of an aminoglycoside with clindamycin in preventing infection after penetrating abdominal trauma.[22–24] Newer, third-generation cephalosporins have also proven effective.

With penetrating abdominal trauma, some investigators have examined key questions related to antimicrobials used to prevent infection, namely, the necessary duration and timing of antimicrobial therapy. Oresovich et al[25] and Stone et al[26] demonstrated that a short course of antimicrobial agents (12 to 24 hours) was as valuable in preventing infection after abdominal trauma as a course lasting 5 to 7 days. In another investigation, Fullen et al[27] determined that an antimicrobial given very soon after traumatic injury, before an operation was performed, was much more likely to prevent infection than an antimicrobial begun intraoperatively or postoperatively. So, after acute intraabdominal bacterial contamination of the abdomen, antimicrobial agents should be given as soon as possible after injury; a duration of therapy of 24 hours should suffice.

A number of studies have been conducted in patients with established intraabdominal infections. A compilation of the more notable studies is provided in Table 82.5. Generally, these studies do not demonstrate clinical differences between agents, although it is doubtful that many of the studies would have detected clinically significant differences in patient outcome, as the numbers of patients studied were often too few.

Comparative trials of antimicrobials for intraabdominal infection have either compared one of the components of two combination drug regimens or compared single-drug regimens with combination regimens. In a few trials the anaerobic components of combination drug regimens have been compared.[29,34,40] These studies indicate that clindamycin or metronidazole is effective against anaerobic bacteria involved in intraabdominal infections.

Other studies have compared single-agent regimens (using cephalosporins or penicillins) with combination regimens, and in these studies the $\beta$-lactams have produced results similar to those for the combination regimens. In one well-controlled trial, where relatively high-risk patients were studied (all over age 40 years and no patients with acute trauma), moxalactam was as effective as the combination of tobramycin and clindamycin[35]; however, it was observed that the pattern of adverse reactions was considerably different between groups. Hematologic toxicity (rise in prothrombin time) occurred more frequently with moxalactam (45% versus 16%), while renal toxicity (rise in serum creatinine) occurred more frequently in the tobramycin/clindamycin group (18% versus 4%).

Intraabdominal infection presents in many different ways and with a wide spectrum of severity. The regimen employed and duration of treatment depend on the specific clinical circumstances (i.e., the nature of the underlying disease process and the condition of the patient). Compromised patients require more aggressive therapies than otherwise healthy patients who experience the same intraabdominal infection.

### Recommendations

For most intraabdominal infections, the antimicrobial regimen should be effective against both aerobic and anaerobic bacteria. Although it is impossible to provide antimicrobial activity against every possible pathogen, agents with activity against enteric gram-negative bacilli, such as *E. coli* and *Klebsiella*, and anaerobes such as *B. fragilis* and *Clostridia* spp. should be administered. If most of the organisms can be eliminated, the synergistic effect may be removed and the

**Table 82.5** Some Comparative Studies of Intraabdominal Infection

| *Investigator* | *Agent tested* | *Number of patients studied* | *% Patients with satisfactory outcome* |
|---|---|---|---|
| Harding, 1980[28] | Clindamycin/gentamicin | 42 | 79 |
| | Chloramphenicol/gentamicin | 53 | 81 |
| | Ticarcillin/gentamicin | 39 | 90 |
| Smith, 1980[29] | Metronidazole/tobramycin | 35 | 87 |
| | Clindamycin/tobramycin | 23 | 91 |
| Stone, 1980[30] | Erythromycin/cefamandole | 60 | 95 |
| | Metronidazole/gentamicin | 60 | 93 |
| | Clindamycin/gentamicin | 68 | 96 |
| Tally, 1981[31] | Cefoxitin with or without amikacin | 37 | 65 |
| | Clindamycin/amikacin | 37 | 54 |
| Drusano, 1982[32] | Cefoxitin | 26 | 66 |
| | Clindamycin/aminoglycoside | 21 | 52 |
| Stone, 1982[33] | Cefotaxime | 56 | 82 |
| | Clindamycin/gentamicin | 56 | 82 |
| Canadian Study Group, 1983[34] | Metronidazole/gentamicin | 69 | 83 |
| | Clindamycin/gentamicin | 72 | 84 |
| Schentag, 1983[35] | Moxalactam | 49 | 76 |
| | Clindamycin/tobramycin | 49 | 74 |
| Busuttil, 1984[36] | Cefamandole | 31 | 77 |
| | Clindamycin/gentamicin | 34 | 84 |
| Harding, 1984[38] | Cefoxitin/tobramycin | 28 | 82 |
| | Clindamycin/tobramycin | 27 | 89 |
| | Ceftizoxime | 24 | 87 |
| | Clindamycin/tobramycin | 15 | 87 |
| Tornqvist, 1985[39] | Cefuroxime | 59 | 78 |
| | Ceforoxime/metronidazole | 63 | 83 |
| Lennard, 1985[40] | Clindamycin/gentamicin | 52 | 65 |
| | Chloramphenicol/gentamicin | 41 | 61 |
| Malangoni, 1985[37] | Cefoxitin | 59 | 83 |
| | Tobramycin/clindamycin | 53 | 79 |

patient's defenses may be able to eradicate the remaining organisms.

Table 82.6 presents recommended and alternative regimens for selected situations. These are general guidelines, not rules, as there are many factors that cannot be incorporated into such tables.

Most patients with severe intraabdominal infections (where there is generalized peritonitis or septic shock or where the patient has a high fever and shaking chills) should be placed on an aminoglycoside in combination with an antianaerobic agent. Gentamicin is the aminoglycoside of choice, based on its lower cost. Other aminoglycosides, tobramycin, amikacin, and netilmicin, have few relative advantages in intraabdominal infections and are generally not drugs of first choice.

The dosage for aminoglycosides should be adjusted on the basis of a patient's age, weight, and renal function. Because the enteric gram-negative bacilli are usually very susceptible to aminoglycosides, and because aminoglycosides are well distributed into peritoneal fluid,[41] high serum aminoglycoside concentrations are generally not required. Unless relatively resistant bacteria are suspected, a gentamicin or tobramycin peak concentration of 5–6 $\mu$g/mL will usually be effective. Also, trough concentrations should not be allowed to decrease below 1 $\mu$g/mL for a substantial portion of the dosage interval. To achieve these serum concentrations, gentamicin or tobramycin dosage may range from 1 to 3 mg per dose given as often as every 6 hours, or as infrequently as every 48 hours if the patient has renal failure. For most patients, a loading dose of 2 mg/kg gentamicin or tobramycin should be given and subsequent doses based on the patient's weight and estimations of creatinine clearance, or on measured serum aminoglycoside concentrations after the first dose. Although the usual daily dose of gentamicin or tobramycin is 3–5 mg/d, we have found that young, previously healthy individuals who undergo acute traumatic injuries often require more than 5 mg/kg/d gentamicin or tobramycin. Patients who experience septic or hypovolemic shock after intraabdominal infection are more likely to develop acute renal failure. In this situation, aminoglycosides should be used with even greater caution (more frequent serum concentration determinations), and usually an increase in dosing interval is required.

When used for intraabdominal infection, aminoglycosides

**Table 82.6** Recommendations for Initial Antimicrobial Agents for Intraabdominal Infections

| *Type of infection* | *Recommended agent* | *Comments or alternatives* |
|---|---|---|
| Primary peritonitis | | |
| Cirrhosis | Aminoglycoside plus penicillin or first-generation cephalosporin | 1. Add clindamycin or metronidazole if anaerobes are suspected<br>2. Third-generation cephalosporins, aminoacylpenicillins, aztreonam, and imipenem as alternatives |
| Peritoneal dialysis | Regimen based on organism isolated<br>1. *Staphylococcus:* penicillinase-resistant penicillin or first-generation cephalosporin<br>2. *Streptococcus*: penicillin G<br>3. Aerobic gram-negative bacilli: aminoglycoside<br>4. *Pseudomonas aeruginosa*: aminoglycoside plus antipseudomonal penicillin or ceftazidime | 1. Alternative for staphylococci is vancomycin<br>2. Alternative for *Streptococcus* is a first-generation cephalosporin<br>3. Alternatives for gram-negative bacilli are third-generation cephalosporins and aztreonam |
| Secondary peritonitis | | |
| Perforated peptic ulcer | First-generation cephalosporins | 1. Cefoxitin as alternative<br>2. Possibly add aminoglycoside if patient condition is poor |
| Other | Aminoglycoside with clindamycin or metronidazole | 1. Add ampicillin if patient is immunocompromised or if biliary tract is origin of infection<br>2. Cefoxitin, mezlocillin, piperacillin, or chloramphenicol as alternative antianaerobic agent<br>3. Moxalactam,[a] cefotaxime, ceftizoxime, or imipenem as single agent |
| Abscess | | |
| General | Aminoglycoside with clindamycin or metronidazole | 1. Third-generation cephalosporin or aztreonam with clindamycin or metronidazole, or imipenem alone as alternative |
| Liver | As above but add a first-generation cephalosporin | 2. Use metronidazole if amoebic liver abscess is suspected |
| Spleen | Aminoglycoside plus penicillinase-resistant penicillin | 3. Alternatives for penicillinase-resistant penicillin are first-generation cephalosporins or vancomycin |
| Appendicitis | | |
| Normal or inflamed | Cefoxitin (discontinued immediately postoperation) | 1. Aminoglycoside with clindamycin or metronidazole<br>2. Antianaerobic cephalosporins as single agents (cefotetan, ceftizoxime) |
| Gangrenous or perforated | Aminoglycoside with clindamycin or metronidazole | |
| Acute cholecystitis | First-generation cephalosporin | Aminoglycoside plus ampicillin if severe infection |
| Cholangitis | Aminoglycoside with ampicillin with or without clindamycin or metronidazole | Use vancomycin for ampicillin if patient is allergic to penicillin |
| Acute contamination from intraabdominal trauma (preventive therapy) | Cefoxitin, cefotetan, or a third-generation cephalosporin | Aminoglycoside with one of the following: clindamycin, metronidazole, mezlocillin, piperacillin, cefoxitin, cefotetan, or third-generation cephalosporin |
| Acute salpingitis with peritonitis | Cefoxitin plus doxycycline | 1. Aminoglycoside plus clindamycin<br>2. Doxycycline plus metronidazole |
| Tuboovarian abscess | Aminoglycoside plus clindamycin or metronidazole | |

[a]Moxalactam poses a greater risk of bleeding disorders than other available cephalosporins.

should be combined with agents that are effective against the majority of *B. fragilis*. Clindamycin or metronidazole would be the agents of first choice but others such as cefoxitin, certain third-generation cephalosporins (moxalactam, cefotaxime, ceftizoxime, cefotetan), piperacillin, mezlocillin, and even chloramphenicol would be suitable alternatives. Clindamycin should be administered intravenously in a dosage of 600 mg every 6 hours or 900 mg every 8 hours. Lower dosages may not achieve serum concentrations that exceed the minimum inhibitory concentrations of common anaerobic bacteria such as *B. fragilis* or *Clostridia*. Metronidazole should be given intravenously at a dosage of 500 mg every 6 hours. Patients receiving multiple, broad-spectrum antimicrobial agents, particularly those who are immunocompromised, should receive oral nystatin (swish and swallow) for prevention of fungal overgrowth in the mouth and GI tract.

With intraabdominal contamination from the upper gastrointestinal tract (e.g., perforation of a peptic ulcer or biliary tract disease), *B. fragilis* is an uncommon pathogen and other agents may therefore be substituted for clindamycin or metronidazole. Alternatives would include ampicillin, penicillin, or first-generation cephalosporins.

The necessity of administering agents with antianaerobic activity is still a subject of controversy. Some investigators have demonstrated that agents directed specifically at *B. fragilis* do not result in lower rates of infection after gastrointestinal perforation when compared with agents with poor *B. fragilis* activity. Most studies of intraabdominal infection have included agents with activity against both colonic aerobes and anaerobes, and presently, most clinicians would use an antimicrobial regimen that is active against both groups of bacteria. As *B. fragilis* and *Clostridia* are regularly cultured from intraabdominal infections, are isolated in the bloodstream, and believed to be important participants in mixed bacterial infections, antimicrobial agents effective against them are usually recommended.

Ampicillin may be added to assure antimicrobial coverage for enterococci although this is also controversial.[16] Regimens without activity against enterococci (such as gentamicin with clindamycin) are generally effective in treating these infections; however, there are numerous reports of enterococcal superinfection in immunocompromised patients, particularly after cephalosporin use. Studies of human intraabdominal infections have shown enterococci to be the most common gram-positive isolate.[42]

The failure of host defenses may be a critical factor in the pathogenicity of enterococci. So, in immunocompromised patients there is more justification to provide specific antimicrobial activity against enterococci. Ampicillin or other penicillins that are active against enterococci (i.e., penicillin, piperacillin, mezlocillin) should be used in patients at high risk, patients with persistent or recurrent intraabdominal infection, patients in shock, or patients who are immunosuppressed, such as after organ transplantation. Ampicillin remains the drug of choice for this purpose because it is most active in vitro against enterococci and is relatively inexpensive. For penicillin-allergic patients, vancomycin is a reasonable alternative.

Another continuing controversy is whether third-generation cephalosporins or new penicillin derivatives (i.e., imipenem) should replace aminoglycoside–clindamycin (metronidazole) combinations as first-line therapy for serious intraabdominal infections. Studies in animals and those available in humans (discussed before) suggest that these agents are as effective as the combination regimens. We believe that for the more severe infections the combination regimens are more appropriate; for less severe infections or acute bacterial contamination the single-agent regimens can be justified. New information or clinical studies of third-generation cephalosporins or new penicillin derivatives may alter this approach in the future.

With peritonitis that occurs from chronic peritoneal dialysis, the antimicrobial regimen used should be tailored to the isolated organism. The selection of a specific agent or combination should be based on culture and sensitivity data. If microbiologic data are unavailable, empiric therapy with a first-generation cephalosporin plus an aminoglycoside is recommended. In less severe infections, a first-generation cephalosporin alone may suffice. Infection with staphylococci may be treated with a penicillinase-resistant penicillin (methicillin, nafcillin, oxacillin), first-generation cephalosporins, or vancomycin if the patient is allergic to penicillin. For streptococcal infections, penicillin or ampicillin would be preferable to penicillinase-resistant penicillins. Most aerobic gram-negative bacilli may be effectively treated with an aminoglycoside. For infections caused by *Pseudomonas aeruginosa*, an antipseudomonal penicillin (ticarcillin, piperacillin, mezlocillin, or azlocillin) or ceftazidime may be added.

Patients with peritonitis who are undergoing chronic peritoneal dialysis (CPD) may receive parenteral as well as intraperitoneal antimicrobial agents. Intraperitoneal antimicrobial agents alone are often sufficient, unless severe infection is present. A number of agents may be installed through peritoneal catheters. Recommended concentrations of antimicrobial agents for intraperitoneal irrigation solutions are 8 mg/L for gentamicin and tobramycin, 1–3 mg/L for clindamycin, 50,000 units/L for penicillin G, 125 mg/L for cephalosporins, 100–150 mg/L for ticarcillin or carbenicillin, 50 mg/L for ampicillin, 100 mg/L for methicillin, 30 mg/L for vancomycin, and 3 mg/L for amphotericin B.[43]

The usual duration of therapy for peritonitis associated with CPD is 10–14 days but may extend to 3 weeks. Antimicrobial therapy should be continued until dialysate cultures are negative for 2–3 days and the patient is asymptomatic. When parenteral agents are administered the initial dose would be the same as that for patients with normal renal function, while subsequent doses should be much less for renally excreted agents and should account for possible loss through peritoneal dialysis. For agents where serum concentrations can easily be measured (e.g., aminoglycosides and vancomycin), these assessments should be performed.

After acute bacterial contamination, such as with abdominal trauma where gastrointestinal contents enter the peritoneum, combination antimicrobial regimens are often not required. If the patient is seen soon after injury (within 2 hours) and surgical measures are instituted promptly, then single-agent regimens (e.g., cefoxitin, cefotetan, ceftizoxime) will be effective in preventing most infectious complications. It is important though that antimicrobials be begun as soon as possible after injury.

For appendicitis, the antimicrobial regimen used should depend on the appearance of the appendix at the time of operation, which may be normal, inflamed, gangrenous, or perforated. Since the condition of the appendix is unknown preoperatively, it is advisable to begin antimicrobial agents before the appendectomy is performed. Reasonable regimens would be antianaerobic cephalosporins or, if the patient is seriously ill, a combination of aminoglycoside with clindamycin or metronidazole. If at operation the appendix is found to be normal or inflamed then postoperative antimicrobials would not be required. If the appendix is gangrenous or perforated, a treatment course of 7–10 days with the agents listed in Table 82.6 would be appropriate.

Other than selection of specific agents, additional controversies surround the use of antimicrobials for intraabdominal infection: the timing of antimicrobial administration, the duration of the antimicrobial regimen, and the route of administration. Timing of antimicrobial administration after bacterial entry into the peritoneum appears to be an important factor. With intraabdominal contamination from a disease process or traumatic injury, antibiotic administration obviously cannot precede bacterial entry, but early antimicrobial administration should be more effective.

The necessary duration of treatment for intraabdominal infections is not clearly defined. Acute intraabdominal contamination, such as after a traumatic injury, may be treated with a very short course (24 hours), but in this situation, the goal is prevention of infectious complications, not resolution of an established infection. For established infections (peritonitis or intraabdominal abscess) an antimicrobial course of at least 7 days is justified. This allows eradication of bacteria that may remain in the peritoneum after a surgical procedure or bacteria that may enter the peritoneum through healing suture lines. Comparative studies examining shorter courses of therapy (i.e., 2 or 3 days) have not been conducted, though, to verify that longer courses are essential. Under certain conditions, therapy for longer than 7 days would be justified; for example, if the patient remains febrile or is in poor general condition, when relatively resistant bacteria are isolated, or when a focus of infection in the abdomen may still be present. For some abscesses, such as pyogenic liver abscess, antimicrobials may be required for a month or longer.

Most routes of antimicrobial administration except the oral route have been studied in the treatment of intraabdominal infection. For seriously ill patients, intravenous antimicrobial administration should remain the basis of therapy. Intramuscular administration may not result in reliable systemic absorption if the patient is severely ill and has poor tissue perfusion, as in hypovolemic shock. Outside the initial, critical phase of therapy, intramuscular antimicrobials may be used.

Intraperitoneal irrigation of antimicrobial agents for treatment of intraabdominal infection has often been studied with somewhat conflicting results. Intraoperative antimicrobial irrigation has not been shown to improve patient outcomes in comparison with copious intraoperative irrigation with normal saline. Possibly the most important aspect of peritoneal irrigation is the dilutional effect on bacteria and adjuvants of substances that promote infection (i.e., intestinal contents and hemoglobin). As discussed before, investigators have shown that most systemically administered antimicrobials easily cross the peritoneal membrane so that peritoneal fluid concentrations are similar to serum.[41,44] Confined areas, such as an abscess, could be expected to attain much lower antimicrobial concentrations.

**Response**

Whichever antimicrobial regimen is chosen, the patient should be continually reassessed to determine the success or failure of therapies. The clinician should recognize that there are many reasons for poor outcome of patients with intraabdominal infection; improper antimicrobial administration is only one. The patient may be immunocompromised which decreases the likelihood of successful outcome with any regimen. It is impossible for antimicrobials to totally compensate for nonfunctioning immune systems. There may be surgical reasons for poor patient outcome. Failure to identify all intraabdominal foci of infection or leaks from a gastrointestinal anastomosis may cause continued intraabdominal infection. Even when intraabdominal infection is controlled, accompanying organ system failure, most often renal or respiratory, but possibly hepatic or cardiac, may lead to patient demise.

Once antimicrobials are initiated and other important therapies described before are used, most patients should show improvement within 2 to 3 days. Usually, temperature will return to near normal, vital signs should stabilize, and the patient should not appear in distress with the exception of recognized discomfort and pain from incisions, drains, and nasogastric tube. At 24–48 hours, aerobic bacterial culture results should return. If a suspected pathogen is not sensitive to the antimicrobial agents being given then the regimen should be changed if the patient has not shown sufficient progress. If the isolated pathogen is extremely sensitive to one antimicrobial, and the patient is progressing well, then concurrent antimicrobial therapy may often be discontinued.

With present anaerobic culturing techniques and the slow growth of these organisms, anaerobes are often not identified until 4 to 7 days after culture, and sensitivity information is difficult to obtain. For this reason there are usually few data with which to alter the antianaerobic component of the antimicrobial regimen. A report indicating that anaerobes were not isolated should not be the sole justification for discontinuing antianaerobic drugs, as anaerobic bacteria that were present in the infectious process may not have been properly transported to the microbiology laboratory or other problems may have led to cell death in vitro.

Reasons for antimicrobial failure may not always be apparent. Even when antimicrobial susceptibility tests indicate an organism that is very susceptible to the antimicrobial in vitro, therapeutic failures may occur. Possibly there is poor penetration of the antimicrobial into the focus of infection, or, after initiation of antimicrobial therapy, bacterial resistance may develop. Also, it is possible that an antimicrobial regimen may encourage the development of infection by organisms not susceptible to the regimen being used. Superinfection in patients being treated for intraabdominal infection is often due to *Candida*, but enterococci or opportunistic gram-negative bacilli such as *Pseudomonas* or *Serratia* may be involved.

Treatment regimens for intraabdominal infection can be judged successful if the patient recovers from the infection without recurrent peritonitis or intraabdominal abscess and without the need for additional antimicrobials. A regimen can be considered unsuccessful if a significant adverse drug reaction occurs, if reoperation is necessary, or if patient improvement is delayed beyond 1 or 2 weeks.

## Conclusion

The term *intraabdominal infection* refers to many widely differing processes that require varying therapeutic approaches. For many intraabdominal infections, surgical procedures are the foundation of treatment while antimicrobials are important adjuncts. The microbiology of intraabdominal infection is complex and agents with activity against aerobic gram-negative bacilli and anaerobes (particularly *Bacteroides fragilis*) will be most effective.

The use of newly introduced antimicrobial agents alone will not dramatically improve outcome of patients with intraabdominal infection. Perhaps the greatest potential for improving patient outcome with these infections will come from treatments that improve patient immune function as well as from improved diagnostic techniques for abscesses, more rapid bacterial identification and determination of susceptibility, and better coordination of currently available technologies and procedures.

*Portions of this chapter were originally published in DiPiro JT, Mansberger JA, Davis JB: Current concepts in clinical therapeutics: Intraabdonminal infections. Clin Pharm 1986;5:34–50.* 

## References


1. Finegold SM. Microflora of the gastrointestinal tract, in Wilson SE, Finegold SM, Williams RA (eds): Intraabdominal Infection. New York, McGraw–Hill, 1982, pp 1–21.
2. Ruddell WSJ, Axon ATR, Findlay JM, et al. The effect of cimetidine on gastric bacterial flora. Lancet 1980;1:672–674.
3. Lou MA, Mandal AK, Alexander JL, et al. Bacteriology of the human biliary tract and duodenum. Arch Surg 1977;112:965–967.
4. Keighley MRB. Infection and the biliary tree, in Blumgart LH (ed): The Biliary Tract. New York, Churchill Livingston, 1982, pp 219–235.
5. Lorber B, Swenson RM. The bacteriology of intra-abdominal infections. Surg Clin North Am 1975;55:1249–1355.
6. Conn HO, Fessel JM. Spontaneous bacterial peritonitis in cirrhosis: variations on a theme. Medicine 1971;50:161–197.
7. Rubin J, Rogers WA, Taylor HM, et al. Peritonitis during continuous ambulatory peritoneal dialysis. Ann Intern Med 1980;92:7–13.
8. Altemeier WA, Culbertson WR, Fullen WD, et al. Intra-abdominal abscesses. Am J Surg 1973;125:70–79.
9. Hau T, Ahrenholz DH, Simmons RL. Secondary bacterial peritonitis: The biologic basis of treatment. Curr Probl Surg 1979;16:1–65.
10. Nichols RL. Empiric antibiotic therapy of intraabdominal infections. Rev Infect Dis 1983;5(suppl):590–597.
11. Wilson SE. Secondary bacterial peritonitis, in Wilson SE, Finegold SM, Williams RA (eds): Intraabdominal Infection. New York, McGraw–Hill, 1982, pp 62–88.
12. Golden GT, Shaw A. Primary peritonitis. Surg Gynecol Obstet 1972; 135:513–516.
13. Altemeier WA. Bacterial flora of acute perforated appendicitis with peritonitis. Ann Surg 1938;107:517–528.
14. Bartlett JG. Pathogenesis of intra-abdominal sepsis, in Wilson SE, Finegold SM, Williams RA (eds): Intra-abdominal Infection. New York, McGraw–Hill, 1982, pp 36–51.
15. Stone HH, Kolb LD, Geheber CE. Incidence and significance of intraperitoneal anaerobic bacteria. Ann Surg 1975;181:705–715.
16. Dougherty SH. Role of enterococcus in intraabdominal sepsis. Am J Surg 1984;148:308–312.
17. Bartlett JG, Marien GJR, Dezfulian M, et al. Relative efficacy of beta-lactam antimicrobial agents in two animal models of infections involving *Bacteroides fragilis*. Rev Infect Dis 1983;5 (suppl):S338–S344.
18. Solomkin JS, Meakins JL, Allo MD, et al. Antibiotic trials in intra-abdominal infections: A critical evaluation of study design and outcome reporting. Ann Surg 1984;200:29–39.
19. Thadepalli H. Principles and practice of antibiotic therapy for post-traumatic abdominal injuries. Surg Gynecol Obstet 1979; 148:937–951.
20. Stephen M, Lowenthal J. Generalized infective peritonitis. Surg Gynecol Obstet 1978;147:231–234.
21. Wilson SE. Intra-abdominal abscess: Subphrenic, lesser sac, intermesenteric, and pelvic, in Wilson SE, Finegold SM, Williams RA (eds): Intra-abdominal Infection. New York, McGraw–Hill, 1982, pp 172–206.
22. Nichols RL, Smith JW, Klein DB, et al. Risk of infection after penetrating abdominal injury. N Engl J Med 1984;311:1065–1070.
23. Hofstetter SR, Pachter HL, Bailey AA, et al. A prospective comparison of two regimens of prophylactic antibiotics in abdominal trauma: Cefoxitin versus triple drug. J Trauma 1984; 24:307–310.
24. Jones RC, Thal ER, Johnson NA, et al. Evaluation of antibiotic therapy following penetrating abdominal trauma. Ann Surg 1985;201:576–585.
25. Oresovich MR, Dellinger EP, Lennard ES, et al. Duration of preventive antibiotic administration for penetrating abdominal trauma. Arch Surg 1982;117:200–205.
26. Stone HH, Haney BB, Kolb LD, et al. Prophylactic and preventive antibiotic therapy: Timing, duration and economics. Ann Surg 1979;189:691–699.
27. Fullen WD, Hunt J, Altemeier WA. Prophylactic antibiotics in penetrating wounds of the abdomen. J Trauma 1972;12:282–289.
28. Harding GKM, Buckwold FJ, Ronald AR, et al. Prospective, randomized comparative study of clindamycin, chloramphenicol and ticarcillin, each in combination with gentamicin, in therapy for intra-abdominal and female genital tract sepsis. Rev Infect Dis 1980;142:384–393.
29. Smith JA, Skidmore AG, Forward AD, et al. Prospective, randomized, double-blind comparison of metronidazole and tobramycin with clindamycin and tobramycin in the treatment of intra-abdominal sepsis. Ann Surg 1980;190:213–220.

30. Stone HH, Fabian TC. Clinical comparison of antibiotic combinations in the treatment of peritonitis and related mixed aerobic-anaerobic surgical sepsis. World J Surg 1980;4:415–421.
31. Tally FP, McGowan K, Kellum JM, et al. A randomized comparison of cefoxitin with or without amikacin and clindamycin plus amikacin in surgical sepsis. Ann Surg 1981;193:318–323.
32. Drusano GL, Warren JW, Saah AJ, et al. A prospective randomized controlled trial of cefoxitin versus clindamycin–aminoglycoside in mixed anaerobic–aerobic infections. Surg Gynecol Obstet 1982;154:715–720.
33. Stone HH, Geheber CE, Kolb LD, et al. Clinical comparison of cefotaxime versus the combination of gentamicin plus clindamycin in the treatment of peritonitis and similar polymicrobial soft-tissue surgical sepsis. Clin Ther 1981;4(suppl A):67–80.
34. Canadian Metronidazole–Clindamycin Study Group. Prospective, randomized comparison of metronidazole and clindamycin, each with gentamicin, for the treatment of serious intra-abdominal infection. Surgery 1983;93:221–229.
35. Schentag JJ, Wels PB, Reitberg DP, et al. A randomized clinical trial of moxalactam alone versus tobramycin plus clindamycin in abdominal sepsis. Ann Surg 1983;198:35–41.
36. Busuttil RW, McGrattan MA, Freischlag J. A comparative study of cefamandole versus gentamicin plus clindamycin in the treatment of documented or suspected bacterial peritonitis. Surg Gynecol Obstet 1984;158:1–8.
37. Henning C, Meden-Britth G, Frolander F, et al. Comparative study of netilmicin/tinidazole versus netilmicin/clindamycin in the treatment of severe abdominal infections. Scand J Infect Dis 1984;16:297–303.
38. Harding GKM, Nicolle LE, Haose DA. Prospective randomized, comparative trials in the therapy for intra-abdominal and female genital tract infections. Rev Infect Dis 1984;6:S283–S292.
39. Tornqvist A, Forsgren A, Leandoer L, et al. Antibiotic treatment during surgery for diffuse peritonitis: a prospective randomized study comparing the effects of cefuroxime and of a cefuroxime and metronidazole combination. Br J Surg 1985;72:261–264.
40. Lennard ES, Minshew BH, Dellinger EP, et al. Stratified outcome comparison of clindamycin–gentamicin vs chloramphenicol–gentamicin for treatment of intra-abdominal sepsis. Arch Surg 1985;120:889–898.
41. Gerding DN, Hall WH. The penetration of antibiotics into peritoneal fluid. Bull NY Acad Med 1975;51:1016–1019.
42. Jones RC. Antibiotics in trauma. J Surg Pract 1977;26–30.
43. Levison ME, Pontzer RE. Peritonitis and other intra-abdominal infections, in Mardell GL, Douglas RG, Bennett JE (eds): Principles and Practice of Infectious Diseases. New York, John Wiley and Sons, 1985, p 488.
44. Wittman DH, Schassan HH. Penetration of eight beta-lactam antibiotics into peritoneal fluid. Arch Surg 1983;118:205–213.

# Chapter 83 / Parasitic Diseases

J.V. Anandan, PharmD

Once considered "exotic," parasitic diseases are much nearer home because of the increased mobility of large segments of the population and the speed of international travel. Environmental changes in other parts of the world have brought an increased incidence of parasitic diseases among the local population. The construction of the Aswan Dam and the creation of Lake Nasser resulted in new habitats for the intermediate snail host and increased the incidence of schistosomiasis in Egypt, while the construction of the TransAmazon Highway in Brazil exposed large number of workers to leishmaniasis.[1,2]

To appreciate the prevalence of parasitic disease, one should review Table 83.1, adapted from World Health Organization data for 1975.[2,3] This chapter covers the major parasitic diseases and includes protozoan diseases (amebiasis, malaria, etc.), helminthic infections (ascariasis, enterobiasis, etc.), and ectoparasitic infestations (head and body lice). Emphasis is placed on those diseases or conditions more frequently seen in the United States.

Distribution of parasites over the world is dependent on the presence of suitable hosts and on habitats and environmental conditions that make possible the transfer from host to host.[3] A human parasite that does not utilize an intermediate host is likely to be found in any inhabited region of the world as long as the environmental conditions are suitable. *Ascaris* (the roundworm) and *Trichuris* (the whipworm), which require carelessness of habits for transfer, are limited, as they require some time outside the body to reach the infective stage, and are exposed to heat and dryness. The distribution of the hookworm is more limited, because these are free-living forms, unprotected by resistant shells or cysts. African trypanosomiasis never occurs outside the range of the tsetse fly, malaria beyond the range of the infective *Anopheles*, and schistosomiasis in the absence of a specific water snail. The prevalence of clonorchiasis (Chinese liver fluke) could be cited as an example of the impact of both environmental and geographical factors. Clonorchiasis requires not only simultaneous presence of man, specific snail species, and certain fish, but also unsanitary conditions that make the eggs accessible to the snails, an association of the snail and fish, and the established local habit of eating raw fish. The ability of some parasites to infect hosts other than man may perpetuate an infection, even when human habits preclude the possibility of more than occasional access to the human body. In North America, the broad tapeworm (*Diphyllobothrium latum*) would perish if it were not that dogs and other carnivores, like the brown bear, serve as reservoir hosts.

## Host–Parasite Relationship

The association of two species for the purpose of obtaining food for either is called *symbiosis*. *Parasitism* is defined as a symbiotic relationship in which one species, the host, is injured through the activities of the other animal. Through evolution, parasites have made specific morphologic adaptations to their way of life. Adaptation to the host has taken a number of forms: the loss of locomotor organelles in the protozoan Sporozoa, the partial and complete lack of digestive systems in the trematodes and cestodes, respectively, the elaboration of proteolytic enzymes to penetrate the host intestinal mucosa in *Entamoeba histolytica*, the cercariae of the blood fluke that penetrate the skin of the host by elaborate enzymes, and finally, the ability to infect an intermediate host to increase reproductive capacity as seen among the cestodes and trematodes.[1,2]

Parasites normally inflict some degree of injury to the host, though at times the relationship may be commensal. The extent of injury may be dependent on factors like parasite load, nutritional status, and immunologic competence of the host. *Entamoeba coli* can be considered commensal because it subsists on the bacterial flora of the gut and does not cause any harm to the host. Unlike *Entamoeba coli*, *Fasciolopsis buski*, the giant intestinal fluke, and *Entamoeba histolytica* can produce severe local damage to the intestinal wall. *Ascaris*, the roundworm, can perforate the bowel wall, cause intestinal obstruction, and invade the appendix and bile duct. Malarial parasites destroy red cells by multiplying in them. *Diphyllobothrium latum*, or the broad fishworm, removes vitamin $B_{12}$ from the gastrointestinal tract, resulting in megaloblastic anemia.[1,2]

## Protozoan Diseases

### Amebiasis

Because of its worldwide distribution and serious gastrointestinal manifestations, amebiasis must be ranked as one of the most important parasitic diseases of man.[2–4] The major causative organism in amebiasis is *Entamoeba histolytica*. *E. histolytica*, which inhabits the colon in amebiasis, must be differentiated from the smaller *E. hartmanni* which is considered nonpathogenic.[5] The trophozoite, the mobile infective form of *E. histolytica*, is antigenically distinct from other entamoebas like *Entamoeba coli*. The mobility of the organism is dependent on pseudopod formation. The trophozoite is characterized by its propensity to ingest erythrocytes of the host in active infections.[4–6]

**Table 83.1** Worldwide Prevalence of Parasitic Diseases

| *Disease* | *Population at risk* | *Population currently infected* |
|---|---|---|
| Amebiasis | | 10% of world |
| Malaria | 1.1 billion | 177 million |
| African trypanosomiasis | 35 million | 10,000 new cases/yr |
| American trypanosomiasis | 35 million | 10 million |
| Schistosomiasis | | >200 million |
| *Schistosoma haematobium* | | 100 million |
| *Schistosoma mansoni* | | 60 million |
| *Schistosoma japonicum* | | 100 million |
| Paragonimiasis | | 19 million |
| Fasciolopsiasis | | 10 million |
| Filariasis | | 250 million |
| Ascariasis | | 650 million |
| Hookworm | | 450 million |
| Trichuriasis | | 350 million |
| Strongyloidiasis | | 35 million |
| Cestodiasis | | 65 million |

***Epidemiology*** *E. histolytica* has a very simple life cycle and exists in two forms, cysts and trophozoites. Encystment of the trophozoite occurs prior to its release from the bowel. Ingestion of the cyst and subsequent release of the trophozoites within the colon perpetuate the infection in the new host. The asymptomatic infected host excretes amebic cysts in the stools and can transmit the infection.[4] It is estimated that 10 million cases of invasive disease result each year worldwide, leading to more than 34,000 deaths.[5] In the United States the incidence of amebiasis is estimated to be about 5% in the general population.[5] The highest incidence of amebiasis in the United States is found in the institutionalized mentally retarded population, in sexually active homosexuals, in subjects with the acquired immune deficiency syndrome (AIDS), among the American Indian population, and in new immigrants from endemic areas.[5,6]

***Pathogenesis*** *E. histolytica* invades mucosal cells of colonic epithelium producing the classic flask-shaped ulcer in the submucosa.[7] The trophozoite has a cytolethal effect on cells through a toxin. If the trophozoite gets into the portal circulation, it will be carried to the liver where it produces abscess and periportal fibrosis. Amebic ulcerations can affect the perineum and genitalia, and abscesses may occur in the lung and brain.

*E. histolytica* activates complement by the alternative pathway.[6,7] Immunity seems not to develop even in the presence of humoral antibodies, except with amebic liver abscess. Reinfection does occur in the presence of high antibody titers[4]; however, some preliminary data suggest that cell-mediated immunity may prevent invasive disease, indicating perhaps that immunization with amebic antigens may prevent the disease.[5]

***Clinical Presentation*** The most frequent clinical manifestations of the disease are gastrointestinal, with vague complaints of abdominal discomfort and malaise, to severe abdominal cramps, flatulence, and bloody diarrhea with mucus.[4,5] Painful spasms of the anal sphincter usually indicate the presence of amebic rectal ulceration.[4]

Right upper quadrant pain, hepatomegaly, and liver tenderness, with referred pain to the left or right shoulder, usually suggest an amebic liver abscess. Liver abscesses that are located in the right lobe can spread to the lungs and pleura.[4,5] Pericardial infection, though rare, may be associated with extension of the amebic abscess from the left lobe of the liver.[4,8] Erosion of liver abscesses also presents as peritonitis.[4]

Eosinophilia is usually absent, though it is not unusual to see mild leukocytosis with intestinal amebiasis.[4,5] A patient with liver abscess, however, usually presents with high fever, significant leukocytosis with left shift, elevated alkaline phosphatase, and liver tenderness on palpation.[4,5,8]

Review of the patient's history and recent travel, especially to an endemic area, cannot be overemphasized. Intestinal amebiasis is diagnosed by demonstrating *E. histolytica* cysts or trophozoites either in the stool or from a fresh specimen obtained by sigmoidoscopy. Fresh diarrheal stool specimens should be examined by wet mount within the hour as the trophozoites are destroyed rapidly. Formed stools may be preserved using polyvinyl alcohol (PVA) fixative and formalin kits that are available from most parasitology laboratories. Three stool samples obtained 24 hours apart will produce a 70% yield for *E. histolytica*.[4] The infection may also be detected by immunologic assays, such as enzyme-linked immunosorbent assay (ELISA) and counterimmunoelectrophoresis (CIE).

Where amebic liver abscess is suspected from initial physical examination and history, confirmatory diagnostic procedures include serology and liver scans (utilizing isotopes by ultrasound or computerized tomography).[4,5,8] In rare instances, needle aspiration of the hepatic abscess may be attempted using ultrasound guidance.[4,5]

***Treatment***[4,5,9–11] In amebiasis, the goals of therapy are initially to eradicate the parasite by use of specific amebicides and then to render supportive therapy. A number of different regimens have been suggested, depending on the category of amebiasis: asymptomatic cyst-passers, intestinal amebiasis, and amebic liver abscess.[4,5,7,9] Electrolyte replacement and nutritional support are essential adjunctive treatment modalities to drug therapy. Large hepatic abscess or amebic pericarditis may require needle aspiration or surgery before drug therapy.[4,5,9] Most of the regimens require a combination of drugs administered either concurrently or sequentially.[10]

Careful history should be taken when one of the differential diagnoses is ulcerative colitis, because corticosteroid administration has the potential to unmask amebiasis and produce toxic megacolon.[4,6] All patients diagnosed as having inflammatory bowel disease should have a serologic test for amebiasis to avoid the serious consequences that result from administration of corticosteroids.[5,7]

In the asymptomatic cyst-passer, it is necessary to administer two drugs: one that is effective in the tissue and another that acts as a luminal amebicide. Metronidazole (Flagyl), tetracycline, and chloroquine (Aralen) are tissue-acting agents; iodoquinol (Yodaxin), diloxanide furoate (Furamide), and paramomycin (Humatin) are luminal amebicides. A tissue-acting agent may be so well absorbed that only small amounts of the drug stay in the bowel and, as such, may prove ineffective as a luminal agent.[4] A lumen-acting agent, on the other hand, may be too poorly absorbed to be effective in the tissue. In the cyst-passer, it is necessary to eradicate the causative agent from both tissue and lumen so as to prevent relapses of intestinal amebiasis or the development of amebic liver abscess. Some investigators advocate using a single agent (e.g., metronidazole, diloxanide, or paromomycin); however, the incidence of relapses is higher.[9] Drug effectiveness must be monitored by stool examination, that is, three or more negative specimens from 1 to 3 months after treatment.

In intestinal amebiasis, without liver involvement, treatment is directed toward eradication of *E. histolytica* from the tissue and lumen; therefore, a two-drug regimen is also required. In liver abscess, it is frequently necessary to use two or three drugs. The various drug regimens have been selected on the basis of the eradication rates reported in the literature.[4,5,9–11]

Adult cyst-passers should be treated with oral metronidazole 750 mg three times daily for 10 days, followed by iodoquinol (diiodohydroxyquin) 650 mg three times daily for 20 days. Alternative regimens include combination of metronidazole with either diloxanide furoate or paromomycin. Tetracycline in combination with a luminal agent like iodoquinol or diloxanide may also be used. Tetracycline should be avoided in children under 8 because of its potential to cause discoloration and inadequate calcification of permanent teeth. In the pediatric patient the dose of oral metronidazole is 50 mg/kg/d in divided doses followed by iodoquinol 40 mg/kg/d. Either diloxanide or paramomycin can be used as alternative luminal agents.

Intestinal amebiasis may be treated with the same regimen used for cyst-passers. An alternative regimen is oral metronidazole 2.4 g over 2 to 3 days, followed by either iodoquinol, diloxanide, or paromomycin. Patients who are too ill to take oral metronidazole should receive the drug in equivalent doses by the intravenous route. Dehydroemetine, an investigational agent available from the Centers for Disease Control, Atlanta, Georgia, is recommended in place of metronidazole. A luminal agent must follow the administration of dehydroemetine.

Amebic liver abscess is treated with a regimen identical to that for intestinal amebiasis; however, in patients who are severely ill, it may be necessary to add chloroquine (base) 600 mg daily for 2 days, followed by 300 mg (base) for 2 to 3 weeks. (See Appendix for side effects of drugs and monitoring parameters.)

Travelers and tourists visiting an endemic area should avoid local tap water, ice, salad, and unpeeled fruits. Water can be disinfected by use of iodine (tincture of iodine or Lugol's solution) or strong chlorine (laundry bleach) solution, but boiled water is probably the safest. As food handlers in Asia and Latin America may be a source of amebiasis, travelers should avoid eating at food stalls and open markets.

## *Malaria*

Malaria represents the most devastating disease in terms of human suffering and economic implications, affecting the largest number of people in the world, with deaths in excess of 1 million in tropical Africa.[12]

Malaria is transmitted by the bite of an infected *Anopheles* mosquito, which introduces the sporozoites (tissue parasites) of the *Plasmodium* species (i.e., *P. falciparum*, *P. vivax*, *P. malariae*, *P. ovale*) into the bloodstream. The asexual reproduction stage develops in man, while the sexual stage occurs in the mosquito.[13,14] The sporozoites invade parenchymal hepatocytes, multiply in stages referred to as exoerythrocytic stages, and become hepatic vegetative forms or schizonts. Schizonts rupture to release daughter cells or merozoites which then infect erythrocytes.

*P. falciparum* and *P. malariae* remain in the primary exoerythrocytic stage in the liver for about 4 weeks before invading erythrocytes, while *P. vivax* and *P. ovale* can exist in the liver in the latent exoerythrocytic form for extended periods; therefore, infected subjects can experience relapses. The merozoites that invade the erythrocytes develop sequentially into ring forms, trophozoites, schizonts and finally merozoites, which can invade other erythrocytes, or develop into gametocytes, which undergo the sexual stage in the *Anopheles* vector. Erythrocytic forms never reinvade the liver without developing into sporozoites in the vector; therefore, malarial infections from transfusion never result in the exoerythrocytic or "liver" form.[13,14] *P. falciparum* can result in high levels of parasitemia because of its ability to invade erythrocytes of all ages, unlike *P. vivax* and *P. ovale*, which invade only young cells.

***Epidemiology*** The exact geographic distribution of the various species is not well documented; however, it is reported that *P. vivax* is more prevalent in India, Pakistan, Bangladesh, Sri Lanka, and Central America, while *P. falciparum* is found predominantly in Africa, Haiti, and New Guinea. Both *P. falciparum* and *P. vivax* are prevalent in all of Southeast Asia and South America.[13] Most of the infection with *P. ovale* occurs in Africa and the distribution of *P. malariae* is considered worldwide.

In the United States, most cases of malaria are reported in

immigrants from endemic areas and American travelers. Blood transfusion has also been cited as a cause of malarial infection.[13,14] The Vietnam War brought an increase in the incidence of malaria because of the large numbers of U.S. military personnel in endemic areas. The transmission of malaria from incoming subjects who have traveled to endemic areas and from Vietnamese refugees, is a real threat because of the presence of two mosquito vectors, *Anopheles quadrimaculatus* and *Anopheles freeborni*, in the United States.

***Pathogenesis*** The hallmark of the erythrocytic phase of malaria is fever; however, the reason for this is obscure.[13,14] The malarial paroxysm characterized by fever, chills, and rigor can cause vasodilation and orthostatic hypotension. The high fever, marked diaphoresis, and vomiting can lead to serious fluid and electrolyte abnormalities. The erythrocytic phase causes extensive hemolysis that results in anemia and splenomegaly. The most serious complications are usually associated with *P. falciparum* infections, and include acute renal failure, pulmonary edema, high-output heart failure, and cerebral vascular congestion and hemorrhage.[13–15] It has been postulated that these complications are due to tissue hypoxia resulting from the anemia and alterations in the microcirculation. Hypoxia may be responsible for the loss of capillary endothelial integrity, leading to increased capillary permeability and interstitial edema. *P. malariae* has been implicated in immune-mediated glomerulonephritis and nephrotic syndrome.[13,14]

***Clinical Presentation*** The erythrocytic phase of malaria is usually preceded by a prodrome that includes headache, anorexia, malaise, fatigue, and myalgias. Patients may also have nonspecific complaints like abdominal pain, chest pain, and arthralgias. The prodromal period is usually followed by the paroxysm, manifested as high fever, chills, and rigor.[13] The typical malarial paroxysm is usually followed by a "cold phase," severe pallor, cyanosis of the lips and nail bed, and cutis anserina ("goose flesh").[13,14] These symptoms are replaced by a "hot phase" where the patient's fever may be between 40.5 and 41°C. Other symptoms during this phase include warm dry skin, tachycardia, cough, severe headache, nausea, vomiting, abdominal pain, and delirium. Patients are usually asymptomatic between the malarial paroxysms.

The diagnosis of malaria is made by demonstrating the parasite in peripheral blood smears. To ensure a positive diagnosis, smears should be obtained several times daily for a number of days.[13,14] The presence of parasites in the blood 3 to 5 days after initiation of therapy suggests drug resistance. Serologic tests like indirect fluorescent antibody (IFA) and indirect hemagglutination (IHA), which are available from the Centers for Disease Control, are used to detect infected blood donors.[14]

***Treatment***[10,13,14,16–19] In an adult, the chemoprophylaxis for all species of *Plasmodium* is chloroquine phosphate 300 mg (base) once weekly, beginning 1 week prior to departure and continuing 6 weeks after leaving an endemic area. When visiting or leaving an area endemic for *P. vivax* or *P. ovale*, primaquine phosphate (Primaquine), 15 mg (base) daily for 14 days beginning the last 2 weeks of chloroquine prophylaxis, should be added to the regimen.

In areas where chloroquine-resistant *P. falciparum* strains exist, travelers should receive, in addition to chloroquine, the combination of pyrimethamine and sulfadoxine (Fansidar), one tablet weekly beginning 1 week prior to departure and continuing 6 weeks after leaving the area. Pediatric subjects should receive chloroquine phosphate 5 mg (base)/kg/wk and follow the adult regimen. The pediatric dose of primaquine phosphate is 0.3 mg/kg/wk. The pediatric dose of the combination pyrimethamine–sulfadoxine varies with age:

$\frac{1}{8}$ tablet (6–11 months)
$\frac{1}{4}$ tablet (1–3 years)
$\frac{1}{2}$ tablet (4–8 years)
$\frac{3}{4}$ tablet (9–14 years)

In an uncomplicated attack of malaria (for all plasmodia except chloroquine-resistant *P. falciparum*), chloroquine 600 mg (base) initially, followed by 300 mg (base) 6 hours later and then 300 mg (base) daily for 2 days, is the recommended regimen. In severe illness or when oral therapy is not tolerated, quinine dihydrochloride 600 mg in 250 mL normal saline should be administered over 8 hours or continued until oral therapy can be started. Intravenous quinine is available from the Centers for Disease Control. The maximum recommended dose of intravenous quinine is 1800 mg/d. Chloroquine can be used as an alternative.

In *P. falciparum* (chloroquine-resistant) infections, a combination of oral quinine sulfate 650 mg, pyrimethamine 25 mg, and sulfadiazine 500 mg administrated twice daily for the first two agents and four times daily for sulfadiazine is recommended. Either intravenous quinine dihydrochloride or quinidine gluconate should be administered for severe illness.[17–19] The intravenous dose of quinidine gluconate is 15 mg/kg (base) in 250 mL normal saline over 4 hours, followed by 7.5 mg/kg (base) every 8 hours for 7 days. This is an investigational regimen and requires close monitoring of the electrocardiogram and other vital signs.[19]

Travelers to areas endemic for malaria should be advised to remain in well-screened areas, wear clothes that cover most of the body, and sleep in mosquito-proof nets. It is prudent to carry the insect repellent DEET (*N*, *N*-diethyltoluamide) and insect sprays for use in mosquito-infested areas. Readers are urged to check the publication of the Centers for Disease Control for a list of countries where chloroquine-resistant *P. falciparum* exists. A malaria vaccine is under investigation and may be available in the near future.[20]

### *Giardiasis*

*Giardia lamblia*, a protozoan, is responsible for a significant number of cases of traveler's diarrhea, though the most common cause still remains the enterotoxigenic bacteria *Escherichia coli*.[21] *Giardia* is the most frequently identified intestinal parasite in the United States.

The life cycle of *G. lamblia* includes two stages, the trophozoite and the cyst. *G. lamblia*, which is found in the small intestine, the gallbladder, and the biliary drainage, is a pear-shaped trophozoite with four pairs of flagella. Two nuclei that lie in the area of the sucking disk give the protozoan a characteristic facelike image.

***Epidemiology*** The distribution of giardiasis is worldwide and the prevalence rate has been reported to be as high as 16% in some parts of the United States. Children seem to be more frequently affected than adults.[22]

***Pathogenesis*** Giardiasis results from ingestion of *G. lamblia* cysts in fecally contaminated water or food. The protozoan excysts under the stimulus of low gastric pH to release the trophozoite, which adheres to the gastrointestinal wall, primarily in the jejunum.[22–24] Colonization and multiplication of the trophozoite lead to mucosal invasion, localized edema, and flattening of the villi resulting in malabsorption states in the host. Lactose intolerance precipitated by giardiasis can persist even after eradication of the protozoan.[24] Achlorhydria, hypogammaglobulinemia, or deficiency in secretory IgA are predispositions for giardiasis.[22–24]

***Clinical Presentation*** Following an incubation period of 1 to 2 weeks after ingestion of the *G. lamblia* cysts, symptomatic giardiasis is marked by acute onset of diarrhea, cramplike abdominal pains, bloating, and flatulence.[23] Complaints from patients include malaise, nausea, anorexia, and belching. Chronic diarrhea may continue with foul-smelling, copious, light-colored fatty stools and weight loss.[22–24] Periods of diarrhea may alternate with constipation. Patients complain of malaise, headache, and abdominal and epigastric discomfort frequently exacerbated by eating. Giardiasis can cause steatorrhea and $B_{12}$ and fat-soluble vitamin deficiencies if left untreated.[22–24] White blood cell and eosinophil counts remain normal even during acute illness.

Diagnosis of giardiasis is made by examination of fresh stool or a preserved specimen during the acute diarrheal phase. Fresh stool specimens may show the trophozoites while preserved specimens usually yield the cysts. It may be necessary to examine several specimens. The alternative method is to use the string test or Entero-Test (Hedeco, Palo Alto, CA). The Entero-Test consists of a weighted gelatin capsule secured to a nylon string, the free end of which is secured at the mouth while the capsule is swallowed. The string is removed in 4 to 6 hours and the end, which normally is located in the jejunum, is checked for trophozoites under a microscope.[24] If both the stool exam and string test prove unsuccessful, it may be necessary to attempt duodenal aspiration and biopsy to confirm the diagnosis; however, most clinicians would advocate a clinical trial of the standard therapy before undertaking invasive diagnostic tests.[24]

***Treatment***[9,10,22,23,25,26] As acute episodes of giardiasis can cause a great deal of discomfort and chronic infections lead to nutritional deficiencies, the major objective of therapy is control of symptoms and minimization of complications. All infected adults and children over 8 should be treated with quinacrine 100 mg three times daily for 7 days. Alternative drugs include metronidazole 250 mg three times daily and furazolidone 100 mg four times daily for 1 week. The pediatric dose for quinacrine is 2 mg/kg three times daily for 7 days. Furazolidone suspension (50 mg/15 mL) is an alternative dosage form.

Quinacrine remains the drug of choice in giardiasis and has been shown to provide cure rates in excess of 90%.[9] Metronidazole also produces cure rates between 85% and 95% and may be better tolerated than quinacrine in pediatric patients. Comparative studies in Egypt demonstrate that quinacrine produced cure rates of 100%, metronidazole 95%, and furazolidone 80%.[9] Furazolidone suspension may be an alternative to metronidazole or quinacrine in pediatric patients. (See Appendix for side effects of drugs.)

Giardiasis can be prevented by good personal hygiene and caution in food and drink consumption. When traveling, especially in Third World countries, it is imperative that all drinking water be adequately treated. It may be prudent to have available either water purifier (Halazone: 5 tabs/L/30 min) or iodine preparations to sterilize drinking water.[27] Infection may be minimized by avoiding uncooked foods (fruits, salads, etc.) which may have been washed with contaminated water.

### *Leishmaniasis*

The disease is caused by the protozoan that belongs to the genus *Leishmania* and the three variations of the diseases are visceral leishmaniasis (*kala-azar*, "black fever," or Assam fever), cutaneous leishmaniasis, and mucocutaneous leishmaniasis. The visceral form is caused predominantly by *L. donovani*, while the other two forms are due to other species. Leishmaniasis is a complex disease and space constraints do not justify an extended discussion here; interested readers are urged to consult other sources.[28,29]

*Leishmania* exists in two forms: a flagellated extracellular parasite in the sandfly vector (*Phlebotomus* in the Indian subcontinent and *Lutzomyia* and *Psychodopygus* in North and South America, Africa, or the Middle East), and an aflagellar amastigote (intracellular form) in the host. The major reservoirs for *Leishmania*, depending on geographic location, are dogs, foxes, squirrels, and rodents.[29] The sandflies ingest the parasite when they feed on the reservoir animals. After metamorphosis in the gut of the sandfly, the parasite is transferred to the human host when the infected sandfly takes a blood meal.[28,29]

In the Middle East, Asia, and Africa (Old World), cutaneous leishmaniasis has also been called "oriental sore," the "Bagdad," or the "Delhi" boil.[29] This form is caused by *L. tropica*, while the so-called "New World" type (primarily in Latin America) is caused by either *L. braziliensis* or *L. mexicana*. The disease can range from cutaneous ulcers to the mucocutaneous form affecting the nose, oral cavity, and pharynx. The highest incidence is usually seen in the summer months, especially in subjects working near jungle areas.[28,29]

***Clinical Presentation*** Visceral leishmaniasis usually begins as a papule, which may or may not ulcerate. Subsequently, the amastigote disseminates throughout the reticuloendothelial system to include the spleen, liver, bone marrow, and lymphatic nodes. Hypertrophy of the spleen and liver can take place. Visceral leishmaniasis results in severe anemia (normocytic, normochromic), marked splenomegaly, hemolysis, leukopenia and neutropenia, and thrombocytopenia with bleeding tendencies. Secondary bacterial infections and severe bleeding may be fatal in some of these patients.[28,29]

In the cutaneous disease, the initial lesion after the bite of the infected sandfly appears between 2 and 8 weeks and progresses to a raised ulcer that may persist for months and years.

The mucocutaneous form, which is usually caused by *L. braziliensis*, results in mutilating mucosal infections.[28] Infection affects primarily the nose, soft palate, and trachea. When the nose is involved, perforation and destruction of the septum and collapse of the tip of the nose may result. Secondary aspiration pneumonia is a serious complication of mucosal infections.[28,29]

Presentation of fever, weakness, weight loss, splenomegaly, hepatomegaly, leukopenia, and thrombocytopenia in a patient from an endemic area and subsequent demonstration of the amastigote in tissue or bone marrow confirm the diagnosis of leishmaniasis.

***Treatment***[10,28–30] All three forms of leishmaniasis are treated with stibogluconate sodium (antimony sodium gluconate), which is obtained from the Centers for Disease Control. In the adult, both visceral and mucocutaneous forms are treated with stibogluconate 10 mg/kg/d (maximum 600 mg) for 20 days. The drug may be administered either intravenously or intramuscularly. The cutaneous form is treated with stibogluconate 10–20 mg/kg/d (maximum 1,200 mg) for 10 days. The alternative drug for the visceral and mucocutaneous forms is pentamidine isethionate (Pentam 300) or amphotericin B (Fungizone). Pediatric patients receive the same dose as adults (see Appendix for side effects of drugs).

Patients should also receive hyperalimentation therapy with vitamins. Blood transfusions may be necessary in severe anemia. Presence of dead amastigotes in tissue and bone marrow, resolution of anemia and leukopenia, and disappearance of splenomegaly and hepatomegaly may be used as monitoring parameters for the disease.

Travelers to endemic areas should use insect repellents and sleep in fine-mesh netting to avoid exposure to the sandfly. No effective chemoprophylaxis against leishmaniasis is available.

### *Trypanosomiasis*

Two distinct forms of the genus *Trypanosoma* occur in man, one associated with African trypanosomiasis (sleeping sickness) and the other with American trypanosomiasis (Chagas' disease). *Trypanosoma brucei gambiense* and *T. brucei rhodesiense* are the causative organisms for African trypanosomiasis. In African trypanosomiasis, the parasite occurs as a long slender flagellated form called a trypomastigote in the blood and spinal fluid. In Chagas' disease, the trypomastigote is found in the bloodstream and an ovoid unflagellated intracellular form is found in cardiac and other tissues.[31,32]

*T. cruzi* is the agent that causes American trypanosomiasis. American trypanosomiasis is transmitted by a number of species of a reduviid bug (*Triatoma infestans*, *Rhodrium prolixus*), which live in wall cracks of houses in rural areas of North, Central, and South America. The reduviid bugs are infected from sucking blood from animals (opossums, dogs, and cats) or man infected with circulating trypomastigotes. The trypomastigotes are discharged in bug feces and may be transmitted to humans through mucosal membranes or breaks in the skin.

The two varieties of African trypanosomiasis are caused by *T. brucei gambiense* (West African sleeping sickness) and *T. brucei rhodesiense* (East African sleeping sickness). West African (Gambian) trypanosomiasis and East African (Rhodesian) trypanosomiasis are considered epidemiologically different, because of the distribution, reservoir, disease pathology, and population at risk. The population at risk in the West African disease comprises mainly rural inhabitants of the endemic area, while in the East African disease, the risk group includes tourists to game parks, and other occupational groups besides the local inhabitants.

African trypanosomiasis is transmitted by the blood-sucking fly of the genus *Glossina* (tsetse fly). Trypomastigotes ingested during a blood meal multiply in the fly, and enter the human host through a bite wound made by the vector. The trypomastigotes circulate in the blood and lymphatics, multiply, and invade the central nervous system.

***Clinical Presentation*** Acute infection is frequently seen in children, though Chagas' disease can also present with the acute phase in adults. Unilateral orbital edema (Romana's sign) resulting from local inflammation produced by the multiplying parasite may be seen. A local inoculation granuloma or chagoma appearing as a dusty erythematous lesion may be present, indicating the site of entry of the parasite. Fever, hepatosplenomegaly, and lymphadenopathy may also be present. In chronic disease, patients present with cardiomyopathy and congestive heart failure. Electrocardiograms will usually be abnormal, demonstrating extrasystoles, first-degree heart block, right bundle branch block, and other serious conduction disturbances.[33] Degeneration of the autonomic ganglia in the smooth muscle of the esophagus and the colon lead to uncoordinated peristalsis. The end result has been reported to be "mega syndromes" of affected organs.

One of the differential diagnoses with Chagas' disease is syphilis, because of the many clinical similarities between the diseases.[31] A history to verify the possible exposure to *T. cruzi* should be an important initial diagnostic workup. Recovery of *T. cruzi* would be definitive; however, this is not always possible, especially in chronic disease. Positive serologic tests are done using indirect hemagglutination, indirect fluorescence, and complement fixation.[32,33]

Most patients with African trypanosomiasis present with fever, headache, and tachycardia. Enlargement of the posterior cervical lymph nodes in the West African disease is called "Winterbottom's sign." Hepatosplenomegaly usually occurs after enlargement of lymph glands. The clinical manifestations of central nervous system involvement include alterations in personality, psychosis, tremor, and daytime somnolence alternating with insomnia at night.[33] A large number of central nervous system changes including extrapyramidal signs, cerebellar ataxia, Parkinson's disease symptoms, and seizures may precede the final stage of progressive mental deterioration and classic sleeping sickness, often resulting in death.

Diagnosis of African trypanosomiasis depends on demonstration of the trypanosome in the lesion, blood, lymph nodes, or cerebrospinal fluid (CSF). Elevated levels of IgM in the CSF in African trypanosomiasis have been used as a diagnostic marker.[31]

***Treatment***[10,32,33] Only two drugs have been used to treat *T. cruzi* infections: nifurtimox (Lampit, Bayer 2502) and benzonidazole (Rochagan). Oral nifurtimox is available from the Centers for Disease Control, while benzonidazole is available only in Brazil. The adult dose of nifurtimox is 8–10 mg/kg/d in divided doses for 60 days. As pediatric patients tolerate the drug better than adults, the dose for children is 15–20 mg/kg/d. Symptomatic treatment for heart failure includes digitalis and diuretics, while the gastrointestinal complications require surgical revisions and reconstruction.

The two classes of drugs for treatment of African trypanosomiasis include those useful for the early stages of disease and those effective for the advanced or central nervous system (CNS) stage. Suramin (Bayer 205, Germanin), which is available from the Centers for Disease Control, is indicated for early disease. After a test dose (100–200 mg), adults receive 1 g suramin intravenously on days 1, 3, 7, 14, and 21. Pediatric patients receive suramin 20 mg/kg/d in the same regimen as adults. For late CNS stage complications, melarsoprol (Arsobal), also obtained from the Centers for Disease Control, is administered at 2–3.6 mg/kg/d intravenously for 3 days. Two other similar regimens are administered over a 3-week period. Pediatric patients with CNS stage disease receive melarsoprol 18–25 mg/kg as a total dose over a 1-month period.

Tourists and visitors to East Africa, where there is a risk of infection in game parks, should wear protective clothing (wrist and ankle length), use insect repellents, and sleep in mosquito-proof nets. Pentamidine administered at 4 mg/kg as a single dose every 6 months has been used as a prophylactic measure for African trypanosomiasis in endemic areas.

## Helminthic Diseases

The helminths are classified into two groups: nematodes (roundworms) and platyhelminths (flatworms). For a list of nematodes and platyhelminths see Table 83.2.

The majority of intestinal helminthic infections may not be associated with clearly defined manifestations of disease, but can cause significant pathology. One of the factors that determines the pathogenicity of helminths is their population density. Light infections may be fairly well tolerated, while high populations of intestinal helminths can result in predictable disease presentations. In the United States these infections are most frequently seen in recent immigrants from Southeast Asia, the Caribbean, Mexico, and Central America. There is a higher incidence of helminthic infections in the southern states. Other populations that have a high risk of infestation include institutionalized patients (both young and elderly), preschool children in day-care centers, residents of Indian reservations, and homosexual individuals.[34] Certain conditions and drugs (fever, corticosteroids, anesthesia) can cause atypical localization of worms.[35] Immunocompromised hosts can be overwhelmed by some helminthic infections, such as strongyloidiasis.[36]

**Table 83.2**

| *Helminth* | *Common name* |
|---|---|
| Nematodes | |
| *Ancylostoma duodenale* | Hookworm |
| *Necator americanus* | Hookworm |
| *Ascaris lumbricoides* | Giant roundworm |
| *Enterobius vermicularis* | Pinworm |
| *Strongyloides stercoralis* | Strongyloides |
| *Trichinella spiralis* | Trichinosis |
| *Trichuris trichiura* | Whipworm |
| *Wuchereria bancrofti* | Filariasis |
| Platyhelminthes | |
| Trematodes | |
| *Clonorchis sinensis* | Chinese liver fluke |
| *Fasciola hepatica* | Liver fluke |
| *Fasciolopsis buski* | Intestinal fluke |
| *Paragonimus westermani* | Lung fluke |
| *Schistosoma haematobium* | Blood fluke |
| *Schistosoma japonicum* | Blood fluke |
| *Schistosoma mansoni* | Blood fluke |
| *Schistosoma mekongi* | Blood fluke |
| Cestodes | |
| *Diphyllobothrium latum* | Fish tapeworm |
| *Taenia saginata* | Beef tapeworm |
| *Taenia solium* | Pork tapeworm |

### *Nematodes (Roundworms)*

#### Hookworm Disease

This is an infection of the small intestine caused by either *Ancylostoma duodenale* or *Necator americanus*. *N. americanus* is found in the southeastern United States where the temperature and humidity provide the proper environment. *Ancylostoma* is rarely seen in the United States.

The life cycles of both species of hookworm are similar. The adult worms live in the small intestine attached to the mucosa. Females liberate eggs which are eliminated in the feces and develop into larvae. The site of entry of the infective larva can result in a papular eruption with localized edema and erythema.

In the small intestine where the adult worm lives attached to the mucosa, injury is usually due to mechanical and lytic destruction of tissue. The loss of blood can lead to anemia and hypoproteinemia.[1,2]

***Clinical Presentation*** Major complaints in patients are abdominal pain and diarrhea with or without blood and mucus. Lassitude, shortness of breath, and swelling of the legs may be presenting symptoms.[1,2]

Stool should be examined for eggs and the rhabditiform larvae. Eosinophilia (30%–60%) is present in patients with chronic infection.

***Treatment***[10,37,38] Mebendazole (Vermox), an oral synthetic benzimidazole, is the agent of first choice. It is also effective against ascariasis, enterobiasis, and trichuriasis. The adult dose for treatment of hookworm infestation is 100 mg twice daily for 3 days. Pediatric patients above 2 years of age should receive the same dose as adults.

### Ascariasis

Ascariasis is caused by the giant roundworm, *Ascaris lumbricoides*. Female worms range from 20 to 35 cm in length. The worm is found worldwide, but more commonly in areas where sanitation is poor. In the United States, endemic areas include southeastern parts of the Appalachian range and the Gulf Coast states.[34,39] It is estimated that about four million people in the United States have ascariasis.[34]

The adult worm inhabits the small intestine, especially the jejunum. The female produces millions of eggs during her lifetime, laying about 200,000 per day. The eggs are expelled with feces and, under optimal conditions, become infective. If the eggs are ingested through contaminated food or water, they hatch and liberate the larvae. The larvae penetrate the blood or lymph vessels, and travel to the lungs. The larvae are filtered out by the capillaries in the lung and get into the alveoli, where they molt and grow in size. They then migrate through the respiratory passages to reach the esophagus and finally end up in the small intestine. The larvae grow to adults, and the cycle is repeated.

***Clinical Presentation*** During migration of the larvae through the lungs, patients can present with pneumonitis, fever, cough, eosinophilia, and pulmonary infiltrates.[40] Other symptoms of ascariasis include abdominal discomfort, vomiting, and appendicitis.[39] Diagnosis is made by demonstrating the characteristic egg in the stool.

***Treatment***[10,37,39] In both adults and pediatric subjects over 2 years of age, the treatment for ascariasis is mebendazole (Vermox) 100 mg twice daily for 3 days. Alternative drugs are pyrantel pamoate (Antiminth) and piperazine citrate (Antepar).

### Enterobiasis

Enterobiasis or pinworm infection is caused by *Enterobius vermicularis*. The pinworm is a small threadlike spindle-shaped worm that is about 1 cm long. It is the most widely distributed helminthic infection in the world. It is estimated that there are 42 million cases in the United States.[34] The majority of those infected are children.

Infection occurs by ingestion of the eggs, which reach the mouth on soiled hands or in contaminated food or drink. In an infected host, the intense pruritus ani is an important factor in autoinfection and perpetuation of the infection.

After ingestion, the eggs hatch in the upper intestine and liberate the larvae which may reside in the jejunum and upper ileum. After copulation, the gravid female migrates to the lower bowel. The gravid female migrates at night to the perianal region and, under the stimulus of cooler temperatures and air, deposits eggs in the perianal skin. Rupture of the worm during scratching will shower the eggs which will become "airborne" and deposit on bedding, clothes, and bathroom fixtures. The eggs become infective in about 6 hours.

***Clinical Presentation*** There are no significant pathologic changes with the infection. The most common problem is cutaneous irritation in the perianal region, made by the migrating females or presence of eggs. The intense pruritus and scratching can cause dermatitis and secondary bacterial infections. In children, the itching can cause loss of sleep and restlessness.

The most effective method of diagnosing pinworm infections is by the use of perianal swab with Scotch tape. The Scotch tape, which is applied to the perianal region with a tongue depressor, is microscopically examined for eggs.

***Treatment***[10,37,39,41] The three common agents for treatment include mebendazole, pyranteal, and piperazine. The dose of mebendazole for adults and children over 2 years of age is 100 mg as a single dose; this may be repeated in 2 weeks.

After treatment, all bedding and underclothes should be sterilized by steaming or boiling to eradicate the eggs. Bathroom rugs and toilet accessories should also be sterilized.

### Strongyloidiasis

Strongyloidiasis is caused by the nematode *Strongyloides stercoralis*. The worms are usually found in the small intestine. Though strongyloidiasis occurs primarily in the subtropics and tropics, it is also found in Eastern Europe (Hungary and Romania) and southern regions of the Soviet Union.[42] Because of the ability of *S. stercoralis* to multiply in man (autoinfection), infections can persist up to 40 years or more.[43]

The rhabditiform larvae, which are passed in the stool, are transformed in the soil within 24 hours into infective filariform larvae, which are capable of penetrating the skin and causing infection. The infective filariform larvae, which penetrate the skin of the host, enter capillaries or lymphatics, migrate through the blood to the heart, then proceed to the pulmonary capillaries. The larvae then make their way through respiratory passages to the esophagus, passing down to the stomach. After copulation, the female burrows into the mucosa of the duodenum or jejunum and completes the cycle.

***Clinical Presentation*** Urticaria, wheals, and other linear lesions similar to creeping eruption and usually located around the perianal region or lower trunk may be caused by the filariform larvae.[42] The lesions last from 12 to 48 hours, and disappear without desquamation.[42]

Migrating larvae that reach the pulmonary capillaries can cause hemorrhage and cellular infiltration in the alveoli. The larvae occasionally lodge in bronchial epithelium and develop to maturity; this can produce chronic bronchitis or asthmatic symptoms.[36] Larvae may be found in the sputum. Immunosuppressed hosts are at risk of overwhelming infections. In the immunosuppressed patient who receives corticosteroids or other immunosuppressive drugs, strongyloidiasis can disseminate with massive numbers of larvae in the lungs and the cerebral spinal fluid.[42,44] Migration through the lungs can cause pneumonitis with dyspnea, cyanosis, and cough. The respiratory distress can mimic pulmonary edema.[44] If the central nervous system is involved, progressive lethargy, coma, and death can result. The cause of death could also be related to septicemia secondary to bacteremia caused by the migrating larvae. Thiabendazole, the drug of choice, is usually ineffective in these massive hyperinfections.[44]

Chronic intestinal strongyloidiasis can cause a malabsorption syndrome with edema and peptic ulcer. Small-bowel obstruction, secondary to paralytic ileus and edema, can also result from the infection.

Eosinophilia is a significant feature of the infection, except in patients on glucocorticosteroids. Besides an erythematous rash at the site of penetration, gastrointestinal infection presents with abdominal discomfort, diarrhea, and weight loss.[42] Disseminated strongyloidiasis in the immunosuppressed host (lymphomas, leukemias, and renal transplants) can present with a spectrum of symptoms that include diffuse pulmonary infiltrates, abdominal pain, and septicemia.[44]

If demonstration of the rhabditiform larvae in the stool is not accomplished, the string test (Beal test) should be used, whereby duodenal samples are examined.[45]

***Treatment***[10,39,46] The most effective antihelminthic drug for strongyloidiasis is thiabendazole (Mintezol); however, this only represents a cure rate of 60% to 85%. The dose in both adults and children is 25 mg/kg twice daily for 2 days. Mebendazole is an alternative drug for strongyloidiasis.

### Trichinosis

Trichinosis is caused by *Trichinella spiralis*, and the infection is initiated by the consumption of raw or undercooked meat containing the infective encysted larvae. The intestinal infection may be only transitory, while the migration and encystment of larvae in muscle tissue cause severe myalgia, swelling, and weakness.[47]

When insufficiently cooked meat infected with cysts of *Trichinella* is ingested, larvae are released from the meat by digestive juices. The larvae penetrate intestinal mucosa, undergo molting over 36 hours, and develop into adult worms. After mating and fertilization, the female worm releases more larvae. Production of larvae may continue for about 3 months or until the adult worms are expelled from the intestine. The larvae migrate into lymphatic vessels and are carried to the arterial circulation via the thoracic duct. They then invade striated muscle tissue, coil in a spiral, and are gradually surrounded by muscle sheath. Encysted *Trichinella* may remain viable for many years.[48]

*Trichinella* infects rats, wild boar, bears, and domesticated hogs.[48] Pigs are usually infected from meat scraps that are fed to them. *Trichinella* is found worldwide, and the incidence in the United States is estimated to be about 4%.[47]

***Clinical Presentation*** Diarrhea, abdominal discomfort, and vomiting are usually early manifestations after ingestion of infected meat and are related to mucosal irritation from the worms. Symptoms associated with tissue invasion include periorbital edema and myositis with pain and fever. These symptoms may be seen between the second and third week after infection. Eosinophilia is an important feature of the disease.[47,48]

When the larvae penetrate facial muscles, inflammatory reaction can cause pain so intense as to make chewing, talking, and swallowing difficult.[47] Though the larvae cannot encyst in the central nervous system, migration into the tissue can cause cerebral hemorrhage and simulate meningitis.[48]

Muscle biopsy from either deltoid or gastrocnemius muscle and demonstration of the larvae from the specimen can be considered definitive. The *Trichinella* skin test lacks specificity. The enzyme-linked immunosorbent assay (ELISA) is used to detect antibody titers in the serum.

***Treatment***[10,47,48] The objective of therapy is to eradicate the parasite from the intestine and provide supportive treatment for systemic symptoms. To eradicate the adult parasite from the intestine so that larva production does not take place, thiabendazole 50 mg/kg/d is administered for a total of 5 days. Pyrantel pamoate 10 mg/base/kg/d for 6 days and mebendazole 200 mg/d for 4 days are effective alternatives.

For the fever, myalgia, and allergic reaction, corticosteroids are recommended. Prednisone 40–60 mg/d is administered until fever and allergic symptoms subside. Thiabendazole may be administered concurrently with corticosteroids.

Hunters and trappers should be advised to fully cook the meat of bears or wild boars before consumption. Farmers should be encouraged to boil meat scraps before feeding them to domestic pigs. Pork prepared in a microwave oven may not be fully cooked in the center, and roasting or baking in a traditional oven is preferred.

### Trichuriasis

Trichuriasis (whipworm infection) is caused by *Trichuris trichiura* which is usually found in the ascending colon of man. The distribution is considered worldwide, with a predominance in warm moist regions. It is estimated that its incidence in the world is 755 million.[34,49] Because the anterior portion of the parasite is longer and threadlike and the posterior portion of the worm is broader, it is called whipworm. Adult worms are about 3 to 5 cm long.[1,2]

Infection is acquired when the barrel-shaped eggs of *T. trichiura* are ingested. The eggs need about 10 days outside the body to become infective. In the intestine, the shell in which the larva is imbedded is digested to release it and the larva temporarily attaches to intestinal villi. After a 1-month maturation period, the adult parasite moves to the ascending colon where it remains attached with its whiplike anterior portion. In heavy infestations, the worms may be found in the terminal ileum, appendix, and all of the large bowel extending to the rectum.[1,2] The worm obtains its nourishment by sucking blood. Blood loss is about 0.005 mL per worm per day.[1,2]

Soil contaminated with the infective eggs is the main source of infection. Ingestion of food or drink contaminated with ova can also initiate the infection. Highest incidence is in the age group 5–15 yr. There is very high prevalence (25%–50%) in the populations of Asia, Africa, and Latin America.[34]

***Clinical Presentation*** Light infection of *Trichuris* may be asymptomatic, while heavy infection produces anorexia, bloody diarrhea, abdominal pain, anemia, and weight loss.[1,2] In an undernourished subject, massive infections (greater than 1000 worms) can result in protein/calorie malnourishment.[1,2]

Rectal prolapse, secondary to inflammation of the descending colon and sigmoids, may be present. Whipworm infection can also cause appendicitis and peritonitis occasionally.[1,2] Eosinophilia is present in subjects with trichuriasis.

Diagnosis is made by demonstrating the barrel-shaped eggs in the stool or from a specimen obtained by sigmoidoscopy or colonoscopy.

***Treatment***[10,39,49] In heavy infections, the severe diarrhea may decrease the luminal effects of the drugs used and it is suggested that the diarrhea be symptomatically controlled before therapy is started. The drug of choice is mebendazole 100 mg twice daily for 3 days. Treatment may have to be administered for 6 days for heavy infections. Mebendazole causes a reduction of 20% to 90% in egg production.

### Filariasis

Filariasis is caused by long threadlike roundworms that inhabit the lymphatic system and subcutaneous or deep connective tissues. There are six different species that produce large numbers of microfilariae and are considered pathogenic in man: *Wuchereria bancrofti* (Bancroftian filariasis), *Brugia malayi* (Malayan filariasis), *Brugia timori*, *Loa loa* (loiasis—"eyeworm"), *Onchocerca volvulus*, and *Mansonella streptocerca*.

Space limitations do not allow discussion of all of these species and readers are urged to check other references for details.[1,2,50] Discussion here includes Bancroftian, Malayan, and Timorian filariasis. The other species are rarely seen in the Western Hemisphere.

The human filarial parasites have the same basic life cycle. When the microfilariae are ingested by the insect vector (e.g., *Anopheles* mosquito) they transform into infective larvae over 1 to 2 weeks. When the mosquito vector bites man, the infective larvae are introduced at the site of the bite, and migrate to the nearest lymphatic vessel. Over a period of 1 to 3 months, the microfilariae undergo a number of molts before reaching adult stage. After the male and female worms mate, microfilariae appear in peripheral blood 6 months to 1 year later, and persist even in the absence of reinfection.

*W. bancrofti* has a wide distribution and is considered to infect approximately 250 million persons. Bancroftian filariasis is found throughout the tropics and subtropics.[50] *B. malayi* is endemic in south and southeastern Asia, while *B. timori* is restricted to southeastern Indonesia.[1,2,50]

***Clinical Presentation*** There is some variation among patients, but the pathological presentations include primarily inflammatory reactions, chronic lymphatic obstruction, and filarial abscess with secondary bacterial infections.[50]

Lymphadenitis and lymphangitis of the leg and arms accompanied by fever, chills, headache, malaise, and joint pains are common symptoms with both Bancroftian and Malayan filariasis. Elephantiasis begins with pitting edema, but subsequently the swelling takes on a nonpitting solid firmness, secondary to extensive hypertrophy and hyperplasia of the skin and subcutaneous tissue. Elephantiasis most frequently affects the legs, scrotum, arms, breasts, pelvis, and labia. Although elephantiasis is painless, the swelling can reach massive proportions, causing incapacitation. Secondary infection from trauma and maceration is a major complication of elephantiasis. Patients may present with chyluria or lymph in urine, caused by rupture of abdominal lymphatics into the urinary tract.[50]

The diagnosis is established by identification of the microfilariae in peripheral blood, and clinical evaluation of recurring attacks of lymphangitis related to history of travel or residence in an area endemic for filariasis. Microfilariae may also be isolated in hydrocele fluid or chylous urine.

***Treatment***[10,50,51] The major drug for filariasis is diethylcarbamazine citrate (Hertrazan), which is effective against both adult worms and microfilariae. (Diethylcarbamazine is available from the Lederle Laboratories, Pearl River, NY.) Besides the side effects of diethylcarbamazine itself (see Appendix), rapid destruction of the parasite by the drug causes high fever (over 41°C), headache, pain in muscles and joints, abdominal pain, nausea and vomiting, dizziness, and asthma. These reactions are usually seen within the first 48 hours, and may persist for 2 to 4 days. Patients should be warned accordingly. The reactions can be ameliorated by administering analgesics or antipyretic drugs like aspirin or acetaminophen.

All three species of filariasis (*W. bancrofti*, *B. malayi*, and *B. timori*) are treated with diethylcarbamazine beginning with a test dose of 50 mg, followed on days 2 and 3 by three doses of 50 and 100 mg, respectively. From day 4 through 21, the dose of diethylcarbamazine is 2–6 mg/kg three times daily. Pediatric patients should receive half the adult dose on days 1 and 3, followed by 2 mg/kg three times daily from day 4 through 21.

Adjunctive therapy includes surgical incision and drainage, aspiration of hydroceles, and excision of redundant tissue of elephantiasis. Visitors to areas endemic for filariasis, especially rural areas, should wear protective clothing, use insect repellents, and sleep in mosquito-proof nets.

## *Platyhelminths*

### Trematodes (Flukes)

The trematodes or flukes are leaf-shaped organisms that parasitize the gastrointestinal tract, liver, vascular system, and lungs. Flukes have a very complex life cycle. Some require more than one intermediate host; for example, *Clonorchis sinensis* (Chinese liver fluke) requires a snail and a freshwater fish in addition to the human host.[1,2] Most flukes have two suckers for attachment to the host. Trematode eggs have specific characteristics which are used to identify the species. Most trematodes, with the exception of the schistosome, are capable of self-fertilization.

All flukes have one or more intermediate hosts. A larva develops from the egg laid in the human host or another vertebrate, which is passed through feces or urine. The larva, which is called a miracidium, swims away to enter an intermediate host, normally a specific species of snail or clam, and goes through a number of developmental stages. When released from the intermediate host, the larva, now called a cercaria, can do one of three things: penetrate the skin of the final host, enter another intermediate host like a fish, or encyst to attach to plants and wait to be eaten by the final host.[1,2]

The habits of the human population are primarily responsible for propagating the disease. Bathing and wading in streams where the schistosome cercariae (infective larvae) are present and consumption of raw fish, snails, or vegetables that harbor the intermediate form of the fluke constitute the two sources of trematode infections. Infection with trematodes normally evokes an eosinophilic response in man.

### Liver Flukes

*Clonorchis* and *Fasciola* are two types of liver flukes that infect the human biliary tract. Although mild infestations may be asymptomatic, heavy infestations can produce significant gastrointestinal symptoms: diarrhea, epigastric pain, fever, and hepatic enlargement.[52]

Clonorchiasis is caused by *Clonorchis sinensis* (Chinese liver fluke) and affects primarily the extrahepatic and intrahepatic biliary tract.[2,52,53] This fluke is found predominantly in China, Japan, Korea, and Southeast Asia. Domestic animals like dogs and cats are major reservoirs for the fluke.[1,2] *Fasciola hepatica*, the sheep liver fluke, is found in all sheep-rearing areas in Europe, Africa, China, South America, and Australia.

***Clinical Presentation*** Clinical manifestations range from mild symptoms of abdominal discomfort, anorexia, low-grade fever, and diarrhea, to severe right upper quadrant pain consistent with biliary abscess or pancreatitis.[53,54] The pathologic changes seen with the liver fluke include bile duct thickening and dilatation and subsequently, with chronic infestation, ductal and periductal fibrosis. Biliary stasis can produce cholangitis.[53] Diagnosis is made by demonstrating the characteristic eggs in the stool.

***Treatment***[10,52,55] Praziquantel (Biltricide) is effective against liver flukes. The recommended adult dose is 25 mg/kg three times a day for 1 day.

### Intestinal Fluke

Fasciolopsiasis is caused by *Fasciolopsis buski* (giant intestinal fluke), which may achieve a length of 2 to 7 cm. The fluke is usually found attached to the mucosal layers of duodenum and jejunum.[52,54] Hosts other than man are domestic pigs and dogs. This parasite is found in China, Southeast Asia, eastern India, and Bangladesh.[52,54]

Infected subjects present with diarrhea alternating with constipation, abdominal pain, nausea, vomiting, and edema of the face and body.[52] It is suggested that the edema may be caused by a protein-losing enteropathy. Eosinophilia is present.[52,54]

The intestinal fluke can cause inflammation, ulceration, and abscess in the duodenum, jejunum, or colon. Heavy infection can result in a malabsorption syndrome and hypoalbuminemia.[52,54] Specific diagnosis is made by demonstrating the characteristic eggs in the stool.

### Lung Fluke

Paragonimiasis is caused by *Paragonimus westermani* and though it most frequently affects the lungs, it can be found in other parts of the body.[52,54] Human infection is found in Asia (including Southeast Asia), the Solomon Islands and Samoa in the Pacific, South America, and the Congo Basin and Nigeria in Africa.[52]

***Clinical Presentation*** Primary complaints include chest pains, productive cough with brown sputum, fever, and bronchitis. Eosinophilia is usually present. Patients may also present with hemoptysis, clubbing of fingers, and bronchopneumonia.

The major pathologic conditions that result from infection by the lung fluke are lung abscess, granuloma formation, and pleural effusions. Worms may develop ectopically in other tissues: spinal cord, brain, and lymph nodes.[52] Demonstration of the egg in sputum or stool confirms the diagnosis.

***Treatment***[10,52,55] Praziquantel (Biltricide) is effective for both liver and lung flukes. The recommended adult dose is 25 mg/kg 3 times a day for 1 day.

### Blood Flukes

Schistosomiasis is a parasitic disease caused by one of the species of the digenetic trematode *Schistosoma*. The three major blood flukes are *S. mansoni*, *S. japonicum*, and *S. haematobium*. The eggs of the schistosome are found in the feces, except those of *S. haematobium*, which are usually found in the urine. Blood flukes differ from other trematodes, because the two sexes are distinct and separate. *S. mansoni* and *S. japonicum* are usually located in the portal and mesenteric vessels while *S. haematobium* is found in the venous vessels of the urinary bladder. Schistosomiasis is related to the different developmental stages of the larvae and to the host's granulomatous reaction to the schistosome eggs.[56,57]

Infection is initiated when cercariae, which are released from specific snail intermediate hosts, penetrate the skin of the human host exposed to a contaminated water source. The cercariae migrate to the lungs and then to the liver to mature over 4 to 6 weeks. The mature worms stay in intestinal and bladder venules and mate, and the females lay eggs. While female worms of *S. mansoni* and *S. haematobium* lay about 300 eggs a day, *S. japonicum* produces about 3,000 eggs daily.[56] The eggs lodge in tissues and cause inflammatory reactions and formation of granulomas, primarily in the liver.

***Clinical Presentation*** The dermatological reaction or swimmer's itch of schistosomiasis presents with macules in nonsensitized subjects. The macules can progress to papules, erythema, vesicle formation, and severe pruritus in the sensitized subject who has previously been exposed. Dermatitis caused by bird cercariae is common in the United States in subjects living in the Great Lakes region.[58]

Katayama fever, first identified in the Katayama River Valley in Japan, is seen less frequently these days. Tourists who are exposed to cercaria-infested water in their travels may present with swimmer's itch and subsequently with serum sickness–like disease.[56,57] Presenting symptoms of Katayama fever are acute fever, chills, and headache, with enlargement of the lymph nodes and liver. Significant eosinophilia is present (20%–30% of leukocytes).[56]

Chronic infections with either *S. japonicum* or *S. mansoni* result in complaints of abdominal pain and diarrhea. On physical examination, subjects present with hepatosplenomegaly and abdominal pain. In the late stages, patients with chronic schistosomiasis can present with jaundice, ascites, and impending hepatic failure.[56,57]

Both *S. japonicum* and *S. mansoni* can cause central nervous system infarctions from migration of eggs to cranial and spinal arteries. The major neuropathologic manifestations are severe lumbar pain, sensory loss, and transverse myelitis.[59]

Since *S. haematobium* has a predilection for the urinary system, signs and symptoms include dysuria, hematuria, and azotemia, progressing to uremia. Obstructive uropathy with hydronephrosis, bacteriuria (with or without pyelonephritis), and bladder cancer are all manifestations of urinary schistosomiasis.[56,57] Patient history, urinary analysis where indicated, bladder biopsy, and an intravenous pyelogram usually confirm the diagnosis.[56]

Because of the large number of pathologic complications of schistosomiasis, especially related to the chronic stage, important aspects of diagnosis include careful history of travel and residence in endemic areas, stool for ova with egg quantitation, barium enema, intravenous pyelogram, and rectal or bladder biopsy (i.e., during sigmoidoscopy or cystoscopy, especially when stool examinations are unsatisfactory).[56] Patients from areas endemic for schistosomiasis may sometimes present with persistent *Salmonella* bacteremia. The following serologic tests have been used for the diagnosis: fluorescent antibody test and ELISA.

***Treatment***[10,55–57] After diagnosis of schistosomiasis by identification of the egg in either stool or urine, patients should be given a complete regimen of therapy. Therapy has been vastly simplified with the availability of praziquantel (Biltricide). Praziquantel is uniformly effective against all three species (*S. japonicum*, *S. mansoni*, *S. haematobium*). The recommended dose of praziquantel is 20 mg/kg three times a day for 1 day. At the end of the course of treatment, at least three consecutive stool samples should be taken to verify eradication of the infection.

Dermatitis (swimmer's itch) requires symptomatic treatment and includes local corticosteroid application (hydrocortisone 1% cream) and antihistamines. Most reactions resolve within 7 to 10 days.

American travelers to areas endemic for schistosomiasis should avoid wading or swimming in streams, irrigational canals, or rivers where they may be exposed to the infective cercariae. On returning from an endemic area, it may be prudent to have a stool and urine examination for schistosome eggs. An infectious disease clinician should be consulted to verify if a specific test or other screening procedure is necessary.

**Cestodes (Tapeworms)**

Tapeworm infections are initiated as a result of ingesting inadequately cooked fish, pork, or beef that contain the larval stages of one of these parasites. The larvae, once released in the gastrointestinal tract, mature into adult tapeworms and inhabit the small intestine in man for extended periods of time.

The cestode or tapeworm body consists of an anterior attachment called a scolex to which are attached segments of proglottids. The segments of proglottids are called strobilae, and it is the strobilae that grow continuously. New segments are immature because they do not contain fully developed internal organs. The mature segments in the middle of strobilae contain either one or two sets of both male and female reproductive organs. The terminal end of a strobila contains the gravid segments filled with eggs. The terminal ends of the strobilae of the tapeworm can become detached and can be found in the stool of the host.[2]

Tapeworms attach to the mucosa of the small intestine by the scolex, which usually contains four suckers, except in *Diphyllobothrium latum* (broad or fish tapeworm). Tapeworms do not have digestive organs and obtain all nutrients directly from the host. In some species, the scolex also contains a protrusible structure called a rostellum which may contain hooks. The scolex of each species of tapeworm is distinct and could be used for identification. Expulsion of the scolex usually results from treatment, though the digestive system of the host may alter it and make identification difficult.[2,61]

Tapeworm infection results from two components of the life cycle: the adult worm produces symptoms confined to the gastrointestinal tract of the host; the larva produces cysts in different organs.[60–62]

Diphyllobothriasis, or broad tapeworm disease, is caused by *D. latum* which is the largest tapeworm of man, being 40–50 ft long.[61] This tapeworm is found worldwide, especially in locations where pickled or improperly cooked freshwater fish is eaten. The incidence of diphyllobothriasis is high in Scandinavia, Finland, Alaska, and Canada.[60]

Intestinal infection is caused by adult tapeworms of two species, *Taenia solium* (pork tapeworm) and *Taenia saginata* (beef tapeworm). The beef tapeworm infection is found more frequently in Yugoslavia, Middle Eastern countries, Ethiopia, Kenya, Southeast Asia, and Latin America; pork tapeworm infections are found in Mexico, Latin America, Slavic countries, Southeast Asia, India, China, and Africa.[60,61] The incidence of both of these infections is low in Canada and the United States.

***Clinical Presentation*** Diphyllobothriasis may be asymptomatic; those patients who are symptomatic usually complain of fatigue, weakness, abdominal pain, headache, sore tongue, and weight loss. A low-grade eosinophilia may be present.[60] Megaloblastic anemia (hyperchromic, macrocytic) with thrombocytopenia and mild leukopenia is a specific finding in these patients. The tapeworm competes with the host for vitamin $B_{12}$ and the deficiency may be more pronounced if the scolex is located in the proximal jejunum. Folate absorption can also be retarded by the worm. Deficiency in ascorbic acid, thiamine, and riboflavin may also be present.[60] Though most patients with diphyllobothriasis have low levels of vitamin $B_{12}$, only 2% of the infected have anemia. If anemia is serious, patients can present with glossitis, weakness, paresthesias, sensory disturbances, and other neurologic abnormalities. Anemia and neurologic complications can be treated by replacement of vitamin $B_{12}$.

With both *T. solium* and *T. saginata* infections, the common symptoms in patients include abdominal cramps, nausea, "hunger pains," restless sleep, and weakness.[60,61] Diagnosis is made by identifying the characteristic scolex and configuration of the gravid proglottids.

Two forms of infection affect man: (1) The adult tapeworm

infection is acquired by eating raw or inadequately cooked pork or beef that contains the infective larvae (cysticercus). (2) Man becomes an intermediate host, and acquires the infection by ingesting tapeworm eggs which develop into the larval stage of cysticercosis. When the meat infected with the cysticerci is ingested and digested, the larvae are released, attach to the mucosa by the scoleces, and mature over 2 months.

When man acquires infection by accidentally ingesting the eggs, either in contaminated water or by reverse peristalsis and autoinfection, the intermediate stage (cysticercus cellulosae) is initiated.[62] The embryo, or oncosphere, penetrates the intestinal wall and migrates through the blood to different organs (CNS, pulmonary, and liver) to form cysts.[62] This larval stage of *T. solium* is called the cysticercus or bladder worm. The larva completes development in about 2 months and remains attached by hooklets inside the fluid-filled bladder or cyst. Cysticercosis can also occur with *T. saginata*; however, this is infrequent compared with *T. solium*.[2]

Hydatid disease caused by *Echinococcus granulosus* and *Echinococcus multilocularis* produces multiple cysts in a large number of organs including the liver, spleen, lungs, bone, and brain.[63,64] These infections are most frequently reported in recent immigrants from Mexico and Latin America. For detailed discussions, readers are directed elsewhere.[63–65]

***Treatment***[10,55,60–62,65] The objective in treating tapeworm infections is to eradicate the infections and supplement patients with nutritional replacements to correct deficiencies. All patients should have their stools checked every 3 weeks for 2 months after treatment to verify that the infection has been eradicated.

The drug of choice for diphyllobothriasis (*D. latum*) is niclosamide. The dose is four tablets (2 g) as a single dose on an empty stomach in the morning; patients should be instructed to chew the drug thoroughly before swallowing. Pediatric patients weighing under 34 kg should receive 1.5 g of niclosamide, while those weighing between 11 and 34 kg should be given 1 g as a single dose. Patients should receive supplemental doses of vitamin $B_{12}$ and folic acid until these deficiencies are corrected.

Both *T. solium* and *T. saginata* infections in adults are treated with praziquantel 10–20 mg/kg as a single dose. Retrograde peristalsis, secondary to vomiting from drug treatment, can cause movement of gravid proglottids of *T. solium* into the gastroduodenal area. Digestion and hatching of the eggs, followed by penetration of the gastric wall by the larvae, can result in cysticercosis. To avoid this potential problem, some clinicians recommend that patients receiving either niclosamide or praziquantel for treatment of *T. solium* should be given a purge (either sodium or magnesium sulfate 15–30 g) about 2 hours after, to facilitate the expulsion of the worm and eggs.

Treatment for cysticercosis and hydatid disease is primarily surgical excision, though mebendazole and praziquantel have been used with some success in nonresectable cases.[62,65] The dose of mebendazole is 40 mg/kg/d for 20–30 days and is repeated when necessary. Praziquantel is administered at 50 mg/kg/d in three divided doses for 10 to 14 days.[62,65] This dose of praziquantel is repeated if symptoms persist.

Finally, to avoid tapeworm infections in an endemic area, all fish, pork, and beef should be adequately cooked, or if freezing is used, this should be over 24–48 hours at −10°C.

## Ectoparasites

A parasite that lives on the outside of the body of the host is called an ectoparasite. It is estimated that there are three million cases of pediculosis in the United States.[66–68] Pediculosis is usually associated with poor personal hygiene, and infections are passed from person to person through social and sexual contact. The three types of human lice belong to two genera: *Pediculus*, including head and body lice, and *Phthirus*, with only one species, the crab louse.[1,2] The human louse is detectable to the human naked eye and measures about 2–3 mm long.

### *Lice*

The two species that belong to this group include *Pediculus humanus capitis* (head louse), and *Pediculus humanus corporis* (body louse). Female lice deposit eggs on the hair. The eggs (or nits) remain firmly attached to the hair and in about 10 days the lice hatch to form nymphs which mature in 2 weeks. Using both their piercing mouth parts and a pumping device, the larvae and adults feed on the blood of the host. The body louse and head louse are essentially identical, though they live on different parts of the body. Unlike the head louse, which lives on the hair, the body louse may more frequently be found on clothing of the infected host.

The pubic or crab louse is found on the hairs around the genitals, though they can occur in other areas of the body (e.g., eyelashes, beards, axillae, etc.). The crab louse has powerful legs which allow it to attach to the hairs and lay eggs. The life cycle is between 30 and 40 days. Infection is transmitted by close contact, usually sexual.

***Clinical Presentation*** Patients usually complain of severe pruritus from papular lesions produced by the bite of the louse. Hypersensitivity to foreign material injected by the lice can produce macular swellings and occasionally lead to secondary bacterial infections. As a result of long-standing pediculosis and secondary infections, hyperpigmentation and thickening of the skin can take place, a condition referred to as "vagabond's disease."[66]

***Treatment***[10,66–69] The agent of choice for all three infections (body, head, and crab lice) is 1% γ-benzene hexachloride lotion, cream, or shampoo (Kwell, Lindane). γ-Benzene hexachloride is highly lipid soluble, is readily absorbed through the skin, and has been reported to cause grand mal seizures in children. Neurologic symptoms including nervousness, insomnia, vertigo, stupor, and coma have also been associated with excessive absorption through the skin. Patients should be instructed against excessive or frequent application of the preparation.

The γ-benzene hexachloride 1% cream or lotion is applied in a thin layer all over the body, and should be worked into the affected area, avoiding mucous membranes and eyes. It is left on for about 12 hours and then showered off. If it is intended to be left overnight, the hair may be wrapped loosely with a towel. The hair should be thoroughly shampooed. A fine-toothed comb should be utilized to remove the nits from the hair. The preceding treatments should be repeated in a week to eradicate unhatched organisms. Other members of the family or sexual partners should also be treated. All bedding and clothes should be sterilized by boiling or steaming to avoid reinfections. Seams of clothes should be examined to verify that all organisms are eradicated. A 1% yellow oxide of mercury ophthalmic ointment should be used twice daily for 7 days for crab louse infections of the eyelids.

Another alternative for pediculosis is 0.3% pyrethrin combined with 3% piperonyl butoxide and 1.2% petroleum distillate (R&C, RID).[67] The same directions used for $\gamma$-benzene hexachloride should be followed when applying this preparation. For the relief of pruritus, a soothing lotion of calamine liniment or a lotion with 0.1% menthol may be used.

### *Scabies*

Scabies is caused by the itch mite *Sarcoptes scabei*, which affects not only man, but also animals. Mange in domestic animals is caused by the same organism.[68,69]

The adult mite penetrates the epidermis of the host, forming burrows where eggs are deposited. The eggs hatch to produce larvae which form more burrows. The larvae mature in about 4 days. Infection usually affects the interdigital and popliteal folds, axillary folds, umbilicus, and scrotum.[68]

***Clinical Presentation*** Patients complain of severe itching and inability to sleep and may have excoriations in the interdigital web spaces, wrists, elbows, buttocks, groin, and scalp. Excoriations may lead to secondary bacterial infections. The diagnosis is made by looking for burrows formed by the mite and taking skin scrapings, which will demonstrate the mite on a wet mount.

***Treatment***[10,67–69] The treatment of choice is crotamiton 10% (Eurax) lotion. To initiate the treatment, the skin should be scrubbed thoroughly in a warm soapy bath, using a soft brush to remove all scabs. The lotion is then applied to the whole body, avoiding the face, mucous membranes, and eyes. The application should be left on for at least 12 hours before bathing. This application is repeated on three successive days. All close contacts should be checked for scabies and treated appropriately.[69]

Other agents used to treat scabies are benzyl benzoate 25%, $\gamma$-benzene hexachloride 1% lotion (Kwell, Lindane) and in infants, sulfur ointment (2.5%–20%). All applications should be left on for 12 hours and followed by a warm bath. All regimens should be repeated on three successive days.

**Appendix** Antiparasitic Drugs

| *Drug* | *Side effects* | *Monitoring parameters* | *References* |
|---|---|---|---|
| Amphotericin B (Fungizone) 50-mg vial | IV infusion: Anaphylaxis, flushing, myalgias, chills, fever, headache, phlebitis<br>Renal: Renal tubular acidosis, decreased renal function<br>Other: Hypokalemia, hypomagnesemia, thrombocytopenia | Increased nephrotoxicity if aminoglycosides or cyclosporine is administered concurrently<br>Monitor: Blood pressure, renal function, serum K+, $HCO_3^-$ | 41 |
| Chloroquine phosphate (Aralen, Nivaquine) 250- and 500-mg tablets; 50 mg/mL (as HCl), 5-mL amps | GI: Nausea, vomiting, diarrhea<br>CNS: Dizziness, headache, blurring of vision, confusion, fatigue<br>Derm: Pruritus | Administer oral dose after meals<br>IV route: Recommend ECG monitoring<br>*Contraindication:* Patients with psoriasis or porphyria | 10, 14, 70, 73 |
| Dehydroemetine dihydrochloride[a] 30 mg/mL, 2-mL amp | GI: Nausea, vomiting, diarrhea<br>Card: Hypotension, arrhythmias, cardiac failure<br>Other: Muscular pains, paralysis, death<br>Cumulative toxicity: Doses > 650 mg | Prolongation: QT, PR, QRS, and ST segments on ECG (may be indication to stop therapy)<br>*Contraindication:* Cardiac and renal disease | 9, 10, 70, 73 |
| Diethylcarbamazine citrate (Hetrazan, Banocide) 50-mg tablet | GI: Anorexia, nausea, vomiting<br>CNS: Headache, lassitude, malaise<br>Allergic reaction: Hyperpyrexia, headache, tachycardia, pruritus, joint pains (may be related to protein release from microfilariae) | Allergic reaction can be ameliorated by aspirin | 9, 10, 50, 71, 72 |
| Diloxanide furoate[a] (Furamide) 500-mg tablet | GI: Nausea, flatulence<br>Derm: Pruritis | | 9, 10, 70, 73 |
| Emetine 65 mg/mL, 1-mL amps IM or SC | GI: Nausea, vomiting, diarrhea<br>Card: Hypotension, precordial pain, arrhythmias, tachycardia, dyspnea<br>ECG: Flattening and inversion of T waves and prolongation of QT interval<br>Other: Dizziness, myalgias, stiffness of skeletal muscles, general weakness | Emetine is more cardiotoxic than dehydroemetine; a course of emetine should not continue for more than 5 days; patient should be closely monitored; should *not* be given by the IV route<br>*Contraindication:* Pregnancy, liver, kidney disease | 9, 10, 70, 73 |

| | | | |
|---|---|---|---|
| Furazolidone (Furoxone) 100-mg tablet Suspension: 50 mg/ 5 mL | GI: Nausea, vomiting<br>Hypersensitivity: Hypotension, fever, arthralgia, urticaria<br>Other: Headache | Disulfiram-like reaction with alcohol; avoid in G6PD[b] deficiency (may cause hemolysis); changes color of urine to brown | 9, 25, 26 |
| Iodoquinol (Yodoxin) 210-mg tablet | GI: Abdominal pain, diarrhea<br>Derm: Rash | May interfere with thyroid function test<br>*Contraindication:* Patients with iodine intolerance | 9, 10, 70, 73 |
| Mebendazole (Vermox) 100-mg chewable tablet | GI: Abdominal pain, diarrhea<br>CNS: Headache, dizziness<br>Other: Pyrexia, neutropenia | Should be taken with meals<br>*Contraindication:* Pregnancy<br>*Drug interaction:* Can increase serum levels of theophylline | 10, 37-39, 41, 49, 71, 72 |
| Melarsoprol 3.6%[a] (Mel B, Arsobal) 36 mg/mL, 6-mL amps | Significant toxicity in more than 25% of all patients<br>CNS: Reactive encephalopathy, confusion, slurring of speech, restlessness, hyperkinesis, tremor, epileptic seizures<br>Renal: Albuminuria with casts<br>Card: Hypertension<br>GI: Hepatosplenomegaly, abdominal pain, diarrhea, vomiting | Because of toxicity, should be used after treatment with suramin and only for CNS complications; close monitoring of all vital signs; baseline for liver, renal and hematologic parameters | 10, 70, 73 |
| Metronidazole (Flagyl) Oral: 250 mg, 500-mg tablets IV: 500-mg vial | GI: Nausea, anorexia, vomiting, diarrhea, abdominal cramping, glossitis, metallic taste<br>CNS: Dizziness, vertigo, headache, paresthesias | Alcohol ingestion causes the disulfiram reaction: abdominal distress, vomiting, hypotension<br>*Contraindication:* First trimester of pregnancy | 9, 10, 70, 73 |
| Nifurtimox[a] (Lampit, Bayer 2502) | GI: Anorexia, nausea<br>CNS: Peripheral neuritis, psychosis<br>Hemat: Hemolysis in G6PD deficiency patients | | 10, 31, 32, 70 |
| Oxamniquine (Vansil) 250-mg capsule | GI: Nausea, vomiting, abdominal pain<br>CNS: Drowsiness, dizziness, headache, rarely seizures (in predisposed) | Should be taken after meals; on day 3 or 4, patient may have fever which may be related to parasite death; drug metabolite can cause a darkening of the urine | 10, 56, 60 |

**Appendix** Antiparasitic Drugs (continued)

| *Drug* | *Side effects* | *Monitoring parameters* | *References* |
|---|---|---|---|
| Pentamidine isethionate (Pentam 300) 300 mg/mL | Derm: Skin rash<br>Card: Hypotension, arrhythmias<br>Hemat: Leukopenia, thrombocytopenia<br>Endo: Hypoglycemia, hyperglycemia<br>Renal: Creatinine and BUN | When administered IM, has caused sterile abscesses; if IV route is used, it should not be infused faster than 5 mg/min; patient should be closely monitored for hypotension and ECG abnormalities (e.g., ST segment depression); check serum creatinine and BUN blood glucose, and other electrolyte panel 3 times weekly | 10, 28, 29, 70, 73 |
| Praziquantel (Biltricide) 600-mg tablet | GI: Abdominal discomfort<br>CNS: Malaise, dizziness, headache<br>Derm: Urticaria | | 10, 55–57, 71, 72 |
| Primaquine phosphate 26.3-mg tablet | GI: Nausea, abdominal pain<br>CNS: Mental depression | In G6PD deficiency can cause hemolysis | 9, 10, 13, 14, 16, 70, 73 |
| Pyrantel pamoate (Antiminth) 50 mg/mL suspension | GI: Anorexia, nausea, abdominal cramps, diarrhea<br>CNS: Headache, dizziness | | 10, 39, 71, 72 |
| Pyrimethamine (Daraprim) 25-mg tablet | GI: Abdominal pain, vomiting, glossitis<br>Hemat: Megaloblastic anemia, hemolytic anemia | It is recommended that folinic acid 1–5 mg/d be concurrently administered; can cause hemolysis in patients with G6PD deficiency | 9, 10, 13, 70, 73 |
| Pyrimethamine 25 mg *plus* sulfadoxime 500 mg (Fansidar) | For pyrimethamine, see above<br>GI: Nausea, abdominal pain, stomatitis<br>Hemat: Agranulocytosis, aplastic anemia, leukopenia<br>Hypersensitivity: Erythema multiforme, Stevens–Johnson syndrome, epidermal necrolysis | Combination has recently been reported to cause the Stevens–Johnson syndrome; patients should be advised to call their physician/pharmacist if a skin rash or other reaction is seen | 10, 70, 73 |
| Quinacrine (Atabrine) 100-mg tablet | GI: Nausea, vomiting<br>CNS: Headache, dizziness, toxic psychosis<br>Other: Rash | Can exacerbate psoriasis | 9, 10, 24–26, 70, 73 |
| Quinidine gluconate 500 mg base/mL, 10 mL | GI: Nausea, vomiting, diarrhea<br>Card: Hypotension, widening of QRS and QT on ECG, heart block | Administration of IV quinidine requires close monitoring; should normally monitor ECG and all vital signs | 10, 19 |

| | | | |
|---|---|---|---|
| Quinine sulfate 325 mg, 650-mg tablets IV[a]: 300 mg/mL, 2 mL (dihydrochloride salt) | Cinchonism: Flushing, dizziness, nausea, vomiting, diarrhea (levels over 10 $\mu$g/mL)<br>Card: Hypotension and widening of QRS complex<br>Hemat: Hemolysis, leukopenia, thrombocytopenia | When drug is administered IV it should be by slow infusion (600 mg over 8 h); close monitoring of vitals and ECG<br>*Avoid Use:* IM administration | 10, 17, 18, 70, 73 |
| Sodium stibogluconate (Sodium antimony gluconate) (Pentostam) | GI: Abdominal pain, nausea, vomiting<br>Renal: Albuminuria<br>Other: Fever, epistaxis, sweating, headache, weakness, edema, rash | *Precaution:* Heart, liver, renal disease; T-wave inversion and widening of QT may progress to arrhythmias; close monitoring of vitals and EKG | 10, 28, 70, 73 |
| Suramin[a] (Bayer 205, Germanin, Moranyl) 1 g/vial | Renal: Albuminuria<br>Derm: Rash, pruritus, edema<br>Ocular: Blepharitis, conjunctivitis, photophobia, lacrimation<br>Other: Vascular collapse | Requires very close monitoring of patient; laboratory parameters: CBC, BUN, U/A, creatinine, SGOT | 10, 33, 73 |
| Thiabendazole (Mintezol) 500-mg tablet 500 mg/5 mL suspension | GI: Nausea, vomiting, epigastric pain, diarrhea<br>CNS: Dizziness, tinnitus, paresthesia, drowsiness | Metabolite in urine imparts odor; some patients experience all GI and CNS side effects | 10, 39, 42, 44, 46, 71, 72 |

[a] Investigational agents obtained from the Parasitic Disease Drug Service, Centers for Disease Control, Atlanta, Ga.

[b] Glucose-6-phosphate dehydrogenase.

## References


1. Beaver PC, Jung RC, Cupp EW. Clinical Parasitology. Philadelphia, Lea and Febiger, 1984.
2. Markell EK, Voge M. Medical Parasitology. Philadelphia, W.B. Saunders, 1981.
3. Strickland GT, Weske JT. Geographic distribution of infectious diseases, in Strickland GT (ed): Hunter's Tropical Medicine. Philadelphia, W.B. Saunders, 1984, pp 965–980.
4. Patterson M, Schoppee LE. The presentation of amebiasis. Med Clin North Am 1982;66:689–705.
5. Ravadin JI, Jones TC. *Entamoeba histolytica* (amebiasis), in Mandell GL, Douglas RG, Bennett JE (eds): Principles and Practice of Infectious Diseases. New York, John Wiley and Sons, 1985, pp 1506–1512.
6. Baker RW, Peppercorn MA. Gastrointestinal ailments of homosexual men. Medicine 1982;61:390–405.
7. Tucker PC, Webster PD, Kilpatrick ZM. Amebic colitis mistaken for inflammatory bowel disease. Arch Intern Med 1975;135:681–685.
8. Shabot JM, Patterson M. Amebic liver abscess 1966–1976. Dig Dis Sci 1978;23:110–123.
9. Wolfe MS. The treatment of intestinal protozoan infections. Med Clin North Am 1982;66:707–720.
10. Drugs for parasitic infections. Med Lett 1986;28:9–18.
11. Wolfe MS. Amebiasis, in Strickland GT (ed): Hunter's Tropical Medicine. Philadelphia, W.B. Saunders, 1984, pp 491–492.
12. Wyler DJ. Malaria: resurgence, resistance and research. N Engl J Med 1983;308:875–878; 934–939.
13. Spenser HC, Strickland GT. Malaria, in Strickland GT (ed): Hunter's Tropical Medicine. Philadelphia, W.B. Saunders, 1984, pp 516–552.
14. Wyler DJ. *Plasmodium* species (malaria), in Mandell GL, Douglas RG, Bennett JE (eds): Principles and Practice of Infectious Diseases. New York, John Wiley and Sons, 1985, pp 1514–1522.
15. James MFM. Pulmonary damage associated with falciparum malaria. A report of ten cases: pulmonary edema with features of ARDS seen in a patient. Ann Trop Med Parasitol 1985;79:123–138.
16. Weniger BG, Blumberg RS, Campbell CC, et al. High-level chloroquine resistance of *Plasmodium falciparum* malaria acquired in Kenya. N Engl J Med 1982;307:1560–1562.
17. White NJ, Looareesuwan S, Warrell DA, et al. High-quinine pharmacokinetics and toxicity in cerebral and uncomplicated falciparum malaria. Am J Med 1982;73:564–572.
18. White NJ, Looareesuwan S, Wendell DA, et al. Quinine loading dose in cerebral malaria. Am J Trop Med Hyg 1983;32:1–5.
19. Phillips RE, Warrell DA, White NJ, et al. Intravenous quinidine for the treatment of severe falciparum malaria. N Engl J Med 1985;312:1273–1278.
20. Ballou WR, Sherwood JA, Chulay JD, et al. Safety and efficacy of a recumbent DNA *Plasmodium falciparum* sporozoite vaccine. Lancet 1987;2:1277.
21. Barrett-Connor E. Traveler's diarrhea. Calif Med 1973;118:1–4.
22. Meyer AE, Jarroll EL. Giardiasis. Am J Epidemiol 1980;111:1–12.
23. Wright SG, Tomkins AM, Ridley DS. Giardiasis: clinical and therapeutic aspects. Gut 1977;18:343–350.
24. Hill DR. *Giardia lamblia*, in Mandell GL, Douglas RG, Bennett JE (eds): Principles and Practice of Infectious Diseases. John Wiley and Sons, New York, 1985, pp 1552–1555.
25. Bassily S, Farid A, Mikhail JW, et al. The treatment of *Giardia lamblia* infections with mepacrine, metronidazole and furazolidone. Am J Trop Med Hyg 1970;73:15–18.
26. Craft JC, Murphy T, Nelson JD. Furazolidone and quinacrine: comparative study of therapy for giardiasis in children. Am J Dis Child 1981;135:164–167.
27. Jarroll EL, Bingham AK, Meyer EA. Giardia cyst destruction: effectiveness of six small quantity water disinfection methods. Am J Trop Med Hyg 1980;29:8–11.
28. Pearson RD, De Queiroz SA. *Leishmania* species (Kala-Azar, cutaneous and mucocutaneous leishmaniasis), in Mandell GL, Douglas RG, Bennett JE (eds): Principles and Practice of Infectious Diseases. John Wiley and Sons, New York, 1985, pp 1522–1530.
29. Chulay JD, Manson-Bahr PEC. Leishmaniasis, in Strickland GT (ed): Hunter's Tropical Medicine. Philadelphia, W.B. Saunders, 1984, pp 574–592.
30. Sampaio SAT, Castro RM, Dillon NL, et al. Treatment of mucocutaneous (American) leishmaniasis with amphotericin B. Report of 70 cases. Int J Dermatol 1971;10:179–181.
31. Marsden PD. American trypanosomiasis, in Strickland GT (ed): Hunter's Tropical Medicine. Philadelphia, W.B. Saunders, 1984, pp 565–573.
32. Kirchhoff LV, Neva FA. *Trypanosoma* species (Chagas' disease), in Mandell GL, Douglas RG, Bennett JE (eds): Principles and Practice of Infectious Diseases. New York, John Wiley and Sons, 1985, pp 1531–1537.
33. Spenser HC. Trypanosomiasis, in Strickland GT (ed): Hunter's Tropical Medicine. Philadelphia, W.B. Saunders, 1984, pp 552–565.
34. Warren KS. Helminthic disease endemic in the United States. Am J Trop Med Hyg 1974;23:723–730.
35. Ihekwaba FN. *Ascaris lumbricoides* and perforation of the ileum: a critical review. Br J Surg 1979;66:132–134.
36. Smith B, Verghese A, Berk SL, et al. Pulmonary strongyloidiasis: diagnosis by sputum Gram stain. Am J Med 1985;79:663–666.
37. Keystone JS, Merdock JK. Mebendazole. Ann Int Med 1979;91:582–586.
38. Muttalib MA, Khan MU, Haq JA. Single dose regimen of mebendazole in the treatment of polyparasitism in children. Am J Trop Med Hyg 1981;84:159–162.
39. Cline BL. Current drug regimens for treatment of intestinal helminth infections. Med Clin North Am 1982;66:721–741.
40. Gelpi AP, Mustapha A. *Ascaris* pneumonia. Am J Med 1968;44:377–379.
41. Brugmans JP, Theinpont DC, Van Wigngaarden I, et al. Mebendazole in enterobiasis. JAMA 1971;217:313–316.
42. Gilles HM. Intestinal nematode infections: strongyloidiasis, in Strickland GT (ed): Hunter's Tropical Medicine. Philadelphia, W.B. Saunders, 1984, pp 642–645.
43. Gill GV, Bell DR. *Strongyloides stercoralis* infections in former Far East prisoners of war. Br Med J 1979;2:572–574.
44. Bradley ST, Dines DE, Brewer NS. Disseminated *Strongyloides stercoralis* in an immunosuppressed host. Mayo Clin Proc 1978;53:332–335.
45. Beal CB, Veins P, Grant R, et al. Technique for sampling duodenal contents. Am J Trop Med Hyg 1970;19:349–352.
46. Shumaker JD, Band JD, Lensmeyer GL, et al. Thiabendazole treatment of severe strongyloidiasis in a hemodialyzed patient. Ann Int Med 1978;89:644–645.
47. Wand M, Lyman D. Trichinosis from bear meat: Clinical and laboratory feature. JAMA 1972;220:245–246.

48. Davis MJ, Cilo M, Yahr MD, et al. Trichinosis: Severe myopathic involvement with recovery. Neurology 1976;25:37–40.
49. Rossignol JF, Maisonneuve H. Benzimidazoles in the treatment of trichuriasis. A review. Ann Trop Med Parasitol 1984;78:135–144.
50. Nelson GS, Dennis DT, Connor DH, et al. Filarial infections, in Strickland GT (ed): Hunter's Tropical Medicine. Philadelphia, W.B. Saunders, 1984, pp 647–686.
51. Hawking F. Diethylcarbamazine and new compounds for treatment of filariasis. Adv Pharmacol Chemother 1979;16:129–194.
52. Markell EK, Goldsmith R. Trematode infections exclusive of schistosomiasis, in Strickland GT (ed): Hunter's Tropical Medicine. Philadelphia, W.B. Saunders, 1984, pp 740–758.
53. Sullivan WG, Keop LJ. Common bile duct obstruction and cholangiohepatitis in clonorchiasis. JAMA 1980;243:2060–2061.
54. Mahmood AAF. Trematodes (schistosomiasis, other flukes), in Mandell GL, Douglas RG, Bennett JE (eds): Principles and Practice of Infectious Diseases. New York, John Wiley and Sons, 1985, pp 1573–1578.
55. Pearson RD, Guerrant RL. Praziquantel: A major advance in antihelminthic therapy. Ann Intern Med 1983;99:195–198.
56. Laughlion LW. Schistosomiasis, in Strickland GT (ed): Hunter's Tropical Medicine. Philadelphia, W.B. Saunders, 1984, pp 708–740.
57. Cook JA. Schistosome infections in humans: Perspectives and recent findings. Ann Intern Med 1982;97:740–754.
58. Hoeffler DF. Cercarial dermatitis. Its etiology, epidemiology, and clinical aspects. Arch Environ Health 1974;29:225–229.
59. Lechtenberg R, Viada GA. Schistosomiasis of the spinal cord. Neurology 1977;27:55–59.
60. Jones TC. Cestodes (tapeworms), in Mandell GL, Douglas RG, Bennett JE (eds): Principles and Practice of Infectious Diseases. New York, John Wiley and Sons, 1985, pp 1579–1583.
61. Goldsmith R, Markell EK. Cestode infections, in Strickland GT (ed): Hunter's Tropical Medicine. Philadelphia, W.B. Saunders, 1984, pp 758–780.
62. Sotelo J, Escobedo F, Rodreguez-Carbajal J, et al. Therapy of parenchymal brain cysticercosis with praziquantel. N Engl J Med 1984;310:1001–1007.
63. Amir-Hahed AK, Fardin R, Farzad A, et al. Clinical echinococcosis. Ann Surg 1975;182:541–546.
64. Wilson JF, Rausch RL. Alveolar hydatid disease: A review of clinical features of 33 indigenous cases of *Echinococcus multilocularis* infection in Alaskan Eskimos. Am J Trop Med Hyg 1980;29:1340–1355.
65. Bekhtia A, Schaaps JP, Capnon M, et al. Treatment of hepatic hydatid disease with mebendazole: Preliminary results in four cases. Br Med J 1977;1:1047–1048.
66. Weary PE. Lice (pediculosis), in Mandell GL, Douglas RG, Bennett JE (eds): Principles and Practice of Infectious Diseases. New York, John Wiley and Sons, 1985, pp 1590–1592.
67. Kastrup EK, Olin BR, Schwach GH (eds). Facts and Comparisons: Drug Information. St. Louis, J.B. Lippincott, 1987.
68. Orkin M, Epstein E, Mailbach HI. Treatment of today's scabies and pediculosis. JAMA 1976;235:1135–1139.
69. Cohen HB. Scabies continues. Int J Dermatol 1982;21:134–135.
70. Catchpool JF. Antiprotozoal drugs, in Katzung BG (ed): Basic and Clinical Pharmacology. Los Altos, CA, Lange Medical Publishers, 1982, pp 570–596.
71. Goldsmith RS. Antihelminth drugs, in Katzung BG (ed): Basic and Clinical Pharmacology. Los Altos, CA, Lange Medical Publishers, 1982, pp 597–628.
72. Webster LT. Drugs used in the chemotherapy of helminthiasis, in Gilman AG, Goodman LS, Rall TW, et al. (eds): The Pharmacological Basis of Therapeutics. New York, Macmillan, 1985, pp 1009–1028.
73. Webster LT. Drugs used in the chemotherapy of protozoal infections, in Gilman AG, Goodman LS, Rall TW, et al. (eds): The Pharmacological Basis of Therapeutics. New York, Macmillan, 1985, pp 1029–1065.

# Chapter 84 / Urinary Tract Infections and Prostatitis

Randall A. Prince, PharmD, Timothy Mullenix, MS, and Ed Casabar, PharmD

## Urinary Tract Infections

The classification of urinary tract infections (UTIs) is varied and sometimes complex. Although UTIs may be caused by yeasts, fungi, and microorganisms other than bacteria, only bacterial causes are discussed in this chapter.

In general, UTIs may be classified by site of infection, such as lower and upper tract. Lower tract infections are referred to as cystitis when the bladder is the site of infection and the symptoms of dysuria, frequency, and urgency are present. Upper tract infections are often referred to as acute pyelonephritis when infection involves the kidney and the patient has fever with flank pain and tenderness. By definition UTI indicates the presence of bacteria in the urine (bacteriuria). Although urine is generally sterile, bacteria may be present without causing infection and significant bacteriuria is generally considered to be $\geq 10^5$ bacteria per milliliter of urine.

Urinary tract infections may be designated as uncomplicated or complicated. Uncomplicated UTIs are not associated with structural or neurologic abnormalities of the urinary tract, which interfere with the normal flow of urine or voiding mechanism. Uncomplicated infections usually occur in females of childbearing age who are otherwise healthy, normal individuals. Males are not classified as having uncomplicated UTI because their infections are most often associated with a structural or neurologic abnormality.

Complicated UTI is the result of a predisposing lesion in the urinary tract, such as a congenital abnormality or distortion of the tract, stone, indwelling catheter, prostatic hypertrophy, or neurologic deficit, that interferes with basic urinary tract defenses. Complicated UTIs may occur in females and males and may be located in the lower or upper tract. Although many cases of acute pyelonephritis could be classified as uncomplicated UTI, many clinicians consider upper tract infection as complicated because of their concern for renal damage.

Some UTIs may be referred to as recurrent. Recurrent infections are characterized by multiple symptomatic episodes with asymptomatic periods occurring throughout. Recurrent infections are due either to reinfection or to relapse. Reinfection is the presence of a new organism in subsequent infections and accounts for the majority of recurrent infections. Relapse is the development of repeated infection caused by the initial infecting organism(s).

Asymptomatic bacteriuria is a common finding, particularly in elderly females, when there are $10^5$ or more bacteria per milliliter of urine but the patient is without symptoms. Symptomatic abacteriuria or acute urethral syndrome occurs in those patients who have symptoms of UTI (frequency, urgency, dysuria), but who fail to have significant bacteriuria.

Treatment of urinary tract infection is necessary because of the possible complications that may arise from no treatment. In children, there is risk of scarring and renal damage. Renal damage is not necessarily caused by bacteriuria alone, but is probably the result of vesicoureteral reflux (reflux of urine from the bladder into the ureters) and bacteriuria. Long-term effects of bacteriuria are not well defined in the adult. Certainly, acute renal damage from upper tract infection may occur in the adult, but the serious concern is the possibility of bacteremia as a result of the bacteriuria. Death may be the final outcome in gram-negative sepsis as a result of a UTI.

### *Epidemiology*

The prevalence of urinary tract infections varies with age and gender. In the neonate, the prevalence of bacteriuria is about 1% and is more common in males.[1] During the preschool years, prevalence of significant bacteriuria is 4.5% for females and 0.5% for males.[2] It is thought that much of the renal damage associated with UTIs occurs at this age.[3] Through grade school and before puberty, the prevalence of UTIs is probably less than 1%. After puberty, possibly related to the onset of increased sexual activity, the prevalence in females increases to 2% to 3% between the ages of 15 and 24. At least 10% to 20% and possibly as many as 50% of all women experience a UTI at some time during their life span.[4,5] Up to 6% of women experience greater than one UTI annually. Conversely, the prevalence of bacteriuria in adult males is low (<0.1%).[6]

In contrast to young adults, the prevalence of UTIs (10%–30%) in those over the age of 65 is approximately equal in males and females.[7] Most of these infections are asymptomatic. The prevalence rises further for those elderly in nursing homes and for those who are frequently hospitalized. The increased incidence in older males is related to prostatic hypertrophy and impaired urine flow, which is common in this age group.

## Pathogenesis

In general, urinary tract infection can be acquired via three possible routes—the ascending or retrograde route (where bacteria ascend the urethra into the bladder), the hematogenous or descending route (where bacteria enter through the bloodstream), and the lymphatic route. Of these routes, the ascending route is the most common.

The female urethra is usually colonized with bacteria believed to originate from the rectal flora, because it is short and is close to perirectal areas making contamination likely.[8] The bacteria can ascend the urethra into the bladder and then pass via the ureters to the kidneys. On the other hand, the male urethra is not in close proximity to the rectum and, because of its length, it is difficult for bacteria to successfully ascend to the bladder. Also, prostatic secretions play a role in the prevention of UTI as the secretions are antibacterial. These differences between males and females, coupled with the observation that urinary tract infections occur more often in adult females than males, lend support to the ascending route of infection as the primary route of infection acquisition.

Infection of the kidney by hematogenous spread of organisms can occur; however, it appears that UTIs via the descending route rarely occur in humans. A possible example is staphylococcal renal abscesses where organisms are known to be spread through blood from another infected site. Also, there is little evidence that the lymphatic route plays a significant role in the pathogenesis of urinary tract infections.[9] Thus, it appears that the ascending pathway of infection is the most important.

Host factors play an important role in the pathogenesis of urinary tract infections. Several defense mechanisms make the lower urinary tract resistant to colonization by bacteria. The normal urinary tract rapidly and efficiently eliminates bacteria that reach the bladder, thereby hindering bacterial growth. It has been shown that an acid pH ($pH < 6$), high or very low osmolality, and high urea and organic acid content in the urine create an environment that inhibits the growth of organisms common to the urethral flora.[10] It appears that individuals with one or more of these aforementioned urine factors are at less risk of bacterial growth in the urine. In addition, a main mechanism for prevention of UTI is the bladder's ability to spontaneously clear bacteria via a flushing mechanism, coupled with the urine's diluting capabilities. Also, any bacteria that adhere to the mucosal surface may be removed by leukocytes and phagocytosis.[11]

Several abnormalities of the urinary tract may interfere with the aforementioned normal host defense mechanisms. The most common anomaly is urinary obstruction. Obstruction inhibits the normal flow of urine and results in stasis, thereby promoting bacterial growth. Residual urine may also result from neurologic abnormalities, vesicoureteral reflux, and congenital abnormalities. Other factors that affect host defenses are pregnancy, immunosuppression, metabolic disorders (diabetes mellitus, gout, hyperparathyroidism), urinary tract instrumentation, and renal disease. These diseases or structural abnormalities "break down" the normal host defense mechanisms for the prevention of bacterial growth in the urine after contamination occurs, which leads to an increased risk of UTI development.

### *Etiology*

By far, gram-negative bacilli are the organisms most frequently isolated from the urinary tract. *Escherichia coli* is primarily responsible for most acute infections, accounting for over 80% of community-acquired infections. *Klebsiella pneumoniae*, *Enterobacter aerogenes*, *Enterobacter cloacae*, *Proteus* sp., *Providencia* sp., and *Pseudomonas aeruginosa* also occur in about 5% to 10% of community-acquired infections.

Gram-positive cocci are the second most common pathogens isolated and account for about 10% of all urinary tract infections. *Staphylococcus saprophyticus* is the primary gram-positive pathogen, most often occurring in young, sexually active females.[12] Group B and group D streptococci account for 1% to 2% of UTIs. *Staphylococcus epidermidis* is frequently isolated, but should be considered a contaminant until proven otherwise.

The prevalence of urinary pathogens is dramatically different in the hospital environment. The prevalence of *E. coli* is substantially lower, while species of *Proteus*, *Klebsiella*, *Pseudomonas*, *Providencia*, *Serratia*, and enterococci are isolated more frequently. Although uncommon, urinary tract infections caused by *S. aureus* most often invade the kidney from the hematogenous route as a result of bacteremia.

Each institution has a different prioritized listing of common pathogens; however, *E. coli* is probably responsible for less than 50% of hospital-acquired UTIs. Clinicians are aware that most UTIs in the hospital environment are due to gram-negative bacilli, but they do not have a clear indication, prior to culture, as to what specific pathogen(s) may be causing a given UTI; this is in contrast to community-acquired UTIs.

Most UTIs, particularly uncomplicated UTI, are caused by a single bacterium; however, complicated UTIs may be caused by two or more bacteria. The presence of multiple organisms is not always indicative of true infection, and may in fact represent contamination of the specimen from outside sources.

### *Clinical Presentation*

The presenting signs and symptoms of lower urinary tract infections in adults are dysuria, urgency, frequency, nocturia, and complaint of suprapubic discomfort; however, elderly patients with lower tract infections may be asymptomatic or the usual symptoms may not be diagnostic because noninfected elderly commonly experience similar symptoms. The manifestations of lower tract infections may also be present in upper tract infections in conjunction with fever, chills, flank pain, or costovertebral angle tenderness. Pain can radiate down the ureter or toward the epigastrium. If infection is confined to the lower tract, fever, when it appears, rarely exceeds 38°C. Attempts at differentiating upper tract from lower tract infection on the basis of symptoms are not reliable.

Symptoms alone are unreliable for the diagnosis of bacterial urinary tract infections. Thus, the diagnosis of UTI is based upon the finding of significant bacteriuria (ie, $\geq 10^5$ bacteria/mL of a midstream, clean-catch urine specimen).

An easy-to-perform and reliable method that correlates well with significant bacteriuria is microscopic examination of a Gram-stained, uncentrifuged urine specimen. The finding of a single bacterium per high-power, oil-immersion field is at least 80% sensitive in relating to significant bacteriuria. Some clinicians increase the sensitivity of this method by using the criterion of at least five organisms per oil-immersion field. The most sensitive microscopic method that correlates with significant bacteriuria appears to be the finding of a single bacterium in a Gram-stained, centrifuged urine specimen.[13]

It is extremely important to emphasize that the urine specimen must be collected in a proper manner, to minimize contamination by noninfecting bacteria. Urine in the bladder is *normally* sterile; therefore, it is statistically possible to differentiate contamination from infection by quantifying the number of bacteria present. Patients with bacterial counts equal to or greater than 100,000/mL have significant bacteriuria and usually infection.[14] If the sample is collected properly, voided urine with fewer than 10,000 bacteria per milliliter is without infection. It is important to remember that as many as one in five *actual* UTIs may have fewer than 100,000 bacteria per milliliter of urine.[15] Controversy exists as to the proper criterion for significant bacteriuria. It appears that the time-honored ≥ 100,000/mL will remain as an overall criterion. It is apparent though that certain patients have infection with fewer than 100,000 organisms per milliliter of urine. Acutely, dysuric women may have infection at a bacterial count greater than 100/mL.[16,17]

Other acceptable methods of urine collection include catheterization and suprapubic aspiration. In patients who are uncooperative or who are unable to void urine, catheterization may be necessary. If performed carefully and with aseptic technique, this method yields reliable results; however, infections from the introduction of bacteria into the bladder via the procedure may result in 1% to 2% of patients.

Contamination is least likely to occur when urine samples are collected by suprapubic bladder aspiration. This method is a safe and painless procedure and is the procedure of choice in newborns, in paraplegics, in seriously ill patients, and in adults when infection is suspected and routine procedures have provided confusing or equivocal results. If the urine is collected by these latter techniques, particularly suprapubic aspiration, the number of bacteria may be far less than 100,000/mL and still represent significant bacteriuria because of the markedly reduced chance of contamination.

The most reliable method of diagnosing urinary tract infections is by urine culture. In the bacteriology laboratory, urine cultures are most accurately performed using the pour plate technique. Unfortunately, this technique is unsuitable for a high-volume laboratory because of its expense and time consumption. An alternative method would be the use of a calibrated loop technique, which is easy to perform and less costly for the laboratory.

A number of methods are available for office use that are reliable and simple to perform. These methods include the filter-paper method, the dip-slide method, and the pad-culture method. The filter-paper method is relatively inexpensive, but provides only an estimate of the bacterial count. The dip-slide and the pad-culture methods are inexpensive, are highly accurate, and allow differentiation of bacteria. Their major drawbacks are lack of specific bacteria identification and sensitivity information.[18]

Bacterial susceptibility testing in the laboratory may be accomplished by several methods. Two of the more popular methods are the Kirby–Bauer method and the tube-dilution method for minimum inhibitory concentration (MIC) testing. With the Kirby–Bauer, or disk sensitivity, method, the organism is plated on a suitable medium and disks impregnated with an antibiotic are applied to the medium. The concentrations of antibiotics in the disks represent achievable serum concentrations for most antibiotics used in the test. The plates containing the antibiotic disks are incubated and the zones of inhibition measured at the end of the incubation period. The size of the zone for each antibiotic on the plate is compared with a standardized chart allowing for the organism to be classified as sensitive (S), intermediate in sensitivity (I), or resistant (R) to the particular antibiotic tested. Unfortunately, the clinician does not get an indication of the extent of sensitivity or resistance for a particular organism(s) when the results are reported as S or R, respectively. Additionally, most of the antibiotics tested achieve concentrations in the *urine* manyfold those in the serum; therefore, this method cannot directly relate to the action of the antibiotic at the site of infection.

A preferred method for indicating organism sensitivity would be the reporting of MICs via a tube-dilution method, for example. Many laboratories have automated systems to determine MICs for the myriad of antibiotics available today. The tube-dilution method determines the minimal concentration of the antibiotic necessary to inhibit the growth of the organism. Knowing the achievable urine concentration for the antibiotics, the clinician is now in a better position to select an appropriate agent to combat the UTI. Many experts differ on how much above the MIC the achievable site concentration should be in treating infections; however, concentrations of at least the MIC should be achieved to maximize the likelihood of therapeutic success. Also, patient conditions, such as renal function, play an important role in the attainment of urine concentrations of many antimicrobials. One cannot simply use a "literature" outlook to the expected urine concentrations. The clinician must always take into account patient and dose regimen factors that will affect the achievable urine concentration in the patient's therapy.

A variety of methods can be utilized to differentiate upper from lower urinary tract infections. The indications for using these localization studies include presence of infection in males less than 50 years of age, females who have multiple recurrences, and anyone in whom a structural abnormality is suspected. The most reliable method is ureteral catheterization for quantitative cultures; however, this is an invasive procedure that carries some risk and is not a desirable routine procedure.

Noninvasive methods of localization may be more acceptable for routine use; however, they may be of limited clinical value. The most promising method is the antibody-coated bacteria (ACB) test, an immunofluorescent method that detects ACB present in the urine. A positive test indicates upper tract infection. The test appears to be reliable and sensitive in detecting renal bacteriuria. Unfortunately, several studies have reported high false-positive and false-negative results.[19,20] These discrepancies may have resulted from lack of standardized criteria for determining positive test results. Fortunately, it is not necessary in the clinical setting to localize the site of infection to direct the management of the patient. Localization studies that are easy to perform and noninvasive are desirable for research studies, for example, efficacy studies, and for those limited number of clinical cases that require site differentiation.

### *Treatment*

The selection of an antimicrobial agent for the treatment of urinary tract infections is based primarily on the severity of the presenting signs and symptoms, the site of the infection, and whether the infection is determined to be complicated or uncomplicated. Other considerations include side effect potential, cost, and the comparative inconvenience of different therapies. Ideally, the antimicrobial agent chosen should be well tolerated, well absorbed, achieve high urine concentrations, and have a spectrum of antibacterial activity limited to the known or suspected pathogen(s). There is insufficient evidence to support any advantage of using bactericidal over bacteriostatic agents in the treatment of lower UTIs; however, in upper tract or recurrent UTIs, it may be advantageous to use a bactericidal agent. Table 84.1 outlines the treatments that may be used in UTI. This listing is by no means exhaustive, but does represent a practical approach.

**Table 84.1** Recommended Drug Regimens for Urinary Tract Infections in Ambulatory Patients

| | |
|---|---|
| Single-dose therapy | |
| Amoxicillin | 3.0 g |
| Trimethoprim–sulfamethoxazole | 2 double-strength tablets |
| Sulfisoxazole | 2 g |
| Short-term therapy | (7–14 days) |
| Sulfisoxazole | 1 g 4 times daily |
| Ampicillin | 0.5 g 4 times daily |
| Amoxicillin | 0.5 g 3 or 4 times daily |
| Trimethoprim–sulfamethoxazole | 1 double-strength tablet daily |
| Nitrofurantoin | 100 mg 4 times daily |
| Tetracycline | 0.5 mg 4 times daily[a] |
| Cephalexin or cephradine | 0.5 g 4 times daily[b] |
| Norfloxacin | 400 mg twice daily |
| Long-term therapy (6 weeks–6 months)[c] | |
| Ampicillin or amoxicillin | |
| Sulfisoxazole | |
| Trimethoprim | |
| Trimethoprim–sulfamethoxazole | |
| Cephalexin or cephradine[b] | |
| Nitrofurantoin | Half the above dose after first week |
| Nalidixic acid | 1.0 g 4 times daily |
| Carbenicillin indanyl sodium | 2 tablets 4 times daily (for *Pseudomonas* only) |
| Methenamine mandelate | 1.0 g 4 times daily[d] |
| Long-term suppression (6 months–2 years) | |
| Trimethoprim–sulfamethoxazole | 1 regular tablet twice daily |
| Sulfisoxazole | 0.5 g 4 times daily |
| Nitrofurantoin | 50 mg 4 times daily |
| Methenamine mandelate | 1.0 g 4 times daily |
| Long-term prophylaxis (6 months–2 years)[e] | |
| Trimethoprim–sulfamethoxazole | $\frac{1}{2}$ regular tablet |
| Trimethoprim | 100 mg |
| Nitrofurantoin | 50 or 100 mg |

[a] Should not be used by pregnant patients.
[b] These agents are much more expensive than alternatives.
[c] Dosage as above unless indicated.
[d] Urine acidifier must be used to keep pH < 5.5.
[e] Single daily dose at bedtime.

Adapted from Farrar WE: Med Clin North Am 1983;67:187–201, with permission.

#### Acute Uncomplicated Urinary Tract Infection

Acute, uncomplicated lower urinary tract infections are the most common and simplest form of infection. These infections are caused predominantly by *E. coli*, and antimicrobials should be directed against this organism. Many antimicrobials are effective against *E. coli* with sulfonamides, tetracycline, and ampicillin or amoxicillin being very popular choices for initial therapy. The choice of therapies is virtually endless because of the plethora of antimicrobials effective against *E. coli*. Conventional therapy has been a treatment of 7 to 14 days, although a variety of treatment lengths have been utilized clinically.

Single-dose antibiotic regimens have become popular in many regions as initial therapy of uncomplicated lower tract infection. Single-dose therapy is based upon the premise that lower tract infection is a superficial mucosal infection and that the urine can be sterilized in 24 to 48 hours. Single-dose therapy achieves high urinary concentrations that are elevated for 12 to 24 hours. Cure rates with this regimen have ranged from 82% to 100% in women with symptomatic lower tract infection.[21–24] The most widely used antimicrobial agents shown to be effective as single-dose oral therapies include sulfisoxazole (2 g), amoxicillin (3 g), and trimethoprim–sulfamethoxazole (2 DS tabs [double-strength tablets]). When compared with conventional therapy, these regimens were equally effective and in studies where the ACB test was used, negative results correlated well with clinical cure.[16] It should not be assumed that all antimicrobial agents will be effective as single-dose agents. For example, a 2-g oral dose of cefaclor produced a 57% failure rate in lower tract infections.[25]

The potential advantages of single-dose therapy include less expense, greater compliance, fewer side effects, and less development of resistance. It also allows women with multiple recurrences to become more involved in their own management and helps identify those women with renal infection because the infecting organism will reappear in a few days. Some clinicians feel that nonresponse of a patient to single-dose therapy indicates possible upper tract infection and warrants further investigation. At present, single-dose therapy appears to be safe and effective for the treatment of lower tract infection in women. It should not be used when symptoms of upper tract infection are present or suspected, stones or other urologic abnormalities are present, or there is a previous history of antibiotic resistance. Follow-up cultures should be obtained 2 weeks after therapy to detect relapses.

Controversy abounds as to the true "benefit" of single-dose therapy of uncomplicated UTI. Philbrick and Braci-

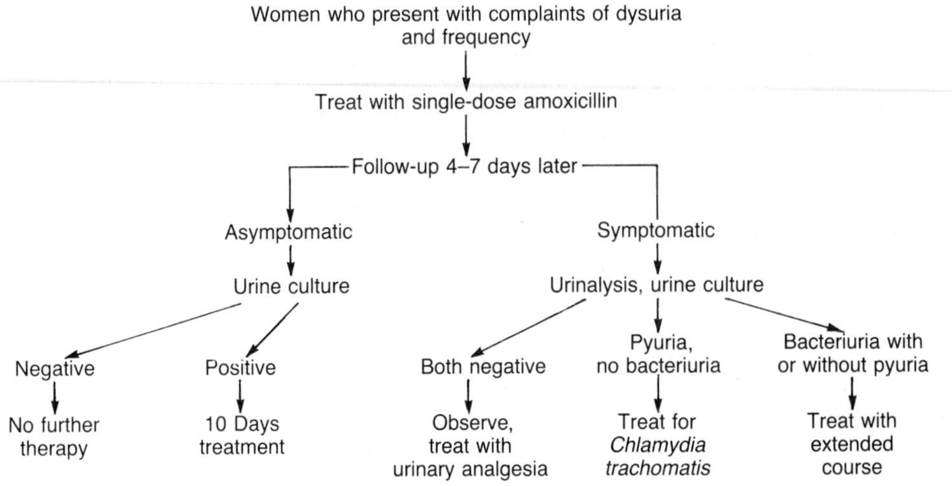


**Figure 84.1** Schematic outline of the therapeutic approach to women who present with symptoms of lower urinary tract inflammation. *(From Tolkoff-Rubin NE, Wilson ME, Zuromskis P, et al: Single-dose amoxicillin therapy of acute uncomplicated urinary tract infection in women. Antimicrob Agents Chemother 984;25:626–629, with permission.)*

kowski have raised the question as to whether the data really suggest that patients get less for less.[26] It appears that of the single-dose regimens, trimethoprim–sulfamethoxazole therapy is comparable to multiple-dose regimens, but the data are preliminary. More recent data suggest that of the short-therapy regimens for uncomplicated UTI, a 3-day regimen of trimethoprim–sulfamethoxazole may be comparable to the conventional 7- to 10-day regimens.[27] As some patients experience side effects or are allergic to the sulfa component of the aforementioned regimen, additional studies comparing several antimicrobials in a variety of treatment lengths are warranted.

Figure 84.1 outlines a systematic and practical approach to the therapy of lower tract infections in women.

### Acute Pyelonephritis

The presentation of high-grade fever and severe flank pain in a patient should be treated as acute pyelonephritis and aggressive management is warranted. Although mild cases of acute pyelonephritis may be managed with orally administered antibiotics in an outpatient setting, severely ill patients require hospitalization and intravenous drugs at least initially.

At the time of presentation, a Gram stain of the urine should be performed, as well as urinalysis and culture and sensitivities. The Gram stain should indicate the morphology of the infecting organism(s) and direct the selection of an appropriate antibiotic. If the Gram stain is not helpful, antibiotic selection should provide a broad spectrum of coverage, including gram-negative organisms. Standard practice suggests that initial therapy include an aminoglycoside in combination with a broad-spectrum penicillin or cephalosporin, such as ampicillin or cefazolin. If the avoidance of an aminoglycoside is desirable, a third-generation cephalosporin or extended-spectrum penicillin as single-agent therapy may also be a reasonable alternative. Within 48 hours, once the organism is identified and susceptibility patterns are known, appropriate therapy changes can be instituted. With the advent of newer quinolone antibiotics, for example, ciprofloxacin, combination parenteral and oral therapy with a single agent is possible for the entire course of therapy, and some, more severe infections may possibly be treated with oral ciprofloxacin alone.

Effective therapy should stabilize the patient within 12 to 24 hours. If sterilization of the urine has not occurred after 48 hours, further investigation is appropriate to exclude bacterial resistance, possible obstruction, papillary necrosis, or some other disease process. Usually, by the third day of therapy, the patient is afebrile and much less symptomatic. The best way to assess therapy is to examine the urine. There should be no or very small numbers of bacteria in the urine. In general, parenteral therapy should be continued until the patient has been afebrile for at least 24 hours. The patient usually can then be discharged from the hospital on appropriate oral therapy for at least a 14-day total treatment. Follow-up cultures should be obtained 2 weeks after completion of therapy to ensure a satisfactory cure and to detect possible relapse. Repeat culture is important because 20% of patients have a relapse with the initial pathogen during this time.

### Complicated Urinary Tract Infection

In complicated UTIs, as in acute pyelonephritis, it is essential to obtain an initial culture of the urine to direct specific antibiotic therapy. With complicated UTIs, the standard, first-line agents may not be effective and a culture and sensitivity report can help the clinician make an appropriate therapy choice.

Single-dose therapy should not be used in complicated UTIs. Conventional therapy of 7 to 14 days is appropriate in this setting. In some situations, however, as with complicated UTIs in adult males, a longer course of therapy (up to 6–12 weeks) may be required.[28] Some cases may warrant hospitalization and intravenous antibiotics may be required.

Often, as in acute pyelonephritis, an aminoglycoside is chosen. Although the aminoglycosides are associated with serious toxicities, they are consistently effective against most gram-negative organisms. A less toxic agent may be selected after the culture and sensitivity results are known. Newer quinolones, for example, norfloxacin and ciprofloxacin, may be of particular benefit in complicated UTI treatment because of their apparent efficacy as single agents when compared with combination antimicrobial therapy.

**Asymptomatic Bacteriuria**

Most patients with asymptomatic bacteriuria are older women and pregnant women. Relapse and reinfection are very common in this group and chronic asymptomatic bacteriuria is very difficult to eradicate.

In the nonpregnant female, treatment is controversial. Most clinicians feel that asymptomatic bacteriuria in the elderly is a benign disease and does not warrant treatment, as most data indicate that the patient is not destined to develop progressive renal damage.[5] After two cultures have been obtained confirming the presence of bacteriuria, an attempt to eradicate such infections with a short course of a nontoxic antimicrobial agent may be reasonable; however, more aggressive treatment should not be attempted. Children with asymptomatic bacteriuria should be treated with conventional courses of therapy, as in symptomatic infections, because of the possibility of renal damage.

In pregnant women, it is generally agreed that aggressive therapy is warranted in asymptomatic bacteriuria.[29] It has been demonstrated that untreated asymptomatic bacteriuria in the pregnant patient is associated with approximately a 40% incidence of acute pyelonephritis.[30] Increased prematurity and fetal wastage are also possible outcomes.[31] Thus, it is recommended that all pregnant women be cultured early in pregnancy and those with bacteriuria be treated for 7 to 14 days with a relatively nontoxic antimicrobial, such as ampicillin, amoxicillin, or cephalexin. Tetracycline should be avoided throughout pregnancy, and sulfonamides should not be prescribed during the third trimester of pregnancy because of the attendant side effects to the fetus.

**Symptomatic Abacteriuria**

Approximately 70% of women with symptomatic abacteriuria have pyuria, but have fewer than $10^5$ bacteria per milliliter of urine.[32] Usually coliforms, staphylococci, or *Chlamydia trachomatis* are isolated from the urine.[33] The remainder of patients present without pyuria or demonstrated infection and the etiology of the problem is unknown.

Most patients that present with pyuria will, in fact, have infection caused by coliforms or staphylococci, rather than *Chlamydia*, but will have a less than "significant" number of bacteria. Single-dose therapy has been shown to be effective and prolonged courses of therapy are not required for most patients.[34] Single-dose therapy is not effective for *Chlamydia* infection; therefore, those patients with dysuria and pyuria who fail single-dose therapy should be treated with a 2-week course of therapy, such as doxycycline or trimethoprim–sulfamethoxazole, directed against *C. trachomatis*. Often, concomitant treatment of any sexual partners is also required to cure *Chlamydia* infections and prevent reacquisition.

**Recurrent Infections**

Recurrent attacks account for about 10% of all UTIs. Of those patients suffering from recurrent UTI, 80% can be considered reinfections, that is recurrence of infection by an organism different from the preceding isolated UTI. With infrequent reinfections (less than two or three episodes per year), each episode should be treated as a separate infection. Single-dose therapy is very useful, especially in women with lower tract symptoms. If reinfection occurs more frequently, then long-term prophylaxis may be instituted. In some women, symptomatic reinfections are associated with sexual activity and the administration of a single dose of antibiotics before or after intercourse effectively decreased the number of episodes with minimal risk of side effects and expense.[35]

The remaining 20% of recurrent UTIs are relapses, that is, persistence of infection with the same organism after therapy for an isolated UTI. Relapse after therapy usually indicates renal involvement, structural abnormalities, or chronic bacterial prostatitis. Most relapses occur within 2 to 4 weeks of completion of antibiotic therapy. Patients with nonobstructive renal infection who relapse after a trial of single-dose therapy should receive a full 2-week course of therapy. About 50% of women are not cured after 2 weeks and require 6 weeks of therapy.[36,37] For those patients who fail a 6-week course, especially children or adults with non–surgically correctable obstructions, a longer course of therapy of 6 months or longer may be of benefit. All patients should be followed with urine cultures monthly, while on therapy. In males, relapse is frequently associated with a prostatic focus of infection.

As an alternative to the acute management of recurrent episodes of UTI, chronic antimicrobial prophylactic therapy using lower dose regimens is available. Prior to chronic prophylaxis, the patient should receive a full course of therapy to eradicate any existing infection. After a negative culture is obtained, prophylactic therapy is started and continued for 6 months. Therapy is then discontinued and the patient is observed for recurrences. If UTI recurs, therapy is reinstituted for 1 to 2 years. A urine culture should be performed every 1 to 2 months, while on prophylactic therapy, to detect bacteriuria. If bacteriuria is present, conventional therapy should be instituted.

A number of prospective studies have documented the efficacy of 50 to 100 mg of nitrofurantoin daily, 40 mg trimethoprim (TMP) plus 200 mg sulfamethoxazole (SMX) daily ($\frac{1}{2}$ tablet), and 50 to 100 mg of trimethoprim alone once daily, as prophylactic therapy.[38] Full-dose therapy is unnecessary for prophylaxis. These regimens prevent more than 90% of recurrences during prophylactic therapy. There is some evidence that long-term use of nitrofurantoin is associated with a large number of adverse effects, including interstitial pneumonitis, blood dyscrasias, neuropathies, liver damage, and acute hypersensitivity reactions.[39] Neither nitrofurantoin or TMP–SMX is likely to allow the development of antimicrobial resistance with prolonged use. These regimens also have little effect on fecal flora.[38] The limited experience with trimethoprim alone, coupled with the possibility of frequent adverse effects, makes this treatment modality an alternative regimen for those patients unable to take a sulfonamide or nitrofurantoin.

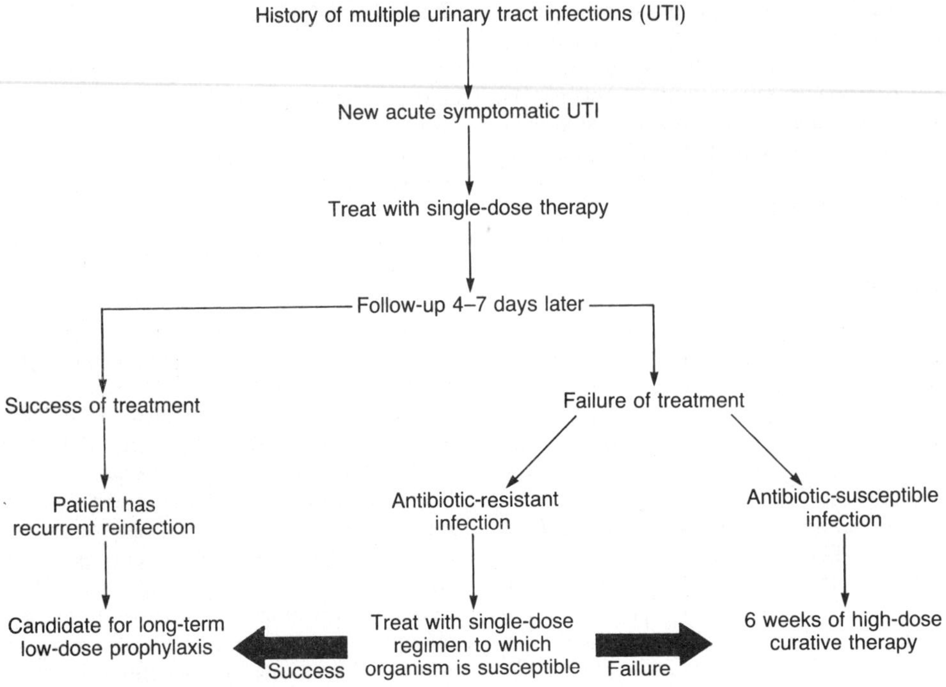


**Figure 84.2** Schematic outline of therapeutic approach to women who present with recurrent urinary tract infections. *(From Tolkoff-Rubin NE, Rubin RH: Urinary tract infection: Significance and management. Bull NY Acad Med 1986;62:142, with permission.)*

Figure 84.2 shows a logical therapeutic approach to the treatment of recurrent UTI.

**Catheterized Patients**

The use of an indwelling catheter is frequently associated with urinary tract infection and represents the most common type of hospital-acquired infection.[40] The incidence of catheter-associated infection is related to a variety of factors: method and duration of catheterization; the catheter system; the care of that system; susceptibility of the patient; and the health care personnel inserting the catheter (see Fig. 84.3). The incidence of infection from a single catheterization in a healthy ambulatory patient is 1%.[41]

Infection may occur by the entry of bacteria into the bladder at the time of catheterization. This probably occurs because the urethral meatus and the distal third of the urethra are normally colonized with bacteria. To minimize infection prior to catheterization, the periurethral area should be cleaned thoroughly and an antiseptic applied (e.g., povidone–iodine).

The use of an open drainage system, where the urine is collected in an unenclosed receptacle, causes infection in virtually all patients in 4 days.[42] With the introduction of the closed sterile drainage system, where the catheter leads to a enclosed, sterile collection receptacle, the incidence of infection has been dramatically reduced; however, even with the closed system, the risk of infection after 14 days is 50%.[43]

When bacteriuria occurs in the asymptomatic catheterized patient, therapy should be withheld, as bacteriuria is inevitable with long-term catheterization. Administration of sys-

**Figure 84.3** Entry points for bacteria. (1) Urethral meatus and around catheter; (2) junction between catheter and collection tube; (3) connection to drainage bag and reflux from bag to tubing; (4) mouth of the spigot. *(From Kunin CM: Urinary tract infections. Med Clin North Am 1980;60:223–231, with permission.)*

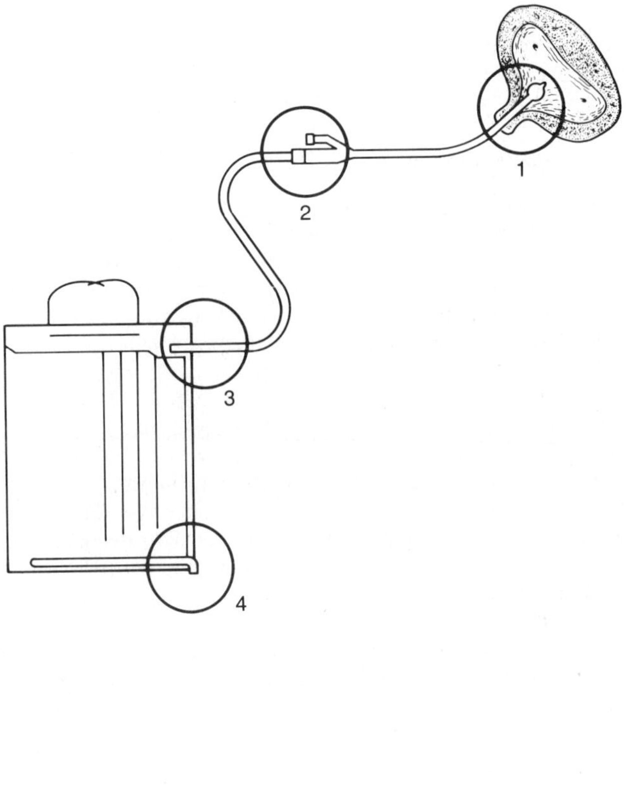

temic antibiotic therapy effective against the infecting organism will sterilize the urine; however, reinfection occurs rapidly in over 50% of patients and often results in the recolonization of the urine with resistant organisms. Removal of the catheter, as soon as possible, is the most effective treatment. Follow-up cultures should be obtained after catheter removal and therapy initiated as necessary.

Symptomatic patients with indwelling catheters must be treated. These patients are at high risk of developing pyelonephritis and bacteremia. If contamination of the catheter is suspected, recatheterization with a new, sterile unit is required.

Various methods have been promoted as preventing infection in the patient with an indwelling catheter. One method is the use of constant bladder irrigation with antiseptic or antibacterial solutions, for example, acetic acid 0.25% and the combination of neomycin and polymyxin. Use of these irrigation solutions has been shown to reduce the incidence of infection in the open drainage system[43]; however, prospective comparisons in the closed drainage system have not shown any advantage.[44]

The use of prophylactic systemic antibiotics in these patients is controversial. Although studies using closed drainage systems indicate that systemic antibiotics reduce the incidence of infection for the first 4 to 7 days, the emergence of resistant organisms is of particular concern.[45]

### *Summary*

Urinary tract infections vary in presentation and therapy. The clinician must have a predetermined therapeutic approach to the diagnosis and treatment of UTI. A well thought out therapeutic plan will minimize patient problems, while hopefully maximizing therapeutic success.

Many antimicrobials are available to treat UTIs, but their use is not without problems. Indiscriminate use of these antimicrobials may adversely affect patient outcomes and add to the "cost" of therapy.

Bacterial sensitivity patterns change and new pathogens continue to be "discovered" in certain patient groups. With the advent of multiply resistant bacteria, coupled with the toxicities of many antimicrobials, new agents will be needed to combat urinary tract infections. One promising class of compounds is the quinolones and we look with anticipation to these antimicrobials for assistance in treating complicated urinary tract infections.

## Prostatitis

Prostatitis includes several types of prostatic syndromes: acute bacterial prostatitis, chronic bacterial prostatitis (CBP), nonbacterial prostatitis, and prostatodynia.[46] It is a disease characterized by inflammation of the prostate gland and surrounding tissue. The exact cause of prostatitis is unknown. It is estimated that 4% to 5% of all males have some form of prostatitis during their life.

Both acute and chronic forms of prostatitis are characterized by the presence of common urinary bacteria and signs of inflammation. Further differentiation of entities is presented in the following sections. In nonbacterial prostatitis, signs of inflammation are present; however, common urinary pathogens are not found. Several sexually transmitted organisms, including *Chlamydia*, *Ureaplasma*, and *Trichomonas*, have been implicated in nonbacterial prostatitis.[47] Prostatodynia is a syndrome in which patients present with symptoms of prostatitis, but lack any evidence of infection or inflammation.

### *Pathogenesis/Etiology*

The manner by which bacteria reach the prostate is unknown. Possible mechanisms include (1) ascending infection from the urethra, (2) reflux of infected urine into prostatic ducts, (3) hematogenous spread, and (4) direct extension or lymphatic spread of rectal bacteria. Known causes of prostatitis include urethral instrumentation and prostatic surgery.[48]

Prostatic fluid obtained from normal males contains a potent antibacterial factor. This factor is a heat-stable, low-molecular-weight cationic substance in the form of a zinc-complexed polypeptide.[49] The antibacterial activity of the substance is directly related to the zinc content of the prostatic fluid.[49] Patients with chronic prostatitis have reduced levels of zinc in prostatic fluid and decreased activity of prostatic antibacterial factor. The actual relationship of this finding to infection is not known.

The pH of prostatic secretions in patients with prostatitis has also been reported to be altered.[50] Normal prostatic secretions have a pH in the range 6.6 to 7.6. With increasing age, the pH tends to become more alkaline. In patients with inflammation of the prostate, prostatic secretions have been reported to have an alkaline pH in the range 7 to 9. These changes suggest a generalized secretory dysfunction of the prostate, which not only may affect the pathogenesis of prostatitis, but may also influence the mode of therapy.[51]

Gram-negative, enteric organisms are the most frequent pathogens in prostatitis.[52] *Escherichia coli* is the predominate organism, occurring in 75% of cases. Other gram-negative organisms, including *Klebsiella pneumoniae*, *Proteus mirabilis*, and species of *Pseudomonas*, *Enterobacter*, and *Serratia*, are also commonly isolated. Occasionally, cases of gonococcal and staphylococcal prostatitis occur, but are unusual.

Chronic bacterial prostatitis is most commonly caused by *E. coli* with other gram-negative organisms isolated much less often.[52] *Staphylococcus epidermidis*, *Staphylococcus aureus*, and diphtheroids have also been isolated in some studies.[53]

### *Clinical Presentation*

Acute bacterial prostatitis is characterized by high fever, chills, perineal and back pain, urinary tract symptoms (frequency, urgency, dysuria, nocturia, retention), and general malaise and myalgia. The prostate is inflamed with marked cellular infiltrates, diffuse edema, and is extremely tender. Prostatic massage is not recommended because of the risk of bacterial sepsis.[52] Most patients will have bacteriuria after the development of acute bacterial prostatitis and the infecting pathogen can be isolated from a midstream specimen. Because of the danger associated with prostatic massage, quantitative lower tract localization studies are usually not performed.

In contrast to acute bacterial prostatitis, chronic bacterial prostatitis is difficult to diagnosis and treat. CBP is characterized by recurrent urinary tract infections with the same pathogen. CBP is the most common cause of recurrent UTI in males. The prostate is usually normal by examination and the clinical presentation can vary widely. Patients usually present with vague symptoms of voiding difficulties including frequency, urgency, and dysuria, along with low back pain and perineal and suprapubic discomfort. Many patients, however, may be asymptomatic.

The diagnosis of acute bacterial prostatitis is easily made from the clinical presentation and the finding of significant bacteriuria. Differentiating chronic prostatitis from nonbacterial prostatitis and prostatodynia, however, is more difficult. Symptoms and physical examination alone cannot distinguish chronic prostatitis from the latter two categories. The diagnosis of chronic prostatitis can be made only by culturing bacteria from the prostatic secretions.

In the diagnosis of chronic prostatitis, the clinician must be able to distinguish urethral from prostatic infection. The method of quantitative localization culture as described by Meares and Stamey is the most accurate for this purpose.[54] The first 10 mL of voided urine is collected (VB1) and constitutes urethral urine. After approximately 200 mL of urine has been voided, a 10-mL midstream urine sample is collected (VB2). This specimen represents bladder urine. After the patient voids, the prostate is massaged and expressed prostatic secretions (EPS) are collected. After massage, the patient voids again and the first 10 mL of urine is retained (VB3).

The diagnosis is made by comparing the quantitative bacterial counts of the various specimens. In chronic prostatitis, the number of bacteria in EPS is 10 times that in the urethral sample (VB1) and the midstream sample (VB2). If there is no EPS available, the urine sample following massage (VB3) should contain a bacterial count 10-fold greater than that of VB1 and VB2.

If the bladder urine is infected with greater than 100,000 bacteria per milliliter, then the site of infection cannot be localized. The urine should be sterilized with an appropriate antimicrobial agent that does not diffuse into the prostate (e.g., nitrofurantoin, penicillin G). After 4 to 5 days, the localization study should be repeated.

The diagnosis of CBP is made by an accurately performed lower tract localization study as described previously. Because of the focal nature of CBP, needle biopsy of the prostate gland is unreliable.[55] Microscopic examination of expressed prostatic fluid reveals an increased number of white blood cells and inflammatory cells, as in acute bacterial prostatitis, and is not specific.

### *Treatment*

Acute bacterial prostatitis responds well to appropriate antimicrobial therapy. Most antibiotics diffuse well into the acutely inflamed prostate and antibiotics that normally do not diffuse into prostatic fluid from the bloodstream are effective. Prostatic penetration of antimicrobials occurs because the acute inflammatory reaction alters the cellular membrane barrier between the bloodstream and the prostate.

Most patients respond to empiric treatment with broad-spectrum antibiotics specifically covering gram-negative organisms. Usual therapy includes an aminoglycoside and a $\beta$-lactam antibiotic upon initial diagnosis. Therapy can be refined when the results of culture and sensitivity studies are known. Parenteral therapy is usually maintained until the patient is afebrile and less symptomatic. The total course of therapy should be 4 weeks. An appropriate oral antibiotic can be initiated usually after 5 to 7 days of intravenous therapy.

Chronic bacterial prostatitis is very difficult to cure. In the past, it was recognized that despite high serum concentrations of bactericidal drugs in excess of the MICs of the infecting organisms, bacteria (sensitive to the administered antibiotic) persisted in the prostatic fluid. The failure to eradicate the sensitive bacteria was thought to be related to the inability of antibiotics to reach sufficient concentrations in the prostatic fluid and cross the prostatic epithelium.

In a series of experiments in dogs, Winningham and colleagues[56] assessed the characteristics of diffusion of various antibiotics from plasma to canine prostatic fluid. The results showed that most antibiotics commonly used in the treatment of UTI did not achieve effective concentrations in the prostatic fluid, even when plasma levels were exceedingly elevated. The only group of antibiotics found to concentrate in the prostatic fluid was the macrolides (erythromycin, oleandomycin, rosamicin), trimethoprim, and clindamycin. The concentrations of these antibiotics were found to be several times that found in the plasma. From these experiments, it was apparent that most antibiotics could not cross the prostatic epithelium.

Several factors that determine antibiotic diffusion into prostatic secretions were delineated from the canine model. Lipid solubility is a major determinant because only lipid-soluble drugs can diffuse from plasma across epithelial membranes. The degree of ionization in plasma also affects the diffusion of drugs. Only un-ionized molecules can cross the lipid barrier of prostatic cells and the drug's $pK_a$ directly determines the fraction of unchanged drug.

The pH gradient across the membrane has an influence on tissue penetration as well. A pH gradient of at least 1 pH unit between separate compartments allows for ion trapping. As un-ionized drug crosses the epithelial barrier into prostatic fluid, it becomes ionized, thus allowing less drug to diffuse back across the lipid barrier. In early studies with the canine model, the prostatic pH was reported to be acidic, 6.4. More recent studies in man, however, have reported that the pH of prostatic secretions from the inflamed prostate is actually basic, 8.1 to 8.3.[50] This is dramatically different from that found in the canine model and affects the diffusing ability of antibiotics.

The choice of antibiotics in chronic bacterial prostatitis should include those agents that are capable of crossing the prostatic epithelium into the prostatic fluid in therapeutic concentrations and possess the spectrum of activity to be effective. Trimethoprim was considered the ideal drug based on its favorable chemical characteristics and its ability to concentrate well in the canine prostate. The rate of cure has been only 32% to 71% among patients receiving TMP 160 mg + SMX 800 mg twice daily for 4 to 16 weeks.[57–60] The low cure rates observed question the current recommendation that TMP–SMX is the drug of choice for CBP. The low cure rates may best be explained by the finding that the pH of prostatic fluid in humans with an inflammatory process is actually alkaline. This pH difference may impede the passage of TMP across the prostatic epithelium. The sulfonamide portion of TMP–SMX probably contributes very little to the activity of TMP in CBP.

Carbenicillin indanyl sodium has proven effective in the treatment of CBP, even though carbenicillin was found not to concentrate in the canine prostate. It has been demonstrated, however, that the esterified form of carbenicillin diffuses well into prostatic interstitial fluid and prostatic tissue.[61] Cure rates have been reported to be 60% to 74% in clinical trials.[62,63] Although carbenicillin is quite costly, it appears to be the most effective agent available at this time.

Other agents, including clindamycin, erythromycin, and tetracycline, are of limited value in the treatment of CBP because of their lack of activity against gram-negative organisms, even though they achieve therapeutic concentrations in the prostate. The one exception may be erythromycin. The activity of erythromycin has been shown to be greatly enhanced against gram-negative organisms in an alkaline environment. Since the inflamed prostatic fluid has an alkaline pH, erythromycin was examined in CBP patients with gram-negative organisms and achieved a cure rate of 88%.[64] Further examination is required; however, erythromycin may be useful in some patients when the infecting organism is sensitive.

Studies for the treatment of prostatitis are presently underway with various new quinolone antibiotics (e.g., enoxacin, ciprofloxacin). It is possible that these newer antimicrobials will play a major role in the treatment of prostatitis in the future.

## Summary

The treatment of prostatitis, particularly chronic prostatitis, continues to be a challenge for the clinician. Fortunately, acute prostatitis is very amenable to therapy. A main issue for future research is the need to assess the comparative efficacy of antimicrobials in the treatment of chronic prostatitis. The issue of prostatic penetration and its relevance to therapeutic outcome remains unanswered. For now, the clinician must await the outcome of research to provide better insight into the care of patients with prostatitis.

## References

1. Boineau FG, Lewy JE. Urinary tract infection in children: An overview. Pediatr Ann 1975;64:515–526.
2. Kunin CM, Deutscher R, Paquin AJ. Urinary tract infection in school children: An epidemiologic, clinical and laboratory study. Medicine 1964;43:91–130.
3. Smellie JM, Normand ICS. Bacteriuria, reflux and renal scarring. Arch Dis Child 1975;50:581–585.
4. Cattel WR. Urinary infection in adults—1985. Postgrad Med J 1985;61:907–913.
5. Sanford JP. Urinary tract symptoms and infections. Annu Rev Med 1975;26:485–498.
6. Kunin CM. An overview of urinary tract infections, in Kunin CM (ed): Detection, Prevention and Management of Urinary Tract Infections, 3rd ed. Philadelphia, Lea and Febiger, 1979, p 42.
7. Kaye D. Urinary tract infection in the elderly. Bull NY Acad Med 1980;56:209–220.
8. Stamey TA, Timothy M, Miller M, et al. Recurrent urinary infections in adult women: the role of introital enterobacteria. Calif Med 1971;3:115:1–19.
9. Sobel JD, Kaye D. Urinary tract infections, in Mandell GL, Douglas RG, Bennett JE (eds): Principles and Practice of Infectious Diseases, 2nd ed. New York, John Wiley and Sons, 1985, pp 426–452.
10. Kaye D. Antibacterial activity of human urine. J Clin Invest 1968;47:2374–2390.
11. Bryant RE, Sutcliffe MC, McGee ZA. Human polymorphonuclear leukocyte function in urine. Yale J Biol Med 1973;46: 113–124.
12. Marrie T, Kwan C, Noble M, et al. *Staphylococcus saprophyticus* as a cause of urinary tract infections. J Clin Microbiol 1982;16:427–431.
13. Jenkins RD, Fenn JP, Matsen JM. Review of urine microscopy for bacteriuria. JAMA 1986;255:3397–3403.
14. Sanford JP, Favour CB, Mao FH, et al. Evaluation of the "positive" urine culture. Am J Med 1956;20:88–93.
15. Stamey TA. Pathogenesis and Treatment of Urinary Tract Infections. Baltimore, Williams and Wilkins, 1980.
16. Stamm WE, Counts GW, Running KR, et al. Diagnosis of coliform infection in acutely dysuric women. N Engl J Med 1982;307:463–468.
17. Platt R. Quantitative definition of bacteriuria. Am J Med 1983; 75:44–52.
18. Kunin CM. New methods in detecting urinary tract infections. Urol Clin North Am 1975;2:423–432.
19. Thomas VL, Forland M. Antibody coated bacteria in urinary tract infections. Kidney Int 1982;21:1–7.
20. Merritt JL, Keys TF. Limitations of the antibody-coated bacteria test in patients with neurogenic bladders. JAMA 1982;247: 1723–1725.
21. Fang LT, Tolkoff-Rubin NE, Rubin RH. Efficacy of single-dose and conventional amoxicillin therapy in urinary tract infection localized by the antibody-coated bacteria technique. N Engl J Med 1978;298:413–416.
22. Gruneberg RN, Brumfitt W. Single-dose treatment of acute urinary tract infection: a controlled trial. Br Med J 1967;3: 649–651.
23. Rubin RH, Fang LST, Jones SR, et al. Single-dose amoxicillin therapy for urinary tract infections: multicenter trial using antibody-coated bacteria localization technique. JAMA 1980; 244:561–564.
24. Souney P, Polk BF. Single-dose antimicrobial therapy for urinary tract infection in women. Rev Infect Dis 1982;4:29–34.
25. Greenberg RN, Sanders CV, Marier R, et al. Single dose therapy of urinary tract infection with cefaclor (abstract 232). Presented at the 20th Interscience Conference on Antimicrobial Agents and Chemotherapy, New Orleans, 1980. Washington DC, American Society for Microbiology.
26. Philbrick JT, Bracikowski JP. Single-dose antibiotic treatment for uncomplicated urinary tract infections: less for less? Arch Intern Med 1985;145:1672–1678.

27. Greenberg RN, Reilly PM, Luppen KL, et al. Randomized study of single-dose, three-day, and seven-day treatment of cystitis in women. J Infect Dis 1986;153:277–282.
28. Smith JW, Jones SR, Reed WP, et al. Recurrent urinary tract infections in men. Characteristics and response to therapy. Ann Intern Med 1979;91:544–548.
29. Andriole VT. Urinary tract infection in pregnancy. Urol Clin North Am 1975;2:485–498.
30. Kass EH. Bacteriuria and pyelonephritis of pregnancy. Trans Assoc Am Physicians 1959;72:257–264.
31. Gruneberg R, Leigh D, Brumfitt W. Relationship of bacteriuria in pregnancy to acute pyelonephritis, prematurity and fetal mortality. Lancet 1969;2:1–3.
32. Gallagher DJA, Montgomerie JZ, North JDK. Acute infections of the urinary tract and the urethral syndrome in general practice. Br Med J 1965;1:622–626.
33. Stamm WE, Wagner KF, Amsel R, et al. Causes of the acute urethral syndrome in women. N Engl J Med 1980;303:409–415.
34. Stamm WE, Running K, McKevitt M, et al. Treatment of the acute urethral syndrome. N Engl J Med 1981;304:956–958.
35. Vosti KL. Recurrent urinary tract infections: prevention by prophylactic antibiotics after sexual intercourse. JAMA 1975; 231:934–940.
36. Turck M, Anderson KN, Petersdorf RG. Relapse and reinfection in chronic bacteriuria. N Engl J Med 1966;275:70–73.
37. Turck M, Ronald AR, Petersdorf RG. Relapse and reinfection in chronic bacteriuria. II. The correlation between site of infection and pattern of recurrence in chronic bacteriuria. N Engl J Med 1968;278:422–427
38. Ronald AR, Harding GKM. Urinary infection prophylaxis in women. Ann Intern Med 1981;94:268–270.
39. Holmberg L, Bowman G, Bottiger LE, et al. Adverse reactions to nitrofurantoin: analysis of 921 reports. Am J Med 1980;69: 733–738.
40. Turck M, Stamm W. Nosocomial infection of the urinary tract. Am J. Med 1981;70:651–654.
41. Turck M, Goffe B, Petersdorf RG. The urethral catheter and urinary tract infection. J Urol 1962;88:834–837.
42. Kass EH. Asymptomatic infections of the urinary tract. Trans Assoc Am Physicians 1956;69:56–64.
43. Andriole VT. Hospital acquired urinary tract infections and the indwelling catheter. Urol Clin North Am 1975;2:451–469.
44. Warren JW, Platt R, Thomas RJ, et al. Antibiotic irrigation and catheter-associated urinary-tract infections. N Engl J Med 1978; 299:570–573.
45. Garibaldi RA, Burke JP, Dickman ML, et al. Factors predisposing to bacteriuria during indwelling urethral catheterization. N Engl J Med 1974;291:215–219.
46. Drach GW, Meares EM Jr, Fair WR, et al. Classification of benign diseases associated with prostatic pain: prostatitis or prostatodynia? J Urol 1978;120:266.
47. Drach GW. Sexuality and prostatitis. A hypothesis. J Am Vener Dis Assoc 1976;3:87.
48. Meares EM Jr, Barbalias GA. Prostatitis: bacterial, non-bacterial and prostatodynia. Semin Urol 1983;1:146–154.
49. Fair WR, Couch J. Wehner N. Prostatic antibacterial factor: identity and significance. Urology 1976;7:169–177.
50. Pfau A, Perlberg S, Shapiro A. The pH of prostatic fluid in health and disease: implications of treatment in chronic bacterial prostatitis. J Urol 1978;119:384–387.
51. Fair WR, Crane DB, Schiller N, et al. A re-appraisal of treatment in chronic bacterial prostatitis. J Urol 1979;121: 437–441.
52. Meares EM. Prostatitis: a review. Urol Clin North Am 1975;2: 3–27.
53. Drach GW. Prostatitis: man's hidden infection. Urol Clin North Am 1975;2:499–520.
54. Meares EM Jr, Stamey TA. Bacteriologic localization patterns in bacterial prostatitis and urethritis. Invest Urol 1968;5: 492–518.
55. Schmidt JD, Patterson MC. Needle biopsy study of chronic prostatitis. J Urol 1966;96:519–533.
56. Winningham DC, Nemoy NJ, Stamey TA. Diffusion of antibiotics from plasma into prostatic fluid. Nature 1968;219:139–143.
57. Paulson DF, White RD. Trimethoprim–sulfamethoxazole and minocycline hydrochloride in the treatment of culture-proved bacterial prostatitis. J Urol 1978;120:184–185.
58. Meares EM. Long-term therapy of chronic bacterial prostatitis with trimethoprim–sulfamethoxazole. Can Med Assoc J 1975; 112(suppl):22s–25s.
59. Drach GW. Trimethoprim/sulfamethoxazole therapy of chronic bacterial prostatitis. J Urol 1974;111:637–639.
60. McGuire EJ, Lytton B. Bacterial prostatitis: treatment with trimethoprim–sulfamethoxazole. Urology 1976;7:499–500.
61. Madsen PO, Baumueller A, Hoyme U. Experimental models for determination of antimicrobials in prostatic tissue, interstitial fluid and secretion. Scand J Infect Dis 1978;14(suppl):145–150.
62. Oliveri RA, Sachs RM, Caste PG. Clinical experience with Geocillin in the treatment of bacterial prostatitis. Curr Ther Res 1979;25:415–421.
63. Mobley DF. Bacterial prostatitis: treatment with carbenicillin indanyl sodium. Invest Urol 1981;19:31–33.
64. Mobley DF. Erythromycin plus sodium bicarbonate in chronic bacterial prostatitis. Urology 1974;3:60–62.

# Chapter 85 / Sexually Transmitted Diseases

Leroy C. Knodel, PharmD

Through the centuries, sexually transmitted diseases (STDs) have been included among the great scourges of mankind. The lives and careers of numerous historical figures including Henry VIII, Napoleon Bonaparte, and Christopher Columbus are known to have been affected by these diseases. Today, as a result of their epidemic nature and potential for significant morbidity, STDs are recognized as a serious public health problem both in the United States and worldwide.

Over the years the spectrum of STDs has broadened from the classic venereal diseases—gonorrhea, syphilis, chancroid, lymphogranuloma venereum, and granuloma inguinale—to include a variety of pathogens known to be spread by sexual contact (Table 85.1).[1,2] *Chlamydia trachomatis* infections, genital herpes, cytomegalovirus infections, genital mycoplasmas, group B streptococcal infections, hepatitis, nonspecific vaginitis, enteric infections, genital warts, ectoparasitic diseases, and the acquired immune deficiency syndrome (AIDS) are now recognized as diseases for which sexual contact is epidemiologically important. Although most of these conditions have probably existed since antiquity, improvement in diagnostic capabilities and epidemiologic investigations has increased their recognition. Because of the large number of infected individuals, the diversity of clinical manifestations, and the high frequency of multiple STDs occurring simultaneously in infected individuals, the diagnosis and management of patients with STDs are much more complex than even a decade ago.

Advances in the diagnosis and treatment of STDs have coincided with increased recognition of the complications of these diseases. Despite a higher reported incidence of all major STDs in men, the complications of STDs generally are more frequent and severe in women. In particular, serious effects on maternal and infant health during pregnancy are well documented. Damage to reproductive organs, increased risk of cancer, and complications associated with pregnancy such as ectopic pregnancy, spontaneous abortion, stillbirth, prematurity, and transmission of disease to the fetus or newborn are associated with several common STDs.

As a result of the physiologic, psychosocial, and economic consequences of STDs, and because of the increasing incidence of STDs such as AIDS and genital herpes, for which curative therapy is not available, there has been a resurgence of interest in STD research and the primary prevention of these diseases.[3]

The most frequently occurring STDs in the United States are reviewed in this chapter. For other less common STDs, only recommended treatment regimens are presented. Because of the increasing incidence of AIDS in the United States and Europe and our rapidly developing understanding of its epidemiology, pathophysiology, clinical presentation, and diagnosis, this syndrome is discussed in a separate chapter (Chapter 91).

## Epidemiology

Numerous interrelated factors have been shown to contribute to the epidemic nature of sexually transmitted diseases. Sociocultural, demographic, and economic factors together with patterns of sexual behavior, host susceptibility to infection, changing properties of the causative pathogens, and environmental factors are important determinants of the frequency and distribution of STDs in the United States and worldwide. In the United States, accurate data on the incidence and distribution of STDs are incomplete because many of these diseases are not reportable. Even for those that are required to be reported, such as gonorrhea and syphilis, surveys indicate that gross underreporting occurs.[2,3]

Because of the heterogeneous nature of STDs, factors influencing their incidence or spread are not always consistent among the individual diseases. Some uniformity is seen for the major STDs, however, when various demographic factors are evaluated.

Age is one of the most important demographic determinants of STD incidence. Overall, STDs are more common in persons in their twenties and middle to late teens, the peak years of sexual activity. With increasing age, the incidence of most STDs decreases exponentially. In sexually active teenagers, STD rates are highest in the youngest, suggesting that physiologic differences may contribute to their susceptibility. For some STDs such as gonorrhea, changing age demographics in the United States appear to have contributed to recent declines in their incidence.[2,4]

Age-specific rates of STDs are higher in men than in women; however, reported rates may not represent true gender differences, but rather may reflect greater ease of detection in men. For many STDs the clinical manifestations are more obvious in men, resulting in a greater percentage seeking confirmatory diagnosis and treatment. In recent years, the ratio of male to female cases for most STDs except syphilis has declined. Major reasons proposed for this change appear to be improvement in diagnosis of STDs in asymptomatic women and changes in female sexual behavior following the availability of improved methods of contraception. Although quite common in homosexual men, STDs are rare in homosexual women.[2,4]

Rates for many STDs including gonorrhea and syphilis are higher in blacks than whites, and are lowest in Orientals; however, herpes genitalis is a common STD that has a disproportionately higher incidence in whites than blacks.

**Table 85.1** Sexually Transmitted Diseases

| *Disease* | *Pathogen* |
|---|---|
| Bacterial | |
| Gonorrhea | *Neisseria gonorrhoeae* |
| Syphilis | *Treponema pallidum* |
| Chancroid | *Hemophilus ducreyi* |
| Granuloma inguinale (donovanosis) | *Calymmatobacterium granulomatis* |
| Salmonellosis | *Salmonella* sp. |
| Shigellosis | *Shigella* sp. |
| *Campylobacter* infection | *Campylobacter jejuni* |
| Nonspecific vaginitis | *Trichomonas vaginalis* |
| Group B streptococcal infections | Group B streptococcus |
| Chlamydial | |
| Nongonococcal urethritis | *Chlamydia trachomatis* |
| Lymphogranuloma venereum | *Chlamydia trachomatis* |
| Viral | |
| Herpes genitalis | Herpes simplex |
| Hepatitis B | Hepatitis B virus |
| Condylomata acuminata | Human papilloma virus |
| Molluscum contagiosum | Poxvirus |
| Cytomegalovirus infection | Cytomegalovirus |
| Mycoplasmal | |
| Nongonococcal urethritis | *Ureaplasma urealyticum* |
| Protozoal | |
| Trichomoniasis | T. vaginalis |
| Amebiasis | *Entamoeba histolytica* |
| Giardiasis | *Giardia lamblia* |
| Fungal | |
| Candidiasis | *Candida albicans* |
| Parasitic | |
| Scabies | *Sarcoptes scabiei* |
| Pediculosis | *Pediculus pubis* |
| Enterobiasis | *Enterobius vermicularis* |

Although not well studied, it is possible that race/ethnic disparities are related to socioeconomic differences.[2,4]

Sexual preference also plays a major role in the transmission of STDs. For all major STDs, rates are disproportionately greater in homosexual men than in heterosexuals. Also, a number of less common STDs, including several caused by enteric protozoans and bacterial pathogens, occur primarily in homosexual men. The major risk factors for homosexual men appear to be related to the greater number of sexual partners and the sexual practices of anal–genital and oral–anal intercourse.[2,4]

Marital status, socioeconomic status, and place of residence are also epidemiologically important when considering STDs. STDs are more common among single, separated, and divorced persons than among married individuals. Also, morbidity rates are highest among individuals of the lowest socioeconomic status and among urban populations.[2,4]

## Common Clinical Syndromes Caused by Sexually Transmitted Diseases

The varied spectrum of clinical syndromes produced by common STDs is determined not only by the etiologic pathogen(s) but also by differences in male and female anatomy and reproductive physiology. For many STDs the signs and symptoms overlap sufficiently to prevent accurate diagnosis without microbiologic confirmation. Frequently, symptoms are minimal or absent despite the presence of infection. Common clinical syndromes associated with STDs are listed in Table 85.2.

### *Lower Urogenital Infections*

In men, urethritis, characterized by urethral discharge and dysuria, is the most common presenting symptom of STD. Discharges are broadly categorized as either gonococcal or nongonococcal. The most common causes of nongonococcal urethritis are *Chlamydia trachomatis* and *Ureaplasma urealyticum*, although intraurethral herpes simplex and syphilitic lesions also can produce a urethral discharge. Frequently, gonococcal and nongonococcal urethral infections are asymptomatic, producing little if any discharge. Complications that are infrequently associated with sexually transmitted urogenital pathogens are epididymitis and acute and chronic prostatitis. In men under 35 years of age, STD is the most common cause of epididymitis.

Symptoms of lower urogenital tract infection are more variable in women than in men and, therefore, are difficult to attribute to a particular anatomic site without a comprehen-

**Table 85.2** Selected Syndromes Associated With Common Sexually Transmitted Pathogens

| *Syndrome* | *Pathogen* |
|---|---|
| Lower urogenital tract infections in men | |
| Urethritis | *Chlamydia trachomatis*, herpes simplex virus, *Neisseria gonorrhoeae*, *Trichomonas vaginalis*, *Ureaplasma urealyticum* |
| Epididymitis | *C. trachomatis*, *N. gonorrhoeae* |
| Lower urogenital tract infections in women | |
| Cervicitis | *C. trachomatis*, herpes simplex virus, *N. gonorrhoeae* |
| Urethritis | *C. trachomatis*, herpes simplex virus, *N. gonorrhoeae* |
| Vulvitis/vaginitis | Herpes simplex virus, *T. vaginalis* |
| Genital ulcers | Herpes simplex virus, *Treponema pallidum* |
| Pharyngitis | *C. trachomatis* (?), herpes simplex virus, *N. gonorrhoeae* |
| Proctitis | *C. trachomatis*, *N. gonorrhoeae*, herpes simplex virus |
| Salpingitis | *C. trachomatis*, *N. gonorrhoeae* |
| Congenital or neonatal infections | *C. trachomatis*, herpes simplex virus, *N. gonorrhoeae*, *T. pallidum*, *U. urealyticum* |
| Torche's syndrome | Herpes simplex virus, *T. pallidum* |

sive pelvic examination. Symptoms such as dysuria are seen with cystitis, urethritis, or vulvovaginitis and vaginal discharge can be secondary to infection of the uterus, cervix, or vagina.

### Genital Ulcers

Genital ulceration is a common symptom of several STDs. In men the ulcers are more easily recognized because of their external location; in women visualization frequently requires internal examination. In the United States the two most common causes of genital ulceration are herpes simplex virus infections and syphilis. Herpes simplex lesions are commonly multiple and painful, while ulcers associated with syphilis are usually painless and single. In both diseases enlargement of inguinal lymph nodes commonly occurs. If secondarily infected, more extensive ulceration can result. In the absence of secondary infections the ulcers of syphilis and herpes genitalis spontaneously heal with little or no scarring; however, recurrence of lesions is common in genital herpes infections.

### Pharyngitis

Pharyngitis after orogenital contact with infected individuals is not uncommon and the incidence is particularly high in male homosexuals. The majority of cases of gonococcal pharyngitis are asymptomatic and resolve spontaneously, while herpes simplex virus infections usually produce moderate to severe pharyngitis.

### Proctitis

In recent years, the anorectal region has been recognized increasingly as a common site of infection for some sexually transmitted pathogens. Genital–anal contact and oral–anal contact are implicated most frequently in homosexual males. In women, a high percentage of anorectal infections probably result from contiguous spread from the genitalia. For some pathogens such as *Neisseria gonorrhoeae* and *C. trachomatis*, anorectal infections are frequently asymptomatic. If present, symptoms may range from mild to very severe constipation, anorectal discomfort, tenesmus, and mucopurulent rectal discharge.

### Salpingitis

Some pathogens ascend the lower genital tract to the endometrium, endosalpinx, perimetrial tissues, and peritoneal cavity, producing an infectious syndrome referred to as *salpingitis* or *pelvic inflammatory disease*. Chlamydial and gonorrheal infections are the most common etiologies. In some cases a sexually transmitted pathogen is implicated directly as the cause of infection; in others it may only initiate an inflammatory process that allows secondary infection by other microorganisms. Common presenting symptoms include abdominal pain, vaginal bleeding, and fever. Tissue damage and scarring increase with each episode of salpingitis, making it a leading cause of infertility, ectopic pregnancy, and chronic pelvic pain in women.

### Congenital and Perinatal Infections

Some of the most serious adverse effects of STDs are associated with congenital or perinatal infections. The majority of neonatal infections are acquired at birth, after infant passage through an infected cervix or vagina. Neonatal *C. trachomatis*, *N. gonorrhoeae*, and herpes simplex virus infections are associated with this type of spread. For pregnant women with syphilis, infection is usually transmitted transplacentally, producing a congenital infection. Depending on the organism, neonatal infections can manifest in a variety of ways. Ophthalmia neonatorum can result from chlamydial or gonorrheal infections, while syphilis and herpes infections can produce more severe complications including neurologic impairment. Neonatal herpes infections are also associated with a high mortality.

### *Syndromes Affecting Multiple Sites*

On rare occasions some STDs produce serious complications associated with multiple anatomic sites. Evidence is strong that genital inflammation, sexually or nonsexually transmitted, is involved in the pathogenesis of Reiter's syndrome.[5] In up to 50% of cases of Reiter's syndrome, *C. trachomatis* has been implicated as the initiating factor. In addition to urethritis, this syndrome is characterized by polyarthropathy, mucous membrane lesions of the mouth and penis, and nonspecific symptoms of fever, malaise, and anorexia. Conjunctivitis is seen in up to 50% of cases. Although most cases resolve within 6 to 12 months, relapses occur.

In 1% to 3% of patients with genital gonorrhea, a disseminated form of the disease develops. It is more common in women than in men and typically produces arthralgias, arthritis, tenosynovitis, and rash. More serious complications such as endocarditis, myocarditis, hepatitis, and meningitis occur rarely.

## Gonorrhea

Galen first used the term *gonorrhea* (Greek for "flow of seed") in 130 AD to describe a urethral discharge he mistakenly believed to be composed of semen. Today, the term is applied to disease caused by the gram-negative diplococcus *Neisseria gonorrhoeae*. Man is the only known natural host of this intracellular parasite.[6–9]

Because of its rapid incubation period and the large number of infected individuals with asymptomatic disease, gonorrhea is difficult to control. Since 1965, gonorrhea has represented the most frequently reported communicable disease in the United States. Although the incidence of gonorrhea has been on a general decline in the United States since 1975, almost 1 million cases are reported annually and it is estimated that twice as many cases are treated.[6–9]

The risk of a male acquiring urethral infection after a single episode of vaginal intercourse with an infected female is approximately 20% to 35% and increases dramatically with multiple exposure. It is thought that the risk of transmission is greater from males to females than females to males. No data are available on the risk of transmission after other types of sexual contact.[6–9]

On contact with a mucosal surface, the gonococci attach to cell membranes by means of surface pili. The virulence of the organism is mediated primarily by the presence of pili and other outer membrane proteins. Several methods of classifying infecting strains of *N. gonorrhoeae* have been developed including serotyping and auxotyping. Serotyping is based on identification of major outer membrane proteins of the gonococcus. Auxotyping, based on differential nutritional requirements of the gonococci, has been used most extensively in epidemiologic studies. One auxotype requiring arginine, hypoxanthine, and uracil (AHU) is implicated most frequently with disseminated infections and in a high percentage of asymptomatic urethral infections. This strain is particularly sensitive to penicillin and tetracycline. The prevalence of different auxotypes varies based on geographic location, race, and sexual preference. In male homosexuals, the AHU auxotype is less frequently the etiologic strain and this may account for the higher incidence of penicillin treatment failures in these individuals.[10]

### *Clinical Presentation*

The clinical presentation of gonorrheal infections is varied. Infected individuals may be symptomatic or asymptomatic, have complicated or uncomplicated infections, and have infections involving several anatomic sites.[6–9]

Urethritis is the most common presenting manifestation in males, and usually develops within 2–8 days of exposure. Dysuria and frequency of urination are seen initially, followed in 1–2 days by a profuse, purulent urethral discharge. In approximately 25%, the discharge is scant and only minimally purulent, making it almost indistinguishable from nongonococcal urethritis. The majority of symptomatic patients who are not treated become asymptomatic within 6 months, with only a few becoming asymptomatic carriers of the disease. Complications resulting from extensions of the infection in males, such as epididymitis, prostatitis, inguinal lymphadenopathy, and urethral stricture, rarely are seen today.[6–9]

The most common site of gonococcal infection in women is the endocervical canal. Anterior spread of infected vaginal secretions produces urethritis. The incubation period is more variable in females but symptoms typically appear within 10 days of exposure. Symptoms are relatively nonspecific and include dysuria, increased frequency of urination, abnormal vaginal discharge, and abnormal uterine bleeding. Diagnosis based on symptoms alone is confounded because infection with other organisms may produce similar manifestations. Most gonococcal urethral and cervical infections in females either are asymptomatic or produce minimal symptoms.[6–9]

Other sites of gonococcal infection include the rectum, oropharynx, and eye. Anorectal gonococcal infections are common in females and in homosexual males. In homosexuals rectal intercourse is the primary cause, whereas most infections in women are due to perineal contamination with vaginal discharge. Many patients with anorectal gonorrhea have minimal if any symptoms. When present, symptoms range from mild pruritis to severe rectal pain, tenesmus, and a mucopurulent rectal discharge.[6–9]

Like rectal infections, pharyngeal infections are more common in females and homosexual males. Symptoms can mimic pharyngitis or tonsillitis, although patients are typically asymptomatic. Gonococcal conjunctivitis is rare and usually results from autoinoculation via the fingers from an anogenital infection.[6–9]

Gonococcal infections in newborns result primarily from passage through an infected birth canal but may also be transmitted in utero. The most common form of infection in neonates is ophthalmia neonatorum, although membranes of the vagina, pharynx, or rectum also can become colonized. Conjunctival involvement usually develops within 1–7 days of delivery and is characterized by intense, bilateral conjunctival inflammation with chemosis. If not promptly treated, corneal ulceration and blindness can develop. Because of routine neonatal ocular prophylaxis, gonococcal ophthalmia neonatorum is uncommon in the United States. Disseminated gonorrhea in infants rarely is seen today, but when it does occur it often presents as infectious arthritis.[6–9,11]

Other complications associated with gonococcal infections include pelvic inflammatory disease and disseminated gonococcal infections. Approximately 15% of women with gonorrhea develop pelvic inflammatory disease, with its attendant tissue damage. In 1% to 3% of patients with gonorrhea, the gonococci invade the bloodstream and produce disseminated disease. Disseminated gonorrhea infections (DGIs) are three times more common in women than in men. The usual clinical manifestations of DGI are skin lesions, tenosynovitis, and monoarticular arthritis. Occasionally, mild hepatitis, myocarditis, and endocarditis occur; very rarely, gonococcal meningitis is reported. The majority of cases of DGI are due to the AHU gonococcus auxotype which is very susceptible to penicillin therapy.[6–9,10]

### *Diagnosis*

Diagnosis of gonococcal infections can be made by Gram-stained smears, culture, or newer methods based on the detection of cellular components of the gonococcus (enzymes, antigens, DNA, or lipopolysaccharide) in clinical specimens.

Various stains have been used to identify gonococci microscopically, with the Gram stain most widely used in clinical practice. Gram-stained smears are positive for gonococci when gram-negative diplococci of typical kidney bean morphology are identified within polymorphonuclear leukocytes. In the presence of equivocal smears (e.g., extracellular gonococcal forms that can be nonpathogenic, commensal *Neisseria*, or gram-negative diplococci of atypical morphology), a culture is mandatory. In urethral smears from men with symptomatic urethritis, the smear is highly sensitive and specific and culture is considered optional. Gram-stained smears are specific but insensitive for endocervical, rectal, cutaneous, and asymptomatic male urethral infections. In these situations culture is the most reliable means of diagnosis. Because of the presence of nonpathogenic *Neisseria* in the pharynx of most people, Gram stain is not useful in the diagnosis of pharyngeal infection.[6–9]

Culture is considered the most reliable means of diagnosing gonococcal infections. Various antibiotic-containing media such as modified Thayer–Martin medium or New York City medium are used. Anatomic sites to be cultured depend on the individual's sexual preferences and body areas exposed. In women, because the urethra and other sites are rarely the sole locus of infection, cervical cultures give the highest yield and are frequently performed in conjunction with rectal cultures. Urethral cultures are recommended in women who have had hysterectomies. In homosexual males, anorectal cultures generally give the highest yields and pharyngeal and urethral cultures are considered optional.[6–9]

Because technical constraints and cost preclude the use of culture techniques in most office settings and clinics, alternative methods of diagnosis have been developed that do not require convenient accessibility to a microbiology laboratory. These rapid diagnostic tests, which can be performed easily in an office, are based on detection of gonococcal antigens, enzymes, DNA, endotoxin, or lipopolysaccharride in clinical specimens. In most cases the tests have not been shown to have increased sensitivity or specificity over either Gram stain for symptomatic gonococcal urethritis in men or culture in women with endocervical infections. For gonococcal infections other than symptomatic urethritis in males, the tests may prove to offer more rapid means of diagnosis than culture.[6–9]

Various serologic tests are available to detect antibody to *N. gonorrhoeae* or its components, but most are not sufficiently sensitive or specific to be clinically useful at present.

In areas where penicillinase-producing strains of *N. gonorrhoeae* are prevalent, $\beta$-lactamase testing is an important consideration once the diagnosis of gonococcal infection is established. Testing is usually done using iodometric, acidometric, or chromogenic cephalosporin disk testing.[6–9]

### *Treatment*

In vitro, a number of antimicrobial agents exhibit good activity against most strains of *N. gonorrhoeae*. These include the penicillins, cephalosporins, tetracyclines, macrolides, and rifampin. In the 1930s sulfonamides were widely used in the treatment of gonorrhea but within a few years widespread resistance was reported. In 1943 Mahoney and colleagues were the first to report the efficacy of penicillin in the treatment of gonorrhea. Soon after, single-dose penicillin became standard therapy. In the 1950s partial resistance to penicillins became apparent and by the 1970s a high percentage of chromosomally mediated resistant *N. gonorrhoeae* (CMRNG) strains had developed that exhibited low-level penicillin resistance. Similar trends were also noted with tetracyclines, spectinomycin, and other antibiotics. To circumvent this low-level resistance, higher doses of antibiotics and the concomitant use of probenecid with penicillin became standard.[6–8,12]

In early 1976, penicillinase-producing strains of *N. gonorrhoeae* that demonstrated absolute resistance to penicillins secondary to plasmid-mediated production of $\beta$-lactamase were isolated. Today, penicillinase-producing strains are widespread throughout the world, constituting a significant percentage of all strains in the Philippines, Southeast Asia, and parts of Africa. Although these strains are responsible for less than 1% of all cases of gonorrhea in the United States, they constitute a much higher percentage of all gonococcal infections in certain areas of the country, and their isolation is increasing dramatically. Many PPNG strains are also highly resistant to tetracycline, as are some penicillin-sensitive strains.[6–8,12,13]

Many antimicrobial regimens are effective in treating uncomplicated gonorrhea; however, no single therapeutic regimen can be recommended as optimal because of regional differences in susceptibility and the high incidence of coexistent infections (particularly *Chlamydia trachomatis*) in certain populations. Recommendations of the Centers for Disease Control for the treatment of gonorrhea are given in Table 85.3.[14]

For uncomplicated infections, treatment with amoxicillin, ampicillin, or aqueous procaine penicillin G (APPG)—plus probenecid—or ceftriaxone is recommended, as these agents

**Table 85.3** Treatment for Gonorrhea

| *Type of Infection* | *Regimen of choice* | *Alternative regimen* |
|---|---|---|
| Uncomplicated urethral, endocervical, or rectal infection | Amoxicillin 3.0 g or ampicillin 3.5 g PO or aqueous procaine penicillin G (APPG) 4.8 million units IM or ceftriaxone 250 mg IM (amoxicillin, ampicillin, and penicillin are accompanied by probenecid 1.0 g PO)[b] | [a] |
| | *plus* | |
| | Tetracycline HCl 500 mg PO 4 times daily for 7 days or doxycycline 100 mg PO twice daily for 7 days | Erythromycin base or stearate 500 mg PO 4 times daily for 7 days or erythromycin ethyl succinate 800 mg PO 4 times daily for 7 days |
| Penicillin-resistant infection | | |
| Penicillinase-producing *Neisseria gonorrhoeae* (PPNG) | Spectinomycin 2.0 g IM or ceftriaxone 250 mg IM[c] | |
| | *plus* | |
| | Tetracycline or doxycycline (as outlined above) | Erythromycin (as outlined above) |
| Chromosomally mediated resistant *N. gonorrhoeae*[d] | Spectinomycin 2.0 g or ceftriaxone 250 mg IM | |
| Gonococcal infections in pregnancy | Amoxicillin 3.0 g or ampicillin 3.5 g PO or ceftriaxone 250 mg IM or APPG 4.8 million units IM (amoxicillin, ampicillin, and penicillin regimens are accompanied by probenecid 1.0 g PO) | Spectinomycin 2.0 g IM |
| | *plus* | *plus* |
| | Erythromycin base 500 mg or erythromycin ethyl succinate 800 mg PO 4 times daily for 7 days | Erythromycin |
| Disseminated gonococcal infection[e,f] | Aqueous crystalline penicillin G 10 million units IV daily for at least 3 days followed by amoxicillin or ampicillin 500 mg PO 4 times daily to complete at least 7 days of therapy *or* Amoxicillin 3.0 g or ampicillin 3.5 g each with probenecid 1.0 g PO followed by amoxicillin or ampicillin 500 mg PO 4 times daily for at least 7 days *or* Cefoxitin 1.0 g IV 4 times daily for at least 7 days *or* Cefotaxime 500 mg IV 4 times daily for 7 days *or* Ceftriaxone 1.0 g IV once daily for 7 days | Tetracycline HCl 500 mg PO 4 times daily for at least 7 days *or* Doxycycline 100 mg PO twice daily for at least 7 days |
| Gonococcal ophthalmia | | |
| Adults | Aqueous crystalline penicillin G 10 million units IV daily for 5 days | |

**Table 85.3** (Continued)

| *Type of infection* | *Regimen of choice* | *Alternative regimen* |
|---|---|---|
| | For PPNG, either cefoxitin 1.0 g IV 4 times daily for 5 days, or cefotaxime 500 mg IV 4 times daily for 5 days, or ceftriaxone 1.0 g IM daily for 5 days | |
| Neonates | Aqueous crystalline penicillin G 100,000 units/kg/d IV in 4 divided doses for 7 days | |
| | For PPNG, cefotaxime or gentamicin in appropriate neonatal doses | |
| Infants born to mothers with gonococcal infection | For full-term infants, aqueous crystalline penicillin G 50,000 units IM or IV as a single dose[g] | |
| | For low-birth-weight infants, aqueous crystalline penicillin G 20,000 units IM or IV as a single dose[g] | |

[a] Patients allergic to penicillins, cephalosporins, or probenecid should be treated with tetracycline or doxycycline for 7 days. Patients not tolerating tetracyclines can be treated with spectinomycin 2.0 g IM followed by erythromycin (except homosexual men with rectal infections).

[b] Homosexual men with rectal gonorrhea should be treated with ceftriaxone or APPG plus probenecid. For those allergic to penicillin, spectinomycin 2.0 g IM should be used. Spectinomycin is not recommended for pharyngeal gonococcal infections. Routine additional tetracycline treatment is not recommended, as homosexual men are less likely than heterosexual men to have coexisting chlamydia.

[c] Pharyngeal infections from PPNG should be treated with ceftriaxone 250 mg IM or nine tablets of trimethoprim–sulfamethoxazole (720 mg/3,600 mg) in one daily dose for 5 days.

[d] For patients who fail standard treatment for gonorrhea or who have infection with penicillin strains that do not produce $\beta$-lactamase.

[e] Except for homosexual men, patients treated with one of the recommended regimens should be treated with tetracycline, doxycycline, or erythromycin for an additional 7 days for possible coexistent chlamydial infection.

[f] For disseminated infections caused by PPNG the cefoxitin, cefotaxime, or ceftriaxone regimen is recommended.

[g] Clinical illness requires additional treatment.

Recommendations are those of the CDC.[14]

are effective in single doses. Because coexisting chlamydial infection is documented in up to 45% of individuals with gonorrhea and is the major cause of postgonococcal urethritis in men and postgonococcal cervicitis and salpingitis in women, concomitant treatment with tetracycline, doxycycline, or erythromycin is also recommended in heterosexual adults.[14] None of the single-dose regimens recommended for gonorrhea is effective against chlamydia. While the tetracycline regimen in general has good activity against *N. gonorrhoeae*, *C. trachomatis*, and some strains of *Ureaplasma urealyticum*, concerns about patient compliance with multiple-day regimens and the recent increase in gonococcal resistance to tetracycline have been raised. Therefore, single-dose penicillins/cephalosporins are still the preferred treatment of gonorrhea. Also, tetracyclines are significantly less effective than either APPG or trimethoprim–sulfamethoxazole for gonorrhea in women.[6,12–15]

APPG offers the advantage of being the most effective antimicrobial for pharyngeal and rectal infections. It is the only antimicrobial listed in CDC recommendations that is effective against incubating syphilis; however, it requires two moderately painful intramuscular injections and has the potential to cause allergic and procaine-related reactions. Approximately 0.1% to 0.3% of patients develop procaine toxicity. Manifestations can include extreme anxiety, violent behavior, disorientation, hallucinations, psychosis, and seizures. The reaction is self-limited, lasting 15–30 minutes, but can be more severe in patients inadvertently given the drug intravenously. Ampicillin and amoxicillin offer the advantages of ease of oral administration and lower cost, while avoiding the potential for procaine reactions.[6,12–15]

For *N. gonorrhoeae* resistant to penicillin and tetracycline, spectinomycin or ceftriaxone in single doses is recommended. Neither is effective against coexisting chlamydia and some strains of PPNG resistant to spectinomycin have been reported; however, the resistance to spectinomycin appears to be chromosomally mediated rather than plasmid mediated, and can be overcome with higher doses. Side effects of spectinomycin are minimal; discomfort at the site of injection is most frequently reported. Like the penicillins and cephalosporins, spectinomycin can be safely administered during pregnancy. Newer cephalosporins such as cefotaxime and cefoxitin in single doses are effective against PPNG and PPNG resistant to spectinomycin, but have been less well studied. Among the newer cephalosporins shown to be effective in single doses, ceftriaxone offers the advantage of a longer half-life and greater in vitro activity against *N. gonorrhoeae*.[6,12–15]

In general, single-dose regimens for treatment of gonorrhea followed by a 7-day course of tetracyclines or erythromycin are advocated. APPG plus probenecid is preferred in homosexual males because of its efficacy in rectal, pharyngeal, and urethral gonorrhea and incubating syphilis. Incubating syphilis is seen more often in homosexual than heterosexual men. Treatment failure rates are unacceptable for ampicillin and tetracycline regimens in treating rectal infections and for spectinomycin and ampicillin in treating pharyngeal infections. For penicillin or spectinomycin treatment failures, gonococcal isolates should be tested for $\beta$-lactamase production or spectinomycin resistance, respectively.[6,12–15]

Strains of *N. gonorrhoeae* found in most cases of disseminated gonorrhea are highly susceptible to penicillins. A few cases of disseminated gonorrhea are due to PPNG and are effectively treated with ceftriaxone, cefoxitin, cefotaxime, or spectinomycin. Although marked improvement is usually noted within 48 hours of initiation of therapy, therapy should be continued for 7–10 days. Analgesics may be necessary in patients with joint involvement.[6,12–15]

Gonococcal ophthalmia is highly contagious in adults and neonates and requires intravenous penicillin G therapy. Topical antibiotics are not sufficiently effective when used alone, and are not necessary with appropriate systemic therapy. For PPNG infections, cefoxitin, cefotaxime, and ceftriaxone have been shown to be effective; in neonates, cefotaxime or gentamicin is recommended.[6,12–15]

Prevention of ophthalmia neonatorum is a primary goal in the medical care of newborns. Therefore, prevention or treatment of gonorrhea in the mother is most desirable. As a precaution, however, neonatal prophylaxis with topical ocular antimicrobials is required by law in most states. The American Academy of Pediatrics recommends that either silver nitrate (1%), tetracycline (1%), or erythromycin (0.5%) be instilled in each conjunctival sac immediately postpartum. Treatment failures have been reported for each agent. In the past silver nitrate has been used most commonly; however, tetracycline and erythromycin are being used more frequently today because of their activity against chlamydia, another important cause of ophthalmia neonatorum. Also, silver nitrate produces a chemical conjunctivitis that may make assessment of therapeutic efficacy difficult.[6,12–16]

Patients treated for gonorrhea should have follow-up cultures of all known infected sites performed at least 3 days after treatment. If tetracycline is used, repeat cultures should not be performed until 4–5 days after the last dose, because of persistence of tetracycline in the serum.[6,14]

Although penicillin has been the mainstay in the treatment of gonorrhea for the past 40 years, the increasing incidence of penicillin resistance has resulted in the evaluation of many newer antibiotics. Second- and third-generation cephalosporins including cefoxitin, cefuroxime, moxalactam, cefoperazone, ceftizoxime, cefonicid, cefotaxime, and ceftriaxone have shown good activity against penicillin-sensitive *N. gonorrhoeae* and PPNG; however, increased penicillin resistance demonstrated by CMRNG appears to correlate with increased resistance to other $\beta$-lactam antibiotics such as the cephalosporins.[6,12,14,17]

Sulfamethoxazole–trimethoprim in doses of 6–10 tablets once daily for 3–5 days has been demonstrated to have efficacy in the treatment of PPNG and non-PPNG infections and produces acceptable cure rates for coexisting *C. trachomatis*; however, these regimens have been associated with a high incidence of neurologic side effects. In preliminary trials the $\beta$-lactamase inhibitors sodium clavulanate and sulbactam in combination with penicillin, ampicillin, or amoxicillin have been used successfully in treating PPNG. Aztreonam, the first monobactam antibiotic approved for use in the United States, also has been shown to be effective in PPNG and non-PPNG infections.[12,14,18]

Norfloxacin and rosoxacin (investigational), two quinolone antibiotics, are highly effective in treating most strains of gonorrhea including PPNG when given in a two-dose schedule. Other antibiotics of proven efficacy in gonococcal infections are carbenicillin, rifampin, chloramphenicol, and some aminoglycosides; however, none of these antibiotics offers important advantages over other more commonly used agents.[12]

Initial trials using vaccines prepared from gonococcal pili have been disappointing. Because of the heterogenicity of gonococcal pili it is unlikely that vaccines of this type will ever be clinically useful; however, other cell surface antigens common to all gonococci offer some hope that an effective vaccine can be developed in the future.[3,6,10,12,14]

## Syphilis

Among diseases for which reporting to the U.S. Public Health Service Centers for Disease Control is required, syphilis is the third most frequently reported communicable disease in the United States. Since 1977 the incidence has been increasing and over 80,000 cases are reported annually. Syphilis is more common in men than women, a reflection of the high incidence among male homosexuals and bisexuals. In addition to being highly contagious, syphilis is of major concern because untreated, it can progress to a chronic systemic disease which can be fatal or seriously disabling.[19,20]

Syphilis is usually acquired by sexual contact with infected mucous membranes or cutaneous lesions, although on rare occasions it can be acquired by nonsexual personal contact, accidental inoculation, or blood transfusion. The causative organism of syphilis is *Treponema pallidum*, a spirochete. The risk of acquiring syphilis from an infected individual after a single exposure is approximately 30%. After sexual contact the organism penetrates the intact mucous membrane or a break in the cornified epithelium and spirochetemia occurs.[19,20]

### *Clinical Presentation*

#### Primary Syphilis

After exposure and an incubation period of 10–90 days (average 21 days), a painless lesion or chancre appears at the site of treponemal penetrance. If several spirochetes penetrate simultaneously, multiple lesions can develop. Classically the chancre is single and begins as a dull red macule. Subsequently it develops into a papule which erodes and ulcerates. Although chancres vary markedly in appearance, most are rounded or oval in shape, indurated, and well marginated. Oral and anorectal chancres are common in homosexual males and frequently have an atypical appearance. All chancres are highly infectious, although they are generally painless lesions unless secondarily infected or located at extragenital sites. Even without treatment, chancres persist only for 1 to 8 weeks before spontaneously disappearing. Because syphilitic chancres can be confused with other infectious etiologies, appropriate diagnostic testing is important.[19,20]

**Secondary Syphilis**

The secondary stage of syphilis develops 2 to 6 weeks after onset of the primary stage in untreated or inadequately treated patients. This stage is characterized by a variety of mucocutaneous eruptions, resulting from widespread hematogenous and lymphatic spread of *T. pallidum*. Skin lesions can either be generalized or localize to a small portion of the body and, with the exception of follicular lesions, are nonpruritic. Often lesions appear on the palms of the hands and the soles of the feet. As few dermatologic conditions are characterized by palm and sole manifestations, involvement of these areas is highly suggestive of syphilis. In addition to the skin lesions, mild and transitory malaise, fever, pharyngitis, headache, anorexia, and arthralgia are common. Generalized lymphadenopathy is also seen in the majority of patients. With or without treatment, signs and symptoms of secondary syphilis disappear in 4 to 10 weeks; however, in untreated patients, lesions may recur at any time within 4 years.[19,20]

**Late Syphilis**

Depending on the clinical manifestations and results of serologic testing, late syphilis is categorized as either latent syphilis or tertiary syphilis. By definition, persons with a positive serologic test for syphilis but without any signs or symptoms have latent syphilis. Latent syphilis is further divided into early and late latency. During early latency the patient is considered potentially infectious because of the risk of spontaneous mucocutaneous relapses. The U.S. Public Health Service defines early latency as 1 year from the onset of infection, although a longer interval such as 2–4 years is proposed by others. With the exception of pregnancy where the mother may pass the disease to the fetus, late latency is considered noninfectious although the patient remains a host.[19,20]

A large percentage of untreated patients with late latent syphilis have no further sequelae; however, approximately 25% to 30% progress to the tertiary stage. Treatment of all patients with latent syphilis is essential, as there is no way to predict which patients will develop tertiary disease.[19,20]

Tertiary syphilis is a slowly progressing, inflammatory manifestation of the disease that can affect any organ in the body. The principal morbidity and mortality of syphilis relate to organ system involvement that can develop 2–30 years after the onset of syphilis.[19,20]

The most common manifestations of tertiary syphilis are the benign gumma, neurosyphilis, and cardiovascular syphilis. The gumma, a nonspecific granulomatous lesion, is the classic lesion of late benign syphilis and develops in 50% of patients with tertiary syphilis. These chronic, destructive lesions characteristically involve the skin, bone, and upper respiratory tract, but may be found in any organ or tissue. Gummas of critical organs such as the heart or brain can be fatal.[19,20]

Neurosyphilis, found in approximately 20% of patients with tertiary diseases, can produce general paresis, eighth cranial nerve deafness, optic atrophy and blindness, progressive dementia, meningovascular complications, and tabes dorsalis. Thirty percent of patients with tertiary disease develop cardiovascular syphilis, characterized by aortitis and aortic insufficiency. Syphilitic aortic aneurysms are also common.[19,20]

**Congenital Syphilis**

In pregnant women with syphilis, *T. pallidum* can cross the placenta and infect the fetus after the 18th week of pregnancy. Fetal death, prematurity, and congenital syphilis are potential sequelae of transplacental infections. Symptoms can be seen during the first months of life (early congenital syphilis) or later in childhood or adolescence (late congenital syphilis). Manifestations of early congenital syphilis resemble those of secondary syphilis, while those of late congenital syphilis correspond to the tertiary stage in adults.[19,20]

## *Diagnosis*

Because *T. pallidum* is difficult to culture in vitro, diagnosis is based primarily on microscopic examination of serous material from a suspected syphilitic lesion or on serologic testing. In primary syphilis, diagnosis is established by the presence of *T. pallidum* on dark-field microscopic examination. Motile treponemes can also be found in cutaneous lesions and enlarged lymph nodes in patients with secondary syphilis. In incubating syphilis, confirmation is frequently by dark-field microscopic examination, as serologic tests can be unreactive early in the disease.[19–23]

Serologic tests used in the diagnosis of syphilis are categorized as nontreponemal and treponemal. Commonly used nontreponemal tests include the Venereal Disease Research Laboratory (VDRL) slide test, rapid plasma reagin (RPR) card test, reagin screen test (RST), unheated serum reagin (USR) test, and automated reagin test (ART). Nontreponemal tests rely on the detection of reagin, a heterogenous group of antibodies. Most laboratories perform either the RPR card test or the VDRL slide test. These tests are inexpensive and easily performed. A positive nontreponemal test can indicate the presence of any stage of syphilis or congenital syphilis, although incubating syphilis and very early primary syphilis produce a negative reaction; however, because they are nonspecific tests, false-positive reactions occur, making them inappropriate alone to confirm the diagnosis. Transiently positive results can be seen in patients with acute febrile illnesses, after immunizations, and during pregnancy. Chronic false-positive results are commonly associated with heroin addiction, aging, chronic infections, connective tissue diseases, and malignant disease. In some cases false-positive reactions are familial and are related to abnormal serum globulin levels.[19,23]

Nontreponemal tests are used primarily as screening tests; however, because reaginic antibody titers also can be quantitated by testing serial dilutions of the patient's serum for reactivity, they are useful in following progression of the disease, recovery after therapy, and possible reinfection. In patients successfully treated for primary and secondary syphilis, the VDRL will almost always return to seronegativity. If the VDRL is going to return to negative in patients with early latent syphilis, it will do so within the first 4 years after adequate therapy. Patients treated for late latent syphilis or tertiary syphilis usually remain seropositive for life. The VDRL also can return to seronegativity in untreated patients, although this is uncommon and occurs more slowly than following adequate treatment.[19–24]

In some patients with secondary syphilis, a prozone phenomenon occurs that produces a negative VDRL despite the presence of high reaginic antibody titers. Because the agglutination reaction occurs only within fixed limits of antibody and antigen, a relative excess of antibody results in a nonreactive or weakly reactive test. This is corrected by diluting the patient's serum prior to testing.[19–23]

In diagnosing all stages of syphilis, treponemal tests are more sensitive than nontreponemal tests. The fluorescent treponemal antibody absorption (FTAABS) test is the most frequently used treponemal test. In the FTAABS test, *T. pallidum* antigen is used to detect specific antibodies to treponemal organisms; however, because it requires fluorescence microscopy and is relatively difficult and expensive to perform, the FTAABS test is used primarily as a confirmatory rather than a screening test. The FTAABS test becomes positive earlier in primary syphilis and tends to remain positive in more patients with latent syphilis than the VDRL. After adequate antibiotic therapy for any stage of syphilis, the FTAABS test usually remains reactive for life, and therefore, is not useful in assessing serologic response to therapy, relapse, or reinfection. False-positive reactions are reported in 1% to 2% of healthy persons. These reactions are usually transitory and the cause is unknown. Although the FTAABS test measures treponemal antibodies, it does not differentiate between syphilis and other nonvenereal treponemal diseases such as yaws and pinta. Two other specific treponemal antibody tests are the microhemagglutination assay for antibodies to *T. pallidum* (MHATP) and the hemagglutination treponemal test for syphilis (HATTS).[19–23]

### *Treatment*

Treatment recommendations from the CDC are presented in Table 85.4.[14] Parenteral penicillin G is the treatment of choice for all stages of syphilis. Because *T. pallidum* multiplies slowly, single doses of short- or intermediate-acting penicillins do not provide prolonged, low-level exposure to penicillin which is required for eradication of the treponememe. Benzathine penicillin G is the only penicillin effective for single-dose therapy.[13–15,19,20]

The recommended treatment for syphilis of less than 1 year's duration is benzathine penicillin G 2.4 million units as a single dose. Although the relapse rate for this regimen is less than 3%, some advocate that 2.4 million units be administered once a week for two consecutive weeks; however, comparative studies of the two dosage regimens have not been conducted. In patients with syphilis of greater than 1 year's duration and normal cerebrospinal fluid examination, benzathine penicillin G is administered weekly for three successive doses. Patients with abnormal CSF findings should be treated as having neurosyphilis. Preferred regimens for the treatment of neurosyphilis provide a total dose of 6–9 million units of penicillin G over a 3- to 4-week period. Benzathine penicillin G in standard doses or procaine penicillin G in doses under 2.4 million units do not consistently provide treponemicidal levels in the CSF and have resulted in treatment failures.[25] Specific treatment regimens for congenital syphilis are given in Table 85.4.[13–15,19,20]

At present, *T. pallidum* resistance to penicillin has not emerged. Therefore, the primary need for alternative drugs in treating syphilis is for penicillin-allergic patients. An alternative regimen recommended for penicillin-allergic patients is tetracycline or erythromycin (stearate, ethyl succinate, or base) 500 mg orally four times daily for 15–30 days, depending on the duration of syphilis. Neither tetracycline nor the erythromycins have been evaluated as extensively as penicillin G in the treatment of syphilis and, therefore, they should be used only in cases of documented penicillin allergy. In addition, alternative regimens involve multiple doses that can adversely affect patient compliance and subsequent therapeutic efficacy. In these cases, follow-up serologic testing is of particular importance.[13–15,19,20]

Other antibiotics that have been used successfully in treating syphilis include chloramphenicol, doxycycline, and various cephalosporins such as cephalexin, cephaloridine, and cephalothin; however, as they are more expensive and require administration of multiple doses, none offers significant advantages over penicillin G.[12–15,18–20,26]

For pregnant patients, penicillin is the treatment of choice. Erythromycin is the drug of choice in pregnant patients who are allergic to penicillin, if compliance and serologic follow-up can be assured. Infants born to mothers treated during pregnancy with erythromycin should receive penicillin at birth because erythromycin levels in fetal blood are probably too low to be consistently effective.[13–15,19,20]

CDC recommendations for serologic follow-up of patients treated for syphilis are given in Table 85.4. Quantitative nontreponemal tests should be performed at 3, 6, and 12 months in all patients treated for syphilis. As the time to reach seronegativity is generally proportional to the duration of the disease, additional testing is recommended in patients with syphilis of greater than 1 year's duration, neurosyphilis, and congenital syphilis. Despite adequate therapy, some patients may remain seropositive. In these cases stabilization of low reaginic titers is indicative of adequate therapy. In addition to serologic testing, patients with neurosyphilis and congenital syphilis should have periodic clinical evaluations at 6-month intervals and serial CSF examinations until findings return to normal or stabilize. For women treated during pregnancy, monthly quantitative nontreponemal tests are recommended throughout pregnancy. Women who do not demonstrate a fourfold decrease in titer over a 3-month period or who show a fourfold increase in titer between tests should be retreated.[13,14,19,20]

The majority of patients treated for primary and secondary syphilis experience the Jarisch–Herxheimer reaction after treatment. This benign, self-limiting reaction is characterized by symptoms of endotoxemia such as transient fever, chills, malaise, arthralgia, myalgia, tachypnea, peripheral vasodilation, and aggravation of syphilitic lesions. The exact mechanism of the reaction is unknown although various

**Table 85.4** Drug Therapy and Follow-Up of Syphilis

| *Stage/type of syphilis* | *Recommended regimen* | *Follow-up serology* |
|---|---|---|
| Primary, secondary, or latent syphilis of less than 1 year's duration | Benzathine penicillin G 2.4 million units IM at a single session | Quantitative nontreponemal tests at 3, 6, and 12 months |
| Syphilis of more than 1 year's duration (except neurosyphilis) | Benzathine penicillin G 2.4 million units IM once a week for 3 successive weeks | Quantitative nontreponemal tests at 3, 6, 12, and 24 months |
| Neurosyphilis | Aqueous crystalline penicillin G 12–24 million units IV (2–4 million units every 4 hours) for 10 days, followed by benzathine penicillin G 2.4 million units IM weekly for 3 doses<br>*or*<br>Aqueous procaine penicillin G 2.4 million units IM daily plus probenecid 500 mg PO 4 times daily, both for 10 days, followed by benzathine penicillin G 2.4 million units IM weekly for 3 doses<br>*or*<br>Benzathine penicillin G 2.4 million units IM weekly for 3 doses | Nontreponemal testing at 6 and 12 months, then yearly for at least 3 years |
| Congenital syphilis | | |
| CSF Abnormal | Aqueous crystalline penicillin G 50,000 units/kg IM or IV daily in 2 divided doses for a minimum of 10 days<br>*or*<br>Aqueous procaine penicillin G 50,000 units/kg IM for a minimum of 10 days | Nontreponemal tests at birth, 1 month, and every 3 months for first 15 months; then every 6 months until negative or until stable at low titer |
| CSF Normal | Benzathine penicillin G 50,000 units/kg IM in a single dose | Same as for abnormal CSF |
| Penicillin-allergic patients | | |
| Primary, secondary or latent syphilis of less than 1 year's duration | Tetracycline 500 mg PO 4 times daily for 15 days<br>*or*<br>Erythromycin 500 mg PO 4 times daily for 15 days | Same as for non-penicillin allergic patients |
| Syphilis of more than 1 year's duration (except neurosyphilis) | Tetracycline 500 mg PO 4 times daily for 30 days<br>*or*<br>Erythromycin 500 mg PO 4 times daily for 30 days | Same as for non-penicillin allergic patients |

Recommendations are those of the CDC.[14]

etiologies, including immunologic mechanisms and release of endotoxin or other toxic treponemal products, are proposed.[19,20]

The Jarisch–Herxheimer reaction is independent of the drug and dose used and should not be confused with penicillin allergy. It usually begins within 2–4 hours of initiation of therapy, peaks at 8 hours, and is complete within 12–24 hours. Most reactions can be managed symptomatically with analgesics, antipyretics, and rest. Steroids and antihistamines have been administered prior to initiation of syphilitic therapy but are of limited value.[19,20]

## Chlamydia

Infections caused by *Chlamydia trachomatis* are now recognized as the most common sexually transmitted disease in the United States and the most common cause of nongonococcal urethritis (NGU). Although reporting is not required officially and microbiologic confirmation is frequently not performed in the United States, it is estimated that 3 to 4 million Americans contract chlamydial infections each year. Precise diagnosis of chlamydia infections has been hampered because of the high percentage of infected individuals who have asymptomatic disease and because culture of the organism is both difficult and expensive.[27]

*C. trachomatis* is an obligate intracellular parasite that shares properties of both viruses and bacteria. Like viruses, chlamydiae require cellular material from host cells for replication; however, unlike viruses, chlamydiae maintain their cellular identity throughout development. Fifteen serovars (subspecies) of *C. trachomatis* exist, of which only the lymphogranuloma venereum strains produce potentially invasive infections. The remaining serovars are involved primarily with superficial infection of epithelial cells.[28–31]

Specific data on risk of transmissibility after exposure are not available. It is estimated that coinfection with chlamydia occurs in up to 45% of individuals with gonorrhea. As a result, chlamydia is the most common cause of postgonococcal urethritis in heterosexuals.[13]

### Clinical Presentation

In males, the most common symptoms of chlamydial genital tract infections are dysuria, urinary frequency, and a mucoid urethral discharge occurring 7–21 days after exposure. The discharge is usually less profuse and more mucoid or watery than the urethral discharge associated with gonorrhea. Typically, it is more obvious in the morning. In many cases the discharge is not noticeable, and crusting of the meatus or staining of undergarments may be the only sign. In approximately 25% of men with chlamydial infections, no signs or symptoms are present. *C. trachomatis* is responsible for approximately 50% of all cases of acute epididymitis reported in the United States annually.[28–31]

The majority of women with chlamydial infections are asymptomatic. In women with urethral infections, dysuria and frequency are uncommon. When symptomatic, the most common manifestation of infection is endocervicitis with a mucopurulent discharge. In recent years, chlamydia has become recognized as a major cause of pelvic inflammatory disease and its associated complications. It also is suggested that women with active chlamydial infections or antichlamydial antibody in their serum have an increased risk of cervical dysplasia.[28–31]

Similar to gonorrhea, chlamydia may be transmitted to an infant during contact with infected cervicovaginal secretions. Up to 70% of infants acquire chlamydial infection after endocervical exposure, with the primary morbidity associated with seeding of the infant's eyes, nasopharynx, rectum, or vagina. Chlamydia is the most common cause of neonatal eye infections and of afebrile interstitial pneumonia in infants less than 6 months. Inclusion conjunctivitis in newborns is usually self-limited but can result in scarring and micropannus of the cornea. Interstitial pneumonitis, occurring secondary to carriage in the nasopharynx, is typically mild, but can be severe and require hospitalization.[11,28–32]

### Diagnosis

Because of the high rate of asymptomatic disease and the relative lack of specificity of symptoms when present, laboratory confirmation of chlamydial infection is important. Prior to the availability of antigen detection methods, diagnosis commonly was based on the presence of greater than four polymorphonuclear leukocytes per high-power field in a smear of urethral secretions and the exclusion of gonorrhea. This indirect means of diagnosis is neither sensitive nor specific.[27–30]

Cytologic techniques are of little practical value in the diagnosis of chlamydial genital tract infections because of their poor sensitivity. As chlamydiae are intracellular parasites, Giemsa-stained smears must be prepared from epithelial cell scrapings rather than urine or urethral discharges. Such evaluation is most useful in screening patients to eliminate the possibility of gonorrhea. Although highly specific, tissue culture techniques are not widely used for diagnostic purposes because they are time consuming, technically demanding, and expensive.[27–30]

Serologic tests also are of limited benefit in diagnosing chlamydial infections and are used primarily as a research tool. The presence of antibody in a blood sample does not differentiate an active infection from previous exposure, and the baseline prevalence of antibody in populations that are sexually active and at greatest risk is high.[27–30]

Recently, two tests that allow rapid identification of chlamydial antigens in genital secretions have become available. The direct-smear fluorescent antibody (DFA) test utilizes fluorescein-conjugated monoclonal antibody that is incubated with specimen material on a slide and examined under a fluorescent microscope. This test is highly specific and sensitive and takes less than 1 hour to perform. Another test used for rapid detection of *C. trachomatis* is the enzyme immunoassay. This enzyme-linked immunoabsorbent assay (ELISA) measures antigen–antibody reactions using a spectrophotometer. Based on limited comparative data, both tests have similar mean sensitivities and specificities in the range 90% to 100% when properly performed. Although it takes approximately 4 hours to perform, the ELISA is less complicated and can be used to test large numbers of specimens at the same time. For both antigen detection methods, questions remain concerning their reliability in screening low-prevalence populations. Other antigen tests are expected to be marketed in the near future.[27,33]

### Treatment

Rifampin, tetracyclines, macrolides, and sulfonamides display good in vitro and in vivo activity against *C. trachomatis*, while penicillin, ampicillin, amoxicillin, pivampicillin, piperacillin, azlocillin, mezlocillin, cefoperazone, ceftriaxone, and clindamycin have some activity against chlamydia in vitro, but are of marginal clinical efficacy. Aminoglycosides, metronidazole, aztreonam, and most cephalosporin antibiotics are not active in vitro against chlamydia.[18,27–36]

In clinical trials, tetracycline hydrochloride, minocycline, erythromycin, trimethoprim–sulfamethoxazole, and rosaramicin have produced comparable cure rates of 85% to 95% in men with chlamydial urethritis. Although fewer studies have been conducted to assess the effectiveness of antibiotic therapy of uncomplicated cervical or urethral infection in women, cure rates appear to be similar to those reported in males; however, sulfonamides have no significant activity against *Ureaplasma urealyticum*, and would not be useful in the treatment of *C. trachomatis*-negative NGU. In limited testing, high-dose amoxicillin therapy (750 mg three times daily for 7 days) also has been effective in the treatment of chlamydial urethral infections in men. Because of its effectiveness, low cost, and limited side effects, tetracycline has been most extensively evaluated and is the treatment of choice. In vitro resistance to tetracyclines has not been demonstrated but has been reported for sulfonamides and rifampin. Recently, a relative resistance to erythromycin has been reported.[27–36]

The recommended therapy for uncomplicated urogenital chlamydial infections is tetracycline hydrochloride 500 mg by mouth four times daily for 7 days (Table 85.5).[27] Although some clinicians advocate a longer regimen of 14–21 days, no clear evidence exists that longer regimens are more effective; however, in patients experiencing relapses, a 14- or 21-day tetracycline regimen is recommended. Longer regimens also can be useful in patients for whom compliance is a concern, as these regimens may increase the chances of cure. Minocycline and doxycycline offer a more convenient twice-daily dosage regimen but are more expensive. In clinical testing minocycline has also produced a high incidence of dizziness and light-headedness. Single-dose studies using doxycycline have shown high failure rates.[13,27–36]

In pregnant women with chlamydial urogenital infections, treatment during pregnancy can significantly reduce the risk of transmission to the newborn. Erythromycin base or erythromycin ethyl succinate are the recommended treatments (Table 85.5). Erythromycin stearate is probably also effective although it has not been adequately evaluated. Patients intolerant of the recommended dosage should be treated with half of the recommended daily dose for 2 weeks instead of 1 week. In one study, amoxicillin 1.5 g daily for 7 days also produced acceptable cure rates.[13,27–36]

The treatment of chlamydial ophthalmia neonatorum is controversial. Some experts recommend only topical treatment with sulfonamides, tetracyclines, or erythromycin four times daily for 2–3 weeks; however, treatment failures are reported. The CDC recommends systemic therapy with oral erythromycin 50 mg/kg/d in four divided doses for 2 weeks, because of treatment failures with topical therapy alone. For prophylaxis of ophthalmia neonatorum, various groups have proposed the use of erythromycin (0.5%) or tetracycline (1%) ophthalmic ointment in lieu of silver nitrate. These treatments are effective against both chlamydial and gonococcal ophthalmia neonatorum, whereas silver nitrate is not effective for chlamydial disease and may cause a chemical conjunctivitis; however, neither topical erythromycin nor tetracycline has any effect on nasal carriage of chlamydia so the potential for pneumonitis remains. Oral erythromycin is the treatment of choice for chlamydial pneumonitis.[16,27–32]

Treatment of chlamydial infections with the recommended regimens is highly effective. Therefore, posttreatment cultures are not routinely recommended. When positive, posttreatment cultures usually represent noncompliance, failure to treat sexual partners, or laboratory error, rather than inadequate therapy.[27]

Because coexisting chlamydial infections occur in a high percentage of patients with gonorrhea, use of treatment

**Table 85.5** Treatment of Chlamydial Infections

| *Infection* | *Regimen of choice* | *Alternative regimen* |
|---|---|---|
| Uncomplicated urethral, endocervical, or rectal infection in adults | Tetracycline hydrochloride 500 mg PO 4 times daily for 7 days<br>*or*<br>Doxycycline hyclate 100 mg PO 2 times daily for 7 days | Erythromycin base or stearate 500 mg PO 4 times daily for 7 days<br>*or*<br>Erythromycin ethyl succinate 800 mg PO 4 times daily for 7 days |
| Urogenital infections during pregnancy | Erythromycin base 500 mg PO 4 times daily for 7 days<br>*or*<br>Erythromycin ethyl succinate 800 mg PO 4 times daily for 7 days | Erythromycin base 250 mg PO 4 times daily for 14 days |
| Conjunctivitis of the newborn | Erythromycin suspension 50 mg/kg/d PO in 4 divided doses for 14 days | |
| Pneumonia in infants | Erythromycin suspension 50 mg/kg/d PO in 4 divided doses for 14 days | |
| Acute epididymo-orchitis | Amoxicillin 3.0 g PO, or ampicillin 3.5 g PO, or aqueous procaine penicillin G 4.8 million units IM at 2 sites (each along with probenecid 1.0 g PO), or spectinomycin 2.0 g IM or ceftriaxone 250 mg IM<br>*followed by*<br>Tetracycline hydrochloride 500 mg PO 4 times daily for 10 days<br>*or*<br>Doxycycline 100 mg PO 2 times daily for 10 days | Alternatives for tetracycline only: same as for uncomplicated infections |

Recommendations are those of the CDC.[27]

regimens that are effective for both infections is important. Tetracycline regimens, or standard single-dose gonococcal regimens followed by tetracycline, are recommended. Trimethoprim alone has some efficacy in treating gonorrhea, but has minimal activity against chlamydia. The combination of trimethoprim and sulfamethoxazole, however, expands the spectrum of activity to include both *C. trachomatis* and *N. gonorrhoeae*. In the future, short-course therapy with quinolone antibiotics such as rosoxacin and ciprofloxacin that have activity against *C. trachomatis*, *N. gonorrhoeae*, and *U. urealyticum* may prove clinically useful for treating combination gonococcal and nongonococcal urethritis and cervicitis.[36]

## Genital Herpes

It is estimated that 5 to 20 million persons in the United States have genital herpes, and this number is increasing by up to 500,000 persons each year.[37] Whether these figures represent increased prevalence or greater recognition as a result of improved diagnostic capabilities is uncertain. Because of their morbidity, frequent recurrences, and potential for complications, genital herpes infections have received increasing attention in recent years.

*Herpes* comes from the Greek "to creep" and is used to describe two distinct but antigenically related serotypes of herpes simplex virus. Herpes simplex virus type 1 (HSV-1) is most commonly associated with oropharyngeal disease and herpes simplex virus type 2 (HSV-2) is most closely associated with genital disease; however, each virus is capable of causing infections that are clinically indistinguishable in both anatomic areas.[38–42]

Humans are the sole known reservoir for HSV. Infection is transmitted via inoculation of virus from infected secretions onto mucosal surfaces (urethra, oropharynx, cervix, conjunctivae) or through abraded skin. On the basis of a recent retrospective study, the risk of developing herpes genitalis after sexual exposure to a person with an active infection is estimated to be 60%. Evidence that the virus survives for a limited time on environmental surfaces suggests the possibility of fomitic transfer as a nonvenereal route of transmission.[38–42]

The cycle of HSV infection occurs in five stages: primary mucocutaneous infection, infection of the ganglia, establishment of latency, reactivation, and recurrent infection. After viral inoculation, HSV infection is associated with cytoplasmic granulation, ballooning degeneration of cells, and production of mononucleated giant cells. Initially, the cellular response is predominantly polymorphonuclear, followed by a lymphocytic response. Replication occurs with viral spread to contiguous cells and peripheral sensory nerves. Latency then is established in sensory or autonomic nerve root ganglia. Latency appears to be lifelong, interrupted only by reactivation of the viral infection. It is unclear what factors are important in maintaining latency, but immune responses and emotional and physical stresses appear to be important in reactivating latent virus.[38–44]

### *Clinical Presentation*

The clinical manifestations of first episodes of genital herpes appear within 1–45 days of inoculation. The signs and symptoms are influenced by many factors including previous exposure to HSV, previous genital herpes infection, viral type, and host factors such as age and site of infection. On the basis of retrospective studies, it is estimated that up to 50% of HSV-2 infections are asymptomatic. As HSV can be transmitted during both symptomatic and asymptomatic infections, asymptomatic shedding of virus poses a significant problem in controlling its spread.[38–40,42,43,45]

In terms of the natural history of genital herpes infections and their treatment, it is important to distinguish between first-episode primary, first-episode nonprimary, and recurrent infections. Primary infections are classified as infections occurring in persons lacking antibody to either type of HSV. These infections are characterized by a prolonged duration of systemic and local symptoms. Over 50% of patients with primary infections experience flulike symptoms of fever, headache, malaise, and myalgias. Systemic symptoms gradually resolve over the course of a week. Local symptoms include development of pustular or ulcerative lesions on the external genitalia. Lesions usually begin as papules or vesicles which rapidly spread over the genitalia. Clusters of the lesions coalesce into large areas of ulceration which, over 2 to 3 weeks, crust and/or reepithelialize. Genital lesions are described as painful by more than 90% of infected men and women. Development of new lesions is fairly common during the first 10 days of a primary infection. Pain from the lesions tends to be most intense during the first 7–11 days of their appearance and gradually recedes. Other local symptoms can include itching, dysuria, vaginal or urethral discharge, and tender inguinal adenopathy. Inguinal adenopathy is usually the last symptom to resolve. Viral shedding usually lasts about 12 days.[39,40,42,43]

First-episode nonprimary herpes genitalis is defined as an infection in individuals who have clinical or serologic evidence of prior HSV (usually HSV-1) infection at another body site. These infections tend to be milder than true primary infections, with a lower incidence of constitutional symptoms and a shorter duration of disease reported.[39,40,42]

In contrast to first-episode primary and first-episode nonprimary infections, recurrent infections are infrequently associated with systemic manifestations. Recurrent infection is localized to the genital area and is milder and of a shorter duration (approximately 8–12 days). Approximately 50% of patients with genital herpes experience a prodrome prior to the appearance of recurrent lesions. This typically consists of a mild tingling or itching sensation hours to a few days prior to the appearance of vesicles. In a few patients symptoms of sacral neuralgia are seen.[39,40,42]

As with first-episode infection, symptoms of recurrent infection tend to be more severe in women, primarily as a result of the greater genital surface area involved. About 80% of patients with a first-episode HSV-2 genital infection experience a recurrence within 12 months. The median number of recurrences is estimated at five to eight per year.[39,40,42]

Complications from genital herpes infection result from both genital spread and autoinoculation of the virus. Lesions at extragenital sites such as the eye, rectum, pharynx, and fingers are not uncommon. Central nervous system involvement is occasionally seen and may take several forms including an aseptic meningitis, transverse myelitis, or a sacral radiculopathy syndrome.[38–40,42,43]

Symptoms of first-episode and recurrent infections tend to be more severe and prolonged in immunocompromised patients than in noncompromised patients. Additionally, immunocompromised patients are more susceptible to initial infection and subsequent recurrences.

A major concern with genital herpes is its effect on pregnancy and the neonate. Neonatal herpes is associated with high mortality and morbidity. It is transmitted to the newborn primarily through exposure to HSV in the birth canal but in rare cases is also transmitted transplacentally. The risk of transmission during birth appears to be much greater for first-episode primary infections than for recurrent infections. Neonatal herpes infection has a case-fatality rate of approximately 50%.[11,39,40,42,43,46]

### *Diagnosis*

Confirmation of a genital herpes infection can be made only with laboratory testing. The nonspecific systemic symptoms seen with primary infection and even the lesions of genital herpes may be difficult to differentiate from other infectious and noninfectious etiologies. Typically, however, genital herpes lesions are painful to touch, in contrast to syphilitic chancres.

Tissue culture is the most specific and sensitive method of confirming the diagnosis of genital herpes; however, viral culture is expensive and time consuming. Also, improper collection or transport of specimens can result in false-negative results. In most situations, HSV isolation on tissue culture takes 48–96 hours. In instances in which rapid detection is necessary (impending birth), other detection methods may be more useful.[38–40,42,43]

The Tzanck test is a rapid detection method in which cells from suspected lesions are stained and examined for the presence of characteristic multinucleated giant cells. While easy to perform and inexpensive, the specificity and sensitivity are low. Other detection methods with acceptable specificities and sensitivities that provide more rapid results than tissue culture also have been evaluated. Immunologic methods such as immunofluorescence, immunoperoxidase, and enzyme-linked immunosorbent assay have sensitivities of 70% to 90% compared with viral culture. A method combining cell culture for 24 hours and specific labeling using antibodies to HSV has sensitivities and specificities only slightly less than those of culture.[38–40,42,43]

The majority of patients infected with either HSV-1 or HSV-2 develop circulating antibody to HSV antigens; however, serologic assays for detection of HSV antibodies are often overutilized and have only limited utility in the diagnosis of genital herpes. The cross-reactivity of antibodies to HSV-1 and HSV-2, coupled with the high prevalence of HSV-1 antibody in the adult population, makes it difficult to interpret the results. A negative antibody titer early in the course of a herpes infection followed by a fourfold or greater rise in the titer after the episode is diagnostic of a primary infection. A rise in antibody titer also can be seen after a first-episode nonprimary infection, but changes in antibody titer are extremely uncommon in patients with recurrent episodes.[38–40,42,43]

While the diagnosis of genital herpes can be confirmed only by laboratory tests such as cell culture, less stringent diagnostic criteria (e.g., characteristic physical findings or clinical history) frequently are used in clinical practice. A presumptive diagnosis of genital herpes commonly is made based on the presence of darkfield–negative, vesicular, or ulcerative genital lesions. A prior history of similar lesions or recent sexual contact with an individual with similar lesions also is useful in making the diagnosis. Other STDs, including chancroid, lymphogranuloma venereum, and granuloma inguinale, and causes such as trauma, allergic reactions, and bacterial or fungal infections are considered in the differential diagnosis.

### *Treatment*

Palliative and supportive measures are the cornerstone of therapy for patients with genital herpes. To prevent bacterial superinfection lesions must be kept clean and dry. The use of analgesics, antipyretics, and antipruritics may be warranted based on symptomatology. Although many therapeutic approaches have been used over the years, few have been subjected to sound scientific evaluation and fewer have demonstrated therapeutic effectiveness.[40–47]

The goals of therapy in genital herpes infection are to shorten the clinical course, prevent complications, prevent the development of latency and/or subsequent recurrences, decrease the transmission of disease, and eliminate established latency. Current research has focused primarily on the treatment of first-episode infections and recurrences and the suppression of recurrences.

Specific chemotherapeutic approaches to treating genital herpes fall into six major areas: antiviral compounds, topical surfactants, photodynamic dyes, immune modulators, vaccines, and interferons (Table 85.6); however, few have undergone extensive evaluation and even fewer have demonstrated any significant clinical effects. To date, antiviral agents, in particular acyclovir, have been the most successful in promoting healing and resolution of symptoms.[38,40,43,48]

Acyclovir, a guanosine analogue available in intravenous, oral, and topical dosage forms, is the first antiviral agent to demonstrate significant efficacy in the treatment of genital herpes and it is the first agent approved in the United States for the treatment of mucocutaneous herpes simplex infections. Specific dosage recommendations are given in Table 85.7.[14] Selective phosphorylation of acyclovir in HSV-infected cells by HSV-specified thymidine kinase is the first step in the conversion of acyclovir triphosphate, the active moiety. Acyclovir triphosphate is a selective substrate and inhibitor of herpesvirus DNA polymerase. As acyclovir is preferentially taken up and converted to its active form by HSV-infected cells, it has a low potential for toxicity in normal, uninfected cells.[49–51]

Oral and intravenous formulations of acyclovir have demonstrated efficacy in reducing viral shedding, duration of symptoms, and time to healing of first-episode genital herpes infections. While local symptoms improve with topical application, this effect is not as pronounced as with oral and intravenous therapy and systemic symptoms are not af-

**Table 85.6** Agents Studied in the Treatment of Herpes Genitalis

| | |
|---|---|
| Antiviral compounds | Immune modulators |
| Acyclovir | Inosiplex |
| Vidarabine | Levamisole |
| Idoxuridine | Transfer factor |
| 2-Deoxy-D-glucose | Vaccines |
| Lithium | BCG |
| L-Lysine | Influenza |
| Phosphonoformate | Polio |
| Ribavirin | Smallpox |
| (*E*)-5-(2-Bromovinyl)-2′-deoxyuridine (BVdU) | Interferons |
| 2′-Fluoro-5-iodoarabinosylcytosine | Leukocyte interferon |
| 1-(2′-Fluoro-2′-deoxy-β-D-arabinofuranosyl)-thymidine | Photodynamic dyes |
| Topical surfactants | Neutral red |
| Chloroform | Acridine red |
| Ether | Proflavine |
| Nonoxynol-9 | Others |
| Povidone–iodine | Butylated hydroxytoluene (BHT) |
| Intervir-A | |

fected. In humans none of the regimens prevents latency or alters the subsequent frequency and severity of recurrences. Oral acyclovir is the treatment of choice for outpatients with first-episode genital herpes. In patients with severe symptoms or complications necessitating hospitalization, parenteral acyclovir may be beneficial; however, the intravenous regimen has been associated with renal, gastrointestinal, bone marrow, and central nervous system toxicity, especially in patients with renal dysfunction.[39,40,42,43,47,49–53]

The role of acyclovir in treatment of recurrent episodes of genital herpes is controversial. Because of the self-limiting nature of recurrent infection in normal hosts, demonstration

**Table 85.7** Treatment of Herpes Genitalis

| *Type of infection* | *Recommended regimen* | *Alternative regimen* |
|---|---|---|
| First clinical episode of genital herpes or proctitis[a] | Acyclovir 200 mg PO 5 times daily for 7–10 days, initiated within 6 days of onset of lesions | Acyclovir 5 mg/kg IV every 8 hours for 5–7 days[b] *or* Acyclovir ointment applied to all lesions 6 times daily for 7 days[c] |
| Recurrent infection | | |
| Treatment | Acyclovir 200 mg PO 5 times daily for 5 days, initiated within 2 days of onset[d] | |
| Suppression | Acyclovir 200 mg PO 2–5 times daily[e] | |

[a] Primary or nonprimary first episode.

[b] Only for patients with severe symptoms or complications that necessitate hospitalization.

[c] Topical acyclovir may be beneficial in patients without cervical, urethral, or pharyngeal involvement. It is of marginal benefit in decreasing viral shedding and has no significant effect on symptoms or healing time.

[d] Treatment should be limited to patients with severe symptoms. Treatment is most beneficial when instituted at the earliest sign of recurrence (i.e., prodrome); therapy initiated 48 hours or more after the onset of symptoms has no effect.

[e] Indicated only for patients with frequent and/or severe recurrences; long-term safety beyond 6 months is unknown.

Recommendations are those of the CDC.[14]

of therapeutic effects is difficult. Also, there is no evidence that shortening the duration of recurrent episodes has any effect on the subsequent recurrence rate. In most instances, treatment with topical acyclovir, whether physician initiated (within 48 hours of onset) or patient initiated (at prodrome or earliest sign of recurrence), has shown minimal effects on symptomatology and duration of viral shedding and time to healing. Oral acyclovir, however, reduces the duration of viral shedding and slightly diminishes the time to crusting and healing of lesions, particularly when initiated early. Appreciable effects on symptomatology are not seen. Patients with prolonged episodes of recurrent infection, in particular, may benefit from oral therapy instituted at the earliest sign of recurrence. Because of the relative mildness and brevity of recurrent infections, parenteral administration of acyclovir is not justifiable.[39,40,42,43,47,49–54]

Acyclovir treatment of first-episode genital herpes has not been shown to prevent later recurrences; however, chronic oral therapy suppresses the frequency and the severity of recurrences in 60% to 90% of patients experiencing frequent recurrences. In some patients experiencing breakthrough recurrences, HSV isolates resistant to acyclovir have been identified. Consideration must be given to the side effects of long-term administration of acyclovir to healthy young adults and the possibility of selection of acyclovir-resistant HSV during suppressive therapy. Patients receiving suppressive therapy should be monitored closely for adverse drug effects; also, therapy should be withdrawn periodically to observe any changes in the patient's intrinsic pattern of recurrence. Presently there is no evidence that suppressive therapy has any effect on ganglionic latency. As a result, recurrence rates after discontinuation of acyclovir are similar to pretreatment rates. Although not yet demonstrated, it is possible that acyclovir prophylaxis may decrease or eliminate periods of asymptomatic virus shedding and reduce transmission of genital herpes. Trials are currently underway to evaluate the comparative efficacy of continuous acyclovir suppression for 1 year versus intermittent suppressive therapy.[39,40,42,43,45,54]

Patients with frequent and physically or psychologically distressing recurrences are candidates for suppressive therapy with oral acyclovir (200 mg three to fives times a day). When recurrences are less severe, patients may benefit from physician- or patient-initiated intermittent therapy (200 mg five times a day for 5 days at the earliest sign of recurrence). Because of its cost and potential for side effects, oral acyclovir is not recommended for routine use in all patients with recurrent genital herpes. Topical acyclovir has no established role in the treatment or prophylaxis of recurrent infections.[52–54]

Immunocompromised patients, who are at greatest risk for severe and recurrent HSV infections, have demonstrated beneficial effects from all three formulations of acyclovir. As with the immunocompetent host, effects are more pronounced with the intravenous and oral dosage forms. Both intravenous and oral acyclovir have been used to prevent reactivation of infection in patients seropositive for HSV who undergo transplantation procedures or induction chemotherapy for acute leukemia.[39,42,52]

With the increasing prevalence of genital herpes worldwide, the potential exists for widespread use and misuse of acyclovir, resulting in development of acyclovir-resistant HSV. In vitro resistance to acyclovir is shown to be mediated by alterations in either viral thymidine kinase or viral DNA polymerase. Clinically, the majority of resistant isolates have been thymidine kinase deficient. Studies in animals suggest that these mutants have reduced virulence and have greater difficulty in establishing latency than parent strains. As the thymidine kinase–deficient mutants rapidly disappear with or without continued therapy, it is likely that they are eliminated by normal host defense mechanisms. Although less common than thymidine kinase–deficient mutants, other resistant strains maintain virulency and can establish latency. The incidence and the clinical implications of acyclovir resistance require further study, particularly with respect to low-dose suppressive therapy, which can provide an environment for emergence of resistant isolates.[40,42,52,53,55]

Numerous agents for the prophylaxis and treatment of genital herpes infections are being studied. Advances in antiviral research have stimulated the development and testing of several antiviral compounds such as ribavirin and phosphonoformate. The immune modulators levamisole and transfer factor also are being evaluated. For both the new antivirals and immune modulators, data are too preliminary to draw any conclusions concerning their efficacy and safety.[38,40,43]

At best, antiviral compounds such as acyclovir provide effective symptomatic and prophylactic therapy; however, antivirals are not curative. Agents that can eliminate ganglionic latency and prevent recurrent infections are not expected to be available in the near future. Therefore, homologous HSV vaccines hold the most promise in prevention of infection and establishment of latency; however, development of safe and effective vaccines for clinical use is only in the initial stages. Administration of various experimental HSV vaccines to persons with established genital herpes has been shown to reduce the incidence of recurrent infections. In comparative, placebo-controlled trials, however, significant reductions in recurrence rates are also reported for placebo. Stimulation of the immune response by repeated injection of heterologous vaccines (e.g., BCG and influenza vaccines) in patients with recurrent genital herpes is of no benefit in reducing the recurrence rate.[38–40,42,43]

## Trichomoniasis

Trichomoniasis is a common STD caused by *Trichomonas vaginalis*, a flagellated, motile protozoan. Humans are host to two other *Trichomonas* species, *T. tenax* and *T. hominis*, but *T. vaginalis* is the only species thought to be pathogenic. *Trichomonas* species are highly site specific and *T. vaginalis* is not known to infect either the oropharynx or rectum.[56,57]

It is estimated that 2.5 to 3 million cases of vaginal trichomoniasis occur annually in the United States. The peak incidence in women occurs between the ages of 16 and 35, although there is a high prevalence between ages 35 and 45. Age-incidence figures in men are less clear because of the difficulty in diagnosis, the high incidence of asymptomatic disease, and the high spontaneous cure rate.[56]

Although infection by nonsexual contact is reported, it is uncommon. *T. vaginalis* can survive for short periods on moist surfaces, so the possibility of contamination of inanimate objects by body discharges exists. Infections can be spread by communal bathing or contact with infected bath or toilet articles. Neonatal infections also represent nonvenereal transmission of the disease.[56,57]

In infected women, trichomonads are isolated most commonly from the vagina, followed by the urethra and Skene's glands. Infrequently they are recovered from the endocervix. Extragenital sites are epidemiologically important, as infection can persist if local therapy alone is used to treat vaginal infections, resulting in reinfection of the vagina. This may account for the higher relapse rates reported for local versus systemic therapy. After attachment to the vaginal or urethral mucosa, trichomonads usually elicit an inflammatory response which manifests as a discharge containing large numbers of polymorphonuclear leukocytes.[56,57]

### *Clinical Presentation*

Trichomonal infections are much more common in women than in men. The incubation period of trichomoniasis is 4–20 days. Approximately 25% of infected women are asymptomatic. When symptomatic, females can present with mild to severe vaginal discharge, vulvar pruritis, and dysuria. Symptoms frequently worsen during menstruation when the pH of the vagina is optimal for growth of trichomonads. Vaginal discharge is noted in approximately 50% to 75% of infected women and classically has been described as malodorous, foamy, and greenish yellow in color; however, more typically the discharge is grayish and only mildly odoriferous. In up to 50% of women, pruritis is noted which is often severe.[56,57]

On examination of symptomatic women, the vulva and surrounding areas may be diffusely erythematous and excoriated as a result of scratching. Secondary infection of excoriated areas is not uncommon. The vagina is often erythematous; surface erosions of the cervix are seen in up to 90% of women. Tender inguinal lymphadenopathy and lower abdominal pain occur infrequently. In a small percentage of patients there may be no abnormal findings on vaginal examination. There is no evidence that trichomonads spread beyond the cervix to cause pelvic inflammatory disease or disseminated disease; however, it is suggested that cervical erosion secondary to trichomoniasis may contribute to malignant transformation.[56,57]

Trichomoniasis may be transmitted to neonates after passage through an infected birth canal. The risk is low and most cases of neonatal infections are self-limited; however, persistent vaginal or urethral infections should be treated.[56,57]

In men, the majority of trichomonal infections are asymptomatic. The most common site of infection is the urethra. It is likely that differences in pathogenicity of trichomonads in men and women are dependent on differences in the microenvironment of the vagina and urethra. In symptomatic males, urethral discharge is seen most commonly, followed by pruritis and dysuria. The discharge may range from mucoid to purulent. *T. vaginalis* has been established as one cause of treatment failure in patients with presumed nongonococcal urethritis treated with tetracycline or erythromycin. For most men, trichomonal urethritis is apparently self-limited. *T. vaginalis* has been implicated in some cases of prostatitis and epididymitis.[56,57]

### *Diagnosis*

Because *T. vaginalis* produces nonspecific symptoms consistent with other causes of vaginitis, laboratory diagnosis is required. The simplest and most reliable means of diagnosis is a wet mount examination of the vaginal discharge. Trichomoniasis is confirmed if characteristic pear-shaped, flagellating organisms are observed. Because the wet mount is only about 75% to 80% sensitive, other means of diagnosis are necessary if no organisms are observed microscopically.[56,57]

Stained smears of cervical specimens have been used in diagnosis but appear to be less sensitive and more time consuming than the wet mount. Culture techniques for trichomonads are highly specific and more sensitive than the wet mount; however, because up to 78 hours or longer may be necessary for growth, cultures are not useful in rapid diagnosis.[56,57]

In males, demonstration of trichomonads in urethral specimens by wet mount is difficult, and diagnosis depends largely on culture. Specimens from males should be taken prior to first voiding, as the small number of trichomonads in males may be reduced by micturition.[56,57]

### *Treatment*

Metronidazole is the only antimicrobial agent available in the United States consistently effective in *T. vaginalis* infections. In only a few cases have *T. vaginalis* isolates been resistant to standard metronidazole doses. In these instances, doses of metronidazole much higher than recommended may be necessary to achieve a cure.[13,15,56–58]

Treatment recommendations for *Trichomonas* infections are given in Table 85.8.[13–15] Until recent years, the standard therapy for trichomoniasis was metronidazole 250 mg three times daily for 7–10 days; however, numerous studies have documented similar efficacy with smaller amounts of metronidazole given as a single dose. When sexual partners are treated simultaneously, cure rates greater than 95% are reported with metronidazole 2 g in a single dose. If sexual partners are not treated concurrently, cure rates are in the range 80% to 90%. In limited clinical testing, single 1- and 1.5-g doses of metronidazole have been shown to produce high cure rates, also. Follow-up laboratory or clinical evaluation is frequently performed 48–72 hours after treatment.[13,14,56–58]

Advantages of single-dose therapy include better patient compliance, lower total dose, lower cost, and shorter exposure of the patient's gastrointestinal and urogenital anaerobic bacterial flora to the drug. As a result of the latter, the likelihood of developing pseudomembranous colitis or symptomatic candidal vulvovaginitis is decreased. Because high doses of metronidazole have metagenic effects in bacteria and oncogenic effects in mice, a reduced time of exposure in humans may be beneficial. At present there is no conclusive clinical evidence for either of these effects in humans after short-term, low-dose metronidazole therapy. Gastrointestinal complaints (anorexia, nausea, vomiting, diarrhea) are

**Table 85.8** Treatment of Trichomoniasis

| *Type* | *Recommended regimen* | *Alternative regimen* |
|---|---|---|
| Symptomatic and asymptomatic infections | Metronidazole 2.0 g PO in a single dose[a] | Metronidazole 250 mg PO 3 times daily for 7 days |
| Treatment in pregnancy | No treatment recommended unless symptoms are severe[b] | Clotrimazole 100 mg intravaginally at bedtime for 7 days[c] |
| Neonatal infections[d] | Metronidazole 10–30 mg/kg daily for 5–8 days | |

[a] Treatment failures should be treated with the same regimen. Persistent failures should be managed in consultation with an expert. Metronidazole 2 g PO daily for 3 days has been effective in patients infected with *T. vaginalis* strains mildly resistant to metronidazole, but experience is limited; higher doses also have been used.

[b] Metronidazole is contraindicated in the first trimester of pregnancy and should be avoided throughout pregnancy.

[c] Clotrimazole may produce symptomatic improvement and some cures.

[d] Only infants with symptomatic trichomoniasis or with urogenital trichomonal colonization that persists beyond the fourth week of life.

Recommendations are those of the CDC.[14]

more common with the single 2-g dose, occurring in 5% to 10% of treated patients. Some patients complain of a bitter metallic taste in the mouth. In patients intolerant of the single 2-g dose because of gastrointestinal side effects, a 7-day course of therapy is recommended.[57]

To achieve maximal cure rates and prevent relapse with the single 2-g dose of metronidazole, simultaneous treatment of infected sexual partners is necessary. In women treated with the 7-day course, however, relapse rates are not appreciably different regardless of whether or not sexual partners are treated. It is speculated that spontaneous resolution of trichomonal infection in many men or reduction in the number of trichomonads below the inoculum necessary to transmit disease may occur during the 7 days of the female's therapy.[56–58]

Frequently, patients who fail to respond to a course of metronidazole respond to re-treatment with the same regimen. In these cases sexual partners also should be retreated. For some *T. vaginalis* strains, higher dosages (2–7.5 g daily for 3–5 days) are usually effective. Good response rates also are reported for metronidazole 2–3 g orally plus a single 500-mg tablet administered intravaginally for 7–14 days. Use of intravenous metronidazole may be warranted for rare cases of intolerance to oral medication.[57,58]

Patients taking metronidazole should be instructed to avoid alcohol ingestion during therapy and for 1–2 days after completion of therapy because of a possible disulfiram-like effect. Metronidazole can potentiate the hypoprothrombinemic effects of warfarin, but a clinically significant effect is unlikely with single-dose regimens. Because metronidazole is secreted in breast milk, it is recommended that breast-feeding be interrupted for at least 24 hours after maternal ingestion of a single 2-g dose.[14,56–58]

At present, no satisfactory treatment is available for pregnant women with *Trichomonas* infections. Metronidazole is contraindicated during the first trimester of pregnancy and many experts recommend avoiding its use throughout pregnancy. Metronidazole easily crosses the placenta and fetal blood levels are comparable to maternal levels. A clear association between teratogenic effects and maternal ingestion during pregnancy has not been shown; on the basis of limited data, short courses of metronidazole administered during the second and third trimesters do not appear to increase the incidence of teratogenicity, prematurity, or fetal death. In pregnant patients with severe symptoms who do not respond to local palliative treatment, metronidazole may be required.[13–15,56–58]

Various local therapies for trichomoniasis also have been proposed for pregnant patients. Clotrimazole vaginal suppositories, 100 mg at bedtime for 6–8 days, relieve symptoms in many women and produce cure rates of 50% or greater.[59] An alternative therapy is gentle douching with 2 tablespoons of vinegar in a quart of warm water once or twice daily until symptoms improve, then less frequently thereafter. This therapy generally provides some symptomatic improvement but few cures. Although once recommended, povidone–iodine douches should be avoided during pregnancy because of the risk of fetal thyroid suppression.[56–57]

Several 5-nitroimidazole antibiotics related to metronidazole (tinidazole, nimorazole, ornidazole, carnidazole) are being investigated worldwide in the treatment of trichomoniasis. None appears to be superior to metronidazole in treating susceptible strains of *T. vaginalis*. Some of these antibiotics, however, may prove beneficial in infections exhibiting resistance to metronidazole.[56,58]

## Other Sexually Transmitted Diseases

Several STDs other than those previously discussed occur with varying frequency in the United States and throughout the world. While an in-depth discussion of these diseases is beyond the scope of this chapter, recommended treatment regimens are given in Table 85.9.[14]

**Table 85.9** Treatment Regimens for Miscellaneous Sexually Transmitted Diseases

| *Infection* | *Regimen of choice* | *Alternative regimen* |
|---|---|---|
| Chancroid (*Hemophilus ducreyi*) | Erythromycin 500 mg PO 4 times daily for 7 days *or* Ceftriaxone 250 mg IM in a single dose | Trimethoprim–sulfamethoxazole 160 mg/800 mg PO twice daily for 7 days, or 640 mg/3,200 mg PO in a single dose[a] *or* Amoxicillin 500 mg plus clavulanic acid 125 mg 3 times daily for 7 days |
| Lymphogranuloma venereum | Tetracycline 500 mg PO 4 times daily for at least 14 days | Doxycycline 100 mg PO twice daily for at least 14 days *or* Erythromycin 500 mg PO 4 times daily for at least 14 days *or* Sulfamethoxazole 1.0 g PO twice daily for at least 14 days |
| Condylomata acuminata | | |
| External genital/perianal warts | Cryotherapy (e.g., liquid nitrogen or carbon dioxide) *or* Podophyllin 10% in compound tincture of benzoin; applications washed off warts after 1–4 hours and repeated once or twice weekly | Electrosurgery *or* Surgical removal |
| Vaginal/cervical warts | Cryotherapy *or* 5-Fluorouracil cream | [b] |
| Enteric infections | | |
| *Campylobacter jejuni* | Erythromycin 500 mg PO 4 times daily for 7 days | |
| *Shigella* species | Trimethoprim–sulfamethoxazole 160 mg/800 mg PO twice daily for 7 days | Ampicillin 500 mg PO 4 times daily for 7 days[c] |
| Amebiasis | Metronidazole 750 mg PO 3 times daily for 5–10 days *plus* Iodoquinol (diiodohydroxyquin) 650 mg PO 3 times daily for 20 days | Metronidazole 750 mg PO 3 times daily for 5–10 days alone[d] *or* Paromomycin 25–30 mg/kg/d in 3 divided doses for 7 days |
| Giardiasis | Quinacrine 100 mg PO 3 times daily for 7 days | Metronidazole 250 mg PO 3 times daily for 7 days |

[a] Susceptibility of *H. ducreyi* varies widely.
[b] Podophyllin 10% in compound tincture of benzoin may be used for vaginal warts only if great care is taken to ensure that the treated area is dried before the speculum is removed. Because podophyllin is systemically absorbed and toxic, use of large amounts should be avoided. Podophyllin is **not recommended** for cervical warts.
[c] Resistance of shigellae to ampicillin is seen in many areas.
[d] Follow with luminal amebicide (e.g., iodoquinol) if clinical cure is not achieved.

Recommendations are those of the CDC.[14]

## Summary

More than 20 different diseases for which sexual transmission is epidemiologically important are identified. In the United States gonorrhea and chlamydia have reached epidemic proportions and the incidence of several other STDs such as genital herpes, syphilis, and AIDS is on the rise. For most STDs effective drug therapies are available; however, current therapeutic approaches to genital herpes and AIDS are not curative and, for herpes infections, provide only palliation and suppression of symptoms. Recently, treatment of gonorrhea and other STDs has been complicated by the emergence of strains resistant to such standard therapies as penicillin and tetracycline. Technologic advances in laboratory medicine during the past 5–10 years have resulted in improved and more rapid diagnostic capabilities for many STDs. For STDs such as gonorrhea and chlamydia, which are associated with a high incidence of asymptomatic cases, these new diagnostic tests may hold particular significance. Asymptomatic patients constitute a large reservoir for transmission of disease and also are potential candidates for development of long-term complications of untreated disease.

As a result of the increasing problem of STDs, greater emphasis today is being placed on primary prevention of STDs. Sexually active persons can minimize their risk of transmitting or acquiring some STDs by avoidance of certain sexual practices and proper use of physical and chemical barriers during intercourse. In the future, vaccines providing protection from gonorrhea, genital herpes, and AIDS also may have a significant effect on reducing the incidence of these infections.

## References

1. Krieger JN. Biology of sexually transmitted diseases. Urol Clin North Am 1984;11:15–25.
2. Holmes KK, Bell TA, Berger RE. Epidemiology of sexually transmitted diseases. Urol Clin North Am 1984;11:3–13.
3. Stone KM, Grimes DA, Magder LS. Primary prevention of sexually transmitted diseases. JAMA 1986;255:1763–1766.
4. Aral S, Holmes KK. Epidemiology of sexually transmitted diseases, in Holmes KK, Mardh P, Sparling PF, Wiesner PJ, (eds): Sexually Transmitted Diseases. New York, McGraw-Hill, 1984, pp 127–141.
5. Keat A. Reiter's syndrome and reactive arthritis in perspective. N Engl J Med 1983;309:1606–1615.
6. Hook EW III, Holmes KK. Gonococcal infections. Ann Intern Med 1985;102:229–243.
7. Duncan WC. Gonorrhea 1983. Dermatol Clin 1983;1:43–51.
8. Harrison WO. Gonococcal urethritis. Urol Clin North Am 1984;11:45–53.
9. Carmen JC. Gonorrhea. US Pharmacist 1983;8(7):53–63.
10. Britigan BE, Cohen MS, Sparling PF. Gonococcal infection: A model of molecular pathogenesis, N Engl J Med 1985;312:1683–1694.
11. Alexander ER. Maternal and infant sexually transmitted diseases. Urol Clin North Am 1984;11:131–139.
12. Rice RJ, Thompson SE. Treatment of uncomplicated infections due to *Neisseria gonorrhoeae*. JAMA 1986;255.1739–1746.
13. Washington AE. Preventing complications of sexually transmitted disease. Drugs 1984;28:355–370.
14. Centers for Disease Control. 1985 STD treatment guidelines. MMWR 1985;34(4S):75S–108S.
15. Anonymous. Treatment of sexually transmitted diseases. Med Lett Drugs Ther 1986;28:23–28.
16. Zola EM. Evaluation of drugs used in the prophylaxis of neonatal conjunctivitis. Drug Intell Clin Pharm 1984;18:692–696.
17. Kunimoto D, Brunham R, Ronald A. Beta-lactams in sexually transmitted diseases: rationale for selection and dosing regimens. Eur J Clin Microbiol 1984;3:605–611.
18. Stamm WE, Guinan ME, Johnson C, et al. Effect of treatment regimens for *Neisseria gonorrhoeae* on simultaneous infection with *Chlamydia trachomatis*. N Engl J Med 1984;310:545–549.
19. Fiumara NJ. Infectious syphilis. Dermatol Clin 1983;1:3–21.
20. Drusin LM. Syphilis: clinical manifestations, diagnosis, and treatment. Urol Clin North Am 1984;11:121–129.
21. Hart G. Syphilis tests in diagnostic and therapeutic decision making. Ann Intern Med 1986;104:368–376.
22. Poirier TI. Use and interpretation of tests for syphilis. Hosp Pharm 1980;15:204–209.
23. Feldman YM, Nikitas JA. Syphilis serology today. Arch Dermatol 1980;116:84–89.
24. Brown ST, Zaidi A, Larsen SA, et al. Serological response to syphilis treatment. JAMA 1985;253:1296–1299.
25. Markovitz DM, Beutner KR, Maggio RP, et al. Failure of recommended treatment of secondary syphilis. JAMA 1986; 255:1767–1768.
26. Stapleton JT, Stamm LV, Bassford PJ Jr. Potential for development of antibiotic resistance in pathogenic treponemes. Rev Infect Dis 1985;7(suppl 2):S314–S317.
27. Centers for Disease Control. Chlamydia trachomatis infections: policy guidelines for prevention and control. MMWR 1985;34 (3S):53S–74S.
28. Bowie WR. Nongonococcal urethritis. Urol Clin North Am 1984;11:55–64.
29. Bowie WR. Epidemiology and therapy of *Chlamydia trachomatis* infections. Drugs 1984;27:459–468.
30. Bowie WR. Nongonococcal urethritis. Dermatol Clin 1983;1: 53–64.
31. Felman YM, Nikitas JA. Nongonococcal urethritis. JAMA 1981;245:381–386.
32. Schachter J, Grossman M, Sweet RL, et al. Prospective study of perinatal transmission of *Chlamydia trachomatis*. JAMA 1986;255:3374–3377.
33. Rapoza PA, Quinn TC, Kiessling LA, et al. Assessment of neonatal conjunctivitis with a direct immunofluorescent monoclonal antibody stain for *Chlamydia*. JAMA 1986;255:3369–3373.
34. Jaffe HW. Nongonococcal urethritis: treatment of men and their sexual partners. Rev Infect Dis 1982;4(suppl):S772–S777.
35. Schachter J, Sweet RL, Grossman M, et al. Experience with the routine use of erythromycin for chlamydial infections in pregnancy. N Engl J Med 1986;276–279.
36. Sanders LL, Harrison HR, Washington AE. Treatment of sexually transmitted chlamydial infections. JAMA 1986;255: 1750–1756.

37. Marlowe SI. Medical management of genital herpes, editorial. Arch Dermatol 1985;121:467–470.
38. Steiner JF, Johnson RB, Driggers DA. Genital herpes simplex: diagnosis, treatment, prevention. US Pharmacist 1984;9:37–49.
39. Corey L, Spear PG. Infections with herpes simplex viruses (second of two parts). N Engl J Med 1986;314:749–757.
40. Straus SE, moderator. Herpes simplex virus infection: biology, treatment, and prevention. Ann Intern Med 1985;103:404–419.
41. Corey L, Spear PG. Infections with herpes simplex viruses (first of two parts). N Engl J Med 1986;314:686–691.
42. Mertz G, Corey L. Genital herpes simplex virus infections in adults. Urol Clin North Am 1984;11:103–119.
43. Corey L, Holmes KK. Genital herpes simplex virus infections: current concepts in diagnosis, therapy, and prevention. Ann Intern Med 1983;98:973–983.
44. Jordan MC, moderator. Latent herpesviruses of humans. Ann Intern Med 1984;100:866–880.
45. Rooney JF, Felser JM, Ostrove JM, et al. Acquisition of genital herpes from an asymptomatic partner. N Engl J Med 1986;314: 1561–1564.
46. Stagno S, Whitley RJ. Herpesvirus infections of pregnancy. Part II. Herpes simplex virus and varicella-zoster virus infections. N Engl J Med 1985;313:1327–1330.
47. Straus SE, Seidlin M, Takiff H. Management of mucocutaneous herpes simplex virus infections. Drugs 1984;27:364–372.
48. Guinan ME. Therapy for symptomatic genital herpes simplex virus infection: a review. Rev Infect Dis 1982;4(suppl): S819–S828.
49. Richards DM, Carmine AA, Brogden RN, et al. Acyclovir: a review of its pharmacodynamic properties and therapeutic efficacy. Drugs 1983;26:378–438.
50. Laskin OL. Acyclovir: pharmacology and clinical experience. Arch Intern Med 1984;144:1241–1246.
51. Gnann JW Jr, Barton NH, Whitley RJ. Acyclovir: mechanism of action, pharmacokinetics, safety and clinical applications. Pharmacotherapy 1983;3:275–283.
52. True BL, Carter BL. Update on acyclovir: oral therapy for herpesvirus infections. Clin Pharm 1984;3:607–613.
53. Guinan ME. Oral acyclovir for treatment and suppression of genital herpes simplex virus infection. JAMA 1986;255:1747–1749.
54. Lehrman SN, Douglas JM, Corey L, et al. Recurrent genital herpes and suppressive oral acyclovir therapy. Ann Intern Med 1986;104:786–790.
55. Crumpacker C. Resistance of herpes simplex virus to antiviral agents: is it clinically important? Drugs 1983;26:373–377.
56. Hume JC. Trichomoniasis, candidiasis and *Gardnerella vaginalis* vaginitis as sexually transmitted diseases. Dermatol Clin 1983;1:137–141.
57. Rein MF, Muller M. *Trichomonas vaginalis*, in Holmes KK, Mardh P, Sparling PF, Wiesner PJ (eds): Sexually Transmitted Diseases. New York, McGraw–Hill, 1984, pp 525–536.
58. Lossick JG. Treatment of *Trichomonas vaginalis* infections. Rev Infect Dis 1982;4(suppl):S801–S818.
59. Schnell JD. The incidence of vaginal candida and trichomonas infections and treatment of trichomonas vaginitis with clotrimazole. Postgrad Med J 1974;50(suppl 1):79–81.

# *Chapter 86* / Bone and Joint Infections

Edward P. Armstrong, PharmD

Osteomyelitis and septic arthritis are infections that continue to cause considerable morbidity. Fortunately, improved antibiotic and surgical therapies have greatly reduced the mortality, but residual damage and chronic relapsing infections may still occur. Recent challenges to clinicians include the emergence of new causative organisms and new precipitating factors. Improved nuclear medicine scanning techniques have decreased the delay in making a diagnosis, and the current emphasis on the rapid initiation of treatment has reduced the residual complications.

## Epidemiology

Osteomyelitis cases may be separated according to the mechanism by which the infecting organism reaches the bone:

- Hematogenous spread (through the bloodstream)
- Contiguous spread of an adjoining soft tissue infection
- Direct inoculation of the bone by a puncture wound, open fracture, or surgery

Because many patients who develop osteomyelitis also have diabetes mellitus, patients are also commonly divided into those patients with and those without peripheral vascular disease.

Osteomyelitis is not an uncommon disease. One case series noted that 247 patients had osteomyelitis over a 4-year period.[1] It is estimated that acute hematogenous osteomyelitis has an annual incidence of 4.5 per 100,000 population.[2] Approximately 19% of osteomyelitis patients developed their infections from hematogenous origin. Infections caused by a contiguous focus of infection (including postoperative, direct puncture, and associated soft tissue infections) constitute 47% of infections. Osteomyelitis occurring in the subgroup of patients with vascular insufficiency constitutes 34% of infections.

Another means of classifying osteomyelitis is according to whether the disease is acute or chronic in nature. Acute osteomyelitis accounts for 56% of patients; chronic infections, defined as those for which a previous hospital admission for the same infection was necessary, account for 44% of patients.

Infectious arthritis continues to be a common problem. An inflammatory reaction in the joint space (arthritis) occurs with infections from many different microorganisms. Infectious arthritis has been shown to be one of the most common causes of new cases of arthritis.[3] One study reported 97 cases of nongonococcal infections over an 18-year period and a slightly higher incidence of gonococcal infections.[4] Infections may involve single or multiple joints and may be caused by a variety of infecting organisms. Joint infections may be categorized according to the entrance route of the infecting organism. Infectious arthritis may arise from hematogenous spread, as a result of direct contamination of the joint space, or from the spread of an adjacent bone infection. Hematogenous disease by far constitutes the majority of cases.[5] Infections occurring from direct inoculation and spread from osteomyelitis are less common. Infectious arthritis frequently occurs in patients over 30 years of age.[3] Approximately 20% of cases occur in children.[6]

## Pathophysiology

### *Hematogenous Osteomyelitis*

Hematogenous osteomyelitis most commonly occurs in children less than 16 years of age. Infections may occur in adults, but these are less common. The vascular structure within the long bones appears to predispose for hematogenous infections within the metaphyses (Fig. 86.1). In this area, the nutrient arteries end in hairpin turns near the growth plate and flow into veins of much wider diameter. This causes considerable slowing of blood flow within the metaphyses, allowing bacteria within the bloodstream to settle and initiate an inflammatory response. In addition, the metaphyseal capillaries have impaired phagocytic function, which also contributes to a predisposition to infection within this area. After bacterial seeding occurs and leads to an infection, avascular necrosis within the bone may develop from occlusion of the nutrient vessels and release of bacterial enzymes.

The exudate within the bone continues to increase as the infection develops, causing increased pressure. The resultant effects of this pressure differ with the patient's age. During childhood, the infection is contained by the growth plate, and thus the exudate pushes out on the periosteum. As the cortex is thin and the periosteum is not tightly bound to the bone in this age group, the exudate may push through the cortex and raise the periosteum, producing a subperiosteal abscess. Impairment of blood flow to the outer portion of cortical bone may then occur, producing sequestra (dead bone, separated from sound bone).

In adults, the periosteum is tightly bound and the cortex is thick. This structure generally causes the infection to remain intramedullary. The infection may spread to adjacent bone structures through the Haversian and Volkmann canals. Chronic osteomyelitis may occur if large segments of avascular bone are involved. In infants, not only can the infection spread to involve the periosteum and the shaft as in children,

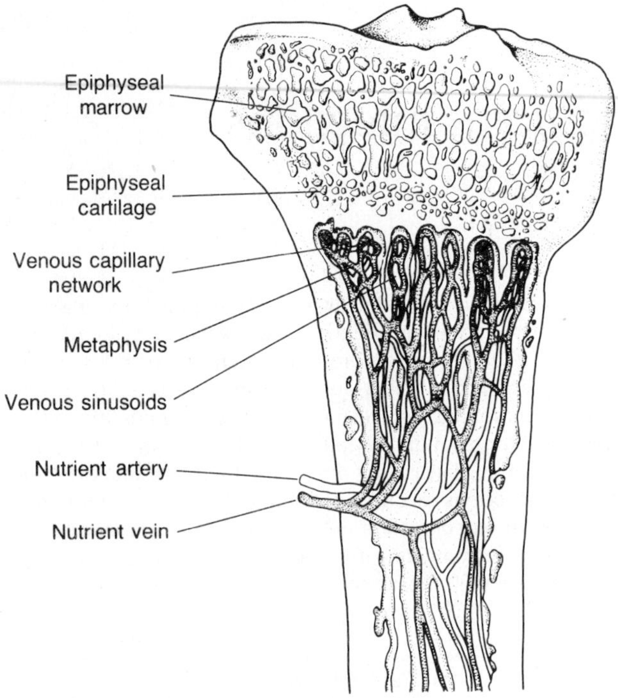


**Figure 86.1.** Cross section of normal bone.

but the infection may also spread to infect the joint space as their capillary loops still penetrate the epiphyseal growth plate.

Within hematogenous osteomyelitis, the specific bones infected are usually age dependent. Infections located within the long bones such as the femur, tibia, and humerus usually occur in children. Vertebral infections are more common in individuals over 50 years of age. Multiple-bone involvement occurs commonly in neonatal infections.

The bacteriology of hematogenous osteomyelitis is unique in that it is most commonly caused by a single organism. *Staphylococcus aureus* constitutes 60% to 90% of the infections in children. *Streptococcus* and gram-negative infections do occur, but these agents are less common. In hematogenous neonatal osteomyelitis, the infecting bacteria are usually *S. aureus*, group B streptococcus, and *Escherichia coli*. *E. coli* and *S. aureus* infections more commonly have multiple-bone involvement and are associated with complications during pregnancy or delivery.

Pyogenic vertebral osteomyelitis from hematogenous spread seems to occur in the vascular areas near the subchondral plate region of the vertebral body. As previously mentioned, this type of infection usually occurs in adults; the highest incidence is in the fifth and sixth decades of life, and the lumbar and thoracic regions are the most commonly involved sites. The most common infecting organisms in vertebral infections are staphylococcal organisms, which constitute at least 60% of infections; however, gram-negative organisms are playing an increasingly important role. *E. coli* is the most common of the gram-negative organisms, and, as one might expect, it often causes osteomyelitis after a urinary tract infection, positive urine culture, or gram-negative bacteremia. Skin and respiratory tract infections are other common sources for septicemias that lead to vertebral infections.

Intravenous drug abusers are another group of patients who appear to be more likely to develop osteomyelitis. Over 50% of the osteomyelitis infections in these patients arise in the vertebral column, with less than 20% occurring in either the pelvic girdle or sternoarticular structures. Infections are seen less commonly in the extremities. A feature unique to intravenous drug abusers is the infecting organism responsible for osteomyelitis: aerobic gram-negative organisms cause 88% of these infections.[7] *Pseudomonas aeruginosa*, either alone or in combination with other organisms, is isolated in approximately 78% of all patients. The organisms *Klebsiella*, *Enterobacter*, and *Serratia* are not infrequent, and staphylococcal and streptococcal infections may also occur. Intravenous abusers of pentazocine hydrochloride and pyribenzamine appear to have a higher incidence of pyogenic infections of the pubic symphysis secondary to *P. aeruginosa*.

Another unusual infecting organism causing osteomyelitis is *Salmonella*. Although uncommon in most patients, patients with sickle cell anemia and related hemoglobinopathy have a predilection for infections from these organisms. *Salmonella* species account for two thirds of the infections in these patients. These infections may occur after bowel infarctions common in sickle cell disease that subsequently allow *Salmonella* to leave the colon and spread hematogenously to the bone. Infections in these patients may occur in any bone; however, they are most common in the medullary cavity of long or tubular bones. Infections in these patients may become quite advanced because of the difficulty of distinguishing the pain of a sickle cell crisis from that of osteomyelitis. Staphylococcal and other gram-positive infections do occur but less commonly.

### *Contiguous-Spread Osteomyelitis*

Osteomyelitis secondary to a contiguous focus of infection is another large category of infections. This group includes those infections caused by direct entrance of organisms from a source outside the body or by progressive spread of infection from tissue adjacent to the bone. Direct inoculation may occur from penetrating wounds (e.g., trauma), open fractures, or various invasive orthopedic procedures. Although postoperative infections may occur with many different types of procedures, more than 80% of infections are caused by open reductions of fractures. Specifically, these infections most commonly occur after an internal fixation of a hip fracture or a femoral or tibial shaft fracture. Osteomyelitis is much less common secondary to craniotomies, disk surgery, and repair of degenerative arthritis. In contrast, open fractures are more likely to become infected because they are contaminated by a wide range of bacteria.

Osteomyelitis occurring secondary to the direct spread of an adjoining soft tissue infection is another important group of infections. Infections involving the fingers and toes constitute the largest number of cases. Less commonly, infections may spread from infected teeth to involve the mandible. In addition, osteomyelitis may occur secondary to sinus infections by spreading through the mucosal lining of the sinuses into the vascular system surrounding the bone.

In great contrast to hematogenous osteomyelitis, which is

most common in children, contiguous-spread osteomyelitis most commonly occurs in patients over the age of 50. Predisposing factors (such as hip fractures, which are common in this older age group) apparently are related to the incidence of osteomyelitis in this group.

In addition, the bacteriology of contiguous-spread osteomyelitis is very different from that found in hematogenous osteomyelitis. Although *S. aureus* is still the most common infecting organism, very often there is gram-negative and multiple-organism involvement. *P. aeruginosa*, *Proteus*, *Streptococcus*, *E. coli*, *Staphylococcus epidermidis*, and anaerobes may all be found. An exception appears to be infections occurring secondary to puncture wounds of the foot; there is a strong association between puncture wounds of the foot and gram-negative osteomyelitis, especially infections caused by *P. aeruginosa*.

Osteomyelitis occurring in association with vascular insufficiency is extremely difficult to manage. Most of these patients have diabetes mellitus or severe atherosclerosis, and these infections usually occur in patients 50–70 years of age. Typically, their infections involve the toes or small bones of the feet. Frequently, the osteomyelitis is contiguous with overlaying areas of cellulitis or ulcers. Diabetic patients who develop osteomyelitis may also have other diabetic complications such as neuropathy and nephropathy.

Infections occurring in patients with concomitant vascular insufficiency almost always result from mixed floral infections. Over half of the cultures obtained from these patients' bones or wounds contain either the combination of *Staphylococcus* and *Streptococcus* or the combination of *Staphylococcus*, *Streptococcus*, and Enterobacteriaceae.

Anaerobic organisms may also play an important role in osteomyelitis. Traditionally, anaerobic involvement was thought to be uncommon; this may in part result from the technical difficulty in obtaining and growing adequate anaerobic cultures. With improved culture techniques, anaerobic organisms are being isolated more frequently. When anaerobic bacteria are the etiological agents of infection, they are often found in association with other organisms, including aerobic bacteria. The most common predisposing factors in patients who have anaerobic osteomyelitis are previous fractures (48%) and diabetes mellitus (11%).[8] The infections associated with diabetes mellitus occur almost exclusively within the foot. *Bacteroides fragilis* and *Bacteroides melaninogenicus* constitute the majority of anaerobic bone isolates.

### *Infectious Arthritis*

In contrast to many cases of osteomyelitis, infectious arthritis is usually hematogenously acquired.[9] The synovial tissue is very vascular and does not have a basement membrane; this provides organisms in the blood convenient access to the synovial fluid. Some organisms, such as *Neisseria gonorrhoeae*, are especially likely to infect a joint during a bacteremia. Organisms may also infect a joint from a deep penetrating wound, intraarticular steroid injection, arthroscopy, prosthetic-joint surgery, and contiguous osteomyelitis rupture into the joint.[4]

Overall, *S. aureus* is the most common infecting organism, accounting for approximately 40% of cases.[4] Streptococcal infections constitute 33% and gram-negative organisms account for 23% of patients. *E. coli* is the most common gram-negative organism; however, *P. aeruginosa* is the most frequent offending agent in intravenous drug abusers.[10] A wide range of organisms may cause septic arthritis in infants under 1 month of age including streptococcus, gram-negative organisms, and *S. aureus*. *Hemophilus influenzae* is a frequent pathogen in children less than 5 years of age. *S. aureus* is the primary organism responsible for infections within adults. In contrast, patients with disseminated gonococcal infection are usually young, healthy adults. *N. gonorrhoeae* is the most common cause of bacterial arthritis in adults under 30. The disease is most common in women.[11]

After entrance into the joint, the bacteria multiply and cause a persistent purulent effusion to develop. Chronic and sometimes irreversible changes may occur in the joint if the effusion is present after 7 days. A hot, swollen, painful joint usually occurs concomitantly with the effusion. Cartilage and bone damage result from the release of proteolytic enzymes and pressure necrosis.

Patients who are more likely to develop joint infections include immunocompromised patients (those with cancer, diabetes mellitus, and chronic liver disease).[6] Intravenous drug abusers are also prone to develop septic arthritis. Arthritis, joint trauma, and surgery are other very important risk factors, as chronic inflammation or trauma makes the joint more likely to become infected. In addition, rheumatoid arthritis patients may be prone to bacterial infection because of an inherent phagocytic defect and because of concomitant corticosteroid therapy. Women are more prone to disseminated gonococcal infections than men and are especially likely to develop gonococcal bacteremias during pregnancy or just after menses.

## Clinical Presentation

### *Signs and Symptoms*

The signs and symptoms of osteomyelitis vary depending on the mechanism by which the infection occurs. The presenting symptoms in hematogenous osteomyelitis vary widely. Some patients complain of tenderness, pain, swelling, fever, chills, decreased motion, and malaise, while other patients may only have a mild fever. Although hematogenous neonatal osteomyelitis infections may spread rapidly to cross the epiphyseal plate and involve the joint, there may be very few systemic symptoms present. A joint effusion, which is seen in 60% to 70% of patients, or decreased limb motion and edema may be the only signs on which to base a diagnosis.

Patients with pyogenic vertebral osteomyelitis may also vary in their presentation. Many complain of severe back pain, fever or night sweats, and weight loss. Others may report a more gradual onset of symptoms with a possible low-grade fever and complaints of a continuous back pain. The pain is usually present at rest but may increase with movement. If the infection extends and compresses the spinal cord, neurologic symptoms may develop.

Signs and symptoms of contiguous-spread osteomyelitis depend on the precipitating event. Symptoms in this type of osteomyelitis usually are apparent within 1 month of the precipitating trauma or surgery. Some patients may develop a fever and leukocytosis, but the most frequent symptom is pain in the area of infection. The physical examination may demonstrate localized tenderness, warmth, edema, and erythema. Patients with vascular insufficiency may complain of systemic manifestations, but usually local symptoms (such as pain, swelling, and redness) predominate. These patients frequently present with cellulitis or ulcers on their toes or feet.

Because of the differences in the clinical presentation and microbiologic characteristics, it is important to separate infectious arthritis into nongonococcal and gonococcal bacterial arthritis. Patients with nongonococcal bacterial arthritis almost always present with hot, swollen, painful joints. Nongonococcal bacterial arthritis patients usually present with elevated temperatures, although only half of the patients have an elevated white blood cell count on initial presentation. The average initial synovial white blood cell count is 100,000/mm$^3$ or greater in these patients.

Nongonococcal bacterial arthritis is usually monoarticular, with the knee being most commonly involved.[12] Other frequently infected joints include the shoulder, wrist, hip, ankle, interphalangeal, and elbow. The initial source of bacteremia leading to the infected joint can be located in most patients. Respiratory tract, skin, and urinary tract are common routes for bacterial entrance. Blood cultures are positive in 50% of patients.

The most frequent initial sign of disseminated gonococcal infection is a migratory polyarthralgia. Fever, dermatitis, and tenosynovitis (inflammation of the tendon sheath) are all found in the presentation of two thirds of patients. Half of these patients have polyarthritis. Small papules on the trunk or extremities are the most frequent skin lesions seen in these patients, but only 30% to 40% of patients with disseminated gonococcal infection present with the classic hot, swollen, purulent joint. The mean synovial white blood cell count is usually 50,000/mm$^3$ or more.

Joint infections occurring after insertion of a prosthetic joint have become a more frequent problem. The infection rate after joint replacement surgery is usually less than 5%; however, infections are more common after surgical revision of prosthetic joints. As expected, these patients are usually elderly and have a history of either osteoarthritis or rheumatoid arthritis. Often, patients state they have had some pain in the area, which may have been present for a period of months. Although the white blood cell count is usually normal in these patients, their erythrocyte sedimentation rate is often elevated. Intraoperative contamination is thought to result in infections within the first year after joint replacement. Infections occurring after this time period most likely result from hematogenous spread. Staphylococci are the most common infecting organisms. *S. epidermidis* accounts for 40% of prosthetic-joint infections, and *S. aureus* is responsible for 20% of infections.[13] Multiple organisms and anaerobic bacteria may also be involved.

### *Radiologic and Laboratory Tests*

In evaluation of a patient who may have osteomyelitis, radiologic examination may be difficult to interpret in the early stages of the disease because the roentgenogram findings are still normal. Most patients with hematogenous osteomyelitis will have no changes in roentgenogram films until 10 days after the onset of the illness because more than 50% of bone matrix must be removed before the lesions can be detected. Radionuclide scanning techniques may allow earlier examination of the focus of infection. Technetium phosphate and gallium scans may be positive as early as 1 day after the onset of symptoms and 10–14 days before any radiographic changes may be seen; however, tumor, bone repair, and other inflammatory processes may produce false-positive scans.

In spite of the seriousness of osteomyelitis, frequently there are minimal laboratory abnormalities; the sedimentation rate and white blood cell count may be the only abnormal findings. The degree of abnormality of these two laboratory findings does not correlate with prediction of the disease outcome.

Accurate culture information is especially important laboratory data in osteomyelitis. To provide appropriate antibiotic therapy, it is essential to establish a definitive bacteriologic diagnosis. Blood cultures, which may be positive in up to 50% of patients with hematogenous osteomyelitis infections, are very important. Aspirates of subperiosteal pus or metaphyseal fluid yield a pathogen in 70% of cases. Cultures should be done for both aerobic and anaerobic bacteria. A needle aspiration at the point of maximal tenderness should be done whenever osteomyelitis is suspected. If subperiosteal pus is not found, the needle should be inserted into the bone to obtain additional culture material. Surgical debridement may be required if pus is found. A Gram stain of the aspirate may be very useful in initiating appropriate antibiotic therapy. This allows a more appropriate choice of antibiotics from the first day of therapy rather than waiting several days while culture results are pending.

If a specimen is obtained from a previously undrained or unopened wound abscess, the pathogen can usually be identified. In chronic osteomyelitis, however, identification can be more difficult. Open wounds and draining sinuses are frequently contaminated with other organisms and thus provide inaccurate culture information. A comparison between sinus-tract cultures and cultures obtained during surgery from 40 patients with chronic osteomyelitis showed that less than half the sinus-tract cultures contained the operative pathogen.[14] Therefore, because of the inaccuracies with sinus-tract cultures, they cannot be relied upon to reflect the bacteriology of the osteomyelitis. On the other hand, cultures of orthopedic devices removed from infected bone or aspirates of loculated pus in the area can be trusted to identify the infecting organism. The preferable time to obtain culture material in a patient with a chronic draining sinus is at the time of open surgical debridement.

In evaluating the possibility of a patient having infectious arthritis, immediate joint aspiration with subsequent analysis of the synovial fluid is extremely important. The presence of purulent fluid usually indicates the presence of a septic joint. The synovial fluid white blood cell count is usually 50,000–200,000/mm$^3$ when an infection is present. Approximately half of the patients with an infected joint will have a low synovial glucose level, usually less than 40 mg/dL.

Gram stains of joint fluid demonstrate bacteria in approximately 50% of patients with septic arthritis, although such stains may be positive in only 25% of patients with gonococcal infections. Synovial fluid cultures are usually positive in patients with nongonococcal infections. Both blood and joint fluid should be cultured aerobically and anaerobically for a patient suspected of having an infected joint. Blood cultures are positive in one half of patients with nongonococcal infections but in only 20% of those with gonococcal infections. Pharyngeal, rectal, and cervical or urethral smears and cultures should be done if a disseminated gonococcal infection is considered. As with osteomyelitis, most patients will have an elevated erythrocyte sedimentation rate.

Roentgenograms of infected joints often reveal distension of the joint capsule with soft tissue swelling in the adjacent space. Magnetic resonance imaging may be helpful in identifying an infected hip. In patients who have developed an infected prosthetic joint, loosening of the prosthesis may be seen radiographically.

### *Prognosis*

The prognosis or ultimate outcome of osteomyelitis depends upon the acute or chronic nature of the disease and how rapidly appropriate therapy is instituted.

Patients with acute osteomyelitis have the best prognosis. One study of 50 patients who had surgery if needed and received injectable antibiotics for a median duration of 12 weeks had a cure rate of 84%.[15] Similar studies have shown cure rates of 80% to 94.7%.[16,17]

Patients with chronic osteomyelitis, on the other hand, have a much poorer prognosis. Dead bone (necrotic material from the infection) acts as a bacterial reservoir and makes the infection very difficult to eliminate. Adequate surgical debridement to remove all the dead bone and prolonged administration of antibiotics provide the best chance to obtain a cure. The inability to remove all the dead bone may allow residual infection and require suppressive antibiotics to keep the infection under control.

Many patients who now develop infectious arthritis recover with no long-term defects. Gonococcal arthritis usually resolves rapidly with antibiotics; however, patients with staphylococcal arthritis have a higher incidence of joint damage. Individuals at greatest risk for long-term sequelae are those in whom (1) symptoms are present for more than 7 days before treatment is started, (2) infections occur in the hip joint, and (3) infections are caused by gram-negative organisms. Death rates are highest among patients with underlying cancer and liver failure. Common long-term residual effects are limited joint motion and persistent joint pain.[3] Shortening of the affected extremity may also occur. One study noted that over half of the children who subsequently developed residual joint damage were believed to be normal at the time of hospital discharge.[18]

## Treatment

After identification of the infecting organism, the cornerstone of therapy in acute osteomyelitis is the administration of appropriate antibiotics in adequate doses. Early antibiotic therapy may avoid the need for surgery but a delay in treatment may allow bone necrosis to occur and make elimination of the infection more difficult. If all necrotic tissue is not removed surgically, microorganisms may remain and cause recurrent exacerbations of the infection.

If a patient with hematogenous osteomyelitis does not respond to intensive antibiotic therapy within 48–72 hours with a decrease in fever, local swelling, redness, and pain, the patient should undergo surgical debridement of the infection. It is very important to emphasize the importance of starting antibiotics as soon as the cultures have been taken. One study found no failures in eliminating the infection if injectable antibiotics were started within 48 hours from the onset of symptoms in children with osteomyelitis.[19]

Antibiotics used in the management of acute osteomyelitis are generally given intravenously in high doses so that adequate drug concentrations are reached within the infected bone. Empirically, 8–12 g daily of a penicillinase-resistant penicillin (such as nafcillin or oxacillin), ampicillin, or cephalosporin or a similar dose of another antibiotic is used in the management of adults with osteomyelitis; however, the specific dose of antibiotic required and its resultant concentration within the infected bone are largely unknown.

Semisynthetic penicillins, cephalosporins, clindamycin, and the aminoglycosides can all be detected in bone homogenates soon after their administration. Studies of bone concentrations of antibiotics have shown a wide range of measured concentrations. Antibiotics most likely enter the bone by passive diffusion, which relies on blood flow to the area.

A great deal of the nonuniformity in antibiotic bone concentration data results from varied techniques of sampling and measuring bone antibiotic concentrations. Much of the data providing bone concentration information have been determined in patients who did not have infections but were undergoing an orthopedic procedure such as a total hip replacement. In these studies, after the patient received the antibiotic, bone biopsies were obtained. The bone fragments were typically washed, allowed to dry, pulverized, and mixed with buffer. The supernatant fluid was used for assay procedures and the measured antibiotic concentration was related to the weight of the original bone sample. This technique does not separate different bone layers nor does it estimate the concentrations within infected bone. Newer techniques with animal models are attempting to provide more meaningful results.

The specific length of antibiotic therapy needed in the management of osteomyelitis is also not clearly defined. Dich et al observed a failure rate of 19% in children who were treated with injectable antibiotics for 3 weeks or less[20]; however, it was noted that only one of 48 children who had received injectable antibiotics for more than 3 weeks relapsed. It has also been shown that the same results are achieved in patients treated for longer than 3 weeks regardless of whether they received subsequent oral antibiotics after injectable doses.

Thus, because there appears to be no additional benefit from follow-up oral therapy, the standard treatment for acute osteomyelitis in all patients should be injectable antibiotic therapy for 4 to 6 weeks without subsequent oral antibiotics.

Glover conducted a retrospective analysis of 58 patients who had acute osteomyelitis.[15] Symptoms (bone pain, tenderness) were present less than 7 days in 30 patients (52%) and for 8–14 days in 8 patients (14%). Forty-four of the patients required surgical drainage. Thirty patients were treated with clindamycin, 16 patients received cloxacillin, and the remaining patients received various other antibiotics according to their culture and sensitivity data. The median duration of antibiotic therapy was 12 weeks. Forty-eight of the patients were cured, 9 patients developed chronic osteomyelitis, and 1 patient died from unclear causes.

Recently, Sheftel and Mader reported the results of a randomized comparison of ceftazidime versus the combination of ticarcillin and tobramycin for the treatment of gram-negative bacterial osteomyelitis.[21] Patients received either ceftazidime 2 g every 12 hours or ticarcillin 3 g every 4 hours plus tobramycin 1.5 mg/kg every 8 hours. The tobramycin dose was adjusted to achieve a peak serum level between 4 and 5 mg/mL and a trough serum level less than 2 mg/mL. Both regimens were administered for at least 4 weeks after the last major surgical debridement (mean duration of therapy was 45 days). Eighteen patients completed the study (nine in each group). Six of nine ceftazidime patients were cured of their infections, and three were ceftazidime failures. All nine patients receiving the combination of ticarcillin and tobramycin were cured of their infections. No patients were noted to have nephrotoxicity from the aminoglycoside; one patient receiving ceftazidime had a mild increase in serum glutamic–oxalacetic transaminase and serum glutamic–pyruvic transaminase levels during therapy.

### *Oral Antibiotic Therapy*

Treatment with oral antibiotics may be appropriate in certain circumstances. Osteomyelitis in children has been treated successfully with oral agents.

Several recent studies have been published.[22–32] Two studies used injectable antibiotics initially and then switched to oral antibiotics when there was a decrease in the clinical signs of inflammation and the erythrocyte sedimentation rate or when the patient was afebrile for 3 days.[22,23] If pus was obtained on the initial needle aspirate or if a reduction in fever, local swelling, and tenderness did not occur despite adequate rest, immobilization, and intensive antibiotic therapy, the patients underwent surgical drainage. Very importantly, in using oral antibiotic therapy, these researchers monitored the patients very closely. In addition to following the clinical and radiographic course of the patients, some studies included the measurement of serum antibiotic concentrations and others included bactericidal titers.[22–27] One group of researchers[24] adjusted the oral doses and added probenecid to regimens to raise the peak serum bactericidal titer to greater than 1:16 and to maintain a trough serum bactericidal titer greater than 1:2. Serum bactericidal titers were used in two other studies with the goal of achieving a peak titer greater than 1:8.[22,28] Serum bactericidal activity may be helpful in verifying the likelihood of success with an antibiotic, as well as in determining the adequacy of oral therapy.[28,31] Studies in which oral therapy followed initial treatment with injectable antibiotics demonstrate that this method is very useful in children with osteomyelitis (Table 86.1).

Patients enrolled in these studies generally had disease of recent onset, identification of the infecting organism, enforced compliance, and surgery if needed. Many studies used microbiologic titers in monitoring the antibiotic regimens. In patients who meet these criteria, oral antibiotics appear to offer a great advantage in the treatment of osteomyelitis. Patients not meeting these criteria are more likely to develop chronic osteomyelitis with the resultant recurrent exacerbations of the infection. For example, because of the vascular compromise and impaired immunologic mechanisms present in patients with long-standing diabetes mellitus, these patients appear to be a very poor choice for oral antibiotic therapy.

A major advance in the oral antibiotic therapy of osteomyelitis has occurred with the availability of ciprofloxacin. Ciprofloxacin is effective in the treatment of osteomyelitis caused by *E. cloacae*, *S. marcescens*, and *P. aeruginosa*. Its activity against gram-negative bacilli allows patients to be treated orally and avoid the potential toxic complications of 4 to 6 weeks of aminoglycoside therapy. However, because ciprofloxacin may cause cartilage damage, it should not be used in children or pregnant women.

### *Selection of Antibiotics*

A critical feature in the management of acute osteomyelitis is the selection of appropriate antibiotics. Often, empiric therapy must be selected on the basis of the most likely infecting organism while the results of culture and sensitivity data are pending. Empiric therapy recommendations are summarized in Table 86.2.

As *S. aureus* is the most common infecting organism in children, a dosage of 150 mg/kg/d of a penicillinase-resistant penicillin, such as nafcillin or oxacillin, is appropriate. Because of the risk of interstitial nephritis, methicillin is not preferred. If patients are allergic to penicillin, a first-generation cephalosporin, vancomycin, or clindamycin may be used. Children with osteomyelitis can usually be treated adequately with 4 weeks of injectable therapy.

Children in whom the infecting organism is identified, and who have undergone surgery if needed, may be candidates for the alternative oral antibiotic regimen. It is currently recommended that injectable antibiotic therapy be continued until there has been a resolution in the erythema, swelling, and tenderness and until the patient is afebrile. Dicloxacillin, cloxacillin, and cephalexin (100 mg/kg/d) are effective oral agents. Because of erratic absorption, nafcillin is not recommended for oral antibiotic use. If peak serum bactericidal titers are used in monitoring oral therapy, the antibiotic dose may be increased or probenecid may be added if the titer is not at least 1:8. Patients should be monitored closely with periodic white blood cell counts, erythrocyte sedimentation rates, and roentgenograms. When oral antibiotics are used, the total duration of oral and injectable therapy is usually 4 to 6 weeks or longer until the signs and symptoms of infection have resolved.

Hematogenous osteomyelitis in an adult is most frequently caused by *S. aureus* and thus is appropriately treated with 8–12 g/d of a penicillinase-resistant penicillin such as oxacillin or nafcillin. A similar dose of a first-generation cephalosporin, clindamycin, 2.4 g/d, or vancomycin, 2 g/d (with normal renal function) may be used in those individuals allergic to penicillin; however, if the infection is located within the vertebrae, *E. coli* must be considered and thus, depending upon the culture and sensitivity data, a switch to ampicillin may be needed. After institution of appropriate antibiotic therapy, the antimicrobial agent should be continued for 4 to 6 weeks.

**Table 86.1** Oral Treatment of Osteomyelitis

| *Reference* | *Number of patients* | *Patient age* | *Antibiotic* | *Duration* | *Serum bactericidal titer* | *Number of patients requiring surgical drainage* | *Outcome* |
|---|---|---|---|---|---|---|---|
| 22 | 22 | 1 mo–14 yr | Methicillin or cefazolin IV | 5–13 d | Yes | 15 | 21 cures, 1 chronic osteomyelitis |
| | | | Cephalexin or penicillin or ampicillin PO | 14–42 d | | | |
| 23 | 18 | 17 mo–16 yr | Oxacillin or methicillin IV | 5–14 d | No | 9 | 18 excellent |
| | | | Dicloxacillin PO | 4–8 wk | | | |
| 24 | 22 | 1–15 yr | Nafcillin or methicillin IV | 4–28 d | Yes | 3 | No recurrences |
| | | | Dicloxacillin and probenecid PO | To complete 6 wk therapy | | | |
| 25 | 29 | 5 wk–15 yr | Clindamycin IV | 3–4 wk | No | — | 28 recovered or healing |
| | | | Clindamycin PO | 4–6 wk | | | 1 had roentgenogram abnormality |
| 26 | 24 | 1 mo–13 yr | Clindamycin IV | 3–17 d | No | — | 19 excellent, 4 fair, and 1 poor |
| | | | Clindamycin PO | At least 6 wk total for acute and 3 mo for chronic | | | |
| 27 | 25 | 1–14 yr | Nafcillin or methicillin IV | 14–38 d | Yes | 12 | 9 excellent, 4 complications |
| | | | ± Dicloxacillin PO | 0–8 wk | | | |
| | | | *or* | | | | |
| | | | Clindamycin IV, then clindamycin PO | Afebrile 3 d<br>3–9 wk | | | 11 excellent, 1 complication |
| 28 | 217 | 1 mo–12 yr | Lincomycin, cloxacillin, ampicillin, benzylpenicillin, fusidic acid, or gentamicin | To complete 6–8 wk of total therapy | No | 69 | 208 successes, 9 failures |
| 30 | 28 | 3–16 yr | Cefadroxil PO | Unknown | No | 22 | 23 excellent, 4 good, 1 failure |
| | 24 | 17–80 yr | Cefadroxil PO | 35 d | No | 37 | 23 excellent, 1 failure |
| | | | *or* | | | | |
| | | | Oxacillin IV, then dicloxacillin PO | 7 d<br>28 d | No | 0 | 22 excellent, 2 failures |
| 31 | 29 | Children | Cefamandole IV | 2–21 d | Yes | 22 | 28 cures<br>1 failure |
| | | | Cefaclor PO | At least 3 wk | | | |
| | | | Cefuroxime IV | 2–21 d | | | |
| | | | Cefaclor or cephalexin PO | At least 3 wk | | | |
| 32 | 10 | 2–15 yr | Cephradine IV | ≤72 h or 4 wk | Yes | 0 | All cured |
| | | | Amoxicillin or cephradine or cloxacillin or penicillin V PO | To complete at least 6 wk | | | |

**Table 86.2** Empiric Treatment of Osteomyelitis

| *Patient subtype* | *Likely infecting organism* | *Antibiotic* |
|---|---|---|
| Children | *Staphylococcus aureus* | Penicillinase-resistant penicillin |
| Adults | *S. aureus* | Penicillinase-resistant penicillin |
| Newborn | *S. aureus,* streptococci, *Escherichia coli* | Penicillinase-resistant penicillin plus aminoglycoside |
| Sickle cell anemia patients | *Salmonella, S. aureus* | Penicillinase-resistant penicillin plus ampicillin |
| IV drug abusers | *Pseudomonas* | Aminoglycoside |
| Postoperative patients | Gram-positive and gram-negative organisms | Penicillinase-resistant penicillin plus aminoglycoside |
| Patients with vascular insufficiency | Gram-positive and gram-negative organisms | Penicillinase-resistant penicillin plus aminoglycoside |

Newborn infants developing osteomyelitis must be covered for the most likely pathogens including *S. aureus*, group B streptococci, and *E. coli*. Therapy with a penicillinase-resistant penicillin such as oxacillin or nafcillin at 150 mg/kg/d and either an aminoglycoside or ampicillin at 150 mg/kg/d may be initiated. The dosage for the aminoglycosides should be adjusted to the patient's age, weight, and renal function. Usually a peak gentamicin or tobramycin concentration of 5 μg/mL is effective. Depending on the results of culture and sensitivity data, a first-generation cephalosporin may be an alternative in these patients. As with children, neonates should receive at least 4 weeks of therapy.

Osteomyelitis in a patient with a hemoglobinopathy, such as sickle cell anemia, may be complicated by either *Salmonella* or *S. aureus* infections. Thus, the empiric antibiotics of first choice are a penicillinase-resistant penicillin and ampicillin. If the patient has a history of a penicillin allergy, chloramphenicol may be substituted for the ampicillin. Bone infections in patients with a history of intravenous drug abuse require coverage for gram-negative organisms; treatment with an aminoglycoside is indicated. The addition of either carbenicillin or ticarcillin is recommended in documented pseudomonal infections. Newer antibiotics with improved antipseudomonal activity may be useful in resistant strains. Antibiotic therapy in these patients should be continued for at least 4 to 6 weeks.

Several microorganisms may cause bone infections postoperatively or from contiguous spread of an adjacent soft tissue infection. *S. aureus* is the single most common organism, but multiple organisms may be involved. To provide the required broad-spectrum coverage, a penicillinase-resistant penicillin and an aminoglycoside should be used as initial therapy. The antibiotic regimen may require modification after culture and sensitivity information is available. Frequently, the antibiotics must be continued for 6 weeks to obtain a cure and surgery is often required to remove any infected or devitalized tissue.

Patients with established vascular insufficiency who subsequently develop osteomyelitis are extremely difficult to manage. Impaired blood flow to the extremities impedes the healing process. Infections in these patients include a wide range of organisms including *S. aureus*, *Streptococcus*, anaerobes, and gram-negative organisms. Broad-spectrum therapy with a penicillinase-resistant penicillin in combination with an aminoglycoside is the preferred initial therapy; however, in spite of aggressive antibiotic therapy along with surgical debridement, these patients continue to have very low cure rates. Amputation of the involved area may be required to obtain a cure of the infection.

## *Controversies in Therapy*

As the management of bone and joint infections frequently requires prolonged injectable antibiotics, newer antibiotic regimens are currently being evaluated. Administration of antibiotics in the home environment as well as the use of antibiotics with extended elimination half-lives is being studied.

### Acute Osteomyelitis

Although acute osteomyelitis is one of the more common infectious diseases that may be treated with outpatient antibiotics, not all patients with osteomyelitis meet the criteria to receive home antibiotic therapy. Initially, patients must be screened to include those patients who are receiving a stable treatment program, those who are interested in participating and are motivated, those with good venous access, those who have support from family members or neighbors, and those who have adequate home facilities for storage and refrigeration.[33] Young, otherwise healthy patients may be able to use a peripheral intravenous catheter; however, a central intravenous catheter may be required if venous access difficulties occur. Certain exclusion criteria must also be considered. Complications of other preexisting diseases such as diabetic retinopathy, intention tremor, disabling inflammatory or degenerative joint disease, coagulopathies, or various neurologic disorders may prevent individuals from receiving home antibiotics.[34] Histories of alcoholism and intravenous drug abuse are also important exclusion criteria. Patients who are fluent in only a foreign language, are illiterate, or are hard of hearing may have to be excluded if a qualified guardian is unavailable. In addition to meeting these initial screening criteria, patients must successfully complete a thorough training program before hospital discharge. Aseptic technique, proper catheter care, and correct administration techniques must be documented. Once a patient is receiving therapy in the home environment, continued monitoring of their antimicrobial therapy is important. It is vital to ensure compliance with the antimicrobial regimen.

In addition, the specific antibiotic regimen characteristics must be considered in evaluating a patient for home antibiotics. Some features that may be important include microbiologic culture and sensitivity data, number of required daily antimicrobial doses, antibiotic stability data, and requirements for unique monitoring for the specific antimicrobial regimen (such as serum creatinines and peak and trough level measurements with aminoglycosides).[35] Although an organism may be sensitive to several antimicrobial agents, one antibiotic may provide practical benefits over other agents.

Newer cephalosporins have received a great deal of attention for use in patients with osteomyelitis. Benefits emphasized include their safety spectrum and less frequent dosing requirements with some agents. For example, an every-4-hour dosing regimen of nafcillin may be very effective within a hospital environment; however, this regimen may be very difficult to follow on an outpatient basis. Long-acting cephalosporins (i.e., cefonicid, ceftriaxone), although more expensive, may allow patients to receive a regimen that is easier to administer.

An uncontrolled trial with cefotaxime demonstrated that an average of 9.1 g per day for an average of 31 days was effective in obtaining a cure in 15 of 16 patients with acute osteomyelitis.[36] The failure occurred in a patient who had an infection caused by *P. aeruginosa*. Another uncontrolled trial was conducted with cefonicid in 15 patients with osteomyelitis.[37] Patients received 1 g of cefonicid once daily for an average of 40.4 days. Patients were hospitalized for an average of 10.9 days and received their subsequent antibiotic doses on an outpatient basis. Three of the 15 patients were withdrawn from the study because they developed adverse reactions (urticaria, high fever, myalgia, and hepatitis). The 12 patients completing the antibiotics had satisfactory clinical responses.

Ceftriaxone was administered in either single- or twice-daily doses for an average of 37 days in 76 patients with either initial or recurrent osteomyelitis.[38] Of 85 causative organisms, 76 were eradicated in 68 of the 76 patients. Cure was achieved in 39 of 76 patients; improvement was observed in 27 patients. Two isolates of *Enterobacter cloacae* and one isolate of *P. aeruginosa* developed resistance to ceftriaxone during therapy, a disconcerting finding. In addition, there were two cases of superinfection, one with *B. fragilis* and one with *Streptococcus faecalis*.

Thus, selected patients who have an infecting organism that is sensitive to one of the less frequently dosed cephalosporins and that is resistant to less expensive agents (e.g., cefazolin) may benefit from the newer antibiotics; however, concern is raised with the development of resistant strains and superinfections following the use of these agents. Certainly, patients receiving these agents should be monitored closely.

**Chronic Osteomyelitis**

Chronic osteomyelitis is much more difficult to treat than the acute form of the disease. Adequate surgical debridement is extremely important. All devitalized tissue, sequestra, and sinus tracts should be removed. Recurrences of infection are common and the disease is seldom cured without the combination of debridement and extensive antibiotic therapy.

Currently, there are no trials comparing different antibiotic regimens in the management of chronic osteomyelitis. Initially, antibiotics must be selected empirically as outlined under the management of acute osteomyelitis. Once definitive culture and sensitivity data are obtained, the specific antibiotics may require modification. The general recommendations for the management of chronic osteomyelitis are to initiate therapy with injectable antibiotics before surgical debridement and to continue therapy for at least 4 to 6 weeks. After completion of the injectable therapy, oral antibiotics are continued, generally for 1 to 2 months.

Uncontrolled trials have demonstrated that high-dose oral antibiotic therapy for an extended period of time in conjunction with adequate surgical debridement may be effective in the management of chronic osteomyelitis in some patients.[39–41] Of 41 patients in one study, 29 had no further recurrences[39]; 90 of 136 patients were symptom free after removal of bone abscesses and sequestra along with oral antibiotic therapy for 6–12 months in another trial.[40]

Wagner et al recently reported a study on the use of long-term intravenous antibiotic therapy in 10 chronic osteomyelitis patients.[42] The patients had had symptoms of chronic osteomyelitis for 3 months to 58 years. There was an average of 2.7 organisms per patient obtained on bone biopsy. *P. aeruginosa*, *S. aureus*, and *S. faecalis* were the most common organisms. Surgery was performed on all but two patients. The intravenous antibiotics were administered on an inpatient basis for an average of 33 days and followed by outpatient therapy for an average of 111 days. Eight of the ten patients were cured of their infections.

It is difficult to establish treatment recommendations based on these data and the previously established guidelines. The importance of surgery and appropriate antibiotic therapy must be emphasized. Injectable antibiotic therapy must be used for initial therapy. Continuation of this therapy for 4 to 6 weeks is preferred, but a shorter course followed by oral antibiotics may be effective in some patients. Peak serum bactericidal titers may prove useful in monitoring the antibiotic therapy in these patients. In individuals who are unable to have all the dead bone surgically removed, long-term suppressive therapy may control the infection.

**Infectious Arthritis**

The three most important therapeutic maneuvers in the management of infectious arthritis are appropriate antibiotics, joint drainage, and joint rest. As previously mentioned, initial smears of the synovial fluid may be very useful in initially selecting appropriate antibiotic therapy. If bacteria are not observed on the Gram stain in a patient who has a purulent joint effusion, antibiotics should still be initiated because of the high risk of an infection being present. A delay in initiating antibiotics significantly increases the likelihood for long-term complications.[6]

The specific antibiotic selected depends on the most likely infecting organism. In infants less than 1 month, the infecting organisms vary widely and thus empiric therapy must provide broad-spectrum coverage. A penicillinase-resistant penicillin (150 mg/kg/d) such as nafcillin or oxacillin plus an aminoglycoside is appropriate. As children less than 5 years of age may be infected with *Hemophilus influenzae*, ampicillin therapy is indicated. The addition of chloramphenicol may be required if the patient is located in a geographic area with a high level of ampicillin resistance.

In children over 5 and in adults, initial therapy with a penicillinase-resistant penicillin is appropriate to provide the necessary coverage against *S. aureus*. As with osteomyelitis, intravenous drug abusers require *P. aeruginosa* coverage and, therefore, an aminoglycoside such as tobramycin is needed. The antibiotics selected are usually administered by injection. Antibiotics administered by this route are able to achieve sufficient concentrations within the synovial fluid, and thus intraarticular antibiotic injections are not necessary.[43] Although studies that clearly define the appropriate length of therapy have not been conducted, 2 to 3 weeks of antibiotics is generally adequate in nongonococcal infections. Joint fluid cultures are usually no longer positive after 7 days of antibiotics.

Because disseminated gonococcal infections readily respond to antibiotics, appropriate therapy may consist of several agents. Intravenous penicillin G (10 million units/d) for 3 days followed by amoxicillin 500 mg orally four times daily for 4 days is the treatment of first choice. Ceftriaxone, cefotaxime, oral erythromycin (2 g/d) and oral tetracycline (2 g/d) for 7 days are also effective agents. Erythromycin is especially useful in pregnant penicillin-allergic patients. Clinical resolution is usually rapid.

Closed-needle aspiration is recommended for all infected joints except the hip. Purulent effusions may promote cartilage destruction by increasing leukocyte enzyme activity. Joint drainage is often repeated daily for 5 to 7 days or until the effusions no longer reaccumulate. Open drainage may be required in hip infections. During the initial phase of the infection, weight bearing (such as walking) on the joint should be avoided. Passive range-of-motion exercises should be initiated when the pain begins to subside to maintain joint mobility.

### *Monitoring*

Patients with bone and joint infections must be monitored closely. The clinical signs of inflammation such as swelling, tenderness, pain, redness, and fever will hopefully resolve with appropriate therapy. Elevations in white blood cell count should also gradually decline.

Elevations in the erythrocyte sedimentation rate may not resolve for several weeks after therapy. If a patient fails to have a resolution in the clinical signs and symptoms of inflammation after appropriate empiric antibiotics, surgical debridement may be needed. In addition, the patient may have a resistant infecting organism which may require a modification in the patient's antibiotic regimen. Follow-up cultures at subsequent debridements may be useful to assess the antibiotic therapy.

## Summary

Osteomyelitis and infectious arthritis are two very important infections that require special attention. As the infecting organisms may vary, careful attention must be placed on adequate culture collection. Because of the difficulty in eliminating these infections, patients must receive antibiotics for an extensive period of time and may require surgical drainage. Injectable antibiotics continue to be the standard therapy of first choice. Recent studies have demonstrated that children with acute osteomyelitis may be treated adequately with a carefully monitored oral antibiotic regimen. It is important to emphasize that osteomyelitis and septic arthritis are infections that require rapid initiation of therapy to prevent extensive tissue damage and to have the best chance to obtain a cure.

## References

1. Waldvogel FA, Medoff G, Swartz MN. Osteomyelitis: A review of clinical features, therapeutic considerations and unusual aspects. N Engl J Med 1970;282:198–206, 260–266, 316–322.
2. Peltola H, Vahuanen V. A comparative study of osteomyelitis and purulent arthritis with special reference to aetiology and recovery. Infection 1984;12:75–79.
3. Sharp JT, Lidsky MD, Duffy J, et al. Infectious arthritis. Arch Intern Med 1979;139:1125–1130.
4. Goldenberg DL, Reed JI. Bacterial arthritis. N Engl J Med 1985;312:764–771.
5. Schmid FR. Routine drug treatment of septic arthritis. Clin Rheum Dis 1984;10:293–311.
6. Goldenberg DK, Cohen AS. Acute infectious arthritis: a review of patients with nongonococcal joint infections (with emphasis on therapy and prognosis). Am J Med 1976;60:369–377.
7. Roca RP, Yoshikawa TT. Primary skeletal infections in heroin users: a clinical characterization, diagnosis and therapy. Clin Orthop 1979;144:238–248.
8. Raff MJ, Melo JC. Anaerobic osteomyelitis. Medicine 1978;57: 83–103.
9. Ward JR, Atcheson SG. Infectious arthritis. Med Clin North Am 1977;61:313–329.
10. Gifford DB, Patzakis M, Ivler D, et al. Septic arthritis due to pseudomonas in heroin addicts. J Bone Joint Surg (Am) 1975;57:631–635.
11. Holmes KK, Counts GW, Beaty HN. Disseminated gonococcal infection. Ann Intern Med 1971;74:979–993.
12. Ho G, Su EY. Therapy for septic arthritis. JAMA 1982;247:797–800.
13. Inman RD, Gallegos RV, Brause BD, et al. Clinical and microbial features of prosthetic joint infection. Am J Med 1984;77:47–53.

14. Mackowiak PA, Jones SR, Smith JW. Diagnostic value of sinus tract cultures in chronic osteomyelitis. JAMA 1978;239:2772–2775.
15. Glover SL, McKendrick MW, Padfield C, et al. Acute osteomyelitis in a district general hospital. Lancet 1982;1:609–611.
16. Gillespie WJ, Mayo KM. The management of acute haematogenous osteomyelitis in the antibiotic era: a study of the outcome. J Bone Joint Surg (Br) 1981;63:126–131.
17. Khazenifar M, Weighill FH, Stanley JK. The management of childhood osteomyelitis. Postgrad Med J 1978;54:541–544.
18. Howard JB, Highgenboten CL, Nelson JD. Residual effects of septic arthritis in infancy and childhood. JAMA 1976;236:932–935.
19. Jacobs JC. Acute osteomyelitis medical management in children. NY State J Med 1978;78:910–912.
20. Dich VQ, Nelson JD, Haltalin KC. Osteomyelitis in infants and children. Am J Dis Child 1975;129:1273–1278.
21. Sheftel TG, Mader JT. Randomized evaluation of ceftazidime or ticarcillin and tobramycin for the treatment of osteomyelitis caused by gram-negative bacilli. Antimicrob Agents Chemother 1986;29:112–115.
22. Tetzlaff TR, McCracken GH, Nelson JD. Oral antibiotic therapy for skeletal infections of children. J Pediatr 1978;92:485–490.
23. Bryson YJ, Connor JD, LeClerc M, et al. High-dose oral dicloxacillin treatment of acute staphylococcal osteomyelitis in children. J Pediatr 1979;94:673–675.
24. Prober CG, Yeager AS. Use of the serum bactericidal titer to assess the adequacy of oral antibiotic therapy in the treatment of acute hematogenous osteomyelitis. J Pediatr 1979;95:131–135.
25. Rodriquez W, Ross S, Khan W, et al. Clindamycin in the treatment of osteomyelitis in children: a report of 29 cases. Am J Dis Child 1977;131:1088–1093.
26. Feigin RD, Pickering LR, Anderson D, èt al. Clindamycin treatment of osteomyelitis and septic arthritis in children. Pediatrics 1975;55:213–223.
27. Kaplan SL, Mason EO, Feigin RD. Clindamycin versus nafcillin or methacillin in the treatment of staphylococcus aureus osteomyelitis in children. South Med J 1982;75:138–142.
28. Jordan GW, Kawachi MM. Analysis of serum bactericidal activity in endocarditis, osteomyelitis, and other bacterial infections. Medicine 1981;60:49–61.
29. Anderson JR, Scobie WG, Watt B. The treatment of acute osteomyelitis in children: a 10-year experience. J Antimicrob Chemother 1981;7(suppl A):43–50.
30. Jimenez-Shehab M, Barragan A. Oral cefadroxil in the treatment of bone and joint infections in children and adults. J Antimicrob Chemother 1982;10(suppl B):149–152.
31. Nelson JD, Bucholz RW, Kusmiesz H, et al. Benefits and risks of sequential parenteral–oral cephalosporin therapy for suppurative bone and joint infections. J Pediatr Orthop 1982; 2:255–262.
32. Kolyvas E, Ahronheim G, Marks MI, et al. Oral antibiotic therapy of skeletal infections in children. Pediatrics 1980;65: 867–871.
33. McAllister JC. The role of the pharmacist in home health care. Drug Intell Clin Pharm 1985;19:282–284.
34. Goldenberg RI. Pitfalls in the delivery of outpatient intravenous therapy. Drug Intell Clin Pharm 1985;19:293–296.
35. Reed MD. Evaluation of antibiotics for home care programs. Drug Intell Clin Pharm 1985;19:288–290.
36. Mader JT, LeFrock JL, Hyams KC, et al. Cefotaxime therapy for patients with osteomyelitis and septic arthritis. Rev Infect Dis 1982;4(suppl):S472–S480.
37. Kunkel MJ, Iannini PB. Cefonicid in a once-daily regimen for treatment of osteomyelitis in an ambulatory setting. Rev Infect Dis 1984;6(suppl 4):S865–S869.
38. Eron LJ, Goldenberg RI, Poretz DM. Combined ceftriaxone and surgical therapy for osteomyelitis in hospital and outpatient settings. Am J Surg 1984;148(4A):1–4.
39. Hedstrom SA. The prognosis of chronic staphylococcal osteomyelitis after long-term antibiotic treatment. Scand J Infect Dis 1974;6:33–38.
40. Bell SM. Further observations on the value of oral penicillins in chronic staphylococcal osteomyelitis. Med J Aust 1976;2:591–593.
41. Hodgin UG. Antibiotics in the treatment of chronic staphylococcal osteomyelitis. South Med J 1975;68:817–823.
42. Wagner DR, Collier D, Rytel MW. Long-term intravenous antibiotic therapy in chronic osteomyelitis. Arch Intern Med 1985;145:1073–1078.
43. Nelson JD. Antibiotic concentrations in septic joint effusions. N Engl J Med 1971;284:349–353.

# Chapter 87 / Gram-Negative Sepsis and Septic Shock

Kenneth E. Record, PharmD

Bacteremia caused by gram-negative bacilli represents an important infectious disease challenge to modern medicine. Bloodborne bacteria usually originate from localized sites such as skin or skin structures, respiratory tract, gastrointestinal tract, urinary tract, and mucous membranes. Bacteremia may manifest itself as a self-limited process of little importance to the continued well-being of the host or may encompass a constellation of hemodynamic and metabolic imbalances that constitutes a true medical emergency. Successful therapeutic intervention of the latter demands early recognition and aggressive treatment focused on termination of the bacterial invasion and correction of any pathophysiologic sequelae.

*Sepsis* suggests a bloodstream invasion by bacteria or the toxic materials produced by bacteria, resulting in overt and severe clinical signs and symptoms characteristic of systemic toxicity. Virtually any bloodstream invader is capable of producing "septic shock," but the association of severe infection with circulatory failure, hypotension, and poor tissue perfusion is most frequently the manifestation of the Enterobacteriaceae and Pseudomonadaceae.

This association of symptomatology with etiologic source of bacterial sepsis may be traced to Osler, who in 1892 noted that "organisms of suppuration" (i.e., staphylococci and streptococci) were the major offenders in producing septicemia.[1] Prior to the introduction of sulfonamides, Felty and Keefer reported a 32% mortality rate for patients with *Escherichia coli* bacteremia.[2] Others recognized that the bacilli need not be viable to produce hypotension when injected intravenously.[3,4] These observations led to the discovery that a severe and prolonged hypotension followed the administration of a "tumor necrotizing polysaccharide" derived from *Serratia marcescens*.[5] This concept of bacterial products having cardiovascular effects was put to therapeutic use in 1949 when malignant hypertension was treated with a pyrogen derived from *Pseudomonas aeruginosa*.[6]

By the early 1950s, a number of uniformly fatal infectious diseases were on the decline, presumably because of the modern antibiotic era, but a fourfold increase in the frequency of gram-negative infections had occurred in 1947 compared with 1941.[7] Concurrent with this increase in frequency, it became sufficiently clear that gram-negative bacilli were capable of producing fatal hypotension as a result of bacteremia acquired from other infected body sites.[8,9] Thus, the ability of man's natural microbial flora to demonstrate "opportunism" when defense mechanisms were depressed became a hallmark of gram-negative sepsis.

By 1972, Boston City Hospital had reported nearly a tenfold increase in the frequency of gram-negative infections since 1941.[7] Although this is probably an overestimation of the true frequency of gram-negative bacteremias, considering community hospitals probably have a lower rate, the magnitude of the problem generated considerable concern. The incidence of gram-negative infection was particularly worrisome in consideration of the more recent reports of 20% to 32% mortality associated with gram-negative bacteremias.[10–12] These studies suggested that despite the advances in antimicrobial therapy and cardiovascular and respiratory support, the mortality from gram-negative bacteremia had not significantly changed. This may be expected if we consider that the hemodynamic changes associated with septic shock occur as a result of cellular injury. Thus, the associated circulatory abnormalities of septic shock are late findings when injury is difficult to reverse. Clearly, early recognition and aggressive intervention of septic shock are of paramount importance.

The 10 years from the mid-1970s to the mid-1980s witnessed a rapid proliferation of antimicrobials directed at the organisms of gram-negative sepsis including a few aminoglycosides and numerous $\beta$-lactam compounds. It is tempting to ascribe the use, misuse, and overuse of antibiotics to the continued increase in gram-negative infections, but we must also consider the paralleling advances in medical and surgical practice. Increasing immunosuppressive therapy and aggressive surgical intervention have left us with many nosocomial infectious challenges. Thus, gram-negative infections are appropriately considered an inevitable consequence of medical progress.

## Epidemiology

As previously stated, the major offenders in gram-negative sepsis are the members of the families Enterobacteriaceae (*Escherichia*, *Klebsiella*, *Enterobacter*, *Serratia*, and *Proteus*) and Pseudomonadaceae. The enteric or coliform bacteria are part of the normal endogenous flora within the lower gastrointestinal tract. The pseudomonads, along with other gram-negative organisms, are ubiquitous in the environment. *E. coli* is the most abundant gram-negative aerobic bacillus and, in the normal individual, is sensitive to most penicillins and cephalosporins. These organisms are usually devoid of plasmids that produce $\beta$-lactamases. On the other hand, a less predictable pattern of antimicrobial resistance is encountered in "hospital-acquired" gram-negative infections because of the prevalence of plasmids. A distinction is made between the circumstances by which a bacteremia is acquired and treated. Recognition of the widespread presence of $\beta$-lactamase–producing plasmids in the hospital setting has certainly made a major impact on the search for enzyme-stable and nontoxic antimicrobials.

A principle important to the epidemiology of gram-negative bacteremia is the host's loss of colonization immunity. That is, the normal flora may extend beyond normal sites of colonization or actually invade the host. Loss of colonization immunity increases the risk of gram-negative bacteremia and a number of factors have augmented this phenomenon. The administration of antimicrobial agents presumably decreases the protective flora and allows for overgrowth of other virulent species. The severity of illness and loss of natural protective barriers such as skin, the cough reflex, or neutropenia all contribute to an increased gram-negative load for the host to bear.[13,14]

Community-acquired gram-negative bacteremia usually arises from the endogenous flora in the biliary, urinary, or genital tract. Environmental or exogenous aerobic gram-negative bacilli, which comprise coliforms and pseudomonads, represent a serious threat to the institutionalized patient. These organisms have the ability to colonize and invade directly through devices intended for supportive care of the patient (i.e., respiratory equipment, urinary catheters, feeding tubes).

Numerous studies describe the outcome of gram-negative bacteremias with respect to host susceptibility and organism virulence. The most important host factor determinant is the severity of underlying disease. McCabe outlined a useful classification of disease based on the time sequence to a fatal event.[15] Patients with "rapidly fatal" diseases, such as acute leukemia, blastic relapses of chronic leukemia, aplastic anemias, and burns greater than 70%, demonstrated a 91% fatality rate from gram-negative bacteremia. Patients with "ultimately fatal" diseases, with an expected fatality within 4 years, showed a death rate from bacteremia of 66%. Examples of such diseases included chronic leukemia, lymphoma, metastatic carcinoma, cirrhosis with hepatic coma or bleeding varices, and chronic renal disease with blood urea nitrogen levels greater than 70 mg%. Finally, patients with "nonfatal" diseases, such as diabetes mellitus and various obstetric conditions, demonstrated an 11% fatality rate from bacteremias. It is interesting that age or bacterial species was not a significant independent determinant of bacteremic fatality. Subsequent studies have confirmed McCabe's analysis of host factor risks. These data have played a major role in the further evaluation of risk factors and treatments.[16,17]

Other important studies have refined our understanding of the relationship among host, organism, and therapeutic interventions. For example, Bryan and associates noted that in patients with nonfatal diseases, mortality was higher in hospital-acquired bacteremia.[12] This was largely attributed to the observation that *E. coli* bacteremia was associated with a mortality of 13%, while *P. aeruginosa* bacteremia was associated with a mortality of 39%. A part of this disparity may be reflective of underlying diseases. They also noted that when compared with incorrect or no therapy, correct antimicrobial therapy made a significant impact on the mortality rate from bacteremia. Not surprisingly, this was more important in the ultimately fatal and nonfatal groups. As mentioned earlier, the problem of gram-negative bacteremia leading to septic shock and the inherently high mortality (i.e., gram-negative bacteremias had a fatality rate eight times greater than gram-positive bacteremias) stimulated the Subcommittee on Health of the United States Senate to appoint a Special Study Group on Gram-Negative Rod Bacteremia. The role of antibiotic overuse in the increased incidence of gram-negative infections was a major focus. It was concluded that antibiotics were an important factor, but quantitative assessment of the relationship between overuse and incidence was impossible.[10]

Finally, some major observations regarding gram-negative septic shock have been published. First, the incidence is estimated to be about 1% of hospital admissions in university-type hospitals and appears to be 0.2% to 0.5% in community hospitals.[18] Overall mortality from gram-negative bacteremia is approximately 20%. Septic shock occurs in 15% of bacteremic patients, with an associated 50% mortality.[18] Second, as endogenous or exogenous (or both) sources are involved, epidemiology is complex and diverse.[18] Third, therapeutic intervention must consider underlying diseases present and risk factors involved. Lastly, prevention is a foremost priority and every effort should be utilized in reducing the risk of a gram-negative bacteremia. Treatment usually suggests failure of prevention.[18]

## Pathophysiology/Clinical Presentation

The pathophysiologic sequelae resulting from the interaction between the gram-negative bacillus and the human host are diverse, complex, and poorly understood. In studies in humans, it is difficult to demonstrate definitive relationships between complications of bacteremia and septic shock. Furthermore, clinical and histopathologic changes are difficult to attribute to intervening infection or underlying disease that may have similar effects. Finally, much of the work in animals has been difficult to adapt to humans because of marked differences in response to gram-negative stimuli.

The pathophysiologic focus of gram-negative bacteremia has been the lipopolysaccharide component of the gram-negative cell wall. Commonly referred to as endotoxin, this substance is present in the gram-negative cell wall but absent in the gram-positive cell. The role of endotoxin appears to involve the activation of at least four humoral systems that are capable of inducing the circulatory and hemodynamic alterations seen in gram-negative bacteremias. A second major focus of attention has been on the metabolic and physiologic disorders that occur during a septic state.[19] This multivariant approach in the analysis of clinically measurable hemodynamic and metabolic parameters has helped to quantify the compensatory nature of the disease. It has also provided a valuable prognostic and therapeutic tool. This discussion focuses on these two areas.

It is well known that when a substantial amount of endotoxin gains access to the bloodstream, many changes occur.[20] These changes may continue and, if left unchecked, are potentially disastrous. Lipopolysaccharides vary in structure among bacterial species, but the major pathogenic effects appear to be constant. Endotoxin is pyrogenic, but fever typically does not occur until 60 to 90 minutes after it enters the circulation. This lag time may be the reason why many blood cultures drawn when a patient is febrile are sterile, even though the fever was caused by gram-negative bacilli. That is, the patient's host defenses may have had adequate time to clear the bacteria from the circulation. Endotoxin is not a pyrogen, but when taken up by the host's

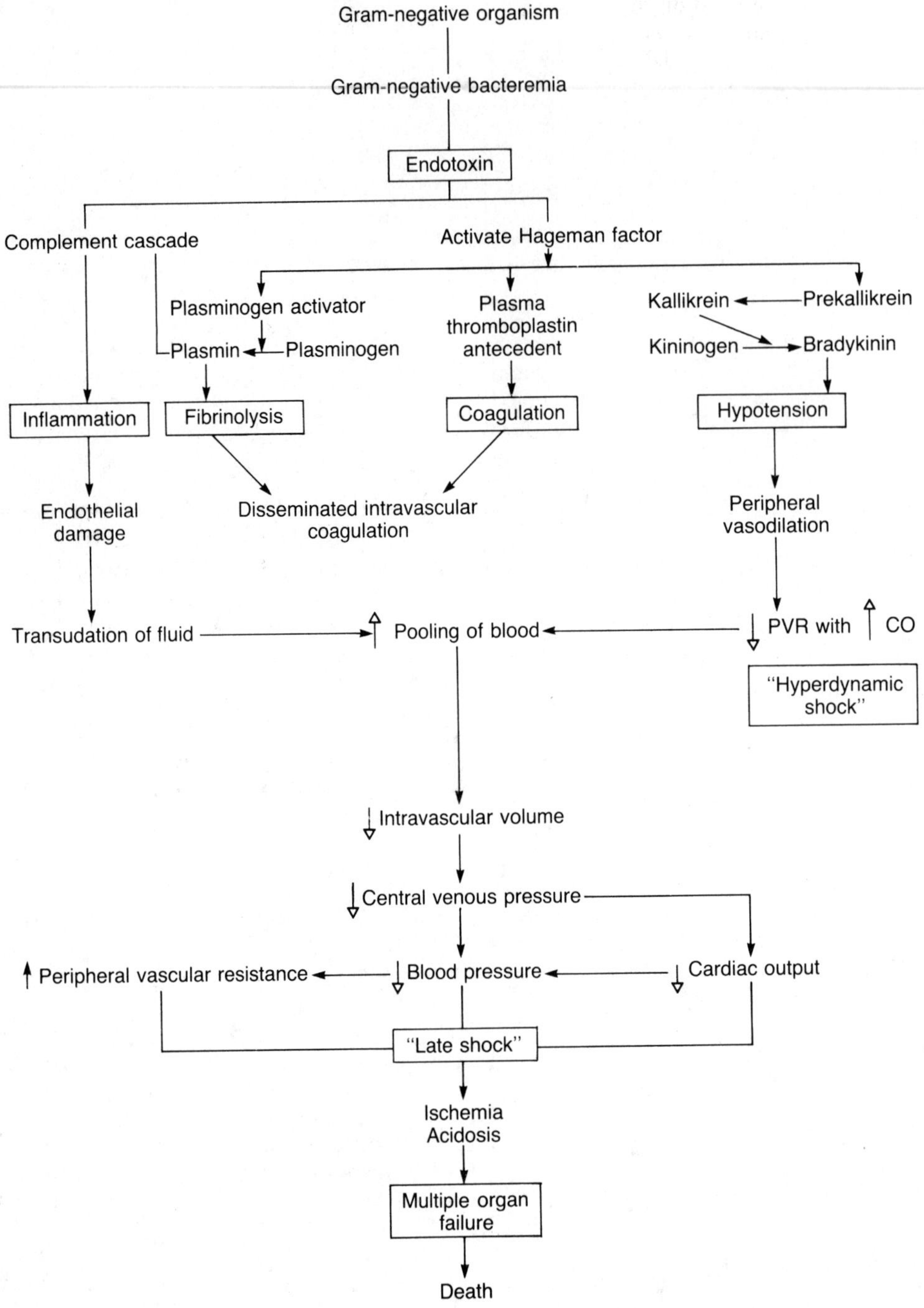


**Figure 87.1** Pathophysiology of septic shock.

polymorphonuclear leukocytes and mononuclear phagocytes, an endogenous pyrogen is released that has a direct effect on the hypothalamus. "Tolerance" to the pyrogenic effect of endotoxin develops upon repeated exposure and is attributed to blockade of the macrophage system (RES) and to the synthesis of IgM antibodies. Many researchers today feel that the response of the macrophage to a lipopolysaccharide stimulus through release of polypeptides (e.g., interleukin-1) is the key to the lethal effects on the host. The reader is referred to several excellent reviews of the topic for further discussion.[21,22]

Other clinical signs and symptoms of the endotoxin's effects are inferred through the activation of complement and direct activation of the Hageman factor. The Hageman factor then activates coagulation and fibrinolysis and release of vasoactive peptides, as shown schematically in Figure 87.1. Hypotension appears to result, in part, from the release of vasosactive peptides like the kinins (bradykinin and serotonin). Activation of complement can occur by both the classical (antigen–antibody activation) pathway and, especially, the alternate pathway. The pathophysiologic consequence of the activation of complement is the generation of chemotactic factors, anaphylatoxins, and other substances that augment or exaggerate the inflammatory response. This ultimately results in deleterious effects on cell membranes.

Disseminated intravascular coagulation (DIC) is mostly attributed to the activation of factor XII (Hageman factor) by endotoxin. The subsequent activation and use of coagulation factors II, V, and VIII and platelets far exceed the rate of synthesis, resulting in levels inadequate for maintenance of hemostasis. Paradoxical bleeding may occur because of the consumption of clotting factors. As plasminogen (fibrinolytic system) is activated simultaneously, newly formed clots undergo rapid lysis. Fibrin breakdown results in circulating soluble peptides called fibrin split products. This may explain why autopsies fail to uncover thrombi when thrombosis has been clinically evident. Every patient with gram-negative bacteremia by virtue of laboratory studies exhibits disseminated intravascular coagulation. Complications are varied and depend on the target organ affected and the severity of the coagulopathy. Severe clinical bleeding, thrombosis, tissue ischemia and necrosis, hemolysis, and major organ failure may result from disturbances induced by gram-negative bacteria on the coagulation systems.

Finally, the diagnosis of DIC requires a careful assessment of the pattern of abnormalities. A suggested guideline for the diagnosis of DIC in a patient without liver disease includes the presence of thrombocytopenia and fibrin split products, and reduction of one or more coagulation factors (II, V, VIII).[22] If hepatic disease is present, suggesting a vitamin K deficiency, then reduction of the non–vitamin K-dependent clotting factor VIII becomes specific as the third criterion.[22]

Shock is the most ominous complication associated with gram-negative bacteremia. In 1951, Waisbren's classic description of a "shocklike picture" associated with gram-negative bacteremia suggested two clinically distinct syndromes.[8] Approximately one half of the patients evaluated exhibited hypotension with cold, clammy skin and lethargy (i.e., low cardiac output, peripheral vasocontrictive state). In contrast, the other group exhibited manifestations of acute bacterial infections (fever, bounding pulses, wide pulse pressure, warm flushed skin, hypotension). This state is characterized by high cardiac output and peripheral vasodilation. It is important to realize that "shock" and "gram-negative bacteremia" are not synonymous. The reason bacteria cause hypotensive changes is unclear, but it does not appear to be a direct effect of endotoxin. The most accepted mechanism by which gram-negative bacteremia induces hypotensive sequelae is through the release of vasoactive peptides such as bradykinin.[23] Activation of the Hageman factor by endotoxin converts prekallikrein to kallikrein. Kallikrein catalyzes the conversion of kininogen to bradykinin. The most significant effects of circulating bradykinin are vasodilation and increased vascular permeability. Thus, a rapid shift of intravascular fluid is the result of smooth muscle relaxation and decreased peripheral resistance, as well as endothelial tissue damage resulting from the margination of leukocytes and leakage of fluid into interstitial spaces. Hypoperfusion of major organs is the ultimate result of this intravascular embarrassment. If hypoperfusion is not effectively corrected, multiple organ failure becomes the hallmark of the unresolved septic process.

To understand the management of sepsis, the cardiovascular response to sepsis in humans must be appreciated. The collective observations of Weil and associates,[24] MacLean et al,[25] Clowes et al,[26,27] and Siegel et al[28,29] showed that the initial response to sepsis in humans is a hyperdynamic process, where increase in cardiac output occurs in the face of falling vascular resistance; however, examination of the pressure–flow relationships indicates that the cardiac output is not completely compensatory. That is, the septic patient has lower vascular resistance for the same body flow than the traumatized patient. This contrasts with the cardiogenic or hypovolemic shock states, in which the vascular resistance is increased. The hyperdynamic state of sepsis may progress to a hypodynamic state characterized by low cardiac output and high peripheral vascular resistance. It appears that the hyperdynamic state of septic shock is due to a failure of the peripheral vasculature. Progression to the hypodynamic state of septic shock is probably due to myocardial failure and carries a far more grim prognosis.

Another fundamental observation relevant to the septic process in humans is that there are changes in intermediary metabolism. In most septic patients oxygen consumption is increased, but in the most seriously ill hyperdynamic patients, the decreased vascular tone relationship was associated with decreasing oxygen consumption and metabolic acidosis. The decrease in oxygen consumption was determined through the observation that oxygen content would rise in venous blood during septic shock. This was initially interpreted to be caused by a physiologic arteriovenous shunt where capillary beds were bypassed. It was unclear why this might occur but the popular theory maintained that a "pathologic shunt," or an increased blood flow to areas of inflammation, may be operating. Subsequent studies using xenon washout techniques in skeletal muscle demonstrated an increase in capillary blood flow and an increase in microvascular blood flow away from the source of sepsis.[30] In addition, very little precapillary shunting took place.

Further studies elucidated that transition from high oxygen consumption states into low oxygen consumption states could occur and that such oscillations occurred until the patient either recovered or succumbed as a result of multiple organ failure.[29–32]

## Treatment

Gram-negative septicemia is an exaggerated inflammatory response to the presence of bacteria in the bloodstream. Epidemiologic and pathophysiologic information repeatedly stresses the importance of early recognition and rigorous therapeutic intervention if mortality is to be avoided. The detection and elimination of all septic sources, aggressive and appropriate antimicrobial therapy, and comprehensive supportive care are the goals in the management of septic shock.

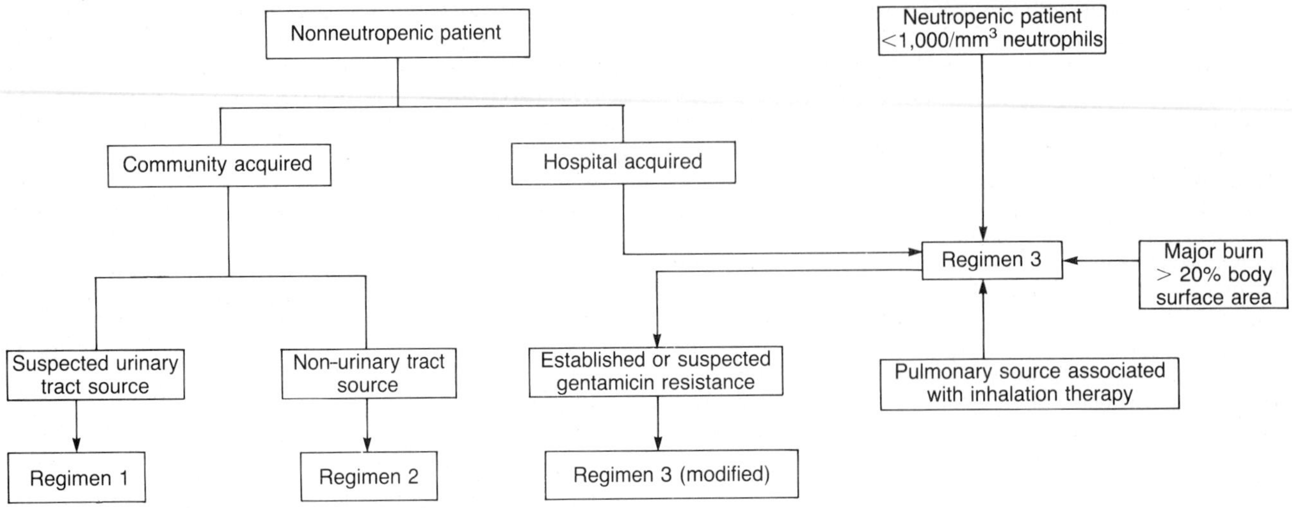


**Figure 87.2** Recommended antimicrobial regimens for presumptive therapy for gram-negative bacteremias.

Regimen 1: First- or second-generation cephalosporin or an aminoglycoside or ampicillin
Regimen 2: A β-lactum agent, or a cephalosporin plus an aminoglycoside
Regimen 3: An antipseudomonal penicillin plus an aminoglycoside or an antipseudomonal third-generation cephalosporin plus aminoglycoside
Regimen 3 (modified): Use amikacin as the aminoglycoside

### *Antimicrobial Therapy*

Assuming that one has done all he or she can to diagnose and eliminate the septic source, antimicrobial therapy becomes a major priority in therapy. Because of the problems inherent in identification of the offending organism or organisms and the similar pathophysiologic pictures that gram-positive and gram-negative organisms present in established shock, the following principles are useful guidelines in initiating antimicrobial therapy.

First, empiric therapy must be comprehensive. An attempt should be made to cover all likely pathogens in the context of the clinical setting. Second, therapy should be initiated rapidly. Clearing the bloodstream before development of the complications of sepsis is a widely accepted mandate. Third, a seriously ill patient or one who is in shock should be treated only with intravenous antibiotics. Absorption from intramuscular and oral sites may be erratic because of changes in regional blood flow. Fourth, bactericidal agents are preferred and combinations with bacteriostatic agents should be avoided. Fifth, for empiric therapy, or treatment of the immunocompromised patient, antimicrobial combinations that are likely to be synergistic are encouraged. Sixth, loading doses, particularly with aminoglycosides, should be given to maximize initial effect. Seventh, patients should be monitored carefully, particularly with respect to the aminoglycosides, for potential nephrotoxicity. Aminoglycoside doses should be adjusted according to serum levels and functional state of the kidneys. Finally, when the patient stabilizes, and if the pathogen is known, specific therapy with cost and safety kept in mind should become a primary concern.[33]

The choice of antimicrobial agents has been a subject of considerable debate over the last 5 years because of the availability of new antibiotics with expanded and enhanced activities in vitro. Mostly β-lactams, these compounds offer the potential advantage of less renal toxicity and ototoxicity compared with the proven effective aminoglycosides; however, they may not be reliably effective against important organisms, namely *Enterobacter cloacae* and *Pseudomonas aeruginosa*. Very few well-controlled, clinical trials in humans are available to assess the value of the new agents or regimens as empiric choices for the treatment of gram-negative bacteremias.[32,34]

Figure 87.2 is an algorithm for the selection of antimicrobial regimens for the initial treatment of gram-negative bacteremias. In the nonneutropenic patient with a community-acquired bacteremia from the urinary tract, a first- or second-generation cephalosporin may be appropriate because *E. coli* and *Klebsiella* are the major concerns. In the same patient, if the source of infection is nonurinary, a combination of a penicillinase-resistant penicillin or a cephalosporin and an aminoglycoside would provide excellent coverage of *E. coli*, *Klebsiella*, and *Proteus* as well as of gram-positive bacteria (*Pneumococcus*, *Staphylococcus aureus*). The traditional regimen for the patient who has acquired a nosocomial infection consists of an aminoglycoside and a β-lactam agent. If the patient is nonneutropenic, a first- or second-generation cephalosporin is preferred, because *Klebsiella* is much more likely than *P. aeruginosa*. Finally, the combination of an aminoglycoside and an antipseudomonal penicillin or an antipseudomonal cephalosporin is preferred in the neutropenic patient, the patient receiving assisted ventilation, or the patient with a major thermal injury.

Amikacin offers a potential advantage over gentamicin and tobramycin. It is less susceptible to plasmid-mediated exoenzyme inactivation and has proven to be a valuable alternative in situations of suspected or established resistance to gentamicin and tobramycin. A few differences with respect to microbiologic activity exist among gentamicin, tobramycin, and amikacin. Tobramycin appears to be somewhat more active (based on an achievable serum level) than gentamicin against *P. aeruginosa*. On the other hand, gentamicin is more active than tobramycin against *Serratia*. Using an inhibitory index that accounts for the higher blood levels achieved with amikacin compared with minimum inhibitory concentrations, this drug appears to be more active against the *Klebsiella–Enterobacter–Serratia* group. It is not clear whether these differences have clinical significance.

The clinical pharmacist has the opportunity to impact significantly the effectiveness of aminoglycoside therapy in gram-negative sepsis. These agents have narrow therapeutic windows and there is a marked variability in individual peak blood levels. Some studies suggest that breakthrough bacteremias are associated with subtherapeutic blood aminoglycoside levels. Thus, the frequent monitoring of blood aminoglycoside levels becomes imperative. Gentamicin, netilmicin, and tobramycin peak levels in the range 5.0 to 10.0 μg/mL are generally associated with optimal response. Amikacin peak levels of 20 to 40 μg/mL are likewise considered optimal. Another advantage to monitoring blood levels is the possible avoidance of some toxic effects, because accumulating levels alert the clinician to changes in renal function earlier than serum creatinines and overdosing errors.

The carboxy- and ureidopenicillins make up the group known as antipseudomonal penicillins. Although there are major enhancements in activity of the ureidopenicillins (azlocillin, mezlocillin, and piperacillin) over the carboxypenicillins (carbenicillin and ticarcillin), their major role in antimicrobial therapy is in combination with an aminoglycoside for potential infections caused by *P. aeruginosa*. Azlocillin and piperacillin are the most active against *Pseudomonas*, whereas ticarcillin and mezlocillin are comparably less active, and carbenicillin is least active. Unfortunately, there is no conclusive evidence from clinical trials to suggest that the more active agents are any more effective than the less active agents when combined with an aminoglycoside against *P. aeruginosa*. It is interesting to note that the enhanced activity of the more recently introduced antipseudomonal penicillins is due to an increase in cell wall permeability and affinity for penicillin-binding proteins. They are very susceptible to inactivation by β-lactamases. It appears that all of these agents would benefit in combination with the β-lactamase inhibitors.

The development of new cephalosporins (third generation), moxalactam, the carbapenems (imipenem), and the monobactams (aztreonam) has added tremendously active agents to the antimicrobial arsenal. These agents have exceptional in vitro activity against the Enterobacteriaceae but highly variable activity against *P. aeruginosa*. Agents such as cefotaxime, ceftizoxime, ceftriaxone, and moxalactam easily achieve blood levels 100 times greater than their minimum inhibitory concentrations against *E. coli* and *Klebsiella*, suggesting that monotherapy directed against those bacteria may be successful; however, resistance among *Pseudomonas*, *Serratia*, and *Enterobacter* is a concern and has limited their singular use.

The first studies reporting the efficacy of monotherapy over combination therapy employed cefoperazone and moxalactam.[35,36] Both agents demonstrated antipseudomonal activity in addition to an enhanced activity against the Enterobacteriaceae. Both studies suggested similar efficacy of monotherapy compared with conventional regimens, but the numbers of neutropenic patients were small and very few patients had *P. aeruginosa* bacteremias. Currently, broadly active agents, notably, ceftazidime and imipenem, are undergoing comparative trials against multidrug combinations. On the basis of their intrinsic activity, these drugs appear to be the front runners if monotherapy is to receive universal acceptance.

Available evidence shows that the combination of an antipseudomonal third-generation cephalosporin with an aminoglycoside is as efficacious as the combination of an antipseudomonal penicillin with an aminoglycoside.[37] There is no convincing evidence that an aminoglycoside–penicillin–cephalosporin combination is superior to an aminoglycoside–β-lactam combination.

### *Fluid Therapy*

The goal of fluid replacement in the gram-negative bacteremic patient is the maintenance of adequate tissue perfusion to vital organs. The changing nature of the hemodynamics of sepsis and septic shock requires that vital signs be monitored adequately and that hemodynamic changes be corrected immediately. The Swan–Ganz catheter has become a useful tool in defining the limits of therapeutic intervention. That is, a falling blood pressure with a normal or low central venous pressure and pulmonary wedge pressure indicates that further volume replacement is needed; however, simple volume replacement, which is usually accomplished with crystalloid solutions, may not be adequate to restore arterial perfusion as pulmonary wedge pressures may rise dangerously high. If cardiac failure is encountered, cautious digitalization is indicated for its inotropic effects. Care must be taken in dosing digoxin in this setting as renal function may be poor or deteriorating, thus reducing the major elimination pathway. Concurrent use of sympathomimetics for arterial pressure support may further exacerbate poor renal function.

The availability of different solutions to expand intravascular volume enables the clinician to address concurrent therapeutic problems. For example, a patient may be hypotensive with anemia and thrombocytopenia. Whole blood would provide the volume, erythrocytes, and platelets. If the patient did not need the red cells, the plasma fractions would be indicated. An important tool to reestablish control of bleeding and DIC is the augmentation of clotting factors with fresh-frozen plasma. In the setting of septic shock, the dextrans are usually avoided because of associated bleeding.

### *Sympathomimetic Amine Therapy*

The role of sympathomimetic amines in the management of septic shock is to augment fluid replacement to maintain tissue perfusion. Historically, norepinephrine and epinephrine have been mainstays in the management of the hemodynamic changes in shock. The observation of local tissue necrosis at a site of norepinephrine extravasation concerned clinicians with regard to denying blood flow to major organs.

Also, both norepinephrine and epinephrine increase myocardial irritability.

Isoproterenol, dopamine, and dobutamine have been used, as they may have some advantage for the management of sepsis. All are beneficial by virtue of their positive inotropic effect on myocardial function. Their $\beta$ activity also enhances peripheral tissue perfusion. Isoproterenol increases cardiac index but not mean arterial pressure which is not desirable in sepsis. Dopamine, at low infusion rates, causes vasodilation of renal, splanchnic, coronary, and cerebral vessels. It also increases heart rate and systolic blood pressure while decreasing blood supply to skeletal muscle. Dobutamine is similar to dopamine but may be less irritable to the myocardium because of less chronotropic effect.

It is important to remember that sympathomimetic therapy should not be undertaken in the presence of inadequate fluid replacement. In this setting, vasodilation may occur as a result of $\beta$ stimulation, causing a precipitous drop in blood pressure. Thus, fluid replacement should be maintained at the upper range of normal limits. If hypotension persists, sympathomimetics are indicated.

## Controversies in the Pharmacologic Management of Septic Shock

The corticosteroids have been the subject of controversy in the management of the septic process. Because corticosteroids have a suppressive effect on the inflammatory and hormonal systems responsible for the early phase of septic shock, their short-term administration has resulted in defervescence, leaving an impression of improvement. It is unknown whether steroid use reduces mortality or even hastens recovery. When this is counterbalanced by the well-known adverse effects on the host immune system, the decision to use steroids becomes more difficult. In 1981, the Food and Drug Administration decided to remove the indications for the use of corticosteroids in septic shock after a review failed to find convincing clinical evidence of their benefits in humans.[38] Regardless, some clinicians still believe corticosteroids are beneficial and continue to use them.

Heparinization for the treatment of DIC is an interesting concept because the paradox of bleeding is caused by the "hypercoagulable state." Heparin has been shown to control this coagulopathy; however, there is little clinical evidence that heparin prolongs survival. It is also unclear whether abolishing the "consumption" has any direct clinical benefits. Heparin therapy for DIC is discouraged by most clinicians. Hemorrhage is usually managed with the replacement of clotting factor and platelets, and appropriate supportive care.

Naloxone, through its antagonistic effects on opiates and $\beta$-endorphins, has been shown to raise systolic blood pressure and sustain it in animals. Trials in humans are not available and are unlikely, because most patients with septic shock are managed with narcotic analgesics for pain and the high doses of naloxone required to maintain blood pressure would surely abate the beneficial effects of the opiates.

Diuretics are widely used in sepsis, particularly when renal function appears to be failing. It is not clear whether the aggressive use of diuretics in the early oliguric phase of acute renal failure avoids the failure or makes the ensuing failure less severe. It appears that most clinicians have abandoned the large doses of loop diuretics because of fear of causing deafness. Prudent doses of diuretics are beneficial when volume expansion fails to maintain adequate urine output.

## Developments on the Horizon

Recently, considerable interest has been focused on the effects of peptides released from macrophages stimulated by lipopolysaccharide. One peptide, cachectin, is believed to be a "proximal mediator" of the effects of lipopolysaccharide. That is, it appears to orchestrate a large number of events leading to shock, tissue injury, and organ failure. Therefore, methods developed to antagonize or neutralize this peptide may prove beneficial in controlling the cascading events of sepsis. In animals, it has been demonstrated that polyclonal antiserum directed against cachectin induces resistance to the lethal effects of lipopolysaccharide,[39] hence the possibility that neutralizing monoclonal antibodies directed against human cachectin may prove very useful in the treatment of early stages of sepsis.[40]

Gram-negative bacteremia remains a serious problem. It encompasses a complex sequence of events that may arise from seemingly innocuous beginnings. Clearly, management is difficult and reduction of fatal outcomes remains a major medical challenge.

## References


1. Osler W. The Principles and Practice of Medicine. New York, Appleton-Century-Crofts, 1892, p 114.
2. Felty AR, Keefen CS. Bacillus coli sepsis. A clinical study of 28 cases of bloodstream infection by the colon bacillus. JAMA 1924;82:1430–1433.
3. Scully FJ. The reaction after intravenous injections of foreign protein. JAMA 1917;69:20–23.
4. Chasis H, Goldring W, Smith HW. Reduction of blood pressure associated with the pyrogenic reaction in hypertensive subjects. J Clin Invest 1942;21:369–376.
5. Brues AM, Shear MJ. Reactions of 4 patients with advanced malignant tumors to injections of a polysaccharide from *Serratia marcescens* culture filtrate. J Natl Clin Inst 1944, 1945; 5:195.
6. Page IH, Taylor RD. Pyrogens in the treatment of malignant hypertension. Mod Concepts Cardiovasc Dis 1949;18:51–52.
7. McGowan JE Jr, Barnes MW, Finland M. Bacteremia at Boston City Hospital: Occurrence and mortality during 12 selected years (1935–1972) with special reference to hospital-acquired cases. J Infect Dis 1975;132:316–335.
8. Waisbren BA. Bacteremia due to gram negative bacilli other than the salmonella. Arch Intern Med 1951;88:467–488.
9. Braude AI, Siemienski J, Williams D, Sanford JP. Overwhelm-

ing bacteremic shock produced by gram negative bacilli: Report of four cases with one recovery. Univ Mich Med Bull 1953; 19:23.
10. Wolff SM, Bennett JV. Gram-negative-rod bacteremia. N Engl J Med 1974;291:733–734.
11. Scheckler WE. Septicemia and nosocomial infections in a community hospital. Ann Intern Med 1978; 89(pt 2):754–756.
12. Bryan CS, Reynolds KL, Brenner ER. Analysis of 1,186 episodes of gram negative bacteremia in non-university hospitals: The effect of antimicrobial therapy. Rev Infect Dis 1983; 5:629–638.
13. Johnson WG, Pierce AK, Sanford JP. Changing pharyngeal bacterial flora of hospitalized patients: Emergence of gram negative bacilli. N Engl J Med 1969; 281:1137–1140.
14. Johnson WG, Pierce AK, Sandford JP. Nosocomial respiratory infections with gram negative bacilli. Intern Med 1972; 77:701.
15. McCabe WR, Jackson GG. Gram negative bacteremia. I. Etiology and ecology. Arch Intern Med 1962; 110:847–855.
16. Fried MA, Vasti KL. The importance of underlying disease in patients with gram negative bacteremia. Arch Intern Med 1968; 121:418–423.
17. Bryant RE, Hood AF, Hood CE, Koenig MG. Factors effecting mortality of gram negative bacteremia. Arch Intern Med 1971; 127:120–128.
18. Sanford JP. Epidemiology and overview of the problem, in Rook RK, Sande MA (eds): Contemporary Issues in Infectious Diseases: Septic Shock. London, Churchill Livingstone, 1985, vol 4, p 10.
19. Siegel JH, Cerra FB, Coleman B, Giovannini I, Shetge M, Border JR, McMenamy RH. Physiological and metabolic correlation in human sepsis. Surgery 1979; 86:163–193.
20. Morrison DC, Ulevitch RJ. The effect of bacterial endotoxins on host mediation systems. Am J Pathol 1978; 93:527–617.
21. Morrison DC, Ryan JL. Bacterial endotoxins and host immune responses. Adv Immunol 1979; 28:293–450.
22. Corrigan JJ. Heparin therapy in bacterial septicemia. J Pediatr 1977;91:695–700.
23. Miller RL, Reichgott MS, Melmon KL. Biochemical mechanisms of generation of bradykinin by endotoxin. J Infect Dis 1973; 128(suppl):S144–S156.
24. Weil MH, Shubin H, Biddle M. Shock caused by gram negative microorganisms: Analysis of 169 cases. Ann Intern Med 1964; 60:384–400.
25. MacLean LD, Mulligan WG, MacLean APH, Duff JM. Patterns of septic shock in man—a detailed study of 56 patients. Ann Surg 1967; 166:543–562.
26. Clowes GHA, Vucinie M, Weidner MG. Circulatory and metabolic alterations associated with survival or death in peritonitis. Ann Surg 1966; 163:866–885.
27. Clowes GHA, O'Donnell TF, Ryan NT, Blackburn GL. Energy metabolism in sepsis: Treatment based on different patterns in shock and high output stage. Ann Surg 1974; 179:684–696.
28. Siegel JH, Greenspan M, DelGuercio LRM. Abnormal vascular tone, defective oxygen transport, and myocardial failure in human septic shock. Ann Surg 1967; 165:504–517.
29. Siegel JH, Goldwyn RM, DelGuercio LRM. Patterns of cardiovascular response in septic shock, in Hershey SG, DelGuercio LRM, McCann R (eds): Septic Shock in Man. Boston, Little Brown, 1971, pp 173–189.
30. Wright CJ, Duff JH, MacLean APH, MacLean LD. Regional capillary blood flow and oxygen uptake in severe sepsis. Surg Gyn Obstet 1971; 132:637–644.
31. Siegel JH, Farrell EJ, Miller M, Goldwyn RM, Friedman HP. Cardiorespiratory interactions as determinants of surgery and the need for respiratory support in human shock state. J Trauma 1973; 13:602–619.
32. Pizzo PA, Hathorn JW, Hiemenz J, et al. A randomized trial comparing ceftazidime alone with combination antibiotic therapy in cancer patients with fever and neutropenia. N Engl J Med 1986; 315:552–558.
33. Young LS. Empirical antimicrobial therapy in the neutropenic host. N Engl J Med 1986; 315:580–581.
34. Klastersky J, Glauser MP, Schimpff SC, Zinner SH, Gaya H, and The European Organizations for Research and Treatment of Cancer Antimicrobial Therapy Project Group. Prospective randomized comparison of three antibiotic regimens for empirical therapy of suspected bacteremic infection in febrile granulocytopenic patients. Antimicrob Agents Chemother 1986; 29: 263–270.
35. Oblinger MJ, Bowers JT, Sande MA, et al. Moxalactam therapy versus standard therapy for selected infections. Rev Infect Dis 1983; 4(suppl):S181.
36. Bolivar R, Fainstein V, Elting L, et al. Cefoperazone for treatment of infections in patients with cancer. Rev Infect Dis 1983; 5(suppl 2):S181–S187.
37. DeJohgn C, Wade JC, Schimpff SC, et al. Empiric antibiotic therapy for suspected infection in granulocytopenic cancer patients. Am J Med 1982; 73:89–96.
38. Sheagren JN. Septic shock and corticosteroids. N Engl J Med 1981; 305:456–458.
39. Buetler B, Milsark IW, Cerami AC. Passive immunization against cachetin/tumor necrosis factor protects mice from lethal effect of endotoxin. Science 1985; 229:869–871.
40. Buetler B, Cerami A. Cachetin: More than a tumor necrosis factor. N Engl J Med 1987;316:379–385.

# Chapter 88 / Systemic Fungal Diseases

Jeanne Hawkins Van Tyle, PharmD, MS

Fungal infections are generally classified either as superficial or as systemic (see Table 88.1). The superficial fungal infections are usually dermatophytosis; chronic fungal infection of the skin, nails, or hair; or tinea, including tinea pedis, tinea cruris, tinea corporis, and tinea versicolor (pityriasis versicolor). The systemic fungal infections are caused by fungi that are usually *dimorphic* (two distinct forms, as yeast or mycelial forms). In addition, systemic fungal infections are almost always caused by soil *saprophytes* (any organism living upon dead or decaying organic matter) where the airborne spores are inhaled and the infection is acquired, or by the opportunistic fungi in compromised hosts (see Table 88.2). In these patients, fungal infections are an important cause of morbidity and mortality.

Many patients currently receive treatment regimens that include extended-spectrum antibiotics, corticosteroids, and antineoplastic agents and the widespread use of these agents has resulted in many serious fungal infections in immunocompromised patients. In addition, patients with prosthetic heart valves, patients receiving intravenous hyperalimentation, and drug abusers are at increased risk of fungal infection.[1] There are data to suggest that fungal episodes during hospitalization are increasing. A comparative study[2] of fungemia at Memorial Sloan–Kettering Cancer Center examined frequency, onset, and therapeutic outcome in 200 fungal episodes. The study compared the years 1978 through 1982 with 1974 through 1977[3] and concluded that the total number of episodes of fungemia per year increased by more than 30% between the two study periods. The study found that fungemia also occurred earlier in the hospitalization. The overall mortality of the patients in the study was greater than 70%.

Fungal illnesses caused by the true pathogenic fungi (histoplasmosis, blastomycosis, coccidioidomycosis, and paracoccidioidomycosis) are related to definite geographic areas of the country, whereas the opportunistic fungi (e.g., *Candida* species, *Aspergillus*, *Cryptococcus*) are ubiquitous in their distribution. Clinical practitioners need to become aware of the organisms found in their area. As examples, 85% to 90% of the population in the geographic area bounded by the Mississippi and Ohio river valleys have positive skin tests for histoplasmin,[4] and an equally high percentage of patients in the southwestern United States have positive skin tests for coccidioidin.[5] More than 99% of these patients have had asymptomatic or mild infections that cleared spontaneously. After resolution, the individual is left with a strong specific immunity to reinfection. Blastomycosis occurs most frequently in the central and south-central areas of the Midwest.[6]

Systemic mycoses fall into two distinct categories, depending on the interaction of two major factors: (1) the inherent virulence of the fungus and (2) the immunocompetence of the host. Histoplasmosis, blastomycosis, coccidioidomycosis, and paracoccidioidomycosis are caused by the true pathogenic fungi. True pathogenic fungi are defined as those species that are capable of producing an infectious process in a normal host.

Opportunistic fungi may also cause systemic fungal infections but these causative agents do not have enough inherent virulence to infect a normal host. They are capable of infecting individuals whose immune defense mechanism is depressed. These include common types of mycoses such as (1) aspergillosis, (2) cryptococcosis, and (3) systemic candidiasis.

This chapter discusses systemic mycotic diseases and diseases caused by *Candida* species that affect patients residing in the United States. Many other fungal diseases occur in other areas of the world and are not covered in this discussion.

## Diagnosis

The diagnosis of a mycosis requires demonstration of the pathogenic fungus in patient specimens. Accurate diagnosis is dependent on prompt and careful identification of the fungus. Skin testing with fungal antigens has little diagnostic value in patients with active fungal disease. Serologic testing can be very helpful in diagnosing aspergillosis, histoplasmosis, cryptococcosis, coccidioidomycosis, and paracoccidioidomycosis as well as monitoring the response to therapy of these mycoses.

In 1985, the American Thoracic Society published a statement on the laboratory diagnosis of mycotic and specific fungal infections[7] in which recommendations for the selection and culturing of a specimen were made. Cultures of *Histoplasma capsulatum*, *Blastomyces dermatitidis*, and *Coccidioides immitis* are very slow growing, usually requiring 2 to 6 weeks. Optimal recovery rate of these organisms is obtained if testing occurs within 3 days of obtaining the specimen. Freezing injures dimorphic fungi and should be avoided.[7]

Two types of serologic tests are useful in the diagnosis of fungal infections: detection of specific antibodies against fungal antigens and detection of specific fungal antigens circulating in the body fluids of infected patients. Testing for antibodies is the most common approach to the diagnosis of fungal infection. Immunoglobulin M (IgM) antibodies are detectable about 2 weeks after infection and generally disappear within 6 months. Detection of IgM antibody strongly

**Table 88.1** Classification of Fungal Diseases

| | Systemic | |
|---|---|---|
| **Superficial** | **Pathogenic** | **Opportunistic** |
| Candidiasis (opportunistic) | Blastomycosis[b] | Aspergillosis |
| Dermatophytosis | Coccidioidomycosis[b] | Cryptococcosis[b] |
| Tinea[a] | Paracoccidioidomycosis[b] | Candidiasis (systemic) |
| | Histoplasmosis[b] | |

[a] Includes tinea corporis, tinea cruris, tinea pedis, and tinea versicolor.
[b] Also referred to as the deep mycoses.

implies recent infection. Immunoglobulin G (IgG) antibody levels take considerably longer to peak (6–12 weeks) and may remain elevated for many months or even a few years after the fungal infection.

Serologic procedures have been developed for aspergillosis, blastomycosis, coccidioidomycosis, and histoplasmosis. In these diseases, one tests for the presence of antibodies to the fungus in the patient's serum. In testing for the antibody, two general methods are used: the complement fixation (CF) test and the immunodiffusion (ID) test. The CF test detects the presence of complement-fixing antibodies in the serum and the results are expressed as a serum dilution (the reported value indicates the most dilute sample in which significant lysis of the target red blood cells can still be prevented). Because IgG antibodies persist a long time, a single complement fixation titer cannot differentiate between recent or remote infections.

The immunodiffusion test is much easier to perform than the CF test and can identify antibody even when the serum is anticomplementary, which makes interpretation of the CF test impossible. A major drawback to the ID test is that it is sometimes less sensitive than CF. Immunodiffusion is performed with a double-diffusion gel plate. The patient's serum is placed in one well (see Fig. 88.1) and antigen from the fungus is placed in the other well. A precipitin band forms between the wells if antibodies to the fungal antigen are present in the patient's serum. A band of identity with a known positive control is indicative of patient antibody against the antigen in question. Partial identity reactions are regarded as positive for antibody against the antigen only if no other identity reaction is present on the plate. Nonidentity reactions are regarded as negative.

**Table 88.2** Patients at Increased Risk of Fungal Infection

| |
|---|
| Compromised hosts |
| Long-term corticosteroid use |
| Cancer patients (antineoplastic use) |
| Extended-spectrum antibiotic use |
| Granulocytopenic patients |
| Diabetics |
| Patients with prosthetic heart valves |
| Patients receiving total parenteral nutrition |
| Intravenous drug abusers |
| Genetic predisposition (chronic mucocutaneous candidiasis) |

## Infections Caused by True Pathogenic Fungi

### *Histoplasmosis*

Histoplasmosis[4] may appear in a number of forms in humans. It is caused by the fungus *Histoplasma capsulatum*, a facultative intracellular parasite. Pulmonary histoplasmosis is usually a benign disease, whereas disseminated histoplasmosis in the adult is frequently associated with defects of the immune system mechanisms.[8] Histoplasmosis occurs most frequently in the midwestern and south-central regions of the United States where it is endemic. Cultures of soil specimens have shown that the organism is more prevalent at sites where bat or bird excrement have collected for several years. Birds are not themselves infected because of high body temperature. Bird roosts, pigeon roosts, chicken houses, and sites frequented by bats such as caves, attics, and old buildings are most likely to be point sources. Mechanical disturbances of such sites can greatly increase the number of airborne spores. Treatment is indicated for all patients with disseminated histoplasmosis or those who are severely immunocompromised.

Infection is initiated by the inhalation of conidia or spores. The conidia convert to yeastlike cells and result in a wide variety of clinical manifestations. Ninety-five percent or more of infections are asymptomatic and completely benign and the illness clears spontaneously. In acute infection the symptoms are nonspecific and rather variable. Fever and headache occur in almost all cases; chills, cough, and chest pain occur in approximately two thirds of patients. Less frequently the patient may experience weakness, weight loss, myalgias, fatigue, and gastrointestinal symptoms such as nausea, vomiting, or diarrhea. Disseminated histoplasmo-

**Figure 88.1** Patterns obtained in immunodiffusion assays. Well 1, reference antiserum (positive control); Well 2, patient test serum; Well 3, reference fungal antigen.

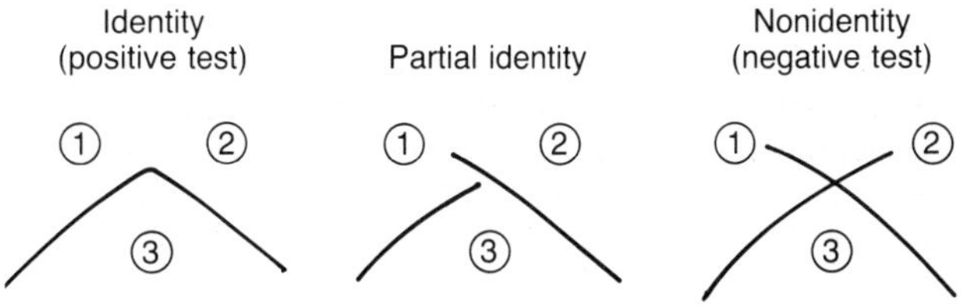

sis may occur if the infection does not resolve spontaneously. If untreated after dissemination, the disease is usually fatal.[9]

The laboratory diagnosis of fungal infection is most easily accomplished by direct microscopic examination of affected area scrapings in a 10% KOH slide mount. The KOH clears the specimen by digesting proteinaceous debris, bleaching pigment, and loosening the sclerotic material without damaging the fungus. *H. capsulatum* is extremely difficult to observe in sputum using the standard KOH preparation because of its small size and intracellular location.[7] The fungus grows on nutrient medium at 25°C as a fluffy, white mycelial colony, but at 37°C it grows as a small budding yeastlike cell.

Serologic tests are useful in the diagnosis and monitoring of response to therapy. The CF test with both yeast and mycelial antigens is most widely used.[7] A titer of 1:8 or greater is considered positive. The CF test becomes positive 21 to 28 days after primary exposure and approximately 70% of patients develop titers within 6 weeks. Fungal immunodiffusion can also be used to diagnose the illness and monitor the course of infection. Two precipitin bands, designated H and M, may be present during active infection. These usually appear later than a positive CF test. Newer, more sensitive serologic tests for *H. capsulatum* antibodies are radioimmunoassay (RIA) and enzyme immunoassay (EIA) but they are not yet available for routine use.

Acute histoplasmosis does not ordinarily require any specific treatment. Traditionally, treatment of disseminated histoplasmosis requires full dosages and courses of amphotericin B such as 40 to 50 mg daily intravenously for 2 or 3 weeks of therapy. Progressive infections in patients whose immune status is depressed, disseminated histoplasmosis, and chronic active pulmonary forms of the disease require prolonged treatment with relatively high doses of amphotericin B. The optimal total dose for disseminated disease was found to be 38 mg/kg body weight in one cooperative study.[6] At this point, no authors have addressed dosage adjustment based on ideal or actual weights. For chronic active pulmonary histoplasmosis, low-dose regimens may be used. When the low-dose (500 mg total) regimen is given, the relapse rate is approximately 25% within 3 years. With the high-dose regimen (2,500 mg total), the relapse rate is nearly zero.[6] Recently, ketoconazole has been investigated in a number of trials. In a multicenter prospective randomized trial, the efficacy and toxicity of low-dose (400 mg/d) and high-dose (800 mg/d) oral ketoconazole were compared in 80 patients with blastomycosis and 54 patients with histoplasmosis.[10] The success rate for all patients with histoplasmosis treated for 6 months or longer was 85%. Adverse effects such as nausea with or without vomiting, abdominal pain, diarrhea, and pruritus occurred in 60% and were more common with the high-dose regimen. Because of the higher frequency of side effects associated with high-dose therapy, ketoconazole should be initiated with the low dose. Ketoconazole appears safe and effective in the treatment of disseminated or progressive cavitary histoplasmosis in the normal host.[11] In the compromised host with disseminated histoplasmosis, ketoconazole does not appear to be effective and conventional therapy with amphotericin B appears warranted.[11]

### *Blastomycosis*

North American blastomycosis, or Gilchrist's disease, is a chronic, granulomatous, suppurative disease involving primarily the lungs, skin, bones, and genitourinary tract.[12] The causative agent is *Blastomyces dermatitidis*. The disease is seen primarily in patients who live east of the Mississippi River. It is endemic in the eastern United States and in Canada, up to the mouth of the St. Lawrence River. Blastomycosis at the present time is an uncommon infection.[12] It is not a reportable illness in most states, making estimates of incidence and prevalence difficult. A complete understanding of the incidence and epidemiology of blastomycosis has been hindered by the lack of a sensitive, specific skin test reagent and the inability to isolate the organism in its natural habitat. The portal of entry for blastomycosis appears to be the lung.

Blastomycosis is a systemic disease with a wide variety of pulmonary and extrapulmonary manifestations. Symptoms of acute pulmonary infection are nonspecific and tend to mimic influenza or bacterial infection in presentation. Blastomycosis usually begins insidiously from a lung site and produces symptoms such as malaise, arthralgias, chills, fever, cough, and weight loss. Pleuritic chest pain may be a prominent symptom but is usually transient. The pulmonary lesions may resolve and the disease may reappear in another organ system such as cutaneous sites or bones.

The definitive diagnosis of blastomycosis may be made by observing the characteristic yeast cells in clinical specimens or histopathological sections of tissue. The complement fixation test is the test most widely used for serologic diagnosis of blastomycosis; however, its clinical value is limited because it is not very sensitive. Fewer than 25% of the culture-proved cases are detected with this method. Recently, an immunodiffusion procedure has become available and is positive in approximately 80% of the culturally provable cases.

All patients with blastomycosis require therapy. Most patients with culture-proved blastomycosis have progressive disease that can be reversed only with specific treatment. Surgical treatment has little role except in the incision and drainage of large abscesses. Intravenous amphotericin B at a daily dose of 0.6 mg/kg body weight up to a total dose of 1 to 3 g is the usual course. The total dose of amphotericin B should be not less than 1.5 g for an adult, and many clinicians advise a total dose of 2 g.[6] Relapse occurs in 10% to 20% of the patients within 5 years; in these cases, re-treatment with amphotericin B is indicated.

### *Coccidioidomycosis*

Coccidioidomycosis (valley fever) is caused by the fungus *Coccidioides immitis*.[5] Coccidioidomycosis is endemic in certain areas of South, Central, and North America. Of the estimated 100,000 annual cases in the United States, almost all occur in seven southwestern states. Understanding of the natural history of the coccidioidomycosis infection is nearly complete. The fungus exists in the soil in the mycelial phase. As it matures, spores are formed which become airborne. These spores may be inhaled by the host. In the host, the spores swell, become spherical, and develop a thick wall. The primary lesion is usually pulmonary, and clinical symptoms of fever, chills, night sweats, malaise, arthralgias, anorexia, slight dry cough, and chest pain occur after an incubation of 7 to 8 days. Chest x-rays show minimal changes, infiltrates, frank pneumonia, or a pleural effusion. Sixty percent of those infected have asymptomatic infections or illness indistinguishable from ordinary upper respiratory infections. Forty percent develop symptoms of a primary infection 1 to 3 weeks after exposure. The disease is usually self-limited but 5% of the patients develop residual cavitary disease or pulmonary abscesses. Progressive disseminated coccidioidomycosis, occurring in less than 1%, develops only in those hosts whose capacity to resist infections or to develop immunity has been compromised.

*C. immitis* may be readily demonstrated in sputum or other clinical specimens using the standard KOH preparation. Cultures of *C. immitis* represent a major biohazard and suspected isolates should be handled only by experienced laboratories. Serologic tests are useful. The hyphal (mycelial) form antigen, coccidioidin, is most useful in detecting humoral antibody. Serum IgM precipitating antibody may be demonstrated by tube precipitation, latex agglutination, or immunodiffusion methods. These antibodies are first detected 1 to 3 weeks after onset of symptoms of primary infection in 75% of cases, and usually disappear within 4 to 6 months. Titers as low as 1:2 or 1:4 by CF may be seen in patients with active primary infection. Titers greater than 1:16 strongly suggest the presence of disseminated disease. The latex agglutination test appears to be the most sensitive test for detection of precipitating antibody.

Coccidioidomycosis is one of those diseases in which significant improvement rather than cure is a more realistic goal of therapy.[13] It is generally agreed that severe primary infections should receive chemotherapy with intravenous amphotericin B to a total dose of 0.5 to 1.5 g.[14] Criteria used to determine the need for treatment are persistent fever (longer than 6 weeks); prostration; extensive, enlarging, or persistent pulmonary involvement; persistent precipitins and negative skin tests.[14] Amphotericin B, although less effective for coccidioidomycosis than for other systemic mycoses, remains the drug of choice in initial treatment.[6] Treatment is indicated in patients with systemic dissemination or meningitis, and when persisting or progressive pulmonary involvement occurs in infants, pregnant women, patients with diabetes mellitus, and members of racial groups most susceptible to the infection, such as blacks and Filipinos.[6]

Treatment should be considered in patients with progressive pulmonary disease and in patients with preexisting debilitation or immune system impairment. In most cases, stable pulmonary lesions require no treatment, as most patients with primary pulmonary coccidioidomycosis recover spontaneously.

When therapy is indicated, the treatment of choice for primary coccidioidomycosis is intravenous amphotericin B.[15] An increasing CF titer is an indicator of possible dissemination and a poor prognostic sign. A total dose of 0.5 to 2.0 g is called for in this situation. Disseminated disease always requires prompt and aggressive amphotericin B therapy in total doses of 2.5 to 3.0 g. Prolonged courses may require 4.0 to 5.0 g if remission is not achieved.[6] Duration of therapy may be as important as, or more important than, the total dose.[14] Intrathecal treatment with amphotericin B is required for coccidioidomycosis meningitis. (See Meningitis in Chapter 75.)

Graybill and associates recommend[16] beginning oral ketoconazole treatment of coccidioidomycosis with 400 mg/d after their initial studies[17] suggested that 200 mg/d is not an adequate dosage for effective treatment. The optimum dose and duration of ketoconazole therapy have not yet been defined.[18] Graybill commented that coccidioidomycosis responds slowly to antifungal therapy. The role of miconazole in the treatment of coccidioidomycosis remains unsettled.[19]

## Infections Caused by Opportunistic Fungi

The species involved in opportunistic infections share few common attributes. *Aspergillus*, *Candida*, and *Cryptococcus* appear to have a greater capacity to adapt to a tissue environment than related species. The pathogenic potential of these fungi falls just short of the capacity to induce spontaneous infection in a normal host. Some impairment of host immune defenses is usually necessary for infection to occur; however, in sufficient numbers, these organisms can invade a healthy individual. To a certain extent, the nature of host debilitation determines the form and the causative agent of the infection. In the setting of reduced host defense mechanisms, fewer organisms and lower virulence are necessary to induce infection. When one is trying to determine a plan of action regarding diagnosis and management of a fungal infection in a compromised host it is reasonable to first consider the potential predisposing factors in the patient. One can then develop an effective plan for initial therapeutic management.

### *Aspergillosis*

Aspergillosis is a collection of distinct clinical entities that have in common an *Aspergillus* species as the causative agent. *Aspergillus* is a ubiquitous mold. The fungus grows well on a variety of substrates, including stored hay or grain, decaying vegetation, and soil. Aspergillosis is usually acquired by inhalation of airborne spores. These spores are small enough to reach alveoli or to gain entrance to the paranasal sinuses. The portal of entry and immune status of the host influence the course of events. Massive inhalation of spores by normal children may be followed within 24 hours by fever, dyspnea, and a miliary infiltrate in chest x-ray. Improvement often begins spontaneously in 2 to 4 weeks, leading to cure. Immunosuppressed patients are prone to an acute and usually fatal pneumonia caused by *Aspergillus*. Illness begins with high fever, followed in a few days by one or more areas of consolidation on chest x-ray.

The most reliable method for the diagnosis of aspergillosis is the recovery of the organism from an infected patient together with the demonstration of the organism in tissue. The detection of precipitating antibodies by immunodiffusion tests appears to be the most readily available and reliable of the serologic tests for the diagnosis of aspergillosis.[7]

Surgical excision of the infected areas is advised and pleural aspergillosis often responds well to surgical drainage alone.[20] Systemic antifungal agents play no role in the treatment of allergic bronchopulmonary aspergillosis or in the management of intracavitary aspergillomas. Intravenous amphotericin B is the drug of choice for invasive aspergillosis. The drug is most effective when diagnosis is made early, immunosuppression is not massive, and amphotericin B doses are advanced rapidly to therapeutic levels.[21] In recent years, favorable outcome has been achieved when aggressive diagnostic methods were used early and therapy with amphotericin B was started within 96 hours of onset of clinical infection.[6] A common maintenance dose would be 0.5 to 0.6 mg/kg/d. 5-Fluorocytosine has been used alone or in combination with amphotericin B with inconsistent success.

## *Cryptococcosis*

Cryptococcosis is a systemic infection caused by the yeast-like fungus *Cryptococcus neoformans*, an encapsulated organism that reproduces by budding.[22] *C. neoformans* is a ubiquitous organism that is distributed worldwide rather than in any defined endemic area. The organism is found in a variety of natural sites, particularly pigeon droppings. Circumstantial evidence suggests that disease occurs after the organisms are aerosolized and inhaled. There must be a high natural resistance to infection because new cases are relatively rare, possibly approximating 300 per year in the United States as a gross estimate. A review by Littman and Walter published in 1968 of a large series of cases of cryptococcosis indicates a threefold preponderance of males over females, with whites more commonly affected than nonwhites.[23] Cryptococcosis has been noted as one of the infections that frequently occur in association with AIDS. In only approximately half of the patients can an underlying defect or predisposing factor be determined.

Cryptococcosis may involve the central nervous system or the respiratory system as well as produce lesions on the face or scalp or in bone. Pulmonary cryptococcosis may be asymptomatic or may cause production of only scant, sometimes blood-streaked, sputum along with a dull ache in the chest. The onset of CNS cryptococcosis is usually insidious, although the manifestations may be more acute, especially in the immunosuppressed. Symptoms are usually present for weeks or months with a typical waxing and waning course. Complaints may be referable to the CNS such as headache, nausea, dizziness, irritability, somnolence, and clumsiness. If present, seizures usually occur only late in the course.

The organism may be recovered from the sputum of patients without serious infection as well as from patients with widespread dissemination of disease. The clinical significance of an isolate must be determined for each patient. Currently, the serologic test of choice for the diagnosis of cryptococcosis is the latex agglutination test for antigen.[7]

Treatment is not indicated for all patients in whom the organism is isolated, such as a positive sputum culture without evidence of pulmonary or systemic involvement or in patients with pneumonitis where spontaneous resolution may occur during a period of a few weeks. In these patients, a lumbar puncture to rule out meningitis is required when *C. neoformans* is isolated from any organ.

Treatment is indicated for pulmonary lesions that persist or progress, particularly in the presence of coexisting diseases such as lymphoma, leukemia, diabetes mellitus, sarcoidosis, or for patients receiving corticosteroids or immunosuppressive therapy.[6] Amphotericin B is the most effective antifungal agent for the treatment of cryptococcosis.[24]

## *Superficial or Systemic Infection with Candida albicans*

### Systemic and Disseminated Candidiasis

Systemic candidiasis is seen increasingly in debilitated patients and those with lymphoreticular or hematologic malignancies or disseminated carcinomas. In addition, patients can be predisposed to systemic candidiasis by other disease such as diabetes, polyendocrine deficiencies, or immunodeficiency diseases, or by certain drug therapies such as high-dose corticosteroids, immunosuppressants, antineoplastics, or broad-spectrum antibiotics. Candidiasis may involve mucocutaneous and gastrointestinal sites or deep organ systems. It is seen with endocarditis, arthritis, peritonitis, as well as diseases of the central nervous system and respiratory system.

There are more than 80 species of *Candida* but only 8 are regarded as important pathogens for humans. Of these, *C. albicans*, *C. parapsilosis*, *C. tropicalis*, and *C. glabrata* are seen most commonly. The organisms are normal flora of man and are commonly found on diseased skin, throughout the gastrointestinal tract, in the female genital tract, and in the urine of patients with transurethral bladder catheters. The defense mechanism of intact integument is of importance in maintaining resistance to cutaneous candidiasis; any process causing skin maceration leaves the involved site susceptible to *Candida* invasion, even in healthy individuals.[25]

Species of *Candida* are commonly observed in the oropharynx and respiratory secretions of normal subjects; therefore, the mere presence of *Candida* species in respiratory tract specimens is not diagnostic of pulmonary disease. The presence of pseudohyphae is unrelated to the presence of active infection. Tissue invasion seen on biopsy of involved areas is diagnostic.[7]

### Fungemia and Candidemia

Fungemia is the term used to describe fungi found in blood and it is noted with increasing frequency in hospitals that have a high proportion of patients who are immunocompromised, in patients where prolonged intravenous therapy or total parenteral nutrition is used, and in cardiac surgery patients.[1] It is also seen in intravenous narcotic abusers. Fungemia is mainly a nosocomial infection. The predominant organism found in blood cultures of fungemic patients is *Candida*. Risk factors predisposing to systemic candidiasis were studied by Klein and Watanakunakorn[26] and were found to be prior antibiotic therapy, indwelling intravenous and bladder catheters, concomitant bacterial infections, recent surgery, and total parenteral nutrition. The clinical picture of candidemia is indistinguishable from sepsis of a bacterial origin and the laboratory data are nonspecific. Diagnosis is usually made by blood culture. Physical examination at the onset of fungemia revealed no characteristic features beyond the nonspecific signs of sepsis. In this study, the authors[26] suggest that fungemia longer than 72 hours, evidence of endophthalmitis, or critically ill clinical status are reasons for instituting amphotericin B therapy.

Once fungemia is verified by positive blood cultures, the decision whether or not to treat with amphotericin B must be individualized in each case. If the patient is critically ill, it would appear wise to immediately begin treatment with therapeutic doses of amphotericin B as well as to remove as many predisposing factors as possible. Amphotericin B should be administered at 0.25 mg/kg/d and increased as tolerated to a maximum intravenous dosage of 0.5 to 1.0 mg/kg/d.

In granulocytopenic patients, empiric antifungal therapy may be necessary to control clinically undetected fungal invasion. Pizzo et al[27] evaluated empiric amphotericin B therapy in patients with fever and granulocytopenia (defined as polymorphonuclear leukocytes $<500$ mm$^3$) whose initial evaluation revealed an infectious etiology with fungal colonization but in whom fever and granulocytopenia remained despite at least 7 days of therapy with cephalothin plus gentamicin and carbenicillin. Their data suggest that empiric antifungal therapy is necessary to prevent fungal superinfections and to control clinically undetected fungal invasion.

**Chronic Mucocutaneous Candidiasis**

Chronic mucocutaneous candidiasis (CMC) is a heterogeneous group of cellular immunodeficiency states that result in chronic infection when the skin and nails as well as oral, esophageal, and genital mucosa become chronically infected with *C. albicans*. Several forms of CMC are associated with endocrinopathies, autoimmune phenomenon, or thymoma. Patients may have a variety of other associated disorders such as recurrent bacterial, viral, and fungal infections, chronic keratitis, alopecia totalis, and the dental enamel dysplasia syndrome.

Most forms of CMC begin in infancy or within the first two decades of life; only rarely is the onset after age 30. Endocrinopathy tends to follow, not precede, CMC, often after an interval of several years.

A skin scraping from mucosal or cutaneous lesions can be treated with KOH and examined under the microscope to identify fungi. *C. albicans* can easily be isolated on a variety of laboratory media. Within 48 hours, a creamy, white, pasty colony develops.

Intravenous amphotericin B has been used effectively in CMC, but nearly all patients relapse. CMC may be treated with topical application of nystatin or miconazole. Long-term suppressive therapy with ketoconazole has been successful.[28] Therapy for months or years may be necessary to prevent relapse.

**Oral Thrush**

Oral candidiasis or oral thrush results when *C. albicans* (normal oral cavity flora) overgrow and cause creamy white lesions called plaques or patches. This condition is most likely to occur in young children, in the elderly, in persons with poor nutrition, and in those receiving broad-spectrum antibiotics, corticosteroids, or immunosuppressants. Patients who take oral inhalation steroids are more predisposed to oral thrush than those receiving systemic corticosteroid therapy. Patients with malignancies may be predisposed to oral thrush as a result of chemotherapy or radiation therapy.

The term *thrush* is applied to a specific form of oral candidiasis characterized by creamy white, curdlike patches on the tongue and on other oral mucosal surfaces, which are removable by scraping and leave a raw, bleeding, and painful surface. Since the introduction of inhaled steroids for the treatment of asthma, especially in children, oral thrush has been more frequently reported. The incidence of thrush has ranged from 0% to 77%[29] in patients using inhalation steroids.

The diagnosis of oral thrush can be made by the clinical appearance of the lesion and by scraping, then using either a KOH smear or Gram's stain to show masses of hyphae, pseudohyphae, and yeast forms.

Standard therapy for oral thrush is nystatin suspension or oral use of vaginal suppositories.[30] The usual adult dose of nystatin is 5 mL (500,000 units) four times daily (every 6 hours).[31] Therapeutic success can be obtained as long as the medication is held in the mouth for 5 minutes and then swallowed. Therapy is usually continued for 7 to 10 days or at least 48 hours after becoming asymptomatic (up to several weeks may be necessary in some patients). The major problem with nystatin has been its unpleasant bitter taste. Thrush in patients on inhaled steroids usually resolves spontaneously but nystatin can be used if desired.

Oral ketoconazole has been effective in adult patients with oral candidiasis given 200 mg daily for 7 to 14 days. In a double-blind comparison study[32] in 56 immunocompromised cancer patients, ketoconazole achieved regression of visible lesions in 26 of the 36 patients (or 72%).

The use of clotrimazole troches has been found to be most effective in adult patients with refractory oral thrush. The troche is held in the mouth until dissolved at which time it is expectorated. The usual adult oral dosage is 10 mg, given five times daily at 3-hour intervals for 14 consecutive days.

**Vaginal Candidiasis**

Vulvovaginal candidiasis (moniliasis) is a common infection of the genital tract in women. Approximately one fourth of women in their childbearing years develop vaginitis. Several factors may predispose a woman to vaginal candidiasis: use of hormonal contraceptives, pregnancy, obesity, general debilitation, diabetes, endocrinopathies, and drug therapy with corticosteroids, antineoplastics, systemic antibiotics, or agents that suppress ovulation.

*Candida*-induced vaginitis is usually accompanied by a thick, curdlike discharge, with intense pruritis of the vulva almost always present. The thick discharge consists of epithelial cells and masses of hyphae and pseudohyphae. The vagina and labia are usually erythematous.[25] A smear may be taken from the vaginal discharge and examined microscopically in a KOH preparation for the presence of pseudohyphae.

Successful treatment of recurrent vaginal candidiasis may be difficult. Currently, topical medications such as miconazole, clotrimazole, econazole, or nystatin appear to be the primary mode of therapy. The intravaginal dosage of clotrimazole is a 100-mg vaginal tablet at bedtime for 7 nights or an applicatorful of cream at bedtime for 7 to 14 days. If the patient is not pregnant, an increased dosage of 2 tablets at bedtime for 3 consecutive nights may be used. Likewise, miconazole as either the cream or vaginal suppositories may be used. Suppositories containing 100 mg of miconazole are used for 7 consecutive days or 200-mg suppositories are used for 3 consecutive days. A vaginal preparation of econazole is not marketed in the United States yet.

Ketoconazole at a dose of 200 to 400 mg daily by the oral route for 5 days appears to be very effective.[33] Many patients prefer oral to topical therapy in the treatment of vaginal infections.

### Candiduria

Urinary tract candidiasis can occur in both men and women. In men, urethral candidiasis results from sexual contact with women with *Candida* vaginitis. In women, it is generally thought to be acquired from an extension of *Candida* vaginitis. Candiduria often follows catheterization and is usually managed without specific antifungal therapy, as in the majority of patients it will clear spontaneously. Antibiotics and bladder catheters have also been associated with acquisition of candiduria. *Candida* cystitis[34] is most commonly a complication of an indwelling bladder catheter and occurs relatively frequently. Within the urinary tract, the most common lesions are either hematogenously disseminated renal abscesses or bladder thrush. *Candida* bladder invasion usually follows catheterization or instrumentation of a patient with diabetes or a patient who is receiving broad-spectrum antibiotics; it generally is asymptomatic and benign. Symptoms may be absent or may be essentially identical to those of bacterial cystitis.

Because of the frequency of candidal urethral colonization in normal individuals, the presence of *Candida* yeast cells or even pseudohyphae in voided urine does not establish the diagnosis of genitourinary (GU) tract candidiasis. While urine colony counts have been used[35] to separate infection from colonization, this procedure is of questionable usefulness. Presence of the organism in any concentration in a specimen obtained by suprapubic aspiration is suggestive of *Candida* infection. The recovery of $\geq$10,000 organisms or visualization of both yeast and pseudohyphae from fresh midstream urine or from bladder urine obtained by single catheterization (not indwelling) is suggestive of GU candidiasis. Antibody coating techniques are not helpful in localizing the source of the GU candidiasis.[7] At present, reliable, validated, routine serologic tests for the detection of *Candida* antigen or antibody are not available to the clinical laboratory.[7]

The initial treatment of candidal cystitis should focus on the removal of precipitating factors. When true urinary candidal cystitis is present, local irrigation with amphotericin B should be undertaken. An irrigation solution containing 50 to 100 mg of amphotericin B in 500 mL of sterile water is instilled into the bladder twice daily.[36] If cultures continue to yield positive candidal growth, treatment with oral flucytosine should be considered.[36] The combination of 5-flucytosine and amphotericin B has shown synergism and increased efficacy when the individual agents have failed. If fungus balls form, they require surgical removal. 5-Flucytosine (5-FC) may be used orally but may have serious hematopoietic side effects and requires dosage modification in renal impairment. Also, *Candida* may develop resistance to 5-FC. The role of miconazole and ketaconazole in urinary candidiasis remains unclear. Neither ketoconazole (only 2%–4% excreted unchanged in urine)[33] nor miconazole is excreted into the urine as active compound. Graybill and Galgiani[37] examined the therapeutic efficacy of 200 mg daily of oral ketoconazole in 12 fungal urinary infections. In this study, resolution of the candiduria often occurred with 200 mg ketoconazole per day despite relatively low urine concentrations (usually <0.4 $\mu$g/mL). The results suggest that ketoconazole may be effective in cases where the organisms are highly sensitive. Overall, there have been insufficient data to evaluate the role of ketoconazole in candiduria.

### Candida Endocarditis

Of all the forms of fungal endocarditis, *Candida* is by far the most common. *Candida*-induced endocarditis occurs in association with five clinical factors: (1) heroin addiction, (2) cancer chemotherapy, (3) prosthetic valve implantation, (4) prolonged use of intravenous catheters, or (5) fungal endocarditis superimposed upon preexisting bacterial endocarditis. Postoperative cardiac surgery alone accounts for approximately one half of the cases of *Candida* endocarditis.

*Candida* endocarditis is associated with large emboli that occlude major arteries and may involve the coronary arteries. The most common valves involed in *Candida* endocarditis are the mitral and the aortic. Complications of *Candida* endocarditis include valve perforation, myocarditis, major emboli, and congestive heart failure.[25]

The diagnosis of *Candida* endocarditis may be difficult as one fourth of patients may have negative blood cultures. Echocardiography is becoming increasingly more helpful, as large vegetations may be detected using this technique.[25]

The primary mode of therapy for *Candida* endocarditis is surgery and amphotericin B remains an adjunct to the surgical procedures. Before the introduction of surgical procedures for the management of *Candida* endocarditis, the mortality rate from this disease was approximately 90%. The mortality rate is lowest with combined surgical and medical therapies. After surgery, amphotericin B should be given for 6 to 10 weeks. These patients should be monitored for a minimum of 2 years postoperatively.

## Therapeutic Management

Deciding whether to treat the fungal illness is easy in some cases and difficult and even controversial in others. There are no general rules for complex cases; each patient has to be evaluated on an individual basis, with all available clinical data considered.[38]

### *Amphotericin B*

First marketed in 1957, amphotericin B has been the principal chemotherapeutic agent used to treat systemic mycoses, yet much is not known about the drug. Amphotericin B is a large polyene macrolide compound (molecular weight 924) that is poorly soluble in water. The commercially available intravenous form (Fungizone, Squibb) utilizes deoxycholate bile salts to achieve a micellar suspension. Orally administered amphotericin B is poorly tolerated and less than 5% is systemically absorbed. After intravenous administration, tissue distribution is initially widespread, including liver, spleen, lungs, kidney, muscle, and skin, but excluding fat and brain.[39] Highest concentrations of amphotericin B are found in the liver.[39] Greater than 90% of the drug is protein bound.[40] No evidence of metabolism of the drug was observed by Christiansen et al[39] even though the highest concentrations of the drug are found in liver. The terminal phase of amphotericin B elimination becomes apparent only when therapy is stopped. The terminal elimination phase has a half-life of approximately 15 days.[41] Previous estimates of a 24- to 48-hour elimination half-life for amphotericin B have largely reflected the initially rapid elimination of amphotericin B from the central and rapidly equilibrating peripheral compartments. The long terminal elimination half-life of amphotericin B is of major clinical importance because it implies that a long time is required to attain pharmacokinetic steady-state conditions with repeated doses of this drug. The large total volume of distribution (4 L/kg) also contributes to the long elimination half-life of this drug.[41] Renal excretion appears to be a relatively minor pathway for the elimination of amphotericin B, accounting for approximately 3% of total drug elimination.[41] Renal impairment does not appear to affect clearance of amphotericin B[42] nor does hemodialysis appreciably alter amphotericin B clearance.[40] Dosage reduction is not required with renal dysfunction.

Recommendations for starting amphotericin B therapy represent an empiric attempt to provide effective therapy reasonably promptly while minimizing toxicity by administering an initial test dose followed by stepwise incremental doses on subsequent days.[40] Because an occasional patient may have an anaphylactic reaction[43] to amphotericin B, an intravenous test dose of 1 mg is recommended by some sources[44]; however, most physicians begin administration with 5 or 10 mg on the first day, increasing the daily dose by 10 mg until the desired dosage level is reached (usually not more than 50 mg/d).[6] Temperature, pulse, respiratory rate, and blood pressure should be recorded every 30 minutes for 4 hours after the test dose. Fever and chills (50%–90% of patients), nausea, vomiting, anorexia, headache, myalgias, and arthralgias occur with early infusions in many patients.

The initial starting dose of amphotericin B is 0.25 to 0.5 mg/kg/d up to 1.0 mg/kg/d or 1.5 mg/kg every other day. No authors have addressed dosage on the basis of ideal or actual body weight. The manufacturer recommends that a total daily dose of 1.5 mg/kg should not be exceeded. The usual daily dose is about 50 mg/d except in severe infections. The total dose of amphotericin B given to children should be decreased according to the body weight of the child. Amphotericin B may also be used intrathecally, intraventricularly, or intracisternally.

Amphotericin B is associated with nephrotoxicity, anemia, phlebitis, and a possible pulmonary toxicity when combined with leukocyte infusions. Impairment of renal function is the most commonly occurring side effect of amphotericin B therapy; it has occurred in over 80% of the patients treated. In most patients, nephrotoxicity develops after a few weeks of therapy. Renal abnormalities may persist long after cessation of the therapy and the degree of renal impairment is related to the total dose of the drug received. Amphotericin B is reported to cause a decline in glomerular filtration rate (GFR), renal tubular acidosis, decreased serum potassium, and diminished renal concentrating ability. The decrease in GFR appears to be related to decreased renal blood flow leading to cortical ischemia. Amphotericin B–induced renal tubular acidosis[45] is characterized by hypokalemia, an inability to excrete an acid load, and occasional nephrocalcinosis, generally without induction of systemic acidosis. Although the mechanism remains unclear, it is thought that this toxicity occurs primarily in the distal tubule. Amphotericin B interacts with membrane-bound sterols to increase passive permeability to sodium, potassium, hydrogen ion, water, and low-molecular-weight solutes such as urea. Renal tubular acidosis (RTA) during amphotericin B therapy is considered to be a dose-related phenomenon, probably occurring most frequently in patients who have received a total dose of 0.5 to 1.0 g or more. RTA may be treated with alkali therapy. If systemic acidosis is present, the bicarbonate deficit may be estimated as follows:

$$\text{bicarbonate deficit} = (\text{normal } HCO_3 - \text{observed } HCO_3) \times 0.5\ (\text{kg body weight})$$

One half of the estimated deficit may be administered and the patient reevaluated. Hypokalemia, if severe enough, should be corrected by the administration of potassium supplements. Amphotericin B therapy should be discontinued for several days if BUN levels are greater than 100 mg/dL and/or serum creatinine levels are higher than 2.0 mg/dL. It is the practice of some[44] to accept serum creatinine concentrations of up to 3 mg/dL while on amphotericin B. The azotemia that develops during treatment is reversible but when more than 4 g (total) amphotericin B is given, persistent renal damage may occur.

Solomkin et al[46,47] studied the dose requirements in patients with acute *Candida* infections in 47 general surgical patients. Their study supports the use of early systemic antifungal therapy in surgical patients based on the presence of three or more sites positive for *Candida*. Negative blood cultures did not rule out the presence of serious fungal infections. An accumulated amphotericin B dosage of approximately 6 to 8 mg/kg total dose appears sufficient to rid the fungemic patients of infection. Infusion rates of 0.5 mg/kg/d were not associated with extraordinary nephrotoxicity. The clinically relevant determinant of organ failure in their study population was uncontrolled infection, not amphotericin B therapy. Solomkin et al[46,47] recommend 0.5 mg/kg/d for 2 weeks as a low-dose amphotericin course for fungemia; it is associated with a lower incidence of nephrotoxicity.

Amphotericin B can severely depress red cell production, resulting in a normochromic, normocytic anemia.[48] The anemia is usually reversible upon discontinuation of therapy, with a return of hematocrit to pretreatment levels within several months. Generally, blood transfusions are neither necessary nor beneficial, as the anemia is apparently well tolerated by most patients.

Phlebitis[49] may be minimized with slower infusion rates (over 4–6 hours). Heparin (500–1,000 units) is often added to the amphotericin B solution to reduce phlebitis.

Wright and associates[50] reported respiratory deterioration in 14 of 22 patients (64%) receiving amphotericin B concurrently with leukocyte transfusions. Respiratory deterioration was defined as an unexplained acute development or worsening of hypoxia, the appearance of new interstitial infiltrates on chest x-ray, or an episode of acute dyspnea. In five patients, respiratory deterioration precipitated death. It was most common when amphotericin B was begun with or after the institution of daily leukocyte transfusions. The mecha-

**Table 88.3** Parameters to Be Monitored in Patients on Amphotericin B

| |
|---|
| Dose of amphotericin B for the day |
| Cumulative total dose for the course of therapy |
| Serum creatinine (or creatinine clearance) |
| Hemoglobin |
| Serum potassium |
| Serum magnesium |

nism proposed by Wright and associates suggests that the leukocyte transfusions may cause changes in the lungs that amplify the acute toxicity of amphotericin B, thereby permitting severe pulmonary reactions.

Therapy should be monitored (see Table 88.3) with the following: dose for the day, total accumulated amount of amphotericin B given, serum creatinine, hemoglobin, potassium, and magnesium.

### *Liposomal Amphotericin B*

At present, liposomal amphotericin B (L-Amp B) is not available as a commercial product, but the use of liposomes as drug carriers for amphotericin B illustrates the successful development of a tool to enhance the therapeutic action of a known active drug. Because of its lipophilic properties, amphotericin B is a good candidate for a liposomal drug carrier (diameters 0.5–6.0 $\mu$m). The liposomal amphotericin B preparation was shown to enhance the therapeutic index of amphotericin B by more than 20-fold in vitro and in animal studies. Liposomal amphotericin B enhanced the delivery of amphotericin B to the liver, spleen, and lungs of mice. Lopez-Berestein et al[51,52] used liposomal amphotericin B as an investigational new drug in 17 patients whose systemic fungal infections were not responding to conventional antifungal medications including amphotericin B. The liposomal amphotericin B was administered intravenously in a 15- to 45-minute infusion, with doses repeated every 24 hours. Five patients were cured, seven responded partially, and five showed no effect. These responses were seen even in the presence of persistent neutropenia (<1,000 cells/mm$^3$). No acute or chronic side effects were observed. Even for patients with impaired renal function at the onset of treatment, administration of the liposomal preparation was achieved without any further deterioration of kidney function. Liposomal amphotericin B has the additional advantages of a short infusion period (10–15 minutes versus 3–6 hours), a low fluid volume (40 mL versus 500 mL), and no need for premedication.[51] At present, liposomal amphotericin B is not available as a commercial product.

### *Flucytosine*

Flucytosine (5-fluorocytosine, 5-FC; Ancobon, Roche) is a synthetic, orally active, antimycotic agent. Its antifungal properties result from its conversion to the antimetabolite 5-fluorouracil (5-FU) in the yeast cell. Flucytosine is indicated in serious fungal infections caused by susceptible strains of *Candida* and/or *Cryptococcus*. The drug has low toxicity in patients, as the enzyme cytosine deaminase, which catalyzes 5-FC to 5-FU in yeast, is absent or in very low concentrations in humans. Flucytosine is readily absorbed from the GI tract ($F > 85\%$).[53] Approximately 90% is excreted unchanged in the urine.[54] Serum half-life is approximately 4 hours in normal subjects.[53] Clearance of flucytosine during hemodialysis approximates that of creatinine.[40] In patients with end-stage renal disease on dialysis, substantial amounts of 5-FC are removed and reloading must be done after dialysis. Flucytosine is generally combined with amphotericin B when used because resistant organisms emerge frequently during therapy.[55] The usual dosage is 150 mg/kg/d in four divided doses. Because the drug is excreted in the urine and may accumulate in renal impairment, the dosage must be lowered. Cutler and associates[53] found the relationship between serum creatinine and the half-life of flucytosine to be approximated by five times the serum creatinine (mg/dL) [flucytosine half-life = 0.4 + (5.2 × serum creatinine)]. This means that in renal failure a patient should receive an initial loading dose of 20 mg/kg followed by a maintenance dose of 10 mg/kg at an interval equal to the patient's individual half-life (as estimated from the serum creatinine). Ultimately, the clinician is advised to use such data for initial therapy estimates only and then to monitor plasma concentrations and adjust as therapy proceeds. Flucytosine can cause rash, hepatitis, severe diarrhea, and fatal bone marrow depression.[56]

### *Miconazole*

Miconazole (Monistat, Janssen) has a broad spectrum of activity with little resistance and is used intravenously as well as topically and vaginally.[57] Intravenous miconazole is indicated in coccidioidomycosis, cryptococcosis, candidiasis and chronic mucocutaneous candidiasis, and paracoccidioidomycosis. Dosages are 600 to 3600 mg per day in an intravenous infusion of 30 to 60 minutes either as a single daily dose or as three divided doses usually for 8 to 16 weeks (see specific dosages and suggested duration of therapy for each indication). Miconazole is considered adjunctive therapy for fungal meningitis and urinary bladder mycoses. Miconazole causes a number of adverse reactions such as hyponatremia which occurs in as many as 50% of the patients receiving it.[58] Phlebitis is an almost universal problem with the intravenous therapy, many times necessitating the use of a central venous line.[59] Miconazole has been suggested to interact with the coumarin anticoagulants, resulting in enhancement of the anticoagulant effect. Miconazole readily penetrates the stratum corneum of the skin and persists there for more than 4 days after application. Miconazole is considered safe for use during pregnancy.

### *Ketoconazole*

Ketoconazole (Nizoral, Janssen)[60] is a well-tolerated oral antifungal agent with a broad spectrum of activity. Ketoconazole has demonstrated efficacy in a wide variety of fungal infections such as in candidiasis, chronic mucocutaneous candidiasis, oral thrush, candiduria, blastomycosis, coccidioidomycosis, histoplasmosis, chromomycosis, and paracoccidioidomycosis. Ketoconazole[35] is normally well absorbed from the gastrointestinal tract,[61] achieving peak serum concentrations within 2 hours of a 200-mg dose. Ketoconazole has several reported drug interactions, including lower bioavailability with cimetidine and antacids, accumulation of cyclosporin during concurrent therapy, and a possible disulfiram-like reaction with alcohol.[62] Because the drug is marketed as the free base form of the drug, it must depend upon stomach hydrochloric acid for solubilization. Any treatment that will raise stomach pH is likely to decrease the bioavailability of ketoconazole. It is highly protein bound to albumin (93%–99%)[35] and is extensively metabolized. Dosage adjustment is not necessary in renal failure. The main side effects are gastrointestinal and occur in 5% to 10% of all patients. Rare side effects include gynecomastia and hepatotoxicity (occurs in 1 in 12,000 patients). Ketaconazole blocks testosterone synthesis.[63] Testosterone blockade occurs from 4 to 16 hours after a dose and is reversed by 24 hours. Therefore it is recommended that administration more than once daily be avoided in men. The usual dosage is 200 to 400 mg once daily. The optimum dosage and duration of therapy are not established. The increasing concern with hepatitis and the effects on testosterone synthesis may limit its place in therapy. The drug is not indicated in the most common cases of candidiasis.[64]

## References


1. Edwards JE, Lehrer RL, Stiehm ER, et al. Severe candidal infections: Clinical perspective, immune defense mechanisms and current concepts of therapy. Ann Intern Med 1978;89:91–106.
2. Horn R, Wong B, Kiehn TE, et al. Fungemia in a cancer hospital: changing frequency, earlier onset and results of therapy. Rev Infect Dis 1985;7:646–655.
3. Meunier-Carpentier F, Kiehn TE, Armstrong D. Fungemia in the immunocompromised host. Changing patterns, antigenemia, high mortality. Am J Med 1981;71:363–370.
4. Goodwin RA, DesPrez RM. Histoplasmosis. Am Rev Resp Dis 1978;117:929–956.
5. Drutz DJ, Catanzaro A. Coccidioidomycosis. Am Rev Resp Dis 1978;117:559–585; 727–771.
6. American Thoracic Society. Statement on treatment of fungal diseases. Am Rev Resp Dis 1979;120:1393–1397.
7. American Thoracic Society. Statement on laboratory diagnosis of mycotic and specific fungal infections. Am Rev Resp Dis 1985;132:1373–1379.
8. Wheat LJ, Slama TG, Norton JA, et al. Risk factors for disseminated or fatal histoplasmosis. Ann Intern Med 1982; 96:159–163.
9. Sathapatayavongs B, Batteiger BE, Wheat LJ, et al. Clinical and laboratory features of disseminated histoplasmosis during two large urban outbreaks. Medicine 1983;62:263–270.
10. National Institute of Allergy and Infectious Diseases Mycoses Study Group. Treatment of blastomycosis and histoplasmosis with ketoconazole. Ann Intern Med 1985;103:861–872.
11. Slama TG. Treatment of disseminated and progressive cavitary histoplasmosis with ketaconazole. Am J Med 1983;74[1B]:70–73.
12. Sarosi GA, Davies SF. Blastomycosis. Am Rev Resp Dis 1979;120:911–938.
13. Dismukes WE, Bennett JE, Drutz DJ, et al. Criteria for evaluation of therapeutic response to antifungal drugs. Rev Infect Dis 1980;2:535–545.
14. Stevens DA. Coccidioidomycosis and the indications for chemotherapy. Drugs 1983;26:334–336.
15. Drutz DJ. Amphotericin B in the treatment of coccidioidomycosis. Drugs 1983;26:337–346.
16. Graybill JR, Craven PC, Donovan W, et al. Ketoconazole therapy for systemic fungal infections: inadequacy of standard dosage regimens. Am Rev Resp Dis 1982;126:171–174.
17. Graybill JR, Lundberg D, Donovan W, et al. Treatment of coccidioidomycosis with ketoconazole: Clinical and laboratory studies of 18 patients. Rev Infect Dis 1980;2:661–673.
18. Galgiani JN. Amphotericin B in the treatment of coccidioidomycosis. Drugs 1983;26:355–363.
19. Stevens DA. Miconazole in the treatment of coccidioidomycosis. Drugs 1983;26:334–336.
20. Bennett JE. *Aspergillus* species, in Mandel GL, Douglas RG, Bennett JE (eds): Principles and Practice of Infectious Diseases, 2nd ed. New York, John Wiley and Sons, 1985, pp 1447–1451.
21. Aisner J, Schimpff SC, Wiernik PH. Treatment of invasive aspergillosis: Relation of early diagnosis and treatment to response. Ann Intern Med 1977;86:539–543.
22. Diamond RD. *Cryptococcus neoformans*, in Mandel GL, Douglas RG, Bennett JE (eds): Principles and Practice of Infectious Diseases, 2nd ed. New York, John Wiley and Sons, 1985, pp 1460–1468.
23. Littman ML, Walter JE. Cryptococcosis: Current status. Am J Med 1968;45:922–932.
24. Bennett JE, Dismukes WE. A comparison of amphotericin B alone and in combination with 5-flucytosine in cryptococcosis. N Engl J Med 1979;301:126–131.
25. Edwards JE Jr. *Candida* species, in Mandel GL, Douglas RG, Bennett JE (eds): Principles and Practice of Infectious Diseases, 2nd ed. New York, John Wiley and Sons, 1985, pp 1435–1447.
26. Klein JJ, Watanakunakorn C. Hospital-acquired fungemia: Its natural course and clinical significance. Am J Med 1979;67:51–58.
27. Pizzo PA, Robichaud KJ, Gill FA, et al. Empiric antibiotic and antifungal therapy for cancer patients with prolonged fever and granulocytopenia. Am J Med 1982;72:101–111.
28. Rosenblatt HM, Stiehm ER. Therapy of chronic mucocutaneous candidiasis. Am J Med 1983;74(1B):20–22.
29. Vogt FC. The incidence of oral candidiasis with use of inhaled corticosteroids. Ann Allergy 1979;43:205–210.
30. Quintiliani R, Owens NJ, Quercia RA, et al. Treatment and prevention of oropharyngeal candidiasis. Am J Med 1984;(suppl 4D):44–48.
31. Jones HE. Therapy of superficial fungal infection. Med Clin North Am 1982;66:873–893.
32. Hughes WT, Bartley DL, Patterson GG, et al. Ketoconazole and candidiasis: A controlled study. J Infect Dis 1983;147: 1060–1063.
33. Van Tyle JH. Ketoconazole. Mechanism of action, spectrum of activity, pharmacokinetics, drug interactions, adverse reactions and therapeutic use. Pharmacotherapy 1984;4:343–373.
34. Rohner TJ, Juliszewski RM. Fungal cystitis: Awareness, diagnosis and treatment. J Urol 1980;124:142–144.
35. Goldberg PK, Kozinn PJ, Wise GJ, et al. Incidence and significance of candiduria. JAMA 1979;241:582–584.
36. Paladino JA, Crass RA. Amphotericin B and flucytosine in the treatment of cystitis. Clin Pharm 1982;1:349–352.

37. Graybill JR, Galgiani JN. Ketoconazole therapy for fungal urinary tract infections. J Urol 1983;129:68–70.
38. Medoff G, Kobayashi GS. Strategies in the treatment of systemic fungal infections. N Engl J Med 1980;302:145–155.
39. Christiansen KJ, Bernard EM, Gold JWM, et al. Distribution and activity of amphotericin B in humans. J Infect Dis 1985; 152:1037–1043.
40. Block ER, Bennett JE, Livoti LG, et al. Flucytosine and amphotericin B: Hemodialysis effects on the plasma concentration and clearance, studies in man. Ann Intern Med 1974;80: 613–617.
41. Atkinson AJ, Bennett JE. Amphotericin B pharmacokinetics in humans. Antimicrob Agents Chemother 1978;13:271–276.
42. Graybill JR, Craven PC. Antifungal agents used in systemic mycoses: activity and therapeutic use. Drugs 1983;24:41–62.
43. Murray HE. Allergic reactions to amphotericin B. N Engl J Med 1974;290:693.
44. Hermans PE, Keys TF. Antifungal agents used for deep-seated mycotic infections. Mayo Clin Proc 1983;58:223–231.
45. Maddux MS, Barriere SL. A review of complications of amphotericin B therapy: Recommendations for prevention and management. Drug Intell Clin Pharm 1980;14:177–181.
46. Solomkin JS, Flohr A, Simmons RL. *Candida* infections in surgical patients; Dose requirements and toxicity of amphotericin B. Ann Surg 1982;195:177–185.
47. Solomkin JS, Flohr A, Simmons RL. Indications for therapy for fungemia in postoperative patients. Arch Surg 1982;117: 1272–1275.
48. MacGregor RR, Bennett JE, Erster AJ. Erythropoietin concentrations in amphotericin-B–induced anemia. Antimicrob Agents Chemother 1978;14:270–273.
49. Arbuthnot R, Dulleea A, Rippel S. Controlling thrombophlebitis from amphotericin-B. Am J Hosp Pharm 1978;35:129.
50. Wright DG, Robichaud KJ, Pizzo PA, et al. Lethal pulmonary reactions associated with the combined use of amphotericin-B and leukocyte transfusions. N Engl J Med 1981;304:1185–1189.
51. Lopez-Berestein G, Fainstein V, Hopfer R, et al. Liposomal amphotericin B for the treatment of systemic fungal infections in patients with cancer: A preliminary study. J Infect Dis 1985;151: 704–710.
52. Lopez-Berestein G. Liposomal amphotericin B in the treatment of fungal infections. Ann Intern Med 1986;105:130–131.
53. Cutler RE, Kelly MR. Flucytosine kinetics in subjects with normal and impaired renal function. Clin Pharmacol Ther 1978;24:334–342.
54. Bennett JE. Flucytosine. Ann Intern Med 1977;86:319–322.
55. Anonymous. Drugs for the treatment of systemic fungal infections. Med Lett 1986;23(711):41–44.
56. Kauffman CA, Frame PT. Bone marrow toxicity associated with 5-flucytosine therapy. Antimicrob Agents Chemother 1977; 11:244–247.
57. Heel RC, Brogden RN, Pakes GE, et al. Miconazole: A preliminary review of its therapeutic efficacy in systemic fungal infections. Drugs 1980;19:7–30.
58. Stevens DA. Miconazole in the treatment of systemic fungal infections. Am Rev Respir Dis 1977;116:801–806.
59. Stranz MC. Miconazole. Drug Intell Clin Pharm 1980;14:86–95.
60. Heel RC, Brogden RN, Carmine A, et al. Ketoconazole: A review of its therapeutic efficacy in superficial and systemic fungal infections. Drugs 1982;23:1–36.
61. Daneshmend TK, Warnock DW, Turner A, et al. Pharmacokinetics of ketoconazole in normal subjects. J Antimicrob Chemother 1981;8:299–304.
62. Fazio RA, Wickremesinghe PC, Arsura EL. Ketoconazole therapy of candida esophagitis—a prospective study of 12 cases. Am J Gastroenterol 1983;79:261–264.
63. Pont A, Williams PL, Azhar S, et al. Ketoconazole impairs testosterone synthesis. Arch Intern Med 1982;142:2137–2140.
64. Smith EB, Henry JC. Ketoconazole: An orally effective antifungal agent. Mechanism of action, pharmacology, clinical efficacy, and adverse effects. Pharmacotherapy 1984;4:199–204.

# Chapter 89 / Antimicrobial Prophylaxis in Surgery

Katherine A. Michael, PharmD, and Joseph T. DiPiro, PharmD

Infection remains a significant problem in surgical practice. Although the actual incidence of surgery-related infections remains controversial, estimates indicate that approximately 30% of hospitalized surgical patients either have established infections at the time of admission or develop some type of infection during their hospital stay. Infections in surgical patients account for up to 70% of all nosocomial infections in some institutions.[1,2] The cost of these infections is striking, not only in the monetary sense, but also in their effect on morbidity, mortality, and the overall quality of life. Prevention of infection remains one of the foremost concerns in modern surgical practice. This chapter discusses the prevention of postoperative wound infection.

## Types of Infection

Many types of infections occur after operations, not all of which are directly related to the surgical incision and manipulation. Postoperative infections are generally grouped into those related to the wound and those at distant sites such as the urinary tract and respiratory tract. Prevention of surgical infection refers only to infections of the surgical wound or sites of internal manipulations. The development of distant-site infections is related to the duration of catheterization of the urinary tract and the use of mechanical ventilation. Seeding of the lungs from the circulation, aspiration during intubation or tracheal suction, and poor pulmonary toilet may contribute to postoperative pneumonia. Bacteremia can result from coexisting urinary, respiratory, or wound infection as well as from infected intravenous catheters.[3] Urinary tract and respiratory tract infections are most readily prevented not by use of prophylactic antimicrobials but by avoidance of bladder catheters or by adherence to proper techniques for catheter use. Encouraging deep inspiration and coughing helps to prevent postoperative pneumonia.

Surgical site infections account for about 30% of all infections in surgical patients and can be divided into those related to (1) the incisional wound and (2) structures adjacent to the wound that were entered, exposed, or manipulated during an operation. The latter are sometimes called deep infections. Some 60% to 80% of wound infections involve the incision. The rest are at adjacent sites (i.e., intraabdominal, retroperitoneal, or in deep soft tissue). Sometimes an abscess may form. If an abscess forms superficially the wound may drain purulent material. The diagnosis of surgical wound infection is usually readily apparent; however, deep-seated infections may be very indolent. Most clinicians would consider a wound obviously infected if it drains pus. Infection may also be diagnosed by drainage of pus from an abscess. In either case, the isolation of organisms from purulent material is helpful in choosing antimicrobial therapy; however, a microbiologic report of "no bacterial growth" does not rule out the presence of infection. Wounds may also be considered infected if nonpurulent drainage is noted where the fluid yields bacteria. Some bacteria, such as streptococci, may produce wide areas of erythema and inflammation around a wound edge.[4,5]

Microbial patterns of surgical wound infections have been the focus of many studies in the past several decades, and these studies have demonstrated a significant change in the prevalence of organisms during this time period. A landmark study of factors influencing the development of surgical wound infections was conducted by the National Academy of Sciences–National Research Council (NAS–NRC) from 1960 to 1964.[6] Analysis of the incidence of microorganisms in 390 postoperatively infected wounds in a total of 1,388 cultured showed *Staphylococcus* species to be the most frequent, being isolated in 52% of patients. *Escherichia* species, the second most frequent organisms, were isolated in 15.1% of the wounds. Other studies during this time period similarly implicated *Staphylococcus aureus* as the pathogen most frequently isolated from surgical wound infections. The first National Nosocomial Infection Study from 1970 to 1973 indicated probable changes in this pattern with the incidence of *Escherichia coli* approaching that of *S. aureus*.[7] This increasing prevalence of gram-negative bacilli was confirmed in the recently published Centers for Disease Control Nosocomial Infection Surveillance Study. While *S. aureus* was still the single most frequently isolated pathogen in surgical wound infections (19.1%), gram-negative organisms including *E. coli, Pseudomonas aeruginosa, Enterobacter* species, *Proteus* species, and *Serratia* species collectively accounted for more than 35% of all isolates (Table 89.1).[2]

## Risk Factors for Postoperative Infections

Because the wound is common to all surgical patients, prevention of postoperative wound infection has received the primary attention of researchers concerned with the prevention of infections in surgical patients; however, as distant-site infections and wound infections are frequently interrelated, many of the principles applied to the prevention of surgical wound infection readily pertain to all infections in surgical patients.

The risk of postoperative wound infections is increased in direct proportion with the dose of bacterial contamination

**Table 89.1** Pathogens Isolated From Surgical Wound Infections

| *Pathogen* | *Percentage of total isolates* |
|---|---|
| *Staphylococcus aureus* | 19.0 |
| *Escherichia coli* | 11.4 |
| Enterococci | 11.4 |
| Coagulase-negative staphylococci | 8.4 |
| *Pseudomonas aeruginosa* | 8.1 |
| *Enterobacter* spp. | 6.9 |
| *Proteus* spp. | 5.0 |
| *Klebsiella* spp. | 4.8 |
| *Bacteroides* spp. | 4.4 |
| *Serratia* spp. | 2.0 |
| Group B streptococci | 1.8 |
| *Candida* spp. | 1.4 |

From Jarvis WR, White JW, Munn VP, et al. Nosocomial infection surveillance, 1983. MMWR Surveillance Summaries 1984;33:955–2155, with permission.

and the virulence of the organism and is decreased by the resistance of the host. These variables are influenced by factors related to the host as well as operative techniques.

### *Dose of Bacterial Contamination*

Contaminating bacteria can enter the wound from exogenous environmental sources or the patient's own endogenous flora (Table 89.2). Infections in some operations are almost always associated with environmental contamination. Possible sources of exogenous contamination are limitless, but organisms shed from the operative team and airborne organisms constitute the majority of identifiable pathogens. Infections attributable to the resident flora of the surgical team reflect inattentiveness to personal cleanliness and dress requirements.[4] Inadequate ventilation and excessive operating room traffic contribute to the risk of exogenous contamination from airborne bacteria. Although the use of ultraviolet lighting in the operating suite decreases the numbers of airborne organisms, it does not lower the rate of wound infection.[6] Multimicrobial infection in a case with no risk for endogenous contamination strongly suggests a major break in sterile technique, failure to properly sterilize instruments and equipment, or improper ventilation in the surgical suite.[4]

Contamination by the patient's endogenous flora occurs more frequently than contamination from exogenous sources. The NAS–NRC study classified surgical procedures into categories according to risk for endogenous bacterial contamination, and the study by Cruse and Foord of 62,939 wounds demonstrated the relationship of the incidence of wound infections to these categories (Table 89.3).[6,8] While the overall rate of wound infection was 4.7%, the incidence of postoperative wound infection increased when the genitourinary, gastrointestinal, or respiratory tract was entered (clean–contaminated, contaminated). When pus was encountered in the wound (dirty) the rate of infection was 25 times higher than that for wounds where no hollow muscular organ was opened and no infection was encountered (clean). The results of this study not only served to clarify the discrepancy in overall wound infection rates observed by different researchers, but also laid the foundation for the use of prophylactic antibiotics as discussed later in this chapter.

**Table 89.2** Sources of Bacterial Contamination

| *Exogenous* | *Endogenous* |
|---|---|
| Surgical team | Skin |
| Instruments and equipment | Respiratory tract |
| Operating room surfaces | Gastrointestinal system |
| Airborne contaminants | Genitourinary tract |

Endogenous contamination from the patient's skin is also an important source of bacterial contamination. Cruse and Foord[9] demonstrated the importance of a preoperative hexachlorophene shower in lowering the rate of wound infection from 2.3% in those who did not shower and 2.1% in those who showered with plain soap. The rate decreased to 1.3% when hexachlorophene was used in the shower. Chlorhexidine scrubs have also been shown effective for preoperative cleansing and have become popular since hexachlorophene was shown to be systemically absorbed. Shaving the operative site, with associated nicking of the skin, also increases the incidence of infection as does the use of surgical drains.[9,10]

### *Virulence*

The pathogenicity of bacteria depends on their ability to invade host tissue, inhibit host defense mechanisms, and destroy host tissues. For example, encapsulated bacteria (such as some streptococci) are resistant to phagocytosis and lysis. Additionally, some bacteria produce exotoxins, endotoxins, and other toxic compounds that enhance their virulence. Synergy between two organisms is important for enhancing pathogenicity in some surgical infections, most importantly the reaction between aerobic and anaerobic organisms in intraabdominal infections.

### *Host Resistance*

Host resistance involves those defense mechanisms that work to prevent bacterial contamination of most surgical incisions from causing clinical wound infection. Modern surgical techniques and advances in anesthesia and medical care have greatly increased the ability to perform potentially curative operations on severely ill and injured patients; however, these advances have also led to the problems of infections in patients with impaired host defenses. Although the problem of dealing with severely immunocompromised hosts is a very recent development, numerous factors influencing host resistance that were identified several years ago remain pertinent to modern surgical care.

Wound infection is related to age, with higher infection rates found at the extremes of age; the lowest rate occurs in the age group 15–24. Postoperative infection rate rises steadily with increasing age and peaks at 10.7% in the age

**Table 89.3** Wound Classification

| *Surgical category* | *Definition* | *Approximate percentage of all operations* | *Infection rate (%)* |
|---|---|---|---|
| Clean | No entry into hollow muscular organs, oropharyngeal cavity, or gastrointestinal, respiratory, or genitourinary tract. No inflammation encountered. No break in sterile technique occurs. Wounds are usually closed primarily and not drained. (Cholecystectomy, incidental appendectomy, and abdominal hysterectomy are included in this category if no inflammation is present.) | 75 | 5 |
| Clean–contaminated | Gastrointestinal, respiratory, biliary, or genitourinary tract is entered under controlled conditions without significant spillage. Clean wounds are included in this category when there is a major break in sterile technique. | 15 | 10–15 |
| Contaminated | Fresh traumatic wounds (less than 4 hours old), gross spillage from the gastrointestinal tract, operations with a major break in sterile technique or in which acute, nonpurulent inflammation is encountered. | 5 | 15–20 |
| Dirty | Traumatic wounds and perforated viscera untreated for more than 4 hours, and operations in which pus, devitalized tissue, or obvious infection is encountered are included in this category. | 5 | 30–40 |

group 65–74. An exception is a slightly higher incidence in those less than 1 year old, and a slightly lower incidence in those older than 74.[6,9,10]

Severe obesity was associated with an infection rate of 18.1% compared with an overall rate of 7.4% in the NAS–NRC study. Although operative procedures in these patients tended to be longer, adjustment for length of operation dropped the infection rate for obese patients only slightly to 16.5%.[6]

For the severely malnourished patient, improvement of the patient's state of nutrition is mandatory prior to elective surgery, as host resistance to infection may be impaired by starvation and by vitamin and protein deficiencies. In 67 severely malnourished patients who underwent surgery in the NAS–NRC study, 22.4% developed wound infections compared with the overall rate of 7.4%. Possibly contributing to this high incidence was the fact that many of these patients were older, had longer operations, or had operations associated with higher-than-average rates of contamination.[6,10]

Patients who harbor infections remote from the operative incision (such as a urinary tract infection, respiratory infection, or infected foot ulcer) have been found to be at higher risk for the development of postoperative wound infections. In the NAS–NRC study the infection rate was 18.4% in this group of patients, compared with 6.7% in those without remote infection.[6]

The NAS–NRC study reported a wound infection rate of 10.4% in 356 diabetic patients.[6] While this increased incidence may have been related in part to a larger number of elderly patients in this group, it is important to remember the effects of diabetes and impaired circulation on wound healing. Other chronic debilitating diseases would be expected to have similar effects on host defenses.

The infection rate for 119 patients in the NAS–NRC study receiving steroid therapy was 16%. Although the patients in this group tended to have additional risk factors, the deleterious effects of steroids as well as other immunosuppressive agents on host defenses appear obvious.[6]

### *Miscellaneous Risk Factors*

Several other factors have been implicated as increasing the risk for postoperative infections. These miscellaneous factors interrelate the principles of bacterial contamination, virulence, and host resistance.

Longer preoperative hospital stays are known to be associated with a greater risk of postoperative infection. Cruse and Foord[9] demonstrated an increase in postoperative wound infection rates from 1.2% to 3.4% when the preoperative hospitalization was extended from 1 day to 2 weeks. These results were confirmed in the NAS–NRC study where the trend remained, even when infection rates were corrected for other potentially contributing factors such as age and underlying disease state. Colonization with hospital flora likely explains this increase in infection rate.[6,9]

The rate of wound infection also increases in direct proportion to the duration of the procedure. This is not explained by the fact that contaminated procedures are generally more complicated, as the same relationship of infection to duration is seen with clean procedures. The higher infection rates seen with longer procedures are probably due to multiple factors including increased endogenous and exogenous contamination, exposure of more tissue, greater tissue damage from prolonged retraction, and finally, greater systemic insult to the patient likely resulting in impaired host defenses.[6,9,10]

## Prevention of Postoperative Infection

The beginning of the modern antibiotic era, marked by the introduction of sulfonamides in the late 1930s, had a revolutionary effect on the treatment of previously often fatal infections; however, after nearly half a century of use, antibiotics alone have failed to decrease the overall incidence of surgical infections. An important consideration, however, is that many types of infections are now preventable and modern medical care now allows for successful surgery in patients who previously were too debilitated to survive an operative procedure. Unfortunately, overuse and misuse of prophylactic antibiotics in surgical patients have contributed to an unwarranted overdependence on their effectiveness and a deemphasis on nonantibiotic factors for the prevention of postoperative infection.[1]

The practice of infection control is too often based on tradition and not on objective data. A set of recommendations for the control of surgical infection, developed from the most objective data available, was established in 1983 by a group of experts (Working Group to Develop Guidelines for Prevention of Surgical Infection, Centers for Disease Control, Atlanta) with a special interest in the control of surgical infections.[11] These recommendations provide useful guidelines and add perspective to many controversial subjects.

The specific guidelines developed by this group are categorized according to the objectivity of the data supporting each and are outlined in Table 89.4. Measures in category I (strongly recommended) are either supported by well-designed, controlled, clinical studies or viewed by the majority of experts to be useful in reducing the risk of nosocomial infections. Category I recommendations are applicable to the majority of hospitals and are considered practical to implement. Measures in category II (moderately recommended) are supported by strongly suggestive clinical data or by definitive studies with limited application to all types of hospitals. Included in this category are measures supported by strong theoretical rationale but limited objective data. Category II measures are not considered a standard of practice for every hospital. Category III measures (weakly recommended) are supported only by anecdotal data and opinions by some authorities or organizations. Although these practices may be useful in some hospitals, they lack both supportive data and strong theoretical rationale.

The important issues for the use of prophylactic antimicrobials are (1) the relative effectiveness of antimicrobial regimens in preventing infection, (2) the costs of the regimens, and (3) the risks that are incurred in the use of these regimens. The generally accepted principles of antimicrobial use in surgery involve five areas:

1. Surgical procedures for which prophylactic antimicrobials are beneficial
2. Proper timing of antimicrobial administration
3. Duration of the antimicrobial regimen
4. Route of antimicrobial administration
5. Selection of a particular antimicrobial agent

Consideration of these principles should result in the use of prophylactic regimens that have the greatest likelihood of preventing postoperative infection at the least possible cost (risk). Each principle is discussed here.

### *Surgical Procedures*

Prophylactic antimicrobials are likely to be beneficial in situations where there is either a high rate of infection or a low rate of postoperative infection with associated significant morbidity and/or mortality (e.g., endocarditis) (Table 89.5). For most clean operations, the rate of postoperative infection is very low, as discussed before, and the prophylactic use of antimicrobials is usually not justified; however, in some situations where prosthetic materials are placed

**Table 89.4** Guidelines for Prevention of Surgical Infection

| *Guidelines* | *Category*[a] |
|---|---|
| **Surveillance** | |
| All procedures should be classified and infection rates calculated for each category | I |
| Data should be available for use by surgeons and infection control committee | I, II |
| **Patient Preparation** | |
| Eliminate coexisting infections | I |
| Shorten preop hospitalization; diagnostic workup as outpatient | III |
| Preoperative nutritional repletion | II |
| Antiseptic bath/shower night before surgery | III |
| Hair removal only if necessary; shaving immediately before surgery | II |
| Operative site should be scrubbed with a detergent solution and covered with an antiseptic; solutions should be chlorhexidine or iodophors | I |
| Patient should be covered with sterile drapes so that only the operative site and those body parts necessary for the administration of anesthesia are exposed | I |
| **Surgical Team** | |
| All persons who enter the OR must wear a mask, cap or hood, and shoe covers | I |
| Surgical team should scrub before each case with chlorhexidine, iodophors, or hexachlorophene | I |
| Surgical team should wear gowns nearly impermeable to bacteria | II |
| Surgical team should wear sterile gloves; gloves should be promptly replaced if punctured | I |
| **Operating Room** | |
| Traffic flow in the OR should be minimal; all air should be filtered | I |
| The OR should be cleaned between procedures, daily and weekly | I |
| **Operative Technique and Wound Care** | |
| The surgical team should work as efficiently as possible to handle tissues gently, prevent bleeding, eradicate dead space, and minimize devitalized tissue and foreign material in the wound | I |
| Dirty and infected wounds should not be closed primarily | I |
| Drains for uninfected wounds should be a closed suction system brought out through a separate stab wound | I |
| Personnel should wash their hands before and after wound care, and should wear sterile gloves to touch an open wound | I |
| Dressing over closed wounds should be removed when wet or if the patient shows signs of infection, and the wound should be inspected for infection and cultured if suspect | I |

[a] Category I—strongly recommended, Category II—moderately recommended, Category III—weakly recommended.

From the Working Group to Develop Guidelines for Prevention of Surgical Infection—Polk et al,[11] with permission.

**Table 89.5** Examples of Operations in Which Prophylactic Antimicrobials Are Justified

| | |
|---|---|
| Clean operations | |
| Cardiac | Open-heart operations |
| Orthopedic | Joint replacements or use of other prosthetic materials |
| | Hip fracture repairs |
| Vascular | Use of prosthetic grafts |
| | Procedures in the abdomen or groin |
| Neurologic | Microneurosurgery |
| Clean–contaminated operations | |
| Gastrointestinal | Any resection of or entry into gastrointestinal tract |
| Obstetric | Cesarean section (with labor or rupture of membranes) |
| Gynecologic | Vaginal hysterectomies |
| | Abdominal hysterectomies (not conclusive) |
| Thoracic | Lung resections |
| Head and neck | Entry into oropharyngeal cavity |
| Urologic | When there is infected urine |
| Biliary tract | When there is risk of bactobilia |

(e.g., open-heart operations, vascular procedures, total hip replacements, hip fracture repairs) the results of the few infections that do occur can be disastrous and prophylactic use of antimicrobials is justified. For some clean procedures (aortic resections, total hip replacements, hip fracture repairs) the value of prophylactic antimicrobials has been demonstrated in placebo-controlled trials. In one of the largest prophylactic antimicrobial trials, Hill and associates[12] studied more than 2,000 patients undergoing total hip replacement and found that cefazolin was significantly more effective than placebo in reducing postoperative infection rate (0.9% versus 3.3%, respectively).

Prophylactic antimicrobials have proven beneficial in operations classified as "clean–contaminated." This group includes most obstetric and gynecologic operations (e.g., cesarean section, vaginal hysterectomy); operations in which the gastrointestinal tract is entered; biliary tract operations in patients who are likely to have bacteria in their bile; lung resection; and urologic procedures in the presence of infected urine. With each of these procedures there is entry into an area that has a resident bacterial flora. For most of these types of operations there are numerous published, placebo-controlled trials that have demonstrated the benefit of prophylactic antimicrobials.[13] Prophylactic antimicrobials are generally not applicable to contaminated or dirty procedures because a treatment course of antibiotics is usually required with these wounds.

Somewhat uncertain is the place of prophylactic antimicrobials in wounds created by traumatic injury. In many of these (such as gunshot wounds to the abdomen) infection is not yet established if the wound is less than 4 hours old, yet bacteria have entered the tissues. Short courses of antimicrobials are effective in preventing infection in previously healthy patients who have surgery within a few hours after injury.

### *Timing of Antimicrobial Administration*

The timing of antimicrobial administration is the most important factor affecting prophylactic antimicrobial efficacy. Antimicrobials given at inappropriate times can be ineffective for surgical prophylaxis. To be most effective in preventing postoperative infection the antimicrobial must be present in the potentially contaminated tissue *before* the bacteria enter the site (i.e., before the surgical incision). When antimicrobials are given after bacterial contamination, the likelihood of preventing infection is much reduced.

The time-dependent nature of the effectiveness of prophylactic antimicrobials was first noted by Miles and associates in the late 1950s.[14,15] They described a guinea pig model of staphylococcal infection where bacteria were introduced subcutaneously. Twenty-four hours after bacterial contamination, a skin lesion was evident and its diameter could be measured. The diameter of the skin lesion was then used as a measure of the severity of infection. These investigators found that if penicillin (to which the organisms were sensitive) was administered at the same time the bacteria were introduced, the dermal lesion measured 24 hours later was equal in size to that produced by killed organisms. Animals who received penicillin from 1 to 3 hours after contamination had increasingly larger lesions. Finally, when the penicillin was administered 3 or more hours after the bacteria were introduced, the dermal lesion seen at 24 hours was the same size as in animals that received no antimicrobials.

The same time-dependent effect was found for substances that were detrimental to wound healing. Epinephrine, which inhibits local immunodefenses by causing vasoconstriction, was injected at various times into the area where bacteria were introduced. It was found to increase the size of the dermal lesion measured at 24 hours. If epinephrine was administered as soon as 3 hours after bacterial contamination the lesion size was not increased.

From these studies the investigators defined the "effective" period for penicillin, when the wound was most susceptible to the positive influence of penicillin (Fig. 89.1). This period lasted only 2 to 3 hours after bacterial contamination. Coincident with this time period, the wound was most susceptible to negative influences that might increase the severity of the infection. As the first few hours after bacterial contamination were the most crucial, with the greatest chance for positive or negative influences to be felt, it was referred to as the "decisive" period. This "decisive" period applies to other antimicrobials and to other models of infection. With surgical procedures, the time at which bacteria are most likely to enter tissue is while the wound is open. These few short hours while the wound is open constitute the "decisive" period for infections that manifest postoperatively.

It was not until the late 1960s that the first studies in humans on this time-dependent effect of prophylactic antimicrobials appeared in the literature. Studies prior to this

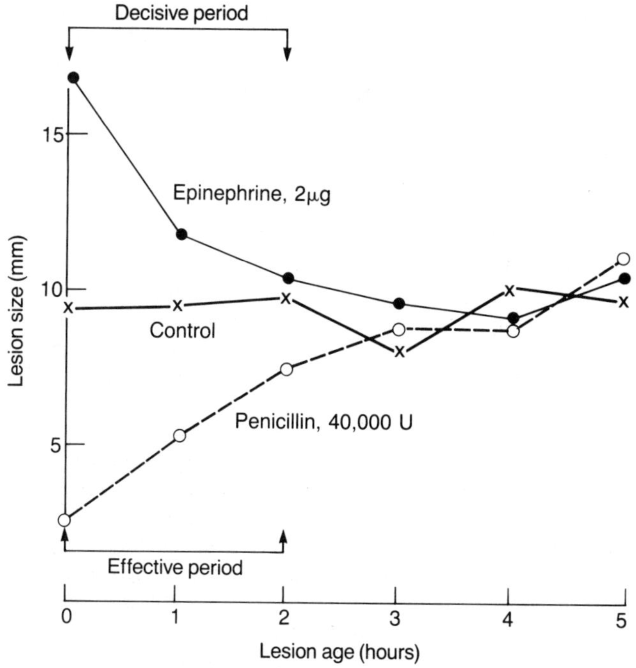


**Figure 89.1** Lesion size after inoculation of bacteria as a function of systemic antibiotic administration or epinephrine-induced ischemia. *(From Howard RJ, Simmons RL, eds: Surgical Infectious Diseases, 2nd ed. Morwalk, Conn, Appleton & Lange, 1987, with permission.)*

time failed to show any benefit of "prophylactic" antibiotics administered *after* the operation. In 1969 Polk and Lopez-Mayor[16] reported one of the first studies to demonstrate that a preoperatively administered antimicrobial (cephaloridine) could reduce the rate of postoperative wound infection after gastrointestinal operations. In a later trial, Stone et al[17] studied cefazolin administered in conjunction with gastric, biliary, or colonic operations. For each procedure there were four groups of patients. Three groups received three doses of cefazolin at varying times while one group received only placebo. For the groups receiving antimicrobials, the doses were administered either (1) as two preoperative and one postoperative dose, (2) as one preoperative and two postoperative doses, or (3) as three postoperative doses. The two groups that received preoperative cefazolin had postoperative infection rates significantly lower than those of the group that received no cefazolin, with no significant difference between one and two preoperative doses. Furthermore, the group that received only postoperative cefazolin had infection rates similar to those of the group that received no cefazolin. This trial substantiated Miles' finding in animal studies that antimicrobials introduced after bacterial contamination are of no benefit in preventing postoperative infection.

### *Duration of Antimicrobial Prophylaxis*

The appropriate duration of postoperative prophylactic antimicrobial use is often debated. A decade ago it was common for antimicrobials to be administered up to 10 days after an operation for the purpose of preventing infection. Now, most surgeons prefer to use antimicrobials no longer than 24 hours after an operation and some do not use any postoperative antimicrobials. The shortest duration of antimicrobial administration that will be effective in preventing postoperative infection is not absolutely known; however, recent studies document that *postoperative* antimicrobial administration is usually not necessary.

Very few studies have compared the effectiveness of antimicrobial regimens of varying duration. Of those that have, all concluded that regimens continuing less than 24 hours after an operation are as effective as those continuing up to 5 days.[18–21] In addition, a number of placebo-controlled studies have been published where patients received only preoperative antimicrobial agents. In all of these studies, involving biliary tract operations, appendectomies, colorectal operations, cesarean sections, and vaginal hysterectomies, single doses were judged to be effective for prophylaxis.[22]

A few new cephalosporins (cefonicid, cefotaxime, ceftriaxone, and cefotetan) have demonstrated benefits for surgical prophylaxis when administered in a single preoperative dose. The long duration of action of some agents and the potent antimicrobial effects of others are believed to allow this single dose to be effective. Clinicians should recognize, however, that older cephalosporins, when studied in single-dose regimens, have shown similar benefits in preventing postoperative infection. In fact, cefazolin is effective in a single preoperative dose for most operations. For long procedures (over 4 hours), a second dose of antimicrobial should be administered intraoperatively, if cephalosporins with short half-lives (cephalothin, cephapirin, cefamandole, cefoxitin) are used.

### *Route of Antimicrobial Administration*

Antimicrobials used for surgical prophylaxis have been administered intravenously, intramuscularly, orally, rectally, and topically (into the surgical wound). The preference for route of administration varies among surgeons, with intravenous and intramuscular administration used most often. Oral antimicrobials (neomycin sulfate and erythromycin base) are used for elective colorectal operations.

For most elective operations, intramuscular administration and intravenous administration are equivalent in terms of antimicrobial delivery to wound tissues. Intramuscular administration results in peak serum and tissue antimicrobial concentrations that can occur as much as 30 to 60 minutes later with intravenous infusion but obviously is more painful. Also, in patients with poor muscle perfusion or in morbidly obese patients, adequate drug absorption may be significantly delayed after intramuscular injection. The antimicrobial agent should be given intravenously if the patient has an intravenous catheter in place. Alternatively, it is reasonable to wait to administer the agent until an intravenous line is placed in the operating room.

Generally, orally administered antimicrobial agents are not recommended for surgical prophylaxis. In situations where general anesthesia will interrupt bowel function, or where nasogastric tubes may be placed, the absorption of orally administered antimicrobials will be unreliable. One situation in which oral antimicrobial agents are routinely used for prophylaxis is colorectal surgery, where the antimicrobials are given the day before surgery with the intended effects being limited to the lumen of the gastrointestinal tract.

Oral antimicrobials have often been used[13] to decrease bacterial counts in the bowel. Many oral antimicrobial regimens have been found to decrease wound infection rates after colorectal surgery, including (1) neomycin sulfate with erythromycin base, (2) kanamycin sulfate with erythromycin base, (3) neomycin sulfate with metronidazole, (4) metronidazole alone, and (5) doxycycline.

Most often, neomycin sulfate with erythromycin base is used. Neomycin sulfate effectively decreases the concentrations of intestinal aerobes and erythromycin base decreases the concentrations of anaerobes.[23] One gram of each agent should be administered 19, 18, and 9 hours prior to the start of the operation. The high-dose, short-duration regimen produces a maximum effect on the fecal flora in a period of time sufficiently short to hinder the development of resistance.

More important for elective colorectal operations than oral antimicrobials, however, is the use of preoperative mechanical bowel preparation. The value of mechanical preparation of the colon (with vigorous use of cathartics, whole-bowel irrigation, and/or enemas) before elective colon surgery is well established. Up to one third the weight of feces may be bacteria; therefore, it is desirable to reduce the numbers of intraluminal bacteria, as they pose a significant threat of infection.

The combination of parenteral antimicrobials with oral agents in elective colorectal operations is controversial. Condon and associates[24] have demonstrated that parenteral cephalothin was of no added benefit when added to an oral regimen of neomycin sulfate and erythromycin base. In another study by Coppa and associates,[25] the addition of cefoxitin to the standard neomycin/erythromycin oral regimen significantly reduced postoperative infection rates. In our institution, parenteral and oral antimicrobials are combined for elective colorectal operations, as contact of oral antimicrobials with all segments of the involved area cannot be assured by use of the oral agents alone.

Many investigators have examined the use of topical antimicrobials for surgical prophylaxis. A wide variety of agents have been mixed with sterile normal saline or sterile water and poured directly into the surgical wound. At present the use of topical antimicrobials remains controversial.[26] In most studies in which topical agents have been used, they have been shown to be as valuable as parenteral agents and more effective than placebo. Other trials have demonstrated that topical agents provide no added benefit when given with parenteral agents.

The advantages of using topically applied antimicrobials are that the surgeon can control the exact time and site of application, and the resulting wound antimicrobial concentrations are very high. Potential disadvantages of topical antimicrobials are that additional maneuvers are required in the surgical procedure, antimicrobials delivered in this manner may have a relatively short duration of activity, and application potentially occurs after bacterial contamination of the wound tissue. Any area with adequate blood supply is likely to be reached by parenterally administered antimicrobials; this is not necessarily true for topically administered agents. In most institutions, topical antimicrobials are generally not applied to surgical wounds.

### *Selection of Antimicrobial Agents*

The selection of antimicrobial agents for surgical prophylaxis is certainly a controversial area as the concern for patient recovery and antimicrobial costs mix and result in many differing opinions. Also, promotion from pharmaceutical manufacturers suggests that there are benefits to adopting new antimicrobials for surgical prophylaxis. To date, there is little evidence to suggest that newer antimicrobials with broader in vitro antibacterial spectra result in a lower rate of postoperative wound infection when compared with older, less active agents.[27]

Generally, the agent chosen should have good antibacterial activity against the most common surgical wound pathogens. For clean–contaminated operations this includes common pathogens found in the gastrointestinal or genitourinary tracts (e.g., *E. coli, Klebsiella, Bacteroides fragilis*). For clean operations gram-positive cocci (staphylococci and streptococci) predominate.

To date over 50 studies in which different parenteral antimicrobial regimens are compared in a controlled fashion have appeared in the literature. In almost every report, no significant differences are demonstrated between agents, possibly because the patient populations are too small. This has also been observed for those studies focusing on cephalosporins.[25] Second- and third-generation cephalosporins have not demonstrated lower postoperative infection rates than have been achieved with first-generation cephalosporins. So, where parenteral cephalosporins are recommended for surgical prophylaxis, an inexpensive, first-generation agent will suffice.[27]

The authors acknowledge that some clinicians have concern for the use of antimicrobials with poor coverage against *B. fragilis* in situations such as colorectal surgery or obstetric/gynecologic surgery where this organism is a potential pathogen. First-generation cephalosporins are relatively inactive against *B. fragilis*, while cefoxitin, cefotetan, and ceftizoxime are very active. Although the advantages of these agents over first-generation cephalosporins, such as cefazolin, are not established, it would be reasonable at present to use any of these agents, particularly when oral neomycin sulfate and erythromycin base are used in conjunction.

The pharmacokinetic properties of antimicrobials used for surgical prophylaxis may be important in selection of an agent.[28] These properties, particularly half-life, determine the presence or absence of the agent at the time bacteria enter the tissue and throughout the length of the procedure. Agents with very short half-lives have a short duration of action, and therefore, if given in a single preoperative dose, may not be present throughout an operation. This would be true for first-generation cephalosporins such as cephalothin, cephapirin, or cephradine and second-generation cephalosporins such as cefamandole, cefuroxime, and cefoxitin. Single doses of longer acting agents, such as cefazolin, cefotetan, cefonicid, and ceforanide, are likely to provide serum antimicrobial activity for the duration of most procedures.

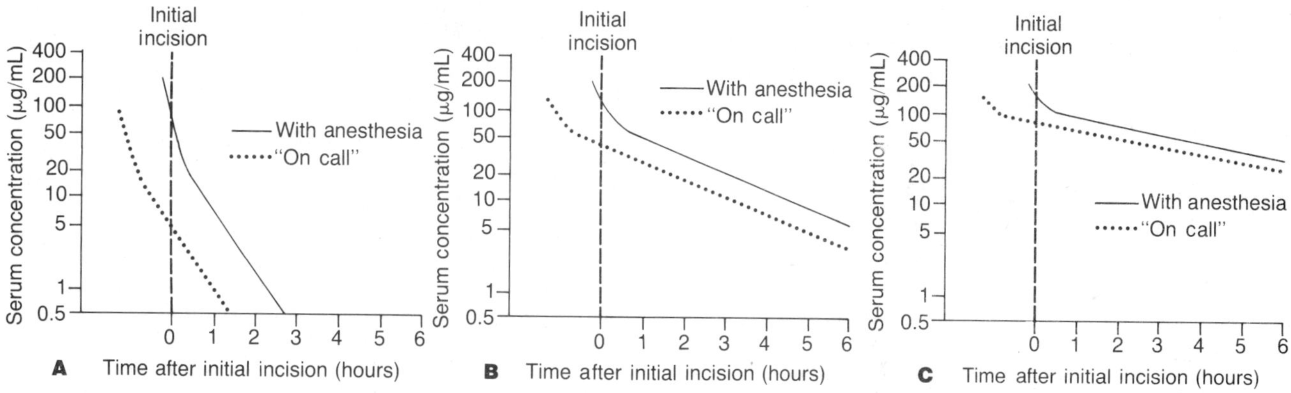


**Figure 89.2** Serum concentrations of cephalosporins administered either "on call" to operating room (30-minute infusion) or at the time of anesthesia induction (5-minute infusion). (A) Cephalothin; dose = 2 g. (B) Cefazolin; dose = 1 g. (C) Cefonicid; dose = 1 g. *(From Nix DE, et al: South Med J 1985;78:962–6, with permission.)*

The relative influence of pharmacokinetic properties of cephalosporins on intraoperative serum concentration can be seen in Figure 89.2. Agents with short half-lives should be administered at the time that anesthesia is induced. Longer acting agents, including cefazolin, may be administered "on call" to surgery, which is generally about 1 hour before initial incision. If short-acting agents are administered, they should be readministered if the operation extends beyond 3 to 4 hours. If an operation is expected to last over 6 or 8 hours then it would be reasonable to administer a cephalosporin with very long duration of action, such as cefonicid or cefotetan.

Specific recommendations for the selection of prophylactic antimicrobials are provided in Table 89.6 for various surgical procedures. A first-generation cephalosporin, cefazolin, is most often recommended because of its relatively low cost and long duration of action and because it has activity against most common pathogens in clean and clean–contaminated operations. For clean operations where staphylococci are common pathogens, penicillinase-resistant penicillins (oxacillin, naficillin) may be suitable alternatives. Vancomycin may sometimes be required in penicillin/cephalosporin–allergic patients.

### *Unintended Effects of Prophylactic Antimicrobials*

The decision to use prophylactic antimicrobials should be taken with the knowledge that some risk accompanies their potential benefit. In some situations the risk of their use outweighs the benefit. With the use of prophylactic antimicrobials, there is risk not only to the individual patient for the occurrence of adverse reactions or superinfections, but also to the hospitalized population as a whole with the potential for development of bacterial resistance.

Adverse effects do not commonly result from prophylactic antimicrobial administration; however, if these agents are used in operations with a very low rate of infection, the rate of adverse effects may exceed the rate of infection. Most commonly, hypersensitivity reactions result from antimicrobial use; however, more serious reactions, such as pseudomembranous colitis, have been reported.[29]

The routine use of prophylactic antimicrobials may increase the selection pressure for resistant strains of bacteria. Archer and associates[30] have shown that in cardiothoracic surgery patients, the isolation of methicillin-resistant coagulase-negative staphylococci occurs much more frequently after cardiac surgery with exposure to prophylactic antimicrobials than in patients preoperatively. The full extent of this problem is not well appreciated. Because of the threat of development of resistance it is reasonable not to routinely use agents for prophylaxis that are commonly used to treat infections in seriously ill patients (e.g., third-generation cephalosporins or parenteral aminoglycosides).

## Summary

Postoperative wound infections continue to be a common occurrence. The rate of postoperative wound infection is influenced by many factors including the type of operation, the surgical techniques used, and the underlying host resistance of the patient. For some operations, mostly clean–contaminated procedures, administration of prophylactic antimicrobials decreases the rate of wound infection.

The use of prophylactic antimicrobials in surgery should conform to specific guidelines:

1. Antimicrobials should be used in operations in which postoperative infections occur frequently or in which infections occur infrequently but result in significant morbidity or mortality.
2. The agents used should be relatively safe, should have activity against common wound pathogens, and should not be the agents routinely used to treat serious infections. In general, older, less expensive agents such as first-generation cephalosporins are adequate.
3. The agent should be administered preoperatively, close enough to the operation so that the antimicrobial will be present in serum and wound tissue during the operation. If short-acting antimicrobials are used for long operations then intraoperative doses should be given.
4. Postoperative antimicrobial administration is not required unless sources of continued bacterial seeding are present.
5. Antimicrobials should be given intravenously or intramuscularly, except for oral neomycin and erythromycin used for elective colorectal operations.

**Table 89.6** Recommendations for Surgical Prophylaxis

| *Procedure* | *High-risk groups* | *Recommended regimen*[a] | *Comments* |
|---|---|---|---|
| Gastroduodenal | Gastric ulcer or carcinoma<br>Impaired gastric motility or acid secretion | 1 | Routine use for duodenal ulcer not recommended |
| Biliary tract | Age 70 years<br>Biliary obstruction<br>Common bile duct stone<br>Acute cholecystitis | 1 or 2 | Recommended where bacteria are likely to be present in the bile tract |
| Appendectomy | Perforated or gangrenous appendix | 3 | High-risk patients may require 5- to 10-day treatment course |
| Colorectal | Emergency operations<br>Colonic obstruction | 4 for nonemergency procedures<br>Possibly add 1 or 3 | All colorectal operations are at relatively high risk of infection; with obstruction, fistulas or emergency operations or where there are discontinuous segments of bowel, use of parenteral agents is justified |
| Vaginal hysterectomy | Premenopausal | 1 | Recommended in all cases |
| Abdominal hysterectomy | None well identified | 1 | Prophylaxis not routinely recommended |
| Cesarean section | Primary cesarean section, labor, or premature rupture of membranes | 1 | Recommended in all high-risk patients but not routinely for elective repeat cesarean sections; antimicrobial may be given after umbilical cord clamping |
| Neurosurgery | Microneurosurgical procedures over 6 hours<br>Shunts placed | 1 | Prophylaxis not routinely recommended |
| Vascular (peripheral) | Aortic resections<br>Prosthetic material used<br>Anastomotic site in groin | 1 | Not recommended for brachial or carotid procedures |
| Thoracic (noncardiac) | Pulmonary resection or transection of the bronchial tree | 1 | Not recommended in thoracotomy without lung resection |
| Cardiac | Open-heart procedures<br>Cardiopulmonary bypass | 1 | Continue regimen if source of contamination persists |
| Orthopedic | Total hip replacement<br>Prosthetic material used<br>Hip fracture repair | 1 | Not recommended routinely for other clean procedures |
| Head and neck | Resection of oropharyngeal or laryngeal carcinoma | 1 | Not recommended for otologic or nasopharyngeal procedures |

[a] 1. Cefazolin 1 g IM or IV 0.5 to 1 hour preoperatively or IV with induction of anesthesia. For operations lasting over 6 hours a second intraoperative dose should be given.
2. Ampicillin 1 g IV with induction of anesthesia. Readminister if operation exceeds 4 hours.
3. Cefoxitin 2 g IV with induction of anesthesia. Readminister every 3 hours intraoperatively.
4. Neomycin sulfate and erythromycin base: 1 g each PO 19, 18, and 9 hours prior to scheduled operation (preceded by mechanical bowel preparation).

## References


1. Altemeier WA, Burke JF, Pruitt BA, Sandusky WR (eds): Manual on Control of Infections in Surgical Patients, 2nd ed. Philadelphia, J.B. Lippincott, 1984.
2. Jarvis WR, White JW, Munn VP, et al. Nosocomial infection surveillance, 1983. MMWR Surveillance Summaries 1984;33: 955–2155.
3. Conte JE, Jacob LS, Polk HC. Antibiotic Prophylaxis in Surgery. Philadelphia, J.B. Lippincott, 1984.

4. Polk HC. Prevention of surgical wound infection. Ann Intern Med 1978;89:770–773.
5. Farber BF, Wenzel RP. Postoperative wound infection rates: Results of prospective statewide surveillance. Am J Surg 1980;140:343–346.
6. Barker WF, Longmire W, Altemeier WA. Postoperative wound infections: the influence of ultraviolet irradiation of the operating room and of various other factors. Ann Surg 1964;160 (suppl):1–192.
7. Centers for Disease Control. National Nosocomial Infections Study Report: Annual Summary. Atlanta, Centers for Disease Control, November, 1979.
8. Altemeier WA, Culbertson WR. Surgical infection, in Moyer C, et al (eds): Surgery, Principles and Practice, 3rd ed. Philadelphia, J.B. Lippincott, 1965.
9. Cruse PE, Foord R. The epidemiology of wound infection: A 10-year prospective study of 62,939 wounds. Surg Clin North Am 1980;60:27–40.
10. Mead PB, Pories SE, Hall P, et al. Decreasing the incidence of surgical wound infections. Arch Surg 1986;121:458–461.
11. Polk HC, Simpson CJ, Simmons BP, et al. Guidelines for prevention of surgical wound infections. Arch Surg 1983;118:1213–1217.
12. Hill C, Mazas F, Flamant R, et al. Prophylactic cefazolin versus placebo in total hip replacement. Lancet 1981;1:795–797.
13. DiPiro JT, Bivins BA, Record KE, et al. The prophylactic use of antimicrobials in surgery. Curr Probl Surg 1983;20:69–132.
14. Miles AA, Miles EM, Burke J. The valve and duration of defense reactions of the skin to the primary lodgement of bacteria. Br J Exp Pathol 1957;38:79–96.
15. Burke JF. The effective period of preventive antibiotic action in experimental incisions and dermal lesions. Surgery 1961;50: 161–168.
16. Polk HC, Lopez-Mayor JF. Postoperative wound infection: A prospective study of determinant factors and prevention. Surgery 1969;66:97–103.
17. Stone HH, Hooper CA, Kolb LA, et al. Antibiotic prophylaxis in gastric, biliary and colonic surgery. Am J Surg 1979;138: 640–643.
18. Strachan CJS, Black J, Powis SJA, et al. Prophylactic use of cefazolin against wound sepsis after cholecystectomy. Br Med J 1977;1:1254–1256.
19. Giercksky KE, Danielson S, Garberg O, et al. A single dose tinidazole and doxycycline prophylaxis in elective surgery of the colon and rectum. Ann Surg 1982;195:227–231.
20. Stone HH, Haney BB, Kolb LD, et al. Prophylactic and preventive antibiotic therapy. Ann Surg 1979;189:691–699.
21. Downing R, McLeish AR, Burdon DW, et al. Duration of systemic prophylactic antibiotic cover against anaerobic sepsis in intestinal surgery. Dis Colon Rectum 1977;20:401–404.
22. DiPiro JT, Cheung RPF, Bowden TA, et al. Single dose systemic antibiotic prophylaxis of surgical wound infections. Am J Surg 1986;152:552–559.
23. Bartlett JG, Condon RE, Gorbach SL, et al. Veterans Administration cooperative study on bowel preparation for elective colorectal operations. Ann Surg 1978;188:249–254.
24. Condon RE, Bartlett JG, Nichols RL, et al. Preoperative prophylactic cephalothin fails to control septic complications of colorectal operations: Results of a controlled clinical trial. Am J Surg 1979;137:68–74.
25. Coppa GF, Eng K, Gouge TH, et al. Parenteral and oral antibiotics in elective colon and rectal surgery. Am J Surg 1983;145:62–65.
26. Roth RM, Gleckman RA, Gantz NM, et al. Antibiotic irrigations: A plea for controlled clinical trials. Pharmacotherapy 1985;5:222–227.
27. DiPiro JT, Bowden TA, Hooks VH. Cephalosporins for prevention of surgical infection: Are the newer agents better? JAMA 1985;252:3277–3279.
28. Nix DA, DiPiro JT, Bowden TA, et al. Cephalosporins for surgical prophylaxis: computer projections of intraoperative availability. South Med J 1985;78:962–966.
29. Block BS, Mercer LJ, Ismail MA, et al. *Clostridium difficile*–associated diarrhea follows perioperative prophylaxis with cefoxitin. Am J Obstet Gynecol 1985;153:835–838.
30. Archer GL, Armstrong BC. Alterations of staphylococcal flora in cardiac surgery patients receiving antibiotic prophylaxis. J Infect Dis 1983;147:642–649.

# Chapter 90 / Vaccines, Toxoids, and Other Immunobiologics

Joseph S. Bertino, Jr, PharmD, and Linda A. Chiarello, BS, RN, CIC

The discovery and introduction of vaccines, toxoids, and immunoglobulins have resulted in significant declines in worldwide morbidity and mortality from their respective diseases. In addition, they have been shown to be generally safe and cost effective.[1,2] This chapter is aimed at introducing the reader to three groups of agents: vaccines, toxoids, and immune sera. These groups are defined and related agents dealt with concurrently in an attempt to illustrate total immunotherapy. Obscure agents have been eliminated from discussion in the interest of brevity.

## Principles of Immunization

Vaccines and toxoids are separate and distinct products. Both types of products, however, act to induce active immunity, that is, immunity generated by a natural immunologic response to an antigen. Vaccines are derived from the infecting organism itself. Viral vaccines can be either live attenuated or killed. Killed viral vaccines may consist of whole or split viral particles or specific viral fragments (subunits) as in the case of hepatitis B vaccine. Bacterial vaccines are generally killed whole bacteria or specific bacterial wall antigens. Live attenuated vaccines induce an immunologic response more consistent with that occurring with natural infection. As the organisms in live attenuated vaccines multiply in the body after injection, they normally confer lifelong immunity with one dose (as does a primary natural infection). Killed vaccines, on the other hand, do not induce permanent immunity and require additional doses at varying time intervals.

Toxoids are inactivated bacterial toxins that are generally combined with aluminum salts (i.e., alum) to enhance their antigenicity by prolonging antigen absorption. These adjuvants also increase local tissue irritation when injected.

Immune sera are sterile solutions containing antibody derived from human or equine sources. These sera are indicated for induction of passive immunity (temporary immunity to infection as a result of the administration of antibodies not produced by the host). Human immune serum is preferred because of the lower incidence of serum sickness and other allergic reactions as compared with equine (horse) derived sera (see Other Immunobiologics).

In general, vaccines and toxoids must be kept refrigerated as breaking the "cold chain" results in loss of potency. Certain vaccines such as measles–mumps–rubella (MMR) may also be frozen. Immune sera generally should be kept refrigerated and not frozen except for lyophilized intravenous human immune globulin which can be stored at room temperature.

Various factors are known to affect response to vaccines and toxoids. Viability of the antigen is an important factor (i.e., live attenuated versus killed) as previously discussed. Total dose is also important, as there seems to exist a threshold dose above which no further increase in antibody titer is seen.[3] The route and site of administration are also important. This is best illustrated by the hepatitis B vaccine, which elicits a satisfactory antibody response when injected into the deltoid muscle but not consistently when administered in the gluteal area.[4]

The age of the recipient is another important determining factor in vaccine/toxoid response. In the first few months of life, passive immunity (temporary immunity to infection as a result of the acquisition of antibodies via maternal–fetal passage) acquired from the mother both protects an infant and prevents adequate vaccine/toxoid response to certain agents. At the other end of the spectrum, response to antigens may be blunted in the elderly individual, requiring larger and/or more frequent doses.

Vaccines in general are very stable, with the exception of live attenuated viral vaccines, which are sensitive to heat and light and must be stored and handled properly. While some vaccines may be stored below 0°C, toxoids in general tend to aggregate upon freezing, leading to increased adverse local effects.

Vaccine administration is via intramuscular, subcutaneous, or intradermal injection, oral administration, or intranasal application. In general, for intramuscular injection in adults, the deltoid and not the gluteus muscle should be used. Dosages should be administered as directed with no dosage reductions recommended.

Questions often arise concerning the simultaneous administration of vaccines. In general, inactivated vaccines can be simultaneously administered at separate sites, while simultaneous administration of live attenuated vaccines should be avoided if possible unless specified (i.e., measles, mumps, and rubella). The data on simultaneous administration of live attenuated viral vaccines should be prefaced with the knowledge that simultaneous administration of these vaccines has been performed with no resultant decrease in immunity to any of the agents used, when compared with single-vaccine administration alone. Live attenuated and killed vaccines may be simultaneously administered at separate sites.

The simultaneous administration of immune globulin (general or disease specific) and live attenuated vaccines (but not inactivated vaccines) may inhibit host antibody response because of impairment of viral replication. The general guidelines are that parenterally administered live vaccines should not be given for at least 6 weeks, and preferably 3 months, after immune globulin administration. These points are discussed further in separate sections.

Pregnant women present a particularly difficult problem in deciding on vaccination. In general, administration of live attenuated vaccines should *not be* done during pregnancy, and inactivated vaccines should not be given until the second trimester (however, inactivated vaccines have not been shown to be teratogenic during the first trimester).[5,6]

While all women of childbearing age should be immunized to poliomyelitis, measles, mumps, rubella, tetanus, and diphtheria, those who are not and become pregnant should be immunized to the latter two agents during pregnancy, and to the others postpartum.

Vaccination in compromised hosts (i.e., those with chronic disease such as diabetes, those with connective tissue disease, alcoholics, or those with cancer) must be individualized based on the disease state and its treatment. Patients with chronic pulmonary, renal, hepatic, or metabolic disease who are not receiving immunosuppressants may be administered both live attenuated and killed vaccines and toxoids to induce active immunity. Those patients with active malignant disease may receive killed vaccines or toxoids but should not be given live vaccines. Those patients with solid tumors (even in the presence of cachexia) will usually have a normal response to killed vaccines and toxoids as will those patients with acute leukemias and lymphomas. Patients with multiple myeloma will in general have a lesser response to killed vaccines. Those individuals receiving chemotherapy, radiotherapy, corticosteroids, or a combination of these should not receive live attenuated vaccines. While killed vaccines may be administered to these patients, the impairment in response depends on the type of therapy. Impairment of response may last for years and necessitate revaccination.

The response to vaccines is often measured in terms of antibody levels. While for diseases such as measles, rubella, and influenza, the presence of sufficient antibody correlates with immunity, other vaccines/toxoids do not have such correlation, and success or failure must be assessed on the basis of clinical results.[7,8]

Finally, adverse reactions to vaccines/toxoids are extremely variable. Mild reactions such as fever, malaise, chills, and local injection site tenderness are not uncommon. Other more serious reactions, including Guillain–Barré syndrome, have shown a temporal relationship to certain vaccines. Overall, however, vaccines/toxoids have respectable safety records.

## Use of Vaccines and Toxoids

The recommended schedules for routine immunization of children and adults are shown in Appendixes 90.1 and 90.2. Children should be fully immunized before 6 years of age. This is a legal requirement in many states. Adults should be fully immunized against diphtheria, tetanus, measles, mumps, and rubella. If this is not the case, a complete series of immunizations should be given. Certain high-risk individuals should be vaccinated against other agents as outlined in Appendix 90.2.

## Toxoids and Their Immunobiologics

### *Diphtheria Toxoid Adsorbed and Diphtheria Antitoxin*

Diphtheria toxoid adsorbed (DTA) is a sterile suspension of toxoids of *Corynebacterium diphtheriae*, which induce immunity against the exotoxin of *C. diphtheriae*. The use of diphtheria toxoid adsorbed (DTA) has essentially eliminated diphtheria from the United States.

Primary immunization with DTA is indicated for children over 6 weeks of age.[1] The usual dose is 0.5 mL intramuscularly at rotating sites. Generally, DTA is given with pertussis and tetanus vaccines at 2, 4, and 6–12 months of age. Additional doses are given at 18 months and 4–6 years. Three doses of DTA induce immunity in 90% of persons for at least 10 years. Booster doses of DTA should be given every 10 years. Immunization prior to 6 weeks of age should not be given because of the possible inhibiting effect of maternal antibodies. If primary immunization is given to an immunosuppressed patient, an additional dose of DTA should be administered 1 month after the return to normal immune status. DTA may be administered to persons with mild febrile illnesses and with other live or killed vaccines.[9]

Adverse effects of DTA include mild to moderate tenderness, erythema, and induration at the injection site. Rarely do systemic reactions occur.[10]

Diphtheria antitoxin (DA) is a sterile antitoxin derived from hyperimmunized horses. It should be stored at 2–8°C but may be frozen.

Diphtheria antitoxin is indicated for immediate use in patients with diphtheria. It is rarely indicated for diphtheria prophylaxis. DA is given intramuscularly or intravenously in a dosage related to the site and size of the diphtheric membrane, degree of toxicity, and duration of illness. The usual doses are 20,000–40,000 units for pharyngeal disease, 40,000–60,000 units for nasopharyngeal lesions, and 80,000–120,000 units for extensive disease of 3 or more days. When given intravenously, the dose should be diluted 1:20 in 0.9% saline or 5% dextrose in water and infused at 1 mL/min after being warmed to 32–34°C.

Adverse reactions to DA include anaphylactic reactions in 7% of patients and/or serum sickness occurring 12 days postadministration. Serum sickness may be accelerated (7–12 days) in persons previously sensitized. Fortunately, the widespread use of diphtheria toxoid adsorbed vaccine has greatly reduced the incidence of the disease and thus the use of DA.

### *Tetanus Toxoid, Tetanus Toxoid Adsorbed, and Tetanus Immune Globulin*

Tetanus toxoid (TT) and tetanus toxoid adsorbed (TTA) (adsorbed onto aluminum hydroxide, phosphate, or potassium sulfate to increase antigenicity) are sterile suspensions of the toxoid from *Clostridium tetani*.

Both toxoids are used to promote immunization against tetanus; however, TTA is the preferred agent. While single doses in a nonimmunized individual do not produce sufficient antibody response, three 0.5-mL doses of TTA or four doses of TT produce protection in 90% of vaccinees over 6 weeks of age. Additional doses of TTA are recommended as

**Table 90.1** Summary Guide to Tetanus Prophylaxis in Routine Wound Management[a]

| History of tetanus immunization | Clean minor wounds | | All other wounds | |
|---|---|---|---|---|
| | Td[a] | TIG | Td[a] | TIG |
| Uncertain | Yes | No | Yes | Yes |
| 0–1 dose | Yes | No | Yes | Yes |
| 2 doses | Yes | No | Yes | No[b] |
| 3 or more doses | No[c] | No | No[d] | No |

[a] For persons age 7 and older, combined tetanus–diphtheria (Td) toxoid is preferred to tetanus toxoid alone.
[b] Yes, if wound is more than 24 hours old.
[c] Yes, if more than 10 years has passed since the last dose.
[d] Yes, if more than 5 years has passed since the last dose. More frequent boosters are not needed and can accentuate side effects.

Data from Reference 9.

part of traumatic wound management. These recommendations are summarized in Table 90.1. In certain situations (see Table 90.1), tetanus immune globulin (TIG) should also be given. TIG should be used with TTA.

In children, primary immunization against tetanus is usually done in conjunction with diphtheria and pertussis vaccination. The trivalent vaccine DPT (diphtheria–pertussis–tetanus), containing TTA, is given intramuscularly at a dose of 0.5 mL at 2, 4, 6, and 18 months of age.[9,11] In adults or children where primary immunization against tetanus alone is needed, a series of three 0.5-mL doses of TTA are administered intramuscularly initially, followed by repeat doses at 4–8 weeks and 6–12 months. Boosters are recommended every 10 years. TT and TTA should not be routinely given to immunosuppressed patients. If they are, one additional dose should be given 1 month after stopping the immunosuppressive agent. TT or TTA may be simultaneously given with other killed and live vaccines.

Adverse reactions to TT and TTA include mild to moderate local reactions at the injection site such as warmth, erythema, and induration. Rarely, fever, malaise, aches, and pains or neurologic disorders have been reported. In general, major local reactions occur within 2–8 hours after administration to patients with high serum tetanus antitoxin levels. While safe use during pregnancy has not been definitely established, TT and TTA have been administered to pregnant women in the prevention of neonatal tetanus.

TIG is a sterile, concentrated, nonpyrogenic solution of immunoglobulins prepared from hyperimmunized humans. TIG is used to provide passive tetanus immunization after traumatic wounds in nonimmunized or suboptimally immunized persons (see Table 90.1) and is preferred over tetanus antitoxin. A dose of 250–500 units should be administered intramuscularly. TIG is also used for the treatment of tetanus. In this setting a single dose of 3,000–6,000 units is administered intramuscularly.

Adverse effects of TIG include pain, tenderness, erythema, and muscle stiffness at the injection site which may persist for several hours. Rarely do systemic reactions occur. Intravenous administration has been associated with severe adverse reactions and is not recommended.

## Vaccines and Their Immunobiologics

### *B-CAPSA I Vaccine* (Hemophilus influenzae *Vaccine*)

B-CAPSA I vaccine is a polysaccharide agent designed to protect against *Hemophilus influenzae* type B disease (HIB). Ten to twenty thousand cases of HIB meningitis occur yearly in children under the age of 5, with 5% to 10% mortality and 2% to 40% neurologic morbidity. The vaccine was developed primarily for this target population.

A single 0.5-mL dose of vaccine is indicated for all children between 24 months and 6 years (or 18 months if at high risk).[12,13] While the vaccine does induce antibody in children less than 24 months of age, 78% show a decline below the protective level of 1 μg/mL over the ensuing 18 months.[14,15] Widespread immunization of children in the United States is expected to prevent 40% of HIB disease if given at 18 months of age and confers protection on 90% of children immunized at 24 months of age or older. Children vaccinated before 24 months of age should receive an additional 0.5-mL dose 18 months later. Repeat doses of B-CAPSA I vaccine do not produce the T-cell memory and booster effect, but do raise antibody levels significantly. DPT and B-CAPSA I vaccines may be given simultaneously at different sites. B-CAPSA I vaccine when combined with diphtheria toxoid produces a heat-stable vaccine that is immunologically superior to B-CAPSA I alone.[16] This combination vaccine is currently available.

High-risk groups for HIB include children at day-care centers, those with anatomic or functional asplenia, and immunosuppressed children. While few data exist documenting HIB vaccine efficacy in asplenic or immunosuppressed patients, the vaccine is recommended for these individuals. Additionally, the vaccine has been suggested for use in high-risk adults; however, data to support this are sparse. In summary, current recommendations are for universal vaccination of children at 24 months, with vaccination for those high-risk patients at 18 months along with an additional dose at 36 months. Vaccination of low-risk children before 18 months is currently not recommended.[12,13]

Adverse reactions to HIB vaccine are uncommon. Fever, erythema, and induration at the injection site occur in approximately 2% of children and resolve within 24 hours.[17] Anaphylaxis has been reported rarely.

### *Bacillus Calmette–Guérin Vaccine*

BCG vaccine is derived from a live attenuated strain of *Mycobacterium bovis*, and is used for vaccination against tuberculosis. While the use of the vaccine has been shown to result in a positive tuberculin skin test in the majority of recipients, field trails in India have led to doubts concerning its efficacy.[5,18] The vaccine is considered to be approximately 50% to 77% effective over a 10- to 20-year period in some populations.[19,20] No data are available as to the total duration of protection, however.

As the incidence of tuberculosis in the United States is low, the indications for this vaccine are few. The vaccine is recommended for (1) health care workers with an annual attack rate of greater than 1% in the face of other tuberculosis control measures, (2) groups with an excessive new infection rate in whom surveillance and treatment cannot be accomplished or have failed, and (3) individuals in close contact with infected patients who have been ineffectually treated.

Within 6 weeks of vaccine administration (either before or after vaccination), a negative Mantoux skin test should be assured. It is difficult to distinguish active disease from vaccine effect in patients with positive skin tests who have received BCG; thus, any patient with a positive PPD should be considered to have active infection unless previously negative.

The vaccine is administered in a dose of 0.1 mL for patients over 1 month of age, and 0.05 mL for those children less than 1 month of age. The vaccine may be administered either intradermally or percutaneously using a bifurcated needle. When it is administered percutaneously, 0.1 mL of the vaccine is placed on the skin and then at least 20 punctures are made to administer the agent. In neonates (less than 1 month of age), if the 0.05-mL dose does not produce a positive PPD and if still indicated, an additional 0.1-mL dose should be administered after 1 year of age. Repeat vaccination is not recommended and does not seem to be guided by the use of skin tests.

After correct intradermal or percutaneous vaccination, a small red papule should appear within 7–10 days. This lesion may reach 8 mm in size within 5 weeks. Within the next 6 months, the lesion should ulcerate and scar.

The agent is contraindicated in immunosuppressed individuals regardless of the cause as it is a live vaccine. The vaccine should not be given to burn patients, patients with new smallpox vaccines, or patients on isoniazid because of inhibition of bacterial replication. The use of the vaccine in pregnant women is discouraged unless there is an excessive risk of exposure. Even then, the vaccine should not be used in the first trimester.

Adverse effects to BCG vaccine have been noted with varying frequencies. Excessive skin ulceration, disseminated *M. bovis* infection, and generalized adenitis have been reported, but for the most part are unusual. Disseminated infection occurs in 1–10 per million doses. Localized or limited adenitis and ulceration may occur in 1% to 10% of patients receiving the vaccine. These effects probably occur in patients who have previously received the vaccine and are transient. Late-onset adverse reactions are usually in the form of granulomas, which may occur 4–6 weeks after injection. These granulomas may persist for months and often go on to form keloid scars.

While the major use of BCG vaccine has been as immunoprophylaxis of tuberculosis, other uses of the agent in neoplastic disease have been studied. In these circumstances, the agent has been used in various dosages and routes of administration. Specific protocols are generally followed. This form of immunotherapy in neoplastic disease has been met with limited success.

### *Hepatitis B Vaccine*

In 1981, a safe, immunogenic vaccine for the prevention of hepatitis B was licensed. The hepatitis B vaccine (Heptavax) is derived from plasma of carefully screened and monitored human, high-titer hepatitis B carriers/donors. The vaccine consists of inactivated hepatitis B surface antigen (HBsAg) subunit particles which are collected by double ultracentrifugation and subjected to a complex inactivation process, including pepsin digestion at pH 2, 8 M urea and formalin treatment which renders the product noninfectious for all known bacteria and viruses, including human immunodeficiency virus.The vaccine induces only hepatitis B surface antibody in recipients.[21] In 1986 a recombinant strain of hepatitis B vaccine (Recombivax) was introduced in the United States. It has been proven as effective as the human-derived vaccine and is expected eventually to be the sole vaccine of this type available. The information presented here pertains to either form.

Clinical trials in healthy individuals have demonstrated antibody conversion rates of 90% after completion of the three-dose series and a protective effect in vaccinees subsequently exposed to hepatitis B virus (HBV).[21] A normal immune response has also been seen in patients with Down's syndrome.[22] Response rates in hemodialysis and immunocompromised patients have been lower, requiring higher vaccine dosages to achieve protective levels.[23,24] The vaccine protects against all hepatitis B serotypes but does not cross-react with other hepatitis viruses.

The high cost of the vaccine and inadequate supplies for widespread distribution have led to recommendations for use directed at individuals and groups who are occupationally, socially, or geographically at significant risk for exposure to hepatitis B and as part of postexposure prophylaxis. In the preexposure setting, the vaccine has been recommended for health care personnel who have frequent contact with blood (e.g., physicians, nurses, dentists, laboratory workers), homosexual/bisexual men, users of illicit injectable drugs, household and sexual contacts of hepatitis B carriers, residents and staff of institutions for the mentally handicapped, hemodialysis and oncology patients, factor VIII and IX recipients, morticians and their assistants, inmates in some prisons, and travelers to high-risk areas who may have sexual or occupational exposure to the population.[21]

The hepatitis B vaccine is also used with hepatitis B immune globulin (HBIG) in the postexposure setting. Persons for whom this regimen is recommended include susceptible individuals having percutaneous or permucosal exposure to blood containing HBsAg, sexual contacts of HBsAg carriers who will continue to be exposed, and infants born of mothers who are HBsAg carriers.[21,24–27] HBIG does not interfere with induction of neutralizing antibody and the combination has been shown to be more protective than two doses of HBIG alone (85% to 90% efficacy versus 70% to 75%).[21]

The primary vaccination series consists of three intramuscular doses of vaccine with a second and third dose given 1 and 6 months, respectively, after the first. Adults and children age 10 and older should receive 20 $\mu$g (1.0 mL) Heptavax or 10 $\mu$g Recombivax, hemodialysis and immunocompromised patients 40 μg (2.0 mL) Heptavax, and infants and children under 10 years 10 μg (0.5 mL) Heptavax or 5 μg Recombivax at each injection. The preferred site of administration is the deltoid muscle in adults (immunogenicity is significantly lower in adults who receive injection in the buttock)[4] and the anterolateral thigh in infants. The need for booster doses of vaccine has not been established. Of persons who develop protective antibody (≧10 or more sample ratio units by radioimmunoassay or positive antibody by enzyme immunoassay), 10% to 15% lose detectable antibody within 4 years but protection against infection and liver inflammation appears to persist.[21,24]

The same dose used for primary immunization is used in the postexposure setting. The hepatitis B vaccine series should be initiated as soon as possible after HBIG administration. In the neonate or an infected mother, HBIG should be given within 12 hours of birth and the first dose of hepatitis B vaccine within 7 days. When this regimen is followed, the second dose of HBIG need not be given.

Side effects of vaccine administration have been minimal, with soreness at the injection site being the primary complaint in approximately 25% of vaccinees. Arthralgias and neurologic side effects are exceedingly rare.[3] The incidence of Guillain–Barré syndrome temporally related to administration of the vaccine does not appear to be above the expected case rate in adults and no etiologic association with the vaccine has been made. The vaccine does not adversely or therapeutically affect hepatitis B carriers or persons who are already antibody positive.[28]

Hepatitis B is a disease of major public health significance, particularly in underdeveloped areas of the world. Worldwide, there are more than 200 million carriers, and complications including chronic liver disease and primary cancer of the liver are common. The present vaccine, because of its expense and limited availability for worldwide distribution, has failed to reach the population at highest risk.

### *Hepatitis B Immune Globulin*

HBIG is used for postexposure, and rarely preexposure, prophylaxis for hepatitis B infection. The product is prepared from pooled plasma obtained from a small group of healthy donors who have high titers of hepatitis B surface antibody as a result of hyperimmunization with hepatitis B vaccine.

Indications for the use of HBIG include passive immunization after exposure to hepatitis B virus via percutaneous, permucosal, or oral ingestion routes (e.g., needle-sticks, accidental splash, sexual contact, mouth pipetting) and for infants born to mothers who are hepatitis B carriers. HBIG has also been used for preexposure prophylaxis in the dialysis setting; however, with the advent of hepatitis B vaccine and a decline in the incidence of hepatitis B in dialysis units, it is not generally recommended.

Reports on the use of HBIG have confirmed a significant protective effect of this product (70%–75% efficacy) and, in general, superior efficacy when compared with standard immune globulin[21,22,29–32]; however, there is evidence that HBIG may prolong the incubation period in situations where protective efficacy is not achieved.[33]

The timing of HBIG prophylaxis regarding both frequency of dosing and proximity to the time of exposure has not been completely defined. It is currently recommended by the Centers for Disease Control (CDC) that HBIG be given as soon as possible after acute exposures (percutaneous, permucosal, oral ingestion), preferably within 24 hours. It is not recommended that HBIG be given beyond 7 days after acute exposure. For infants born of HBsAg-positive mothers, the recommended timing is within 12 hours of birth; for sexual contacts, a single dose of HBIG within 14 days of the last exposure. Variations in the recommendations reflect the relative risk associated with the type of exposure that exists.[34]

Until recently, a second dose of HBIG 1 month after exposure was recommended to provide extended immunity; however, because HBIG has not been found to be 100% effective in preventing hepatitis B, recent CDC recommen-

**Table 90.2** Recommendations for Hepatitis B Virus Postexposure Prophylaxis

| | *HBIG* | | *Hepatitis B vaccine* | |
|---|---|---|---|---|
| **Exposure** | **Dose** | **Recommended timing** | **Dose** | **Recommended timing** |
| Perinatal | 0.5 mL IM | Within 12 h of birth | 0.5 mL (10 μg) IM | Within 7 d[a]; repeat at 1 and 6 mo |
| Percutaneous | 0.06 mL/kg IM or 5 mL for adults | Single dose within 24 h | 1.0 mL (20 μg) IM[b] | Within 7 d[a]; repeat at 1 and 6 mo |
| | *or* | | | |
| | 0.06 mL/kg IM or 5 mL for adults | Within 24 h; repeat at 1 mo[c] | | |
| Sexual | 0.06 mL/kg IM or 5 mL for adults | Within 14 d of sexual contact | Vaccine is recommended for homosexually active males and for regular sexual contacts of chronic HBV carriers. | |

[a] The first dose can be given at the same time as the HBIG dose but at a separate site.
[b] For persons under 10 years of age, use 0.5 mL (10 μg).
[c] For those who choose not to receive hepatitis B vaccine.

Data from Reference 113.

dations include the simultaneous initiation of the hepatitis B vaccine series, particularly for persons at risk for subsequent exposure. (See Hepatitis B Vaccine). When this is done, the second dose of HBIG should not be given.

Table 90.2 contains the recommendations for dosing of HBIG for hepatitis B virus postexposure prophylaxis.

### *Influenza Virus Vaccine*

Influenza virus vaccine (IVV) was first introduced in 1945. Currently, IVV is an inactivated (killed), trivalent whole or split virus vaccine. The virus is grown in antibiotic-free chick embryos and is formaldehyde inactivated for use. Currently available preparations generally contain 45 μg of antigen, in 15-μg trivalent units per 0.1 mL.

Influenza is classified as type A or B, with influenza A further subtyped based on hemagglutinin (H) and neuraminadase (N) antigens. Influenza A causes significant disease in humans and the virus is subject to mutation by a phenomenon known as antigenic drift and shift, resulting in the development of different influenza strains. Influenza B, also a significant cause of human disease, is less likely to mutate. Development of IVV from year to year is determined by the predominant circulating strains worldwide and may change on a yearly basis.

Issues pertaining to dose, composition, number of doses, route of administration, reactogenicity (adverse effects), antibody response, and efficacy have been debated. IVV efficacy and reactogenicity may be related to the dose of the antigen and the immune status of the individual.[35] Split virus vaccine is felt to be less reactogenic than whole virus vaccine, particularly in children.[36] Antigenic superiority of whole versus split virus vaccine is controversial. In patients who are immunologically "unprimed" (previously unexposed to the antigen), whole and split virus vaccines are likely to induce equal rises in antibody titer[37,38]; however, in "primed" individuals, split virus vaccine may be more effective than whole.[39]

Response to IVV is generally measured in terms of antibody response and, more importantly, efficacy. Generally, an antibody titer of ≧1:40 is considered protective.[37,38,40,41] Efficacy in a high-risk nursing home population has been proven; vaccinated individuals are significantly less likely to develop influenza, be hospitalized, develop radiologically proven pneumonia, or die.[42] It must be noted that while IVV has been shown to be cost effective,[43] not all individuals respond with a significant antibody titer rise and thus acquire protection. Generally, sufficient titer rises (greater than fourfold) are determined by the age of the patient and whether or not they have been previously exposed to the antigen.[39] Younger individuals (ages 16–25) generally have a lower response to a single dose than those 26 or older.[39] These differences have led to vaccine dose standardization to facilitate response in the majority of subjects. Antibody titers that generally decline at least twofold by 6 months postvaccination are not changed significantly by the use of booster doses.[44]

Indications for current split and whole virus influenza vaccine are as follows: (1) adults with chronic cardiovascular or pulmonary diseases, (2) residents of nursing home facilities, (3) health care personnel dealing with high-risk patients, (4) healthy adults over age 65, (5) adults with chronic metabolic disease, and (6) children with chronic metabolic or cardiopulmonary diseases.

IVV (split or whole virus) is given as a single 0.5-mL intramuscular injection to persons over 12 years of age. Because split virus vaccine is more available, it is the more commonly used vaccine. In persons 12 or younger, or in persons in whom no prior exposure to influenza virus of the type contained in the vaccine is suspected, two 0.5-mL doses of split virus vaccine given 1 month apart are recommended.

Adverse reactions to the vaccine include local tenderness or low-grade fever in 3% to 5% beginning 6–12 hours postimmunization and lasting 1–2 days. Treatment with salicylates or acetaminophen is recommended. Immediate allergic reactions are rare but may occur in patients with hypersensitivity to eggs. Guillain–Barré syndrome was associated only with the 1976 swine influenza vaccine, not with subsequent vaccines.

### *Measles Vaccine*

Measles vaccine is a live attenuated virus vaccine that produces a subclinical, noncommunicable infection providing a 95% lifetime protection rate.[45] The vaccine is available as a lyophilized powder derived from virus grown in chick embryo cell cultures.

Measles vaccine is administered in the arm (or in the thigh if the patient is younger than 15 months), via subcutaneous injection only, as a single 0.5-mL dose. The vaccine is administered for primary immunization to persons 15 months or older usually as MMR. The vaccine should not be given to immunosuppressed patients, pregnant women, or patients with a history of egg allergy. In addition, the vaccine should not be given within 6 weeks (preferably 3 months) of immune globulin administration. It is recommended that the vaccine not be given within 1 month of any other live vaccine except mumps, rubella, and oral polio vaccines. In allergic patients with a history of anaphylaxis to eggs, skin testing and desensitization are recommended (see Fig. 90.1). Allergy to chickens or feathers is not a contraindication to use.

**Figure 90.1** Algorithm for using measles and/or mumps vaccine in egg-allergic patients.

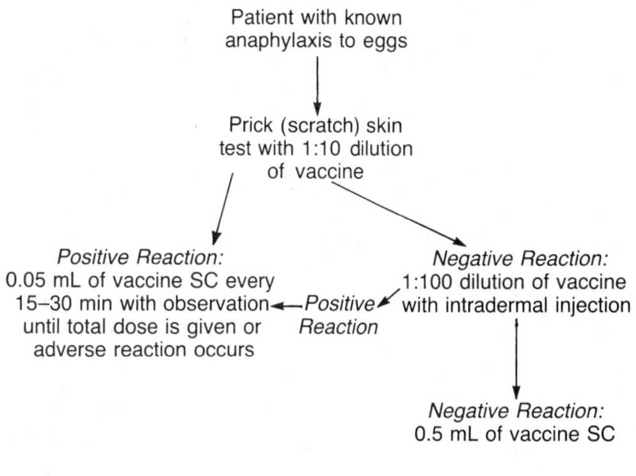

Additionally, these patients are not at increased risk for anaphylaxis. Finally, mild febrile illness is not a contraindication to vaccination. Known neomycin sensitivity is a contraindication to use, as each 0.5-mL dose contains 25 μg of neomycin.

Measles vaccine is indicated in all persons born after 1956 or in those who lack documentation of wild virus infection either by history or by antibody titers. Persons who received killed measles vaccine alone, who were given live vaccine within 3 months of receiving killed vaccine, or who received a vaccine of unknown type between 1963 and 1967 should be revaccinated. After vaccination, antibodies may be detected within 2 to 3 weeks in patients 15 months or older.

For postexposure prophylaxis, the vaccine is effective if given within 72 hours of exposure. In addition, immune globulin may be administered intramuscularly at a dose of 0.25 mg/kg (maximum dose, 15 mL), if given within 6 days of exposure. In children under 1 year, postexposure vaccination may be given as early as 6 months, but should be repeated at 15 months.[45,46]

Adverse effects to measles vaccine are limited. Febrile reactions (rarely above 39.4°C) may occur in the month following immunization. Transient rash (generalized) may also occur. These reactions generally appear 5–12 days postvaccination and last 2–5 days. Febrile seizures rarely occur. Other adverse effects such as headache, cough, sore throat, eye pain, malaise, and transient thrombocytopenia may occur. Local reactions at the injection site, while rare, may occur in subjects who have previously been vaccinated with killed vaccine. The vaccine may suppress a positive tuberculin skin test up to 6 weeks postadministration.

Measles vaccine has nearly eradicated the disease in the United States; however, the need for the vaccine continues because of the importation of cases of measles to this country.

### *Meningococcal Polysaccharide Vaccine*

Meningococcal polysaccharide vaccine (MPV) containing purified capsular antigen from *Neisseria meningitidis* is licensed for use in the United States. Serotypes currently available include groups A, C, Y, and W 135. MPV is available for use as a bivalent (50 μg each of serotypes A and C) or quadrivalent preparation. MPV vaccination produces antibody response for an unknown duration.

MPV is indicated in high-risk populations such as those exposed to the disease, those in the midst of uncontrolled outbreaks, or travelers to an area with epidemic or hyperendemic meningococcal disease. In the United States, serotype B, a strain not contained in the current vaccine, causes the majority of disease; thus routine vaccination is not recommended. The vaccine should not be given to pregnant women unless there is a substantial risk of infection.

MPV (bivalent or quadrivalent) is administered subcutaneously as a single 0.5-mL dose. Subjects should be over 2 years of age[47,48]; however, younger children can produce sufficient antibody levels if given two doses 3 months apart.[47] Antibody levels are attained within 10–14 days.[49] Revaccination may be reconsidered in 2–3 years in children who on initial vaccination were less than 4 years old.[48,50] Antibody decline is more rapid in infants and children.[48] The vaccine shows documented effectiveness in preventing meningococcal disease in 85% to 95% of recipients for serotypes A and C.[49,50] Efficacy of the vaccine for serotypes Y and W 135 is presumed but not documented.

Adverse effects of MPV include fever and erythema at the injection site lasting 1–2 days. Occasionally, headache occurs.

### *Mumps Vaccine*

The current mumps vaccine is a lyophilized live attenuated vaccine prepared from chick embryo cultures. Each 0.5-mL dose of the vaccine also contains 25 μg of neomycin. The vaccine is available alone or in combination with measles and rubella.

Mumps vaccine is used to produce active immunity while producing a subclinical, noncommunicable infection. A single dose induces antibody formation in 97% of children older than 12 months and in 93% of adults. Clinical efficacy approaches 75% to 90%.[51,52] Protection may last a lifetime; however, as the vaccine has been available less than 20 years this is not known for certain.[51]

The vaccine (usually given in conjunction with measles and rubella at 15 months of age) is given as a single 0.5-mL subcutaneous dose in the upper arm to children older than 12 months. It is also indicated in previously unvaccinated adults and in those in whom a poor history of wild virus infection or previous administration of killed mumps exists. If the vaccine is given before 12 months of age, revaccination is necessary and should be given after reaching 1 year of age.[51] Postexposure vaccination is of no benefit.

The vaccine should not be given to pregnant women or immunosuppressed patients. Additionally, conception should be avoided for 3 months after vaccination. In patients with a history of anaphylaxis to eggs, the same schema as in the case of measles should be used (Fig. 90.1). The vaccine should not be given within 6 weeks (preferably 3 months) of administration of immune globulin. Finally, the vaccine should not be given to neomycin-sensitive individuals.

Serious adverse reactions to the vaccine are rarely reported. Parotitis, rash, pruritis, and purpura rarely occur. Local reactions including soreness, burning, and stinging may occur at the injection site.

### *Pertussis Vaccine*

Vaccines for the prevention of pertussis (whooping cough) have been available since 1948. Pertussis vaccine is a suspension of killed whole *Bordetella pertussis* organisms and is usually administered in combination with diphtheria and tetanus toxoids (DPT). A course of primary immunization consists of four 0.5-mL intramuscular doses given at ages 2, 4, 6, and 18 months with a booster dose at 4–6 years. Rotation of injection sites is recommended, with no site being used more than once. After age 7, the risk of pertussis disease diminishes and the incidence of vaccine side effects increases; thus, vaccine use after this age is not recommended.

Pertussis vaccine use has stimulated significant controversy in recent years, as adverse effects are greater with pertussis vaccine than with other vaccines.[9] Adverse effects of pertussis vaccine include local reactions or fever (60%), prolonged crying (3%), unusual high-pitched cry (1 in 1,000), convulsions (1 in 1,750), and acute neurologic illness with a 33% rate of sequelae (1 in 110,000).[53,54] Other authors have reported mortality in 0.05% to 0.1% and permanent brain damage in 0.005% of vaccine recipients.[55,56] No toxicity data are available for the vaccine currently licensed in the United States[53]; available data are derived from foreign vaccine use.

Advocates of pertussis vaccine cite the increased incidence of pertussis in Great Britain following decreased use of vaccine after 1975. Vaccination levels decreased from 70%–90% in 1975 to 30% by 1978,[57–59] while pertussis disease reached epidemic proportions in 1977–1979 and 1982–1983.[57–59] These advocates also stress the decline in mortality from pertussis in the United States and England prior to and after vaccine institution. Between 1926 and 1930, there were 36,013 whooping cough deaths in the United States. Between 1979 and 1981, however, only 7 deaths were reported in the United States.[60] Finally, 1984 data suggest a significant decrease in pertussis among household contacts ages 6 months to 9 years vaccinated with three or more doses of the vaccine versus nonvaccinated individuals.[61]

These data have led the American Academy of Pediatrics and the Immunization Practices Advisory Committee to continue to recommend routine pertussis vaccine. The vaccine is not recommended in persons with a history of seizures temporally associated with pertussis vaccine.[11] A history of a seizure disorder is not itself a contraindication. If seizures occur, vaccine should be withheld until it is determined whether a neurologic disorder is evolving; if not, pertussis vaccine may be continued.[62]

### *Pneumococcal Vaccine*

Pneumococcal vaccine is a mixture of highly purified capsular polysaccharides from 23 of the 83 most prevalent or invasive types of *Streptococcus pneumoniae* seen in the United States. These 23 types represent 90% of all blood isolates and 85% of pneumococcal isolates from other generally sterile sites seen in the United States. Each 0.5-mL dose of vaccine contains 25 μg of each polysaccharide type dissolved in isotonic saline solution, for a total of 575 μg of polysaccharide, and contains 0.25% phenol as preservative. Cross-reactivity with other pneumococcal capsular antigens does not occur.

The pneumococcal vaccine is recommended for persons at high risk of acquiring the disease. Data have demonstrated an increased incidence of serious pneumococcal infection in patients who are immunosuppressed (e.g., Hodgkin's disease and other lymphoproliferative disorders, multiple myeloma, renal failure) and those with splenic dysfunction or anatomic asplenia. Patients with chronic illnesses of the cardiovascular and pulmonary systems, alcoholics, and the elderly, particularly those who are institutionalized, are also felt to be at increased risk.[1–4] Previous hospitalization can help define high-risk individuals, as two thirds of patients with serious disease have been hospitalized within the previous 5 years, generally with an underlying condition that would predispose to pneumococcal disease.[60] Recommendations for pneumococcal vaccine include adults and children over the age of 2 who are at high risk for pneumococcal disease and otherwise healthy adults over the age of 65.[5,6,63,64]

Two parameters are often used to assess the efficacy of a vaccine: its ability to generate an antibody response and its ability to reduce the incidence of disease in target populations. An antibody rise of 1.4- to 2-fold or 200 to 300 ng of antibody nitrogen per milliliter is often used to define an adequate immune response to this vaccine.[65–67] Most immunocompetent groups of patients have demonstrated at least a twofold rise in antibody within 2 to 3 weeks of immunization. Children over 2 and young adults with sickle cell anemia and splenectomy have also had adequate responses; however, certain groups have not demonstrated an adequate response, including children under 2, asplenic Hodgkin's disease patients on chemotherapy, and persons with impaired immunoglobulin synthesis and multiple myeloma.[67,68]

Studies demonstrating decreases in the incidence of pneumococcal disease are more difficult to carry out because of low and variable attack rates and the need for large study populations. In controlled studies of African goldminers, immunization resulted in a 76% to 78.5% reduction in pneumonia and an 82.3% to 92% reduction in bacteremia.[65] In patients with sickle cell disease and patients with splenectomy, a protective effect against vaccine-specific organisms has been suggested.[69,70] An octavalent vaccine was demonstrated to reduce the incidence of otitis media in immunized black children ages 6 to 11 months, but had no effect on a similar white population.[71] Efficacy studies in both noninstitutionalized and institutionalized elderly patients and those in a psychiatric facility were inconclusive .[72,73] Conflicting opinions also exist with regard to the use of the vaccines in patients with chronic lung disease. It is not clear if this group is at significant risk of pneumococcal disease, or if preexisting high antibody levels in these patients affect vaccine response.[74] As a result, considerable controversy exists over widespread use of the vaccine, particularly in healthy elderly populations.

Pneumococcal vaccine safety is well documented. Local reactions occur frequently and are generally mild. Local erythema and induration (30%), local discomfort (40%), and local swelling (3%) are the side effects most commonly observed. Rarely, severe systemic reactions can occur and consist of weakness, myalgia, headache, photophobia, chills, and fever. Revaccination is not recommended, regardless of previous vaccine used, as immune complex and systemic reactions have been observed when booster doses are given.[65]

### *Poliovirus Vaccines*

Two types of trivalent poliovirus vaccines are currently licensed for distribution in the United States. An inactivated vaccine (IPV), developed by Salk was licensed for use in 1955. Since 1962, a live attenuated, oral vaccine (OPV), developed by Sabin, has been available and is currently the primary immunizing agent for poliovirus infection. Both vaccines are produced from three approved, attenuated, Sabin seed strains of poliovirus: type I Mahoney, type II MEF, and type III Saukett.

Primary immunization with IPV consists of a series of three 1-mL subcutaneous injections given 4 to 8 weeks apart with a similar booster dose 6 to 12 months after the third injection. If interruption of the series occurs, a sufficient immune response can be obtained by administration of only those doses that have been omitted. After immunization, humoral antibodies are induced in 95% of recipients. The duration of protection after immunization has not been definitively determined but current recommendations include a booster dose every 5 years up to the age of 18.

There are no serious side effects or contraindications to IPV except pregnancy where IPV should be given only if clearly needed (e.g., women will be traveling or living in an area with endemic or epidemic poliovirus).

OPV is administered in a series of three oral 0.5-mL doses with a second dose given 6 to 8 weeks after the first and the third dose 8 to 12 months after the second. In children, OPV immunization generally begins at 6 to 12 weeks of age, commonly with the first DPT immunization.

OPV closely parallels natural infection, stimulating humoral antibody and secretory IgA in lymphatic tissues surrounding the intestinal tract within 7 to 10 days of ingestion. It replicates and can be found in pharyngeal secretions and is excreted in stool for several weeks, resulting in immunization of some contacts of vaccinees. Immunity is achieved in 95% of vaccine recipients.[75]

There are no immediate side effects of OPV. Rarely, vaccine-associated poliomyelitis develops in vaccinees (1 out of 9 million doses) or contacts (1 out of 7 million doses).[6] Individuals with primary immune deficiency are at increased risk for this adverse reaction and for this reason OPV is not recommended for persons who are immunodeficient or for normal individuals who reside in a household where another person is immunodeficient. The vaccine should not be given during pregnancy because of the small but theoretical risk to the fetus.

Primary poliomyelitis immunization is recommended for all children and young adults up to age 18. OPV is the vaccine of choice in this age group unless an immunodeficiency state exists in the patient or a household contact, in which case IPV is recommended. Primary immunization of adults over 18 is not routinely recommended as a high level of immunity already exists in this age group and the risk of exposure in developed countries is small; however, unimmunized adults who are at increased risk for exposure because of travel, residence, or occupation should receive primary immunization with IPV as there is a small but increased risk of vaccine-induced paralysis after OPV administration in adults.

Incompletely immunized adults or children should complete the series of IPV or OPV regardless of the interval since initiation of primary immunization. Booster doses of OPV or IPV are recommended for children before entering school. Children who received IPV as a primary series should receive subsequent doses every 5 years through age 17 unless a primary series with OPV is administered. In adults, booster doses are not routinely recommended unless an increased risk of exposure (e.g., travel) exists, in which case a single dose of OPV or IPV should be given.

### *Rabies Vaccine*

Human diploid cell vaccine (HDCV) is a killed vaccine used for pre- and postexposure rabies virus prophylaxis. It is a successor to previous vaccines, including duck embryo vaccine, is more immunogenic, and has fewer side effects than its predecessors.

Transmission of rabies can occur via percutaneous, permucosal, or airborne exposure to the rabies virus. Circumstances favoring such transmission include animal bites or attacks, and contamination of scratches, cuts, abrasions, or mucous membranes with saliva or other infectious material (e.g., brain tissue). Airborne acquisition in laboratories and in bat-infested caves has been reported. Unprovoked attacks and daytime attacks by nocturnal animals are considered highly suspect. Common wild animal transmitters include skunks, foxes, and raccoons. Rabies in domestic animals in the United States varies among regions. Dog rabies is very common in certain foreign countries (e.g., India, African nations). Rodents, rabbits, and hares are rarely infected. There have been four reports of person-to-person transmission via corneal transplant.[76]

Preexposure indications for using HDCV include persons whose vocation or avocation places them at high risk for rabies exposure, for example, veterinarians, animal handlers, and field personnel (trappers, hunters, cave explorers). Travelers who will be in a country or area of a country where there is a constant threat of rabies, whose stay is likely to extend beyond 1 month, and who may not have readily available medical services (e.g., Peace Corps workers, missionaries) should also be considered for preexposure prophylaxis.

Postexposure prophylaxis should be given after percutaneous or permucosal exposure to saliva or other infectious material from a high-risk source. Each case needs to be handled individually. Consideration needs to be given to the geographic area, species of animal, circumstances of the incident, and type of exposure. Local or state health departments may be able to provide guidelines.

HDCV for preexposure prophylaxis is administered intramuscularly in three doses of 1.0 mL IM or 0.1 mL intradermally on day 0, day 7, and between days 21 and 28. Pregnancy is not a contraindication if the risk is great. The vaccine is not recommended for persons who are immunocompromised. A booster dose every year is recommended for persons who will have continued exposure; however, if antibody titers are adequate, immunization may be deferred. Suboptimal responses have been documented in persons receiving chloroquine chemoprophylaxis for malaria.[77–79] Thus the vaccine should be administered 1 month before chloroquine therapy begins.

Preexposure prophylaxis does not eliminate the need for postexposure prophylaxis. The regimen for postexposure prophylaxis is determined by whether a person has previously received HDCV. Persons previously immunized with HDCV should receive two 1.0-mL intramuscular doses of HDCV on postexposure days 0 and 3. Rabies immune globulin should not be given to this group. Persons who have not been previously immunized should receive the recommended regimen of rabies immune globulin (see next section) and five doses of HDCV—1.0 mL intramuscularly on days 0, 3, 7, 14, and 28 after exposure.[5,6,76] The intradermal route should not be used.

Adverse reactions to HDCV are not uncommon. Approximately 20% experience pain, erythema, swelling, and itching at the injection site. Another 20% may have headache, nausea, abdominal pain, muscle aches, and/or dizziness.[5] Systemic allergic reactions ranging from hives to anaphylaxis occur in an estimated 11/10,000 vaccinees.[80] It is recommended that persons exposed to rabies who do have adverse reactions continue the vaccine series in a setting with medical support services. In persons receiving booster doses of HDCV, an immune complex–like disease has been seen in up to 7% of vaccinees.[80]

Antibody conversion occurs in virtually 100% of HDCV recipients; however, recent data suggest that persons who are concurrently receiving chloroquine may exhibit a reduced antibody response.[81] The CDC considers titers of 5 by rapid fluorescent focus inhibition testing as being protective. The World Health Organization uses a value of 0.5 IU/mL as evidence of protective antibody. Persons who are receiving corticosteroids or other immunosuppressant agents and who receive postexposure prophylaxis should have their antibody status determined.

### *Rabies Immune Globulin*

Human rabies immune globulin is an immunoglobulin used in conjunction with rabies vaccine as part of postexposure rabies management. The product is derived from plasma obtained from donors who have been hyperimmunized with rabies vaccine and have high titers of circulating antibody.

In persons who have not been previously immunized against rabies, rabies immune globulin is given simultaneously with HDCV to provide optimal coverage in the interval before immune response to the vaccine occurs. The efficacy of this regimen has been clearly demonstrated. In situations where vaccine has been used alone, mortality rates of 50% to 60% have been observed. Mortality after the combination vaccine/rabies immune globulin regimen is an exceedingly rare event.[5,82,83]

Rabies immune globulin does not interfere with vaccine-induced antibody formation; however, its use is not recommended beyond 8 days after initiation of the vaccine series nor in persons previously immunized to rabies.

Human rabies immune globulin is administered in a dose of 20 IU/kg (0.133 mL/kg), half to be given intramuscularly and the other half infiltrated around the wound site. This product should never be administered by the intravenous route. Because other antibodies in the rabies immune globulin may interfere with the response to live virus vaccines (e.g., measles–mumps–rubella), it is recommended that these immunizations be delayed for 3 months.

Side effects are rare, but may include local soreness at the wound or intramuscular injection site and mild temperature elevations. Caution is advised when administering this product to persons with known systemic allergies to immune globulin or thimerosal. Pregnancy is not a contraindication for its use.

### *Rubella Vaccine*

Rubella vaccine contains lyophilized live attenuated rubella (German measles) virus grown in human diploid cell culture. The vaccine is available alone or in combination with measles and/or mumps vaccine. Each 0.5-mL dose also contains 25 $\mu$g of neomycin.

Rubella vaccine induces antibodies to the virus that are thought to be protective against wild virus infection.[84] After a single 0.5-mL subcutaneous dose, 95% of children 1 year old become rubella antibody positive within 2–6 weeks.[85,86] The duration of immunity has not been established; however, booster doses are not recommended. The vaccine is indicated for children older than 1 year, persons 12 years or older without evidence of wild virus infection, women of childbearing potential for whom serologic testing is unavailable, and persons at a substantial risk for exposure.[86,87] The vaccine should not be given to immunosuppressed individuals nor used within 6 weeks (preferably 3 months) of immune globulin administration. Additional immune globulin should not be given within 14 days of vaccine. The vaccine should not be given to neomycin-sensitive patients.

Adverse effects of rubella virus vaccine tend to increase with the age of the recipient. Symptoms are similar to those of wild virus infection and include lymphadenopathy, rash, urticaria, fever, malaise, sore throat, headache, myalgias, and paresthesias of the extremities. These occur 11–20 days after vaccination and last 1–5 days. Joint symptoms occur at 1–10 weeks in 20% to 40% of adult women and their incidence is greater in adolescent women than in children.[88] Frank arthritis occurs in fewer than 1% of recipients. Symptoms last 1–3 days and rarely recur. The vaccine may cause suppression of tuberculin skin tests up to 6 weeks postvaccination. Although the vaccine virus may be excreted in nose and throat secretions, it is not contagious.

While the vaccine has been shown to be safe to the fetus, its use in pregnancy is discouraged.[88] Women should be counseled not to become pregnant for 3 weeks after vaccination. Termination of pregnancy is not indicated in women who are accidentally given the vaccine.[4]

### *Smallpox Vaccine*

Smallpox vaccine is a lyophilized live unattenuated preparation of vaccinia (cowpox) virus that induces protection against smallpox (variola virus) vaccinia and other orthopox viruses in 95% or more of recipients. Since May 1980, when the world was declared to be free of smallpox by the World Health Organization (WHO), routine smallpox vaccination has not been recommended. The only current indication for the vaccine is in persons working with orthopox viruses.[89] The vaccine is not commercially available and should be obtained through the CDC.

Antibodies appear within 4–5 days of vaccination, peak at 4 weeks, and persist up to 20 years. Adequate antibody response rarely occurs without the characteristic skin lesion at the vaccination site. The vaccine is given as a single, intradermal injection into the deltoid region using a supplied bifurcated needle and making a 30-mm circle via repeated pricks at the site. The vaccine should not be given to immunosuppressed patients. The vaccine may be given with other live vaccines if necessary. Booster doses are recommended every 3 years.

Adverse reactions associated with the vaccine include skin necrosis and eczema (particularly in those with a history of eczema), erythema and tenderness at the site of injection, fever, and regional adenopathy. Rarely, encephalitis and related neurologic complications or disseminated vaccinia occur. Occasional false-positive serologic tests for syphilis may occur within 2–4 weeks of vaccination and persist for 2 months.

### *Varicella Vaccine*

Live attenuated varicella vaccines are currently being tested in field trials in Japan and the United States. Takahashi, in 1974, developed a vaccine using an OKA strain of varicella zoster (VZ) virus. Most subsequent vaccines have used the OKA strain but a KMcC strain has also been studied. It is only recently that the existence of multiple VZ strains has been recognized and no comparison of the strains has been made; however, there is evidence that the OKA strain may not be cross-protective against some other wild virus strains. Preliminary studies indicate that OKA VZ vaccine is safe and immunogenic in healthy adults and children as well as severely immunocompromised patients.[90–92] The target group for varicella vaccine is VZ-susceptible immunocompromised children in whom infection may be a life-threatening event. In this population, seroconversion after vaccination with OKA vaccine occurs in 90% to 100% of vaccinees. The reported incidence of clinical infection in vaccinees after exposure to VZ is low (18%) and usually mild. In similar unvaccinated populations attack rates after exposure have averaged 87%. Antibody can persist for at least 5–7 years. The incidence of secondary spread of virus after vaccination is 0% to 3% and secondary infections have been mild, confirming attenuation of the virus.[2] A study of the KMcC strain vaccine in healthy children has produced similar results and studies are underway to determine its efficacy in immunosuppressed patients.[93]

Varicella vaccine has been shown to boost VZ-specific immunologic response in the elderly, but its potential effectiveness in reducing clinical zoster infection has yet to be shown.[94]

No severe side effects to the vaccine have been reported. Mild to moderate delayed-onset rashes have occurred, as have local swelling and erythema at the injection site, fever, and mild upper respiratory symptoms.

The future for commercial production of varicella vaccine is promising. In addition to its use in immunocompromised children, benefit may be derived from vaccination of susceptible healthy children and health care workers in pediatric, obstetrical, or oncology areas.[95]

### *Varicella Zoster Immune Globulin*

Varicella zoster immune globulin (VZIG) is used for passive immunization of susceptible immunodeficient patients exposed to VZ infection. It is prepared by Cohn cold ethanol fractionation from plasma found in routine screening of normal volunteer blood donors to contain high titers of VZ antibody.[96,97] On the average, VZIG has been found to contain 10 to 20 times more VZ antibody than immune globulin (IG).[98]

Use of VZIG should be considered in exposed children and certain adults who are immunocompromised and susceptible to VZ. Criteria for its use in children are listed in Table 90.3 and take into consideration underlying disease, type of exposure, prior varicella history, age, and interval since exposure. Criteria for its use in immunocompromised adults are less clear because of difficulties in determining susceptibility status. A positive history eliminates the need for VZIG; however, a negative history is not a valid indicator as 85% to 95% of persons with negative or unknown histories are serologically positive for VZ antibodies. Individuals with a previous household exposure (siblings or children) and those who have attended an urban school or have had previous occupational exposure (e.g., nursery school, kindergarten) are likely to be immune.[98] Positive serologic tests on immunocompromised patients can be misleading as VZ antibody may be transiently acquired from blood products. In such cases it is best to consult with the regional Red Cross Blood Distribution Center regarding the appropriate course of action.

Varicella can cause congenital malformation early and, rarely, late in pregnancy. While VZIG may attenuate maternal infection, its efficacy in preventing intrauterine infection has not been demonstrated. There is an increased risk of serious infection and an associated 30% mortality in infants whose mothers develop varicella 4 days prior to or 2 days after delivery or whose onset of infection is between 5 and 10 days of age. Normal, full-term infants exposed postnatally are not at increased risk for complications. Use of VZIG perinatally is therefore aimed at the critical period for complications (see Table 90.3).[97]

The efficacy of VZIG has been measured by three parameters: clinical attack rates, severity of illness, and incidence of subclinical disease. Clinical attack rates after VZIG have varied from 20% to 65%, as compared with normal attack rates of 80% to 90% after household exposures without prophylaxis; however, the severity of illness has been significantly affected with VZIG, and the majority of cases have been mild, with complications occurring in only 7%. Subclinical infections commonly occur after VZIG. In one study, 33% of leukemic patients had evidence of subclinical infection after VZIG as compared with 5% after natural infections.[99–101]

**Table 90.3** Criteria for Use of VZIG

Patients should meet all four criteria.

1. Susceptible to varicella zoster infection
2. Significant exposure within 96 h
   a. Household contact
   b. Playmate contact (1 h play indoors)
   c. Hospital contact (in adjacent beds or same 2- to 4-bed room)
   d. School contact (adjacent desks in same classroom or same carpool)
   e. Newborn contact (newborn whose mother developed varicella less than 5 d prior to or 48 h after delivery)
3. Age <15, with administration to immunocompromised adolescents, adults and other older patients on an individual basis
4. One of the following underlying illnesses or conditions
   a. Leukemia or lymphoma
   b. Congenital or acquired immunodeficiency
   c. Immunosuppressive treatment
   d. Newborn of mother with varicella (2e above)
   e. Premature infant (≧28 wk gestation) whose mother lacks a prior history of chicken pox
   f. Premature infants (<28 wk gestation or ≦1000 g) regardless of maternal history

Data from Reference 6.

For maximum effectiveness, VZIG must be given within 48 hours and not more than 96 hours after exposure. As this agent may only attenuate infection, patients who receive VZIG may still have a period of communicability. VZIG may prolong the incubation period to 28 days.

VZIG is distributed by the American Red Cross Services. Contact with the distribution centers must be made within 72 hours of exposure and specific criteria must be met for the product to be released.

Administration of VZIG is by the intramuscular route (never intravenously) at doses of 125 units/10 kg body weight up to 625 units (5 vials). The dose for newborn infants is one-half vial, or 1.25 mL. Side effects include local soreness at the site of injection. VZIG should be avoided in persons with bleeding diathesis. There are no other contraindications for the use of this product. Duration of antibody protection is not known, but is felt to be at least one half-life of the immune globulin, approximately 3 weeks.

**Table 90.4** Indications and Dosage of Immune Globulin in Infectious Diseases

| | |
|---|---|
| Hepatitis A exposure | 0.02 mL/kg IM within 2 wk |
| Hepatitis A prophylaxis | 0.05–0.06 mL/kg IM every 4–6 mo |
| Hepatitis B | 0.06 mL/kg IM (HBIG is preferred in known exposures) as soon as possible |
| Non-A/non-B hepatitis | 0.06 mL/kg IM as soon as possible |
| Measles | 0.25 mL/kg IM within 6 d |
| Rubella | 20 mL IM as one dose |
| Immunodeficiency states | 1.2 mL/kg IM, then 0.6 mL/kg IM every 2–4 wk *or* 2 mL/kg (100 mg/kg) IV up to 300 mg/kg monthly |

Data from Reference 6.

## Other Immunobiologics

### *Immune Globulin*

Immune globulin (IG) is available as both intramuscular and intravenous preparations. Intramuscular IG or the Cohn fraction II is prepared from pooled plasma of several thousand donors by cold ethanol fractionation.[102] Intramuscular IG typically contains greater than 95% IgG and trace amounts of IgM, IgA, and other plasma proteins. As IG is harvested from a large donor pool, it contains a wide spectrum of IgG antibodies to the pathogens prevalent in the area from which the donors were obtained. In the fractionation process, high-molecular-weight IgG aggregates are formed, which can activate complement in the absence of antigen and precipate anaphylactoid reactions. For this reason, intramuscular IG is unsuitable for intravenous administration. Intramuscular IG typically contains 15% to 18% protein.

Three intravenous preparations of IG are commercially available in the United States. These agents are rendered suitable for intravenous use, as their anticomplement activity is removed either by selective reduction and alkylation of interchain disulfide bonds or by treatment at low pH in the presence of small amounts of pepsin which removes the IgG aggregates.

When administered either intravenously or intramuscularly, IG distributes in approximately 10% of the body weight of the recipient.[103] The plasma half-life of IG averages 20 to 30 days. Peak serum concentrations occur relatively immediately with intravenous IG, whereas intramuscular IG produces peak concentrations within 1 to 4 days. After the initial period of equilibration, circulating IgG levels are superimposable between intravenous and intramuscular equivalent dosages. No dosage adjustment is necessary in patients with renal and/or hepatic insufficiency, in dialysis patients, or in geriatric patients. Serum IgG levels increase approximately 250 mg% for each 100 mg/kg in intravenous IG infused.[104,105]

IG is indicated in a wide variety of circumstances to provide passive immunity to individuals. It is also used in the treatment of certain other disease states. The indications and dosages of IG are shown in Tables 90.4 and 90.5.

Adverse effects of IG vary with the route of administration. After intramuscular IG, pain, tenderness, and muscle stiffness persisting for hours or days are seen. Repeat courses may cause sensitization with resultant allergic reactions. With intravenous IG, adverse effects are seen in fewer than 1% of patients. Most adverse effects are related to the rate of the infusion. Infusion should be given at 0.01–0.02 mL/kg/min for 30 minutes and then, if no reactions occur, increased to 0.02–0.04 mL/kg/min. While infusion rate recommendations vary slightly depending on the preparation, the guidelines presented can be followed for either intravenous preparation.

### *Lymphocyte Immune Globulin*

Lymphocyte IG (antithymocyte globulin, ATG) is an equine-derived $\gamma$-globulin directed against human thymocytes and is used to reduce the number of circulating thymus-dependent lymphocytes. The reduction of these cells results in immunosuppression. The preparation is given intravenously diluted in 0.9% saline.

The indications for ATG are limited mainly to the prevention and treatment of renal transplant rejection.[106,107] As a preventative agent, ATG when combined with standard immunosuppressive therapy results in significantly fewer rejection episodes.[107] In acute renal transplant rejection, ATG is also effective when used along with conventional therapy.[108] Additionally, ATG has been used successfully in

**Table 90.5** Indications and Dosage of Immune Globulin in Diseases Other Than Infectious Diseases

| | |
|---|---|
| Idiopathic thrombocytopenia purpura | 400 mg/kg (8 mL/kg) IV daily for 5 d |
| Autoimmune neutropenia | 400 mg/kg (8 mL/kg) IV daily for 3 d |

Data from Reference 105.

**Table 90.6** Adverse Reactions to Antithymocyte Globulin

| *Adverse reaction* | *Incidence (%)* | *Treatment* |
|---|---|---|
| Leukopenia | 14 | Discontinue agent if unremitting |
| Thrombocytopenia | 11 | Discontinue agent if unremitting |
| Back/chest pain | 1–5 | Analgesics |
| Hypotension | 1–5 | Supportive |
| Hypertension | <1 | Supportive |
| Fever | 33 | Antipyretics |
| Chills | 14 | Supportive |
| Diarrhea | 1–5 | Supportive |
| Dyspnea | 1–5 | Slow infusion rate |
| Dermatologic reactions | 12.5 | Slow infusion, monitor carefully |
| Intravenous site pain | 1–5 | — |
| Arthralgia | 1–5 | Analgesics |
| Anaphylaxis | Rare | Discontinue agent, give epinephrine and steroids |

the treatment of myasthenia gravis[109] and multiple sclerosis.[110]

ATG is available as a 50 mg/mL solution. The normal adult dose is 10–30 mg/kg/d infused over a minimum of 4 hours. For rejection prophylaxis, 15–30 mg/kg/d for 14 days has been used or 15 mg/kg/d for 14 days followed by 15 mg/kg every other day for seven doses. Therapy should be instituted within 24 hours of transplant. In acute transplant rejection, 10–15 mg/kg/d for 14–21 days is recommended.

A 0.1-mL intradermal test dose of a 1:1,000 dilution (5 μg equine ATG) is recommended prior to the first infusion of ATG along with a saline control. If systemic reactions occur, no ATG should be administered. If a wheal or erythema greater than 10 mm occurs, ATG may be given with caution.

Adverse effects of ATG are numerous. These are listed in Table 90.6. The concurrent use of steroids may reduce allergic reactions.

### *$Rh_0$(D) Immune Globulin*

$Rh_0$(D) immune globulin (RDIG) is a sterile solution of immunoglobulins prepared from human sera with high titers of $Rh_0$(D) antibody. Plasma or serum used to prepare RDIG is negative for hepatitis B surface antigen.

RDIG suppresses the antibody response and formation of anti-$Rh_0$(D) in $Rh_0$(D)-negative, $D^u$-negative women exposed to $Rh_0$(D)-positive blood. Administration of RDIG prevents the occurrence of erythroblastosis fetalis in subsequent pregnancies with an $Rh_0$(D)-positive fetus. When administered within 72 hours of delivery of a full-term infant, RDIG reduces active antibody formation from 12% to 1%–2%. The reduction of antibody formation is less when RDIG is given after 72 hours postpartum. Additionally, smaller doses of RDIG are used after abortion, miscarriage, amniocentesis, or abdominal trauma. RDIG is also used in premenopausal women who are $Rh_0$(D)-negative or $D^u$-negative and have inadvertently received $Rh_0$(D)- or $D^u$-positive blood or blood products.

The dosage of RDIG varies with the indication. A standard dose of 300 μg is given within 72 hours of a term delivery. Occasionally, where the fetus is known to be $Rh_0$(D)-positive, a 300-μg dose is given at 28 weeks gestations and within 72 hours of delivery. After pregnancy termination occurring up to 13 weeks gestation, one microdose (50 μg) vial is given within 72 hours. For pregnancy termination after 13 weeks, one standard dose (300 μg) is given within 72 hours. In other circumstances such as in abdominal trauma, amniocentesis, or transfusion accidents, the dosage (number of standard dose vials) is based on the estimated packed red blood cell volume of the fetal/maternal hemorrhage divided by 15. RDIG is administered intramuscularly only.

When considering RDIG for use, one must be certain of the mother's $Rh_0$(D) and $D^u$ antigen status. RDIG should not be given to individuals positive for either of these antigens or to those with anti-$Rh_0$(D) antibodies. Occasionally, a large fetal bleed of $Rh_0$(D)- or $D^u$-positive blood may make cross-matching of the mother difficult. In those cases, RDIG should be given only if previous tests have shown the mother to be $Rh_0$(D)-negative and $D^u$-negative with no anti-$Rh_0$(D) antibody.

Adverse reactions to RDIG include injection site tenderness and fever.

## Vaccines for Travel

Persons who are planning travel to underdeveloped parts of the world where unsanitary conditions or unusual diseases exist need to be evaluated for additional vaccines or immunobiologics. The yearly publication *Health Information for International Travel*,[111] published by the CDC, provides country-specific information on required and recommended immunization for travel. This section reviews three vaccines commonly used for foreign travel: cholera, typhoid, and yellow fever. Based on the nature of the travel, other vaccines previously discussed may need to be considered. These include polio, tetanus, rabies, hepatitis B, measles, and meningococcal vaccines. Also, immune globulin is frequently administered for hepatitis A prophylaxis.

### *Cholera Vaccine*

The currently available vaccine for cholera consists of a suspension of killed whole cell *Vibrio cholerae* bacteria from two bacterial strains: Ogawa and Inaba.

Cholera vaccine is approximately 50% effective in reducing the incidence of disease but does not prevent transmission of infection. The vaccine provides greater efficacy in persons who have previously had the disease. The duration of antibody after vaccination is 3–6 months, as compared with 3 years after natural infection. Frequent booster doses (every 6 months) are therefore needed to sustain protection.

The primary use of cholera vaccine is in travelers who will be visiting countries that require health department validation of cholera vaccination. Some clinicians also administer it to persons who will be traveling in endemic areas; however, the risk of cholera to tourists is exceedingly low and therefore does not warrant routine vaccination.

The primary immunization series in adults consists of two 0.5-mL intramuscular or subcutaneous doses or two 0.2-mL intradermal doses administered 1 week to 1 month apart. Intramuscular doses in children under 10 years are modified accordingly (0.2 mL for 6 months–4 years, 0.3 mL for 5–10 years). Similar booster doses are recommended every 6 months.

Side effects are common and consist of local reactions (pain, erythema, induration, tenderness), fever, malaise, and headache. Serious reactions, including neurologic complications, are rare. No data are available on its use in pregnancy but it is not felt to be contraindicated. The only contraindication is a history of previous severe systemic reaction to the vaccine. A 3-week interval between administrations of cholera and yellow fever vaccines is recommended because of reported decreased antibody response with their simultaneous administration; however, there is no evidence that protection is affected by simultaneous administration and when necessary may be done.[5,6]

### *Typhoid Vaccine*

Typhoid vaccine consists of a saline suspension of killed *Salmonella typhi* bacteria. It is recommended for travelers to underdeveloped areas where there is poor sanitation and where typhoid is often endemic. It is also recommended for use in household contacts of *S. typhi* carriers. The vaccine is 50% to 90% effective, depending in part on levels of existing natural immunity and size of inoculum exposures.[5,112] Hence, careful selection of food and water is still a very important part of disease prevention.

The recommended primary immunization schedule for adults is two 0.5-mL subcutaneous doses given 4 or more weeks apart or, where time does not permit, three 0.5-mL doses given weekly. A single booster dose (0.5 mL SC or 0.1 mL IM) is recommended every 3 years for persons traveling to or remaining in endemic areas. The intradermal dose is not recommended for primary immunization nor is it recommended if an acetone or dried vaccine is used (as occurs in military population).[6]

Side effects are common and include local reactions (pain, induration, and erythema at the injection site), malaise, headache, and fever which start within 24 hours of receiving the vaccine, last 1 to 2 days, and are usually responsive to mild analgesia. No studies have been done during pregnancy but, as the vaccine is composed of killed bacteria, it is not felt to pose any fetal risk. The vaccine should not be given during acute viral respiratory infections nor to persons who have a known hypersensitivity to the vaccine.

### *Yellow Fever Vaccine*

Live, attenuated, yellow fever virus vaccine is recommended for persons who will be traveling or living in areas where yellow fever infection occurs (currently, parts of Africa and South America), and is required for entry into certain countries.[5] Vaccination should also be considered for laboratory workers who may be exposed to the virus. The WHO approves the vaccine which is administered only at approved Yellow Fever Vaccination Centers. The reconstituted vaccine is thermolabile and unused portions must be discarded within 1 hour.

The recommended dose is 0.5 mL SC given once with similar booster doses recommended every 10 years; however, the vaccine has been shown to be highly immunogenic, with antibodies persisting at least 40 years and perhaps for life. Mild side effects, consisting of headache, myalgias, and low-grade fever 1 to 2 weeks after vaccination, occur in less than 10% of vaccinees; treatment should be symptomatic. Immediate hypersensitivity reactions are rare (1 per 1 million doses) and occur primarily in persons who have anaphylactic reactions to eggs. Neurologic accidents are rare (20 cases to date) and have occurred primarily in infants younger than 6 months in whom the vaccine is not recommended. The French Neurotropic Vaccine (Dakar strain) was associated with meningoencephalitis in children and is no longer manufactured. This has not occurred with the 17D strain.

On theoretical grounds, the vaccine should be avoided during pregnancy unless travel to a high-risk area is imperative. It is also not recommended for persons who are immunocompromised or immunosuppressed. Additionally, it should not be given to infants less than 6 months. It is contraindicated in persons with a history of anaphylactic reaction to eggs. Where the history is in question, intradermal testing consisting of 0.02 to 0.03-mL doses of vaccine and normal saline control applied to the volar surface of the forearm should be done. The demonstration of an erythematous, urticarial wheal and negative control constitutes a positive response and contraindicates vaccination.

Yellow fever vaccine may be simultaneously administered with all other vaccines except cholera, with which a 3-week interval is recommended. Simultaneous administration of immune globulin does not interfere with the immune response to this agent.

**Appendix 90.1** Recommendations for Immunization of Infants and Children

| *Age* | *DPT/OPV*[a] | *MMR*[b] | *H Flu*[c] |
|---|---|---|---|
| 2 mo | * | | |
| 4 mo | * | | |
| 6 mo | *[d] | | |
| 15 mo | | * | |
| 18 mo | * | | *[e] |
| 24 mo | | | * |
| 36 mo | | | *[e] |
| 4–6 yr | * | | |

[a] Diphtheria–pertussis–tetanus/oral polio vaccine.
[b] Measles–mumps–rubella vaccine.
[c] *Hemophilus influenzae* vaccine.
[d] OPV may be omitted.
[e] If H Flu is given at 18 months, do not repeat at 24 months; repeat at 36 months.

Compiled from Behrman RE, Vaughan VC III (Eds): Nelson's Handbook of Pediatrics, 12th ed. Philadelphia, W. B. Saunders, 1983, pp 189–192.

**Appendix 90.2** Recommendations for Immunization of Adults (18 years or Older)

| *Patient group* | *TD*[a] | *MMR*[b] | *Polio* | *Flu*[c] | *Pneumo*[d] | *HepB*[e] |
|---|---|---|---|---|---|---|
| I. Healthy adults | | | | | | |
| A. 18–24 | × | [f] | [g] | | | |
| B. 25–64 | × | [h] | [g] | | | |
| C. ≧65 | × | | | × | × | |
| II. Special groups | | | | | | |
| A. Pregnancy | | [i] | [g] | | | [j] |
| B. Occupational | | | | | | |
| College | | [f] | | | | |
| Health care | | [f] | | × | | × |
| Essential community services | | | | × | | |
| Day-care | | × | × | × | | |
| C. Lifestyles | | | | | | |
| Homosexual males | | | | | | × |
| Illicit drug users | × | | | | | × |
| D. Environmental situations | | | | | | |
| Prisons | | | | | | |
| Institutionalized mentally retarded | | | | | | × |
| E. Compromised hosts | | | | | | |
| Systemic disease | | | | × | × | |
| Immunocompromised | | | | [k] | [k] | [l] |

[a] Tetanus–diphtheria.
[b] Measles–mumps–rubella.
[c] Influenza.
[d] Pneumococcal.
[e] Hepatitis B.
[f] Documentation of receipt of rubella vaccine or antibody titer is essential.
[g] Killed polio vaccine may be given to nonimmune parents of children scheduled to receive live oral polio vaccine.
[h] Indicated for women up to age 45; check rubella antibody titer. Mumps indicated for susceptible males. Measles indicated for persons born after 1956.
[i] MMR contraindicated during pregnancy.
[j] If mother is a chronic carrier of HBsAg, newborn should be protected by perinatal administration of hepatitis B immune globulin and hepatitis B vaccine.
[k] Response unpredictable.
[l] Chronic dialysis patients.

From the American College of Physicians[5] and the Centers for Disease Control,[6] with permission.

## References


1. Willems JS, Sanders CR. Cost–effectiveness and cost–benefits analysis of vaccines. J Infect Dis 1981;144:486–493.
2. Koplan JP, Axnick MW. Benefits, risks and costs of viral vaccines. Prog Med Virol 1982;28:180–191.
3. Edsall G. Immunoprophylaxis of bacterial diseases, in Gell PGH, Coombs RRA, Lachmann PJ (eds): Clinical Aspects of Immunology. Oxford, Blackwell Scientific, 1975, p 1601–1630.
4. Centers for Disease Control. Suboptimal response to hepatitis B vaccine given by injection into the buttock. MMWR 1985; 34:105–113.
5. American College of Physicians. Guide for Adult Immunization 1985, 1st ed. Philadelphia, American College of Physicians 1985, 72–76.
6. Centers for Disease Control. Adult immunization. Recommendations of the Immunization Practices Advisory Committee. MMWR 1984;33(15):265–285.
7. Milgrom F, Abeyounis CJ, Kano K. Principles of Immunological diagnosis in Medicine. Philadelphia, Lea and Febiger, 1981.
8. Beal AJ. Immunoprophylaxis of viral disease, in Gell PGH, Coombs RRA, Lachmann PJ (eds): Clinical Aspects of Immunology. Oxford, Blackwell Scientific, 1975, p 1631–1642.
9. Centers for Disease Control. Recommendation of the Immunization Practices Advisory Committee: diphtheria tetanus and pertussis. Guidelines for vaccine prophylaxis and other preventive measures. MMWR 1981;30:392–396, 401–407.
10. Middaugh JP. Side effects of diphtheria–tetanus toxoid in adults. Am J Public Health 1979;69:246–249.

11. Eckmann L. Active and passive tetanus immunization. N Engl J Med 1964;271:1087–1090.
12. American Academy of Pediatrics Committee on Infectious Disease. Hemophilus type B polysaccharide vaccine. Pediatrics 1985;76:322–324.
13. Centers for Disease Control. Polysaccharide vaccine for prevention of hemophilus influenza type B disease. MMWR 1985;34:201–205.
14. Kayhty H, Karanko V, Peltola H, et al. Serum antibodies after vaccination with hemophilus influenza type B capsular polysaccharide and responses to reimmunization: no evidence of immunologic tolerance or memory. Pediatrics 1984;74: 857–865.
15. Anderson P. The protective level of serum antibodies to the capsular polysaccharide of hemophilus influenza type B. J Infect Dis 1984;149:1034.
16. Lepow ML, Peter G, Glade M, et al. Response of infants to hemophilus influenza type B polysaccharide and diphtheria–tetanus–pertussis vaccines in combination. J Infect Dis 1984; 149:950–955.
17. Mead Johnson Nutrition Division. B-CAPSA I Vaccine product literature. Evansville, IN, April 1985.
18. Clemens JD, Chuong JJH, Feinstein AR. The BCG controversy: A methodological and statistical reappraisal. JAMA 1983;249:2362–2369.
19. Hart PDA, Sutherland I. BCG and the role of bacillus vaccines in the prevention of tuberculosis in adolescence and early adult life. Br Med J 1977;2:293–295.
20. U.S. Department of Health, Education, and Welfare. Status of immunization in tuberculosis in 1971: Report of a conference on progress to date, future trends and research needs. DHEW Publication No (NIH) 72–68, 1971.
21. Centers for Disease Control. Recommendations for protection against viral hepatitis. MMWR 1985;34:313–315.
22. Troisi C, Heiberg D, Hollinger F. Normal immune response to hepatitis B vaccine in patients with Down's syndrome: A basis for immunization guidelines. JAMA 1985;254:3196–3199.
23. Stevens C, Ater H, Taylor P, et al. Hepatitis B vaccine in patients receiving hemodialysis: Immunogenicity and efficacy. N Engl J Med 1984;311:496–501.
24. Barin F, Denis F, Cheron JP, et al. Immune response in neonates to hepatitis B vaccine. Lancet 1982;1:251–253.
25. Seeff L, Koff J. Passive and active immunoprophylaxis of hepatitis B. Gastroenterology 1984;86:958–981.
26. Tada H, Mosohiko Y, Mishira J, et al. Combined passive and active immunization for preventing perinatal transmission of hepatitis B virus carrier state. Pediatrics 1982;70:613–619.
27. Beasley R, Hwang L, Lee G, et al. Prevention of perinatally transmitted hepatitis B virus infections with hepatitis B immune globulin and hepatitis B vaccine. Lancet 1983;2:1099–1102.
28. Dienstag JL, Stevens CO, Bhan AK, et al. Hepatitis B vaccine administered to chronic carrier of hepatitis B surface antigen. Ann Intern Med 1982;96:575–579.
29. Prince AM, Semunness W, Mann M, et al. Hepatitis B immune globulin: Final report of a controlled multicenter trial of efficacy in prevention of dialysis-associated hepatitis. J Infect Dis 1978;137:131–144.
30. Seeff LB, Wright EC, Zimmerman H, et al. Type B hepatitis after needle-stick exposure: Prevention with hepatitis B immune globulin. Ann Intern Med 1978;88:285–293.
31. Frosner G, Frosner H, Dienhardt F, et al. Failure of hyperimmune serum globulin, given several days after exposure, to protect against hepatitis B. Lancet 1977;2:1023.
32. Masuko K, Mitsui T, Iwano K, et al. Factors influencing postexposure immunoprophylaxis of hepatitis B virus infection with hepatitis B immune globulin. Gastroenterology 1985;88: 151–155.
33. Grady GF, Lee VA. Hepatitis B immune globulin—prevention of hepatitis from accidental exposure among medical personnel. N Engl J Med 1975;293:1067–1070.
34. Perillo R, Campbell C, Strang S, et al. Immune globulin and hepatitis B immune globulin: Prophylactic measures for intimate contacts exposed to acute type B hepatitis. Arch Intern Med 1984;144:81–85.
35. LaMontagne JR, Noble GR, Quinnan GV, et al. Summary of clinical trials of inactivated influenza vaccine—1978. Rev Infect Dis 1983;5:723–736.
36. Gross RA, Ennis FA. Influenza vaccine: Split product versus whole virus types—how do they differ? N Engl J Med 1977; 296:567–568.
37. Waldman RH, Mann JJ, Small PA Jr. Immunization against influenza. Prevention of illness in man by aerosolized inactivated vaccine. JAMA 1969;207:520–524.
38. Hobson D, Curry RL, Beare AS. Hemagglutinin-inhibiting antibody titers as a measure of protection against influenza in man, in Perkins FT, Regamey RH (eds): Symposia Series in Immunological Standardization No. 20. Basel, S. Karger AG, 1973, pp 164–168.
39. Quinnan GV, Schooley R, Dolin R, et al. Serologic responses and systemic reactions in adults after vaccination with monovalent A/USSR/77 and trivalent A/USSR/77, A/Texas/77, B/Hong Kong/72 influenza vaccines. Rev Infect Dis 1983; 5:748–757.
40. Feery BJ, Evered MG, Morrison EI. Different protection rates in various groups of volunteers given subunit influenza virus vaccine in 1976. J Infect Dis 1979;139:237–241.
41. Monto AS, Davenport FM, Napier JA, et al. Modification of an outbreak of influenza in Tecumseh, Michigan by vaccination of schoolchildren. J Infect Dis 1970;122:16–25.
42. Patriarca PA, Weber JA, Parker RA, et al. Efficacy of influenza vaccine in nursing homes, reduction in illness and complications during an influenza B (H3N2) epidemic. JAMA 1985; 253:1136–1139.
43. Riddiough MA, Sisk JE, Bell JC. Influenza vaccination cost–effectiveness and public policy. JAMA 1983;249:3189–3195.
44. Cate TR, Caulh RB, Parker D, et al. Reactogenicity, immunogenicity, and antibody persistence in adults given inactivated influenza virus vaccines—1978. J Infect Dis 1983;5:737–747.
45. Centers for Disease Control: Recommendations of the Immunization Practices Advisory Committee (ACIP). Measles prevention. MMWR 1982;31:217–224, 229–231.
46. Linnemann CC, Dine MS, Roselle GH, et al. Measles immunity after revaccination: results in children vaccinated before 10 months of age. Pediatrics 1982;69:332–335.
47. Gold R, Lepow ML, Goldschneider I, et al. Kinetics of antibody production to group A and group C meningococcal polysaccharide vaccines administered during first 6 years of life: prospects for routine immunization of infants and children. J Infect Dis 1979;140:690–697.
48. Centers for Disease Control. Recommendations of the Immunization Practices Advisory Committee (ACIP). Meningococcal vaccines. MMWR 1985;34:255–256.
49. Binkin N, Bond J. Epidemic of meningococcal meningitis in Banako, Mali: epidemiological features and analysis of vaccine's efficacy. Lancet 1982;2:315–318.
50. Reingold A, Broome CV, Hightower AW, et al. Age-specific

differences in duration of clinical protection after vaccination with meningococcal polysaccharide A vaccine. Lancet 1985; 2:114–118.

51. Centers for Disease Control: Recommendations of the Immunization Practices Advisory Committee (ACIP). Mumps vaccine: Recommendation of the Immunization Practices Advisory Committee. MMWR 1982;31:617–620, 625.
52. Brunell PA, Brickman H, Steinberg S. Evaluation of a live attenuated mumps vaccine. Am J Dis Child 1969;118:435–440.
53. Cody CL, Baraff IJ, Cherry JD, et al. The nature and rate of adverse reactions associated with DTP and DT immunization in infants and children. Pediatrics 1981;68:650–660.
54. Miller DL, Ross EM, Alderslade R, et al. Pertussis immunization and serious acute neurological illness in children. Br Med J 1981;282:1595–1599.
55. Cherry JD. The epidemiology of pertussis and pertussis immunization in the United Kingdom and the U.S.: A comparative study. Curr Probl Pediatr 1984;14:7–77.
56. Leung A. Pertussis vaccine production. (Lett) Am J Dis Child 1985;139:9.
57. Johnstone T. Whooping cough in the United States and Britain. (Lett) N Engl J Med 1983;309:108–109.
58. Fulginitti VA. Pertussis vaccine. (Lett) Am J Dis Child 1984;183:890–891.
59. Centers for Disease Control. Pertussis surveillance, 1979–1981. MMWR 1982;31:333–335.
60. Fedson D, Chiarello L. Previous hospital care and pneumococcal bacteremia: Importance for pneumococcal immunization. Arch Intern Med 1983;143:885–889.
61. Centers for Disease Control. Pertussis—United States, 1982–1983. MMWR 1984;33:573–575.
62. Centers for Disease Control. Supplementary statement of contraindications to receipt of pertussis vaccine. MMWR 1984;33:169–171.
63. Hirschman J, Lipsky B. Pneumococcal vaccine in the United States. JAMA 1981;246:1428–1431.
64. American Academy of Pediatrics. Recommendations for using pneumococcal vaccine in children. Pediatrics 1985;75:1153–1157.
65. Smit P, Oberholzer D, Hayden-Smith S, et al. Protective efficacy of pneumococcal polysaccharide vaccines. JAMA 1977;238:2613–2616.
66. Hilleman M, Carlson A, McLean A, et al. *Streptococcus pneumoniae* polysaccharide vaccine: Age and dose responses, safety, persistence of antibody, revaccination, and simultaneous administration of pneumococcal and influenza vaccines. Rev Infect Dis 1981;3:S31–S42.
67. Schwartz JS. Pneumococcal vaccine: Clinical efficacy and effectiveness. Ann Intern Med 1982;96:208–220.
68. Broome C. Efficacy of pneumococcal polysaccharide vaccines. Infect Dis 1981;3(suppl):S82–S96.
69. Bolan G, Broome C, Facklam R, et al. Pneumococcal vaccine efficacy in selected populations in the United States. Ann Intern Med 1986;104:1–6.
70. Ammann A, Addiego J, Wara D, et al. Polyvalent pneumococcal-polysaccharide immunization of patients with sickle cell anemia and patients with splenectomy. N Engl J Med 1977; 297:897–900.
71. Howie V, Ploussard J, Sloyer J, et al. Use of pneumococcal polysaccharide vaccine in preventing otitis media in infants: Different results between racial groups. Pediatrics 1984; 73:79–81.
72. Bentley D, Ha K, Mamot K, et al. Pneumococcal vaccine in the institutionalized elderly: Design of a nonrandomized trial and preliminary results. Rev Infect Dis 1981;3(suppl):S71–S81.
73. Bentley D. Pneumococcal vaccine in the institutionalized elderly: Review of past and recent studies. Rev Infect Dis 1981;3:S61–S70.
74. Williams J, Moser K. Pneumococcal vaccine and patients with chronic lung disease. Ann Intern Med 1986;104:106–109.
75. American Hospital Formulary Service Drug Information '86. Bethesda, MD, American Society of Hospital Pharmacists, pp 1714–1718.
76. Centers for Disease Control: Recommendations of the Immunization Practices Advisory Committee (ACIP). Rabies prevention—United States, 1984. MMWR 1984;33:393–402, 407–408.
77. Ajjan M, Soulebat JP, Triau R, et al. Intradermal immunization with rabies vaccine: Inactivated Wistar strain cultivated in human diploid cells. JAMA 1980;244:2528–2531.
78. Bernhard KW, Roberts MA, Samner J, et al. Human diploid cell rabies vaccine: Effectiveness of immunization with small intradermal or subcutaneous doses. JAMA 1982;247:1138–1142.
79. Centers for Disease Control. Field evaluation of pre-exposure use of human diploid cell rabies vaccine. MMWR 1983;32: 601–603.
80. Centers for Disease Control. Systemic allergic reactions following immunization with human diploid cell rabies vaccine. MMWR 1984;33:185–187.
81. Pappaioanou M, Fishbein D, Dreesen D, et al. Antibody response to pre-exposure human diploid cell rabies vaccine given concurrently with chloroquine. N Engl J Med 1986; 314:280–284.
82. Nicholson KG, Turner GS, Aoki EY. Immunization with a human diploid cell strain of rabies virus vaccine: Two-year results. J Infect Dis 1978;137:783–788.
83. Bahmanyar M, Fayaz A, Nour-Salehi S, et al. Successful protection of humans exposed to rabies infection: Post-exposure treatment with the new human diploid cell rabies vaccine and antirabies serum. JAMA 1976;236:2751–2754.
84. Greaves WI, Orenstein WA, Hinman AZ, et al. Clinical efficacy of rubella vaccine. Pediatr Infect Dis 1983;2:284–286.
85. Centers for Disease Control: Recommendations of the Immunization Practices Advisory Committee (ACIP). Rubella prevention. MMWR 1984;33:301–310.
86. Centers for Disease Control: Recommendations of the Immunization Practices Advisory Committee (ACIP). Rubella prevention. MMWR 1984;33:315–318.
87. Centers for Disease Control. Rubella vaccination during pregnancy—United States, 1971–82. MMWR 1983;32:429–432.
88. Polk EF, Madlen JR, White JA, et al. A controlled comparison of joint reactions among women receiving one or two rubella vaccines. Am J Epidemiol 1982;115:19–25.
89. Centers for Disease Control. Recommendation of the Immunization Practices Advisory Committee: Smallpox vaccine. MMWR 1980;29:35.
90. Gershon A. Immunoprophylaxis of varicella-zoster infections. Am J Med 1984;76:672–677.
91. Gershon A, Steinberg S, Geld L, et al. Live attenuated varicella vaccine: Efficacy for children with leukemia in remission. JAMA 1984;252:355–362.
92. Weibel R, Neff B, Kuter B, et al. Live attenuated varicella vaccine: Efficacy trial in healthy children. N Engl J Med 1984;310:1409–1415.
93. Arbeter A, Starr S, Weibel R, et al. Live attenuated varicella vaccine: The KMcC strain in healthy children. Pediatrics 1983;71:307–312.
94. Berger R, Leuscher D, Just M. Enhancement of varicella-

zoster–specific immune responses in the elderly by boosting with varicella vaccine. J Infect Dis 1984;149:647.

**95.** McIntosh K. Varicella vaccine: Decisions a little nearer. N Engl J Med 1984;310:1456–1457.

**96.** Zaia JA, Lewis MJ, Wright GG, et al. A practical method for preparation of varicella-zoster immune globulin. J Infect Dis 1978;137:601–604.

**97.** Centers for Disease Control. Recommendations of the Immunization Practices Advisory Committee (ACIP). Varicella-zoster immune globulin for the prevention of chicken pox. MMWR 1984;33:84–90.

**98.** Committee on Infectious Diseases. Expanded guidelines for use of varicella-zoster immune globulin. Pediatrics 1983; 72:886–889.

**99.** Zaia JA, Levin NJ, Preblud SR, et al. Evaluation of varicella-zoster immune globulin: Protection of immunosuppressed children after household exposure to varicella. J Infect Dis 1983;147:737–743.

**100.** Gershon AA. Immunoprophylaxis of varicella-zoster infection. Am J Med 1984;76:672–677.

**101.** Orenstein WA, Heyman D, Ellis R. Prophylaxis of varicella in high-risk children: Dose–response effect of zoster immune globulin. J Pediatr 1981;98:368–373.

**102.** Cohn E, Strong L, Hues W. Preparation and properties of serum plasma proteins. IV: A system for the separation into fractions of the protein and lipoprotein components of biological tissues and fluids. J Am Chem Soc 1946;68:459–675.

**103.** Smith GM, Mollison D, Griffiths B, et al. Uptake of IgG after intramuscular and subcutaneous injection. Lancet 1972;1: 1208–1212.

**104.** Morell A, Schurch B, Ryser D, et al. In vivo behavior of gammaglobulin preparations. Vox Sang 1980;38:272–283.

**105.** Ochs HD, Fischer SH, Wedgwood RJ, et al. Comparison of high-dose and low-dose intravenous immunoglobulin therapy in patients with primary immunodeficiency diseases. Am J Med 1984;76:78–82.

**106.** Cosimi AB. The clinical value of antilymphocyte antibodies. Transplant Proc 1981;13:462–468.

**107.** Butt KMH, Zielinski CM, Parsa I, et al. Trends in immunosuppression for kidney transplantation. Kidney Int 1978; 13(suppl 8):595–598.

**108.** Hardy MD, Nowygrod R, Elberg A, et al. Use of ATG in treatment of steroid-resistant rejection. Transplantation 1980; 29:162–164.

**109.** Pirofsky B, Reid R, Bardana E. Myasthenia gravis treated with purified antithymocyte antiserum. Neurology 1979;29:112–116.

**110.** Mertin J, Knight S, Rudge P. Double-blinded controlled trial of immunosuppression in treatment of multiple sclerosis. Lancet 1980;2:949–951.

**111.** Centers for Disease Control. Health Information for International Travel, Atlanta, GA, CDC, 1985.

**112.** Hook E. *Salmonella* species (including typhoid fever), in Mandell GL, Douglas RG, Bennett JE (eds): Principles and Practice of Infectious Diseases, New York, John Wiley and Sons, 1985, p 1265.

**113.** Centers for Disease Control. Postexposure prophylaxis of hepatitis B. MMWR 1984;33:285.

# Chapter 91 / Principles and Management of the Acquired Immunodeficiency Syndrome

Teresa A. Tartaglione, PharmD, and Ann C. Collier, MD

The acquired immunodeficiency syndrome (AIDS) was initially recognized in the late seventies but formally introduced to the medical community as a distinct clinical entity in 1981. AIDS affects previously healthy individuals and is characterized by profound immunologic deficiencies, multiple opportunistic infections, and uncommon forms of malignant neoplasms.[1–4] Over the last 5 years, more than 50,000 individuals in the United States have been diagnosed with AIDS, with the number still increasing and projected to reach 196,000 by 1991.[5] Much concern and alarm have been generated, as the disease appears to be approaching epidemic proportions, no cure has been found, and there is a high mortality rate. A retrovirus related to the human T-cell leukemia/lymphoma virus, human immunodeficiency virus (HIV) [originally called human T lymphotropic virus type III (HTLV-III) or lymphadenopathy-associated virus (LAV)], has been firmly implicated as the cause of AIDS.[6–8] Various means are now used to characterize patients with manifestations of HIV infection, and to describe their signs, symptoms, and laboratory phenomena. A large number of persons with serologic evidence of HIV infection may not manifest symptoms. Others may develop persistent generalized lymphadenopathy, constitutional symptoms, neurologic disease, or overt AIDS (defined by the appearance of an opportunistic infection or related malignancy). Several populations at risk for HIV infection have been identified, including homosexual males, intravenous drug abusers, hemophiliacs, and sexual partners of persons in these groups. Evidence strongly suggests that this retrovirus is transmitted by sexual contact and by contact with contaminated blood or blood-related products. Transmission of HIV between heterosexuals has been observed.[9] The number of sexual partners may be an important factor in the identification of either male or female patients at risk for HIV infection. Unfortunately, fear of catching AIDS and a lack of understanding of the disease have precipitated a general alarm throughout the United States, both in the general population and in medical communities. The availability of blood tests to detect the presence of antibodies to HIV is a major advancement. The terminologies and criteria for diagnosis of HIV infection are changing; consequently, caution should be used when a patient is given a diagnosis of HIV infection. It must be emphasized that not all patients with HIV infection have AIDS or will develop the disease in future years.

All treatments to date have been unsuccessful in eradicating HIV, although a few therapies have been able to suppress viral replication in vivo and one treatment, zidovudine (formerly azidothymidine, AZT), has been shown to prolong survival in patients with AIDS. Current treatments are being directed at four areas: HIV infection, associated opportunistic infections and neoplasms, and immune reconstitution. Research has concentrated on finding agents to eradicate HIV and to counteract the immunodeficiency caused by HIV. This chapter provides a thorough discussion of treatment modalities, with emphasis placed on management of infectious diseases secondary to infection with HIV.

## Epidemiology

The number of cases of overt AIDS in the United States (meeting the surveillance definition of the Centers for Disease Control) has continued to increase, with greater than 50,000 reported as of March, 1988.[10] Initial mortality following diagnosis of AIDS is about 50%, although the ultimate mortality approaches 100%.[11] The CDC estimates that up to one million persons in the United States were infected by HIV as of mid-1985, and it is likely that this number will continue to increase.[12]

Seroepidemiologic studies have demonstrated increasing prevalence of antibodies to HIV in homosexual men and other high-risk populations in the United States and elsewhere.[13] Studies have indicated that of homosexual men infected with HIV, approximately 5% to 20% will develop AIDS within 2 to 5 years after initial infection, whereas a much larger percentage will remain asymptomatic during this time.[14,15] Ongoing studies of homosexual men with persistent generalized lymphadenopathy (PGL) suggest that 5% to 30% may develop overt AIDS within 2 to 3 years.[14,16] Among a large cohort of homosexual men not selected for AIDS-related conditions, 6.4% of the seropositive subjects had developed overt AIDS and 26% had developed signs attributable to HIV during a median follow-up interval of 61 months.[13] During the first few years after infection, the ratio of infected individuals to AIDS patients may be at least 100:1. In ongoing cohort studies, the development of overt AIDS in HIV-infected persons was highly correlated with the duration of seropositivity.[17] This lengthy lag phase between infection with HIV and diagnosis of AIDS has worrisome implications for people with antibodies against HIV. Equal numbers of cases were diagnosed in 1986 as were from 1978 to 1985.

Every state in the United States has reported at least one case of AIDS, although the majority of cases have been reported from New York City, San Francisco, Los Angeles, Miami, and Newark. Most recently, the number of cases being reported outside of these major cities has increased. It has been suggested that there are three major endemic areas for AIDS including the United States, Equatorial Africa, and Haiti. The syndrome has also been reported in most European countries,[18] as well as in China and Japan.

It must be assumed that any sexual practice involving exchange of body fluids could potentially transmit HIV. Explanations for the higher prevalence of HIV infection and AIDS among homosexual males include the practices of anonymous sex with large number of sexual partners and frequent receptive anal intercourse and "fisting." A number of other risk factors may be associated with the increased incidence in this group including the increased risk of other sexually transmitted diseases (e.g., herpes virus and cytomegalovirus) which are associated with subclinical immunologic alterations.[19] Seminal plasma is a likely means of transmission of the retrovirus.[20,21] The likelihood of contracting HIV infection through contact with only tears or saliva appears to be minimal.

In the United States, persons developing overt AIDS have been mostly males (90%) and frequently homosexual/bisexual (71%) or drug abusers (17%).[22] The majority of AIDS patients are 20–50 years old, and most patients are in the third decade of life. Fewer than 10% of cases are women, 52% of whom are known drug abusers. Cases have been reported in all racial groups; 60% have been reported in Caucasians, 25% in blacks, and 15% in Hispanics. The relative risk appears to be highest in blacks. Approximately 10% of patients in the United States, including Haitians with no other risk factors, fall into none of the aforementioned groups. A list of expanded risk groups is shown in Table 91.1. AIDS has also been reported in at least 750 infants and children. Approximately 75% of children with AIDS had a parent in a high-risk group. The racial and sexual distribution of pediatric AIDS cases is different from that of adult cases: 50% of pediatric patients are black; the remainder are equally divided between Caucasian and Hispanic races.[23] Approximately half of children with AIDS are females. The implicated routes of transmission for pediatric AIDS include congenital and perinatal contact and contaminated transfusions. Increasing evidence suggests that infants contract the disease in utero.[24–26] The vaginal canal may be a source of HIV transmission. Transmission of HIV through artificial insemination has also been reported.[27]

Drug abusers (particularly of cocaine and heroin) who have no other concomitant risk factors are at high risk for AIDS. The practice of sharing blood-contaminated needles and syringes is the presumed mode of transmission. Other risk groups include the heterosexual partners of HIV-infected bisexual males, and hemophiliacs or recipients of HIV-contaminated blood products. Few female prostitutes have developed AIDS thus far in the United States.

Approximately 4% of reported cases of AIDS are presumed to be caused by heterosexual transmission, with the majority of these in women who have contracted the virus from infected men. Among the few men who have thus far contracted HIV from women, there appears to be a high incidence of association with prostitutes.[28]

Casual contact with AIDS patients (e.g., as occurs with household contacts, health care personnel) does not appear to be a significant risk factor. A number of studies have shown the lack of nonsexual household transmission of HIV infection among adults, children, and friends in close contact with AIDS or AIDS-related complex (ARC) patients.[29]

**Table 91.1** Risk Factors for Seropositivity to Human Immunodeficiency Virus (HIV)

| *Risk group and factors* | *Direction of association with HIV seropositivity* |
|---|---|
| Homosexual men | |
| Number of partners | ↑ |
| Receptive anal intercourse | ↑ |
| Homosexual contact in high-risk area | ↑ |
| Parenteral drug user | |
| Proximity to endemic region | ↑ |
| Frequent injections | ↑ |
| Hemophiliacs | |
| Dose of factor concentrate | ↑ |
| Noncommercial plasma product | ↓ |
| Blood recipients | |
| Number of blood transfusions | ↑ |
| Donor from risk group | ↑ |
| Other groups[a] | |
| Heterosexual contact with risk group member | ↑ |
| Number of heterosexual contacts | ↑ |
| Frequent prostitute contact | ↑ |
| Blood transfusion | ↑ |
| Needle-stick exposure | ↑ |
| Parent from risk group | ↑ |

[a] Haitians, Africans, heterosexual patients from the United States, and family members.

From Blatner WA et al: Ann Intern Med 1985;103:665–670, with permission.

Since August 1983, the CDC has been following prospectively health care workers with documented parenteral or mucous membrane exposure to blood or other body fluids of patients with definite or suspected AIDS. More than 2,500 health care workers have been enrolled (76% needle-stick injuries) and are to be followed for at least 3 years.[30] Thus far, 15 health care workers in non–high risk groups have become seropositive for HIV and 1 participant has developed AIDS; all had occupational exposure to blood.[10] Several other studies assessing over 1,100 health care workers have also shown low transmission rates; only one homosexual male worker seroconverted during follow-up.[31,32]

Guidelines to be followed by health care workers have been adopted by the CDC.[33]

## Etiology

AIDS has been recognized by different research groups to be caused by a novel retrovirus, known variously as human T lymphotropic virus type III (HTLV-III), lymphadenopathy-associated virus (LAV), and AIDS-associated retrovirus (ARV).[6–8] Characterization of the genomes of HTLV-III,

LAV, and ARV by nucleotide sequencing and restriction enzyme analysis has demonstrated that they are variants of the same virus.[34–37] The term *HIV* has now been adopted as the official name for this virus.

The pathogenesis of this disease is not completely understood, although our understanding is increasing. It would appear that HIV begins its assault on the host's immune system through direct attachment to specific receptors on a subpopulation of T lymphocytes (T4).[38,39] Monocytes/macrophages may also become infected. Upon entering the lymphocyte, the virus is uncoated and viral RNA is acted on by reverse transcriptase, an enzyme found in the core of the virus, and a single-stranded DNA is formed (see Fig. 91.1). This is a reversal of classic dogma in which the process of transferring genetic information is unidirectional from DNA to RNA. Single-stranded DNA is then copied into a double-stranded DNA. The virus DNA genome either becomes integrated into the cell genome or remains extrachromosomal. The virus may remain latent, or the DNA may subsequently be transcribed to messenger RNA and translated into viral proteins. All infected cells may not produce infectious virus. When the DNA is transcribed and proteins are produced the completed virus, after assembly in the cytoplasm, buds off the modified cell membrane and becomes coated with a lipid envelope. The virus may infect another cell. The discovery of the heterogenicity of certain parts of the viral genome implies a rapid mutation rate which may increase the challenge of vaccine development.[40]

Once a cell is infected, the cell may lyse/die or replicate with the latent viral genes present within the normal cell genes. The viral (HIV) infected cells may evolve into cancer cells or lead to changes in the expression of other cellular genes resulting in the pathologic effects of the virus.[41] There may be other mechanisms by which retroviruses induce disease (e.g., autoimmune).

Gallo and associates originally isolated the virus from 30% to 48% of peripheral blood lymphocytes in patients with the full-blown syndrome and 86% of patients with ARC who were seropositive.[6] The low isolation rate in the former group was attributed to very low T-cell counts (specifically T4), thus making isolation difficult. More recent work has suggested that virtually 100% of patients with documented AIDS and ARC have HIV infection.[42]

HIV has been cultured from a variety of body fluids and tissues, including blood, lymphocytes, plasma, cerebrospinal fluid, semen, saliva, tears, urine, cervical secretions, and breast milk.[6–8,20,21,43–48] Although limited data regarding culture positivity in seropositive persons have been reported, HIV has been isolated from the blood of 50% to 80% of persons with AIDS, ARC, and PGL, and asymptomatic seropositive homosexual men.[6,8,49–50]

In summary, several significant findings strongly suggest that HIV is causally associated with the acquired immunodeficiency syndrome and its related complex: (1) its absolute connection with these diseases despite its relatively rare occurrence in nature, (2) its in vitro biologic effect on immune cells, and (3) consistent isolation of the virus from patients with AIDS or ARC and from high-risk donors. Based upon analogies with known animal retroviruses and limited data in humans, it is suspected that infection with this virus is lifelong.

With the viral etiology of AIDS established and the availability of screening tests to detect antibodies against HIV, there has been much controversy over screening outside the blood bank setting. Of critical importance is the development of a test that is both sensitive and specific so as to minimize false-negative and false-positive results, respectively. The current commercial enzyme-linked immunosorbent assays (ELISAs) are excellent for detecting HIV antibody, although there will be occasional false-negative and false-positive results.[51] Currently licensed tests (including Abbott, Electro-Nucleonics, Litton) to detect antibody to HIV range in sensitivity from 93% to 99%, and are all above 99% in specificity.[51] The Western blot or radioimmunoprecipitation assay (RIP) is useful as a confirmatory assay. One problem in the development of a screening test surrounds the widely variable prevalence of HIV in different populations. Some have suggested that different cutoffs of the ELISA be used in populations with greatly differing disease prevalence. The lack of wide availability of the HIV culture against which to evaluate a positive antibody test coupled with the long "incubation period" makes it very difficult to determine which patients among those who are seropositive will develop clinical disease.

## Clinical Presentation

### *Immunologic Alterations and Laboratory Abnormalities*

HIV is an infection that attacks the immune system, and a wide number of immunologic abnormalities have been described in persons with full-blown AIDS (Table 91.2).[52–53] Although the diagnosis of AIDS cannot be made solely on immunologic evidence, a distinct immunologic pattern has emerged, especially in patients with the full-blown syndrome. A persistent quantitative decrease in the T4-lymphocyte subpopulation and functional depression in other lymphocyte populations have been observed. The cell surface of the T4 molecule is a receptor for HIV.[38,39]

Before discussion of the details of the immunologic abnormalities, a review of T-cell differentiation and function is useful. In the initial developmental stages of T cells, both T4 and T8 antigens are expressed simultaneously on the same cell. Later in development, T cells express either the T4 or the T8 antigen; occasionally, neither or both are expressed. Functionally speaking, T4 cells have been commonly called "helper" cells, whereas T8 cells are associated with suppressor activity; however, more correctly it must be recognized that T4 cells are heterogeneous and may be cytotoxic cells as well as suppressor inducer and effector cells. Accordingly, T8 cells occasionally "help" or amplify the interaction of T4 cells with B cells. Abnormalities in the number of either T4 or T8 cells can be associated with abnormalities in the cognitive functions of T cells and may be associated with in vitro evidence of immuno-incompetence. Patients with HIV infection show decreased numbers of T4 cells, increased T8 cells, and decreased T4:T8 ratios. The absolute number of T4 cells is often negligible. Usually there are twice as many T8 cells as T4 cells. HIV may reduce the number of detectable T4 cells either through direct lysis or by blocking the CD4 receptor (on the T cell) such that the cell becomes unrecognizable.

**Table 91.2** Immunologic Abnormalities in AIDS

I. Abnormalities that characterize the syndrome
 1. Lymphopenia
 2. Selective T-cell deficiency based on a quantitative reduction within the antigenic subset designated by T4 or Leu 3 monoclonal antibodies
 3. Decreased or absent delayed-type cutaneous hypersensitivity to both recall and new antigens
 4. Elevated serum immunoglobulins, predominantly IgG and IgA in adults and including IgM in children
 5. Increased spontaneous immunoglobulin secretion by individual B lymphocytes

II. Consistently observed abnormalities
 1. Decreased in vitro lymphocyte proliferative responses
  a. Mitogens
  b. Antigens
  c. Alloantigens; autoantigens
 2. Decreased cytotoxic responses
  a. Natural killer cells
  b. Cell-mediated cytotoxicity (T-cell)
 3. Decreased ability to mount a de novo antibody response to a new antigen
 4. Altered monocyte function
 5. Elevated serum levels of immune complexes

III. Other reported abnormalities
 1. Increased levels of acid-labile $\alpha$-interferon
 2. Antilymphocyte antibodies
 3. Suppressor factors
 4. Increased levels of $\beta_2$-microglobulin and $\alpha_1$-thymosin; decreased serum thymulin levels

From Seligmann M et al: N Engl J Med 1984;311:1286–1292, with permission.

Functional abnormalities of T lymphocytes in HIV-infected patients with AIDS are numerous. Pure T-cell mitogens, pure B-cell stimuli, and mixed T- and B-cell stimuli are depressed.[54–59] T4 cells are markedly deficient in their ability to alter pokeweed mitogen–induced immunoglobulin secretion. Decreased responses to soluble protein antigens (e.g., tetanus toxoid) are the result of quantitative and qualitative deficiencies within this lymphocyte subset. Natural killer cell activity, cytomegalovirus-specific cytotoxicity, and cytotoxic T-cell responses are frequently abnormal. Diminished lymphokine production and decreased ability to provide help to B lymphocytes for immunoglobulin production have also been reported.[53]

B-cell lymphocytes also do not function normally in AIDS patients. There is often a depressed response to pure B-cell mitogens, as well as an inability to mount a response to new antigens.[59] There is spontaneous secretion of immunoglobulin, increased spontaneous proliferation, elevated circulatory immune complexes, and numerous autoimmune phenomena. Finally, monocyte and macrophage function (e.g., chemotaxis) is also abnormal in AIDS patients.[60]

Of more clinical relevance is the observation that most patients with AIDS are anergic. Regardless of the mechanism, the patient with AIDS has inadequate immune responsiveness to specific antigens. Characteristically, they present with a moderate anemia (hemoglobin of 7–12 g/dL), moderate leukopenia (1,000–3,000/mm$^3$), and moderate thrombocytopenia.[53] Antiplatelet antibodies can sometimes be found regardless of the platelet count. Lymphocyte counts are frequently less than 1,200/mm$^3$ with a disproportionate decrease in T lymphocytes compared with B lymphocytes; the ratio of T4 to T8 cells is less than 1.2 and often is close to zero.

The clinical manifestations of AIDS stem from an immune system that has been critically impaired because of a selective infection of the T4-cell subset by HIV and the multiple subsequent immunologic changes just described. The deficiencies discussed before appear to be most pronounced in patients who have had opportunistic infections, whereas immunologic abnormalities are often minimal in patients at diagnosis of Kaposi's sarcoma.[52] Maintaining immunoregulation appears to be critical in the prevention of clinical manifestations of HIV infection. Several approaches are currently under investigation in an attempt to restore the immune system in AIDS patients: wholesale immune replacement, biologics intended to boost immune function, and anti-retroviral therapy. A complete review of immunologic treatment will not be addressed in this chapter but may be found elsewhere.[61] Anti-HIV agents are discussed later.

### *Manifestations*

The clinical manifestations of infection with HIV are now recognized to include a broad spectrum of conditions, including an asymptomatic state, an acute mononucleosis-like syndrome, PGL, and severe cellular immunodeficiency complicated by multiple infections and malignancies.[6–8,16,21,42] AIDS-related complex has been used to describe individuals with HIV infection who have constitutional symptoms or signs (e.g., persistent fever, night sweats, weight loss, or PGL) and immunodeficiency without documented systemic opportunistic infection or related malignancies. Some of the AIDS-associated opportunistic infections are infections of the central nervous system (CNS), but CNS complications attributable to HIV may also occur,[62,63] and increasing evidence suggests that HIV may be neurotropic as well as lymphotropic.[64]

The explanation for the diversity of clinical symptoms and signs found in persons infected with HIV is unknown. Hypotheses have implicated possible roles for repeated exposure to HIV or other infectious cofactors (e.g., cytomegalovirus, Epstein–Barr virus, hepatitis B virus), noninfectious cofactors (e.g., anal exposure to semen), the state of the immune system at the time of exposure to HIV, and variations intrinsic to the virus itself. The natural history of these various clinical states is not yet completely characterized.

The signs and symptoms in the patient with AIDS are often nonspecific, but are often due to infectious or neoplastic complications in addition to the virus itself. Clinical presentation of HIV infection varies. A patient may appear to be asymptomatic but may demonstrate lymphopenia, a depressed T4:T8 cell ratio, cutaneous anergy, and reduced in vitro immunologic responses to various antigens and mitogens. Another patient may present with respiratory failure from *P. carinii* infection or with disseminated Kaposi's sarcoma. Other patients complain of ill-defined persistent constitutional symptoms suggestive of a chronic viral illness, or a variety of symptoms involving the pulmonary, gastrointestinal, or central nervous systems. Some individuals develop generalized lymphadenopathy (usually anterior or posterior cervical, and axillary) with or without constitutional symptoms. Another presentation may be that of a single mucocutaneous lesion of Kaposi's sarcoma in the absence of any systemic symptoms. Of patients reported to the CDC, *P. carinii* pneumonia accounts for 51% of primary AIDS diagnoses; 26% of patients have Kaposi's sarcoma; 8% have both the pneumonia and Kaposi's sarcoma; and 15% have other opportunistic infections without *P. carinii* pneumonia or Kaposi's sarcoma.[75] Although the varied clinical presentations of HIV infection in children are similar in many respects to those in adults, a separate discussion of presenting manifestations is warranted.

Virtually all reported cases of HIV-related illnesses in children have presented with unexplained physical signs (presented in order of their reported frequency): hepatomegaly, failure to thrive and weight loss, unexplained fever, splenomegaly, unexplained lymphadenopathy, low birth weight (in prenatally exposed infants), eczema, and parotitis.[66,67] Unexplained laboratory findings have included anemia, a high frequency of hypergammaglobulinemia, altered mononuclear cell function, and altered T-cell subset ratios. Many children with HIV infections have an unexplained lymphocytic interstitial pneumonitis without evidence of *P. carinii* or other pathogens on lung biopsy.[66–68] Some children have presented with progressive, unexplained, neurologic deterioration, including late-onset seizures, loss of developmental milestones, cessation of brain growth, and diffuse, unexplained encephalopathy.[67] A history of recurrent or persistent bacterial, viral, or fungal infections, including some children who have presented with chronic, subclinical infections with a slowly progressive course, has been observed. Included in this group are children with recurrent bacterial sepsis, meningitis, and chronic otitis media, and children with chronic oral candidiasis and possibly disseminated histoplasmosis.[66–68] The current pediatric AIDS definition excludes children with congenital or perinatally acquired cytomegalovirus. Other children have presented with unexplained immune thrombocytopenia and neutropenia.[69] A few children with transfusion-associated infections have been reported to have had a recognizable, acute clinical syndrome (compatible with a neonatal "viral" infection in infants and a "mononucleosis-like syndrome" in older children) in the immediate posttransfusion period, as has been reported in adults.[69] In part, because of reporting bias, the majority of children reported with HIV infections have had opportunistic infections with the organisms seen most often in adults, especially *P. carinii* and *Mycobacterium avium-intracellulare*.[67] Bacterial infections, including *Streptococcus pneumoniae*, *Salmonella* sp., and *Mycobacterium tuberculosis* may be more prevalent in children with AIDS than in adults with the disease. Kaposi's sarcoma is rare in children.

**Table 91.3** Summary of Classification System for Human Immunodeficiency Virus Infection

| | |
|---|---|
| Group I | Acute infection |
| Group II | Asymptomatic infection[a] |
| Group III | Persistent generalized lymphadenopathy[a] |
| Group IV | Other disease |
| Subgroup A | Constitutional disease |
| Subgroup B | Neurologic disease |
| Subgroup C | Secondary infectious diseases |
| Category C-1 | Specified secondary infectious diseases listed in the CDC surveillance definition for AIDS[b] |
| Category C-2 | Other specified secondary infectious diseases |
| Subgroup D | Secondary cancers[b] |
| Subgroup E | Other conditions |

[a] Patients in groups II and III may be subclassified on the basis of a laboratory evaluation.

[b] Includes those patients whose clinical presentation fulfills the definition of the acquired immunodeficiency syndrome (AIDS) used by the Centers for Disease Control (CDC) for national reporting.

Several schemes have been proposed to stratify HIV infection into different categories, some of which are subdivided further.[70–72] One such scheme characterizing adult HIV infection is illustrated in Table 91.3.

### *Infectious Complications*

The spectrum of infectious diseases and the etiologic agents commonly observed in AIDS patients are shown in Table 91.4. Most of the pathogens listed have been associated with other immunosuppressed populations, although the frequency and pattern of infection are quite unique within the AIDS group. The prevalence of *P. carinii* in AIDS is probably 35% to 60% per year compared with less than 2% in childhood acute lymphocytic leukemia.[73] Disseminated *Mycobacterium avium-intracellulare* is common, although its pathogenicity is controversial. Oral candidiasis and esophagitis are almost universal in this patient population. Disseminated cytomegalovirus, especially with retinitis, has been

**Table 91.4** Microorganisms Causing Opportunistic Infections in Patients With AIDS

| | *Syndrome* | *Comments* |
|---|---|---|
| Viruses | | |
| Cytomegalovirus | Encephalitis, chorioretinitis, pneumonia, hepatitis, colitis, adrenalitis, disseminated infection | Found in almost all patients; liver, lungs, and colon frequent sites of severe disease; and biopsy usually needed to document. Responsible for clinical adrenal insufficiency. Characteristic chorioretinitis. |
| Herpes simplex virus | Persistent, recurrent, or disseminated skin ulcers | Herpes simplex virus type-2 perineal lesions are frequently an early occurrence; respond to antiviral therapy but recur. |
| Varicella zoster | Local, severe, or disseminated infection | Tends to recur. |
| Epstein–Barr virus | Lymphoma | Aggressive B-cell lymphomas seen, including central nervous system lesions. |
| Papovavirus-JC | Central nervous system infection | Progressive multifocal leukoencephalopathy is one of the major central nervous system diseases. |
| Adenoviruses | Colonization<br>Disseminated infection | Regularly isolated, rarely cause symptomatic disease; high serotypes similar to those of bone marrow transplant recipients. |
| Bacteria | | |
| Commonly taking advantage of T-cell defects | | |
| *Mycobacterium avium-intracellulare* | Disseminated infection, severe gastrointestinal disease, massive intraabdominal lymphadenopathy | Usually serovar 4, remarkably heavy infection. Isolated regularly from blood and seen on acid-fast stain of stool. Portal of entry appears to be gastrointestinal tract. Poor response to therapy. |
| *Mycobacterium tuberculosis* | Adenitis, pulmonary infection, meningitis | Variable presentation. Responds to therapy. Some strains may be resistant. |
| *Mycobacterium species* | Disseminated infection | Usually accompanies other life-threatening infection. |
| *Nocardia asteroides* | Pulmonary–pericardial infection, brain abscess | Accompanies other opportunistic infection. |
| *Salmonella* species | Typhoidal syndrome, severe gastroenteritis with bacteremia | Recurs. |
| *Listeria monocytogenes* | Bacteremia | Responds promptly to therapy. |
| *Legionella* species | Pneumonias, cellulitis | Especially severe. |
| Commonly taking advantage of B-cell defects | | |
| *Streptococcus pneumoniae* | Pneumonia, bacteremia | Responds promptly to therapy. |
| *Hemophilus influenzae* | Pneumonia, bacteremia | May cause diffuse infiltrates resembling pneumocystosis. |
| Reasons uncertain | | |
| *Staphylococcus aureus* | Bacteremia, skin infections, pneumonia | Pneumonias complicate pneumocystosis in patients with Kaposi's sarcoma. |
| *Clostridium perfringens* | Bacteremia | Mild abdominal complaints. Transient. Secondary to Kaposi's sarcoma lesions of bowel? |
| *Shigella* species | Diarrhea, bacteremia | Persistent and recurrent. |
| Parasites | | |
| *Pneumocystis carinii* | Pneumonia | Often large numbers of organisms seen, toluidine blue on bronchoalveolar lavage fluid an effective stain in our experience; prolonged therapy advisable ($\geq$ 3 wk). |
| *Toxoplasma gondii* | Encephalitis, brain abscess | Brain abscess and encephalitis common; antibody response may be poor, especially IgM; prolonged therapy necessary. |
| *Cryptosporidium* species | Gastroenteritis | Illness varies from mild, self-limited diarrhea to cholera-like syndrome, unresponsive to any therapy; organisms seen by acid-fast stain or sucrose flotation. |

**Table 91.4** Microorganisms Causing Opportunistic Infections in Patients With AIDS (*Continued*)

| | *Syndrome* | *Comments* |
|---|---|---|
| Fungi | | |
| *Candida* species | Oropharyngitis, esophagitis, vaginitis | Most disease is of the mucous membranes and esophagus; most isolates are *C. albicans*, but *C. tropicalis* has been identified. |
| *Cryptococcus neoformans* | Meningitis, disseminated infection, pneumonia | Pneumonias as well as meningitis seen; should look for antigen in serum as well as cerebrospinal fluid. |
| *Histoplasma capsulatum* | Disseminated infection | Seen in nonendemic areas in persons with residence in endemic areas in the past; should stain and culture marrow and peripheral blood buffy coat. |
| *Aspergillus* species | Pneumonia | Reported, but apparently very uncommon. |

From Armstrong D, Gold JWM, Dryjanski J, et al. Treatment of infections in patients with the acquired immunodeficiency syndrome. Ann Intern Med 1985;103:738–743, with permission.

recognized with increasing frequency. In addition, *Toxoplasma gondii* cerebral lesions and cryptococcal meningitis occur frequently in this immunodeficiency syndrome. Surprisingly, other opportunistic pathogens, such as *Aspergillus* and *Nocardia*, have been infrequently identified in AIDS patients, compared with some other immunocompromised populations (e.g., leukemics, bone marrow transplants).

Bacteremia, especially with encapsulated organisms, and fungemia have been reported with increasing frequency in patients with AIDS. Infections commonly associated with T-cell immunodeficiency (e.g., *Salmonella* sp., *Listeria monocytogenes*, and *Histoplasma capsulatum*) and B-cell deficiencies (*S. pneumoniae* and *Hemophilus influenzae*) have been reported.[74] *M. tuberculosis* bacteremia has also been observed in AIDS patients.[75]

Of particular significance concerning opportunistic infections in AIDS is the observation that these patients may recover from one infectious episode, only to become reinfected with the same organism or another unusual pathogen. Furthermore, infections from multiple organisms are extremely common. Many organisms that cause infections in AIDS patients can result in multisystem manifestations. Throughout the remainder of this chapter, each pathogen is discussed under the most frequent manifestation or organ system in which it causes disease (Table 91.5).

## Pulmonary Infection

Pulmonary symptoms observed frequently in AIDS patients include high fevers (>102°F), dypsnea on exertion, nonproductive cough, and vague, nonpleuritic chest pain. Respiratory symptoms are often insidious in onset and have been present 2 to 12 weeks prior to presentation. Approximately 30% of patients present with a rapidly progressive pulmonary disorder. The etiology of pneumonia is usually *P. carinii*, although pulmonary cryptococcosis, *M. avium-intracellulare*, cytomegalovirus, Legionnaire's disease, *M. tuberculosis*, and Kaposi's sarcoma have been reported.[76] Severe and unusual presentations of overwhelming extrapulmonary and disseminated tuberculosis have been noted recently among patients with AIDS.[77] Several of these pathogens that have unique or controversial treatments are discussed in this section.

### *Pneumocystis carinii*

The most common pulmonary infection occurring in AIDS patients is *Pneumocystis carinii* pneumonia (PCP). This organism is regarded as a protozoan because of its structure and sensitivity to antiparasitic drugs. Epidemiologic data suggest that there is widespread exposure to PCP in childhood (>75%). *P. carinii* is believed to reside in the human lung without consequence unless the host becomes immunologically compromised. In this circumstance, *P. carinii* may multiply and cause disease. Approximately 60% of AIDS patients develop PCP as their initial illness or in association with other severe infections or malignancies.[78]

PCP in AIDS differs in clinical presentation from the disease seen in patients with malignant neoplasms. In AIDS patients, the presentation is often chronic in nature with milder symptoms. The onset in the AIDS patient is frequently insidious, over a period of weeks. Chest radiographs may show subtle infiltrates or even be normal, and arterial blood gases may show minimal hypoxia (e.g., $Pao_2$ 80–95 mm Hg); however, patients with PCP and AIDS may have fulminant respiratory failure, and for patients who require ventilatory assistance, the chance of survival decreases sharply.[79] Histologic improvement has been noted to lag behind clinical improvement, as biopsies obtained 2 to 3 weeks after commencement of therapy often show little improvement. Current mortality from PCP after the first episode has decreased since the early 1980s; most patients (e.g., >70%) survive the first episode but are subject to relapses and/or recurrences.

Much controversy exists concerning whether trimethoprim–sulfamethoxazole (TMP–SMX) or pentamidine should be the first-line treatment for PCP.[73,78,80] Although pentamidine had been used for many years in the treatment of the previously infrequent cases of PCP, TMP–SMX replaced pentamidine in the 1970s as the drug of choice because of its apparently lower incidence of adverse effects. Hughes et al compared the efficacy and tolerance of TMP–SMX and pentamidine in children with PCP and found TMP–SMX to be less toxic, although both agents were found to be equally efficacious.[81] The San Francisco group recently compared TMP–SMX and pentamidine for first-episode PCP in 40 patients with AIDS.[82] Both groups were similar with respect to the severity of their pulmonary disease. During the 21-day

**Table 91.5** Drugs Used to Treat the Infectious Complications of AIDS and Their Common Adverse Effects

| *Disease* | *Drug regimen* | *Common adverse effects* |
|---|---|---|
| Mycobacterial Infections | | |
| *Mycobacterium avium-intracellulare*[a] | Isoniazid 300 mg PO daily | Peripheral neuropathy, central nervous system manifestations |
| | Rifampin 600 mg PO daily | Gastrointestinal irritation, drug fever pruritus |
| | Ethambutol hydrochloride 25 mg/kg/d PO for 6 weeks, then 15/mg/kg/d | Optic neuritis, peripheral neuritis, headache |
| | Streptomycin 0.75–1.0 g (as the sulfate salt) daily IM for 2 months, then 2–3 times a week | Vertigo, paresthesias, nausea, tinnitus |
| | Capreomycin 1 g (as the sulfate salt) daily IM (alternative to streptomycin) | Nephrotoxicity, ototoxicity, eosinophilia |
| | Ethionamide 500–1000 mg PO daily in 1–3 divided doses | Gastrointestinal irritation, goiter, rashes |
| | Cycloserine 750–1000 mg PO daily in 2–4 divided doses | Convulsions, headaches, psychoses |
| | Pyridoxine hydrochloride 100 mg PO daily | |
| | Pyrazinamide 25 mg/kg/d PO (alternative if toxicity develops) | Arthralgias, hyperuricemia |
| Resistant *M. avium-intracellulare*[a] | Ansamycin 150–300 mg PO daily (for rifampin-resistant cases) | Minimal information; adverse effects appear similar to rifampin |
| | Clofazimine 300 mg PO daily in 3 divided doses | Skin discoloration, pigmentation (skin and ocular), ichthyosis, gastrointestinal |
| Protozoal infections | | |
| *Pneumocystis carinii* pneumonia | Trimethoprim–sulfamethoxazole (TMP–SMZ) IV/PO: 20 mg/kg/d TMP + 100 mg/kg/d SMZ in 4 divided doses | Crystalluria, skin rash, leukopenia, gastrointestinal disorders, fever |
| | *or* | |
| | Pentamidine isethionate 4 mg/kg/d IM or IV | Intramuscular: pain on injection, swelling, sterile abscesses<br>Intravenous: thrombophlebitis, facial flushing, tachycardia, hypotension, metallic taste, nephrotoxicity, glycosuria |
| *Toxoplasma gondii* | Sulfadiazine 1 g PO 4 times daily | Allergy, rash, drug fever, neurotoxicity |
| | *and* | |
| | Pyrimethamine 25 mg PO daily | Bone marrow suppression, blood dyscrasias |
| *Giardia lamblia* | Quinacrine hydrochloride 100 mg PO 3 times daily | Dizziness, headache, fever, jaundiced appearance |
| | *or* | |
| | Metronidazole 250–500 mg PO 3 times daily (alternative) | Nausea, headache, metallic taste, disulfiram-like reactions |
| *Isospora belli* | Trimethoprim 160 mg–sulfamethoxazole 800 mg orally 4 times daily | Anemia, rash, gastrointestinal irritation, central nervous system toxicity |
| *Cryptosporidium muris* | Spiramycin 1 g PO 3–4 times daily | Diarrhea, nausea, vomiting, epigastric pain, giddiness |
| Fungal Infections | | |
| *Candida albicans* | | |
| Oral thrush | Nystatin 500,000 units, swish in mouth 4–6 times daily | Nontoxic, rare topical sensitization |
| | *or* | |
| | Clotrimazole 10 mg (1 troche) PO 5 times daily | Nontoxic |

Table 91.5 Drugs Used to Treat the Infectious Complications of AIDS and Their Common Adverse Effects (*Continued*)

| *Disease* | *Drug regimen* | *Common adverse effects* |
|---|---|---|
| Esophagitis | Ketoconazole 400 mg PO daily | Elevated liver function test results, nausea, vomiting, abdominal pain |
| Transient fungemia | Amphotericin B 0.3 mg/kg/d IV | Fever, chills, nausea, thrombophlebitis, anemia, impaired renal function, hypokalemia |
| Disseminated disease with or without pneumonia | Amphotericin B 0.6 mg/kg/d IV | Same effects as listed above |
| *Cryptococcus neoformans* | | |
| Meningeal | Amphotericin B 0.3 mg/kg/d IV | Same effects as listed above |
| | *plus* | |
| | Flucytosine 150 mg/kg/d PO in 4 divided doses | Occasional nausea, vomiting, diarrhea, bone marrow depression, elevated liver function tests |
| | *or* | |
| | Amphotericin B 0.5 mg/kg/d IV | Same effects as listed above |
| *Asperigillus* | Amphotericin B 0.6 mg/kg/d IV | Same effects as listed above |
| | *or* | |
| | Amphotericin B 0.3 mg/kg/d IV | Same effects as listed above |
| | *and* | |
| | Flucytosine 150 mg/kg/d PO in 4 divided doses | Same effects as listed above |
| *Coccidioides immitis* | Amphotericin B 0.6 mg/kg/d IV | Same effects as listed above |
| | Ketoconazole 400 mg PO daily (for the treatment failures) | |
| Viral infections | | |
| Cytomegalovirus | DHPG[b] 5 mg/kg IV every 12 h for 14–21 d, followed by maintenance doses 5 d per week | Bone marrow suppression, gastrointestinal disturbances, skin rash, increased SGOT and SGPT concentrations, headache and disorientation |
| Herpes simplex | Acyclovir 500 mg/m$^2$ IV every 8 h for 7 d | Bone marrow suppression, increased creatinine, increased SGOT and SGPT concentrations, CNS manifestations |
| | *or* | |
| | Vidarabine 15 mg/kg/d IV over 12 h for 10 d | Gastrointestinal (nausea, vomiting, diarrhea), skin rash, hallucinations |
| Herpes zoster | Acyclovir 500 mg/m$^2$ IV every 8 h for 7 d[b] | Same effects as listed above |
| | *or* | |
| | Vidarabine 10 mg/kg/d IV over 12 h for 10 d | Same effects as listed above |

[a] A five- or six-drug combination is used for disseminated *M. intracellulare* infections. For immunocompromised patients, ansamycin and clofazimine are included in the regimen. Rifampin is not used with ansamycin. Initial regimen for AIDS patients should include enthambutol, streptomycin, clofazimine, ethionamide, and rifampin or ansamycin.

[b] Not approved by FDA for this dose and indication.

[c] Will probably not be effective.

From Furio MM, Wardell CJ. Treatment of infectious complications of acquired immunodeficiency syndrome. Clin Pharm 1985;4:539–554, with permission Copyright 1985 American Society of Hospital Phasmacists.

treatment period, 5 patients treated initially with TMP–SMX and 1 patient treated initially with pentamidine died. Adverse reactions that required a change of therapy occurred in 10 and 11 patients in the TMP–SMX and pentamidine groups, respectively. Neutropenia (<1,000/mL) occurred with approximately the same frequency in each group, whereas severe rash was more common in the TMP–SMX group. In another study, TMP–SMX and pentamidine were randomly administered for the treatment of PCP to 66 patients with AIDS. There was no difference in outcome; change in therapy because of drug toxicity was not associated with a worsened survival rate in contrast to change resulting from failure to respond.[83] Nevertheless, in association with AIDS and PCP, TMP–SMX has generally been used as first-line treatment. Recommended doses are high, 20 mg/kg/d for the trimethoprim component divided into three or four doses for 3 weeks. TMP–SMX is usually administered by the intravenous route, although oral therapy may suffice in mildly ill, reliable patients, as percentage absorption is high; however, gastrointestinal disturbances or a malabsorption syndrome in AIDS patients may prevent complete bioavailability of the oral form, and intravenous administration is generally preferred. Experience with treatment of moderate to severe cases of PCP with oral TMP–SMX is limited at this time. Regardless of which agent is initiated first, an alternative agent must be started if the patient has not improved by day 4 or 5 of treatment.

The low incidence of adverse effects and high degree of effectiveness observed for TMP–SMX in other immunocompromised groups are not consistently seen with AIDS patients. In fact, for unknown reasons AIDS patients appear to have a higher prevalence of significant toxicity. Bowden and colleagues documented, in seven AIDS patients, high SMX serum concentrations following multiple doses of intravenous or oral TMP–SMX (20 mg/kg/d TMP).[84] High serum SMX levels may be a factor contributing to the high incidence of adverse reactions, although this hypothesis needs further study. Gordin et al compared TMP–SMX with pentamidine in a retrospective chart review of 38 AIDS patients who were treated for PCP.[85] Only 5 of 37 patients started on TMP–SMX (20 mg/kg/d) were able to complete a course of treatment on this drug. Treatment had to be changed in 30 patients because of adverse effects such as rash, neutropenia (leukocyte count < 2,200), thrombocytopenia (platelet count < 80,000), and transaminase elevation. The most common side effect was a total body rash, usually erythematous and maculopapular in appearance.

Limited data are available regarding the management of hypersensitivity reactions induced by TMP–SMX in AIDS patients. Two patients, one with an erythematous, macular rash and the other with a severe reaction including tachycardia, hypertension, and bronchospasm, received diphenhydramine either alone or with subcutaneous epinephrine with each TMP–SMX dose.[86] Several days after these ameliorative therapies no further hypersensitivity reactions occurred, even though TMP–SMX was continued and diphenhydramine and/or epinephrine was terminated. A short course with diphenhydramine may be attempted before switching to pentamidine.

Pentamidine isethionate, an aromatic diamidine, was first used to treat PCP in infants in the United States in 1958 and was shown to decrease mortality from 50% to <4% in the period from 1958 to 1962.[87] The mechanisms of pentamidine's antiprotozoal effects remain uncertain.

The pharmacokinetics of pentamidine have been poorly understood because of poor assay technology, but this has recently improved.[88] Mean peak serum concentrations after IM and IV 4 mg/kg doses were 209 ng/mL and 612 ng/mL, respectively.[88] The majority of drug excretion in humans is handled by the kidney, with approximately 20% excreted unchanged in the urine. The elimination half-life ranges from 6 to 10 hours depending on route of administration. The recommended human dose is 4 mg/kg/d for the isethionate salt, given by slow intravenous infusion or intramuscularly. The dose should be adjusted in those who have moderate to severe renal impairment (creatinine clearance <35 mL/min).[89] Hemodialysis did not appear to significantly affect plasma concentrations.[89] Bennett et al.[90] suggested extending the dosing interval to 24–36 hours if the creatinine clearance is 10–50 mL/min, and to 48 hours if the creatinine clearance is less than 10 mL/min.

Approximately 50% of patients treated with pentamidine have side effects, which may include hypotension, tachycardia, nausea and vomiting, facial flushing, urticarial eruptions (generalized or localized), azotemia, severe hypoglycemia, elevation of liver enzymes, irreversible diabetes mellitus, thrombophlebitis after intravenous administration, cardiac arrythmia, hypocalcemia, and even sudden death.[73] Severe hemorrhagic acute pancreatitis has been reported in one AIDS patient and was fatal despite drug discontinuation.[91] When intramuscular injections are used, pain, swelling, and sterile abscesses are common.[92] It is unknown whether AIDS patients have a higher incidence of adverse reactions to pentamidine than other immunocompromised individuals. Several reactions (e.g., hypotension, tachycardia, nausea, vomiting, and hypoglycemia) have been associated with rapid intravenous infusions. Patients given pentamidine by slow intravenous infusion (over 60 minutes) have few side effects, namely transient elevations in serum creatinine (36%) and rashes (18%).[92] A recent study showed no difference in cardiovascular toxicity when pentamidine was administered as a slow intravenous infusion and intramuscularly.[93] The overall incidence of side effects appears similar for intramuscular and intravenous administration. The mechanism of the hypotensive effect is uncertain; direct vasodilatory effects or drug-induced histamine release has been proposed.

Hypoglycemic reactions have been reported to occur during pentamidine therapy in 6.2% to 9% of patients treated in the United States.[73,87] Reactions may be observed as early as 2 hours after therapy commences, although a severe, life-threatening hypoglycemia has been noted after completion of pentamidine therapy.[94] Some non-AIDS immunocompromised patients have developed diabetes mellitus subsequent to the hypoglycemia, as early as 6 days after abnormally low serum glucose levels, but often several weeks into therapy.[95] It should be noted that hypoglycemia does not always precede the diagnosis of diabetes mellitus. One mechanism has been suggested to explain these observations: pentamidine may stimulate an acute release of insulin, followed by inhibition of insulin release and ultimately cytolysis of insulinoma cells.[96] Diazoxide may aid in controlling the severe hypoglycemia, although experience is limited.[97] Unfortunately, there are no predictive factors that identify patients at risk for dysglycemia. Close monitoring of serum glucose is recommended.

Impaired renal function as measured by elevations in serum creatinine occurs in about 25% of patients receiving pentamidine, including patients with normal pretreatment renal function.[73] The impairment is usually mild and reversible. Although severe renal impairment has been reported, it is difficult to attribute the reaction solely to pentamidine in the face of other concurrent nephrotoxins and associated disease states.

One adverse effect that is theoretically attributable to either TMP–SMX or pentamidine is leukopenia caused by folic acid inhibition. Data reported to the CDC revealed that 14.5% of pentamidine-treated AIDS patients had a 50%

reduction in total leukocyte count.[98] In fewer than 10% of these cases, pentamidine was discontinued because of leukopenia. A direct causal relationship was often difficult to establish, as many patients had received other medications, including TMP–SMX. Controversy exists over whether to coadminister folinic acid with TMP–SMX and pentamidine to prevent leukopenia.[87,99] Recommended prophylactic doses of folinic acid range from 60 $\mu$g daily to 15 mg daily.[100,101] In the patient with existing hematotoxicity, 15 mg every 6 hours has been suggested.[100]

Alternative therapies for PCP are limited. In February 1988, trimetrexate was approved as an investigational new drug for the treatment of PCP. Trimetrexate is a potent inhibitor of the protozoan dihydrofolate reductase, about 1,500 times more active than trimethoprim. However, the use of this agent is complicated by myelosuppression. Consequently, simultaneous treatment with leukovorin is required to protect host cells while maintaining trimetrexate's effectiveness. Trimetrexate has been shown to be equally efficacious compared to trimethoprim/sulfamethoxazole and pentamadine for the treatment of PCP.

Allegra and co-workers randomly studied three groups of patients (N = 49) with 21 days of IV trimetrexate/leukovorin.[102] The trimetrexate dose was given as 30 mg/$M^2$ as a daily bolus. Response and survival rates were not significantly different among patients who had not tolerated or who had failed conventional therapy, or in those with sulfonamide allergies as initial therapy combined with sulfadiazine. Trimetrexate was associated with minimal toxicity although transient neutropenia or thrombocytopenia was observed in 25% of patients; only one patient had to be withdrawn from therapy. Mean peak and trough levels measured in these patients were $11.8 \pm 6$ $\mu$M and $1.9 \pm 1.4$ $\mu$M, respectively. There was no association between these levels and clinical outcomes. Accumulation of drug was not observed following repeated doses. The terminal half-life was estimated at 11 hours. Unpublished data indicate that trimetrexate glucuronate is 40% to 50% orally bioavailable. Outpatient oral regimens will ultimately be available.

Dapsone (diaminodiphenylsulfone) and difluoromethylornithine (DFMO), have been studied as alternatives for the treatment of PCP.[103–105] In a small group of patients (41) who did not respond to (or were allergic to) TMP–SMX or pentamidine, DFMO was given intravenously (400 mg/kg/d) for approximately 2 weeks and followed by oral drug (75–350 mg/kg/d) for an additional 4 weeks.[102,106] Fewer than 50% of patients with a poor prognosis responded and were cured. Many of the failures occurred in patients requiring mechanical ventilation. Significant side effects included thrombocytopenia, leukopenia, and hepatitis. The value of DFMO as an alternative agent is unclear. The use of oral dapsone alone (100 mg daily for 3 weeks) was found to be less effective than standard therapy for first-episode PCP among 18 AIDS patients.[107] Side effects with dapsone are significant (e.g., hemolytic anemia, methemoglobinemia, nausea, vomiting). It has been suggested that treatment with a combination of dapsone and trimethoprim may provide synergy while allowing the dose of dapsone to be decreased to minimize toxicities. Leoung and colleagues studied the efficacy and safety of oral dapsone (100 mg/d) plus trimethoprim (20 mg/kg/d) in 15 AIDS patients with first-episode PCP.[104] Clinical and radiographic improvement was observed in all patients within 3 to 10 days after initiation of treatment. Side effects occurred in 14 patients, but only 2 required discontinuation of therapy. The use of dapsone alone in the treatment of PCP cannot be recommended.

Inhaled pentamidine is currently under evaluation for both treatment and prophylaxis of PCP. Limited data exists to prove the efficacy of this treatment, however, many studies are underway. Pharmacokinetic studies have documented good bronchial alveolar concentrations and minimal systemic absorption.[108] Montgomery and co-workers have reported successful first PCP episode outcomes in 13 of 15 patients following 21 days of aerosolized pentamidine.[109] Six hundred milligrams of pentamidine isethionate was dissolved in 6 mL of sterile water and administered through a specially designed nebulizer system over 20 minutes.[110] Systemic side effects were not observed; the only local side effect was cough in 12 patients. Conte and co-workers evaluated inhaled pentamidine in nine patients with first episode PCP.[108] Pentamidine was given as a 4 mg/kg aerosolized dose over 30 to 60 minutes. A satisfactory response was seen in 90% of patients. Two patients developed neutropenia during therapy but both were receiving zidovudine. Reversible bronchospasms were associated with inhalation in five patients. The most effective dose, dosing interval, and type of nebulizer are uncertain; many regimens are being evaluated. The advantages of this route proven beneficial include directed therapy, minimal systemic toxicity, and the possibility of home care. Disadvantages may include airway toxicity, ineffectiveness outside the lung (some clinicians have suggested that *Pneumocystis carinii* may reside outside the lungs), and high cost. Other problems include the need for patient coordination, potential for pseudomonal contamination, need for bronchodilators, and reimbursement issues. Although this is an exciting new treatment/prophylaxis option, it must be emphasized that the benefits are unclear.

Because of the high relapse rate of PCP seen in AIDS patients, the need for prophylactic treatment after the initial infection has resolved or in those at high risk has been discussed but is controversial.[85] Hughes et al conducted a randomized, double-blind, placebo-controlled study in which pediatric cancer patients (non-AIDS) at high risk for PCP were randomized to receive 150 mg TMP and 750 mg SMX/$m^2$ per day or placebo.[111] Twenty-one percent of placebo patients contracted PCP, as compared with none on TMP–SMX; however, mortality was not affected by TMP–SMX prophylaxis in either group. Other studies have documented the value of TMP–SMX prophylaxis.[112] Because of the high rate of adverse reaction to TMP–SMX in AIDS, the use of secondary prophylaxis is still controversial but has been used from two to seven days each week. The Sloan–Kettering group has examined the prophylactic benefits of aerosolized pentamidine in 120 patients.[113] Weekly doses from 30 to 60 mg were studied. Eight cases of PCP occurred during the 14 months surveillance period; mean prophylaxis period was 5 months. No adverse reactions were noted. Pyrimethamine–sulfadoxine (Fansidar) and monthly IM pentamidine have also been utilized.[114] The Fansidar dose (500 mg sulfadoxine plus 25 mg pyrimethamine) has been administered weekly to small numbers of patients for 3–12 months without toxicity or recurrence of PCP.[115] However, Navin and co-workers have reported four cases of Stevens-Johnson syndrome associated with pyrimethamine–sulfadoxine prophylaxis.[116] Additionally, a recent case of fatal hepatic necrosis has been reported in a non-AIDS patient.[117] Prospective studies to evaluate the efficacy and toxicity of long-term administration of pyrimethamine–sulfadoxine in AIDS patients is warranted.

### *Mycobacterium avium-intracellulare*

*Mycobacterium avium-intracellulare* (MAI), a complex of two strains of *Mycobacterium*, was rarely recognized to cause disseminated disease until the identification of AIDS. The Memorial Sloan–Kettering Cancer Center has reported that 50% of AIDS patients in their institution have disseminated MAI at autopsy.[118] Other investigators have questioned the pathogenicity of MAI. The organism has been isolated from multiple sites including the lung, lymph nodes, gastrointestinal tract, spleen, bone marrow, brain, and blood. Isolation of MAI from the blood, using radiolabeled liquid medium is a practical, sensitive diagnostic test.[119] Stool smears positive for acid-fact bacilli have also been a useful marker for MAI in AIDS patients. These findings have correlated with invasive MAI infection in the majority of cases.[119]

Symptoms of MAI gastrointestinal infection range from mild indigestion to persistent diarrhea, and may be associated with disabling abdominal pain and a malabsorption syndrome. In other patients, no symptoms are apparent even in the presence of positive blood cultures for MAI. Other patients have nonspecific signs of intermittent fever and progressive weight loss. It may be difficult to differentiate MAI infection from *M. tuberculosis*. Racial, geographic, and socioeconomic factors may be helpful in differentiating MAI from *M. tuberculosis* in AIDS patients. White, middle-class homosexual males appear more likely to contract MAI, and inner-city intravenous drug abusers or Haitian immigrants are more likely to have *M. tuberculosis*.

Unfortunately, MAI has marked resistance to conventional antituberculosis agents, including rifampin, streptomycin, ethambutol, cycloserine, ethionamide, *para*-aminosalicylic acid, and isoniazid (INH).[120,121] Although many combinations of these agents have been prescribed for the treatment of MAI, few bacteriologic or clinical cures have been achieved. Two investigational drugs have been demonstrated to have in vitro activity against MAI: ansamycin is a rifampin derivative, and clofazamine has been used to treat leprosy. These agents have been used together with other traditional antituberculous drugs in the hope of attaining bactericidal synergy. Multidrug combinations are commonly prescribed.[122] In one study, cycloserine included as part of the drug regimen was more frequently associated with responders, and the use of INH and cycloserine produced an even greater response rate. Also, most responders received clofazamine. These authors concluded by recommending the use of INH, ethambutol, cycloserine, clofazamine, ethionamide, and rifampin or ansamycin initially.[122]

Ansamycin is a semisynthetic rifamycin compound which is available from the CDC in the United States.[123] It has good activity in vitro against *M. avium-intracellulare* and rifampin-sensitive *M. tuberculosis* organisms, as well as one third of the rifampin-resistant strains.[123,124] Ansamycin is probably more active than rifampin against MAI because of its higher degree of lipophilicity, thereby allowing for better absorption into the bacteria.

Dosage recommendations for ansamycin range from 150 to 300 mg as one single daily oral dose. For patients with creatinine clearance below 50 mL/min, the recommended dose of ansamycin is 150 mg/d, and for creatinine clearance below 10 mL/min, 75 mg every 3 days. If hepatic impairment is present, the recommended dose is 150 mg/d. Intermittent administration of ansamycin (e.g., biweekly) is recommended in the following situations: (1) renal insufficiency, (2) after suspected bone marrow toxicity, (3) following evidence of hepatotoxicity, or (4) for maintenance treatment of patients who are in apparent remission. Duration of treatment should be lifelong in AIDS patients.

With normal doses, ansamycin may cause a slight elevation of liver function tests as well as moderate, reversible decreases in hematopoietic cells and mild transient decreases in platelets. The patient should be monitored closely if the platelet count falls below 150,000/mm$^3$ and the white blood cell count is less than 4,000/mm$^3$ (or falls 50%). The dose should be reduced to 150 mg/d and discontinued if the platelet and white blood cell counts fall below 50,000/mm$^3$ and 1,000/mm$^3$, respectively. Experience with ansamycin in humans is limited, but it appears to have a relatively low toxic potential.

Clofazamine is an agent that was originally used for the treatment of leprosy, specifically for dapsone-resistant strains. At present, clofazamine is available from National Jewish Hospital in Denver, Colorado, and from the FDA. Its postulated mechanism of action is prevention of mycobacterial growth through inhibition of aerobic respiration, and possibly via inhibition of DNA function.[125]

Clofazamine is hepatically metabolized to two polar metabolites; therefore no dosage adjustment is needed in renal failure. Nearly 100% of the drug is absorbed, yet less than 1% is excreted each day, indicating that the drug has a very long half-life (reported to be about 70 days).[126] The recommended dose for treatment of MAI infections is 300 mg, given orally once daily. There are few controlled published studies in the literature that examine the benefit of treating AIDS patients with clofazamine.

Associated toxicities are dependent on both duration of treatment and dose utilized.[127] Skin discoloration resulting from deposition of drug in the reticuloendothelial cells and subcutaneous fat has been noted. During the first months of therapy, the initial hyperpigmentation appears red. In later months, a black-brown skin discoloration has been observed in patients treated for leprosy.[128] Patients receiving clofazamine may also complain of dry skin. Pigmentation of the conjunctiva is a common adverse reaction. Other reversible ocular toxicities include the appearance of fine brown lines in the cornea and pigment deposits in the macular area of the fundus. Gastrointestinal effects include abdominal pain, nausea, vomiting, and diarrhea. Deposits of drug crystals have been found in the small bowel.[126,127] These reactions appear to be cumulatively dose related and usually appear late in treatment.

Clofazamine and ansamycin have been used to treat disseminated MAI in some AIDS patients;[129–131] however, despite in vitro susceptibility to ansamycin, clofazamine, ethionamide, and ethambutol, sustained remissions have rarely been observed in the treated patients.[129,130] Among 26

AIDS patients with disseminated MAI infection who were treated with two or more drugs for a mean of 6 weeks, bacteremia persisted in 24 of 26 patients.[131] Most patients received ansamycin, clofazamine, ethionamide, or ethambutol. Clinical improvement was not documented in any patient. Treatment may have been ineffective because of severity of infection at the time of diagnosis, a short duration of therapy, ineffective antimicrobial therapy, and underlying immunodeficiency in the patients. Earlier diagnosis and more active agents or drug combinations are definitely needed.

There are a number of important considerations regarding the treatment of disseminated MAI disease including whom and when to treat, which drugs to employ, how long to treat, and how to assess response to therapy. It is often difficult to discern in AIDS patients whether MAI or another concomitant pathogen is causing their pulmonary disease. As most AIDS patients present with disseminated MAI, management, if one decides to treat, has consisted of a five- or six-drug regimen including (1) rifampin (600 mg PO per day) if the organism is sensitive or ansamycin (150–300 mg PO per day) if the organism is rifampin-resistant; (2) clofazamine (100 mg PO three times per day); (3) ethambutol (150 mg/kg PO per day); (4) ethionamide (250 mg PO two to four times daily); and (5) streptomycin (15 mg/kg IM daily for 2–6 months, if renal function is normal). Occasionally, other agents have been added depending on susceptibility and tolerance. Total duration of therapy probably should be lifelong. Unfortunately, experience with these agents has not shown any clear benefit, and AIDS patients often succumb to other complications before an adequate response can be assessed.

## Neurologic Infection

Central nervous disease is a common affliction in AIDS patients. Problems observed include progressive idiopathic encephalopathy, mass lesions caused by *Toxoplasma gondii*, cryptococcal meningitis, CNS lymphoma, and progressive multifocal leukoencephalopathy.[118] Numerous pathogens may cause opportunistic CNS infections including *T. gondii*, *Cryptococcus neoformans*, cytomegalovirus, papovavirus-JC, *Mycobacterium tuberculosis*, *Nocardia* sp., and herpes simplex virus. Signs and symptoms are often nonspecific. Sensory disturbances, aphasia, paresia, and/or seizures have been observed. Other patients may develop symptoms consistent with a chronic meningitis (e.g., headache, photophobia) or complain of memory loss and an inability to concentrate which may progress to a dementia that is incapacitating. Increased evidence associates this syndrome with HIV infection, rather than its associated infection or malignant complications.

### *Toxoplasma gondii*

*T. gondii* is a protozoan that seroepidemiologic studies suggest infects up to one third of the general population; however, most individuals do not have symptoms of disease. In patients with AIDS, *T. gondii* has become an important pathogen in the differential diagnosis if neurologic symptoms occur or deficits are noted. Although this infection is not observed as frequently as PCP in AIDS patients, the morbidity and mortality may be higher. Toxoplasmosis most commonly manifests itself in patients with AIDS as a mass lesion in the CNS,[132] however, it may cause diffuse neurologic dysfunction, either with focal signs or as a diffuse encephalopathy. A meningoencephalitic presentation has also been observed.[133] In AIDS patients, it is thought that toxoplasmosis results from reactivation of a chronic, latent infection rather than as an acute, recently acquired infection. Once reactivation occurs, this opportunistic pathogen can disseminate quickly and may invade any organ system; however, it has predilection for the central nervous system.

As clinical signs and symptoms are nonspecific, special diagnostic measures are required. On computerized tomography (CT) or magnetic resonance (MR), single or multiple ring-enhancing lesions are often found in the basal ganglia. Examination of cerebrospinal fluid may reveal elevated protein and low glucose, but does not provide a definitive diagnosis. Brain biopsy is usually required to make a definitive diagnosis, with the finding of trophozoites on histology and *T. gondii* on culture.[134] Unfortunately, biopsy is not always feasible because of the potential morbidity, location of the lesion, or thrombocytopenia. A recent study suggested that approximately 30% of patients with serologic evidence of previous toxoplasmosis infection would develop CNS disease.[135] Early therapy may be essential to increase the patient's chance of survival. Empiric treatment for toxoplasmosis in patients with AIDS who have CNS mass lesions is probably warranted. If patients do not respond to this, biopsy should be undertaken. Some suggest treatment for 2 to 3 weeks prior to biopsy to decrease the risk of dissemination with biopsy.

First-line treatment of AIDS-related CNS toxoplasmosis includes a combination of sulfadiazine (1.5–2 g every 6 hours) or another sulfonamide and pyrimethamine (25 mg/d, after a 75-mg loading dose). If not biopsy confirmed, a response within 7–10 days will help confirm an empiric diagnosis.[134] These agents work together by inhibiting sequential steps in the synthesis of folic acid, similar to TMP–SMX. Therapy is given orally and must be continued indefinitely because of frequency of recurrence. Adverse effects of these drugs are similar to those seen with TMP–SMX as discussed earlier: leukopenia, rash, fever, and crystalluria.[134,136] As with TMP–SMX, leukopenia may limit the use of sulfadiazine and pyrimethamine in this patient population. Folinic acid (10 mg PO or IV) may reserve bone marrow suppression, although experience is limited.[133,136] If neutropenia occurs, 50 mg of pyrimethamine may be administered alone each day. Second-line therapy is controversial, as few effective alternatives have been identified.

Other drug treatment alternatives include clindamycin[137] and spiramycin, an erythromycin derivative, widely used in Europe and Canada.[134,136] Clindamycin may be used to eradicate extra-CNS toxoplasma cysts. Although clindamycin is not considered to penetrate into the CSF reliably, this combination may offer an alternative for patients with allergies to sulfonamides.[138] Spiramycin is a macrolide antibiotic with an antimicrobial spectrum similar to that of erythromycin and is usually administered in doses of 2–3 g (PO) daily in divided doses.[136]

### *Cryptococcus neoformans*

Disseminated cryptococcal disease, including meningeal involvement, is not uncommon in AIDS patients. It has been estimated that approximately 5% of patients with AIDS are infected with this organism.[139] Infections are probably originally contracted through inhalation, and the respiratory tract is believed to be the primary infected site. Central nervous system infections with *C. neoformans* are the most important manifestation, and are fatal if not treated appropriately. The presenting signs and symptoms are similar to those observed in other immunocompromised hosts. Initially, meningitis may be manifested as subtle personality changes, as alterations in level of consciousness, or as a debilitating illness. Often there is no nuchal rigidity. CSF fluid samples frequently exhibit many organisms, and only a few leukocytes. Antigen titers in both serum and CSF are usually ≥1:10,000.[118] As with other individuals, the AIDS patient with a cryptococcal meningitis responds slowly to antimicrobial therapy and may often experience a relapse.

Standard treatment for cryptococcal meningitis consists of intravenous low-dose amphotericin B (0.3–0.5 mg/kg/d) in combination with oral flucytosine (150 mg/kg/d in four divided doses), for a period of 6 weeks.[140] This combination appears to be associated with fewer relapses and treatment failures, more rapid sterilization of the cerebral spinal fluid, and less nephrotoxicity than treatment with amphotericin B alone (0.5 mg/kg/d); however, in cases in which there is significant impairment of bone marrow function, liver disease, or the presence of gastrointestinal disorders that may impair absorption from oral therapy, amphotericin B alone is the preferred treatment. AIDS patients often do not tolerate flucytosine because of their concurrent multiorgan diseases. There is no indication for administration of intraventricular amphotericin B in AIDS patients at this time.[141] Ketoconazole (400 mg daily) has been used as an alternative therapy in AIDS patients,[142] but is not recommended routinely as long-term follow-up data are limited. Because relapse appears to be common in AIDS patients, early aggressive treatment is necessary with close follow-up. Lifelong therapy is probably necessary. Maintenance amphotericin B (100 mg/wk) for periods up to 12 months has been used.[139]

Toxicities associated with amphotericin B and flucytosine have been thoroughly discussed elsewhere.[143] There does not appear to be any major differences in side effects in AIDS patients.

### *Herpes Simplex Virus*

Herpes simplex virus (HSV) has been described to cause meningitis and encephalitis in AIDS patients.[144] HSV meningitis has been estimated to occur in up to 5% to 15% of non-AIDS patients at the time of the initial episode of genital infection.[145] Herpes encephalitis is considered the most common cause of sporadic fatal encephalitis in the United States. The clinical presentation of herpes encephalitis includes fever, headache, alterations of consciousness, and focal neurologic signs. Untreated, the outcome is fatal in approximately 70% of cases while causing severe neurologic sequelae in the surviving 30%.

Acyclovir (10 mg/kg IV every 8 hours) or vidarabine (15 mg/kg/d IM) have been used to treat HSV encephalitis. Whitley and the NIAID collaborative antiviral study group recently documented that acyclovir is clearly the drug of choice.[146] Among 69 non-AIDS patients with HSV encephalitis randomized to either therapy, mortality was lower in the acyclovir-treated group (28%) than in the vidarabine-treated group (54%). In addition, at 6-month follow-up the acyclovir group had significantly less debility compared with vidarabine-treated patients. AIDS patients with biopsy-proven HSV encephalitis should receive intravenous acyclovir treatment for 10 days.

### *Cytomegalovirus Retinitis*

Chorioretinitis caused by cytomegalovirus (CMV) has recently been recognized in the AIDS patient.[147–149] Clinical diagnosis is suspected on the basis of progressive decrease in vision. The retina becomes inflamed with areas of white, fluffy lesions, often with associated hemorrhages and a vascular pattern of distribution. A positive blood culture for CMV confirms the presence of systemic disease, whereas positive cultures at other sites provide supportive but not diagnostic evidence.

Antiviral therapy for serious CMV disease has previously been unsuccessful. A guanosine analog related to acyclovir, 9-(1,3-dihydroxy-2-propoxymethyl)guanine (DHPG), has been shown to inhibit CMV in vitro. This nucleoside is 10 to 100 times more active than acyclovir for CMV.[150,151] Within CMV-infected cells, DHPG is converted to DHPG triphosphate, which competitively inhibits binding of deoxyguanosine triphosphate to DNA polymerase, inhibiting DNA synthesis.

DHPG's pharmacokinetic properties have been evaluated. A 5 mg/kg intravenous dose has produced peak serum levels ranging from 19.6 to 30.6 μmol/L with corresponding trough concentrations from 2.2 to 4.4 μmol/L 8 hours postdose.[147] No accumulation was observed after multiple doses. Elimination half-life averaged 2 hours and 78% of the unchanged drug was eliminated in the urine over 24 hours.

Several groups have reported favorable although transient improvement after DHPG treatment for CMV retinitis.[147–149,152] Most patients experience recurrence of the disease within 30 days of discontinuing DHPG. Maintenance therapy is not consistently effective. Neutropenia developed or worsened in 20% of those treated. Other adverse reactions included eosinophilia, increased liver transaminases, myalgias, and headaches as well as disorientation and hallucinations. Relapse also occurred after discontinuation of therapy; several patients responded to a second DHPG course.

The results with DHPG are encouraging; however, it must be emphasized that current experience is limited. If a patient responds to an initial course (15 mg/kg/d for 10–30 days) and does not develop leukopenias, maintenance therapy is recommended (e.g., 5–7 times per week). Even if hematologic and other toxicities are minimal, long-term cures have not been observed.

## Gastrointestinal Infections

Gastrointestinal complaints are a major problem encountered with AIDS patients and are attributable to multiple causes. Diarrhea may be voluminous (e.g., 10–15 L/d) and/or persistent. The patient may present in a cachexic state complaining of frequent loose stools without fever or may seek medical attention after symptoms of fever and tenesmus. Multiple enteric organisms, including *Cryptosporidium*, *Isospora belli*, *Giardia lamblia*, *Campylobacter*, *Salmonella* sp., and *Shigella* sp., have been reported in patients with AIDS.[153] *Entamoeba histolytica*, the parasite responsible for amebiasis, rarely causes clinical disease in homosexual males, although it is detected frequently. Antimicrobial therapy may eliminate most of these pathogens, but frequently fails to ameliorate the copious watery diarrhea. Many patients, however, have persistent diarrhea without identifiable pathogens.

### *Candida albicans*

Superficial candidal infections (e.g., oral thrush) are very common and may be one of the first signs to indicate HIV-associated immunodeficiency. The most frequent candidal species involved in human disease are *C. albicans* and *C. tropicalis*. Oral candidiasis has been shown to be an early predictor of the development of overt AIDS in patients at high risk. Candidal oropharyngitis does not meet the CDC's surveillance definition for AIDS, whereas documented esophageal candidiasis is included. Candidal infections can be found throughout the alimentary tract and frequently persist after diagnosis.

Local candidal infections of the oropharynx can be treated with either nystatin suspension (swish and swallow) or clotrimazole troches four to six times daily. The troches must be dissolved (not chewed) in the mouth. Both regimens are equally effective and probably need to be given indefinitely or as needed. Twice-daily administration has shown some success.[154] Ketoconazole (200–400 mg daily for 10 days) may provide some benefit in refractory cases.[155]

Candidal esophagitis may occur in the presence or absence of oral thrush. Dysphagia and retrosternal pain are symptoms that suggest esophageal involvement. Recurrent fever (<101°F) may also be observed. If the patient is symptomatic, systemic antifungal therapy may be indicated to reduce the risks of perforation and hemorrhage.[156] Low-dose amphotericin B (5–10 mg daily for 5–14 days) or ketoconazole (400 mg daily) may be used.[155] Again, as with oral candidiasis, esophageal infections can recur. A dose of 200 mg ketoconazole once daily has been effective in prophylaxis.[156] Although esophagitis is common in AIDS patients, dissemination does not appear to occur frequently in this population compared with other immunocompromised groups.

### *Salmonella typhimurium*

*Salmonella typhimurium* causes most cases of nontyphoidal salmonella bacteremia in patients with defects in their cell-mediated immunity.[157] The prevalence of bacteremia among patients with *Salmonella* appears higher in AIDS patients than in patients with *Salmonella* who do not have underlying disease (1%–4% prevalence rate).[158] In patients with impaired T-cell function and frequent gastrointestinal membrane interruptions, such as AIDS patients, salmonellosis can be unusually severe.

The drugs of choice for the treatment of disseminated salmonellosis or of other patients who are severely ill include chloramphenicol, ampicillin, amoxicillin, TMP–SMX, and norfloxacin. Intravenous ampicillin (2 g every 4 hours) has been used most often, in some cases for up to 3 weeks.[157,158] Armstrong et al have recommended treatment for at least 6 weeks and perhaps indefinitely, as relapse is common.[118] Chronic prophylaxis is indicated; TMP–SMX has been used in non-AIDS patients. Because of the high frequency of adverse reactions in these patients,[80,85] ampicillin or amoxicillin may be the drug of choice. Currently, we would not recommend treatment of patients with mild salmonellosis limited to the gastrointestinal tract.

### *Cryptosporidium* sp. and *Isospora belli*

Two coccidian infections that may be seen in patients with AIDS are cryptosporidia and coccidiosis. *Cryptosporidium* sp. is a coccidian parasite that infects the brush border of the mammalian gastrointestinal tract. In the immunocompetent patient, the infection causes self-limited diarrhea that resolves in approximately 2 weeks; however, in patients who are immunocompromised, cryptosporidiosis may cause protracted diarrhea (up to 11 L/d) that leads to anorexia, malabsorption, and weight loss.[153] No drug therapy has proven consistently effective in treating this parasite. Hyperalimentation is often used to maintain nutritional support.

In the past, the CDC has recommended trial therapies of TMP–SMX, metronidazole, tetracycline, and furazolidone; however, the failure rates with these agents are very high.[159,160] Spiramycin has elicited some response in the treatment of cryptosporidiosis but no controlled trials have been done.[161,162]

*I. belli* is the infecting agent in coccidiosis. This rare parasite presents in a similar manner to cryptosporidiosis, with chronic, watery diarrhea, weight loss, malabsorption, and long-term fever, and is more common in immunocompromised patients than in patients without any underlying disease. This pathogen may be sexually transmitted.[163] Isosporiasis had been observed in fewer than 0.2% of patients with AIDS in the United States as of November 1985.[164] In normal hosts the disease may be self-limited; however, in the immunocompromised patient, the illness is often protracted. Possible drugs of choice include furazolidine, TMP–SMX and pyrimethamine–sulfadoxine. Prophylaxis with daily doses of TMP–SMX or weekly doses of pyrimethamine–sulfadoxine may be needed indefinitely.

## Disseminated Viral Diseases

### *Herpes Simplex and Varicella Zoster Viruses*

Herpes simplex virus (HSV) and varicella zoster virus (VZV) are frequent causes of infection in AIDS patients, as well as in other immunocompromised patients such as bone marrow transplant patients. HSV and VZV have been observed in approximately 90% and 30% of these patients, respectively.[144]

HSV occasionally is the presenting opportunistic infection in patients with AIDS, but also frequently appears later in the course of the disease. The usual presentation is the appearance of large ulcerative mucocutaneous lesions in the perirectal area.[3] Proctitis and esophagitis resulting from HSV have been reported. Lesions are frequently persistent and do not resolve spontaneously. Local progression usually occurs if treatment is not given.

Acyclovir is indicated for the treatment of both initial and recurrent mucosal and cutaneous HSV infections (types 1 and 2) in immunocompromised patients, as well as in the treatment of early initial genital HSV infection in immunocompetent patients. Significant benefit with the intravenous or oral form, but not topical acyclovir, has been shown in the treatment of primary genital HSV infection. Acyclovir decreases the formation of new lesions, the average healing time, the duration of symptoms, and the duration of viral shedding.[165,166] The dose used for intravenous treatment is 5 mg/kg (250 mg/m$^2$) every 8 hours for 10 days; the oral dose is 200–400 mg five times per day. Doses are adjusted as needed in the presence of renal impairment. Vidarabine has shown inconsistent results in the treatment of HSV and is considered more toxic than acyclovir.[166,167]

Unfortunately, the traditional 7- to 10-day treatment course with intravenous acyclovir does not prevent the high incidence of recurrent HSV infections following discontinuation of therapy in the immunocompromised host. Oral acyclovir has been used chronically for prophylaxis of recurrent mucocutaneous HSV.[166] In a small study of immunosuppressed non-AIDS patients, doses from 200 mg five times daily tapered down to twice daily were effective in decreasing duration of viral shedding and reducing symptoms and signs of acute recurrences.[168] More prolonged or repeated courses may be necessary. The role of chronic prophylaxis requires further evaluation. Currently, we use oral acyclovir 200 mg (for genital) or 400 mg (for rectal) every 8 hours as a prophylaxis regimen.

Varicella zoster virus infections appear to be occurring more frequently in patients at risk for AIDS and may precede diagnosis of the syndrome.[118] Often, VZV infection is only severe locally, but it can disseminate if local lesions are left untreated. Extensive cutaneous dissemination develops in 20% to 50% of cases in other patients with immunodeficiency states. VZV may be treated with vidarabine or acyclovir, although acyclovir is probably less toxic.[166] In clinical studies in immunosuppressed (non-AIDS) patients, the use of vidarabine has been shown to decrease acute pain, decrease the rate of new vesicle formation, and increase clearance of the virus from the patient. Treatment with vidarabine 10 mg/kg/d as a 12-hour intravenous infusion for 5 days within 3 days of onset was associated with a more rapid healing of lesions, a decreased rate of cutaneous dissemination and visceral complications, and a decreased duration of post-herpetic neuralgia when compared with placebo.[169] Intravenous acyclovir (1500 mg/m$^2$/d for 7 days) has also been successful in halting the progression of localized or disseminated herpes zoster.[170] Other studies suggest that intravenous acyclovir produces only modest benefit in herpes zoster infections and does not improve post-herpetic neuralgia.[171] Experience is still limited in the treatment of AIDS patients with disseminated herpes zoster.

### *Cytomegalovirus*

Cytomegalovirus (CMV) infection is very common in patients with AIDS, third in frequency to PCP and HSV infections.[118] Previous to the recognition of AIDS, CMV infection was known to be a major cause of morbidity and mortality in patients undergoing renal, bone marrow, or cardiac transplantations.[172] In AIDS patients, disseminated infection may involve multiple organs, including the liver, lungs, heart, pancreas, adrenals, and brain. Manifestations of CMV infection include fevers, granulocytopenia, lymphocytopenia, thrombocytopenia pupura, maculopapular rashes, interstitial pneumonia, encephalitis, and ulcerative gastrointestinal lesions. As discussed before, chorioretinitis is the most clinically significant cited CMV infection in AIDS patients. Biopsy showing characteristic inclusion bodies is necessary to diagnose CMV pneumonia, colitis, or liver disease. Effective treatment for most manifestations of CMV is unknown. Acyclovir, vidarabine, cytarabine, and idoxuridine have been tried without success.[166] Newer agents, like DHPG (see earlier text) may offer some hope for suppression of this virus.

### *Epstein–Barr Virus*

Epstein–Barr virus (EBV) causes widespread asymptomatic disease (i.e., high antibody prevalence in individuals without disease) and is associated with Burkitt's lymphoma, infectious mononucleosis, and nasopharyngeal carcinoma.[173] The virus reactivates with immunosuppressive states. Although some reports seem to suggest that acyclovir has potential in the treatment of EBV,[173] most of the evidence indicates that there is no currently effective treatment.[145] EBV has been associated with B-cell lymphoma following bone marrow transplants. An association between B-cell lymphomas and EBV among persons at risk for AIDS has been described. If so, antiviral therapy directed at EBV may play an important role in reducing the hyperplasia that may predate the malignancy.

### *Hepatitis B Virus*

Antibodies to the hepatitis B virus (HBV) surface and core antigens are detectable in more than 80% of patients with AIDS.[174] Also, studies have shown a high rate of HBV infection among homosexual men.[175] This virus is transmitted through contact with contaminated needles, blood transfusions, and contact with infected blood and/or mucous membrane secretions during sexual intercourse.[174–176]

There is no proven effective treatment for acute HBV infections, although a variety of agents for chronic HBV infection are now under investigation. Combinations of vidarabine and interferon have been studied in the treatment of chronic active hepatitis with some promising results.[177] The relationship between HBV and AIDS is still unclear, although some have suggested that HBV may be a cofactor in the development of AIDS.[175,178]

## AIDS-Related Malignancies

Several types of cancers have been shown to be associated with HIV infection and are at least moderately indicative of a defect in cell-mediated immunity. These cancers include Kaposi's sarcoma, non-Hodgkin's lymphoma (small noncleaved lymphomas or immunoblastic sarcoma), or primary lymphoma of the brain. A patient with one or more of the forementioned cancers who is known to have HIV infection would be classified as having AIDS.

### *Kaposi's Sarcoma*

Prior to the advent of AIDS, Kaposi's sarcoma was considered a rare tumor occurring in individuals with immune dysfunction or genetic predisposition. In the spring of 1981, the CDC reported a sudden increase in the incidence of Kaposi's sarcoma among homosexual men in New York City and San Francisco.[179] Kaposi's sarcoma now accounts for approximately 30% of initially diagnosed cases of AIDS, with the vast majority occurring in homosexual males with AIDS.

Moric and Kaposi first described the neoplasm in 1872 as an "idiopathic, multiple pigmented sarcoma of the skin."[180] Fifteen years later, Kaposi described the disseminated form of the disease. The sarcoma usually occurred in elderly men (fifth to eighth decades) of Mediterranean background (mostly Italian and Jewish men). In the United States the incidence is very low in patients without AIDS (<1%—0.03 cases per 100,000 people). The etiology of Kaposi's sarcoma is probably multifactorial, although CMV has been hypothesized to have a role in its development.

Kaposi's sarcoma is believed to be an endothelial malignancy. It usually manifests itself as an asymptomatic macule, papule, or nodule.[180] Patients initially present with a single or multiple red to violet lesions. Eventually there is progression from the macular/papular stage to plaques and nodules. In older men of Mediterranean extraction, lesions characteristically develop on the lower extremities (75%), but patients with AIDS may have lesions anywhere on the skin. The course of the disease in North American and European (non-AIDS) patients is usually chronic and progressive. The average survival time in American reported cases ranges from 8 to 13 years, but has often been observed to be considerably longer. These patients generally succumb to a second malignancy or another disease, rather than dying of Kaposi's sarcoma.

In contrast to the cutaneous lesions of the "classical" patients, those in homosexual males tend to be smaller, pink and located on the upper trunk, arms, head, and neck. The tip of the nose is a common site for these lesions. Some have observed that elongated lesions may follow the lines of cleavage. In addition to skin lesions, purple nodules on the oral mucosa, as well as visceral organ involvement particularly of the lymph nodes and gastrointestinal tract, are observed frequently. In addition to the differences in skin lesion presentation, patients with AIDS often present with systemic symptoms including fever, malaise, anorexia, and diarrhea. These symptoms may be secondary to HIV, other infection, or visceral involvement. Finally, some AIDS patients with Kaposi's sarcoma have abnormal cytopenias and immune studies; however, patients with Kaposi's sarcoma tend to have much more normal lymphocyte counts and numbers of the helper cells than AIDS patients who present with opportunistic infections.

The AIDS patient with Kaposi's sarcoma usually develops progressive disease over several months with gradual debilitation. Homosexual men with Kaposi's sarcoma may develop a second primary malignancy; however, more frequently they contract one of the opportunistic infections associated with AIDS. Median survival is 18 months, although some patients are still alive 3 to 4 years after their Kaposi's sarcoma diagnosis.

Kaposi's sarcoma is sensitive to both radiation and chemotherapy.[181] Cautious observation is warranted if the patient is asymptomatic and has limited skin involvement. When progressive local disease is present, radiation or single-agent chemotherapy (vincristine, vinblastine, etoposide) is the treatment of choice. Single-agent or combination chemotherapy is utilized for disseminated diseases. A major disadvantage in treating Kaposi's sarcoma in patients with AIDS with chemotherapeutic agents is the potential additional immune suppression that may result. Survival may be decreasing because of occurrences of opportunistic infections.

Many single chemotherapeutic agents have been administered to non-AIDS patients with Kaposi's sarcoma, including vincristine, vinblastine, DTIC, actinomycin D, BCNU, and cyclophosphamide.[180,182,183] In general, these agents have shown 60% initial "effectiveness" ratios. Vincristine has most often been used in combination with actinomycin D in patients with advanced Kaposi's sarcoma; antitumor activity was observed with regression of some lesions.[184–186] Vinblastine is considered to have some limited activity in the treatment of Kaposi's sarcoma. Its use should be restricted to patients who do not have anemia or significant leukopenia.

Etoposide (VP-16) has shown some activity against Kaposi's sarcoma. In one series of 22 homosexual males with early-stage, disseminated Kaposi's sarcoma, an 86% objective benefit was achieved, with approximately one half of these being complete remissions at 15 months follow-up[183]; however, patients entered into this trial did not have constitutional symptoms (i.e., fever, night sweats, weight loss), which may be a poor prognostic sign. Fewer than 15% developed opportunistic infections throughout the 10-month observation period.

Combination chemotherapeutic regimens are also being investigated. The New York and San Francisco groups have reported a response rate of approximately 80% to doxorubicin-bleomycin-vinblastine (ABV) therapy in patients with AIDS-related Kaposi's sarcoma.[182] The patients tested had rapidly progressive, widespread disease. Most responses (75%), however, were partial and not complete. Futhermore, toxicities and rate of opportunistic infections were higher with combination therapy than single-therapy studies.

Several investigators have used $\alpha$-interferon in the treatment of AIDS-related Kaposi's sarcoma because of its antiviral, antiproliferative, and immune modulatory activities.[180,187,188] Although recombinant $\alpha$-interferon has shown promise in stabilizing or reversing Kaposi's sarcoma, it has not proven beneficial in preventing opportunistic infections or in boosting the immune systems. $\alpha$-Interferon is now approved for use in the treatment of Kaposi's sarcoma in the United States. Other forms of interferon (lymphoblastoid) have been administered to patients with AIDS-related Kaposi's sarcoma with limited success.[189,190]

### *Lymphomas*

Hodgkin's disease and non-Hodgkin's lymphomas have become increasingly recognized in young adult males who are homosexual or intravenous drug abusers.[191] The appearance of non-Hodgkin's lymphoma is probably related to immunodeficiencies as have been noted among the other immunosuppressed groups (e.g., renal/cardiac transplants). The lymphomas observed in AIDS patients differ in many aspects from those seen in the general population.[192] Young males in the second and third decades of life usually acquire Hodgkin's lymphoma rather than the non-Hodgkin's variety.

Patients at risk for AIDS have been observed to have predominantly non-Hodgkin's lymphomas. Another striking difference is the ratio of nodal to extranodal location of non-Hodgkin's lymphoma. For most of the AIDS patients, lymphomas originated outside the lymph nodes, including the gastrointestinal tract and bone marrow. Nonneoplastic lymphadenopathies precede the lymphomas in many patients. Involvement of the CNS appears to be another characteristic feature of non-Hodgkin's lymphomas in AIDS.[193] Usually no more than 2% of non-Hodgkin's lymphomas involve the brain primarily and very rarely even as a secondary presentation.

The lymphomas in AIDS patients are highly aggressive (high-grade) and consistently involve multiple organs. Histology has revealed that many are of diffuse pattern and of large cell or undifferentiated cytology, thus indicative of poor response to treatment and short survival. Most drug regimens used to treat these lymphomas have contained cyclophosphamide, doxorubicin, vincristine, and prednisone (CHOP). Methotrexate, etoposide, and bleomycin were incorporated in some cases.[194] The mortality rate of AIDS patients with lymphomas appears to be much higher than that of the general population.

## Anti–Human Immunodeficiency Virus Agents

There is sufficient evidence now to accept that HIV is the cause of AIDS. Strategies are needed to inhibit the active replication of the virus and to eradicate the latent form in affected cells. There are multiple potential sites at which antivirals might attack, inhibit, or kill HIV. One possible antiviral mechanism would be interference with the HIV receptor site on the cell, thereby decreasing viral absorption and penetration into the target cell (see Fig. 91.1). The target cell that HIV attacks usually has surface T4 antigens.[38,39] Monoclonal antibodies directed against these antigens may prevent HIV attachment and penetration, and are one potential antiviral treatment. Prevention of uncoating of HIV is another step in which HIV may be inhibited. Reverse transcriptase (RT), an enzyme essential to HIV replication, is a prime target against which antivirals are being developed. Prevention of posttranscription processing, assembly, and release of new HIV are other potential processes for which anti-HIV agents are being developed.

In addition to antiviral regimens, a variety of immunomodulating agents, including interleukin-2, inosine pranobex, γ-interferon, and levamisole have been used in vivo for treatment of persons with AIDS and ARC.[195–198] Bone marrow transplantation and thymus transplants have been performed without sustained clinical or immunologic change.[199] It has been suggested that the combination of agents with anti-HIV activity and immunoregulatory properties may prove to be more effective therapy for HIV infection than either alone. Similarly, the use of two antivirals may be an especially useful approach if the drugs have different mechanisms of action and appear additive or synergistic in vitro and/or in any animal model.

A variety of agents have been reported to have antiretroviral activity in vitro. The majority of these have been

**Figure 91.1** Schematic diagram indicating possible sites of action of antiviral agents against the human immunodeficiency virus type III. *(Adapted from Gallo RC, Wong-Staal F. A human T-lymphotropic retrovirus (HTLV-III) as the cause of the acquired immunodeficiency syndrome. Ann Intern Med 1985;103:679–689; Tartaglione T, Collier A. Development of antiviral agents for the treatment of human immunodeficiency virus infection. Clin Pharm 1987;6:929, with permission. Copyright 1987 American Society of Hospital Pharmacists.)*

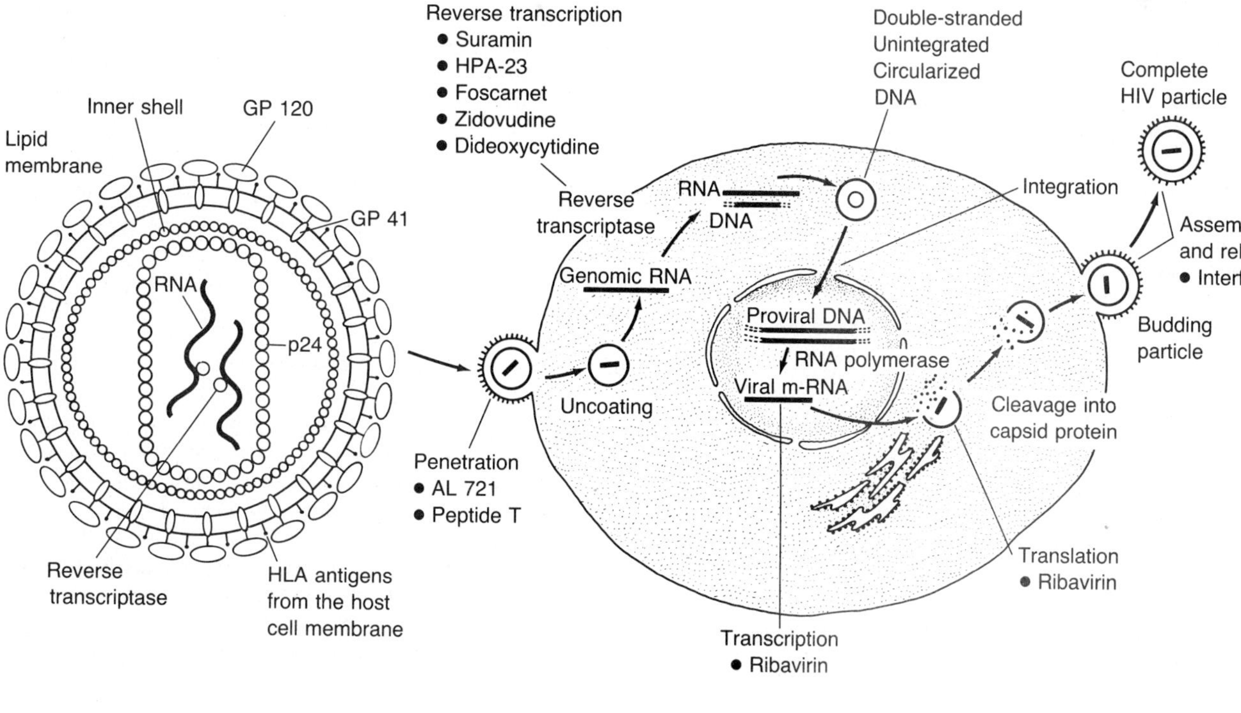

**Table 91.6** Drug Concentrations and Mechanisms of Action for In Vitro Inhibition of HIV

| *Agent* | *Anti-HIV concentration* | *Achievable serum concentration* | *Action* |
|---|---|---|---|
| Suramin[202] | Suppression, 50 μg/mL; inhibition, 100–1000 μg/mL | >100 μg/mL with 1-g IV dose | RT[a] inhibition |
| Ribavirin[203] | Suppression, 50–100 μg/mL | 1–3 μg/mL | RT inhibition |
| HPA-23[204] | $ID_{50}$,[b] 30 μg/mL | ... | RT inhibition |
| Interferon alpha[205] | Suppression, 4–64 U/mL; inhibition, 256–1064 U/mL | 50–300 U/mL | Inhibits viral release |
| Foscarnet[206] | Suppression, 132 μM; inhibition, 680 μM | 100–450 μM | RT inhibition |
| Zidovudine[207,208] | Inhibition, <0.13–2.7 μg/mL | 0.5–3 μg/mL | RT inhibition; DNA chain termination |
| AL 721[212] | $ED_{50}$,[c] 100 μg/mL; $ED_{90}$,[d] 1000 μg/mL | ... | Alteration of viral envelope |
| Inosine pranobex[209] | Suppression, 100–200 μg/mL | Theoretically 200–400 μg/mL achievable with 6–8 g/d | RT inhibition |
| Rifabutine[210] | Suppression, 0.1–0.5 μg/mL | 0.2–0.5 μg/mL | RT inhibition |
| Dideoxycytidine[211] | Inhibition, 0.1–0.5 μg/mL | 0.02–0.4 μg/mL | RT inhibition; DNA chain termination |

[a] RT = reverse transcriptase.
[b] $ID_{50}$ = median initial dose (a measure of the amount of pathogenic organisms that will produce infection in 50% of test subjects).
[c] $ED_{50}$ = median effective dose (the dose that produces effects in 50% of the population).
[d] $ED_{90}$ = median effective dose (the dose that produces effects in 90% of the population).

Adapted from Tartaglione TA, Collier AC. Development of antiviral agents for the treatment of human immunodeficiency virus infection. Clin Pharm 1987;6:931, with permission. Copyright 1987 American Society of Hospital Pharmacists.

shown to inhibit reverse transcriptase, an enzyme characteristic of both animal and human retroviruses.[200,201] The agents that have been shown to inhibit the reverse transcriptase of HIV in vitro include suramin, ribavirin, ammonium 21-tungsto-9-antimoniate (HPA-23), recombinant α-interferon (INF), phosphonoformate (PFA), ansamycin (rifabutine), zidovudine (formerly azidothymidine, AZT, BW A509U), sodium diethyldithiocarbamate ("imuthiol"), and inosine pranobex (isoprinosine).[202–208,209,210] Two nucleoside analogs (relatives of AZT), dideoxycytidine and dideoxyadenosine, have recently been shown to inhibit the cytopathic effect and replication of HIV.[211] In addition to agents with this mechanism of action, AL 721, a lipid compound that extracts cholesterol from cellular membranes, has been shown to inhibit HIV replication in vitro.[212] Preliminary reports of a phase 1 trial have been published.[213] Peptide T, a 10-amino-acid peptide binds to the CD-4 receptor in vitro and appears to prevent HIV from entering cells.[214] Table 91.6 summarizes the published information regarding in vitro inhibition of HIV replication.

Although the published in vivo experience with agents having in vitro anti-HIV activity is limited, the demonstration of suppression of HIV viremia is an encouraging preliminary result. The first drug reported to have in vitro activity against HIV was suramin.[202] Previously, this drug was used for the treatment of East African trypanosomiasis. Treatment of patients with AIDS or ARC with suramin (6.2 g IV over 5–6 weeks) has been reported[215–217] to transiently suppress detectable HIV in blood cultures. Pharmacokinetic paramaters can be found in Table 91.7. Side effects, including proteinuria, fever, rash, and elevation of hepatic transaminases occurred in the majority of patients; however, no consistent clinical or immunologic improvement was noted. A number of additional studies discussed at the 1986 International Conference on AIDS provided similar findings following suramin treatment including (1) confirmation of suramin's in vivo inhibition of HIV; (2) lack of significant clinical improvement; (3) lack of immunologic improvements; and (4) considerable, yet reversible, toxicity.[218–223] In one study, adrenal insufficiency occurred in 27 of 63 evaluable patients and neutropenia was noted in 36%.[218] Suramin did not prevent the development of recurrent or new opportunistic infections. These data support the belief that suramin does not have a role as a single agent in the treatment of HIV disease.

The published experience with HPA-23 is also limited to small numbers of patients, but intravenous administration (1–3.3 mg/kg per dose in two courses over 4 months in one patient and 200 mg/d for 15 days in three patients) inhibited HIV replication in all four patients during therapy.[223] Thrombocytopenia and elevations in hepatic transaminases occurred in three patients, but returned to pretreatment levels after therapy was stopped. By the time of the AIDS Antiviral Workshop, 47 patients had been treated in France with intravenous doses of HPA-23 ranging from 50 to 200 mg/d with similar results (viral suppression, moderate side effects, and little observable clinical improvement). Thrombocytopenia was observed in 33 of the 47 patients. Limited pharmacokinetic data indicate that HPA-23 may be seques-

**Table 91.7** Pharmacokinetic Properties of Several Anti-HIV Agents

| *Agent* | *Dose (route)* | *Peak serum concentration* | *Bioavailability* | *Elimination half-life with normal renal function* | *Mode of elimination* | *Cerebrospinal fluid penetration* |
|---|---|---|---|---|---|---|
| Suramin[218] | 1 g (IV) | >100 μg/mL | Poor | 44–54 d | Renal | Minimal |
| Ribavirin[226] | 600–2400 mg (IV) | 10–40 μg/mL | 10% | 2 h (beta) | Extensively metabolized | Yes |
| | 600–2400 mg (PO) | 1–3 μg/mL | | 36 h (gamma) | | |
| HPA-23[224] | 1–3.3 mg/kg (IV) | | Poor | 2–3 h | Renal (15–50%) | Unknown |
| Foscarnet[231] | 20 mg/kg/24 hr (IV) | 250–500 μM | Poor | 6 hr | Renal | Yes |
| Zidovudine[232,235] | 200–250 mg every 4 hr (IV) | 1.5–3 μg/mL | 70% | 1.1 h | Hepatic (75%) | Yes |
| | 200–250 mg every 4 hr (PO) | 1–2 μg/mL | | | | |
| Dideoxycytidine[242] | 0.03 mg/kg (IV) | 0.02–0.06 μg/mL | 100% | 1.0 h | Renal | Yes |
| | 0.25 mg/kg (IV) | 0.2–0.4 μg/mL | | | | |

Adapted from Tartaglione TA, Collier AC. Development of antiviral agents for the treatment of human immunodeficiency virus infection. Clin Pharm 1987;6:932, with permission. Copyright 1987 American Society of Hospital Pharmacists.

tered outside of the plasma (Table 91.7). The role of HPA-23 in treating HIV infection remains unclear.[224]

Ribavirin is a synthetic purine nucleoside that has shown in vitro activity against a broad spectrum of DNA and RNA viruses. Its mechanism of action may be twofold: competitive inhibition of reverse transcriptase and interference with the GTP-dependent capping of the 5′ end of viral mRNA.[203,225] Partial suppression of HIV replication has been observed at concentrations of 50 to 100 μg/mL.

Ribavirin has been administered orally and intravenously. Oral bioavailability is approximately 10% (Table 91.7).[226] Peak serum concentrations after the 600- to 2400-mg doses ranged from 1 to 3 μg/mL and 10 to 40 μg/mL for oral and intravenous administration, respectively. Of importance is its excellent cerebrospinal fluid penetration. Ribavirin is metabolized extensively to inactive compounds with a beta elimination half-life of 2 hours and a gamma half-life of approximately 36 hours.

Phase I-II studies, initiated in early 1985, indicated that ribavirin was well tolerated with its major toxic effect being a reversible reduction in hemoglobin. Results of a placebo-controlled trial of 163 patients with persistent generalized lymphadenopathy were recently reported; 107 patients received either 600 or 800 mg of ribavirin orally once daily.[227] Initial reports indicated that 18% of placebo recipients developed AIDS compared with 11% and 0% of the 600-mg and 800-mg ribavirin recipients, respectively. However, the number of subjects with very low T4 cell counts were not equally distributed between placebo and treatment groups. The FDA recently ruled that no substantial evidence exists of ribavirin's effectiveness in decreasing the number of patients with HIV-associated lymphadenopathy who develop AIDS.

A similar trial of ribavirin therapy in ARC patients has also been conducted.[228] Treatment with oral ribavirin for 12 weeks did not alter serum concentrations of the p24 core antigen. In vitro, ribavirin and zidovudine are antagonistic, and these two agents should not be coadministered.[229] Further clinical trials will be required to determine if ribavirin offers any promise as an HIV antiviral agent.

Foscarnet sodium (trisodium phosphonoformate hexahydrate, PFA) is a selective agent that inhibits reverse transcriptase and inhibits a wide range of DNA and RNA polymerases.[206] Specifically, foscarnet appears to interact with nucleic acid polymerases at the site where pyrophosphate is released during elongation of the DNA or RNA chain.[230] The cell-free reverse transcriptase of HIV is inhibited by 50% at a concentration of approximately 1 μM foscarnet.[206]

Foscarnet is currently available only as an intravenous product. Most studies have used a dosage of 20 mg/kg over 24 hours as a continuous infusion. Plasma concentrations ranged from 250 to 500 μM (75–150 μg/mL) during the infusion period (Table 91.7).[231] Most of the drug is eliminated unchanged in the urine, with an estimated serum elimination half-life of 6 hours. Foscarnet appears to penetrate the cerebrospinal fluid in patients with and without meningeal inflammation, although concentrations were significantly higher during meningitis.

Pilot studies with foscarnet in patients with AIDS and ARC and cytomegalovirus retinitis are under way in both the United States and Europe. Preliminary results with patients who have AIDS or ARC indicate some clinical improvement, return of delayed-type hypersensitivity, and inability to isolate HIV after initiation of therapy in several patients.[232,233]

Isoprinosine has also been tested on a limited basis among immunosuppressed homosexual males and clinical manifestations and symptoms associated with early HIV infection and ARC.[234] Clinical improvement has been documented in one half of subjects receiving a 3-g treatment compared with 10% in the placebo group. Also, a variety of immunologic improvements such as increases in natural killer cells, total T lymphocytes, and T4 cells were observed.

Zidovudine is a thymidine analog in which the 3′ hydroxy group is replaced by an azido ($N_3$) group (Fig. 91.2). At

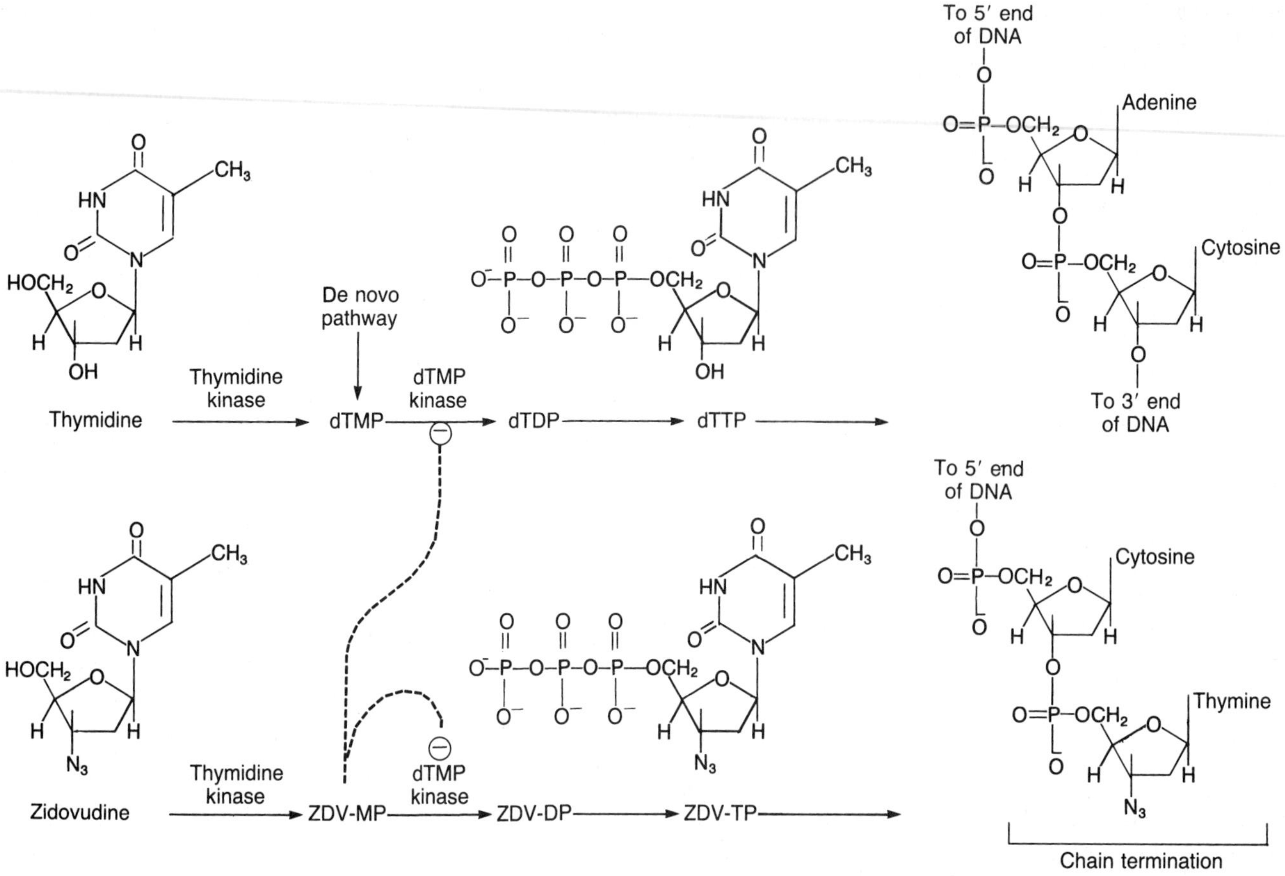


**Figure 91.2** Intracellular metabolism of zidovudine and thymidine and postulated mechanism of inhibition of HIV replication by dideoxynucleoside triphosphates. dTMP = deoxythymidylic acid, dTDP = thymidine 5′-diphosphate. dTTP = thymidine 5′-triphosphate, ZDV-MP = zidovudine monophosphate, ZDV-DP = zidovudine diphosphate, and ZDV-TP = zidovudine triphosphate. *(Adapted from Mitsuya H, Broder S. Development of antiretroviral therapy for the acquired immunodeficiency syndrome and related disorders N Engl J Med 1987; 31:557–564; Tartaglione T, Collier A. Development of antiviral agents for the treatment of human immunodeficiency virus infection. Clin Pharm 1987;6:934, with permission. Copyright 1987 American Society of Hospital Pharmacists.)*

concentrations of less than 0.13 ug/mL, zidovudine inhibits 90% of detectable HIV in vitro. In vivo, zidovudine is converted by cellular enzymes to a triphosphate form, which is subsequently used by HIV reverse-transcriptase (Fig. 91.2). Incorporation of zidovudine-triphosphate in the HIV-DNA chain results in chain termination for DNA synthesis.

A phase I trial in ARC/AIDS patients has been completed by Blum and colleagues at Burroughs–Wellcome Research Laboratories.[235] In these initial dose-finding trials, zidovudine was shown to have good oral bioavailability and to be well tolerated. Additionally, some positive immunologic and/or clinical responses (e.g., induced remission of KS) were observed, although several patients developed non-life-threatening infections in therapy. Zidovudine's pharmacokinetics are summarized in Table 91.7. Of note is zidovudine's ability to penetrate the blood–brain barrier.[236]

A phase II study (as part of a multicenter trial sponsored by the Burroughs–Wellcome Company) to evaluate the antiviral efficacy of zidovudine was performed in 281 patients with AIDS or ARC.[237,238] Half of the patients were assigned to receive zidovudine at a dose of 250 mg every 4 hours (1.5 g daily) and half received placebo. Many patients on zidovudine required a reduction in dosage or interruption of treatment, primarily because of anemia. The groups were comparable at entry for a variety of variables including age, sex, race, weight, mean Karnofsky score, and severity of illness. On September 18, 1986, the study was prematurely terminated because of the marked imbalance in mortality, primarily in AIDS patients secondary to opportunistic infection. Patients had received between $3\frac{1}{2}$ and 7 months of therapy (median of 4.5 months) at the time the placebo group was discontinued. Twenty-three percent of zidovudine-treated patients showed a significantly reduced risk of acquiring an AIDS-defining opportunistic infection after 6 weeks of treatment compared with 43% of placebo-treated patients. A modest increase in mean T4 cell counts was seen in the zidovudine-treated group at 12 weeks, but the importance of this finding is unclear because the T4 cell counts declined later in therapy in some patients. Preliminary findings in 22 patients (19 AIDS, 3 ARC) treated with either placebo or zidovudine for 16 to 20 weeks revealed a significant decrease in HIV core antigen in zidovudine-patients.[239] This marker may be a significant serologic tool for the monitoring of disease progression and effectiveness of antiviral drug therapy.

Zidovudine administration was associated with a significant degree of neutropenia and anemia.[238] Forty-seven of 145 patients receiving zidovudine experienced greater than 25% reduction in hemoglobin, compared with 13 or 137 patients receiving placebo. Blood transfusions were required for 31% of the patients receiving zidovudine (all patients, including AIDS and ARC) and for 11% of those on placebo. Blood transfusions were required for 46% of the patients with AIDS who received zidovudine, compared with 15% of those on placebo. Neutropenia (<750 granulocytes) developed in 39% of all patients receiving zidovudine and 7% of those of placebo. Neutropenia (<500 granulocytes) developed in 15% of all patients receiving zidovudine and 2% of those on placebo. In patients with AIDS who received zidovudine, neutropenia (<750 granulocytes) occurred in 48% while neutropenia (<500 granulocytes) occurred in 18% of the patients. The respective degrees of neutropenia in AIDS patients receiving placebo were 9% and 3%. In general, decreases in hemoglobin and neutrophils occurred during the second month of therapy and appeared to be reversible if the dose was decreased or the drug discontinued.

Other side effects reported with zidovudine include rashes, pruritis, nausea, headache, and mild confusion. Recently, a case of central nervous system toxicity contributing to death was reported in an AIDS patient treated with zidovudine.[240] Complaints of headache or confusion may precede severe neurotoxicity and should be monitored closely. Some patients may require reduction of their zidovudine dose or complete discontinuation of the drug.

On the basis of this information, zidovudine was approved by the FDA during March 1987 and is indicated for the management of adult patients with symptomatic HIV infection (AIDS and advanced ARC) who have a history of cytologically confirmed *Pneumocystis carinii* pneumonia or an absolute T4, lymphocyte count of fewer than 200 cells/mm$^3$ in the peripheral blood.[241] For eligible patients, the recommended starting dosage of zidovudine is 200 mg orally every 4 hours around the clock. Dosage adjustment may be needed in some patients if toxicity develops. Careful monitoring of hematologic variables is recommended at least every 2 weeks. Reductions in hemoglobin may occur as early as 2 to 4 weeks after starting therapy, whereas granulocytopenia often is not observed until weeks 6 through 8. If anemia (hemoglobin of <7.5 g/dL or a reduction of >25% from baseline) or granulocytopenia (granulocyte count of <750 cells/mm$^3$ or a reduction of >50% from baseline) occurs, zidovudine may need to be temporarily discontinued. Many practitioners favor continuing zidovudine at a reduced dosage if the only adverse effect is anemia and providing transfusions when necessary. For less severe bone marrow suppression, dosage modification alone may reverse the effects; if bone marrow recovery occurs, gradual increases in dosage may be attempted.

Limited information is available on the interaction of other drugs with zidovudine. Coadministration of zidovudine with agents that produce hematologic, nephrotoxic, or cytotoxic effects (e.g., dapsone, pentamidine, amphotericin B, flucytosine, vincristine, vinblastine, doxorubicin, interferon) may increase the risk of toxicity. Acetaminophen, rifampin, cimetidine, ranitidine, flurazepam, indomethacin, probenecid, and other drugs that may competitively inhibit glucuronidation should be avoided. Little information on additive toxicity is available for trimethoprim–sulfamethoxazole, pyrimethamine, or other drugs commonly taken by patients with AIDS. Long-term administration of other medications with zidovudine has not been systematically studied and should be avoided if possible.

2′,3′-Dideoxycytidine is another nucleoside analogue similar in structure to zidovudine. In some in vitro systems dideoxycytidine appears to be a more potent inhibitor of the replication and cytopathic effect of HIV than zidovudine. Concentrations ranging from 0.5 $\mu$M (0.1 $\mu$g/mL) to 2 $\mu$M (0.425 $\mu$g/mL) of dideoxycytidine have been shown to inhibit HIV growth and to prevent the expression of the p24 core protein in T cell lines.[211] Preliminary pharmacokinetic data from a phase I trial at the National Institutes of Health is outlined in Table 91.7. Patients with AIDS or ARC are currently being enrolled in phase I clinical trials.[242] Adverse effects observed so far include peripheral neuropathy, rashes, fever, aphthous stomatitis, thrombocytopenia, lactate dehydrogenase elevation, and anemia. The relationship of these reactions to drug administration is unclear. Other trials to establish the most appropriate dosage regimens and to further explore the pharmacokinetics and bioavailability of dideoxycytidine are under way.

Many newer agents are now being considered as potential therapies for HIV infection including ampligen, castanospermine, tumor necrosis factor (TNF gamma), and granulocyte macrophage colony stimulating factor (GMCSF).[243–245] Combinations of antivirals are also under consideration, such as zidovudine plus acyclovir. The establishment of the AIDS Clinical Trials Group (formerly the AIDS Treatment Evaluation Unit) by the National Institutes of Health will hopefully expedite controlled clinical trials with anti-retroviral agents and facilitate the rate to which a cure for AIDS is found.

## References


1. Gottlieb MS, Schroff R, Schauber HM, et al. *Pneumocystis carinii* pneumonia and mucosal candidiasis in previously healthy homosexual men. N Engl J Med 1981;305:1425–1431.
2. Masur H, Michelis MA, Greene JB, et al. An outbreak of community acquired *Pneumocystis carinii* pneumonia—initial manifestation of cellular immune dysfunction. N Engl J Med 1981;305:1431–1438.
3. Siegal FP, Lopez C, Hammer GS, et al. Severe acquired immunodeficiency in male homosexuals manifested by chronic perianal ulcerative herpes simplex lesions. N Engl J Med 1981;305:1439–1444.
4. Friedman-Kien AE, Laubenstein LJ, Rubinstein P, et al. Disseminated Kaposi's sarcoma in homosexual men. Ann Intern Med 1982;96:693–700.

5. Barnes DM. Grim projection of AIDS epidemic. Science 1986;232:1589–1590.
6. Gallo RC, Salahuddin SZ, Popovic M, et al. Frequent detection and isolation of cytopathic retroviruses (HTLV-III) from patients with AIDS and at risk for AIDS. Science 1984;224: 500–503.
7. Barre-Sinoussi F, Chermann JC, Rey F, et al. Isolation of a T-lymphotropic retrovirus from a patient at risk for acquired immune deficiency syndrome (AIDS). Science 1983;220:868–871.
8. Levy JA, Hoffman AD, Kramer SM, et al. Isolation of lymphocytopathic retroviruses from San Francisco patients with AIDS. Science 1984;225:840–842.
9. Chamberland ME, Castro KG, Haverkos HW, et al. Acquired immunodeficiency syndrome in the United States: an analysis of cases outside high-incidence groups. Ann Intern Med 1984; 101:617–623.
10. Centers for Disease Control. Update: acquired immunodeficiency syndrome and human immunodeficiency virus infection in health care workers. MMWR 1988;37:229–239.
11. Centers for Disease Control. Update: acquired immunodeficiency syndrome (AIDS)—United States. MMWR 1984;33: 661–664.
12. Curran JW, Morgan WM, Hardy AM, et al. The epidemiology of AIDS: current status and future prospects. Science 1985; 229:1352–1357.
13. Jaffe HW, Darrow WW, Echenberg DF, et al. The acquired immunodeficiency syndrome in a cohort of homosexual men: a six year follow-up study. Ann Intern Med 1985;103:210–214.
14. Collier AC, Meyers JD, Roberts PL, et al. Relationship between antibody to LAV/HTLV-III and the natural course of subclinical cellular immune dysfunction in homosexual men. Sex Transmitt Dis 1987;14:1–8.
15. Melbye M, Biggar RJ, Ebbesen P, et al. Long-term seropositivity for human T-lymphotropic virus type III in homosexual men without the acquired immunodeficiency syndrome: development of immunologic and clinical abnormalities. Ann Intern Med 1986;104:496–500.
16. Abrams DI, Lewis BJ, Beckstead JH, et al. Persistent diffuse lymphodenopathy in homosexual men: endpoint or prodrome? Ann Intern Med 1984;100:801–808.
17. Jaffe H, O'Malley P, Rulherford G, et al. Natural history of HTLV-III/LAV infection in a cohort of gay men. Twenty-sixth Interscience Conference on Antimicrobial Agents and Chemotherapy, 1986. Washington, DC, American Society of Microbiology. Abstract 1, p 97.
18. Brunet JB, Ancelle RA. International occurrence of the acquired immunodeficiency syndrome. Ann Intern Med 1985; 103:670–674.
19. Polk BF, Fox R, Brookmeyer R, et al. Predictors of the acquired immunodeficiency syndrome developing in a cohort of seropositive homosexual men. N Engl J Med 1987;316:61–66.
20. Zagury D, Bernard J, Leibowitch J, et al. HTLV-III in cells cultured from semen of two patients with AIDS. Science 1984; 226:449–451.
21. Ho DD, Schooley RT, Rota T, et al. HTLV-III in the semen and blood of a healthy homosexual man. Science 1984;226: 451–453.
22. Report of the Centers for Disease Control Task Force on Kaposi's Sarcoma and Opportunistic Infections. Epidemiologic aspects of the current outbreak of Kaposi's sarcoma and opportunistic infections. N Engl J Med 1982;306:248–252.
23. Centers for Disease Control. World Health Organization workshop: conclusions and recommendations on acquired immunodeficiency syndrome. MMWR 1985;253:3385–3391.
24. Lapointe N, Michaud J, Pekovic D, et al. Transplacental transmission of HTLV-III virus. N Engl J Med 1985;312:1325–1326.
25. Cowan MJ, Hellmann D, Chudwin D, et al. Maternal transmission of acquired immune deficiency syndrome. Pediatrics 1984;73:382–386.
26. DiMakia H, Courpotin C, Rouzioux C, et al. Transplacental transmission of human immunodeficiency virus. Lancet 1986;2:215–216.
27. Wofsky CB, Cohen JB, Hauer LB, et al. Isolation of AIDS-associated retrovirus from genital secretion of women with antibodies to the virus. Lancet 1986;1:527–529.
28. Centers for Disease Control. Heterosexual transmission of human T-lymphotropic virus type III/lymphadenopathy-associated virus. MMWR 1985;34:561–563.
29. Friedland GH, Saltzman BR, Rogers MF, et al. Lack of transmission of HTLV-III/LAV infection to household contacts of patients with AIDS or AIDS-related complex with oral candidiasis. N Engl J Med 1986;314:344–349.
30. Centers for Disease Control. Update: Human immunodeficiency virus infection in health care workers exposed to blood of infected patients. MMWR 1987;36:285–289.
31. Gerberding JL, Bryant CE, Moss A, et al. Risk of acquired immunodeficiency syndrome (AIDS) virus transmission to health care workers (HCW): Results of a prospective cohort study. Paper presented to Second International Conference on AIDS. Paris, June 23–25, 1986, p 124.
32. Kuhls TL, Viker S, Parris NB, et al. A prospective cohort study of the occupational risk of AIDS and AIDS-related infections in health care personnel. Paper presented to Second International Conference on AIDS. Paris, June 23–25, 1986, p 117.
33. Centers for Disease Control. Recommendations for preventing transmission of infection with human T-lymphotropic virus type III/lymphadenopathy-associated virus during invasive procedures. Ann Intern Med 1986;104:824–825.
34. Ratner L, Gallo RC, Wong-Staal F. HTLV-III, LAV, ARV are variants of the same AIDS virus. Nature 1985;313:636–637.
35. Wain-Hobson S, Alizon M, Montagnier S. Relationship of AIDS to other retroviruses. (Lett) Nature 1985;313:743.
36. Wong-Staal F, Shaw GM, Hahn BH, et al. Genomic diversity of human T-lymphotropic virus type III (HTLV-III). Science 1985;229:759–762.
37. Benn S, Rutledge R, Folks T, et al. Genomic heterogeneity of AIDS retroviral isolates from North America and Zaire. Science 1985;230:949–951.
38. Dalgleish AG, Beverley PCL, Clapham PR, et al. The CD4 (T4) antigen is an essential component of the receptor for the AIDS retrovirus. Nature 1984;312:763–767.
39. Klatzmann D, Champagne E, Chamaret S, et al. The lymphocyte T4 molecule behaves as the receptor for human retrovirus LAV. Nature 1984;312:767–768.
40. Shaw GM, Hahn BH, Arya SK, et al. Molecular characterization of human T-cell leukemia (lymphotropic) virus type III in the acquired immunodeficiency syndrome. Science 1984;226: 1165–1171.
41. Gallo RC, Wong-Staal F. A human T-lymphotropic retrovirus (HTLV-III) as the cause of the acquired immunodeficiency syndrome. Ann Intern Med 1985;103:679–689.
42. Sarngadharan MG, Popovic M, Bruch L, et al. Antibodies reactive with human T-lymphotropic retroviruses (HTLV-III) in the serum of patients with AIDS. Science 1984;224:506–508.
43. Vogt MW, Witt DJ, Craven DE, et al. Pattern of HTLV-III

isolation from cervical secretions during the menstrual cycle of women at risk for AIDS. Twenty-Sixth Interscience Conference on Antimicrobial Agents and Chemotherapy. Washington DC, American Society for Microbiology. 1986, Abstract 179, p 128.

44. Fujikawa LS, Salahuddin SZ, Palestine AG, et al. Isolation of human T-lymphotropic virus type III from the tears of a patient with the acquired immunodeficiency syndrome. Lancet 1985;2: 529–530.
45. Levy JA, Shimabukuro J, Hollander H, et al. Isolation of AIDS associated retroviruses from cerebrospinal fluid and brain of patients with neurological symptoms. Lancet 1985;2: 586–588.
46. Groopman JE, Salahuddin SZ, Sarngaharan MG, et al. HTLV-III in saliva of people with AIDS-related complex and healthy homosexual men at risk for AIDS. Science 1984;226:447–449.
47. Zagury D, Fouchard M, Vol JC, et al. Detection of infectious HTLV-III/LAV virus in cell-free plasma from AIDS patients. (Lett) Lancet 1985;2:505–506.
48. Thiry L, Sprecher-Goldbergger S, Jondkheer T, et al. Isolation of AIDS virus from cell-free breast milk of three healthy virus carriers. (Lett) Lancet 1985;2:891–892.
49. Jaffe HW, Feorino PM, Darrow WW, et al. Persistent infection with human T-lymphotropic virus type III/lymphadenopathy-associated virus in apparently healthy homosexual men. Ann Intern Med 1985;102:627–628.
50. Kaplan JE, Spira TJ, Feorino PM, et al. HTLV-III viremia in homosexual men with generalized lymphadenopathy. (Lett) N Engl J Med 1985;312:1572–1573.
51. Petricciani JC. Licensed tests for antibody to human T-lymphotropic virus type III: sensitivity and specificity. Ann Intern Med 1985;103:726–729.
52. Seligmann M, Chess L, Fahey JL, et al. AIDS—an immunologic reevaluation. N Engl J Med 1984;311:1286–1292.
53. Bowen DL, Lane HC, Fauci AS. Immunopathogenesis of the acquired immunodeficiency syndrome. Ann Intern Med 1985; 103:704–709.
54. Ciobanu N, Welk K, Kruger G, et al. Defective T-cell response to PHA and mitogenic monoclonal antibodies in male homosexuals with acquired immunodeficiency syndrome and its in vitro correction by interleukin 2. J Clin Immunol 1983;3:332–340.
55. Gupta S, Safai B. Deficient autologous mixed lymphocyte reaction in cells. J Clin Invest 1983;71:296–300.
56. Murray H, Rubin BY, Masur H, et al. Impaired production of lymphokines and immune (gamma) interferon in the acquired immunodeficiency syndrome. N Engl J Med 1984;310:883–889.
57. Cunningham-Rundles S, Michelis MA, Masur H. Serum suppression of lymphocyte activation in vitro in acquired immunodeficiency disease. J Clin Immunol 1983;3:156–165.
58. Rook RH, Masur H, Lane HC, et al. Interleukin-2 enhances the depressed natural killer and cytomegalovirus-specific cytotoxic activities of lymphocytes from patients with the acquired immunodeficiency syndrome. J Clin Invest 1983;72:398–403.
59. Lane HC, Masur H, Edgar LC, et al. Abnormalities of B-cell activation and immunoregulation in patients with the acquired immunodeficiency syndrome. N Engl J Med 1983;309:453–458.
60. Smith P, Ohura K, Masur H, et al. Monocyte function in the acquired immune deficiency syndrome: defective chemotaxis. J Clin Invest 1984;74:2121–2128.
61. Purdy BD, Plaisance KI. Current concepts in clinical therapeutics: Immunologic treatment of human immunodeficiency virus infections. Clin Pharm 1987;6:851–865.
62. Carne CA, Tedder RS, Smith A, et al. Acute encephalitis coincident with seroconversion for anti-HTLV-III. Lancet 1985;2:1206–1208.
63. Ho DD, Sarngadharan MG, Resnick L, et al. Primary human T-lymphotropic virus type III infection. Ann Intern Med 1985; 103:880–883.
64. Black PH. HTLV-III, AIDS, and the brain, editorial. N Engl J Med 1985;313:1538–1540.
65. Gottlieb MS, Groopman JE, Weinstein WM, et al. The acquired immunodeficiency syndrome. Ann Intern Med 1983;99: 208–220.
66. Rubinstein A, Sicklick M, Gupta A, et al. Acquired immunodeficiency with reversed T4/T8 ratios in infants born to promiscuous and drug-addicted mothers. JAMA 1983;249:2350–2356.
67. Scott GB, Buck BE, Leterman JG, et al. Acquired immunodeficiency syndrome in infants. N Engl J Med 1985;310:76–81.
68. Shannon KM, Ammann AJ. Acquired immune deficiency syndrome in childhood. J Pediatr 1985;106:332–342.
69. Wykoff RF, Pearl ER, Saulsbury FT. Immunologic dysfunction in infants infected through transfusions with HTLV-III. N Engl J Med 1985;312:294–296.
70. Haverkos HW, Gottlieb MS, Killen JY, et al. (Lett) J Infect Dis 1985;152:1095.
71. Redfield RR, Wright DC, Tramont EC. The Walter Reed staging classification for HTLV-III/LAV infection. N Engl J Med 1986;314:131–132.
72. Centers for Disease Control. Classification system for human T-lymphotropic virus type III/lymphadenopathy-associated virus infections. Ann Intern Med 1986;105:234–237.
73. Walzer PD, Perl DP, Krogstad DJ, et al. *Pneumocystis carinii* pneumonia in the United States—epidemiologic, diagnostic and clinical features. Ann Intern Med 1974;80:83–93.
74. Whimbey E, Gold JWM, Polsky B, et al. Bacteremia and fungemia in patients with the acquired immunodeficiency syndrome. Ann Intern Med 1986;104:511–514.
75. Saltzman BR, Motyl MR, Friedland GH, et al. *Mycobacterium tuberculosis* bacteremia in the acquired immunodeficiency syndrome. JAMA 1986;256:390–391.
76. Polsky B, Gold JWM, Whimbey E, et al. Bacterial pneumonia in patients with the acquired immunodeficiency syndrome. Ann Intern Med 1986;104:38–41.
77. Sunderam G, McDonald RJ, Maniatis T, et al. Tuberculosis as a manifestation of the acquired immunodeficiency syndrome (AIDS). JAMA 1986;256:362–366.
78. Fauci AS, Masur H, Gelmann EP, et al. The acquired immunodeficiency syndrome: an update. Ann Intern Med 1985;102: 800–813.
79. Murray JF, Felton CP, Garray SM, et al. Pulmonary complications of the acquired immunodeficiency syndrome: report of a National Heart, Lung and Blood Institute workshop. N Engl J Med 1984;310:1682–1688.
80. Jaffe HS, Ammann A, Abrams D, et al. Complications of co-trimoxazole in treatment of AIDS-associated *Pneumocystis carinii* pneumonia in homosexual men. Lancet 1983;2:1109–1111.
81. Hughes WT, Feldman S, Chaudhary S, et al. Comparison of pentamidine isethionate and trimethoprim–sulfamethoxazole in the treatment of *Pneumocystis carinii* pneumonia. J Pediatr 1978;92:285–291.
82. Wharton JM, Coleman DL, Wofsky CB, et al. Trimethoprim–sulfamethoxazole or pentamidine for *Pneumocystis carinii* pneumonia in the acquired immunodeficiency syndrome. Ann Intern Med 1986;105:37–44.
83. Klein NC, Duncanson FP, Lenox TH, et al. Prospective randomized treatment for *Pneumocystis carinii* pneumonia

(PCP) in AIDS patients. Paper presented to Second International Conference on AIDS. Paris, June 23–25, 1986, p 52.

**84.** Bowden FJ, Harman PJ, Lucas CR. Serum trimethoprim and sulfamethoxazole levels in AIDS. Lancet 1986;2:853.

**85.** Gordin FM, Simon GL, Wofsy CB, et al. Adverse reactions to trimethoprim–sulfamethoxazole in patients with acquired immunodeficiency syndrome. Ann Intern Med 1984;100:495–499.

**86.** Gibbons RB, Lindauer JA. Successful treatment of *Pneumocystis carinii* pneumonia with trimethoprim–sulfamethoxazole in hypersensitive AIDS patients (Lett) JAMA 1985;253:1259–1260.

**87.** Western KA, Perera DR, Schultz MG. Pentamidine isethionate in the treatment of *Pneumocystis carinii* pneumonia. Ann Intern Med 1970;73:695–702.

**88.** Conte, JE, Upton RA, Phelps RT, et al. Use of a specific and sensitive assay to determine pentamidine pharmacokinetics in patients with AIDS. J Infec Dis 1986;154:923–929.

**89.** Conte JE, Upton RA, Lin ET. Pentamidine pharmacokinetics in patients with AIDS with impaired renal function. J Infec Dis 1987;156:885–890.

**90.** Bennett WM, Muther RS, Parker RA, et al. Drug therapy in renal failure: dosing guidelines for adults. Ann Intern Med 1980;93:62–89.

**91.** Zuger A, Wolf BZ, El-Sadr W, et al. Pentamidine associated fatal acute pancreatitis. JAMA 1986;256:2383–2385.

**92.** Navin TR, Fontaine RE, Intravenous versus intramuscular administration of pentamidine. (Lett) N Engl J Med 1984;311:1701–1702.

**93.** Mallory DL, Bailey KR, Parrillo JE, et al. Cardiovascular effects of intravenous and intra-muscular pentamidine. Twenty-Sixth Interscience Conference on Antimicrobial Agents and Chemotherapy, Washington D.C., American Society for Microbiology, 1986, Abstract 35, p 102.

**94.** Pearson RD, Hewlett EL. Pentamidine for the treatment of *Pneumocystis carinii* pneumonia and other protozoal diseases. Ann Intern Med 1985;103:782–786.

**95.** Bouchard P, Sai P, Reach G, et al. Diabetes mellitus following pentamidine-induced hypoglycemia in humans. Diabetes 1982; 31:40–45.

**96.** Osei F, Falsko JM, Nelson KP, et al. Diabetogenic effect of pentamidine: in vitro and in vivo studies in a patient with malignant insulinoma. Am J Med 1984;77:41–46.

**97.** Fitzgerald DB, Young IS. Reversal of pentamidine-induced hypoglycemia with oral diazoxide. J Trop Med Hyg 1984; 87:15–19.

**98.** Centers for Disease Control. Severe neutropenia during pentamidine treatment of *Pneumocystis carinii* pneumonia in patients with acquired immunodeficiency syndrome—New York City. MMWR 1984;33:65–67.

**99.** Hollander H. Leukopenia, trimethoprim–sulfamethoxazole, and folinic acid. (Lett.) Ann Intern Med 1985;102:138.

**100.** Kinzie BJ, Taylor JW. Trimethoprim and folinic acid. (Lett) Ann Intern Med 1984;101:565.

**101.** Stock C. Trimethoprim–sulfamethoxazole and folinic acid. (Lett) Ann Intern Med 1985;102:277.

**102.** Allegra CJ, Drake J, Swan J, et al. Preliminary results of a phase I-II trial for the treatment of *Pneumocystis carinii* pneumonia (PCP) using a potent lipid-soluble dihydrofolate reductase (DHFR) inhibitor, trimetrexate (TMTX). Twenty-Sixth Interscience Conference on Antimicrobial Agents and Chemotherapy. Washington DC, American Society of Microbiology, 1986, Abstract 691, p 224.

**103.** Hughes WT, Smith BL. Efficacy of diaminodiphenylsulfone and other drugs in murine *Pneumocystis carinii* pneumonitis. Antimicrob Agents Chemother 1984;26:436–440.

**104.** Leoung GS, Mills J, Hopewell PC, et al. Dapsone–trimethoprim for *Pneumocystis carinii* pneumonia in the acquired immunodeficiency syndrome. Ann Intern Med 1986;105:45–48.

**105.** Golden JA, Sjoerdsma A, Santi DV. *Pneumocystis carinii* pneumonia treated with α-difluoromethylornithine. West J Med 1984;141:613–623.

**106.** Neibart E, Sacks HS, Hammer G, et al. Difluoromethylornithine (DFMO) in the treatment of *Pneumocystis carinii* pneumonia (PCP). Twenty-Sixth Interscience Conference on Antimicrobial Agents and Chemotherapy. Washington, DC, American Society for Microbiology, 1986, Abstract 693, p 224.

**107.** Mills J, Leoung G. Medina I, et al. Dapsone is ineffective therapy for *Pneumocystis* pneumonia in patients with AIDS. Clin Res 1986;34:101A.

**108.** Conte JE, Hollander H, Golden JA. Inhaled or reduced-dose intravenous pentamidine for *Pneumocystis carinii* pneumonia. Ann Intern Med 1987;107:495–498.

**109.** Montgomery AB, Debs RJ, Luce JM, et al. Aerosolized pentamidine as sole therapy for *Pneumocystis carinii* pneumonia in patients with acquired immunodeficiency syndrome. Lancet 1987;2:480–482.

**110.** Montgomery AB, Debs RJ, Luce JM, et al. Concentration of pentamidine in bronchoalveolar lavage fluid after aerosol and intravenous administration. Am Rev Respir Dis 1987;135: A167.

**111.** Hughes WT, Kuhn S, Chadhary S, et al. Successful chemoprophylaxis for *Pneumocystis carinii* pneumonia. N Engl J Med 1977;297:1419–1426.

**112.** Fischl MA, Dickenson GM, LaVoie L. Safety and efficacy of sulfamethoxazole and trimethoprim chemoprophylaxis for *Pneumocystis carinii* pneumonia in AIDS. JAMA 1988;259:1185–1189.

**113.** Bernard E, Schmitth H, Pagel L, et al. Safety and effectiveness of aerosol pentamidine for prevention of PCP in patients with AIDS. Twenty-Sixth Interscience Conference on Antimicrobial Agents and Chemotherapy, Washington DC, American Society of Microbiology, 1986, Abstract.

**114.** Karaffa C, Rehm S, Calabreses L, et al. Efficacy of monthly pentamidine infusions in preventing recurrent *Pneumocystis carinii* pneumonia (PCP) in the AIDS patient. Twenty-Sixth Interscience Conference on Antimicrobial Agents and Chemotherapy. Washington DC, American Society for Microbiology, 1986, Abstract 690, p 224.

**115.** Gottlieb MS, Knight S, Weisman J. Prophylaxis of *Pneumocystis carinii* infection in AIDS with pyrimethamine–sulfadoxine. (Lett) Lancet 1984;2:398.

**116.** Navin TR, Miller KD, Satriale RF, et al. Adverse reactions associated with pyrimethamine-sulfadoxine prophylaxis for *Pneumocystis carinii* infections in AIDS. Lancet 1985;1:1332.

**117.** Zitelli BJ, Alexander J, Taylor S, et al. Fatal hepatic necrosis due to pyrimethamine-sulfadoxine (Fansidar). Ann Intern Med 1987;106:393–395.

**118.** Armstrong D, Gold JWM, Dryjanski J, et al. Treatment of infections in patients with the acquired immunodeficiency syndrome. Ann Intern Med 1985;103:738–743.

**119.** Gold JWM, Hierholzer J, Armstrong D. Adenoviruses in patients with acquired immune deficiency syndrome (Abstr), in The International Conference on the Acquired Immunodeficiency Syndrome: Abstracts, Philadelphia, American College of Physicians, 1985.

**120.** Bass JB, Hawkins EL. Treatment of disease caused by nontuberculous mycobacteria. Arch Intern Med 1983;143:1439–1441.

**121.** Greene JB, Sidhu GS, Lewin S, et al. *Mycobacterium avium-intracellulare*: A cause of disseminated life-threatening infection in homosexuals and drug abusers. Ann Intern Med 1982; 97:539–546.

**122.** Horsburgh CR, Mason UG, Farhi DC, et al. Disseminated infection with *Mycobacterium avium-intracellulare*. Medicine 1985;64:36–48.

**123.** Woodley CL, Kilburn JO. In vitro susceptibility of *Mycobacterium avium* complex and mycobacterium tuberculosis strains to a spiro-piperidyl rifamycin. Am Rev Respir Dis 1982;126: 586–587.

**124.** Hawkins JE, Gross WM, Vadney FS. Ansamycin LM 427 activity against mycobacteria in vitro. (Abstr) Am Rev Respir Dis 1984;129:A187.

**125.** Morrison NE, Marley GM. Clofazimine binding studies with deoxyribonucleic acid. Int J Lepr 1976;44:475–481.

**126.** Levy, L. Pharmacologic studies of clofazimine. Am J Trop Med Hyg 1974;23:1097–1109.

**127.** Moore VJ. A review of side-effects experienced by patients taking clofazamine. Lepr Rev 1983;54:327–335.

**128.** Granstein RD, Sorber AJ. Drug- and heavy metal-induced hyperpigmentation. J Am Acad Dermatol 1981;5:1–18.

**129.** Masur H, Tuazon C, Gill V, et al. Effect of combined clofazamine and ansamycin therapy on *Mycobacterium avium–Mycobacterium intracellulare* bacteremia in patients with AIDS. J Infect Dis 1987;155:127–129.

**130.** Kiehn TE, Edwards FF, Brannon P, et al. Infections caused by *Mycobacterium avium* complex in immunocompromised patients: diagnosis by blood culture and fecal examination, antimicrobial susceptibility tests, and morphological and seroagglutination characteristics. J Clin Microbiol 1985;21:168–173.

**131.** Hawkins CC, Gold JWM, Whimbey E, et al. *Mycobacterium avium* complex infections in patients with the acquired immunodeficiency syndrome. Ann Intern Med 1986;105:184–188.

**132.** Ryning FW, Mills J. *Pneumocystis carinii*, *Toxoplasma gondii*, cytomegalovirus, and the compromised host. West J Med 1979;130:18–34.

**133.** Navia BA, Petito CK, Gold JVM, et al. Cerebral toxoplasmosis complicating the acquired immune deficiency syndrome: Clinical and neuropathologic findings in 27 patients. Ann Neurol 1986;19:224–238.

**134.** Luft BJ, Brooks RG, Conley FK, et al. Toxoplasmic encephalitis in patients with acquired immune deficiency syndrome. JAMA 1984;252:913–917.

**135.** Grant IH, Gold JWM, and Armstrong D. Risk of CNS toxoplasmosis in patients with acquired immune deficiency syndrome. Twenty-Sixth Interscience Conference on Antimicrobial Agents and Chemotherapy. American Society for Microbiology, Washington DC, 1986, Abstract 441, p 177.

**136.** Tuazon CU. How would you treat central nervous system toxoplasmosis? Drug Ther 1984;74–75.

**137.** Araujo FG, Remington JS. Effect of clindamycin on acute and chronic toxoplasmosis in mice. Antimicrob Agents Chemother 1974;5:647–651.

**138.** Rolston KVI, Hoy J. Role of clindamycin in the treatment of central nervous system toxoplasmosis. Am J Med 1987;83:551–554.

**139.** Zuger A, Louie E, Holzman RS, et al. Cryptococcal disease in patients with the acquired immunodeficiency syndrome. Ann Intern Med 1986;104:234–240.

**140.** Bennett JE, Dismukes WE, Duma RJ, et al. A comparison of amphotericin B alone and combined with flucytosine in the treatment of cryptococcal meningitis. N Engl J Med 1979;301: 126–131.

**141.** Kovacs JA, Kovacs AA, Polis M, et al. Cryptococcosis in the acquired immunodeficiency syndrome. Ann Intern Med 1985; 103:533–538.

**142.** Dismukes WE, Stamm AM, Graybill JR, et al. Treatment of systemic mycoses with ketoconazole: emphasis on toxicity and clinical response in 52 patients. Ann Intern Med 1983;98:13–20.

**143.** Utz JP. Chemotherapy of the systemic mycoses. Med Clin North Am 1982;66:221–233.

**144.** Quinnan GV Masur H, Rook AH, et al. Herpesvirus infections in the acquired immune deficiency syndrome. JAMA 1984;252: 72–77.

**145.** Powers RD, Hayden RG. Herpesvirus infections: current antiviral therapy. Hosp Formul 1984;19:1040–1054.

**146.** Whitley RJ, Alford CA, Hirsch MS, et al. Vidarabine versus acyclovir therapy in herpes simplex encephalitis. N Engl J Med 1986;314:144–149.

**147.** Felsenstein D, D'Amico DJ, Hirsch MS, et al. Treatment of cytomegalovirus retinitis with 9-[2-hydroxy-1-(hydroxymethyl) ethoxymethyl] guanine. Ann Intern Med 1985;103:377–380.

**148.** Bach MC, Bagwell SP, Knapp NP, et al. 3-(1-3-Dihydroxy-2-propoxymethyl) guanine for cytomegalovirus infections in patients with the acquired immunodeficiency syndrome. Ann Intern Med 1985;103:381–384.

**149.** Masur H, Lane HC, Palestine A, et al. Effect of 9-(1,3-dihydroxy-2-propoxymethyl) guanine on serious cytomegalovirus disease in eight immunosuppressed homosexual men. Ann Intern Med 1986;104:41–44.

**150.** Elion GB, Furman PA, Fyfe JA, et al. Selectivity of action of an antiherpetic agent, 9-(2-hydroxy-ethoxymethyl)guanine. Proc Natl Acad Sci USA 1977;74:5716–5720.

**151.** Tocci MJ, Livelli TJ, Perry HC, et al. Effects of the nucleoside analog 2′-nor-2′-deoxyguanosine on human cytomegalovirus replication. Antimicrob Agents Chemother 1984;25:247–252.

**152.** Collaborative DHPG Treatment Study Group. Treatment of serious cytomegalovirus infections with 9-(1,3-dihydroxy-2-propoxymethyl)guanine in patients with AIDS and other immunodeficiencies. N Engl J Med 1986;314:801–805.

**153.** Current WL, Reese NC, Ernst JC, et al. Human cryptosporidiosis in immunocompetent and immunodeficient persons—studies of an outbreak and experimental transmission. N Engl J Med 1983;308:1252–1257.

**154.** Owens NJ, Nightingale CH, Schweizer RT, et al. Prophylaxis of oral candidiasis with clotrimazole troches. Arch Intern Med 1984;144:290–293.

**155.** Furio MM, Wardell CJ. Treatment of infectious complications of acquired immunodeficiency syndrome. Clin Pharm 1985;4: 539–554.

**156.** Jones PG, Kauffman CA, McAuliffe LS, et al. Efficacy of ketoconazole versus nystatin in prevention of fungal infections in neutropenic patients. Arch Intern Med 1984;144:549–551.

**157.** Glaser JB, Morton-Kute L, Berger SR, et al. Recurrent *Salmonella typhimurium* bacteremia associated with the acquired immunodeficiency syndrome. Ann Intern Med 1985;102:189–193.

**158.** Jacobs JL, Gold JWM, Murray HW, et al. Salmonella infections in patients with the acquired immunodeficiency syndrome. Ann Intern Med 1985;102:186–188.

**159.** Soave R, Danner RL, Honig CL. Cryptosporidiosis in homosexual men. Ann Intern Med 1984;100:504–511.

**160.** Hart A, Baxby O. Management of cryptosporidiosis. J Antimicrob Chemother 1985;15:3–4.

**161.** Portnoy D, Whiteside ME, Buckley E, et al. Treatment of intestinal cryptosporidiosis with spiramycin. Ann Intern Med 1984;101:202–204.

**162.** Centers for Disease Control. Update: Treatment of cryptosporidiosis in patients with acquired immunodeficiency syndrome (AIDS). MMWR 1984;33:117–119.

**163.** Whiteside ME, Barkin JS, May RG, et al. Enteric coccidiosis among patients with the acquired immunodeficiency syndrome. Am J Trop Med Hyg 1984;33:1065–1072.

**164.** DeHovitz JA, Pope JW, Boncy M, et al. Clinical manifestations and therapy of *Isospora belli* infection in patients with the acquired immunodeficiency syndrome. N Engl J Med 1986; 315:87–90.

**165.** Mitchell CD, Gentry SR, Bean B, et al. Acyclovir therapy for mucocutaneous herpes simplex infections in immunocompromised patients. Lancet 1981;1:1389–1392.

**166.** Nicholson KG. Antiviral therapy. Varicella-zoster virus infections, herpes labialis, and mucocutaneous herpes, and cytomegalovirus infections. Lancet 1984;2:677–682.

**167.** Whitley RJ, Spruance S, Hayden FG, et al. Vidarabine therapy for mucocutaneous herpes simplex virus infections in the immunocompromised host. J Infect Dis 1984;149:1–8.

**168.** Straus SE, Seidlin M, Takiff H, et al. Oral acyclovir to suppress recurring herpes simplex virus infections in immunodeficient patients. Ann Intern Med 1984;100:522–524.

**169.** Whitley RJ, Soong S, Dolin R. Early vidarabine therapy to control the complications of herpes zoster in immunosuppressed patients. N Engl J Med 1982;307:971–975.

**170.** Balfour HH, Bean B, Laskin OL, et al. Acyclovir halts progression of herpes zoster in immunocompromised patients. N Engl J Med 1983;308:1448–1453.

**171.** Purtillo DT. Immune deficiency predisposing to Epstein–Barr virus induced lymphoproliferative diseases. The X-linked lymphoproliferative syndrome as a model, in Klein G, Winehouse S (eds): Advances in Cancer Research. New York, Academic Press, vol 34, 1981, pp 279–312.

**172.** Meyers JD, Flournoy N, Thomas ED. Non-bacterial pneumonia after allogeneic marrow transplantation: A review of 10 years experience. Rev Infec Dis 1982;4:1119–1132.

**173.** Hanto DW, Frizzera G, Gajl-Peczaiska KJ, et al. Epstein-Barr virus-induced B cell lymphoma after renal transplantation: Acyclovir therapy and transition from polyclonal to monoclonal B cell proliferation. N Engl J Med 1982;306:913–918.

**174.** McDonald MI, Hamilton JD, Durack DT. Hepatitis B surface antigen could harbour the infective agent of AIDS. Lancet 1983;2:882–884.

**175.** Ravenholt RT. Role of hepatitis B virus in acquired immunodeficiency syndrome. Lancet 1983;2:885–886.

**176.** Reiner NE, Judson FN, Bond WW et al. Asymptomatic rectal mucosal lesions and hepatitis B surface antigen at sites of sexual contact in homosexual men with persistent hepatitis B virus: Evidence for de facto parenteral transmission. Ann Intern Med 1982;96:170–173.

**177.** Cahill K. The AIDS Epidemic, New York, St. Martin's Press, 1983, pp 1–178.

**178.** Laure F, Zagury D, Saimot AG, et al. Hepatitis B virus DNA sequences in lymphoid cells from patients with AIDS and AIDS-related complex. Science 1985;229:561–563.

**179.** Centers for Disease Control. Kaposi's sarcoma and *Pneumocystis pneumoniae* among homosexual men—New York City and California. MMWR 1981;25:305–308.

**180.** Volberding P. Therapy of Kaposi's sarcoma in AIDS. Semin Oncol 1984;11:60–67.

**181.** Safai B, Johnson KG, Myskowski PL, et al. The natural history of Kaposi's sarcoma in the acquired immunodeficiency syndrome. Ann Intern Med 1985;103:744–750.

**182.** Mintzer DM, Real FX, Jovino L, et al. Treatment of Kaposi's sarcoma and thrombocytopenia with vincristine in patients with the acquired immunodeficiency syndrome. Ann Intern Med 1985;102:200–202.

**183.** Laubenstein LJ, Krigel RL, Hymes KB, et al. Treatment of epidemic Kaposi's sarcoma with VP 16-213 (etoposide) and a combination of doxorubicin, bleomycin, and vinblastine (ABV). Proc Am Soc Clin Oncol 1983;2:228.

**184.** Olweny C, Toya T, Katongole-MBiddle E, et al. Treatment of Kaposi's sarcoma by combination of actinomycin-D, vincristine and imidazole carboxamide (NSC-45388): results of a randomized clinical trial. Int J Cancer 1974;14:649–656.

**185.** Vogel CL, Primack A, Dhru D, et al. Treatment of Kaposi's sarcoma with a combination of actinomycin D and vincristine: results of a randomized clinical trial. Cancer 1973;31:1382–1391.

**186.** Lanzotti VJ, Campos LT, Sinkovics JG, et al. Chemotherapy for advanced Kaposi's sarcoma. Arch Dermatol 1975;111: 1331–1333.

**187.** Groopman JE, Gottlieb MS, Goodman J, et al. Recombinant alpha-2 interferon therapy for Kaposi's sarcoma associated with the acquired immunodeficiency syndrome. Ann Intern Med 1984;100:671–676.

**188.** Volberding P, Moran T, Abrams D, et al. Recombinant alpha interferon therapy of Kaposi's sarcoma in the acquired immunodeficiency syndrome. (Abstr) Blood 1983;62(suppl 1):118a.

**189.** Gelmann EP, Preble OT, Steis R, et al. Human lymphoblastoid interferon treatment of Kaposi's sarcoma in the acquired immune deficiency syndrome. Ann J Med 1985;78:737–741.

**190.** Krigel RL, Odajnyk CM, Laubenstein LJ, et al. Therapeutic trial of Interferon-$\gamma$ in patients with epidemic Kaposi's sarcoma. J Biological Response Modifiers 1985;4:358–364.

**191.** Boring CC, Brynes RK, Chan WC, et al. Increase in high-grade lymphomas in young men. Lancet 1985;1:857–859.

**192.** Ioachim HL, Cooper MC, Hellman GC. Lymphoma in men at high risk for acquired immune deficiency syndrome (AIDS). Cancer 1985;56:2831–2842.

**193.** Hochberg FH, Miller G, Schooley RT, et al. Central-nervous system lymphoma related to Epstein–Barr virus. N Engl J Med 1983;309:745–748.

**194.** Ziegler JL, Beckstead JA, Volberding PA, et al. Non-Hodgkin's lymphoma in 90 homosexual men. N Engl J Med 1984; 311:565–570.

**195.** Frederick WR, Epstein JS, Gelmann EP, et al. Viral infections and cell-mediated immunity in immunodeficient homosexual men with Kaposi's sarcoma treated with human lymphoblastoid interferon. J Infect Dis 1985;152:162–170.

**196.** Parkin JM, Eales LJ, Moshtael O, et al. Results of a trial of recombinant interferon-gamma (biogen) in patients with the acquired immune deficiency syndrome. Paper presented to Second International Conference on AIDS, Paris, June 23–25, 1986, p 76.

**197.** Kern P, Toy J, Dietrich M. Preliminary clinical observations with recombinant interleukin-2 in patients with AIDS or LAS. Blut 1985;50:1–6.

**198.** Surapaneni N, Raghunathan R, Beall GN, et al. Levamisole, immunostimulation, and the acquired immunodeficiency syndrome. (Lett) Ann Intern Med 1985;102:137.

**199.** Ciobanu B, Paietta E, Karten M, et al. Thymus fragment transplantation in the acquired immunodeficiency syndrome. (Lett) Ann Intern Med 1985;103:479.

**200.** Baltimore D. Viral RNA–dependent DNA polymerase. Nature 1970;226:1209–1211.

**201.** Temin HM, Mizutani S. RNA-dependent DNA polymerase in virions of rous sarcoma virus. Nature 1970;226:1211–1213.

**202.** Mitsuya H, Popovic M, Yarchoan R, et al. Suramin protection of T cells in vitro against infectivity and cytopathic effect of HTLV-III. Science 1984;226:172–174.

**203.** McCormick JB, Getchell JP, Mitchell SW, et al. Ribavirin suppresses replication of lymphadenopathy-associated virus in culture of human adult T-lymphocytes. Lancet 1984;2:1367–1369.

**204.** Dormont D, Spire B, Barre-Sinoussi F, et al. Inhibition of RNA-dependent DNA polymerases of AIDS and SAIDS retroviruses by HPA-23 (ammonium-21-tungsto-9-antimoniate). Ann Virol 1985;136E:75–83.

**205.** Ho DD, Hartshorn KL, Rota TR, et al. Recombinant human interferon alfa-A suppresses HTLV-III replication in vitro. Lancet 1985;1:602–604.

**206.** Sandstrom EG, Kaplan JC, Byington RE, et al. Inhibition of human T-cell lymphotropic virus type III in vitro by phosphonoformate. Lancet 1985;1:1480–1482.

**207.** Mitsuya H, Barry DW, Nusinoff-Lehrman S, et al. Interscience Conference on Antimicrobial Agents and Chemotherapy (XXV), Minneapolis, MN, September 29–October 2, 1985. Washington DC, American Society for Microbiology, Abstract 437.

**208.** Furman PA, St Clair M, Wernhold K, et al. Interscience Conference on Antimicrobial Agents and Chemotherapy (XXV), Minneapolis, Mn, September 29–October 2, 1985, Abstract 440.

**209.** Pompidou A, Zagury D, Gaool RC, et al. In-vitro inhibition of LAV/HTLV-III infected lymphocytes by dithiocarb and inosine pranobex. (Lett) Lancet 1985;2:1423.

**210.** Anand R, Moore J, Feorino P, et al. Rifabutine inhibits HTLV-III. Lancet 1986;1:97–98.

**211.** Mitsuya H, Broder S. Inhibition of the in vitro infectivity and cytoplathic effect of HTLV-III/LAV by 2′,3′-dideoxynucleosides. Proc Natl Acad Sci USA 1986;83:1911–1915.

**212.** Sarin PS, Gallo RC, Scheer DI, et al. Effect of a novel compound (AL 721) on HTLV-III infectivity in vitro (Lett) N Engl J Med 1985;313:1289–1290.

**213.** Grieco MH, Lange M, Klein EB, et al. Open study of AL 721 treatment of HIV-infected subjects with generalized lymphadenopathy syndrome. Paper presented to the Third International Conference on AIDS. Washington DC, June 2, 1987.

**214.** Wetterberg L, Alexius B, Sääf J, et al. Peptide T in treatment of AIDS. Lancet 1987;1:159.

**215.** Broder S, Yarchoan R, Collins JM, et al. Effects of suramin on HTLV-III/LAV infection presenting as Kaposi's sarcoma or AIDS-related complex: clinical pharmacology and suppression of virus replication in vivo. Lancet 1985;2:627–630.

**216.** Rouvroy D, Bogairts J, Habyarimana JB, et al. Short term results with suramin for AIDS-related conditions. (Lett) Lancet 1985;1:878–879.

**217.** Busch W, Brodt R, Ganser A, et al. Suramin treatment for AIDS. (Lett) Lancet 1985;2:1247.

**218.** Cheson BD, Levine AM, Mildvan D, et al. Suramin therapy in AIDS and related disorders. Report of the U.S. Suramin Working Group. JAMA 1987;258:1347–1351.

**219.** Saimot AG, Matheron S, Leport C, et al. Long-term administration of suramin to AIDS patients: Effects on LAV/HTLV III replication and clinical outcome. Paper presented to Second International Conference on AIDS. Paris, June 23–25, 1986, p 34.

**220.** Mildvan D, Poiesoz B, Matheir-Wagh V, et al. Suramin treatment in AIDS complicated by opportunistic infections (AIDS-OI). Paper presented to Second International Conference on AIDS. Paris, June 23–25, 1986, p 67.

**221.** Wolfe PR, Gottlieb MF, Hardy WD, et al. Suramin in AIDS and ARC: Results of a pilot toxicity/efficacy study. Paper presented to Second International Conference on AIDS. Paris, June 23–25, 1986, p 67.

**222.** Kaplan LD, Abrams DA, Wong R, et al. Failure of suramin as treatment for AIDS. Paper presented to Second International Conference on AIDS. Paris, June 23–25, 1986, p. 68.

**223.** Rozenbaum W, Dormont D, Spire B, et al. Antimoniotungstate (HPA 23) treatment of three patients with AIDS and one with prodrome. Lancet 1985;1:450–451.

**224.** Kornhauser DM, Petty BG, Chan DW, et al. Pharmacokinetics of Intravenous HPA-23. Twenty-Sixth Interscience Conference on Antimicrobial Agents and Chemotherapy. Washington DC, American Society for Microbiology, 1986, Abstract 1098, p 297.

**225.** Gilbert BE, Knight V. Biochemistry and clinical application of ribavirin. Antimicrob Agents Chemother 1986;30:201–205.

**226.** Catlin OH, Smith AR, Samuels AI. $^{14}$C-ribavirin: distribution and pharmacokinetics studies in rats, baboons and man, in Smith NA, Kirkpatrick W (eds): Ribavirin: A Broad Spectrum Antiviral Agent. New York, Academic Press, 1980, pp 83–98.

**227.** Mansell PWA, Haseltine PNR, Roberts RB, et al. Ribavirin delays progression of the lymphadenopathy syndrome (LAS) to the acquired immune deficiency syndrome (AIDS). Paper presented to the Third International Conference on AIDS. Washington DC, June 2, 1987.

**228.** Vernon A, Schulof RS. Serum HIV core antigen in symptomatic ARC patients taking oral ribavirin or placebo. Paper presented to the Third International Conference on AIDS. Washington DC, June 2, 1987.

**229.** Vogt MW, Hatshorn KL, Furman PA, et al. Ribavirin antagonizes the effect of azidothymidine on HIV replication. Science 1987;235:1376–1379.

**230.** Öberg B. Antiviral effects of phosphonoformate (FPA, foscarnet sodium). Pharmacol Ther 1983;19:387–415.

**231.** Ringden O, Lönnquist B, Paulin T, et al. Pharmacokinetics safety and preliminary clinical experiences using foscarnet in treatment of cytomegalovirus infections in bone marrow and renal transplant recipients. J Antimicrob Chemother 1986;17: 373–387.

**232.** Farthing CF, Dalgleish AG, Clark A, et al. Phosphonoformate (forscarnet): A pilot study in AIDS and AIDS-related complex. AIDS 1987;1:21–25.

**233.** Gaub J, Pedersen C, Poulsen AG, et al. The effect of foscarnet (phosphonoformate) on human immunodeficiency virus isolation, T-cell subsets and lymphocyte function in AIDS patients. AIDS 1987;1:27–33.

**234.** Wallace JI, Bekeski JG. A double-blind clinical trial of the effects of inosine pranobex in immunodepressed patients with prolonged generalized lymphodenopathy. Clin Immunol Immunopathol 1986;39:179–186.

**235.** Blum MR, Liao S, Good SS, et al. Pharmacokinetics of azidothymidine following intravenous and oral administration. Paper presented to Second International Conference on AIDS. Paris, June 23–25, 1986, p 26.

**236.** Yarchoan R, Klecker RW, Weinhold KJ, et al. Administration of 3′-azido-3′-deoxythymidine, an inhibitor of HTLV-III replication, to patients with AIDS or AIDS-related complex. Lancet 1986;1:575–580.

**237.** Fischl MA, Richman DD, Grieco MH. The efficacy of azidothymidine (AZT) in the treatment of patients with AIDS and AIDS-related complex. N Engl J Med 1987;317:185–191.

**238.** Richman DD, Fischl MA, Grieco MH, et al. The toxicity of azidothymidine (AZT) in the treatment of patients with AIDS and AIDS-related complex. N Engl J Med 1987;307:192–197.

**239.** Chaisson RE, Allain JP, Volberding PA. Significant changes in HIV antigen level in the serum of patients treated with azidothymidine. N Engl J Med 1986;315:1611–1612.

**240.** Hagler DN, Frame PT. Azidothymidine neurotoxicity. Lancet 1986;2:1392–1393.

**241.** Burroughs Wellcome. Retrovir (Zidovudine) package insert. Research Triangle Park, NC, March, 1987.

**242.** Yarchoan R, Perno CF, Thomas RV, et al. Phase I studies of 2′, 3′-dideoxycytidine in severe human immunodeficiency virus infections as a single agent and alternating with zidovudine (AZT). Lancet 1988;1:76–81.

**243.** Mitchell WM, Montefiori DC, Robinson WE, et al. Mismatched double-stranded RNA (ampligen) protects target cells from HIV infection and reduces the concentration of 3′-azido-3′ deoxythymidine (AZT) required for virus-static activity. Paper presented to the Third-International Conference on AIDS. Washington DC, June 2, 1987.

**244.** Henrigues HF, Simon GL, Strayer DR, et al. Ampligen therapy for HIV-related immunodeficiency. Paper presented to the Third International Conference on AIDS. Washington DC, June 2, 1987.

**245.** Walker BD, Kowalski M, Goh WC, et al. Anti-HIV properties of castanospermine. Paper presented to the Third International Conference on AIDS. Washington DC, June 2, 1987.

# Chapter 92 / Nosocomial Infections

Robert P. Rapp, PharmD

## Definition

Infections that occur in an institutional setting are known as *nosocomial infections*. Institutional refers to any health care facility where patients are housed for a period of time such as hospitals, nursing homes, or convalescent care centers. Most epidemiologic studies exclude infections that occur in the first 48–72 hours after admission to the institution, as such infections were most likely acquired before admission. On the other hand, infections that become apparent months after discharge are considered "nosocomial" and will be missed unless there is sufficient follow-up after discharge. During the midnineteenth century, Semmelweiss in Austria and Holmes in the United States were the first to describe the tremendously high rates of puerperal fever occurring in obstetrical hospitals as caused by group A streptococci transferred from the hands of physicians and nurses from patient to patient.

## Historic Overview

Before the days of Joseph Lister and Louis Pasteur the rate of infection in both traumatic and surgical wounds was virtually 100%. Because of high mortality rates, modern medicine and surgery gained slow acceptance during the first half of the nineteenth century. During his tenure at the Royal Infirmary in Glasgow from 1861 to 1869, Joseph Lister developed the principles and practice of antisepsis. Using "carbolic acid," Lister sprayed operating room suites, instruments, and wounds and noted a significant reduction in postoperative infection rates. Unfortunately, instruments dropped on floors, hands wiped on dirty aprons, and other less-than-acceptable practices continued to lead to an unacceptably high rate of fatal infections in patients.

Lister, during the latter part of his work on antiseptic surgery, gave full credit to the work of Louis Pasteur, a French scientist who worked out the germ theory of disease. Using the groundwork laid by both Lister and Pasteur in the 1880s German physicians and scientists developed the ritual of aseptic surgery as a logical extension of antiseptic surgery. Surgical gowns and instruments were sterilized prior to use. Wound infections, urinary tract infections, and septicemia continued to occur, however, and as surgeons operated on older patients or more debilitated patients and entered areas of the body containing natural endogenous flora, postoperative and posttraumatic infections remained a problem between 1900 and the 1930s.

Prior to the antibiotic era (1940) the cause of most nosocomial infections remained relatively constant, with gram-positive aerobic cocci constituting the majority of infections. Commonly encountered organisms included coagulase-positive staphylococci, β-hemolytic non–group D streptococci, and *Streptococcus pneumoniae*. Prior to the late 1950s the only important gram-negative aerobic bacilli were *Escherichia coli* and a few infections caused by *Salmonella*.[1] The scarcity of nosocomial infections caused by fungal species, other Enterobacteriaceae (*Klebsiella*, *Enterobacter*, *Serratia* species), enterococcal group D streptococci, and coagulase-negative staphylococci should be noted and duly appreciated by every student and practitioner with an interest in infectious disease.

The antibiotic era ushered in major changes in the species of bacteria causing nosocomial infections. Other major factors in the changing etiology of hospital-acquired infections were the development of intensive care units, specialized critical care units, life support systems with respirators, arterial catheters, access to the central veins, immunosuppressive therapy, and organ transplant surgery as well as the aging of the U.S. population. Many organisms including bacteria, fungus, and viral species have recently been observed to play an important part in modern hospitalization, with some organisms that are either not treatable or treatable only with difficulty or with toxic chemotherapeutic agents. For a complete review of the changing face of infectious disease the reader is referred to reviews of this area and to studies of the incidence and etiology of nosocomial bacteremia and fungemia in hospital populations over extended periods of time.[2–4]

## The Antibiotic Era

Coagulase-positive staphylococci (*S. aureus*) were the most important pathogens encountered in U.S. hospitals in the 1940s and became epidemic in the 1950s and early 1960s. Introduction of the penicillinase-resistant penicillin (methicillin) and the first-generation cephalosporins was responsible for the decreasing importance of this bacteria in the 1970s. *S. aureus* continues to be the great "true pathogen" and is still responsible for some 10% to 20% of nosocomial infections. The recent isolation of methicillin-resistant *S. aureus* (MRSA), which is not susceptible to cephalosporin antibiotics, represents one of the major events in infectious disease research in the twentieth century.[5,6] Instead of producing an enzyme that destroys the antibiotic, MRSA is generally not inhibited by virtue of alterations in its penicillin-binding protein characteristics. This feature has also been found in penicillin-resistant *Streptococcus pneumoniae* in the past 10 years.

One of the most interesting infectious disease events of the past several years has been the emergence of coagulase-negative staphylococci (*S. epidermidis*) as a significant pathogen in selected groups of patients. Studies of nosocomial bacteremias in hospitals before 1970 usually ignored blood cultures that grew *S. epidermidis*. For surgical patients with implanted foreign devices on cardiac, orthopedic, neurosurgical, and urology services, this organism is now recognized as a significant cause of postoperative infections. The same holds true for renal and bone marrow transplant services, and in the 1980s infectious disease specialists feel compelled to place the febrile neutropenic patient on therapy effective against *S. epidermidis* as well as gram-negative bacilli.

With the exception of *E. coli*, few gram-negative organisms appeared in nosocomial infection surveys prior to the mid-1950s. With the introduction of the penicillins and the first-generation cephalosporins, gram-negative organisms became important pathogens. Common isolates included species of *Klebsiella*, *Enterobacter*, *Serratia*, and indole-positive *Proteus*; *Pseudomonas aeruginosa*; and nonfermenting bacteria such as *Citrobacter* and *Acinetobacter*. During the 1970s anaerobic culture techniques were further developed and refined, leading to the recognition that specific anaerobes were an important component of polymicrobial pelvic and peritoneal infections. The *Bacteroides fragilis* group of organisms and *Clostridium* species were the most prominent pathogens recognized. In the late 1970s the disease pseudomembranous colitis was recognized after therapy with many antibiotics. This disease was subsequently found to result from overgrowth of the anaerobic bacteria *Clostridum difficile* in the lumen of the large intestine.[7]

Prior to the antibiotic era fungi caused few significant infections in hospitalized patients and virtually no cases of fungemia are found in bacteremia/fungemia surveys prior to 1953. Today, as a result of broad-spectrum antibiotic therapy and suppression of anaerobic gut flora, fungi (primarily *Candida albicans*) are responsible for 7% to 8% of cases of septicemia with positive blood cultures.[8]

## Common Nosocomial Infections

Approximately 5% of all general medical and surgical patients admitted to U.S. hospitals suffer a nosocomial infection (over 1 million patients per year). Further, some 18% of patients with nosocomial infections have more than one infection.

The most common site of nosocomial infections is the urinary tract, which accounts for 40.1% of reported infections (Table 92.1); 17% are surgical wound infections, 16.8% pneumonias, and 7.3% bacteremias. For differences in nosocomial infections between surgical and medical patients see Table 92.2. Although surgical patients constitute only about 42% of hospital admissions they have 71% of all nosocomial infections. Nosocomial infections generally increase with increasing age at all sites of infection; patients older than 84 have two to five times the risk of infection of 18- to 24-year-old patients. Sexual differences are also noted, with women being more susceptible to surgical wound infections, pneumonia, and bacteremia.

Surgical specialty has a predictable effect on the site of nosocomial infections: neurosurgical and urology patients have high rates of urinary tract infection (indwelling Foley catheters); surgical wound infection rates are highest for general surgery and obstetrics; and bacteremias are highest for cardiothoracic surgery patients. Many other factors have major effects on the occurrence of nosocomial infections. Factors known to increase risk include immunosuppressive therapy, longer hospital stay, previous infections, longer duration of surgery, and mechanical ventilatory support.

Nosocomial infections are caused by a wide variety of microorganisms but about one-half dozen are most prevalent (Table 92.3). *E. coli* is the most common pathogen in most hospitals, causing approximately 18% to 20% of all nosocomial infections. Enterococci, *S. aureus*, and *P. aeruginosa* each cause about 10% of all nosocomial infections followed by *Proteus* species and *Klebsiella* species (8% each). These "endemic" hospital infections are quite different from epidemic infections that occur in clusters from a

**Table 92.1** Nosocomial Infections by Site: All Patients

| *Site* | % |
|---|---|
| Urinary tract | 40.1 |
| Surgical wound | 17.8 |
| Pneumonia | 16.8 |
| Bacteremia | 7.3 |
| Other sites | 18.0 |

Data from Reference 45.

**Table 92.2** Nosocomial Infections by Site: Medical Versus Surgical Patients

| *Site* | % *Medical* | % *Surgical* |
|---|---|---|
| Urinary tract | 55.0 | 41.4 |
| Surgical wound | 1.4 | 27.7 |
| Pneumonia | 20.1 | 15.8 |
| Bacteremia | 7.9 | 4.0 |
| Other sites | 15.6 | 11.1 |

Data from Reference 45.

**Table 92.3** Pathogens Causing Nosocomial Endemic Infections

| *Pathogen* | % |
|---|---|
| *Escherichia coli* | 19 |
| *Staphylococcus aureus* | 10 |
| Enterococci | 10 |
| *Pseudomonas aeruginosa* | 9 |
| *Proteus* species | 8 |
| *Klebsiella* | 8 |
| *Enterobacter* | 4 |
| Other | 32 |

Data from Reference 46.

definable reservoir. Reports of epidemic infections show that *S. aureus* is the most common organism, (19%), followed by *Salmonella* (13%), tribe Klebsielleae (12%), and hepatitis B (8%).

## New Nosocomial Organisms

### *Viral Infections*

Nosocomial viral infections are now recognized as an increasing and significant problem in hospitals. Viruses are particularly important on transplant services where treatment includes immunosuppressive therapy. Cytomegalovirus, varicella, herpes zoster, rotavirus, herpes simplex, and hepatitis virus are seen with increasing frequency.[9–11] In immunocompromised patients cytomegalovirus acquired either exogenously (from a transplanted organ, granulocyte transfusions, etc.) or by activation of endogenous latent viruses can involve the liver and lungs and be rapidly associated with a fatal outcome. Better diagnostic methods and viral chemotherapeutic agents will play important roles in transplant centers in the future.

### *Methicillin-Resistant Staphylococcus aureus*

Resistant *S. aureus* has been a clinical problem since the early 1960s. Since 1980 MRSA has reached epidemic proportions in some large U.S. hospitals.[12] Recent work, primarily by Tomasz et al, has attributed the resistance to alteration of the penicillin-binding proteins, which have a low affinity for methicillin and cephalosporins.[13] This organism (MRSA) has significant clinical and financial implications for the hospital pharmacy. Even though standard sensitivity tests might indicate that MRSA is sensitive to cephalosporin antibiotics, therapeutic failures are common.[14] The drug of choice for MRSA is vancomycin.[15] Vancomycin is the only agent presently available for MRSA and is a very expensive antibiotic. Hospitals with widespread epidemics of MRSA not only face therapeutic problems but suffer serious financial problems with the drug budget as well. MRSA can cause a variety of serious infections including bacteremia, pneumonia, endocarditis, and wound infections.

### *Increasing Role of the Enterococcus*

Enterococci (group D streptococci) reside as normal inhabitants of the gastrointestinal tract and thus are isolated from sites where fecal contamination occurs. Frequent sites of isolation include the urinary tract, abdominal and pelvic surgical wounds, and bacteremias. When isolated from the blood, infective endocarditis must be suspected.[16] Surveys of causative organisms in endocarditis show that the enterococcus is responsible for 15% of such cases. Even excluding endocarditis, enterococcus bacteremia is associated with a high mortality. The usual source of most enterococcal bacteremia is the genitourinary area. *Streptococcus faecalis* is the most common enterococcus isolated from clinical specimens. *Streptococcus faecium* is infrequently isolated.

All cephalosporin antibiotics exhibit either total resistance or poor activity against the enterococcus; thus, when these agents are used prophylactically or therapeutically the enterococcus frequently colonizes or less frequently infects the patient. In a recent study in which either a second- or third-generation cephalosporin was used in either a one- or three-dose regimen as prophylaxis in vaginal hysterectomy, the enterococcus colonized the vaginal cuff in over 60% of patients.[17] This selection process may explain why the rate of superinfection has increased since cephalosporins were introduced in the 1960s. When serious infections, especially bacteremia, occur with the enterococcus, treatment is difficult; combinations of penicillins or vancomycin with an aminoglycoside are used to achieve a synergistic killing effect. For urinary tract infections (uncomplicated) the use of ampicillin alone may be effective in eradicating the organism.

### *Continuing Role of Enterobacteriaceae*

*E. coli* has always been an important nosocomial pathogen but it was not until the late 1960s and early 1970s that other members of this group of organisms were recognized as prominent pathogens. In many hospitals, *Klebsiella*[18] *pneumoniae*, *Enterobacter* species,[19] and *Serratia marcescens*[20] are now among the most frequent causes of "gram-negative sepsis." Fever, hypotension, complement activation, and disseminated intravascular coagulation (activation of factor XII) are seen when these organisms invade the bloodstream. Antibiotic resistance of hospital-associated Enterobacteriaceae is an ever increasing problem. In major teaching hospitals resistance to aminoglycosides and first-, second-, and even third-generation cephalosporins is common. Methods of resistance include both plasmid-mediated and chromosomally mediated β-lactamases, cell wall permeability barriers, and the production of aminoglycoside-altering enzymes.[21] Recent reviews indicate the Enterobacteriaceae cause greater than 50% of all nosocomial infections in the United States. See Table 92.4 for a classification of the Enterobacteriaceae.

**Table 92.4** Classification of the Enterobacteriaceae

| | |
|---|---|
| Tribe Klebsielleae | Tribe Proteeae |
| *Klebsiella pneumoniae* | *Proteus mirabilis* (indole-negative) |
| *Klebsiella oxytoca* | *Proteus vulgaris* |
| *Enterobacter aerogenes* | *Proteus morganii* |
| *Enterobacter cloacae* | *Providencia rettgeri* |
| *Enterobacter agglomerans* | *Providencia stuartii* |
| *Serratia marcescens* | |
| *Serratia liquefaciens* | |
| Tribe Escherichieae | Tribe Salmonelleae |
| *Escherichia coli* | *Citrobacter freundii* |
| *Shigella dysenteriae* | *Citrobacter diversus* |
| | *Salmonella typhi* |
| | *Salmonella paratyphi* |
| | *Salmonella arizona* |

### *Pseudomonas Species*

*Pseudomonas aeruginosa* is a major nosocomial pathogen in trauma, immunocompromised, and cystic fibrosis patients. As with the enterococcus, the differentiation between colonization and infection with *P. aeruginosa* is sometimes difficult. Many respirator-dependent patients who are receiving antibiotics colonize their bronchial–tracheal secretions with *P. aeruginosa*. When actual pneumonia does occur, usually with lower lobe infiltrates, the organisms must be treated with vigorous antibiotic therapy (usually aminoglycoside/antipseudomonal penicillin combinations). In patients with pneumonia who develop bacteremia the sequela is grave, with some reports of mortality approaching 100%.[22] One of the pathologic features of *P. aeruginosa* infections is the ability to invade the walls of blood vessels, leading to ecthyma gangrenosum, a grave clinical sign with massive tissue infection. *P. aeruginosa* is a notorious antibiotic-resistant organism producing both chromosomally and plasmid-mediated $\beta$-lactamases.[23] Present in the environment of many hospitals are *P. aeruginosa* which are resistant to the aminoglycosides, especially gentamicin. Aminoglycoside resistance can result from enzymatic alteration or from an inability of the antibiotic to penetrate the cell wall.

Aminoglycoside antibiotics continue to be required in a majority of life-threatening *P. aeruginosa* infections. Even the newer cephalosporins such as ceftazidime, and the carbapenems such as imipenem, are not totally reliable when used as single agents against *P. aeruginosa*, and monotherapy continues to be a subject of great debate among infectious disease physicians. An unusual feature of *P. aeruginosa* is its ability to flourish in a variety of environments and supposedly bactericidal solutions. Hospital soap dispensers and benzalkonium chloride and povidone–iodine solutions have been found to be contaminated with this organism.

*Pseudomonas maltophilia* and *Pseudomonas cepacia* are becoming more frequently encountered nosocomial pathogens. They have been reported in association with contaminated hospital products such as disinfectants,[24] blood components, and arterial pressure transducers. Both organisms are resistant to many currently available antibiotics. *P. maltophilia* is usually resistant to all aminoglycosides and has even been found to be resistant to newer agents such as imipenem.[25]

### *Staphylococcus epidermidis*

*S. epidermidis* organisms are contaminants in about 1% of all positive blood cultures obtained in adults. If *S. epidermidis* is indeed causing invasive disease this usually occurs in a specific number of clinical situations in patients who are granulocytopenic,[26] and in patients with prosthetic heart valves, intravenous or intraarterial catheters, ventriculoperitoneal shunts, or other implantable devices.[27] Persistent recovery of *S. epidermidis* from multiple blood cultures must lead the clinician to suspect infection and not contamination. Methicillin-resistant *S. epidermidis* constitutes 25% to 50% of all isolates of this organism in larger hospitals. Further, 70% to 85% of *S. epidermidis* organisms causing prosthetic valve endocarditis are methicillin resistant. Like MRSA the drug of choice for this organism when found to be methicillin resistant is vancomycin.[28]

### *Legionella pneumophilia*

Legionnaire's disease is now considered in cases of unresponsive nosocomial pneumonia. The prevalence of this organism depends on its presence in the hospital's water supply.[29] The organism can grow and proliferate in standing water such as cooling or holding tanks. *Legionella* spreads through aerosolization of the contaminated water supply and inhalation by patients. Parenteral erythromycin is presently the suggested drug for Legionnaire's disease.

### *Atypical Mycobacterium*

Prior to 1970 *Mycobacterium fortuitium* and *Mycobacterium chelonei* caused only an occasional nosocomial infection. Since 1970 there has been a significant increase in infections caused by these organisms. Wound infections are reported in increasing frequency after cardiac surgery, vascular surgery, and breast implants.[30,31] Severe disseminated infection is seen most frequently in the immunocompromised host. Unfortunately, the antimicrobial drugs presently available are for the most part ineffective against the atypical mycobacterium, and a satisfactory response requires a combination of drugs. Imipenem may prove useful against these two organisms in the future.

### *Increasing Role of Fungi*

Hospital-acquired fungemia now accounts for about 5% of all positive blood cultures. Patients at risk include those who receive parenteral nutrition, have indwelling urinary catheters or intravascular catheters, or are dialysis patients, particularly when broad-spectrum antimicrobial agents are used. Substantial alteration of the intestinal flora may occur when broad-spectrum antibiotics are prescribed, leading to a marked increase in *Candida albicans* in the stool flora.[32] This phenomenon is particularly seen for drugs with a high degree of biliary elimination such as cefoperazone and ceftriaxone where *C. albicans* becomes the predominant aerobic flora. It is reasonable to expect that as more broad-spectrum drugs are used, fungi will play an increasing role, with *C. albicans* being the most frequently encountered pathogen.[33]

## Infusion-Related Nosocomial Bacteremias

During 1970–1971 hospitals using a certain company's intravenous fluids experienced a significant occurrence of primary bacteremia caused by *Enterobacter* species.[34] Subsequent studies indicated that members of the tribe Klebsielleae are responsible for over 90% of infusion-related bacteremias. *Klebsiella pneumoniae Enterobacter cloacae*, *Enterobacter agglomerans*, and *Serratia marcescens* are uniquely capable of growing in crystalloid intravenous fluids containing dextrose.[35] These organisms do well because they can (1) fix atmospheric nitrogen for use as a protein

**Table 92.5** Microorganisms Associated With Infusion-Related Infections

| *Source* | *Microorganism* |
|---|---|
| Contaminated IV fluids | *Klebsiella* spp.<br>*Enterobacter* spp.<br>*Serratia* spp.<br>*Citrobacter* spp.<br>*Pseudomonas cepacia* |
| Parenteral nutrition (synthetic amino acids as protein source) | *Candida albicans* (most septicemia related to catheter sepsis; solutions with synthetic amino acids—poor growth medium) |

source, (2) grow at room temperature, and (3) survive the low acidity of dextrose-containing intravenous fluids. Interestingly, even though these organisms can survive in intravenous fluids they reach a concentration of only $10^5$ to $10^6$ organisms per 1 mL of fluid, which is below the concentration necessary to cause turbidity; thus, heavily contaminated solutions are usually crystal clear by visual inspection. Reviews of world literature between 1965 and 1978 show 97 epidemics of hospital-acquired bacteremia; one third of these resulted from some aspect of infusion therapy.[36] *Pseudomonas cepacia* has also been implicated in infusion-related bacteremia in recent years (see Table 92.5).

When total parenteral nutrition (TPN) solutions were manufactured using protein hydrolysates as the nitrogen source, the incidence of primary bacteremia/fungemia from use of these TPN solutions increased.[37] Most bacteria and fungi could grow to turbidity in these solutions in 48–72 hours with inocula greater than $10^7$ CFU/mL of fluid.[38] In the late 1970s and early 1980s, TPN fluids contained, as the nitrogen source, mainly synthetic amino acids that were solubilized as the acetate salts. The high concentration of acetate ion in the final solution acts as a "bacteriostatic" agent in synthetic amino acid/dextrose TPN fluids, as most bacteria and fungal organisms do not grow well or at all in these fluids. The failure of these fluids to support microbiologic growth has resulted in a significant decrease in primary infusate-related sepsis in patients receiving TPN.

Pharmacy-run intravenous admixture programs have been responsible for a number of infusion-related infections in the past 10 years.[39,40] All instances of contamination resulted from poor or nonexistent quality control procedures in the pharmacy department.[41] Errors included (1) failure to include a preservative in a multiple-dose vial stored at room temperature, leading to fungal infection; (2) failure to clean the vacuum system used in preparing TPN solutions, leading to contaminated solutions; and (3) failure to follow aseptic practice in preparing large-volume potassium chloride admixtures, leading to septicemia.

To avoid such catastrophes the hospital pharmacist must have a broad knowledge of microbiology and infectious diseases.

## Control of Nosocomial Infections in the Hospital

The Joint Commission on the Accreditation of Hospitals states, as a principle, "There shall be an effective infection control program within the hospital."[42] The program includes the following basic elements:

1. The definition of nosocomial infections
2. A system of reporting, evaluating, and maintaining a record of nosocomial infections
3. Ongoing review and evaluation of all aseptic, isolation, and sanitation techniques employed in the hospital
4. Written policies defining the specific indications for isolation requirements (this usually includes a category of isolation for patients with infections caused by antibiotic-resistant bacteria)
5. Control procedures relating to the inanimate hospital environment including sterilization and disinfection practices
6. Provision of necessary microbiologic laboratory support
7. Orientation programs for new employees about infection control procedures
8. Coordination with the medical staff on a regular review of the clinical use of antibiotics in the hospital

The pharmacist is a key individual in aiding the Hospital Infection Committee to implement many of the preceding elements. A member of the pharmacy clinical staff who is familiar with the practice of infectious disease should represent the pharmacy department on the Committee. In addition, the pharmacy department must have written policies and procedures relating to infection control for all areas where aseptic technique, sterilization, or manufacture of parenteral solutions occurs.

## Antibiotic Use and Nosocomial Infections

Hospitalized patients become colonized with a variety of bacteria during any admission period. Surveillance studies indicate that inpatients acquire new organisms at the rate of 0.5 organism per patient per week. Most of these organisms are gram-negative bacilli of the type most likely to cause nosocomial infections. Colonizing bacteria or fungi in patients receiving antibiotics are frequently resistant to the drug or drugs the patient is receiving. Examples are easy to identify: *C. albicans* colonizes the vaginal tract, urinary tract, and bronchial tree of patients receiving broad-spectrum antibiotics. Enterococci frequently colonize the vaginal cuff in patients receiving cephalosporin antibiotics as prophylaxis for vaginal hysterectomy. *P. aeruginosa* colonizes bronchial secretions in patients receiving cephalosporins not effective against this organism. Third-generation cephalosporins are capable of inducing β-lactamase production in members of the Enterobacteriaceae.[43] These enzymes accumulate in the periplasmic space of the organism and can cause slow hydrolysis of even the most β-lactamase-stable cephalosporins.[44] Recent evidence indicates that this process may also cause a "nonhydrolytic" resistance by acting as a barrier to the penetration of other drugs so they cannot reach their site of action. The use of antibiotics can of course save a patient's life; by the same token, the misuse of antibiotics can have a devastating effect on both the patient and the hospital environment.It is mandatory that antimicrobial drugs be prescribed with both knowledge and restraint if therapy is to be maximized and adverse effects are to be minimized.

## References


1. McGowan JE. Changing etiology of nosocomial bacteremia and fungemia and other hospital-acquired infections. Rev Infect Dis 1985;7(suppl 3):5357–5379.
2. Eickhoff TC. Nosocomial infections—a 1980 view: Progress, priorities and prognosis, in Dixon RE (ed): Nosocomial Infections. New York, Yorke Medical Books, 1981, pp 1–9.
3. Finegold SM, Kirby WM. Changing pattern of hospital infections: Implications for therapy. Am J Med 1984;77:1–2.
4. Neu HC. Changing mechanisms of bacterial resistance. Am J Med 1984;77:11–23.
5. Dunkle LM, Naqvi SH, Callum R, et al. Eradication of epidemic methicillin–gentamicin-resistant *Staphylococcus aureus* in an intensive care nursery. Am J Med 1981;70:455–458.
6. Boyce JM, White RL, Spruell EY. Impact of methicillin-resistant *Staphylococcus aureus* on the incidence of nosocomial staphylococcal infections. J Infect Dis 1983;148:763.
7. Riley TV, Bowman RA, Carroll SM. Diarrhea associated with *Clostridium difficile* in a hospital population. Med J Aust 1983; 19:166–169.
8. McGowan JE, Barrer MW, Fireland M. Bacteremia at Boston City Hospital: occurrence and mortality during 12 selected years (1935–1972) with special reference to hospital acquired cases. J Infect Dis 1975;132:316–335.
9. Dworsky ME, Welch K, Cassady G, et al. Occupational risk for primary cytomegalovirus infection among pediatric health care workers. N Engl J Med 1983;309:950–953.
10. Hammerberg O, Watts J, Chernesky M, et al. An outbreak of herpes simplex virus type I in an intensive care nursery. Pediatr Infect Dis 1983;2:290–294.
11. Hall CB. The nosocomial spread of respiratory syncytial viral infection. Ann Rev Med 1983;34:311–319.
12. Haley RW, Hightower AW, Khobbaz RF, et al. The emergence of methicillin-resistant *Staphylococcus aureus* infections in United States hospitals. Ann Intern Med 1982;97:297–308.
13. Hartman B, Tomasz A. Altered penicillin binding protein in methicillin resistant strains of *Staphylococcus aureus*. Antimicrob Agents Chemother 1981;19:726–735.
14. Sabath LD, Wallace SJ. Factors influencing methicillin resistance in staphylococci. Ann NY Acad Sci 1971;182:258–266.
15. Sorrell TC, Packman DR, Shanker S, et al. Vancomycin therapy for methicillin-resistant *Staphylococcus aureus*. Ann Intern Med 1983;97:344–350.
16. Mandell GL, Kaye D, Levison ME, et al. Enterococcal endocarditis: an analysis of 38 patients. Arch Intern Med 1970; 125:258–264.
17. Rapp RP, Connors JE, Hager WD, et al. Comparison of single-dose moxalactam and a three-dose regimen of cefoxitin for prophylaxis in vaginal hysterectomy. Clin Pharm 1986; 5:988–993.
18. Montgomerie JZ. Epidemiology of *Klebsiella* and hospital associated infections. Rev Infect Dis 1983;148:795–801.
19. John JF, Sharbaugh RJ, Bannister ER. *Enterobacter cloacae* bacteremia; epidemiology and antibiotic resistance. Rev Infect Dis 1982;4:13–28.
20. Marrie TJ, Noble MA, Holdave EV, et al. *Serratia marcescens*—a marker for an infection control program. Infect Control 1982;3:134–142.
21. Neu HC. Current mechanisms of resistance to antimicrobial agents in microorganisms causing infection in the patient at risk for infection. Am J Med 1984;76(5A):11–27.
22. Cross A, Allen JR, Burke J, et al. Nosocomial infections due to *Pseudomonas aeruginosa*: Review of recent trends. Rev Infect Dis 1983;5(suppl):5837–5845.
23. Neu HC. Changing mechanisms of bacterial resistance. Am J Med 1984;77(1B):11–23.
24. Newman KA, Tenney JH, Oken HA, et al. Persistent isolation of an unusual *Pseudomonas* species from a phenolic disinfectant system. Infect Control 1984;5:219–222.
25. Krapp H, Gerchens L, Sundelof JG, et al. Antibacterial activity of imipenem: The first thienamycin antibiotic. Rev Infect Dis 1985;7(suppl 3):S389–S410.
26. Wade JC, Schempff SC, Newman KA, et al. *Staphylococcus epidermidis*: An increasing cause of infection in patients with granulocytopenia. Ann Intern Med 1982;97:503–508.
27. Karchmer AW, Archer GL, Dismukes WE. *Staphylococcus epidermidis* causing prosthetic valve endocarditis: Microbiologic and clinical observations as guides to therapy. Ann Intern Med 1983;98:447–455.
28. Lowy FD, Chang D, Lash P. Synergy studies using combinations of vancomycin, gentamicin or rifampin against methicillin-resistant coagulase negative staphylococci. Antimicrob Agents Chemother 1983;23:932–934.
29. Meyer RD. Legionnaires' disease: Aspects of nosocomial infection. Am J Med 1984;76:657–663.
30. Hand WL, Sanford JP. *Mycobacterium fortuitum*—a human pathogen. Ann Intern Med 1970;73:971–977.
31. Levy C, Curtin JA, Watkins A, et al. *Mycobacterium chelanei* infection of porcine heart valves. N Engl J Med 1977; 197:667–668.
32. Guggenbichler JP, Kofler J, Allerberger F. The influence of third-generation cephalosporins on the aerobic intestinal flora. Infections 1985;13(suppl 1):S137–S139.
33. Mulligan ME, Citron DM, McNamara BT, et al. Impact of cefoperazone therapy on fecal flora. Antimicrob Agents Chemother 1982;22:222–230.
34. Maki DG, Rhame FS, Mackel DC, et al. Nationwide epidemic of septicemia caused by contaminated intravenous products. I. Epidemiologic and clinical features. Am J Med 1976;60:471–485.
35. Goldman DA, Fuederson CC, Dixon RE, et al. Nationwide epidemic of septicemia caused by contaminated intravenous products. II. Assessment of the problem by a national nosocomial infection surveillance system. Am J Epidemiol 1978; 108:207–213.
36. Maki DG, Nosocomial bacteremia, an epidemiologic overview, in Dixon RE (ed): Nosocomial Infections. New York, Yorke Medical Books, 1981, pp 183–196.
37. Ashcroft KW, Leape LL. Candida sepsis complicating parenteral feeding. JAMA 1970;212:454–456.
38. Goldman DA, Martin WT, Worthington JW. Growth of bacteriaand fungi in total parenteral nutrition solutions. Am J Surg 1973;126:314–318.

39. Plouffe JF, Brown DG, Silva J, et al. Nosocomial outbreak of *Candida parapsilosis* fungemia related to intravenous infusion. Arch Intern Med 1977;137:1686–1689.
40. Anonymous. Primary bacteremia—Illinois. MMWR 1976;April 16.
41. Zellmer W. Quality control in admixture services. Am J Hosp Pharm 1978;35:527.
42. Anonymous. Accreditation manual for Hospitals. Chicago, Joint Commission on Accreditation of Hospitals. 1983, p 72.
43. Sanders CC. Novel resistance selected by the new expanded spectrum cephalosporins: A concern. J Infect Dis 1983;147: 585–589.
44. Livermore DM. Do beta-lactamases "trap" cephalosporins? J Antimicrob Chemother 1985;14:511–521.
45. Jarvis WR, White JW, Munn VP, et al. Nosocomial infection surveillance, 1983. MMWR 1984;33(255):9–21.
46. Stamm WE, Weinstein RA, Dixon RE. Comparison of endemic and epidemic nosocomial infections, in Dixon RE (ed): Nosocomial Infections. New York, Yorke Medical Books, 1981, pp 9–13.

# 4 Oncologic Disorders

# Chapter 93 / Breast Cancer

Timothy R. McGuire, PharmD, and Nicky Dozier, PharmD

In 1987, an estimated 127,000 new cases of breast cancer were diagnosed in the United States.[1] One out of every 11 American women, or about 9%, develops breast cancer during her lifetime. Breast cancer accounts for nearly 40,000 deaths and, along with lung cancer, is the leading cause of cancer deaths among women. Although the mortality rate from breast cancer has remained nearly unchanged from that for 1950 to 1982,[2] there have been significant gains in disease-free survival and quality of life.

## Epidemiology/Etiology

In the United States, breast cancer is uncommon before the age of 30; the incidence rises sharply between the ages of 30 and 45, reaching a plateau in the perimenopausal years.[1]

The cause of breast cancer is not known but environmental, endocrine, genetic, viral, and immunologic factors have been implicated (Table 93.1). There are no significant racial differences in the incidence of breast cancer among American-born whites, blacks, and Asians[3]; however, the incidence of breast cancer in North America and Northern Europe is five times higher than that in Asia and Africa. This is probably the result of some environmental difference as opposed to racial differences between the populations. Support for an environmental cause comes from Asian immigrant populations, where the offspring of North American immigrants have the same incidence of breast cancer as the general North American population.

Because animal studies have shown that dietary fat can act as a promoter in the development of breast cancer and certain epidemiologic studies have demonstrated a relationship between dietary fat and breast cancer in humans, the high-fat diet of North Americans and Northern Europeans has been implicated as an environmental cause of breast cancer.[4] Other studies, however, have failed to show a definite association between fatty diet and breast cancer.[5,6] In one study, nearly 90,000 nurses from the United States were questioned regarding dietary fat intake and asked to keep a record of dietary consumption. After 4 years of follow-up, 601 study subjects developed breast cancer with no correlation being found between risk of developing breast cancer and dietary fat intake. This was true for both pre- and postmenopausal breast cancer.[6]

As endogenous estrogen is important in the pathogenesis of breast cancer,[7] reproductive history and family history are important determinants for the development of breast cancer. Women with early menarche and women with late menopause are at higher risk of developing breast cancer.[8,9] Conversely, women without functioning ovaries have a decreased risk of breast cancer, particularly if ovarian dysfunction occurred before age 35.[10] The age at which a women bears her first child is also important; those bearing children before the age of 18 have one third the risk of breast cancer compared with those having their first child after age 30. Women who have a first-degree relative with breast cancer are at two to three times the risk of the general population. This risk increases if the relative had bilateral disease or if the cancer developed at an early age. For example, the risk of developing breast cancer in a woman with a first-degree relative who developed bilateral breast cancer at an early age is about nine times higher than that of the general population.[11]

Although endogenous estrogen is important in the pathogenesis of breast cancer, estrogen replacement therapy in postmenopausal patients has not been shown to increase the risk of breast cancer.[12] The risk associated with oral contraceptives remains controversial. A recent case–control study in 4,711 newly diagnosed breast cancer patients showed no increased risk of breast cancer in contraceptive users[13]; however, another study showed an association between oral contraceptive usage for at least 7 years and subsequent development of breast cancer.[14] Currently, the predominance of evidence suggests that estrogen replacement therapy or oral contraceptive usage does not increase the risk of developing breast cancer.

Benign breast disease increases the risk of developing breast cancer. In a prospective study of 747 women with benign breast disease, the age-adjusted incidence of breast cancer was two to three times higher than that of a matched control group.[15]

Ionizing radiation at the levels of exposure produced by the Hiroshima bombing, multiple fluoroscopies in women with pulmonary tuberculosis, and treatment with radiation for postpartum mastitis have been shown to increase the risk of breast cancer.[16] The risk associated with the much smaller doses used in mammography remains controversial and is discussed under Diagnosis.

Cigarette smokers may have a slightly lower risk of breast cancer because of an earlier onset of menopause[17]; however, this small benefit does not offset the increased risk of death from lung cancer, cardiovascular disease, and chronic pulmonary disease caused by cigarette smoking.

Alcohol consumption, even in moderation, appears to significantly increase the risk of breast cancer. Of 17 cohort and case–control studies, 14 concluded that moderate alcohol consumption is associated with an increased risk of breast cancer. In a recent study of 90,000 nurses, of whom 70% were premenopausal, one or more drinks per day increased the risk of developing breast cancer by 60% compared with nondrinkers.[18]

**Table 93.1** Risk Factors Associated With Breast Cancer

| *Increased risk* | *Decreased risk* |
|---|---|
| Alcohol | Castration < 35 yr of age |
| Reproductive history | First child < 18 yr of age |
| Early menarche | Cigarette smoking? |
| Late menopause | |
| Radiation | |
| Family history | |
| Benign breast disease | |
| Oral contraceptives? | |
| Fatty diet? | |

## Diagnosis

Early diagnosis of breast cancer is crucial because of the tendency of the disease to spread systemically and the high mortality rate in patients with disseminated disease. The methods of early diagnosis currently being recommended are monthly self-examination with occasional physical examination by a physician (Table 93.2). In addition, as mammography is substantially more sensitive than physical examination, particularly with lesions less that 1 cm, a baseline mammogram at ages 35 to 40 with periodic mammograms thereafter is also recommended.[19]

Patients diagnosed with breast cancer seldom have characteristic signs or symptoms of metastatic disease at the time of diagnosis. In a series of 100 consecutive patients with breast cancer, the most common presenting sign was a painless lump.[20] Most breast lesions are not malignant. In one large series of 5,604 breast operations performed at New York Medical College between 1960 and 1975, 73% were found to be benign lesions while 27% were malignant.[21] The characteristics of the breast mass can help to differentiate malignant from benign lesions. Solid or hard fixed lesions with irregular borders are more likely to be cancerous than movable soft or cystic lesions with regular borders; however, because it is not possible to differentiate between benign and malignant lesions by physical examination, a biopsy is required to determine cytology.

The role of mammography in the detection of breast cancer has become better defined because of two large prospective studies. In the first study, The Health Insurance Plan of Greater New York randomized 62,000 women, 40–64 years old, either to mammography and clinical examination or to no intervention. After a 10-year follow-up in women older than 50 there was a 33% reduction in mortality compared with the control group.[22] In a second study sponsored by the Breast Cancer Detection Demonstration Project (BCDDP), 280,000 women enrolled throughout the United States were screened with physical examination and mammography. They were also taught the appropriate method of self-examination. Of the 4,443 cancers diagnosed over an 8-year period, about 30% were less than 1 cm in size and of these 57% could be detected only by mammography. Importantly, less than 20% of the cancers detected had axillary node metastases compared with the 50% reported in other studies not using mammography. It was also observed that the use of mammography in the screening process allowed physicians to diagnose tumors at an earlier stage.[23]

Despite its high sensitivity, 10% to 15% of palpable masses are not well imaged by mammography. Physical examination of the breast should therefore remain an important element in any screening program for breast cancer.[24] The risk of cancer from the small doses of radiation used in mammography is low. To date there have been no documented cases of breast cancer as a result of mammography. In the BCDDP study, exposure levels ranged from 0.04 to 0.37 rads per mammogram. It is estimated that 1 rad given to the breast of a million women would produce six cancers per year after a latency period of 6 to 10 years. For comparison, it is estimated that appropriate use of mammography in screening programs can reduce the death rate by one third, saving an estimated 12,000 lives per year. Thus, over a 30-year period, the lives of 360,000 women could be saved by mammography at the cost of 120 lives from radiation-induced breast cancer. The economic cost of screening with mammography is substantial; with 40 million women at risk and each mammogram costing $90, baseline mammograms in these 40 million women would cost $3.6 billion.[25]

Other methods for breast imaging include ultrasound and thermography but both methods have important limitations.[25,26]

**Table 93.2** American Cancer Society Guidelines for Breast Cancer Screening

| *Age group* | *Screening procedure* |
|---|---|
| 20–40 | Monthly breast self-examination<br>Physical examination every 3 years<br>Baseline mammogram at age 35–40 |
| 40–49 | Monthly breast self-examination<br>Physical examination every year<br>Mammogram every 2 years |
| > 50 | Monthly breast self-examination<br>Physical examination every year<br>Mammogram every year |

## Staging

Although several different staging procedures have been devised for breast cancer, the most widely accepted staging system is the TNM classification, based on characteristics of the primary tumor (T), extent of nodal involvement (N), and presence or absence of metastatic disease (M). Table 93.3 is a summary of the TNM system for the staging of breast cancer.

## Prognostic Factors

The most important prognostic factors in breast cancer are extent of axillary node involvement, size of the primary tumor, and estrogen and progesterone receptor status. Other

**Table 93.3** Clinical Staging of Breast Cancer

| | |
|---|---|
| Stage I<br>Tumor < 2 cm in diameter<br>Negative axillary nodes<br>No distant metastases | Stage III<br>Tumor > 5 cm or any size with skin or chest wall invasion<br>No distant metastases |
| Stage II<br>Tumor < 5 cm in diameter<br>Positive axillary nodes<br>No distant metastases | Stage IV<br>Distant metastases |

From American Joint Committee for Cancer Staging of Breast Cancer, Chicago, 1977, p 104, with permission.

prognostic factors include age at diagnosis, histologic grade, and thymidine labeling index.[27]

At the time of diagnosis, evidence of breast cancer spread to the axillary lymph nodes is found in 40% to 50% of patients.[28] Five-year survival in untreated patients is related to the number of axillary nodes that are positive for tumor. Five-year survival in node-negative patients is 60% to 80% while those with one to three or more than three positive nodes have 50% and 20% 5-year survival rates, respectively[29] (Table 93.4). Recent studies have shown that patients with more than three positive axillary nodes have a variable course depending upon how many nodes are positive. Therefore, many recent protocols further subdivide patients with more than three positive nodes into those with four to nine and those with ten or more positive nodes.[30]

Larger tumors are more likely to have axillary node metastasis than smaller tumors.[31] Lesions less than 1.5 cm have axillary node involvement in 38% of cases versus 70% of cases for tumors greater than 5 cm. The size of the primary tumor is an important prognostic factor, regardless of axillary node involvement, with tumors less than 2 cm considered to have a good prognosis.

Estrogen receptors (ERs) and progesterone receptors (PRs) are indicators of tumor differentiation.[32] In general, patients with tumors positive for these steroid receptors have a better 5-year survival than receptor-negative patients, which may be related to a slower growth rate as measured by a low thymidine labeling index. Receptor status has major implications in the treatment of breast cancer which are discussed under Chemotherapy/Hormonal Therapy.

Age as an indicator of prognosis remains controversial; however, there is evidence that women between ages 45 and 49 have better survival rates compared with other age groups.[33]

**Table 93.4** Disease-Free Survival 5 and 10 Years After Mastectomy

| *Nodal status* | *Number of patients* | *Survival (%)* 5 yr | 10 yr |
|---|---|---|---|
| Node negative | 198 | 82 | 76 |
| Node positive | 172 | 35 | 24 |
| 1–3 | 82 | 50 | 35 |
| > 3 | 90 | 21 | 14 |

## Estrogen Receptors

The introduction of reliable laboratory assays for estrogen receptors in human breast tissue represents a major advance in the knowledge and treatment of breast cancer.[34] Binding capacity of ERs is expressed as femtomoles of [$^3$H]estradiol bound per milligram of cytosol protein. Values above 10 fmol/mg are usually considered positive, whereas values less than 3 fmol/mg are considered negative; values in between are considered borderline.

About 50% to 70% of patients with primary or metastatic breast cancer have ER+ tumors. The median level and frequency of ER+ tumors are higher in postmenopausal patients compared with premenopausal patients, presumably because greater amounts of endogenous estrogens occupy a proportion of the available binding sites in premenopausal patients.[34,35]

ER status may correlate with certain clinical characteristics of the patient. Axillary node spread at the time of mastectomy has been reported to be more frequent in patients with ER− tumors.[35,36] Several investigators have observed that lack of ERs may serve as a predictor of early recurrence.[37–39] Patients with ER− tumors tended to have a shorter disease-free interval (time from mastectomy to metastases) than patients with ER+ tumors.[40] This relationship appears to be independent of the size of the tumor or the extent of nodal involvement.

The major importance of ER status is its ability to predict for response to endocrine therapy. In unselected patients, about one third of patients have an objective response to endocrine therapy; however, of patients with ER+ tumors, 50% to 60% can be expected to achieve an objective response to endocrine therapy, whereas only 5% to 10% of patients with ER− tumors respond.[40] The predictive value of ER status on response rate appears to be independent of other known clinical factors that influence response to endocrine therapy.[41] Estrogen receptor status does not appear to correlate with the duration of remission. The routine use of ER assays can spare some patients from unnecessary major ablative surgical procedures, and can save others valuable time by earlier institution of combination chemotherapy.

The high incidence of unresponsive ER+ tumors has prompted a search for additional predictors of response to endocrine therapy. The absolute ER level may be helpful. In one series, response rates of 9%, 30%, 63%, and 77% were reported in patients with ER values of <10, 10–20, 20–50, and >50 fmol/mg cytosol protein, respectively.[42] Various studies have reported that the use of progesterone receptors (PRs) improves the predicted response rate from 50%–60% to 80%–90% in patients who have ER+/PR+ tumors.[32,43]

The role of ER status in predicting response to chemotherapy in patients with metastatic disease is controversial. An early study suggested that patients with ER− tumors were more likely to respond to combination chemotherapy than those with ER+ tumors[44]; however, other studies have reported that ER status does not correlate with antitumor response to chemotherapy or that patients with ER− tumors are less likely to respond to chemotherapy.[45] The reasons for the divergent results are unclear. Studies that have reported a higher response rate for ER− tumors are supported by cell kinetic studies demonstrating that tumors with high turnover rates are associated with absence of ERs.

## Treatment of Primary Breast Cancer

Until recently, the major treatment for breast cancer was radical mastectomy. The rationale for this approach was that because breast cancer spreads contiguously from the localized lesion, the use of radical surgery would eliminate the cancer. In the view of many surgeons, the extent of resection was limited only by the ability to support the patient postsurgically.[46]

Nevertheless, more recent data show that breast cancer remains localized only briefly and the ability to cure the patient with surgery or radiation is lost early in the disease.[47] At the time of diagnosis, breast cancer has often already spread to axillary lymph nodes. Although evidence of distant metastases is seldom found at diagnosis, a number of observations support the concept that breast cancer has usually metastasized to distant sites at the time of diagnosis. First, even in patients with as few as three positive axillary lymph nodes, about one half will die of metastatic breast cancer within 5 years (Table 93.4). This high death rate is not significantly influenced by local irradiation, which shows that lymph nodes are not adequate barriers to tumor spread. Second, it has been observed that the most common initial sign of tumor recurrence after "curative" surgery is distant metastases. Third, it is estimated that by the time a malignant breast lesion is detected by physical exam (1 cm), the tumor has undergone 30 doublings and may have been present for 15 years.[48] Finally, studies have shown that the metastatic spread of breast cancer is not through direct invasion of tissue by the primary tumor, but through embolization of cancer cells into the lymphatics and bloodstream. It is therefore not surprising that most breast cancers have metastasized before diagnosis has occurred and that most patients cannot be treated by local therapy alone.

### *Surgery*

Radical mastectomy involves removal of the breast and both major and minor pectoralis muscles. The axillary nodes on the same side (ipsilateral) as the breast lesion are also removed. There can be substantial morbidity from the procedure; muscle resection decreases strength and range of motion, and removal of axillary lymph nodes can produce edema of the arm and resected breast area. The swelling and chronic edema around the resected breast tissue can make it difficult to perform reconstructive surgery.

Over the past 15 years, radical mastectomy has been nearly replaced by modified radical mastectomy and many surgeons do not feel that radical mastectomy is an appropriate method for surgical management of breast cancer.[49] Modified radical mastectomy spares the pectoralis muscles and higher level axillary nodes. It is a less disfiguring operation and improves the chances of successful breast reconstruction. As the axillary nodes are partially dissected, it allows for adequate evaluation of axillary metastasis.

Total mastectomy is similar to a modified radical mastectomy but axillary nodes are preserved. The major disadvantage of this procedure is that it reduces the accuracy of axillary node staging. Many surgeons use this procedure in patients without palpable axillary nodes (stage I), because it leaves functioning lymph nodes that theoretically can mount an immunologic response to residual tumor.

Partial mastectomy is surgery that preserves the breast and includes segmental mastectomy, local excision, and lumpectomy. These procedures are gaining in popularity because of the obvious cosmetic advantages over radical or modified radical procedures. The criteria used to select patients for partial mastectomy are breast size and size of the primary tumor. The procedure is usually combined with radiation and axillary node dissection.

The studies sponsored by NSABP were designed to answer some important questions regarding the use of these conservative procedures (total mastectomy and partial mastectomy). After 8 years of follow-up in 1,765 patients no difference in survival or incidence or site of recurrence has been seen in clinically node-negative patients treated with radical mastectomy, total mastectomy plus radiation, or total mastectomy alone.[50] Partial mastectomy is compared with total mastectomy in the most recent NSABP study. Patients were enrolled from 1976 to 1984 and the 5-year results were published in 1985. A total of 1,843 patients were randomized to total mastectomy or partial mastectomy with or without radiation. All patients underwent axillary node dissection, with all node-positive patients receiving adjuvant chemotherapy. Disease-free survival was significantly longer in patients treated with partial mastectomy and radiation.[51]

### *Radiation*

Radiation is usually given after surgery to reduce the incidence of local relapse. Despite even the most aggressive surgical procedures, about 20% of axillary node-positive patients and 10% of node-negative patients have local relapse of their disease.[52] Also, at the time of diagnosis, metastatic disease can often be found in the internal mammary and supraclavicular lymph nodes, which are not removed with any of the current surgical methods. In one study, local relapse was reduced to less than 5% with moderate-dose radiotherapy (4,500–5,000 rads over 4 weeks).[53] This improvement in local relapse rates did not translate into improved survival, supporting the concept that patients with local spread to the axillary, internal mammary, or supraclavicular nodes already have distant spread of the disease. Because of the lack of survival benefit, the use of supraclavicular or internal mammary node irradiation is controversial and should not be considered routine therapy.

An increasing number of surgeons are performing conservative surgery (lumpectomy) with axillary node dissection and postsurgical radiation in patients with stage I or stage II disease. The amount of radiation delivered depends on the extent of axillary dissection and the amount of healthy tissue around the margins of the excised tumor. Radiation to the area of axillary dissection is not recommended because of the high incidence of chronic edema on the irradiated side.[54]

### *Chemotherapy/Hormonal Therapy*

As just discussed, the rationale for chemotherapy shortly *after* surgery ("*adjuvant* chemotherapy") is based on the concept that the disease has usually spread to distant sites at the time of diagnosis; however, some protocols are evaluating the use of chemotherapy *before* surgery; this approach is referred to as *neoadjuvant* chemotherapy. The rationale for neoadjuvant chemotherapy is based on the observation that cytotoxic therapy is most effective in patients with small tumor burdens. The fewer the number of cells, the less likely resistant clones are to develop during therapy and the more likely are effective drug concentrations to reach sensitive cancer cells. Although the ultimate goal of neoadjuvant chemotherapy is to prolong disease-free survival, another benefit of this form of therapy is its ability to "debulk" large primary tumors before surgical removal.[55,56] Several years will be required before the efficacy of this approach is known.

A number of cytotoxic drugs have been used alone and in combination as adjuvant therapy in breast cancer, including doxorubicin, cyclophosphamide, methotrexate, 5-fluorouracil, L-phenylalanine mustard (L-PAM), prednisone, and vincristine. Newer agents that have shown some activity include mitoxantrone, epirubicin, etoposide, and vindesine. Early adjuvant chemotherapy regimens usually contained a single drug or a low-dose combination but the current trend is to treat aggressively with multiple-drug regimens at high doses in an attempt to increase long-term survival.[57] Table 93.5 summarizes the single-agent activity of the chemotherapeutic agents used in breast cancer.

The optimal duration of adjuvant chemotherapy is not known. Most studies have administered chemotherapy for 6 months to 2 years. Several studies have randomized patients to two different drug regimens differing only in the duration of treatment. Most of the trials have shown a trend toward improved survival with the *short*-duration therapy, which suggests that any benefit from additional cycles of chemotherapy is more than offset by the acute and chronic toxic effects of the treatment.[58] Of concern is the preliminary report of an increased risk of leukemia in patients treated with adjuvant chemotherapy.[59] Until longer durations of chemotherapy are clearly shown to be superior to shorter durations, adjuvant chemotherapy should be given for 6 months to 1 year in most patients. In some high-risk patient groups (i.e., those with more than ten positive lymph nodes), however, the potential benefit from a longer duration of adjuvant chemotherapy may exceed the risk of secondary malignancy.

The other major type of treatment in primary breast cancer is endocrine therapy. Hormonal therapies that have been studied in the treatment of primary breast cancer include oophorectomy, ovarian irradiation, and most recently tamoxifen. As discussed earlier, endocrine therapy takes advantage of the estrogen dependence of breast tumors that are positive for ER. Overall, about 60% of patients with ER+ tumors respond to endocrine therapy. If the patient is also positive for the progesterone receptor (PR), the response rate is improved to 80%. This increased response rate in ER+ and PR+ patients is not surprising as PR concentration is dependent on ER function. Also, patients with higher ER concentrations are more likely to respond to hormonal therapy. Table 93.6 summarizes the endocrine and cytotoxic adjuvant treatments in pre- and postmenopausal patients with known estrogen receptor status.

**Table 93.5** Antitumor Activity of Single Agents in Breast Cancer [a]

| *Drug class* | *Response rate (%)* |
|---|---|
| Anthracycline antibiotics | |
| Doxorubicin | 33 |
| Epirubicin | 31 |
| Mitoxantrone | 20 |
| Alkylating agents | |
| Cyclophosphamide | 34 |
| Mitomycin C | 22 |
| Melphalan (L-PAM)[b] | 23 |
| *cis*-Platinum | 8 |
| Antimetabolites | |
| 5-Fluorouracil | 26 |
| Methotrexate | 25 |
| Vinca alkaloids | |
| Vincristine | 21 |
| Vindesine | 31 |
| Vinblastine[c] | 40 |

[a] Complete and partial response in patients previously treated for metastatic disease.
[b] L-Phenylalanine mustard.
[c] With 5-day continuous infusion.

Compiled from References 57 and 73.

The following discussion of adjuvant treatment for breast cancer is divided into four patient groups: premenopausal node-positive patients, premenopausal node-negative patients, postmenopausal node-positive patients, and postmenopausal node-negative patients.

#### Premenopausal Node-Positive Patients

The greatest improvements in disease-free survival and overall survival from adjuvant chemotherapy have been in this group of patients. Early studies using L-PAM (melphalan) alone demonstrated a significant improvement in disease-free and overall survival in premenopausal patients with one to three positive nodes when compared with placebo (Table 93.7). This benefit was not observed in patients over 50 years of age or in those with more than three positive axillary nodes.[60] In another study, the Milan group reported that premenopausal patients treated with a combination of cyclophosphamide, methotrexate, and 5-fluorouracil (CMF) had significantly longer disease-free and overall survival than untreated patients.[61] Unlike the L-PAM study, the Milan trial showed a significant improvement in disease-free survival in premenopausal women with more than three positive nodes treated with CMF (Table 93.7)

A number of studies have demonstrated a significant benefit of combination chemotherapy over single-agent

**Table 93.6** Summary of Initial Systemic Therapy of Breast Cancer

| *Disease severity* | *Receptor status*[a] | *Treatment* |
|---|---|---|
| **Premenopausal Patients** | | |
| Stage I | ER+ | No treatment |
| | ER− | No treatment or adjuvant chemotherapy[b] |
| Stage II/III | ER+ | Adjuvant Chemotherapy or adjuvant chemotherapy combined with endocrine therapy[b] |
| | ER− | Adjuvant chemotherapy |
| Stage IV | ER+ | Oophorectomy, tamoxifen; or other hormonal treatments |
| | ER− | Combination chemotherapy |
| **Postmenopausal Patients** | | |
| Stage I | ER+ | No treatment |
| | ER− | No treatment or adjuvant chemotherapy[b] |
| Stage II/III | ER+ | Endocrine therapy either alone or combined with adjuvant chemotherapy[b] |
| | ER− | Adjuvant chemotherapy[b] |
| Stage IV | ER+ | Endocrine therapy |
| | ER− | Combination chemotherapy |

[a] ER, estrogen receptor.
[b] These treatments should be considered investigational.

chemotherapy.[28] In a recent SWOG study, with a median follow-up of 6 years, treatment failure rates were 48% for L-PAM alone and 31% for the combination of cyclophosphamide, methotrexate, 5-fluorouracil, vincristine, and prednisone (CMFVP).[62]

The use of neoadjuvant chemotherapy is most likely to be beneficial in this subgroup of patients. The use of high-dose combination chemotherapy prior to surgery has been shown to be safe and preliminary data support its effectiveness.[54,63]

Currently, the use of endocrine therapy for the management of primary breast cancer in premenopausal patients is controversial. The earliest studies, conducted between 1948 and 1973, suggest that adjuvant oophorectomy or ovarian irradiation can prolong disease-free and overall survival in premenopausal patients[58]; however, the differences in survival were not statistically significant in most of the studies. It is important to emphasize that these studies were conducted before the importance of ER status was recognized. Therefore, one possible reason for the lack of a survival benefit is the inclusion of women with ER− tumors, who are

**Table 93.7** 10-Year Results of Randomized Adjuvant Chemotherapy Trials

| | *NSABP*[a] | | *Milan* | |
|---|---|---|---|---|
| *Patient group* | **Control** | **L-PAM** | **Control** | **CMF**[a] |
| **Disease-Free Survival (%)** | | | | |
| Postmenopausal | 28 | 34 | 32 | 38 |
| Premenopausal | 29 | 46[b] | 31 | 48[b] |
| 1–3 Positive nodes | 41 | 66[b] | 40 | 61[b] |
| > 3 Positive nodes | 17 | 22 | 15 | 26[b] |
| **Overall Survival (%)** | | | | |
| Postmenopausal | 43 | 41 | 50 | 52 |
| Premenopausal | 37 | 61[b] | 45 | 59[b] |
| 1–3 Positive nodes | 48 | 81[b] | 51 | 68[b] |
| > 3 Positive nodes | 26 | 35 | 30 | 42 |

[a] NSABP, National Surgical Adjuvant Breast Project; L-PAM, L-phenylalanine mustard (melphalan); CMF, cyclophosphamide, methotrexate, and 5-fluorouracil.
[b] Statistically significant difference between control and treatment at $P < 0.05$.

not likely to respond to any form of hormonal therapy. More recently, tamoxifen has been used either alone or combined with chemotherapy in some studies.[64] Preliminary analysis of these studies indicates that the major benefit of hormonal or chemohormonal therapy is seen in postmenopausal women, particularly those who are ER+.[64,65] The benefit, if any, in premenopausal women is likely to be marginal.

In summary, as adjuvant chemotherapy has clearly been shown to prolong disease-free and overall survival in this patient group, it should be offered to every premenopausal patient with axillary node involvement. The optimal regimen and duration of therapy are not known. While hormonal therapy may prove to be beneficial in premenopausal patients with ER+ tumors, this form of therapy should currently be reserved as treatment for tumor recurrence.

### Premenopausal Node-Negative Patients

In general, this group of patients has a good prognosis with local therapy alone, 5-year survival being in the area of 70%[66]; however, certain subgroups of these patients, such as those having tumors with a high thymidine labeling index or those younger than 35, appear to have a high risk of tumor recurrence. Similarly, preliminary results show that node-negative ER− patients randomized to receive CMF have a significant improvement in disease-free and overall survival compared with a control group given no systemic therapy.[67] Therefore, these data suggest that ER status may help to select a group of node-negative patients who have a high risk of tumor recurrence and who therefore are most likely to benefit from adjuvant chemotherapy.

### Postmenopausal Node-Positive Patients

The use of adjuvant chemotherapy in this category of patients is controversial. Ten-year results of both the NSABP and the Milan studies show that single-agent (L-PAM) or combination chemotherapy (CMF) does not significantly prolong disease-free or overall survival in postmenopausal node-positive patients.[60,61] In both studies, however, patients randomized to receive chemotherapy tended to survive longer than untreated patients. As most patients did not have their tumor assayed for ER status, survival of patients according to ER status was not analyzed.

The reasons for the lack of efficacy in postmenopausal patients are not completely understood. Some investigators have proposed that the survival benefit in premenopausal patients is due to a chemotherapy-induced ("chemical") oophorectomy; however, measurement of follicle-stimulating hormone, luteinizing hormone, and estradiol shows that ovarian function and menses do not correlate with response to adjuvant chemotherapy. For example, although amenorrhea was common in women 40 to 49 years old, the group that has shown the greatest benefit of adjuvant chemotherapy has been women younger than 40.[68] Alternatively, postmenopausal patients may have less aggressive tumors that are less responsive to chemotherapy. Results of one study suggest that postmenopausal patients do worse than premenopausal patients because of the more frequent dosage reductions resulting from more severe drug-related toxicity.[61] In that study, patients who received more than 85% of their prescribed CMF dosage had a similar improvement in survival, regardless of menopausal status.

Although adjuvant chemotherapy has not been shown to be beneficial in unselected postmenopausal node-positive patients, it is possible that certain subgroups will benefit from adjuvant therapy. With the advent of knowledge concerning ER status, it is also possible that the type of adjuvant therapy (chemotherapy versus hormonal therapy) can be tailored according to ER status.

***Estrogen-Receptor Positive*** Based on the poor results of adjuvant chemotherapy in postmenopausal patients, many studies have evaluated the role of adjuvant hormonal therapy, either alone or combined with chemotherapy. In most of these studies, tamoxifen was used because of its low toxicity. In every study, patients who received tamoxifen alone had a significant increase in disease-free survival compared with untreated patients; overall survival also tended to be longer but the difference was not always statistically significant.[58,69] When postmenopausal patients were analyzed according to ER status, patients with ER+ tumors had a significantly longer disease-free and overall survival. In contrast, no effect of tamoxifen was usually observed in patients with ER− tumors. Because progesterone receptor concentration is directly related to estrogen receptor function, the survival benefit in patients with ER+/PR+ tumors is even more dramatic; 5-year survival in patients with ER+/PR+ tumors was 92% compared with 49% in the control group.[70]

Tamoxifen has also been added to a number of chemotherapeutic regimens in an attempt to improve clinical response ("chemohormonal therapy"). Although chemohormonal therapy appears to prolong disease-free survival in unselected patients compared with tamoxifen or chemotherapy alone, no significant difference in overall survival has been noted. For example, preliminary results of a recent NSABP study comparing chemotherapy (L-PAM and 5-fluorouracil) with chemohormonal therapy (the same two agents plus tamoxifen) show that patients with ER+ or ER+/PR+ tumors are most likely to benefit from chemohormonal therapy.[64] In some subgroups of patients, chemohormonal therapy appeared to have a detrimental effect on disease-free survival compared with chemotherapy alone. The reasons for this are unclear but may result from drug interactions between tamoxifen and all or part of the cytotoxic regimen or from less favorable cytokinetics caused by tamoxifen's inhibition of tumor growth.[71]

***Estrogen-Receptor Negative*** Although adjuvant chemotherapy for this subgroup of patients cannot be recommended at this time, there are data to support its use and this group of patients continues to be a subject of active clinical investigation. In one trial, adjuvant CMF and prednisone treatment resulted in a significant improvement in disease-free survival in patients with ER− tumors compared with no treatment.[72] As discussed under Estrogen Receptors, the use of chemotherapy in these patients is supported by observations that ER status correlates with the degree of tumor differentiation. In general, tumors that are ER− are usually more rapidly growing and more poorly differentiated than ER+ tumors, characteristics that are associated with a response to chemotherapy.

### Postmenopausal Node-Negative Patients

Although these patients have no evidence of metastatic spread to the lymph nodes at diagnosis, about one third of them ultimately die of breast cancer. While adjuvant treatment is not currently recommended in this group of patients, many believe that tamoxifen should be given to patients with ER+ tumors and that adjuvant chemotherapy should be given to patients with ER− tumors.[60] One small study has reported that CMF improves disease-free and overall survival in node-negative patients, regardless of menopausal status.[67]

## Treatment of Advanced Breast Cancer

Despite adjuvant therapy, many patients with breast cancer develop metastatic disease. Once there are signs or symptoms that the disease has spread beyond the primary breast lesion and axillary nodes, the disease is rarely cured. The goal of therapy in advanced breast cancer is therefore to relieve symptoms and to prolong survival.

### *Endocrine Therapy*

Endocrine therapy takes advantage of the estrogen dependence of breast cancer and includes both surgical (i.e., oophorectomy, adrenalectomy) and medical (i.e., tamoxifen, estrogen, progestins) approaches. About one third of unselected patients with metastatic breast cancer have an objective response to endocrine therapy. Responses are almost always partial rather than complete and are usually short, lasting 9 to 18 months. Some patients, however, have prolonged responses that last several years.[73]

Several clinical and laboratory characteristics correlate with response to endocrine therapy. As ER status is an indicator of the estrogen dependence of breast cancer, it is the most important prognostic factor for response to any endocrine therapy (see Estrogen Receptors). In general, 50% to 60% of patients with ER+ tumors respond to endocrine therapy, whereas the response rate in patients with ER− tumors is only 5% to 10%. If the patient has a ER+/PR+ tumor, the response rate increases to 80% to 90%.[32] The chronologic age and menstrual status of the patient influence response. Younger premenopausal or postmenopausal patients usually have a lower response rate than older women within each menopausal group. Postmenopausal women also tend to respond more often than premenopausal women. The site of metastatic disease also influences the likelihood of response; breast, skin, and lymphatic metastases respond more favorably than bone or visceral (i.e., brain, liver) metastases. Patients with a short disease-free interval, usually defined as less than 2 years from diagnosis to recurrence, are less likely to respond than patients with longer disease-free intervals. Finally, patients who have a durable response to one hormonal therapy are more likely to have a second response to another hormonal treatment.[74]

Endocrine therapy is the treatment of choice in most women with ER+ tumors. As women with ER− tumors are not likely to benefit from endocrine therapy, they should be treated with cytotoxic chemotherapy. The type of initial endocrine therapy depends on menopausal status. If the patient experiences a good response to initial endocrine therapy and does not have rapidly progressing disease, second-line endocrine therapy is usually given. Patients are sequentially treated with endocrine therapy until they have progressive symptoms resulting from rapidly growing metastatic disease, at which time cytotoxic chemotherapy can be given.

#### Surgery

Surgical management of metastatic breast cancer is becoming less common and is gradually being replaced by noninvasive medical treatment with tamoxifen, aminoglutethemide, progesterones, trilostane, and luteinizing hormone–releasing hormone (LHRH) agonists.[73]

Bilateral oophorectomy remains the endocrine treatment of choice for *premenopausal* patients with metastatic breast cancer.[74] Oophorectomy removes the major source of estrogen in premenopausal patients. Castration is of little value in truly postmenopausal women.

Sources of estrogen outside of the ovaries must be considered when treating a hormonally responsive tumor in the castrated or *postmenopausal* woman. As androstenedione from the adrenal gland is converted to estrone and estradiol in extraadrenal tissues and is the major source of estrogen in these patients, adrenalectomy is an effective endocrine treatment for breast cancer.[75] Adrenalectomized patients require replacement therapy and cortisone acetate is adequate for most patients. Mineralocorticoid replacement may also be necessary, particularly in the summer months.

Hypophysectomy indirectly removes estrogen in *postmenopausal* patients by surgically removing the source of pituitary-derived releasing hormones. The choice between adrenalectomy and hypophysectomy often depends on the expertise of the surgeons at the particular institution. Hypophysectomized patients require cortisone acetate and thyroid replacement therapy, and patients with symptomatic diabetes insipidus require maintenance vasopressin therapy.[76]

#### Drug Therapy

***Tamoxifen*** Tamoxifen is an antiestrogen given as adjuvant hormonal therapy or as palliative hormonal therapy in *postmenopausal* patients with ER+ tumors. The drug binds to intracytosolic estrogen receptors, thereby blocking the effects of endogenous estrogens.[77] Tamoxifen is usually given two or three times daily at dosages ranging from 20 to 80 mg daily[78] and is very well tolerated. Symptoms of estrogen withdrawal (hot flashes) are the most troublesome but decrease in frequency and intensity with time. At higher doses, tamoxifen has mild estrogen activity and tumor stimulation can occur.[79] A flare of bone pain and hypercalcemia rarely occurs in patients with bony metastases, but with continued therapy, regression of the tumor and improvement of pain and hypercalcemia usually result.

***Aminoglutethemide*** Aminoglutethemide decreases peripheral estrogen concentrations by inhibiting the cytochrome $P_{450}$-dependent conversion of androstenedione to estrone in target tissues.[80] At higher doses, it also inhibits the adrenal conversion of cholesterol to pregnenolone, resulting in a decrease in androstenedione. Although aminoglutethemide elicits about the same response rate as tamoxifen, the drug is less well tolerated and is therefore used as a second-line agent in the palliative treatment of metastatic breast cancer in *postmenopausal* women with ER+ tumors. The common side effects of aminoglutethemide are dose related and include nystagmus, ataxia, lethargy, dizziness, and nausea. A generalized, macular, pruritic skin rash, often associated with mild fever, has been noted in 30% to 40% of treated patients. The usual doses of aminoglutethemide are 750–1,000 mg per day. Hydrocortisone at doses of 30–40 mg/d has been added to avoid Addisonian symptoms and to suppress the compensatory rise in adrenocorticotropin (ACTH) caused by the inhibition of adrenal steroid synthesis.[81] Aminoglutethemide doses as low as 250 mg/d have been effective in metastatic breast cancer. As low-dose aminoglutethemide may selectively inhibit peripheral conversion of androstenedione to estrone without significantly inhibiting adrenal function, it may not be necessary to add hydrocortisone; however, in one study of low-dose aminoglutethemide (250 mg/d) without hydrocortisone the authors implicated the drug in four deaths secondary to Addisonian crisis.[82] Currently, low-dose aminoglutethemide without hydrocortisone cannot be recommended.

***Estrogens*** Paradoxically, high-dose estrogens can induce an objective response in patients with metastatic breast cancer. The mechanism of action of high-dose estrogens is not known, although there are data to support a direct inhibitory effect on malignant cells. The most commonly used estrogen is diethylstilbestrol (DES), given initially as a 5-mg non–enteric-coated tablet at night and gradually increased to three times daily. One large cooperative study evaluated DES at dosages ranging from 1.5 to 1,500 mg and showed an increasing response rate with escalating doses; however, the duration of response was similar regardless of the dosage used.[83] Diethylstilbestrol is not given routinely at dosages greater than 15 mg/d because of bothersome side effects. At a dosage of 15 mg/d 25% to 50% of patients experience initial anorexia, nausea, vomiting, and fluid retention, which tend to decrease in severity with continued therapy. Less common side effects include possible areolar hyperpigmentation, breast tenderness and engorgement, vaginal discharge, incontinence, hot flashes, and phlebitis.

***Trilostane*** Trilostane inhibits 3$\beta$-ol-hydroxysteroid dehydrogenase and, along with small doses of corticosteroids can produce a medical adrenalectomy. It is as effective as aminoglutethemide but is less well tolerated with significant diarrhea and nausea and vomiting. The usual dose in metastatic breast cancer is 960 mg/d.[84]

***Progestins*** Megesterol acetate (MA) and medroxyprogesterone acetate (MPA) are the two progestins currently used as palliative therapy in widely metastatic breast cancer. MA has antiestrogenic activity; MPA has androgenic and anabolic properties. The mechanism of action of these drugs in breast cancer is unknown, although both have direct cytotoxic effects and an antiestrogen effect has been demonstrated in cell culture.[85]

The common dose used for MA is 160 mg/d but doses as high as 1,600 mg/d have been used. The response rate is similar to that of tamoxifen. There is evidence that higher doses increase the response rate and can produce a second response in patients who relapse after low-dose MA.[86] MPA doses ranged from 500 mg intramuscularly twice weekly to 4 g orally daily. The higher doses seem to be more effective than the lower doses (33% versus 15%). In a group of patients refractory to other hormonal therapies, high-dose MPA produced a 23% response.[87]

Side effects of these agents are minor. The common side effects are weight gain, edema, and hot flashes. Less commonly, these drugs can cause glucose intolerance, hypertension, and vaginal bleeding. In 10% to 15% of patients, adrenocortical side effects are seen with high-dose MPA.[88]

***LHRH Agonists*** The LHRH agonists leuprolide and buserlin have been used in metastatic breast cancer. Their mechanism of action in breast cancer is thought to result from downregulation of LHRH receptors in the pituitary with decreased circulating levels of luteinizing hormone and, subsequently, a decrease in estrogen to castrate levels. Recent information suggests an additional direct cytotoxic effect on cancer cells.

Leuprolide is commercially available in the United States and is used in doses of 1 mg subcutaneously daily. Toxic effects are minimal, usually consisting of menopausal symptoms. Also, tumor flare may occur in the first 2 to 3 weeks of therapy corresponding to an initial increase in estrogen levels prior to LHRH receptor downregulation.[89]

Buserlin is currently not available in the United States and is equivalent in activity to leuprolide with the advantage of intranasal administration.[90]

### *Cytotoxic Chemotherapy*

Cytotoxic chemotherapy will eventually be required in most patients with evidence of axillary node spread or distant metastases. Patients with ER− tumors usually require chemotherapy at the first sign of metastatic disease. In most patients with ER+ tumors, however, various endocrine therapies can be tried before chemotherapy is given. With present chemotherapeutic regimens, the goal is to prolong quality survival.

In general, combination chemotherapy is significantly more effective than single-agent therapy in metastatic breast cancer. Single-agent therapy with drugs active against breast cancer produce an objective response in 20% to 30% of patients (Table 93.5); the duration of response is usually less than 6 months.

#### Single Agents

***Doxorubicin*** Doxorubicin is the drug used most frequently as a single agent in metastatic breast cancer, although response rates and duration of response are improved when it is part of combination therapy. Doxorubicin-containing combination regimens usually produce the best overall response. For example, the combination of cyclophosphamide, doxorubicin, and 5-fluorouracil (CAF) produces a higher initial response than cyclophosphamide, methotrexate, and 5-fluorouracil (CMF)[91]; however, patients treated with CAF did not have a longer duration of response and experienced more drug-related toxic effects than CMF-treated patients. Although the substitution of newer an-

**Table 93.8** Selected Combination Chemotherapy Regimens in Metastatic Breast Cancer

| *Drug regimen* | *Drug* | *Dosage* |
|---|---|---|
| CMFVP (Cooper) | Cyclophosphamide | 2 mg/kg/d PO |
| | Methotrexate | 0.7 mg/kg/wk IV for 8 wk |
| | 5-Fluorouracil | 12 mg/kg/wk IV every other week |
| | Vincristine | 35 μg/kg/wk IV for 4–5 wk |
| | Prednisone | 0.75 mg/kg/d PO with 50% decrease every 10 d |
| CMF (Milan) | Cyclophosphamide | 100 mg/m$^2$/d PO days 1–14 |
| | Methotrexate | 30–40 mg/m$^2$ IV days 1 and 8 |
| | 5-Fluorouracil | 400–600 mg/m$^2$ IV days 1 and 8 |
| CAF | Cyclophosphamide | 400 mg/m$^2$ day 1 |
| | Doxorubicin | 40 mg/m$^2$ day 1 |
| | 5-Fluorouracil | 400 mg/m$^2$ days 1 and 8 |

thracycline drugs such as *mitoxantrone* reduces the severity of drug-related toxic effects, it also reduces the antitumor effect.[92] The dose of doxorubicin usually used is 40–75 mg/m$^2$ every 3 to 4 weeks. The major toxic effects are dose-limiting myelosuppression, stomatitis, nausea and vomiting, alopecia, and cardiotoxicity.

Doxorubicin is often given by short intravenous infusion. The severity of nausea and vomiting and cardiotoxicity has been reported to be significantly reduced by using continuous intravenous infusions over 72 to 96 hours or by giving the drug in equally divided doses over several days.[93,94] In patients given doxorubicin by continuous intravenous infusion, cumulative doses as high as 1,000 mg/m$^2$ have been tolerated without major decreases in ejection fraction. The effectiveness of the drug is apparently not decreased with these different dosage schedules.

### Cyclophosphamide

Cyclophosphamide is probably the second most active agent in the treatment of breast cancer and is usually a part of cytotoxic combinations. The major toxic effect of this drug is myelosuppression but, unlike doxorubicin, it does not cause profound thrombocytopenia. A unique and potentially serious toxic effect of cyclophosphamide is hemorrhagic cystitis, which is probably mediated by toxic metabolites of the drug. Cyclophosphamide is often administered orally in breast cancer regimens. For example, some of the CMF regimens include oral cyclophosphamide at a dosage of 100 mg/m$^2$ for the first 14 days of the cycle. At these doses, the drug is well tolerated, although many patients experience nausea and vomiting. High fluid intake must be maintained to reduce the risk of hemorrhagic cystitis. Cyclophosphamide has also been used in high intravenous doses in metastatic breast cancer prior to autologous marrow transplant.[95] The procedure was usually well tolerated in these heavily pretreated patients. Although the response rate was higher than that observed with standard-dose therapy, most of the responses were partial and the duration of response was short.

### Other Agents

It was a logical step in early investigations of combination chemotherapy in the treatment of breast cancer to add two drugs with proven activity against adenocarcinomas of other organs. Methotrexate and 5-fluorouracil are two of these drugs. The usual dose of methotrexate is in the range of 30–40 mg/m$^2$ intravenously twice during the 28-day cycle. As with methotrexate, 5-fluorouracil is administered intravenously twice during the cycle at doses of 400–600 mg/m$^2$. These drugs are well tolerated and can be administered on an outpatient basis.

The use of vincristine has become less popular because of the significant neurotoxic effects produced when it is added to CMF regimens.[96]

### Combinations

The use of combination chemotherapy in the management of breast cancer was first reported in 1966 and was followed in 1969 by the description of the "Cooper regimen," which was a five-drug combination of cyclophosphamide, methotrexate, 5-fluorouracil, vincristine, prednisone (CMFVP) (Table 93.8).[97] Cooper et al reported an impressive 90% response rate in a group of 60 hormone-resistant patients with advanced breast cancer. Although these results could not be confirmed by other studies, an analysis of 11 clinical trials involving 529 patients treated with the same five drugs shows that the regimen is active, with a cumulative response rate of 47%.[98]

Many trials have been conducted to delineate which of the five chemotherapeutic agents in the "Cooper regimen" could be eliminated or substituted and still achieve objective remission in at least 50% of patients with advanced disease. Nonrandomized studies and one randomized study have shown that three- and four-drug regimens are equivalent to Cooper's five-drug regimen.[98–101] In the randomized study, the response rate of the CMF regimen was found to be comparable to that of the CMFVP regimen.[102] Another study found that the addition of vincristine to cyclophosphamide, 5-fluorouracil, and prednisone (CFP) did not increase the response rate and resulted only in greater neurotoxicity.[103]

The efficacy of doxorubicin as a single agent has led to its inclusion in many combination regimens. Results from nonrandomized and randomized studies have shown that doxorubicin-containing regimens have response rates equal to or higher than those achieved with non–doxorubicin-containing regimens.[74] As discussed earlier, however, doxorubicin-containing regimens do not prolong the duration of survival and are associated with more drug-related toxic effects. Although most doxorubicin-containing combination regimens include at least three drugs (i.e., CAF), the contribution of a third or fourth drug to the combination of cyclophosphamide and doxorubicin is probably minimal.

The importance of chemotherapy dose in the treatment of breast cancer is not clear. In one randomized study, patients who received high-dose 5-fluorouracil, doxorubicin, and cyclophosphamide (FAC) entered into response more rapidly than those treated with low-dose FAC[104]; however, the eventual response rate, duration of response, and survival were similar for both groups. Furthermore, patients treated with low-dose CMF have similar duration of response and survival as those treated with standard-dose CMF.[101] Until newer high-dose combination regimens are shown to prolong survival, these data suggest that standard-dose combination chemotherapy should be given to most patients.

As the duration of response is usually short, lasting only 6 to 12 months, some investigators have studied the benefit of sequentially giving non–cross-resistant combination chemotherapy.[105] The rationale for this approach is to delay or prevent the emergence of resistant cells by the use of non–cross-resistant chemotherapeutic drugs. Although this approach is theoretically attractive, no significant improvement in duration of response and survival has been observed in patients treated with alternating non–cross-resistant regimens compared with those continued on the same initial regimen. This type of approach, however, may be beneficial in patients who experience severe drug-related toxic effects from a specific combination regimen.

Nearly all patients experience tumor recurrence after first-line combination chemotherapy; many of these patients require second-line chemotherapy. If doxorubicin has not been previously given, many patients will respond to single-agent doxorubicin.[106] Another novel approach is high-dose therapy with autologous or allogeneic marrow rescue. In most of these studies, high-dose therapy with cyclophosphamide, amsacrine, L-PAM, mitomycin C, cisplatin, or BCNU, either alone or in combination, was given.[73] Although the toxicity of this approach can be severe, some complete and partial responses have been noted. Finally, some investigators have studied the efficacy and toxicity of active single agents given by continuous intravenous infusion. This approach is attractive because if a drug was found to be more active or less toxic when given by continuous intravenous infusion, then it could be incorporated into combination regimens. Drugs that have been studied include doxorubicin, vinblastine, and mitomycin C. Preliminary results of these studies show encouraging antitumor activity with vinblastine and less cardiotoxicity with doxorubicin.[92,107]

In summary, although combination chemotherapy can induce an objective response in 50% to 80% of patients, most responses are partial and the duration of response is usually 6 to 12 months. Predictors for response are not well identified. There is some conflicting evidence that patients with ER− tumors are more likely to respond to chemotherapy than those with ER+ tumors. In advanced breast cancer, there is no correlation between age, menopausal status, size of the primary tumor, or extent of axillary node involvement and the likelihood of response to chemotherapy. Thus far, attempts to improve the duration of response or survival have not been successful.

## Summary

Although the age-adjusted mortality from breast cancer has not changed from 1950 to 1982, there have been recent gains in disease-free survival and quality of life, primarily because of increasing acceptance of adjuvant chemotherapy or chemohormonal therapy.

The role of surgery in the treatment of breast cancer has changed. Early treatment of breast cancer consisted of radical mastectomy, which involved removal of the breast, the underlying muscles, and the axillary lymph nodes. In the midseventies, it was observed that at the time of diagnosis, most patients already had involvement of axillary nodes and that most of these patients would develop distant metastases and die of their disease. As a result, it is now generally accepted that the goal of local therapies, such as surgery and irradiation, is removal of the primary tumor and inhibition of local recurrence. More conservative methods of surgery (partial mastectomy) are now preferred over radical mastectomy, which has lifted some of the psychologic burden of breast cancer.

A number of prognostic factors affect outcome of patients with breast cancer, but the two that have had a significant impact on therapy are axillary node status and ER status. The observation that most patients with positive axillary nodes develop distant metastases led to two randomized studies of cytotoxic chemotherapy in these high-risk patients. In both studies, chemotherapy was started shortly after surgery and given for 1 to 2 years ("adjuvant chemotherapy"). Although the two studies differed in their choice of chemotherapeutic regimen (L-PAM versus CMF), the results were remarkably similar. After 10 years of follow-up, both studies showed improved disease-free and overall survival in patients receiving adjuvant chemotherapy. Further analysis showed that the survival benefit was restricted primarily to premenopausal patients. It is not clear why postmenopausal patients have a poorer response to adjuvant chemotherapy.

The use of ER status and, more recently, PR status has allowed oncologists to predict which patients with metastatic breast cancer are likely to respond to endocrine therapy. The predictive accuracy is quite good; patients with ER+/PR+ tumors have a 80% to 90% response rate while those with ER−/PR− tumors have a 5% to 10% response rate. Recent adjuvant therapy studies have used ER status to identify patients who may benefit from hormonal therapy (i.e., tamoxifen), either alone or with combination chemotherapy. Some of the early results of these adjuvant studies are encouraging.

Recognition of the importance of axillary node status and ER status has changed the treatment of breast cancer. Adjuvant chemotherapy is now standard therapy for premenopausal patients with positive axillary nodes. Adjuvant chemotherapy in postmenopausal patients and those without positive nodes is an area of active clinical research but should not be considered as standard therapy. Similarly, the use of chemohormonal therapy in patients with ER+ tumors should also be considered investigational.

After patients have experienced tumor recurrence, the type of further therapy depends on ER status. Patients with ER+ tumors are treated with either oophorectomy or tamoxifen, depending on their menopausal status. Major second-line endocrine therapies include adrenalectomy, hypophysectomy, high-dose estrogens, progestins, and aminoglutethimide. Responses with all of the endocrine therapies are usually short, lasting 9 to 18 months. Patients with ER− tumors or those with rapidly progressive ER+ tumors are treated with combination chemotherapy. The optimal combination regimen for metastatic breast cancer is not known; two common regimens are CMF and CAF. Although the response rates with these combination regimens are 50% to 80%, most responses are partial and the duration of response is generally less than 1 year. Patients who fail first- and second-line chemotherapy are often treated with experimental protocols of new cytotoxic agents or immunotherapy.

The demonstration that adjuvant chemotherapy or chemohormonal therapy can increase disease-free and overall survival in certain subgroups of patients provides reason for cautious optimism. It is possible that 10 years from now, a decrease in age-adjusted mortality will be demonstrated for breast cancer. As treatment of breast cancer continues to evolve, it is important for clinicans in oncology to carefully weigh the benefits and risks of a given treatment.

## References


1. Silverberg E. Cancer statistics, 1987. CA 1986;36:9–25.
2. Bailar JC, Smith EM. Progress against cancer? N Engl J Med 1986;314:1226–1232.
3. Waterhouse J, et al (eds): Cancer Incidence in Five Continents. Lyon, IARC Scientific Publications, vol III, no 15, 1976.
4. Wynder EL. Dietary factors related to breast cancer. Cancer 1980;46:899–904.
5. Hirohara T, Nomura AM, Hankin JH, et al. An epidemiologic study on the association between diet and breast cancer. J Natl Cancer Inst 1987;78:595–600.
6. Willett WC, Stamper MJ, Golditt GA, et al. Dietary fat and the risk of breast cancer. N Engl J Med 1987;316:22–28.
7. Santen RJ. Determinants of tissue oestradiol levels in human breast cancer. Cancer Surveys 1986;5:597–616.
8. Moore JW, Thomas BS, Wang DY. Endocrine status and the epidemiology and clinical course of breast cancer. Cancer Surveys 1986;5:537–549.
9. Vihko RK, Apter DL. The epidemiology and endocrinology of menarche in relation to breast cancer. Cancer Surveys 1986;5: 561–571.
10. Trichopoulos D, MacMahon B, Cole P. Menopause and breast cancer risk. J Natl Cancer Inst 1968;41:315–329.
11. Anderson DE. A genetic study of human breast cancer. J Natl Cancer Inst 1972;48:1069.
12. Wingo PA, Layde PM, Lee NC, et al. The risk of breast cancer in postmenopausal women who have used estrogen replacement therapy. JAMA 1987;257:209–215.
13. Cancer and Steroid Hormone Study of CDC and NICH. Oral contraceptive use and risk of breast cancer. N Engl J Med 1986;315:405–411.
14. Meirik O, Lund E, Adami HO, et al. Oral contraceptive use and breast cancer in young women. Lancet 1986;2:650–654.
15. Coombs J, Lilienfeld AM, Bross ID, et al. A prospective study of the relationship between benign breast diseases and breast carcinoma. Prev Med 1979;8:40.
16. Baker LH. The Breast Cancer Detection Demonstration Project: Five year summary report. CA 1982;32:194–230.
17. IARC Working Group on the Evaluation of the Carcinogenic Risk of Chemical to Humans: Tobacco Smoking. Epidemiology studies of cancer in humans. IARC Monographs 1986;38: 294–297.
18. Willett WC, Stamper MJ, Colditz GA, et al. Moderate alcohol consumption and the risk of breast cancer. N Engl J Med 1987; 316:1174–1180.
19. Tabar L, Gad A, Holmberg LH, et al. Reduction in mortality from breast cancer after mass screening with mammography. Lancet 1985;1:829–832.
20. Delregato JA, Spjut HJ. Cancer: Diagnosis, Treatment and Prognosis, 5th ed. St. Louis, C.V. Mosby, 1977.
21. Leis HP. The diagnosis of breast cancer. CA 1977;27:209.
22. Stark P. Evaluation of screening programs for the early diagnosis of breast cancer. Surg Clin North Am 1978;58:667–679.
23. Chin TD, Wagner KV. Progress in screening for early breast cancer. J Surg Oncol 1985;30:96–102.
24. Newsome JF, McLelland R. A word of caution concerning mammography. JAMA 1986;255:528.
25. Peters PN. Screening for breast cancer. What, when, how? Cancer Bull 1986;38:170–175.
26. Mushlin AI. Diagnostic tests in breast cancer. Ann Intern Med 1985;103:79–85.
27. McGuire WL. Prognostic factors in primary breast cancer. CA 1986;5:527–536.
28. Bonadonna G, Valagussa P. Current status of adjuvant chemotherapy for breast cancer. Semin Oncol 1987;14:8–22.
29. Fisher B, Slack N, Katrych D, et al. Ten year follow-up results of patients with carcinoma of the breast in a cooperative clinical trial evaluating surgical adjuvant chemotherapy. Surg Gynecol Obstet 1975;140:528.
30. Fisher B, Bauer M, Wickerham L, et al. Relation of number of positive axillary nodes to prognosis of patients with primary breast cancer. Cancer 1983;52:1551–1557.
31. Feldman JG, Carter AC, Nicastri AD, et al. Breast self-examination: Relationship to stage of breast cancer at diagnosis. Cancer 1981;47:2740–2745.
32. Clark GM, McGuire WL, Hubay CA, et al. Progesterone receptors as a prognostic factor in stage II breast cancer. N Engl J Med 1983;309:1343–1346.
33. Hans-Olov A, Malker B, Holmberg L, et al. The relation between survival and age at diagnosis in breast cancer. N Engl J Med 1986;315:559–563.
34. Rich MA, Furmanski P, Brooks SC, et al. Prognostic value to estrogen receptor determinants in patients with breast cancer. Cancer Res 1978;38:4296–4298.
35. Kiang DT, Kennedy BJ. Factors affecting estrogen receptors in breast cancer. Cancer 1977;40:1571–1576.

36. Allegra JC, Lippman ME, Thompson ED, et al. Distribution, frequency, and quantitative analysis of estrogen, progesterone, androgens, and glucocorticoid receptors in human breast cancer. Cancer Res 1979;39:1447–1454.
37. Furmanski P, Saunders DE, Brooks SC, et al. The prognostic value of estrogen receptor determinants in patients with primary breast cancer. Cancer 1980;46:2794–2796.
38. Allegra JC, Lippman ME, Simon R, et al. Association between steroid hormone receptor status and disease-free interval in breast cancer. Cancer Treat Rep 1979;63:1271–1277.
39. Knight MA, Livingston RB, Gregory EJ, et al. Estrogen receptor as an independent prognostic factor for early recurrence in breast cancer. Cancer Res 1977;37:4669–4671.
40. Allegra JC, Lippman ME, Thompson EB, et al. Estrogen receptor status: An important variable in predicting response to endocrine therapy in metastatic breast cancer. Eur J Cancer 1980;16:323–332.
41. Byer DP, Sears ME, McGuire WL, et al. Relationship between estrogen receptor values and clinical data in predicting the response to endocrine therapy for patients with advanced breast cancer. Eur J Cancer 1979;15:299.
42. Lippman ME, Allegra JC. Quantitative estrogen receptor analysis: The response to endocrine and cytotoxic chemotherapy in human breast cancer and the disease-free interval. Cancer 1980;46:2829–2834.
43. Deganshein GA, Bloom M, Tobin E. The value of progesterone receptor assays in the management of advanced breast cancer. Cancer 1980;46:2789–2793.
44. Lippman ME, Allegra JC, Thompson EB, et al. The relation between estrogen receptors and response rates to cytotoxic chemotherapy in metastatic breast cancer. N Engl J Med 1978;298:1223–1228.
45. Walmark N, Fisher B. Adjuvant therapy in primary breast cancer. Surg Clin North Am 1985;65:161–180.
46. Robinson JO. Treatment of breast cancer through the ages. Am J Surg 1986;151:317–333.
47. Fisher B, Redmond C, Wolmark N, et al. Disease free survival at intervals during and following completion of adjuvant chemotherapy: The NSABP experiences from 3 breast protocols. Cancer 1981;48:1273–1280.
48. Sheckney SE, McCormack GW, Cuchural GJ. Growth rate patterns of solid tumors and their relation to responsiveness to therapy. Ann Intern Med 1978;89:107–121.
49. Bluming AZ. Treatment of primary breast cancer without mastectomy. Am J Med 1982;72:820–828.
50. Fisher B, Redmond C, Fisher ER, et al. Ten-year results of a randomized clinical trial comparing radical mastectomy and total mastectomy with or without radiation. N Engl J Med 1985;312:674–681.
51. Fisher B, Bauer M, Margolese R, et al. Five-year results of a randomized clinical trial comparing total mastectomy and segmental mastectomy with or without radiation in the treatment of breast cancer. N Engl J Med 1985;312:666–672.
52. Fletcher GH. Local results of irradiation in the primary management of localized breast cancer. Cancer 1972;29:545–552.
53. Weichselbaum RR, March A, Hellman S. The role of postoperative irradiation in carcinoma of the breast. Cancer 1976; 37:2682–2690.
54. Harris JR, Hellman S, Kinne DW. Limited surgery and radiotherapy for early breast cancer. N Engl J Med 1985;313:1365–1368.
55. Ragaz J. Emerging modalities for adjuvant therapy of breast cancer: Neoadjuvant chemotherapy. NCI Monographs 1986;1: 145–152.
56. Goldie JH. Scientific basis for adjuvant and primary (neoadjuvant) chemotherapy. Semin Oncol 1987;14:1–7.
57. Harris JR, Hellman S, Canellos GP, et al. Cancer of the breast, in Devita VR (ed): Cancer Principles and Practice of Oncology. Philadelphia, J.B. Lippincott, 1985, pp 1119–1177.
58. Henderson CI. Adjuvant systemic therapy for early breast cancer. Curr Probl Cancer 1987;11:129–207.
59. Fisher B, Rockette H, Fisher ER, et al. Leukemia in breast cancer patients following adjuvant chemotherapy or postoperative radiation: The NSABP experience. J Clin Oncol 1985;3:1640–1658.
60. Fisher B, Fisher ER, Redmond C, et al. Ten-year results from the NSABP clinical trials evaluating the use of L-phenylalanine mustard (L-PAM) in the management of primary breast cancer. J Clin Oncol 1986;4:929–941.
61. Bonadonna G, Valagussa P, Rossi A, et al. Ten-year experience with CMF based adjuvant chemotherapy in resectable breast cancer. Breast Cancer Res Treat 1985;5:95–115.
62. Osborne CK, Rivkin SE, McDivitt RW, et al. Adjuvant therapy of breast cancer: Southwest Oncology Group Studies. NCI Monographs 1986;1:71–76.
63. Lippman ME, Edwards BK, Findlay P, et al. Influence of definitive radiation therapy for primary breast cancer on ability to deliver adjuvant chemotherapy. NCI Monographs 1986;1: 99–104.
64. Fisher B, Redmond C, Brown A, et al. Adjuvant chemotherapy with and without tamoxifen in the treatment of primary breast cancer: 5 year results from the National Surgical Adjuvant Breast and Bowel Project Trial. J Clin Oncol 1986;4:459–471.
65. Ludwig Breast Cancer Study Group. Chemotherapy with or without oophorectomy in high risk premenopausal patients with operable breast cancer. J Clin Oncol 1985;3:1059–1067.
66. Lippman ME. The NIH Consensus Development Conference on adjuvant chemotherapy for breast cancer—A commentary. Breast Cancer Res Treat 1985;6:195–200.
67. Bonadonna G, Valagussa P, Tancini G, et al. Current status of Milan adjuvant chemotherapy trials for node-positive and node-negative breast cancer. NCI Monographs 1986;3:35–38.
68. Padmanabhan N, Howell A, Rubens RD. Mechanism of action of adjuvant chemotherapy in early breast cancer. Lancet 1986; 2:411–414.
69. Baum M. Nolvadex Adjuvant Trial Organization: Controlled trial of tamoxifen as single adjuvant agent in management of early breast cancer; analysis at 6 years. Lancet 1985;1:836–839.
70. Delozier T, Julien J, Juret P, et al. Adjuvant tamoxifen in postmenopausal breast cancer: Preliminary results of a randomized trial. Breast Cancer Res Treat 1986;7:105–110.
71. Hug BV, Hortobagyi GN, Drewinko B, et al. Tamoxifen citrate counteracts the antitumor effects of cytotoxic drugs in vitro. J Clin Oncol 1985;3:1672–1677.
72. Taylor SG, Kalish LA, Olson JE, et al. Adjuvant CMFP versus CMFP plus tamoxifen versus observation alone in postmenopausal node positive breast cancer patients: 3 year results of an ECOG study. J Clin Oncol 1985;3:144–154.
73. Henderson CI, Hayes DF, Cone S, et al. New agents and new medical treatments for advanced breast cancer. Semin Oncol 1987;14:34–64.
74. Paridaens RJ. Salvage therapy in advanced breast cancer. Eur J Cancer Clin Oncol 1985;21:1443–1447.
75. Newsome HH, Brown PW, Terz JJ, et al. Medical and surgical adrenalectomy in patients with advanced breast cancinoma. Cancer 1977;39:542–546.
76. Fracchia AA, Farrow JH, Miller TR, et al. Hypophysectomy as compared with adrenalectomy in the treatment of advanced carcinoma of the breast. Surg Gynecol Obstet 1971;133:241.

77. Kiang DT, Kennedy BJ. Tamoxifen (antiestrogen) therapy in advanced breast cancer. Ann Intern Med 1977;87:687–690.
78. Ward HW. Antiestrogen therapy for breast cancer—a trial of tamoxifen at 2 dose levels. Br Med J 1973;1:13–14.
79. Plotkin D, Lechner JJ, June WE, et al. Tamoxifen flare in advanced breast cancer. JAMA 1978;240:2644–2646.
80. Santen RJ, Santner S, Davis B, et al. Aminoglutethemide inhibits extraglandular estrogen production in postmenopausal women with breast carcinoma. J Clin Endocrinol Metab 1978; 47:1257–1265.
81. Smith IE, Fitzharris BM, McKinna JA, et al. Aminoglutethemide in treatment in metastatic breast cancer. Lancet 1978;2: 646–649.
82. Murray R, Pitt P. Low-dose aminoglutethemide without steroid replacement in the treatment of postmenopausal women with advanced breast cancer. Eur J Cancer Clin Oncol 1985;21:19–22.
83. Carter AC, Sedransk N, Kelley RM, et al. Diethylstilbestrol: Recommended dosages for different categories of breast cancer patients. JAMA 1977;237:2079–2083.
84. Buzdar AU, Hortobagyi GN, Marcus CE, et al. Evaluation of trilostane in treatment of metastatic breast cancer—a phase II study. (Abstr) Proc Assoc Can Res 1986;27:218.
85. Haller DG, Glick JH. Progestational agents in advanced breast cancer—an overview. Semin Oncol 1986;13:2–8.
86. Tchekmedgian SN, Tait N, Aisner J. High-dose megesterol acetate in the treatment of postmenopausal women with advanced breast cancer. Semin Oncol 1986;13:20–25.
87. Canalli F, Goldhirsch A, Surgi F. Randomized trial of low versus high-dose medroxyprogesterone acetate in the induction treatment of postmenopausal patients with advanced breast cancer. J Clin Oncol 1984;2:414–419.
88. Mattsson W. Current status of high dose progestin treatment in advanced breast cancer. Breast Cancer Res Treat 1983;3:231–235.
89. Harvey HA, Lipton A, Max DT, et al. Medical castration produced by GNRH analogue leuprolide to treat metastatic breast cancer. J Clin Oncol 1985;3:1068–1072.
90. Kiljn JG, DeJong FH. Treatment with a luteinising hormone releasing hormone analogue. Lancet 1982;1:1213–1216.
91. Bull JM, Tormey DC, Li SH, et al. A randomized comparative trial of adriamycin versus methotrexate in combination drug therapy. Cancer 1978;41:1649.
92. Steward DJ, Maroun JA, Hirte W, et al. A randomized comparison of cyclophosphamide–mitoxantrone–5-fluorouracil vs. cyclosphosphamide–doxorubicin–5-fluorouracil in advanced breast cancer. Preliminary observations. Semin Oncol 1984;11:23–27.
93. Legha SS, Benjamin RS, Mackay B, et al. Adriamycin therapy by continuous intravenous infusion in patients with metastatic breast cancer. Cancer 1982;49:1762–1766.
94. Weiss A, Manthel RW. Experience with the use of adriamycin in combination with other anticancer agents using a weekly schedule with particular reference to lack of cardiac toxicity. Cancer 1977;40:2046–2052.
95. Stewart PS. Autologous bone marrow transplantation in metastatic breast cancer. Breast Cancer Res Treat 1982;2:85–92.
96. Hopkins JO, Jackson DV, White DR, et al. Vincristine by continuous infusion in refractory breast cancer: A phase II study. Am J Clin Oncol 1983;6:529–532.
97. Cooper RG. Combination chemotherapy in hormone resistant breast cancer. Proc Am Assoc Cancer Res 1969;10:15.
98. Henderson IC. Chemotherapy for advanced disease, in Bonadonna G (ed): Breast Cancer: Diagnosis and Management. New York, John Wiley, 1984, pp 247–280.
99. Carbone PP, Bauer M, Band P, et al. Chemotherapy of disseminated breast cancer. Cancer 1977;39:2916–2922.
100. Canellos GP, Devita VT, Gold GL, et al. Combination chemotherapy for advanced breast cancer: Response and effect on survival. Ann Intern Med 1976;84:389–392.
101. Creech RH, Catalano RB, Mastrangelo MJ, et al. An effective low-dose intermittent cyclophosphamide, methotrexate, and 5-fluorouracil treatment regimen for metastatic breast cancer. Cancer 1975;35:1101.
102. Muss HB, White DR, Cooper MA, et al. Combination chemotherapy in advanced breast cancer. Arch Intern Med 1977;137: 1711–1714.
103. Ahmann DL, Bisel HF, Hahn RG, et al. An analysis of a multiple-drug program in the treatment of patients with advanced breast cancer utilizing 5-fluorouracil, cyclophosphamide, and prednisone with or without vincristine. Cancer 1975;36:1925.
104. Malik R, Blumenschein GR, Legha SS, et al. A randomized trial of high dose 5-fluorouracil, doxorubicin, and cyclophosphamide versus conventional FAC regimens in metastatic breast cancer. Proc Am Soc Clin Oncol 1982;1:79.
105. Vogel CL, Smalley RV, Raney M, et al. Randomized trial of cylophosphamide, doxorubicin, and 5-fluorouracil alone or alternating with a "cycle active" non–cross-resistant combination in women with visceral metastatic breast cancer. J Clin Oncol 1984;2:1260–1265.
106. Nemoto T, Rosner D, Diaz R, et al. Combination chemotherapy for metastatic breast cancer. Cancer 1978;41:2073–2077.
107. Franschini G, Yap HY, Hortobagyi GN, et al. Five-day continuous infusion vinblastine in the treatment of breast cancer. Cancer 1985;56:225–229.

# Chapter 94 / Lung Cancer

Rebecca S. Finley, PharmD, MS

Lung cancer is a significant cause of morbidity and mortality that has reached epidemic proportions in many industrialized countries. The American Cancer Society estimated that 150,000 new cases of lung cancer were diagnosed in the United States during 1987 and 136,000 deaths were attributed to this disease during the same year.[1] Despite major advances in the understanding and management of the disease, the overall 5-year survival rate for all types of lung cancer remains 13%.[1]

Lung cancer accounts for 22% of all cancer in men and 10% of all cancer in women.[1] It is the leading cause of cancer death in men aged 35 years and older (accounting for 35% of all cancer deaths in men) and the leading cause of cancer death in women (20% of all cancer deaths)[2]. It is estimated that lung cancer now surpasses breast cancer as the primary cause of cancer death among American women.[2] The incidence of lung cancer increases with age; the average age of onset is about 60 years.[3] Among patients 40 years of age and older, the likelihood that a solitary pulmonary nodule seen on chest x-ray is a carcinoma is high and this probability increases proportionally with age.[4]

## Etiology

The natural history of lung cancer begins with exposure of a susceptible host to carcinogens that eventually leads to cytologic changes and progression to carcinoma.[5] Numerous studies have established the relationship between tobacco exposure and lung cancer. The American Cancer Society estimates that cigarette smoking is responsible for about 83% of all lung cancer cases.[1] The increased rate of lung cancer deaths among women has also been attributed to increased smoking.[1] Cessation of smoking is associated with a gradual decrease in the risk, but a long time (more than 6 years) is necessary before an appreciable diminution of the risk occurs.[6] Industrial or occupational exposure to asbestos,[7] chloromethyl ethers,[8] and various heavy metals[3] has also been associated with the development of lung cancer. In addition, the incidence of lung cancer is higher in urban than in rural areas and air pollution has been implicated as a possible causative agent.[9]

## Histologic Classification

In 1981 the World Health Organization published the currently accepted lung cancer classification (Table 94.1).[10] Four major cell type of carcinomas (i.e., squamous cell carcinoma, adenocarcinoma, and large and small cell carcinomas) account for more than 90% of all lung tumors.[11] Histologic confirmation of cell type is usually made by light microscopy and is essential in treatment planning because of differences in the natural histories, clinical features, and response to therapy of the various types. In terms of management strategy and overall prognosis, adenocarcinoma and squamous cell and large cell carcinomas are frequently grouped together and referred to as non–small cell lung cancers.

Squamous cell (or epidermoid) carcinoma is the most common type of lung cancer, accounting for 30% to 35% of all lung cancers,[12] and is distinguished histologically by evidence of squamous differentiation.[11] This tumor tends to be central in origin, arising from metaplastic bronchial epithelium, and frequently extends into the bronchial lumen resulting in obstruction.[12] Squamous cell carcinomas (along with small cell lung cancers) have a much higher incidence among smokers.[13] Many squamous cell carcinomas are confined to the lungs (especially early in the disease course); however, such tumors may metastasize to the hilar and mediastinal lymph nodes, liver, adrenal glands, kidneys, bone, and gastrointestinal tract.[11]

Adenocarcinomas are usually located in the peripheral sections of the lung and are distinguished pathologically by a glandular or papillary pattern.[11] These tumors account for 25% to 29% of all lung cancers.[12] Adenocarcinomas are likely to metastasize at an early stage and spread widely to distant sites including the contralateral lung, liver, bone, adrenal glands, kidneys, and central nervous system.[11]

Large cell carcinomas are anaplastic tumors that show no evidence of differentiation.[11] These tumors account for 14% to 19% of all lung cancers.[12] The large cell carcinomas tend to be large and bulky tumors arising in the periphery of the lung and to have a propensity to metastasize in a pattern quite similar to that of adenocarcinomas.[11]

Small cell carcinomas account for about 25% of all lung tumors[12] and are distinguished by a proliferation of neoplastic cells with round to oval nucleii.[11] These tumors tend to arise in the central portion of the lung but may also be found in the lung periphery. Small cell lung carcinoma is a very aggressive and rapidly growing tumor, with about 70% of patients initally presenting with disseminated disease.[14] This disease has a propensity to metastasize to the lymph nodes, opposite lung, liver, adrenal glands, bone, bone marrow, and central nervous system.[11]

## Clinical Presentation

Location and extent of the tumor determine the presenting signs and symptoms. The most common initial signs and symptoms include cough, dyspnea, chest pain, sputum pro-

**Table 94.1** World Health Organization's Classification of Lung Cancer

| | | | |
|---|---|---|---|
| I. | Epidermoid carcinoma (squamous cell) | VII. | Bronchial gland tumors |
| II. | Small cell carcinoma | VIII. | Papillary tumors of the surface epithelium |
| III. | Adenocarcinoma | IX. | "Mixed" tumors and carcinosarcomas |
| IV. | Large cell carcinoma | X. | Sarcomas |
| V. | Combined epidermoid and adenocarcinomas | XI. | Unclassified tumors |
| VI. | Carcinoid tumors | XII. | Melanoma |

From Sobin LH: The World Health Organization's Histological Classification of Lung Tumors: A comparison of the first and second editions. Cancer Detect Prev 1982;5:392–393, with permission.

duction, and hemoptysis.[15] Unfortunately, many patients with lung cancer also have chronic pulmonary and/or cardiovascular diseases (usually related to smoking) and such symptoms may go unnoticed or be attributed to the concomitant disease. Many patients also exhibit systemic symptoms such as anorexia, weight loss and fatigue that are suggestive of a malignancy.[5] Other signs and symptoms that may be associated with the primary tumor or its spread within the thorax are listed in Table 94.2. Such symptomatology may occur at the tumor's initial presentation or at any point during its recurrence or progression.

Disseminated disease may also be responsible for extrapulmonary signs and symptoms such as neurologic deficits resulting from central nervous system metastases, bone pain or pathologic fractures secondary to bone metastases, or liver dysfunction resulting from tumor involvement in the liver.

Paraneoplastic syndromes are signs and symptoms that occur at sites away from the primary tumor or its metastases and are not associated with "direct" tumor involvement. These syndromes may be the first sign of a tumor and may prompt the search for an underlying malignancy. Paraneoplastic syndromes that commonly occur in association with lung cancers include cachexia, hypercalcemia, syndrome of inappropriate hormone secretion, and Cushing's syndrome.[5]

**Table 94.2** Common Signs and Symptoms of Lung Cancer

| |
|---|
| Local signs and symptoms associated with primary tumor |
| Cough |
| Hemoptysis |
| Dyspnea |
| Rust-streaked or purulent sputum |
| Chest, shoulder, or arm pain |
| Superior vena caval obstruction |
| Pleural effusion or pneumonitis |
| Dysphagia (secondary to esophageal compression) |
| Hoarseness (secondary to laryngeal nerve paralysis) |
| Extrapulmonary signs and symptoms associated with metastatic involvement |
| Bone pain and/or pathologic fractures |
| Liver dysfunction |
| Neurologic deficits |
| Spinal cord compression |
| Paraneoplastic syndromes |
| Weight loss |
| Cushing's syndrome |
| Hypercalcemia |
| Syndrome of inappropriate antidiuretic hormone (SIADH) |
| Pulmonary hypertrophic osteoarthropathy |
| Anemia |
| Eaton–Lambert syndrome |

## Diagnosis

Once signs and symptoms of lung cancer have been recognized, chest x-rays are the most valuable diagnostic test. When there is radiologic evidence of a tumor, pathologic confirmation must be established. This may be accomplished by examination of sputum cytology and/or tumor biopsy by fiber-optic bronchoscopy, percutaneous needle biopsy, or open-lung biopsy. All patients must also have a thorough history and physical examination with emphasis on detecting signs and symptoms of the primary tumor, regional spread of the tumor, distant metastases, and paraneoplastic syndromes.

Unfortunately, by the time the tumor is diagnosed, dissemination has already occurred in many patients. Determination of the extent (or stage) of tumor involvement is important because it will aid in the selection of treatment, estimate the probability of cure and survival, and facilitate comparison of the individual patient with large-scale clinical trials.

## Staging

### *Non–Small Cell Lung Cancer*

The American Joint Committee[16] has established a TNM staging classification for lung cancer based on primary tumor size and extent (T), regional lymph node involvement (N), and presence or absence of distant metastases (M). Table 94.3 outlines this staging system. For comparison of various therapeutic modalities, a more simple stage grouping system is also used in which stage I refers to tumors confined to the lung without lymphatic spread, stage II refers to large tumors with peribronchial or hilar lymph node involvement, and stage III includes all advanced cancers.[16]

The primary tumor is assessed using chest x-rays and fiber-optic bronchoscopy while lymphatic spread is usually assessed by mediastinoscopy, gallium-67 citrate scanning, or computerized tomography (CT).[5] At the time of diagnosis, distant metastases are found in less than 15% of patients with

**Table 94.3** Tumor (T), Node (N), Metastasis (M) Staging for Lung Cancer

| | |
|---|---|
| $T_1$ | 3 cm with no invasion |
| $T_2$ | 3 cm/extension to hilar region |
| $T_3$ | Gross extension/effusion/atelectasis |
| $N_0$ | No lymph node involvement |
| $N_1$ | Hilar lymph node involvement |
| $N_2$ | Mediastinal lymph node involvement |
| $M_0$ | No distant metastases |
| $M_1$ | Distant metastases present |
| **Stage Groupings** | |
| Stage I | $T_1$, $N_0$, $M_0$ |
| | $T_1$, $N_1$, $M_0$ |
| | $T_2$, $N_0$, $M_0$ |
| Stage II | $T_2$, $N_1$, $M_0$ |
| Stage III | $T_3$, Any N, Any M |
| | Any T, $N_2$, Any M |
| | Any T, Any N, $M_1$ |

From American Joint Committee for Cancer Staging and End-Results Reporting Task Force on Lung: Staging of Lung Cancer. Philadelphia, JB Lippincott, 1983, pp 100–101, with permission.

non–small cell lung cancer.[5,17] Therefore, it is recommended that special scans (e.g., bone, brain, or liver) or biopsies (e.g., bone marrow or liver) be carried out only if the physical examination or other clinical evidence suggests the possibility of metastatic disease.[5]

### *Small Cell Lung Cancer*

A two-stage classification established by the Veterans Administration Lung Cancer Study Group is currently widely used in the United States to stage small cell lung cancer (SCLC).[18] Limited disease is classified as disease confined to one hemithorax and to the regional lymph nodes. All other disease is classified as extensive. Approximately 70% of patients initially present with extensive disease. Because of this high frequency of disseminated disease at diagnosis (bone 38%, liver 22%–28%, bone marrow 17%–23%, CNS 8%–14%), radionuclide scans of the bone and liver, CT scans of the brain, and bone marrow biopsies are generally recommended prior to initiation of therapy.In addition any suspicious signs or symptoms detected during the physical examination should be carefully investigated.

## Treatment

### *Non–Small Cell Lung Cancer*

Currently, only surgery (and, to a lesser extent, radiation therapy) offers an opportunity for long-term survival in a significant percentage of patients; however, only about 15% of unselected patients have localized disease that is amenable to local therapy.[2,21] Curative therapy in this disease is determined by the anatomic stage of the disease (it must be localized with no evidence of distant metastases) and the ability of the patient to withstand the therapy. If untreated, most patients die within 1 year of diagnosis.[4]

#### Surgery

Surgical resection is the treatment of choice for patients with clinical stage I and II disease (disease that by all evidence is stage I or II before surgical dissection of mediastinal lymph nodes).[4] Overall, approximately 30% of all patients who are resected for cure survive 5 years.[5] The single most important prognostic factor in patients undergoing curative resection is the presence or absence of lymph node involvement. In one series of 216 patients who had clinical stage I disease before surgery only 125 patients were found to have stage I disease after surgery and lymph node dissection.[21] Therefore, it is apparent that mediastinal lymph node dissection at the time of surgery is of great importance. In patients with clinical stage I or II disease Paulson et al reported a 5-year survival rate of 46% in patients without lymph node involvement ($N_0$), 33% in patients with peribronchial or hilar nodal involvement ($N_1$), and only 8% in patients with mediastinal involvement ($N_2$).[22] Patients found to have mediastinal lymph node involvement at the time of surgery may benefit from postoperative radiation therapy.[4] Even if no residual disease is evident at surgery, 50% of patients die within 2 years as a result of recurrent disease.[5]

The size of the tumor in stage I and II disease also has prognostic importance[14] and patients with stage I disease tend to have a better overall survival than patients with stage II disease.[5] In patients with stage I disease, Martini et al reported a 5-year survival rate of 80% when the primary tumor was 3 cm but only 50% when the tumor was greater than 3 cm.[21]

#### Radiation

Radiation therapy is considered an alternative modality of therapy in patients with stage I or II disease who decline surgery or are considered high surgical risks because of concomitant illness or restrictive pulmonary reserve.[5] In addition, radiation therapy may also be utilized when the tumor is not resectable because of fixation to a major blood vessel, the trachea, or the esophagus. Local control of tumor growth may be achieved in up to 80% of patients with stage I or II disease; however, the overall 5-year survival is only about 6%.[5]

#### Chemotherapy

As many patients with non–small cell lung cancer (NSCLC) are inoperable at diagnosis, and as systemic dissemination occurs in the majority of patients who are surgically resected or radiated for potential cure, there is a definite need for effective systemic therapy (i.e., chemotherapy) in this disease. Unfortunately, the response rates for chemotherapy in NSCLC have been disappointingly low and overall survival benefits have not been clearly demonstrated; however, it does appear that patients who respond to chemotherapy are likely to have a survival benefit over nonresponders.[24,25] In addition, several factors have been suggested as having prognostic importance in terms of response and survival in patients receiving chemotherapy. These factors include the patient's initial performance status, weight loss, and extent of disease.[23,26] Among these factors, an initial favorable performance status of the patient appears to be the most consistent factor predicting a better response and improved survival.[23]

Direct comparison of response rates between clinical trials is difficult and interpretation of the results requires careful analysis of the methodology. Two factors that must be considered are the method of patient selection and the criteria for response. As previously mentioned, several factors are believed to have prognostic significance and it is necessary to know the status of such factors (i.e., performance status, extent of disease) in the study population when comparing clinical trials. Likewise, it is important to know if patients with an unfavorable prognosis were excluded from the trial. In addition, to compare results of clinical trials it is imperative that both trials utilize the same response criteria. In most series a complete response is defined as the complete disappearance of all evidence of the tumor while a partial response is defined as a reduction in measurable tumor mass of greater than 50% lasting longer than 1 month. Because many lung tumors do not have definite margins to measure, the term "objective response" is used to describe disease where there has been a definite decrease in the size of the lesion without appearance of any new lesions.[5]

Single-agent chemotherapy has generally demonstrated objective response rates of 5% to 15% with no significant effect on overall survival.[24] When responses do occur after single-agent chemotherapy the duration of the response is usually quite brief (2–4 months) and complete responses are rare.[5] Among the most active single agents in NSCLC are cisplatin, doxorubicin, etoposide, and mitomycin.

Combination chemotherapy has been utilized in the management of NSCLC since the late 1960s and although response rates for combination therapy have generally been better than those for single-agent therapy, consistent improvement in overall survival rates has been more difficult to demonstrate. Therefore, the use of combination chemotherapy in advanced NSCLC remains controversial.

Early regimens utilized in NSCLC frequently incorporated such agents as cyclophosphamide, methotrexate, lomustine, vincristine, and bleomycin. Overall response rates for such regimens were in the range 5% to 59%, with median survivals similar to those for single-agent therapy[27–31]; however, the results of many of these trials are difficult to compare because of inconsistencies in the methods of evaluation.

After reports of significant activity as a single agent, doxorubicin was incorporated into many regimens. The regimens often combined doxorubicin with an alkylating agent (e.g., cyclophosphamide) and methotrexate. One of the most widely studied regimens was the "CAMP" regimen, which combined cyclophosphamide (C), doxorubicin (A), methotrexate (M), and procarbazine (P). Rates of response to the CAMP regimen reported by various investigators ranged from 17% to 44%[32–38] and responders to therapy have generally survived longer than nonresponders (approximately 12 months versus 2–4 months).[32,34,35] Examples of doxorubicin-containing regimens are listed in Table 94.4.

The introduction of cisplatin hailed another new generation of combination therapy in NSCLC. Cisplatin is a heavy compound that exerts its cytotoxic effects primarily by forming intrastrand DNA crosslinks.[63,64] The formation of crosslinks is a slow process that continues hours after drug exposure.[63] It appears that some cells are most sensitive to cisplatin when exposed during the $G_1$ phase of the cell cycle, possibly because of the delay in crosslink formation, which would then be maximal during the following S phase.[65] Twenty percent to 75% of administered drug is excreted in urine as the result of glomerular filtration of unbound platinum in the 24 hours after administration. The remainder is bound to tissues or plasma protein[66] and is excreted much more slowly.

The usual dose of cisplatin is 40 to 120 mg/m$^2$ per course of therapy depending on the frequency of cycles, the other agents in the combination, and the patient's renal function; however, dosages of up to 200 mg/m$^2$ have been advocated in some refractory tumors.[67]

Nephrotoxicity is the usual dose-limiting toxic effect of cisplatin. The primary pathologic finding is necrosis of the distal tubular epithelium and collecting ducts.[68] Without hydration, the incidence of nephrotoxicity reaches 30% in patients treated with 50–75 mg/m$^2$ per course.[69] Aggressive hydration and mannitol or furosemide diuresis have been advocated for the prevention of cisplatin nephrotoxicity.[70] Administration in hypertonic saline[67] and careful circadian timing of infusions have also been suggested to attenuate the nephrotoxic effects of cisplatin.[71]

Cisplatin is generally considered to be the most emetogenic cytotoxic agent. Indeed, this effect may represent the dose-limiting toxic effect in some patients. Division of the total dosage over 5 consecutive days (e.g., 20 mg/m$^2$ per day for 5 days) and combinations of high-dose antiemetic agents have been used to lessen cisplatin nausea and vomiting. Other toxic effects associated with cisplatin therapy include hypomagnesemia, progressive high-frequency hearing loss, distal sensory neuropathy, and hypersensitivity.[63]

Table 94.4 describes some of the cisplatin-containing regimens studied in NSCLC. Among the most studied combinations are the CAP regimen (cyclophosphamide [C] + doxorubicin [A] + cisplatin [P]) and various cisplatin–etoposide regimens. In general, response rates have been in the range 20% to 40%, with responders surviving longer than nonresponders and complete responses occurring only rarely.

Other active agents commonly included in NSCLC regimens include mitomycin, vindesine (an investigational vinca alkoloid), and vincristine. Table 94.4 describes some of these combinations; however, at the present time no single regimen is considered standard therapy for NSCLC. Because of the questionable benefits of chemotherapy in terms of overall survival advantage in NSCLC and the toxic effects associated with its use, it is common practice to reserve chemotherapy for patients with a good performance status and otherwise favorable prognosis. Patients with an unfavorable prognosis (weight loss, poor performance status) and/or significant concomitant diseases should be given supportive care and palliative radiation if necessary.

In patients receiving chemotherapy, a minimum of two courses of therapy are usually given before evaluating the patient for response. If no objective response is seen, the regimen should be discontinued. Patients responding to chemotherapy should continue therapy until disease progression has been documented.

**Table 94.4** Combination Chemotherapy in Non–Small Cell Lung Cancer

| *Combination* | *Dosage* | *Schedule* | *Overall response rate (%)* | *Reference* |
|---|---|---|---|---|
| CAMP | | | | |
| CTX[a] | 300 mg/m$^2$ IV days 1 and 8 | | | |
| ADR | 20 mg/m$^2$ IV days 1 and 8 | Repeat course every 4 wk | 17–44 | 32–37 |
| MTX | 15 mg/m$^2$ IV days 1 and 8 | | | |
| PRO | 100 mg/m$^2$ PO days 1–10 | | | |
| BACON | | | | |
| BLE | 30 units IV day 2 | | | |
| ADR | 40 mg/m$^2$ IV day 1 | | | |
| CCNU | 65 mg/m$^2$ PO day 1 | Repeat course every 4 wk | 21–42 | 39–40 |
| ONC | 0.75–1 mg IV day 2 | | | |
| $HN_2$ | 8 mg/m$^2$ IV day 1 | | | |
| MACC | | | | |
| MTX | 30–40 mg/m$^2$ IV day 1 | | | |
| ADR | 30–40 mg/m$^2$ IV day 1 | Repeat course every 3 wk | 12–44 | 41–43 |
| CTX | 400 mg/m$^2$ IV day 1 | | | |
| CCNU | 30 mg/m$^2$ PO day 1 | | | |
| CAP | | | | |
| CTX | 400 mg/m$^2$ IV day 1 | | | |
| ADR | 40 mg/m$^2$ IV day 1 | Repeat course every 4 wk | 6–39 | 44–51 |
| DDP | 40 mg/m$^2$ IV day 1 | | | |
| DDP/VP-16 | | | | |
| DDP | 60–100 mg/m$^2$ IV day 1 | | | |
| ETO | 80–120 mg/m$^2$ IV days 1–3 or 4, 6, and 8 | Repeat course every 3–4 wk | 19–38 | 52–55 |
| CAVP | | | | |
| CTX | 400 mg/m$^2$ IV day 3 | | | |
| ADR | 40 mg/m$^2$ IV day 2 | Repeat course every 4 wk | 46 | 56 |
| ETO | 50 mg/m$^2$ IV days 1–3 | | | |
| DDP | 20 mg/m$^2$ IV days 1–3 | | | |
| **or** | | | | |
| CTX | 800 mg/m$^2$ IV day 1 | | | |
| ADR | 45 mg/m$^2$ IV day 1 | Repeat course every 3 wk | 28 | 57 |
| ETO | 100 mg/m$^2$ IV days 1, 3, and 5 | | | |
| DDP | 40 mg/m$^2$ IV day 1 | | | |
| PEV | | | | |
| DDP | 60 mg/m$^2$ IV day 1 | | | |
| ETO | 120 mg/m$^2$ IV days 3, 5, and 7 | Repeat course every 3 wk | 40 | 58 |
| VCR | 1.5 mg/m$^2$ IV days 1 and 7 | | | |
| DDP/VIND | | | | |
| DDP | 120 mg/m$^2$ IV days 1 and 29 | Then repeat every 6 wk | 40 | 59 |
| VIN | 3 mg/m$^2$ IV every week × 6 wk | Then every 2 wk | | |
| **or** | | | | |
| DDP | 60 mg/m$^2$ IV days 1 and 29 | Then repeat every 6 wk | 46 | 59 |
| VIN | 3 mg/m$^2$ IV every week × 6 wk | Then every 2 wk | | |
| MVP | | | | |
| MIT | 10 mg/m$^2$ day 1 | | | |
| VIN | 6 mg/m$^2$ day 1 | Repeat course every 3 wk | 53 | 60–61 |
| DDP | 40 mg/m$^2$ day 1 | | | |
| MV | | | | |
| MIT | 15–20 mg/m$^2$ day 1 | Every 6 wk | 36 | 62 |
| VIN | 3 mg/m$^2$ every week × 6 wk | Then every 2 wk | | |

[a] CTX, cyclophosphamide; ADR, Adriamycin (doxorubicin); MTX, methotrexate; PRO, procarbazine; BLE, bleomycin; CCNU, lomustine; VCR or ONC, vincristine or Oncovin; $HN_2$, mechlorethamine; DDP, cisplatin; ETO, etoposide; VIN, vindesine; MIT, mitomycin.

## *Small Cell Lung Cancer*

### Chemotherapy

In contrast to NSCLC, the use of aggressive combination chemotherapy regimens in SCLC has demonstrated a four- to fivefold increase in median survival.[72] Because SCLC has the propensity to disseminate early in the disease, surgery is almost never indicated, except possibly in the rare patient who presents with a small, isolated lesion.[73]

A number of factors have been identified that appear to have prognostic importance in SCLC. Patients who initially present with limited disease and are treated with aggressive chemotherapy regimens demonstrate a significantly longer median survival than patients presenting with extensive disease treated with the same regimens.[19,72,74] Patients presenting with a better performance status[18,19,72,74] and no weight loss[72] also appear to have an improved prognosis. Females appear to have a better prognosis than males as do patients under age 60 as opposed to patients over age 60.[72]

A number of cytotoxic agents have demonstrated significant single-agent activity in SCLC. Cyclophosphamide was the first single agent to demonstrate that chemotherapy could positively affect the survival of patients with SCLC.[75] On the basis of this early documented activity, cyclophosphamide has been included in many widely used combination regimens. After systemic administration, cyclophosphamide is activated by hepatic microsomal metabolism, in the plasma and within the target cell, through several intermediate processes to the final active alkylating compound, phosphoramide mustard, and a side product, acrolein.[63,76] The alkylating effect of the active compound prevents cell division primarily by crosslinking DNA strands. As a class, alkylating agents exert cytotoxic effects on cells throughout all phases of the cell cycle but have quantitatively greater activity against rapidly dividing cells.[63]

The pharmacokinetics of cyclophosphamide and its metabolites has been studied; however, because the active metabolites are generated intracellularly, it is difficult to relate these studies to clinical toxicity.[63] In patients with renal failure, the serum half-life is prolonged, which correlates with increased myelosuppression.[77]

Cyclophosphamide is widely used in the management of many malignant as well as nonmalignant diseases and is commonly employed in combination with other cytotoxic drugs and/or radiation therapy. Therefore, a variety of doses and schedules have been utilized. In the treatment of lung cancer single intravenous dosages of 500 to 2,000 mg/m$^2$ of body surface area per treatment course have most commonly been used.[5,62,72–74,78–87] Higher doses of cyclophosphamide (to 8 g/m$^2$) have also been used in combination with autologous bone marrow support.[88,89]

Bone marrow supression is the usual dose-limiting toxic effect of cyclophosphamide. Leukopenia is generally more significant than thrombocytopenia. Nausea and vomiting are common after cyclophosphamide therapy and may be severe and prolonged after high-dose therapy. Acute sterile hemorrhagic cystitis is an infrequent toxic manifestation but may be dose limiting.[90–92] The investigational analogue ifosfamide is more commonly associated with this toxic effect. The cystitis is believed to result from local irritation by the acrolein in the urine and is more common in poorly hydrated or renally compromised patients.[93] Adequate hydration and frequent voiding appear to offer protection. Instillation of thiol compounds into the bladder or systemic administration of *N*-acetylcysteine or sodium 2-mercaptoethanesulfonate (MESNA) mitigates this toxic effect.[94] Other toxic effects reported with cyclophosphamide include alopecia, a syndrome of inappropriate antidiuretic hormone (SIADH), sterility, and interstitial pulmonary fibrosis.

Among the other active agents are doxorubicin, etoposide, vincristine, vindesine, lomustine, cisplatin, procarbazine, and methotrexate with response rates ranging from 15% to 45%.[79] Combination chemotherapy is clearly superior to single-agent therapy and the best results are generally observed when three or more active agents are combined.[80] In recent years it has been observed that aggressive chemotherapy regimens appear to produce higher response rates, longer median survivals, and a higher percentage of long-term survivals.[72] Among some of the more frequently used regimens are CAV—cyclophosphamide (*C*) + doxorubicin (*A*) + vincristine (*V*), CAE—C + A + etoposide (*E*), and CMCc—C + methotrexate (*M*) + lomustine (*Cc*). These regimens are described in Table 94.5. Cisplatin has also been incorporated into similar regimens; however, its role in SCLC remains uncertain. Use of such aggressive regimens generally results in complete response rates of 40% to 50% in patients with limited disease and 15% to 20% in patients with extensive disease.[72] The median survival among patients with limited disease is approximately 14 months as opposed to about 8 months in patients with extensive disease[72]; however, it should be noted that such aggressive regimens may be associated with a significant degree of toxicity, especially granulocytopenia, which may increase the risk of serious infections.

Restaging to determine the effects of chemotherapy is usually done after three courses of therapy. At this point therapy is continued in patients responding to therapy and discontinued or changed in patients demonstrating evidence of disease progression. In patients achieving a complete response the optimal duration to continue therapy remains unknown, with recommendations ranging from 6 to 24 months.[72]

### Radiation

SCLC is a very radiosensitive tumor and radiotherapy has been used in combination with chemotherapy to treat tumors limited to the thoracic cavity. The rationale for combined-modality therapy is for radiotherapy and chemotherapy together to deal with bulk disease in the chest primary site and for chemotherapy to take care of systemic metastases.[5] This combined-modality therapy may decrease the incidence and delay the onset of local tumor recurrences[95]; however, its ability to improve the overall duration of survival over that achieved with chemotherapy alone has not been firmly established. Although most studies have not demonstrated an improvement in median survival[95–97] several studies have shown an advantage of the combined modality. One study reported by Perez et al has demonstrated a significant survival advantage (13.9 versus 11.4 months) for patients receiving chemotherapy (CAV) followed by radiotherapy.[98] Likewise, the Cancer and Leukemia Group B and the NCI-VA Group have also demonstrated significantly higher

**Table 94.5** Combination Chemotherapy in Small Cell Lung Cancer

| *Combination* | *Dosage* | *Schedule* | *Overall response rate (%)* | *Reference* |
|---|---|---|---|---|
| CAV | | | | |
| CTX[a] | 750–1,500 mg/m² IV day 1 | | | |
| ADR | 45–50 mg/m² IV day 1 | Repeat course every 3 wk | 63–100 | 83, 84 |
| VCR | 2 mg IV day 1 | | | |
| CAE | | | | |
| CTX | 1,000 mg/m² IV day 1 | | | |
| ADR | 45 mg/m² IV day 1 | | | |
| ETO | 50 mg/m² IV days 1–5 **or** 80 mg/m² IV days 1–3 | Repeat course every 3 wk | 63–100 | 62, 72–74, 78–85 |
| CMCc | | | | |
| CTX | 700 mg/m² IV day 1 | | | |
| MTX | 20 mg/m² PO days 18–21 | Repeat course every 3 wk | 75 | 86 |
| CCNU | 70 mg/m² PO day 1 | | | |
| CEV | | | | |
| CTX | 1,000 mg/m² IV day 1 | | | |
| ETO | 50 mg/m² IV day 1, then 100 mg/m² PO days 2–5 | Repeat course every 3 wk | 80 | 87 |
| VCR | 1.4 mg/m² IV day 1 | | | |

[a] CTX, cyclophosphamide; ADR, Adriamycin (doxorubicin); VCR, vincristine; ETO, etoposide; MTX, methotrexate; CCNU, lomustine.

complete response rates and 2-year survival rates for combined-modality regimens compared with chemotherapy alone.[99,100] Combined-modality therapy has also been associated with increased morbidity.[101] When radiation therapy is combined with radiosensitizing drugs like doxorubicin the incidence of radiation esophagitis and pneumonitis may increase.[102] Clinical trials currently underway are evaluating various dosages and schedules of radiation therapy in combination with a variety of chemotherapeutic agents in an attempt to maximize tumor control with an acceptable degree of toxicity.

Central nervous system metastases are present in about 10% of patients initially and occur at some point in the disease process in greater than 50% of patients.[103] For this reason, prophylactic cranial irradiation is currently recommended in all patients achieving a complete response to chemotherapy.[72] In a review of randomized trials evaluating prophylactic whole-brain irradiation, Bleehen et al reported that the incidence of brain metastases was 20% in patients not receiving prophylactic whole-brain irradiation compared with 6% in patients who did receive it.[104] In patients with persistent disease the tumor may continue to seed the CNS, therefore negating any effects of prophylactic irradiation.[105] In patients with intracranial metastases, therapeutic cranial irradiation usually controls the CNS disease and patients generally die from progressive systemic disease.[103] Adrenocorticosteroids (to decrease intracranial pressure) and anticonvulsants (to prevent seizures) are routinely administered to patients with CNS metastases.

Although SCLC is highly responsive to combination chemotherapy the low rate of long-term survival (about 8%–10% of patients survive 3 years) is disappointing. Currently, the major emphasis of research in SCLC is to extend the median survival and improve the cure rate.

Because the duration of response is usually brief (<1 year) in patients achieving a complete response it appears that drug-resistant cells continue to grow during treatment and eventually constitute a major portion of the tumor. The Goldie–Coldman theory[106] predicts that the cycling of two separate active chemotherapeutic regimens may overcome this problem. (Although theoretically it would seem ideal to administer all the drugs simultaneously, the treatment-related toxic effects would be prohibitive.) A number of trials have employed the use of alternating, non–cross-resistant regimens in the management of SCLC; however, thus far any improvement with this approach appears to be modest.[72] Examples of such regimens include cyclophosphamide, methotrexate, and lomustine alternating with vincristine, doxorubicin, and procarbazine; vincristine, doxorubicin, and cyclophosphamide alternating with etoposide; and cyclophosphamide, doxorubicin, and etoposide alternating with vincristine, methotrexate, lomustine, and procarbazine. It should be noted, however, that in many of these trials the second regimen was not cross-resistant and subtherapeutic doses were administered.[107]

Other modalities that are also under investigation include total-body irradiation[108] or high-dose chemotherapy followed by autologous bone marrow transplantation. Because there exists a small, but definite, cure rate in SCLC, such extensive research efforts are warranted in the hope that this rate will improve.

### *Complications and Supportive Care*

Patients with lung cancer frequently have many medical problems. Such problems may be related to the primary tumor and its metastases (see Clinical Presentation), the antitumor therapy, or concomitant diseases.

Many of the chemotherapy regimens used in the management of lung cancer are very intense (Tables 94.4 and 94.5) and are associated with a wide variety of toxic effects. Nausea and vomiting may be severe (especially in the cisplatin-containing regimens) and require aggressive antiemetic regimens. Patients experiencing protracted nausea and vomiting may require intravenous hydration (and nutritional support). Myelosuppression is often the dose-limiting toxic effect associated with these combinations and granulocytopenia following many of the more aggressive regimens places patients at high risk of serious infections. Other toxic effects associated with these regimens include mucositis, peripheral neuropathies, nephrotoxicity, and ototoxicity.

Likewise, patients receiving radiation therapy may experience complications including esophagitis, pulmonary insufficiency, and cardiac toxicity.

As previously mentioned, patients with lung cancer frequently suffer from concomitant medical problems including chronic obstructive pulmonary diseases and cardiovascular disorders (probably related to smoking) that require pharmacologic interventions.

It is apparent that many patients with lung cancer often receive complex pharmacologic regimens that may include chemotherapeutic agents, antiemetics, antibiotics, analgesics, bronchodilators, corticosteroids, anticonvulsants and cardiovascular agents. Such regimens necessitate intensive therapeutic monitoring to avoid drug-related toxic effects and to optimize patient management.

## Summary

Lung cancer is currently the leading cause of cancer death in the United States although the American Cancer Society has estimated that up to 83% of all cases could be prevented if cigarette smoking were eliminated.

Surgery (and radiation therapy to a lesser extent) offers the only chance of cure in patients with NSCLC; however, the majority of patients are inoperable at diagnosis. Unfortunately, the response rates to combination chemotherapy in this disease are disappointingly low and it is controversial whether such therapy offers significant benefit to the patient in terms of quality of life or survival. Research endeavors continue to look for new effective agents and regimens in NSCLC in the hope of improving response rates and survival.

In contrast, combination chemotherapy has demonstrated dramatic response rates and clearly improved survival in patients with SCLC; however, the percentage of long-term survivors remains low. Research endeavors in SCLC continue to look for new agents, improved combinations, and new modalities that will enhance the cure rate.

Despite progress over the last decade in the management of advanced lung cancer the only clear-cut hope for control of this devastating disease lies in the elimination of cigarette smoking.

## References

1. American Cancer Society. 1987 Cancer Facts and Figures.
2. Silverberg E. Cancer statistics. CA 1988;38:5–27.
3. Van Houtte P, Salazar OM, Phillips CE, et al. Lung cancer, in Rubin P (ed): Clinical Oncology for Medical Students and Physicians, 6th ed. American Cancer Society 1983, pp 142–152.
4. Martini N. Preoperative staging and surgery for non-small cell lung cancer, in Aisner JA (ed): Lung Cancer. New York, Churchill Livingston, 1985, pp 101–130.
5. Minna JD, Higgins GA, Glatstein EJ. Cancer of the lung, in Devita V, Hellman S, Rosenberg S (eds): Cancer—Principles and Practice of Oncology, 2nd ed. Philadelphia, J.B. Lippincott, 1985, pp 507–597.
6. Wynder EL. Etiology of lung cancer: Reflections on 2 decades of research. Cancer 1972;30:1332–1339.
7. Selikoff IJ, Hammond EC. Asbestos-associated diseases in United States shipyards. CA 1978;28:87–99.
8. Strauss MJ (ed): Lung Cancer: Clinical Diagnosis and Treatment. New York, Grune and Stratton, 1977.
9. Menck HR, Casagrande JT, Henderson BE. Industrial air pollution. Possible effect on lung cancer. Science 1974;183: 210–212.
10. Sobin LH. The World Health Organization's histological classification of lung tumors: A comparison of the first and second editions. Cancer Detect Prev 1982;5:391–406.
11. Aisner SC, Matthews MJ. The pathology of lung cancer, in Aisner JA (ed): Lung Cancer. New York, Churchill Livingston, 1985, pp 1–23.
12. Matthews MJ, Gordon PR. Morphology of pulmonary and pleural malignancies, in Strauss MJ (ed): Lung Cancer: Clinical Diagnosis and Treatment. New York, Grune and Stratton, 1977, pp 49–69.
13. Rosenow EC, Carr DT. Bronchogenic carcinoma. CA 1979;29:233–246.
14. Cohen MH, Matthews MJ. Small cell carcinoma of the lung. A distinct clinicopathologic entity. Semin Oncol 1978;5:234–243.
15. Cohen MH. Signs and symptoms of bronchogenic carcinoma, in Strauss MJ (ed): Lung Cancer: Clinical Diagnosis and Treatment. New York, Grune and Stratton, 1977, pp 85–94.
16. American Joint Committee for Cancer Staging and End-Results Reporting Task Force on Lung: Staging of Lung Cancer. Chicago, IL, 1979;1–23.
17. Ramsdell JW, Peters RM, Taylor AT, et al. Multiorgan scans for staging lung cancer: Correlation with clinical evaluation. J Thorac Cardiovasc Surg 1977;73:653–659.
18. Zelen M. Keynote address on biostatistics and data retrieval. Cancer Chemother Rep 1973;4:31–42.
19. Ihde DC, Makuch RW, Carney DN, et al. Prognostic implication of sites of metastases in patients with small cell carcinoma of the lung given intensive combination chemotherapy. Am Rev Respir Dis Chest 1981;123:500–507.
20. Hansen HH, Dombernowsky P, Hirsch FR. Staging procedures and prognostic features in small cell anaplastic bronchogenic carcinoma. Semin Oncol 1978;5:280–287.
21. Martini R, Beattie EJ. Results of surgical treatment in stage I lung cancer. J Thorac Cardiovasc Surg 1977;74:499–506.
22. Paulson DL, Reisch JS. Long-term survival after resection for bronchogenic carcinoma. Ann Surg 1976;184:324–332.

23. Stanley KE. Prognostic factors for survival in patients with inoperable lung cancer. J Natl Cancer Inst 1980;65:25–32.
24. Livingston RB. Combination chemotherapy of bronchogenic carcinoma. Cancer Treat Rev 1977;4:154–165.
25. Aisner J, Hansen HH. Commentary: Current status of chemotherapy for non–small cell lung cancer. Cancer Treat Rep 1981;65:979–986.
26. Stanley KE. Prognostic factors in lung cancer, in Aisner JA (ed): Lung Cancer. New York, Churchill Livingston, 1985, pp 41–66.
27. Bodey GP, Lagakos SW, Gutierrez AC. Therapy of advanced squamous carcinoma of the lung: Cyclophosphamide vs "COMB." Cancer 1976;39:1026–1031.
28. Livingston RB, Einhorm LH, Bodey GP. COMB (cyclophosphamide, oncovin, methyl-CCNU, and bleomycin) a four-drug combination in solid tumors. Cancer 1975;36:327–332.
29. Vincent RG, Mehta CR, Tucker RD, et al. Chemotherapy of extensive large cell and adenocarcinoma of the lung. Cancer 1980;46:256–260.
30. Strauss MJ. Cytokinetic chemotherapy design for the treatment of advanced lung cancer. Cancer Treat Rep 1979;63:767–773.
31. Hansen HH, Selawy OS, Simon RS. Combination chemotherapy of advanced lung cancer. Cancer 1976;38:2201–2207.
32. Shepard KV, Golomb HM, Bitran ID, et al. CAMP chemotherapy for metastatic non-oat cell bronchogenic carcinoma: A seven-year experience (1975–1981) with 160 patients. Cancer 1985;56:2385–2390.
33. Vogelzang NJ, Bonomi PD, Rossof AH, et al. Cyclophosphamide, adriamycin, methotrexate, and procarbazine (CAMP) treatment of non–oat cell bronchogenic carcinoma. Cancer Treat Rep 1978;62:1595–1597.
34. Ruckdeschel JC, Mehta CR, Salazar OM, et al. Chemotherapy for metastatic non–small cell bronchogenic carcinoma: EST 2575, generation 111, HAM versus CAMP. Cancer Treat Rep 1981;65:959–963.
35. Lad T, Sarma PR, Diekamp U, et al. "CAMP" combination chemotherapy for unresectable non–oat cell bronchogenic carcinoma. Cancer Clin Trials 1970;2:321–326.
36. Lad TE, Nelson RB, Diekamp U, et al. Immediate versus postponed combination chemotherapy (CAMP) for unresectable non–small cell lung cancer: A randomized trial. Cancer Treat Rep 1981;65:973–978.
37. Cambareri RJ, Smith FP, MacDonald JS, et al. CAMP (cyclophosphamide, doxorubicin, methotrexate and procarbazine) for epidermoid and large cell anaplastic carcinoma of the lung. Cancer Treat Rep 1981;65:317–320.
38. Bitran JD, Desser RK, DeMeester T, et al. Metastatic non–oat cell bronchogenic carcinoma therapy with cyclophosphamide, doxorubicin, methotrexate, and procarbazine (CAMP). JAMA 1978;240:2743–2746.
39. Livingston RB, Fee WH, Einhorn LH. BACON (bleomycin, adriamycin, CCNU, oncovin, and nitrogen mustard) in squamous lung cancer. Cancer 1976;37:1237–1242.
40. Livingston RB, Heilbrun L, Lehane D, et al. Comparative trial of combination chemotherapy in extensive squamous carcinoma of the lung: A Southwest Oncology Group study. Cancer Treat Rep 1977;61:1623–1629.
41. Chahinian AP, Mandel EM, Holland JF, et al. MACC (methotrexate, adriamycin, cyclphosphamide and CCNU) in advanced lung cancer. Cancer 1979;43:1590–1597.
42. Vogl JE, Mehta CR, Cohen MH. MACC chemotherapy for adenocarcinoma and epidermoid carcinoma of the lung. Cancer 1979;44:864–868.
43. Milstein D, Robinson E. Four-drug combination chemotherapy in advanced lung cancer: Methotrexate, doxorubicin, cyclophosphamide, and CCNU. Cancer 1981;48:2358–2363.
44. Eagan RT, Ingle JN, Frytak S, et al. Platinum-based polychemotherapy versus dianhydrogalactitol in advanced non–small cell lung cancer. Cancer Treat Rep 1977;61:1339–1345.
45. Ruckdeschel JC, Mason B, Ettinger D, et al. Chemotherapy of metastatic non–oat cell bronchogenic carcinoma: The Eastern Cooperative Group experience, in The III World Conference on Lung Cancer. 1978;1207–1210.
46. Krook JE, Fleming TR, Eagen RT, et al. Comparison of combination chemotherapy programs in advanced adenocarcinoma–large cell carcinoma of the lung: A North Central Cancer Treatment Group study. Cancer Treat Rep 1984;68:493–498.
47. Knost JA, Greco FA, Hande KR, et al. Cyclophosphamide, doxorubicin and cisplatin in the treatment of advanced non–small cell lung cancer. Cancer Treat Rep 1981;65:941–945.
48. Britell JC, Eagan RT, Ingle JN, et al. *cis*-Dichlorodiammineplatinum(II) alone followed by Adriamycin plus cyclophosphamide at progression versus *cis*-dichlorodiammineplatinum(II), Adriamycin, and cyclophosphamide in combination for adenocarcinoma of the lung. Cancer Treat Rep 1978;62:1207–1210.
49. Evans WK, Feld R, DeBoer G, et al. Cyclophosphamide, doxorubicin and cisplatin in the treatment of non–small cell bronchogenic carcinoma. Cancer Treat Rep 1981;65:947–954.
50. Gralla RJ, Cvitkovic E, Goldberg RB, et al. *cis*-Dichlorodiammineplatinum (II) in non–small cell carcinoma of the lung. Cancer Treat Rep 1979;63:1585–1588.
51. Davis S, Rambotti P, Park YK. Combination cyclophosphamide, doxorubicin and cisplatin (CAP) chemotherapy for extensive non–small cell carcinomas of the lung. Cancer Treat Rep 1981;65:955–958.
52. Longeval E, Klastersky J. Combination chemotherapy with cisplatin and etoposide in bronchogenic squamous cell carcinoma and adenocarcinoma: A study by the EORTC Lung Cancer Working Party. Cancer 1982;50:2751–2756.
53. Dhingra HM, Valdivieso M, Booser DJ, et al. Chemotherapy for advanced adenocarcinoma and squamous cell carcinoma of the lung with etoposide and cisplatin. Cancer Treat Rep 1984;671–673.
54. Dhingra HM, Valdivieso M, Carr DT, et al. Randomized trial of three combinations of cisplatin with vindesine or VP-16-213 in the treatment of advanced non–small-cell lung cancer. J Clin Oncol 1985;3:176–183.
55. Cavalli F, Goldhirsch A, Joss R. *cis*-Dichlorodiammineplatinum(II) and VP-16-213 combination chemotherapy for non–small cell lung cancer. Chemoterapia 1982;1:164–167.
56. Eagan RT, Frytak S, Nichols WC, et al. Evaluation of VP-16-213, cyclophosphamide, doxorubicin and cisplatin (V-CAP) in advanced large cell lung cancer. Cancer Treat Rep 1981;65: 715–717.
57. Fuks JZ, Aisner JA, VanEcho DA, et al. Randomized study of cyclophosphamide, doxorubicin and etoposide (VP-16-213) with or without cisplatinum in non–small cell lung cancer. J Clin Oncol 1983;1:295–301.
58. Klastersky J, Sculier JP, Nicaise C, et al. Combination chemotherapy with cisplatin, etoposide, and vindesine in non–small cell lung carcinoma: A clinical trial of the EORTC Lung Cancer Working Party. Cancer Treat Rep 1983;67:727–730.
59. Gralla RJ, Casper ES, Kelsen DP, et al. Cisplatin and vindesine combination chemotherapy for advanced carcinoma of the lung: A randomized trial investigating two dosage schedules. Ann Intern Med 1981;95:414–420.
60. Ruckdeschel JC, Finkelstein FM, Mason BA, et al. Chemo-

therapy for metastatic non–small cell bronchogenic carcinoma: EST 2575, generation V—A randomized comparison of four cisplatin-containing regimens. J Clin Oncol 1985;3:72–79.
61. Mason BA, Catalano RB. Mitomycin, vinblastine and cisplatin combination chemotherapy in non–small cell lung cancer. Proc ASCO/AACR 1980;21:447.
62. Luedke D, Luedke S, Martello O, et al. Response of non–small cell lung cancer to vindesine and mitomycin: A Southeastern Cancer Study Group Pilot Study. (Abstr) Proc ASCO 1983;2:190.
63. Chabner BA, Myers CE. Clinical pharmacology of cancer chemotherapy, in DeVita VT, Hellman S, Rosenberg SA (eds): Cancer. Principles and Practice of Oncology, 2nd ed. Philadelphia, J.B. Lippincott, 1985, pp 287–350.
64. Zwelling LA, Kohn KW. Mechanism of action of *cis*-dichlorodiammineplatinum (II). Cancer Treat Rep 1979;63:1439–1444.
65. Fraval HNA, Roberts JJ. $G_1$ phase Chinese hamster V79-379A cells are inherently more sensitive to platinum bound to their DNA than mid S phase or asynchronously treated cells. Biochem Pharmacol 1979;28:1575–1580.
66. Patton TF, Himmelstein KJ, Belt R, et al. Plasma levels and urinary excretion of filterable platinum species following bolus injection and i.v. infusion of *cis*-dichlorodiammineplatinum(II) in man. Cancer Treat Rep 1979;63:1359–1361.
67. Ozols RF, Corden BJ, Jacob J, et al. High-dose cisplatin in hypertonic saline. Ann Intern Med 1984;100:19–24.
68. Gonzalez-Vitale JC, Hayes DM, Cvitkovic E, et al. The renal pathology in clinical trials of *cis*-platinum(II)diamminedichloride. Cancer 1977;39:1362–1371.
69. Madias NE, Harrington JT. Platinum nephrotoxicity. Am J Med 1978;65:307–314.
70. Al-Sarraf M, Fletcher W, Oishi N, et al. Cisplatin hydration with and without mannitol diuresis in refractory disseminated malignant melanoma: A Southwest Oncology Group study. Cancer Treat Rep 1982;66:31–35.
71. Hrushesky WJM. Chemotherapy timing: An important variable in toxicity and response, in Perry MC, Yarbro JW (eds): Toxicity of Chemotherapy. Orlando, Grune and Stratton, 1984, pp 449–477.
72. Hansen HH, Rorth M, Aisner JA. Management of small-cell carcinoma of the lung, in Aisner JA (ed): Lung Cancer. New York, Churchill Livingston, 1985, pp 269–285.
73. Higgins GA, Shields TW, Matthews MJ. The role of surgery in small cell carcinoma. III World Conference on Lung Cancer. 1982;165.
74. Bunn PA, Cohen MH, Ihde DC, et al. Advances in small cell bronchogenic carcinoma. Cancer Treat Rep 1977;61:333–342.
75. Green RA, Humphrey E, Close H, et al. Alkylating agents in bronchogenic carcinoma. Am J Med 1969;46:516.
76. Colvin M. A review of the pharmacology and clinical use of cyclophosphamide, in Pinedo HM (ed): Clinical Pharmacology of Antineoplastic Drugs. Amsterdam, Elsevier, 1978, pp 245–261.
77. Juma FD, Rogers HJ, Trounce JR. Effect of renal insufficiency on the pharmacokinetics of cyclophosphamide and some of its metabolites. Eur J Clin Pharmacol 1981;19:443.
78. Broder LE, Cohen MH, Selawry OS. Treatment of bronchogenic carcinoma. II. Small cell. Cancer Treat Rev 1977;4:219–260.
79. Aisner J, Alberto P, Comis R, et al. Role of chemotherapy in small cell lung cancer. A consensus report of the IASLC Workshop. Cancer Treat Rep 1983;67:37–43.
80. Johnson RE, Brereton HD, Kent CH. 'Total' therapy for small cell carcinoma of the lung. Ann Thorac Surg 1978;25:510–515.
81. Greco FA, Richardson RL, Snell JD, et al. Small cell lung cancer: Complete remission and improved survival. Am J Med 1979;66:625–630.
82. Mandelbaum I, Williams SD, Hornback NB, et al. Combined therapy for small cell undifferentiated carcinoma of the lung. J Thorac Cardiovasc Surg 1978;76:292–296.
83. Aisner J, Wiernik PH. Chemotherapy versus chemoimmunotherapy for small-cell undifferentiated carcinoma of the lung. Cancer 1980;46:2543–2549.
84. Klastersky J, Sculier JP, Weerts D. Combination chemotherapy with cyclophosphamide, adriamycin and etoposide for small cell carcinoma of the lung. Proc ASCO 1983;2:188.
85. Hansen HH, Dombernowsky P, Hansen M. Chemotherapy of advanced small-cell anaplastic carcinoma: Superiority of a four-drug combination to a three-drug combination. Ann Intern Med 1978;89:177–181.
86. Bunn PA, Ihde DC. Small cell bronchogenic carcinoma: A review of therapeutic results, in Livingston RB (ed): Lung Cancer: Advances in Research and Treatment. The Hague, Martinus Nijhoff, 1981, pp 169–208.
87. Issell B, Rudolph A, Lawson R, et al. The substitution of etoposide for doxorubicin in small cell lung cancer combination chemotherapy. Proceedings of the Thirteenth International Congress of Chemotherapy, 1983.
88. Souhami RL, Harper PG, Linch D, et al. High-dose cyclophosphamide with autologous bone marrow transplantation as initial treatment of small cell carcinoma of the lung. Cancer Chemother Pharmacol 1982;8:31.
89. Souhami RL, Fin G, Gregory WM, et al. High-dose cyclophosphamide in small-cell carcinoma of the lung. J Clin Oncol 1985;3:958.
90. Berkson GM, Lome LG, Shapiro I. Severe cystitis induced by cyclophosphamide. JAMA 1973;225:605–606.
91. Hutter AM, Bauman AW, Frank IN. Cyclophosphamide and severe hemorrhagic cystitis. NY State J Med 1969;69:305–309.
92. Pearlman CK. Cystitis due to cytoxan: Case report. J Urol 1966;95:713–715.
93. Cox PJ. Cyclophosphamide cystitis. Identification of acrolein as the causative agent. Biochem Pharmacol 1979;28:2045–2049.
94. Brock N, Pohl J, Stekar J. Detoxification of urotoxic oxazaphosphorines by sulfhydryl compounds. J Cancer Res Clin Oncol 1981;100:311.
95. Wilson HE, Stanley K, Vincent RG, et al. Comparison of chemotherapy alone versus chemotherapy and radiation therapy of extensive small cell carcinoma of the lung. J Surg Oncol 1983;23:181–184.
96. Livingston RB, Moore TN, Heilbrum L, et al. Small cell carcinoma of the lung: Combined chemotherapy and radiation. A Southwest Oncology Group study. Ann Intern Med 1978;88:194–199.
97. McCracken JD, Chen T, White J, et al. Combination chemotherapy, radiotherapy and BCG immunotherapy in limited small cell carcinoma of the lung. Cancer 1982;49:2252–2258.
98. Perez CA, Einhorn L, Oldham RK, et al. Randomized trial of radiotherapy to the thorax in limited small-cell and elective brain irradiation: A preliminary report. J Clin Oncol 1984;2:1200–1208.
99. Perry MC, Eaton WL, Chahinian P, et al. Chemotherapy (CTH) with or without radiation therapy (RT) in limited small cell cancer of the lung. (Abstr) Proc Am Soc Clin Oncol 1986;5:173.
100. Idhe DC, Deisseroth AB, Lichter AS, et al. Late intensive combined modality therapy followed by autologous bone marrow infusion in extensive stage small-cell lung cancer. J Clin Oncol 1986;4:1443.
101. Nugent JL, Bunn PA, Matthews MJ, et al. CNS metastases in

small cell bronchogenic carcinoma: Increasing frequency and changing pattern with lengthening survival. Cancer 1979;44: 1885–1893.

**102.** Phillips TL, Fu KK. Acute and late effects of multimodal therapy on normal tissues. Cancer 1977;40:489–494.

**103.** Bunn PA, Rosen ST. Central nervous system manifestations of small cell lung cancer, in Aisner JA (ed): Lung Cancer. New York, Churchill Livingston, 1985, 287–305.

**104.** Bleehen NM, Bunn PA, Cox JD et al. Role of radiation therapy in small anaplastic carcinoma of the lung. Cancer Treat Rep 1983;67:11–19.

**105.** Qasim MM. Combined total body irradiation and local radiation therapy in oat cell carcinoma of the bronchus. Clin Radiol 1979;30:161–163.

**106.** Goldie JH, Coldman AJ, Gudauskas GA. Rationale for the use of alternating non–cross resistant chemotherapy. Cancer Treat Rep 1982;66:439–449.

**107.** Greco FA, Johnson DH, Hainsworth JD, et al. Chemotherapy of small-cell lung cancer. Semin Oncol 1985;4(suppl 6):31–37.

**108.** Spitzer G, Dicke KA, Litam J, et al. High-dose combination chemotherapy with autologous bone marrow transplantation in adult solid tumors. Cancer 1980;45:3075–3085.

# Chapter 95 / Squamous Head and Neck Cancer

Paul R. Hutson, PharmD, and Melody A. Cobleigh, MD

## Epidemiology/Etiology

Cancers of the head and neck constitute about 6% of new cancers in males and 2% in females in the United States.[1] Approximately 42,000 new cases are expected in 1987.[1] Head and neck cancer is a physically, mentally, and socially debilitating disease that relies on an integrated therapeutic strategy for any hope of cure.

Head and neck cancer in the United States is almost entirely preventable by avoiding the combined use of ethanol and tobacco.[2] Less than 4% of the reported cases of head and neck cancer occur in people who do not use tobacco.[3] Although alcohol or tobacco alone may elicit neoplastic transformation of the mucosa of the lungs or esophagus, it is their concurrent use that greatly increases the risk of cancer. Ethanol may promote head or neck cancer by (1) solubilizing tobacco-associated carcinogens, (2) contributing to poor nutrition, (3) inhibiting detoxification of carcinogens by a diseased liver, or (4) decreasing immunocompetence.[2] Patients with head and neck cancer also have a higher incidence of esophageal and lung cancer.[4] The increased risk of second primary malignancies is thought to be a result of the ingestion or inhalation of carcinogens, but the possibility of a predisposition to oncogenesis in such individuals exists.[5]

Head and neck cancer is the most common malignancy among men, and the second most common tumor among women, in southern India. This is due to the widespread chewing of a mixture of tobacco, lime, and betel nuts. The increasing use of smokeless tobacco products by Americans and Europeans has resulted in an increased incidence of oral cancers, particularly among oral snuff users.[6,7] Other factors associated with an increased risk of head and neck cancer are iron deficiency (Plummer–Vinson syndrome), wood dust, and Epstein–Barr virus.

Epstein–Barr virus (EBV) can be isolated from the tumor cells of most patients with nasopharyngeal cancer.[5] The EBV DNA genome has been identified within nasopharyngeal tumor cells, but a cause-and-effect relationship between the virus and tumor has not yet been established. The Plummer–Vinson syndrome is an acquired, reversible nutritional deficiency of iron resulting in dysphagia from postcricoid membranous webs. These individuals are at an increased risk of developing head and neck cancer and should be followed closely for signs or symptoms of carcinoma.[8]

## Clinical Presentation

### *Primary Site*

Symptoms of head and neck cancer depend greatly upon the primary site of disease. Common signs and symptoms are sore throat, oropharyngeal swelling, pain on chewing, odynophagia, otitis media, slow-healing ulcer, dysphagia, referred otalgia, bloody nasal discharge, voice changes, facial pain or palsies, and chronic sinusitis.[9,10] Lip cancer is usually visualized or palpated at an early stage. Tumor in the oral cavity may present as a painless, slow-healing lesion. Advanced lesions of the oropharynx and hypopharynx may be painful, particularly during swallowing, but early disease may be asymptomatic or present as a chronic sore throat. Nasopharyngeal or maxillary sinus cancer can present with nasal discharges, facial pain or swelling, or nasal blockage. Involvement of cranial nerves by these latter tumors may lead to diplopia, Horner's syndrome, facial pain, hoarseness, or referred otalgia. Referred otalgia is also an occasional manifestation of tumors that arise in more inferior sites, such as the tongue or hypopharynx. The pain impulse in the afferent fifth, ninth, or tenth cranial nerve may cross into afferent nerves from the outer, middle, and inner ear canal and tympanic membrane, causing referred ear pain.[9]

Tumors of the glottic larynx are often discovered at an early stage because of hoarseness; however, disease above or below the vocal cords may remain asymptomatic until late in the course.

The histology of most head and neck neoplasms is squamous carcinoma.[11] Surface lesions may be hard with rolled, indurated borders, or may present as more advanced surface ulcerations with indurated edges. Surface lesions may also be verrucous (wartlike) in appearance. Chronic oropharyngeal irritation may give rise to precancerous white plaques (leukoplakia) or velvety red patches (erythroplakia). The likelihood of cancerous transformation is much greater for erythroplakia, but its incidence is much less than that of leukoplakia.[9,11] These lesions often regress and disappear when the source of local irritation is removed.

### *Cervical Lymphatic System*

An estimated 150 to 350 lymph nodes are located above the clavicle, constituting roughly one third of all lymph nodes in the body. The risk of lymph node metastases is determined by the site and size of the primary tumor, the degree of histologic differentiation (more poorly differentiated histologies spread more rapidly), and the density of the capillary lymphatics that drain the region of the primary tumor.[12] Nasopharyngeal and pyriform sinus tumors have a profuse network of capillary lymphatics and a high rate of regional lymph node metastases. Regional lymph node involvement is found at diagnosis in 75% to 85% of patients with primary disease at these sites.[12] The vocal cords have poorer lymphatic drainage and a much lower incidence of regional lymphatic spread. Tumors arising on one side of the neck tend to spread to the ipsilateral lymphatics. Midline tumors and tumors of the tongue or nasopharynx are more likely to cross to the contralateral side, particularly in patients with obstructed ipsilateral lymphatics resulting from surgery or radiation damage.

### *Distant Metastases*

The incidence of distant metastases after treatment with surgery or radiation averages 11%.[13] The risk of distant metastases is largely influenced by site of the primary tumor, use of surgery and/or radiation for "definitive therapy," and size and local spread of the initial tumor.[14] Patients with primary disease in the nasopharynx or hypopharynx are most likely to develop distant metastases. The most common metastatic sites are the lung, bone, and liver. Almost 12% of patients who have a complete response after chemotherapy, surgery, and radiation relapse in a distant site.[14] An additional 14% of complete responders develop recurrent disease at both primary and distant sites.

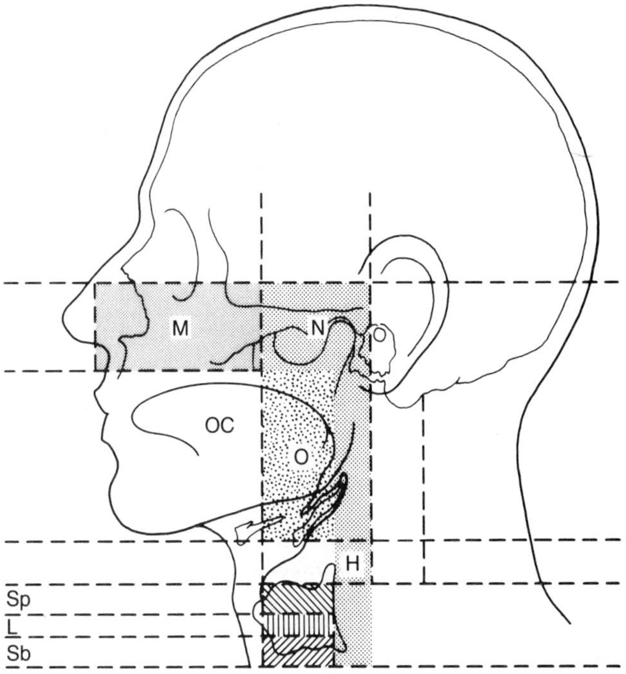


**Figure 95.1** Anatomy of head and neck area. M, maxillary sinus; N, nasopharynx; O, oropharynx; H, hypopharynx; SP, supraglottic larynx; L, glottic larynx; Sb, subglottic larynx; OC, oral cavity. (From Zagars G, Norante JD: Head and neck tumors. In Rubin P (Ed): Clinical Oncology—A Multidisciplinary Approach, 6th ed. New York, American Cancer Society, 1983, p 243, with permission.

## Diagnosis/Staging

The diagnostic workup of a patient with possible head and neck cancer emphasizes a thorough visual inspection of the entire aerodigestive tract and palpation of regional lymph node chains. Computed axial tomography (CAT) scans of the head and neck often reveal more extensive disease than is appreciated on physical examination. Magnetic resonance imaging (MRI) scans will probably replace CAT scans as the imaging modality of choice. MRI scans provide excellent delineation between tumors and surrounding normal soft tissue.

Chest roentgenograms are obtained to check for possible metastatic disease or a second primary (lung) cancer. A "triple endoscopy" is usually performed to visualize the posterior and lower pharynx for head and neck cancer, the bronchi for possible lung cancer, and the esophagus for possible cancer at this site.[4] Patients with signs or symptoms of metastatic disease to lung, bone, liver, or brain will also receive diagnostic imaging of these regions.

Head and neck cancers are categorized by their primary site. The anatomic divisions are oral cavity, nasopharynx, oropharynx, hypopharynx, larynx, and maxillary or paranasal sinus (Fig. 95.1). The site of origin is important because it affects how quickly the tumor is diagnosed, how readily the tumor spreads to regional lymph nodes or distant metastatic sites, and how accessible the tumor is to curative therapy (surgery and/or radiation). For example, patients with lip cancer have a far lower mortality rate (4%) than patients with pharyngeal cancer (50%), largely because of the early detection and surgical accessibility of tumors of the lip.[1]

In addition to the primary site, other factors have been used to identify subsets of patients with a similar prognosis. The TNM staging of disease incorporates the size and degree of local extension of the tumor ("T"), the size, number, and distribution of locoregional lymph nodes ("N"), and the presence and location of any distant metastases ("M").[15] An example of the TNM staging of oropharyngeal cancer is given in Table 95.1. Cancer of the nasopharynx or hypopharynx is more difficult to measure, and the "T" classification for tumors at these sites is based upon the extent and degree of fixation to surrounding normal tissue.

Historically, the staging of head and neck cancer has emphasized surgical resection or curative irradiation of small, solitary lesions ($T_1$, $T_2$). Bulky, unresectable primary tumors, spread to regional lymph nodes ($N_1$–$N_3$), and/or metastasis to distant sites ($M_1$) predicts a poorer cure rate with surgery or radiation.

## Treatment

Patients who present with small cancers with solitary enlarged ($\leq$ 3 cm) lymph nodes or no lymph node involvement ($T_1$–$T_2$, $N_0$–$N_1$) are treated with curative intent with either

**Table 95.1** TNM Staging for Oropharyngeal Cancer

| | |
|---|---|
| **Primary Tumor ("T")** | |
| $T_X$ | Tumor that cannot be assessed by the rules |
| $T_0$ | No evidence of the primary tumor |
| $T_{IS}$ | Carcinoma in situ |
| $T_1$ | Tumor 2 cm or less in greatest diameter |
| $T_2$ | Tumor greater than 2 cm but less than or equal to 4 cm in greatest diameter |
| $T_3$ | Tumor greater than 4 cm in greatest diameter |
| $T_4$ | Massive tumor greater than 4 cm with extensive soft tissue invasion |
| **Nodal Involvement** | |
| $N_X$ | Nodes cannot be assessed |
| $N_0$ | No clinically positive node |
| $N_1$ | Single clinically positive homolateral node, less than or equal to 3 cm |
| $N_2$ | One or more homolateral nodes, greater than 3 cm but less than or equal to 6 cm |
| $N_3$ | Bilateral, contralateral, or massive homolateral nodes, greater than 6 cm |
| **Distant Metastases** | |
| $M_X$ | Not assessed |
| $M_0$ | No distant metastases |
| $M_1$ | Distant metastases present (site specified) |
| **Stage Grouping** | |
| Stage I | $T_1$, $N_0$, $M_0$ |
| Stage II | $T_2$, $N_0$, $M_0$ |
| Stage III | $T_3$, $N_0$, $M_0$, any T, $N_1$, $M_0$ |
| Stage IV | $T_4$; any T, $N_2$–$N_3$, $M_0$; any T, any N, $M_1$ |

surgery or radiation. The decision to use surgery or radiation as the definitive therapy for small cancers is determined by multiple practical and personal factors (Table 95.2). Patients who fail either form of "curative" therapy can often be salvaged with additional therapy. The cumulative toxic effect of radiation upon normal tissues in the irradiated area limits the amount of radiation that can be given. Patients with advanced tumors usually require both surgery and radiation therapy. If this initial planned combined therapy does not cure the patient of the tumor, salvage with additional therapy is only occasionally successful.

**Table 95.2** Radiation Versus Surgery as Primary Treatment for Early Head and Neck Squamous Cell Cancer

| |
|---|
| Practical considerations |
| Availability and expertise of personnel and equipment |
| Cost |
| Prior history of radiation treatments |
| Resectability of tumor |
| Radiocurability of tumor |
| Number of tumor sites (radiation therapy better for multiple sites) |
| Personal considerations |
| Length of treatment |
| Compliance and transportation for daily radiotherapy |
| State of health |
| Preference |
| Prior experience |
| Surgical consent (1%–2% mortality rate) |

From Hill JH: Personal communication, Department of Surgery, University of Illinois at Chicago, 1987.

Chemotherapy is reserved for patients with advanced or metastatic disease that is unlikely to be cured with surgery and/or radiation alone. Chemotherapy can palliate symptoms of the cancer for varying time periods, but to date there is no evidence that chemotherapy, in any form, prolongs survival in patients with head and neck cancer. Reports of extended survival with the addition of chemotherapy in patients with resectable head and neck cancer have not included patients concurrently treated without chemotherapy.

The internal location of many tumors makes direct measurement difficult. Responses of head and neck cancers are often difficult to objectively assess visually or by palpation. In assessing response at our institution, we accept only those primary tumor or lymph node measurements that are directly obtained by physical examination or occasionally by CAT scan. Other interior cancers must also demonstrate stabilization or regression to allow the directly measured site(s) to be called a response. Complete response (CR) to therapy is defined as complete disappearance of tumor for a period of at least 1 month. Partial response (PR) is defined as a $\geq$50% reduction in the sum of the product of the largest perpendicular axes of the measured tumor sites. Overall response is the sum of complete and partial responses. Stabilization of the disease (responses less than 50%) may occasionally be considered "objective" or "clinical" responses but should not be included in the overall response rate.

### *Surgery*

Removal of all malignant tissues with appropriate margins of normal tissue is the optimal treatment for small, accessible cancers of the head and neck. Details of surgical management of the primary tumor depend upon the cancer site and size. For example, oral cavity and oropharyngeal tumors are treated with wide excision, with or without mandible excision (composite resection). Reconstruction is applied at the time of original resection and/or in subsequent surgical procedures. Laryngeal cancers are removed with either total laryngectomy or one of the conservative laryngeal procedures that preserve speech. Multiple procedures are described for resection of tumors of specific sites and stages.[16,17]

The ability to detect local nodal metastases depends on the number and size of the involved lymph nodes, the shape and muscular development of the neck, and the skill of the examiner. The incidence of failure to clinically detect involved cervical lymph nodes has been shown by subsequent pathologic examination to be 10% to 50%.[16] Elective, empiric resection of the cervical lymph nodes at risk is usually indicated when the historic risk of undetected nodal metastasis for the specific tumor site and stage exceeds 15%.[16]

The standard radical neck dissection is frequently performed for treatment of palpable cervical metastases. The superficial and deep cervical fascia with its enclosed lymph nodes is removed in continuity with the sternocleidomastoid and omohyoid muscles, the internal and external jugular veins, the spinal accessory nerve (XI), and the contents of the submandibular triangle. The accessory nerve, internal jugular vein, and sternocleidomastoid muscle may be spared in modifications of this procedure. A unilateral resection is performed unless bilateral disease is present or suspected.[9]

### *Radiotherapy*

Radiation therapy alone is often curative for patients with small ($T_1$ and $T_2$) head and neck cancers.[18,19] Radiation doses of 6,500 to 7,000 rads (or centigray units, cGy) are common and are usually administered in daily 200-rad fractions over 6.5 to 7 weeks. The decision to irradiate clinically uninvolved regions of the neck is based upon the histology of the tumor, its primary site, and the corresponding likelihood of subclinical metastases to the regional lymph nodes.

### *Radiotherapy/Surgery*

Moderate doses of radiation (5,000–6,000 rads) are used for advanced tumors before or after surgical resection. Presurgical irradiation (5,000–6,000 rads) avoids the delay in treatment resulting from postoperative convalescence, but it substantially increases the risk of delayed wound healing after surgery. In a randomized study by the Radiation Therapy Oncology Group (RTOG), no difference in survival between pre- and postoperative radiation therapy groups was found; however, preoperatively irradiated patients had up to a 2.5 times greater risk of surgical complications than did postoperatively radiated patients.[20] Radiation therapy is therefore most frequently used postoperatively, and should be initiated within 6 weeks of surgery.

### *Brachytherapy*

The implantation of radioactive isotopes (brachytherapy) has been used with good results in small, localized, accessible tumors. The dosimetry of the intended radiation exposure is first modeled with plane films and CAT scans. Under general anesthesia, hollow metal or plastic tubes are placed into or passed through the tumor. After surgery, these tubes are loaded with radioisotope "seeds" that either are permanent or are removed on a daily schedule to divide the total radiation dose. This "afterloading" technique has the advantage of preventing exposure of operating room personnel to radiation during the initial insertion of tubes into the tumor. The removable seeds have the added advantage of allowing rapid removal of the radiation source if necessary.

The most popular radioisotopes are iridium-192 and iodine-125 for temporary implants and iodine-125 for permanent implants. The amount of radiation to which the tissue surrounding the implants is exposed is very high, causing a greater local exposure of the tumor compared with surrounding normal tissues. In practice, radioisotope implants are usually combined with a moderate dose of external beam irradiation to treat the broader tumor field.[21]

### *Chemotherapy*

Chemotherapy is used in surgically resectable disease with a high likelihood of recurrence, unresectable advanced disease, and local or distant recurrence of disease.

Usually, antineoplastic agents for head and neck cancer are initially clinically tested in heavily pretreated patients that have refractory or advanced, unresectable disease. These patients are less likely to respond to a new drug because of the increased likelihood of pleiomorphic drug resistance or disruption of the structure and perfusion of the affected sites. Table 95.3 summarizes results from single-agent studies of the drugs most commonly incorporated into combination chemotherapy regimens for head and neck cancer. An overall response rate of 20% to 30% is seen with many of the single-agent studies. Increasing the dose of methotrexate offers no benefit. Administering 5-fluorouracil as a 4- to 5-day infusion increases the response rate over intravenous boluses, but has no proven effect on overall survival.

Patients with good performance status (ECOG 0–2) have a higher response rate than do those with poor performance status (ECOG 3–4).[22–24] The relationship between response and performance status may reflect malnutrition, immunodeficiency, concurrent diseases, and ability to tolerate full doses of antineoplastic drugs. A small primary tumor predicts a better response rate to chemotherapy.[24,25] Patients with disseminated, metastatic disease are unlikely to achieve a complete response, and their prognosis is dismal.

**Table 95.3** Results of Single-Agent Chemotherapy for Head and Neck Cancer[a]

| *Drug* | *Dose and schedule* | *N* | *CR + PR (%)* | *Reference* |
|---|---|---|---|---|
| MTX | 40–60 mg/m²/wk | 304 | 26 | 24, 26–29 |
| HDMTX | 240–1,500 mg/m² every 7–14 d | 99 | 26 | 27, 30 |
| Bleomycin | 15 U/m²/wk | 158 | 15 | 31 |
| Cisplatin | 80–120 mg/m² | 100 | 32 | 32 |
| 5-FU | (IVP) 15 mg/kg/d for 5 d then 7.5 mg/kg every 2–3 d | 118 | 15 | 29, 33, 34 |
| | (IV INF) 1 g/m²/d for 4–5 d | 11 | 72 | 34 |
| Vinblastine | 0.1–0.3 mg/kg/wk | 35 | 29 | 35 |

[a] MTX, methotrexate; HDMTX, high-dose methotrexate; 5-FU, 5-fluorouracil; IVP, intravenous bolus; INF, continuous infusion.

### Chemotherapy Concurrent With Radiotherapy

The rationale for use of chemotherapy concurrent with radiotherapy is based upon in vitro data that indicate a potentiation of radiation cytotoxicity by chemotherapy.[36–39] Although randomized trials have shown that combined drug and radiation treatment may provide a local response rate higher than that obtained with radiation treatment alone,[40,41] there is little or no survival benefit for patients treated with single-agent chemotherapy combined with radiation therapy.[42,43] For example, one randomized study found an increase in survival of only 1 to 4 months with adjunctive methotrexate.[44] In other studies, the survival benefit from addition of bleomycin or 5-fluorouracil (5-FU) to radiation appears limited to certain subsets of patients, such as those with primary disease of the oral cavity.[40,42] A large controlled study of radiation with or without 5-FU showed that combined therapy significantly improved the local response rate, but did not decrease the incidence of distant metastases.[42] Many patients receiving this combined therapy required hospitalization for severe mucosal reactions.

Cisplatin and 5-FU with radiation have been shown in an uncontrolled study to provide a 100% response rate in patients with advanced, unresectable head and neck cancer,[45] but the toxic effects (mucositis) were severe, with 52% of patients losing more than 10% of their body weight from inanition. The lack of controls and the wide variation in chemotherapy and radiation treatment schedules make such studies difficult to evaluate and compare. At present, the combination of radiation and chemotherapy has not been shown to prolong survival of head and neck cancer patients.

### Multimodality Therapy

Induction or ''neoadjuvant'' chemotherapy is the systemic administration of drugs to previously untreated patients prior to, rather than concurrent with, such definitive therapy as surgery and radiation. Alternatively, chemotherapy may be administered after definitive local therapy (''adjuvant treatment'') to eradicate subclinical regional or distant metastatic disease. Regardless of the sequence, the intent of this multimodal treatment is cure, in contrast to the palliative treatment given patients with recurrent or metastatic disease. Current induction chemotherapy can yield complete and partial responses in the majority of patients, but the duration of response is short unless surgery and/or radiation follow.[46]

Despite providing overall response rates of up to 100% in uncontrolled trials, induction chemotherapy has not been proven in randomized studies to prolong survival as compared with surgery and/or radiation.[47] Most trials of chemotherapy for head and neck cancer have not incorporated a control for surgery and/or radiation alone. Toxic effects are common with chemotherapy and are potentially lethal. Induction chemotherapy should therefore be considered an unproven, experimental treatment modality that should not be used in the routine management of patients with head and neck cancer.

Patients who completely or partially respond to induction chemotherapy should receive subsequent surgery plus radiation. If the tumor is unresectable or the patient is a poor surgical risk, radiation alone can be given. One study evaluated the effect of surgery after two induction courses of cisplatin and bleomycin.[48] At surgery, three of four complete clinical responders were found to have gross residual disease at the primary site. The same number of complete clinical responders were found to have tumor involvement of local lymph nodes after dissection and microscopic evaluation. These findings suggest that preoperative chemotherapy did not reliably eradicate primary or metastatic disease[48]; however, a small pilot study suggests that patients with biopsy-proven complete response after chemotherapy be treated with radiation alone.[49] Additional follow-up and larger studies are needed to confirm these results.

Despite a recent pilot study with a short follow-up showing no difference in survival, there are few data to establish the proper sequence for administration of chemotherapy relative to surgery or radiation.[50] Patients who undergo surgery must usually recuperate for several weeks before chemotherapy is instituted. This delay may allow residual tumor cells to grow or disseminate to distant sites; however, as surgical dissection after response to chemotherapy must include adequate margins beyond the original perimeter of the tumor, induction chemotherapy may impair identification of the initial extent of disease at the time of surgical dissection.

In addition, up to one third of patients experiencing a response to induction chemotherapy refuse surgery.[50] Disfigurement from surgery and relief of symptoms after che-

**Table 95.4** Results of Induction Chemotherapy for Head and Neck Cancer[a]

| *Reference* | *Regimen* | *N* | *Overall response (CR + PR, %)* | *% CR before surgery* | *Median duration of survival (mo)* CR | PR | R | NR | All |
|---|---|---|---|---|---|---|---|---|---|
| 18 | Surgery and/or RT | | — | — | | | | | |
| 54 | Surgery and/or RT | | | | | 38%–50% 3-year survival | | | |
| 55 | Surgery and/or RT | 27 | — | — | NG | NG | NG | NG | 40 |
| 55 | MTX | 28 | 73 | 5 | NG | NG | NG | NG | 40 |
| 54 | HDMTX with LV rescue | 30 | 77 | NG | NG | NG | NG | NG | NG |
| 44 | MTX + RT | 312 | NG | NG | | (12.4–19.2 all patients) | | | |
| 44 | RT only | 326 | | | | (9.7–17.2 all patients) | | | |
| 52 | CDDP + Bleo | 29 | 48 | 0 | >13 | NG | NG | NG | NG |
| 53 | CDDP + Bleo | 21 | 71 | 19 | >12 | >10 | >11 | 4 | 9 |
| 48 | CDDP + Bleo | 40 | 76 | 20 | >9.5 | 8 | 8 | 7.5 | 8 |
| 56 | CDDP + MTX + Bleo | 22 | 73 | 18 | NG | NG | NG | NG | >6 |
| 57 | CDDP + MTX + Bleo | 114 | 78 | 26 | NG | NG | NG | NG | NG |
| 58 | CDDP + VBL + Bleo | 63 | 65 | 22 | 52 | 12 | NG | 10 | NG |
| 59 | CDDP + VBL + Bleo | 23 | 74 | 22 | >10 | NG | NG | NG | NG |
| 60 | "COB" CDDP + VCR + Bleo | 77 | 79 | 29 | >19 | 19 | 19 | 35 | 77 |
| 61 | | 37 | 67 | 5 | NG | NG | >16 | NG | >16 |
| 62 | | 48 | 88 | 22 | NG | NG | NG | NG | >40 |
| 51 | CDDP + 5-FU | 19 | 84 | 26 | >14 | NG | NG | 6 | >8 |
| 63 | CDDP + 5-FU | 61 | 93 | 54 | NG | NG | NG | NG | >18 |
| 64 | CDDP + 5-FU | 31 | 84 | 23 | >5 | NG | NG | NG | >22 |
| 65 | CDDP + 5-FU | 60 | 87 | 37 | NG | NG | NG | NG | 23 |
| 66[b] | CDDP + Bleo + MTX + 5-FU (IVP) | 167 | 65 | 7 III IV | 64–>96 | NG | 22–38 | 8–19 | 17–38 |

[a] CR, complete response; PR, partial response; R, all responders; NR, nonresponders; HDMTX, high-dose methotrexate; N, number of evaluable patients; NG, not given; CDDP, cisplatin; Bleo, bleomycin; LV, leucovorin; RT, radiation therapy; VBL, vinblastine; VCR, vincristine; 5-FU, 5-fluorouracil; IVP, intravenous push.

[b] Survival reported for stages III and IV.

motherapy affect the patient's decision to refuse definitive treatment. Most of these patients experience a locoregional relapse of their disease.[14,51] Although in most of the recent, uncontrolled studies chemotherapy has been administered before surgery, additional controlled studies are needed to decide the optimal sequence.

Current induction chemotherapy in patients with stage III or IV head and neck cancer can be expected to yield a complete response rate of 25% to 50%, with an overall response rate of 48% to 93%. The 2-year disease-free survival is approximately 80% for patients achieving a complete response to chemotherapy with subsequent surgical dissection and/or radiation therapy. Most patients with stage III or IV head and neck cancer who achieve a partial response to current chemotherapy regimens can be rendered disease free with surgery and radiation or with radiation treatment alone.[51] Despite encouraging response rates, there is no consistent evidence that chemotherapy increases the survival of patients with advanced head and neck cancer compared with surgery and radiation alone.

***Cisplatin and Bleomycin*** Induction chemotherapy with bleomycin and cisplatin is effective in obtaining responses in advanced head and neck cancer.[48,50,52] In most trials bleomycin has been used as a 5- to 7-day continuous infusion of 10–15 U/m$^2$ per day after an initial intravenous bolus of 10–15 /U/m$^2$. The dose of cisplatin varied from 80 to 120 mg/m$^2$ as a 20-minute bolus or a 24-hour infusion.[48,50,52] Overall response rates ranged from 48% to 76% and complete responses varied from 0% to 20% (Table 95.4). Although the response to chemotherapy varied among studies, there was no significant difference in complete response rate after completion of subsequent surgery and/or radiation.[52,53]

***Cisplatin and 5-Fluorouracil*** 5-Fluorouracil has been substituted for bleomycin in an effort to avoid pulmonary toxicity and because of evidence of synergy with cisplatin in animal models. Increasing the duration of 5-FU infusion from 4 to 5 days (1,000 mg/in$^2$ per day) increased the overall response rate from 70% to 93%.[63] The 54% complete response rate obtained by this group has not been confirmed in studies of comparable patients receiving similar 5-day infusions of 5-FU (Table 95.5).

Intravenous bolus doses of 5-FU on days 1 and 8 were tried in an effort to make the cisplatin/fluorouracil infusion combination more amenable to outpatient administration. The change from 5-day infusion to bolus 5-FU resulted in significantly lower response rates (20% versus 72%).[23] The moderate mucositis observed with infusion regimens was replaced by severe, life-threatening myelosuppression.[23]

In contrast with the favorable results initially reported with cisplatin and 5-FU, a randomized study of 50 patients

**Table 95.5** Results of Induction Therapy With Cisplatin and 5-Fluorouracil[a]

| | *Cisplatin* | | | | |
|---|---|---|---|---|---|
| *Reference* | **Dose (mg/m²)** | **Infusion rate (h)** | *CR (%)* | *PR (%)* | *CR + PR (%)* |
| Kish (Wayne State[23]) | 100 | IV bolus | 54 | 39 | 93 |
| Dasmahaptra[51] | 100 | 1–2 | 26 | 58 | 84 |
| Amrein[64] | 80 | 24 | 22 | 61 | 83 |
| Kies[65] | 100 | 1–2 | 37 | 50 | 87 |

[a] Results from rapid versus 24-hour infusion of cisplatin.

indicated that treatment with cisplatin and 5-FU does not improve the clinical results of surgery and radiation therapy.[67] This and other small negative trials emphasize the lack of convincing evidence that chemotherapy affects the prognosis of patients with advanced or recurrent head and neck cancer. A prospective, randomized study has been initiated to compare surgery + radiation with surgery + chemotherapy (cisplatin + 5-FU) + radiation. This controlled study will help define the efficacy of adjuvant cisplatin and 5-FU in operable, advanced head and neck cancer.

***Multiple Drugs*** Common additions to the cisplatin + bleomycin and cisplatin + 5-FU infusion regimens are vincristine and methotrexate. The addition of a third or fourth agent has not provided consistent, significant improvements in overall response, complete response rate, or duration of remission or survival (Table 95.4).

### Chemotherapy for Recurrent or Disseminated Disease

Patients with recurrent or disseminated head and neck cancer have a grim prognosis. If possible, recurrent disease should be excised and/or irradiated. In recent multimodal salvage regimens, disease was surgically resected after a partial or complete response to preoperative chemotherapy. Unresectable recurrences are common, however, and previous radiotherapy may limit additional doses to subcurative levels. Patients treated with single-agent chemotherapy have a median survival of 5 months, which is not significantly longer than that for untreated patients (Table 95.6).

Cisplatin and bleomycin have been combined in several trials with overall response rates of 24% to 61%.[26,48,53,59,61,69] The increased response rate over weekly methotrexate has not led to any increase in the duration of survival. The use of bleomycin in patients previously irradiated in the head and neck region has resulted in a high incidence of mucositis.

The median duration of survival for patients treated with cisplatin and a 5-day infusion of 5-FU was 6 months, because of the short survival of nonresponding patients or of nonresectable, partially responding patients; however, the median survival of post-surgical complete responders had not been reached at 28 weeks.[23] Another group using a similar regimen reported a 17% complete response rate to chemotherapy, with four of the five complete responders alive at 12 months.[64] These trials suggest that the combination of cisplatin and 5-fluorouracil by infusion can produce durable remissions in the limited number (20%) of patients with recurrent or disseminated disease who achieve a complete response after chemotherapy and subsequent surgery and/or radiotherapy. The short follow-up in these reports precludes predictions of the actual duration of response or survival. No controlled study has demonstrated a benefit from the addition of chemotherapy over salvage surgery and radiation alone.[24,26,28]

## Future Directions

### *Intraarterial Infusions*

Investigators have explored the use of intraarterial infusions in the treatment of head and neck cancer.[71] Most early work utilized transcutaneous arterial catheters to deliver such drugs as methotrexate, bleomycin, 5-fluorouracil, and more recently cisplatin.[29,72,73] Although, theoretically, intraarterial delivery should provide increased concentrations of cytotoxic drugs in the blood perfusing the tumor, no drug given by intraarterial infusion has been shown to have a clinically significant dose–response effect for head and neck cancer. Local toxicity can be more severe than with intravenous administration. Nonrandomized, clinical trials of intraarterial infusions in head and neck cancer patients have not demonstrated a clear response advantage for this route of administration.[74,75] For these reasons, intraarterial infusions cannot be recommended for the routine treatment of patients with head and neck cancer.[74]

### *Radiation Sensitizers and Heavy Particle Irradiation*

Drugs have been studied for use as radiation sensitizers, to enhance the cytotoxicity of radiation in large, poorly vascularized and hypoxic tumors.[76] The most extensively studied drug is the metronidazole congener misonidazole. The mechanism by which it potentiates the effect of radiation on hypoxic cells is not known.[77] An increased response rate was seen in 68 patients given 11 g/m² in either 8 or 20 fractions before the corresponding radiation treatments; however, overall survival was not significantly extended by the use of this sensitizing agent and dose-limiting neurotoxic effects were common.[76,78] Two cooperative oncology groups have initiated separate prospective, randomized trials evaluating the benefit of misonidazole with radiation in the treatment of head and neck cancer. Less neurotoxic drugs

**Table 95.6** Treatment of Recurrent or Disseminated Head and Neck Cancer[a]

| *Reference* | *Regimen* | *N* | *CR (%)* | *CR + PR (%)* | *Median duration of survival (mo)* | | | | |
|---|---|---|---|---|---|---|---|---|---|
| | | | | | **CR** | **PR** | **CR + PR** | **NR** | **All** |
| 14 | No treatment | 30 | — | — | | | | | 5–6 |
| 30 | | 81 | 7 | 26 | NG | NG | 7 | 4 | 5 |
| 26 | MTX (standard dose) | 98 | NG | 16 | NG | NG | 9 | 6 | 7 |
| 24 | (40–60 mg/m² IV | 83 | 8 | 35 | 10 | 8 | 10 | 5 | 6 |
| 28 | weekly) | 24 | 8 | 33 | NG | NG | 9 | 3 | 6 |
| 27 | | 18 | 0 | 22 | NG | NG | NG | NG | 4 |
| 30 | MTX (high dose with | 80 | 3 | 24 | NG | NG | 5 | 4 | 4 |
| 27 | rescue) | 19 | 5 | 32 | NG | NG | NG | NG | 4 |
| 53 | CDDP + Bleo | 12 | 0 | 33 | NG | NG | NG | NG | NG |
| 24 | CDDP + MTX + Bleo | 85 | 16 | 48 | 10 | 8 | 10 | 5 | 6 |
| 26 | CDDP + VBL + Bleo | 92 | NG | 24 | NG | NG | 9 | 6 | 7 |
| 28 | | 27 | 11 | 41 | NG | NG | 9 | 3 | 4 |
| 59 | CDDP + VCR + Bleo | 22 | 9 | 45 | NG | NG | NG | NG | NG |
| 61 | | 33 | 3 | 30 | NG | NG | 12 | 5 | 6 |
| 69 | | 26 | 23 | 61 | >6 | 3 | NG | 4 | 4 |
| 68[b] | CDDP + 5-FU (96 h) | 30 | 27 | 70 | 11[c] | 7[c] | 8 | 3 | 6 |
| 64 | CDDP + 5-FU (120 h) | 39 | 17 | 46 | >12 | 9 | NG | 8 | 9 |
| 23[b] | CDDP + 5-FU (96 h) | 18 | 22 | 72 | >28 | 7 | NG | 5 | 6 |

[a] CR, complete response; PR, partial response; MTX, methotrexate; LV, leucovorin; CDDP, cisplatin; Bleo, bleomycin; VBL, vinblastine; VCR, vincristine; 5-FU, 5-fluorouracil; NG, not given.
[b] Serial studies by same group.
[c] Average survival duration.

such as SR-2508 are also being evaluated as possible radiation sensitizers.[79]

The use of nuclear particles such as neutrons or pions in the treatment of head and neck cancer is presently under study. Theoretically, these beams provide a higher cytotoxic effect for a given amount of normal tissue damage than current radiation sources, particularly in large tumors that may be hypoxic.[80] The role of radiation sensitizers or nuclear particle therapy in the treatment of head and neck cancer patients remains to be established in phase III clinical trials.

## Minimization of Antineoplastic Toxicity

Nephrotoxicity remains the dose-limiting toxic effect of cisplatin and can be minimized with adequate hydration and diuresis. Diuresis should be maintained for at least 4 hours after completion of a cisplatin infusion.[81] Regimens utilizing lower cisplatin doses of 60–80 mg/m² have successfully been applied to outpatients,[69] but most clinicians hospitalize patients for the high-dose cisplatin (100 mg/m²) used in some head and neck cancer protocols.[23,64] This caution arises in part from concerns about the patient's ability to comply with pretreatment oral fluid loading at home.

Cumulative cisplatin doses greater than 200 mg/m² appear to increase the likelihood of a hearing deficit, but this attenuation of high-frequency hearing often does not interfere with conversation and may go unnoticed in adults.[82] Audiograms are not necessary for all adult patients, but pretreatment audiograms are prudent for patients in whom there may be a preexisting hearing loss.

Nausea and vomiting are common and often severe. All patients receiving cisplatin should receive prophylactic antiemetic medications. (See Chapter 29).

Mucositis is the acute dose-limiting toxic effect of bleomycin in head and neck cancer patients and may be particularly severe if the patient is receiving local radiotherapy concurrently. Rashes and skin changes are seen in up to 50% of patients, but these effects rarely restrict use of the drug.[31] The dose of bleomycin should be decreased or eliminated in patients with moderate to severe renal dysfunction.

Hypersensitivity and anaphylaxis are seen in less than 1% of head and neck cancer patients. Test doses of bleomycin are not routinely used for head and neck cancer patients, but emergency drug and resuscitative equipment should always be available. Up to 50% of patients may experience a transient fever during and/or shortly after the administration of bleomycin.

Pulmonary fibrosis is seen in approximately 4% of head and neck cancer patients.[83,84] It may present as a dry, nonproductive cough with dyspnea or as fine, cellophane rales at lung bases. Risk factors that may predispose a patient to this adverse effect include cumulative dose greater than 200 mg/m², age (≥ 70 years), preexisting lung disease (common in patients with head and neck cancer), irradiation of the lungs, exposure to high concentrations of inspired oxygen ($Fio_2 \geq 35\%$). Renal dysfunction may also increase the risk.[84]

Bleomycin-induced pulmonary fibrosis is not usually reversible, but may stabilize if no additional drug is administered. Progression of the fibrosis and hypoxia is frequent and the overall mortality is approximately 50%.[83] Anecdotal reports suggest that corticosteroids may allow some subjective and objective improvement, particularly in cases with a possible hypersensitivity component.[85]

Mucositis is a common problem in patients with head and neck cancer undergoing chemotherapy. It is caused by the cytotoxic action of antineoplastic drugs upon the epithelial cells of the gatrointestinal tract. It can be associated with severe pain, anorexia, and reduced oral intake. Bleomycin, methotrexate, and 5-FU are commonly associated with mucositis. Drug-induced mucositis is potentiated by previous or concurrent radiation therapy.

Recommendations for the treatment of mucositis are empiric. Salty or acidic foods or fluids (e.g., potassium chloride, orange juice) may irritate the raw mucosa. Oral pain can be attenuated by rinsing the mouth with viscous lidocaine (2%) or a 0.5% to 1.0% solution of dyclomine. Although they often blunt taste, when given before meals such anesthetics may enhance food and fluid ingestion by decreasing the discomfort of chewing and swallowing. It is important to instruct the patient to spit out the excess lidocaine to minimize the risk of central nervous system toxicity, particularly if the patient has liver disease or is allowed to freely self-medicate.[86] Some patients find that a mixture of 15–30 mL of an antacid or kaolin/pectin suspension and diphenhydramine decreases oral pain and provides a coating that extends the relief. An intravenous formulation of diphenhydramine may be used to avoid possible irritation from the ethanol used in the elixir. A suspension of sucralfate may decrease the duration and severity of mucositis.[87]

Irradiation of the mandible or maxilla can lead to dental and periodontal disease, mucositis, dental necrosis, and, less commonly, osteonecrosis of the underlying bone. These complications are more common in patients who do not maintain good oral hygeine.[88] Irradiation of the salivary glands decreases saliva volume and increases its viscosity and acidity. Frequent rinses with solutions of sodium bicarbonate and sodium chloride help to neutralize and remove the tenacious saliva; occasionally, hydrogen peroxide may be added to the regimen to loosen scales and decrease bacterial overgrowth.

Xerostomia (dryness of the mouth and throat) is a common long-term effect of irradiation of the salivary glands.[88] The lack of saliva impairs taste, chewing, and swallowing, and increases the incidence of periodontal disease. Several artificial saliva products containing electrolytes in a carboxymethylcellulose base for viscosity and durability are commercially available: Saliva Substitute (Roxane), Orex (Young Dental), Xero-Lube (Scherer), Moi-Stir (Kingswood), Salivart (Westport Pharmaceutical). While helpful and nontoxic, these products require frequent administration. Less expensive and more readily available alternatives to commercial products include sugarless candies, ice chips, and ample fluid made available for sipping during mealtime.

Inanition is common in head and neck cancer patients and is caused by a loss of appetite, dental pain (periodontal disease, radiation-induced osteonecrosis, carious teeth), difficulty in chewing because of radiation-induced xerostomia, or pain or stricture when swallowing. Percutaneous placement of a gastrostomy ("G") tube is a common intervention in patients who have significant pharyngeal (or esophageal) restriction, extended anorexia, or an incompetent swallowing process that makes the risk of aspiration prohibitive. Gastrostomy tubes and enteral nutrition are covered in greater detail in Chapter 110.

Patients with advanced, ulcerating or fungating head and neck cancer may have a "smelly tumor." These foul odors may be caused by anaerobic bacteria despite a lack of microbiological evidence of infection. Anecdotal experience and reports of treating advanced breast cancer patients have found that chronic oral metronidazole therapy (250 mg twice to three times daily) is helpful in suppressing this noncritical but bothersome problem.[89] Some head and neck cancer patients experienced a decrease in local pain when administered an oral penicillin or first-generation cephalosporin.[90] It was suggested that even in the absence of classic signs of infection such as fever or leukocytosis, secondary bacterial infections may exacerbate the pain experienced by some patients with head and neck cancer. An empiric trial of oral antibiotics can be considered for head and neck cancer patients who experience an unexplained, rapidly changing pain pattern.[90] In addition, it is prudent to immunize head and neck cancer patients with annual influenza vaccinations.

## Summary

Few diseases require such an integration of treatment modalities and cooperation between medical disciplines as does head and neck cancer. Despite a general lack of proven effect on overall patient survival, drug therapy for head and neck cancer is increasingly aggressive and requires careful supervision to minimize life-threatening or debilitating adverse effects. Careful attention to supportive treatment and preventative measures such as hydration, antiemetic prophylaxis, oral care, and pain control maximizes the therapeutic index of combined treatment of head and neck cancer and provides maximal comfort for the patient.

## Acknowledgments

The authors acknowledge the contributions of Dr. James H. Hill, MD, Assistant Professor, Department of Otolaryngology–Head and Neck Surgery, University of Illinois College of Medicine, Chicago, and Chief of Otolaryngology–Head and Neck Surgery, West Side Veterans Administration Medical Center, Chicago.

## References

1. Silverberg E, Lubera J. Cancer statistics, 1986. CA 1986;36: 9–25.
2. Schottenfeld D, Bergad BM. Epidemiology of cancers of the oral cavity, pharynx, and larynx, in Wittes RE (ed): Head and Neck Cancer. New York, John Wiley and Sons, 1985.
3. Hodge KM, Flynn MB, Drury T. Squamous cell carcinoma of the upper aerodigestive tract in non-users of tobacco. Cancer 1985;55:1232–1235.

4. Atkinson D, Fleming S, Weaver A. Triple endoscopy: A valuable procedure in head and neck cancer surgery. Am J Surg 1982;144:416–419.
5. Decker J, Goldstein JC. Risk factors in head and neck cancer. N Engl J Med 1982;306:1151–1155.
6. Vainio H, Heseltine E. Tobacco and cancer. Cancer Res 1986;46:444–447.
7. Anonymous. Health effects of smokeless tobacco. JAMA 1986;255:1038–1044.
8. Jesse RH. General considerations, in Suen JY, Myers EN (eds): Cancer of the Head and Neck. New York, Churchill Livingstone, 1981, pp 1–11.
9. Million RR, Cassisi NJ, Wittes RE. Cancer in the head and neck, in DeVita VT, Hellman S, Rosenberg SA (eds): Cancer: Principles and Practice of Oncology, lst ed. Philadelphia, J.B. Lippincott, 1982, pp. 407–506.
10. Lingeman RE, Singer MI. Evaluation of the patient with head and neck cancer, in Suen JY, Myers EN (eds): Cancer of the Head and Neck. New York, Churchill Livingstone, 1981; pp 12–24.
11. Strong EW, Spiro RH. Cancer of the oral cavity, in Suen JY, Myers EN (eds): Cancer of the Head and Neck. New York, Churchill Livingstone, 1981, pp 301–341.
12. Lindberg R. Distribution of cervical lymph node metastases from squamous cell carcinoma of the upper respiratory and digestive tracts. Cancer 1972;29:1446–1449.
13. Merino OR, Lindberg RD, Fletcher GH. An analysis of distant metastases from squamous cell carcinoma of the upper respiratory and digestive tracts. Cancer 1977;40:145–151.
14. Hong WK, Bromer RH, Amato DA, et al. Patterns of relapse in locally advanced head and neck cancer patients who achieved complete remission after combined modality therapy. Cancer 1985;56:1242–1245.
15. American Joint Committee on Cancer. Beahrs OH, Myers MH (eds): Manual for staging of cancer, 2nd ed. Philadelphia, J. B. Lippincott, 1983.
16. Shedd DP. Surgical treatment of head and neck cancer, in Hamner JE III (ed): The Management of Head and Neck Cancer. New York, Springer Verlag, 1984, pp. 192–206.
17. DeSanto LW. Treatment options in early cancers of the larynx, in Chretien PB, Johns ME, Shedd DP, et al. (eds): Head and Neck Cancer. St. Louis, C.V. Mosby, 1985, pp. 203–213.
18. Marcial VA, Pajak TF. Radiation therapy alone or in combination with surgery in head and neck cancer. Cancer 1985;55: 2259–2265.
19. Fletcher GH. Place of irradiation in the management of head and neck cancers. Semin Oncol 1977;4:375–385.
20. Snow JB, Gelber RDE, Kramer S, et al. Comparison of preoperative and postoperative radiation therapy for patients with carcinoma of the head and neck. Acta Otolaryngol 1981;91:611–626.
21. Vikram B. Brachytherapy, in Wittes RE (ed): Head and Neck Cancer. New York, John Wiley and Sons, 1985, pp 121–136.
22. Oken MM, Creech RH, Tormey DC, et al. Toxicity and response criteria of the Eastern Cooperative Oncology Group, Am J Clin Oncol 1982;5:649–655.
23. Kish JA, Ensley JF, Jacobs J, et al. A randomized trial of cisplatin (CACP) + 5-fluorouracil (5-FU) infusion and CACP + 5-FU bolus for recurrent and advanced squamous cell carcinoma of the head and neck. Cancer 1985;56:2740–2744.
24. Vogl SE, Schoenfeld DA, Kaplan BH, et al. A randomized prospective comparison of methotrexate with a combination of methotrexate, bleomycin, and cisplatin in head and neck cancer. Cancer 1985;56:432–442.
25. Wolf GT, Makuch RW, Baker SR. Predictive factors of tumor response to preoperative chemotherapy in patients with head and neck squamous carcinoma. Cancer 1984;54:2869–2877.
26. Williams SD, Velez-Garcia E, Essessee I, et al. Chemotherapy for head and neck cancer: Comparison of cisplatin + vinblastine + bleomycin versus methotrexate. Cancer 1986;57:18–23.
27. Taylor SG, McGuire WP, Hauck WW, et al. A randomized comparison of high-dose methotrexate versus standard-dose weekly therapy in head and neck squamous cancer. J Clin Oncol 1984;2:1006–1011.
28. Drelichman, A, Cummings G, Al-Sarraf M. A randomized trial of the combination of cis-platinum, Oncovin, and bleomycin (COB) versus methotrexate in patients with advanced squamous cell carcinoma of the head and neck. Cancer 1983;52:399–403.
29. Carter SK. The chemotherapy of head and neck cancer. Semin Oncol 1977;4:413–424.
30. DeConti RC, Schoenfeld D. A randomized prospective comparison of intermittent methotrexate, methotrexate with leucovorin, and a methotrexate combination in head and neck cancer. Cancer 1981;48:1061–1072.
31. Blum RH, Carter S, Agre K. A clinical review of bleomycin—a new antineoplastic agent. Cancer 1973;31:903–914.
32. Goldsmith MA, Greenspan EM. Chemotherapy for head and neck cancer, in Greenspan EM (ed): Clinical Interpretation and Practice of Cancer Chemotherapy. New York, Raven, 1982, pp 361–372.
33. Amer MH, Al-Sarraf M, Vaitkevicius VK. Factors that affect response to chemotherapy and survival of patients with advanced head and neck cancer. Cancer 1979;43:2202–2206.
34. Tapazoglou E, Kish J, Ensley J, et al. The activity of a single-agent 5-fluorouracil infusion in advanced and recurrent head and neck cancer. Cancer 1986;57:1105–1109.
35. Smart CR, Rochlin DB, Nahum AM, et al. Clinical experience with vinblastine sulfate (NSC-49842) in squamous cell carcinoma and other malignancies. Cancer Chemother Rep 1964;34: 31–45.
36. Fu KK. Concurrent radiotherapy and chemotherapy, in Wittes RE (ed): Head and Neck Cancer. New York, John Wiley and Sons, 1985, pp 221–248.
37. Vietti T, Eggerding F, Valeriote F. Combined effect of x-radiation and 5-fluorouracil on survival of transplanted leukemic cells. J Natl Cancer Inst 1971;47:865–870.
38. Sinclair WK. The combined effect of hydroxyurea and x-rays on Chinese hamster cells in vitro. Cancer Res 1968;28:190–206.
39. Terasima T, Takabe Y, Yasukawa M. Combined effect of x-ray and bleomycin on cultured mammalian cells. Gann 1975;66:701–703.
40. Shanta V, Krishnamurthi S. Combined bleomycin and radiotherapy in oral cancer. Clin Radiol 1980;31:617–620.
41. Condit PT. Treatment of carcinoma with radiation therapy and methotrexate. Mo Med 1968;65:832–835.
42. Lo TC, Wiley Jr AL, Ansfield FJ, et al. Combined radiation therapy and 5-fluorouracil for advanced squamous cell carcinoma of the oral cavity and oropharynx: A randomized study. Am J Roentgenol 1976;126:229–235.
43. Stefani S, Eells RW, Abbate J. Hydroxyurea and radiotherapy in head and neck cancer. Radiology 1971;101:391–396.
44. Fazecas J, Sommer C, Kramer S. Adjuvant intravenous methotrexate or definitive radiotherapy alone for advanced squamous cancers of the oral cavity, oropharynx, supraglottic larynx, or hypopharynx. Int J Radiat Oncol Biol Phys 1980;6:533–541.
45. Taylor SG, Murthy AK, Showel JL, et al. Improved control in advanced head and neck cancer with simultaneous radiation and cisplatin/5-fluorouracil chemotherapy. Cancer Treat Rep 1985; 69:933.
46. Glick JH, Taylor SG. Integration of chemotherapy into a

combined modality treatment plan for head and neck cancer: A review. Int J Radiat Oncol Biol Phys 1981;7:229–242.

47. Tannaock IF, Browman G. Lack of evidence for a role of chemotherapy in the routine management of locally advanced head and neck cancer. J Clin Oncol 1986;4:1121–1126.

48. Hong WK, Shapshay SM, Bhutani R, et al. Induction chemotherapy in advanced squamous head and neck carcinoma with high dose *cis*-platinum and bleomycin infusion. Cancer 1979;44: 19–25.

49. Jacobs C, Goffinet D, Fee W, et al. Chemotherapy as a substitute for surgery in the treatment of advanced operable head and neck cancer: An NCOG pilot. Proc Am Soc Clin Oncol 1985;4:137(C-534).

50. Al-Sarraf M, Pajak T, Laramore G. Timing of chemotherapy as part of definitive treatment for patients with advanced head and neck cancer: An RTOG study. Proc Am Soc Clin Oncol 1985;4: 141(C-550).

51. Dasmahaptra KS, Citrin P, Hill GJ, et al. A prospective evaluation of 5-fluorouracil plus cisplatin in advanced squamous-cell cancer of the head and neck. J Clin Oncol 1985;3: 1486–1489.

52. Glick JH, Marcial V, Richter M, et al. The adjuvant treatment of inoperable stage III-IV epidermoid carcinoma of the head and neck with platinum and bleomycin infusions prior to definitive radiotherapy: An RTOG pilot study. Cancer 1980;46:1919–1924.

53. Randolph VL, Vallejo A, Spiro RH, et al. Combination therapy of advanced head and neck cancer: Induction of remissions with diamminedichloroplatinum (II), bleomycin, and radiation therapy. Cancer 1978;41:460–467.

54. Tarpley JL, Chretien PB, Alexander JC, et al. High dose methotrexate as a preoperative adjuvant in the treatment of epidermoid carcinoma of the head and neck: A feasibility study and clinical trial. Am J Surg 1975;130:481–486.

55. Rentschler RE, Wilbur DW, Petti GH, et al. Adjuvant methotrexate escalated to toxicity for resectable stage III and IV squamous head and neck carcinoma—a prospective, randomized study. J Clin Oncol 1987;5:278–285.

56. Elias EG, Chretien PB, Monnard E, et al. Chemotherapy prior to local therapy in advanced squamous cell carcinoma of the head and neck: Preliminary assessment of an intensive drug regimen. Cancer 1979;43:1025–1031.

57. Weichselbaum RR, Miller D, Pitman SW, et al. Initial adjuvant weekly high dose methotrexate with leucovorin rescue in advanced squamous carcinoma of the head and neck. Int J Radiat Oncol Biol Phys 1978;4:671–674.

58. Perry DJ, Davis RK, Zajtchuk JR, et al. Vinblastine, bleomycin, and cisplatin in the treatment of squamous carcinoma of the head and neck, in Jones SE, Salmon SE (eds): Adjuvant Therapy of Cancer IV. Proceedings of the Fourth International Conference on the Adjuvant Therapy of Cancer. New York, Grune and Stratton, 1984, pp 135–143.

59. Brown AW, Blom J, Butler WM. Combination chemotherapy with vinblastine, bleomycin, and *cis*-diamminedichloroplatinum (II) in squamous cell carcinoma of the head and neck. Cancer 1980;45:2830–2835.

60. Al-Sarraf M, Drelichman A, Jacobs J, et al. Adjuvant chemotherapy with *cis*-platinum, Oncovin, and bleomycin followed by surgery and/or radiotherapy in patients with advanced previously untreated head and neck cancer: Final report, in Jones SE, Salmon SE (eds): Adjuvant Therapy of Cancer. New York, Grune and Stratton, 1981; Vol 3, pp 145–152.

61. Amrein PC, Fingert H, Weitzman SA. Cisplatin–vincristine–bleomycin therapy in squamous cell carcinoma of the head and neck. J Clin Oncol 1983;1:421–427.

62. Spaulding SE, Kahn A, De Los Santos R, et al. Adjuvant chemotherapy in advanced head and neck cancer: An update. Am J Surg 1982;144:432–436.

63. Rooney M, Kish J, Jacobs J, et al. Improved complete response rate and survival in advanced head and neck cancer after three-course induction therapy with 120-hour and 5-FU infusion and cisplatin. Cancer 1985;55:1123–1128.

64. Amrein PC, Weitzman SA. Treatment of squamous cell carcinoma of the head and neck with cisplatin and 5-fluorouracil. J Clin Oncol 1985;3:1632–1639.

65. Kies MS, Lester EP, Gordon LI, et al. Cisplatin and infusion 5-fluorouracil (5-FU) in stage III and IV squamous cancer of the head and neck. Proc Am Soc Clin Oncol 1985;4:139(C-540).

66. Price LA, Hill BL. Impact of primary site of stage III and IV squamous cell carcinomas, in Ragaz J, Band PR, Goldie JH (eds): Preoperative (Neoadjuvant) Chemotherapy. Recent Results in Cancer Research. New York, Springer-Verlag, 1986, pp 124–134.

67. Haas C, Byhardt R, Cox J, et al. Randomized study of 5-fluorouracil and *cis*-platinum as initial therapy of locally advanced squamous carcinoma of the head and neck. Proc Am Soc Clin Oncol 1985;4:143(C-557).

68. Kish JA, Weaver A, Jacobs J, et al. Cisplatin and 5-fluorouracil infusion in patients with recurrent and disseminated epidermoid cancer of the head and neck. Cancer 1984;53:1819–1824.

69. Vogl SE, Kaplan BH. Chemotherapy of advanced head and neck cancer with methotrexate, bleomycin, and *cis*-diamminedichloroplatinum II in an effective outpatient schedule. Cancer 1979;44:26–31.

70. Spaulding M, Ziegler P, Sundquist N, et al. Induction therapy in head and neck cancer: A comparison of two regimens. Cancer 1986;57:1110–1114.

71. Baker SR, Wheeler R. Intraarterial chemotherapy for head and neck cancer. Part 1: Theoretical considerations and drug delivery systems. Head Neck Surg 1983;6:664–682.

72. Baker SR, Wheeler R. Intraarterial chemotherapy for head and neck cancer. Part 2: Clinical experience. Head Neck Surg 1983;6:751–760.

73. Frustaci S, Barzan L, Tumolo S, et al. Intra-arterial continuous infusion of *cis*-diamminedichloroplatinum in untreated head and neck cancer patients. Cancer 1986;57:1118–1123.

74. Zielke-Temme BC, Stevens KR, Everts EC, et al. Combined intraarterial chemotherapy, radiation therapy, and surgery for advanced squamous cell carcinoma of the head and neck. Cancer 1980;45:1527–1532.

75. Nervi C, Arcangeli G, Badaracco G, et al. The relevance of tumor size and cell kinetics as predictors of radiation response in head and neck cancer. Cancer 1978;41:900–906.

76. Alexander GA, Pistenmaa DA. Hypoxic cell radiation sensitizers, in Wittes RE (ed): Head and Neck Cancer. New York, John Wiley and Sons, 1985, pp 137–150.

77. Phillips TL. Sensitizers and protectors in clinical oncology. Semin Oncol 1981;8:65–82.

78. Overgaard J, Anderson AP, Jensen RH, et al. Misonidazole combined with split-course radiotherapy in the treatment of invasive carcinoma of the larynx and pharynx. Acta Otolaryngol 1982;386(suppl):215–220.

79. Brown JM. Clinical perspectives for the use of new hypoxic cell sensitizers. Int J Radiat Oncol Biol Phys 1982;8:1491–1497.

80. Maor MH, Hussey DH, Fletcher GH, et al. Fast neutron therapy for locally advanced head and neck tumors. Int J Radiat Oncol Biol Phys 1981;7:155–163.

81. Vermorken JB, van der Vijgh WJF, Klein I, et al. Pharmacokinetics of free and total platinum species after rapid and prolonged infusions of cisplatin. Clin Pharmacol Ther 1986;39:136–144.

**82.** Reddel RR, Kefford RF, Grant JM, et al. Ototoxicity in patients receiving cisplatin: Importance of dose and method of drug administration. Cancer Treat Rep 1982;66:19–23.
**83.** Ginsberg SJ, Comis RL. The pulmonary toxicity of antineoplastic agents. Semin Oncol 1982;9:34–51.
**84.** Cooper JAD, White DA, Matthay RA. Drug-induced pulmonary disease. Part 1: Cytotoxic drugs. Am Rev Respir Dis 1986;133: 321–340.
**85.** White DA, Stover DE. Severe bleomycin-induced pneumonitis: Clinical features and response to corticosteroids. Chest 1984;86: 723–728.
**86.** Fruncillo RJ, Gibbons W, Bowman SM. CNS toxicity after ingestion of topical lidocaine. N Engl J Med 1982;306:426–427.
**87.** Solomon MA. Oral sucralfate suspension for mucositis. N Engl J Med 1986;315:459–460.
**88.** Carl W. Dental management of head and neck cancer patients. J Surg Oncol 1980;15:265–281.
**89.** Ashford RFU, Plant GT, Maher J. Metronidazole in smelly tumours. Lancet 1980;1:874–875.
**90.** Bruera E, MacDonald N. Intractable pain in patients with advanced head and neck tumors: A possible role of local infection. Cancer Treat Rep 1986;70:691–692.

# Chapter 96 / Gastrointestinal Cancers

Judy L. Chase, PharmD, Robert J. Ignoffo, PharmD, and Robert J. Stagg, PharmD

Gastrointestinal tumors are a major health problem in the United States, accounting for 23% of all cancers and 25% of all cancer-related deaths. A gastrointestinal malignancy may arise from the esophagus, stomach, small intestine, colon, rectum, liver, biliary tract, or pancreas. Table 96.1 lists the annual incidences and mortality rates of the various gastrointestinal tumors in the United States.[1]

Unfortunately, gastrointestinal malignancies are often asymptomatic, making early diagnosis difficult. Symptoms of advanced gastrointestinal tumors include pain, bleeding, gastrointestinal obstruction, weight loss, fever, jaundice, and anemia. Radiographic, endoscopic, and serologic tests are all used in the diagnosis of gastrointestinal tumors.

In general, the prognosis of gastrointestinal cancers is poor. Surgical resection is the treatment of choice for early-stage locally confined tumors, as it is the only modality that offers a potential for cure. Unfortunately, because most gastrointestinal cancers are not discovered until there is locally advanced and/or metastatic disease, curative surgical resection is impossible. Nevertheless, with the exception of the hepatobiliary tumors, palliative resection of the primary tumor is usually performed to prevent complications, such as gastrointestinal obstruction. Locally advanced and metastatic disease is not curable and is usually treated with radiation and/or systemic chemotherapy.New methods of early detection and innovative treatments for gastrointestinal tumors are needed.

In this chapter we discuss the four most common gastrointestinal tumors in the United States: colorectal, pancreatic, gastric, and hepatocellular carcinoma.

## Colorectal Cancer

Colorectal cancer is the second most common malignancy in the United States, with about 145,000 new cases and 60,000 deaths occurring annually. It is estimated that about 6% of females and 5% of males will develop colorectal cancer in their lifetime. It is a disease primarily of the elderly, but 8% of cases occur in patients under the age of 40 and rare cases have been reported under the age of 20.

### *Epidemiology/Etiology*

Geographically, there are wide variations in the incidence of colorectal cancer, with low rates in Japan and Black Africa and high rates in the United States and Western Europe. Immigrants from Japan and Africa to the United States acquire an incidence of colorectal cancer similar to that of Americans, suggesting that environmental and dietary factors are involved in the etiology of this tumor.

The low incidence of colorectal cancer in Africa is thought to result from a high intake of dietary fiber, which increases the bulk of the stool, facilitating its transit through the gut.[2] This may be beneficial because it decreases the exposure time of the gastrointestinal epithelium to carcinogens present in the stool. Additionally, fiber appears to interfere with the production of carcinogens by bacteria. Diets high in fiber content have been effective in preventing chemically induced colorectal cancer in rats.[3] Conversely, diets high in fat, particularly saturated fat, may increase the risk of colorectal cancer. Saturated fat is metabolized to bile acid, which is a carcinogen promoter. In the past, the American diet was higher in saturated fat than the Japanese diet, but recently, the fat content of the Japanese diet has increased, coinciding with a rise in the incidence of colorectal cancer.[4]

Populations living in geographic areas with a high soil content of selenium, such as the Western Plains region, have a lower rate of colorectal cancer than people in other regions. Selenium is an essential dietary trace element that protects normal tissues from oxidation. Additional study is needed to determine if selenium truly protects against colorectal cancer.

Familial polyposis or a family history of polyps increases the risk of colorectal cancer severalfold. About 10% of colonic polyps eventually transform into colorectal malignancies.[5] There are three histologic types of polyps: adenomatous, villoglandular, and villous. The greatest risk of colorectal cancer occurs in patients with polyps of the villous type, polyps greater than 2 cm in size, and multiple polyps. For example, about 35% of patients with villous polyps larger than 2 cm eventually develop colorectal cancer. Prophylactic polypectomy decreases the risk of colorectal cancer and therefore should always be performed.

Ulcerative colitis and Crohn's disease are also strongly associated with colorectal cancer. The incidence is 5 to 10 times higher than normal in patients having either of these diseases longer than 10 years.[6,7] Other conditions that appear to be associated with colorectal cancer are Gardner's syndrome, radiation proctocolitis, and ureterosigmoidoscopy.[8]

### *Pathophysiology*

The anatomic distribution of colorectal cancer is shown in Table 96.2.[9] There are several histologic types of colorectal cancers. Most cases are adenocarcinoma; mucinous adenocarcinoma, signet ring adenocarcinoma, and carcinoma simplex are less common. About 60% of patients with colorectal cancer have metastatic disease at the time of surgery. Spread

**Table 96.1** Estimated Annual Incidence of and Deaths From Gastrointestinal Cancers in 1987

| *Tumor* | *New cases* | *Deaths* |
|---|---|---|
| Esophagus | 9,700 | 8,800 |
| Stomach | 24,600 | 14,200 |
| Small intestine | 2,500 | 800 |
| Colon | 102,000 | 52,000 |
| Rectum | 43,000 | 8,000 |
| Liver and biliary | 14,000 | 10,600 |
| Pancreas | 26,200 | 24,300 |
| Other unspecified | 2,400 | 1,200 |
| Total | 224,400 | 119,900 |

may occur by direct invasion of adjacent tissues or metastases via the lymphatic or hematogenous route. The liver is the most common metastatic site, followed by the lung, although metastases may occur at virtually any site. Colorectal cancer is generally a slow-growing malignancy. The primary lesion has a doubling time of about 600 days; metastases have a much shorter doubling time, about 100 days.[10–12]

### *Clinical Presentation*

The symptoms of colorectal cancer are often quite subtle and include a change in bowel habits (diarrhea, constipation, and/or narrow stools), melena, and vague abdominal distress. Carcinomas of the ascending and transverse colon usually present with vague abdominal pain and occult bleeding rather than gastrointestinal obstruction. In contrast, carcinomas of the descending colon are most often associated with obstructive symptoms. Cancers of the rectum most often present with rectal bleeding. In advanced cases of colorectal cancer, a palpable abdominal mass may be detected on physical examination.[13,14]

### *Diagnosis*

Colorectal carcinoma should be suspected in any patient presenting with a change in bowel habits, abdominal pain, hematochezia, or unexplained anemia. Blood in the stool should not be attributed to hemorrhoids or diverticulosis until the possibility of a malignancy has been excluded. Initially, the patient should have a digital rectal examination and a hemoccult test to detect occult blood in the stool. While the rectal exam is useful only for detecting lesions below the rectosigmoid, it is simple to perform. Sigmoidoscopy is often the next test performed, as it can be done in the physician's office and will detect approximately one half of all colorectal tumors; however, sigmoidoscopy is useful only for examining the lower 25 cm of the colorectum; thus, a normal exam does not exclude the possibility of a malignancy. The two methods of examining the entire bowel are the double-contrast barium enema and the colonoscopy. A barium enema is less expensive than colonoscopy and identifies most lesions. Many clinicians prefer the colonoscopy, which enables direct visualization of the entire bowel and allows a biopsy specimen to be obtained.

Certain laboratory tests are also useful in the diagnosis of colorectal cancer. A low hematocrit is often the first sign that leads to the discovery of the colorectal tumor. Liver function tests may be elevated if the patient has hepatic metastases. Lastly, the carcinoembryonic antigen (CEA) level is often elevated[14]; however, the CEA level is elevated in several other malignant epithelial tumors (adenocarcinomas) and thus is not specific for colorectal cancer. The major utility of the CEA level is in monitoring of patients after resection of the primary tumor, as an elevated value is consistent with residual disease.[15]

Abdominal computerized axial tomography (CAT), abdominal magnetic resonance imaging (MRI), or liver–spleen scanning is often performed to determine if hepatic metastases are present. A chest x-ray should also be obtained, as the lung is a common site of metastatic disease.

**Table 96.2** Anatomic Distribution of Colorectal Cancers

| *Site* | *Distribution of large-bowel cancers (%)* |
|---|---|
| Rectum | 23 |
| Rectosigmoid junction | 10 |
| Sigmoid | 24 |
| Descending colon | 7 |
| Transverse colon | 12 |
| Ascending colon | 10 |
| Cecum | 13 |
| Appendix | 1 |

### *Staging/Prognosis*

The original staging system for colorectal cancer, developed by Duke, classified tumors by the depth of local invasion and the degree of regional lymph node involvement. Currently, a modification of Duke's system, developed by Turnbull, is used; it divides patients into six basic clinicopathologic stages—A, $B_1$, $B_2$, $C_1$, $C_2$, and D.[16] The various stages and associated 5-year survival rates are listed in Table 96.3. The prognosis for early-stage malignancies is generally good, as surgery is often curative; however, advanced-stage tumors have a very poor prognosis. Certain histopathologic features also associated with a poor prognosis include the presence of lymphatic, vascular, or perineural invasion and tumors of the mucinous or signet ring variety.

### *Treatment*

The three major treatment modalities for colorectal cancer are surgery, radiotherapy, and chemotherapy.

***Surgery*** Surgical resection of the primary tumor is almost always performed. Removal of the primary malignancy is often curative in patients with stage A, $B_1$, and $B_2$ tumors and is occasionally curative in patients with stage $C_1$ and $C_2$ tumors. Surgical resection of the primary tumor in patients with stage D malignancies, while not curative, is usually performed to prevent future complications, such as gastrointestinal obstruction and anemia. Additionally, after re-

**Table 96.3** Staging and Survival of Colorectal Cancer

| *Stage* | *Extent of invasion* | *5-yr survival (%)* |
|---|---|---|
| A | Mucosa | 75–100 |
| $B_1$ | Muscularis propria | 65 |
| $B_2$ | Serosa or pericolic fat | 50 |
| $C_1$ | Stage A or $B_1$ + positive lymph nodes | 40 |
| $C_2$ | Stage $B_2$ + positive lymph nodes | 15 |
| D | Distant metastases | <5 |

moval of the primary tumor, surgical resection of an isolated metastasis, such as a unilobar liver lesion, may occasionally be curative.

***Radiotherapy*** Radiotherapy is used postoperatively in patients with rectal cancer to decrease the incidence of local recurrence.[17] Radiotherapy is also occasionally used for the palliation of metastatic colorectal lesions that are obstructing vital organs, such as the stomach or ureters.

***Chemotherapy*** For patients with unresectable metastatic disease, the only viable treatment option is systemic chemotherapy. As single agents, 5-fluorouracil (5-FU), floxuridine (FUDR), lomustine, and mitomycin C produce about a 15% to 20% partial response rate; complete remissions are rare.[13,18] 5-Fluorouracil is the least toxic of the agents and is usually the drug of choice. Several dosage schedules of 5-FU have been employed. The most common is an intravenous bolus injection of 12–15 mg/kg administered weekly.[19] A loading dose schedule of 15 mg/kg/d administered by intravenous bolus for 5 days followed by weekly injections of 12–15 mg/kg has also been used, but produces significant neutropenia and mucositis.[20] Additionally, 5-FU has been administered by continuous intravenous infusion.[21,22] FUDR is given as a continuous intravenous infusion of 0.05–0.1 mg/kg/d for 14 days, repeated every 28 days. Mitomycin C is reserved primarily as a second-line drug because of cumulative myelosuppression. It is administered by intravenous bolus injection at a dose of 15–20 mg/m$^2$ every 6 to 8 weeks. Lomustine is taken orally, but is usually reserved for 5-FU and mitomycin C failures. Combination regimens have been extensively studied, but offer no advantage over single-agent 5-FU.[23–27]

***Hepatic Intraarterial Chemotherapy*** About 60% of patients with colorectal cancer ultimately develop liver metastases. Hepatic metastases derive 90% of their blood supply from the hepatic artery; thus, hepatic intraarterial administration of chemotherapeutic agents is often used to treat patients with disease confined to the liver. This route allows delivery of higher drug concentrations within the tumor than intravenous administration. In addition, as normal liver tissue receives its blood supply predominantly by the portal vein, the hepatic parenchyma is relatively spared of the effects of intraarterial chemotherapy. Drugs with high hepatic extractions are best suited for intraarterial administration, because only a small fraction of the dosage reaches the systemic circulation; thus, systemic toxic effects are minimized. Chemotherapeutic agents with high hepatic extractions include FUDR, doxorubicin, and 5-FU.

Hepatic intraarterial chemotherapy requires placement of a catheter into the hepatic artery. Until recently, the most common technique of drug delivery was via a radiographically placed percutaneous intraarterial catheter. Unfortunately, this requires 7 to 10 days of hospitalization for each treatment course and is associated with significant morbidity, including arterial thrombosis, infection, and catheter migration resulting in drug misperfusion. Percutaneous intraarterial catheters can also be placed operatively, which eliminates some of the problems seen with radiographically placed catheters, but the disadvantages of a percutaneous system remain. A totally implantable infusion pump and implanted ports are now available that are associated with fewer complications than percutaneously placed catheters.

Hepatic intraarterial 5-FU or FUDR produces an objective response in about 60% of patients with liver metastases from colorectal cancer and a median survival of approximately 18 months.[28,29] In one nonrandomized trial of 30 patients, hepatic intraarterial cisplatin also produced a 60% response rate, including three complete remissions.[30] Intraarterial mitomycin C has been used in combination with other agents, but has not been studied as a single agent. Recently, a randomized trial of intraarterial versus intravenous FUDR demonstrated a significantly higher response rate and longer time to hepatic progression for the patients receiving intraarterial therapy.[31] In experienced hands, hepatic intraarterial chemotherapy appears to be the optimal treatment for patients with metastatic colorectal cancer confined to the liver.

### *Summary*

Colorectal cancer remains a major health problem in the United States. Surgical resection of the primary tumor is often curative for patients with early-stage locally confined tumors, but, unfortunately, most patients have advanced disease at the time of presentation. After removal of the primary tumor, resection of isolated liver metastases may also occasionally be curative. Radiation therapy is used postoperatively in patients with rectal cancer to minimize the risk of local recurrence and occasionally for palliation of lesions that are obstructing vital organs. Systemic chemotherapy is the only viable treatment for patients with widely metastatic disease, but produces response rates of only 15% to 20%. Patients with liver-only metastases should be considered for hepatic intraarterial chemotherapy, which produces a response rate of about 60%.

## Cancer of the Pancreas

Pancreatic cancer is a relatively uncommon malignancy, with approximately 26,000 new cases diagnosed annually in the United States. The reported incidence of pancreatic cancer has increased over the last few decades, probably as a result of an increased awareness of this malignancy and advances in diagnostic technology. It is one of the most aggressive solid tumors, with only 1% of patients surviving 5 years or longer from the time of diagnosis.[32] It is currently the fourth most common cause of cancer death behind lung, colon, and breast cancer.

### *Epidemiology/Etiology*

The majority of patients diagnosed are between 30 and 70 years old, with a rapid increase in incidence seen among aging populations. The male:female ratio is about 1.7:1.[33] The incidence is higher in urban than in rural areas, and higher in industrialized countries than in underdeveloped nations, implying that environmental factors play a role in the etiology of this disease. Employees of the petroleum and chemical industries appear to be at especially high risk. Workers exposed to industrial solvents or petroleum products for 10 years or longer have up to a fivefold increase in incidence of pancreatic cancer.[3]

Dietary factors such as excessive fat, coffee, and/or alcohol consumption have been associated with the development of pancreatic cancer, but a causal relationship has not been definitively established.[33] Cigarette smoking appears to be associated with pancreatic cancer, increasing the incidence of the disease two- to threefold.[33] There also appears to be an increased incidence in patients with chronic pancreatitis.[33] No association has been found between cholecystitis or biliary lithiasis and pancreatic cancer.[34]

A possible association may exist between diabetes and pancreatic cancer, as 15% of patients with a pancreatic malignancy have a history of diabetes.[35] Because diabetes may be present before or after the diagnosis of cancer, it is difficult to determine whether the malignancy produced the diabetic state or the diabetes increased the risk of pancreatic cancer.[33,36] Presently, there is no firmly established etiologic relationship.

### *Pathophysiology*

The pancreas is made up of two functionally separate organs: the exocrine pancreas and the endocrine pancreas. Neoplasms may involve either the parenchyma of the exocrine pancreas or the islets of the endocrine pancreas, but most (95%) pancreatic tumors involve the exocrine portion of the pancreas. Tumors can arise from the pancreatic ductal epithelial cells, acinar cells, connective tissue, or lymphatics. By far the most common histologic type of malignancy of the pancreas is ductal adenocarcinoma, which accounts for greater than 80% of pancreatic neoplasms. The head of the pancreas is the site for approximately 70% of pancreatic tumors, with 20% occurring in the body and 10% in the tail.[37]

### *Clinical Presentation*

At the time of presentation, pancreatic tumors tend to be large (average of 5 cm in diameter) and approximately 90% of patients have locally invasive or metastatic disease. This is due to the insidious nature of pancreatic cancer, which usually remains asymptomatic until advanced stages of the malignancy. Pain in the upper abdomen is the single most common presenting symptom. Other symptoms include weight loss, anorexia, nausea, vomiting, and weakness. Gastrointestinal bleeding is commonly associated with tumors of the head of the pancreas, but is rare in tumors of the body or tail. Because of the vague nature of the majority of these symptoms, most patients have complaints for greater than 2 months before the diagnosis of pancreatic cancer is made. As most tumors arise in the ductal system, obstruction of the pancreatic duct is common. Obstructive jaundice occurs in approximately 50% of all patients with pancreatic cancer and in up to 90% of patients with tumors in the head of the pancreas.

Pancreatic cancer may spread by direct invasion of surrounding tissues or by metastasizing to distant sites. Commonly, direct invasion into the lymph nodes, liver, and gastroduodenum occurs, accounting for the high incidence of locally advanced disease seen at diagnosis. In addition, pancreatic cancer often metastasizes to the peritoneum, and less frequently to the lungs, abdominal viscera, adrenals, kidneys, bone, brain, and skin.[37]

### *Diagnosis*

A high index of suspicion for pancreatic cancer should be present in any patient who presents with obstructive jaundice, unexplained pancreatitis, weight loss, or recent onset of upper abdominal or back pain. The goals of evaluating a patient with possible pancreatic cancer are to establish the presence or absence of a primary tumor and, if present, to determine the extent of local and metastatic spread. The diagnostic evaluation usually begins with noninvasive radiologic studies, then proceeds to more invasive radiologic and endoscopic procedures, and eventually to tissue biopsy.

Ultrasonography of the upper abdomen is commonly used as a screening procedure in patients suspected of having pancreatic cancer. This test has the advantages of being noninvasive and inexpensive, but the diagnostic yield depends on the interpretive skills of the ultrasonographer. Ultrasound patterns can differentiate pancreatic carcinoma from acute pancreatitis, pseudocysts, or abscesses, but cannot distinguish between chronic pancreatitis and cancer of the pancreas. Computerized axial tomograms and magnetic resonance images of the upper abdomen are probably the most sensitive means of detecting neoplastic disease of the pancreas. The most common CAT and MRI findings in pancreatic carcinoma include enlargement of the pancreas, a pancreatic mass, dilatation of the biliary tree and pancreatic duct, hepatic metastases, and retroperitoneal adenopathy. While more expensive than ultrasound, CAT and MRI offer the advantages of producing a superior image and visualizing the entire abdomen.

More invasive procedures used to visualize the pancreas and biliary tree include transhepatic cholangiography, endoscopic retrograde cholangiopancreatography, and arteriography of the pancreas. The diagnostic accuracy of these procedures varies and depends on the experience of the radiologist performing the procedure. Frequently, the evaluation of patients with suspected pancreatic cancer progresses to an exploratory laparotomy. At surgery, biopsies of the pancreas, lymph nodes, and liver are obtained to confirm the diagnosis.

Several serum enzymes may be elevated in carcinoma of the pancreas, including amylase, lipase, alkaline phosphatase, leucine aminopeptidase, and pancreatic ribonuclease. If the tumor involves the liver, levels of lactic dehydrogenase and the transaminases may also be elevated.[38,39]

A variety of biologic substances have been identified in the serum of some patients with pancreatic cancer and have been suggested as possible tumor markers for the disease.[38] Carcinoembryonic antigen, pancreatic oncofetal antigen, and $\alpha$-fetoprotein (AFP) have all been reported to be elevated in some patients with pancreatic cancer; however, these tumor markers lack sensitivity and specificity for pancreatic carcinoma. At the present time tumor markers have not proven to be clinically helpful in identifying patients with pancreatic cancer.

### *Staging/Prognosis*

Pancreatic cancer is surgically staged using the TNM system in Table 96.4. Tumor status (T) is defined by the degree of tumor extension through the pancreatic capsule; nodal status (N) is defined by the presence of regional lymph node involvement; and metastatic status (M) is defined by the presence of distant nodal, peritoneal, or visceral involvement. Stage I disease is limited to the pancreas and is surgically resectable. Stage II disease represents locally advanced disease, not involving regional lymph nodes, and is not surgically resectable. Stage III disease involves the regional lymph nodes without clinical evidence of distant metastases. Stage IV disease indicates metastatic spread. Obviously, patients with stage I disease have the best prognosis, whereas those with stage IV disease have the worst prognosis.

### *Treatment*

#### Stage I Disease

Surgical resection of stage I pancreatic cancer (confined to the pancreas) offers a potential cure and is the treatment of choice whenever feasible. The Whipple procedure (pancreaticoduodenectomy) is the most frequently performed operation for carcinoma of the pancreas. This entails en bloc removal of the head and neck of the pancreas, duodenum, a variable portion of the distal stomach and upper jejunum, gallbladder, common bile duct, and regional lymphatic nodes. Pancreaticoduodenal resections carry an operative mortality rate of approximately 20% and a complication rate of greater than 50%. The most common complications encountered are fistula formation, hemorrhage, and infection. The 5-year survival rate for pancreaticoduodenal resection is less than 10%.[40] Patients with stage I disease who undergo pancreatic resection and are found to have clear margins of resection may be followed clinically without further therapy until recurrence develops. Often, laparotomy reveals that the malignancy is not completely resectable; however, surgical resection may still be attempted, as patients often obtain some palliation of symptoms.[34,37,40]

**Table 96.4** TMN Staging System for Pancreatic Cancer

| | |
|---|---|
| Stage 1 | $T_1$–$T_2$, $N_0$, $M_0$: No direct extension or limited extension of tumor with no regional nodal involvement; resectable with curative intent |
| Stage 2 | $T_3$, $N_0$, $M_0$: Direct extension of tumor into adjacent tissue with no lymph node involvement; not resectable with curative intent |
| Stage 3 | $T_1$–$T_3$, $N_1$, $M_0$: Regional lymph node involvement with or without direct tumor extension, but without distant metastases |
| Stage 4 | $T_1$–$T_3$, $N_0$–$N_1$, $M_1$: Distant metastases present |
| $T_1$ | No direct extension of the primary tumor beyond the pancreas |
| $T_2$ | Limited direct extension to duodenum, bile ducts, or stomach |
| $T_3$ | Advanced direct extension (not surgically resectable) |
| $T_X$ | Direct extension of tumor not assessed |
| $N_0$ | Regional lymph nodes not involved |
| $N_1$ | Regional lymph nodes involved |
| $N_X$ | Regional lymph nodes not assessed |
| $M_0$ | No known distant metastases |
| $M_1$ | Distant metastases present |
| $M_X$ | Distant metastases not assessed |

Adjuvant therapy for stage I pancreatic cancer is currently experimental, but recent studies suggest some benefit over surgery alone. A small number of patients have been treated with pre- or postoperative radiation in an attempt to enhance the survival rate. The current data suggest that adjuvant radiotherapy may prolong survival; however, randomized controlled trials have not been done.[41,42] Adjuvant chemotherapy has not been studied alone, but has been used postoperatively in combination with radiotherapy. In a comparative trial, 49 patients were randomized to surgical resection alone or surgical resection plus two courses of postoperative 5-FU 500 mg/m$^2$ daily for 3 days and 2,000 rads of external radiation.[43,44] An increase in median survival was observed in the combined modality group compared with the surgery-alone group (20 months versus 11 months). In a retrospective review, 11 patients treated with pancreatectomy alone were compared with 8 patients who received postoperative radiotherapy (4,500 rads) plus 5-FU. There appeared to be a slight increase in the 1-year survival rate with combined modality therapy when compared with patients treated with pancreatectomy alone (75% versus 64%). These results suggest an improved survival in patients receiving surgical resection plus adjuvant chemotherapy and radiation, although the available data are limited.

#### Advanced-Stage Disease

Unfortunately, 80% to 90% of patients present with advanced pancreatic cancer (stages II, III, and IV) for which curative surgical resection is impossible. Treatment of these patients is directed at the palliation of symptoms and the prolongation of survival.

***Surgery*** Surgery is performed in patients with advanced pancreatic cancer to alleviate biliary and/or gastric outlet obstruction as well as to determine the extent of disease. This is usually accomplished by choledochojejunostomy or cholecystojejunostomy. In patients with severe pain, 50% ethyl alcohol or 6% phenol can be injected into the splanchnic nerve and celiac ganglia at the time of surgery and may offer some pain relief.[34,37,45]

***Radiotherapy*** Radiotherapy often provides effective palliation of symptoms in patients with advanced-stage disease. Patients suitable for aggressive external beam irradiation should have locally advanced, surgically unresectable disease, an adequate nutritional status, and no evidence of metastatic disease. Total doses of approximately 6,000–7,000 rads are administered in fractions of 180–200 rads/d.[46] Radiotherapy provides local tumor control in up to 50% of patients, but only a few patients survive 5 years or longer.[47–49] Although the use of radiotherapy has not substantially altered survival, it does provide symptomatic palliation for some patients with locally advanced pancreatic carcinoma.

***Chemotherapy*** Approximately 10% to 20% of patients with advanced pancreatic cancer achieve a partial response with single-agent chemotherapy and approximately 30% of patients respond to combination chemotherapy. An improved duration of survival is observed in those patients who respond to chemotherapy; therefore, a limited trial of chemotherapy is usually warranted to assess tumor responsiveness. In stage II and III disease, chemotherapy is often combined with radiotherapy. For metastatic disease (stage IV), systemic chemotherapy is the only treatment option.

Only three drugs have significant activity in patients with pancreatic carcinoma: 5-FU, mitomycin C, and streptozocin.[50–52] 5-FU has been the most extensively studied agent and has a response rate of about 25%.[50] The 5-FU regimen commonly used is a weekly intravenous bolus of 15 mg/kg. Mitomycin C, an antitumor antibiotic, is the second most widely used drug in the treatment of pancreatic cancer and has a response rate comparable to that of 5-FU. In a collected series from the literature, 12 of 44 patients (27%) treated with mitomycin C achieved a partial response. It is usually administered intravenously in a dose of 10–15 $mg/m^2$ every 6 to 8 weeks.[53] Streptozocin, a naturally occurring nitrosourea, is toxic to pancreatic beta cells and also has independent activity against adenocarcinomas of the exocrine pancreas.[52,54] It produces a partial response rate of 31% to 50% and is given weekly in doses of 1.0–1.5 $g/m^2$ intravenously for 6 consecutive weeks, followed by a 4-week rest period.[55,56] Nephrotoxicity occurs in 45% to 65% of patients and is dose limiting and occasionally irreversible.[57] Streptozotocin may also cause severe nausea and vomiting. The drug causes only mild myelosuppression, making it an attractive agent for inclusion into combination drug regimens.

A number of combination regimens have been employed in an attempt to increase the dismal results obtained with single-agent chemotherapy. No single combination regimen has emerged that produces uniformly high response rates or a significant survival advantage. However, encouraging results have been obtained with the SMF (streptozotocin, methotrexate, 5-FU) and FAM (5-FU, doxorubicin, methotrexate) regimens (Table 96.5). Initially, these regimens were reported to have a response rate of 37% to 43%; however, subsequent trials have suggested that response rates for both SMF and FAM regimens are less than 30%.[58–62] Recently, investigators incorporated the four individual drugs in the FAM and SMF regimens into the FAM-S regimen in the hope of producing an improved response rate.[63] Partial or complete responses were observed in 12 of 25 (48%) patients and responders had a median survival of 10 months. Randomized prospective trials are now under way to determine whether FAM-S is superior to SMF or FAM.

**Table 96.5** Combination Chemotherapy Regimens for Pancreatic Cancer

| |
|---|
| FAM |
| 5-Fluorouracil 600 $mg/m^2$ IV bolus on days 1, 8, 29, and 36 |
| Adriamycin 30 $mg/m^2$ IV bolus on days 1 and 29 |
| Mitomycin C 10 $mg/m^2$ IV bolus on day 1 |
| Repeat cycle every 6–8 weeks |
| SMF |
| Streptozocin 1 $g/m^2$ IV over 1 to 2 h on days 1, 8, 29, and 36 |
| Mitomycin C 10 $mg/m^2$ IV bolus on day 1 |
| 5-Fluorouracil 600 $mg/m^2$ IV bolus on days 1, 8, 29, and 36 |
| Repeat cycle every 6–8 weeks |

***Combined Modality Treatment*** The combination of chemotherapy and radiotherapy may offer a survival benefit over the use of radiotherapy alone in locally advanced unresectable pancreatic cancer. The optimal chemotherapy regimen for use with radiotherapy has not yet been determined. 5-FU plus high-dose (6,000 rads) or low-dose (4,000 rads) radiation had been compared with high-dose (6,000 rads) radiation alone in a prospective randomized trial. The median survival time for patients given 6,000 rads alone was 23 weeks, compared with median survival times of 40 and 42 weeks in patients given combined modality therapy.[64] Trials of SMF or FAM plus radiation therapy are currently under way.

### *Summary*

Pancreatic cancer is a relatively rare, but highly lethal, malignancy that results in the death of over 99% of patients within 5 years of diagnosis. The symptoms of pancreatic cancer are usually vague until advanced stages are present. Less than 10% of patients have locally confined disease (stage I) at the time of diagnosis. For this minority of patients, surgical resection with and without adjuvant radiation and/or chemotherapy offers a potential cure and is the treatment of choice. For patients with advanced pancreatic cancer (stages II, III, and IV) curative resection is not feasible; however, palliative surgical resection may still be performed to alleviate obstructions. Some patients with locally advanced disease (stages II and III) may benefit from combined radiation and chemotherapy. Patients with metastatic disease (stage IV) have the poorest prognosis, but up to 30% obtain a partial response with combination chemotherapy.

## Gastric Cancer

About 25,000 new cases of gastric cancer and 14,000 deaths from gastric cancer occur annually in the United States.[1] Both the incidence and mortality rate of gastric cancer have declined significantly in the last several decades. This decline, which has not been adequately explained, has occurred predominantly in older persons, women, and whites.

### *Epidemiology/Etiology*

The incidence of gastric cancer varies considerably depending on geographic location and socioeconomic group. High-incidence countries include Japan, Chile, Costa Rica, Iceland, and Finland. Mortality in these countries is about five times that in low-risk countries like the United States, Australia, New Zealand, Thailand, and the Dominican Republic.[1] Immigrants from high- to low-incidence countries show a significant decrease in the occurrence of gastric cancer, suggesting that environmental factors contribute to the development of this cancer.

Gastric cancer is a disease primarily of people over the age of 60, but may occur in younger people and rarely in teenagers. The male:female ratio is 3:2, except in patients under 30, where female cases predominate. In the United States and Western Europe, gastric cancer is more common in low economic groups, as well as, in particular working groups such as coal miners, Japanese farmers, Russian nickel refinery workers, and asbestos workers. It is unclear whether the high incidence in these groups is related to their occupation or socioeconomic situation.[65] Other populations with a high incidence include blacks and individuals with type A blood.

Several factors may predispose a patient to gastric cancer, including gastric polyposis–achlorhydria syndrome, pernicious anemia, gastric calcifications, atrophic gastritis, and Menetriere's disease. It is postulated that the achlorhydria induced by these conditions allows carcinogen-forming organisms to grow in the stomach. The intake of some foods, such as red meats, cabbage, spices, fish, and salt-preserved or smoked foods, may also predispose individuals to gastric cancer because of the formation of nitrosoamines during the cooking process.

### *Pathophysiology*

Gastric cancers are primarily adenocarcinomas, although 5% are leimyosarcomas or lymphomas. The tumor originates in the pylorus or antrum in 50%, the lesser curvature in 20%, the body in 20%, the cardia in 7%, and the greater curvature in 3% of cases.[66] About 2% of patients with gastric cancer have multiple gastric lesions.[67]

Gastric cancer is an aggressive tumor, often directly infiltrating adjacent tissues and metastasizing to distant sites. Tumors that extend into the gastric serosa frequently lead to widespread peritoneal seeding.[68] Distant metastases may result from lymphatic or hematogenous spread of tumor cells. Metastases to regional lymph nodes are observed in almost 90% of patients at laparotomy. In addition, approximately 60% of patients have distant metastases discovered at the time of surgery. Common metastatic sites include the liver and lung, although virtually any site can be involved. Other sites of metastases include the adrenal gland, pancreas, retroperitoneum, ovary, bone, uterus, and kidney.

### *Clinical Presentation*

The common presenting symptoms of gastric cancer are vague abdominal discomfort, fatigue, weight loss, "coffee ground" vomitus, melena, change in bowel habits, and gastric ulceration.[69] Other symptoms include persistent nausea and vomiting or dysphagia. The mean duration of symptoms prior to diagnosis is about 7 months.

### *Diagnosis*

Initially, a physical examination is performed, including palpation of the lymph nodes and liver. The earliest evidence of lymph node metastases is the finding of either a firm left supraclavicular (Virchow's) node, a periumbilical (Sister Mary Joseph) node, or a left axillary lymph node. Tissue diagnosis is possible from any of these sites. The finding likely to lead to early diagnosis is occult blood identified in the stool. The stomach should be evaluated using an upper gastrointestinal contrast study to detect any gastric lesions. A definitive diagnosis is determined by fiberoptic endoscopy with biopsies of gastric lesions.

Ancillary diagnostic procedures are sometimes useful, including CAT, MRI, ultrasonography, and plasma tumor markers. CAT or MRI provides the greatest amount of information regarding the extent of extragastric extension. Plasma tumor markers are of limited benefit in gastric cancer. While CEA is elevated in about 60% of patients, it is not specific to gastric cancer, as several other conditions may cause an elevation.

### *Staging/Prognosis*

Traditionally, gastric cancer has been informally staged as being completely resectable, locally unresectable, or unresectable with disseminated disease. More recently, the TNM classification (Table 96.6), which more accurately classifies lesions, has been established. Tumors are also histologically graded into well-differentiated, moderately well-differentiated, and poorly differentiated types. Clinical staging is based on grouping of tumor, nodal, and metastatic involvement. In general, gastric cancer carries a poor prognosis with an overall 5-year survival of only 7%.[70] The extent of

**Table 96.6** TNM Classification of Gastric Cancer

| | |
|---|---|
| **Primary Tumor (T)** | |
| $T_0$ | No evidence of disease |
| $T_1$ | Limited to the mucosa |
| $T_2$ | Involves the mucosa and extends to the serosa |
| $T_3$ | Penetrates serosa without invading surrounding contiguous structures |
| $T_4$ | Penetrates serosa, invading adjacent tissues ($T_{4a}$) or major organs ($T_{4b}$) |
| **Nodal Involvement (N)** | |
| $N_0$ | No evidence of disease |
| $N_1$ | Involvement of perigastric lymph nodes within 3 cm of the primary tumor |
| $N_2$ | Involvement of perigastric lymph nodes more than 3 cm from the primary tumor |
| $N_3$ | Involvement of intraabdominal lymph nodes |
| **Distant Metastases (M)** | |
| $M_0$ | No evidence of metastases |
| $M_1$ | Distant metastases present |

disease at presentation is an important determinant of survival, as those with locally confined disease have a 5-year survival rate of 30%.

### *Treatment*

Gastric cancer is treated with surgery, radiation, and/or chemotherapy depending on the stage of disease.

***Surgery*** Surgery is the only potentially curative treatment for gastric carcinoma. Resection is performed in about 90% of patients, but only about 10% of the patients have disease confined only to stomach. Lesions of the distal stomach are treated with a subtotal radical gastrectomy, which includes removal of 80% of the stomach, omentum, first portion of the duodenum, and node-bearing region of the hepatoduodenal pedicle. Lesions of the pylorus and antrum are usually treated with subtotal gastrectomy and splenectomy. The overall 5-year survival of surgically resected patients ranges from 25% to 45%.[70,71]

***Radiotherapy*** Radiotherapy is used to palliate symptoms and to prevent obstruction of vital organs, such as the ureter or large bowel. The usual dose is 4,000–5,000 rads fractionated over a 4- to 5-week period of 170–200 rads daily. A boost to 5,500 rads for unresected or residual disease may be given. Radiation sensitizers such as 5-FU are sometimes coadministered to enhance the local radiation effect.[72]

***Chemotherapy*** Chemotherapy is frequently used to treat advanced gastric cancer. The most active single agent is doxorubicin, which has a partial response rate of about 25%; complete responses are uncommon with single-agent therapy.[73] The median duration of response is 4 months. Other active single agents are mitomycin C, 5-FU, and carmustine.

Combination chemotherapy is the mainstay of treatment for advanced disease. FAM produces responses in about 45% of patients, with about 5% having a complete response.[74,75] Survival appears to be longer in responding than in nonresponding patients. 5-Fluorouracil plus carmustine produces responses in about 35% of patients, with several complete responses.[76] Recently, in a small study of 17 patients, treatment with 5-FU/doxorubicin/cisplatin produced a response rate of 53%, including three complete remissions.[77] Further study of cisplatin-containing regimens is needed to confirm these preliminary results. While palliation of symptoms is probably best achieved with combination treatment, a clear survival benefit has not been demonstrated in a randomized trial.

### *Summary*

Gastric cancer is usually at an advanced stage at the time of diagnosis. Surgery is performed initially, but most patients relapse or have metastatic disease at the time of presentation. Combination chemotherapy is the primary treatment for advanced stages and produces responses in about 40% of patients, with a small number of complete remissions. Radiotherapy is used primarily to palliate symptoms or prevent obstruction of vital organs.

## Hepatocellular Carcinoma

Hepatocellular carcinoma (HCC), also known as hepatoma, accounts for approximately 90% of all primary liver cancers. The majority of the remaining cases are intrahepatic cholangiocarcinomas—tumors arising from the bile ducts. Other rare types of primary liver cancer include hemangioendothelioma, hepatoblastoma, angiosarcoma, and undifferentiated sarcomas. As HCC is the most prevalent primary tumor of the liver, it is the major focus of this section.

### *Epidemiology/Etiology*

The worldwide annual incidence of HCC is estimated to be 300,000 to 1,200,000 cases per year.[1] There are marked geographic variations in the incidence. In the United States, HCC is a relatively rare tumor, with 3,000 to 4,000 cases diagnosed annually, whereas the annual incidence in Africa, Southeast Asia, Taiwan, and China is as high as 130 per 100,000 population. HCC is more common in males than in females. Patients diagnosed with HCC from high-incidence areas tend to be younger than those from low-incidence areas.

HCC is frequently associated with preexisting liver disease. In the United States, 50% of patients with HCC have cirrhosis. Overall, it is estimated that approximately 5% of all patients with cirrhosis eventually develop HCC.[78]

Worldwide exposure to the hepatitis B virus (HBV) appears to play a major etiologic role in the pathogenesis of HCC. Approximately 80% of all HCC cases appear to result from prior hepatitis B infection. Two theories have been proposed to explain the mechanism by which HBV causes HCC. The first is that the liver injury caused by the HBV leads directly to the development of HCC. The second theory postulates that the HBV DNA is integrated into the hepatocyte DNA and that the altered DNA subsequently causes malignant transformation of the cell.[79,80] Hepatitis B vaccines are now available (Heptavax-B and Recombivax, Merck Sharp & Dohme) and their use in hepatitis endemic areas should decrease the incidence of HCC in the future.[79] There is no evidence to suggest that prior infection with hepatitis A or non-A, non-B hepatitis predisposes patients to HCC.

Aflatoxin, a naturally occurring carcinogen (produced by the food-spoiling fungus *Aspergillus flavus*), is prevalent in the food supply of HCC endemic areas. In humans, epidemiologic data correlate the amount of aflatoxin found in food with the incidence of HCC in a given region; however, this finding is complicated by the fact that areas with high aflatoxin ingestion are also endemic for hepatitis infections. Therefore, a cocarcinogenic effect has been postulated, but further study is needed to verify this suggestion.[81]

Recently, steroids have been implicated as possible etiologic agents in HCC. A few cases of HCC have been reported in patients taking oral contraceptives.[82] In addition, there have been a few reports of males taking androgens who developed hepatoma.[83] Because of the small number of reports, it remains unclear whether steroid ingestion increases the risk of HCC.

It has been suggested that malnutrition might be a risk

factor for development of HCC; however, in many areas of the world where malnutrition is epidemic, such as India, the incidence of HCC is low.

### Pathophysiology

Primary hepatocellular cancer is classified into three major categories based on its macroscopic appearance: a nodular form, with multiple often widely dispersed nodules; a massive form, with one dominant mass, but possibly smaller satellite lesions in the surrounding parenchyma; and a diffuse form, with extensive small nodules throughout the liver. The nodular form accounts for approximately 65%, the massive form 30%, and the diffuse form 5% of the cases of HCC. The diffuse form always occurs in association with cirrhosis. It is not known whether the widespread pattern of the diffuse and nodular forms is secondary to metastases or to multiple sites of neoplastic formation. Occasionally, HCC presents as an encapsulated form where a fibrous tissue surrounds the tumor. This variety of HCC is less aggressive and is associated with a longer survival than typical HCC.[84]

Hepatocellular carcinoma commonly invades adjacent tissues (such as the diaphragm and stomach) and the portal vein. At autopsy, over 50% of patients are found to have metastatic disease. The most common sites of metastases are the regional lymph nodes and lungs.

### Clinical Presentation

Unfortunately, the vague and subtle nature of most of the presenting symptoms of HCC delays the diagnosis until advanced disease is present. The most common presenting symptoms of HCC include weakness, anorexia, abdominal fullness, and a dull aching upper abdominal pain. If the hepatic or portal vein is obstructed by tumor, portal hypertension, bleeding esophageal varices, and hemoperitoneum may also be presenting symptoms or may occur later in the course of the disease.

Patients often present with significant abnormalities in their laboratory values, particularly liver function tests. The transaminases and alkaline phosphatase are almost always elevated; approximately 50% of patients also have an elevated serum bilirubin. As the disease progresses and liver function deteriorates, the synthetic ability of the liver decreases, causing the albumin level to fall and the prothrombin and partial thromboplastin times to rise.

A number of paraneoplastic syndromes have been reported to occur in patients with HCC. These symptoms are infrequently seen at presentation, but the practitioner needs to be aware of the possibility of their occurrence. HCC occasionally synthesizes excess erythropoietin or erythropoietin precursors, leading to erythrocytosis.[85] Tumor production of a parathormone-like substance may cause hypercalcemia. Approximately 10% to 15% of patients with HCC are found to have elevated serum cholesterol and triglyceride levels. Hypoglycemia may occur as a result of an acquired form of glycogen storage disease or impaired hepatic gluconeogenesis.[85,86] Other paraneoplastic syndromes include dysfibrinogenemia with prolonged prothrombin and thrombin times, thrombocytosis, and ectopic adrenocorticotropic and gonadotropin hormone production.

### Diagnosis

The clinician should have a high index of suspicion for HCC when a patient complains of unexplained right upper quadrant pain and abdominal fullness. Rapid clinical deterioration of patients with a history of cirrhosis or hepatitis should alert the clinician to the possibility of HCC.

As mentioned earlier, liver function tests are frequently elevated, but are not diagnostic of HCC. The most valuable laboratory test consistent with a diagnosis of HCC is the AFP test. AFP is a glycoprotein synthesized by fetal liver and intestinal yolk sac cells. Levels are very high in utero and fall to adult levels of less than 10 ng/mL after birth. AFP is strongly associated with HCC and approximately 75% to 90% of patients have elevated levels.[87] Serial AFP determinations are used in patients with confirmed HCC to aid in the evaluation of response to treatment: AFP levels rise with tumor progression and fall with response to therapy.[88]

Several radiologic tests are useful in making the diagnosis of HCC. A radionuclide liver–spleen scan with technetium sulfur colloid may be used to initially detect a hepatic mass. This procedure has the advantages of being simple to perform, relatively inexpensive, and associated with no major morbidity; however, it is limited by the inability to visualize the entire abdomen. Ultrasound may also be used and has advantages similar to those of liver–spleen scanning. The disadvantage of ultrasound is that abdominal gas or overlying ribs may interfere with imaging and make interpretation difficult. CAT and MRI are also useful in the diagnosis of HCC. Although they are more expensive, they may provide a superior image and allow visualization of the entire abdomen.

Arteriography may be a useful adjunct in the diagnosis of patients with HCC when the previously discussed radiologic techniques provide equivocal results. HCC has a characteristic arteriographic appearance, with a dilated feeding artery and multiple vessels running throughout the lesion; however, unlike the other procedures, arteriography is an invasive technique and may increase patient morbidity.

All of these radiologic techniques may indicate the presence of a hepatic mass; however, no radiologic procedure can provide a definitive diagnosis of HCC. A definitive diagnosis of HCC can be made only by pathologic examination of a tissue sample. Tissue specimens may be obtained by percutaneous biopsy, peritoneoscopy with directed needle biopsy, or open biopsy at laparotomy.

### Staging/Prognosis

There is no generally accepted staging system for HCC. Numerous authors cite personal staging systems, but no one system is universally used. The overall prognosis for patients with HCC is poor. Survival is usually measured in weeks to months. The reported median survival time of untreated patients is 1 to 8 months from the time of diagnosis.[89–91] Several prognostic factors can influence the duration of survival. The surgical resectability of the tumor is the most important prognostic factor, as it affords the only potential cure for HCC. Other factors that appear to have an important and favorable influence on survival time include the absence of cirrhosis, normal liver function, no metastatic disease, a good performance status, and an age of less than

45 years.[91–93] Those patients who respond to therapy have a longer survival than nonresponders.[92–95]

Women with HCC have been reported to have a median survival time of 24 weeks versus 9 weeks for their male counterparts.[92] In addition, patients with HCC who reside in North America have a significantly longer median survival time than those patients residing in Africa or Asia.

### *Treatment*

***Surgery*** Surgical resection represents the only possibility for cure or long-term survival in patients with HCC. In general, resection is feasible only when the tumor is confined to a single lobe of the liver, thus allowing removal by wedge resection, segmentectomy, or unilobar hepatectomy. Small bilateral tumors or unsuspected metastatic disease may be found at surgery. Therefore, the final decision regarding resectability is always made at the time of surgery. Because of their poor prognosis, patients with jaundice, portal hypertension, severe coagulopathy, or ascites should not be considered for resection. Approximately 10% of patients with HCC are surgically resectable, and only 30% of these patients are cured.[96]

***Radiotherapy*** External irradiation is ineffective for patients with primary HCC, yielding no significant prolongation of survival. This is due primarily to the inherent sensitivity of the normal liver tissue to radiation, which limits the total dose that can be delivered to the tumor. Doses greater than 3,000 rads cause hepatitis. Some patients have been treated with doses in the range 2,000–2,500 rads, but only minimal efficacy is achieved at this dosage.

***Chemotherapy*** Doxorubicin is the most active single agent for treatment of HCC; the response rate is approximately 25%. The usual dose is 60–75 mg/m$^2$ administered intravenously every 3 to 4 weeks. Numerous studies have employed 5-FU either orally or intravenously; however, it has been found to possess only minimal activity, with an overall response rate of less than 10%. Occasional responses have also been reported in patients receiving dichloromethotrexate, neocarzinostatin, or etoposide, but overall response rates have been low.

In an attempt to improve upon the results with single-agent chemotherapy various combination regimens have been tried. Unfortunately, combination chemotherapy has not proven to be superior to single-agent doxorubicin.

***Intraarterial Chemotherapy*** As systemic chemotherapy appears to be of limited benefit in patients with HCC, investigators have attempted to enhance the efficacy by administering drugs intraarterially. Intraarterial administration of 5-FU has produced an overall response rate of approximately 50%. Small numbers of hepatoma patients have received intraarterial doxorubicin or cisplatin, with partial response rates of 43% and 19%, respectively.[97,98] High response rates have also been observed with combination intraarterial chemotherapy. A combination of mitomycin C, 5-FU, vinblastine, vincristine, and doxorubicin produced responses in 8 of 15 (53%) patients.[99] In addition, responses were reported in 8 of 12 (67%) patients receiving intraarterial FUDR, doxorubicin, and mitomycin C.[100] Because of the small number of patients treated with combination intraarterial chemotherapy, it is not possible compare the results with single-agent intraarterial infusion. Although the current experience with intraarterial chemotherapy for HCC is limited, the results have been encouraging and warrant further research.

***Hepatic Artery Ligation*** Hepatic artery ligation, with or without concomitant chemotherapy, has been performed in patients with HCC in an attempt to produce tumor necrosis secondary to ischemia. Although initial responses are seen, collateral vessels, which revascularize the tumor, develop rapidly. Hepatic artery ligation also makes the patient ineligible for other forms of regional therapy (i.e., hepatic artery infusion or chemoembolization). Toxic effects associated with ligation of the hepatic artery include high fever, right upper quadrant pain, leukocytosis, and transient worsening of the liver function tests.

***Embolization and Chemoembolization*** Embolization and chemoembolization are relatively new modalities for treating HCC. Embolization involves the injection of small particles into the hepatic artery (via a percutaneous catheter) that occlude the tumor capillary bed and block blood flow to the tumor. The advantages of embolization over surgical ligation are that it is a nonsurgical technique and that occlusion with embolization minimizes the development of collateral flow to the tumor. The size, concentration, and nature of the particles used determine the site and duration of the vascular block.

Only a few studies of embolization therapy for HCC have been reported. In one report, 6 of 9 (67%) patients responded to embolization, with median survival of 17.4 months.[101] In Japan, 120 patients with HCC were embolized, resulting in a 90% response rate. The 1-, 2-, and 3-year survival rates were 44%, 29%, and 15%, respectively.[102]

Chemoembolization combines the ischemic effects of embolization with the delivery of high concentrations of chemotherapeutic drugs within the tumor bed. This can be accomplished by injection of specially prepared particles that encapsulate the chemotherapeutic drug or simply by mixing highly concentrated chemotherapeutic agents with the embolization particles. The embolization agent holds the chemotherapeutic drug within the tumor bed, providing high local drug concentrations for a prolonged period. Additionally, systemic toxic effects from the chemotherapy are minimized, compared with systemic administration, because of the hepatic extraction of some agents and the slow release of drug into the systemic circulation. In two studies, chemoembolization with mitomycin C microspheres produced at least a 25% reduction in tumor size and clinical improvement in 4 of 7 (57%) and 15 of 20 (75%) patients with HCC.[103,104] In a recent study, gelfoam chemoembolization with mitomycin C, doxorubicin, and cisplatin produced an objective response in 9 of 20 (45%) patients with HCC.[105]

Both embolization and chemoembolization are generally well tolerated and have toxic effects similar to those of hepatic artery ligation (liver pain, fever, and elevated liver function tests).

### *Summary*

The overall worldwide incidence of HCC is high, but it is a relatively rare tumor in the United States, with only 3,000 to 4,000 cases diagnosed annually. HCC has a poor prognosis; less than 5% of patients survive 5 years from the time of diagnosis. Unfortunately, the symptoms associated with HCC are often vague, precluding early diagnosis. Surgical resection is the only treatment modality that offers a potential cure, but is feasible only for tumors confined to a single hepatic lobe. In patients with unresectable HCC, systemic chemotherapy or radiation therapy is of limited benefit, but the former is the only viable treatment option for widely metastatic disease. Intraarterial chemotherapy produces approximately a 50% partial response rate in patients with locally confined disease. In addition, preliminary results with new modalities, such as chemoembolization, appear encouraging and warrant further investigation.


## References


1. Silverberg E, Lubera J. Cancer statistics 1987. CA 1987;37:2–19.
2. Burkitt DP. Epidemiology of cancer of the colon and rectum. Cancer 1971;28:3–13.
3. Reedy BS, Wynder EL. Large bowel carcinogenesis: Fecal constituents of populations with diverse incidence rates of colon cancer. J Natl Cancer Inst 1973;50:1437–1442.
4. Lee JAH. Recent trends of large bowel cancer in Japan compared to United States, England and Wales. Int J Epidemiol 1976;5:187–194.
5. Muto T, Bussey HJR, Morson BC. The evolution of cancer of the colon and rectum. Cancer 1975;36:2251–2270.
6. Morson BC. Cancer in ulcerative colitis. Gut 1966;7:425–426.
7. Hinton JM. Risk of malignant changes in ulcerative colitis. Gut 1966;7:427–432.
8. Connor A, Altorski N, Moosa AR. Tumors of the colon, rectum, and anus, in Moosa AR, Robson MC, Schimpff SC (eds): Comprehensive Textbook of Oncology. Baltimore, Williams and Wilkins, 1986, pp 1063–1086.
9. Berk JE, Haubrich WS. Benign tumors of the colon and rectum; malignant tumors of the colon and rectum, in Bockus HL (ed): Gastroenterology. Philadelphia, W.B. Saunders, 1964, vol 2, pp 954–1033.
10. Welin S, Youker J, Spratt JS, et al. The rates and patterns of growth of 375 tumors of the large intestine and rectum observed serially by double contrast enema study (Malbo technique). Am J Roentgenol Rad Ther Nucl Med 1963;90:673–687.
11. Collins VP, Loeffler RK, Tivey H. Observations on growth of human tumors. Am J Roentgenol 1956;76:988–1000.
12. Havelaar I, Sugarbaker PH, Vermess M, et al. Rate of growth of intraabdominal metastases from colo-rectal cancer. Cancer 1984;65:163–171.
13. Moertel CG. Large bowel, in Holland JH, Frei EJ III (eds): Cancer Medicine. Philadelphia, Lea and Febiger, 1974, pp 1597–1626.
14. Sugarbaker PH, Gunderson LL, Wittes RE. Colorectal cancer (chapter 25), in DeVita VT, Hellman S, Rosenberg SA (eds): Cancer: Principles and Practice of Oncology. Philadelphia, J.B. Lippincott, 1985, pp 795–884.
15. Sugarbaker PH, Zamcheck N, Moore FD. Assessment of serial carcinoembryonic antigen (CEA) assays in postoperative detection of recurrent colorectal cancer. Cancer 1976;38:2310–2315.
16. Turnbull RB, Kyle K, Watson FR, et al. Cancer of the colon: The influence of the no-touch isolation technique on survival rates. Ann Surg 1967;166:420–427.
17. Gunderson LL, Dosoretz DE, Hedberg SE, et al. Low-dose preoperative irradiation, surgery, and elective postoperative radiation therapy for resectable rectum and rectosigmoid carcinoma. Cancer 1983;52:446–451.
18. Moertel CG, Thynne GS. Large bowel, in Holland JF, Frei E III (eds): Cancer Medicine. Philadelphia, Lea and Febiger, 1982, pp 1830–1859.
19. Moertel CG, Reitemeier RJ, Hahn RG. A controlled comparison of 5-fluoro-2-deoxyuridine therapy administered by rapid intravenous injection and by continuous intravenous infusion. Cancer Res 1967;27:549–552.
20. Jacobs EM, Reeves WJ, Wood DA, et al. Treatment of colon cancer with weekly intravenous 5-fluorouracil. Cancer 1971; 27:1302–1305.
21. Seifert P, Baker LH, Reed ML, et al. Comparison of continuously infused 5-fluorouracil with bolus injection in treatment for colorectal adenocarcinoma. Cancer 1975;36:123–128.
22. Lokich JJ, Perri J, Bothe A, et al. Cancer chemotherapy via ambulatory infusion pump. Am J Clin Oncol 1983;6:355–363.
23. Moertel CG. Chemotherapy of gastrointestinal cancer. N Engl J Med 1978;229:1049–1052.
24. Loehrer PJ, Einhorn LH. Chemotherapy of colorectal cancer. Adv Oncol 1986;2:21–29.
25. Benz C, Degregorio M, Sambol N, et al. Sequential infusions of methotrexate and 5-fluorouracil in advanced cancer: Pharmacology, toxicology, and response. Cancer Res 1985;45: 3354–3358.
26. Valone FH, Kohler M, Fisher K, et al. A NCOG randomized trial of 5-FU vs high dose leucovorin (LV) plus 5-FU vs sequential MTX, 5-FU, leucovorin for patients with advanced colorectal carcinoma. Proc Am Soc Clin Oncol 1986;5:89.
27. Greene H, Desai A, Levich S, et al. Combined 5-fluorouracil infusion plus high dose folinic acid in the treatment of metastatic gastrointestinal cancer. Proc Am Soc Clin Oncol 1986;5: 89.
28. Wanebo H. A staging system for liver metastases from colorectal cancer. Proc Am Soc Clin Oncol 1984;3:143.
29. Stagg RJ, Lewis BJ, Friedman MA, et al. Hepatic arterial chemotherapy for colorectal cancer metastatic to the liver. Ann Intern Med 1984;100:736–743.
30. Lehane DE, Zubler MA, Lawe M, et al. Intraarterial cisplatin in metastatic or recurrent colon cancer. Proc Am Soc Clin Oncol 1982;1:94.
31. Hohn DC, Stagg RJ, Friedman MA, et al. The NCOG randomized trial of intravenous (IV) vs hepatic arterial (IA) FUDR for colorectal cancer metastatic to the liver. Proc Am Soc Clin Oncol 1987;6:85.
32. Malagelada JR. Pancreatic cancer. An overview of epidemiology, clinical presentation, and diagnosis. Mayo Clin Proc 1979; 54:459–467.
33. Buncher CR. Epidemiology of pancreatic cancer, in Moossa AR (ed): Tumors of the Pancreas. Baltimore, Williams and Wilkins, 1980, pp 415–427.
34. Brooks JR. Cancer of the pancreas, in Brooks JR (ed): Surgery

of the Pancreas. Philadelphia, W.B. Saunders, 1983, pp 263–298.

**35.** Clark CG, Mitchell PEG. Diabetes mellitus and primary carcinoma of the pancreas. Br Med J 1961;2:1259–1262.

**36.** Schwartz SS, Zeidler A, Moossa AR, et al. A prospective study of glucose tolerance, insulin, C-peptide, and glucagon responses in patients with pancreatic carcinoma. Am J Dig Dis 1978;23:1107–1114.

**37.** Howard JM, Jordan GL. Cancer of the pancreas. Curr Probl Cancer 1977;2:1–52.

**38.** Moossa AR, Mackie CR, Gelder FB, et al. The value of tumor markers in the diagnosis and management of nonendocrine tumors of the pancreas, in Moossa AR (ed): Tumors of the Pancreas. Baltimore, Williams and Wilkins, 1980, pp 397–414.

**39.** Fitzgerald PJ, Fortner JG, Watson RC, et al. The value of diagnostic aids in detecting pancreas cancer. Cancer 1978;41: 868–879.

**40.** Sindelar WE, Kinsella TJ, Mayer RJ. Cancer of the pancreas, in DeVita VT (ed): Cancer: Principles and Practice, 2nd ed. Philadelphia, J.B. Lippincott, 1985, pp 691–739.

**41.** Pilepich MV, Miller HH. Preoperative irradiation in carcinoma of the pancreas. Cancer 1980;46:1945–1949.

**42.** Kopelson G. Curative surgery for adenocarcinoma of the pancreas/ampulla of Vater: The role of adjuvant pre or post-operative radiation therapy. Int J Radiat Oncol Biol Phys 1983;9:911–915.

**43.** Appelqvist P, Viren M, Minkkinen J, et al. Operative finding, treatment, and prognosis of carcinoma of the pancreas: An analysis of 267 cases. J Surg Oncol 1983;23:143–150.

**44.** Kalser MH, Ellenberg S. Pancreatic cancer: Adjuvant combined radiation and chemotherapy following curative resection. Arch Surg 1985;120:899–903.

**45.** Moertel CG. Exocrine pancreas, in Holland JF, Frei E (eds): Cancer Medicine, 2nd ed. Philadelphia, Lea and Febiger, 1982, pp 1792–1804.

**46.** Edis AJ, Kiernan PD, Taylor WF. Attempted curative resection of ductal carcinoma of the pancreas. Review of the Mayo Clinic experience, 1951–1975. Mayo Clin Proc 1980;55:531–536.

**47.** Haslam JB, Cavanaugh PJ, Stroup SL. Radiation therapy in the treatment of irresectable adenocarcinoma of the pancreas. Cancer 1973;32:1341–1345.

**48.** Dobelbower RR, Borgelt BB, Strubler KA, et al. Precision radiotherapy for cancer of the pancreas: Technique and results. Int J Radiat Oncol Biol Phys 1980;6:1127–1133.

**49.** Whittington R, Dobelbower RR, Mohiuddin M, et al. Radiotherapy of unresectable pancreatic carcinoma: A six year experience with 104 patients. Int J Radiat Oncol Biol Phys 1981;7:1639–1644.

**50.** Carter SK, Comis RL. The integration of chemotherapy into a combined modality approach for cancer treatment: VI. Pancreatic adenocarcinoma. Cancer Treat Rev 1975;2:193–214.

**51.** Crooke ST, Bradner WT. Mitomycin C: A review. Cancer Treat Rev 1976;3:121–139.

**52.** Smith FP, Schein PS. Chemotherapy of pancreatic cancer. Semin Oncol 1979;6:368–377.

**53.** Schein PS. The role of chemotherapy in the management of gastric and pancreatic carcinomas. Semin Oncol 1985;12:49–60.

**54.** Schein PS, O'Connell MJ, Blom J, et al. Clinical antitumor activity and toxicity of streptozotocin (NSC-85998). Cancer 1974;34:993–1000.

**55.** Stolinsky DC, Sadoff L, Braunwald J, et al. Streptozotocin in the treatment of cancer. Cancer 1972;30:61–69.

**56.** DuPriest RW, Huntington MC, Massey WH, et al. Streptozotocin therapy in 22 cancer patients. Cancer 1975;25:358–367.

**57.** Broder LE, Carter SK. Pancreatic islet cell carcinoma. II. Results of therapy with streptozotocin in 52 patients. Ann Intern Med 1973;79:108–118.

**58.** Wiggans RG, Woolley PV, Macdonald JS, et al. Phase II trial of streptozotocin, mitomycin C and 5-fluorouracil (SMF) in the treatment of advanced pancreatic cancer. Cancer 1978;41:387–391.

**59.** Smith FP, Hoth DF, Levin B, et al. 5-Fluorouracil, adriamycin, and mitomycin-C (FAM) chemotherapy for advanced carcinoma of the pancreas. Cancer 1980;46:2014–2018.

**60.** Bukowski RM, Abderhalden RT, Hewlett JS, et al. Phase II trial of streptozotocin, mitomycin C, and 5-fluorouracil in adenocarcinoma of the pancreas. Cancer Clin Trials 1980;3: 321–324.

**61.** Bitran JD, Desser RK, Kozloff MF, et al. Treatment of metastatic pancreatic and gastric adenocarcinomas with 5-fluorouracil, Adriamycin, and mitomycin-C (FAM). Cancer Treat Rep 1979;63:2049–2051.

**62.** Mallinson CN, Rake MO, Cocking JE, et al. Chemotherapy in pancreatic cancer: Results of a controlled prospective, randomized multicentre trial. Br Med J 1980;281:1589–1591.

**63.** Bukowski RM, Schacter LP, Groppe CW, et al. Phase II trial of 5-fluorouracil, Adriamycin, mitomycin C, and streptozotocin (FAM-S) in pancreatic carcinoma. Cancer 1982;50:197–200.

**64.** Moertel GC, Frytak S, Hahn RG, et al. Therapy of locally unresectable pancreatic carcinoma: A randomized comparison of high dose (6000 rads) radiation alone, moderate dose radiation (4000 rads + 5-fluorouracil), and high dose radiation + 5-fluorouracil. The Gastrointestinal Tumor Study Group. Cancer 1981;48:1705–1710.

**65.** Macdonald JS, Cohn Jr I, Gunderson LL. Cancer of the stomach, in DeVita VT, Hellman S, Rosenberg SA (eds): Cancer: Principles and Practice of Cancer. Philadelphia, J.B. Lippincott, 1985, pp 659–690.

**66.** Cady B, Ramsden DA, Stein A. Gastric cancer: Contemporary aspects. Am J Surg 1977;133:423–429.

**67.** Moertel CG. The stomach, in Holland JH, Frei E III (eds): Cancer Medicine. Philadelphia, Lea and Febiger, 1982, pp 1527–1541.

**68.** Dupont Jr JB, Cohn Jr I. Gastric adenocarcinoma. Curr Probl Cancer 1980;4:1–46.

**69.** LaDue JS, Murison PJ, McNeer G, et al. Symptomatology and diagnosis of gastric cancer. Arch Surg 1950;60:305–335.

**70.** Dupont Jr JB, Lee JR, Burton GR, et al. Adenocarcinoma of the stomach: Review of 1497 cases. Cancer 1978;41:941–947.

**71.** Remine WH, Priestley JT, Berkson J. Cancer of the Stomach. Philadelphia, W.B. Saunders, 1964, pp 255–285.

**72.** Childs DS, Moertel CG, Holbrook MA, et al. Treatment of unresectable adenocarcinomas of the stomach with a combination of 5-fluorouracil and radiation. Am J Roentgenol 1968;102:541–544.

**73.** Moertel CG, Lavin PT. Phase I–II chemotherapy studies in advanced gastric cancer. Cancer Treat Rep 1979;63:1863–1869.

**74.** MacDonald JS, Schein PS, Woolley PV, et al. 5-Fluorouracil, mitomycin C, and adriamycin (FAM): A new combination chemotherapy program for advanced gastric carcinoma. Ann Intern Med 1980;93:533–536.

**75.** Douglass H, Lavin PT, Goudsmit A, et al. An ECOG evaluation of combinations of methyl-CCNU, mitomycin C, adriamycin, and 5-fluorouracil in advanced measurable cancer (EST-2277). J Clin Oncol 1984;2:1372–1381.

**76.** Baker LH, Talley RW, Lehane DG, et al. Phase III comparison of the treatment of advanced gastrointestinal cancer with

bolus weekly 5-FU vs methyl-CCNU plus bolus weekly 5-FU. Cancer 1976;38:1–7.
77. Moertel CG, Fleming T, O'Connell M, et al. A phase II trial of combined intensive course 5FU, Adriamycin and *cis*-platinum in advanced gastric and pancreatic cancer. Proc Am Soc Clin Oncol 1984;3:137.
78. Moertel CG. The liver, in Holland JF, Frei E III (eds): Cancer Medicine. Philadelphia, Lea and Febiger, 1973, pp 1541–1547.
79. Blumberg BS, London WT. Hepatitis B virus and the prevention of hepatocellular carcinoma. N Engl J Med 1981;304:782–784.
80. Fisher RL, Schever PJ, Sherlock S. Primary liver cell carcinoma in the presence or absence of hepatitis antigen. Cancer 1976;38:901–905.
81. Knop RH, Berg CD, Ihde DC. Primary liver cancer in the adult, in Moosa AR, Robson MC, Schimpff SC (eds): Comprehensive Textbook of Oncology. Baltimore, Williams and Wilkins, 1986, pp 1087–1096.
82. Mays ET, Christopherson WM, Mahr MM, et al. Hepatic changes in young women ingesting contraceptive steroids. JAMA 1976;235:730–732.
83. Farrell GC, Uren RF, Perkins RW, et al. Androgen induced hepatoma. Lancet 1975;1:430–431.
84. Okuda K, Musha H, Nakajima Y, et al. Clinicopathologic features of encapsulated hepatocellular carcinoma. Cancer 1977;40:1240–1245.
85. Margolis S, Homey C. Systemic manifestations of hepatoma. Medicine (Baltimore) 1972;51:381–391.
86. Ihde DC, Sherlock P, Winawer SJ, et al. Clinical manifestations of hepatoma. Am J Med 1974;56:83–91.
87. Waldman TA, McIntire KR. The use of radioimmunoassay for alpha-fetoprotein in the diagnosis of malignancy. Cancer 1974;34:1510–1515.
88. McIntire KR, Vogel CL, Primack A. Effect of surgical and chemotherapeutic treatment on alpha-fetoprotein levels in patients with hepatocellular carcinoma. Cancer 1976;37:677–683.
89. Okuda K, Obata H, Hakajima Y, et al. Prognosis of primary hepatocellular carcinoma. Hepatology 1984;4:3S–6S.
90. Primack A, Vogel CL, Kyalwazi SK, et al. A staging system for hepatocellular carcinoma: Prognostic factors in Ugandan patients. Cancer 1975;35:1357–1364.
91. Falkson G, Moertel CG, Lavin P, et al. Chemotherapy studies in primary liver cancer. Cancer 1978;42:2149–2156.
92. Olweny CLM, Katorgol-Moidde E, Bahendeka S, et al. Further experience in treating patients with hepatocellular carcinoma in Uganda. Cancer 1980;46:2717–2722.
93. Ihde DC, Kane RC, Cohen MH, et al. Adriamycin therapy in American patients with hepatocellular carcinoma. Cancer Treat Rep 1977;61:1385–1387.
94. Vogel CL, Bayley AC, Brockes RJ. A phase II study of adriamycin in patients with hepatocellular carcinoma from Zambia and the United States. Cancer 1977;39:1923–1929.
95. Chlebowski RT, Tong M, Weissman J, et al. Hepatocellular carcinoma: Diagnostic and prognostic features in North American patients. Cancer 1984;53:2701–2706.
96. Cady B, Macdonald JS, Gunderson LL. Cancer of the hepatobiliary system, in DeVita VT (ed): Cancer: Principles and Practice. Philadelphia, J.B. Lippincott, 1985, pp 741–770.
97. Bern MM, McDermott W, Cady B, et al. Intraarterial hepatic infusion and intravenous adriamycin for treatment of hepatocellular cancer. Cancer 1978;42:399–405.
98. Cheng E, Watson RC, Fortner J, et al. Regional intraarterial infusion of cisplatin in primary liver cancer. Proc Am Soc Clin Oncol 1982;1:179.
99. Douglass CC. Prolongation of survival with periodic percutaneous multidrug arterial infusions in patients with primary and metastatic gastrointestinal carcinoma to liver. Proc Am Soc Clin Oncol 1980;21:416.
100. Patt YZ, Chuang VP, Wallace S, et al. Hepatic arterial infusion of floxuridine, adriamycin and mitomycin C (FAM) for hepatoma confined to the liver. Proc Am Soc Clin Oncol 1981;22:450.
101. Wallace S, Charnsangavej C, Carrasco H, et al. Infusion-embolization. Cancer 1983;51:2751–2765.
102. Yamada R, Sato M, Kawabata M, et al. Hepatic artery embolization in 120 patients with unresectable hepatoma. Radiology 1983;148:397–401.
103. Fujimoto R, Miyazaki M, Endoh F, et al. Biodegradable mitomycin-C microspheres given intra-arterially for inoperable hepatic cancer. Cancer 1985;56:2404–2410.
104. Ohnishi K, Tsuchiya S, Nakayama T, et al. Arterial chemoembolization of hepatocellular carcinoma with mitomycin C microcapsules. Radiology 1984;152:51–55.
105. Hohn D, Chase J, Stagg R, et al. A phase I–II trial of gelfoam chemoembolization in patients with primary liver tumors. Proc Am Soc Clin Oncol 1987;6:85.

# Chapter 97 / Malignant Lymphomas

Jim Koeller, MS, and Christopher P. Murphy, PharmD

## Hodgkin's Disease

Thomas Hodgkin first described the mysterious disease of the lymph system that bears his name over 150 years ago. Hodgkin's disease is a form of lymphoma, the cause of which is still unknown, and is invariably fatal if left untreated. Studies have demonstrated the orderly spread of this disease. Hodgkin's disease is classified into four histologic subtypes that differ somewhat in their natural history and treatment. The stage of Hodgkin's disease influences prognosis as well as therapy. The pathologic stage represents the best approximation of extent of disease and is based on histopathologic examination of the specimen obtained from biopsy of appropriate tissue or during staging laparotomy. Dramatic advances have been made in the understanding and treatment of Hodgkin's disease over the past two decades. Today, the majority of newly diagnosed patients with Hodgkin's disease are cured. The overall survival rates for Hodgkin's disease are listed in Table 97.1.[1] This extraordinary success has not been without cost. The programs are intense and technically demanding and are associated with significant acute toxicity and several long-term effects. The latent effects are only now becoming apparent and may have a major impact on treatment in the future.

### *Incidence/Epidemiology/Etiology*

Hodgkin's disease represents nearly 1% of all cancers; an estimated 6,900 new cases were diagnosed in 1986 (56% male and 44% female).[2] It is estimated that during this same period, only 1,500 people will have died of Hodgkin's disease.[2] Although Hodgkin's disease is considered a disease of the young, with an average age of 32 years, there appears to be a bimodal incidence curve that peaks between 15 and 34 years of age and again in those over 50.[3]

The etiology of Hodgkin's disease remains a mystery. It is known that untreated patients have varying degrees of impaired cellular immunity. Hodgkin's disease has been associated with defective T-lymphocyte function and may be a malignancy of a special monocyte–macrophage lineage that presents antigen to a T cell called the interdigitating dendritic cell (IDC).[4] Viruses have long been implicated in the etiology of Hodgkin's disease. This association is of interest in view of the presence of Sternberg–Reed cells in some patients with infectious mononucleosis and the presence of high titers of antibodies to Epstein–Barr virus antigen.[5,6] To date, there is still no direct linkage between Epstein–Barr virus and Hodgkin's disease. The human T-cell leukemia/lymphoma viruses (HTLVs) constitute a new class of viruses that have also been implicated in Hodgkin's disease.[7] Bacterial organisms, including *Mycobacterium tuberculosis* and *Brucella,* have also been implicated but have not withstood careful evaluation. Other possible etiologic factors include ionizing radiation, genetic predisposition, and environmental factors.

### *Biology/Histopathology/Classification*

Lymphocytes, the principal cellular component of lymphoid tissue, are widely distributed throughout the body and in aggregated centers. The bone marrow and thymus are the primary organs of lymphopoiesis, with secondary sites being the lymph nodes, spleen, lamina propria of the gastrointestinal tract, and Waldeyer's ring.

Hodgkin's disease is unique among the lymphomas because only a very small percent of cells from the involved tissue actually contain malignant cells; the vast majority are normal reactive hemopoietic cells. The exact cellular origin of the malignant cell has yet to be determined. Many believe that it is derived from either a T-lymphocyte or a macrophage/reticulum cell line. It is generally accepted that the Sternberg–Reed cell (or a variant of it) is the actual malignant cell. Recent evidence suggests that it may be derived from the interdigitating reticulum cell found in the paracortex of the lymph node.[4,8]

Lukes, Hicks, and Butler introduced a histopathologic classification of Hodgkin's disease (known as the Lukes–Butler classification) that was modified at the Rye conference in 1965 and is today called the Rye classification.[9,10] This classification is still widely accepted by both pathologists and clinicians. The Rye classification divides Hodgkin's disease into four subtypes: lymphocyte-predominant, nodular sclerosis, mixed cellularity, and lymphocyte-depleted (Table 97.2). The subtypes in this classification are based on characteristics of the Sternberg–Reed cell and the surrounding cells and connective tissue. They differ somewhat in natural history and response to treatment. With the introduction of extensive staging, sophisticated megavolt radiotherapy, and high-dose intermittent chemotherapy, the true prognostic value of these subtypes has become less clear.

#### Lymphocyte-Predominant

Lymphocyte-predominant Hodgkin's disease has characteristic benign-appearing lymphocytes that have a more diffuse growth pattern. The lymph nodes are usually partially to completely destroyed. Sternberg–Reed cells are uncommon, but a lymphocyte-predominant variant may be more important. Fibrosis is also uncommon. This subtype can account

**Table 97.1** 10-Year Hodgkin's Disease Survival

| *Stage* | *Survival (%)*[a] |
|---|---|
| I | 84 |
| II | 78 |
| III | 62 |
| IV | 42 |

[a] Based on deaths due only to the Hodgkin's disease. Overall survival = 65%.

Compiled from Kennedy BJ, Loeb V, Peterson VM, et al. National survey of patterns of care for Hodgkin's disease. Cancer 1985;56:2547–2556, with permission.

for 5% to 15% of all Hodgkin's disease, is slightly more common in males than females, and represents a more favorable prognosis.

**Nodular Sclerosis**

Nodular sclerosis Hodgkin's disease has two features that distinguish it from all other forms: the presence of the lacunar cell, which is a variant of the Sternberg–Reed cell, and the presence of a capsule that divides the lymphoid tissue into distinct nodules. Actual Sternberg–Reed cells are rare. This subtype can represent 30% to 60% of all Hodgkin's disease, is usually more localized, is slightly more common in females than males, and again is associated with a more favorable prognosis.

**Mixed Cellularity**

Mixed cellularity Hodgkin's disease occupies a position between the lymphocyte-predominant and lymphocyte-depleted subtypes with regard to the number of neoplastic cells present. It can be mistaken for diffuse histiocytic lymphoma and other non-Hodgkin's lymphomas. Sternberg–Reed cells are more common in this subtype. Diffuse fibrosis is uncommon. This subtype can account for 20% to 40% of all Hodgkin's disease, is slightly more common in males than females, and is associated with an intermediate prognosis.

**Table 97.2** The Rye (Lukes–Butler) Classification

| *Histologic subtype* | *Incidence (%)* |
|---|---|
| Lymphocyte-predominant | 5–15 |
| Nodular sclerosis | 30–60 |
| Mixed cellularity | 20–40 |
| Lymphocyte-depleted | < 5 |

Compiled from Lukes RJ, Craver LF, Hall TC, et al. Report of the nomenclature committee. Cancer Res 1966;26:1311, with permission.

**Lymphocyte-Depleted**

Lymphocyte-depleted Hodgkin's disease is associated with an abundance of Sternberg–Reed cells and their variants. It also can be easily mistaken for diffuse histiocytic lymphoma. Diffuse fibrosis and necrosis are commonly seen. This subtype can account for up to 5% of all Hodgkin's disease, is more common in males than females, is often widespread at the time of diagnosis, and is associated with a less favorable prognosis.

### *Clinical Presentation*

Most patients with lymphomas present with some form of adenopathy. The clinical presentations of Hodgkin's disease and the non-Hodgkin's lymphomas have some striking differences (Table 97.3). It is generally not possible to differentiate the various lymphomas by the physical characteristics of the lymph node itself, but the distribution can offer useful information.

Patients with Hodgkin's disease may have adenopathy that waxes and wanes for an average of 5 months before diagnosis. This adenopathy is usually localized to the cervical region and is painless and rubbery. Adenopathies of the inguinal and axillary regions may be present at diagnosis but are less common, whereas involvement of Waldeyer's ring and the epitrochlear nodes occurs in roughly 1% of patients (see Figure 97.1).[11] Other common sites of nodal involvement include the mediastinal, hilar, and retroperitoneal regions. Up to 40% of patients with Hodgkin's disease may

**Table 97.3** Clinical Features of the Lymphomas

| | *Hodgkin's disease* | *Non-Hodgkin's lymphoma* |
|---|---|---|
| Lymph node disease | Centripetal | Centrifugal |
| Contiguous spread | Common | Uncommon |
| Mediastinal disease | 50% | 20%[a] |
| Abdominal disease | Uncommon | Common |
| Bone marrow involvement | Uncommon | Common |
| Liver involvement | Uncommon (if present, spleen usually involved) | Common in follicular, uncommon in diffuse |
| Extranodal disease | Uncommon | Gastrointestinal tract, Waldeyer's ring, testes, epitrochlear nodes, brain |
| Systemic "B" symptoms | 40% | 20% |

[a] With the exception of T-cell lymphoblastic lymphoma.

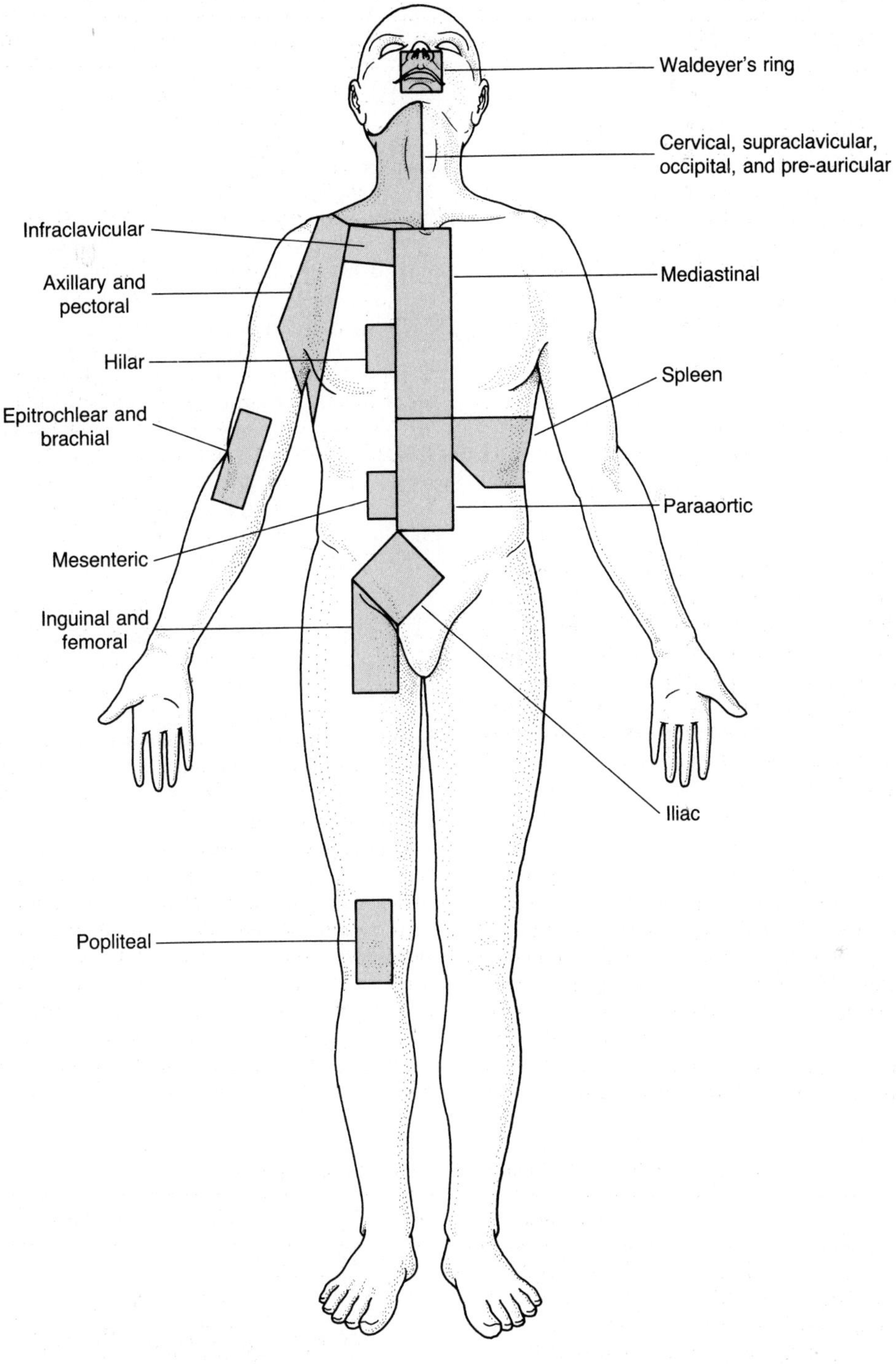


**Figure 97.1** Schematic representation of the anatomic regions used in the staging of Hodgkin's disease. *(From Rosenberg SA: The staging of Hodgkin's disease. [Letter to the Editor] Radiology 1966;87:145, with permission.)*

also present with constitutional symptoms including fever, night sweats, weight loss, and pruritis.[11] Hodgkin's disease, similar to most lymphomas, can also present as superior vena cava syndrome, acute spinal cord compression, a solitary thyroid nodule, a tumor nodule of the skin, or an unexplained anemia.

### *Diagnosis/Staging*

The diagnosis and pathologic classification of Hodgkin's disease can be made only by biopsy of the enlarged node and histopathologic examination under a microscope. There are four major reasons why a full evaluation for extent of disease

**Table 97.4** Features that Imply a Poor Prognosis

| |
|---|
| Hodgkin's disease |
| Advanced age |
| Male sex |
| Presence of "B" symptoms |
| Lymphocyte-depleted histology |
| Large mediastinal or abdominal involvement |
| Three to five involved sites |
| Extranodal extension |
| Subdiaphragmatic, lower abdominal, mesenteric, or pelvic lymph node involvement |
| Non-Hodgkin's lymphoma |
| Stage II disease or greater |
| Large-cell or Burkitt's lymphoma |
| Advanced age |
| Male sex |
| Presence of "B" symptoms |
| Bone marrow and gastrointestinal involvement |
| Richter's syndrome (conversion of low-grade to high-grade lymphoma) |

is necessary with Hodgkin's disease. First, the information is necessary for making an accurate diagnosis. Because of the toxic effects associated with the treatment (chemotherapy and radiotherapy), it is important to avoid unnecessary treatment if possible. Second, it is still believed by many that certain patterns of organ involvement have prognostic implications. Third, staging is based on the diagnostic evaluation. Fourth, specific knowledge of the involved sites can be used to determine response. As mentioned earlier, certain features may imply a poor prognosis for a given patient. These specific features are listed in Table 97.4.

The Ann Arbor staging classification, which was developed at the 1970 Ann Arbor conference, has proven to be a good workable scheme.[12] The Ann Arbor version modified the Rye staging classification of 1965 and is outlined in Table 97.5. After careful staging, roughly half the patients have localized disease (stages I, II, and IIE) and the remainder have advanced disease, of which 10% to 15% is stage IV. One of the most important factors to remember is that Hodgkin's disease appears to follow a predictable pattern of nodal spread that is not seen with the non-Hodgkin's lymphomas.

The appropriate diagnostic and staging procedures are shown in Table 97.6. These are based on recommendations made at the Ann Arbor conference. Clinical staging begins with a thorough history to evaluate possible symptoms including fever, night sweats, and weight loss; greater than 10% weight loss has been associated with a poor prognosis. A complete physical exam is done to determine nodal and extranodal involvement. Laboratory tests assess bone marrow, renal, and hepatic function. As stated previously, a true diagnosis can be made only with an adequate surgical biopsy. A chest roentgenogram and bipedal lymphangiography are necessary as part of the staging process. A bone marrow biopsy is especially helpful in patients that are symptomatic or have an elevated alkaline phosphatase, hypercalcemia, or unexplained anemia.

Over the past several years, considerable attention has

**Table 97.5** Ann Arbor Staging Classification for Hodgkin's Disease

| | |
|---|---|
| Stage I | Involvement of single lymph node region (I) or single extralymphatic organ or site ($I_E$) |
| Stage II | Involvement of two or more lymph node regions on one side of the diaphragm (II), or localized involvement of an extralymphatic organ or site ($II_E$) |
| Stage III | Involvement of lymph node regions on both sides of the diaphragm (III), or localized involvement of an extralymphatic site ($III_E$), or spleen ($III_S$), or both ($III_{SE}$) |
| Stage IV | Diffuse of disseminated involvement of one or more extralymphatic organs with or without associated bone marrow involvement |
| | A—Asymptomatic |
| | B—Fever (greater than 38°C for 3 consecutive days), sweats, weight loss (greater than 10%). |

From Kaplan HS. Hodgkin's Disease, 2nd ed. Cambridge, Harvard University Press, 1980, with permission.

been focused on new methods used for the assessment of Hodgkin's disease. It must be realized that a majority of these new techniques should be used only in specific circumstances. Mediastinal and hilar adenopathies are best evaluated with a standard chest x-ray. Whole-lung tomography or computerized axial tomography (CAT) of the thorax generally do not modify treatment plans. Lymphangiography (LAG) remains the most accurate method for evaluating disease below the diaphragm. Abdominal CAT, pelvic CAT,

**Table 97.6** Diagnosis and Staging Procedures

| |
|---|
| Required |
| Thorough history |
| Complete physical examination |
| Laboratory studies |
| Complete blood count |
| Serum chemistries |
| Renal and liver function |
| Adequate surgical biopsy |
| Radiologic studies |
| Chest roentgenogram (paraaortic and lateral) |
| Bilateral lower extremity lymphangiogram |
| Bone marrow biopsy (needle or open) |
| May be required in specific circumstances |
| Abdominal computerized tomography |
| Thoracic computerized tomography |
| Intravenous pyelogram |
| Skeletal survey |
| Whole-lung tomography |
| Pelvic computerized tomography |
| Exploratory laparotomy |
| Gallium whole-body scan |

intravenous pyelogram, and gallium scanning should be reserved for special situations.

Staging can be based on clinical or pathologic findings. Clinical staging is based on the history, physical exam, initial diagnostic biopsy, laboratory tests, and radiologic findings. Pathologic staging is based on the biopsy findings of strategic sites (muscle, bone, skin, spleen, abdominal nodes) using an invasive procedure such as a laparoscopy or laparotomy. These patients with extranodal disease (muscle, skin, bone, Waldeyer's ring) contiguous to involved nodes are classified with the subscript "E" in the Rye staging system. An example would be a patient who was clinically classified as stage II without symptoms but, at laparotomy, was found to have a positive spleen and paraaortic nodes. This patient would then be classified as a PS $IIIA_{SE}$. These patients have a more favorable prognosis than those with frank disseminated disease.

One of the most controversial areas in staging continues to be the role of laparotomy in the diagnosis and treatment of Hodgkin's disease. The sole purpose of the laparotomy is to determine the extent of disease in the abdomen. It has been used to remove the spleen. Unfortunately, splenectomy has not demonstrated any survival advantage.[13] The true value of the laparotomy is realized when the improved accuracy of the staging permits selection of the most effective method of treatment. Laparotomy itself is not without risk; the overall mortality rate can range from 0.5% to as high as 6%, with morbidity rates as high as 27%.[14,15] Controversy over the use of staging laparotomy will continue until a clear survival advantage can be shown. Until that time, staging laparotomy should be reserved for those instances where the treatment plan would be altered by the information obtained or should be considered a research tool to correlate outcome of therapy. Staging laparotomy should generally not be used in the private practice setting.

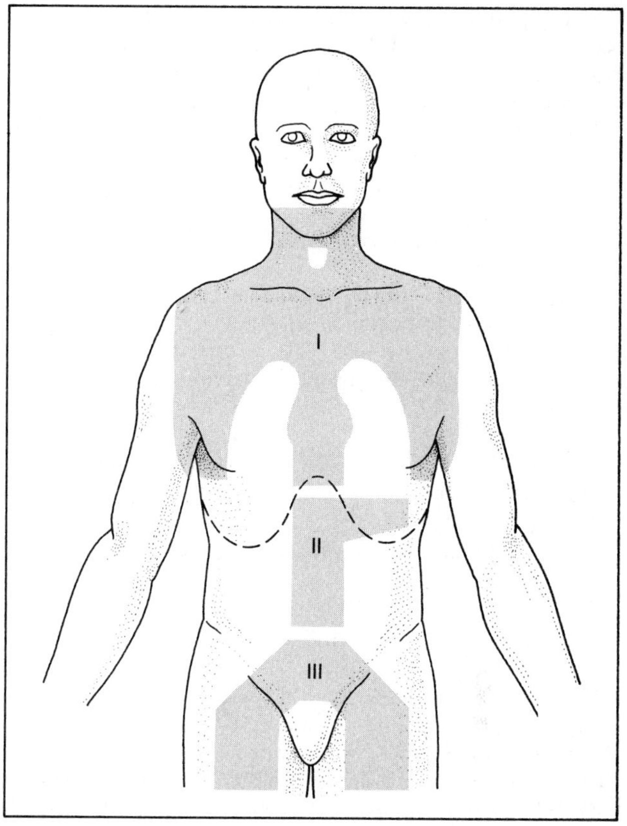


**Figure 97.2** Radiation fields (shaded) commonly employed in Hodgkin's disease. I = mantle, II = paraaortic–splenic pedicle, III = pelvic, I + II = subtotal nodal irradiation (STNI), I + III = total nodal irradiation (TNI). *(From Rubin P (Ed): Clinical Oncology, 6th ed. Washington, D.C., American Society, 1983, p. 352, with permission.)*

### *Treatment*

The current goal in the treatment of Hodgkin's disease is to maximize curability while minimizing treatment-related complications. The development of effective therapies for all stages of Hodgkin's disease remains one of the most remarkable achievements and success stories in modern cancer treatment. This has been brought about by the introduction of modern linear accelerators providing radiation beams in the range 4–8 MeV, effective combination chemotherapy regimens, and new methods of combining these two modalities.

#### Radiation Therapy

Radiation therapy alone is still the cornerstone of treatment for patients with localized Hodgkin's disease. In stages IA and IIA, extended-field radiotherapy (mantle plus paraaortic irradiation) is the current treatment of choice (see Fig. 97.2). This produces disease-free survival rates ranging from 65% to 85% and overall survival rates of 75% to 90%.[16–19] The survival rates remain high because of excellent salvage chemotherapy. These studies also revealed pelvic relapse rates ranging from only 3% to 8%. Treatment of patients with stage IB and IIB (constitutional symptoms) disease is less clear. Studies have shown disease-free survival rates near 75% for symptomatic stage I and II disease.[17,18] Another trial compared extended-field with involved-field radiation plus six cycles of involved-field radiation plus six cycles of MOPP (Table 97.7) therapy and found a significant increase in disease-free survival for the combined treatment group[20]; however, no overall survival advantage could be shown. Because of such high salvage rates from current chemotherapy regimens, extended-field or total nodal irradiation is still considered the therapy of choice.

**Table 97.7** MOPP Regimen[a]

| *Drug* | *Full dose ($mg/m^2$)* | *Route* | *Days* |
|---|---|---|---|
| Mechlorethamine (nitrogen mustard) | 6 | IV | 1, 8 |
| Vincristine (Oncovin) | 1.4 | IV | 1, 8 |
| Procarbazine | 100 | PO | 1–14 |
| Prednisone | 40 | PO | 1–14 |

[a] One cycle is 28 days. Prednisone is given in cycle 1 and every subsequent third cycle.

There appears to be a separate subgroup of stage I and II patients with a much higher likelihood of relapse. These are patients with large mediastinal masses that are greater than one third the thoracic diameter. Studies have shown that relapse-free survival is as low as 45% in this subgroup of patients.[17,21–23] Because of the significant difference, this subgroup of patients is discussed later.

For patients with pathologic stage IIIA disease treated with total nodal or extended-field irradiation, disease-free survival rates range from 35% to 65%.[18,24–27] Overall, 50% of stage IIIA patients treated with these types of radiation therapy relapse. From these studies[18,24–27] was isolated a subgroup of patients with stage $III_1A$ disease (spleen, celiac, splenic, or portal nodes) who did not have significantly lower disease-free survival rates compared with other early staged patients. This subgroup should probably be treated with extended-field or total nodal irradiation and monitored closely. The other subtypes of stage III disease patients are also discussed later.

### Chemotherapy

In 1963, the first pilot study to use four drugs in combination (mechlorethamine, vincristine, methotrexate, prednisone) was carried out in patients with Hodgkin's disease.[28] In 1964, by substituting procarbazine for methotrexate, the four-drug combination of MOPP was formed. MOPP chemotherapy has been the mainstay of treatment for patients with stage IIIB and IV advanced Hodgkin's disease. The MOPP regimen is shown in Table 97.7. MOPP produces complete remissions (disappearance of all measurable disease) in 80% of patients and has a 10-year cure rate of 54%,[29] in contrast with single-agent therapy, where remissions occur less rapidly and are not as durable. Several other trials reviewed by Coltman have reported similar results, with complete response rates ranging from 60% to 80% and survival rates ranging from 54% to 80%.[30] These studies indicate that patients should receive two cycles of therapy beyond that required to produce a complete response; a minimum of six cycles should be administered. Maintenance therapy has not been shown to increase survival. Delivering full or nearly full doses of chemotherapy is extremely important. Dose reduction within the various studies is probably the single most important factor explaining the differences in response rates between institutions administering seemingly similar regimens. Dosage reductions based on toxicity can be made, but significant reductions can alter response and survival.[31]

***Comparative Trials With MOPP Variations*** Many variations of the MOPP regimen have been tested over the years, with the goals of improving efficacy and decreasing both acute and long-term complications of MOPP. The results of these trials are given in Table 97.8. Behrens and colleagues have written an excellent in-depth review of these trials.[32] These trials have not proven the variations to be superior in response rate, duration, or survival to the original MOPP. Complete responses to treatment with MOPP variants range from 60% to 80% in previously untreated patients as compared with 70% to 100% for MOPP. Additionally, 10-year follow-up data are available only for MOPP. Several of these trials have shown less acute toxicity, although long-term complications are less well defined and difficult to assess because of the shorter follow-up periods. Toxicity is addressed later.

***Alternating Non–Cross-Resistant Regimens*** The Goldie–Coldman hypothesis concerning spontaneous mutation rates and the development of resistant clones can explain many clinical findings related to cancer chemotherapy including chemotherapy failure.[33] Their findings have led to the investigation of non–cross-resistant drug combinations.[34] One of the key requirements in such a concept is that each alternating regimen possess equal activity. The Milan Cancer Institute was one of the first groups to apply the Goldie–Coldman hypothesis to the treatment of Hodgkin's disease. They began a prospective randomized trial of MOPP versus

**Table 97.8** Results of Treatment With Variants of MOPP

| *Regimen*[a] | *N* | *Complete response rate (%)* | *Restaged* | *Median disease-free interval (yr)* | *Author* |
|---|---|---|---|---|---|
| MOPP | 54 | 77.8 | No | >5 | Jacobs |
| BOPP | 103 | 69 | No | 4 | Nissen |
| COPP | 138 | 66 | No | 4 | Morgenfield |
| CVPP | 157 | 71 | Yes | >4 | Morgenfield |
| BVCPP | 324 | 68 | No | N/A | Durant |
| MOPP-Bleo | 156 | 82 | No | N/A | Coltman |

[a] MOP=mechlorethamine, vincristine, procarbazine
BOPP=BCNU, vincristine, procarbazine, prednisone
COPP=Cyclophosphamide, vincristine, procarbazine, prednisone
CVPP=Cyclophosphamide, vinblastine, procarbazine, prednisone
BVCPP=BCNU, vinblastine, cyclophosphamide, procarbazine, prednisone
MOPP-Bleo=Mechlorethamine, vincristine, procarbazine, prednisone, bleomycin

Data from References 28 and 29.

ABVD (doxorubicin, bleomycin, vinblastine, dacarbazine).[35] Their results indicated that both regimens were equally effective and that the crossover treatment in patients resistant to either combination revealed no cross-resistance between the two regimens. From these data several alternating programs using MOPP/ABVD were initiated. The Milan group has reported 7-year follow-up data on a randomized trial comparing MOPP with MOPP/ABVD given for 12 cycles to 88 patients with stage IV disease.[36] The results indicate a statistically significant increase in disease-free survival (44.4% versus 76.8%) and overall survival (61.1% versus 82.3%) for the alternating regimen. Another group has used alternating MOPP/ABVD for 24 cycles plus radiation therapy in 57 patients, with a disease-free survival at 4 years of 88%.[37] The National Cancer Institute has randomized 79 patients to a trial comparing MOPP with alternating MOPP/SCAB (streptozocin, lomustine, doxorubicin, bleomycin).[38] Initial complete remission rates of nearly 85% were seen with both regimens, and median survival for both groups at 4 years exceeded 80%.

#### Combined Modality Treatment

As mentioned earlier, there are several instances in which combined modality treatment for Hodgkin's disease may be indicated, such as in early-stage disease with large mediastinal involvement, bulky disease, nodular sclerosis subtype, or stage $III_2A$ disease.

In patients with limited disease, but large mediastinal involvement (roughly 20% of these patients), relapse rates range from 45% to 75% when radiation therapy is used alone.[17,21–23] The rationale for combined modality therapy in patients with massive mediastinal involvement is clear. Neither radiation therapy nor chemotherapy alone is particularly successful in this group of patients. The Stanford group has collected the largest series of early staged patients with mediastinal involvement. The 5-year disease-free survival was prolonged in patients treated with combined modality therapy (86% versus 73%), but there was no overall survival gain.[17] Other trials have shown similar advantages in treating mediastinal involvement in early-stage disease.[22,23,39] Chemotherapy alone has failed to show significant responses in these patients.[40]

In stage IIIA disease, only subgroup $III_1A$ appears to do well with radiation therapy alone. Patients with stage $III_2A$ (involvement of paraaortic or iliac nodes plus or minus the nodes involved in $III_1A$ disease) have a much lower disease-free and overall survival when treated with radiation therapy alone.[24] A collaborative university report compared combined modality treatment with radiation alone in stage $III_1A$ and $III_2A$ patients.[25] The combined modality group showed an advantage in both disease-free and overall survival (94% versus 65% and 74% versus 46%). Another trial evaluated 120 patients with stage IIIA and IIIB disease treated with either total nodal irradiation or combined MOPP/radiation therapy.[41] The 12-year disease-free and actual survival rates were 83% versus 40% and 80% versus 64% respectively. In the subset of patients with stage $III_2A$ disease, survival was improved from 44% to 66% using combined modality therapy. In contrast, a Stanford trial involving 117 patients failed to show this type of advantage with combined modality therapy.[27] Part of the discrepancy may be explained by differences in radiation technique. It is also recommended that patients with nodular sclerosis Hodgkin's disease receive combined modality therapy and not combination chemotherapy alone.[42]

Various studies have evaluated the usefulness of combined modality therapy in advanced disease (stages IIIB and IV). The Yale group has tested stage III, IVA, and IVB patients with 6 months of combination chemotherapy followed by 1,500–2,000 rads of radiation to involved sites, followed then by 4 more months of combination chemotherapy.[43] The 5-year disease-free and overall survival rates were 74% and 80%. These data are quite similar to those reported with combination chemotherapy alone and may not offer a true advantage in the treatment of advanced disease.

Combined modality therapy can produce significant disease-free and overall survival in certain subsets of Hodgkin's patients. The true role that it plays in the overall management of patients with Hodgkin's disease has yet to be determined. One must weigh the increased acute toxic effects and potential long-term complications against the use of effective initial or salvage chemotherapy.

#### Salvage Chemotherapy

Despite the large success of MOPP therapy in producing complete responses in a majority of patients treated, 50% of these patients with advanced disease ultimately are not cured (20%–40% will not respond initially to MOPP therapy, and an additional 30% of responders relapse after achieving a complete response).[31] For patients who relapse after an initial complete response to MOPP, reinduction is possible. One trial reported a 59% complete response rate in 32 patients retreated with MOPP after relapse.[44] The median duration of remission was 21 months. Reinduction was more successful if relapse occurred more than 12 months after the original therapy was administered. In patients who cannot be successfully reinduced or who failed MOPP originally, salvage therapy is required. Numerous salvage regimens have been tested and several examples are given in Table 97.9. These salvage regimens produce complete remission rates ranging from 25% to 60%, as reported in two excellent reviews.[31,45]

The Milan group has evaluated the potentially non–cross-resistant combination of ABVD in 70 patients who failed MOPP.[46] They reported a complete response rate of 54%, with a median duration of response of 34 months and a median survival for complete responders of 55 months. Constitutional symptoms and extranodal involvement were poor prognostic indicators in this group of patients. These data are similar to those reported by Papa and colleagues,[47] but several other trials reviewed by Longo et al[48] have shown much lower response rates.

Salvage therapy can effectively produce complete remissions in up to 50% of patients who fail MOPP. Unfortunately, many of these patients relapse at some point. Single-agent palliative therapy may be useful in truly refractory patients.[49]

**Table 97.9** Salvage Therapy for MOPP Failures

| *Regimen*[a] | *N* | *Complete response rate (%)* | *Disease-free survival (mo)* | *Author* |
|---|---|---|---|---|
| ABVD | 70 | 54 | 34 | Santoro |
| VABCD | 18 | 44 | >36 | Einhorn |
| B-CAVe | 52 | 40 | — | Harker |
| CEP | 58 | 40 | >15 | Santoro |
| CBVD | 20 | 45 | 10 | Weiss |
| SCAB | 17 | 35 | >8 | Levi |
| ADBIC | 29 | 35 | >28 | Rogers |

[a] ABVD=doxorubicin, bleomycin, vinblastine, dacarbazine
VABCD=vinblastine, doxorubicin, bleomycin, lomustine, dacarbazine
B-CAVe=bleomycin, lomustine, doxorubicin, vinblastine
CEP=lomustine, etoposide, prednimustine
CBVD=lomustine, bleomycin, vinblastine, dacarbazine
SCAB=streptozotocin, lomustine, doxorubicin, bleomycin
ADBIC=doxorubicin, dacarbazine, bleomycin, lomustine, prednisone

Data from References 28 and 29.

## Complications

The various treatment programs outlined in this review can be quite complicated and may be associated with various acute and long-term toxic effects that can lead to significant morbidity. For an in-depth review of the general complications associated with the treatment of Hodgkin's disease, two recent reviews may be of assistance.[11,50]

A variety of side effects can occur during radiation therapy for Hodgkin's disease. Most are transient and seldom produce significant morbidity. Anorexia, xerostomia, odynophagia, skin burns, and changes in taste perception are quite common. Myelosuppression can also be seen.

More serious toxic effects can occur during radiation therapy for Hodgkin's disease involving the mantle and the heart. Paramediastinal pulmonary densities, radiation pneumonitis and fibrosis, pericardial complications, and abnormal ventricular function have been reported.

The most common neurologic complication seen as a result of radiation therapy for Hodgkin's disease is L'hermitte's syndrome, which occurs in up to 15% of patients.[10] This syndrome consists of numbness and tingling caused by head flexion. Spinal cord transections have been reported with overlap of mantle and paraaortic fields.

As the techniques for radiation therapy improve, the significant complications associated with its use will continue to be reduced.

Side effects of chemotherapy can be acute or long term. Acute toxic effects seen with the treatment of Hodgkin's disease are similar to those seen with most combination regimens. Myelosuppression is the major dose-limiting toxic effect of most of these regimens. Nausea and vomiting are frequently seen with the use of dacarbazine, doxorubicin, and mechlorethamine. A significant number of patients experience neurotoxicity secondary to the vincristine used in MOPP therapy. Other acute toxic effects are alopecia, dermatitis, mucositis, phlebitis, malaise and fatigue, pulmonary reactions, cardiomyopathy, and renal dysfunction.

The achievement of cures in Hodgkin's disease with chemotherapy or combined modality programs has provided the unique opportunity to observe long-term complications of cancer treatment in patients. The mutagenic, carcinogenic, and teratogenic potential of chemotherapy has been long recognized.

Gonadal dysfunction and secondary malignancies have become important considerations in the treatment of Hodgkin's disease. It is now recognized that these are major long-term complications.

The effects of cancer chemotherapy on gonadal function have recently been reviewed.[51] Almost all men treated with MOPP and some of those treated with ABVD become sterile.[44,52] Chemotherapy can cause ovarian failure in up to 50% of premenopausal women and premature menopause in others.[53] Gonadal dysfunction in men and women is more common as the age of the patient increases.

As 10- and 15-year survival data for treated Hodgkin's patients become more common, the appearance of preleukemias and leukemias will also become more common. The overall risk of developing leukemia ranges from 6% to 9% and in certain subsets of patients may be as high as 20%.[54–57] The chance of developing leukemia is greater after chemotherapy than after radiation therapy, for older patients, those requiring salvage treatment, and especially those receiving combined modality therapy. Various solid tumors and other non-Hodgkin's lymphomas may also occur after combined modality therapy. The drugs most often implicated in this phenomenon are the alkylating agents and procarbazine. These drugs in combination with radiation therapy seem especially dangerous.

## Current Recommendations

A large number of patients with Hodgkin's disease can be cured with currently available therapy. Although specific treatment recommendations are influenced by special circumstances and available resources, general recommendations for the treatment of Hodgkin's disease can be made (see Table 97.10).

Patients with supradiaphragmatic stage I or IIA disease are best treated with extended-field radiation therapy (mantle plus paraaortic fields). This treatment is associated with high overall survival and minimal complications.

Patients with stage IIB and $III_1A$ disease should receive either total nodal or extended-field irradiation. Combination chemotherapy by itself may prove to be just as effective.

Patients with stage I and II disease and large mediastinal involvement may be treated in very special instances with entended-field irradiation and special mantle treatment. Otherwise, combined modality therapy is considered the treatment of choice.

Excluding the subset of patients with stage $III_1A$, all other patients with stage IIIA Hodgkin's disease should not receive radiation therapy alone. The optimal therapy for these patients still needs to be determined. Either chemotherapy alone or combined modality therapy is generally used.

**Table 97.10** Current Recommendations for the Treatment of Hodgkin's Disease

| *Stage* | *Treatment* |
|---|---|
| IA or IIA | Extended-field irradiation (mantle + paraaortic) |
| IIB or $III_1A$ | Extended-field irradiation or total nodal irradiation<br>Combination chemotherapy may also be effective |
| I or II with large mediastinal disease | Combined modality therapy (radiation therapy + combination chemotherapy)<br>Extended-field irradiation + special mantle treatment may be used in select patients |
| IIIA (excluding $III_2A$) | Combined modality therapy (total nodal irradiation + chemotherapy) or combination chemotherapy alone |
| IIIB or IV | Combination chemotherapy (MOPP alone or MOPP/ABVD) |

Patients with stage IIIB or IV disease should receive combination chemotherapy. MOPP remains the current treatment of choice, although alternating MOPP/ABVD may become the standard.

### *Future Directions*

Although great strides have been made in the treatment of Hodgkin's disease, there remain areas where much progress can still be made. Several areas of controversy also need to be clarified.

One area under evaluation is the use of chemotherapy in early-stage disease. It is realized that effective radiation therapy requires the technical expertise and sophisticated equipment that are usually available only in large treatment centers. Such treatment, therefore, is not available to all patients. Results for patients treated without this expertise and sophisticated equipment are inferior to those reported by the successful larger institutions. Standardization of effective therapy is needed. Combination chemotherapy may play a role in this setting and is currently being tested.

Areas of debate still exist in the treatment of Hodgkin's disease. The treatment of large mediastinal disease and stage IIIA disease remains unclear. For patients with large mediastinal disease it is now realized that radiation therapy or chemotherapy alone results in significant relapse rates. Currently, agressive treatment including alternating MOPP/ABVD and radiation therapy to the original disease plus a boost to the mediastinum is being evaluated. Treatment of stage IIIA disease also remains unclear. Radiation therapy alone is probably acceptable for only a small subset of these patients. Trials involving either chemotherapy alone or combined modality therapy are being tested.

Further progress for advanced disease is needed. Continued evaluation of non–cross-resistant alternating regimens is needed. Additionally, more effective salvage therapy must be developed.

Another issue that needs to be addressed is the occurrence of secondary malignancy after curative therapy. Less carcinogenic, equally effective combinations need to be found. Unfortunately, research of this type requires many years for full evaluation.

Finally, some very preliminary data suggest the use of allogeneic bone marrow transplantation in MOPP-resistant Hodgkin's disease.[58] Out of eight patients treated, two remain in complete remission more than 38 months. This may prove to be another alternative treatment method for selected patients.

## Non-Hodgkin's Lymphoma

The non-Hodgkin's lymphomas are a heterogeneous group of lymphoproliferative disorders involving the lymphatic and immune systems. Non-Hodgkin's lymphomas represent a complex group of neoplastic diseases with a variable morphologic appearance, natural history, and clinical presentation and divergent patterns of response to treatment. The classification of non-Hodgkin's lymphoma, which traditionally has been based on morphology, is now based on prognostic factors such as morphology, biologic aggressiveness, and functional and immunologic characteristics. A multidisciplinary approach to treatment has become increasingly important as new data from therapeutic programs become available. The use of extensive combination chemotherapeutic regimens has shown dramatic improvement in survival and cure in patients with a disease that was considered incurable only a decade ago.

### *Incidence/Epidemiology/Etiology*

Non-Hodgkin's lymphomas are the eight most common cause of newly diagnosed cancer in the United States; an estimated 27,200 new cases were diagnosed in 1986, and it is claimed that nearly 14,600 people will have died during this same period.[2] The incidence of non-Hodgkin's lymphoma steadily increases with advancing age from childhood through age 80, and is more common in males (8.1 per 100,000) than in females (5.7 per 100,000).[59]

The etiology of non-Hodgkin's lymphoma is unknown in most cases. A hereditary influence is suggested as a possible cause, as patients with inherited immunodeficiency diseases and patients from families immunologic disorders show an increased incidence of non-Hodgkin's lymphoma.[60] A mechanism for this cause includes chronic antigenic stimulation for either infection or defective immunoregulation. Likewise, patients with the acquired immunodeficiency syndrome or with other disorders of immunity, such as Sjögren's syndrome, systemic lupus erythematosus, and disorders caused by chronic pharmacologic immunosuppression, especially that associated with renal allografts, have a

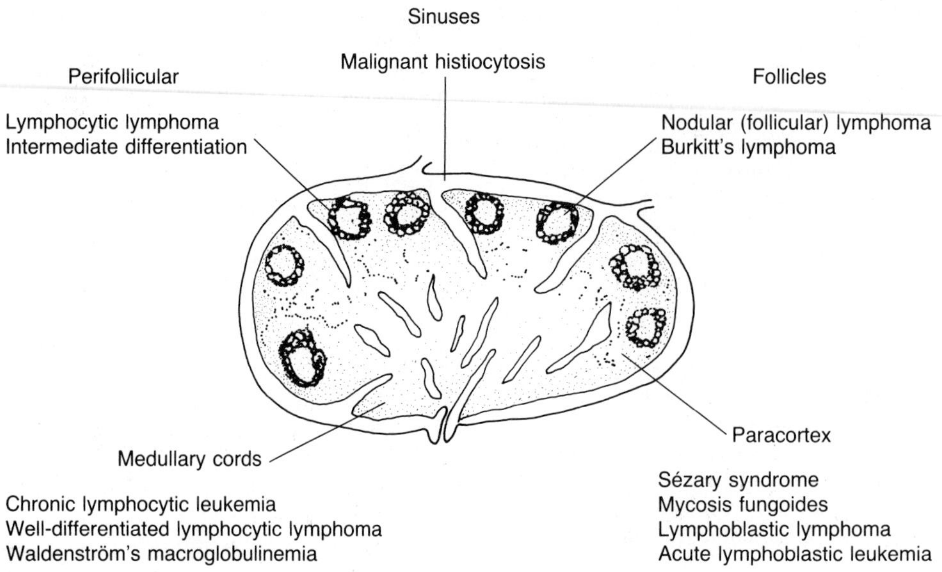


**Figure 97.3** Classification on non-Hodgkin's lymphomas according to functional anatomy. *(From Mann RB, Jaffe ES, Berard CW: Am J Pathol 1979;94:103–192, with permission.)*

greater incidence of non-Hodgkin's lymphomas. Other diseases with a predisposition to develop lymphomas include ataxia telangiectasia, Wiskott–Aldrich syndrome, Kleinfelter's syndrome, and acquired hypogammaglobulinemia.[60] Other possible etiologic factors include exposure to ionizing radiation; occupational hazards such as persistent exposure to asbestos, organic solvents, and herbicides; and infectious agents such as the Epstein–Barr virus, which is associated with Burkitt's lymphoma.[60] As the non-Hodgkin's lymphomas comprise a heterogeneous group of neoplastic disorders, it should be no surprise that diverse etiologies exist.

### *Histopathology/Classification*

Most non-Hodgkin's lymphomas are derived from monoclonal proliferation of B lymphocytes; neoplasms of T-lymphocyte origin are much less common. The non-Hodgkin's lymphomas are also described by different developmental and functional subclasses, nodular (follicular) and diffuse.

Nodular or follicular lymphomas are neoplasms of the proliferative regions of the B-lymphocyte system, the lymphoid follicle (see Fig. 97.3). These neoplasms form circumscribed aggregates that may involve only a portion of the node or the entire lymph node, causing total effacement of nodal architecture. In contrast, the diffuse non-Hodgkin's lymphomas develop from the medullary cord region of the lymph node, which relates to the secretory compartment of the B-lymphocyte system.

Lymphoid neoplasma derived from T lymphocytes are much less common. Malignant transformation of T lymphocytes, found predominantly in the paracortical region of the lymph node, gives rise to mycosis fungoides/Sézary syndrome and approximately one quarter of the diffuse aggressive non-Hodgkin's lymphomas.

The lymphomatous lymph node or marrow usually shows replacement of normal cells and architecture by a relatively uniform population of lymphoid cells. This infiltration may be nodular, when the tumor arises from the follicular centers of the lymph node, or diffuse.

The classification of lymphomas is in evolution. There are currently at least six different pathologic classification systems (modified Rappaport, Dorfman, Lukes and Collins, Bennett, Kiel, and WHO) for non-Hodgkin's lymphoma in use worldwide, posing much controversy and confusion among clinicians. The classification by Rappaport, which characterizes lymphomas by architecture and cytologic differentiation, has been the most widely used and valuable scheme for clinicopathologic studies. This system, however, includes some imprecise classification (''histiocytic'' lymphomas and lymphoid in nature) and lacks immunologic classification. A Working Formulation for non-Hodgkin's lymphoma has been devised to serve as common language for the comparison of clinical trials.[61] A comparison of the Working Formulation and the Rappaport classification is found in Table 97.10. Non-Hodgkin's lymphomas can be divided into three major subtypes: low, intermediate, and high grade.

***Low-Grade Lymphomas*** Malignant lymphoma, small lymphocytic (diffuse, well-differentiated lymphocytic), is the solid tumor counterpart of chronic lymphocytic leukemia (CLL). At presentation, bone marrow, liver, and other visceral organ involvement along with generalized asymptomatic lymphadenopathy is seen. This lymphoma appears if an arrest in the process of lymphocyte transformation has occurred at the level of site A in Figure 97.4.[62] The natural history of this monoclonal B-lymphocyte disease is one that progresses to CLL. Only a very small number of patients show an emergence and proliferation of larger lymphoid cells, indicating a progression to a diffuse large-cell lymphoma. This transformation is known as Richter's syndrome.

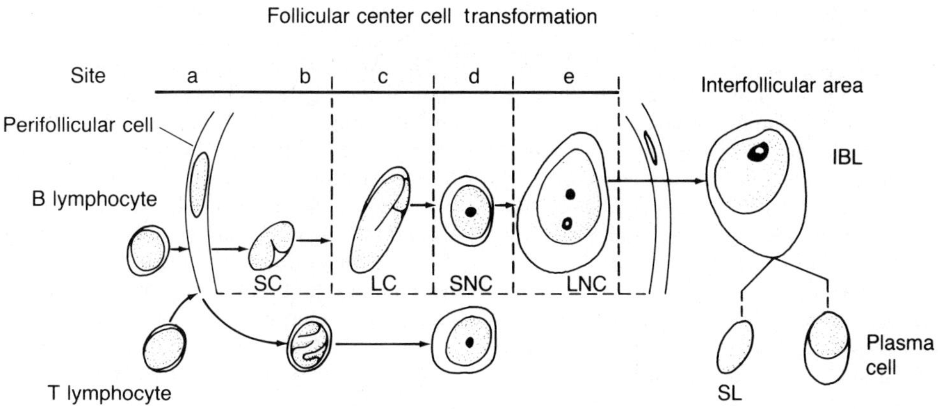


**Figure 97.4** Process of lymphocyte transformation and theoretical sites for development of non-Hodgkin's lymphoma. SNC, small noncleaved cell; LNC, large noncleaved cell; SC, small cleaved cell; LC, large cleaved cell; IBL, immunoblast; SL, small lymphocyte—often with plasmacytoid features. *(Modified from Lukes RJ: Am J Clin Path 1979;72:657, with permission.)*

Malignant lymphoma, follicular, predominantly small cleaved cell (nodular poorly differentiated lymphyocytic), occurs if transformation was arrested at site B in Figure 97.4 and accounts for approximately 50% of all cases of nodular lymphoma.[60] This lymphoma is also notable, because in up to 30% of cases, a spontaneous regression may occur.[63]

Malignant lymphoma, follicular mixed (nodular mixed lymphocytic–histiocytic), is composed of equal numbers of large and small cells. In follicular lymphomas, the nodular-growth pattern may be seen only in parts of the nodes, with coexistent diffuse patterns. If a diffuse growth component within diseased lymph nodes exceeds one half of the node, the tumor usually will behave in a much more aggressive pattern.

***Intermediate-Grade Lymphomas*** Malignant lymphoma, follicular predominantly large cell (nodular histiocytic), is the least common of the follicular lymphomas and usually is found in an earlier clinical stage at diagnosis. Prognosis for this lymphoma is worse than for the other follicular lymphoma and actually is similar to that of the diffuse lymphomas if even a focal diffuse component is present. An arrest at site C would result in accumulation of these large cleaved cells (see Fig. 97.4).

Malignant lymphoma, diffuse small cleaved (diffuse poorly differentiated lymphocytic), may arise de novo or as a consequence of progression of a follicular lymphoma. Its natural history is rather indolent, with a continuous relapse rate over time.

Malignant lymphoma, diffuse mixed (diffuse mixed lymphocytic–histiocytic), is probably a diffuse transformation of the follicular mixed lesion, and as such is more aggressive. Atypical binucleated large lymphocytes may be present and may simulate Sternberg–Reed cells, resulting in the possibility of a misdiagnosis of Hodgkin's disease.

Malignant lymphoma, diffuse large cell (diffuse histiocytic), results from a block in lymphocyte transformation at site E in Figure 97.2, producing a metabolically active and rapidly dividing tumor.

**High-Grade Lymphomas**

Malignant lymphoma, large cell immunoblastic (diffuse histiocytic), is subtyped into clear cell, plasmacytoid, epithelioid, and polymorphous categories and occurs with an apparent arrest at the level of the immunoblast. Immunologically, these lymphomas may arise from either B or T lymphocytes. The prognosis of patients with this aggressive lymphoma is unfavorable.

Malignant lymphoma, lymphoblastic (diffuse lymphoblastic), generally has T-cell markers and terminal deoxynucleotidyl transferase (TdT) present and frequently progresses into acute lymphoblastic leukemia.[60] Notable about this lymphoma is its frequent occurrence in young adults and adolescents, predominantly in males, and its tendency to involve the meninges.

Malignant lymphoma, small noncleaved (diffuse, undifferentiated), includes Burkitt's and non-Burkitt's subtypes which are very aggressive tumors with a dismal median survival. A block at site D in Figure 97.4 results in expression of these two tumor subtypes. Endemic Burkitt's lymphomas are usually associated with Epstein–Barr virus genome and complement receptors and chromosomal abnormalities. Non-Burkitt's cells are more variable in size and shape and show immunologic heterogeneity.

### *Clinical Presentation*

Patients with non-Hodgkin's lymphoma present with a wide variety of symptoms, which depend on the site of involvement and whether tumor involvement is nodal or extranodal. Patients may have either localized or generalized adenopathy, with the involved nodes being painless, rubbery, and discrete and usually located in the cervical and supraclavicular regions as in Hodgkin's disease. The liver or spleen may be enlarged in patients with generalized adenopathy. Patients with mesenteric or gastrointestinal involvement may present with signs and symptoms of nausea, vomiting, obstruction, abdominal pain, a palpable abdominal mass, or gastrointestinal bleeding. Patients with bone marrow involvement may have symptoms related to anemia (fatigue, pallor, tachycardia, dyspnea on exertion), neutropenia (recurrent infections), or thrombocytopenia (easy bruising, epistaxis, petechiae). Non-Hodgkin's lymphoma has a greater tendency to involve the testicles, epitrochlear nodes, and Waldeyer's ring than Hodgkin's disease. The incidence of solitary brain lymphomas is increasing, especially in patients with the acquired immune deficiency syndrome. Infrequently, patients with non-Hodgkin's lymphoma may present with acute renal failure from retroperitoneal adenopathy causing ureteral obstruction or from metabolic abnormalities such as hyperuricemia with uric acid nephropathy.

In contrast to Hodgkin's disease, about 20% of patients with non-Hodgkin's lymphoma have the constitutional symptoms of fevers, night sweats, and weight loss of greater than 10%. The clinical features of Hodgkin's disease and non-Hodgkin's lymphomas are compared in Table 97.3.

### *Diagnosis/Staging*

As with Hodgkin's disease, the diagnosis of non-Hodgkin's lymphoma must be established by an appropriate biopsy to provide tissue for pathologic review. An entire involved lymph node should be removed carefully for evaluation to preserve its architecture and prevent distortional artifact of the architecture, which could lead to an inaccurate diagnosis. Likewise, needle biopsy of the node prevents architecture evaluation and is not adequate in the diagnosis of non-Hodgkin's lymphoma. When adenopathy is not present, diagnosis may be established by biopsy of cutaneous lesions; bone marrow biopsy and aspiration in patients with unexplained myelosuppression; liver biopsy in patients with hepatomegaly or elevated liver function tests; or biopsy of involved extranodal organs, such as bone, Waldeyer's ring, lung, and testicles.

In patients whose age or underlying medical problems limit treatment to local palliation, further diagnostic procedures and staging are not indicated. Otherwise, the extent of the investigative workup required prior to therapy is determined by the histopathology and available treatment for the subtype of non-Hodgkin's lymphoma. Table 97.6 outlines evaluation and staging procedures for non-Hodgkin's lymphoma. At a minimum, all patients should have a complete blood count, serum chemistries including liver and kidney profiles, a chest x-ray, and bone marrow aspiration and biopsy. Bone marrow biopsy from each posterior iliac crest should be performed early in the evaluation of all patients, because a positive result given further confirmation of the diagnosis, establishes stage IV disease, and eliminates the need for more extensive and invasive tests.

Radiologic studies utilized in the staging of non-Hodgkin's lymphoma include CAT of the abdomen (to evaluate upper abdominal, mesenteric, splenic, and hepatic nodes) and chest; lymphangiogram to evaluate the lower aortic, iliac, and retroperitoneal nodes; liver–spleen scan, bone scan, upper gastrointestinal series, and intravenous pyelogram in patients with organ symptomatology or serum chemistry abnormalities.

Staging laparotomy is reserved for patients with clinical stage I disease, where the discovery of intraabdominal disease would mandate a change in therapy from localized radiation therapy to combination chemotherapy directed against intraabdominal disease.

The Ann Arbor Staging Classification developed for the clinical staging of Hodgkin's disease is also useful in staging and defining patient composition in non-Hodgkin's lymphoma (see Table 97.5); however, stage is more important prognostically in Hodgkin's disease than in non-Hodgkin's lymphomas. As an example, the distinction between stage III and IV non-Hodgkin's lymphoma is of little importance in the determination of treatment, as stage III non-Hodgkin's lymphoma is not commonly treatable with total nodal irradiation as it is in Hodgkin's disease.

Several factors have been identified that indicate a poorer prognosis for non-Hodgkin's lymphomas. These are outlined in Table 97.4.

#### Treatment

The primary goals of the treatment of non-Hodgkin's lymphoma are to relieve symptoms and eradicate disease whenever possible and to do this with acceptable toxicity. The treatment strategy depends upon many factors including patient age, coexistence of significant other disease, and histologic subtype and stage of the disease. With the introduction, development, and improvement of megavoltage radiotherapy and combination chemotherapy regimens, complete remission and cure can be achieved in a number of patients, including those with high-grade, aggressive unfavorable lymphomas.

Traditionally, the non-Hodgkin's lymphomas have been classified by the clinical behavior and degree of aggression they exhibit. The terms *good-risk, favorable, indolent,* and *low grade* have been applied to certain lymphomas by virtue of their relatively indolent behavior, as compared with high-grade lymphomas; however, some unfavorable characteristics of these lymphomas have emerged, including their tendency to show a constant rate of relapse over time, with no evidence of a survival curve. They also have the ability to transform over time into higher grade malignant lymphomas.

The unfavorable, high-grade, aggressive lymphomas, in contrast, are less differentiated and highly malignant diseases that have a relatively short natural history if left untreated. Because of their high growth fractions and rapid tumor doubling times, these high-grade lymphomas can be cured with intensive combination chemotherapeutic regimens. Thus, the terminology for the non-Hodgkin's lymphomas represents a paradox, where "good" is bad and "bad" is good. In other words, the favorable (good) lymphomas are relatively indolent tumors that respond to chemotherapy but cannot be cured. On the other hand, the unfavorable (bad) lymphomas generally are much more aggressive and in certain instances can be cured.

#### Radiation Therapy

The role of radiation therapy in the treatment of non-Hodgkin's lymphoma is different from the role already discussed for Hodgkin's disease. Although the disease is responsive to radiation therapy, only a small percentage of patients with non-Hodgkin's lymphoma are amenable to remission induction and cure with local or regional irradiation. This is because truly localized disease at diagnosis is rare.

**Chemotherapy**

Effective chemotherapy for the malignant lymphomas ranges from single-agent therapy in the low- and intermediate-grade lymphomas to aggressive, complex combination chemotherapeutic regimens in the high-grade lymphomas. The rationale for intensive combination chemotherapeutic regimens is based, in part, on the somatic mutation theory of Goldie and Coldman. This model and the rational for its use have been previously discussed.

**Limited Disease (Stages I and II)**

***Low-Grade Lymphomas*** It is very uncommon for patients with the nodular lymphomas to present with localized disease. Most patients with low-grade lymphomas have painless, and many times waxing and waning, lymph node enlargement and tolerate the disease despite its usual widespread dissemination. As stated earlier, these lymphomas demonstrate spontaneous regression in up to 30% of cases.

The primary role of radiation therapy in non-Hodgkin's lymphoma is in the treatment of localized disease. Involved-field, extended-field, and total nodal irradiation have been used. Carefully staged patients with either state I or contiguous stage II disease treated with radiation therapy can achieve up to a 90% relapse-free survival that can exceed 10 years.[60] Unlike treatment for Hodgkin's disease, there are no data to support the use of extended-field irradiation to clinically uninvolved contiguous lymph node chains. This is because in non-Hodgkin's lymphoma, the spread of disease is less certain than the usual contiguous spread seen in Hodgkin's disease.

Total-body irradiation (TBI), in total doses of 100–250 rads, has been administered in fractions of 5–15 rads per dose three to five times weekly. In a study at Stanford, no significant difference in survival was noted among involved-field, extended-field, and total body irradiation.[60] Total-body irradiation, however, causes marked myelosuppression, which affects primarily the platelets. Because combination chemotherapy can cure a significant percentage of diffuse lymphomas but not nodular lymphomas, total-body irradiation should be reserved for the palliative treatment of nodular disease. Even though only 10% of patients with follicular lymphoma have early-stage disease, it is important to identify these patients in view of the high likelihood of cure with radiation therapy, in contrast to the much poorer prognosis for patients with advanced disease.

In the small percentage of patients who present with localized stage I or II disease, single alkylating agent therapy is rarely used, as a true benefit of chemotherapy over radiation therapy has yet to be demonstrated.

***Intermediate-Grade Lymphomas*** It is relatively uncommon for patients with intermediate-grade non-Hodgkin's lymphoma to present with limited stage I or II disease. Additionally, they have a less indolent disease than patients with low-grade lymphomas and, as such, usually have slightly worse 5-year survival rates. Although radiation therapy is the mainstay of localized stage I and contiguous stage II disease, combination chemotherapy, with or without radiation therapy, is the primary therapy for stage II–IV disease. Prior to the advent of combination chemotherapy, overall survival of patients with intermediate-grade lymphomas was 50% at 2 years. Through development of combination chemotherapeutic regimens, it has become apparent that the incorporation of doxorubicin into these regimens has resulted in increased complete response rates (58%–69% versus 13%–43%) over non–doxorubicin-containing regimens.[64] Patients with follicular, large-cell lymphoma (nodular histiocytic) treated with various multiagent regimens have demonstrated a median survival of 31 to 47 months associated with a plateau on the survival curve suggesting long-term disease-free survival and cure.[65,66]

***High-Grade Lymphomas*** Among the heterogeneous group of non-Hodgkin's lymphomas, the most important therapeutic advances have been made with intensive chemotherapeutic regimens for the high-grade lymphomas. There are several important points to consider in the treatment of these lymphomas. First, the high-grade non-Hodgkin's lymphomas are curable diseases, even when they are widely metastatic. Therefore, unlike the patient with a low-grade non-Hodgkin's lymphoma, "no treatment" is not an option. These tumors, when left untreated, are almost universally fatal within 2 years. Second, as it is uncommon to achieve a complete remission with single-agent therapy and long-term survival is not possible without induction of a complete remission, intensive combination chemotherapeutic regimens should be used. Third, administration schedules for these intensive regimens, which are oftentimes accompanied by severe toxic effects, must be rigidly adhered to. Prolongation of the interval between cycles can be associated with rapid regrowth of the tumor and the inability to produce cure.

Controversy exists over the treatment of stage I and II diffuse large-cell (diffuse histiocytic) lymphoma. The extent of clinical evaluation prior to therapy is determined by the therapy being considered. Radiation therapy alone has been shown to provide an 11-year actuarial disease-free survival rate of 93% in stage I disease.[67] When radiation therapy is used alone, however, pathologic stage must be established by pretreatment laparotomy. Therefore, early initiation of chemotherapy has been suggested, as it carries the advantage of eliminating the need for staging laparotomy. This obviates the potential complications of surgery and allows for earlier treatment, which is an important point when dealing with aggressive tumors that have the potential for rapid growth and dissemination.

Using various chemotherapeutic regimens, Cabanillas demonstrated 89% and 66% relapse-free complete response rates in stage I and II disease, respectively.[68] While chemotherapy alone appears to be effective for stage I disease, combined modality therapy may be useful in improving the complete response rate. A trial of three courses of either CVP or BACOP on both sides of extended-field irradiation in stage I and II disease has yielded complete response rates of 94% and 97% for the CVP and BACOP therapies, respectively.[44] Relapse-free survival was shown to be significantly longer for the group of patients receiving radiation therapy and BACOP.

**Advanced Disease (Stages III and IV)**

***Low-Grade Lymphomas*** Therapeutic options for the patient with Stage III or IV low-grade lymphomas are diverse, ranging from no therapy to combination chemotherapy combined with radiation. Total lymphoid irradiation in doses of 3,500 to 5,000 rads has been used as the sole modality for stage III low-grade lymphomas, with 40% relapse-free survival at 10 years.[69] Most patients who relapsed in this study had disease in nonirradiated sites, suggesting that extended treatment fields might have produced increased disease-free survival. Total-body irradiation therefore has been investigated; however, results have not been superior to those for chemotherapy.[69,70] In addition, a 12% incidence of secondary acute nonlymphocytic leukemia was noted in the irradiated group. Several randomized trials have shown equivalent efficacy of single alkylating agents (chlorambucil or cyclophosphamide) versus CVP[71] and CVP versus CVP plus total lymphoid irradiation.[72] Regardless of treatment modality, the majority of patients respond but relapse at a rate of 10% to 15% per year. Use of more intensive regimens, such as BACOP,[73] CHOP-Bleo,[74] or CHOP versus CHOP–levamisole versus CHOP–levamisole–BCG,[75] again shows high response rates but no significant survival advantage.

As chemotherapeutic regimens have not produced convincing data supporting improved survival, it has been suggested that therapy be withheld from patients who are asymptomatic. At Stanford, 83 selected patients have been followed without initial therapy.[64] Fifty percent of patients required some form of therapy by 3 years and had a median survival of 11 years. Survival was not significantly different among concurrently studied patients treated with radiation therapy, chemotherapy, or both.

Advantages of treatment deferral include the following: exposure to agents that may induce drug resistance is prevented; drug-induced toxicity is prevented; a spontaneous regression may occur; administration of appropriate palliative therapy can occur when the disease progresses; and the disease may evolve to a potentially curable lymphoma. Potential disadvantages of withholding treatment include disease progression in threatening sites, which may compromise palliative therapy, and evolution of the disease to a lymphoma that is more aggressive and more resistant to therapy.

***Intermediate-Grade Lymphomas*** Patients with diffuse mixed and small-cleaved-cell (diffuse poorly differentiated) lymphomas have shown complete response rates ranging from 60%–74% for the CTX (L2) and NHL-5 protocols[76] to 60% for the COPP/COPA regimens.[77] Most relapses with these regimens occur within the first year of therapy.

The M-BACOD regimen developed at the Dana Farber Cancer Institute resulted in a 57% complete response rate in 44 patients with advanced, symptomatic, bulky intermediate-grade non-Hodgkin's lymphoma.[78] They showed a 5-year disease-free survival for complete responders of 43%, suggesting a survival plateau. Although intensive chemotherapeutic regimens are having an impact on improving survival from intermediate-grade non-Hodgkin's lymphoma, the toxicity attributed to chemotherapy is also increasing. For example, the M-BACOD regimen resulted in a treatment-associated mortality rate of 4%, plus other adverse effects such as profound myelosuppression, bleomycin-induced pulmonary fibrosis, and methotrexate-induced renal compromise.[78] One must balance the potential toxic effects and benefits of each regimen before using it in selected individuals.

As with the low-grade lymphomas, the optimal management of most intermediate-grade lymphomas remains controversial. With a few exceptions, most studies to date have failed to demonstrate curative treatments.

***High-Grade Lymphomas*** Advanced-stage large-cell lymphoma was considered an incurable disease some 15 to 20 years ago. Initial combination regimens using CVP produced a plateau on the survival curve of just 10%, with a median survival less than 1 year. During this same period, DeVita and colleagues demonstrated improved responses, survival, and cure in treatment of patients with Hodgkin's disease with MOPP. As an outgrowth of this trial, DeVita et al developed with C-MOPP regimen and demonstrated complete remission rates of approximately 40% in the large-cell lymphomas.[79] Because of their rapid growth rate, high thymidine labeling index, and large growth fraction, large-cell lymphomas are usually associated with an early relapse after therapy, usually within 2 years. These investigators found that few patients relapsed 2 years after achieving a complete response without maintenance chemotherapy, which suggested that more intensive regimens could induce a substantial number of cures. Introduction of the antineoplastic agents bleomycin and doxorubicin in the middle 1970s was an important advance in the treatment of large-cell lymphomas. Many first-generation chemotherapeutic regimens were then developed (CHOP,[64] BACOP,[80] and COMLA[81]). All of these regimens produced complete response rates in the range of 48% to 58% and long-term disease-free survival rates of 30% to 48% (Table 97.11). None of these early trials clearly demonstrated a superior regimen.[82]

Application of the theories of Goldie and Coldman led to development of "second-generation" regimens. These regimens are characterized by the use of six or more antineoplastic agents; the myelosuppressive agents are cycled more frequently, generally every 3 weeks, and the nonmyelosuppressive agents are administered during weeks of cytopenias. These nonmyelosuppressive agents are marrow sparing, are generally non–cross-resistant to the myelosuppressive agents, and provide continuous tumor suppression even during periods of cytopenia. COP-BLAM,[83] M-BACOD,[84] and ProMACE-MOPP[85] are examples of these second-generation regimens. These regimens have produced complete response rates of greater than 70% with long-term survival of 60% to 65% (Table 97.11).

The success of these regimens has led to the evolution of even more intense regimens—MACOP-B,[86] ProMACE-CytaBOM,[87] COP-BLAM III,[88] and F-MACHOP.[89] Complete response rates for these regimens exceed 80%, with long-term disease-free survival ranging from 63% to 76% (Table 97.11). In the MACOP-B regimen, combinations of myelosuppressive and nonmyelosuppressive agents are alternated and administered weekly. The efficacy of this regimen is due to a variety of factors including a high rate of drug dose delivery, more continuous exposure of the tumor to cytotoxic agents, early introduction of non–cross-resistant agents, and minimization of toxic effects from myelosuppression which tends to cause treatment delays and the chance for tumor regrowth and development of resistance.[86]

The COP-BLAM III regimen is unique among other regimens in that it allows for escalation of dosages of the

**Table 97.11** Chemotherapeutic Regimens for Advanced High-Grade Lymphomas

| *Regimen*[a] | *N* | *Complete response (%)* | *Long-term*[b] *survival (%)* |
|---|---|---|---|
| CHOP[c64] | 112 | 58 | 30 |
| C-MOPP[79] | 24 | 41 | 37 |
| BACOP[80] | 32 | 48 | 37 |
| COMLA[81] | 42 | 55 | 48 |
| COP-BLAM I[83] | 33 | 73 | 60 |
| M-BACOD[84] | 101 | 72 | 59 |
| ProMACE-MOPP[85] | 79 | 73 | 65 |
| MACOP-B[86] | 61 | 84 | 75 |
| ProMACE-CytaBOM[87] | 28 | 89 | TE[b] |
| COP-BLAM III[88] | 34 | 85 | TE |
| F-MACHOP[89] | 44 | 81 | 73 |

[a] CHOP=cyclophosphamide, doxorubicin, vincristine, prednisone
C-MOPP=cyclophosphamide, vincristine, prednisone, procarbazine
BACOP=bleomycin, doxorubicin, cyclophosphamide, vincristine, prednisone
COMLA=cyclophosphamide, vincristine, methotrexate, leucovorin, cytarabine
COP-BLAM I/III=cyclophosphamide, vincristine, prednisone, bleomycin, doxorubicin, procarbazine
M-BACOD=methotrexate, bleomycin, doxorubicin, cyclophosphamide, vincristine, dexamethasone
ProMACE–MOPP=prednisone, methotrexate, doxorubicin, cyclophosphamide, etoposide, MOPP
MACOP-B=methotrexate, doxorubicin, cyclophosphamide, vincristine, prednisone, bleomycin
Pro-MACE-CytaBOM=proMACE (as above) plus cytarabine, bleomycin, vincristine
F-MACHOP=fluorouracil, methotrexate, cytarabine, cyclophosphamide, doxorubicin, vincristine, prednisone

[b] More than 3 years.

[c] Too early to evaluate.

antineoplastic agents appropriate to patient tolerance. This is an important provision, as many antineoplastic agents appear to have a steep dose–response relationship. Response rates for these regimens are outlined in Table 97.12.

Some observations can be made concerning the treatment of advanced high-grade lymphomas: (1) the incidence of complete remission and of long-term survivorship has greatly been improved with the use of intensive chemotherapeutic regimens; (2) relapse usually occurs within the first 2 years of induction of a complete remission, such that the vast majority of disease-free survivors are probably cured; and (3) while the best regimen has not yet been identified, the currently available regimens stress the importance of delivering, up front and in different sequences, full doses of effective cytotoxic agents. Ongoing randomized, multiarmed trials at the National Cancer Institute (ProMACE-MOPP versus ProMACE-CytaBOM) and the Southwest Oncology Group (CHOP versus MACOP-B versus M-BACOD versus ProMACE-CytaBOM) should better define the optimal regimen and alternating schedule to be used in patients with the advanced high-grade lymphomas.

Central nervous system (CNS) relapse is a major problem in patients with high-grade lymphomas who have achieved a complete response, occurring with an incidence between 7% and 40%.[90,91] Risk factors for CNS relapse include advanced diseases, and bone marrow, peripheral blood, or spinal cord involvement. Use of regimens containing high-dose methotrexate has reduced the incidence of CNS relapse to less than 5%.[84,85] The optimal prophylaxis for CNS relapse has yet to be determined, though various modalities, including high-dose methotrexate with leucovorin rescue, high-dose cytarabine, intrathecal methotrexate or cytarabine, or whole-brain irradiation, have been used.

### Salvage Therapy

While long-term remissions for non-Hodgkin's lymphomas are now possible with newer intensive treatment regimens, 20% to 30% of patients do not enter a complete remission

**Table 97.12** Comparison of Systems of Classification of Non-Hodgkin's Lymphomas: The Working Formulation and the Rappaport Scheme

| *Working formulation* | *Rappaport classification* | |
|---|---|---|
| Low grade | | |
| A. Small lymphocytic (SL) | Diffuse well-differentiated lymphocytic (DWDL) | 5% |
| B. Follicular, small-cleaved-cell (FSC) | Nodular poorly differnetiated lymphocytic (NPDL) | 25% |
| C. Follicular mixed, small-cleaved- and large-cell (FM) | Nodular mixed, lymphocytic–histiocytic (NM) | 10% |
| Intermediate Grade | | |
| D. Follicular large-cell (FL) | Nodular histiocytic (NH) | 4% |
| E. Diffuse small-cleaved-cell (DSC) | Diffuse poorly differentiated lymphocytic (DPDL) | 8% |
| F. Diffuse mixed, small-cleaved- and large-cell (DM) | Diffuse mixed lymphocytic–histiocytic (DM) | 8% |
| G. Diffuse large-cell (DL) | Diffuse histiocytic (DH) | 20% |
| High Grade | | |
| H. Immunoblastic, large-cell | Diffuse histiocytic (DH) | 10% |
| I. Lymphoblastic | Diffuse lymphoblastic (DL) | 5% |
| J. Small-noncleaved-cell (SNC) | Diffuse undifferentiated (DU) (Burkitt's and non-Burkitt's) | 5% |

with these therapies. Of those patients achieving a complete response, 20% to 40% subsequently relapse and die within a few months. Unfortunately, there do not appear to be second-line salvage therapies capable of consistently inducing remission from non-Hodgkin's lymphoma, in contrast to the effective salvage regimens available for Hodgkin's disease. A possible reason for the failure of salvage regimens might be the use of nearly all effective agents in the primary treatment regimens in the hope of improving the chance for cure. Many clinical trials are now evaluating the utility of newer investigational agents, alone and in combination, or the use of commercially available agents in high doses, with or without bone marrow rescue.

As doxorubicin has contributed substantially to the efficacy of treatment regimens for non-Hodgkin's lymphoma, much interest has focused on newly synthesized anthracycline-like compounds. In phase II clinical trials, mitoxantrone, a bis-substituted anthraquinone, has demonstrated some activity against refractory non-Hodgkin's lymphoma. Coltman and co-workers administered doses of 12 $mg/m^2$ every 3 weeks and noted 2 complete responses and 7 partial responses in 37 patients; the median duration of response was 231 days.[92] Similarly, 4 complete and 26 partial responses were achieved in 69 patients treated with 14 $mg/m^2$ every 3 weeks by Gams and his associates.[93] Myelosuppression and gastrointestinal complaints were the primary toxic effects noted, although one patient who had previously received doxorubicin 450 $mg/m^2$ developed congestive heart failure after mitoxantrone 240 $mg/m^2$.[92] Other intercalators, such as bisantrene[94] and amsacrine[95] have shown limited activity in refractory non-Hodgkin's lymphoma. Other investigators[96] have noted a more significant activity for amsacrine, with a 30% response rate in 46 patients; however, median duration of response was only 3 months.

The epipodophyllotoxin teniposide (VM-26) has activity in non-Hodgkin's lymphoma as both a first-line and a salvage agent.[97] One group utilizing doses of 10 $mg/m^2$/wk demonstrated response rates of 50% in 22 elderly previously untreated patients and 36% in 31 pretreated patients; the median duration of complete response was greater than 7 months.[96] Toxicity in this study was minimal, with only mild to moderate myelosuppression.

As tumor cell resistance to conventional-dose chemotherapy may be overcome with increased doses, agents that have demonstrated efficacy in non-Hodgkin's lymphoma, such as cytarabine, have been studied at high doses.[98–100] Cytarabine, 3–4.5/$g/m^2$ every 12 hours for 4 to 12 doses, has demonstrated complete response rates of 17% to 35%; however, the median duration of response has been only approximately 3 months. Primary toxic effects of these regimens include profound myelosuppression and CNS effects.

The use of high-dose chemotherapy with autologous bone marrow transplantation (ABMT) has been shown to be an effective salvage therapy in many patients with non-Hodgkin's lymphoma. In the middle 1970s, Appelbaum and colleagues reported complete remission in 10 of 22 patients with non-Hodgkin's lymphoma with BACT (BCNU, cytarabine, cyclophosphamide, 6-thioguanine) therapy and autologous bone marrow transplantation.[101] Four of those patients, all with Burkitt's lymphoma, have disease-free survival at greater than 3 years. Hartmann and associates treated 16 patients with BACT therapy and noted a 68% complete response rate, with five patients in unmaintained remission 96+ to 177+ weeks after high-dose treatment.[102] Using total-body irradiation in combination with high-dose cyclophosphamide with or without doxorubicin, Braine and his associates induced continuous complete remission in 10 of 18 patients, with a median survival of 528 days (range, 39–2,657+ days).[103] Kaplan–Meier plot analysis revealed a 2-year disease-free survival probability of 73%, which is extremely promising with respect to cure in refractory patients.

A preliminary report by the European Bone Marrow Transplant Group of 112 patients with non-Hodgkin's lymphoma noted a complete response rate of 79% after treatment with various high-dose regimens and autologous bone marrow transplantation.[104] Of those patients achieving a complete response, 61% are in a continuous complete remission. It is difficult to evaluate the usefulness of autologous bone marrow transplantation carried out in this group of patients, as 10% and 21% of these patients underwent autologous bone marrow transplantation at diagnosis and as a part of consolidation, respectively, and many of these patients would be expected to be cured by conventional therapy. Excluding the patients in these two groups, complete remission was induced in 76% of 77 patients, with 50% of these patients in continuous complete remission.

These results confirm the possibility of producing durable responses in some patients who respond poorly to conventional therapy. It must be noted, however, that these procedures carry a 10% to 18% mortality rate.[102,104]

## Summary

Twenty years ago, the lymphomas were considered fatal cancers. Today, over 60% of all patients with Hodgkin's disease and nearly half of all patients with non-Hodgkin's lymphoma are cured. This drop in mortality is the result of innovations in treatment, including megavoltage radiotherapy, combination chemotherapy, and multimodality techniques.

There are still plenty of advances to be made. The cure rate for advanced disease needs to be improved. We also need to find less toxic, equally effective regimens. This type of progress will be made only with intensive clinical research.

## References

1. Kennedy BJ, Loeb V, Peterson VM, et al. National survey of patterns of care for Hodgkin's disease. Cancer 1985;56:2547–2556.
2. Silverberg E, Lubera J. Cancer statistics, 1986. CA 1986;36:9–25.
3. Gutensohn NM. Social class and age at diagnosis of Hodgkin's disease: New epidemiologic evidence for the "two-disease hypothesis." Cancer Treat Rep 1982;66:689–695.
4. Kadin ME. Possible origin of the Reed–Sternberg cell from an interdigitating reticulum cell. Cancer Treat Rep 1982;66:601–608.

5. Lukes RJ, Tindle BH, Parket JW. Reed–Sternberg-like cells in infectious mononucleosis. Lancet 1969;2:1000–1004.
6. Shope TC, Khalifa AS, Smith ST, et al. Epstein–Barr virus antibody in childhood Hodgkin's disease. Am J Dis Child 1982;136:701–703.
7. Gallo RC, Gelman EP. In search of the Hodgkin's disease virus. N Engl J Med 1981;340:169–170.
8. Beckstead JH, Warnke R, Bainton DF. Histochemistry of Hodgkin's disease. Cancer Treat Rep 1982;66:609–613.
9. Lukes RF, Butler JJ, Hicks ED. Natural history of Hodgkin's disease as related to its pathological picture. Cancer 1966;19:319.
10. Lukes RJ, Craver LF, Hall TC, et al. Report of the nomenclature committee. Cancer Res 1966;26:1311.
11. Kaplan HS. Hodgkin's Disease, 2nd ed. Cambridge, Harvard University Press, 1980.
12. Carbone PP, Kaplan HS, Musshoff K, et al. Report of the committee on Hodgkin's disease staging classification. Cancer Res 1970;31:1860–1861.
13. Panettiere FJ, Coltman CA, Delaney FC. Splenectomy, chemotherapy and survival in Hodgkin's disease. Arch Intern Med 1977;137:341–343.
14. Dresser RL, Ultmann JE. Risk of severe infection in patients with Hodgkin's disease or lymphoma after diagnostic laparotomy and splenectomy. Ann Intern Med 1972;77:143–147.
15. Meeker WR, Richardson JD, West W, et al. Critical evaluation of laparotomy and splenectomy in Hodgkin's disease. Arch Surg 1972;105:222.
16. Goodman RL, Piro AJ, Hellman S. Can pelvic irradiation be omitted in patients with pathologic stage IA and IIA Hodgkin's disease? Cancer 1976;37:2834–2839.
17. Hoppe RT, Coleman CN, Cox RS, et al. The management of stage I–II Hodgkin's disease with irradiation alone or in combined modality therapy: The Stanford experience. Blood 1982;59:455–465.
18. Hellman S, Mauch P. Role of radiation therapy in the treatment of Hodgkin's disease. Cancer Treat Rep 1982;66:915–923.
19. Zagars G, Rubin P. Hodgkin's disease stage IA and IIA: A long-term follow-up study on the gains achieved by modern therapy. Cancer 1985;56:1905–1912.
20. Coltman CA, Myers JW, Montague E, et al. The role of combined radiotherapy and chemotherapy in the primary management of Hodgkin's disease: Southwest Oncology Group Studies, in Rosenberg SA, Kaplan HS (eds): Malignant Lymphomas: Etiology, Immunology, Pathology, Treatment. New York, Academic, 1982, vol 3, pp 523–535.
21. Mauch P, Goodman R, Hellman S. The significance of mediastinal involvement in early stage Hodgkin's disease. Cancer 1978;42:1039–1045.
22. Hagemeister FB, Fuller LM, Sullivan JA, et al. Prognostic classification of Hodgkin's disease. Radiology 1981;141:783–789.
23. Mauch P, Ryback ME, Rosenthal P, et al. The influence of initial pathologic stage on the survival of patients who relapse from Hodgkin's disease. Blood 1980;56:892–897.
24. Desser RK, Golomb HM, Ultman JE, et al. Prognostic classification of Hodgkin's disease in pathologic stage III based on anatomic considerations. Blood 1977;49:883–893.
25. Stein RS, Golomb HM, Diggs CH, et al. Anatomic substaging of stage III-A Hodgkin's disease. Ann Intern Med 1980;92:159–165.
26. Prosnitz LR, Montalvo RL, Fischer DB, et al. Treatment of stage IIIA Hodgkin's disease: Is radiotherapy alone adequate? Int J Radiat Oncol Biol Phys 1978;4:781–787.
27. Hoppe RT, Rosenberg SA, Kaplan HS, et al. Prognostic factors in pathologic stage IIIA Hodgkin's disease. Cancer 1980;46:1240–1246.
28. DeVita VT, Moxley JH, Brance K, et al. Intensive combination chemotherapy and x-irradiation in the treatment of Hodgkin's disease. Proc Am Assoc Cancer Res 1965;6:15.
29. DeVita VT, Simon RM, Hubbard SM, et al. Curability of advanced Hodgkin's disease with chemotherapy: Long-term follow-up of MOPP-treated patients at the National Cancer Institute. Ann Intern Med 1980;92:587–595.
30. Coltman CA. Chemotherapy of advanced Hodgkin's disease. Semin Oncol 1980;7:155–173.
31. Carde P, MacKintosh FR, Rosenburg SA. A dose and time response analysis of the treatment of Hodgkin's disease with MOPP chemotherapy. J Clin Oncol 1983;1:146–153.
32. Behrens BC, Young RC, DeVita VT. Current management of Hodgkin's disease. Drugs 1985;30:355–367.
33. Goldie JH, Coldman AJ. The genetic origin of drug resistance in neoplasms, implications for systemic therapy. Cancer Res 1984;44:3643–3653.
34. Goldie JH, Coldman AJ, Gudauskas GA. Rationale for the use of alternating non–cross-resistant chemotherapy. Cancer Treat Rep 1982;66:439–450.
35. Bonadonna G. Chemotherapy strategies to improve the control of Hodgkin's disease. Cancer Res 1982;42:4309–4320.
36. Bonadonna G, Santoro A, Valagussa P, et al. Current status of the Milan trials of Hodgkin's disease in adults, in Rozencweig M, Cavalli R, Bonadonna G (eds): Second International Conference on Malignant Lymphomas. Boston, Martinus Nijhoff, 1985, pp 299-307.
37. Young CW, Straus DJ, Myers J, et al. Multidisciplinary treatment of advanced Hodgkin's disease by an alternating chemotherapeutic regimen of MOPP/ABVD and low-dose radiation therapy restricted to originally bulky disease. Cancer Treat Rep 1982;66:907–914.
38. Young RC, Longo DL, Glatstein E, et al. The current status of NCI trials in Hodgkin's disease, in Rozencweig M, Cavalli F, Bonadonna G (eds): Second International Conference on Malignant Lymphomas. Boston, Martinus Nijhoff, 1985, pp 293–298.
39. Hagemeister FB, Fuller LM, Velasquez WS, et al. Stage I and II Hodgkin's disease: Involved-field radiotherapy versus extended-field radiotherapy versus involved-field radiotherapy followed by six cycles of MOPP. Cancer Treat Rep 1982;66: 789–798.
40. DeVita VT, Young RC, Chabner BA. Unpublished data.
41. Mauch P, Goffman T, Rosenthal DS, et al. Stage III Hodgkin's disease: Improved survival with combined modality therapy as compared with radiation therapy alone. J Clin Oncol 1985;3:1166–1173.
42. Bloomfield CD, Pajak TF, Glicksman AS, et al. Chemotherapy and combined modality therapy for Hodgkin's disease: A progress report on cancer and leukemia group B studies. Cancer Treat Rep 1982;66:835–846.
43. Farber LR, Prosnitz LR, Cadman EC. Curative potential of combined modality therapy for advanced Hodgkin's disease. Cancer 1980;46:1509–1517.
44. Fisher RI, DeVita VT, Hubbard SP, et al. Prolonged disease-free survival in Hodgkin's disease with MOPP reinduction after first relapse. Ann Intern Med 1979;90:761–763.
45. Bonadonna G. Chemotherapy of malignant lymphomas. Semin Oncol 1985;6(suppl 6):1–14.
46. Santoro A, Bonfante V, Vivianidi S, et al. Salvage chemotherapy in relapsing Hodgkin's disease. Proc Am Soc Clin Oncol 1984;3:254.
47. Papa G, Mandell F, Anselmo AP, et al. Treatment of MOPP-resistant Hodgkin's disease with adriamycin, bleomycin, vin-

blastine and dacarbazine (ABVD). Eur J Cancer Clin Oncol 1982;18:803–806.
48. Longo DL, Young RC, DeVita VT. Chemotherapy for Hodgkin's disease: The remaining challenges. Cancer Treat Rep 1982;66:925–936.
49. Mead GM, Harker WG, Kushlan P, et al. Single-agent palliative chemotherapy for end-stage Hodgkin's disease. Cancer 1982;50:829–835.
50. Gams RA. Complications of chemotherapy in the treatment of Hodgkin's disease. Semin Oncol 1980;7:184–186.
51. Chapman RM. Effect of cytotoxic therapy on sexuality and gonadal function. Semin Oncol 1982;9:84–94.
52. DeVita VT. The consequences of the chemotherapy of Hodgkin's disease. The 10th David A. Karnofsky memorial lecture. Cancer 1981;47:1–13.
53. Whitehead E, Shalit SM, Blackledge G, et al. The effect of combination chemotherapy on ovarian function in women treated for Hodgkin's disease. Cancer 1983;52:988–993.
54. Pedersen-Bjergaard J, Larsen SO. Evidence of acute nonlymphocytic leukemia, preleukemia and acute myeloproliferative syndromes up to 10 years after treatment of Hodgkin's disease. N Engl J Med 1982;307:965–971.
55. Valagussa P, Santoro A, Kendra R, et al. Second malignancies in Hodgkin's disease: A complication of certain forms of therapy. Br Med J 1980;280:216–219.
56. Coltman CA, Dixon DO. Second malignancies complicating Hodgkin's disease: A Southwest Oncology Group 10-year follow-up. Cancer Treat Rep 1982;66:1023–1034.
57. Aisenberg AC. Acute non-lymphocytic leukemia after treatment of Hodgkin's disease. Am J Med 1983;75:449–454.
58. Applebaum FR, Sullivan KM, Thomas ED, et al. Allogeneic marrow transplantation in the treatment of MOPP-resistant Hodgkin's disease. J Clin Oncol 1985;3:1490–1494.
59. Cantor KP, Fraumini JF. Distribution of non-Hodgkin's lymphoma in the United States between 1950 and 1975. Cancer Res 1980;40:2645–2652.
60. DeVita VT, Jaffe ES, Hellman S. Hodgkin's disease and the non-Hodgkin's lymphomas, in DeVita VT, Hellman S, Rosenberg SA (eds): Cancer—Principles and Practice of Oncology, 2nd ed. Philadelphia, J.P. Lippincott, 1985; pp 1623–1710.
61. Berard CW, Green MH, Jaffe ES, et al. A multidisciplinary approach to non-Hodgkin's lymphomas. Ann Intern Med 1981;93:218–235.
62. Hait WN, Farber L, Cadman E. Non-Hodgkin's lymphoma for the non-oncologist. JAMA 1985;253:1431–1435.
63. Rosenberg SA. The low grade non-Hodgkin's lymphomas: Current approaches to therapy, in Cavalli F, Bonadonna G, Rozencweig M (eds): Malignant Lymphomas and Hodgkin's Disease: Experimental and Therapeutic Advances. Boston, Martinus Nijhoff, 1985.
64. Jones SE, Grozea PN, Metz EN, et al. Superiority of adriamycin containing combination chemotherapy in the treatment of diffuse lymphomas: A Southwest Oncology Group study. Cancer 1979;43:417–425.
65. Osborne CK, Norton L, Young RL, et al. Nodular histiocytic lymphoma: An aggressive nodular lymphoma with potential for prolonged disease free survival. Blood 1980;56:98–103.
66. Glick JH, McFadden E, Costello W, et al. Nodular histiocytic lymphoma: Factors influencing prognosis and implications for aggressive chemotherapy. Cancer 1982;49:840–845.
67. Sweet DL, Kinzie J, Gaske ME, et al. Survival of patients with localized diffuse histiocytic lymphoma. Blood 1981;58:1218–1223.
68. Cabanillas F. Chemotherapy as definitive treatment of stage I–II large cell and diffuse mixed lymphomas. Hematol Oncol 1985;3:25–31.
69. Paryani SB, Hoppe RT, Cox RS, et al. The role of radiation therapy in the management of stage III follicular lymphomas. J Clin Oncol 1984;2:841–848.
70. Hancock SL, Young R, Longo D, et al. Advanced lymphoma: Update of a randomized comparison of chemotherapy and radiotherapy. Proc Am Soc Clin Oncol 1985;4:203.
71. Lister TA, Cullen MH, Beard MEJ, et al. Comparison of combined and single agent chemotherapy in non-Hodgkin's lymphoma of favorable histologic type. Br Med J 1978;1:533–537.
72. Portlock CS, Rosenberg SA, Glatstein E, et al. Treatment of advanced non-Hodgkin's lymphomas with favorable histologies: Preliminary results of a prospective trial. Blood 1976;47:474–476.
73. Skarin AT, Rosenthal DS, Maloney WC, et al. Combination chemotherapy of advanced non-Hodgkin's lymphoma with bleomycin, adriamycin, cyclophosphamide, vincristine and prednisone (BACOP). Blood 1977;49:759–770.
74. Rodriguez V, Cabanillas F, Burgess MA, et al. Combination chemotherapy (CHOP-Bleo) in advanced non-Hodgkin's malignant lymphoma. Blood 1977;49:325–333.
75. Jones SE, Grozea PN, Miller TP, et al. Chemotherapy with cyclophosphamide, doxorubicin, vincristine and prednisone alone or with levamisole or with levamisole plus BCG for malignant lymphoma: A Southwest Oncology Group study. J Clin Oncol 1985;3:1318–1324.
76. Al-Katib A, Koziner B, Kurland E, et al. Treatment of diffuse poorly differentiated lymphocytic lymphoma. Cancer 1984;53:2404–2412.
77. Bitran JC, Golomb HM, Ultmann J, et al. Non-Hodgkin's lymphoma, poorly differentiated lymphocytic and mixed cell types: Results of sequential staging procedures, response to therapy and survival of 100 patients. Cancer 1978;42:88–95.
78. Anderson KC, Skarin AT, Rosenthal DS, et al. Combination chemotherapy for advanced non-Hodgkin's lymphomas other than diffuse histiocytic or undifferentiated histologies. Cancer Treat Rep 1984;68:1343–1350.
79. DeVita VT, Cannelos GP, Chabner BA, et al. Advanced diffuse histiocytic lymphoma, a potentially curable disease. Lancet 1975;1:248–250.
80. Schein PS, DeVita VT, Hubbard S, et al. Bleomycin, adriamycin, cyclophosphamide, vincristine and prednisone (BACOP) combination chemotherapy in the treatment of advanced diffuse histiocytic lymphomas. Ann Intern Med 1976;85:417–422.
81. Sweet DL, Golomb HM, Ultmann JE, et al. Cyclophosphamide, vincristine, methotrexate with leucovorin rescue and cytarabine (COMLA) combination sequential chemotherapy for advance diffuse histiocytic lymphoma. Ann Intern Med 1980;92:785–790.
82. DuPont J, Caray G, Scaglione C, et al. A randomized comparison of two chemotherapy regimens: BACOP vs COPP in the treatment of diffuse histiocytic and mixed lymphoma, in Cavalli F, Bonadonna G, Rozencweig M (eds): Malignant Lymphomas and Hodgkin's Disease: Experimental and Therapeutic Advances. Boston, Martinus Nijhoff, 1985, pp 475–483.
83. Laurence J, Coleman M, Allen SL, et al. Combination chemotherapy of advanced diffuse histiocytic lymphoma with the six drug COP-BLAM regimen. Ann Intern Med 1976;85:417–422.
84. Skarin AT, Canellos GP, Rosenthal DS, et al. Improved prognosis of diffuse histiocytic and undifferentiated lymphoma by use of high dose methotrexate alternating with standard agents (M-BACOD). Clin Oncol 1983;1:91–97.
85. Fisher RI, DeVita VT, Hubbard SM, et al. Diffuse aggressive

lymphomas: Increased survival after alternating flexible sequences of ProMACE and MOPP chemotherapy. Ann Intern Med 1983;98:304–309.

**86.** Klimo P, Connors JM. MACOP-B chemotherapy for the treatment of diffuse large cell lymphoma. Ann Intern Med 1985;102:596–602.

**87.** Fisher RI, DeVita VT, Hubbard SM, et al. Randomized trial of ProMACE-MOPP vs ProMACE-CytaBOM in previously untreated advanced stage diffuse aggressive lymphomas. Proc Am Soc Clin Oncol 1984;3:C-945.

**88.** Coleman M, Boyd DB, Bernhardt B, et al. COP-BLAM III: Combination chemotherapy for diffuse large cell lymphoma with cyclophosphamide, infusional Oncovin, prednisone, infusional bleomycin, adriamycin and matulane. Proc Am Soc Clin Oncol 1984;3:C-964.

**89.** Amadori S, Gugliemi C, Anselmo AP, et al. Treatment of diffuse aggressive non-Hodgkin's lymphomas with an intensive multi-drug regimen including high dose cytosine arabinoside (F-MACHOP). Semin Oncol 1985;12:218–222.

**90.** Herman TS, Hammond N, Jones SE, et al. Involvement of the central nervous system by non-Hodgkin's lymphoma. Cancer 1979;43:390–397.

**91.** Mackintosh FT, Colby TV, Podolsky WJ, et al. Central nervous system involvement in non-Hodgkin's lymphoma: An analysis of 105 cases. Cancer 1982;49:586–595.

**92.** Coltman CA, Coltman TM, Balcerzak SP, et al. Mitoxantrone in refractory non-Hodgkin's lymphoma. A Southwest Oncology Group study. Semin Oncol 1984;3(suppl 1):50–53.

**93.** Gams RA, Bryan S, Dukart G, et al. Mitoxantrone in malignant lymphomas. Invest New Drugs 1985;3:219–222.

**94.** Miller TP, Cowan JD, Neilan BA, et al. A phase II study of bisantrene in malignant lymphomas. A Southwest Oncology Group study. Cancer Chemother Pharmacol 1986;16:67–69.

**95.** Bramwell VH, Holdener EE, Siegenthaler P, et al. Phase II study of amsacrine in refractory lymphomas. A report of the EORTC early clinical trials group. Eur J Cancer Clin Oncol 1984;20:753–759.

**96.** Bajetta E, Buzzoni R, Viviani S, et al. Phase II study with amsacrines (m-AMSA and m-AMSA lactate) in refractory lymphomas. Cancer Treat Rep 1985;69:965–969.

**97.** Tirelli U, Carbone A, Crivellari D, et al. A phase II trial of teniposide (VM-26) in advanced non-Hodgkin's lymphoma, with emphasis on the treatment of elderly patients. Cancer 1984;54:393–396.

**98.** Richards MA, Barnett MJ, Waxman J, et al. The use of high dose cytosine arabinoside for non-Hodgkin's lymphoma. Semin Oncol 1985;12(suppl 3):223–226.

**99.** Shipp MA, Takvorian RC, Canellos GP. High dose cytosine arabinoside. Active agent in treatment of non-Hodgkin's lymphoma. Am J Med 1984;77:845–850.

**100.** Adelstein DJ, Lazarus HM, Hines JD, et al. High dose cytosine arabinoside in previously treated patients with poor-prognosis non-Hodgkin's lymphoma. Cancer 1985;56:1493–1496.

**101.** Appelbaum FR, Diesseroth AB, Graw RG, et al. Prolonged complete remission following high dose chemotherapy of Burkitt's lymphoma in relapse. Cancer 1978;41:1059–1063.

**102.** Hartmann O, Pein F, Beaujean F, et al. High dose polychemotherapy with autologous bone marrow transplantation in children with relapsed lymphomas. J Clin Oncol 1984;2:979–985.

**103.** Braine HG, Kaizer H, Yeager AM, et al. Treatment of refractory non-Hodgkin's lymphoma with intensive chemoradiotherapy and autologous bone marrow transplantation, in Cavalli F, Bonadonna G, Rozencweig M (eds): Malignant Lymphoma and Hodgkin's Disease: Experimental and Therapeutic Advances. Boston, Martinus Nijhoff, 1985, pp 529–536.

**104.** Goldstone AH. Autologous bone marrow transplantation for non-Hodgkin's lymphomas: The preliminary European experience, in Dicke KA, Spitzer G, Zander AR (eds): Autologous Bone Marrow Transplantation. Houston, The University of Texas Press, 1985, pp 67–74.

# *Chapter 98* / Pediatric Solid Tumors and Childhood Leukemias

Anne M. Glynn-Barnhart, PharmD, Mary E. Teresi, PharmD, and William R. Crom, PharmD

Unlike adult tumors, which often are environmentally induced, pediatric cancers (see Table 98.1) tend to be embryonic in nature; more than 40% of pediatric tumors occur in the age range 0 to 4 years. Treatment and prognosis of pediatric tumors have progressed with the improvement of surgical and diagnostic procedures and the advent of megavoltage radiotherapy and chemotherapy. For the most part, radical surgical procedures have been replaced with multimodal treatment. Treatment goals are total elimination of tumor with minimal acute and chronic toxic effects. Staging of tumors has a prominent function in establishing prognosis and treatment, as more favorable low-stage disease often does not require intensive radiotherapy and chemotherapy. New methods of drug delivery and administration are under investigation to improve drug penetration of the tumor, especially for brain and bone tumors. Significant advances have already been made and, with the development of a better understanding of the disease processes themselves, further improvements in treatment and prognosis are likely.[1]

## Solid Tumors

### *Central Nervous System Tumors*

Brain tumors are the most common nonhematopoietic malignancy of childhood, accounting for approximately 20% of all childhood malignancies.[2] Improvements in diagnostic, surgical, and radiation techniques have produced an improvement in survival from 20% to approximately 50%. The age of the child and the type, location, and extent of tumor have a significant effect on the consequences of therapy—survival and long-term sequelae. Reported peak age of occurrence ranges from 0 to 9 years with a slight male predominance (1.3:1).[3]

### *Etiology/Pathology*

The precise etiology of central nervous system (CNS) tumors remains unknown. The early age at which some tumors occur indicates primitive neuronal cell precursors that had been "misplaced" during early embryonic development. These cells maintain their ability to proliferate, yet never mature. The occurrence of brain tumors in older children and adults postulates a role for environmental factors causing mutations. One of the difficulties in evaluating the etiology and pathology is the lack of consistency for pathologic labeling of tumors. Many are of mixed cellularity, reported as a "mixture" in some reports and according to the most prevalent type in others. The more common neoplasms are astrocytomas, medulloblastomas, ependymomas, and brain stem tumors.

#### Clinical Presentation

The presenting signs and symptoms depend on the age of the child and the type, size, extension, and location of the tumor.[4,5] With the exception of localized brain stem tumors, the most frequent presenting signs result from increased intracranial pressure (ICP) (Table 98.2). Unfortunately, these signs are ambiguous and can be accounted for by a less serious diagnosis (i.e., influenza). Other presentations depend on tumor location: dysmetria, strabismus, nystagmus, ataxia, gait disturbances, cranial nerve dysfunctions, abnormal reflexes, and seizures. Shunt placement to decrease ICP, although generally effective, is discouraged, as its use has caused herniation and increased incidence of tumor seeding. Steroids effectively decrease cerebral edema, allowing for better diagnosis and treatment planning.

#### Diagnosis

An ophthalmologic exam showing papilledema is indicative of increased ICP and warrants an extensive workup. Computerized axial tomography (CAT) with contrast enhancement is the diagnostic method of choice. The size, location, and tumor density obtained from CAT aid in diagnosis and treatment planning. Angiography studies, to determine the blood supply to the tumor, also aid in assessing surgical procedures. Radionuclide brain scans also provide insight into the location and extent of tumor.

#### Treatment

To date, the available staging methods have not been completely validated. Some methods are based on presurgical assessment of tumor size, histology, and location; other methods are based on postsurgical excision or debulking, which some investigators believe correlates more accurately with survival. Variation in the criteria used to determine response also limits comparison of study results and evaluation of toxicity.[6] Surgical removal of the total tumor mass and margins is optimal, but not always possible. Surgical debulking in these cases may enhance the effectiveness of radiotherapy and chemotherapy, treatment modalities that are based on log cell kill. Hence, radiation or drug therapy should be initiated immediately after surgery, when the number of tumor cells is small and the growth fraction is high.

**Table 98.1** Incidence of Malignant Tumors in U.S. Children

| *Diagnosis* | *Male* | *Female* | *Total* | *Rate per million white children per year* |
|---|---|---|---|---|
| Leukemia | 377 | 274 | 651 | 42.1 |
| Acute lymphocytic | 223 | 157 | 380 | |
| Acute granulocytic | 54 | 48 | 102 | |
| Acute monocytic | 1 | 4 | 5 | |
| Acute, unclassified | 52 | 36 | 88 | |
| Lymphoma | 137 | 67 | 204 | 13.2 |
| Hodgkin's disease | 54 | 35 | 89 | |
| Burkitt's lymphoma | 6 | 2 | 8 | |
| Lymphoma, unclassified | 13 | 4 | 17 | |
| Central nervous system | 202 | 168 | 370 | 23.9 |
| Ependymoma | 9 | 11 | 20 | |
| Medulloblastoma | 50 | 24 | 74 | |
| Glioma, unclassified | 38 | 29 | 67 | |
| Glioblastoma | 24 | 27 | 51 | |
| Astrocytoma | 40 | 40 | 80 | |
| Astroblastoma | 26 | 20 | 46 | |
| Oligodendroglioma | 1 | 3 | 4 | |
| Sympathetic nervous system | 83 | 65 | 148 | 9.6 |
| Neuroblastoma | 72 | 51 | 123 | |
| Retinoblastoma | 25 | 27 | 52 | 3.4 |
| Bone tumors | 46 | 40 | 86 | 5.6 |
| Osteosarcoma | 26 | 25 | 51 | |
| Ewing's tumor | 15 | 11 | 26 | |
| Soft tissue | 71 | 59 | 130 | 8.4 |
| Rhabdomyosarcoma | 40 | 29 | 69 | |

From Young JL, Miller RW: Incidence of malignant tumors in U.S. children. J Pediatr 1975;86:255, with permission.

***Radiotherapy*** Although radiotherapy remains a secondary treatment modality, the extent and dose of radiation are controversial. Astrocytomas that are totally excised do not need to be irradiated. On the other hand, medulloblastomas, which are highly metastatic, spreading through the CNS in the cerebrospinal fluid, are generally treated with total craniospinal radiation.[5] The maximum tolerated dosage is 4,500 to 6,000 rads, given in divided fractions over 4 to 6 weeks.[7] The dose-limiting critical tissue for radiotherapy to the brain appears to be the cerebral vasculature, which develops a late (1–3 years) small-vessel fibrosis; however, arteriosclerotic changes and occlusive disease, intellectual deficits, bone malformations, dermatitis, and personality changes are other neurotoxic effects that can affect the quality of life for the patient after therapy is completed.[7] Radiation treatment has been reported to enhance the toxicity of chemotherapy.

**Table 98.2** Symptoms of Increased Intracranial Pressure

| | |
|---|---|
| Headache | Separation of cranial sutures (young children) |
| Vomiting (usually early morning) | Papilledema |
| Bulging fontanelle | Lethargy |
| Diplopia | Irritability |
| Blurred vision | Seizures |

***Chemotherapy*** Drug therapy for brain tumors presents some unique problems. The foremost problem is the inability of the drug to cross the blood–brain barrier (BBB).[8] Generally, physicochemical properties of drugs that cross the BBB include small molecular size, low protein binding, weak ionization, and good lipid solubility. Because the nitrosoureas (BCNU and CCNU), procarbazine, and, to a minor extent, the nitrogen mustards possess these characteristics, they are the mainstay of therapy for brain tumors.[4,6] The effects of the tumor, surgery, and irradiation on the permeability of the BBB complicates assessment of treatment. Another dilemma is the brain-adjacent tumor (BAT). Cells at the edge of the tumor that have the greatest growth fraction tend to have an intact BBB, whereas the necrotic, central point of the tumor tends to have increased BBB permeability. Drugs have little effect on this dead or slowly dividing tissue. Drugs demonstrating minimal effectiveness are vincristine, teniposide, etoposide, and methotrexate (MTX).[5,6,9] Triethylinemelamine (TEM), one of the first drugs used to treat medulloblastoma, is no longer recommended for therapy, as no efficacy has been demonstrated.[5] New drug delivery systems, such as intraarterial[4,10] or intrathecal administration[5] and incorporation of drugs into liposomes with or without monoclonal antibodies, are being investigated. Membrane-modifying drugs such as 6-thioguanine improve the activity of the nitrosoureas and warrant further studies.[11] Preliminary studies with thermochemotherapy indicate a "selective inability" of the tumor to dissipate heat that may potentiate intravenous therapy.[12]

## *Neuroblastoma*

Neuroblastoma, a malignant tumor arising from the primitive neural crest cells that form the adrenal medulla and the sympathetic nervous system, is third in incidence among pediatric tumors, affecting approximately 1 in 100,000 children.[2] Eighty-five percent of affected children are less than 6 years, the peak incidence occurring at age 2.[2] The tumor may occur wherever sympathetic neural tissue exists, with approximately 45% originating in the adrenal gland, 24% in the retroperitoneal ganglia, 15% to 20% in the mediastinum, and 4% in the pelvic area.[13] Location of the primary site not only determines the presenting signs and symptoms, but also has prognostic significance. Patients with abdominal primary tumors tend to have poorer survival, with metastases often present in the liver, bone marrow, bone, lymph nodes, skin, and orbits at diagnosis. Other clinical features include urinary and respiratory problems, weakness or paralysis, Horner's syndrome, bone pain (caused by bone metastases), diarrhea, and hypertension secondary to tumor production of catecholamines.[10,14]

### Prognosis

Only two factors have been reported to independently influence outcome: the stage of disease at diagnosis and the patient's age at diagnosis.[13] Although various staging systems are available (Evans,[15] SJCRH, POG), the general strategy behind all methods is differentiation between favorable (localized, resectable tumors) and unfavorable (disseminated disease) prognosis. Children younger than 1 year have a better response to therapy and a lower incidence of relapse once remission is attained.[13] Other reported prognostic factors are tumor location (higher incidence of metastases with abdominal tumors), site of metastases (worse prognosis with bone metastases), and histology.[16] The histologic composition of neural crest tumors varies from entirely primitive cells (neuroblastoma) to entirely mature neural tissue (ganglioneuroma). More highly differentiated tumors, such as ganglioneuromas, have a better prognosis.

### Diagnosis

Physical exam should include a check for spinal cord compression and hypertension. Laboratory workup should include a complete blood count, liver and renal function tests, and a urinalysis including urinary catecholamine concentrations. Chest x-ray, pyelogram, skeletal survey, liver scan, and bone marrow aspirate should also be obtained to determine the location, size, extent, and possible metastasis of the disease.[16]

### Treatment

Combinations of surgery, radiation therapy, and chemotherapy may be used, depending on age and stage of disease.[13,16] Children with totally resectable tumors generally receive surgery only. Partially resected tumors may receive radiation to the tumor bed, while patients with systemic involvement are treated with chemotherapy. Local and regional neuroblastoma is curable with combined therapy in a high proportion of patients, but disseminated neuroblastoma remains a usually fatal disease.[16,17] Various combinations of drugs have been explored.[13,15,16,18,19] Cyclophosphamide (CTX), one of the first effective agents to be identified, appears in most combination therapies. Sequential administration of cyclophosphamide and doxorubicin increased the response rate from 22% to 55% in children with disseminated disease.[17] This therapy is based on consideration of cell cycle kinetics. A cell cycle nonspecific drug (CTX) is administered for 7 days. As tumor cells are killed, additional cells in the resting phase ($G_0$) are recruited into the cell cycle, resulting in an increase in the labeling and mitotic indices (LI, MI). This improves the effectiveness of a cell cycle–specific drug such as doxorubicin. A similar concept underlies the administration of cisplatin (CDDP), which increases the LI and decreases the MI, indicating accumulation of cells in the S phase, followed by teniposide (VM-26), which kills cells in the S phase.[18,19] Other drugs used in various combination regimens include *v*incristine, doxorubicin (*A*driamycin), nitrogen *m*ustard (VAM), ± *d*acarbazine; nitrogen *m*ustard, doxorubicin (*A*driamycin), *d*acarbazine, cisplatin (cis-*d*iamminedichloroplatinum), vincristine (*On*covin), *c*yclophosphamide (MADDOC)[13]; and vincristine (*O*ncovin), cisplatin (*p*latinum), *e*pipodophyllotoxin, *c*yclophosphamide (OPEC).[19] Melphalan combined with total-body irradiation has also been investigated with promising results.[20]

## *Rhabdomyosarcoma*

The most common soft tissue sarcoma is rhabdomyosarcoma, a malignant tumor of the embryonic mesenchyme that gives rise to striated skeletal muscle. Because of its origin, rhabdomyosarcoma may arise in multiple areas: 36% occur in the head and neck, 18% in the genitourinary area, and 21% in the extremities.[21] The site of the primary tumor often dictates the presentation, treatment, and prognosis. Most present as a mass or swelling with or without pain. Seventy percent of affected children are less than 10 years old, with the peak incidence occurring in 2- to 5-year-olds.[21]

### Prognosis

Factors reported to have prognostic significance include staging, tumor location, histology, and age.[22] Most of these factors are interrelated and individual effects are difficult to determine. Staging is currently based on amount of tumor excised and degree of dissemination.[22] Younger children tend to have localized tumor and, therefore, lower staging. In addition, younger children tend to have embryonal histology while older children have alveolar, which has a greater tendency to disseminate or metastasize. Location affects the surgeon's ability to excise the tumor and margins, thus influencing staging. Tumors arising in the orbit, prostate, head, neck, or trunk have a 50% or greater 2-year disease-free survival, probably because they usually exhibit symptoms early and are discovered before dissemination. Controversy exists over the efficacy of the current staging guidelines, which place primary emphasis on surgical excision,[21,23,24] because treatment with radiation therapy and chemotherapy has reduced the size of some tumors necessitating less radical surgery. The regional lymph nodes are the most common site of metastasis. Whether grossly negative nodes should be irradiated remains controversial. Rhabdomyosarcoma also metastasizes via the blood to the lungs, liver, bone marrow, bones, and brain.

**Treatment**

Historically, treatment for rhabdomyosarcoma has involved radical and invasive surgical procedures, because of the tumor's tendency to infiltrate surrounding tissues.[22] The location of the primary tumor often meant such surgery would result in cosmetic and functional deformities. The advent of megavoltage irradiation reduced the need for invasive surgery.[25,26] Sites such as the orbit, parameningeal and prostate could be biopsied, staged, and treated with irradiation. Drug therapy was also evaluated, for both local and systemic control of disease. Vincristine (V), cyclophosphamide (C), and dactinomycin (A) were found to be effective as single agents and in combination (VA ± C).[23,24,27] Investigators next looked at developing optimal combinations of surgery, radiation therapy, and chemotherapy for the various stages of the disease. The first Intergroup Rhabdomyosarcoma Study (IRS1) attempted to determine if all stages needed radiation, if VA was as effective as VAC in controlling lower stage disease, and if VAC plus doxorubicin was better than VAC in higher stages.[21] The results indicated that patients with localized, completely resected tumors did not need irradiation if treated with VAC. VAC was no more effective than VA in stage II patients when postoperative radiation was administered. Neither stage III nor stage IV patients had a better response with VAC plus doxorubicin over VAC when routine radiation therapy was also used.[21,28] IRS2 is currently assessing reduction of chemotherapy in the favorable stages and application of more aggressive therapy in the higher, unfavorable stages.[29] Other agents are also under investigation for possible efficacy. Melphalan is non–cross-resistant with VAC and doxorubicin and has demonstrated antitumor activity in tumor xenograft animal models.[30] Dacarbazine is also reported to be active in animal models and may prove effective in treating human disease.

### *Osteosarcoma*

Osteosarcoma, a malignant tumor of the bone consisting of spindle-cell sarcomatous stroma, is the most frequently encountered bone tumor. The majority of the tumors occur in the metaphyses of long bones, such as the femur, tibia, and humerus, during periods of rapid growth.[31] There is rapid invasion and destruction of bone cortex with spread of tumor into the adjacent tissue. The frequency of occurrence in long bones is proportional to the growth potential of that bone. The peak age of diagnosis correlates with the age of peak growth rates, 13–15 years. Osteosarcoma is a highly malignant disease, and gross or microscopic metastases are often present at diagnosis or develop within the first year thereafter. Although other bones may become involved, the primary site of metastases is the lungs.[31] The extent of pulmonary involvement varies from a single nodule to bilateral involvement with multiple nodes. The etiology of osteosarcoma remains unknown, though some cases have been associated with Paget's disease or radiation exposure (i.e., therapeutic radiation for retinoblastoma[32]).

**Clinical Presentation**

Patients generally present with an insidious onset of pain and swelling at the site of the tumor. If untreated, the tumor continues to enlarge, and the skin surrounding the mass becomes taut and thin with a glossy sheen as it is stretched. When weight-bearing bones are involved, the presence of a limp may indicate destruction of the cortex of the involved bone, and pathologic fractures may develop. Trauma or injury to the involved bone often draws attention to the tumor, but has not been shown to cause the disease.

**Diagnosis**

After a physical exam, roentgenograms of the affected area, bone scan, tumor biopsy, chest x-ray, and CAT scan should be obtained. Prior to routine use of CAT, many lung lesions were not detected on regular chest x-ray. Laboratory diagnostic tests should include a total blood count, renal and liver function tests, and serum alkaline phosphatase determination. An increase in serum alkaline phosphatase has been observed in osteosarcoma, probably secondary to osteoblastic activity. The concentrations generally return to normal after surgery, but may increase with subsequent pulmonary metastases or local recurrence.

**Treatment**

The goal of treatment is to eradicate all tumor and prevent metastases. Depending on the age of the patient, the site and size of the primary tumor, and the presence of metastatic disease, various surgical options are available. Amputation is generally recommended for patients who have not reached at least 75% of their expected growth to avoid limb dyssymmetry. Newer "limb-salvage" techniques have been developed that consist of en bloc resections of the affected bone.[33,34] The cosmetic and psychologic benefits of en bloc resections make it an appealing alternative to amputation; however, metal fatigue and breakage of the rods inserted to replace the resected bone, infections, and local recurrence may later necessitate amputation.

At diagnosis, pulmonary metastases are present in 80% of patients. Thoracotomies for single or easily resectable pulmonary metastases are effective in controlling or (in selected cases) eradicating metastatic disease. For multiple unresectable nodules, systemic chemotherapy has been evaluated for possible benefit. Initial trials were of single agents: vinca alkaloids (VCR), cyclophosphamide (CTX), melphalan (MEL), mitomycin (MTM), dacarbazine, and dactinomycin (D) produced disappointing response rates of less than 15%.[35] In the early 1970s, high-dose methotrexate with leucovorin rescue (HDMTX) and doxorubicin (A) were reported to achieve response rates (complete + partial responses) of 40%[36] and 31%,[37] respectively. Cisplatin (C) also showed promising results, with an overall response rate as a single agent of about 19% to 36%.[35,38]

Combinations of chemotherapy (A + CTX + HDMTX[39];

A + C[40]; bleomycin + CTX + D[41]) were evaluated in the adjuvant setting to eradicate undetectable micrometastases, after a definitive surgical procedure and removal of all detectable disease. These trials demonstrated 40% to 60% long-term disease-free survival, compared with the historical experience of less than 25% 2-year and less than 20% 5-year disease-free survival after surgery alone[31]; however, the Mayo Clinic reported a disease-free survival approaching 40% with surgery alone, suggesting that with modern diagnostic and surgical techniques, adjuvant chemotherapy offers little additional benefit to offset the toxic effects, costs, and inconvenience associated with up to 1 year of chemotherapy.[42] At about the same time, Rosen and colleagues at Memorial Sloan–Kettering Hospital demonstrated survival of nearly 90% of patients treated with an intense year-long adjuvant drug regimen.[43] To better evaluate the role of adjuvant chemotherapy, the Multi-institutional Osteosarcoma Study was initiated, which randomized patients to surgery alone or surgery plus an adjuvant chemotherapy regimen similar to that used by Rosen et al. At 2 years, the actuarial relapse-free survival was 17% in the surgery-alone group versus 66% in the adjuvant chemotherapy group.[44] Therefore, adjuvant chemotherapy is recommended for all children with osteosarcoma. One third of these patients, however, can be expected to relapse.[44] Other therapeutic approaches include presurgery chemotherapy to allow objective evaluation of the drug effect on the primary tumor and lung metastases,[43,45,46] and because of the limited ability of drugs to penetrate the relatively avascular, osteoid enclosed tumor, direct intraarterial administration of doxorubicin[45] and cisplatin[47] is being evaluated with promising results. New drugs are also being studied, such as ifosfamide, an alkylating agent that appears to be active in osteosarcoma.[31,48]

Radiation therapy has little role in osteosarcoma because normal tissue, especially lung, is more sensitive than the tumor. It has been used for palliation, to relieve pain from uncontrolled tumor.

## *Ewing's Sarcoma*

The second most common bone tumor in children, Ewing's sarcoma, is composed of small round cells of marked vascularity, often with hemorrhagic areas and without osteoid formation. Unlike osteosarcoma, these tumors occur in the midshaft of long bones or in the flat bones, with more than half the lesions originating in the axial skeleton. Metastasis occurs primarily via the blood to the lungs, bones, and bone marrow. The lung is the primary site of relapse.

### Clinical Presentation

The exact presentation depends on the location and extent of metastasis. Generally, most patients present with pain and swelling over the tumor area. The area may be warm as a result of the vascular nature of the tumor. Weight loss, fever, and malaise may be present, especially in patients with disseminated disease. Elevated lactate dehydrogenase (LDH) and erythocyte sedimentation rate have been associated with poorer treatment outcomes[49]; however, these features may also be indicative of larger tumor size which is known to have a poorer prognosis.[50]

### Prognosis

The site of the primary tumor markedly influences the outcome, with pelvic, humeral, and femoral primaries having a more unfavorable prognosis.[49–52] This may be related to the larger tumor size and significant soft tissue extension of these tumors by the time they are diagnosed.[50] Patients presenting with metastases tend to develop recurrences more often, despite an apparent response to therapy.[52] Other unfavorable prognostic factors that have been reported included male sex[49] and elevated LDH or erythrocyte sedimentation rate.[49,50]

### Treatment

No universal staging system exists. Most centers consider size, location, and metastasis in planning therapy. Primary goals of therapy are to control the primary tumor and to eliminate microscopic or macroscopic deposits of tumor while maintaining the functional ability of the tumor site. Prior to the introduction of systemic chemotherapy and megavoltage radiotherapy, the prognosis for Ewing's sarcoma at all sites was dismal, with surgical therapy having long-term survival rates below 10%. The primary reason for failure has been distant metastases.

Unlike osteosarcoma, Ewing's is highly sensitive to radiotherapy. Generally, local doses of at least 4,000 rads control 44% to 86% of the cases, but the tumor often recurs.[52,53] Therefore, radiation may replace or supplement surgery as the primary treatment for Ewing's sarcoma, though surgery is preferred in cases where the lesion is an expendable bone, if the primary tumor is very large, if there is an unmanageable pathologic fracture, or if the tumor occurs in a young child in whom radiation therapy could result in a major functional deformity.

Single-agent chemotherapy trials were initiated in the 1960s with encouraging results. Cyclophosphamide and doxorubicin were the most effective single agents, but vincristine, dactinomycin, lomustine, etoposide, and cisplatin have shown promising results. In 1973, the first Intergroup Ewing's Sarcoma Study (IESS1) was started to evaluate the effect of VAC versus VAC plus doxorubicin versus VAC plus bilateral pulmonary irradiation. The survival rate at 172 weeks median survival time for the entire group was 58%.[52] The addition of doxorubicin to VAC improved the 3-year survival from 38% to 78%.[52] VAC plus bilateral pulmonary irradiation was better than VAC alone, but not as effective as VAC plus doxorubicin, with a 55% 3-year survival.[52] Rosen et al[51] have reported a 2-year disease-free survival of 79% for patients treated with adjuvant chemotherapy plus radiation or surgery. They report dramatic shrinkage of primary tumors with the combination of doxorubicin, methotrexate, and cyclophosphamide,[52] but vincristine, dactinomycin, and bleomycin were also included in this treatment regimen. Current studies are attempting to define optimal radiation doses and chemotherapy schedules and regimens. Rosen et al[51] report good results with chemotherapy before radiation or surgery. Not only did the tumor size decrease, but the affected bone was able to begin healing. This may increase the tolerance to radiation therapy and chemotherapy and decrease the extent of surgery. Other areas of investigation include sequential half-body irradiation and bone marrow transplantation.[49]

### *Retinoblastoma*

Retinoblastoma is the most common primary malignant intraocular tumor of childhood. It arises in the retina of one or both eyes, and is often multicentric.

#### Incidence

In the United States, retinoblastoma occurs in approximately 1 in 15,000 to 30,000 live births.[54] Males and females are equally affected, as are whites and nonwhites; however, the mortality for nonwhites affected with the disease is two to three times greater than that for whites.[54,55] A longer delay in diagnosis and treatment in the nonwhite population may be responsible for this difference. The majority of the cases are reported in children less than 3 years old, and although retinoblastoma has been reported in adults, occurrence after 6 years of age is rare.

#### Genetics

Unlike other childhood tumors, genetic factors are known to play an important role in the occurrence of retinoblastoma. Approximately 40% of all retinoblastomas are inherited via an autosomal dominant gene. All bilateral cases and approximately 20% of unilateral tumors are considered congenital. An affected parent has a 50% chance of passing the gene to offspring; however, some people who inherit the gene never develop the tumor, but may transmit the gene to their offspring, who may be affected. This skipped-generation event has led some investigators to postulate that two mutational events are needed for retinoblastoma. In the acquired type, it is postulated that two somatic mutations must occur to induce the disease.[56]

Although the precise incidence has not been determined, a specific chromosome abnormality, the D-deletion syndrome involving chromosome 13, has been found to be associated with retinoblastoma.[54] Some characteristics of this syndrome are cleft palate, malformed ears, skeletal deformities, and mental deficiency.

#### Pathology

The tumor consists of closely packed, round, undifferentiated small cells with darkly stained nuclei and scant cytoplasm. Some cells may form rosettes, which are thought to be derivations of the early rods and cones. Degenerative changes, patchy mineralization, and hemorrhage may occur within the tumor. Within the globe, two tumor types have been described. The more common, endophytic type arises from the inner nuclear area, the nerve fiber layer, or the ganglion cell layer of the retina, and has a chalky white appearance. These tumors may seed into the vitreous humor, are associated with large tumors, and are a negative prognostic sign. The other tumor type is exophytic; it arises from the external nuclear layer and grows into the subretinal space, detaching from the retina in the process. Exophytic types are more difficult to diagnose as the tumor itself is hidden.

#### Metastasis

Three main pathways of tumor extension exist.[51] Transecteral extension into the orbit occurs along the perivascular spaces of the vessels that perforate the globe. As the tumor fills the cavity, proptosis may develop. Intraocular extension is manifested by a nodule or plaque forming in the plane of the retina, which can invade the vitreous or subretinal space, producing implants on the other parts of the retina, choroid, or iris. Extraocular extension occurs via three mechanisms: through the subarachnoid space to the brain; through the lamina cribrosa to the optic nerve; and via direct infiltration of veins to distant organs such as the liver, lungs, kidney, testes, viscera, lymph nodes, and skeletal bones. Deaths from retinoblastoma generally are due to intracranial spread or distant metastases.[57]

#### Clinical Presentation

The majority of the cases present with leukokosia (cat's-eye reflex), a white pupillary reflex caused by the reflection of light from the surface of the white fundus of the tumor.[58] Other pupillary reflex changes have also been noted, and any abnormality should raise suspicion. Inequality of pupils, changes in the iris color, prominence of the vessels over the conjunctiva, and strabismus are other possible presentations. If the tumor has extended beyond the globe, proptosis, eyelid edema, headaches, bony discomfort, vomiting, and seizures may occur.

#### Diagnosis

Funduscopic exams, performed under anesthesia by an ophthalmologist, should confirm the diagnosis of retinoblastoma. CAT scans of the skull and orbital views, along with a skeletal survey or bone scan and bone marrow and cerebrospinal fluid evaluation, aid in determining the location and extent of the tumor. Liver and kidney function tests should be obtained along with a hemogram and urinalysis. Increases in urine catecholamine concentrations may occur secondary to tumor secretion. Facial photographs are needed for evaluation of response and later to detect treatment-induced abnormalities.

#### Staging

The treatment goals of retinoblastoma are to preserve life and maintain sight. In an attempt to optimize therapy, predict prognosis, and allow for interstudy comparisons, methods of classifying retinoblastoma have been established. The first classification, the Reese–Ellsworth (RE) grouping, introduced in 1963, was designed to assess the likelihood of local tumor control and preservation of vision, but lacks correlation with patient survival (Table 98.3).[59] Patients are divided according to tumor size, number and location of lesions, and presence of vitreous seeding. Although this staging system is widely used, a more detailed grouping introduced by St. Jude Children's Research Hospital (Table 98.4)[60] considers intra- and extraocular extension and correlates with patient survival, thus permitting the integration of multimodal treatment planning for patients with advanced local disease.

#### Treatment

The major factors determining therapy include involvement (unilateral or bilateral); the size, number, and location of tumors; site and extent of tumor extension; and evidence of extraocular or distant spread of disease. Localized disease

**Table 98.3** Reese-Ellsworth Clinical Grouping System for Retinoblastoma

| |
|---|
| Group I: very favorable |
| 1. Solitary tumor, less than 4 disc diameters[a] in size, at or beyond equator |
| 2. Multiple tumors, none over 4 disc diameters in size, all at or behind equator |
| Group II: favorable |
| 1. Solitary tumor, 4 to 10 disc diameters in size, at or behind equator |
| 2. Multiple tumors, 4 to 10 disc diameters in size, at or behind equator |
| Group III: doubtful |
| 1. Any lesion anterior to equator |
| 2. Solitary tumors larger than 10 disc diameters behind equator |
| Group IV: unfavorable |
| 1. Multiple tumors, some larger than 10 disc diameters |
| 2. Any lesion extending anteriorly to ora serrata |
| Group V: very unfavorable |
| 1. Massive tumors involving over half the retina |
| 2. Vitreous seeding |

[a] 1 Disc diameter = 1.6 mm.

From Reese AB, Ellsworth RM: The evaluation and current concepts of retinoblastoma therapy. Trans Am Acad Ophthalmol Otolaryngol 1963; 67:164–172, with permission.

**Table 98.4** Treatment of Retinoblastoma According to Extent of Tumor

| *Stage* | *Clinical staging of retinoblastoma (unilateral or bilateral tumor; unifocal or multifocal tumor)* |
|---|---|
| I | Tumor confined to retina |
| | A. One quadrant or less |
| | B. Two quadrants or less |
| | C. More than 50% of retinal surface |
| II | Tumor confined to globe |
| | A. Vitreous seeding |
| | B. Extension to optic nerve head |
| | C. Extension to choroid |
| | D. Extension to choroid and optic nerve head |
| | E. Extension to emissaries |
| III | Extraocular extension of tumor—regional |
| | A. Extension beyond cut end of optic nerve |
| | B. Extension through sclera into orbital contents |
| | C. Extension to choroid and beyond cut end of optic nerve (including subarachnoid extension) |
| | D. Extension through sclera into orbital contents and beyond cut end of optic nerve (including subarachnoid extension) |
| IV | Distant metastases—generalized |
| | A. Extension via optic nerve to brain |
| | B. Bloodborne metastases to soft tissue, bone, and viscera |
| | C. Bone marrow metastasis |

From Pratt CB: Management of malignant solid tumors in children. Pediatr Clin North Am 1972;19:1152, with permission.

(RE stages I and II; St. Jude stages I, IIA, and IIB) is controlled with surgery or irradiation, while advanced disease may necessitate combined modalities.

***Surgery*** The exact surgical procedure is determined by the extent and location of the tumor(s). If the tumor is localized to the globe, and the lesion(s) can be treated with radiation or cryotherapy, no surgery may be necessary. In bilateral involvement, both eyes should receive treatment and then the least responsive globe removed.

***Radiotherapy*** The location and extent of tumor at the start of therapy determine the port size and dosage. The port(s) should extent beyond the known borders of the tumor, and the treatment dose should be delivered over 2 to 6 weeks. The general dosage range is 3,500–4,500 rads.[57] Skull irradiation should be performed when there is evidence of tumor extension beyond the cut end of the optic nerve or into the subarachnoid space around the optic nerve. Sedation of infants and small children may be required prior to treatment. Patients with unilateral disease[61] with no evidence of optic nerve or orbital involvement can be treated surgically, without radiation therapy.

Short-term effects of radiation treatment include dermatitis, mucositis, and conjunctivitis.[57] Cataract formation may occur after irradiation through anterior ports.[61] Long-term effects include radiation retinopathy, retardation of bone growth, and secondary malignancies.[57]

***Cryotherapy*** Cryotherapy is the freezing and thawing of tumors with an external probe. Tumors involving the periphery of the globe have been successfully treated with cryotherapy. Its use is expected to increase, as it maintains useful vision, lacks the complications of irradiation, and has been successful in treating large tumors (10 dd) and tumors in the periphery of the globe.[61]

***Light Coagulation*** Laser treatment is used to destroy the vascular supply of the tumor, thus leading to tumor regression. New tumors or recurrent tumors have been associated with its use, thus limiting its application. An experimental approach now being explored at several institutions in the United States is the use of high-frequency external light sources after hematoporphyrin administration.

***Chemotherapy*** As effective local control and survival are achieved in 90% of patients with surgery and radiation, chemotherapy is generally reserved for patients with locally extensive, regional, or distant disease.[62] Metastatic extension of retinoblastoma to the cerebrospinal fluid has been treated with intrathecal methotrexate with minimal response. Cyclophosphamide and ifosfamide have shown effectiveness,[62] while doxorubicin,[63] dactinomycin, and vincristine[64] have minimal effect. Increased antitumor effects have been demonstrated with the use of two- or three-drug combinations (VC, VAC, cisplatin/teniposide).[62,63]

**Prognosis**

Deaths from retinoblastoma are generally due to intracranial or distant spread.[57] A study done at the Harkness Eye Institute from 1965 to 1972 reported 5-year survival rates of 86% for unilateral tumors and 88% for bilateral tumors. A 92% overall survival has been reported by Howarth et al.[61] With the Reese–Ellsworth staging scheme, a range from 29% for 5-year survival for stage V to 91% for stage I was observed.

## *Wilms' Tumor*

Wilms' tumor, or nephroblastoma, arises from renal parenchyma, separated from normal tissue by a fibrotic pseudocapsule. Areas of hemorrhage and necrosis may be present. The tumor displaces and infiltrates normal renal structures and can extend beyond the capsule, invading the adrenal gland, colon, and renal vein. Metastases most commonly occur in the lungs.[65] The general age of presentation is 6 months to 5 years, and approximately 7.8 of every million children in the United States are affected. Bilateral Wilms' tumor occurs in 4% to 13% of reported cases.

**Clinical Presentation**

Wilms' tumor frequently presents as a palpable asymptomatic abdominal mass. Seventy-five to ninety percent of affected children have increased plasma renin concentrations with subsequent elevation in blood pressure. Fever, pain, and hematuria are other associated features. Congenital abnormalities associated with Wilms' tumor are aniridia, genitourinary anomalies (ectopic or horseshoe kidney), and hemihypertrophy.[65] These anomalies may be associated with a chromosomal abnormality of the short arm (p) of chromosome 11, including band 11p13.

**Diagnosis**

Physical assessment should provide a description of the mass, presenting blood pressure, eyes, external genitalia, and facial and extremity symmetry. Laboratory workup should include a complete blood count, liver and renal function tests, and a urinalysis. The most helpful diagnostic tool is the pyelogram, which differentiates intrarenal versus extrarenal and nonmalignant causes of a flank mass. Abdominal flat plates should also be obtained to aid in the differential diagnosis. If calcifications are present, the mass is probably not Wilms' tumor. Chest x-rays should also be obtained to evaluate pulmonary metastasis.

**Prognosis**

The first National Wilms' Tumor Study (NWTS) identified characteristics of patients who responded poorly to treatment.[66,67] The most significant predictor of a poor treatment outcome is histology.[68] Wilms' tumor is composed of a variety of mesenchymal and epithelial cells in various stages of development. Anaplastic or sarcomatous histology is significantly related to greater relapse rates and poorer overall survival, having an 88% mortality compared with 17% mortality for a more favorable histology.[68] Positive regional lymph nodes also indicate a considerably poorer outlook.[66] Age below 2 years has a better prognosis,[65] and if a favorable histology type is present, radiation therapy is not necessary. Tumor weight (thought to correlate with tumor size) less than 250 g is associated with fewer abdominal relapses and deaths.[66]

**Staging**

The NWTS devised a grading system for its first two studies. Based on the results of these studies, a staging system was developed utilizing histology, lymph node involvement, and tumor extension.[69] The treatment plan in the third NWTS is based on this staging system, with the intent to optimize therapy at each stage.

**Treatment**

The current results of treatment for Wilms' tumor constitute one of the success stories of pediatric oncology. From a 32% survival rate with surgery alone and a 47% rate with the addition of radiation therapy, the disease-free survival rate has increased to 80% to 90% with the addition of chemotherapy.[65] Surgery remains the primary treatment. Complete excision of the tumor and affected kidney, collection of any free fluid in the abdomen for cytology, and biopsy of adjacent lymph nodes and suspicious areas confirm the diagnosis, determine the stage of disease, and establish subsequent therapy.

***Radiotherapy*** Not all patients must receive radiation therapy. NWTS1 determined that children less than 2 years of age with favorable histology (group I) did not need radiation therapy.[65] Retrospective analysis of the dosages and time between surgery and radiation indicated that there was not a significant difference between relapse patterns whether 1,000 or 4,000 rads was used, or if delays as long as 10 days between surgery and radiation therapy occurred. Controversy still exists over port size and the exact doses of radiation that are optimal.

***Chemotherapy*** Dactinomycin was the first agent to demonstrate efficacy for Wilms' tumor. In NWTS1, 55% of patients treated with vincristine alone were disease free at 2 years. The combination of dactinomycin and vincristine was more efficacious than either drug alone, with 80% of patients disease free at 2 years (groups II and III).[65] NWTS2 reported increased benefit with the addition of doxorubicin to this regimen.[70] NWTS3 is attempting to determine what effect addition of cyclophosphamide to these three drugs will have on stage IV patients. Because of doxorubicin's cardiotoxicity, NWTS3 will also evaluate a regimen that includes increased dactinomycin and vincristine dosages but omits doxorubicin in patients with stages II and III disease.[67]

Because overall treatment results are very good today, future goals will be the reduction of both radiation therapy and chemotherapy for lower stage disease, to avoid unnecessary toxic effects. At the same time, more effective therapy for advanced disease is needed.

## Leukemias and Lymphomas

Acute lymphocytic leukemia (ALL) and acute nonlymphocytic leukemia (ANLL) are the most common childhood leukemias. Each has its own subclassifications, characteristics, and prognoses.

Description of the disease leukemia is relatively recent. The clinical disease was first described in the early nineteenth century by Velpean. The term *leukemia* was first used in the middle of that century by Virchow, who also clearly described the pathology of the disease. In 1857, Friedreich reported the first case of acute leukemia. Ehrlich, in 1891, discovered cell-staining techniques that allowed detailed study of cellular structure.

The natural history of the acute leukemias was at first dismal. No drug treatment was available prior to 1945, although blood transfusions were performed, and all patients were dead approximately 9 months after diagnosis. Death was caused by general bone marrow failure; as a result, infection or bleeding complications occurred.

Antibiotics and antifolates became available at about the same time in the mid-1940s. A study at this time showed that antibiotics and blood transfusions improved survival more than either transfusion or irradiation alone (average survival: 6–9 months), demonstrating the important role of infection in morbidity rates. Antifolates increased survival time, although all children in one study were dead by 24 months. Use of ACTH and cortisone also improved remission rates.

### *Acute Lymphocytic Leukemia*

#### Incidence

According to the National Cancer Institute's Surveillance, Epidemiology, and End Results (SEER) program, the incidence of ALL in white children less than 15 years of age is 2.5 per 100,000, and has remained stable since national surveys began tabulating such incidences in 1950.[71] The incidence is slightly higher in boys than girls. It is not clear if these incidence figures are also true of nonwhites, as the numbers in this population are too small to analyze statistically. The incidence of ALL appears to peak at ages 0–4, followed by 5–9 and 10–14.

#### Etiology

The cause of the acute leukemias is not known. An infectious etiology in some animal models (e.g., feline leukemia) implicates a viral cause.[72] In humans, the Epstein–Barr virus has been implicated as the cause of both African Burkitt's lymphoma and some types of nasopharyngeal carcinoma. Of most current interest is the isolation of the human T-cell leukemia virus (HTLV) from a human lymphoma.[72]

There is a strong relationship between prior radiation or chemotherapy and leukemia. There are three plausible explanations. First, it is possible that either treatment may cause genetic damage, producing cells with malignant, uncontrolled-growth characteristics. Second, these therapies suppress the immune system. As the immune system is responsible for recognition of self versus non-self cells and destruction of those cells it recognizes as foreign, it is conceivable that abnormal cells (malignant cells or virally infected cells) may be allowed to grow unchecked. Third, it is possible that patients who have received prior chemotherapy or radiation may be genetically predisposed to malignancy, and the second malignancy (leukemia) is actually part of the natural history of the disease.[73,74] Illustrative of these last two points is the high occurrence of acute leukemias in patients previously treated for Hodgkin's disease.

There is an increase in the occurrence of leukemia in children with genetic derangements such as Down's syndrome.[75] These children not only have a much higher incidence of acute leukemias than age-matched controls, but have lower remission rates for ALL, and a much higher incidence of adverse and toxic effects from chemotherapy. The reason is not known.

#### Prognosis

In the SEER survey of 1973–1979, white children less than 15 with ALL were found to have a 3-year survival rate of 59% when diagnosed in 1973–1975, compared with 74% when diagnosed in 1976–1978. Five-year survival rates for the same periods were 49% and 62% (projected), respectively, showing a marked improvement in disease treatment. This may be compared with the earliest survey years, 1950–1954, when both 3- and 5-year survival rates for all age groups were zero.[71] In more recent years, mortality was slightly higher in males than females for all age groups, although this difference was not statistically significant.

The importance of various prognostic variables differs from center to center; some of the most common ones are listed in Table 98.5. Age at diagnosis is very important. Children diagnosed between ages 2 and 10 typically have a lower mortality rate than those diagnosed either before or after these ages. A white blood cell count over 20,000, representing a larger tumor burden, generally signifies a poorer prognosis. White blood cell (WBC) count is correlated with the type of lymphoblast manifested, as children with high WBC counts are more likely to have T-cell ALL, which in itself is a poor prognostic indicator. Nonwhite children also have a poorer prognosis, although this may be related to lower socioeconomic status, leading to delays in diagnosis and treatment rather than disease characteristics.[76] Male children, on average, have a slightly poorer prognosis than female children. The reason for this is not entirely clear. Relapses in pharmacologic sanctuaries, such as the testes, have been thought to explain the difference, but testicular relapses do not completely explain this sex-related difference. Presence of a mediastinal mass on chest x-ray is a factor indicating a poor prognosis, and closely correlates with other high-risk factors such as high WBC count and T-cell ALL. Although in use for only the past decade, morphologic cell classification has become an im-

**Table 98.5** Patient Characteristics With Prognostic Importance in Acute Lymphocytic Leukemia

| | |
|---|---|
| Age | DNA index |
| Sex | Cell type/cell markers |
| Race | Mediastinal mass |
| White blood cell count | Cytogenetics/translocation |

portant factor in determining prognosis. Table 100.2 lists the characteristics of the three types of lymphocytic leukemia cells.

### Immunologic Markers

The classification of leukemias by immunologic markers is the most recent advance in the subclassification of this disease (see Table 100.2). Both T and B lymphocytes may be found in various degrees of maturity in the body. As cells become more mature, or differentiated, their surfaces change, and new "antigens" express themselves.

It is traditionally felt that one parent stem cell produces leukemic cells fixed at one stage of differentiation. Theoretically, all leukemic cells should therefore have the same differentiation antigens on their surfaces. B lymphocytes, which normally produce antibodies, express surface immunoglobulins. Precursors of B cells (pre-B cells) contain immunoglobulin in their cytoplasm. T cells and their precursors also have cell surface antigens specific to their degree of maturity and function. The most common form of ALL, called common ALL, expresses an antigen called the common ALL antigen (cALLa), felt to be of pre-pre-B-cell origin.

### Biochemical Markers

Altered concentrations of some enzymes have been noted in various forms of leukemia. Myeloperoxidase, for example, is found only in nonlymphocytic forms of leukemia. Other enzymes are present in only B- or T-cell types of ALL.[77]

Rather than analyzing cells for quantities of enzyme, stains that visually quantitate enzyme concentrations can be used. These stains can, like biochemical markers, differentiate between lymphocytic and nonlymphocytic cell forms and between B- and T-cell types of ALL.

In summary, the use of biochemical markers is relatively new. There is no clear relationship between cell morphology and immunologic markers, except that L3 morphology correlates with B-cell leukemia. Prognostically, L1 has the best survival outcome, and is frequently associated with the common ALL antigen (85%). Cells may, however, express both B- and T-cell antigens.[78,79]

### Pathology/Clinical Presentation

The pathology and clinical presentation of ALL are closely related. Because of the leukemic infiltration of the marrow and crowding out of normal marrow components, thrombocytopenia, resulting in bleeding, is a common feature. Bone pain and pathologic fractures may occur, secondary to infiltration of bone. As the immature leukemic cells are not able to fight invading organisms, infection and inability to heal are common. Leukemic cells may also infiltrate the spleen, liver, kidneys, and other organs, causing enlargement. Renal failure as a result of leukemic cell infiltration of the kidneys may occur.

The peripheral WBC count may be high, low, or normal. Lymphoblasts accounting for more than 5% of the circulating WBCs indicate the possibility of leukemia. Other bizarre, immature forms may be seen, reflecting the overcrowded condition of the marrow. Thrombocytopenia (less than 150,000 platelets/$\mu$L) is common.

A bone marrow biopsy and aspirate are necessary to confirm the diagnosis of leukemia. The biopsy demonstrates the architecture of the marrow (empty or packed), whereas the aspirate provides a blast count. A lumbar puncture is also done at the time of diagnosis to assess degree of CNS infiltration. A clean tap (no red blood cells) with five or more blasts indicates CNS involvement.

### Treatment

Chemotherapy is the primary treatment for ALL. Although treatment regimens vary among institutions, it is agreed that chemotherapy should be adjusted for the projected risk of relapse; that is, those patients with more "high-risk" factors are treated more intensively (more different drugs and higher dosages) than those with "standard-risk" factors.

Treatment regimens are typically divided into segments of induction, intensification, and maintenance (see Figure 100.3). The goal of induction therapy is to induce a complete remission, defined as a state in which no leukemic cells can be found, either circulating or in the bone marrow, and the patient looks and feels clinically well. Presence of leukemic cells in the CNS is common in this disease, especially in the T-cell form. Systemic chemotherapy generally penetrates the CNS very poorly, so standard "CNS prophylaxis" regimens have been developed to kill leukemic cells in the CNS. The regimens consist of both drugs and irradiation. Maintenance or continuation treatment refers to treatment given to maintain remission; almost all patients relapse if further treatment is not given after induction, despite the lack of evidence of disease at that time.

Many different drug regimens are being evaluated; however, some general treatment concepts can be discussed. Overall, about 85% to 95% of patients achieve a complete remission on a combination of prednisone and vincristine.[80] Either drug alone induces remission in about 50% of patients. Although initial remission induction with this combination is good, the subsequent relapse rate is high. Therefore, a third agent, usually L-asparaginase or an anthracycline (doxorubicin or daunorubicin), has been added to prolong remission duration and increase the likelihood of cure. Addition of a fourth agent increases toxicity and may or may not improve remission duration. Children who fail this induction treatment may be treated with a combination of cytarabine and teniposide.[81]

As only about 50% of standard-risk patients (and fewer high-risk patients) will be long-term survivors, attention has focused on maintenance therapy. The major cause of treatment failure is leukemic relapse, probably as a result of acquired resistance of leukemic cells to the administered chemotherapy. Methotrexate and mercaptopurine are the most effective single agents available to maintain remission. Use of other drugs and different schedules, such as rotation of pairs of drugs, has been successfully evaluated. For example, in the Total X Study at St. Jude, addition of teniposide and cytarabine to standard therapy increased the 2-year continuous complete remission rate from 30% to 50% in high-risk patients.[82]

The CNS is treated prophylactically after remission has been achieved. The CNS, as well as the testes, are known pharmacologic sanctuaries; most drugs are unable to enter these areas in sufficient amounts to be effective. Leukemic cells in these areas are thus protected from antineoplastic drugs. Prior to CNS prophylaxis, 50% or more of patients had their first relapse in the CNS.[83] CNS "prophylaxis" is provided in three forms: craniospinal irradiation (CI); cranial irradiation and intrathecal chemotherapy consisting of methotrexate alone or combined with cytarabine or hydrocortisone or both; and systemic intermediate-dose methotrexate without cranial irradiation. Intermediate-dose methotrexate in this context is the administration of dosages greater than 50 mg/m$^2$ infused over 24 hours. This long infusion time allows for equilibration of methotrexate into the CNS to produce cytocidal concentrations.

In a restrospective study combining single-institution and cooperative groups, intrathecal methotrexate 12 mg/m$^2$ was compared with intermediate-dose methotrexate (500 mg/m$^2$ as a 24-hour infusion) plus intrathecal methotrexate 12 mg/m$^2$, and with 2,400 rads cranial irradiation and intrathecal methotrexate. Standard-risk patients had a higher disease-free survival when treated with intermediate-dose plus intrathecal methotrexate than with the other regimens. Higher-risk patients had a longer disease-free survival when treated with cranial irradiation plus intrathecal methotrexate.[84]

Radiotherapy is directed at two locations, the cranium or the cranium and the spinal column. In a study by the CCSG, a dose of 1,800 rads of cranial irradiation was found to be as effective as 2,400 rads for most children for prevention of CNS relapse.[85]

Few anticancer drugs can be injected directly into the CNS because of their toxicity; three drugs that can be administered in this fashion are methotrexate, cytarabine, and hydrocortisone. To determine whether it was better to give two or three together, the Southwest Oncology Group compared intrathecal methotrexate/hydrocortisone with intrathecal methotrexate/hydrocortisone/cytarabine in patients with meningeal leukemia. There was no difference in remission rate or in length of remission.[86]

Intrathecal therapy has been found to be effective for CNS prophylaxis and treatment of CNS disease. Sullivan et al[86] treated 91 patients with meningeal leukemia. Forty-three children were randomized to receive methotrexate and hydrocortisone, and 48 to receive these two drugs plus cytarabine. No statistical difference in CNS remission length (47 weeks versus 65 weeks) was seen.

Intrathecal therapy is not completely benign. Leakage of drug from the lumbar space can damage spinal nerves, producing pain and paralysis. Leukoencephalopathy (damage to the white matter) and chemical arachnoiditis also occur. Actual penetration of drug into the ventricles is unpredictable and poor. Intraventricular administration can overcome this problem.[87]

Intermediate-dose methotrexate has been used for CNS prophylaxis and treatment of CNS disease. The first study using this approach[88] included 41 children of unclear risk status with newly diagnosed ALL and 5 children with overt CNS leukemia. Forty of forty-one achieved complete remission (CR) and have remained in CR for 1–44 months as of this report. Methotrexate concentrations in the cerebrospinal fluid remained approximately $10^{-7}$ M; the serum concentration achieved from use of intravenous drug alone was $10^{-5}$ M. Addition of intrathecal methotrexate increased the lumbar concentrations to $5 \times 10^{-5}$ M, which remained above $10^{-6}$ M for 24 hours. Improvement was seen in 3 of the 5 children with CNS leukemia, both clinically and pathologically.

The preceding methods have been compared at several institutions. Green et al[84] restrospectively compared intrathecal methotrexate, CI/intrathecal methotrexate, and intermediate-dose methotrexate/intrathecal methotrexate, at three institutions, in both high- and standard-risk patients. For standard-risk patients, intermediate-dose methotrexate/intrathecal methotrexate provided the best disease-free and overall survival, while CI/intrathecal methotrexate gave the best protection against meningeal relapse. For high-risk patients, CI/intrathecal methotrexate provided the best results for disease survival, meningeal relapse, and overall survival.

A prospective trial (Total X for standard-risk patients) of intermediate-dose methotrexate/intrathecal methotrexate versus CI/intrathecal methotrexate was performed at St. Jude starting in 1979. After a median follow-up of 2 years, the CI/intrathecal methotrexate group showed slightly fewer CNS relapses, while the intermediate-dose methotrexate/intrathecal methotrexate group had slightly more children in continuous complete remission.

**Relapse**

Relapse may occur while the patient is receiving chemotherapy or after therapy is stopped. Relapse within 6 months of the final treatment is considered relapse on therapy. Relapse on therapy carries a very poor prognosis; median survival is usually less than 1 year. Leukemic cells that grow in the presence of anticancer drugs are resistant to these drugs and are difficult to treat. Treatment regimens for on-therapy relapses must therefore contain new drugs or different combinations of previously used drugs. Patients who relapse off therapy are frequently sensitive to the drugs they previously received. This latter group has a median survival of 2.5 years or longer, although long-term prognosis is poor.[89]

Another treatment alternative for some relapse patients is bone marrow transplantation (BMT). This procedure involves removal of marrow from the iliac crest from either the patient in remission (autologous), an identical twin (syngeneic), or an HLA-matched donor (allogeneic). The patient is then given total-body irradiation and very-high-dose chemotherapy, usually including cyclophosphamide, to kill residual leukemic cells (see Figure 100.4). The harvested donor marrow is then intravenously infused into the patient. Engraftment usually occurs in approximately 3 weeks.

Hazards of BMT include, first, the possibility that the allogeneic marrow will not engraft. However, in addition to killing leukemic cells, the high-dose conditioning regimen also inhibits proliferation of the T lymphocytes that are responsible for transplant rejection. Second, autologous marrow may contain tumor cells. To avoid this, monoclonal antibodies that selectively kill tumor cells or chemotherapeutic agents (e.g., 4-hydroperoxycyclophosphamide) are added to the marrow preparation. Third, immunosuppression from radiation, chemotherapy, or agents used to suppress rejection reduces the patient's ability to fight infection. Viral and fungal infections are especially common in this group. Fourth, graft-versus-host disease (GVHD) may occur. Acute GVHD results when T lymphocytes from donor marrow react against host tissue, usually skin, liver, and gastrointestinal tract. Moderate to severe acute GVHD occurs in 30% to 60% of allogeneic transplants, develops 1 to 3 months posttransplant, and is fatal in 50% of affected patients.[90] Incidence increases directly with increasing age. To reduce the severity of acute GVHD, prophylaxis or treatment includes high-dose glucocorticoids, antithymocyte globulin, cyclosporine, and methotrexate. Chronic GVHD develops more than 3 months after transplantation. This disease consists of immune-related immunodeficiency syndromes and may result in infections, especially fungal and viral. Interstitial pneumonitis, caused by *Pneumocystis carinii*, cytomegalovirus, or other viruses, occurs in 25% to 60% of patients.

The benefit of BMT is increased chance of long-term survival. Long-term survival depends in part on age and the number of remissions the patient has previously achieved. Older patients and those in a second or later remission tend to have a poorer chance of long-term survival.

### *Acute Nonlymphocytic Leukemia*

As reported by the SEER program, the incidence of acute nonlymphocytic leukemia (ANLL) is approximately 7.8 per million white children under 15 years of age, or about one third the incidence of ALL. Of these cases of ANLL, about 80% are of the acute myelogenous leukemia (AML) type.[91] Therefore, about 15% of all leukemias are of the AML type. In contrast to ALL, there is no pattern of peak age incidence in ANLL, and there is no increased incidence in male children.

#### Prognosis

Advances in the treatment of ANLL do not parallel those of ALL. Children diagnosed with AML in 1976–1978 had 3- and 5-year survivals of 29% and 22%, respectively. These survival figures are slightly (but not statistically significantly) higher than those for 1973–1975; however, these figures are significantly higher than the survival statistics generated in 1950–1953, when both 3- and 5-year survival rates were approximately 1%.

As most children are not long-term survivors of ANLL, prognostic variables have been difficult to define. In a study conducted by the Children's Cancer Study Group,[92] age at diagnosis and time to achieve remission from the start of treatment were found to be of importance in predicting long-term outcome. Children who were 3 to 10 years of age at diagnosis or who achieved remission more quickly, for example, at day 14 rather than day 25 or 42, had an improved prognosis.

#### Morphology/Cytochemistry/Immunology

Seven types of ANLL have been described morphologically, both by cell type and by degree of maturation (see Table 98.6).[93, 94] Surface antigens, loosely correlating with stages of differentiation, have been identified for $M_1$ to $M_6$ forms of ANLL[95] and for $M_7$.[96] As with the morphologic and immunologic classifications for ALL, there is incomplete correlation between morphology and cell surface antigens. Currently, there is no prognostic relationship between cell type and disease outcome (life span, response to treatment, duration of remission).

**Table 98.6** French–American–British Morphologic Classification of ANLL

| | |
|---|---|
| $M_1$ | Myeloblastic leukemia without differentiation |
| $M_2$ | Myeloblastic leukemia with maturation to or beyond the promyelocyte stage |
| $M_3$ | Hypergranula promyelocytic leukemia—many abnormal promyelocytes with heavy granulation |
| $M_4$ | Myelomonocytic leukemia—cells with both granulocytic and monocytic differentiation |
| $M_5$ | Monocytic leukemia—subtypes: poorly differentiated-large blasts differentiated |
| $M_6$ | Erythroleukemia—erythropoietic cells constitute more than 50% of nucleated cells in the bone marrow |
| $M_7$ | Megakaryoblastic leukemia |

#### Treatment

The optimal approach to treatment of ALL is still unknown. Remission is achieved by producing marrow hypoplasia (see Figure 100.3). Conventional induction regimens, which produce severe prolonged periods of aplasia, commonly consist of daunorubicin, 5-azacytidine, cytarabine, and an epipodophyllotoxin. As single agents, these drugs produce complete remissions in about one third of patients.[96] Combinations, such as that of daunorubicin and cytarabine, can induce remissions in 70% to 80% of patients. Combination regimens, including other agents that are not highly effective alone, such as thioguanine, mercaptopurine, vincristine, prednisone, and cyclophosphamide, significantly increase the percentage of patients able to attain a complete response. Various doses and schedules have been evaluated. Two of the most successful regimens are the Berlin–Frankfort–Munster (BFM) protocol,[97] developed by a group in West Germany, and the VAPA protocol[98] developed by the Dana Farber group in Boston (see Fig. 98.1 and Table 98.7). The BFM protocol produced a complete response in 79% of children (119/151). Probability of disease-free survival was 41%; probability of survival was 45% at 57 months. The VAPA protocol induced an initial complete remission in 74% of patients up to 17 years old. Nineteen subsequently relapsed. Probability of 5-year survival was 44% for all patients. Median follow-up was 43 months.

In patients refractory to various induction regimens, Look et al[99] found a 29% (11/38) complete remission rate using a combination of etoposide and azacytidine. Five of eleven patients stayed in unmaintained remissions for a median of 19 weeks. Four of eleven received the combination monthly and remained in CR a median of 10 weeks. The other two subjects had bone marrow transplants.

The usefulness of CNS prophylaxis in the treatment of ANLL is not as apparent as it is in ALL therapy. Maintaining marrow remission has been the primary problem, and most patients do not survive long enough in marrow remission for CNS disease to have an effect on long-term survival. The West German group, as well as the St. Jude group,[100] has used cranial irradiation plus intrathecal methotrexate as CNS prophylaxis. The Boston group did not use CNS

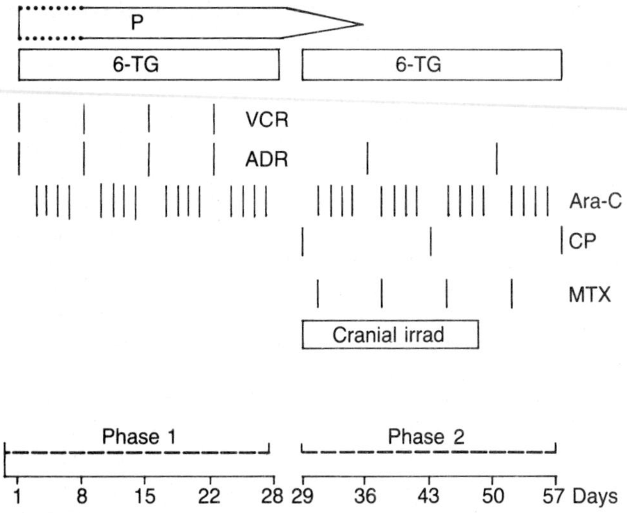


**Figure 98.1** Induction/consolidation regimen of German Cooperative Study AML-BFM-78. P, prednisone (60 mg/m$^2$ orally daily in three divided doses for 28 days, tapering in three 3-day stages at one half, one fourth, and one eighth of starting dose); TG, thioguanine (60 mg/m$^2$ orally for 28 days); VC, vincristine (1.5 mg/m$^2$ IV × 4; maximal single VC dose, 2 mg); ADR, Adriamycin (25 mg/m$^2$ IV × 4); Ara-c, cytarabine (75 mg/m$^2$ IV × 16); CP, cyclophosphamide (500 mg/m$^2$ × 3); MTX, methotrexate (12.5 mg/m$^2$ ith × 4); Cranial irrad, whole-brain irradiation with focal dose in first year of life, 12 Gy, in second year of life, 18 Gy. *(From Creutzig U, Ritler J, Riehm H, et al: Improved treatment results in childhood acute myelogenous leukemia: A report of the German Cooperative Study AML-BFM-78. Blood 1985;65:29.9, with permission.)*

prophylaxis but survival was the same for patients in the Boston and West German groups because hematologic relapse was the major cause of treatment failure.

Death in early therapy is not uncommon, approaching 20% of all children in some studies, and is frequently due to bleeding and infection. The protocols employed for remission induction produce severe, prolonged marrow hypoplasia. Considerable support measures, including antibiotics for bacterial, fungal, and viral infections, availability of large amounts of blood products, and parenteral nutrition support, are necessary to sustain these patients through induction. Long hospitalizations are the rule rather than the exception. This therapy must be given in a setting able to support the patient.

Because of the short duration of unmaintained remission, continuation of therapy after achievement of remission has become routine. Maintenance therapy, consisting of high or low doses of effective agents, is used after remission induction for variable lengths of time. The best drugs and the best schedules remain still unknown. Intensification therapy, which is the use of maximum tolerated dosages of the induction chemotherapy, has been evaluated. Intensification may be termed "early" or "late," depending on the time during maintenance at which it is given. The purpose of this "reinduction" is to eradicate any residual undetectable cells that may have become resistant to maintenance therapy.

Bone marrow transplantation may have a more clear role in the treatment of ANLL[101] than in ALL,[102] as ANLL at present is less curable with chemotherapy. Outcome has been best in patients in first remission with an HLA-matched donor. Survival in first complete remission is approximately 50% in patients less than 21 years old.[103] Side effects include both acute and chronic GVHD; disseminated fungal, viral, and bacterial infections can also occur, caused in part by the immunosuppressive agents used to treat the GVHD.

## *Non-Hodgkin's Lymphoma*

### Incidence

In the nationwide survey completed for the years 1969–1971, the incidence of lymphomas for white children less than 15 years of age was 13.2 per million. Forty-four percent of these lymphomas were Hodgkin's disease (HD) and 56%, non-Hodgkin's lymphoma (NHL). In the NHL group, 72% of children were male.[91] Incidence peaks between 7 and 9 years of age.

**Table 98.7** VAPA Protocol for Maintenance of Remission of AML

| *Sequence I* | *Sequence II* | *Sequence III* | *Sequence IV* |
|---|---|---|---|
| Adriamycin, 45 mg/m$^2$/d, day, 1, IV<br>Cytarabine, 200 mg/m$^2$/d, days 1–5, continuous IV infusion | Adriamycin, 30 mg/m$^2$/d, day 1, IV<br>Azacytidine, 150 mg/m$^2$/d, days 1–5, continuous IV infusion | Vincristine, 1.5 mg/m$^2$/d, day 1, IV<br>Methylprednisolone, 800 mg/m$^2$/day, days 1–5, IV | Cytarabine, 200 mg/m$^2$/day, days 1–5, continuous IV infusion |
| | | 6-Mercaptopurine, 500 mg/m$^2$/d, days 1–5, IV<br>Methotrexate, 7.5 mg/m$^2$/d, days 1–5, intravenous | |
| Given 4 times at 3- to 4-wk intervals | Given 4 times at 4-wk intervals | Given 4 times at 3-wk intervals | Given 4 times 3- to 4-wk intervals |

From Weinstein HJ, Mayer RJ, Rosenthal DS, et al: Chemotherapy for acute myelogenous leukemia in children and adults: VAPA update. Blood 1983;62:316, with permission.

**Table 98.8** Staging Scheme for Non-Hodgkin's Lymphoma

| | |
|---|---|
| Stage I | Single tumor (extranodal) or single anatomic area (nodal) with the exclusion of mediastinum or abdomen. |
| Stage II | Single tumor (extranodal) with regional node involvement. Two or more nodal areas on the same side of the diaphragm. Two single (extranodal) tumors with or without regional nodal involvement on the same side of the diaphragm. A primary gastrointestinal tract tumor, usually in the ileocecal area, with or without involvement of associated mesenteric nodes only. |
| Stage III | Two single tumors (extranodal) on opposite sides of the diaphragm. Two or more nodal areas above and below the diaphragm. All primary intrathoracic tumors (mediastinal, pleural, thymic). All extensive primary intraabdominal disease. All paraspinal or epidural tumors, regardless of other tumor site(s). |
| Stage IV | Any of the above with initial CNS and/or bone marrow involvement. |

From Murphy SB: Classification, staging and end results of treatment of childhood non-Hodgkin's lymphomas: Dissimilarities from lymphomas in adults. Semin Oncol 1980;7:336, with permission.

### Staging

Pediatric NHL is typically high grade and disseminated at diagnosis. Although the Ann Arbor clinical staging system for Hodgkin's disease has been used for non-Hodgkin's lymphoma, NHL does not behave in the same manner. A clinical staging system has been formulated for pediatric NHL at St. Jude Children's Research Hospital to establish prognosis and guide therapy (Table 98.8).

### Prognosis

Each histologic subtype of the non-Hodgkin's lymphomas behaves differently with its own metastatic characteristics and sensitivity to chemotherapy. Each is discussed separately.

***Lymphoblastic Lymphoma*** Lymphoblastic lymphoma is the lymphomatous presentation of T-cell ALL, as the cells are identical. Lymphoblastic lymphoma frequently presents with mediastinal mass, and has a tendency to spread to the central nervous system and bone marrow. By St. Jude staging, this tumor typically presents as stage III (mediastinal involvement) or stage IV (CNS disease). Typical signs and symptoms include coughing and dyspnea as the result of pleural fluid accumulation. Overall survival has improved considerably with more intensive chemotherapy regimens. In a study performed at the NCI, children with lymphoblastic lymphoma had an estimated 3-year survival rate of 60%,[104] with median follow-up of 3 years. Prognostic indicators in their study were stage, tumor burden, marrow involvement, and CNS involvement. Patients who were older did worse, but this was related to stage (i.e., older patients had a higher stage).

***Undifferentiated Lymphomas*** There are two major subclassifications of undifferentiated lymphomas, Burkitt and non-Burkitt pleomorphic types. Both are B-cell malignancies. Burkitt's lymphoma in the United States is also known as nonendemic Burkitt's, to differentiate it from the endemic form, or African Burkitt's. African Burkitt's lymphoma is caused by the Epstein–Barr virus (EBV); viral particles have been isolated in all cases of African Burkitt's studied, and all children have high titers of antibody to EBV. The causative agent of nonendemic Burkitt's has not been identified. Some children have antibody titers to EBV but most do not. Rarely, viral particles of EBV have been located. Morphologically and immunologically, the cells are identical, but, clinically, the diseases behave quite differently. African Burkitt's has a strong predisposition to present in the maxillomandibular area. The first symptoms are often loosening of the teeth or exophthalmia. American Burkitt's generally presents in the abdomen. Areas typically include the ileocecal region, mesentery, ovaries, or retroperitoneum. Common symptoms are abdominal pain and vomiting. Ascites is a common sign in these children, and large masses may be felt. Only a small percentage of these patients show marrow involvement at diagnosis, and a leukemic phase is unusual (unlike lymphoblastic lymphoma). Relapse frequently occurs locally. Like the lymphoblastic lymphomas, survival has improved with intensive chemotherapy, although survival is still not high and relapse is common. In a study performed at the NCI, overall 2-year survival was 54%; those whose disease was resected had a longer survival than those whose disease was not surgically treatable (82% versus 41% 2-year survival). Unfortunately, most patients do not have surgically resectable disease.[105] Burkitt's lymphomas have a labeling index (LI) higher than any other known tumor,[106] consistent with their high degree of aggressiveness and sensitivity to chemotherapy.

Undifferentiated, non-Burkitt's lymphomas are similar to Burkitt-type lymphomas, except that they have a greater tendency to present in peripheral areas. Their sensitivities to chemotherapy are similar. The difference between the two types of undifferentiated lymphoma is their cellular appearance. Although frequently difficult to differentiate, the non-Burkitt type has a larger and more pleomorphic nucleus.

***Large-Cell Lymphomas*** The last type of NHL has been erroneously termed "histiocytic" because of the cellular resemblance to normal histiocytes. Upon closer observation, it has been found that these cells are not malignant histiocytes, and the more appropriate "large lymphoid cell" is in current use. This group of lymphomas is very heterogeneous. Presenting sites are variable, including both nodal and extranodal areas. The mediastinum is not one of these extranodal sites.[107] The presenting symptoms of large-cell lymphoma are nonspecific. Survival in this group of patients is about the same as that for the lymphoblastic lymphomas. In one study, 11 of 28 children had large-cell histology. The treatment used in this study resulted in long-term survival for all patients.[108]

Unlike Hodgkin's disease, NHL cannot be treated with

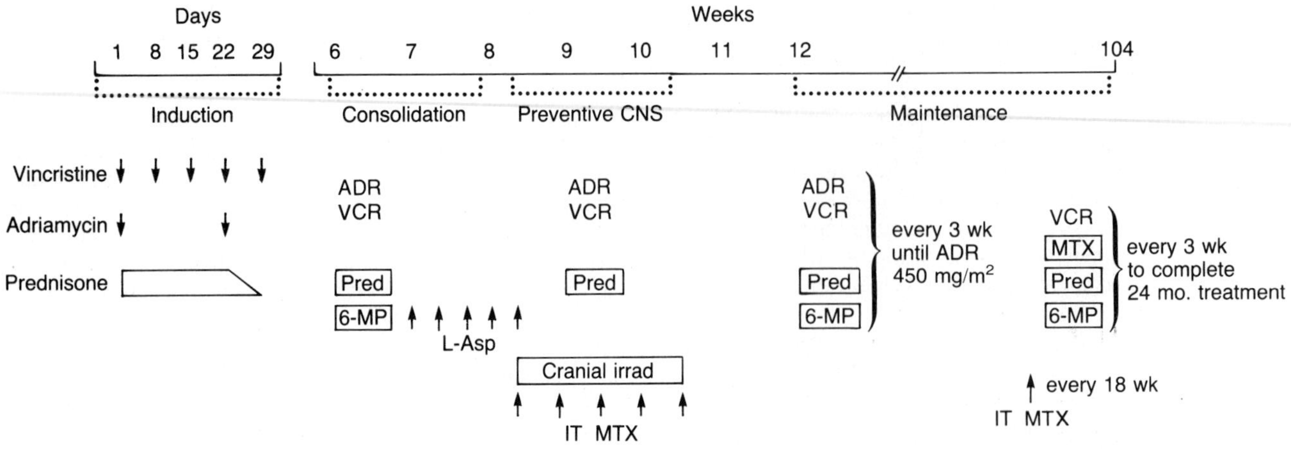


**Figure 98.2** APO protocol for treatment of non-Hodgkin's lymphoma. *Induction*: vincristine (VC) 1.5 mg/m$^2$ IV, Adriamycin (ADR) 75 mg/m$^2$ IV, prednisone (Pred) 40 mg/m$^2$ PO. *Consolidation*: ADR 30 mg/m$^2$ IV, VCR 2 mg/m$^2$ IV, Pred 120 mg/m$^2$ PO, 6-mercaptopurine (6-MP) 225 mg/m$^2$ PO,L-asparaginase (L-Asp) 56,000 IU/m$^2$ if > 6 years old, 28,000 IU/m$^2$ if < 6 years old, IV or IM. *Maintenance*: ADR 30 mg/m$^2$ IV, VCR 2 mg/m$^2$ IV, Pred 120 mg/m$^2$ PO, 6-MP 225 mg/m$^2$ PO to cumulative ADR dose 450 mg/m$^2$. Then methotrexate MTX, substituted for ADR, 7.5 mg/m$^2$ IV on day 1, IM days 2–5. *CNS prophylaxis*: intrathacal (IT) MTX 12 mg/m$^2$, cranial irradiation 2,400 rads. *(From Weinstein HJ, Cassady JR, Lavey R: Long-term results of the APO protocol (vincristine, doxorubicin [Adriamycin], and prednisone) for treatment of mediastinal lymphoblastic lymphoma. J Clin Oncol 1983;1:538,with permission.)*

radiation alone, as it is usually high grade and disseminated in children. Therefore, chemotherapy is always used, and extensive staging laparotomy procedures are unnecessary. Laparotomy may be useful in providing markers of disease or removing bulky obstructive disease. Radiographic scans likewise may be used to monitor the disease.

Protocols have been developed for treatment of both lymphoblastic and undifferentiated forms of lymphoma. The group at the Dana Farber Cancer Institute have tested the combination of doxorubicin, prednisone, and vincristine—the APO protocol (*A*driamycin, *p*rednisone, *O*ncovin) (see Fig. 98.2)—in children with mediastinal lymphoblastic lymphoma.[109] Complete responses were achieved in 20 of 21 patients. Six patients have since relapsed, and two died in complete remission. Five-year estimated survival for all 21 patients is 69%. A protocol designed by Magrath[104] (see Fig. 98.3) for both lymphoblastic and undifferentiated forms consists of cyclophosphamide, doxorubicin, vincristine, and prednisone plus 42-hour methotrexate infusions. Ninety-seven percent of children achieved complete response; the estimated 3-year survival was 60% with a median follow-up of 3 years.

The COMP (*C*yclophosphamide, vincristine [*O*ncovin], *m*ethotrexate, *p*rednisone) regimen was compared with Sloan–Kettering's LSA$_2$-L$_2$ protocol (cyclophosphamide, vincristine, prednisone, daunomycin, methotrexate, cytarabine, thioguanine, asparaginase, carmustine) (see Fig. 98.4) in treatment of NHL[110] Two hundred thirty-four patients were treated. Overall survival was 74% at 12 months and 66% at 24 months. Disease-free survival was 84% for those with localized disease and 47% for those with nonlocalized disease at diagnosis. Patients with lymphoblastic lymphoma treated with LSA$_2$-L$_2$ had a better disease-free survival rate (76% versus 26%). Patients with nonlymphoblastic lymphoma fared better on COMP (57% versus 28% disease-free survival at 2 years).

Murphy et al have designed a protocol for children with localized disease that is both less intensive and shorter.[108] An induction regimen (vincristine, methotrexate, prednisone) plus involved-field radiation (2,000 rads) and maintenance therapy (mercaptopurine daily, methotrexate weekly) were used. Twenty-eight of twenty-eight attained complete remission, and 24 of 28 are disease free a median of greater than 24 months. The four failures were undifferentiated types.

The major challenge lies in treatment of nonlocalized Burkitt's lymphomas. These tumors grow rapidly and respond well to chemotherapy initially; however, resistance occurs equally rapidly. Murphy et al[111] have developed a treatment protocol for B-cell leukemia–lymphomas, designed to deliver maximum amounts of chemotherapy to which tumors are susceptible (cytarabine, cyclophosphamide, methotrexate) in a short amount of time (6 months). Of 29 stage III and IV patients, 86% achieved complete remission. Overall survival was 14 of 18 with stage III, 0 of 3 with stage IV, and 1 of 8 with B-cell ALL, showing that marrow and CNS involvement is associated with a poor prognosis.

### *Hodgkin's Disease*

The annual incidence of Hodgkin's disease (HD) is approximately 5.6 per million white children under the age of 15. The disease is very rare in children under 5. Sixty percent of the affected children are male.[91] This male predominance ends at the start of puberty: the male:female ratio then inverts, and may be as low as 1:2.

Clinical stage (see Table 98.9) is the chief prognostic indicator. The staging procedure is one of the most important components of the treatment process; patients with local disease can be treated with irradiation alone.

There is controversy regarding treatment of pediatric HD. Because of the side effects of chemotherapy, possible male

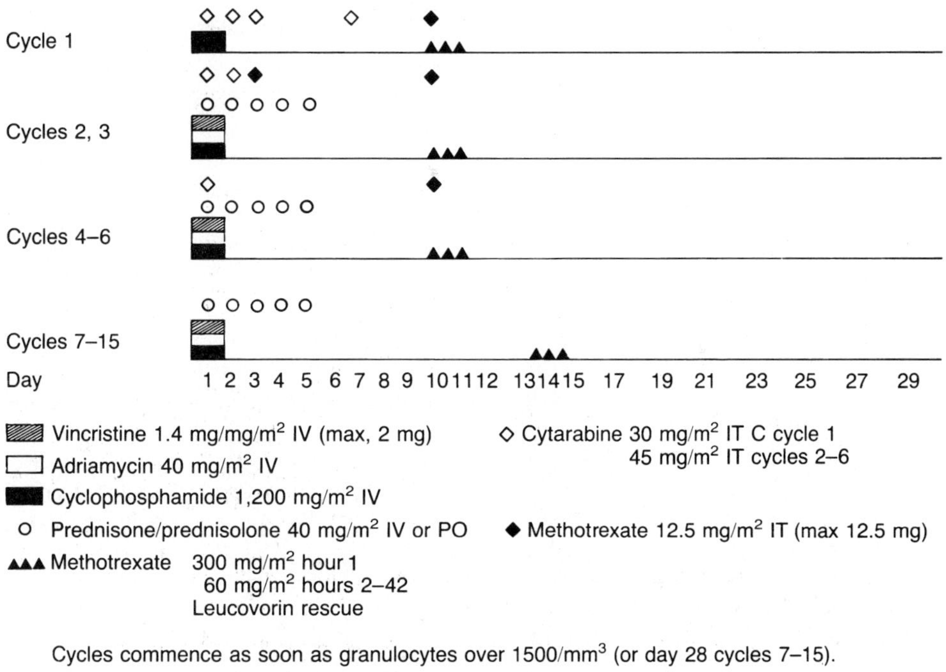


**Figure 98.3** Treatment scheme for non-Hodgkin's lymphoma. *(From Magrath ET, Janus C, Edwards BK, et al: An effective therapy for both undifferentiated (including Burkitt's) lymphomas and lymphoblastic lymphomas in children and young adults. Blood 1984;63:1102–1111, with permission.)*

sterility in particular, an attempt has been made to use radiotherapy to treat children with low stages (IA and IIA) of disease and to use chemotherapy as salvage treatment in cases of relapse.[112]

The other alternative is combined radiotherapy and chemotherapy in low-stage disease.[113] This provides a higher relapse-free survival rate (92% versus 88%), yet exposes children to chemotherapy, which may produce long-term side effects. Both methods of treatment provide initial complete remission rates that approach 100%. Patients presenting with higher stages or symptoms are generally treated with chemotherapy plus extended-field irradiation.

Chemotherapy typically consists of two regimens. The MOPP regimen (*m*echlorethamine, vincristine [*O*ncovin], *p*rocarbazine, *p*rednisone[113] is the "gold standard" of therapy. A more recently developed regimen, ABVD[114] (doxorubicin [*A*driamycin], *b*leomycin, *v*inblastine, *d*acarbazine), is used either in place of MOPP or as salvage treatment in the case of relapse.

As the alkylating agents are responsible for sterility (i.e., mechlorethamine), the ABVD regimen may be a better alternative for pediatric patients. Cyclophosphamide is sometimes substituted for mechlorethamine; in boys treated for nephrotic syndrome with cyclophosphamide for short times, transient but reversible decreases in sperm production have been seen. It is therefore hoped that cyclophosphamide is as effective as mechlorethamine, but will cause less infertility.

Several studies have compared treatment of stage III and IV HD patients with either radiation or radiation plus chemotherapy. Radiation plus chemotherapy has been the most effective regimen. Lange et al[115] showed an 86% overall survival and 60% disease-free survival at 5 years with cyclophosphamide, vincristine (Oncovin), prednisone, and procarbazine (COPP) plus 2,000–3,600 rads to the involved field. This is compared with 60% and 0%, respectively, for 3,600–4,000 rads of radiation alone. Jenkin et al[116] treated stages IB and II-IV with MOPP and low-dose radiation (2,000–3,500 rads in 20 fractions). For stage III patients, 5-year survival and disease-free survival were 92% and 88%; for stage IV, these figures were 85% and 65%, respectively.

## Long-Term Consequences of Treatment

### *Intellectual Function*

Cranial irradiation appears to play a major role in deterioration of intellectual function in leukemic children. A neuropsychologic evaluation[117] of three groups of children who received intrathecal methotrexate, intrathecal methotrexate plus 2,400 rads of cranial irradiation, or intrathecal methotrexate plus intravenous methotrexate for CNS prophylaxis was performed 6.3, 4.7, and 3.2 years, respectively, after CNS treatment. Children who received 2,400 rads of cranial irradiation performed significantly worse on various tests of neuropsychologic function.

Moss et al[118] found a statistically significant difference in IQs of patients receiving cranial irradiation as compared with a group of children with ALL who did not receive CNS therapy and with siblings. These differences continued at 1 year.

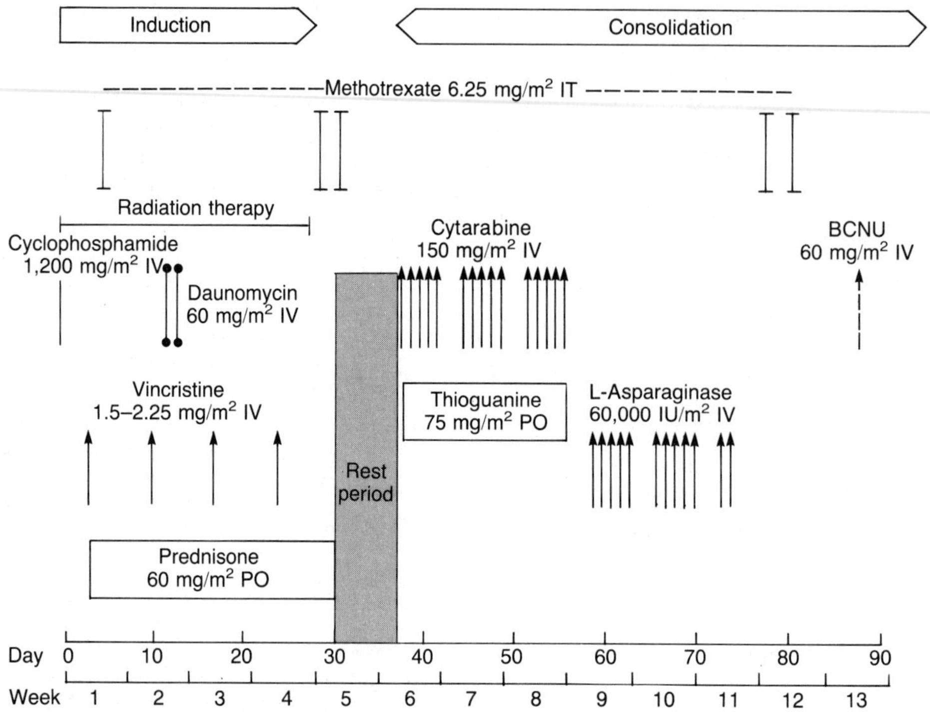


**Figure 98.4** LSA$_2$-L$_2$ protocol for non-Hodgkin's lymphoma. *(From Wollner N, Burchenal JH, Lieberman PH, Exelby PR, D'Angio GJ, Murphy ML: Non-Hodgkin's lymphoma in children. Med Pediatr Oncol 1975;1:23:237, with permission.)*

Prophylactic treatment of the CNS may also cause seizures and dementia. The wide range of effects may in part result from the combination and order of CNS prophylactic treatment.[119] For example, children receiving intermediate- or high-dose methotrexate infusions after cranial irradiation experience a higher incidence of systemic side effects. It has been proposed that the blood–brain barrier is damaged by radiation, allowing more methotrexate to enter the CNS and cause damage.[120]

Children under 2 years of age appear to sustain more CNS damage from cranial irradiation than older children.[121] Cranial irradiation is therefore often avoided as CNS prophylaxis in this age group.

**Table 98.9** Ann Arbor Staging Classification for Hodgkin's Disease[a]

| | |
|---|---|
| Stage I | Involvement of a single lymph node region (I) or a single extralymphatic organ or site (I$_E$) |
| Stage II | Involvement of two or more lymph node regions on the same side of the diaphragm (II) or localized involvement of an extralymphatic organ or site (II$_E$). |
| Stage III | Involvement of lymph node regions on both sides of the diaphragm (III) or localized involvement of an extralymphatic organ or site (III$_E$) or spleen (III$_S$) or both (III$_{SE}$). |
| Stage IV | Diffuse or disseminated involvement of one or more extralymphatic organs with or without associated lymph node involvement |

[a] A = asymptomatic; B = fever, sweats, or weight loss greater than 10% body weight.

### *Growth Retardation*

Abnormalities in the function of hypothalamus resulting from cranial irradiation can lead to decreased production of growth hormone and to growth retardation.[122] Irradiation can cause early fusion of the growing bones.[123]

### *Hypothyroidism*

Hypothalamic irradiation may also result in decreased release of thyrotropin releasing hormone,[124] producing either clinical or subclinical hypothyroidism.

### *Infertility*

Gonadal irradiation is a frequent cause of infertility in males and females who received radiation before puberty.[125] Females do not commonly experience ovarian leukemic infiltration as a site of relapse; the testes, however, are a pharmacologic sanctuary and are irradiated in cases of leukemic infiltration.

In cases of lymphoma, abdominal disease is frequent. In females, an attempt is made to move the ovaries out of the way of the radiation port to decrease the dosage given to the ovaries. This is sometimes effective in maintaining normal ovarian function.

Alkylating agents are administered to most lymphoma patients. These drugs may be a primary cause of infertility in patients who receive them prior to the onset of puberty.

### *Birth Defects*

With limited information available, there appears to be no increased incidence of birth defects in children of parents treated for acute leukemia as children. As more children become long-term survivors, the true incidence of birth defects will become apparent.

## References


1. Miller RW, McKay FW. Decline in US childhood cancer mortality 1950 through 1980. JAMA 1984;251:1567–1570.
2. Young JL, Miller RW. Incidence of malignant tumors in U.S. children. J Pediatr 1975;86:254–258.
3. Farwell JR, Dohrmann GJ, Flannery JT. Central nervous system tumors in children. Cancer 1977;40:3123–3132.
4. Levin VA. Chemotherapy of primary brain tumors. Neurol Clin 1985;3:855–866.
5. Shapiro WR. Chemotherapy of primary malignant brain tumors in children. Cancer 1975;35:965–972.
6. Edwards MS, Levin VA, Wilson CB. Brain tumor chemotherapy: An evaluation of agents in current use for phase II & III trials. Cancer Treat Rep 1980;64:1179–1205.
7. Sheline GE. Radiation therapy of tumors of the central nervous system in childhood. Cancer 1975;35:957–964.
8. Levin VA, Landahl HD, Patlak CS. Drug delivery to CNS tumors. Cancer Treat Rep 1981;65(suppl 2):19–25.
9. Djerassi I, Kim JS, Reggev A. Response of astrocytoma to high-dose methotrexate with citrovorum factor rescue. Cancer 1985;55:2741–2747.
10. Kimmel DW, Shapiro, WR. Brain tumors, in Pinedo HM, Chabner BA (eds): Cancer Chemotherapy 7. New York, Elsevier Science Publishers, 1985, pp 439–455.
11. Dobell WJ, Morgan WF, Rasmussen J, et al. Potentiation of 1,3-bis(2-chlorethyl)1-nitrosurea (BCNU)-induced cytotoxicity in 9L cells by pretreatment with 6-thioguanine. Biochem Pharmacol 1985;34:515–520.
12. Silberman AW, Rand RW, Storm K, et al. Phase I trial of thermochemotherapy for brain malignancy. Cancer 1985;56: 48–56.
13. Rosen EM, Cassady JR, Frantz CN, et al. Neuroblastoma: The Joint Center for Radiation Therapy/Dana-Farber Cancer Institute/Children's Hospital experience. J Clin Oncol 1984;2:719–732.
14. Graham-Pole J, Salmi T, Anton AH, et al. Tumor and urine catecholamines (CATs) in neurogenic tumors. Cancer 1983;51: 834–839.
15. Evans AE, D'Angio GJ, Randolph J. A proposed staging for children with neuroblastoma. Cancer 1971;27:374–378.
16. Evans A. Staging and treatment of neuroblastoma. Cancer 1980;45:1799–1802.
17. Green AA, Hayes FA, Hustu HO. Sequential cyclophosphamide and doxorubicin for induction of complete remission in children with disseminated neuroblastoma. Cancer 1981;48: 2310–2317.
18. Hayes FA, Green AA, Casper J, et al. Clinical evaluation of sequentially scheduled cisplatin and VM26 in neuroblastoma: Response and toxicity. Cancer 1981;48:1715–1718.
19. Shafford EA, Rogers DW, Pritchard J. Advanced neuroblastoma: Improved response rate using a multiagent regimen (OPEC) including sequential cisplatin and VM-26. J Clin Oncol 1984;2:742–747.
20. August CS, Schlesinger H, D'Angio GJ, et al. Bone marrow transplantation (BMT) for relapsed stage IV neuroblastoma (NBL/IV). Pediatr Res 1983;17:228A.
21. Maurer HM, Moon T, Donaldson M, et al. The Intergroup Rhabdomyosarcoma Study (a preliminary report). Cancer 1977;40:2015–2026.
22. Donaldson SS. The value of adjuvant chemotherapy in the management of sarcomas in children. Cancer 1985;55:2184–2197.
23. Donaldson SS, Castro JR, Wilbur JR, et al. Rhabdomyosarcoma of head and neck in children. Cancer 1973;31:26–35.
24. Pratt CB. Response of childhood rhabdomyosarcoma to combination chemotherapy. J Pediatr 1969;74:791–794.
25. Tefft M, Fernandez CH, Moon TE. Rhabdomyosarcoma: Response with chemotherapy prior to radiation in patients with gross residual disease. Cancer 1977;39:665–670.
26. Tepper JE, Suit HD. Radiation therapy of soft tissue sarcomas. Cancer 1985;55:2273–2277.
27. Pratt CB, Hustu HO, Fleming ID, et al. Coordinated treatment of childhood rhabdomyosarcoma with surgery, radiotherapy, and combination chemotherapy. Cancer Res 1972;32:606–610.
28. Maurer H, Foulkes M, Grehan E. Intergroup Rhabdomyosarcoma Study (IRS). II: Preliminary report. (Abstr) Proc Am Soc Clin Oncol 1983;2:70.
29. Flamant F, Hill C. The improvement in survival associated with combined chemotherapy in childhood rhabdomyosarcoma. Cancer 1984;53:2417–2421.
30. Houghton JA, Cook RL, Lutz PJ, et al. Melphalan: A potential new agent in the treatment of childhood rhabdomyosarcoma. Cancer Treat Rep 1985;69:91–96.
31. Goorin AM, Abelson HT, Frei E. Osteosarcoma: 15 years later. N Engl J Med 1985;313:1637–1643.
32. Meadows AT, Strong LC, Li FP, et al. Bone sarcoma as a second malignant neoplasm in children: Influence of radiation and genetic predisposition. Cancer 1980;46:2603–2606.
33. Marcove RC, Rosen G. En bloc resections for osteogenic sarcoma. Cancer 1980;45:3040–3044.
34. Rosen G, Murphy ML, Huvos AG. Chemotherapy, en bloc resection, and prosthetic bone replacement in the treatment of osteogenic sarcoma. Cancer 1976;37:1–11.
35. Tichler TE, Am YB, Brenner HJ. Chemotherapy in osteosarcoma, in Osteosarcoma: New Trends in Diagnosis and Treatment. New York, Alan R. Liss, 1982, pp 49–75.
36. Jaffe N, Paed D. Recent advances in the chemotherapy of metastatic osteogenic sarcoma. Cancer 1972;30:1627–1631.
37. Cortes EP, Holland JF, Wang JJ, et al. Doxorubicin in disseminated osteosarcoma. JAMA 1972;221:1132–1138.
38. Gasparini M, Rouesse J, van Oosterom A, et al. Phase II study

of cisplatin in advanced osteogenic sarcoma. Cancer Treat Rep 1985;69:211–213.

39. Pratt CB, Rivera G, Shanks E, et al. Combination chemotherapy for osteosarcoma. Cancer Treat Rep 1978;62:251–257.
40. Ettinger LJ, Douglas HO, Mindell ER, et al. Adjuvant adriamycin and cisplatin in newly diagnosed, nonmetastatic osteosarcoma of the extremity. J Clin Oncol 1986;4:353–362.
41. Mosende C, Gutierrez M, Caparros B, et al. Combination chemotherapy with bleomycin, cyclophosphamide and dactinomycin for the treatment of osteogenic sarcoma. Cancer 1977;40:2779–2786.
42. Taylor WF, Ivins JC, Pritchard DJ, et al. Trends and variability in survival among patients with osteosarcoma: A 7-year update. Mayo Clin Proc 1985;60:91–104.
43. Rosen G, Caparros B, Huvos AG, et al. Preoperative chemotherapy for osteogenic sarcoma: Selection of postoperative adjuvant chemotherapy based on the response of the primary tumor to preoperative chemotherapy. Cancer 1982;49:1221–1230.
44. Link MP, Goorin AM, Miser AW, et al. The effect of adjuvant chemotherapy on relapse-free survival in patients with osteosarcoma of the extremity. N Engl J Med 1986;314:1600–1606.
45. Eilber FR, Grant T, Morton DL. Adjuvant therapy for osteosarcoma: Preoperative and postoperative treatment. Cancer Treat Rep 1978;62:213–216.
46. Rosen G, Marcove RC, Caparros B, et al. Primary osteogenic sarcoma. Cancer 1979;43:2163–2177.
47. Jaffe N, Robertson R, Ayala A, et al. Comparison of intraarterial *cis*-diamminedichloroplatinum II with high-dose methotrexate and citrovorum factor rescue in the treatment of primary osteosarcoma. J Clin Oncol 1985;3:1101–1104.
48. Marti C, Kronver T, Remagan W, et al. High-dose ifosfamide in advanced osteosarcoma. Cancer Treat Rep 1985;69:115–117.
49. Berry MP, Jenkin RDT, Harwood AR, et al. Ewing's sarcoma: A trial of adjuvant chemotherapy and sequential half-body irradiation. Int J Rad Oncol Biol Phys 1986;12:19–24.
50. Mendenhall CM, Marcus RB, Enneking WF, et al. The prognostic significance of soft tissue extension in Ewing's sarcoma. Cancer 1983;51:913–917.
51. Rosen G, Caparros B, Nirenberg A, et al. Ewing's sarcoma: Ten-year experience with adjuvant chemotherapy. Cancer 1981;41:888–899.
52. Pilepich MV, Vietti TJ, Nesbit ME, et al. Radiotherapy and combination chemotherapy in advanced Ewings's sarcoma—Interstudy Group. Cancer 1981;47:1930–1936.
53. Razek A, Perez CA, Tefft M, et al. Intergroup Ewing's Sarcoma Study: Local control related to radiation dose, volume and site of primary lesions in Ewing's sarcoma. Cancer 1980;46:516–521.
54. Jensen RD, Miller RW. Retinoblastoma: Epidemiologic characteristics. N Engl J Med 1971;285:307–311.
55. Newell GR, Roberts JD, Baranovsky A. Retinoblastoma: Presentation and survival in Negro children compared with whites. J Natl Cancer Inst 1972;49:989–992.
56. Knudson AG. Mutation and cancer: Statistical study of retinoblastoma. Proc Natl Acad Sci USA 1971;68:820–823.
57. Freeman CR, Esseltine DL, Whitehead VM, et al. Retinoblastoma: The case for radiotherapy and adjuvant chemotherapy. Cancer 1980;46:1913–1918.
58. Lennox EL, Draper GJ, Sanders BM. Retinoblastoma: A study of natural history and prognosis of 268 cases. Br Med J 1975;3:731–734.
59. Reese AB, Ellsworth RM. The evaluation and current concept of retinoblastoma therapy. Trans Am Acad Ophthalmol Otolaryngol 1963;67:169–172.
60. Pratt CB. Management of malignant solid tumors in children. Pediatr Clin North Am 1972;19:1141–1155.
61. Howarth C, Meyer D, Hustu O, et al. Stage-related combined modality treatment of retinoblastoma. Cancer 1980;45:851–858.
62. Pratt CB, Crom DB, Howarth C. The use of chemotherapy for extraocular retinoblastoma. Med Pediatr Oncol 1985;13:330–333.
63. Tan C, Rosen G, Ghavimi F, et al. Adriamycin (NSC-123127) in pediatric malignancies. Cancer Chemother Rep 1975;68:259–266.
64. Southwest Cancer Chemotherapy Study Group. Chemotherapeutic trials in patients with metastatic retinoblastoma. Cancer Chemother Rep 1968;52:631–634.
65. D'Angio GJ, Evans AE, Breslow N, et al. The treatment of Wilms' tumor. Cancer 1976;38:633–646.
66. Breslow NE, Palmer NF, Hill LR, et al. Wilms' tumor prognostic factors for patients without metastases at diagnosis. Cancer 1978;41:1577–1589.
67. D'Angio GJ, Evans A, Breslow N, et al. The treatment of Wilms' tumor: Results of the Second National Wilms' Tumor Study. Cancer 1981;47:2302–2311.
68. Beckwith JB, Palmer NF. Histopathology and prognosis of Wilms' tumor. Cancer 1978;41:1937–1948.
69. D'Angio GJ, Beckwith JB, Breslow NE, et al. Wilms' tumor: An update. Cancer 1980;45:1791–1798.
70. Breslow N, Churchill G, Beckwith JB, et al. Prognosis for Wilms' tumor patients with nonmetastatic disease at diagnosis—results of the Second National Wilms' Tumor Study. J Clin Oncol 1985;3:521–531.
71. Steinhorn SC, Myers MH. Progress in the treatment of childhood acute leukemia: A review. Med Pediatr Oncol 1981;9:333–346.
72. Gallo RC, Wong-Staal F. Retroviruses as etiologic agents of some animal and human leukemias and lymphomas and as tools for elucidating the molecular mechanism of leukemogenesis. Blood 1982;60:545–556.
73. Penn P. Second malignant neoplasms associated with immunosuppressive medications. Cancer 1976;37:1024–1032.
74. Rosner F. Acute leukemia as a delayed consequence of cancer chemotherapy. Cancer 1976;37:1033–1036.
75. Robison LL, Nesbit ME, Sather HN, et al. Down syndrome and acute leukemia in children: A 10-year retrospective survey from Children's Cancer Study Group. J Pediatr 1984;105:235–242.
76. Pendergrass TW, Hoover R, Godwin JD. Prognosis of black children with acute lymphocytic leukemia. Med Pediatr Oncol 1975;1:143.
77. Blaff J, Reaman G, Poplack DG. Biochemical markers in lymphoid malignancy. N Engl J Med 1980;303:918–922.
78. Aisenberg AC, Wilkes BM. The genotype and phenotype of T cell and non-T, non-B acute lymphoblastic leukemia. Blood 1985;66:1215–1218.
79. Mirro J, Zipf TF, Pui C-H, et al. Acute mixed lineage leukemia: Clinicopathologic correlations and prognostic significance. Blood 1985;66:1115–1123.
80. Simone JV, Aur RJA, Dahl GV, et al. Combined modality therapy of acute lymphocytic leukemia. Cancer 1975;305:25–35.
81. Rivera G, Aur RJA, Dahl GV, et al. Combined VM-26 and cytosine arabinoside in treatment of refractory childhood lymphocytic leukemia. Cancer 1980;45:1281–1288.
82. Murphy SB, Dahl GV, Look AT, et al. Recent results from total therapy Study X for standard and high-risk acute lymphoblastic leukemia in children: Recognition of new clinical and

biologic risk features. Hematol Blood Transfusion 1985;29:78–81.

83. Evans AE, Gilbert EG, Sandistra R. The increasing incidence of central nervous system leukemia in children. Cancer 1970; 26:404–409.
84. Green DM, Freeman EI, Sather HN, et al. Comparison of three methods of central nervous system prophylaxis in childhood acute lymphoblastic leukemia. Lancet 1980;1:1398–1402.
85. Nesbit ME, Sather HN, Robison LL, et al. Presymptomatic central nervous system therapy in previously untreated childhood acute lymphoblastic leukemia: Comparison of 1800 rad and 2400 rad. A report for Children's Cancer Study Group. Lancet 1981;1:461–466.
86. Sullivan MP, Moon TE, Trueworthy B, et al. Combination intrathecal therapy for meningeal leukemia: Two versus three drugs. Blood 1977;50:471–479.
87. Shapiro WB, Young DF, Wehta BM. Methotrexate: Distribution in cerebrospinal fluid after intravenous, ventricular and lumbar infections. N Engl J Med 1975;293:161–166.
88. Freeman AI, Wang JJ, Sinks LF. High-dose methotrexate in acute lymphocytic leukemia. Cancer Treat Rep 1977;61:727–731.
89. Chessells J, Leper A, Rogers D. Outcome following late marrow relapse in childhood acute lymphoblastic leukemia. J Clin Oncol 1984;2:1088–1091.
90. Champlin RE, Gale RG. Role of bone marrow transplantation in the treatment of hematologic malignancies and solid tumors: Critical review of syngeneic, autologous, and allogeneic transplants. Cancer Treat Rep 1984;68:145–161.
91. Young JL, Miller RW. Incidence of malignant tumors in U.S. children. J Pediatr 1975;86:254–258.
92. Bachner RL, Kennedy A, Sather H, et al. Characteristics of children with acute nonlymphocytic leukemia in long-term continuous remission: A report for Children's Cancer Study Group. Med Pediatr Oncol 1981;9:393–403.
93. Bennett JM, Catorsky D, Daniel MT, et al. Proposals for the classification of the acute leukemias. Br J Haematol 1976;33: 451–458.
94. Bennett JM, Catorsky D, Daniel MT, et al. Criteria for the diagnosis of acute leukemia of megakaryocytic lineage (M7): A report of the French–American–British Cooperative Group. Ann Intern Med 1985;103:460–462.
95. Griffen JD, Mayer RJ, Weinstein HJ, et al. Surface marker analysis of acute myeloblastic leukemia: Identification of differentiation-associated phenotypes. Blood 1983;62:557–563.
96. Gale RP. Advances in the treatment of acute myelogenous leukemia. N Engl J Med 1979;300:1189–1199.
97. Creutzig U, Ritter J, Riehm H, et al. Improved treatment results in childhood acute myelogenous leukemia: A report of the German Cooperative Study AML-BFM-78. Blood 1985;65: 298–304.
98. Weinstein HJ, Mayer RJ, Rosenthal DS, et al. Chemotherapy for acute myelogenous leukemia in children and adults: VAPA update. Blood 1983;62:315–319.
99. Look TA, Dahl GV, Kalwinsky D, et al. Effective remission induction of refractory childhood acute nonlymphocytic leukemia by VP-16-213 plus azacytidine. Cancer Treat Rep 1981;65: 995–999.
100. Pui C-H, Dahl GV, Kalwinsky DK, et al. Central nervous system leukemia in children with acute nonlymphoblastic leukemia. Blood 1985;66:1062–1067.
101. Sanders JE, Thomas ED, Seattle Marrow Transplant Group. Marrow transplantation for children with acute nonlymphoblastic leukemia in first remission. Med Pediatr Oncol 1981;9:423–427.
102. Thomas DE, Sanders JE, Flournoy N, et al. Marrow transplantation for patients with acute lymphoblastic leukemia: A long-term follow-up. Blood 1983;62:1139–1141.
103. Thomas DE. Marrow transplant for acute non-lymphoblastic leukemia in first remission: A follow-up. N Engl J Med 1983; 308:1539–1540.
104. Magrath ET, Janus C, Edwards BK, et al. An effective therapy for both undifferentiated (including Burkitt's) lymphomas and lymphoblastic lymphomas in children and young adults. Blood 1984;63:1102–1111.
105. Ziegler JL. Treatment results of 54 American patients with Burkitt's lymphoma are similar to the African experience. N Engl J Med 1977;297:75–80.
106. Murphy SB, Melvin SL, Mauer AM. Correlation of tumor cell kinetic studies with surface marker results in childhood non-Hodgkin's lymphomas. Cancer Res 1979;39:1534–1538.
107. Murphy SB. Classification, staging and end results of treatment of childhood non-Hodgkin's lymphomas: Dissimilarities from lymphomas in adults. Semin Oncol 1980;7:332–339.
108. Murphy SB, Hustu HO, Rivera G, et al. End results of treating children with localized non-Hodgkin's lymphomas with a combined modality approach of lessened intensity. J Clin Oncol 1983;1:326–330.
109. Weinstein HJ, Cassady JR, Lavey R. Long-term results of the APO protocol (vincristine, doxorubicin [Adriamycin], and prednisone) for treatment of mediastinal lymphoblastic lymphoma. J Clin Oncol 1983;1:537–541.
110. Anderson JR, Wilson JF, Jenkin DT, et al. The results of a randomized therapeutic trial comparing a 4-drug regimen (COMP) with a 10-drug regimen ($LSA_2$-$L_2$). N Engl J Med 1983;308:559–565.
111. Murphy SB, Bowman WP, Hustu HO, et al. Advanced stage (III-IV) Burkitt's lymphoma and B-cell acute lymphoblastic leukemia in children: Kinetics and pharmacology rationale for treatment and recent results (1979–1983). IARC Sci Pub 1985;60:405–418.
112. Mauch PM, Weinstein H, Botnick L, et al. An evaluation of long-term survival and treatment complications in children with Hodgkin's disease. Cancer 1983;51:925–932.
113. Cramer P, Andrien JM. Hodgkin's disease in children and adolescence: Results of chemotherapy–radiotherapy in clinical stages IA–IIB. J Clin Oncol 1985;3:1495–1502.
114. Bonadonna G, Santore A. ABVD in the treatment of Hodgkin's disease. Cancer Treat Rev 1983;9:21–35.
115. Lange B, Littman P. Management of Hodgkin's disease in children and adolescents. Cancer 1983;51:1371–1377.
116. Jenkin D, Chan H, Freedman M, et al. Hodgkin's disease in children: Treatment results with MOPP and low-dose, extended-field irradiation. Cancer Treat Rep 1982;66:949–959.
117. Rowland JH, Glidewell OJ, Sibley RF, et al. Effects of different forms of central nervous system prophylaxis on neuropsychologic function in childhood leukemia. J Clin Oncol 1984;2:1327–1335.
118. Moss HA, Nannis ED, Poplack DG. The effects of prophylactic treatment of the central nervous system on the intellectual functioning of children with acute lymphocytic leukemia. Am J Med 1981;71:47–52.
119. Abelson HT. Methotrexate and central nervous system toxicity. Cancer Treat Rep 1978;62:1999–2001.
120. Bleyer WA. Neurologic sequelae of methotrexate and ionizing radiation: A new classification. Cancer Treat Rep 1981;65:89–98.
121. Meadows AT, Gordon J, Massari DJ, et al. Decline in IQ scores and cognitive dysfunctions in children with acute lymphocytic leukemia treated with cranial irradiation. Lancet 1981;2:1015–1018.

122. Oliff A, Bode U, Beran B, et al. Hypothalamic–pituitary dysfunction following CNS prophylaxis in acute lymphocytic leukemia: Correlation with CT scan abnormalities. Med Pediatr Oncol 1979;7:141–151.
123. Tefft M, Radiation effect on growing bone and cartilage. Frontiers Rad Ther Oncol 1972;6:289–311.
124. Shalet SM, Beardwell CG, Twomey JA, et al. Endocrine function following the treatment of acute leukemia in childhood. J Pediatr 1977;90:920–923.
125. Siris ES, Leventhal BG, Vaitukaitis JL, Effects of childhood leukemia and chemotherapy on puberty and reproductive function in girls. N Engl J Med 1976;294:1143–1146.

# Chapter 99 / Prostate Cancer

Barry R. Goldspiel, PharmD, and John G. Kuhn, PharmD, FCCP

Cancer of the prostate gland is the second most frequent cancer among American males and represents the third leading cause of cancer-related deaths in elderly males.[1] In the United States alone, it was estimated that 90,000 new cases of prostatic carcinoma would be diagnosed and more than 30,000 males would die from this disease in 1986.[1] The endocrine dependence of this tumor is well documented and hormonal manipulation to decrease circulating androgens remains the basis of the treatment for advanced disease.

## Epidemiology/Etiology

The occurrence of prostate cancer is influenced by both age and race.[2] The disease is infrequent under the age of 50, but the incidence sharply increases with each subsequent decade.[2] The mean age at presentation is 70 years. Geographically, prostate cancer is relatively uncommon in the Far East and common in the Scandinavian countries (Fig. 99.1). Black Americans have one of the highest incidence rates worldwide.[3] Although there appears to be a 10% survival rate difference between whites and blacks, the current national figures indicate an improved 5-year survival for both groups (Table 99.1).

The etiology of prostatic carcinoma is unknown. Several causative factors have been implicated; however, these remain speculative at present. Table 99.2 summarizes the possible factors associated with development of prostate cancer.[4] Hormonal influence appears to have the strongest etiological association. The precise relationship between prostatic hyperplasia and development of prostate cancer is unclear, although some evidence suggests a three-fold higher incidence rate. Smoking has not been associated with prostate cancer.

## Pathophysiology

The prostate gland is a solid, rounded, heart-shaped organ positioned between the neck of the bladder and the urogenital diaphragm (Fig. 99.2). The organ consists of single anterior, posterior, and median lobes with two lateral lobes. The posterior lobe is palpable by anterior rectal exam at 2 to 5 cm from the anal verge. Within the four morphologically defined areas of the prostate gland, 95% of the carcinomas arise from the glandular epithelium of the peripheral zone.[5] In contrast, benign prostatic hyperplasia arises from the central or periurethral regions of the prostate gland.

Normal growth and differentiation of the prostate depend on the presence of androgens, specifically dihydrotestosterone.[6,7] The testes and the adrenal glands are the major sources of circulating androgens. Hormonal regulation of androgen synthesis is mediated through a series of biochemical interactions among the hypothalamus, pituitary, adrenal glands, and testes (Fig. 99.3). Luteinizing hormone–releasing hormone (LH-RH) released from the hypothalamus stimulates the release of luteinizing hormone (LH) and follicle-stimulating hormone (FSH) from the anterior pituitary gland. Luteinizing hormone complexes with receptors on the Leydig cell testicular membrane and stimulates the production of testosterone and small amounts of estrogen. FSH acts on the Sertoli cell within the testis to promote the maturation of LH receptors and to produce an androgen-binding protein. Circulating testosterone and estradiol influence the synthesis of LH-RH, LH, and FSH by a negative-feedback loop operating at the hypothalamic and pituitary levels.[6–8] Prolactin, growth hormone, and estradiol appear to be important accessory regulators for prostatic tissue permeability, receptor binding, and testosterone synthesis; however, a precise relationship between these hormones and prostate growth has not been defined.[6–8]

Testosterone, the major androgenic hormone, accounts for 95% of the androgen concentration. The primary source of testosterone is the testes; however, 3% to 5% of the testosterone concentration is derived from direct adrenal cortical secretion of testosterone or $C_{19}$ steroids.[9] Androstenedione, a $C_{19}$ steroid, can be converted to testosterone in peripheral tissues.

Only 2% of total plasma testosterone is present in the physiologically active unbound state. The remaining testosterone is reversibly bound to a steroid hormone–binding globulin. The unbound testosterone or androgen precursors penetrate the prostatic cell by passive diffusion where conversion to dihydrotestosterone by 5$\alpha$-reductase occurs.[9,10] Dihydrotestosterone subsequently binds with a specific cytoplasmic receptor. This dihydrotestosterone–receptor complex is then transported to the nucleus of the cell, where transcription and ultimately translation of stored genetic material occurs.[9,10]

## Pathology

The normal prostate is composed of acinar secretory cells arranged radially and surrounded by a foundation of supporting tissue. The size, shape, or presence of acini is almost always altered in the gland that has been invaded by prostatic carcinoma. Adenocarcinoma, the major pathologic cell type, accounts for more than 95% of prostate cancer cases.[2,11] Rare tumor types include sarcomas and transitional cell carcinomas.

Prostate cancer can be systematically graded according to

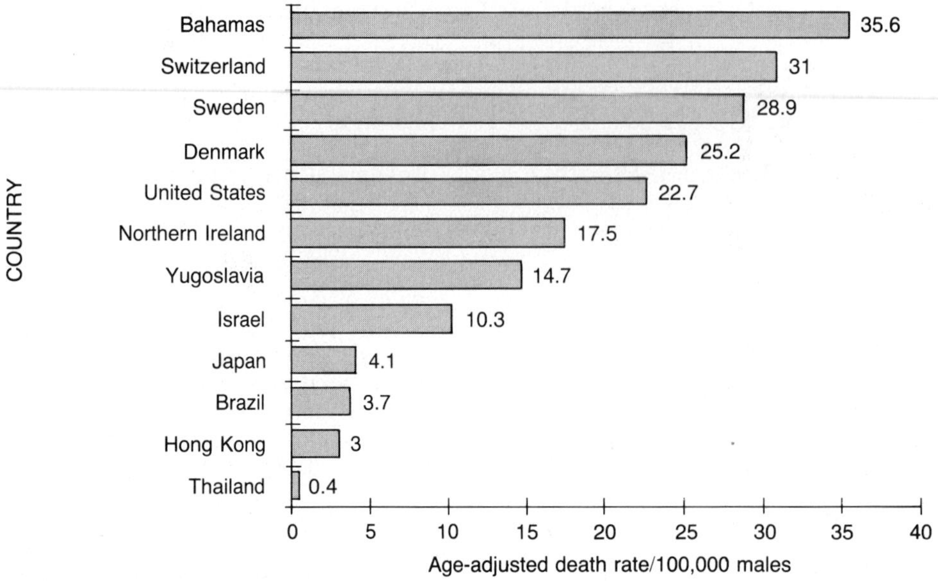


**Figure 99.1** Regional variations in prostate cancer, 1980–1981. *(From Silverberg E, Lubera J: Cancer statistics: 1986. CA 1986;36:21, with permission.)*

the histologic appearance of the malignant cell and then grouped into highly, moderately, or poorly differentiated grades.[12] Depending on the grade of the malignancy, prostatic carcinoma has a marked variability in biologic behavior.[2,12]

Metastatic spread can occur by local extension, lymphatic drainage, or hematogenous dissemination.[11] Lymph node metastases are more common in patients with large, undifferentiated tumors that invade the seminal vesicles. The pelvic and abdominal lymph node groups are the most common sites of lymph node involvement (Fig. 99.2). Skeletal metastases from hematogenous spread represent the most common site of distant spread. Typically, the bone lesions are osteoblastic or a combination of osteoblastic and osteolytic. The most common site of bone involvement is the lumbar spine. Other sites of bone involvement include the proximal femurs, pelvis, thoracic spine, ribs, sternum, skull, and humerus. The lung, liver, brain, and adrenal glands are the most common site of visceral involvement; however, these organs are not usually involved initially. Twenty-five to thirty-five percent of patients have evidence of lymphangitic or nodular pulmonary infiltrates at autopsy. The prostate is a rare site for metastatic involvement from other solid tumors.

**Table 99.1** Prostate Cancer: 5-Year Survival Rates

| *Period* | % Survival: **Blacks** | **Whites** |
|---|---|---|
| 1960–1963 | 35 | 50 |
| 1970–1973 | 55 | 63 |
| 1973–1976 | 57 | 67 |
| 1977–1982 | 62 | 72 |

From Silverberg E, Lubera J: Cancer statistics: 1986. CA 1986;36:25, with permission.

## Clinical Presentation

Although prostatic carcinoma may be asymptomatic in patients with localized disease, most patients with signs and symptoms have advanced disease at presentation.[2,13] In patients with locally invasive disease, the most common complaints arise from ureteral dysfunction or impingement. Patients complain of alterations in micturation manifested by urinary frequency, hesitancy, and dribbling.[2,11] Most commonly, patients with advanced disease present with back pain and stiffness caused by osseous metastases. Eventually,

**Table 99.2** Etiologic Factors Associated with Prostate Cancer

| *Factor* | *Possible relationship* |
|---|---|
| Environmental | Regional variations in incidence worldwide for both clinical and latent carcinoma |
| | Nationalized males adopt incidence rates intermediate to those of United States and their native country |
| Occupational | Increased risk associated with cadmium exposure |
| Genetic | Case reports of familial association |
| Diet | Increased risk associated with high-meat and -fat diets |
| Venereal | Higher frequency associated with prior venereal disease |
| Hormonal | Does not occur in eunuchs |
| | Up to 80% are hormonally dependent |

From Flanders WD: Review: Prostate cancer epidemiology. Prostate 1984; 5:621–629, with permission.

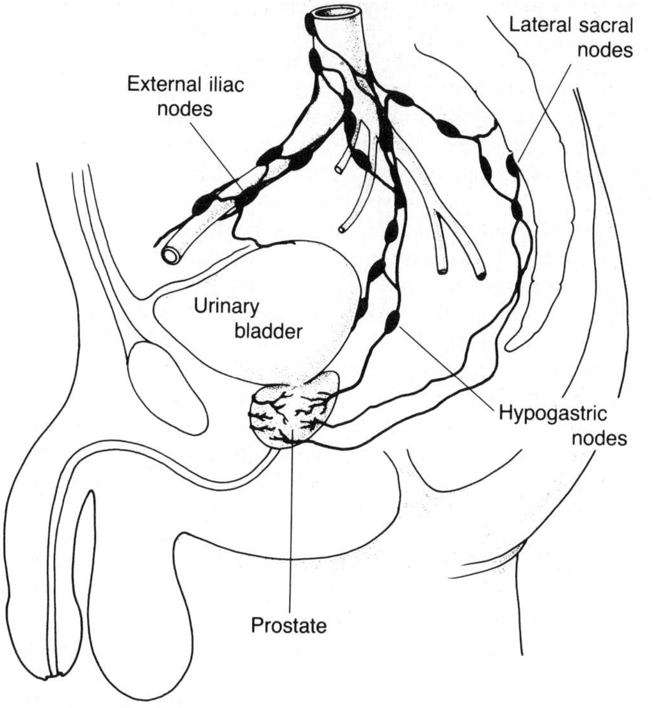


**Figure 99.2** The prostate gland. *(From Spirnak JP, Kesnick MI: Urol Clin N Am 1984;11:224, with permission.)*

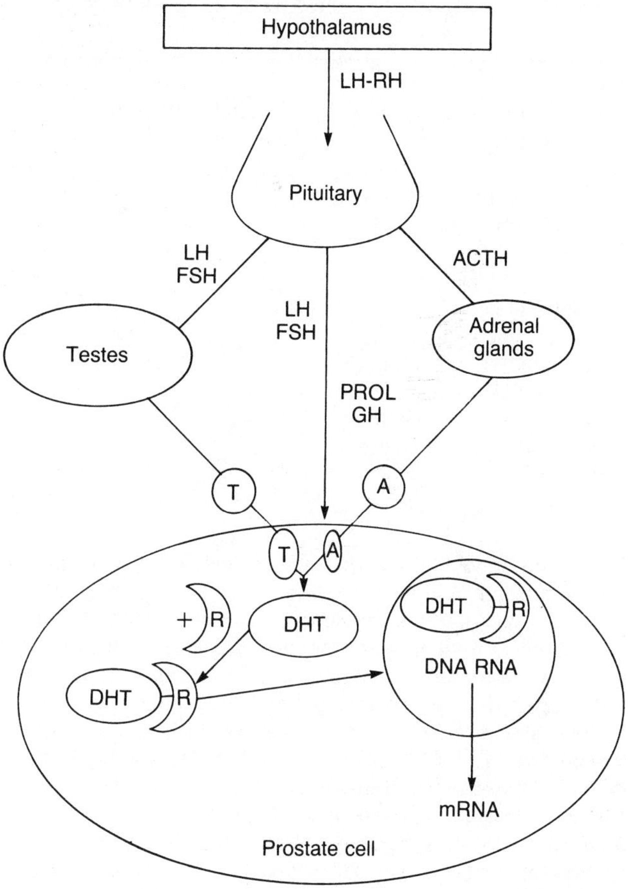


**Figure 99.3** Hormonal regulation of the prostate gland. LH-RH, luteinizing hormone–releasing hormone; LH, luteinizing hormone; FSH, follicle-stimulating hormone; PROL prolactin; ACTH, adrenocorticotropic hormone; GH, growth hormone; A, androgens; T, testosterone; R, receptor; DHT, dihydrotestosterone.

spinal cord lesions may lead to cord compression if not properly treated. Rarely, pathologic fractures can occur. Lower extremity edema can occur as a result of lymphatic obstruction. Anemia and weight loss are nonspecific signs of advanced disease.

Laboratory abnormalities include an elevated serum acid phosphatase in greater than 60% of patients with metastatic spread. Alkaline phosphatase is elevated in patients with bone metastases.

## Diagnosis/Staging

The diagnostic workup should include a thorough history and physical examination. Physical examination should include careful digital inspection of the rectum and palpation of regional lymph nodes, abdomen, and spine. The lower extremities should be tested for strength and reflex symmetry. Initial laboratory tests should include a complete blood chemistry, liver function tests, serum creatinine, serum acid and alkaline phosphatase, and urinalysis.

Digital rectal palpation is the fundamental method for both screening and recognition of prostatic disease.[11] The posterior lobe of the prostate is palpated for size, configuration, and consistency. Classically, prostatic carcinoma is characterized by a rock-hard nodule or mass in the gland. This contrasts the findings in benign prostatic hypertrophy, where the gland is smooth and rubbery. Approximately, 50% of prostate nodules found on rectal exam are confirmed to be malignant.[2,11] When considered as a screening mechanism for prostate cancer, the digital rectal exam has the highest overall efficiency.[11,14,15] The American Cancer Society recommends that males over the age of 50 receive a rectal examination concurrently with their annual physical examination.

Although rectal examination remains the best method for detecting prostate cancer, the actual diagnosis and histologic grading can be established only by biopsy. The transperianal or transrectal routes for needle biopsy are the most common approaches. Fine-needle aspiration of the prostate gland to determine cytology is gaining popularity as a diagnostic procedure. This relatively simple procedure can be performed in an outpatient setting without anesthesia. In the hands of an experienced cytologist, the results from fine-needle aspiration compare favorably with those from needle biopsy.

Table 99.3 outlines the recommended procedures for clinical staging of prostate cancer. Prostatic acid phosphatase, measured by radioimmunoassay or enzymatic methods, is not a useful biologic marker for routine screening because of its low sensitivity and high false-positive rate.[11,15] Traditionally, serum acid phosphatase levels have been used for staging. There is high correlation between an elevated serum acid phosphatase and the probability of disease extending beyond the prostate gland; however,

**Table 99.3** Diagnostic and Staging Workup for Prostate Cancer

| | |
|---|---|
| Routine tests | |
| | Physical examination with digital rectal palpation |
| | Excretory urogram |
| | Chest x-ray |
| | Serum phosphatases (acid/alkaline) |
| | Liver function tests |
| | Bone scan |
| Additional tests for staging | |
| | Skeletal films |
| | Lymph node evaluation |
| | Bipedal lymphangiogram |
| | Pelvic CAT scan |
| | Pelvic lymphadenectomy |
| | Transrectal ultrasonography |

because up to 40% of patients with metastatic disease may have a normal acid phosphatase, its value in staging is limited. A major clinical use for acid phosphatase is in measurement of treatment response. Patients with an elevated acid phosphatase that does not decline after treatment or that rises after an initial response have a poor prognosis. Acid phosphatase measurements can be falsely elevated in patients within 24 to 48 hours of rectal examination, prostatic resection, or urethral instrumentation.

Alkaline phosphatase is frequently increased in prostate cancer because of the metabolic activity of the bone surrounding the bone metastases.[11] The source of an elevated alkaline phosphatase can be determined by the reaction of the sample to heat. Alkaline phosphatase derived from bone is heat labile, whereas the fraction derived from liver is heat stable.

The bone scan is more sensitive than a skeletal survey in detecting early metastatic disease.[11,15] Thirty to fifty percent of bone must be replaced by tumor before it can be detected by routine radiologic procedures. Up to 50% of patients with a positive bone scan can have a normal skeletal radiograph.[11,15] The bone scan is highly sensitive, but also detects other bone abnormalities. Because of its low specificity, the bone scan should be reviewed along with skeletal films or tomograms directed at the radioisotope positive areas.[11,15]

Several techniques are used to evaluate lymph node involvement.[11,13,15] Bipedal lymphangiography determines the extent of periaortic and pelvic node involvement. This technique is associated with a false-negative rate of 40% to 50% because all places of metastatic involvement are not opacified by the contrast medium.

Pelvic computerized tomography scanning is useful in determining the local extension of the tumor and the appearance of the seminal vesicles.[11] This scan fails to discriminate lesions within the lymph nodes unless the lymph nodes are greater than 2 cm in diameter.

Pelvic lymph node dissection is used in conjunction with definitive radiation therapy or as a staging procedure prior to radical prostatectomy. Pelvic lymph node dissection is associated with a high morbidity and this procedure is reserved for patients in whom the information obtained will directly affect treatment decisions.[15,16]

Prostatic carcinoma produces a specific hypoechogenic pattern by ultrasound imaging.[17] Sagittal and axial imaging by transrectal ultrasound is able to identify the prostatic capsule, seminal vesicles, and intraprostatic extent of disease. This provides both a method for determining the precise local extent of disease and a parameter to follow for treatment outcome.[17] Recent evidence suggests that prostatic ultrasound may become a primary screening and diagnostic test. The value of magnetic imaging techniques as a means of diagnosis and staging of prostate cancer is currently under investigation in a number of institutions.

The information obtained from the diagnostic tests is applied to the staging procedure. There are two commonly recognized staging classification systems (Table 99.4). The formal international classification system (TNM) adopted by the International Union Against Cancer in 1974 is not routinely used to stage prostate cancer in the United States; however, this system is used in clinical trials to further delineate the various prognostic groups on the basis of precise disease involvement. The most commonly used staging system in the United States assigns patients to stages A through D according to size of the tumor, local or regional extension, presence of involved lymph node groups, and presence of metastases.[11,16] An additional subclassification system has been proposed that further divides each of the major stages into subcategories.[2,16] Stage A patients constitute 5% to 10% of the cases and stage B patients account for 10% to 15% of cases. Stages C and D account for the majority of patients with prostate cancer. Each of these latter stages represents 40% of the cases of newly diagnosed prostatic carcinoma.[2]

## Prognosis

The prognosis for patients with prostate cancer depends on histologic grade, tumor size, and local extent of the primary tumor.[2,11] The most important prognostic criterion appears to be histologic grade, as the degree of differentiation ultimately determines the stage of disease. Poorly differentiated tumors are highly associated with both regional lymph node involvement and distant metastases.[11,15] For stages B and C, poorly differentiated tumors are associated with a 5-year survival of approximately 40% and highly differentiated tumors carry an 80% 5-year survival rate.[18] With treatment, the 5-year survival rates for patients with stages A, B, C, and D are 77%, 65%, 48%, and 21%.[11,18]

## Treatment

The treatment for prostate cancer depends on the stage of the disease (Table 99.5). Patients with incidental carcinoma found at the time of a transurethral resection for benign prostatic hypertrophy (stage $A_1$) require only careful observation because of slow progression of the disease to more advanced stages.[2,15] The 10-year mortality rate for these patients is less than 1%.[11] The treatment of patients with stage $A_2$, B, or C disease remains controversial. In select patients, surgical extirpation by radical prostatectomy with staging pelvic lymphadenectomy can be performed [2,11];

**Table 99.4** Staging and Classification Systems for Prostate Cancer

| *AUS[a] stage (A–D)* | *AJC—UICC[b] classification (TNM)* |
|---|---|
| A (occult, nonpalpable) | $T_0N_0M_0$ (Nonpalpable) |
| $A_1$ Focal | $T_0$ Focal or diffuse |
| $A_2$ Diffuse | $T_1N_0M_0$; $T_2N_0M_0$ |
| B (confined to prostate) | $T_1$ Intracapsular, surrounded by normal gland |
| $B_1$ Single nodule in one lobe, <1.5 cm | $T_2$ Intraglandular, contour deformed |
| $B_2$ Diffuse involvement of whole gland, >1.5 cm | $T_3N_0M_0$; $T_4N_0M_0$ |
| C (localized to periprostatic area) | $T_3$ Tumor beyond capsule, with or without seminal vesicle or lateral sulcus involvement, or both |
| $C_1$ No seminal vesicle involvement, <70 g | $T_4$ Tumor fixed or invading adjacent structures |
| $C_2$ Seminal vesicle involvement, >70 g | Any T, $N_1$–$N_4$, $M_0$; any T, $N_0$–$N_4$, $M_1$ |
| D (metastatic disease) | $N_1$–$N_3$ Regional lymph nodes |
| $D_1$ Pelvic lymph nodes or ureteral obstruction | $N_4$ Juxtaregional lymph node |
| $D_2$ Bone, distant lymph node, organ, or soft tissue metastases | $M_1$ Distant metastases |

[a] American Urologic System.
[b] American Joint Committee—International Union Against Cancer.

From Jones GW: Diagnosis and management of prostate cancer. Cancer 1983;51:2458, with permission.

however, this procedure is associated with complications that include stricture formation, incontinence, and impotence. Impotence can occur in as many as 90% of patients. This high complication rate has prompted an increased interest in the use of radiation therapy for these patients. Both external beam radiation and radioactive interstitial implants of iodine-125 or gold-198 have produced response rates equivalent to those for surgery.[2] Complications from radiation therapy include cystitis, proctitis, and impotence. In contrast to surgery, impotence occurs only in 30% of patients treated with radiation therapy for locally advanced prostate cancer. Local radiation therapy is commonly used to palliate painful skeletal metastases in patients who have relapsed after endocrine therapy. The major treatment modality for advanced prostate cancer (stage D) is pharmacotherapy in the form of hormonal manipulation or cytotoxic chemotherapy.[19–26]

**Table 99.5** Treatment of Prostate Cancer by Stage of Disease

| *Stage* | *Treatment* |
|---|---|
| $A_1$ | Observation |
| $A_2$, B | Radical prostatectomy[a] |
| | Interstitial irradiation[a] |
| $A_2$, B, C | External beam irradiation |
| D | Pharmacotherapy |
| | Hormonal manipulation |
| | Combination hormonal therapy |
| | Cytotoxic chemotherapy |
| | Combination hormonal therapy/chemotherapy |

[a] For select patients only.

## *Pharmacotherapy of Advanced Prostate Cancer*

### Hormonal Manipulation

The observation by Huggins and Hodges that both normal tissue and malignant prostatic tissue contain a high level of acid phosphatase suggests that prostatic malignancy represents an overgrowth of prostate tissue.[27] Both Huggins and Hodges[27] and Nesbit and Baum[28] demonstrated that a decrease in serum acid phosphatase along with symptomatic relief occurred in patients with metastatic prostate cancer treated with either estrogens or orchiectomy, therapy known to reduce circulating androgens. The use of hormonal manipulation in the treatment of advanced prostate cancer is based on the observation that prostatic epithelium undergoes atrophy when the normal physiologic effect of androgens is reduced[6,7]. Therefore, the purpose of hormonal manipulation in both the treatment and palliation of advanced prostate cancer is ablation of androgenic stimuli.[6,22,24]

Several hormonal manipulations ablate or reduce circulating androgens (Table 99.6). Surgical ablation of androgen sources is achieved by removal of the organs responsible for androgen production. Hormonal pathways that modulate prostatic growth can be interrupted at several steps (Fig. 99.3). Interference with LH-RH or LH reduces testosterone secretion by the testes. Androgen synthesis can be inhibited at the level of the testes or the adrenal gland. Finally, direct interference at the target tissue level by antiandrogens offers another treatment alternative.

***Ablation of Androgen Sources*** Bilateral orchiectomy, adrenalectomy, and hypophysectomy can reduce circulating androgens. Removing the major androgen source by orchiectomy is still the preferred ablative procedure[2,11,19]. Unfortunately, many patients are not surgical candidates because of advanced age, and other patients find this procedure psychologically unacceptable[23,24]. The subcapsular orchiectomy approach promptly produces castration levels of

**Table 99.6** Hormonal Manipulations in Advanced Prostate Cancer

| |
|---|
| Ablation of androgen sources |
| Orchiectomy |
| Adrenalectomy |
| Hypophysectomy |
| Inhibition of LH-RH or LH |
| Estrogens |
| LH-RH agonists |
| Progestogens[a] |
| Cyproterone acetate[a] |
| Inhibition of androgen synthesis |
| Aminoglutethimide |
| Ketoconazole |
| Progestogens[a] |
| Antiandrogens |
| Progestogens |
| Cyproterone acetate |
| Flutamide |

[a] Minor mechanisms of action.

testosterone (<50 ng/dL), yet preserves the outer integrity of the testicles. Adrenalectomy and hypophysectomy remove extratesticular sources of androgens; however, these androgens account for less than 5% of the circulating androgen concentration. Therefore, these procedures should be used only after testicular-derived androgens are diminished. Presently, adrenalectomy and hypophysectomy are reserved for patients refractory to either estrogen therapy or orchiectomy. These surgical procedures are associated with high mortality rates and since suitable pharmacologic alternatives are available, they are not commonly performed today.

***Inhibition of LH-RH or LH*** Several pharmacologic agents suppress the release of LH from the pituitary gland, resulting in reduced testosterone production.[8,21,22] These agents include estrogens, LH-RH agonists, progestogens, and cyproterone acetate.

Estrogen administration causes androgen ablation by either direct inhibition of LH release, interference with hormone synthesis, or direct action on the prostate cell. Further information suggests that estrogens increase the steroid-binding globulin level, thereby reducing the amount of free circulating androgens.[11] The onset of response is usually 1 to 2 weeks after initiation of therapy. Several Veterans Administration Cooperative Urological Research Group (VACURG) trials have assessed the role of estrogen therapy in the treatment of advanced prostate cancer.[29,30] In one trial, patients were randomized to receive either diethylstilbestrol (DES) 5 mg per day, orchiectomy, both treatments simultaneously, or placebo.[29] Fewer deaths from cancer were observed in patients treated with estrogens, but there was an increased incidence of death from cardiovascular complications. The excess mortality from cardiovascular-related deaths offset any therapeutic advantage of estrogen administration. The cardiovascular deaths were more common in patients older than 75 and those with a prior history of cardiovascular disease.

In a second VACURG trial,[30] DES doses of 5, 1, and 0.2 mg daily were compared with placebo. Compared with the 0.2-mg dose or placebo, both the 1- and 5-mg doses reduced cancer-related deaths. The 5-mg dose was superior to the 1-mg dose in suppressing acid phosphatase and testosterone levels. Nevertheless, the clinical responses observed with either of these doses were similar, suggesting that the lower estrogen dose (1 mg) maintains antitumor activity. Again, cardiovascular-related deaths occurred more frequently in patients treated with DES 5 mg per day. The incidence of cardiovascular-related deaths in the group given DES 1 mg was not different from that in the placebo-treated group. Other complications from DES therapy include fluid retention, nausea, vomiting, impotence, and painful gynecomastia. Gynecomastia can be attenuated with bilateral breast irradiation if instituted prior to estrogen therapy.

The results of the VACURG trials demonstrated that estrogen therapy should be withheld from a patient with advanced prostate cancer until he becomes symptomatic from the disease. Several investigators argue that treatment should be initiated early in the course of the disease when the suspected tumor burden is low.[26] Estrogen therapy provides symptomatic relief in 60% to 80% of previously untreated patients.[22,24] The response is manifested by decreased bone pain and relief of urinary symptoms. The usual duration of response is 1 to 2 years and almost all patients progress and present with bone pain as a result of metastatic disease.[23,26] DES 3 mg per day in three divided doses is the current recommended dose because castration levels of testosterone are uniformly produced; however, the relative incidence of cardiovascular complications from 3 mg compared with 1 or 5 mg has not been assessed in clinical trials.

Ethinyl estradiol, conjugated estrogens, chlorotrianisene, and polyestradiol phosphate have been used as alternatives to DES.[24,26] In general, no therapeutic advantage over DES can be expected with any of the alternate estrogen products, and all of the these products are considerably more expensive than DES. These estrogenic substances can be used, however, if patients cannot tolerate DES administration.

Isolation of the naturally occurring hypothalamic decapeptide hormones, gonadotropin hormone–releasing hormone and LH-RH, has provided a new class of effective agents for the treatment of advanced prostate cancer.[8,31] The physiological response to LH-RH depends not only on the dose, but also the mode of administration. Intermittent pulsed LH-RH administration, which mimics the endogenous release pattern, causes sustained release of both LH and FSH[31]; however, high-dose or continuous intravenous administration of LH-RH inhibits gonadotropin release because of a decrease in both the number and the sensitivity of pituitary receptors, a physiological process termed downregulation.[8,31,32] Structural modification of the naturally occurring LH-RH at the sixth and tenth positions has produced a series of LH-RH agonist analogues that possess supraphysiologic potency and longer plasma half-lives.[8,31] The longer duration of action provided by these analogues causes a similar downregulation of pituitary receptors and a decrease in testosterone production. Leuprolide is the first LH-RH agonist analogue approved by the FDA for the treatment of advanced prostate cancer.

In the first multicenter leuprolide trial, 94 evaluable patients with stage $D_2$ prostate cancer received either 1 or 10 mg of leuprolide as a daily subcutaneous injection.[33] Initially, leuprolide stimulates both LH and FSH release within 4 hours of the first dose; however, with continued administration, serum levels of LH and FSH decline significantly within 14 days. Serum testosterone concentration falls to castration levels within 4 weeks. During the first week of treatment, 10% of patients reported a "flare-up" in their disease manifested by increased bone pain. This drug-induced disease flare corresponds to the initial increase in both LH and FHS and resolves by the second week of continued therapy. While no patient has required modification of treatment for this exacerbation, care should be taken in initiating leuprolide therapy in patients with widely metastatic disease involving the spinal cord.

The clinical responses reported in this trial were similar to those seen with estrogen administration. Of the 47 previously untreated patients, 76% responded favorably, with 36% experiencing a complete or partial response and an additional 40% remaining with stable disease. Of the 47 patients who had prior endocrine therapy, only 48% of patients previously treated with estrogen and 23% of patients who had had an orchiectomy responded favorably to leuprolide. There was no difference in response or toxicity between patients treated with 1 and 10 mg of leuprolide. The current recommended dose is 1 mg given subcutaneously daily.

The adverse effects noted in this trial include the initial disease "flare-up" and hot flashes reported in 61% of patients. Sexual dysfunction manifested by erectile impotence and decreased libido occurred in most patients who had been sexually active prior to study entry. Several patients experienced minor irritation at the injection site.

In a multicenter randomized trial of untreated patients with stage $D_2$ prostate cancer, leuprolide 1 mg subcutaneously daily was compared with DES 3 mg daily.[34] Responses evaluated according to National Prostatic Cancer Project (NPCP) criteria were similar for both groups. Of 92 evaluable patients in the leuprolide group, the total response rate was 86%, with 38% of patients experiencing a complete or partial response. In the DES-treated group, 85% of 94 evaluable patients responded favorably, with 46% obtaining a complete or partial response. Neither the median time to disease progression nor the median survial time was significantly different between the two groups.

Substantial differences in drug-related toxicity were demonstrated in this trial. Patients assigned to the leuprolide group had a significantly higher incidence of hot flashes, and 7% experienced a transient exacerbation of their disease during the first week of therapy. Patients in the DES group had a higher incidence of gynecomastia and breast tenderness despite pretreatment breast irradiation in 50% of patients. Cardiovascular complications, which included peripheral edema, thrombosis, phlebitis, and pulmonary embolus, were more common in estrogen-treated patients. These findings suggest that leuprolide is a suitable alternative to estrogen administration. Similar response rates can be expected with a lower incidence of cardiovascular-related adverse effects. A limitation to leuprolide use is a cost of greater than $300 per month compared with only a few dollars for DES therapy. This relatively high cost may be offset by the lower incidence of serious adverse effects associated with leuprolide treatment.

Several other LH-RH analogues (Buserelin, Naferelin, ICI-118630, AY-25650), currently under clinical investigation, differ with respect to route of administration and duration of action.[8,31] Several LH-RH congeners are being tested that can be administered intranasally or that provide a sustained duration of action because of their depot nature. If these agents become available, they may provide attractive alternatives to leuprolide therapy.

Both megestrol acetate, a progestational agent, and cyproterone acetate, a progestagenic antiandrogen, inhibit the release of LH from the pituitary in addition to their antiandrogen action at the target tissue level.[9,22]

***Inhibition of Androgen Synthesis*** Several compounds interfere with the synthesis of androgens by the testes or adrenal gland. These agents include aminoglutethimide, ketoconazole, and the progestational agents.

As the majority of patients with advanced prostate cancer progress after initial hormonal therapy, surgical adrenalectomy has been used to reduce extratesticular sources of androgens. Response rates observed with surgical adrenalectomy range from 20% to 40%[26]; however, the operative morbidity and mortality with this procedure are high. Medical adrenalectomy using aminoglutethimide is now the preferred alternative to surgery.

Aminoglutethimide inhibits the desmolase enzyme complex in the adrenal gland, thereby preventing the conversion of cholesterol to pregnenolone. Pregnenolone is the precursor substrate for all adrenal-derived steroids, including androgens, glucocorticoids, and mineralocorticoids.[21,23] Concurrent glucocorticoid administration is necessary to prevent negative-feedback increases in ACTH production that could competitively overcome the adrenal blockade. Mineralocorticoid replacement may be necessary in select patients.

In clinical trials, aminoglutethimide can delay disease progression and produce symptomatic relief for a short time in up to 50% of patients with progressive disease despite previous estrogen administration or orchiectomy.[35–37] If the patient is currently taking an estrogen, it is continued so as to suppress the testicular source of androgen production. Because of central nervous system–related adverse effects, therapy is usually initiated with aminoglutethimide 250 mg orally twice daily and increased gradually to 250 mg orally three or four times daily depending on patient tolerance. Supplementation with physiologic doses of hydrocortisone or cortisone acetate is begun concomitantly. Dexamethasone should be avoided because of the variability in dexamethasone metabolism induced by aminoglutethimide.[38] Care should be taken in patients already on oral anticoagulants, as aminoglutethimide increases the rate of warfarin clearance. The duration of therapy should be at least 4 to 6 weeks to properly assess the efficacy of aminoglutethimide.

Adverse effects during aminoglutethimide therapy occur in approximately 50% of patients.[35–37] Central nervous system effects, which include lethargy, ataxia, and dizziness, are the major adverse reactions. A generalized morbilliform pruritic rash has been reported in up to 30% of patients treated. The rash is usually self-limiting and resolves within 5 to 8 days with continued therapy.

Ketoconazole, an imidazole antifungal agent, has been used in the treatment of advanced prostate cancer based on the observation that this drug produces gynecomastia in select individuals. Subsequent investigations have determined that ketoconazole administration results in a dose-related, reversible reduction in serum cortisol and testosterone concentrations[39,40] At high doses, ketoconazole blunts the response to exogenous ACTH administration and suppresses secretion of testosterone, suggesting that this agent may interfere with both adrenal and testicular steroidogenesis.[40] At doses of 400 to 600 mg, ketoconazole causes a significant reduction in testosterone and cortisol concentrations that persists 8 to 12 hours after the dose.[39,41] In contrast, 200 mg of ketoconazole produces only a modest reduction of androgens. Levels of both cortisol and testosterone return to normal within 4 to 16 hours of a 200-mg dose, suggesting that clinical hypoadrenalism should not occur with conventional doses of ketoconazole, but may occur with increased doses.

In several uncontrolled nonrandomized trials, ketoconazole 400 mg given orally every 8 hours produced symptomatic relief in 20 previously untreated patients with stage D prostate cancer.[41–43] Responses were manifested by a rapid diminution of pain and discontinuation of narcotic analgesics, decrease in prostatic acid phosphatase, and decrease in prostate size. The rapidity of response appears to be the major therapeutic advantage and is similar to that seen after orchiectomy. Adverse effects included gastrointestinal intolerance and transient increases in liver and renal function tests. Two elderly patients (83 and 84 years old) reported weakness and lethargy and developed skin pigmentation suggestive of hypocortisolism. Supplementation with prednisone was necessary despite reductions in the ketoconazole dose.

Secondary to its antiandrogen action, megestrol acetate inhibits the synthesis of androgens. This inhibition appears to occur at the adrenal level, but circulating levels of testosterone are also reduced, suggesting that inhibition may also occur at the testicular level.[9,24]

***Antiandrogens*** Antiandrogens inhibit the formation of the dihydrotestosterone–receptor complex and thereby interfere with androgen-mediated action at the cellular level. Currently, megestrol acetate is the only commercially available agent with antiandrogen actions. Cyproterone acetate and flutamide are both under clinical investigation.

Megestrol acetate, a progestational antiandrogen, blocks both androgen production and androgen action at doses of 120 to 160 mg orally per day.[9,44] The possible mechanisms of action for megestrol include weak competition with dihydrotestosterone, inhibition of nuclear and cytosol androgen receptor formation, and moderate inhibition of 5$\alpha$-reductase.[9] At doses of 80 mg per day, megestrol can maintain castration levels of testosterone up to 5 months.[9]

As a single agent, megestrol 120 mg orally per day produced subjective responses in 85% of 25 patients.[44] The duration of response was 10 months and more than 60% of initial responders progressed despite continued megestrol therapy. Of those patients who relapsed, all responded to subsequent orchiectomy, suggesting that androgen deprivation equivalent to either DES or orchiectomy cannot be achieved with megestrol alone at these doses.

Two other antiandrogens, cyproterone acetate and flutamide, act primarily by inhibiting the formation of the dihydrotestosterone–receptor complex.[21,23,26,45,46] While cyproterone, a synthetic $C_{21}$ steroid, decreases testosterone production,[21,26] flutamide, a nonsteroidal analide, either maintains or causes an increase in testosterone secretion.[45,46]

In a study of 72 previously untreated patients with advanced prostate cancer, flutamide 250 mg orally three times a day produced a favorable response in 88% of patients.[45] Response was manifested by improvement in bone pain, decrease in prostate size, or improvement in performance status. Adverse effects were minimal. Gynecomastia was the major adverse reaction and occurred in 72% of patients. Of 37 patients who claimed sexual potency prior to study entry, 32 patients (86%) were able to maintain potency during treatment.

Preliminary results with cyproterone also demonstrate an 80% response rate for previously untreated patients[26]; however, less than 40% of patients respond to either cyproterone or flutamide if they have relapsed after previous treatment with estrogens.[21,26] Gynecomastia is the main adverse effect associated with cyproterone.

**Combination Hormonal Therapy**

Although up to 80% of patients with advanced prostate cancer respond to initial hormonal manipulation, almost all patients relapse within 2 years of initiation of therapy. Two mechanisms have been proposed to explain this tumor resistance.[9,26] The tumor may be heterogeneously composed of cells that are hormone dependent and hormone independent, or the tumor may be stimulated by extratesticular androgens that are converted intracellularly to dihydrotestosterone. The rationale for combination hormonal therapy is that interference with multiple hormonal pathways completely ablates androgen action. In clinical trials, combination hormonal therapy has included an agent that suppresses testosterone synthesis and an agent that either interferes with androgen synthesis or blocks androgen action. Combinations of low-dose estrogen with megestrol, an LH-RH analogue with ketoconazole, and an LH-RH analogue with flutamide are examples of this approach.

Low-dose estrogen has been combined with megestrol acetate to prolong the duration of testosterone suppression.[9] In seven patients tested, DES 0.1 to 0.2 mg daily plus megestrol 80 to 120 mg produced castration levels of testosterone for greater than 12 months. With the combination of low-dose estrogen and megestrol, edema and thromboembolism have not been reported and gynecomastia was mild.

Ketoconazole, an inhibitor of adrenal androgen synthesis at high doses, has been added to therapy for two patients who progressed during treatment with an LH-RH analogue.[47] Serum prostatic acid phosphatase declined significantly after the addition of ketoconazole. Although this combination represents a second rational alternative, more clinical trials are necessary before this therapy is adopted.

The combination of an LH-RH analogue and flutamide is the most novel combination hormonal therapy. LH-RH analogues produce castration levels of testosterone and flutamide interferes with androgen-mediated action at the cellular level. This combination could attenuate the initial disease flare produced by the LH-RH analogues and provide total androgen ablation. In the initial reports, response rates have been greater than 95% in previously untreated patients[48]; however, response rates less than 35% have been observed with this combination in patients previously treated with initial hormonal manipulation. Several oncology groups are evaluating the combination of leuprolide with or without the investigational antiandrogen flutamide in randomized double-blind trials. The results of this multi-institution trial should help to establish the role of combination hormonal therapy in advanced prostate cancer.

Although combination hormonal therapy represents a rational and interesting approach to the patient with advanced prostate cancer, clinical trials have not demonstrated a significant survival advantage. This supports the hypothesis that the tumor is composed of a heterogeneous group of both hormone-responsive and hormone-independent cells. Treatment alternatives that eradicate these hormone-independent cells need to be explored if a cure for prostate cancer is to be achieved.

### Cytotoxic Chemotherapy

Although cytotoxic agents for other malignancies have been extensively tested over the past four decades, the use of nonhormonal cytotoxic chemotherapy for the management of prostate cancer emerged only in the last 10 years. Several factors have contributed to this delay. Endocrine manipulation often benefits patients initially and is relatively nontoxic compared with chemotherapy. Most patients with prostate cancer are elderly and those with advanced disease usually have osteoblastic bone involvement, thus lowering their threshold for chemotherapy-related adverse reactions. In addition, clinical trials that attempt to evaluate the role of chemotherapy often lack adequate response criteria.

In an effort to standardize the response criteria, the NPCP and other organizations have formulated specific guidelines.[49] These guidelines recognize that there are few marker lesions with which to evaluate an objective response. Thus, parameters that measure subjective responses are also included in the response criteria. The objective parameters include assessment of the primary tumor size, evaluation of involved lymph nodes, and response of tumor markers to treatment. Subjective parameters include a scale for activity grading, an assessment of weight change, alterations in analgesic requirement, and general patient symptoms. After each criterion is evaluated, the response is then judged to be a complete objective response, partial objective response, stable disease, objective progression, or subjective response. Inclusion of stable disease as a favorable response is controversial. Some investigators argue that halting cancer progression is a meaningful response; however, the significance of delaying disease progression in a tumor that progresses slowly is questionable. As a summary, Yagoda and colleagues demonstrated the importance of considering response criteria by determining that the objective response rate to cisplatin can vary from 4% to 23% depending on the system of evaluation used.[50]

In addition to response criteria, the rationale for exclusion of patients who did not complete treatment must be considered in evaluation of a clinial trial. This is especially important when comparing treatments that have differing toxic effects. Also, studies that use survival as the treatment outcome should include age-adjusted survival rates because the patients are elderly.

A variety of trials have assessed the role of single-agent and combination therapy in the treatment of stage D prostate cancer (Table 99.7). Most of these trials have evaluated the use of chemotherapeutic agents in patients with progressive disease after hormonal therapy, a situation in which the expected response based on cell kinetic principles should be low. Nevertheless, chemotherapy appears to be effective in a limited number of patients with metastatic disease.

**Table 99.7** Chemotherapy for Advanced Prostate Cancer

| *Agent* | *Number of patients* | *Number (%) of responses* |
|---|---|---|
| Cyclophosphamide | 119 | 43 (36) |
| + 5-FU | 72 | 14 (19) |
| + Doxorubicin | 145 | 57 (39) |
| + 5-FU + doxorubicin | 21 | 12 (57) |
| + 5-FU + methotrexate | 20 | 7 (35) |
| + Doxorubicin + methotrexate | 20 | 7 (35) |
| Cisplatin | 100 | 24 (24) |
| + Cyclophosphamide | 17 | 12 (70) |
| + Doxorubicin | 38 | 19 (50) |
| Doxorubicin | 75 | 14 (19) |
| + 5-FU + methotrexate | 92 | 46 (50) |
| 5-FU | 106 | 27 (25) |
| Hydroxyurea | 58 | 19 (33) |
| Methotrexate | 58 | 24 (41) |
| Methyl-CCNU | 27 | 8 (30) |
| Nitrogen mustard | 31 | 12 (39) |
| Streptozotocin | 38 | 12 (32) |

[a] Includes stable disease.

Compiled from References 53, 54, and 56.

***Single Agents*** Several chemotherapeutic agents have demonstrated modest activity in prostate cancer.[51–56] These agents include cyclophosphamide, 5-fluorouracil, methotrexate, DTIC, doxorubicin, and cisplatin. Cisplatin and doxorubicin appear to be the most active agents at present; objective responses occur in 10% to 30% of patients; an additional 20% to 30% achieve disease stabilization. Cyclophosphamide is used as the standard agent for comparison in NPCP trials. The reported response range is 26% to 41% if stable disease is included as a favorable response. Less than 5% of patients achieve objective partial regression with cyclophosphamide. 5-Fluorouracil has an objective partial response rate of 8% to 12%. Although evaluated in a limited number of patients, hydroxyurea, streptozotocin, and methyl-CCNU appear to be active agents. Of the investigational agents evaluated in phase II trials, only mitoguanazone (MGBG) and vindestine produced objective regression of disease in 25% to 30% of patients.[56]

***Combinations*** Several trials have evaluated the use of combination therapy containing the single agents that demonstrate activity.[51–56] Combination regimens that include doxorubicin appear to have the highest response rate, with 32% to 60% of patients demonstrating an objective response.

In NPCP-sponsored trials, however, randomized comparison of single agents versus combination therapy failed to demonstrate a marked difference in response rates, although the intensity of combination treatment as measured by nadir leukocyte count was questioned.[56] These studies justify the use of single-agent therapy as the control arm in clinical trials and suggest a need for development of more active single agents.

### Combination Cytotoxic Chemotherapy/Hormonal Therapy

Although the results observed with chemotherapy seem promising, few complete responses are observed. As prostate cancer is a heterogeneous disease based on response, it is likely that the tumor is composed of cells that are sensitive to hormonal therapy, to chemotherapy, to both therapies, or to neither therapy. It would then seem rational to combine endocrine therapy and chemotherapy to produce an additive effect.

In an NPCP-sponsored prospective randomized trial, standard therapy (DES or orchiectomy) and combined therapy (DES plus cyclophosphamide) were compared in newly diagnosed patients with stage D prostate cancer.[57] The response rate, median survival, and time to progressive disease for the two treatment groups were similar. Other trials have failed to demonstrate a significant advantage of combination hormonal therapy/chemotherapy over hormonal therapy or chemotherapy alone.[55]

Estramustine phosphate, a novel compound that is a nitrogen mustard conjugated with estradiol phosphate, can be considered a form of combined hormonal therapy/chemotherapy. This agent was designed to take advantage of the site-specific action of estradiol by allowing the estrogen moiety to carry the akylating agent directly to sites of metastatic disease.[58] Clinical trials with this agent have shown response rates similar to those for DES therapy in previously untreated patients and no significant advantage in patients with refractory disease. Several investigators question whether the alkylating agent in this compound provides any additional therapeutic effect and suggest that the main action of this compound is through estrogenic mechanisms.

As androgenic hormones cause growth of prostate malignancies, it is possible that stimulation of the tumor prior to administration of chemotherapy would produce better results. This relies on the hypothesis that chemotherapeutic agents have greater cytotoxicity in the more rapidly growing cells. In several studies, androgen priming with fluoxymesterone before chemotherapy produced variable results. While objective and subjective responses have been reported in a small number of patients, fatal tumor stimulation resulting in spinal cord compression has occurred. The preliminary results suggest that the risks of androgen priming outweigh the benefits.

### *Approach to the Patient With Advanced Prostate Cancer*

The patient with stage D prostate cancer should be offered hormonal manipulation when symptoms appear. Hormonal therapy should be instituted before the development of symptoms only in the context of a clinical trial, as data are limited in this area. The initial hormonal manipulation should be orchiectomy, especially in the patient with cardiovascular disease. If the patient refuses orchiectomy or is not a surgical candidate, DES 1 mg three times a day and leuprolide 1 mg subcutaneously daily are suitable alternatives. Lower doses of DES (1 mg daily) can be used if serum testosterone levels are followed to ensure that castration levels are achieved. The combination of leuprolide and an antiandrogen is currently being investigated as an initial hormonal manipulation. When disease progresses, a second hormonal manipulation can be attempted, although the response rates are lower. Chemotherapy can be instituted at this point and, if possible, should be done as part of a research protocol. Also, earlier institution of chemotherapy or the use of combined chemotherapy/hormonal therapy should be done as part of a clinical trial. Adjunctive therapy for palliation of bone pain includes reassessment of current therapy, radiation therapy, and analgesics.

## Summary

Prostate cancer occurs in older males and is curable when local disease is present. Efforts to properly stage the patient at presentation are important because the intensity of therapy depends on the stage of disease. With the newer staging methods, it is anticipated that more patients with suspected localized disease will be proven to have more advanced disease than expected. For patients with advanced disease, only a few treatment options exist. Although hormonal manipulations to decrease circulating androgen concentrations are very effective for symptom palliation, no treatment modality prolongs survival. The LH-RH agonists are the most interesting addition to the various methods for hormonal manipulation and appear to produce fewer serious toxic effects than conventional DES administration. Antiandrogens offer another treatment alternative and are currently under clinical investigation. The role of chemotherapy is undefined. Single-agent therapy is as effective as combination therapy and neither produces many complete objective responses.

Several areas still require further research. The appropriate time to institute both hormonal therapy and chemotherapy should be identified. Chemotherapeutic agents with better activity than the presently available agents are needed. A better relationship between the steroid receptor content of the tumor and selection of patient treatment needs to be defined. When these and other questions are resolved, it is likely that a cure for prostate cancer will be in reach.

## References

1. Silverberg E, Lubera J. Cancer Statistics: 1986. CA 1986;36:9–25.
2. Klein LA. Prostatic carcinoma. N Engl J Med 1979; 300:824–833.
3. Jackson MA, Ahluwalia BS, Herson J. Characterization of prostate carcinoma among blacks: A continuation report. Cancer Treat Rep 1977;61:167–172.
4. Flanders WD. Review: Prostate cancer epidemiology. Prostate 4;5:621–629.

5. McNeal JE. The prostate gland. Monogr Urol 1983;4:3–33.
6. Walsh PC. Physiologic basis for hormonal therapy in carcinoma of the prostate. Urol Clin North Am 1975;2:125–140.
7. Sanberg AA. Endocrine control and physiology of the prostate. Prostate 1980;1:169–184.
8. Eisenberger MA, O'Dwyer PJ, Friedman MA. Gonadotropin hormone–releasing hormone analogues: A new therapeutic approach for prostatic carcinoma. J Clin Oncol 1986;4:414–424.
9. Geller J. Rationale for blockade of adrenal as well as testicular androgens in the treatment of advanced prostate cancer. Semin Oncol 1985;12(suppl 1):28–35.
10. Aumuller G. Morphologic and endocrine aspects of prostatic function. Prostate 1983;4:195–214.
11. Murphy GP. Prostate cancer: Continuing progress. CA 1981;31: 96–110.
12. Murphy GP, Whitmore WF. A report of the workshops on the current status of the histologic grading of prostate cancer. Cancer 1979;44:1490–1494.
13. Slack NH, Lane WW, Priore RL, et al. Prostate cancer. Urology 1986;27:205–213.
14. Guinan P, Bush I, Ray V, et al. The accuracy of the rectal examination in the diagnosis of prostate carcinoma. N Engl J Med 1980;303:499–503.
15. Jones GW. Diagnosis and management of prostate cancer. Cancer 1983;51:2456–2459.
16. Murphy GP, Gaeta JF, Pickren J, et al. Current status of classification and staging of prostate cancer. Cancer 1980;45: 1889–1895.
17. Lee F, Gray JM, McLeary RD, et al. Transrectal ultrasound in the diagnosis of prostate cancer: Location, echogenicity, histopathology, and staging. Prostate 1985;7:117–129.
18. Perez CA. Carcinoma of the prostate: A vexing biological and clinical enigma. Int J Radiat Oncol Biol Phys 1983;9:1427–1438.
19. Scott WW, Menon M, Walsh PC. Hormonal therapy of prostatic cancer. Cancer 1980;45:1929–1936.
20. Elder JS, Catalona WJ. Management of newly diagnosed metastatic carcinoma of the prostate. Urol Clin North Am 1984;11: 283–295.
21. Creaven PJ, Madajewicz S, Mittelman A. New potential treatment modalities for disseminated prostatic cancer. Urol Clin North Am 1984;11:343–356.
22. Resnick MI. Hormonal therapy in prostatic carcinoma. Urology 1984;24:18–23.
23. Soloway MS. Newer methods of hormonal therapy for prostate cancer. Urology 1984;24:30–39.
24. Waxman J. Hormonal aspects of prostatic cancer: A review. J R Soc Med 1985;78:129–135.
25. Paulson DF. Management of metastatic prostatic cancer. Urology 1985;25:49–52.
26. Chisolm GD. Treatment of advanced cancer of the prostate. Semin Surg Oncol 1985;1:38–55.
27. Huggins C, Hodges CV. Studies on prostatic cancer: 1. The effect of castration, of estrogen and of androgen injection on serum phosphatases in metastatic carcinoma of the prostate. Cancer Res 1941;1:293–297.
28. Nesbit RM, Baum WC. Endocrine control of prostatic carcinoma: Clinical and statistical survey of 1818 cases. JAMA 1950; 143:1317–1320.
29. The Veterans Administration Cooperative Urological Research Group. Carcinoma of the prostate: Treatment comparisons. J Urol 1967;98:516–522.
30. Blackard CE. The Veterans Administration Cooperative Urological Research Group studies of carcinoma of the prostate: A review. Cancer Chemother Rep 1975;59:225–227.
31. Cutler Jr GB, moderator. Therapeutic applications of luteinizing-hormone–releasing hormone and its analogs. Ann Intern Med 1985;102:643–657.
32. Santen RJ, Warner B. Evaluation of synthetic agonist analogue of gonadotropin-releasing hormone (leuprolide) on testicular androgen production in patients with carcinoma of the prostate. Urology 1985;25:53–59.
33. Smith JA, Glode LM, Max DT, et al. Clinical effects of gonadotropin-releasing hormone analogue in metastatic carcinoma of the prostate. Urology 1985;25:112–114.
34. Garnick MR, Glode LM, et al. Leuprolide versus diethylstilbestrol for metastatic prostate cancer. N Engl J Med 1984;311: 1281–1286.
35. Ponder BAJ, Shearer RJ, Pocock RD, et al. Response to aminoglutethimide and cortisone acetate in advanced prostate cancer. Br J Cancer 1984;50:757–763.
36. Murray R, Pitt P. Treatment of advanced prostatic cancer, resistant to conventional therapy, with aminoglutethimide. Eur J Can Clin Oncol 1985;21:453–458.
37. Drago Jr, Santen RJ, Lipton A, et al. Clinical effect of aminoglutethimide, medical adrenalectomy, in treatment of 43 patients with advanced prostatic carcinoma. Cancer 1984;53:1447–1450.
38. Sanford EJ, Drago JR, Rohner TJ, et al. Aminoglutethimide medical adrenalectomy for advanced prostatic carcinoma. J Urol 1976;115:170–172.
39. Heyns, W, Drochmans A, van der Schueren E, et al. Endocrine effects of high-dose ketoconazole therapy in advanced prostatic cancer. Acta Endocrinol 1985;110:276–283.
40. English HF, Santner SJ, Levine HB, et al. Inhibition of testosterone production with ketoconazole alone and in combination with a gonadotropin releasing hormone analogue in the rat. Cancer Res 1986;46:38–42.
41. Trachtenberg J, Halpern N, Pont A. Ketoconazole: A novel and rapid treatment for advanced prostatic cancer. J Urol 1983;130: 152–153.
42. Trachtenberg J. Ketoconazole therapy in advanced prostatic cancer. J Urol 1984;132:61–63.
43. Trachtenberg J, Pont A. Ketoconazole therapy for advanced prostate cancer. Lancet 1984;2:433–435.
44. Bonomi P, Pessis D, Bunting N, et al. Megestrol acetate used as primary hormonal therapy in stage D prostate cancer. Semin Oncol 1985;12(suppl 1):36–39.
45. Sogani PC, Vagaiwala MR, Whitmore WF. Experience with flutamide in patients with advanced prostatic cancer without prior endocrine therapy. Cancer 1984;54:744–750.
46. MacFarlane JR, Tolley DA. Flutamide therapy for advanced prostatic cancer: A phase II study. Br J Urol 1985;57:172–174.
47. Allen JM, Kerle DJ, Ware H, et al. Combined treatment with ketoconazole and luteinizing hormone releasing hormone analogue: A novel approach to resistant progressive prostate cancer. Br Med J 1983;287:1766.
48. Labrie F, Dupont A, Belanger A, et al. Simultaneous administration of pure antiandrogens, a combination necessary for the use of luteinizing hormone–releasing hormone agonists in the treatment of prostate cancer. Proc Natl Acad Sci USA 1984;81: 3861–3863.
49. Slack NH, Murphy GP, et al. Criteria for evaluating patient responses to treatment modalities for prostatic cancer. Urol Clin North Am 1984;11:337–342.
50. Yagoda A, Watson RC, Natale RB, et al. A critical analysis of response criteria in patients with prostatic cancer treated with *cis*-diamminedichloride, II. Cancer 1979;44:1553–1562.
51. Torti FM, Carter SK. The chemotherapy of prostatic adenocarcinoma. Ann Intern Med 1980;92:681–689.

52. Murphy GP. Chemotherapy: Is it effective in treatment of prostate cancer? Urol 1984;24:41–47.
53. Slack NH, Murphy GP. A decade of experience with chemotherapy for prostate cancer. Urology 1983;22:1–7.
54. Tannock IF. Is there evidence that chemotherapy is of benefit to patients with carcinoma of the prostate? J Clin Oncol 1985;3:1013–1021.
55. deKernion JB, Lindner A. Chemotherapy of hormonally unresponsive prostatic carcinoma. Urol Clin North Am 1984;11:319–326.
56. Eisenberger MA, Simon R, O'Dwyer PJ, et al. A reevaluation of nonhormonal cytotoxic chemotherapy in the treatment of prostatic carcinoma. J Clin Oncol 1985;3:827–841.
57. Murphy GP, Beckley S, Brady MF, et al. Treatment of newly diagnosed metastatic prostate cancer patients with chemotherapy agents in combination with hormones versus hormones alone. Cancer 1983;51:1264–1272.
58. Walzer Y, Oswalt J, Soloway MS. Estramustine phosphate—hormone, chemotherapeutic agent, or both? Urology 1984;24:53–58.

# Chapter 100 / Adult Acute Leukemia

Thomas P. Lennon, PharmD, and Gary C. Yee, PharmD

Leukemia is a hematologic malignancy characterized by unregulated proliferation of neoplastic cells. These immature proliferating leukemic cells (blasts) physically "crowd out" or inhibit normal cellular maturation in bone marrow, resulting in anemia, granulocytopenia, and thrombocytopenia. Leukemic blasts may also leave the bone marrow and infiltrate a variety of tissues such as lymph nodes, skin, liver, spleen, and central nervous system.

Symptoms associated with leukemia have been reported since the time of Hippocrates, although the disease was not described as a separate clinical entity until the middle nineteenth century. At that time, Virchow, noting that the blood of some patients was whitish in color, named the disease *leukemia* (white blood).[1] In 1877, Ehrlich developed cellular staining techniques that led to Naegeli's classification of the disease into lymphocytic and myelocytic types.[2] Historically, leukemia has also been classified as acute or chronic based on differences in life expectancy and rapidity of progression of the untreated disease. As age plays a significant role in prognosis and response to treatment, acute leukemia is discussed in two chapters. In this chapter, we consider adult acute leukemia, which includes acute nonlymphocytic leukemia (ANLL) and acute lymphocytic leukemia (ALL). When subclassified on the basis of morphologic, immunologic, and histochemical differences, adult acute leukemia comprises a heterogenous group of diseases (Tables 100.1 and 100.2) Chronic leukemia (Chapter 101) and childhood acute leukemia (Chapter 98) are discussed elsewhere.

As the median survival of untreated acute leukemia is only 2 to 3 months without hope of long-term survival, the disease has previously been regarded as uniformly fatal. After the development of the antimetabolite drug methotrexate, rapid progress was made in the treatment of acute leukemia. Nearly all children with acute leukemia achieve a complete remission from their disease, and many are actually considered cured (Chapter 98). Although the prognosis of adult acute leukemia is generally worse than that of childhood leukemia, survival has gradually improved, with 20% to 40% of patients becoming long-term survivors.

About 25,600 new cases of leukemia are diagnosed per year in the United States, accounting for about 3% of the total cancer incidence.[3,4] More than 90% of these cases (23,600) occur in adults, of which ANLL and ALL account for about 33% and 13% of all cases, respectively. Chronic leukemia accounts for the remaining 54% (Fig. 100.1). In children, ALL is more common than ANLL; the opposite is true in adults. Among adults, the incidence of both ALL and ANLL increases with increasing age.

Leukemia accounts for an estimated 17,400 deaths per year, or about 7 people per 100,000 population.[5] Acute leukemia is slightly more common in males than in females. In the United States, leukemia is slightly more common in whites than in blacks.

## Etiology

A number of environmental and genetic factors have been associated with an increased risk of acute leukemia but in most patients who develop leukemia, a causative agent cannot be identified.

### *Chemicals and Drugs*

Several chemicals and drugs, most of which cause marrow suppression, have been associated with an increased risk of leukemia. Data from workers chronically exposed to benzene clearly demonstrate its leukemogenic potential.[6] Other drugs associated with an increased risk of leukemia include Bacillus Calmette–Guerin (BCG) vaccine,[7,8] chloramphenicol[9], arsenic,[10] and phenylbutazone.[11] Many antineoplastic agents cause marrow suppression and are potent carcinogens. It is therefore not surprising that cytotoxic therapy has been associated with the development of "secondary" leukemia. An increased risk of developing secondary ANLL has been reported in patients treated with alkylating agents for Hodgkin's disease,[12] non-Hodgkin's lymphoma,[13] multiple myeloma,[14] breast cancer,[15] ovarian cancer,[16] and other malignancies.[17,18]

### *Nonneoplastic Diseases and Immunosuppression*

Many congenital diseases, most of which are associated with chromosomal abnormalities or instability, have been associated with an increased risk of leukemia. Patients with Down's syndrome have a 20-fold increased risk of acute leukemia.[1] Other congenital diseases associated with an increased risk of ANLL include Bloom's syndrome, Fanconi's anemia, Kleinfelter's syndrome, ataxia telangiectasia, and Wiskott–Aldrich syndrome.[1]

Immunosuppression, whether caused by underlying disease, infection, or drug therapy, has also been associated with an increased risk of ANLL and lymphomas.[1]

### *Ionizing Radiation*

Large radiation doses have been clearly associated with an increased risk of a variety of tumors, including chronic and acute nonlymphocytic leukemia.[2] Survivors of the nuclear explosions in Japan, depending on their proximity to the hypocenter, have up to a 20-fold increased incidence of

Table 100.1 Classification of Acute Nonlymphocytic Leukemia[a]

| *Designation* | *Name* | *Predominant cell type* |
|---|---|---|
| $M_1$ | Undifferentiated myelocytic | Myeloblasts |
| $M_2$ | Myelocytic | Myeloblasts, promyelocytes, myelocytes |
| $M_3$ | Promyelocytic | Hypergranular promyelocytes |
| $M_4$ | Myelomonocytic | Promyelocytes, myelocytes, promonocytes, monocytes |
| $M_{5a}$ | Monoblastic | Monoblasts |
| $M_{5b}$ | Differentiated monocytic | Monoblasts, promonocytes, monocytes |
| $M_6$ | Erythroleukemia | Erythroblasts |
| $M_7$ | Megakaryocytic | Megakaryocytes |

[a] FAB: French–American–British classification.

From Gale RP, Foon KA: Therapy of acute myelogenous leukemia. Semin Hematol 1987;24:41, with permission.

leukemia.[2] An increased risk of leukemia has been noted in patients who had received therapeutic radiation for polycythemia vera, ankylosing spondylitis, and malignant disease.[1] Before the risks associated with radiation exposure were widely known, radiologists also had an increased risk of leukemia.[19] With the use of protective measures and lower radiologic doses for diagnostic purposes, however, the current risk of malignancies in radiologists is similar to that in the general population.

The small doses of radiation associated with diagnostic radiologic procedures have not been associated with an increased risk of leukemia. In the United States, over 200 million diagnostic radiologic examinations are performed each year, with the average dose being 0.08 rad.[20] Animal experiments have shown a linear relationship between radiation dose and risk of subsequent leukemia. Although a linear relationship between radiation dose and risk of cancer has not been conclusively demonstrated in humans,[20] studies after the atomic blast in Japan suggest that the risk of leukemia is highest in survivors who were exposed to more than 50 rads.[20]

Paradoxically, the risk of leukemia may actually decline with larger radiation doses ( > 150–200 rads).[20] This lower risk is probably due to cell death from larger doses of radiation. The minimum radiation dose associated with an increased risk of leukemia is unknown, although an increased risk of leukemia has not been observed in Japanese atomic blast survivors who were exposed to less than 5 rads.[1]

The minimum latency period after radiation exposure varies greatly with age and individual characteristics, but is generally assumed to be about 2 years for leukemia.[20]

### *Viruses*

RNA tumor viruses have frequently been isolated from a variety of animals with leukemia, clearly implicating these oncogenic viruses in the development of the disease. RNA-dependent DNA polymerase, which is found only in some types of oncogenic viruses, and intracytoplasmic virus-like particles have occasionally been found in human leukemic cells but not in normal blood cells.[21]

## Pathogenesis

A basic understanding of normal hematopoiesis is needed before one can understand the pathogenesis of leukemia. Normal hematopoiesis may be divided into five levels,

Table 100.2 Classification of Acute Lymphocytic Leukemia

| *Morphologic*[a] | | *Immunologic* | |
|---|---|---|---|
| Group | Cell type | Classification | Marker |
| $L_1$ | Microlymphoblast | CALLA | Common ALL antigen |
| $L_2$ | Pleomorphic lymphoblast and prolymphocyte | T-cell | Forms rosettes with sheep erythrocytes or reacts with anti–T-cell monoclonal antibodies |
| $L_3$ | Morphologically identical to Burkitt's lymphoma cells | B-cell | Presence of surface membrane or cytoplasmic immunoglobulin or reacts with anti–B-cell monoclonal antibodies |
| | | Null-cell | No identifiable surface antigen |

[a] FAB: French–American–British classification.

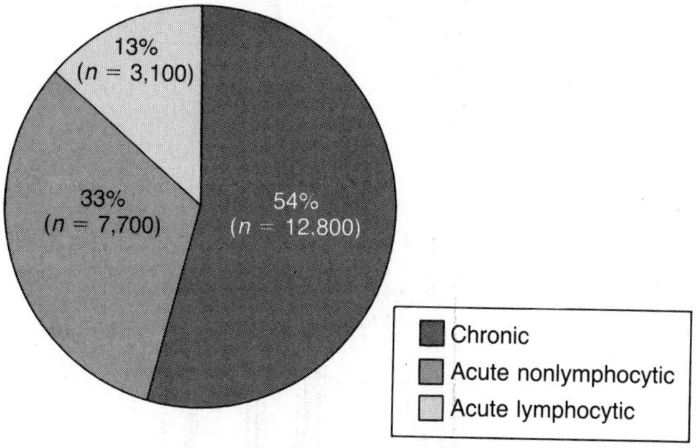


**Figure 100.1** Annual occurrence of adult leukemia by type ($n$ = 23,600). Estimates from the American Cancer Society.[4]

beginning from a pool of pluripotent stem cells capable of differentiating to form mature blood cells (Figure 100.2).[22] These pluripotent stem cells differentiate to form two distinct stem cell pools. The first stem cell pool gives rise to the six types of blood cells (erythrocytes, megakaryocytes, monocytes, basophils, neutrophils, eosinophils); the second pool differentiates to form circulating lymphocytes.

ANLL affects the hematopoietic cell population and probably arises from a defect in the pluripotent (level 1) or hematopoietic stem cell (level 2), resulting in partial differentiation and proliferation of immature precursors of the blood-forming cells.[22] One cell type usually predominates and results in the different morphologic and histochemical classifications of ANLL (Table 100.1)

ALL is a disease characterized by proliferation of immature lymphoblasts. In this type of acute leukemia, the defect is probably at the level of the lymphopoietic stem cell (level 2).[22] As with ANLL, one cell type usually predominates. Markers on the cell surface or membrane of the lymphoblast can be used to classify ALL (Table 100.2).

Leukemic cells have a growth advantage over normal cells, leading to a "crowding out" phenomenon in the bone marrow. This growth advantage is not due to more rapid proliferation as compared with normal cells,[23] but is probably due to a factor produced by leukemic cells that inhibits normal cellular proliferation and differentiation or to a lower rate of leukemic cell loss compared with normal blood cells.[24]

## Clinical Presentation

### *Signs and Symptoms*

The signs and symptoms of acute leukemia are nonspecific and can be attributed to replacement of normal functional blood cells with immature dysfunctional leukemic cells and to leukemic infiltration of a specific organ or site.[2] *Anemia* often manifests as lassitude, malaise, and pallor. Fatigue is the most common symptom, and is usually worse than expected for the degree of anemia. Less commonly, palpitations or dyspnea on exertion may be noted. *Granulocytopenia* may present as fever with or without frank infection. *Thrombocytopenia* may manifest as bleeding or bruising, often involving the gums, skin, or gastrointestinal tract. As leukemic infiltrates may involve any organ, unusual presenting symptoms such as seizures, gum hypertrophy, loss of vision, the presence of an abnormal mass, or bone pain may also be observed. As is frequently seen with many types of cancer, mild weight loss may be present. Patients with acute leukemia can occasionally be diagnosed by routine blood analysis without any significant history or physical findings.

### *Physical and Laboratory Findings*

Physical findings are compatible with anemia (pallor, tachycardia, cardiac murmurs), granulocytopenia (infection, fever), thrombocytopenia (bruising, frank bleeding, petechiae, ecchymoses, purpura), and leukemic infiltration (lymphadenopathy, splenomegaly, hepatomegaly, sternal tenderness). Other physical findings related to leukemia cell infiltration include cervical lymphadenopathy, gingival hypertrophy, cranial palsies, and skin infiltration.

Anemia and decreased reticulocytes are nearly always present because of decreased red blood cell production. The anemia is usually normocytic and normochromic. The hematocrit is usually reduced to about 30% to 35%, with a proportional fall in hemoglobin.[2] The platelet count is reduced in nearly all patients; about 30% of patients with ALL have a platelet count below 50,000/$\mu$L, while a platelet count below 20,000/$\mu$L is more common in patients with ANLL. As a result, patients with ANLL are more likely to have physical evidence of significant hemorrhage. The white blood cell count is normal or elevated in about 85% of patients with ALL; in some patients, the white blood cell count is greatly elevated ($>$ 50,000/$\mu$L).[1] A high white blood cell count is often associated with T-cell ALL. In adults with ANLL, the white blood cell count at the time of diagnosis will be elevated in one third, normal in one third, and low in one third.[2] The peripheral blood smear usually demonstrates a decrease in granulocytes, with an increase in blasts.

Serum uric acid is mildly elevated in about one half of patients with adult leukemia. Occasionally, patients may present with renal failure secondary to uric acid nephropathy. Serum calcium imbalances may be noted. In patients with mild renal failure, hypocalcemia may be seen and is usually accompanied by hyperphosphatemia. Hypercalcemia is often due to ectopic parathyroid hormone production by leukemic cells, or rapid destruction of large numbers of leukemic cells. Serum albumin, usually normal at diagnosis, may decrease as the disease progresses. Diffuse hypergammaglobulinemia is also present in some patients.

As many as two thirds of adults with ALL have leukemic cell chromosomal abnormalities, including the presence of the Philadelphia chromosome ($Ph^1$).[25] A majority of patients with ANLL also have chromosomal abnormalities.[26] These chromosomal abnormalities appear to be of prognostic importance in both ALL[25] and ANLL[26] (see Risk Factors).

Marrow biopsy is necessary to establish a diagnosis and follow disease progression and response to therapy. At diagnosis, the marrow is usually hypercellular with a predominance of blasts. Myelofibrosis is occasionally seen.

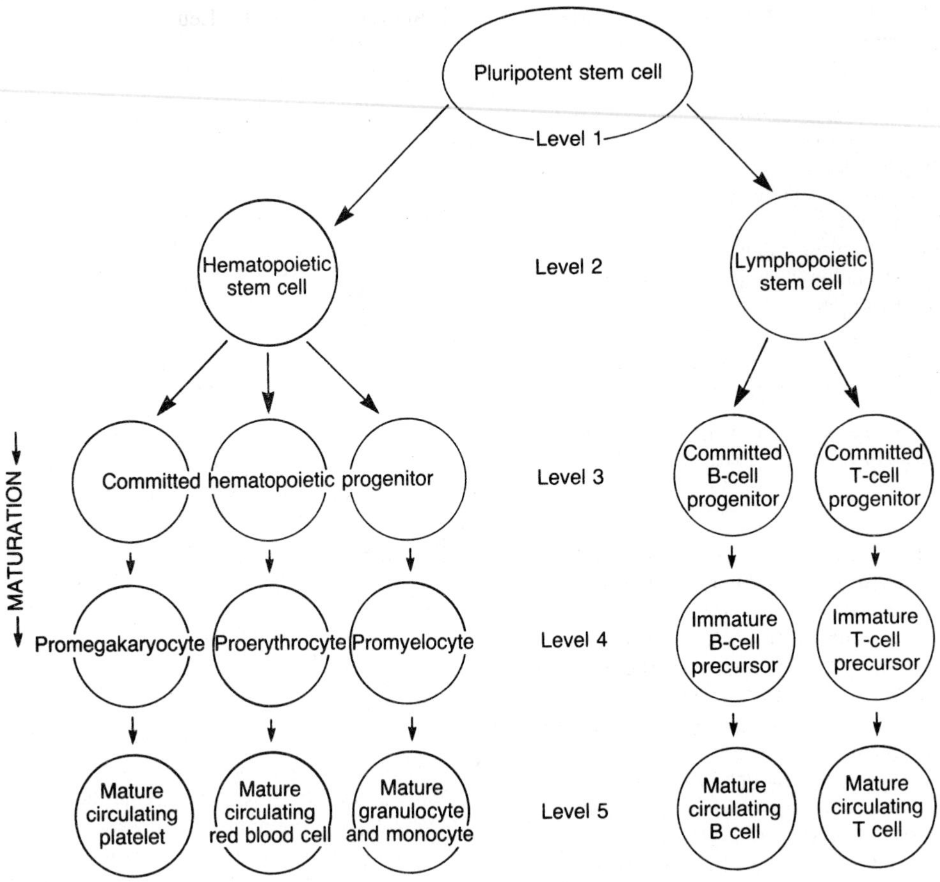


**Figure 100.2** Normal hematopoiesis. Normal hematopoiesis probably arises from a pool of pluripotent stem cells (level 1), which differentiate to form the hematopoietic and lymphopoietic stem cell pools (level 2). Further differentiation leads to committed progenitor cells (level 3) that are responsive to specific cytopoietic hormones including erythropoietin, thrombopoietin, and neutropoietin. These hormones mediate further maturation and proliferation (level 4). At level 4, morphologically identifiable precursors are present, which ultimately differentiate to form functional circulating blood cells (level 5). *(Modified from Lichtman MA, Segel GB: The leukemias. In Rubin P [ed]: Clinical Oncology, 6th ed. Washington, D.C., American Cancer Society, 1983, with permission.)*

## Risk Factors

Many clinical and laboratory features at diagnosis have been associated with response to treatment. Identification of these risk factors may allow the oncologist to better understand the disease and to tailor treatment according to the predicted response. For example, if a patient has many clinical and laboratory features that are associated with a good response to chemotherapy ("good risk"), then the oncologist may choose to give less intensive therapy to reduce the risk of long-term toxic effects. Conversely, if a patient is not likely to respond well to therapy ("high or poor risk"), then the oncologist may choose to give more intensive chemotherapy. This approach has been particularly helpful in the treatment of childhood ALL (see chapter 98).

In adults with ALL, recent studies have identified several risk factors that correlate with prognosis (Table 100.3).[25,27] As most patients with ALL achieve a complete clinical remission, these factors refer to the risk of leukemic relapse rather than the risk of not achieving a complete remission.

Prognostic factors in ANLL have not been as well defined, but several patient- and disease-related factors have been reported to influence prognosis.[28] The most important patient factor is age, with younger patients more likely to achieve a complete remission than elderly patients. The low complete remission rate in elderly patients appears to result from increased frequency of fatal infectious and bleeding complications rather than chemotherapy failure.[29] Once a complete remission is achieved, however, the duration of remission is similar in young and elderly patients. Disease-related factors include histologic subtype, presence of a preleukemic syndrome, evidence of extramedullary disease, and presence of cytogenetic abnormalities. High-resolution chromosomal analysis, surface marker analysis, cell cycle characteristic analysis, and in vitro leukemic cell growth and sensitivity studies have shown recently that the percentage of blast cells actively synthesizing DNA, the growth of

**Table 100.3** Prognostic Factors in Adult Acute Lymphocytic Leukemia

| *Factor* | *Risk for leukemic relapse* | |
|---|---|---|
| | Low | High |
| Morphology | $L_1$ and $L_2$ | $L_3$ |
| Immunologic phenotype | CALLA | Null-cell, T-cell, B-cell |
| Patient age | Risk increases with increasing age | |
| WBC count at diagnosis | Risk increases with increasing WBC count | |
| Time to achieve complete remission | ≤ 4 wk | > 4 wk |
| Cytogenetics | Normal karyotype | Abnormal karyotype |
| Patient sex | Female sex | Male sex |
| Central nervous system involvement | No | Yes |
| Hepatosplenomegaly | No | Yes |

Based on Hoelzer D, Gale RP: Acute lymphoblastic leukemia in adults: Recent progress, future directions. Semin Hematol 1987;24:2739, with permission.

the leukemic cells in culture, and the chromosomal pattern of the blast cells may also have prognostic significance.[26,30–33] In addition, patients who develop a "secondary" leukemia after treatment of another malignancy have a very poor response to further chemotherapy, with less than 10% achieving a complete remission.[16]

In childhood ALL, prognostic factors are routinely used to categorize patients according to their likelihood of cure from chemotherapy. Although this approach is not routinely used in adult acute leukemia, some investigators are prospectively using known prognostic factors to individualize chemotherapeutic regimens,[32,34,35] but it is too early to determine if this novel approach is superior to conventional approaches.

## Treatment

### *Chemotherapy*

The short-term goal of treatment for adult acute leukemia is to rapidly achieve a complete clinical and hematologic remission. In the absence of a complete remission, a rapid and fatal outcome is inevitable. Complete remission is defined as the disappearance of all clinical and bone marrow evidence (normal cellularity with < 5% blasts) of leukemia, with restoration of normal hematopoiesis. Partial remission is a significant response to treatment, although evidence of residual disease (5%–25% blasts) in the bone marrow remains.

After a complete remission is achieved, the goal is to maintain the patient in continuous complete remission. As discussed later, the occurrence of leukemic relapse in the bone marrow usually removes any hope of cure of the disease. Patients are considered "cured" of their leukemia when they have been in continuous complete remission for an extended period (i.e., more than 5 years).

#### Acute Lymphocytic Leukemia

Because most children with ALL can be cured with current chemotherapeutic regimens (see Chapter 98), treatment of adult ALL has been modeled after treatment of childhood ALL. Although treatment results with adult ALL are worse than those with childhood ALL, recent use of aggressive therapy in adult ALL has increased the proportion of 5-year disease-free survivors to 20% to 30%.[25,27,36–40] Therapy for adult ALL has been designed after treatment for childhood ALL and is divided into four phases: (1) remission induction, (2) central nervous system prophylaxis, (3) consolidation therapy, and (4) maintenance therapy (Fig. 100.3). Table 100.4 shows several representative treatment regimens for adult ALL.

***Remission Induction Therapy*** The goal of remission induction is to rapidly induce a complete clinical and hematologic remission. As single agents, daunomycin, prednisone, vincristine, and L-asparaginase induce remission in about 25%, 35%, 40%, and 50% of adults, respectively.[41] The combination of vincristine and prednisone induces complete remission in about 50% of adults with ALL. The addition of a third or fourth agent (daunorubicin, doxorubicin, or L-asparaginase) to vincristine and prednisone increases the complete remission rate to about 75% in adults.[25,36–41] Most oncologists currently give prednisone, vincristine, daunorubicin or doxorubicin, and L-asparaginase as remission induction therapy. Similar results have been reported with the combination of low-dose methotrexate, high-dose prednisone (350 mg/m$^2$), and vincristine.[42] Other agents that are sometimes included in remission induction regimens are cyclophosphamide, cytosine arabinoside, dexamethasone, mercaptopurine, and 6-thioguanine, although it is uncertain whether they significantly contribute to the efficacy of the remission induction regimen.

Few prospective studies have compared remission induction regimens. In one trial, patients who were randomized to receive remission induction that included daunorubicin had a higher complete remission rate than those who received three-drug remission induction without daunorubicin (83% versus 47%).[37] Although the most active regimen has not been defined, remission induction regiments in adult ALL should include at least three drugs: vincristine, prednisone, and either daunomycin, doxorubicin, or L-asparaginase. Higher doses of the standard three or four-drug regimen or

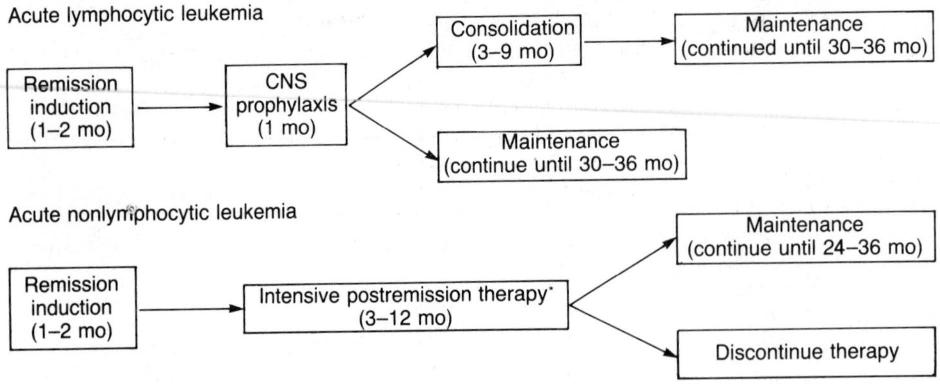


**Figure 100.3** Therapy for acute lymphocytic and nonlymphocytic leukemias. *Also referred to as consolidation or intensification.

addition of other chemotherapeutic agents should be considered for patients with poor prognostic features.

***Central Nervous System Prophylaxis*** After patients achieve complete remission, they usually receive central nervous system (CNS) prophylaxis. The rationale for CNS prophylaxis is based on two observations. First, many chemotherapeutic agents do not readily cross the blood–brain barrier. Second, 20% to 30% of patients with ALL who had no evidence of CNS involvement at diagnosis experience a relapse of their leukemia in the CNS.[25] These observations indicate that the CNS is a potential sanctuary for leukemic cells and that undetectable leukemic cells are present in the CNS in many patients. CNS involvement is more common in ALL than ANLL, and is also more common in children than adults. CNS involvement at the time of diagnosis is relatively uncommon (<10%) in adult ALL.[25] Factors that have been associated with an increased risk of CNS involvement at diagnosis include an initially high white blood cell count, T-cell phenotype, and $L_3$ morphology.[25]

The goal of CNS prophylaxis is to eradicate residual but undetectable leukemic cells present in the CNS after remission induction. Once CNS relapse has occurred, patients are at increased risk of bone marrow relapse and death from refractory leukemia. In childhood ALL, effective CNS prophylaxis has decreased CNS relapse rates from about 50% to less than 10% and has increased long-term survival (see Chapter 98). It is important to note that the benefit of CNS prophylaxis became apparent only after 2 years of continu-

**Table 100.4** Representative Chemotherapy Regimens for Adult Acute Lymphocytic Leukemia[a]

| *Remission induction* | *CNS prophylaxis* | *Consolidation* | *Maintenance* |
|---|---|---|---|
| **Memorial Sloan–Kettering Cancer Center[38]** | | | |
| VCR, ADR, Pred for 4 wk, followed by ADR and CTX | IT or Ommaya Reservoir MTX beginning during remission induction and continued during maintenance | Six alternating cycles of MTX or 6-TG with Ara-C and one additional cycle of VCR and Pred, ending with one cycle and ASP and CTX | VCR, Pred, 6-MP, MTX, DACT and either (1) ADR or (2) BCNU and CTX continued for 3 yr |
| **Federal Republic of Germany[39]** | | | |
| Phase I (4 wk) VCR, DNR, Pred, ASP | Cranial irradiation and IT MTX | Phase I (starting at week 20) DEX, VCR, ADR | 6-MP and MTX continued until 30 mo |
| Phase II (4 wk)CTX, Ara-C, 6-MP | | Phase II CTX, Ara-C, 6-TG | |
| **University of California San Francisco; Stanford University; and City of Hope Medical Center[40]** | | | |
| VCR, DNR, ASP, Pred | Cranial irradiation and IT MTX | Alternating cycles of treatments A (cycles 1,3,5,7)—VCR, DNR, ASP, Pred B (cycles 2,4,6,8)—VM-26, Ara-C C (cycle 9)—IMD MTX | 6-MP and MTX continued until 30 mo |

[a] ADR, doxorubicin; Ara-C, cytosine arabinoside; ASP, L-asparaginase; BCNU, carmustine; CNS, central nervous system; CTX, cyclophosphamide; DAC, dactinomycin; DEX, dexamethasone; DNR, daunorubicin; IMD MTX, intermediate-dose methotrexate; IT MTX, intrathecal methotrexate; 6-MP, 6-mercaptopurine; MTX, methotrexate; Pred, prednisone; 6-TG, 6-thioguanine; VCR, vincristine.

ous complete remission. Although CNS prophylaxis has been shown to significantly decrease the risk of CNS relapse in adults (from 32% to 11%), survival in the CNS prophylaxis group was not significantly longer compared with patients not given CNS prophylaxis.[42,43] This difference in treatment results between adult and childhood ALL is probably due to the lower risk of CNS relapse in adults and the smaller proportion of adults who survive longer than 2 years.

Although CNS prophylaxis has not been shown to improve survival in adults with ALL, some form of CNS prophylaxis is usually included in ALL treatment protocols.[25,36–41] CNS prophylaxis usually includes cranial irradiation and intrathecal methotrexate to eradicate undetectable leukemia in the cranial region and spinal column, respectively. Cranial irradiation is typically given in 2-Gy fractions to a total dose of 18–24 Gy. Methotrexate 10 mg/m$^2$ (12–15 mg maximum) is given intrathecally once or twice weekly for five to six doses. In some protocols, intrathecal cytosine arabinoside (30–100 mg) and methotrexate are given with cranial irradiation for CNS prophylaxis.[25]

Cranial irradiation has been associated with significant acute and chronic neurotoxic effects, ranging from mild neuropsychologic deficits and learning disabilities to a life-threatening syndrome called leukoencephalopathy.[44,45] Cranial irradiation can also limit the amount of subsequent systemic chemotherapy that can be given because of an increased incidence of CNS side effects.[46] This presumably occurs because cranial irradiation increases permeability of the blood–brain barrier to toxic chemotherapeutic agents.[47] In an effort to reduce the neurotoxicity of CNS prophylaxis, several trials have examined the use of systemic chemotherapy, continuous intravenous infusions of intermediate-dose methotrexate, or intrathecal methotrexate alone without cranial irradiation as CNS prophylaxis.[38,48,49] Preliminary results show that these approaches are effective in preventing CNS leukemia.

The selection of a CNS prophylaxis regimen must therefore consider both efficacy and toxicity. Because few randomized studies have compared different CNS regimens in adult ALL, it is not possible to recommend any one regimen over another; however, based largely on the experience with childhood ALL, CNS prophylaxis should be included in treatment protocols for adult ALL and should include intrathecal methotrexate either alone or combined with cranial radiation or continuous intravenous infusions of intermediate-dose methotrexate.

***Consolidation Therapy*** Consolidation therapy is started after a complete remission has been achieved and refers to continued intensive chemotherapy in an attempt to eradicate clinically undetectable disease. Though most adults with ALL achieve complete remission, median remission duration and survival (15–30 months) have been short in most studies.[25,31] Several studies suggest that the addition of consolidation therapy may prolong remission duration and survival.[38–40] For example, a recent study conducted at Memorial Sloan–Kettering Cancer Center reported median remission and survival durations of 51 and 53 months, respectively, in patients treated with a complicated and intensive remission induction and consolidation regimen (Table 100.4).[38] Another study that included a consolidation phase with nine alternating cycles of non–cross-resistant chemotherapy reported a median remission duration greater than 36 months[40]; however, in a large German multicenter trial, the addition of consolidation therapy did not appear to significantly prolong the duration of remission (median 25 months).[38] In each of these studies, survival at 5 years is projected to be 35% to 45%, which suggests that the addition of an intensive consolidation phase in adult ALL increases the proportion of long-term survivors.

***Maintenance Therapy*** Many patients relapse shortly after completion of remission induction and consolidation therapy, presumably because of residual disease. The goal of maintenance therapy is therefore to further eradicate residual leukemic cells and prolong remission duration. While maintenance therapy is clearly beneficial in childhood ALL, the benefit in adults is less well defined, particularly in patients receiving intensive remission induction and consolidation regimens. As with childhood ALL, maintenance therapy usually consists of mercaptopurine and methotrexate, at doses that produce minimal myelosuppression, with or without intermittent "pulses" of vincristine and prednisone.[25] Some of the best results have been reported with a complicated treatment program that includes intensive consolidation and maintenance phases[38]; however, similar results were reported with two other treatment protocols that included standard mercaptopurine and low-dose methotrexate as maintenance therapy.[39,40] As discussed previously, both of those treatment programs differed from most other treatment programs by the addition of an intensive consolidation phase, suggesting that standard low-dose maintenance therapy may be adequate when an intensive consolidation phase is included.

The optimal duration of maintenance therapy in adults is unknown, but most treatment programs continue maintenance therapy for at least 30 months.

### Acute Nonlymphocytic Leukemia

ANLL accounts for the majority of acute leukemia in adults and occurs with increasing frequency in elderly patients. Until recently, only about 40% to 60% of adults with ANLL achieved complete remission and very few were long-term survivors. With recent advances in chemotherapy and supportive care, however, 60% to 80% achieve complete remission and 20% to 30% become long-term survivors.[28,33,50] In contrast to ALL, all of the active drugs in ANLL are marrow suppressive. Therefore, patients with ANLL, particularly elderly (>60) patients, are at greater risk for treatment-related fatal infectious and bleeding complications.

Treatment of ANLL was initially designed after successful treatment of childhood ALL and can be divided into remission induction, intensive postremission therapy, and maintenance therapy (Fig. 100.3). Central nervous system prophylaxis is not routinely given for ANLL because the risk of CNS relapse is lower than in patients with ALL.[28,33,50] Several representative chemotherapeutic regimens for treatment of ANLL are presented in Table 100.5.

***Remission Induction Therapy*** As with ALL, the goal of remission induction for ANLL is to rapidly induce a complete remission. Compared with ALL, fewer adults with

**Table 100.5** Representative Chemotherapy Regimens for Adult Acute Nonlymphocytic Leukemia

| *Remission induction* | *Intensive postremission therapy* | *Maintenance therapy* |
|---|---|---|
| **Dana Farber Cancer Institute and Harvard Medical School**[56] | | |
| Ara-C and ADR | Alternating cycles of sequences<br>I—AZA and ADR<br>II—VCR, Pred, 6-MP, MTX<br>III—Ara-C | None |
| **University of Washington and Fred Hutchinson Cancer Research Center**[60] | | |
| Ara-C and DNR (7 + 3), 6-TG, VCR, Pred | Alternating cycles of regimens<br>A (cycle 2)—HD Ara-C and ASP<br>B (cycles 3 and 5)—same as remission induction<br>C (cycles 4)—AMSA and VP-16<br>D (cycle 6)—VCR, Pred, 6-MP, MTX | None |
| **Roswell Park Memorial Hospital and Other Institutions**[62] | | |
| Ara-C and ADR (10 + 3) | Alternating cycles of regimens<br>A (cycles 1 and 3)—Ara-C and ADR (7 + 3)<br>B (cycles 2 and 4)—Ara-C and AMSA or HD Ara-C | None |

[a] ADR, doxorubicin; AMSA, amasacrine; Ara-C, cytosine arabinoside; ASP, L-asparaginase; AZA, azacytidine; DNR, daunorubicin; HD Ara-C, high-dose cytosine arabinoside; 6-MP, 6-mercaptopurine; MTX, methotrexate; Pred, prednisone; 6-TG, 6-thioguanine; VCR, vincristine; VP-16, etoposide.

ANLL achieve complete remission. The lower complete remission rate in ANLL is related in part to differences in the toxicity of the drugs in remission induction regimens. In ALL, several active agents are relatively nonmyelosuppressive (prednisone, vincristine, L-asparaginase), whereas in ANLL, every active agent is myelosuppressive. As a result, patients with ALL may achieve complete remission without severe marrow hypoplasia. However, since the complete remission rate in ANLL is related to the intensity of the remission induction regimen, the drugs used in ANLL are given at doses that uniformly cause severe marrow hypoplasia. Thus, one reason for the lower complete remission rate in ANLL compared with ALL is the inability to give optimal doses of chemotherapy because of marrow toxicity. With continued improvement of supportive care for patients undergoing chemotherapy, more intensive treatment regimens are being given in an effort to reduce the high rate of leukemic relapse and increase the proportion of long-term survivors.

The most active single agents in ANLL, the anthracycline antibiotics (daunorubicin and doxorubicin) and cytosine arabinoside (Ara-C), can induce complete remission in about 50% and 25% of patients, respectively.[33,50] The complete remission rate with combination of Ara-C and an anthracycline is 60% to 80%.[37] Because daunorubicin has similar antileukemic activity but causes less gastrointestinal toxicity than doxorubicin, daunorubicin is the preferred anthracycline for remission induction regimens.[51] The optimal dosage schedules for daunorubicin and Ara-C are not known, but one randomized study showed that patients who received 7 days of Ara-C by continuous intravenous infusion and 3 days of daunorubicin (7 + 3) had a significantly higher complete remission rate than patients who received 5 days of ARA-C and 2 days of daunorubicin (5 + 2).[52] This study also showed that patients who received Ara-C by continuous intravenous infusion had a higher response rate than those who received Ara-C by intravenous bolus. Pharmacologic considerations, dosage selection, and toxic effects of Ara-C and the anthracyclines are discussed in detail under Drug Monitoring and Supportive Care. Vincristine, prednisone, 6-thioguanine, 6-mercaptopurine, 5-azacytidine, etoposide, cyclophosphamide, amsacrine, and CCNU are often added to the remission induction regimen but they probably do not significantly improve the complete remission rate. These drugs may be beneficial, however, when given as intensive postremission therapy.

The major cause of remission induction failure is not resistant leukemia but death from infection and bleeding.[29] As elderly patients are more likely to develop these complications, it is not clear how these individuals should be treated. Based on observations that elderly ($\geq$ 60) patients have the same complete remission rate after an intensive remission induction regimen as younger patients, Foon et al suggested that the same remission induction regimen should be given regardless of age.[53] In a study of elderly ($\geq$ 70) patients with ANLL, however, survival in patients randomized to receive attenuated doses of chemotherapy was significantly better than that in patients who received full doses of chemotherapy.[54] The improved survival was due to fewer early deaths from infection or bleeding.

Most patients achieve a complete remission after one or two courses of chemotherapy. Patients who require additional chemotherapy to achieve a complete remission have been reported to have a poor prognosis, even if remission is ultimately achieved.[28]

*Intensive Postremission Therapy* Although most adults with ANLL achieve a complete remission, the duration of remission is short if no further treatment is given. Relapse is presumably due to the presence of residual but clinically undetectable leukemic cells after remission induction therapy. The goal of intensive postremission therapy (IPRT) is to eradicate these residual leukemic cells and prevent the emergence of drug-resistant disease. The need for IPRT is based on postmortem analysis and cell kinetic data suggesting that nearly $10^8$ to $10^9$ residual leukemic cells remain after effective remission induction therapy[55] and on the low relapse rates observed after intensive chemoradiotherapy with marrow rescue (see later).

In the treatment of ANLL, IPRT is often referred to as consolidation or intensification. Consolidation therapy is defined as the administration of one or two courses of high doses of the same drugs used for remission induction, immediately after a complete remission is achieved.[50] Intensification is also instituted after a complete remission is achieved but involves the administration of drugs that the patient has not previously received.[50] Intensification may be started early (within a few months of achievement of remission) or late (complete remission longer than 6–12 months). As consolidation and intensification are sometimes defined differently by different investigators, we refer to both phases as IPRT throughout this section. IPRT may be defined as the administration of high-dose combination chemotherapy to a patient in complete remission in an attempt to eradicate clinically undetectable disease.

The benefit of IPRT is controversial, but the results of several uncontrolled trials suggest that several cycles of IPRT, when given immediately after remission induction, prolong remission duration and survival.[28,33,50,55–61] For example, in a large German trial, patients who received IPRT (termed consolidation in this trial) had a significantly longer complete remission duration than patients who received no postremission therapy.[58] It is not clear whether the same agents given for remission induction (Ara-C and an anthracycline) or different agents should be given in IPRT. One recent randomized study suggests that IPRT regimens that include drugs different from those used in remission induction may further prolong remission duration and survival than regimens that include the same drugs in both remission induction and IPRT.[59] Furthermore, treatment programs that introduce different drugs during IPRT have reported that 25% to 30% of patients are alive disease free at 3 years.[56,59–62] IPRT regimens that include four courses [56,60,62] or high-dose Ara-C[60–62] appear to be particularly efficacious. Toxicity of IPRT regimens can be severe; in some studies, 15% to 20% of patients could not complete their four courses of IPRT because of the severe toxic effects.[60,62]

Other investigators have given IPRT after months to years of continuous complete remission (often called late intensification).[56,63] In one of these studies, early IPRT was also given.[56] In that study, 45% of patients 18 to 50 years old are estimated to be alive disease free at 3 years; however, treatment programs that do not include late IPRT have reported similar results,[62] suggesting that late IPRT may not further improve treatment results. In summary, IPRT given after intensive remission induction probably decreases relapse rates and prolongs survival. Future randomized studies are needed to define the optimal timing and duration of IPRT and the most effective drug combinations.

*Maintenance Therapy* Historically, maintenance chemotherapy for acute leukemia has involved the use of relatively low-dose chemotherapy in an effort to further eradicate residual disease while minimizing toxicity. As the antileukemic efficacy of active drugs is related to the intensity of treatment, the benefit of prolonged maintenance therapy with repeated cycles of low-dose chemotherapy is questionable. Several controlled studies have reported that conventional low-dose maintenance therapy does not prolong remission duration and survival in patients treated with intensive remission induction followed by IPRT.[57,64] This is supported by uncontrolled studies that have reported excellent results with no maintenance therapy.[56,61,62] Two large randomized studies, however, have reported that maintenance therapy prolongs disease-free survival.[58,59] In both studies, the maintenance regimen consisted of 5 days of Ara-C combined with 2 days of daunorubicin. Although this therapy was referred to as maintenance therapy, it should more appropriately be considered IPRT because of its intensity.[59] When maintenance therapy is given, it is usually continued for 1 to 3 years.[50]

In summary, in patients who receive adequate IPRT, maintenance therapy with low-dose chemotherapy is not effective in treating ANLL and may actually contribute to development of drug resistance. Maintenance therapy with intensive chemotherapy, however, can be considered another form of IPRT and may therefore be beneficial, particularly in patients who do not receive adequate IPRT.

**Relapse**

Most adult patients with acute leukemia who achieve complete remission eventually experience a leukemic relapse. Relapse usually occurs in the bone marrow, but may also occur in the CNS or other extramedullary sites. Treatment and outcome depend primarily on whether relapse occurred during or after completion of treatment.

About one half of patients with ALL or ANLL who experience a leukemic relapse while receiving chemotherapy may achieve a second complete remission with chemotherapy, but remission duration usually lasts only several months and long-term survivors are uncommon. Some patients with ALL who relapse after chemotherapy is discontinued, however, can experience prolonged survival with chemotherapy. Bone marrow transplantation may be undertaken if the patient is a suitable candidate (see later).

Several agents, including high-dose Ara-C, etoposide, intermediate- or high-dose methotrexate, L-asparaginase, 5-azacytidine, amsacrine, and mitoxantrone have been useful in the treatment of relapsed or resistant disease. The pharmacology of Ara-C and L-asparaginase is discussed later. 5-Azacytidine is an antimetabolite that interferes with nucleic acid metabolism. It appears to induce remission in about 20% of patients with relapsed ANLL refractory to other therapy.[65] Toxic effects are primarily gastrointestinal (nausea, vomiting, diarrhea) and hematologic (leukopenia). Amsacrine is an acridine derivative that probably exerts its antitumor activity by DNA intercalation and subsequent inhibition of DNA synthesis. Amsacrine has been reported to cause myelosuppression, nausea and vomiting, stomatitis, alopecia, and hyperbilirubinemia.[66] The agent is also cardiotoxic, and life-threatening arrhythmias and cardiomyopathy may occur.[67] The complete remission rate for amsacrine in refractory acute leukemia is about 25%.[66] In one randomized study, amsacrine and high-dose Ara-C had similar complete remission rates.[68] Because of its significant antileukemic activity, amsacrine has been included in some remission induction[34] and IPRT[60,62] regimens. Mitoxantrone is a member of a new class of antineoplastics called the anthracenediones. It appears to act by intercalation with DNA, interfering with nucleic acid synthesis. It is active in ALL and ANLL, and may induce complete remission in up to 25% of patients refractory to other chemotherapy.[69] Toxic effects of mitoxantrone are similar to those of other chemotherapeutic agents, and like the anthracyclines, mitoxantrone may cause dose-related congestive heart failure and some transient ECG alterations.[70]

Several drug combinations are effective in refractory leukemia. Intermediate to high-dose methotrexate and L-asparaginase have induced complete remission rates of 30% to 70% in resistant ALL.[25] High-dose Ara-C combined with amsacrine is also active, with a complete remission rate of 60% to 70% in patients with refractory ALL or ANLL.[71,72] The combination of high-dose Ara-C and doxorubicin or daunorubicin[73] and the combination of amsacrine and etoposide are also effective in refractory ANLL.

### *Drug Monitoring and Supportive Care*

The most common and significant toxic effect of antileukemic agents is marrow suppression. With the exception of prednisone, L-asparaginase, and vincristine, antineoplastic agents used to treat adult leukemias cause a rapid fall in peripheral platelet and white blood cell counts. During remission induction therapy, daily monitoring of the complete blood count and the absolute granulocyte count is necessary. Marrow hypoplasia usually reaches its lowest point (nadir) after 1 to 2 weeks of beginning therapy and lasts for another 1 to 2 weeks. During this period of hypoplasia, infectious and bleeding complications are major causes of death in leukemic patients. As signs and symptoms of infection may be absent in the neutropenic host, frequent monitoring of vital signs and daily physical examination are important. Infection control strategies include routine hand washing, fungal and bacterial prophylaxis, gut decontamination, prophylactic granulocyte transfusions, dietary restriction, reverse isolation and laminar-airflow rooms, routine surveillance cultures, and the empiric use of broad-spectrum antibiotics (see Chapter 91).

Acute leukemia patients, particularly those with an initial elevated white blood cell count, should receive allopurinol prior to and during chemotherapy to prevent the development of urate nephropathy from rapid destruction of white cells. In adults, 300 mg of allopurinol once daily, started 1 to 2 days prior to chemotherapy, is usually adequate. Once marrow hypoplasia ensues, allopurinol may be discontinued.

Hematologic support consists primarily of platelet and packed red cell transfusions. Platelet transfusions are often given for peripheral counts below 20,000/$\mu$L or clinical signs of bleeding. Transfusions of packed red cells for low hematocrits may also be indicated. Because of the gastrointestinal toxic effects of chemotherapy, parenteral nutrition should be used liberally.

While all chemotherapeutic agents used to treat adult leukemia are toxic and require careful monitoring by experienced health care professionals, several agents require special consideration regarding dosage, toxic effects, and pharmacologic effects. These agents are discussed in detail here.

***Cytosine Arabinoside*** Cytosine arabinoside is an antimetabolite that acts as an inhibitor of DNA polymerase. A variety of dose schedules have been employed for Ara-C. Selection of the appropriate dosage, route, and infusion duration should be based on the observations that as a cycle-specific agent (S phase, DNA synthesis), Ara-C is probably more effective when given by intravenous infusion rather than bolus injection.[52] Second, as with most anticancer drugs, Ara-C exhibits a steep dose–response relationship.[75] In one large randomized study of patients with ANLL, remission induction regimens that included 7-day continuous infusions of Ara-C (100 mg/m$^2$/d) had a higher complete remission rate (59%) compared with 5-day continuous infusion (45%), twice-daily bolus dosing (200 mg/m$^2$/d) for 5 days (36%), and twice-daily bolus dosing (200 mg/m$^2$/d) for 7 days (51%).[52] Other studies suggest that Ara-C 200 mg/m$^2$/d, given twice daily as an intravenous bolus injection for 7 to 10 days, is as efficacious as 100 mg/m$^2$/d over 7 days as a continuous infusion.[50] Prolonging the duration of the Ara-C infusion from 7 to 10 days probably does not increase the complete remission rate, but may increase gastrointestinal toxicity.[50] These data suggest that continuous infusion of Ara-C is more effective than by bolus administration of equal doses, but increasing the bolus dose may make the two routes of administration similar in efficacy.

Nearly 75% of patients have some degree of resistance to Ara-C prior to treatment and most responding patients develop resistance during treatment. In an effort to overcome this resistance, several investigators have increased the dosage of Ara-C (2–3 g/m$^2$/d for 5–8 days) therapy.[76,77] Preliminary studies have reported complete remission rates of 25% to 50% in refractory ANLL with single-agent therapy. Combinations of high-dose Ara-C and other agents are also very active in refractory acute leukemia.[71–73] These encouraging results have led to the addition of high-dose Ara-C as part of remission induction [78,79] and IPRT [60–62] for ANLL.

The most significant toxic effect of Ara-C is profound myelosuppression with a nadir of 7 to 10 days. The incidence and types of other toxic effects seen with Ara-C vary according to the dosage schedule and route. When Ara-C is given as a continuous infusion for more than 7 days at 200 mg/m$^2$/d or more than 10 days at 100 mg/m$^2$/d, the gastrointestinal toxicity is often dose limiting. Ara-C has been reported to cause less gastrointestinal toxicity when given twice daily as an intravenous bolus rather than continuous infusion,[33] although no difference was observed in a randomized trial.[52] High-dose Ara-C has been associated with several types of toxicity not observed after standard-dose Ara-C, including central nervous system toxicity, conjuctivitis, erythroderma, and pulmonary toxicity.[76,77,80]

***Anthracyclines*** The precise mechanism of action for the anthracyclines is unknown, but it is known that these drugs intercalate DNA. Both daunorubicin and doxorubicin have been used in the treatment of adult acute leukemia. A recent large clinical trial compared the efficacy and toxicity of doxorubicin (30 mg/m$^2$/d) and daunorubicin (30 and 45 mg/m$^2$/d) combined with Ara-C in patients with ANLL.[51] The results of this study demonstrate the similar efficacy of the two agents, but a higher incidence of gastrointestinal toxicity (i.e., mucositis and lethal necrotizing colitis) with doxorubicin compared with daunorubicin. As the gastrointestinal tract serves as a barrier to bacterial or fungal invasion, the increased gastrointestinal toxicity may increase the risk of infection in patients treated with doxorubicin. Therefore, the results of this study suggest that daunorubicin may be the preferred agent for treating ANLL because of less gastrointestinal toxicity. Based on phase II studies,[33] daunorubicin has been administered by short intravenous infusion for 3 days at a dose of 30–60 mg/m$^2$/d when combined with Ara-C for treatment of acute leukemia.

The chronic and cululative dose-limiting toxic effect of the anthracycline antibiotics is cardiotoxicity.[81] Cardiotoxicity associated with daunorubicin and doxorubicin may be acute, subacute, or chronic. Acute toxicity occurs during or shortly after infusion of the drug and is characterized by asymptomatic supraventricular arrhythmias or premature ventricular contractions. Subacute toxic effects including transient left ventricular dysfunction or pericarditis/myocarditis may rarely occur. In a retrospective study of 4,018 patients, Von Hoff et al estimated that the overall incidence of chronic congestive cardiomyopathy associated with doxorubicin was 2.2% and that the risk increased with increasing total dose.[82] A cumulative maximum doxorubicin dose of 550 mg/m$^2$ is associated with a 0.07 probability of developing subsequent heart failure.[82] Modifications in the dosage schedule, including low-dose weekly or continuous infusion administration, have reduced the chronic cardiotoxicity of doxorubicin in a variety of malignancies,[83] but this approach has not been examined in patients with adult leukemia. The effect of potential cardioprotective agents such as vitamin E, *N*-acetylcysteine, digitalis, carnitine, and calcium channel blockers is being investigated, but cannot be routinely recommended at this time. Currently, treatment goals to avoid anthracycline cardiotoxicity should include limitation of the cumulative dose to 450–550 mg/m$^2$ in all patients and routine screening for patients with risk factors in whom a lower total cumulative dose might be appropriate. Risk factors include prior cardiac irradiation, age greater than 70 years, and underlying heart disease or hypertension. In these high-risk patients, routine cardiac monitoring, including baseline and routine radionuclide ejection fractions or biopsy catheterization, should be performed.

While cardiotoxicity is the chronic dose-limiting toxic effect of the anthracyclines, marrow suppression is the acute dose-limiting toxic effect. Drug infiltration may cause severe local ulceration, necessitating the use of bolus or short-infusion administration with careful monitoring during drug administration. Several agents including low doses of corticosteriods, $\beta$-adrenergic compounds, adenosine, and vitamine E in dimethylsulfoxide have demonstrated limited protection against local ulceration after extravasation.[84] Recent data in mice suggest that local hypothermia may decrease intradermal toxicity in contrast to heat, which may actually enhance skin toxicity.[85] Other local effects that occur frequently during venous administration include pruritis, rash, and erythematous streaking of the vein. Nausea and vomiting, diarrhea, and alopecia occur frequently. Other side effects include dose-related stomatitis, fever and chills, and red urine, which is related to drug excretion and not hematuria.

***L-Asparaginase*** L-Asparaginase is an enzyme produced by several species of bacteria. This enzyme acts as an anticancer drug by depleting circulating pools of L-asparagine. As sensitive tumor cells lack the enzyme to replace this amino acid, protein synthesis ceases and the cell dies. Most of the commercially available drug is isolated from *Escherichia coli* and, to a lesser degree, *Erwinia caratovora*. Most toxic effects may be attributed to hypersensitivity reactions and inhibition of protein synthesis.[86] Hypersensitivity reactions range from mild urticarial skin eruptions to life-threatening anaphylaxis. Risk factors for development of L-asparaginase hypersensitivity include previous drug exposure, infrequent administration, high doses, intravenous administration, and use as a single agent.[86] If a severe hypersensitivity reaction to *E. coli* L-asparaginase occurs, the *Erwinia* preparation may be used, as the two preparations are not usually cross-reactive.

Unlike many other chemotherapeutic agents, L-asparaginase usually does not cause severe marrow suppression, alopecia, or mucosal damage. Hepatic and pancreatic toxicity, typically manifest as liver function abnormalities or abdominal pain, is quite common.[86,87] Hyperosmolar nonketotic hyperglycemia, responsive to insulin and hydration, may occur presumably because of defective insulin release or a decrease in insulin receptors.

## *Alternate Therapy*

### Bone Marrow Transplantation

Although survival has improved with advances in chemotherapy, most adults with acute leukemia experience a leukemic relapse and die of their disease. In an effort to further increase antileukemic activity, many investigators are exploring the use of bone marrow transplantation as another form of intensification therapy. Bone marrow transplantation allows the administration of otherwise lethal doses of preparative chemoradiotherapy by rescuing the patient with intravenous infusion of donor bone marrow. Marrow transplantation has two potential advantages over the standard chemotherapeutic approach in treating acute leukemia.[88] First, the high-dose chemotherapeutic regimen increases leukemic cell kill. Second, immunoregulation following transplantation may provide some protection against disease relapse (i.e., graft-versus-leukemia effect).

Marrow transplantation may be performed between identical monozygous twins (syngeneic) or genetically dissimilar but immunologically compatible (allogeneic) individuals. Additionally, some patients are transplanted with their own previously treated and stored marrow (autologous). Donor and recipient compatibility is determined by study of the histocompatibility complex, called the human leukocyte antigen (HLA) complex.[89] The ideal donor for allogeneic

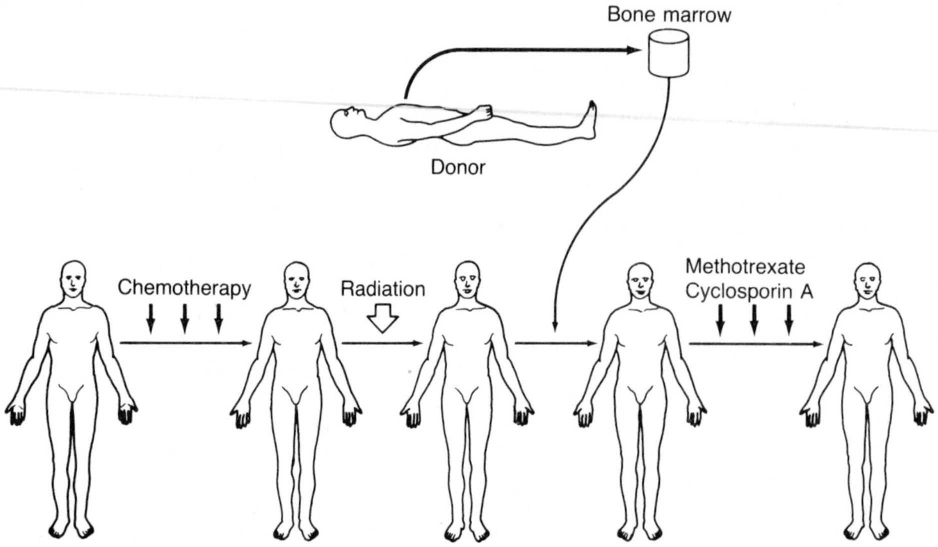


**Figure 100.4** Scheme for allogeneic bone marrow transplantation in the treatment of hematologic malignancies. Most preparative regimens include cyclophosphamide and total-body irradiation; patients with aplastic anemia are usually prepared with cyclophosphamide alone. *(From Champlin RE, Gale RP: Cancer Treat Rep 1984;68:146, with permission.)*

marrow transplantation is an HLA-identical sibling but only about 30% to 40% of patients with at least one sibling have an HLA-identical sibling donor. In an effort to increase the number of marrow transplant candidates, current research has focused on autologous marrow transplantation[90] and on the use of non–HLA-identical related donors for allogeneic marrow transplantation.[91] Marrow transplantation is also generally limited to patients less than 50 years old because of the unacceptably high transplant-related morbidity and mortality in older patients.

Prior to transplantation, the patient is ''prepared'' or ''conditioned'' with high-dose chemotherapy, either alone or combined with total-body irradiation. The purpose of the preparative regimen is to suppress the immune system of the recipient so that the marrow graft is not rejected and to eradicate all residual leukemic cells. One advantage of total-body irradiation is its ability to penetrate pharmacologic sanctuaries. One widely used conditioning regimen includes cyclophosphamide (60 mg/kg × 2) and total-body irradiation (12–15 Gy in fractionated doses).[88,89] Other conditioning regimens include busulfan, high-dose Ara-C, and etoposide.

The technique of bone marrow aspiration is described in detail elsewhere.[89] Briefly, bone marrow is obtained from the donor by aspirations from the anterior and posterior iliac crests. The procedure takes less than 2 hours and yields 200–1200 mL of bone marrow, depending on the size of the donor. After fat and bone particles are removed, the marrow is given intravenously over several hours like a blood transfusion (Fig. 100.4).

Allogeneic marrow transplantation is now accepted as a therapeutic alternative to standard chemotherapy in ANLL. Recent studies show that about 50% of adults with ANLL transplanted in first remission or early first relapse become long-term disease-free survivors.[92,93] When transplantation is delayed until the second or subsequent remission, the proportion of long-term survivors decreases to 10% to 40%.[92,93] The actuarial leukemic relapse rate is between 10% and 40% for patients with ANLL transplanted in first remission and about 50% for patients transplanted in second or subsequent remission. These encouraging results have led to several prospective comparisons of allogeneic marrow transplantation with chemotherapy in adults with ANLL.[64,93,94] Patients who received marrow transplantation while in first remission tended to have better 5-year survival (40%–47%) than those who continued to receive chemotherapy (20%–27%).[64] The risk of early death (within 6 months) was greater in the marrow transplant patients because of transplant-related complications, whereas leukemic relapse was significantly less in the bone marrow transplant group compared with the chemotherapy group.

As many adults with ALL achieve long-term disease-free survival with chemotherapy, marrow transplantation is usually not performed in patients during first remission but is delayed until after the patient relapses.[93,95] Most patients are transplanted while in second or subsequent remission and about 25% to 40% of these patients become long-term survivors. Leukemic relapse is the major cause of treatment failure. Two prospective comparisons of allogeneic marrow transplantation with chemotherapy in children and young adults with ALL in second or subsequent remission show that marrow transplantation offers the best chance for long-term survival when compared with continued chemotherapy.[96,97]

Although marrow transplantation is an effective treatment of leukemia, several transplant-related complications occur, resulting in a high incidence of early morbidity and mortality. A detailed discussion of these complications is beyond the scope of this chapter, but some of the major complications deserve comment. After the preparative regimen, a period of severe marrow aplasia occurs and may last several weeks. During this time, the patient is at risk of opportunistic infection. Although improvements in supportive care, antibiotic treatment and prophylaxis, and the use of reverse isolation of laminar-airflow rooms have significantly decreased infectious complications in marrow transplant recipients, nearly all patients experience fever during this neutropenic period (see Chapter 91).

Graft-versus-host disease, resulting from immunocompetent donor cells reacting against antigens on host tissue, is also a major cause of postransplant morbidity. Graft-versus-host disease is divided into acute (usually occurring within 6 weeks of grafting) or chronic (more than 100 days postransplant) syndromes. The acute disease usually manifests itself initially as skin rash, and may progress to gastrointestinal tract and liver involvement.[98] The overall incidence of moderate to severe acute graft-versus-host disease is about 30% to 50% after allogeneic marrow grafting, and increases with advancing age. As treatment of established acute graft-versus-host disease is poor, early prophylaxis with combinations of immunosuppressive agents is necessary. Most prophylactic regimens include methotrexate, cyclosporine, antithymocyte globulin, or steroids. Graft-versus-host disease has also been shown to decrease the incidence of leukemic relapse, presumably because of the effect of immunocompetent donor cells on leukemic host cells.[99]

Interstitial pneumonia occurs in about 40% of patients and remains a major cause of posttransplant mortality.[100] Cytomegalovirus is the most common infectious cause, although many cases are idiopathic. The prognosis of interstitial pneumonia after marrow transplantation is poor, with a 60% to 90% mortality rate. Major risk factors for interstitial pneumonia include age, severe graft-versus-host disease, and the use of total-body irradiation. As treatment of established cytomegaloviral pneumonia has not significantly reduced the high mortality rate, current research efforts have focused on the prevention of cytomegaloviral infection through the administration of blood products from cytomegalovirus-seronegative donors, passive immunoprophylaxis with cytomegalovirus immune globulin, and prophylaxis with antiviral drugs.[101]

In summary, although the procedure is associated with significant acute and chronic toxicity, marrow transplantation is a valuable treatment modality for many patients; however, as marrow transplantation is currently limited to younger patients with a suitable donor, aggressive chemotherapy remains the major treatment option for most adults with acute leukemia.

### Immunotherapy

The rationale for immunotherapy is to take advantage of the immunogenic and antigenic differences between host and tumor cells. Stimulation of the host immune system may result in destruction of leukemic cells, such as that postulated to occur in marrow transplant patients with graft-versus-host disease. To date, specific and nonspecific immunotherapy (bacillus Calmette–Guerin and interferon) used alone[102] or combined with chemotherapy[103] has not been shown to be useful in the treatment of adult acute leukemia. Continued research into the use of monoclonal antibodies[104] and lymphokine-activated killer (LAK) cells[105] holds promise for future clinical utility of immunotherapy in treating leukemia.

## References


1. Wintrobe WM. Clinical Hematology, 8th ed. Philadelphia, Lea and Febiger, 1981, pp 1449–1564.
2. Wiernik PH. Acute leukemias of adults, in Devita VT, Hellman S, Rosenberg SA (eds): Cancer. Principles and Practice of Oncology, 2nd ed. Philadelphia, J.B. Lippincott, 1985.
3. Brincker H. Estimate of overall treatment results in acute nonlymphocytic leukemia based on age-specific rates of incidence and of complete remission. Cancer Treat Rep 1985; 69:5–11.
4. American Cancer Society. Cancer facts and figures: 1986. New York, American Cancer Society, 1986.
5. U.S. Department of Health and Human Services, Public Health Service, National Institute of Health. Cancer Rates and Risks, 3rd ed. NIH publication no. 85–691, 1985.
6. Aksoy M, Erdem S, DinCol G. Leukemia in shoe-workers exposed chronically to benzene. Blood 1974;44:837–841.
7. Rosenthal SR, Crispen RG, Thorne MD, et al. BCG vaccination and leukemia mortality. JAMA 1972;222:1543–1544.
8. Comstock GW. Leukemia and BCG. Lancet 1971;2:1062–1063.
9. Cohen T, Creger WP. Acute myeloid leukemia following seven years of aplastic anemia induced by chloramphenicol. Am J Med 1967;43:762–770.
10. Kjeldsberg CR, Ward HP. Leukemia in arsenic poisoning. Ann Intern Med 1972;77:935–937.
11. Jensen MK, Roll K. Phenylbutazone and leukemia. Acta Med Scand 1965;178:505–513.
12. Aisenberg AC. Acute nonlymphocytic leukemia after treatment for Hodgkin's disease. Am J Med 1983;75:449–454.
13. Pedersen-Bjergaard J, Ersboll J, Sorenson HM, et al. Risk of acute nonlymphocytic leukemia and preleukemia in patients treated with cyclophosphamide for non-Hodgkin's lymphomas. Ann Intern Med 1985;103:195–200.
14. Rosner R, Grunwald HW. Multiple myeloma terminating in acute leukemia. Report of 12 cases and review of the literature. Am J Med 1974;57:927–939.
15. Fisher B, Rockette H, Fisher ER, et al. Leukemia in breast cancer patients following adjuvant chemotherapy and postoperative radiation: The NSABP experience. J Clin Oncol 1985; 3:1640–1658.
16. Reimer RR, Hoover R, Fraumeni JF, et al. Acute leukemia after alkylating-agent therapy of ovarian cancer. N Engl J Med 1977;297:117–181.
17. Zarrabi MH, Rosner F. Acute myeloblastic leukemia following treatment for non-hematopoietic cancers: Report of 19 cases and review of the literature. Am J Hematol 1979;7:357–367.
18. Casciato DA, Scott JL. Acute leukemia following prolonged cytotoxic agent therapy. Medicine 1979;58:32–47.
19. Lawrence JS. Irradiation leukemogenesis. JAMA 1964;190:93–98.
20. Kohn HI, Fry RJM. Radiation carcinogenesis. N Engl J Med 1984;310:504–511.
21. Gallo RC, Meyskens FL. Advances in the viral etiology of leukemia and lymphoma. Semin Oncol 1978;15:379–398.
22. Lichtman MA, Segel GB. The leukemias, in Rubin P (ed): Clinical Oncology, 6th ed. American Cancer Society, 1983.
23. Kantarjian HM, Barlogie B, Keating MJ, et al. Pretreatment

cytokinetics in acute myelogenous leukemia. Age-related prognostic implications. J Clin Invest 1985;76:319–324.
24. Broxmeyer HE, Grossbard E, Jacobsen N, et al. Persistence of inhibitory activity against normal bone marrow cells during remission of acute leukemia. N Engl J Med 1979;30:346–351.
25. Hoelzer D, Gale RP. Acute lymphoblastic leukemia in adults: Recent progress, future directions. Semin Hematol 1987;24: 2739.
26. Yunis JJ, Brunning RD, Howe RB, et al. High-resolution chromosomes as an independent prognostic indicator in adult acute nonlymphocytic leukemia. N Engl J Med 1984;311:812–818.
27. Clarkson B, Ellis S, Little C, et al. Acute lymphoblastic leukemia in adults. Semin Oncol 1985;12:160–179.
28. Champlin R, Gale RP. Acute myelogenous leukemia: Recent advances in therapy. Blood 1987;69:1551–1562.
29. Estey EH, Keating MJ, McCredie KB, et al. Causes of initial remission induction failure in acute myelogenous leukemia. Blood 1982;60:309–315.
30. Griffin JD, Mayer RJ, Weinstein HJ. Surface marker analysis of acute myeloblastic leukemia: Identification of differentiation-associated phenotypes. Blood 1983;62:557–563.
31. Preisler HD, Azarnia N, Raza A, et al. Relationship between the percent of marrow cells in S phase and the outcome of remission-induced therapy for acute nonlymphocytic leukaemia. Br J Haematol 1984;56:399–407.
32. Preisler HD. Prediction of response to chemotherapy in acute myelocytic leukemia. Blood 1980;56:361–367.
33. Lister TA, Rohatiner AZS. The treatment of acute myelogenous leukemia in adults. Semin Oncol 1982;19:172–192.
34. Keating MJ, Gehan EA, Smith TL, et al. A strategy for evaluation of new treatments in untreated patients: Application to a clinical trial of AMSA for acute leukemia. J Clin Oncol 1987;5:710–721.
35. Reizenstein P, Giannoulis NE, Johansson NO. Predicting response to combination chemotherapy in acute myeloblastic leukemia—a way to individualize treatment. Acta Med Scand 1980;207:321–325.
36. Gottlieb AJ, Weinberg V, Ellison RR, et al. Efficacy of daunorubicin in the therapy of adult acute lymphocytic leukemia: A prospective randomized trail by Cancer and Leukemia Group B. Blood 1984;64:267–274.
37. Gingrich RD, Burns CP, Armitage JO, et al. Long-term relapse-free survival in adult acute lymphoblastic leukemia. Cancer Treat Rep 1985;69:153–160.
38. Schauer P, Arlin ZA, Mertelsmann R, et al. Treatment of acute lymphoblastic leukemia in adults: Results of L-10 and L-10M protocols. J Clin Oncol 1983;1:462–470.
39. Hoelzer D, Thiel E, Loffler H, et al. Intensified therapy of acute lymphoblastic and acute undifferentiated leukemia in adults. Blood 1984;64:38–47.
40. Linker CA, Levitt LJ, O'Donnell M, et al. Improved results of treatment of adult acute lymphoblastic leukemia. Blood 1987; 69:1242–1248.
41. Woodruff R. The management of adult lymphoblastic leukemia. Cancer Treat Rev 1978;5:95–113.
42. Omura GA, Moffitt S, Vogler WR, et al. Combination chemotherapy of adult acute lymphoblastic leukemia with randomized central nervous system prophylaxis. Blood 1980;55:199–204.
43. Omura GA, Raney M. Long-term survival in adult acute lymphoblastic leukemia: Follow-up of a Southeastern Cancer Study Group Trial. J Clin Oncol 1985;3:1053–1058.
44. Goldberg ID, Bloomer WD, Dawson DM. Nervous system toxic effects of cancer therapy. JAMA 1982;247:1437–1441.
45. Byrd R. Late effects of treatment of cancer in children. Pediatr Clin North Am 1985;32:835–857.
46. Aur RJA, Simone JV, Verzosa MS, et al. Childhood acute lymphocytic leukemia. Study VIII. Cancer 1978;42:2123–2134.
47. Storm AJ, Van Der Kogel AJ, Nooter K. Effect of x-irradiation on the pharmacokinetics of methotrexate in rats: Alteration of the blood–brain barrier. Eur J Cancer Clin Oncol 1985;21:759–764.
48. Esterhay RJ, Wiernik PH, Grove WR, et al. Moderate dose methotrexate, vincristine, asparaginase, and dexamethasone for treatment of adult acute lymphoblastic leukemia. Blood 1982;59:334–345.
49. Evans WE, Crom WR, Abromowitch M, et al. Clinical pharmacodynamics of high-dose methotrexate in acute lymphocytic leukemia: Identification of a relation between concentration and effect. N Engl J Med 1986;314:471–477.
50. Gale RP, Foon KA. Therapy of acute myelogenous leukemia. Semin Hematol 1987;24:40–54.
51. Yates J, Glidewell O, Wiernik P, et al. Cytosine arabinoside with daunorubicin or Adriamycin for therapy of acute myelocytic leukemia: A CALBG study. Blood 1982;60:454–462.
52. Rai KR, Holland JF, Glidewell OJ, et al. Treatment of acute myelocytic leukemia: A study by Cancer and Leukemia Group B. Blood 1981;58:1203–1211.
53. Foon KA, Zighelboim J, Yale C, et al. Intensive chemotherapy is the treatment of choice for elderly patients with acute myelogenous leukemia. Blood 1981;58:467–470.
54. Kahn SB, Begg CB, Mazza JJ, et al. Full dose versus attenuated dose daunorubicin, cytosine arabinoside, and 6-thioguanine in the treatment of acute nonlymphocytic leukemia in the elderly. J Clin Oncol 1984;2:865–870.
55. Mayer RJ, Weinstein HJ, Coral FS, et al. The role of intensive postinduction chemotherapy in the management of patients with acute myelogenous leukemia. Cancer Treat Rep 1982;66: 1455–1462.
56. Weinstein HJ, Mayer RJ, Rosenthal DS, et al. Chemotherapy for acute myelogenous leukemia in children and adults: VAPA update. Blood 1983;62:315–319.
57. Champlin R, Gale RP, Elashoff R, et al. Prolonged survival in acute myelogenous leukemia without maintenance chemotherapy. Lancet 1984;1:894–896.
58. Buchner T, Urbanitz D, Hiddemana W, et al. Intensified induction and consolidation with or without maintenance chemotherapy for acute myeloid leukemia (AML): Two multicenter studies of the German AML Cooperative Group. J Clin Oncol 1985;3:1583–1589.
59. Vogler WR, Winton EF, Gordon DS, et al. A randomized comparison of postremission therapy in acute myelogenous leukemia: A Southeastern Cancer Study Group trial. Blood 1984;63:1039–1045.
60. Tallman MS, Appelbaum FR, Amos D, et al. Evaluation of intensive postremission chemotherapy for adults with acute nonlymphocytic leukemia using high-dose cytosine arabinoside with L-asparaginase and amsacrine with etoposide. J Clin Oncol 1987;5:918–926.
61. Cassileth PA, Begg CB, Silber R, et al. Prolonged unmaintained remission after intensive consolidation therapy in adult acute nonlymphocytic leukemia. Cancer Treat Rep 1987;71: 137–140.
62. Preisler HD, Raza A, Early A, et al. Intensive remission consolidation therapy in the treatment of acute nonlymphocytic leukemia. J Clin Oncol 1987;5:722–730.
63. Glucksberg H, Cheever MA, Farewell VT, et al. Intensification therapy for acute nonlymphoblastic leukemia in adults. Cancer 1983;52:198–205.

64. Appelbaum FR, Dahlberg S. Thomas ED, et al. Bone marrow transplantation or chemotherapy after remission induction for adults with acute nonlymphoblastic leukemia. A prospective comparison. Ann Intern Med 1984;101:581–588.
65. Von Hoff DD, Slavik M, Muggia FM. 5-Azacyticine. A new anticancer drug with effectiveness in acute myelogenous leukemia. Ann Intern Med 1976;85:237–245.
66. Legha SS, Keating MJ, McCredie KB, et al. Evaluation of AMSA in previously treated patients with acute leukemia: Results of therapy in 109 adults. Blood 1982;60:484–490.
67. Steinherz LJ, Steinherz PG, Mangiacasale D, et al. Cardiac abnormalities after AMSA administration. Cancer Treat Rep 1982;66:483–488.
68. Vogler WR, Preisler HD, Winton EF, et al. Randomized trial of high-dose cytarabine versus amsacrine in acute myelogenous leukemia in relapse: A leukemia intergroup study. Cancer Treat Rep 1986;70:455–459.
69. Paciucci PA, Cuttner J, Holland JF. Mitoxantrone as a single agent and in combination chemotherapy in patients with refractory acute leukemia. Semin Oncol 1984;11(suppl 1):36–40.
70. Crossley RJ. Clinical safety and tolerance of mitoxantrone. Semin Oncol 1984;11(suppl 1):54–58.
71. Hines JD, Oken MM, Mazza JJ, et al. High-dose cytosine arabinoside and m-AMSA is effective therapy in relapsed acute nonlymphocytic leukemia. J Clin Oncol 1984;2:545–549.
72. Arlin ZA, Ahmed T, Mittelman A, et al. A new regimen of amsacrine with high-dose cytarabine is safe and effective therapy for acute leukemia. J Clin Oncol 1987;5:371–375.
73. Herzig RH, Lazarus HM, Wolff SN, et al. High-dose cytosine arabinoside with and without anthracycline antibiotics for remission reinduction of acute nonlymphoblastic leukemia. J Clin Oncol 1985;3:992–997.
74. Tschopp L, von Fliedner VE, Sauter C, et al. Efficacy and clinical cross-resistance of a new combination therapy (AMSA/VP16) in previously treated patients with acute nonlymphocytic leukemia. J Clin Oncol 1986;4:318–324.
75. Skipper HE, Schabel FM, Wilcox WS. Experimental evaluation of potential anticancer agents. XXI. Scheduling of arabinosylcytosine to take advantage of its S-phase specificity against leukemic cells. Cancer Chemother Rep 1967;51:125–141.
76. Herzig RH, Wolff SN, Lazarus HM, et al. High-dose cytosine arabinoside for refractory leukemia. Blood 1983;62:361–369.
77. Kantarjian HM, Estey EH, Plunkett W, et al. Phase I–II clinical and pharmacologic studies of high-dose cytosine arabinoside in refractory leukemia. Am J Med 1986;81:387–394.
78. Forman SJ, Nademanee AP, O'Donnell MR, et al. High-dose cytosine arabinoside and daunomycin as primary therapy for adults with acute nonlymphoblastic leukemia: A pilot study. Semin Oncol 1985;12(suppl 3):114–116.
79. Hines JD, Mazza JJ, Oken MM, et al. High-dose cytosine arabinoside and mAMSA induction and consolidation in patients with previously untreated de novo acute nonlymphocytic leukemia: Phase I pilot study for the Eastern Cooperative Oncology Group. Semin Oncol 1985;12(suppl 3):117–119.
80. Herzig RH, Hines JD, Herzig GP, et al. Cerebellar toxicity with high-dose cytosine arabinoside. J Clin Oncol 1987;5:927–932.
81. Kantrowitz NE, Bristow MR. Cardiotoxicity of antitumor agents. Prog Cardiovasc Dis 1984;27:195–200.
82. Von Hoff DD, Layard MW, Busa P, et al. Risk factors for doxorubicin-induced congestive heart failure. Ann Intern Med 1979;91:710–717.
83. Torti FM, Bristow MR, Howes AE, et al. Reduced cardiotoxicity of doxorubicin delivered on a weekly schedule. Ann Intern Med 1983;99:745–749.
84. Harwood KV, Aisner J. Treatment of chemotherapy extravasation: Current status. Cancer Treat Rep 1984;68:939–945.
85. Dorr RT, Alberts DS, Stone A. Cold protection and heat enhancement of doxorubicin skin toxicity in the mouse. Cancer Treat Rep 1985;69:431–437.
86. Haskell CM. L-Asparaginase: Human toxicology and single agent activity in nonleukemic neoplasms. Cancer Treat Rep 1981;65(suppl 4):57–59.
87. Zubrod CG. The clinical toxicities of L-asparaginase in treatment of leukemia and lymphoma. Pediatrics 1970;45:555–559.
88. Santos GW, Kaizer H. Bone marrow transplantation in acute leukemia. Semin Hematol 1982;19:227–239.
89. Thomas ED, Storb R, Clift RA, et al. Bone-marrow transplantation. N Engl J Med 1975;292:832–843; 895–902.
90. Appelbaum FR, Buckner CD. Overview of the clinical relevance of autologous bone marrow transplantation. Clin Haematol 1986;15:1–18.
91. Beatty PG, Clift RA, Mickelson EM, et al. Marrow transplantation from related donors other than HLA-identical siblings. N Engl J Med 1985;313-765–771.
92. Zwann FE, Jansen J. Bone marrow transplantation in acute nonlymphoblastic leukemia. Semin Hematol 1984;21:36–42.
93. Champlin R, Gale RP. Bone marrow transplantation for acute leukemia: Recent advances and comparison with alternative therapies. Semin Hematol 1987;24:55–67.
94. Champlin RE, Ho WG, Gale RP, et al. Treatment of acute myelogenous leukemia. A prospective controlled trial of bone marrow transplantation versus consolidation chemotherapy. Ann Intern Med 1985;102:285–291.
95. Buckner CD, Clift RA. Marrow transplantation for acute lymphoblastic leukemia. Semin Oncol 1984;21:43–47.
96. Woods WG, Nesbit ME, Ramsay NKC, et al. Intensive therapy followed by bone marrow transplantation for patients with acute lymphocytic leukemia in second or subsequent remission: Determination of prognostic factors. Blood 1983;61:1182–1189.
97. Johnson FL, Thomas ED, Clark BS, et al. A comparison of marrow transplantation with chemotherapy for children with acute lymphoblastic leukemia in second or subsequent remission. N Engl J Med 1981;305:846–851.
98. Sullivan KM, Parkman R. The pathophysiology and treatment of graft-versus-host disease. Clin Hematol 1983;12:775–789.
99. Weiden PL, Sullivan KM, Flournoy N, et al. Antileukemic effect of graft versus host disease in human recipients of allogeneic marrow grafts. N Engl J Med 1979;304:1529–1533.
100. Meyers JD, Flournoy N, Thomas ED. Nonbacterial pneumonia after allogeneic marrow transplantation: A review of ten years' experience. Rev Infect Dis 1982;4:1119–1132.
101. Meyers JD, Flournoy N, Thomas ED. Risk factors for cytomegalovirus after human marrow transplantation. J Infect Dis 1986;153:478–488.
102. Lutz D. Immunotherapy of cancer: A critical review. Int J Clin Pharmacol Ther Toxicol 1983;21:118–129.
103. Hewlett JS, Chen T, Balcerzak SP. High rate of long-term survival in adult acute leukemia following ten-day chemotherapy (OAP) induction. Arch Intern Med 1985;145:1006–1012.
104. Carter PW. Monoclonal antibodies and the biological approach to cancer. J Biol Response Mod 1985;4:325–339.
105. Mule JJ, Ettinghausen SE, Spiess PJ, et al. Antitumor efficacy of lymphokine-activated killer cells and recombinant interleukin-2 in vivo: Survival benefit and mechanisms of tumor escape in mice undergoing immunotherapy. Cancer Res 1986;46:676–683.

# *Chapter 101* / Chronic Leukemia

Clinton F. Stewart, PharmD

Chronic leukemia is characterized by unregulated proliferation of mature, differentiated leukemic cells resulting in an elevated white cell count. Within the broad classification of chronic leukemias two general categories are recognized: chronic myelogenous leukemia (CML) and chronic lymphocytic leukemia (CLL). CML is also referred to as chronic granulocytic leukemia. In this chapter, we discuss only CML and CLL; the reader is referred to excellent reviews for more information about other forms of chronic leukemia.[1–5]

Unlike the acute leukemias, where much progress has been made in the area of therapy, progress in the area of treatment for chronic leukemia has been poor; however, there have been major advances in the understanding of the biology of these diseases that may ultimately be translated into improved treatment and increased survival.[5]

## Chronic Myelogenous Leukemia

CML is a disease of unknown etiology characterized by an abnormality in the hematopoietic stem cell pool.[6] This abnormality results in a marked increase in proliferating granulocytes and megakaryocytes and, usually, an impairment in erythropoiesis. The increased granulopoiesis is not due to an accelerated proliferative rate as measured by doubling time or labeling index. Instead, the disease is characterized by a massive expansion of the pools of committed myeloid progenitors.[7,8] Although a majority of the red blood cells, white blood cells, and platelets are derived from the leukemic cell clone, these cells are still able to carry out their physiologic functions.

### *Epidemiology*

It was expected that 25,600 new cases of leukemia would occur in 1986, half of which would be chronic leukemia.[9] Previous reports have indicated that CML constitutes 15% to 20% of all cases of leukemia reported in the United States.[10] The death rate has been reported to be 1 per 100,000 per year.[11,12] Incidence of disease and death rate have not changed in the last 25 years.

CML is a disease that affects middle-aged adults. The majority of patients are 25 to 60 years old; incidence peaks between the ages of 40 and 49. Between 50 and 80, there is little change in incidence.[13] As is the case with all types of leukemia, there is a slight male predominance with a male: female ratio of 1.3:1. The course of disease is the same regardless of sex. There is no evidence of case clustering or of case-to-case transmission of CML.

### *Pathophysiology*

Ionizing radiation enhances the likelihood of developing CML in a dose-related manner.[14] The only chemical that has been clearly identified as one that increases the incidence of CML in humans is heavy occupational exposure to benzene[15]; however, neither radiation nor chemical exposure alone can explain the observed incidence of CML. There are no data at present that support a viral etiology for CML.

CML is one of the few neoplasias that regularly show a chromosomal abnormality, the Philadelphia chromosome ($Ph^1$). In 1960, Nowell and Hungerford first described a small chromosome 22 ($Ph^1$) in myeloid cells from two patients with CML.[16] $Ph^1$ is an acquired or induced karyotypic abnormality that is present in 90% to 95% of cases of typical CML. The abnormal karyotype is also found in erythroid precursors and megakaryocytes, but the karyotype in somatic cells, fibroblasts, and the majority of lymphocytes is normal. This suggests that CML is a clonal disorder that has arisen from a single pluripotent hematopoietic stem cell.[17,18]

$Ph^1$-negative CML is rare[13] and is associated with a poor prognosis. Recently, the reported incidence of $Ph^1$-negative CML has decreased, which can be attributed in part to improved cytogenetic studies and stricter diagnostic criteria for CML.

In summary, $Ph^1$ is clinically significant because it allows better definition of CML and recognition of atypical disorders or neoplasms other than CML. More precise definition of the disease, and the resultant more homogeneous patient groups, will allow comparison of clinical and hematologic findings and therapeutic responses and enable the identification of prognostic factors.[6]

### *Clinical Presentation*

The clinical features of CML seen at diagnosis vary with the stage of disease. Patients with CML usually present one of two ways. First, a patient may present with nonspecific signs and symptoms that are seen in many other diseases (see Table 101.1). As these signs and symptoms are nonspecific, the diagnosis of CML should not be made on the basis of clinical features alone.[19] Second, an asymptomatic patient with CML may be identified by an abnormal blood test during a routine physical.

The diagnosis of CML is based almost solely on a complete blood count with differential and examination of the bone marrow. Table 101.1 lists typical values for a complete blood count and differential for a patient with moderately advanced CML. Examination of the bone marrow usually shows granulocytic and often megakaryocytic hyperplasia.

**Table 101.1** Signs, Symptoms, and Laboratory Findings in Patients With Chronic Myelogenous Leukemia

| | | | |
|---|---|---|---|
| **Signs and Symptoms** | | | |
| Malaise | Dyspnea | | |
| Fatigue | Pallor | | |
| Heat intolerance | Weight Loss | | |
| Splenic enlargement | | | |
| **Laboratory** | | | |
| Hemoglobin (g/dL) | 9–12 (12–16)[a] | | |
| RBCs ($\times 10^6/\mu L$) | 3–4.5 (3.8–6) | | |
| Platelets ($\times 10^3/\mu L$) | 250–1,000 (150–440) | | |
| WBCs ($\times 10^3/\mu L$) | 50–250 (3.5–11) | | |
| **Differential White Blood Cell Count** (%)[13] | | | |
| Polymorphonuclear neutrophils | 20–35 (3–11) | Myeloblasts | 1–4 (0–5) |
| Nonsegmented bands | 25–30 (9–15) | Eosinophils | 3–4 (1–5) |
| Metamyelocytes | 10–18 (9–25) | Basophils | 4–5 (0–1) |
| Myelocytes | 10–20 (8–16) | Lymphocytes | 1–5 (11–23) |
| Promyelocytes | 2–4 (1–8) | Monocytes | 1–3 (0–1) |

[a] Normal range is given in parentheses.

The proportion of cells at each level of maturation is approximately normal.

Increased production of uric acid with hyperuricosuria and hyperuricemia occurs in untreated CML. These patients have adapted to the increased load of uric acid and may excrete two or three times the normal amount of uric acid. If aggressive therapy leads to rapid cell lysis, excretion of additional purine load may result in urinary tract obstruction.

### *Clinical Course*

Two distinct courses (or phases) characterize CML—chronic and acute. After a relatively benign chronic course, which lasts a median of 36 months, the disease will progress in the majority of patients to an accelerated phase ultimately leading to an acute phase. The most prominent feature of the acute phase of CML is the relative ineffectiveness of current treatment modalities.[11,12] Table 101.2 lists the characteristics of the acute course of CML. Although chemotherapy can control the signs and symptoms of the chronic phase of CML, the disease uniformly metamorphoses into an accelerated phase. It is important for the reader to distinguish between this phase and the more commonly known "blast crisis" phase of CML.[20]

**Table 101.2** Characteristics of the Acute Course of Chronic Myelogenous Leukemia

- Accelerated phase
  - Anemia and thrombocytopenia present during the chronic phase worsen
  - The number of basophils increases
  - Spleen size increases and splenic infarctions are more common
  - Fever and bone pain may be present
  - Extramedullary myeloblastic tumors may develop in skin, paranasal sinuses, or epidural space
- Blast phase
  - Disease develops into an acute myelogenous leukemia
  - Blast cells in marrow increase markedly
  - Severe cytopenias develop

In the most severe form of metamorphosis the disease may rapidly develop into a picture of acute leukemia, or the blast crisis phase, although there is no specific sequence of phases. The clinical symptoms and hematologic picture for a patient in blast crisis and a patient in the accelerated phase are similar. The patient in blast crisis may have more symptoms, depending upon the severity of the hematologic picture (see Table 101.2). In the blast phase, cells no longer differentiate as they did in the chronic phase of CML. In general, blast crisis can be divided into two general forms, lymphoid and myeloid, although erythroid and megakaryocytic variants of blast crisis also occur. Approximately 70% of patients in blast crisis have blast cells with myeloid characteristics and 30% have lymphoid blast cells.

Although various staging systems have been proposed, no system is currently accepted for classification of CML.[21] Thus, plans for treatment and estimates of prognosis based on clinical and hematologic parameters determined at the time of diagnosis cannot be made. Furthermore, the lack of an accepted staging system makes comparisons of survival estimates among various treatment regimens difficult.

### *Treatment*

The two major objectives of therapy are to postpone the onset of blast crisis and to control the signs and symptoms associated with the disease. These are usually accomplished by controlling abnormal white cell proliferation with as much selectivity as possible. No study has determined the exact extent of control of the white blood cell count that is optimal for CML.

At present there is no chemotherapy regimen that can "cure" CML. With the exception of bone marrow transplantation, none of the numerous efforts to eradicate the malignant clone from bone marrow cells have been successful.[22–24] Thus, although a patient may respond or achieve "clinical remission" (i.e., reduction of blood counts to normal range and control of signs and symptoms), Ph[1]-positive cells persist in the bone marrow of most patients. Although the survival duration for patients receiving chemotherapy is the same as for untreated patients, the true impact of chemotherapy on the survival duration in CML is difficult to assess accurately because of the lack of prospective, randomized trials of no therapy versus chemotherapy.[25]

As compared with the acute leukemias, CML rarely requires any emergency therapy. The only potentially life-threatening complication that might require immediate therapy is hyperleukocytosis. If the initial white blood cell count is greater than 200,000 and symptoms exist, leukapheresis is combined with transfusion of packed red blood cells (to replace volume). At the same time, treatment with allopurinol (300 mg/m$^2$/d) and hydroxyurea (1,000 mg/m$^2$ every 8 hours) is begun. If the white blood count falls below 100,000 and symptoms abate, the leukapheresis is discontinued and chemotherapy is continued.

### Chronic Phase

***Chemotherapy*** Numerous chemotherapeutic agents have been used to treat patients with chronic-phase CML. Table 101.3 summarizes the commonly used chemotherapeutic regimens. At present, the major chemotherapeutic agents used to treat CML are busulfan and hydroxyurea.

Busulfan was one of the first chemotherapeutic agents used successfully in CML, and still leads to normalization of blood counts in about 90% of patients in the chronic phase.[30] A typical dosage regimen for busulfan is presented in Table 101.3. Once the white blood cell count is reduced, therapy can gradually be tapered and stopped until the count begins to rise again. Maintenance therapy with busulfan has not been reported to affect survival once a patient has achieved a response.

Hydroxyurea is frequently used when rapid reduction of white cell and platelet counts is desired. After a "clinical remission" is achieved, maintenance dosing (i.e., 20 mg/kg) is recommended to avoid recurrent leukocytosis. This dose may have to be increased gradually to maintain control of the white cell count. The dosage regimen for hydroxyurea is also presented in Table 101.3.

As summarized in Table 101.3, other drugs have been used with varying degrees of success to treat chronic-phase CML. None of these agents has proved superior to busulfan, but they do have therapeutic advantages in select patients. For example, the effect of melphalan on platelets may be particularly beneficial in patients with severe thrombocytosis and a relatively low white cell count.[6] Leukocyte interferon has been shown to be effective in chronic-phase CML. Interferon has antiproliferative activity and also affects cellular differentiation.[31] Another innovative approach to therapy for chronic-phase CML is the clinical use of agents (e.g., retinoids) to induce cellular differentiation in vitro in an attempt to prevent or delay the development of blast crisis.[22]

More intensive chemotherapy regimens have been used to prolong the chronic phase and to prevent the onset of the accelerated and blast phases (see Table 101.4); however, because these regimens have been unable to eradicate the clone of Ph[1]-positive leukemic cells or prolong median survival, this treatment modality cannot be routinely recommended.

***Surgery*** The rationale for splenectomy in patients with CML is based on the observation that blastic transformation may originate in the spleen.[38] To date, there are no convincing data to show that splenectomy prolongs the chronic phase of CML, increases survival, or enhances the response to chemotherapy. Splenectomy should be reserved for patients with painful splenomegaly or hypersplenism associated with life-threatening anemia or thrombocytopenia.

***Radiotherapy*** Splenic radiotherapy was considered an effective form of treatment prior to the advent of chemotherapy and busulfan. Currently, radiation is rarely used, except

**Table 101.3** Summary of Chemotherapeutic Regimens Commonly Used to Treat Chronic Myelogenous Leukemia

| *Agent* | *Regimen*[a] | *Response rate* |
|---|---|---|
| Busulfan[26] | Start with 2–4 mg/d for approximately 3 wk; if WBC count has not decreased, dose can be increased to 4–6 mg/d and continued for another 3 wk<br>Once WBC count falls below 20,000, stop busulfan<br>Pulse doses may be necessary to control WBC count | 41 |
| Hydroxyurea[27] | Start with 1,000 mg orally every 8 h; cut dose in half when the WBC count falls below 20,000 and then again when the WBC count is less than 10,000<br>Maintenance dosage is 500–2,000 mg/d | 43–50 |
| Other alkylating agents[28,29] | Melphalan 0.25 mg/kg/d for 4–7 d, repeated at 4- to 6-wk intervals<br>Dibromomannitol 250 mg/d, decreased to 250 mg given every 2 to 3 d | 29–43 |

[a] Also begin allopurinol 300 mg/d.

**Table 101.4** Summary of Studies Designed to Prevent the Onset of the Accelerated and Blast Phases

| *Treatment*[a] | *Number of patients* | *Median survival (mo)* |
|---|---|---|
| HU + MY alternating monthly | | |
| With splenectomy[32] | 56 | 50 |
| Without splenectomy[32] | 83 | 50 |
| MY vs HU[33] | 55 | 41 (MY)<br>57 (HU)[c] |
| MY vs HU[34,b] | 44 | 41 (MY)<br>150 (HU)[d] |
| Splenic RT ± HU; splenectomy + DAT × 3, Ara-C + HU; Ara-C + MTX; Ara-C + TG; Ara-C + VCR + CTX + Pred + DAT[35,36] | 37 | 50 (34 mo in 27 patients with no reduction in Ph[1]-positive cells; 7 yr in 12 patients with significant reduction; older patients excluded from study) |
| ROAP[37] | | 52 |

[a] HU, hydroxyurea; MY, busulfan; Ara-C, cytosine arabinoside; VCR, vincristine; Pred, prednisone, DAT, daunorubicin/cytosine/arabinoside/thioguanine; MTX, methotrexate; CTX, cyclophosphamide; TG, 6-thioguanine.
[b] Retrospective study.
[c] Not significant.
[d] $P < 0.001$.

Adapted from Wiernik PH: The current status of therapy for and prevention of blast crisis of chronic myelogenous leukemia. J Clin Oncol 1984;2:333, with permission.

for granulocytic sarcomas of soft tissue, brain, and paranasal sinuses, and osseous involvement that may require localized radiation therapy.

**Accelerated Phase and Blast Crisis**

The clinical management of the accelerated phase is different from that of the blastic phase. Many patients in the accelerated phase of CML may have a relatively indolent disease process, and conservative management is recommended.[13]

The current treatment for blast crisis is poor. Only a few new agents—vindesine, razoxane, mitoxantrone, and 5-azacytidine—have shown enough activity to prompt additional clinical trials.[23] Description of the lymphoid blast cell on only a morphologic basis, variability in the diagnosis of blast crisis, and lack of a uniform definition of complete response make evaluation of the results of studies describing the treatment of blast crisis difficult.

The results of selected clinical trials of the treatment of blast crisis are summarized in Table 101.5. A major advance in blast crisis treatment is the recognition that 50% to 60% of patients with lymphoid blast cells respond to a regimen of vincristine (2 mg intravenously each week) and prednisone (usually 60 mg/m$^2$ orally daily).[6] Most clinicians agree that treatment should be continued at least 2 or 3 weeks before the patient is considered a treatment failure. The duration of remission is often brief (usually 5–7 months, with less than 20% alive at 1 year) and maintenance therapy is usually ineffective.[46]

**Table 101.5** Treatment of Blast Crisis Phase in Chronic Myelogenous Leukemia

| *Regimen*[a] | *Number of patients* | *Median survival (mo)* | |
|---|---|---|---|
| | | **Responder** | **Nonresponder** |
| VCR/Pred[24,39–41,b] | >40 | 7 | 5 |
| TRAMPCOL[42] | 19 | 7 | — |
| Ara-C + anthracycline (and other agents)[43,44] | >100 | 4–6 | 2–3 |
| VP-16 + 5-AZA[45] | 27 | 7.5 | 1.5 |

[a] VCR, vincristine; Pred, prednisone; TRAMPCOL, 6-thioguanine, daunorubicin, cytarabine, methotrexate, prednisone, cyclophosamide, vincristine, L-asparaginase; Ara-C, cytarabine; VP-16, etoposide; 5-AZA, 5-azacytidine.
[b] Complete remission: lymphoid type, 60%; myeloid type, 0%–18%.

In patients with myeloid blast crisis, the use of vincristine and prednisone to induce remission is not usually effective. Instead, these patients, similar to those with acute nonlymphocytic leukemia, usually are treated with intensive combination chemotherapy. Unfortunately, less than 30% of patients achieve remission, and remissions are usually brief. Because these aggressive regimens are associated with significant toxic effects, many patients, especially patients with a low performance status, experience morbidity and even mortality as a result of the therapy. A number of clinical trials are now evaluating less toxic palliative regimens for patients with acute-phase CML. Many of these regimens include hydroxyurea, 6-mercaptopurine, and prednisone and can be administered on an outpatient basis. This approach is unlikely to induce complete remission, but may result in survival comparable with that for more intensive chemotherapy.[19]

**Bone Marrow Transplantation**

The lack of improved survival for patients with CML during the last several decades has prompted investigators to pursue new avenues of treatment. One very promising approach to restore normal hematopoiesis is bone marrow transplantation (BMT).[47] The sources of stem cells used for bone marrow transplantation include autologous (obtained from the patient during the chronic phase), syngeneic (from an identical twin), or allogeneic (usually from a HLA-identical sibling). To perform a transplant using autologous stem cells, large amounts of bone marrow cells are collected from patients during the chronic phase of the disease. When the disease enters the acute or blast phase the patient is subjected to intensive "marrow-ablative" chemoradiotherapy. Then, the cryopreserved cells are reinfused; however, because $Ph^1$-positive cells are reinfused, patients usually relapse within 4 months and less than 20% to 30% survive 1 year.[5] In a recent review, Champlin and Golde stated that autologous bone marrow transplantation is marginally beneficial and cannot routinely be recommended.[22]

The use of syngeneic or allogeneic bone marrow transplantation in patients with CML is much more encouraging. The goal in this approach is to eradicate $Ph^1$ with intensive chemoradiotherapy, and then restore hematopoiesis with cells from a normal donor. Syngeneic or allogeneic bone marrow transplantation done during the chronic phase results in a disease-free survival of 3 to greater than 5 years in approximately 50% to 70% of patients. These results are significantly better than those for transplantation done during the acute phase, where approximately 10% to 30% survived 3 to 7 years without recurrence. The major side effects of this treatment approach are graft-versus-host disease (only in allogeneic bone marrow transplantation) and interstitial pneumonitis.

Recent studies suggest that transplantation early in the chronic phase provides the best chance for long-term survival[48]; however, this potential benefit must be weighed against the possible risks of such a procedure and the fact that many patients can be maintained with relatively nontoxic chemotherapy in the chronic phase for months before the onset of the acute phase. At present, none of the currently identified prognostic features of CML (see Table 101.6) allow prediction of the onset of the acute phase.[49,50]

**Table 101.6** Prognostic Features in Philadelphia Chromosome–Positive Chronic Myelogenous Leukemia

| *Factors known at diagnosis* | *Factors known after initial therapy* |
|---|---|
| Spleen size | Response of WBC count to treatment |
| Hemoglobin | Cytogenetic analysis |
| Liver size | Myelofibrosis |
| WBC count | Cytokinetic studies |
| Platelet count | |

Compiled from References 49 and 50.

## Chronic Lymphocytic Leukemia

Chronic lymphocytic leukemia (CLL) is a disease in which malfunctioning lymphocytes progressively accumulate in bone marrow, blood, lymph nodes, and sometimes tissues. CLL is typically a clonal disorder of the B lymphocyte, although T-cell CLL may also occur. Special marker studies may serve to distinguish the CLL population from other lymphocytes. Variability in presenting symptoms, physical findings, progress of the disease, and response to therapy has hindered complete understanding of the natural history of CLL and evaluation of the efficacy of therapeutic management.

### *Epidemiology*

CLL is the most common leukemia in the United States. Like CML, CLL occurs more often in men than women (2:1 to 3:1), but black and white populations are equally affected. The median age of onset is in the sixties. Incidence increases markedly with advancing age. The reported age-adjusted incidence for men at ages 50 to 54 is 2.7 per 100,000. This increases to 53 per 100,000 at age 85 and older. CLL is uncommon before the age of 30. A familial tendency, as well as concordance in several identical twins, has been suggested, but no pattern of inheritance has been reported.[51]

### *Pathophysiology*

In contrast to CML, ionizing radiation has not been shown to play a role in the etiology of CLL. This disease is considered to result from monoclonal expansion of B cells; thus, an infectious etiology, in which many cell lines would be affected, seems unlikely. As with other forms of cancer, an interaction between heredity and environment may be required.[52]

*Lymphocyte* is now known to be a general term that describes many different subsets of cells. Recognition of these different subsets has allowed investigators to classify CLL as four major leukemic disorders: B-cell CLL (the classic type), T-cell CLL, prolymphocytic leukemia, and malignant lymphoma leukemia. The major features of B- and T-cell CLL are listed in Table 101.7. About 95% of the cases of CLL demonstrate leukemic lymphocytes, the phenotype of which is that of a B lymphocyte.[53] (The reader is referred

**Table 101.7** Features of the Two Major Forms of Chronic Lymphocytic Leukemia

| *Feature* | *B-cell* | *T-cell* |
|---|---|---|
| Age at diagnosis | >40 | Any |
| Male:female ratio | 2:1 | 1:1 |
| Peripheral lymphadenopathy | Common | Rare |
| Splenomegaly | Frequent | Usually large |
| Skin lesions | Rare | Common |
| Lymphocyte count | >10,000 | 3,000–300,000 |
| Immunologic markers | IgM, IgD | None |
| Response to therapy | Very good | Partial, variable |
| Survival | Long, related to initial stage of disease | 6–12 mo |

Compiled from References 52 and 53.

to many recent reviews of the molecular biology of CLL for a more detailed discussion of the pathophysiology.[54–56])

The exact level of differentiation at which the leukemic lesion originates is unknown. Despite a dominant phenotypic expression of B-cell markers (e.g., surface immunoglobulin, complement receptors, etc.) a large number of CLL cells have a T-cell surface antigen present, suggesting that the CLL lesion is at the level of the common lymphopoietic progenitor cell.[12]

The ratio of helper/inducer T cells to suppressor T cells is lower in patients with CLL (< 2) than in normal patients (~ 2). The decreased ratio is attributed to the increased proportion of suppressor T cells. It has been suggested that the excessive suppressor activity observed may limit the immunoglobulin response of residual normal B cells in CLL, eventually leading to hypogammaglobulinemia. In the later stages of the disease, T-cell function may be depressed by large accumulations of B cells or by an intrinsic defect.[52]

The toxic effects of the massive accumulation of lymphocytes in the marrow indirectly impair normal hematopoietic cell development, resulting in anemia, neutropenia, and thrombocytopenia. As mentioned before, hypogammaglobulinemia is present in 50% to 75% of patients, and becomes more severe as the disease progresses. Neutropenia combined with hypogammaglobulinemia predisposes CLL patients to infection (especially with encapsulated organisms), which accounts for about one half of deaths in these patients.[57]

### *Clinical Presentation*

The earliest clinical manifestations of CLL generally are insidious onset of fatigue and reduced exercise tolerance, weight loss, or abdominal discomfort or distension from organomegaly. Physical findings include enlargement of lymph nodes, splenomegaly, and hepatomegaly; occasionally, nodular skin infiltrates or other cutaneous lesions occur.[58] A large proportion of the patients are asymptomatic at diagnosis, and the disorder is discovered during a routine physical examination.

The characteristic finding in CLL is a persistently increased number of immature or abnormal lymphocytes in the peripheral blood. The total white blood cell count at diagnosis ranges from 15,000 to 200,000 per milliliter, with 70% to 90% lymphocytes. These lymphocytes are generally small with scant cytoplasm, although large lymphocytes are occasionally observed. Upon light microscopy, CLL lymphocytes appear mature and are indistinguishable from normal lymphocytes, except that they tend to smudge on slides (and are often referred to as "smudge cells") and seem to be more fragile than normal lymphocytes.[52]

Bone marrow examination is usually not necessary to establish a diagnosis of CLL, but aspiration and needle biopsies are often performed to confirm the diagnosis or to evaluate the need for therapy. The marrow aspirate or biopsy demonstrates a diffuse infiltration with small, well-differentiated lymphocytes. These cells account for 25% to 90% of the marrow nucleated cells.[59]

Red blood cell and platelet counts are generally reduced at diagnosis, which can be attributed to bone marrow infiltration, hypersplenism, or autoimmune mechanisms. Approximately 10% to 20% of patients with CLL develop a Coombs-positive test, but only half of these have an autoimmune hemolytic anemia. Conversely, in some patients with clinically apparent immune hemolytic anemia, both direct and indirect Coombs' tests may be negative.[10] Thrombocytopenia may also be caused by an autoimmune mechanism, but antiplatelet antibodies usually cannot be demonstrated.[52]

In contrast to CML and the Philadelphia chromosome, there is no characteristic chromosomal abnormality in CLL. Routine chemistries are normal except for an occasional increased level of lactic dehydrogenase.

### *Staging/Prognosis*

A major problem in the clinical management of CLL is determination of the optimal therapeutic strategy for each patient. One approach is to classify or stage patients on the basis of certain clinical features. Table 101.8 summarizes two systems that have been proposed. The major limitation to both systems is that even though subgroups have been proposed, no staging system has been prospectively validated in a clinical trial.[60]

### *Treatment*

Evaluation of results from therapeutic trials in patients with CLL is complicated by the lack of uniform response criteria. Response to therapy for any leukemia is generally defined as normalization of white blood cell count and differential, hemoglobin, platelet count, and bone marrow aspirate and biopsy, and improvement of signs and symptoms (e.g., resolution of enlarged lymph nodes, spleen, or liver). These subjective criteria describe only a complete clinical response and not a complete remission (or an absence of leukemic cells). Other more objective indicators of complete remission have been proposed, but thus far, there are no uniformly accepted criteria. The definition of partial response has also varied between studies.

It is not clear when to initiate treatment in patients with CLL, particularly those who have no or mild symptoms (stage I or II).[57] Despite marked increases in lymphocyte

**Table 101.8** Clinical Staging Criteria Used in Rai and Binet Procedures

| *Stage* | *Rai* | *Binet* |
|---|---|---|
| 0 | Blood and marrow lymphocytosis | Same |
| 1 | Lymphocytosis + lymphadenopathy, no splenomegaly | Same |
| 2 | Lymphocytosis + splenomegaly or hepatomegaly (with or without lymph nodes) | Lymphocytosis + splenomegaly (without lymph node enlargement) |
| 3 | Lymphocytosis + anemia (Hb < 11 g/dL) | Stage 1 + stage 2 |
| 4 | Lymphocytosis + thrombocytopenia (platelet count < 100,000/mm$^3$) | Lymphocytosis with anemia (Hb < 10 g/dL) or thrombocytopenia (platelet count < 100,000/mm$^3$) |

Adapted from Skinnider LF, Tan L, Schmidt J, et al: G: Chronic lymphocytic leukemia. A review of 745 cases and assessment of clinical staging. Cancer 1982;50:2952, with permission.

counts in the blood and marrow, and moderate lymph node and splenic enlargement, many patients maintain adequate numbers of red blood cells, neutrophils, and platelets. Most clinicians start cytotoxic drug therapy in patients with active disease (stage III or IV), if anemia, thrombocytopenia, hypermetabolism, or symptomatic lymph node or spleen enlargement is present.

***Radiotherapy*** Total-body irradiation is reported to have improved symptoms, physical signs, peripheral blood counts, and bone marrow infiltration in a study of selected patients with advanced disease[61]; however, because of the toxic effects observed and the specialized nature of this treatment modality, total-body irradiation has limited usefulness.

Local radiation is very effective in controlling symptoms resulting from enlarged lymph nodes or bone lesions. Splenic irradiation has also been used to treat painful splenomegaly, progressive lymphoytosis, anemia, and thrombocytopenia. Mediastinal irradiation has shown beneficial effects, but with a high incidence of toxicity.[62]

***Single-Agent Chemotherapy*** Chlorambucil is the alkylating agent most frequently used in the treatment of CLL.[63] The dosage schedule, monitoring criteria, and response rates are listed in Table 101.9. In addition to daily administration, chlorambucil can be administered on an intermittent schedule, which may cause less hematologic toxicity.[65] Cyclophosphamide is considered as effective as chlorambucil in the treatment of CLL and can be given intravenously as well as orally (see Table 101.9). Busulfan also has activity in CLL but less than that of chlorambucil or cyclosphosphamide.[10]

Steroids are used as single agents or in combination chemotherapy regimens.[71] A clear indication for the use of steroids is the presence of Coombs' test–positive hemolytic anemia or immune thrombocytopenia. In some patients, initial chemotherapy is begun with a short course of steroids, followed by an alkylating agent either alone or combined with steroids. Their well-known side effects must be considered when steroids are used to treat patients with CLL.

***Combination Chemotherapy*** As indicated in Table 101.9, the combination of a steroid and an alkylating agent may yield a small increase in the response rate compared with a single-agent alkylating agent. Although this combination is widely used clinically, its superiority in terms of increased response rate has not been proven in a large prospective randomized trial.

Other combination chemotherapy regimens that have been used are summarized in Table 101.9. These regimens are generally reserved for patients with advanced-stage disease or those patients who are refractory to other therapeutic approaches. The morbidity and mortality are greater with these regimens than with alkylator therapy with or without steroids. One major concern in the use of these combination chemotherapy regimens is the secondary development of acute myelogenous leukemia.[57]

***Other Therapeutic Modalities*** Although splenectomy has been useful in the management of hemolytic anemia, thrombocytopenia, pancytopenia, and painful splenomegaly, there is no curative role for splenectomy in CLL.[72] Leukapheresis also may be beneficial in select patients unresponsive to other therapies.[73] Two new promising therapeutic approaches to treatment of CLL are monoclonal antibodies and $\alpha$- and $\gamma$-interferon.[57]

## Summary

Although little progress has been made recently in the treatment of chronic leukemia, much progress has been made in understanding the molecular biology of these disorders. This knowledge can hopefully be translated into more effective and less toxic therapies capable of achieving selective eradication of malignant cells. With the improved supportive care now available, trials of more aggressive chemotherapy may be possible. Newer approaches such as the biologic therapies (i.e., interferons, monoclonal antibodies) and bone marrow transplantation may also prove useful in the treatment of chronic leukemias.

**Table 101.9** Summary of Chemotherapy Regimens Used to Treat Chronic Lymphocytic Leukemia

| ***Regimen***[a] | | ***Response rate***[b] |
|---|---|---|
| Single agent | | |
| Chlorambucil | Start with 0.1–0.2 mg/kg/d until disease responds or toxic effects occur; then reduce dose or stop drug[64] | 45 |
| | Start with 0.4–0.6 mg/kg every 2–4 wk until disease responds or toxic effects occur; then reduce dose or stop drug[65] | 60 |
| Cyclophosphamide | Start with 2–3 mg/kg/d or 20 mg/kg every 2–3 wk[66] | 40 |
| Combination | | |
| Chlorambucil | Start with 0.6 mg/kg on day 1 and every 28 d thereafter; prednisone 0.8 mg/kg/d for 2 wk, then 0.4 mg/kg/d for 2 wk, then stop[67] | 50 |
| COP[68,69] | Repeat cycle every three weeks:<br>CTX 400 mg/m$^2$/d PO days 1–5<br>VCR 1.4 mg/m$^2$ (max dose 2 mg) IV<br>Pred 100 mg/m$^2$/d PO | 68 |
| M-2[70] | Repeat cycle every 6 wk<br>Day 1<br>VCR 1 mg/m$^2$ (max 2 mg) IV, BCNU 0.5 mg/kg IV (or CCNU PO), CTX 10 mg/kg IV, melphalan 0.25 mg/kg/d PO × 4 d, Pred 1 mg/kg/d PO<br>Day 7<br>Pred 0.5 mg/kg/d<br>Day 14<br>Pred stopped | 61 |

[a] VCR, vincristine; Pred, prednisone; CTX, cyclophosphamide; BCNU, carmustine; ADR, adriamycin.

[b] Response expressed as total remissions (partial + complete).

Compiled from References 57 and 58.

## References


1. Miescher PA, Farquet JJ. Chronic myelomonocytic leukemia in adults. Semin Hematol 1974;11:129–139.
2. Golomb HM, Catovsky D, Golde DW. Hairy cell leukemia—A clinical review based on 71 cases. Ann Intern Med 1978;89:677–683.
3. Greenberg PL. The smoldering myeloid leukemic states: Clinical and biologic features. Blood 1983;61:1035–1044.
4. Jansen J, den Ottolander GJ, Schuit HRE, et al. Hairy cell leukemia: Its place among the chronic B cell leukemias. Semin Oncol 1984;11:386–393.
5. Champlin R, Gale RP, Foon KA, et al. Chronic leukemias: Oncogenes, chromosomes, and advances in therapy. Ann Intern Med 1986;104:671–688.
6. Hellriegel KP. Management of chronic myelogenous leukemia and blastic crisis. Recent Results Cancer Res 1984;93:259–268.
7. Chervenick PA, Boggs DR. Granulocyte kinetics in chronic myelocytic leukemia. Semin Hematol 1968;1:24.
8. Galbraith PR, Abu-Zahra HT. Granulopoiesis in chronic granulocytic leukaemia. Br J Haematol 1972;22:135.
9. American Cancer Society. 1986 Cancer Facts and Figures. New York, American Cancer Society, 1986.
10. Koeffler HP, Golde DW. Chronic leukemia, in Haskell CM (ed): Cancer Treatment. Philadelphia, W.B. Saunders, 1980;pp 832–852.
11. Liepman MK. The chronic leukemias. Med Clin North Am 1980;64:705–727.
12. Rundles RW. Chronic myelogenous leukemia, in Williams WJ, Beutler E, Erslev AJ, et al (eds): Hematology. New York, McGraw-Hill, 1983, pp 196–214.
13. Spiers ASD. Chronic granulocytic leukemia. Med Clin North Am 1984;68:713–727.
14. Moloney WC. Leukemia in survivors of atomic bombing. N Engl J Med 1955;253:88.
15. Vigliani EC, Saita G. Benzene and leukemia. N Engl J Med 1964;271:872.
16. Nowell PC, Hungerford DA. A minute chromosome in human chronic granulocytic leukemia. Science 1960;132:1497.
17. Fialkow PJ, Martin PJ, Najfeld V, et al. Evidence for a

multistep pathogenesis of chronic granulocytic leukemia. Blood 1981;58:158–163.
18. Gale RP, Cannani E. The molecular biology of chronic myelogenous leukaemia. Br J Haematol 1985;60:395–408.
19. Silver RT, Gale RP. Chronic myeloid leukemia. Am J Med 1986; 80:1137–1148.
20. Muehleck SD, McKenna RW, Arthur DC, et al. Transformation of chronic myelogenous leukemia: Clinical, morphologic, and cytogenetic features. Am J Clin Pathol 1984;82:1–14.
21. Goldman JM, Lu D. New approaches in chronic granulocytic leukemia–origin, prognosis, and treatment. Semin Hematol 1982;19:241–256.
22. Champlin RE, Golde DW. Chronic myelogenous leukemia: Recent advances. Blood 1985;65:1039–1047.
23. Clarkson B. Chronic myelogenous leukemia: Is aggressive treatment indicated. J Clin Oncol 1985.3:135–139.
24. Wiernik PH. The current status of therapy for and prevention of blast crisis of chronic myelogenous leukemia. J Clin Oncol 1984; 2:329–335.
25. Shimkin MB, Mettier SR, Bierman HR. Myelocytic leukemia: An analysis of incidence, distribution and fatality 1910–1948. Ann Intern Med 1951;35:194–212.
26. Haut A, Abbott WS, Wintrobe MM, et al. Busulfan in the treatment of chronic myelocytic leukemia: The effect of long term intermittent therapy. Blood 1961;17:1–19.
27. Kennedy BJ. Hydroxyurea therapy in chronic myelogenous leukemia. Cancer 1972;29:1052–1056.
28. Hauch T, Logue G, Laszlo J, et al. Treatment of chronic granulocytic leukemia with melphalan. Blood 1978;51:571–577.
29. Dibromomannitol Cooperative Study Group. Survival of chronic myeloid leukemia patients treated by dibromomannitol. Eur J Cancer 1973;9:583–589.
30. Galton DAG. Myleran in chronic myeloid leukaemia. Lancet 1953;1:208.
31. Talpaz M, McCredie K, Mavligit GM, et al. Leukocyte interferon–induced myeloid cytoreduction in chronic myelogenous leukemia. Blood 1983;62:689.
32. Baccarani M, Corbelli G, Tura S, et al. Early splenectomy and polychemotherapy versus polychemotherapy alone in chronic myeloid leukemia. Leuk Res 1981;5:149–157.
33. Lamar S, Sanjuan I, Zabala P, et al. Chronic myeloid leukemia. Clinical study and analysis of therapeutical results in 55 cases. Sangre (Barc) 1982;27:493–507.
34. Bolin RW, Robinson WA, Sutherland J, et al. Busulfan versus hydroxyurea in the long term therapy of chronic myelogenous leukemia. Cancer 1982;50:1683–1686.
35. Cunningham I, Gee T, Dowling M, et al. Results of treatment of $Ph^1$+ chronic myelogenous leukemia with an intensive treatment regimen (L-5 protocol). Blood 1979;53:375–395.
36. Goto T, Nishikoii M, Arlin Z, et al. Growth characteristics of leukemic and normal hematopoietic cells in $Ph^1$+ chronic myelogenous leukemia and effects of intensive treatment. Blood 1982;59:793–808.
37. Kantarjian HM, Vellekoop L, McCredie KB, et al. Intensive combination chemotherapy (ROAP 10) and splenectomy in the management of chronic myelogenous leukemia. J Clin Oncol 1985;3:192–200.
38. Wolf DJ, Silver RT, Coleman M. Splenectomy in chronic myeloid leukemia. Ann Intern Med 1978;89:684–689.
39. Rosenthal S, Canellos GP, DeVita VT, et al. Blast crisis of chronic granulocytic leukemia morphologic variants and therapeutic implications. Am J Med 1977;63:542.
40. Janossy G, Woodrugg RK, Pippard MJ, et al. Relation of "lymphoid" phenotype and response to chemotherapy incorporating vincristine–prednisone in the acute phase of $Ph^1$ positive leukemia. Cancer 1979;43:426.
41. Marks SM, Baltimore D, McCaffrey R. Terminal transferase as a predictor of initial responsiveness to vincristine and prednisone in blastic crisis myelogenous leukemia: A co-operative study. N Engl J Med 1978;298:812.
42. Spiers ASD, Goldman JM, Catovsky D, et al. Multiple-drug chemotherapy for acute leukemia: The TRAMPCOL regimen. Results in 86 patients. Cancer 1977;40:20.
43. Theologides A. Unfavorable signs in patients with chronic myelocytic leukemia. Ann Intern Med 1972;76:95.
44. Winton EF, Miller D, Vagler WR. Intensive chemotherapy with daunorubicin, 5-azacytidine, 6-thioguanine, and cytarabine (DATA) for the blastic transformation of chronic granulocytic leukemia. Cancer Treat Rep 1981;64:389.
45. Schiffer CA, DeBellis R, Kasdorf H, et al. Treatment of the blast crisis of chronic myelogenous leukemia with 5-azacytidine, and VP-16-213. Cancer Treat Rep 1982;66:267.
46. Lichtman MA, Segel GB. The leukemias, in Rubin P (ed): Clinical Oncology—For Medical Students and Physicians—A Multidisciplinary Approach. Rochester, NY, American Cancer Society, 1983, pp 370–390.
47. Speck B, Gratwhol A, Osterwalder B, et al. Bone marrow transplantation for chronic myeloid leukemia. Semin Hematol 1984;21:48–52.
48. Thomas ED, Clift RA, Fefer A, et al. Marrow transplantation for the treatment of chronic myelogenous leukemia. Ann Intern Med 1986;104:155–163.
49. Medical Research Council's Working Party for Therapeutic Trials in Leukemia. Randomized trial of splenectomy in $Ph^1$-positive chronic granulocytic leukaemia, including an analysis of prognostic features. Br J Haematol 1983;54:415–430.
50. Cervantes F, Rozman C. A multivariate analysis of prognostic factors in chronic myeloid leukemia. Blood 1982;60:1298–1304.
51. Bloomfield CD, Hurd DD, Peterson BA. Leukemias, in Calabresi P, Schein PS, Rosenberg SA (eds): Medical Oncology—Basic Principles and Clinical Management of Cancer. New York, Macmillan, 1986, pp 523–575.
52. Silber R. Chronic lymphocytic leukemia in the elderly. Hosp Pract 1982;17:131–141.
53. Frenkel EP. Clinical forms of chronic lymphocytic leukemia—implications for prognosis and therapy. Postgrad Med 1984;75: 101–110.
54. Caligaris-Cappio F, Janossy G. Surface markers in chronic lymphoid leukemias of B cell type. Semin Hematol 1985;22:1–12.
55. Foon KA, Schroff RW, Gale RP. Surface markers of leukemia and lymphoma cells: Recent advances. Blood 1982;60:1.
56. Theml H, Ziegler-Heitbrock HWL. Management of CLL and allied disorders with reference to their immunology and proliferation kinetics. Recent Results Cancer Res 1984;93:240–258.
57. Gale RP, Foon KA. Chronic lymphocytic leukemia. Recent advances in biology and treatment. Ann Intern Med 1985;103: 101–120.
58. Rai KR, Sawitsky A, Jagathambal K, et al. Chronic lymphocytic leukemia. Med Clin North Am 1984;68:697–711.
59. Rundles RW. Chronic lymphocytic leukemia, in Williams WJ, Beutler E, Erslev AJ, et al (eds): Hematology. New York McGraw-Hill, 1983, pp 981–999.
60. Skinnider LF, Tan L, Schmidt J, et al. Chronic lymphocytic leukemia. A review of 745 cases and assessment of clinical staging. Cancer 1982;50:2951–2955.

**61.** Byhardt RW, Brace KC, Wiernik PH. The role of splenic irradiation in chronic lymphocytic leukemia. Cancer 1976;35: 1621–1625.

**62.** Richards F, Spurr CL, Ferree C, et al. The control of chronic lymphocytic leukemia with mediastinal irradiation. Am J Med 1978;64:947–954.

**63.** Foon KA, Gale RP. Chronic lymphocytic leukemia, in Gale RP (ed): Leukemia Therapy. Boston, Blackwell Scientific, 1986, pp 165–181.

**64.** Han T, Ezdinli EZ, Shimaoka KS, et al. Chlorambucil vs. combined chlorambucil–corticosteroid therapy in chronic lymphocytic leukemia. Cancer 1973;31:502–508.

**65.** Knospe WH, Loeb V, Huguley CM. Bi-weekly chlorambucil treatment of chronic lymphocytic leukemia. Cancer 1974;33: 555–562.

**66.** Huguley CM. Treatment of chronic lymphocytic leukemia. Cancer Treat Rev 1977;4:261–273.

**67.** Sawitsky A, Rai KR, Glidewell O, et al. Comparison of daily versus intermittent chlorambucil and prednisone therapy in the treatment of patients with chronic lymphocytic leukemia. Blood 1977;50:1049.

**68.** Oken MM, Kaplan ME. Combination chemotherapy with cyclophosphamide, vincristine, and prednisone in the treatment of refractory chronic lymphocytic leukemia. Cancer Treat Rep 1979;63:441.

**69.** Liepman M, Votaw ML. The treatment of chronic lymphocytic leukemia with COP chemotherapy. Cancer 1978;41:1664.

**70.** Kempin BS, Lee BJ, Thaler HT, et al. Combination chemotherapy of advanced chronic lymphocytic leukemia: The M-2 protocol (vincristine, BCNU, cyclophosphamide, melphalan, and prednisone). Blood 1982;60:1110–1121.

**71.** Panesar NS, Bird CC, Roberts BE, et al. Prednisolone levels in plasma and leukemia cells during therapy of chronic lymphocytic leukemia. J Pharm Sci 1984;73:66–68.

**72.** Merl SA, Theodorakis ME, Goldberg J, et al. Splenectomy for thrombocytopenia in chronic lymphocytic leukemia. Am J Hematol 1983;15:253–259.

**73.** Marti GE, Folks T, Longo DL, et al. Therapeutic cytapheresis in chronic lymphocyte leukemia. J Clin Apheresis 1983;1:243–248.

# 5 Electrolyte and Nutritional Disorders

# Section One
# Fluid and Electrolyte Disorders

## Chapter 102 / Body Electrolyte Homeostasis

Nathan J. Schultz, PharmD, and David M. Angaran, MS

Electrolyte disorders are associated with many disease states and are thus frequently encountered in the acute care setting. A basic understanding of the pathophysiology of these disorders is necessary to determine etiology of, properly classify, and adequately treat these syndromes. As iatrogenic electrolyte disorders are not infrequent, it is important that the pharmacist be cognizant of the electrolyte content of medicinals as well as the drugs most frequently causing these disorders. In this chapter, we review the etiology, classification, symptomatology, and therapy of disorders of sodium, potassium, calcium, magnesium, and phosphorus homeostasis.

### Disorders of Sodium Homeostasis

Sodium metabolism and water metabolism are intimately coupled. Sodium is actively excluded from the intracellular milieu, creating an osmotic gradient that maintains water distribution between the intracellular fluid (ICF) and extracellular fluid (ECF). Sodium, accompanied by chloride and bicarbonate, accounts for more than 90% of the osmolality of the extracellular compartment, while potassium is the major osmotic force within the cell.[1]

The kidney has the remarkable ability to maintain body homeostasis over a wide range of dietary intake. A change in effective circulating volume promotes an afferent response from pressure receptors in the renal juxtaglomerular apparatus. This causes an efferent response in which glomerular filtration rate (GFR), aldosterone, oncotic pressure, adrenergic activity, renal hormones, and atrial natriuretic factor contribute to volume expansion through both water and sodium retention.[1] These processes result in the maintenance of adequate extracellular fluid volume.

The kidney possesses the ability to effectively conserve sodium even in the presence of markedly reduced intake. The patient placed on a 10-mEq sodium-restricted diet is capable of reducing urinary excretion to an equivalent amount in 3 to 4 days. This is in contrast to potassium where continued urinary loss occurs even in the presence of severe hypokalemia. A change in tonicity of only 1% to 2% stimulates the production of antidiuretic hormone (ADH), stimulating free water retention and normalization of tonicity (sodium concentration). The maintenance of an effective extracellular fluid volume, however, takes precedence over the control of tonicity. A decrease in effective circulating volume of 10% or greater will promote fluid retention despite concurrent hypotonic hyponatremia. This partially explains why a patient with hyponatremia and a decreased effective intravascular volume (e.g., congestive heart failure, CHF) continues to have a concentrated urine and poor free water excretion even within a severe edematous state.

The proper assessment of serum sodium requires recognition that the serum sodium concentration may bear no relationship to total body sodium content. The serum sodium concentration is equal to the amount of total body sodium divided by the amount of ECF water, with normal concentrations ranging from 135 to 145 mEq/L.[2] Hypernatremia and hyponatremia may be associated with conditions of high, low, or normal ECF water and high, low, or normal total body sodium. As sodium is the major determinant of ECF osmolality, disorders of sodium homeostasis result in disorders of plasma tonicity.

#### *Hyponatremia*

Hyponatremia (serum sodium < 135 mEq/L) is the most common electrolyte abnormality in hospitalized patients. In one study, hyponatremia was present in 15.2% of a hospitalized population.[3] In another study, the incidence of hyponatremia in a hospitalized population was reported as 0.97%, with a prevalence of 2.48%.[4] Thirty-three percent of these patients were hyponatremic on admission and 67% developed hyponatremia during their stay. The mortality of patients with hyponatremia was 60-fold greater than the mortality of those without, but was attributed to the progression of their underlying disease. Patient morbidity and mortality directly attributable to hyponatremia depend upon patient age, rate of fall of sodium concentration, absolute level of serum sodium, and concurrent disease states. Hyponatremia may serve as a marker for patients with a poor prognosis, but is not usually the direct cause of death.[4]

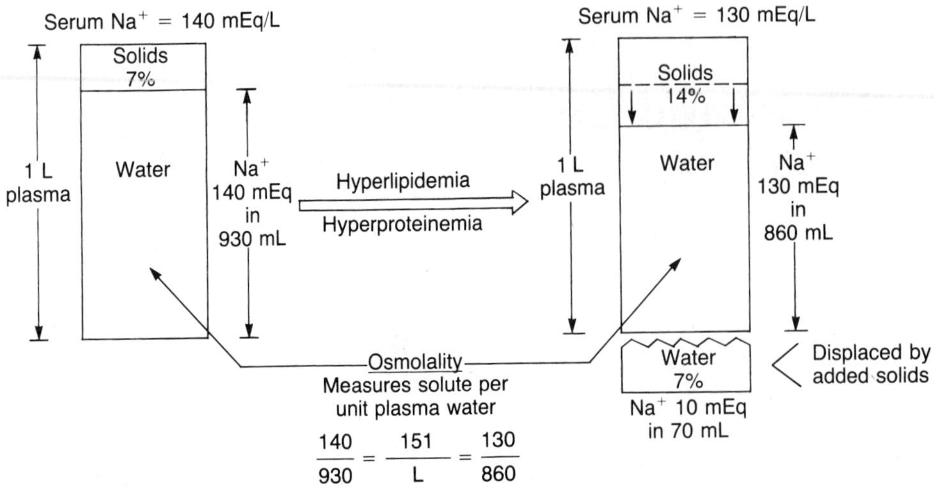


**Figure 102.1** Isotonic hyponatremia. The manner by which sodium-free lipid and protein displace sodium-rich serum water from each liter of serum; the concentration of sodium in remaining serum water is unchanged, but each liter of serum contains less water and sodium. *(From Narins RG, Lazarus JM: The renal system, in Vandam LD (Ed): To Make the Patient Ready for Anesthesia. Menlo Park, CA, Addison–Wesley, 1980, with permission.)*

### Etiology

***Isotonic Hyponatremia*** The first step in the proper assessment of hyponatremia is to measure serum osmolality. Hyponatremia associated with normal serum osmolality (isotonic hyponatremia) may be observed in patients with hyperlipidemia or hyperproteinemia. Sodium-free lipid or protein displaces sodium-rich serum water. While the concentration of sodium in serum water remains normal, the laboratory assessment assumes normal plasma solid content, resulting in a falsely decreased serum sodium concentration, termed pseudohyponatremia[5] (Fig. 102.1).

Isotonic hyponatremia may also occur during intravenous infusion of isotonic, sodium-free solutions. Initially, these solutions (e.g., glucose, mannitol, glycerol) are restricted to the intravascular space, where they dilute serum sodium and result in isotonic hyponatremia.[5] Hyponatremia caused by isotonic fluids is usually mild and readily reversible with the addition of sodium-containing fluids.

***Hypertonic Hyponatremia*** Hyponatremia in the presence of elevated serum osmolality suggests the presence of excess measured or unmeasured osmoles in the serum. This is most frequently encountered in the settings of hyperglycemia or the administration of hyperosmolar glycerin or mannitol solutions. These effective osmoles create an osmotic gradient between the isotonic ICF and the hyperosmolar ECF, drawing sodium-free water into the ECF, diluting the serum sodium, and resulting in hyponatremia.[5] The presence of a milliosmolar gap (measured mosm/L − calculated mosm/L > 10 mosm) suggests the presence of hyperosmolar compounds not normally measured and can hint at the cause of hyponatremia. Serum sodium falls by 1.6 mEq/L for each 100 mg/dL increase in blood glucose.[5]

***Hypotonic Hyponatremia*** The second step in determining the cause of hyponatremia is the clinical assessment of extracellular fluid volume. Hypotonic hyponatremia may be classified as (1) hypovolemic hyponatremia, (2) hypervolemic hyponatremia, or (3) isovolemic hyponatremia (Fig. 102.2).

*Hypovolemic hyponatremia* is associated with a deficit of ECF volume and sodium with a proportionally greater deficit of sodium than water. Replacement of sodium-rich fluid losses with sodium-free fluids results in hyponatremia. Hypovolemia is clinically detected by the presence of poor skin turgor, tachycardia, orthostatic hypotension, oliguria, and azotemia. The ECF volume contraction stimulates the activation of the renin–angiotensin, aldosterone, and ADH systems, and also changes certain aspects of renal hemodynamics.[6] In patients with extrarenal sodium losses, these changes result in a low urinary sodium concentration (<20 mEq/L). Sodium losses through the kidney are associated with high urinary sodium concentration (>20 mEq/L).[6] In all of these conditions, the hypovolemic state is associated with an impairment of water excretion as a result of the body's attempt to maintain volume even at the expense of tonicity.[6] Extrarenal causes include gastrointestinal and skin losses and third-spacing of plasma volume; renal causes include renal diseases, diuretic therapy, and adrenal insufficiency[5] (Table 102.1).

Diuretic-induced hypovolemic hyponatremia is one of the most common causes of drug-induced hyponatremia. Diuretic action causes a decrease in free water excretion by (1) blocking sodium reabsorption in the thick ascending loop of Henle, thereby decreasing the kidney's ability to dilute urine; (2) causing ECF volume depletion, which decreases sodium delivery to the proximal tubule and stimulates ADH secretion; (3) causing magnesium and potassium losses in the urine, which decreases renal sensitivity to ADH; and (4) causing urinary sodium excretion.[7] Diuretic-induced hyponatremia may have a quick onset, particularly in elderly females, and may occur as soon as 3 to 15 days after the start

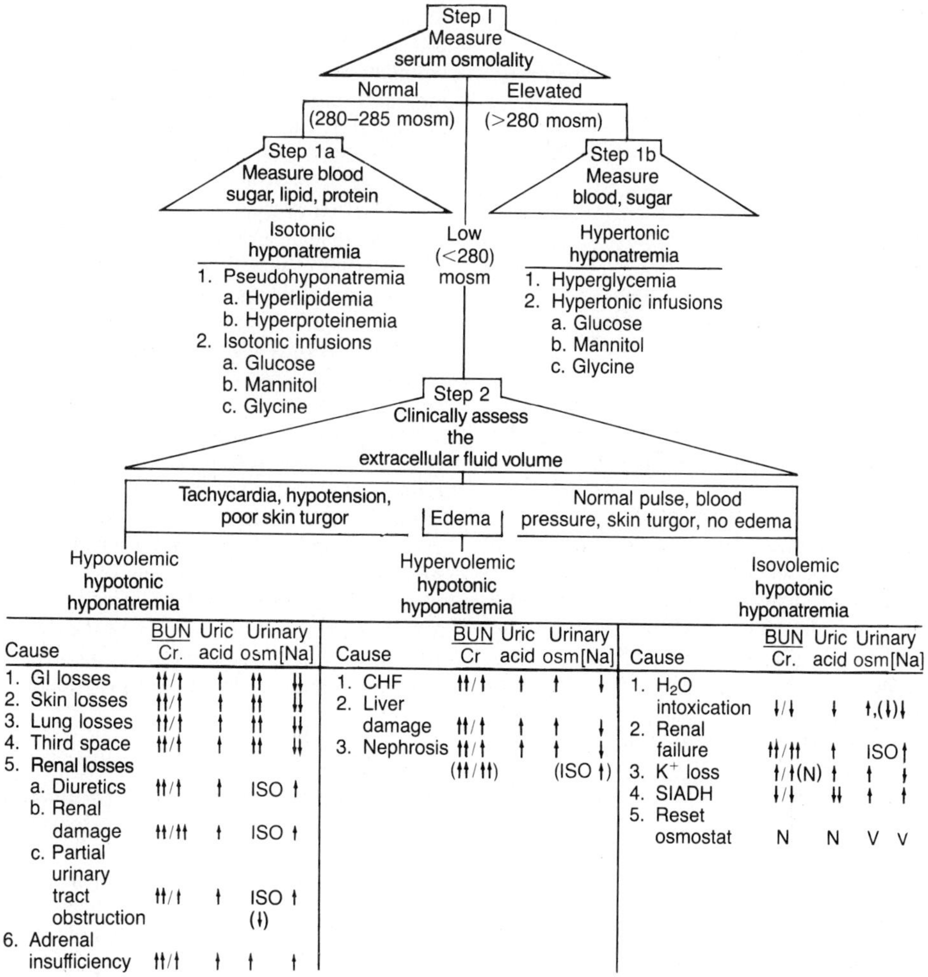


**Figure 102.2** Diagnostic approach to hyponatremia. Arrows indicate direction of change. Single and double arrows define the magnitude of change. Iso, isotonic; N, normal; V, variable. *(From Narins RG, Jones RE, Stom MC, et al: Diagnostic strategies and disorders of fluid, electrolyte and acid base homeostasis. Am J Med 1982;72:498, with permission.)*

of therapy. Diuretic-induced hyponatremia is commonly associated with hypokalemia as well.

*Isovolemic hyponatremia* is associated with a normal total body sodium content and with small increases in ECF volume. Fluid gains are usually no greater than 4–5 L, and evidence of edema is lacking because the excess water is distributed throughout total body water. In the setting of normal renal function, the body's ability to totally suppress ADH secretion can result in excretion of up to 14–28 L of free water in 24 hours.[8] Therefore, the retention of free water present in the setting of isovolemic hyponatremia is always the result of an imbalance of water intake and excretion.[5] Isovolemic hyponatremia is thus due to combinations of altered thirst, ADH secretion, and defective renal diluting mechanisms causing water retention and hyponatremia in patients who appear clinically envolemic. Conditions associated with isovolemic hyponatremia are listed in Table 102.2.

The most common cause of isovolemic hyponatremia is the syndrome of inappropriate antidiuretic hormone secretion (SIADH). SIADH is defined as a sustained or intermittently elevated level of ADH that is inappropriate in the face of osmotic and volume stimuli that normally inhibit ADH secretion.[6] SIADH has been found to be the most common cause of hyponatremia in hospitalized patients.[4] SIADH

**Table 102.1** Conditions Associated With Hypovolemic Hyponatremia

| |
|---|
| Extrarenal sodium loss |
| Gastrointestinal losses (vomiting, diarrhea, ostomy drainage, nasogastric suction) |
| Skin losses (sweating, burns) |
| Lung losses (bronchorrhea) |
| "Third-space" losses (pancreatitis, peritonitis, trauma, ileus) |
| Renal sodium loss |
| Diuretics |
| Adrenal insufficiency |
| Sodium-losing renal disease |
| Proximal renal tubular acidosis |

**Table 102.2** Conditions Associated With Isovolemic Hyponatremia

| |
|---|
| Rapid water administration |
| Water intoxication |
| Syndrome of inappropriate antidiuretic hormone secretion (SIADH) |
| Reset osmostat |
| Glucocorticoid deficiency |
| Severe hypokalemia |
| Renal disease |

may occur in a wide variety of clinical diseases (Table 102.3). Drugs are an important cause of SIADH and act by either (1) sensitizing the kidney to ADH or (2) stimulating the release of ADH[5] (Table 102.4).

*Hypervolemic hyponatremia* is associated with an elevated total body sodium content and an expanded ECF volume, clinically apparent as edema and weight gain. Diseases such as congestive heart failure and the hypoalbuminemic syndromes (cirrhosis, nephrotic syndrome, malnutrition, etc.) are associated with a decreased effective circulating plasma volume, resulting in secretion of renin, angiotensin, aldosterone, and ADH, causing sodium and water retention.[5] Even though total body sodium is elevated, the disproportionate accumulation of water results in hyponatremia. Hypervolemic hyponatremia is thus often termed *dilutional hyponatremia*.

### Clinical Presentation

In hypovolemic hyponatremia, most of the clinical manifestations are due to hypovolemia and not hypotonicity. In contrast, the hypotonicity associated with isovolemic and hypervolemic hyponatremia may result in symptoms. Symptoms of hypotonicity can be related to the development of cellular swelling, with CNS symptoms of cerebral edema and increased intracranial pressure being most severe. While the degree of hyponatremia appears to be related to the severity of symptoms, there is no consistent relationship.[8] The severity of symptoms is also a function of the rapidity of development of hyponatremia.

A decrease in serum sodium concentration from 140 to 130 mEq/L over a period of minutes to hours may be accompanied by moderate symptoms, such as bloating, headache, anorexia, muscle cramps, nausea, and vomiting.[6] A more dramatic decrease of greater than 10 mEq/L over a period of minutes to hours may be associated with more severe syndromes such as headache, lethargy, and disorientation which may progress to seizures and coma.[6] There is considerable overlap between serum sodium values and symptomatology; this may be partially related to the ECF volume status of the patient and its role in the development of cerebral edema. Patients with serum sodium concentrations of 115–120 mEq/L may be free of symptoms, particularly in chronic cases in which the hyponatremia developed slowly. While there is a wide overlap in the serum sodium concentration at which symptoms appear, the occurrence of seizures and coma carries grave prognostic significance.[6]

**Table 102.3** Disorders Associated With the Syndrome of Inappropriate Antidiuretic Hormone Secretion

| |
|---|
| Carcinomas |
| Lung |
| Duodenum |
| Pancreas |
| Pulmonary disorders |
| Viral pneumonia |
| Bacterial pneumonia |
| Pulmonary abscess |
| Tuberculosis |
| Aspergillosis |
| Central nervous system disorders |
| Encephalitis, viral or bacterial |
| Meningitis, viral, bacterial, or tuberculosis |
| Acute psychosis |
| Stroke (cerebral thrombosis or hemorrhage) |
| Acute intermittent porphyria |
| Brain tumors |
| Brain abscess |
| Subdural or subarachnoid hematoma or hemorrhage |
| Guillain–Barré syndrome |
| Head trauma |

### Treatment

The appropriate treatment of hyponatremia is dependent upon the correct classification of hyponatremia, severity of symptoms, concurrent disease states, ECF volume, rate of decline of serum sodium concentration, and degree of hyponatremia. Treatment begins with attention to possible reversible causes of hyponatremia and treatment of underlying disorders. Specific therapies are then determined by the type of hyponatremia present in the patient.

As hypovolemic hyponatremia is rarely associated with hypotonic symptoms, therapy is directed at replacing the sodium and volume losses with normal saline over a period of 6 to 12 hours.[6] It is rarely necessary to infuse hypertonic saline (3% or 5% NaCl), as isotonic saline corrects the pathophysiologic factors that lead to impaired free water excretion.[6] Ongoing sodium losses must be accounted for by appropriate maintenance fluid adjustments.

Isovolemic hyponatremia associated with nonacute reduction of serum sodium concentration to values not less than 115 mEq/L and an absence of symptoms may be treated by water restriction. Fluids are provided to allow for mandatory urinary solute excretion, allowing insensible water loss to correct the hyponatremia. As the kidney can concentrate urine up to an osmolality of 1,200 mosm/kg, and the average solute load excreted per day is 600 mosm, a minimum of 500 mL/d is necessary to meet obligatory urine excretion. Fluid restrictions of 500 mL/d or less may be necessary to correct hyponatremia. This is usually accomplished gradually over 3 to 5 days.[6]

Isovolemic hyponatremia resulting from chronic SIADH may require pharmacologic intervention in addition to water restriction. Demeclocycline, a tetracyline antibiotic, interferes with the action of ADH at the renal collecting duct, resulting in a nephrogenic diabetes insipidus–like picture. Demeclocycline is effective chronic therapy for isovolemic

**Table 102.4** Drugs Causing Hyponatremia

| *Drugs* | *Mechanism of action* Sensitize kidney to ADH | Stimulate release of ADH | Other | *Comments* |
|---|---|---|---|---|
| Hypoglycemic agents | | | | |
| Chlorpropamide | + | +(?) | | Hyponatremia found in 3% to 4% of patients taking chlorpropamide |
| Tolbutamide | + | | | Tolbutamide rarely causes hyponatremia |
| Antineoplastic drugs | | | | |
| Cyclophosphamide | | + | ? Direct ADH effect of cyclophosphamide metabolite | Cystitis and uric acid lithiasis demand $H_2O$ intake |
| Vincristine | | | | Associated with vincristine neurotoxicity |
| Sedatives | | | | |
| Barbiturates | | + | | |
| Morphine | | + | | |
| Psychotropic agents | | | | |
| Thioridazine | | | Thirst | SIADH associated with psychosis without drugs; role of drugs is tenuous |
| Thiothixine | | | Thirst | |
| Amitriptyline | | | | |
| Fluphenazine | | | Thirst | |
| Diuretics | | + | | All diuretics may cause hyponatremia; volume contraction stimulates ADH release; furosemide, ethacrynic acid, and thiazides block diluting mechanisms |
| Miscellaneous | | | | |
| Indomethacin | + | | | Hyponatremia not yet described with indomethacin and acetaminophen |
| Acetaminophen | + | | | |
| Clofibrate | | + | | Clofibrate is useful in partial central diabetes insipidus |
| Nicotine | | + | | |
| Oxytocin | | | Direct ADH effect | Leads to hyponatremia when pregnant woman receives oxytocin with excess water |

From Narins RG, Jones RE, Stom MC, et al: Diagnostic strategies and disorders of fluid, electrolyte and acid base homeostasis. Am J Med 1982;72:500, with permission.

hyponatremia when SIADH is not self-limiting and when the underlying cause cannot be corrected. Hyponatremia should clearly be due to an inability to excrete free water (salt overload or depletion should be corrected before considering demeclocycline therapy) and should generally be severe (<125 mEq/L) and symptomatic, and rigorous fluid restriction should have been proven unsuccessful or impossible because of other management requirements.[9] Demeclocycline doses of 600–1,200 mg/d have been effective, with the onset of action ranging from 5 to 8 days.[10] Because of the delay in onset of action, demeclocycline has no role in the acute treatment of severe hyponatremia. Demeclocycline has been found to be superior to lithium in the therapy of SIADH and hyponatremia.[11] Adverse effects of demeclocycline include photosensitivity, antianabolic effect, and nephrotoxicity. The antianabolic effect has caused worsening azotemia in patients with underlying renal disease.[11] Direct nephrotoxicity has occurred, and is of greatest risk in patients with cirrhosis or CHF.[10] Nephrotoxicity has been suggested to occur as a result of accumulation of excessively high serum concentrations of drug in liver disease patients.[10]

Acute, severe (sodium < 115 mEq/L), symptomatic hyponatremia is a medical emergency and is most efficiently treated by the concurrent administration of a loop diuretic and hypertonic saline (3% NaCl 513 mEq/L or 5% NaCl 855 mEq/L).[6] The loop diuretic elicits a free water loss; urinary sodium and potassium losses should then be replaced with hypertonic saline and potassium supplements. This method requires frequent measurement of both serum and urinary sodium and potassium concentrations. The goals of therapy are an increase in the sodium concentration to 120–125 mEq/L and the cessation of symptoms.[6] The rate of sodium concentration correction has been the subject of controversy. Retrospective uncontrolled studies have stated that correction of serum sodium at a rate grater than 12 mEq/L/24 h may result in an osmotic demyelination syndrome resulting in neurologic complications[12,13]; however, these studies have been criticized on the basis of their retrospective, uncontrolled nature and the rarity with which the demyelination syndrome is encountered in the clinical setting.[14] While very rapid correction of severe hyponatremia may be dangerous, most experts believe that increasing the serum sodium concentration no faster than 2 mEq/L/h to a level of 120–130 mEq/L is not excessive.[14]

Treatment of hypervolemic hyponatremia is centered on the correction of the underlying disease and the restriction of both water and salt.[6] Loop diuretics may be necessary to elicit a loss of free water. Improvement of hemodynamics and renal plasma flow and GFR may also promote a water and sodium diuresis. Therapy for hypervolemic hyponatremia is often difficult secondary to the severity of the associated illness (i.e., CHF, cirrhosis, nephrotic syndrome).

## *Hypernatremia*

Hypernatremia (serum sodium > 150 mEq/L) is always associated with hypertonicity, resulting from a state of relative water deficit.[15] Because the thirst mechanism is so effective in correcting the hypertonic state, hypernatremia results only when hypotonic fluid loss occurs in combination with a disturbance of water intake.[7] Therefore, patients who cannot express their thirst (infants, unconscious patients) or who are unable to ambulate (elderly and disabled patients) may not be able to obtain fluids, and are thus at the highest risk for developing hypernatremia. Hypernatremia occurs less frequently than does hyponatremia. Mortality from acute hypernatremia in children ranges from 10% to 70% (mean 45%), while chronic hypernatremia in children has a mortality rate of 10%.[7] An acute increase in serum sodium to more than 160 mEq/L in adults is associated with a 75% mortality rate, with chronic cases resulting in a 60% mortality rate.[7] Hypernatremia in adults is often associated with serious underlying illness, which may contribute to the high mortality rates.

### Etiology

An approach to the assessment of hypernatremia is shown in Figure 102.3. Hypernatremia may be classified according to the status of the ECF volume. Unlike hyponatremia, which may be associated with low, normal, or even high osmolality, hypernatremia is always associated with hyperosmolality.[5]

**Figure 102.3** Diagnostic approach to hypernatremia. Arrows indicate direction of change. Single and double arrows define the magnitude of change. Iso, isotonic; N, normal; V, variable. *(From Narins RG, Jones RE, Stom MC, et al: Diagnostic strategies and disorders of fluid, electrolyte and acid base homeostasis. Am J Med 1982;72:496–520, with permission.)*

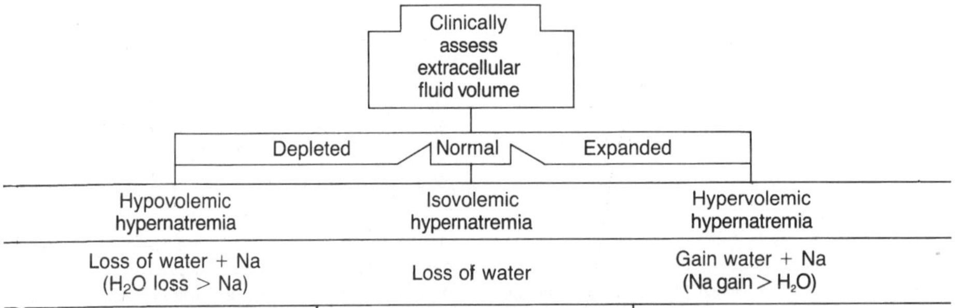

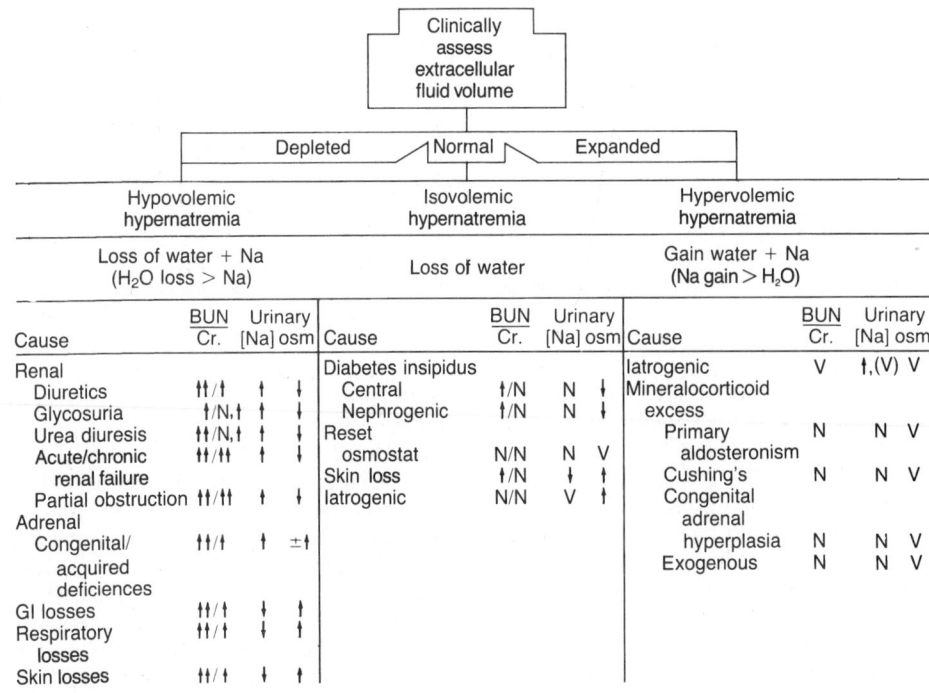

Hypovolemic hypernatremia — Loss of water + Na ($H_2O$ loss > Na)

| Cause | BUN/Cr. | Urinary [Na] | Urinary osm |
|---|---|---|---|
| Renal | | | |
| Diuretics | ↑↑/↑ | ↑ | ↓ |
| Glycosuria | ↑/N,↑ | ↑ | ↓ |
| Urea diuresis | ↑↑/N,↑ | ↑ | ↓ |
| Acute/chronic renal failure | ↑↑/↑↑ | ↑ | ↓ |
| Partial obstruction | ↑↑/↑↑ | ↑ | ↓ |
| Adrenal | | | |
| Congenital/acquired deficiences | ↑↑/↑ | ↑ | ±↑ |
| GI losses | ↑↑/↑ | ↓ | ↑ |
| Respiratory losses | ↑↑/↑ | ↓ | ↑ |
| Skin losses | ↑↑/↑ | ↓ | ↑ |

Isovolemic hypernatremia — Loss of water

| Cause | BUN/Cr. | Urinary [Na] | Urinary osm |
|---|---|---|---|
| Diabetes insipidus | | | |
| Central | ↑/N | N | ↓ |
| Nephrogenic | ↑/N | N | ↓ |
| Reset osmostat | N/N | N | V |
| Skin loss | ↑/N | ↓ | ↑ |
| Iatrogenic | N/N | V | ↑ |

Hypervolemic hypernatremia — Gain water + Na (Na gain > $H_2O$)

| Cause | BUN/Cr. | Urinary [Na] | Urinary osm |
|---|---|---|---|
| Iatrogenic | V | ↑,(V) | V |
| Mineralocorticoid excess | | | |
| Primary aldosteronism | N | N | V |
| Cushing's | N | N | V |
| Congenital adrenal hyperplasia | N | N | V |
| Exogenous | N | N | V |

***Hypovolemic Hypernatremia*** Hypernatremia that occurs in the setting of ECF volume depletion is termed *hypovolemic hypernatremia*. This disease is caused by losses of both sodium and water, with water deficit being of a greater magnitude. Hypovolemic hypernatremia is probably the most common cause of hypernatremia.[16] Loss of sodium and water from renal and extrarenal sources, when replaced with fluids containing more sodium than present in the fluid lost, will result in the development of hypernatremia (Fig. 102.3). Important drug-induced causes include osmotic diuresis with mannitol, diuretics, and laxative-induced diarrhea.

***Isovolemic Hypernatremia*** Isovolemic hypernatremia is associated with an isolated pure water loss. As pure water loss is shared equally across total body water the ratio of ICF to ECF is not changed; thus, signs of ECF volume depletion are rare unless water losses are massive (serum sodium 160–170 mEq/L).[5] Total body sodium content is normal in patients with isovolemic hypernatremia.[15] Mechanisms of pure water loss are listed in Figure 102.3. Iatrogenic causes include failure to replace insensible water loss or the replacement of insensible water losses with relatively hypertonic solutions. Excessive insensible water loss may occur with fever or high ambient temperatures. Insufficient fluid intake may result from lack of access to water such as in elderly patients with decreased levels of consciousness. Nursing home patients are especially at risk.

Isovolemic hypernatremia associated with the production of large amounts of hypotonic urine characterizes diabetes insipidus (DI). Severe, life-threatening hypernatremia may develop if free water intake is not maintained. DI may be categorized as central DI, characterized by low levels of circulating ADH and an inability to produce a maximally concentrated urine, and nephrogenic DI, characterized by an ADH-resistant defect in the renal concentrating mechanism.[15] The causes of both central and nephrogenic DI are listed in Table 102.5. Central DI and nephrogenic DI can be distinguished by characteristic responses to water deprivation and exogenous ADH administration.

Central DI is associated with (1) an initial diuretic phase, (2) an antidiuretic phase in which urine output normalizes because of the release of ADH from injured axons, and (3) resumption of the polyuric phase.[7] The amount of polyuria may range from 3 to 15 L per 24 hours; serum sodium is increased only if water intake is inhibited.[7]

Nephrogenic DI is usually associated with less severe polyuria (3–4 L/24 h) than is central DI, especially in the acquired causes of nephrogenic DI (underlying renal disease and drugs).[7] Drugs causing nephrogenic DI include democlocycline, lithium, methoxyflurane, colchicine, phenytoin, vinblastine, and amphotericin B.[7] While maximal urine concentrating ability is impaired in nephrogenic DI, a hypertonic urine may still be produced; thus the risk of hypernatremia is considerably less than in central DI.[7]

***Hypervolemic Hypernatremia*** Hypervolemic hypernatremia results from an increase in total body sodium and water, with the gain of sodium exceeding the water gain. The gain in sodium results in an expansion of the ECF and the intravascular space, concurrent with a decrease in ICF volume.[15] In patients with renal failure, the inability to diurese the expanded ECF may result in vascular overload and pulmonary edema. Hypervolemic hypernatremia is commonly iatrogenic, because of excessive sodium administration.[15] Some examples include sodium bicarbonate therapy, intraamniotic hypertonic saline for therapeutic abortion inadvertently administered intravenously, and inadvertent use of salt instead of sugar in preparation of infant formulas. Patients with conditions associated with primary mineralocorticoid excess may also develop hypervolemic hypernatremia, usually of less severity than that caused iatrogenically.

**Clinical Presentation**

Most of the signs and symptoms of hypernatremia represent central nervous system dysfunction, and can be attributed to the effect of hypertonicity on brain cells. Cellular dehydration may lead to the symptoms of thirst, restlessness, irritability, tremulousness, spasticity, hyperreflexia, ataxia, seizures, coma, and death.[8] In addition, the shrinking effect of hypernatremia may result in the tearing of cerebral blood vessels, leading to intracranial bleeding.[7] The severity of symptoms is related to both the degree and the rate of rise of serum osmolality; thus, acute hypernatremia is more dangerous than chronic hypernatremia.[15] In an attempt to preserve intracellular volume, brain cells form new intracellular solutes, called idiogenic osmoles. Idiogenic osmoles are effective in restoring intracellular brain water to normal over a 7-day period in the presence of chronic hypernatremia.[15] The presence of idiogenic osmoles has important implications in the rate of correction of serum hypertonicity, as discussed later.

**Treatment**

The goal of therapy for hypernatremia is the normalization of serum tonicity. The approach to therapy is dependent upon correction of reversible causes of hypernatremia, attention to underlying disorders, and the patient's ECF volume status.

In patients with hypovolemic hypernatremia, restoration of intravascular volume with isotonic 0.9% NaCl solution over 30 to 45 minutes should be accomplished to reverse hemodynamic alteration.[17] It should be noted that 0.9% NaCl solution will be hypotonic relative to the hypernatremic plasma and thus will aid in correcting hypertonicity as well as intravascular volume. Once intravascular volume is replaced, the water deficit can begin to be replaced. Total water deficit can be estimated by the following formula[15]: Water deficit = normal TBW − current TBW, where TBW = total body water, normal TBW = 0.60 × normal body weight in kilograms, and current TBW = normal TBW × 140/current measured Na concentration. The free water deficit can be replaced with 5% dextrose or 0.45% NaCl solution. Serum sodium must be replaced slowly to avoid the development of cerebral edema, seizures, permanent neurologic damage, or even death.[8] The presence of idiogenic osmoles inside brain cells causes an osmotic gradient to develop between the brain and plasma, and rapid lowering of plasma osmolality may result in the rapid movement of water from plasma into the intracellular space, leading to cerebral edema and increased intracranial pressure. An acceptable rate of decrease in osmolality is 2 mosm/h (1 mEq/L Na per hour) over a period of 48 to 72 hours.[8,17] Hypernatremia

**Table 102.5** Causes of Diabetes Insipidus

| *Cause* | *Character of urine* Volume (L/24 h) | Tonicity | *Comments* |
|---|---|---|---|
| Central diabetes insipidus (CDI) | | | "Complete" defects: highest volume and lowest osmolarity; "partial" defects: relatively normal volume with mildly hypertonic urine |
| Primary | | | |
| Familial | Variable (<3 to >10) | Variable, usually hypotonic | Less than 1% of cases |
| Idiopathic | Variable | Variable, usually hypotonic | 50% of all cases |
| Secondary | | | |
| Trauma | Variable | Variable | Neoplasm and trauma account for vast majority of secondary causes; other secondary causes are quite rare |
| Neoplasms: lung, breast most common | Variable | Variable | |
| Granulomatous diseases: lues, tuberculosis, sarcoid | Variable | Variable | Sarcoid may also cause NDI |
| Eosinophilic granuloma, Hand–Schuller–Christian disease | Variable | Variable | |
| Cardiovascular: aneurysm, thrombosis, Sheehan syndrome | Variable | Variable | Sheehan syndrome more commonly affects anterior pituitary function |
| Nephrogenic diabetes insipidus (NDI) | | | |
| Primary | | | |
| Congenital | >3–5 | Hypotonic | NDI usually associated with mild polyuria but for congenital NDI; seen in Nova Scotia Scottish |
| Secondary | | | |
| Electrolyte disorders: Hypercalcemia, Hypokalemia | 2–4 | Isotonic | $K^+$ depletion of >200 mEq required |
| Renal: ATN, postobstruction partial obstruction, posttransplantation | Variable, usually <2–4 | Isotonic | Excretion of retained fluid and urea diuresis play important roles in diuretic phase of ATN and postobstruction diuresis |
| Hematologic: sickle cell trait and disease | Variable, usually 2–3 | Isotonic | |
| Drugs: lithium, demeclocycline, methoxyflurane | Variable, usually 2–3 | Isotonic to hypotonic | Lithium also causes distal RTA; methoxyflurane causes calcium oxalate crystalluria |
| Miscellaneous: amyloid, myeloma, Sjögren syndrome, malnutrition | Variable, usually 2–4 | Variable, usually isotonic | |

From Narins RG, Jones RE, Stom MC, et al: Diagnostic strategies and disorders of fluid, electrolyte and acid base homeostasis. Am J Med 1982;72:502, with permission. ATN, acute tubular necrosis; RTA, renal tubular acidosis.

greater than 175 mEq/L should not be corrected by more than 15 mEq/L during the first 24 hours.[8]

Treatment of isovolemic hypernatremia is targeted at replacing water deficit, as outlined earlier, with 5% dextrose or 0.45% NaCl solutions. Initial therapy with 0.9% NaCl is not necessary, as ECF volume is usually not decreased. In addition, potentially reversible or treatable underlying conditions must be addressed. Patients with central DI will respond to administration of natural and synthetic ADH (vasopressin) preparations (Table 102.6). Parenteral products are usually used for acute management; intranasally administered agents are utilized for long-term management. Drugs with antidiuretic properties such as chlorpropamide, carbamazepine, and clofibrate have also been successfully used to manage patients with partial central DI.[18]

Hypervolemic hypernatremia should be treated by replacement of water deficit in conjunction with diuretics to eliminate sodium excess. Patients with hypervolemic hyper-

**Table 102.6** Comparison of Antidiuretic Agents

| | *Desmopressin (DDAVP)* | *Vasopressin (ADH, AVP)* | *Lypressin (DIAPID)* |
|---|---|---|---|
| Pharmacology | | | |
| Vasoconstriction/ADH ratio | + | +++ | ± |
| ACTH release | – | ++++ | – |
| Oxytocicity | + | ++++ | + |
| ADH activity | +++ (IV 10 × nasal) | + | +++ |
| Factor VIII | +++ | – | ? |
| Pharmacokinetics | (nasal) | (parenteral) | (nasal) |
| Onset | 1 h | | Minutes |
| Peak | 1–5 h | | 0.5–2 h |
| Duration | 8–20 h | Aqueous 2–8 h; oil IM 48–72 h | 3–8 h |
| Route of administration | | | |
| Parenteral | IV/SC | Oil IM/SC Aqueous IM/IV/SQ | – |
| Intranasal | + | – | + |
| Dose | Nasal: 0.05–0.4 mL (0.01% solution); 5–40 g in 1–3 doses<br>Parenteral: 2–4 g/d in 2 doses | Aqueous: 5–10 units SC/IM 2–4 × day prn<br>Oil: 1.5–5 units IM every 2–3 d | 1–2 sprays QID |

natremia and renal failure may be treated by hemodialysis against a relatively hypotonic dialysate.[7] The rate of correction of hypernatremia is the same as previously mentioned for hypervolemic and isovolemic hypernatremias.

## Disorders of Potassium Homeostasis

Potassium has two major physiologic functions: (1) cell metabolism, participating in such processes as protein and glycogen synthesis; and (2) determination of the resting potential across cell membranes from its concentration ratio inside the cell versus the ECF.[19] Potassium disorders can thus be expected to adversely influence cellular metabolism and neural and muscular function.

Potassium is the primary intracellular cation at a concentration of approximately 150–160 mEq/L, while the ECF contains 3.5–5 mEq/L. There is approximately 50–75 mEq of potassium per liter of ECF, in contrast to 3,400 mEq per liter of ICF.[20] Muscle tissue represents the major site of intracellular potassium and varies with age (decreased in elderly), sex (males > females), and muscle mass.[20] Even though the serum potassium represents only a small percentage of total body potassium, it is the ratio of intracellular potassium to serum potassium that is important in maintaining the resting membrane potential, responsible for normal action potential generation in cardiovascular and noncardiovascular tissue.[19] This ratio is approximately 30:1, and any alterations can have significant physiologic implications.[21] It becomes evident that the maintenance of a stable serum potassium is vital to life.

Potassium homeostasis and the maintenance of normal serum potassium concentration (3.5–5.0 mEq/L) depend upon complex extrarenal and renal factors. As only 2% of total body potassium resides in the serum (ECF), and as the serum potassium level is influenced by shifts between the intracellular and extracellular fluids in addition to potassium balance, estimation of the magnitude of an excess or deficit of total body potassium extrapolated from the serum potassium concentration is imprecise.[22] Figure 102.4 depicts the approximate relationship between serum potassium concentration and total body potassium. A 1 mEq/L decrease in serum potassium approximates a 200-mEq deficit, a 2 mEq/L decrease approximates a deficit of 300–500 mEq, and a 3 mEq/L decrease approximates a deficit of 500–800 mEq. In addition, it can be seen that relatively small incremental increases in total body potassium may result in fatal increases in serum potassium concentration. Thus, the evaluation of serum potassium concentration requires the consideration of factors influencing redistribution of potassium across cell membranes, as well as factors influencing total body potassium balance (intake and excretion).

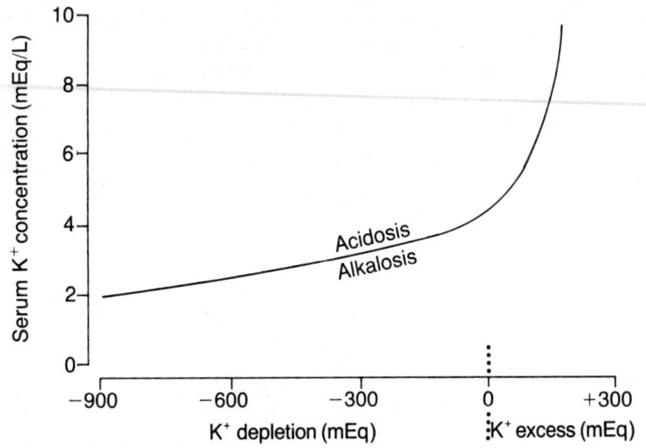


**Figure 102.4** Approximate relationship between changes in total body potassium and serum potassium concentration in an adult. The graph depicts a rough gauge of the degree of negative or positive potassium balance with hypokalemia or hyperkalemia and the effect of acidosis to raise, and alkalosis to lower, the serum potassium concentration. *(From Brown RS: Potassium homeostasis and clinical implications. Am J Med 1984;77 (5A):4, with permission.)*

Factors influencing the intracellular–extracellular movement of potassium are listed in Table 102.7. The $Na^+,K^+$-ATPase pump is responsible for maintaining the basal intracellular-to-extracellular gradients of both sodium and potassium. The importance of this homeostatic mechanism is dramatically evident in massive digitalis overdose, which inhibits the $Na^+,K^+$-ATPase pump, resulting in severe hyperkalemia.

Changes in arterial pH may have important effects on the plasma potassium concentration. During the acidotic state, hydrogen ions enter the cell and obligate sodium and potassium exit to preserve electrical neutrality. A commonly quoted estimate of the pH effect is that for every decrease of 0.1 unit of pH there is an increase in potassium of 0.6 mEq/L. This rule of thumb was generated from data derived from nine observations in five patients, and the potassium increase to acidosis ranged from 0.4 to 1.3 mEq/L.[23] This estimate is only a rough guess and should be interpreted as such. Only metabolic acids, for example, hydrochloric acid, cause this increase in serum potassium. Organic acids, for example, lactic acid, do not produce a change in potassium concentration because with $H^+$ ion entry, lactate follows, thereby preserving electroneutrality and not affecting potassium movement.[23] Respiratory acidosis does not produce large changes in serum potassium concentration.[19]

Metabolic alkalosis causes a shift of potassium inside cells; however, this effect is considerably less prominent than the opposite effect produced by metabolic acidosis.[19] The potassium shift of alkalosis may not be entirely pH dependent. Experimental work in animals has documented that increases in serum bicarbonate with no change in pH also move potassium intracellularly.[23] Respiratory alkalosis does not appreciably influence serum potassium.[23]

$\beta_2$ stimulation by epinephrine lowers serum potassium by stimulation of the $Na^+,K^+$-ATPase pump.[24] $\alpha$-Adrenergic stimulation has the opposite effect and inhibits potassium movement into the cell. The mechanism of $\alpha$-mediated inhibition of intracellular potassium movement is not known.[25] The use of nonselective $\beta$-blockers, such as propranolol, may inhibit the $\beta_2$-mediated catecholamine-induced intracellular redistribution of potassium. These agents may offer better antiarrhythmic potential than $\beta_1$-selective $\beta$-blockers because of their ability to prevent a decrease in serum potassium in the setting of myocardial infarction, which is associated with a hyperadrenergic state.[26]

Insulin increases potassium uptake by both skeletal muscle and hepatic cells by stimulating the $Na^+,K^+$-ATPase pump.[19,27] Insulin release is stimulated by hyperkalemia and serves as a primary defense against pathologic potassium elevations. Hyperkalemia also causes a concurrent release in glucagon as protection from insulin-associated hypoglycemia. Hypokalemia inhibits insulin release and accounts for the hyperglycemia associated with diuretic use.[27]

Osmolality increases of 10 mosm/kg can raise serum potassium 0.3–0.6 mEq/L.[23] Potassium leaves the cell to lower the intracellular osmolality caused by water loss. This hypertonic movement of potassium and possible hyperkalemia are more likely in diabetics who lack insulin and who develop an inadequate aldosterone response.[23]

In addition to the intracellular–extracellular redistribution of potassium, the regulation of serum potassium by renally controlled potassium excretion is paramount in the pathogenesis of potassium disorders. Almost all of the potassium that is filtered in the glomerulus is reabsorbed in the proximal tubule and ascending loop of Henle.[19] Potassium is

**Table 102.7** Factors Influencing Redistribution of Potassium

| | *Serum $K^+$ concentration* |
|---|---|
| Serum pH | |
| Metabolic acidosis (mineral acids) | ↑ |
| Metabolic alkalosis | ↓ |
| Respiratory acidosis | ↔ |
| Respiratory alkalosis | ↔ |
| Adrenergic system | |
| $\beta_2$ agonists (epinephrine, terbutaline) | ↓ |
| $\beta_2$-blockade (propranolol) | ↑ |
| $\alpha_1$ agonists (phenylephrine) | ↑ |
| $\alpha_1$-blockade (phentolamine) | ↓ |
| Insulin | |
| Excess | ↓ |
| Deficit | ↑ |
| Hyperosmolarity | ↑ |
| Cellular disruption | ↑ |
| Trauma/injury | |
| Nutrition | |
| Anbabolism | ↓ |
| Catabolism | ↑ |
| Exercise | ↑ |
| $Na^+$, $K^+$-ATPase pump | |
| Stimulate (catecholamines) | ↓ |
| Inhibit (digitalis toxicity) | ↑ |

excreted into the urine by secretion from the distal tubule and collecting duct.[19] Potassium secretion is regulated primarily by aldosterone and plasma potassium concentration.[19] These regulators act to increase tubular intracellular potassium concentration, resulting in increased secretion. Distal tubule urine flow may also influence potassium secretion; increased distal flow results in a reduced concentration gradient, thus increasing potassium secretion; conversely, decreased tubular flow results in decreasing potassium secretion.[19] The transepithelial potential difference across tubular cell membranes is influenced by sodium reabsorption. Sodium reabsorption makes the tubular lumen relatively electronegative. The enhanced electronegativity favors the movement of positively charged potassium from the cell into the lumen.[19] Alterations of the mechanisms of potassium homeostasis result in hyperkalemia or hypokalemia.

## *Hypokalemia*

Abnormalities that affect any of the factors that may influence serum potassium concentration may result in hypokalemia. Hypokalemia may be classified as moderate (serum potassium 2.5–3.5 mEq/L) or severe (serum potassium less than 2 mEq/L). Hypokalemia is a common disorder, and occurs with greater frequency than does hyperkalemia. The clinical significance of moderate hypokalemia has been a matter of some controversy, and is discussed here. An approach to evaluation of the hypokalemic patient is depicted in Figure 102.5.

### Etiology

The multifactorial causes of hypokalemia can be classified as occurring with normal body stores (laboratory error, redistribution) or decreased total body stores (gastrointestinal loss, renal loss, other) (Table 102.8). The most frequent causes of hypokalemia are gastrointestinal and diuretic-induced renal losses.[19] Gastrointestinal causes resulting in hypokalemia are (1) direct loss of potassium from gastrointestinal fluids (vomiting, diarrhea, draining fistulas, etc.); (2) metabolic alkalosis from hydrogen ion loss (vomiting, nasogastric suction), resulting in intracellular potassium shift; and (3) plasma volume contraction, leading to secondary

**Figure 102.5** Diagnostic approach to hypokalemia. PRA, plasma renin activity; RTA, renal tubular acidosis. *(From Narins RG, Jones RE, Stom MC, et al: Diagnostic strategies and disorders of fluid, electrolyte, and acid base homeostasis. Am J Med 1982;72:496–520, with permission.)*

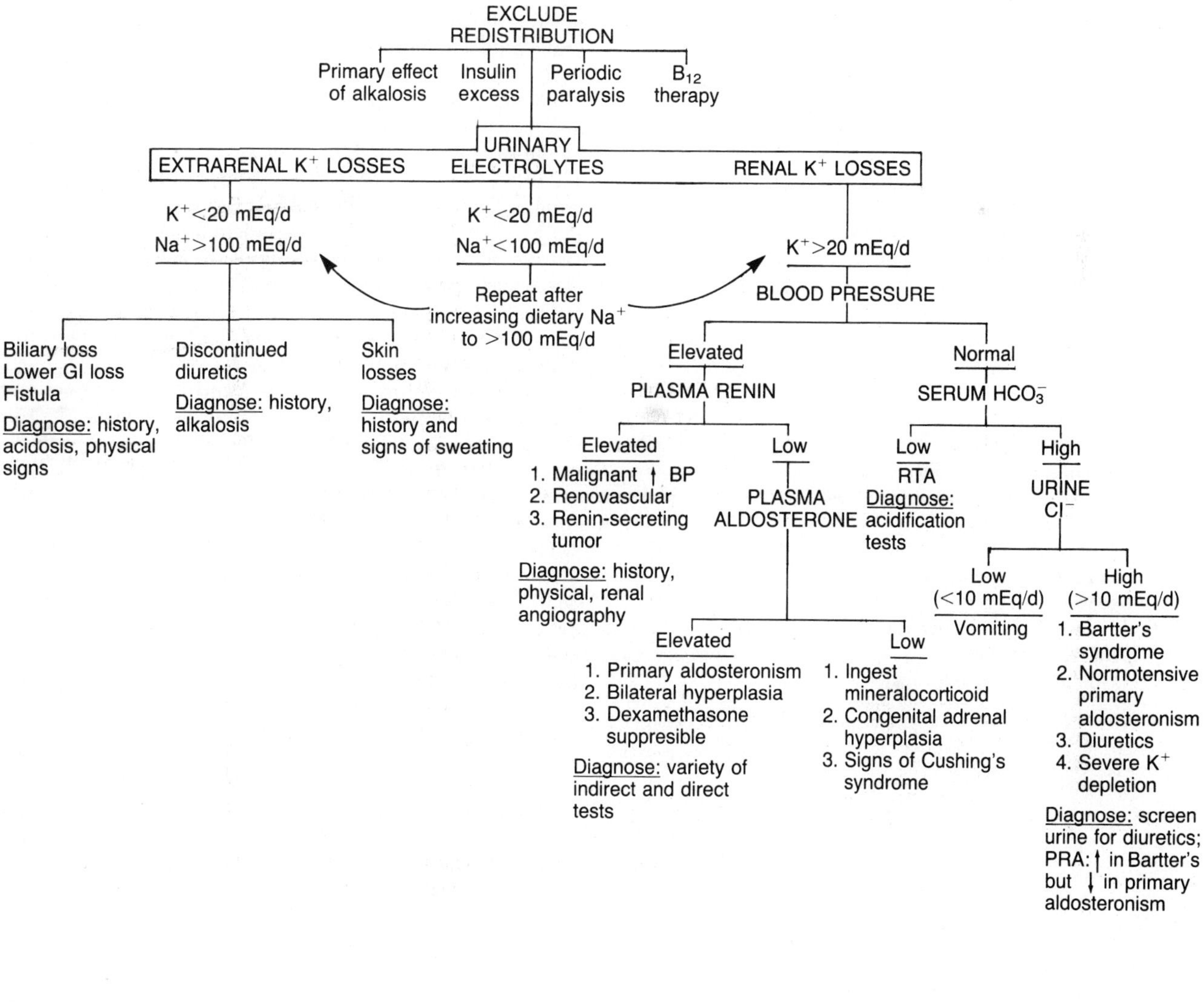

**Table 102.8** Syndromes of Hypokalemia

| |
|---|
| **Normal Body $K^+$** |
| Laboratory error |
| Redistribution |
| Metabolic alkalosis |
| Insulin |
| $\beta_2$-Adrenergic agonists |
| $B_{12}$ therapy |
| Barium poisoning |
| Periodic paralysis |
| Athletes (exercise) |
| **Low Body $K^+$** |
| Gastrointestinal losses |
| Nasogastric drainage |
| Poor dietary intake |
| Protracted vomiting |
| Diarrhea (laxative abuse) |
| Ureterosigmoidostomy |
| Biliary drainage |
| Skin losses |
| Sweat |
| Renal losses associated with normal blood pressure |
| Hypomagnesemia |
| Bartter's syndrome |
| Renal tubular acidosis (proximal and distal) |
| Vomiting (metabolic alkalosis and volume depletion) |
| Drugs |
| Diuretics (acetazolamide, loop diuretics, thiazides) |
| Amphotericin B |
| Carbenicillin, ticarcillin (nonreabsorbable anion) |
| Aminoglycosides |
| Renal losses associated with increased blood pressure |
| Hyperreninemic |
| Renovascular hypertension |
| Renin tumor |
| Malignant essential hypertension |
| Hyporeninemic steroid dependent |
| Exogenous mineralocorticoid |
| Licorice |
| Desoxycorticosterone |
| Fludrocortisone |
| Chewing tobacco |
| Carbenoxolone |
| Endogenous mineralocorticoid |
| Adrenal adenoma |
| Adrenal glomerulosa hyperplasia |
| Enzyme deficiency (17-hydroxylase, 11-hydroxylase) |
| Liddle's syndrome |
| Exogenous glucocorticoid |
| Endogenous glucocorticoid |
| Excessive ACTH |
| Cushing's syndrome |

Adapted from Narins RG, Jones RC, Stom MC, et al: Diagnostic strategies and disorders of fluid, electrolyte and acid base homeostasis. Am J Med 1982;72:496–520, with permission.

increase in aldosterone. Diuretics cause hypokalemia by increasing distal tubular flow, resulting in potassium loss down its concentration gradient.[19]

### Clinical Presentation

Hypokalemia may cause a wide variety of physiologic abnormalities, resulting in a symptomatology involving several organ systems (Table 102.9). The severity of symptoms is generally regarded to be related to the degree and acuteness of hypokalemia, although substantial interindividual variability does exist.[19] Marked symptoms are unusual unless serum potassium concentration is less than 2.5–3.0 mEq/L.[19,29]

The most serious effects, such as paralysis, rhabdomyolysis with myoglobinuria, elevated serum enzymes (aspartate transaminase), and orthostatic hypotension usually occur only when serum potassium is less than 2.5 mEq/L.[29] The association between serum potassium and arrhythmias can be explained by the effect of potassium on resting membrane potential (RMP). The RMP is proportional to the log of the ratio of extracellular to intracellular potassium; therefore, small changes in external potassium can have a significant effect on this ratio. Excitability is the degree of difficulty in initiating an action potential, defined as the difference between the membrane potential and the threshold potential. Potassium affects the membrane potential but not the threshold potential. Hypokalemia makes the membrane potential more negative and therefore moves it farther away from the threshold potential. This means that initiation of depolarization requires a stronger stimulus, with a resultant decrease in excitability.[21]

The cardiovascular effects of hypokalemia shown (Fig. 102.6) are characterized by a decrease in ST segment lowering or flattening, inversion of the T wave, and elevation of the U wave. A widening of the PR interval, an increase in P-wave amplitude, and widening of the QRS complex may also occur, most frequently when serum potassium concentration is less than 2.7 mEq/L.[30] Hypokalemia-associated arrhythmias include bradyarrhythmias, heart block, atrial flutter, paroxysmal atrial tachycardia with block, atrioventricular dissociation, premature ventricular contractions, and ventricular fibrillation. That hypokalemia lowers the threshold for digitalis cardiotoxic arrhythmias is well accepted; however, the association of hypokalemia and arrhythmias in the nondigitalized patient is the subject of some controversy, and is discussed here.

The neuromuscular effects of hypokalemia can be attributed to decreased muscular excitability, as a result of decreased resting membrane potential. As it is the ratio of extracellular to intracellular potassium that determines membrane potential, acute reduction of serum potassium would be expected to be associated with more severe neuromuscular changes.[20] Both smooth muscle and skeletal muscle may be affected, resulting in the symptoms listed in Table 102.9. The pattern of muscle weakness is relatively characteristic, first involving the lower extremities and subsequently ascending to the trunk, upper extremities, and muscles of respiration.[19,20] Smooth muscle involvement is commonly related to gastrointestinal tract, resulting in paralytic ileus.[19,20]

**Table 102.9** Clinical Problems Associated With Potassium Deficiency

| *Cardiovascular* | *Muscular* | *Metabolic* | *Renal* |
|---|---|---|---|
| Arrhythmias<br>  Reentry phenomena<br>  Delayed conductance<br>  Ventricular escape rhythms<br>Increased risk of digitalis toxicity<br>Increased risk of complications after myocardial infarction<br>  Ventricular tachycardia or fibrillation<br>  Increased ischemia<br>Orthostatic hypotension<br>  Impaired pressor responsiveness to catecholamine or angiotensin infusions<br>  Decreased cardioacceleration in response to postural change | Myalgia<br>Weakness<br>Cramps<br>Akathisia<br>Paralysis<br>Rhabdomyolysis with myoglobinuria<br>Hypodynamic ileus<br>Decreased ureteral peristalsis<br>Elevated serum enzymes<br>Creatine kinase (MM isoenzyme)<br>AST<br>Aldolase | Abnormal carbohydrate metabolism<br>  Reduced muscle glycogen content and synthesis<br>  Precipitation of overt diabetes mellitus<br>  Increased glucose intolerance in diabetes mellitus<br>  Reduced normal insulin release during hyperglycemia<br>Increased risk of complications from electrolyte abnormalities<br>  Hypercalcemia<br>  Hypomagnesemia<br>Achlorhydria<br>Hyperlipidemia<br>Impotence | Increased production of ammonia by the kidneys<br>  Decreased protein synthesis<br>  Negative nitrogen balance<br>  Growth retardation<br>  Hepatic encephalopathy or coma in susceptible patients with end-stage liver disease<br>Nephrogenic diabetes insipidus<br>Increased risk of pyelonephritis |

From Knochel JP: Diuretic-induced hypokalemia. Am J Med 1984;77 (5A):18–26, with permission.

**Treatment**

There seems to be universal agreement that serum potassium levels less than 3.5 mEq/L in the digitalized patient or when associated with symptoms require treatment. The indications for the treatment of moderate to mild hypokalemia in the asymptomatic, nondigitalized patient have been the subject of much controversy.[28,31] In favor of potassium replacement therapy are studies suggesting that diuretic therapy for hypertension may be associated with an increase in sudden death, attributable to ventricular arrhythmias, perhaps mediated by stress-induced intracellular potassium shifts on top of diuretic-induced hypokalemia.[32,33] Arguing against the routine treatment of mild hypokalemia in nondigitalized patients are the criticisms of the published reports of ventricular ectopy associated with hypokalemia.[28] These criticisms include (1) the lack of a firm temporal relationship between the serum potassium level and the observation of ventricular ectopy, (2) the possibility of spontaneous variation of ventricular ectopic activity influencing study results, and (3) the influence of alternative causes of ventricular ectopic activity on study results.[28] The possibility of life-threatening hyperkalemia in certain at-risk groups may outweigh the benefits of therapy.[34] Further controlled clinical trials are necessary to solve this controversy. Indications for prudent prophylaxis and replacement therapy of hypokalemia are depicted in Tables 102.10 and 102.11 and in Figure 102.7.[35]

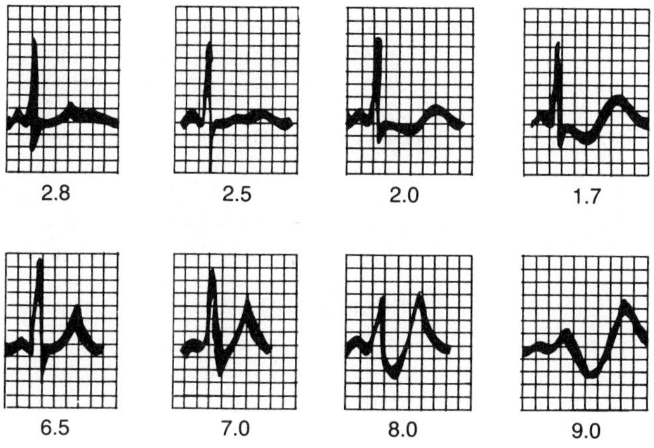


**Figure 102.6** ECG patterns in hypokalemia (top) and in hyperkalemia (bottom). Serum potassium in mEq/L. *(From The Merck Manual, 10th ed, Rahway, NJ, Merck & Co., 1972, Figure 48, with permission.)*

A variety of salts of potassium are available for replacement and prophylactic therapy. Potassium salts include chloride, bicarbonate (acetate and citrate are rapidly metabolized to bicarbonate), phosphate, and gluconate. The most frequently utilized potassium salt is potassium chloride. Metabolic alkalosis is often associated with hypokalemia, and as the causes of metabolic alkalosis (vomiting and diuretics) also cause chloride depletion, the administration of chloride is essential for correction of both the alkalosis and the potassium deficit.[19] Nonchloride salts of potassium are indicated in the potassium depletion associated with metabolic acidosis (e.g., renal tubular acidosis).

The route of administration in potassium replacement therapy depends upon feasibility, severity of hypokalemia, and presence of symptoms. Intravenous potassium is indicated when the oral route is not feasible and/or in the presence of life-threatening hypokalemia (paralysis, arrhythmias). The primary concerns regarding the intravenous administration of potassium are concentration of parenteral potassium-containing fluids and rate of parenteral potassium

**Table 102.10** Indications for Potassium Replacement and Prophylactic Potassium Therapy

| |
|---|
| Replacement |
| Symptoms of hypokalemia or serum potassium consistently <3 mEq/L |
| Surgical conditions accompanied by nitrogen loss or suction drainage |
| Starvation and debilitation |
| Potassium loss associated with vomiting or diarrhea |
| Increased renal excretion of potassium resulting from acidosis |
| Diabetic ketoacidosis treated with insulin |
| Adrenocortical hyperactivity |
| Cardiac arrhythmias resulting from digitalis intoxication |
| Hypokalemic familial periodic paralysis |
| Myocardial infarction with low serum potassium |
| Prophylaxis |
| High-risk patients treated with loop or thiazide diuretics, including those with |
| Heart failure managed with digitalis glycosides |
| High risk for myocardial infarction (angina, coronary artery disease, prior myocardial infarction) |
| Severe hepatic disease |
| Diabetes mellitus |
| Aldosterone excess with normal renal function |
| Potassium-losing nephropathy |
| Chronic diarrhea conditions |

From Stanaszek WF, Romankiewicz JA: Current approaches to management of potassium deficiency. Drug Intell Clin Pharm 1985;19:176–184, with permission.

**Table 102.11** Proposed Guidelines for Potassium Administration to Patients on Diuretic Therapy

| |
|---|
| Nonedematous patients |
| Monitor serum potassium concentration prior to and at 1- to 2-mo intervals during diuretic therapy until a pattern emerges |
| If serum potassium remains > 3.0 mEq/L, do not treat unless clear symptoms of hypokalemia develop |
| If serum potassium falls < 3.0 mEq/L, use 50–60 mEq/d oral KCl solution or wax matrix KCl if oral solutions not tolerated |
| Monitor serum potassium carefully if potassium-sparing diuretics are used; use with great caution in renal impairment |
| Edematous patients[a] |
| Value of restoring potassium balance appears to outweigh risk of treatment with potassium salts or potassium-sparing diuretics |
| Oral therapy to correct mild deficits: 40–80 mEq/d; with more severe deficits use up to 100–120 mEq/d with careful monitoring of serum potassium |
| Use potassium-sparing diuretic if serum potassium does not increase with oral therapy |

[a] For example congestive heart failure, cirrhosis with ascites, severe aldosteronism.

From Stanaszek WF, Romankiewicz JA: Current approaches to management of potassium deficiency. Drug Intell Clin Pharm 1985;19:176–184, with permission.

**Figure 102.7** Approach to the treatment and prevention of potassium deficiencies. *(From Stanaszek WF, Romankiewicz JA: Current approaches to management of potassium deficiency. Drug Intell Clin Pharm 1985;19:176–184, with permission.)*

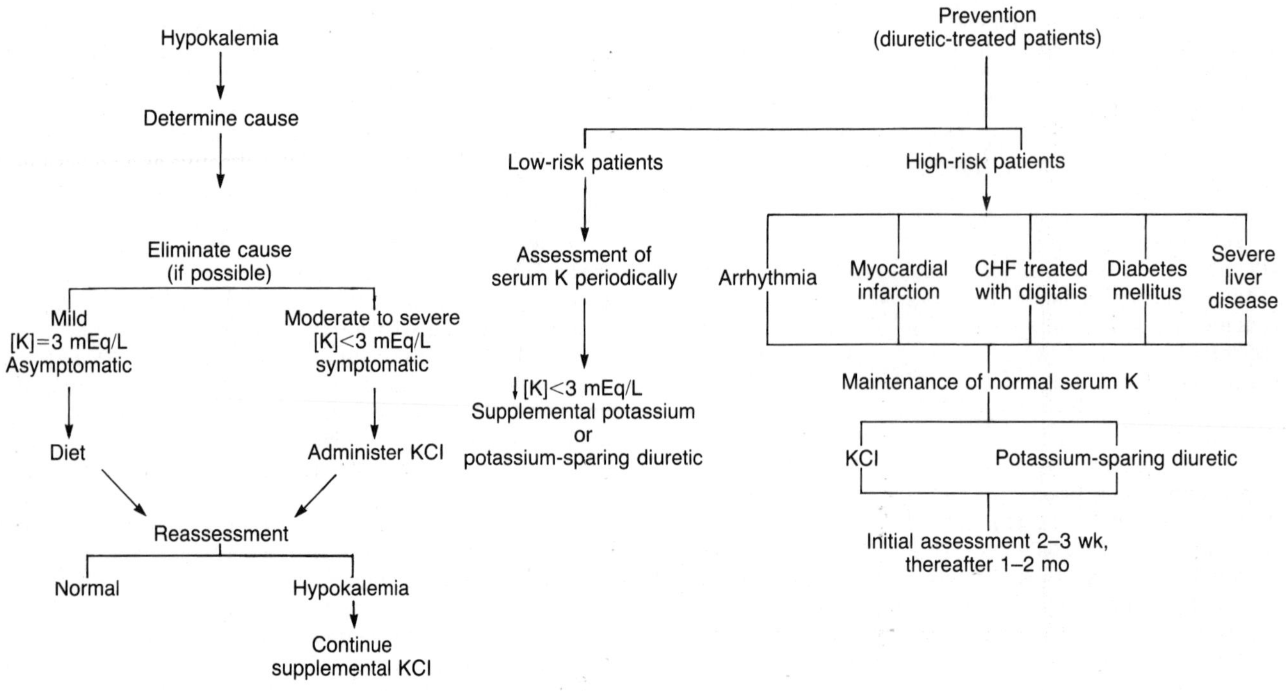

replacement. Because of the many factors influencing the internal distribution of potassium, rapid administration of potassium directly into the plasma can potentially result in hyperkalemia. In general, potassium can be intravenously administered safely at a rate of 10–20 mEq/h.[19] Potassium administration at rates greater than 10 mEq/h should be accompanied by electrocardiographic monitoring for the signs of hyperkalemia (see later). In rare instances, severe hypokalemia associated with paralysis or life-threatening arrhythmias has been treated by the administration of parenteral potassium 40–100 mEq/h, necessitating careful electrocardiographic monitoring and frequent serum potassium determinations.[36–38] Limiting the utility of peripheral-vein intravenous potassium replacement is the generally accepted maximally tolerated potassium concentration of 40–60 mEq/L.[19,39] Potassium concentrations greater than 50–60 mEq/L are often not tolerated by patients because of burning pain and peripheral venous sclerosis. Thus, more centrally located, larger veins have been suggested as more appropriate sites of administration for large potassium doses. The femoral veins have been advocated as the preferred site of administration of large potassium doses.[19,39] The use of central venous lines emptying directly into the right atrium has been discouraged by some authors, because of the potential for adverse cardiac effects of locally high potassium concentrations.[19,39] Data supporting these warnings are scarce, however, and many institutions use central line access for the administration over 1 hour of potassium 10–20 mEq/L mixed in 100 mL of dextrose or saline solution. These concentrated solutions have been employed to avoid the necessity of administration of large volumes of fluid to patients who may be at risk for fluid overload and yet avoid excessively rapid potassium replacement.

Subcutaneous infiltration of potassium is another potential problem resulting from intravenous potassium administration. High local concentrations extravasated under the skin can cause vasoconstriction of both pre- and postcapillary sphincters, resulting in significant ischemic damage. Local infiltration of the site of infiltration with hyaluronidase subcutaneously has been reported to increase local potassium absorption and limit tissue damage.[40]

Because the rate of intracellular movement and the total body deficit of potassium are unpredictable, caution is advised when parenteral potassium therapy is deemed necessary.

Oral administration, when feasible, is the preferred route for potassium replacement in hypokalemia not associated with life-threatening symptoms and for prophylaxis of diuretic-induced hypokalemia. Oral potassium products are available in a wide variety of dosage forms and preparations. Factors influencing the choice of an oral potassium chloride dosage form include product effectiveness, adverse effects, cost, and ability to comply with the prescribed regimen, as no comprehensive study has shown that any one dosage form is more effective than another.[35] Liquid potassium preparations are inexpensive, but are often poorly tolerated by patients because of unpleasant taste, aftertaste, nausea, heartburn, and diarrhea.[19,35] Enteric-coated tablets should be avoided, because a high incidence of small-bowel ulceration and scarring is associated with their use.[41,42] Because of poor patient acceptance of liquid potassium preparations and the small-bowel toxicity of enteric-coated potassium products, sustained-release potassium products have enjoyed an immense popularity. Potassium crystals embedded in a wax matrix or microencapsulated in polymers result in dosage forms releasing potassium in the gut in a sustained, gradual manner, thereby minimizing gastric irritation and ulceration. Studies in healthy volunteers have shown that these products may cause endoscopically evident mild gastric irritation and bleeding, especially when gastric motility is artificially impaired.[43,44] Adverse gastrointestinal effects of slow-release potassium chloride have occurred in patients with delayed gastrointestinal transit or impaired esophageal or intestinal motility.[35] The 1983 Cardio–Renal and Gastrointestinal Drugs Advisory Committee of the FDA reviewed the data regarding slow-release potassium products and concluded that (1) there are upper gastrointestinal lesions associated with all solid potassium chloride preparations that apparently disappear with time, despite continued use of the product, and their relationship to significant disease is unknown; (2) no dosage form is superior to any other with regard to reduced irritative effects on gastrointestinal mucosa; and (3) whether acute studies in healthy volunteers have clinical relevance to the population being chronically treated remains to be determined, although evidence suggests that gastric lesions are generally mild and not clinically important.[45] Because of their palatability and low side effect profile, the sustained-release potassium chloride products are excellent alternative dosage forms for potassium therapy.

Alternatives to pharmaceutical dosage forms of potassium chloride include salt substitutes and potassium-rich food sources (i.e., bananas, orange juice). Salt substitutes are an effective, inexpensive potassium supplement, usually better tolerated by patients than liquid potassium chloride products.[19] Food sources of potassium are generally not recommended for chronic potassium supplementation because they often contain less chloride than other potassium sources, and may add unwanted calories to the diets of patients who may benefit from caloric restriction.[19]

An alternative to exogenous potassium supplementation during diuretic therapy is the potassium-sparing diuretics. Potassium-sparing diuretics are widely used in combination with thiazide diuretics. Spironolactone antagonizes aldosterone and thereby reduces potassium exchange in the distal tubule. Spironolactone is especially effective as a potassium-sparing agent in conditions associated with primary and secondary hyperaldosteronism. Spironolactone is converted to the long-acting active metabolite canrenone with a duration of onset of 2 to 3 days. Triamterene and amiloride act by an aldosterone-independent but unknown method of reducing potassium excretion.[46] The combination of triamterene and hydrochlorothiazide is the most commonly prescribed combination product in this country. Potassium-sparing diuretics may enjoy a resurgence of interest because they prevent not only hypokalemia, but hypomagnesemia as well. Some studies suggest that cardiac arrhythmias may be exacerbated not only by hypokalemia, but by diuretic-induced hypomagnesemia as well, and potassium-sparing diuretics would be expected to be beneficial because of their ability to prevent diuretic-induced hypokalemia and hypomagnesemia.[47]

Combined use of potassium chloride supplements and potassium-sparing diuretics is generally contraindicated, except during the initial phase of therapy for disorders requiring replenishment of total body potassium stores along with prevention of ongoing potassium losses. The risk of hyperkalemia with combined use is significant, especially in patients with renal dysfunction or diabetes mellitus or the elderly.[35]

A report from the Boston Collaborative Drug Surveillance Program highlights the dangers of spironolactone use with concurrent potassium replacement and/or decreased renal function. Patients receiving both KCl and spironolactone had a 15.8% incidence of hyperkalemia compared with a 5.7% rate for patients administered spironolactone alone. When this combined administration occurred in patients with a BUN greater than 50 mg/dL, the hyperkalemic rate was 42.1%.[48]

### *Hyperkalemia*

Hyperkalemia is defined as serum potassium greater than 5.5 mEq/L. Hyperkalemia may be classified as mild (serum potassium > 5.5–6.5 mEq/L without electrocardiographic changes), moderate (> 6.5–8.0 mEq/L), and severe (> 8.0 mEq/L).[49] The incidence of hyperkalemia in hospitalized patients is 3% to 8%, with probably greater prevalence in elderly patients, most likely because of the frequency in this population of diseases and conditions associated with hyperkalemia.[50]

#### Etiology

Hyperkalemia may be associated with normal or elevated total body stores of potassium (Table 102.12). Hyperkalemia associated with normal total body stores includes redistribution of potassium and "pseudohyperkalemia." Pseudohyperkalemia is an in vitro phenomenon in which the measured serum potassium level is falsely elevated compared with the actual in vivo level, usually as a result of release from RBCs, WBCs, or platelets, as may occur in myeloproliferative or hemolytic disorders.[49] Redistribution of potassium from the intracellular to the extracellular space may occur in vivo. Acidosis and insulin deficiency may result in ECF movement of potassium as previously discussed. Release of potassium from ischemic, injured, or lysed cells may occur secondary to crush injury, rhabdomyolysis, burns, and chemotherapy (tumor lysis syndrome).[19] Drugs may cause redistribution of potassium by (1) disruption of the $Na^+,K^+$-ATPase pump (digitalis intoxication),[51] (2) depolarizing muscle relaxants (succinylcholine),[52] (3) $\beta_2$-blockade (propranolol),[53] and (4) positively charged molecules entering cells to displace potassium (lysine and arginine).[54]

Hyperkalemia associated with excessive total body potassium stores is due to excessive potassium ingestion, limitation of potassium excretion, or both (Table 102.12). Any of the potassium supplements may cause hyperkalemia, with the intravenous route of administration associated with a higher risk than the oral route. Hyperkalemia resulting from the administration of potassium supplements is rare unless severe overdose or rapid intravenous administration occurs, or severe kidney dysfunction or inhibition of renal tubular secretion or the renin–angiotensin–aldosterone axis coexists.[5] Exogenous administration of potassium to patients receiving concomitant potassium-sparing diuretics or angiotensin-converting enzyme inhibitors should be undertaken with extreme caution and close monitoring. Diabetic patients are especially at risk for development of hyperkalemia because of lack of insulin and its vital role in potassium redistribution. Diabetics also have a tendency toward hyporeninemic hypoaldosteronism, which decreases the kidney's ability to excrete potassium. The combination of insulin deficiency and attenuated aldosterone response places the diabetic at greater risk for the development of hyperkalemia.[51] In summary, excessive potassium intake, alteration of intracellular potassium movement, and alteration of

**Table 102.12** Syndromes of Hyperkalemia

| *Normal body $K^+$* | *Elevated body $K^+$* |
|---|---|
| "Pseudohyperkalemia" | Excessive $K^+$ ingestion with compromised excretion; hidden sources of potassium include |
| Leukocytosis (>5 × $10^5$/mm$^3$) | K-penicillin (1.7 mEq/$10^6$ units) |
| Thrombocytosis (>7.5 × $10^5$/mm$^3$) | Low-salt diet ($K^+$ rich) |
| Test tube hemolysis | Salt substitutes (contain KCl) |
| Ischemic blood drawing | Stored blood |
| Redistribution | Syndromes of limited $K^+$ excretion associated with defects in renin–angiotensin–aldosterone–renal axis |
| Acidosis | |
| Insulin deficiency | |
| Tissue necrosis | |
| Periodic paralysis | |
| Drugs/toxins | |
| Digitalis | |
| Arginine | |
| Succinylcholine | |
| $\beta$-Adrenergic blockers | |

From Narins RG, Jones RE, Stom MC, et al: Diagnostic strategies and disorders of fluid, electrolyte and acid base homeostasis. Am J Med 1982;72:496–520, with permission.

potassium excretion, alone or in concert, may lead to hyperkalemia. It should be noted that chronic hyperkalemia is always associated with impairment in renal potassium excretion.

### Clinical Presentation

The clinical presentation of hyperkalemia is limited primarily to muscle weakness and abnormalities of cardiac conduction, in addition to the symptoms associated with underlying disease. Muscle weakness is attributed to reductions in resting membrane potential resulting from a decrease in the ratio of intracellular to extracellular potassium. As the resting potential falls to or below the threshold potential, the cell is unable to sustain an action potential, and weakness or paralysis results.[19] Symptoms often begin in the lower extremities, ascending to the trunk and upper extremities.[19] Muscle weakness does not usually develop unless serum potassium concentration exceeds 8 mEq/L.[55] Life-threatening cardiac arrhythmias generally occur before the onset of complete paralysis.[56]

The cardiac rhythm disturbances associated with hyperkalemia pose the greatest danger to the patient, as they may lead to ventricular fibrillation or cardiac standstill (asystole). Electrocardiographic changes occur that are characteristic of hyperkalemia, and are related to degree of hyperkalemia (Fig. 102.6). The earliest ECG changes are peaked T waves and shortening of the QT interval, reflecting increased rate of repolarization, because the increased permeability of the cell membrane to potassium allows a more rapid intracellular potassium exit.[19] These repolarization changes are seen typically when serum potassium concentration exceeds 6 mEq/L. When serum concentration exceeds 7–8 mEq/L, electrocardiographic manifestations of delayed depolarization occur, resulting in slowed cardiac conduction, and appearing as widening of the QRS complex and decreased amplitude, widening, and eventual loss of the P wave.[19] As serum concentrations exceed 9–10 mEq/L, the QRS complex merges with the T wave, resulting in a sine wave pattern, which may deteriorate to ventricular fibrillation or asystole.[19] Depolarization slowing is the result of a slowing of sodium permeability into the cell, caused by hyperkalemia-induced reduction of resting membrane potential.[19] It should be noted that the serum concentrations at which the characteristic electrocardiographic changes occur are variable because of the influence of other factors. Hypocalcemia, acidosis, hyponatremia, and rapid elevation of serum potassium all may enhance the cardiotoxicity of hyperkalemia.[19] The rapidity of development of hyperkalemia is an important factor in determining cardiac effects. Acute hyperkalemia is generally potentially more dangerous than chronic hyperkalemia, because the protective mechanisms for rapid intracellular movement of potassium may be overwhelmed, resulting in acute, dramatic changes of the intracellular to extracellular potassium ratio. Chronic hyperkalemia, where hyperkalemia develops gradually, may not produce electrocardiographic changes until serum potassium levels exceed 7–7.5 mEq/L.[53] Ventricular fibrillation usually results from rapidly progressive hyperkalemia, while asystole is most often observed in patients with slow progression to severe hyperkalemia.[54]

### Treatment

Severe hyperkalemia (> 8 mEq/L) or moderate hypokalemia (> 6.5–8 mEq/L), when associated with clinical symptoms or electrocardiographic changes, requires immediate treatment. Treatment of hyperkalemia is achieved by (1) antagonism of the membrane actions of hyperkalemia (calcium); (2) decrease in extracellular potassium concentration by promotion of intracellular movement of the cation (glucose, insulin, bicarbonate); and (3) removal of potassium from the body (hemodialysis, cation-exchange resins)[57] (Table 102.13). Exogenous potassium must be withheld, and potentially reversible causes of hyperkalemia must be reversed as well.

Calcium administration is an effective, rapidly acting, but short-lived therapy that dramatically reverses the electrocardiographic manifestations and arrhythmias of hyperkalemia.[57] Calcium changes the relationship between membrane potential and threshold potential, restoring normal conduction in the heart.[19] Calcium administration does not in any way lower serum potassium concentration and, be-

**Table 102.13** Treatment of Hyperkalemia

| *Medication* | *Dose* | *Route of administration* | *Mechanism of action* | *Expected result* | *Onset/duration* |
|---|---|---|---|---|---|
| Calcium chloride | 1 g (13.5 mEq) | IV over 5–10 min | Raises threshold potential and reestablishes cardiac excitability | Reverses ECG effects | 1–2 min/10–30 min |
| Dextrose 50% | 50 mL (25 g) | IV over 5 min | Increases insulin release | Redistribution of $K^+$ into the cell | 30 min/2–6 h |
| Dextrose 10% | 1,000 mL (100 g) | IV over 1–2 h | | | |
| Sodium bicarbonate | 50–100 mEq | IV over 2–5 min | Increases serum pH | Redistribution of $K^+$ into the cell | 30 min/2–6 h |
| Insulin (regular) | 1 unit per 3–5 g dextrose | IV with 10% dextrose SC | Potassium intracellular uptake | Redistribution of $K^+$ into the cell | 30 min/2–6 h |
| Sodium polystyrene sulfonate | 15–60 g | Orally or rectally | Exchanges resin $Na^+$ for $K^+$ | Increase in $K^+$ elimination | 1 h/variable |
| Hemodialysis | 2–4 h | — | Removal from plasma | Increase in $K^+$ elimination | Immediate/variable |

cause it is so short-acting, must be repeated if symptoms recur, until serum potassium can be lowered.

Promoting intracellular movement of potassium is an effective mechanism for lowering serum concentration. Intravenous glucose enhances endogenous insulin release in nondiabetics, promoting intracellular uptake of potassium. Insulin is often administered with glucose to facilitate the glucose effect.[57] Glucose administration may be omitted and insulin alone administered to the hyperglycemic patient. Sodium bicarbonate also promotes the intracellular movement of potassium, by increasing extracellular pH and also by a direct action of the bicarbonate anion itself.[19] Sodium bicarbonate may be given directly intravenously, then added to parenteral glucose infusions. It should be remembered that glucose, insulin, and sodium bicarbonate do not reduce total body potassium stores; thus, therapy directed at reducing the potassium is necessary.

Total body potassium stores can be decreased by hemodialysis and cation-exchange resins. Peritoneal dialysis and hemodialysis are effective, but are generally too slow to be useful in the treatment of acute hyperkalemia. Dialysis is useful when other measures fail, or when hyperkalemia is due to ongoing potassium release from tissues in the setting of renal failure.[19] Sodium polysterene sulfonate, a cation-exchange resin, is effective, when given orally or rectally, in removing potassium from the body. Each gram of resin may bind as much as 1 mEq of potassium and release 1–2 mEq of sodium.[19] The resin remains in the gastrointestinal tract and must be removed to be effective. Sodium polysterene sulfonate should be administered with sorbitol to prevent constipation and retention of the resin. Prepackaged suspensions in sorbitol are commercially available. Each sodium polysterene sulfonate dose may decrease serum potassium concentrations by as much as 0.5–1.0 mEq/L.[11] Repeated doses every 3 to 6 hours may be necessary; caution is advised in patients at risk for sodium overload, as sodium release from the resin is available for intestinal absorption.

## Disorders of Calcium Homeostasis

The control and maintenance of calcium concentration in the intracellular and extracellular spaces is vital for the normal functioning of many important biologic systems. Calcium is important in the preservation and function of cell membranes, propagation of neuromuscular activity, regulation of endocrine and exocrine secretory functions, blood coagulation cascade, platelet adhesion process, bone metabolism, muscle cell excitation/contraction coupling, and mediation of the electrophysiologic slow channel response in cardiac and smooth muscle tissue. Because of the biologic importance of calcium, concentration of this cation is closely regulated by a complex system involving parathyroid hormone, vitamin D, calcitonin, and their target organs (Figs. 102.8–102.10). Disruption of these homeostatic mechanisms results in the clinical manifestations of hypercalcemia or hypocalcemia.

The disorders of calcium homeostasis are related to the calcium content of the extracellular fluid, which contains less than 0.5% of the total body stores of calcium. Skeletal bone contains over 99.5% of total body calcium stores.

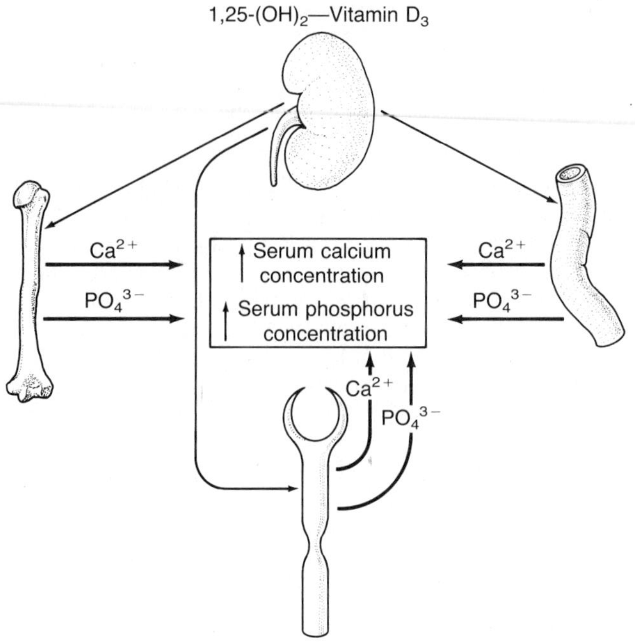


**Figure 102.8** Hypercalcemic and hyperphosphatemic effects of 1,25-(OH)$_2$-vitamin D$_3$. Its actions are (1) mobilization of mineral from bone, (2) enhanced intestinal absorption of calcium and phosphorus, and (3) augmented tubular absorption of phosphorus and calcium. The net physiologic effect is the maintenance of a normal serum calcium and phosphorus product, which allows mineralization of bone. *(From Popovtzer MM, Knochel JP: Disorders of calcium, phosphorus, vitamin D, and parathyroid hormone activity. In Schreier RW (Ed): Renal and Electrolyte Disorders, 2nd ed. Boston, Little, Brown, 1980, p 235, with permission.)*

Extracellular fluid calcium is bound to plasma proteins to an extent of about 46%, with albumin being the primary binding protein. Unbound ionized calcium constitutes about 44% of extracellular fluid calcium. It is the only physiologically active form and is the fraction that is homeostatically regulated. Extracellular calcium is most commonly measured as the total serum calcium level, which includes both bound and unbound calcium.[58] The normal total calcium serum concentration is 8.5–10.5 mg/dL.[2]

Any factor that alters the albumin binding of calcium may be expected to change the fraction of total serum calcium in the ionized form. Alterations in serum albumin concentrations affect the total and ionized calcium concentrations as well. The most significant cause of alteration in extent of calcium binding to albumin occurs in the setting of changing extracellular fluid pH. Metabolic alkalosis and respiratory alkalosis favor an increased binding of calcium to albumin, thus lowering the ionized free calcium fraction while leaving total serum calcium unchanged. This may result in clinically evident, symptomatic hypocalcemia.[58] Conversely, metabolic or respiratory acidosis decreases calcium–protein binding and results in increased ionized calcium. Changes in plasma protein content may also affect free ionized calcium concentration. Hypoalbuminemic states are probably the most common cause of low laboratory values of serum calcium. Because of the decreased protein content, how-

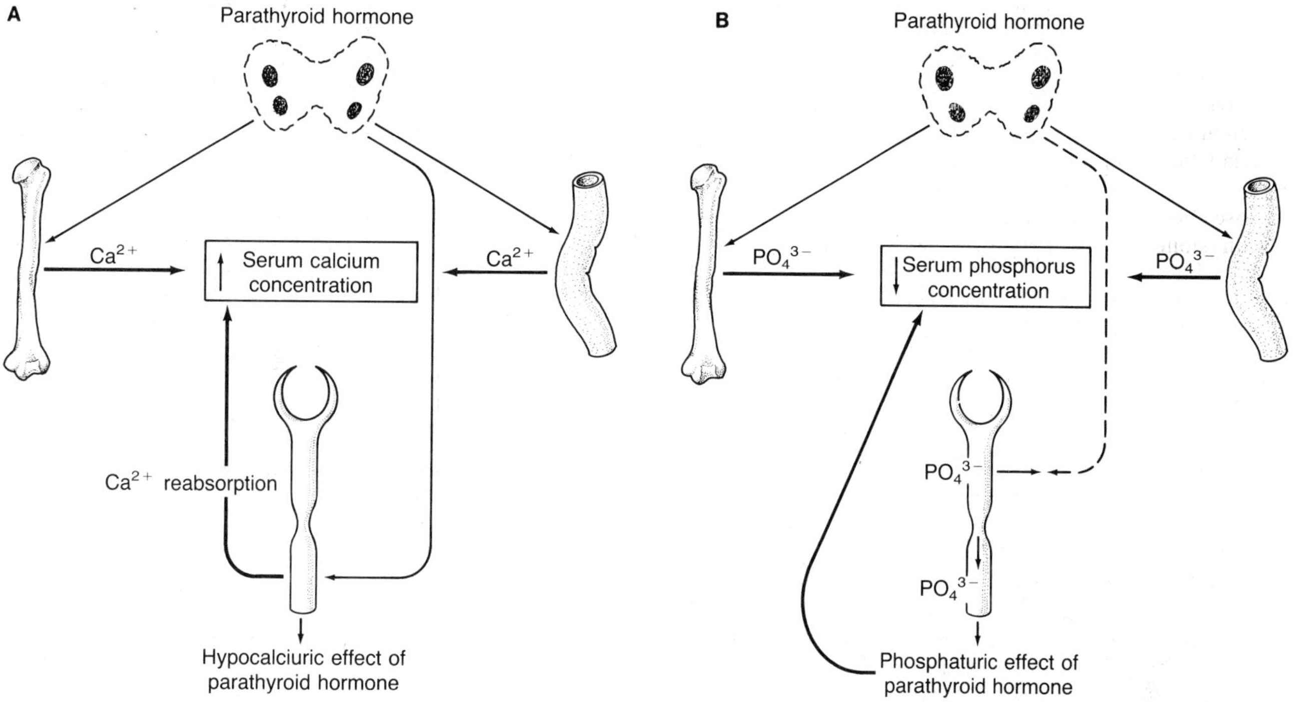


**Figure 102.9** (*A*) The hypercalcemic effect of parathyroid hormone is a summation of mineral mobilization from bone, calcium absorption from the bowel, and distal tubular reabsorption of calcium in the kidney. The effect on the bowel is probably related to parathyroid hormone–induced renal production of 1,25-$(OH)_2$-vitamin $D_3$. (*B*) The hypophosphatemic effect of parathyroid hormone is based on its phosphaturic action, which supersedes its effect of mobilizing phosphorus from bone and enhancing phosphate absorption from the intestine. (Solid lines represent an enhancement of action; broken line represents an inhibition of action.) *(From Popovtzer MM, Knochel JP: Disorders of calcium phosphorus, vitamin D, and parathyroid hormone activity. In Schrier RW (Ed): Renal and Electrolyte Disorders, 2nd ed. Boston, Little, Brown, 1980, pp 223–297, with permission.)*

ever, ionized calcium concentration is normal. Thus, total serum calcium concentration must be evaluated in light of the serum albumin concentration. A general rule of thumb is that for each 1 g/dL that the serum albumin concentration is below 4 g/dL, total serum calcium concentration decreases by 0.8 mg/dL.[58,59]

### *Hypercalcemia*

Hypercalcemia (total serum calcium > 10.5 mg/dL) may have a multitude of causes (Table 102.14). In a large Swedish study, the incidence of asymptomatic hypercalcemia in the general population was 3.9%.[60] The most common causes of hypercalcemia are cancer and primary hyperparathyroidism. The incidence of hypercalcemia of cancer is 150 new cases per million persons per year, compared with an incidence of approximately 250 new cases of primary hyperparathyroidism per million persons per year[61]; however, cancer-associated hypercalcemia is the most common variety of hypercalcemia encountered in hospitalized patients, as many patients with primary hyperparathyroidism are asymptomatic and ambulatory when first diagnosed.[61,62]

#### Etiology

***Hypercalcemia of Malignancy*** About 10% of cancer patients develop hypercalcemia.[63] The most frequent causes of malignancy-associated hypercalcemia are carcinomas of the lung and breast.[61] The most common example of a hematologic cancer associated with hypercalcemia is multiple myeloma, with 20% to 30% of patients developing hypercalcemia.[61]

Tumors cause hypercalcemia by stimulating osteoclastic bone resorption.[61,62,64] Polyuria and the resultant dehydration result in an increased renal tubular reabsorption of sodium and, concomitantly, an increased reabsorption of calcium. The decrease in renal excretion of calcium is an additive mechanism of potentiating hypercalcemia.[62,64] The gastrointestinal tract does not appear to play a significant role in the development of hypercalcemia of malignancy, as calcium absorption is reduced.[65]

***Hyperparathyroidism*** Hyperparathyroidism is the most common cause of hypercalcemia in the general population. Increased levels of circulating parathyroid hormone are associated with increased gastrointestinal calcium absorption, renal tubular calcium reabsorption, and calcium reabsorption from bone, resulting in hypercalcemia. Primary hyperparathyroidism is the result of parathyroid carcinoma in only 5% of cases. Benign parathyroid adenomas account for 70% to 85% of cases of hyperparathyroidism, with parathyroid hyperplasia accounting for the remaining 15%.[58,66] Other causes of hypercalcemia are listed in Table 102.14.

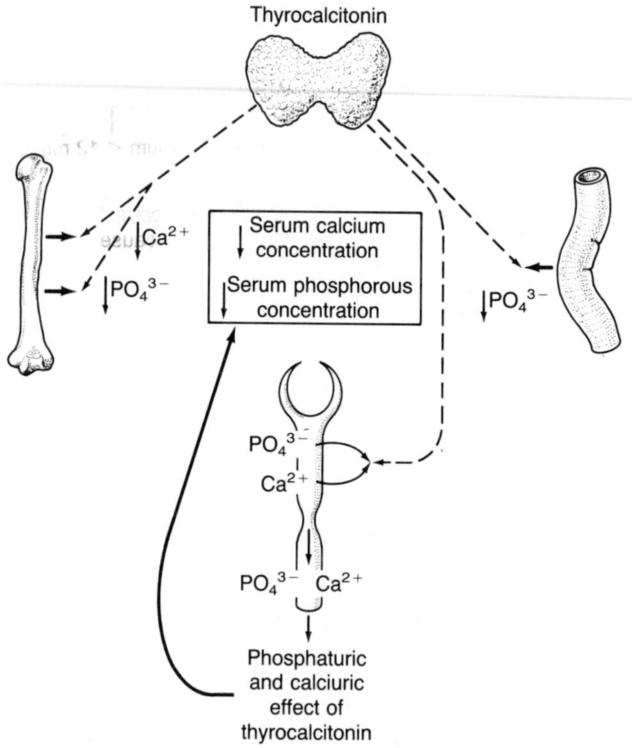


**Figure 102.10** The hypocalcemic and hypophosphatemic actions of thyrocalcitonin are based on inhibition of mineral mobilization from the bone, decreased tubular reabsorption and increased urinary excretion of calcium and phosphorus, and decreased intestinal absorption of phosphorus. (Solid lines represent an enhancement of action; broken lines represent an inhibition of action.) *(From Popovtzer MM, Knochel JP: Disorders of calcium, phosphorus, vitamin D, and parathyroid hormone activity. In Schreier RW (Ed): Renal and Electrolyte Disorders, 2nd ed. Boston, Little, Brown, 1980, p 241, with permission.)*

**Table 102.14.** Causes of Hypercalcemia

| | |
|---|---|
| Neoplasms | Granulomatous disease |
| Bone metastasis | Sarcoidosis |
| Breast | Tuberculosis |
| Multiple myeloma | Berylliosis |
| Lymphoma | Histoplasmosis |
| Leukemia | Coccidioidomycosis |
| Humoral induced | Endocrine disorders |
| Ovary | Hyperthyroidism |
| Kidney | Adrenal insufficiency |
| Lung | Miscellaneous |
| Head and neck | Immobilization |
| Esophagus | Paget's disease |
| Cervix | Familial hypocalciuric |
| Lymphoproliferative disease | hypercalcemia |
| Multiple endocrine neoplasia | |
| Pheochromocytoma | |
| Hyperparathyroidism | |
| Primary | |
| Tertiary | |
| After renal transplant | |
| Drug induced | |
| Thiazides | |
| Lithium | |
| Vitamin A toxicity | |
| Vitamin D toxicity | |
| Milk–alkali syndrome | |
| Calcium supplements | |

### Clinical Presentation

The signs and symptoms of hypercalcemia generally occur along with the symptoms of the underlying disease state. Mild to moderate hypercalcemia with serum calcium concentrations less than 13 mg/dL may often be asymptomatic, as is usually the case in drug-induced hypercalcemia and the vast majority of patients with hyperparathyroidism.[58] The signs and symptoms of hypercalcemia may differ depending upon the acuteness of onset of elevated serum calcium levels.[67] Symptoms of hypercalcemia associated with malignancy usually have an acute presentation, as onset of hypercalcemia is often very rapid. Patients with hypercalcemia of malignancy may infrequently present in hypercalcemic crisis, manifested by the acute onset of severe hypercalcemia, acute renal failure, and obtundation.[58] If untreated, acute hypercalcemic crisis may progress to oliguric renal failure, coma, and malignant ventricular arrhythmias, which may result in death.[58] Hypercalcemia more frequently presents with a symptom complex characterized by anorexia, nausea and vomiting, constipation, polyuria and polydypsia, and nocturia.[58] Polyuria and polydypsia secondary to a urinary concentrating defect constitute one of the most frequent renal effects of hypercalcemia.[58] Disorders associated with long-standing hypercalcemia (i.e., hyperparathyroidism) are more likely to present with metastatic calcification, nephrolithiasis, and chronic renal insufficiency caused by deposition of calcium phosphate in soft tissue.[58]

The electrocardiographic changes associated with hypercalcemia include shortening of the QT interval, and coving of the ST-T wave.[58] Very high serum calcium concentrations may cause T-wave widening, indicating a repolarization defect that may be associated with spontaneous ventricular tachyarrhythmias.[58] Increased sensitivity to the pharmacologic and toxic actions of digitalis may be enhanced in the setting of hypercalcemia.[68]

### Treatment

The indications for treatment of hypercalcemia are dependent upon degree of hypercalcemia, acuteness of development of hypercalcemia, and presence or absence of symptoms. Patients with acute hypercalcemic crisis or symptomatic hypercalcemia should be immediately treated. Asymptomatic patients with serum calcium levels greater than 12–13 mg/dL should also be treated to avoid the consequences that chronic hypercalcemia may have on gastrointestinal, renal, cardiovascular, and other systems.[69] In assessing serum calcium concentrations, determination of the patient's acid–base status and measurement of the serum albumin concentration are necessary for proper interpretation of total serum calcium concentration.

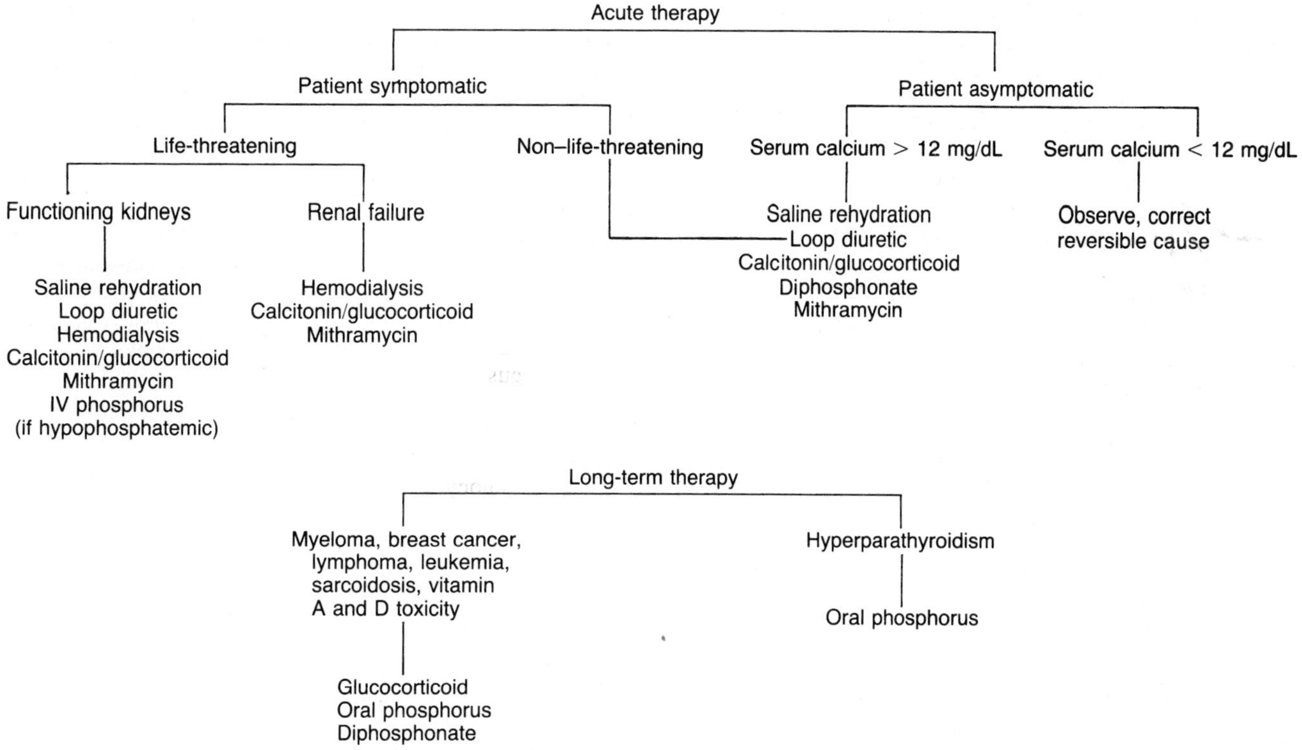


**Figure 102.11** Approach to the hypercalcemic patient.

Figure 102.11 describes a rational treatment approach to therapy for hypercalcemia. Effective treatment begins with attention to the underlying disorder. Patients with primary hyperparathyroidism often require surgery, patients with malignancy often require reduction of tumor load, and patients with drug-associated hypercalcemia should have the agent(s) discontinued. The pharmacologic therapy for hypercalcemia should be individualized according to the patient's presentation, symptoms, and underlying disease.

Few comparative studies of the different agents available for treatment of hypercalcemia exist; thus, treatment modalities vary from center to center. Modalities for hypercalcemia can be classified by mechanism of action (Table 102.15). In patients with functioning kidneys, the cornerstone of treatment is rehydration with normal saline. Patients with symptomatic hypercalcemia often are dehydrated secondary to vomiting and polyuria; thus, rehydration with saline-containing fluids is necessary to interrupt the stimulus for sodium and calcium reabsorption in the kidney tubule. Loop diuretics such as furosemide block calcium reabsorption in the thick ascending loop of Henle and augment the calciuric effect of saline alone.[70] Loop diuretics should be employed only after the patient has been fully rehydrated, as use of a diuretic may lead to further reduction in glomerular filtration rate and a consequential reduction in clearance of calcium.[62,67] Rehydration can be accomplished by the infusion of normal saline at rates of 200–300 mL/h, checking for continued dehydration or fluid overload by monitoring fluid intake and output or by central venous pressure monitoring. Once rehydration has been accomplished, loop diuretics such as furosemide (40–80 mg intravenously every 1–4 hours) are instituted to increase urine output to a goal of 200–250 mL/h.[67] Potassium chloride should be added to the saline solution after rehydration is accomplished to maintain normokalemia. Serum magnesium levels should also be monitored, and magnesium replacement should be instituted if diuretic-induced hypomagnesemia occurs. Rehydration with saline and administration of furosemide often lead to decreases of 2–3 mg/dL in total serum calcium within 24 to 48 hours.[62]

Patients with acute life-threatening hypercalcemia crisis

**Table 102.15** Classification of Agents Used in the Therapy of Hypercalcemia

| |
|---|
| Agents that increase urinary calcium excretion |
| Saline infusion |
| Loop diuretics |
| Agents that decrease intestinal calcium absorption |
| Oral phosphorus |
| Glucocorticoids |
| Agents that decrease ionized calcium concentration |
| EDTA |
| Intravenous phosphorus |
| Hemodialysis |
| Agents that decrease bone resorption |
| Calcitonin |
| Mithramycin |
| Glucocorticoids |
| Diphosphonates |

require rapid reduction of serum calcium concentration. The chelating agent ethylenediaminetetraacetate (EDTA) reduces ionized calcium immediately; however, use of this agent is not recommended because of the possibility of renal tubular damage.[64,67] Intravenous phosphate may rapidly reduce ionized calcium concentrations through the formation of insoluble calcium phosphate salts. Intravenous phosphate is extremely hazardous, because extraskeletal precipitation of calcium phosphate may result in metastatic calcification, hypotension, acute renal failure, or death.[58,63,64] Intravenous phosphates should be reserved for the extraordinary patient with severe hypercalcemia and hypophosphatemia unresponsive to other measures. If employed, doses of intravenous phosphorus should be initiated at 400–800 mg of elemental phosphorus infused over 12 to 24 hours. Therapy must be monitored carefully with measurement of calcium, phosphorus, and creatinine on a daily basis; therapy should be withheld when serum phosphorus values reach a mid-normal range.[62] If rapid reduction of ionized calcium levels is indicated, hemodialysis with calcium-free dialysate solutions may rapidly reduce serum calcium concentrations.[62]

Fortunately, life-threatening hypercalcemic crisis is rare; thus, agents that decrease bone resorption or decrease intestinal calcium absorption are preferred over the more toxic EDTA and intravenous phosphorus therapies. Therapy can be subdivided into agents employed in the acute situation versus those utilized chronically. Acute, short-term therapy with calcitonin is effective in rapidly reducing serum calcium concentration. Calcitonin may be administered subcutaneously or intramuscularly in doses of 4 Medical Research Council (MRC) units/kg every 12 hours, or intravenously by a constant infusion at rates of 10–12 MRC units per hour. Adverse effects of calcitonin administration, including nausea and allergic reaction, occur infrequently.[62] Calcitonin has a rapid onset of action (within 1–2 hours); however, the degree and extent of serum calcium level reduction are often unpredictable and show a great degree of variability between patients.[62,67] Calcitonin therapy is frequently associated with the development of resistance of the osteoclasts to the calcitonin-induced inhibition of bone resorption.[71] Combination of corticosteroid therapy with calcitonin may attenuate this escape phenomenon.[72]

Mithramycin, a potent cytotoxic antibiotic, inhibits osteoclast-mediated bone resorption by inhibition of DNA-directed RNA synthesis of proteins.[67] Mithramycin is the only available, uniformly effective drug for treatment of hypercalcemia.[73] Mithramycin is administered in doses of 25 μg/kg via intravenous infusion over 1 to 3 hours in saline or 5% dextrose solution.[62,67] Serum calcium levels begin to fall within 12 hours of a mithramycin dose and peak effect generally occurs within 48 to 96 hours.[62] Mithramycin is a potentially toxic compound. The most common abnormalities produced by mithramycin are thrombocytopenia, inhibition of platelet function, renal toxicity, and hepatotoxicity.[62] Toxicity has not been reported with single antihypercalcemic doses in patients with normal bone marrow, renal, and hepatic function, however.[62] Mithramycin should probably be limited to short-term therapy in patients who have not responded to hydration and diuretics.[63] Safe long-term therapy with mithramycin has been reported; however, therapy should probably be limited to a period of 2 to 3 weeks to minimize toxicity.[62,74] Repeated doses may be given every 3 to 4 days as needed, along with frequent determinations of complete blood count, liver function tests, and renal function tests. Mithramycin should be avoided in patients with thrombocytopenia, liver disease, or renal disease.

Glucocorticoids are usually effective in the treatment of hypercalcemia resulting from multiple myeloma, leukemia, lymphoma, sarcoidosis, and hypervitaminoses A and D.[58,62,64] Mechanisms of action of glucocorticoids include direct tumor lysing effect, interference in production of osteoclast-activating factor, and interference in metabolism of vitamin $D_2$ to calcitriol.[58,62] Daily doses of 40–60 mg of prednisone or the equivalent have been effective. The disadvantages of glucocorticoid therapy are (1) a lag time of 5 to 10 days before onset of hypercalcemic effect, (2) potential immunosuppressive and catabolic effects, and (3) skeletal demineralization and osteolysis.[62] Treatment of hypercalcemia with inhibitors of prostaglandin synthesis, such as indomethacin, is rarely effective and thus not recommended.[75]

The administration of oral phosphorus may be especially effective in the treatment of chronic hypercalcemia associated with hyperparathyroidism and malignancy. Oral phosphorus in doses of 1–3 g of elemental phosphorus per day inhibits intestinal absorption of calcium and may stimulate osteoblastic activity, leading to deposition of calcium in bone.[75] Oral phosphorus is systemically absorbed and therefore should be avoided in the presence of hyperphosphatemia or renal failure. Oral phosphorus may also result in diarrhea, which may necessitate withdrawal of the drug.[76] Long-term administration of oral phosphorus may lead to calcification of the kidneys or other major organs; thus serum calcium, phosphorus, and creatinine should be monitored closely.

An exciting new class of agents undergoing investigational use for the treatment of hypercalcemia is the diphosphonates. Diphosphonates block bone resorption very efficiently. Diphosphonates render the hydroxyapatite crystal of bone mineral resistant to hydrolysis by phosphatases and also appear to inhibit osteoclasts and their precursors via an intracellular mechanism.[62,77] Three diphosphonates have been used in human trials: ethane-1-hydroxy-1,1-diphosphonic acid (EHDP, etidronate); aminohydroxypropylidine diphosphonate (APD); and dichloromethylene diphosphonate ($Cl_2$MDP, clodronate). EHDP is currently available in the United States in oral form for the treatment of Paget's disease. EHDP, the least potent diphosphonate, has been shown to be effective when administered intravenously in the treatment of malignancy-associated hypercalcemia[78]; however, the use of this agent seems limited by the development of osteomalacia with long-term use.[62] The newer diphosphonates clodronate and APD appear to have less effect on the mineralization process of bone. Both agents have been used orally and intravenously in patients with hypercalcemia associated with malignancy.[78–82] These agents have shown to be very effective in controlling hypercalcemia associated with malignancy. Adverse effects of the diphosphonates appear minimal, with transient fever having been associated with APD and mild gastrointestinal discomfort associated with clodronate in preliminary clinical trials.[62] Further studies will define the ultimate role of diphosphonates in the treatment of hypercalcemia of malignancy.

### *Hypocalcemia*

Hypocalcemia (total serum calcium less than 8.5 mg/dL) occurs when the normal homeostatic mechanisms are disrupted. The incidence of hypocalcemia in the general population was reported to be 0.6% in 15,000 persons undergoing a health screen program.[83]

#### Etiology

The causes of hypocalcemia are listed in Table 102.16. Hypocalcemia results from alteration of the effect of parathyroid hormone and vitamin D on the target end organs (bone, gut, and kidney). The majority of cases of hypocalcemia can be classified as caused by vitamin D deficiency states and hypoparathyroidism.

***Hypoalbuminemia*** Proper assessment of total serum calcium levels includes measurement of serum albumin concentrations; however, hypoalbuminemia, which may be associated with many disease states, is probably the most common cause of laboratory hypocalcemia. Patients remain asymptomatic because the ionized fraction of serum calcium remains normal. Thus, measurement of serum albumin is paramount in the assessment of the cause of hypocalcemia.

**Table 102.16** Causes of Hypocalcemia

| |
|---|
| Hypoalbuminemia |
| Hypoparathyroidism |
|   Surgical |
|   Infiltrative |
|   Idiopathic |
|   Pseudohypoparathyroidism |
|   Pseudoidiopathic |
| Hypomagnesemia |
| Hyperphosphatemia |
| Pancreatitis |
| Intestinal malabsorption |
| Drugs |
|   Oral phosphorus |
|   Furosemide |
|   Calcitonin |
|   Mithramycin |
|   Drugs causing hypomagnesemia |
|   Phenytoin |
|   Barbiturates |
| Hungry bone syndrome |
|   Recovery from parathyroid surgery |
| Vitamin D deficiency |
|   Nutritional |
|   Malabsorption |
|   Liver disease |
|     Decreased production of 25-OH-vitamin $D_3$ |
|   Increased metabolism of 25-OH-vitamin $D_3$ |
|     Phenytoin, barbiturates |
|     Accelerated loss of 25-OH-vitamin $D_3$ |
|     Nephrotic syndrome |
|   Decreased production of 1,25-$(OH)_2$-vitamin $D_3$ |
|     Renal disease |
|     Hereditary vitamin D–dependent rickets |
|   Decreased end-organ response of 1,25-$(OH)_2$-vitamin $D_3$ |
|     Hereditary |

***Hypoparathyroidism*** Symptomatic hypocalcemia most commonly occurs because of parathyroid gland dysfunction secondary to surgical procedures involving the thyroid, parathyroid, and neck, with a reported incidence of 1% to 4% depending on the type of surgery and experience of the surgeon.[84–86] Hypocalcemia in these postsurgical patients is transient in nature in 50% of cases. Serum calcium concentration should be monitored carefully during the first 24 hours.

Hypomagnesemia of any cause may be associated with severe symptomatic hypocalcemia that is unresponsive to calcium replacement therapy (see Disorders of Magnesium Homeostasis). The magnesium cation plays an important role in the secretion of and skeletal response to parathyroid hormone. Serum magnesium levels are important in determining the cause of hypocalcemia.

***Vitamin D Deficiency States*** Vitamin D and its metabolites play an important role in the maintenance of extracellular calcium concentrations, and in normal skeletal structure and mineralization. On a worldwide basis, the most common cause of hypocalcemia is nutritional vitamin D deficiency. In malnourished populations this is manifested by rickets and osteomalacia.

Nutritional vitamin D deficiency is uncommon in Western societies because of the supplementation of milk with ergocalciferol.[86] The most common cause of vitamin D deficiency is related to gastrointestinal disease resulting in vitamin D and calcium malabsorption.[87] Gastric surgery, chronic pancreatitis, small-bowel disease, and intestinal resection and bypass surgery have all been associated with decreased levels of vitamin D and metabolites.[58]

Decreased production of 1,25-dihydroxyvitamin $D_3$ may occur as a result of a hereditary defect resulting in vitamin D–dependent rickets. It also can occur secondary to chronic renal insufficiency where insufficient $1\alpha$-hydroxylase enzyme is available for the production of the most active metabolite.[88,89] Treatment for hypocalcemia associated with chronic renal failure by the use of oral calcitriol is reviewed in Chapter 35.

#### Clinical Presentation

The manifestations of hypocalcemia are listed in Table 102.17. The clinical manifestations of hypocalcemia are characterized by a large degree of individual variability. In general, individual tolerance to subnormal serum calcium levels varies inversely with the rapidity with which hypocalcemia develops.[67] The acuteness of the development of hypocalcemia also plays a large role in determination of whether or not symptoms will occur.[86] The more acute the drop in ionic calcium concentration, the more likely the development of symptoms. It should be recalled that symptomatic hypocalcemia is dependent upon a decrease in unbound ionic calcium concentration. Thus, acid–base bal-

**Table 102.17** Signs and Symptoms of Hypocalcemia

| | |
|---|---|
| Central nervous system | Ocular |
| Fatigue | Cataracts |
| Irritability | Cardiovascular |
| Memory loss | Prolonged QT interval |
| Depression | Acute myocardial failure |
| Confusion | Hypotension |
| Delusion | Skin |
| Hallucinations | Hair loss |
| Areflexia | Brittle, grooved nails |
| Seizures | Eczema |
| Neuromuscular tetany | Psoriasis |
| Perioral paresthesias | Hyperpigmentation with dermatitis |
| Carpopedal spasm | |
| Muscle spasms | |
| Cramps | |
| Latent tetany | |
| Positive Chvostek's sign | |
| Positive Trousseau's sign | |
| Weakness | |

ance plays a significant role in the likelihood of development of hypocalcemic symptoms, with alkalosis predisposing and acidosis inhibiting symptom development.

Hypocalcemia may manifest as neuromuscular, psychiatric, dermatologic, and cardiac sequelae.[58] Acute hypocalcemia is more likely to manifest as neuromuscular and cardiovascular symptoms, while chronic hypocalcemia may often present as psychiatric and dermatologic symptoms associated with an underlying chronic disease (i.e., hypoparathyroidism). The hallmark sign of acute hypocalcemia is tetany, which represents an enhanced peripheral neuromuscular irritability.[58] Tetany manifests as paresthesias around the mouth and in the extremities, muscle spasms and cramps, carpopedal spasms, and rarely as laryngospasm and bronchospasm.[58,86]

The cardiovascular manifestations of hypocalcemia result in electrocardiographic changes characterized by a prolonged QT interval and symptoms of decreased myocardial contractility often associated with congestive heart failure.[90] Both acute and chronic hypocalcemia may result in a reversible syndrome characterized by acute myocardial failure. Chronic hypoparathyroidism and acute hypocalcemia associated with rapid transfusion of citrated blood have been reported as reversible causes of acute myocardial failure.[59,91,92] Refractory congestive heart failure has been reported to be precipitated by hypocalcemia associated with hypoparathyroidism.[93]

### *Treatment*

Treatment of hypocalcemia revolves around identification of the pathophysiologic genesis of the disorder, acuteness of onset, and presence and severity of symptoms. Hypocalcemia associated with hypoalbuminemia requires no treatment, as ionized plasma calcium concentrations are normal. Acute, symptomatic hypocalcemia requires parenteral administration of soluble calcium salts. The initial goal of therapy is to provide 200–300 mg of parenteral elemental calcium until symptoms (i.e., tetany) are fully controlled.[58] This may be provided by the administration of 1 g of calcium chloride or 2–3 g of calcium gluconate. Calcium gluconate is generally preferred over calcium chloride for peripheral venous administration because extravasation of calcium chloride may result in tissue necrosis.[58] Disadvantages to the use of calcium gluconate are the small amounts of elemental calcium per volume and a less predictable, slightly smaller increase in plasma ionic calcium compared with calcium chloride. It is hypothesized that the gluconate and gluceptate salts of calcium may require metabolism of the organic anion to liberate elemental calcium, thus resulting in poorer systemic availability.[94] Intravenous calcium should be administered no faster than 30 to 60 mg per minute. Rapid administration may be associated with hypotension, bradycardia, or cardiac asystole. Calcium should not be added to bicarbonate-containing solutions because of the possibility of precipitation. If symptoms recur after initial intravenous calcium replacement, a slow intravenous infusion of 15 mg/kg of elemental calcium over 4 to 6 hours may be administered.[58] Intravenous calcium administration should be used with caution in patients receiving digitalis glycosides, because of the possibility of cardiac arrhythmias.

Once acute hypocalcemia is corrected by parenteral administration, further treatment modalities should be individualized according to the cause of hypocalcemia. If hypomagnesemia is present, magnesium supplementation is indicated (see Disorders of Magnesium Homeostasis). Chronic hypocalcemia associated with hypoparathyroidism and vitamin D–deficient states may be managed by oral calcium supplementation and vitamin D administration. In chronic hypoparathyroidism, hypocalcemia is usually managed by increasing intestinal absorption of calcium with oral calcium and vitamin D supplementation. Therapy is begun with elemental calcium 2–4 g/d.[58] Elemental calcium content differs among the available oral calcium salts. Some common oral calcium supplements are listed in Table 102.18. Fla-

**Table 102.18** Calcium Preparations

| | *Elemental calcium per gram of salt* | | |
|---|---|---|---|
| *Calcium salt* | mg | mEq | *Route* |
| Calcium carbonate | 400 | 20.0 | PO |
| Calcium chloride | 270 | 13.5 | IV |
| Calcium citrate | 211 | 10.6 | PO |
| Calcium glubionate | 64 | 3.2 | PO |
| Calcium gluceptate | 82 | 4.1 | IV |
| Calcium gluconate | 90 | 4.5 | IV/PO |
| Calcium glycerophosphate | 191 | 9.6 | IV |
| Calcium lactate | 130 | 6.5 | PO |
| Calcium phosphate (dibasic anhydrous) | 290 | 14.5 | PO |
| Calcium phosphate (dibasic dihydrate) | 230 | 11.5 | PO |
| Calcium phosphate (tribasic) | 400 | 20.0 | PO |

**Table 102.19** Comparison of Various Vitamin D Preparations

| | *Vitamin $D_2$ (ergocalciferol)* | *Dihydro-tachysterol* | *25-Hydroxy-vitamin $D_3$ (calcifediol)* | *1,25-Dihydroxy-vitamin $D_3$ (calcitriol)* |
|---|---|---|---|---|
| Physiologic dose ($\mu$g/d) | 10 | 20 | 5 | 0.5 |
| Pharmacologic dose ($\mu$g/d)[a] | 1,250 | 400 | 50 | 1 |
| Onset of maximal effect (d) | 30 | 15 | 15 | 3 |
| How administered | 1,250 $\mu$g Capsules Tablets | 125 $\mu$g 200 $\mu$g 400 $\mu$g Tablets | 20 $\mu$g 50 $\mu$g Capsules | 0.25 $\mu$g 0.5 $\mu$g Capsules |

[a] Usual dose for treating hypoparathyroidism, osteomalacia resulting from vitamin D malabsorption or resistance, and renal osteodystrophy. Smaller doses may be adequate when combined with calcium supplements or when treating anticonvulsant-induced hypovitaminosis D. 1 $\mu$g of ergocalciferol has an activity of 40 IU; 1,250 $\mu$g is approximately 50,000 IU.

vored calcium carbonate antacids such as Tums are often preferred as calcium supplements. These products contain a higher elemental calcium content compared with other salts and flavoring that may increase palatability.[95] If serum calcium does not normalize, a vitamin D preparation should be added. A comparison of vitamin D preparations is found in Table 102.19.

Treatment for hypocalcemia associated with vitamin D–deficient states should be individualized.[58] In patients with malabsorption, vitamin D requirements vary markedly, and large doses may be required. In contrast, vitamin D deficiency associated with anticonvulsant medication may be corrected with smaller doses of vitamin D (e.g, 5,000–10,000 units of ergocalciferol per day).[58] The treatment for vitamin D deficiency associated with 1$\alpha$-hydroxylase deficiency (i.e., renal failure) is discussed in Chapter 35. Situations in which 25-hydroxylase activity is reduced (e.g., hepatic disease) may require treatment with calcitriol (1,25-dihydroxyvitamin $D_3$). In selected cases, calcium supplementation may be required if vitamin D replacement alone is ineffective in returning calcium concentrations to normal.

Adverse effects of oral calcium and vitamin D supplementation include hypercalcemia and hypercalciuria, especially in the hypoparathyroid patient, where the renal calcium-sparing effect of parathyroid hormone is absent. Hypercalciuria may increase the risk of calcium stone formation and nephrolithiasis in susceptible patients. Addition of thiazide diuretics in patients at risk for stone formation may result in reduction of both urinary calcium excretion and vitamin D requirement.[96]

## Disorders of Magnesium Homeostasis

The biologic importance of magnesium is immense. Magnesium is ionically bound to the center of chlorophyll molecules; thus, the entire food chain and transfer of energy in biologic systems are dependent on its presence. Magnesium is an important cofactor for hundreds of enzyme systems, including all phosphate transfer reactions involving ATP.[97] Recent research has focused on the complex relationship between magnesium and calcium. Magnesium appears to modulate the neuromuscular activity of the calcium ion; indeed, magnesium has been called ''nature's physiologic calcium blocker.''[98] Magnesium is the fourth most plentiful cation and the second most abundant intracellular cation behind potassium. As the clinical significance of magnesium disorders becomes more clearly defined, the need for an understanding of the appropriate therapy for these disorders becomes vital.

As only about 1% of total body magnesium resides in the extracellular fluid space, serum magnesium concentration provides only a rough index of total body magnesium stores. Magnesium is bound to albumin to an extent of 30%. In contrast to calcium, changes in albumin concentration have much less effect on serum magnesium concentration. Normal serum magnesium concentration is 1.5–2.0 mEq/L (1.8–2.4 mg/dL).[2]

The kidney is the primary regulator of magnesium balance in the body. Magnesium homeostasis is maintained by a process of glomerular filtration and tubular reabsorption. Renal handling of magnesium seems to follow a tubular maximum mechanism similar to the renal handling of glucose. This tubular maximum is set very close to the filtered load of magnesium that is present at normal serum concentrations. Thus, small increases in serum magnesium concentration are associated with a rise in magnesium excretion.[99] Conversely, decreases in serum magnesium concentration result in the near disappearance of magnesium from the urine.

### *Hypermagnesemia*

Hypermagnesemia results when magnesium intake exceeds the elimination capacity of the kidneys. Because of the tubular maximum threshhold mechanism, hypermagnesemia occurs only in the setting of renal dysfunction or excessive exogenous administration of magnesium. The prevalence of hypermagnesemia (serum magnesium > 2 mEq/L) has been reported as 4% to 9.3% among hospitalized patients.[100,101] Fortunately, symptomatic hypermagnesemia is an uncommon clinical problem.[102]

**Table 102.20** Causes of Hypermagnesemia

| | |
|---|---|
| Decreased renal excretion | Other |
| Acute renal failure | Lithium therapy |
| Chronic renal failure with exogenous intake | Hypothyroidism |
| Excessive Intake | Milk-alkali syndrome |
| Treatment of toxemia of pregnancy | Addison's disease |
| Ureteral irrigants (hemiacidrin) | Viral hepatitis |
| Cathartics | Acute diabetic ketoacidosis |

### Etiology

Hypermagnesemia most commonly occurs in the setting of renal insufficiency, when glomerular filtration rates are less than 30 mL/min.[58] Hypermagnesemia is usually a preventable phenomenon, as most causes are iatrogenic. Acute renal failure may result in hypermagnesemia even without exogenous magnesium administration and usually peaks in the early diuretic phase.[103] Drug-induced, iatrogenic hypermagnesemia most frequently occurs with the use of magnesium-containing antacids in patients with renal insufficiency.[104] Patients in the intensive care unit with multiple-system organ failure receiving magnesium-containing antacids for stress ulcer prophylaxis or magnesium-containing parenteral fluids (i.e., TPN) constitute a population of patients particularly at risk for developing hypermagnesemia. Parenteral treatment of eclampsia with magnesium sulfate has caused symptomatic hypermagnesemia in both mother and neonate.[105,106] Other causes of hypermagnesemia are listed in Table 102.20. They are uncommon and produce only mild increases in magnesium concentration.

### Clinical Presentation

Hypermagnesemia manifests as neuromuscular, cardiovascular, and endocrine effects (Table 102.21). Signs and symptoms of hypermagnesemia occur when plasma magnesium concentration exceeds 4 mEq/L. The severity of neuromuscular and cardiovascular symptoms is magnesium concentration related. The neuromuscular manifestations of hypermagnesemia can be ascribed to neuromuscular blockade. Hypermagnesemia may cause hypotonic, diminished, or absent deep tendon reflexes, varying degrees of muscle weakness, and complete flaccid paralysis with resultant respiratory depression, depending upon the serum concentration of magnesium attained.[58,97,102] Because deep tendon reflexes disappear before the appearance of paralysis of voluntary muscle, monitoring of the deep tendon reflex is a useful tool to assess magnesium therapy for toxicity. Central nervous system depression may result in varying degrees of lethargy and sedation which may progress to stupor and coma, especially at high serum magnesium concentrations.[58]

Excessively high magnesium concentrations may affect heart rate, cardiac conduction, and blood pressure. Hypotension and cutaneous vasodilation may occur above serum levels of 3 mEq/L.[58,104] A variety of mechanisms have been implicated, including vascular smooth muscle relaxation and sympathetic blockade.[97] Sinus bradycardia, first-degree heart block, nodal rhythms, or bundle branch block may occur at serum magnesium concentrations of 4.5 mEq/L or greater.[107] Complete heart block progressing to asystole and cardiac arrest may occur at serum concentrations greater than 14–15 mEq/L.[102,104]

**Table 102.21** Clinical Findings Associated With Hypermagnesemia

| *Serum magnesium level (mEq/L)* | *Cardiovascular* | *Neuromuscular* | *Other* |
|---|---|---|---|
| > 3 | Hypotension | | Nausea |
| | Cutaneous vasodilation | | Vomiting |
| > 4 | QT interval prolongation | | Skin warmth |
| > 4.5 | Bradycardia | | |
| | First-degree heart block | | |
| | Nodal rhythms | | |
| | Bundle branch block | | |
| > 5 | QRS interval prolongation | Sedation | |
| | PR interval prolongation | Hypotonia | |
| | | Hyporeflexia | |
| > 7 | | Somnolence | |
| > 10 | | Coma | |
| | | Muscle paralysis | |
| | | Respiratory depression | |
| > 14 | Complete heart block | | |
| > 15 | Asystole | | |

### Treatment

Because the large majority of instances of hypermagnesemia are iatrogenic in nature, treatment begins with prevention. Therapeutic guidelines for the treatment of hypermagnesemia are based on clinical signs and symptoms and degree of elevation of serum magnesium level. Treatment is indicated in symptomatic patients with serum magnesium levels of 5–8 mEq/L, and in all patients whose serum level is greater than 8 mEq/L regardless of symptoms.[104] As calcium directly antagonizes the neuromuscular and cardiovascular effects of magnesium, intravenous administration of calcium in doses of 100–200 mg of elemental calcium is indicated.[104] Reversal of symptomatic hypermagnesemia after calcium administration is rapid but transient in nature; thus, repeated doses of calcium may be necessary in life-threatening situations. When symptoms persist or when serum magnesium concentration is greater than 8 mEq/L in the absence of symptoms, rapid reduction in serum magnesium concentration may be accomplished by peritoneal dialysis or hemodialysis. Dialysis is the treatment of choice in all patients with renal dysfunction.[102] Supportive care with mechanical ventilation, pressors, and cardiac pacemakers may be necessary until serum magnesium concentrations are lowered. In patients with adequate renal function and non–life-threatening hypermagnesemia, promotion of renal magnesium excretion may be accomplished by administering intravenous saline and furosemide.

## *Hypomagnesemia*

Hypomagnesemia occurs when magnesium intake is less than renal excretion, or when the renal magnesium-conserving mechanisms fail, resulting in magnesium excretion exceeding intake. Hypomagnesemia (serum magnesium $< 1$ mEq/L) is a common clinical disorder but is frequently overlooked because of the typically complex clinical setting in which it occurs.[58] The prevalence of hypomagnesemia has been found to be 9% to 11% among patients hospitalized in acute care facilities.[99,100] Hypomagnesemia is much more common in the intensive care unit patient population. In one study, hypomagnesemia occurred in 20% of medical intensive care unit patients and was the most common electrolyte disorder observed.[108] As less than 1% of total body magnesium is extracellular, serum magnesium concentration may not be an accurate measure of total body magnesium deficiency.[102,109] In a study in intensive cardiac care unit patients, serum magnesium was normal in over 90% of patients while intracellular magnesium concentration in mononuclear cells was abnormally low in 53% of these patients.[110] This study indicates that the incidence of intracellular magnesium deficiency may be much higher than the serum magnesium concentration indicates.

### Etiology

Magnesium depletion is almost always secondary to disturbances of either the intestinal tract or the kidney. Table 102.22 illustrates the many causes of hypomagnesemia.

***Gastrointestinal*** Magnesium conservation in normal subjects is extremely effective; therefore, dietary magnesium deprivation rarely leads to significant magnesium depletion unless it is prolonged.[58] Generalized malabsorption syndromes associated with hypomagnesemia occur in various intestinal mucosal diseases (e.g., coeliac sprue, Whipple's disease, radiation enteritis), massive intestinal resection, and pancreatic insufficiency.[58,102,111] Magnesium losses exceeding intake may produce hypomagnesemia. Gastrointestinal disorders may result in hypomagnesemia, secondary to the loss of intestinal fluids (magnesium 14 mEq/L) or biliary, gastric, and pancreatic fluids (0.4–1.1 mEq/L).[58]

***Renal*** The causes of renal magnesium wasting may be differentiated into intrinsic tubular disorders and drug-induced, hormone-induced, and ion- or nutrient-induced renal tubular magnesium losses. Intrinsic tubular disorders are listed in Table 102.22. Particularly severe hypomagnesemia may occur with diuresis associated with the recovery phase of acute tubular necrosis, the postobstructive period, and the post–renal transplantation period.[112]

The most frequent cause of renal magnesium wasting is long-term diuretic therapy.[58] Of patients receiving long-term diuretic therapy, 50% develop hypomagnesemia.[113] Patients at highest risk for development of hypomagnesemia from chronic diuretic therapy include elderly patients, alcohol abusers, and patients consuming diets low in magnesium.[113] Potassium-sparing diuretics such as triamterene and amiloride are also magnesium sparing; thus, combination therapy with distal tubular diuretics may limit magnesium depletion.[114] It has also been suggested that the use of the lowest effective dose of diuretic may be important in limiting diuretic-induced renal magnesium loss.[114]

Cisplatin therapy is another drug-induced cause of renal magnesium wasting.[115] Hypomagnesemia has been reported to occur in up to 88% of patients receiving cisplatin; thus, this disorder should be suspected in all patients receiving cisplatin chemotherapy.[116] The cause of hypomagnesemia associated with cisplatin is unrelated to the recurrence of classic cisplatin-induced renal toxicity.[58] Renal magnesium wasting resulting in hypomagnesemia has also been associated with amphotericin B therapy for systemic fungal infections.[117] Renal magnesium wasting and mild to moderate hypomagnesemia can be demonstrated by the second week of therapy after relatively small cumulative dosages of amphotericin B, and the lowest serum levels of magnesium appear by the fourth week of therapy.[118] Renal magnesium wasting appears to plateau after 4 weeks of amphotericin B therapy and appears to be reversible.[118] Other drugs causing hypomagnesemia are listed in Table 102.22.

The most common clincial setting for hypomagnesemia is acute and chronic alcoholism.[58,109] The causes of hypomagnesemia in the alcoholic are multifactorial and include malnutrition, dietary magnesium deficiency, vomiting and diarrhea, increased urinary magnesium excretion, hypophosphatemia, hyperaldosteronism, and pancreatic insufficiency.[109] In addition, upon entry of alcoholic patients into the hospital, acute ethanol withdrawal and intravenous glucose therapy may lead to further reductions in extracellular fluid magnesium levels.[58] It appears likely that magnesium deficiency along with other metabolic disorders associated with alcoholism and alcohol withdrawal contribute to the delirium tremens associated with alcohol withdrawal.[58,109] Monitoring of serum magnesium concentration

**Table 102.22** Causes of Hypomagnesemia

**Gastrointestinal**
Reduced intake
- Protein-calorie malnutrition
- Total parenteral nutrition without magnesium
- Prolonged parenteral fluid administration without magnesium
- Alcoholism

Reduced absorption
- Primary hypomagnesemia
- Malabsorption syndromes (e.g., tropical sprue, celiac disease, radiation enteritis, intestinal lymphectasia)
- Short-bowel syndrome (e.g., small-bowel resection, ileal bypass)
- Pancreatic insufficiency

Increased loss
- Excessive vomiting
- Prolonged nasogastric suction
- Excessive laxative use
- Intestinal and biliary fistulas
- Prolonged diarrhea (ulcerative colitis, Crohn's disease, cancer of the colon)

**Renal**
Primary tubular disorders
- Primary renal magnesium wasting
- Bartter's syndrome
- Renal tubular acidosis
- Diuretic phase of acute tubular necrosis
- Postobstructive diuresis
- Post–renal transplant diuresis
- Glomerulonephritis
- Pyelonephritis
- Nephrotic syndrome

Drug-induced renal losses
- Aminoglycosides
- Amphotericin B
- Cyclosporine
- Diuretics
- Digitalis
- Cisplatin
- Alcohol

Hormone-induced renal losses
- Hyperparathyroidism
- Hyperthyroidism
- Aldosteronism
- Hypoparathyroidism
- "Hungry bone syndrome" after parathyroidectomy

**Internal Redistribution**
- Diabetic ketoacidosis
- Glucose, amino acid, insulin administration
- Massive blood transfusion (citrate)
- Pancreatitis with lipidemia (magnesium soap)

**Other**
- Excessive sweating and lactation
- Hypercalcemia and hypercalciuria
- Phosphate depletion
- Chronic alcoholism
- ECF volume expansion

is indicated in alcoholic patients, and supplementation is recommended in all patients undergoing acute alcohol withdrawal.[109]

### Clinical Presentation

Clinical manifestations of hypomagnesemia are illustrated in Table 102.23. Symptoms of magnesium depletion are generally not seen until serum magnesium concentrations approach 1 mEq/L.[8] Patients with magnesium depletion may develop symptoms suddenly and without warning, even if hypomagnesemia has been chronic.[119] Magnesium deficiency can result in various nonspecific neuromuscular signs and symptoms. Concomitant hypocalcemia and hypokalemia may contribute as well. Neuromuscular signs and symptoms of hypomagnesemia are the converse of those for hypermagnesemia. Neuromuscular hyperactivity is predominant, as magnesium deficiency increases neuronal excitability in neuromuscular transmission.[120]

The cardiovascular manifestations of magnesium deficiency have gained recent attention. Several studies have suggested an association between dietary magnesium deficiency from drinking water with decreased magnesium content ("soft water") and sudden death from coronary artery disease.[121–123] Myocardial magnesium content in accident victims in cities having "soft water" has been found to be reduced by 7% compared with those in "hard water"

**Table 102.23** Clinical Manifestations of Hypomagnesemia

| | |
|---|---|
| Neuromuscular | Cardiac |
| Muscle twitching and tremor | Premature ventricular beats |
| Muscle weakness | Ventricular fibrillation |
| Hyperreflexia | Ventricular tachycardia |
| Paresthesias | Torsades de pointes |
| Positive Chvostek's and Trousseau's signs | Predisposition to digitalis-mediated arrhythmias |
| Tetany | Supraventricular tachycardia |
| Seizures | Electrocardiographic changes (PR, QT prolongation, widened QRS) |
| Coma | Coronary artery spasm |
| Nystagmus, ataxia, vertigo | Calcium and potassium |
| Choreoathetoid movements | Refractory hypocalcemia |
| Psychiatric | Refractory hypokalemia |
| Apathy | |
| Depression | |
| Delirium | |
| Agitation | |
| Confusion | |
| Hallucinations | |

areas.[121] Numerous reports of patients with ventricular tachycardia and fibrillation associated with hypomagnesemia and responding to magnesium replacement exist in the literature.[124–127] Magnesium may play an important etiologic role in atypical ventricular tachycardia (i.e., Torsades de pointes), and successful therapy of this potentially lethal arrhythmia with magnesium has been reported.[128] Of equal importance is the well-known finding that hypomagnesemia may exacerbate digitalis toxicity–induced arrhythmias. The finding of a 19% frequency of hypomagnesemia in hospitalized patients receiving digitalis combined with the potential life-threatening manifestations of digitalis toxicity has prompted several recommendations for routine monitoring and supplementation of both potassium and magnesium in patients receiving digitalis.[129]

The electrocardiographic changes associated with hypomagnesemia are nonspecific and include wide QRS complexes and tall, peaked T waves in moderate magnesium deficiency, and prolonged PR, QRS, and QT intervals, ST-segment depression, and flat, broad T waves with prominent U waves in severe magnesium deficiency.[111] These electrocardiographic changes probably reflect alterations in intracellular potassium and calcium in the myocardium.

Magnesium is important in regulating intracellular potassium content.[129] Movement of these intracellular cations appears to be closely linked, as attempts to replace potassium deficits in the presence of magnesium deficiency are difficult. Magnesium deficiency impairs the $Na^+$,$K^+$-ATPase pump and allows potassium to escape from the cell.[109] It is estimated that the incidence of hypomagnesemia in hypokalemic patients ranges from 38% to 42%.[130]

Hypocalcemia is a prominent manifestation of magnesium deficiency. Mechanisms postulated to explain the hypocalcemia of magnesium deficiency include altered equilibrium between calcium in extracellular fluid and bone, impaired release of parathyroid hormone, impaired formation of parathyroid hormone, and end-organ resistance to parathyroid hormone.[109] Serum calcium concentration should be assessed if hypomagnesemia is discovered.

### Treatment

Treatment guidelines for magnesium deficiency are outlined in Table 102.24. Route of administration depends upon severity of hypomagnesemia, presence of symptoms, and patient tolerance. Magnesium supplementation may be administered via the intravenous, intramuscular, or oral route (Table 102.25). Patients with nonsymptomatic hypomagnesemia with levels greater than 1 mEq/L (1.2 mg/dL) may be treated with oral magnesium supplements. Diarrhea may be a limiting factor for oral magnesium therapy. Patients who have magnesium levels less than 1 mEq/L (1.2 mg/dL) or who are symptomatic should receive parenteral magnesium therapy. Regardless of route of administration, assessment of renal function is indicated, as patients with renal insufficiency should be treated with lower doses and must be monitored by measuring serum or plasma levels frequently.[117] Even if severe magnesium deficiency is present, approximately 50% of an administered dose is excreted in the urine.[58,131] Magnesium replacement must thus be accomplished over 3 to 5 days, and subsequent maintenance magnesium administration should continue in patients who are unable to eat or with continuing magnesium losses. Magnesium therapy should be monitored by measuring serum magnesium levels. Rapid intravenous injection of magnesium may be associated with flushing, sweating, and a sensation of warmth; thus, rapid bolus injection of magnesium should be avoided.[124] Excessively high doses of magnesium in patients with renal dysfunction may lead to hypermagnesemia and its subsequent symptoms. During administration of intravenous magnesium, parenteral calcium chloride should be available should overdose or symp-

**Table 102.24** Guidelines for Treatment of Magnesium Deficiency in Adults

1. Serum magnesium < 1 mEq/L (1.2 mg/dL) with life-threatening symptoms (seizure, arrhythmia)
   **Day 1**
   a. 2 g MgSO4[a] mixed with 6 mL 0.9% NaCl in 10-mL syringe and administer IV push over 1 min
   b. Follow with 0.5 mEq $Mg^{2+}$/kg lean body weight IV infusion over 5–6 h, then 0.5 mEq $Mg^{2+}$/kg lean body weight IV infusion over 17–18 h
   **Days 2–5**
   0.5 mEq $Mg^{2+}$/kg lean body weight per day divided in maintenance IV fluids
2. Serum magnesium < 1 mEq/L (1.2 mg/dL) without life-threatening symptoms
   **Day 1**
   Total of 1 mEq $Mg^{2+}$/kg lean body weight per day as continuous IV infusion, or divided and given IM every 4 h for five doses
   **Days 2–5**
   Total of 0.5 mEq $Mg^{2+}$/kg lean body weight IV infusion per day as continuous IV infusion or divided and given IM every 6–8 h
3. Serum magnesium > 1 mEq/L (1.2 mg/dL) and < 1.5 mEq/L (1.8 mg/dL) without symptoms
   As in No. 2, or
   a. Milk of Magnesia 5 mL four times daily as tolerated
   b. Magnesium-containing antacid 15 mL three times daily as tolerated
   c. Magnesium oxide tablets 300 mg four times daily, increase to two tablets four times daily as tolerated

[a] 1 g $MgSO_4$ = 8.1 mEq $Mg^{2+}$.

toms of hypermagnesemia occur. Direct intravenous administration of 50% magnesium sulfate may produce pain and venosclerosis; therefore, it should be diluted to 20% before administration. As intramuscular injections are painful, involve multiple punctures, and have no therapeutic advantage over the intravenous route, intramuscular therapy should be reserved for situations in which peripheral venous access is impossible.

## Disorders of Phosphorus Homeostasis

Phosphorus is an important element of all body tissues, and its presence is critical for many aspects of cellular structure and function. Phosphorus is an essential element in phospholipid cell membranes, nucleic acids, and phosphoproteins required for mitochondrial function.[132] Phosphorus regulates the intermediary metabolism of carbohydrates, fats, and proteins. Phosphorus also regulates enzymatic reactions including glycolysis, ammoniogenesis, and the 1-hydroxylation of 25-hydroxyvitamin D.[132–135] In red blood cells, 2,3-diphosphoglycerate (2,3-DPG) modulates the oxygen-carrying capacity of hemoglobin. This critical enzymatic process is closely regulated by phosphorus.[136] Phosphorus is the source of the high-energy bonds of ATP, thus fueling a wide variety of physiologic processes, including muscle contractibility, electrolyte transport, neurologic function, and other important biochemical reactions.[132] Considering its diverse biologic importance, it is not difficult to appreciate the clinical implications of disorders of phosphorus homeostasis.

Phosphorus is present in living organisms mainly as inorganic phosphate and organic phosphate esters. The total body distribution of phosphorus is depicted in Table 102.26. As potassium is the major intracellular cation, phosphorus is the major intracellular anion. The majority of intracellular phosphorus exists as organic esters, mainly 2,3-DPG, adenosine and guanosine triphosphate, and fructose 1,6-diphosphate.[137] Only a small fraction of intracellular phosphorus exists as inorganic phosphate; however, this fraction is critical as it is the source from which ATP is resynthesized.[137] The majority of inorganic phosphate is located in

**Table 102.25** Magnesium Salt Forms and Their Respective Amounts of Elemental Magnesium

| | *Elemental magnesium* | |
|---|---|---|
| *Salt form*[a] | **mmol** | **mEq** |
| Oxide (heavy) | 24.80 | 49.60 |
| Hydroxide | 17.00 | 34.00 |
| Carbonate | 10.50 | 21.00 |
| Chloride | 4.42 | 9.80 |
| Acetate | 4.66 | 9.32 |
| Sulfate | 4.06 | 8.11 |

[a] All mmol and mEq amounts are stated to be equivalent to 1 g of the salt form.

From Gums JG: Clinical significance of magnesium: A review. Drug Intell Clin Pharm 1987; 21:245, with permission.

**Table 102.26** Body Distribution of Phosphorus

| | *mM* | *% Total* |
|---|---|---|
| Bone | 19,000 | 85.0 |
| Skeletal muscle | 1,900 | 9.0 |
| Extracellular fluid | 17 | 0.08 |
| Red blood cells | 40 | 0.2 |
| Other | 1,200 | 5.2 |

**Table 102.27** Serum Distribution of Phosphorus

| | *mmol/L* | *mg/dL* | *% Total* |
|---|---|---|---|
| $HPO_4^{2-}$ | 0.81 | 2.53 | 68 |
| $H_2PO_4^-$ | 0.20 | 0.63 | 17 |
| Complexed | 0.07 | 0.19 | 5 |
| $CaPO_4$ | 0.04 | 0.11 | 3 |
| $MgPO_4$ | 0.03 | 0.08 | 2 |
| Protein bound | 0.12 | 0.37 | 10 |
| Total diffusible | 1.08 | 3.35 | 90 |
| Total | 1.20 | 3.72 | 100 |

the extracellular space (Table 102.27). Normal serum phosphorus concentration in the adult is 3.0–4.5 mg/100 mL.[2] Extracellular inorganic phosphate is the prime determinant of intracellular phosphate; thus, small increments in the organic phosphate pool can profoundly alter both the extracellular and intracellular phosphate pools. Metabolic disturbances, hydrogen ion shifts, and hormones all can cause important syndromes. Because of these phenomena, the serum phosphorus level does not accurately reflect total body stores.[138] The regulation of phosphorus excretion by the kidney is the single most important regulator of steady-state serum phosphorus levels. Renal excretion of phosphorus is regulated by glomerular filtration and active tubular reabsorption. Under normal conditions, 85% to 90% of filtered phosphate is reabsorbed, the majority in the early proximal tubule. Renal tubular reabsorption of phosphorus is inhibited by parathyroid hormone and 1,25-dihydroxyvitamin $D_3$.[132] Conversely, phosphorus reabsorption is increased by growth hormone and thyroxine.[139,140] Internal phosphorus balance (transcellular phosphate distribution) is also of importance in the maintenance of normal serum phosphorus. Normal serum phosphorus levels may vary by as much as 2 mg/dL throughout the day, reflecting acute changes in transcellular distribution of phosphate influenced primarily by carbohydrate intake and insulin secretion.[312]

### *Hyperphosphatemia*

Hyperphosphatemia (serum phosphorus concentration greater than 4.5 mg/dL) occurs much less frequently than hypophosphatemia. Serum phosphorus concentration is so closely regulated by the kidneys that it is unusual for hyperphosphatemia to develop in patients with normal renal function. The most frequent causes of hyperphosphatemia are increase in phosphate entrance into the extracellular fluid via either exogenous administration or endogenous intracellular phosphate release, and decreased renal excretion of phosphate (Table 102.28).

#### Etiology

***Decreased Renal Phosphorus Excretion*** The most common cause of hyperphosphatemia is a decrease in urinary phosphorus excretion secondary to acute and chronic renal failure.[141] Patients with excessive exogenous phosphorus

**Table 102.28** Causes of Hyperphosphatemia

| |
|---|
| Decreased renal phosphorus excretion |
| Acute renal failure |
| Chronic renal insufficiency |
| Increased renal tubular phosphorus reabsorption |
| Hypoparathyroidism |
| Growth hormone excess |
| Hyperthyroidism |
| Etidronate disodium |
| Tumoral calcinosis |
| Exogenous phosphorus loads |
| Phosphate enema |
| Phosphate laxatives |
| Parenteral phosphorus administration |
| Oral phosphorus replacement |
| Endogenous phosphorus loads |
| Rhabdomyolysis |
| Tumor lysis syndrome |
| Leukemias |
| Lymphomas |
| Diabetic ketoacidosis |

administration or endogenous intracellular phosphorus release in the setting of acute renal failure may develop profound hyperphosphatemia. In patients with chronic progressive renal insufficiency, severe hyperphosphatemia is usually encountered only in patients with advanced disease, when the glomerular filtration rate is less than 25 mL/min.[142] Patients with renal dysfunction are at greatest risk for developing hyperphosphatemia of any cause.

***Increased Renal Tubular Reabsorption*** Hypoparathyroidism results in increased renal tubular reabsorption of phosphorus and may result in hyperphosphatemia. Hyperphosphatemia associated with hypoparathyroidism is usually less severe than that associated with severe renal failure or excessive exogenous or endogenous introduction of phosphorus into the extracellular fluid space. Hypoparathyroidism is the most important cause of increased tubular reabsorption. Other causes are listed in Table 102.28.

***Exogenous Phosphorus Loads*** Iatrogenic causes of hyperphosphatemia have been widely reported, and awareness of the phosphorus content of intravenously, orally and rectally administered phosphorus-containing drugs can aid in the prevention of this cause of hyperphosphatemia. Sodium phosphate enemas may cause severe symptomatic hyperphosphatemia when administered to children.[143–150] In adults, hyperphosphatemia has been observed in patients ingesting laxatives containing phosphate salts.[151–157] Administration and retention of phosphate-containing enemas in patients with moderate and severe renal insufficiency has also been reported to cause severe hyperphosphatemia with severe symptoms.[154,155] Retention of significant amounts of sodium phosphate enema occurs even in normal subjects.[153,156]

Intravenous phosphorus administration has also been reported to cause hyperphosphatemia.[157–159] Large doses of phosphorus administered intravenously to treat hypercalcemic patients have been reported to cause severe life-threatening hyperphosphatemia.[158]

***Endogenous Phosphorus Loads*** Any disorder that causes disruption of skeletal muscle cells can release large amounts of phosphorus into the systemic circulation and cause hyperphosphatemia. Rhabdomyolysis (destruction of skeletal muscle) of any cause may result in the release from intracellular stores of large amounts of phosphorus. This condition is frequently associated with acute renal failure as well; thus, hyperphosphatemia of a severe degree may result.

Endogenous hyperphosphatemia is not uncommonly observed in patients undergoing treatment for acute leukemia and lymphomas.[160–162] Chemotherapeutic treatment of acute lymphoblastic leukemia may result in the release of large amounts of phosphorus into the systemic circulation as lysis of lymphoblasts occurs. Initiation of chemotherapy for Burkitt's lymphoma may result in a rapid lysis of malignant cells, resulting in hyperphosphatemia, hyperuricemia, hyperkalemia, and hypocalcemia (tumor lysis syndrome).[163,164]

Diabetic ketoacidosis is an unappreciated but common cause of hyperphosphatemia. In one study, hyperphosphatemia was present in 94.7% of patients with diabetic ketoacidosis prior to the initiation of treatment.[165] With the institution of treatment, serum phosphorus levels decrease and may ultimately result in hypophosphatemia; however, prior to the initiation of therapy in diabetic ketoacidotic patients, hyperphosphatemia is very common.[165]

### Clinical Presentation

Signs and symptoms of hyperphosphatemia can be related to the solubility of phosphorus and calcium. It has been estimated that the in vivo solubility product of calcium phosphate in mg/dL is about 58.[166] In vivo calcium phosphate solubility products greater than 58 pose a significant risk of calcium phosphate precipitation. Because of this relationship, the major effect of hyperphosphatemia is related to the development of hypocalcemia with its consequences and damage resulting from the deposition of calcium phosphate precipitate. The calcium phosphate solubility relationship may be influenced by the acid–base status of the patient. An alkaline environment would be predicted to decrease the solubility product; conversely, an acidic environment would increase the solubility product of calcium phosphate.

Hypocalcemia associated with hyperphosphatemia is thought to be caused by deposition of calcium phosphate in the bone, in soft tissues, or possibly both.[59] Acute renal failure secondary to calcium phosphate precipitation in the kidney is well described, especially in patients with hyperphosphatemia secondary to tumor lysis.[160,161] In patients with severe longstanding hyperphosphatemia, metastatic calcification may occur in the hip, shoulder, wrist, and finger joints.[160,161] Ocular and vascular calcification may also occur.[141]

Hyperphosphatemia associated with chronic renal disease may result in azotemic osteodystrophy (osteitis fibrosis cystica and osteomalacia) and is discussed in Chapter 34.

### Treatment

The treatment of hyperphosphatemia should initially be directed at the correction of reversible factors and the treatment of the disease states associated with its development. Severe symptomatic hyperphosphatemia manifesting as hypocalcemia and tetany should be treated by the intravenous administration of calcium salts. In general, the most effective way to treat hyperphosphatemia itself is to decrease phosphate absorption in the lumen of the gastrointestinal tract by the use of phosphate binders.[141] Antacids containing divalent cations are the agents most frequently used in the prevention and treatment of hyperphosphatemia. As magnesium salts should be avoided in patients with renal failure, aluminum hydroxide and aluminum carbonate gels have been most frequently utilized.[141] Short-term therapy with these agents is effective, the most frequent adverse effect being constipation; however, long-term treatment and prevention of hyperphosphatemia with aluminum-containing antacids in patients with chronic renal failure have led to concern over the toxic effects of aluminum accumulation (see Chapter 35).

## *Hypophosphatemia*

Hypophosphatemia has been classified clinically on the basis of severity: moderate hypophosphatemia is defined as serum phosphorus concentrations from 1 to 2.5 mg/dL, and severe hypophosphatemia as serum phosphorus concentrations less than 1 mg/dL. Hypophosphatemia is an extremely common finding. Different studies have reported the incidence of hypophosphatemia to range from 2% to 30% among inpatients.[167,168] Hypophosphatemia has been reported to be present in 42% of patients admitted with acute alcoholism.[169] Fortunately, moderate hypophosphatemia is much more common than severe hypophosphatemia, and thus seldom causes recognizable effects.[170] Certain patient populations are at increased risk for the development of severe hypophosphatemia, however, and an awareness of these select groups of patients is important in preventing the severe life-threatening symptoms associated with severe hypophosphatemia.

### Etiology

The causes of hypophosphatemia are many, but can be divided among those associated with phosphate depletion, such as decreased intake or excess renal excretion; those associated with transcellular shifts, resulting in a redistribution of phosphate; or a combination of both[132] (Tables 102.29 and 102.30). While patients with moderate hypophosphatemia generally lack significant symptomatology, severe hypophosphatemia can be associated with life-threatening symptoms. While the causes of severe hypophosphatemia are relatively few (Table 102.30), these conditions are frequently seen in patients in the acute care setting.

***Pharmacologic Phosphate Binding*** Phosphate-binding substances such as sucralfate, calcium carbonate, and aluminum/magnesium-containing antacids have the potential to bind large amounts of phosphorus in the gut. If phosphate-binding agents are ingested on a chronic basis in conjunction with a dietary phosphorus deficiency, severe hypophosphatemia may result.[133,138,170] Patients who are receiving long-term phosphate-binding agents (peptic ulcer disease or chronic renal failure) and who may already possess moderate hypophosphatemia (alcoholics) are at highest risk for the development of severe hypophosphatemia.

**Table 102.29** Conditions Causing Moderate Hypophosphatemia

| | |
|---|---|
| Inadequate intake | Rapid tumor growth |
| Starvation | Increased excretion |
| Diet deficiency | Glucagon |
| Malabsorption | Diuretics |
| Vitamin D deficiency | Volume expansion |
| Vomiting | Hypomagnesemia |
| Gastrectomy | Hyperparathyroidism |
| Phosphate-binding drugs | Recovery from hypothermia |
| Antacids | Diabetic keoacidosis |
| Sulcralfate | Acute gout |
| Intracellular shifts | Renal tubular defects |
| Moderate respiratory alkalosis | Heavy metal toxicity |
| Gram-negative bacteremia | Fanconi syndrome |
| Salicylate poisoning | Nephrotic syndrome |
| Hepatic coma | Multiple myeloma |
| Heat Stroke | Amyloidosis |
| Throtoxicosis | Aldosteronism |
| Primary hyperventilation | |
| Administration of | |
| Glucose | |
| Fructose | |
| Insulin | |
| Glycerol | |
| Epinephrine | |
| Gastrin | |
| Corticosteroids | |
| Lactate | |

***Burn Recovery*** The healing process associated with recovery from extensive third-degree burns is associated with a marked diuretic phase. This marked diuresis may be associated with an impressive loss of phosphate through the urine.[137,138,170] This recovery may also be associated with the development of an anabolic state as stress levels decrease and nutritional therapies take effect. Phosphorus is rapidly taken up by the new cells and severe hypophosphatemia may result.

***Nutritional Recovery Syndrome*** In World War II, a syndrome associated with peripheral edema, ascites, hydrothorax, and death was associated with refeeding protein-calorie malnourished prisoners with simple carbohydrate diets.[170]

**Table 102.30** Conditions Causing Severe Hypophosphatemia

| |
|---|
| Diabetic ketoacidosis |
| Respiratory alkalosis |
| Hyperalimentation |
| Alcohol withdrawal |
| Pharmacologic phosphate binding |
| Nutritional recovery syndrome |
| Recovery from severe burns |
| Recovery from acute respiratory acidosis |
| Reactivation of hematologic malignancy |
| Hypothermia |

Refeeding these patients with skim milk was associated with less morbidity, suggesting that the potassium and phosphorus content of skim milk might have been important in the decline in morbidity in the treatment of severe protein-calorie malnutrition. That this syndrome may be reproduced in experimental animal studies supports the credence of this phenomenon.[171]

***Hyperalimentation*** A modern-day version of the nutritional recovery syndrome has been described in patients receiving hyperalimentation, through both oral and intravenous routs.[137,172,173] Rapid refeeding of malnourished patients with high-carbohydrate, high-calorie nutritional diets with inadequate amounts of supplemental phosphorus may result in severe symptomatic hypophosphatemia. This phenomenon is especially significant in patients with other underlying risk factors for the development of hypophosphatemia such as alcoholism.[174] The etiology of severe hypophosphatemia associated with hyperalimentation and nutritional recovery may be separated into (1) the development of acute, rapid hypophosphatemia secondary to intracellular shifts of phosphorus resulting from glucose-induced insulin secretion and transcellular shift, and (2) the more gradual decrease in serum phosphorus concentration over 5 to 10 days secondary to tissue repair in the presence of phosphorus deprivation.[137] The development of severe hypophosphatemia secondary to hyperalimentation can be prevented by the administration of 12–15 mmol of phosphorus per liter of hyperalimentation solution or 15 mmol per 1,000 Cal of dextrose administered.[175]

**Table 102.31** Manifestations of Severe Hypophosphatemia

| | |
|---|---|
| Central nervous system | Gastrointestinal |
| Irritability | Anorexia |
| Apprehension | Nausea |
| Weakness | Emesis |
| Numbness | Skeletal/muscle |
| Paresthesias | Weakness |
| Dysarthria | Myalgia |
| Confusion | Rhabdomyolysis |
| Obtundation | Osteomalacia |
| Seizures | Hematologic |
| Coma | Decreased RBC 2,3-diphosphoglycerate |
| Pulmonary | Hemolysis |
| Acute respiratory failure | WBC dysfunction |
| Slow weaning from ventilator | Platelet dysfunction |
| Respiratory muscle fatigue | Renal |
| Cardiac | Acute tubular necrosis if myoglobinemia and rhabdomyolysis are present |
| Congestive cardiomyopathy | Bicarbonate and glucose wasting |
| Decreased contractility | |
| Hepatic | |
| Exacerbation of underlying hepatic insufficiency | |
| Hepatocellular dysfunction | |

***Respiratory Alkalosis*** Severe and prolonged respiratory alkalosis may cause profound hypophosphatemia, with values as low as 0.3 mg/dL reported.[176] The mechanism of hypophosphatemia associated with respiratory alkalosis is thought to be secondary to intracellular shifts of phosphorus. Respiratory alkalosis is thought to significantly contribute to the hypophosphatemia observed during alcohol withdrawal.

***Diabetic Ketoacidosis*** Patients with diabetic ketoacidosis may present with hyperphosphatemia. With the institution of therapy, however, serum phosphorus levels may rapidly drop as phosphorus shifts back into the intracellular compartment. As the acidosis associated with the diabetic ketoacidotic state causes decomposition of organic compounds inside the cell, inorganic phosphorus is released into the plasma and subsequently excreted into the urine.[137] The combination of intracellular phosphorus loss and intracellular shift of phosphorus upon initiation of treatment may cause severe hypophosphatemia.

***Alcoholism*** Chronic ethanol abusers are prone to a variety of serum electrolyte disorders including hypocalcemia, hypomagnesemia, hypokalemia, and hypophosphatemia. The etiology of hypophosphatemia in the alcoholic patient is multifactorial. Malnutrition, poor dietary intake, diarrhea, vomiting, and the use of phosphate-binding antacids may contribute to the hypophosphatemia of alcoholism.[137,138,170] In addition, serum phosphorus levels may decrease after 2 or 3 days of hospitalization in the alcoholic patient with the institution of dextrose-containing intravenous fluids, as a result of an intracellular shift of phosphorus.[138] Hyperventilation associated with the alcohol withdrawal syndrome may also contribute to the development of hypophosphatemia in the alcoholic patient.[177] Alcoholic patients are particularly susceptible to the complications of hypophosphatemia such as rhabdomyolysis, which occurs with great frequency in these patients.[177] As this complication can be prevented by the administration of phosphorus, particular awareness of serum phosphorus concentration is indicated when dealing with the alcoholic patient.

**Clinical Presentation**

The clinical manifestations of severe hypophosphatemia are diverse and may affect many major organ systems (Table 102.31). It is likely that two primary biochemical abnormalities are responsible for most of the clinical manifestations of severe hypophosphatemia.[132] Intracellular energy stores may be decreased secondary to depletion of intracellular ATP, which in itself is dependent upon inorganic intracellular phosphate. Phosphate is also vital in the formation of red blood cell 2,3-diphosphoglycerate, a substance vitally important in the promotion of release of oxygen from oxyhemoglobin.[137] Reduced red blood cell 2,3-diphosphoglycerate levels are associated with a shift to the left of the oxyhemoglobin saturation curve. This shift to the left is associated with a decrease in the release of oxygen to peripheral tissues, and may result in tissue hypoxia.[170] These metabolic disorders have been best characterized in studies of erythrocyte metabolism, but their implications can be seen in the wide variety of organ systems affected.[178]

Central nervous system manifestations of severe hypophosphatemia are compatible with a syndrome of metabolic encephalopathy.[137] A progressive syndrome of irritability, apprehension, weakness, numbness, paresthesias, dysarthria, confusion, obtundation, seizures, and coma has been described in patients with severe hypophosphatemia secondary to parenteral nutrition lacking phosphorus.[179,180]

Severe hypophosphatemia may result in significant dysfunction of skeletal and cardiac muscle. Skeletal muscle dysfunction may range from myalgia and weakness, associated with chronic hypophosphatemia, to potentially fatal rhabdomyolysis, associated with severe, acute hypophosphatemia.[181–183]

Hypophosphatemia has resulted in acute respiratory failure secondary to respiratory muscle weakness.[184] Diaphragmatic contractile dysfunction has been demonstrated in patients with acute respiratory failure associated with concomitant hypophosphatemia.[185] Correction of serum phosphorus with replacement therapy has been demonstrated to result in an increase in diaphragmatic function and reversal of acute respiratory failure.[184] Close assessment of serum phosphorus concentration is indicated in patients at risk for respiratory failure to potentially prevent this complication. Treatment of hypophosphatemia in respiratory failure patients may aid in achieving successful weaning from the ventilator.

Cardiac muscle function has also been reported to be impaired in the setting of hypophosphatemia, and has resulted in reversible congestive cardiomyopathy.[186] Hypophosphatemia is a potentially reversible cause of heart failure and thus should be considered in patients with acute deterioration in ventricular function.

The hematologic abnormalities of hypophosphatemia constitute a major manifestation of the syndrome.[132] Red blood cell manifestations of hypophosphatemia include decreased levels of 2,3-diphosphoglycerate, decreased red blood cell ATP, and alteration of red blood cell structure.[132,127,138,170] When red blood cell ATP decreases to below 15% of normal, cells become spherocytic and rigid and are trapped and destroyed in the spleen.[137,138,187] Therefore, hemolysis may be a manifestation of severe hypophosphatemia.

Reduction in ATP content of white blood cells may cause dysfunction of white blood cell mobility, chemotaxis, phagocytosis, and bacteria-killing ability.[132,137,138,170] White blood cell dysfunction may contribute to an increased risk of gram-negative sepsis in hypophosphatemia patients.[188] Animal studies have demonstrated thrombocytopenia, shortened platelet survival time, alteration of clot retraction, and hemorrhage as manifestations of platelet dysfunction in the setting of hypophosphatemia.[138] The implications of hypophosphatemia on human platelet function have not been determined.

It is clear that severe hypophosphatemia may result in a variety of symptoms and syndromes. These manifestations emphasize the vital importance of phosphorus in the biologic system.

**Treatment**

Treatment is guided by the presence or absence of symptoms and the severity of hypophosphatemia. Awareness of the clinical situations in which hypophosphatemia may be anticipated (alcoholism, diabetic ketoacidosis, glucose infusion) is of vital importance in preventing iatrogenic hypophosphatemia. Frequent serum phosphorus determinations should be made in patients at risk. The routine addition of phosphorus in concentrations of 12–15 mmol/L of intravenous hyperalimentation solution is of utmost importance for the prevention of severe hypophosphatemia which may be associated with phosphorus-free hyperalimentation solutions.

Mild to moderate asymptomatic hypophosphatemia can be treated orally by the administration of oral phosphorus salts (Table 102.32). The dose-limiting adverse effect associated with oral phosphorus replacement is the development of an osmotic diarrhea. Patients with moderate hypophosphatemia and concomitant renal dysfunction should receive reduced daily oral doses (i.e., 1 g or approximately 30 mmol of phosphorus) and careful monitoring of serum phosphorus concentration.

Severe symptomatic hypophosphatemia should be treated with parenteral phosphorus replacement. Similar to potassium, estimation of total body phosphorus deficit is extremely difficult as phosphorus is an intracellular element as well. Recommendations for parenteral phosphorus replacement have evolved from recommendations based on theoretical grounds to recommendations based on patient experience.[189–192] Response to intravenous serum phosphorus supplementation is highly variable. Infusion of 9–15 mmol of phosphorus (0.15–0.25 mmol/kg) over 4 to 12 hours has been shown to be safe and effective treatment for severe hypophosphatemia.[189,190]

Parenteral phosphorus supplementation is associated with the risks of hyperphosphatemia, metastatic soft tissue deposition of calcium phosphate, hypocalcemia, and hyperkalemia or hypernatremia, depending upon the salt employed. Inappropriate administration of large doses of parenteral phosphorus administered over relatively short time periods has resulted in symptomatic hypocalcemia and soft tissue calcification.[160] Rate of infusion and choice of initial dosage

**Table 102.32** Phosphorus Replacement Therapy

| |
|---|
| Moderate hypophosphatemia (serum phosphorus 1.0–2.5 mg/dL) |
| Oral therapy |
| 1.5–2 g (50–60 mmol) phosphorus per day, divided into three or four doses |
| Parenteral therapy |
| 0.15 mmol/kg lean body weight infused in 250–1,000 mL $D_5W$ over 12 h; repeat until serum phosphorus > 2 mg/dL |
| Severe hypophosphatemia (serum phosphorus < 1 mg/dL) |
| Parenteral therapy |
| 0.25 mmol/kg lean body weight infused in 250–500 mL $D_5W$ by infusion pump over 4–6 h; repeat until serum phosphorus > 2 mg/dL |

should therefore be based on severity of hypophosphatemia and presence of symptoms. Patients should be closely monitored with frequent serum phosphorus determinations. Monitoring should also include assessment of serum calcium concentrations, and therapy with parenteral phosphorus should be undertaken with great caution and at reduced dosage with patients with baseline hypercalcemia, renal dysfunction, or evidence of tissue injury.[137]

## References


1. Schrier RW, Anderson RJ. Renal sodium excretion, edematous disorders and diuretic use, in, Schier RW (ed): Renal and Electrolyte Disorders, 2nd ed. Boston, Little Brown and Company, 1980, pp 65–114.
2. Scully RE, McNeely BV, Mark EJ. Normal reference laboratory values. N Engl J Med 1986;314:39–49.
3. Flear CT, Gill GV, Burn J. Hyponatremia: Mechanisms and management. Lancet 1981;1:26–31.
4. Anderson RJ, Chung HM, Kluge R, et al. Hyponatremia: A prospective analysis of its epidemiology and the pathogenic role of vasopressin. Ann Intern Med 1985;102:164–168.
5. Narins RG, Jones RE, Stom MC, et al. Diagnostic strategies and disorders of fluid, electrolyte and acid base homeostasis. Am J Med 1982;72:496–520.
6. Goldberg M. Hypotnatremia. Med Clin North Am 1981;65: 251–269.
7. Schier RW, Berl T. Disorders of water metabolism, in Schier RW (ed): Renal and Electrolyte Disorders, 2nd ed. Boston, Little, Brown, 1980, pp 1–69.
8. Rose BD. Clinical Physiology of Acid Base and Electrolyte Disorders. New York, McGraw–Hill, 1984, pp 515–547.
9. Trump DL. Serious hyponatremia in patients with cancer: Management with demeclocycline. Cancer 1981;47:2908–2912.
10. Forrest JN, Cox M, Hong C, et al. Superiority of demeclocycline over lithium in the treatment of chronic syndrome of inappropriate secretion of antidiuretic hormone. N Engl J Med 1978;298:173–177.
11. De Troyer A. Demeclocycline: Treatment of syndrome of inappropriate antidiuretic hormone secretion. JAMA 1977;237: 2723–2726.
12. Arieff AI. Hyponatremia, convulsions, respiratory arrest and permanent brain damage after elective surgery in healthy women. N Engl J Med 1986;314:1529–1535.
13. Sterns RH, Riggs JE, Schochet SS Jr. Osmotic demyelination syndrome following correction of hyponatremia. N Engl J Med 1986;314:1535–1542.
14. Narins RG. Therapy of hyponatremia, does haste make waste? N Engl J Med 1986;314:1573–1575.
15. Feig PU. Hypernatremia and hypertonic syndromes. Med Clin North Am 1981;65:271–290.
16. Baylis PH. Hyponatremia and hypernatremia: Disorders of tonicity. Clin Endocrinol Metab 1980;9:625–637.
17. Gabow PA. Fluids and Electrolytes: Clinical Problems and Their Solutions. Boston, Little Brown, 1983, pp 69–75.
18. Weitzman RE, Kleeman CR. The clinical physiology of water metabolism. II. Renal mechanisms for urinary concentration: Diabetes insipidus. West J Med 1979;131:486–515.
19. Rose BD. Clinical Physiology of Acid–Base and Electrolyte Disorders. New York, McGraw–Hill, 1984, pp. 248–268.
20. Gabow AP, Peterson LN. Disorders of potassium metabolism, Schrier RW (ed): Renal and Electrolyte Disorders, 2nd ed. Boston, Little, Brown, 1980, pp 183–222.
21. Schultz RG, Nissenson AR. Potassium, in Maxwell MH, Kleeman CR (eds): Clinical Disorders of Fluid and Electrolyte Metabolism, 3rd ed. New York, McGraw–Hill, 1980 pp 113–144.
22. Brown RS. Potassium homeostasis and clinical implications. Am J Med 1984;77(5A):3–10.
23. Stearns RH, Cox M, Feig PU. Internal potassium balance and the control of the plasma potassium concentration. Medicine 1981;60:339–354.
24. Brown MJ, Murphy MB. Hypokalemia from beta 2-receptor stimulation by circulating epinephrine. N Engl J Med 1983;309: 1414–1419.
25. Williams ME, Rosa RM, Silva P, et al. Impairment of extrarenal potassium disposal by alpha adrenergic stimulation. N Engl J Med 1984;311:145–149.
26. Hampton JR. Should every survivor of a heart attack be given a beta blocker? I. Evidence from clinical trials. Br Med J 1982;285:33–36.
27. Knochel JP. Role of glucoregulatory hormones in potassium homeostasis. Kidney Int 1977;11:443–452.
28. Harrington JT, Isner JM, Kasirer JP. Our national obsession with potassium. Am J Med 1982;73:155–159.
29. Knochel JP. Diuretic-induced hypokalemia. Am J Med 1984;77(5A):18–26.
30. Surawicz B. Relationship between electrocardiogram and electrolytes. Am Heart J 1967;73:814–834.
31. Kaplan NM. Our appropriate concern about hypokalemia. Am J Med 1984;77:1–4.
32. Helgeland A. Treatment of mild hypertension: A five year controlled drug trial. Am J Med 1980;69:725–732.
33. Multiple Risk Factor Intervention Trial Research Group. Multiple risk factor intervention trial: Risk factor changes and mortality results. JAMA 1982;248:1465–1477.
34. Lawson DH. Adverse reactions to potassium chloride. Q J Med 1974;63:433–440.
35. Stanaszek WF, Romankiewicz JA. Current approaches to management of potassium deficiency. Drug Intel Clin Pharm 1985;19:176–183.
36. Pullen HM, Doig A, Lambie AT. Intensive intravenous potassium replacement therapy. Lancet 1967;2:809–811.
37. Seftel HC, Kew MC. Early and intensive potassium replacement in diabetic acidosis. Diabetes 1966;15:694–696.
38. Abramson E, Arky R. Diabetic acidosis with initial hypokalemia. JAMA 1966;196:401–403.
39. Bia MJ, Defronzo RA. Potassium chloride therapy. JAMA 1981;246:2501.
40. Zenk K. Management of intravenous extravasations. Infusion 1981;5:77–79.
41. Boley SJ, Allen AC, Schultz L, et al. Potassium induced lesions of the small bowel: I. Clinical aspects. JAMA 1965;193: 997–1000.
42. Allen AC, Boley SJ, Schultz L, et al. Potassium-induced lesions of the small bowel: II. Pathology and pathogenesis. JAMA 1965;193:1001–1006.
43. Barkin J, Harary A, Shambler C, et al. Potassium chloride and gastrointestinal injury. Ann Intern Med 1983;98:261–262.
44. Patterson D, Jeffries G. Spectrum of mucosal injury from oral potassium chloride supplements in normal volunteers. (Abstr) Gastroenterology 1983;84:1271.
45. Sherlock P. Cardiovascular and Renal Drugs and Gastrointes-

tinal Drugs Advisory Committee Meeting. Bethesda, Food and Drug Administration, 1983, pp 1–273.

46. Mudge GH. Chapter 36, Diuretics, in Gilman AG, Goodman LS, Gilman A (eds): Goodman and Gilman's The Pharmacologic Basis of Therapeutics. New York, Macmillan, 1980, pp 892–915.
47. Hollifield JW. Potassium and magnesium abnormalities, diuretics and arrhythmias in hypertension. Am J Med 1984;77(5A): 28–32.
48. Greenblatt DJ, Koch-Weser J. Adverse reactions to spironolactone. A report from the Boston Collaborative Drug Surveillance Program. JAMA 1973;225:40–43.
49. Martin ML, Hamilton R, West MF. Potassium. Emerg Med Clin North Am 1986;4:131–144.
50. Walmsley RN, White GH, Cain M, et al. Hyperkalemia in the elderly. Clin Chem 1984;30:1409–1412.
51. DeFronzo RA, Ria M, Smith D. Clinical disorders of hyperkalemia. Annu Rev Med 1982;33:521–554.
52. Kunis CL, Lowenstein J. The emergency treatment of hyperkalemia. Med Clin North Am 1981;65:165–176.
53. Smith JD, Bia MJ, DeFronza RA. Clinical disorders of potassium metabolism, in Arieff AI, DeFronzo RA (eds): Fluid, Electrolyte, and Acid–Base Disorders. New York, Churchill Livingstone, 1985, vol 1, pp 413–510.
54. Janson CL. Fluid and electrolyte balance, in Rosen P (ed): Emergency Medicine: Concepts and Clinical Practice. St. Louis, C.V. Mosby, 1983, vol 2, pp 1419–1465.
55. Finch CA, Sawyer CG, Flynn JM. Clinical syndrome of potassium intoxication. Am J Med 1946;1:337–357.
56. Dubois GD, Arieff AI. Clinical manifestations of electrolyte disorders, in Arieff AI, DeFronzo RA (eds): Fluid, Electrolyte, and Acid–Base Disorders. New York, Churchill Livingstone, 1985, vol 2, pp 1987–2144.
57. Newmark SR, Dluhy RG. Hyperkalemia and hypokalemia. JAMA 1975;231:631–633.
58. Agus ZS, Wasserstein A, Goldfarb S. Disorders of calcium and magnesium homeostasis. Am J Med 1982;72:473–488.
59. Popovtzer MM, Knochel JP. Disorders of calcium, phosphorus, vitamin D, and parathyroid hormone activity, in Schreier RW (ed): Renal and Electrolyte Disorders, 2nd ed. Boston, Little Brown, 1980, pp 223–297.
60. Christenson T, et al. Prevalence of hypercalcemia in a health screening in Stockholm. Acta Med Scand 1976;200:131–137.
61. Mundy GR, Ibbotson KJ, D'Souze SM, et al. The hypercalcemia of cancer, clinical implications and pathogenic mechanisms. N Engl J Med 1984;310:1718–1727.
62. Stewart AF. Therapy of malignancy-associated hypercalcemia: 1983. Am J Med 1983;74:475–480.
63. Burt ME, Brennan MF. Incidence of hypercalcemia in malignant neoplasm. Arch Surg 1980;115:704–707.
64. Body JJ. Cancer hypercalcemia: Recent advances in understanding and treatment. Eur J Cancer Clin Oncol 1984;20:865–869.
65. Coombs RC, Wood MK, Greenberg PB, et al. Calcium metabolism in cancer. Cancer 1976;38:2111–2120.
66. Mallette LE, Bilezikian JP, Heath DA, et al. Primary hyperparathyroidism: Clinical and biochemical features. Medicine 1974;53:127–146.
67. Purnell DC, VanHoerden JA. Management of symptomatic hypercalcemia and hypocalcemia. World J Surg 1982;6:702–709.
68. Bronsky D, Dubin A, Waldstein SS, et al. Calcium and electrocardiogram. II. The electrocardiogram manifestations of hyperparathyroidism and of marked hypercalcemia from various etiologies. Am J Cardiol 1961;7:833–839.
69. Potts JT. Disorders of parathyroid gland, in Isselbacher KJ, Adams RO, Brunwald E, et al (eds): Harrison's Principles of Internal Medicine. New York, McGraw–Hill, 1980, pp 1929–1943.
70. Suki WN, Wyum JJ, VonMinden M, et al. Acute treatment of hypercalcemia with furosemide. N Engl J Med 1970;283:836–840.
71. Hosking OJ. Treatment of severe hypercalcemia with calcitonin. Metab Bone Dis Rel Res 1980;2:207–212.
72. Binstock ML, Mundy GR. Effect of calcitonin and glucocorticoids in combination in the hypercalcemia of malignancy. Ann Intern Med 1980;93:269–272.
73. Perlia CP, Gubisch NG, Wolter J, et al. Mithramycin treatment of hypercalcemia. Cancer 1970;25:389–394.
74. Lebbin D, Ryan WG, Schwartz TB. Outpatient treatment of Paget's disease of bone with mithramycin. Ann Intern Med 1984;81:635–637.
75. Brenner DE, Harvey HA, Lipton A, et al. A study of prostaglandin $E_2$, parathyroid hormone, and response to indomethacin in patients with hypercalcemia of malignancy. Cancer 1982;44:556–561.
76. Mundy GR, Wilkinson R, Heath DA. Comparative study of available medical therapy for hypercalcemia of malignancy. Am J Med 1983;74:421–432.
77. Reitsma PH, Teitelbaum SL, Bijvoet OLM, et al. Differential action of the biphosphonates (3-amino-1-hydroxypropylidene)-1,1-biphosphonate (APD) and disodium dichloromethylidene biphosphonate (C12MDP) on rat macrophage-mediated bone resorption in vitro. J Clin Invest 1982;70:927–933.
78. Jung A. Comparison of two parenteral diphosphonates in hypercalcemia of malignancy. Am J Med 1982;72:221–226.
79. Percival RC, Paterson AD, Yates AJP, et al. Treatment of malignant hypercalcemia with clodronate. Br J Cancer 1985; 51:665–669.
80. Sleeboom HP, Bijvoet OLM, VanOosterom AT, et al. Comparison of intravenous (3-amino-1-hydroxypropylidene)-1,1-biphosphonate and volume repletion in tumor-induced hypercalcemia. Lancet 1983;2:239–243.
81. Jung A, Chentraine A, Donerth A, et al. Use of dichloromethylene diphosphonate in metastatic bone disease. N Engl J Med 1983;308:1499–1501.
82. Ralston SH, Gardner MD, Dryburgh FA, et al. Comparison of aminohydroxypropylidene diphosphonate, mithramycin and corticosteroids–calcitonin in treatment of cancer-associated hypercalcemia. Lancet 1985;2:907–910 (Letter to the Editor: Lancet 1985;Dec 7;1299).
83. Philipson B, Angelin B, Christenson T, et al. Hypocalcemia with zonular cataract due to idiopathic hypoparathyroidism. Acta Med Scand 1978;203:223–226.
84. Davis RH, Forman P, Smith JWG. Prevalence of parathyroid insufficiency after thyroidectomy. Lancet 1963;2:121–124.
85. Michie W, Duncan T, Hamer-Hodges DW, et al. Mechanism of hypocalcemia after thyroidectomy for thyrotoxicosis. Lancet 1971;1:508–514.
86. Juan D. Hypocalcemia: Differential diagnosis and mechanisms. Arch Intern Med 1979;139:1166–1171.
87. Sitrin M, Meredith S, Rosenberg IH. Vitamin D deficiency and bone disease in gastrointestinal disorders. Arch Intern Med 1978;138:886–888.
88. Fraser D, Kooh SW, Kind HP, et al. Pathogenesis of hereditary vitamin D–dependent rickets: An inborn error of vitamin D metabolism involving defective conversion of 25-hydroxy vitamin D to 1-alpha,25-dihydroxy vitamin D. N Engl J Med 1973;289:817–822.
89. Coburn JW, Hartenbower DL, Brickman AS. Advances in

vitamin D metabolism as they pertain to chronic renal disease. Am J Clin Nutr 1976;29:1293–1299.
90. Surawicz B. Relationship between electrocardiogram and electrolytes. Am Heart J 1967;73:814–834.
91. Rimalho A, Bouchard P, Schaison G, et al. Improvement of hypocalcemic cardiomyopathy by correction of serum calcium level. Am Heart J 1985;109:611–613.
92. Bashour TT, Ryan C, Kabbani SS, et al. Hypocalcemic acute myocardial failure secondary to rapid transfusion of citrated blood. Am Heart J 1984;108:1040–1042.
93. Connor TB, Rosen BL, Blaustein MP, et al. Hypocalcemia precipitating congestive heart failure. N Engl J Med 1982;307: 869–872.
94. White RD, Goldsmith RS, Rodriguez R, et al. Plasma ionic calcium levels following injection of chloride, gluconate, and glyceptate salts of calcium. J Thorac Cardiovasc Surg 1976;71: 609–613.
95. Keyler D, Peterson CD. Oral calcium supplements. How much of what, for whom, and why? Postgrad Med 1985;78:123–125.
96. Porter RH, Cox BA, Heaney D. Treatment of hypoparathyroid patients with chlorthalidone. N Engl J Med 1978;298:577–581.
97. Graber TW, Yee AS, Baker FJ. Magnesium: Physiology, clincial disorders, and therapy. Ann Emerg Med 1981;10:49–57.
98. Iseri LT, French JH. Magnesium: Nature's physiologic calcium blocker. Am Heart J 1984;108:188–193.
99. Alfrey, AC. Disorders of magnesium metabolism, in Schreier RW (ed): Renal and Electrolyte Disorders, 2nd ed. Boston, Little, Brown, 1980, pp 299–318.
100. Whang R, Aikawa JK, Oei TO, et al. The need for routine serum magnesium determination. (Abstr) Clin Res 1977;25: 154.
101. Wong ET, Rude RK, Singer FR, et al. A high prevalence of hypomagnesemia and hypermagnesemia in hospitalized patients. Am J Clin Pathol 1983;79:348–352.
102. Rude RK, Singer FR. Magnesium deficiency and excess. Ann Rev Med 1981;32:245–259.
103. Wacker WE, Vallee BL. A study of magnesium metabolism in acute renal failure employing a multichannel flame spectrometer. N Engl J Med 1957;257:1254–1262.
104. Mordes JP, Waker WC. Excess magnesium. Pharmacol Rev 1978;29:273–300.
105. Eisenbud E, Lobac CC. Hypocalcemia after therapeutic use of magnesium sulfate. Arch Intern Med 1976;136:688–691.
106. Lipsitz PJ, English IC. Hypermagnesemia in the newborn infant. Pediatrics 1967;40:856–862.
107. Randall RE, Cohen MD, Spray CC, et al. Hypermagnesemia in renal failure. Etiology and toxic manifestations. Ann Intern Med 1964;61:73–76.
108. Reinhart RA, Desbiens MA. Hypomagnesemia in patients entering the ICU. Crit Care Med 1985;13(6):506–507.
109. Cronin RE, Knochel JP. Magnesium deficiency. Adv Intern Med 1983;28:509–533.
110. Ryzen E, Elkayam U, Rude RK. Low blood mononuclear cell magnesium in intensive cardiac care patients. Am Heart J 1986;111:475–480.
111. Berkelhammer C, Benir RA. A clinical approach to common electrolyte problems. 4. Hypomagnesemia. Can Med Assoc J 1985;1321:360–368.
112. Davis BB, Preuss HG, Murdaugh JV Jr. Hypomagnesemia following the diuresis of post-renal obstruction and renal transplant. Nephron 1975;14:275–280.
113. Sheehan J, White A. Diuretic-associated hypomagnesemia. Br Med J 1982;285:1157–1159.
114. Leary WP, Reyes AJ. Prophylaxis and treatment of magnesium depletion. S Afr Med J 1983;64:281–282.
115. Lyman MW, Hemalathe C, Viscuso RL, et al. Cisplatin-induced hypocalcemia and hypomagnesemia. Arch Intern Med 1980;140:1513–1514.
116. Stewart AF, Keuting T, Schwartz PE. Magnesium homeostasis following chemotherapy with cisplatin: A prospective study. Am J Obstet Gynecol 1985;153:660–665.
117. Flink EB. Nutritional aspects of magnesium metabolism. West J Med 1980;144:304–312.
118. Barton CH, Pahl M, Vaziri ND, et al. Renal magnesium wasting associated with amphotericin B therapy. Am J Med 1984;77:471–474.
119. Flink EB. Magnesium deficiency. Etiology and clinical spectrum. Acta Med Scand 1980;647(suppl):125–137.
120. Birch GE, Giled TD. The importance of magnesium deficiency in cardiovascular disease. Am Heart J 1977;94:649–657.
121. Anderson TW, Neri LC, Schreiber GB, et al. Ischemic heart disease, water hardness and myocardial magnesium. Can Med Assoc J 1975;113:199–203.
122. Turlapaty PDMV, Altura BM. Magnesium deficiency produces spasm of coronary arteries: Relationship of sudden death ischemic heart disease. Science 1980:208:198–200.
123. Johnson CJ, Peterson DR, Smith EK. Myocardial tissue concentrations of magnesium and potassium in men dying suddenly from ischemic heart disease. Am J Clin Nutr 1979;32: 967–970.
124. Iseri LT, Freed J, Bures AR. Magnesium deficiency in cardiac disorders. Am J Med 1975;58:837–845.
125. Loeb HS, Pietras RP, Gunnar RM, et al. Paroxysmal ventricular fibrillation in two patients with hypomagnesemia. Circulation 1968;37:210–215.
126. Chadda KD, Lichstein E, Gupta P. Hypomagnesemia and refractory cardiac arrhythmia in a non-digitalized patient. Am J Cardiol 1973;31:98–100.
127. Isin LT, Chung P, Tobis J. Magnesium therapy for intractable ventricular tachyarrhythmias in normomagnesemic patients. West J Med 1983;138:823–828.
128. Topac EJ, Lerman EB. Hypomagnesemic torsades de pointes. Am J Cardiol 1983;52:1367–1368.
129. Webb S, Schade DS. Hypomagnesemia as a cause of persistent hypokalemia. JAMA 1975;233:23–24.
130. Whang R, Oei TO, Watanabe. Frequency of hypomagnesemia in hospitalized patients receiving digitalis. Arch Intern Med 1985;145:655–656.
131. Flink EB. Therapy of magnesium deficiency. Ann NY Acad Sci 1969;162:901–905.
132. Stoff JS. Phosphate homeostasis and hypophosphatemia. Am J Med 1982;72:489–495.
133. Tsuboi KK, Fukungo K. Inorganic phosphate and enhanced glucose degradation by the intact erythrocyte. J Biol Chem 1965;240:2806–2810.
134. O'Donovan DJ, Lotspeich WD. Activation of kidney mitochondrial glutaminase by inorganic phosphate and organic acids. Nature 1966;212:930–932.
135. Tanaka Y, DeLuca HF. The control of 25-hydroxy vitamin D metabolism by inorganic phosphorus. Arch Biochem Biophys 1973;154:566–574.
136. Lichtman MA, Miller DR, Cohen J. Reduced red cell glycolysis, 2,3-diphosphoglycerate and adenosine triphosphate concentration and increased hemoglobin–oxygen affinity caused by hypophosphatemia. Ann Intern Med 1971;74:562–568.
137. Knochel JP. The pathophysiology and clinical characteristics

of severe hypophosphatemia. Arch Intern Med 1977;137:203–220.

**138.** Janson C, Birnbaum G, Baker FJ. Hypophosphatemia. Ann Emerg Med 1983;12:107–116.

**139.** Corvilain J, Abramow M. Effect of growth hormone on tubular transport of phosphate in normal and parathyroidectomized dogs. J Clin Invest 1964;34:1608–1612.

**140.** Bommer J, Bonjour JP, Ritze, et al. Parathyroid independent changes in renal handling of phosphate in hyperthyroid rats. Kidney Int 1979;15:325.

**141.** Slatopolsky E, Rutherford WE, Rosenbaum R, et al. Hyperphosphatemia. Clin Nephrol 1977;7:138–146.

**142.** Goldman R, Basset SH. Phosphorus excretion in renal failure. J Clin Invest 1954;33:1623–1628.

**143.** Moseley PK, Segar WE. Fluid and serum electrolyte disturbances as a complication of enemas in Hirschprung's disease. Am J Dis Child 1968;115:714–718.

**144.** Chesney RW, Houghton PB. Tetany following phosphate enemas in chronic renal disease. Am J Dis Child 1974;127:584–586.

**145.** Oxnard SA, O'Bell J, Grupp WE. Severe tetany in an azotemic child related to a sodium phosphate enema. Pediatrics 1974;53:105–106.

**146.** Swerdlow DB, Labow S, D'Anna FJ. Tetany in enemas: Report of a case. Dis Colon Rectum 1974;17:786–787.

**147.** Honig PJ, Holtzapple PG. Hypocalcemic tetany following hypertonic phosphate enemas. Clin Pediatr 1975;14:678–679.

**148.** Sotos JF, Cutler EA, Finkel MA, et al. Hypocalcemic coma following two pediatric phosphate enemas. Pediatrics 1977;60:305–307.

**149.** Loughnan P, Mullins GC. Brain damage following a hypertonic phosphate enema. Am J Dis Child 1977;131:1032.

**150.** Davis RF, Eichner JM, Bleyer WA, et al. Hypocalcemia, hyperphosphatemia and dehydration following a single hypertonic phosphate enema. J Pediatr 1977;90:484–485.

**151.** McConnell TH. Fatal hypocalcemia from phosphate absorption from laxative preparation. JAMA 1971;216:147–148.

**152.** Goldfinger P. Hypokalemia, metabolic acidosis and hypocalcemic tetany in a patient taking laxatives: A case report. J Mt Sinai Hosp 1969;36:113–116.

**153.** Wiberg JJ, Turner GG, Nuttall FQ. Effect of phosphate or magnesium cathartics on serum calcium. Arch Intern Med 1978;138:1114–1116.

**154.** Haldimann B, Vogt K. Hyperphosphatemietic tetanie apres clystere au phosphate. Schweiz Med Wochenschr 1983;113:1231–1233.

**155.** Biberstein M, Parker BA. Enema-induced hyperphosphatemia. Am J Med 1985;79:645–646.

**156.** Flentie EH, Cherkin A. Electrolyte effects of sodium phosphate enema. Dis Colon Rectum 1958;1:295–299.

**157.** Goldsmith RS, Ingbar SH. Inorganic phosphate treatment of hypercalcemia of diverse etiologies. N Engl J Med 1966;274:1–7.

**158.** Breuer RI, LeBauer J. Caution in the use of phosphates in the treatment of severe hypercalcemia. J Clin Endocrinol 1967;27:695–698.

**159.** Chernow B, Raimey TG, Georges LP, et al. Iatrogenic hyperphosphatemia: A metabolic consideration in critical care medicine. Crit Care Med 1981;9:772–774.

**160.** Boles JM, Dutel JL, Briere J, et al. Acute renal failure caused by extreme hyperphosphatemia after chemotherapy of an acute lymphoblastic leukemia. Cancer 1984;53:2424–2429.

**161.** Ettinger DS, Harker WG, Gerry HW, et al. Hyperphosphatemia, hypocalcemia, and transient renal failure. Results of cytotoxic treatment of acute lymphoblastic leukemia. JAMA 1978;239:2472–2474.

**162.** Zusman J, Brown DM, Nesbit ME. Hyperphosphatemia, hyperphosphaturia, and hypocalcemia in acute lymphoblastic leukemia. N Engl J Med 1973;289:1335–1340.

**163.** Monballyu J, Zachee P, Verberckmoes R, et al. Transient acute renal failure due to tumor-lysis–induced severe phosphate load in a patient with Burkitt's lymphoma. Clin Nephrol 1984;22:47–50.

**164.** Brerereton HD, Anderson T, Johnson RE, et al. Hyperphosphatemia and hypocalcemia in Burkitt lymphoma. Arch Intern Med 1975;135:307–309.

**165.** Kebler R, McDonald FD, Cadnapaphornchai P. Dynamic changes in serum phosphorus levels in diabetic ketoacidosis. Am J Med 1985;79:571–576.

**166.** Herbert LA, Lemann J Jr, Petersen JR, et al. Studies of the mechanism by which phosphate infusion lowers serum calcium concentration. J Clin Invest 1966;45:1886–1894.

**167.** Betro MG, Pain WR. Hypophosphatemia and hyperphosphatemia in a hospital population. Br Med J 1972;1:273–276.

**168.** Gilbert FR, Casey AB, Downey EL, et al. Admission inorganic phosphorus correlated with discharge diagnoses and other metabolic profile components. Ala J Med Sci 1970;3:343–349.

**169.** Stein JH, Smith WO, Ginn HE. Hypophosphatemia in acute alcoholism. Am J Med Sci 1969;252:78–83.

**170.** Knochel JP. Hypophosphatemia. Clin Nephrol 1977;4:131–137.

**171.** Smith GS, Smith JL, Maneesch MS, et al. Hypertension and cardiovascular abnormalities in starved–refed swine. J Nutr 1964;82:173.

**172.** Martin BK, Slingerland AW, Jenks JS. Severe hypophosphatemia associated with nutritional support. Nutr Support Services 1985;5:34–38.

**173.** Weinsier RL, Krumdieck CL. Death resulting from overzealous total parenteral nutrition: The refeeding syndrome revisited. Am J Gastroenterol 1980;73:215–222.

**174.** Silvis SE, DiBartolomeo AG, Aaker HM. Hypophosphatemia and neurological changes secondary to oral caloric intake. Am J Gastroentrol 1980;73:215–222.

**175.** Berkelhammer C, Bear RA. A clinical approach to common electrolyte problems. 3. Hypophosphatemia. Can Med Assoc J 1984;130:17–23.

**176.** Okel BB, Hurst JW. Prolonged hyperventilation in man: Associated electrolyte changes and subjective symptoms. Arch Intern Med 1961;108:757–762.

**177.** Knochel JP. Hypophosphatemia in the alcoholic. Arch Intern Med 1980;140:613–615.

**178.** Lichtman MA, Miller TR, Cohen J, et al. Reduced red cell glycolysis, 2,3-diphosphoglycerate and adenosine triphosphate concentration, and increased hemoglobin–oxygen affinity caused by hypophosphatemia. Ann Intern Med 1981;74:562–568.

**179.** Silvis SE, Paragas PD. Paresthesias, weakness, seizures and hypophosphatemia in patients receiving hyperalimentation. Gastroentrology 1972;62:513–520.

**180.** Travis SF, Sugerman HJ, Ruberg RL, et al. Alterations of red cell glycolytic intermediates and oxygen transport as a consequence of hypophosphatemia in patients receiving intravenous hyperalimentation. N Engl J Med 1971;285:763–768.

**181.** Ravid M, Robson M. Proximal myopathy caused by iatrogenic phosphate depletion. JAMA 1976;236:1380–1381.

**182.** Knochel JP. Skeletal muscle in hypophosphatemia and phosphorus deficiency. Adv Exp Med Biol 1978;103:357–366.

**183.** Knochel JP, Barcenas C, Cotten JR, et al. Hypophosphatemia and rhabdomyolysis. J Clin Invest 1978;62:1240–1246.

184. Newman JH, Neff TA, Ziporin P. Acute respiratory failure associated with hypophosphatemia. N Engl J Med 1977;296:1101–1103.
185. Aubier M, Murciano D, Lecocguic Y, et al. Effect of hypophosphatemia on diaphragmatic contractility in patients with acute respiratory failure. N Engl J Med 1985;313:420–424.
186. Darsee JR, Nutter DO. Reversible severe congestive cardiomyopathy in three cases of hypophosphatemia. Ann Intern Med 1978;89:867–870.
187. Jacob HS, Amsden T. Acute hemolytic anemia with rigid red cells in hypophosphatemia. N Engl J Med 1971;285:1446–1450.
188. Riedler GF, Scheitlin WA. Hypophosphatemia in septicemia: Higher incidence in gram negative than in gram positive infections. Br Med J 1969;1:753–756.
189. Vannatta JB, Whang R, Papper S. Efficacy of intravenous phosphorus therapy in severely hypophosphatemic patients. Arch Intern Med 1981;141:885–887.
190. Kingston M, Badawi Al-Sibai M. Treatment of severe hypophosphatemia. Crit Care Med 1985;13:16–18.
191. Andress DL, Vannatta JB, Whang R. Treatment of refractory hypophosphatemia. South Med J 1982;75:767–7.
192. Wilson HK, Keuer SP, Lea AS, et al. Phosphate therapy in diabetic ketoacidosis. Arch Intern Med 1982;142:517–520.

# Chapter 103 / Hypovolemic Shock

David M. Angaran, MS

Hypovolemic shock is a condition characterized by hypotension resulting from acute intravascular volume deficiency. This volume deficiency is associated either with external losses from acute hemorrhage, burns, diarrhea, vomiting, insensible water loss, or Addison's disease or with internal redistribution of extracellular water resulting from septic systemic vasodilation and increased microvascular permeability. Neurogenic and anaphylactic shock may also cause this redistribution phenomenon.

The loss of intravascular volume is accompanied by a decrease and redistribution of cardiac output that may decrease oxygen delivery to a critical point. The resuscitation goal is restoration of oxygen delivery to meet the demands of the body. It is fortunate that the most efficient way to increase cardiac output and achieve normal distribution is by restoring plasma volume.

There are two conflicting philosophies over the replacement of fluids in hypovolemic shock: colloid use (5% albumin, plasma protein fraction, hetastarch) and crystalloid use (lactated Ringer's, normal saline). This controversy has existed for more than 20 years. In this chapter, we attempt to provide the physiologic basis for each side of the controversy. We are not able to declare which is "correct," but we hope that the reader will be able to understand and work with proponents of both philosophies.

## Body Water Distribution

Total body water (TBW) varies from 50% to 70% of body weight. The variation in TBW depends on the lean body mass:fat ratio. Fat water content is 10% compared with 75% for muscle mass. An obese person, therefore, has a lower percentage of TBW by weight than does a slender person.[1]

TBW is divided into two compartments: intracellular water (ICW) and extracellular water (ECW). ICW and ECW represent 55% and 35% of TBW, respectively. The remaining 10% is located in bone and transcellular water (Fig. 103.1). In addition, ECW is subdivided further into plasma volume (PV, 7.5%) and interstitial fluid (ISF, 27.5%).

The distribution of TBW between ICW and ECW is maintained primarily by the balancing of osmotic forces into and out of the cell. The osmostic solutes within the cell are potassium (major), magnesium, protein, and organic phosphorus. The major osmotic solutes in ECW are sodium and its anions, chloride and bicarbonate. Sodium chloride and bicarbonate are relatively impermeable to the cell membrane and move intracellularly with great difficulty. Therefore, sodium chloride is the primary ion contributing to the 285 mosM/L osmotic gradient found in ECW.[2] The division of ECW between PV and ISF is discussed at length with respect to Starling's law (see later). The formula

$$2 \times \text{Na (mEq/L)} + \frac{\text{blood glucose}}{18} + \frac{\text{blood urea nitrogen}}{2.8}$$

(latter two values in mg/dL) is handy to estimate the serum osmolarity at the patient's bedside. The BUN is included in the calculation but distributes equally between ECW and ICW and does not move water into or out of the cell. Alcohol is another compound that distributes equally and the presence of alcohol can create a situation in which the calculated or measured serum osmolarity is greater than the "effective" osmolarity because alcohol is present in equal concentrations on both sides of the cell membrane.

TBW is clinically assessed primarily by physical examination, except for PV, which is estimated by the central venous pressure (CVP) and pulmonary artery wedge pressure (PAWP). These are not volumes, but pressures, and are functions of plasma volume, the area inside the blood vessels, ventricular compliance, and cardiac output. These pressures may be altered without changes in PV by constriction or dilation of blood vessels or by a disease that changes ventricular compliance, such as myocardial infarction. For example, a stiff noncompliant ventricle provides a higher PAWP with a smaller end-diastolic volume. Such clinical assessments as skin turgor, blood pressure, and changes in weight are even more indirect and an accurate documentation of the decrease or increase in PV, ISF, or TBW is imprecise at the patient's bedside.

The maintenance of proper fluid distribution among the various body spaces is necessary for homeostasis. *Starling's law of fluid movement* describes the major forces that maintain an adequate plasma volume. These forces are dynamic and remain the subject of great controversy because some can be measured only experimentally and with little confidence.

The Starling equation[3] governing fluid movement is

$$J_v = K_{F,c}\,[(P_c - P_T) - \sigma_c\,(\pi_c - \pi_T)]$$

where

$J_v$ = rate of fluid movement into or out of capillary (mL/min/100 g)
$J_v>0$ = fluid movement out of the capillary
$J_v<0$ = fluid movement into the capillary

$K_{F,c}$ = capillary filtration coefficient (mL/mm Hg/min/100 g); normal, 0.1

$P_c$ = capillary hydrostatic pressure (mm Hg); normal, 6

$P_T$ = tissue fluid hydrostatic pressure (mm Hg); normal, −7,

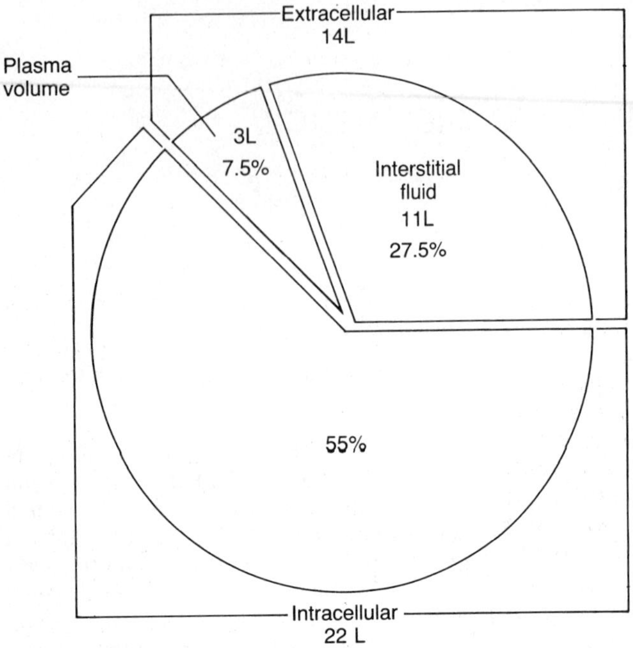


**Figure 103.1** Diagrammatic representation of fluid distribution in the body, showing intracellular fluid (55%) and extracellular fluid (35%) with its components, plasma volume (7.5%) and interstitial fluid (27.5%). *(From Ross AD, Angaran DM: Drug Intell Clin Pharm 1984;18:203, with permission.)*

$\sigma_c$ = capillary membrane permeability coefficient to proteins; range 0–1

$\pi_c$ = plasma oncotic pressure (colloid osmotic pressure)(mm Hg); normal, 26

$\pi_T$ = tissue fluid oncotic pressure (tissue colloid osmotic pressure)(mm Hg); normal, 14

Figure 103.2 details the normal values presumed to exist on the arterial side of the human lung. At the venous side, the hydrostatic pressure ($P_c$) drops from 7 to 4, and $J_v$ decreases below zero with flow going into the capillary.[4]

The capillary filtration coefficient ($K_{F,c}$) represents variations in the capillary membrane's permeability to small solutes and water. This value depends on the porosity and surface area of the endothelium and varies in different organs with different disease states.[5] An increase in $K_{F,c}$ may occur during PV overexpansion such as that accompanying congestive heart failure (CHF).

Capillary hydrostatic pressure ($P_c$) is the outward pushing force created by the mechnical pressure of the heart. It is the primary force pushing fluid out of the capillaries. Pulmonary $P_c$ is approximated clinically by the PAWP. The $P_c$ values of various organs differ. In the lung $P_c$ is 7 mm Hg[6]; in skeletal muscle, 15–20 mm Hg[7]; and in the liver, 5–6 mm Hg.[8]

Plasma colloid osmotic pressure ($\pi_c$) is the inward pulling force exerted across the capillary membrane by the intravascular proteins. The term *colloid osmotic pressure* is used to distinguish the osmotic pressure at the capillary from the pressure exerted at the cell membrane by such salts as sodium. Oncotic pressure is synonymous with colloid osmotic pressure.

$\pi_c$ is the only parameter in the Starling equation that can be measured directly in the clinical setting. All plasma proteins are active oncotically, but albumin, which represents only 50% of the total gram amount of serum protein, accounts for 65% to 75% of the $\pi_c$. Globulins can be important in some unusual circumstances such as multiple myeloma, but are not discussed in this chapter.[1]

Albumin (300 g) is found throughout the body, with only 30% to 40% located in the plasma compartment. The remaining portion is found in extravascular sites such as the interstitial fluid of skin, muscle, lungs, and lymph.[9] The plasma concentration of albumin is a function of hepatic synthesis, metabolic breakdown, and rate of flow into and out of the plasma from extravascular sites. The normal half-life of albumin from the vascular space is 16 hours, but may be as low as 2 to 3 hours in pathologic states. The elimination half-life of albumin from the body is 17 to 19 days.[10]

Albumin movement from the vascular space of capillaries to the lymph, and vice versa, is a normal physiologic process. The rate of movement may be altered by a change not only in $\sigma$ (reflection coefficient) but also by variations in plasma volume caused by shock. Liver function and nutritional status also play a vital role in maintaining albumin stores.[10]

The normal $\pi_c$ is 25–28 mm Hg and declines to 21 mm Hg in the recumbent position. This value is 1–2 mm Hg lower in older patients (>50 years) and 2 mm Hg lower in females.[11] Oncotic pressure can be approximated from the total plasma protein (TPP) concentration (g/dL) by the formula[12]

**Figure 103.2** Currently perceived normal values for the forces that govern fluid exchange across the pulmonary capillary. These approximate values can be substituted into the Starling equation, resulting in a 1-mm Hg imbalance in forces favoring the extravascular movement of fluid. The $K_{F,c}$ for the normal lung, 0.1 mL/torr/min/100 g, defines the resultant flow across the membrane caused by the 1-mm Hg imbalance to be 0.1 mL/min/100 g. The normal pulmonary lymph flow rate is in the range of 0.1 mL/min/100 g. Thus, under normal conditions, lymph flow compensates for the small imbalances in forces that govern fluid exchange across the pulmonary capillary membrane and lung weight remains stable; the lung is in an isogravimetric state. *(From Gabel JC, Drake RE: Pulmonary capillary pressure and permeability. Crit Care Med 1979;7:92–97, with permission.)*

$$J_V = K_{F,c}\,[(P_c - P_T) - \sigma_c(\pi_c - \pi_T)]$$

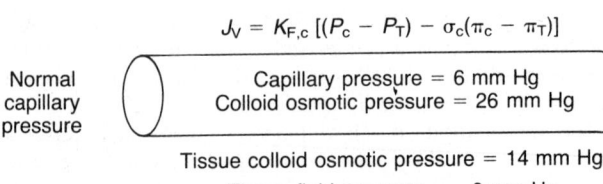

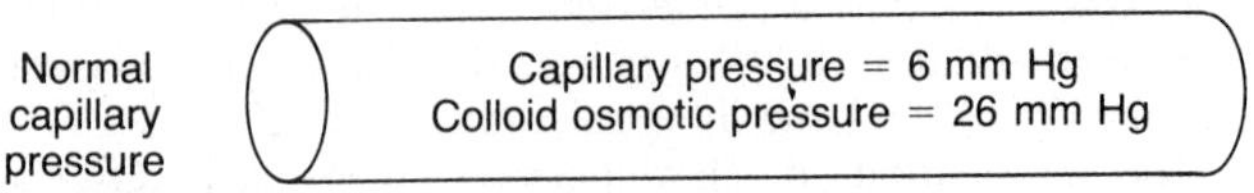


Tissue colloid osmotic pressure = 14 mm Hg

Tissue fluid pressure = −6 mm Hg

$(P_c - P_T) - \sigma_c(\pi_c - \pi_T)$

$(6 - -6) - 0.9\ (26 - 14)$

12 mm Hg    11 mm Hg

1 mm Hg imbalance

Lymph flow = 0.1 mL/min/100 g

$K_{F,c}$ = 0.1 mL/mm Hg/min/100 g

$$\pi_c = 2.1(\text{TPP}) + 0.16(\text{TPP})^2 + 0.009\,(\text{TPP})^3$$

Such clinical conditions as elevated temperature, changes in blood pH, and liver disease or treatment with albumin can affect the actual $\pi_c$; therefore, a poor correlation may exist between the calculated $\pi_c$ and the actual $\pi_c$.[13]

Some studies have evaluated $\pi_c$ in the clinical setting and found that a $\pi_c$ less than 10 mm Hg was associated with an increase in pulmonary edema and mortality. Weil et al[14] proposed that the parameter $\pi_c - P_c$ can be useful in predicting the development of pulmonary edema. The normal difference is 18 mm Hg ($\pi_c[25] - P_c[7]$) and a gradient of less than 3 mm Hg for 12 hours or longer is considered dangerous.[15] As might be expected, there is considerable disagreement about the utility and clinical usefulness of both $\pi_c$ and the $\pi_c - P_c$ gradient, with some investigators being unable to reproduce the previously quoted works.[16,17] It does not necessarily follow that elevating the $\pi_c$ to some minimum value is beneficial. Grundmann and Heistermann conducted a prospective trial of albumin in 220 patients to keep their $\pi c$ at either 19 or 24 mm Hg and could find no difference in outcome.[18]

### *Reflection Coefficient*

The reflection coefficient ($\sigma$) is the ability of capillary membranes to prevent plasma proteins and other molecules (>60,000 molecular weight) from crossing into the interstitium. The value of $\sigma$ varies from 1 (impermeable) to 0 (completely permeable) and differs among vascular beds. Although absolute values are not known, certain capillaries have a very low reflection (hepatic microcirculation, 0.2), whereas the lungs are higher (0.8) and skeletal muscle is virtually impermeable (1.0).[19] The normal $\pi_c - P_c$ pressure gradient is confounded when conditions, such as sepsis, increase the permeability of the capillary membrane (0.8 to 0.4), allowing more protein to leak out. An albumin-containing solution, for example, might aggravate this type of pulmonary edema. The beneficial impact of increasing $\pi_c$ is lost secondary to the increased permeability of the capillary. The effective gradient to pull necessary water out of the lung interstitium is no longer present. The $\sigma$ of pulmonary capillaries changes as a result of adult respiratory distress syndrome, but returns to normal after some unknown time. Therapy that might be harmful in the early "leaky" phase of the disease process may be beneficial later.[20]

### *Interstitium*

Plasma volume and content are most useful in evaluating the clinical effects of colloids and crystalloids because this compartment is assessed readily by intravascular pressures and the other parameters of adequate perfusion (i.e., blood pressure, urine output, central nervous system function). The interstitium, the space between plasma volume and cells, is vital to fluid homeostasis, yet is assessed imprecisely in clinical practice.

The interstitium serves as a reservoir of fluid. It is composed primarily of hyaluronic acid, a mucopolysaccharide that has the ability to sequester fluid or release it into the plasma volume. The normal amount of water sequestered in the interstitium is two to three times the plasma volume and is the source of fluid for the transcapillary refill phenomenon seen after any fluid loss.

Hypovolemic shock, with the resultant reduction in plasma volume, is accompanied by a process called transcapillary refill (TCR). TCR is a physiologic process that is activated by a reduction in volume and loss of oncotic pressure, as a result of pressure receptors located in the atrium. The response to this reduction in pressure is an increase in ECW osmolarity and movement of protein and water from the interstitium into the capillary to maintain an adequate plasma volume.[21] A drop in hematocrit occurs because fluid with a 40% hematocrit is replaced by interstitial fluid not containing red cells. The resultant hemodilution has two effects: (1) reduction of the hemoglobin and, therefore, the oxygen-carrying capacity; (2) a contrasting beneficial effect—decrease in blood viscosity that promotes better flow through small vasoconstricted capillaries. The response to TCR is variable depending on the patient's underlying physiologic and hydration status and amount, rate, and type of fluid loss. Schwartzkopff et al[22] bled 940 mL from normal subjects in 19 minutes and reported that 40% of lost volume, 38% of lost total protein, and 30% of albumin were replenished within 19 minutes. Skillman et al[23] reported that the rate of TCR varied from 40 to 100 mL/h depending on the speed at which blood was lost and hours postbleed. The TCR replacement rate was greatest in the first 6 hours after rapid (20 minute) blood loss. TCR is capable of meeting blood volume deficits of 10% to 15% (500–750 mL), equivalent to a class I hemorrhage.[23] Table 103.1 lists the changes that take place during TCR and the resultant time frames in which replacement occurs.

Tissue hydrostatic pressure ($P_T$) of the interstitium is negative (−7 mm Hg) because of lymphatic drainage of the interstitium and fluid movement into the capillaries. Tissue fluid oncotic pressure ($\pi_T$) approximates its albumin concentration and normally is 40% of the $\pi_c$.

### *Lymphatic Flow and Organ Resistance to Edema*

There are two remaining influences on fluid distribution: lymphatic flow and organ tissue resistance. As fluid flows out of the capillaries into the interstitium, the body provides for removal by lymph, which drains away excess interstitial fluid. Crandall et al[24] relate that lymphatic flow is the primary protection against pulmonary edema because it can increase to 20 times normal. Organs that are tightly covered provide physical resistance against the development of edema.[24]

The following statements summarize important basic physiologic points:

1. The Starling equation and the movement of fluid still are not understood completely, but are more complex than what we measure clinically, $P_c$ and $\pi_c$.
2. This complexity and lack of understanding are even greater in the various pathologic states.
3. The human body has wide tolerance and can withstand a variety of insults.[25]

To understand how maintenance of plasma volume and Starling's law relate to the pathophysiology of hypovolemic shock we must now discuss the body's response to a loss of intravascular volume.

**Table 103.1** The Crystalloid–Colloid Controversy

| Crystalloid View | Colloid View |
|---|---|
| 1. Interstitial fluid is decreased after shock and must be replaced to reestablish normal physiology. | 1. Interstitial fluid increases in traumatic and septic states or in typical malnourished postsurgical patients. |
| 2. The Starling law is more sensitive to an increase in $P_c$ than a decrease in $\pi_c$. | 2. Restoration of PV with increased perfusion and adequate oxygen delivery is the highest priority. |
| 3. Peripheral edema associated with crystalloid resuscitation (two to three times the colloid volume) is not harmful. | 3. Colloid is the most effective way to restore PV. |
| 4. Colloids leak out into the interstitium during ARDs, worsening the situation. | 4. A low $\pi_c$ (<10 mm Hg) has been associated with increased mortality. |
| 5. Colloids are more expensive than crystalloid solutions. | |

**Agreement**

Proponents of crystalloid and colloid use do have some areas of agreement:

1. Blood is needed to maintain hemoglobin and hematocrit of at least 10 g% and 30%, respectively.
2. Administration of whole blood or fresh-frozen plasma eliminates the need for concurrent colloid.
3. Crystalloid administration often requires two to three times the amount of colloid to resuscitate a patient.
4. Colloid administration still requires crystalloid to meet the normal daily maintenance requirements and other documented water and salt losses, such as diarrhea or nasogastric suction.

## Hemodynamic Consequences of Hypovolemic Shock

The hemodynamic consequences of hypovolemic shock are best discussed in terms of the equation BP = CO × SVR. The relationship among blood pressure (BP), cardiac output (CO), and systemic vascular resistance (SVR) is the key to understanding the overall physiologic response of the body to loss of blood volume (BV). Cardiac output is the product of stroke volume (SV) and heart rate (HR). The body has developed survival mechanisms that maintain blood flow to the heart and brain at all costs by protecting CO and BP. This is accomplished in two major ways: increased HR—with a loss of PV the milliliters per heart beat (SV) falls and to maintain the same liters per minute, the heart must increase its rate and ejection fraction; and as CO falls, SVR is also increased. The purpose of this elevated SVR is to maintain an adequate preload and diastolic pressure for coronary filling and CNS perfusion. Blood flow is redirected from "nonessential" areas, such as the skin, skeletal muscle, and gut, by selective vasoconstriction to the heart, brain, pituitary, and adrenals, where vasodilation has occurred. Concurrently, interstitial fluid is mobilized to the capillary by TCR.

There is a limit to this compensatory response and after a 15% to 20% loss of BV, BP decreases significantly. Even without a noticeable decrease in BP, the loss of BV has set into play a cascade of hormonal consequences in response to this diminution in CO (see Table 103.2).

A class I hemorrhage (see Table 103.2) involves loss of 15% of blood volume (750 mL or less). In the normal, healthy individual, this kind of blood loss over hours to minutes is tolerated without a great deal of distress or apparent physiologic damage. Complete recovery of volume and plasma proteins and clotting factors takes only a few hours. Red blood cell replacement requires weeks. TCR response depends in part on the previous hydration status, cardiovascular function, and general state of health of the patient; older, sicker, dehydrated patients cannot be counted on to compensate even such mild losses.[26]

Class II, III, and IV hemorrhages depict the worsening clinical status as blood loss increases. Class IV is profound shock and the pulse may be found only in the carotid artery. This can quickly lead to loss of arterial pressure and consciousness, pulselessness, and cardiovascular arrest. The usual cardiac arrest from exsanguination occurs in the form of electromechanical dissociation which then progresses to asystole. The heart's response to resuscitation is usually satisfactory if accomplished within 10 minutes of being pulseless.[27]

Not all fluid losses are outside the body. The loss of intravascular blood or plasma to areas within the body is termed "third spacing." Technically, any edema is third spacing, but clinically this term is applied to blood or plasma sequestered in the chest, retroperitoneal areas, buttocks, shoulder girdle, or pelvis. Up to 6 L of extravascular volume may be sequestered in the abdomen with only a 2-cm change in apparent length and radius. During peritonitis, fluid may accumulate for 24 to 48 hours and then return to the vascular system. This remobilization can increase urine output and lead the unsuspecting clinician to increase intravenous fluids to keep up with the output, thereby creating a vicious cycle.[28]

The loss of hypotonic fluid from the body results in a distribution of water loss different from that seen with hemorrhage. Blood loss involves only the blood volume. Crystalloid losses affect blood volume, ECW, and ICW. A 4-L hypotonic loss, resulting from either diarrhea or osmotic diuresis, typically contains approximately 77 mEq of sodium per liter. This 4-L loss could be evaluated as 2 L of pure water from the TBW and 2 L of isotonic saline from ECW. The 2 L of saline reduces PV approximately 500 mL (PV = 0.25 × ECW 2 L), with another 160-mL decrease (PV = 0.08 × TBW 2 L) because of the 2-L pure water loss, for a total of 660 mL. A patient with a 4-L hypotonic fluid loss would have the hemodynamics of a class I hemorrhage.[2]

**Table 103.2** Hypovolemic Classes

| *Blood loss* | *Blood pressure (approximately)* | *Vascular response* | *Temperature* | *Color* | *Circulation (response to blanching)* | *Endocrine response* | *Metabolic response* | *Signs and symptoms* |
|---|---|---|---|---|---|---|---|---|
| Class I (< 15%) 750 mL | Normal to 20% decrease | Contraction of great veins; recruitment of ECF | Cool | Pale | Definite slowing | Slight | Slight | Usually transient |
| Class II (20%–25%) 1,000–1,250 mL | Decreased systolic; increased diastolic; narrow pulse pressure | Mild tachycardia; all of the above; arteriolar constriction with reduced flow to skin, muscle, kidney, liver; tachycardia; decreased cardiac output | Cool | Pale | Definite slowing | Increase in aldosterone, ADH,[a] growth hormone, beta endorphins. Variable increase in cortisol, catecholamine, clotting factor. No increase in insulin | Increased glycolysis and mild hyperglycemia; increased lipolysis and free fatty acid levels; small increase in lactate levels; hyperventilation with alkalemia; $O_2$ consumption may be increased; decreased urinary sodium and volume | Thirst; orthostatic hypotension; apprehension; weakness; pallor; cool skin |
| Class III (30%–35%) 1,500–1,750 mL | Frank hypotension 20%–40% | | Cold | Pale | Definite slowing | | | |
| Class IV (40%–45%) 2,000–2,500 mL | Decreased 40% to nonrecordable | All of the above; CO < 50% of normal; most CO to heart and brain. Agonal rhythm bradycardia to asystole or V. fib | Cold | Ashen to cyanotic (mottling) | Very sluggish | All of the above; marked increase in catechol-amines | Severe lactic acidosis; severe oliguria; mixed venous $O_2$; approx 20 mm Hg or less | Air hunger; apathetic to comatose; little distress, except thirst |

[a] Antidiuretic hormone.

Compiled from References 34 and 50.

**Table 103.3** Priorities for Critically Ill Patients

1. Control hemorrhage and restore blood volumes, maintain arterial pressures, and then volume load to about 500–1,000 mL in excess of predicted norms, unless CVP is greater than 15 cm $H_2O$ or wedge pressure is greater than 19 mm Hg.
2. Maintain patent upper airway and provide adequate ventilation.
3. Respiratory care, including chest physical therapy, encourage coughing, endotracheal suction, turn patient side to side every 2 h, postural drainage, humidification of inspired air, avoid salt and water overload, oxygen via mask or nasopharyngeal catheter, trachael intubation with mechanical ventilation when $Pao_2$ falls below 50–60 torr or $Paco_2$ rises above 60 torr, enriched concentrations of inspired oxygen as needed to maintain $Pao_2$ above 70 torr but less than 120 torr.
4. Correct acid–base alterations: (a) metabolic acidosis with sodium bicarbonate administration, fluids, improvement of blood flow; (b) respiratory acidosis with endotracheal suction, bronchodilators, and mechanical ventilation; (c) respiratory alkalosis by sedation, proper adjustment of the mechanical ventilation, and increase in dead space; addition of $CO_2$ to the inspired air; (d) metabolic alkalosis (when appreciable) with HCl or acetazolamide 250–500 mg IV. Goal: pH 7.25–7.50.
5. Use cardiotonic agents for cardiac failure with pulmonary edema: inotropic agents (digitalis, isoproterenol, calcium, (dopamine); fluid and salt restriction; diuretics; glucagon and glucose; antiarrhythmic agents; blocking agents such as nitroprusside, nitroglycerin, phentolamine, and chlorpromazine when fluid overload occurs; phlebotomy, ultrafiltration, or dialysis for large fluid overloads unresponsive to other therapy.
6. Resort to vasopressors when all other measures to correct hypotension have been ineffective.
7. Prevent or correct fluid maldistribution (i.e., excess ICW with deficient plasma volume) by adequate plasma expansion with oncotically active agents, and avoidance of salt and water overload from excessive volumes of sodium-rich solutions. After hemodynamic stability is achieved, correct ECW overload by restriction of salt and water, and diuretics such as furosemide, ethacrynic acid, or mannitol; if these are ineffective, resort to dialysis.
8. Control infections: culture all potentially infected body fluids, drain abscesses or fluid collections, provide wound care, and give appropriate antibiotics.
9. Provide for nutritional needs: 2,000 or 3,000 cal/d with hypertonic glucose, amino acids, and IV fat solution.
10. For coma or semiconsciousness, which may be associated with cerebral edema, give high doses of steroids, mannitol, or urea; use fluid and salt restriction, diuretics, and adequate parenteral alimentation.
11. Provide for psychologic and social needs.

Adapted from Shoemaker WC, Thompson WL, Holbrook PR (eds): Textbook of Critical Care. Philadelphia, W.B. Saunders, 1984, p 68.

## Hypovolemic Shock Therapy

The primary goal of therapy is to ensure adequate oxygen delivery to meet demand. This is clearly indicated in Table 103.3, where the first four goals deal with the maintenance of adequate oxygen delivery. The cornerstone of all therapy for the patient in hypotensive shock is assurance of adequate preload. For a more detailed discussion on tissue oxygenation the reader is referred to Snyder and Carroll.[29]

The components of oxygen delivery are summarized by the equation

$$Do_2 = Cao_2 \times CI \times 10 \text{ mL/min/m}^2$$
$$Cao_2 = Hg_b \times 1.36 \times Sao_2 + Pao_2 \times 0.003$$

$Cao_2$ is a function of the percentage oxygen saturation and the hemoglobin content of the blood ($Hg_b$). The normal $Hg_b$ for men is 13–15 g/dL, but the resuscitation recommendations are for $Hg_b$ of 10–12 g/dL (Hct 30%–36%) because of the increasing viscosity that occurs as the hemoglobin increases. The best combination of $Cao_2$, viscosity, flow characteristics, distribution of flow to organs, and cardiac work is found at a Hct of 25% to 35%.

When the patient's $Cao_2$ is optimized, the only remaining way to increase oxygen delivery is by raising the cardiac output. Ideally, this should be accomplished at the lowest possible energy expenditure for the heart. The major determinants of myocardial oxygen ($MVo_2$) demands are intramyocardial tension (blood pressure, ventricular volume); myocardial contractility; and heart rate. Increases in blood pressure, ventricular volume, contractility, and heart rate all increase $MVo_2$. Heart rate not only increases $MVo_2$ but decreases diastolic filling time with a potential reduction in coronary artery blood flow. The goal is oxygen delivery to meet demand at the lowest cardiovascular work, maintaining the lowest optimal blood pressure, with just enough preload to achieve the proper cardiac output at a heart rate between 60 and 100, without use of cardiotonic agents. That is the ideal but there are times when there is no choice but to increase contractility, blood pressure, or heart rate through pharmacologic means in an attempt to preserve life. Note that cardiotonic agents are listed as priority 5 in Table 103.3, and vasopressors are priority 6, after manipulations of plasma volume, oxygenation, and pH.

## Preload Alteration

We have discussed that preload alteration is the most efficient way to ensure adequate cardiac output and oxygen delivery. The ideal relationship between PAWP and CI is shown in Figure 103.3. Please note that in this figure, three Starling curves depict the relationship of PAWP to CI. The analogy of preload to gasoline is very useful in understanding this relationship. Think of cardiac index as the speed of a

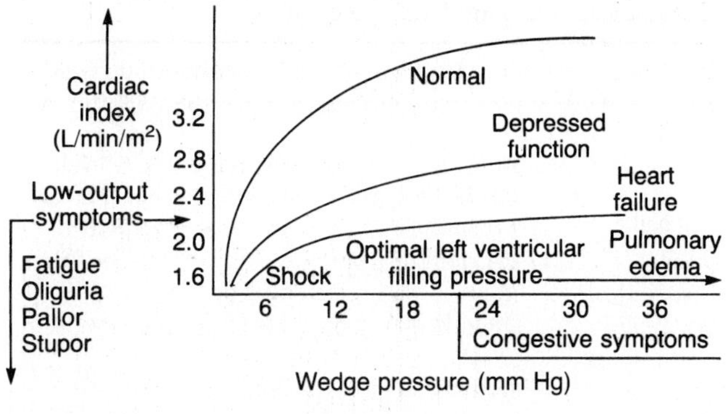


**Figure 103.3** Idealized relationship between PAWP and CI.

car; regardless of how well the car is tuned, if there is no gasoline (very low or absent preload), it will not run. Administration of inotropic agents in a low-preload situation makes about as much sense as tuning up a car because it is out of gas. The top curve is a well-tuned car and requires only a little gas (preload) to travel very fast (increased CI). The middle curve is the car that is not as well tuned. To achieve the same speed (cardiac index) it must be given more gasoline; this heart has borderline function but does not need cardiotonic agents and is typtical of the elderly patient with a mild degree of heart failure. The lowest curve is heart failure or a car that needs a tune-up. No matter how much gasoline you supply, it can never achieve an adequate rate of speed (i.e., CI) without the continuing symptoms of inadequate CI. The tune-up is the inotropic agents or vasodilators. Please note that like an automobile, you can actually give too much gas (preload) and flood it. In the human being, this flooding is called pulmonary edema and typically occurs at a PAWP somewhere between 20 and 30 mm Hg.

Because the wedge pressure is a function not only of volume but of vascular tone, the actual value may not reflect true PV. As the intravascular volume drops, vascular tone increases, maintaining the PAWP in the normal range. Therefore, the response of both PAWP and CVP to a fluid challenge is as important as the actual value. Please note that

**Figure 103.4** Responses of PCWP to controlled fluid challenge. *(Adapted from Majerus TC: A Practical Guide for the Administration of Dobutrex$^R$. Indianapolis, Eli Lilly & Co., 1983, p 12.)*

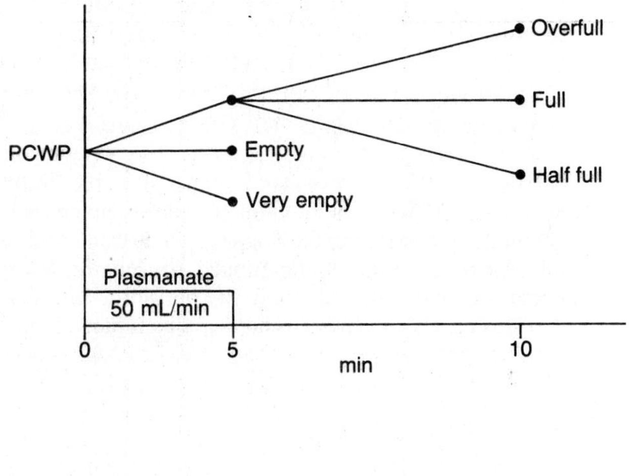


| | | |
|---|---|---|
| 1. Baseline PCWP | <12 mm Hg | 200 mL over 10 min |
| | <16 mm Hg | 100 mL over 10 min |
| | ≥16 mm Hg | 50 mL over 10 min |
| 2. During infusion | Δ>7 mm Hg | Stop fluid challenge |
| 3. After infusion | Δ>3 but <7 mm Hg | Wait |
| | Δ>3 mm Hg | Wait |
| | Δ≤3 mm Hg | Repeat fluid challenge |

**Figure 103.5** "7–3" rule for PCWP measurements with fluid challenge. *(Adapted from Majerus TC: A Practical Guide for the Administration of Dobutrex$^R$. Indianapolis, Eli Lilly & Co., 1983, p 12.)*

Figure 103.4 indicates the three different responses to a controlled fluid challenge of the PAWP. As fluid is added, the SVR declines and the PAWP may actually increase, decrease, or stay the same. A decrease indicates that the system was very empty; no change, moderately empty; and an increase, almost full.

The fluid challenge itself can be accomplished by many different methods. Weil and Henning[30] described a commonly quoted method that is detailed in Figure 103.5. It is sometimes called the "7–3" rule. Note that the higher the baseline PAWP, the smaller the fluid challenge. This intuitively makes sense because the higher the PAWP, the smaller the tolerance limits are to possible overload of the patient. The relationship between volume and pressure is not linear. As the optimal volume is approached, the pressure rises at an ever-increasing rate. It is like filling up a car's gasoline tank; as you approach full, you must slow down the entry rate to prevent spillover.

During the initial 10-minute challenge, if the PAWP rises above 7 or exceeds 20 mm Hg, fluid administration should be stopped and the patient observed for 10 minutes. If PAWP decreases after 10 minutes but adequate perfusion is not achieved, then another fluid challenge may be instituted with a new baseline PAWP. The full 10-minute infusion is completed when the increase in PAWP is greater than a change of 3 but less than a change of 7 and has not exceeded 20 mm Hg. The patient should then be monitored for adequate perfusion. If PAWP changed less than 3 mm Hg during the 10-minute infusion, perfusion should be continued for another 10 minutes per step 1.

The parameters commonly used for successfully monitoring resuscitation of the hypovolemic patient are listed in Table 103.4. The normal values are given and the goals described by Shoemaker[31] are listed in the far right-hand column. Shoemaker's goals were derived from a study of 113 postsurgical patients and statistically analyzed to determine what value predicted the best chance of survival. These goals are not universally accepted, but they are the first to be backed by study.

## Treatment

There are two treatments for the hypovolemic patient: crystalloids and colloids. Table 103.1 summarizes the contrasting views and areas of agreement.

**Table 103.4** Cardiovascular and Respiratory Parameters (Measured and Calculated)

| *Parameter* | *Abbreviation* | *Formula* | *Unit* | *Normal* | *Goal* |
|---|---|---|---|---|---|
| Volume-related variables | | | | | |
| Mean arterial pressure | MAP | DP + 1/3 pp | mm Hg | 82–102 | >84 |
| Central venous pressure | CVP | Measured | cm $H_2O$ | 1–9 | <5 |
| Stroke volume | SV | SV = (CO/HR) × 1,000 | mL/min | 70 | 70 |
| Stroke index | SI | SI = (CI/HR) × 1,000 | mL/min/$m^2$ | 30–50 | >48 |
| Hemoglobin | Hg | Measured | g% | 12–16 | >12 |
| Mean pulmonary arterial pressure | MPAP | Measured | mm Hg | 11–15 | <19 |
| Pulmonary capillary wedge pressure | PCWP | Measured | mm Hg | 0–12 | >9.5 |
| Flow-related variables | | | | | |
| Cardiac output | CO | Measured | L/min | 4.5–6.5 | >7.5 |
| Cardiac index | CI | CO/BSA | L/min/$m^2$ | 2.8–3.6 | >4.5 |
| Left ventricular stroke work index | LVSWI | SI × MAP × 0.0136 | g-m/$m^2$/beat | 44–68 | >55 |
| Left cardiac work index | LCWI | CI × MAP × 0.0136 | kg-m/$m^2$/beat | 3–4.6 | >5 |
| Right ventricular stroke work index | RVSWI | SI × MPAP × 0.0136 | g-m/$m^2$/beat | 4–18 | >13 |
| Right cardiac work index | RCWI | CI × MPAP × 0.0136 | kg-m/$m^2$/beat | 0.4–0.6 | >1.1 |
| Stress-related variables | | | | | |
| Systemic vascular resistance index | SVRI | [(MAP-CVP)/CI] × 79.92 | dynes-s/$cm^5$ | 1,760–2,600 | <1,450 |
| Pulmonary vascular resistance index | PVRI | [(MPAP-PCWP)/CI] × 79.92 | dynes-s/$cm^5$ | 45–225 | <226 |
| Heart rate | HR | Measured | bpm | 72–88 | <100 |
| Rectal temperature | Temp | Measured | °F | 97.8–98.6 | >100.4 |
| Oxygen transport | | | | | |
| Arterial pH | pH | Measured | — | 7.36–7.44 | >7.47 |
| Arterial $CO_2$ tension | $Paco_2$ | Measured | mm Hg | 36–44 | >30 |
| Mixed venous $O_2$ tension | $Pvo_2$ | Measured | mm Hg | 33–53 | >36 |
| Arterial Hg[b] saturation | $Sao_2$ | Measured | % | 95–99 | >95 |
| Arterial–venous $O_2$ content difference | a–$vDo_2$ | $Cao_2$ - $Cvo_2$ | ml% | 4–5.5 | <3.5 |
| $O_2$ availability | $O_2$ avail | $Cao_2$ × CI × 10 | mL/min/$m^2$ | 520–720 | >550 |
| $O_2$ consumption | $Vo_2$ | a–$vDo_2$ × CI × 10 | mL/min/$m^2$ | 100–180 | >167 |
| $O_2$ extraction | $O_2$ ext | ($Cao_2$-$Cvo_2$)/$Cao_2$ | % | 22–30 | <31 |
| Rate–pressure product | RPP | HR × SBP | — | 12,000 | 12,000 |

Adapted from Shoemaker WC et al: Therapy of critically ill postoperative patients based on outcome prediction and prospective clinical trials. Surg Clin North Am 1985;65:814–815.

The treatment algorithms for emergency room admission and postoperative ICU patients are found in Figures 103.6 and 103.7. Some general comments on the use of these algorithms are necessary.

1. The emergency room algorithm (Figure 103.6) is designed to be completed in less than 1 hour; most patients respond to 2 L of fluid. Shoemaker's belief in colloids is evident from his recommendation in step 3.
2. Because hemorrhagic shock can reduce the body's temperature, the use of warmed fluids (40°C lactated Ringer's) and blood is recommended by some authorities.[32]
3. The proper, optimal, or maximum PAWP must be determined for each patient. The common goal of 14–18 mm Hg was arrived at in postmyocardial infarction patients; young trauma patients with normal cardiovascular systems may require a PAWP of only 6–10 mm Hg.[33] A PAWP of 12 mm Hg was reported to be optimal in a group of septic patients by Packman and Rackow.[34] Because of abnormalities in left ventricular compliance the relationship between PAWP and left ventricular end diastolic pressure may be different not only between patients and disease states but in a single patient over the course of disease.[35] Trunkey et al recommend keeping the PAWP between 3 and 8 mm Hg if the patient has ARDs or other capillary leak syndromes.[26]
4. Adequate intravenous fluid access is crucial and a function of (a) bore of the tubing, (b) length of the tubing, (c) catheter site, and (d) pressure. Moore[27] provides an excellent discussion on this topic.

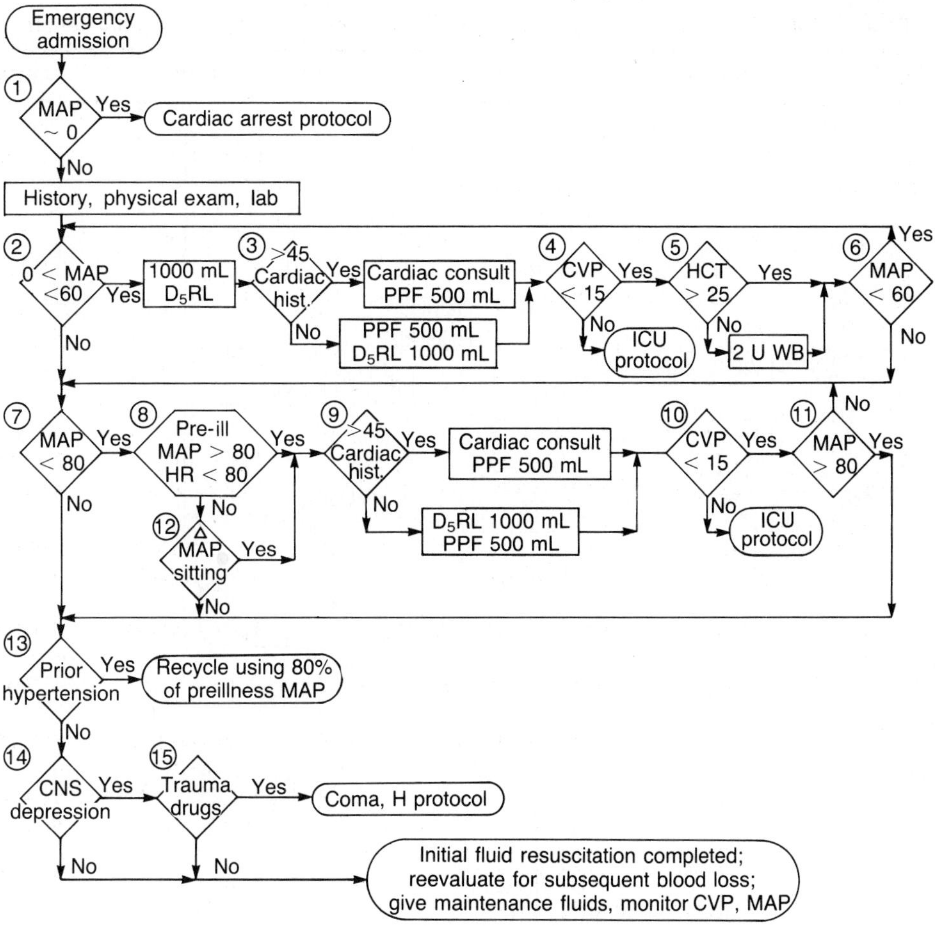


**Figure 103.6** Clinical algorithm for initial (first-hour) resuscitation of emergency admissions. This algorithm was designed for resuscitation of the acute emergency patient to restore circulatory integrity as rapidly as possible without producing fluid overload. **Step 1.** If the MAP is 0 or nearly 0, determine that there is a cardiac arrest and begin CPR imediately. If the patient has a MAP < 20 mm Hg, alert personnel for a possible cardiac arrest. **Step 2.** If MAP < 60 mm Hg, immediately start $D_5$ lactated Ringer's solution 1,000 mL and run as rapidly as possible, especially if MAP < 50 mm Hg. **Step 3.** If the patient is less than 45 years old and does not have a cardiac history, place a CVP line and start another $D_5$ lactated Ringer's solution 1,000 mL plus 500 mL plasma protein factor (PPF) or artificial colloid through a third IV line. **Step 4.** Monitor the CVP at frequent intervals during the rapid infusion of these three solutions so as not to exceed 15 cm $H_2O$. If CVP > 15 cm $H_2O$, go directly to the ICU protocol (Fig. 103.7). **Step 5.** If Hct < 25%, give 2 units of O-negative, type-specific blood. When cross-matched blood becomes available, transfusions of whole blood or packed red cells should be given to maintain Hct > 33%. **Step 6.** Rapid restoration of the MAP to 60 mm Hg is the titration endpoint for fluids in this section. If MAP < 60 mm Hg, recycle from steps 2 through 6. If MAP > 60 mm Hg has been achieved, proceed to step 7. **Step 7.** If MAP < 80 mm Hg, go to step 8, if not, proceed to step 13. **Step 8.** If MAP < 80 mm Hg, inquire from the patient, the patient's family, or a previous hospital record to evaluate the patient's "normal" preillness control MAP. If MAP < 80 mm Hg and heart rate > 80 beats per mnute, measure orthostatic blood pressure (step 12). **Step 9.** As in step 3, the cardiac patient requires less salt and water but more colloid. If the patient is more than 45 years old or if there is a cardiac history, give 500 mL colloid; if the patient is less than 45 years old and there is no cardiac history, give 1,000 mL $D_5$ lactated Ringer's solution plus 500 mL colloid. **Step 10.** Fluids may be given safely if CVP < 15 cm $H_2O$; if the latter is exceeded, go to the ICU protocol (Fig. 103.7) and continue to give fluids as needed to restore circulatory integrity provided wedge pressures of 18 mm Hg are not exceeded. **Step 11.** If MAP > 80 mm Hg without exceeding CVP > 15 cm $H_2O$, the objective of this cycle has been achieved. If MAP < 80 mm Hg, recycle steps 7 through 11. **Step 12.** Orthostatic blood pressure is measured. If there is a change in the MAP > 10 mm Hg on sitting or standing, this is presumptive evidence of at least 1,000-mL blood volume deficit. **Step 13.** After MAP has been restored to the normal value (> 80 mm Hg), it is still necessary to be sure that the preillness blood pressure was normal. If a prior hypertension was observed, the patient should be recycled from steps 7 through 13 using 80% of the preillness value as the criterion for the adequacy of resuscitation. **Step 14.** Examine the patient for evidence of central nervous system depression, drug poisoning, or drug abuse. **Step 15.** Examine the patient for evidence of head injury or other trauma. If positive, the patient should be treated in accordance with a coma–head injury (H) protocol. *(Adapted from Shoemaker WC, Flemming AW: Ann Emerg Med 1986;15:1438.)*

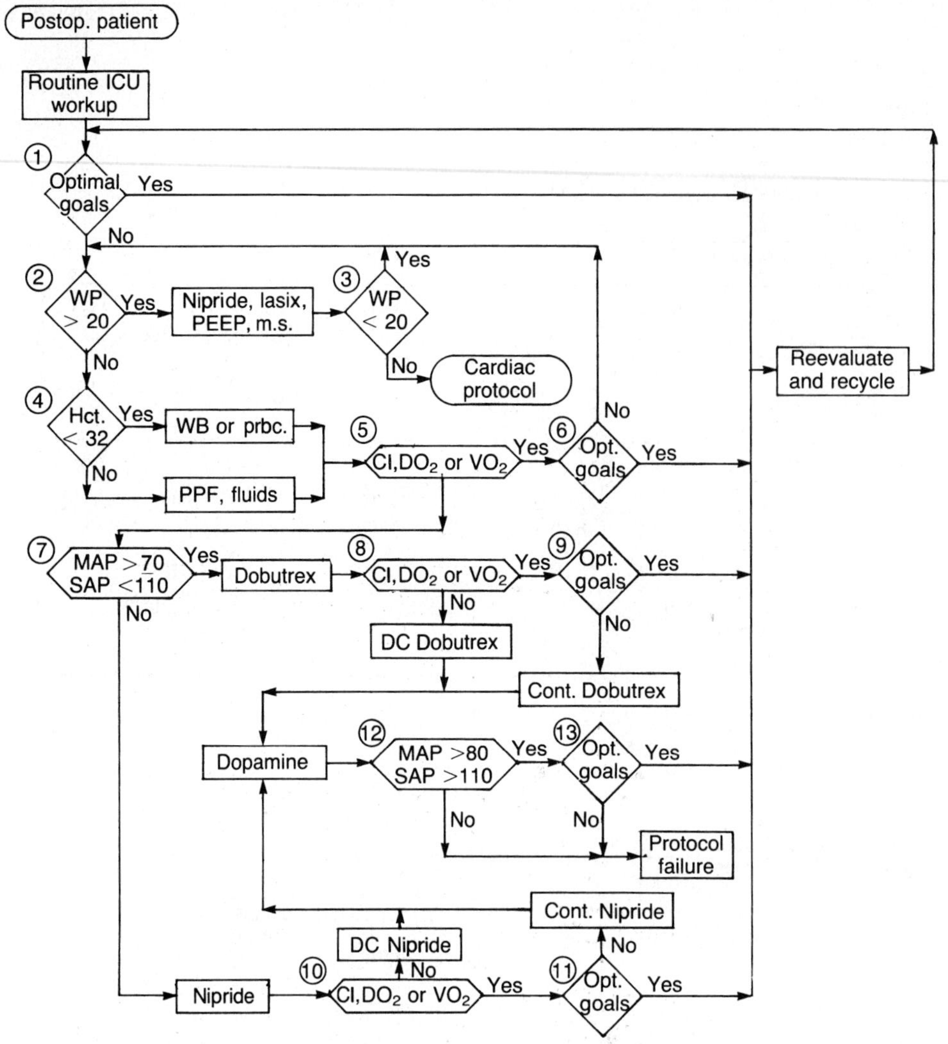


**Figure 103.7** Decision tree for management of critically ill patients. Preliminary evaluation by routine ICU work up that includes arterial blood gases, chest x-ray, routine blood chemistries, ECG, and coagulation studies. These tests should be either performed or in process and the observed defects corrected. For example, if $Pa_{O_2} < 70$ torr, $7.3 > pH > 7.5$, $Pa_{CO_2} > 55$ torr, or respiration rate (RR) > 30 breaths per minute, place on the respiratory protocol. If none of these is present, proceed to step 1. **Step 1.** Determine if the patient has reached the optimal goals. Measure CI, $\dot{D}_{O_2}$, $\dot{V}_{O_2}$, and blood volume (BV). If CI < 4.5 L/min·m$^2$, $\dot{D}_{O_2}$ < 600 mL/min·m$^2$, $\dot{V}_{O_2}$ < 170 mL/min·m$^2$ for men or 2.7 L/min·m$^2$ for women, take Hct. If any of the preceding optimal values have not been reached, proceed to step 2. If the goals are reached, the objective of the algorithm has been achieved. Reevaluate and recycle at intervals to maintain these goals. **Step 2.** Take pulmonary wedge pressure (WP). If WP > 20 mm Hg, proceed to step 3; if WP < 20, proceed to step 4. **Step 3.** If WP >20, give furosemide (Lasix) IV at increasing dose levels (20, 40, 80, 160 mg) if there is clinical or x-ray evidence of salt and water overload or clinical findings of pulmonary congestion. If not, consider vasodilators, nitroprusside, or nitroglycerin if MAP > 80 mm Hg and systolic pressure > 100 mm Hg. Recycle up to 5 times to titrate the dose needed to reduce WP < 20 but maintain MAP > 80 mm Hg. If unsuccessul, place on cardiac procotol. **Step 4.** If Hct < 32%, give 1 unit of whole blood (WB) or 2 units of packed red blood cells (Prbc). If Hct > 32%, give a fluid load (volume challenge) consisting of one of the following (depending on clinical indications of plasma volume deficit or hydration): 5% PPF, 500 mL; 5% albumin, 500 mL; 25% albumin (25 g), 100 mL; 6% hydroxyethyl starch, 500 mL; 6% dextran 60, 500 mL; D5RL, 1,000 mL. **Step 5.** If the blood or fluid load improved any of the optimal therapeutic goals defined in step 1, proceed to step 6; if none are improved, proceed to step 7. **Step 6.** If goals are not reached, recycle steps 2 through 6 until these goals are met or WP > 20 mm Hg. **Step 7.** If MAP > 70 or systolic arterial pressure (SAP) < 100 mm Hg, give dobutamine (Dobutrex) by constant IV infusion in increasing doses. **Step 8.** Titrate dobutamine beginning with 1 to 2 $\mu$g/min·kg and gradually increasing doses up to 20 $\mu$g/min·kg provided there is improvement in CI, $\dot{D}_{O_2}$ or $\dot{V}_{O_2}$ without further lowering of arterial pressure until goals are met. **Step 9.** If goals are reached, reevaluate and recycle. If goals are not reached or it becomes evident that higher doses of the drug are not more effective or that they produce hypotension and tachycardia, continue dobutamine at its most effective dose range. **Step 10.** If MAP > 80 mm Hg and SAP > 110 mm Hg, give sodium nitroprusside or nitroglycerin in gradually increasing doses. If the arterial pressures are lower than MAP 80 mm Hg and SAP 110 mm Hg, give vasopressors. **Step 11.** If there is no improvement in CI, $\dot{D}_{O_2}$, or $\dot{V}_{O_2}$, titrate vasodilator to its maximum effect consistent with satisfactory pressures. **Step 12.** If optimal goals are reached, reevaluate and recycle at intervals. If these goals are not reached and MAP < 80 mm Hg, SAP < 110 mm Hg, give vasopressor. **Step 13.** Titrate doses of vasopressor (dopamine) in the lowest doses possible to maintain arterial pressures, MAP > 80 mm Hg, SAP > 110 mm Hg. If pressures cannot be maintained, the patient is considered to be a protocol failure. *(Adapted from Shoemaker WC et al: Surg Clin North Am 1985;65:828–29.)*

**Table 103.5** Colloid and Crystalloid Preparations

| *Contents* | *Albumin 25%* | *Albumin 5%* | *Plasma protein fraction 5%* | *Dextran-40, 10% in NS or $D_5W$* | *Dextran-70, 6% in NS or $D_5W$* | *Hetastarch 6% in NS* | *Lactated Ringer's* |
|---|---|---|---|---|---|---|---|
| Albumin (g/L) | ~250 | ~50 | ~44 | | | | |
| Globulin (g/L) | | | ~6 | | | | |
| Other | | | | Glucose polysaccharides average molecular weight 40,000 (10,000–90,000) | Average molecular weight 70,000 (20,000–200,000) | Hydroxyethyl starch average molecular weight 450,000 (10,000–1,000,000)[a] | Lactate 28 mEq/L, calcium 3.0 mEq/L, potassium 4 mEq/L |
| Sodium (mEq/L) | 130–160 | 130–160 | 130–160 | NS 154 | NS 154 | 154 | 130 |
| Chloride (mEq/L) | | | | NS 154 | NS 154 | 154 | 109 |
| Osmolarity (mOsm/L) | 1,500 | 300 | 290 | NS 308, $D_5W$ 277 | NS 308, $D_5W$ 277 | 310 | 273 |
| Plasma volume (mL) expansion per 500 mL infused | 1,500–2,000 | 500 | 500 | 500–1,000 | 500–700 | 500–700 | 100 mL |
| Duration of volume expansion[b] | ≤24 h | ≤24 h | ≤24 h | Normal, 1 h Severely ill, 4–6 h | ≤24 h | ≤36 h | |
| Half-life in body[c] | 21 d | 21 d | 27 d | 10–40 h | 24–48 h | ≤2 mo | |
| Metabolism | Liver to free amino acids | Liver to free amino acids | Liver to free amino acids | 70–90 mg/kg/d to glucose, then $CO_2$ and $H_2O$ | 70–90 mg/kg/d to glucose, then $CO_2$ and $H_2O$ | Amylase to hydroxyethylated glucose | Lactate to bicarbonate |
| Distribution | Albumin (see text) | Albumin (see text) | Albumin (see text) | Reticuloendothelial system | See Dextran-40 | Liver, kidney, spleen, pancreas, lymph nodes, lungs, testes | ECW and ICW |
| Excretion[d] | | | | Renal—70% unchanged in 24 h | Renal—50% unchanged in 24 h | Renal—40% unchanged in 24 h | Renal |

**Table 103.5** Colloid and Crystalloid Preparations (continued)

| *Contents* | *Albumin 25%* | *Albumin 5%* | *Plasma protein fraction 5%* | *Dextran-40, 10% in NS or $D_5W$* | *Dextran-70, 6% in NS or $D_5W$* | *Hetastarch 6% in NS* | *Lactated Ringer's* |
|---|---|---|---|---|---|---|---|
| Cautions | CHF, pulmonary edema, active bleeding, thrombocytopenia, hypofibrinogenemia, dehydration | See Albumin 25% | See Albumin 25% | See Albumin 25%: greater effect on coagulation | See Albumin 25%: greater effect on coagulation | See Albumin 25%: greater effect on coagulation | May need 3–5 L for each L of blood loss |
| | | | | Oliguria and anuria | Oliguria and anuria | Serum amylase > 2× normal, 2–4 d | |
| Adverse reactions | | | | | | | |
| Allergy (%)[e] | All albumin solutions combined | | 0.011 | All dextrans | 0.03–4.7 | 0.085 | |
| Anaphylaxis (%)[f] | | | 0.003 | | 0.008–0.6 | 0.006 | |
| Others | | | Hypotension rates >10 mL/min | Osmotic nephrosis, bleeding | Osmotic nephrosis, bleeding | Bleeding | |
| Acquisition cost/500 mL[g] | $260 | $52.00 | $52.00 | $13.84 | $12.99 | $29.37 | $0.97 |
| Dose | 25 g up to 125 g/d, maximum 250 g/48 h, rate not to exceed 1 mL/min | Rate not to exceed 2–4 mL/min | Rate not to exceed 10 mL/min | Rate not to exceed 2 g/kg (20 mL—10%) in 24 h; beyond 24 h, 1 g/kg/d up to 5 d | Rate not to exceed 1.2 g/kg (20 ml—6%) 24 h; beyond 24 h, 600 mg/kg (10 mL of 6%) up to 5 d; rate up to 20–40 mL/min to shock | Recommended maximum 1,500 mL/d, 20 mL/kg rates up to 20 mL/kg/h may be used | |

[a] Average molecular weight = 70,000.
[b] Duration of expansion—this is a function of the patient's volume status, serum protein concentration, heart function, perfusion, and kidney function.
[c] Half-life in body—dextrans and hetastarch have multiphasic half-lives. Smaller molecules (<50,000) are filtered by the kidney; the remainder are metabolized and excreted. Hetastarch $t_{1/2}$ increased with time—17 d up to 6 wk, 48 d after 6 wk.
[d] Excretion—smaller molecules (<50,000 molecular weight) are filtered first.
[e] Allergy—all allergic reactions.
[f] Anaphylaxis—life-threatening allergic reactions: bronchospasm with hypotension and shock.
[g] Acquisition cost does not necessarily equal cost to the patient.

Adapted from Ross AD, Angaran DM: Colloids vs. crystalloids: A continuing controversy. Drug Intelligence Clin Pharm 1984;18:208, with permission.

### *Colloid Therapy*

The colloids and crystalloids currently in use are summarized in Table 103.5. The ideal colloid should have an oncotic pressure comparable with that of plasma and a reasonable duration of intravascular volume expansion; should not rely on renal excretion alone for elimination; should not have antigenic, allergenic, or pyretic properties; should not interfere with typing or cross-matching of blood; should be easily sterilized and pharmacologically inert; and should be inexpensive but easy to manufacture. We review only selected topics such as volume expansion characteristics, uses, and volume-induced coagulopathy.

The reported volume expansion capability of 5% albumin, plasma protein fraction (PPF), dextrans, and hydroxyethyl starch is 1 mL per milliliter infused over 4 to 24 hours. The extent and duration of volume expansion achieved are a function of the dose, rate, volume status of the patient, baseline plasma oncotic pressure, cardiovascular function, renal function, and degree of capillary integrity (reflection coefficient). Schwartzkopff et al[22] gave 500 mL of a 5% albumin solution over 1 hour to three groups: normovolemic patients, patients with acute blood loss, and patients with both hypoproteinemia and hypovolemia. The normovolemic patients retained the total amount of 5% albumin infused in the intravascular space during that 1 hour; the acutely bled patients lost 22% and the hypoproteinemic hypovolemic patients lost 38% from the intravascular space. At 4 hours after the infusion, the normovolemic patients still retained 40%, the acutely bled patients retained 43%, and the hypoproteinemic hypovolemic patients retained only 10% to 20% of the infused albumin. The TCR response may be the reason for greater albumin retention in the acutely bled patients than in those with hypoproteinemia hypovolemia.

Thompson,[36] using a hetastarch slightly different from the commercially available preparation (molecular weight 85,000, substitution 0.75), compared its volume expansion properties with dextran 70 and 5% albumin. He found that hypoalbuminemic patients had only 25% to 33% ($P$ = 0.00005) of the intravascular volume retention of each colloid compared with healthy subjects.

A patient with periperal or pulmonary edema and reduced serum albumin (<2.5 g%) might benefit from the 25% albumin hyperoncotic form. When used in this situation, the 25% albumin pulls fluid from the interstitium into the PV, 3–4 mL for every milliliter infused. If not given in conjunction with a diuretic in the cardiovascular-compromised patient, it may precipitate CHF.[5] This hyperoncotic form is not useful in the treatment of hypovolemic states.

Albumin solutions have also been used in the following situations: in ARDS, as an adjunct to hemodilution therapy in cardiopulmonary bypass, during exchange transfusion, after ascites removal, in acute nephrosis with a loop diuretic to enhance diuresis for short periods (7–10 days), and in postrenal dialysis in certain patients prone to shock. The use of albumin for hypoalbuminemia in malnutrition is not warranted. Albumin has poor content of essential amino acids and is an unsatisfactory source of amino acids. The overuse of albumin may increase its own catabolism. Albumin supplementation for chronic nephrosis and cirrhosis is not an appropriate use.[37]

Hetastarch has been used successfully in postoperative patients,[38] during bypass,[39] after bypass,[40] and posttrauma.[41]

Dextran is the only colloid that is currently FDA approved for prevention of thromboembolic disease in high-risk surgical patients.

There is a general decrease in all clotting factors and platelets during hypovolemic shock. The net result is an increase in partial thromboplastin time (PTT) and prothrombin time (PT). This may result from the transfusion of massive amounts of blood (>10 units) with ineffective clotting factors or the use of solutions not containing clotting factors, producing a hemodilution.[27] But it may also be associated with impaired production, disseminated intravascular coagulation, and internal shifts related to the hypotension itself. A recent retrospective study by Hewson et al indicated that the PTT was better correlated with the duration of hypotension than it was with treatment.[42]

The effects of hetastarch on the blood coagulation system have been of concern to many practitioners. In vitro, the effects are minimal and primarily reflect dilution. In vivo, however, when hydroxyethyl starch is infused in massive amounts to dogs (>25% of blood volume), overt bleeding is observed regularly, with laboratory abnormalities in all aspects of hemostasis. When hydroxyethyl starch was investigated in humans or animals after moderate replacement (hydroxyethyl starch volume < 20 mL/kg or 1,500 mL total volume), minor effects on coagulation were detected, including prolonged PTT and PT.

### *Crystalloid Therapy*

#### Lactated Ringer's, Normal Saline

With lactate added in place of bicarbonate, the chemical composition of lactated Ringer's (LR) solution closely approximates the electrolyte concentration of ECW. Lactate is metabolized to bicarbonate and is both more stable and more compatible than bicarbonate in solution. The advantage of LR over NaCl is more theoretical than documented. Lowery et al[43] resuscitated 26 LR patients compared with 27 NS patients suffering from hemorrhagic shock and could detect no difference in lactate disposition or outcome.

A reasonable question is if the use of lactated Ringer's increases lactate acidosis in shock. McClelland et al found that replacement of shed blood plus lactated Ringer's alleviated poor tissue perfusion and anaerobic metabolism, thus reversing lactic acidosis.[44] Canizaro et al[45] also reported the same results in 69 patients (56 with hemorrhagic shock, 8 with sepsis, and 5 with cardiogenic shock) who all responded to LR administration with a decrease in lactate and an increase in pH to 7.4.

Administration of the volumes necessary to maintain perfusion may exacerbate certain preexisting medical conditions, such as CHF, in the compromised patient. Unless appropriate patient parameters are monitored, there is a tendency to underresuscitate when crystalloid is used.

#### Hypertonic Solutions

The use of hypertonic sodium solutions (HSSs) ranging from 514 to 2,400 mOsm/L has been investigated in both animals and humans.[46–48] These HSSs have been either the chloride or lactate salt and in one report were combined with albumin 12.5 g/L (HALFD).[49]

Shackford et al[48] compared sodium lactate solution 514 mOsm/L to LR mOsm/L in the resuscitation of 58 randomly assigned patients undergoing major aortic resection. The HSS group required significantly less fluid both intraoperatively and the first day postoperatively to maintain adequate perfusion, with less weight gain and smaller positive fluid balance compared with the LR group. Although the LR patients had a greater pulmonary shunt than the HSS group, all patients were extubated at the same time.

The HSS solution is not without potential complications as demonstrated by Prough et al, who documented a significant drop in intracranial pressure and speculated on the possibility of subdural hematoma formation in dogs given 7.5% NaCl[47]; Shackford et al[48] had to interrupt HSS administration when serum osmolarity exceeded 330 mOsm/L in two patients. These solutions seem to hold promise but more detailed investigations with larger populations are needed.

### *Blood and Blood Product Transfusions*

Tables 103.6 and 103.7 summarize the indications, contents, and major complications associated with the use of blood and blood products.

The complications of massive, greater-than-one-blood volume (10–12 units in 12 hours), transfusions are summarized in Table 103.8.[50]

Hemolytic transfusion reactions are divided into two types, acute and delayed. The acute reaction is almost always associated with a clinical error leading to mismatching. Signs and symptoms vary from fever, chills, hypotension, and flushing to dyspnea, chest pain, shock, and generalized bleeding. Therapy consists of stopping the transfusion, replacing it with saline, and maintaining adequate volume to prevent or treat hypotension and the potential renal failure resulting from shock and hemoglobinuria.[51]

The delayed reaction occurs most often in patients who have been previously transfused or pregnant and have antibodies to antigens not screened in the ABO system. The signs and symptoms may be subtle or as apparent as in the acute reaction and occur 7 to 10 days after the transfusion but are rarely dangerous.[52]

The transfusion of blood stored in either acid citrate dextrose (ACD) or citrate phosphate dextrose (CPD) is accompanied by a reduced $P_{50}$ or affinity of hemoglobin for oxygen. The delivery of oxygen to the cells and its subsequent release from red blood cells to tissue constitute a complex topic that involves RBC oxygen pressure, 2-diphosphoglycerate concentration, temperature, and pH.[52]

Urticarial reactions are limited to the skin (hives, itching, erythema) and are not accompanied by fever. The transfusion may be continued and antihistamines administered.

Metabolic alkalosis is the most common acid–base disturbance associated with blood administration as the citrate is metabolized to bicarbonate. Citrate toxicity itself is rare and administration of up to one unit every 5 minutes in adults is safe.

Hyperkalemia and hypocalcemia have proven not to be serious problems associated with massive blood replacement.

Coagulation problems are associated primarily with dilution of the percentage of clotting factors and platelets and the low levels of clotting factors in stored blood. These factors should be checked in patients undergoing replacement of 0.5 to 1 more blood volume in 12 to 24 hours. The reduction in ionized calcium is thought not to play an important part.

Blood is usually administered through a filter to remove microaggregates and with a NS to-keep-open solution. $D_5W$, $D_5L$, and LR are incompatible and may cause clumping or hemolysis. The usual duration is over 1 hour and administration times greater than 4 hours are not recommended because of bacterial proliferation and temperature-induced hemolysis. Volume-expanded patients should receive packed cells (RBCs without plasma). Faster rates, for exam-

**Table 103.6** Indications for Blood Products

| *Indications* | *First choice* | *Alternatives* |
|---|---|---|
| Severe anemia with hypovolemia (acute hemorrhage) | Whole blood | Red blood cells plus a plasma expander |
| Severe anemia without hypovolemia | Red blood cells | Washed or frozen red cells if high risk of febrile or allergic reaction |
| Severe anemia with hypervolemia or diminished cardiac reserve | Slow infusion of red cells | Red cells with plasmapheresis; exchange transfusion |
| Severe thrombocytopenia | Platelet concentrate | |
| Coagulation defects | | |
| Hemophilia (factor VIII deficiency) | Cryoprecipitate or antihemophilic factor concentrate | Fresh-frozen plasma |
| Von Willebrand's disease | Cryoprecipitate | Fresh-frozen plasma |
| Parahemophilia (factor V deficiency) | Fresh-frozen plasma | Fresh single-donor plasma |
| Factor II, VII, IX, or X deficiency | Factor IX complex | Single-donor plasma |
| Congenital hypofibrinogenemia | Cryoprecipitate | Any preparation of plasma |

From Blood Products. Med Lett 1979;21:96, with permission.

**Table 103.7** Blood and Blood Components

| *Material* | *Usual package* | *Content* | *Major complications* |
|---|---|---|---|
| Whole blood | unit | 450 mL blood | Hepatitis; fever; chills; allergic reactions; circulatory overload; rare hemolytic reactions; HIV[a] |
| Red blood cells | unit | 220–300 mL RBCs—yield from one unit whole blood | Same as for whole blood but with reduced risk of circulatory overload |
| Washed or frozen | | Same | Same as for RBCs but fewer febrile and allergic reactions |
| Platelet concentrate | unit | 5.5–10.0 × $10^{10}$ platelets in 30–50 mL plasma | Hepatitis; fever; chills; allergic reactions; development of antiplatelet antibodies; graft-versus-host disease; HIV |
| Granulocyte concentrate | unit | 10–20 × $10^9$ granulocytes in 500 mL plasma | Hepatitis; fever; chills; allergic reactions; pulmonary infiltrates; graft-versus-host disease; HIV |
| Fresh-frozen plasma | unit | 200–250 mL plasma—yield from 1 unit whole blood[b] | Hepatitis; fever; chills; allergic reactions; HIV |
| Cryoprecipitate | unit | 80–120 units factor VIII in 15–25 mL plasma | Hepatitis; fever; chills; allergic reactions; hemolysis from anti-A or anti-B; HIV |

[a] Estimated 1:200,000 administrations—American Red Cross, 1988.
[b] Contains stable coagulation factors, albumin, complement and other plasma proteins.

From Blood Products. Med Lett, 1979;21:96, with permission.

ple, 500 mL in 5 minutes, can be achieved by using pressure, multiple infusion sites, and large-diameter catheters. Massive transfusions can also contribute to the hypothermia accompanying hypovolemic shock. Warmed blood should be used when greater than 5 units are administered.[53]

**Table 103.8** Some Potentially Deleterious Effects of the Massive Transfusion of Stored Blood

| |
|---|
| Volume related |
| Transmission of disease |
| Immunologic mismatch |
| Immunization of recipient |
| Rate and volume related |
| Altered hemoglobin affinity for oxygen |
| Coagulation abnormalities |
| Acid–base imbalance |
| Citrate toxicity |
| Hypothermia |
| Microembolization |
| Impaired red cell deformability |
| Infusion of plasticizers |
| Infusion of denatured proteins |
| Infusion of vasoactive substances |
| Elevated potassium, phosphate, ammonia levels |
| Hemolyzed blood products |
| Impaired antibacterial defenses |
| Graft-versus-host reactions |
| Toxicity of new additives |

From Collins JA: Problems associated with massive transfusion of stored blood. Surgery 1974;75:274–295, with permission.

### *Fresh-Frozen Plasma*

An NIH consensus panel reported that there is no justification for the use of fresh-frozen plasma (FFP) as a volume expander or as a nutritional source. The NIH panel stated that FFP is indicated for documented coagulation protein deficiencies, for selected patients who require massive (>5 L in 12 hours) transfusions, for patients with multiple coagulation-related defects as in liver disease, in combination with therapeutic plasma exchange for thrombotic thrombocytopenic purpura, for infants with protein-losing enteropathy, and for selected patients with other immunodeficiencies.[54]

### *Flurocarbon, Stroma-Free Hemoglobin*

These two red cell–free alternatives are able to maintain normal oxygen consumption. They are experimental agents resulting from attempts to find replacements for blood replenishment that are less expensive, have fewer potential complications, and are in line with the religious preference preventing patients from receiving blood transfusions.[55]

### *Naloxone*

Faden and Holaday[56] were the first to postulate the hypothesis that endogenous opiates play a role in the pathophysiology of hypovolemic shock after their studies in rats. They found that in their rat shock model, naloxone produced a significant improvement in mean arterial pressure and survival after 24 hours compared with those rats resuscitated with sodium chloride. Vargish et al[57] confirmed this hypothesis with their work in dogs, in which hemorrhagic shock had been induced. Vargish et al indicated a significant increase in mean arterial pressure, most likely attributable to an increase in cardiac output associated with increased left ventricular contractility, with no change in preload or afterload. Survival was also enhanced by increasing the dose of naloxone to approximately 2 mg/kg. It was noted that there was no response in the nonshock, nonstressed dog to the administration of naloxone.

Although there have been reports of the successful use of naloxone in the treatment of both hemorrhage and septic shock, the outcomes have not been entirely uniform or without side effects, including pulmonary edema, cardiac failure, and hypotension.[58]

The results of studies to date on the use of naloxone in either septic or hemorrhagic shock have been variable. They have consisted of small groups of mixed types of patients with varying degrees of shock. Therefore, it is not surprising that mixed results should have occurred. Naloxone's potential role and usefulness compared with its potential side effects and adverse effects are unknown but bear further study.

### *Military Antishock Trousers (MAST)*

The MAST suit is a three-compartment suit that fits over the legs and abdomen of the patient. When inflated with air the suit compresses blood vessels with a resultant increase in systemic vascular resistance that can increase preload in the hypovolemic patient and aid hemostasis in case of a leg wound. Pressure in the MAST suit is adjusted according to the patient's response. Contraindications include normovolemic cardiogenic shock, cardiac tamponade, and evisceration of abdominal contents. Rapid deflation of the MAST suit can produce hypovolemic shock as a result of rapid vasodilation.

## References


1. Guyton AC. Textbook of Medical Physiology. Philadelphia, W.B. Saunders, 1976, p 392.
2. Feig UP, McCurdy DK. The hypertonic state. N Engl J Med 1977;297:1444–1454.
3. Civetta JM. A new look at the Starling equation. Crit Care Med 1979;7:84–91.
4. Gabel JC, Drake RE. Pulmonary capillary pressure and permeability. Crit Care Med 1979;7:92–97
5. Lewis RT. Albumin: Role and discriminative use in surgery. Can J Surg 1980;23:322–333.
6. Gaar KA, Taylor AE, Owens LJ, et al. Pulmonary capillary pressure and filtration coefficients in the isolated perfused lung. Am J Physiol 1967;23:910–914.
7. Staub NC. Pulmonary edema. Physiol Rev 1971;54:678–811.
8. Landis EM. Capillary pressure and capillary permeability. Physiol Rev 1934;14:404–481.
9. Rothschild MA, Oratz M, Schreiber SS. Albumin synthesis (first of two parts). N Engl J Med 1972;286:748–757.
10. Tullis JL. Albumin. 1. Background and use. JAMA 1977;237: 355–360.
11. Morisette MP. Colloid osmotic pressure: Its measurement and clinical value. Can Med Assoc J 1977;116:897–900.
12. Landis EM, Pappenheimer JR. Exchange of substances through the capillary walls, in: Handbook of Physiology and Circulation. Sect. 2. Washington DC, American Physiology Society, 1963, vol 2, p 961.
13. Weil MH, Henning RJ, Puri VK. Colloid oncotic pressure: Clinical significance. Crit Care Med 1979;3:113–116.
14. Weil MH, Henning RJ, Morisette M, et al. Relationship between colloid osmotic pressure and pulmonary artery wedge pressure in patients with acute respiratory failure. Am J Med 1978;64:643–650.
15. Weil MH, Henning RJ. New concepts in the diagnosis and fluid treatment of circulatory shock. Anesth Analg 1979;58:124–132.
16. Feeley TW, Mihm FG, Halperin BD, et al. Failure of the colloid oncotic–pulmonary artery wedge pressure gradient to predict changes in extravascular lung water. Crit Care Med 1985;13: 1025–1028.
17. Rafferty TD, Ljungquist R, Firestone L, et al. Plasma colloid oncotic pressure–pulmonary artery occlusion pressure gradient. Arch Surg 1983;118:841–843.
18. Grundmann R, Heistermann S. Post operative albumin infusion therapy based on colloid osmotic pressure. Arch Surg 1985;120: 911–915.
19. Granger DN, Gabel JC, Drake RE, et al. Physiologic basis for the clinical use of albumin solutions. Surg Gynecol Obstet 1978; 146:97–104.
20. Loyd JE, Newman JH, Brigham KL. Permeability pulmonary edema, diagnosis and management. Arch Intern Med 1984;144: 143–147.
21. Gann DS, Amaral JF. Pathophysiology of trauma and shock, in Zuidema GD, Rutherford RB, Bellinger WF (eds): The Management of Trauma, 4th ed. Philadelphia, W.B. Saunders, 1985, pp 37–103.
22. Schwartzkopff W, Schwartzkopff B, Wurm W, et al. Physiological aspects of the role of human albumin in the treatment of chronic and acute blood loss. Dev Biol Stand 1980;48:7–30.
23. Skillman JJ, Awwad HK, Moore FD. Plasma protein kinetics on the early transcapillary refill after hemorrhage in man. Surg Gynecol Obstet 1967;125:983–996.
24. Crandall ED, Staub NC, Goldberg HS, et al. UCLA conference: Recent developments in pulmonary edema. Ann Intern Med 1983;99:808–822.
25. Granger HJ. Role of interstitial matrix and lymphatic pump in regulation of transcapillary fluid balance. Microvasc Res 1979; 18:209–216.
26. Trunkey DD, Sheldon GF, Collins JA. The treatment of shock, in Zuidema GD, Rutherford RB, Bellinger WF (eds): The Management of Trauma, 4th ed. Philadelphia, W.B. Saunders, 1985, pp 105–125.
27. Moore EE. Resuscitation and evaluation of the injured patient, in Zuidema GD, Rutherford RB, Bellinger WF (eds): The Management of Trauma, 4th ed. Philadelphia, W.B. Saunders, 1985, pp 1–26.
28. Etheredge EE, Hruska KA. Acute renal failure in the surgical patient, in Zuidema GD, Rutherford RB, Bellinger WF (eds): The Management of Trauma, 4th ed. Phladelphia, W.B. Saunders, 1985, pp 169–205.
29. Snyder JC, Carroll GC. Tissue oxygenation: A physiological approach to a clinical problem. Curr Probl Surg 1982;650–717.
30. Weil MH, Henning RH. Early treatment of circulatory shock. Hosp Physician 1977;13:20–28.
31. Shoemaker WC, Bland RD, Appel PL: Therapy of critically ill

postoperative patients based on outcome prediction and prospective clinical trials. Surg Clin North Am 1985;65:811–834.

**32.** Calvin JE, Dreideger AA, Sibbald WJ. The hemodynamic effect of rapid fluid infusion in critically ill patients. Surgery 1981;90: 61–76.

**33.** Crexal SC, Chatterjee K, Forrester J, et al. Optimum level of filling pressure in the left sided heart in acute myocardial infarction. N Engl J Med 1973;289:1264.

**34.** Packman MI, Rackow EC. Optimum left heart filling pressure during fluid resuscitation of patients with hypovolemic and septic shock. Crit Care Med 1983;11:165–169.

**35.** Calvin JE, Dreideger AA, Sibbald WJ. Does the pulmonary capillary wedge pressure predict left ventricular preload in critically ill patients? Crit Care Med 1981;9:437–443.

**36.** Thompson WL. Hydroxyethyl starch. Dev Biol Stand 1980;48: 259–266.

**37.** Tullis JL. Albumin. 2. Guidelines for clinical use. JAMA 1977; 237:460–463.

**38.** Lazrove S, Waxman K, Shippy C, et al. Hemodynamic, blood volume, and oxygen transport responses to albumin and hydroxyethyl starch infusions in critically ill post-operative patients. Crit Care Med 1980;8:302–305.

**39.** Hicks GL, Jensen LA, Norsen LH, et al. Platelet inhibitors in hydroxyethyl starch: Safe and cost-effective interventions in coronary artery surgery. Ann Thorac Surg 1985;40:422–426.

**40.** Diehl JT, Lester JL, Cosgrove DM. Clinical comparison of hetastarch and albumin in post-operative cardiac patients. Ann Thorac Surg 1982;34:674–679.

**41.** Shatney CH, Deepika K, Militello PR, et al. Efficacy of hetastarch in the resuscitation of patients with multisystem trauma and shock. Arch Surg 1983;118:804–809.

**42.** Hewson JR, Neame PB, Kumar N, et al. Coagulopathy related to dilution and hypotension during massive transfusion. Crit Care Med 1985;13:387–391.

**43.** Lowery BD, Cloutier CT, Carey LC. Electrolyte solutions in resuscitation in human hemorrhagic shock. Surg Gynecol Obstet 1971;133:273–284.

**44.** McClelland RN, Shives GT, Baxter CR, et al. Balanced salt solution in the treatment of hemorrhagic shock. JAMA 1967; 199:830–834.

**45.** Canizaro PC, Prager MD, Shires TG. The infusion of Ringer's lactate during shock. Am J Surg 1971;122:494–501.

**46.** De Felippe Jr J, Timoner J. Treatment of refractory hypovolemic shock by 7.5% sodium chloride injections. Lancet 1980;2: 1002–1004.

**47.** Prough DS, Johnson JC, Stullken EH, et al. Effects on cerebral hemodynamics of resuscitation from endotoxic shock with hypertonic saline versus lactated Ringer's solution. Crit Care Med 1985;13:1040–1044.

**48.** Shackford SR, Sise JM, Friedlund PH, et al. Hypertonic sodium lactate versus lactated Ringer's solution for intravenous fluid therapy in operations on the abdominal aorta. Surgery 1983;94: 41–51.

**49.** Jelenko C, Williams JB, Wheeler ML, et al. Studies in shock and resuscitation. I: Use of a hypertonic albumin-containing, fluid demand regimen (HALFD) in resuscitation. Crit Care Med 1979;7:157–167.

**50.** Collins JA. Problems associated with massive transfusion of stored blood. Surgery 1974;75:274–295.

**51.** Goldfinger D. Adverse reactions to blood transfusion, in Barnes Jr A, Nelson IF (eds): Safe Transfusion, A Technical Workshop. Chicago, Committee on Technical Workshops, American Association of Blood Banks, 1981, pp 137–154.

**52.** Barnes A. Complications of transfusion, in Mayer K (ed): Guidelines to Transfusion Practices, 1st ed. Washington DC, American Association of Blood Banks, 1980, pp 63–76.

**53.** Wilson JN, Marshall SB, Beresford V, et al. Experimental hemorrhage: Deleterious effect of hypothermia on survival and a comparative evaluation of plasma volume changes. Ann Surg 1956;144:696–714.

**54.** Consensus conference: Fresh-frozen plasma, indications and risk. JAMA 1985;253:551–553.

**55.** Gould SA, Rosen AL, Sehgal LR, et al. Red cell substitutes: Hemoglobin solution or flurocarbon? J Trauma 1982;22:736–740.

**56.** Faden AL, Holaday JW. Opiate antagonists: A role in treatment of hypovolemic shock. Science 1979;205:317–318.

**57.** Vargish T, Reynolds DG, Gurll NJ. Naloxone reversal of hypovolemic shock in dogs. Circ Shock 1980;7:31–38.

**58.** Rock P, Silverman H, Plumb D, et al. Efficacy and safety of naloxone in septic shock. Crit Care Med 1985;13:28–33.

# Chapter 104 / Acid–Base Disorders

Mary Jane Watson, PharmD, and David M. Angaran, MS

In acid–base chemistry, an *acid* is defined as the substance that can donate hydrogen ions, $H^+$, for example,

$$\underset{\text{(acid)}}{HCl} \rightarrow H^+ + Cl^-$$

A *base* is a substance that can accept hydrogen ions, for example,

$$\underset{\text{(base)}}{NH_3} + H^+ \rightarrow NH_4^+$$

Table 104.1 shows acid–base pairs commonly encountered in the body. A substance capable of accepting and donating hydrogen ions is a buffer. Buffering refers to the ability of a solution containing a weak acid and its anion (a base) to resist a change in pH upon addition of a strong acid or base. Examples of buffer systems utilized by the body are shown in Table 104.2.

The degree of acidity of body fluids is expressed in terms of the hydrogen ion concentration. The normal concentration of hydrogen ions in blood is 0.00004 mEq/L or $40 \times 10^{-9}$ Eq/L.[1] By convention, the degree of acidity is often expressed as pH, or the negative logarithm (base 10) of the hydrogen ion concentration. Normally, the pH of blood is maintained at 7.40, with a range of 7.35–7.45. A pH less than 6.8 or greater than 7.8 is considered incompatible with life.[1] pH and hydrogen ion concentration are inversely related. Low pH values, below 7.40, are associated with higher-than-normal hydrogen ion concentration; high pH values, greater than 7.40, indicate lower-than-normal hydrogen ion concentration. Figure 104.1 shows the nonlinear relationship between pH and hydrogen ion concentration.

The hydrogen ion concentration in blood may not be indicative of that in other areas of the body. For example, the pH within cells, within cerebrospinal fluid, and on the surface of bone may all be altered without causing an alteration in blood pH.[2] The blood pH is still important in determining acid–base status within the body and in diagnosing acid–base disorders.

The relationship among pH, acid, and base in the body is described by the Henderson–Hasselbach equation:

$$pH = pK + \log \frac{[\text{base}]}{[\text{acid}]} \qquad (2)$$

## Buffers

Because the carbonic acid/bicarbonate buffer system is the body's most abundant and measurable buffer, bicarbonate and carbonic acid are most commonly used to assess acid–base status. The equation describing the dissociation of carbonic acid is

$$\text{dissolved } CO_2\ (P_{CO_2}) + H_2O \underset{\text{anhydrase}}{\overset{\text{carbonic}}{\rightleftharpoons}} H_2CO_3 \rightarrow H^+ + HCO_3^- \qquad (1)$$

$$\frac{[H^+][HCO_3^-]}{[H_2CO_3]} = K \qquad (2)$$

where $K$ is the dissociation constant for the buffer system. Rearrangement of Equation 2 gives

$$[H^+] = K \frac{[H_2CO_3]}{[HCO_3^-]} \qquad (3)$$

By taking the negative logarithm of each term, Equation 3 appears in the form of the Henderson–Hasselbach equation,

$$pH = pK + \log\ ([HCO_3^-]/[H_2CO_3]) \qquad (4)$$

The concentration of carbonic acid is directly proportional to the amount of $CO_2$ dissolved in blood, which is directly proportional to the partial pressure of $CO_2$ gas, $P_{CO_2}$. The dissolved $CO_2$, $P_{CO_2}$, can be substituted into Equation 4, as it is more readily measurable than carbonic acid, giving

$$pH = pK + \log([HCO_3^-]/P_{CO_2}) \qquad (5)$$

Substitution of the appropriate values for p$K$ (6.1) and 0.03, the solubility constant for $CO_2$ in blood, into the equation results in

$$pH = 6.1 + \log([HCO_3^-]/\ 0.03\ P_{CO_2}) \qquad (6)$$

Equation 6 demonstrates that pH and $H^+$ concentration are determined not by absolute amounts of bicarbonate and $P_{CO_2}$, but by their ratio.[2] Examples of calculations using the Henderson–Hasselbach equation are shown in Figure 104.2.

Normally, the body's acid–base balance is maintained despite daily acid and alkali loads. Cellular metabolism of neutral dietary and tissue components results in the production of hydrogen ions and fixed acid anions, both of which need to be excreted to maintain acid–base balance. Small amounts of acid and alkali are presented as such to the body through the diet. On the average, 0.8 mEq/kg/d or 50–100 mEq of acid is consumed as part of our normal American diet.[3] Neutral substances such as glucose are metabolized to intermediates, lactic and pyruvic acids, with the production of hydrogen ion.[4] These intermediates are normally metabolized to $H_2O$ and $CO_2$. Other organic anions, such as citrate and acetoacetate, are metabolized to $CO_2$. When respiratory function is normal, the blood $CO_2$ concentration remains constant, and the amount of $CO_2$ produced metabolically is equal to the amount lost by respiration. The average adult produces 15,000–20,000 mmol of $CO_2$ each day.

Digestion of dietary substances and tissue metabolism also result in the production of nonvolatile acids. These acids are derived primarily from the sulfur-containing amino acids,

**Table 104.1** Acid–Base Pairs

| | |
|---|---|
| Carbonic acid/bicarbonate | $H_2CO_3/HCO_3$ |
| Monobasic/dibasic phosphate | $H_2PO_4/HPO_4$ |
| Ammonium/ammonia | $NH^+/NH_3$ |
| Lactic acid/lactate | |

From Broughton JO: Understanding Blood Gases. Ohio Medical Products, with permission.

cysteine and methionine, as well as from ingested sulfur. Additionally, phosphate is produced from metabolism of proteins and phospholipids.

Three mechanisms collectively maintain acid–base balance: extracellular buffering, renal regulation of hydrogen ion and bicarbonate, and ventilatory regulation of carbon dioxide elimination.

Extracellular buffering is the body's first defense against an increase in hydrogen ion concentration. The body's buffering system can be broken down into three components: bicarbonate/carbonic acid, proteins, and phosphates. The bicarbonate buffer is the most important of the body's buffers, because (1) there is more bicarbonate present in the extracellular fluid than any other buffer component, (2) the supply of carbon dioxide is unlimited, and (3) the acidity of extracellular fluid can be regulated by controlling either the bicarbonate concentration or the $Pco_2$.

Carbonic acid represents the respiratory component of the buffer pair because its concentration is directly proportional to the partial pressure of $CO_2$ ($Pco_2$), which is determined by ventilation. Bicarbonate represents the metabolic component because the kidney may alter its concentration by reabsorption, generating new bicarbonate, or elimination. The bicarbonate buffer system easily adapts to changes in acid–base status by alterations in ventilatory elimination of acid ($Pco_2$) and renal elimination of base ($HCO_3$).[3]

The phosphate buffer system consists of serum inorganic phosphate (3.5–5.0 mg/dL), intracellular organic phosphate, and calcium phosphate in bone. Extracellular phosphate is present only in low concentrations so that its usefulness as a buffer is limited; however, as an intracellular buffer, phosphate is more useful. Calcium phosphate in bone is relatively inaccessible as a buffer, but prolonged metabolic acidosis will result in the release of phosphate from bone.

Intracellular and extracellular proteins also act as buffering systems. The charged side chains of amino acids provide the buffering action. Because the concentration of protein is much greater intracellularly than extracellularly, protein is much more important as an intracellular buffer.

**Table 104.2** Body Buffer Systems

| *$H^+$* | ***Buffer (base)*** |
|---|---|
| $H^+$ | $HCO_3$ (Bicarbonate) |
| $H^+$ | $HPO_4$ (Phosphate) |
| $H^+$ | HB (Hemoglobin) |
| $H^+$ | Protein |

From Broughton JO: Understanding Blood Gases. Ohio Medical Products, with permission.

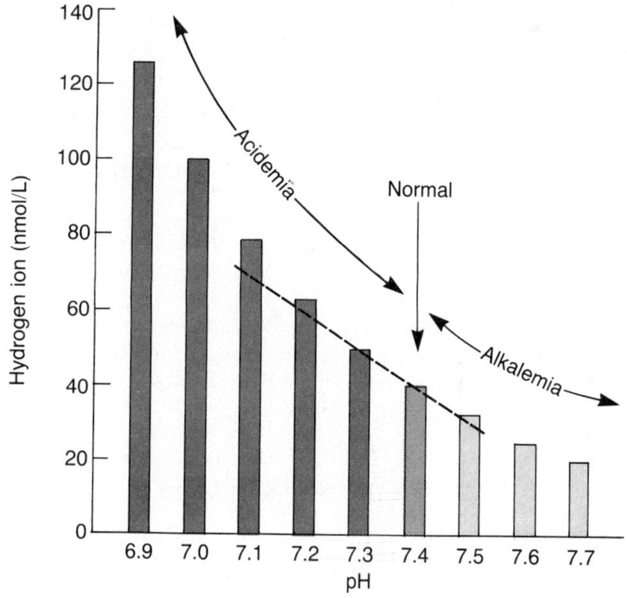


**Figure 104.1** Relationship of pH to hydrogen ion concentration. *(From Narins RG, Emmett M: Simple and mixed acid–base disorders: A practical approach. Medicine 1980;59:161–187, with permission.)*

Renal regulation of $H^+$ and $HCO^-_3$ is a second mechanism by which the body maintains acid–base balance. The kidney is responsible for reabsorption of filtered $HCO^-_3$ and elimination of $H^+$ to regulate the daily acid load.[5] Essentially all of the approximately 4000 mEq of $HCO^-_3$ filtered daily is reabsorbed, primarily in the proximal tubule. The filtered bicarbonate is reabsorbed in combination with secreted $H^+$. The $HCO^-_3$ and $H^+$ combine to form $H_2CO_3$, which later dissociates to $HCO^-_3$ and $H^+$. The hydrogen ion is secreted back into the tubule.

The final mechanism of acid–base balance is ventilation. Both the rate and depth of ventilation can be varied to allow for excretion of $CO_2$ generated by diet and tissue metabolism. Medullary chemoreceptors sense changes in $Pco_2$ or in

**Figure 104.2** Examples of the Henderson–Hasselbach equation.

1. $Pco_2$ = 40 mm Hg, $HCO_3$ = 24 mEq/L (normal)

$$pH = 6.1 + \frac{24}{\log (0.03)\ (40)}$$

$$= 6.1 + 1.30$$

$$= 7.40$$

2. $Pco_2$ = 60 mm Hg, $HCO_3$ = 24 mm Hg (uncompensated respiratory acidosis)

$$pH = 6.1 + \frac{24}{\log (0.03)\ (60)}$$

$$= 6.1 + 1.12$$

$$= 7.22$$

pH condition after ventilation. This system rapidly adjusts, within minutes, to changes in acid–base balances so that ventilation can be altered.

## Laboratory Assessment of Acid–Base Status

Several pieces of information must be considered in determining the desired treatment for a patient with an abnormal acid–base status. Initially, arterial blood gases indicate an acid–base abnormality. Serum electrolytes, medical history, medication history, and the clinical condition of the patient are all needed to determine the cause of the disorder and to design a course of therapy.

### *Obtaining Arterial Blood Gases*

Arterial blood gases are measured to determine the patient's oxygenation and acid–base status. Blood gases are most commonly measured on arterial blood rather than venous blood for two reasons.[2] First, arterial blood is a mixture of blood from all parts of the body. Venous blood obtained from an extremity provides information only about that extremity. Extrapolating the information from that extremity to the entire body can be misleading if the metabolism in the extremity is altered by hypoperfusion, exercise, infection, or some other cause. Second, arterial blood provides the added information of how well the lungs are oxygenating the blood. A low venous oxygen concentration may mean the heart, lungs, or both, are at fault.

The most accessible sites for direct arterial puncture are the brachial, radial, and femoral arteries. The brachial artery is most preferred, though the radial is also used.[2] The femoral should be avoided if possible, but it is sometimes used in hypotensive patients.

All methods of arterial blood gas analysis currently used in hospital laboratories are similar and measure pH, $Pco_2$, and $Po_2$ of the sample directly. The bicarbonate and $O_2$ saturation are calculated. The apparatus for measuring blood gases consists of a pH electrode for measuring the hydrogen ion concentration of the sample, an electrode designed for measuring the partial pressure or tension of carbon dioxide ($Pco_2$), and an electrode that measures the partial pressure of oxygen ($Po_2$) in the sample.

The temperature of the blood has an effect on pH. For this reason, the analyzer warms the samples to 37°C. Most systems also allow for corrections in temperature when the patient's body temperature differs from 37°C (e.g., during hypothermia in coronary artery bypass).

**Table 104.3** Normal Blood Gas Values

| | *Arterial blood* | *Mixed venous blood* |
|---|---|---|
| pH | 7.40 (7.35–7.45) | 7.38 (7.33–7.43) |
| $Po_2$ | 80–100 mm Hg | 35–40 mm Hg |
| $Sao_2$ | ≥95% | 70%–75% |
| $Pco_2$ | 35–45 mm Hg | 41–51 mm Hg |
| $HCO_3$ | 22–26 mEq/L | 24–28 mEq/L |

From Broughton JO: Understanding Blood Gases. Ohio Medical Products, with permission.

Certain samples cannot be used to obtain blood gas measurements and should be discarded and new samples obtained. These include clotted samples, samples with air bubbles, and small samples. Clotted samples may provide misleading information and damage the machinery. Samples that contain air bubbles also provide distorted blood gas information. Inadequate samples, less than 1 mL, may also provide distorted information because of the concentration of heparin, an acid that is added to anticoagulate the sample. The normal values for arterial and venous blood gases are shown in Table 104.3.

### *Evaluating Arterial Blood Gases*

To evaluate a set of arterial blood gas values, one must first examine the pH. The pH determines if the body is in an acidotic, alkalotic, or normal stage. Low pH values (below 7.35) indicate an acidemia, and high pH values (above 7.45) indicate an alkalemia (see Figure 104.3).

Next, one looks at the $Pco_2$ value to determine if there is a respiratory abnormality. Two conditions are associated with an abnormal $Pco_2$: respiratory acidosis and respiratory alkalosis. In respiratory acidosis, the $Pco_2$ is elevated with compensatory increase in bicarbonate concentration. In respiratory alkalosis, the $Pco_2$ is decreased with a compensatory decrease in bicarbonate concentration. Next, one examines the bicarbonate concentration to determine if there is a metabolic abnormality. The two conditions that occur with altered bicarbonate concentration are metabolic acidosis and metabolic alkalosis. With metabolic acidosis, there is a decrease in bicarbonate concentration and a compensatory decrease in $Pco_2$. An increase in bicarbonate concentration

**Figure 104.3** Analysis of arterial blood gases.

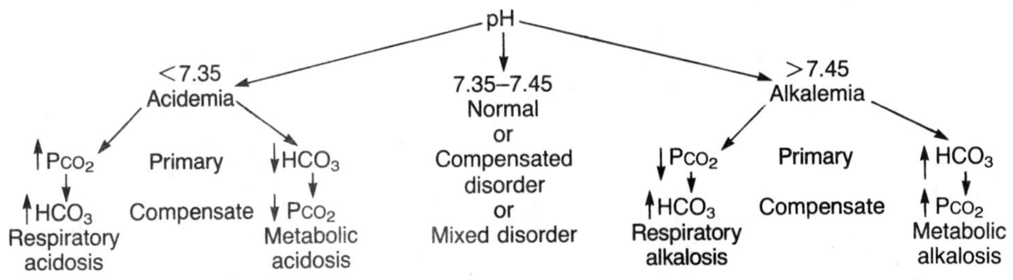

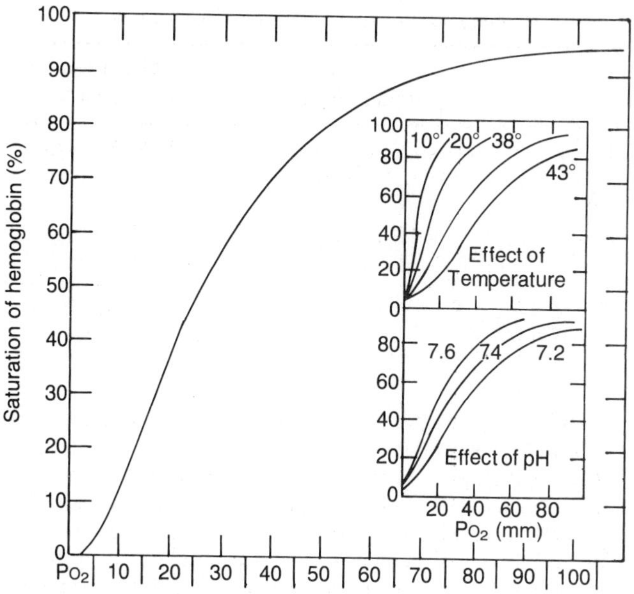


**Figure 104.4** Oxyhemoglobin dissociation curve.

and compensatory increase in $P_{CO_2}$ occur in metabolic alkalosis.

The $P_{O_2}$ value is used to measure oxygen in blood. The majority of oxygen in blood is carried by hemoglobin and a small amount is dissolved in the plasma. The $P_{O_2}$ measurement tells only the pressure exerted by the small amount of $O_2$ dissolved in plasma, whereas the percentage saturation with oxygen (or amount of $O_2$ that hemoglobin is carrying compared with the amount it is capable of carrying) gives a close estimate of the total amount of $O_2$ carried in blood; however, the $P_{O_2}$ measurement is useful because it and oxygen saturation of hemoglobin are related. This relationship is described by the oxyhemoglobin dissociation curve (Fig. 104.4). The dissociation curve shows the nonlinear relationship between $P_{O_2}$ and percentage saturation. When $P_{O_2}$ is high, the percentage saturation of hemoglobin with oxygen is also high (e.g., $P_{O_2}$ is high in such areas as lung capillaries, where hemoglobin combines with $O_2$ and carries a large percentage of the total $O_2$ it is capable of carrying). When $P_{O_2}$ is low, the percentage saturation of hemoglobin is also low. This occurs in tissue capillaries, where hemoglobin carries a small percentage of the total $O_2$ it is capable of carrying, thereby giving up $O_2$ for use by tissues. The smaller graphs in Figure 104.4 show how temperature and pH affect the oxyhemoglobin dissociation curve. With acidosis or fever, the curve is shifted to the right so that for a given $O_2$ saturation the $P_{O_2}$ is greater and more oxygen is available to tissue. With alkalosis or hypothermia, the $P_{O_2}$ is lower than usual at a given $O_2$ saturation and less oxygen is available to tissues.

Occasionally, acid–base reports may be significantly different from those expected on the basis of the patient's clinical condition and previous laboratory determinations. For this reason, it is a good idea, when drawing blood for blood gas studies, to draw additional blood for electrolyte determinations. Then, the bicarbonate associated with the patient's $P_{CO_2}$ and pH can be compared with the bicarbonate value estimated from the total $CO_2$ content (the amount of $CO_2$ gas extractable from plasma, consisting of $HCO_3^-$, $H_2CO_3$, and $P_{CO_2}$). Ordinarily, the bicarbonate estimated from the pH and $P_{CO_2}$ will be approximately 1.0–2.0 mEq/L less than $CO_2$ content.

## Acid–Base Disturbances

Two types of physiologic force can cause primary alterations in pH: metabolic and respiratory. Metabolic acid–base disturbances result from processes that alter pH primarily by changing the plasma bicarbonate concentration ($HCO_3^-$), the metabolic component of the Henderson–Hasselbach equation. Respiratory acid–base disturbances result from primary changes in the arterial carbon dioxide tension ($P_{CO_2}$), the respiratory component of the Henderson–Hasselbach equation. The changes in pH resulting from these metabolic and respiratory disturbances are dictated by the $P_{CO_2}$:$HCO_3^-$ ratio.[6]

The remainder of this chapter focuses on the pathophysiology and treatment of these acid–base disturbances.

A nomogram such as that shown in Figure 104.5 can be used to differentiate among the various acid–base disorders. In this nomogram, each pathologic acid–base disorder, together with the appropriate range of in vivo physiologic compensation, is represented as a shaded band. Acid–base values falling within a band usually represent a single disturbance; however, such values may represent a combination of acid–base disorders, a mixed disturbance. On the other hand, acid–base values falling outside any band almost certainly represent at least two acid–base disturbances.

Serum electrolyte concentrations are also useful when evaluating a patient with an acid–base abnormality. If possible, blood for determination of serum electrolytes, including sodium, potassium, chloride, and $CO_2$ content, should be drawn at the same time as that for arterial blood gases. If a metabolic acidosis is suspected, then calculation of the anion gap will be useful in determining the cause and deciding on the proper treatment. The anion gap is calculated by subtracting the sum of the chloride and bicarbonate concentrations from the sodium concentration. An increase in anion gap indicates the presence of organic acids.

## Respiratory Acid–Base Disorders

There are two types of simple respiratory acid–base disturbances: acidosis and alkalosis. These disorders are generated by a primary alteration in carbon dioxide excretion, which changes the concentration of carbon dioxide and therefore the carbonic acid concentration in body fluids. A primary reduction in $P_{CO_2}$ causes a rise in pH (respiratory alkalosis) and a primary increase in $P_{CO_2}$ causes a decrease in pH (respiratory acidosis) (Table 104.4).[7]

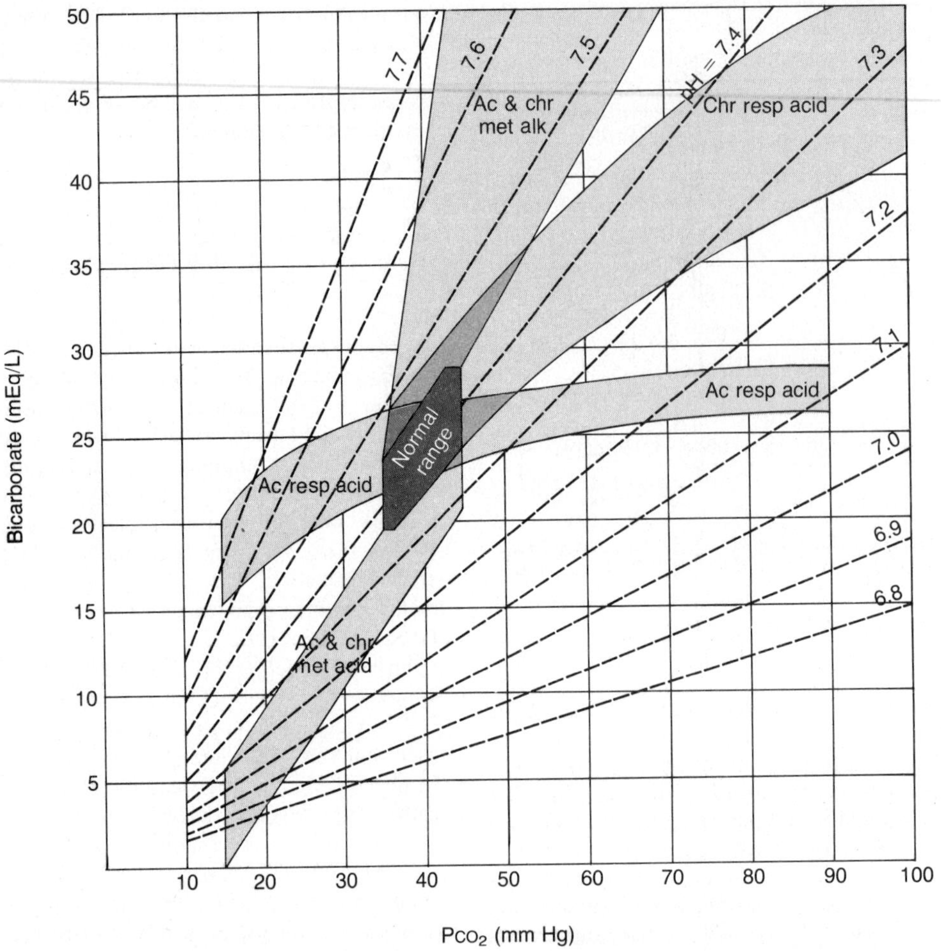


**Figure 104.5** Acid–base nomogram. Chr Resp Acid, chronic respiratory acidosis; Ac & Chr Met Alk, acute and chronic metabolic acidosis; Ac Resp Acid, acute respiratory acidosis; Ac Resp Alk, acute respiratory alkalosis; Ac & Chr Met Acid, acute and chronic metabolic acidosis *(From Mazzara JR, Ayers SM, Grace WJ: Extreme hypocapnia in the critically ill patient. Am J Med 1974;56: 450–456, with permission.)*

## *Respiratory Alkalosis*

### Pathophysiology

Respiratory alkalosis is an acid–base disorder characterized by a primary decrease in $Pco_2$, hypocapnia, that raises pH and produces a secondary decrease in plasma bicarbonate concentration. This disorder is one of the most commonly found acid–base disturbances among hospitalized patients.[8] Mazarra et al[9] reviewed 8,607 blood gas samples from critically ill patients. Respiratory alkalosis, defined as pH greater than or equal to 7.45 and $Pco_2$ less than 35 mm Hg without metabolic alkalosis was observed in 46% of patients. The incidence of shock and sepsis was significantly higher in patients with spontaneous extreme hypocapnia ($Pco_2 \leq 15$ mm Hg). Mortality from sepsis and shock correlated inversely with the $Pco_2$ concentration and a $Pco_2$ concentra-

**Table 104.4** Respiratory Abnormalities

| *Parameter* | *Condition* | *Mechanism* | |
|---|---|---|---|
| ↑ $PCO_2$ | Respiratory acidosis | Decreased elimination by lungs of $CO_2$ gas | Hypoventilation |
| ↑ $PCO_2$ | Respiratory alkalosis | Increased elimination by lungs of $CO_2$ gas | Hypoventilation |

From Broughton JO: Understanding Blood Gases. Ohio Medical Products, with permission.

**Table 104.5** Causes of Respiratory Alkalosis

| | |
|---|---|
| Central stimulation of respiration | Physical stimuli |
| Anxiety | Mechanical ventilation |
| Pain | Stiff lungs |
| Fever | Irritative lesions of the air conduits, e.g., tumor, spasm, inflammation |
| Injury, inflammation | |
| Brain tumors, vascular accidents | Miscellaneous |
| Head trauma | Drugs or hormones |
| Voluntary | Salicylate |
| Peripheral stimulation of respiration | Nicotine |
| Hypoxemia | Thyroid hormone |
| Altitude | Progesterone |
| Pulmonary shunts | Catecholamines |
| Pulmonary ventilation–perfusion imbalance | Xanthines (e.g., Aminophylline) |
| Pulmonary diffusion defects | Conditions |
| Hypotension | Liver cirrhosis |
| Pulmonary emboli | Gram-negative sepsis |
| Congestive heart failure | Pregnancy |
| Pneumonia | Hyponatremia |
| | Heat exposure |
| | Recovery from metabolic acidosis |

From Kaehny WD: Respiratory acid–base disorders. Med Clin N Am 1983;67:915–929, with permission.

tion of 15 mm Hg or less was a morbid prognostic sign. While respiratory alkalosis occurs in a significant number of critically ill patients, treatment of the alkalosis itself has not been shown to produce a change in mortality.

A decrease in $P_{CO_2}$ occurs when ventilatory excretion exceeds metabolic production. An increase in ventilatory excretion of $P_{CO_2}$, hyperventilation, is responsible for the decrease, as the metabolic production of $P_{CO_2}$ remains relatively constant except during periods of stress or carbohydrate administration (i.e., parenteral nutrition) when it may be increased.[10] Two processes can cause hyperventilation: an increase in neurochemical stimulation via central or peripheral mechanisms, or a physical increase in ventilation either voluntarily or artificially by means of mechanical ventilation.[6] Specific causes of respiratory alkalosis are listed in Table 104.5.

Stimulation of the medullary respiratory center occurs in such conditions as anxiety, pain, or fever. Head trauma, brain tumors, or other lesions can also stimulate the respiratory center. Peripheral stimulation of respiration occurs secondary to pulmonary or cardiovascular disorders that cause hypoxemia. These include pulmonary emboli, congestive heart failure, and others. A decrease in $P_{CO_2}$ may occur secondary to hypotension in such conditions as cardiogenic, hypovolemic, or septic shock.[11] During hypotension, oxygen delivered to the carotid and aortic chemoreceptors is reduced and thus stimulates an increase in ventilation. Hyperventilation-induced respiratory alkalosis with an elevation in cardiac index and hypotension without peripheral vasoconstriction may be an early sign of sepsis.[10]

### Signs/Symptoms

Respiratory alkalosis may cause adverse effects in the neuromuscular, cardiovascular, and gastrointestinal systems. During periods of decreased $P_{CO_2}$, there is a decrease in cerebral blood flow.[12] This may be responsible for symptoms of lightheadedness, confusion, decreased intellectual functioning, syncope, and seizures. Nausea and vomiting may occur, probably as a result of cerebral hypoxia. In severe respiratory alkalosis, cardiac arrhythmias may occur. Lawson et al[12] studied nine posttraumatic patients who developed cardiac arrhythmias during periods of inadvertent severe alkalosis. Four of the patients had a simple respiratory alkalosis and the remaining five had a mixed respiratory and metabolic alkalosis. They concluded that the development of arrhythmias in the presence of alkalosis was independent of preexisting heart disease, although patients with heart disease and those taking digitalis were at an increased risk. The increased risk of arrhythmias is thought to result from the shift of potassium from extracellular fluid to intracellular fluid that occurs during alkalosis. Arrhythmias occurring during alkalosis were generally resistant to antiarrhythmic therapy and required correction of the alkalosis. Correction of the alkalosis itself resulted in conversion of these arrhythmias to sinus rhythm without additional drug therapy. The arrhythmia mechanism is unknown, but may result from an enhancement of automaticity by hypoxia or hypokalemia. Alkalosis may also sensitize the myocardium to the arrhythmogenic effects of circulating catecholamines.

Alkalosis, either metabolic or respiratory, may cause an increase in cardiac output, an increase in heart rate, and a decrease in peripheral vascular resistance. McElroy et al[13] studied the effects of altering the $P_{CO_2}$ and bicarbonate concentrations in a solution used to perfuse guinea pig hearts. They reported an increase in heart rate and contractility as the carbon dioxide tension was decreased. Burnum et al[14] measured cardiac output, forearm blood flow, and arterial pressure during hyperventilation in normal patients and in patients with sympathetic paresis. They noted a doubling of forearm blood flow, a 30% increase in cardiac output, and a 70% increase in heart rate, at a carbon dioxide pressure of 20 mm Hg.

The concentration of serum electrolytes may also be altered in respiratory alkalosis. The serum chloride concentration is slightly increased and serum potassium concentration may be slightly decreased. Clinically significant hypokalemia has been reported as a consequence of extreme respiratory alkalosis, although most studies of both acute and chronic respiratory alkalosis report very small or negligible effects on plasma potassium concentration.[15] Serum phosphorus concentration may decrease by as much as 1.5–2.0 mg/dL to a concentration of 0.3 mg/dL at pH 7.7 because of the movement of inorganic phosphate into cells.[16] The amount of ionized calcium is reduced in respiratory alkalosis, which may be responsible for such symptoms as muscle cramps, tetany, and decreased deep-tendon reflexes.[11] Approximately 50% of calcium is bound to albumin and an increase in pH results in an increase in binding. This may result from conformational changes in the albumin molecule. The amount of free, ionized calcium decreases by about 0.04 mM/L for each 0.1-unit increase in pH.[2]

### Compensation

The initial response of the body to acute respiratory alkalosis during the first 6 hours is to chemically buffer excess bicarbonate. Hydrogen ions from intracellular proteins, phosphates, and hemoglobin move extracellularly to titrate bicarbonate.[5] Acutely, the bicarbonate concentration is decreased by a maximum of no more than 3.5 mEq/L for each 10 mm Hg decrease in $Pco_2$.

The second, or compensatory, phase of the body's response to the increase in pH occurs when respiratory alkalosis is prolonged beyond 6 hours. During this stage, the renal system compensates for the decrease in the respiratory acid component, $Pco_2$, by increasing bicarbonate elimination. This compensation consists of a decrease in both reclamation of filtered bicarbonate and net acid excretion.[6] In general, the bicarbonate concentration can be reduced by up to 5 mEq/L for each 10 mm Hg drop in $Pco_2$.[5] For example, a sustained decrease in $Pco_2$ of 20 mm Hg will lower serum bicarbonate from 24 to 14 mEq/L with a pH of 7.46. Bicarbonate concentrations differing from those anticipated using the preceding guideline would suggest a mixed acid–base disorder (refer to nomogram, Fig. 104.5).

### Treatment

The first consideration in the treatment of respiratory alkalosis is correction of the underlying cause. Relief of pain, correction of hypovolemia with volume, treatment of fever or infection, treatment of salicylate overdose, and other direct measures may prove effective.[11] A rebreathing device, for example, a paper bag, may be useful in controlling hyperventilation in some patients. Oxygen therapy should be initiated in patients with severe hypoxemia. In cases of life-threatening alkalosis (pH $>$ 7.55) with complications such as arrhythmia or seizures, patients may require mechanical ventilation. These patients may also require sedation and paralysis to control hyperventilation.[11] Simple respiratory alkalosis rarely requires such aggressive therapy, but it may be required in mixed respiratory and metabolic alkalosis. Respiratory alkalosis in patients on mechanical ventilators may be treated by increasing the length of dead space tubing. This involves placing a known length of tubing between the artificial airway and the "Y" piece of the ventilator. This results in "rebreathing" of expired gas and, therefore, an increase in the inspired carbon dioxide concentration. This should increase the carbon dioxide tension of the patient and thereby correct the respiratory alkalosis.

## *Respiratory Acidosis*

### Pathophysiology

The second of the simple respiratory acid–base disorders is respiratory acidosis. This disorder is caused by a primary retention of carbon dioxide that lowers the pH and produces a compensatory increase in plasma bicarbonate concentration. Respiratory acidosis was found to occur in 14% and 22% of critically ill hospitalized patients in two large reviews.[9,17]

Respiratory acidosis results from a failure of carbon dioxide excretion secondary to a disorder that restricts ventilation or an increase in $CO_2$ production, such as those listed in Table 104.6. With acute respiratory acidosis, hypoxemia, hypercarbia, and acidosis are life-threatening. Those disorders that produce an increase in $Pco_2$ and hypoxemia to a degree compatible with life, with or without oxygen therapy, produce a chronic respiratory acidosis (Table 104.7). The most common cause of chronic respiratory acidosis is chronic obstructive pulmonary disease. These patients can function normally without noticeable neurologic defects with $Pco_2$ concentration chronically in the range 90–100 mm Hg (normal 40 mm Hg), provided adequate oxygenation is maintained.

### Signs/Symptoms

The signs and symptoms of respiratory acidosis are primarily those related to the underlying cause. Neuromuscular and cardiovascular symptoms may also occur. Neuromuscular symptoms include altered mental status, abnormal behavior,

**Table 104.6** Causes of Acute Respiratory Acidosis

| |
|---|
| Perfusion |
|   Massive pulmonary embolism |
|   Cardiac arrest |
| Ventilation |
|   Severe pulmonary edema |
|   Severe pneumonia |
|   Adult respiratory distress syndrome |
|   Airway obstruction |
| Central nervous system |
|   Anesthesia |
|   Drugs |
|   Trauma, stroke |
| Spinal cord and peripheral nerves |
|   Cervical cord injury |
|   Drugs |
| Failure of mechanical ventilator |

From Kaehny WD: Respiratory acid–base disorders. Med Clin N Am 1983;67:915–929, with permission.

**Table 104.7** Causes of Chronic Respiratory Acidosis

| |
|---|
| Ventilation |
| Chronic obstructive pulmonary disease |
| Thorax, chest wall, muscular problems |
| Central nervous system |
| Obesity–hypoventilation syndrome |
| Tumors |
| Brain stem infarcts |
| Spinal cord and peripheral nerves |
| Poliomyelitis |
| Multiple sclerosis |

From Kaehny WD: Respiratory acid–base disorders. Med Clin N Am 1983;67:915–929, with permission.

stupor, and coma.[18] Hypercapnia may mimic stroke or central nervous system tumor by producing headache, papilledema, focal paresis, and abnormal reflexes. Carbon dioxide acts as a vasodilator in the brain, thus causing an increase in cerebral blood flow. This increase in cerebral blood flow is thought to be responsible for the central nervous system symptoms of respiratory acidosis. These central nervous system effects of hypercapnia may be worsened in patients with chronic respiratory acidosis who are given oxygen therapy. The drive for respiration in these patients is hypoxemia rather than hypercapnia. Oxygen administration will cause a decrease in respiratory drive and an acute increase in $Pco_2$, which rapidly distributes into the central nervous system. This may result in the syndrome of carbon dioxide narcosis, characterized by extreme stupor and coma.[7]

The degree to which cardiac contractility and heart rate are decreased depends upon the severity of acidosis whether metabolic or respiratory and the rapidity with which acidosis develops.[19] Acidosis may also cause a decrease in myocardial responsiveness to catecholamines. It has been shown that both the heart and peripheral vessels are less responsive to catecholamines at a pH below 7.1 than at a pH of 7.4.[20]

In respiratory acidosis serum concentrations of sodium and chloride remain normal or increase slightly. The effect of respiratory acidosis on serum potassium concentration depends upon the duration of the disturbance. The effect after only 1 hour is negligible.

**Compensation**

The body responds to acute respiratory acidosis with chemical buffering. Nonbicarbonate buffers (i.e., proteins, phosphate, and hemoglobin) take up the hydrogen ions from the carbonic acid formed from the increase in $Pco_2$ and allow the bicarbonate concentration to increase. Buffering begins almost immediately after an acute increase in $Pco_2$. In general the bicarbonate concentration increases by 1 mmol/L above 24 for each 10 mm Hg increase in $Pco_2$ above 40 in acute respiratory acidosis.[6]

When respiratory acidosis is prolonged beyond 12 to 24 hours or becomes chronic, renal excretion of hydrogen ion increases to compensate for acidosis. The kidneys excrete hydrogen ion which generates new bicarbonate and raises the pH toward normal. A new steady state in acid–base values occurs within 5 days of the onset of hypercapnia in dogs.[6] The time to steady state has not been established in humans. A guideline for renal compensation for chronic hypercapnia is that the plasma bicarbonate concentration increases by 4 mmol/L above 24 for each 10 mm Hg increase in $Pco_2$ above 40 in compensated respiratory acidosis.[6]

**Treatment**

The treatment of respiratory acidosis may be divided into three categories: acute respiratory acidosis, acute respiratory acidosis superimposed on chronic respiratory acidosis, and chronic respiratory acidosis.

***Acute Respiratory Acidosis*** There is apparent failure of carbon dioxide excretion and life-threatening hypoxia, and the immediate therapeutic goal is to provide adequate ventilation in acute respiratory acidosis. This involves maintenance of a patent airway, which may necessitate emergency tracheotomy, bronchoscopy, or intubation. In addition, excessive secretions must be cleared from the airway. Oxygen should be administered to restore adequate oxygenation. Mechanical ventilation may be required in cases of life-threatening hypoxia.

Attempts should be made at correcting the underlying cause of the acidosis (i.e., bronchodilators for treatment of severe bronchospasm). Bicarbonate administration is rarely necessary in the treatment of acute respiratory acidosis. Rapid correction of acidosis with bicarbonate may eliminate the drive to breathe or precipitate a metabolic alkalosis. Arterial blood gases should be monitored closely to ensure that the respiratory acidosis is resolving without creating a metabolic alkalosis caused by an elevated $HCO_3^-$ and decreasing $Pco_2$. Arterial blood gases should be obtained every 2 to 4 hours during the acute phase and less frequently (every 12–24 hours) as the acidosis improves.

***Acute Respiratory Acidosis in a Compensated Chronic Respiratory Acidosis Patient*** Patients with a history of chronic respiratory acidosis caused by conditions such as chronic obstructive pulmonary disease may experience an acute worsening of their acidosis. This may result in severe life-threatening hypoxemia. As with acute respiratory acidosis, the goals of therapy are maintenance of a patent airway and adequate oxygenation. Individuals with chronic respiratory acidosis are routinely able to tolerate a low $Po_2$ and an elevated $Pco_2$ because of compensation (increased red blood cells, hemoglobin, and 2,3-diphosphoglycerate). The drive to breathe in these patients is dependent on hypoxemia rather hypercarbia. Administration of oxygen to a patient with chronic respiratory acidosis can eliminate this drive to breathe and result in the syndrome of carbon dioxide narcosis. In this case, if the $Po_2$ is greater than or equal to 50 mm Hg, no oxygen treatment is necessary. If the $Po_2$ is less than 50 mm Hg, oxygen therapy should be initiated carefully.

Arterial blood gases should be checked periodically to ensure adequate oxygenation. If the $Pco_2$ is increasing during oxygen therapy, it may be a sign of impending carbon dioxide narcosis and oxygen therapy may need to be discontinued. If the pH remains less than 7.2 and the $Pco_2$ remains elevated and/or the patient develops symptoms of acidosis, bicarbonate may be given. The amount of bicarbonate given should increase the pH to no more than 7.3 (see Metabolic

Acidosis). Arterial blood gases should be monitored to avoid precipitation of metabolic alkalosis.

Measures should be taken to treat the underlying cause of the acute exacerbation. Pulmonary infections should be treated with the appropriate antibiotics and with bronchodilators and steroids as necessary. Excess secretions should be cleared from the airway to allow proper gas exchange. This may involve increasing oral fluid intake to decrease secretion viscosity, deep breathing and postural drainage, suctioning, or bronchoscopy.

*Chronic Respiratory Acidosis* The need for treatment of the acidosis in these patients is dependent upon their ability to maintain an adequate $Po_2$. Oxygen therapy is not indicated for all patients with chronic respiratory acidosis; some patients with chronic obstructive pulmonary disease can remain ambulatory with a $Po_2$ of 40 mm Hg and a $Pco_2$ of 50 mm Hg or higher. Oxygen treatment is indicated when hypoxemia becomes symptomatic—the patient can no longer function without symptoms of dyspnea and shortness of breath or experiences central nervous system or cardiac symptoms. Oxygen should be administered cautiously as in the case of an acute exacerbation of chronic respiratory acidosis. Infections and bronchospasm should be treated and excessive secretions should be removed from the airway.

## Metabolic Acid–Base Disorders

The two metabolic acid–base disorders, acidosis and alkalosis, are generated by a primary change in bicarbonate concentration. Table 104.8 demonstrates the differences between these two disorders.

### *Metabolic Acidosis*

#### Pathophysiology

Metabolic acidosis is the acid–base disorder characterized by a decrease in pH, a low serum bicarbonate concentration, and a compensatory decrease in $Pco_2$. This can result from addition of organic acid to the extracellular fluid (e.g., lactic acid, ketoacids), loss of bicarbonate stores (e.g., in diarrhea), or progressive accumulation of endogenous acids secondary to impaired renal function (e.g., phosphates, sulfates).[3] Metabolic acidosis can be one of two types, depending on the value of the anion gap: (1) elevated anion gap and (2) normal anion gap (or hyperchloremic metabolic acidosis).

**Table 104.8** Metabolic Abnormalities

| *Disorder* | *Mechanism* | *Compensation* |
|---|---|---|
| Metabolic acidosis | 1. Nonvolatile acid is added<br>2. $HCO_3$ is lost | $Pco_2$ |
| Metabolic alkalosis | 1. Nonvolatile acid is lost<br>2. $HCO_3$ is gained | $Pco_2$ |

From Broughton JO: Understanding Blood Gases. Ohio Medical Products, with permission.

The anion gap is calculated using the formula

$$\text{anion gap} = Na^+ - (Cl^- + HCO_3^-)$$

In the serum, the total concentration of cations must equal the total concentration of anions. The cation concentration is equal to the sodium concentration plus the concentration of the unmeasured cations (UC)—magnesium, calcium, and potassium—which is 11 mEq/L. The anion concentration is equal to the concentration of chloride and bicarbonate and the unmeasured anions (UA)—proteins, sulfates, phosphate, and organic acid—which total 23 mEq/L. Therefore,

$$Na^+ + UC = (Cl^- + HCO_3^-) + UA$$
$$Na^+ - (Cl^- + HCO_3^-) = UA - UC$$

The normal value for the anion gap is approximately 12 mEq/L with a range of 8–16 mEq/L.[21] The potassium concentration may be included with the sodium concentration in the calculation of the anion gap, in which case the normal range is 12–16 mEq/L. As the potassium concentration varies over a narrow range, it rarely increases the accuracy of the equation and therefore may be excluded from the calculation. In most clinical situations, an increase in the anion gap can be equated with accumulation of unmeasured anions in extracellular fluid. The increase in unmeasured anions may result from accumulation of endogenous organic acids, such as lactic acid, acetoacetic acid, or β-hydroxybutyric acid, or from ingestion of such toxins as methanol or ethylene glycol. Addition of an organic acid to the extracellular fluid decreases the bicarbonate concentration and increases the anion gap.

The metabolic acidosis results from the decrease in bicarbonate concentration and not from the accumulation of organic acids. In chronic renal failure, the metabolic acidosis is caused by the inability of the kidney to secrete hydrogen ion. The increase in the anion gap is caused by the inability of the kidney to excrete unmeasured anions, such as sulfate and phosphate.

Metabolic acidosis with a normal anion gap occurs when bicarbonate losses from the extracellular fluid are replaced by chloride. This decrease in bicarbonate may result from losses from the gastrointestinal tract, dilution of bicarbonate in the extracellular fluid space by the addition of sodium chloride solution, or addition of chloride-containing acids to the extracellular fluid, which titrates the bicarbonate and replaces it with chloride. Specific causes of an increased anion gap and normal anion gap metabolic acidosis are listed in Table 104.9.

Gastrointestinal disorders such as diarrhea and pancreatic fistula can result in hyperchloremic metabolic acidosis. Diarrhea is by far the most common cause.[6] Severe diarrhea can lead to a daily loss of 5–10 L of fluid. Each liter of stool contains 100–140 mEq of sodium, 20–40 mEq of potassium, 80–100 mEq of chloride, and 30–50 mEq of bicarbonate.[2]

Those patients with disease of the lower urinary tract who require removal of the bladder and urinary diversion into the sigmoid colon may also develop a hyperchloremic metabolic acidosis. While urine is retained in the colon, water reabsorption, passive chloride reabsorption, and active bicarbonate secretion occur, resulting in a net loss of bicarbonate.[6]

Renal tubular acidosis (RTA) causes a metabolic acidosis

**Table 104.9** Causes of Metabolic Acidosis

| *Increased anion gap* | *Normal anion gap* |
|---|---|
| Ketoacidosis | Gastrointestinal disorders |
| Diabetic | Diarrhea |
| Alcoholic | Pancreatic fistula |
| Starvation | Ureterosigmoidostomy, ileostomy |
| Lactic acidosis | Acid ingestion |
| Chronic renal failure | Dilutional acidosis |
| Methanol ingestion | Carbonic anhydrase inhibitors |
| Ethylene glycol ingestion | Renal acidification defects |
| Paraldehyde ingestion | Renal tubular acidosis |
| Salicylate overdose | |

From Bleigh HL, Schwartz WB: Tris buffer (THAM): An appraisal of its physiologic effects and clinical usefulness. N Engl J Med 1966;274:782–787, with permission.

with a normal anion gap because the kidneys fail to excrete sufficient hydrogen ion to generate the new bicarbonate that must replace the bicarbonate lost in titrating the daily acid load.[3,6] There are two major types of RTA: type I, classic, distal or gradient limited; and type II, proximal or quantity limited.

In type I, a defect in the distal nephron prevents the kidney from acidifying the urine to a pH less than 5.4. A mild to moderate metabolic acidosis results from failure to excrete the endogenous acid load and from the bicarbonate leak. In the presence of metabolic acidosis, up to 3% to 5% of the filtered load of bicarbonate may be excreted in the urine when the plasma bicarbonate is normal. Hypokalemia may occur because of an increase in potassium excretion.

The defect in type II RTA is in the proximal tubule. Normally, 85% of the filtered load of bicarbonate is reabsorbed here, but in type II RTA, the bicarbonate is shunted to the distal nephron, which has a limited capacity for bicarbonate reabsorption. Up to 15% of the filtered bicarbonate load may be lost in the urine when plasma bicarbonate concentration is normal, resulting in a metabolic acidosis. The bicarbonaturia also leads to hypovolemia and hypokalemia secondary to sodium and potassium losses.

Both type I and type II RTA are treated with the administration of alkali; in type I RTA, 1–3 mEq/kg/d may be needed to correct the metabolic acidosis.[6] Potassium supplementation may also be necessary (e.g., potassium citrate, which would provide both potassium and alkali). In type II RTA, 10–25 mEq of alkali per kilogram per day may be needed to maintain the bicarbonate concentration in the normal range. Potassium supplementation is also necessary because of urinary potassium losses that increase with the increasing bicarbonaturia following alkali treatment.

#### Elevated Anion Gap Metabolic Acidosis

Metabolic acidosis with an increased anion gap occurs when bicarbonate losses are replaced by an anion other than chloride. This type of acidosis is commonly caused by increased endogenous acid production, as occurs in diabetic ketoacidosis or lactic acidosis.

Lactic acidosis is one of the most common causes of metabolic acidosis. Lactic acid is the end product of anaerobic metabolism of glucose (glycolysis). In normal individuals, lactic acid, derived from pyruvate, enters the circulation in small amounts that are promptly removed by the liver. In the liver, lactic acid is reoxidized to pyruvic acid, which is then metabolized to $CO_2$ and $H_2O$.[2] Plasma lactate concentration in normal, healthy subjects is approximately 1 mEq/L.[1]

Normally, the concentration of lactate in blood is 10 times the concentration of pyruvate (L/P ratio).[22] If pyruvate is elevated (e.g., by increased glucose intake), lactate increases, but the L/P ratio remains unchanged. If anaerobic glycolysis increases (e.g., because of tissue hypoxia) and sufficient NAD is not available to reconvert lactate to pyruvate, lactate will increase more than pyruvate and an increase in L/P ratio will result. This increase in L/P ratio is associated with metabolic acidosis. The basic cause of lactic acid overproduction seems to lie either in the failure of adequate oxygen delivery to cells or the inability of the cells to utilize oxygen.

The definitive diagnosis of lactic acidosis is made by measuring serum lactate concentrations. The serum lactate threshold necessary for a diagnosis of lactic acidosis has not been defined, although lactate concentrations of 4.0–5.0 mEq/L or greater and a simultaneous decrease in bicarbonate and arterial pH would indicate lactic acidosis.[23] Each 1 mEq/L increase in plasma lactate causes an equivalent decrease in serum bicarbonate, so that the severity of elevated lactate concentrations depends upon the patient's prevailing serum bicarbonate concentration.

The causes of lactic acidosis can be divided into two types: those associated with tissue hypoxia, type A; and those associated primarily with systemic disorders, type B (Table 104.10).

The most frequent form of lactic acidosis is type A. Cardiovascular collapse with resultant tissue underperfusion is the most common cause of type A lactic acidosis. Poor tissue perfusion and hypoxia influence enzymatic pyruvate and lactate metabolism to stimulate anaerobic glycolysis and decrease lactate utilization. This leads to hyperlactatemia and lactic acidosis. The rate of mortality from type A lactic acidosis may be as great as 80% and appears to be related to blood lactate concentrations. In a review of patients with

**Table 104.10** Causes of Lactic Acidosis

| |
|---|
| Type A (associated with tissue hypoxia) |
| Shock |
| Cardiogenic |
| Endotoxic |
| Hypovolemic |
| Severe anemia |
| Congestive heart failure |
| Asphyxia |
| Carbon monoxide poisoning |
| Type B (associated with systemic disorders) |
| Diabetes mellitus |
| Neoplastic disease |
| Liver failure |
| Sepsis |
| Convulsions |
| Abnormal gut flora |
| Type B1 |
| Biguanides (phenformin, buformin, metformin) |
| Fructose, sorbitol, xylitol |
| Ethanol |
| Methanol, ethylene glycol |
| Salicylates |
| Type B3 (associated with inborn errors of metabolism) |
| Glucose-6-phosphatase deficiency (type 1 glycogen storage disease) |
| Fructose-6-diphosphatase deficiency |
| Pyruvate dehydrogenase and carboxylase deficiency |
| Defective oxidative phosphorylation |

From Frommer JP: Lactic acidosis. Med Clin North Am 1983;67:815–829, with permission.

septic shock and type A lactic acidosis, a 73% mortality with lactate concentrations of 4.4–8.9 mEq/L and an 18% death rate with lactate concentrations between 1.3 and 4.4 mEq/L were reported.[22]

Type B lactic acidosis may result from a variety of causes, including drugs, toxins, and congenital enzyme deficiency. The exact role of diabetes mellitus in the induction of lactic acidosis is not clear. It may involve a decrease in pyruvate dehydrogenase activity, the enzyme responsible for pyruvate metabolism. Lactic acidosis in neoplastic disease is uncommon and reported mostly in patients with myeloproliferative disorders. Leukocytes and neoplastic cells in general have high rates of glycolysis. In the case of a large tumor or tightly packed bone marrow, oxygenation can be decreased, favoring the accumulation of lactate. Lactic acidosis has been reported in patients with massive liver replacement tumors, and it has been postulated that the liver uptake of lactate is decreased in these patients.[22] Type B lactic acidosis associated with seizures is usually transient and no treatment is necessary. Lactate overproduction occurs because of excessive muscle activity. Generally, no treatment is necessary.

### Signs/Symptoms

Adverse effects of metabolic acidosis can occur in the cardiovascular, gastrointestinal, and central nervous systems. Often, hyperventilation is the first sign of metabolic acidosis. At a pH of 7.2, pulmonary ventilation increases about four times; at a pH of 7.0, about eight times.[2] In extremely severe acidosis (pH $< 6.8$), the function of the central nervous system is disrupted to such a degree that the respiratory center is depressed. Respiratory compensation may occur as Kussmaul's respirations—deep, rapid respirations—seen commonly in diabetic ketoacidosis.

Central nervous system signs, including stupor and coma, may appear. Central nervous system (CNS) depression has been found to relate more closely with spinal fluid pH than with blood pH. For this reason, neurologic symptoms are found to occur more frequently and to a greater degree in patients with respiratory acidosis, as the $CO_2$ accumulated in the respiratory form readily crosses the blood–brain barrier to cause acidosis in the CNS and blood.[2] Because of the slow penetration of administered bicarbonate into the CNS, the CNS pH fails to normalize as rapidly as blood pH. Therefore, patients continue to hyperventilate because of sustained CNS acidity, and severe respiratory alkalosis may occur. Sustained lowering of $P_{CO_2}$ within 12 to 36 hours is to be anticipated during the correction of any metabolic acidosis period.[2]

Systemic acidosis causes peripheral vasodilation, characterized by flushing, a rapid heart rate, and a wide pulse pressure. Initially, cardiac output may be increased, but as acidosis becomes more severe, it falls as the hypotension becomes more pronounced. In experimental animals, cardiac contractility decreased as pH was decreased to less than 7.0 by infusion of lactic acid.[24] Cardiac function may be depressed because of the decrease in myocardial responsiveness that occurs in acidosis. Increases in heart rate and contractile force in response to catecholamines appear to be markedly less at pH 7.1 than at pH 7.4.[25] In contrast, the effects of vagostimulation are enhanced at pH below 7.1, probably as a consequence of inhibition of acetylcholinesterase. This increases the danger of vagally mediated bradycardia or arrest during acidosis.

Gastrointestinal symptoms of metabolic acidosis include loss of appetite, nausea, and vomiting. These symptoms occur commonly in patients with renal insufficiency who experience a mild acidosis.[1] Severe acidosis (pH $< 7.1$) interferes with carbohydrate metabolism and insulin utilization with a resultant hyperglycemia.

The effects of metabolic acidosis on serum potassium depends upon the type of acidosis: the effects of mineral acids (e.g., hydrochloric acid) differ from those of organic acids (e.g., lactic acid). In dogs, during a steady-state metabolic acidosis produced by the infusion of hydrochloric acid, the change in plasma potassium concentration per 0.1-unit change in pH was a rather consistent increase, averaging 0.6 mEq/L. In contrast, the experimental infusion of organic acid (acetic, lactic, or $\beta$-hydroxybutyric acid) into animals produces much smaller increments in the plasma potassium concentrations.[15]

### Compensation

The body attempts to compensate for metabolic acidosis by hyperventilating. This causes an increase in carbon dioxide excretion and a decrease in $P_{CO_2}$. This ventilatory compensation is initiated by the stimulation of the respiratory center by the changes in cerebral bicarbonate concentration and pH.[2] Arterial blood compensation begins rapidly, but does not reach a steady state for 12 to 24 hours after the onset of metabolic acidosis. For every 1 mEq/L decrease in bicarbonate concentration below the average normal of 24 mEq/L, the $P_{CO_2}$ decreases by 1.0–1.5 mm Hg from the normal value of 40 mm Hg.

### Treatment

***Sodium Bicarbonate*** In an acute situation (e.g., treatment of metabolic acidosis in cardiac arrest), sodium bicarbonate administration may be necessary (Fig. 104.6). The standards and guidelines from the National Conference on Cardiopulmonary and Emergency Cardiac Care state that sodium bicarbonate is useful in cardiac life support when combined with ventilation in an attempt to maintain near-normal arterial pH during an arrest.[26] It has become apparent that less sodium bicarbonate is needed to provide adequate acid–base control during an arrest than had previously been assumed.

By ensuring adequate ventilation, a major component of depressed pH (respiratory acidosis) can be managed without sodium bicarbonate. It must be kept in mind that administration of sodium bicarbonate is followed by release of carbon dioxide, which requires adequate alveolar activity to ensure continued excretion of this source of potential acid. Thus, the importance of adequate ventilation in the control of pH must be emphasized, as well as the need for repeated arterial measurements of blood pH and $P_{CO_2}$. Excessive sodium bicarbonate administration during resuscitation may result in (1) metabolic alkalosis and subsequent impairment of oxygen release from hemoglobin to tissues and (2) sodium and water overload with subsequent hypernatremia and hyperosmolality.[27]

During a cardiac arrest, sodium bicarbonate may be administered by rapid, direct intravenous injection when initial immediate injection of the drug is considered necessary (e.g., unwitnessed arrest). A sodium bicarbonate dose of 1 mEq/kg is administered initially with subsequent doses of 0.5 mEq/kg given at 10-minute intervals. Ideally, subsequent doses of sodium bicarbonate should be based on measurements of arterial blood pH and $P_{CO_2}$.

**Figure 104.6** Treatment of metabolic acidosis. *See Chapter 54.

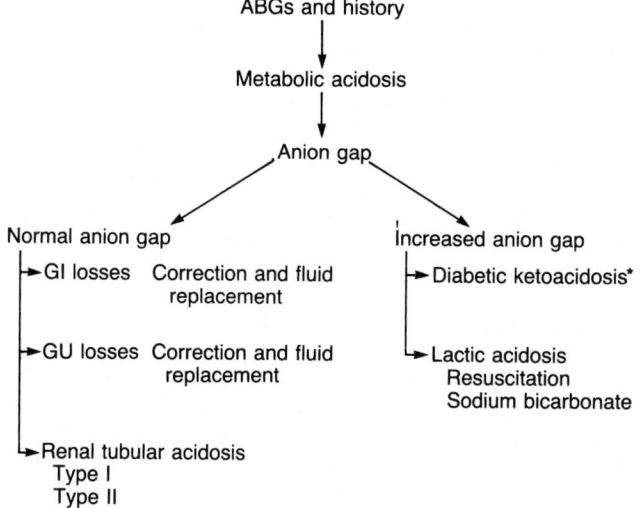

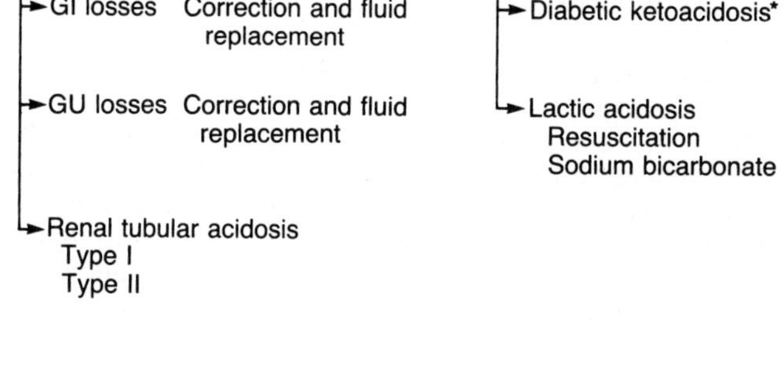


It has been recommended that sodium bicarbonate be administered to raise the arterial pH to about 7.15–7.20; however, there are no controlled clinical trials demonstrating that sodium bicarbonate administration is significantly better than general supportive care in reducing morbidity and mortality in these patients. Bicarbonate administration may actually have detrimental effects.

In theory, sodium bicarbonate administration provides the fluid and electrolyte replacement and increases arterial pH, thereby improving cardiac function, perfusion and oxygenation of peripheral tissues, intracellular pH, and therefore lactate metabolism[27]; however, sodium bicarbonate administration can actually have an adverse effect on intracellular pH. When bicarbonate is given by intravenous infusion, the carbon dioxide generated diffuses more readily than bicarbonate across cell membranes and into cerebrospinal fluid. Therefore, the intracellular pH can actually be decreased by administration of bicarbonate.

In the case of an endogenous source of bicarbonate, a bicarbonate "overshoot" may develop. This may occur in the ketoacidosis of lactic acidosis. The ketoacids (acetoacetic acid and $\beta$-hydroxybutyric) or lactic acid can be biologically converted in the liver to bicarbonate once the underlying cause of acidosis is corrected. Serum bicarbonate is then increased as regenerated bicarbonate adds to exogenous bicarbonate and an alkalosis may result. Bicarbonate should be administered cautiously in these patients, with frequent monitoring of blood gases and serum electrolytes.

Other alkalinizing agents include lactate, acetate, and citrate ions. These agents are converted in the liver to bicarbonate and may have an advantage over bicarbonate because of their compatibility and stability in the solutions. In patients already receiving total parenteral nutrition (TPN), sodium or potassium acetate may be substituted for the usual chloride salts in the TPN to provide a source of bicarbonate. Ringer's lactate solution has been found to be useful in the resuscitation period of patients in shock. In theory, it would appear that Ringer's lactate solution would be contraindicated for two reasons: (1) the level of excess lactate may increase and compound the lactic acidosis already present; (2) blood pH may be decreased because the pH of Ringer's lactate is 6–6.5. Canizaro et al[28] studied 69 patients with hemorrhagic, septic, cardiogenic, or neurogenic shock and 15 injured patients not in shock, all of whom received Ringer's lactate solution during resuscitation. Initial lactate concentrations correlated well with the clinical impression of the depth of shock. These concentrations rapidly returned to normal after successful resuscitation. This was attributed to reestablishment of tissue perfusion resulting in cessation of excess production of lactate. The remaining lactate would then be rapidly metabolized by the liver after restoration of adequate hepatic blood flow.

***Tromethamine*** Tromethamine (THAM, Tris) has also been used to correct metabolic acidosis. It is a highly alkaline, sodium-free organic amine that acts as a proton acceptor to prevent or correct acidosis. Tromethamine combines with hydrogen ions from carbonic acid to form bicarbonate and a cationic buffer. THAM also acts as an osmotic diuretic to increase urine flow, increase urine pH, and increase excretion of fixed acids, $CO_2$, and electrolytes. At pH 7.4, 30% of THAM is not ionized and therefore is capable of reaching equilibrium with total body water.[29] This portion may penetrate into cells and may neutralize acidic anions of the intracellular fluid. Intracellular pH increases within 1 hour of the infusion of THAM. There is no clinical or physiologic evidence that this action is beneficial and there are theoretical reasons for believing that it may be undesirable.

When THAM is used, it must be administered slowly and with careful monitoring to avoid alkalosis. Large doses may cause respiratory depression because of a decrease in ventilation secondary to an increase in blood pH and decrease in $P_{CO_2}$ concentration. Tromethamine solution is highly alkaline and may cause severe inflammation, vascular spasm, or tissue damage (necrosis, sloughing, pain, chemical phlebitis, thrombosis) if infiltration occurs.

In theory, THAM would be useful in fluid-overloaded patients because it contains no sodium. In practice, it has no proven advantage over sodium bicarbonate because it delivers the same osmotic load and is more expensive.[5]

Vasodilators have been used in the treatment of metabolic acidosis. Theoretically, these drugs would be of value in decreasing peripheral vascular resistance and improving tissue perfusion. Methylene blue has also been used experimentally in animals and humans to treat lactic acidosis.[30] In theory, methylene blue should act as an oxidizing agent to oxidize nicotinamide adenine dinucleotide (NADH), which should then oxidize lactate to pyruvate. In animals, methylene blue was found to have an unpredictable effect on serum lactate concentrations. In humans, methylene blue has not been shown to influence mortality from lactic acidosis.[31]

## *Metabolic Alkalosis*

### Pathophysiology

The second type of simple nonrespiratory, or metabolic, acid–base disorder is metabolic alkalosis. This disorder is characterized by a primary increase in bicarbonate concentration leading to an elevation in plasma pH and a compensatory hypoventilation that increases $P_{CO_2}$. Metabolic alkalosis is a common acid–base disturbance among hospitalized patients. Wilson et al[30] reported that among 1,415 critically ill patients, 33% of the patients with acid–base disturbances experienced metabolic alkalosis. Forty-one percent of the patients who had pH values between 7.54 and 7.56 died and more than 80% of those with pH values greater than 7.56 died. The mortality was highest among those patients experiencing severe sepsis with metabolic alkalosis and respiratory alkalosis. Although they reported a significant correlation between degree of alkalosis and incidence of mortality, this does not suggest that reversal of the alkalosis would have altered the mortality rate.

A primary elevation of bicarbonate concentration can be generated by three mechanisms: (1) a net loss of hydrogen ion from the extracellular fluid space; (2) a net addition of bicarbonate or its precursors (i.e., carbonate, citrate, acetate) to the extracellular fluid space; or (3) loss of chloride-rich, bicarbonate-poor fluid. Disturbances that initiate metabolic alkalosis can be divided into two categories by their response to treatment with saline volume expansion. Those categories are sodium chloride–responsive disorders and sodium chloride–resistant disorders. Causes of metabolic alkalosis are listed in Table 104.11.

**Table 104.11** Causes of Metabolic Alkalosis

| |
|---|
| Sodium chloride responsive (urinary chloride concentration <10 mmol/L) |
| Gastrointestinal disorders |
| Vomiting |
| Gastric drainage |
| Villous adenoma of the colon |
| Chloride diarrhea |
| Diuretic therapy |
| Correction of chronic hypercapnia |
| Cystic fibrosis |
| Sodium chloride resistant (urinary chloride concentration >20 mmol/L) |
| Excess mineralocorticoid activity |
| Hyperaldosteronism |
| Cushing's syndrome |
| Bartter's syndrome |
| Excessive licorice intake |
| Profound potassium depletion |
| Unclassified |
| Alkali administration |
| Milk-alkali syndrome |
| Massive blood or plasmanate transfusion |
| Nonparathyroid hypercalcemia |
| Glucose ingestion after starvation |
| Large doses of carbenicillin or penicillin |

From Navins RG, Emmett M: Medicine 1980;59:161–187, with permission.

The most common initiating event for metabolic alkalosis is the loss of chloride-rich, bicarbonate-poor fluid from the body as seen with diuretic use, nasogastric suctioning, or vomiting.[5] Gastric secretory volume is usually less than 50 mL/h in the basal state but may increase fivefold with stimulation.[2] One, two, or more liters of gastric fluid may be lost daily with persistent vomiting. The 24-hour gastric juice output of a 70-kg adult includes 1–2 L of fluid, 40–160 mEq of sodium, 10 mEq of potassium, 200 mEq of chloride, and 25–100 mEq of hydrogen ion. Hydrogen ion and bicarbonate are formed from $CO_2$ and water by gastric parietal cells:

$$H_2O + CO_2 \rightarrow H_2CO_3 \rightarrow H + HCO_3$$

The hydrogen ion is secreted into gastric fluid and the bicarbonate is retained in the extracellular fluid. Normally, an amount of bicarbonate equal to the bicarbonate generated in the stomach is eliminated in the alkaline pancreatic and small-bowel secretions, maintaining hydrogen ion balance. With vomiting and nasogastric suctioning, hydrogen ion is lost externally. Bicarbonate is not eliminated and metabolic alkalosis is generated.

Diuretic therapy with agents acting on the cortical and medullary ascending limb of the loop of Henle (e.g., furosemide, ethacrynic acid, and thiazides) is a common cause of metabolic alkalosis. These agents promote the excretion of sodium and potassium almost exclusively in association with chloride without a proportionate increase in bicarbonate excretion.[32] Net acid excretion is also frequently increased during the diuresis because of both the disproportionate loss of chloride and the loss of hydrogen ion in the urine by increasing tubular flow and sodium delivery to the distal tubule for sodium–hydrogen exchange. Patients at risk from metabolic alkalosis are those with a combined risk depletion, in which the distal tubule exchange sites are stimulated to reabsorb sodium; those on a low-salt diet that limits the sodium chloride available for reabsorption; and those on diuretics, which continue to deliver sodium to the distal exchange site.[5] Alkalosis caused by diuretic use is usually mild, but the accompanying hypokalemia may be serious.

Other causes of metabolic alkalosis are those that are resistant to sodium chloride administration. Many of these are associated with excess mineralocorticoid activity. Increased mineralocorticoid activity may result from (1) primary adrenal overproduction, as in primary hyperaldosteronism, or oversupply of endogenous mineralocorticoids, as in licorice ingestion; and (2) oversecretion of mineralocorticoid secondary to increased renin activity. In the sodium chloride–resistant group, renin secretion is driven by stimuli other than extracellular fluid depletion. Stimuli include renal artery stenosis, magnesium deficiency, or Bartter's syndrome, a renal tubular reabsorptive defect. Mineralocorticoids act on the distal segment of the renal tubule where they increase sodium reabsorption and enhance secretion of potassium and hydrogen ion into the tubular lumen. For example, in hyperaldosteronism, an increase in aldosterone leads to stimulation of distal renal tubular exchange of sodium for hydrogen. The increased hydrogen ion secreted into the renal tubule causes the generation of new bicarbonate or the reclamation of filtered bicarbonate.

Miscellaneous causes of metabolic alkalosis include large doses of penicillins (e.g., carbenicillin).[33] Carbenicillin is thought to act as a nonreabsorbable anion. High concentrations of the poorly reabsorbable anion act on the distal renal tubule to increase the flow rate and electrical negativity within the tubular lumen. Changes in flow and electrochemical gradient across the tubular cells enhance the secretion of potassium and hydrogen ion, producing increased plasma bicarbonate concentration and hypokalemia.

No matter which condition initiated the metabolic alkalosis, the kidney is responsible for its maintenance. Normally, the kidneys are capable of excreting all bicarbonate presented to them, even during periods of increased bicarbonate loads.[5] The kidney senses changes in the blood bicarbonate concentration and excess bicarbonate is excreted in the urine to return the blood bicarbonate concentration back to normal. If the kidneys are working properly, excess bicarbonate is excreted and metabolic alkalosis does not occur.

There are several mechanisms by which elimination of excess bicarbonate by the kidney is prevented, thereby maintaining a metabolic alkalosis. The combination of decreased extracellular fluid volume, hypochloremia, and hypokalemia associated with diuretic use or nasogastric suction can maintain a metabolic alkalosis.[5] During periods of decreased extracellular fluid volume, sodium reabsorption is enhanced in the proximal and distal tubules. This reabsorption from the renal tubule must be associated with an ion with a negative charge, such as chloride, or it must be exchanged for an ion in the tubular cell that has a positive charge, such as potassium or hydrogen. Normally, 80% of sodium is reabsorbed while accompanied by chloride and 20% is exchanged for hydrogen or potassium.[7] In hypochloremia, there is less chloride available for reabsorption with sodium and more sodium must be exchanged for potassium or hydrogen. Only a small amount of potassium is available for exchange with sodium and when the patient becomes hypokalemic, hydrogen is exchanged instead. This loss of hydrogen ions results in hypochloremic metabolic alkalosis.

Metabolic alkalosis may also be maintained by persistent hypokalemia, independent of hypovolemia.[5] Such hypokalemic metabolic alkalosis is frequently associated with excess mineralocorticoid activity. As stated before, mineralocorticoids promote sodium reabsorption and enhance potassium and hydrogen ion excretion in the urine.

### Signs/Symptoms

Patients with metabolic alkalosis may complain of symptoms related to the underlying cause of the disorder (e.g., muscle weakness with hypokalemia or postural dizziness with volume depletion). They may have a history of vomiting, gastric drainage, or diuretic use leading to the metabolic alkalosis. Neuromuscular irritability may be present with signs of tetany of hyperactive reflexes possibly caused by the decreased ionized calcium concentration that occurs secondary to an increase in pH. This decrease in ionized calcium may be caused by a conformational change in the albumin molecules, to which the calcium is bound, resulting in increased binding, or by decreased competition from hydrogen ions for binding sites on the albumin molecule. Mental confusion, muscle cramping, and paresthesias may occur. Severe alkalemia (blood pH $> 7.55$) has been associated with cardiac arrhythmias in patients with normal hearts, but particularly in those with heart disease (see Respiratory Alkalosis).[12]

### Compensation

Once the plasma bicarbonate has been elevated by one of the three basic mechanisms that generate metabolic alkalosis, the body attempts to restore the pH to normal.

The immediate response to elevated bicarbonate is chemical buffering. This buffering involves the movement of hydrogen ions from within the cells to the extracellular fluid in exchange for potassium and sodium. This system is immediate in onset but limited in its capacity to protect the body from sudden life-threatening changes in extracellular pH.

The second phase of the body's attempt to return the pH toward normal is respiratory compensation. The body compensates for a nonrespiratory, or metabolic, alkalosis with the respiratory system by hypoventilating to raise the $P_{CO_2}$.[7] Using the Henderson–Hasselbach equation, one can see that an increase in the $P_{CO_2}$ will return the $P_{CO_2}$/bicarbonate ratio, and therefore the pH, toward normal. Respiratory compensation is initiated when central and peripheral chemoreceptors sense an increase in pH and occurs over one to several hours.[7] Hypoventilation allows the $P_{CO_2}$ to rise only to a maximum of 50–60 mm Hg before hypoxia sensors react to prevent further hypoventilation. The $P_{CO_2}$ increases 6–7 mm Hg for each 10 mEq/L increase in bicarbonate, up to a $P_{CO_2}$ of about 50–60 mm Hg[5]; however, the respiratory response to metabolic alkalosis is variable. If the $P_{CO_2}$ is normal, less than normal, or slightly increased, one should investigate for a condition that may be a respiratory stimulant, for example, fever gram-negative sepsis or a restrictive lung disease.

### Treatment

Once the underlying cause of the metabolic alkalosis has been identified, treatment is aimed at correcting that cause. Although the original cause of the elevated plasma bicarbonate may have disappeared, metabolic alkalosis may persist until the renal mechanism responsible for maintaining the disorder is eliminated.[10] For example, hypovolemia must be treated with sodium chloride in certain cases (i.e., diuretic abuse, nasogastric suction) to allow excretion of bicarbonate by the kidney. Therapy for metabolic alkalosis is divided into two treatment categories: sodium chloride–responsive disorders and sodium chloride–resistant disorders (Fig. 104.7).

Sodium chloride–responsive disorders are those resulting from volume depletion and chloride loss as in severe vomiting or nasogastric suction. Initially, therapy is directed at expanding intravascular volume and replenishing chloride stores. Sodium chloride and potassium solutions are administered to patients who can tolerate the administration of fluid and sodium.[5]

Patients with a metabolic alkalosis who are volume expanded or intolerant to sodium volume loads, as in congestive heart failure, may benefit from the carbonic anhydrase inhibitor acetazolamide. This agent inhibits the action of carbonic anhydrase in the kidney tubule cell and promotes renal bicarbonate and potassium excretion, resulting in a decreased concentration of bicarbonate in the extracellular fluid. Administration of one or two doses of acetazolamide, 250 or 500 mg, may promote a sufficient bicarbonate diuresis to return the pH toward normal. Fraley et al[34] reported resolution of a severe metabolic alkalosis in a 63-year-old man using a combination of intravenous acetazolamide and saline with mechanical ventilation to induce hypercarbia. The patient's pH fell from 7.63 to 7.39 within 1 hour of a 500-mg dose of acetazolamide and remained stable after a repeat dose 12 hours later.

Other agents used to treat sodium chloride–responsive metabolic alkalosis include hydrochloric acid, ammonium chloride, and arginine monohydrochloride. Indications for the use of hydrochloric acid include severe metabolic alkalosis (pH > 7.55) or symptoms of alkalotic toxicity unresponsive to fluid and electrolyte administration and inability to tolerate a large sodium and fluid load (i.e., decompensated CHF or renal failure with oliguria).[35] The dosing of hydrochloric acid may be used on an estimate of the chloride deficit:

$$\text{dose of HCl (mEq)} = [0.2\ \text{L/kg} \times \text{body weight (kg)}] \times [130 - \text{observed serum chloride}].$$

The estimated chloride space is 0.2 times the body weight. The average serum chloride is 103 mEq/L. The duration of infusion of hydrochloric acid has ranged from 4 to 24 hours, although the total dose is usually administered over 12 to 24 hours.[35] Improvement is usually seen within 24 hours of initiating therapy. Arterial blood gases and serum electrolytes should be drawn every 4 to 12 hours to evaluate and adjust therapy. If the $P_{CO_2}$ is markedly elevated because of respiratory compensation, the estimated dose of hydrochloric acid should be infused over at least 24 hours. Otherwise, a severe transient respiratory acidosis may occur because of the slower reduction of the elevated bicarbonate concentration in the cerebrospinal fluid than in the extracellular fluid.[36]

Solutions of hydrochloric acid are generally prepared at 0.1 or 0.2 N with the higher concentration (0.2 N) reserved for patients who cannot tolerate additional volume. The solution should be prepared with aseptic technique.[37–39]

The hydrochloric acid solution should be administered via a large central vein.[33] Mirtallo et al[40] demonstrated that hydrochloric acid may also be added to parenteral nutrient solutions and administered via a central line without serious degradation of proteins.

Ammonium chloride is available as a 2.14% solution containing 400 mEq of ammonium ion and 400 mEq of chloride per liter.[35] Metabolic alkalosis is corrected indirectly by ammonium chloride, which is converted by the liver to urea and free hydrochloric acid:

$$2NH_4Cl \rightarrow CON_2H_4 + H_2O + 2HCl$$

Improvement in metabolic status is usually seen within 24 hours of ammonium chloride administration. It may be administered by peripheral vein and the rate of infusion should not exceed 20 g per 24 hours (approximately 1 L/24 h of 2.14% solution). Central nervous system toxicity, marked by confusion, irritability, seizures, and coma, is associated with faster rates of administration. It must be administered cautiously to patients with renal or hepatic impairment.[5] Ammonia may accumulate and lead to encephalopathy in patients with hepatic dysfunction because of impaired conversion of ammonia to urea. In renal impairment, urea may accumulate.

Arginine monohydrochloride is available as a 300-mL 10% solution containing 142.5 mg of both hydrogen and chloride ions.[35] The FDA has approved this product only for evalu-

**Figure 104.7** Treatment of metabolic alkalosis.

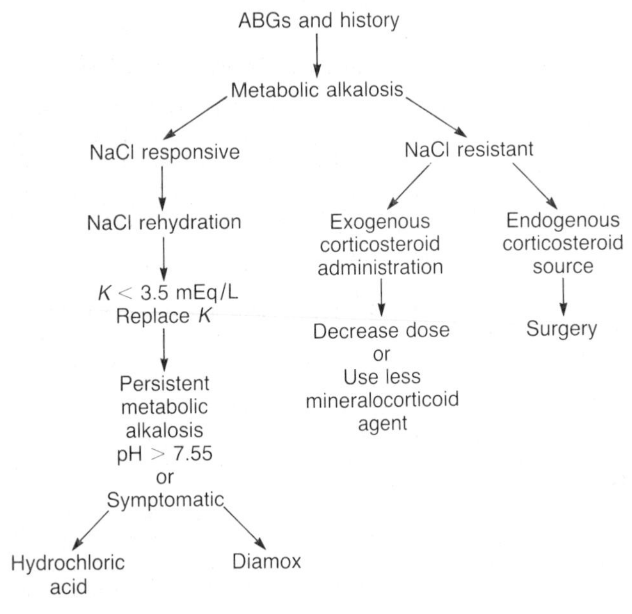

ation of pituitary function; thus, use of this product to treat metabolic alkalosis must be considered investigational. A dose of 10 g/h given intravenously has been used to treat metabolic alkalosis. Like ammonium chloride, arginine must undergo metabolism by the liver to produce hydrogen ions. Unlike ammonium chloride, arginine combines with ammonia in the body to synthesize urea; thus, it may be used in patients with relative hepatic insufficiency. In renal failure patients, arginine monohydrochloride may elevate blood urea nitrogen and has been associated with severe hyperkalemia.[35] The increase in potassium is caused by arginine-induced shifts of potassium from the intracellular to the extracellular state. Rapid infusion may result in nausea and vomiting.

In patients with metabolic alkalosis caused by nasogastric suction, histamine $H_2$-receptor antagonists have been used to decrease the volume of and hydrogen ion content in gastric fluids. Rowlands et al[38] administered intravenous cimetidine 200 mg to suppress gastric secretion in two patients with Zollinger–Ellison syndrome. This produced a marked reduction in volume of gastric aspirate and acid production in both patients within 4 hours.

Sodium chloride–resistant disorders are those commonly associated with hypermineralocorticoidism. Unlike sodium chloride–responsive disorders, these are associated with plasma volume expansion, hypertension, and a high urinary chloride concentration.[10] Treatment of these disorders involves the removal of the source of excess mineralocorticoid activity. Patients who are taking corticosteroids may have to have their dose decreased or may need to be switched to a corticosteroid with less mineralocorticoid activity. Patients with an endogenous source of excess mineralocorticoid activity may require surgery. Restriction of dietary sodium also helps prevent metabolic alkalosis.

## Mixed Acid–Base Disorders

Two simple acid–base disturbances occurring simultaneously are called a mixed acid–base disorder. A mixed disturbance can be suspected from the clinical setting and medical history and can be diagnosed with this information together with arterial blood gases and electrolytes.

### *Diagnosis*

The diagnosis of a mixed disorder depends upon an understanding of the appropriate quantitative response of the defense mechanisms in the primary, uncomplicated acid–base disorders. To diagnose mixed disorders, one must know how each of the four simple disorders alters pH, $Pco_2$, and $HCO_3$. If a given set of blood gases does not fall within the range of expected responses for a simple acid–base disorder, a mixed disorder should be suspected. In addition to laboratory information, a clinical evaluation of the patient is important. A thorough history and physical examination often lead to the diagnosis, even before the laboratory data are available. Examples of common mixed disorders follow.

**Table 104.12** Mixed Respiratory and Metabolic Acidosis

| | *Normal* | *Uncompensated metabolic acidosis* | *Mixed* | |
|---|---|---|---|---|
| | | | **Severe** | **Mild** |
| $HCO_3$ | 25 | 15 | 17 | 16 |
| $Pco_2$ | 40 | 30 | 50 | 37 |
| pH | 7.40 | 7.32 | 7.15 | 7.26 |
| Anion gap | 10 | 20 | 20 | 21 |

From Navins RG, Emmett M: Medicine 1980;59:161–187, with permission.

### *Respiratory Acidosis and Metabolic Acidosis*

A compensatory increase in $HCO_3$ concentration occurs in response to a primary respiratory acidosis. When acute or chronic respiratory acidosis is associated with an inappropriate response in $HCO_3$ concentration, a mixed respiratory and metabolic acidosis may be diagnosed. Likewise, when a patient with metabolic acidosis has an inappropriately high $Pco_2$, a complicating respiratory acidosis may be diagnosed.

In mixed respiratory and metabolic acidosis there is a failure of compensation. The respiratory disorder prevents the compensatory decrease in $Pco_2$ expected in the defense against metabolic acidosis. The metabolic disorder prevents the buffering and renal mechanisms from raising the bicarbonate concentration as expected in the defense against respiratory acidosis. In the absence of compensatory mechanisms, the pH decreases markedly (Table 104.12).

A mixed respiratory and metabolic acidosis may develop in patients in cardiorespiratory arrest, in chronic lung disease patients who are in shock, and in metabolic acidosis patients who develop respiratory failure. This mixed disorder should be treated by responding to both the respiratory and the metabolic acidosis. Improved oxygen delivery must be initiated to improve hypercarbia and hypoxia. Mechanical ventilation may be needed to reduce $Pco_2$. During the initial stage of therapy appropriate amounts of $NaHCO_3$ should be given to reverse the metabolic acidosis (see Treatment under Metabolic Acidosis).

### *Respiratory Alkalosis and Metabolic Alkalosis*

In mixed respiratory and metabolic alkalosis, there is also a failure of compensation. The compensatory decrease in bicarbonate concentration that occurs in respiratory alkalosis is prevented by the complicating metabolic alkalosis. Likewise, the increase in $Pco_2$ expected to compensate for

**Table 104.13** Mixed respiratory and metabolic alkalosis

| | *Normal* | *Uncompensated* | | *Mixed* | |
|---|---|---|---|---|---|
| | | **Metabolic alkalosis** | **Respiratory alkalosis** | **Severe** | **Mild** |
| $HCO_3$ | 24 | 35 | 17 | 32 | 32 |
| $Pco_2$ | 40 | 47 | 25 | 39 | 30 |
| pH | 7.40 | 7.49 | 7.45 | 7.53 | 7.63 |

From Navins RG, Emmett M: Medicine 1980;59:161–187, with permission.

**Table 104.14** Mixed Respiratory Alkalosis and Metabolic Acidosis

| | Normal | Uncomplicated metabolic acidosis | Mixed: Severe | Mixed: Mild |
|---|---|---|---|---|
| $HCO_3$ | 24 | 15 | 13 | 14 |
| $Pco_2$ | 40 | 30 | 15 | 24 |
| pH | 7.40 | 7.32 | 7.56 | 7.39 |

From Navins RG, Emmett M: Medicine 1980;59:161–187, with permission.

**Table 104.15** Mixed Metabolic Alkalosis and Respiratory Acidosis

| | Normal | Uncomplicated respiratory acidosis | Mixed disorder |
|---|---|---|---|
| $HCO_3$ | 24 | 36 | 40 |
| $Pco_2$ | 40 | 70 | 67 |
| pH | 7.40 | 7.49 | 7.40 |

From Navins RG, Emmett M: Medicine 1980;59:161–187, with permission.

metabolic alkalosis is prevented by primary respiratory alkalosis. Sample laboratory values found in mixed respiratory and metabolic alkalosis are listed in Table 104.13. The failure of compensation that occurs on the mixed respiratory and metabolic alkalosis may result in a severe alkalosis.

The combination of respiratory and metabolic alkalosis is the most common mixed acid–base disorder. This mixed disorder occurs frequently in critically ill surgical patients with respiratory alkalosis caused by mechanical ventilation, hypoxia, sepsis, hypotension, neurologic damage, pain, or drugs, and with metabolic alkalosis caused by vomiting or nasogastric suction and massive blood transfusions. It may also occur in patients with hepatic cirrhosis, hyperventilation, diuretic use, or vomiting, and in patients with chronic respiratory acidosis and an elevated plasma bicarbonate concentration who are placed on mechanical ventilation and undergo a rapid fall in $Pco_2$ to hypocapnic levels.

Correction of the metabolic component by administration of sodium chloride and potassium chloride solutions should be undertaken, and readjustment of the ventilator or treatment of an underlying disorder causing hyperventilation may correct or ameliorate the respiratory disorder.

### *Metabolic Acidosis and Respiratory Alkalosis*

The combination of respiratory alkalosis and metabolic acidosis is a disorder of excessive compensation. The respiratory alkalosis decreases the $Pco_2$ beyond the appropriate range of the respiratory compensation for metabolic acidosis. The plasma bicarbonate concentration also falls below the level expected in simple respiratory alkalosis. In a sense, the defense of pH for either disorder alone is enhanced; thus, the pH may be normal or close to normal, with a low $Pco_2$ and a low $HCO_3$ (Table 104.14).

This mixed disorder may be seen in patients with advanced liver disease, salicylate intoxication, and pulmonary–renal syndromes. Treatment of this disorder should be directed at the underlying cause. Because of the enhanced compensation, the pH is usually closer to normal than in either of the two simple disorders.

### *Metabolic Alkalosis and Respiratory Acidosis*

When acute and chronic respiratory acidosis is associated with an inappropriately elevated $HCO_3$ concentration, mixed respiratory acidosis and metabolic alkalosis may be diagnosed. Conversely, when a patient with a known metabolic alkalosis has inappropriately elevated $Pco_2$, a complicating respiratory acidosis may be diagnosed (Table 104.15).

This mixed disorder may occur in patients with chronic obstructive pulmonary disease and respiratory acidosis who are treated with salt restrictions, diuretics, and possibly glucocorticoids. Renal bicarbonate production and reabsorption are increased in this situation, providing mechanisms for both generating and maintaining metabolic alkalosis. The elevated pH diminishes respiratory drive and may therefore worsen the pulmonary disease.

Although the pH may not deviate significantly from normal, treatment may need to be initiated to maintain $Pco_2$ at an acceptable level. Treatment should be aimed at decreasing plasma bicarbonate (see Treatment under Metabolic Alkalosis).

## References


1. Narins RG, Emmett M. Simple and mixed acid–base disorders; A practical approach. Medicine 1980;59:161–187.
2. Maxwell MH, Kleeman R (eds). Clinical Disorders of Fluid and Electrolyte Metabolism, 3rd ed. New York, McGraw–Hill.
3. Laske ME. Normal regulation of acid–base balance. Med Clin North Am 1983;67:771–780.
4. Goofhart RS, Shils ME (eds). Modern Nutrition in Health and Disease, 6th ed. Philadelphia, Lea and Febiger.
5. Hyneck ML. Simple acid–base disorders. Am J Hosp Pharm 1985;42:1992–2003.
6. Schrier RW (ed). Renal and Electrolyte Disorders, 2nd ed. Boston, Little Brown.
7. Broughton JO. Understanding Blood Gases, Ohio Medical Products.
8. Arbus GS. An in-vivo acid–base nomogram for clinical use. Can Med Assoc J 1973;109:291–293.
9. Mazzara JR, Ayers SM, Grace WJ. Extreme hypocapnia in the critically ill patient. Am J Med 1974;56:450–456.
10. Cogan MG, Liu FY, Berger BE, et al. Metabolic alkalosis. Med Clin North Am 1983;67:903–913.
11. Kaehny WD. Respiratory acid–base disorders. Med Clin North Am 1983;67:915–929.
12. Lawson NW, Butler GH, Ray CT. Alkalosis and cardiac arrhythmias. Anesth Analg 1973;52:951–964.

13. McElroy WT, Gerdes AS, Brown EB. Effects of $CO_2$, bicarbonate, and pH on the performance of isolated perfused guinea pig hearts. Am J Physiol 1958;195:412–416.
14. Burnum JF, Hickman JB, McIntosh HD. Effect of hypocapnia on arterial blood pressure. Circulation 1954;9–89.
15. Stearns RH, Cox M, Feig PU, et al. Internal potassium balance and the control of the plasma potassium concentration. Medicine 1981;60:339–354.
16. Weiner MW, Epstein FH. Signs and symptoms of electrolyte disorders, in Maxwell MH, Kleeman CR, (eds): Clinical Disorders of Fluid and Electrolyte Metabolism. New York, McGraw–Hill,
17. Wilson RF, Gibson D, Percinel AK, et al. Severe alkalosis in critically ill patients. Arch Surg 1972;105:197–203.
18. Kilburn KH. Neurologic manifestations of respiratory failure. Arch Intern Med 1965;116:409.
19. Mitchell JH, Wildenthal K, Johnson RL. The effects of acid–base disturbances of cardiovascular and pulmonary function. Kidney Int 1972;1:375–389.
20. Monroe RG, French G, Whittenberger JL. Effects of hypocapnia and hypercapnia on myocardial contractility. Am J Physiol 1960;199:1121–1124.
21. Smithline N, Gardner K. Gaps–anionic and osmolar. JAMA 1976;236:1594–1597.
22. Frommer JP. Lactic acidosis. Med Clin North Am 1983;67:815–829.
23. Alberti KG, Nattrass M. Lactic acidosis. Lancet 1977;25–29.
24. Thrower WB, Barby TD, Aldinger EE. Acid–base derangements and myocardial contractility. Arch Surg 1961;82:56–65.
25. Mitchell JH, Wildenthal K, Johnson RL. The effects of acid–base disturbance on cardiovascular and pulmonary function. Kidney Int 1972;1:375–389.
26. Drug Information. American Hospital Formulary Service 1985.
27. Stacpoole PW. Lactic acidosis: The case against bicarbonate therapy. Ann Intern Med 1986;105:276–278.
28. Canizaro PC, Prager MD, Shires GT. The infusion of Ringer's lactate solution during shock. Surg Forum 1971;122:494–501.
29. Bleigh HL, Schwartz WB. TRIS buffer (THAM): An appraisal of its physiologic effects and clinical usefulness. N Engl J Med 1966;274:782–787.
30. Wilson RF, Gibson D, Percinel AK, et al. Severe alkalosis in critically ill patients. Arch Surg 1972;105:197–203.
31. Harken AH. Lactic acidosis. Surg Gynecol Obstet 1972;142: 593–606.
32. Goodman LS, Gilman A (eds). The Pharmacological Basis of Therapeutics. New York, Macmillan,
33. Lipner HI, Ruzany F, Dasgupta M, et al. The behavior of carbenicillin as a nonreabsorbable anion. J Lab Clin Med 1975; 86:183.
34. Fraley DS, Adler S, Bruns F. Life-threatening metabolic alkalosis in a comatose patient. South Med J 1979;72:1024–1025.
35. Martin WJ, Matzke GR. Treating severe metabolic alkalosis. Clin Pharm 1982;1:42–48.
36. Harken AH, Gabel RA, Fencl A, et al. Hydrochloric acid in the correction of metabolic alkalosis. Arch Surg 1975;110:819–821.
37. Brimoulle S, Vincent JL, Dufaye P, et al. Hydrochloric acid infusion for treatment of metabolic alkalosis: Effects on acid–base balance and oxygenation. Crit Care Med 1985;13:738–742.
38. Rowlands BJ, Tindall SF, Elliot DJ. The use of dilute hydrochloric acid and cimetidine to reverse severe metabolic alkalosis. Postgrad Med J 1978;54:118–123.
39. Pilla S, Muller RJ. The use of intravenous hydrochloric acid in severe metabolic alkalosis. Hosp Pharm 1985;20:725–729.
40. Mirtallo JM, Rogers KR, Johnson JA, et al. Stability of amino acids and the availability of acid in total parenteral nutrition solutions containing hydrochloric acid. Am J Hosp Pharm 1981;38:1729–1731.

# Section Two
# Clinical Nutrition

## Chapter 105 / Nutrient Metabolism in Health and Disease

Jay M. Mirtallo, MS

Nutrition is defined as a function of living plants and animals, consisting of the taking in and assimilation of material through chemical changes (metabolism) whereby tissue is built up and energy liberated. Its successive stages, that is, metabolism, are known as digestion, absorption, assimilation, and excretion. In humans, digestion is preceded by mastication and deglutition. Excretion is effected by expiration, perspiration, urination, and defecation.[1] Not all of the materials involved with human metabolism can be synthesized by the body. Therefore, these essential materials—nutrients—must be provided by the diet.

Malnutrition is either primary (lack of food) or conditioned (potentially adequate diet but inefficient nutrient utilization related to chronic or acute disease and its treatment).[2] As a result of the presence of the variables causing conditioned malnutrition, this form is more complicated to manage successfully but, unfortunately, is the most common type of malnutrition encountered in clinical practice. Nutritional therapeutics is defined as management of the nutritional state of the patient. The purpose of nutritional therapeutics is the successful prevention, recognition, and management of malnutrition during the course of medical and pharmacologic management of disease.

The information required to practice nutritional therapeutics is not easily retained by most, even by those specializing in this area of professional practice. This chapter summarizes those principles of nutrient metabolism most frequently encountered by the clinical pharmacist and is intended to be comprehensive but not totally inclusive. As such, this chapter provides a scientific and biochemical basis for the clinically oriented chapters that follow. It is organized as energy metabolism, normal metabolism, and malnutrition including starvation, stress, and altered metabolism of nutrients in specific diseases.

### Energy Metabolism

Metabolism includes the absorption, digestion (preparation of foodstuffs in the alimentary tract for optimal absorption), distribution, metabolism, and excretion of nutrients. This discussion emphasises metabolism or assimilation; other components are considered only when clinical problems frequently occur requiring this knowledge for appropriate nutritional therapeutics.

The body needs a constant source of fuel (energy) for growth and maintenance. The major function of metabolic pathways is to process this fuel into energy that can be used for synthetic reactions, for locomotion, for pumping ions or molecules against concentration gradients, and for other cell processes.[3] Energy is most commonly stored and provided by the high-energy phosphate bond, that is, adenosine triphosphate (ATP, Fig. 105.1). Energy is stored in the two terminal high-energy phosphate bonds and is released or transferred to support reactions requiring energy. Most of the high-energy phosphate available to the cells is produced in the mitochondria[3] via the citric acid cycle, also known as the trichloroacetic acid (TCA) or Krebs cycle. The production of ATP requires adequate amounts of oxygen, acetyl coenzyme A (Fig. 105.2), and the presence of adenosine diphosphate (ADP) as a stimulus to the body for the need of high-energy phosphate. Thus, the presence of ADP in the mitochondria increases oxygen consumption, with the production of 3 ATP molecules per molecule of oxygen consumed. This is accomplished via the citric acid cycle as illustrated in Figure 105.3. During the complete oxidation of the acetyl group of acetyl coenzyme A, the high-energy yield is 12 molecules of ATP. The source of ATP is the conversion of acetyl coenzyme A to oxaloacetate (1 ATP), three NADH via oxidative phosphorylation (9 ATP), and oxidative phosphorylation of ubiquinone (2 ATP).[4] Note that one NADH yields three molecules of ATP during oxidative phosphorylation. This occurs when there is a perfect coupling of oxidation and phosphorylation, and consumes four molecules of oxygen.[4] "Uncoupled" oxidative phosphorylation occurs when the electron transfers in the mitochondria are dissociated from phosphorylation, thereby impairing the supply of ATP. This causes an increased oxygen consumption without a further increase in ATP production or utilization.[3]

High-energy bonds are not all from the citric acid cycle

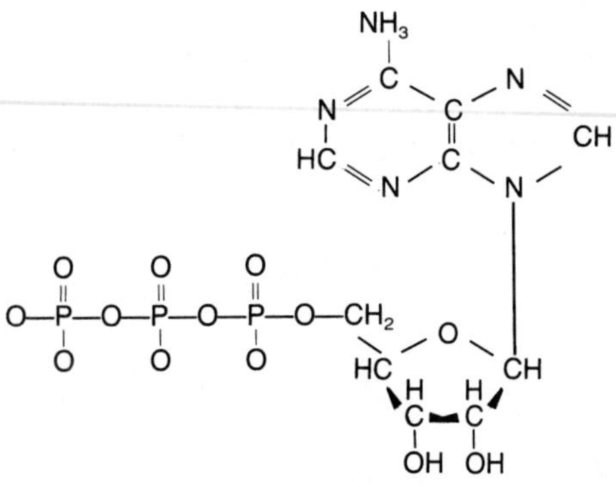


**Figure 105.1** Structure of adenosine triphosphate (ATP).

within the cell. The conversion of glucose to pyruvate during oxidation reactions is a source of cellular ATP, as are anaerobic sources via the Cori cycle[3] as discussed later. Nutrient sources of fuel for energy metabolism (production of ATP) are fat, carbohydrate, and protein. The biochemical processes by which these fuel sources are used by the body to produce ATP are discussed in the next sections.

***Fat Metabolism*** The major storage form of energy in the body is adipose (fat) tissue.[5] This endogenous source of energy is of significance during periods of starvation and stress, when it is used as a major fuel for the preservation of life.

Fat oxidation occurs when free fatty acids (FFAs) are present within the cell. Rapid uptake of FFAs by various cells occurs by diffusion across cell membranes. Another source of intracellular FFAs is the hydrolysis of triglycerides (Fig. 105.4). Once within the cell cytosol, FFAs are converted to long-chain acyl coenzyme A and transported into the mitochondria along with carnitine.[6] Acyl coenzyme A (Fig. 105.5) differs from acetyl coenzyme A in that an acyl (derived from the fatty acid) group, rather than an acetyl group, is attached to the coenzyme A molecule. Once formed within the cell, acyl coenzyme A requires transport into the mitochondria for β-oxidation and ultimately ATP production. As the mitochondrial membrane is nearly impermeable to coenzyme A (CoA) and its derivatives, carnitine is required to facilitate transport of acyl CoA into the mitochondrial matrix in the following manner (Fig. 105.6). Carnitine at the outer surface of the mitochondrial membrane picks up the acyl groups of acyl CoA and transports these to the mitochondrial matrix, where acyl carnitine equilibrates with CoA to form acyl CoA within the mitochondria. The transfer of acyl groups is governed by carnitine palmitoyl transferase and is facilitated by a carnitine–*o*–acylcarnitine antiport carrier.[6] An antiport carrier facilitates the movement of two compounds, in opposite direction to each other (see Fig. 105.6). This carnitine-dependent transport is required only for long-chain fatty acids, because shorter chain (4–12 carbons) fatty acids are sufficiently water soluble to pass freely across membranes.[5] The short-chain fatty acids

**Figure 105.2** Structure of acetyl coenzyme A with its constituents. Phosphopantetheine is the combination of pantothenic acid and β-mercaptoethylamine. *(From McGilvery RW [Ed]: Biochemistry, a Functional Approach, 3rd ed. Philadelphia, W.B. Saunders, 1983, pp 423, with permission.)*

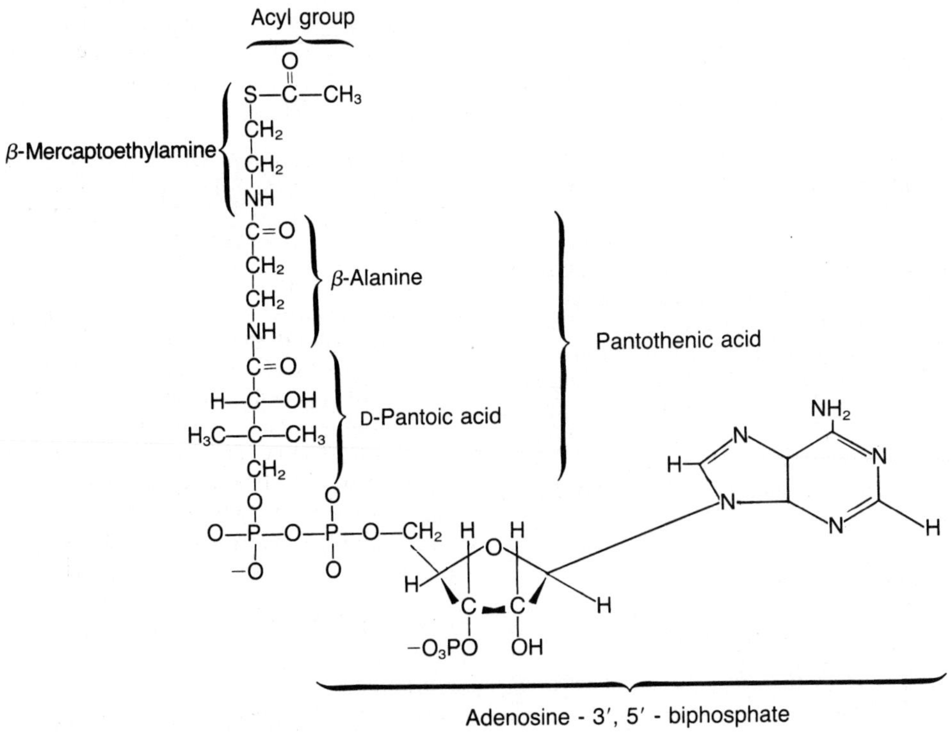

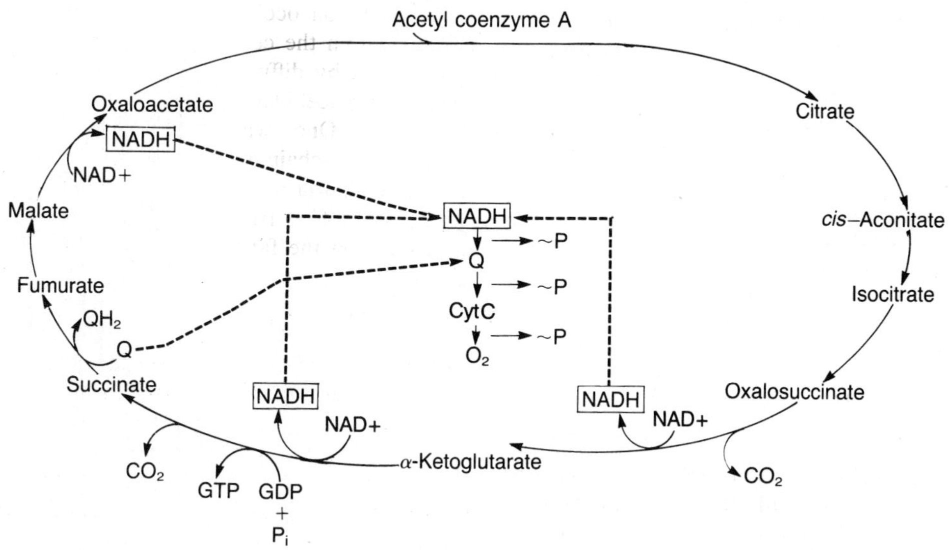


**Figure 105.3** The citric acid cycle. The enzymes required for the citric acid cycle are present in the aqueous phase of the mitochondria and are responsible for transfer of the energy of the carbon–hydrogen bonds from acetyl CoA to specific carriers; NADH enters the solid phase of the mitochondria in which the energy is converted into high-energy phosphate through the process of oxidative phosphorylation. In the oxidation of succinate to fumurate, flavin adenine dinucleotide is a coenzyme that transfers electrons directly to ubiquinone (Q), thereby bypassing the first phosphorylation site of oxidative phosphorylation. *(Compiled from References 3 and 4.)*

are then acted upon by butyl CoA synthetase for further oxidation within the mitochondria.

Once inside the mitochondrial matrix, β-oxidation, the process by which acyl CoA is reduced by two carbons to form acetyl CoA, occurs. Each acetyl CoA molecule may then enter the citric acid cycle. For palmitate, the most abundantly used fatty acid for oxidation, a total of five high-energy phosphate bonds are generated per molecule of acetyl CoA cleaved through β-oxidation of the fatty acid (acyl) CoA and its residual parts. This occurs before energy (ATP) production by the acetyl CoA via the citric acid cycle.[5] Oxidation of fatty acids differs for the following:

1. Saturated fatty acids. Carbons are cleaved two at a time until the entire fatty acid is used to produce acetyl CoA.
2. Odd-numbered fatty acids. Oxidation results in a three-carbon fragment (proprionyl CoA), which does not yield substantial energy when metabolized.
3. Unsaturated fatty acids. Oxidation follows the general route of saturated fatty acids, with the addition of two more reactions: isomerization of the double bond and racematization of a D-isomer product of unsaturated fatty acid oxidation to its metabolically active L-isomer.

**Figure 105.4** Chemical structure of triglycerides. $R_1$, $R_2$, and $R_3$ are fatty acids. Mono- and diglycerides contain one and two fatty acids, respectively.

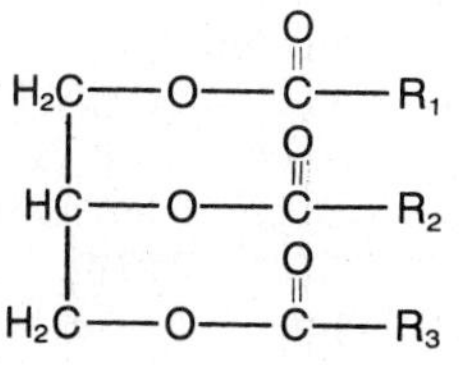

Glycerol, which is released by the hydrolysis of fats, is another source of energy derived from fat. It may be taken up by the liver and converted to glycerol 3-phosphate by a reaction catalyzed by a glycerokinase. This glycerol 3-phosphate may then be used to form new triglycerides or add to the dihydroxyacetone phosphate supply and either be converted to glucose or be used as a fuel (Figure 105.7).[6]

***Carbohydrate Metabolism*** Glucose is the major source of fuel for most tissues; especially important is its support of the central nervous system. Glucose oxidation (Fig. 105.7) is considered in four parts[7,8]:

1. Transport into cells, which occurs via a concentration gradient across the plasma membrane. Transport is by facilitated diffusion into muscles and adipose tissue in a reaction that is governed by insulin.
2. Glucose phosphorylation, a process that uses one mole of ATP, is regulated by the enzyme, hexokinase. The phosphorylated glucose, fructose 1,6-phosphate, then splits to yield two triose phosphates.
3. Conversion of triose phosphate to pyruvate.
4. Oxidation of pyruvate in the mitochondria.

**Figure 105.5** Acyl coenzyme A.

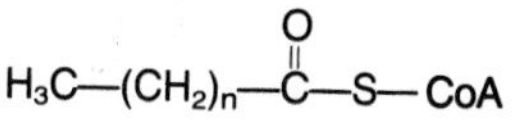

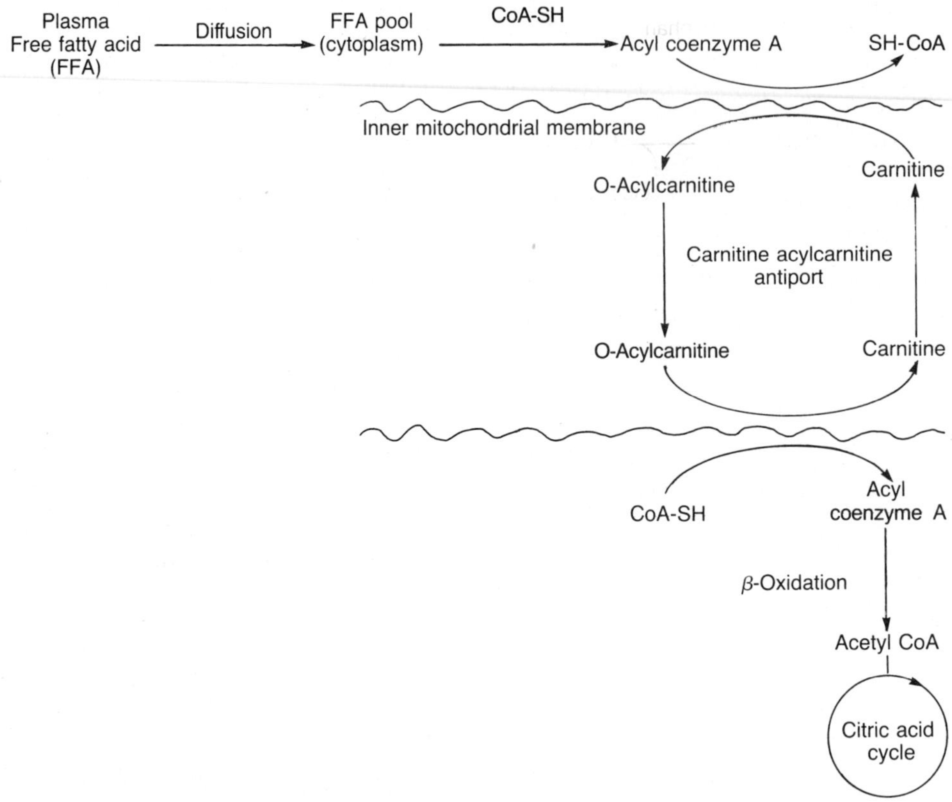


**Figure 105.6** Schematic representation of fatty acid oxidation.

Nondextrose carbohydrates are also available for energy use by the body.[9] Carbohydrates such as fructose, sorbitol, and xylitol have had considerable use as a fuel in parenteral nutrition regimens outside the United States and have had somewhat limited use in this country. Fructose is readily converted to fructose 1-phosphate, which may be split by aldolase into dihydroxyacetone phosphate and glyceraldehyde. Dihydroxyacetone phosphate may follow the glycolytic pathway in the production of energy (Fig. 105.7). Glyceraldehyde may either be reduced to glycerol or be phosphorylated and enter the glycolytic pathway as glyceraldehyde 3-phosphate (Fig. 105.7). Sorbitol can be converted into both glucose and fructose, with reactions for conversion favoring oxidation of sorbitol to fructose and reduction of glucose to sorbitol. Therefore, the thrust of sorbitol oxidation is via the same pathway as fructose.[7] Finally, xylitol is oxidized to D-xylulose and subsequently phosphorylated to D-xylulose 5-phosphate, an intermediate in the pentose phosphate pathway. This intermediate, when catalyzed by transketolase, is converted to glyceraldehyde 3-phosphate and may then be oxidized via the glycolytic pathway previously described.[7]

**Figure 105.7** Glucose oxidation via glycolysis, with the production of pyruvate (Embden–Meyerhof pathway) for entry into the citric acid cycle or as a precursor to lactate under anaerobic conditions. Glycerol oxidation, also depicted, is a reaction that occurs only within the liver.

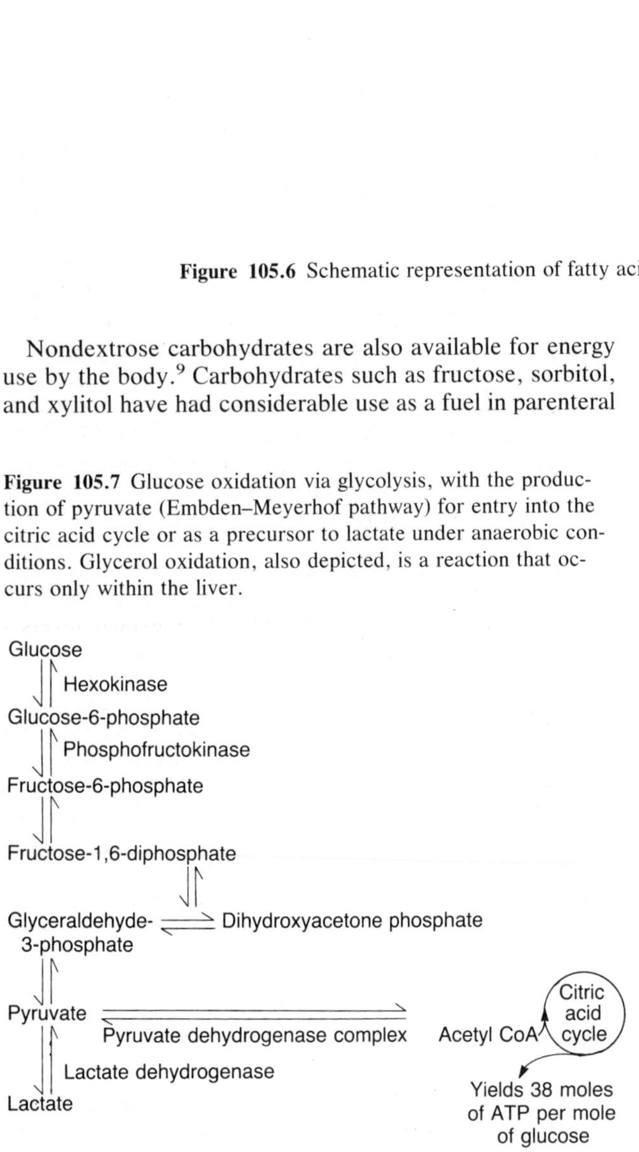


***Protein as a Fuel*** Protein is usually an insignificant fuel source as compared with fat and carbohydrate sources, but in some conditions it is very important. In general, humans obtain only one tenth of high-energy phosphate by oxidizing amino acids (protein).[10] When used as a fuel, the nitrogen of amino acids is transferred to α-keto acids by aminotransferases. Much of this nitrogen later appears as glutamate, which may undergo oxidative deamination, in a reaction catalyzed by glutamate dihydrogenase. Carbon atoms of the

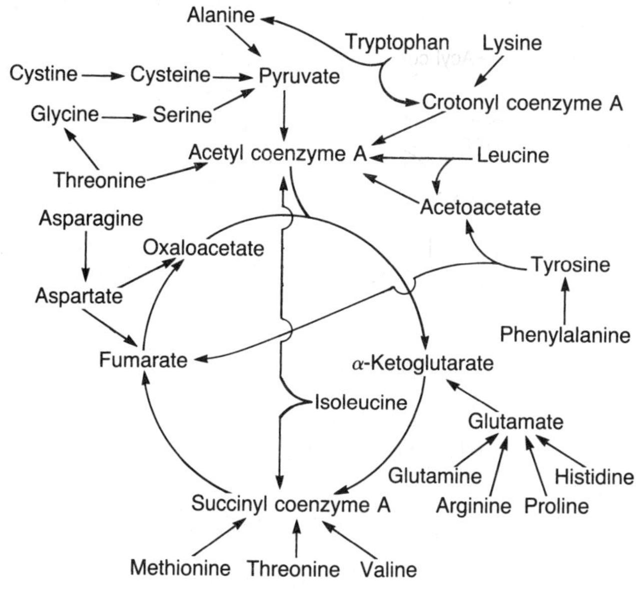


**Figure 105.8** Outline of the fate of the carbon skeletons of the amino acids used as fuels.

amino acids are processed to make other constituents and appear either as carbon dioxide or as eight familiar intermediates of fuel metabolism (Fig. 105.8).[11]

## Normal Metabolism

In fed humans, the availability of substrate (nutrients) for cellular reactions is accomplished by the enteral or parenteral intake of nutrients. The metabolic fate of these nutrients depends on nutrient needs of individual cells or tissues; the body's recognition and normal reaction to these needs; nervous system and hormonal regulatory mechanisms; substrate (nutrient) availability; and the appropriate ratio of nutrients in the diet.[12] The net result of these factors could be that the nutrient becomes a component of cellular material, influences synthetic reactions, is used as energy, is stored for use as a fuel or substrate during periods of excess need or nutrient deprivation (starvation), or is metabolized and subsequently disposed of by the body. Discussion of normal metabolism deals with the source and assimilation of nutrients by the body with consideration of carbohydrates, fats, proteins, trace elements, and vitamins. Electrolytes and water are considered elsewhere.

*Nutrient Absorption* For an oral diet, foodstuffs are presented to the alimentary tract where they are processed for absorption. Through chewing, enzymes, and neurochemical control of organ function and enzyme secretion, foodstuffs are broken down to substrates that can be absorbed via either active or passive processes in the small intestine. Subsequently, these water-soluble substrates pass into the circulation via the portal vein. Fat-soluble molecules are taken up by the lymphatics and made available to the circulation where the lymph channels join the blood vessels in the thoracic duct.[13] The major sites of absorption of nutrients are shown in Figure 105.9.[14]

After absorption, nutrients are available for metabolism or assimilation in the body. A discussion of the metabolism of major nutrients follows.

*Carbohydrate Metabolism* Starch is the principal source of carbohydrate from the diet. It is digested to monosaccharides such as dextrose and fructose and oligosaccharides such as sucrose, maltose, dextrin, lactose.[13] Clinical nutrition is concerned primarily with glucose or dextrose metabolism. Glucose is absorbed either by diffusion or by active processes. Use of oral rehydration solutions prescribed for the treatment of acute diarrhea for improved electrolyte balance in the body for patients with short-bowel syndrome relies on active absorption of glucose.[15] In these cases, active uptake of glucose creates a solvent drag that facilitates fluid and electrolyte absorption in the small bowel proximal to the diseased area of the bowel.

The use of glucose as a fuel has been discussed previously. The major storage form of glucose is glycogen. Normally, glycogen stores in the liver are 65 g (or 400 mol) per kilogram of tissue, whereas skeletal muscle contains 14 g (or 85 mol) per kilogram of tissue. In the synthesis of glycogen, glucose 6-phosphate is converted to uridine diphosphate glucose (UDP-glucose) under the regulation of phosphoglucomutase, and UDP-glucose glucosyl units are then transferred to amylose chains under the regulation of glycogen synthase, with final creation of branches of glycogen under the influence of glycosyl-4:6-transferases.

Glycogen synthesis is dependent on the balance of the levels of insulin and glucagon in various tissues. In the liver, insulin produces glycogenesis and glucagon causes glycogenolysis. In the muscle, receptors for glucagon are absent,[16] and the hormone therefore exerts no regulatory effect in this tissue. Glycogen synthesis in the muscle is favored when insulin as well as glucose is available. In this setting, glycogen synthase and pyruvate dehydrogenase activity is increased and phosphorylation of glycogen is suppressed. This results in net glycogen synthesis and increased conversion of pyruvate to acetyl CoA. Contrarily, phosphorylation of glycogen and subsequent glycogenolysis are facilitated by catecholamines that activate phosphorylase *a* via the second messenger cyclic AMP.[16] Elevated levels of ionized calcium in the skeletal muscle cell may also activate phosphorylase *a*.[16]

As there is a limit to the storage of glucose as glycogen in the body, any excess glucose not oxidized or stored as glycogen is converted to and stored as fat. In this process, glucose is converted to acetyl CoA, which may then be processed into fatty acids (described in next section). Also, if glucose intake exceeds the body's ability to transport it intracellularly, increased extracellular levels in excess of the renal threshold for glucose reabsorption will result in glucosuria and, if left unrecognized, could lead to excessive free water losses and hyperosmolar coma.[17]

Endogenous sources of glucose via gluconeogenesis (Fig. 105.10) are available from lactate, protein, and sorbitol. The Cori cycle provides a cyclical turnover of glucose[18] whereby 6.5 mol of ATP is consumed for each mole of glucose produced from 2 mol of lactate. Lactate is the end product of glycolysis under anaerobic conditions; it is released from the

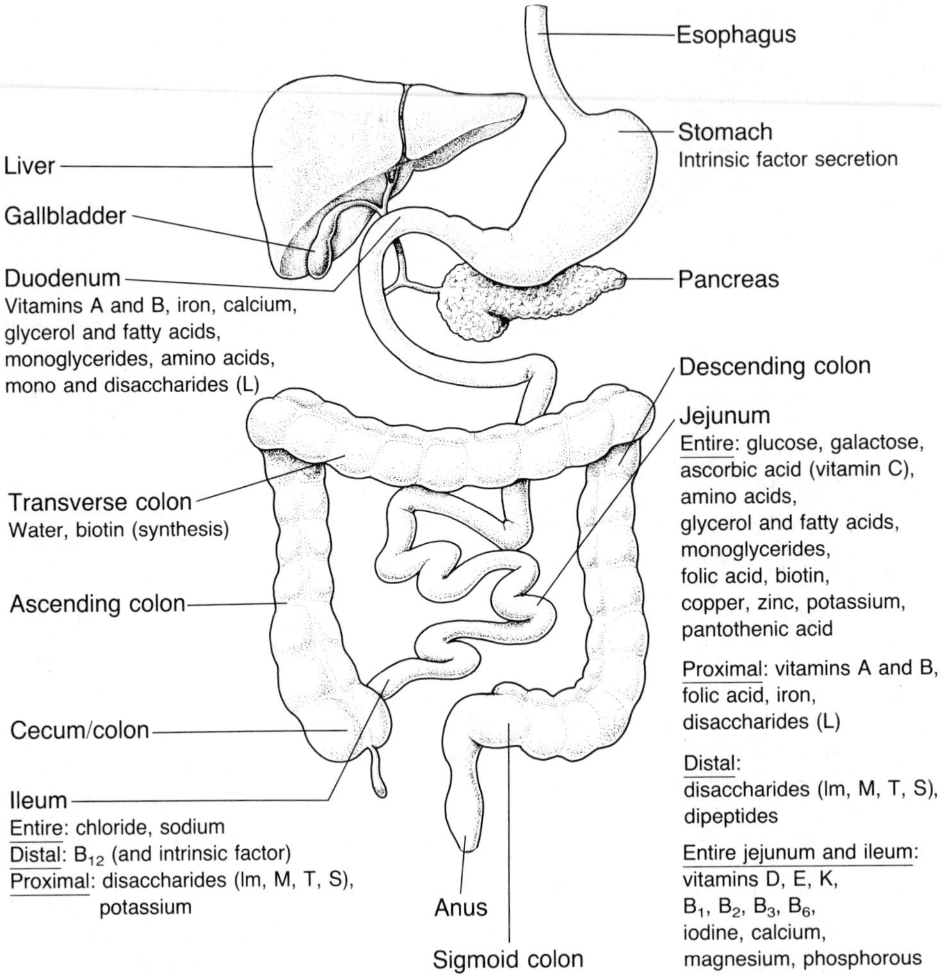


**Figure 105.9** The sites of absorption of nutrients are shown. The exact sites for absorption of manganese, cobalt, selenium, chromium, molybdenum, and cadmium are unknown. L, lactose; Im, isomaltase; M, maltase; T, trehalase; S, sucrase.

muscle and carried by the bloodstream to the liver where it is available for conversion to glucose.

In general, amino acids are gluconeogenic during periods of starvation[11] (Fig. 105.8), but one of the most important protein sources of glucose is the glucose–alanine cycle (Fig. 105.11).[19] Alanine and glutamine serve as nitrogen carriers in the body. Uptake of glutamine occurs in the small bowel, where it is metabolized. It then appears in the liver as either ammonium ions, alanine, and citrulline. Contrarily, alanine produced in the muscle from the nitrogen of branched-chain amino acids and pyruvate is taken up by the liver. The nitrogen of alanine is transferred to glutamate, in a reaction catalyzed by alanine aminotransferase to yield glutamine plus pyruvate. Pyruvate may then be converted to glucose. The glutamine, in the presence of aspartate aminotransferase, is converted to aspartate, which may enter either the urea cycle (discussed later) or the citric acid cycle (requires aminotransferase activity) as either oxaloacetate or fumurate (Fig. 105.3).

The oxidation of sorbitol produces glucose in a process that allows fructose to become a glucose source as well.[20] As discussed previously though, enzymes in the body do not favor this metabolic process. Side effects of this process include increased production of lactate and uric acid in addition to loss of body water and electrolytes. These effects have limited the usefulness of sorbitol as an energy source in clinical practice.

***Fat Metabolism*** Dietary lipids, as the major source of fat to the body, are ingested as long-chain triglycerides, phospholipids (lecithin predominantly), and cholesterol.[5] Long-chain triglycerides are fatty acid esters of glycerol, the hydroxyl groups of which are esterified with either one, two, or three fatty acids to form monoglycerides, diglycerides, or triglycerides, respectively. Triglycerides are the predominant dietary, storage, and transport forms of lipid.

The fatty acids of the triglyceride molecule are the precursors to cholesterol and therefore to prostaglandins, glucocorticoids, mineralocorticoids, androgens, estrogens, and bile acids. Fatty acids consist of carboxyl groups with hydrocarbon chains (R-COOH). Saturated fatty acids have no double bonds present, whereas unsaturated fatty acids

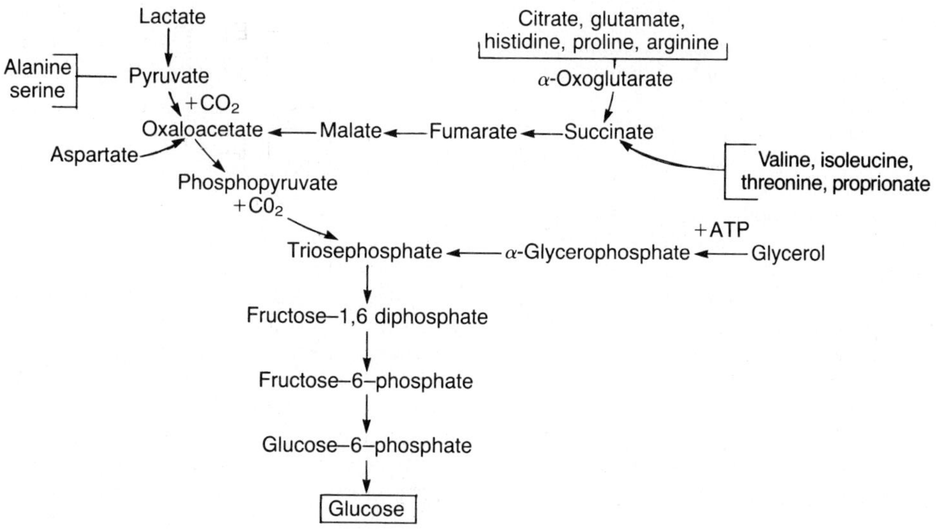


**Figure 105.10** Pathways of gluconeogenesis from various precursors.

have one or more double bonds present in the hydrocarbon chains. The human body is not capable of synthesizing fatty acids with a double bond between the ninth and terminal carbons of the fatty acid chain.[5] Therefore, linoleic acid and linolenic acid are essential fatty acids in man. Arachidonic acid may be synthesized from linoleic acid and is therefore conditionally essential to the human body.

Phospholipids have both hydrophobic (fatty acids) and hydrophilic (phosphoryl) ends, which allow for interaction with both water- and fat-soluble surfaces.[5] These serve the body as emulsifying agents and as essential components of the cell membrane. As such, phospholipids are not generally used as an energy source and are preserved, even in severe cases of malnutrition, such that cell membrane integrity is

**Figure 105.11** The glucose–alanine cycle. A major gluconeogenic pathway from protein.

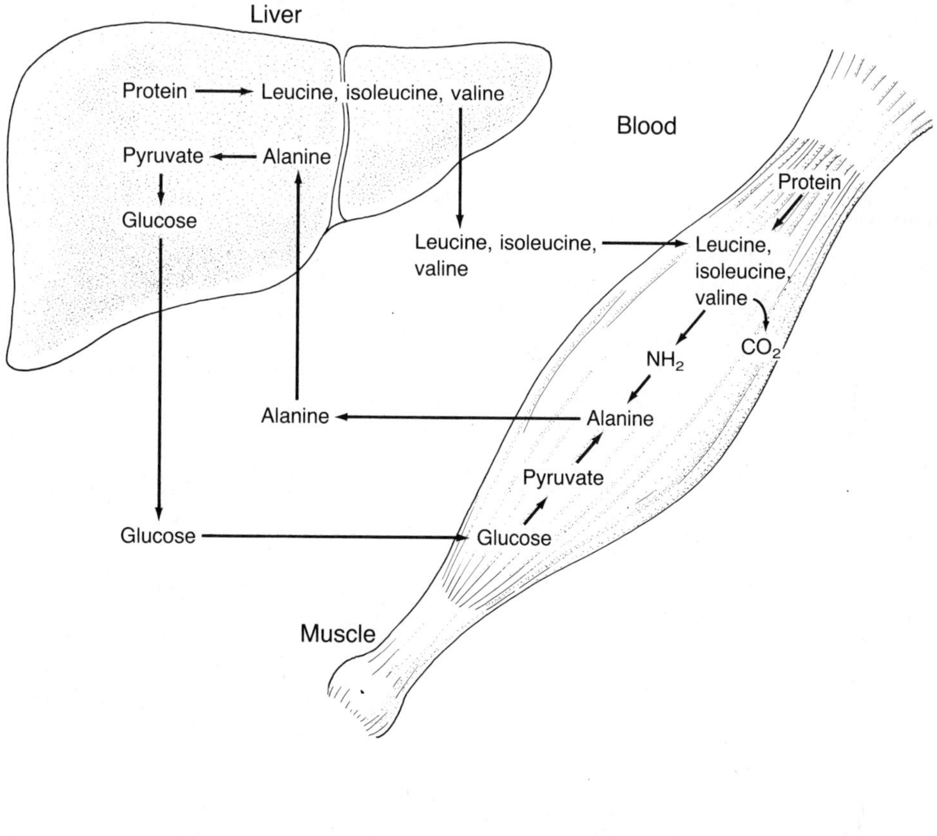

maintained.[5] Phospholipids consist of glycerol, two fatty acids, and phosphoric acid with esterification of phosphoric acid to a nitrogen-containing moiety such as serine, ethanolamine, or choline (lecithin).

Oral lipids are acted upon by gastric lipase, pancreatic enzymes, biliary lecithin, and bile salts. This results in the hydrolysis and emulsification of the lipids for absorption.[13] Hydrolysis by gastrointestinal lipase yields medium-chain triglycerides that are available for absorption via passive diffusion across the gastrointestinal mucosa in the jejunum (Fig. 105.9). Long-chain triglycerides require hydrolysis and emulsification with lecithin and bile salts for gastrointestinal mucosal uptake. Once within the mucosal cell, fatty acids are recombined with glycerol to form triglycerides, which are then packaged in a chylomicron consisting of a triglyceride (80%), cholesterol (9%), and phospholipid (7%) and coated with lipoprotein (4%).[21] Lipoproteins have a triglyceride as a hydrophobic core and a cholesterol ester surrounded by a surface coat of apoproteins, phospholipids, and free cholesterol.[5] Lipoproteins serve as solubilizing agents for lipid transport through an aqueous medium.[5] These are classified as chylomicrons, very low density lipoproteins (VLDLs), low-density lipoproteins (LDLs), and high-density lipoproteins (HDLs) with each having a specific protein or apoprotein that may direct the lipoprotein's metabolism via interaction with key enzymes and receptors.[22] In the final process of lipid absorption, chylomicrons are secreted into the lymph and transported into the blood via the thoracic duct.

Fatty acids are made available to the liver via the enterohepatic circulation for medium-chain triglycerides or the systemic circulation for long-chain fatty acids and remnants of chylomicrons. Once in the liver, the triglyceride may enter the hepatocyte and be available for hydrolysis to its glycerol and fatty acid components.[21] The fate of glycerol is either oxidation as a carbohydrate or in the synthesis of a new triglyceride molecule, whereas the fatty acid may become a triglyceride or phospholipid or undergo β-oxidation. Excess fatty acids have various metabolic fates including synthesis of phospholipids, resynthesis of triglycerides, complete degradation with the production of energy, or ketogenesis (the production of ketones for use as energy substrates in the muscle).

Cellular deposition of fat occurs from chylomicrons made available from the small intestine or from VLDLs released by the liver.[21] Fatty acids are removed from chylomicrons and VLDLs circulating in the bloodstream by lipoprotein lipase, which is present in muscle and adipose tissue. The fatty acids normally move freely into the cell, but they are converted to triglycerides in preparation for storage in situations of excess for the muscle and normally in adipose tissue. Lipoprotein lipase is activated by contact with specific proteins present in the chylomicron or VLDLs and is also activated by heparin.

Fat is mobilized and released (lipolysis) from adipose tissue by a hormone-sensitive lipase that hydrolyzes any and all bonds in the triglyceride molecule. The fatty acids are then bound to albumin for transport and the glycerol is transported to the liver for processing. Lipolysis is regulated by insulin and catecholamine levels. Insulin favors fat storage, blocks fat release, favors fat synthesis from glucose in the liver, and permits the use of glucose as a fuel in skeletal muscle rather than fat. Simply, insulin promotes fat storage and use of glucose as the principal fuel. In contrast, catecholamines mediate the release of fatty acids from the adipocyte. Subsequently increased levels of fatty acids in the blood increase their utilization by muscle tissue as an energy source. In addition, hepatic uptake of fatty acids is increased. The diet is the major source of fatty acids, but fatty acids may be made available and synthesized from endogenous (glucose and amino acids) sources.[21]

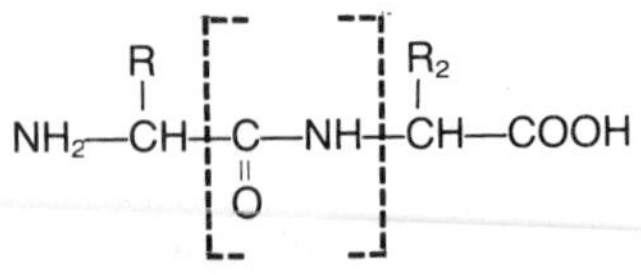

**Figure 105.12** Peptide linkage of two amino acids.

***Protein Metabolism*** Proteins are complex polymers of α-amino acids joined by a peptide linkage (Fig. 105.12) from the amino group of one amino acid to a carboxyl group of another. Proteins consist elementally of carbon, hydrogen, oxygen, nitrogen, and sometimes sulfur.[23] Proteins function as structural components and in regulatory, movement, immunologic, transport, and repair processes. Protein is an essential component of the nucleus, cytoplasm, and membrane of the cell.[24] Proteins are the "machinery" of the body and as such are vital to life-sustaining processes.[25] Alterations in protein metabolism are common and may be partially responsible for the determination of death in some common diseases.[23] Protein metabolism is discussed with respect to dietary sources, the amino acid pool, and protein flux in the body.

Dietary protein is hydrolyzed to amino acids, dipeptides, and tripeptides before absorption into the portal system. No intact protein enters the human body; therefore, all body protein is synthesized de novo.[23] Most amino acids entering the liver from the portal vein are extracted by this organ, except the branched-chain amino acids, which become available to the systemic circulation. The metabolic fate of amino acids is determined by the nutritional state and clinical condition of the patient. Metabolic processes are present for protein catabolism in which the carbon skeleton (ketoacid) of the amino acid is removed and used for energy. The ammonia component of the amino acid may be either transaminated to a new ketoacid, producing another amino acid, or discarded as urea. Also, protein synthetic processes are available to make use of the amino acids in the production of structural, enzymatic, and transport proteins.

Amino acids released into the circulation from the liver or from "endogenous" sources (protein breakdown) are rapidly taken up by metabolically active tissues (kidney, pancreas, and intestinal mucosa). Uptake by the skeletal muscle is slow but the large mass of this tissue makes it the largest reservoir or pool of "labile" amino acids.[23] This "labile" or "free" amino acid pool is only about 1% of total body amino acids, provides for movement of amino acids between various organs, and supports the dynamic state of protein metabolism. The dynamic state of protein metabolism is referred to as "protein flux,"[25] meaning that the quantities of amino acids entering the pool (from either exogenous or

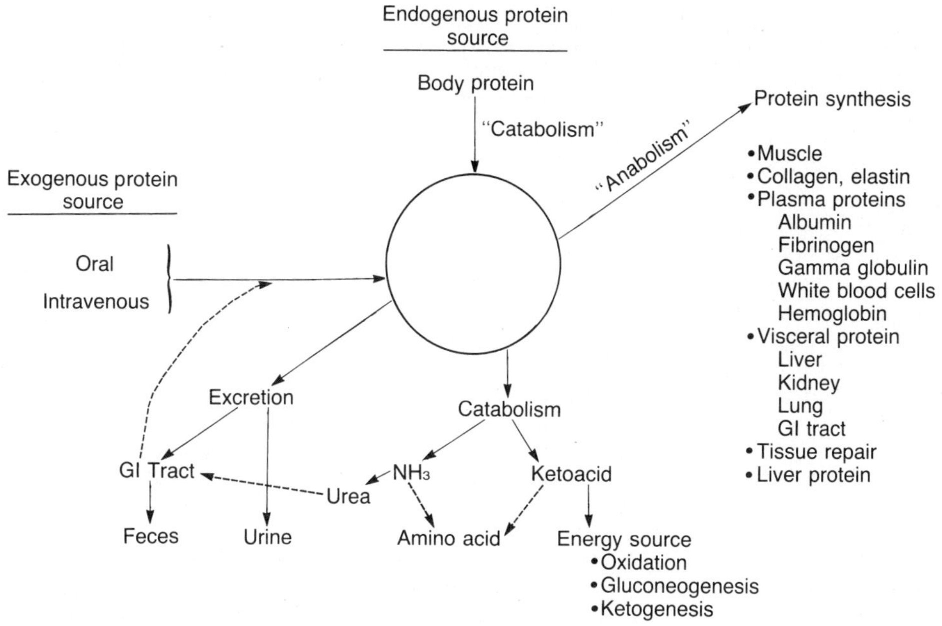


**Figure 105.13** Body protein dynamics. Under normal homeostatic conditions, anabolic and catabolic protein processes are in equilibrium (''protein flux''), leaving the size of the free amino acid pool constant.

endogenous sources) or leaving the pool (via synthesis or catabolism and excretion of protein) are in equilibrium. This leaves the amino acid pool constant in quantity. Thus, protein flux refers to the turnover of protein such that a balance exists between synthetic and catabolic processes (Fig. 105.13). The state of this dynamic equilibrium determines the state of the overall protein balance of the body.

Whether an amino acid is incorporated into new protein or is catabolized is determined by a number of factors. These factors include the amino acid supply, hormonal milieu present in the body, and state of protein deprivation. Essential amino acids (EAAs) are those that the body is incapable of producing in sufficient quantities to prevent deficiency symptoms in healthy individuals when exogenous sources of the amino acid are absent. The essential amino acids in man are isoleucine (Iso), leucine (Leu), lysine (Lys), methionine (Meth), phenylalanine (Phe), threonine (Thr), tryptophan (Trp), and valine (Val) (Table 105.1). Histidine (His) and arginine (Arg) are ''semiessential'' or conditionally essential in some clinical states involving impaired function of the kidney or liver.[26]

Important classifications of amino acids are provided in Table 105.1[27] and the chemical structures of selected amino acids important to nutritional therapeutics are in Figure 105.14. As noted previously, branched-chain amino acids (BCAAs) are used by muscle for energy and are the only amino acids that are not metabolized by the liver. The ammonia from BCAAs may become a precursor along with pyruvate for alanine and also glutamine, both of which are nitrogen carriers in the body and gluconeogenic precursors. The aromatic amino acids (AAAs), metabolized by the liver, may accumulate in patients with liver disease and contribute to encephalopathic symptoms. Important to the disulfide bridges providing for the configuration and structure of protein are the sulfur-containing amino acids: cysteine (Cys) and methionine (Meth). The semiessential amino acid arginine (Arg) is an essential component of the urea cycle and thus nitrogen disposal by the body. Specific to collagen synthesis is proline, which provides a source of hydroxyproline and is a major component of collagen along with glycine. Glutamic acid and lysine are also important to collagen synthesis.[28] In the classification of amino acids, gluconeogenic refers to glucose precursors while ketogenic is the precursor to fatty acids and ketones. Cationic and anionic amino acids are included, particularly for their contribution in parenteral nutrition to acid–base disorders reported in early experiences with synthesized amino acid products. This classification refers to the release of acid (cationic) or base (anionic) during metabolism.

In anabolic pathways, amino acids are linked by peptide bonds in a predetermined sequence involving a complex interaction with nucleic acids in the ribosome and result in the synthesis of a specific protein.[23] Steps in protein synthesis may be outlined as follows[29]:

1. The DNA molecule is unwound to provide a template on one of its strands to direct the formation of heterogenous nuclear RNA (hnRNA).
2. Messenger RNA (mRNA) molecules are then synthesized in the nucleoplasm using hnRNA as a template. mRNA passes into the cytoplasm.
3. Concurrently, amino acids in the cytoplasm combine with specific molecules of transfer RNA (tRNA). This reaction involves the use of an ATP molecule.

**Table 105.1** Important Classifications of Amino Acids

| *Amino acid* | *Essential* | *Gluconeogenic* | *Ketogenic* | *Cationic* | *Anionic* |
|---|---|---|---|---|---|
| Iso | ● | ● | ● | | |
| Leu | ● | | ● | | |
| Lys | ● | ● | ● | ● | |
| Met | ● | ● | | | |
| Phe | ● | ● | ● | | |
| Thr | ● | | | | |
| Trp | ● | ● | ● | | |
| Val | ● | ● | | | |
| His | | | | ● | |
| Arg | | ● | | ● | |
| Cys | | ● | | | |
| Pro | | ● | | | |
| Gln[a] | | | | ● | |
| Ala | | ● | | | |
| Asp | | ● | | | ● |
| Asn | | | | | ● |
| Gly | | ● | | | |
| Glu[a] | | | | | ● |
| Hyp | | ● | | | |
| Ser | | ● | | | |
| Tyr | | ● | ● | | |
| Citr | | | | ● | |
| Orn | | | | ● | |

[a] Glu, glutamate; Gln, glutamine.

The following steps are repeated in sequence on the same ribosome. The successive ribosomes create longer and longer polypeptide chains as they move down a molecule of mRNA.

4. tRNA carrying amino acid acyl groups has a sequence of nucleotides allowing for attachment to mRNA on the ribosome.
5. In the presence of the proper alignment, the polypeptide transfers onto the amino acid group of the new residue.
6. Dissociation of the bound tRNA (free of amino acid) follows and returns the tRNA to the cytoplasm of the cell, while the ribosome moves to position on mRNA for the next amino acid transfer.
7. Steps 4, 5, and 6 are repeated until the ribosome reaches a specific terminator sequence in mRNA. Then, the completed polypeptide is detached into the soluble cytoplasm, freeing the ribosomes for detachment and availability for new attachment to mRNA.

Protein metabolism occurs by removal of amino groups, decarboxylation, or transmethylation.[30] The primary site of amino group removal is the liver, although other tissues may participate. One type of amino group removal is transamination, a process that transfers an amino group to another $\alpha$-ketoacid, forming a new amino acid plus the keto acid residue of the original amino acid. This reaction requires a transaminase enzyme, which exerts its activity only in the presence of pyridoxal phosphate and a metal ion.[30] The most active exchange of transamination occurs between glutamate and aspartate. More than one half of total nitrogen in amino acids passes through glutamate which undergoes transamination to aspartate or oxidative deamination to ammonia that goes into either the production of urea, pyrimidines, or glutamine. Most ketoacids of amino acids are available in the body for transamination except for lysine and methionine.[31] Oxidative deamination has been previously described; oxidases required for this reaction are available in the liver and kidney and catalyze the oxidation of all amino acids except serine, threonine, and di- and tricarboxylic acids. Finally, amino groups may be removed from amino acids by pyridoxal-dependent dehydrases and desulfurases that are responsible for the deamination of threonine, serine, and cysteine.

Protein metabolism via decarboxylation involves the conversion of amino acids to a corresponding amine such as histamine from histidine, tyramine from tyrosine, and norepinephrine and epinephrine from phenylalanine. This reaction requires pyridoxal phosphate as a coenzyme and a specific decarboxylase for each amino acid.[30]

Finally, certain methyl donors such as methionine and choline have a ''labile'' methyl group attached to the sulfur or nitrogen group that allows for transmethylation as a means of protein metabolism. The primary methyl donor is *S*-adenosyl methionine, the transfer of which is regulated by the enzyme methyl transferase. The methyl transfers of importance include the formation of phosphatidylcholine, a component of the cell membrane, and the synthesis of creatine, used for energy transfer in the muscle.[30]

***Trace Elements and Vitamins*** The discussion of nutrient metabolism thus far has been restricted to the macronu-

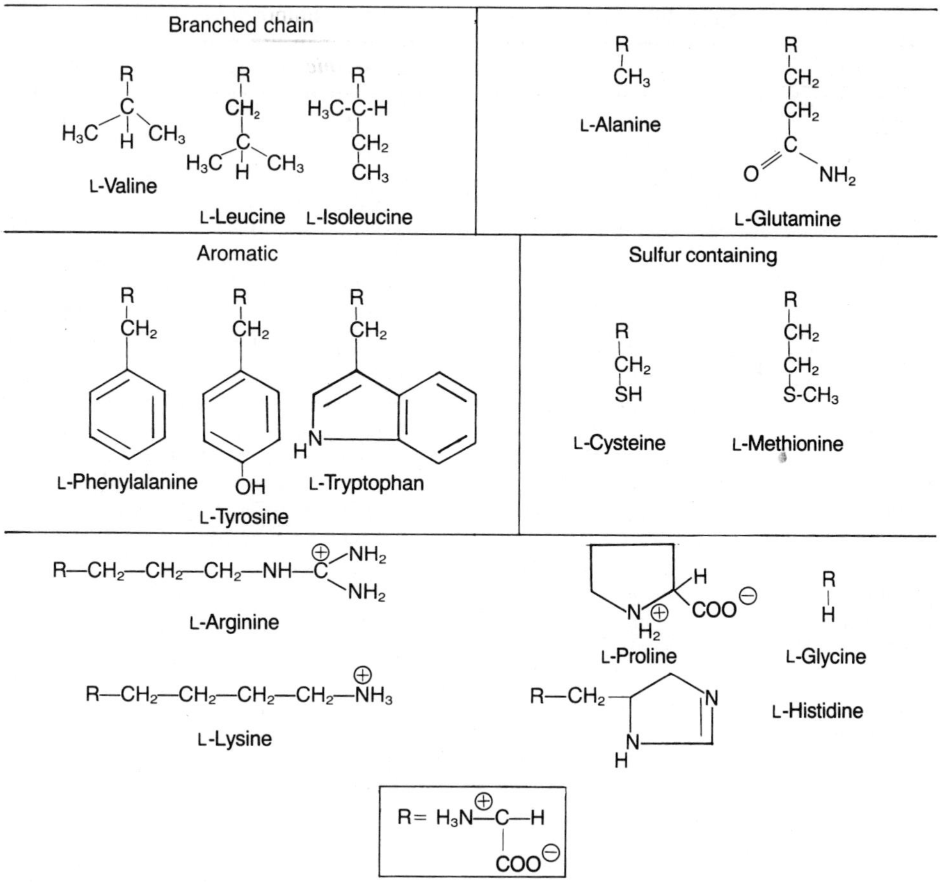


**Figure 105.14** Chemical structures of selected amino acids important to nutritional therapeutics.

trients, but micronutrients such as trace elements and vitamins serve several important functions in the regulatory mechanisms of normal homeostasis of the body. The metabolism of trace elements and vitamins is an extensive topic covered in many texts. The purpose of this section is to provide an overview of the essential functions of trace elements and vitamins and, specifically, the enzymatic processes in which these elements are involved important to energy and macronutrient metabolism.

Trace elements are substances present in human tissue in minute amounts and constitute microgram or even picogram amounts of wet tissue weight.[32] Trace elements function as nonprotein cofactors in metalloenzymes required for proper catalytic activity, cofactors in protein and nucleic acid synthesis, and structural stabilizers of some proteins. Essential trace elements are chromium, manganese, selenium, molybdenum, vanadium, nickel, tin, silicon, fluorine, and arsenic. Four trace elements with functional roles in metabolism are cobalt, iodine, zinc, and copper. The trace elements and their associated metalloenzymes of importance to nutritional therapeutics are provided in Table 105.2.[32]

Vitamins are organic compounds that are neither carbohydrate, protein, nor fat that are necessary in minute quantities for the maintenance of normal biologic activity. Vitamins function primarily as coenzymes in the metabolism of energy-yielding nutrients. In this manner, they coordinate growth and maintenance as well as assist in storage and utilization of energy. Vitamins cannot be synthesized by the body, making dietary supplementation necessary. The 13 vitamins may be classified as either fat or water soluble and serve many coenzyme functions (Table 105.3).[33]

**Table 105.2** Trace Elements and Associated Coenzymes

| *Trace element* | *Metalloenzyme* |
|---|---|
| Zinc | Carbonic anhydrase, alcohol dehydrogenase, alkaline phosphatase, lactic dehydrogenase |
| Copper | Cytochrome c oxidase, tyrosinase, monoamine oxidase, ascorbic acid oxidase |
| Chromium | Glucose tolerance factor |
| Manganese | Pyruvate carboxylase; activates alkaline phosphatase, arginase, carboxylase, and cholinesterase |
| Selenium | Glutathione peroxidase |
| Molybdenum | Aldehyde oxidase, sulfite oxidase, xanthine oxidase |

**Table 105.3** Coenzyme Functions of Vitamins

| *Vitamin* | *Coenzyme function* |
|---|---|
| Fat soluble | |
| A, retinol | Rhodopsin, visual cycle, night vision |
| K, menadiol | Blood clotting factors II, VII, IX, X |
| D, calciferol | Calcium and phosphorus homeostasis |
| E, tocopherol | Antioxidant, glutathione oxidase |
| Water soluble | |
| C, ascorbate | Antioxidant, regulation of intracellular oxidation–reduction potentials, certain hydroxylation reactions that require copper or iron, i.e., hydroxylation of proline in collagen synthesis |
| $B_1$, thiamine | Oxidative decarboxylation of amino acids, transketolase |
| $B_2$, riboflavin | Flavin mononucleotide and flavin adenine dinucleotide, essential for oxidative systems and oxygen transport |
| $B_3$ pantothenic acid | As coenzyme A precursor, necessary for acyl transfers |
| $B_5$, niacin | Endogenous source is tryptophan; component of nicotinamide adenine dinucleotide (NAD) and its phosphorylate (NADP); assists in hydrogen transfer of glycolysis, fatty acid synthesis, and tissue respiration |
| $B_6$, pyridoxine | Nitrogen metabolism: transamination, racemization, decarboxylation, cleavage, synthesis, dehydration, and desulfhydration |
| $B_{12}$, cyanocobalamin | Methylation of homocysteine to methionine, conversion of methyl malonyl coenzyme A to succinyl coenzyme A |
| Biotin | Cofactor for some carboxylases: acetyl COA carboxylase, pyruvate carboxylase, β-methylcrotonyl carboxylase, and methyl malonyl carboxylase |
| Folic acid | Transport of single carbon fragments, especially in nucleic acid synthesis and metabolism of some amino acids |

## Malnutrition

Malnutrition is the impaired nutrient utilization that results from malassimilation, poor diet, overeating, or altered metabolism by disease. Types of malnutrition discussed in this section are starvation, stress metabolism, and obesity. Included in the section on stress metabolism is the presentation of altered metabolism caused by some common diseases (i.e., renal and hepatic failure).

### *Starvation*

Humans have the ability to go without food for sustained periods with minimal impairment of mobility and thus survival. The change in the availability of substrate elicits a metabolic response involving changes in hormonal concentrations in an attempt to maintain glucose homeostasis during acute stages of starvation and a gradual adaptation to fat as the primary fuel for the purposes of preserving body protein mass during prolonged periods of a fast.[34] The stages of starvation are summarized as brief, uncomplicated starvation; prolonged starvation; and stressed starvation. During starvation, the body calls upon its body stores of energy and protein (Table 105.4)[24,34] for the maintenance of vital body functions. Significant adaptations occur during a fast to minimize losses of vital body elements, a process regulated by the balance of hormones in the plasma of starved patients. This hormonal milieu alters the metabolism of protein, glucose, and fat.

***Protein Metabolism*** The initial response to a fast is a decrease in protein synthetic rate with either no change or a slight increase in protein catabolism. The protein catabolism is via oxidative deamination and gluconeogenesis as a mechanism to preserve glucose levels in the circulation via the alanine cycle. With prolonged starvation, an adaptation to fat as an energy source occurs and the need for glucose and therefore gluconeogenesis from protein is reduced. Protein catabolism then decreases accordingly (Table 105.4). The clinical observation of this process is the decrease in appearance of urea nitrogen in the urine of fasting subjects from 12 g/d in the first 3 to 5 days of starvation to a minimal level of 3–4 g/d in 1 to 2 weeks.[34] This energy interrelation of adaptation to fat as a fuel is depicted by the use of 2 g of fat per gram of protein catabolized early in starvation to a level of 7.5 g of fat per gram of protein in late stages of starvation.[35]

***Glucose Metabolism*** During a fast, insulin concentrations are depressed favoring glycogenolysis, and glycogen stores are rapidly depleted.[36] Key organs that usually use glucose as a primary energy source are the brain, central nervous system, red blood cells, white blood cells, active fibroblasts, and certain phagocytes.[37] This need for glucose is met by gluconeogenesis from protein after glycogen stores are depleted. The source of alanine is muscle (only 8% of muscle protein is alanine) with the remainder being synthesized from pyruvate (muscle glycogen), incomplete oxidation of blood glucose, and other amino acids, especially the branched-chain amino acids. Under the hormonal influence of decreased insulin and increased glucagon concentrations

**Table 105.4** Energy Stores (kcal), expenditure, and protein metabolism during periods of starvation

| | *Overnight* | | *8 d* | | *40 d* | |
|---|---|---|---|---|---|---|
| | **Stores** | **Daily loss** | **Stores** | **Daily loss** | **Stores** | **Daily loss** |
| Total | 125,000 | 1,700 | 111,380 | 1,600 | 60,380 | 1,425 |
| Fat | 100,000 | 1,200 | 88,000 | 1,400 | 42,000 | 1,350 |
| Carbohydrate | 680 | 300 | 380 | 0 | 300 | 0 |
| Protein | 25,000 | 200 | 23,000 | 200 | 18,500 | 75 |
| Energy Expendutre (kcal/h) | | | | | | |
| Total | 70 | | 65 | | 60 | |
| Fat | 50 | | 58 | | 56 | |
| Glucose[a] | 20 | | 7 | | 4 | |
| Protein metabolism (g/kg/d) | | | | | | |
| Synthesis | 300 | | 150 | | 150 | |
| Catabolism | 300 | | 170 | | 150 | |

[a] Includes glycogen and gluconeogenic sources of glucose.

in the circulation, glycogenolysis, hepatic glucose release, gluconeogenesis from amino acids, breakdown of ketogenic amino acids with an increase in peripheral FFAs, enhanced fatty acid oxidation, and ketone body production occur.

***Fat Metabolism*** FFAs are released from triglycerides in the presence of low insulin concentrations and transported to the remainder of the body to be consumed as a fuel. Fat provides the greater proportion of calories for the human body during starvation (Table 105.4). The oxidation of fatty acids in the liver leads to ketone body production and release into the circulation. This is important, as fatty acids are not available to the central nervous system as an energy source, whereas ketone bodies are capable of passage across the blood–brain barrier and are available as a source of fuel for the brain.

In summary, the metabolic adaptation in acute starvation is for (1) the conservation of protein mass by decreasing proteolysis, increasing the availability and use of ketone bodies as an energy source, with subsequent decreased levels of amino acids in the plasma, a decline in amino acid efflux in the muscle, and a decreased splanchnic uptake of amino acids; and (2) a gradual decrease in energy expenditure (Table 105.4). With prolonged starvation, there is an enhanced oxidation of fat, and the use of ketones as primary fuels by the brain with a decreased need and production of glucose by the body and the kidney increases its production of glucose to equal that synthesized by the liver. The substrate source for gluconeogenesis as protein decreases but remains the same for lactate and glycerol. Hopefully, the loss of nitrogen is minimized for preservation of life-sustaining processes, but, if more than 30% to 50% of body nitrogen stores (Table 105.4) are lost, death will ensue.[38]

An important consideration in early starvation is that the liver is geared for fatty acid oxidation and gluconeogenesis, because the enzymes required for these processes are preserved at this time. Concurrently, urea cycle enzymes are decreased. Therefore, the ammonia generated from the alanine–glucose cycle does not necessarily appear in urea and may need to be eliminated by the kidney. The other major source of ammonia in the kidney is glutamine, which facilitates acid elimination by the kidney by producing ammonia under regulation of the enzyme glutaminase. The ammonia thus produced may accept a hydrogen molecule, thereby neutralizing the acidic products of metabolism. This is important in starvation because ketones produced by the body at this time in excess of body need will be eliminated in the kidney and be required to be neutralized by the ammonia of glutamine. At this time, urine urea nitrogen excretion may decrease to 1–2 g/d while ammonia nitrogen excretion increases from 0.5 to 2.5 g/d.[38] Therefore, the protein conservation of adapted starvation is compromised to the extent that body protein (via proteolysis of muscle) is made available to provide for sufficient synthesis of glutamine in the kidney, which will be used for renal ammoniagenesis that is required for the disposal of ketones.

### *Stress Metabolism*

Injury or stress generates a vigorous metabolic response designed to establish the metabolic priorities required for the repair of injured tissues.[39] The hormones secreted in response to stress elicit various metabolic effects (Table 105.5). Cuthbertson has described two metabolic periods after acute stress: (1) the "ebb" phase almost immediately after the injury, which is a period of diminished vitality or shock; and (2) the "flow" phase, the subsequent period of increased metabolism or traumatic inflammation that facilitates the healing process.[39] Both anabolic and catabolic processes increase after injury as mediated by the hormonal milieau present. Catabolism occurs predominantly in the carcass (as opposed to vital organ muscle such as liver, kidney, heart, lungs, etc), with skeletal muscle being the major source of extra nitrogen excreted in the urine after injury. Anabolism occurs predominantly in the liver at this time.[39] With this elevated turnover and disposal of nitrogen, only 12% to 22% of total body energy expenditure is from protein while 80% to 90% is from fat oxidation.[40]

The overall effects of stress metabolism is the appearance of hyperglycemia with insulin resistance; increased protein synthesis, breakdown, and catabolism; mobilization and utilization of FFAs for energy; increased energy expendi-

**Table 105.5** Metabolic Effects of Hormones Secreted in Response to Stress

| *Hormone* | *Metabolic effect* |
|---|---|
| Catecholamines | Increased glycogenolysis, inhibition of pancreatic release of insulin, increased fatty acid oxidation |
| Corticosteroids | Increased gluconeogenesis, inhibition of insulin activity, increased muscle catabolism, inhibition of protein synthesis, mobilization of fatty acids, increased protein turnover in the liver and kidney, increased amino acid released from muscle |
| Growth hormone | Increased gluconeogenesis, inhibition of insulin activity, mobilization of fatty acids |
| Glucagon | Increased glycogenolysis, inhibition of insulin activity, increased muscle protein catabolism (proteolysis), inhibition of protein synthesis, mobilization of fatty acids, increased hepatic fatty acid oxidation |

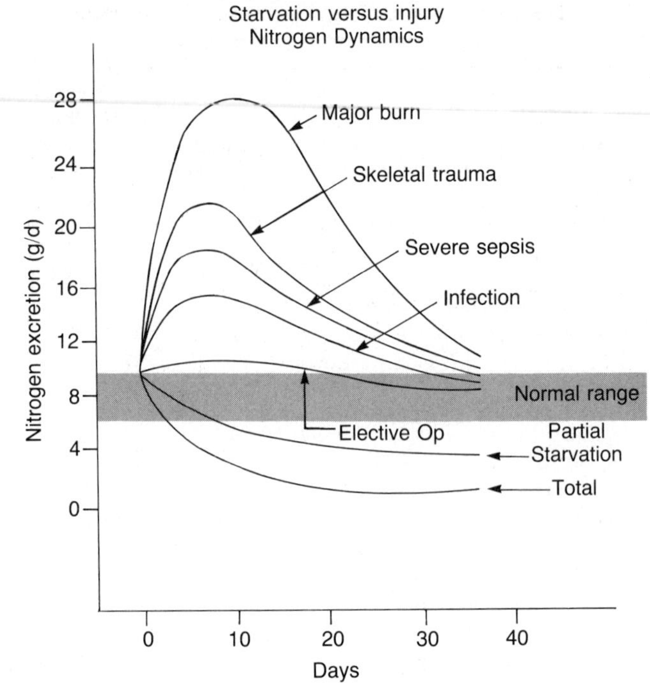


**Figure 105.15** Increase in urinary nitrogen losses in the six patient groups with time.

ture; and urinary nitrogen losses as urea that are quantitatively proportional to the extent of injury.[39] Gluconeogenesis occurs via the glucose–alanine cycle and contributes to lactate production under the anaerobic metabolism occurring in hypoxic tissues. Hypoxia may further contribute to increases in $\beta$-hydroxybutyrate levels, ketone bodies, and the lactate/pyruvate ratio. Energy expenditure (as nitrogen losses[41]) is increased in proportion to the severity of illness (Fig. 105.15).[42] The nitrogen loss during stress is increased not just from disposal of injured or infected tissue but from skeletal muscle (proteolysis) as well.[43]

### Starvation During Stress

Injury blocks the normal adaptation to starvation and its protein conservation effect. Therefore, the protein catabolism of stress is unaltered,[44] hastening protein losses of the body and substantially decreasing the lethal starvation period. In stress, injured tissue, the brain, and kidneys use glucose as a fuel, while the skeletal muscle uses fatty acids for energy. In the injured tissue or wound, glucose undergoes anaerobic metabolism resulting in lactate production. The lactate then becomes a gluconeogenic precursor via the Cori cycle in the liver. The source of the nitrogen loss in injury is the result of an imbalance of protein catabolism and anabolism. Some evidence exists that during stress there may be a decrease in protein synthesis with no change in catabolic rates,[45,46] while others have found an increase in both synthetic and catabolic protein processes.[47,48] These processes are mediated by increased circulating concentrations of catecholamines, glucocorticoids, and glucagon and an inappropriately low insulin concentration in relation to serum glucose concentration.[49] With sepsis as the source of injury, the response is mediated by the release of endogenous pyrogens. Leukocyte endogenous mediator has a direct action on organ metabolism and an indirect effect on CNS and neuroendocrine responses. In contrast to starvation, gluconeogenesis is not turned off by the exogenous administration of glucose in infection and sepsis.[50]

### Hormonal Regulation

Periods of starvation and stress are hormonally mediated. The specific effects of hormones such as catecholamines, glucagon, glucocorticoids, growth hormone, and insulin have been tabulated (Table 105.5). Catecholamines increase hepatic gluconeogenesis, stimulate glycogenolysis, and stimulate the conversion of three-carbon precursors such as lactate and pyruvate to glucose. In skeletal muscle, the mobilization of glycogen stores with subsequent lactate production is stimulated, while in adipose tissue, FFAs are mobilized. Meanwhile, glucagon release is stimulated and insulin secretion by the pancreas is suppressed. The release of glucagon accentuates glycogenolysis, gluconeogenesis, and ureagenesis in the liver and has little effect on skeletal muscle. Glucocorticoids and growth hormone have a permissive effect on the metabolic response to injury. Glucotorticoids potentiate hepatic and skeletal muscle effects of catecholamines by stimulating intracellular enzymes, while growth hormone increases FFA release from adipose tissue and increases peripheral insulin resistance.[28] Insulin concentrations in the circulation are elevated in stress, as the major storage hormone of the body facilitates glycogenesis, lipogenesis, and protein synthesis; however, the differential resistance of adipose and muscle tissue to elevated insulin concentration results in inadequate insulin activity to re-

**Table 105.6** Percentage Loss of Muscle Mass[a] During Starvation and Trauma

| *Condition* | *Duration (d)* | *% Muscle lost* |
|---|---|---|
| Starvation | 1 | 0.6 |
| Starvation | 5 | 3.1 |
| Mild trauma | 5 | 4.1 |
| Severe trauma | 10 | 12.4 |
| Severe trauma | 30 | 36.8 |

[a] Assumes all nitrogen loss is from muscle mass as explained in text.

verse the muscle breakdown and might possibly inhibit lipolysis while allowing the release of amino acids into the bloodstream.

In summary, the hormonal profile of injury produces a rapid lysis of body protein and a quick and maximal rate of fat oxidation. The body favors endogenous stores of fuel while a "biologic importance of the wound" prevails whereby net negative nitrogen balance occurs for the body in toto and positive nitrogen balance exists in the injured tissue.[28] This adaptation of body protein turnover is well tolerated for short periods (Table 105.6), but with extension of this period along with starvation, significant decreases in body cell mass (BCM) could occur (Table 105.6).

### Biological Importance of the Wound

The composite process of wound healing is made up of various components including epithelialization, contraction, establishment of full-thickness continuity, and restoration of tensile strength through collagen synthesis.[28] The biochemical events of collagen synthesis are sensitive to certain nutritional deficiencies.[51,52] Protein deficiency causes a decrease in proteoglycan and collagen synthesis. Methionine is essential for the reversal of the negative influence on collagen production by protein deficiency. Its conversion to cysteine allows for appropriate cofactor activity in the presence of a cation or provides a disulfide bond essential for alignment and triple helix formation of tropocollagen. Vitamins have various effects on collagen synthesis. Ascorbic acid is required for hydroxylation of proline and lysine while vitamin A is reported to counteract the inhibitory action of corticosteroids on collagen synthesis and may be a cofactor for collagen synthesis and crosslinkage. Vitamin E interferes with collagen synthesis and wound repair; the vitamins pyridoxine, riboflavin, and thiamine may act as cofactors in collagen crosslinking reactions.

The major components of collagen are glycine, proline, alanine, and hydroxyproline. Hydroxyproline and hydroxylysine are not found in significant quantities in any other protein than collagen. Approximately every third amino acid in collagen is glycine and 25% of collagen is hydroxyproline. Collagen is low in content of tyrosine and tryptophan (aromatic amino acids). The amino acid sequence of collagen is highly repetitive, with alternating polar (glutamic acid, lysine) and nonpolar compounds. The fibroblast is the active cell of collagen formation.[28]

### Sepsis

Sepsis is a severe metabolic derangement culminating in multiorgan failure and death, apparently as a result of the inhibition of ATP production.[53] The metabolic response is mediated by a leukocyte endogenous mediator, resulting in a fuel deficit appearing as resistance to insulin, carnitine deficiency, and possibly intracellular metabolic blocks that lead to decreased substrate utilization and low oxygen consumption.[54] On muscle biopsy, decreased ATP and increase ADP concentrations have been reported, suggesting an inhibition of substrate entry into the citric acid cycle in muscle during sepsis.[55] This decreased oxygen consumption results in physiologic and hemodynamic abnormalities characteristic of sepsis. The cause of these metabolic blocks may be an alteration in the redox potential and alteration of processes that require oxidized NAD at the mitochondrial level.[54] In comparison to other forms of stress, sepsis is intermediate in magnitude of injury response to traumatic injuries, such as multiple fractures and severe burns.[50]

### Renal Failure

Renal failure patients have impaired ability to excrete nitrogenous waste products or regulate fluid, electrolyte, or acid–base balance. The accumulation of these waste products along with fluid, electrolyte, and acid–base disturbances creates alterations in normal nutrient metabolism. It is important to consider though the difference between chronic and acute renal failure conditions. In chronic renal failure, alterations in fat, carbohydrate, and protein metabolism alter the patient's nutritional status during the course of a chronic and debilitating disease. Acute renal failure is usually associated with other, sometimes critical, diseases; therefore, nutrient metabolism may be the combined effect of altered nutrient metabolism related to renal failure and uremic toxins in addition to stress, sepsis, or other metabolic alterations.

Renal failure influences the hormonal effects of insulin and glucagon. Insulin concentrations are increased, but insulin activity may be reduced, resulting in variable glucose homeostasis. In animals, gluconeogenesis from protein is increased with the recognition of increased alanine synthesis and release from skeletal muscle.[56] Glucose production is increased threefold, an effect directly related to an increase in alanine and glucose turnover. Hemodialysis influences these effects by decreasing gluconeogenesis and possibly improving insulin responsiveness of the peripheral tissue.[57] Glucagon concentrations are elevated in renal disease, an effect that is not influenced by dialytic therapy. In relation to fat metabolism, the decreased insulin effect and impaired lipolytic activity may cause a decrease in triglyceride removal from the blood.

Altered protein metabolism and the renal disease may lead to an intolerance (characterized by uremic symptoms and accumulation of nitrogenous waste) of normal or necessary doses of protein intake for maintaining the dynamic state of body protein. It has been noted that the rate of appearance of urea nitrogen in the body differs depending on the patient's condition; the rate was 12 g/d in patients with acute renal failure after episodes of hypotension and sepsis and only 4 g/d in patients with acute renal failure from nonhypermetabolic illness.[28] Rate of urea nitrogen accumulation and

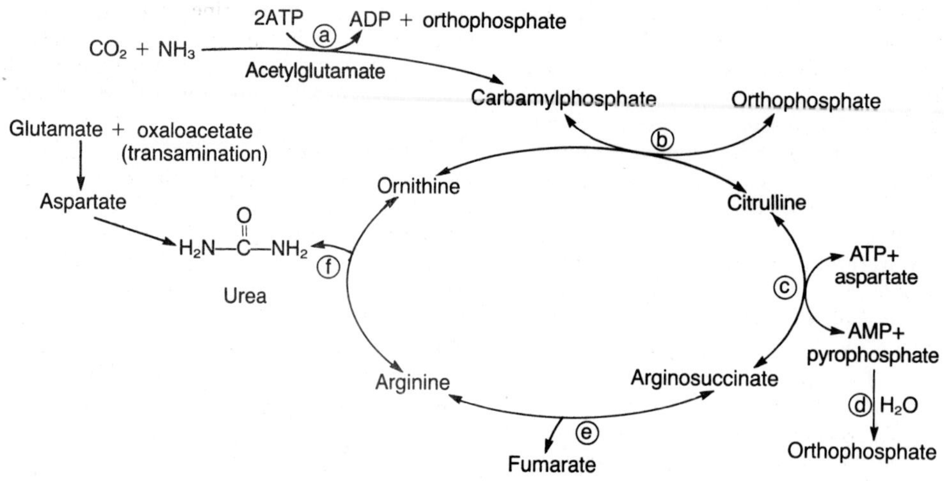


**Figure 105.16** Schematic representation of the urea cycle. (a) carbamoylphosphate synthase, (b) ornithine carbamoyltransferase, (c) arginosuccinate synthetase, (d) pyrophosphatase, (e) arginosuccinate lypase, (f) arginase.

uremic symptoms can be reduced in renal failure patients by the administration of restricted protein doses of high biologic value (high content of essential amino acids).[58] Urea nitrogen in the body can be recycled into new amino acids and protein normally; however, during normal functioning of the urea cycle (Fig. 105.16 and 105.17) in the liver, any ammonia made available from urea metabolism in the gastrointestinal tract returns to the urea pool.[59] Urea cycle activity has been reported to be abnormal in a renal failure patient receiving parenteral nutrition.[60] The clinical effect observed was hyperammonemic encephalopathy. The elevated ammonia levels were believed to be the consequence of inadequate arginine intake even though essential amino acids were provided.[60]

Protein dynamics in renal failure may be altered by dialytic therapy. About 9–12 g of amino acids is lost per hemodialysis procedure.[61] Larger protein losses of up to 13 g albumin, 6 g amino acids, and 22 g of total protein in 36 hours are caused by peritoneal dialysis.[62]

In summary, disorders of amino acid protein synthesis, degradation (proteolysis), and catabolism (such as oxidative deamination) may be attributed to the accumulation of toxic products in renal failure patients. Further deterioration in protein metabolism is related to inadequate intake caused by anorexia, unpalatable diet, and a semifunctional or nonfunctional gastrointestinal tract.[63]

In evaluating intracellular abnormalities occurring in renal disease, Freund[63] has reported a decreased muscle glycogen content, increased glycogenolysis, decreased glycogen synthesis, and increased gluconeogenesis. This leads to increased protein degradation, with the release of intracellular substances such as potassium, phosphorus, and products of nitrogen metabolism to the extracellular water and plasma. The net protein degradation at this point may reach losses of

**Figure 105.17** Aspartate biosynthesis and utilization in urea synthesis.

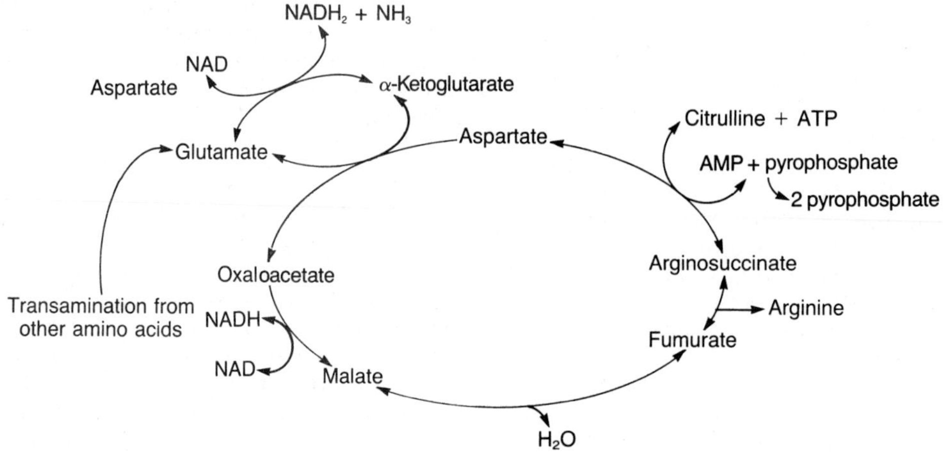

150–250 g/d.[63] Correction of the extracellular accumulation of these cellular products has been attempted by using the absorptive capacity of the peritoneum for both glucose and amino acid instillation. Use of this combination in peritoneal dialysis produces an increase in plasma amino acid concentrations similar to that observed after a protein meal.[63] Normalization of the plasma amino acid profile may correct some of the disturbances in renal failure protein metabolism. Increased levels of urea in renal failure patients result not only from dietary nitrogen intake but more likely from increased protein breakdown (cellular catabolism), impaired protein synthesis (dysanabolism), or increased urea synthetic activity.[64] Proteolysis is increased in renal failure patients as a result of inadequate intake of both calories and protein, coexistent catabolic conditions, circulating proteolytic enzymes, increased levels of catabolic hormones, insulin resistance, and increased nutrient loss during dialysis.[65] Also, urea synthesis may be increased but the protein synthetic rate overall may be unchanged, except for an altered uptake of amino acids by muscle tissue and a decreased hepatic albumin synthesis.[65]

### Liver Disease

The hepatic dysfunction and necrosis that occur during liver disease shunt portal blood flow and decrease the delivery of nutrients to this organ. The liver is the main regulatory organ for metabolism in the body, serving more than 1,500 functions.[66] Injury to this organ markedly impairs nutrient metabolism.

***Carbohydrate Metabolism*** Liver failure causes a sustained gluconeogenesis related to an improper ratio of insulin to glucagon. Decreased hepatic degradation of epinephrine and cortisol may also contribute to abnormal glucose metabolism, resulting in hyperglycemia. In severe cirrhosis, though, hepatic gluconeogenesis may be impaired, leading to severe hypoglycemia.[67]

***Fat Metabolism*** The incomplete metabolism of long-chain fatty acids in liver leads to the accumulation of intermediate metabolites and short-chain fatty acids. Therefore, there is an increased dependency on gluconeogenesis for energy substrate.

***Protein Metabolism*** An intolerance of dietary protein of multiple etiologies is commonly found in liver disease. Increased catabolism for gluconeogenesis[68,69] via the alanine cycle results in increased skeletal muscle utilization of branched-chain amino acids (BCAAs). Plasma concentrations of branched-chain amino acids (BCAAs) are subsequently depressed. Concurrently, the uptake and metabolism of aromatic amino acids (AAAs) and methionine are decreased, resulting in plasma accumulation of these amino acids. The improper profile thus created—a decreased BCAA to AAA and methionine ratio—is associated with hepatic encephalopathy.[70] Hepatic encephalopathy is the result of a preferential CNS uptake of AAAs over BCAAs because of concentration-dependent competition for CNS uptake of these classes of amino acids. With the increased AAA concentrations in the CNS, an imbalance of aminergic substances (norepinephrine, dopamine, and serotonin) occurs and results in the accumulation of false neurotransmitters such as octopamine and other phenylethylamines that may be etiologic factors in hepatic encephalopathy.[71]

***Miscellaneous Effects*** Other nutritional considerations are that malabsorption occurs in 50% of cirrhotic patients, which may affect the availability of fat and thus fat-soluble vitamins[72]; however, medium-chain triglycerides may be absorbed normally. Vitamin deficiencies are due to decreased intake, malabsorption of fat, abnormal hepatic conversion to the active form, or impaired storage for fat-soluble vitamins in the liver. Also, depending on the cause of the liver disease, folic acid, vitamin C, and the B complex vitamins may be deficient.[72]

Alcohol alters the redox state of the liver and decreases gluconeogenesis from lactate by shifting the equilibrium of lactase dehydrogenase toward lactate.[73] The enhanced demand for oxygen that ensues precipitates hepatocellular hypoxia and aggravates hepatic cellular injury. In addition, acetaldehyde, a metabolic product of alcohol metabolism via alcohol dehydrogenase activity is 10 to 30 times more hepatotoxic than alcohol.[73]

The resultant intermediary metabolism of liver disease may be summarized as follows: (1) lactic acidosis leading to decreased uric acid excretion and increased hepatic collagen synthesis and accumulation; (2) alterations in gluconeogenesis depending on stage of disease resulting in either hypoglycemia or hyperglycemia; (3) decreased urea formation with ammonia accumulation or increased renal excretion; (4) increased $\alpha$-glycerophosphate and hepatic triglyceride content; (5) decreased fatty acid oxidation; and (6) decreased protein synthesis possibly related to the altered redox state influencing ribosomal synthesis directly.[74]

### Cardiopulmonary Disease

Cardiopulmonary dysfunction affects the nutritional state and metabolism indirectly. Organ failure affects tolerance of nutrients through impaired expiration of metabolic products (carbon dioxide in the lungs) or reduced capacity to transport nutrients in the circulatory system (cardiac failure). In addition, the increased work or effort exerted by these diseased organs may result in increased or ineffective energy consumption. In heart disease, a decreased nutrient intake may be related to an epigastric fullness caused by chronic hepatic congestion and portal hypertension and an unpalatable low-salt diet. Low cardiac output also causes poor delivery of nutrients to peripheral tissues, leading to "tissue starvation."

### Cancer

There are many nutrient metabolic abnormalities in cancer patients. Anorexia related to an altered taste-and-smell sensation is common.[75] Metabolic abnormalities may also be created by the stress of cancer treatment, be it surgery, chemotherapy, radiation therapy, or their combined complications. Altered metabolism includes increased energy metabolism, glucose intolerance, change in fatty acid metabolism with increased oxidation and lipolysis, and increased protein breakdown and gluconeogenesis from protein as well as lactate.[76] The cancer cell creates a demand for glucose as a fuel at a high rate of anaerobic metabolism. This elevated gluconeogenic activity drains the body's ATP, as 6 mol of ATP is required per mole of synthesized glucose, while anaerobic metabolism of glucose to lactate consumes a further 2 mol of ATP. Per mole of glucose recycled, the body loses 8 mol of ATP. In contrast, the complete oxidation of glucose via the citric acid cycle forms 30 mol of ATP.

The cancer cell depends on glucose as a fuel, even though fatty acids are available from lipolysis created by a deranged insulin-to-glucagon ratio. (Lipolysis will, however, make fat available as an energy source for normal tissues.[77]) Protein turnover and synthesis increase, with an increase in hepatic synthesis, but skeletal muscle synthesis declines.[78] Also, cancer tissue may act as a "nitrogen trap," as protein taken up by the cancer cell may not be influenced by hormonal and neuroendocrine protein control and therefore not be available to support the dynamic protein state that normally exists.

## Obesity

Obesity, a common condition, is the excessive accumulation of fat in the storage areas of the body. Adipose cell enlargement, hyperplasia of the cell, or both may lead to fat accumulation. Obese individuals have a higher likelihood of mortality than lighter individuals.

Obesity is difficult to define, and is usually based on weight, percentage over normal or as weight relates to Metropolitan Life Table definitions of ideal weight. An accepted definition is a body mass index greater than 25 $kg/m^2$. Gross obesity is a body mass greater than 40 $kg/m^2$.[79]

Metabolic abnormalities during obesity relate to insulin homeostasis.[79] Insulin secretion is increased while growth hormone is decreased. Also, cortisol secretion and turnover are increased, which, combined with the insulin status, lead to increased lipogenesis and decreased lipolysis. The pathogenesis of this abnormality may be related to beta cell hypersensitivity to carbohydrate loading to a postprandial hyperinsulinism, hypoglycemia, and hypercorticism. Tissue resistance to insulin along with the resultant hyperglycemia will then cause beta cell hyperplasia. This energy imbalance, along with an excessive energy intake, results in an intensive lipogenesis caused by the hyperinsulin state.[79]

Excess caloric intake also can result in fat accumulation in the liver (fatty infiltration). This fatty liver is the result of increased fatty acid synthesis, accumulation of acetyl CoA from glucose metabolism, and fat storage. This rate of fat synthesis may exceed the liver's normal capacity to mobilize newly synthesized fat, leading to hepatic steatosis.[80] Also, excess energy intake and the resultant lipogenesis may exceed the pulmonary capacity to expire the carbon dioxide produced during lipogenesis.

**Table 105.7** Some Effects of Drugs in Relation to Vitamins

| *Drug* | *Possible vitamin effect* |
|---|---|
| Antacids | Thiamine deficiency |
| Antibiotics | Vitamin K deficiency |
| Antineoplastics | Folic acid antagonism and malabsorption |
| Cathartics | Increased requirements for vitamins D and C and pyridoxine |
| Anticonvulsants | Impaired absorption of vitamin D and folic acid |
| Isonizid | Pyridoxine deficiency |

## Drug Effects on Nutrient Metabolism

The pharmacologic management of disease leads to various abnormalities in nutrient metabolism. Drug effects on appetite and taste-and-smell sensations may impair nutrient intake. Also, gastrointestinal disturbances caused by appropriate or toxic doses of drugs may interfere with nutrient intake or gastrointestinal absorption (Table 105.7). Altered metabolism may result, especially from steroids or other hormones used to control the progression of disease. Finally, increased losses of nutrients may be induced by drugs that affect renal excretion of electrolytes, such as diuretics. Cancer chemotherapeutic agents in particular have many effects on nutrient metabolism that may affect nutrient intake, absorption, assimilation, and excretion.

## Summary

Nutrition affects every metabolic and organ process in the body. As such, the provision of nutrients by either the oral or parenteral route makes available essential nutrients for metabolic purposes; however, it is the capability of the organ, tissue, or cell and the influences of the regulatory systems present at the time of nutrient availability that dictate the metabolic fate of that nutrient. This discussion presents the various possible metabolic fates that a nutrient may undergo after ingestion during both health and disease. Normal metabolism and, therefore, the treatment of malnutrition during disease processes are impaired. As a result, rehabilitation of the malnourished patient requires the stabilization of disease as well. Simply, the provision of nutrients to the body does not necessarily effect a cure for malnutrition unless a favorable metabolic status exists for efficient nutrient utilization.

## References

1. Stedman's Medical Dictionary, 22nd ed. Baltimore, Williams and Wilkins, 1972, p 865.
2. Van Itallie TB. Malnutrition: Concepts of pathogenesis and treatment, in Thorn GW, Adams RO, Braunwald E, et al (eds): Harrison's Principles of Internal Medicine, 8th ed. New York, McGraw-Hill, 1977, pp 442–445.

3. Cahill GF. Intermediary metabolism of protein, fat, and carbohydrate, in Thorn GW, Adams RO, Braunwald E, et al (eds): Harrison's Principles of Internal Medicine, 8th ed. New York, McGraw-Hill, 1977, pp 352–363.
4. The citric acid cycle, in McGilvery RW (ed): Biochemistry, A Functional Approach, 3rd ed. Philadelphia, W.B. Saunders, 1983, pp 421–439.
5. Wolfe BM, Ney DM. Lipid metabolism in parenteral nutrition, in Rombeau JL, Caldwell MD (eds): Clinical Nutrition. Philadelphia, W.B. Saunders, 1986, vol 2: Parenteral Nutrition, pp 72–99
6. The oxidation of fatty acids, in McGilvery RW (ed): Biochemistry, A Functional Approach, 3rd ed. Philadelphia, W.B. Saunders, 1983, pp 440–458.
7. The oxidation of glucose, in McGilvery RW (ed): Biochemistry, A Functional Approach, 3rd ed. Philadelphia, W.B. Saunders, 1983, pp 459–483.
8. Wolfe RR. Carbohydrate metabolism and requirements, in Rombeau JL, Caldwell MD (eds): Clinical Nutrition. Philadelphia, W.B. Saunders, 1986, vol 2: Parenteral Nutrition, pp 53–71.
9. Van Eys J. Nonglucose carbohydrates in parenteral nutrition, in Rombeau JL, Caldwell MD (eds): Clinical Nutrition. Philadelphia, W.B. Saunders, 1986, vol. 2: Parenteral Nutrition, pp 198–209.
10. Amino acids: Disposal of nitrogen, in McGilvery RW (ed): Biochemistry, A Functional Approach, 3rd ed. Philadelphia, W.B. Saunders, 1983, pp 572–592.
11. Amino acids: Disposal of the carbon skeletons, in McGilvery RW (ed): Biochemistry: A Functional Approach, 3rd ed. Philadelphia, W.B. Saunders, 1983, pp 593–617.
12. Rudman D, Millikan WJ, Richardson TJ, et al. Elemental balances during intravenous hyperalimentation of underweight adult subjects. J Clin Invest 1975;55:99–104.
13. Digestion, absorption and metabolism of food, in Hui YH (ed): Human Nutrition and Diet Therapy. Monterey, CA, Wadsworth Health Sciences Division, 1983, pp 193–226.
14. Caldwell MD, Kennedy-Caldwell C. Normal nutritional requirements. Surg Clin North Am 1981;61:489–508.
15. MacMahon RA. The use of the World Health Organization's oral rehydration solution in patients on home parenteral nutrition. J Parenter Enter Nutr 1984;8:720–721.
16. Storage of glucose as glycogen, in McGilvery RW (ed): Biochemistry, A Functional Approach, 3rd ed. Philadelphia, W.B. Saunders, 1983, pp 500–526.
17. Bivins BA, Hyde BL, Sachatello CR, et al. Physiopathology and management of hyperosmolar hyperglycemic nonketotic dehydration. Surg Gynecol Obstet 1982;154:434–440.
18. Glycolysis and gluconeogenesis, in McGilvery RW (ed): Biochemistry. A Functional Approach, 3rd ed. Philadelphia, W.B. Saunders, 1983, pp 484–499.
19. Felig P. The glucose–alanine cycle. Metabolism 1973; 22:179.
20. Zollner N. Evaluation of non-glucose carbohydrates in parenteral nutrition, in Johnston ID (ed): Advances in Parenteral Nutrition. Baltimore, University Park, 1978, p 64.
21. Kirkpatrick JR. Fat and energy metabolism, in Kirkpatrick JR (ed): Nutrition and Metabolism in the Surgical Patient. Mount Kisco, Futura Publishing, 1983, pp 3–28.
22. Mahley RW. Atherogenic hyperlipoproteinemia—the cellular and molecular biology of plasma lipoproteins altered by dietary fat and cholesterol. Med Clin North Am 1982;66:375–403.
23. Stein TP, Buzby GP. Protein metabolism in surgical patients. Surg Clin North Am 1981;61:519–528.
24. Stein TP. Protein metabolism and parenteral nutrition, in Rombeau JL, Caldwell MD (eds): Clinical Nutrition. Philadelphia, W.B. Saunders, 1986, vol 2: Parenteral Nutrition, pp 100–134.
25. Blackburn GL, Bistrian BR, Hemsy FN. Protein metabolism in the surgical patient, in Kirkpatrick JR (ed): Nutrition and Metabolism in the Surgical Patient. Mount Kisco, Futura Publishing, 1983, pp 59–88.
26. Wolfe BM, Ruderman RL. Pollard A. Basic principles of surgical nutrition: Metabolic response to starvation, trauma, and sepsis, in Dietel M (ed): Nutrition in Clinical Surgery, 2nd ed. Baltimore, Williams and Wilkins, 1985, pp 14–23.
27. Amino acids and peptides, in McGilvery RW. Biochemistry, A Functional Approach, 3rd ed. Philadelphia, W.B. Saunders, 1983, pp 3–23.
28. Moore FD, Brennan MF. Surgical injury: Body composition, protein metabolism and neuroendocrinology, in Billinger WF, Collins JA, Saucker WR, et al (eds): Manual of Surgical Nutrition. Philadelphia, W.B. Saunders, 1975, pp 169–222.
29. Ribonucleic acids and formation and function, in McGilvery RW (ed): Biochemistry, A Functional Approach, 3rd ed. Philadelphia, W.B. Saunders, 1983, pp 60–99.
30. Coon WW, Kowalczyk RS. Protein metabolism, in Ballinger WF, Collins JA, Drucker WR, et al (eds): Manual of Surgical Nutrition. Philadelphia, W.B. Saunders, 1975, pp 50–72.
31. Jackson AA. Amino acids: Essential and non-essential? Lancet 1983;1:1034–1037.
32. Minerals, in Alpers DA, Clouse RE, Starson WF (eds): Manual of Nutritional Therapeutics, 1st ed. Boston, Little Brown, 1983, pp 53–110.
33. Gann DS, Robinson HB. Salt, water and vitamins, in Ballinger WF, Collins JA, Drucker WR, et al (eds): Manual of Surgical Nutrition. Philadelphia, W.B. Saunders, 1975, pp 73–92.
34. Mequid MM, Collin MP, Howard LJ. Uncomplicated and stressed starvation. Surg Clin North Am 1981;61:529–544.
35. Aoki TT, Finley RJ. The metabolic response to fasting, in Rombeau JL, Caldwell MD (eds): Clinical Nutrition. Philadelphia, W.B. Saunders, 1986, vol 2: Parenteral Nutrition, pp 9–28.
36. Cahill GF. Starvation in man. N Engl J Med 1978;282:668–675.
37. Levenson SM, Crowley LV, Seifter E. Starvation, in Ballinger WF, Collins JA, Drucker WR, et al (eds): Manual of Surgical Nutrition. Philadelphia, W.B. Saunders, 1975, pp 236–266.
38. Felig P, Owen OE, Wahren J, et al. Amino acid metabolism during prolonged starvation. J Clin Invest 1969;48:584–594.
39. Cuthberton DP. Alterations in metabolism following injury: Part 1. Injury 1979;11:175–89.
40. Duke JG, Jorgenson SB, Broell JR, et al. The contribution of protein to caloric expenditure following injury. Surgery 1970;68:168.
41. Long CL, Kinney JM, Broell JR, et al. Contribution of protein to caloric expenditure. Surgery 1970;68:168–174.
42. Long CL, Schaffel N, Geiger JW, et al. Metabolic response to injury and illness: Estimation of energy and protein needs from indirect calorimetry and nitrogen balance. J Parenter Enter Nutr 1979;3:452–456.
43. Airlick LH, Wilmore DW. Increased peripheral amino acid release following burn injury. Surgery 1979;85:560–565.
44. Gann DS. Endocrine and metabolic response to injury, in Schwartz SI (ed): Principles of Surgery, 3rd ed. New York, McGraw-Hill, 1979, pp 1–63.
45. O'Keefe SJD, Sculler PM, James WPT. "Catabolic" loss of body nitrogen in response to surgery. Lancet 1974;2:1035–1037.
46. Crane CW, Pilou D, Smith R, et al. Protein turnover in patients before and after elective orthopedic operations. Br J Surg 1977; 64:129–33.
47. Kien CL, Young VR, Rohrbaugh DK, et al. Increased rates of

whole body protein synthesis and breakdown in children recovering from burns. Ann Surg 1978;187:383–391.
48. Wolfe RR, Goodenough RD, Burke JF, et al. Response of protein and urea kinetics in burn patients to different levels of protein intake. Ann Surg 1983;197:163–171.
49. Kudsk KA, Mirtallo JM. Nutritional support of the critically ill patient. Drug Intell Clin Pharm 1983;17:501–506.
50. Long CL. Energy balance and carbohydrate metabolism in infection and sepsis. Am J Clin Nutr 1977;30:1301–1310.
51. Ruberg RL. Role of nutrition and wound healing. Surg Clin North Am 1984;64:705–714.
52. Kanke Y, Bashey RI, Mori Y. Biochemistry of collagen. NY State Med J 1981;81:1045–1052.
53. Freund HR. Parenteral nutrition in the septic patient, in Rombeau JL, Caldwell MD (eds): Clinical Nutrition. Philadelphia, W.B. Saunders, 1986, vol 2: Parenteral Nutrition, pp 533–554.
54. Cerra FB, Caprioli J, Siegel JH, et al. Proline metabolism in sepsis, cirrhosis and general surgery. Ann Surg 1979;190:577–581.
55. Bergstrom J, Bostrous H, Furst R, et al. Pulmonary studies of energy rich phosphorus in critically ill patients. Crit Care Med 1976;4:197–204.
56. Maillet C, Garber SJ. Skeletal muscle amino acid metabolism in chronic uremia. Am J Clin Nutr 1980;33:1343–1353.
57. Furannini E, Pilo A, Navalise A, et al. Insulin kinetics and glucose-induced insulin delivery in chronically dialyzed subjects: Acute effects of dialysis. J Clin Endocrinol Metab 1979; 49:15–22.
58. Feistein EL, Blumenkrantz MJ, Healy H, et al. Clinical and metabolic responses to parenteral nutrition in acute renal failure: A controlled double blind study. Medicine 1981;60:124–137.
59. Mirtallo JM, Kudsk KA, Ebbert ML. Nutritional support of patients with renal disease. Clin Pharm 1984;3:253–263.
60. Rapp RD, Bivins BA, McRoberts JW. Hyperammonemia encephalopathy in a patient receiving essential amino acid/dextrose parenteral nutrition. Clin Pharm 1982;1:276–280.
61. Kopple JD, Cianciaruso B. Nutritional management of acute renal failure, in Fischer JE (ed): Surgical Nutrition. Boston, Little Brown, 1983, pp 567–589.
62. Blumenkrantz MJ, Gahl GM, Kopple JD, et al. Protein loss during peritoneal dialysis. Kidney Int 1981;19:593–602.
63. Freund HR. Acute renal failure, in Dietel M (ed): Nutrition in Clinical Surgery, 2nd ed. Baltimore, Williams and Wilkins, 1985, pp 348–356.
64. Steffee WP. Nutritional support in renal failure. Surg Clin North Am 1978;61:661–670.
65. Feinstein EZ. Nutrition in acute renal failure, in Rombeau JL, Caldwell MD (eds): Clinical Nutrition. Philadelphia, W.B. Saunders, 1986, vol 2: Parenteral Nutrition, pp 586–601.
66. Metabolism-Detoxication Mechanisms: Synthesis of urea. Documenta Geigy, Scientific Tables, in Diem K, Lenter C (eds): 7th ed. 1970, pp 443–444.
67. Owen OE, Richle FA, Mozzoli MA, et al. Hepatic, gut, and renal substrate flux rates in patients with hepatic cirrhosis. J Clin Invest 1981;68:240–252.
68. Morgan MY, Milson JP, Sherlock S. Plasma ratio of valine, leucine and isoleucine to phenylalanine and tyrosine in liver disease. Gut 1978;19:1068–1073.
69. Cascino A, Cangiano C, Calcaterra V, et al. Plasma amino acids imbalances in patients with liver disease. Dig Dis 1978;23:591–598.
70. Fischer JE, Fumovics JM, Aquierre A, et al. The role of plasma amino acids in hepatic encephalopathy. Surgery 1978; 80:77–91.
71. Nachbauer CT, Fischer JE. Nutritional support in hepatic failure, in Fischer JE (ed): Surgical Nutrition. Boston, Little Brown, 1983, pp 551–565.
72. Reilly JJ, Gerhardt AL. Modern surgical nutrition. Curr Probl Surg 1985;22:1–81.
73. Geokas ML, Lieber CS, French S, et al. Ethanol, the liver, and the gastrointestinal tract. Ann Intern Med 1981;95:198–211.
74. Lieber CS. Alcohol, protein metabolism, and liver injury. Gastroenterology 1980;79:373–390.
75. Brennan MF. Total parenteral nutrition in the cancer patient. N Engl J Med 1981;305:375–382.
76. Wesdorp RIC, Krause R, Von Meyenfeldt MF. Cancer cachexia and its nutritional implications. Br J Surg 1983;70:352–355.
77. Harris BA, Probert JC. Nutrition and metabolism in cancer patients: A review. NZ Med J 1981;94:227–229.
78. Lowry SF, Brennan MF. Intravenous feeding of the cancer patient, in Rombeau JL, Caldwell MD (eds): Clinical Nutrition. Philadelphia, W.B. Saunders, 1986, vol 2: Parenteral Nutrition, pp 445–470.
79. Mazansky H. A review of obesity and its management in 203 cases. S Afr Med J 1975;49:1955–1962.
80. Wolfe BM, Chock E. Energy sources, stores and hormonal controls. Surg Clin North Am 1981;61:509–518.

# Chapter 106 / Assessment, Prevalence, and Clinical Significance of Malnutrition

Kathleen M. Teasley, MS

The scientific basis for nutritional assessment is rapidly developing and changing. Old parameters are being applied to new patient populations (e.g., patients with organ failure or high-level metabolic stress, the elderly) and require new interpretations. New parameters, such as plasma amino acid profiles and neutron activation analysis, are being evaluated for validity and clinical applicability. The interpretation of each parameter currently available for use in the nutritional assessment of a hospitalized patient requires a combination of clinical skills and a knowledge of patient-specific factors which may effect each parameter. The significance of the nutritional assessment must then be determined relative to the clinical outcome of the patient.

This chapter is a critical review of the current parameters used for nutritional assessment of the hospitalized patient. Nutritional diagnoses are defined both generally and in terms of specific nutritional assessment parameters. The prevalence of hospital malnutrition as defined by selected parameters is documented, and the significance of observed abnormalities in these nutritional assessment parameters is evaluated relative to morbidity and mortality. It is the purpose of this chapter to present information that enables the clinician to develop a scheme for accurate, relevant, and cost-effective nutritional assessment of the hospitalized patient.

## Diagnosis of Nutritional Disease

Malnutrition, or more specifically undernutrition, results from starvation or altered metabolism. In starvation states the problem is one of not getting adequate amounts of the appropriate nutrition to the cells. A metabolic alteration exists when the cell has altered substrate demands or utilization characteristics. The outcome of malnutrition is an inappropriate reduction in lean body mass resulting in loss of structure and/or function (Table 106.1). A clinically useful definition of malnutrition, therefore, is a state induced by alterations in dietary intake or nutrient utilization resulting in changes in subcellular, cellular, and/or organ function that expose the individual to increased risks of morbidity and mortality and that can be reversed by appropriate nutritional support.[1]

In general, deficiency states can be grouped into those involving protein and calories (protein-calorie malnutrition, PCM) and those stemming from single nutrients such as individual vitamins or trace minerals. Three terms are used to describe PCM[2,3]:

1. *Marasmus* is a chronic condition resulting from a deficiency in total energy intake. Consequently, the individual's reserves of protein and energy are depleted. There is wasting of both somatic protein (skeletal muscle) and adipose stores, but visceral protein production is preserved. When severe, cell-mediated immunity (measured by delayed hypersensitivity) and muscle function are impaired. Patients with wasting diseases such as cancer commonly have marasmus and a starved, cachectic appearance. The relative weight loss threshold for marasmus is 85% of ideal body weight.
2. *Kwashiorkor* is common in patients who have adequate calorie intake but a relative protein deficiency and who are catabolic, usually with trauma, infection, or burns. There is depletion of visceral (and to some degree somatic) protein pools with relative preservation of adipose tissue. Kwashiorkor is classically characterized by hypoalbuminemia and edema. This condition may develop rapidly in response to protein deprivation in the setting of metabolic stress and may be accompanied by impaired immunofunction.
3. *Mixed kwashiorkor/marasmus* is a form of severe PCM in chronically ill, starved patients who are undergoing hypermetabolic stress. It manifests as reduced visceral protein synthesis superimposed on wasting of somatic protein and energy (adipose tissue) stores. Immunocompetence is lowered, the incidence of infection is increased, and there is poor wound healing.

Single-nutrient deficiencies can occur in combination with any of the preceding diagnoses and commonly do. Depletion of individual nutrients leads to symptoms related to that nutrient's function. Therefore, recognition and treatment of nutritional deficiency states must be inclusive of all nutrients to facilitate metabolic processes and allow for repletion.

## Assessment of Nutritional Status

### *Clinical Evaluation*

Clinical evaluation with history and physical examination remains the oldest, simplest, and probably most widely used method of evaluating nutritional status. Clinical evaluation of nutritional status has been well-correlated with objective evaluations (e.g., laboratory parameters, anthropometric measurements).[4] Laboratory parameters confirm the diagnosis, quantify the degree of malnutrition, and reflect the end-organ changes that occur with malnutrition. These ob-

Table 106.1 End-Organ Responses in Malnutrition

| *Organ* | *Anatomical responses* | *Physiological responses* |
|---|---|---|
| Heart | Four-chamber dilation; atrophic degeneration with necrosis and fibrosis; myofibrillar disruption | QT prolongation, low voltage, bradycardia; decreased cardiac output, stroke volume, and contractility; preload intolerance; diminished responsiveness to drugs |
| Lung | Emphysematous changes; pulmonary infarcts; reduced bacterial clearance; muscle atrophy | Pneumonia; decreases in functional residual capacity, vital capacity, and maximum breathing capacity; depressed hypoxic/hypercarbic drives |
| Hematologic system | Failure of stem cell production; depressed erythropoietin synthesis; decreased PMN chemotaxis; decreased lymphocyte count with reduced helper T and increased suppressor T and killer cells; decreased blastogenesis to phytohemagglutinin; depressed erythropoietin synthesis | Anemia; anergy; decreased granuloma formation; impaired response to chemotherapy; increased infection rate |
| Renal system | Epithelial swelling; atrophy; mild cortical calcification | Reduced glomerular filtration rate and inability to handle sodium loads; polyuria; metabolic acidosis |
| Gastrointestinal tract | Disproportionate mass loss; hypoplastic and atrophic changes; decrease in total mucosal height | Depressed enzymatic activity; shortened transit time; impaired motility, propensity for bacterial overgrowth; maldigestion and malabsorption |
| Liver | Mass loss; periportal fat accumulation | Decreased visceral protein synthesis; depressed microsomal activity; eventual hepatic insufficiency |

From Cerra FB: Manual of Surgical Nutrition. St. Louis, C.V. Mosby, 1984, p 6, with permission.

jective parameters also provide a baseline for the nutritional therapies that follow.

The clinical evaluation consists of a routine history and a physical examination. The medical history provides information about factors that predispose the patient to developing malnutrition (e.g., chronic disease, gastrointestinal malfunction, alcohol abuse). The medical history should emphasize weight loss, anorexia, vomiting, diarrhea, and decreased or unusual food intake (Table 106.2). The physical examination focuses on an assessment of lean body mass and the physical findings of vitamin, trace element, and essential fatty acid deficiency. The assessment should emphasize muscle wasting, edema, loss of subcutaneous fat, dermatitis, glossitis, cheilosis, and jaundice (Table 106.3).

### *Anthropometric Measurements*

Anthropometric measurements are gross measurements of body cell mass. The most common measurements are height, weight, and measurements of limb size, such as midarm muscle circumference, skinfold thickness, and wrist circumference. These parameters are used in two ways—to compare an individual with a population and as repeated measurements to indicate the response of an individual to changes in nutritional environment. Nutrition-related changes in anthropometric measurements are long term; weeks are required for detectable changes to occur. Acute changes in anthropometric measurements, specifically weight and skinfold thickness, usually reflect changes in fluid status, and fluid must be considered in the interpretation of these parameters.

Body weight is a nonspecific measure of body cell mass, representing skeletal mass, body fat, and the energy-utilizing component referred to as the "lean body mass."[5] Changes in weight over time, particularly in the absence of edema, ascites, and voluntary losses, are an important indicator of altered lean body mass. Interpretation of any actual body weight (ABW) measurement should take into consideration: ideal weight for height, usual body weight, fluid status, and age.

The ideal body weight for height (IBW) provides a population reference standard against which the ABW can be compared. The ideal weight for a given height is that weight correlating with maximum longevity. Numerous reference tables exist based on various population statistics.[6–8] The most commonly accepted table of ideal weight for height is that from the 1959 Metropolitan Life Insurance's Data (Table 106.4).[9] The percentage IBW is derived from the equation %IBW = (ABW/IBW) × 100. A more accurate reflection of clinically and nutritionally significant change in weight makes use of the patient's usual body weight (UBW) as a reference point. Determining a patient's UBW, however, usually depends on recall which may be inaccurate.[10] The percentage UBW is derived with the formula %UBW = (ABW/UBW) × 100. This method avoids the problems of normative tables and documents comparative changes in body weight. The change in weight must be interpreted relative to time (Table 106.5). An absolute unintentional weight loss of more than 10 pounds in less than 6 months has

**Table 106.2** Pertinent Historical Data for Nutritional Assessment

A. Nutrition intake/diet history
1. Anorexia; change in taste
2. Actual intake; special diets
3. Supplemental vitamin or mineral intake
4. Food allergies or intolerance

B. Underlying pathology with nutritional effects
1. Chronic infections or inflammatory states
2. Neoplastic diseases
3. Endocrine disorders
4. Chronic illnesses including pulmonary disease, cirrhosis, renal failure
5. Hypermetabolic states—trauma, burns, sepsis
6. Digestive or absorptive diseases
7. Hyperlipidemia

C. End-organ effects
1. Weight changes
2. Skin or hair changes
3. Exercise tolerance, fatigue
4. Obesity
5. Muscle mass relative to exercise status
6. Gastrointestinal tract symptoms—diarrhea, vomiting, constipation

D. Miscellaneous
1. Catabolic medications or therapies: steroids, immunosuppressive agents, radiation, or chemotherapy
2. Genetic background: body habitus of parents, siblings, and family
3. Other medications: diuretics, laxatives
4. Alcohol or drug abuse

been correlated with an increased incidence of mortality in adult surgical patients.[11]

Interpretation of a body weight measurement is also dependent on knowledge of the patient's hydrational status. Dehydration from nausea, vomiting, or other fluid losses results in a decreased body weight but not a loss in body cell mass. The presence of edema or ascites indicates excess total body water, which will increase body weight. More subtle changes in fluid status may be detected by monitoring the patient's daily fluid intake and output and should be evaluated coincident with weight changes.

Skinfold thickness measurement provides an estimate of subcutaneous fat. More than half of the total body fat is subcutaneous, and changes in subcutaneous fat have been assumed to reflect changes in body fat.[12] The measurement of skinfold thickness is relatively insensitive to short-term changes in tissue composition, but serial measurements in a given patient performed by the same trained observer on the same body side are reproducible.[13] Triceps-skinfold thickness (TSF) is the most common site of measurement, although reference standards also exist for subscapular and iliac sites. Careful technique and the use of pressure-regulated calipers (Lange, Halipern) are essential for reproducibility and reliability in measuring TSF[14]:

1. Position the patient sitting, with nondominant arm hanging freely at the side, or supine, with the nondominant arm flexed at the shoulder to the vertical position with the forearm crossing the chest.
2. Mark the midpoint between the acromion (bony point of the shoulder) and the olecranon (bony prominence of the elbow) posteriorly over the triceps muscle.
3. Gently pinch the skin and subcutaneous tissue at the midpoint and apply the caliper for 3 seconds before taking the reading.
4. Perform the procedure three times, taking an average of the values obtained.

**Table 106.3** Physical Findings Suggestive of Malnutrition

A. General appearance
1. Edema
2. Cachexia or obesity
3. Ascites
4. Signs and symptoms of dehydration—skin turgor, sunken eyes, orthostasis, dry mucous membranes

B. Skin and mucous membranes
1. Thin, shiny, or scaling skin
2. Decubitus ulcers
3. Ecchymoses, perifollicular petechiae
4. Poorly healing surgical or traumatic wounds
5. Pallor or redness of gums, fissures at mouth edges
6. Glossitis; stomatitis; cheilosis

C. Musculoskeletal
1. Retarded growth
2. Bone pain or tenderness, epiphyseal swelling
3. Muscle mass less than expected for habitus, genetic history, and level of exercise

D. Neurologic
1. Ataxia, positive Romberg test, decreased vibratory or position sense
2. Nystagmus
3. Convulsions, paralysis
4. Encephalopathy

E. Hepatic
1. Jaundice
2. Hepatomegaly

The value measured is compared with population standards (Table 106.6). Values between the 35th and 40th percentiles indicate mild depletion, between the 25th and 35th percentiles, moderate depletion, and below the 25th percentile, severe depletion.[15]

Interpretation of results must include consideration of differences in body build, particularly extremes such as obesity or muscle hypertrophy associated with weight training. Fat-reserve measurements do not necessarily correlate with muscle mass and body protein status.

Midarm-muscle assessment is based on the measurement of midarm circumference (MAC). This value is used to calculate midarm-muscle circumference (MAMC) and was designed as a noninvasive, easy, inexpensive method of assessing skeletal muscle mass. Triceps MAC is measured at the same midpoint as triceps-skinfold thickness. MAMC is calculated with the equation[16]

$$\text{MAMC (cm)} = \text{MAC (cm)} - \text{TSF (mm)}/10$$

**Table 106.4** Ideal Weight for Height[a]

| *Height (cm)* | *Weight (kg)* | *Height (cm)* | *Weight (kg)* | *Height (cm)* | *Weight (kg)* |
|---|---|---|---|---|---|
| **Males** | | | | | |
| 157 | 58.6 | 167 | 64.6 | 177 | 71.6 |
| 158 | 59.3 | 168 | 65.2 | 178 | 72.4 |
| 159 | 59.9 | 169 | 65.9 | 179 | 73.3 |
| 160 | 60.5 | 170 | 66.6 | 180 | 74.2 |
| 161 | 61.1 | 171 | 67.3 | 181 | 75.0 |
| 162 | 61.7 | 172 | 68.0 | 182 | 75.8 |
| 163 | 62.3 | 173 | 68.7 | 183 | 76.5 |
| 164 | 62.9 | 174 | 69.4 | 184 | 77.3 |
| 165 | 63.5 | 175 | 70.1 | 185 | 78.1 |
| 166 | 64.0 | 176 | 70.8 | 186 | 78.9 |
| **Females** | | | | | |
| 140 | 44.9 | 150 | 50.4 | 160 | 56.2 |
| 141 | 45.4 | 151 | 51.0 | 161 | 56.9 |
| 142 | 45.9 | 152 | 51.5 | 162 | 57.6 |
| 143 | 46.4 | 153 | 52.0 | 163 | 58.3 |
| 144 | 47.0 | 154 | 52.5 | 164 | 58.9 |
| 145 | 47.5 | 155 | 53.1 | 165 | 59.5 |
| 146 | 48.0 | 156 | 53.7 | 166 | 60.1 |
| 147 | 48.6 | 157 | 54.3 | 167 | 60.7 |
| 148 | 49.2 | 158 | 54.9 | 168 | 61.4 |
| 149 | 49.8 | 159 | 55.5 | 169 | 62.1 |

[a] This table represents Metropolitan Life Insurance's 1959 data corrected to nude weight and height without shoes.

From Metropolitan Life Insurance Company: Statistical Bulletin, New Weights and Standards for Men and Women 1959;40:Nov–Dec, with permission.

This calculation assumes the compartment is round, that TSF is accurate and consistent about the circumference, and that the bone is of constant cross-sectional area. The calculated value for MAMC is compared with population standards (Table 106.7). A decrease from the expected value at the 20th percentile suggests a significant reduction in somatic protein mass.[15]

General considerations for the interpretation of both triceps-skinfold thickness and midarm-muscle circumference are the following:

1. Standards do not account for individual variations in bone size, hydrational status, or skin compressibility.
2. Technique is critical and interobserver error may be as high as 30%.
3. These parameters are slow to change, often requiring weeks before significant alterations from baseline can be observed.
4. These are excellent tests for both population analysis and individual long-term monitoring.

**Table 106.5** Weight Changes Reflecting Significant Loss of Body Mass

| *Time* | *Significant weight loss (%)* | *Severe weight loss (%)* |
|---|---|---|
| 1 wk | 1–2 | >2 |
| 1 mo | 5 | >5 |
| 3 mo | 7.5 | >7.5 |
| 6 mo | 10 | >10 |

From Blackburn GL, Bistrian BR, Maini BS, et al: Nutritional and metabolic assessment of the hospitalized patient. J Parenter Enter Nutr 1977;1:17, with permission.

### *Biochemical Parameters of Lean Body Mass*

The lean body mass is represented by both structural proteins (skeletal muscle somatic protein compartment) and functional proteins (circulating proteins, visceral protein compartment). The somatic protein compartment, which has thus far been quantified by body weight and midarm-muscle circumference measurements, can be further assessed by creatinine–height index and visceral protein levels.

Creatinine–height index (CHI) is based on creatinine, which is the metabolic end product of creatine, a complex molecule synthesized in the liver and concentrated mainly in body muscle. Creatinine is excreted unchanged in the urine; therefore, collection of a timed urine with measurement of total creatinine excreted indirectly reflects on the total muscle mass.[17] For clinical assessment, the creatinine production of an individual patient is compared with expected excretion by a healthy individual of similar height and ideal weight. Expected creatinine excretion is derived from the product of the mean creatinine excretion in healthy young

**Table 106.6** Percentiles for Triceps Skinfold Thickness[a] of Adults in the United States

| | *Population percentile* | | | | | | |
|---|---|---|---|---|---|---|---|
| ***Age (yr)*** | **5** | **10** | **25** | **50** | **75** | **90** | **95** |
| Men | | | | | | | |
| 18–24 | 4.0 | 5.0 | 7.0 | 9.5 | 14.0 | 20.0 | 21.0 |
| 25–34 | 4.5 | 5.5 | 8.0 | 12.0 | 16.0 | 21.5 | 24.0 |
| 35–44 | 5.0 | 6.0 | 8.5 | 12.0 | 15.5 | 20.0 | 23.0 |
| 45–54 | 5.0 | 6.0 | 8.0 | 11.0 | 15.0 | 20.0 | 25.5 |
| 55–64 | 5.0 | 6.0 | 8.0 | 11.0 | 14.0 | 18.0 | 21.5 |
| 65–74 | 4.5 | 5.5 | 8.0 | 11.0 | 15.0 | 19.0 | 22.0 |
| Women | | | | | | | |
| 18–24 | 9.4 | 11.0 | 14.0 | 18.0 | 24.0 | 30.0 | 34.0 |
| 25–34 | 10.5 | 12.0 | 16.0 | 21.0 | 26.5 | 31.5 | 37.0 |
| 35–44 | 12.0 | 14.0 | 18.0 | 23.0 | 29.5 | 39.5 | 39.0 |
| 45–54 | 13.0 | 15.0 | 20.0 | 25.0 | 30.0 | 36.0 | 40.0 |
| 55–64 | 11.0 | 14.0 | 19.0 | 25.0 | 30.5 | 35.0 | 39.0 |
| 65–74 | 11.5 | 14.0 | 18.0 | 23.0 | 28.0 | 33.0 | 36.0 |

[a] Triceps skinfold thickness in millimeters.

From Bishop CW, Bower PE, Ritchey SJ: Norms for nutritional assessment of American adults by upper arm anthropometry. Am J Clin Nutr 1981;34:2533, with permission.

men (23 mg/kg/d) and women (18 mg/kg/d) and the ideal weight for height (Table 106.8).[18] The CHI is the percentage the actual 24-hour creatinine represents of the expected value.

$$\text{CHI} = \frac{\text{actual 24-hour creatinine excretion}}{\text{ideal 24-hour creatinine excretion}} \times 100\%$$

A CHI of 80% or greater indicates no or mild somatic muscle depletion, a CHI of 60% to 80% indicates moderate depletion, and a CHI less than 60% represents severe depletion.[19] The CHI does not accurately reflect muscle mass in patients with impaired renal function and dehydration and may be affected by a high dietary protein intake, steroids, age, or stress. It is also dependent on the accuracy of the 24-hour urine collection and the appropriateness of the ideal weight for height standards.

The visceral protein compartment is assessed by measuring the concentration of serum transport proteins synthesized in the liver. It is assumed that a low serum protein

**Table 106.7** Percentiles for Midarm Muscle Circumferences[a] of Adults in the United States

| | *Population percentile* | | | | | | |
|---|---|---|---|---|---|---|---|
| ***Age (yr)*** | **5** | **10** | **25** | **50** | **75** | **90** | **95** |
| Men | | | | | | | |
| 18–24 | 235 | 244 | 258 | 272 | 289 | 308 | 323 |
| 25–34 | 242 | 253 | 265 | 280 | 300 | 317 | 329 |
| 35–44 | 250 | 256 | 271 | 287 | 303 | 321 | 330 |
| 45–54 | 240 | 249 | 265 | 281 | 298 | 315 | 326 |
| 55–64 | 228 | 244 | 262 | 279 | 296 | 310 | 318 |
| 65–74 | 225 | 237 | 253 | 268 | 285 | 299 | 307 |
| Women | | | | | | | |
| 18–24 | 177 | 185 | 194 | 206 | 221 | 236 | 249 |
| 25–34 | 183 | 189 | 200 | 214 | 229 | 249 | 266 |
| 35–44 | 185 | 192 | 206 | 220 | 240 | 261 | 274 |
| 45–54 | 188 | 195 | 207 | 222 | 243 | 266 | 278 |
| 55–64 | 186 | 195 | 208 | 226 | 244 | 263 | 281 |
| 65–74 | 186 | 195 | 208 | 225 | 244 | 265 | 281 |

[a] Midarm muscle circumference in millimeters.

From Bishop CW, Bowen PE, Ritchey SJ: Norms for nutritional assessment of American adults by upper arm anthropometry. Am J Clin Nutr 1981;34:2533–2534, with permission.

**Table 106.8** Ideal 24-Hour Urinary Creatinine Excretion by Adults of Various Heights (for Use in Calculation of the Creatinine–Height Index)

| *Height* | | *Ideal creatinine excretion (mg)* | |
|---|---|---|---|
| **in.** | **cm** | **Adult women**[a] | **Adult men**[b] |
| 58 | 147.3 | 830 | — |
| 59 | 149.9 | 851 | — |
| 60 | 152.4 | 875 | — |
| 61 | 154.9 | 900 | — |
| 62 | 157.5 | 925 | 1,288 |
| 63 | 160.0 | 949 | 1,325 |
| 64 | 162.6 | 977 | 1,359 |
| 65 | 165.1 | 1,006 | 1,386 |
| 66 | 167.6 | 1,044 | 1,426 |
| 67 | 170.2 | 1,076 | 1,467 |
| 68 | 172.7 | 1,109 | 1,513 |
| 69 | 175.3 | 1,141 | 1,555 |
| 70 | 177.8 | 1,174 | 1,596 |
| 71 | 180.3 | 1,206 | 1,642 |
| 72 | 182.9 | 1,240 | 1,691 |
| 73 | 185.4 | — | 1,739 |
| 74 | 188.0 | — | 1,785 |
| 75 | 190.5 | — | 1,831 |
| 76 | 193.0 | — | 1,891 |

[a] Creatinine coefficient (women) = 18 mg/kg of ideal body weight.
[b] Creatinine coefficient (men) = 23 mg/kg of ideal body weight.

From Blackburn GL, Bistrian RB, Maini BS, et al: Nutritional and metabolic assessment of the hospitalized patient. J Parenter Enter Nutr 1977;1:12, with permission.

concentration in states of malnutrition reflects the hepatic protein synthetic mass[20] and, therefore, indirectly the functional protein mass of other organs such as heart, lung, kidney, and intestines. The visceral proteins that are currently thought to be of greatest relevance for nutritional assessment are serum albumin, transferrin, retinol-binding protein, and thyroxine-binding prealbumin. Many factors besides nutrition affect the serum concentration of these proteins, such as abnormal losses via the kidney (e.g., nephrotic syndrome) or gastrointestinal tract (e.g., protein-losing enteropathy), hydrational status (dehydration may result in hemoconcentration, overhydration in hemodilution), and hepatic function. Therefore, visceral protein data must be interpreted relative to the clinical status of the individual (Table 106.9).

Albumin was one of the first biochemical markers of malnutrition and has long been used in population studies. Because of a large body pool size (4–5 g/kg body weight), a high extravascular distribution (60%), and a long biologic half-life (20 days), albumin is a relatively insensitive index of early protein malnutrition; however, chronic protein deficiency in the setting of adequate nonprotein caloric intake leads to marked hypoalbuminemia because of a net loss of albumin from the intravascular and extravascular pools (Kwashiorkor malnutrition). Serum albumin concentrations are also affected by zinc deficiency, caloric deficiency, hepatic disease, renal disease, and infection. Although interpretation of serum albumin concentrations is difficult, data consistently indicate a positive correlation between depressed albumin levels and poor clinical outcome.[21–25]

Transferrin is the glycoprotein that binds and transports ferric iron. It is more likely to respond to protein depletion before alterations in albumin are manifest because of its

**Table 106.9** Summary of Visceral Proteins Used for Assessment of Lean Body Mass

| | | *Values during malnutrition* | | | | |
|---|---|---|---|---|---|---|
| *Laboratory test* | *Normal values* | **Mild malnutrition** | **Moderate malnutrition** | **Severe malnutrition** | *Factors resulting in increased values* | *Factors resulting in decreased values* |
| Albumin (g/dL) | 3.5 | 2.8–3.5 | 2.1–2.7 | 2.1 | Dehydration, anabolic steroids, insulin, infection | Overhydration, edema, renal insufficiency, nephrotic syndrome, poor intake, impaired digestion, burns, congestive heart failure, cirrhosis, thyroid/adrenal/pituitary hormones |
| Transferrin (mg/dL) | 200–400 | 150–200 | 100–150 | 100 | Iron deficiency, pregnancy, hypoxia, chronic blood loss, estrogens | Chronic infection, cirrhosis, iron overdose, enteropathies, nephrotic syndrome, burns, cortisone, testosterone |
| Thyroxin-binding prealbumin (mg/dL) | 10–40 | 10–15 | 5–10 | 5 | Renal dysfunction | Cirrhosis, hepatitis, stress, inflammation, surgery, hyperthyroidism, cystic fibrosis, renal dysfunction |
| Retinol-binding protein (mg/dL) | 2.7–7.6 | Not defined | Not defined | Not defined | Renal dysfunction, vitamin A supplementation | See prealbumin, vitamin A deficiency |

shorter biologic half-life (8–10 days) and smaller body pool (less than 100 mg/kg body weight).[26] Transferrin concentrations may be determined by direct measurement or can be estimated indirectly from measurement of total iron-binding capacity (TIBC). Several formulas using TIBC have been proposed, but it is recommended that each laboratory establish its own formula relating its measurement of TIBC to the results of immunodiffusion radioassay for transferrin.[19,27] The serum transferrin concentration is affected by the same factors affecting serum albumin and by serum iron stores. In iron deficiency, transferrin concentrations are elevated, and in iron excess, transferrin concentrations are depressed.

Thyroxine-binding prealbumin (TBPA), the transport protein for thyroxine, is a carrier protein for retinol-binding protein. It has a short biologic half-life (2 days) and a small body pool size (10 mg/kg body weight). TBPA is sensitive to dietary intake and may show response to a decreased intake in as few as 3 days[26,28,29]; however, TBPA concentrations also rapidly decline in acute stress, such as trauma or sepsis, in which there is increased protein catabolism. As with albumin and transferrin, TBPA concentrations are depressed with hepatitis and cirrhosis because of decreased hepatic synthesis. Increased TBPA concentrations have been noted in renal disease patients and are thought to result from impaired degradation of TBPA by the kidney.[30]

Retinol-binding protein (RBP) is a specific protein for vitamin A alcohol (retinol) transport. It is filtered by the glomeruli and is metabolized by the kidney. RBP has a very short biologic half-life (12 hours) and a small body pool size (2 mg/kg body weight). As a nutritional assessment parameter it has the same deficiencies as TBPA, reacting to acute stress and being dependent on hepatic and renal function. Vitamin A deficiency results in depressed RBP concentrations, whereas vitamin A supplementation may result in elevated amounts in the serum.[31,32]

These four serum proteins (albumin, transferrin, TBPA, RBP) are of greatest value in assessing uncomplicated semistarvation and recovery. Other serum proteins, such as fibronectin (an opsonic protein), have been suggested as indicators of nutritional status[2]; however, sensitive assays for these proteins are not yet available, and the relevance to the nutritional status and outcome of hospitalization has not been determined.

Plasma amino acid concentrations have also been used to assess lean body mass. Altered amino acid patterns have been identified in the setting of PCM and are characterized by small amounts of essential amino acids and an increase or no change in the nonessential amino acid concentrations.[6,33–35] Consequently, the ratio of essential to nonessential amino acid concentrations decreases and has been used to characterize PCM; however, unless the nutritional depletion is severe, plasma amino acid concentrations are maintained fairly constant by the body's homeostatic mechanisms. The depletion state is clinically apparent before changes in amino acid concentrations become significant. Furthermore, plasma amino acid concentrations are altered in various disease states such as hepatic failure, renal failure, and sepsis. In addition to the lack of sensitivity and specificity, the measurement of plasma amino acid concentrations is not widely available and is very expensive. Therefore, plasma amino acid concentrations are of limited usefulness in the assessment of lean body mass.

### *Indices of Immune Function*

The frequency with which immunocompetence is impaired and the high incidence of infection in malnutrition led to the suggestion that tests of immune function be used as indices of nutritional status.[36] Alterations in the immune system represent an end-organ or functional response to malnutrition and may reflect a decline in lean body mass as well as a deficiency in specific nutrients such as zinc. The manner in which nutritional factors interact with immune status may be either direct, affecting primarily the lymphoid system, or indirect, affecting cellular metabolism or another organ system that is in turn involved with the regulation of immunocompetence.

The immune response is highly complex and involves interaction of three major interrelated systems: (1) B-cell immunity, representing the humoral component and consisting of antibody response by an antigen-stimulated B lymphocyte, is apparently bone marrow dependent: (2) T-cell-mediated immunity, comprising such antigen-specific responses as cell-mediated immunity; and (3) nonspecific responses including phagocytosis, opsonization, complement system, lysozyme, and others. Specific immune function parameters have been correlated with nutritional deficiency states, such as total lymphocyte count, lymphocyte transformation, delayed cutaneous hypersensitivity reaction, T-cell count, mitogen-stimulated T-cell response, serum immunoglobulin concentrations, complement levels, leukocyte chemotaxis, and bactericidal capacity (Table 106.10).[37–50] Those most frequently used in the hospital setting are total lymphocyte count (TLC) and delayed cutaneous hypersensitivity (DCH) reaction. These are simple, readily available, and inexpensive, but both TLC and DCH may be affected by nonnutritional factors and, therefore, at best are nonspecific indicators of malnutrition.

Total lymphocyte count reflects the number of circulating lymphocytes, most of which are T cells. Tissues generating

**Table 106.10** Immune Function in Malnutrition

| *Parameter* | *Observation in malnutrition* |
|---|---|
| Cell-mediated immunity | |
| Delayed cutaneous hypersensitivity | Decreased |
| Total lymphocyte count | Decreased |
| Lymphocyte transformation | Decreased |
| Humoral immunity | |
| Serum immunoglobulins | Normal |
| Complement activity ($CH_{50}$) | Decreased |
| Serum complement | Decreased or normal |
| Serum opsonization | Normal |
| Polymorphonuclear leukocyte function | |
| Phagocytosis | Normal |
| Metabolism | Decreased |
| Bacterial capacity | Decreased |
| Chemotaxis | Decreased |

**Table 106.11** Nonnutritional Influences on Skin-Test Response

| | |
|---|---|
| Technical | Immune alterations |
| Antigen source and batch | Congenital |
| Preparation and storage | DiGeorge's syndrome |
| Method of administration | Thymic aplasia |
| Site of test | Acquired |
| Booster effect | Systemic lupus erythematosus |
| Criteria of positivity | Rheumatoid arthritis |
| Reader variability | Trauma, burns, hemorrhage |
| Patient factors | Diseases—malignant |
| Age | Most solid tumors, especially advancing stages |
| Race | Lymphomas |
| Geographic location | Leukemias |
| Prior exposure to antigen | |
| Circadian rhythm | |
| Psychologic state | Prior malignancy, especially squamous cancer, lymphoma |
| Diseases—nonmalignant | Iatrogenic |
| Infectious | Drugs |
| Viral | Immunosuppressants |
| Bacterial | Most antineoplastics |
| Fungal | Anti-inflammatory agents |
| Metabolic | Anticoagulants |
| Uremia | $H_2$-receptor antagonists |
| Liver diseases | ? Aspirin |
| Inflammatory | x-ray therapy |
| Crohn's disease | General anesthesia |
| Ulcerative colitis | Surgery |

From Twomey P, Siegler D, Rombeau J: Utility of skin testing in nutritional assessment: A critical review. J Parenter Enter Nutr 1982; 6:51, with permission.

T-cells are very sensitive to malnutrition and undergo involution with a decrease in the production of T cells.[44] This eventually leads to lymphopenia. The circulating lymphocyte count can be calculated from the peripheral white blood cell (WBC) count and differential:

$$\text{total lymphocyte count (cells/mm}^3) = \text{WBC (cells/mm}^3) \times \frac{\%\ \text{lymphocytes}}{100}$$

A TLC of 1,200–2,000/mm³ correlates with mild malnutrition, 800–1,200/mm³ with moderate malnutrition, and 800/mm³ with severe malnutrition.[15] Nonnutritional factors that affect TLC include infection, immunosuppressant drugs, steroids, and the presence of neoplasia.

DCH reactions represent an in vivo test of cell-mediated immunity. DCH may be assessed as a primary response to new antigens using a chemical irritant such as dinitrochlorobenzene (DCNB), but is more commonly assessed as a secondary response using antigens to which the patient has been previously sensitized. The recall antigens used in nutritional assessment are mumps, *Candida albicans*, streptokinase–streptodornase (SKSD), *Trichophyton*, coccidioidin, and purified protein derivative (PPD). There is no standardized, uniformly accepted protocol used for testing DCH, but usually a battery of three to five antigens is applied. The inflammatory reaction, marked by dermal erytherma and induration, is evaluated at 24 and 48 hours. A positive response is defined as induration at the site of antigen injection of at least 5 mm at 24 to 48 hours.[15] Interpretation of the degree of anergy or failure of DCH response, varies somewhat with different investigators.[51, 52] If three of five tests are nonresponsive, the individual is generally considered anergic. Numerous studies have correlated anergy with malnutrition in hospitalized patients,[38,42,53] and with aggressive nutritional support a positive DCH response has been restored[42]; however, anergy may not be specifically indicative of nutritional depletion as multiple factors such as fever, stress, surgery, and drugs affect DCH (Table 106.11).

## Specific Nutrient Deficiencies

The assessment of nutritional status should include an evaluation of possible trace mineral, vitamin, and essential fatty acid deficiencies. Because of their key role in metabolic processing (e.g., as coenzymes and cofactors), the deficiency of any single nutrient may result in altered metabolism and cell dysfunction and may interfere with process necessary for repletion of PCM. As with PCM, single-nutrient-deficiency states are assessed by an accurate history to evaluate symptoms and the existence of factors predisposing the patient to developing a deficiency state, a physical examination for signs of deficiencies, and biochemical assessment to confirm the diagnosis.

**Table 106.12** Assessment of Trace Mineral Status

| *Trace mineral* | *Signs of deficiency* | *Normal serum value* | *Factors resulting in altered serum concentrations* |
|---|---|---|---|
| Zinc | Dermatitis, hypogeusia, alopecia, diarrhea, apathy, depression | 55–150 μg/dL | Decreased: infection, hypoalbuminemia, corticosteroid therapy, stress<br>Increased: tissue injury, hemolysis, contaminated hemolysis, contaminated collection tubes |
| Copper | Neutropenia, hypochromic anemia, osteoporosis, decreased hair and skin pigmentation; dermatitis, anorexia, diarrhea | 70–150 μg/dL | Decreased: ceruloplasmin levels, corticosteroid therapy, Wilson's disease infection, rheumatoid arthritis, liver disease, leukemia, lymphoma, myocardial infarction |
| Chromium | Glucose intolerance, peripheral neuropathy, increased free fatty acid levels, low respiratory quotient | 1–3 mg/mL | Not known |
| Manganese | Nausea, vomiting, dermatitis, color changes in hair, hypocholesterolemia, growth retardation | 2–3 μg/dL | Not known |
| Selenium | Muscle weakness and pain, cardiomyopathy | 0.10–0.34 μg/mL | Not known |
| Molybdenum | Tachycardia, tachypnea, altered mental status, visual changes, headache, nausea, vomiting | 0.4–0.5 mg/mL (by neutron activation) | Varies with assay method used |

### *Trace Minerals*

The trace minerals identified as essential to humans and for which deficiency states have been described are zinc, copper, manganese, selenium, chromium, molybdenum (Table 106.12), and iron. Each of these minerals participates in a variety of biologic functions and is necessary for normal metabolism (see Chapter 107). Other trace minerals that are essential to humans but for which deficiency states have not been recognized include nickel, vanadium, cobalt, and silicon.

Zinc deficiency is clinically characterized by the development of a moist eczematous dermatitis most apparent in the nasolabial folds and around orifices. Other presenting signs and symptoms may include hypogeusia, alopecia, diarrhea, rash (which may vary from papular, scaly lesions to weeping, open erosions), apathy, and depression. Clinical zinc deficiency occurs most frequently in the setting of abnormal losses, such as in Crohn's disease, malabsorption states, and fistula losses, or from prolonged inadequate intake, such as with zinc-free parenteral nutrition. Zinc deficiency can be documented with low serum zinc concentrations, but many other factors may affect zinc concentrations (Table 106.12). Zinc status can also be assessed by red cell zinc content, urinary zinc concentration, or zinc content in hair, but these assays are not widely available.

Copper deficiency presents with hematologic changes (anemia, leukopenia, and neutropenia) and skeletal demineralization. In severe cases, as in Menkes' syndrome, copper deficiency is further manifest as hypothermia, depigmentation of hair and skin, progressive mental deterioration, and growth retardation. Factors predisposing to copper deficiency include malabsorption states, protein-losing enteropathy, nephrotic syndrome, and copper-free parenteral nutrition. Laboratory diagnosis of copper deficiency is made most frequently on the basis of serum concentrations, although urinary concentrations may also be assessed. As with zinc, serum copper concentrations may be altered by a variety of conditions and, therefore, may not accurately reflect copper nutrition (Table 106.13).

Chromium deficiency is characterized by glucose intolerance but may also include neuropathy, increased free fatty acid concentrations, and a low respiratory quotient.[54] Chromium deficiency has been identified in the setting of long-term, copper-free parenteral nutrition. Serum chromium concentrations do not reflect chromium nutrition, presumably because the biologically active form of chromium is an organic chromium-containing substance known as glucose tolerance factor. Currently, urinary chromium concentrations are considered the best laboratory marker of chromium status.[55]

Manganese deficiency has no specific syndrome and has been reported only in association with clinically defined manganese-deficient oral diets.[55] The symptoms include nausea, vomiting, dermatitis, color changes in hair, hypocholesterolemia, and growth retardation. Serum concentrations are difficult to measure. The effect of other specific diseases on serum manganese concentrations is unknown.

Selenium deficiency has been described in long-term selenium-free total parenteral nutrition.[56–58] Myopathy and abnormal glutathione peroxidase concentrations are most frequently observed. In one case a fatal cardiomyopathy was seen.[58] Selenium status may be assessed by plasma or red blood cell concentrations. Reduced plasma concentrations may indicate selenium deficiency, but reduced amounts have also been observed in patients with malignancies, cirrhosis, or renal failure. Measurement of the activity of the selenium-containing enzyme glutathione peroxidase in platelets is a

**Table 106.13** Indirect Assessment of Body Iron Stores

| *Parameter* | *Normal values (adult)* Women | Men | *Value in iron deficiency* | *Value in specific medical states* |
|---|---|---|---|---|
| Hemoglobin (mg/dL) | 14.5 | 15.5 | Decreased | Decreased value in chronic illness |
| Serum iron ($\mu$g/dL) | 90 ± 40 | 100 ± 35 | Decreased | Decreased value in infection, nephrosis<br>Increased value in hemolytic disorders, hemochromatosis, oral contraceptive use, acute liver disease |
| Total iron-binding capacity ($\mu$g/dL) | ⟨200–400⟩ | | Increased | Decreased value in chronic disease, protein deficiency, liver disease<br>Increased value in pregnancy |
| Serum ferritin (mg/mL) | 3–200 | 10–400 | 15 | Decreased value in reticuloendothelium cell damage<br>Increased value in inflammation |

more sensitive measure of selenium status, although not widely available.

Molybdenum deficiency in humans has only recently been reported.[59] The presenting symptoms included tachycardia, tachypnea, headache, night blindness, nausea, vomiting, central scotomas, lethargy, disorientation, and ultimately coma. Biochemical assessment has revealed amino acid intolerance, particularly of methionine, and low serum uric acid concentrations. Serum molybdenum concentrations were not assessed. Predisposing factors to molybdenum deficiency appear to be excessive loss via the gastrointestinal tract, as with short-bowel syndrome, and long-term inadequate intake, as with molybdenum-free parenteral nutrition.

Patients with iron deficiency anemia present with fatigue, weakness, and pallor and possibly also with glossitis, cheilosis, dysphagia, fingernail changes, gastric atrophy, and paresthesias. Inadequate intake of iron, malabsorption, and blood loss from any origin are the principal causes of iron deficiency anemia. Iron deficiency is confirmed on the basis of an assessment of body iron stores as reflected indirectly by measurement of hemoglobin, serum iron, iron-binding capacity, and serum ferritin or directly by marrow staining and liver biopsy. The direct methods are the most accurate but are invasive; therefore, the indirect measurements are more commonly used (see Chapter 69). Each indirect parameter may be altered by chronic illness independent of iron stores; thus, concomitant illness must be considered in their interpretation (Table 106.13).

### *Vitamins*

A carefully performed history and physical examination may be the most valuable means of screening patients for risk factors as well as of identifying symptoms that suggest physical findings of vitamin deficiency (Table 106.14). Laboratory assessment is useful in confirming clinical suspicions. Laboratory assessment also identifies subclinical vitamin deficiencies; the first step in deficiency is usually a fall in circulating amounts of the vitamin or its coenzyme. Subsequently, there is a decrease in urinary excretion of the vitamin, which in turn is followed by diminished concentrations of the vitamin in tissue.

The most common measurements of vitamin status are assays of circulating amounts in plasma or serum. Assays may also be performed to determine biochemical or metabolic function of the vitamin and are more likely to reflect body stores than are serum assays. Most of these functional assays use extracts of erythrocytes or leukocytes to determine activity of an apoenzyme, which is dependent on the vitamin coenzyme, in the presence or absence of added coenzyme. Vitamin assays are summarized in Table 106.14.

### *Essential Fatty Acids*

In general, essential fatty acid (EFA) deficiency, or more specifically linoleic acid deficiency, is rare but can occur during prolonged use of continuously infused parenteral nutrition that does not include long-chain fatty acids. It may also occur with severe PCM. Symptoms of EFA deficiency include dermatitis (dry, cracked, scaly skin), alopecia, and impaired wound healing. In severe cases neurologic deficits, abnormal liver function, respiratory insufficiency, cardiac arrhythmias, and hemolysis may occur. A deficiency may appear as early as within 1 week of fat-free parenteral nutrition.

Laboratory assessment of EFA deficiency is expensive and not readily available. Fatty acid composition of plasma may be measured; 5,8,11-eicosatrienoic acid and arachidonic acid are the primary fatty acids of interest. Eicosatrienoic acid is not normally present. With a deficiency of linoleic acid, and hence decreased synthesis of arachidonic acid from linoleic acid, oleic acid metabolism to 5,8,11-eicosatrienoic acid becomes the primary metabolic pathway. The ratio of 5,8,11-eicosatrienoic (triene) acid to arachidonic acid (tetraene) reflects this derangement in metabolism. Normally, this ratio of triene to tetraene is less than 0.4; values of 0.5 or greater define a deficiency state.

## Metabolic Assessment and Stress Stratification

Just as important as the need for assessment of nutritional status is the need to evaluate the patient's metabolic status relative to stress level. The metabolic response to high levels

**Table 106.14** Assessment of Vitamin Status

| *Vitamin* | *Signs of deficiency* | *Laboratory assay* | *Normal values* | *Comments* |
|---|---|---|---|---|
| Niacin ($B_5$) | Pellagra: dermatitis, dementia, glossitis, diarrhea, loss of memory, and headaches | Urinary niacin metabolites | >1.6 mg/g creatinine | Vary with age, sex, pregnancy; blood levels not done |
| Folate ($B_9$) | Megaloblastic anemia, diarrhea, and glossitis | Serum folate | >6.0 ng/mL | Levels may be decreased in cases of increased cellular or tissue turnover (pregnancy, malignancy, hemolytic anemia) |
| Cyanocobalamin ($B_{12}$) | Pernicious anemia, glossitis, spinal cord degeneration, and peripheral neuropathy | Serum $B_{12}$ | >150 pg/mL | |
| Thiamine | Paresthesias, nystagmus, impaired memory, congestive heart failure, and Wernicke–Korsakoff syndrome | Urinary thiamine | >60 $\mu$g/g creatinine | Varies with age; blood levels difficult, not sensitive |
| Riboflavin ($B_2$) | Mucositis, dermatitis, cheilosis; vascularization of cornea, photophobia, lacrimation, and decreased vision, impaired wound healing | Urinary riboflavin | ≥80 $\mu$g/g creatinine | Varies with age, pregnancy, exercise, nitrogen balance |
| Pyridoxine ($B_6$) | Dermatitis, neuritis, and convulsions | Plasma $B_6$ | >50 ng/mL | Varies with age, sex |
| Pantothenic acid | Fatigue, malaise, headache, insomnia, vomiting, and abdominal cramps | Urinary pantothenic acid | >1 mg/d | |
| Biotin | Dermatitis, depression, alopecia, lassitude, somnolence | Serum biotin | 0.5–2.7 ng/mL | |
| Ascorbic acid (C) | Enlargement and keratosis of hair follicles; impaired wound healing; anemia, lethargy, depression, bleeding, and ecchymosis | Serum ascorbic acid | >0.30 mg/dL | |
| A | Dermatitis, night blindness, keratomalacia, and xerophthalmia | Plasma vitamin A | >20 $\mu$g/dL | |
| D | Rickets and osteomalacia | Plasma 25-hydroxyvitamin D | 29.4 ± 15.7 ng/mL | Decreased in uremia, in cirrhosis, in individuals greater than 60 years old; may be decreased in winter |
| E | Hemolysis | Plasma $\alpha$-tocopherol | >0.5 mg/dL | Decreased with low blood lipoprotein concentrations |
| K | Bleeding | Prothrombin time | Clotting within 1 s of laboratory control | Decreased with hepatic disease, anticoagulants |

**Table 106.15** The Stratification of Stress

| | *Stress level and clinical example (mean ± SD)* | | | |
|---|---|---|---|---|
| | **0 (nonstressed starvation)** | **1 (elective surgery)** | **2 (polytrauma)** | **3 (sepsis)** |
| Urinary nitrogen loss (g/d) | 5 | 5 –10 | 10 –15 | 15 |
| Plasma lactate (μmol/L) | 100 ± 50 | 1,200 ± 200 | 1,200 ± 200 | 2,500 ± 500 |
| Plasma glucose (mg/dL) | 100 ± 20 | 150 ± 25 | 150 ± 25 | 250 ± 50 |
| Oxygen consumption index (mL/m$^2$) | 90 ± 10 | 130 ± 6 | 140 ± 6 | 160 ± 10 |
| Glucagon/insulin | 2 ± 0.5 | 2.5 ± 0.8 | 3.0 ± 0.7 | 8 ± 1.5 |
| Insulin resistance | –[a] | –[a] | ±[a] | +[a] |

[a] –, absent; ±, may be present; +, present.

of stress, as seen in sepsis, major trauma, and burns, is manifest by accelerated catabolism and may result in a rapidly progressive, severe form of acquired protein-calorie malnutrition. Therefore, a patient with a baseline nutritional assessment within normal limits who experiences major trauma is at risk for developing PCM. The patient who is nutritionally depleted at the outset will have limited nutritional reserve and will rapidly develop severe PCM. An assessment of the patient's metabolic status also provides useful information regarding substrate utilization and provides a basis for determining protein and energy requirements, designing a nutrition support regimen, and anticipating potential complications of nutrition support.

The metabolic response to stress or injury is a complex, dynamic process involving many neuroendocrine factors and the activation of mediators such as endotoxin, complement, and prostaglandin (see Chapter 107). Numerous parameters, including plasma amino acid concentrations, β-hydroxybutyrate and acetoacetate concentrations, and urinary 3-methylhistidine, have been used in the development of a stress stratification scheme to characterize the different levels of metabolic stress.[60,61] For routine clinical use, the most useful characteristics are urinary nitrogen excretion, blood glucose concentration and its response to insulin, plasma lactate concentration, and the oxygen consumption index (Table 106.15).

## Clinical Research Parameters and Newer Methods of Nutritional Assessment

More precise methods for the measurement of body cell mass as well as specific body compartments have been developed recently. These methods are complex, require expensive technology, and at present are limited mainly to experimental studies; however, some of these techniques, particularly noninvasive methods such as measurement of total body electrical conductivity, may become available for routine clinical use in the future.

Isotope dilution employs the use of naturally occurring radioactive isotopes of sodium, hydrogen, and potassium to measure total body water, body cell mass, body fat mass, and lean body mass.[62,63] These measurements, therefore, provide information about the "metabolic size" of the body or the part of the body that performs oxidative metabolism. Shizgal[64] has developed a modification of this technique in which exchangeable sodium ($Na_e$) and potassium ($K_e$) are calculated relative to total body water. The $Na_e/K_e$ ratio, termed the "Shizgal index," is a marker of body cell mass and has been shown to correlate with a malnutrition-associated decrease in body cell mass; however, because it involves radiation exposure to the patient and may be altered by nonnutritional disease, it has not gained wide clinical use.

Neutron activation analysis has been used to derive body composition parameters such as total body fat, separation of total body water into intracellular and extracellular components, and separation of body protein into muscle and nonmuscle mass.[65,66] For total body nitrogen determination the technique involves bombardment of the patient with a uniform neutron flux through the body to create a short-lived isotope of nitrogen that can be counted subsequently in a whole body counter. It is used for investigational purposes only because it is technically difficult, exposes the patient to radiation, and is expensive.

Radiography and computed tomography can be used to estimate the volume of specific organs or tissues such as liver, spleen, fat, muscle, and brain and, therefore, may be used for quantification of PCM[67,68]; however, the cost of the procedure and the radiation exposure to the patient may limit its use for nutritional assessment.

Total body electrical conductivity measurement is one of the newest and perhaps most promising methods of nutritional assessment.[69] It has been used to measure lean body mass on the basis of lean tissue that has a higher electrical conductivity because of its greater electrolyte content. It is a simple, noninvasive technique. The potential limitations of the use of electrical conductivity measurements include variability with electrolyte imbalance, interference by large fat masses, and the need for standards that reflect variations in individual body sizes.

Urinary 3-methylhistidine and $^{15}N$ whole body protein turnover have been used clinically to determine the rates of protein catabolism and synthesis.[70,71] The data provided are more a reflection of protein metabolic status than of overall nutritional status; therefore, these parameters have greater utility in metabolic assessment or in evaluating the response to nutritional therapy. 3-Methylhistidine is the amino acid by-product of histidine degradation. Histidine is found mainly in myofibrillar protein. 3-Methylhistidine cannot be reutilized and is rapidly and quantitatively excreted in the urine. The measurement of urinary 3-methylhistidine is expensive and not widely available.

Whole body protein turnover is measured with the stable, radioactive isotope of nitrogen, $^{15}N$, usually as $[^{15}N]$glycine, which must be administered orally or intravenously to the patient. The enrichment of $^{15}N$ into by-products of protein metabolism such as urea and ammonia is determined by isotope ratio mass spectrometry. The methodology is complex, the equipment is expensive, and there is controversy about the assumptions upon which the procedure is based.

## Hospital Malnutrition

The value of any given parameter or group of parameters used for nutritional assessment is only as great as its ability to accurately identify the patient with malnutrition and to correlate with malnutrition-associated complications. Most of the currently available indices of nutritional status were first used in epidemiologic studies to define large populations suffering from malnutrition caused by famine. The recognition of hospital malnutrition initially required astute clinical observation of the association between complications and the clinically debilitated patient. Loss of weight was one of the earliest recognized nutritional factors associated with increased morbidity and mortality in surgical patients.[72]

The systematic application of nutritional assessment techniques to populations of hospitalized individuals has only come about in recent years. Surveys of patients from varying socioeconomic backgrounds hospitalized in a variety of institutions on numerous specialty services have detected a high prevalence (25%–50%) of previously unrecognized malnutrition.[24,73–78]

Coincident with the recognition of this substantial prevalence of hospital malnutrition was definition of the risks associated with abnormalities in specific parameters of nutritional status. Mullen et al[24] examined the values of 16 nutritional and immunologic variables in predicting subsequent morbidity and mortality in surgical patients. Serum transferrin, albumin, and delayed cutaneous hypersensitivity reaction were the most reliable predictors of outcome. These factors have been shown by several authors to correlate with morbidity and mortality.[79–81] A more comprehensive study by Buzby et al[82] confirmed the findings of their initial study about the usefulness of these markers and also about the usefulness of measuring triceps skinfold thickness. A linear predictive model, the prognostic nutritional index (PNI), was developed from these data that correlated baseline nutritional status with risk of morbidity and mortality after surgery as a quantitative measure:

$$\text{PNI}\ (\%) = 158 - 1.66\ (\text{ALB}) - 0.78\ (\text{TSF}) - 0.02\ (\text{TFN}) - 5.8\ (\text{DH})$$

where ALB is serum albumin concentration (g/dL), TSF is triceps skinfold thickness (mm), TFN is serum transferrin concentration (mg/dL), and DH is maximal skin test reactivity (graded 0 for nonreactive, 1 for 5-mm reactivity, and 2 for 5-mm reactivity). High-risk patients were defined as those with a PNI greater than 50%. Using this model, they accurately identified 87% of the patients who developed significant complications and 96% of the postoperative deaths. This predictive model has been validated in prospective studies of different patient groups by comparing the risk of morbidity and mortality predicted by the model with actual outcome.[83–85]

This increased awareness of the prevalence and significance of untreated protein-calorie malnutrition has provided a strong clinical incentive for the nutritional support of malnourished patients. The response of the various indices of nutritional status to nutritional therapy and the correlation between improvement in these indices and decreased morbidity and mortality further support the validity of specific indices. For example, preoperative total parenteral nutrition in patients with malnutrition, particularly when associated with a low albumin concentration, has been demonstrated to reduce the incidence of major postoperative complications in several patient populations.[79,86–89] Furthermore, early postoperative parenteral nutrition has been shown to improve convalescence coincident with improvement in nutritional status after esophagogastrectomy[90] and radical bladder cystectomy.[91]

## Practical Guidelines for Nutritional Assessment

An "ideal" test for nutritional assessment should be highly sensitive and specific, be unaffected by factors unrelated to nutrition, and correlate with response to nutritional repletion. Given the lack of sensitivity, specificity, and independence of most of the aforementioned parameters, devising a clinically useful, cost-effective approach to the nutritional assessment of an individual hospitalized patient is challenging. The value of the history and physical examination cannot be overemphasized. The least amount of objective data that can further substantiate the clinical impression and provide a baseline for subsequent monitoring are those parameters that show the best correlation with outcome: weight, serum albumin and transferrin, and delayed cutaneous hypersensitivity reaction. The cost-effectiveness of the addition of further biochemical parameters, such as creatinine–height index, or serum thyroxine-binding prealbumin, is questionable. The assessment of anthropometric measures is probably most useful in the setting of anticipated long-term nutritional support in which these indices will serve as a longitudinal marker of the individual response to therapy.

Better indices of nutritional status are definitely needed. Functional tests and simple, noninvasive tests for body composition analysis hold promise for the future; however, the currently available battery of tests used in support of clinical evaluation continues to be the mainstay of nutritional assessment until better methods of assessment become available.

## References


1. Grant JP. Nutritional assessment in clinical practice. Nutr Clin Pract 1986;1:3–11
2. Haider M, Haider SQ. Assessment of protein-calorie malnutrition. Clin Chem 1984;30:1286–1299.
3. Coward WA, Lunn PG. The biochemistery and physiology of kwashiorkor and marasmus. Br Med Bull 1981;37:19–24.
4. Baker JP, Detsky AS, Wesson DE, et al. Nutritional assessment: A comparison of clinical judgment and objective measurement. N Engl J Med 1982;306:969-972.
5. Goode AW. The scientific basis of nutritional assessment. Br J Anaesth 1981;53:161–167.
6. Jeliffe DB. The Assessment of Nutritional Status of the Community. World Health Organization Monograph No. 53. Geneva, World Health Organization, 1966.
7. Weight by Height and Age of Adults 18–74 Years: United States, 1971–74. Atlanta GA, National Center for Health Statistics, 1979, Series II, No. 9.
8. Bishop CW, Bowen PE, Ritchey SJ. Norms for nutritional assessment of American adults by upper arm anthropometry. Am J Clin Nutr 1981;31:2530–2539.
9. Metropolitan Life Insurance Company. Statistical Bulletin, New Weights and Standards for Men and Women. Chicago, Metropolitan Life, 1959, vol 40, November–December.
10. Morgan DB, Hill GL, Burkinshaw L. The assessment of weight loss from a single measurement of body weight: The problems and limitations. Am J Clin Nutr 1980;33:2101–2105.
11. Seltzer MH, Slocum BA, Cataldi-Betcher EL, et al. Instant nutritional assessment; absolute weight loss and surgical morbidity. J Parenter Enter Nutr 1982;6:218–221.
12. Bastow MD. Anthropometrics revisited. Proc Nutr Soc 1982;41: 381–388.
13. Edwards DAW, Hammond WH, Healey MJR, et al. Design and accuracy of calipers for measuring subcutaneous tissue thickness. Br J Nutr 1955;9:133–143.
14. Jensen TG, Dudrick SJ, Johnston DA. A comparison of triceps skinfold and upper arm circumference measurements taken in standard and supine positions. J Parenter Enter Nutr 1981;5: 519–521.
15. Grant JP, Custer PB, Thurlow J. Current techniques of nutritional assessment. Surg Clin North Am 1981;61:437–463.
16. Buzby GP, Mullen JL. Nutritional assessment, in Rombeau J, Caldwell MD (eds): Clinical Nutrition, Philadelphia, W.B. Saunders, 1984, vol 1, pp 127–128.
17. Forbes GB, Bruining GJ. Urinary creatinine excretion and lean body mass. Am J Clin Nutr 1976; 29:1359–1366.
18. Bistrian BR, Blackburn GL, Sherman M, et al. Therapeutic index of nutritional depletion in hospital patients. Surg Gynecol Obstet 1975;141:512–516.
19. Blackburn GL, Bistrian BR, Maini BS, et al. Nutritional and metabolic assessment of the hospitalized patient. J Parenter Enter Nutr 1977;1:11–22.
20. Travill AS. The synthesis and degradation of liver-produced proteins. Gut 1972;13:225–241.
21. Seltzer MH, Bastidas JA, Cooper DM, et al. Instant nutritional assessment. J Parenter Enter Nutr 1979;3:157–159.
22. Mullen JL, Gertner MH, Buzby GP, et al. Implications of malnutrition in the surgical patient. Arch Surg 1979;114:121–125.
23. Rainey-Macdonald CG, Holliday RL, Wells GA, et al. Validity of a two-variable nutritional index for use in selecting candidates for nutritional support. J Parenter Enter Nutr 1983;7:15–20.
24. Bienia R, Ratcliff S, Barbour GL, et al. Malnutrition and hospital prognosis in the alcoholic patient. J Parenter Enter Nutr 1982;6:301–303.
25. Anderson CF, Wochos DN. The utility of serum albumin values in nutritional assessment of hospitalized patients. Mayo Clin Proc 1982;57:181–184.
26. Ingenbleek Y, Van Den Schriek HG, DeNayer P, et al. Albumin, transferrin, and thyroxine-binding prealbumin/retinol-binding protein (TBPA–RBP) complex in assessment of malnutrition. Clin Chim Acta 1975;63:61–67.
27. Weisberg HF. Evaluation of nutritional status. Ann Clin Lab Sci 1983;13:95–106.
28. Ingenbleek Y, Van Den Schriek HC, DeNayer P, et al. The role of retinol-binding protein in protein calorie malnutrition. Metabolism 1975;24:633–641.
29. Fischer JE. Plasma proteins as indicators of nutritional status, in Levenson SM (ed): Nutritional Assessment—Present Status, Future Direction and Prospects. Report of the Second Ross Conference on Medical Research. Columbus OH, Ross Laboratories, 1981.
30. Smith FR, Goodman DS, Zaklama MS, et al. Serum vitamin A, retinol-binding protein, and prealbumin concentrations in protein calorie malnutrition. I. A functional defect in hepatic retinol release. Am J Clin Nutr 1973;26:973–981.
31. Large S, Neal G, Glover J, et al. The early changes in retinol-binding protein and prealbumin concentrations in plasma of protein energy malnourished children after treatment with retinol and an improved diet. Br J Nutr 1980;43:393–402.
32. Muhilal H, Glover J. Effects of dietary deficiencies of protein and retinol on the plasma level of retinol-binding protein in the rat. Br J Nutr 1974;32:549–558.
33. Arroyave G, Wilson D, de Funes C, et al. The free amino acids in blood plasma of children with kwashiorkor and marasmus. Am J Clin Nutr 1962;11:517–524.
34. Edozien JC, Phillips EJ, Collis WRF. The free amino acids of plasma and urine in kwashiorkor. Lancet 1960;1:615–618.
35. Holt LE, Snyderman SE, Norton PM, et al. The plasma aminogram in kwashiorkor. Lancet 1963;2:1343–1348.
36. Chandra RK. Immunocompetence as a functional index of nutritional status. Br Med Bull 1981;37:89–94.
37. Balch HH, Spencer MT. Phagocytosis by human leukocytes. II. Relation of nutritional deficiency in man to phagocytosis. J Clin Invest 1954;33:1321–1328.
38. Bistrian BR, Blackburn GL, Scrimshaw NS, et al. Cellular immunity in semi-starved states in hospitalized adults. Am J Clin Nutr 1975;28:1148–1155.
39. Bistrian BR, Blackburn GL, Marshall R, et al. Cellular immunity in adult marasmus. Arch Intern Med 1977;137:1408–1411.
40. Chandra RK. Immunocompetence in undernutrition. J Pediatr 1972;81:1194–1200.
41. Geefhuysen J, Rose EU, Katz J, et al. Impaired cellular immunity in kwashiorkor with improvement after therapy. Br Med J 1971;4:527–529.
42. Law DK, Dudrick SJ, Abdou NI. Immunocompetence of patients with protein-calorie malnutrition. The effects of nutritional repletion. Ann Intern Med 1973;79:545–550.
43. Newmann CG, Lawlor GJ, Stiehm ER, et al. Immunologic responses in malnourished children. Am J Clin Nutr 1975;28:89–104.
44. Smythe PM, Schonland M, Brereton-Stiles GC, et al. Thymolytic deficiency and depression of cell-mediated immunity in protein-calorie malnutrition. Lancet 1971;2:939–943.
45. Keat MP, Thorn H. Serum immunoglobulins in kwashiorkor. Arch Dis Child 1969;44:600–603.
46. Nahani J, Nik-Aeen A, Rafii M, et al. Effect of malnutrition on several parameters of the immune system of children. Nutr Metab 1976;20:302–306.

47. Selvaraj RJ, Seetharam Bhat K. Metabolic and bactericidal activities of leukocytes in protein-calorie malnutrition. Am J Clin Nutr 1972;25:166–174.
48. Seth V, Chandra RK. Opsonic activity, phagocytosis, and bactericidal capacity of polymorphs in undernutrition. Arch Dis Child 1972;47:282–284.
49. Sirisinha S, Suskind R, Edelman R, et al. Complement and C3-proactivator levels in children with protein-calorie malnutrition and effect of dietary treatment. Lancet 1973;1:1016–1018.
50. Chandra RK, Chandra S, Chai OP. Chemotaxis, random mobility and mobilization of polymorphonuclear leukocytes in malnutrition. J Clin Pathol 1976;29:224–227.
51. Twoney R, Ziegler D, Rombeau J. Utility of skin testing in nutritional assessment: A critical review. J Parenter Enter Nutr 1982;6:50–58.
52. Miller CL. Immunologic assays as measurements of nutritional status: A review. J Parenter Enter Nutr 1978;2:554–566.
53. Jensen TG, Englert DM, Dudrick SJ, et al. Delayed hypersensitivity skin testing: Response rates in a surgical population. J Am Diet Assoc 1983;82:17–23.
54. Jeejeebhoy KW, Chu RC, Marliss EB. Chromium deficiency, glucose intolerance, and neuropathy reversed by chromium supplementation in a patient receiving long-term total parenteral nutrition. Am J Clin Nutr 1977;30:531–538.
55. Lindeman RD. Assessment of trace element depletion, in Wright RA, Heymsfield S (eds): Nutritional Assessment. Boston, Blackwell Scientific, 1984, pp 239–261.
56. Johnson RA. An occidental case of cardiomyopathy and selenium deficiency. N Engl J Med 1981;304:1210–1212.
57. King WW. Reversal of selenium deficiency with oral selenium. N Engl J Med 1981;304:1304–1305.
58. Fleming CR. Selenium deficiency and fatal cardiomyopathy in a patient on home parenteral nutrition. Gastroenterology 1982;83: 689–693.
59. Abumrad NN, Schneider AJ, Steel D, et al. Amino acid intolerance during prolonged parenteral nutrition reversed by molybdate therapy. Am J Clin Nutr 1981;34:2551–2559.
60. Border JR, Chenier R, McMenamy RH, et al. Multiple systems organ failure: Muscle fuel deficit with visceral protein malnutrition. Surg Clin North Am 1976;56:1147–1167.
61. Cerra FB, Siegel JH, Border JR, et al. Correlations between metabolic and cardiopulmonary measurements in patients after trauma, general surgery, and sepsis. J Trauma 1979;19:621–629.
62. Shizgal HM. Total body potassium and nutritional status. Surg Clin North Am 1976;56:1185–1194.
63. Shizgal HM, Spanier AH, Kurtz RS. Effect of parenteral nutrition on body composition in the critically ill patient. Am J Surg 1976;131:156–161.
64. Shizgal HM. Body composition by multiple isotope dilution, in Levenson SM (ed): Nutritional Assessment—Present Status, Future Directions and Prospects. Report of the Second Ross Conference on Medical Research. Columbus OH, Ross Laboratories, 1982, pp 94–98.
65. Anderson J, Osborn SB, Tomlinson RWS, et al. Neutron activation analysis in man in vivo: A new technique in medical investigation. Lancet 1964;2:1201–1205.
66. Beddoe AH, Hill GL. Clinical measurement of body composition using in vivo neutron activation. J Parenter Enter Nutr 1985;9:504–520.
67. Heymsfield SB, Fulenwider T, Nordlinger B, et al. Accurate measurement of liver, kidney, and spleen volume and mass by computerized axial tomography. Ann Intern Med 1979;90:185–187.
68. Heymsfield SB, Olafson RP, Kutner MH, et al. A radiographic method of quantifying protein calorie malnutrition. Am J Clin Nutr 1972;32:693–702.
69. Presta E, Wang J, Harrison GG, et al. Measurement of total body electrical conductivity: A new method for estimation of body composition. Am J Clin Nutr 1983;37:735–739.
70. Young VR, Munro HN. $N^{T}$-Methylhistidine (3-methylhistidine) and muscle protein turnover. An overview. Fed Proc Fed Am Soc Exp Biol 1978;37:2291–2300.
71. Fern EB, Garlick PJ, Waterlow JC. The concept of the single body pool of metabolic nitrogen in determining the rate of whole-body nitrogen turnover. Hum Nutr Clin Nutr 1985;39C:85–99.
72. Studley HO. Percentage of weight loss: A basic indicator of surgical risk in patients with chronic peptic ulcer. JAMA 1936;106:458–460.
73. Bistrian BR, Blackburn GL. Hallowell E, et al. Protein status of general surgical patients. JAMA 1974;230:858–860.
74. Weinsier RL, Hunker EM, Krumdieck CL, et al. Hospital malnutrition: A prospective evaluation of general medical patients during the course of hospitalization. Am J Clin Nutr 1979;32:418–426.
75. Bistrian BR, Blackburn GL, Vitale J, et al. Prevalence of malnutrition in general medical patients. JAMA 1976; 235:1567–1570.
76. O'Leary JP, Dunn GD, Basil S, et al. Incidence of malnutrition among patients admitted to a VA hospital. South Med J 1982;75:1095–1098.
77. Willard MD, Gilsdorf RB, Price RA. Protein-calorie malnutrition in a community hospital. JAMA 1980;243:1720–1722.
78. Merritt RJ, Suskind RM. Nutritional survey of hospitalized pediatric patients. Am J Clin Nutr 1979;32:1320–1325.
79. Meakins JL, Pietsch JB, Bubenick O, et al. Delayed hypersensitivity: An indicator of acquired failure of host defenses in sepsis and trauma. Ann Surg 1977;186:241–250.
80. Harvey KB, Ruggiero JA, Regan CS, et al. Hospital morbidity–mortality risk factors using nutritional assessment. J Clin Nutr 1978;26:251–257.
81. Kaminsky MV, Fitzgerald MJ, Murphy RJ, et al. Correlation of mortality with serum transferrin and anergy. J Parenter Enter Nutr 1977;1(4):27A.
82. Buzby GP, Mullen JL, Mathews DC, et al. Prognostic nutritional index in gastrointestinal surgery. Am J Surg 1980;139:160–166.
83. Buzby GP, Mullen JL, Mathews DC, et al. Prognostic nutritional index in gastrointestinal surgery. Am J Surg 1980;139:160–167.
84. Smale BF, Mullen JL, Buzby GP, et al. The efficacy of nutritional assessment and support in cancer surgery. Cancer 1981;47:2375–2381.
85. Dempsey DT, Buzby GP, Mullen JL. Nutritional assessment in the seriously ill patient. J Am Coll Nutr 1983;2:15–23.
86. Holler AR, Fischer JE. The effects of perioperative hyperalimentation on complications in patients with carcinoma and weight loss. J Surg Res 1977;23:31–34.
87. Mullen JL, Buzby GP, Mathews DC, et al. Reduction of operative morbidity and mortality by combined preoperative and postoperative nutritional support. Ann Surg 1981;192:604–613.
88. Mullen JM, Brenner U, Dienot C, et al. Preoperative parenteral feeding in patients with gastrointestinal carcinoma. Lancet 1982;1: 68–71.
89. Starker PM, Lasala PA, Askanazi J, et al. The response to TPN–A form of nutritional assessment. Ann Surg 1983;198:720–724.
90. Moghissi K, Hornshaw J, Teasdale PR, et al. Parenteral nutrition in carcinoma of the oesophagus treated by surgery: Nitrogen balance and clinical studies. Br J Surg 1977;64:125–128.
91. Askanazi J, Starker PM, Olsson C, et al. Effect of immediate postoperative nutritional support on length of hospitalization. Ann Surg 1986;203:236–239.

# *Chapter 107* / Nutritional Requirements in Health and Disease

Maria G. Hegland, PharmD

## Recommended Dietary Allowances

The need for standard dietary recommendations was first recognized in the late eighteenth century when the British introduced lemon juice into the rations of the British Navy for the prevention of scurvy.[1] In the midnineteenth century, Gerrit Mulder made recommendations for daily protein intake in the general population, based on his studies of the dietary habits of the Dutch army.[1] From these modest beginnings, more comprehensive dietary guidelines gradually evolved to include most known nutrients.

In 1933, Hazel Stiebling of the U.S. Department of Agriculture made recommendations of daily needs for protein, calories, several vitamins, minerals, calcium, phosphorus, and iron for the purpose of maintaining health in various age and activity groups.[1] Motivation for these first U.S. dietary recommendations stemmed from the period of the Great Depression when the food supply for the general population was critical. In 1940 the U.S. federal government founded a permanent Committee on Food and Nutrition under the National Research Council of the National Academy of Sciences in Washington, D.C. Established to advise the government on problems concerning defense, the committee produced the first U.S. standard table of Recommended Dietary Allowances (RDAs) in 1940 (published in 1943).[1,2]

Since 1940, every 5 years a new Committee on Dietary Allowances (under the Food and Nutrition Board) has been chosen, and the members are entrusted with the task of revising the U.S. RDAs.*

### *Determination*

RDAs are defined as "the levels of intake of essential nutrients considered, in the judgment of the Committee on Dietary Allowances of the Food and Nutrition Board on the basis of available scientific knowledge, to be adequate to meet the known nutritional needs of practically all healthy persons."[3] Determination of RDAs is a complex process and may be accomplished by various methods, including (1) collection of data on nutrient intake from the food supply of apparently normal, healthy people; (2) review of epidemiologic observations when clinical consequences of nutrient deficiencies are found to be correctable by dietary improvement; (3) biochemical measurements that assess degree of tissue saturation or adequacy of molecular function in relation to nutrient intake; (4) nutrient balance studies that measure nutritional status in relation to intake; (5) studies of subjects maintained on diets containing marginally low or deficient levels of a nutrient, followed by correction of the deficit with measured amounts of that nutrient (such studies are undertaken in humans only when the risk is minimal); and (6) in some few instances, extrapolation from animal experiments in which deficiencies have been produced by the exclusion of a single nutrient from the diet.[2–5] Once data are interpreted to estimate the average requirement of a population, the required value is assumed to follow a Gaussian distribution and is increased by two standard deviations to meet the needs of 97% to 98% of all individuals, and is increased to account for inefficient utilization by the body, for example, poor absorption, poor conversion of precursor to active forms.[2–5] The only exception is energy requirement, which is not increased by two standard deviations.

### *Interpretation*

Emphasis must be placed on proper interpretation of the RDAs.[3–5]

1. RDAs are the average daily amounts of nutrients that *population groups* should consume over a period of time; individual needs may vary.
2. RDAs were established for *healthy* populations; they are not intended for use in patients in depleted states, in patients with illness or metabolic disorders, or in premature infants.
3. RDAs do not take into account altered needs of healthy individuals secondary to increased physical activity, extreme climate, or aging (recommendations for adults older than 51 years are extrapolations from nutrient needs of younger adults).
4. RDAs have not been established for all essential nutrients.
5. RDAs do not compensate for nutrient–nutrient or nutrient–drug interactions, which may alter nutrient bioavailability.

### *U.S. Recommended Dietary Allowances*

Tables 107.1 and 107.2 cite the RDAs for energy and most nutrients. The following discussion encompasses nutrients not found on these two tables.

***Carbohydrate*** No specific dietary requirement for carbohydrate exists because of the human ability to convert amino acids and glycerol derived from fats to glucose; however, to

*Publication of the 1985 U.S. RDAs has been delayed because of review committee discussion.

**Table 107.1** Mean Heights and Weights and U.S. Recommended Daily Energy Intake[a]

| | *Age (yr)* | *Weight* kg | lb | *Height* cm | in. | *Energy needs [kcal (range)]* | |
|---|---|---|---|---|---|---|---|
| Infants | 0–0.5 | 6 | 13 | 60 | 24 | kg × 115 | (95–145) |
| | 0.5–1.0 | 9 | 20 | 71 | 28 | kg × 105 | (80–135) |
| Children | 1–3 | 13 | 29 | 60 | 24 | 1,300 | (900–1,800) |
| | 4–6 | 20 | 44 | 112 | 44 | 1,700 | (1,300–2,300) |
| | 7–10 | 28 | 62 | 132 | 52 | 2,400 | (1,650–3,300) |
| Males | 11–14 | 45 | 99 | 157 | 62 | 2,700 | (2,000–3,700) |
| | 15–18 | 66 | 145 | 176 | 69 | 2,800 | (2,100–3,900) |
| | 19–22 | 70 | 154 | 178 | 70 | 2,900 | (2,500–3,300) |
| | 23–50 | 70 | 154 | 178 | 70 | 2,700 | (2,300–3,100) |
| | 51–75 | 70 | 154 | 178 | 70 | 2,400 | (2,000–2,800) |
| | 76+ | 70 | 154 | 178 | 70 | 2,050 | (1,650–2,450) |
| Females | 11–14 | 46 | 101 | 157 | 62 | 2,200 | (1,500–3,000) |
| | 15–18 | 55 | 120 | 163 | 64 | 2,100 | (1,200–3,000) |
| | 19–22 | 55 | 120 | 163 | 64 | 2,100 | (1,700–2,500) |
| | 23–50 | 55 | 120 | 163 | 64 | 2,000 | (1,600–2,400) |
| | 51–75 | 55 | 120 | 163 | 64 | 1,800 | (1,400–2,200) |
| | 76+ | 55 | 120 | 163 | 64 | 1,600 | (1,200–2,000) |
| Pregnancy | | | | | | +300 | |
| Lactation | | | | | | +500 | |

[a] Energy allowances for children through age 18 are based on median energy intakes of children followed in longitudinal growth studies. The values in parentheses are the 10% and 90% percentiles of energy intake for children in these age groups. The energy allowances for young adult men and women reflect the activity of light work. Allowances for the two older adult age groups allow a 2% decrease in basal (resting) metabolic rate per decade and a reduction in activity of 200 kcal/d for men and women between 51 and 75, 500 kcal/d for men over 75, and 400 kcal/d for women over 75. The range of energy output is shown in parentheses for adults and is based on a variation in energy needs of ± 400 kcal at any age.

From Food and Nutrition Board, National Research Council: Recommended Dietary Allowances, 9th ed. Washington DC, National Academy of Sciences, 1980, p 23, with permission.

avoid ketosis, muscle catabolism, loss of cations, and involuntary dehydration, a minimum of 50–100 g of digestible carbohydrate per day is recommended.[3] Excellent enteral sources of carbohydrate include fruits, vegetables, and whole grain cereals.

***Essential Fatty Acids*** For the general population to avoid essential fatty acid deficiency, 3% of total daily caloric intake should be as linoleic acid.[3]

***Protein*** The adult allowance for protein, including a 75% correction factor to correct for inefficiency of mixed protein utilization, is 0.8 g/kg/d. During pregnancy, an additional 30 g/d is recommended to compensate for fetal growth and development along with uncertain protein storage and efficiency during gestation. The dietary protein allowance for lactating women is an additional 20 g over the allowance for a nonpregnant woman.[3]

***Vitamin K*** A specific recommended allowance for vitamin K does not exist because approximately one half of a person's vitamin K source is synthesized by intestinal bacteria; however, the RDA committee has recommended an intake range based on a 2 μg/kg requirement (Table 107.3). The low end of the range assumes that 1 μg/kg is supplied via intestinal flora, and the high end assumes that the full 2 μg/kg is supplied by the diet.[3,5]

***Pantothenic Acid and Biotin*** Biotin and pantothenic acid, like vitamin K, are synthesized by intestinal microflora that contribute a large part of the body's daily needs. Therefore, the dietary allowances for biotin and pantothenic acid are unknown. Based upon dietary intake and urinary excretion studies, recommended ranges have been developed for biotin and pantothenic acid (Table 107.3).[3]

***Trace Elements*** Copper, manganese, fluoride, chromium, selenium, and molybdenum are trace elements. Because of the danger of toxicity and lack of complete information on which to base recommendations, these trace elements are not included in the main RDA table. Daily dietary intake ranges are given, with the advice that the upper level of the range should not be habitually exceeded to avoid toxic effects (Table 107.4).[3]

***Water*** Water requirements vary greatly with environmental temperature and humidity and an individual's level of activity and state of health. The minimal water intake recommended is 1 mL/kcal for adults and 1.5 mL/kcal for infants[3]; however, altered water needs secondary to fever,

**Table 107.2** Recommended Daily Dietary Allowances

| | Weight | | Height | | | Fat-soluble vitamins | | | Water-soluble vitamins | | | | | | | Minerals | | | | | |
|---|---|---|---|---|---|---|---|---|---|---|---|---|---|---|---|---|---|---|---|---|---|
| *Age (yr)* | kg | lb | cm | in. | *Protein (g)* | Vitamin A ($\mu g$ RE)[a] | Vitamin D ($\mu g$)[b] | Vitamin E (mg $\alpha$-TE)[c] | Vitamin C (mg) | Thiamine (mg) | Riboflavin (mg) | Niacin (mg NE)[d] | Vitamin $B_6$ (mg) | Folacin[e] ($\mu g$) | Vitamin $B_{12}$ ($\mu g$)[f] | Calcium (mg) | Phosphorus (mg) | Magnesium (mg) | Iron[g] (mg) | Zinc (mg) | Iodine ($\mu g$) |
| Infants | | | | | | | | | | | | | | | | | | | | | |
| 0.0–0.5 | 6 | 13 | 60 | 24 | kg × 2.2 | 420 | 10 | 3 | 35 | 0.3 | 0.4 | 6 | 0.3 | 30 | 0.5 | 360 | 240 | 50 | 10 | 3 | 40 |
| 0.5–1.0 | 9 | 20 | 71 | 28 | kg × 2.0 | 400 | 10 | 4 | 35 | 0.5 | 0.6 | 8 | 0.6 | 45 | 1.5 | 540 | 360 | 70 | 15 | 5 | 50 |
| Children | | | | | | | | | | | | | | | | | | | | | |
| 1–3 | 13 | 29 | 90 | 35 | 23 | 400 | 10 | 5 | 45 | 0.7 | 0.8 | 9 | 0.9 | 100 | 2.0 | 800 | 800 | 150 | 15 | 10 | 70 |
| 4–6 | 20 | 44 | 112 | 44 | 30 | 500 | 10 | 6 | 45 | 0.9 | 1.0 | 11 | 1.3 | 200 | 2.5 | 800 | 800 | 200 | 10 | 10 | 90 |
| 7–10 | 28 | 62 | 132 | 52 | 34 | 700 | 10 | 7 | 45 | 1.2 | 1.4 | 16 | 1.6 | 300 | 3.0 | 800 | 800 | 250 | 10 | 10 | 120 |
| Males | | | | | | | | | | | | | | | | | | | | | |
| 11–14 | 45 | 99 | 157 | 62 | 45 | 1000 | 10 | 8 | 50 | 1.4 | 1.6 | 18 | 1.8 | 400 | 3.0 | 1,200 | 1,200 | 350 | 18 | 15 | 150 |
| 15–18 | 66 | 145 | 176 | 69 | 45 | 1000 | 10 | 8 | 60 | 1.4 | 1.7 | 18 | 2.0 | 400 | 3.0 | 1,200 | 1,200 | 400 | 18 | 15 | 150 |
| 19–22 | 70 | 154 | 177 | 70 | 56 | 1000 | 7.5 | 10 | 60 | 1.5 | 1.7 | 19 | 2.2 | 400 | 3.0 | 800 | 800 | 350 | 10 | 15 | 150 |
| 23–50 | 70 | 154 | 178 | 70 | 56 | 1000 | 5 | 10 | 60 | 1.4 | 1.6 | 18 | 2.2 | 400 | 3.0 | 800 | 800 | 350 | 10 | 15 | 150 |
| 51+ | 70 | 154 | 178 | 70 | 56 | 1000 | 5 | 10 | 60 | 1.2 | 1.4 | 16 | 2.2 | 400 | 3.0 | 800 | 800 | 350 | 10 | 15 | 150 |
| Females | | | | | | | | | | | | | | | | | | | | | |
| 11–14 | 46 | 101 | 157 | 62 | 46 | 800 | 10 | 8 | 50 | 1.1 | 1.3 | 15 | 1.8 | 400 | 3.0 | 1,200 | 1,200 | 300 | 18 | 15 | 150 |
| 15–18 | 55 | 120 | 163 | 64 | 46 | 800 | 10 | 8 | 60 | 1.1 | 1.3 | 14 | 2.0 | 400 | 3.0 | 1,200 | 1,200 | 300 | 18 | 15 | 150 |
| 19–22 | 55 | 120 | 163 | 64 | 44 | 800 | 7.5 | 8 | 60 | 1.1 | 1.3 | 14 | 2.0 | 400 | 3.0 | 800 | 800 | 300 | 18 | 15 | 150 |
| 23–50 | 55 | 120 | 163 | 64 | 44 | 800 | 5 | 8 | 60 | 1.0 | 1.2 | 13 | 2.0 | 400 | 3.0 | 800 | 800 | 300 | 18 | 15 | 150 |
| 51+ | 55 | 120 | 163 | 64 | 44 | 800 | 5 | 8 | 60 | 1.0 | 1.2 | 13 | 2.0 | 400 | 3.0 | 800 | 800 | 300 | 10 | 15 | 150 |
| Pregnant | | | | | +30 | +200 | +5 | +2 | +20 | +0.4 | +0.3 | +2 | +0.6 | +400 | +1.0 | +400 | +400 | +150 | +8 | +5 | +25 |
| Lactating | | | | | +20 | +400 | +5 | +3 | +40 | +0.5 | +0.5 | +5 | +0.5 | +100 | +1.0 | +400 | +400 | +150 | +9 | +10 | +50 |

[a] One retinol equivalent (RE) = 1 $\mu g$ retinol or 6 $\mu g$ $\beta$-carotene.

[b] As cholecalciferol. 10 $\mu g$ cholecalciferol = 400 IU of vitamin D.

[c] One $\alpha$-tocopherol equivalent ($\alpha$-TE) = 1 mg D-$\alpha$-tocopherol.

[d] One niacin equivalent (NE) = 1 mg niacin or 60 mg of dietary tryptophan.

[e] The folacin allowances refer to dietary sources as determined by *Lactobacillus casei* assay after treatment with enzymes (conjugases) to make polyglutamyl forms of the vitamin available to the test organism.

[f] RDA for $B_{12}$ in infants is based on average concentrations in human milk. The allowances after weaning are based on energy intake and consideration of other factors such as intestinal absorption.

[g] Increased iron requirements during pregnancy cannot be met by the average U.S. diet nor by the existing iron stores of many women; therefore, the use of 30–60 mg of supplemental iron is recommended. Iron needs during lactation are not substantially different from those of nonpregnant women, but continued supplementation 2 to 3 months postparturition is advised to replete stores depleted by pregnancy.

From Food and Nutrition Board, National Research Council: Recommended Dietary Allowances, 9th ed. Washington DC, National Academy of Sciences, 1980, p 180, with permission.

**Table 107.3** Ranges of Estimated Safe and Adequate Daily Dietary Intakes for Vitamins With Undetermined RDAs

| *Age (yr)* | *Vitamin K (μg)* | *Biotin (μg)* | *Pantothenic acid (mg)* |
|---|---|---|---|
| Infants | | | |
| 0–0.5 | 12 | 35 | 2 |
| 0.5–1.0 | 10–20 | 50 | 3 |
| Children | | | |
| 1–3 | 15–30 | 65 | 3 |
| 4–6 | 20–40 | 85 | 3–4 |
| 7–10 | 30–60 | 120 | 4–5 |
| 11+ | 50–100 | 100–200 | 4–7 |
| Adults | 70–140 | 100–200 | 4–7 |

From Food and Nutrition Board, National Research Council: Recommended Dietary Allowances, 9th ed. Washington DC, National Academy of Sciences, 1980, p 178, with permission.

vomiting, diarrhea, high-protein diets, diuretics, and hot environments must be given proper consideration.

***Sodium, Potassium, and Chloride*** Recommendations of safe dietary intakes of these three electrolytes are listed in Table 107.5.[3] Values for the young infant (0–6 months) are based upon breast milk for the low end of the range and formula feeding for the high end. Recommendations for older infants, children, and adults at the low end of the range are based upon young infants' breast milk consumption data extrapolated to correct for body surface area. The high end of the range is simply three times greater than the low end.[3]

***Miscellaneous Substances*** Many substances are consumed daily for which there is no or little proof of dietary essentiality. Trace elements in particular are difficult to determine because of the minute amounts ingested. Although the essentiality of the following substances in man is yet unknown, these nutrients are essential for certain higher animals: cobalt (ingested with vitamin $B_{12}$); nickel, vanadium, and silicon (essential in more than two higher animal species, but more study is required in humans); tin, arsenic, and cadmium (deficiency syndromes reported in animals, but more study is required in humans).[3]

## Nutritional Requirements in Disease

Nutritional requirements can vary greatly depending on an individual's disease state. Repletional needs are greater than those of maintenance; increased energy needs exist in situations of elevated metabolic states such as surgical stress, trauma, and sepsis; protein needs vary with renal function, hepatic function, metabolic stress, and depletion. Carbohydrate tolerance is affected by pancreatic function, respiratory status, and neurohumoral metabolic effects in stress. Electrolyte requirements are dictated largely by renal function, presence of congestive heart failure, vomiting, diarrhea, gastric output, and high-output fistula losses. Fat-soluble vitamin dosage is usually increased secondary to disease states associated with intestinal malabsorption (e.g., cystic fibrosis, short-bowel syndrome, steatorrhea). Normal water-soluble vitamin requirements may be increased in specialized cases (i.e., $B_{12}$ deficiency secondary to inadequate intrinsic factor, increased oral vitamin needs secondary to drug–nutrient interactions result in decreased bioavailability, or increased needs secondary to losses during hemodialysis). Other than in states of documented deficiency, increased trace element needs are present during

**Table 107.4** Ranges of Estimated Safe and Adequate Daily Dietary Intakes of Trace Elements

| *Age (yr)* | *Copper (mg)* | *Manganese (mg)* | *Fluoride (mg)* | *Chromium (mg)* | *Selenium (mg)* | *Molybdenum (mg)* |
|---|---|---|---|---|---|---|
| Infants | | | | | | |
| 0–0.5 | 0.5–0.7 | 0.5–0.7 | 0.1–0.5 | 0.01–0.04 | 0.01–0.04 | 0.03–0.06 |
| 0.5–1.0 | 0.7–1.0 | 0.7–1.0 | 0.2–1.0 | 0.02–0.06 | 0.02–0.06 | 0.04–0.08 |
| Children | | | | | | |
| 1–3 | 1.0–1.5 | 1.0–1.5 | 0.5–1.5 | 0.02–0.08 | 0.02–0.08 | 0.05–0.1 |
| 4–6 | 1.5–2.0 | 1.5–2.0 | 1.0–2.5 | 0.03–0.12 | 0.03–0.12 | 0.06–0.15 |
| 7–10 | 2.0–2.5 | 2.0–3.0 | 1.5–2.5 | 0.05–0.20 | 0.05–0.20 | 0.10–0.30 |
| 11+ | 2.0–3.0 | 2.5–5.0 | 1.5–2.5 | 0.05–0.20 | 0.05–0.20 | 0.15–0.50 |
| Adults | 2.0–3.0 | 2.5–5.0 | 1.5–4.0 | 0.05–0.20 | 0.05–0.20 | 0.15–0.50 |

From Food and Nutrition Board, National Research Council: Recommended Dietary Allowances, 9th ed. Washington DC, National Academy of Sciences, 1980, p 178, with permission.

**Table 107.5** Estimated Safe and Adequate Daily Dietary Intakes of Sodium, Potassium, and Chloride

| *Age (yr)* | *Sodium (mg)* | *Potassium (mg)* | *Chloride (mg)* |
|---|---|---|---|
| Infants | | | |
| 0–0.5 | 115–350 | 350–925 | 275–700 |
| 0.5–1.0 | 250–750 | 425–1,275 | 400–1,200 |
| Children | | | |
| 1–3 | 325–975 | 550–1,650 | 500–1,500 |
| 4–6 | 450–1,350 | 775–2,325 | 700–2,100 |
| 7–10 | 600–1,800 | 1,000–3,000 | 925–2,775 |
| 11+ | 900–2,700 | 1,525–4,575 | 1,400–4,200 |
| Adults | 1,100–3,300 | 1,875–5,625 | 1,700–5,100 |

From Food and Nutrition Board, National Research Council: Recommended Dietary Allowances, 9th ed. Washington DC, National Academy of Sciences, 1980, p 178, with permission.

times of increased intestinal output, when substantial amounts of zinc and chromium may be lost.

The following guidelines are meant to be a general overview of nutritional needs in various disease states; more comprehensive discussions may be found in other chapters dealing primarily with special consideration in nutritional support, including parenteral and enteral nutrition.

### *Energy*

Individuals require energy for metabolic processes such as maintenance of bodily functions, growth, repair, and physical activity. Energy requirements are calculated as kilocalories (kcal) and vary with age, sex, height, weight, activity, and disease state. One method commonly used to calculate energy requirements is the Harris–Benedict equation of basal energy expenditure (BEE). In 1919, Harris and Benedict studied the oxygen consumption of 239 healthy men and women to determine metabolic energy requirements for normal men and women.[6–8] Their efforts resulted in the equations

$$\text{BEE (men)} = 66.4730 + 13.7516\ \text{Wt} + 5.0033\ \text{Ht} - 6.7550\ \text{Age}$$

$$\text{BEE (women)} = 655.0950 + 9.5630\ \text{Wt} + 1.8496\ \text{Ht} - 4.6756\ \text{Age}$$

where BEE is in kilocalories per day, Wt is in kilograms, Ht is in centimeters, and Age is in years. BEE reflects estimated basal energy requirements, and, to accommodate states of activity or illness, it is multiplied by a correction factor. Based on indirect calorimetry studies by Long et al[6] the method in Table 107.6 can be used.

A more individualized approach to measuring metabolic requirements is the resting energy expenditure (REE). To calculate REE, indirect calorimetry is employed with a metabolic measuring cart or apparatus. A metabolic measurement cart analyzes a subject's inspired and expired air to calculate oxygen consumption, carbon dioxide production, expired volume, breaths per minute, breath temperature, and pressure.[8–10] Urinary nitrogen data may or may not be included. Indirect calorimetry is based on the principle that at steady state, oxygen consumption and carbon dioxide production are directly related to the production of energy in the body.[8,9,11] Thus, the quantities of oxygen consumed and carbon dioxide produced by an individual are measured through analysis of respiratory gases. The Weir equation is employed to calculate the REE from the measured data[8–10,12]

$$\text{REE} = (3.941\ V_{O_2} + 1.106\ V_{CO_2})\ 1.44 - 2.14\ \text{UN}$$

REE is kilocalories per day, $V_{O_2}$ ($O_2$ consumption) is in milliliters per minute, $V_{CO_2}$ ($CO_2$ production) is in milliliters per minute, and UN (urinary nitrogen excretion) is in grams per 24 hours. Often, the urinary nitrogen excretion data are omitted because of collection inconvenience and the abbreviated Weir equation is used.[12] By ignoring the effects of protein metabolism an error, usually of less than 1%, is introduced into the final value of measured REE.[12]

$$\text{REE} = (3.941\ V_{O_2} + 1.106\ V_{CO_2})\ 1.44$$

Although indirect calorimetry measures the individual's needs whatever level of stress the patient may be experiencing, additional kilocalories must be supplied if malnutrition is present and repletion is a goal.

**Table 107.6** BEE Correction Factors for Activity and Injury

| *Activity factor* | *Use* | *Injury factor* | *Use* |
|---|---|---|---|
| Confined to bed | 1.20 | Minor operation | 1.20 |
| Out of bed | 1.30 | Skeletal trauma | 1.35 |
| | | Major sepsis | 1.60 |
| | | Severe thermal burns | 2.10 |

From Long CL, Scheffel N, Geiger JW, et al: Metabolic response to injury and illness: Estimation of energy and protein needs from indirect calorimetry and nitrogen balance. J Parenter Enter Nutr 1979;3(6):455, with permission.

### Protein

In healthy, well-nourished individuals, the RDA for protein should adequately provide sufficient amounts of amino acids necessary for synthesis of all human proteins. In addition, amino acids may normally be metabolized to nitrogenous compounds such as purines, pyrimidines, and catecholamines as well as oxidized to carbon dioxide as an energy source[13]; however, during periods of inadequate protein or energy intake, muscle catabolism occurs so that amino acids are precursors for liver gluconeogenesis and energy production.[14]

Eventually, lean body mass diminishes, and, if not reversed, could lead to seriously impaired organ function. Shaw et al[15] found that repletion of nonstressed malnourished patients with nitrogen 364 mg/kg/d and approximately 33 kcal/kg/d allowed a markedly positive nitrogen balance without excessive energy intake.

Protein needs during high levels of stress are greatly elevated. Metabolically there is increased nitrogen excretion, increased basal oxygen consumption, and altered substrate metabolism.[7,9–11,16–19] Accelerated skeletal muscle breakdown occurs to meet energy needs. Controversy exists as to the appropriate amino acid mix in high levels of stress. Clinical trials using amino acids containing 45% to 50% branched-chain amino acids have yielded preliminary data indicating possibly better nitrogen retention[20–22]; however, generally 2.0–2.5 g protein per kilogram per day are required in hypermetabolic, high-stress patients.[7,19,23]

In renal failure patients, protein dosage depends on degree of renal dysfunction and presence of dialysis. A common nutritional problem in this population is depletion of protein reserves. Therefore, effort must be made to provide adequate protein. Traditional guidelines state that when the glomerular filtration rate (GFR) is greater than 25 mL/min, protein should be restricted to 0.4–0.5 g/kg/d.[10] During dialysis, protein is lost in the dialysate; also the patient's protein tolerance improves. Therefore, 1.0–1.5 g/kg dry body weight per day during dialysis is recommended.[24]

Protein intolerance in liver failure patients is secondary to the liver's inability to metabolize amino acids such as the aromatic amino acids (AAAs), methionine and glutamine.[25,26] Branched-chain amino acids (BCAAs), however, are metabolized primarily in peripheral muscle for energy.[27] Typically, the plasma amino acid profile of end-stage hepatic failure shows increased concentrations of aromatic amino acids, methionine and glutamine, along with decreased concentrations of branched-chain amino acids. Fischer has traditionally recommended a limited protein intake of 20–25 g/d to prevent encephalopathy[28]; however, recent studies with parenteral amino acid mixtures containing 35.5% BCAAs and only 1.25% AAAs have successfully improved encephalopathy.[29,30] Use of parenteral high-BCAA/low-AAA mixtures is based upon the false neurotransmitter hypothesis. Guidelines for use are as follows[31]:

1. Hepatic encephalopathy more severe than or equal to grade 2
2. Or abnormal plasma amino acid profile with a plasma molar ratio of BCAA:AAA of 2 or less
3. Or hepatic encephalopathy associated with total parenteral nutrition solutions containing standard amino acid solutions in doses needed for nutritional support

This specialized solution should be initiated at 0.5–0.75 g/kg/d and increased by 0.25–0.5 g/kg/d to a goal of 1.5 g/kg/d.[32] This therapy is still controversial.

Burn patients represent a nutritional challenge because of their increased protein and energy needs. Both energy and protein needs are dependent upon magnitude of burn size and closure of the burn wound. General recommendations for large burns are 20–25 g nitrogen per day for the first 13 days followed by 15 g nitrogen per day for the next 25 days.[19,33]

### Carbohydrate

The minimal amount of carbohydrate necessary to avoid ketosis and provide necessary carbohydrate to neural and hematopoietic tissue is 100–150 g/d[34]; however, a normal person can oxidize glucose at 2–4 mg/kg/min.[35] Stressed patients with increased energy needs can oxidize glucose at a rate up to 3–5 mg/kg/min.[36] As the patient's level of stress increases there is increased production of catecholamines, cortisol, and glucagon; insulin concentrations may be relatively normal, though inappropriately low in relation to blood glucose.[19,23,37–39] In such an elevated level of stress hyperglycemia exists along with insulin resistance. The picture is complicated by increased energy needs, which are difficult to meet in the face of glucose intolerance. Attempts to provide the patient with adequate kilocalories to meet energy needs may be disastrous. Hypermetabolic patients preferentially metabolize greater proportions of glucose than fat as compared with normal patients.[23,29,40] This results in increased carbon dioxide production, which can precipitate respiratory distress.[23,40] Critically ill patients have some impairment of the ratio of dead space to tidal volume associated with increased resting levels of minute ventilation.[16,23] The increased carbon dioxide load from carbohydrate may lead to respiratory failure. Therefore, glucose intake should be restricted to one half or less of the resting energy expenditure in this patient population, and higher doses of lipid should be provided in the short term.[23]

### Electrolytes and Minerals

Electrolyte and mineral requirements are dependent upon organ function and vary considerably with organ dysfunction and disease state. Table 107.7 lists instances of abnormal electrolyte and mineral requirements.

### Trace Elements

***Zinc*[40,43]** The major route of excretion from the body is via pancreatic and intestinal secretions; however, increased urinary zinc losses are found in alcoholic, fasting obese, renal disease, diabetic, liver disease, porphyric, proteinuric, trauma, and sickle cell disease patients. Zinc supplementation in acute catabolic states ranges from 4.5 to 6.0 mg using the parenteral route. In intestinal losses, supplementation of 12.1 mg/L of small-bowel fluid output and 17.1 mg/L of diarrhea or ileostomy output via the parenteral route should be adequate.

***Copper*[40,44]** Absorption of copper occurs primarily in the stomach and duodenum, but some absorption in all parts of the small intestine is possible. The major routes of excretion are biliary and intestinal. Deficiency is uncommon but is more likely in patients with shortened intestines. Copper

**Table 107.7** States of Altered Electrolyte and Mineral Requirements

| | *Increased needs* | *Decreased needs* |
|---|---|---|
| Sodium | Increased intestinal losses | Congestive heart failure<br>Renal dysfunction<br>Circulatory insufficiency |
| Potassium | Increased gastric losses<br>Increased intestinal losses<br>Excessive renal losses, e.g., diabetic ketoacidosis, diuretics | Renal dysfunction<br>Congestive heart failure<br>Possibly untreated Addison's disease<br>Patients possibly taking potassium-sparing diuretics |
| Chloride | Increased gastric losses | |
| Magnesium | Malabsorption syndromes<br>Possibly with diuretics or alcohol | Renal dysfunction |
| Calcium | Malabsorption syndromes<br>Hypoparathyroidism | |
| Phosphorous | Malabsorption syndromes<br>Nutrition recovery syndrome | Renal dysfunction |

Compiled from References 40–42.

intake should be decreased to 0.2 mg/d, parenterally, in patients with liver dysfunction or cholestatic liver disease.

***Selenium***[40,41,45] Selenium requirements are decreased in renal failure patients, as the primary route of excretion is renal. Deficiencies may be seen in patients receiving long-term, unsupplemented total parenteral nutrition. Parenteral recommendations are 150 $\mu$g/d.

***Manganese***[40,41,46] Manganese is excreted primarily in the bile; therefore, exogenous requirements are decreased in patients with cholestatic liver disease.

***Chromium***[40,41,47] Mechanisms of chromium absorption and metabolism are poorly understood. Excretion is primarily in the urine, though feces contain predominantly nonabsorbed dietary chromium. Increased chromium excretion is associated with diabetes mellitus, burns, trauma, glucose load, and insulin injection. Parenteral chromium supplementation with increased intestinal losses is 20 $\mu$g/d. Normal intake may need to be decreased in renal dysfunction.

***Iron***[40,41] Iron is absorbed predominantly in the duodenum and lost via skin, hair, urine, intestinal desquamation, and bleeding (e.g., menstrual losses). Acute and chronic blood loss and impaired absorption (such as seen with achlorhydria) may lead to iron deficiency. A formula commonly used to calculate total body iron deficiency is

$$\text{mg iron} = (0.3 \times \text{pounds body weight}) \times [100 - (100 \times \text{g/dL hemoglobin}/14.8)]$$

When repleting adults parenterally, the maximal daily amount to be administered is 20 mg iron–dextran for patients under 110 pounds and 50 mg iron–dextran for patients over 110 pounds. Injections should be administered daily until the total calculated dose has been given. Caution should be exhibited in administering iron to septic patients, as iron sequesteration in this population is thought to be a protective mechanism, depriving certain gram-negative bacteria of the iron necessary for their proliferation.

## Summary

The purpose of this chapter was not only to summarize the U.S. RDA guidelines but also to emphasize that these recommendations have definite limitations. Recognition of these limitations is vital to the interpretation and proper use of the RDAs. It is important to consider that the RDAs are oral dietary intake guidelines for normal populations and are not applicable to the intravenous route or to sick individuals.

Nutritional requirements in disease states may vary greatly from normal needs. Depending on the organ system involved, requirements for energy, macronutrients, and micronutrients can vary such that an imprudent decision in determining needs may result in a disastrous outcome. Therefore, recognizing that each nutritional entity is a separate pharmacologic compound that should be determined in an individual manner is imperative to providing the patient with the most efficacious nutritional therapy in their current state of health.

## References

1. Harper AE. Origin of recommended dietary allowances—an historic overview. Am J Clin Nutr 1985;41:140–148.
2. Kamin H. Status of the 10th edition of the recommended dietary allowances—Prospects for the future. Am J Clin Nutr 1985;41:165–170.
3. Food and Nutrition Board, National Research Council. Recom-

mended Dietary Allowances, 9th ed. Washington DC, National Academy of Sciences, 1980.

4. Beaton GH. Uses and limits of the use of the recommended dietary allowances for evaluating dietary intake data. Am J Clin Nutr 1985;41:155–164.
5. Munro HN. Evolving scientific basis for the recommended dietary allowances—A critical look at methodologies. Am J Clin Nutr 1985;41:149–154.
6. Long CL, Scheffel N, Geiger JW, et al. Metabolic responses to injury and illness: Estimation of energy and protein needs from indirect calorimetry and nitrogen balance. J Parenter Enter Nutr 1979;3:452–456.
7. Wilmore DW. The Metabolic Management of the Critically Ill. New York, Plenum, 1977.
8. Beckman Electronic Instruments Division, Beckman Instruments Division. Assessment of Energy Expenditure and Nutritional Requirements by Indirect Calorimetry. Schiller Park, IL, 1981.
9. Hunker FD, Bruton CW, Hunker EM, et al. Metabolic and nutritional evaluation of patients supported with mechanical ventilation. Crit Care Med 1980;8:628–634.
10. Silberman H, Eisenberg D. Parenteral and Enteral Nutrition for the Hospitalized Patient. Norwalk, CT, Appleton-Century-Crofts, 1982.
11. Knox LS, Crosby LO, Feurer ID, et al. Energy expenditure of malnourished cancer patients. Ann Surg 1983;197:152–162.
12. Weir JB de V. New methods for calculating metabolic rate with special reference to protein metabolism. J Physiol 1949;109:1–9.
13. Munro HN, Crim MC. The proteins and amino acids, in Goodman RS, Shils ME (eds): Modern Nutrition in Health and Disease. Philadelphia, Lea and Febiger, 1980, pp 51–98.
14. Young VR, Munro HN. *N*-Methylhistidine (3-methylhistidine) and muscle protein turnover: An overview. Fed Proc 1978;37:2291–2300.
15. Shaw SN, Elwyn DH, Askanazi J, et al. Effects of increasing nitrogen intake on nitrogen balance and energy expenditure in nutritionally depleted adult patients receiving parenteral nutrition. Am J Clin Nutr 1983;37:930–940.
16. Askanazi J, Nordenstrom J, Rosenbaum SH, et al. Nutrition for the patient with respiratory failure: Glucose vs. fat. Anesthesiology 1981;54:373–377.
17. Askanazi J, Rosenbaum J, Hyman AI, et al. Respiratory changes induced by the large glucose loads of parenteral nutrition. JAMA 1980;243:1444–1447.
18. Barrocas A, Tretola R, Alanso A. Nutrition and the critically ill pulmonary patient. Resp Care 1983;28:50–61.
19. Cerra FB. Pocket Manual of Clinical Nutrition. St. Louis, C.V. Mosby, 1984.
20. Cerra FB, Mazuski J, Teasley K, et al. Nitrogen retention in critically ill patients is proportional to the branched chain amino acid load. Crit Care Med 1983;11:775–778.
21. Cerra FB, Mazuski J, Chute E, et al. Branched chain metabolic support. Ann Surg 1984;199:286–291.
22. Freund HR, Ryan JA, Fischer J. Amino acid derangements in patients with sepsis: Treatment with branched chain amino acid rich solutions. Ann Surg 1978;188:423–430.
23. Elwyn DH. Nutritional requirements of adult surgical patients. Crit Care Med 1980;8:9–20.
24. Kopple JD. Nutritional therapy in kidney failure, in Olson RE (ed): Nutrition Review's Present Knowledge in Nutrition, 5th ed. Washington DC, Nutrition Foundation, 1984.
25. Morgan MY, Milson JP, Sherlock S. Plasma ratio of valine, leucine and isoleucine to phenylalanine and tyrosine in liver disease. Gut 1978;19:1068–1073.
26. Cascino A, Cangiano C, Calcaterra V. Plasma amino acid imbalance in patients with liver disease. Am J Dig Dis 1978;23:591–598.
27. Felig P. Amino acid metabolism in man. Ann Rev Biochem 1975;44:936–955.
28. Fischer JE, Yoshimura N, Aguirre A, et al. Plasma amino acids in patients with hepatic encephalopathy: Effects of amino acid infusion. Am J Surg 1974;127:40–47.
29. Cerra FB, Cheung NK, Fischer JE, et al. Disease specific amino acid infusion (F080) in hepatic encephalopathy: A prospective, randomized, double-blind, controlled trial. J Parenter Enter Nutr 1985;9:288–295.
30. Egberts EH, Schomerus H, Hamster W, et al. Branched chain amino acids in the treatment of latent portosystemic encephalopathy: A double-blind placebo controlled crossover study. Gastroenterology 1985;88:887–895.
31. Barber JR, Teasley KT. Nutritional support of patients with severe hepatic failure. Clin Pharm 1984;3:245–253.
32. Nachbauer CA, Fischer JE. Nutritional support in hepatic failure, in Fischer JE (ed): Surgical Nutrition. Boston, Little Brown, 1983.
33. Shires TG. Second conference on supportive therapy in burn care. J Trauma 1981;21:666–749.
34. Cahill GF. Starvation in man. N Engl J Med 1970;282:668–675.
35. Jacot E, Defronzo RA, Jequier E, et al. The effect of hyperglycemia, hyperinsulinemia, and route of glucose administration on glucose oxidation and glucose storage. Metabolism 1982;31:922–930.
36. Burke JF, Wolfe RR, Mullany CJ, et al. Glucose requirements following burn injury. Ann Surg 1979;190:274–285.
37. Askanazi J, Carpentier YA, Elwyn DH, et al. Influence of total parenteral nutrition on fuel utilization in injury and sepsis. Ann Surg 1980;191:40–46.
38. Elwyn DH, Kinney JM, Askanazi J. Energy expenditures in surgical patients. Surg Clin North Am 1981;61:545–556.
39. Cerra FB. Sepsis, metabolic failure and total parenteral nutrition. Nutr Sup Serv 1981;1:26–29.
40. Tuckerman MM, Turco SJ (eds): Human Nutrition. Philadelphia, Lea & Febiger, 1983.
41. Reilly JJ, Gerhardt AL. Modern surgical nutrition. Curr Probl Surg 1985;12(10):3–81.
42. Knochel JP. The Pathophysiology and Clinical Characteristics of Severe Hypophosphatemia. Ann Intern Med 1977;137:203–220.
43. Solomons N. Nutrition chart number one—Zinc. Nutr Sup Serv 1984;4(4):8.
44. Askan A. Nutrition chart number five—Copper. Nutr Sup Serv 1984;4(9):35.
45. Whitney A. Nutrition chart number six—Selenium. Nutr Sup Serv 1984;4(10):31.
46. Betzhold J. Nutrition chart number eight—Manganese. Nutr Sup Serv 1985;5(1):49.
47. Danford DE, Anderson RA. Nutrition chart number nine—Chromium. Nutr Sup Serv 1985;5(2):21.

# Chapter 108 / Pediatric Parenteral Nutrition

Sharon L. Young, PharmD

Total parenteral nutrition (TPN) has become an important factor in the improved outcome of infants and children who are unable to meet their nutritional requirements with enteral nutrition. The majority of these infants and children have disease states that complicate their nutritional intake, such as premature birth, chronic diarrhea, short-bowel syndrome, cystic fibrosis, malignancies, and gastrointestinal surgical procedures. With the development of TPN therapy, infants and children have been able to maintain adequate growth when the gastrointestinal tract is not functioning.

In 1944 Helfrick and Abelson described the first successful trial of total parenteral nutrition in a child.[1] They treated a 5-month-old male infant with Hirschsprung's disease and marasmus for a 5-day period with total parenteral nutrition using an infusate of 50% glucose, 10% solution of amino acids and electrolytes alternating with a 10% fat emulsion consisting of olive oil and lecithin. While this therapy was complicated by thrombophlebitis, its partial success provided incentive for others to pursue this therapeutic modality. For over 20 years efforts to duplicate these results were unsuccessful. The many failures were attributed to the inability of peripheral veins to tolerate the hyperosmolarity of the infusates. Some tried to reduce the hyperosmolarity by diluting the solutions, but this resulted in complications related to fluid overload. Others tried substituting dextrose with ethanol to reduce the osmolarity; however, the toxicity associated with ethanol has limited its utility. The development of intravenous fat emulsions has reduced the complications associated with hyperosmolarity.

Another major advancement in TPN therapy has been the utilization of central venous catheters. Increased concentrations of dextrose and protein may be administered through central venous catheters without the complication of thrombophlebitis. The first such case was by Wilmore and Dedrick in 1968 who administered a 25% glucose and 5% fibrin hydrolysate infusate containing electrolytes and vitamins to a 1-month-old female infant with short-bowel syndrome.[2] By administering the infusate through a catheter in the superior vena cava, the patient was successfully treated with TPN for 44 days before beginning gradual enteral feedings. Of significance was the positive nitrogen balance and continual weight gain sustained throughout the treatment period.

Today total parenteral nutrition has become a significant component of nutritional support therapy. Techniques have been developed that allow patients to receive TPN therapy for an extended period of time; however, TPN therapy is not without complications and is reserved for those patients in whom the gastrointestinal tract as a route of nutritional intake is not feasible or is unable to meet the patient's nutritional requirements.

## Indications

Total parenteral nutrition is an important component of the management of the critically ill child. In the low-birth-weight infant TPN has become a mainstay of therapy. TPN therapy has been identified as a principal factor in the improved survival rate of low-birth-weight infants over the past 15 years. The low-birth-weight infant is often unable to tolerate enteral feedings. Malnutrition develops quickly without adequate nutritional intake in these infants because of the limited endogenous stores of essential nutrients. Studies have demonstrated the ability to maintain adequate weight gain and positive nitrogen balance in low-birth-weight infants utilizing TPN therapy.[3–6] In a recent survey of 269 neonatal intensive care units in the United States parenteral nutrition was used during the first week of life in 80% of those neonates weighing less than 1,000 g.[7]

Infants with congenital anomalies of the gastrointestinal tract, such as gastroschisis, bowel fistulas, malrotation, intestinal obstructions, and atresias, frequently require prolonged TPN support after surgical correction. Studies have shown the ability to attain a positive nitrogen balance and weight gain in these infants with TPN therapy.[8,9] In a recent study of 13 children with very small short bowel, the improved survival rate of 69% as compared to 23% in such patients reported in 1972 was attributed to the improved techniques of TPN therapy.[10,11]

Prolonged or recurrent diarrhea in the young child may quickly lead to a state of protein-calorie malnutrition which may compromise the patient.[12] Studies have documented a cessation of diarrhea within a few days of initiation of TPN therapy.[13,14] In addition to reducing the amount of diarrhea, TPN therapy has corrected the protein-calorie malnutrition common in infants with intractable diarrhea.[13,15–17] Children with inflammatory bowel disease have also benefited from the bowel rest provided by TPN therapy. TPN therapy may effectively induce remission of clinical symptoms and improve the nutritional status in children with severe Crohn's disease and chronic inflammatory bowel disease.[18–20] Growth arrest, a common manifestation of protein-calorie malnutrition in children with inflammatory bowel disease, has been reversed and catchup linear growth documented with TPN therapy.[20–22]

Children with cystic fibrosis often have pancreatic insufficiency as a component of their disease. Pancreatic insufficiency frequently results in malnutrition in the child with cystic fibrosis.[23] While the prognosis of cystic fibrosis is most directly related to pulmonary function, there appears to be a relationship between declining nutritional status and declining pulmonary function.[24] Studies evaluating the effect

**Table 108.1** Recommended Daily Caloric and Protein Needs for Infants and Children

| *Age* | *kcal/kg/d (range)* | | *kcal/d* | *Protein (g/kg/d)* |
|---|---|---|---|---|
| 0–6 mo | 115 (95–145) | | | 2.2 |
| 6–12 mo | 105 (80–135) | | | 2.0 |
| 1–3 yr | 100 (69–138) | | 900–1,800 | 1.8 |
| 4–6 yr | 85 (65–115) | | 1,300–2,300 | 1.5 |
| 7–10 yr | 85 (59–118) | | 1,650–3,300 | 1.2 |
| 11–14 yr | 50–60 (33–82) | Female | 2,100–3,500 | 1.0 |
| | | Male | 2,000–3,700 | 1.0 |
| 15–18 yr | 40 (22–56) | Female | 1,200–3,000 | 0.9 |
| | | Male | 2,100–3,500 | 0.9 |

From Food and Nutrition Board, National Research Council: Recommended Dietary Allowances, 9th ed. Washington DC, National Academy of Sciences, 1980, p. 23, with permission.

of intravenous nutritional supplementation and clinical status have demonstrated a less rapid deterioration in respiratory status with improvement in nutritional status.[24–26]

The child with cancer frequently develops some degree of malnutrition during the course of their disease. The impact of malnutrition may be reflected in tumor response tolerance to chemotherapy, incidence of complications, and general survival.[27,28] Filler et al demonstrated an improvement in general nutrition and in appearance in 41 children with various childhood cancers receiving TPN therapy.[29] Reversal of anergy associated with protein-energy malnutrition was attributed to TPN therapy in 5 children with Wilms' tumor.[30]

Anorexia nervosa is another disease state seen in childhood that may lead to a state of severe protein-calorie malnutrition. In several case reports TPN therapy has been beneficial in reversing malnutrition associated with extremes of this disease.[31–33] Not only has TPN benefited the child in a state of malnutrition, but children with metabolic disturbances such as in acute renal failure and inborn errors of metabolism have benefited as well.[34–38]

Children suffering from severe trauma or burns are frequently in a hypermetabolic state. Without adequate nutritional support, protein-calorie malnutrition may quickly develop and further compromise the patient.[39,40] Popp et al demonstrated an improvement in clinical and nutritional status in 26 children with severe burns with the utilization of TPN therapy.[41]

## Nutritional Requirements

Nutritional requirements in children vary with respect to age, size, physical activity, and disease state. Recommended daily caloric intakes have been estimated on the basis of longitudinal growth studies of children (Table 108.1).[42] Infants have greater caloric requirements (kcal/kg body weight/d) than children and adults because of increased activity and growth. They also have increased heat losses because of a larger body surface area in proportion to body weight.

Daily caloric requirements may be partitioned into those required for basal metabolism, specific dynamic action of foods, fecal and urinary losses, growth, and activity. The basal metabolic rate is the energy required to support life in a fasting and relaxed state. It represents the greatest proportion of total daily caloric requirements, ranging from approximately 50% (40–60 kcal/kg/d) in infants to 66% (25–30 kcal/kg/d) in adults. The specific dynamic action of foods refers to the 5 kcal/kg/d increase in caloric expenditure over the basal metabolic rate after the ingestion of food. This increase has been associated with the digestion and absorption of nutrients; however, it has also been observed with parenteral administration of nutrients.[43] Fecal and urinary losses of calories generally remain constant throughout life at 5–10 kcal/kg/d.[44] The caloric requirement for tissue growth in children has been shown to range from 4 to 6 kcal for each gram of body weight gained.[45–49] Physical activity represents the greatest variable in daily patient caloric requirements.[45] A reduction in physical activity associated with disease often decreases this energy requirement as compared with the healthy child.[43]

The importance of adequate nutrition in the low-birth-weight infant is well accepted; however, the goal of nutrition in this patient population is less well defined. The current approach is to achieve a postnatal growth rate that approximates in utero growth rates of a normal fetus at the same postconceptional age.[46] In the third trimester these growth rates are between 10 and 15 g/kg/d.[46,48,50] The partition of caloric requirements has been evaluated in the low-birth-weight infant (Table 108.2).[47–51] In addition to the caloric

**Table 108.2** Estimated Caloric Requirements of a Growing Premature Infant

| | *kcal/kg/d* |
|---|---|
| Resting caloric expenditure | 50 |
| Intermittent activity | 15 |
| Occasional cold stress | 10 |
| Specific dynamic action | 8 |
| Fecal loss of calories | 12 |
| Growth allowance | 25 |
| Total | 120 |

From American Academy of Pediatrics, Committee on Nutrition: Nutritional needs of low-birth weight infants. Pediatrics 1985;75:976–986, with permission.

requirements for basal metabolism, specific dynamic action of foods, fecal and urinary losses, growth, and activity, the low-birth-weight infant has an additional requirement of approximately 10 kcal/kg/d to respond to occasional cold stress.[46,51] Therefore, the low-birth-weight infant requires 40–60 kcal/kg/d to meet maintenance caloric requirements. To achieve a weight gain of 10–15 g/kg/d an additional 50–75 kcal/kg/d is required for a total caloric requirement of 90–135 kcal/kg/d in the low-birth-weight infant.

Caloric requirements in ill children are based upon their growth status, the state of their reserves, and the degree of stress from illness.[45] Basal energy requirements take priority over growth. Disease-related stress has been associated with an increase in the basal metabolic rate. The magnitude of the increase in the basal metabolic rate correlates with the severity of the disease state (Table 108.3).[52] For example, in adult patients skeletal trauma has been associated with a 32% increase in the basal metabolic rate, whereas severe burns have been associated with a 130% increase.[52]

Protein is essential for growth and other anabolic processes. Recommended daily protein intakes have been estimated by longitudinal growth and nitrogen balance studies in children (Table 108.1).[42] As with calorie requirements, infants and children have greater protein requirements (g/kg/d) than adolescents and adults primarily because of increased growth rates. Protein will be utilized as a caloric source to meet energy requirements rather than anabolic processes if adequate nonprotein calories are not provided. Therefore, to utilize protein efficiently for anabolic processes, the patient must receive an adequate amount of nonprotein calories. This requirement has been identified as the nitrogen (grams)-to-nonprotein calorie ratio (N:NPC). Early studies demonstrated an optimal N:NPC ratio of 1:300–350 in healthy active adults[53]; however, changes in the basal metabolic rate associated with disease states have been shown to alter the optimal N:NPC ratio.[54,55] Studies evaluating the optimal N:NPC ratio in pediatric patients are lacking. In studies of adult patients in gastrointestinal disease states requiring prolonged parenteral nutrition, the optimal N:NPC ratio has ranged from 1:148 to 1:163.[54,55] It is currently accepted that a N:NPC ratio of 1:150–200 should provide adequate nonprotein calories for appropriate utilization of protein in infants and children requiring total parenteral nutrition.[56,57]

**Table 108.3** Effects of Disease-Related Stress on Resting Metabolism

| | *Percentage increase* |
|---|---|
| Fever | 10 for each °C rise in temperature |
| Elective surgery | 24 |
| Skeletal trauma | 32 |
| Blunt trauma | 37 |
| Trauma with steroids | 61 |
| Sepsis | 79 |
| Burns | 131 |

Adapted from Long CL, Schaffel N, Geiger JW: Metabolic response to injury and illness. Estimation of energy and protein needs from indirect calorimetry and nitrogen balance. J Parenter Enter Nutr 1979;3:453, with permission.

Kanaya et al achieved a positive nitrogen balance in seven infants receiving TPN with a N:NPC ratio of 1:216.[58]

There are also qualitative requirements for the amino acid composition of protein. Amino acids that are not synthesized in vivo in adequate quantities and must be provided nutritionally are termed essential amino acids. Eight amino acids are considered essential in healthy adults; these include isoleucine, leucine, lysine, methionine, phenylalanine, threonine, tryptophan, and valine. In addition, cysteine, histidine, tyrosine, and taurine may also be essential amino acids in the neonate and young infant.[59–63] Decreased plasma concentrations of cysteine, histidine, tyrosine, and taurine have been observed in infants receiving diets free of these amino acids.[62,63] Impaired growth rates have been described in infants receiving cysteine-free and histidine-free diets.[60,61] Retinal changes have been described in children receiving taurine-free TPN therapy that corrected with the addition of taurine to nutritional therapy.[62,63]

Fat provides 35% to 45% of the daily caloric intake in the average American diet. As with amino acids, there are fatty acids that are not synthesized in vivo and must be provided nutritionally. Linoleic acid is the primary essential fatty acid in humans. Some consider linolenic acid and arachidonic acid also to be essential as they are synthesized from linoleic acid.[64–67] Essential fatty acids are involved in a multitude of physiologic functions such as prostaglandin synthesis, platelet function, immune function, neurologic tissue growth, wound healing, and integrity of cell membranes, skin, and hair.[64,67] Essential fatty acid deficiency has been well described in infants and children receiving fat-free enteral and parenteral diets.[68–71] The laboratory findings associated with essential fatty acid deficiency include decreased serum concentrations of linoleic acid and arachidonic acid, increased serum concentrations of 5,8,11-eicosatrienoic acid, and a triene fatty acid-to-tetraene fatty acid ratio greater than 0.4:1.[64,68,71] The clinical manifestations of essential fatty acid deficiency in children include a scaly dermatitis, sparse hair growth, thrombocytopenia, failure to thrive, poor wound healing, and increased susceptibility to infection.[69–71] Both the laboratory findings and the clinical manifestations of essential fatty acid deficiency are readily reversible by enteral or parenteral administration of linoleic acid.[68–71] To prevent the development of essential fatty acid deficiency a minimum daily linoleic acid intake equal to 1% of the total calories is required, with an optimum intake of 4%.[72] The American Academy of Pediatrics recommends that infant formulas contain a minimum of 3.3 g of fat for each 100 kcal (30% of total calories) and 300 mg as linoleic acid (2.7% of total calories).[73]

Commonly referred to as the micronutrients, electrolytes, minerals, trace elements, and vitamins play vital roles in metabolic processes and are considered essential nutrients. The major electrolytes and minerals include sodium, potassium, chloride, calcium, phosphorus, and magnesium. Physiologic serum concentrations of these elements are well defined with age-related ranges (Table 108.4). Serum concentrations outside these ranges are associated with acute life-threatening reactions.

The average daily requirements for the major electrolytes and minerals are listed in Table 108.5.[42] Actual patient requirements may vary with disease state; therefore, adjustments may be needed to maintain serum concentrations

**Table 108.4** Normal Serum Concentrations of Electrolytes and Minerals According to Age

| | *Neonates* | | | | |
|---|---|---|---|---|---|
| | **Premature** | **Term** | ***Infants*** | ***Children*** | ***Adults*** |
| Sodium (mEq/L) | 128–148 | 133–144 | 138–146 | 138–146 | 135–148 |
| Potassium (mEq/L) | 3.0–6.0 | 3.7–5.0 | 4.1–5.3 | 3.5–5.5 | 3.5–5.3 |
| Chloride (mEq/L) | 95–110 | 96–107 | 95–108 | 95–108 | 95–108 |
| Calcium (mg/dL) | 6–10 | 7.3–12.0 | 10–12 | 9–11.5 | 9–11 |
| Phosphorus (mg/dL) | 5.6–8.0 | 5.0–10.0 | 4.0–7.0 | 4.0–6.0 | 3.5–5.0 |
| Magnesium (mEq/L) | | 1.5–2.1 | 1.5–2.1 | 1.5–2.1 | 1.5–2.1 |

within the accepted age-related ranges. Sodium requirements are frequently increased in children with increased gastric losses such as those associated with diarrhea, irritable bowel disease, or short-bowel syndrome.[74,75] Children with cystic fibrosis have increased sodium excretion in sweat and may require increased sodium intakes especially during the warm summer months. Premature infants may require additional sodium because of increased renal losses resulting from renal tubular immaturity.[75] To prevent fluid overload in children with congenital heart disease or pulmonary disease, sodium intakes are often restricted.[76]

Potassium requirements are often increased in children recovering from major trauma resulting from utilization of potassium in tissue synthesis.[74] Increased renal losses of potassium, such as that observed with renal tubular immaturity in the premature infant or diuretic therapy, also increase patient requirements for potassium.[75] Decreased potassium requirements may develop in children with significant renal dysfunction.

Calcium and phosphorus are required for bone growth and maintenance of bone integrity as well as other metabolic processes. Increased nutritional requirements for calcium and phosphorus in infants and children are due primarily to rapid bone growth. Premature infants have minimal body stores of calcium and are at increased risk for the development of osteopenia and rickets.[46,77] Increased renal losses of calcium are associated with nephrotic syndrome and drug therapy (e.g., glucocorticoids and loop diuretics). Children with significant renal dysfunction have reduced renal clearance of phosphorus and magnesium, resulting in decreased nutritional requirements of these elements.

The trace elements, iron, iodine, zinc, copper, manganese, fluoride, chromium, selenium, and molybdenum, are called such because they constitute less than 0.01% of the total body weight. The major functions of these elements are to act as cofactors for metal ion–activated enzymes or to complex with protein to form metalloenzymes. They also function as components of proteins and hormones.[78,79] The nutritional importance of iron and iodine is well documented; the other trace elements have only recently been recognized as essential nutrients. The widespread distribution of these elements in food sources and relatively small nutritional requirements may account for the low incidence of nutritional deficiencies. The Food and Nutrition Board of the National Research Council has established recommended daily nutritional intake of these elements (Table 108.5).[42] Children appear to have increased nutritional requirements for the trace elements because of their rapid growth rates.[78–81] Premature infants have the greatest trace element nutritional requirements because of reduced body stores in combination with rapid growth rates.[46] Deficiency states have been associated with nutritional intakes lacking in the various trace elements. Patients receiving long-term TPN therapy and premature infants are at particular risk for trace element deficiencies.[82–85]

Iron is a component of hemoglobin, myoglobin, cytochromes, and a number of metalloenzymes. The nutritional importance of iron is related to its role in the transportation and utilization of oxygen. The common causes of iron deficiency are inadequate dietary iron intake, rapid growth, and blood loss. Iron deficiency is most common in infants and young children between the ages 6 months and 3 years. There is also an increased incidence of iron deficiency in adolescents and menopausal females. Iron deficiency is not common prior to 4 months of age as a result of the substantial iron stores present at birth. Premature infants have reduced iron stores that may be depleted by 2 months postnatal age.[86] The American Academy of Pediatrics recommends 1–3 mg/kg/d of elemental iron be provided nutritionally to prevent iron deficiency in children.[86]

The primary function of iodine is its role in the synthesis of the thyroid hormones thyroxine and triiodothyronine. Iodine deficiency in children is associated with the clinical manifestations of hypothyroidism (goiter, myxedema, growth failure, and delayed sexual maturation).[79] The utilization of iodized salt in the United States has reduced the incidence of endemic goiter; however, infants and children receiving TPN therapy lack this nutritional source, placing them at risk for iodine deficiency. In infants and children receiving TPN therapy, 3–5 μg/kg added daily to the infusate prevents iodine deficiency.[78]

Zinc is involved in a number of diverse enzymatic pro-

**Table 108.5** Recommended Daily Dietary Intakes of Electrolytes, Minerals, Trace Elements, and Vitamins

| | *0–1 yr* | *1–10 yr* | *Over 10 yr* |
|---|---|---|---|
| Electrolytes | | | |
| Sodium (mg) | 115–750 | 325–1,800 | 900–2,700 |
| Potassium (mg) | 350–1,275 | 550–3,000 | 1,525–4,575 |
| Chloride (mg) | 275–1,200 | 500–2,775 | 1,400–4,200 |
| Minerals | | | |
| Calcium (mg) | 360–540 | 800 | 1,200 |
| Phosphorus (mg) | 240–360 | 800 | 1,200 |
| Magnesium (mg) | 50–70 | 150–200 | 350 |
| Iron (mg) | 10–15 | 10–15 | 18 |
| Zinc (mg) | 3–5 | 10 | 15 |
| Iodine (ug) | 40–50 | 70–90 | 150 |
| Trace elements | | | |
| Copper (mg) | 0.5–1.0 | 1.0–2.5 | 2.0–3.0 |
| Manganese (mg) | 0.5–1.0 | 1.0–3.0 | 2.5–5.0 |
| Fluoride (mg) | 0.1–1.0 | 0.5–2.5 | 1.5–2.5 |
| Chromium (mg) | 0.01–0.06 | 0.02–0.2 | 0.05–0.2 |
| Selenium (mg) | 0.01–0.06 | 0.02–0.2 | 0.05–0.2 |
| Molybdenum (mg) | 0.03–0.08 | 0.03–0.3 | 0.15–0.5 |
| Vitamins | | | |
| Vitamin A (μg RE)[a] | 400–420 | 400–700 | 800–1,000 |
| Vitamin D (μg) | 10 | 10 | 5–10 |
| Vitamin E (mg α-TE)[b] | 3–4 | 5–7 | 8–10 |
| Vitamin K (μg) | 10–20 | 15–60 | 50–140 |
| Ascorbic acid (mg) | 35 | 45 | 50–60 |
| Thiamine (mg) | 0.3–0.5 | 0.7–1.2 | 1.0–1.5 |
| Riboflavin (mg) | 0.4–0.6 | 0.8–1.4 | 1.2–1.6 |
| Pyridoxine (mg) | 0.3–0.6 | 0.9–1.6 | 1.8–2.2 |
| Niacin (mg) | 6–8 | 9–16 | 13–19 |
| Folacin (μg) | 30–45 | 100–300 | 400 |
| Cyanocobalamin (μg) | 0.5–1.5 | 2.0–3.0 | 3.0 |
| Biotin (μg) | 35–50 | 65–120 | 100–200 |
| Pantothenic acid (mg) | 2–3 | 3–5 | 4–7 |

[a] One retinol equivalent (RE) = 1 μg retinol or 6 μg β-carotene.
[b] One α-tocopherol equivalent (α-TE) = 1 mg D-α-tocopherol.

From Food and Nutrition Board, National Research Council: Recommended Dietary Allowances, 9th ed. Washington DC, National Academy of Sciences, 1980, with permission.

cesses. Premature infants lack body stores of zinc and are at high risk for deficiencies.[78,79] Zlotkin et al recently reported that supplemental zinc 438 μg/kg/d is required in premature infants to achieve accumulation rates equal to that in utero.[87] To prevent zinc deficiency in premature infants the American Medical Association currently recommends that zinc 300 μg/kg be added to the daily infusate.[88] The nutritional requirements for zinc in infants and children are less than that for premature infants because of endogenous stores; however, to prevent zinc deficiency in infants and children receiving TPN therapy, the American Medical Association recommends that 100 μg/kg be added to the daily infusate.[86]

Copper is a structural component of several metalloenzymes involved in oxidative metabolism. To prevent copper deficiency in infants and children receiving TPN therapy, the American Medical Association recommends that copper 20 μg/kg be added to the daily infusate.[88] Like zinc, the fetus accumulates copper during the third trimester of pregnancy; therefore, premature infants lack body stores of copper and are at high risk for deficiencies.[78,79,81] Premature neonates may require up to 60 μg/kg/d to meet in utero accumulation rates of copper.[87]

Clinical syndromes of chromium or manganese deficiency have not been described in children receiving long-term TPN therapy. Dahlstrom et al reported low serum concentrations of these elements in nine children on long-term TPN therapy without supplementation.[89] While none had symptoms of chromium or manganese deficiency, these elements should be added to TPN infusates to prevent deficiencies. The American Medical Association recommends chromium 0.14–0.20 μg/kg and manganese 2–10 μg/kg be added daily to the TPN infusate.[87]

Selenium has antioxidant actions similar to those of vitamin E and may have a sparing effect on vitamin E requirements. Selenium deficiency has been described in a child receiving TPN therapy.[85] To prevent selenium deficiency in infants and children receiving TPN therapy selenium 2–3 μg/kg should be added to the infusate daily.[85]

Vitamins function primarily as cofactors in a variety of metabolic processes. As with trace elements, the serum concentrations of vitamins do not reflect tissue concentrations or biologic activity. Assays utilizing vitamin-dependent enzymes provide a more accurate measure of vitamin activity.[90] Vitamin deficiency syndromes are well described and the nutritional need for vitamins has long been recognized. The nutritional requirements for vitamins are not well defined; however, recommended daily intakes have been established (Table 108.5) and are the basis of use of vitamins in TPN therapy.[42]

Because of their rapid growth rates, infants and children have greater nutritional requirements for the fat-soluble vitamins (vitamins A,D,E, and K) than adolescents and adults. Fat-soluble vitamins are stored in body tissues; therefore, short periods without nutritional intake generally do not result in deficiencies. Premature infants are at risk for deficiencies as accumulation of body stores occurs during the last trimester of pregnancy.[66] Children with fat-malabsorption syndromes are also at risk for deficiencies. Fat-soluble vitamins may accumulate with excessive intakes and result in toxic effects.

Vitamin D is commonly referred to as the antirachitic vitamin as it is involved in the absorption of calcium from the gastrointestinal tract and the retention and mobilization of calcium in bones. Deficiencies of vitamin D are associated with osteopenia and rickets in growing infants and children and osteomalacia in adolescents and adults.[91] The increased incidence of osteopenia and rickets in premature infants may result from reduced metabolism of vitamin D to its active forms as well as increased requirements of calcium and phosphorus.[46] The American Academy of Pediatrics recommends that infants receiving either enteral or parenteral nutrition should be supplemented with 400 IU (10 μg) vitamin D daily.[46] On the contrary, the addition of vitamin D to long-term TPN therapy in adults is controversial. Metabolic bone disease has been associated with vitamin D supplementation in adults receiving long-term TPN therapy. Characterized by bone pain, hypercalciuria, low serum parathyroid hormone levels, and bone changes consistent with osteomalacia, these symptoms resolved with the removal of vitamin D from TPN therapy.[92]

Vitamin E functions primarily as an antioxidant. It may also function in selenium and sulfur amino acid metabolism and in the liver microsomal enzyme system. An important function of vitamin E is the inhibition of lipid peroxidation. The nutritional requirement for vitamin E is related to the dietary intake of polyunsaturated fatty acids. The American Academy of Pediatrics recommends that infants receive 0.7 IU vitamin E per gram of linoleic acid and premature infants receive 1.0 IU vitamin E per gram of linoleic acid.[46] The current commercially available pediatric parenteral multivitamin preparation provides 7 IU of vitamin E per 5 mL. A high intake of iron may increase the vitamin E requirement. Infants are born with a relative deficiency of vitamin E that has been associated with hemolytic anemia and generalized edema.[46] As an antioxidant, vitamin E may reduce the peroxidation of membrane lipids and increase the lifespan of fetal red blood cells; however, in a recent study in premature infants Zipursky et al found no evidence to support vitamin E supplementation to prevent anemia of prematurity.[93] Some investigators have suggested that relatively high doses of vitamin E are protective against the development of retinopathy of prematurity and bronchopulmonary dysplasia in premature infants.[94,95] Recent studies have not substantiated these findings.[96,97] Several adverse effects have been associated with vitamin E supplementation. An increased incidence of sepsis and necrotizing enterocolitis in premature infants has been associated with vitamin E supplementation.[98] A series of neonatal deaths after a syndrome characterized by hepatomegaly, direct hyperbilirubinemia, azotemia, ascites, and thrombocytopenia was associated with the administration of a parenteral vitamin E formulation (E-Ferol) in premature infants.[99] It is not known if the syndrome was the result of excessive vitamin E levels, the polysorbate used to solubilize the vitamin E, or other factors.

Vitamin A is involved in immune function, vision, and growth. The clinical manifestations of vitamin A deficiency include thickening and dryness of the skin, night blindness, xerophthalmia, growth retardation, and increased susceptibility to infection. To prevent vitamin A deficiency in infants and children 400–700 μg retinol equivalents (2,000–3,300 IU retinol) is recommended daily.[42,90] The toxic effects associated with excessive intake of vitamin A include dry skin, painful joints, hepatomegaly, and jaundice.

Vitamin K is essential for the hepatic synthesis of clotting factors II, VII, IX, and X. The primary sources of vitamin K are the diet and the normal bacterial flora of the gastrointestinal tract. Vitamin K deficiency manifests as a prolongation of the prothrombin time and, rarely, hemorrhagic events. Neonates are at risk for hemorrhagic complications because they lack bacterial flora in the gastrointestinal tract at birth as well as body stores of vitamin K. To prevent these complications neonates are administered an intramuscular injection of vitamin K at birth. The premature infant receiving TPN therapy and antibiotics is at increased risk for vitamin K deficiency and should receive vitamin K supplementation.[46,90] The current commercially available pediatric parenteral multivitamin preparation provides 200 μg of vitamin K per 15 mL, which should eliminate the need for weekly intramuscular vitamin K injections.

The water-soluble vitamins include vitamin C and the B vitamins. As with the fat-soluble vitamins, infants and growing children have increased nutritional requirements for the water-soluble vitamins because of their rapid growth rates. They differ from the fat-soluble vitamins in that they are not stored in body tissues (with the exception of cyanocobalamin) and must be supplied daily to prevent deficiency syndromes. Toxic effects associated with excessive intakes are uncommon because of the body's ability to eliminate excess quantities. Similarly, the requirements for the water-soluble vitamins are increased two- to threefold when administered intravenously because of concurrent renal elimination.[90,100,101]

Ascorbic acid (vitamin C) is involved in collagen synthesis, amino acid catabolism, and hematopoiesis.[101] Without nutritional intake, deficiency of vitamin C may develop quickly and is characterized by anorexia, tenderness of the extremities, and hemorrhages of the gums, mucous membranes, skin, and periosteum of the long bones.

The B vitamins include thiamine, riboflavin, pyridoxine,

niacin, folate, cyanocobalamin, pantothenic acid, and biotin. They are involved in a number of metabolic processes, functioning primarily as enzyme cofactors.[100,101] Deficiency syndromes of the B vitamins are well described in children; the symptoms of beriberi, pellagra, and other B vitamin deficiency syndromes are similar to those in adults.[100,101] Seizures resulting from pyridoxine deficiency are rare but occur most often in infants; they are usually refractory to standard anticonvulsant therapy but resolve with the administration of 50–100 mg of pyridoxine.[102] Pantothenic acid and biotin are synthesized by the normal bacterial flora of the gastrointestinal tract; therefore, deficiency is uncommon. Children lacking the normal gastrointestinal bacterial flora, such as in short-bowel syndrome or premature infants who have been administered broad-spectrum antibiotics for an extended period, are at risk for deficiencies.[103,104]

Several substances possess biologic activity but have yet to be considered essential nutrients in the human diet. These include choline, inositol and carnitine.[101] Choline, the precursor of acetylcholine, forms the base for lecithin and sphingomyelin. It is present in large quantities in a variety of food sources and is also synthesized endogenously from methionine. Choline is not considered an essential nutrient in adults and is not currently included in TPN therapeutic regimens; however, premature infants may have a nutritional requirement for choline. The American Academy of Pediatrics recommends that choline be added to commercial milk-based formulas.[73]

The biologic function of inositol is unknown; however, it is found in large quantities primarily as a component of phospholipids and glycoprotein complexes. In humans, inositol is synthesized from glucose. The nutritional requirement of inositol is unknown at this time. As with choline, inositol is not currently included in TPN therapy for infants and children; however, the American Academy of Pediatrics recommends that it be added to commercial milk-based formulas.[73]

Carnitine is involved in the oxidation of long-chain fatty acids. As acylcarnitine it functions as a carrier molecule in the transfer of long-chain fatty acid across mitochondrial membranes. The nutritional requirement of carnitine is not well defined at this time. It is present in a variety of food sources and is also synthesized in the liver from lysine and methionine. A relative carnitine deficiency has been shown to develop in low-birth-weight infants receiving TPN therapy without carnitine supplementation.[105] Carnitine deficiency may be attributed to the decreased ability of the infants to metabolize intravenous fat emulsions. Recent studies have shown an increase in the hydrolysis of fatty acids with carnitine supplementation in infants receiving intravenous fat emulsions.[106,107]

## Composition of Total Parenteral Nutrition Solutions

To meet the nutritional requirements of the child who is unable to take adequate enteral nutrition, combinations of carbohydrates, protein, and fat as dextrose, crystalline amino acids, and fat emulsions, respectively, are utilized in TPN therapy. Carbohydrates constitute the main source of calories (35–45%) provided by TPN therapy. Dextrose, the monohydrate form of glucose and primary carbohydrate used in TPN solutions, provides 3.4 cal per gram. Other carbohydrate sources, such as fructose, galactose, sorbitol, and ethanol, offer no advantages over dextrose and are rarely used. A minor additional source of carbohydrate is contributed by the glycerol contained in fat emulsions (0.2 cal/mL of fat emulsion).

The primary limitations to providing optimal carbohydrate calories in TPN therapy are patient glucose intolerance and hyperosmolarity of the infusate. To minimize glucose intolerance, the TPN infusion should be initiated at a homeostatic rate of 6–8 mg glucose/kg/min and gradually increased over several days to an optimum rate of 15 mg/kg/min.[57,72] Premature neonates and severely stressed patients have a reduced glucose tolerance. In these patients, glucose infusions should be initiated at a lower rate (3–6 mg/kg/min) to minimize hyperglycemia.[76]

The amount of glucose supplied by TPN therapy is also limited by the osmolarity of the infusate and the route of administration. The major factor determining the osmolarity of a TPN solution is the dextrose concentration. Amino acids, electrolytes, minerals, as well as vitamin additives also contribute to the osmolarity of TPN solutions (Table 108.6). Solutions with an osmolarity of 300–900 mOsm/L (a dextrose concentration of 10% or less) may be infused through peripheral veins. Solutions with an osmolarity exceeding 900 mOsm/L (12.5% dextrose) must be infused through a central venous catheter to avoid venous sclerosis and phlebitis.[72] Occasionally, TPN solutions with 12.5% dextrose are administered through peripheral veins, but are associated with a high incidence of phlebitis.

Hydrolysates of fibrin or casein were the first source of protein utilized in TPN solutions. They were effective in maintaining a positive nitrogen balance and provided a majority of the essential amino acids; however, several disadvantages have been identified.[108] The amino acid composition is relatively fixed by the structure of the protein

**Table 108.6** Osmolarity of Various Solutions

| *Solution* | *Calculated Osmolarity (mOsm/L)* |
|---|---|
| Dextrose | |
| 5% | 252 |
| 10% | 505 |
| 12.5% | 631 |
| 20% | 1,010 |
| 25% | 1,263 |
| 30% | 1,515 |
| 10% Dextrose[a] | |
| + 1% Amino acids | 800 |
| + 2% Amino acids | 900 |
| 12.5% Dextrose[a] | |
| + 1% Amino acids | 925 |
| + 2% Amino acids | 1,025 |
| 20% Dextrose[a] | |
| + 2% Amino acids | 1,400 |
| + 3% Amino acids | 1,500 |

[a] Includes standard electrolytes, minerals, and vitamins which contribute approximately 200 mOsm/L.

**Table 108.7** Amino Acid Composition of Solutions in Use in the United States

| | *Standard solutions* | | | *Pediatric solutions* | | |
|---|---|---|---|---|---|---|
| | **Aminosyn** | **Novamine** | **Travasol** | **FraAmineIII** | **TrophAmine** | **Aminosyn PF** |
| Amino acid concentration (%) | 8.5 | 8.5 | 8.5 | 8.5 | 6 | 7 |
| Nitrogen (g/100 mL) | 1.34 | 1.35 | 1.42 | 1.42 | | |
| Essential (mg/100 mL) | | | | | | |
| Isoleucine | 620 | 420 | 406 | 590 | 490 | 534 |
| Leucine | 810 | 590 | 526 | 770 | 840 | 831 |
| Lysine | 624 | 673 | 492 | 620 | 490 | 475 |
| Methionine | 340 | 420 | 492 | 450 | 200 | 125 |
| Phenylalanine | 380 | 590 | 526 | 480 | 290 | 300 |
| Threonine | 460 | 420 | 356 | 340 | 250 | 360 |
| Tryptophan | 150 | 140 | 152 | 130 | 120 | 125 |
| Valine | 680 | 550 | 390 | 560 | 470 | 452 |
| Nonessential (mg/100 mL) | | | | | | |
| Alanine | 1,100 | 1,200 | 1,760 | 600 | 320 | 490 |
| Arginine | 850 | 840 | 880 | 810 | 730 | 861 |
| Histidine | 260 | 500 | 372 | 240 | 290 | 220 |
| Proline | 750 | 500 | 356 | 950 | 410 | 570 |
| Serine | 370 | 340 | | 500 | 230 | 347 |
| Tyrosine | 44 | 20 | 34 | | 140 | 44 |
| Glycine | 1,100 | 590 | 1,760 | 1,190 | | 270 |
| Glutamine | | 420 | | | 300 | 576 |
| Aspartate | | 250 | | | 190 | 370 |
| Cysteine | | 40 | | <20 | <20 | |
| Taurine | | | | | 150 | 50 |
| Aminoacetate | | | | | 220 | |

prior to hydrolysis. The hydrolysis process is incomplete, resulting in dipeptides and tripeptides that require further in vivo metabolism to their component amino acids. The process also produces large amounts of ammonia which increases the risk for hyperammonemia.

Crystalline amino acids have largely replaced protein hydrolysates. They offer the advantage of providing flexibility in their formulation to meet specific amino acid needs, such as in renal or hepatic failure and in the low-birth-weight infant. The initial crystalline amino acid solutions used were associated with metabolic acidosis in infants.[109] This complication has been corrected by the replacement of the hydrochloride salt of lysine with its acetate equivalent and the use of basic salts of histidine.

There is a wide variety in the amino acid composition of the standard amino acid solutions currently available in the United States (Table 108.7). All contain a combination of the L-stereoisomers of the eight essential amino acids (40%–50%) and nonessential amino acids (50%–60%). The most notable difference between these solutions is the nonessential amino acid compositions, which differ in both the types and the amounts of amino acids contained. They are similar, however, in that the dispensible amino acid nitrogen content is provided by glycine and alanine. These solutions also contain varying amounts of electrolytes from the salts of the amino acids.

Several techniques have been used to determine nutritional protein requirements. In addition to growth assessments and nitrogen balance studies, plasma amino acid concentrations (plasma aminograms) are being used with increased frequency. Normal plasma amino acid concentrations have been established in healthy adults, children, infants, and full-term neonates.[110,111] The differences in the amino acid content of the standard amino acid solutions do not appear to be clinically significant in adults without significant renal or hepatic disease. Abnormal plasma aminograms have been documented in neonates receiving the standard amino acid solutions.[58,112–116] On the basis of these findings two pediatric amino acid solutions have been developed to meet the unique amino acid requirements of infants less than 6 months of age. These special solutions (Table 108.7) differ in composition from the standard amino acid solutions in that they contain reduced amounts of methionine, tryptophan, alanine, and glycine and increased amounts of tyrosine. They also contain glutamate, aspartate, cysteine, and taurine, which are not contained in the standard amino acid solutions. Clinical studies with these formulations have demonstrated more normal plasma aminograms in neonates.[115]

There are several approaches to initiating crystalline amino acids in pediatric TPN solutions. Because of the recognized hepatic dysfunction in the neonate and the associated risk of hepatic toxicity, amino acids are generally started at a low dose (0.5–1.0 g/kg/d) and gradually increased over several days. In older infants and children, amino acids may be initiated at a higher dose (1.0–1.5 g/kg/d) and increased over a shorter period of time.[56] Some institutions are beginning amino acids at an optimal regimen (Table 108.1) providing there is no significant renal or hepatic

**Table 108.8** Composition of Fat Emulsions

| | *10% Emulsion* | *20% Emulsion* |
|---|---|---|
| Calories/mL | 1.1 | 2.0 |
| Osmolarity (mOsm/L) | 260–300 | 268–340 |
| | *Soybean oil* | *Safflower oil* |
| Fatty acids (%) | | |
| Linoleic acid | 50–60 | 77 |
| Oleic acid | 21–23 | 13 |
| Palmitic acid | 9–13 | 7 |
| Linolenic acid | 6–9 | 0.1 |
| Stearic acid | 0–5 | 2.5 |
| Egg yolk phospholipids (%) | 1.2 | 1.2 |
| Glycerin (%) | 2.21–2.25 | 2.5 |

disease and adequate nonprotein calories are also being provided.

The development of a parenteral form of fat has been a major step in the evolution of TPN therapy. It was identified early that fat could be administered parenterally as an emulsion resembling natural chylomicrons.[117] It was not until 1960 that the first commercial fat emulsion prepared from cottonseed oil was available; however, it was removed from the market because of the high incidence of a toxic effect described as a "fat overloading syndrome." The syndrome was characterized by a sudden onset of high fever, rigors, hemolytic anemia with increased fat deposition in the bone marrow, thrombocytopenia, and hypoproteinemia.[118] In addition patients experienced headache, sore throat or tender neck muscles, anorexia, and malaise. The current commercially available parenteral fat emulsions are prepared from soybean oil and safflower oil. While the fat overloading syndrome has been reported with these preparations, the incidence has been less than that seen with the cottonseed oil fat emulsion.[117]

The combination of fat emulsions and dextrose solutions in TPN therapy has improved the intake of nonprotein calories without the associated problem of hyperosmolarity. Fat supplies 9.0 kcal/g, whereas the 10% and 20% intravenous fat emulsions provide 1.1 and 2.0 kcal/mL, respectively (Table 108.8). This difference results from the small amount of glycerol added to fat emulsions that provides 0.2 kcal/mL in both the 10% and 20% emulsions. Glycerol is added to make the emulsion isotonic (260–340 mOsm/L). Egg yolk phospholipids are added as emulsifying agents. The fatty acid composition of the fat emulsion varies with the oil used. Safflower oil emulsions contain a larger amount of linoleic acid (77%), but are almost void of linolenic acid (0.1%). Soybean oil emulsions contain less linoleic acid (50%–60%), but also contain linolenic acid (6%–9%). The significance of these differences is not evident at this time. A dose of 0.5–1.0 g/kg/d of intravenous fat emulsion provides a sufficient intake of linoleic acid to prevent essential fatty acid deficiency. To optimize calorie intake intravenous fat emulsions should provide 30% to 50% of the daily calorie intake, but should not exceed 60%.

The fat particles of parenteral fat emulsions are similar to natural chylomicrons in size (0.4–0.5 $\mu$m) and composition, and are cleared from the circulation by similar mechanisms.[119–121] Lipoprotein lipase, an enzyme bound to capillary endothelial walls by heparin sulfate, hydrolyzes the fat particles to free fatty acids and monoglycerides. Hepatic lipase found in the endothelium of the liver capillaries also hydrolyzes fat particles to free fatty acids and monoglycerides. Free fatty acids are then carried to adipose tissue for storage, to muscle tissue for oxidation, or to the liver bound to albumin where they are converted to very low density lipoproteins (VLDLs) which are released into the circulation.

Because of the associated toxic effects, hyperlipidemia is a major factor limiting the utilization of parenteral fat emulsions in TPN therapy. Hyperlipidemia or fat intolerance results when the rate of the fat emulsion infusion exceeds the plasma lipid clearance rate. Infants and children have plasma lipid clearance rates similar to those of adults. Premature neonates have reduced clearance rates which correlate with gestational age.[122–124] Plasma lipid clearance rates have been shown to increase with increasing doses of fat emulsion.[125] Therefore, parenteral fat emulsion therapy should be initiated at a low dose (0.5–1.0 g/kg/d) and gradually increased by 0.5 g/kg increments over several days to an optimal dose (2–3 g/kg/d).[66,126] An additional means of minimizing hyperlipidemia is to administer the fat emulsion infusions as long as possible throughout the 24-hour period.[127] The American Academy of Pediatrics recommends that fat emulsions should be administered at a rate not greater than 0.25 g/kg/h in the low-birth-weight infant.[46]

Immediate adverse reactions have been associated with parenteral fat emulsion infusions and include dyspnea, cyanosis, flushing, fever, chills, shivering, nausea, vomiting, and allergic reactions.[66,119] To minimize these reactions a test dose should be administered to the patient prior to the initial dose of fat emulsion. In the infant less than 5 kg, a test dose of 1 ml/kg over 1 hour is used. Infants and children weighing 5 kg or more may be given a test dose of 0.1 mL/min for 10 to 15 minutes.

With the exception of bicarbonate, the salts of the major electrolytes, minerals, and trace elements are added to the TPN infusate to meet the nutritional requirements for these

**Table 108.9** Recommended Daily Intakes of Electrolytes, Minerals, and Trace Elements in Pediatric TPN Solutions

| | *Premature infants* | *Infants and children* |
|---|---|---|
| Electrolytes | | |
| Sodium (mEq/kg) | 2–5 | 2–4 |
| Potassium (mEq/kg) | 2–4 | 2–4 |
| Chloride (mEq/kg) | 2–3 | 2–3 |
| Minerals | | |
| Calcium (mg/kg) | 20–60 | 10–40 |
| Phosphorus (mmol/kg) | 0.5–2.0 | 0.4–0.8 |
| Magnesium (mEq/kg) | 0.25–0.5 | 0.25–0.5 |
| Trace elements | | |
| Iron (mg/kg) | 0.1–0.2 | 0.1–0.2 |
| Iodine (μg/kg) | 3–5 | 3.5 |
| Zinc (μg/kg) | 300–500 | 100 |
| Copper (μg/kg) | 20–60 | 20 |
| Chromium (μg/kg) | 0.14–0.2 | 0.14–0.2 |
| Manganese (μg/kg) | 2–10 | 2–10 |
| Selenium (μg/kg) | 2–3 | 2–3 |

elements. The recommended daily intakes of these elements in TPN solutions are listed in Table 108.9. Bicarbonate salts cannot be added to TPN solutions containing calcium as a precipitate of calcium carbonate will form. Acetate and lactate salts are utilized in place of bicarbonate salts. Both acetate and lactate are metabolized in vivo to bicarbonate in equal molar ratios.

Infants and growing children require relatively large amounts of calcium and phosphorus. Providing adequate amounts of these minerals in TPN solutions is complicated by the solubility of calcium phosphate. The formation of calcium phosphate is dependent on a complex interrelationship among pH, temperature, amino acid product, amino acid concentration, dextrose concentration, calcium salt, order of calcium and phosphorus addition to TPN solution, and contact with intravenous fat emulsion.[128] Solubility curves based on amino acid product, amino acid concentration, and pH have been developed that help determine whether calcium phosphate will precipitate.[129–131]

Iron has not routinely been added to TPN solutions because of potential incompatibility problems and anaphylaxis associated with intravenous iron–dextran administration. To prevent iron deficiency in patients receiving long-term TPN therapy periodic intramuscular injections of iron–dextran have been used. This may not be the preferred route of administration in infants and children because of reduced muscle mass as well as the pain associated with deep intramuscular injections. The use of intravenous iron–dextran infusions has been shown to be safe and effective in the treatment of iron deficiency in infants and children receiving TPN therapy.[132,133] The addition of iron–dextran to TPN solutions daily in low doses has been evaluated in adults and no adverse effects have been noted.[134] Stability studies on the compatibility of iron–dextran in TPN solutions are limited, but to date no physiochemical incompatibilities have been described.[135]

Vitamins are traditionally added to TPN solutions as commercial multivitamin preparations. Until recently, parenteral multivitamin preparations were formulated to meet the nutritional needs of the adult patient. A new formulation is now available that is designed to meet the vitamin requirements of infants and children (Table 108.10). It differs from other intravenous multivitamin preparations in the quantities of the vitamins and also contains vitamin K, which is not included in the other preparations. The pediatric dosing recommendation for this preparation is 5 mL daily in infants weighing over 3 kg through children 11 years of age. Infants weighing 1 to 3 kg should receive 65% of the daily pediatric dose (3.25 mL). Infants weighing less than 1 kg should receive 30% of the daily pediatric dose (1.5 mL). In a clinical trial of this preparation blood vitamin activity of the water-soluble and fat-soluble vitamins was maintained within the reference ranges in term infants and children throughout the

**Table 108.10** Composition of Parenteral Multivitamin Solutions

| | *Standard solutions* | | |
|---|---|---|---|
| | **MVI Concentrate (in 5 mL)** | **Berocca (in 2 mL)** | ***Pediatric MVI (in 5 mL)*** |
| Vitamin A (IU) | 10,000 | 3,300 | 2,300 |
| Vitamin D (IU) | 1,000 | 200 | 400 |
| Vitamin E (IU) | 5 | 10 | 7 |
| Vitamin K (μg) | | | 200 |
| Ascorbic acid (mg) | 500 | 100 | 80 |
| Thiamine (mg) | 50 | 3 | 1.2 |
| Riboflavin (mg) | 10 | 3.6 | 1.4 |
| Niacin (mg) | 100 | 40 | 17 |
| Pantothenic acid (mg) | 25 | 15 | 5 |
| Pyridoxine (mg) | 15 | 4 | 1 |
| Cyanocobalamin (μg) | | 5 | 1 |
| Folate (μg) | | 400 | 140 |
| Biotin (μg) | | 60 | 20 |

study period.[136,137] In premature infants ascorbic acid, pantothenic acid, and biotin were noted to accumulate to levels above the reference ranges during the study period, whereas vitamin A was below the reference range and did not increase throughout the study period.[136,137] The inability to achieve normal vitamin A levels may have been related to its loss in the delivery system. Vitamin A will absorb onto the plastic matrix of the intravenous administration sets, rendering it unavailable.[128]

Heparin sulfate is frequently added to TPN infusates being administered through central vein catheters to prevent thrombus formation at the catheter tip. The incidence of clinical manifestations of thrombosis of the subclavian vein in adults receiving central TPN therapy is reported as 0.2% to 0.3%.[138] The incidence in infants and children has been reported to range from 1% to 7%.[139,140] Thrombosis of the subclavian vein has been associated with significant morbidity and mortality in infants and children.[140,141] The addition of heparin (1 U/mL) to the TPN infusate in infants and children has been shown to decrease the incidence of thrombus formation at the catheter tip without significantly interfering with the normal clotting mechanisms.[141,142]

The addition of heparin to TPN infusates being administered through peripheral vein catheters is more controversial. Heparin may minimize phlebitis, prevent venous thrombosis, and therefore increase the duration of patency of the vein. In a controlled study of 26 premature infants receiving peripheral TPN therapy, the patency of the infusion site was maintained for a significantly longer period in the heparin group (1 U/mL) than in the nonheparin group.[143] In the same study, Alpan et al also reported a significant reduction in the incidence of phlebitis in the heparin group; however, there was no difference in the incidence of tissue sloughs caused by extravasations.[143] As with the administration of heparin (1 U/mL) through central veins, changes in the normal clotting mechanisms were not observed.

Heparin administration has also been shown to increase plasma lipoprotein lipase activity. Described as postheparin lipolytic activity, heparin is thought to stimulate the release and subsequent synthesis of lipoprotein and hepatic lipase.[65] The use of low-dose heparin (1 U/mL) in TPN infusates to minimize intravascular clotting has been shown to increase serum lipolytic activity.[144] An associated decrease in serum triglycerides and an increase in serum free fatty acids were also shown.[144] Until further studies are able to better define the role of exogenous heparin on fat metabolism the addition of heparin to TPN infusates as a means to facilitate fat emulsion clearance is not recommended.[67]

## Route of Administration

Total parenteral nutrition may be administered through a peripheral vein catheter or central vein catheter. The choice between these routes of administration is based upon a number of factors, such as the extent of the patient's nutritional depletion and the anticipated duration of TPN therapy. Pediatric TPN therapy is often initiated through the peripheral venous route. The amount of calories provided by this route is restricted by the osmolarity of the infusate and the volume that can be tolerated by the infant or child. The duration of TPN therapy by the peripheral route is often limited by the ability to maintain continuous venous access. Periodic interruptions in peripheral TPN administration frequently occur because of loss of venous access.

Central TPN therapy should be considered for the infant or child who is expected to require TPN therapy for longer than 2 weeks or who is nutritionally depleted prior to the initiation of TPN therapy.[43,73] The major deterrent to central TPN therapy in infants and children is the risks associated with catheter placement; these include general anesthesia, catheter placement, and loss of the sterile field during catheter placement. The most common venous access used in infants and children is percutaneous cannulation of the subclavian vein, as it may be done at the bedside with local anesthesia and sedation, eliminating the risks associated with general anesthesia.[73] The use of the femoral vein for central venous access is avoided if possible because of an associated increased incidence of sepsis in infants and children.[145]

Another method of central venous access is through the use of peripherally inserted central venous catheters. These catheters are placed into the basilic or cephalic vein and extend into the superior vena cava. They have the advantage of peripheral vein catheters with bedside placement using local anesthesia. Because they are a central vein catheter, hypertonic solutions may be infused through them with a relatively low incidence of phlebitis. Bottino et al reported an average life of 30 days for these catheters.[146]

## Complications

Central TPN therapy has been associated with a greater rate of complications than peripheral TPN therapy. In a clinical study of 585 infants and children receiving either central or peripheral TPN therapy the overall complication rate was highest in those patients receiving central TPN therapy (20.0% versus 9.08%)[139]; however, when compared on a per diem basis, there was no difference between the complication rate in those receiving central versus peripheral TPN therapy, 0.604% and 0.797% respectively.

Sepsis, a major complication of TPN therapy, is associated with a high incidence of morbidity and mortality. Infants and children receiving TPN therapy are at increased risk for sepsis as compared with adults. Conditions that predispose infants and children to infection include prematurity, malnutrition, and immunosuppression. The reported incidence of sepsis in infants and children receiving TPN therapy varies greatly. In a small study of 15 infants and children receiving long-term TPN therapy, eight episodes of bacterial sepsis and eight episodes of fungal sepsis were documented in 12 patients (80% incidence).[147] Ziegler et al reported a 10.5% incidence of sepsis in 200 infants and children receiving long-term TPN therapy.[139]

In addition to the general status of the patient, the risk of sepsis associated with TPN therapy is also related to the route of administration, aseptic technique during solution preparation, catheter care, and duration of therapy. The incidence of sepsis is increased with TPN administration through a central venous catheter versus a peripheral venous catheter. In a study evaluating the route of TPN administration, 21 of 200 infants and children receiving central TPN therapy through a central venous catheter developed sepsis versus none of 385 infants and children receiving TPN therapy through a peripheral venous catheter.[139]

The catheter is the most common source of infection associated with TPN therapy. Another potential source of infection is the TPN solution itself, which provides a favorable environment for bacterial and fungal growth. Strict aseptic technique must be adhered to during solution preparation and administration. Early TPN solutions were prepared in patient care areas without the use of sterile laminar-airflow hoods, which increased the risk of contamination by microorganisms. Saunders et al reported a decrease in the incidence of septic complications from 28.6% to 4.7% over a 5-year period with the initiation of a TPN service that included an intravenous additive center maintained by pharmacists and nursing inservice training programs on administration techniques and catheter care.[148]

The pathogens associated with sepsis during TPN therapy include both bacteria and fungi. The most prevalent pathogens are *Staphylococcus epidermidis* and *Staphylococcus aureus* which are normal flora of the skin. Other common bacteria include *Streptococcus* sp., *Escherichia coli*, *Klebsiella* sp., *Pseudomonas* sp., and *Enterococcus* sp. The most common fungus associated with sepsis during TPN therapy is *Candida* sp. which is associated with significant morbidity and mortality. Boeckman et al reported a 50% mortality rate in six infants and children receiving long-term TPN therapy who developed candidiasis.[147]

The symptoms of sepsis in the pediatric population are variable and depend upon the patient's age. The symptoms associated with septicemia generally include fever, leukocytosis, and hyperglycemia with glucosuria; however, in the neonate the symptoms may include hypothermia, leukopenia, and glucose intolerance. When sepsis is suspected in a patient receiving TPN therapy, blood cultures should be drawn from the TPN catheter and a peripheral site. Cultures of the catheter site, urine, sputum, and other sites and other studies which may identify the site of infection should be done at this time. A positive blood culture drawn from the TPN catheter is a strong indication that the catheter is the source of infection. The catheter may also be suspect when another site of infection is not identified and the patient remains symptomatic.

After the evaluation for infection, empiric antibiotic therapy should be initiated. When the site of infection and/or pathogen are identified, antibiotic therapy is adjusted accordingly. If the patient remains clinically stable and becomes afebrile with the initiation of antibiotic therapy, the catheter may be left in place throughout therapy. Removal of the catheter should be considered if the patient remains symptomatic after the initiation of antibiotic therapy. The catheter tip should be sent for both bacterial and fungal cultures upon removal.

Other complications associated with the central venous catheters during TPN therapy include thrombosis formation, resulting in pulmonary emboli or superior vena cava syndrome, pneumothorax, malposition of the catheter resulting in the infusion of TPN solution into pleural and pericardial spaces, and malposition of the catheter in the right atrium resulting in cardiac arrhythmias. The most frequent complications associated with peripheral venous catheters are thrombophlebitis and extravasations. Extravasation of the hypertonic TPN infusate may cause both partial-thickness and full-thickness tissue loss.[149] In 385 infants and children receiving peripheral TPN therapy tissue loss associated with extravasation of the infusate occurred in 8.3%.[139] Close monitoring of the infusion site should prevent the development of severe tissue necrosis from extravasations.

The metabolic complications associated with pediatric TPN therapy result from incorrect formulation or incorrect administration of the TPN infusate as well as the inability of some infants and children to metabolize the components of the TPN infusate. The majority of these complications can be prevented with close patient monitoring (Table 108.11). Infants and children receiving TPN therapy require more frequent monitoring during any period of metabolic instability and during the initial period of TPN therapy before reaching optimal dosages of dextrose, crystalline amino acids, and intravenous fat emulsions. When the patient is metabolically stable less frequent monitoring is required.[73]

Hyperglycemia results from the administration of glucose at a rate that exceeds the patient's ability to utilize the glucose. Premature infants are at increase risk of developing hyperglycemia.[76,150] Sepsis can cause hyperglycemia as a result of decreased glucose utilization. Decreased glucose tolerance has also been associated with intravenous fat infusions.[151] The major complications associated with hyperglycemia include serum hyperosmolarity and osmotic diuresis. Monitoring of the serum glucose and adjusting the concentration of dextrose in the TPN infusate prevent the development of severe hyperglycemia and its associated complications. Interruption of the TPN infusion can result in hypoglycemia. If the TPN infusion must be temporarily interrupted it is essential that an alternative source of glucose, such as 10% dextrose, be administered to the patient to prevent hypoglycemia. When TPN therapy is discontinued, the infusion should be tapered and the patient closely monitored to prevent hypoglycemia.

Electrolyte and mineral imbalances can result if the formulation of the TPN infusate does not meet or exceeds the patient's requirements. Monitoring of the patient's serum electrolytes and minerals should prevent the development of severe electrolyte and mineral imbalances (Table 108.11). During the initial period or if the patient becomes metabolically unstable, these parameters should be monitored three to four times per week. In the child receiving long-term TPN therapy who is metabolically stable, less frequent monitoring is adequate.

TPN therapy has been identified as one of the many potential causes of metabolic bone disease in infants and children as well as adults. In infants and growing children metabolic bone disease is characterized by osteopenia and rickets. Because of the solubility problems associated with calcium and phosphorus in TPN infusates, providing adequate amounts of these minerals is often difficult. Another potential cause of metabolic bone disease in premature infants is aluminum toxicity. Aluminum is a common contaminate of many intravenous additives used in TPN infusates. In children with normal renal function aluminum is excreted renally without accumulation or toxicity. Sedman et al described aluminum accumulation and toxicity in 18 premature infants receiving intravenous therapy.[152] Prema-

**Table 108.11** Suggested Monitoring Schedule During Pediatric Total Parenteral Nutrition

| | *Initial period*[a] | *Later period*[b] |
|---|---|---|
| Growth parameters | | |
| Weight | Daily | Daily |
| Height | Weekly | Weekly |
| Head circumference | Weekly | Weekly |
| Clinical observations | | |
| Activity, vital signs, temperature, etc | Daily | Daily |
| Laboratory parameters | | |
| Urine glucose | Daily | Daily |
| Serum glucose | As needed[c] | As needed[c] |
| Serum electrolytes | 3–4 times/wk | 2–3 times/wk |
| Serum acid–base status | 3–4 times/wk | 2–3 times/wk |
| Serum calcium, magnesium, and phosphorus | 3 times/wk | 2 times/wk |
| Hemoglobin | 2 times/wk | 2 times/wk |
| Serum urea nitrogen | 3 times/wk | 2 times/wk |
| Serum ammonia | 2 times/wk | Weekly |
| Serum protein | Weekly | Weekly |
| Serum triglyceride and cholesterol | 2 times/wk | Weekly |
| Serum bilirubin and hepatic enzymes | Weekly | Weekly |

[a] The period before optimal dosages of dextrose, amino acids, and intravenous fats are reached, or any period of metabolic instability.
[b] The period in which the patient is metabolically stable.
[c] Serum glucose should be monitored closely (two or three times daily) during periods of glucosuria and during the discontinuation of TPN therapy. Dextrostix may provide adequate screening in the stable patient during discontinuation of TPN therapy.

From AAP Committee on Nutrition: Pediatrics 1983;71:548, with permission.

ture infants may be at risk for aluminum accumulation because of decreased renal function.

Metabolic acidosis was a frequent problem with the use of protein hydrolysates and early crystalline amino acid solutions.[109] Adjustments in the salts of the amino acids utilized in the current crystalline amino acid solutions have largely corrected this complication; however, metabolic acidosis remains a complication in the premature infant. The use of the acetate and lactate salts of sodium and potassium in the infusate may correct the metabolic acidosis that develops in infants and children during TPN therapy.

Hyperammonemia in infants and children receiving TPN therapy has been attributed to the high ammonia content of protein hydrolysates.[108,153] The use of crystalline amino acid solutions with neglible quantities of ammonia has minimized this complication; however, hyperammonemia has been described in infants receiving crystalline amino acid solutions. The suggested mechanisms of hyperammonemia with the crystalline amino acid solutions have included hepatic immaturity in the infant and amino acid imbalances.[154] The administration of arginine 0.5–1.0 mmol/kg to the infusate resulted in a correction in the serum ammonia in three infants who developed hyperammonemia while receiving protein 2.5 g/kg/d.[154]

The major metabolic complication associated with TPN therapy in infants and children is liver dysfunction characterized by cholestatic jaundice with an increase in direct bilirubin and mild to moderate elevations in liver enzymes (serum glutamic–oxalacetic and glutamic–pyruvic transaminases).[155] Liver biopsies have universally described both intracellular and intracanalicular cholestasis with varying degrees of portal fibrosis, portal–portal bridging, bile duct proliferation, biliary cirrhosis, and extramedullary hematopoiesis.[156–159] The primary pathology of TPN-associated liver dysfunction is cholestasis, with the more severe hepatic changes resulting from prolonged cholestasis.[156,157] The cause of cholestasis is unknown and many possible etiologies have been suggested. At this time the amino acid component of the infusate is the most likely etiology. Infants receiving greater than 2.5 g/kg appear to have a higher incidence of liver dysfunction.[159,160] Prematurity also appears to increase the risk of liver dysfunction associated with TPN therapy.[158]

Severe liver dysfunction associated with TPN therapy may be prevented by monitoring of the serum bilirubin and hepatic enzymes. Changes in these laboratory parameters do not develop rapidly and should be monitored on a weekly basis throughout TPN therapy. The clinical manifestations of TPN-associated liver dysfunction resolve spontaneously with discontinuation of TPN therapy in the majority of the infants and children. Direct bilirubin and hepatic enzymes usually decrease significantly by 14 days after discontinuation and return to baseline by 4 to 6 weeks.[157–159] Repeat liver biopsies have also shown resolution of the pathologic findings in those patients with mild to moderate liver dysfunction. In those children with severe liver dysfunction some pathologic findings, such as portal fibrosis, have persisted.[156–159]

Despite the complications associated with intravenous fat emulsions, they are widely used in pediatric TPN therapy. Hyperlipidemia is a common complication of intravenous fat emulsion therapy. Premature infants have decreased plasma lipid clearance rates and are at risk for hyperlipidemia.[122–124] Serum concentrations of triglyceride, cholesterol, and phospholipid have been shown to increase with intravenous fat emulsion therapy in infants and children.[123,125,127,161,162] A potential complication of hyperlipidemia is intravascular lipid accumulation. Pulmonary vascular lipid deposits have been described in infants receiving intravenous fat emulsions.[163–165] Premature infants are at risk for pulmonary disease; pulmonary diffusion abnormalities and increased pulmonary vascular resistance have been associated with hyperlipidemia in premature infants.[166–168]

Hydrolysis of intravenous fat emulsions produces free fatty acids and monoglycerides. Elevations in serum free fatty acids have been described in infants receiving intravenous fat emulsions.[155,156] Free fatty acids alter the binding of bilirubin on serum albumin. When the molar ratio of free fatty acids to albumin is greater than 6:1 the binding of bilirubin to albumin is decreased.[169] Hyperbilirubinemia is common in newborn infants. The primary complication associated with hyperbilirubinemia in the newborn is kernicterus, which results from the deposition of bilirubin in brain tissues. Kernicterus is associated with neurologic deficits such as cerebral palsy and mental retardation and, in severe cases, death. The risk of kernicterus increases with the displacement of bilirubin from albumin binding sites. Spear et al evaluated the effect of varying dosage of intravenous fat infusions on bilirubin binding in premature infants with hyperbilirubinemia.[170] They concluded that intravenous fat emulsions of 1 g/kg/d infused over 15 hours had a minimal risk of decreasing bilirubin binding.

Thrombocytopenia has been associated with intravenous fat emulsions in several case reports.[171,172] Goulet et al reported thrombocytopenia in seven children receiving long-term TPN therapy for short-bowel syndrome.[171] Each child experienced one to five episodes of thrombocytopenia that appeared related to intravenous fat emulsion infusions. Laboratory studies in these children suggest hyperactivation of the histiocyte macrophage system, causing thrombocytopenia.

In vitro studies have shown an impairment in neutrophil function by intravenous fat emulsions.[173,174] From these findings it was inferred that immune function would be impaired in patients receiving intravenous fat emulsions. More recent in vitro and in vivo studies were unable to demonstrate an impairment in immune function by intravenous fat emulsions.[175,176] Further studies are needed to better define the effect of intravenous fat emulsions on immune function.

Little is known about the long-term effects of TPN therapy on the gastrointestinal tract. Animal studies have described pancreatic hyposecretion and intestinal mucosal atrophy which reversed with enteral feeding.[177] Kotler et al described gastric and pancreatic hyposecretion in adults receiving long-term TPN therapy.[178] Similar studies in infants and children are limited; however, gastrointestinal tract function appears to normalize over time with the institution of enteral feeds.

## References


1. Helfrick FW, Abelson NM. Intravenous feeding of a complete diet in a child: Report of a case. J Pediatr 1944;25:400–403.
2. Wilmore DW Dudrick SV. Growth and development of an infant receiving all nutrients exclusively by vein. JAMA 1963;203:140–144.
3. Driscoll JM, Heird WC, Schullinger JN, et al. Total intravenous alimentation in low birth weight infants: A preliminary report. J Pediatr 1972;81:145–153.
4. Peden VH, Karpel JT. Total parenteral nutrition in premature infants. J Pediatr 1972;81:137–144.
5. Gunn T, Reaman G, Outerbridge EW, et al. Peripheral total parenteral nutrition for premature infants with the respiratory distress syndrome: A controlled study. J Pediatr 1978;92: 608–613.
6. Yu VYH, Hendry BJP, MacMahon RA. Total parenteral nutrition in very low birthweight infants: A controlled trial. Arch Dis Child 1979;54:652–661.
7. Churella HR, Bachhuber BS, MacLean WC. Survey: Methods of feeding low birth weight infants. Pediatrics 1985;76:243–249.
8. Filler RM, Eraklis AJ, Rubin VG, et al. Long-term total parenteral nutrition in infants. N Engl J Med 1969;281:589–594.
9. Meurling S, Grotte G. Complete parenteral nutrition in the surgery of the newborn infant. Acta Chir Scand 1981;147: 465–473.
10. Dorney SFA, Ament ME, Berquist WE, et al. Improved survival in very short small bowel of infancy with use of long-term parenteral nutrition. J Pediatr 1985;107:521–525.
11. Wilmore DW. Factors correlating with successful outcome following extensive intestinal resection in newborn infants. J Pediatr 1972;80:88–95.
12. Ament ME. Management of chronic diarrhea with parenteral nutrition and enteral infusion techniques. Pediatr Ann 1985; 14:53–60.
13. Lloyd-Still JD, Shwachman H, Filler RM. Protracted diarrhea in infancy treated by intravenous alimentation. I. Clinical studies of 16 infants. Am J Dis Child 1973;125:358–364.
14. Green HL, McCabe DR, Merenstein GB. Protracted diarrhea and malnutrition in infancy: Changes in intestinal morphology and disaccharidase activities during treatment with total intravenous nutrition or oral elemental diets. J Pediatr 1975;87:695–704.
15. Hyman CJ, Reiter J, Rodnan J, et al. Parenteral and oral alimentation in the treatment of the nonspecific protracted diarrheal syndrome of infancy. J Pediatr 1971;78:17–29.
16. Keating JP, Ternberg JL. Amino acid–hypertonic glucose treatment for intractable diarrhea in infants. Am J Dis Child 1971;122:226–228.
17. Gunn T, Brown RS, Pencharz P, et al. Total parenteral nutrition in malnourished infants with intractable diarrhea. Can Med Assoc J 1977;117:357–360.

18. Cohen MI, Boley SJ, Daum F, et al. The role and effect of parenteral nutrition on the liver and its use in chronic inflammatory bowel disease in childhood. Adv Exp Med Biol 1974;46:214–224.
19. Layden T, Rosenberg J, Nemchausky B, et al. Reversal of growth arrest in adolescents with Crohn's disease after parenteral alimentation. Gastroenterology 1976;70:1017–1021.
20. Strobel CT, Byrne WJ, Ament ME. Home parenteral nutrition in children with Crohn's disease: An effective management alternative. Gastroenterology 1979;77:272–279.
21. Grand RJ, Shen G, Werlin SL, et al. Reversal of growth arrest in Crohn's disease: A new approach. Pediatr Res 1977;11:444.
22. Lake AM, Kim S, Mathis RK, et al. Influence of preoperative parenteral alimentation on postoperative growth in adolescent Crohn's disease. J Pediatr Gastroenterol Nutr 1985;4:182–186.
23. Lester LA, Rothberg RM, Dawson G, et al. Supplemental parenteral nutrition in cystic fibrosis. J Parenter Enter Nutr 1986;10:289–295.
24. Mansell AL, Andersen JC, Muttart CR, et al. Short-term pulmonary effect of total parenteral nutrition in children with cystic fibrosis. J Pediatr 1984;104:700–705.
25. Shepherd R, Cooksley WGE, Domville-Cooke WD. Improved growth and clinical, nutritional, and respiratory changes in response to nutritional therapy in cystic fibrosis. J Pediatr 1980;97:351–357.
26. Kusoffsky E, Straduick B, Troell S. Prospective study of fatty acid supplementation over 3 years in patients with cystic fibrosis. J Pediatr Gastroenterol Nutr 1983;2:434–438.
27. Rickard KA, Baehner RL, Coates TD, et al. Supportive nutritional intervention in pediatric cancer. Cancer Res 1982; 42(suppl):766s–773s.
28. Van Eys J. Nutritional therapy in children with cancer. Cancer Res 1977;37:2457–2461.
29. Filler RM, Jaffe N, Cassady JR, et al. Parenteral nutrition support in children with cancer. Cancer 1977;39:2665–2669.
30. Rickard KA, Kirksey A, Baehner RL, et al. Effectiveness of enteral and parenteral nutrition in the nutritional management of children with Wilms' tumors. Am J Clin Nutr 1980;33: 2622–2629.
31. Hirschman GH, Ras DD, Chan JCM. Anorexia nervosa with acute tubular necrosis treated with parenteral nutrition. Nutr Metab 1977;21:341–348.
32. Maloney MJ, Farrell MK. Treatment of severe weight loss in anorexia nervosa with hyperalimentation and psychotherapy. Am J Psychiat 1980;137:310–314.
33. Pertschuk MJ, Forster J, Buzby G, et al. The treatment of anorexia nervosa with total parenteral nutrition. Biol Psychiat 1981;16:539–550.
34. Arturson G. Metabolic changes and nutrition in children with severe burns. Prog Pediatr Surg 1981;14:81–109.
35. Derganc M. Parenteral nutrition in severely burned children. Scand J Plast Reconstr Surg 1979;13:195–200.
36. Popp MD, Law EJ, MacMillan BG. Parenteral nutrition in children with burns. Experience in the Shriners Burns Institute in Cincinnati. Adv Exp Med Biol 1974;46:240–246.
37. Fischer JE. Parenteral nutrition of renal disease. Adv Exp Med Biol 1974;46:225–230.
38. Holliday MA, Wassner S, Ramirez J. Intravenous nutrition in uremic children with protein-energy malnutrition. Am J Clin Nutr 1978;31:1854–1860.
39. Motil KJ, Harmon WE, Grupe WE. Complications of essential amino acid hyperalimentation in children with acute renal failure. J Parenter Enter Nutr 1980;4:32–35.
40. Townsend I, Kerr DS. Total parenteral nutrition therapy of toxic maple syrup urine disease. Am J Clin Nutr 1982;36: 359–365.
41. Cole DE, Landry DA. Parenteral nutrition in a premature infant with phenylketonuria. J Parenter Enter Nutr 1984;8: 42–44.
42. Food and Nutrition Board, National Research Council. Recommended Dietary Allowances, 9th ed. Washington DC, National Academy of Sciences, 1980.
43. Kanarek KS, Williams PR, Curran JS. Total parenteral nutrition in infants and children. Adv Pediatr 1982;29:151–181.
44. Vaughan VC, McKay RJ (eds): Nelson's Textbook of Pediatrics, 12th ed. Philadelphia, W.B. Saunders, 1983, pp 136–139.
45. Getchell EL. Estimating energy and protein needs for the hospitalized child. Am J Intraven Ther Clin Nutr 1983;10:7–15.
46. American Academy of Pediatrics, Committee on Nutrition. Nutritional needs of low-birth weight infants. Pediatrics 1985;75:976–986.
47. Brooke OG, Alvear J, Arnold M. Energy retention, energy expenditure, and growth in healthy immature infants. Pediatr Res 1979;13:215–220.
48. Reichman BL, Chessex P, Putet G, et al. Partition of energy metabolism and energy cost of growth in the very low-birth-weight infant. Pediatrics 1982;69:446–451.
49. Sauer PJJ, Dane HJ, Visser HKA. Longitudinal studies on metabolic rate, heat loss, and energy cost of growth in low birth weight infants. Pediatr Res 1984;18:254–259.
50. Catzeflis C, Schutz Y, Micheli JL, et al. Whole body protein synthesis and energy expenditure in very low birth weight infants. Pediatr Res 1985;19:679–687.
51. Sinclair JC, Driscoll JM, Hard WC, et al. Supportive management of the sick neonate. Pediatr Clin North Am 1970;17: 863–893.
52. Long CL, Schaffel N, Geiger JW. Metabolic response to injury and illness. Estimation of energy and protein needs from indirect calorimetry and nitrogen balance. J Parenter Enter Nutr 1979;3:452–456.
53. Wilmore DW. Energy requirements for maximum nitrogen retention, in Green HC, Holliday MA, Munro HN (eds): Proceedings of a Symposium on Amino Acids. American Medical Association, 1977, pp 47–57.
54. Smith RC, Burkinshaw L, Hill GL. Optimal energy and nitrogen intake for gastroenterological patients requiring intravenous nutrition. Gastroenterology 1982;82:445–452.
55. Peters C, Fischer JE. Studies on calorie to nitrogen ratio for total parenteral nutrition. Surg Gynecol Obstet 1980;151:1–8.
56. Kerner JA. Protein requirements, in Kerner JA (ed): Manual of Pediatric Parenteral Nutrition. New York, John Wiley, 1983, pp 89–99.
57. Pereira GR, Glassman M. Parenteral nutrition in the neonate, in Rombeau JL, Caldwell MD (eds): Parenteral Nutrition. Philadelphia, W.B. Saunders, 1986, pp 702–720.
58. Kanaya S, Nose O, Harada T, et al. Total parenteral nutrition with a new amino acid solution for infants. J Pediatr Gastroenterol Nutr 1984;3:440–445.
59. Raiha NCR. Biochemical basis for nutritional management of preterm infants. Pediatrics 1975;53:147–156.
60. Pohlandt F. Cystine: A semi-essential amino acid in the newborn infant. Acta Pediatr Scand 1974;63:801–804.
61. Synderman SE, Boyer A, Roitman E, et al. The histidine requirement of the infant. Pediatrics 1963;31:786–801.
62. Geggel HS, Ament ME, Heckenlively JR, et al. Nutritional requirement for taurine in patients receiving long-term parenteral nutrition. N Engl J Med 1985;312:142–146.
63. Vinton NE, Geggel HS, Ament ME, et al. Taurine deficiency in a child on total parenteral nutrition. Nutr Rev 1985;43:81–83.

64. Friedman Z. Essential fatty acids revisited. Am J Dis Child 1980;134:397–403.
65. Stahl GE, Spear ML, Hamosh M. Intravenous administration of lipid emulsions to preterm infants. Perinat Nutr 1986;13: 133–162.
66. Kennedy-Caldwell C, Caldwell MD. Developmental considerations in neonatal TPN, in Rombeau JL, Caldwell MD (eds): Parenteral Nutrition. Philadelphia, W.B. Saunders, 1986, pp 680–701.
67. Kerner JA. Fat requirements, in Kerner JA (ed): Manual of Pediatric Parenteral Nutrition. New York, John Wiley, 1983, pp 103–127.
68. Friedman Z, Danon A, Stahlman MT, et al. Rapid onset of essential fatty acid deficiency in the newborn. Pediatrics 1976;58:640–649.
69. Caldwell MD, Jonsson HT, Othersen HB. Essential fatty acid deficiency in an infant receiving prolonged parenteral alimentation. J Pediatr 1972;81:894–898.
70. Postuma R, Pease PWB, Watts R, et al. Essential fatty acid deficiency in infants receiving parenteral nutrition. J Pediatr Surg 1978;13:393–398.
71. Hansen AE, Wiese HF, Boelsche AN, et al. Role of linoleic acid in infant nutrition. Pediatrics 1963;31:171–192.
72. American Academy of Pediatrics Committee on Nutrition. Commentary on breast-feeding and infant formulas including proposed standards for formulas. Pediatrics 1976;57:278–285.
73. American Academy of Pediatrics, Committee on Nutrition. Commentary on parenteral nutrition. Pediatrics 1983;71:547–552.
74. Weil WB. Nutrition-specific dietary needs, in Rudolph AM, Hoffman JIE (eds): Pediatrics, 17th ed. Norwalk, CT, Appleton-Century-Crofts, 1982, pp 181–197.
75. Nash MA. The management of fluid and electrolyte disorders in the neonate. Clin Perinatol 1981;8:257–262.
76. Baumgart S, Langman CB, Sosulski R, et al. Fluid, electrolyte, and glucose maintenance in the very low birth weight infant. Clin Pediatr 1982;21:199–205.
77. Steichen JJ, Gratton TL, Tsang RC. Osteopenia of prematurity: The cause and possible treatment. J Pediatr 1980;96:528–534.
78. Hambridge KM. Trace elements in pediatric nutrition. Adv Pediatr 1977;24:191–230.
79. Solomons NW. Trace minerals, in Rombeau JL, Caldwell MD (eds): Parenteral Nutrition. Philadelphia, W.B. Saunders, 1986, pp 169–197.
80. Shaw JCL. Trace elements in the fetus and young infants. I. Zinc. Am J Dis Child 1979;133:1260–1268.
81. Shaw JCL. Trace elements in the fetus and young infant. II. Copper, manganese, selenium, and chromium. Am J Dis Child 1980;134:74–81.
82. Weber TR, Sears N, Davies B, et al. Clinical spectrum of zinc deficiency in pediatric patients receiving total parenteral nutrition. J Pediatr Surg 1981;16:236–240.
83. Joffe G, Etzione A, Levy J. A patient with copper deficiency anemia while on prolonged intravenous feeding. Clin Pediatr 1981;20:226–228.
84. Heller RM, Kirchner SG, O'Neill JA, et al. Skeletal changes of copper deficiency in infants receiving prolonged total parenteral nutrition. J Pediatr 1978;92:947–949.
85. Kein CL, Ganther HE. Manifestations of chronic selenium deficiency in a child receiving total parenteral nutrition. Am J Clin Nutr 1983;37:319–328.
86. American Academy of Pediatrics. Pediatric Nutrition Handbook, 2nd ed. Elk Grove, American Academy of Pediatrics, 1985, pp 213–220.
87. American Medical Association, Department of Foods and Nutrition. Guidelines for essential trace element preparations for parenteral use. JAMA 1979;241:2051–2054.
88. Zlotkin SH, Buchanan BE. Meeting zinc and copper intake requirements in the parenterally fed preterm and full-term infant. J Pediatr 1983;103:441–446.
89. Dahlstrom KA, Ament ME, Medhin MG, et al. Serum trace elements in children receiving long-term parenteral nutrition. J Pediatr 1986;109:625–630.
90. Kerner JA. Vitamin requirements, in Kerner JA (ed): Manual of Pediatric Parenteral Nutrition. New York, John Wiley, 1983, pp 137–155.
91. Dempsey D, Hodges RE. Parenteral vitamin therapy in hospital patients, in Rombeau JL, Caldwell MD (eds): Parenteral Nutrition. Philadelphia, W.B. Saunders, 1986, pp 154–168.
92. Shike M, Sturtridge WC, Cherk ST, et al. A possible role of vitamin D in the genesis of parenteral-nutrition-induced metabolic bone disease. Ann Intern Med 1981;95:560–568.
93. Zipursky A, Brown EJ, Watts J, et al. Oral vitamin E supplementation for the prevention of anemia in premature infants: A controlled trial. Pediatrics 1987;79:61–68.
94. Hittner HM, Gadio LB, Rudolph AJ, et al. Retrolental fibroplasia: Efficacy of vitamin E in a double-blind clinical study of preterm infants. N Engl J Med 1981;305:1365–1371.
95. Ehrenkranz RA, Ablow RC, Warshaw JB. Prevention of bronchopulmonary dysplasia with vitamin E administration during acute stages of respiratory distress syndrome. J Pediatr 1979;95:873–878.
96. Phelps DL, Rosenbaum AL, Isenberg SJ, et al. Tocopherol efficacy and safety for preventing retinopathy in prematurity: A randomized, controlled, double-blind trial. Pediatrics 1987; 79:489–500.
97. Saldanha RL, Cepeda EE, Poland RL. The effect of vitamin E prophylaxis on the incidence and severity of bronchopulmonary dysplasia. J Pediatr 1982;101:89–93.
98. Johnson L, Bowen FW, Abbasi S, et al. Relationship of prolonged pharmacologic serum levels of vitamin E to incidence of sepsis and necrotizing enterocolitis in infants with birth weight 1500 grams or less. Pediatrics 1985;75:619–638.
99. Martone WJ, Williams WW, Mortensen ML, et al. Illness with fatalities in premature infants. Association with an intravenous vitamin E preparation, E-Ferol. Pediatrics 1986;78:591–600.
100. Moran JR, Greene HL. The B vitamins and vitamin C in human nutrition. I. General considerations and 'obligatory' B vitamins. Am J Dis Child 1979;133:192–199.
101. Moran JR, Greene HL. The B vitamins and vitamin C in human nutrition. II. 'Conditional' B vitamins and vitamin C. Am J Dis Child 1979;133:308–314.
102. Clarke TA, Saunders BS, Feldman B. Pyridoxine-dependent seizures requiring high doses of pyridoxine for control. Am J Dis Child 1979;133:963–965.
103. Mock DM, DeLorimer AA, Leibman WM, et al. Biotin deficiency: An unusual complication of parenteral alimentation. N Engl J Med 1981;304:820–822.
104. Gillis J, Murphy FR, Boxall LBH, et al. Biotin deficiency in a child on long-term TPN. J Parenter Enter Nutr 1982;6:308–310.
105. Schiff D, Chan G, Seccombe D, et al. Plasma carnitine levels during intravenous feeding of the neonate. J Pediatr 1979;95:1043–1046.
106. Schmidt-Sommerfeld E, Penn D, Wolf H. Carnitine deficiency in premature infants receiving total parenteral nutrition: Effect of L-carnitine supplementation. J Pediatr 1983;102:931–935.
107. Orazli A, Donzelli F, Enzi G, et al. Effect of carnitine on lipid metabolism in the newborn. Biol Neonate 1983;43:186–190.

108. Stegink LD. Amino acids in pediatric parenteral nutrition. Am J Dis Child 1983;137:1008–1016.
109. Heird WC, Dell RB, Driscoll JM, et al. Metabolic acidosis resulting from intravenous alimentation mixtures containing synthetic amino acids. N Engl J Med 1972;287:943–948.
110. Cohn RM, Jezyk P. Metabolic screening, in Hicks JM, Boeck RL (eds): Pediatric Clinical Chemistry. Philadelphia, W.B. Saunders, 1984, pp 657–689.
111. Wu PYK, Edwards N, Storm MC. Plasma amino acid pattern in normal term breast-fed infants. J Pediatr 1986;109:347–349.
112. Das JB, Filler RM. Amino acid utilization during total parenteral nutrition in the surgical neonate. J Pediatr Surg 1973;8: 793–799.
113. Dale G, Pander-Brick M, Wagget J, et al. Plasma amino acid changes in the postsurgical newborn during intravenous nutrition with a synthetic amino acid solution. J Pediatr Surg 1974;11:17–22.
114. Anderson GE, Bucher D, Friis-hansen B, et al. Plasma amino acid concentrations in newborn infants during parenteral nutrition. J Parenter Enter Nutr 1983;7:369–373.
115. Chessex P, Zebiche H, Pineault M, et al. Effect of amino acid composition of parenteral solutions on nitrogen retention and metabolic response in very low birth weight infants. J Pediatr 1985;106:111–117.
116. Helms RA, Chrisensen ML, Mauer EC, et al. Comparison of a pediatric versus standard amino acid formulation in preterm neonates requiring parenteral nutrition. J Pediatr 1987;110: 466–470.
117. Wretlind A. Development of fat emulsions. J Parenter Enter Nutr 1981;5:230–235.
118. Alexander CS, Zieve L. Fat infusions. Arch Intern Med 1961;107:514–528.
119. Pelham LD. Rational use of intravenous fat emulsions. Am J Hosp Pharm 1981;38:198–208.
120. Wolfe BM, Ney DM. Lipid metabolism in parenteral nutrition, in Rombeau JL, Caldwell MD (eds): Parenteral Nutrition. Philadelphia, W.B. Saunders, 1986, pp 72–99.
121. Stahel GE, Spear ML, Hamosh M. Intravenous administration of lipid emulsions to premature infants. Clin Perinatal 1986;13: 133–162.
122. Gustaffson A, Kjellmer I, Olegard R, et al. Nutrition in low-birth-weight infants. II. Repeated intravenous injections of fat emulsion. Acta Pediatr Scand 1974;63:177–182.
123. Andrew G, Chan G, Schiff D. Lipid metabolism in the neonate. I. The effects of intralipid on plasma triglyceride and free fatty acid concentrations in the neonate. J Pediatr 1976;88:273–278.
124. Shennan AT, Bryan MH, Angel A. The effect of gestational age on intralipid tolerance in the newborn infant. J Pediatr 1977;91:134–137.
125. Forget PP, Fernandes J, Haverkamp PB. Utilization of fat emulsion during parenteral nutrition in children. Acta Pediatr Scand 1975;64:377–384.
126. American Academy of Pediatrics Committee on Nutrition. Use of intravenous fat emulsions in pediatric patients. Pediatrics 1981;68:738–743.
127. Hillard JL, Shannon DL, Hunter MA, et al. Plasma lipid levels in preterm neonates receiving parenteral fat emulsions. Arch Dis Child 1983;58:29–33.
128. Niemiec PW, Vanderveen TW. Compatibility considerations in parenteral nutrient solutions. Am J Hosp Pharm 1984;41: 893–911.
129. Eggert LD, Rusho WJ, MacKay MW, et al. Calcium and phosphorus compatibility in parenteral nutrition solutions for neonates. Am J Hosp Pharm 1982;39:49–53.
130. Poole RL, Rupp CA, Kerner JA. Calcium and phosphorus in neonatal parenteral nutrition solutions. J Parenter Enter Nutr 1983;7:358–360.
131. Fitzgerald KA, MacKay MW. Calcium and phosphate solubility in neonatal parenteral nutrient solutions containing TrophAmine. Am J Hosp Pharm 1986;43:88–93.
132. Reed MD, Bertino JS, Halpen TC. Use of intravenous iron dextran injection in children receiving total parenteral nutrition. Am J Dis Child 1981;135:829–831.
133. Halpin TC, Bertino JS, Rothstein FC, et al. Iron-deficiency anemia in childhood inflammatory bowel disease: Treatment with intravenous iron–dextran. J Parenter Enter Nutr 1982;6: 9–11.
134. Norton JA, Peters ML, Wesley R, et al. Iron supplemention of total parenteral nutrition: A prospective study. J Parenter Enter Nutr 1983;7:457–461.
135. Wan KK, Tsallas G. Dilute iron dextran formulation for addition to parenteral nutrient solutions. Am J Hosp Pharm 1980;37:206–210.
136. Moore MC, Greene HL, Phillips B, et al. Evaluation of a pediatric multiple vitamin preparation for total parenteral nutrition in infants and children. I. Blood levels of water-soluble vitamins. Pediatrics 1986;77:530–538.
137. Greene HL, Moore ME, Phillips B, et al. Evaluation of a pediatric multiple vitamin preparation for total parenteral nutrition. II. Blood levels of vitamins A, D, and E. Pediatrics 1986;77:539–547.
138. Bozzetti F, Scarpa D, Terno G, et al. Subclavian venous thrombosis due to indwelling catheters: A prospective study on 52 patients. J Parenter Enter Nutr 1983;7:560–562.
139. Ziegler M, Jakobowski D, Hoelzer D, et al. Route of pediatric parenteral nutrition: Proposed criteria revision. J Pediatr Surg 1980;15:472–476.
140. Mollitt DL, Golladay ES. Complications of TPN catheter-induced vena caval thrombosis in children less than one year of age. J Pediatr Surg 1983;18:462–467.
141. Wesley JR, Keens TG, Miller SW, et al. Pulmonary embolism during the course of total parenteral nutrition. J Pediatr 1978;93:113–115.
142. Mendeza GJB, Soto A, Brown EG, et al. Intracardiac thrombi complicating central total parenteral nutrition: Resolution without surgery or thrombolysis. J Pediatr 1986;108:610–613.
143. Alpan G, Eyal F, Springer C, et al. Heparinization of alimentation solutions administered through peripheral veins in premature infants: A controlled study. Peidatrics 1984;74:375–378.
144. Zaidan H, Dhanireddy R, Hamosh M, et al. Effect of continuous heparin administration on intralipid clearing in very low-birth-weight infants. J Pediatr 1982;101:599–602.
145. Grant JP. Catheter access, in Rombeau JL, Caldwell MD (eds): Parenteral Nutrition. Philadelphia, W.B. Saunders, 1986, pp 306–315.
146. Bottino J, McCredie KB, Groschel DHM, et al. Long-term intravenous therapy with peripherally inserted silicone elastomer central venous catheters in patients with malignant diseases. Cancer 1979;43:1937–1943.
147. Boeckman CR, Krill CE. Bacterial and fungal infections complicating parenteral alimentation in infants and children. J Pediatr Surg 1970;5:117–126.
148. Sanders RA, Sheldon GF. Septic complications of total parenteral nutrition. Am J Surg 1976;132:214–220.
149. Brown AS, Hoelzer DH, Piercy SA. Skin necrosis from extravasation of intravenous fluids in children. Plast Reconstr Surg 1979;64:146–150.
150. Seashore JH. Metabolic complications of parenteral nutrition

in infants and children. Surg Clin North Am 1980;60:1239–1252.

151. Vileisis RA, Cowett RM, Oh W. Glycemic response to lipid infusion in the premature neonate. J Pediatr 1982;100:108–112.
152. Sedman AB, Klein GL, Merritt RJ, et al. Evidence of aluminum loading in infants receiving intravenous therapy. N Engl J Med 1985;312:1337–1343.
153. Johnson JD, Albritton WL, Sunshine P. Hyperammonemia accompanying parenteral nutrition in newborn infants. J Pediatr 1972;81:154–161.
154. Heird WC, Nicholson JF, Driscoll JM, et al. Hyperammonemia resulting from alimentation using a mixture of synthetic L-amino acids: A preliminary report. J Pediatr 1972;81:162–165.
155. Vileisis RA, Inwood RJ, Hunt CE. Laboratory monitoring of parenteral nutrition–associated hepatic dysfunction in infants. J Parenter Enter Nutr 1981;5:67–69.
156. Benjamin DR. Hepatobiliary dysfunction in infants and children associated with long-term total parenteral nutrition. A clinico-pathologic study. Am J Clin Pathol 1981;76:276–283.
157. Dahms BB, Halpin TC. Serial liver biopsies in parenteral nutrition–associated cholestasis of early infancy. Gastroenterology 1981;81:136–144.
158. Pereira GR, Sherman MS, DiGiacomo J, et al. Hyperalimentation-induced cholestasis. Am J Dis Child 1981;135:842–845.
159. Beale EF, Nelson RM, Bucciarelli RL, et al. Intrahepatic cholestasis associated with parenteral nutrition in premature infants. Pediatrics 1979;64:342–347.
160. Sankaran K, Berscheid B, Verma V, et al. An evaluation of total parenteral nutrition using Vamin and Aminosyn as protein base in critically ill preterm infants. J Parenter Enter Nutr 1985;9:439–442.
161. Cooke RJ, Burckhart GJ. Hypertriglyceridemia during the intravenous infusion of a safflower oil–based fat emulsion. J Pediatr 1983;103:959–961.
162. Kao LC, Cheng MH, Warburton D. Triglycerides, free fatty acids, free fatty acids/albumin molar ratio, and cholesterol levels in serum of neonates receiving long-term lipid infusions: Controlled trial of continuous and intermittent regimens. J Pediatr 1984;104:429–435.
163. Shulman RJ, Langston C, Schanler RJ. Pulmonary vascular lipid deposition after administration of intravenous fat to infants. Pediatrics 1987;79:99–102.
164. Hertel J, Tygstrup I, Andersen GE. Intravascular fat accumulation after intralipid infusion in the very low-birth-weight infant. J Pediatr 1982;100:975–976.
165. Levene MI, Wigglesworth JS, Desai R. Pulmonary fat accumulation after intralipid infusion in the preterm infant. Lancet 1980;2:815–819.
166. Pereira GR, Fox WW, Stanley CA, et al. Decreased oxygenation and hyperlipidemia during intravenous fat infusions in premature infants. Pediatrics 1980;66:26–30.
167. Stahe GE, Spear ML, Egler JM, et al. Effect of lipid infusion rate on oxygenation in premature infants. Pediatr Res 1984;18:406A.
168. Lloyd TR, Boucek MM. Effect of intralipid on the neonatal pulmonary bed: An echographic study. J Pediatr 1986;108:100–103.
169. Andrew G, Chan G, Schiff D. Lipid metabolism in the neonate. II. The effect of intralipid on bilirubin binding in vitro and in vivo. J Pediatr 1976;88:279–284.
170. Spear ML, Stahl GE, Paul MH, et al. The effect of 15-hour fat infusions of varying dosage on bilirubin binding to albumin. J Parenter Enter Nutr 1985;9:144–147.
171. Goulet O, Girot R, Maier-Redelsperger M, et al. Hematologic disorders following prolonged use of intravenous fat emulsions in children. J Parenter Enter Nutr 1986;10:284–288.
172. Lipson AH, Pritchard J, Thomas G. Thrombocytopenia after intralipid infusion in a neonate. Lancet 1974;2:1462–1463.
173. Nordenstrom J, Jarstrand C, Wiernik A. Decreased chemotactic and random migration of leukocytes during intralipid infusion. Am J Clin Nutr 1979;32:2416–2422.
174. Fischer GW, Hunter KW, Wilson SR, et al. Diminished bacterial defences with intralipid. Lancet 1980;2:819–820.
175. English D, Roloff JS, Lukens JN, et al. Intravenous lipid emulsions and human neutrophil function. J Pediatr 1981;99:913–916.
176. Usmani SS, Harper RG, Sia CG, et al. In vitro effect of intralipid on polymorphonuclear leukocyte function in the neonate. J Pediatr 1986;109:710–712.
177. Feldman EJ, Dowling RH, McNaughton J, et al. Effects of oral versus intravenous nutrition on intestinal adaptation after small bowel resection in the dog. Gastroenterology 1976;70:712–719.
178. Kotler DP, Levine GM. Reversible gastric and pancreatic hyposecretion after long-term total parenteral nutrition. N Engl J Med 1979;300:241–242.

# Chapter 109 / Parenteral Nutrition

Jacqueline R. Barber, PharmD

In recent years, nutrition has been recognized to play an important role in promoting maximal response to therapeutic measures, resistance to sepsis, and recovery of wounds whether sustained traumatically, created surgically, or caused by a chronically debilitating disease.[1–6] Frequently, aggressive nutritional support may be necessary in certain hospitalized as well as ambulatory patients, often for prolonged periods of time.[7,8] Whenever feasible, the optimal route for providing nutrients is the gastrointestinal tract, but where use of this route is precluded, parenteral nutrition must be employed.[9]

In the early 1960s, nutritional support utilized dilute nutrient solutions infused peripherally along with early forms of intravenous fat emulsions to provide adequate calories. Because of the side effects associated with cottonseed oil fat emulsions, however, these products were removed from the market in the United States in 1964. For the next several years, larger volumes of dilute dextrose and protein hydrolysate solutions were given via peripheral vein along with diuretics. Problems with fluid overload and electrolyte imbalance using such techniques prompted investigators to begin using larger central veins for infusion of hypertonic nutrient solutions, thus decreasing the fluid volume required and avoiding the phlebitis that commonly occurred with hypertonic infusions given peripherally.[10]

By the late 1960s, Dudrick and colleagues had documented success in maintaining growth and positive nutritional status using intravenous nutrition techniques first in beagle puppies and soon after in humans for several months at a time.[9] In subsequent years, these methods were enthusiastically received,[11,12] but as a result of the early lack of experience and consistency in application of the meticulous protocols required for successful use, complications were reported. This fostered improvements in techniques and practice, allowing for greater success and safety in the use of this form of nutritional therapy.[13] Today, it is widely accepted that parenteral nutrition, if properly managed, may be used to replete and sustain certain populations of patients in better nutritional status than ever previously possible.[10]

Technology in nutritional support has advanced rapidly in the past two decades, offering the clinician a sophisticated array of products, techniques, and equipment, as well as vastly expanding practical experience with this form of nutritional therapy considered by many to be a major breakthrough in medicine. This chapter addresses indications for parenteral nutrition, components of formulations, routes of administration and design of regimens, and practical aspects of solution preparation, stability, and compatibility. Also discussed are management of patients receiving parenteral nutrition, complications and monitoring considerations, and the growing area of home parenteral nutrition.

## Definition/Indications

Parenteral nutrition (PN) allows the provision of required nutrients by intravenous routes. It is also commonly referred to as total parenteral nutrition (TPN), or hyperalimentation. Goals of parenteral nutrition therapy include maintenance or restoration of nutritional integrity in the face of disease, injury, or inability to consume adequate nutrients by other means. In certain instances, parenteral nutrition may also improve the outcome of the illness, or may add to quality of life for the patient.[14]

While *absolute* criteria have not been defined for use of this (relatively) new and costly method of therapy in various patient populations, clinical judgment coupled with practical experience has led to recommendations for use in specific circumstances where benefits outweigh the risks.[15–18]

It is generally accepted that parenteral nutrition should be considered only when oral or enteral support is impossible, or when the gastrointestinal absorptive or functional capacity is not sufficient to meet the nutritional needs of the patient. This is especially critical in the malnourished patient who may otherwise have little or no nutritional intake for prolonged periods of time. As recently outlined by the Board of Directors of the American Society for Parenteral and Enteral Nutrition (ASPEN), Table 109.1 lists specific instances in which administration of parenteral nutrition should be considered.[16] Table 109.2 continues with clinical settings in which parenteral nutrition is often beneficial; however, these patients should receive thorough evaluation of condition, diagnoses, and clinical course on an individual basis to determine the advisability of this therapy.[16]

In addition to the indications already outlined, PN is often beneficial for intensive support of low-birth-weight infants, intractable diarrhea of infancy, alimentary diseases or disorders, and other conditions such as burns or trauma in pediatric patients.[14,15,19]

## Design of Parenteral Nutrition Regimen

To meet the specific nutritional needs of the patient (discussed in Chapter 107), the PN regimen can be designed to provide, in addition to fluid (water), six essential categories of nutrients necessary for tissue synthesis and energy balance: nitrogen, energy, essential fatty acids, electrolytes, vitamins, and trace elements. Table 109.3 lists the nutrient components of PN solutions along with their commercially available forms.[20,21]

Nitrogen is provided as protein in the form of crystalline amino acids (CAAs) available commercially from a variety of manufacturers. Such products contain a physiologic ratio

**Table 109.1** Indications for Parenteral Nutrition

| |
|---|
| Inability to absorb adequate nutrients enterally |
| Massive small-bowel resection |
| Diseases of the small intestine |
| Radiation enteritis |
| Severe diarrhea |
| Intractable vomiting |
| Patients receiving chemotherapy, radiation, and bone marrow transplantation |
| Moderate to severe pancreatitis |
| Severe malnutrition with nonfunctional gastrointestinal tract |
| Severe catabolism when gastrointestinal tract not usable for longer than 5–7 days |

Data from Reference 16.

of essential to nonessential biologically utilizable amino acids as substrates for protein synthesis. Products differ by concentration, amino acid profile, electrolyte profile (some with maintenance levels of electrolytes premixed into the stock solution), and other specific characteristics such as pH. The majority of CAA formulations are considered general or standard solutions and differ in composition only slightly from one manufacturer to the next. They are essentially equivalent for general PN use. Certain products, however, are designed with modified amino acid profiles having specific indications for use in renal failure, hepatic disease, stress or trauma, or in neonates and pediatric patients. Representative CAA solutions from various manufacturers are included in Table 109.4.[21]

Energy in PN solutions is most commonly provided as the carbohydrate dextrose monohydrate, which is relatively inexpensive, readily available, and efficiently utilized by most patients. Dextrose solutions for admixture are commercially available in stock concentrations ranging from 5% to 70%. One gram of dextrose provides approximately 3.4 kcal; therefore, 1 L of 10% dextrose contains 340 kcal. Dextrose in concentrations less than 10% (approximately 500 mOsm/L, or 50 mOsm/1% dextrose) may be given peripherally, but higher concentrations are considered too hypertonic for peripheral administration and may only be used centrally. Other carbohydrate sources such as glycerol,[22,23] fructose, invert sugar, alcohol, sorbitol, and xylitol have been employed in PN solutions but are not widely used or accepted in the United States at present.[20,24]

**Table 109.2** Settings in Which Parenteral Nutrition May Be Beneficial

| |
|---|
| Major surgery |
| Moderate stress |
| Enterocutaneous fistulae |
| Inflammatory bowel disease |
| Hyperemesis gravidarum |
| Moderate malnutrition with intensive medical/surgical intervention |
| Enteral nutrition not feasible within 7–10 days |
| Inflammatory adhesions with small-bowel obstruction |
| Intensive cancer chemotherapy |

Data from Reference 16.

**Table 109.3** Nutrient Components of Parenteral Nutrition Solutions

| *Nutrient* | *Intravenous source* |
|---|---|
| Fluid | Sterile water for injection, USP |
| Nitrogen | Crystalline amino acids |
| Energy (carbohydrate and/or fat) | Dextrose, IV fat emulsions |
| Essential fatty acids | Linoleic acid, linolenic acid |
| Electrolytes | Salts |
| | Sodium |
| | Potassium |
| | Calcium |
| | Magnesium |
| | Phosphate |
| | Chloride |
| | Acetate |
| Vitamins | Fat-soluble vitamins (A, D, E, K) |
| | Water-soluble vitamins |
| | Thiamine |
| | Riboflavin |
| | Pyridoxine |
| | Cyanocobalamin |
| | Ascorbic acid |
| | Folic acid |
| | Nicotinic acid |
| | Pantothenic acid |
| | Biotin |
| Trace elements | Zinc |
| | Copper |
| | Chromium |
| | Manganese |
| | Iodine |
| | Selenium |
| | Molybdenum |

Compiled from References 20 and 21.

Intravenous fat emulsion may also be used to provide a concentrated source of energy or calories in the PN regimen (9 kcal/g), as well as a source of essential fatty acids. Several products are commercially available in either 10% (1.1 kcal/mL) or 20% (2.0 kcal/mL) concentrations of safflower or soybean oil emulsion, incorporating egg yolk phospholipid to stabilize the emulsion. Table 109.5 lists commercially available fat emulsions for intravenous use.[25,26] Glycerin is added to fat emulsions to render them isotonic and, as such, they may be administered either peripherally or centrally. It is recommended that no greater than 60% of total infused calories be provided as intravenous fat emulsion each day, or a maximum of 2.5 g/kg/d for adults and 4 g/kg/d in pediatric patients.[27–29] The remaining calories would be supplied as protein or carbohydrate (dextrose). As little as 500 mL of 10% fat emulsion two or three times weekly is considered adequate to prevent essential fatty acid deficiency in an adult patient receiving parenteral nutrition.[30,31]

Electrolytes must be provided to patients receiving PN for

**Table 109.4** Commercially Available Crystalline Amino Acid Products

| *Standard CAA solution* | *Manufacturer* | |
|---|---|---|
| Aminosyn | Abbott | |
| FreAmine | McGaw | |
| Travasol | Travenol | |
| Novamine | KabiVitrum | |
| ***Specialized CAA solution*** | ***Indication*** | ***Manufacturer*** |
| Hepatamine | Liver disease | McGaw |
| Aminosyn RF | Renal failure | Abbott |
| NephrAmine | Renal failure | McGaw |
| RenAmin | Renal failure | Travenol |
| Aminosyn HBC | Stress | Abbott |
| FreAmine HBC | Stress | McGaw |
| BranchAmin | Stress | Travenol |
| Aminosyn PF | Pediatrics | Abbott |
| TrophAmine | Pediatrics | McGaw |

Data from Reference 26.

maintenance or for correction of deficiency. Doses may be based on many factors including cardiovascular, renal, hepatic, and fluid status, in conjunction with monitoring of specific serum laboratory parameters. Requirements may differ greatly from one patient to the next, with changes in clinical course, and from day to day. For these reasons, solutions of electrolyte salts for intravenous use are available as single- or multiple-entity products for admixture with other nutrient substrates, or they may be provided premixed in the CAA product in maintenance concentrations.[26] Electrolyte salt forms are listed in Table 109.6.

Vitamins are essential components for the maintenance of normal metabolism and cellular function. General maintenance guidelines for vitamin supplementation have been established by the American Medical Association Nutrition Advisory Group (AMA/NAG) for adults and pediatric patients receiving parenteral nutrition.[32] Several commercially available adult and pediatric multiple vitamin products have been formulated to specifically comply with these guidelines and are widely used in PN regimens.[26]

Adult multiple vitamin products do not contain vitamin K,

**Table 109.5** Commercially Available Intravenous Fat Emulsions

| *Product* | *Oil source* | *Manufacturer* |
|---|---|---|
| Intralipid 10%, 20% | Soybean | KabiVitrum |
| Liposyn II 10%, 20% | Soybean/safflower | Abbott |
| Soyacal 10%, 20% | Soybean | Alpha Therapeutics |
| Travamulsion 10%, 20% | Soybean | Travenol |

Data from Reference 26.

**Table 109.6** Electrolyte Salts for Parenteral Nutrition Solutions

| | |
|---|---|
| Sodium | Magnesium |
| Acetate | Sulfate |
| Chloride | |
| Lactate | |
| Phosphate | |
| Bicarbonate (see text) | |
| Potassium | Calcium |
| Acetate | Chloride |
| Chloride | Gluceptate |
| Phosphate | Gluconate |

which must be given (most commonly) intramuscularly in addition to the PN vitamin protocol.[21] Vitamin requirements in specific disease states or with certain drug therapies may be altered. Individual and combination products are available to provide for additional and/or tailored supplementation as needed. The reader is referred to current drug references for detailed lists of commercially available vitamin products for parenteral use.[26]

Trace elements for PN admixture are also available as single entities or in various combinations. The AMA/NAG has issued guidelines for trace element supplementation of zinc, copper, chromium, and manganese.[33] Products incorporating these four trace elements are readily available; newer products containing additional trace elements such as selenium, molybdenum, and iodine for which no specific guidelines currently exist have been developed, though they too appear significant in long-term PN administration.[21,26] Detailed information regarding individual micronutrients (vitamins, electrolytes, and trace elements) in parenteral nutrition is available in the literature and may be consulted for specific questions regarding use.[10,21,26,34]

## Preparation of Parenteral Nutrition Solutions

### *Aseptic Admixture*

Assurance of solution sterility during compounding and handling is of paramount importance in reducing the risk of sepsis and related complications in parenteral nutrition patients.[35] Nutrient solutions by definition offer a potentially fertile growth medium for microorganisms. Extensive evaluation of solutions and risk factors for this occurrence has allowed for the development of guidelines designed to minimize the probability of microbial growth, thereby lessening the risk of microbial contaminant–induced septicemia.

Although commercially available solutions, by virtue of their acidity and hypertonicity, are not ideal media for microbial proliferation, certain pathogens may grow very rapidly in solutions kept at room temperature. Proliferation of *Candida albicans* can be reduced by cooling the solution to 4°C.[36,37] Thus, the National Coordinating Committee on Large Volume Parenterals (NCCLVP) recommends that admixed solutions be refrigerated immediately if not to be administered soon after admixing, and that they be used within 24 hours of final admixture.[38] Albumin as an additive to PN solutions increases the potential for fungal and bacterial growth.[39] Intravenous fat emulsions are also supportive of substantial microbial growth of certain bacteria and fungi under the right conditions, especially for example, when allowed to have expiration times longer than 12 hours.[40,41]

Aseptic handling during all phases of compounding and administration is a prerequisite for assuring that the patient receives an uncontaminated PN solution. Solutions should be prepared in the aseptic environment provided by a properly maintained laminar flow hood. The hood should be situated such that the contaminant potential of normal work traffic and air currents is minimized. Personnel must be adequately trained and must practice strict aseptic technique. Supervision by a hospital pharmacist experienced in handling solutions and additives and familiar with stability, compatibility, and storage considerations is also necessary. Pharmacy-based admixture programs following specific guidelines developed to assure proper handling of PN solutions can greatly lessen the potential risk of sepsis associated with solution contamination in parenteral nutrition.[35,42–44]

### *Stability and Compatibility*

As a result of their complex compositions, PN solutions are prone to problems with stability and compatibility. Reports of such compatibility interactions (most often formation of a precipitate) and stability problems abound in the literature. Several reference books and comprehensive reviews exist, as well as numerous tables and charts, all of which can be quite confusing. Often, the exact answer to a compatibility question is not readily available, and one must resolve the situation on the basis of some objective data but largely practical judgment and experience. It may be necessary to review the primary literature in specific circumstances to determine the appropriate application of study results.[45,46]

Admixed dextrose/CAA solutions are referred to as base solutions. Without further additives, they are generally accepted as stable for 2 weeks under refrigeration, although recent data are suggestive of stability of base solutions plus electrolytes for up to 30 days under refrigeration.[47] If used according to NCCLVP guidelines, final admixed PN solutions containing the usual nutrient additives are generally stable after compounding for at least 24 hours (if stored under refrigeration and protected from freezing and strong light).[21,38] Vitamins that are known to be less stable may require special consideration. Certain vitamins may be adversely affected by changes in pH, presence of other additives, and storage factors of time, temperature, and light exposure.[21,48] Specific reports in the literature address variable but significant loss of vitamin A resulting from adsorption to the plastics in intravenous administration sets or to polyvinyl chloride intravenous bags. In patients with severe vitamin A deficiency, oral or intramuscular dosing should be considered where feasible.[21,45] Thiamine may be subject to degradation in solutions containing bisulfite. Patients predisposed to thiamine deficiency should be monitored carefully and should receive appropriate supplementation if necessary.[21,45]

Electrolytes and trace elements in their usual salt forms and amounts are generally compatible in PN solutions with the exception of sodium bicarbonate. Because of its basic pH, it *may* form carbon dioxide gas or insoluble calcium or magnesium carbonates upon addition to the acidic PN solution. It may also have adverse effects on the stability of certain vitamins in the PN solution. For these reasons, bicarbonate precursor salts such as acetate or lactate, which are bioavailable as well as compatible, are preferred for PN admixture.[21,45,49,50]

Compatibility of calcium and phosphorus in PN solutions has been a concern, especially in solutions for neonatal use where complex factors interact to create a high likelihood of incompatibility. Factors that enhance the risk of precipitate formation include higher molar concentrations necessary for appropriate supplementation, alkalinity of solutions, additives, or piggybacked medications, decreased amino acid concentration, increased environmental temperature, improper mixing sequence, long standing time or slow infusion rates, and use of chloride as the calcium salt.[45] Once a precipitate forms, the solution is no longer suitable for patient use and must be discarded. Reports and guidelines relating to this problem are available in the literature in common use in hospital pharmacy practice.[46,50–55]

### *Medication Admixture*

Although addition of medications to PN solutions is generally discouraged because of potential instability, questions of therapeutic efficacy, risk of contamination, and increased potential for wastage with changes in dose, certain medications are often added or considered for addition to PN solutions. Insulin, albumin, and heparin are often used in PN solutions and are considered to be compatible. Conflicting reports exist, however, regarding the availability of insulin because of variable adsorption to glass or plastic containers and tubing; there is great controversy surrounding the indications and logistics of albumin administered via PN solution, and debate exists concerning appropriate amounts of heparin to add to PN regimens. Numerous other medications are variably compatible or incompatible for admixture or administration with PN solutions. The reader is urged to consult appropriate references and literature for information specific to each situation.[21,45,46,50,51,56]

### *Total Nutrient Admixtures*

Numerous recent reports attest to the growing use of a new method, the total nutrient admixture (TNA), for delivering PN.[57–62] In this system, all standard components of the PN solution (dextrose, crystalline amino acids, electrolytes, vitamins, and trace elements) are combined *along with* the fat emulsion in one large container usually of 3-L capacity. Thus, the total parenteral nutrient supply for a 24-hour period can be admixed at one time and hung for administration once daily. This confers potential advantages in terms of reduced inventory, savings in personnel time for compounding and administration, and decreased need for multiple manipulations of the central line (thus reducing the risk of sepsis), and it may preclude the need for a peripheral catheter solely to administer intravenous fat emulsion.[59] TNAs also require less training time and offer the potential for improved compliance in home patients.[60]

In addition, TNAs appear to be well tolerated and clinically safe and effective when properly managed,[63] and to allow for delivery of a mixed-fuel substrate load. This may reduce PN-induced hepatic fat accumulation and the exacerbation of respiratory pathology sometimes aggravated by metabolism of large dextrose loads.[57,59,62]

Disadvantages and controversies regarding use of the TNA system include the issues of wastage with changes in daily formulation, enhanced microbial growth potential with extended hanging time (although TNAs appear to be of intermediate risk in microbial growth potential when compared with standard dextrose/CAA solutions alone versus fat emulsion, which poses the highest risk).[64–66] Constraints on ability to filter the formulation, accuracy of delivery with certain pump systems, inability to visually detect particulate matter in the opaque admixture,[58] and questions of stability of the fat emulsion–containing admixture when using varying concentrations of drugs, nutrients, or other additives are also yet to be resolved.[57,61,67–69] In light, however, of the significant potential advantages of the TNA system it is probable that its use will increase, although further study and clinical experience are necessary to better address these partially defined issues to utilize this system safely and effectively.[70]

## Ordering the Parenteral Nutrition Solution

Because of the relative complexity of the PN regimen, many institutions have elected to simplify the ordering process by development and implementation of order forms specifically for parenteral nutrition. In an attempt to foster completeness, to improve "prescription" communication, and often to standardize PN prescription where feasible, these forms are designed to meet the unique needs of the practitioners and patient population of the institution. The format may be simple and specify only the PN solution itself, or it may be comprehensive and offer the options of ordering certain related procedures, laboratory monitoring, protocols for patient management, and even multidisciplinary services related to the patient's nutritional support.[21] Figure 109.1 is an example of an order form for adult parenteral nutrition.

Note that even preprinted forms and standardized ordering procedures must be used appropriately, especially with the current emphasis on cost containment in health care. Both over- and underutilization of established services and procedures for PN therapy should be discouraged where not indicated or of little potential benefit in assuring continued therapeutic and cost-effective patient care.[21]

## Implementation of Parenteral Nutrition

### *Route of Administration*

Parenteral nutrition may be administered via either central or peripheral vein. Each route has specific characteristics, indications, advantages, and potential disadvantages associated with its use; therefore, each is addressed individually.

Considerations that are important in determining the appropriate route of administration for the patient are listed in Table 109.7. Each issue must be evaluated in determining the best approach to parenteral nutrition for a given patient. A discussion follows.

#### Peripheral Vein

Peripheral vein parenteral nutrition involves administration of 2–3 L per day of a 5% to 10% dextrose plus 3% to 5% amino acid solution into any suitable peripheral vein. This is generally accompanied by intravenous fat emulsion which is necessary to provide the majority of calories in this regimen. It may also confer some protective dilutional effect on the infusion that may lessen the chance of phlebitis. (The phlebitis/lipid issue, however, remains unresolved at present.) When accompanied by intravenous fat emulsion, it is referred to as the "lipid" system and generally provides around 2,000 kcal and 60–90 g protein per day. Electrolytes, vitamins, and trace elements are added to the solution and adjusted according to the needs of the patient.

A variation of this peripheral regimen may employ amino acids only. This is known as "protein-sparing" therapy, and its use is based on the finding that appropriate amounts of such a solution are effective in decreasing a negative nitrogen balance by reducing the metabolic requirement for gluconeogenesis in a starving patient.[71] This approach was used more commonly some years ago prior to the "reintroduction" of safer intravenous fat emulsions now available in the United States.

Advantages of using any form of peripheral PN generally center around the lesser risks of the peripheral mode of access when compared with the technical hazards and metabolic problems associated with a central line utilizing hypertonic dextrose.[72,73]

Disadvantages of peripheral PN are more significant in that the prerequisite suitable peripheral veins may not be available, especially in patients with an illness of long duration who have already been subjected to multiple venous accesses for administration of fluids and medications. Complicating this situation is the reality that peripheral veins are susceptible to phlebitis at osmolarities greater than 600 mOsm/L (easily possible with many peripheral regimens), and thus may be viable only for 1 to 2 weeks, even accounting for the questionable (as yet unresolved)[74] protective effects of concurrently administered intravenous fat emulsion.[75] (Other efforts to minimize the incidence of phlebitis include addition of subtherapeutic doses of heparin and hydrocortisone to the infusion.[71,72,75]) Large volumes of fluid are necessary to meet full nutritional requirements by this route, and such fluid loads are often contraindicated in many patients. In addition, use of lipid (intravenous fat emulsion) to provide calories increases the complexity of care by adding a second bottle and intravenous set that must be piggybacked into the main PN line. Finally, overall costs of the peripheral system may approach that of the central PN system owing to the necessity of using fat emulsion, though this will vary with the institution.[73]

In summary, peripheral parenteral nutrition is a relatively safe and simple method of nutritional support, and is valuable primarily in patients who do not have large nutritional needs, who can tolerate moderately large fluid loads, and in whom the necessity of such therapy is only of temporary duration (less than 2 weeks).[71,72,75]

MEDICAL UNIVERSITY OF SOUTH CAROLINA
ADULT PARENTERAL NUTRITION ORDERS

ADDRESSOGRAPH

PLEASE NOTE:
1) All orders must be in the pharmacy by 1:00 P.M.
2) Hyperalimentation orders must be written daily.
3) Use continuous bottle numbering.
4) Use Regular Physician's order sheet to continue current hyperalimentation, to change rate, or to discontinue bottles.
5) All hyperalimentation content changes will require a new Parenteral Nutrition Order Form.

I. STANDARD FORMULAS: Final Concentrations (per liter)**

| ☐ Central Formula I | | ☐ Central Formula II | | ☐ Peripheral Formula | |
|---|---|---|---|---|---|
| Dextrose | 25% | Dextrose | 20% | Dextrose | 5% |
| Amino acids | 4.25% | Amino acids | 7% | Amino acids | 4.25% |
| Nonprotein calories | 850 | Nonprotein calories | 680 | Nonprotein calories | 170 |
| Total calories | 1020 | Total calories | 960 | Total calories | 340 |
| Grams protein | 42.5 | Grams protein | 70 | Grams protein | 42.5 |
| Approx volume | 1,000 mL | Approx volume | 1,000 mL | Approx volume | 1,000 mL |

**All Standard Formulas contain the following added electrolytes per liter: Na 40 mEq, K 40.5 mEq, Acetate 40.6 mEq, Cl 33.5 mEq, Phos 11.22 mMol, Ca 5 mEq, Mg 8 mEq. (Amino Acid stock solution contains 8.7mEq Acetate and 4.0mEq Chloride per 1%).

Rate____mL/h Bottle No.____,____,____(24-h supply)

II. MODIFIED FORMULA: 1,000 mL

☐ *Dextrose ____ %
Amino acids ____ %
Sodium ____ mEq/L
Potassium ____ mEq/L
Magnesium ____ mEq/L
Calcium ____ mEq/L
Phosphorus ____ mmol/L

ACETATE/CHLORIDE
Acetate and chloride will be added to balance cations ($Na^+$ $K^+$) ordered.
If desired, indicate preference below (check one) OR (specify amount)
____Maximum acetate ____mEq acetate
____Maximum chloride ____mEq chloride

*Maximum dextrose concentration for peripheral administration is 10%

Rate____mL/h Bottle No.____,____,____(24 hr supply)

III. DAILY VITAMIN AND TRACE ELEMENT SUPPLEMENTS

____MVI–12 (10 mL/d)
____Vitamin K (1 mg/d)
____Standard trace elements: (per day)

Zn 3 mg Mn 0.3 mg
Cu 1.2 mg Cr 12 μg

Other (specify additive, per liter or per day)
Additional zinc____ mg per____
Vitamin C ____ g per ____

IV. OTHER ADDITIVES (per liter)

____Regular insulin____units
____Heparain*____units
____Other (specify)

*Heparin is no longer routinely added. Must be specifically ordered.

V. IV FAT EMULSION

____mL 10% (1.1 kcal/mL)
____mL 20% (2 kcal/mL)

Available as:
100, 250, 500 mL
250, 500 mL

Note: Fat emulsions may also be ordered separately on Regular Physician's order sheet.

Rate____mL/h Infusion time:____hrs

VI. HYPERALIMENTATION ACCESS: Must be noted
____Peripheral
____Center

VII. SPECIAL INSTRUCTIONS

| Physician's Signature | Date | Time |
|---|---|---|
| CS NO 410153 (4/87) | | |

**Figure 109.1** Adult parenteral nutrition order form.

**Table 109.7** Selecting the Route of Administration for Parenteral Nutrition

| | *Characteristics* | |
|---|---|---|
| *Considerations* | **Peripheral** | **Central** |
| Goal of nutrition therapy<br>Total versus supplemental | Supplemental or total if moderate or low needs | May achieve total needs |
| Nutritional requirements | Low or moderate | High or large |
| Viability of peripheral vein | Good | Poor or NA |
| Length of therapy | Short-term (<2 wk) | Long term |
| Fluid tolerance | Must be high | Can be fluid restricted |
| Risk of central line | NA | Greater risk |
| Cost | Varies | Varies |

Data from Reference 76.

### Central Vein

Central parenteral nutrition utilizes hypertonic dextrose and amino acid solutions along with electrolytes, vitamins, trace elements, and fat emulsion to provide 2,000–4,000 kcal/d. Because of the hypertonicity of such PN solutions (often in excess of 2,000 mOsm/L), they must be administered through a large central vein having a high blood flow to ensure rapid dilution and thereby avoid the phlebitis and thrombosis that would occur using a smaller (peripheral) vein.[13,76,77] Access is most commonly through percutaneous insertion of a catheter into the subclavian vein, then advancement of the catheter to the superior vena cava. If, for anatomic reasons, this approach is not possible, the internal jugular vein may also be used. X-ray verification of correct placement is necessary prior to infusion of the PN solution. Catheterization may be accomplished either in the operating suite or in the patient's hospital room, and complications are few, assuming that strict adherence to established procedures is enforced.[77]

Numerous catheters are commercially available for different purposes. They vary in terms of composition, lumen size, number of injection ports, and other special features. With recent advances in catheter technology (double- and triple-lumen catheters in addition to standard single-lumen designs such as the Hickman and Broviac catheters), much greater flexibility is possible in intravenous administration of nutritional solutions, medications, and blood products and in serum sampling for monitoring purposes.[77–79]

Central hyperalimentation provides for more options in designing the regimen, as there are fewer constraints regarding allowed concentrations of solutions for infusion. As an example, dextrose concentrations *may* range from 10% to 50%; however, most central PN regimens employ dextrose in the range 15% to 35%. Amino acid concentrations also vary, but most regimens commonly fall between 3% and 7% CAA. Either 10% or 20% fat emulsion may be used with central PN on a daily basis to provide a certain portion of the caloric load, or intermittently to prevent essential fatty acid deficiency.[25] Use of the large central vein in most instances permits infusion of a sufficiently concentrated dextrose/CAA solution plus additives to meet full nutritional requirements without the necessity of daily fat emulsion to make up for caloric deficit.[80,81]

With the ability to concentrate the PN solution and thereby provide high levels of nutrients in a smaller volume of fluid, central PN is useful in patients who must be fluid restricted (as in renal failure), those who have large nutritional requirements (metabolic stress/hypermetabolism resulting from trauma, surgery, infection, malignancy, or chemotherapy), and those for whom intravenous nutritional support is indicated for prolonged periods (greater than 7–10 days). The central route of administration is also employed in patients sent home with parenteral nutritional support.[76,77,81]

Relative disadvantages of central vein parenteral nutrition center mainly around the risks associated with insertion, use, and maintenance of the central line access for administration of solutions. There is greater potential for infection, more serious catheter-induced trauma and related sequelae, metabolic aberrations, and other technical or mechanical problems than with peripheral administration.[77,80,81] Complications are reviewed later.

## Administration/Management

Infusion of PN regimens, both peripheral and central, is accomplished using an intravenous pump set to a specific rate of flow expressed in milliliters per hour. The pump is necessary to ensure proper metered delivery of nutrients and to prevent excessive delivery of highly concentrated dextrose and electrolyte solutions that could precipitate metabolic disturbances. The solution is infused using special tubing for intravenous administration that leads from the bottle or bag of solution directly to the catheter. PN solution administration includes final in-line filtration at a point prior to the solution's entrance into the catheter. This is done to remove particulate matter, air, and microorganisms that may be present from prior manipulation of solutions, containers, and intravenous lines. Fat emulsions may not be filtered, as the fat particles would clog filters of conventional (bacteria eliminating) 0.22-$\mu$m pore size; therefore, in the standard PN setup, any fat emulsion must be added through a separate intravenous line piggybacked into the main intravenous line at a site beyond the location of the in-line filter as it approaches the catheter.[82]

The primary concern with initiation and advancement of

**Table 109.8** Infusion Guidelines for Parenteral Nutrition[a]

| | *Initiation* | *Discontinuation* |
|---|---|---|
| Peripheral PN | May begin at maximum desired rate | May discontinue without tapering |
| Central PN | Begin slowly; increase rate over 48–72 h to maximum desired rate | Gradually taper rate over 24 h, or may rapidly taper by decreasing rate to 40 mL/h for 2–4 h, then discontinue |
| IV fat emulsions (peripheral or central) | Test dose: infuse at 1 mL/min for 30 min; if no adverse effects, advance to desired rate<br>Maximum rate<br>10% 125 mL/h<br>20% 60 mL/h | May discontinue without tapering |

[a] Intermittent or cyclic PN may be infused over 10–18 h/d with initiation and discontinuation over 1–2 h of infusion at one half the desired final rate.

Data from Reference 76.

PN infusions is to avoid metabolic imbalances (fluid and electrolyte disturbance, acid–base aberrations) and adverse reactions. With hypertonic dextrose solutions (central vein PN), the standard of practice is to begin at a low rate of infusion and work up gradually to the final desired rate to avoid hyperglycemia. Conversely, the rate is lowered in a stepwise fashion upon discontinuation to avoid hypoglycemic reactions. This is of much less concern with peripheral administration of low concentrations of dextrose, and does not apply to intravenous fat emulsions. It is important that these *general* rules be followed to provide for safe delivery of PN by either route.[76,77,82] Basic infusion guidelines are specific to each route and are summarized in Table 109.8. General guidelines for intravenous administration of fat emulsion are also listed.

## *Monitoring*

Thorough and consistent monitoring of the patient receiving parenteral nutrition is necessary to ensure that goals for nutritional therapy are met and to prevent the occurrence of adverse effects or complications. Routine evaluation should include attention to nutritional and metabolic effects of the PN regimen as well as an awareness of the sequence of development for potential complications. As nutritional requirements are estimated for a patient upon initiation of nutritional support, it is important to routinely assess and document progress on a particular regimen, with adjustments made as necessary.

Monitoring should include accurate serial recording of vital signs, weight, serum levels of electrolytes, nutritional parameters, liver function tests, hematologic indices, nutritional intake, and losses. Not all serum parameters are drawn every day. Table 109.9 outlines the monitoring parameters important for patients receiving parenteral nutrition, along with the suggested frequency of collection. Appropriate assessment and evaluation of patient data can identify impending complications, such that further development and sequelae might be avoided, and are critical to the success of the nutritional therapy.[76]

## *Complications*

Parenteral nutrition therapy can be safe and effective in maintaining or restoring nutritional status in patients who are unable to meet their nutritional needs by enteral means; however, it is complex in nature and its use carries the risk of numerous complications, some of which are potentially life-threatening. Complications may be divided into four categories: mechanical or technical, infectious, metabolic, and nutritional. Awareness of their potential for development as well as timely recognition of warning signs can help to ensure a successful course of nutritional therapy.[80]

Mechanical or technical complications include malfunctions in the system for intravenous delivery of the solution. This includes pump failure, problems with lines and tubing, administration sets, and the catheter itself. Of particular concern are catheter-related complications as they often have serious implications for the immediate well-being of the patient. Pneumothorax, catheter misdirection (into the wrong vein or ill-positioned within the cardiac chambers), arterial puncture, bleeding, and hematoma formation may all occur during surgical placement of the catheter, although their incidence is reportedly rare when performed by experienced operators.[77] Many of these same complications, along with venous thrombosis and air embolism, may be seen postinsertion as well. Catheters occasionally occlude or break during use. If these problems cannot be easily rectified, the catheter may need to be removed and surgically reinserted.[78,83,84]

Infectious complications can be a major hazard in patients receiving parenteral nutrition through a central catheter. Often, these patients are predisposed to infection as a result of concomitant infections already present in the urinary tract, wounds, or lungs, frequent use of broad-spectrum antibiotic therapy, and malnutrition.[82] Infection *may* develop secondary to solution contamination; however, strict adherence to modern protocols for preparation of large-volume parenterals has minimized this occurrence. More common is catheter sepsis, which may occur in several ways, for example, through multiple manipulations of the intravenous PN line (as for administration of other infusions

**Table 109.9** Routine Monitoring Data for Parenteral Nutrition

| *Every day* | *2–3 times/week* | *Every week* |
|---|---|---|
| Weight | Complete blood count | Nitrogen balance |
| Vital signs (temperature, pulse, respirations) | Clotting studies (PT/PTT,[a] platelets) | Total protein |
| Fluid | Creatinine | Albumin |
| Nutritional intake (kCal), protein, fat | Calcium | Transferrin |
| Electrolytes, vitamins | Phosphorus | Prealbumin |
| Trace elements | Magnesium | Liver function tests |
| Serum electrolytes | | Alkaline phosphatase |
| Sodium | | SGOT[b] |
| Potassium | | SGPT[c] |
| Chloride | | LDH[d] |
| Bicarbonate | | Bilirubin |
| Glucose | | Other tests as warranted |
| BUN | | |
| Urine glucose, acetone (every 6 h) | | |
| Output | | |
| Urine | | |
| Gastrointestinal | | |
| Other losses | | |

[a] PT, prothrombin time; PTT, partial thromboplastin time.
[b] Serum glutamic–oxalacetic transaminase.
[c] Serum glutamic–pyruvic transaminase.
[d] Lactate dehydrogenase.

via that line), failure of bacterial filters, and through contamination during catheter placement and subsequent routine maintenance procedures.[82–84]

Catheter sepsis involves a septic episode (e.g., fever, shaking chills, glucose intolerance) in which no other site of infection can be identified, the fever resolves when the catheter is removed, and cultures of blood and catheter tip produce the same organism. If catheter sepsis is suspected, the PN solution is generally discontinued until culture results are obtained and a diagnosis is made. If the catheter is implicated, the central line may be removed; however, if the fever resolves of its own accord, the PN infusion may be resumed. Frequently, no specific definitive cause for an episode of catheter sepsis can be identified; however, as many PN patients have multiple complicating factors or concurrent conditions, this comes as no great surprise.[80,82,84]

In addition to proper techniques of solution preparation, proper care of the catheter and site of insertion, as well as maintenance of the central line for PN *only*, greatly minimize the incidence of catheter sepsis.[80,82]

Metabolic complications associated with PN therapy are numerous and, if left untreated, potentially serious. Common metabolic abnormalities related to substrate intolerance and fluid, electrolyte, and acid–base disturbances are presented in Tables 109.10 and 109.11. Predisposing factors and general strategies for intervention are also included.[76]

Hepatic dysfunction, as detected by elevations in serum liver function parameters, is well documented in the literature. It may take several forms, most commonly fatty liver, cholelithiasis and cholestasis.[85,86] Over the usual duration of PN therapy these complications are generally reversible by manipulations in substrate intake; however, there is concern for the development of progressive liver injury in patients who may require lifelong total parenteral nutrition therapy.[87]

Detailed discussions of etiology, mechanisms, and implications regarding individual metabolic abnormalities are available in standard references and in the literature.[76,82,88–92]

Nutritional complications of parenteral nutrition therapy generally develop over a prolonged course of therapy (weeks to months) as a result of inappropriate intake of a particular nutrient. Certain conditions, such as stress in a previously malnourished patient, may elicit symptoms of deficiency much earlier if a nutrient is not appropriately provided. For this reason, at least maintenance doses (as currently defined) of vitamins,[32] trace elements,[33] and essential fatty acids[30,31] should be provided to all patients receiving parenteral nutrition.

Trace element deficiencies, although rare, do occur. Chromium deficiency presents as a diabetes-like syndrome, while copper deficiency may appear as a hypochromic, normocytic anemia with neutropenia. More common is development of zinc deficiency in both children and adults on long-term PN.

**Table 109.10** Substrate Intolerance in Parenteral Nutrition

| *Complication* | *Possible causes* | *Intervention* |
|---|---|---|
| Hyperglycemia | Stress, infection, corticosteroids, pancreatitis, diabetes mellitus, peritoneal dialysis, excessive dextrose administration | Decrease dextrose load by decreasing infusion rate or dextrose concentration (may substitute fat calories); administer insulin |
| Hypoglycemia (rare) | Abrupt withdrawal of dextrose, insulin overdose | Increase dextrose intake; decrease exogenous insulin |
| Excess of carbon dioxide production | Excess dextrose intake | Decrease dextrose intake; balance calories from fat and dextrose |
| Hyperlipidemia (elevated cholesterol and triglyceride) | Stress, familial hyperlipidemia, pancreatitis | Decrease intake of fat or discontinue if indicated |
| Serum amino acid imbalance | Stress, hepatic failure | Modify amino acid intake if possible or decrease intake of amino acids |
| Abnormal liver function tests (elevated SGOT, alkaline phosphatase, and bilirubin) | Stress, infection, cancer, excess carbohydrate intake, excess caloric intake, essential fatty acid deficiency | Decrease dextrose load (substitute fat); decrease total calories; provide essential fatty acids |

[a] Serum glutamic–oxalacetic transaminase.

Adapted from Cerra FB: Pocket Manual of Surgical Nutrition. St. Louis, C. V. Mosby, 1984, p 158, with permission.

This is usually found in patients with high ostomy losses or severe or chronic diarrhea. It may be suspected in the presence of such signs as hair loss, periorbital seborrheic dermatitis, dysgeusia, and sometimes ileus.[89,91]

Essential fatty acid deficiency likewise may occur in PN patients, especially after weeks to months of fat-free PN. Symptoms include malabsorption and diarrhea resulting from changes in intestinal mucosa, dryness of the skin, hair loss, brittle nails, impaired wound healing, and increased susceptibility to infection.[30,31]

Occasionally, patients may develop nutrient-induced toxic effects, most commonly as a result of accumulation of fat-soluble vitamins or trace elements. This accumulation may be caused by either excessive intake or decreased

**Table 109.11** Fluid, Electrolyte, and Acid–Base Abnormalities

| *Problem* | *Possible causes* | *Intervention* |
|---|---|---|
| Hypovolemia | Gastrointestinal fluid losses, osmotic diuresis | Increase fluid intake |
| Hypervolemia | Renal failure, excess influid intake | Decrease fluid intake and diuretics |
| Hyponatremia | Gastrointestinal losses, fluid overload, diuretics | Varies with cause |
| Hypernatremia | Dehydration | Increase fluid intake |
| Hypokalemia | Gastrointestinal losses, diuretics, anabolism | Increase potassium intake |
| Hyperkalemia | Renal failure | Decrease potassium intake |
| Hypophosphatemia | Phosphate-binding antacids, anabolism, phosphate-free dialysate | Discontinue phosphate binders; increase phosphorus intake |
| Hyperphosphatemia | Renal failure | Decrease phosphorus intake |
| Hypomagnesemia | Diarrhea, malabsorption, anabolism | Increase magnesium intake |
| Hypermagnesemia | Renal failure | Decrease magnesium intake |
| Hypocalcemia | Hypoalbuminemia, chronic renal failure | Increase calcium intake (with chronic renal failure only) |
| Hypercalcemia | Rare | Decrease calcium intake |
| Metabolic acidosis | Diarrhea, high-output fistulae, renal failure, excess amino acid intake | Treat underlying causes; increase acetate and decrease Cl in TPN solution; decrease amino acid intake |
| Metabolic alkalosis | Gastric losses | Treat underlying cause; increase Cl and decrease acetate in TPN solution |

Adapted from Cerra FB: Pocket Manual of Surgical Nutrition. St. Louis, C. V. Mosby, 1984, p 161, with permission.

excretion. Certain disease states, for example renal failure, may necessitate reduction in trace element intake.[76,91]

Patients receiving parenteral nutrition should be monitored closely by clinical observation and serum levels, if indicated, to detect developing symptoms of deficiency or excess of nutrients, and appropriate supplementation or reduction in dose should be effected.

## Home Parenteral Nutrition

Widespread acceptance and successful utilization of techniques for provision of full nutritional requirements parenterally have allowed a population of patients with permanent nutritional disability to be maintained indefinitely on intravenous nutrition. As the delivery of PN has become increasingly sophisticated in recent years, and greater emphasis is being placed on cost considerations, programs have been developed for nutritional support in the home setting. Numerous programs are now available to support patients with various long-term or permanent conditions outside the traditional health care settings. Home health care programs involving parenteral nutrition services may be coordinated and administered through a hospital, by a commercially run corporation, or through a joint venture relationship between the two.[92–95]

Many factors are considered in selecting candidates for home PN therapy. Significant benefit must be expected from placing a patient into the program. Additionally, the patient and family must be willing to assume certain responsibility, successfully undergo training, and be capable of managing the daily routine in the home setting. Other logistics such as funding, procurement of solutions and supplies, and clinical management and follow-up must be evaluated, resolved, and implemented for each patient for a program to be successful.[93,95,96]

Patients with a variety of conditions may be considered for home parenteral nutrition (HPN). Examples of indications for HPN include severe short-bowel syndrome, severe Crohn's disease, chronic radiation enteritis, extensive intestinal obstruction, enterocutaneous fistulae, and certain malignancies.[92,95–98]

HPN is provided by "permanent" venous access through a central vein catheter. Solutions may be provided largely premixed from the hospital or commercial vendor (but requiring addition of vitamins prior to administration), or the patient and family may be trained to mix solutions in the home setting. The solution is generally administered at night by infusion pump using a cycle of 10 to 18 hours. This allows for time away from the pump during the day to allow the patient and family some semblance of a normal daily routine. Clinical management and follow-up are done periodically according to the needs of the patient and the services of the program, and involve a coordinated effort among physician, pharmacist, nurse, social worker, patient (family), and suppliers.[92,93,96–98]

HPN programs are a further advance in the science of nutritional support. They are able to provide the patient the potential for an ambulatory lifestyle while maintaining an intravenous feeding regimen previously only available in the hospital setting at substantial cost. With appropriate training, patients are able to maintain adequate nutrition in the home, utilizing self-care and assistance from family members, but with qualified medical and administrative personnel providing monitoring, periodic reevaluation, adjustment of the formula, and provision of supplies. The availability of such options benefits the patient medically, financially, and psychologically, and continued growth of home health care programs is expected in this era of concern over ever-rising hospital costs.[93,96]

## Summary

Over the past 20 years parenteral nutrition has become an integral component of the array of options for managing the patient unable to maintain adequate nutritional intake via the gastrointestinal tract. Parenteral nutrition is not without risks. Specific precautions must be taken and protocols must be followed in the administration and monitoring of PN, all of which are crucial to achieving successful nutritional therapy and preventing unnecessary complications or harm to the patient. Pharmacists have been involved in the provision of parenteral nutrition at many levels since its development. Their contribution is expected to continue as techniques are further refined and the field of nutritional support grows through knowledge and experience toward even greater sophistication.

Two recently published bibliographies may serve useful in locating further detailed information regarding special aspects of parenteral nutrition.[99,100]

## References

1. Butterworth Jr CE. The skeleton in the hospital closet. Nutr Today 1974;9:4–8.
2. Dudrick SJ, Ruberg RL. Principles and practice of parenteral nutrition. Gastroenterology 1971;61:901–910.
3. Law DK, Dudrick SJ, Abdou NI. Immunocompetence of patients with protein-calorie malnutrition—The effects of nutritional repletion. Ann Intern Med 1973;79:545–550.
4. Mullen JL, Gertner MH, Buzby GP, et al. Implications of malnutrition in the surgical patient. Arch Surg 1979;114: 121–125.
5. Weinsier RL, Hunker EM, Krumdiek CL, et al. A prospective evaluation of general medical patients during the course of hospitalization. Am J Clin Nutr 1979;32:418–426.
6. Buzby GP, Mullen JL, Matthews DC, et al. Prognostic nutritional index in gastrointestinal surgery. Am J Surg 1980;139: 160–167.
7. Mullen JL, Buzby GP, Matthews DC, et al. Reduction of operative morbidity and mortality by combined preoperative and postoperative nutritional support. Ann Surg 1980;192: 604–613.

8. Starker PM, LaSala PA, Askanazi J, et al. The influence of preoperative total parenteral nutrition upon morbidity and mortality. Surg Gynecol Obstet 1986;162:569–574.
9. Dudrick SJ, Wilmore DW, Vars HM, et al. Long-term total parenteral nutrition with growth, development and positive nitrogen balance. Surgery 1968;64:134–142.
10. Sanderson I, Basi SS, Deitel M. History of nutrition in surgery, in Deitel M (ed): Nutrition in Clinical Surgery, 2nd ed. Baltimore, Williams and Wilkins, 1985, pp 3–13.
11. Dudrick SJ, Rhoads JE. Total intravenous feeding. Sci Am 1972;226:73–80.
12. Law DH. Total parenteral nutrition. N Engl J Med 1977;297: 1104–1107.
13. Shils ME. Guidelines for total parenteral nutrition. JAMA 1972;220:1721–1729.
14. Zlotkin SH, Stallings VA, Pencharz PB. Total parenteral nutrition in children. Pediatr Clin North Am 1985;32:381–401.
15. Goodgame Jr T. Critical assessment of the indications for total parenteral nutrition. Surg Gynecol Obstet 1980;151:433–441.
16. American Society for Parenteral and Enteral Nutrition, Board of Directors. Guidelines for use of total parenteral nutrition in the hospitalized adult patient. J Parenter Enter Nutr 1986;10: 441–445.
17. Health and Public Policy Committee, American College of Physicians. Perioperative parenteral nutrition. Ann Intern Med 1987;107:252–253.
18. Detsky AS, Baker JP, O'Rourke K, et al. Perioperative parenteral nutrition: A meta analysis. Ann Intern Med 1987;107: 195–203.
19. Kerner Jr JA. Indications for parenteral nutrition in children, in Kerner Jr JA (ed): Manual of Pediatric Parenteral Nutrition. New York, John Wiley, 1983, pp 3–18.
20. Phillips GD, Odgers CL. Parenteral nutrition: Current status and concepts. Drugs 1982;23:276–323.
21. Louie N, Niemiec PW. Parenteral nutrition solutions, in Rombeau JL, Caldwell MD (eds): Parenteral Nutrition. Philadelphia, W. B. Saunders, 1986, pp 272–305.
22. Freeman JB, Fairfull-Smith R, Rodman GH, et al. Safety and efficacy of a new peripheral intravenously administered amino acid solution containing glycerol and electrolytes. Surg Gynecol Obstet 1983;156:625–631.
23. Tao RC, Kelley RE, Yoshimura NN, et al. Glycerol: Its metabolism and use as an intravenous energy source. J Parenter Enter Nutr 1983;7:479–488.
24. Wretlind A. Evaluation of carbohydrates in parenteral nutrition. Nutr Metab 1975;18:(suppl 1):242–255.
25. Pelham LD. Rational use of intravenous fat emulsions. Am J Hosp Pharm 1981;38:198–208.
26. Kastrup EK, Olin BR (eds): Facts and Comparisons. Philadelphia, J. B. Lippincott, 1987.
27. Hansen LM, Hardie WR, Hidalgo J. Fat emulsion for intravenous administration: Clinical experience with intralipid 10%. Ann Surg 1976;184:80–88.
28. Silberman H, Freehauf M, Fong G. Parenteral nutrition with lipids. JAMA 1977;238:1380–1382.
29. Wretlind A. Parenteral nutrition. Surg Clin North Am 1978;58:1055–1070.
30. Reilla MC, Broviac JW, Wells M, et al. Essential fatty acid deficiency in human adults during total parenteral nutrition. Ann Intern Med 1975;83:786–789.
31. Faulkner WJ, Flint LM. Essential fatty acid deficiency associated with total parenteral nutrition. Surg Gynecol Obstet 1977;144:665–667.
32. American Medical Association, Department of Foods and Nutrition. Multivitamin preparations for parenteral use—A statement by the Nutrition Advisory Group. J Parenter Enter Nutr 1979;3:253–262.
33. American Medical Association, Department of Foods and Nutrition. Guidelines for essential trace element preparations for parenteral use—A statement by the Nutrition Advisory Group. J Parenter Enter Nutr 1979;3:263–267.
34. Baumgartner TG (ed): Clinical Guide to Parenteral Micronutrition, 1st ed. Melrose Park, IL, Educational Publishers, 1984.
35. Goldmann DA, Maki DG. Infection control in total parenteral nutrition. JAMA 1973;223:1360–1364.
36. Goldmann DA, Martin WR, Worthington JW. Growth of bacteria and fungi in total parenteral nutrition solutions. Am J Surg 1973;126:314–318.
37. Wilkinson WR, Flores LL, Pagones JN. Growth of microorganisms in parenteral nutritional fluids. Drug Intell Clin Pharm 1973;7:226–231.
38. National Coordinating Committee on Large Volume Parenterals. Recommendations to pharmacists for solving problems with large-volume parenterals. Am J Hosp Pharm 1976;33: 231–236.
39. Mirtallo JM, Caryer K, Schneider PJ, et al. Growth of bacteria and fungi in parenteral nutrition solutions containing albumin. Am J Hosp Pharm 1981;38:1907–1910.
40. Keammerer D, Marshall CG, Hall GO, et al. Microbial growth patterns in intravenous fat emulsions. Am J Hosp Pharm 1983:40;1650–1653.
41. Crocker KS, Noga R, Filibeck DJ, et al. Microbial growth comparisons of five commercial parenteral lipid emulsions. J Parenter Enter Nutr 1984;8:391–395.
42. National Coordinating Committee on Large Volume Parenterals. Recommended methods for compounding intravenous admixtures in hospitals. Am J Hosp Pharm 1975;32:261–270.
43. Stolar MH. Assuring the quality of intravenous admixture programs. Am J Hosp Pharm 1979;36:605–608.
44. National Coordinating Committee on Large Volume Parenterals. Recommended guidelines for quality assurance in hospital centralized intravenous admixture services. Am J Hosp Pharm 1980;37:645–655, 660–663, 663–667.
45. Niemiec Jr PW, Vanderveen TW. Compatibility considerations in parenteral nutrient solutions. Am J Hosp Pharm 1984;41:893–911.
46. Bergman HD. Incompatibilities in large volume parenterals. Drug Intell Clin Pharm 1977;11:345–360.
47. Parr MD, Bertch KE, Rapp RP. Amino acid stability in total parenteral nutrient solutions. Am J Hosp Pharm 1985;42: 2688–2691.
48. Das Gupta V, Allwood MC, Louie N. Stability of vitamins in total parenteral nutrition. Am J Hosp Pharm 1986;43:2132, 2138, 2143.
49. Henann NE, Jacks Jr TT. Compatibility and availability of sodium bicarbonate in total parenteral nutrient solutions. Am J Hosp Pharm 1985;42:2718–2720.
50. Trissel LA. Handbook of Injectable Drugs, 4th ed. Washington, DC, American Society of Hospital Pharmacists, 1986.
51. King J. Guide to Parenteral Admixtures. St. Louis, KabiVitrum, 1986.
52. Eggert LD, Rusho WJ, MacKay MW, et al. Calcium and phosphorus compatibility in parenteral nutrition solutions for neonates. Am J Hosp Pharm 1982;39:49–53.
53. Poole RL, Rupp CA, Kerner JA. Calcium and phosphorus in neonatal parenteral nutrition solutions. J Parenter Enter Nutr 1983;7:358–360.
54. Fitzgerald KA, MacKay MW. Calcium and phosphate solubility in neonatal parenteral nutrient solutions containing TrophAmine. Am J Hosp Pharm 1986;43:88–93.

55. Fitzgerald KA, MacKay MW. Calcium and phosphate solubility in neonatal parenteral nutrient solutions containing Aminosyn PF. Am J Hosp Pharm 1987;44:1396–1400.
56. Newton DW. Physicochemical determinants of incompatibility and instability in injectable drug solutions and admixtures. Am J Hosp Pharm 1978;35:1213–1222.
57. Ang SC, Canham JE, Daly JM. Parenteral infusion with an admixture of amino acids, dextrose and fat emulsion solution: Compatibility and clinical safety. J Parenter Enter Nutr 1987;11:23–27.
58. Brown R, Quercia RA, Sigman R. Total nutrient admixture: A review. J Parenter Enter Nutr 1986;10:650–658.
59. Driscoll DF, Baptista RJ, Bistrian BR, et al. Practical considerations regarding the use of total nutrient admixtures. Am J Hosp Pharm 1986;43:416–419.
60. Epps DR, Knutsen CV, Kaminski Jr MV, et al. Clinical results with total nutrient admixture for intravenous infusion. Clin Pharm 1983;2:268–270.
61. Knutsen CV, Epps DR, McCormick DS, et al. Total nutrient admixture guidelines. Drug Intell Clin Pharm 1984;18:253–254.
62. O'Keefe SJD, Bean E, Symmonds K, et al. Clinical evaluation of a "3-in-1" intravenous nutrient solution. S Afr Med J 1985;68:82–86.
63. Gilbert M, Gallagher SC, Eads M, et al. Microbial growth patterns in a total parenteral nutrition formulation containing lipid emulsion. J Parenter Enter Nutr 1986;10:494–497.
64. D'Angio R, Quercia RA, Treiber NK, et al. The growth of microorganisms in total parenteral nutrition admixtures. J Parenter Enter Nutr 1987;11:394–397.
65. Mershon J, Nogami W, Williams JM, et al. Bacterial/fungal growth in a combined parenteral nutrition solution. J Parenter Enter Nutr 1986;10:498–502.
66. Scheckelhoff DJ, Mirtallo JM, Ayers LW, et al. Growth of bacteria and fungi in total nutrient admixtures. Am J Hosp Pharm 1986;43:73–77.
67. Parry VA, Harrie KR, McIntosh-Lowe NL. Effect of various nutrient ratios on the emulsion stability of total nutrient admixtures. Am J Hosp Pharm 1986;43:3017–3022.
68. Sayeed FA, Johnson HW, Sukumaran KB, et al. Stability of Liposyn II fat emulsion in total nutrient admixtures. Am J Hosp Pharm 1986;43:1230–1235.
69. Baptista RJ, Lawrence RW. Compatibility of total nutrient admixtures and secondary antibiotic infusions. Am J Hosp Pharm 1985;42:362–363.
70. Dolin BJ, Davis PD, Holland TA, et al. Contamination rates of 3-in-1 total parenteral nutrition in a clinical setting. J Parenter Enter Nutr 1987;11:403–405.
71. Fong WL, Grimley GW. Peripheral intravenous infusion of amino acids. Am J Hosp Pharm 1981;38:652–659.
72. Fairfull-Smith RJ, Freeman JB. Peripheral parenteral nutrition, in Deitel M (ed): Nutrition in Clinical Surgery, 2nd ed. Baltimore, Williams and Wilkins, 1985, pp 200–205.
73. Watters JM, Freeman JB. Parenteral nutrition by peripheral vein. Surg Clin North Am 1981;61:593–604.
74. Daly JM, Masser E, Hansen L, et al. Peripheral vein infusion of dextrose/amino acid solutions +/− 20% fat emulsion. J Parenter Enter Nutr 1985;296–299.
75. Chipponi JX, Blier JC, Rudman D. Current status of peripheral alimentation. Ann Intern Med 1981;95:114–115.
76. Cerra FB. Pocket Manual of Surgical Nutrition. St. Louis, C. V. Mosby, 1984.
77. Steiger E, Grundfest-Broniatowski S, Misny TJ. Intravenous hyperalimentation: Temporary and permanent vascular access and administration, in Deitel M (ed): Nutrition in Clinical Surgery, 2nd ed. Baltimore, Williams and Wilkins, 1985, pp 88–104.
78. Crocker KS, Pine RW, Steffee WP. The triple lumen central venous catheter. Nutr Clin Pract 1986;1:90–96.
79. Kaufman JL, Rodriquez JL, McFadden JA, et al. Clinical experience with the multiple lumen central venous catheter. J Parenter Enter Nutr 1986;10:487–489.
80. Teasley KM, Shronts EP, Lysne J, et al. Nutritional/metabolic support: Parenteral and enteral, in Higby DJ (ed): Supportive Care in Cancer Therapy. Boston, Martinus Nijhoff, 1983, pp 93–123.
81. Fischer JE, Freund HR. Central hyperalimentation, in Fischer JE (ed): Surgical Nutrition. Boston, Little Brown, 1983, pp 663–702.
82. Grant JP. Handbook of Total Parenteral Nutrition. Philadelphia, W. B. Saunders, 1980.
83. Benotti PN, Bistrian BR. Practical aspects and complications of total parenteral nutrition. Crit Care Clin 1987;3:115–131.
84. Pessa ME, Howard RJ. Complications of Hickman–Broviac catheters. Surg Gynecol Obstet 1985;161:257–260.
85. Sheldon GF, Petersen SR, Sanders S. Hepatic dysfunction during hyperalimentation Arch Surg 1978;113:504–508.
86. Pitt HA, King W, Mann LL, et al. Increased risk of cholelithiasis with prolonged total parenteral nutrition. Am J Surg 1983;145:106–112.
87. Baker AL, Rosenberg IH. Hepatic complications of total parenteral nutrition. Am J Med 1987;82:489–497.
88. Ang SD, Daly JM. Potential complications and monitoring of patients receiving total parenteral nutrition, in Rombeau JL, Caldwell MD (eds): Parenteral Nutrition. Philadelphia, W. B. Saunders, 1986, pp 331–343.
89. Wolk R. Metabolic complications and deficiencies of parenteral nutrition. Compr Ther 1985;11:67–75.
90. Giner M, Curtas S. Adverse metabolic consequences of nutritional support: Macronutrients. Surg Clin North Am 1986;66: 1025–1047.
91. Husami T, Abumrad NN. Adverse metabolic consequences of nutritional support: Micronutrients. Surg Clin North Am 1986;66:1049–1069.
92. Steiger E, Srp F, Helbley MI, et al. Home parenteral nutrition, in Rombeau JL, Caldwell MD (eds): Parenteral Nutrition. Philadelphia, W. B. Saunders, 1986, pp 654–679.
93. Gaffron RE, Fleming CR, Berkner S, et al. Organization and operation of a home parenteral nutrition program with emphasis on the pharmacist's role. Mayo Clin Proc 1980;55:94–98.
94. Scheckelhoff DJ, Mirtallo JM. Hospital-based home health care. US Pharm 1985;10:H4-H20.
95. American Society for Parenteral and Enteral Nutrition, Board of Directors. Guidelines for use of home total parenteral nutrition. J Parenter Enter Nutr 1987;11:342–344.
96. Dudrick SJ, O'Donnell JJ, Englert DM, et al. 100 Patient-years of ambulatory total parenteral nutrition. Ann Surg 1984;199:770–781.
97. Fleming CR, Beart RW, Berkner S, et al. Home parenteral nutrition for management of the severely malnourished adult patient. Gastroenterology 1980;79:11–18.
98. Wolfe, BM, Beer WH, Hayashi JT, et al. Experience with home parenteral nutrition. Am J Surg 1983;146:7–14.
99. Mirtallo JM. A key to the literature of total parenteral nutrition. Drug Intell Clin Pharm 1983;17:189–200.
100. Mirtallo JM, Oh T. A key to the literature of total parenteral nutrition: Update 1987. Drug Intell Clin Pharm 1987;21: 594–606.

# Chapter 110 / Enteral Nutrition

Mary Lou Ebbert-Sauer, PharmD

Enteral nutrition support is defined as provision of food or nutrients via the gastrointestinal tract. In its broadest sense, the term includes normal eating; however, it is often distinguished from normal eating by the special formulas, delivery techniques, and equipment available to administer the nourishment. Patients with abnormal esophageal or stomach peristalsis, altered anatomy secondary to surgery, depressed consciousness, or impaired digestive capacity all may benefit by receiving their nutrients by methods discussed in this chapter.

In this chapter the principles and practices related to the successful use of enteral nutrition support are described. Included herein are evidence to support the use of the enteral feeding route whenever possible, a description of the various access routes, characteristics of commercially available products, and information regarding modular compounding. In addition, drug/product compatibilities are discussed as are complications that can be anticipated and their treatment.

## Importance of Supplying Nutrients Enterally

The gastrointestinal tract is the body's primary organ of nutrient absorption and digestion. Small intestinal villi are structural units that increase the surface area through which such nutrients enter the bloodstream. They also contain enzymes to metabolize various food components. Therefore, maintenance of their functional capacity is vital to health preservation. Studies in rats support this concept. One investigator[1] showed that feeding rats a known nutrient composition orally as opposed to intravenously yielded a higher intestinal mass. The higher mass correlated with more mucosal protein and enzymatic activity, indicative of a higher functional level. A second researcher[2] noted that something in addition to good nutritional intake was necessary to prevent intestinal wasting. He reported that oral food intake was needed in conjunction with intravenous feeding; his data revealed that intravenous nutrition support alone resulted in hypotrophic intestinal tissues.

Human evidence is not as convincing, possibly because most studies in humans have been conducted in cancer patients. Such patients may have altered intestinal function that is not correctable by nutritional intervention as a result of their disease state. Consequently, several authors[3] have concluded that parenteral nutrition is actually preferable for cancer patients. It appears to yield a more positive nitrogen balance and better weight gain. In addition, parenteral nutrition may be better tolerated, allowing for a more consistent nutrient intake. Cancer patients often suffer from nausea, vomiting, and malabsorption, all of which limit oral intake. Further study in a different patient population is warranted.

The site of nutrient introduction to the gastrointestinal tract as well as nutrient complexity may also affect intestinal response to the food. Research in this area, again, has been done with rats. The study designs are quite elegant, however, and may provide the groundwork for future investigation in humans. For instance, Young and co-workers[4] fed four different diets to rats via the gastric or oral route. In every case, animals fed orally gained more weight. They also found that diets containing simplified (i.e., partially digested) nutrients produced less weight gain. These and other data support several hypotheses of intestinal and body mass preservation, including the following: (1) Dietary fiber has some growth-stimulating effect and may stimulate release of growth-promoting factors. (2) Defined formula diets either lack a growth-stimulating factor or may contain a growth-inhibiting factor. (3) The location of nutrient delivery into the gastrointestinal tract may stimulate different responses for growth. The work of Levine et al[1] and Young et al[4] raises the possibility of varied response to nutrition support depending on content and route of delivery. The impact of such variability on human outcome has not yet been determined.

The intestine is an organ of protein synthesis as well as one of digestion and absorption. It therefore utilizes nutritional substrates directly. Glucose, glutamine, and L-leucine are examples of fuels used more efficiently when given via the enteral route as opposed to parenterally.[5,6] L-Leucine yields greater protein synthesis when given orally and is incorporated into the intestinal structure differently depending on the route of ingestion. Serum glutamine levels fall during stress, while intestinal uptake rises.[7] Glutamine and ketones are absent from parenteral solutions and may account for some of the intestinal structural deterioration seen with parenteral nutrition.

Hormones also help maintain structural integrity in the stomach and small intestine. Gastrin is a hormone released during eating that causes hyperplasia evident primarily in the stomach and less so in the duodenum and ileum. Its influence is virtually void in the remaining intestine.[8] Pentagastrin, a synthetic gastrin analog, actually prevents the characteristic atrophy seen in starved animals receiving total parenteral nutrition (TPN) when administered exogenously.[9] Cholecystokinin is another hormone resembling gastrin. It has been found to prevent pancreatic atrophy in animals,[10] but its role in maintaining intestinal structure is not as clear as gastrin's.[11] All of these hormones are found in humans, but have not been studied as intensively in humans as they have been in animal models.

One last significant reason for maintaining the functionality of the gastrointestinal tract is for the immunologic function it serves. Hydrochloric acid secreted by the stomach kills a majority of the bacteria ingested with food. Specific immunoglobulins are then secreted by intact intestinal tissues to kill any remaining organisms and neutralize any toxins they may produce.

Two studies[12,13] in rats illustrate statistically higher survival in postoperative and malnourished animals fed enterally versus parenterally when each group was challenged with an infectious insult. Such results could be explained by the fact that substances involved in fighting infections are produced in the gastrointestinal tract. One study[14] shows that depressed production of these substances can occur even after only 3 days, putting a body at increased risk for infectious morbidity. A second study[15] documents that animals being fed via the gastrointestinal tract produce more immunoglobulins than those fed intravenously. Therefore, it appears that enteral feeding better prepares a body to combat infectious insults.

Even though the preceding studies were not performed in humans, the results generated deserve consideration when providing nutritional support to humans until studies in humans are performed. Preservation of intestinal mass, functionality, and immunologic capabilities is a worthwhile goal. Therefore, it is reasonable to feed patients enterally whenever clinical circumstances allow.

## Administration Routes and Techniques

As mentioned in the introduction, enteral nutrition support is distinguished in part from normal eating by the routes of nutrient intake and the equipment needed to administer it. As the conditions necessitating specialized nutrition support are varied, multiple options are available to provide the therapy. All routes involve placement of a tube through which a liquid formula is infused. As the site of nutrient delivery moves further away from the mouth, the tube insertion becomes more difficult and invasive but, at the same time, more permanent. The available routes for nutrient delivery have been delineated in Table 110.1.

The most frequently used enteral feeding routes are those accessed by inserting a tube through the nose and threading it into the stomach or upper small bowel. The names of these routes are nasogastric (NG), nasoduodenal (ND), and nasojejunal (NJ), indicating both the tube insertion point and the termination point. They do not require surgical intervention and, therefore, are the least invasive of all. They are also temporary, as the tubes are held in place, at most, by a piece of tape on the nose. They can easily be pulled out during routine patient care.

The NG route may employ a large-bore rubber tube. In contrast, the ND and NJ routes always use small-bore, very flexible tubes. These tubes are very lightweight and are very comfortable for the patient. Their weighted ends help facilitate successful tube passage through the pylorus and into the small intestine after entering the stomach. Often, the passage is achieved as stomach peristalsis moves the tube. If peristalsis alone does not achieve the desired placement, metoclopromide may help. Its use, however, is most successful when given prior to tube insertion.[16] Alternatively, it may be necessary to physically move the tube through the pylorus with an endoscope under fluoroscopic guidance.[17] Lastly, some physicians[18] have increased the chance of successful small-bowel intubation by carefully positioning the patient after tube insertion to maximize peristaltic tube propulsion.

Dobbie and Hoffmeister[19] were the first to describe feeding through a flexible, weighted tube. Prior to their report, all enteral feedings were infused through heavy, rigid rubber tubes, causing loss of lower esophageal sphincter tone, otitis media, esophagitis, esophageal perforations, and mucosal injury.[20] Modern tubes patterned after Dr. Dobbie's prototype are fashioned from pliable silicone rubber, polyvinyl, or polyurethane substances and have tungsten- or mercury-weighted tips mentioned above (see Fig. 110.1). Even though these newer products are safer, they are not without problems. Their small lumen size makes them particularly susceptible to clogging when medications are given through them. When used with an infusion device, they are more prone to rupture. They can also be dislodged by vomiting, coughing, or inadvertent tugging. Easy dislodgement necessitating tube replacement is time consuming and expensive. Several methods of tube anchoring have been described to help decrease this problem.[21,22] A problem not reported with the older, more rigid tubes is that of inadvertent bronchial intubation,[23] especially when tube placement is not radiographically verified. This complication is most important in the patient who has an impaired cough reflex, or depressed mental status and is intubated. The less rigid, more modern tubes occasionally do not stimulate the gag or cough reflex to indicate tube misplacement. This can lead to formula infusion into the lungs and development of a pneumothorax or pleural effusion.

More invasive, yet more permanent enteral feeding accesses include esophagostomy or pharyngostomy, gastrostomy, and jejunostomy placement. Esophagostomy, pharyngostomy, and gastrostomy are similar in several ways.[20] First, they all require surgery but can be created while employing either local or general anesthesia. This is beneficial, as the population requiring long-term enteral nutrition support is usually debilitated by age, disease, or both. Therefore, general anesthesia can be risky. Second, the tubing used tends to be of larger bore than that used for the nasal routes. This allows for noncontinuous or bolus nutrient administration. Bolus feedings are given by infusion of 200 mL or more of formula over a few minutes several times a day. They are often tolerated well, as these routes deliver food to the stomach and do not require the use of an infusion pump, as do continuous feedings. Large-bore tubes also become clogged less often than small-bore ones. Lastly, after the entry point to the body is well granulated and healed, the tubes can be changed as necessary without employing another surgical procedure.

Pharyngostomies and esophagostomies are indicated in patients with head and neck malignancies or maxillofacial anomalies; both are contraindicated in patients with distal alimentary tract obstructions or perforations. Complications of these routes, though infrequent, include recurrent laryngeal nerve damage, aspiration, and infection. Gastrostomies are used for patients with esophageal obstruction or impaired swallowing. Gastrostomy placement in the past was a significant surgical procedure requiring general anesthesia. Currently, methods are becoming popular that can be per-

**Table 110.1** Enteral Nutrition Routes

| *Route* | *Surgery required* | *Permanent* | *Advantages* | *Disadvantages* |
|---|---|---|---|---|
| Oral (PO) | No | — | Ad libitum consumption<br>Physiologic | Cannot ensure adequate intake<br>Requires cooperative, alert patient |
| Nasogastric (NG) | No | No | Can be used for patients in whom eating is not desirable | Aspiration risk<br>Use of large-bore tubes causes nasopharyngeal irritation and/or ulceration<br>Tubes easily malpositioned |
| Esophagostomy | Yes | Yes | Does not require laparotomy<br>Tube can be replaced easily as needed<br>Patient may feed without loosening clothing<br>Large-tube lumen permits use of blenderized diets | Cannot be hidden by clothes<br>Uncomfortable<br>Aspiration risk |
| Nasoduodenal (ND) or nasojejunal (NJ) | No | No | Small, pliable tubing relatively comfortable<br>Decreased aspiration risk | Transpyloric passage difficult<br>Tubes easily clogged<br>Tubes easily malpositioned<br>Often requires flow controller to increase tolerance |
| Gastrostomy | Yes[a] | Yes | Conducive to bolus feeding<br>Offers access for passage of duodenal or jejunal tubes endoscopically<br>May be placed endoscopically<br>Concealed by clothing | Aspiration risk<br>Possible peritonitis<br>Leakage of gastric contents<br>Cellulitis |
| Jejunostomy | Yes | Yes | Low aspiration risk<br>Early postoperative feeding | Requires meticulous infusion rate control<br>Easily clogged<br>Easily dislodged<br>Fistula formation<br>Intestinal obstruction<br>Requires laparotomy |

[a] Gastrostomy tubes may be inserted surgically with general anesthesia or with endoscopic guidance under local anesthesia.

formed safely and cost-effectively using local anesthesia. The primary procedure is called a percutaneous endoscopic gastrostomy. If necessary, a gastrostomy may be modified to a jejunostomy by endoscopic passage of a nasoenteric tube through the gastrostomy and then the pylorus. Complications of either placement include aspiration, peritonitis, leaking, infection, and fistula development.[24,25] Jejunostomies require a laparotomy for placement, and are used instead of gastrostomies in cases of stomach or duodenal obstruction, or in the same instances as a gastrostomy. Many times jejunostomies are placed during a surgical procedure when the small bowel is readily accessible. This is because early postoperative feeding can be initiated soon after surgery. Small-bowel function is least affected by

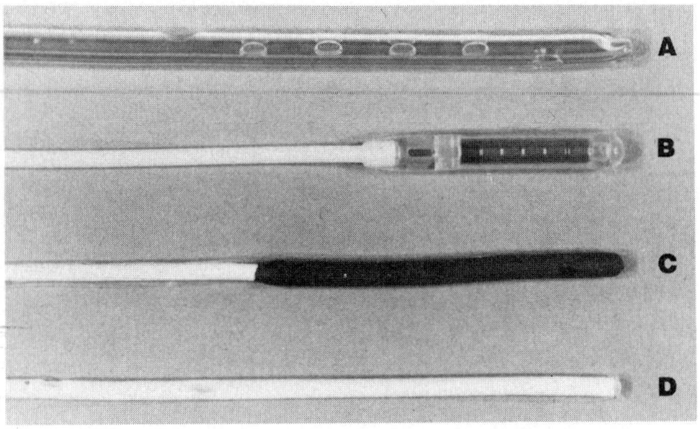


**Figure 110.1** Examples of feeding tubes. (A) Levine tube (multiple manufacturers; large rigid), (B) Dobbhoff tube (Biosearch), (C) Flexiflo tube (Ross Laboratories), (D) Keofeed tube (IVAC).

surgical manipulation, whereas stomach atony and large-bowel ileus may persist for long periods of time. Additionally, the risk of aspiration is substantially reduced, as the feeding solutions are not often regurgitated. Jejunostomy complications include infection, hemorrhage, and intraperitoneal feeding infusion in addition to the disadvantages listed in Table 110.1.

## Bolus Feeding

As defined before, bolus feeding is the administration of 200 mL or more over a few minutes; it is used primarily for esophagostomy, pharyngostomy, or gastrostomy patients. Note that such large volumes as these should be instilled only into patients who have intact stomachs. The stomach then regulates the flow of food into the small intestine which is sensitive to both high volume and osmolality. Bolus feedings have the advantage of requiring little administration time and minimal equipment. Many times, only a syringe is needed to instill the feedings into the appropriate tube. Alternatively, they can be infused via a complete infusion system consisting of an infusion bottle, tubing, and possibly a feeding pump. Unfortunately, bolus feedings may not be tolerated well and may result in cramping, nausea, vomiting, aspiration, and diarrhea.

## Intermittent Feeding

This method can be used for any enteral route and is similar to bolus feeding, except that the infusion time is increased to 20 to 30 minutes.[26] The administration system includes a feeding reservoir (bottle or bag) attached to an extension set that may or may not connect to a pump infusion set. All of this is attached to the patient's enteral access tube. Intermittent infusion may be better tolerated than bolus administration, but often produces the same complications. It does, however, give the patient more freedom to be mobile than continuous administration.

## Continuous Feeding

This method is self-explanatory. It utilizes the same infusion system as intermittent feeding to administer food over 18 to 24 hours a day. The 18-hour infusion interval is sometimes preferred in patients at risk of aspiration, because feeding can be stopped for a few hours at night when aspiration is most likely to occur. Even though continuous infusion consumes much nursing time, it does provide maximal tolerance by minimizing bloating and diarrhea, thereby facilitating optimal nutrient infusion. Continuous feeding is almost always necessary for jejunostomy, nasoduodenal, or nasojejunal routes or in critically ill patients.

## Initiation of Enteral Feedings

Protocols for initiating enteral feeding regimens vary between institutions and prescribers. Generally, most recommendations suggest starting with a half-strength dilution of the chosen feeding solution or formula to infuse at 30–50 mL/h, regardless of the actual route or formula employed. This practice is used to prevent possible well-known gastrointestinal complications of enteral feeds. With tolerance, the rate is increased every 6 to 24 hours until the desired maximal rate is achieved. Next, the formula concentration is advanced until either full-strength concentrations or the appropriate caloric intake is achieved. Many authors advocate pump-assisted rate control, as roller clamps used to manually adjust the rate are known to be inaccurate and some patients may be acutely sensitive to even small volume variances.[26] In small-bowel feedings, a small infusion volume is important regardless of the osmolality. Slow, continuous, pump-assisted infusion is always strongly recommended.[27] Gastric instillation, though, may not require such meticulous titration, as long as gastric motility and the pyloric sphincter are intact. Recall that the stomach is the natural nutrient reservoir that controls the volume and osmolality reaching the small intestine, thus preventing the dumping syndrome. The dumping syndrome occurs when a large quantity of a hyperosmolar solution is introduced too rapidly into the small bowel. Clinically, the syndrome manifests as nausea, cramping, lightheadedness, and diarrhea—all of which may be associated with enteral nutrition support.

## Feeding Equipment

Little information is available to aid in choosing an enteral feeding infusion system for institutional use.[28] Feeding containers, administration tubing, and pumps must all be evaluated carefully. Feeding containers should be at least leakproof, unbreakable, and easy to clean; they should be equipped with a reliable closure and have easy-to-read volume markings. Freezable containers might be desirable if a hospital prepares large batches of solutions and freezes them until they are needed. The containers' adaptability to multiple infusion sets, volume capacity, and distinguishability from an intravenous container may also be examined.

**Table 110.2** Enteral Nutrient Component Complexity

| *Nutrient* | *Intact entities* | *Partially digested* | *Simple* |
|---|---|---|---|
| Carbohydrate | Corn syrup solids<br>Cornstarch<br>Fruit, vegetable, cereal solids<br>Glucose polymers | Maltodextrins<br>Lactose<br>Sucrose<br>Oligosaccharides | Glucose<br>Galactose |
| Fat | Butterfat<br>Corn oil<br>Safflower oil | Medium-chain triglycerides<br>Diglycerides | Fatty acids |
| Protein | Milk<br>Eggs<br>Meat<br>Sodium caseinate<br>Calcium caseinate | Soy protein isolate<br>Dipeptides<br>Tripeptides<br>Oligopeptides<br>Lactalbumin | Amino acids |

Administration sets consist of the tubing that connects the feeding container with the feeding tube. These sets should not be easily mistaken for intravenous sets. They should be adaptable to many feeding containers and feeding tubes. In addition, they should be long enough to easily connect the feeding container and the patient. Lastly, the administration set should be equipped with an infusion control device that allows a reasonably accurate flow rate, thus often eliminating the need for an electronic feeding pump. ''Reasonably accurate'' has been defined as consistent delivery of within 20% of the expected volume per time period.[28]

Pharmacists are sometimes asked to assist in evaluating enteral feeding pumps because of their familiarity with intravenous infusion pumps. Many considerations are the same for both types of pumps. They should be lightweight, easy to operate, have a reasonably long battery life, and have few maintenance requirements. The pump should have a useful alarm system that indicates when the bottle is dry or the pressure in the set is rising. Rising pressure indicates set occlusion. Lastly, the pump should be easy to operate by hospital or nursing home personnel and patients alike.

At first glance, feeding tubes may appear to be very similar. Choice of features for the products may be more subtle than for pumps and feeding containers. Most of these tubes are very pliable, which increases patient comfort. Pliability, however, may make tube insertion difficult; so a wire stylet may be a useful feature. Extreme pliability also impairs aspiration of gastric contents through the tube. The tube should have markings to help in determining proper placement as well as be radioopaque to make radiographic confirmation possible. Weighted capsules on the tube ends should be narrow to facilitate movement through the nares and down the throat. Lastly, the feeding tube should be compatible with multiple enteral feeding administration sets, but incompatible with intravenous sets.

## Formula Selection

Enteral feeding product selection should involve the consideration of several aspects. First, a knowledge of the patient's medical history should be obtained, as small-bowel length and functional capacity help determine the appropriate formula complexity.

Viscosity is an important consideration when using small-bore feeding tubes. Thick formulas flow slowly through tiny passages and may impair the attainment of the proper infusion rate. Most commercially prepared products contain electrolytes, vitamins, and trace elements, making them nutritionally complete. Such a predetermined nutrient complement may not fit an individual's needs and require alteration. Caloric density should be part of the formula selection process, as more concentrated formulas require less volume to provide one's daily caloric requirement.

Protein, carbohydrate, and fat are all available as intact, partially digested, and simple entities; examples of nutrients from each category may be found in Table 110.2. Caloric contents are listed in Table 110.3.

Protein is possibly the most important nutrient, as it is the only source of nitrogen. Intact protein molecules such as meat, milk, eggs, and caseinates begin their digestion in the stomach when acted upon by hydrochloric acid and specific protein enzymes. Further breakdown occurs in the duodenum by pancreatic enzymes.[29] The resultant dipeptides, tripeptides, and oligopeptides are absorbed via specific carriers located in the small intestinal wall. These carriers do not depend upon sodium to function properly and have proven to be very efficient. Free amino acids, on the other hand, are absorbed via sodium-dependent mechanisms that appear to be slower and less efficient than peptide ones.[30] Therefore, partially digested protein entities are in general the most readily absorbable form of nitrogen substrate. Whenever a digestion or absorption deficiency is suspected, a partially digested protein source should be tried before simple amino acids. If intolerance is detected, then simple amino acids are an alternative. Protein molecule simplifica-

**Table 110.3** Caloric Content of Nutrients[a]

| | |
|---|---|
| Carbohydrates | 4 kcal/g |
| Fat | 9 kcal/g |
| Protein | 4 kcal/g |

[a] Electrolytes, trace elements, vitamins, and water do not contribute to caloric content.

tion increases the prevalence of amino acids containing free sulfur, which in turn imparts a bitter flavor and foul odor to feeding solutions, making them undesirable for oral consumption.[31] Simplified protein products are thus suited best for tube feedings.

Carbohydrate metabolism begins in the mouth, where starch is hydrolyzed to a small extent.[32] Further starch digestion occurs in the small intestine, where pancreatic enzymes function; however, the majority of disaccharide and oligosaccharide breakdown is performed by enzymes located in the intestinal brush border, before the carbohydrates are transported across the villous surface. Three major carbohydrate-specific, brush-border enzymes are maltase, sucrase, and lactase. Maltase and sucrase activity can be reduced by small intestinal resection or reduced dietary intake of maltose and sucrose. Fortunately, dietary challenge increases their activity.[33] Lactase activity, on the other hand, although in part determined by dietary concentration, is also determined by genetic influence. Specifically, black, Indian, Jewish, and Oriental populations have a high incidence of genetically determined lactase deficiency, making them intolerant to milk and other lactose-containing products. This is why most commercially available enteral formulas are lactose free.

Simple carbohydrate molecules such as glucose and galactose contribute significantly to osmolality. High osmolality is thought to be directly correlated to enteral feeding intolerance; therefore, partially digested entities should be the choice for inclusion in enteral formulas. Glucose polymers provide an especially useful carbohydrate source that is tolerated by most individuals. The polymers are large chains that provide a minimal osmotic load, yet are easily absorbed in the small intestine.[31] Hence, they can be used to provide large concentrations of calories for most patients. The one shortcoming of glucose polymers is that they are not as sweet as simple glucose, and may decrease the palatability of orally consumed products.

Fat is an important constituent in the diet and provides a concentrated calorie source, essential fatty acids for tissue integrity, and a carrier for fat-soluble vitamins. Its digestion and absorption are more complicated than those of either protein or carbohydrates. Long-chain triglycerides (LCTs) are the major fat source in standard enteral diets. Their digestion begins when stomach contractions begin to emulsify the fat. Emulsification increases the particle surface area so the pancreatic lipases can form monoglycerides or free fatty acids. Bile salts then work to form micelles, or water-soluble fat spheres that facilitate absorption. In the presence of any lipase deficiency or absorption defect such as pancreatic insufficiency, medium-chain triglycerides (MCTs) should be used as the major fat source. These are more easily digested and can be absorbed without bile salts, as they do not need to form micelles. MCT oil does not, however, provide the only known essential fatty acid, linoleic acid. Essential fatty acids should be provided in a dose of 1% to 3%[34] of the total caloric intake to prevent a deficiency.

Formula viscosity is an important consideration when administering nutrition through a tube. High-viscosity formulas are sometimes difficult to infuse through the narrow lumens of the small, pliable nasoenteric tubes of needle catheter jejunostomies. As a general rule, viscosity increases with caloric density, but no index exists for classifying formula thickness by a standardized number. Blenderized diets of intact foods tend to be very thick and, therefore, not useful for many access routes. One commercially available blenderized product has recently been modified to decrease its thickness, making it a candidate for administration through small-bore tubes.

A formula's electrolyte content may be a concern in the choice of an enteral diet. Electrolytes may contribute significantly to osmolality. Therefore, they may also contribute to the bloating and diarrhea commonly associated with intolerance; however, electrolyte quantities are fixed, and cannot be subtracted from. The electrolyte profiles contained in prepared formulas closely resemble the complement thought to be necessary for optimal nutrient utilization. Decrease in any ion, then, could result in decreased benefit from the enteral nutrition and therefore would not be desirable.

One fairly common electrolyte abnormality occurring with enteral nutrition is hyponatremia.[35] Most formulas are made to mimic a low-salt diet so hyponatremia could arise from such a limited sodium concentration. A low-salt intake appears reasonable, as many patients who receive enteral nutrition are elderly and may have compromised cardiac function.

Specialized products for renal and hepatic insufficiency do not contain adequate electrolyte profiles. Travasorb Renal, Amin-Aid, and Hepatic-Aid II are completely devoid of electrolytes, because requirements for renal and hepatic patients are not easily defined and also fluctuate with treatment.

Vitamins, zinc, iodine, iron, copper, and manganese are present in most formulas in maintenance doses. Amin-Aid and Hepatic-Aid have no vitamins. Travasorb Renal is devoid of fat-soluble vitamins (A,D,E,K) as well as vitamin $B_{12}$. Concentrations of selenium, chromium, and molybdenum are usually not available from product literature. Vitamin and trace element concentrations are calculated such that when caloric needs are met, so are the micronutrient requirements.

It is important to have a feel for the electrolyte, vitamin, and trace element composition of commercially available enteral feedings. Of course, the quantities administered per day can best be altered by compounding an individual formula from modular ingredients. Fortunately, most patients can be managed well with commercially marketed products.

Lastly, caloric density should be considered in product selection. It influences the volume of formula needed to meet daily nutritional requirements. Therefore, caloric density preference may be influenced by a patient's fluid needs and tolerance. Anywhere from 0.66 to 2.0 kcal may be provided per milliliter of enteral product. As caloric density increases, the free water content per volume decreases. Dilute formulas contain approximately 80% free water; more concentrated formulas contain only about 50%. Daily fluid requirements are actually water requirements. Therefore, water must be instilled through the enteral access device to prevent deficits that may be caused by high solute loads of concentrated formulas, thereby preventing dehydration and the hyperosmolar state. Dehydration may be clinically detected as thirst, dry mucous membranes, depressed skin turgor, or an increased serum BUN or sodium level.

All products containing protein, carbohydrate, fat, vitamins, electrolytes, and trace elements are considered to be nutritionally complete. As such, they are designed to maintain most patients for long periods of time without causing nutritional deficiencies. Some products, however, are referred to specifically as supplements. If used in addition to a meal and consumed orally as desired, an enteral product is termed a *supplement*.

Success of supplement use depends upon its appeal to the patient. Individual preference is particularly important; it is also highly variable and subjective. As such, it is impossible to predict a product's desirability as an enteral formulary item without detailed patient evaluation. One attempt has been made to more objectively determine a product's overall acceptance by the use of a wine-tasting scale composed of several product variables.[36] The variables include appearance, bouquet (aroma), body, sweetness, flavor, and aftertaste; the scale has been found to be useful. Remember that such a scale is not infallible and that true overall product success must also depend upon other parameters such as avoidance of bloating, diarrhea, or cramping with use.

Specific guidelines do not exist to help a clinician choose with certainty the perfect product for an individual. Most products contain a combination of intact and partially digested components, and will adequately support a majority of patients, including those receiving jejunostomy feedings. Simple nutrients should be reserved for those with diarrhea from malabsorption or short-bowel syndrome and patients who do not tolerate isosmolar products containing more intact nutrients. Remember that when nutrient components become simpler, osmolality rises and so does cost. Simple proteins are unpalatable to most individuals, whereas simple sugars are very sweet.

Infant formulas are significantly different from adult enteral nutrition products. Babies are sensitive to both deficiency and toxicity development because their body's compensatory mechanisms are immature. Therefore, infant products must be formulated according to strict guidelines, and tend to mimic human milk. Protein content of these products, however, is never exactly the same as human protein, because cow's milk contains a slight variation of the lactalbumin found in human milk. Most infant formulas are cow milk protein based.[37] Soy protein is used for infants who are lactose intolerant.[38,39] Soy-containing products must contain DL-methionine to meet the guidelines established by the Infant Formula Act which determined the necessary content of infant formulas.[40]

Lactose is the primary carbohydrate in formulas designed for normal infants,[37] as it is also the major carbohydrate in human milk. Lactase activity is usually functional at birth[41]; it develops during the last 8 weeks of gestation and may increase when lactose-containing nutrition is instituted. In infant formulas for lactose-intolerant babies, dextrose substitutes for a portion of the usual lactose content.

Infant formulas contain vegetable oils[38] as their fat source because babies do not absorb animal fat efficiently. The fat from cow's milk is especially difficult to absorb. Cholesterol is contained in these products, but to a lower extent than in human milk. Like their adult counterparts, infants have the capacity to synthesize endogenous cholesterol. MCT may be used for preterm infants to increase fat absorption, but must be supplemented with LCT to provide essential fatty acids. Improved fat absorption with MCT has also been shown to contribute to improved calcium and nitrogen balance.

Industry has supplied the medical community with multiple products specifically designed to compensate for many digestive, absorptive, and metabolic problems seen with some infants. A detailed description of these products is beyond the scope of this chapter.[42]

## Formulary Consideration

Product selection may be restricted in the institutional setting if a formulary is utilized. Formulary development is important to ensure that product duplication is avoided. A formulary should be developed allowing dietetic, pharmacy, and medical staff input with consideration being given to points outlined previously. In addition, such administrative concerns as cost, shelf life, ordering policies, and contract opportunities should be taken into account. Suggestions for formulary development have been described elsewhere.[43,44] Suggestions for formulary classification are listed in Table 110.4.

## The Modular Concept

Despite the array of ready-to-use enteral nutrition products, it is occasionally desirable or necessary to achieve a nutrient mix not supplied by any single available product. Single nutrient components such as carbohydrate, protein, and fat are marketed for the purpose of altering a readily available solution or preparing a new one conforming to different specifications. Such single nutrient admixture is known as modular compounding. Primary utilization of the modular concept occurs in institutions that feel that enteral nutrition deserves the same individualization as parenteral nutrition. Special care must be used in designing individual formulas to ensure that the minimum requirements for vitamins, trace elements, and electrolytes are met.

## Available Products

Protein modules are marketed in powder form and may contain free amino acids, caseinates, or whole proteins such as egg white solids or whey. The module chosen for inclusion in a compounded formula should be based upon the patient's digestive capacity. Palatability of the final formula is improved when intact proteins are used; simple amino acids impart a bitter taste that is difficult to mask; consequently, it is preferable to deliver the feeding via a tube when an amino acid protein source is indicated.[31] Protein modules may be singularly added to ready-made formulas where a higher nitrogen dose is desired.

Carbohydrate modules are marketed in multiple complexities, as are their protein counterparts. As with protein, the simpler the additive composition, the higher its contribution to the overall formula osmolality. Simpler components are also more sweet than more complex ones. Carbohydrate products are available in either solid or liquid forms and their

**Table 110.4** Suggested Enteral Formula Categories and Products[a]

| | |
|---|---|
| Blenderized diets | Compleat B, Compleat B Modified |
| Defined-formula diets | Criticare HN, Stresstein, Vital, Vivonex |
| High-calorie tube feedings (calorically dense) | Ensure Plus, Magnacal, Sustacal HC, TwoCal HN |
| High-calorie/high-nitrogen tube feedings | Ensure Plus HN, Isocal HCN, TwoCal HN |
| High-nitrogen tube feedings | Ensure HN, Osmolite HN, Travasorb HN, TwoCal HN |
| Isosmolar diets | Compleat B Modified, Isocal, Isotein HN, Osmolite |
| Lactose-free diets | All products except Meritene and Sustacal Powder |
| Modular additives | MCT oil, Polycose, RDP |
| Oral supplements | Ensure, Meritene, Sustacal |
| Special-use products (disease specific) | AminAid, HepaticAid II, Pulmocare, Travasorb Hepatic, Travasorb Renal |

[a] Only representative products and categories are listed, so the table may not include all products for each category. Not all categories are included in each formulary.

caloric content varies with the product. Therefore, each should be closely examined prior to use to ensure the appropriate caloric content of the final preparation.

Fat modules are available as liquids or solids of two types, either triglycerides with medium-chain fatty acids or triglycerides with long-chain fatty acids.[31] Long-chain triglycerides are preferred for most patients because they contain the essential fatty acid, linoleic acid. Medium-chain triglycerides (derived from coconut oil) are beneficial for patients who are intolerant of or unable to utilize LCT. MCT use, however, should be supplemented with LCT (10%–22% of the total fat) to provide sufficient linoleic acid. The caloric contents of fat additive products vary, so they should be examined to ensure adequate caloric content of the final formula.

Equipment requirements necessary to provide adequate modular compounding capabilities vary with the volume of workload. A suggested minimal equipment expenditure should include a top loading balance, a standard laboratory graduated cylinder, and a large-capacity commercial blender that is easy to clean and sanitize.[31] Refrigeration is necessary for solution storage after compounding and prior to administration. Because solution contamination is a large concern, all ingredient manipulation should be performed in a sanitary area designated for this purpose.

## Special Considerations

Because of the relatively limited modular product line, compounding an acceptable product could be difficult. For instance, protein products may contain a high concentration of electrolytes which is variable between the protein source and product. Proteins may be difficult to solubilize depending upon the final solution pH. Casein-based modules are more soluble than whey-based ones, but whey becomes more soluble when mixed at a concentration less than 12%. Whey is sensitive to pH ranges and is most soluble in the pH range 3.5–7.0. Casein, on the other hand, is more soluble at neutral pH.

Carbohydrates are sensitive to heat-induced reactions when mixed with amino acids. Therefore, it is best that compounded nutrient mixtures containing carbohydrates and proteins not be heated.

Fats may be difficult to mix with the other components because of their amicability with aqueous solutions, but commercially available fat modules contain emulsifiers to help alleviate this problem. Protein, as opposed to amino acids, stabilizes fat components better; so do complex carbohydrates as opposed to simple ones. In general, the lower the fat content, the more stable the solution.

Overall formula stability is influenced by final moisture content, temperature, and mixing procedure in addition to the concerns noted thus far.[31] Dry products are much more stable than liquid ones. This consideration is probably most important when purchasing the modules, especially if the use is low. Liquid formulations or reconstituted dry products should generally be used within 24 hours. Mixing should always be done with a commercial blender rather than with a utensil, such as a wire whisk. Blenders create a smaller fat particle size, increasing stability and homogeneity.

Modular formula preparation requires meticulous attention to detail, as omission or misdosing of a single nutrient component could cause deficiencies, side effects (i.e., from increased osmolality), or solution instability.

### *Noncommercial Enteral Nutrients*

In some cases, it may be advantageous to use blenderized foods to provide nutritional support in lieu of commercial preparations. The major advantage of this is cost control for patients at home. Disadvantages, however, are numerous, including the following: (1) There is no guarantee that adequate nutrients are being administered. (2) Blenderized foods are too viscous to flow through small-lumen feeding tubes. (3) Sanitized preparation areas may not be available. The cost eventually incurred from possible nutrient depletion, clogged tubes, and rehospitalization may far outweigh the cost of more convenient, prepared nutrients.

### *Miscellaneous Products/Additives*

A few products are marketed for direct admixture to enteral formulas that supply vitamins and minerals. One product in particular is the only vitamin module available (NutriSource vitamin, Sandoz). It is available as a powder packet and contains the RDA for vitamins. Such an addition should be necessary only when modular formulas are employed or when the disease-specific formulas, which are devoid of most vitamins (Amin-Aid, Hepatic-Aid II, Travasorb Renal), are used. Specific vitamin deficiencies may be supplemented with crushed tablets or intravenous preparations, as single-entity oral vitamin liquids are not always available. Four mineral modules are available to supply a fixed electrolyte and trace element profile. Again, these products would be for primary use with modular compounds. Aside from the specifically designed commercially available preparations, additions to enteral products should be made with caution to avoid incompatibilities or tube clogging.

### *Special Compounding and Contamination*

Institutions with large enteral feeding programs as well as those using standardized modular formulations may be interested in using bulk manufacturing techniques to simplify staffing and storage requirements. Alternatively, one author has described a method by which enteral additives are distributed in unit-dose packaging to ensure proper additive content.[45]

Formula manipulation dictates that care be taken to guarantee ingredient stability and integrity. Manipulation may be defined as combination of two or more components or dilution of a commercial product with water. Stability has been investigated in one enteral product's vitamin A, E, and $B_2$ (riboflavin) content after freezing and thawing. The authors concluded that vitamin stability was not affected by temperature changes; it also appeared that the storage container material did not influence the results.[46]

Bacterial contamination, however, has been studied in much greater detail. The gastrointestinal tract may serve as a port of entry of bacteria into the systemic circulation, especially in patients who are receiving multiple antibiotics or who have undergone a surgical procedure. Sterile or semisterile diets have been correlated to decreased infectious complications in immunocompromised patients.[47] Diarrhea can have a bacterial origin. In addition, formulas subjected to manipulation have been positively associated with increased bacterial concentration. Therefore, controlling bacteria populations found in enteral feedings could decrease tolerance problems and perhaps avoid serious infectious complications.

Current practices of mixing products in areas not maintained as "clean" work areas could significantly increase the risk of inoculating products that were sterile initially. Improperly cleaned blenders may also cause bacterial contamination. Once a pathogen has been introduced to a medium, such as feeding formulas, rapid population increases may occur. As much as a 1,000-fold increase over a 10-hour hang time has been reported. One study[48] revealed low contamination after 12 hours of hanging, yet "solid" bacterial growth could be noted after 24 hours. Therefore, it appears that hang times should be as short as possible, or less than 12 hours. No guidelines exist for safe bacterial levels in enteral feeding solutions; however, as diarrhea is a common problem with tube feedings and seriously ill patients are often managed with them, it seems prudent to keep bacterial contamination at a minimum.

## Medication Compatibility With Enteral Products

Surprisingly, the compatibility of medication with enteral feeding products has not been studied to a great extent. One group[49,50] has studied a total of seven commercially available, ready-to-use products with a variety of pharmaceuticals. As outlined in these publications, the recommended dose of a drug was mixed with various amounts of an enteral product, then examined for pH or viscosity changes as well as clumping. Failure of small-volume mixing led to large-volume testing, or trial of a solid dosage form. Table 110.5 which is extrapolated from both of these articles, lists the detected incompatibilities. Note that the drugs that required vigorous mixing have been classified in this table as "conditionally incompatible," as vigorous mixing or agitation cannot be guaranteed in the clinical setting. In its absence, feeding tube clogging from particulate matter could become a problem. Methods to avoid physical incompatibility problems between drugs and enteral products are available.[49,50] The most prudent recommendations include avoiding combination of these substances whenever possible, especially the nonaqueous preparations and syrups. Substitution of solid dosage forms or granules may prove to be a viable alternative when liquids form unacceptable mixtures. Powders and tablets should always be completely dispersed before administration so tube clogging is prevented.

Enteral nutrition products have been implicated in decreasing the pharmacologic effect of warfarin[51,52] and phenytoin.[53] Warfarin resistance has been contributed to the high vitamin K contents of some products in the past. Before October 1980, some products had particularly high vitamin K concentrations equaling as much as 1,330 $\mu$g per 1,000 kcal. The usual dietary intake of this vitamin has been estimated at 300–500 $\mu$g daily. In addition, the gastrointestinal flora synthesize vitamin K. Consequently, these products were reformulated to contain less than 200 $\mu$g of vitamin K per 1,000 kcal. Other enteral products contain between zero and 1,013 $\mu$g per 1,000 kcal. Warfarin resistance has continued to be reported[54] despite reductions in vitamin K content. Therefore, it should be kept in mind that physical interference can also decrease a drug's pharmaceutical efficacy.

Why tube feedings affect phenytoin is unclear, but subtherapeutic drug levels do result when phenytoin suspension is administered to a patient receiving continuous nasoenteric feeding. Failure to achieve therapeutic concentrations when phenytoin therapy is initiated and a decline in therapeutic phenytoin concentrations upon institution of tube feeding have been documented.[53] Perhaps the phenytoin is being adsorbed to the tube feeding components. A method proposed to decrease this interaction is to discontinue the tube feedings for 2 hours, administer the drug, flush the feeding tube, then restart the feeding infusion 2 hours later. Note, however, that such a regimen would result in significant reduction in tube feeding intake. It is an impractical alternative.

**Table 110.5** Drugs Found to Be Physically Incompatible With Enteral Nutrient Products[a]

| *Drug* | *Product tested* |
|---|---|
| **Absolutely Incompatible** | |
| Cibalith-S, 5 mL | E, EHN, EP, EPHN, O, OHN, V |
| Dimetane elixir, 10 mL | E, EHN, EP, EPHN, O, OHN, V |
| Dimetapp elixir, 10 mL | E, EHN, EP, EPHN, O, OHN, V |
| Feosol elixir, 5 mL | E, EHN, EP, EPHN, O, OHN, V |
| KC1 elixir, Barre 15 mL (10% and 20%) | E, EHN, EP, EPHN, O, OHN, V |
| Klorvess syrup, 15 mL | E, EHN, EP, EPHN, O, OHN, V |
| MCT oil, 10 mL | E, EHN, EP, EPHN, O, OHN, V |
| Mandelamine Suspension Forte, 10 mL | E, EHN, EP, EPHN, O, OHN, V |
| Mellaril Oral Solution, 5 mL | E, EHN, EP, EPHN, O, OHN, V |
| Neo-Calglucon syrup, 5 mL | E, EHN, EP, EPHN, O, OHN, V |
| Robitussin expectorant, 10 mL | E, EHN, EP, EPHN, O, OHN, V |
| Sudafed syrup, 10 mL | E, EHN, EP, EPHN, O, OHN, V |
| Thorazine concentrate, 1 mL | E, EHN, EP, EPHN, O, OHN, V |
| **Conditionally Incompatible** | |
| Achromycin syrup, 5 mL | EH, EPHN, OHN, V[b] |
| Decadron elixir, 5 mL | E, EHN, EP, EPHN, O, OHN, V[b] |
| Elixophyllin, 15 mL | E, EHN, EP, EPHN, O, OHN, V[b] |
| Furadantin suspension, 10 mL | E, EHN, EP, EPHN, O, OHN, V[b] |
| Haldol drops, 10 mL | E, EHN, EP, EPHN, O, OHN, V[b] |
| Isuprel elixir, 15 mL | E, EHN, EP, EPHN, O, OHN, V[b] |
| Keflex suspension, 5 mL | E, EHN, EP, EPHN, O, OHN, V[b] |
| Lomotil liquid, 5 mL | E, EHN, EP, EPHN, O, OHN, V[b] |
| Navane concentrate, 2 mL | E, EHN, EP, EPHN, O, OHN, V[b] |
| Slo-phyllin syrup, 15 mL | E, EHN, EPHN, OHN, V[b] |
| Sumycin syrup, 5 mL | E, EP, O[b] |
| Theolair liquid, 15 mL | E, EP, O[b] |
| Lanoxin elixir, 1 mL | E, EHN, EP, EPHN, O, OHN, V[b,c] |

[a] E, Ensure; EHN, Ensure High Nitrogen; EP, Ensure Plus; EPHN, Ensure Plus High Nitrogen; O, Osmolite; OHN, Osmolite High Nitrogen; V, Vital.
[b] Combine drugs slowly with vigorous mixing.
[c] Becomes rubbery after 24–48 hours.

## Tube Feeding Complications and Monitoring

Tube feeding complications may arise from the tube itself, the feeding formula, or bacterial contamination. In addition, there may be more than one complication. Those related to the tube itself include esophagitis, otitis media, esophageal erosion, esophageal perforation, and pneumothorax, and large tube size may cause esophageal irritation which may progress to ulceration and then perforation[21] as the tube rubs against the mucosal tissue. These problems can be avoided by inserting one of the more modern tubes mentioned before. These products are small and pliable. Therefore, they are less prone to cause mucosal damage. They are, however, more difficult to place properly, may be inserted into the lung instead of the stomach,[23] and can cause lung perforation or pneumothorax.[55] The small-lumen tubes may not trigger the gag reflex which indicates improper placement, so their position should always be verified with an x-ray to minimize the chance of infusion into the lung.

A second way for tube feeding liquids to enter the lung is by aspiration of gastric contents. Nasogastric tubes destroy the lower esophageal sphincter tone so that it does not close properly. This makes it relatively easy for the gastric contents to reflux up the esophagus to the lungs. Small tubes preserve the sphincter integrity and are less prone to allow reflux. Aspiration can be minimized further by not allowing a large volume to accumulate in the stomach. The amount of liquid residing in the stomach is called the "gastric residual" and can be checked by attaching a syringe to the open end of the tube and filling it with the liquid. In adults, the residual should be less than 150 mL. Small tubes often collapse easily when back-pressure is applied, making it difficult to measure residuals. Additionally, aspiration can be minimized by keeping the patient's head elevated 30–45° during feeding and for 30 to 60 minutes after intermittent infusion. This makes it more difficult for fluid to migrate up the esophagus against gravity. Lastly, aspiration can be minimized by infusing the feedings into the small intestine instead of the stomach. Physical complications in gastrostomy, jejunostomy, and pharyngostomy patients have been outlined in Table 110.1 under Disadvantages. Alleviation or prevention of these involves meticulous tube insertion and site care.

**Table 110.6** Composition of World Health Organization's Oral Rehydration Solution

| | |
|---|---|
| Glucose | 20.0 g |
| Sodium chloride | 3.5 g (60 mEq) |
| Sodium bicarbonate | 2.5 g (30 mEq) |
| Potassium chloride | 1.5 g (20 mEq) |
| Water | 1.0 L |

Feeding-induced diarrhea may be of infectious or osmolar origin. It is defined as an increased frequency or volume of stool and may be accompanied with increased water content. Infectious diarrhea may be inherent to a patient's disease state, but may also be caused by contaminated enteral formulas. A complete diarrhea workup, therefore, should include stool and formula cultures to rule out an iatrogenic etiology. Feeding preparation is best performed in a clean environment by conscientious personnel who are knowledgeable in infection control procedures such as handwashing. Feeding containers and tubing should be changed every 24 hours, and enteral products should not hang at the bedside for longer than 8 to 12 hours to reduce bacterial multiplication. Osmolality-induced diarrhea might be generated by hyperosmolar feedings, lactase deficiency, or fat malabsorption. Appropriate treatment, therefore, should follow determination of the etiology. Hyperosmolar feedings are particularly offensive in patients receiving small-bowel infusion, because the small intestine is especially sensitive to hyperosmolar loads. In these patients, the solution should be diluted to at least an isosmolar strength and infused slowly, preferably with the aid of an infusion device. Many institutions avoid lactose-induced diarrhea by stocking only lactose-free products. Fat malabsorption is determined only with an in-depth knowledge of the patient; it can be alleviated by using elemental formulas or supplying fat primarily as medium-chain triglycerides.

Occasionally, pharmacologic intervention is indicated to control diarrheal severity. The primary agents employed are opiates, diphenoxylate, and loperamide.[56] Diphenoxylate acts by the same mechanism as the opiates, by decreasing gastrointestinal motility and secretions. These actions decrease the amount of fluid to be reabsorbed in the small intestine and colon and increase the transit time to allow more absorption of exogenous fluids. A newer agent, loperamide, produces decreased gastrointestinal motility and decreases small-bowel output via ileostomy. It is two to three times as potent as diphenoxylate and may be administered less frequently. Use of these agents should be limited, as overuse may produce constipation and paralytic ileus.

Oral rehydration solutions may be used in dehydrated patients to reverse diarrheal sequelae from the previously described causes or replenish ostomy drainage fluid and electrolyte losses. Such formulas do not require intravenous access, are economical, and can be either purchased commercially or extemporaneously compounded.

The World Health Organization's solution contains the components shown in Table 110.6. It has been used successfully in mild to moderate dehydration in both children and adults. Treatment of severe dehydration, however, should be initiated with intravenous fluids.[57] The oral rehydration solution is successful because of its glucose content. Glucose stimulates active transport systems which in turn stimulate passive sodium and water uptake simultaneously with the glucose. Therefore, oral administration of several liters may actually decrease fecal water loss and generate a positive electrolyte balance.

The three most common electrolyte abnormalities seen with enteral feeding are hyperkalemia, hypophosphatemia, and hyponatremia.[39] Hyperkalemia and hyponatremia might be suspected upon examination of the enteral product's contents. Many products contain large potassium loads that may alone generate elevated serum levels. If metabolic acidosis develops (i.e., secondary to diarrhea and bicarbonate losses), these levels could go even higher. Potassium intake can be minimized by diluting certain concentrated, high-calorie formulas. Product information should be evaluated closely for actual electrolyte content on a per calorie or per volume basis. Hyponatremia can inherently be generated with extended use because of the low sodium concentrations found in commercial feeding preparations. Additional sodium may be prescribed in the form of salt tablets or simple table salt when necessary. Hypophosphatemia has been reported with initiation of parenteral as well as enteral nutrition support. It is generated when insulin administration drives phosphate intracellularly with the glucose.

Patients receiving enteral nutrition should be monitored closely for any of the potential complications previously described. Physicians are responsible for detecting complications arising with insertion of the surgically placed tubes. Nurses and pharmacists sometimes insert tubes nasally and must know how to verify tube placement in these cases. Anyone can examine the insertion site to detect tissue breakdown. As mentioned, diarrhea should be worked up with cultures to rule out an infectious etiology. Pharmacists may suggest a culture be performed on both the stool and the feeding formula. Familiarity with enteral feeding composition can help pharmacists and other health professionals determine the cause of fluid and electrolyte abnormalities and how to correct them by manipulation of the feeding solution. It is difficult to recommend a specific monitoring schedule for tube feeding complications, as actual need varies so significantly between patients. Most organized nutritional support services insist on accurate intake and output records daily and patient weights three or more times weekly. Electrolyte monitoring profiles should include at least sodium, potassium, chloride, bicarbonate, calcium, phosphorus, and magnesium determinations weekly. The frequency decreases as a patient is judged to be stable. Albumin should be measured one to two times monthly. Enteral nutrition support does not seem to affect hepatic enzymes as does parenteral nutrition. Therefore, they require monitoring every month or less.

## Summary

Quality control measures are best included in all aspects of feeding administration. Tubes should be placed and maintained carefully. Nutritional products should be chosen with each patient's disease state and personal preference in mind. Provision of enteral nutrition therapy is not without potential for complications. Therefore, patient monitoring for mechanical, infectious, or metabolic sequelae should be an important part of each patient's nutritional regimen. Metabolic abnormalities should be detected with laboratory serum analysis. Serum electrolytes and glucose should be assayed frequently during feeding initiation. The monitoring interval can then be increased once tolerance is determined. Lastly, the patient's nutritional status should improve as a result of therapy.

## References


1. Levine GM, Deren JJ, Steiger E, et al. Role of oral intake in maintenance of gut mass and disaccharide activity. Gastroenterology 1974;67:975–982.
2. Johnson LR, Copeland EM, Dudrick SJ, et al. Structural and hormonal alterations in the gastrointestinal tract of parenterally fed rats. Gastroenterology 1975;68:1177–1183.
3. Muggia-Sollam M, Bower RH, Murphy RF, et al. Posteroperative enteral versus parenteral nutritional support in gastrointestinal surgery. Am J Surg 1985;149:106–112.
4. Young EA, Cioletti LA, Traylor JB, et al. Gastrointestinal response to oral versus gastric feeding of defined formula diets. Am J Clin Nutr 1982;35:715–726.
5. Adibi SA. Leucine absorption rate and net movements of sodium and water in human jejunum. J Appl Phys 1970;28: 753–757.
6. Souba WW, Scott TE, Wilmore DW. Intestinal consumption of intravenously administered fuels. J Parenter Enter Nutr 1985;9:18–22.
7. Souba WW, Wilmore DW. Postoperative alteration of arteriovenous exchange of amino acids across the gastrointestinal tract. Surgery 1983;94:342–350.
8. Lichtenberger L, Welsh JD, Johnson LR. Relationship between the changes in gastrin levels and intestinal properties in the starved rat. Dig Dis 1976;21:33–38.
9. Johnson LR, Lichtenberg LM, Copeland EM, et al. Action of gastrin on gastrointestinal structure and function. Gastroenterology 1975;68:1184–1192.
10. Johnson LR, Guthrie P. Effect of cholecystokinin and 16,16-dimethyl prostaglandin $E_2$ on DNA and RNA of gastric and duodenal mucosa. Gastroenterology 1976;70:59–65.
11. Weser E, Bell D, Tawil T. Effect of octapeptide-cholecystokinin, secretin, and glucagon on intestinal mucosal growth in parenterally nourished rats. Dig Dis Sci 1981;26:409–416.
12. Kudsk KA, Stone JM, Carpenter G, et al. Enteral and parenteral feeding influences mortality after hemoglobin–*E. coli* peritonitis in normal rats. J Trauma 1983;23:605–609.
13. Kudsk KA, Carpenter G, Peterson SR, et al. Effect of enteral and parenteral feeding in malnourished rats with hemoglobin–*E. coli* adjuvant peritonitis. J Surg Res 1981;31:105–110.
14. Nohr CW, Tchervenkov JI, Meakis JL, et al. Malnutrition and humoral immunity: Short term acute nutritional deprivation. Surgery 1985;98:769–776.
15. Alverdy J, Chi HS, Sheldon GF. The effect of parenteral nutrition on gastrointestinal immunity. Ann Surg 1985;202:681–684.
16. Whatley K, Turner WW, Dey M, et al. When does metoclopramide facilitate transpyloric intubation? J Parenter Enter Nutr 1984;8:679–681.
17. Shipps FC, Sayler CB, Egan JF, et al. Fluoroscopic placement of intestinal tubes. Radiology 1979;132:226–227.
18. Ramos SM, Lindine P. Inexpensive, safe and simple nasoenteral intubation—An alternative for the cost conscious. J Parenter Enter Nutr 1986;10:78–81.
19. Dobbie RP, Hoffmeister JA. Continuous pump-tube enteric hyperalimentation. Surg Gynecol Obstet 1976;143:273–276.
20. Torosian MH, Rombeau JL. Feeding by tube enterostomy. Surg Gynecol Obstet 1980;150:918–927.
21. Levenson R, Dyson A, Turner WW. Feeding tube anchor. Nutr Supp Serv 1985;5(8):40–41.
22. Armstrong C, Luther W, Sykes T. A technique for preventing extubation of feeding tubes. "The bridle." J Parenter Enter Nutr 1980;4:603.
23. Lipman TO, Kessler T, Arabian A. Nasopulmonary intubation with feeding tubes: Case reports and review of the literature. J Parenter Enter Nutr 1985;9:618–620.
24. Glaser D, de Tarnowsky GO. Percutaneous endoscopic gastrostomy: A nonoperative technique for alternative placement of a gastrostomy tube. Nutr Supp Serv 1983;3(3):11–12.
25. Kirby DF, Craig RM, Tsang T, et al. Percutaneous endoscopic gastrostomies: A prospective evaluation and review of the literature. J Parenter Enter Nutr 1986;10:155–159.
26. Leider Z, Sullivan L, Mullen MA, et al. Intermittent tube feedings: Pros and cons. Nutr Supp Serv 1984;4(3):59–62.
27. Randall HT. Osmolality and its relationship to GI tolerance, in: Current Concepts in Nutritional Support: Monograph I. 1983.
28. Orvieto A, Kirsch J, Goldberger J. Evaluation of enteral delivery systems. Nutr Supp Serv 1983;3(4):44–48.
29. Gray G, Cooper H. Protein digestion and absorption. Gastroenterology 1971;61:535–544.
30. Adibi SA. Intestinal phase of protein assimilation in man. Am J Clin Nutr 1976;29:205–215.
31. Smith JL, Heymsfield SB. Enteral nutrition support: Formula preparation from modular ingredients. J Parenter Enter Nutr 1983;7:280–288.
32. Roberts P, Whelan W. The mechanism of carbohydrase action: Action of human salivary alpha-amylase on amylopectin and glycogen. Biochem J 1960;76:246–253.
33. Rosenweig NS, Herman RH. Control of jejunal sucrase and maltase activity by dietary sucrose or fructose in man. A model for the study of enzyme regulation in man. J Clin Invest 1968;47:2253–2262.
34. Mead J. Nutrients with special functions: Essential fatty acids, in Alfin-Slater R, Kritchervsky D (eds): Human Nutrition. New York, Plenum, vol 3A, 1980.
35. Vanlandingham S, Simpson S, Daniel P, et al. Metabolic abnormalities in patients supported with enteral tube feeding. J Parenter Enter Nutr 1981;5:322–324.
36. Brown RO, Hall NH, Elkordy M, et al. Use of wine-tasting scale to evaluate enteral nutritional supplements. Nutr Supp Serv 1985;5(6):21–24.
37. Fomon S, Filer L, Anderson T. Recommendations for feeding normal infants. Pediatrics 1979;63:52–59.
38. Committee on Nutrition. Soy–protein formulas: Recommendations for use in infant feeding. Pediatrics 1983;72:359–364.
39. Santosham M, Foster S, Reid R, et al. Role of soy-based, lactose-free formula during treatment of acute diarrhea. Pediatrics 1985;76:292–298.
40. United States Congress Infant Formula Act of 1980. Washington DC, Public Law 96-359, September 26, 1980.
41. Mobassaleh M, Montgomery R, Biller J, et al. Development of

carbohydrate absorption in the fetus and neonate. Pediatrics 1985;75(suppl):160–166.
42. McKenzie M, Bender K, Seals A. Infant formula products, in: Handbook of Nonprescription Drugs, 7th ed. Washington DC, American Pharmaceutical Association, 1982, pp 305–330.
43. Maratese LE. Standardized enteral nutritional support. Nutr Supp Serv 1983;3(8):27–30.
44. Hopefl AW, Herrmann VM. Developing a formulary for enteral nutrition products. Am J Hosp Pharm 1982;39:1514–1517.
45. Berry DT, Summerfield MR, Wiggins PA. Unit dose distribution of pediatric enteral formulas. Am J Hosp Pharm 1985;42: 2218–2219.
46. Fagerman KE, Dean RE. Bulk production and freezing of elemental enteral feedings. Nutr Supp Serv 1983;3(4):8–10.
47. Pizzo PA, Levine AS. The utility of protected-environment regimens for the compromised host. Prog Hematol 1977;10:331.
48. Schroeder P, Fisher D, Volz M, et al. Microbial contamination of enteral feeding solutions in a community hospital. J Parenter Enter Nutr 1983;7:364–368.
49. Cutie AJ, Altman E, Lenkel L. Compatibility of enteral products with commonly employed drug additives. J Parenter Enter Nutr 1983;7:186–191.
50. Altman E, Cutie AJ. Compatibility of enteral products with commonly employed drug additives. Nutr Supp Serv 1984;4(12): 8–17.
51. Lader E, Yang L, Clarke A. Warfarin dosage and vitamin K in Osmolite. (Lett) Ann Intern Med 1980;93:373–374.
52. Lee M, Schwartz RN, Sharifi R. Warfarin resistance and vitamin K. (Lett) Ann Intern Med 1981;94:140–141.
53. Bauer LA. Interference of oral phenytoin absorption by continuous nasogastric feedings. Neurology 1982;32:570–572.
54. Parr MD, Record KE, Griffith GL. Effect of enteral nutrition on warfarin therapy. Clin Pharm 1982;1:274–276.
55. Valentine RJ, Turner WW. Pleural complications of nasoenteric feeding tubes. J Parenter Enter Nutr 1985;9:605–607.
56. Mirtallo JM, Fabri PJ. Concurrent therapy for complications of enteral nutrition support. Hosp Form 1982;17(July):945–953.
57. Sack DA. Treatment of acute diarrhoea with oral rehydration solution. Drugs 1982;23:150–157.

# Chapter 111 / Nutritional Considerations in Major Organ Failure

Rex O. Brown, PharmD

Organ failure may alter the absorption, utilization, and excretion of essential nutrients. Therefore, administration of conventional or standard nutrient formulas to patients with significant organ dysfunction may be inappropriate or harmful. Formulation of a nutrition-care plan for these patients often requires a carefully planned, disease-specific approach. The monitoring of these patients may require different laboratory markers and tests or more frequent use of traditional markers to ensure that the nutrients are being administered in utilizable forms. Also, close assessment of the patient with compromised organ dysfunction is needed to ensure that the nutrition formula is not causing harm. Monitoring the efficacy of nutrition support in patients with organ failure may also be very difficult. For example, it would be impossible to collect a 24-hour urine specimen for urea nitrogen measurement to calculate nitrogen balance in an anuric patient. An alternative that estimates nitrogen appearance or protein breakdown is required in this situation.

Alterations in the metabolism or excretion of macronutrients can have a major impact on the preparation of an appropriate nutrition support formula, while altered homeostasis of a micronutrient may require little adjustment in the nutrition support formula. In this chapter, we discuss specific nutritional alterations in hepatic, renal, pulmonary, cardiac, and gastrointestinal failure and a rational approach to ensuring delivery of safe and efficacious nutrition support, of macronutrients as well as micronutrients, to patients with these disorders.

## Hepatic Failure

The liver is the primary organ involved in the digestion, metabolism, and storage of nutrients. It contains many enzymes and receives, processes, and prepares nutrients for the periphery. Therefore, when functional capacity is depressed, profound macronutrient and micronutrient intolerance may result. Other sequelae that may accompany the failing liver are fluid and electrolyte imbalances,[1] vitamin deficiencies,[2] and undernutrition.[3] The challenge of providing nutritional support in utilizable forms during severe liver failure is formidable. A comprehensive review of this subject contains additional information.[4]

### *Macronutrient Considerations*

#### Carbohydrate

The liver is of critical importance in carbohydrate homeostasis because of its ability to remove and release glucose into the circulatory system. In health, approximately 60% of absorbed glucose is taken up by the liver for glycogen synthesis, triglyceride synthesis, and glycolysis.[2] In general, glycogen synthesis and glycolysis are enhanced by insulin, while gluconeogenesis and glycogen breakdown are controlled by glucagon.

Hyperglycemia is quite common in patients with cirrhosis, most likely as a result of peripheral insulin resistance.[5] It has been suggested that this disorder is mediated by a reduction of insulin receptor concentration in the monocyte, one of the leukocytes in the circulation. Plasma concentrations of insulin are usually elevated with or without a glucose stimulus. This may make administration of large doses of glucose questionable, as administration of insulin to control hyperglycemia may not improve utilization substantially.

Patients with fulminant hepatitis are prone to hypoglycemia. There is depressed hepatic glucose production secondary to decreased glycogen stores and diminished gluconeogenesis. Also, impaired degradation of insulin by the damaged liver may contribute to this disorder. A continuous intravenous infusion of glucose usually prevents hypoglycemia in acute hepatitis, but concentrations greater than 10% glucose in water may be needed in the more severe forms of this disease.

#### Fat

The liver is responsible for synthesis of cholesterol, high-density lipoproteins, and very low density lipoproteins. The enzymes hepatic lipoprotein lipase and lecithin–cholesterol acyltransferase (LCAT) are also synthesized in this organ. Increased serum triglyceride and free fatty acid concentrations are often encountered in patients with hepatic dysfunction or failure. Alcohol ingestion has been shown to increase circulating triglycerides, and chronic intake has caused fatty infiltration of the liver. The patient with liver failure is often lipid intolerant. Monitoring serum triglyceride concentration and free fatty acid oxidation (using carbon-labeled fat emulsion experimentally) to ensure that administered intravenous lipid is both cleared from the bloodstream and oxidized appropriately has been suggested. Most institutions are not able to measure free fatty acid oxidation, leaving serum triglyceride concentrations as the most available monitoring marker. Although not an indicator of utilization, this can help prevent marked hypertriglyceridemia and associated disorders (e.g., pancreatitis) if followed closely. During parenteral nutrition in patients with liver failure, intravenous fat should be used only to prevent essential fatty acid deficiency when serum triglyceride concentrations exceed 300 mg/dL.

Steatorrhea is very common in patients with hepatic

cholestasis because inadequate bile acids or pancreatic enzymes are secreted into the gastrointestinal tract lumen. Micelle formation is impeded and the long-chain fatty acids pass through the colon, resulting in a foul-smelling, soapy diarrhea. Therefore, assessment of the gastrointestinal tract is necessary before large amounts of lipid are administered by the oral route. Oral medium-chain triglycerides have been occasionally used with success because they do not require pancreatic enzymes or micelle formation before absorption. These products do not, however, provide essential fatty acids.

### Protein

Nitrogen requirements for the patient with liver failure are not unlike those of normal subjects,[6] but intolerance to protein is well described in patients with cirrhosis and protein restriction has been used rather successfully as part of the therapy. A dilemma arises when the diet becomes so restrictive that undernutrition inevitably results and the patient becomes susceptible to infection and other complications. Overzealous use of protein to correct nutritional deficits invariably results in hepatic encephalopathy because the diseased liver cannot process and metabolize the aromatic amino acids and excess ammonia may be liberated. Therefore, careful monitoring and recognition that a therapeutic window for protein intake exists (40–80 g/d) are essential. During stress, the patient with liver failure has a decreased insulin-to-glucagon ratio, which results in protein catabolism by gluconeogenesis.

Because the liver metabolizes the aromatic amino acids (phenylalanine, tyrosine, tryptophan) and methionine, the plasma concentrations of these amino acids are often elevated in cirrhotic patients. Plasma concentrations of the branched-chain amino acids (valine, leucine, isoleucine) are often depressed because these amino acids are metabolized by the skeletal muscle. This altered plasma aminogram is thought to be involved in the etiology of hepatic encephalopathy. In health the ratio of branched-chain amino acids to aromatic amino acids is 3–3.5:1, but ratios of 1.0 have been associated with hepatic encephalopathy.[7]

Therapy directed at the normalization of this altered plasma aminogram has prompted the clinical testing and marketing of both parenteral and enteral nutrition products with modified amino acid profiles.[8] Modified amino acid products also may suppress protein breakdown and stimulate protein synthesis.[9] While altered plasma amino acid concentrations have been normalized with these products, improvement in encephalopathy or outcome has not been universal. These conflicting results may be explained in part by the complexity of the disease process.

Other etiologies of hepatic encephalopathy include excessive ammonia production from conversion of protein or amino acids in the gastrointestinal tract and increased concentrations of glutamine, free tryptophan, or $\gamma$-aminobutyric acid in the central nervous system.[10] Most likely, hepatic encephalopathy is a multifactorial disorder that includes several of these etiologies.

In most cases, parenteral nutritional support in the patient with liver failure can be administered with standard amino acids (Fig. 111.1). If the gastrointestinal tract is functioning, the enteral route can be used. In those patients who have grade III or IV encephalopathy (Table 111.1) or who have decompensated or have not attained nitrogen equilibrium while receiving moderate doses of standard amino acids, use of a modified amino acid should be considered. This provides amino acid nitrogen in high concentrations of branched-

**Figure 111.1** Nutritional support approach to the patient with liver failure (selection of amino acid).

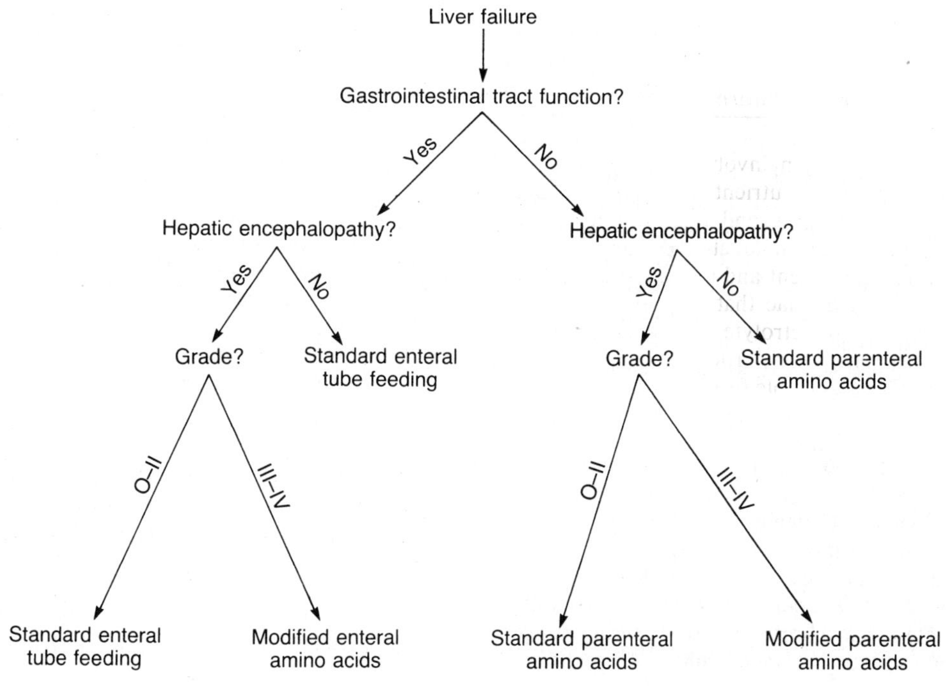

**Table 111.1** Grades of Hepatic Encephalopathy

| | |
|---|---|
| Grade 0 | No encephalopathy |
| Grade 1 | Fluctuant confusion |
| Grade 2 | Impending stupor |
| Grade 3 | Stupor |
| Grade 4 | Coma, unresponsive to pain |

chain amino acids and low concentrations of aromatic amino acids and methionine. Because this modified amino acid product costs considerably more than standard amino acids, the strict criteria described before should be used to prevent inappropriate use leading to unnecessary expense.

**Sodium and Water**

Patients with severe cirrhosis often have ascites and peripheral edema.[4] This represents excess total body sodium with an even greater excess in total body water. Hyponatremia invariably results from this disorder. Increased sympathetic activity has been shown to correlate well with the impaired sodium and water excretion in cirrhosis patients.[11] Stimulation of arginine vasopressin secretion secondary to a decrease in effective blood volume has also been demonstrated.[12] Generally, salt and fluid restriction is required so as not to exacerbate this overhydrated state. It would not be uncommon for these patients who require parenteral nutrition to have sodium eliminated from the formula. Severe sodium and fluid restriction during intravascular depletion may cause or exacerbate hepatic encephalopathy.[10] Therefore, during fluid and salt restriction, symptoms of volume depletion (↑ pulse rate, ↓ blood pressure, dry mucous membranes) should be watched closely. Recently, hypernatremia has been reported to be associated with lactulose therapy in patients with portal-systemic encephalopathy.[13]

**Potassium**

Hypokalemia is very common in the patient with liver failure who has normal renal function. Poor intake and frequent vomiting may cause this disorder. If vomiting is severe enough, contraction alkalosis may occur, which results in increased renal excretion of potassium. Secondary hyperaldosteronism, which is frequently seen in the liver failure patient with intravascular depletion, also increases renal excretion of potassium. Loop-diuretic therapy can increase renal excretion of potassium, while diarrhea secondary to lactulose or antacid therapy may increase fecal excretion of it. All these conditions can lead to profound hypokalemia. Therefore, potassium requirements in the liver failure patient receiving nutritional support are often supranormal.

**Phosphorus**

Treating patients with upper gastrointestinal hemorrhages with vigorous antacid therapy can lead to hypophosphatemia and, potentially, phosphate depletion.[14] During nutritional support, requirements for intracellular ions such as phosphorus may be supranormal as new synthesis of lean body mass takes place (refeeding). Recent data show that sucralfate may also bind dietary phosphorus and lower serum concentrations in patients with chronic renal failure.[15] Patients with liver failure are very susceptible to upper gastrointestinal hemorrhage and frequently are treated with these drugs. Therefore, this patient population is at increased risk of developing hypophosphatemia from refeeding.

**Magnesium**

Poor intake and increased excretion of magnesium secondary to diuretic therapy or alcohol ingestion contribute to depletion of magnesium and hypomagnesemia in the liver failure patient.[16,17] Magnesium repletion is usually part of standard care of the alcoholic patient with liver failure early in the hospital course; however, needs may become supranormal during aggressive nutritional support. Doses of magnesium to maintain serum concentrations in the normal range should be administered during nutritional support.

**Acid–Base Disorders**

Liver failure patients who have excessive diarrhea will lose considerable quantities of bicarbonate in the stool leading to metabolic acidosis. Replacement therapy with bicarbonate, acetate, or citrate may be required.

Excessive losses of gastrointestinal fluid by vomiting or nasogastric suction result in considerable loss of acid, resulting in metabolic alkalosis. Replacement therapy in these patients should include volume, potassium, and chloride.

### *Micronutrient Considerations*

**Trace Elements**

The Nutrition Advisory Group of the American Medical Association (NAG-AMA)[18] has recommended that zinc, copper, manganese, and chromium be given daily in parenteral nutrition solutions (Table 111.2). Since these recommendations were made, considerable evidence that selenium is essential has accumulated.[19,20] Data addressing appropriate administration of trace elements and monitoring frequency in patients with organ dysfunction who are receiving parenteral nutrition are relatively scarce. Patients with liver failure who have reduced bile acid synthesis or pancreatic insufficiency have considerable malabsorption and diarrhea. Chronic diarrhea has been shown to cause zinc deficiency because stool contains substantial quantities of zinc.[21] Considering the importance of zinc in metalloenzyme reactions, immunocompetence, and the senses of taste and smell, patients with chronic diarrhea or large ostomy losses should be suspected of having zinc deficiency if replacement therapy has not been administered. This may be very difficult in a patient receiving a protein-restricted diet because substantial amounts of zinc are found in red meat. Oral supplementation of zinc as zinc sulfate capsules could be used to prevent deficiency or correct deficits.

**Table 111.2** Suggested Daily Intravenous Intake of Essential Trace Elements in Adults

| | |
|---|---|
| Zinc | 2.5–4.0 mg |
| Copper | 0.5–1.5 mg |
| Chromium | 10–15 $\mu$g |
| Manganese | 150–800 $\mu$g |

Because copper and manganese are excreted in the bile, it has been recommended that these two trace elements not be administered or be administered in reduced dose to patients with serious cholestasis.[18] Although manganese toxicity is rare, copper overload or toxicity causes serious symptoms. Appropriate administration of copper should, therefore, be addressed in the long-term TPN patient with cholestasis.

Recently, an association between alcoholism and low serum selenium concentrations has been reported.[22,23] The lowest selenium concentrations were reported in patients who had decompensated alcoholic cirrhosis. Because selenium is important in maintaining the enzyme glutathione perioxidase, a deficiency of this trace element is being implicated as a cause of hepatic injury in the alcoholic patient. Therefore, consideration of supplementation with selenium should be an early priority during nutritional rehabilitation in this patient population.

### Vitamins

Deficiencies of vitamins are common in patients with chronic liver disease. Poor intake and malabsorption are the principal causes of these nutrient disorders.[2] Depletion of hepatic stores of vitamin A, pyridoxine, folic acid, riboflavin, pantothenic acid, vitamin $B_{12}$, and thiamine have been reported in patients with hepatic failure; folate deficiency is the most common.[24] Folic acid deficiency may lead to megaloblastic anemia, while thiamine deficiency may result in Wernicke's encephalopathy after rehydration with intravenous glucose. If dextrose-based TPN is started in these patients, additional thiamine may be needed to prevent Wernicke's encephalopathy.

Recent evidence shows that hepatic stores of vitamin A are depleted in the patient with alcoholic liver injury.[25] Because vitamin D is metabolized to the active form, 25-hydroxyvitamin D, in the liver, low concentrations of this vitamin are seen in patients with biliary cirrhosis. Impaired absorption of dietary vitamin D may also contribute to these low serum concentrations. It is unclear whether vigorous supplementation of fat-soluble vitamins should be given to these patients during nutritional support, but therapeutic doses are indicated when a deficiency has been documented.

## *Administration Routes and Products*

### Parenteral Therapy

Generally, the indications for parenteral nutrition in the patient with liver failure would be similar to those for general hospitalized patients. If the gastrointestinal tract is functioning and accessible, enteral nutrition support should be attempted. Patients with liver failure may have periods of acute malabsorption and maldigestion requiring parenteral nutrition or specialized enteral nutrition support. Concomitant sepsis causing a prolonged ileus would also require the parenteral route for nutrient administration.

The major controversy in nutritional support of the patient with liver failure has centered around the use of protein products. The package insert of intravenous standard amino acids lists hepatic coma as a contraindication, but these products have been cautiously administered for years fairly successfully. A modified amino acid solution for parenteral nutrition (Hepatamine, Kendall McGaw) is now marketed for patients with liver failure and hepatic encephalopathy. It is enriched with branched-chain amino acids (BCAAs) and has reduced amounts of aromatic amino acids (AAAs) and methionine. The product was formulated on the basis of the false neurotransmitter hypothesis where AAAs become elevated in the serum and pass into the central nervous system.

Administration of the product during TPN has normalized plasma profiles of amino acids, which correlated with improved encephalopathy in some studies. One prospective, randomized clinical trial involved comparison of neomycin/glucose with modified amino acids/glucose and found decreased encephalopathy score and mortality in the amino acid group.[26] Currently, this is the best controlled study available in evaluating amino acids in liver failure. Some investigators in this field are stating that a controlled study comparing standard amino acids with modified amino acids needs to be done. Interestingly, a study from France failed to show improvement in hepatic encephalopathy when modified amino acids were compared with standard amino acids during TPN in cirrhotic patients.[27]

Other studies with modified amino acids in liver failure have shown efficacy comparable with that of lactulose,[28] improvement in plasma aminograms without improvement in encephalopathy,[29,30] and very low tyrosine and cystine concentrations without improvement in encephalopathy.[31] These studies either had few subjects, used an intravenous formula with only BCAAs (i.e., not a complete nutritional formula), or attempted comparison of this nutritional product to standard pharmacologic therapy. Therefore, these and future studies need to be evaluated very closely. Cost also precludes use of the modified amino acid product in all patients with liver failure.

Table 111.3 gives an example of a central TPN formula for a patient in liver failure. These patients need a very individualized approach based on fluid and electrolyte balance, acid–base status, grade of encephalopathy, and concurrent drug therapy.

### Enteral Therapy

Currently, there are two products marketed as a food supplement for patients with hepatic encephalopathy (Hepatic-Aid II, Kendall McGaw; Travasorb Hepatic, Travenol). These supplements also have increased amounts of BCAAs and reduced amounts of AAAs and methionine. Although these products can be used in enteral tube feeding, they are virtually electrolyte and vitamin free, necessitating supplementation in appropriate amounts if the tube feeding is used as the sole source of nutrient intake. Like the clinical trials with the intravenous amino acids in liver failure, results with these products have been inconsistent. Uncontrolled and comparative studies (dietary protein versus dietary protein/BCAA supplement) have demonstrated benefit by improving nitrogen balance and improving encephalopathy grade.[32–34] A recent cooperative study demonstrated improved nutritional status in patients with alcoholic hepatitis who were given BCAA supplementation with their normal hospital diet.[35] Other studies have also demonstrated improved nitrogen balance but no improvement in encephalopathy grade when these modified amino acids were compared with standard casein protein.[36,37] Restriction of these

**Table 111.3** Examples of TPN Formulas for Patients With Organ Failure

| | *Hepatic failure* | *Acute renal failure* | *Chronic renal failure* | *Respiratory failure* | *Cardiac failure* | *Short-bowel syndrome* |
|---|---|---|---|---|---|---|
| Dextrose, mL (%) | 500 (50) | 500 (70) | 500 (70) | 500 (40) | 500 (70) | 500 (50) |
| CAAs,[a] mL (%) | 500 (8.5)[b] | 250 (10) | 500 (10) | 500 (10) | 500 (10) | 500 (8.5) |
| Lipid, mL (%) | — | — | — | 500 (10) | — | 500 (10) |
| 0.45% Sodium chloride injection, mL | | | | | | 500 |
| Sodium, mEq/L | 20 | 0 | 30 | 50 | 0 | 100[c] |
| Potassium, mEq/L | 50 | 0 | 20 | 50 | 50 | 60 |
| Chloride, mEq/L | 50 | 10 | 20 | 40 | 50 | 120 |
| Phosphorus, mmol/L | 15 | 0 | 7.5 | 15 | 15 | 15 |
| Acetate, mEq/L | 50 | 20 | 80 | 60 | 40 | 40 |
| Magnesium, mEq/L | 12 | 0 | 0 | 8 | 8 | 16 |
| Sulfate, mEq/L | 12 | 0 | 0 | 8 | 8 | 16 |
| Calcium, mEq/L | 5 | 0 | 5 | 5 | 5 | 10 |
| Gluconate, mEq/L | 5 | 0 | 5 | 5 | 5 | 10 |
| Multivitamins, mL/d | 10 | 10 | 10 | 10 | 10 | 10 |
| Zinc, mg/d | 3 | 3 | 3 | 3 | 3 | 10 |
| Copper, mg/d | 1.2 | 1.2 | 1.2 | 1.2 | 1.2 | 1.2 |
| Manganese, μg/d | 300 | 300 | 300 | 300 | 300 | 300 |
| Chromium, μg/d | 12 | 12 | 12 | 12 | 12 | 20 |
| Selenium, μg/d | 40 | — | — | — | 40 | 40 |

[a] Crystalline amino acids.
[b] Hepatamine 8% when criteria for use are met.
[c] Does not include 0.45% sodium chloride injection or lipid.

modified amino acid supplements is suggested as outlined in Figure 111.1.

Recently, there has been considerable interest in the use of vegetable-protein diets in the chronic management of patients with cirrhosis and hepatic encephalopathy.[38,39] Enthusiasm for this therapy is based on the reduced amounts of phenylalanine, tyrosine, methionine, and tryptophan in vegetable protein. Dried beans are an example of a vegetable high in protein. Although these diets are somewhat more difficult to adhere to, preliminary results justify further study of this concept.

### *Future Directions*

Some work has been completed in patients with hepatic encephalopathy who received keto-analogues of essential or branched-chain amino acids.[40,41] Benefit from this therapy has been marginal at best and interest in this theory may be waning somewhat. Certainly, more studies demonstrating which patients with liver failure need modified amino acids for optimal therapy should be done.

## Renal Failure

The kidney is responsible primarily for excretion of water, nonmetabolized solute from the diet, and the end products of nitrogen metabolism. Impairment of these processes results in overhydration, urea nitrogen accumulation, and impaired protein synthesis. Patients who have chronic renal failure (CRF) and receive dialysis therapy have impaired host-defense mechanisms and increased risk of infection.[42,43] Undernourished patients with CRF have decreased skeletal muscle function.[44] Renal failure may be acute or chronic and oliguric or nonoliguric, making provision of appropriate nutritional support very challenging. As in hepatic failure, nutritional support in renal failure requires provision of substrate in utilizable forms in an appropriate volume while limiting accumulation of nitrogen waste. Major differences in the nutritional management of acute renal failure (ARF) and CRF exist and are discussed separately where appropriate. Excellent reviews are available on the nutritional management of acute and chronic renal failure patients.[45–47]

### *Macronutrient Considerations*

#### Carbohydrate

More than one half of patients with renal failure have insulin resistance and hyperglycemia.[48] This is related in part to an abnormal increased glucagon:insulin ratio, resulting in protein breakdown and gluconeogenesis. As glucagon and insulin are both degraded by the kidney, their levels are elevated in uremia.[49] In assessment of carbohydrate homeostasis, the type of renal failure (chronic versus acute) and the dialytic therapies must be considered. The patient with ARF usually has a superimposed illness (sepsis, hypotension), which in itself may cause glucose intolerance and insulin resistance. Patients who have CRF and are being treated with continuous ambulatory peritoneal dialysis (CAPD) absorb a substantial amount of glucose from the dialysis fluid. This can worsen existing hyperglycemia and contribute significantly to the patient's energy intake. One study found that more than 180 g of glucose (approximately 600 kcal) was absorbed per day during CAPD.[50] This provided 12% to 34% of these patients' energy intake. It is, therefore, not uncommon for these patients to have Kwashiorkor-type malnutrition.

Occasionally, patients with ARF are treated with intermittent peritoneal dialysis (IPD), which may exacerbate glucose intolerance already present from the stress of illness. Addition of regular insulin to the dialysate has been advocated during IPD and CAPD to prevent or minimize hyperglycemia.[51] This may be particularly beneficial in the diabetic nephropathy patient, as it may prevent frequent intravenous or subcutaneous dosing of insulin during dialysis therapy. As in plastic bags used for intravenous solutions, insulin adsorbs to bags used for CAPD, which needs to be considered when dosing a CRF patient.[52] During hemodialysis there may be some carbohydrate loss but it is not clinically important.

### Fat

Type IV hypertriglyceridemia is present in more than one half of all renal failure patients.[53] This is thought to be caused mainly by decreased catabolism of triglycerides secondary to decreased hepatic lipoprotein lipase activity. For this reason, currently marketed fat emulsions must be administered cautiously in both ARF and CRF. Serum triglyceride concentrations have been advocated as markers for fat intolerance in this patient population.[45] Most patients receiving hemodialysis should receive heparin, which should activate lipoprotein lipase and convert triglycerides to free fatty acids and glycerol. If free fatty acids are not utilized by the body properly (e.g., as in carnitine deficiency), serum triglyceride measurements will not identify this defect. Also, patients receiving long-term dialysis treatment have been shown to accumulate remnants of triglyceride-rich lipoproteins.[54] Currently, intravenous fat emulsions containing medium-chain triglycerides are undergoing clinical trials in the United States. Potentially, these fat emulsions could be utilized more efficiently than currently available products.

### Protein

Urea, the end product of nitrogen metabolism, accumulates in both patients with ARF and patients with CRF. The composition and dose of protein during nutrition support in renal failure have been the subject of considerable investigation and controversy. The appropriate nitrogen intake is determined by the type of renal failure and the interventions being used (e.g., dialysis). Even the type of dialysis has an influence on the appropriate amount of nitrogen to administer. Nitrogen metabolism differs substantially in patients with acute and chronic renal failure.

In early acute renal failure, the nutritional support formula needs to be protein restricted (20–30 g/d) while the patient is being evaluated for etiologic factors. A low protein intake during ARF minimizes urea nitrogen accumulation from exogenous protein. Urea nitrogen appearance is also determined by endogenous breakdown of protein, which is very important in a stressed patient with sepsis. Therefore, in this type of patient, endogenous catabolism certainly contributes more to nitrogen accumulation when a restricted dose of exogenous protein is given. If dialysis is instituted, the protein intake can be liberalized somewhat. Generally, the patient receiving hemodialysis can tolerate 1–1.2 g of protein per kilogram per day.[46] If IPD is used, the protein intake may be liberalized to 1.2–1.5 g/kg/d.[55] Frequency and effectiveness of dialytic therapy are the final determinants of use of these protein-infusion ranges.

Some investigations have suggested that dialysis therapy be instituted early in ARF so that aggressive nutritional support can be started.[56] In patients with severe injury or sepsis plus ARF, attainment of protein requirements (1.5–2.5 g/kg/d) may not be possible, even with early institution of dialysis. Three commercially available intravenous preparations of essential amino acids are marketed for nutritional support of ARF, as is discussed later in this chapter.

With respect to nitrogen requirements in CRF, patients should be divided into two groups: those receiving dialysis and those not receiving it. Protein intake can be liberalized to approximately 1 g/kg/d when patients are receiving hemodialysis and 1.2–1.3 g/kg/d for CAPD.[57] When nutritional status is adequate, 1 g/kg/d usually maintains nitrogen equilibrium with either method of dialysis.[58] The original studies on protein losses during CAPD were conducted during the day's first exchange. As protein losses during this exchange are higher than subsequent exchanges,[59] total daily losses were somewhat overestimated and protein doses may have been too liberal.

Patients with chronic renal dysfunction who are not yet candidates for dialysis need a protein-restricted diet.[60,61] There are substantial data demonstrating that this approach preserves residual renal function and prolongs the period before dialytic therapy is begun.[62] Some investigators have advocated that this beneficial effect results from concurrent phosphorus restriction during protein restriction.[63] Others have recommended an essential amino acid supplement plus a low-protein diet and found similar results.[64] Currently, a protein dose of 0.6 g/kg/d is recommended for these patients before dialysis is started. This has been shown to maintain nutritional status and preserve residual renal function.

### Sodium and Water

The patient with oliguric renal failure will have impaired excretion of sodium and water. In these situations, the nutritional support formula should be concentrated in as small a volume as possible and contain little or no sodium. In the patient with nonoliguric ARF, considerable quantities of sodium may be lost in the urine, necessitating replacement to maintain sodium balance. This may also apply to the patient who is losing considerable quantities of gastric fluid from suction. Sodium and chloride losses will be large if more than 1,000 mL is lost per day.

Hyponatremia is very common in the dialysis patient, usually reflecting overhydration, but does not require additional administration of sodium. Regular dialysis eliminates excess body water and serum sodium concentration increases. Generally, sodium should be administered to renal failure patients during nutritional support only to replace losses.

#### Potassium

Hyperkalemia may be frequent in both patients with ARF and patients with CRF. In ARF, there is considerable protein catabolism and intracellular potassium release. Hyperkalemia may result from impaired secretion and excretion of potassium by the kidney. If this disorder is severe enough, emergency dialysis may need to be instituted. TPN formulas in patients with ARF and hyperkalemia should not contain potassium salts. After several days of feeding, the serum potassium concentration decreases, often necessitating cautious addition of this electrolyte to the TPN formula. If the enteral route can be used for nutritional support, formulas void of potassium may need to be used initially.

Patients with CRF who develop hyperkalemia have usually ingested potassium in excess of what the kidneys or dialysis can handle. The malnourished CRF patient who is receiving TPN may require considerable potassium as new lean body tissue is synthesized. When inappropriate amounts of potassium are given during refeeding, hypokalemia may develop. Overzealous use of potassium salt supplements may result in hyperkalemia in patients with CRF.

#### Phosphorus

Because phosphorus is excreted renally, hyperphosphatemia is very common in patients with ARF and CRF. Like potassium, large amounts of phosphorus may be released into the circulation secondary to tissue breakdown during ARF. Control of hyperphosphatemia is extremely important during ARF because when the product of serum phosphorus (in mg/dL) and serum calcium (in mg/dL) exceeds 70, metastatic calcification of the renal tubules can occur. Therefore, for patients with ARF, phosphorus should be omitted from the nutrition formula until serum concentrations have normalized.

Patients with CRF are often treated for hyperphosphatemia with aluminum-containing antacids or phosphorus-restricted diets.When these patients receive aggressive nutritional support, the combination of refeeding (cellular uptake of phosphorus for synthesis of lean body mass) and vigorous antacid therapy can result in hypophosphatemia. Therefore, conservative amounts of phosphorus usually need to be administered during TPN. If the CRF patient is being dialyzed and has a functioning gastrointestinal tract, concentrated complete enteral formulas containing phosphorus can be used.

#### Magnesium

Magnesium is also excreted by the kidney and excessive intake results in hypermagnesemia. Therefore, magnesium is usually not added to the TPN formula until a low serum concentration of this electrolyte is encountered. Magnesium is rarely needed during short-term TPN in patients with ARF or CRF.

#### Acid–Base Disorders

The patient with renal failure has a metabolic acidosis because of problems with excretion of waste products and organic acids. If potassium and sodium additions are needed for the patient with renal failure who is receiving TPN, they should be added as acetate salts. This may help treat or at least not worsen the acid–base disorder by giving excessive chloride salts (hyperchloremic metabolic acidosis).

### *Micronutrient Considerations*

#### Trace Elements

The requirements for trace elements during nutritional support of ARF are not well established. Zinc and chromium are excreted mainly by the kidney in the absence of ostomy output or diarrhea. Some authors have advocated elimination of trace elements from the TPN formula of patients with ARF.[65] Because manganese and copper are excreted in the bile and zinc may be lost in the dialysis bath, patients with ARF receiving TPN should be treated according to the NAG-AMA guidelines for trace elements.[18]

There are considerably more data involving trace element nutriture in patients with CRF.[66–69] One group found that total body stores of zinc in CRF were increased, but skeletal muscle and serum concentrations of zinc were both decreased. This suggests a translocation of zinc or increased need to maintain normal enzymatic function. It appears that most patients with CRF who are being hemodialyzed have depressed serum concentrations of zinc and elevated concentrations of copper.[68] The clinical relevance of these disorders is difficult to interpret; however, universal zinc supplementation of CRF patients cannot be recommended at this time. Interestingly, zinc absorption has been reported to be impaired in patients with uremia, especially in those receiving hemodialysis.[70]

The most severe trace element disorder in patients with CRF is aluminum toxicity.[71,72] This has been caused by aluminum in the dialysate or excessive use of aluminum-containing antacids. Consequently, significant quantities of aluminum have been removed from currently available dialysis solutions. Also, the aluminum content of human serum albumin has recently been decreased. This may have contributed to aluminum toxicity in the CRF patient as this product is used frequently in dialysis hypotension. The older protein solutions for TPN (protein hydrolysates) contained considerable aluminum, but the crystalline amino acid products have eliminated that problem.

#### Vitamins

There are very few data concerning vitamin requirements in patients with ARF who are receiving TPN. Currently, it seems prudent to administer vitamins as recommended by the NAG-AMA. If the enteral route can be used for nutritional support during ARF, vitamin administration to meet the RDAs is reasonable.

Patients with CRF are very prone to develop water-soluble vitamin deficiencies because foods that are restricted because of their potassium content also contain these vitamins. Specifically, CRF patients should receive ascorbic acid 70–100 mg/d, pyridoxine 5–10 mg/d, and folic acid I mg/d in addition to the other essential vitamins. During short-term TPN in patients with CRF, elimination or reduction of the dose of vitamins A and D has been recommended. Vitamin A concentrations are often elevated in CRF patients and vitamin D administration has been associated with metabolic bone disease and osteomalacia, especially in this patient population.

**Table 111.4** Studies Comparing EAAs and MAAs in Nutritional Support for Acute Renal Failure Patients

| *Authors* | *Study design* | *Patients* | *Nutritional regimen* | *Results* |
|---|---|---|---|---|
| Blackburn et al[76] | Prospective | 19<br>(11 unstressed)<br>(8 stressed) | EAAs + 37% glucose<br>MAAs + 37% glucose<br>MAAs + 52% glucose | No significant difference in decreased BUN in the unstressed patients; 5/8 died in the stressed group |
| Freund et al[77] | Retrospective | 50 | EAAs + 46% glucose<br>MAAs + 46% glucose | 91% mortality in the group receiving MAAs vs. 25% in the group receiving EAAs |
| Feinstein et al[78] | Prospective<br>Double-blind | 30 | 46% glucose[a]<br>EAAs + 46% glucose<br>MAAs + 46% glucose | No significant difference in mortality and return of renal function in the amino acid groups |
| Mirtallo et al[79] | Prospective<br>Double-blind<br>Randomized | 45 | EAAs + 46% glucose[b]<br>MAAs + 46% glucose[b] | No significant difference in mortality, urea nitrogen appearance, and nitrogen balance |

[a] 70% glucose and 20% glucose were used to deliver 2,050 or 2,800 kcal/d.
[b] 70% glucose was used to administer 1.75 × basal energy expenditures.

## *Administration Routes and Products*

### Parenteral Therapy

Most patients with ARF have a superimposed illness (septic shock, hypotension, ileus) that requires nutritional support by the parenteral route. An early study by Abel et al[73] showed both improved survival rate and return of renal function when essential amino acids (EAAs) plus glucose were compared with glucose alone in patients with ARF. Consequently, intravenous amino acids containing only EAAs (Nephramine, Kendall McGaw; RenAmin, Travenol, Aminosyn-RF, Abbott) were marketed on the basis of such studies. These products are usually mixed with concentrated dextrose 70%. These products were formulated on the hypothesis that substantial nitrogen reutilization occurs during ARF (i.e., circulating urea can be used to synthesize nonessential amino acids). This reutilization of nitrogen does not occur in patients with uremia.[74,75] Thereafter, investigators began to question whether EAAs were any more effective than general mixed amino acids (MAAs). This led to several controlled and uncontrolled studies comparing these different amino acid products in patients with ARF.[76–79] A summary of these studies appears in Table 111.4.

The studies by Feinstein et al[78] and Mirtallo et al[79] were prospective and well controlled. Freund et al[77] studied a group of very ill patients with ARF who received TPN with MAAs. These patients were compared with a group of retrospective controls who had ARF and received TPN with EAAs.[73] The patients in the Freund et al study had concomitant trauma, burns, or cardiac disease. These disease states were exclusions in the control group. The poor study design makes any conclusions from these data very questionable. The type of intravenous protein for TPN in ARF remains somewhat controversial, but the well-controlled studies do not indicate clinically significant disadvantages when MAAs are used. See Table 111.3 for an example of TPN in ARF. Note that dextrose 70% is the energy substrate of choice when fluid restriction is required. Some investigators advocate the use of EAAs in ARF when the creatinine clearance is less than 10 mL/min *and* dialysis will not be instituted or there is a contraindication to administer nonessential amino acids. This would severely restrict the indications for EAAs.

Patients with CRF who require nutritional support rarely need parenteral nutrition because their gastrointestinal tract is functioning. If there is superimposed illness that prevents enteral administration of nutrients, parenteral nutrition is indicated. As many of these patients are already receiving hemodialysis or peritoneal dialysis, MAAs can be used (Table 111.3).

### Enteral Therapy

Continuous pump-tube feeding should be used when patients with ARF or CRF have functioning gastrointestinal tracts and will not or cannot ingest sufficient nutrients. The products used most frequently during enteral nutritional support of renal failure appear in Table 111.5. The electrolyte-free formulas are useful in patients with hyperkalemia, hyperphosphatemia, or hypermagnesemia. The calorically dense, low-electrolyte formulas are used when fluid restriction is needed and serum concentrations of electrolytes are normal. All of these products are hyperosmolar and may require dilution with water during initial administration.

## *Future Directions*

There are some data available that support infusion of glucose/amino acid solutions during hemodialysis.[80] This was shown to maintain plasma amino acid concentrations and prevent a net loss of nitrogen during the dialytic period. This approach is particularly appealing when used in the undernourished patient with CRF receiving dialysis therapy.

**Table 111.5** Enteral Nutrition Products Used in Renal Failure

| *Product* | *AminAid (Kendall McGaw)* | *Travasorb Renal (Travenol)* | *Isocal-HCN (Mead Johnson)* | *Magnacal (Sherwood Medical)* |
|---|---|---|---|---|
| Caloric density (kcal/mL) | 2.0 | 1.3 | 2.0 | 2.0 |
| Electrolytes | None | None | Low | Low |
| Vitamins | None | Water soluble only | Yes | Yes |
| Osmolality (mOsm/kg $H_2O$) | 1,095 | 590 | 690 | 590 |

Studies documenting this potential benefit are needed to justify the increased expense.

Keto-analogues of EAAs have been given with a phosphorus-restricted diet (20–30 g protein per day) to patients with chronic renal dysfunction and either slowed or halted the progression of renal insufficiency.[81] More work in this area is certainly justified.

Because urine collections for assessing nitrogen balance are often impossible (anuria) in patients with renal failure, a method for determination of nitrogen balance that estimates urea nitrogen appearance has been developed. This method estimates protein catabolism by measuring losses in the urine and/or the dialysate fluid and the nitrogen that remains in the body.[82,83] When nitrogen intake is known, an estimated nitrogen balance can be calculated:

$$\text{ENB} = \text{Ni} - (\text{UUN} + 4 + \text{UNA} + \text{N dialysate})$$

where ENB = estimated nitrogen balance, Ni = nitrogen intake for 24 hours, UUN = urea nitrogen collected in urine over 24 hours, N dialysate = urea nitrogen lost in dialysate fluid during 24 hours, and UNA = urea nitrogen remaining in the body produced over the last 24 hours (calculated from changes in weight and BUN). These calculations may be very helpful in adjusting nitrogen and caloric doses during nutritional support in patients with ARF or CRF and are appearing more frequently in studies of nutritional support of this patient population.

## Pulmonary Failure

The lung is responsible primarily for gas exchange. Oxygen is inhaled into the body through the lung and is absorbed into the circulatory system while carbon dioxide is exhaled. Recently, substantial information has become available emphasizing the interaction between nutrition and respiratory function.[84–88] For example, decreased inspiratory muscle strength,[85] increased tracheobronchial bacterial colonization,[86] and lung dysfunction have all been reported in patients with respiratory disease and poor nutritional status. Also, preliminary data suggest that enteral tube feedings may help prevent stress ulcers in patients who are receiving mechanical ventilation.[89] The deleterious effects of overfeeding the patient with pulmonary compromise have received a great amount of the attention, but other substrates and electrolytes need to be considered during nutritional support in these patients. Although patients with pulmonary disease do not have the metabolic alterations seen in patients with renal or hepatic disease, there is substantial information to aid the practitioner in providing safe and efficacious nutritional support. The reader is also referred to several in-depth reviews of nutritional support in patients with respiratory disease.[90–92]

### *Macronutrient Considerations*

**Carbohydrate**

Semistarvation in normal subjects (500 kcal of carbohydrate per day) has been shown to blunt the normal response to hypoxia, and refeeding restored this response to normal.[93] Depression in the hypoxic ventilatory response correlated well with decreases in all of the following: body weight, oxygen consumption ($V_{O_2}$), carbon dioxide production ($V_{CO_2}$), resting minute ventilation, and heart rate. These data suggest early feeding of the mechanically ventilated patient may improve the hypoxic response.

Oxidation of the major nutritional substrates can be represented by a respiratory quotient (RQ) determined by dividing $V_{CO_2}$ by $V_{O_2}$. The respiratory quotients for oxidation of the major substrates and synthesis of fat appear in Table 111.6.

Much interest has been generated from reports of the inability to wean mechanically ventilated patients because of overfeeding with glucose-based TPN.[94–96] It is presumed that excessive infused carbohydrate is used for fat synthesis, resulting in substantial liberation of carbon dioxide. This made weaning impossible secondary to respiratory acidosis; however, the percentage of spontaneous ventilation does increase as calories are increased in mechanically ventilated patients.[97] One group has reported significant increases in $V_{CO_2}$ and RQ when glucose-based TPN was administered to both depleted and severely stressed patients at approximately 50% above measured energy expenditure.[98] From these data and the case reports of overfeeding with carbohydrate, glucose-based TPN should be administered in moderate doses to patients with respiratory disease or mechanical ventilation.

**Table 111.6** Respiratory Quotients for Oxidation of the Major Substrates and Fat Synthesis

| *Substrate* | *RQ* |
|---|---|
| Carbohydrate oxidation | 1.0 |
| Protein oxidation | 0.8 |
| Fat oxidation | 0.7 |
| Fat synthesis from carbohydrate | 8.0 |

### Fat

Because fat is oxidized at a lower RQ than glucose, intravenous fat emulsion at 30% to 50% of the nonprotein calories has been suggested in patients with respiratory failure who require TPN.[98] As discussed before, patients who are overfed with glucose synthesize fat, which increases carbon dioxide production. Decreases of 18% and 24% in $V_{CO_2}$ were recorded when ventilated patients were switched from glucose-based TPN to TPN containing 33% and 50% intravenous fat emulsion, respectively.[99] These data are supported by other investigations.[100,101] There has been some concern with a reduction in pulmonary membrane diffusion capacity and intravenous fat emulsion administration[102]; however, clearance and oxidation of these infusions are actually accelerated in critically ill patients.[103,104] Although it is now clear that TPN with glucose as a sole nonprotein caloric source substantially increases carbon dioxide production in both unstressed and severely ill patients, the full clinical significance of these findings remains to be shown. Nevertheless, overfeeding should be avoided and intravenous fat emulsions may have a role in the provision of nutritional support in selected patients with respiratory failure.

### Protein

Recent studies have demonstrated a blunted response to hypercapnia in undernourished patients and an improved response after 1 week of adequate nutrition support.[105] This response was thought to result from protein administration as measured by decreased $P_{CO_2}$, increased minute ventilation, and improved breathing patterns. It may be caused by increased metabolism[106] or an increase in neuromuscular ventilatory drive.[107] It appears that increasing protein intake beyond normal significantly improves this response.[108] Even though increased neuromuscular drive from protein administration can be beneficial, it can also be detrimental in patients who are unable to increase their minute ventilation. In other words, excessive protein intake might increase pulmonary workload, resulting in muscle fatigue and respiratory failure. Therefore, only moderate doses of protein (1.0–1.5 g/kg/d) can be recommended for the patient with stable COPD. Patients who are mechanically ventilated with superimposed illness (e.g., sepsis) may require higher doses of protein (1.5–2.5 g/kg/d).

### Sodium and Water

Ill patients with chronic obstructive pulmonary disease (COPD) or patients with pneumonia receiving mechanical ventilation should have intake and output recorded daily. In most cases, it is desirable to keep these patients slightly "dry." Therefore, excessive infusions of salt and water should be avoided as these may exacerbate already compromised pulmonary function, and parenteral and enteral formulas should be relatively low in sodium. Losses of sodium from nasogastric suction or abdominal drains should, of course, be replaced.

### Phosphorus

The incidence of hypophosphatemia is higher in patients with pulmonary disease than in the general hospitalized population.[109] This is particularly true in patients with pneumonia. It is well known that phosphorus is essential for adenosine triphosphate (ATP) and 2,3-diphosphoglycerate (2,3-DPG). Hypophosphatemia can cause reduced erythrocyte concentrations of these two compounds.[110] Hemoglobin does not release oxygen during hypoxia appropriately without adequate 2,3-DPG, and respiratory muscles may be weakened without adequate stores of ATP. Recently, it was shown that hypophosphatemia impairs diaphragmatic contractibility in patients with acute respiratory failure.[111] Correction of this disorder with intravenous potassium phosphate improved diaphragmatic contractility significantly. These data combined with the problems of hypophosphatemia from refeeding emphasize the importance of phosphorus homeostasis in this patient population during nutritional support.

### Acid–Base Disorders

Ventilator-dependent patients and those with stable COPD often have respiratory acidosis. As mentioned earlier, excessive administration of carbohydrate results in net fat synthesis and liberalization of large quantities of carbon dioxide. This can make weaning from the ventilator extremely difficult and even induce respiratory failure in a stable COPD patient. The acid–base status of the patient with pulmonary compromise who is receiving nutrition support should be monitored very closely.

## *Micronutrient Considerations*

There are no known significant alterations in trace element and vitamin metabolism in patients with pulmonary disease. Patients who are receiving TPN should receive vitamins and trace elements as recommended by the NAG-AMA. Patients receiving enteral nutrition should receive the RDAs for vitamins and zinc and the recommended amounts for the other trace elements.

## *Administration Routes and Products*

### Parenteral Therapy

Patients with pulmonary failure should receive nutritional support by the enteral route unless the gastrointestinal tract is not functional or accessible. Patients with pulmonary failure from severe pneumonia or septicemia may have a prolonged ileus, necessitating TPN for nutritional support. As there are no major substrate alterations in pulmonary failure, moderate doses of intravenous carbohydrate, fat, and protein are appropriate in most clinical conditions. As emphasized earlier, excessive carbohydrate administration increases carbon dioxide production, which may impair weaning of patients from the ventilator. As a result of this well-published concept, many investigators are advocating the use of lipid as a daily caloric source in TPN regimens. The availability of three-in-one administration systems for glucose, fat, and crystalline amino acids has made it very convenient to administer intravenous lipid to patients on a daily basis. Table 111.3 gives an example of a parenteral nutrition formula using lipid as a caloric source. While intravenous fat emulsions are certainly not reserved for only the patient with pulmonary failure, their use as a daily caloric source is being advocated.

**Table 111.7** Formulas Used to Calculate Energy Expenditure From Indirect Calorimetry[a]

| *Formula* | *Reference* |
|---|---|
| $(V_{O_2} \times 4.83)\ (1.44)$ | 122 |
| $(V_{CO_2} \times 5.52)\ (1.44)$ | 123 |
| $[(V_{O_2} \times 3.9) + (V_{CO_2} \times 1.11)]\ (1.44)$ | 124 |

[a] Energy expenditure in kcal/d.

### Enteral Therapy

Most general tube feeding products contain a balance of nonprotein energy between carbohydrate and fat. Elemental or chemically defined products would be the exception because they are intended to be high-carbohydrate, low-fat formulas. Comparison of high-carbohydrate with high-fat enteral tube feeding in undernourished patients revealed a significant increase in minute ventilation, heat production, and carbon dioxide production when the high-carbohydrate formula was infused.[112] Also, outpatients with COPD and hypercapnia demonstrated a significant decrease in $V_{CO_2}$, RQ, and $Pa_{CO_2}$ when changed from a high-carbohydrate, low-fat to a low-carbohydrate, high-fat liquid diet.[113] It appears that the principles of energy expenditure calculated from $V_{CO_2}$ and $V_{O_2}$ also apply during enteral nutrition support. Because most general formulas contain balanced nonprotein calories, moderate doses of these products are appropriate in most patients with pulmonary disease.

Recently, an enteral product (Pulmocare, Ross Laboratories) was marketed for the patient with pulmonary failure that contains a substantial amount of fat (55% fat, 31% carbohydrate, 14% protein). A formula similar in composition can be prepared by adding a fat module to a general complete formula or by using a modular enteral formulation system. Further studies with enteral nutrition in pulmonary failure patients are needed before high-fat formulas can be recommended universally.

### *Future Directions*

Sophisticated methods for assessing energy expenditure of hospitalized patients have become commercially available. Techniques of indirect calorimetry are employed by collecting expired air from the patient. This can be done by placing a canopy over the patient's head or by collecting expired air from the mechanically ventilated patient. $V_{CO_2}$ and $V_{O_2}$ can be used to calculate energy expenditure (Table 111.7).[114–116] These instruments are very expensive, precluding most hospitals from purchasing them for use in nutritional support, but their use in research protocols is becoming more essential.

## Cardiac Failure

The major function of the heart is to circulate the blood throughout the body, providing needed oxygen and nutrients. Heart failure can result in ischemia. A significant relationship exists between cardiac function and protein-calorie deprivation.[117] In starvation, cardiac muscle is not spared and the loss roughly parallels loss of lean body mass. Cardiac output and stroke volume are reduced in undernutrition, resulting in hypotension and bradycardia. This allows the heart to function at a reduced oxygen consumption.

Refeeding the starved patient disrupts the cardiovascular dynamics of starvation. There is usually a marked increase in metabolic rate and only gradual restoration of myocardial contractile proteins with refeeding.[118] Consequently, excessive administration of nutrients or fluid volume could overwhelm the heart, resulting in failure. The goal of nutritional support in the patient with cardiac disease should be to gradually improve or maintain nutritional status. Also, improvement in serum albumin concentrations should decrease edema in this patient population.

### *Macronutrient Considerations*

#### Carbohydrate/Fat/Protein

Patients with cardiac failure should be able to handle the major substrates without problem. It is usually beneficial to restrict intake in these patients, making the most concentrated substrates very desirable during nutrition support.

#### Sodium and Water

Generally, the patient with cardiac disease is at risk of developing congestive heart failure (CHF). Salt and water restriction continues to be an important part of the management of these patients and the nutrition formula should reflect these restrictions. Overzealous addition of sodium to the TPN formula can exacerbate CHF and worsen edema. Hyponatremia in this patient population usually signifies fluid and sodium overload and should be treated with restriction. Loop-diuretic therapy is frequently used to increase excretion of salt and water.

#### Potassium

It is well known that loop-diuretic therapy increases the urinary excretion of potassium, often resulting in hypokalemia. This can be particularly significant in the undernourished patient receiving nutritional support because potassium requirements increase as lean body mass is synthesized. Patients receiving concomitant digoxin therapy need to have serum potassium concentrations maintained in the normal range.

#### Phosphorus

Hypophosphatemia and cardiopulmonary decompensation have been associated with refeeding the undernourished patient.[119] Phosphorus shifts from the serum to the intracellular space as new lean body mass is synthesized. Energy is shifted from fat metabolism (which does not require phosphate-containing intermediates) to glucose (which does). There is also an association between profound hypophosphatemia and severe congestive cardiomyopathy.[120] It would seem prudent to treat the severely undernourished patient conservatively by increasing the nutrient infusion slowly, administering a portion of the energy as fat, checking heart rate regularly, and assessing the patient for edema or rales.

#### Magnesium

Homeostasis of magnesium may be affected by aggressive loop-diuretic therapy in that renal excretion of this cation is markedly enhanced. Poor magnesium intake secondary to anorexia of CHF coupled with increased excretion from diuretic therapy may compound existing hypomagnesemia. Serum concentrations need to be checked frequently during nutritional support of these patients.

### *Micronutrient Considerations*

Patients with cardiac failure who are receiving TPN should receive the vitamins and trace elements as recommended by the NAG-AMA. Those receiving enteral nutrition support should receive the RDAs for vitamins and zinc. Theoretically, urinary excretion of zinc may be increased by vigorous loop-diuretic therapy, but routine supplementation above suggested intake is not recommended.

Selenium deficiency has been shown to cause Keshan's disease, a dilated congestive cardiomyopathy, in geographic areas where the selenium content of the soil is extremely low (e.g., China). There are now several cases of selenium deficiency that have been reported in patients on long-term TPN without selenium supplementation.[121–124] Some of these case studies reported deaths from cardiomyopathy, presumed to be secondary to selenium deficiency. Because this cardiomyopathy is irreversible, selenium supplementation of 40–60 $\mu$g/d should be considered in long-term TPN patients. A recent study in long-term TPN patients demonstrated improvement in serum concentrations of selenium after supplementation but not in functional activity as measured by erythrocyte glutathione perioxidase.[125]

### *Administration Routes*

#### Parenteral Therapy

Patients with cardiac disease need parenteral nutrition only when there is superimposed illness preventing use of the gastrointestinal tract. Currently, there are no disease-specific products marketed for this patient population. An example of a TPN formula for this patient type is given in Table 111.3.

#### Enteral Therapy

Most patients with cardiac failure have functioning gastrointestinal tracts so that enteral nutrition support can be used. Both poor palatability of a salt-restricted diet and anorexia secondary to CHF may impede adequate ingestion of nutrients. If dietary intervention with oral liquid supplements is unsuccessful and the patient is either undernourished or at risk of becoming so, enteral tube feeding should be strongly considered. Because fluid restriction is often desirable in cardiac failure, enteral products delivering 1.5–2.0 kcal/mL may be indicated. Also, most commercially available enteral formulas are relatively low in sodium (20–50 mEq/L).

## Short-Bowel Syndrome

Because the gastrointestinal tract is essential for absorption and digestion of nutrients, dysfunction or malabsorption can have a significant impact on nutritional status.[126,127] Gastrointestinal failure secondary to the short-bowel syndrome (SBS) is a disease state in which morbidity and mortality have been significantly improved by parenteral nutrition. TPN has also had a major impact on the treatment of patients with severe inflammatory bowel disease,[128] enterocutaneous fistulas,[129] and radiation enteritis.[130]

The goal of nutritional support in patients with gastrointestinal failure (SBS) should be to maintain nutritional status or correct nutritional deficiencies by the appropriate route. Both parenteral and enteral nutrition support are used extensively in patients with gastrointestinal disease.

### *Macronutrient Considerations*

#### Carbohydrate/Fat/Protein

Once absorbed, the macronutrients should be processed normally in patients with gastrointestinal failure. If enteral nutrients cannot be absorbed appropriately, parenteral nutrition will need to be used temporarily or, in patients with extreme SBS, indefinitely. Occasionally, the enteral route can be used for provision of part of the required nutrients, with parenteral nutrition supplying the balance.

Generally, fat malabsorption is the disorder most often manifested in SBS because this process is very complex (pancreatic enzymes, bile acids). Some patients with fat malabsorption have been treated with medium-chain triglycerides that do not require pancreatic enzymes or bile acids for absorption. This product, however, does not provide essential fatty acids, which could lead to essential fatty acid deficiency. Long-chain fatty acids would need to be given orally or parenterally.

Traditionally, nitrogen in its simplest form (free amino acids) has been recommended in patients with moderate to severe SBS because it was assumed that this absorptive pathway was most efficient. Recent studies have demonstrated that enteral formulas containing partially hydrolyzed protein were absorbed better than formulas containing nitrogen only as free amino acids.[131–133] These studies suggest an alternative pathway for nitrogen absorption that may even be superior to that of free amino acids. There remains much needed research to determine which pathway for nitrogen absorption is superior and would theoretically be optimal for the patient with SBS.

#### Sodium and Water

Fluid and sodium balance are extremely important in the patient with gastrointestinal failure because of potential extrarenal losses. Often, the appropriate TPN or enteral nutrition regimen includes extra fluid to meet needs and maintain urine output. Substantial losses of any body fluids (e.g., from jejunostomy or colostomy) need to be considered when preparing the nutritional formula. Diarrhea is a hallmark disorder of SBS and losses may be difficult to measure. Stool frequency and consistency may aid in the amount of replacement needed. Serum sodium concentration may not reflect sodium and fluid status, especially in the dehydrated state in which hypernatremia can result.

### Potassium

Losses of potassium from an ostomy in the SBS can be considerable. If these losses are stable, they can be replaced by adding supplemental potassium into the TPN formula. Metabolic alkalosis, which occurs when a patient becomes dehydrated, can accelerate the renal excretion of potassium, as all hydrogen ions will be conserved to correct the acid–base disorder. As bicarbonate ions are excreted renally, potassium is taken with them to maintain osmotic balance. Diarrheal fluid is also concentrated in potassium and requires fluid and potassium replacement if it cannot be controlled.

### Calcium

Patients with severe SBS invariably have fat malabsorption. Complexation of both dietary and secreted calcium in the remaining bowel by unabsorbed free fatty acids renders the ion unabsorbable, leading to negative calcium balance. Patients on long-term TPN will need calcium added to their nutrition formula to maintain calcium balance. Also, long-term TPN has been associated with metabolic bone disease resulting in osteomalacia and osteoporosis. Excessive aluminum loading from protein hydrolysates (no longer used), parenteral vitamin D, and excessive infusion of protein have all been shown to cause hypercalciuria, which is a potential etiology of this disorder. It therefore appears reasonable to assay a 24-hour urine collection for calcium before a patient is sent home with TPN. This will help identify patients who may have trouble maintaining calcium balance. For patients with SBS who are able to maintain nutritional status on oral nutrition, calcium supplementation as the gluconate salt is often required.

### Magnesium

Considerable losses of magnesium occur with diarrhea and ostomy losses. Like the other electrolytes above, magnesium is usually replaced in the TPN formula in patients with severe SBS. Oral replacement of magnesium with gluconate or oxide salts may be used in less severe cases of SBS, but excessive use of oral magnesium results in diarrhea and may exacerbate a magnesium deficit.

### Acid–Base Disorders

Patients with severe SBS are at great risk of developing dehydration and metabolic alkalosis. They can lose substantial amounts of chloride (60–140 mEq/L) and sodium (80–160 mEq/L) from ostomies and daily losses may vary from 0.5 to 10 L. Dehydration occurs when there are stable losses from an ostomy that are not replaced or when the patient is noncompliant with a restricted diet. Patients who have SBS complicated by a pancreatic fistula lose considerable bicarbonate and may develop metabolic acidosis. Quantifying fluid losses with particular attention to the sources of loss will aid in the acid–base management of these complex patients.

## *Micronutrient Considerations*

### Trace Elements

Much of the information that has been gained about trace element nutriture during nutritional support has come from patients on long-term TPN. This can, in part, be explained by the length of time required for a deficiency in trace elements to develop or be recognized (months to years). Also, signs or symptoms of deficiency may not be appreciated and biochemical analysis is not available in all hospitals.

Zinc is the trace element that has been studied most often during TPN. Wolman et al[21] reported on 24 patients with gastrointestinal disease who were receiving central TPN. These patients were given three separate doses of parenteral zinc during three 1-week periods while zinc balance was done. It was shown that small-bowel fluid, colostomy fluid, and diarrheal fluid contained considerable quantities of zinc. An equation to estimate zinc requirements was developed:

$$\text{Zn replacement (mg/d)} = 2.0 + 17.1a + 12.2b$$

where $a$ = kilograms of stool or ileostomy output and $b$ = liters of small-bowel fluid lost. Zinc deficiency has been reported in a patient receiving this trace element in the TPN formula.[134] In this case, it appears that the zinc contained in the trace element solution did not meet the needs of this critically ill patient as supplementation improved symptoms and normalized biochemical abnormalities. Therefore, patients who have SBS and require TPN should clearly have zinc added to their formula. Doses above the NAG-AMA recommendations should be given when excessive losses of gastrointestinal fluids occur.[21]

Because copper is excreted primarily in the bile, excessive losses of gastrointestinal fluid can have a substantial impact on copper balance. Copper balance during TPN has also been studied in a group of patients with gastrointestinal disease.[135] Although requirements for patients with excessive gastrointestinal losses were higher (0.4–0.5 mg/d) than those for patients with normal gastrointestinal losses (0.3 mg/d), recommendations by the NAG-AMA exceed both of these doses. It is clear, however, that administration of TPN without copper will result in depressed serum copper concentrations[136] and eventually copper deficiency.[137,138]

Two of the three patients reported in the literature who have developed chromium deficiency during long-term TPN had excessive gastrointestinal fluid losses after enterectomy.[139,140] It was suggested that these losses contributed to the chromium deficiency and glucose intolerance experienced by these patients. These data, although scant, suggest that patients with excessive gastrointestinal fluid losses need a supplemental dose of chromium (20 $\mu$g/d).[139]

### Vitamins

Most water-soluble vitamins (except vitamin B-12) are absorbed in the jejunum, so unless the patient has severe SBS, these can be maintained with an oral diet. Because patients with resection of the distal ileum cannot absorb vitamin $B_{12}$, the parenteral form of this vitamin has to be administered. Patients with SBS who have fat malabsorption are prone to malabsorb the fat-soluble vitamins (A, D, E, and K). These vitamins can often be orally supplemented if there is sufficient gastrointestinal tract left. The patient with severe SBS will be receiving TPN with parenteral vitamins in most cases.

### *Administration Routes and Products*

#### Parenteral Therapy

Patients who have had a major resection of the gastrointestinal tract usually require a period of central TPN to maintain nutritional status while the remaining small bowel is undergoing hypertrophy.[141] There are usually no substrate alterations in these patients, so standard crystalline amino acids, glucose, and intravenous lipids may be used in conventional doses either to maintain nutritional status or to correct nutritional deficits in these patients. An example of a TPN formula for the patient with SBS is given in Table 111.3. If the patient has had major enterectomy, home TPN may be needed for the rest of the patient's life. A recent report suggests that most patients with severe SBS can be converted to enteral nutrition therapy.[142] If other studies verify these data, the need for home TPN would be reduced markedly.

#### Enteral Therapy

After major gastrointestinal resection, enteral therapy should be introduced soon, as food is the stimulus for secretion of pancreatic enzymes and other trophic hormones that are thought to be essential for small-bowel hyperplasia. Elemental diets or chemically defined formulas have been used initially during enteral therapy in selected patients because the substrates are in the simplest or an easily digestible form. Other investigators have used enteral glucose polymer solutions to replace fluid and electrolyte losses, but this method is not used often.[143]

Traditionally, patients with SBS who can maintain nutritional status by the oral route have been prescribed low-fat diets because fat malabsorption is a common disorder in these patients. Recent studies have challenged this traditional approach and the patients were given regular diets.[144,145] Five end jejunostomy patients who were studied on three diets with different percentages of fat demonstrated no significant increases in loss of ostomy volume or monovalent cations with the high-fat diet.[144] In this study, only divalent cations (copper, zinc, calcium, magnesium) were lost in significantly greater quantities when the high-fat diet was used. Likewise, other investigators found no difference in ostomy volume, blood chemistry, or stool volume in patients with SBS who were switched from a low-fat to high-fat diet.[145]

### *Future Directions*

Further study of this population will identify other essential trace elements needed in patients who are receiving long-term TPN. If the surgical procedure for small-bowel transplantation in humans becomes a reality, many patients with severe SBS will be potential candidates for this operation.

## References


1. Satta A, Chiandussi L, Faedda R, et al. Fluid and electrolytes in liver disease. Postgrad Med J 1983;59:64–72.
2. Mezey E. Liver disease and nutrition. Gastroenterology 1978; 74:770–783.
3. Medenhall CL, Anderson S, Weesner RE, et al. Protein-calorie malnutrition associated with alcoholic hepatitis. Am J Med 1984;76:211–222.
4. Barber JR, Teasley KM. Nutritional support of patients with severe hepatic failure. Clin Pharm 1984;3:245–253.
5. Blei AT, Robbins DC, Drobny E, et al. Insulin resistance and insulin receptors in hepatic cirrhosis. Gastroenterology 1982; 83:1191–1199.
6. Gabuzda GJ, Shear L. Metabolism of dietary protein in hepatic cirrhosis. Am J Clin Nutr 1970;23:479–487.
7. Fischer JE, Rosen HM, Ebeid AM, et al. The effect of normalization of plasma amino acids on hepatic encephalopathy in man. Surgery 1976;80:77–91.
8. Mizock BA. Branched-chain amino acids in sepsis and hepatic failure. Arch Intern Med 1985;145:1284–1288.
9. Marchesini G, Zoli M, Dondi C, et al. Anticatabolic effect of branched-chain amino acid–enriched solutions in patients with liver cirrhosis. Hepatology 1982;2:420–424.
10. Fraser CL, Arieff AI. Hepatic encephalopathy. N Engl J Med 1985;313:865–873.
11. Bichet DG, Van Putten VJ, Schrier RW. Potential role of increased sympathetic activity in impaired sodium and water excretion in cirrhosis. N Engl J Med 1982;307:1552–1557.
12. Bichet D, Szatalowicz V, Chaimovitz C, et al. Role of vasopressin in abnormal water excretion in cirrhotic patients. Ann Intern Med 1982;96:413–417.
13. Nelson DC, McGrew WR, Hoyumpa AM. Hypernatremia and lactulose therapy. JAMA 1983;249:1295–1298.
14. Lotz M, Zisman E, Bartter FC. Evidence for a phosphorus-depletion syndrome in man. N Engl J Med 1968;278:409–415.
15. Sherman RA, Hwang ER, Walker JA, et al. Reduction in serum phosphorus due to sucralfate. Am J Gastroenterol 1983; 78:210–211.
16. Dickerson RN, Brown RO. Hypomagnesemia in hospitalized patients receiving nutritional support. Heart Lung 1985;14: 561–569.
17. Agus ZS, Wasserstein A, Goldfarb S. Disorders of calcium and magnesium homeostasis. Am J Med 1982;72:473–488.
18. Anonymous. Guidelines for essential trace element preparations for parenteral use. JAMA 1979;241:2051–2054.
19. Baptista RJ, Bistrian BR, Blackburn GL, et al. Suboptimal selenium status in home parenteral nutrition patients with small bowel resections. J Parenter Enter Nutr 1984;8:542–545.
20. Baker SS, King WW, Michel L, et al. Reversal of biochemical and functional abnormalities in erythrocytes secondary to selenium deficiency. J Parenter Enter Nutr 1983;7:293–295.
21. Wolman SL, Anderson H, Marliss EB, et al. Zinc in total parenteral nutrition: Requirements and metabolic effects. Gastroenterology 1979;76:458–467.
22. Dworkin B, Rosenthal WS, Jankowski RH, et al. Low blood selenium levels in alcoholics with and without advanced liver disease. Dig Dis Sci 1985;30:838–844.

23. Korpela H, Kumpulainen J, Luoma PV, et al. Decreased serum selenium in alcoholics as related to liver structure and function. Am J Clin Nutr 1985;42:147–151.
24. Leevy CM, Thompson A, Baker H. Vitamins and liver injury. Am J Clin Nutr 1970;23:493–498.
25. Leo MA, Lieber CS. Hepatic vitamin A depletion in alcoholic liver injury. N Engl J Med 1982;307:597–601.
26. Cerra FB, Cheung NK, Fischer JE, et al. Disease-specific amino acid infusion (F080) in hepatic encephalopathy: A prospective, randomized, double-blind, controlled trial. J Parenter Enter Nutr 1985;9:288–295.
27. Michel H, Bories P, Aubin JP, et al. Treatment of acute hepatic encephalopathy in cirrhotics with a branched-chain amino acids enriched versus a conventional amino acids mixture. Liver 1985;5:282–289.
28. Rossi-Fanelli F, Riggio O, Cangiano C, et al. Branched-chain amino acids vs. lactulose in the treatment of hepatic coma. Dig Dis Sci 1982;27:929–935.
29. Wahren J, Denis J, Desurmont P, et al. Is intravenous administration of branched chain amino acids effective in the treatment of hepatic encephalopathy? A multicenter study. Hepatology 1983;3:475–480.
30. Millikan WJ, Henderson JM, Warren WD, et al. Total parenteral nutrition with F080 in cirrhotics with subclinical encephalopathy. Ann Surg 1983;197:294–304.
31. Rudman D, Kutner M, Ansley J, et al. Hypotyrosinemia, hypocystinemia, and failure to retain nitrogen during total parenteral nutrition of cirrhotic patients. Gastroenterology 1981;81:1025–1035.
32. Keohane PP, Attrill SR, Grimble G, et al. Enteral nutrition in malnourished patients with hepatic cirrhosis and acute encephalopathy. J Parenter Enter Nutr 1983;7:346–350.
33. Horst D, Grace ND, Conn HO, et al. Comparison of dietary protein with an oral, branched chain–enriched amino acid supplement in chronic portal-systemic encephalopathy: A randomized controlled trial. Hepatology 1984;4:279–287.
34. Egberts EH, Schomerus H, Hamster W, et al. Branched chain amino acids in the treatment of latent portosystemic encephalopathy. Gastroenterology 1985;88:887–895.
35. Medenhall C, Bongiovanni G, Goldberg S, et al. VA cooperative study on alcoholic hepatitis. III: Changes in protein-calorie malnutrition associated with 30 days of hospitalization with and without enteral nutritional therapy. J Parenter Enter Nutr 1985;9:590–596.
36. McGhee A, Henderson JM, Millikan WJ, et al. Comparison of the effects of hepatic-acid and a casein modular diet on encephalopathy, plasma amino acids, and nitrogen balance in cirrhotic patients. Ann Surg 1983;197:288–293.
37. Christie ML, Sack DM, Pomposelli J. Enriched branched chain amino acid formula versus a casein-based supplement in the treatment of cirrhosis. J Parenter Enter Nutr 1985;9:671–678.
38. Uribe M, Dibildox M, Malpica S, et al. Beneficial effect of vegetable protein diet supplemented with *Psyllium plantago* in patients with hepatic encephalopathy and diabetes mellitus. Gastroenterology 1985;88:901–907.
39. Weber FL, Minco D, Fresard KM, et al. Effects of vegetable diets on nitrogen metabolism in cirrhotic subjects. Gastroenterology 1985;89:538–544.
40. Maddrey WC, Weber FL,Coulter AW, et al. Effects of keto analogues of essential amino acids in portal-systemic encephalopathy. Gastroenterology 1976;71:190–195.
41. Herlong HF, Maddrey WC, Walser M. The use of ornithine salts of branched-chain ketoacids in portal-systemic encephalopathy. Ann Intern Med 1980;93:545–550.
42. Goldblum SE, Reed WP. Host defenses and immunologic alterations associated with chronic hemodialysis. Ann Intern Med 1980;93:597–613.
43. Mattern WD, Hak LJ, LaManna RW, et al. Malnutrition, altered immune function, and the risk of infection in maintenance hemodialysis patients. Am J Kidney Dis 1982;1:206–218.
44. Berkelhammer CH, Leiter LA, Jeejeebhoy KN, et al. Skeletal muscle function in chronic renal failure: An index of nutritional status. Am J Clin Nutr 1985;42:845–854.
45. Mirtallo JM, Kudsk KA, Ebbert ML. Nutritional support of patients with renal disease. Clin Pharm 1984;3:253–263.
46. Kopple JD. Nutritional therapy in kidney failure. Nutr Rev 1981;5:193–206.
47. Walser M. Nutritional management of chronic renal failure. Am J Kidney Dis 1982;1:261–275.
48. Hutchings RH, Hengstrom RM, Scribner BH. Glucose intolerance in patients with long term intermittent dialysis. Ann Intern Med 1966;66:275–285.
49. DeFronzo RA. Pathogenesis of glucose intolerance in uremia. Metabolism 1978;27:1866–1880.
50. Grodstein GP, Blumenkrantz MJ, Kopple JD, et al. Glucose absorption during continuous ambulatory peritoneal dialysis. Kidney Int 1981;19:564–567.
51. Wideroe TE, Smeby LC, Berg KJ, et al. Intraperitoneal insulin absorption during intermittent and continuous peritoneal dialysis. Kidney Int 1983;23:22–28.
52. Kanke M, Jay M, DeLuca PP. Binding of insulin to a continuous ambulatory peritoneal dialysis system. Am J Hosp Pharm 1986;43:81–88.
53. Bagdade JD, Porte D, Bierman EL. Hypertriglyceridemia: A metabolic consequence of chronic renal failure. N Engl J Med 1968;279:181–185.
54. Nestel PJ, Fidge NH, Tan MH. Increased lipoprotein-remnant formation in chronic renal failure. N Engl J Med 1982;307:329–333.
55. Blumenkrantz MJ, Gahl GM, Kopple JD, et al. Protein losses during peritoneal dialysis. Kidney Int 1981;19:593–602.
56. Steffee WP. Nutritional support in renal failure. Surg Clin North Am 1981;61:661–670.
57. Blumenkrantz MJ, Kopple JD, Moran JK, et al. Metabolic balance studies and dietary protein requirements in patients undergoing continuous ambulatory peritoneal dialysis. Kidney Int 1982;21:849–861.
58. Gahl GM, Baeyer RV, Averdunk R, et al. Outpatient evaluation of dietary intake and nitrogen removal in continuous ambulatory peritoneal dialysis. Ann Intern Med 1981;94:643–646.
59. Miller FN, Nolph KD, Sorkin MI, et al. The influence of solution composition on protein loss during peritoneal dialysis. Kidney Int 1983;23:35–39.
60. Giordano C. Protein restriction in chronic renal failure. Kidney Int 1982;22:401–408.
61. Giovannetti S. Dietary treatment of chronic renal failure: Why is it not used more frequently? Nephron 1985;40:1–12.
62. Rosman JB, Meijer S, Sluiter WJ, et al. Prospective randomized trial of early dietary protein restriction in chronic renal failure. Lancet 1984;2:1291–1295.
63. Maschio G, Oldrizzi L, Tessitore N, et al. Effects of dietary protein and phosphorus restriction on the progression of early renal failure. Kidney Int 1982;22:371–376.
64. Alvestrand A, Ahlberg M, Furst P, et al. Clinical results of long-term treatment with a low protein diet and a new amino acid preparation in patients with chronic uremia. Clin Nephrol 1983;19:67–73.

**65.** Hak LJ, Teasley KM. Total parenteral nutrition in acute renal failure. US Pharm 1981;5:H-6–H-9, H-12, H-13, H-16.

**66.** Smythe WR, Alfrey AC, Craswell PW, et al. Trace element abnormalities in chronic uremia. Ann Intern Med 1982;96:302–310.

**67.** Zumkley H, Bertram HP, Lison A, et al. Aluminum, zinc, and copper concentrations in plasma in chronic renal insufficiency. Clin Nephrol 1979;12:18–21.

**68.** Tsukamoto Y, Iwanami S, Marumo F. Disturbances of trace element concentrations in plasma of patients with chronic renal failure. Nephron 1980;26:174–179.

**69.** Mahajan SK, Prasad AS, Rabbani P, et al. Zinc deficiency: A reversible complication of uremia. Am J Clin Nutr 1982;36:1177–1183.

**70.** Grekas D, Nicolaides P, Tsakalos N, et al. Pharmacokinetics of zinc in chronic renal failure patients. Trace Elements Med 1985;4:139–142.

**71.** Thomson NM, Stevens BJ, Humphrey TJ, et al. Comparison of trace elements in peritoneal dialysis, hemodialysis, and uremia. Kidney Int 1983;23:9–14.

**72.** Alfrey AC, Hegg A, Craswell P. Metabolism and toxicity of aluminum in renal failure. Am J Clin Nutr 1980;33:1509–1516.

**73.** Abel RM, Beck CH, Abbott WM, et al. Improved survival from acute renal failure after treatment with intravenous essential L-amino acids and glucose. N Engl J Med 1973;288:695–699.

**74.** Varcoe R, Halliday D, Carson ER. Efficiency of utilization of urea nitrogen for albumin synthesis by chronically uremic and normal man. Clin Sci Mol Med 1975;48:379–390.

**75.** Long CL, Jeovanandam M, Kinney JM. Metabolism and recycling of urea in man. Am J Clin Nutr 1978;31:1367–1382.

**76.** Blackburn GL, Etter G, Mackenzie T. Criteria for choosing amino acid therapy in acute renal failure. Am J Clin Nutr 1978;31:1841–1853.

**77.** Freund H, Atamian S, Fischer JE. Comparative study of parenteral nutrition in renal failure using essential and nonessential amino acid containing solutions. Surg Gynecol Obstet 1980;151:652–656.

**78.** Feinstein EI, Blumenkrantz MJ, Healy M, et al. Clinical and metabolic responses to parenteral nutrition in acute renal failure. Medicine 1981;60:124–137.

**79.** Mirtallo JM, Schneider PJ, Mavko K, et al. A comparison of essential and general amino acid infusions in the nutritional support of patients with compromised renal function. J Parenter Enter Nutr 1982;6:109–113.

**80.** Wolfson M, Jones MR, Kopple JD. Amino acid losses during hemodialysis with infusion of amino acids and glucose. Kidney Int 1982;21:500–506.

**81.** Mitch WE, Walser M, Steinman TI, et al. The effect of a keto acid–amino acid supplement to a restricted diet on the progression of chronic renal failure. N Engl J Med 1984;311:623–629.

**82.** Mirtallo JM, Schneider PJ, Ruberg RL, et al. Monitoring protein requirements of the patient receiving hemodialysis and total parenteral nutrition. Am J Hosp Pharm 1981;38:1483–1486.

**83.** Maroni BJ, Steinman TI, Mitch WE. A method for estimating nitrogen intake of patients with chronic renal failure. Kidney Int 1985;27:58–65.

**84.** Braun SR, Dixon RM, Keim NL, et al. Predictive clinical value of nutritional assessment factors in COPD. Chest 1984;85:353–357.

**85.** Kelly SM, Rosa A, Field S, et al. Inspiratory muscle strength and body composition in patients receiving total parenteral nutrition therapy. Am Rev Resp Dis 1984;130:33–37.

**86.** Niederman MS, Merrill WW, Ferranti RD, et al. Nutritional status and bacterial binding in the lower respiratory tract in patients with chronic tracheostomy. Ann Intern Med 1984;100:795–800.

**87.** Driver AG, LeBrun M. Iatrogenic malnutrition in patients receiving ventilatory support. JAMA 1980;244:2195–2196.

**88.** Driver AG, McAlevy MT, Smith JL. Nutritional assessment of patients with chronic obstructive pulmonary disease and acute respiratory failure. Chest 1982;82:568–571.

**89.** Pingleton SK, Hadzima SK. Enteral alimentation and gastrointestinal bleeding in mechanically ventilated patients. Crit Care Med 1983;11:13–16.

**90.** Askanazi J, Weissman C, Rosenbaum SH, et al. Nutrition and the respiratory system. Crit Care Med 1982;10:163–172.

**91.** Brown RO, Heizer WD. Nutrition and respiratory disease. Clin Pharm 1984;3:152–161.

**92.** Barrocas A, Tretola R, Alonso A. Nutrition and the critically ill pulmonary patient. Resp Care 1983;28:50–61.

**93.** Doekel RC, Zwillich CW, Scoggin CH, et al. Clinical semistarvation. Depression of hypoxic ventilatory response. N Engl J Med 1976;295:358–361.

**94.** Askanazi J, Elwyn DH, Silverberg PA, et al. Respiratory distress secondary to a high carbohydrate load: A case report. Surgery 1980;87:596–598.

**95.** Covelli HD, Black JW, Olsen MS, et al. Respiratory failure precipitated by high carbohydrate loads. Ann Intern Med 1981;95:579–581.

**96.** Dark DS, Pingleton SK, Kerby GR. Hypercapnia during weaning. A complication of nutritional support. Chest 1985;88:141–143.

**97.** Laaban JP, Lemaire F, Baron JF, et al. Influence of caloric intake on the respiratory mode during mandatory minute volume ventilation. Chest 1985;87:67–72.

**98.** Askanazi J, Rosenbaum SH, Hyman AI, et al. Respiratory changes induced by the large glucose loads of total parenteral nutrition. JAMA 1980;243:1444–1447.

**99.** Askanazi J, Nordenstrom J, Rosenbaum SH, et al. Nutrition for the patient with respiratory failure: Glucose vs. fat. Anesthesiology 1981;54:373–377.

**100.** Macfie J, Holmfield JH, King RF, et al. Effect of the energy source on changes in energy expenditure and respiratory quotient during total parenteral nutrition. J Parenter Enter Nutr 1983;7:1–5.

**101.** Herve P, Simonneau G, Girard P, et al. Hypercapnic acidosis induced by nutrition in mechanically ventilated patients: Glucose vs. fat. Crit Care Med 1985;13:537–540.

**102.** Greene HL, Haglett S, Demaree R. Relationship between intralipid-induced hyperlipemia and pulmonary function. Am J Clin Nutr 1976;29:127–135.

**103.** Jarnberg PO, Lindholm M, Eklund J. Lipid infusion in critically ill patients. Crit Care Med 1981;9:27–31.

**104.** Van Deyk K, Hempel V, Munch F, et al. Influence of parenteral fat administration on the pulmonary vascular system in man. Intensive Care Med 1983;9:73–77.

**105.** Askanazi J, Rosenbaum SH, Hyman AI, et al. Effects of parenteral nutrition on ventilatory drive. (Abstr) Anesthesiology 1980;53:S185.

**106.** Zwillich CW, Sahn SA, Weil JV. Effects of hypermetabolism on ventilation and chemosensitivity. J Clin Invest 1977;60:900–906.

**107.** Weissman C, Askanazi J, Rosenbaum S, et al. Amino acids and respiration. Ann Intern Med 1983;98:41–44.

**108.** Askanazi J, Weissman C, LaSala PA, et al. Effect of protein intake on ventilatory drive. Anesthesiology 1984;60:106–110.

**109.** Fisher J, Magid N, Kallman C, et al. Respiratory illness and hypophosphatemia. Chest 1983;83:504–508.

110. Lichtman MA, Miller DR, Cohen J, et al. Reduced red cell glycolysis, 2,3-diphosphoglycerate and adenosine triphosphate concentration, and increased hemoglobin–oxygen affinity caused by hypophosphatemia. Ann Intern Med 1971;74:562–568.
111. Aubier M, Murciano D, Lecocguic Y, et al. Effect of hypophosphatemia on diaphragmatic contractility in patients with acute respiratory failure. N Engl J Med 1985;313:420–424.
112. Heymsfield SB, Head A, McManus CB, et al. Respiratory, cardiovascular, and metabolic effects of enteral hyperalimentation: Influence of formula dose and composition. Am J Clin Nutr 1984;40:116–130.
113. Angelillo VA, Sukhdarshan B, Durfee D, et al. Effects of low and high carbohydrate feedings in ambulatory patients with chronic obstructive pulmonary disease and chronic hypercapnia. Ann Intern Med 1985;103:883–885
114. Wilmore DW. Metabolic Management of the Critically Ill. New York, Plenum, 1977, p 9.
115. McCamish MA, Dean RE, Quellette TR. Assessing energy requirements of patients on respirators. J Parenter Enter Nutr 1981;5:513–516.
116. Weir JB. New methods for calculating metabolic rate with special reference to protein metabolism. J Physiol 1949;109:1–9.
117. Heymsfield SB, Smith J, Redd S, et al. Nutritional support in cardiac failure. Surg Clin North Am 1981;61:635–652.
118. Sheldon GF, Petersen SR. Malnutrition and cardiopulmonary function: Relation to oxygen transport. J Parenter Enter Nutr 1980;4:376–383.
119. Silvis SE, Paragas PD. Paresthesias, weakness, seizures and hypophosphatemia in patients receiving hyperalimentation. Gastroenterology 1972;62:513–520.
120. O'Connor LR, Wheeler WS, Bethune JE. Effect of hypophosphatemia on myocardial performance in man. N Engl J Med 1977;297:901–903.
121. Lane HW, Barroso AO, Englert D, et al. Selenium status of seven chronic intravenous hyperalimentation patients. J Parenter Enter Nutr 1982;6:426–431.
122. Baker SS, King WW, Michel L, et al. Reversal of biochemical and functional abnormalities in erythrocytes secondary to selenium deficiency. J Parenter Enter Nutr 1983;7:293–295.
123. Fleming CR, Lie JT, McCall JT, et al. Selenium deficiency and fatal cardiomyopathy in a patient on home parenteral nutrition. Gastroenterology 1982;83:689–693.
124. Johnson RA, Baker SS, Fallon JT, et al. An occidental case of cardiomyopathy and selenium deficiency. N Engl J Med 1981; 304:1210–1212.
125. Baptista RJ, Bistrian BR, Blackburn GL, et al. Utilizing selenious acid to reverse selenium deficiency in total parenteral nutrition patients. Am J Clin Nutr 1984;39:816–820.
126. Heizer WD. Nutritional problems in gastrointestinal diseases. Compr Ther 1981;7:59–64.
127. MacFadyen BV. The use of intravenous hyperalimentation in gastrointestinal diseases. Nutr Supp Serv 1982;2:6–10.
128. Kushner RF, Craig RM. Intense nutritional support in inflammatory bowel disease: A review. J Clin Gastroenterol 1982;4: 511–520.
129. Soeters PB, Ebeid AM, Fischer JE. Review of 404 patients with gastrointestinal fistulas: Impact of parenteral nutrition. Ann Surg 1979;190:189–202.
130. Donaldson SS. Nutritional support as an adjunct to radiation therapy. J Parenter Enter Nutr 1984;8:302–310.
131. Smith JL, Arteaga C, Heymsfield SB. Increased ureagenesis and impaired nitrogen use during infusion of a synthetic amino acid formula. N Engl J Med 1982;306:1013–1018.
132. Jones BJ, Lees R, Andrews J, et al. Comparison of an elemental and polymeric enteral diet in patients with normal gastrointestinal function. Gut 1983;24:74–84.
133. Nasrallah SM, Martin DM. Comparative effects of Criticare HN and Vivonex HN in the treatment of malnutrition due to pancreatic insufficiency. Am J Clin Nutr 1984;39:251–254.
134. Moran DM, Russo J, Bell LV. Zinc deficiency dermatitis accompanying parenteral nutrition supplemented with trace elements. Clin Pharm 1982;1:169–176.
135. Shike M, Roulet M, Kurian R, et al. Copper metabolism and requirements in total parenteral nutrition. Gastroenterology 1981;81:290–297.
136. Solomons NW, Layden TJ, Rosenberg IH, et al. Plasma trace metals during total parenteral nutrition. Gastroenterology 1977;70:1022–1025.
137. Bernard LZ, Shadduck RK, Zeigler Z, et al. Observations on the anemia and neutropenia of human copper deficiency. Am J Hematol 1977;3:177–185.
138. Vilter RW, Bozian RC, Hess EV. Manifestations of copper deficiency in a patient with systemic sclerosis on intravenous hyperalimentation. N Engl J Med 1974;291:188–191.
139. Jeejeebhoy KN, Chu RC, Marliss EB, et al. Chromium deficiency, glucose intolerance, and neuropathy revised by chromium supplementation, in a patient receiving long-term total parenteral nutrition. Am J Clin Nutr 1977;30:531–538.
140. Brown RO, Forloines-Lynn S, Cross RE, et al. Chromium deficiency after long-term total parenteral nutrition. Dig Dis Sci 1986;31:661–664.
141. Wilmore DW, Dudrick SJ, Daly JM, et al. The role of nutrition in the adaption of the small intestine after massive resection. Surg Gynecol Obstet 1971;673–680.
142. Cosnes J, Gendre JP, Evard D, et al. Compensatory enteral hyperalimentation for management of patients with severe short bowel syndrome. Am J Clin Nutr 1985;41:1002–1009.
143. Griffin GE, Fagan EF, Hodgson HJ, et al. Enteral therapy in the management of massive gut resection complicated by chronic fluid and electrolyte depletion. Dig Dis Sci 1982;27: 902–908.
144. Ovesen L, Chu R, Howard L. The influence of dietary fat on jejunostomy output in patients with severe short bowel syndrome. Am J Clin Nutr 1983;38:270–277.
145. Woolf GM, Miller C, Kurian R, et al. Diet for patients with a short bowel: High fat or high carbohydrate? Gastroenterology 1983;84:823–828.

# Index

## G

## N

## P

## Q



## R